2017 HCPCS Leve

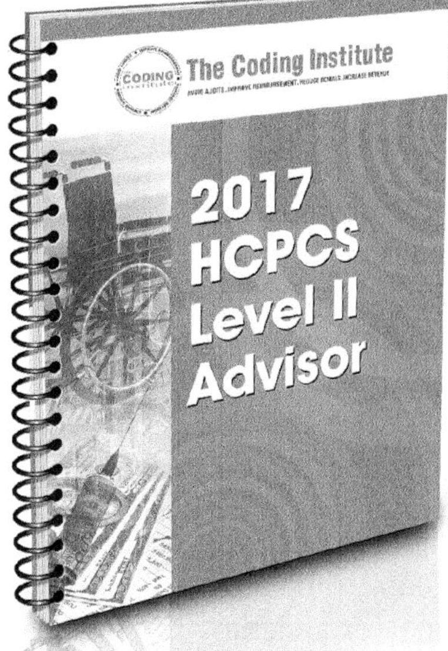

Improve Your HCPCS Coding for Services, Supplies, Drugs, and DME with the 2017 Expanded HCPCS Coding Manual.

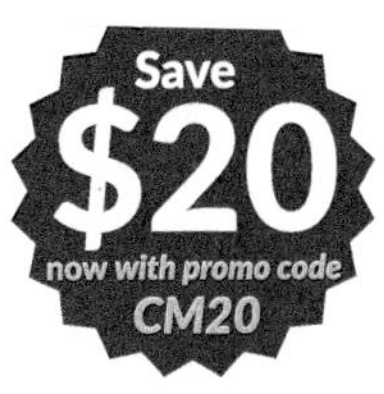

Don't miss out on one penny of reimbursement - rely on the ***2017 HCPCS Level II Advisor*** for the latest code updates to bill supplies, equipment, and drugs to Medicare and many other payers. Bonus features include a fold-out cover with 2017 HCPCS modifiers and anesthesia, ambulatory, and ambulance modifiers – plus, a HCPCS coding procedures tutorial.

Customized essential features shore up your reimbursement:

- ✓ Newly-expanded alphabetic index with hundreds of additional entries
- ✓ Over 5,000 HCPCS codes with full code descriptors
- ✓ New/Revised/Deleted codes for 2017 with a deleted codes crosswalk
- ✓ HCPCS G Codes to CPT® crosswalk
- ✓ Table of Drugs and Biologicals ***including brand-name drugs and generic drugs***
- ✓ Colored anatomical illustrations
- ✓ Pub 100 references
- ✓ Place of service and type of service lists
- ✓ Medicare Unlikely Edits (MUEs)
- ✓ PQRS Table with HCPCS Code Numerator and Corresponding Denominator

***Plus, our coding educators added even more benefits beyond the basic features:**

- ✓ Column 1 and column 2 CCI edits
- ✓ General correct coding policies
- ✓ Dictionary-style headers and color-coded bleed tabs, including the first and last code on each page
- ✓ Color coding and symbols throughout the Tabular List for:
- ✓ *Male only/Female only/Age*
- ✓ *APC status indicators*
- ✓ *ASC approved procedure/ ASC payment indicator*
- ✓ *Special coverage instructions apply*
- ✓ *Not payable by Medicare/Noncovered by Medicare/ Noncovered by Medicare statute/Paid under the DME fee schedule/Carrier judgement*
- ✓ *AHA Coding Clinic® article references*
- ✓ *New code/Revised code*
- ✓ *PQRS code*

To order call 1-800-508-2582
or visit (https://www.codinginstitute.com/books/hcpcs-level-ii-advisor.html)

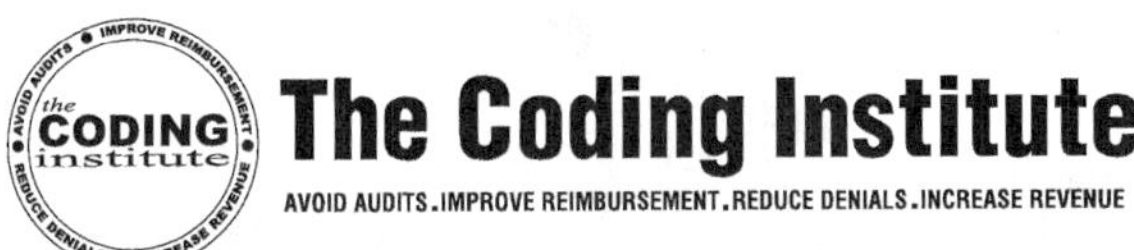

Call us: 800-508-2582 | www.codinginstitute.com
The Coding Institute LLC
2222 Sedwick Drive Durham, NC 27713

AMA CPT® PROFESSIONAL EDITION 2017

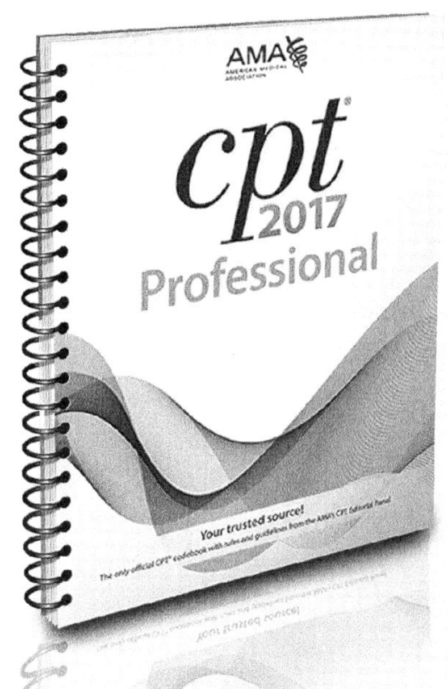

Complete CPT® Code Details to Help You Correctly Report and Bill Procedures and Services in 2017.

Rely on the most updated ***AMA CPT® Professional Edition*** to guide you to accurate reporting of your 2017 claims. This AMA-authored resource covers the official 2017 CPT® coding rules and guidelines and all of the updated code/guideline/text changes.

The AMA guide includes:

- ✓ Summary of new and revised CPT® code changes for 2017 – no need to look up previous editions
- ✓ Reliable cross-reference guidance on *CPT® code usage from* ***CPT® Assistant, CPT® Changes, Clinical Examples in Radiology Citations***, and more
- ✓ Tabular listing of most analytes in the pathology and lab section to simplify your code search – Find more relevant molecular pathology codes based on a specific analyte
- ✓ More granularity in molecular pathology that enhances your ability to report the correct code for a lab procedure
- ✓ Detailed index that helps in quickly locating codes related to a specific procedure, service, anatomic site, condition, synonym, and more
- ✓ Clear illustrations to enhance your coding accuracy and understanding of the anatomy and procedures under consideration
- ✓ Valuable coding tips in each section to boost your understanding of the intricacies of the code set
- ✓ Enhanced table of contents that allows you to conduct a quick search of the manual without being in a specific section
- ✓ Additional information – Get key insight on topics such as modifiers, add-on codes, clinical examples, and vascular families
- ✓ Supplemental information of multianalyte assays with algorithmic analyses – gets you an administrative code set of single-sourced tests

To order call 1-800-508-2582
or visit (https://www.codinginstitute.com/books/ama-cpt-professional-edition.html)

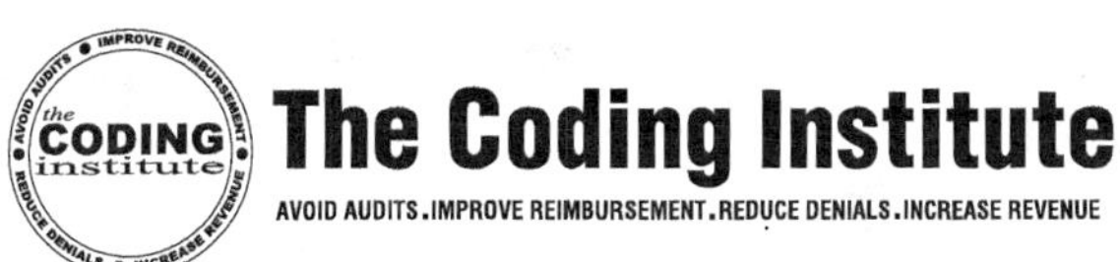

Call us: 800-508-2582 | www.codinginstitute.com
The Coding Institute LLC
2222 Sedwick Drive Durham, NC 27713

Modifier Coding Handbook Bundle

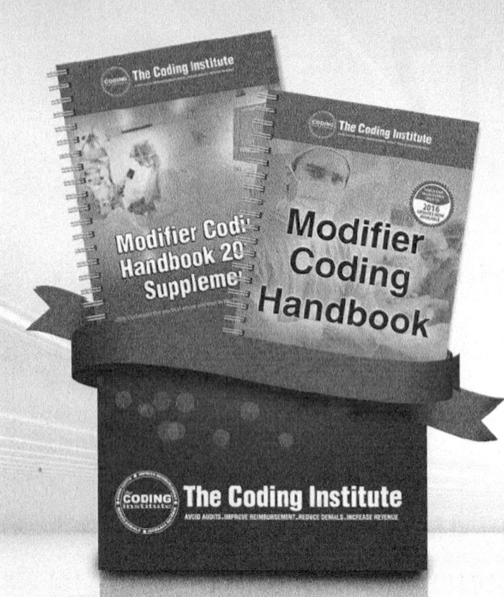

You're Go-to Source for All Your Modifier Coding Needs: HCPCS, Lab, E/M, Surgical, Anesthesia & More.

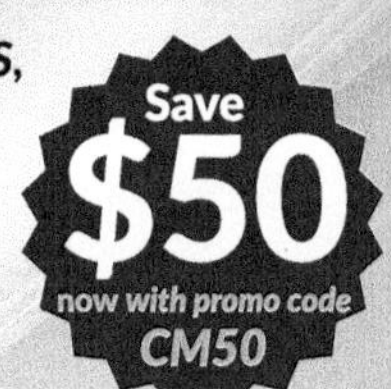

Don't make the crucial mistake of assigning the wrong modifiers to CPT® and HCPCS codes. Clear up modifier confusion to avoid claim denials and partial payments, and earn the reimbursement you deserve.

Are you wondering how to use E/M modifiers 24, 25, or 27, when to assign 33 for screenings, or the differences between 51 or 59? Are you hoping to capture more reimbursement for modifier 22? Do you know when to use assistant surgeon modifiers 80, 81, and 82?

The ***Modifier Coding Handbook*** has all the answers you need! Brought to you by The Coding Institute, our how-to modifier guide is packed with critical information you need to decide when to use specific modifiers. Plus you'll get expert answers to common readers' questions and learn how to assign the most challenging modifiers.

Here are some of the hot topics included in the *Modifier Coding Handbook:*

- ✓ Look for opportunities to use X modifiers in place of 59
- ✓ Surprise! Modifier 59 for repeat procedures may not fly
- ✓ Brush up on 5 coronary modifiers
- ✓ Use severity modifiers with physiotherapy treatment to complete coding
- ✓ Reduce denials with correct use of modifier 50
- ✓ Dispel 5 modifier 24 myths
- ✓ Replace confusion with expertise when using modifier 57
- ✓ Explore these modifier 78 possibilities when addressing surgical complications
- ✓ Use this 4 step plan to justify reporting modifier 23
- ✓ Recognize 2 lab modifiers to capture same-day test payment
- ✓ Grab modifier GG for mammogram screening and diagnostic in same day

That's not all! To help you keep abreast of the latest modifier changes, we have an all-new **2016 Supplement** for your **Modifier Coding handbook,** which comes with over 30 articles and readers' questions covering the ins and outs of using E/M modifiers for postop and prolonged services, decisions for surgery, team surgeries, and multiple outpatient E/M services. Find out when to report the modifier for mandated services and the latest news on reporting modifiers for radiology and lab.

Check out some of the hot topics in **2016 Supplement:**

- ✓ Use modifier 27 on multiple outpatient E/Ms
- ✓ CPT® 2016: Learn new prolonged services codes, and master 'team' coding
- ✓ Coding return E/Ms for similar injuries
- ✓ Multiple procedures: Focus on debridement types before adding 59
- ✓ Consider finger/toe, 51 modifiers when provider fixes cut, or splints finger
- ✓ Flu testing: Include 59 when providers test for 2 flu strains
- ✓ HCPCS modifiers new for 2016
- ✓ Put post-op surgeries into focus with 78, 79
- ✓ Catastrophe/disasters: Prepare for the worst with modifier CR smarts
- ✓ Note new POS to nail 'off-campus' coding
- ✓ And much more

Simplify modifier use and stay on track for correct reimbursement in 2016 using our comprehensive ***Modifier Coding Handbook.***

To order call 1-800-508-2582
or visit (https://www.codinginstitute.com/books/2016-modifier-coding-handbook-bundle.html)

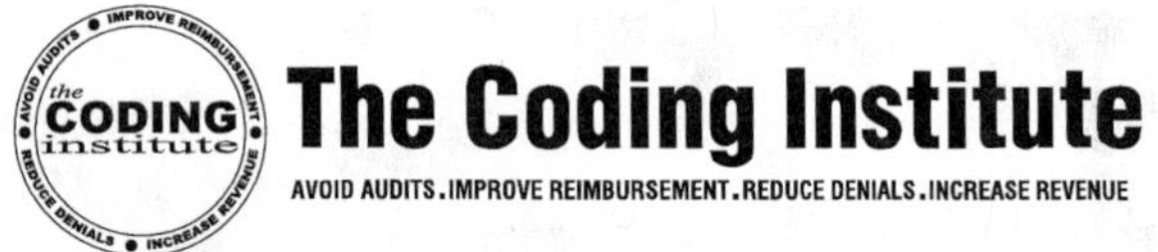

Call us: 800-508-2582 | www.codinginstitute.com
The Coding Institute LLC
2222 Sedwick Drive Durham, NC 27713

2017 ICD~10~CM For Physicians and Hospitals

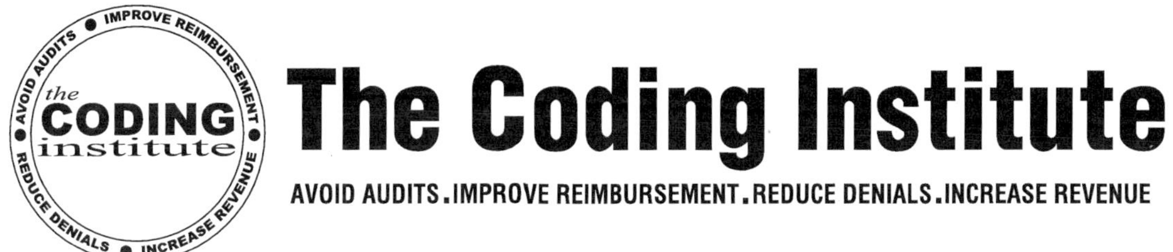

PUBLISHER'S NOTICE

Coding, billing, and reimbursement decisions should not be made based solely upon information within this book. Application of the information in this book does not imply or guarantee claims payment. Inquiries of your local carrier(s)' bulletins, policy announcements, etc., should be made to resolve local billing requirements. Finally, the law, applicable regulations, payers' instructions, interpretations, enforcement, etc., of the codes in this book may change at any time in any particular area. Information in this book is solely based on coding rules and regulations.

Codes in this book are designed to be an accurate and authoritative source regarding coding, and every reasonable effort has been made to ensure accuracy and completeness of content. However, the publisher makes no guarantee, warranty, or representation that this publication is complete, accurate, or without errors. It is understood that the publisher is not rendering any legal or professional services or advice in this code book and bears no liability for any results or consequences arising from use of this book.

This book contains IPPS FY 2017 proposed rule data for CMS which was the latest information available at the time of printing. Visit the CMS website at www.cms.gov for further updates.

THE PUBLISHER'S COMMITMENT TO ACCURACY

The publisher is committed to providing you with accurate and reliable materials. However, codes and the guidelines by which they are applied change or are reinterpreted through the year. Check www.SuperCoder.com periodically for updates. To report corrections and updates, please contact TCI Customer Service via 1-800-508-2582 or via email to service@codinginstitute.com.

Images/Illustrations by the following artists at shutterstock.com
miucci - 119473492 | ducu59us - 104022683, 125200733 | Alila Medical Media - 228843262, 155445686, 101696095, 96426923, 97755608, 97755611, 147943922, 125899358, 147943910, 155445662, 147943874, 108567068, 106263593, 106263560 | BlueRingMedia - 141162229, 141161560, 141161404 , 149006000, 145028440 | snapgalleria - 142194094 | okili77 - 156466463 | Designua - 180938618, 135935735, 186535475, 165084413 | stockshoppe - 99671552, 180896807, 180896810, 187162247, 187162193, 187162175, 187162163, 187162142, 187162118, 187162106, 187162070, 180896873, 180896855, 180896738, 180896720, 177791516, 177790997 | lotan - 186878060 | sciencepics - 199873508| Blamb - 24129706 | joshya - 226909492, 261971498 | Della_Liner - 324447776 | Marochkina Anastasiia - 414103342 | Alexander_P - 404964388

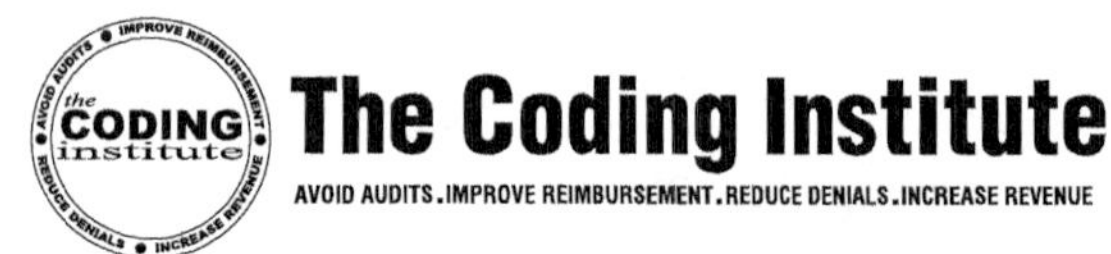

ISBN: 978-1-63012-921-7

Table of Contents
ICD-10-CM for Physicians and Hospitals

Preface

ICD-10-CM Official Preface

This FY 2017 update of the International Statistical Classification of Diseases and Related Health Problems, 10th revision, Clinical Modification (ICD-10-CM) is being published by the United States Government in recognition of its responsibility to promulgate this classification throughout the United States for morbidity coding. The International Statistical Classification of Diseases and Related Health Problems, 10th Revision (ICD-10), published by the World Health Organization (WHO), is the foundation of ICD-10-CM. ICD-10 continues to be the classification used in cause-of-death coding in the United States. The ICD-10-CM is comparable with the ICD-10. The WHO Collaborating Center for the Family of International Classifications in North America, housed at the Centers for Disease Control and Prevention's National Center for Health Statistics (NCHS), has responsibility for the implementation of ICD and other WHO-FIC classifications and serves as a liaison with the WHO, fulfilling international obligations for comparable classifications and the national health data needs of the United States. The historical background of ICD and ICD-10 can be found in the Introduction to the International Classification of Diseases and Related Health Problems (ICD-10), 2010, World Health Organization, Geneva, Switzerland.

ICD-10-CM is the United States' clinical modification of the World Health Organization's ICD-10. The term "clinical" is used to emphasize the modification's intent: to serve as a useful tool in the area of classification of morbidity data for indexing of health records, medical care review, and ambulatory and other health care programs, as well as for basic health statistics. To describe the clinical picture of the patient the codes must be more precise than those needed only for statistical groupings and trend analysis.

Characteristics of ICD-10-CM

ICD-10-CM far exceeds its predecessors in the number of concepts and codes provided. The disease classification has been expanded to include health-related conditions and to provide greater specificity at the sixth and seventh character level.

The sixth and seventh characters are not optional and are intended for use in recording the information documented in the clinical record. ICD-10-CM extensions, interpretations, modifications, addenda, or errata other than those approved by the Centers for Disease Control and Prevention are not to be considered official and should not be utilized. Continuous maintenance of the ICD-10-CM is the responsibility of the aforementioned agencies. However, because the ICD-10-CM represents the best in contemporary thinking of clinicians, nosologists, epidemiologists, and statisticians from both public and private sectors, when future modifications are considered, advice will be sought from all stakeholders. All official authorized addenda since the last complete update (October 1, 2013) have been included in this revision. For more detailed information please see the complete official authorized addenda to ICD-10-CM, including the "ICD-10-CM Official Guidelines for Coding and Reporting," and a description of the ICD-10-CM updating and maintenance process.

2017 ICD-10-CM for Physicians and Hospitals

This *2017 ICD-10-CM for Physicians and Hospitals* edition includes the following features, designed in consultation with coding consultants and ICD-10 trainers, to provide a comprehensive and easy-to-use reference manual:

- A table of contents page
- The complete 2017 ICD-10-CM code set
- Full code descriptions
- Special color coding throughout to highlight instructional notes, bilateral and unilateral indicators, and other features
- Color coding and symbols for Medicare code edits to highlight age, sex, manifestation, other specified and unspecified codes
- Illustrations at the beginning of the book and throughout the Tabular List
- ICD-10-CM conventions
- ICD-10-CM Official Coding Guidelines
- Official Index to Diseases and Injuries
- Official Index to External Causes of Injuries
- Table of Drugs and Chemicals
- Table of Neoplasms
- Extension "X" alert symbol to alert readers to the ICD-10-CM placeholder "x" convention
- Anatomy and physiology for various body systems, including illustrations and pathologies
- Trimester icon for applicable codes

List of Features

ICD-10-CM is essential to documenting medical necessity for services rendered, and accurate codes mean better outcomes for the patient, your claims, and your practice or facility.

Count on this manual to help you choose and report the right ICD-10-CM code. Unique features, intuitive design, and expert features that coders developed assure this manual will keep your coding on target.

This manual includes the ICD-10-CM complete code set for 2017, including the Tabular List, Alphabetic Index to Diseases and Injuries, Table of Neoplasms, Table of Drugs and Chemicals, and Index to External Causes of Injuries, effective October 1, 2016.

To help you make the most of *2017 ICD-10-CM for Physicians and Hospitals*, this manual also includes the following features:

- ICD-10-CM Official Guidelines for Coding and Reporting for FY 2017. Visit the CMS website at www.cms.gov for further updates. The Health Insurance Portability and Accountability Act (HIPAA) requires all entities assigning ICD-10-CM codes to follow these guidelines.
- Summaries before each chapter of the relevant ICD-10-CM Official Guidelines in easy-to-understand lay language
- Anatomy and physiology descriptions before Tabular List chapters containing codes pertaining to specific body anatomy
- Full illustrations of body systems at the front of the book so you don't have to search the manual for these large color images of body systems
- Illustrations of anatomy and conditions throughout the Tabular List to help you to better understand how to assign specific codes
- AHA's *Coding Clinic®* article references
- Symbols indicating "Additional character required" so you know when a code requires an additional character for code specificity and validity (provided in both the Alphabetic Index and Tabular List)
- Age and sex edits showing which codes have restrictions on use based on age or sex of the patient
- Highlighted coding instructional and informational notes help you recognize important code usage guidance for specific sections including Includes, Excludes1, and Excludes2 notes
- Z code as first-listed diagnosis symbol to alert you when you can only assign a Z code as the first-listed diagnosis
- Intuitive color-coded symbols and alerts identify critical coding and reimbursement issues quickly, such as "Other Specified" and "Unspecified" diagnosis alerts
- Manifestation code alerts so you properly use codes that represent manifestations of an underlying disease and know when you must use two codes
- A user-friendly page design, including dictionary-style headers, color bleed tabs, and legend keys
- Key word green font is used to differentiate key words that appear in similar code descriptions in a given category.
- Symbols indicating new code, revised code, or revised text

Practical Steps for Using the ICD-10-CM Manual

This manual includes the diagnosis code set from the International Classification of Diseases, Tenth Revision, Clinical Modification (ICD-10-CM) 2017.

Understand Code Structure to Choose the Most Specific Code

ICD-10-CM codes are made up of a minimum of three characters and a maximum of seven characters:

- Character 1 – capital letter A-Z, except the letter U, which is not used
- Character 2 – number
- Character 3 – number
- Character 4 – number or letter – capital or lowercase
- Character 5 – number or letter – capital or lowercase
- Character 6 – number or letter – capital or lowercase
- Character 7 – number or letter – capital or lowercase; character 7 is only used in specific chapters, including pregnancy, musculoskeletal, injuries, and external causes of morbidity

Each Tabular List chapter is divided into subchapters, which are also called blocks. Subchapters are divided into groups of categories (3 characters).

Subchapters are divided into:

Categories (3 characters) – Represents one disease or a group of diseases or related conditions. If a category does not have a further subdivision, it is called a code.

Categories are divided into:

Subcategories (4-5 characters) – Represents greater specificity of one disease or a group of diseases.

Subcategories are divided into:

Codes (4-7 characters) – Codes are the final level which cannot be subdivided further. Codes that are 7 characters are always called "codes" because 7 is the maximum number of characters in a code.

Review the ICD-10-CM Volumes Included in This Manual

This manual includes:

- Tabular List, includes diagnosis codes in numerical order and their official descriptors in 21 chapters
- Alphabetic Index, includes three sections:
  - o Index to Diseases and Injuries, which you'll use to search for the vast majority of codes
  - o Two tables you'll find at the end of the Index to Diseases:
    - Table of Neoplasms
    - Table of Drugs and Chemicals
  - o Alphabetic Index to External Cause of Injuries

This manual follows the industry standard of placing the Alphabetic Index before the Tabular List because when you search for a code, you should always check the Index first to make a preliminary code choice and then check the Tabular List for confirmation.

Code Diagnoses With Confidence Following This Approach

➢ The first step in choosing the proper ICD-10-CM code is reading the medical documentation to identify the diagnosis the provider documents and confirms. If there is no confirmed diagnosis, look for the sign or symptom that brought the patient in or other reason for the encounter.

- Be sure to check online or hard copy references, such as medical dictionaries and anatomy resources to look up unfamiliar terms.

➢ Next, decide which main term you will search in the Index based on the patient's specific case. ICD-10-CM doesn't use body sites as main terms. Instead, look for the disease, sign, symptom, etc. You can find the body site as a subterm. For neoplasm diagnoses, review the Table of Neoplasms for the appropriate diagnosis. Search for the neoplasm histology as a main term (carcinoma, leukemia, glioblastoma) and the body site as a subterm. The histology will take you to a code to cross-reference to the Tabular or direct you to the Table of Neoplasms. If you cannot find the histology as a main term, or cannot find a code to cross-reference for the histology and body site, then go directly to the Table of Neoplasms to search for the body site of the neoplasm. You will also need to go directly to the Table of Neoplasms if the provider does not document the histology..

➢ Once you find the main term in the Index, note the recommended code. Start with the main term and review any available subterms. Also note whether the Index offers any other clues to proper coding, such as the need for additional characters or the need for an additional code.

➢ Turn to that code in the Tabular List, and read the full code descriptor. Keep in mind that you may need to read the subcategory and category titles as well as the code descriptor to get the full meaning of the code.

➢ Check to see whether ICD-10-CM requires additional characters for that code. If so, review the code definitions of any available categories and subcategories.

- Remember, if a code has seven characters available, you must report all seven characters, both to comply with coding rules and to prevent insurers from denying your claim. Similarly, if a code has four characters, with no fifth character available, you must report all four characters rather than a three-character code. This manual will alert you to the need for an additional character using easily identifiable symbols.

➢ If the Index points you to a code that includes the terms other, unspecified, NOS (not otherwise specified), or NEC (not elsewhere classifiable), double check that a more specific code isn't available. Always report the most specific code the medical record supports.

➢ Before making your final code decision, review all applicable notes and instructions to be sure they don't affect your choice. You'll find these notes and instructions on every level, from the chapter to the code itself. You will find many notes highlighted and color coded for easy reference in the Tabular List. You can find the meaning of the highlights in the legend at the bottom of each page in the Tabular List. Also review the surrounding codes to be sure there isn't a more appropriate code available.

➢ Finally, take a moment to confirm that your code choice complies with the philosophy of ethical coding. Never report an ICD-10-CM code simply because it will support reimbursement from a payer. Report only those codes the documentation supports.

Factor In the Other Resources in This Manual

In addition to the Alphabetic Index and Tabular List, you'll find the following materials in this manual:

Conventions Specific to This ICD-10-CM Manual: To be sure you make the most of all of the resources and instructional symbols this manual includes, read this section.

ICD-10-CM Official Guidelines for Coding and Reporting: No coder should let a year go by without reviewing the Official Guidelines. These authoritative rules provide many instructions not available in the Tabular List.

Additional Content in Tabular List Chapters: At the beginning of specific Tabular List chapters, you'll find anatomy descriptions and a useful breakdown of the relevant Official Guidelines specific to codes in that chapter.

ICD-10-CM Official Conventions

The conventions for the ICD-10-CM are the general rules for use of the classification independent of the guidelines. These conventions are incorporated within the Alphabetic Index and Tabular List of the ICD-10-CM as instructional notes.

Format and Structure

The ICD-10-CM Tabular List contains categories, subcategories and codes. Characters for categories, subcategories and codes may be either a letter or a number. All categories are 3 characters. A three-character category that has no further subdivision is equivalent to a code. Subcategories are either 4 or 5 characters. Codes may be 3, 4, 5, 6 or 7 characters. That is, each level of subdivision after a category is a subcategory. The final level of subdivision is a code. Codes that have applicable 7th characters are still referred to as codes, not subcategories. A code that has an applicable 7th character is considered invalid without the 7th character.

The ICD-10-CM uses an indented format for ease in reference.

Codes for reporting purposes

For reporting purposes only codes are permissible, not categories or subcategories, and any applicable 7th character is required.

Placeholder Character

The ICD-10-CM utilizes a placeholder character "X". The "X" is used as a placeholder at certain codes to allow for future expansion. An example of this is at the poisoning, adverse effect and underdosing codes, categories T36-T50.

Where a placeholder exists, the X must be used in order for the code to be considered a valid code.

7th Characters

Certain ICD-10-CM categories have applicable 7th characters. The applicable 7th character is required for all codes within the category, or as the notes in the Tabular List instruct. The 7th character must always be the 7th character in the data field. If a code that requires a 7th character is not 6 characters, a placeholder X must be used to fill in the empty characters.

Abbreviations

a. Alphabetic Index abbreviations

NEC "Not elsewhere classifiable"

This abbreviation in the Alphabetic Index represents "other specified". When a specific code is not available for a condition, the Alphabetic Index directs the coder to the "other specified" code in the Tabular List.

NOS "Not otherwise specified"

This abbreviation is the equivalent of unspecified.

b. Tabular List abbreviations

NEC "Not elsewhere classifiable"

This abbreviation in the Tabular List represents "other specified". When a specific code is not available for a condition the Tabular List includes an NEC entry under a code to identify the code as the "other specified" code.

NOS "Not otherwise specified"

This abbreviation is the equivalent of unspecified.

Punctuation

[ ] Brackets are used in the Tabular List to enclose synonyms, alternative wording or explanatory phrases. Brackets are used in the Alphabetic Index to identify manifestation codes.

( ) Parentheses are used in both the Alphabetic Index and Tabular List to enclose supplementary words that may be present or absent in the statement of a disease or procedure without affecting the code number to which it is assigned. The terms within the parentheses are referred to as nonessential modifiers.

: Colons are used in the Tabular List after an incomplete term which needs one or more of the modifiers following the colon to make it assignable to a given category.

Notes

Other and Unspecified codes

a. "Other" codes

Codes titled "other" or "other specified" are for use when the information in the medical record provides detail for which a specific code does not exist. Alphabetic Index entries with NEC in the line designate "other" codes in the Tabular List. These Alphabetic Index entries represent specific disease entities for which no specific code exists so the term is included within an "other" code.

b. "Unspecified" codes

Codes titled "unspecified" are for use when the information in the medical record is insufficient to assign a more specific code. For those categories for which an unspecified code is not provided, the "other specified" code may represent both other and unspecified.

Includes Notes

This note appears immediately under a three character code title to further define, or give examples of, the content of the category.

Inclusion Terms

A list of terms is included under some codes. These terms are the conditions for which that code is to be used. The terms may be synonyms of the code title, or, in the case of "other specified" codes, the terms are a list of the various conditions assigned to that code. The inclusion terms are not necessarily exhaustive. Additional terms found only in the Alphabetic Index may also be assigned to a code.

Excludes Notes

The ICD-10-CM has two types of excludes notes. Each type of note has a different definition for use but they are all similar in that they indicate that codes excluded from each other are independent of each other.

a. **Excludes1**

   A type 1 Excludes note is a pure excludes note. It means "NOT CODED HERE!" An Excludes1 note indicates that the code excluded should never be used at the same time as the code above the Excludes1 note. An Excludes1 is used when two conditions cannot occur together, such as a congenital form versus an acquired form of the same condition.

b. **Excludes2**

   A type 2 Excludes note represents "Not included here". An Excludes2 note indicates that the condition excluded is not part of the condition represented by the code, but a patient may have both conditions at the same time. When an Excludes2 note appears under a code, it is acceptable to use both the code and the excluded code together, when appropriate.

Etiology/Manifestation Codes

Etiology/manifestation convention ("code first", "use additional code" and "in diseases classified elsewhere" notes)

Certain conditions have both an underlying etiology and multiple body system manifestations due to the underlying etiology. For such conditions, the ICD-10-CM has a coding convention that requires the underlying condition be sequenced first followed by the manifestation. Wherever such a combination exists, there is a "use additional code" note at the etiology code, and a "code first" note at the manifestation code. These instructional notes indicate the proper sequencing order of the codes, etiology followed by manifestation.

In most cases the manifestation codes will have in the code title, "in diseases classified elsewhere." Codes with this title are a component of the etiology/ manifestation convention. The code title indicates that it is a manifestation code. "In diseases classified elsewhere" codes are never permitted to be used as first-listed or principal diagnosis codes. They must be used in conjunction with an underlying condition code and they must be listed following the underlying condition.

There are manifestation codes that do not have "in diseases classified elsewhere" in the title. For such codes, there is a "use additional code" note at the etiology code and a "code first" note at the manifestation code and the rules for sequencing apply.

In addition to the notes in the Tabular List, these conditions also have a specific Alphabetic Index entry structure. In the Alphabetic Index both conditions are listed together with the etiology code first followed by the manifestation codes in brackets. The code in brackets is always to be sequenced second.

An example of the etiology/manifestation convention is dementia in Parkinson's disease. In the Alphabetic Index, code G20 is listed first, followed by code F02.80 or F02.81 in brackets. Code G20 represents the underlying etiology, Parkinson's disease, and must be sequenced first, whereas codes F02.80 and F02.81 represent the manifestation of dementia in diseases classified elsewhere, with or without behavioral disturbance.

"Code first" and "Use additional code" notes are also used as sequencing rules in the classification for certain codes that are not part of an etiology/ manifestation combination.

And/With/See Also

a. "And"

   The word "and" should be interpreted to mean either "and" or "or" when it appears in a title.

   For example, cases of "tuberculosis of bones", "tuberculosis of joints" and "tuberculosis of bones and joints" are classified to subcategory A18.0, Tuberculosis of bones and joints.

b. "With"

   The word "with" should be interpreted to mean "associated with" or "due to" when it appears in a code title, the Alphabetic Index, or an instructional note in the Tabular List.

   The word "with" in the Alphabetic Index is sequenced immediately following the main term, not in alphabetical order.

c. "See" and "See Also"

   The "see" instruction following a main term in the Alphabetic Index indicates that another term should be referenced. It is necessary to go to the main term referenced with the "see" note to locate the correct code.

   A "see also" instruction following a main term in the Alphabetic Index instructs that there is another main term that may also be referenced that may provide additional Alphabetic Index entries that may be useful. It is not necessary to follow the "see also" note when the original main term provides the necessary code.

Code Also

A "code also" note instructs that two codes may be required to fully describe a condition, but this note does not provide sequencing direction.

Default Codes

A code listed next to a main term in the ICD-10-CM Alphabetic Index is referred to as a default code. The default code represents that condition that is most commonly associated with the main term, or is the unspecified code for the condition. If a condition is documented in a medical record (for example, appendicitis) without any additional information, such as acute or chronic, the default code should be assigned.

Symbols and Conventions

Additional Characters Required

- This red symbol cautions that the code requires an additional fourth character.
- This red symbol cautions that the code requires an additional fifth character.
- This red symbol cautions that the code requires an additional sixth character.
- This red symbol cautions that the code requires an additional seventh character.

Extension "X" Alert

- This blue symbol cautions that the code requires an additional seventh character following the placeholder X.

Medicare Code Edits Symbols and Colors

Code edit symbols and colors in this manual are based on the Medicare Code Editor (MCE) and Medicare's Integrated Outpatient Code Editor (I/OCE). The code edit information in this manual is based on MCE v33 with the addition of FY 2017 Inpatient Prospective Payment System (IPPS) Proposed Rule updates and I/OCE v16.2, the most current information available at the time of printing.

Age Conflict

Medicare's MCE and I/OCE code editors detect inconsistencies between a patient's age and any diagnosis on the patient's record. Examples include: a five-year-old patient with benign prostatic hypertrophy or a 78-year-old patient coded with a delivery.

N Newborn	Age of 0 years; a subset of diagnoses intended only for newborns and neonates (e.g., fetal distress, perinatal jaundice).
P Pediatric	Age range is 0–17 years inclusive (e.g., Reye's syndrome, routine child health exam).
M Maternity	Age range is 12–55 years inclusive (e.g., diabetes in pregnancy, antepartum pulmonary complication).
A Adult	Age range is 18–124 years inclusive (e.g., senile delirium, mature cataract).

Sex Conflict

Medicare's MCE and I/OCE code editors detect inconsistencies between a patient's sex and any diagnosis or procedure on the patient's record. Examples include: a male patient with cervical cancer (diagnosis) or a female patient with a prostatectomy (procedure).

In both instances, the indicated diagnosis or the procedure conflicts with the stated sex of the patient. Therefore, either the patient's diagnosis, procedure or sex is presumed to be incorrect.

- ♂ Male code symbol
- ♀ Female code symbol

Manifestation Codes

The code description is highlighted with a light blue color. Manifestation codes describe the manifestation of an underlying disease, not the disease itself, and therefore should not be used as a primary diagnosis.

Other Symbols and Color Coding

Key Terms

Bold green font is used in code descriptions throughout the Tabular List to quickly identify key terms in a given category.

Other Specified Codes

The code description is highlighted with gray color. These codes are assigned when the documentation indicates a specified diagnosis, but the ICD-10-CM code set does not have a specific code that describes the condition.

Unspecified Codes

The code description is highlighted with yellow color. These codes are assigned when neither the diagnostic statement nor the documentation provides enough information to assign a more specific code.

Sequencing, Admission, Complication, and Comorbidity

When relevant, you'll see the following symbols to the right of the code descriptor:

PDx	Unacceptable principal diagnosis; based on Medicare code edits
POA	Code exempt from diagnosis present on admission requirement; based on ICD-10-CM Official Guidelines
CC	Complication or comorbidity; based on CMS data
MCC	Major complication or comorbidity; based on CMS data
CC/MCC Exc	Complications or comorbidities/Major complications or comorbidities (CC/MCC) exclusions; based on CMS data
HAC	Hospital-acquired condition; based on CMS data
PDx CC	Principal diagnosis as its own complication or comorbidity; based on CMS data
PDx MCC	Principal diagnosis as its own major complication or comorbidity; based on CMS data
?	Questionable admission when used as principal diagnosis symbol; based on Medicare code edits

Z Code as First-listed Diagnosis

Certain codes may only be reported as the primary/first-listed diagnosis, except when there are multiple encounters on the same day and the medical records for the encounters are combined.

EXCLUDES 1 Not coded here
Excludes1 notes are highlighted in black to alert you to NEVER assign codes listed under Excludes1 along with the code that you cross-referenced.

EXCLUDES 2 Not included here
Excludes2 notes are highlighted in gray to alert you that you most likely will not assign codes listed under Excludes2 along with the code that you cross-referenced. However, you could assign both an Excludes2 code with the cross-referenced code, as long as the provider documents both conditions.

INCLUDES The word "Includes" appears immediately under certain categories to further define, or give examples of, the content of the category

1st The 1st trimester symbol appears with applicable codes that apply to the first trimester.

2nd The 2nd trimester symbol appears with applicable codes that apply to the second trimester.

3rd 3rd trimester symbol appears with applicable codes that apply to the third trimester.

● New Code The new code symbol appears with a code that is new for the current year.

▲ Revised Code Title A revised code title symbol appears with a code title that is revised for the current year.

►◄ Revised Text The revised text facing triangles symbol appears before and after text that is revised for the current year.

Citations to AHA's Coding Clinic® for ICD-10-CM

AHA's Coding Clinic®, a quarterly newsletter, is the official publication for coding guidelines and advice as designated by the four Cooperating Parties (American Hospital Association, American Health Information Management Association, Centers for Medicare and Medicaid Services (CMS), and National Center for Health Statistics) and the Editorial Advisory Board.

AHA We've marked codes with related *Coding Clinic®* articles with a citation that includes the quarter and year of the issue.

This page intentionally left blank

ICD-10-CM Official Guidelines for Coding and Reporting FY 2017

Narrative changes appear in **bold** text

Items underlined have been moved within the guidelines since the FY 2016 version

Italics are used to indicate revisions to heading changes

The Centers for Medicare and Medicaid Services (CMS) and the National Center for Health Statistics (NCHS), two departments within the U.S. Federal Government's Department of Health and Human Services (DHHS) provide the following guidelines for coding and reporting using the International Classification of Diseases, 10th Revision, Clinical Modification (ICD-10-CM). These guidelines should be used as a companion document to the official version of the ICD-10- CM as published on the NCHS website. The ICD-10-CM is a morbidity classification published by the United States for classifying diagnoses and reason for visits in all health care settings. The ICD-10-CM is based on the ICD-10, the statistical classification of disease published by the World Health Organization (WHO).

These guidelines have been approved by the four organizations that make up the Cooperating Parties for the ICD-10-CM: the American Hospital Association (AHA), the American Health Information Management Association (AHIMA), CMS, and NCHS.

These guidelines are a set of rules that have been developed to accompany and complement the official conventions and instructions provided within the ICD-10-CM itself. The instructions and conventions of the classification take precedence over guidelines. These guidelines are based on the coding and sequencing instructions in the Tabular List and Alphabetic Index of ICD-10-CM, but provide additional instruction. Adherence to these guidelines when assigning ICD-10-CM diagnosis codes is required under the Health Insurance Portability and Accountability Act (HIPAA). The diagnosis codes (Tabular List and Alphabetic Index) have been adopted under HIPAA for all healthcare settings. A joint effort between the healthcare provider and the coder is essential to achieve complete and accurate documentation, code assignment, and reporting of diagnoses and procedures. These guidelines have been developed to assist both the healthcare provider and the coder in identifying those diagnoses that are to be reported. The importance of consistent, complete documentation in the medical record cannot be overemphasized. Without such documentation accurate coding cannot be achieved. The entire record should be reviewed to determine the specific reason for the encounter and the conditions treated.

The term encounter is used for all settings, including hospital admissions. In the context of these guidelines, the term provider is used throughout the guidelines to mean physician or any qualified health care practitioner who is legally accountable for establishing the patient's diagnosis. Only this set of guidelines, approved by the Cooperating Parties, is official.

The guidelines are organized into sections. Section I includes the structure and conventions of the classification and general guidelines that apply to the entire classification, and chapter-specific guidelines that correspond to the chapters as they are arranged in the classification. Section II includes guidelines for selection of principal diagnosis for non-outpatient settings. Section III includes guidelines for reporting additional diagnoses in non-outpatient settings. Section IV is for outpatient coding and reporting. It is necessary to review all sections of the guidelines to fully understand all of the rules and instructions needed to code properly.

Section I. Conventions, general coding guidelines and chapter specific guidelines

The conventions, general guidelines and chapter-specific guidelines are applicable to all health care settings unless otherwise indicated. The conventions and instructions of the classification take precedence over guidelines.

A. Conventions for the ICD-10-CM

The conventions for the ICD-10-CM are the general rules for use of the classification independent of the guidelines. These conventions are incorporated within the Alphabetic Index and Tabular List of the ICD-10-CM as instructional notes.

1. The Alphabetic Index and Tabular List

The ICD-10-CM is divided into the Alphabetic Index, an alphabetical list of terms and their corresponding code, and the Tabular List, a structured list of codes divided into chapters based on body system or condition. The Alphabetic Index consists of the following parts: the Index of Diseases and Injury, the Index of External Causes of Injury, the Table of Neoplasms and the Table of Drugs and Chemicals.

See Section I.C2. General guidelines

See Section I.C.19. Adverse effects, poisoning, underdosing and toxic effects

2. Format and Structure

The ICD-10-CM Tabular List contains categories, subcategories and codes. Characters for categories, subcategories and codes may be either a letter or a number. All categories are 3 characters. A three-character category that has no further subdivision is equivalent to a code. Subcategories are either 4 or 5 characters. Codes may be 3, 4, 5, 6 or 7 characters. That is, each level of subdivision after a category is a subcategory. The final level of subdivision is a code. Codes that have applicable 7th characters are still referred to as codes, not subcategories. A code that has an applicable 7th character is considered invalid without the 7th character.

The ICD-10-CM uses an indented format for ease in reference.

3. Use of codes for reporting purposes

For reporting purposes only codes are permissible, not categories or subcategories, and any applicable 7th character is required.

4. Placeholder character

The ICD-10-CM utilizes a placeholder character "X". The "X" is used as a placeholder at certain codes to allow for future expansion. An example of this is at the poisoning, adverse effect and underdosing codes, categories T36-T50. Where a placeholder exists, the X must be used in order for the code to be considered a valid code.

5. 7th characters

Certain ICD-10-CM categories have applicable 7th characters. The applicable 7th character is required for all codes within the category, or as the notes in the Tabular List instruct. The 7th character must always be the 7th character in the data field. If a code that requires a 7th character is not 6 characters, a placeholder X must be used to fill in the empty characters.

6. Abbreviations

a. Alphabetic Index abbreviations

NEC "Not elsewhere classifiable"

This abbreviation in the Alphabetic Index represents "other specified." When a specific code is not available for a condition, the Alphabetic Index directs the coder to the "other specified" code in the Tabular List.

NOS "Not otherwise specified"

This abbreviation is the equivalent of unspecified.

b. Tabular List abbreviations

NEC "Not elsewhere classifiable"

This abbreviation in the Tabular List represents "other specified". When a specific code is not available for a condition, the Tabular List includes an NEC entry under a code to identify the code as the "other specified" code.

NOS "Not otherwise specified"

This abbreviation is the equivalent of unspecified.

7. Punctuation

[ ] Brackets are used in the Tabular List to enclose synonyms, alternative wording or explanatory phrases. Brackets are used in the Alphabetic Index to identify manifestation codes.

( ) Parentheses are used in both the Alphabetic Index and Tabular List to enclose supplementary words that may be present or absent in the statement of a disease or procedure without affecting the code number to which it is assigned. The terms within the parentheses are referred to as nonessential modifiers. The nonessential modifiers in the Alphabetic Index to Diseases apply to subterms following a main term except when a nonessential modifier and a subentry are mutually exclusive, the subentry takes precedence. For example, in the ICD-10-CM Alphabetic Index under the main term Enteritis, "acute" is a nonessential modifier and "chronic" is a subentry. In this case, the nonessential modifier "acute" does not apply to the subentry "chronic".

: Colons are used in the Tabular List after an incomplete term which needs one or more of the modifiers following the colon to make it assignable to a given category.

8. Use of "and"

See Section I.A.14. Use of the term "And"

9. Other and Unspecified codes

a. " Other " codes

Codes titled "other" or "other specified" are for use when the information in the medical record provides detail for which a specific code does not exist. Alphabetic Index entries with NEC in the line designate "other" codes in the Tabular List. These Alphabetic Index entries represent specific disease entities for which no specific code exists so the term is included within an "other" code.

b. " Unspecified" codes

Codes titled "unspecified" are for use when the information in the medical record is insufficient to assign a more specific code. For those categories for which an unspecified code is not provided, the "other specified" code may represent both other and unspecified.

See Section I.B.18 Use of Signs/Symptom/Unspecified Codes

10. Includes Notes

This note appears immediately under a three character code title to further define, or give examples of, the content of the category.

11. Inclusion terms

List of terms is included under some codes. These terms are the conditions for which that code is to be used. The terms may be synonyms of the code title, or, in the case of "other specified" codes, the terms are a list of the various conditions assigned to that code. The inclusion terms are not necessarily exhaustive. Additional terms found only in the Alphabetic Index may also be assigned to a code.

12. Excludes Notes

The ICD-10-CM has two types of excludes notes. Each type of note has a different definition for use but they are all similar in that they indicate that codes excluded from each other are independent of each other.

a. Excludes1

A type 1 Excludes note is a pure excludes note. It means "NOT CODED HERE!" An Excludes1 note indicates that the code excluded should never be used at the same time as the code above the Excludes1 note. An Excludes1 is used when two conditions cannot occur together, such as a congenital form versus an acquired form of the same condition.

An exception to the Excludes1 definition is the circumstance when the two conditions are unrelated to each other. If it is not clear whether the two conditions involving an Excludes1 note are related or not, query the provider. For example, code F45.8, Other somatoform disorders, has an Excludes1 note for "sleep related teeth grinding (G47.63)," because "teeth grinding" is an inclusion term under F45.8. Only one of these two codes should be assigned for teeth grinding. However psychogenic dysmenorrhea is also an inclusion term under F45.8, and a patient could have both this condition and sleep related teeth grinding. In this case, the two conditions are clearly unrelated to each other, and so it would be appropriate to report F45.8 and G47.63 together.

b. Excludes2

A type 2 Excludes note represents "Not included here." An excludes2 note indicates that the condition excluded is not part of the condition represented by the code, but a patient may have both conditions at the same time. When an Excludes2 note appears under a code, it is acceptable to use both the code and the excluded code together, when appropriate.

13. Etiology/manifestation convention ("code first", "use additional code" and "in diseases classified elsewhere" notes)

Certain conditions have both an underlying etiology and multiple body system manifestations due to the underlying etiology. For such conditions, the ICD-10-CM has a coding convention that requires the underlying condition be sequenced first, **if applicable,** followed by the manifestation. Wherever such a combination exists, there is a "use additional code" note at the etiology code, and a "code first" note at the manifestation code. These instructional notes indicate the proper sequencing order of the codes, etiology followed by manifestation.

In most cases the manifestation codes will have in the code title, "in diseases classified elsewhere." Codes with this title are a component of the etiology/ manifestation convention. The code title indicates that it is a manifestation code. "In diseases classified elsewhere" codes are never permitted to be used as first-listed or principal diagnosis codes. They must be used in conjunction with an underlying condition code and they must be listed following the underlying condition. See category F02, Dementia in other diseases classified elsewhere, for an example of this convention.

There are manifestation codes that do not have "in diseases classified elsewhere" in the title. For such codes, there is a "use additional code" note at the etiology code and a "code first" note at the manifestation code, and the rules for sequencing apply.

In addition to the notes in the Tabular List, these conditions also have a specific Alphabetic Index entry structure. In the Alphabetic Index both conditions are listed together with the etiology code first followed by the manifestation codes in brackets. The code in brackets is always to be sequenced second.

An example of the etiology/manifestation convention is dementia in Parkinson's disease. In the Alphabetic Index, code G20 is listed first, followed by code F02.80 or F02.81 in brackets. Code G20 represents the underlying etiology, Parkinson's disease, and must be sequenced first, whereas codes F02.80 and F02.81 represent the manifestation of dementia in diseases classified elsewhere, with or without behavioral disturbance.

"Code first" and "Use additional code" notes are also used as sequencing rules in the classification for certain codes that are not part of an etiology/ manifestation combination.

See Section I.B.7. Multiple coding for a single condition.

14. "And"

The word "and" should be interpreted to mean either "and" or "or" when it appears in a title.

For example, cases of "tuberculosis of bones", "tuberculosis of joints" and "tuberculosis of bones and joints" are classified to subcategory A18.0, Tuberculosis of bones and joints.

15. "With"

The word "with" should be interpreted to mean "associated with" or "due to" when it appears in a code title, the Alphabetic Index, or an instructional note in the Tabular List. **The classification presumes a causal relationship between the two conditions linked by these terms in the Alphabetic Index or Tabular List. These conditions should be coded as related even in the absence of provider documentation explicitly linking them, unless the documentation clearly states the conditions are unrelated. For conditions not specifically linked by these relational terms in the classification, provider documentation must link the conditions in order to code them as related.**

The word "with" in the Alphabetic Index is sequenced immediately following the main term, not in alphabetical order.

16. "See" and "See Also"

The "see" instruction following a main term in the Alphabetic Index indicates that another term should be referenced. It is necessary to go to the main term referenced with the "see" note to locate the correct code.

A "see also" instruction following a main term in the Alphabetic Index instructs that there is another main term that may also be referenced that may provide additional Alphabetic Index entries that may be useful. It is not necessary to follow the "see also" note when the original main term provides the necessary code.

17. "Code also" note

A "code also" note instructs that two codes may be required to fully describe a condition, but this note does not provide sequencing direction.

18. Default codes

A code listed next to a main term in the ICD-10-CM Alphabetic Index is referred to as a default code. The default code represents that condition that is most commonly associated with the main term, or is the unspecified code for the condition. If a condition is documented in a medical record (for example, appendicitis) without any additional information, such as acute or chronic, the default code should be assigned.

19. Code assignment and clinical criteria

The assignment of a diagnosis code is based on the provider's diagnostic statement that the condition exists. The provider's statement that the patient has a particular condition is sufficient. Code assignment is not based on clinical criteria used by the provider to establish the diagnosis.

B. General Coding Guidelines

1. Locating a code in the ICD-10-CM

To select a code in the classification that corresponds to a diagnosis or reason for visit documented in a medical record, first locate the term in the Alphabetic Index, and then verify the code in the Tabular List. Read and be guided by instructional notations that appear in both the Alphabetic Index and the Tabular List.

It is essential to use both the Alphabetic Index and Tabular List when locating and assigning a code. The Alphabetic Index does not always provide the full code. Selection of the full code, including laterality and any applicable 7th character can only be done in the Tabular List. A dash (-) at the end of an Alphabetic Index entry indicates that additional characters are required. Even if a dash is not included at the Alphabetic Index entry, it is necessary to refer to the Tabular List to verify that no 7th character is required.

2. Level of Detail in Coding

Diagnosis codes are to be used and reported at their highest number of characters available.

ICD-10-CM diagnosis codes are composed of codes with 3, 4, 5, 6 or 7 characters. Codes with three characters are included in ICD-10-CM as the heading of a category of codes that may be further subdivided by the use of fourth and/or fifth characters and/or sixth characters, which provide greater detail.

A three-character code is to be used only if it is not further subdivided. A code is invalid if it has not been coded to the full number of characters required for that code, including the 7th character, if applicable.

3. Code or codes from A00.0 through T88.9, Z00-Z99.8

The appropriate code or codes from A00.0 through T88.9, Z00-Z99.8 must be used to identify diagnoses, symptoms, conditions, problems, complaints or other reason(s) for the encounter/visit.

4. Signs and symptoms

Codes that describe symptoms and signs, as opposed to diagnoses, are acceptable for reporting purposes when a related definitive diagnosis has not been established (confirmed) by the provider. Chapter 18 of ICD-10-CM, Symptoms, Signs, and Abnormal Clinical and Laboratory Findings, Not Elsewhere Classified (codes R00.0 - R99) contains many, but not all, codes for symptoms.

See Section I.B.18 Use of Signs/Symptom/Unspecified Codes

5. Conditions that are an integral part of a disease process

Signs and symptoms that are associated routinely with a disease process should not be assigned as additional codes, unless otherwise instructed by the classification.

6. Conditions that are not an integral part of a disease process

Additional signs and symptoms that may not be associated routinely with a disease process should be coded when present.

7. Multiple coding for a single condition

In addition to the etiology/manifestation convention that requires two codes to fully describe a single condition that affects multiple body systems, there are other single conditions that also require more than one code. "Use additional code" notes are found in the Tabular List at codes that are not part of an etiology/manifestation pair where a secondary code is useful to fully describe a condition. The sequencing rule is the same as the etiology/manifestation pair, "use additional code" indicates that a secondary code should be added.

For example, for bacterial infections that are not included in chapter 1, a secondary code from category B95, Streptococcus, Staphylococcus, and Enterococcus, as the cause of diseases classified elsewhere, or B96, Other bacterial agents as the cause of diseases classified elsewhere, may be required to identify the bacterial organism causing the infection. A "use additional code" note will normally be found at the infectious disease code, indicating a need for the organism code to be added as a secondary code.

"Code first" notes are also under certain codes that are not specifically manifestation codes but may be due to an underlying cause. When there is a "code first" note and an underlying condition is present, the underlying condition should be sequenced first.

"Code, if applicable, any causal condition first" notes indicate that this code may be assigned as a principal diagnosis when the causal condition is unknown or not applicable. If a causal condition is known, then the code for that condition should be sequenced as the principal or first-listed diagnosis.

Multiple codes may be needed for sequela, complication codes and obstetric codes to more fully describe a condition. See the specific guidelines for these conditions for further instruction.

8. Acute and Chronic Conditions

If the same condition is described as both acute (subacute) and chronic, and separate subentries exist in the Alphabetic Index at the same indentation level, code both and sequence the acute (subacute) code first.

9. Combination Code

A combination code is a single code used to classify:

Two diagnoses, or

A diagnosis with an associated secondary process (manifestation)

A diagnosis with an associated complication

Combination codes are identified by referring to subterm entries in the Alphabetic Index and by reading the inclusion and exclusion notes in the Tabular List.

Assign only the combination code when that code fully identifies the diagnostic conditions involved or when the Alphabetic Index so directs. Multiple coding should not be used when the classification provides a combination code that clearly identifies all of the elements documented in the diagnosis. When the combination code lacks necessary specificity in describing the manifestation or complication, an additional code should be used as a secondary code.

10. Sequela (Late Effects)

A sequela is the residual effect (condition produced) after the acute phase of an illness or injury has terminated. There is no time limit on when a sequela code can be used. The residual may be apparent early, such as in cerebral infarction, or it may occur months or years later, such as that due to a previous injury. Examples of sequela include: scar formation resulting from a burn, deviated septum due to a nasal fracture, and infertility due to tubal occlusion from old tuberculosis. Coding of sequela generally requires two codes sequenced in the following order: the condition or nature of the sequela is sequenced first. The sequela code is sequenced second.

An exception to the above guidelines are those instances where the code for the sequela is followed by a manifestation code identified in the Tabular List and title, or the sequela code has been expanded (at the fourth, fifth or sixth character levels) to include the manifestation(s). The code for the acute phase of an illness or injury that led to the sequela is never used with a code for the late effect.

See Section I.C.9. Sequelae of cerebrovascular disease

See Section I.C.15. Sequelae of complication of pregnancy, childbirth and the puerperium

See Section I.C.19. Application of 7th characters for Chapter 19

11. Impending or Threatened Condition

Code any condition described at the time of discharge as "impending" or "threatened" as follows:

If it did occur, code as confirmed diagnosis.

If it did not occur, reference the Alphabetic Index to determine if the condition has a subentry term for "impending" or "threatened" and also reference main term entries for "Impending" and for "Threatened."

If the subterms are listed, assign the given code.

If the subterms are not listed, code the existing underlying condition(s) and not the condition described as impending or threatened.

12. Reporting Same Diagnosis Code More than Once

Each unique ICD-10-CM diagnosis code may be reported only once for an encounter. This applies to bilateral conditions when there are no distinct codes identifying laterality or two different conditions classified to the same ICD-10- CM diagnosis code.

13. Laterality

Some ICD-10-CM codes indicate laterality, specifying whether the condition occurs on the left, right or is bilateral. If no bilateral code is provided and the condition is bilateral, assign separate codes for both the left and right side. If the side is not identified in the medical record, assign the code for the unspecified side.

When a patient has a bilateral condition and each side is treated during separate encounters, assign the "bilateral" code (as the condition still exists on both sides), including for the encounter to treat the first side. For the second encounter for treatment after one side has previously been treated and the condition no longer exists on that side, assign the appropriate unilateral code for the side where the condition still exists (e.g., cataract surgery performed on each eye in separate encounters). The bilateral code would not be assigned for the subsequent encounter, as the patient no longer has the condition in the previously-treated site. If the treatment on the first side did not completely resolve the condition, then the bilateral code would still be appropriate.

14. Documentation for BMI, *Depth of* Non-pressure ulcers, Pressure Ulcer Stages, Coma Scale, *and NIH Stroke Scale*

For the Body Mass Index (BMI), depth of non-pressure chronic ulcers, pressure ulcer stage, **coma scale, and NIH stroke scale (NIHSS) codes**, code assignment may be based on medical record documentation from clinicians who are not the patient's provider (i.e., physician or other qualified healthcare practitioner legally accountable for establishing the patient's diagnosis), since this information is typically documented by other clinicians involved in the care of the patient (e.g., a dietitian often documents the BMI, a nurse often documents the pressure ulcer stages, **and an emergency medical technician often documents the coma scale**). However, the associated diagnosis (such as overweight, obesity, **acute stroke**, or pressure ulcer) must be documented by the patient's provider. If there is conflicting medical record documentation, either from the same clinician or different clinicians, the patient's attending provider should be queried for clarification.

The BMI, **coma scale, and NIHSS** codes should only be reported as secondary diagnoses.

15. Syndromes

Follow the Alphabetic Index guidance when coding syndromes. In the absence of Alphabetic Index guidance, assign codes for the documented manifestations of the syndrome. Additional codes for manifestations that are not an integral part of the disease process may also be assigned when the condition does not have a unique code.

16. Documentation of Complications of Care

Code assignment is based on the provider's documentation of the relationship between the condition and the care or procedure, **unless otherwise instructed by the classification**. The guideline extends to any complications of care, regardless of the chapter the code is located in. It is important to note that not all conditions that occur during or following medical care or surgery are classified as complications. There must be a cause-and-effect relationship between the care provided and the condition, and an indication in the documentation that it is a complication. Query the provider for clarification, if the complication is not clearly documented.

17. Borderline Diagnosis

If the provider documents a "borderline" diagnosis at the time of discharge, the diagnosis is coded as confirmed, unless the classification provides a specific entry (e.g., borderline diabetes). If a borderline condition has a specific index entry in ICD-10-CM, it should be coded as such. Since borderline conditions are not uncertain diagnoses, no distinction is made between the care setting (inpatient versus outpatient). Whenever the documentation is unclear regarding a borderline condition, coders are encouraged to query for clarification.

18. Use of Sign/Symptom/Unspecified Codes

Sign/symptom and "unspecified" codes have acceptable, even necessary, uses. While specific diagnosis codes should be reported when they are supported by the available medical record documentation and clinical knowledge of the patient's health condition, there are instances when signs/symptoms or unspecified codes are the best choices for accurately reflecting the healthcare encounter. Each healthcare encounter should be coded to the level of certainty known for that encounter.

If a definitive diagnosis has not been established by the end of the encounter, it is appropriate to report codes for sign(s) and/or symptom(s) in lieu of a definitive diagnosis. When sufficient clinical information isn't known or available about a particular health condition to assign a more specific code, it is acceptable to report the appropriate "unspecified" code (e.g., a diagnosis of pneumonia has been determined, but not the specific type). Unspecified codes should be reported when they are the codes that most accurately reflect what is known about the patient's condition at the time of that particular encounter. It would be inappropriate to select a specific code that is not supported by the medical record documentation or conduct medically unnecessary diagnostic testing in order to determine a more specific code.

C. Chapter-Specific Coding Guidelines

In addition to general coding guidelines, there are guidelines for specific diagnoses and/or conditions in the classification. Unless otherwise indicated, these guidelines apply to all health care settings. Please refer to Section II for guidelines on the selection of principal diagnosis.

1. Chapter 1: Certain Infectious and Parasitic Diseases (A00-B99)

a. Human Immunodeficiency Virus (HIV) Infections

1) Code only confirmed cases

Code only confirmed cases of HIV infection/illness. This is an exception to the hospital inpatient guideline Section II, H.

In this context, "confirmation" does not require documentation of positive serology or culture for HIV; the provider's diagnostic statement that the patient is HIV positive, or has an HIV-related illness is sufficient.

2) Selection and sequencing of HIV codes

(a) Patient admitted for HIV-related condition

If a patient is admitted for an HIV-related condition, the principal diagnosis should be B20, Human immunodeficiency virus [HIV] disease followed by additional diagnosis codes for all reported HIV-related conditions.

(b) Patient with HIV disease admitted for unrelated condition

If a patient with HIV disease is admitted for an unrelated condition (such as a traumatic injury), the code for the unrelated condition (e.g., the nature of injury code) should be the principal diagnosis. Other diagnoses would be B20 followed by additional diagnosis codes for all reported HIV-related conditions.

(c) Whether the patient is newly diagnosed

Whether the patient is newly diagnosed or has had previous admissions/encounters for HIV conditions is irrelevant to the sequencing decision.

(d) Asymptomatic human immunodeficiency virus

Z21, Asymptomatic human immunodeficiency virus [HIV] infection status, is to be applied when the patient without any documentation of symptoms is listed as being "HIV positive," "known HIV," "HIV test positive," or similar terminology. Do not use this code if the term "AIDS" is used or if the patient is treated for any HIV-related illness or is described as having any condition(s) resulting from his/her HIV positive status; use B20 in these cases.

(e) Patients with inconclusive HIV serology

Patients with inconclusive HIV serology, but no definitive diagnosis or manifestations of the illness, may be assigned code R75, Inconclusive laboratory evidence of human immunodeficiency virus [HIV].

(f) Previously diagnosed HIV-related illness

Patients with any known prior diagnosis of an HIV-related illness should be coded to B20. Once a patient has developed an HIV-related illness, the patient should always be assigned code B20 on every subsequent admission/encounter. Patients previously diagnosed with any HIV illness (B20) should never be assigned to R75 or Z21, Asymptomatic human immunodeficiency virus [HIV] infection status.

(g) HIV Infection in Pregnancy, Childbirth and the Puerperium

During pregnancy, childbirth or the puerperium, a patient admitted (or presenting for a health care encounter) because of an HIV-related illness should receive a principal diagnosis code of O98.7-, Human immunodeficiency [HIV] disease complicating pregnancy, childbirth and the puerperium, followed by B20 and the code(s) for the HIV-related illness(es). Codes from Chapter 15 always take sequencing priority.

Patients with asymptomatic HIV infection status admitted (or presenting for a health care encounter) during pregnancy, childbirth, or the puerperium should receive codes of O98.7- and Z21.

(h) Encounters for testing for HIV

If a patient is being seen to determine his/her HIV status, use code Z11.4, Encounter for screening for human immunodeficiency virus [HIV]. Use additional codes for any associated high risk behavior.

If a patient with signs or symptoms is being seen for HIV testing, code the signs and symptoms. An additional counseling code Z71.7, Human immunodeficiency virus [HIV] counseling, may be used if counseling is provided during the encounter for the test.

When a patient returns to be informed of his/her HIV test results and the test result is negative, use code Z71.7, Human immunodeficiency virus [HIV] counseling.

If the results are positive, see previous guidelines and assign codes as appropriate.

b. Infectious agents as the cause of diseases classified to other chapters

Certain infections are classified in chapters other than Chapter 1 and no organism is identified as part of the infection code. In these instances, it is necessary to use an additional code from Chapter 1 to identify the organism. A code from category B95, Streptococcus, Staphylococcus, and Enterococcus as the cause of diseases classified to other chapters, B96, Other bacterial agents as the cause of diseases classified to other chapters, or B97, Viral agents as the cause of diseases classified to other chapters, is to be used as an additional code to identify the organism. An instructional note will be found at the infection code advising that an additional organism code is required.

c. Infections resistant to antibiotics

Many bacterial infections are resistant to current antibiotics. It is necessary to identify all infections documented as antibiotic resistant. Assign a code from category Z16, Resistance to antimicrobial drugs, following the infection code only if the infection code does not identify drug resistance.

d. Sepsis, Severe Sepsis, and Septic Shock

1) Coding of Sepsis and Severe Sepsis

(a) Sepsis

For a diagnosis of sepsis, assign the appropriate code for the underlying systemic infection. If the type of infection or causal organism is not further specified, assign code A41.9, Sepsis, unspecified organism.

A code from subcategory R65.2, Severe sepsis, should not be assigned unless severe sepsis or an associated acute organ dysfunction is documented.

(i) Negative or inconclusive blood cultures and sepsis

Negative or inconclusive blood cultures do not preclude a diagnosis of sepsis in patients with clinical evidence of the condition; however, the provider should be queried.

(ii) Urosepsis

The term urosepsis is a nonspecific term. It is not to be considered synonymous with sepsis. It has no default code in the Alphabetic Index.

Should a provider use this term, he/she must be queried for clarification.

(iii) Sepsis with organ dysfunction

If a patient has sepsis and associated acute organ dysfunction or multiple organ dysfunction (MOD), follow the instructions for coding severe sepsis.

(iv) Acute organ dysfunction that is not clearly associated with the sepsis

If a patient has sepsis and an acute organ dysfunction, but the medical record documentation indicates that the acute organ dysfunction is related to a medical condition other than the sepsis, do not assign a code from subcategory R65.2, Severe sepsis. An acute organ dysfunction must be associated with the sepsis in order to assign the severe sepsis code. If the documentation is not clear as to whether an acute organ dysfunction is related to the sepsis or another medical condition, query the provider.

(b) Severe sepsis

The coding of severe sepsis requires a minimum of 2 codes: first a code for the underlying systemic infection, followed by a code from subcategory R65.2, Severe sepsis. If the causal organism is not documented, assign code A41.9, Sepsis, unspecified organism, for the infection. Additional code(s) for the associated acute organ dysfunction are also required.

Due to the complex nature of severe sepsis, some cases may require querying the provider prior to assignment of the codes.

2) Septic shock

(a) Septic shock generally refers to circulatory failure associated with severe sepsis, and therefore, it represents a type of acute organ dysfunction.

For cases of septic shock, the code for the systemic infection should be sequenced first, followed by code R65.21, Severe sepsis with septic shock or code T81.12, Postprocedural septic shock. Any additional codes for the other acute organ dysfunctions should also be assigned. As noted in the sequencing instructions in the Tabular List, the code for septic shock cannot be assigned as a principal diagnosis.

3) Sequencing of severe sepsis

If severe sepsis is present on admission, and meets the definition of principal diagnosis, the underlying systemic infection should be assigned as principal diagnosis followed by the appropriate code from subcategory R65.2 as required by the sequencing rules in the Tabular List. A code from subcategory R65.2 can never be assigned as a principal diagnosis.

When severe sepsis develops during an encounter (it was not present on admission), the underlying systemic infection and the appropriate code from subcategory R65.2 should be assigned as secondary diagnoses.

Severe sepsis may be present on admission, but the diagnosis may not be confirmed until sometime after admission. If the documentation is not clear whether severe sepsis was present on admission, the provider should be queried.

4) Sepsis and severe sepsis with a localized infection

If the reason for admission is both sepsis or severe sepsis and a localized infection, such as pneumonia or cellulitis, a code(s) for the underlying systemic infection should be assigned first and the code for the localized infection should be assigned as a secondary diagnosis. If the patient has severe sepsis, a code from subcategory R65.2 should also be assigned as a secondary diagnosis. If the patient is admitted with a localized infection, such as pneumonia, and sepsis/severe sepsis doesn't develop until after admission, the localized infection should be assigned first, followed by the appropriate sepsis/severe sepsis codes.

5) Sepsis due to a postprocedural infection

(a) Documentation of causal relationship

As with all postprocedural complications, code assignment is based on the provider's documentation of the relationship between the infection and the procedure.

(b) Sepsis due to a postprocedural infection

For such cases, the postprocedural infection code, such as T80.2, Infections following infusion, transfusion, and therapeutic injection, T81.4, Infection following a procedure, T88.0, Infection following immunization, or O86.0, Infection of obstetric surgical wound, should be coded first, followed by the code for the specific infection. If the patient has severe sepsis, the appropriate code from subcategory R65.2 should also be assigned with the additional code(s) for any acute organ dysfunction.

(c) Postprocedural infection and postprocedural septic shock

In cases where a postprocedural infection has occurred and has resulted in severe sepsis the code for the precipitating complication such as code T81.4, Infection following a procedure, or O86.0, Infection of obstetrical surgical wound should be coded first followed by code R65.20, Severe sepsis without septic shock. A code for the systemic infection should also be assigned.

If a postprocedural infection has resulted in postprocedural septic shock, the code for the precipitating complication such as code T81.4, Infection following a procedure, or O86.0, Infection of obstetrical surgical wound should be coded first followed by code T81.12-, Postprocedural septic shock. A code for the systemic infection should also be assigned.

6) Sepsis and severe sepsis associated with a noninfectious process (condition)

In some cases a noninfectious process (condition), such as trauma, may lead to an infection which can result in sepsis or severe sepsis. If sepsis or severe sepsis is documented as associated with a noninfectious condition, such as a burn or serious injury, and this condition meets the definition for principal diagnosis, the code for the noninfectious condition should be sequenced first, followed by the code for the resulting infection. If severe sepsis is present, a code from subcategory R65.2 should also be assigned with any associated organ dysfunction(s) codes. It is not necessary to assign a code from subcategory R65.1, Systemic inflammatory response syndrome (SIRS) of non-infectious origin, for these cases.

If the infection meets the definition of principal diagnosis, it should be sequenced before the non-infectious condition. When both the associated non-infectious condition and the infection meet the definition of principal diagnosis, either may be assigned as principal diagnosis.

Only one code from category R65, Symptoms and signs specifically associated with systemic inflammation and infection, should be assigned. Therefore, when a non-infectious condition leads to an infection resulting in severe sepsis, assign the appropriate code from subcategory R65.2, Severe sepsis. Do not additionally assign a code from subcategory R65.1, Systemic inflammatory response syndrome (SIRS) of non- infectious origin.

See Section I.C.18. SIRS due to non-infectious process

7) Sepsis and septic shock complicating abortion, pregnancy, childbirth, and the puerperium

See Section I.C.15. Sepsis and septic shock complicating abortion, pregnancy, childbirth and the puerperium

8) Newborn sepsis

See Section I.C.16. f. Bacterial sepsis of Newborn

e. Methicillin Resistant *Staphylococcus aureus* (MRSA) Conditions

1) Selection and sequencing of MRSA codes

(a) Combination codes for MRSA infection

When a patient is diagnosed with an infection that is due to methicillin resistant Staphylococcus aureus (MRSA), and that infection has a combination code that includes the causal organism (e.g., sepsis, pneumonia) assign the appropriate combination code for the condition (e.g., code A41.02, Sepsis due to Methicillin resistant Staphylococcus aureus or code J15.212, Pneumonia due to Methicillin resistant Staphylococcus aureus). Do not assign code B95.62, Methicillin resistant Staphylococcus aureus infection as the cause of diseases classified elsewhere, as an additional code, because the combination code includes the type of infection and the MRSA organism. Do not assign a code from subcategory Z16.11, Resistance to penicillins, as an additional diagnosis.

See Section C.1. for instructions on coding and sequencing of sepsis and severe sepsis.

(b) Other codes for MRSA infection

When there is documentation of a current infection (e.g., wound infection, stitch abscess, urinary tract infection) due to MRSA, and that infection does not have a combination code that includes the causal organism, assign the appropriate code to identify the condition along with code B95.62, Methicillin resistant Staphylococcus aureus infection as the cause of diseases classified elsewhere for the MRSA infection. Do not assign a code from subcategory Z16.11, Resistance to penicillins.

(c) Methicillin susceptible Staphylococcus aureus (MSSA) and MRSA colonization

The condition or state of being colonized or carrying MSSA or MRSA is called colonization or carriage, while an individual person is described as being colonized or being a carrier. Colonization means that MSSA or MSRA is present on or in the body without necessarily causing illness. A positive MRSA colonization test might be documented by the provider as "MRSA screen positive" or "MRSA nasal swab positive".

Assign code Z22.322, Carrier or suspected carrier of Methicillin resistant Staphylococcus aureus, for patients documented as having MRSA colonization. Assign code Z22.321, Carrier or suspected carrier of Methicillin susceptible Staphylococcus aureus, for patient documented as having MSSA colonization. Colonization is not necessarily indicative of a disease process or as the cause of a specific condition the patient may have unless documented as such by the provider.

(d) MRSA colonization and infection

If a patient is documented as having both MRSA colonization and infection during a hospital admission, code Z22.322, Carrier or suspected carrier of Methicillin resistant Staphylococcus aureus, and a code for the MRSA infection may both be assigned.

f. Zika virus infections

1) Code only confirmed cases

Code only a confirmed diagnosis of Zika virus (A92.5, Zika virus disease) as documented by the provider. This is an exception to the hospital inpatient guideline Section II, H.

In this context, " confirmation" does not require **documentation of the type of test performed;** the physician' s **diagnostic statement that the condition is confirmed is sufficient. This code should be assigned regardless of the stated mode of transmission.**

If the provider documents "suspected", "possible" or "probable" Zika, do not assign code A92.5. Assign a code(s) explaining the reason for encounter (such as fever, rash, or joint pain) or Z20.828, Contact with and (suspected) exposure to other viral communicable diseases.

2. Chapter 2: Neoplasms (C00-D49)

General guidelines

Chapter 2 of the ICD-10-CM contains the codes for most benign and all malignant neoplasms. Certain benign neoplasms, such as prostatic adenomas, may be found in the specific body system chapters. To properly code a neoplasm it is necessary to determine from the record if the neoplasm is benign, in-situ, malignant, or of uncertain histologic behavior. If malignant, any secondary (metastatic) sites should also be determined.

Primary malignant neoplasms overlapping site boundaries

A primary malignant neoplasm that overlaps two or more contiguous (next to each other) sites should be classified to the subcategory/code .8 ('overlapping lesion'), unless the combination is specifically indexed elsewhere. For multiple neoplasms of the same site that are not contiguous such as tumors in different quadrants of the same breast, codes for each site should be assigned.

Malignant neoplasm of ectopic tissue

Malignant neoplasms of ectopic tissue are to be coded to the site of origin mentioned, e.g., ectopic pancreatic malignant neoplasms involving the stomach are coded to pancreas, unspecified (C25.9).

The neoplasm table in the Alphabetic Index should be referenced first. However, if the histological term is documented, that term should be referenced first, rather than going immediately to the Neoplasm Table, in order to determine which column in the Neoplasm Table is appropriate. For example, if the documentation indicates "adenoma," refer to the term in the Alphabetic Index to review the entries under this term and the instructional note to "see also neoplasm, by site, benign." The table provides the proper code based on the type of neoplasm and the site. It is important to select the proper column in the table that corresponds to the type of neoplasm. The Tabular List should then be referenced to verify that the correct code has been selected from the table and that a more specific site code does not exist.

See Section I.C.21. Factors influencing health status and contact with health services, Status, for information regarding Z15.0, codes for genetic susceptibility to cancer.

a. Treatment directed at the malignancy

If the treatment is directed at the malignancy, designate the malignancy as the principal diagnosis.

The only exception to this guideline is if a patient admission/encounter is solely for the administration of chemotherapy, immunotherapy or radiation therapy, assign the appropriate Z51.-- code as the first-listed or principal diagnosis, and the diagnosis or problem for which the service is being performed as a secondary diagnosis.

b. Treatment of secondary site

When a patient is admitted because of a primary neoplasm with metastasis and treatment is directed toward the secondary site only, the secondary neoplasm is designated as the principal diagnosis even though the primary malignancy is still present.

c. Coding and sequencing of complications

Coding and sequencing of complications associated with the malignancies or with the therapy thereof are subject to the following guidelines:

1) Anemia associated with malignancy

When admission/encounter is for management of an anemia associated with the malignancy, and the treatment is only for anemia, the appropriate code for the malignancy is sequenced as the principal or first-listed diagnosis followed by the appropriate code for the anemia (such as code D63.0, Anemia in neoplastic disease).

2) Anemia associated with chemotherapy, immunotherapy and radiation therapy

When the admission/encounter is for management of an anemia associated with an adverse effect of the administration of chemotherapy or immunotherapy and the only treatment is for the anemia, the anemia code is sequenced first followed by the appropriate codes for the neoplasm and the adverse effect (T45.1X5, Adverse effect of antineoplastic and immunosuppressive drugs).

When the admission/encounter is for management of an anemia associated with an adverse effect of radiotherapy, the anemia code should be sequenced first, followed by the appropriate neoplasm code and code Y84.2, Radiological procedure and radiotherapy as the cause of abnormal reaction of the patient, or of later complication, without mention of misadventure at the time of the procedure.

3) Management of dehydration due to the malignancy

When the admission/encounter is for management of dehydration due to the malignancy and only the dehydration is being treated (intravenous rehydration), the dehydration is sequenced first, followed by the code(s) for the malignancy.

4) Treatment of a complication resulting from a surgical procedure

When the admission/encounter is for treatment of a complication resulting from a surgical procedure, designate the complication as the principal or first-listed diagnosis if treatment is directed at resolving the complication.

d. Primary malignancy previously excised

When a primary malignancy has been previously excised or eradicated from its site and there is no further treatment directed to that site and there is no evidence of any existing primary malignancy, a code from category Z85, Personal history of malignant neoplasm, should be used to indicate the former site of the malignancy. Any mention of extension, invasion, or metastasis to another site is coded as a secondary malignant neoplasm to that site. The secondary site may be the principal or first-listed with the Z85 code used as a secondary code.

e. Admissions/Encounters involving chemotherapy, immunotherapy and radiation therapy

1) Episode of care involves surgical removal of neoplasm

When an episode of care involves the surgical removal of a neoplasm, primary or secondary site, followed by adjunct chemotherapy or radiation treatment during the same episode of care, the code for the neoplasm should be assigned as principal or first-listed diagnosis.

2) Patient admission/encounter solely for administration of chemotherapy, immunotherapy and radiation therapy

If a patient admission/encounter is solely for the administration of chemotherapy, immunotherapy or radiation therapy assign code Z51.0, Encounter for antineoplastic radiation therapy, or Z51.11, Encounter for antineoplastic chemotherapy, or Z51.12, Encounter for antineoplastic immunotherapy as the first-listed or principal diagnosis. If a patient receives more than one of these therapies during the same admission more than one of these codes may be assigned, in any sequence.

The malignancy for which the therapy is being administered should be assigned as a secondary diagnosis.

3) Patient admitted for radiation therapy, chemotherapy or immunotherapy and develops complications

When a patient is admitted for the purpose of radiotherapy, immunotherapy or chemotherapy and develops complications such as uncontrolled nausea and vomiting or dehydration, the principal or first-listed diagnosis is Z51.0, Encounter for antineoplastic radiation therapy, or Z51.11, Encounter for antineoplastic chemotherapy, or Z51.12, Encounter for antineoplastic immunotherapy followed by any codes for the complications.

f. Admission/encounter to determine extent of malignancy

When the reason for admission/encounter is to determine the extent of the malignancy, or for a procedure such as paracentesis or thoracentesis, the primary malignancy or appropriate metastatic site is designated as the principal or first-listed diagnosis, even though chemotherapy or radiotherapy is administered.

g. Symptoms, signs, and abnormal findings listed in Chapter 18 associated with neoplasms

Symptoms, signs, and ill-defined conditions listed in Chapter 18 characteristic of, or associated with, an existing primary or secondary site malignancy cannot be used to replace the malignancy as principal or first-listed diagnosis, regardless of the number of admissions or encounters for treatment and care of the neoplasm.

See section I.C.21. Factors influencing health status and contact with health services, Encounter for prophylactic organ removal.

h. Admission/encounter for pain control/management

See Section I.C.6. for information on coding admission/encounter for pain control/management.

i. Malignancy in two or more noncontiguous sites

A patient may have more than one malignant tumor in the same organ. These tumors may represent different primaries or metastatic disease, depending on the site. Should the documentation be unclear, the provider should be queried as to the status of each tumor so that the correct codes can be assigned.

j. Disseminated malignant neoplasm, unspecified

Code C80.0, Disseminated malignant neoplasm, unspecified, is for use only in those cases where the patient has advanced metastatic disease and no known primary or secondary sites are specified. It should not be used in place of assigning codes for the primary site and all known secondary sites.

k. Malignant neoplasm without specification of site

Code C80.1, Malignant (primary) neoplasm, unspecified, equates to Cancer, unspecified. This code should only be used when no determination can be made as to the primary site of a malignancy. This code should rarely be used in the inpatient setting.

l. Sequencing of neoplasm codes

1) Encounter for treatment of primary malignancy

If the reason for the encounter is for treatment of a primary malignancy, assign the malignancy as the principal/first-listed diagnosis. The primary site is to be sequenced first, followed by any metastatic sites.

2) Encounter for treatment of secondary malignancy

When an encounter is for a primary malignancy with metastasis and treatment is directed toward the metastatic (secondary) site(s) only, the metastatic site(s) is designated as the principal/first-listed diagnosis. The primary malignancy is coded as an additional code.

3) Malignant neoplasm in a pregnant patient

When a pregnant woman has a malignant neoplasm, a code from subcategory O9A.1-, Malignant neoplasm complicating pregnancy, childbirth, and the puerperium, should be sequenced first, followed by the appropriate code from Chapter 2 to indicate the type of neoplasm.

4) Encounter for complication associated with a neoplasm

When an encounter is for management of a complication associated with a neoplasm, such as dehydration, and the treatment is only for the complication, the complication is coded first, followed by the appropriate code(s) for the neoplasm.

The exception to this guideline is anemia. When the admission/encounter is for management of an anemia associated with the malignancy, and the treatment is only for anemia, the appropriate code for the malignancy is sequenced as the principal or first-listed diagnosis followed by code D63.0, Anemia in neoplastic disease.

5) Complication from surgical procedure for treatment of a neoplasm

When an encounter is for treatment of a complication resulting from a surgical procedure performed for the treatment of the neoplasm, designate the complication as the principal/first-listed diagnosis. See guideline regarding the coding of a current malignancy versus personal history to determine if the code for the neoplasm should also be assigned.

6) Pathologic fracture due to a neoplasm

When an encounter is for a pathological fracture due to a neoplasm, and the focus of treatment is the fracture, a code from subcategory M84.5, Pathological fracture in neoplastic disease, should be sequenced first, followed by the code for the neoplasm.

If the focus of treatment is the neoplasm with an associated pathological fracture, the neoplasm code should be sequenced first, followed by a code from M84.5 for the pathological fracture.

m. Current malignancy versus personal history of malignancy

When a primary malignancy has been excised but further treatment, such as an additional surgery for the malignancy, radiation therapy or chemotherapy is directed to that site, the primary malignancy code should be used until treatment is completed.

When a primary malignancy has been previously excised or eradicated from its site, there is no further treatment (of the malignancy) directed to that site, and there is no evidence of any existing primary malignancy, a code from category Z85, Personal history of malignant neoplasm, should be used to indicate the former site of the malignancy.

See Section I.C.21. Factors influencing health status and contact with health services, History (of)

n. Leukemia, Multiple Myeloma, and Malignant Plasma Cell Neoplasms in remission versus personal history

The categories for leukemia, and category C90, Multiple myeloma and malignant plasma cell neoplasms, have codes indicating whether or not the leukemia has achieved remission. There are also codes Z85.6, Personal history of leukemia, and Z85.79, Personal history of other malignant neoplasms of lymphoid, hematopoietic and related tissues. If the documentation is unclear as to whether the leukemia has achieved remission, the provider should be queried.

See Section I.C.21. Factors influencing health status and contact with health services, History (of)

o. **Aftercare following surgery for neoplasm**

See Section I.C.21. Factors influencing health status and contact with health services, Aftercare

p. **Follow-up care for completed treatment of a malignancy**

See Section I.C.21. Factors influencing health status and contact with health services, Follow-up

q. **Prophylactic organ removal for prevention of malignancy**

See Section I.C. 21, Factors influencing health status and contact with health services, Prophylactic organ removal

r. **Malignant neoplasm associated with transplanted organ**

A malignant neoplasm of a transplanted organ should be coded as a transplant complication. Assign first the appropriate code from category T86.-, Complications of transplanted organs and tissue, followed by code C80.2, Malignant neoplasm associated with transplanted organ. Use an additional code for the specific malignancy.

3. **Chapter 3: Disease of the Blood and Blood-forming Organs and Certain Disorders Involving the Immune Mechanism (D50-D89)**

Reserved for future guideline expansion

4. **Chapter 4: Endocrine, Nutritional, and Metabolic Diseases (E00-E89)**

a. **Diabetes mellitus**

The diabetes mellitus codes are combination codes that include the type of diabetes mellitus, the body system affected, and the complications affecting that body system. As many codes within a particular category as are necessary to describe all of the complications of the disease may be used. They should be sequenced based on the reason for a particular encounter. Assign as many codes from categories E08 – E13 as needed to identify all of the associated conditions that the patient has.

1) **Type of diabetes**

The age of a patient is not the sole determining factor, though most type 1 diabetics develop the condition before reaching puberty. For this reason type 1 diabetes mellitus is also referred to as juvenile diabetes.

2) **Type of diabetes mellitus not documented**

If the type of diabetes mellitus is not documented in the medical record the default is E11.-, Type 2 diabetes mellitus.

3) **Diabetes mellitus and the use of insulin and oral hypoglycemics**

If the documentation in a medical record does not indicate the type of diabetes but does indicate that the patient uses insulin, code E11, Type 2 diabetes mellitus, should be assigned. Code Z79.4, Long-term (current) use of insulin, **or Z79.84, Long term (current) use of oral hypoglycemic drugs**, should also be assigned to indicate that the patient uses insulin **or hypoglycemic drugs**. Code Z79.4 should not be assigned if insulin is given temporarily to bring a type 2 patient's blood sugar under control during an encounter.

4) **Diabetes mellitus in pregnancy and gestational diabetes**

See Section I.C.15. Diabetes mellitus in pregnancy.

See Section I.C.15. Gestational (pregnancy induced) diabetes

5) **Complications due to insulin pump malfunction**

(a) **Underdose of insulin due to insulin pump failure**

An underdose of insulin due to an insulin pump failure should be assigned to a code from subcategory T85.6, Mechanical complication of other specified internal and external prosthetic devices, implants and grafts, that specifies the type of pump malfunction, as the principal or first-listed code, followed by code T38.3X6-, Underdosing of insulin and oral hypoglycemic [antidiabetic] drugs. Additional codes for the type of diabetes mellitus and any associated complications due to the underdosing should also be assigned.

(b) **Overdose of insulin due to insulin pump failure**

The principal or first-listed code for an encounter due to an insulin pump malfunction resulting in an overdose of insulin, should also be T85.6-, Mechanical complication of other specified internal and external prosthetic devices, implants and grafts, followed by code T38.3X1-, Poisoning by insulin and oral hypoglycemic [antidiabetic] drugs, accidental (unintentional).

6) **Secondary diabetes mellitus**

Codes under categories E08, Diabetes mellitus due to underlying condition, E09, Drug or chemical induced diabetes mellitus, and E13, Other specified diabetes mellitus, identify complications/manifestations associated with secondary diabetes mellitus. Secondary diabetes is always caused by another condition or event (e.g., cystic fibrosis, malignant neoplasm of pancreas, pancreatectomy, adverse effect of drug, or poisoning).

(a) **Secondary diabetes mellitus and the use of insulin or hypoglycemic drugs**

For patients who routinely use insulin **or hypoglycemic drugs**, code Z79.4, Long-term (current) use of insulin, **or Z79.84, Long term (current) use of oral hypoglycemic drugs** should also be assigned. Code Z79.4 should not be assigned if insulin is given temporarily to bring a patient's blood sugar under control during an encounter.

(b) **Assigning and sequencing secondary diabetes codes and its causes**

The sequencing of the secondary diabetes codes in relationship to codes for the cause of the diabetes is based on the Tabular List instructions for categories E08, E09 and E13.

(i) **Secondary diabetes mellitus due to pancreatectomy**

For postpancreatectomy diabetes mellitus (lack of insulin due to the surgical removal of all or part of the pancreas), assign code E89.1, Postprocedural hypoinsulinemia. Assign a code from category E13 and a code from subcategory Z90.41-, Acquired absence of pancreas, as additional codes.

(ii) **Secondary diabetes due to drugs**

Secondary diabetes may be caused by an adverse effect of correctly administered medications, poisoning or sequela of poisoning.

See section I.C.19.e for coding of adverse effects and poisoning, and section I.C.20 for external cause code reporting.

5. **Chapter 5: Mental, Behavioral and Neurodevelopmental Disorders (F01 – F99)**

a. **Pain disorders related to psychological factors**

Assign code F45.41, for pain that is exclusively related to psychological disorders. As indicated by the Excludes 1 note under category G89, a code from category G89 should not be assigned with code F45.41.

Code F45.42, Pain disorders with related psychological factors, should be used with a code from category G89, Pain, not elsewhere classified, if there is documentation of a psychological component for a patient with acute or chronic pain.

See Section I.C.6. Pain

b. **Mental and behavioral disorders due to psychoactive substance use**

1) **In Remission**

Selection of codes for "in remission" for categories F10-F19, Mental and behavioral disorders due to psychoactive substance use (categories F10-F19 with -.21) requires the provider's clinical judgment. The appropriate codes for "in remission" are assigned only on the basis of provider documentation (as defined in the Official Guidelines for Coding and Reporting).

2) **Psychoactive Substance Use, Abuse And Dependence**

When the provider documentation refers to use, abuse and dependence of the same substance (e.g. alcohol, opioid, cannabis, etc.), only one code should be assigned to identify the pattern of use based on the following hierarchy:

- If both use and abuse are documented, assign only the code for abuse
- If both abuse and dependence are documented, assign only the code for dependence
- If use, abuse and dependence are all documented, assign only the code for dependence
- If both use and dependence are documented, assign only the code for dependence.

3) **Psychoactive Substance Use**

As with all other diagnoses, the codes for psychoactive substance use (F10.9-, F11.9-, F12.9-, F13.9-, F14.9-, F15.9-, F16.9-) should only be assigned based on provider documentation and when they meet the definition of a reportable diagnosis (*see Section III, Reporting Additional Diagnoses*). The codes are to be used only when the psychoactive substance use is associated with a mental or behavioral disorder, and such a relationship is documented by the provider.

6. **Chapter 6: Diseases of the Nervous System (G00-G99)**

a. **Dominant/nondominant side**

Codes from category G81, Hemiplegia and hemiparesis, and subcategories G83.1, Monoplegia of lower limb, G83.2, Monoplegia of upper limb, and G83.3, Monoplegia, unspecified, identify whether the dominant or nondominant side is affected. Should the affected side be documented, but not specified as dominant or nondominant, and the classification system does not indicate a default, code selection is as follows:

- For ambidextrous patients, the default should be dominant.
- If the left side is affected, the default is non-dominant.
- If the right side is affected, the default is dominant.

b. Pain - Category G89

1) General coding information

Codes in category G89, Pain, not elsewhere classified, may be used in conjunction with codes from other categories and chapters to provide more detail about acute or chronic pain and neoplasm-related pain, unless otherwise indicated below.

If the pain is not specified as acute or chronic, post- thoracotomy, postprocedural, or neoplasm-related, do not assign codes from category G89.

A code from category G89 should not be assigned if the underlying (definitive) diagnosis is known, unless the reason for the encounter is pain control/ management and not management of the underlying condition.

When an admission or encounter is for a procedure aimed at treating the underlying condition (e.g., spinal fusion, kyphoplasty), a code for the underlying condition (e.g., vertebral fracture, spinal stenosis) should be assigned as the principal diagnosis. No code from category G89 should be assigned.

(a) Category G89 Codes as Principal or First-Listed Diagnosis

Category G89 codes are acceptable as principal diagnosis or the first-listed code:

- ❑ When pain control or pain management is the reason for the admission/encounter (e.g., a patient with displaced intervertebral disc, nerve impingement and severe back pain presents for injection of steroid into the spinal canal). The underlying cause of the pain should be reported as an additional diagnosis, if known.
- ❑ When a patient is admitted for the insertion of a neurostimulator for pain control, assign the appropriate pain code as the principal or first-listed diagnosis. When an admission or encounter is for a procedure aimed at treating the underlying condition and a neurostimulator is inserted for pain control during the same admission/encounter, a code for the underlying condition should be assigned as the principal diagnosis and the appropriate pain code should be assigned as a secondary diagnosis.

(b) Use of Category G89 Codes in Conjunction with Site Specific Pain Codes

(i) Assigning Category G89 and Site-Specific Pain Codes

Codes from category G89 may be used in conjunction with codes that identify the site of pain (including codes from chapter 18) if the category G89 code provides additional information. For example, if the code describes the site of the pain, but does not fully describe whether the pain is acute or chronic, then both codes should be assigned.

(ii) Sequencing of Category G89 Codes with Site- Specific Pain Codes

The sequencing of category G89 codes with site- specific pain codes (including chapter 18 codes), is dependent on the circumstances of the encounter/admission as follows:

- ❑ If the encounter is for pain control or pain management, assign the code from category G89 followed by the code identifying the specific site of pain (e.g., encounter for pain management for acute neck pain from trauma is assigned code G89.11, Acute pain due to trauma, followed by code M54.2, Cervicalgia, to identify the site of pain).
- ❑ If the encounter is for any other reason except pain control or pain management, and a related definitive diagnosis has not been established (confirmed) by the provider, assign the code for the specific site of pain first, followed by the appropriate code from category G89.

2) Pain due to devices, implants and grafts

See Section I.C.19. Pain due to medical devices

3) Postoperative Pain

The provider's documentation should be used to guide the coding of postoperative pain, as well as *Section III. Reporting Additional Diagnoses and Section IV. Diagnostic Coding and Reporting in the Outpatient Setting.*

The default for post-thoracotomy and other postoperative pain not specified as acute or chronic is the code for the acute form.

Routine or expected postoperative pain immediately after surgery should not be coded.

(a) Postoperative pain not associated with specific postoperative complication

Postoperative pain not associated with a specific postoperative complication is assigned to the appropriate postoperative pain code in category G89.

(b) Postoperative pain associated with specific postoperative complication

Postoperative pain associated with a specific postoperative complication (such as painful wire sutures) is assigned to the appropriate code(s) found in Chapter 19, Injury, poisoning, and certain other consequences of external causes. If appropriate, use additional code(s) from category G89 to identify acute or chronic pain (G89.18 or G89.28).

4) Chronic pain

Chronic pain is classified to subcategory G89.2. There is no time frame defining when pain becomes chronic pain. The provider's documentation should be used to guide use of these codes.

5) Neoplasm Related Pain

Code G89.3 is assigned to pain documented as being related, associated or due to cancer, primary or secondary malignancy, or tumor. This code is assigned regardless of whether the pain is acute or chronic.

This code may be assigned as the principal or first-listed code when the stated reason for the admission/encounter is documented as pain control/pain management. The underlying neoplasm should be reported as an additional diagnosis.

When the reason for the admission/encounter is management of the neoplasm and the pain associated with the neoplasm is also documented, code G89.3 may be assigned as an additional diagnosis. It is not necessary to assign an additional code for the site of the pain.

See Section I.C.2 for instructions on the sequencing of neoplasms for all other stated reasons for the admission/encounter (except for pain control/ pain management).

6) Chronic pain syndrome

Central pain syndrome (G89.0) and chronic pain syndrome (G89.4) are different than the term "chronic pain," and therefore codes should only be used when the provider has specifically documented this condition.

See Section I.C.5. Pain disorders related to psychological factors

7. Chapter 7: Diseases of the Eye and Adnexa (H00-H59)

a. Glaucoma

1) Assigning Glaucoma Codes

Assign as many codes from category H40, Glaucoma, as needed to identify the type of glaucoma, the affected eye, and the glaucoma stage.

2) Bilateral glaucoma with same type and stage

When a patient has bilateral glaucoma and both eyes are documented as being the same type and stage, and there is a code for bilateral glaucoma, report only the code for the type of glaucoma, bilateral, with the seventh character for the stage.

When a patient has bilateral glaucoma and both eyes are documented as being the same type and stage, and the classification does not provide a code for bilateral glaucoma (i.e. subcategories H40.10, H40.11 and H40.20) report only one code for the type of glaucoma with the appropriate seventh character for the stage.

3) Bilateral glaucoma stage with different types or stages

When a patient has bilateral glaucoma and each eye is documented as having a different type or stage, and the classification distinguishes laterality, assign the appropriate code for each eye rather than the code for bilateral glaucoma.

When a patient has bilateral glaucoma and each eye is documented as having a different type, and the classification does not distinguish laterality (i.e. subcategories H40.10, H40.11 and H40.20), assign one code for each type of glaucoma with the appropriate seventh character for the stage.

When a patient has bilateral glaucoma and each eye is documented as having the same type, but different stage, and the classification does not distinguish laterality (i.e. subcategories H40.10, H40.11 and H40.20), assign a code for the type of glaucoma for each eye with the seventh character for the specific glaucoma stage documented for each eye.

4) Patient admitted with glaucoma and stage evolves during the admission

If a patient is admitted with glaucoma and the stage progresses during the admission, assign the code for highest stage documented.

5) Indeterminate stage glaucoma

Assignment of the seventh character "4" for "indeterminate stage" should be based on the clinical documentation. The seventh character "4" is used for glaucomas whose stage cannot be clinically determined. This seventh character should not be confused with the seventh character "0", unspecified, which should be assigned when there is no documentation regarding the stage of the glaucoma.

8. **Chapter 8: Diseases of the Ear and Mastoid Process (H60-H95)**

Reserved for future guideline expansion

9. **Chapter 9: Diseases of the Circulatory System (I00-I99)**

a. **Hypertension**

The classification presumes a causal relationship between hypertension and heart involvement and between hypertension and kidney involvement, as the two conditions are linked by the term "with" in the **Alphabetic Index. These conditions should be coded as related even in the absence of provider documentation explicitly linking them, unless the documentation clearly states the conditions are unrelated.**

For hypertension and conditions not specifically linked by relational terms such as "with," "associated with" or "due to" in the classification, **provider documentation must link the conditions in order to code them as related.**

1) **Hypertension with Heart Disease**

Hypertension with heart conditions classified to I50.- or I51.4- I51.9, are assigned to a code from category I11, Hypertensive heart disease. Use an additional code from category I50, Heart failure, to identify the type of heart failure in those patients with heart failure.

The same heart conditions (I50.-, I51.4-I51.9) with hypertension are coded separately **if the provider has specifically documented a different cause**. Sequence according to the circumstances of the admission/encounter.

2) **Hypertensive Chronic Kidney Disease**

Assign codes from category I12, Hypertensive chronic kidney disease, when both hypertension and a condition classifiable to category N18, Chronic kidney disease (CKD), are present. **CKD should not be coded as hypertensive if the physician has specifically documented a different cause.**

The appropriate code from category N18 should be used as a secondary code with a code from category I12 to identify the stage of chronic kidney disease.

See Section I.C.14. Chronic kidney disease.

If a patient has hypertensive chronic kidney disease and acute renal failure, an additional code for the acute renal failure is required.

3) **Hypertensive Heart and Chronic Kidney Disease**

Assign codes from combination category I13, Hypertensive heart and chronic kidney disease, when **there is hypertension with both heart and kidney involvement**. If heart failure is present, assign an additional code from category I50 to identify the type of heart failure.

The appropriate code from category N18, Chronic kidney disease, should be used as a secondary code with a code from category I13 to identify the stage of chronic kidney disease.

See Section I.C.14. Chronic kidney disease.

The codes in category I13, Hypertensive heart and chronic kidney disease, are combination codes that include hypertension, heart disease and chronic kidney disease. The Includes note at I13 specifies that the conditions included at I11 and I12 are included together in I13. If a patient has hypertension, heart disease and chronic kidney disease, then a code from I13 should be used, not individual codes for hypertension, heart disease and chronic kidney disease, or codes from I11 or I12.

For patients with both acute renal failure and chronic kidney disease, an additional code for acute renal failure is required.

4) **Hypertensive Cerebrovascular Disease**

For hypertensive cerebrovascular disease, first assign the appropriate code from categories I60-I69, followed by the appropriate hypertension code.

5) **Hypertensive Retinopathy**

Subcategory H35.0, Background retinopathy and retinal vascular changes, should be used with a code from category I10 – I16, Hypertensive disease to include the systemic hypertension. The sequencing is based on the reason for the encounter.

6) **Hypertension, Secondary**

Secondary hypertension is due to an underlying condition. Two codes are required: one to identify the underlying etiology and one from category I15 to identify the hypertension. Sequencing of codes is determined by the reason for admission/encounter.

7) **Hypertension, Transient**

Assign code R03.0, Elevated blood pressure reading without diagnosis of hypertension, unless patient has an established diagnosis of hypertension. Assign code O13.-, Gestational [pregnancy-induced] hypertension without significant proteinuria, or O14.-, Pre-eclampsia, for transient hypertension of pregnancy.

8) **Hypertension, Controlled**

This diagnostic statement usually refers to an existing state of hypertension under control by therapy. Assign the appropriate code from categories I10-I16, Hypertensive diseases.

9) **Hypertension, Uncontrolled**

Uncontrolled hypertension may refer to untreated hypertension or hypertension not responding to current therapeutic regimen. In either case, assign the appropriate code from categories I10- I16, Hypertensive diseases.

10) **Hypertensive Crisis**

Assign a code from category I16, Hypertensive crisis, for documented hypertensive urgency, hypertensive emergency or unspecified hypertensive crisis. Code also any identified hypertensive disease (I10-I15). The sequencing is based on the reason for the encounter.

b. **Atherosclerotic Coronary Artery Disease and Angina**

ICD-10-CM has combination codes for atherosclerotic heart disease with angina pectoris. The subcategories for these codes are I25.11, Atherosclerotic heart disease of native coronary artery with angina pectoris and I25.7, Atherosclerosis of coronary artery bypass graft(s) and coronary artery of transplanted heart with angina pectoris.

When using one of these combination codes it is not necessary to use an additional code for angina pectoris. A causal relationship can be assumed in a patient with both atherosclerosis and angina pectoris, unless the documentation indicates the angina is due to something other than the atherosclerosis.

If a patient with coronary artery disease is admitted due to an acute myocardial infarction (AMI), the AMI should be sequenced before the coronary artery disease.

See Section I.C.9. Acute myocardial infarction (AMI)

c. **Intraoperative and Postprocedural Cerebrovascular Accident**

Medical record documentation should clearly specify the cause- and- effect relationship between the medical intervention and the cerebrovascular accident in order to assign a code for intraoperative or postprocedural cerebrovascular accident.

Proper code assignment depends on whether it was an infarction or hemorrhage and whether it occurred intraoperatively or postoperatively. If it was a cerebral hemorrhage, code assignment depends on the type of procedure performed.

d. **Sequelae of Cerebrovascular Disease**

1) **Category I69, Sequelae of Cerebrovascular disease**

Category I69 is used to indicate conditions classifiable to categories I60-I67 as the causes of sequela (neurologic deficits), themselves classified elsewhere. These "late effects" include neurologic deficits that persist after initial onset of conditions classifiable to categories I60-I67. The neurologic deficits caused by cerebrovascular disease may be present from the onset or may arise at any time after the onset of the condition classifiable to categories I60-I67.

Codes from category I69, Sequelae of cerebrovascular disease, that specify hemiplegia, hemiparesis and monoplegia identify whether the dominant or nondominant side is affected. Should the affected side be documented, but not specified as dominant or nondominant, and the classification system does not indicate a default, code selection is as follows:

- ❑ For ambidextrous patients, the default should be dominant.
- ❑ If the left side is affected, the default is non-dominant.
- ❑ If the right side is affected, the default is dominant.

2) **Codes from category I69 with codes from I60-I67**

Codes from category I69 may be assigned on a health care record with codes from I60-I67, if the patient has a current cerebrovascular disease and deficits from an old cerebrovascular disease.

3) **Codes from category I69 and Personal history of transient ischemic attack (TIA) and cerebral infarction (Z86.73)**

Codes from category I69 should not be assigned if the patient does not have neurologic deficits.

See Section I.C.21. 4. History (of) for use of personal history codes

e. **Acute myocardial infarction (AMI)**

1) **ST elevation myocardial infarction (STEMI) and non ST elevation myocardial infarction (NSTEMI)**

The ICD-10-CM codes for acute myocardial infarction (AMI) identify the site, such as anterolateral wall or true posterior wall. Subcategories I21.0-I21.2 and code I21.3 are used for ST elevation myocardial infarction (STEMI). Code I21.4, Non-ST elevation (NSTEMI) myocardial infarction, is used for non ST elevation myocardial infarction (NSTEMI) and nontransmural MIs.

If NSTEMI evolves to STEMI, assign the STEMI code. If STEMI converts to NSTEMI due to thrombolytic therapy, it is still coded as STEMI.

For encounters occurring while the myocardial infarction is equal to, or less than, four weeks old, including transfers to another acute setting or a postacute setting, and the myocardial infarction meets the definition for "other diagnoses" (see **Section III, Reporting Additional Diagnoses)**, codes from category I21 may continue to be reported. For encounters after the 4 week time frame and the patient is still receiving care related to the myocardial infarction, the appropriate aftercare code should be assigned, rather than a code from category I21. For old or healed myocardial infarctions not requiring further care, code I25.2, Old myocardial infarction, may be assigned.

2) Acute myocardial infarction, unspecified

Code I21.3, ST elevation (STEMI) myocardial infarction of unspecified site, is the default for unspecified acute myocardial infarction. If only STEMI or transmural MI without the site is documented, assign code I21.3.

3) AMI documented as nontransmural or subendocardial but site provided

If an AMI is documented as nontransmural or subendocardial, but the site is provided, it is still coded as a subendocardial AMI.

See Section I.C.21.3 for information on coding status post administration of tPA in a different facility within the last 24 hours.

4) Subsequent acute myocardial infarction

A code from category I22, Subsequent ST elevation (STEMI) and non ST elevation (NSTEMI) myocardial infarction, is to be used when a patient who has suffered an AMI has a new AMI within the 4 week time frame of the initial AMI. A code from category I22 must be used in conjunction with a code from category I21. The sequencing of the I22 and I21 codes depends on the circumstances of the encounter.

10. Chapter 10: Diseases of the Respiratory System (J00-J99)

a. Chronic Obstructive Pulmonary Disease [COPD] and Asthma

1) Acute exacerbation of chronic obstructive bronchitis and asthma

The codes in categories J44 and J45 distinguish between uncomplicated cases and those in acute exacerbation. An acute exacerbation is a worsening or a decompensation of a chronic condition. An acute exacerbation is not equivalent to an infection superimposed on a chronic condition, though an exacerbation may be triggered by an infection.

b. Acute Respiratory Failure

1) Acute respiratory failure as principal diagnosis

A code from subcategory J96.0, Acute respiratory failure, or subcategory J96.2, Acute and chronic respiratory failure, may be assigned as a principal diagnosis when it is the condition established after study to be chiefly responsible for occasioning the admission to the hospital, and the selection is supported by the Alphabetic Index and Tabular List. However, chapter- specific coding guidelines (such as obstetrics, poisoning, HIV, newborn) that provide sequencing direction take precedence.

2) Acute respiratory failure as secondary diagnosis

Respiratory failure may be listed as a secondary diagnosis if it occurs after admission, or if it is present on admission, but does not meet the definition of principal diagnosis.

3) Sequencing of acute respiratory failure and another acute condition

When a patient is admitted with respiratory failure and another acute condition, (e.g., myocardial infarction, cerebrovascular accident, aspiration pneumonia), the principal diagnosis will not be the same in every situation. This applies whether the other acute condition is a respiratory or nonrespiratory condition. Selection of the principal diagnosis will be dependent on the circumstances of admission. If both the respiratory failure and the other acute condition are equally responsible for occasioning the admission to the hospital, and there are no chapter-specific sequencing rules, the guideline regarding two or more diagnoses that equally meet the definition for principal diagnosis (*Section II, C.*) may be applied in these situations.

If the documentation is not clear as to whether acute respiratory failure and another condition are equally responsible for occasioning the admission, query the provider for clarification.

c. Influenza due to certain identified influenza viruses

Code only confirmed cases of influenza due to certain identified influenza viruses (category J09), and due to other identified influenza virus (category J10). This is an exception to the hospital inpatient guideline Section II, H. (Uncertain Diagnosis).

In this context, "confirmation" does not require documentation of positive laboratory testing specific for avian or other novel influenza A or other identified influenza virus. However, coding should be based on the provider's diagnostic statement that the patient has avian influenza, or other novel influenza A, for category J09, or has another particular identified strain of influenza, such as H1N1 or H3N2, but not identified as novel or variant, for category J10.

If the provider records "suspected" or " possible" or " probable" avian influenza, or novel influenza, or other identified influenza, then the appropriate influenza code from category J11, Influenza due to unidentified influenza virus, should be assigned. A code from category J09, Influenza due to certain identified influenza viruses, should not be assigned nor should a code from category J10, Influenza due to other identified influenza virus.

d. Ventilator associated Pneumonia

1) Documentation of Ventilator associated Pneumonia

As with all procedural or postprocedural complications, code assignment is based on the provider's documentation of the relationship between the condition and the procedure.

Code J95.851, Ventilator associated pneumonia, should be assigned only when the provider has documented ventilator associated pneumonia (VAP). An additional code to identify the organism (e.g., Pseudomonas aeruginosa, code B96.5) should also be assigned. Do not assign an additional code from categories J12-J18 to identify the type of pneumonia.

Code J95.851 should not be assigned for cases where the patient has pneumonia and is on a mechanical ventilator and the provider has not specifically stated that the pneumonia is ventilator-associated pneumonia. If the documentation is unclear as to whether the patient has a pneumonia that is a complication attributable to the mechanical ventilator, query the provider.

2) Ventilator associated Pneumonia Develops after Admission

A patient may be admitted with one type of pneumonia (e.g., code J13, Pneumonia due to Streptococcus pneumonia) and subsequently develop VAP. In this instance, the principal diagnosis would be the appropriate code from categories J12-J18 for the pneumonia diagnosed at the time of admission. Code J95.851, Ventilator associated pneumonia, would be assigned as an additional diagnosis when the provider has also documented the presence of ventilator associated pneumonia.

11. Chapter 11: Diseases of the Digestive System (K00-K95)

Reserved for future guideline expansion

12. Chapter 12: Diseases of the Skin and Subcutaneous Tissue (L00-L99)

a. Pressure ulcer stage codes

1) Pressure ulcer stages

Codes from category L89, Pressure ulcer, identify the site of the pressure ulcer as well as the stage of the ulcer.

The ICD-10-CM classifies pressure ulcer stages based on severity, which is designated by stages 1-4, unspecified stage and unstageable.

Assign as many codes from category L89 as needed to identify all the pressure ulcers the patient has, if applicable.

2) Unstageable pressure ulcers

Assignment of the code for unstageable pressure ulcer (L89.--0) should be based on the clinical documentation. These codes are used for pressure ulcers whose stage cannot be clinically determined (e.g., the ulcer is covered by eschar or has been treated with a skin or muscle graft) and pressure ulcers that are documented as deep tissue injury but not documented as due to trauma. This code should not be confused with the codes for unspecified stage (L89.--9). When there is no documentation regarding the stage of the pressure ulcer, assign the appropriate code for unspecified stage (L89.--9).

3) Documented pressure ulcer stage

Assignment of the pressure ulcer stage code should be guided by clinical documentation of the stage or documentation of the terms found in the Alphabetic Index. For clinical terms describing the stage that are not found in the Alphabetic Index, and there is no documentation of the stage, the provider should be queried.

4) Patients admitted with pressure ulcers documented as healed

No code is assigned if the documentation states that the pressure ulcer is completely healed.

5) Patients admitted with pressure ulcers documented as healing

Pressure ulcers described as healing should be assigned the appropriate pressure ulcer stage code based on the documentation in the medical record. If the documentation does not provide information about the stage of the healing pressure ulcer, assign the appropriate code for unspecified stage.

If the documentation is unclear as to whether the patient has a current (new) pressure ulcer or if the patient is being treated for a healing pressure ulcer, query the provider.

For ulcers that were present on admission but healed at the time of discharge, assign the code for the site and stage of the pressure ulcer at the time of admission.

6) **Patient admitted with pressure ulcer evolving into another stage during the admission**

If a patient is admitted with a pressure ulcer at one stage and it progresses to a higher stage, **two separate codes should be assigned: one code for the site and stage of the ulcer on admission and a second code for the same ulcer site and the highest stage reported during the stay.**

13. **Chapter 13: Diseases of the Musculoskeletal System and Connective Tissue (M00-M99)**

a. **Site and laterality**

Most of the codes within Chapter 13 have site and laterality designations. The site represents the bone, joint or the muscle involved. For some conditions where more than one bone, joint or muscle is usually involved, such as osteoarthritis, there is a "multiple sites" code available. For categories where no multiple site code is provided and more than one bone, joint or muscle is involved, multiple codes should be used to indicate the different sites involved.

1) **Bone versus joint**

For certain conditions, the bone may be affected at the upper or lower end, (e.g., avascular necrosis of bone, M87, Osteoporosis, M80, M81). Though the portion of the bone affected may be at the joint, the site designation will be the bone, not the joint.

b. **Acute traumatic versus chronic or recurrent musculoskeletal conditions**

Many musculoskeletal conditions are a result of previous injury or trauma to a site, or are recurrent conditions. Bone, joint or muscle conditions that are the result of a healed injury are usually found in chapter 13. Recurrent bone, joint or muscle conditions are also usually found in chapter 13. Any current, acute injury should be coded to the appropriate injury code from chapter 19. Chronic or recurrent conditions should generally be coded with a code from chapter 13. If it is difficult to determine from the documentation in the record which code is best to describe a condition, query the provider.

c. **Coding of Pathologic Fractures**

7th character A is for use as long as the patient is receiving active treatment for the fracture. While the patient may be seen by a new or different provider over the course of treatment for a pathological fracture, assignment of the 7th character is based on whether the patient is undergoing active treatment and not whether the provider is seeing the patient for the first time.

7th character D is to be used for encounters after the patient has completed active treatment. The other 7th characters, listed under each subcategory in the Tabular List, are to be used for subsequent encounters **for routine care of fractures during the healing and recovery phase as well as** treatment of problems associated with the healing, such as malunions, nonunions, and sequelae.

Care for complications of surgical treatment for fracture repairs during the healing or recovery phase should be coded with the appropriate complication codes.

See Section I.C.19. Coding of traumatic fractures.

d. **Osteoporosis**

Osteoporosis is a systemic condition, meaning that all bones of the musculoskeletal system are affected. Therefore, site is not a component of the codes under category M81, Osteoporosis without current pathological fracture. The site codes under category M80, Osteoporosis with current pathological fracture, identify the site of the fracture, not the osteoporosis.

1) **Osteoporosis without pathological fracture**

Category M81, Osteoporosis without current pathological fracture, is for use for patients with osteoporosis who do not currently have a pathologic fracture due to the osteoporosis, even if they have had a fracture in the past. For patients with a history of osteoporosis fractures, status code Z87.310, Personal history of (healed) osteoporosis fracture, should follow the code from M81.

2) **Osteoporosis with current pathological fracture**

Category M80, Osteoporosis with current pathological fracture, is for patients who have a current pathologic fracture at the time of an encounter. The codes under M80 identify the site of the fracture. A code from category M80, not a traumatic fracture code, should be used for any patient with known osteoporosis who suffers a fracture, even if the patient had a minor fall or trauma, if that fall or trauma would not usually break a normal, healthy bone.

14. **Chapter 14: Diseases of Genitourinary System (N00-N99)**

a. **Chronic kidney disease**

1) **Stages of chronic kidney disease (CKD)**

The ICD-10-CM classifies CKD based on severity. The severity of CKD is designated by stages 1-5. Stage 2, code N18.2, equates to mild CKD; stage 3, code N18.3, equates to moderate CKD; and stage 4, code N18.4, equates to severe CKD. Code N18.6, End stage renal disease (ESRD), is assigned when the provider has documented end-stage-renal disease (ESRD).

If both a stage of CKD and ESRD are documented, assign code N18.6 only.

2) **Chronic kidney disease and kidney transplant status**

Patients who have undergone kidney transplant may still have some form of chronic kidney disease (CKD) because the kidney transplant may not fully restore kidney function. Therefore, the presence of CKD alone does not constitute a transplant complication. Assign the appropriate N18 code for the patient's stage of CKD and code Z94.0, Kidney transplant status. If a transplant complication such as failure or rejection or other transplant complication is documented, see section I.C.19.g for information on coding complications of a kidney transplant. If the documentation is unclear as to whether the patient has a complication of the transplant, query the provider.

3) **Chronic kidney disease with other conditions**

Patients with CKD may also suffer from other serious conditions, most commonly diabetes mellitus and hypertension. The sequencing of the CKD code in relationship to codes for other contributing conditions is based on the conventions in the Tabular List.

See I.C.9. Hypertensive chronic kidney disease.

See I.C.19. Chronic kidney disease and kidney transplant complications.

15. **Chapter 15: Pregnancy, Childbirth, and the Puerperium (O00-O9A)**

a. **General Rules for Obstetric Cases**

1) **Codes from chapter 15 and sequencing priority**

Obstetric cases require codes from chapter 15, codes in the range O00-O9A, Pregnancy, Childbirth, and the Puerperium. Chapter 15 codes have sequencing priority over codes from other chapters. Additional codes from other chapters may be used in conjunction with chapter 15 codes to further specify conditions. Should the provider document that the pregnancy is incidental to the encounter, then code Z33.1, Pregnant state, incidental, should be used in place of any chapter 15 codes. It is the provider's responsibility to state that the condition being treated is not affecting the pregnancy.

2) **Chapter 15 codes used only on the maternal record**

Chapter 15 codes are to be used only on the maternal record, never on the record of the newborn.

3) **Final character for trimester**

The majority of codes in Chapter 15 have a final character indicating the trimester of pregnancy. The timeframes for the trimesters are indicated at the beginning of the chapter. If trimester is not a component of a code, it is because the condition always occurs in a specific trimester, or the concept of trimester of pregnancy is not applicable. Certain codes have characters for only certain trimesters because the condition does not occur in all trimesters, but it may occur in more than just one.

Assignment of the final character for trimester should be based on the provider's documentation of the trimester (or number of weeks) for the current admission/encounter. This applies to the assignment of trimester for pre-existing conditions as well as those that develop during or are due to the pregnancy. The provider's documentation of the number of weeks may be used to assign the appropriate code identifying the trimester.

Whenever delivery occurs during the current admission, and there is an "in childbirth" option for the obstetric complication being coded, the "in childbirth" code should be assigned.

4) **Selection of trimester for inpatient admissions that encompass more than one trimester**

In instances when a patient is admitted to a hospital for complications of pregnancy during one trimester and remains in the hospital into a subsequent trimester, the trimester character for the antepartum complication code should be assigned on the basis of the trimester when the complication developed, not the trimester of the discharge. If the condition developed prior to the current admission/encounter or represents a pre-existing condition, the trimester character for the trimester at the time of the admission/encounter should be assigned.

5) **Unspecified trimester**

Each category that includes codes for trimester has a code for "unspecified trimester." The "unspecified trimester" code should rarely be used, such as when the documentation in the record is insufficient to determine the trimester and it is not possible to obtain clarification.

6) **7th character for Fetus Identification**

Where applicable, a 7th character is to be assigned for certain categories (O31, O32, O33.3 - O33.6, O35, O36, O40, O41, O60.1, O60.2, O64, and O69) to identify the fetus for which the complication code applies.

Assign 7th character "0":

- ❑ For single gestations
- ❑ When the documentation in the record is insufficient to determine the fetus affected and it is not possible to obtain clarification.
- ❑ When it is not possible to clinically determine which fetus is affected.

b. Selection of OB Principal or First-listed Diagnosis

1) **Routine outpatient prenatal visits**

For routine outpatient prenatal visits when no complications are present, a code from category Z34, Encounter for supervision of normal pregnancy, should be used as the first-listed diagnosis. These codes should not be used in conjunction with chapter 15 codes.

2) ***Supervision of High-Risk Pregnancy***

Codes from category O09, Supervision of high-risk pregnancy, are intended for use only during the prenatal period. For complications during the labor or delivery episode as a result of a high-risk pregnancy, assign the applicable complication codes from Chapter 15. If there are no complications during the labor or delivery episode, assign code O80, Encounter for full-term uncomplicated delivery.

For routine prenatal outpatient visits for patients with high-risk pregnancies, a code from category O09, Supervision of high-risk pregnancy, should be used as the first-listed diagnosis. Secondary chapter 15 codes may be used in conjunction with these codes if appropriate.

3) **Episodes when no delivery occurs**

In episodes when no delivery occurs, the principal diagnosis should correspond to the principal complication of the pregnancy which necessitated the encounter. Should more than one complication exist, all of which are treated or monitored, any of the complications codes may be sequenced first.

4) **When a delivery occurs**

When an obstetric patient is admitted and delivers during that admission, the condition that prompted the admission should be sequenced as the principal diagnosis. If multiple conditions prompted the admission, sequence the one most related to the delivery as the principal diagnosis. A code for any complication of the delivery should be assigned as an additional diagnosis. In cases of cesarean delivery, if the patient was admitted with a condition that resulted in the performance of a cesarean procedure, that condition should be selected as the principal diagnosis. If the reason for the admission was unrelated to the condition resulting in the cesarean delivery, the condition related to the reason for the admission should be selected as the principal diagnosis.

5) **Outcome of delivery**

A code from category Z37, Outcome of delivery, should be included on every maternal record when a delivery has occurred. These codes are not to be used on subsequent records or on the newborn record.

c. Pre-existing conditions versus conditions due to the pregnancy

Certain categories in Chapter 15 distinguish between conditions of the mother that existed prior to pregnancy (pre-existing) and those that are a direct result of pregnancy. When assigning codes from Chapter 15, it is important to assess if a condition was pre-existing prior to pregnancy or developed during or due to the pregnancy in order to assign the correct code.

Categories that do not distinguish between pre-existing and pregnancy-related conditions may be used for either. It is acceptable to use codes specifically for the puerperium with codes complicating pregnancy and childbirth if a condition arises postpartum during the delivery encounter.

d. Pre-existing hypertension in pregnancy

Category O10, Pre-existing hypertension complicating pregnancy, childbirth and the puerperium, includes codes for hypertensive heart and hypertensive chronic kidney disease. When assigning one of the O10 codes that includes hypertensive heart disease or hypertensive chronic kidney disease, it is necessary to add a secondary code from the appropriate hypertension category to specify the type of heart failure or chronic kidney disease.

See Section I.C.9. Hypertension.

e. Fetal Conditions Affecting the Management of the Mother

1) **Codes from categories O35 and O36**

Codes from categories O35, Maternal care for known or suspected fetal abnormality and damage, and O36, Maternal care for other fetal problems, are assigned only when the fetal condition is actually responsible for modifying the management of the mother, i.e., by requiring diagnostic studies, additional observation, special care, or termination of pregnancy. The fact that the fetal condition exists does not justify assigning a code from this series to the mother's record.

2) **In utero surgery**

In cases when surgery is performed on the fetus, a diagnosis code from category O35, Maternal care for known or suspected fetal abnormality and damage, should be assigned identifying the fetal condition. Assign the appropriate procedure code for the procedure performed.

No code from Chapter 16, the perinatal codes, should be used on the mother's record to identify fetal conditions. Surgery performed in utero on a fetus is still to be coded as an obstetric encounter.

f. HIV Infection in Pregnancy, Childbirth and the Puerperium

During pregnancy, childbirth or the puerperium, a patient admitted because of an HIV-related illness should receive a principal diagnosis from subcategory O98.7-, Human immunodeficiency [HIV] disease complicating pregnancy, childbirth and the puerperium, followed by the code(s) for the HIV-related illness(es).

Patients with asymptomatic HIV infection status admitted during pregnancy, childbirth, or the puerperium should receive codes of O98.7- and Z21, Asymptomatic human immunodeficiency virus [HIV] infection status.

g. Diabetes mellitus in pregnancy

Diabetes mellitus is a significant complicating factor in pregnancy. Pregnant women who are diabetic should be assigned a code from category O24, Diabetes mellitus in pregnancy, childbirth, and the puerperium, first, followed by the appropriate diabetes code(s) (E08- E13) from Chapter 4.

h. Long term use of insulin and oral hypoglycemics

Code Z79.4, Long-term (current) use of insulin, or **code Z79.84, Long-term (current) use of oral hypoglycemic drugs**, should also be assigned if the diabetes mellitus is being treated with insulin **or oral medications. If the patient is treated with both oral medications and insulin, only the code for insulin-controlled should be assigned.**

i. Gestational (pregnancy induced) diabetes

Gestational (pregnancy induced) diabetes can occur during the second and third trimester of pregnancy in women who were not diabetic prior to pregnancy. Gestational diabetes can cause complications in the pregnancy similar to those of pre-existing diabetes mellitus. It also puts the woman at greater risk of developing diabetes after the pregnancy. Codes for gestational diabetes are in subcategory O24.4, Gestational diabetes mellitus. No other code from category O24, Diabetes mellitus in pregnancy, childbirth, and the puerperium, should be used with a code from O24.4.

The codes under subcategory O24.4 include diet controlled, insulin controlled, **and controlled by oral hypoglycemic drugs**. If a patient with gestational diabetes is treated with both diet and insulin, only the code for insulin-controlled is required. **If a patient with gestational diabetes is treated with both diet and oral hypoglycemic medications, only the code for "controlled by oral hypoglycemic drugs" is required.** Code Z79.4, Long-term (current) use of insulin **or code Z79.84, Long-term (current) use of oral hypoglycemic drugs**, should not be assigned with codes from subcategory O24.4.

An abnormal glucose tolerance in pregnancy is assigned a code from subcategory O99.81, Abnormal glucose complicating pregnancy, childbirth, and the puerperium.

j. Sepsis and septic shock complicating abortion, pregnancy, childbirth and the puerperium

When assigning a chapter 15 code for sepsis complicating abortion, pregnancy, childbirth, and the puerperium, a code for the specific type of infection should be assigned as an additional diagnosis. If severe sepsis is present, a code from subcategory R65.2, Severe sepsis, and code(s) for associated organ dysfunction(s) should also be assigned as additional diagnoses.

k. Puerperal sepsis

Code O85, Puerperal sepsis, should be assigned with a secondary code to identify the causal organism (e.g., for a bacterial infection, assign a code from category B95-B96, Bacterial infections in conditions classified elsewhere). A code from category A40, Streptococcal sepsis, or A41, Other sepsis, should not be used for puerperal sepsis. If applicable, use additional codes to identify severe sepsis (R65.2-) and any associated acute organ dysfunction.

l. Alcohol and tobacco use during pregnancy, childbirth and the puerperium

1) Alcohol use during pregnancy, childbirth and the puerperium

Codes under subcategory O99.31, Alcohol use complicating pregnancy, childbirth, and the puerperium, should be assigned for any pregnancy case when a mother uses alcohol during the pregnancy or postpartum. A secondary code from category F10, Alcohol related disorders, should also be assigned to identify manifestations of the alcohol use.

2) Tobacco use during pregnancy, childbirth and the puerperium

Codes under subcategory O99.33, Smoking (tobacco) complicating pregnancy, childbirth, and the puerperium, should be assigned for any pregnancy case when a mother uses any type of tobacco product during the pregnancy or postpartum. A secondary code from category F17, Nicotine dependence, should also be assigned to identify the type of nicotine dependence.

m. Poisoning, toxic effects, adverse effects and underdosing in a pregnant patient

A code from subcategory O9A.2, Injury, poisoning and certain other consequences of external causes complicating pregnancy, childbirth, and the puerperium, should be sequenced first, followed by the appropriate injury, poisoning, toxic effect, adverse effect or underdosing code, and then the additional code(s) that specifies the condition caused by the poisoning, toxic effect, adverse effect or underdosing.

See Section I.C.19. Adverse effects, poisoning, underdosing and toxic effects.

n. Normal Delivery, Code O80

1) Encounter for full term uncomplicated delivery

Code O80 should be assigned when a woman is admitted for a full-term normal delivery and delivers a single, healthy infant without any complications antepartum, during the delivery, or postpartum during the delivery episode. Code O80 is always a principal diagnosis. It is not to be used if any other code from chapter 15 is needed to describe a current complication of the antenatal, delivery, or perinatal period. Additional codes from other chapters may be used with code O80 if they are not related to or are in any way complicating the pregnancy.

2) Uncomplicated delivery with resolved antepartum complication

Code O80 may be used if the patient had a complication at some point during the pregnancy, but the complication is not present at the time of the admission for delivery.

3) Outcome of delivery for O80

Z37.0, Single live birth, is the only outcome of delivery code appropriate for use with O80.

o. The Peripartum and Postpartum Periods

1) Peripartum and Postpartum periods

The postpartum period begins immediately after delivery and continues for six weeks following delivery. The peripartum period is defined as the last month of pregnancy to five months postpartum.

2) Peripartum and postpartum complication

A postpartum complication is any complication occurring within the six-week period.

3) Pregnancy-related complications after 6 week period

Chapter 15 codes may also be used to describe pregnancy-related complications after the peripartum or postpartum period if the provider documents that a condition is pregnancy related.

4) Admission for routine postpartum care following delivery outside hospital

When the mother delivers outside the hospital prior to admission and is admitted for routine postpartum care and no complications are noted, code Z39.0, Encounter for care and examination of mother immediately after delivery, should be assigned as the principal diagnosis.

5) Pregnancy associated cardiomyopathy

Pregnancy associated cardiomyopathy, code O90.3, is unique in that it may be diagnosed in the third trimester of pregnancy but may continue to progress months after delivery. For this reason, it is referred to as peripartum cardiomyopathy. Code O90.3 is only for use when the cardiomyopathy develops as a result of pregnancy in a woman who did not have pre-existing heart disease.

p. Code O94, Sequelae of complication of pregnancy, childbirth, and the puerperium

1) Code O94

Code O94, Sequelae of complication of pregnancy, childbirth, and the puerperium, is for use in those cases when an initial complication of a pregnancy develops a sequelae requiring care or treatment at a future date.

2) After the initial postpartum period

This code may be used at any time after the initial postpartum period.

3) Sequencing of Code O94

This code, like all sequela codes, is to be sequenced following the code describing the sequelae of the complication.

q. Termination of Pregnancy and Spontaneous abortions

1) Abortion with Liveborn Fetus

When an attempted termination of pregnancy results in a liveborn fetus, assign code Z33.2, Encounter for elective termination of pregnancy and a code from category Z37, Outcome of Delivery.

2) Retained Products of Conception following an abortion

Subsequent encounters for retained products of conception following a spontaneous abortion or elective termination of pregnancy are assigned the appropriate code from category O03, Spontaneous abortion, or codes O07.4, Failed attempted termination of pregnancy without complication and Z33.2, Encounter for elective termination of pregnancy. This advice is appropriate even when the patient was discharged previously with a discharge diagnosis of complete abortion.

3) Complications leading to abortion

Codes from Chapter 15 may be used as additional codes to identify any documented complications of the pregnancy in conjunction with codes in categories in O07 and O08.

r. Abuse in a pregnant patient

For suspected or confirmed cases of abuse of a pregnant patient, a code(s) from subcategories O9A.3, Physical abuse complicating pregnancy, childbirth, and the puerperium, O9A.4, Sexual abuse complicating pregnancy, childbirth, and the puerperium, and O9A.5, Psychological abuse complicating pregnancy, childbirth, and the puerperium, should be sequenced first, followed by the appropriate codes (if applicable) to identify any associated current injury due to physical abuse, sexual abuse, and the perpetrator of abuse.

See Section I.C.19. Adult and child abuse, neglect and other maltreatment.

16. Chapter 16: Certain Conditions Originating in the Perinatal Period (P00-P96)

For coding and reporting purposes the perinatal period is defined as before birth through the 28th day following birth. The following guidelines are provided for reporting purposes.

a. General Perinatal Rules

1) Use of Chapter 16 Codes

Codes in this chapter are never for use on the maternal record. Codes from Chapter 15, the obstetric chapter, are never permitted on the newborn record. Chapter 16 codes may be used throughout the life of the patient if the condition is still present.

2) Principal Diagnosis for Birth Record

When coding the birth episode in a newborn record, assign a code from category Z38, Liveborn infants according to place of birth and type of delivery, as the principal diagnosis. A code from category Z38 is assigned only once, to a newborn at the time of birth. If a newborn is transferred to another institution, a code from category Z38 should not be used at the receiving hospital.

A code from category Z38 is used only on the newborn record, not on the mother's record.

3) Use of Codes from other Chapters with Codes from Chapter 16

Codes from other chapters may be used with codes from chapter 16 if the codes from the other chapters provide more specific detail. Codes for signs and symptoms may be assigned when a definitive diagnosis has not been established. If the reason for the encounter is a perinatal condition, the code from chapter 16 should be sequenced first.

4) Use of Chapter 16 Codes after the Perinatal

Period Should a condition originate in the perinatal period, and continue throughout the life of the patient, the perinatal code should continue to be used regardless of the patient's age.

5) Birth process or community acquired conditions

If a newborn has a condition that may be either due to the birth process or community acquired and the documentation does not indicate which it is, the default is due to the birth process and the code from Chapter 16 should be used. If the condition is community-acquired, a code from Chapter 16 should not be assigned.

6) Code all clinically significant conditions

All clinically significant conditions noted on routine newborn examination should be coded. A condition is clinically significant if it requires:

- ❑ clinical evaluation; or
- ❑ therapeutic treatment; or

- ☐ diagnostic procedures; or
- ☐ extended length of hospital stay; or
- ☐ increased nursing care and/or monitoring; or
- ☐ has implications for future health care needs

Note: The perinatal guidelines listed above are the same as the general coding guidelines for "additional diagnoses", except for the final point regarding implications for future health care needs. Codes should be assigned for conditions that have been specified by the provider as having implications for future health care needs.

b. Observation and Evaluation of Newborns for Suspected Conditions not Found

1) Assign a code from category Z05, Observation and evaluation of newborns and infants for suspected conditions ruled out, to identify those instances when a healthy newborn is evaluated for a suspected condition that is determined after study not to be present. Do not use a code from category Z05 when the patient has identified signs or symptoms of a suspected problem; in such cases code the sign or symptom.

2) A code from category Z05 may also be assigned as a principal or first-listed code for readmissions or encounters when the code from category Z38 code no longer applies. Codes from category Z05 are for use only for healthy newborns and infants for which no condition after study is found to be present.

3) Z05 on a birth record

A code from category Z05 is to be used as a secondary code after the code from category Z38, Liveborn infants according to place of birth and type of delivery.

c. Coding Additional Perinatal Diagnoses

1) Assigning codes for conditions that require treatment

Assign codes for conditions that require treatment or further investigation, prolong the length of stay, or require resource utilization.

2) Codes for conditions specified as having implications for future health care needs

Assign codes for conditions that have been specified by the provider as having implications for future health care needs.

Note: This guideline should not be used for adult patients.

d. Prematurity and Fetal Growth Retardation

Providers utilize different criteria in determining prematurity. A code for prematurity should not be assigned unless it is documented. Assignment of codes in categories P05, Disorders of newborn related to slow fetal growth and fetal malnutrition, and P07, Disorders of newborn related to short gestation and low birth weight, not elsewhere classified, should be based on the recorded birth weight and estimated gestational age. Codes from category P05 should not be assigned with codes from category P07.

When both birth weight and gestational age are available, two codes from category P07 should be assigned, with the code for birth weight sequenced before the code for gestational age.

e. Low birth weight and immaturity status

Codes from category P07, Disorders of newborn related to short gestation and low birth weight, not elsewhere classified, are for use for a child or adult who was premature or had a low birth weight as a newborn and this is affecting the patient's current health status.

See Section I.C.21. Factors influencing health status and contact with health services, Status.

f. Bacterial Sepsis of Newborn

Category P36, Bacterial sepsis of newborn, includes congenital sepsis. If a perinate is documented as having sepsis without documentation of congenital or community acquired, the default is congenital and a code from category P36 should be assigned. If the P36 code includes the causal organism, an additional code from category B95, Streptococcus, Staphylococcus, and Enterococcus as the cause of diseases classified elsewhere, or B96, Other bacterial agents as the cause of diseases classified elsewhere, should not be assigned. If the P36 code does not include the causal organism, assign an additional code from category B96. If applicable, use additional codes to identify severe sepsis (R65.2-) and any associated acute organ dysfunction.

g. Stillbirth

Code P95, Stillbirth, is only for use in institutions that maintain separate records for stillbirths. No other code should be used with P95. Code P95 should not be used on the mother's record.

17. Chapter 17: Congenital malformations, deformations, and chromosomal abnormalities (Q00-Q99)

Assign an appropriate code(s) from categories Q00-Q99, Congenital malformations, deformations, and chromosomal abnormalities when a malformation/deformation or chromosomal abnormality is documented.

A malformation/deformation/or chromosomal abnormality may be the principal/first-listed diagnosis on a record or a secondary diagnosis.

When a malformation/deformation or chromosomal abnormality does not have a unique code assignment, assign additional code(s) for any manifestations that may be present.

When the code assignment specifically identifies the malformation/ deformation or chromosomal abnormality, manifestations that are an inherent component of the anomaly should not be coded separately. Additional codes should be assigned for manifestations that are not an inherent component.

Codes from Chapter 17 may be used throughout the life of the patient. If a congenital malformation or deformity has been corrected, a personal history code should be used to identify the history of the malformation or deformity. Although present at birth, malformation/deformation/or chromosomal abnormality may not be identified until later in life. Whenever the condition is diagnosed by the physician, it is appropriate to assign a code from codes Q00-Q99.For the birth admission, the appropriate code from category Z38, Liveborn infants, according to place of birth and type of delivery, should be sequenced as the principal diagnosis, followed by any congenital anomaly codes, Q00- Q99.

18. Chapter 18: Symptoms, signs, and abnormal clinical and laboratory findings, not elsewhere classified (R00-R99)

Chapter 18 includes symptoms, signs, abnormal results of clinical or other investigative procedures, and ill-defined conditions regarding which no diagnosis classifiable elsewhere is recorded. Signs and symptoms that point to a specific diagnosis have been assigned to a category in other chapters of the classification.

a. Use of symptom codes

Codes that describe symptoms and signs are acceptable for reporting purposes when a related definitive diagnosis has not been established (confirmed) by the provider.

b. Use of a symptom code with a definitive diagnosis code

Codes for signs and symptoms may be reported in addition to a related definitive diagnosis when the sign or symptom is not routinely associated with that diagnosis, such as the various signs and symptoms associated with complex syndromes. The definitive diagnosis code should be sequenced before the symptom code.

Signs or symptoms that are associated routinely with a disease process should not be assigned as additional codes, unless otherwise instructed by the classification.

c. Combination codes that include symptoms

ICD-10-CM contains a number of combination codes that identify both the definitive diagnosis and common symptoms of that diagnosis. When using one of these combination codes, an additional code should not be assigned for the symptom.

d. Repeated falls

Code R29.6, Repeated falls, is for use for encounters when a patient has recently fallen and the reason for the fall is being investigated.

Code Z91.81, History of falling, is for use when a patient has fallen in the past and is at risk for future falls. When appropriate, both codes R29.6 and Z91.81 may be assigned together.

e. Coma scale

The coma scale codes (R40.2-) can be used in conjunction with traumatic brain injury codes, acute cerebrovascular disease or sequelae of cerebrovascular disease codes. These codes are primarily for use by trauma registries, but they may be used in any setting where this information is collected. **The coma scale may also be used to assess the status of the central nervous system for other non-trauma conditions, such as monitoring patients in the intensive care unit regardless of medical condition.** The coma scale codes should be sequenced after the diagnosis code(s).

These codes, one from each subcategory, are needed to complete the scale. The 7th character indicates when the scale was recorded. The 7th character should match for all three codes.

At a minimum, report the initial score documented on presentation at your facility. This may be a score from the emergency medicine technician (EMT) or in the emergency department. If desired, a facility may choose to capture multiple coma scale scores.

Assign code R40.24, Glasgow coma scale, total score, when only the total score is documented in the medical record and not the individual score(s).

f. Functional quadriplegia

Functional quadriplegia (code R53.2) is the lack of ability to use one's limbs or to ambulate due to extreme debility. It is not associated with neurologic deficit or injury, and code R53.2 should not be used for cases of neurologic quadriplegia. It should only be assigned if functional quadriplegia is specifically documented in the medical record.

g. SIRS due to Non-Infectious Process

The systemic inflammatory response syndrome (SIRS) can develop as a result of certain non-infectious disease processes, such as trauma, malignant neoplasm, or pancreatitis. When SIRS is documented with a noninfectious condition, and no subsequent infection is documented, the code for the underlying condition, such as an injury, should be assigned, followed by code R65.10, Systemic inflammatory response syndrome (SIRS) of non-infectious origin without acute organ dysfunction, or code R65.11, Systemic inflammatory response syndrome (SIRS) of non-infectious origin with acute organ dysfunction. If an associated acute organ dysfunction is documented, the appropriate code(s) for the specific type of organ dysfunction(s) should be assigned in addition to code R65.11. If acute organ dysfunction is documented, but it cannot be determined if the acute organ dysfunction is associated with SIRS or due to another condition (e.g., directly due to the trauma), the provider should be queried.

h. Death NOS

Code R99, Ill-defined and unknown cause of mortality, is only for use in the very limited circumstance when a patient who has already died is brought into an emergency department or other healthcare facility and is pronounced dead upon arrival. It does not represent the discharge disposition of death.

i. NIHSS Stroke Scale

The NIH stroke scale (NIHSS) codes (R29.7- -) can be used in conjunction with acute stroke codes (I63) to identify the patient's neurological status and the severity of the stroke. The stroke scale codes should be sequenced after the acute stroke diagnosis code(s).

At a minimum, report the initial score documented. If desired, a facility may choose to capture multiple stroke scale scores.

See Section I.B.14. for information concerning the medical record documentation that may be used for assignment of the NIHSS codes.

19. Chapter 19: Injury, poisoning, and certain other consequences of external causes (S00-T88)

a. Application of 7th Characters in Chapter 19

Most categories in chapter 19 have a 7th character requirement for each applicable code. Most categories in this chapter have three 7th character values (with the exception of fractures): A, initial encounter, D, subsequent encounter and S, sequela. Categories for traumatic fractures have additional 7th character values. While the patient may be seen by a new or different provider over the course of treatment for an injury, assignment of the 7th character is based on whether the patient is undergoing active treatment and not whether the provider is seeing the patient for the first time.

For complication codes, active treatment refers to treatment for the condition described by the code, even though it may be related to an earlier precipitating problem. For example, code T84.50XA, Infection and inflammatory reaction due to unspecified internal joint prosthesis, initial encounter, is used when active treatment is provided for the infection, even though the condition relates to the prosthetic device, implant or graft that was placed at a previous encounter.

7th character "A", initial encounter is used **for each encounter where** the patient is receiving active treatment for the condition.

7th character "D" subsequent encounter is used for encounters after the patient has **completed** active treatment of the condition and is receiving routine care for the condition during the healing or recovery phase.

The aftercare Z codes should not be used for aftercare for conditions such as injuries or poisonings, where 7th characters are provided to identify subsequent care. For example, for aftercare of an injury, assign the acute injury code with the 7th character "D" (subsequent encounter).

7th character "S", sequela, is for use for complications or conditions that arise as a direct result of a condition, such as scar formation after a burn. The scars are sequelae of the burn. When using 7th character "S", it is necessary to use both the injury code that precipitated the sequela and the code for the sequela itself. The "S" is added only to the injury code, not the sequela code. The 7th character "S" identifies the injury responsible for the sequela. The specific type of sequela (e.g. scar) is sequenced first, followed by the injury code.

See Section I.B.10 Sequelae, (Late Effects)

b. Coding of Injuries

When coding injuries, assign separate codes for each injury unless a combination code is provided, in which case the combination code is assigned. Code T07, Unspecified multiple injuries should not be assigned in the inpatient setting unless information for a more specific code is not available. Traumatic injury codes (S00-T14.9) are not to be used for normal, healing surgical wounds or to identify complications of surgical wounds.

The code for the most serious injury, as determined by the provider and the focus of treatment, is sequenced first.

1) Superficial injuries

Superficial injuries such as abrasions or contusions are not coded when associated with more severe injuries of the same site.

2) Primary injury with damage to nerves/blood vessels

When a primary injury results in minor damage to peripheral nerves or blood vessels, the primary injury is sequenced first with additional code(s) for injuries to nerves and spinal cord (such as category S04), and/or injury to blood vessels (such as category S15). When the primary injury is to the blood vessels or nerves, that injury should be sequenced first.

c. Coding of Traumatic Fractures

The principles of multiple coding of injuries should be followed in coding fractures. Fractures of specified sites are coded individually by site in accordance with both the provisions within categories S02, S12, S22, S32, S42, S49, S52, S59, S62, S72, S79, S82, S89, S92 and the level of detail furnished by medical record content.

A fracture not indicated as open or closed should be coded to closed. A fracture not indicated whether displaced or not displaced should be coded to displaced.

More specific guidelines are as follows:

1) Initial vs. Subsequent Encounter for Fractures

Traumatic fractures are coded using the appropriate 7th character for initial encounter (A, B, C) **for each encounter where** the patient is receiving active treatment for the fracture. The appropriate 7th character for initial encounter should also be assigned for a patient who delayed seeking treatment for the fracture or nonunion.

Fractures are coded using the appropriate 7th character for subsequent care for encounters after the patient has completed active treatment of the fracture and is receiving routine care for the fracture during the healing or recovery phase.

Care for complications of surgical treatment for fracture repairs during the healing or recovery phase should be coded with the appropriate complication codes.

Care of complications of fractures, such as malunion and nonunion, should be reported with the appropriate 7th character for subsequent care with nonunion (K, M, N,) or subsequent care with malunion (P, Q, R).

Malunion/nonunion: The appropriate 7th character for initial encounter should also be assigned for a patient who delayed seeking treatment for the fracture or nonunion.

The open fracture designations in the assignment of the 7th character for fractures of the forearm, femur and lower leg, including ankle are based on the Gustilo open fracture classification. When the Gustilo classification type is not specified for an open fracture, the 7th character for open fracture type I or II should be assigned (B, E, H, M, Q).

A code from category M80, not a traumatic fracture code, should be used for any patient with known osteoporosis who suffers a fracture, even if the patient had a minor fall or trauma, if that fall or trauma would not usually break a normal, healthy bone.

See Section I.C.13. Osteoporosis.

The aftercare Z codes should not be used for aftercare for traumatic fractures. For aftercare of a traumatic fracture, assign the acute fracture code with the appropriate 7th character.

2) Multiple fractures sequencing

Multiple fractures are sequenced in accordance with the severity of the fracture.

d. Coding of Burns and Corrosions

The ICD-10-CM makes a distinction between burns and corrosions. The burn codes are for thermal burns, except sunburns, that come from a heat source, such as a fire or hot appliance. The burn codes are also for burns resulting from electricity and radiation. Corrosions are burns due to chemicals. The guidelines are the same for burns and corrosions.

Current burns (T20-T25) are classified by depth, extent and by agent (X code). Burns are classified by depth as first degree (erythema), second degree (blistering), and third degree (full-thickness involvement).

Burns of the eye and internal organs (T26-T28) are classified by site, but not by degree.

1) Sequencing of burn and related condition codes

Sequence first the code that reflects the highest degree of burn when more than one burn is present.

a. When the reason for the admission or encounter is for treatment of external multiple burns, sequence first the code that reflects the burn of the highest degree.

b. When a patient has both internal and external burns, the circumstances of admission govern the selection of the principal diagnosis or first-listed diagnosis.

c. When a patient is admitted for burn injuries and other related conditions such as smoke inhalation and/or respiratory failure, the circumstances of admission govern the selection of the principal or first-listed diagnosis.

2) **Burns of the same local site**

Classify burns of the same local site (three-character category level, T20-T28) but of different degrees to the subcategory identifying the highest degree recorded in the diagnosis.

3) **Non-healing burns**

Non-healing burns are coded as acute burns.

Necrosis of burned skin should be coded as a non-healed burn.

4) **Infected Burn**

For any documented infected burn site, use an additional code for the infection.

5) **Assign separate codes for each burn site**

When coding burns, assign separate codes for each burn site. Category T30, Burn and corrosion, body region unspecified is extremely vague and should rarely be used.

6) **Burns and Corrosions Classified According to Extent of Body Surface Involved**

Assign codes from category T31, Burns classified according to extent of body surface involved, or T32, Corrosions classified according to extent of body surface involved, when the site of the burn is not specified or when there is a need for additional data. It is advisable to use category T31 as additional coding when needed to provide data for evaluating burn mortality, such as that needed by burn units. It is also advisable to use category T31 as an additional code for reporting purposes when there is mention of a third-degree burn involving 20 percent or more of the body surface.

Categories T31 and T32 are based on the classic "rule of nines" in estimating body surface involved: head and neck are assigned nine percent, each arm nine percent, each leg 18 percent, the anterior trunk 18 percent, posterior trunk 18 percent, and genitalia one percent. Providers may change these percentage assignments where necessary to accommodate infants and children who have proportionately larger heads than adults, and patients who have large buttocks, thighs, or abdomen that involve burns.

7) **Encounters for treatment of sequela of burns**

Encounters for the treatment of the late effects of burns or corrosions (i.e., scars or joint contractures) should be coded with a burn or corrosion code with the 7th character "S" for sequela.

8) **Sequelae with a late effect code and current burn**

When appropriate, both a code for a current burn or corrosion with 7th character "A" or "D" and a burn or corrosion code with 7th character "S" may be assigned on the same record (when both a current burn and sequelae of an old burn exist). Burns and corrosions do not heal at the same rate and a current healing wound may still exist with sequela of a healed burn or corrosion.

See Section I.B.10 Sequela (Late Effects)

9) **Use of an external cause code with burns and corrosions**

An external cause code should be used with burns and corrosions to identify the source and intent of the burn, as well as the place where it occurred.

e. **Adverse Effects, Poisoning, Underdosing and Toxic Effects**

Codes in categories T36-T65 are combination codes that include the substance that was taken as well as the intent. No additional external cause code is required for poisonings, toxic effects, adverse effects and underdosing codes.

1) **Do not code directly from the Table of Drugs**

Do not code directly from the Table of Drugs and Chemicals. Always refer back to the Tabular List.

2) **Use as many codes as necessary to describe**

Use as many codes as necessary to describe completely all drugs, medicinal or biological substances.

3) **If the same code would describe the causative agent**

If the same code would describe the causative agent for more than one adverse reaction, poisoning, toxic effect or underdosing, assign the code only once.

4) **If two or more drugs, medicinal or biological substances**

If two or more drugs, medicinal or biological substances are reported, code each individually unless a combination code is listed in the Table of Drugs and Chemicals.

5) **The occurrence of drug toxicity is classified in ICD-10- CM as follows:**

(a) **Adverse Effect**

When coding an adverse effect of a drug that has been correctly prescribed and properly administered, assign the appropriate code for the nature of the adverse effect followed by the appropriate code for the adverse effect of the drug (T36-T50). The code for the drug should have a 5th or 6th character "5" (for example T36.0X5-) Examples of the nature of an adverse effect are tachycardia, delirium, gastrointestinal hemorrhaging, vomiting, hypokalemia, hepatitis, renal failure, or respiratory failure.

(b) **Poisoning**

When coding a poisoning or reaction to the improper use of a medication (e.g., overdose, wrong substance given or taken in error, wrong route of administration), first assign the appropriate code from categories T36-T50. The poisoning codes have an associated intent as their 5th or 6th character (accidental, intentional self-harm, assault and undetermined. **If the intent of the poisoning is unknown or unspecified, code the intent as accidental intent. The undetermined intent is only for use if the documentation in the record specifies that the intent cannot be determined.** Use additional code(s) for all manifestations of poisonings.

If there is also a diagnosis of abuse or dependence of the substance, the abuse or dependence is assigned as an additional code.

Examples of poisoning include:

(i) Error was made in drug prescription or in the administration of the drug by provider, nurse, patient, or other person.

(ii) Overdose of a drug intentionally taken If an overdose of a drug was intentionally taken or administered and resulted in drug toxicity, it would be coded as a poisoning.

(iii) Nonprescribed drug taken with correctly prescribed and properly administered drug If a nonprescribed drug or medicinal agent was taken in combination with a correctly prescribed and properly administered drug, any drug toxicity or other reaction resulting from the interaction of the two drugs would be classified as a poisoning.

(iv) Interaction of drug(s) and alcohol

When a reaction results from the interaction of a drug(s) and alcohol, this would be classified as poisoning.

See Section I.C.4. if poisoning is the result of insulin pump malfunctions.

(c) **Underdosing**

Underdosing refers to taking less of a medication than is prescribed by a provider or a manufacturer's instruction. For underdosing, assign the code from categories T36- T50 (fifth or sixth character "6").

Codes for underdosing should never be assigned as principal or first-listed codes. If a patient has a relapse or exacerbation of the medical condition for which the drug is prescribed because of the reduction in dose, then the medical condition itself should be coded.

Noncompliance (Z91.12-, Z91.13-) or complication of care (Y63.6-Y63.9) codes are to be used with an underdosing code to indicate intent, if known.

(d) **Toxic Effects**

When a harmful substance is ingested or comes in contact with a person, this is classified as a toxic effect. The toxic effect codes are in categories T51-T65.

Toxic effect codes have an associated intent: accidental, intentional self-harm, assault and undetermined.

f. **Adult and child abuse, neglect and other maltreatment**

Sequence first the appropriate code from categories T74.- (Adult and child abuse, neglect and other maltreatment, confirmed) or T76.- (Adult and child abuse, neglect and other maltreatment, suspected) for abuse, neglect and other maltreatment, followed by any accompanying mental health or injury code(s).

If the documentation in the medical record states abuse or neglect it is coded as confirmed (T74.-). It is coded as suspected if it is documented as suspected (T76.-).

For cases of confirmed abuse or neglect an external cause code from the assault section (X92-**Y09**) should be added to identify the cause of any physical injuries. A perpetrator code (Y07) should be added when the perpetrator of the abuse is known. For suspected cases of abuse or neglect, do not report external cause or perpetrator code.

If a suspected case of abuse, neglect or mistreatment is ruled out during an encounter code Z04.71, Encounter for examination and observation following alleged physical adult abuse, ruled out, or code Z04.72, Encounter for examination and observation following alleged child physical abuse, ruled out, should be used, not a code from T76.

If a suspected case of alleged rape or sexual abuse is ruled out during an encounter code Z04.41, Encounter for examination and observation following alleged **adult rape** or code Z04.42, Encounter for examination and observation following alleged **child** rape, should be used, not a code from T76.

See Section I.C.15. Abuse in a pregnant patient.

g. Complications of care

1) General guidelines for complications of care

(a) Documentation of complications of care

See Section I.B.16. for information on documentation of complications of care.

2) Pain due to medical devices

Pain associated with devices, implants or grafts left in a surgical site (for example painful hip prosthesis) is assigned to the appropriate code(s) found in Chapter 19, Injury, poisoning, and certain other consequences of external causes. Specific codes for pain due to medical devices are found in the T code section of the ICD-10-CM. Use additional code(s) from category G89 to identify acute or chronic pain due to presence of the device, implant or graft (G89.18 or G89.28).

3) Transplant complications

(a) Transplant complications other than kidney

Codes under category T86, Complications of transplanted organs and tissues, are for use for both complications and rejection of transplanted organs. A transplant complication code is only assigned if the complication affects the function of the transplanted organ. Two codes are required to fully describe a transplant complication: the appropriate code from category T86 and a secondary code that identifies the complication.

Pre-existing conditions or conditions that develop after the transplant are not coded as complications unless they affect the function of the transplanted organs.

See I.C.21. for transplant organ removal status

See I.C.2. for malignant neoplasm associated with transplanted organ.

(b) Kidney transplant complications

Patients who have undergone kidney transplant may still have some form of chronic kidney disease (CKD) because the kidney transplant may not fully restore kidney function. Code T86.1- should be assigned for documented complications of a kidney transplant, such as transplant failure or rejection or other transplant complication. Code T86.1- should not be assigned for post kidney transplant patients who have chronic kidney (CKD) unless a transplant complication such as transplant failure or rejection is documented. If the documentation is unclear as to whether the patient has a complication of the transplant, query the provider.

Conditions that affect the function of the transplanted kidney, other than CKD, should be assigned a code from subcategory T86.1, Complications of transplanted organ, Kidney, and a secondary code that identifies the complication.

For patients with CKD following a kidney transplant, but who do not have a complication such as failure or rejection, see section I.C.14. Chronic kidney disease and kidney transplant status.

4) Complication codes that include the external cause

As with certain other T codes, some of the complications of care codes have the external cause included in the code. The code includes the nature of the complication as well as the type of procedure that caused the complication. No external cause code indicating the type of procedure is necessary for these codes.

5) Complications of care codes within the body system chapters

Intraoperative and postprocedural complication codes are found within the body system chapters with codes specific to the organs and structures of that body system. These codes should be sequenced first, followed by a code(s) for the specific complication, if applicable.

20. Chapter 20: External Causes of Morbidity (V00-Y99)

The external causes of morbidity codes should never be sequenced as the first- listed or principal diagnosis.

External cause codes are intended to provide data for injury research and evaluation of injury prevention strategies. These codes capture how the injury or health condition happened (cause), the intent (unintentional or accidental; or intentional, such as suicide or assault), the place where the event occurred the activity of the patient at the time of the event, and the person's status (e.g., civilian, military).

There is no national requirement for mandatory ICD-10-CM external cause code reporting. Unless a provider is subject to a state-based external cause code reporting mandate or these codes are required by a particular payer, reporting of ICD-10-CM codes in Chapter 20, External Causes of Morbidity, is not required. In the absence of a mandatory reporting requirement, providers are encouraged to voluntarily report external cause codes, as they provide valuable data for injury research and evaluation of injury prevention strategies.

a. General External Cause Coding Guidelines

1) Used with any code in the range of A00.0-T88.9, Z00-Z99

An external cause code may be used with any code in the range of A00.0-T88.9, Z00-Z99, classification that is a health condition due to an external cause. Though they are most applicable to injuries, they are also valid for use with such things as infections or diseases due to an external source, and other health conditions, such as a heart attack that occurs during strenuous physical activity.

2) External cause code used for length of treatment

Assign the external cause code, with the appropriate 7th character (initial encounter, subsequent encounter or sequela) for each encounter for which the injury or condition is being treated.

Most categories in chapter 20 have a 7th character requirement for each applicable code. Most categories in this chapter have three 7th character values: A, initial encounter, D, subsequent encounter and S, sequela. While the patient may be seen by a new or different provider over the course of treatment for an injury or condition, assignment of the 7th character for external cause should match the 7th character of the code assigned for the associated injury or condition for the encounter.

3) Use the full range of external cause codes

Use the full range of external cause codes to completely describe the cause, the intent, the place of occurrence, and if applicable, the activity of the patient at the time of the event, and the patient's status, for all injuries, and other health conditions due to an external cause.

4) Assign as many external cause codes as necessary

Assign as many external cause codes as necessary to fully explain each cause. If only one external code can be recorded, assign the code most related to the principal diagnosis.

5) The selection of the appropriate external cause code

The selection of the appropriate external cause code is guided by the Alphabetic Index of External Causes and by Inclusion and Exclusion notes in the Tabular List.

6) External cause code can never be a principal diagnosis

An external cause code can never be a principal (first-listed) diagnosis.

7) Combination external cause codes

Certain of the external cause codes are combination codes that identify sequential events that result in an injury, such as a fall which results in striking against an object. The injury may be due to either event or both. The combination external cause code used should correspond to the sequence of events regardless of which caused the most serious injury.

8) No external cause code needed in certain circumstances

No external cause code from Chapter 20 is needed if the external cause and intent are included in a code from another chapter (e.g. T36.0X1- Poisoning by penicillins, accidental (unintentional)).

b. Place of Occurrence Guideline

Codes from category Y92, Place of occurrence of the external cause, are secondary codes for use after other external cause codes to identify the location of the patient at the time of injury or other condition.

Generally, a place of occurrence code is assigned only once, at the initial encounter for treatment. However, in the rare instance that a new injury occurs during hospitalization, an additional place of occurrence code may be assigned. No 7th characters are used for Y92.

Do not use place of occurrence code Y92.9 if the place is not stated or is not applicable.

c. Activity Code

Assign a code from category Y93, Activity code, to describe the activity of the patient at the time the injury or other health condition occurred.

An activity code is used only once, at the initial encounter for treatment. Only one code from Y93 should be recorded on a medical record.

The activity codes are not applicable to poisonings, adverse effects, misadventures or sequela.

Do not assign Y93.9, Unspecified activity, if the activity is not stated.

A code from category Y93 is appropriate for use with external cause and intent codes if identifying the activity provides additional information about the event.

d. Place of Occurrence, Activity, and Status Codes Used with other External Cause Code

When applicable, place of occurrence, activity, and external cause status codes are sequenced after the main external cause code(s). Regardless of the number of external cause codes assigned, generally there should be only one place of occurrence code, one activity code, and one external cause status code assigned to an encounter. However, in the rare instance that a new injury occurs during hospitalization, an additional place of occurrence code may be assigned.

e. If the Reporting Format Limits the Number of External Cause Codes

If the reporting format limits the number of external cause codes that can be used in reporting clinical data, report the code for the cause/intent most related to the principal diagnosis. If the format permits capture of additional external cause codes, the cause/intent, including medical misadventures, of the additional events should be reported rather than the codes for place, activity, or external status.

f. Multiple External Cause Coding Guidelines

More than one external cause code is required to fully describe the external cause of an illness or injury. The assignment of external cause codes should be sequenced in the following priority:

If two or more events cause separate injuries, an external cause code should be assigned for each cause. The first-listed external cause code will be selected in the following order:

External codes for child and adult abuse take priority over all other external cause codes.

See Section I.C.19., Child and Adult abuse guidelines.

External cause codes for terrorism events take priority over all other external cause codes except child and adult abuse.

External cause codes for cataclysmic events take priority over all other external cause codes except child and adult abuse and terrorism.

External cause codes for transport accidents take priority over all other external cause codes except cataclysmic events, child and adult abuse and terrorism.

Activity and external cause status codes are assigned following all causal (intent) external cause codes.

The first-listed external cause code should correspond to the cause of the most serious diagnosis due to an assault, accident, or self-harm, following the order of hierarchy listed above.

g. Child and Adult Abuse Guideline

Adult and child abuse, neglect and maltreatment are classified as assault. Any of the assault codes may be used to indicate the external cause of any injury resulting from the confirmed abuse.

For confirmed cases of abuse, neglect and maltreatment, when the perpetrator is known, a code from Y07, Perpetrator of maltreatment and neglect, should accompany any other assault codes.

See Section I.C.19. Adult and child abuse, neglect and other maltreatment

h. Unknown or Undetermined Intent Guideline

If the intent (accident, self-harm, assault) of the cause of an injury or other condition is unknown or unspecified, code the intent as accidental intent. All transport accident categories assume accidental intent.

1) Use of undetermined intent

External cause codes for events of undetermined intent are only for use if the documentation in the record specifies that the intent cannot be determined.

i. Sequelae (Late Effects) of External Cause Guidelines

1) Sequelae external cause codes

Sequela are reported using the external cause code with the 7th character "S" for sequela. These codes should be used with any report of a late effect or sequela resulting from a previous injury.

See Section I.B.10 Sequela (Late Effects)

2) Sequela external cause code with a related current injury

A sequela external cause code should never be used with a related current nature of injury code.

3) Use of sequela external cause codes for subsequent visits

Use a late effect external cause code for subsequent visits when a late effect of the initial injury is being treated. Do not use a late effect external cause code for subsequent visits for follow- up care (e.g., to assess healing, to receive rehabilitative therapy) of the injury when no late effect of the injury has been documented.

j. Terrorism Guidelines

1) Cause of injury identified by the Federal Government (FBI) as terrorism

When the cause of an injury is identified by the Federal Government (FBI) as terrorism, the first-listed external cause code should be a code from category Y38, Terrorism. The definition of terrorism employed by the FBI is found at the inclusion note at the beginning of category Y38. Use additional code for place of occurrence (Y92.-). More than one Y38 code may be assigned if the injury is the result of more than one mechanism of terrorism.

2) Cause of an injury is suspected to be the result of terrorism

When the cause of an injury is suspected to be the result of terrorism a code from category Y38 should not be assigned. Suspected cases should be classified as assault.

3) Code Y38.9, Terrorism, secondary effects

Assign code Y38.9, Terrorism, secondary effects, for conditions occurring subsequent to the terrorist event. This code should not be assigned for conditions that are due to the initial terrorist act.

It is acceptable to assign code Y38.9 with another code from Y38 if there is an injury due to the initial terrorist event and an injury that is a subsequent result of the terrorist event.

k. External cause status

A code from category Y99, External cause status, should be assigned whenever any other external cause code is assigned for an encounter, including an Activity code, except for the events noted below. Assign a code from category Y99, External cause status, to indicate the work status of the person at the time the event occurred. The status code indicates whether the event occurred during military activity, whether a non-military person was at work, whether an individual including a student or volunteer was involved in a non-work activity at the time of the causal event.

A code from Y99, External cause status, should be assigned, when applicable, with other external cause codes, such as transport accidents and falls. The external cause status codes are not applicable to poisonings, adverse effects, misadventures or late effects.

Do not assign a code from category Y99 if no other external cause codes (cause, activity) are applicable for the encounter.

An external cause status code is used only once, at the initial encounter for treatment. Only one code from Y99 should be recorded on a medical record.

Do not assign code Y99.9, Unspecified external cause status, if the status is not stated.

21. Chapter 21: Factors influencing health status and contact with health services (Z00-Z99)

Note: The chapter specific guidelines provide additional information about the use of Z codes for specified encounters.

a. Use of Z codes in any healthcare setting

Z codes are for use in any healthcare setting. Z codes may be used as either a first-listed (principal diagnosis code in the inpatient setting) or secondary code, depending on the circumstances of the encounter.

Certain Z codes may only be used as first-listed or principal diagnosis.

b. Z Codes indicate a reason for an encounter

Z codes are not procedure codes. A corresponding procedure code must accompany a Z code to describe any procedure performed.

c. Categories of Z Codes

1) Contact/Exposure

Category Z20 indicates contact with, and suspected exposure to, communicable diseases. These codes are for patients who do not show any sign or symptom of a disease but are suspected to have been exposed to it by close personal contact with an infected individual or are in an area where a disease is epidemic.

Category Z77, Other contact with and (suspected) exposures hazardous to health, indicates contact with and suspected exposures hazardous to health.

Contact/exposure codes may be used as a first-listed code to explain an encounter for testing, or, more commonly, as a secondary code to identify a potential risk.

2) Inoculations and vaccinations

Code Z23 is for encounters for inoculations and vaccinations. It indicates that a patient is being seen to receive a prophylactic inoculation against a disease. Procedure codes are required to identify the actual administration of the injection and the type(s) of immunizations given. Code Z23 may be used as a secondary code if the inoculation is given as a routine part of preventive health care, such as a well-baby visit.

3) Status

Status codes indicate that a patient is either a carrier of a disease or has the sequelae or residual of a past disease or condition.

This includes such things as the presence of prosthetic or mechanical devices resulting from past treatment. A status code is informative, because the status may affect the course of treatment and its outcome. A status code is distinct from a history code. The history code indicates that the patient no longer has the condition.

A status code should not be used with a diagnosis code from one of the body system chapters, if the diagnosis code includes the information provided by the status code. For example, code Z94.1, Heart transplant status, should not be used with a code from subcategory T86.2, Complications of heart transplant. The status code does not provide additional information. The complication code indicates that the patient is a heart transplant patient.

For encounters for weaning from a mechanical ventilator, assign a code from subcategory J96.1, Chronic respiratory failure, followed by code Z99.11, Dependence on respirator [ventilator] status.

The status Z codes/categories are:

Z14 Genetic carrier

Genetic carrier status indicates that a person carries a gene, associated with a particular disease, which may be passed to offspring who may develop that disease. The person does not have the disease and is not at risk of developing the disease.

Z15 Genetic susceptibility to disease

Genetic susceptibility indicates that a person has a gene that increases the risk of that person developing the disease.

Codes from category Z15 should not be used as principal or first-listed codes. If the patient has the condition to which he/she is susceptible, and that condition is the reason for the encounter, the code for the current condition should be sequenced first. If the patient is being seen for follow-up after completed treatment for this condition, and the condition no longer exists, a follow-up code should be sequenced first, followed by the appropriate personal history and genetic susceptibility codes. If the purpose of the encounter is genetic counseling associated with procreative management, code Z31.5, Encounter for genetic counseling, should be assigned as the first-listed code, followed by a code from category Z15. Additional codes should be assigned for any applicable family or personal history.

Z16 Resistance to antimicrobial drugs

This code indicates that a patient has a condition that is resistant to antimicrobial drug treatment. Sequence the infection code first.

Z17 Estrogen receptor status

Z18 Retained foreign body fragments

Z19 Hormone sensitivity malignancy status

Z21 Asymptomatic HIV infection status

This code indicates that a patient has tested positive for HIV but has manifested no signs or symptoms of the disease.

Z22 Carrier of infectious disease

Carrier status indicates that a person harbors the specific organisms of a disease without manifest symptoms and is capable of transmitting the infection.

Z28.3 Underimmunization status

Z33.1 Pregnant state, incidental

This code is a secondary code only for use when the pregnancy is in no way complicating the reason for visit. Otherwise, a code from the obstetric chapter is required.

Z66 Do not resuscitate

This code may be used when it is documented by the provider that a patient is on do not resuscitate status at any time during the stay.

Z67 Blood type

Z68 Body mass index (BMI)

As with all other secondary diagnosis codes, the BMI codes should only be assigned when they meet the definition of a reportable diagnosis (see Section III, Reporting Additional Diagnoses).

Z74.01 Bed confinement status

Z76.82 Awaiting organ transplant status

Z78 Other specified health status

Code Z78.1 Physical restraint status, may be used when it is documented by the provider that a patient has been put in restraints during the current encounter. Please note that this code should not be reported when it is documented by the provider that a patient is temporarily restrained during a procedure.

Z79 Long-term (current) drug therapy

Codes from this category indicate a patient's continuous use of a prescribed drug (including such things as aspirin therapy) for the long-term treatment of a condition or for prophylactic use. It is not for use for patients who have addictions to drugs. This subcategory is not for use of medications for detoxification or maintenance programs to prevent withdrawal symptoms in patients with drug dependence (e.g., methadone maintenance for opiate dependence). Assign the appropriate code for the drug dependence instead.

Assign a code from Z79 if the patient is receiving a medication for an extended period as a prophylactic measure (such as for the prevention of deep vein thrombosis) or as treatment of a chronic condition (such as arthritis) or a disease requiring a lengthy course of treatment (such as cancer). Do not assign a code from category Z79 for medication being administered for a brief period of time to treat an acute illness or injury (such as a course of antibiotics to treat acute bronchitis).

Z88 Allergy status to drugs, medicaments and biological substances

Except: Z88.9, Allergy status to unspecified drugs, medicaments and biological substances status

Z89 Acquired absence of limb

Z90 Acquired absence of organs, not elsewhere classified

Z91.0- Allergy status, other than to drugs and biological substances

Z92.82 Status post administration of tPA (rtPA) in a different facility within the last 24 hours prior to admission to a current facility

Assign code Z92.82, Status post administration of tPA (rtPA) in a different facility within the last 24 hours prior to admission to current facility, as a secondary diagnosis when a patient is received by transfer into a facility and documentation indicates they were administered tissue plasminogen activator (tPA) within the last 24 hours prior to admission to the current facility.

This guideline applies even if the patient is still receiving the tPA at the time they are received into the current facility.

The appropriate code for the condition for which the tPA was administered (such as cerebrovascular disease or myocardial infarction) should be assigned first.

Code Z92.82 is only applicable to the receiving facility record and not to the transferring facility record.

Z93 Artificial opening status

Z94 Transplanted organ and tissue status

Z95 Presence of cardiac and vascular implants and grafts

Z96 Presence of other functional implants

Z97 Presence of other devices

Z98 Other postprocedural states

Assign code Z98.85, Transplanted organ removal status, to indicate that a transplanted organ has been previously removed. This code should not be assigned for the encounter in which the transplanted organ is removed. The complication necessitating removal of the transplant organ should be assigned for that encounter.

See section I.C19. for information on the coding of organ transplant complications.

Z99 Dependence on enabling machines and devices, not elsewhere classified

Note: Categories Z89-Z90 and Z93-Z99 are for use only if there are no complications or malfunctions of the organ or tissue replaced, the amputation site or the equipment on which the patient is dependent.

4) History (of)

There are two types of history Z codes, personal and family. Personal history codes explain a patient's past medical condition that no longer exists and is not receiving any treatment, but that has the potential for recurrence, and therefore may require continued monitoring.

Family history codes are for use when a patient has a family member(s) who has had a particular disease that causes the patient to be at higher risk of also contracting the disease.

Personal history codes may be used in conjunction with follow- up codes and family history codes may be used in conjunction with screening codes to explain the need for a test or procedure. History codes are also acceptable on any medical record regardless of the reason for visit. A history of an illness, even if no longer present, is important information that may alter the type of treatment ordered.

The history Z code categories are:

Z80 Family history of primary malignant neoplasm

Z81 Family history of mental and behavioral disorders

Z82 Family history of certain disabilities and chronic diseases (leading to disablement)

Z83 Family history of other specific disorders

Z84 Family history of other conditions

Z85 Personal history of malignant neoplasm

Z86 Personal history of certain other diseases

Z87 Personal history of other diseases and conditions

Z91.4- Personal history of psychological trauma, not elsewhere classified

Z91.5 Personal history of self-harm

Z91.8- Other specified personal risk factors, not elsewhere classified

Exception:

Z91.83, Wandering in diseases classified elsewhere

Z92 Personal history of medical treatment

Except: Z92.0, Personal history of contraception

Except: Z92.82, Status post administration of tPA (rtPA) in a different facility within the last 24 hours prior to admission to a current facility

5) Screening

Screening is the testing for disease or disease precursors in seemingly well individuals so that early detection and treatment can be provided for those who test positive for the disease (e.g., screening mammogram).

The testing of a person to rule out or confirm a suspected diagnosis because the patient has some sign or symptom is a diagnostic examination, not a screening. In these cases, the sign or symptom is used to explain the reason for the test.

A screening code may be a first-listed code if the reason for the visit is specifically the screening exam. It may also be used as an additional code if the screening is done during an office visit for other health problems. A screening code is not necessary if the screening is inherent to a routine examination, such as a pap smear done during a routine pelvic examination.

Should a condition be discovered during the screening then the code for the condition may be assigned as an additional diagnosis.

The Z code indicates that a screening exam is planned. A procedure code is required to confirm that the screening was performed.

The screening Z codes/categories:

Z11 Encounter for screening for infectious and parasitic diseases

Z12 Encounter for screening for malignant neoplasms

Z13 Encounter for screening for other diseases and disorders

Except: Z13.9, Encounter for screening, unspecified

Z36 Encounter for antenatal screening for mother

6) Observation

There are **three** observation Z code categories. They are for use in very limited circumstances when a person is being observed for a suspected condition that is ruled out. The observation codes are not for use if an injury or illness or any signs or symptoms related to the suspected condition are present. In such cases the diagnosis/symptom code is used with the corresponding external cause code.

The observation codes are to be used as principal diagnosis only. **The only exception to this is when the principal diagnosis is required to be a code from category Z38, Liveborn infants according to place of birth and type of delivery. Then a code from category Z05, Encounter for observation and evaluation of newborn for suspected diseases and conditions ruled out, is sequenced after the Z38 code**. Additional codes may be used in addition to the observation code, but only if they are unrelated to the suspected condition being observed.

Codes from subcategory Z03.7, Encounter for suspected maternal and fetal conditions ruled out, may either be used as a first-listed or as an additional code assignment depending on the case. They are for use in very limited circumstances on a maternal record when an encounter is for a suspected maternal or fetal condition that is ruled out during that encounter (for example, a maternal or fetal condition may be suspected due to an abnormal test result). These codes should not be used when the condition is confirmed. In those cases, the confirmed condition should be coded. In addition, these codes are not for use if an illness or any signs or symptoms related to the suspected condition or problem are present. In such cases the diagnosis/symptom code is used.

Additional codes may be used in addition to the code from subcategory Z03.7, but only if they are unrelated to the suspected condition being evaluated.

Codes from subcategory Z03.7 may not be used for encounters for antenatal screening of mother. *See Section I.C.21.* Screening.

For encounters for suspected fetal condition that are inconclusive following testing and evaluation, assign the appropriate code from category O35, O36, O40 or O41.

The observation Z code categories:

Z03 Encounter for medical observation for suspected diseases and conditions ruled out

Z04 Encounter for examination and observation for other reasons

Except: Z04.9, Encounter for examination and observation for unspecified reason

Z05 Encounter for observation and evaluation of newborn for suspected diseases and conditions ruled out

7) Aftercare

Aftercare visit codes cover situations when the initial treatment of a disease has been performed and the patient requires continued care during the healing or recovery phase, or for the long-term consequences of the disease. The aftercare Z code should not be used if treatment is directed at a current, acute disease. The diagnosis code is to be used in these cases. Exceptions to this rule are codes Z51.0, Encounter for antineoplastic radiation therapy, and codes from subcategory Z51.1, Encounter for antineoplastic chemotherapy and immunotherapy. These codes are to be first-listed, followed by the diagnosis code when a patient's encounter is solely to receive radiation therapy, chemotherapy, or immunotherapy for the treatment of a neoplasm. If the reason for the encounter is more than one type of antineoplastic therapy, code Z51.0 and a code from subcategory Z51.1 may be assigned together, in which case one of these codes would be reported as a secondary diagnosis.

The aftercare Z codes should also not be used for aftercare for injuries. For aftercare of an injury, assign the acute injury code with the appropriate 7th character (for subsequent encounter).

The aftercare codes are generally first-listed to explain the specific reason for the encounter. An aftercare code may be used as an additional code when some type of aftercare is provided in addition to the reason for admission and no diagnosis code is applicable. An example of this would be the closure of a colostomy during an encounter for treatment of another condition.

Aftercare codes should be used in conjunction with other aftercare codes or diagnosis codes to provide better detail on the specifics of an aftercare encounter visit, unless otherwise directed by the classification. Should a patient receive multiple types of antineoplastic therapy during the same encounter, code Z51.0, Encounter for antineoplastic radiation therapy, and codes from subcategory Z51.1, Encounter for antineoplastic chemotherapy and immunotherapy, may be used together on a record. The sequencing of multiple aftercare codes depends on the circumstances of the encounter.

Certain aftercare Z code categories need a secondary diagnosis code to describe the resolving condition or sequelae. For others, the condition is included in the code title.

Additional Z code aftercare category terms include fitting and adjustment, and attention to artificial openings.

Status Z codes may be used with aftercare Z codes to indicate the nature of the aftercare. For example code Z95.1, Presence of aortocoronary bypass graft, may be used with code Z48.812, Encounter for surgical aftercare following surgery on the circulatory system, to indicate the surgery for which the aftercare is being performed. A status code should not be used when the aftercare code indicates the type of status, such as using Z43.0, Encounter for attention to tracheostomy, with Z93.0, Tracheostomy status.

The aftercare Z category/codes:

Z42 Encounter for plastic and reconstructive surgery following medical procedure or healed injury

Z43 Encounter for attention to artificial openings

Z44 Encounter for fitting and adjustment of external prosthetic device

Z45 Encounter for adjustment and management of implanted device

Z46 Encounter for fitting and adjustment of other devices

Z47 Orthopedic aftercare

Z48 Encounter for other postprocedural aftercare

Z49 Encounter for care involving renal dialysis

Z51 Encounter for other aftercare **and medical care**

8) Follow-up

The follow-up codes are used to explain continuing surveillance following completed treatment of a disease, condition, or injury. They imply that the condition has been fully treated and no longer exists. They should not be confused with aftercare codes, or injury codes with a 7th character for subsequent encounter, that explain ongoing care of a healing condition or its sequelae. Follow-up codes may be used in conjunction with history codes to provide the full picture of the healed condition and its treatment. The follow-up code is sequenced first, followed by the history code.

A follow-up code may be used to explain multiple visits. Should a condition be found to have recurred on the follow-up visit, then the diagnosis code for the condition should be assigned in place of the follow-up code.

The follow-up Z code categories:

Z08 Encounter for follow-up examination after completed treatment for malignant neoplasm

Z09 Encounter for follow-up examination after completed treatment for conditions other than malignant neoplasm

Z39 Encounter for maternal postpartum care and examination

9) Donor

Codes in category Z52, Donors of organs and tissues, are used for living individuals who are donating blood or other body tissue. These codes are only for individuals donating for others, not for self-donations. They are not used to identify cadaveric donations.

10) Counseling

Counseling Z codes are used when a patient or family member receives assistance in the aftermath of an illness or injury, or when support is required in coping with family or social problems. They are not used in conjunction with a diagnosis code when the counseling component of care is considered integral to standard treatment.

The counseling Z codes/categories:

Z30.0- Encounter for general counseling and advice on contraception

Z31.5 Encounter for genetic counseling

Z31.6- Encounter for general counseling and advice on procreation

Z32.2 Encounter for childbirth instruction

Z32.3 Encounter for childcare instruction

Z69 Encounter for mental health services for victim and perpetrator of abuse

Z70 Counseling related to sexual attitude, behavior and orientation

Z71 Persons encountering health services for other counseling and medical advice, not elsewhere classified

Z76.81 Expectant mother prebirth pediatrician visit

11) Encounters for Obstetrical and Reproductive Services

See Section I.C.15. Pregnancy, Childbirth, and the Puerperium, for further instruction on the use of these codes.

Z codes for pregnancy are for use in those circumstances when none of the problems or complications included in the codes from the Obstetrics chapter exist (a routine prenatal visit or postpartum care). Codes in category Z34, Encounter for supervision of normal pregnancy, are always first-listed and are not to be used with any other code from the OB chapter.

Codes in category Z3A, Weeks of gestation, may be assigned to provide additional information about the pregnancy. **Category Z3A codes should not be assigned for pregnancies with abortive outcomes (categories O00-O08), elective termination of pregnancy (code Z33.2), nor for postpartum conditions, as category Z3A is not applicable to these conditions.** The date of the admission should be used to determine weeks of gestation for inpatient admissions that encompass more than one gestational week.

The outcome of delivery, category Z37, should be included on all maternal delivery records. It is always a secondary code. Codes in category Z37 should not be used on the newborn record.

Z codes for family planning (contraceptive) or procreative management and counseling should be included on an obstetric record either during the pregnancy or the postpartum stage, if applicable.

Z codes/categories for obstetrical and reproductive services:

Z30 Encounter for contraceptive management

Z31 Encounter for procreative management

Z32.2 Encounter for childbirth instruction

Z32.3 Encounter for childcare instruction

Z33 Pregnant state

Z34 Encounter for supervision of normal pregnancy

Z36 Encounter for antenatal screening of mother

Z3A Weeks of gestation

Z37 Outcome of delivery

Z39 Encounter for maternal postpartum care and examination

Z76.81 Expectant mother prebirth pediatrician visit

12) Newborns and Infants

See Section I.C.16. Newborn (Perinatal) Guidelines, for further instruction on the use of these codes.

Newborn Z codes/categories:

Z76.1 Encounter for health supervision and care of foundling

Z00.1- Encounter for routine child health examination

Z38 Liveborn infants according to place of birth and type of delivery

13) Routine and administrative examinations

The Z codes allow for the description of encounters for routine examinations, such as, a general check-up, or, examinations for administrative purposes, such as, a pre-employment physical. The codes are not to be used if the examination is for diagnosis of a suspected condition or for treatment purposes. In such cases the diagnosis code is used. During a routine exam, should a diagnosis or condition be discovered, it should be coded as an additional code. Pre-existing and chronic conditions and history codes may also be included as additional codes as long as the examination is for administrative purposes and not focused on any particular condition.

Some of the codes for routine health examinations distinguish between "with" and "without" abnormal findings. Code assignment depends on the information that is known at the time the encounter is being coded. For example, if no abnormal findings were found during the examination, but the encounter is being coded before test results are back, it is acceptable to assign the code for "without abnormal findings." When assigning a code for "with abnormal findings," additional code(s) should be assigned to identify the specific abnormal finding(s).

Pre-operative examination and pre-procedural laboratory examination Z codes are for use only in those situations when a patient is being cleared for a procedure or surgery and no treatment is given.

The Z codes/categories for routine and administrative examinations:

Z00 Encounter for general examination without complaint, suspected or reported diagnosis

Z01 Encounter for other special examination without complaint, suspected or reported diagnosis

Z02 Encounter for administrative examination Except: Z02.9, Encounter for administrative examinations, unspecified

Z32.0- Encounter for pregnancy test

14) Miscellaneous Z codes

The miscellaneous Z codes capture a number of other health care encounters that do not fall into one of the other categories. Certain of these codes identify the reason for the encounter; others are for use as additional codes that provide useful information on circumstances that may affect a patient's care and treatment.

Prophylactic Organ Removal

For encounters specifically for prophylactic removal of an organ (such as prophylactic removal of breasts due to a genetic susceptibility to cancer or a family history of cancer), the principal or first-listed code should be a code from category Z40, Encounter for prophylactic surgery, followed by the appropriate codes to identify the associated risk factor (such as genetic susceptibility or family history).

If the patient has a malignancy of one site and is having prophylactic removal at another site to prevent either a new primary malignancy or metastatic disease, a code for the malignancy should also be assigned in addition to a code from subcategory Z40.0, Encounter for prophylactic surgery for risk factors related to malignant neoplasms. A Z40.0 code should not be assigned if the patient is having organ removal for treatment of a malignancy, such as the removal of the testes for the treatment of prostate cancer.

Miscellaneous Z codes/categories:

Z28 Immunization not carried out

Except: Z28.3, Underimmunization status

Z29 Encounter for other prophylactic measures

Z40 Encounter for prophylactic surgery

Z41 Encounter for procedures for purposes other than remedying health state

Except: Z41.9, Encounter for procedure for purposes other than remedying health state, unspecified

Z53 Persons encountering health services for specific procedures and treatment, not carried out

Z55 Problems related to education and literacy

Z56 Problems related to employment and unemployment

Z57 Occupational exposure to risk factors

Z58 Problems related to physical environment

Z59 Problems related to housing and economic circumstances

Z60 Problems related to social environment

Z62 Problems related to upbringing

Z63 Other problems related to primary support group, including family circumstances

Z64 Problems related to certain psychosocial circumstances

Z65 Problems related to other psychosocial circumstances

Z72 Problems related to lifestyle

Note: These codes should be assigned only when the documentation specifies that the patient has an associated problem

Z73 Problems related to life management difficulty

Z74 Problems related to care provider dependency

Except: Z74.01, Bed confinement status

Z75 Problems related to medical facilities and other health care

Z76.0 Encounter for issue of repeat prescription

Z76.3 Healthy person accompanying sick person

Z76.4 Other boarder to healthcare facility

Z76.5 Malingerer [conscious simulation]

Z91.1- Patient's noncompliance with medical treatment and regimen

Z91.83 Wandering in diseases classified elsewhere

Z91.89 Other specified personal risk factors, not elsewhere classified

15) Nonspecific Z codes

Certain Z codes are so non-specific, or potentially redundant with other codes in the classification, that there can be little justification for their use in the inpatient setting. Their use in the outpatient setting should be limited to those instances when there is no further documentation to permit more precise coding. Otherwise, any sign or symptom or any other reason for visit that is captured in another code should be used.

Nonspecific Z codes/categories:

Z02.9 Encounter for administrative examinations, unspecified

Z04.9 Encounter for examination and observation for unspecified reason

Z13.9 Encounter for screening, unspecified

Z41.9 Encounter for procedure for purposes other than remedying health state, unspecified

Z52.9 Donor of unspecified organ or tissue

Z86.59 Personal history of other mental and behavioral disorders

Z88.9 Allergy status to unspecified drugs, medicaments and biological substances status

Z92.0 Personal history of contraception

16) Z Codes That May Only be Principal/First-Listed Diagnosis

The following Z codes/categories may only be reported as the principal/first-listed diagnosis, except when there are multiple encounters on the same day and the medical records for the encounters are combined:

Z00 Encounter for general examination without complaint, suspected or reported diagnosis Except: Z00.6

Z01 Encounter for other special examination without complaint, suspected or reported diagnosis

Z02 Encounter for administrative examination

Z03 Encounter for medical observation for suspected diseases and conditions ruled out

Z04 Encounter for examination and observation for other reasons

Z33.2 Encounter for elective termination of pregnancy

Z31.81 Encounter for male factor infertility in female patient

Z31.83 Encounter for assisted reproductive fertility procedure cycle

Z31.84 Encounter for fertility preservation procedure

Z34 Encounter for supervision of normal pregnancy

Z39 Encounter for maternal postpartum care and examination

Z38 Liveborn infants according to place of birth and type of delivery

Z42 Encounter for plastic and reconstructive surgery following medical procedure or healed injury

Z51.0 Encounter for antineoplastic radiation therapy

Z51.1- Encounter for antineoplastic chemotherapy and immunotherapy

Z52 Donors of organs and tissues

Except: Z52.9, Donor of unspecified organ or tissue

Z76.1 Encounter for health supervision and care of foundling

Z76.2 Encounter for health supervision and care of other healthy infant and child

Z99.12 Encounter for respirator [ventilator] dependence during power failure

Section II. Selection of Principal Diagnosis

The circumstances of inpatient admission always govern the selection of principal diagnosis. The principal diagnosis is defined in the Uniform Hospital Discharge Data Set (UHDDS) as "that condition established after study to be chiefly responsible for occasioning the admission of the patient to the hospital for care."

The UHDDS definitions are used by hospitals to report inpatient data elements in a standardized manner. These data elements and their definitions can be found in the July 31, 1985, Federal Register (Vol. 50, No, 147), pp. 31038-40.

Since that time the application of the UHDDS definitions has been expanded to include all non- outpatient settings (acute care, short term, long term care and psychiatric hospitals; home health agencies; rehab facilities; nursing homes, etc). **The UHDDS definitions also apply to hospice services (all levels of care).**

In determining principal diagnosis, coding conventions in the ICD-10-CM, the Tabular List and Alphabetic Index take precedence over these official coding guidelines.

(See Section I.A., Conventions for the ICD-10-CM)

The importance of consistent, complete documentation in the medical record cannot be overemphasized. Without such documentation the application of all coding guidelines is a difficult, if not impossible, task.

A. Codes for symptoms, signs, and ill-defined conditions

Codes for symptoms, signs, and ill-defined conditions from Chapter 18 are not to be used as principal diagnosis when a related definitive diagnosis has been established.

B. Two or more interrelated conditions, each potentially meeting the definition for principal diagnosis

When there are two or more interrelated conditions (such as diseases in the same ICD- 10-CM chapter or manifestations characteristically associated with a certain disease) potentially meeting the definition of principal diagnosis, either condition may be sequenced first, unless the circumstances of the admission, the therapy provided, the Tabular List, or the Alphabetic Index indicate otherwise.

C. Two or more diagnoses that equally meet the definition for principal diagnosis

In the unusual instance when two or more diagnoses equally meet the criteria for principal diagnosis as determined by the circumstances of admission, diagnostic workup and/or therapy provided, and the Alphabetic Index, Tabular List, or another coding guidelines does not provide sequencing direction, any one of the diagnoses may be sequenced first.

D. Two or more comparative or contrasting conditions

In those rare instances when two or more contrasting or comparative diagnoses are documented as "either/or" (or similar terminology), they are coded as if the diagnoses were confirmed and the diagnoses are sequenced according to the circumstances of the admission. If no further determination can be made as to which diagnosis should be principal, either diagnosis may be sequenced first.

E. A symptom(s) followed by contrasting/comparative diagnoses

GUIDELINE HAS BEEN DELETED EFFECTIVE OCTOBER 1, 2014

F. Original treatment plan not carried out

Sequence as the principal diagnosis the condition, which after study occasioned the admission to the hospital, even though treatment may not have been carried out due to unforeseen circumstances.

G. Complications of surgery and other medical care

When the admission is for treatment of a complication resulting from surgery or other medical care, the complication code is sequenced as the principal diagnosis. If the complication is classified to the T80-T88 series and the code lacks the necessary specificity in describing the complication, an additional code for the specific complication should be assigned.

H. Uncertain Diagnosis

If the diagnosis documented at the time of discharge is qualified as "probable", "suspected", "likely", "questionable", "possible", or "still to be ruled out", or other similar terms indicating uncertainty, code the condition as if it existed or was established. The bases for these guidelines are the diagnostic workup, arrangements for further workup or observation, and initial therapeutic approach that correspond most closely with the established diagnosis.

Note: This guideline is applicable only to inpatient admissions to short-term, acute, long-term care and psychiatric hospitals.

I. Admission from Observation Unit

1. Admission Following Medical Observation

When a patient is admitted to an observation unit for a medical condition, which either worsens or does not improve, and is subsequently admitted as an inpatient of the same hospital for this same medical condition, the principal diagnosis would be the medical condition which led to the hospital admission.

2. Admission Following Post-Operative Observation

When a patient is admitted to an observation unit to monitor a condition (or complication) that develops following outpatient surgery, and then is subsequently admitted as an inpatient of the same hospital, hospitals should apply the Uniform Hospital Discharge Data Set (UHDDS) definition of principal diagnosis as "that condition established after study to be chiefly responsible for occasioning the admission of the patient to the hospital for care."

J. Admission from Outpatient Surgery

When a patient receives surgery in the hospital's outpatient surgery department and is subsequently admitted for continuing inpatient care at the same hospital, the following guidelines should be followed in selecting the principal diagnosis for the inpatient admission:

- ❑ If the reason for the inpatient admission is a complication, assign the complication as the principal diagnosis.
- ❑ If no complication, or other condition, is documented as the reason for the inpatient admission, assign the reason for the outpatient surgery as the principal diagnosis.
- ❑ If the reason for the inpatient admission is another condition unrelated to the surgery, assign the unrelated condition as the principal diagnosis.

K. Admissions/Encounters for Rehabilitation

When the purpose for the admission/encounter is rehabilitation, sequence first the code for the condition for which the service is being performed. For example, for an admission/encounter for rehabilitation for right-sided dominant hemiplegia following a cerebrovascular infarction, report code I69.351, Hemiplegia and hemiparesis following cerebral infarction affecting right dominant side, as the first-listed or principal diagnosis.

If the condition for which the rehabilitation service is no longer present, report the appropriate aftercare code as the first-listed or principal diagnosis. For example, if a patient with severe degenerative osteoarthritis of the hip, underwent hip replacement and the current encounter/admission is for rehabilitation, report code Z47.1, Aftercare following joint replacement surgery, as the first-listed or principal diagnosis.

See Section I.C.21.c.7, Factors influencing health states and contact with health services, Aftercare.

Section III. Reporting Additional Diagnoses

GENERAL RULES FOR OTHER (ADDITIONAL) DIAGNOSES

For reporting purposes the definition for "other diagnoses" is interpreted as additional conditions that affect patient care in terms of requiring:

clinical evaluation; or

therapeutic treatment; or

diagnostic procedures; or

extended length of hospital stay; or

increased nursing care and/or monitoring.

The UHDDS item #11-b defines Other Diagnoses as "all conditions that coexist at the time of admission, that develop subsequently, or that affect the treatment received and/or the length of stay. Diagnoses that relate to an earlier episode which have no bearing on the current hospital stay are to be excluded." UHDDS definitions apply to inpatients in acute care, short-term, long term care and psychiatric hospital setting. The UHDDS definitions are used by acute care short- term hospitals to report inpatient data elements in a standardized manner. These data elements and their definitions can be found in the July 31, 1985, Federal Register (Vol. 50, No, 147), pp. 31038-40.

Since that time the application of the UHDDS definitions has been expanded to include all non- outpatient settings (acute care, short term, long term care and psychiatric hospitals; home health agencies; rehab facilities; nursing homes, etc). **The UHDDS definitions also apply to hospice services (all levels of care).**

The following guidelines are to be applied in designating "other diagnoses" when neither the Alphabetic Index nor the Tabular List in ICD-10-CM provide direction. The listing of the diagnoses in the patient record is the responsibility of the attending provider.

A. Previous conditions

If the provider has included a diagnosis in the final diagnostic statement, such as the discharge summary or the face sheet, it should ordinarily be coded. Some providers include in the diagnostic statement resolved conditions or diagnoses and status-post procedures from previous admission that have no bearing on the current stay. Such conditions are not to be reported and are coded only if required by hospital policy.

However, history codes (categories Z80-Z87) may be used as secondary codes if the historical condition or family history has an impact on current care or influences treatment.

B. Abnormal findings

Abnormal findings (laboratory, x-ray, pathologic, and other diagnostic results) are not coded and reported unless the provider indicates their clinical significance. If the findings are outside the normal range and the attending provider has ordered other tests to evaluate the condition or prescribed treatment, it is appropriate to ask the provider whether the abnormal finding should be added.

Please note: This differs from the coding practices in the outpatient setting for coding encounters for diagnostic tests that have been interpreted by a provider.

C. Uncertain Diagnosis

If the diagnosis documented at the time of discharge is qualified as "probable", "suspected", "likely", "questionable", "possible", or "still to be ruled out" or other similar terms indicating uncertainty, code the condition as if it existed or was established. The bases for these guidelines are the diagnostic workup, arrangements for further workup or observation, and initial therapeutic approach that correspond most closely with the established diagnosis.

Note: This guideline is applicable only to inpatient admissions to short-term, acute, long-term care and psychiatric hospitals.

Section IV. Diagnostic Coding and Reporting Guidelines for Outpatient Services

These coding guidelines for outpatient diagnoses have been approved for use by hospitals/ providers in coding and reporting hospital-based outpatient services and provider-based office visits. **Guidelines in Section I, Conventions, general coding guidelines and chapter-specific guidelines, should also be applied for outpatient services and office visits.**

Information about the use of certain abbreviations, punctuation, symbols, and other conventions used in the ICD-10-CM Tabular List (code numbers and titles), can be found in Section IA of these guidelines, under "Conventions Used in the Tabular List." Section I.B. contains general guidelines that apply to the entire classification. Section I.C. contains chapter-specific guidelines that correspond to the chapters as they are arranged in the classification. Information about the correct sequence to use in finding a code is also described in Section I.

The terms encounter and visit are often used interchangeably in describing outpatient service contacts and, therefore, appear together in these guidelines without distinguishing one from the other.

Though the conventions and general guidelines apply to all settings, coding guidelines for outpatient and provider reporting of diagnoses will vary in a number of instances from those for inpatient diagnoses, recognizing that:

The Uniform Hospital Discharge Data Set (UHDDS) definition of principal diagnosis **does not apply to hospital-based outpatient services and provider-based office visits.**

Coding guidelines for inconclusive diagnoses (probable, suspected, rule out, etc.) were developed for inpatient reporting and do not apply to outpatients.

A. Selection of first-listed condition

In the outpatient setting, the term first-listed diagnosis is used in lieu of principal diagnosis.

In determining the first-listed diagnosis the coding conventions of ICD-10-CM, as well as the general and disease specific guidelines take precedence over the outpatient guidelines.

Diagnoses often are not established at the time of the initial encounter/visit. It may take two or more visits before the diagnosis is confirmed.

The most critical rule involves beginning the search for the correct code assignment through the Alphabetic Index. Never begin searching initially in the Tabular List as this will lead to coding errors.

1. Outpatient Surgery

When a patient presents for outpatient surgery (same day surgery), code the reason for the surgery as the first-listed diagnosis (reason for the encounter), even if the surgery is not performed due to a contraindication.

2. Observation Stay

When a patient is admitted for observation for a medical condition, assign a code for the medical condition as the first-listed diagnosis.

When a patient presents for outpatient surgery and develops complications requiring admission to observation, code the reason for the surgery as the first reported diagnosis (reason for the encounter), followed by codes for the complications as secondary diagnoses.

B. Codes from A00.0 through T88.9, Z00-Z99

The appropriate code(s) from A00.0 through T88.9, Z00-Z99 must be used to identify diagnoses, symptoms, conditions, problems, complaints, or other reason(s) for the encounter/visit.

C. Accurate reporting of ICD-10-CM diagnosis codes

For accurate reporting of ICD-10-CM diagnosis codes, the documentation should describe the patient's condition, using terminology which includes specific diagnoses as well as symptoms, problems, or reasons for the encounter. There are ICD-10-CM codes to describe all of these.

D. Codes that describe symptoms and signs

Codes that describe symptoms and signs, as opposed to diagnoses, are acceptable for reporting purposes when a diagnosis has not been established (confirmed) by the provider. Chapter 18 of ICD-10-CM, Symptoms, Signs, and Abnormal Clinical and Laboratory Findings Not Elsewhere Classified (codes R00-R99) contain many, but not all codes for symptoms.

E. Encounters for circumstances other than a disease or injury

ICD-10-CM provides codes to deal with encounters for circumstances other than a disease or injury. The Factors Influencing Health Status and Contact with Health Services codes (Z00-Z99) are provided to deal with occasions when circumstances other than a disease or injury are recorded as diagnosis or problems.

See Section I.C.21. Factors influencing health status and contact with health services.

F. Level of Detail in Coding

1. ICD-10-CM codes with 3, 4, 5, 6 or 7 characters

ICD-10-CM is composed of codes with 3, 4, 5, 6 or 7 characters. Codes with three characters are included in ICD-10-CM as the heading of a category of codes that may be further subdivided by the use of fourth, fifth, sixth or seventh characters to provide greater specificity.

2. Use of full number of characters required for a code

A three-character code is to be used only if it is not further subdivided. A code is invalid if it has not been coded to the full number of characters required for that code, including the 7th character, if applicable.

G. ICD-10-CM code for the diagnosis, condition, problem, or other reason for encounter/visit

List first the ICD-10-CM code for the diagnosis, condition, problem, or other reason for encounter/visit shown in the medical record to be chiefly responsible for the services provided. List additional codes that describe any coexisting conditions. In some cases the first-listed diagnosis may be a symptom when a diagnosis has not been established (confirmed) by the physician.

H. Uncertain diagnosis

Do not code diagnoses documented as "probable", "suspected," "questionable," "rule out," or "working diagnosis" or other similar terms indicating uncertainty. Rather, code the condition(s) to the highest degree of certainty for that encounter/visit, such as symptoms, signs, abnormal test results, or other reason for the visit.

Please note: This differs from the coding practices used by short-term, acute care, long-term care and psychiatric hospitals.

I. Chronic diseases

Chronic diseases treated on an ongoing basis may be coded and reported as many times as the patient receives treatment and care for the condition(s)

J. Code all documented conditions that coexist

Code all documented conditions that coexist at the time of the encounter/visit, and require or affect patient care treatment or management. Do not code conditions that were previously treated and no longer exist. However, history codes (categories Z80- Z87) may be used as secondary codes if the historical condition or family history has an impact on current care or influences treatment.

K. Patients receiving diagnostic services only

For patients receiving diagnostic services only during an encounter/visit, sequence first the diagnosis, condition, problem, or other reason for encounter/visit shown in the medical record to be chiefly responsible for the outpatient services provided during the encounter/visit. Codes for other diagnoses (e.g., chronic conditions) may be sequenced as additional diagnoses.

For encounters for routine laboratory/radiology testing in the absence of any signs, symptoms, or associated diagnosis, assign Z01.89, Encounter for other specified special examinations. If routine testing is performed during the same encounter as a test to evaluate a sign, symptom, or diagnosis, it is appropriate to assign both the Z code and the code describing the reason for the non-routine test.

For outpatient encounters for diagnostic tests that have been interpreted by a physician, and the final report is available at the time of coding, code any confirmed or definitive diagnosis(es) documented in the interpretation. Do not code related signs and symptoms as additional diagnoses.

Please note: This differs from the coding practice in the hospital inpatient setting regarding abnormal findings on test results.

L. Patients receiving therapeutic services only

For patients receiving therapeutic services only during an encounter/visit, sequence first the diagnosis, condition, problem, or other reason for encounter/visit shown in the medical record to be chiefly responsible for the outpatient services provided during the encounter/visit. Codes for other diagnoses (e.g., chronic conditions) may be sequenced as additional diagnoses.

The only exception to this rule is that when the primary reason for the admission/encounter is chemotherapy or radiation therapy, the appropriate Z code for the service is listed first, and the diagnosis or problem for which the service is being performed listed second.

M. Patients receiving preoperative evaluations only

For patients receiving preoperative evaluations only, sequence first a code from subcategory Z01.81, Encounter for pre-procedural examinations, to describe the pre-op consultations. Assign a code for the condition to describe the reason for the surgery as an additional diagnosis. Code also any findings related to the pre-op evaluation.

N. Ambulatory surgery

For ambulatory surgery, code the diagnosis for which the surgery was performed. If the postoperative diagnosis is known to be different from the preoperative diagnosis at the time the diagnosis is confirmed, select the postoperative diagnosis for coding, since it is the most definitive.

O. Routine outpatient prenatal visits

See Section I.C.15. Routine outpatient prenatal visits.

P. Encounters for general medical examinations with abnormal findings

The subcategories for encounters for general medical examinations, Z00.0-, provide codes for with and without abnormal findings. Should a general medical examination result in an abnormal finding, the code for general medical examination with abnormal finding should be assigned as the first-listed diagnosis. **An examination with abnormal findings refers to a condition/diagnosis that is newly identified or a change in severity of a chronic condition (such as uncontrolled hypertension, or an acute exacerbation of chronic obstructive pulmonary disease) during a routine physical examination.** A secondary code for the abnormal finding should also be coded.

Q. Encounters for routine health screenings

See Section I.C.21. Factors influencing health status and contact with health services, Screening

Appendix I: Present on Admission Reporting Guidelines

Introduction

These guidelines are to be used as a supplement to the *ICD-10-CM Official Guidelines for Coding and Reporting* to facilitate the assignment of the Present on Admission (POA) indicator for each diagnosis and external cause of injury code reported on claim forms (UB-04 and 837 Institutional).

These guidelines are not intended to replace any guidelines in the main body of the *ICD-10-CM Official Guidelines for Coding and Reporting*. The POA guidelines are not intended to provide guidance on when a condition should be coded, but rather, how to apply the POA indicator to the final set of diagnosis codes that have been assigned in accordance with Sections I, II, and III of the official coding guidelines. Subsequent to the assignment of the ICD-10-CM codes, the POA indicator should then be assigned to those conditions that have been coded.

As stated in the Introduction to the ICD-10-CM Official Guidelines for Coding and Reporting, a joint effort between the healthcare provider and the coder is essential to achieve complete and accurate documentation, code assignment, and reporting of diagnoses and procedures. The importance of consistent, complete documentation in the medical record cannot be overemphasized. Medical record documentation from any provider involved in the care and treatment of the patient may be used to support the determination of whether a condition was present on admission or not. In the context of the official coding guidelines, the term "provider" means a physician or any qualified healthcare practitioner who is legally accountable for establishing the patient's diagnosis.

These guidelines are not a substitute for the provider's clinical judgment as to the determination of whether a condition was/was not present on admission. The provider should be queried regarding issues related to the linking of signs/symptoms, timing of test results, and the timing of findings.

Please see the CDC website for the detailed list of ICD-10-CM codes that do not require the use of a POA indicator (ftp://ftp.cdc.gov/pub/Health_Statistics/NCHS/Publications/ICD10CM/2017/). The conditions on this exempt list represent categories and/or codes for circumstances regarding the healthcare encounter or factors influencing health status that do not represent a current disease or injury or are always present on admission.

General Reporting Requirements

All claims involving inpatient admissions to general acute care hospitals or other facilities that are subject to a law or regulation mandating collection of present on admission information.

Present on admission is defined as present at the time the order for inpatient admission occurs -- conditions that develop during an outpatient encounter, including emergency department, observation, or outpatient surgery, are considered as present on admission.

POA indicator is assigned to principal and secondary diagnoses (as defined in Section II of the Official Guidelines for Coding and Reporting) and the external cause of injury codes.

Issues related to inconsistent, missing, conflicting or unclear documentation must still be resolved by the provider.

If a condition would not be coded and reported based on UHDDS definitions and current official coding guidelines, then the POA indicator would not be reported.

Reporting Options

Y - Yes

N - No

U - Unknown

W – Clinically undetermined

Unreported/Not used – (Exempt from POA reporting)

Reporting Definitions

Y = present at the time of inpatient admission

N = not present at the time of inpatient admission

U = documentation is insufficient to determine if condition is present on admission

W = provider is unable to clinically determine whether condition was present on admission or not

Timeframe for POA Identification and Documentation

There is no required timeframe as to when a provider (per the definition of "provider" used in these guidelines) must identify or document a condition to be present on admission. In some clinical situations, it may not be possible for a provider to make a definitive diagnosis (or a condition may not be recognized or reported by the patient) for a period of time after admission. In some cases it may be several days before the provider arrives at a definitive diagnosis. This does not mean that the condition was not present on admission. Determination of whether the condition was present on admission or not will be based on the applicable POA guideline as identified in this document, or on the provider's best clinical judgment.

If at the time of code assignment the documentation is unclear as to whether a condition was present on admission or not, it is appropriate to query the provider for clarification.

Assigning the POA Indicator

Condition is on the "Exempt from Reporting" list

Leave the "present on admission" field blank if the condition is on the list of ICD-10-CM codes for which this field is not applicable. This is the only circumstance in which the field may be left blank.

POA Explicitly Documented

Assign Y for any condition the provider explicitly documents as being present on admission.

Assign N for any condition the provider explicitly documents as not present at the time of admission.

Conditions diagnosed prior to inpatient admission

Assign "Y" for conditions that were diagnosed prior to admission (example: hypertension, diabetes mellitus, asthma)

Conditions diagnosed during the admission but clearly present before admission

Assign "Y" for conditions diagnosed during the admission that were clearly present but not diagnosed until after admission occurred.

Diagnoses subsequently confirmed after admission are considered present on admission if at the time of admission they are documented as suspected, possible, rule out, differential diagnosis, or constitute an underlying cause of a symptom that is present at the time of admission.

Condition develops during outpatient encounter prior to inpatient admission

Assign Y for any condition that develops during an outpatient encounter prior to a written order for inpatient admission.

Documentation does not indicate whether condition was present on admission

Assign "U" when the medical record documentation is unclear as to whether the condition was present on admission. "U" should not be routinely assigned and used only in very limited circumstances. Coders are encouraged to query the providers when the documentation is unclear.

Documentation states that it cannot be determined whether the condition was or was not present on admission

Assign "W" when the medical record documentation indicates that it cannot be clinically determined whether or not the condition was present on admission.

Chronic condition with acute exacerbation during the admission

If a single code identifies both the chronic condition and the acute exacerbation, see POA guidelines pertaining to **codes that contain multiple clinical concepts.**

If a single code only identifies the chronic condition and not the acute exacerbation (e.g., acute exacerbation of chronic leukemia), assign "Y."

Conditions documented as possible, probable, suspected, or rule out at the time of discharge

If the final diagnosis contains a possible, probable, suspected, or rule out diagnosis, and this diagnosis was based on signs, symptoms or clinical findings suspected at the time of inpatient admission, assign "Y."

If the final diagnosis contains a possible, probable, suspected, or rule out diagnosis, and this diagnosis was based on signs, symptoms or clinical findings that were not present on admission, assign "N".

Conditions documented as impending or threatened at the time of discharge

If the final diagnosis contains an impending or threatened diagnosis, and this diagnosis is based on symptoms or clinical findings that were present on admission, assign "Y".

If the final diagnosis contains an impending or threatened diagnosis, and this diagnosis is based on symptoms or clinical findings that were not present on admission, assign "N".

Acute and Chronic Conditions

Assign "Y" for acute conditions that are present at time of admission and N for acute conditions that are not present at time of admission.

Assign "Y" for chronic conditions, even though the condition may not be diagnosed until after admission.

If a single code identifies both an acute and chronic condition, see the POA guidelines for codes **that contain multiple clinical concepts.**

Codes **That Contain Multiple Clinical Concepts**

Assign "N" if at least one of the clinical concepts included in the code was not present on admission (e.g., COPD with acute exacerbation and the exacerbation was not present on admission; gastric ulcer that does not start bleeding until after admission; asthma patient develops status asthmaticus after admission).

Assign "Y" if all of the **clinical concepts included in the code** were present on admission (e.g., **duodenal ulcer that perforates prior to admission**).

For infection codes that include the causal organism, assign "Y" if the infection (or signs of the infection) **were** present on admission, even though the culture results may not be known until after admission (e.g., patient is admitted with pneumonia and the provider documents Pseudomonas as the causal organism a few days later).

Same Diagnosis Code for Two or More Conditions

When the same ICD-10-CM diagnosis code applies to two or more conditions during the same encounter (e.g. two separate conditions classified to the same ICD-10-CM diagnosis code):

Assign "Y" if all conditions represented by the single ICD-10-CM code were present on admission (e.g. bilateral unspecified age-related cataracts).

Assign "N" if any of the conditions represented by the single ICD-10-CM code was not present on admission (e.g. traumatic secondary and recurrent hemorrhage and seroma is assigned to a single code T79.2, but only one of the conditions was present on admission).

Obstetrical conditions

Whether or not the patient delivers during the current hospitalization does not affect assignment of the POA indicator. The determining factor for POA assignment is whether the pregnancy complication or obstetrical condition described by the code was present at the time of admission or not.

If the pregnancy complication or obstetrical condition was present on admission (e.g., patient admitted in preterm labor), assign "Y".

If the pregnancy complication or obstetrical condition was not present on admission (e.g., 2nd degree laceration during delivery, postpartum hemorrhage that occurred during current hospitalization, fetal distress develops after admission), assign "N".

If the obstetrical code includes more than one diagnosis and any of the diagnoses identified by the code were not present on admission assign "N".

(e.g., Category O11, Pre-existing hypertension with pre-eclampsia)

Perinatal conditions

Newborns are not considered to be admitted until after birth. Therefore, any condition present at birth or that developed in utero is considered present at admission and should be assigned "Y". This includes conditions that occur during delivery (e.g., injury during delivery, meconium aspiration, exposure to streptococcus B in the vaginal canal).

Congenital conditions and anomalies

Assign "Y" for congenital conditions and anomalies except for categories Q00- Q99, Congenital anomalies, which are on the exempt list. Congenital conditions are always considered present on admission.

External cause of injury codes

Assign "Y" for any external cause code representing an external cause of morbidity that occurred prior to inpatient admission (e.g., patient fell out of bed at home, patient fell out of bed in emergency room prior to admission)

Assign "N" for any external cause code representing an external cause of morbidity that occurred during inpatient hospitalization (e.g., patient fell out of hospital bed during hospital stay, patient experienced an adverse reaction to a medication administered after inpatient admission)

Anatomical Illustrations

Circulatory System — Arteries and Veins

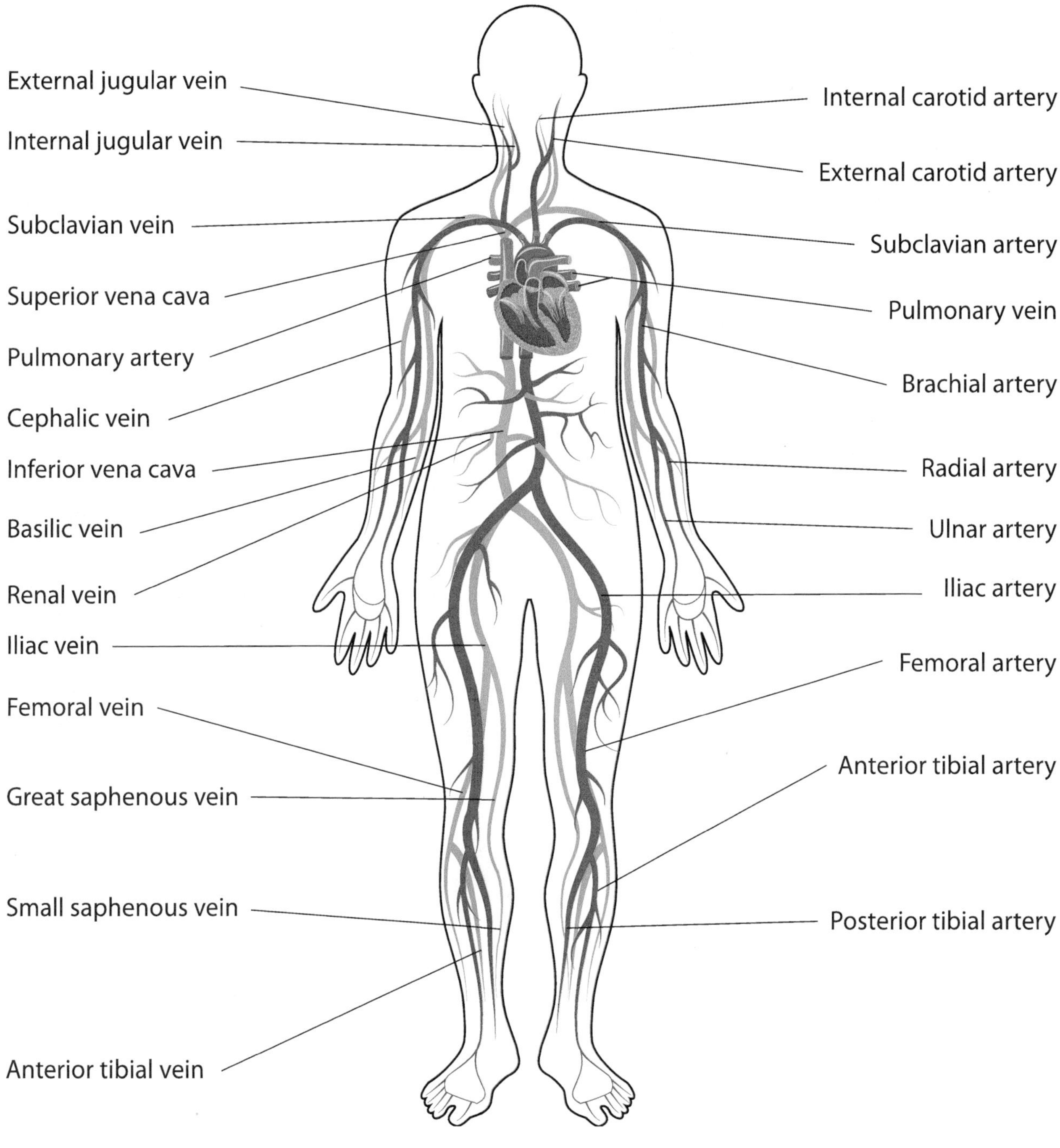

Circulatory System — Artery and Vein Anatomy

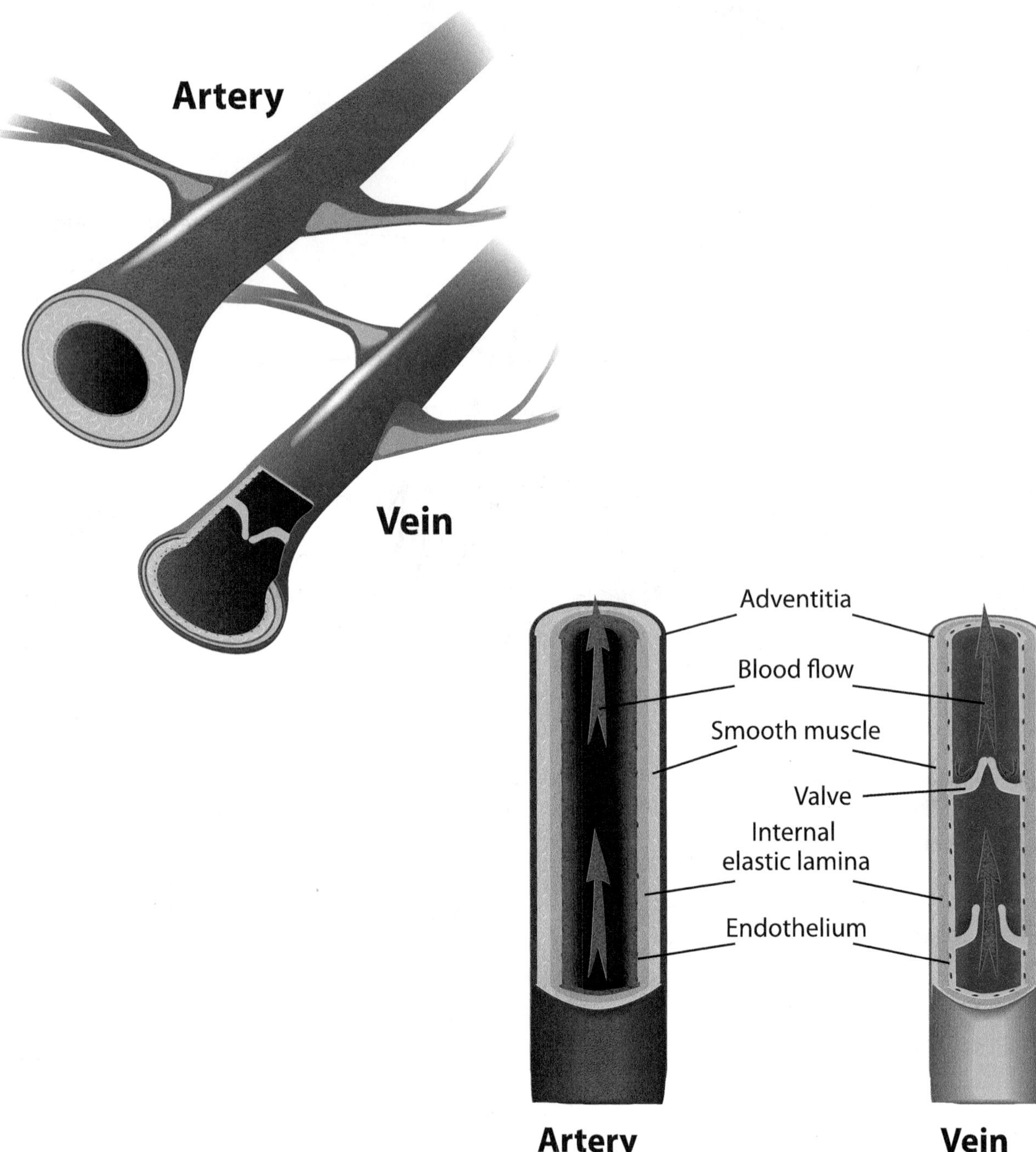

Circulatory System — Heart Anatomy and Cardiac Cycle

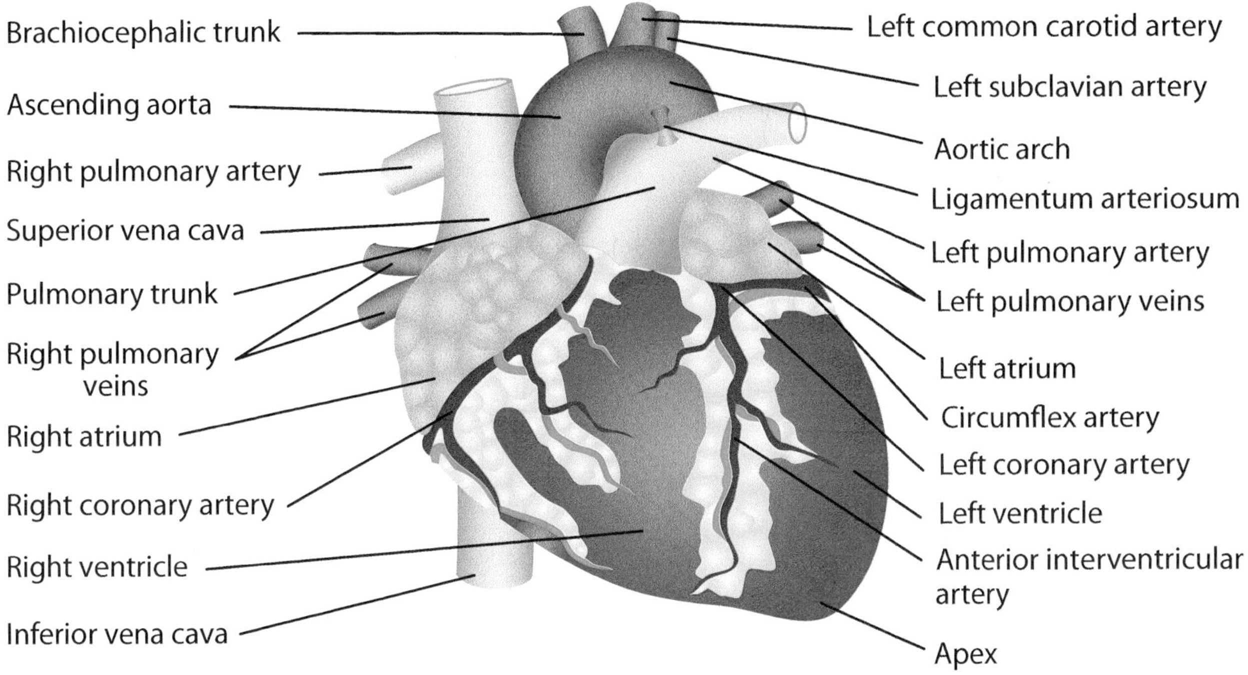

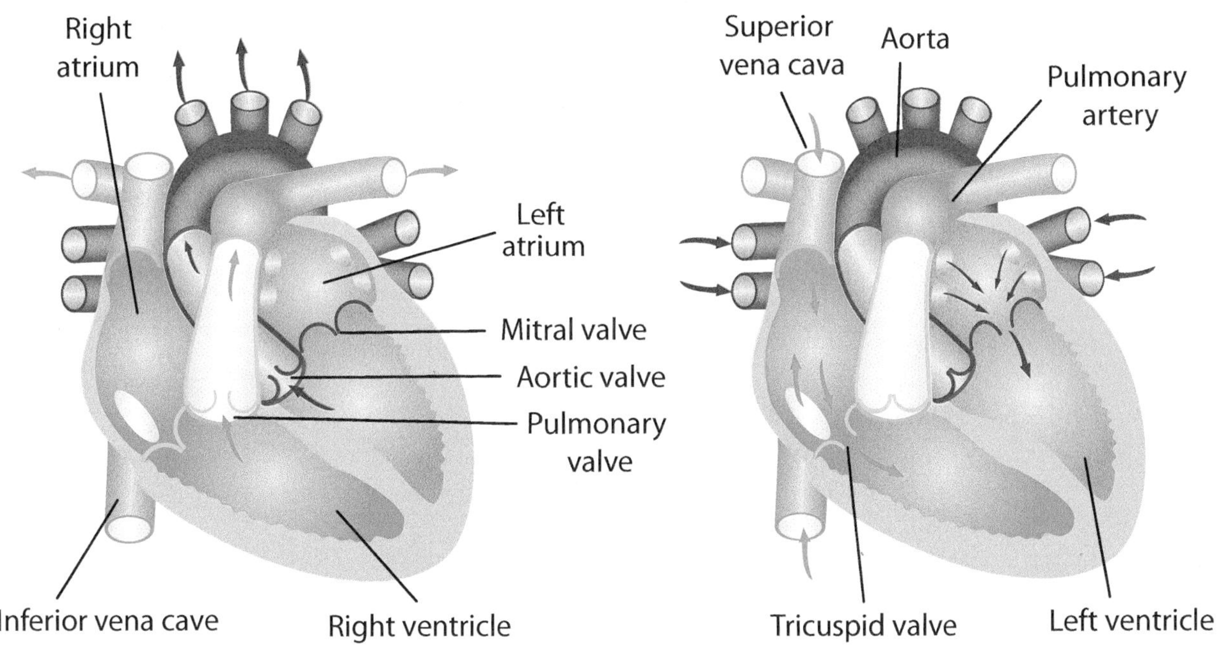

Diastole Ventricular Relaxation and Filling

Systole Ventricular Contraction and Ejection

Digestive System — Digestive Organs

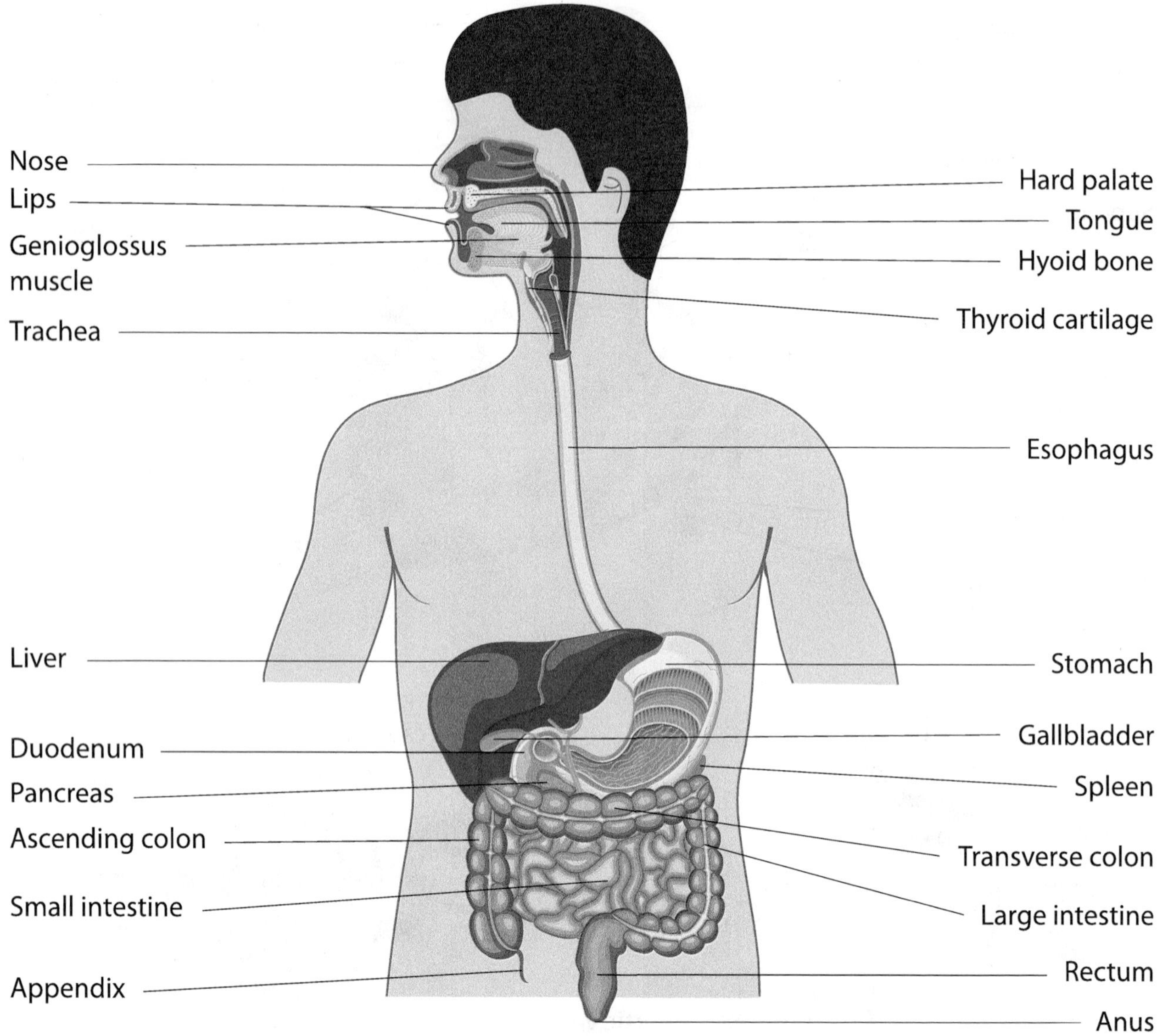

Digestive System — Large Intestine Anatomy

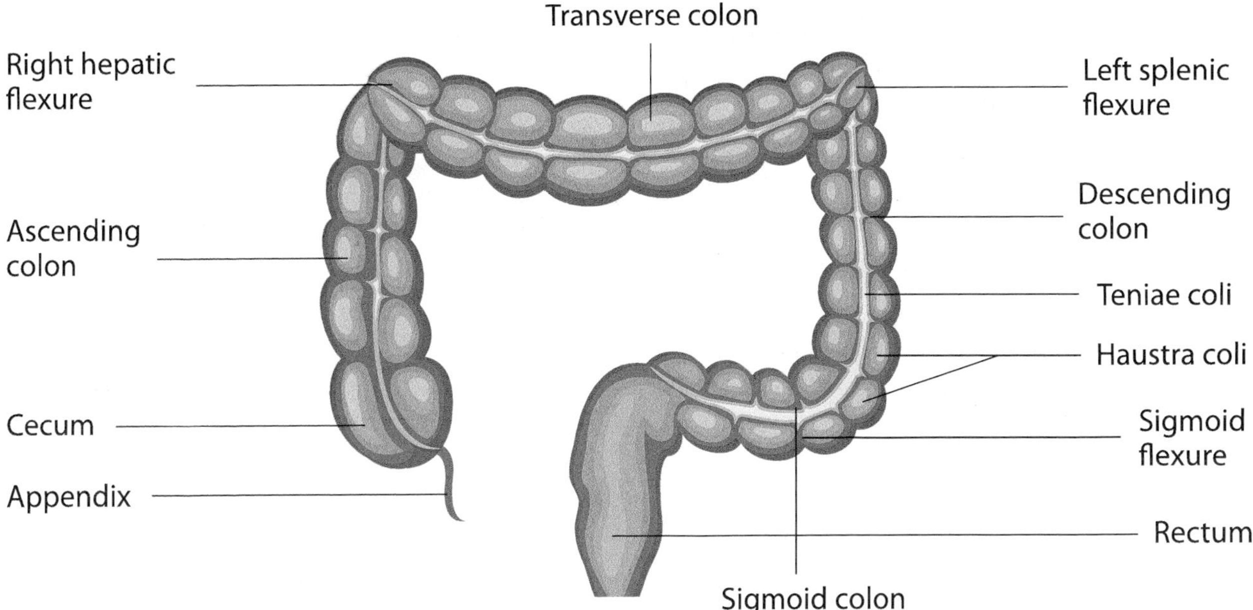

Rectum Anatomy

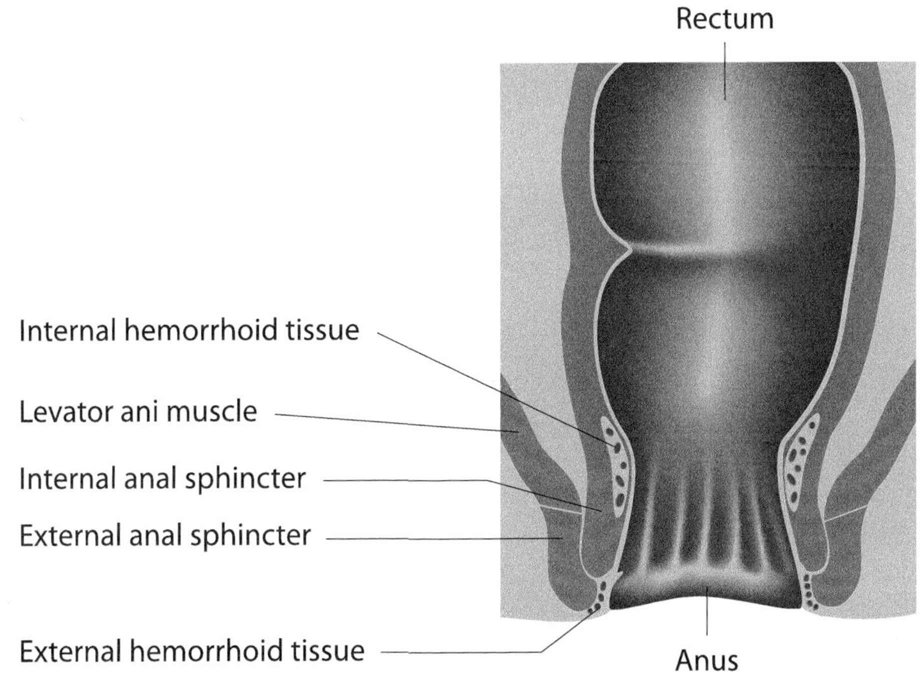

Digestive System — Liver Anatomy

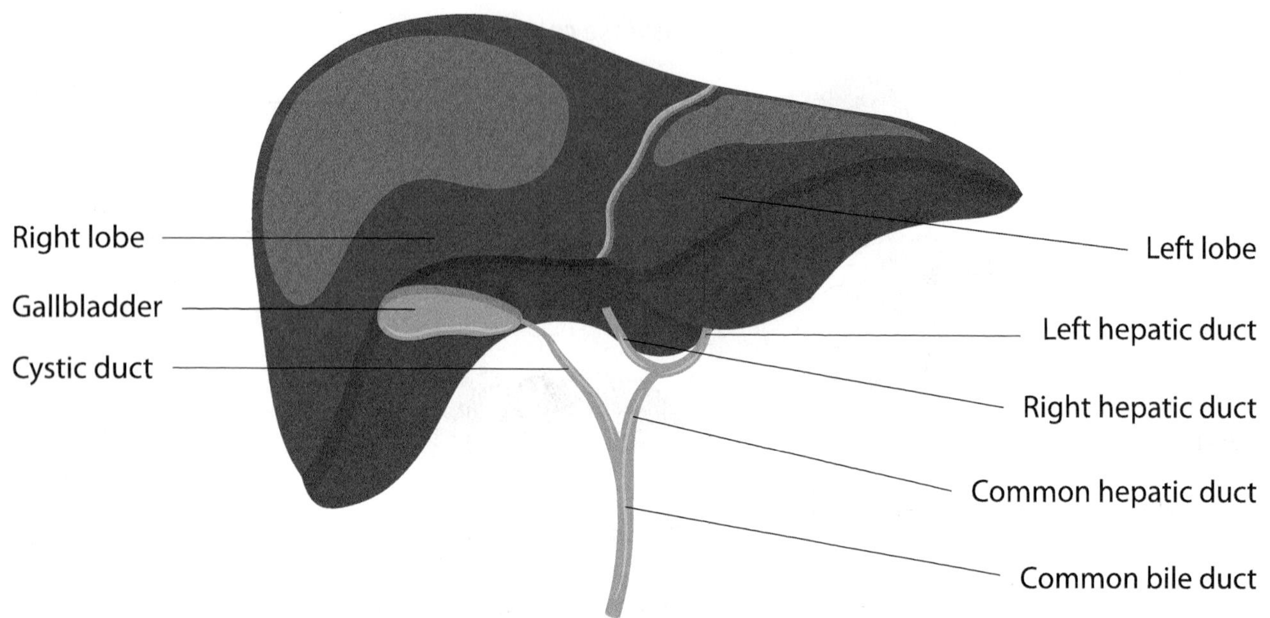

Pancreas Anatomy

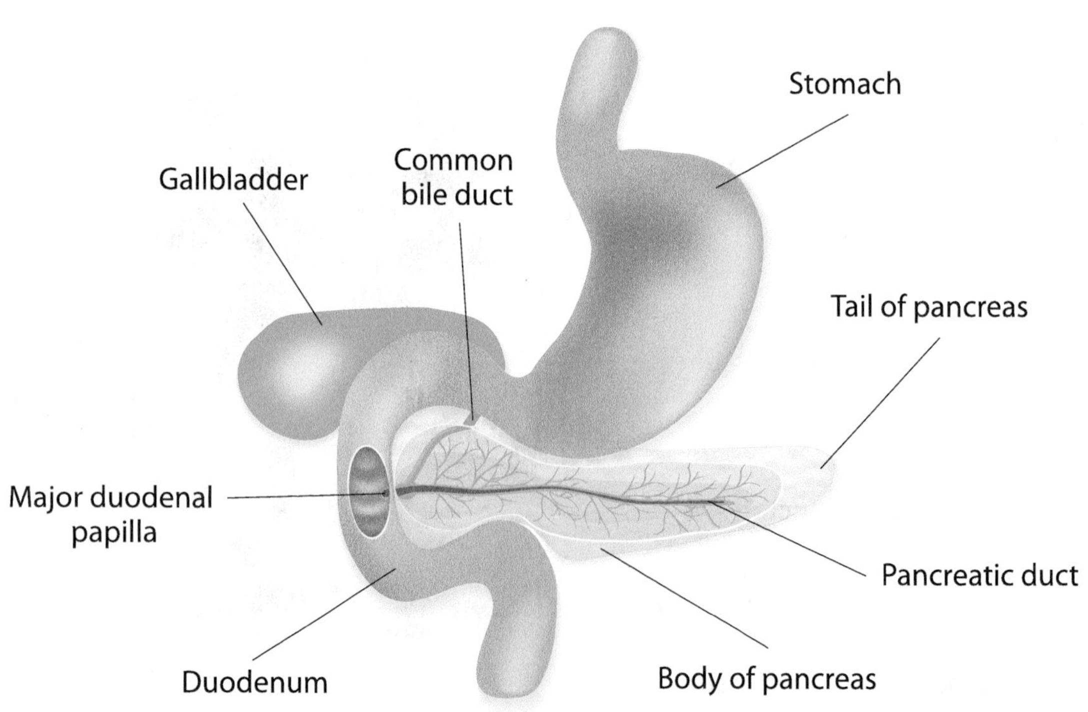

Digestive System — Mouth Anatomy

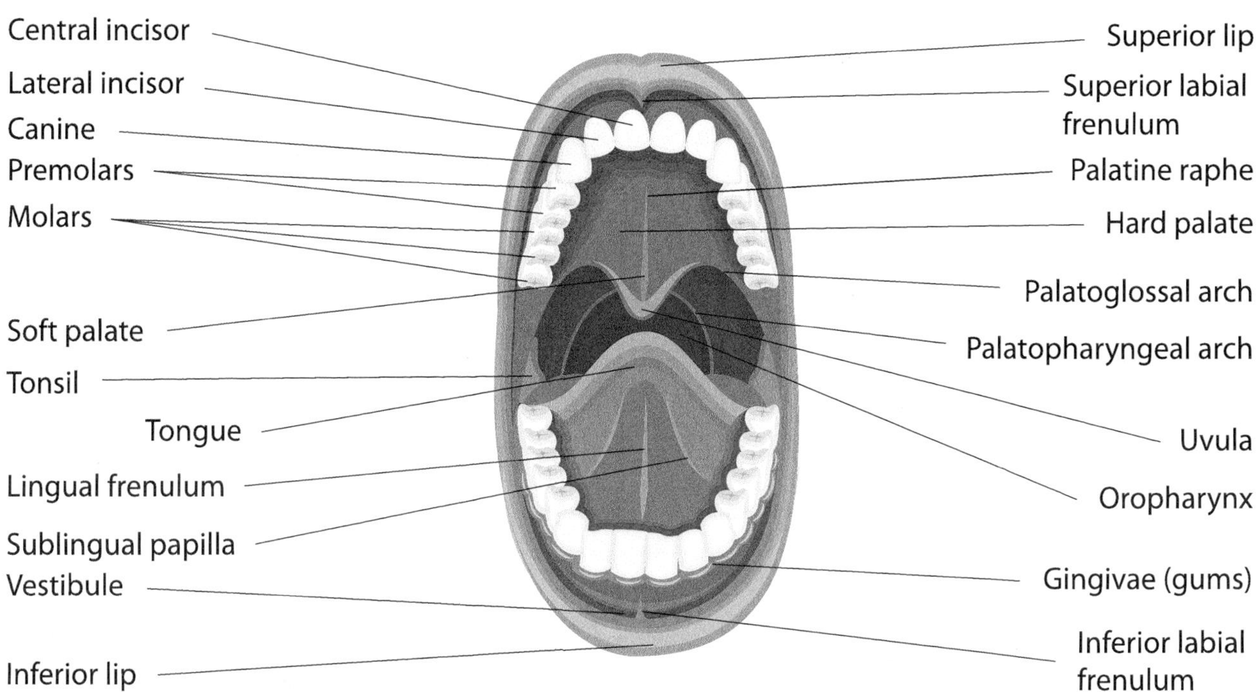
Central incisor
Lateral incisor
Canine
Premolars
Molars
Soft palate
Tonsil
Tongue
Lingual frenulum
Sublingual papilla
Vestibule
Inferior lip
Superior lip
Superior labial frenulum
Palatine raphe
Hard palate
Palatoglossal arch
Palatopharyngeal arch
Uvula
Oropharynx
Gingivae (gums)
Inferior labial frenulum

Tongue Anatomy

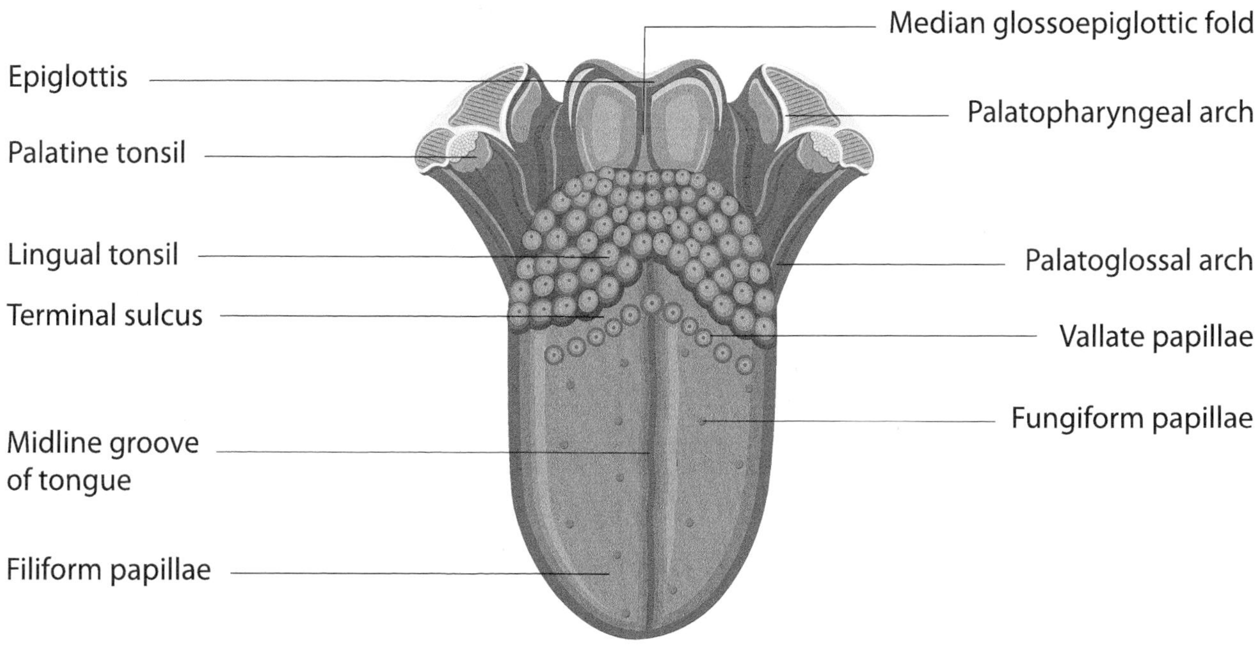
Median glossoepiglottic fold
Epiglottis
Palatine tonsil
Lingual tonsil
Terminal sulcus
Midline groove of tongue
Filiform papillae
Palatopharyngeal arch
Palatoglossal arch
Vallate papillae
Fungiform papillae

Digestive System — Small Intestine Anatomy

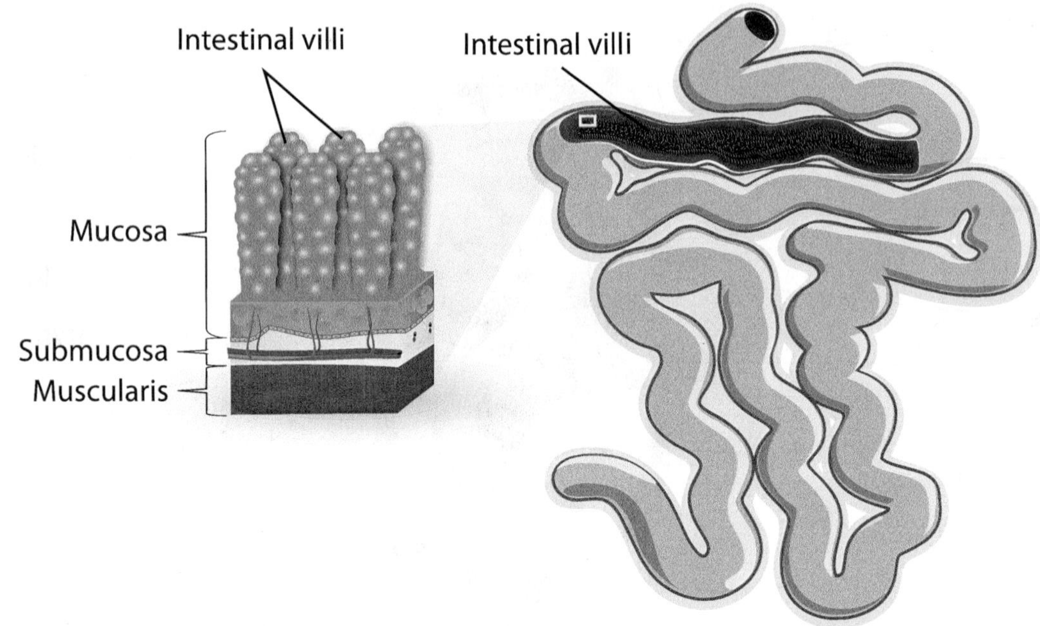

Stomach Anatomy

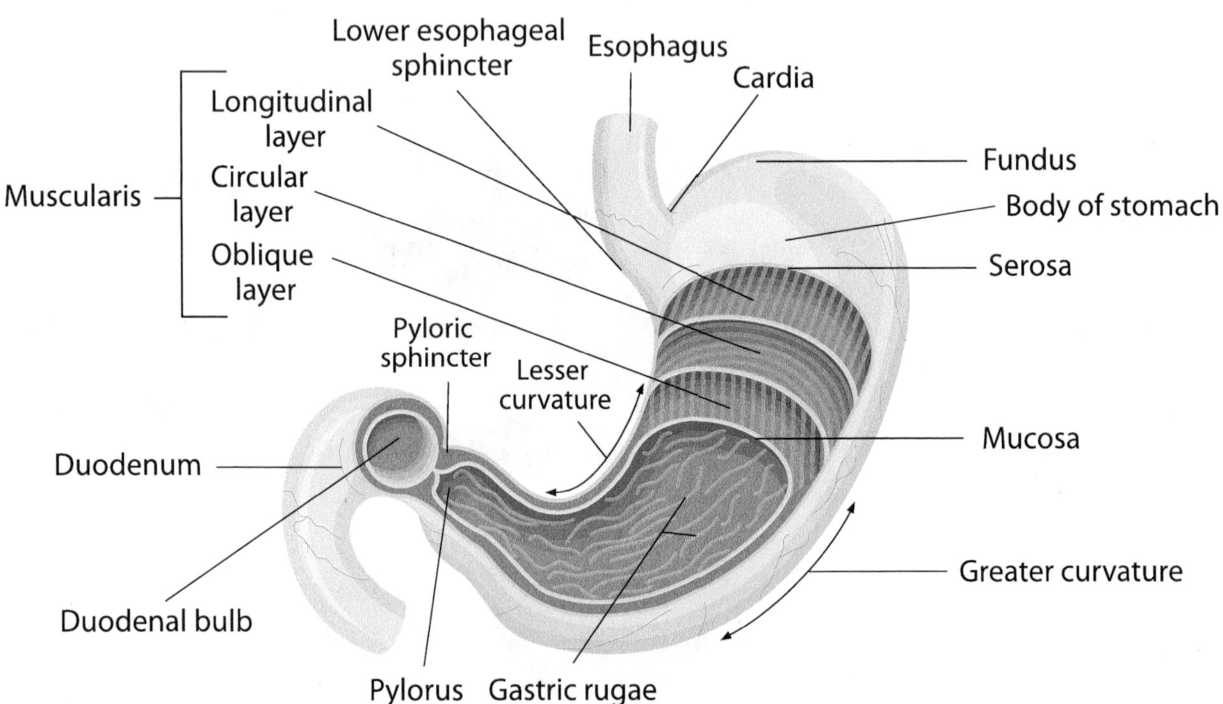

Ear — Ear Anatomy

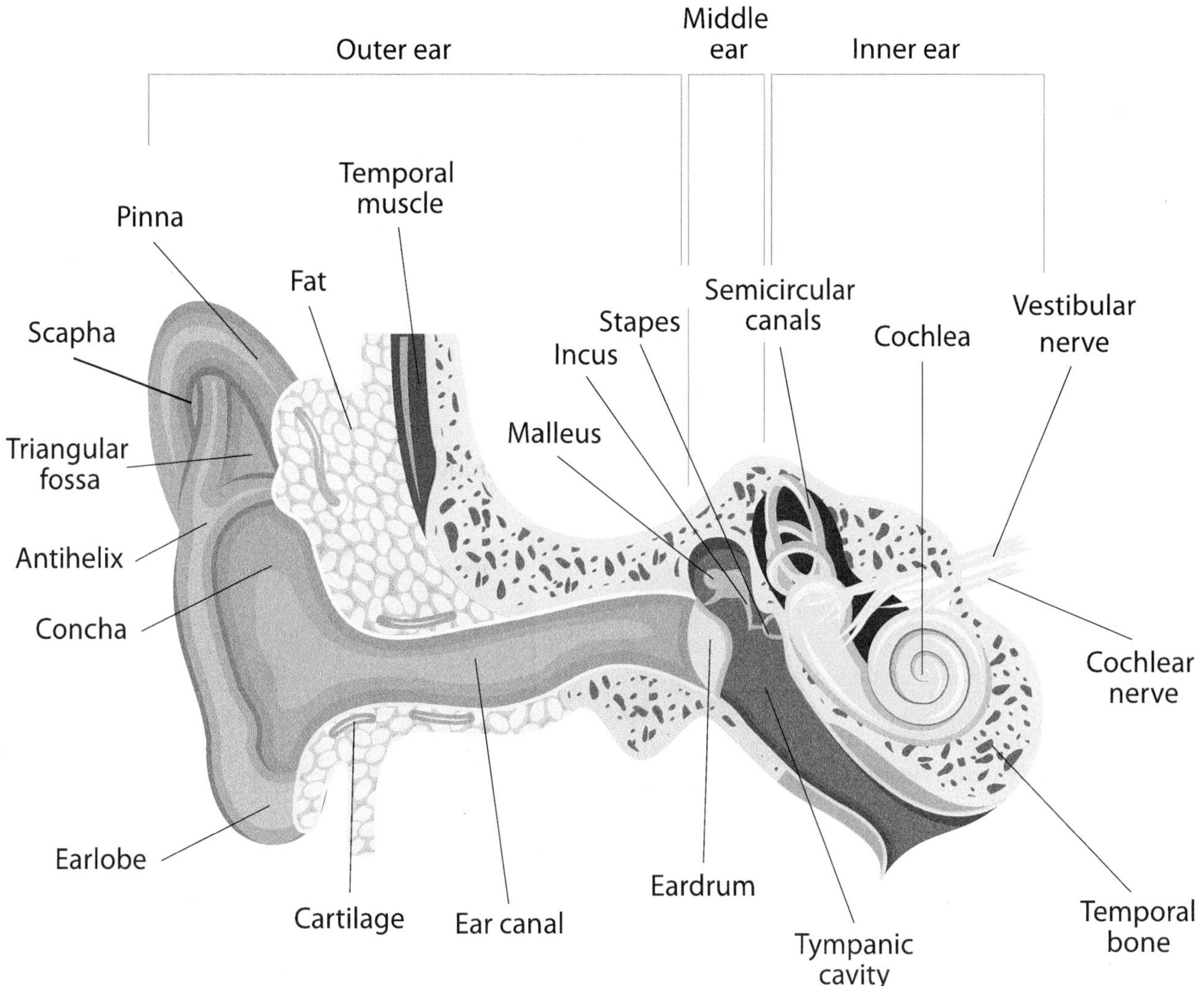

Ear — Cochlea Anatomy (Inner Ear)

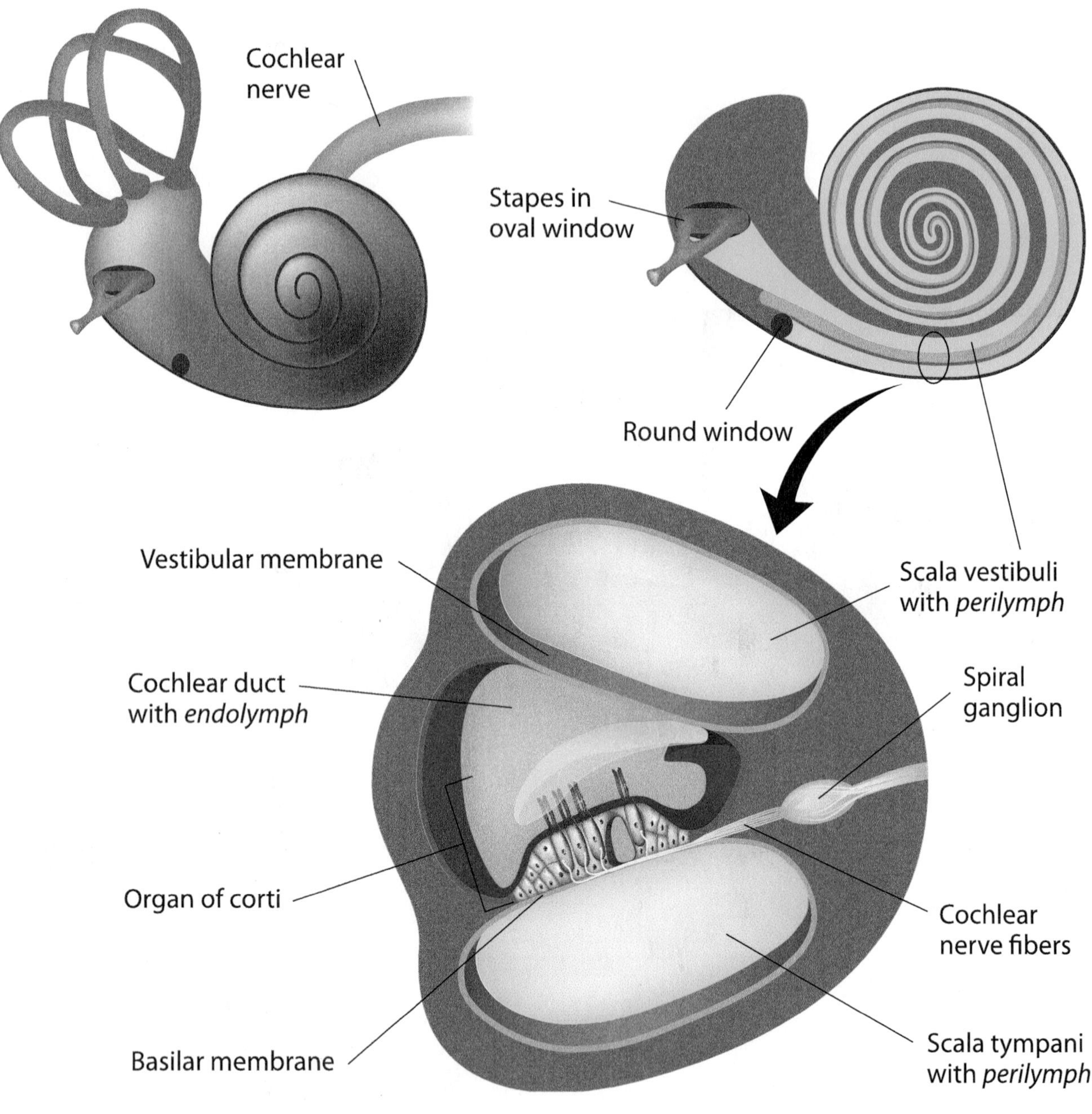

Endocrine System — Endocrine Anatomy

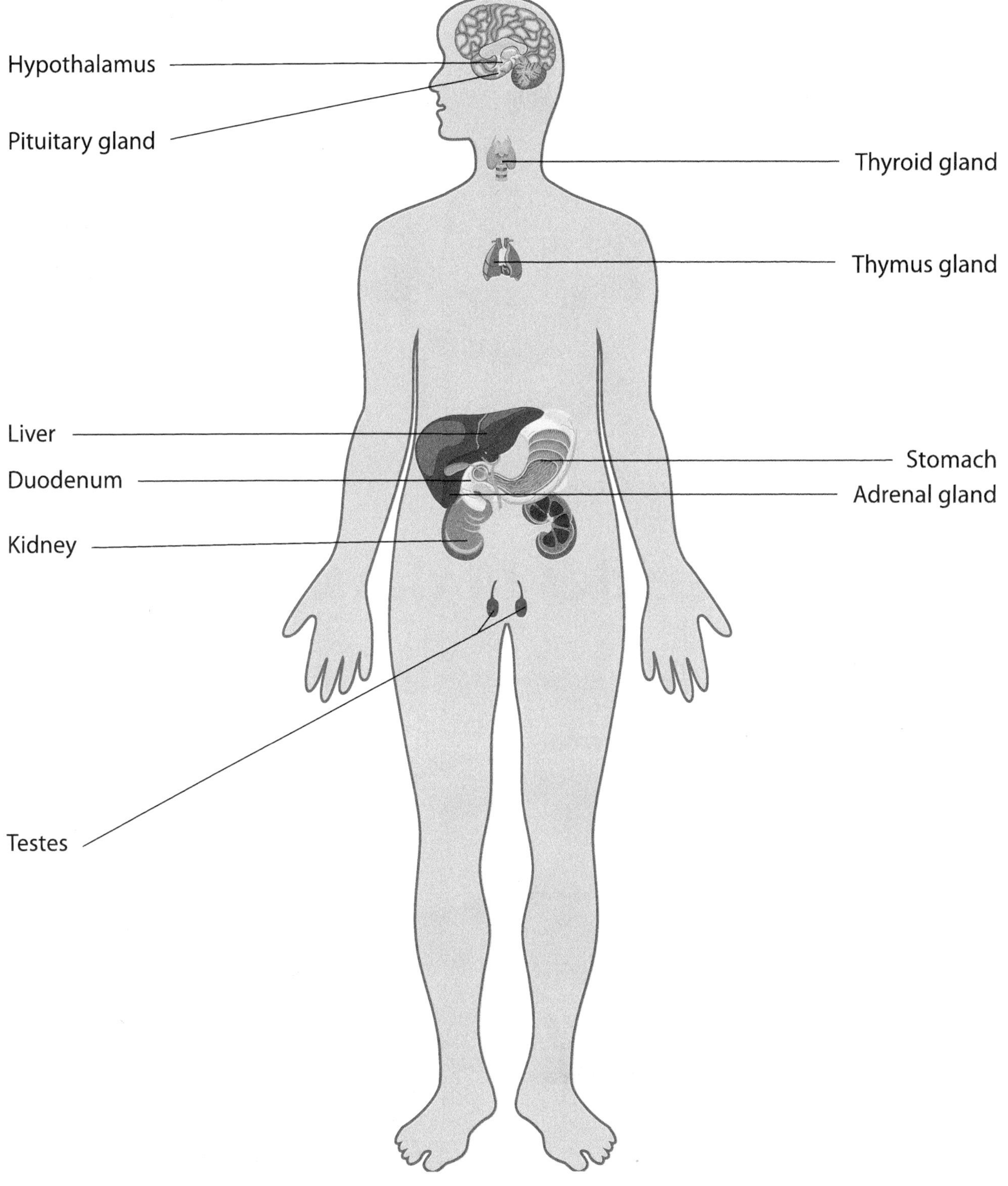

Eye — Eye Anatomy

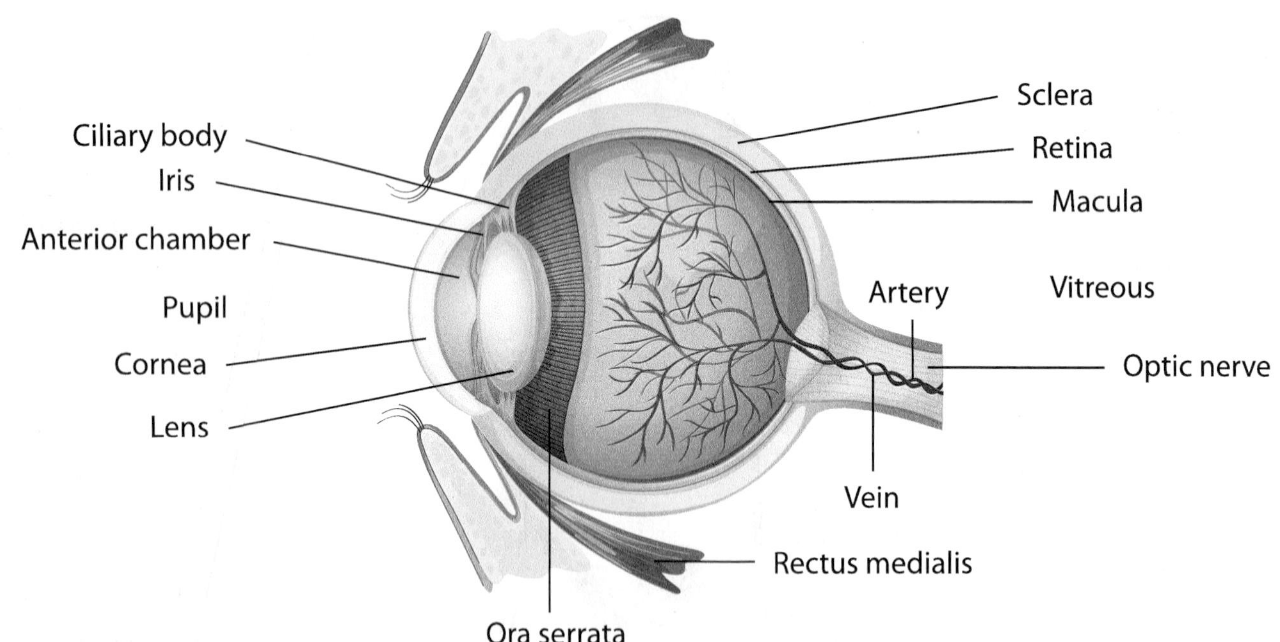
Ciliary body
Iris
Anterior chamber
Pupil
Cornea
Lens
Sclera
Retina
Macula
Artery
Vitreous
Optic nerve
Vein
Rectus medialis
Ora serrata

Muscles of the Eye

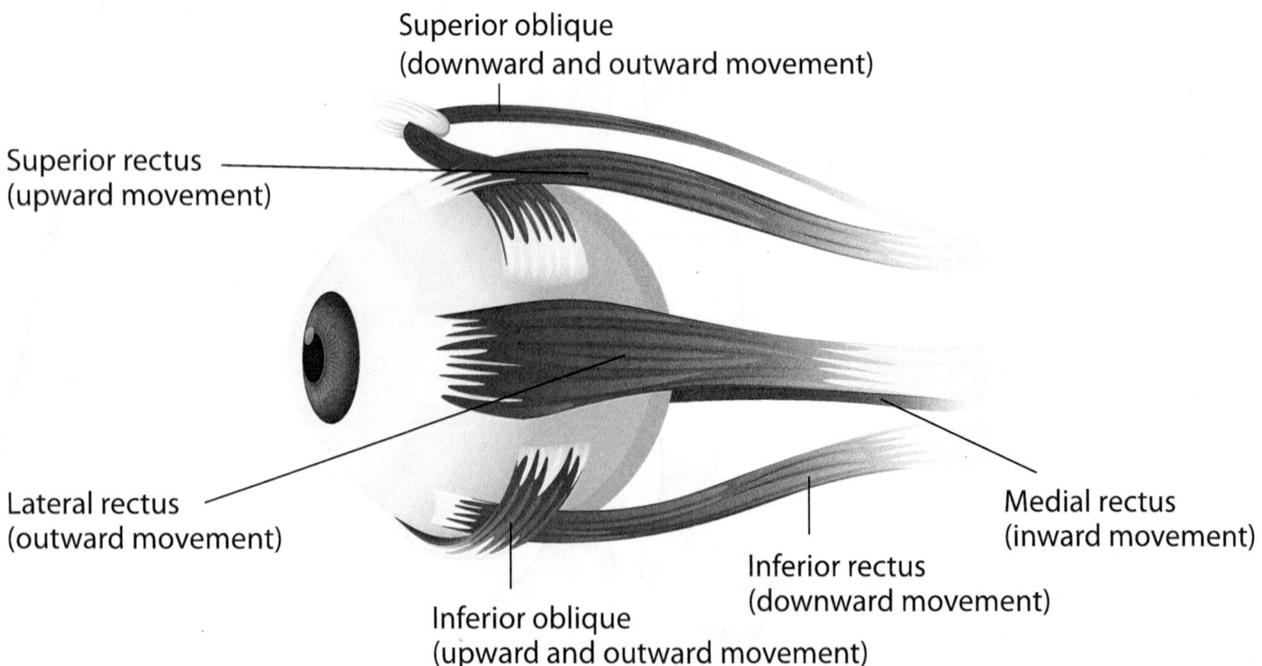
Superior oblique
(downward and outward movement)
Superior rectus
(upward movement)
Lateral rectus
(outward movement)
Medial rectus
(inward movement)
Inferior rectus
(downward movement)
Inferior oblique
(upward and outward movement)

Female Reproductive System — Breast Anatomy

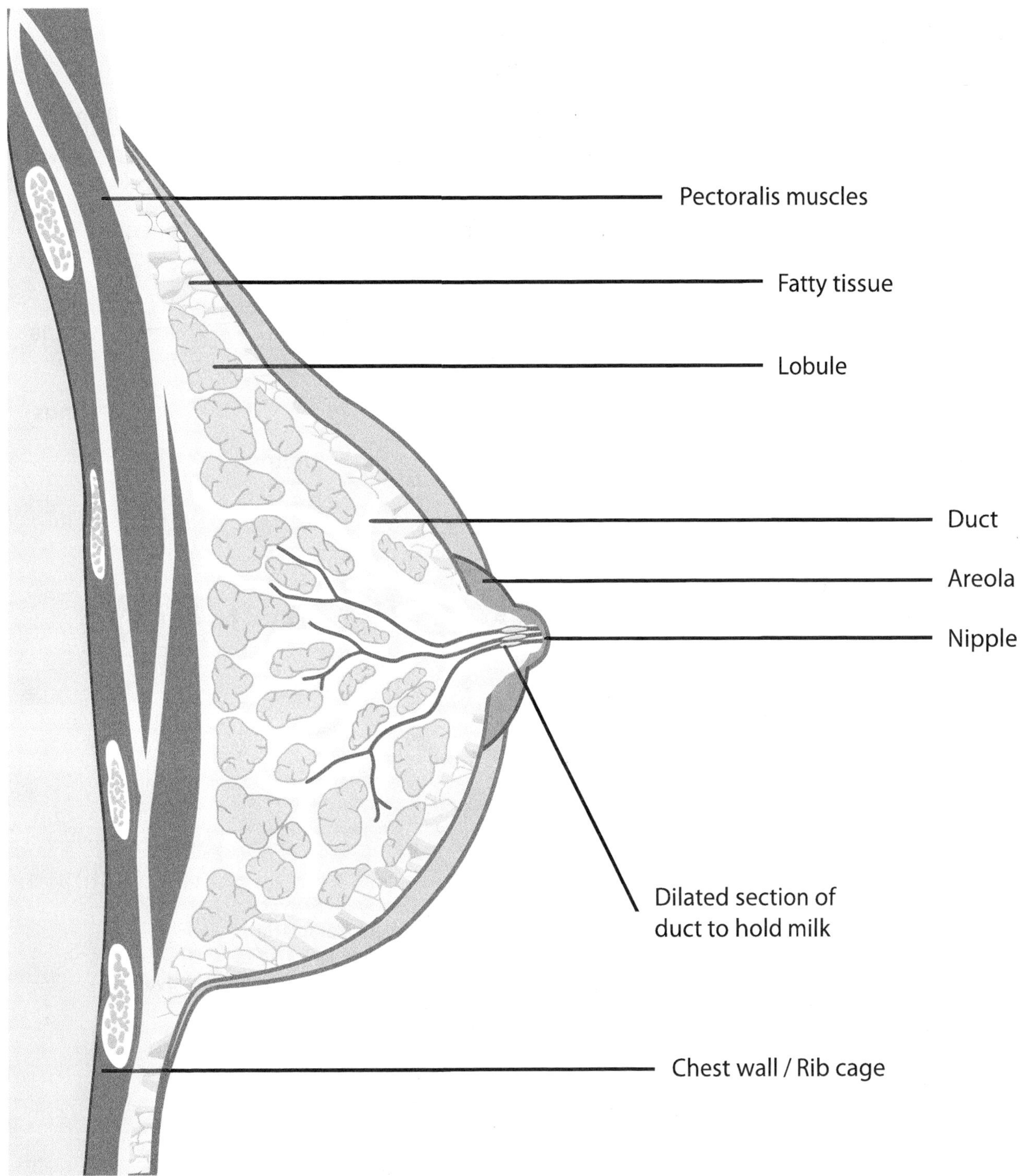

Female Reproductive System — Female Reproductive Anatomy

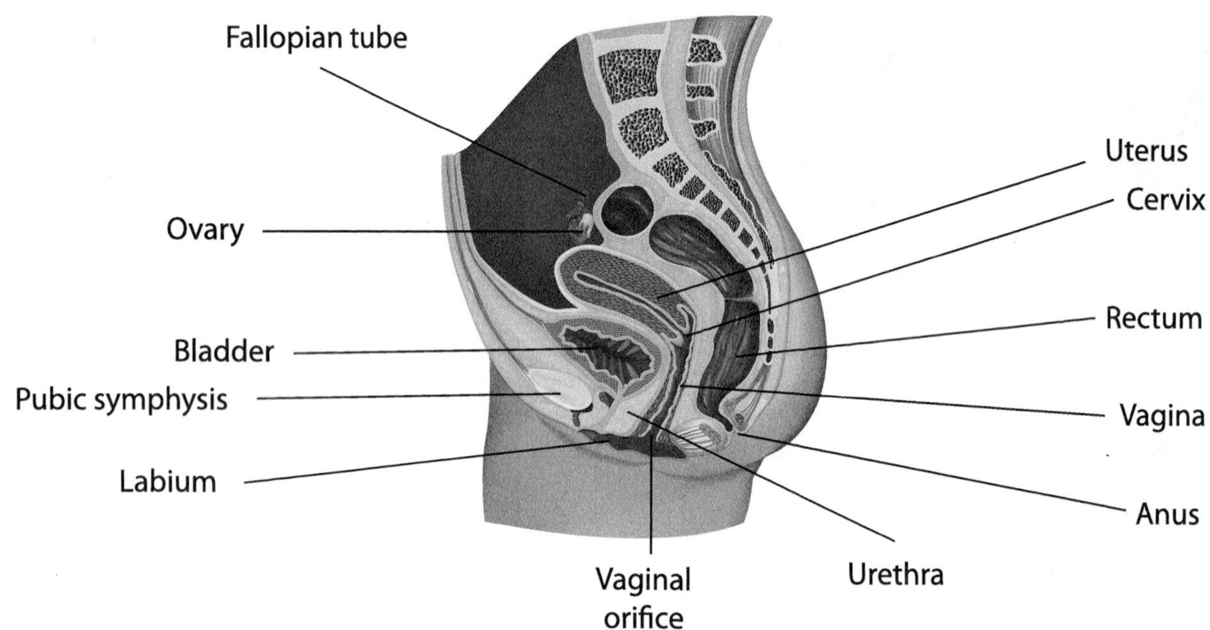

Uterus and Adnexa Anatomy

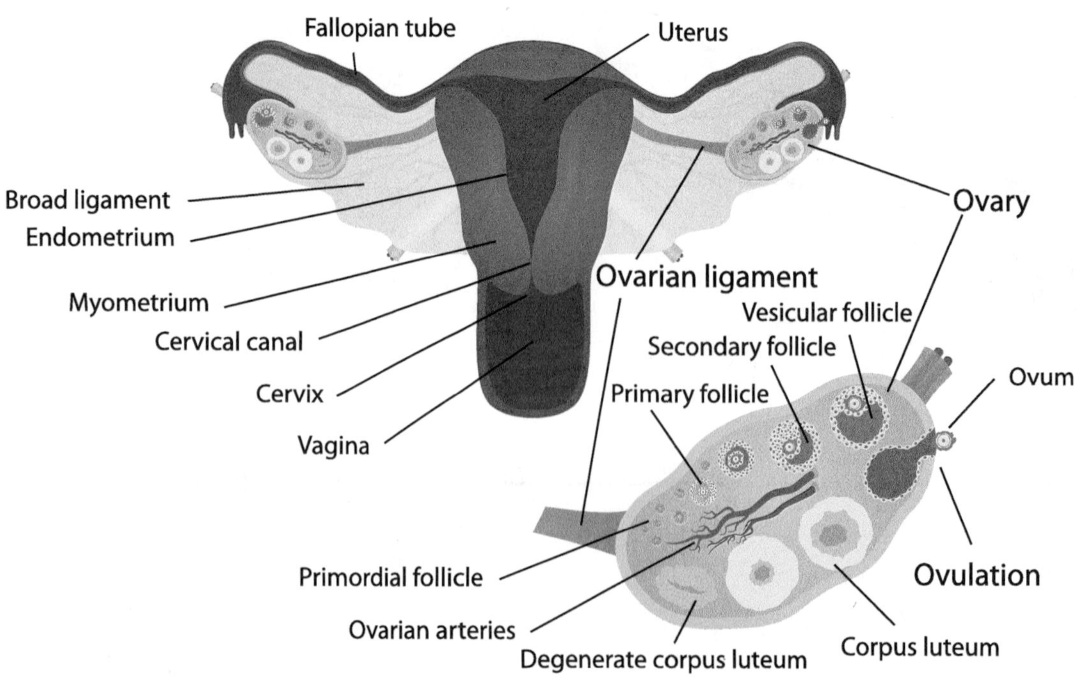

Female Reproductive System — Perineum Anatomy

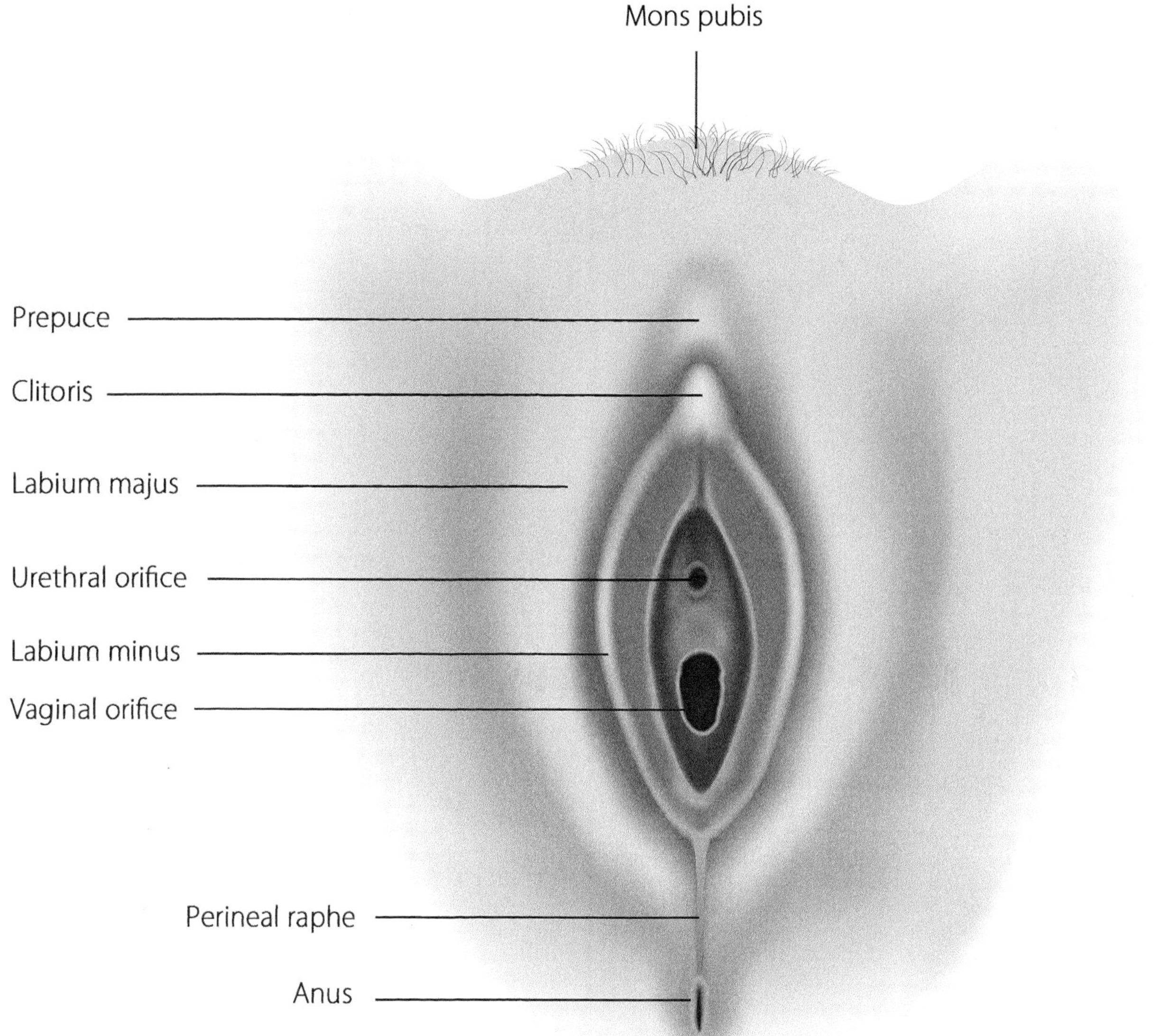

Mons pubis

Prepuce

Clitoris

Labium majus

Urethral orifice

Labium minus

Vaginal orifice

Perineal raphe

Anus

Integumentary System — Skin Anatomy

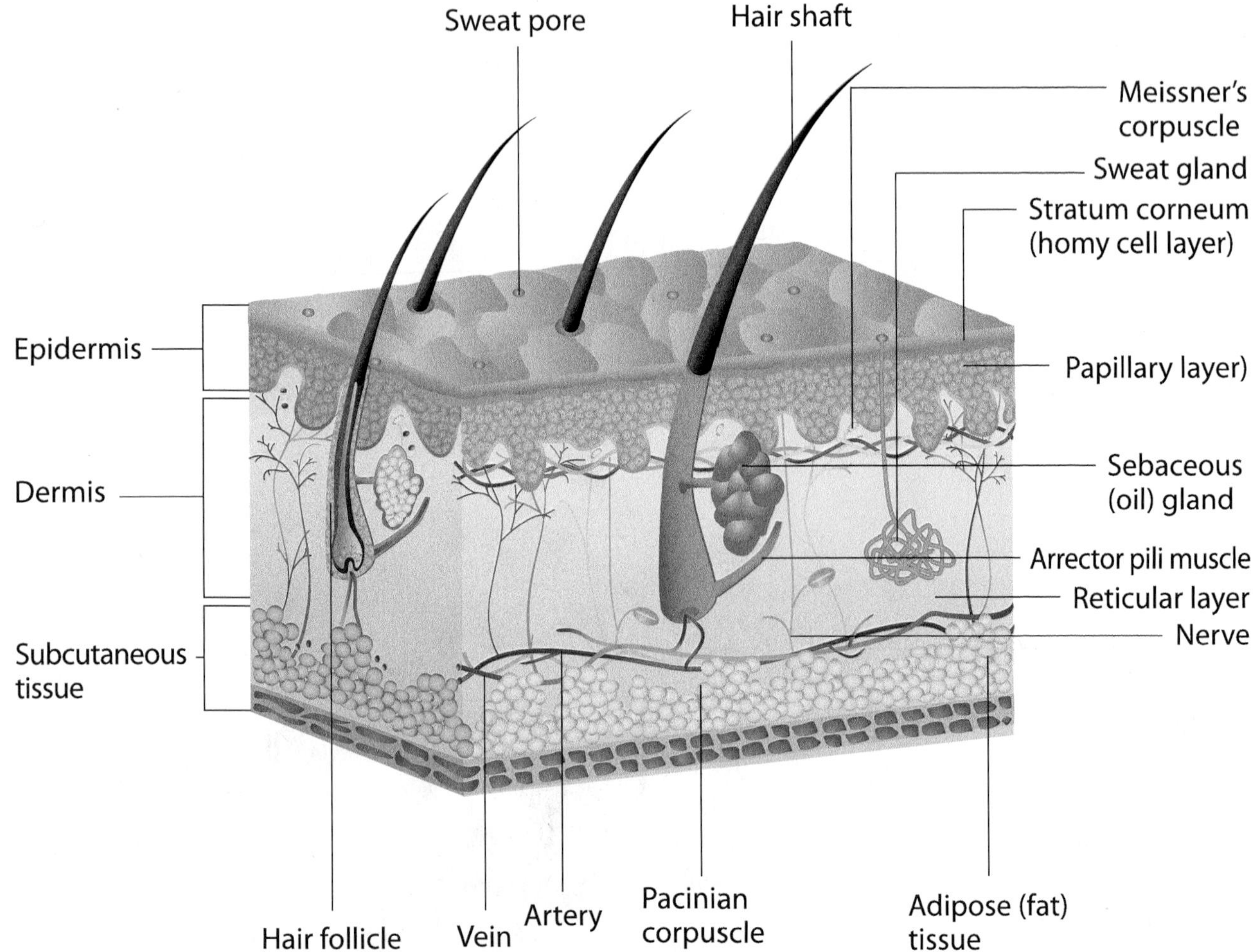

Lymphatic System — Lymphatic Anatomy

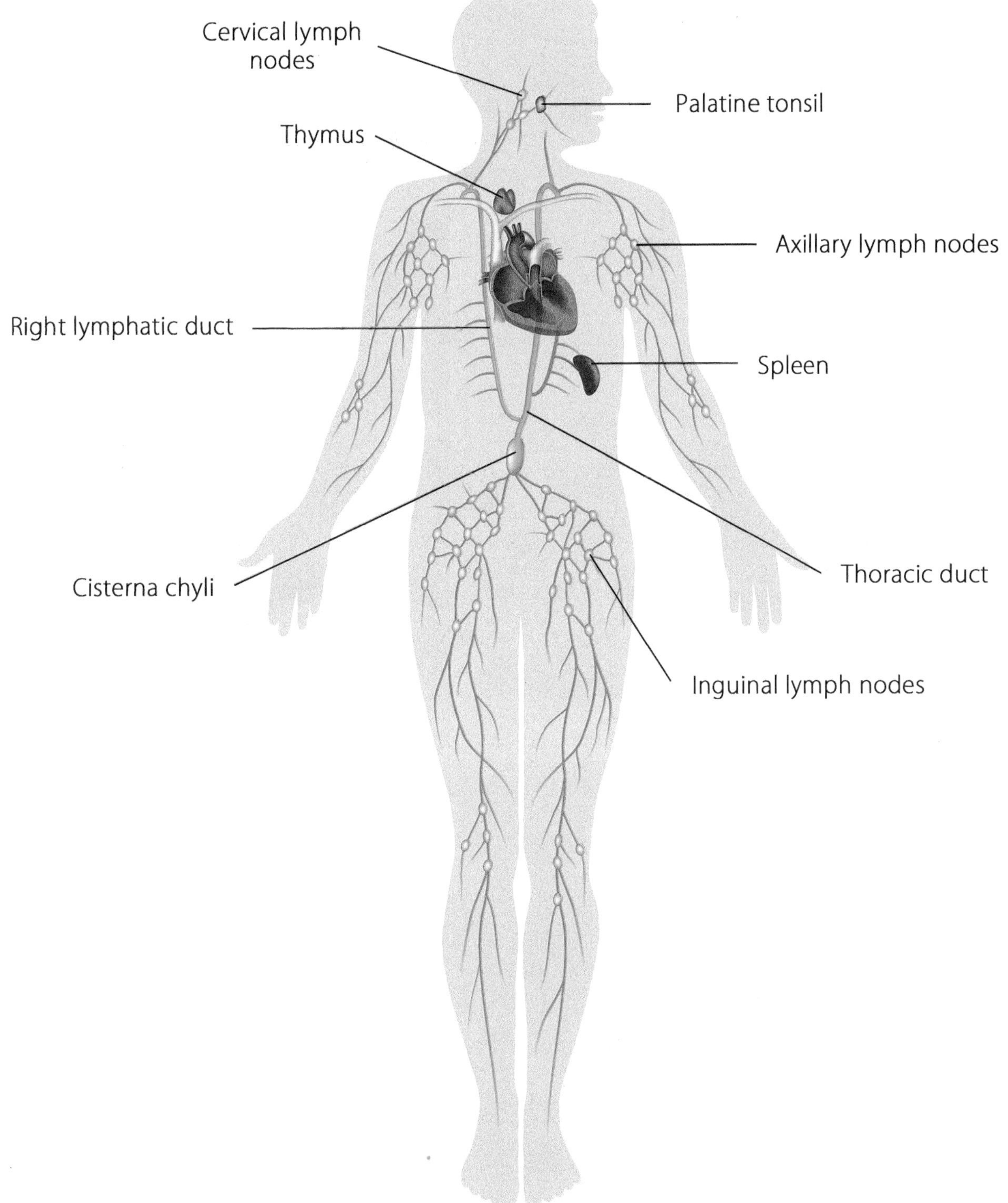

Lymphatic System — Humoral Immunity

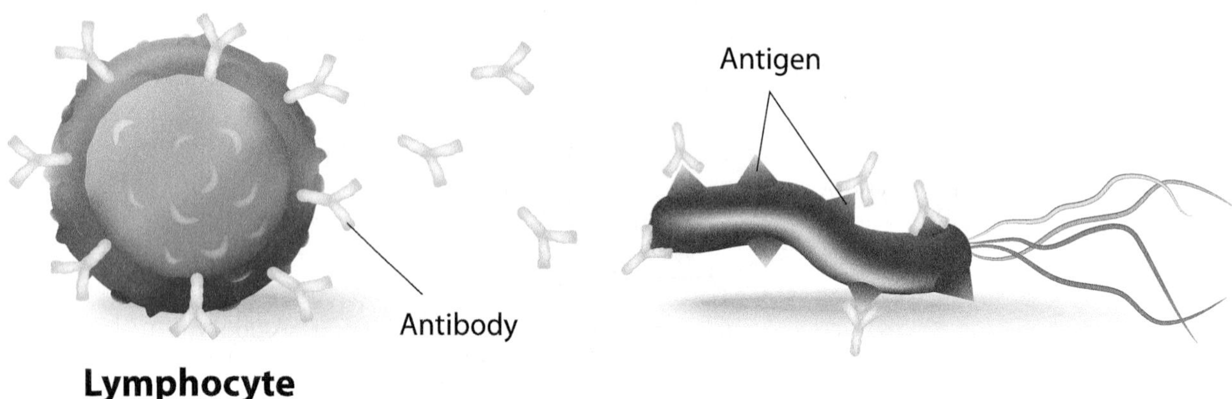

Lymphocyte

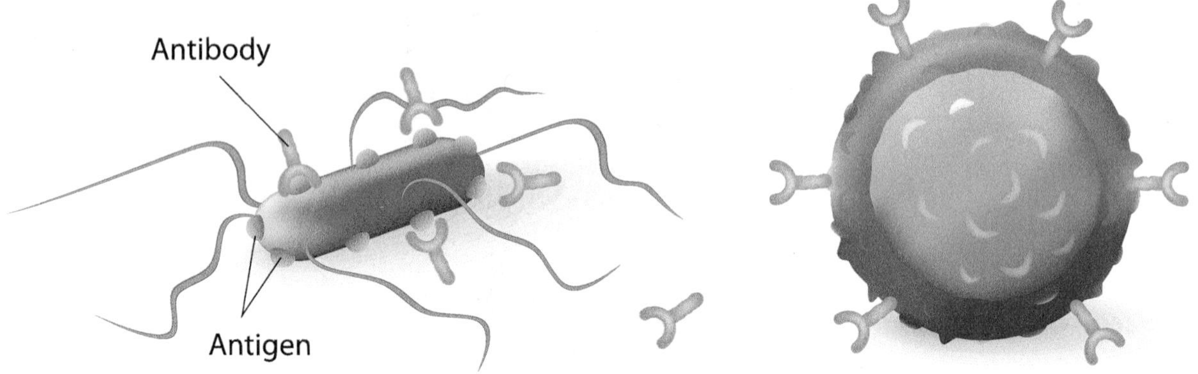

Lymphocyte

Lymphatic System — Lymph Node Anatomy

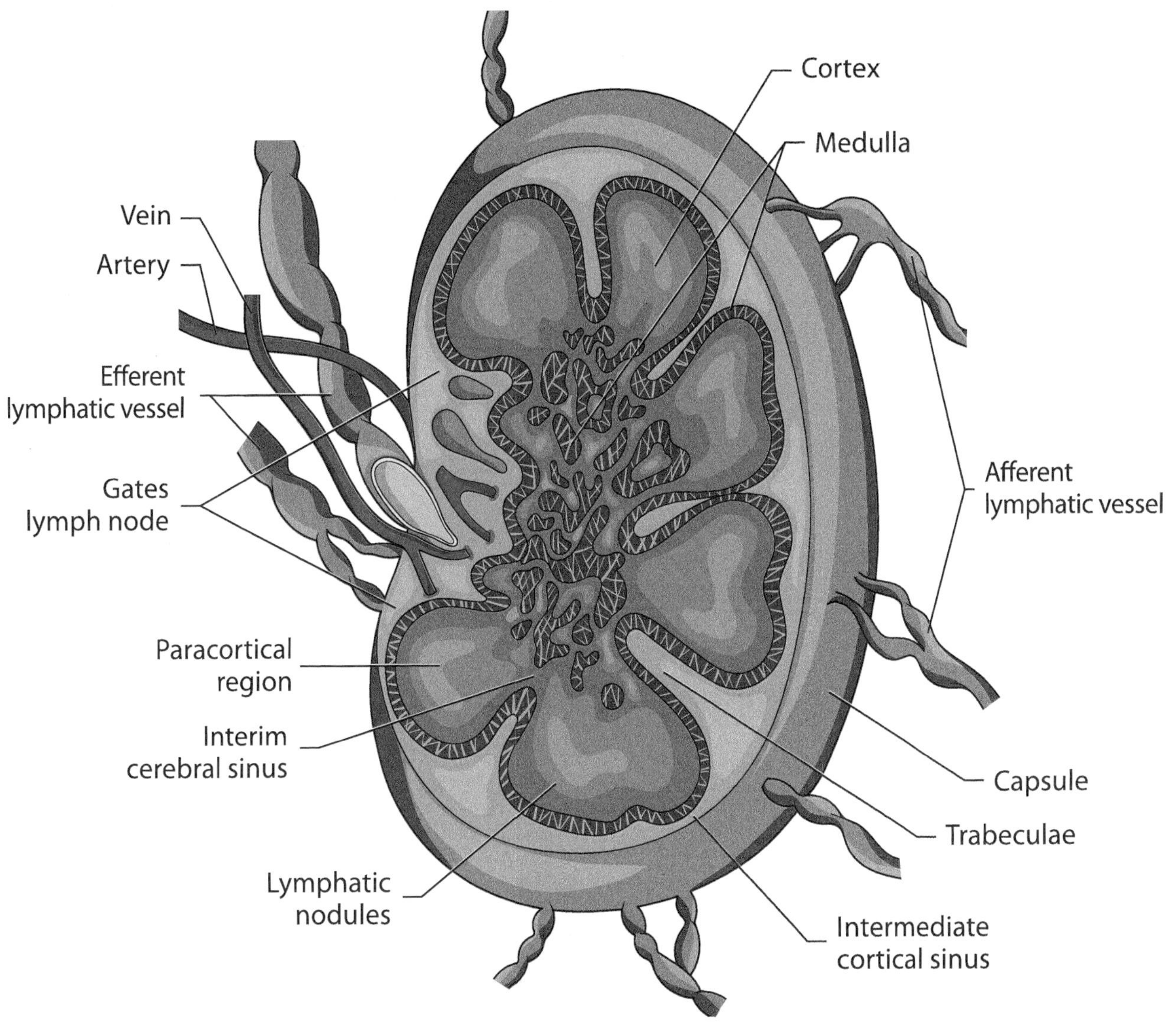

Male Reproductive System — Male Reproductive Anatomy

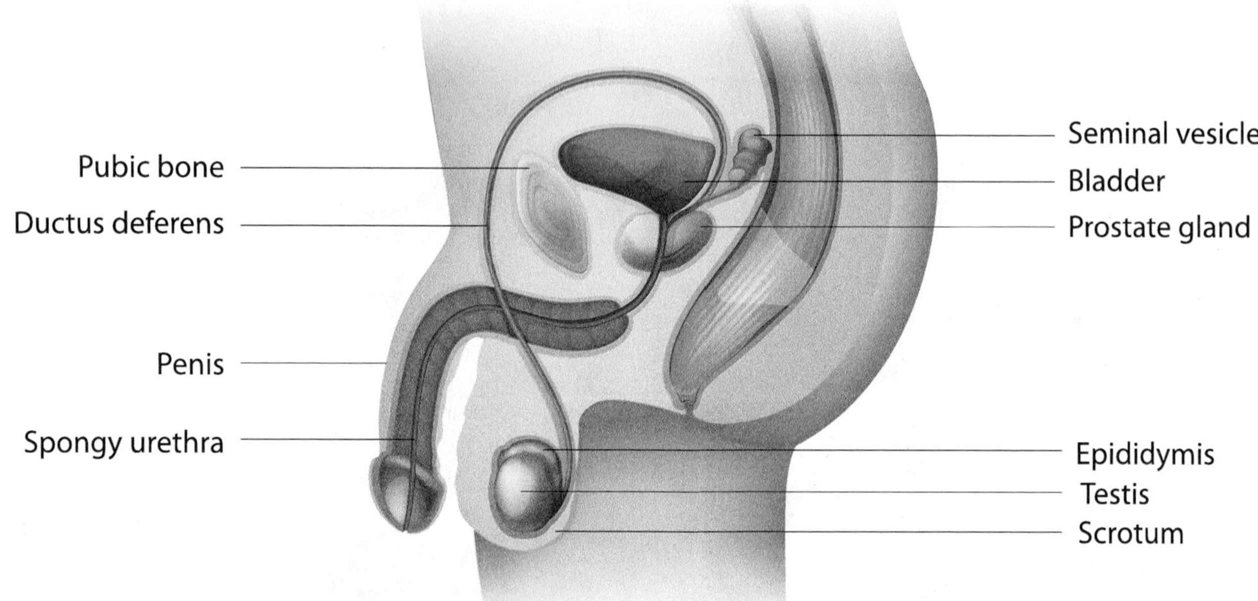

Testicle Anatomy

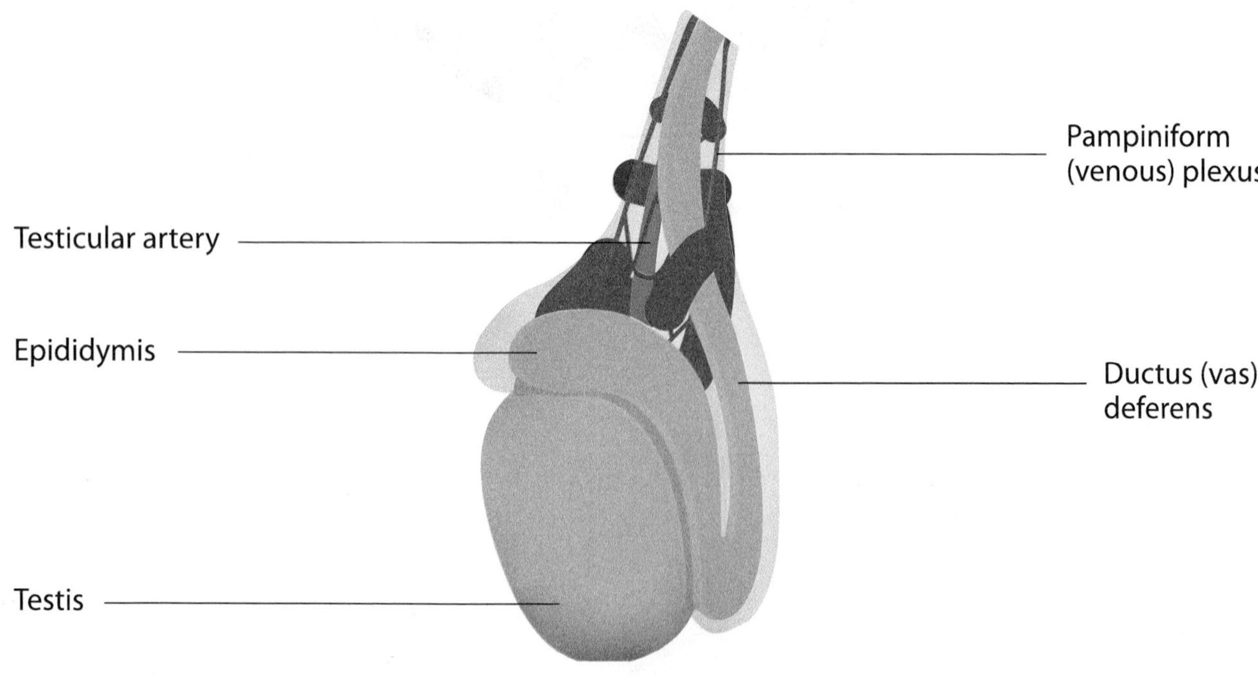

Male Reproductive System — Penis Anatomy

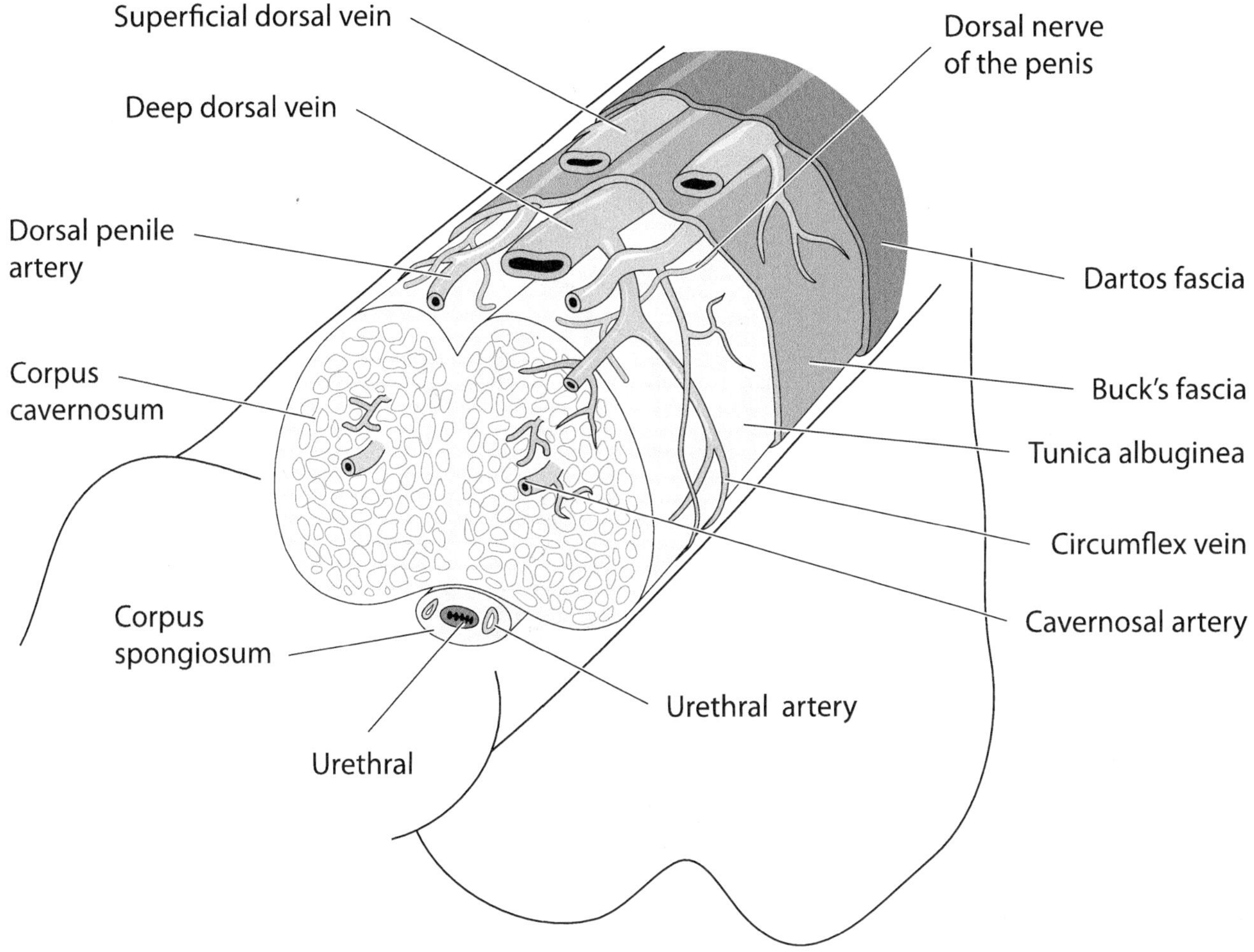

Muscular System — Muscle Anatomy

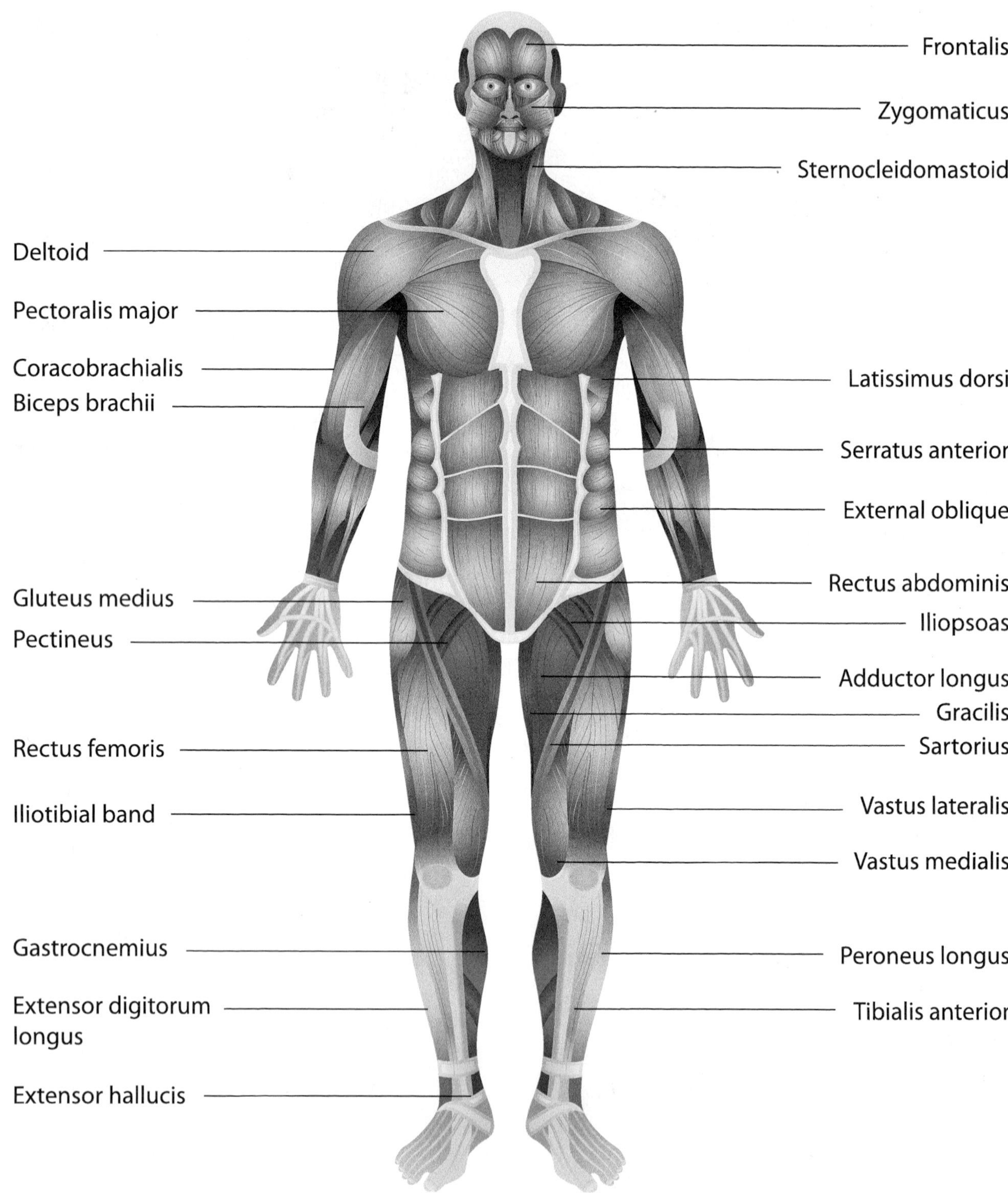
Frontalis
Zygomaticus
Sternocleidomastoid
Deltoid
Pectoralis major
Coracobrachialis
Biceps brachii
Latissimus dorsi
Serratus anterior
External oblique
Gluteus medius
Pectineus
Rectus abdominis
Iliopsoas
Adductor longus
Gracilis
Rectus femoris
Sartorius
Iliotibial band
Vastus lateralis
Vastus medialis
Gastrocnemius
Peroneus longus
Extensor digitorum longus
Tibialis anterior
Extensor hallucis

Muscular System — Forearm Muscles (right arm, posterior compartment)

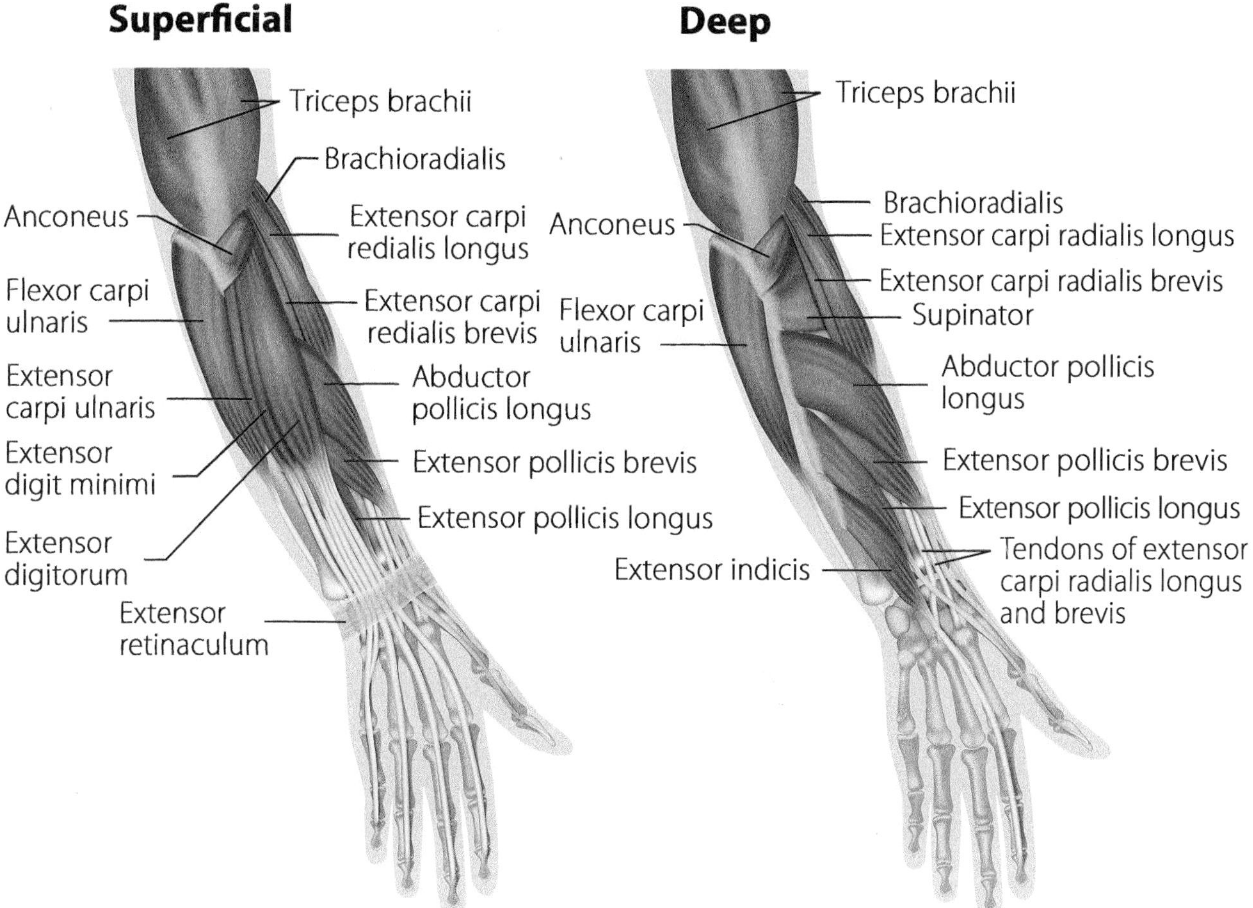
Superficial
Triceps brachii
Brachioradialis
Anconeus
Extensor carpi redialis longus
Flexor carpi ulnaris
Extensor carpi redialis brevis
Extensor carpi ulnaris
Abductor pollicis longus
Extensor digit minimi
Extensor pollicis brevis
Extensor pollicis longus
Extensor digitorum
Extensor retinaculum
Deep
Triceps brachii
Brachioradialis
Anconeus
Extensor carpi radialis longus
Extensor carpi radialis brevis
Flexor carpi ulnaris
Supinator
Abductor pollicis longus
Extensor pollicis brevis
Extensor pollicis longus
Extensor indicis
Tendons of extensor carpi radialis longus and brevis

Muscular System — Knee Joint Anatomy

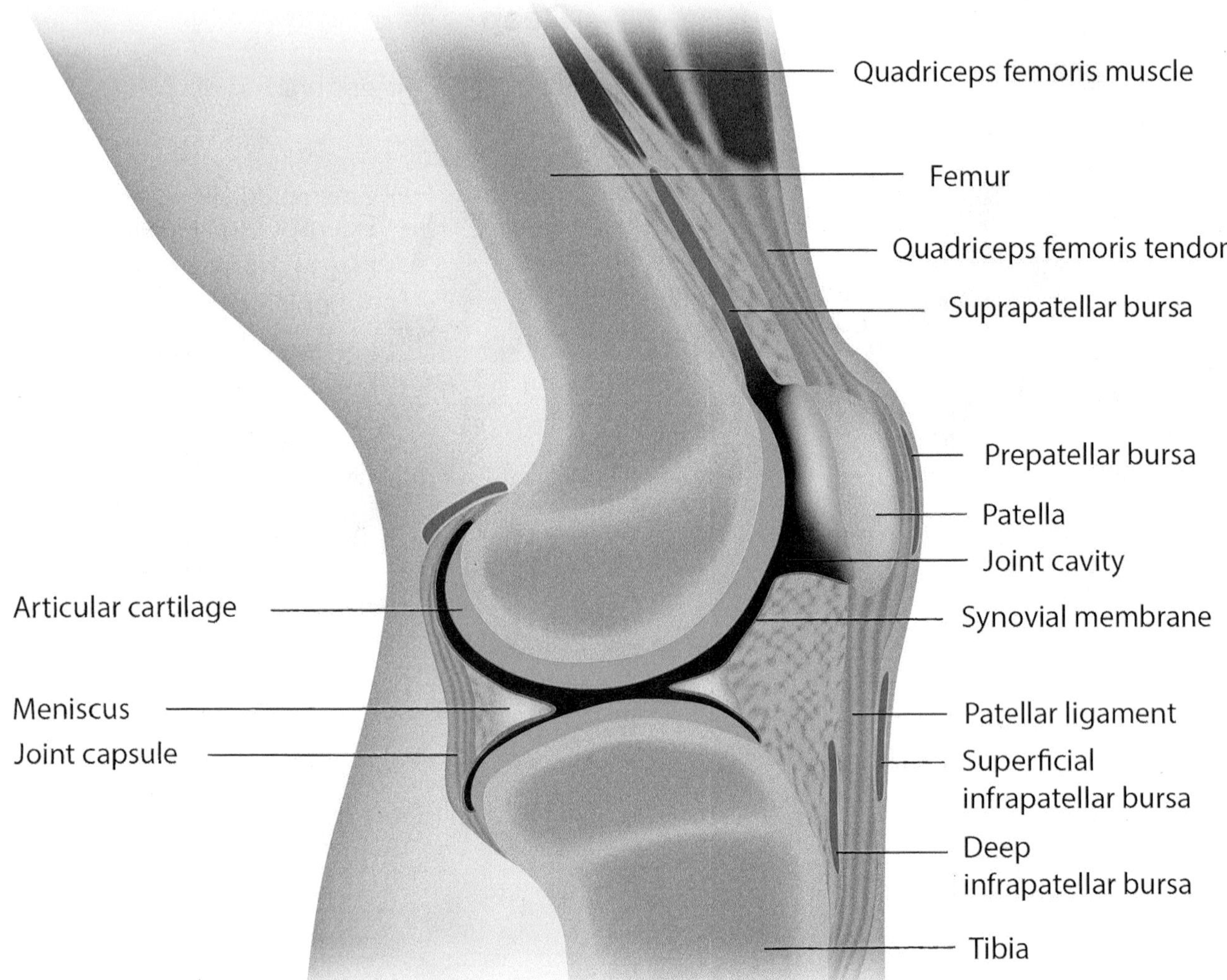

Muscular System — Shoulder (Rotator Cuff) Muscles

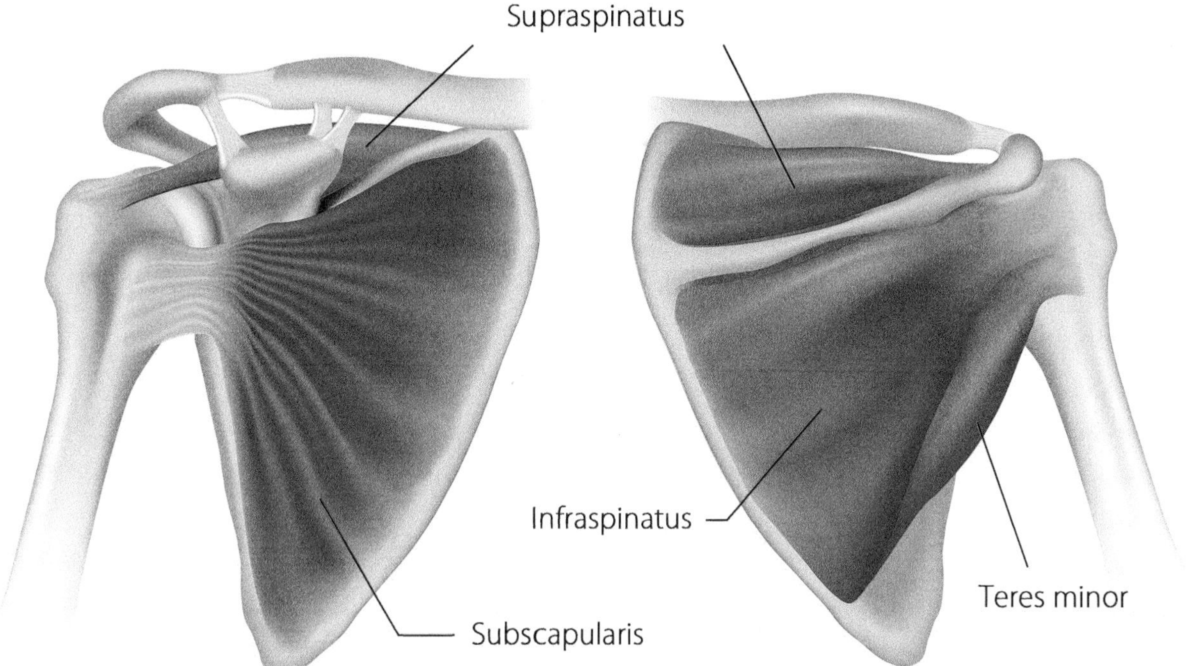

Nervous System — Nervous System Anatomy

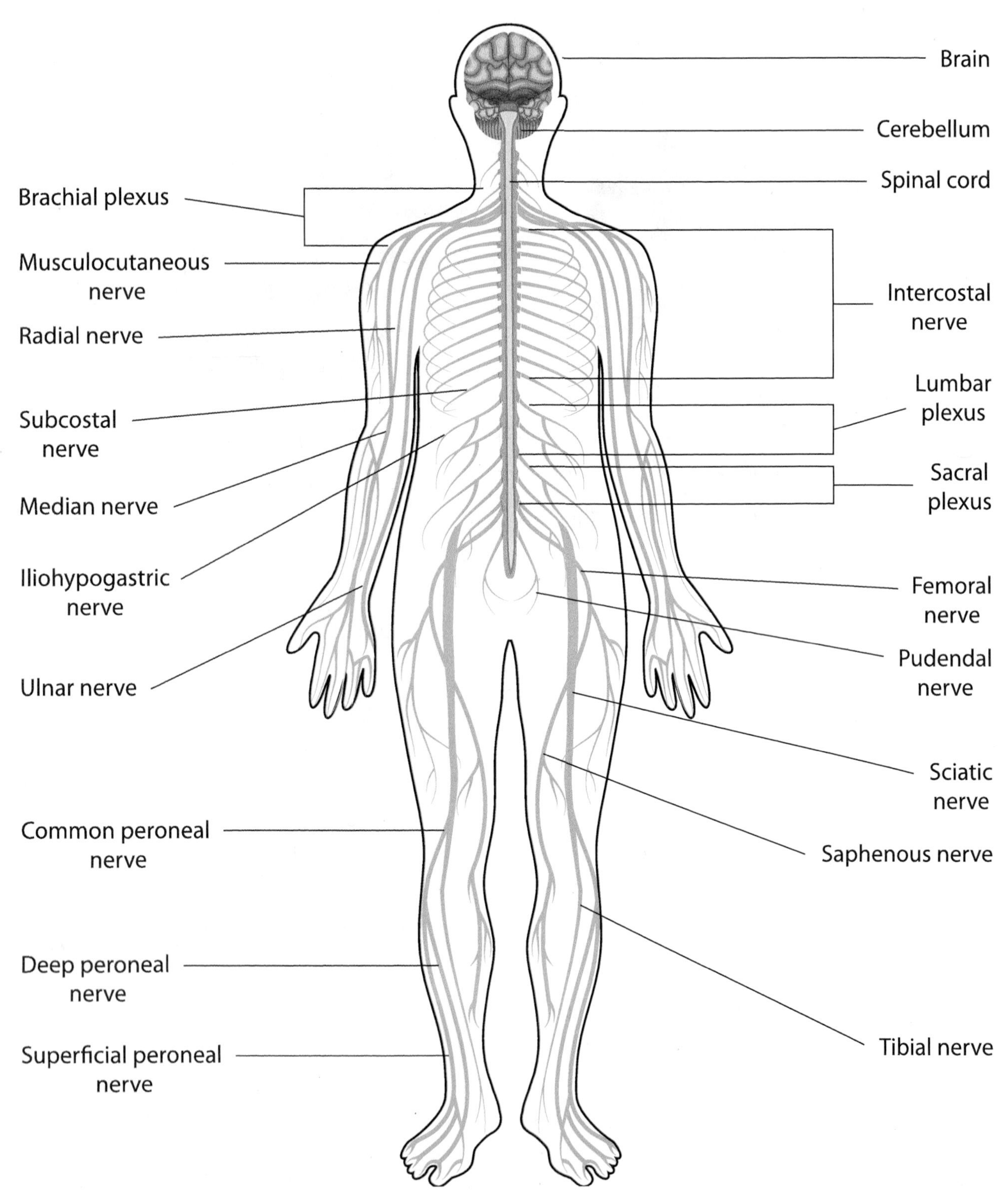

Nervous System — Brain Anatomy

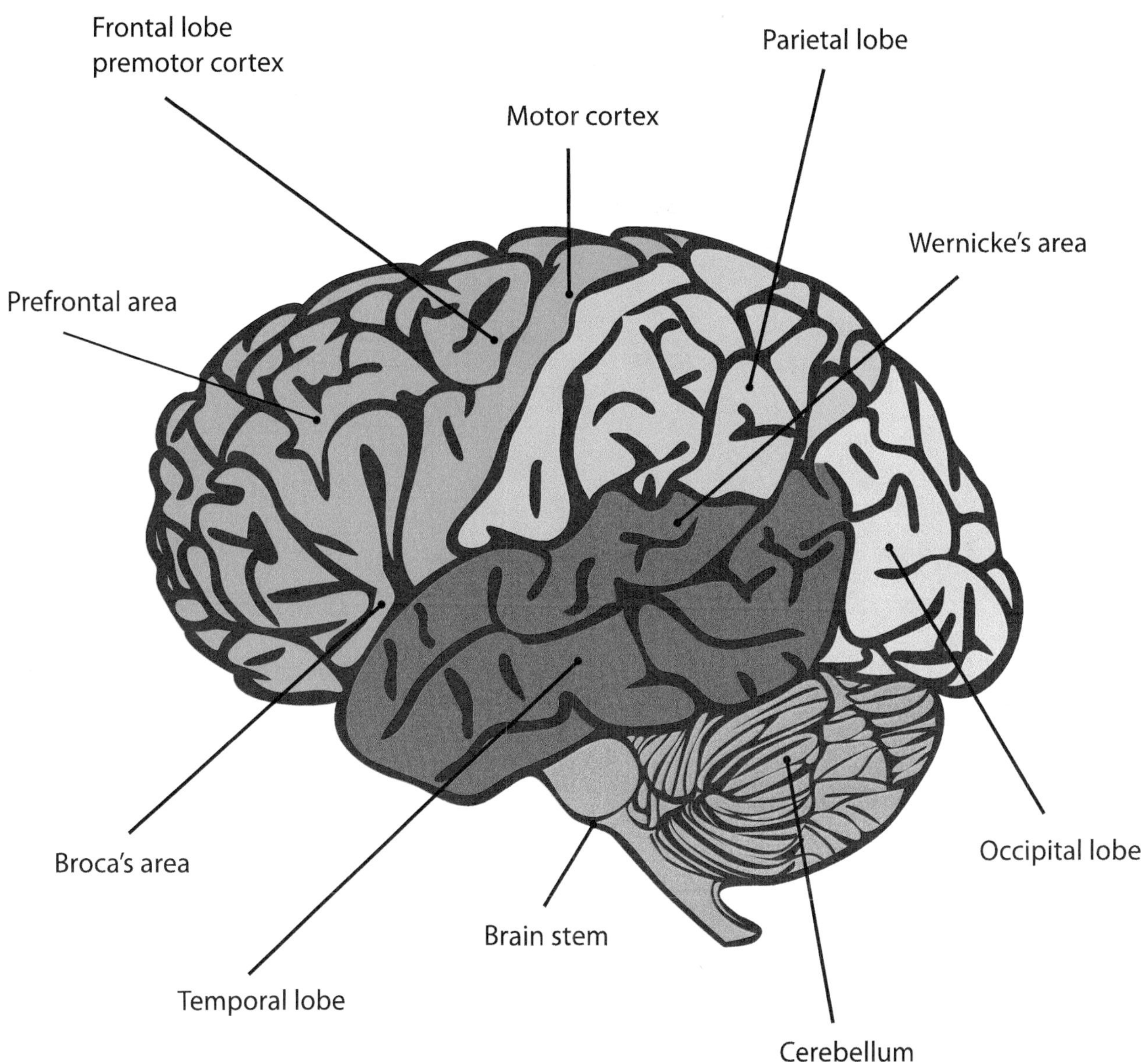

Nervous System — Cranial Nerves

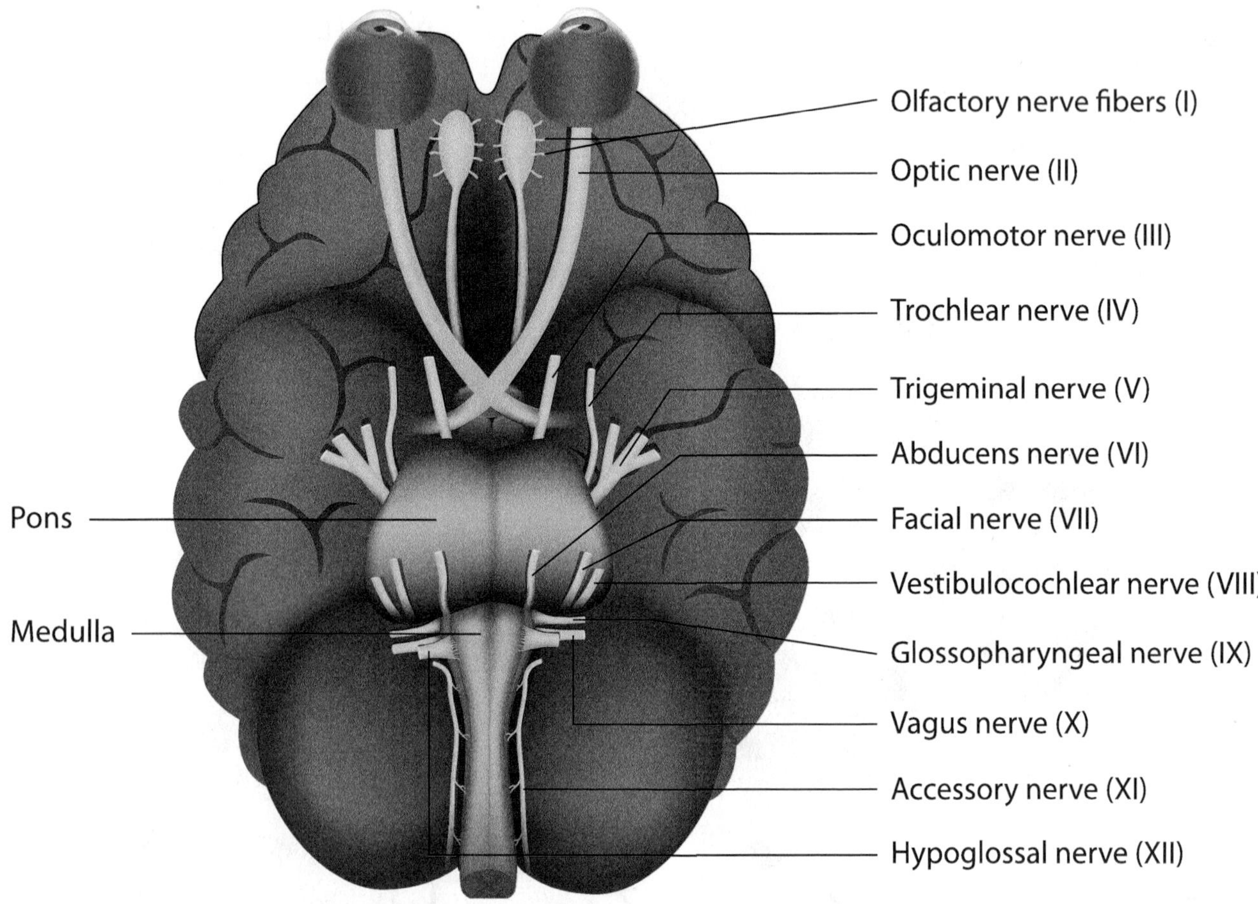

Nervous System — Nerve Anatomy

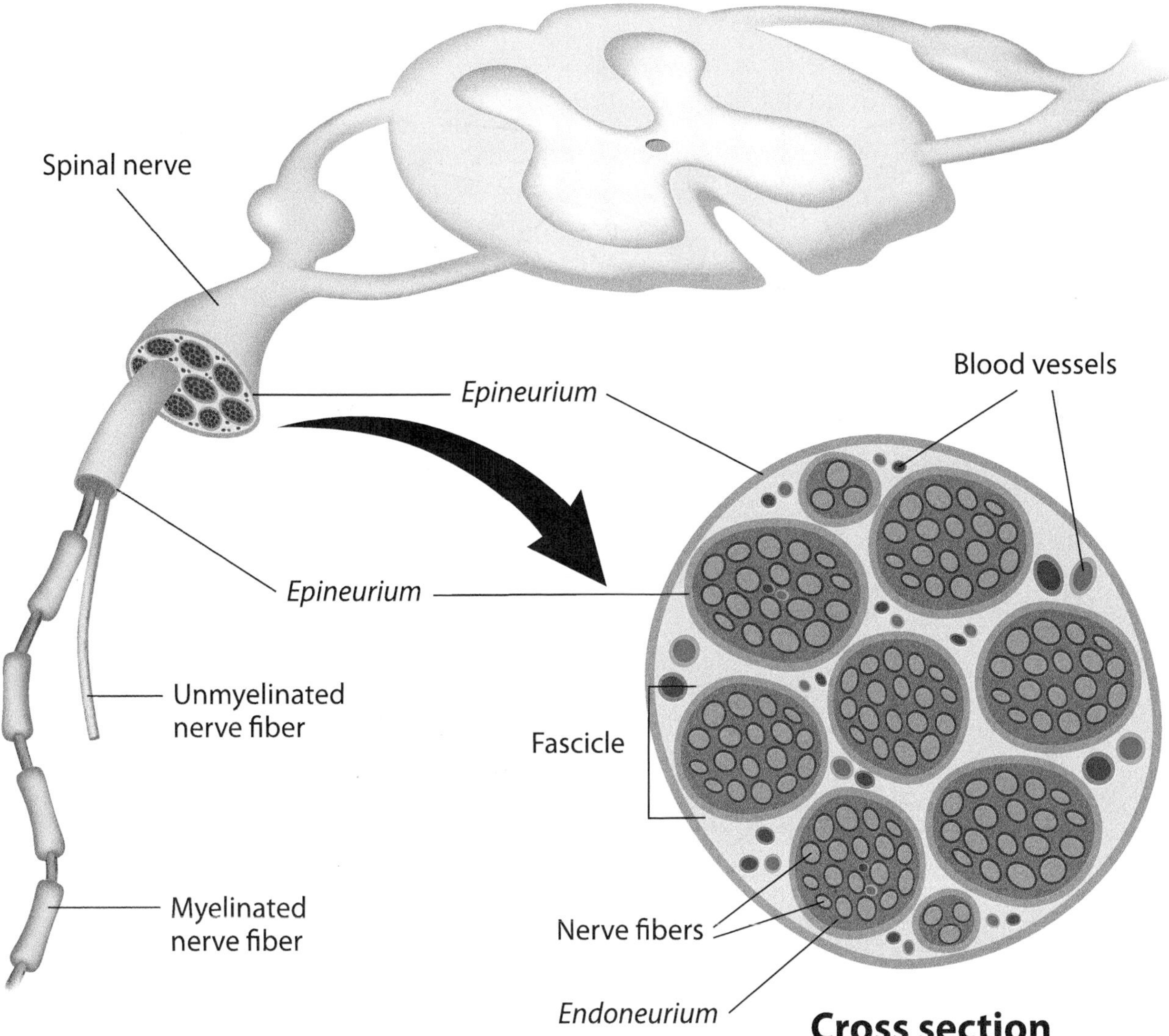

Nervous System — Parasympathetic System Anatomy

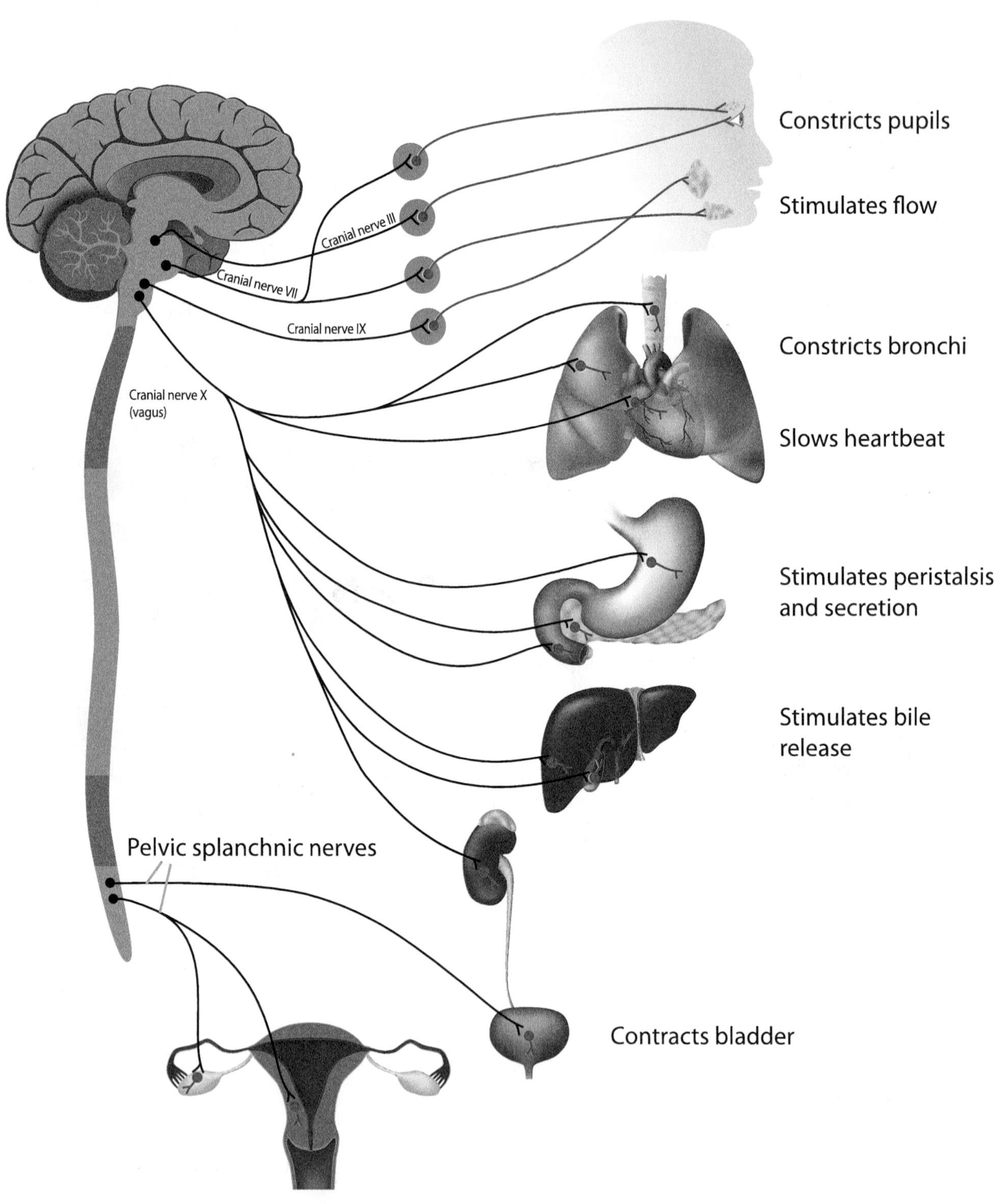

Nervous System — Sympathetic System Anatomy

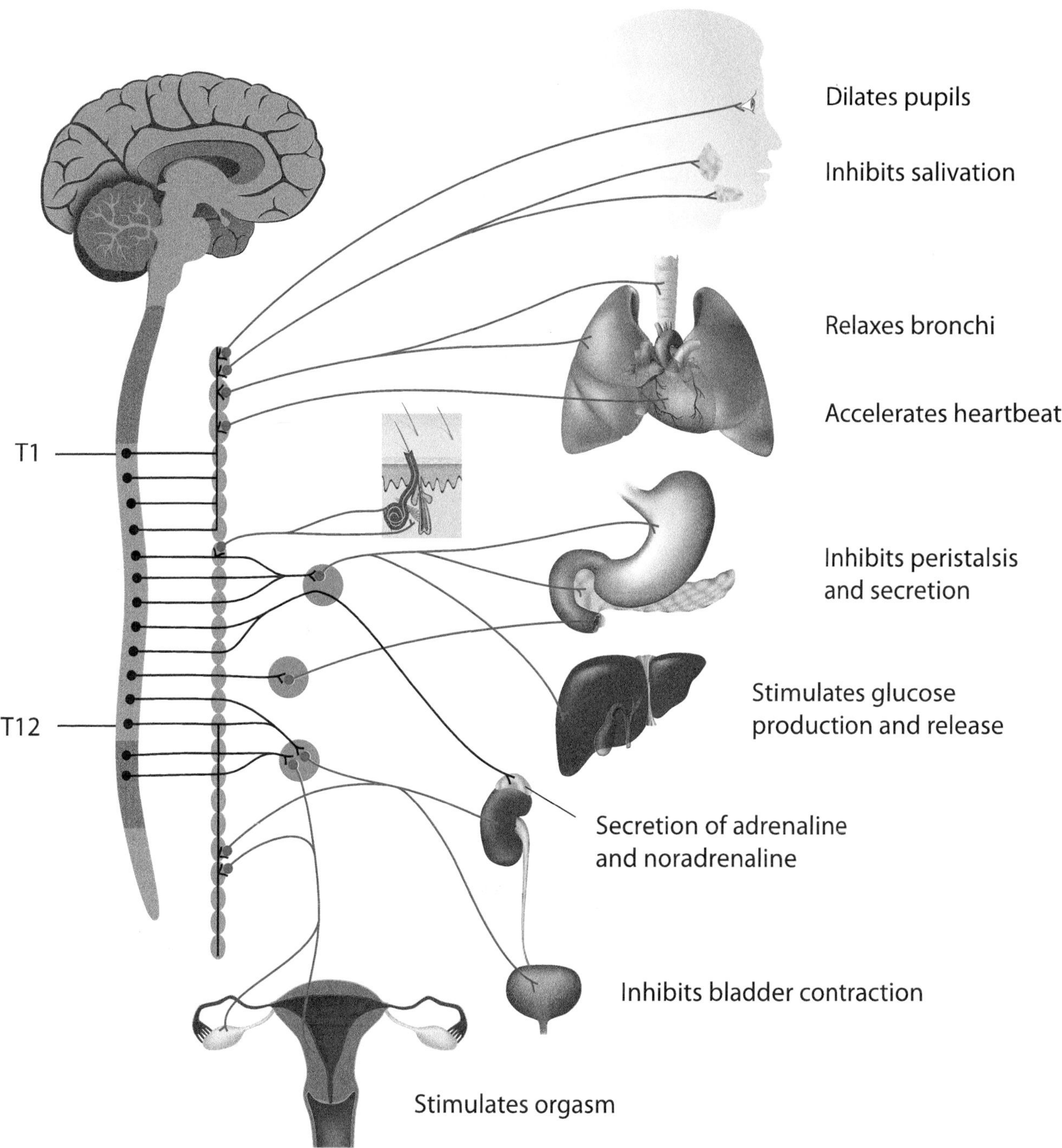

Respiratory System — Respiratory Anatomy

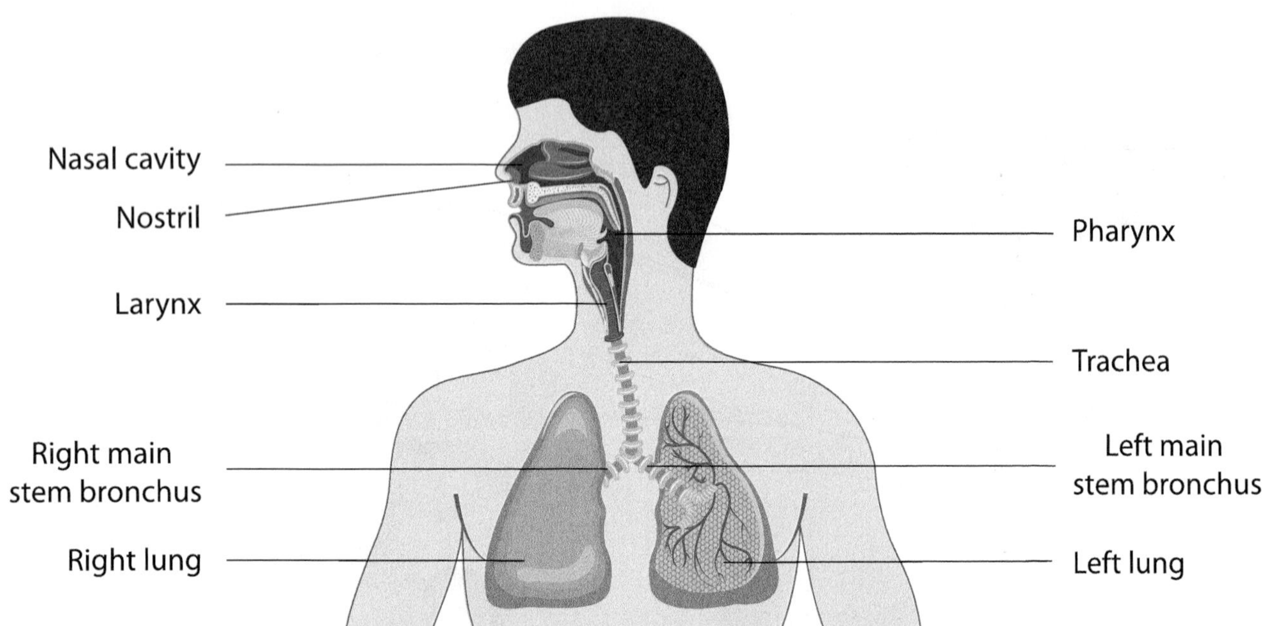

Larynx Anatomy

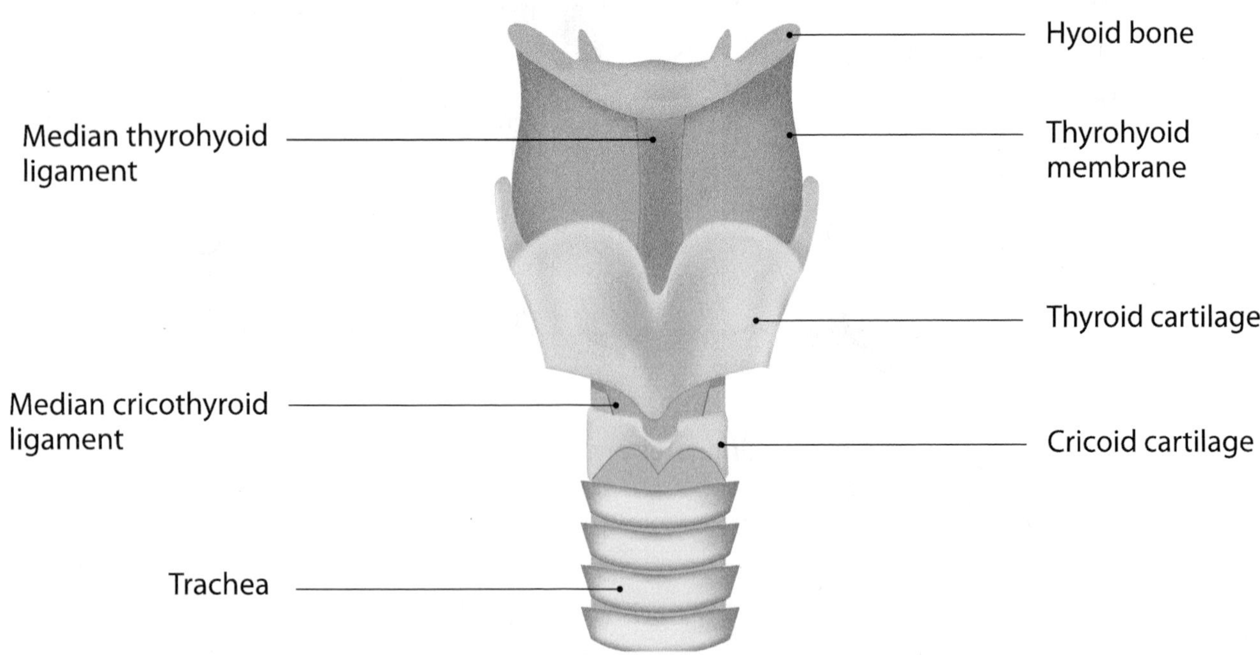

Respiratory System — Lung Anatomy

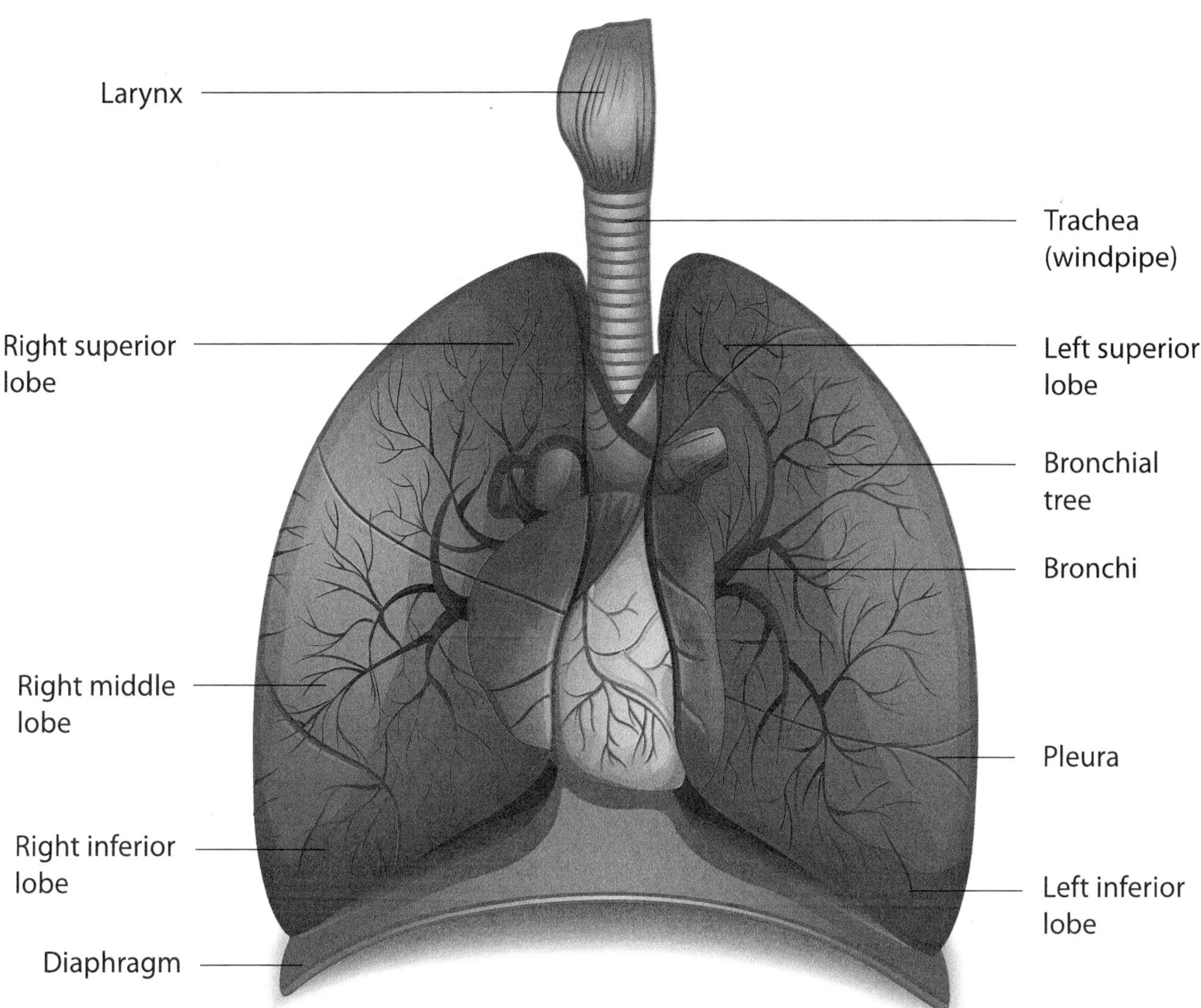

Respiratory System — Lung Anatomy and Function

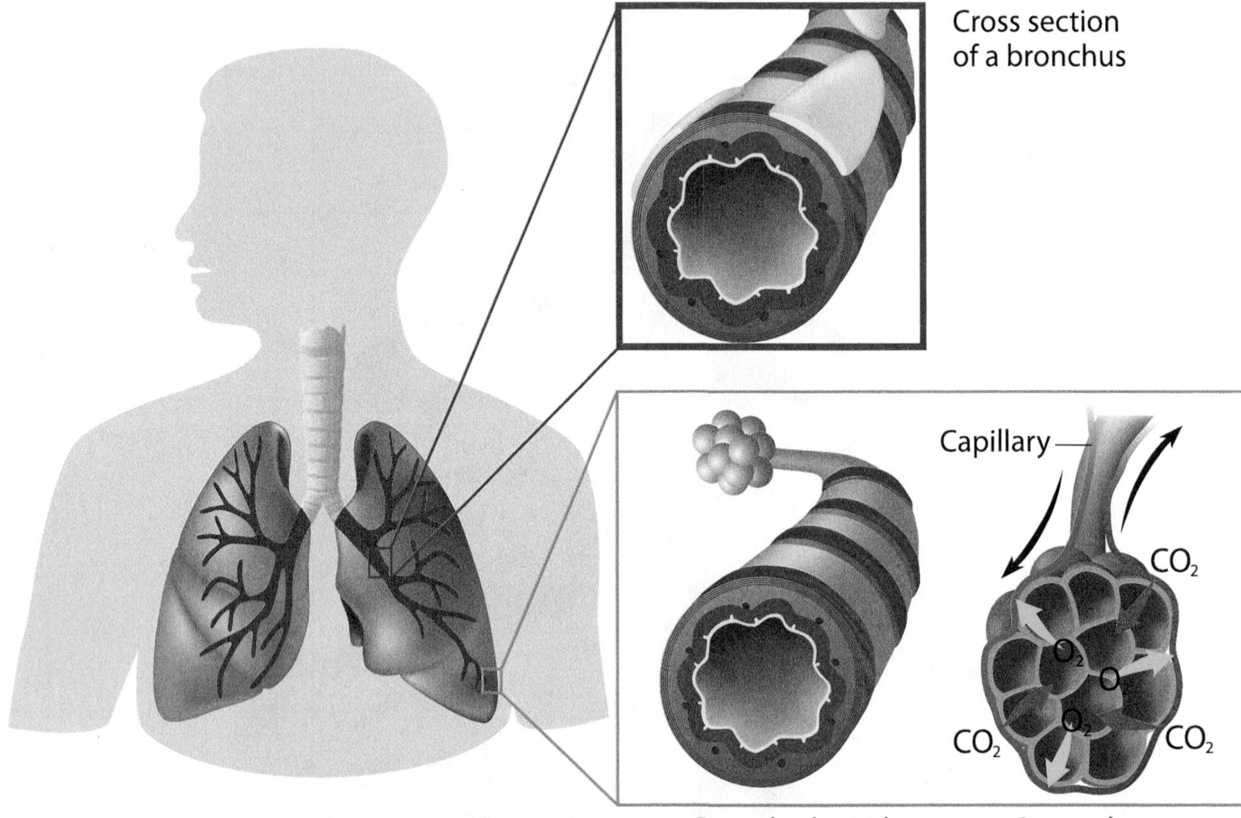

Respiratory System — Nose Anatomy

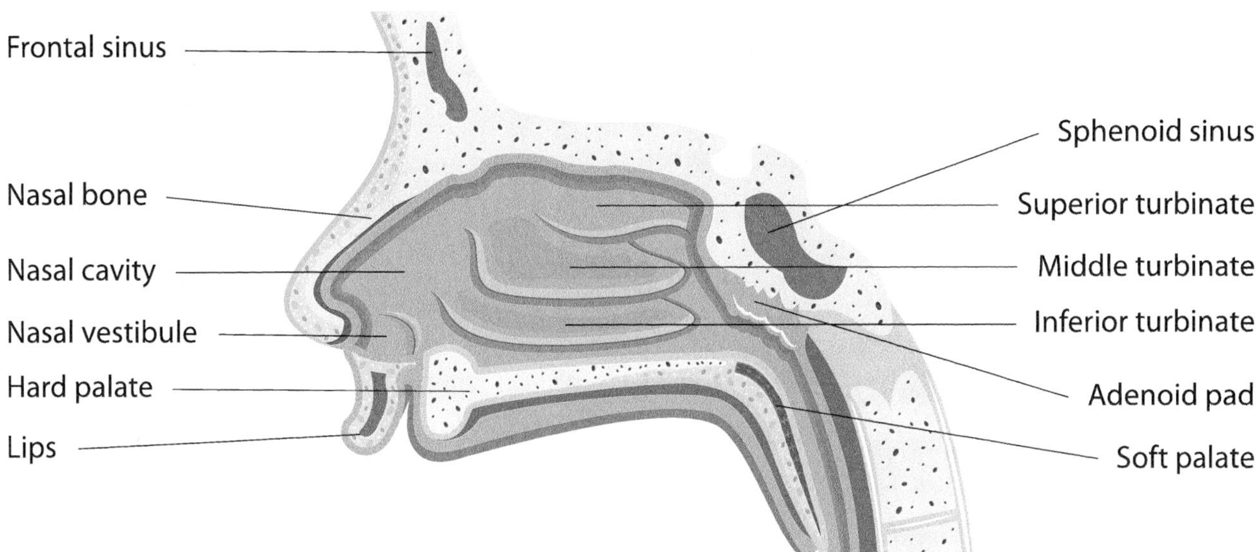

Sinus Anatomy

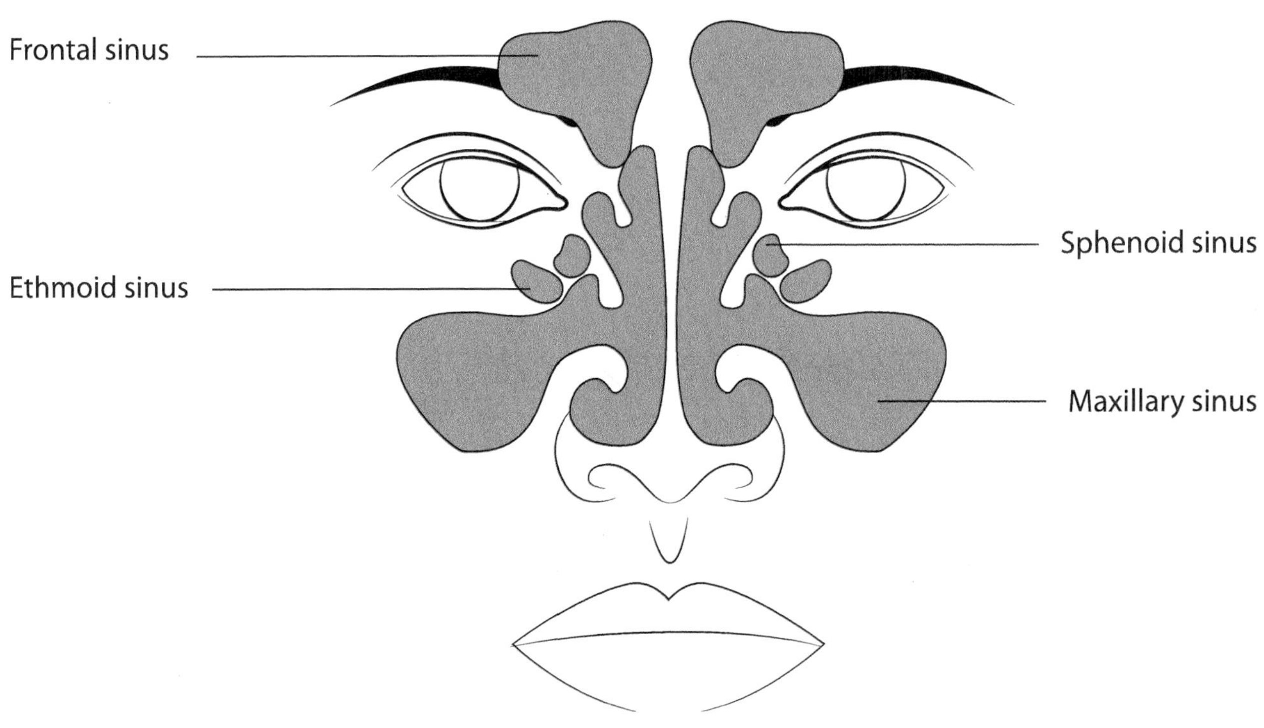

Respiratory System — Throat Anatomy

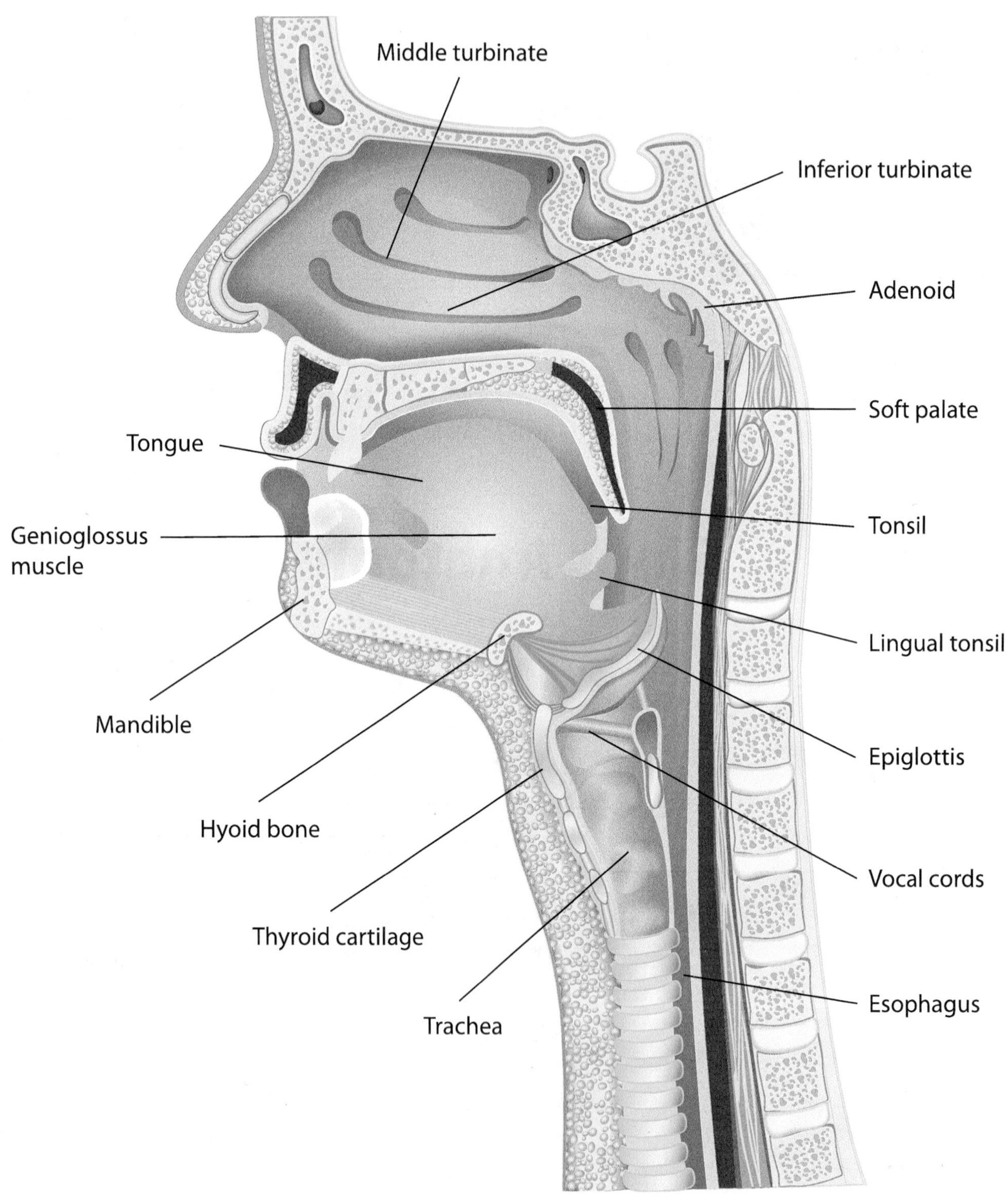

Skeletal System — Skeletal Anatomy

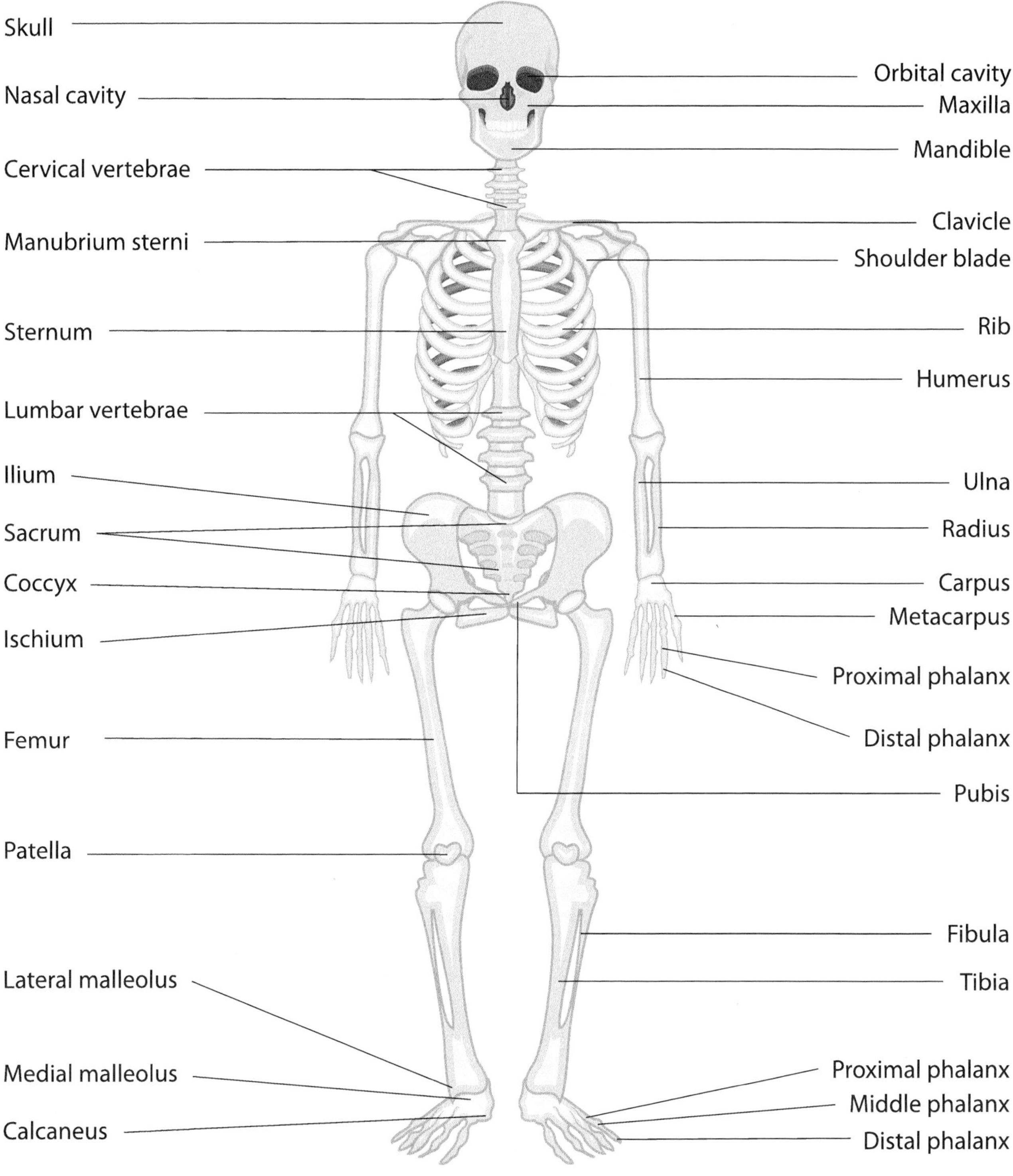
Skull
Nasal cavity
Cervical vertebrae
Manubrium sterni
Sternum
Lumbar vertebrae
Ilium
Sacrum
Coccyx
Ischium
Femur
Patella
Lateral malleolus
Medial malleolus
Calcaneus
Orbital cavity
Maxilla
Mandible
Clavicle
Shoulder blade
Rib
Humerus
Ulna
Radius
Carpus
Metacarpus
Proximal phalanx
Distal phalanx
Pubis
Fibula
Tibia
Proximal phalanx
Middle phalanx
Distal phalanx

Skeletal System — Bone Structure

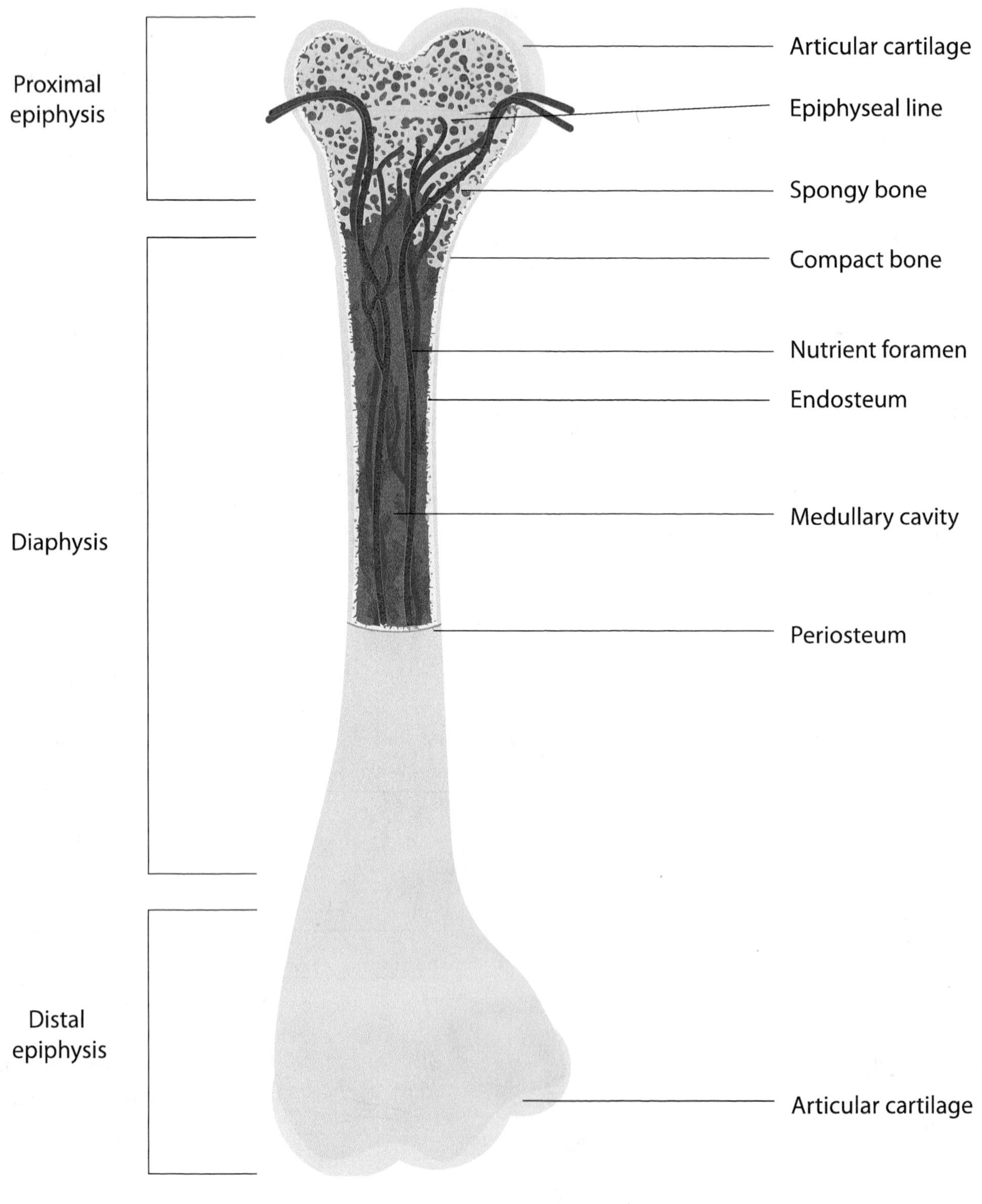

Skeletal System — Cervical, Thoracic, and Lumbar Spine

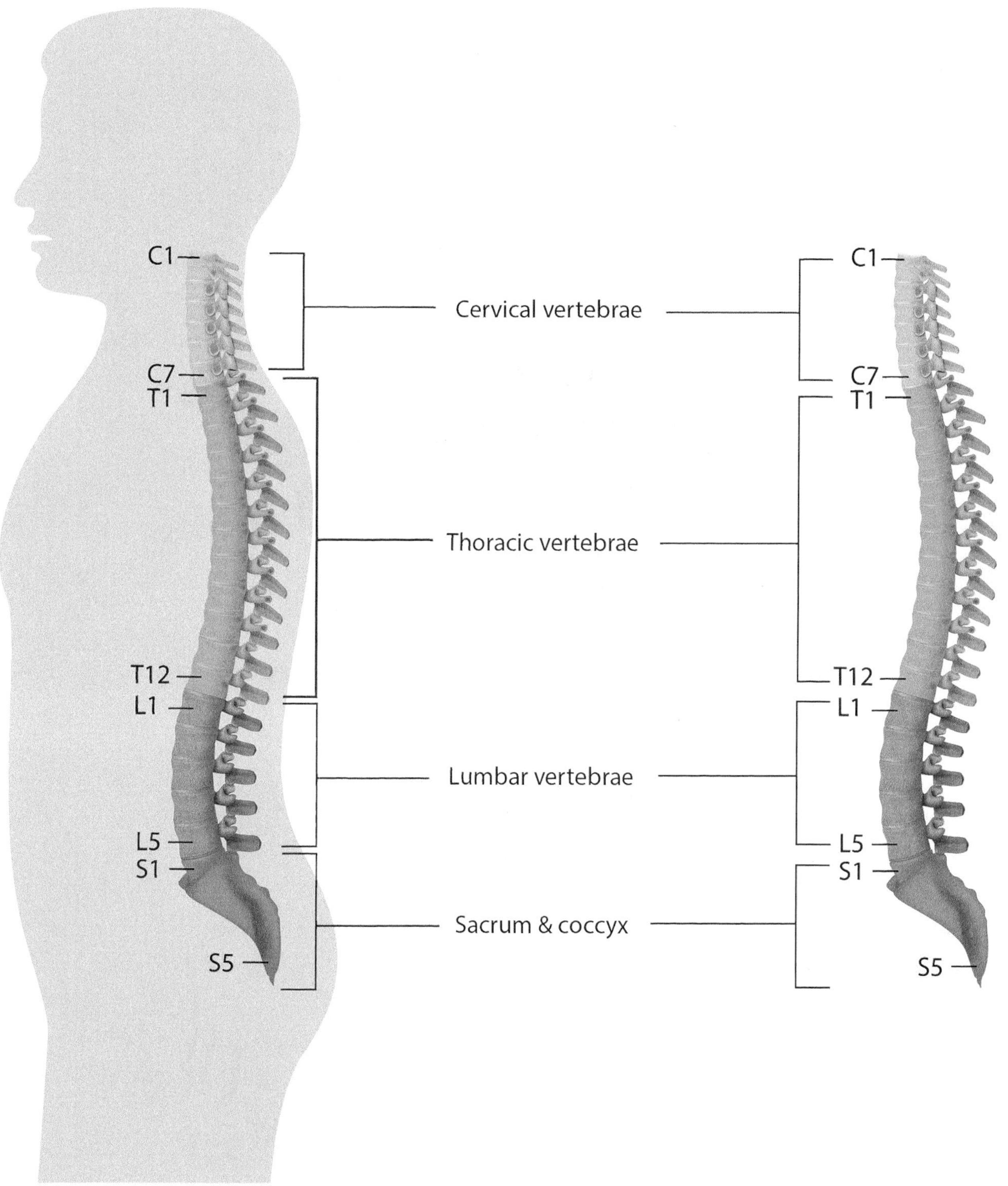

Skeletal System — Foot Bones (right foot, lateral view)

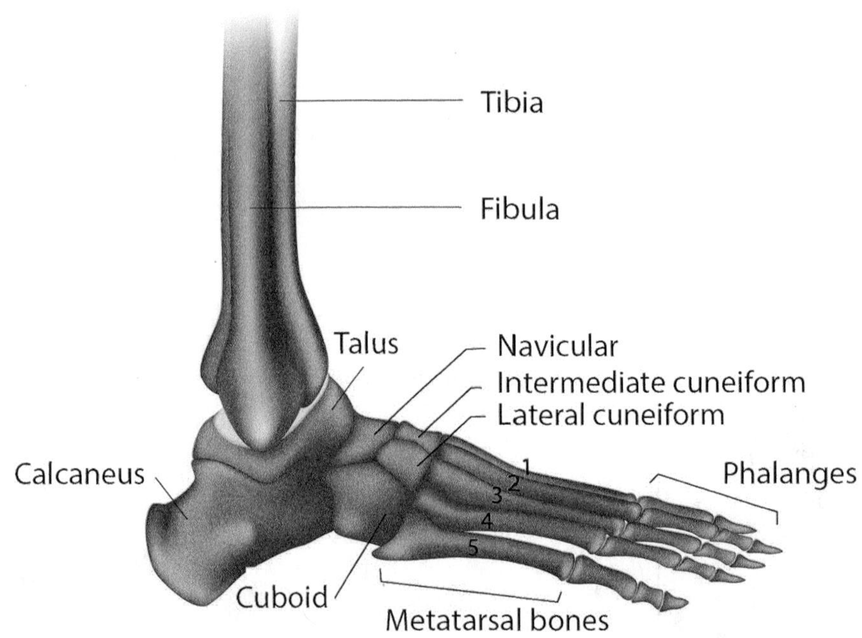

Hand Bones

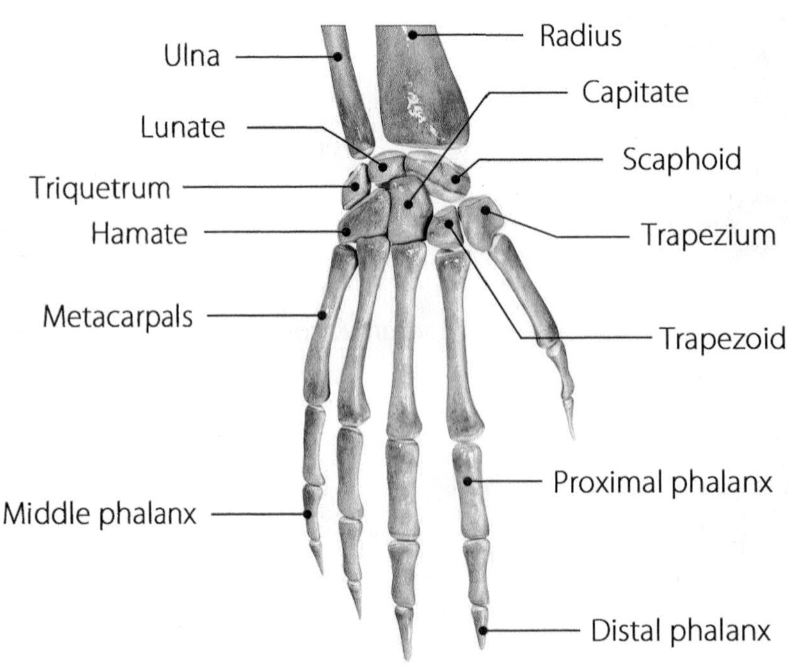

Skeletal System — Skull Anatomy

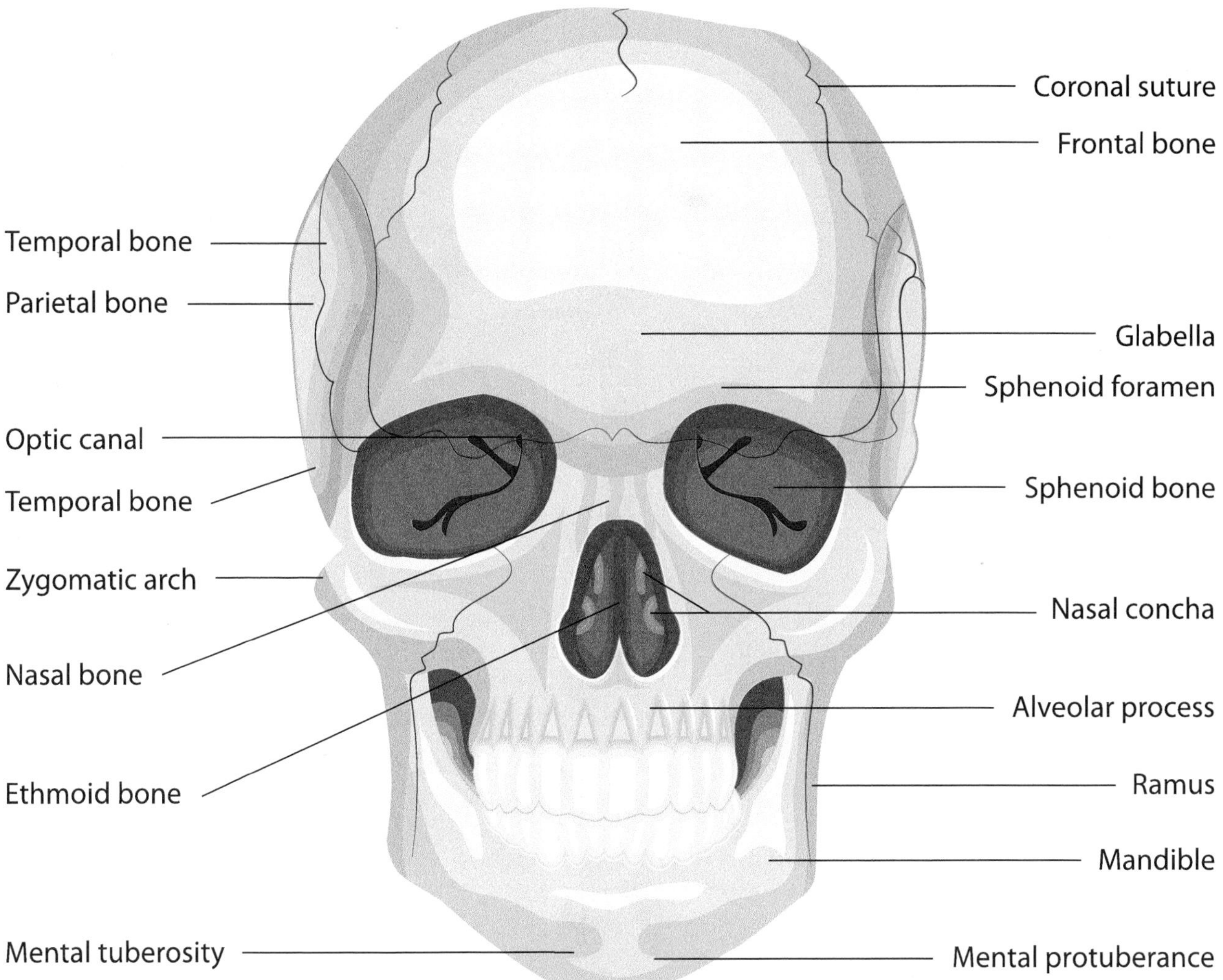

Urinary System — Kidney Anatomy

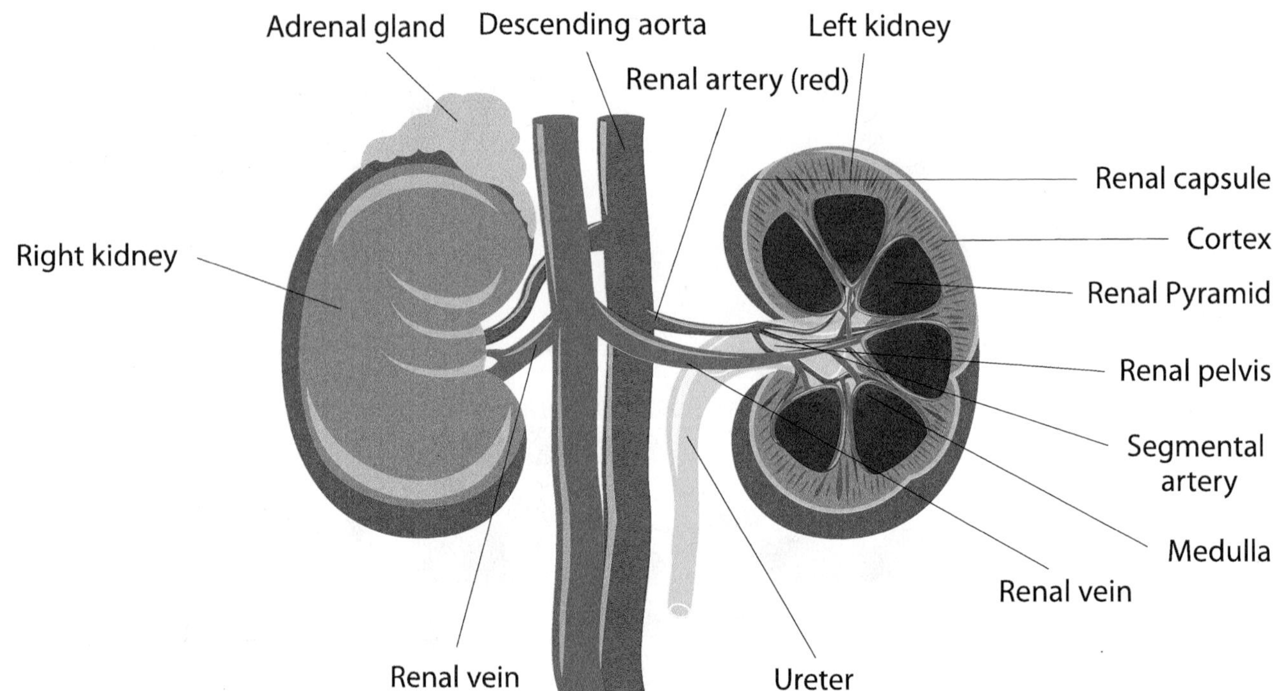

Urinary Organs and Structures

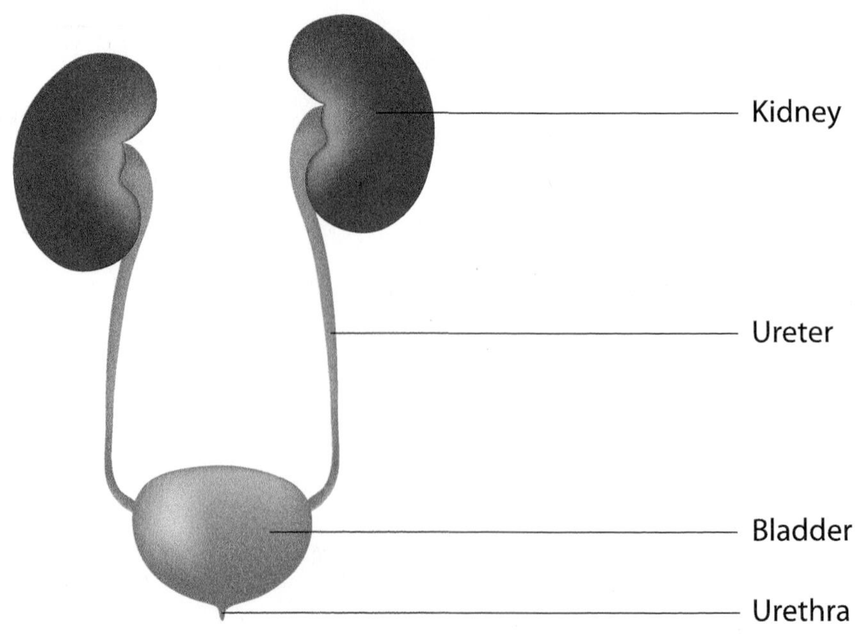

ICD-10-CM Index to Diseases and Injuries

A

- **Abnormal** — *continued*
  - function studies — *continued*
    - placenta R94.8
    - pulmonary R94.2
    - special senses NEC R94.128
    - spleen R94.8
    - thyroid R94.6
    - vestibular R94.121
  - gait — *see* Gait
    - hysterical F44.4
  - gastrin secretion E16.4
  - globulin R77.1
    - cortisol-binding E27.8
    - thyroid-binding E07.89
  - glomerular, minor (*see also* N00-N07 with fourth character .0)N05.0
  - glucagon secretion E16.3
  - glucose tolerance (test) (non-fasting) R73.09
  - gravitational (G) forces or states (effect of) T75.81 ☑
  - hair (color) (shaft) L67.9
    - specified NEC L67.8
  - hard tissue formation in pulp (dental) K04.3
  - head movement R25.0
  - heart
    - rate R00.9
      - specified NEC R00.8
    - shadow R93.1
    - sounds NEC R01.2
  - hemoglobin (disease) (*see also* Disease, hemoglobin)D58.2
    - trait — *see* Trait, hemoglobin, abnormal
  - histology NEC R89.7
  - immunological findings R89.4
    - in serum R76.9
      - specified NEC R76.8
  - increase in appetite R63.2
  - involuntary movement — *see* Abnormal, movement, involuntary
  - jaw closure M26.51
  - karyotype R89.8
  - kidney function test R94.4
  - knee jerk R29.2
  - leukocyte (cell) (differential) NEC D72.9
  - liver — *see* categories
  - loss of
    - height R29.890
    - weight R63.4
  - mammogram NEC R92.8
    - calcification (calculus) R92.1
    - microcalcification R92.0
  - Mantoux test R76.11
  - movement (disorder) (*see also* Disorder, movement)
    - head R25.0
    - involuntary R25.9
      - fasciculation R25.3
      - of head R25.0
      - spasm R25.2
      - specified type NEC R25.8
      - tremor R25.1
  - myoglobin (Aberdeen) (Annapolis) R89.7
  - neonatal screening P09
  - oculomotor study R94.113
  - palmar creases Q82.8
  - Papanicolaou (smear)
    - anus R85.619
      - atypical squamous cells cannot exclude high grade squamous intraepithelial lesion (ASC-H) R85.611
      - atypical squamous cells of undetermined significance (ASC-US) R85.610
      - cytologic evidence of malignancy R85.614
      - high grade squamous intraepithelial lesion (HGSIL) R85.613
      - human papillomavirus (HPV) DNA test
        - high risk positive R85.81
        - low risk positive R85.82
      - inadequate smear R85.615
      - low grade squamous intraepithelial lesion (LGSIL) R85.612
      - satisfactory anal smear but lacking transformation zone R85.616
      - specified NEC R85.618
      - unsatisfactory smear R85.615
    - bronchial washings R84.6
    - cerebrospinal fluid R83.6
    - cervix R87.619
      - atypical squamous cells cannot exclude high grade squamous intraepithelial lesion (ASC-H) R87.611

- **Abnormal** — *continued*
  - Papanicolaou (smear) — *continued*
      - atypical squamous cells of undetermined significance (ASC-US) R87.610
      - cytologic evidence of malignancy R87.614
      - high grade squamous intraepithelial lesion (HGSIL) R87.613
      - inadequate smear R87.615
      - low grade squamous intraepithelial lesion (LGSIL) R87.612
      - non-atypical endometrial cells R87.618
      - satisfactory cervical smear but lacking transformation zone R87.616
      - specified NEC R87.618
      - thin preparation R87.619
      - unsatisfactory smear R87.615
    - nasal secretions R84.6
    - nipple discharge R89.6
    - peritoneal fluid R85.69
    - pleural fluid R84.6
    - prostatic secretions R86.6
    - saliva R85.69
    - seminal fluid R86.6
    - sites NEC R89.6
    - sputum R84.6
    - synovial fluid R89.6
    - throat scrapings R84.6
    - vagina R87.629
      - atypical squamous cells cannot exclude high grade squamous intraepithelial lesion (ASC-H) R87.621
      - atypical squamous cells of undetermined significance (ASC-US) R87.620
      - cytologic evidence of malignancy R87.624
      - high grade squamous intraepithelial lesion (HGSIL) R87.623
      - inadequate smear R87.625
      - low grade squamous intraepithelial lesion (LGSIL) R87.622
      - specified NEC R87.628
      - thin preparation R87.629
      - unsatisfactory smear R87.625
    - vulva R87.69
    - wound secretions R89.6
  - partial thromboplastin time (PTT) R79.1
  - pelvis (bony) — *see* Deformity, pelvis
  - percussion, chest (tympany) R09.89
  - periods (grossly) — *see* Menstruation
  - phonocardiogram R94.39
  - plantar reflex R29.2
  - plasma
    - protein R77.9
      - specified NEC R77.8
    - viscosity R70.1
  - pleural (folds) Q34.0
  - posture R29.3
  - product of conception O02.9
    - specified type NEC O02.89
  - prothrombin time (PT) R79.1
  - pulmonary
    - artery, congenital Q25.79
    - function, newborn P28.89
    - test results R94.2
  - pulsations in neck R00.2
  - pupillary H21.56 ☑
    - function (reaction) (reflex) — *see* Anomaly, pupil, function
  - radiological examination — *see* Abnormal, diagnostic imaging
  - red blood cell (s) (morphology) (volume) R71.8
  - reflex — *see* Reflex
  - renal function test R94.4
  - response to nerve stimulation R94.130
  - retinal correspondence H53.31
  - retinal function study R94.111
  - rhythm, heart (*see also* Arrhythmia)
  - saliva — *see* Abnormal, specimen, digestive organs
  - scan
    - kidney R94.4
    - liver R93.2
    - thyroid R94.6
  - secretion
    - gastrin E16.4
    - glucagon E16.3
  - semen, seminal fluid — *see* Abnormal, specimen, male genital organs
  - serum level (of)
    - acid phosphatase R74.8
    - alkaline phosphatase R74.8
    - amylase R74.8
    - enzymes R74.9

- **Abnormal** — *continued*
  - serum level — *continued*
      - specified NEC R74.8
    - lipase R74.8
    - triacylglycerol lipase R74.8
  - shape
    - gravid uterus — *see* Anomaly, uterus
  - sinus venosus Q21.1
  - size, tooth, teeth K00.2
  - spacing, tooth, teeth, fully erupted M26.30
  - specimen
    - digestive organs (peritoneal fluid) (saliva) R85.9
      - cytology R85.69
      - drug level R85.2
      - enzyme level R85.0
      - histology R85.7
      - hormones R85.1
      - immunology R85.4
      - microbiology R85.5
      - nonmedicinal level R85.3
      - specified type NEC R85.89
    - female genital organs (secretions) (smears) R87.9
      - cytology R87.69
        - cervix R87.619
          - human papillomavirus (HPV) DNA test
            - high risk positive R87.810
            - low risk positive R87.820
          - inadequate (unsatisfactory) smear R87.615
          - non-atypical endometrial cells R87.618
          - specified NEC R87.618
        - vagina R87.629
          - human papillomavirus (HPV) DNA test
            - high risk positive R87.811
            - low risk positive R87.821
          - inadequate (unsatisfactory) smear R87.625
        - vulva R87.69
      - drug level R87.2
      - enzyme level R87.0
      - histological R87.7
      - hormones R87.1
      - immunology R87.4
      - microbiology R87.5
      - nonmedicinal level R87.3
      - specified type NEC R87.89
    - male genital organs (prostatic secretions) (semen) R86.9
      - cytology R86.6
      - drug level R86.2
      - enzyme level R86.0
      - histological R86.7
      - hormones R86.1
      - immunology R86.4
      - microbiology R86.5
      - nonmedicinal level R86.3
      - specified type NEC R86.8
    - nipple discharge — *see* Abnormal, specimen, specified
    - respiratory organs (bronchial washings) (nasal secretions) (pleural fluid) (sputum) R84.9
      - cytology R84.6
      - drug level R84.2
      - enzyme level R84.0
      - histology R84.7
      - hormones R84.1
      - immunology R84.4
      - microbiology R84.5
      - nonmedicinal level R84.3
      - specified type NEC R84.8
    - specified organ, system and tissue NOS R89.9
      - cytology R89.6
      - drug level R89.2
      - enzyme level R89.0
      - histology R89.7
      - hormones R89.1
      - immunology R89.4
      - microbiology R89.5
      - nonmedicinal level R89.3
      - specified type NEC R89.8
    - synovial fluid — *see* Abnormal, specimen, specified
    - thorax (bronchial washings) (pleural fluids) — *see* Abnormal, specimen, respiratory organs
    - vagina (secretion) (smear) R87.629
    - vulva (secretion) (smear) R87.69
    - wound secretion — *see* Abnormal, specimen, specified
  - spermatozoa — *see* Abnormal, specimen, male genital organs

Abrasion - Abscess

- **Abrasion** — *continued*
  - head S00.91 ☑
    - ear — *see* Abrasion, ear
    - eyelid — *see* Abrasion, eyelid
    - lip S00.511 ☑
    - nose S00.31 ☑
    - oral cavity S00.512 ☑
    - scalp S00.01 ☑
    - specified site NEC S00.81 ☑
  - heel — *see* Abrasion, foot
  - hip S70.21 ☑
  - inguinal region S30.811 ☑
  - interscapular region S20.419 ☑
  - jaw S00.81 ☑
  - knee S80.21 ☑
  - labium (majus) (minus) S30.814 ☑
  - larynx S10.11 ☑
  - leg (lower) S80.81 ☑
    - knee — *see* Abrasion, knee
    - upper — *see* Abrasion, thigh
  - lip S00.511 ☑
  - lower back S30.810 ☑
  - lumbar region S30.810 ☑
  - malar region S00.81 ☑
  - mammary — *see* Abrasion, breast
  - mastoid region S00.81 ☑
  - mouth S00.512 ☑
  - nail
    - finger — *see* Abrasion, finger
    - toe — *see* Abrasion, toe
  - nape S10.81 ☑
  - nasal S00.31 ☑
  - neck S10.91 ☑
    - specified site NEC S10.81 ☑
    - throat S10.11 ☑
  - nose S00.31 ☑
  - occipital region S00.01 ☑
  - oral cavity S00.512 ☑
  - orbital region — *see* Abrasion, eyelid
  - palate S00.512 ☑
  - palm — *see* Abrasion, hand
  - parietal region S00.01 ☑
  - pelvis S30.810 ☑
  - penis S30.812 ☑
  - perineum
    - female S30.814 ☑
    - male S30.810 ☑
  - periocular area — *see* Abrasion, eyelid
  - phalanges
    - finger — *see* Abrasion, finger
    - toe — *see* Abrasion, toe
  - pharynx S10.11 ☑
  - pinna — *see* Abrasion, ear
  - popliteal space — *see* Abrasion, knee
  - prepuce S30.812 ☑
  - pubic region S30.810 ☑
  - pudendum
    - female S30.816 ☑
    - male S30.815 ☑
  - sacral region S30.810 ☑
  - scalp S00.01 ☑
  - scapular region — *see* Abrasion, shoulder
  - scrotum S30.813 ☑
  - shin — *see* Abrasion, leg
  - shoulder S40.21 ☑
  - skin NEC T14.8
  - sternal region S20.319 ☑
  - submaxillary region S00.81 ☑
  - submental region S00.81 ☑
  - subungual
    - finger (s) — *see* Abrasion, finger
    - toe (s) — *see* Abrasion, toe
  - supraclavicular fossa S10.81 ☑
  - supraorbital S00.81 ☑
  - temple S00.81 ☑
  - temporal region S00.81 ☑
  - testis S30.813 ☑
  - thigh S70.31 ☑
  - thorax, thoracic (wall) S20.91 ☑
    - back S20.41 ☑
    - front S20.31 ☑
  - throat S10.11 ☑
  - thumb S60.31 ☑
  - toe (s) (lesser) S90.416 ☑
    - great S90.41 ☑
  - tongue S00.512 ☑
  - tooth, teeth (dentifrice) (habitual) (hard tissues) (occupational) (ritual) (traditional) K03.1
  - trachea S10.11 ☑
  - tunica vaginalis S30.813 ☑
  - tympanum, tympanic membrane — *see* Abrasion, ear

- **Abrasion** — *continued*
  - uvula S00.512 ☑
  - vagina S30.814 ☑
  - vocal cords S10.11 ☑
  - vulva S30.814 ☑
  - wrist S60.81 ☑
- **Abrism** — *see* Poisoning, food, noxious, plant
- **Abruptio** placentae O45.9 ☑
  - with
    - afibrinogenemia O45.01 ☑
    - coagulation defect O45.00 ☑
      - specified NEC O45.09 ☑
    - disseminated intravascular coagulation O45.02 ☑
    - hypofibrinogenemia O45.01 ☑
  - specified NEC O45.8 ☑
- **Abruption**, placenta — *see* Abruptio placentae
- **Abscess** (connective tissue) (embolic) (fistulous) (infective) (metastatic) (multiple) (pernicious) (pyogenic) (septic) L02.91
  - with
    - diverticular disease (intestine) K57.80
      - with bleeding K57.81
      - large intestine K57.20
        - with
          - bleeding K57.21
          - small intestine K57.40
            - with bleeding K57.41
      - small intestine K57.00
        - with
          - bleeding K57.01
          - large intestine K57.40
            - with bleeding K57.41
    - lymphangitis - code by site under Abscess
  - abdomen, abdominal
    - cavity K65.1
    - wall L02.211
  - abdominopelvic K65.1
  - accessory sinus — *see* Sinusitis
  - adrenal (capsule) (gland) E27.8
  - alveolar K04.7
    - with sinus K04.6
  - amebic A06.4
    - brain (and liver or lung abscess) A06.6
    - genitourinary tract A06.82
    - liver (without mention of brain or lung abscess) A06.4
    - lung (and liver) (without mention of brain abscess) A06.5
    - specified site NEC A06.89
    - spleen A06.89
  - anaerobic A48.0
  - ankle — *see* Abscess, lower limb
  - anorectal K61.2
  - antecubital space — *see* Abscess, upper limb
  - antrum (chronic) (Highmore) — *see* Sinusitis, maxillary
  - anus K61.0
  - apical (tooth) K04.7
    - with sinus (alveolar) K04.6
  - appendix K35.3
  - areola (acute) (chronic) (nonpuerperal) N61.1
    - puerperal, postpartum or gestational — *see* Infection, nipple
  - arm (any part) — *see* Abscess, upper limb
  - artery (wall) I77.89
  - atheromatous I77.2
  - auricle, ear — *see* Abscess, ear, external
  - axilla (region) L02.41 ☑
    - lymph gland or node L04.2
  - back (any part, except buttock) L02.212
  - Bartholin's gland N75.1
    - with
      - abortion — *see* Abortion, by type complicated by, sepsis
      - ectopic or molar pregnancy O08.0
    - following ectopic or molar pregnancy O08.0
  - Bezold's — *see* Mastoiditis, acute
  - bilharziasis B65.1
  - bladder (wall) — *see* Cystitis, specified type NEC
  - bone (subperiosteal) (*see also* Osteomyelitis, specified type NEC)
    - accessory sinus (chronic) — *see* Sinusitis
    - chronic or old — *see* Osteomyelitis, chronic
    - jaw (lower) (upper) M27.2
    - mastoid — *see* Mastoiditis, acute, subperiosteal
    - petrous — *see* Petrositis
    - spinal (tuberculous) A18.01
      - nontuberculous — *see* Osteomyelitis, vertebra
  - bowel K63.0

- **Abscess** — *continued*
  - brain (any part) (cystic) (otogenic) G06.0
    - amebic (with abscess of any other site) A06.6
    - gonococcal A54.82
    - pheomycotic (chromomycotic) B43.1
    - tuberculous A17.81
  - breast (acute) (chronic) (nonpuerperal) N61.1
    - newborn P39.0
    - puerperal, postpartum, gestational — *see* Mastitis, obstetric, purulent
  - broad ligament N73.2
    - acute N73.0
    - chronic N73.1
  - Brodie's (localized) (chronic) M86.8X ☑
  - bronchi J98.09
  - buccal cavity K12.2
  - bulbourethral gland N34.0
  - bursa M71.00
    - ankle M71.07 ☑
    - elbow M71.02 ☑
    - foot M71.07 ☑
    - hand M71.04 ☑
    - hip M71.05 ☑
    - knee M71.06 ☑
    - multiple sites M71.09
    - pharyngeal J39.1
    - shoulder M71.01 ☑
    - specified site NEC M71.08
    - wrist M71.03 ☑
  - buttock L02.31
  - canthus — *see* Blepharoconjunctivitis
  - cartilage — *see* Disorder, cartilage, specified type NEC
  - cecum K35.3
  - cerebellum, cerebellar G06.0
    - sequelae G09
  - cerebral (embolic) G06.0
    - sequelae G09
  - cervical (meaning neck) L02.11
    - lymph gland or node L04.0
  - cervix (stump) (uteri) — *see* Cervicitis
  - cheek (external) L02.01
    - inner K12.2
  - chest J86.9
    - with fistula J86.0
    - wall L02.213
  - chin L02.01
  - choroid — *see* Inflammation, chorioretinal
  - circumtonsillar J36
  - cold (lung) (tuberculous) (*see also* Tuberculosis, abscess, lung)
    - articular — *see* Tuberculosis, joint
  - colon (wall) K63.0
  - colostomy K94.02
  - conjunctiva — *see* Conjunctivitis, acute
  - cornea H16.31 ☑
  - corpus
    - cavernosum N48.21
    - luteum — *see* Oophoritis
  - Cowper's gland N34.0
  - cranium G06.0
  - cul-de-sac (Douglas') (posterior) — *see* Peritonitis, pelvic, female
  - cutaneous — *see* Abscess, by site
  - dental K04.7
    - with sinus (alveolar) K04.6
  - dentoalveolar K04.7
    - with sinus K04.6
  - diaphragm, diaphragmatic K65.1
  - Douglas' cul-de-sac or pouch — *see* Peritonitis, pelvic, female
  - Dubois A50.59
  - ear (middle) (*see also* Otitis, media, suppurative)
    - acute — *see* Otitis, media, suppurative, acute
    - external H60.0 ☑
  - entamebic — *see* Abscess, amebic
  - enterostomy K94.12
  - epididymis N45.4
  - epidural G06.2
    - brain G06.0
    - spinal cord G06.1
  - epiglottis J38.7
  - epiploon, epiploic K65.1
  - erysipelatous — *see* Erysipelas
  - esophagus K20.8
  - ethmoid (bone) (chronic) (sinus) J32.2
  - external auditory canal — *see* Abscess, ear, external
  - extradural G06.2
    - brain G06.0
      - sequelae G09
    - spinal cord G06.1

Abscess — *continued*
- extraperitoneal K68.19
- eye — *see* Endophthalmitis, purulent
- eyelid H00.03 ☑
- face (any part, except ear, eye and nose) L02.01
- fallopian tube — *see* Salpingitis
- fascia M72.8
- fauces J39.1
- fecal K63.0
- femoral (region) — *see* Abscess, lower limb
- filaria, filarial — *see* Infestation, filarial
- finger (any) (*see also* Abscess, hand)
  - nail — *see* Cellulitis, finger
- foot L02.61 ☑
- forehead L02.01
- frontal sinus (chronic) J32.1
- gallbladder K81.0
- genital organ or tract
  - female (external) N76.4
  - male N49.9
    - multiple sites N49.8
    - specified NEC N49.8
- gestational mammary O91.11 ☑
- gestational subareolar O91.11 ☑
- gingival — *see* Periodontitis, aggressive, localized
- gland, glandular (lymph) (acute) — *see* Lymphadenitis, acute
- gluteal (region) L02.31
- gonorrheal — *see* Gonococcus
- groin L02.214
- gum — *see* Periodontitis, aggressive, localized
- hand L02.51 ☑
- head NEC L02.811
  - face (any part, except ear, eye and nose) L02.01
- heart — *see* Carditis
- heel — *see* Abscess, foot
- helminthic — *see* Infestation, helminth
- hepatic (cholangitic) (hematogenic) (lymphogenic) (pylephlebitic) K75.0
  - amebic A06.4
- hip (region) — *see* Abscess, lower limb
- ileocecal K35.3
- ileostomy (bud) K94.12
- iliac (region) L02.214
  - fossa K35.3
- infraclavicular (fossa) — *see* Abscess, upper limb
- inguinal (region) L02.214
  - lymph gland or node L04.1
- intestine, intestinal NEC K63.0
  - rectal K61.1
- intra-abdominal (*see also* Abscess, peritoneum)K65.1
  - postprocedural T81.43
    - retroperitoneal K68.11
- intracranial G06.0
- intramammary — *see* Abscess, breast
- intra-muscular, postprocedural T81.42
- intraorbital — *see* Abscess, orbit
- intraperitoneal K65.1
- intrasphincteric (anus) K61.4
- intraspinal G06.1
- intratonsillar J36
- ischiorectal (fossa) K61.3
- jaw (bone) (lower) (upper) M27.2
- joint — *see* Arthritis, pyogenic or pyemic
  - spine (tuberculous) A18.01
    - nontuberculous — *see* Spondylopathy, infective
- kidney N15.1
  - with calculus N20.0
    - with hydronephrosis N13.6
  - puerperal (postpartum) O86.21
- knee (*see also* Abscess, lower limb)
  - joint M00.9
- labium (majus) (minus) N76.4
- lacrimal
  - caruncle — *see* Inflammation, lacrimal, passages, acute
  - gland — *see* Dacryoadenitis
  - passages (duct) (sac) — *see* Inflammation, lacrimal, passages, acute
- lacunar N34.0
- larynx J38.7
- lateral (alveolar) K04.7
  - with sinus K04.6
- leg (any part) — *see* Abscess, lower limb
- lens H27.8
- lingual K14.0
  - tonsil J36
- lip K13.0
- Littre's gland N34.0

Abscess — *continued*
- liver (cholangitic) (hematogenic) (lymphogenic) (pylephlebitic) (pyogenic) K75.0
  - amebic (due to Entamoeba histolytica) (dysenteric) (tropical) A06.4
    - with
      - brain abscess (and liver or lung abscess) A06.6
      - lung abscess A06.5
- loin (region) L02.211
- lower limb L02.41 ☑
- lumbar (tuberculous) A18.01
  - nontuberculous L02.212
- lung (miliary) (putrid) J85.2
  - with pneumonia J85.1
    - due to specified organism (see Pneumonia, in (due to))
  - amebic (with liver abscess) A06.5
    - with
      - brain abscess A06.6
      - pneumonia A06.5
- lymph, lymphatic, gland or node (acute) (*see also* Lymphadenitis, acute)
  - mesentery I88.0
- malar M27.2
- mammary gland — *see* Abscess, breast
- marginal, anus K61.0
- mastoid — *see* Mastoiditis, acute
- maxilla, maxillary M27.2
  - molar (tooth) K04.7
    - with sinus K04.6
  - premolar K04.7
  - sinus (chronic) J32.0
- mediastinum J85.3
- meibomian gland — *see* Hordeolum
- meninges G06.2
- mesentery, mesenteric K65.1
- mesosalpinx — *see* Salpingitis
- mons pubis L02.215
- mouth (floor) K12.2
- muscle — *see* Myositis, infective
- myocardium I40.0
- nabothian (follicle) — *see* Cervicitis
- nasal J32.9
- nasopharyngeal J39.1
- navel L02.216
  - newborn P38.9
    - with mild hemorrhage P38.1
    - without hemorrhage P38.9
- neck (region) L02.11
  - lymph gland or node L04.0
- nephritic — *see* Abscess, kidney
- nipple N61.1
  - associated with
    - lactation — *see* Pregnancy, complicated by
    - pregnancy — *see* Pregnancy, complicated by
- nose (external) (fossa) (septum) J34.0
  - sinus (chronic) — *see* Sinusitis
- omentum K65.1
- operative wound T81.40
- orbit, orbital — *see* Cellulitis, orbit
- otogenic G06.0
- ovary, ovarian (corpus luteum) — *see* Oophoritis
- oviduct — *see* Oophoritis
- palate (soft) K12.2
  - hard M27.2
- palmar (space) — *see* Abscess, hand
- pancreas (duct) — *see* Pancreatitis, acute
- parafrenal N48.21
- parametric, parametrium N73.2
  - acute N73.0
  - chronic N73.1
- paranephric N15.1
- parapancreatic — *see* Pancreatitis, acute
- parapharyngeal J39.0
- pararectal K61.1
- parasinus — *see* Sinusitis
- parauterine (*see also* Disease, pelvis, inflammatory)N73.2
- paravaginal — *see* Vaginitis
- parietal region (scalp) L02.811
- parodontal — *see* Periodontitis, aggressive, localized
- parotid (duct) (gland) K11.3
  - region K12.2
- pectoral (region) L02.213
- pelvis, pelvic
  - female — *see* Disease, pelvis, inflammatory
  - male, peritoneal K65.1
- penis N48.21
  - gonococcal (accessory gland) (periurethral) A54.1

Abscess — *continued*
- perianal K61.0
- periapical K04.7
  - with sinus (alveolar) K04.6
- periappendicular K35.3
- pericardial I30.1
- pericecal K35.3
- pericemental — *see* Periodontitis, aggressive, localized
- pericholecystic — *see* Cholecystitis, acute
- pericoronal — *see* Periodontitis, aggressive, localized
- peridental — *see* Periodontitis, aggressive, localized
- perimetric (*see also* Disease, pelvis, inflammatory)N73.2
- perinephric, perinephritic — *see* Abscess, kidney
- perineum, perineal (superficial) L02.215
  - urethra N34.0
- periodontal (parietal) — *see* Periodontitis, aggressive, localized
  - apical K04.7
- periosteum, periosteal (*see also* Osteomyelitis, specified type NEC)
  - with osteomyelitis (*see also* Osteomyelitis, specified type NEC)
    - acute — *see* Osteomyelitis, acute
    - chronic — *see* Osteomyelitis, chronic
- peripharyngeal J39.0
- peripleuritic J86.9
  - with fistula J86.0
- periprostatic N41.2
- perirectal K61.1
- perirenal (tissue) — *see* Abscess, kidney
- perisinuous (nose) — *see* Sinusitis
- peritoneum, peritoneal (perforated) (ruptured) K65.1
  - with appendicitis K35.3
  - pelvic
    - female — *see* Peritonitis, pelvic, female
    - male K65.1
  - postoperative T81.43
  - puerperal, postpartum, childbirth O85
  - tuberculous A18.31
- peritonsillar J36
- perityphlic K35.3
- periureteral N28.89
- periurethral N34.0
  - gonococcal (accessory gland) (periurethral) A54.1
- periuterine (*see also* Disease, pelvis, inflammatory)N73.2
- perivesical — *see* Cystitis, specified type NEC
- petrous bone — *see* Petrositis
- phagedenic NOS L02.91
  - chancroid A57
- pharynx, pharyngeal (lateral) J39.1
- pilonidal L05.01
- pituitary (gland) E23.6
- pleura J86.9
  - with fistula J86.0
- popliteal — *see* Abscess, lower limb
- postcecal K35.3
- postlaryngeal J38.7
- postnasal J34.0
- postoperative (any site) T81.40
  - retroperitoneal K68.11
- postpharyngeal J39.0
- posttonsillar J36
- post-typhoid A01.09
- pouch of Douglas — *see* Peritonitis, pelvic, female
- premammary — *see* Abscess, breast
- prepatellar — *see* Abscess, lower limb
- prostate N41.2
  - gonococcal (acute) (chronic) A54.22
- psoas muscle K68.12
- puerperal - code by site under Puerperal, abscess
- pulmonary — *see* Abscess, lung
- pulp, pulpal (dental) K04.01
  - irreversible K04.02
  - reversible K04.01
- rectovaginal septum K63.0
- rectovesical — *see* Cystitis, specified type NEC
- rectum K61.1
- renal — *see* Abscess, kidney
- retina — *see* Inflammation, chorioretinal
- retrobulbar — *see* Abscess, orbit
- retrocecal K65.1
- retrolaryngeal J38.7
- retromammary — *see* Abscess, breast
- retroperitoneal NEC K68.19
  - postprocedural K68.11

Abscess — *continued*
- retropharyngeal J39.0
- retrouterine — *see* Peritonitis, pelvic, female
- retrovesical — *see* Cystitis, specified type NEC
- root, tooth K04.7
  - with sinus (alveolar) K04.6
- round ligament (*see also* Disease, pelvis, inflammatory)N73.2
- rupture (spontaneous) NOS L02.91
- sacrum (tuberculous) A18.01
  - nontuberculous M46.28
- salivary (duct) (gland) K11.3
- scalp (any part) L02.811
- scapular — *see* Osteomyelitis, specified type NEC
- sclera — *see* Scleritis
- scrofulous (tuberculous) A18.2
- scrotum N49.2
- seminal vesicle N49.0
- septal, dental K04.7
  - with sinus (alveolar) K04.6
- serous — *see* Periostitis
- shoulder (region) — *see* Abscess, upper limb
- sigmoid K63.0
- sinus (accessory) (chronic) (nasal) (*see also* Sinusitis)
  - intracranial venous (any) G06.0
- Skene's duct or gland N34.0
- skin — *see* Abscess, by site
- specified site NEC L02.818
- spermatic cord N49.1
- sphenoidal (sinus) (chronic) J32.3
- spinal cord (any part) (staphylococcal) G06.1
  - tuberculous A17.81
- spine (column) (tuberculous) A18.01
  - epidural G06.1
  - nontuberculous — *see* Osteomyelitis, vertebra
- spleen D73.3
  - amebic A06.89
- stitch T81.48
- subarachnoid G06.2
  - brain G06.0
  - spinal cord G06.1
- subareolar — *see* Abscess, breast
- subcecal K35.3
- subcutaneous (*see also* Abscess, by site)
  - pheomycotic (chromomycotic) B43.2
  - postprocedural T81.41
- subdiaphragmatic K65.1
- subdural G06.2
  - brain G06.0
    - sequelae G09
  - spinal cord G06.1
- subgaleal L02.811
- subhepatic K65.1
- sublingual K12.2
  - gland K11.3
- submammary — *see* Abscess, breast
- submandibular (region) (space) (triangle) K12.2
  - gland K11.3
- submaxillary (region) L02.01
  - gland K11.3
- submental L02.01
  - gland K11.3
- subperiosteal — *see* Osteomyelitis, specified type NEC
- subphrenic K65.1
  - postoperative T81.43
- suburethral N34.0
- sudoriparous L75.8
- supraclavicular (fossa) — *see* Abscess, upper limb
- suprapelvic, acute N73.0
- suprarenal (capsule) (gland) E27.8
- sweat gland L74.8
- tear duct — *see* Inflammation, lacrimal, passages, acute
- temple L02.01
- temporal region L02.01
- temporosphenoidal G06.0
- tendon (sheath) M65.00
  - ankle M65.07 ☑
  - foot M65.07 ☑
  - forearm M65.03 ☑
  - hand M65.04 ☑
  - lower leg M65.06 ☑
  - pelvic region M65.05 ☑
  - shoulder region M65.01 ☑
  - specified site NEC M65.08
  - thigh M65.05 ☑
  - upper arm M65.02 ☑
- testis N45.4
- thigh — *see* Abscess, lower limb
- thorax J86.9
  - with fistula J86.0

Abscess — *continued*
- throat J39.1
- thumb (*see also* Abscess, hand)
  - nail — *see* Cellulitis, finger
- thymus (gland) E32.1
- thyroid (gland) E06.0
- toe (any) (*see also* Abscess, foot)
  - nail — *see* Cellulitis, toe
- tongue (staphylococcal) K14.0
- tonsil (s) (lingual) J36
- tonsillopharyngeal J36
- tooth, teeth (root) K04.7
  - with sinus (alveolar) K04.6
  - supporting structures NEC — *see* Periodontitis, aggressive, localized
- trachea J39.8
- trunk L02.219
  - abdominal wall L02.211
  - back L02.212
  - chest wall L02.213
  - groin L02.214
  - perineum L02.215
  - umbilicus L02.216
- tubal — *see* Salpingitis
- tuberculous — *see* Tuberculosis, abscess
- tubo-ovarian — *see* Salpingo-oophoritis
- tunica vaginalis N49.1
- umbilicus L02.216
- upper
  - limb L02.41 ☑
  - respiratory J39.8
- urethral (gland) N34.0
- urinary N34.0
- uterus, uterine (wall) (*see also* Endometritis)
  - ligament (*see also* Disease, pelvis, inflammatory)N73.2
  - neck — *see* Cervicitis
- uvula K12.2
- vagina (wall) — *see* Vaginitis
- vaginorectal — *see* Vaginitis
- vas deferens N49.1
- vermiform appendix K35.3
- vertebra (column) (tuberculous) A18.01
  - nontuberculous — *see* Osteomyelitis, vertebra
- vesical — *see* Cystitis, specified type NEC
- vesico-uterine pouch — *see* Peritonitis, pelvic, female
- vitreous (humor) — *see* Endophthalmitis, purulent
- vocal cord J38.3
- von Bezold's — *see* Mastoiditis, acute
- vulva N76.4
- vulvovaginal gland N75.1
- web space — *see* Abscess, hand
- wound T81.40
- wrist — *see* Abscess, upper limb

Absence (of) (organ or part) (complete or partial)
- adrenal (gland) (congenital) Q89.1
  - acquired E89.6
- albumin in blood E88.09
- alimentary tract (congenital) Q45.8
  - upper Q40.8
- alveolar process (acquired) — *see* Anomaly, alveolar
- ankle (acquired) Z89.44 ☑
- anus (congenital) Q42.3
  - with fistula Q42.2
- aorta (congenital) Q25.41
- appendix, congenital Q42.8
- arm (acquired) Z89.20 ☑
  - above elbow Z89.22 ☑
    - congenital (with hand present) — *see* Agenesis, arm, with hand present
      - and hand — *see* Agenesis, forearm, and hand
  - below elbow Z89.21 ☑
    - congenital (with hand present) — *see* Agenesis, arm, with hand present
      - and hand — *see* Agenesis, forearm, and hand
  - congenital — *see* Defect, reduction, upper limb
  - shoulder (following explantation of shoulder joint prosthesis) (joint) (with or without presence of antibiotic-impregnated cement spacer) Z89.23 ☑
    - congenital (with hand present) — *see* Agenesis, arm, with hand present
- artery (congenital) (peripheral) Q27.8
  - brain Q28.3
  - coronary Q24.5
  - pulmonary Q25.79
  - specified NEC Q27.8
  - umbilical Q27.0

Absence — *continued*
- atrial septum (congenital) Q21.1
- auditory canal (congenital) (external) Q16.1
- auricle (ear), congenital Q16.0
- bile, biliary duct, congenital Q44.5
- bladder (acquired) Z90.6
  - congenital Q64.5
- bowel sounds R19.11
- brain Q00.0
  - part of Q04.3
- breast (s) (and nipple (s)) (acquired) Z90.1 ☑
  - congenital Q83.8
- broad ligament Q50.6
- bronchus (congenital) Q32.4
- canaliculus lacrimalis, congenital Q10.4
- cerebellum (vermis) Q04.3
- cervix (acquired) (with uterus) Z90.710
  - with remaining uterus Z90.712
  - congenital Q51.5
- chin, congenital Q18.8
- cilia (congenital) Q10.3
  - acquired — *see* Madarosis
- clitoris (congenital) Q52.6
- coccyx, congenital Q76.49
- cold sense R20.8
- congenital
  - lumen — *see* Atresia
  - organ or site NEC — *see* Agenesis
  - septum — *see* Imperfect, closure
- corpus callosum Q04.0
- cricoid cartilage, congenital Q31.8
- diaphragm (with hernia), congenital Q79.1
- digestive organ (s) or tract, congenital Q45.8
  - acquired NEC Z90.49
  - upper Q40.8
- ductus arteriosus Q28.8
- duodenum (acquired) Z90.49
  - congenital Q41.0
- ear, congenital Q16.9
  - acquired H93.8 ☑
  - auricle Q16.0
  - external Q16.0
  - inner Q16.5
  - lobe, lobule Q17.8
  - middle, except ossicles Q16.4
    - ossicles Q16.3
  - ossicles Q16.3
- ejaculatory duct (congenital) Q55.4
- endocrine gland (congenital) NEC Q89.2
  - acquired E89.89
- epididymis (congenital) Q55.4
  - acquired Z90.79
- epiglottis, congenital Q31.8
- esophagus (congenital) Q39.8
  - acquired (partial) Z90.49
- eustachian tube (congenital) Q16.2
- extremity (acquired) Z89.9
  - congenital Q73.0
  - knee (following explantation of knee joint prosthesis) (joint) (with or without presence of antibiotic-impregnated cement spacer) Z89.52 ☑
  - lower (above knee) Z89.619
    - below knee Z89.51 ☑
  - upper — *see* Absence, arm
- eye (acquired) Z90.01
  - congenital Q11.1
  - muscle (congenital) Q10.3
- eyeball (acquired) Z90.01
- eyelid (fold) (congenital) Q10.3
  - acquired Z90.01
- face, specified part NEC Q18.8
- fallopian tube (s) (acquired) Z90.79
  - congenital Q50.6
- family member (causing problem in home) NEC (*see also* Disruption, family)Z63.32
- femur, congenital — *see* Defect, reduction, lower limb, longitudinal, femur
- fibrinogen (congenital) D68.2
  - acquired D65
- finger (s) (acquired) Z89.02 ☑
  - congenital — *see* Agenesis, hand
- foot (acquired) Z89.43 ☑
  - congenital — *see* Agenesis, foot
- forearm (acquired) — *see* Absence, arm, below elbow
- gallbladder (acquired) Z90.49
  - congenital Q44.0
- gamma globulin in blood D80.1
  - hereditary D80.0
- genital organs
  - acquired (female) (male) Z90.79

Absence — *continued*
- genital organs — *continued*
  - female, congenital Q52.8
    - external Q52.71
    - internal NEC Q52.8
  - male, congenital Q55.8
- genitourinary organs, congenital NEC
  - female Q52.8
  - male Q55.8
- globe (acquired) Z90.01
  - congenital Q11.1
- glottis, congenital Q31.8
- hand and wrist (acquired) Z89.11 ☑
  - congenital — *see* Agenesis, hand
- head, part (acquired) NEC Z90.09
- heat sense R20.8
- hip (following explantation of hip joint prosthesis) (joint) (with or without presence of antibiotic-impregnated cement spacer) Z89.62 ☑
- hymen (congenital) Q52.4
- ileum (acquired) Z90.49
  - congenital Q41.2
- immunoglobulin, isolated NEC D80.3
  - IgA D80.2
  - IgG D80.3
  - IgM D80.4
- incus (acquired) — *see* Loss, ossicles, ear
  - congenital Q16.3
- inner ear, congenital Q16.5
- intestine (acquired) (small) Z90.49
  - congenital Q41.9
    - specified NEC Q41.8
  - large Z90.49
    - congenital Q42.9
      - specified NEC Q42.8
- iris, congenital Q13.1
- jejunum (acquired) Z90.49
  - congenital Q41.1
- joint
  - acquired
    - hip (following explantation of hip joint prosthesis) (with or without presence of antibiotic-impregnated cement spacer) Z89.62 ☑
    - knee (following explantation of knee joint prosthesis) (with or without presence of antibiotic-impregnated cement spacer) Z89.52 ☑
    - shoulder (following explantation of shoulder joint prosthesis) (with or without presence of antibiotic-impregnated cement spacer) Z89.23 ☑
  - congenital NEC Q74.8
- kidney (s) (acquired) Z90.5
  - congenital Q60.2
    - bilateral Q60.1
    - unilateral Q60.0
- knee (following explantation of knee joint prosthesis) (joint) (with or without presence of antibiotic-impregnated cement spacer) Z89.52 ☑
- labyrinth, membranous Q16.5
- larynx (congenital) Q31.8
  - acquired Z90.02
- leg (acquired) (above knee) Z89.61 ☑
  - below knee (acquired) Z89.51 ☑
  - congenital — *see* Defect, reduction, lower limb
- lens (acquired) (*see also* Aphakia)
  - congenital Q12.3
  - post cataract extraction Z98.4 ☑
- limb (acquired) — *see* Absence, extremity
- lip Q38.6
- liver (congenital) Q44.7
- lung (fissure) (lobe) (bilateral) (unilateral) (congenital) Q33.3
  - acquired (any part) Z90.2
- menstruation — *see* Amenorrhea
- muscle (congenital) (pectoral) Q79.8
  - ocular Q10.3
- neck, part Q18.8
- neutrophil — *see* Agranulocytosis
- nipple (s) (with breast (s)) (acquired) Z90.1 ☑
  - congenital Q83.2
- nose (congenital) Q30.1
  - acquired Z90.09
- organ
  - of Corti, congenital Q16.5
  - or site, congenital NEC Q89.8
    - acquired NEC Z90.89
- osseous meatus (ear) Q16.4

Absence — *continued*
- ovary (acquired)
  - bilateral Z90.722
  - congenital
    - bilateral Q50.02
    - unilateral Q50.01
  - unilateral Z90.721
- oviduct (acquired)
  - bilateral Z90.722
  - congenital Q50.6
  - unilateral Z90.721
- pancreas (congenital) Q45.0
  - acquired Z90.410
    - complete Z90.410
    - partial Z90.411
    - total Z90.410
- parathyroid gland (acquired) E89.2
  - congenital Q89.2
- patella, congenital Q74.1
- penis (congenital) Q55.5
  - acquired Z90.79
- pericardium (congenital) Q24.8
- pituitary gland (congenital) Q89.2
  - acquired E89.3
- prostate (acquired) Z90.79
  - congenital Q55.4
- pulmonary valve Q22.0
- punctum lacrimale (congenital) Q10.4
- radius, congenital — *see* Defect, reduction, upper limb, longitudinal, radius
- rectum (congenital) Q42.1
  - with fistula Q42.0
  - acquired Z90.49
- respiratory organ NOS Q34.9
- rib (acquired) Z90.89
  - congenital Q76.6
- sacrum, congenital Q76.49
- salivary gland (s), congenital Q38.4
- scrotum, congenital Q55.29
- seminal vesicles (congenital) Q55.4
  - acquired Z90.79
- septum
  - atrial (congenital) Q21.1
  - between aorta and pulmonary artery Q21.4
  - ventricular (congenital) Q20.4
- sex chromosome
  - female phenotype Q97.8
  - male phenotype Q98.8
- skull bone (congenital) Q75.8
  - with
    - anencephaly Q00.0
    - encephalocele — *see* Encephalocele
    - hydrocephalus Q03.9
      - with spina bifida — *see* Spina bifida, by site, with hydrocephalus
    - microcephaly Q02
- spermatic cord, congenital Q55.4
- spine, congenital Q76.49
- spleen (congenital) Q89.01
  - acquired Z90.81
- sternum, congenital Q76.7
- stomach (acquired) (partial) Z90.3
  - congenital Q40.2
- superior vena cava, congenital Q26.8
- teeth, tooth (congenital) K00.0
  - acquired (complete) K08.109
    - class I K08.101
    - class II K08.102
    - class III K08.103
    - class IV K08.104
    - due to
      - caries K08.139
        - class I K08.131
        - class II K08.132
        - class III K08.133
        - class IV K08.134
      - periodontal disease K08.129
        - class I K08.121
        - class II K08.122
        - class III K08.123
        - class IV K08.124
      - specified NEC K08.199
        - class I K08.191
        - class II K08.192
        - class III K08.193
        - class IV K08.194
      - trauma K08.119
        - class I K08.111
        - class II K08.112
        - class III K08.113
        - class IV K08.114
    - partial K08.409

Absence — *continued*
- teeth, tooth — *continued*
      - class I K08.401
      - class II K08.402
      - class III K08.403
      - class IV K08.404
      - due to
        - caries K08.439
          - class I K08.431
          - class II K08.432
          - class III K08.433
          - class IV K08.434
        - periodontal disease K08.429
          - class I K08.421
          - class II K08.422
          - class III K08.423
          - class IV K08.424
        - specified NEC K08.499
          - class I K08.491
          - class II K08.492
          - class III K08.493
          - class IV K08.494
        - trauma K08.419
          - class I K08.411
          - class II K08.412
          - class III K08.413
          - class IV K08.414
- tendon (congenital) Q79.8
- testis (congenital) Q55.0
  - acquired Z90.79
- thumb (acquired) Z89.01 ☑
  - congenital — *see* Agenesis, hand
- thymus gland Q89.2
- thyroid (gland) (acquired) E89.0
  - cartilage, congenital Q31.8
  - congenital E03.1
- toe (s) (acquired) Z89.42 ☑
  - with foot — *see* Absence, foot and ankle
  - congenital — *see* Agenesis, foot
  - great Z89.41 ☑
- tongue, congenital Q38.3
- trachea (cartilage), congenital Q32.1
- transverse aortic arch, congenital Q25.49
- tricuspid valve Q22.4
- umbilical artery, congenital Q27.0
- upper arm and forearm with hand present, congenital — *see* Agenesis, arm, with hand present
- ureter (congenital) Q62.4
  - acquired Z90.6
- urethra, congenital Q64.5
- uterus (acquired) Z90.710
  - with cervix Z90.710
  - with remaining cervical stump Z90.711
  - congenital Q51.0
- uvula, congenital Q38.5
- vagina, congenital Q52.0
- vas deferens (congenital) Q55.4
  - acquired Z90.79
- vein (peripheral) congenital NEC Q27.8
  - cerebral Q28.3
  - digestive system Q27.8
  - great Q26.8
  - lower limb Q27.8
  - portal Q26.5
  - precerebral Q28.1
  - specified site NEC Q27.8
  - upper limb Q27.8
- vena cava (inferior) (superior), congenital Q26.8
- ventricular septum Q20.4
- vertebra, congenital Q76.49
- vulva, congenital Q52.71
- wrist (acquired) Z89.12 ☑

Absorbent system disease I87.8

Absorption
- carbohydrate, disturbance K90.49
- chemical — *see* Table of Drugs and Chemicals
  - through placenta (newborn) P04.9
    - environmental substance P04.6
    - nutritional substance P04.5
    - obstetric anesthetic or analgesic drug P04.0
- drug NEC — *see* Table of Drugs and Chemicals
  - addictive
    - through placenta (newborn) P04.49
      - cocaine P04.41
  - medicinal
    - through placenta (newborn) P04.1
  - through placenta (newborn) P04.1
    - obstetric anesthetic or analgesic drug P04.0
- fat, disturbance K90.49
  - pancreatic K90.3

- **Absorption** — *continued*
  - noxious substance — *see* Table of Drugs and Chemicals
  - protein, disturbance K90.49
  - starch, disturbance K90.49
  - toxic substance — *see* Table of Drugs and Chemicals
  - uremic — *see* Uremia
- **Abstinence** symptoms, syndrome
  - alcohol F10.239
    - with delirium F10.231
  - cocaine F14.23
  - neonatal P96.1
  - nicotine — *see* Dependence, drug, nicotine, with, withdrawal
  - opioid F11.93
    - with dependence F11.23
  - psychoactive NEC F19.939
    - with
      - delirium F19.931
      - dependence F19.239
        - with
          - delirium F19.231
          - perceptual disturbance F19.232
        - uncomplicated F19.230
      - perceptual disturbance F19.932
    - uncomplicated F19.930
  - sedative F13.939
    - with
      - delirium F13.931
      - dependence F13.239
        - with
          - delirium F13.231
          - perceptual disturbance F13.232
        - uncomplicated F13.230
      - perceptual disturbance F13.932
    - uncomplicated F13.930
  - stimulant NEC F15.93
    - with dependence F15.23
- **Abulia** R68.89
- **Abulomania** F60.7
- **Abuse**
  - adult — *see* Maltreatment, adult
    - as reason for
      - couple seeking advice (including offender) Z63.0
  - alcohol (non-dependent) F10.10
    - with
      - anxiety disorder F10.180
      - intoxication F10.129
        - with delirium F10.121
        - uncomplicated F10.120
      - mood disorder F10.14
      - other specified disorder F10.188
      - psychosis F10.159
        - delusions F10.150
        - hallucinations F10.151
      - sexual dysfunction F10.181
      - sleep disorder F10.182
      - unspecified disorder F10.19
    - counseling and surveillance Z71.41
  - amphetamine (or related substance) — *see* Abuse, drug, stimulant NEC
  - analgesics (non-prescribed) (over the counter) F55.8
  - antacids F55.0
  - antidepressants — *see* Abuse, drug, psychoactive NEC
  - anxiolytic — *see* Abuse, drug, sedative
  - barbiturates — *see* Abuse, drug, sedative
  - caffeine — *see* Abuse, drug, stimulant NEC
  - cannabis, cannabinoids — *see* Abuse, drug, cannabis
  - child — *see* Maltreatment, child
  - cocaine — *see* Abuse, drug, cocaine
  - drug NEC (non-dependent) F19.10
    - with sleep disorder F19.182
    - amphetamine type — *see* Abuse, drug, stimulant NEC
    - analgesics (non-prescribed) (over the counter) F55.8
    - antacids F55.0
    - antidepressants — *see* Abuse, drug, psychoactive NEC
    - anxiolytics — *see* Abuse, drug, sedative
    - barbiturates — *see* Abuse, drug, sedative
    - caffeine — *see* Abuse, drug, stimulant NEC
    - cannabis F12.10
      - with
        - anxiety disorder F12.180
        - intoxication F12.129
          - with

- **Abuse** — *continued*
  - drug NEC — *continued*
    - cannabis F12.10 — with — intoxication — with (continued)
            - delirium F12.121
            - perceptual disturbance F12.122
          - uncomplicated F12.120
        - other specified disorder F12.188
        - psychosis F12.159
          - delusions F12.150
          - hallucinations F12.151
        - unspecified disorder F12.19
    - cocaine F14.10
      - with
        - anxiety disorder F14.180
        - intoxication F14.129
          - with
            - delirium F14.121
            - perceptual disturbance F14.122
          - uncomplicated F14.120
        - mood disorder F14.14
        - other specified disorder F14.188
        - psychosis F14.159
          - delusions F14.150
          - hallucinations F14.151
        - sexual dysfunction F14.181
        - sleep disorder F14.182
        - unspecified disorder F14.19
    - counseling and surveillance Z71.51
    - hallucinogen F16.10
      - with
        - anxiety disorder F16.180
        - flashbacks F16.183
        - intoxication F16.129
          - with
            - delirium F16.121
            - perceptual disturbance F16.122
          - uncomplicated F16.120
        - mood disorder F16.14
        - other specified disorder F16.188
        - perception disorder, persisting F16.183
        - psychosis F16.159
          - delusions F16.150
          - hallucinations F16.151
        - unspecified disorder F16.19
    - hashish — *see* Abuse, drug, cannabis
    - herbal or folk remedies F55.1
    - hormones F55.3
    - hypnotics — *see* Abuse, drug, sedative
    - inhalant F18.10
      - with
        - anxiety disorder F18.180
        - dementia, persisting F18.17
        - intoxication F18.129
          - with delirium F18.121
          - uncomplicated F18.120
        - mood disorder F18.14
        - other specified disorder F18.188
        - psychosis F18.159
          - delusions F18.150
          - hallucinations F18.151
        - unspecified disorder F18.19
    - laxatives F55.2
    - LSD — *see* Abuse, drug, hallucinogen
    - marihuana — *see* Abuse, drug, cannabis
    - morphine type (opioids) — *see* Abuse, drug, opioid
    - opioid F11.10
      - with
        - intoxication F11.129
          - with
            - delirium F11.121
            - perceptual disturbance F11.122
          - uncomplicated F11.120
        - mood disorder F11.14
        - other specified disorder F11.188
        - psychosis F11.159
          - delusions F11.150
          - hallucinations F11.151
        - sexual dysfunction F11.181
        - sleep disorder F11.182
        - unspecified disorder F11.19
    - PCP (phencyclidine) (or related substance) — *see* Abuse, drug, hallucinogen
    - psychoactive NEC F19.10
      - with
        - amnestic disorder F19.16
        - anxiety disorder F19.180
        - dementia F19.17
        - intoxication F19.129
          - with
            - delirium F19.121
            - perceptual disturbance F19.122
          - uncomplicated F19.120

- **Abuse** — *continued*
  - drug NEC — *continued*
    - psychoactive NEC F19.10 — with (continued)
        - mood disorder F19.14
        - other specified disorder F19.188
        - psychosis F19.159
          - delusions F19.150
          - hallucinations F19.151
        - sexual dysfunction F19.181
        - sleep disorder F19.182
        - unspecified disorder F19.19
    - sedative, hypnotic or anxiolytic F13.10
      - with
        - anxiety disorder F13.180
        - intoxication F13.129
          - with delirium F13.121
          - uncomplicated F13.120
        - mood disorder F13.14
        - other specified disorder F13.188
        - psychosis F13.159
          - delusions F13.150
          - hallucinations F13.151
        - sexual dysfunction F13.181
        - sleep disorder F13.182
        - unspecified disorder F13.19
    - solvent — *see* Abuse, drug, inhalant
    - steroids F55.3
    - stimulant NEC F15.10
      - with
        - anxiety disorder F15.180
        - intoxication F15.129
          - with
            - delirium F15.121
            - perceptual disturbance F15.122
          - uncomplicated F15.120
        - mood disorder F15.14
        - other specified disorder F15.188
        - psychosis F15.159
          - delusions F15.150
          - hallucinations F15.151
        - sexual dysfunction F15.181
        - sleep disorder F15.182
        - unspecified disorder F15.19
    - tranquilizers — *see* Abuse, drug, sedative
    - vitamins F55.4
  - hallucinogens — *see* Abuse, drug, hallucinogen
  - hashish — *see* Abuse, drug, cannabis
  - herbal or folk remedies F55.1
  - hormones F55.3
  - hypnotic — *see* Abuse, drug, sedative
  - inhalant — *see* Abuse, drug, inhalant
  - laxatives F55.2
  - LSD — *see* Abuse, drug, hallucinogen
  - marihuana — *see* Abuse, drug, cannabis
  - morphine type (opioids) — *see* Abuse, drug, opioid
  - non-psychoactive substance NEC F55.8
    - antacids F55.0
    - folk remedies F55.1
    - herbal remedies F55.1
    - hormones F55.3
    - laxatives F55.2
    - steroids F55.3
    - vitamins F55.4
  - opioids — *see* Abuse, drug, opioid
  - PCP (phencyclidine) (or related substance) — *see* Abuse, drug, hallucinogen
  - physical (adult) (child) — *see* Maltreatment
  - psychoactive substance — *see* Abuse, drug, psychoactive NEC
  - psychological (adult) (child) — *see* Maltreatment
  - sedative — *see* Abuse, drug, sedative
  - sexual — *see* Maltreatment
  - solvent — *see* Abuse, drug, inhalant
  - steroids F55.3
  - vitamins F55.4
- **Acalculia** R48.8
  - developmental F81.2
- **Acanthamebiasis** (with) B60.10
  - conjunctiva B60.12
  - keratoconjunctivitis B60.13
  - meningoencephalitis B60.11
  - other specified B60.19
- **Acanthocephaliasis** B83.8
- **Acanthocheilonemiasis** B74.4
- **Acanthocytosis** E78.6
- **Acantholysis** L11.9
- **Acanthosis** (acquired) (nigricans) L83
  - benign Q82.8
  - congenital Q82.8
  - seborrheic L82.1
    - inflamed L82.0
  - tongue K14.3

Acapnia E87.3
Acarbia E87.2
Acardia, acardius Q89.8
Acardiacus amorphus Q89.8
Acardiotrophia I51.4
Acariasis B88.0
- scabies B86

Acarodermatitis (urticarioides) B88.0
Acarophobia F40.218
Acatalasemia, acatalasia E80.3
Acathisia (drug induced) G25.71
Accelerated atrioventricular conduction I45.6
Accentuation of personality traits (type A) Z73.1
Accessory (congenital)
- adrenal gland Q89.1
- anus Q43.4
- appendix Q43.4
- atrioventricular conduction I45.6
- auditory ossicles Q16.3
- auricle (ear) Q17.0
- biliary duct or passage Q44.5
- bladder Q64.79
- blood vessels NEC Q27.9
  - coronary Q24.5
- bone NEC Q79.8
- breast tissue, axilla Q83.1
- carpal bones Q74.0
- cecum Q43.4
- chromosome (s) NEC (nonsex) Q92.9
  - with complex rearrangements NEC Q92.5
    - seen only at prometaphase Q92.8
  - partial Q92.9
  - sex
    - female phenotype Q97.8
  - 13 — *see* Trisomy, 13
  - 18 — *see* Trisomy, 18
  - 21 — *see* Trisomy, 21
- coronary artery Q24.5
- cusp (s), heart valve NEC Q24.8
  - pulmonary Q22.3
- cystic duct Q44.5
- digit (s) Q69.9
- ear (auricle) (lobe) Q17.0
- endocrine gland NEC Q89.2
- eye muscle Q10.3
- eyelid Q10.3
- face bone (s) Q75.8
- fallopian tube (fimbria) (ostium) Q50.6
- finger (s) Q69.0
- foreskin N47.8
- frontonasal process Q75.8
- gallbladder Q44.1
- genital organ (s)
  - female Q52.8
    - external Q52.79
    - internal NEC Q52.8
  - male Q55.8
- genitourinary organs NEC Q89.8
  - female Q52.8
  - male Q55.8
- hallux Q69.2
- heart Q24.8
  - valve NEC Q24.8
    - pulmonary Q22.3
- hepatic ducts Q44.5
- hymen Q52.4
- intestine (large) (small) Q43.4
- kidney Q63.0
- lacrimal canal Q10.6
- leaflet, heart valve NEC Q24.8
- ligament, broad Q50.6
- liver Q44.7
  - duct Q44.5
- lobule (ear) Q17.0
- lung (lobe) Q33.1
- muscle Q79.8
- navicular of carpus Q74.0
- nervous system, part NEC Q07.8
- nipple Q83.3
- nose Q30.8
- organ or site not listed — *see* Anomaly, by site
- ovary Q50.31
- oviduct Q50.6
- pancreas Q45.3
- parathyroid gland Q89.2
- parotid gland (and duct) Q38.4
- pituitary gland Q89.2
- preauricular appendage Q17.0
- prepuce N47.8
- renal arteries (multiple) Q27.2
- rib Q76.6
  - cervical Q76.5

Accessory — *continued*
- roots (teeth) K00.2
- salivary gland Q38.4
- sesamoid bones Q74.8
  - foot Q74.2
  - hand Q74.0
- skin tags Q82.8
- spleen Q89.09
- sternum Q76.7
- submaxillary gland Q38.4
- tarsal bones Q74.2
- teeth, tooth K00.1
- tendon Q79.8
- thumb Q69.1
- thymus gland Q89.2
- thyroid gland Q89.2
- toes Q69.2
- tongue Q38.3
- tooth, teeth K00.1
- tragus Q17.0
- ureter Q62.5
- urethra Q64.79
- urinary organ or tract NEC Q64.8
- uterus Q51.2
- vagina Q52.10
- valve, heart NEC Q24.8
  - pulmonary Q22.3
- vertebra Q76.49
- vocal cords Q31.8
- vulva Q52.79

Accident
- birth — *see* Birth, injury
- cardiac — *see* Infarct, myocardium
- cerebral I63.9
- cerebrovascular (embolic) (ischemic) (thrombotic) I63.9
  - aborted I63.9
  - hemorrhagic — *see* Hemorrhage, intracranial, intracerebral
  - old (without sequelae) Z86.73
    - with sequelae (of) — *see* Sequelae, infarction, cerebral
- coronary — *see* Infarct, myocardium
- craniovascular I63.9
- vascular, brain I63.9

Accidental — *see* condition
Accommodation (disorder) (*see also* condition)
- hysterical paralysis of F44.89
- insufficiency of H52.4
- paresis — *see* Paresis, of accommodation
- spasm — *see* Spasm, of accommodation

Accouchement — *see* Delivery
Accreta placenta O43.21 ☑
Accretio cordis (nonrheumatic) I31.0
Accretions, tooth, teeth K03.6
Acculturation difficulty Z60.3
Accumulation secretion, prostate N42.89
Acephalia, acephalism, acephalus, acephaly Q00.0
Acephalobrachia monster Q89.8
Acephalochirus monster Q89.8
Acephalogaster Q89.8
Acephalostomus monster Q89.8
Acephalothorax Q89.8
Acerophobia F40.298
Acetonemia R79.89
- in Type 1 diabetes E10.10
  - with coma E10.11

Acetonuria R82.4
Achalasia (cardia) (esophagus) K22.0
- congenital Q39.5
- pylorus Q40.0
- sphincteral NEC K59.8

Ache (s) — *see* Pain
Acheilia Q38.6
Achillobursitis — *see* Tendinitis, Achilles
Achillodynia — *see* Tendinitis, Achilles
Achlorhydria, achlorhydric (neurogenic) K31.83
- anemia D50.8
- diarrhea K31.83
- psychogenic F45.8
- secondary to vagotomy K91.1

Achluophobia F40.228
Acholia K82.8
Acholuric jaundice (familial) (splenomegalic) (*see also* Spherocytosis)
- acquired D59.8

Achondrogenesis Q77.0
Achondroplasia (osteosclerosis congenita) Q77.4
Achroma, cutis L80
Achromat (ism), achromatopsia (acquired) (congenital) H53.51
Achromia, congenital — *see* Albinism
Achromia parasitica B36.0
Achylia gastrica K31.89
- psychogenic F45.8

Acid
- burn — *see* Corrosion
- deficiency
  - amide nicotinic E52
  - ascorbic E54
  - folic E53.8
  - nicotinic E52
  - pantothenic E53.8
- intoxication E87.2
- peptic disease K30
- phosphatase deficiency E83.39
- stomach K30
  - psychogenic F45.8

Acidemia E87.2
- argininosuccinic E72.22
- isovaleric E71.110
- metabolic (newborn) P19.9
  - first noted before onset of labor P19.0
  - first noted during labor P19.1
  - noted at birth P19.2
- methylmalonic E71.120
- pipecolic E72.3
- propionic E71.121

Acidity, gastric (high) K30
- psychogenic F45.8

Acidocytopenia — *see* Agranulocytosis
Acidocytosis D72.1
Acidopenia — *see* Agranulocytosis
Acidosis (lactic) (respiratory) E87.2
- in Type 1 diabetes E10.10
  - with coma E10.11
- kidney, tubular N25.89
- lactic E87.2
- metabolic NEC E87.2
  - with respiratory acidosis E87.4
  - late, of newborn P74.0
- mixed metabolic and respiratory, newborn P84
- newborn P84
- renal (hyperchloremic) (tubular) N25.89
- respiratory E87.2
  - complicated by
    - metabolic
      - acidosis E87.4
      - alkalosis E87.4

Aciduria
- argininosuccinic E72.22
- glutaric (type I) E72.3
  - type II E71.313
  - type III E71.5 ☑
- orotic (congenital) (hereditary) (pyrimidine deficiency) E79.8
  - anemia D53.0

Acladiosis (skin) B36.0
Aclasis, diaphyseal Q78.6
Acleistocardia Q21.1
Aclusion — *see* Anomaly, dentofacial, malocclusion
Acne L70.9
- artificialis L70.8
- atrophica L70.2
- cachecticorum (Hebra) L70.8
- conglobata L70.1
- cystic L70.0
- decalvans L66.2
- excoriée (des jeunes filles) L70.5
- frontalis L70.2
- indurata L70.0
- infantile L70.4
- keloid L73.0
- lupoid L70.2
- necrotic, necrotica (miliaris) L70.2
- neonatal L70.4
- nodular L70.0
- occupational L70.8
- picker's L70.5
- pustular L70.0
- rodens L70.2
- rosacea L71.9
- specified NEC L70.8
- tropica L70.3
- varioliformis L70.2
- vulgaris L70.0

Acnitis (primary) A18.4
Acosta's disease T70.29 ☑
Acoustic — *see* condition
Acousticophobia F40.298
Acquired (*see also* condition)
- immunodeficiency syndrome (AIDS) B20

Acrania Q00.0
Acroangiodermatitis I78.9

- **Acroasphyxia,** chronic I73.89
- **Acrobystitis** N47.7
- **Acrocephalopolysyndactyly** Q87.0
- **Acrocephalosyndactyly** Q87.0
- **Acrocephaly** Q75.0
- **Acrochondrohyperplasia** — *see* Syndrome, Marfan's
- **Acrocyanosis** I73.8 ☑
  - newborn P28.2
    - meaning transient blue hands and feet - omit code
- **Acrodermatitis** L30.8
  - atrophicans (chronica) L90.4
  - continua (Hallopeau) L40.2
  - enteropathica (hereditary) E83.2
  - Hallopeau's L40.2
  - infantile papular L44.4
  - perstans L40.2
  - pustulosa continua L40.2
  - recalcitrant pustular L40.2
- **Acrodynia** — *see* Poisoning, mercury
- **Acromegaly,** acromegalia E22.0
- **Acromelalgia** I73.81
- **Acromicria,** acromikria Q79.8
- **Acronyx** L60.0
- **Acropachy,** thyroid — *see* Thyrotoxicosis
- **Acroparesthesia** (simple) (vasomotor) I73.89
- **Acropathy,** thyroid — *see* Thyrotoxicosis
- **Acrophobia** F40.241
- **Acroposthitis** N47.7
- **Acroscleriasis,** acroscleroderma, acrosclerosis — *see* Sclerosis, systemic
- **Acrosphacelus** I96
- **Acrospiroma,** eccrine — *see* Neoplasm, skin, benign
- **Acrostealgia** — *see* Osteochondropathy
- **Acrotrophodynia** — *see* Immersion
- **ACTH** ectopic syndrome E24.3
- **Actinic** — *see* condition
- **Actinobacillosis,** actinobacillus A28.8
  - mallei A24.0
  - muris A25.1
- **Actinomyces** israelii (infection) — *see* Actinomycosis
- **Actinomycetoma** (foot) B47.1
- **Actinomycosis,** actinomycotic A42.9
  - with pneumonia A42.0
  - abdominal A42.1
  - cervicofacial A42.2
  - cutaneous A42.89
  - gastrointestinal A42.1
  - pulmonary A42.0
  - sepsis A42.7
  - specified site NEC A42.89
- **Actinoneuritis** G62.82
- **Action,** heart
  - disorder I49.9
  - irregular I49.9
    - psychogenic F45.8
- **Activated** protein C resistance D68.51
- **Activation**
  - mast cell (disorder) (syndrome) D89.40 ☑
    - idiopathic D89.42
    - monoclonal D89.41
    - secondary D89.43
    - specified type NEC D89.49
- **Active** — *see* condition
- **Acute** (*see also* condition)
  - abdomen R10.0
  - gallbladder — *see* Cholecystitis, acute
- **Acyanotic** heart disease (congenital) Q24.9
- **Acystia** Q64.5
- **Adair-Dighton** syndrome (brittle bones and blue sclera, deafness) Q78.0
- **Adamantinoblastoma** — *see* Ameloblastoma
- **Adamantinoma** (*see also* Cyst, calcifying odontogenic)
  - long bones C40.90
    - lower limb C40.2 ☑
    - upper limb C40.0 ☑
  - malignant C41.1
    - jaw (bone) (lower) C41.1
      - upper C41.0
  - tibial C40.2 ☑
- **Adamantoblastoma** — *see* Ameloblastoma
- **Adams-Stokes** (-Morgagni) disease or syndrome I45.9
- **Adaption** reaction — *see* Disorder, adjustment
- **Addiction** (*see also* Dependence)F19.20
  - alcohol, alcoholic (ethyl) (methyl) (wood) (without remission) F10.20
    - with remission F10.21
  - drug — *see* Dependence, drug
  - ethyl alcohol (without remission) F10.20
    - with remission F10.21

Addiction — *continued*

  - heroin — *see* Dependence, drug, opioid
  - methyl alcohol (without remission) F10.20
    - with remission F10.21
  - methylated spirit (without remission) F10.20
    - with remission F10.21
  - morphine (-like substances) — *see* Dependence, drug, opioid
  - nicotine — *see* Dependence, drug, nicotine
  - opium and opioids — *see* Dependence, drug, opioid
  - tobacco — *see* Dependence, drug, nicotine
- **Addisonian** crisis E27.2
- **Addison's**
  - anemia (pernicious) D51.0
  - disease (bronze) or syndrome E27.1
    - tuberculous A18.7
  - keloid L94.0
- **Addison-Biermer** anemia (pernicious) D51.0
- **Addison-Schilder** complex E71.528
- **Additional** (*see also* Accessory)
  - chromosome (s) Q99.8
    - sex — *see* Abnormal, chromosome, sex
    - 21 — *see* Trisomy, 21
- **Adduction** contracture, hip or other joint — *see* Contraction, joint
- **Adenitis** (*see also* Lymphadenitis)
  - acute, unspecified site L04.9
  - axillary I88.9
    - acute L04.2
    - chronic or subacute I88.1
  - Bartholin's gland N75.8
  - bulbourethral gland — *see* Urethritis
  - cervical I88.9
    - acute L04.0
    - chronic or subacute I88.1
  - chancroid (Haemophilus ducreyi) A57
  - chronic, unspecified site I88.1
  - Cowper's gland — *see* Urethritis
  - due to Pasteurella multocida (P. septica) A28.0
  - epidemic, acute B27.09
  - gangrenous L04.9
  - gonorrheal NEC A54.89
  - groin I88.9
    - acute L04.1
    - chronic or subacute I88.1
  - infectious (acute) (epidemic) B27.09
  - inguinal I88.9
    - acute L04.1
    - chronic or subacute I88.1
  - lymph gland or node, except mesenteric I88.9
    - acute — *see* Lymphadenitis, acute
    - chronic or subacute I88.1
  - mesenteric (acute) (chronic) (nonspecific) (subacute) I88.0
  - parotid gland (suppurative) — *see* Sialoadenitis
  - salivary gland (any) (suppurative) — *see* Sialoadenitis
  - scrofulous (tuberculous) A18.2
  - Skene's duct or gland — *see* Urethritis
  - strumous, tuberculous A18.2
  - subacute, unspecified site I88.1
  - sublingual gland (suppurative) — *see* Sialoadenitis
  - submandibular gland (suppurative) — *see* Sialoadenitis
  - submaxillary gland (suppurative) — *see* Sialoadenitis
  - tuberculous — *see* Tuberculosis, lymph gland
  - urethral gland — *see* Urethritis
  - Wharton's duct (suppurative) — *see* Sialoadenitis
- **Adenoacanthoma** — *see* Neoplasm, malignant, by site
- **Adenoameloblastoma** — *see* Cyst, calcifying odontogenic
- **Adenocarcinoid** (tumor) — *see* Neoplasm, malignant, by site
- **Adenocarcinoma** (*see also* Neoplasm, malignant, by site)
  - acidophil
    - specified site — *see* Neoplasm, malignant, by site
    - unspecified site C75.1
  - adrenal cortical C74.0 ☑
  - alveolar — *see* Neoplasm, lung, malignant
  - apocrine
    - breast — *see* Neoplasm, breast, malignant
    - in situ
      - breast D05.8 ☑
      - specified site NEC — *see* Neoplasm, skin, in situ
      - unspecified site D04.9

Adenocarcinoma — *continued*

  - apocrine — *continued*
    - specified site NEC — *see* Neoplasm, skin, malignant
    - unspecified site C44.99
  - basal cell
    - specified site — *see* Neoplasm, skin, malignant
    - unspecified site C08.9
  - basophil
    - specified site — *see* Neoplasm, malignant, by site
    - unspecified site C75.1
  - bile duct type C22.1
    - liver C22.1
    - specified site NEC — *see* Neoplasm, malignant, by site
    - unspecified site C22.1
  - bronchiolar — *see* Neoplasm, lung, malignant
  - bronchioloalveolar — *see* Neoplasm, lung, malignant
  - ceruminous C44.29 ☑
  - cervix, in situ (*see also* Carcinoma, cervix uteri, in situ)D06.9
  - chromophobe
    - specified site — *see* Neoplasm, malignant, by site
    - unspecified site C75.1
  - diffuse type
    - specified site — *see* Neoplasm, malignant, by site
    - unspecified site C16.9
  - duct
    - infiltrating
      - with Paget's disease — *see* Neoplasm, breast, malignant
      - specified site — *see* Neoplasm, malignant, by site
      - unspecified site (female) C50.91 ☑
        - male C50.92 ☑
    - specified site — *see* Neoplasm, malignant, by site
    - unspecified site
      - female C56.9
      - male C61
  - eosinophil
    - specified site — *see* Neoplasm, malignant, by site
    - unspecified site C75.1
  - follicular
    - with papillary C73
    - moderately differentiated C73
    - specified site — *see* Neoplasm, malignant, by site
    - trabecular C73
    - unspecified site C73
    - well differentiated C73
  - Hurthle cell C73
  - in
    - adenomatous
      - polyposis coli C18.9
  - infiltrating duct
    - with Paget's disease — *see* Neoplasm, breast, malignant
    - specified site — *see* Neoplasm, by site, malignant
    - unspecified site (female) C50.91 ☑
      - male C50.92 ☑
  - inflammatory
    - specified site — *see* Neoplasm, by site, malignant
    - unspecified site (female) C50.91 ☑
      - male C50.92 ☑
  - intestinal type
    - specified site — *see* Neoplasm, by site, malignant
    - unspecified site C16.9
  - intracystic papillary
  - intraductal
    - breast D05.1 ☑
    - noninfiltrating
      - breast D05.1 ☑
      - papillary
        - with invasion
          - specified site — *see* Neoplasm, by site, malignant
          - unspecified site (female) C50.91 ☑
            - male C50.92 ☑
        - breast D05.1 ☑
        - specified site NEC — *see* Neoplasm, in situ, by site
        - unspecified site D05.1 ☑

- **Adenocarcinoma** — *continued*
  - intraductal — *continued*
    - specified site NEC — *see* Neoplasm, in situ, by site
    - unspecified site D05.1 ☑
    - papillary
      - with invasion
        - specified site — *see* Neoplasm, malignant, by site
        - unspecified site (female) C50.91 ☑
          - male C50.92 ☑
      - breast D05.1 ☑
      - specified site — *see* Neoplasm, in situ, by site
      - unspecified site D05.1 ☑
    - specified site NEC — *see* Neoplasm, in situ, by site
    - unspecified site D05.1 ☑
  - islet cell
    - with exocrine, mixed
      - specified site — *see* Neoplasm, malignant, by site
      - unspecified site C25.9
    - pancreas C25.4
    - specified site NEC — *see* Neoplasm, malignant, by site
    - unspecified site C25.4
  - lobular
    - in situ
      - breast D05.0 ☑
      - specified site NEC — *see* Neoplasm, in situ, by site
      - unspecified site D05.0 ☑
    - specified site — *see* Neoplasm, malignant, by site
    - unspecified site (female) C50.91 ☑
      - male C50.92 ☑
  - mucoid (*see also* Neoplasm, malignant, by site)
    - cell
      - specified site — *see* Neoplasm, malignant, by site
      - unspecified site C75.1
  - nonencapsulated sclerosing C73
  - papillary
    - with follicular C73
    - follicular variant C73
    - intraductal (noninfiltrating)
      - with invasion
        - specified site — *see* Neoplasm, malignant, by site
        - unspecified site (female) C50.91 ☑
          - male C50.92 ☑
      - breast D05.1 ☑
      - specified site NEC — *see* Neoplasm, in situ, by site
      - unspecified site D05.1 ☑
    - serous
      - specified site — *see* Neoplasm, malignant, by site
      - unspecified site C56.9
  - papillocystic
    - specified site — *see* Neoplasm, malignant, by site
    - unspecified site C56.9
  - pseudomucinous
    - specified site — *see* Neoplasm, malignant, by site
    - unspecified site C56.9
  - renal cell C64 ☑
  - sebaceous — *see* Neoplasm, skin, malignant
  - serous (*see also* Neoplasm, malignant, by site)
    - papillary
      - specified site — *see* Neoplasm, malignant, by site
      - unspecified site C56.9
  - sweat gland — *see* Neoplasm, skin, malignant
  - water-clear cell C75.0
- **Adenocarcinoma-in-situ** (*see also* Neoplasm, in situ, by site)
  - breast D05.9 ☑
- **Adenofibroma**
  - clear cell — *see* Neoplasm, benign, by site
  - endometrioid D27.9
    - borderline malignancy D39.10
    - malignant C56 ☑
  - mucinous
    - specified site — *see* Neoplasm, benign, by site
    - unspecified site D27.9
  - papillary
    - specified site — *see* Neoplasm, benign, by site
    - unspecified site D27.9
  - prostate — *see* Enlargement, enlarged, prostate
- **Adenofibroma** — *continued*
  - serous
    - specified site — *see* Neoplasm, benign, by site
    - unspecified site D27.9
  - specified site — *see* Neoplasm, benign, by site
  - unspecified site D27.9
- **Adenofibrosis**
  - breast — *see* Fibroadenosis, breast
  - endometrioid N80.0
- **Adenoiditis** (chronic) J35.02
  - with tonsillitis J35.03
  - acute J03.90
    - recurrent J03.91
    - specified organism NEC J03.80
      - recurrent J03.81
    - staphylococcal J03.80
      - recurrent J03.81
    - streptococcal J03.00
      - recurrent J03.01
- **Adenoids** — *see* condition
- **Adenolipoma** — *see* Neoplasm, benign, by site
- **Adenolipomatosis,** Launois-Bensaude E88.89
- **Adenolymphoma**
  - specified site — *see* Neoplasm, benign, by site
  - unspecified site D11.9
- **Adenoma** (*see also* Neoplasm, benign, by site)
  - acidophil
    - specified site — *see* Neoplasm, benign, by site
    - unspecified site D35.2
  - acidophil-basophil, mixed
    - specified site — *see* Neoplasm, benign, by site
    - unspecified site D35.2
  - adrenal (cortical) D35.00
    - clear cell D35.00
    - compact cell D35.00
    - glomerulosa cell D35.00
    - heavily pigmented variant D35.00
    - mixed cell D35.00
  - alpha-cell
    - pancreas D13.7
    - specified site NEC — *see* Neoplasm, benign, by site
    - unspecified site D13.7
  - alveolar D14.30
  - apocrine
    - breast D24 ☑
    - specified site NEC — *see* Neoplasm, skin, benign, by site
    - unspecified site D23.9
  - basal cell D11.9
  - basophil
    - specified site — *see* Neoplasm, benign, by site
    - unspecified site D35.2
  - basophil-acidophil, mixed
    - specified site — *see* Neoplasm, benign, by site
    - unspecified site D35.2
  - beta-cell
    - pancreas D13.7
    - specified site NEC — *see* Neoplasm, benign, by site
    - unspecified site D13.7
  - bile duct D13.4
    - common D13.5
    - extrahepatic D13.5
    - intrahepatic D13.4
    - specified site NEC — *see* Neoplasm, benign, by site
    - unspecified site D13.4
  - black D35.00
  - bronchial D38.1
    - cylindroid type — *see* Neoplasm, lung, malignant
  - ceruminous D23.2 ☑
  - chief cell D35.1
  - chromophobe
    - specified site — *see* Neoplasm, benign, by site
    - unspecified site D35.2
  - colloid
    - specified site — *see* Neoplasm, benign, by site
    - unspecified site D34
  - duct
  - eccrine, papillary — *see* Neoplasm, skin, benign
  - endocrine, multiple
    - single specified site — *see* Neoplasm, uncertain behavior, by site
    - two or more specified sites D44 ☑
    - unspecified site D44.9
  - endometrioid (*see also* Neoplasm, benign)
    - borderline malignancy — *see* Neoplasm, uncertain behavior, by site
  - eosinophil
    - specified site — *see* Neoplasm, benign, by site
    - unspecified site D35.2
- **Adenoma** — *continued*
  - fetal
    - specified site — *see* Neoplasm, benign, by site
    - unspecified site D34
  - follicular
    - specified site — *see* Neoplasm, benign, by site
    - unspecified site D34
  - hepatocellular D13.4
  - Hurthle cell D34
  - islet cell
    - pancreas D13.7
    - specified site NEC — *see* Neoplasm, benign, by site
    - unspecified site D13.7
  - liver cell D13.4
  - macrofollicular
    - specified site — *see* Neoplasm, benign, by site
    - unspecified site D34
  - malignant, malignum — *see* Neoplasm, malignant, by site
  - microcystic
    - pancreas D13.6
    - specified site NEC — *see* Neoplasm, benign, by site
    - unspecified site D13.6
  - microfollicular
    - specified site — *see* Neoplasm, benign, by site
    - unspecified site D34
  - mucoid cell
    - specified site — *see* Neoplasm, benign, by site
    - unspecified site D35.2
  - multiple endocrine
    - single specified site — *see* Neoplasm, uncertain behavior, by site
    - two or more specified sites D44 ☑
    - unspecified site D44.9
  - nipple D24 ☑
  - papillary (*see also* Neoplasm, benign, by site)
    - eccrine — *see* Neoplasm, skin, benign, by site
  - Pick's tubular
    - specified site — *see* Neoplasm, benign, by site
    - unspecified site
      - female D27.9
      - male D29.20
  - pleomorphic
    - carcinoma in — *see* Neoplasm, salivary gland, malignant
      - specified site — *see* Neoplasm, malignant, by site
      - unspecified site C08.9
  - polypoid (*see also* Neoplasm, benign)
    - adenocarcinoma in — *see* Neoplasm, malignant, by site
    - adenocarcinoma in situ — *see* Neoplasm, in situ, by site
  - prostate — *see* Neoplasm, benign, prostate
  - rete cell D29.20
  - sebaceous — *see* Neoplasm, skin, benign
  - Sertoli cell
    - specified site — *see* Neoplasm, benign, by site
    - unspecified site
      - female D27.9
      - male D29.20
  - skin appendage — *see* Neoplasm, skin, benign
  - sudoriferous gland — *see* Neoplasm, skin, benign
  - sweat gland — *see* Neoplasm, skin, benign
  - testicular
    - specified site — *see* Neoplasm, benign, by site
    - unspecified site
      - female D27.9
      - male D29.20
  - tubular (*see also* Neoplasm, benign, by site)
    - adenocarcinoma in — *see* Neoplasm, malignant, by site
    - adenocarcinoma in situ — *see* Neoplasm, in situ, by site
    - Pick's
      - specified site — *see* Neoplasm, benign, by site
      - unspecified site
        - female D27.9
        - male D29.20
  - tubulovillous (*see also* Neoplasm, benign, by site)
    - adenocarcinoma in — *see* Neoplasm, malignant, by site
    - adenocarcinoma in situ — *see* Neoplasm, in situ, by site
  - villous — *see* Neoplasm, uncertain behavior, by site
    - adenocarcinoma in — *see* Neoplasm, malignant, by site

Adenoma - Admission

Adenoma — *continued*
- villous — *continued*
  - adenocarcinoma in situ — *see* Neoplasm, in situ, by site
- water-clear cell D35.1

Adenomatosis
- endocrine (multiple) E31.20
  - single specified site — *see* Neoplasm, uncertain behavior, by site
- erosive of nipple D24 ☑
- pluriendocrine — *see* Adenomatosis, endocrine
- pulmonary D38.1
  - malignant — *see* Neoplasm, lung, malignant
- specified site — *see* Neoplasm, benign, by site
- unspecified site D12.6

Adenomatous
- goiter (nontoxic) E04.9
  - with hyperthyroidism — *see* Hyperthyroidism, with, goiter, nodular
  - toxic — *see* Hyperthyroidism, with, goiter, nodular

Adenomyoma (*see also* Neoplasm, benign, by site)
- prostate — *see* Enlarged, prostate

Adenomyometritis N80.0

Adenomyosis N80.0

Adenopathy (lymph gland) R59.9
- generalized R59.1
- inguinal R59.0
- localized R59.0
- mediastinal R59.0
- mesentery R59.0
- syphilitic (secondary) A51.49
- tracheobronchial R59.0
  - tuberculous A15.4
    - primary (progressive) A15.7
- tuberculous (*see also* Tuberculosis, lymph gland)
  - tracheobronchial A15.4
    - primary (progressive) A15.7

Adenosalpingitis — *see* Salpingitis

Adenosarcoma — *see* Neoplasm, malignant, by site

Adenosclerosis I88.8

Adenosis (sclerosing) breast — *see* Fibroadenosis, breast

Adenovirus, as cause of disease classified elsewhere B97.0

Adentia (complete) (partial) — *see* Absence, teeth

Adherent (*see also* Adhesions)
- labia (minora) N90.89
- pericardium (nonrheumatic) I31.0
  - rheumatic I09.2
- placenta (with hemorrhage) O72.0
  - without hemorrhage O73.0
- prepuce, newborn N47.0
- scar (skin) L90.5
- tendon in scar L90.5

Adhesions, adhesive (postinfective) K66.0
- with intestinal obstruction K56.5
- abdominal (wall) — *see* Adhesions, peritoneum
- appendix K38.8
- bile duct (common) (hepatic) K83.8
- bladder (sphincter) N32.89
- bowel — *see* Adhesions, peritoneum
- cardiac I31.0
  - rheumatic I09.2
- cecum — *see* Adhesions, peritoneum
- cervicovaginal N88.1
  - congenital Q52.8
  - postpartal O90.89
    - old N88.1
- cervix N88.1
- ciliary body NEC — *see* Adhesions, iris
- clitoris N90.89
- colon — *see* Adhesions, peritoneum
- common duct K83.8
- congenital (*see also* Anomaly, by site)
  - fingers — *see* Syndactylism, complex, fingers
  - omental, anomalous Q43.3
  - peritoneal Q43.3
  - tongue (to gum or roof of mouth) Q38.3
- conjunctiva (acquired) H11.21 ☑
  - congenital Q15.8
- cystic duct K82.8
- diaphragm — *see* Adhesions, peritoneum
- due to foreign body — *see* Foreign body
- duodenum — *see* Adhesions, peritoneum
- ear
  - middle H74.1 ☑
- epididymis N50.89
- epidural — *see* Adhesions, meninges
- epiglottis J38.7
- eyelid H02.59
- female pelvis N73.6

Adhesions — *continued*
- gallbladder K82.8
- globe H44.89
- heart I31.0
  - rheumatic I09.2
- ileocecal (coil) — *see* Adhesions, peritoneum
- ileum — *see* Adhesions, peritoneum
- intestine (*see also* Adhesions, peritoneum)
  - with obstruction K56.5
- intra-abdominal — *see* Adhesions, peritoneum
- iris H21.50 ☑
  - anterior H21.51 ☑
  - goniosynechiae H21.52 ☑
  - posterior H21.54 ☑
  - to corneal graft T85.898 ☑
- joint — *see* Ankylosis
  - knee M23.8X ☑
  - temporomandibular M26.61 ☑
- labium (majus) (minus), congenital Q52.5
- liver — *see* Adhesions, peritoneum
- lung J98.4
- mediastinum J98.59
- meninges (cerebral) (spinal) G96.12
  - congenital Q07.8
  - tuberculous (cerebral) (spinal) A17.0
- mesenteric — *see* Adhesions, peritoneum
- nasal (septum) (to turbinates) J34.89
- ocular muscle — *see* Strabismus, mechanical
- omentum — *see* Adhesions, peritoneum
- ovary N73.6
  - congenital (to cecum, kidney or omentum) Q50.39
- paraovarian N73.6
- pelvic (peritoneal)
  - female N73.6
    - postprocedural N99.4
  - male — *see* Adhesions, peritoneum
  - postpartal (old) N73.6
  - tuberculous A18.17
- penis to scrotum (congenital) Q55.8
- periappendiceal (*see also* Adhesions, peritoneum)
- pericardium (nonrheumatic) I31.0
  - focal I31.8
  - rheumatic I09.2
  - tuberculous A18.84
- pericholecystic K82.8
- perigastric — *see* Adhesions, peritoneum
- periovarian N73.6
- periprostatic N42.89
- perirectal — *see* Adhesions, peritoneum
- perirenal N28.89
- peritoneum, peritoneal (postinfective) (postprocedural) K66.0
  - with obstruction (intestinal) K56.5
  - congenital Q43.3
  - pelvic, female N73.6
    - postprocedural N99.4
  - postpartal, pelvic N73.6
  - to uterus N73.6
- peritubal N73.6
- periureteral N28.89
- periuterine N73.6
- perivesical N32.89
- perivesicular (seminal vesicle) N50.89
- pleura, pleuritic J94.8
  - tuberculous NEC A15.6
- pleuropericardial J94.8
- postoperative (gastrointestinal tract) K66.0
  - with obstruction K91.3
  - due to foreign body accidentally left in wound — *see* Foreign body, accidentally left during a procedure
  - pelvic peritoneal N99.4
  - urethra — *see* Stricture, urethra, postprocedural
  - vagina N99.2
- postpartal, old (vulva or perineum) N90.89
- preputial, prepuce N47.5
- pulmonary J98.4
- pylorus — *see* Adhesions, peritoneum
- sciatic nerve — *see* Lesion, nerve, sciatic
- seminal vesicle N50.89
- shoulder (joint) — *see* Capsulitis, adhesive
- sigmoid flexure — *see* Adhesions, peritoneum
- spermatic cord (acquired) N50.89
  - congenital Q55.4
- spinal canal G96.12
- stomach — *see* Adhesions, peritoneum
- subscapular — *see* Capsulitis, adhesive
- temporomandibular M26.61 ☑
- tendinitis (*see also* Tenosynovitis, specified type NEC)
  - shoulder — *see* Capsulitis, adhesive

Adhesions — *continued*
- testis N44.8
- tongue, congenital (to gum or roof of mouth) Q38.3
  - acquired K14.8
- trachea J39.8
- tubo-ovarian N73.6
- tunica vaginalis N44.8
- uterus N73.6
  - internal N85.6
  - to abdominal wall N73.6
- vagina (chronic) N89.5
  - postoperative N99.2
- vitreomacular H43.82 ☑
- vitreous H43.89
- vulva N90.89

Adiaspiromycosis B48.8

Adie (-Holmes) pupil or syndrome — *see* Anomaly, pupil, function, tonic pupil

Adiponecrosis neonatorum P83.8

Adiposis (*see also* Obesity)
- cerebralis E23.6
- dolorosa E88.2

Adiposity (*see also* Obesity)
- heart — *see* Degeneration, myocardial
- localized E65

Adiposogenital dystrophy E23.6

Adjustment
- disorder — *see* Disorder, adjustment
- implanted device — *see* Encounter (for), adjustment (of)
- prosthesis, external — *see* Fitting
- reaction — *see* Disorder, adjustment

Administration of tPA (rtPA) in a different facility within the last 24 hours prior to admission to current facility Z92.82

Admission (for) (*see also* Encounter (for))
- adjustment (of)
  - artificial
    - arm Z44.00 ☑
      - complete Z44.01 ☑
      - partial Z44.02 ☑
    - eye Z44.2 ☑
    - leg Z44.10 ☑
      - complete Z44.11 ☑
      - partial Z44.12 ☑
  - brain neuropacemaker Z46.2
    - implanted Z45.42
  - breast
    - implant Z45.81 ☑
    - prosthesis (external) Z44.3 ☑
  - colostomy belt Z46.89
  - contact lenses Z46.0
  - cystostomy device Z46.6
  - dental prosthesis Z46.3
  - device NEC
    - abdominal Z46.89
    - implanted Z45.89
      - cardiac Z45.09
        - defibrillator (with synchronous cardiac pacemaker) Z45.02
        - pacemaker (cardiac resynchronization therapy (CRT-P)) Z45.018
          - pulse generator Z45.010
        - resynchronization therapy defibrillator (CRT-D) Z45.02
      - hearing device Z45.328
        - bone conduction Z45.320
        - cochlear Z45.321
      - infusion pump Z45.1
      - nervous system Z45.49
        - CSF drainage Z45.41
        - hearing device — *see* Admission, adjustment, device, implanted, hearing device
        - neuropacemaker Z45.42
        - visual substitution Z45.31
      - specified NEC Z45.89
      - vascular access Z45.2
      - visual substitution Z45.31
    - nervous system Z46.2
      - implanted — *see* Admission, adjustment, device, implanted, nervous system
    - orthodontic Z46.4
    - prosthetic Z44.9
      - arm — *see* Admission, adjustment, artificial, arm
      - breast Z44.3 ☑
      - dental Z46.3
      - eye Z44.2 ☑
      - leg — *see* Admission, adjustment, artificial, leg

African
- sleeping sickness B56.9
- tick fever A68.1
- trypanosomiasis B56.9
  - gambian B56.0
  - rhodesian B56.1

Aftercare (*see also* Care)Z51.89
- following surgery (for) (on)
  - amputation Z47.81
  - attention to
    - drains Z48.03
    - dressings (nonsurgical) Z48.00
      - surgical Z48.01
    - sutures Z48.02
  - circulatory system Z48.812
  - delayed (planned) wound closure Z48.1
  - digestive system Z48.815
  - explantation of joint prosthesis (staged procedure)
    - hip Z47.32
    - knee Z47.33
    - shoulder Z47.31
  - genitourinary system Z48.816
  - joint replacement Z47.1
  - neoplasm Z48.3
  - nervous system Z48.811
  - oral cavity Z48.814
  - organ transplant
    - bone marrow Z48.290
    - heart Z48.21
    - heart-lung Z48.280
    - kidney Z48.22
    - liver Z48.23
    - lung Z48.24
    - multiple organs NEC Z48.288
    - specified NEC Z48.298
  - orthopedic NEC Z47.89
  - planned wound closure Z48.1
  - removal of internal fixation device Z47.2
  - respiratory system Z48.813
  - scoliosis Z47.82
  - sense organs Z48.810
  - skin and subcutaneous tissue Z48.817
  - specified body system
    - circulatory Z48.812
    - digestive Z48.815
    - genitourinary Z48.816
    - nervous Z48.811
    - oral cavity Z48.814
    - respiratory Z48.813
    - sense organs Z48.810
    - skin and subcutaneous tissue Z48.817
    - teeth Z48.814
  - specified NEC Z48.89
  - spinal Z48.89
  - teeth Z48.814
- fracture - code to fracture with seventh character D
- involving
  - removal of
    - drains Z48.03
    - dressings (nonsurgical) Z48.00
    - staples Z48.02
    - surgical dressings Z48.01
    - sutures Z48.02
- neuropacemaker (brain) (peripheral nerve) (spinal cord) Z46.2
  - implanted Z45.42
- orthopedic NEC Z47.89
- postprocedural — *see* Aftercare, following surgery

After-cataract — *see* Cataract, secondary

Agalactia (primary) O92.3
- elective, secondary or therapeutic O92.5

Agammaglobulinemia (acquired (secondary)) (nonfamilial) D80.1
- with
  - immunoglobulin-bearing B-lymphocytes D80.1
  - lymphopenia D81.9
- autosomal recessive (Swiss type) D80.0
- Bruton's X-linked D80.0
- common variable (CVAgamma) D80.1
- congenital sex-linked D80.0
- hereditary D80.0
- lymphopenic D81.9
- Swiss type (autosomal recessive) D80.0
- X-linked (with growth hormone deficiency) (Bruton) D80.0

Aganglionosis (bowel) (colon) Q43.1

Age (old) — *see* Senility

Agenesis
- adrenal (gland) Q89.1
- alimentary tract (complete) (partial) NEC Q45.8
  - upper Q40.8
- anus, anal (canal) Q42.3
  - with fistula Q42.2
- aorta Q25.41
- appendix Q42.8
- arm (complete) Q71.0 ☑
  - with hand present Q71.1 ☑
- artery (peripheral) Q27.9
  - brain Q28.3
  - coronary Q24.5
  - pulmonary Q25.79
  - specified NEC Q27.8
  - umbilical Q27.0
- auditory (canal) (external) Q16.1
- auricle (ear) Q16.0
- bile duct or passage Q44.5
- bladder Q64.5
- bone Q79.9
- brain Q00.0
  - part of Q04.3
- breast (with nipple present) Q83.8
  - with absent nipple Q83.0
- bronchus Q32.4
- canaliculus lacrimalis Q10.4
- carpus — *see* Agenesis, hand
- cartilage Q79.9
- cecum Q42.8
- cerebellum Q04.3
- cervix Q51.5
- chin Q18.8
- cilia Q10.3
- circulatory system, part NOS Q28.9
- clavicle Q74.0
- clitoris Q52.6
- coccyx Q76.49
- colon Q42.9
  - specified NEC Q42.8
- corpus callosum Q04.0
- cricoid cartilage Q31.8
- diaphragm (with hernia) Q79.1
- digestive organ (s) or tract (complete) (partial) NEC Q45.8
  - upper Q40.8
- ductus arteriosus Q28.8
- duodenum Q41.0
- ear Q16.9
  - auricle Q16.0
  - lobe Q17.8
- ejaculatory duct Q55.4
- endocrine (gland) NEC Q89.2
- epiglottis Q31.8
- esophagus Q39.8
- eustachian tube Q16.2
- eye Q11.1
  - adnexa Q15.8
- eyelid (fold) Q10.3
- face
  - bones NEC Q75.8
  - specified part NEC Q18.8
- fallopian tube Q50.6
- femur — *see* Defect, reduction, lower limb, longitudinal, femur
- fibula — *see* Defect, reduction, lower limb, longitudinal, fibula
- finger (complete) (partial) — *see* Agenesis, hand
- foot (and toes) (complete) (partial) Q72.3 ☑
- forearm (with hand present) — *see* Agenesis, arm, with hand present
  - and hand Q71.2 ☑
- gallbladder Q44.0
- gastric Q40.2
- genitalia, genital (organ (s))
  - female Q52.8
    - external Q52.71
    - internal NEC Q52.8
  - male Q55.8
- glottis Q31.8
- hair Q84.0
- hand (and fingers) (complete) (partial) Q71.3 ☑
- heart Q24.8
  - valve NEC Q24.8
    - pulmonary Q22.0
- hepatic Q44.7
- humerus — *see* Defect, reduction, upper limb
- hymen Q52.4
- ileum Q41.2
- incus Q16.3
- intestine (small) Q41.9
  - large Q42.9
    - specified NEC Q42.8

Agenesis — *continued*
- iris (dilator fibers) Q13.1
- jaw M26.09
- jejunum Q41.1
- kidney (s) (partial) Q60.2
  - bilateral Q60.1
  - unilateral Q60.0
- labium (majus) (minus) Q52.71
- labyrinth, membranous Q16.5
- lacrimal apparatus Q10.4
- larynx Q31.8
- leg (complete) Q72.0 ☑
  - with foot present Q72.1 ☑
  - lower leg (with foot present) — *see* Agenesis, leg, with foot present
    - and foot Q72.2 ☑
- lens Q12.3
- limb (complete) Q73.0
  - lower — *see* Agenesis, leg
  - upper — *see* Agenesis, arm
- lip Q38.0
- liver Q44.7
- lung (fissure) (lobe) (bilateral) (unilateral) Q33.3
- mandible, maxilla M26.09
- metacarpus — *see* Agenesis, hand
- metatarsus — *see* Agenesis, foot
- muscle Q79.8
  - eyelid Q10.3
  - ocular Q15.8
- musculoskeletal system NEC Q79.8
- nail (s) Q84.3
- neck, part Q18.8
- nerve Q07.8
- nervous system, part NEC Q07.8
- nipple Q83.2
- nose Q30.1
- nuclear Q07.8
- organ
  - of Corti Q16.5
  - or site not listed — *see* Anomaly, by site
- osseous meatus (ear) Q16.1
- ovary
  - bilateral Q50.02
  - unilateral Q50.01
- oviduct Q50.6
- pancreas Q45.0
- parathyroid (gland) Q89.2
- parotid gland (s) Q38.4
- patella Q74.1
- pelvic girdle (complete) (partial) Q74.2
- penis Q55.5
- pericardium Q24.8
- pituitary (gland) Q89.2
- prostate Q55.4
- punctum lacrimale Q10.4
- radioulnar — *see* Defect, reduction, upper limb
- radius — *see* Defect, reduction, upper limb, longitudinal, radius
- rectum Q42.1
  - with fistula Q42.0
- renal Q60.2
  - bilateral Q60.1
  - unilateral Q60.0
- respiratory organ NEC Q34.8
- rib Q76.6
- roof of orbit Q75.8
- round ligament Q52.8
- sacrum Q76.49
- salivary gland Q38.4
- scapula Q74.0
- scrotum Q55.29
- seminal vesicles Q55.4
- septum
  - atrial Q21.1
  - between aorta and pulmonary artery Q21.4
  - ventricular Q20.4
- shoulder girdle (complete) (partial) Q74.0
- skull (bone) Q75.8
  - with
    - anencephaly Q00.0
    - encephalocele — *see* Encephalocele
    - hydrocephalus Q03.9
      - with spina bifida — *see* Spina bifida, by site, with hydrocephalus
    - microcephaly Q02
- spermatic cord Q55.4
- spinal cord Q06.0
- spine Q76.49
- spleen Q89.01
- sternum Q76.7
- stomach Q40.2
- submaxillary gland (s) (congenital) Q38.4

- **Agenesis** — *continued*
  - tarsus — *see* Agenesis, foot
  - tendon Q79.8
  - testicle Q55.0
  - thymus (gland) Q89.2
  - thyroid (gland) E03.1
    - cartilage Q31.8
  - tibia — *see* Defect, reduction, lower limb, longitudinal, tibia
  - tibiofibular — *see* Defect, reduction, lower limb, specified type NEC
  - toe (and foot) (complete) (partial) — *see* Agenesis, foot
  - tongue Q38.3
  - trachea (cartilage) Q32.1
  - ulna — *see* Defect, reduction, upper limb, longitudinal, ulna
  - upper limb — *see* Agenesis, arm
  - ureter Q62.4
  - urethra Q64.5
  - urinary tract NEC Q64.8
  - uterus Q51.0
  - uvula Q38.5
  - vagina Q52.0
  - vas deferens Q55.4
  - vein(s) (peripheral) Q27.9
    - brain Q28.3
    - great NEC Q26.8
    - portal Q26.5
  - vena cava (inferior) (superior) Q26.8
  - vermis of cerebellum Q04.3
  - vertebra Q76.49
  - vulva Q52.71
- **Ageusia** R43.2
- **Agitated** — *see* condition
- **Agitation** R45.1
- **Aglossia** (congenital) Q38.3
- **Aglossia-adactylia** syndrome Q87.0
- **Aglycogenosis** E74.00
- **Agnosia** (body image) (other senses) (tactile) R48.1
  - developmental F88
  - verbal R48.1
    - auditory R48.1
      - developmental F80.2
    - developmental F80.2
  - visual (object) R48.3
- **Agoraphobia** F40.00
  - with panic disorder F40.01
  - without panic disorder F40.02
- **Agrammatism** R48.8
- **Agranulocytopenia** — *see* Agranulocytosis
- **Agranulocytosis** (chronic) (cyclical) (genetic) (infantile) (periodic) (pernicious) (*see also* Neutropenia)D70.9
  - congenital D70.0
  - cytoreductive cancer chemotherapy sequela D70.1
  - drug-induced D70.2
    - due to cytoreductive cancer chemotherapy D70.1
  - due to infection D70.3
  - secondary D70.4
    - drug-induced D70.2
      - due to cytoreductive cancer chemotherapy D70.1
- **Agraphia** (absolute) R48.8
  - with alexia R48.0
  - developmental F81.81
- **Ague** (dumb) — *see* Malaria
- **Agyria** Q04.3
- **Ahumada-del** Castillo syndrome E23.0
- **Aichmophobia** F40.298
- **AIDS** (related complex) B20
- **Ailment** heart — *see* Disease, heart
- **Ailurophobia** F40.218
- **Ainhum** (disease) L94.6
- **AIN** — *see* Neoplasia, intraepithelial, anal
- **AIPHI** (acute idiopathic pulmonary hemorrhage in infants (over 28 days old)) R04.81
- **Air**
  - anterior mediastinum J98.2
  - compressed, disease T70.3 ☑
  - conditioner lung or pneumonitis J67.7
  - embolism (artery) (cerebral) (any site) T79.0 ☑
    - with ectopic or molar pregnancy O08.2
    - due to implanted device NEC — *see* Complications, by site and type, specified NEC
    - following
      - abortion — *see* Abortion by type, complicated by, embolism
      - ectopic or molar pregnancy O08.2
- **Air** — *continued*
  - embolism — *continued*
      - infusion, therapeutic injection or transfusion T80.0 ☑
    - in pregnancy, childbirth or puerperium — *see* Embolism, obstetric
    - traumatic T79.0 ☑
  - hunger, psychogenic F45.8
  - rarefied, effects of — *see* Effect, adverse, high altitude
  - sickness T75.3 ☑
- **Airplane** sickness T75.3 ☑
- **Akathisia** (drug-induced) (treatment-induced) G25.71
  - neuroleptic induced (acute) G25.71
- **Akinesia** R29.898
- **Akinetic** mutism R41.89
- **Akureyri's** disease G93.3
- **Alactasia,** congenital E73.0
- **Alagille's** syndrome Q44.7
- **Alastrim** B03
- **Albers-Schönberg** syndrome Q78.2
- **Albert's** syndrome — *see* Tendinitis, Achilles
- **Albinism,** albino E70.30
  - with hematologic abnormality E70.339
    - Chédiak-Higashi syndrome E70.330
    - Hermansky-Pudlak syndrome E70.331
    - other specified E70.338
  - I E70.320
  - II E70.321
  - ocular E70.319
    - autosomal recessive E70.311
    - other specified E70.318
    - X-linked E70.310
  - oculocutaneous E70.329
    - other specified E70.328
    - tyrosinase (ty) negative E70.320
    - tyrosinase (ty) positive E70.321
  - other specified E70.39
- **Albinismus** E70.30
- **Albright** (-McCune) (-Sternberg) syndrome Q78.1
- **Albuminous** — *see* condition
- **Albuminuria,** albuminuric (acute) (chronic) (subacute) (*see also* Proteinuria)R80.9
  - complicating pregnancy — *see* Proteinuria, gestational
    - with
      - gestational hypertension — *see* Pre-eclampsia
      - pre-existing hypertension — *see* Hypertension, complicating pregnancy, pre-existing, with, pre-eclampsia
  - gestational — *see* Proteinuria, gestational
    - with
      - gestational hypertension — *see* Pre-eclampsia
      - pre-existing hypertension — *see* Hypertension, complicating pregnancy, pre-existing, with, pre-eclampsia
  - orthostatic R80.2
  - postural R80.2
  - pre-eclamptic — *see* Pre-eclampsia
  - scarlatinal A38.8
- **Albuminurophobia** F40.298
- **Alcaptonuria** E70.29
- **Alcohol,** alcoholic, alcohol-induced
  - addiction (without remission) F10.20
    - with remission F10.21
  - amnestic disorder, persisting F10.96
    - with dependence F10.26
  - anxiety disorder F10.980
  - bipolar and related disorder F10.94
  - depressive disorder F10.94
  - major neurocognitive disorder, amnestic-confabulatory type F10.96
  - major neurocognitive disorder, nonamnestic-confabulatory type F10.97
  - mild neurocognitive disorder F10.988
  - psychotic disorder F10.959
  - sexual dysfunction F10.981
  - sleep disorder F10.982
  - brain syndrome, chronic F10.97
    - with dependence F10.27
  - cardiopathy I42.6
  - counseling and surveillance Z71.41
    - family member Z71.42
  - delirium (acute) (tremens) (withdrawal) F10.231
    - with intoxication F10.921
      - in
        - abuse F10.121
        - dependence F10.221
- **Alcohol** — *continued*
  - dementia F10.97
    - with dependence F10.27
  - deterioration F10.97
    - with dependence F10.27
  - hallucinosis (acute) F10.951
    - in
      - abuse F10.151
      - dependence F10.251
  - insanity F10.959
  - intoxication (acute) (without dependence) F10.129
    - with
      - delirium F10.121
      - dependence F10.229
        - with delirium F10.221
        - uncomplicated F10.220
    - uncomplicated F10.120
  - jealousy F10.988
  - Korsakoff's, Korsakov's, Korsakow's F10.26
  - liver K70.9
    - acute — *see* Disease, liver, alcoholic, hepatitis
  - mania (acute) (chronic) F10.959
  - paranoia, paranoid (type) psychosis F10.950
  - pellagra E52
  - poisoning, accidental (acute) NEC — *see* Table of Drugs and Chemicals, alcohol, poisoning
  - psychosis — *see* Psychosis, alcoholic
  - withdrawal (without convulsions) F10.239
    - with delirium F10.231
- **Alcoholism** (chronic) (without remission) F10.20
  - with
    - psychosis — *see* Psychosis, alcoholic
    - remission F10.21
  - Korsakov's F10.96
    - with dependence F10.26
- **Alder** (-Reilly) anomaly or syndrome (leukocyte granulation) D72.0
- **Aldosteronism** E26.9
  - familial (type I) E26.02
  - glucocorticoid-remediable E26.02
  - primary (due to (bilateral) adrenal hyperplasia) E26.09
  - primary NEC E26.09
  - secondary E26.1
  - specified NEC E26.89
- **Aldosteronoma** D44.10
- **Aldrich** (-Wiskott) syndrome (eczema-thrombocytopenia) D82.0
- **Alektorophobia** F40.218
- **Aleppo** boil B55.1
- **Aleukemic** — *see* condition
- **Aleukia**
  - congenital D70.0
  - hemorrhagica D61.9
    - congenital D61.09
  - splenica D73.1
- **Alexia** R48.0
  - developmental F81.0
  - secondary to organic lesion R48.0
- **Algoneurodystrophy** M89.00
  - ankle M89.07 ☑
  - foot M89.07 ☑
  - forearm M89.03 ☑
  - hand M89.04 ☑
  - lower leg M89.06 ☑
  - multiple sites M89.0 ☑
  - shoulder M89.01 ☑
  - specified site NEC M89.08
  - thigh M89.05 ☑
  - upper arm M89.02 ☑
- **Algophobia** F40.298
- **Alienation,** mental — *see* Psychosis
- **Alkalemia** E87.3
- **Alkalosis** E87.3
  - metabolic E87.3
    - with respiratory acidosis E87.4
  - respiratory E87.3
- **Alkaptonuria** E70.29
- **Allen-Masters** syndrome N83.8
- **Allergy,** allergic (reaction) (to) T78.40 ☑
  - air-borne substance NEC (rhinitis) J30.89
  - alveolitis (extrinsic) J67.9
    - due to
      - Aspergillus clavatus J67.4
      - Cryptostroma corticale J67.6
      - organisms (fungal, thermophilic actinomycete) growing in ventilation (air conditioning) systems J67.7
    - specified type NEC J67.8
  - anaphylactic reaction or shock T78.2 ☑
  - angioneurotic edema T78.3 ☑

- **Allergy** — *continued*
  - animal (dander) (epidermal) (hair) (rhinitis) J30.81
  - bee sting (anaphylactic shock) — *see* Toxicity, venom, arthropod, bee
  - biological — *see* Allergy, drug
  - colitis (*see also* Colitis, allergic)K52.29
  - dander (animal) (rhinitis) J30.81
  - dandruff (rhinitis) J30.81
  - dental restorative material (existing) K08.55
  - dermatitis — *see* Dermatitis, contact, allergic
  - diathesis — *see* History, allergy
  - drug, medicament & biological (any) (external) (internal) T78.40 ☑
    - correct substance properly administered — *see* Table of Drugs and Chemicals, by drug, adverse effect
    - wrong substance given or taken NEC (by accident) — *see* Table of Drugs and Chemicals, by drug, poisoning
  - due to pollen J30.1
  - dust (house) (stock) (rhinitis) J30.89
    - with asthma — *see* Asthma, allergic extrinsic
  - eczema — *see* Dermatitis, contact, allergic
  - epidermal (animal) (rhinitis) J30.81
  - feathers (rhinitis) J30.89
  - food (any) (ingested) NEC T78.1 ☑
    - anaphylactic shock — *see* Shock, anaphylactic, due to food
    - dermatitis — *see* Dermatitis, due to, food
    - dietary counseling and surveillance Z71.3
    - in contact with skin L23.6
    - rhinitis J30.5
    - status (without reaction) Z91.018
      - eggs Z91.012
      - milk products Z91.011
      - peanuts Z91.010
      - seafood Z91.013
      - specified NEC Z91.018
  - gastrointestinal (*see also* specific type of allergic reaction)
    - meaning colitis (*see also* Colitis, allergic)K52.29
    - meaning gastroenteritis (*see also* Gastroenteritis, allergic)K52.29
    - meaning other adverse food reaction not elsewhere classified T78.1 ☑
  - grain J30.1
  - grass (hay fever) (pollen) J30.1
    - asthma — *see* Asthma, allergic extrinsic
  - hair (animal) (rhinitis) J30.81
  - history (of) — *see* History, allergy
  - horse serum — *see* Allergy, serum
  - inhalant (rhinitis) J30.89
    - pollen J30.1
  - kapok (rhinitis) J30.89
  - medicine — *see* Allergy, drug
  - milk protein (*see also* Allergy, food)Z91.011
    - anaphylactic reaction T78.07 ☑
    - dermatitis L27.2
    - enterocolitis syndrome K52.21
    - enteropathy K52.22
    - gastroenteritis K52.29
    - gastroesophageal reflux (*see also* Reaction, adverse, food)K21.9
      - with esophagitis K21.0
    - proctocolitis K52.82
  - nasal, seasonal due to pollen J30.1
  - pneumonia J82
  - pollen (any) (hay fever) J30.1
    - asthma — *see* Asthma, allergic extrinsic
  - primrose J30.1
  - primula J30.1
  - proctocolitis K52.82
  - purpura D69.0
  - ragweed (hay fever) (pollen) J30.1
    - asthma — *see* Asthma, allergic extrinsic
  - rose (pollen) J30.1
  - seasonal NEC J30.2
  - Senecio jacobae (pollen) J30.1
  - serum (*see also* Reaction, serum)T80.69 ☑
    - anaphylactic shock T80.59 ☑
  - shock (anaphylactic) T78.2 ☑
    - due to
      - administration of blood and blood products T80.51 ☑
      - adverse effect of correct medicinal substance properly administered T88.6 ☑
      - immunization T80.52 ☑
      - serum NEC T80.59 ☑
      - vaccination T80.52 ☑
  - specific NEC T78.49 ☑
  - tree (any) (hay fever) (pollen) J30.1
    - asthma — *see* Asthma, allergic extrinsic
  - upper respiratory J30.9
  - urticaria L50.0
  - vaccine — *see* Allergy, serum
  - wheat — *see* Allergy, food
- **Allescheriasis** B48.2
- **Alligator** skin disease Q80.9
- **Allocheiria,** allochiria R20.8
- **Almeida's** disease — *see* Paracoccidioidomycosis
- **Alopecia** (hereditaria) (seborrheica) L65.9
  - androgenic L64.9
    - drug-induced L64.0
    - specified NEC L64.8
  - areata L63.9
    - ophiasis L63.2
    - specified NEC L63.8
    - totalis L63.0
    - universalis L63.1
  - cicatricial L66.9
    - specified NEC L66.8
  - circumscripta L63.9
  - congenital, congenitalis Q84.0
  - due to cytotoxic drugs NEC L65.8
  - mucinosa L65.2
  - postinfective NEC L65.8
  - postpartum L65.0
  - premature L64.8
  - specific (syphilitic) A51.32
  - specified NEC L65.8
  - syphilitic (secondary) A51.32
  - totalis (capitis) L63.0
  - universalis (entire body) L63.1
  - X-ray L58.1
- **Alpers'** disease G31.81
- **Alpine** sickness T70.29 ☑
- **Alport** syndrome Q87.81
- **ALTE** (apparent life threatening event) in newborn and infant R68.13
- **Alteration** (of), Altered
  - awareness
    - transient R40.4
    - unintended under general anesthesia, during procedureT88.53
  - mental status R41.82
  - pattern of family relationships affecting child Z62.898
  - sensation
    - following
      - cerebrovascular disease I69.998
        - cerebral infarction I69.398
        - intracerebral hemorrhage I69.198
        - nontraumatic intracranial hemorrhage NEC I69.298
        - specified disease NEC I69.898
        - subarachnoid hemorrhage I69.098
- **Alternating** — *see* condition
- **Altitude,** high (effects) — *see* Effect, adverse, high altitude
- **Aluminosis** (of lung) J63.0
- **Alveolitis**
  - allergic (extrinsic) — *see* Pneumonitis, hypersensitivity
  - due to
    - Aspergillus clavatus J67.4
    - Cryptostroma corticale J67.6
  - fibrosing (cryptogenic) (idiopathic) J84.112
  - jaw M27.3
  - sicca dolorosa M27.3
- **Alveolus,** alveolar — *see* condition
- **Alymphocytosis** D72.810
  - thymic (with immunodeficiency) D82.1
- **Alymphoplasia,** thymic D82.1
- **Alzheimer's** disease or sclerosis — *see* Disease, Alzheimer's
- **Amastia** (with nipple present) Q83.8
  - with absent nipple Q83.0
- **Amathophobia** F40.228
- **Amaurosis** (acquired) (congenital) (*see also* Blindness)
  - fugax G45.3
  - hysterical F44.6
  - Leber's congenital H35.50
  - uremic — *see* Uremia
- **Amaurotic** idiocy (infantile) (juvenile) (late) E75.4
- **Amaxophobia** F40.248
- **Ambiguous** genitalia Q56.4
- **Amblyopia** (congenital) (ex anopsia) (partial) (suppression) H53.00 ☑
  - anisometropic — *see* Amblyopia, refractive
  - deprivation H53.01 ☑
  - hysterical F44.6
  - nocturnal (*see also* Blindness, night)
    - vitamin A deficiency E50.5
- **Amblyopia** — *continued*
  - refractive H53.02 ☑
  - strabismic H53.03 ☑
  - suspect H53.04 ☑
  - tobacco H53.8
  - toxic NEC H53.8
  - uremic — *see* Uremia
- **Ameba,** amebic (histolytica) (*see also* Amebiasis)
  - abscess (liver) A06.4
- **Amebiasis** A06.9
  - with abscess — *see* Abscess, amebic
  - acute A06.0
  - chronic (intestine) A06.1
    - with abscess — *see* Abscess, amebic
  - cutaneous A06.7
  - cutis A06.7
  - cystitis A06.81
  - genitourinary tract NEC A06.82
  - hepatic — *see* Abscess, liver, amebic
  - intestine A06.0
  - nondysenteric colitis A06.2
  - skin A06.7
  - specified site NEC A06.89
- **Ameboma** (of intestine) A06.3
- **Amelia** Q73.0
  - lower limb — *see* Agenesis, leg
  - upper limb — *see* Agenesis, arm
- **Ameloblastoma** (*see also* Cyst, calcifying odontogenic)
  - long bones C40.9 ☑
    - lower limb C40.2 ☑
    - upper limb C40.0 ☑
  - malignant C41.1
    - jaw (bone) (lower) C41.1
      - upper C41.0
  - tibial C40.2 ☑
- **Amelogenesis** imperfecta K00.5
  - nonhereditaria (segmentalis) K00.4
- **Amenorrhea** N91.2
  - hyperhormonal E28.8
  - primary N91.0
  - secondary N91.1
- **Amentia** — *see* Disability, intellectual
  - Meynert's (nonalcoholic) F04
- **American**
  - leishmaniasis B55.2
  - mountain tick fever A93.2
- **Ametropia** — *see* Disorder, refraction
- **AMH** (asymptomatic microscopic hematuria) R31.21
- **Amianthosis** J61
- **Amimia** R48.8
- **Amino-acid** disorder E72.9
  - anemia D53.0
- **Aminoacidopathy** E72.9
- **Aminoaciduria** E72.9
- **Amnes** (t)ic syndrome (post-traumatic) F04
  - induced by
    - alcohol F10.96
      - with dependence F10.26
    - psychoactive NEC F19.96
      - with
        - abuse F19.16
        - dependence F19.26
    - sedative F13.96
      - with dependence F13.26
- **Amnesia** R41.3
  - anterograde R41.1
  - auditory R48.8
  - dissociative F44.0
    - with dissociative fugue F44.1
  - hysterical F44.0
  - postictal in epilepsy — *see* Epilepsy
  - psychogenic F44.0
  - retrograde R41.2
  - transient global G45.4
- **Amnion,** amniotic — *see* condition
- **Amnionitis** — *see* Pregnancy, complicated by
- **Amok** F68.8
- **Amoral** traits F60.89
- **Amphetamine** (or other stimulant)-induced
  - anxiety disorder F15.980
  - bipolar and related disorder F15.94
  - delirium F15.921
  - depressive disorder F15.94
  - obsessive-compulsive and related disorder F15.988
  - psychotic disorder F15.959
  - sexual dysfunction F15.981
  - sleep disorder F15.982
  - stimulant withdrawal F15.23
- **Ampulla**
  - lower esophagus K22.8
  - phrenic K22.8

- **Amputation** (*see also* Absence, by site, acquired)
  - neuroma (postoperative) (traumatic) — *see* Complications, amputation stump, neuroma
  - stump (surgical)
    - abnormal, painful, or with complication (late) — *see* Complications, amputation stump
    - healed or old NOS Z89.9
  - traumatic (complete) (partial)
    - arm (upper) (complete) S48.91 ☑
      - at
        - elbow S58.01 ☑
          - partial S58.02 ☑
        - shoulder joint (complete) S48.01 ☑
          - partial S48.02 ☑
      - between
        - elbow and wrist (complete) S58.11 ☑
          - partial S58.12 ☑
        - shoulder and elbow (complete) S48.11 ☑
          - partial S48.12 ☑
      - partial S48.92 ☑
    - breast (complete) S28.21 ☑
      - partial S28.22 ☑
    - clitoris (complete) S38.211 ☑
      - partial S38.212 ☑
    - ear (complete) S08.11 ☑
      - partial S08.12 ☑
    - finger (complete) (metacarpophalangeal) S68.11 ☑
      - index S68.11 ☑
      - little S68.11 ☑
      - middle S68.11 ☑
      - partial S68.12 ☑
        - index S68.12 ☑
        - little S68.12 ☑
        - middle S68.12 ☑
        - ring S68.12 ☑
      - ring S68.11 ☑
      - thumb — *see* Amputation, traumatic, thumb
      - transphalangeal (complete) S68.61 ☑
        - index S68.61 ☑
        - little S68.61 ☑
        - middle S68.61 ☑
        - partial S68.62 ☑
          - index S68.62 ☑
          - little S68.62 ☑
          - middle S68.62 ☑
          - ring S68.62 ☑
        - ring S68.61 ☑
    - foot (complete) S98.91 ☑
      - at ankle level S98.01 ☑
        - partial S98.02 ☑
      - midfoot S98.31 ☑
        - partial S98.32 ☑
      - partial S98.92 ☑
    - forearm (complete) S58.91 ☑
      - at elbow level (complete) S58.01 ☑
        - partial S58.02 ☑
      - between elbow and wrist (complete) S58.11 ☑
        - partial S58.12 ☑
      - partial S58.92 ☑
    - genital organ (s) (external)
      - female (complete) S38.211 ☑
        - partial S38.212 ☑
      - male
        - penis (complete) S38.221 ☑
          - partial S38.222 ☑
        - scrotum (complete) S38.231 ☑
          - partial S38.232 ☑
        - testes (complete) S38.231 ☑
          - partial S38.232 ☑
    - hand (complete) (wrist level) S68.41 ☑
      - finger (s) alone — *see* Amputation, traumatic, finger
      - partial S68.42 ☑
      - thumb alone — *see* Amputation, traumatic, thumb
      - transmetacarpal (complete) S68.71 ☑
        - partial S68.72 ☑
    - head
      - ear — *see* Amputation, traumatic, ear
      - nose (partial) S08.812 ☑
        - complete S08.811 ☑
      - part S08.89 ☑
        - scalp S08.0 ☑
    - hip (and thigh) (complete) S78.91 ☑
      - at hip joint (complete) S78.01 ☑
        - partial S78.02 ☑
      - between hip and knee (complete) S78.11 ☑
        - partial S78.12 ☑
      - partial S78.92 ☑
    - labium (majus) (minus) (complete) S38.21 ☑

- **Amputation** — *continued*
  - traumatic — *continued*
      - partial S38.21 ☑
    - leg (lower) S88.91 ☑
      - at knee level S88.01 ☑
        - partial S88.02 ☑
      - between knee and ankle S88.11 ☑
        - partial S88.12 ☑
      - partial S88.92 ☑
    - nose (partial) S08.812 ☑
      - complete S08.811 ☑
    - penis (complete) S38.221 ☑
      - partial S38.222 ☑
    - scrotum (complete) S38.231 ☑
      - partial S38.232 ☑
    - shoulder — *see* Amputation, traumatic, arm
      - at shoulder joint — *see* Amputation, traumatic, arm, at shoulder joint
    - testes (complete) S38.231 ☑
      - partial S38.232 ☑
    - thigh — *see* Amputation, traumatic, hip
    - thorax, part of S28.1 ☑
      - breast — *see* Amputation, traumatic, breast
    - thumb (complete) (metacarpophalangeal) S68.01 ☑
      - partial S68.02 ☑
      - transphalangeal (complete) S68.51 ☑
        - partial S68.52 ☑
    - toe (lesser) S98.13 ☑
      - great S98.11 ☑
        - partial S98.12 ☑
      - more than one S98.21 ☑
        - partial S98.22 ☑
      - partial S98.14 ☑
    - vulva (complete) S38.211 ☑
      - partial S38.212 ☑
- **Amputee** (bilateral) (old) Z89.9
- **Amsterdam** dwarfism Q87.1
- **Amusia** R48.8
  - developmental F80.89
- **Amyelencephalus,** amyelencephaly Q00.0
- **Amyelia** Q06.0
- **Amygdalitis** — *see* Tonsillitis
- **Amygdalolith** J35.8
- **Amyloid** heart (disease) E85.4 *[I43]*
- **Amyloidosis** (generalized) (primary) E85.9
  - with lung involvement E85.4 *[J99]*
  - familial E85.2
  - genetic E85.2
  - heart E85.4 *[I43]*
  - hemodialysis-associated E85.3
  - liver E85.4 *[K77]*
  - localized E85.4
  - neuropathic heredofamilial E85.1
  - non-neuropathic heredofamilial E85.0
  - organ limited E85.4
  - Portuguese E85.1
  - pulmonary E85.4 *[J99]*
  - secondary systemic E85.3
  - skin (lichen) (macular) E85.4 *[L99]*
  - specified NEC E85.8
  - subglottic E85.4 *[J99]*
- **Amylopectinosis** (brancher enzyme deficiency) E74.03
- **Amylophagia** — *see* Pica
- **Amyoplasia** congenita Q79.8
- **Amyotonia** M62.89
  - congenita G70.2
- **Amyotrophia,** amyotrophy, amyotrophic G71.8
  - congenita Q79.8
  - diabetic — *see* Diabetes, amyotrophy
  - lateral sclerosis G12.21
  - neuralgic G54.5
  - spinal progressive G12.21
- **Anacidity,** gastric K31.83
  - psychogenic F45.8
- **Anaerosis** of newborn P28.89
- **Analbuminemia** E88.09
- **Analgesia** — *see* Anesthesia
- **Analphalipoproteinemia** E78.6
- **Anaphylactic**
  - purpura D69.0
  - shock or reaction — *see* Shock, anaphylactic
- **Anaphylactoid** shock or reaction — *see* Shock, anaphylactic
- **Anaphylactoid** syndrome of pregnancy O88.01 ☑
- **Anaphylaxis** — *see* Shock, anaphylactic
- **Anaplasia** cervix (*see also* Dysplasia, cervix)N87.9
- **Anaplasmosis,** human A77.49
- **Anarthria** R47.1
- **Anasarca** R60.1
  - cardiac — *see* Failure, heart, congestive

- **Anasarca** — *continued*
  - lung J18.2
  - newborn P83.2
  - nutritional E43
  - pulmonary J18.2
  - renal N04.9
- **Anastomosis**
  - aneurysmal — *see* Aneurysm
  - arteriovenous ruptured brain I60.8
  - intestinal K63.89
    - complicated NEC K91.89
      - involving urinary tract N99.89
  - retinal and choroidal vessels (congenital) Q14.8
- **Anatomical** narrow angle H40.03 ☑
- **Ancylostoma,** ancylostomiasis (braziliense) (caninum) (ceylanicum) (duodenale) B76.0
  - Necator americanus B76.1
- **Andersen's** disease (glycogen storage) E74.09
- **Anderson-Fabry** disease E75.21
- **Andes** disease T70.29 ☑
- **Andrews'** disease (bacterid) L08.89
- **Androblastoma**
  - benign
    - specified site — *see* Neoplasm, benign, by site
    - unspecified site
      - female D27.9
      - male D29.20
  - malignant
    - specified site — *see* Neoplasm, malignant, by site
    - unspecified site
      - female C56.9
      - male C62.90
  - specified site — *see* Neoplasm, uncertain behavior, by site
  - tubular
    - with lipid storage
      - specified site — *see* Neoplasm, benign, by site
      - unspecified site
        - female D27.9
        - male D29.20
    - specified site — *see* Neoplasm, benign, by site
    - unspecified site
      - female D27.9
      - male D29.20
  - unspecified site
    - female D39.10
    - male D40.10
- **Androgen** insensitivity syndrome (*see also* Syndrome, androgen insensitivity)E34.50
- **Androgen** resistance syndrome (*see also* Syndrome, androgen insensitivity)E34.50
- **Android** pelvis Q74.2
  - with disproportion (fetopelvic) O33.3 ☑
    - causing obstructed labor O65.3
- **Androphobia** F40.290
- **Anectasis,** pulmonary (newborn) — *see* Atelectasis
- **Anemia** (essential) (general) (hemoglobin deficiency) (infantile) (primary) (profound) D64.9
  - with (due to) (in)
    - disorder of
      - anaerobic glycolysis D55.2
      - pentose phosphate pathway D55.1
    - koilonychia D50.9
  - achlorhydric D50.8
  - achrestic D53.1
  - Addison (-Biermer) (pernicious) D51.0
  - agranulocytic — *see* Agranulocytosis
  - amino-acid-deficiency D53.0
  - aplastic D61.9
    - congenital D61.09
    - drug-induced D61.1
    - due to
      - drugs D61.1
      - external agents NEC D61.2
      - infection D61.2
      - radiation D61.2
    - idiopathic D61.3
    - red cell (pure) D60.9
      - chronic D60.0
      - congenital D61.01
      - specified type NEC D60.8
      - transient D60.1
    - specified type NEC D61.89
    - toxic D61.2
  - aregenerative
    - congenital D61.09
  - asiderotic D50.9
  - atypical (primary) D64.9
  - Baghdad spring D55.0
  - Balantidium coli A07.0

Anemia — *continued*
- Biermer's (pernicious) D51.0
- blood loss (chronic) D50.0
  - acute D62
- bothriocephalus B70.0 *[D63.8]*
- brickmaker's B76.9 *[D63.8]*
- cerebral I67.89
- childhood D58.9
- chlorotic D50.8
- chronic
  - blood loss D50.0
  - hemolytic D58.9
    - idiopathic D59.9
  - simple D53.9
- chronica congenita aregenerativa D61.09
- combined system disease NEC D51.0 *[G32.0]*
  - due to dietary vitamin B12 deficiency D51.3 *[G32.0]*
- complicating pregnancy, childbirth or puerperium — *see* Pregnancy, complicated by (management affected by), anemia
- congenital P61.4
  - aplastic D61.09
  - due to isoimmunization NOS P55.9
  - dyserythropoietic, dyshematopoietic D64.4
  - following fetal blood loss P61.3
  - Heinz body D58.2
  - hereditary hemolytic NOS D58.9
  - pernicious D51.0
  - spherocytic D58.0
- Cooley's (erythroblastic) D56.1
- cytogenic D51.0
- deficiency D53.9
  - 2, 3 diphosphoglycurate mutase D55.2
  - 2, 3 PG D55.2
  - 6 phosphogluconate dehydrogenase D55.1
  - 6-PGD D55.1
  - amino-acid D53.0
  - combined B12 and folate D53.1
  - enzyme D55.9
    - drug-induced (hemolytic) D59.2
    - glucose-6-phosphate dehydrogenase (G6PD) D55.0
    - glycolytic D55.2
    - nucleotide metabolism D55.3
    - related to hexose monophosphate (HMP) shunt pathway NEC D55.1
    - specified type NEC D55.8
  - erythrocytic glutathione D55.1
  - folate D52.9
    - dietary D52.0
    - drug-induced D52.1
  - folic acid D52.9
    - dietary D52.0
    - drug-induced D52.1
  - G SH D55.1
  - GGS-R D55.1
  - glucose-6-phosphate dehydrogenase D55.0
  - glutathione reductase D55.1
  - glyceraldehyde phosphate dehydrogenase D55.2
  - G6PD D55.0
  - hexokinase D55.2
  - iron D50.9
    - secondary to blood loss (chronic) D50.0
  - nutritional D53.9
    - with
      - poor iron absorption D50.8
      - specified deficiency NEC D53.8
  - phosphofructo-aldolase D55.2
  - phosphoglycerate kinase D55.2
  - PK D55.2
  - protein D53.0
  - pyruvate kinase D55.2
  - transcobalamin II D51.2
  - triose-phosphate isomerase D55.2
  - vitamin B12 NOS D51.9
    - dietary D51.3
    - due to
      - intrinsic factor deficiency D51.0
      - selective vitamin B12 malabsorption with proteinuria D51.1
    - pernicious D51.0
    - specified type NEC D51.8
- Diamond-Blackfan (congenital hypoplastic) D61.01
- dibothriocephalus B70.0 *[D63.8]*
- dimorphic D53.1
- diphasic D53.1
- Diphyllobothrium (Dibothriocephalus) B70.0 *[D63.8]*

Anemia — *continued*
- due to (in) (with)
  - antineoplastic chemotherapy D64.81
  - blood loss (chronic) D50.0
    - acute D62
  - chemotherapy, antineoplastic D64.81
  - chronic disease classified elsewhere NEC D63.8
  - chronic kidney disease D63.1
  - deficiency
    - amino-acid D53.0
    - copper D53.8
    - folate (folic acid) D52.9
      - dietary D52.0
      - drug-induced D52.1
    - molybdenum D53.8
    - protein D53.0
    - zinc D53.8
  - dietary vitamin B12 deficiency D51.3
  - disorder of
    - glutathione metabolism D55.1
    - nucleotide metabolism D55.3
  - drug — *see* Anemia, by type (*see also* Table of Drugs and Chemicals)
  - end stage renal disease D63.1
  - enzyme disorder D55.9
  - fetal blood loss P61.3
  - fish tapeworm (D. latum) infestation B70.0 *[D63.8]*
  - hemorrhage (chronic) D50.0
    - acute D62
  - impaired absorption D50.9
  - loss of blood (chronic) D50.0
    - acute D62
  - myxedema E03.9 *[D63.8]*
  - Necator americanus B76.1 *[D63.8]*
  - prematurity P61.2
  - selective vitamin B12 malabsorption with proteinuria D51.1
  - transcobalamin II deficiency D51.2
- Dyke-Young type (secondary) (symptomatic) D59.1
- dyserythropoietic (congenital) D64.4
- dyshematopoietic (congenital) D64.4
- Egyptian B76.9 *[D63.8]*
- elliptocytosis — *see* Elliptocytosis
- enzyme-deficiency, drug-induced D59.2
- epidemic (*see also* Ancylostomiasis)B76.9 *[D63.8]*
- erythroblastic
  - familial D56.1
  - newborn (*see also* Disease, hemolytic)P55.9
  - of childhood D56.1
- erythrocytic glutathione deficiency D55.1
- erythropoietin-resistant anemia (EPO resistant anemia) D63.1
- Faber's (achlorhydric anemia) D50.9
- factitious (self-induced blood letting) D50.0
- familial erythroblastic D56.1
- Fanconi's (congenital pancytopenia) D61.09
- favism D55.0
- fish tapeworm (D. latum) infestation B70.0 *[D63.8]*
- folate (folic acid) deficiency D52.9
- glucose-6-phosphate dehydrogenase (G6PD) deficiency D55.0
- glutathione-reductase deficiency D55.1
- goat's milk D52.0
- granulocytic — *see* Agranulocytosis
- Heinz body, congenital D58.2
- hemolytic D58.9
  - acquired D59.9
    - with hemoglobinuria NEC D59.6
    - autoimmune NEC D59.1
    - infectious D59.4
    - specified type NEC D59.8
    - toxic D59.4
  - acute D59.9
    - due to enzyme deficiency specified type NEC D55.8
    - Lederer's D59.1
  - autoimmune D59.1
    - drug-induced D59.0
  - chronic D58.9
    - idiopathic D59.9
  - cold type (secondary) (symptomatic) D59.1
  - congenital (spherocytic) — *see* Spherocytosis
  - due to
    - cardiac conditions D59.4
    - drugs (nonautoimmune) D59.2
      - autoimmune D59.0
    - enzyme disorder D55.9
      - drug-induced D59.2
    - presence of shunt or other internal prosthetic device D59.4

Anemia — *continued*
- hemolytic — *continued*
  - familial D58.9
  - hereditary D58.9
    - due to enzyme disorder D55.9
      - specified type NEC D55.8
    - specified type NEC D58.8
  - idiopathic (chronic) D59.9
  - mechanical D59.4
  - microangiopathic D59.4
  - nonautoimmune D59.4
    - drug-induced D59.2
  - nonspherocytic
    - congenital or hereditary NEC D55.8
      - glucose-6-phosphate dehydrogenase deficiency D55.0
      - pyruvate kinase deficiency D55.2
      - type
        - I D55.1
        - II D55.2
    - type
      - I D55.1
      - II D55.2
  - secondary D59.4
    - autoimmune D59.1
  - specified (hereditary) type NEC D58.8
  - Stransky-Regala type (*see also* Hemoglobinopathy)D58.8
  - symptomatic D59.4
    - autoimmune D59.1
  - toxic D59.4
  - warm type (secondary) (symptomatic) D59.1
- hemorrhagic (chronic) D50.0
  - acute D62
- Herrick's D57.1
- hexokinase deficiency D55.2
- hookworm B76.9 *[D63.8]*
- hypochromic (idiopathic) (microcytic) (normoblastic) D50.9
  - due to blood loss (chronic) D50.0
    - acute D62
  - familial sex-linked D64.0
  - pyridoxine-responsive D64.3
  - sideroblastic, sex-linked D64.0
- hypoplasia, red blood cells D61.9
  - congenital or familial D61.01
- hypoplastic (idiopathic) D61.9
  - congenital or familial (of childhood) D61.01
- hypoproliferative (refractive) D61.9
- idiopathic D64.9
  - aplastic D61.3
  - hemolytic, chronic D59.9
- in (due to) (with)
  - chronic kidney disease D63.1
  - end stage renal disease D63.1
  - failure, kidney (renal) D63.1
  - neoplastic disease (*see also* Neoplasm)D63.0
- intertropical (*see also* Ancylostomiasis)D63.8
- iron deficiency D50.9
  - secondary to blood loss (chronic) D50.0
    - acute D62
  - specified type NEC D50.8
- Joseph-Diamond-Blackfan (congenital hypoplastic) D61.01
- Lederer's (hemolytic) D59.1
- leukoerythroblastic D61.82
- macrocytic D53.9
  - nutritional D52.0
  - tropical D52.8
- malarial (*see also* Malaria)B54 *[D63.8]*
- malignant (progressive) D51.0
- malnutrition D53.9
- marsh (*see also* Malaria)B54 *[D63.8]*
- Mediterranean (with other hemoglobinopathy) D56.9
- megaloblastic D53.1
  - combined B12 and folate deficiency D53.1
  - hereditary D51.1
  - nutritional D52.0
  - orotic aciduria D53.0
  - refractory D53.1
  - specified type NEC D53.1
- megalocytic D53.1
- microcytic (hypochromic) D50.9
  - due to blood loss (chronic) D50.0
    - acute D62
  - familial D56.8
- microdrepanocytosis D57.40
- microelliptopoikilocytic (Rietti-Greppi- Micheli) D56.9
- miner's B76.9 *[D63.8]*
- myelodysplastic D46.9

Anemia — *continued*
- myelofibrosis D75.81
- myelogenous D64.89
- myelopathic D64.89
- myelophthisic D61.82
- myeloproliferative D47.Z9
- newborn P61.4
  - due to
    - ABO (antibodies, isoimmunization, maternal/fetal incompatibility) P55.1
    - Rh (antibodies, isoimmunization, maternal/fetal incompatibility) P55.0
  - following fetal blood loss P61.3
  - posthemorrhagic (fetal) P61.3
- nonspherocytic hemolytic — *see* Anemia, hemolytic, nonspherocytic
- normocytic (infectional) D64.9
  - due to blood loss (chronic) D50.0
    - acute D62
  - myelophthisic D61.82
- nutritional (deficiency) D53.9
  - with
    - poor iron absorption D50.8
    - specified deficiency NEC D53.8
  - megaloblastic D52.0
- of prematurity P61.2
- orotaciduric (congenital) (hereditary) D53.0
- osteosclerotic D64.89
- ovalocytosis (hereditary) — *see* Elliptocytosis
- paludal (*see also* Malaria)B54 *[D63.8]*
- pernicious (congenital) (malignant) (progressive) D51.0
- pleochromic D64.89
  - of sprue D52.8
- posthemorrhagic (chronic) D50.0
  - acute D62
  - newborn P61.3
- postoperative (postprocedural)
  - due to (acute) blood loss D62
    - chronic blood loss D50.0
  - specified NEC D64.9
- postpartum O90.81
- pressure D64.89
- progressive D64.9
  - malignant D51.0
  - pernicious D51.0
- protein-deficiency D53.0
- pseudoleukemica infantum D64.89
- pure red cell D60.9
  - congenital D61.01
- pyridoxine-responsive D64.3
- pyruvate kinase deficiency D55.2
- refractory D46.4
  - with
    - excess of blasts D46.20
      - 1 (RAEB 1) D46.21
      - 2 (RAEB 2) D46.22
      - in transformation (RAEB T) — *see* Leukemia, acute myeloblastic
    - hemochromatosis D46.1
    - sideroblasts (ring) (RARS) D46.1
  - megaloblastic D53.1
  - sideroblastic D46.1
  - sideropenic D50.9
  - without ring sideroblasts, so stated D46.0
  - without sideroblasts without excess of blasts D46.0
- Rietti-Greppi-Micheli D56.9
- scorbutic D53.2
- secondary to
  - blood loss (chronic) D50.0
    - acute D62
  - hemorrhage (chronic) D50.0
    - acute D62
- semiplastic D61.89
- sickle-cell — *see* Disease, sickle-cell
- sideroblastic D64.3
  - hereditary D64.0
  - hypochromic, sex-linked D64.0
  - pyridoxine-responsive NEC D64.3
  - refractory D46.1
  - secondary (due to)
    - disease D64.1
    - drugs and toxins D64.2
  - specified type NEC D64.3
- sideropenic (refractory) D50.9
  - due to blood loss (chronic) D50.0
    - acute D62
- simple chronic D53.9
- specified type NEC D64.89
- spherocytic (hereditary) — *see* Spherocytosis
- splenic D64.89
- splenomegalic D64.89
- stomatocytosis D58.8
- syphilitic (acquired) (late) A52.79 *[D63.8]*
- target cell D64.89
- thalassemia D56.9
- thrombocytopenic — *see* Thrombocytopenia
- toxic D61.2
- tropical B76.9 *[D63.8]*
  - macrocytic D52.8
- tuberculous A18.89 *[D63.8]*
- vegan D51.3
- vitamin
  - B6-responsive D64.3
  - B12 deficiency (dietary) pernicious D51.0
- von Jaksch's D64.89
- Witts' (achlorhydric anemia) D50.8

Anemophobia F40.228

Anencephalus, anencephaly Q00.0

Anergasia — *see* Psychosis, organic

Anesthesia, anesthetic R20.0
- complication or reaction NEC (*see also* Complications, anesthesia)T88.59 ☑
  - due to
    - correct substance properly administered — *see* Table of Drugs and Chemicals, by drug, adverse effect
    - overdose or wrong substance given — *see* Table of Drugs and Chemicals, by drug, poisoning
  - unintended awareness under general anesthesia during procedure T88.53 ☑
  - personal history of Z92.84
- cornea H18.81 ☑
- dissociative F44.6
- functional (hysterical) F44.6
- hyperesthetic, thalamic G89.0
- hysterical F44.6
- local skin lesion R20.0
- sexual (psychogenic) F52.1
- shock (due to) T88.2 ☑
- skin R20.0
- testicular N50.9

Anetoderma (maculosum) (of) L90.8
- Jadassohn-Pellizzari L90.2
- Schweniger-Buzzi L90.1

Aneurin deficiency E51.9

Aneurysm (anastomotic) (artery) (cirsoid) (diffuse) (false) (fusiform) (multiple) (saccular) I72.9
- abdominal (aorta) I71.4
  - ruptured I71.3
  - syphilitic A52.01
- aorta, aortic (nonsyphilitic) I71.9
  - abdominal I71.4
    - ruptured I71.3
  - arch I71.2
    - ruptured I71.1
  - arteriosclerotic I71.9
    - ruptured I71.8
  - ascending I71.2
    - ruptured I71.1
  - congenital Q25.43
  - descending I71.9
    - abdominal I71.4
      - ruptured I71.3
    - ruptured I71.8
    - thoracic I71.2
      - ruptured I71.1
  - root Q25.43
  - ruptured I71.8
  - sinus, congenital Q25.43
  - syphilitic A52.01
  - thoracic I71.2
    - ruptured I71.1
  - thoracoabdominal I71.6
    - ruptured I71.5
  - thorax, thoracic (arch) I71.2
    - ruptured I71.1
  - transverse I71.2
    - ruptured I71.1
  - valve (heart) (*see also* Endocarditis, aortic)I35.8
- arteriosclerotic I72.9
  - cerebral I67.1
    - ruptured — *see* Hemorrhage, intracranial, subarachnoid
- arteriovenous (congenital) (*see also* Malformation, arteriovenous)
  - acquired I77.0
    - brain I67.1
    - coronary I25.41
    - pulmonary I28.0
  - brain Q28.2

Aneurysm — *continued*
- arteriovenous — *continued*
    - ruptured I60.8
  - peripheral — *see* Malformation, arteriovenous, peripheral
  - precerebral vessels Q28.0
  - specified site NEC (*see also* Malformation, arteriovenous)
    - acquired I77.0
- basal — *see* Aneurysm, brain
- basilar (trunk) I72.5
- berry (congenital) (nonruptured) I67.1
  - ruptured I60.7
- brain I67.1
  - arteriosclerotic I67.1
    - ruptured — *see* Hemorrhage, intracranial, subarachnoid
  - arteriovenous (congenital) (nonruptured) Q28.2
    - acquired I67.1
      - ruptured I60.8
    - ruptured I60.8
  - berry (congenital) (nonruptured) I67.1
    - ruptured (*see also* Hemorrhage, intracranial, subarachnoid)I60.7
  - congenital Q28.3
    - ruptured I60.7
  - meninges I67.1
    - ruptured I60.8
  - miliary (congenital) (nonruptured) I67.1
    - ruptured (*see also* Hemorrhage, intracranial, subarachnoid)I60.7
  - mycotic I33.0
  - ruptured — *see* Hemorrhage, intracranial, subarachnoid
  - syphilitic (hemorrhage) A52.05
- cardiac (false) (*see also* Aneurysm, heart)I25.3
- carotid artery (common) (external) I72.0
  - internal (intracranial) I67.1
    - extracranial portion I72.0
  - ruptured into brain I60.0 ☑
  - syphilitic A52.09
    - intracranial A52.05
- cavernous sinus I67.1
  - arteriovenous (congenital) (nonruptured) Q28.3
    - ruptured I60.8
- celiac I72.8
- central nervous system, syphilitic A52.05
- cerebral — *see* Aneurysm, brain
- chest — *see* Aneurysm, thorax
- circle of Willis I67.1
  - congenital Q28.3
    - ruptured I60.6
  - ruptured I60.6
- common iliac artery I72.3
- congenital (peripheral) Q27.8
  - aorta (root) (sinus) Q25.43
  - brain Q28.3
    - ruptured I60.7
  - coronary Q24.5
  - digestive system Q27.8
  - lower limb Q27.8
  - pulmonary Q25.79
  - retina Q14.1
  - specified site NEC Q27.8
  - upper limb Q27.8
- conjunctiva — *see* Abnormality, conjunctiva, vascular
- conus arteriosus — *see* Aneurysm, heart
- coronary (arteriosclerotic) (artery) I25.41
  - arteriovenous, congenital Q24.5
  - congenital Q24.5
  - ruptured — *see* Infarct, myocardium
  - syphilitic A52.06
  - vein I25.89
- cylindroid (aorta) I71.9
  - ruptured I71.8
  - syphilitic A52.01
- ductus arteriosus Q25.0
- endocardial, infective (any valve) I33.0
- femoral (artery) (ruptured) I72.4
- gastroduodenal I72.8
- gastroepiploic I72.8
- heart (wall) (chronic or with a stated duration of over 4 weeks) I25.3
  - valve — *see* Endocarditis
- hepatic I72.8
- iliac (common) (artery) (ruptured) I72.3
- infective I72.9
  - endocardial (any valve) I33.0
- innominate (nonsyphilitic) I72.8
  - syphilitic A52.09

- **Aneurysm** — *continued*
  - interauricular septum — *see* Aneurysm, heart
  - interventricular septum — *see* Aneurysm, heart
  - intrathoracic (nonsyphilitic) I71.2
    - ruptured I71.1
    - syphilitic A52.01
  - lower limb I72.4
  - lung (pulmonary artery) I28.1
  - mediastinal (nonsyphilitic) I72.8
    - syphilitic A52.09
  - miliary (congenital) I67.1
    - ruptured — *see* Hemorrhage, intracerebral, subarachnoid, intracranial
  - mitral (heart) (valve) I34.8
  - mural — *see* Aneurysm, heart
  - mycotic I72.9
    - endocardial (any valve) I33.0
    - ruptured, brain — *see* Hemorrhage, intracerebral, subarachnoid
  - myocardium — *see* Aneurysm, heart
  - neck I72.0
  - pancreaticoduodenal I72.8
  - patent ductus arteriosus Q25.0
  - peripheral NEC I72.8
    - congenital Q27.8
      - digestive system Q27.8
      - lower limb Q27.8
      - specified site NEC Q27.8
      - upper limb Q27.8
  - popliteal (artery) (ruptured) I72.4
  - precerebral
    - congenital (nonruptured) Q28.1
    - specified site, NEC I72.5
  - pulmonary I28.1
    - arteriovenous Q25.72
      - acquired I28.0
    - syphilitic A52.09
    - valve (heart) — *see* Endocarditis, pulmonary
  - racemose (peripheral) I72.9
    - congenital — *see* Aneurysm, congenital
  - radial I72.1
  - Rasmussen NEC A15.0
  - renal (artery) I72.2
  - retina (*see also* Disorder, retina, microaneurysms)
    - congenital Q14.1
    - diabetic — *see* Diabetes, microaneurysms, retinal
  - sinus of Valsalva Q25.49
  - specified NEC I72.8
  - spinal (cord) I72.8
    - syphilitic (hemorrhage) A52.09
  - splenic I72.8
  - subclavian (artery) (ruptured) I72.8
    - syphilitic A52.09
  - superior mesenteric I72.8
  - syphilitic (aorta) A52.01
    - central nervous system A52.05
    - congenital (late) A50.54 *[I79.0]*
    - spine, spinal A52.09
  - thoracoabdominal (aorta) I71.6
    - ruptured I71.5
    - syphilitic A52.01
  - thorax, thoracic (aorta) (arch) (nonsyphilitic) I71.2
    - ruptured I71.1
    - syphilitic A52.01
  - traumatic (complication) (early), specified site — *see* Injury, blood vessel
  - tricuspid (heart) (valve) I07.8
  - ulnar I72.1
  - upper limb (ruptured) I72.1
  - valve, valvular — *see* Endocarditis
  - venous (*see also* Varix)I86.8
    - congenital Q27.8
      - digestive system Q27.8
      - lower limb Q27.8
      - specified site NEC Q27.8
      - upper limb Q27.8
  - ventricle — *see* Aneurysm, heart
  - vertebral artery I72.6
  - visceral NEC I72.8
- **Angelman** syndrome Q93.5
- **Anger** R45.4
- **Angiectasis,** angiectopia I99.8
- **Angiitis** I77.6
  - allergic granulomatous M30.1
  - hypersensitivity M31.0
  - necrotizing M31.9
    - specified NEC M31.8
  - nervous system, granulomatous I67.7
- **Angina** (attack) (cardiac) (chest) (heart) (pectoris) (syndrome) (vasomotor) I20.9
- **Angina** — *continued*
  - with
    - atherosclerotic heart disease — *see* Arteriosclerosis, coronary (artery),
    - documented spasm I20.1
  - abdominal K55.1
  - accelerated — *see* Angina, unstable
  - agranulocytic — *see* Agranulocytosis
  - angiospastic — *see* Angina, with documented spasm
  - aphthous B08.5
  - crescendo — *see* Angina, unstable
  - croupous J05.0
  - cruris I73.9
  - de novo effort — *see* Angina, unstable
  - diphtheritic, membranous A36.0
  - equivalent I20.8
  - exudative, chronic J37.0
  - following acute myocardial infarction I23.7
  - gangrenous diphtheritic A36.0
  - intestinal K55.1
  - Ludovici K12.2
  - Ludwig's K12.2
  - malignant diphtheritic A36.0
  - membranous J05.0
    - diphtheritic A36.0
    - Vincent's A69.1
  - mesenteric K55.1
  - monocytic — *see* Mononucleosis, infectious
  - of effort — *see* Angina, specified NEC
  - phlegmonous J36
    - diphtheritic A36.0
  - post-infarctional I23.7
  - pre-infarctional — *see* Angina, unstable
  - Prinzmetal — *see* Angina, with documented spasm
  - progressive — *see* Angina, unstable
  - pseudomembranous A69.1
  - pultaceous, diphtheritic A36.0
  - spasm-induced — *see* Angina, with documented spasm
  - specified NEC I20.8
  - stable I20.8
  - stenocardia — *see* Angina, specified NEC
  - stridulous, diphtheritic A36.2
  - tonsil J36
  - trachealis J05.0
  - unstable I20.0
  - variant — *see* Angina, with documented spasm
  - Vincent's A69.1
  - worsening effort — *see* Angina, unstable
- **Angioblastoma** — *see* Neoplasm, connective tissue, uncertain behavior
- **Angiocholecystitis** — *see* Cholecystitis, acute
- **Angiocholitis** (*see also* Cholecystitis, acute)K83.0
- **Angiodysgenesis** spinalis G95.19
- **Angiodysplasia** (cecum) (colon) K55.20
  - with bleeding K55.21
  - duodenum (and stomach) K31.819
    - with bleeding K31.811
  - stomach (and duodenum) K31.819
    - with bleeding K31.811
- **Angioedema** (allergic) (any site) (with urticaria) T78.3 ☑
  - hereditary D84.1
- **Angioendothelioma** — *see* Neoplasm, uncertain behavior, by site
  - benign D18.00
    - intra-abdominal D18.03
    - intracranial D18.02
    - skin D18.01
    - specified site NEC D18.09
  - bone — *see* Neoplasm, bone, malignant
  - Ewing's — *see* Neoplasm, bone, malignant
- **Angioendotheliomatosis** C85.8 ☑
- **Angiofibroma** (*see also* Neoplasm, benign, by site)
  - juvenile
    - specified site — *see* Neoplasm, benign, by site
    - unspecified site D10.6
- **Angiohemophilia** (A) (B) D68.0
- **Angioid** streaks (choroid) (macula) (retina) H35.33
- **Angiokeratoma** — *see* Neoplasm, skin, benign
  - corporis diffusum E75.21
- **Angioleiomyoma** — *see* Neoplasm, connective tissue, benign
- **Angiolipoma** (*see also* Lipoma)
  - infiltrating — *see* Lipoma
- **Angioma** (*see also* Hemangioma, by site)
  - capillary I78.1
  - hemorrhagicum hereditaria I78.0
  - intra-abdominal D18.03
  - intracranial D18.02
- **Angioma** — *continued*
  - malignant — *see* Neoplasm, connective tissue, malignant
  - plexiform D18.00
    - intra-abdominal D18.03
    - intracranial D18.02
    - skin D18.01
    - specified site NEC D18.09
  - senile I78.1
  - serpiginosum L81.7
  - skin D18.01
  - specified site NEC D18.09
  - spider I78.1
  - stellate I78.1
  - venous Q28.3
- **Angiomatosis** Q82.8
  - bacillary A79.89
  - encephalotrigeminal Q85.8
  - hemorrhagic familial I78.0
  - hereditary familial I78.0
  - liver K76.4
- **Angiomyolipoma** — *see* Lipoma
- **Angiomyoliposarcoma** — *see* Neoplasm, connective tissue, malignant
- **Angiomyoma** — *see* Neoplasm, connective tissue, benign
- **Angiomyosarcoma** — *see* Neoplasm, connective tissue, malignant
- **Angiomyxoma** — *see* Neoplasm, connective tissue, uncertain behavior
- **Angioneurosis** F45.8
- **Angioneurotic** edema (allergic) (any site) (with urticaria) T78.3 ☑
  - hereditary D84.1
- **Angiopathia,** angiopathy I99.9
  - cerebral I67.9
    - amyloid E85.4 *[I68.0]*
  - diabetic (peripheral) — *see* Diabetes, angiopathy
  - peripheral I73.9
    - diabetic — *see* Diabetes, angiopathy
    - specified type NEC I73.89
  - retinae syphilitica A52.05
  - retinalis (juvenilis)
    - diabetic — *see* Diabetes, retinopathy
    - proliferative — *see* Retinopathy, proliferative
- **Angiosarcoma** (*see also* Neoplasm, connective tissue, malignant)
  - liver C22.3
- **Angiosclerosis** — *see* Arteriosclerosis
- **Angiospasm** (peripheral) (traumatic) (vessel) I73.9
  - brachial plexus G54.0
  - cerebral G45.9
  - cervical plexus G54.2
  - nerve
    - arm — *see* Mononeuropathy, upper limb
      - axillary G54.0
      - median — *see* Lesion, nerve, median
      - ulnar — *see* Lesion, nerve, ulnar
    - axillary G54.0
    - leg — *see* Mononeuropathy, lower limb
    - median — *see* Lesion, nerve, median
    - plantar — *see* Lesion, nerve, plantar
    - ulnar — *see* Lesion, nerve, ulnar
- **Angiospastic** disease or edema I73.9
- **Angiostrongyliasis**
  - due to
    - Parastrongylus
      - cantonensis B83.2
      - costaricensis B81.3
  - intestinal B81.3
- **Anguillulosis** — *see* Strongyloidiasis
- **Angulation**
  - cecum — *see* Obstruction, intestine
  - coccyx (acquired) (*see also* subcategory)M43.8 ☑
    - congenital NEC Q76.49
  - femur (acquired) (*see also* Deformity, limb, specified type NEC, thigh)
    - congenital Q74.2
  - intestine (large) (small) — *see* Obstruction, intestine
  - sacrum (acquired) (*see also* subcategory)M43.8 ☑
    - congenital NEC Q76.49
  - sigmoid (flexure) — *see* Obstruction, intestine
  - spine — *see* Dorsopathy, deforming, specified NEC
  - tibia (acquired) (*see also* Deformity, limb, specified type NEC, lower leg)
    - congenital Q74.2
  - ureter N13.5
    - with infection N13.6
  - wrist (acquired) (*see also* Deformity, limb, specified type NEC, forearm)
    - congenital Q74.0

Anomaly

Anomaly — *continued*
- ear — *continued*
  - inner Q16.5
  - middle (causing impairment of hearing) Q16.4
  - ossicles Q16.3
- Ebstein's (heart) (tricuspid valve) Q22.5
- ectodermal Q82.9
- Eisenmenger's (ventricular septal defect) Q21.8
- ejaculatory duct Q55.4
- elbow Q74.0
- endocrine gland NEC Q89.2
- epididymis Q55.4
- epiglottis Q31.8
- esophagus Q39.9
- eustachian tube Q17.8
- eye Q15.9
  - anterior segment Q13.9
    - specified NEC Q13.89
  - posterior segment Q14.9
    - specified NEC Q14.8
  - ptosis (eyelid) Q10.0
  - specified NEC Q15.8
- eyebrow Q18.8
- eyelid Q10.3
  - ptosis Q10.0
- face Q18.9
  - bone (s) Q75.9
- fallopian tube Q50.6
- fascia Q79.9
- femur NEC Q74.2
- fibula NEC Q74.2
- finger Q74.0
- fixation, intestine Q43.3
- flexion (joint) NOS Q74.9
  - hip or thigh Q65.89
- foot NEC Q74.2
  - varus (congenital) Q66.3
- foramen
  - Botalli Q21.1
  - ovale Q21.1
- forearm Q74.0
- forehead Q75.8
- form, teeth K00.2
- fovea centralis Q14.1
- frontal bone — *see* Anomaly, skull
- gallbladder (position) (shape) (size) Q44.1
- Gartner's duct Q52.4
- gastrointestinal tract Q45.9
- genitalia, genital organ (s) or system
  - female Q52.9
    - external Q52.70
    - internal NOS Q52.9
  - male Q55.9
    - hydrocele P83.5
    - specified NEC Q55.8
- genitourinary NEC
  - female Q52.9
  - male Q55.9
- Gerbode Q21.0
- glottis Q31.8
- granulation or granulocyte, genetic (constitutional) (leukocyte) D72.0
- gum Q38.6
- gyri Q07.9
- hair Q84.2
- hand Q74.0
- hard tissue formation in pulp K04.3
- head — *see* Anomaly, skull
- heart Q24.9
  - auricle Q20.8
  - bands or folds Q24.8
  - fibroelastosis cordis I42.4
  - obstructive NEC Q22.6
  - patent ductus arteriosus (Botalli) Q25.0
  - septum Q21.9
    - auricular Q21.1
    - interatrial Q21.1
    - interventricular Q21.0
      - with pulmonary stenosis or atresia, dextraposition of aorta and hypertrophy of right ventricle Q21.3
    - specified NEC Q21.8
    - ventricular Q21.0
      - with pulmonary stenosis or atresia, dextraposition of aorta and hypertrophy of right ventricle Q21.3
  - tetralogy of Fallot Q21.3
  - valve NEC Q24.8
    - aortic
      - bicuspid valve Q23.1
      - insufficiency Q23.1
      - stenosis Q23.0

Anomaly — *continued*
- heart — *continued*
  - valve NEC — *continued*
    - aortic — *continued*
      - subaortic Q24.4
    - mitral
      - insufficiency Q23.3
      - stenosis Q23.2
    - pulmonary Q22.3
      - atresia Q22.0
      - insufficiency Q22.2
      - stenosis Q22.1
        - infundibular Q24.3
        - subvalvular Q24.3
    - tricuspid
      - atresia Q22.4
      - stenosis Q22.4
  - ventricle Q20.8
- heel NEC Q74.2
- Hegglin's D72.0
- hemianencephaly Q00.0
- hemicephaly Q00.0
- hemicrania Q00.0
- hepatic duct Q44.5
- hip NEC Q74.2
- hourglass stomach Q40.2
- humerus Q74.0
- hydatid of Morgagni
  - female Q50.5
  - male (epididymal) Q55.4
    - testicular Q55.29
- hymen Q52.4
- hypersegmentation of neutrophils, hereditary D72.0
- hypophyseal Q89.2
- ileocecal (coil) (valve) Q43.9
- ileum Q43.9
- ilium NEC Q74.2
- integument Q84.9
  - specified NEC Q84.8
- interarch distance (excessive) (inadequate) M26.25
- intervertebral cartilage or disc Q76.49
- intestine (large) (small) Q43.9
  - with anomalous adhesions, fixation or malrotation Q43.3
- iris Q13.2
- ischium NEC Q74.2
- jaw — *see* Anomaly, dentofacial
  - alveolar — *see* Anomaly, alveolar
- jaw-cranial base relationship — *see* Anomaly, dentofacial, jaw-cranial base relationship
- jejunum Q43.8
- joint Q74.9
  - specified NEC Q74.8
- Jordan's D72.0
- kidney (s) (calyx) (pelvis) Q63.9
  - artery Q27.2
  - specified NEC Q63.8
- Klippel-Feil (brevicollis) Q76.1
- knee Q74.1
- labium (majus) (minus) Q52.70
- labyrinth, membranous Q16.5
- lacrimal apparatus or duct Q10.6
- larynx, laryngeal (muscle) Q31.9
  - web (bed) Q31.0
- lens Q12.9
- leukocytes, genetic D72.0
  - granulation (constitutional) D72.0
- lid (fold) Q10.3
- ligament Q79.9
  - broad Q50.6
  - round Q52.8
- limb Q74.9
  - lower NEC Q74.2
    - reduction deformity — *see* Defect, reduction, lower limb
  - upper Q74.0
- lip Q38.0
- liver Q44.7
  - duct Q44.5
- lower limb NEC Q74.2
- lumbosacral (joint) (region) Q76.49
  - kyphosis — *see* Kyphosis, congenital
  - lordosis — *see* Lordosis, congenital
- lung (fissure) (lobe) Q33.9
- mandible — *see* Anomaly, dentofacial
- maxilla — *see* Anomaly, dentofacial
- May (-Hegglin) D72.0
- meatus urinarius NEC Q64.79
- meningeal bands or folds Q07.9
  - constriction of Q07.8
  - spinal Q06.9

Anomaly — *continued*
- meninges Q07.9
  - cerebral Q04.8
  - spinal Q06.9
- meningocele Q05.9
- mesentery Q45.9
- metacarpus Q74.0
- metatarsus NEC Q74.2
- middle ear Q16.4
  - ossicles Q16.3
- mitral (leaflets) (valve) Q23.9
  - insufficiency Q23.3
  - specified NEC Q23.8
  - stenosis Q23.2
- mouth Q38.6
- Müllerian (*see also* Anomaly, by site)
  - uterus NEC Q51.818
- multiple NEC Q89.7
- muscle Q79.9
  - eyelid Q10.3
- musculoskeletal system, except limbs Q79.9
- myocardium Q24.8
- nail Q84.6
- narrowness, eyelid Q10.3
- nasal sinus (wall) Q30.8
- neck (any part) Q18.9
- nerve Q07.9
  - acoustic Q07.8
  - optic Q07.8
- nervous system (central) Q07.9
- nipple Q83.9
- nose, nasal (bones) (cartilage) (septum) (sinus) Q30.9
  - specified NEC Q30.8
- ocular muscle Q15.8
- omphalomesenteric duct Q43.0
- opening, pulmonary veins Q26.4
- optic
  - disc Q14.2
  - nerve Q07.8
- opticociliary vessels Q13.2
- orbit (eye) Q10.7
- organ Q89.9
  - of Corti Q16.5
- origin
  - artery
    - innominate Q25.8
    - pulmonary Q25.79
    - renal Q27.2
    - subclavian Q25.48
- osseous meatus (ear) Q16.1
- ovary Q50.39
- oviduct Q50.6
- palate (hard) (soft) NEC Q38.5
- pancreas or pancreatic duct Q45.3
- papillary muscles Q24.8
- parathyroid gland Q89.2
- paraurethral ducts Q64.79
- parotid (gland) Q38.4
- patella Q74.1
- Pelger-Huët (hereditary hyposegmentation) D72.0
- pelvic girdle NEC Q74.2
- pelvis (bony) NEC Q74.2
  - rachitic E64.3
- penis (glans) Q55.69
- pericardium Q24.8
- peripheral vascular system Q27.9
- Peter's Q13.4
- pharynx Q38.8
- pigmentation L81.9
  - congenital Q82.8
- pituitary (gland) Q89.2
- pleural (folds) Q34.0
- portal vein Q26.5
  - connection Q26.5
- position, tooth, teeth, fully erupted M26.30
  - specified NEC M26.39
- precerebral vessel Q28.1
- prepuce Q55.69
- prostate Q55.4
- pulmonary Q33.9
  - artery NEC Q25.79
  - valve Q22.3
    - atresia Q22.0
    - insufficiency Q22.2
    - specified type NEC Q22.3
    - stenosis Q22.1
      - infundibular Q24.3
      - subvalvular Q24.3
  - venous connection Q26.4
    - partial Q26.3
    - total Q26.2

Anomaly — *continued*
- pupil Q13.2
  - function H57.00
    - anisocoria H57.02
    - Argyll Robertson pupil H57.01
    - miosis H57.03
    - mydriasis H57.04
    - specified type NEC H57.09
    - tonic pupil H57.05 ☑
- pylorus Q40.3
- radius Q74.0
- rectum Q43.9
- reduction (extremity) (limb)
  - femur (longitudinal) — *see* Defect, reduction, lower limb, longitudinal, femur
  - fibula (longitudinal) — *see* Defect, reduction, lower limb, longitudinal, fibula
  - lower limb — *see* Defect, reduction, lower limb
  - radius (longitudinal) — *see* Defect, reduction, upper limb, longitudinal, radius
  - tibia (longitudinal) — *see* Defect, reduction, lower limb, longitudinal, tibia
  - ulna (longitudinal) — *see* Defect, reduction, upper limb, longitudinal, ulna
  - upper limb — *see* Defect, reduction, upper limb
- refraction — *see* Disorder, refraction
- renal Q63.9
  - artery Q27.2
  - pelvis Q63.9
    - specified NEC Q63.8
- respiratory system Q34.9
  - specified NEC Q34.8
- retina Q14.1
- rib Q76.6
  - cervical Q76.5
- Rieger's Q13.81
- rotation — *see* Malrotation
  - hip or thigh Q65.89
- round ligament Q52.8
- sacroiliac (joint) NEC Q74.2
- sacrum NEC Q76.49
  - kyphosis — *see* Kyphosis, congenital
  - lordosis — *see* Lordosis, congenital
- saddle nose, syphilitic A50.57
- salivary duct or gland Q38.4
- scapula Q74.0
- scrotum — *see* Malformation, testis and scrotum
- sebaceous gland Q82.9
- seminal vesicles Q55.4
- sense organs NEC Q07.8
- sex chromosomes NEC (*see also* Anomaly, chromosomes)
  - female phenotype Q97.8
  - male phenotype Q98.9
- shoulder (girdle) (joint) Q74.0
- sigmoid (flexure) Q43.9
- simian crease Q82.8
- sinus of Valsalva Q25.49
- skeleton generalized Q78.9
- skin (appendage) Q82.9
- skull Q75.9
  - with
    - anencephaly Q00.0
    - encephalocele — *see* Encephalocele
    - hydrocephalus Q03.9
      - with spina bifida — *see* Spina bifida, by site, with hydrocephalus
    - microcephaly Q02
- specified organ or site NEC Q89.8
- spermatic cord Q55.4
- spine, spinal NEC Q76.49
  - column NEC Q76.49
    - kyphosis — *see* Kyphosis, congenital
    - lordosis — *see* Lordosis, congenital
  - cord Q06.9
  - nerve root Q07.8
- spleen Q89.09
  - agenesis Q89.01
- stenonian duct Q38.4
- sternum NEC Q76.7
- stomach Q40.3
- submaxillary gland Q38.4
- tarsus NEC Q74.2
- tendon Q79.9
- testis — *see* Malformation, testis and scrotum
- thigh NEC Q74.2
- thorax (wall) Q67.8
  - bony Q76.9
- throat Q38.8
- thumb Q74.0
- thymus gland Q89.2
- thyroid (gland) Q89.2
  - cartilage Q31.8

Anomaly — *continued*
- tibia NEC Q74.2
  - saber A50.56
- toe Q74.2
- tongue Q38.3
- tooth, teeth K00.9
  - eruption K00.6
  - position, fully erupted M26.30
  - spacing, fully erupted M26.30
- trachea (cartilage) Q32.1
- tragus Q17.9
- tricuspid (leaflet) (valve) Q22.9
  - atresia or stenosis Q22.4
  - Ebstein's Q22.5
- Uhl's (hypoplasia of myocardium, right ventricle) Q24.8
- ulna Q74.0
- umbilical artery Q27.0
- union
  - cricoid cartilage and thyroid cartilage Q31.8
  - thyroid cartilage and hyoid bone Q31.8
  - trachea with larynx Q31.8
- upper limb Q74.0
- urachus Q64.4
- ureter Q62.8
  - obstructive NEC Q62.39
    - cecoureterocele Q62.32
    - orthotopic ureterocele Q62.31
- urethra Q64.70
  - absence Q64.5
  - double Q64.74
  - fistula to rectum Q64.73
  - obstructive Q64.39
    - stricture Q64.32
  - prolapse Q64.71
  - specified type NEC Q64.79
- urinary tract Q64.9
- uterus Q51.9
  - with only one functioning horn Q51.4
- uvula Q38.5
- vagina Q52.4
- valleculae Q31.8
- valve (heart) NEC Q24.8
  - coronary sinus Q24.5
  - inferior vena cava Q24.8
  - pulmonary Q22.3
  - sinus coronario Q24.5
  - venae cavae inferioris Q24.8
- vas deferens Q55.4
- vascular Q27.9
  - brain Q28.3
  - ring Q25.45
- vein (s) (peripheral) Q27.9
  - brain Q28.3
  - cerebral Q28.3
  - coronary Q24.5
  - developmental Q28.3
  - great Q26.9
    - specified NEC Q26.8
- vena cava (inferior) (superior) Q26.9
- venous — *see* Anomaly, vein (s)
- venous return Q26.8
- ventricular
  - bands or folds Q24.8
  - septa Q21.0
- vertebra Q76.49
  - kyphosis — *see* Kyphosis, congenital
  - lordosis — *see* Lordosis, congenital
- vesicourethral orifice Q64.79
- vessel (s) Q27.9
  - optic papilla Q14.2
  - precerebral Q28.1
- vitelline duct Q43.0
- vitreous body or humor Q14.0
- vulva Q52.70
- wrist (joint) Q74.0

Anomia R48.8

Anonychia (congenital) Q84.3
- acquired L60.8

Anophthalmos, anophthalmus (congenital) (globe) Q11.1
- acquired Z90.01

Anopia, anopsia H53.46 ☑
- quadrant H53.46 ☑

Anorchia, anorchism, anorchidism Q55.0

Anorexia R63.0
- hysterical F44.89
- nervosa F50.00
  - atypical F50.9
  - binge-eating type F50.2
    - with purging F50.02
  - restricting type F50.01

Anorgasmy, psychogenic (female) F52.31
- male F52.32

Anosmia R43.0
- hysterical F44.6
- postinfectional J39.8

Anosognosia R41.89

Anosteoplasia Q78.9

Anovulatory cycle N97.0

Anoxemia R09.02
- newborn P84

Anoxia (pathological) R09.02
- altitude T70.29 ☑
- cerebral G93.1
  - complicating
    - anesthesia (general) (local) or other sedation T88.59 ☑
      - in labor and delivery O74.3
      - in pregnancy O29.21 ☑
      - postpartum, puerperal O89.2
    - delivery (cesarean) (instrumental) O75.4
  - during a procedure G97.81
  - newborn P84
  - resulting from a procedure G97.82
- due to
  - drowning T75.1 ☑
  - high altitude T70.29 ☑
- heart — *see* Insufficiency, coronary
- intrauterine P84
- myocardial — *see* Insufficiency, coronary
- newborn P84
- spinal cord G95.11
- systemic (by suffocation) (low content in atmosphere) — *see* Asphyxia, traumatic

Anteflexion — *see* Anteversion

Antenatal
- care (normal pregnancy) Z34.90
- screening (encounter for) of mother Z36

Antepartum — *see* condition

Anterior — *see* condition

Antero-occlusion M26.220

Anteversion
- cervix — *see* Anteversion, uterus
- femur (neck), congenital Q65.89
- uterus, uterine (cervix) (postinfectional) (postpartal, old) N85.4
  - congenital Q51.818
  - in pregnancy or childbirth — *see* Pregnancy, complicated by

Anthophobia F40.228

Anthracosilicosis J60

Anthracosis (lung) (occupational) J60
- lingua K14.3

Anthrax A22.9
- with pneumonia A22.1
- cerebral A22.8
- colitis A22.2
- cutaneous A22.0
- gastrointestinal A22.2
- inhalation A22.1
- intestinal A22.2
- meningitis A22.8
- pulmonary A22.1
- respiratory A22.1
- sepsis A22.7
- specified manifestation NEC A22.8

Anthropoid pelvis Q74.2
- with disproportion (fetopelvic) O33.0

Anthropophobia F40.10
- generalized F40.11

Antibodies, maternal (blood group) — *see* Isoimmunization, affecting management of pregnancy
- anti-D — *see* Isoimmunization, affecting management of pregnancy, Rh
  - newborn P55.0

Antibody
- anticardiolipin R76.0
  - with
    - hemorrhagic disorder D68.312
    - hypercoagulable state D68.61
- antiphosphatidylglycerol R76.0
  - with
    - hemorrhagic disorder D68.312
    - hypercoagulable state D68.61
- antiphosphatidylinositol R76.0
  - with
    - hemorrhagic disorder D68.312
    - hypercoagulable state D68.61
- antiphosphatidylserine R76.0
  - with
    - hemorrhagic disorder D68.312
    - hypercoagulable state D68.61

Antibody - Apraxia

Antibody — *continued*
- antiphospholipid R76.0
  - with
    - hemorrhagic disorder D68.312
    - hypercoagulable state D68.61

Anticardiolipin syndrome D68.61

Anticoagulant, circulating (intrinsic) (*see also* - Disorder, hemorrhagic)D68.318
- drug-induced (extrinsic) (*see also* - Disorder, hemorrhagic)D68.32
- iatrogenic D68.32

Antidiuretic hormone syndrome E22.2

Antimonial cholera — *see* Poisoning, antimony

Antiphospholipid
- antibody
  - with hemorrhagic disorder D68.312
  - syndrome D68.61

Antisocial personality F60.2

Antithrombinemia — *see* Circulating anticoagulants

Antithromboplastinemia D68.318

Antithromboplastinogenemia D68.318

Antitoxin complication or reaction — *see* Complications, vaccination

Antlophobia F40.228

Antritis J32.0
- maxilla J32.0
  - acute J01.00
    - recurrent J01.01
- stomach K29.60
  - with bleeding K29.61

Antrum, antral — *see* condition

Anuria R34
- calculous (impacted) (recurrent) (*see also* Calculus, urinary)N20.9
- following
  - abortion — *see* Abortion by type complicated by, renal failure
  - ectopic or molar pregnancy O08.4
- newborn P96.0
- postprocedural N99.0
- postrenal N13.8
- traumatic (following crushing) T79.5 ☑

Anus, anal — *see* condition

Anusitis K62.89

Anxiety F41.9
- depression F41.8
- episodic paroxysmal F41.0
- generalized F41.1
- hysteria F41.8
- neurosis F41.1
- panic type F41.0
- reaction F41.1
- separation, abnormal (of childhood) F93.0
- specified NEC F41.8
- state F41.1

Aorta, aortic — *see* condition

Aortectasia — *see* Ectasia, aorta
- with aneurysm — *see* Aneurysm, aorta

Aortitis (nonsyphilitic) (calcific) I77.6
- arteriosclerotic I70.0
- Doehle-Heller A52.02
- luetic A52.02
- rheumatic — *see* Endocarditis, acute, rheumatic
- specific (syphilitic) A52.02
- syphilitic A52.02
  - congenital A50.54 *[I79.1]*

Apathetic thyroid storm — *see* Thyrotoxicosis

Apathy R45.3

Apeirophobia F40.228

Apepsia K30
- psychogenic F45.8

Aperistalsis, esophagus K22.0

Apertognathia M26.29

Apert's syndrome Q87.0

Aphagia R13.0
- psychogenic F50.9

Aphakia (acquired) (postoperative) H27.0 ☑
- congenital Q12.3

Aphasia (amnestic) (global) (nominal) (semantic) (syntactic) R47.01
- acquired, with epilepsy (Landau-Kleffner syndrome) — *see* Epilepsy, specified NEC
- auditory (developmental) F80.2
- developmental (receptive type) F80.2
  - expressive type F80.1
  - Wernicke's F80.2
- following
  - cerebrovascular disease I69.920
    - cerebral infarction I69.320
    - intracerebral hemorrhage I69.120
    - nontraumatic intracranial hemorrhage NEC I69.220

Aphasia — *continued*
- following — *continued*
    - specified disease NEC I69.820
    - subarachnoid hemorrhage I69.020
- primary progressive G31.01 *[F02.80]*
  - with behavioral disturbance G31.01 *[F02.81]*
- progressive isolated G31.01 *[F02.80]*
  - with behavioral disturbance G31.01 *[F02.81]*
- sensory F80.2
- syphilis, tertiary A52.19
- Wernicke's (developmental) F80.2

Aphonia (organic) R49.1
- hysterical F44.4
- psychogenic F44.4

Aphthae, aphthous (*see also* condition)
- Bednar's K12.0
- cachectic K14.0
- epizootic B08.8
- fever B08.8
- oral (recurrent) K12.0
- stomatitis (major) (minor) K12.0
- thrush B37.0
- ulcer (oral) (recurrent) K12.0
  - genital organ (s) NEC
    - female N76.6
    - male N50.89
  - larynx J38.7

Apical — *see* condition

Apiphobia F40.218

Aplasia (*see also* Agenesis)
- abdominal muscle syndrome Q79.4
- alveolar process (acquired) — *see* Anomaly, alveolar
  - congenital Q38.6
- aorta (congenital) Q25.41
- axialis extracorticalis (congenita) E75.29
- bone marrow (myeloid) D61.9
  - congenital D61.01
- brain Q00.0
  - part of Q04.3
- bronchus Q32.4
- cementum K00.4
- cerebellum Q04.3
- cervix (congenital) Q51.5
- congenital pure red cell D61.01
- corpus callosum Q04.0
- cutis congenita Q84.8
- erythrocyte congenital D61.01
- extracortical axial E75.29
- eye Q11.1
- fovea centralis (congenital) Q14.1
- gallbladder, congenital Q44.0
- iris Q13.1
- labyrinth, membranous Q16.5
- limb (congenital) Q73.8
  - lower — *see* Defect, reduction, lower limb
  - upper — *see* Agenesis, arm
- lung, congenital (bilateral) (unilateral) Q33.3
- pancreas Q45.0
- parathyroid-thymic D82.1
- Pelizaeus-Merzbacher E75.29
- penis Q55.5
- prostate Q55.4
- red cell (with thymoma) D60.9
  - acquired D60.9
    - due to drugs D60.9
  - adult D60.9
  - chronic D60.0
  - congenital D61.01
  - constitutional D61.01
  - due to drugs D60.9
  - hereditary D61.01
  - of infants D61.01
  - primary D61.01
  - pure D61.01
    - due to drugs D60.9
  - specified type NEC D60.8
  - transient D60.1
- round ligament Q52.8
- skin Q84.8
- spermatic cord Q55.4
- spleen Q89.01
- testicle Q55.0
- thymic, with immunodeficiency D82.1
- thyroid (congenital) (with myxedema) E03.1
- uterus Q51.0
- ventral horn cell Q06.1

Apnea, apneic (of) (spells) R06.81
- newborn NEC P28.4
  - obstructive P28.4
  - sleep (central) (obstructive) (primary) P28.3
- prematurity P28.4

Apnea — *continued*
- sleep G47.30
  - central (primary) G47.31
    - in conditions classified elsewhere G47.37
  - obstructive (adult) (pediatric) G47.33
  - primary central G47.31
  - specified NEC G47.39

Apneumatosis, newborn P28.0

Apocrine metaplasia (breast) — *see* Dysplasia, mammary, specified type NEC

Apophysitis (bone) (*see also* Osteochondropathy)
- calcaneus M92.8
- juvenile M92.9

Apoplectiform convulsions (cerebral ischemia) I67.82

Apoplexia, apoplexy, apoplectic
- adrenal A39.1
- heart (auricle) (ventricle) — *see* Infarct, myocardium
- heat T67.0 ☑
- hemorrhagic (stroke) — *see* Hemorrhage, intracranial
- meninges, hemorrhagic — *see* Hemorrhage, intracranial, subarachnoid
- uremic N18.9 *[I68.8]*

Appearance
- bizarre R46.1
- specified NEC R46.89
- very low level of personal hygiene R46.0

Appendage
- epididymal (organ of Morgagni) Q55.4
- intestine (epiploic) Q43.8
- preauricular Q17.0
- testicular (organ of Morgagni) Q55.29

Appendicitis (pneumococcal) (retrocecal) K37
- with
  - perforation or rupture K35.2
  - peritoneal abscess K35.3
  - peritonitis NEC K35.3
    - generalized (with perforation or rupture) K35.2
    - localized (with perforation or rupture) K35.3
- acute (catarrhal) (fulminating) (gangrenous) (obstructive) (retrocecal) (suppurative) K35.80
  - with
    - peritoneal abscess K35.3
    - peritonitis NEC K35.3
      - generalized (with perforation or rupture) K35.2
      - localized (with perforation or rupture) K35.3
  - specified NEC K35.89
- amebic A06.89
- chronic (recurrent) K36
- exacerbation — *see* Appendicitis, acute
- gangrenous — *see* Appendicitis, acute
- healed (obliterative) K36
- interval K36
- neurogenic K36
- obstructive K36
- recurrent K36
- relapsing K36
- subacute (adhesive) K36
- subsiding K36
- suppurative — *see* Appendicitis, acute
- tuberculous A18.32

Appendicopathia oxyurica B80

Appendix, appendicular (*see also* condition)
- epididymis Q55.4
- Morgagni
  - female Q50.5
  - male (epididymal) Q55.4
    - testicular Q55.29
- testis Q55.29

Appetite
- depraved — *see* Pica
- excessive R63.2
- lack or loss (*see also* Anorexia)R63.0
  - nonorganic origin F50.89
  - psychogenic F50.89
- perverted (hysterical) — *see* Pica

Apple peel syndrome Q41.1

Apprehension state F41.1

Apprehensiveness, abnormal F41.9

Approximal wear K03.0

Apraxia (classic) (ideational) (ideokinetic) (ideomotor) (motor) (verbal) R48.2
- following
  - cerebrovascular disease I69.990
    - cerebral infarction I69.390
    - intracerebral hemorrhage I69.190

- **Apraxia** — *continued*
  - following — *continued*
    - nontraumatic intracranial hemorrhage NEC I69.290
    - specified disease NEC I69.890
    - subarachnoid hemorrhage I69.090
  - oculomotor, congenital H51.8
- **Aptyalism** K11.7
- **Apudoma** — *see* Neoplasm, uncertain behavior, by site
- **Aqueous** misdirection H40.83 ☑
- **Arabicum** elephantiasis — *see* Infestation, filarial
- **Arachnitis** — *see* Meningitis
- **Arachnodactyly** — *see* Syndrome, Marfan's
- **Arachnoiditis** (acute) (adhesive) (basal) (brain) (cerebrospinal) — *see* Meningitis
- **Arachnophobia** F40.210
- **Arboencephalitis,** Australian A83.4
- **Arborization** block (heart) I45.5
- **ARC** (AIDS-related complex) B20
- **Arches** — *see* condition
- **Arcuate** uterus Q51.810
- **Arcuatus** uterus Q51.810
- **Arcus** (cornea) senilis — *see* Degeneration, cornea, senile
- **Arc-welder's** lung J63.4
- **Areflexia** R29.2
- **Areola** — *see* condition
- **Argentaffinoma** (*see also* Neoplasm, uncertain behavior, by site)
  - malignant — *see* Neoplasm, malignant, by site
  - syndrome E34.0
- **Argininemia** E72.21
- **Arginosuccinic** aciduria E72.22
- **Argyll** Robertson phenomenon, pupil or syndrome (syphilitic) A52.19
  - atypical H57.09
  - nonsyphilitic H57.09
- **Argyria,** argyriasis
  - conjunctival H11.13 ☑
  - from drug or medicament — *see* Table of Drugs and Chemicals, by substance
- **Argyrosis,** conjunctival H11.13 ☑
- **Arhinencephaly** Q04.1
- **Ariboflavinosis** E53.0
- **Arm** — *see* condition
- **Arnold-Chiari** disease, obstruction or syndrome (type II) Q07.00
  - with
    - hydrocephalus Q07.02
      - with spina bifida Q07.03
    - spina bifida Q07.01
      - with hydrocephalus Q07.03
  - type III — *see* Encephalocele
  - type IV Q04.8
- **Aromatic** amino-acid metabolism disorder E70.9
  - specified NEC E70.8
- **Arousals,** confusional G47.51
- **Arrest,** arrested
  - cardiac I46.9
    - complicating
      - abortion — *see* Abortion, by type, complicated by, cardiac arrest
      - anesthesia (general) (local) or other sedation — *see* Table of Drugs and Chemicals, by drug,
        - in labor and delivery O74.2
        - in pregnancy O29.11 ☑
        - postpartum, puerperal O89.1
      - delivery (cesarean) (instrumental) O75.4
    - due to
      - cardiac condition I46.2
      - specified condition NEC I46.8
    - intraoperative I97.71 ☑
    - newborn P29.81
    - postprocedural I97.12 ☑
      - obstetric procedure O75.4
  - cardiorespiratory — *see* Arrest, cardiac
  - circulatory — *see* Arrest, cardiac
  - deep transverse O64.0 ☑
  - development or growth
    - bone — *see* Disorder, bone, development or growth
    - child R62.50
    - tracheal rings Q32.1
  - epiphyseal
    - complete
      - femur M89.15 ☑
      - humerus M89.12 ☑
      - tibia M89.16 ☑
      - ulna M89.13 ☑
    - forearm M89.13 ☑
- **Arrest** — *continued*
  - epiphyseal — *continued*
    - specified NEC M89.13 ☑
    - ulna — *see* Arrest, epiphyseal, by type, ulna
    - lower leg M89.16 ☑
      - specified NEC M89.168
      - tibia — *see* Arrest, epiphyseal, by type, tibia
    - partial
      - femur M89.15 ☑
      - humerus M89.12 ☑
      - tibia M89.16 ☑
      - ulna M89.13 ☑
    - specified NEC M89.18
  - granulopoiesis — *see* Agranulocytosis
  - growth plate — *see* Arrest, epiphyseal
  - heart — *see* Arrest, cardiac
  - legal, anxiety concerning Z65.3
  - physeal — *see* Arrest, epiphyseal
  - respiratory R09.2
    - newborn P28.81
  - sinus I45.5
  - spermatogenesis (complete) — *see* Azoospermia
    - incomplete — *see* Oligospermia
  - transverse (deep) O64.0 ☑
- **Arrhenoblastoma**
  - benign
    - specified site — *see* Neoplasm, benign, by site
    - unspecified site
      - female D27.9
      - male D29.20
  - malignant
    - specified site — *see* Neoplasm, malignant, by site
    - unspecified site
      - female C56.9
      - male C62.90
  - specified site — *see* Neoplasm, uncertain behavior, by site
  - unspecified site
    - female D39.10
    - male D40.10
- **Arrhythmia** (auricle) (cardiac) (juvenile) (nodal) (reflex) (sinus) (supraventricular) (transitory) (ventricle) I49.9
  - block I45.9
  - extrasystolic I49.49
  - newborn
    - bradycardia P29.12
    - occurring before birth P03.819
      - before onset of labor P03.810
      - during labor P03.811
    - tachycardia P29.11
  - psychogenic F45.8
  - specified NEC I49.8
  - vagal R55
  - ventricular re-entry I47.0
- **Arrillaga-Ayerza** syndrome (pulmonary sclerosis with pulmonary hypertension) I27.0
- **Arsenical** pigmentation L81.8
  - from drug or medicament — *see* Table of Drugs and Chemicals
- **Arsenism** — *see* Poisoning, arsenic
- **Arterial** — *see* condition
- **Arteriofibrosis** — *see* Arteriosclerosis
- **Arteriolar** sclerosis — *see* Arteriosclerosis
- **Arteriolith** — *see* Arteriosclerosis
- **Arteriolitis** I77.6
  - necrotizing, kidney I77.5
  - renal — *see* Hypertension, kidney
- **Arteriolosclerosis** — *see* Arteriosclerosis
- **Arterionephrosclerosis** — *see* Hypertension, kidney
- **Arteriopathy** I77.9
- **Arteriosclerosis,** arteriosclerotic (diffuse) (obliterans) (of) (senile) (with calcification) I70.90
  - aorta I70.0
  - arteries of extremities — *see* Arteriosclerosis, extremities
  - brain I67.2
  - bypass graft
    - coronary — *see* Arteriosclerosis, coronary, bypass graft
    - extremities — *see* Arteriosclerosis, extremities, bypass graft
  - cardiac — *see* Disease, heart, ischemic, atherosclerotic
  - cardiopathy — *see* Disease, heart, ischemic, atherosclerotic
  - cardiorenal — *see* Hypertension, cardiorenal
  - cardiovascular — *see* Disease, heart, ischemic, atherosclerotic
  - carotid (*see also* Occlusion, artery, carotid)I65.2 ☑
  - central nervous system I67.2
- **Arteriosclerosis** — *continued*
  - cerebral I67.2
  - cerebrovascular I67.2
  - coronary (artery) I25.10
    - due to
      - calcified coronary lesion (severely) I25.84
      - lipid rich plaque I25.83
    - bypass graft I25.810
      - with
        - angina pectoris I25.709
          - with documented spasm I25.701
          - specified type NEC I25.708
          - unstable I25.700
        - ischemic chest pain I25.709
      - autologous artery I25.810
        - with
          - angina pectoris I25.729
            - with documented spasm I25.721
            - specified type I25.728
            - unstable I25.720
          - ischemic chest pain I25.729
      - autologous vein I25.810
        - with
          - angina pectoris I25.719
            - with documented spasm I25.711
            - specified type I25.718
            - unstable I25.710
          - ischemic chest pain I25.719
      - nonautologous biological I25.810
        - with
          - angina pectoris I25.739
            - with documented spasm I25.731
            - specified type I25.738
            - unstable I25.730
          - ischemic chest pain I25.739
      - specified type NEC I25.810
        - with
          - angina pectoris I25.799
            - with documented spasm I25.791
            - specified type I25.798
            - unstable I25.790
          - ischemic chest pain I25.799
    - native vessel
      - with
        - angina pectoris I25.119
          - with documented spasm I25.111
          - specified type NEC I25.118
          - unstable I25.110
        - ischemic chest pain I25.119
    - transplanted heart I25.811
      - bypass graft I25.812
        - with
          - angina pectoris I25.769
            - with documented spasm I25.761
            - specified type I25.768
            - unstable I25.760
          - ischemic chest pain I25.769
      - native coronary artery I25.811
        - with
          - angina pectoris I25.759
            - with documented spasm I25.751
            - specified type I25.758
            - unstable I25.750
          - ischemic chest pain I25.759
  - extremities (native arteries) I70.209
    - bypass graft I70.309
      - autologous vein graft I70.409
        - leg I70.409
          - with
            - gangrene (and intermittent claudication, rest pain and ulcer) I70.469
            - intermittent claudication I70.419
            - rest pain (and intermittent claudication) I70.429
          - bilateral I70.403
            - with
              - gangrene (and intermittent claudication, rest pain and ulcer) I70.463
              - intermittent claudication I70.413
              - rest pain (and intermittent claudication) I70.423
            - specified type NEC I70.493
          - left I70.402
            - with
              - gangrene (and intermittent claudication, rest pain and ulcer) I70.462
              - intermittent claudication I70.412
              - rest pain (and intermittent claudication) I70.422

- **Arteriosclerosis** — *continued*
  - extremities — *continued*
              - ulceration (and intermittent claudication and rest pain) I70.449
                - ankle I70.443
                - calf I70.442
                - foot site NEC I70.445
                - heel I70.444
                - lower leg NEC I70.448
                - midfoot I70.444
                - thigh I70.441
            - specified type NEC I70.492
          - right I70.401
            - with
              - gangrene (and intermittent claudication, rest pain and ulcer) I70.461
              - intermittent claudication I70.411
              - rest pain (and intermittent claudication) I70.421
              - ulceration (and intermittent claudication and rest pain) I70.439
                - ankle I70.433
                - calf I70.432
                - foot site NEC I70.435
                - heel I70.434
                - lower leg NEC I70.438
                - midfoot I70.434
                - thigh I70.431
            - specified type NEC I70.491
          - specified type NEC I70.499
        - specified NEC I70.408
          - with
            - gangrene (and intermittent claudication, rest pain and ulcer) I70.468
            - intermittent claudication I70.418
            - rest pain (and intermittent claudication) I70.428
            - ulceration (and intermittent claudication and rest pain) I70.45
          - specified type NEC I70.498
      - leg I70.309
        - with
          - gangrene (and intermittent claudication, rest pain and ulcer) I70.369
          - intermittent claudication I70.319
          - rest pain (and intermittent claudication) I70.329
        - bilateral I70.303
          - with
            - gangrene (and intermittent claudication, rest pain and ulcer) I70.363
            - intermittent claudication I70.313
            - rest pain (and intermittent claudication) I70.323
          - specified type NEC I70.393
        - left I70.302
          - with
            - gangrene (and intermittent claudication, rest pain and ulcer) I70.362
            - intermittent claudication I70.312
            - rest pain (and intermittent claudication) I70.322
            - ulceration (and intermittent claudication and rest pain) I70.349
              - ankle I70.343
              - calf I70.342
              - foot site NEC I70.345
              - heel I70.344
              - lower leg NEC I70.348
              - midfoot I70.344
              - thigh I70.341
          - specified type NEC I70.392
        - right I70.301
          - with
            - gangrene (and intermittent claudication, rest pain and ulcer) I70.361
            - intermittent claudication I70.311
            - rest pain (and intermittent claudication) I70.321
            - ulceration (and intermittent claudication and rest pain) I70.339
              - ankle I70.333
              - calf I70.332
              - foot site NEC I70.335
              - heel I70.334

- **Arteriosclerosis** — *continued*
  - extremities — *continued*
              - lower leg NEC I70.338
              - midfoot I70.334
              - thigh I70.331
          - specified type NEC I70.391
        - specified type NEC I70.399
      - nonautologous biological graft I70.509
        - leg I70.509
          - with
            - gangrene (and intermittent claudication, rest pain and ulcer) I70.569
            - intermittent claudication I70.519
            - rest pain (and intermittent claudication) I70.529
          - bilateral I70.503
            - with
              - gangrene (and intermittent claudication, rest pain and ulcer) I70.563
              - intermittent claudication I70.513
              - rest pain (and intermittent claudication) I70.523
            - specified type NEC I70.593
          - left I70.502
            - with
              - gangrene (and intermittent claudication, rest pain and ulcer) I70.562
              - intermittent claudication I70.512
              - rest pain (and intermittent claudication) I70.522
              - ulceration (and intermittent claudication and rest pain) I70.549
                - ankle I70.543
                - calf I70.542
                - foot site NEC I70.545
                - heel I70.544
                - lower leg NEC I70.548
                - midfoot I70.544
                - thigh I70.541
            - specified type NEC I70.592
          - right I70.501
            - with
              - gangrene (and intermittent claudication, rest pain and ulcer) I70.561
              - intermittent claudication I70.511
              - rest pain (and intermittent claudication) I70.521
              - ulceration (and intermittent claudication and rest pain) I70.539
                - ankle I70.533
                - calf I70.532
                - foot site NEC I70.535
                - heel I70.534
                - lower leg NEC I70.538
                - midfoot I70.534
                - thigh I70.531
            - specified type NEC I70.591
          - specified type NEC I70.599
        - specified NEC I70.508
          - with
            - gangrene (and intermittent claudication, rest pain and ulcer) I70.568
            - intermittent claudication I70.518
            - rest pain (and intermittent claudication) I70.528
            - ulceration (and intermittent claudication and rest pain) I70.55
          - specified type NEC I70.598
      - nonbiological graft I70.609
        - leg I70.609
          - with
            - gangrene (and intermittent claudication, rest pain and ulcer) I70.669
            - intermittent claudication I70.619
            - rest pain (and intermittent claudication) I70.629
          - bilateral I70.603
            - with
              - gangrene (and intermittent claudication, rest pain and ulcer) I70.663
              - intermittent claudication I70.613
              - rest pain (and intermittent claudication) I70.623

- **Arteriosclerosis** — *continued*
  - extremities — *continued*
            - specified type NEC I70.693
          - left I70.602
            - with
              - gangrene (and intermittent claudication, rest pain and ulcer) I70.662
              - intermittent claudication I70.612
              - rest pain (and intermittent claudication) I70.622
              - ulceration (and intermittent claudication and rest pain) I70.649
                - ankle I70.643
                - calf I70.642
                - foot site NEC I70.645
                - heel I70.644
                - lower leg NEC I70.648
                - midfoot I70.644
                - thigh I70.641
            - specified type NEC I70.692
          - right I70.601
            - with
              - gangrene (and intermittent claudication, rest pain and ulcer) I70.661
              - intermittent claudication I70.611
              - rest pain (and intermittent claudication) I70.621
              - ulceration (and intermittent claudication and rest pain) I70.639
                - ankle I70.633
                - calf I70.632
                - foot site NEC I70.635
                - heel I70.634
                - lower leg NEC I70.638
                - midfoot I70.634
                - thigh I70.631
            - specified type NEC I70.691
          - specified type NEC I70.699
        - specified NEC I70.608
          - with
            - gangrene (and intermittent claudication, rest pain and ulcer) I70.668
            - intermittent claudication I70.618
            - rest pain (and intermittent claudication) I70.628
            - ulceration (and intermittent claudication and rest pain) I70.65
          - specified type NEC I70.698
      - specified graft NEC I70.709
        - leg I70.709
          - with
            - gangrene (and intermittent claudication, rest pain and ulcer) I70.769
            - intermittent claudication I70.719
            - rest pain (and intermittent claudication) I70.729
          - bilateral I70.703
            - with
              - gangrene (and intermittent claudication, rest pain and ulcer) I70.763
              - intermittent claudication I70.713
              - rest pain (and intermittent claudication) I70.723
            - specified type NEC I70.793
          - left I70.702
            - with
              - gangrene (and intermittent claudication, rest pain and ulcer) I70.762
              - intermittent claudication I70.712
              - rest pain (and intermittent claudication) I70.722
              - ulceration (and intermittent claudication and rest pain) I70.749
                - ankle I70.743
                - calf I70.742
                - foot site NEC I70.745
                - heel I70.744
                - lower leg NEC I70.748
                - midfoot I70.744
                - thigh I70.741
            - specified type NEC I70.792
          - right I70.701
            - with

- **Arteriosclerosis** — *continued*
  - extremities — *continued*
              - gangrene (and intermittent claudication, rest pain and ulcer) I70.761
              - intermittent claudication I70.711
              - rest pain (and intermittent claudication) I70.721
              - ulceration (and intermittent claudication and rest pain) I70.739
                - ankle I70.733
                - calf I70.732
                - foot site NEC I70.735
                - heel I70.734
                - lower leg NEC I70.738
                - midfoot I70.734
                - thigh I70.731
            - specified type NEC I70.791
          - specified type NEC I70.799
        - specified NEC I70.708
          - with
            - gangrene (and intermittent claudication, rest pain and ulcer) I70.768
            - intermittent claudication I70.718
            - rest pain (and intermittent claudication) I70.728
            - ulceration (and intermittent claudication and rest pain) I70.75
          - specified type NEC I70.798
      - specified NEC I70.308
        - with
          - gangrene (and intermittent claudication, rest pain and ulcer) I70.368
          - intermittent claudication I70.318
          - rest pain (and intermittent claudication) I70.328
          - ulceration (and intermittent claudication and rest pain) I70.35
        - specified type NEC I70.398
    - leg I70.209
      - with
        - gangrene (and intermittent claudication, rest pain and ulcer) I70.269
        - intermittent claudication I70.219
        - rest pain (and intermittent claudication) I70.229
      - bilateral I70.203
        - with
          - gangrene (and intermittent claudication, rest pain and ulcer) I70.263
          - intermittent claudication I70.213
          - rest pain (and intermittent claudication) I70.223
        - specified type NEC I70.293
      - left I70.202
        - with
          - gangrene (and intermittent claudication, rest pain and ulcer) I70.262
          - intermittent claudication I70.212
          - rest pain (and intermittent claudication) I70.222
          - ulceration (and intermittent claudication and rest pain) I70.249
            - ankle I70.243
            - calf I70.242
            - foot site NEC I70.245
            - heel I70.244
            - lower leg NEC I70.248
            - midfoot I70.244
            - thigh I70.241
        - specified type NEC I70.292
      - right I70.201
        - with
          - gangrene (and intermittent claudication, rest pain and ulcer) I70.261
          - intermittent claudication I70.211
          - rest pain (and intermittent claudication) I70.221
          - ulceration (and intermittent claudication and rest pain) I70.239
            - ankle I70.233
            - calf I70.232
            - foot site NEC I70.235
            - heel I70.234
            - lower leg NEC I70.238
            - midfoot I70.234
            - thigh I70.231
        - specified type NEC I70.291
      - specified type NEC I70.299
    - specified site NEC I70.208

- **Arteriosclerosis** — *continued*
  - extremities — *continued*
    - with
      - gangrene (and intermittent claudication, rest pain and ulcer) I70.268
      - intermittent claudication I70.218
      - rest pain (and intermittent claudication) I70.228
      - ulceration (and intermittent claudication and rest pain) I70.25
    - specified type NEC I70.298
  - generalized I70.91
  - heart (disease) — *see* Arteriosclerosis, coronary (artery),
  - kidney — *see* Hypertension, kidney
  - medial — *see* Arteriosclerosis, extremities
  - mesenteric (artery) K55.1
  - Mönckeberg's — *see* Arteriosclerosis, extremities
  - myocarditis I51.4
  - peripheral (of extremities) — *see* Arteriosclerosis, extremities
  - pulmonary (idiopathic) I27.0
  - renal (arterioles) (*see also* Hypertension, kidney)
    - artery I70.1
  - retina (vascular) I70.8 *[H35.0-]*
  - specified artery NEC I70.8
  - spinal (cord) G95.19
  - vertebral (artery) I67.2
- **Arteriospasm** I73.9
- **Arteriovenous** — *see* condition
- **Arteritis** I77.6
  - allergic M31.0
  - aorta (nonsyphilitic) I77.6
    - syphilitic A52.02
  - aortic arch M31.4
  - brachiocephalic M31.4
  - brain I67.7
    - syphilitic A52.04
  - cerebral I67.7
    - in
      - diseases classified elsewhere I68.2
      - systemic lupus erythematosus M32.19
    - listerial A32.89
    - syphilitic A52.04
    - tuberculous A18.89
  - coronary (artery) I25.89
    - rheumatic I01.8
      - chronic I09.89
    - syphilitic A52.06
  - cranial (left) (right), giant cell M31.6
  - deformans — *see* Arteriosclerosis
  - giant cell NEC M31.6
    - with polymyalgia rheumatica M31.5
  - necrosing or necrotizing M31.9
    - specified NEC M31.8
  - nodosa M30.0
  - obliterans — *see* Arteriosclerosis
  - pulmonary I28.8
  - rheumatic — *see* Fever, rheumatic
  - senile — *see* Arteriosclerosis
  - suppurative I77.2
  - syphilitic (general) A52.09
    - brain A52.04
    - coronary A52.06
    - spinal A52.09
  - temporal, giant cell M31.6
  - young female aortic arch syndrome M31.4
- **Artery, arterial** (*see also* condition)
  - abscess I77.89
  - single umbilical Q27.0
- **Arthralgia** (allergic) (*see also* Pain, joint)
  - in caisson disease T70.3 ☑
  - temporomandibular M26.62 ☑
- **Arthritis**, arthritic (acute) (chronic) (nonpyogenic) (subacute) M19.90
  - allergic — *see* Arthritis, specified form NEC
  - ankylosing (crippling) (spine) (*see also* Spondylitis, ankylosing)
    - sites other than spine — *see* Arthritis, specified form NEC
  - atrophic — *see* Osteoarthritis
    - spine — *see* Spondylitis, ankylosing
  - back — *see* Spondylopathy, inflammatory
  - blennorrhagic (gonococcal) A54.42
  - Charcot's — *see* Arthropathy, neuropathic
    - diabetic — *see* Diabetes, arthropathy, neuropathic
    - syringomyelic G95.0
  - chylous (filarial) (*see also* category M01)B74.9
  - climacteric (any site) NEC — *see* Arthritis, specified form NEC
  - crystal (-induced) — *see* Arthritis, in, crystals

- **Arthritis** — *continued*
  - deformans — *see* Osteoarthritis
  - degenerative — *see* Osteoarthritis
  - due to or associated with
    - acromegaly E22.0
    - brucellosis — *see* Brucellosis
    - caisson disease T70.3 ☑
    - diabetes — *see* Diabetes, arthropathy
    - dracontiasis (*see also* category M01)B72
    - enteritis NEC
      - regional — *see* Enteritis, regional
    - erysipelas (*see also* category M01)A46
    - erythema
      - epidemic A25.1
      - nodosum L52
    - filariasis NOS B74.9
    - glanders A24.0
    - helminthiasis (*see also* category M01)B83.9
    - hemophilia D66 *[M36.2]*
    - Henoch- (Schönlein) purpura D69.0 *[M36.4]*
    - human parvovirus (*see also* category M01)B97.6
    - infectious disease NEC M01
    - leprosy (see also category M01) (*see also* Leprosy)A30.9
    - Lyme disease A69.23
    - mycobacteria (*see also* category M01)A31.8
    - parasitic disease NEC (*see also* category M01)B89
    - paratyphoid fever (see also category M01) (*see also* Fever, paratyphoid)A01.4
    - rat bite fever (*see also* category M01)A25.1
    - regional enteritis — *see* Enteritis, regional
    - respiratory disorder NOS J98.9
    - serum sickness (*see also* Reaction, serum)T80.69 ☑
    - syringomyelia G95.0
    - typhoid fever A01.04
  - epidemic erythema A25.1
  - febrile — *see* Fever, rheumatic
  - gonococcal A54.42
  - gouty (acute) — *see* Gout
  - in (due to)
    - acromegaly (*see also* subcategory M14.8-)E22.0
    - amyloidosis (*see also* subcategory M14.8-)E85.4
    - bacterial disease (*see also* subcategory M01)A49.9
    - Behçet's syndrome M35.2
    - caisson disease (*see also* subcategory M14.8-) T70.3 ☑
    - coliform bacilli (Escherichia coli) — *see* Arthritis, in, pyogenic organism NEC
    - crystals M11.9
      - dicalcium phosphate — *see* Arthritis, in, crystals, specified type NEC
      - hydroxyapatite M11.0 ☑
      - pyrophosphate — *see* Arthritis, in, crystals, specified type NEC
      - specified type NEC M11.80
        - ankle M11.87 ☑
        - elbow M11.82 ☑
        - foot joint M11.87 ☑
        - hand joint M11.84 ☑
        - hip M11.85 ☑
        - knee M11.86 ☑
        - multiple sites M11.8 ☑
        - shoulder M11.81 ☑
        - vertebrae M11.88
        - wrist M11.83 ☑
    - dermatoarthritis, lipoid E78.81
    - dracontiasis (dracunculiasis) (*see also* category M01)B72
    - endocrine disorder NEC (*see also* subcategory M14.8-)E34.9
    - enteritis, infectious NEC (*see also* category M01)A09
      - specified organism NEC (*see also* category M01)A08.8
    - erythema
      - multiforme (*see also* subcategory M14.8-) L51.9
      - nodosum (*see also* subcategory M14.8-)L52
    - gout — *see* Gout
    - helminthiasis NEC (*see also* category M01)B83.9
    - hemochromatosis (*see also* subcategory M14.8-)E83.118
    - hemoglobinopathy NEC D58.2 *[M36.3]*
    - hemophilia NEC D66 *[M36.2]*
    - Hemophilus influenzae M00.8 ☑ *[B96.3]*
    - Henoch (-Schönlein) purpura D69.0 *[M36.4]*
    - hyperparathyroidism NEC (*see also* subcategory M14.8-)E21.3
    - hypersensitivity reaction NEC T78.49 ☑ *[M36.4]*

- **Arthritis** — *continued*
  - in — *continued*
    - hypogammaglobulinemia (*see also* subcategory M14.8-)D80.1
    - hypothyroidism NEC (*see also* subcategory M14.8-)E03.9
    - infection — *see* Arthritis, pyogenic or pyemic
      - spine — *see* Spondylopathy, infective
    - infectious disease NEC M01
    - leprosy (*see also* category M01)A30.9
    - leukemia NEC C95.9 ☑ *[M36.1]*
    - lipoid dermatoarthritis E78.81
    - Lyme disease A69.23
    - Mediterranean fever, familial (*see also* subcategory M14.8-)M04.1
    - Meningococcus A39.83
    - metabolic disorder NEC (*see also* subcategory M14.8-)E88.9
    - multiple myelomatosis C90.0 ☑ *[M36.1]*
    - mumps B26.85
    - mycosis NEC (*see also* category M01)B49
    - myelomatosis (multiple) C90.0 ☑ *[M36.1]*
    - neurological disorder NEC G98.0
    - ochronosis (*see also* subcategory M14.8-)E70.29
    - O'nyong-nyong (*see also* category M01)A92.1
    - parasitic disease NEC (*see also* category M01)B89
    - paratyphoid fever (*see also* category M01)A01.4
    - Pseudomonas — *see* Arthritis, pyogenic, bacterial NEC
    - psoriasis L40.50
    - pyogenic organism NEC — *see* Arthritis, pyogenic, bacterial NEC
    - Reiter's disease — *see* Reiter's disease
    - respiratory disorder NEC (*see also* subcategory M14.8-)J98.9
    - reticulosis, malignant (*see also* subcategory M14.8-)C86.0
    - rubella B06.82
    - Salmonella (arizonae) (cholerae-suis) (enteritidis) (typhimurium) A02.23
    - sarcoidosis D86.86
    - specified bacteria NEC — *see* Arthritis, pyogenic, bacterial NEC
    - sporotrichosis B42.82
    - syringomyelia G95.0
    - thalassemia NEC D56.9 *[M36.3]*
    - tuberculosis — *see* Tuberculosis, arthritis
    - typhoid fever A01.04
    - urethritis, Reiter's — *see* Reiter's disease
    - viral disease NEC (*see also* category M01)B34.9
  - infectious or infective (*see also* Arthritis, pyogenic or pyemic)
    - spine — *see* Spondylopathy, infective
  - juvenile M08.90
    - with systemic onset — *see* Still's disease
    - ankle M08.97 ☑
    - elbow M08.92 ☑
    - foot joint M08.97 ☑
    - hand joint M08.94 ☑
    - hip M08.95 ☑
    - knee M08.96 ☑
    - multiple site M08.99
    - pauciarticular M08.40
      - ankle M08.47 ☑
      - elbow M08.42 ☑
      - foot joint M08.47 ☑
      - hand joint M08.44 ☑
      - hip M08.45 ☑
      - knee M08.46 ☑
      - shoulder M08.41 ☑
      - vertebrae M08.48
      - wrist M08.43 ☑
    - psoriatic L40.54
    - rheumatoid — *see* Arthritis, rheumatoid, juvenile
    - shoulder M08.91 ☑
    - vertebra M08.98
    - specified type NEC M08.80
      - ankle M08.87 ☑
      - elbow M08.82 ☑
      - foot joint M08.87 ☑
      - hand joint M08.84 ☑
      - hip M08.85 ☑
      - knee M08.86 ☑
      - multiple site M08.89
      - shoulder M08.81 ☑
      - specified joint NEC M08.88
      - vertebrae M08.88
      - wrist M08.83 ☑
    - wrist M08.93 ☑
  - meaning osteoarthritis — *see* Osteoarthritis

- **Arthritis** — *continued*
  - meningococcal A39.83
  - menopausal (any site) NEC — *see* Arthritis, specified form NEC
  - mutilans (psoriatic) L40.52
  - mycotic NEC (*see also* category M01)B49
  - neuropathic (Charcot) — *see* Arthropathy, neuropathic
    - diabetic — *see* Diabetes, arthropathy, neuropathic
    - nonsyphilitic NEC G98.0
    - syringomyelic G95.0
  - ochronotic (*see also* subcategory M14.8-)E70.29
  - palindromic (any site) — *see* Rheumatism, palindromic
  - pneumococcal M00.10
    - ankle M00.17 ☑
    - elbow M00.12 ☑
    - foot joint — *see* Arthritis, pneumococcal, ankle
    - hand joint M00.14 ☑
    - hip M00.15 ☑
    - knee M00.16 ☑
    - multiple site M00.19
    - shoulder M00.11 ☑
    - vertebra M00.18
    - wrist M00.13 ☑
  - postdysenteric — *see* Arthropathy, postdysenteric
  - postmeningococcal A39.84
  - postrheumatic, chronic — *see* Arthropathy, postrheumatic, chronic
  - primary progressive (*see also* Arthritis, specified form NEC)
    - spine — *see* Spondylitis, ankylosing
  - psoriatic L40.50
  - purulent (any site except spine) — *see* Arthritis, pyogenic or pyemic
    - spine — *see* Spondylopathy, infective
  - pyogenic or pyemic (any site except spine) M00.9
    - bacterial NEC M00.80
      - ankle M00.87 ☑
      - elbow M00.82 ☑
      - foot joint — *see* Arthritis, pyogenic, bacterial NEC, ankle
      - hand joint M00.84 ☑
      - hip M00.85 ☑
      - knee M00.86 ☑
      - multiple site M00.89
      - shoulder M00.81 ☑
      - vertebra M00.88
      - wrist M00.83 ☑
    - pneumococcal — *see* Arthritis, pneumococcal
    - spine — *see* Spondylopathy, infective
    - staphylococcal — *see* Arthritis, staphylococcal
    - streptococcal — *see* Arthritis, streptococcal NEC
      - pneumococcal — *see* Arthritis, pneumococcal
  - reactive — *see* Reiter's disease
  - rheumatic (*see also* Arthritis, rheumatoid)
    - acute or subacute — *see* Fever, rheumatic
  - rheumatoid M06.9
    - with
      - carditis — *see* Rheumatoid, carditis
      - endocarditis — *see* Rheumatoid, carditis
      - heart involvement NEC — *see* Rheumatoid, carditis
      - lung involvement — *see* Rheumatoid, lung
      - myocarditis — *see* Rheumatoid, carditis
      - myopathy — *see* Rheumatoid, myopathy
      - pericarditis — *see* Rheumatoid, carditis
      - polyneuropathy — *see* Rheumatoid, polyneuropathy
      - rheumatoid factor — *see* Arthritis, rheumatoid, seropositive
      - splenoadenomegaly and leukopenia — *see* Felty's syndrome
      - vasculitis — *see* Rheumatoid, vasculitis
      - visceral involvement NEC — *see* Rheumatoid, arthritis, with involvement of organs NEC
    - juvenile (with or without rheumatoid factor) M08.00
      - ankle M08.07 ☑
      - elbow M08.02 ☑
      - foot joint M08.07 ☑
      - hand joint M08.04 ☑
      - hip M08.05 ☑
      - knee M08.06 ☑
      - multiple site M08.09
      - shoulder M08.01 ☑
      - vertebra M08.08
      - wrist M08.03 ☑

- **Arthritis** — *continued*
  - rheumatoid — *continued*
    - seronegative M06.00
      - ankle M06.07 ☑
      - elbow M06.02 ☑
      - foot joint M06.07 ☑
      - hand joint M06.04 ☑
      - hip M06.05 ☑
      - knee M06.06 ☑
      - multiple site M06.09
      - shoulder M06.01 ☑
      - vertebra M06.08
      - wrist M06.03 ☑
    - seropositive M05.9
      - specified NEC M05.80
        - ankle M05.87 ☑
        - elbow M05.82 ☑
        - foot joint M05.87 ☑
        - hand joint M05.84 ☑
        - hip M05.85 ☑
        - knee M05.86 ☑
        - multiple sites M05.89
        - shoulder M05.81 ☑
        - vertebra — *see* Spondylitis, ankylosing
        - wrist M05.83 ☑
      - without organ involvement M05.70
        - ankle M05.77 ☑
        - elbow M05.72 ☑
        - foot joint M05.77 ☑
        - hand joint M05.74 ☑
        - hip M05.75 ☑
        - knee M05.76 ☑
        - multiple sites M05.79
        - shoulder M05.71 ☑
        - vertebra — *see* Spondylitis, ankylosing
        - wrist M05.73 ☑
    - specified type NEC M06.80
      - ankle M06.87 ☑
      - elbow M06.82 ☑
      - foot joint M06.87 ☑
      - hand joint M06.84 ☑
      - hip M06.85 ☑
      - knee M06.86 ☑
      - multiple site M06.89
      - shoulder M06.81 ☑
      - vertebra M06.88
      - wrist M06.83 ☑
    - spine — *see* Spondylitis, ankylosing
  - rubella B06.82
  - scorbutic (*see also* subcategory M14.8-)E54
  - senile or senescent — *see* Osteoarthritis
  - septic (any site except spine) — *see* Arthritis, pyogenic or pyemic
    - spine — *see* Spondylopathy, infective
  - serum (nontherapeutic) (therapeutic) — *see* Arthropathy, postimmunization
  - specified form NEC M13.80
    - ankle M13.87 ☑
    - elbow M13.82 ☑
    - foot joint M13.87 ☑
    - hand joint M13.84 ☑
    - hip M13.85 ☑
    - knee M13.86 ☑
    - multiple site M13.89
    - shoulder M13.81 ☑
    - specified joint NEC M13.88
    - wrist M13.83 ☑
  - spine (*see also* Spondylopathy, inflammatory)
    - infectious or infective NEC — *see* Spondylopathy, infective
    - Marie-Strümpell — *see* Spondylitis, ankylosing
    - pyogenic — *see* Spondylopathy, infective
    - rheumatoid — *see* Spondylitis, ankylosing
    - traumatic (old) — *see* Spondylopathy, traumatic
    - tuberculous A18.01
  - staphylococcal M00.00
    - ankle M00.07 ☑
    - elbow M00.02 ☑
    - foot joint — *see* Arthritis, staphylococcal, ankle
    - hand joint M00.04 ☑
    - hip M00.05 ☑
    - knee M00.06 ☑
    - multiple site M00.09
    - shoulder M00.01 ☑
    - vertebra M00.08
    - wrist M00.03 ☑
  - streptococcal NEC M00.20
    - ankle M00.27 ☑
    - elbow M00.22 ☑
    - foot joint — *see* Arthritis, streptococcal, ankle
    - hand joint M00.24 ☑

- **Arthritis** — *continued*
  - streptococcal NEC — *continued*
    - hip M00.25 ☑
    - knee M00.26 ☑
    - multiple site M00.29
    - shoulder M00.21 ☑
    - vertebra M00.28
    - wrist M00.23 ☑
  - suppurative — *see* Arthritis, pyogenic or pyemic
  - syphilitic (late) A52.16
    - congenital A50.55 *[M12.80]*
  - syphilitica deformans (Charcot) A52.16
  - temporomandibular M26.69
  - toxic of menopause (any site) — *see* Arthritis, specified form NEC
  - transient — *see* Arthropathy, specified form NEC
  - traumatic (chronic) — *see* Arthropathy, traumatic
  - tuberculous A18.02
    - spine A18.01
  - uratic — *see* Gout
  - urethritica (Reiter's) — *see* Reiter's disease
  - vertebral — *see* Spondylopathy, inflammatory
  - villous (any site) — *see* Arthropathy, specified form NEC
- **Arthrocele** — *see* Effusion, joint
- **Arthrodesis** status Z98.1
- **Arthrodynia** (*see also* Pain, joint)
- **Arthrodysplasia** Q74.9
- **Arthrofibrosis,** joint — *see* Ankylosis
- **Arthrogryposis** (congenital) Q68.8
  - multiplex congenita Q74.3
- **Arthrokatadysis** M24.7
- **Arthropathy** (*see also* Arthritis)M12.9
  - Charcot's — *see* Arthropathy, neuropathic
    - diabetic — *see* Diabetes, arthropathy, neuropathic
    - syringomyelic G95.0
  - cricoarytenoid J38.7
  - crystal (-induced) — *see* Arthritis, in, crystals
  - diabetic NEC — *see* Diabetes, arthropathy
  - distal interphalangeal, psoriatic L40.51
  - enteropathic M07.60
    - ankle M07.67 ☑
    - elbow M07.62 ☑
    - foot joint M07.67 ☑
    - hand joint M07.64 ☑
    - hip M07.65 ☑
    - knee M07.66 ☑
    - multiple site M07.69
    - shoulder M07.61 ☑
    - vertebra M07.68
    - wrist M07.63 ☑
  - following intestinal bypass M02.00
    - ankle M02.07 ☑
    - elbow M02.02 ☑
    - foot joint M02.07 ☑
    - hand joint M02.04 ☑
    - hip M02.05 ☑
    - knee M02.06 ☑
    - multiple site M02.09
    - shoulder M02.01 ☑
    - vertebra M02.08
    - wrist M02.03 ☑
  - gouty (*see also* Gout)
    - in (due to)
      - Lesch-Nyhan syndrome E79.1 *[M14.8-]*
      - sickle-cell disorders D57 ☑ *[M14.8-]*
  - hemophilic NEC D66 *[M36.2]*
    - in (due to)
      - hyperparathyroidism NEC E21.3 *[M14.8-]*
      - metabolic disease NOS E88.9 *[M14.8-]*
  - in (due to)
    - acromegaly E22.0 *[M14.8-]*
    - amyloidosis E85.4 *[M14.8-]*
    - blood disorder NOS D75.9 *[M36.3]*
    - diabetes — *see* Diabetes, arthropathy
    - endocrine disease NOS E34.9 *[M14.8-]*
    - erythema
      - multiforme L51.9 *[M14.8-]*
      - nodosum L52 *[M14.8-]*
    - hemochromatosis E83.118 *[M14.8-]*
    - hemoglobinopathy NEC D58.2 *[M36.3]*
    - hemophilia NEC D66 *[M36.2]*
    - Henoch-Schönlein purpura D69.0 *[M36.4]*
    - hyperthyroidism E05.90 *[M14.8-]*
    - hypothyroidism E03.9 *[M14.8-]*
    - infective endocarditis I33.0 *[M12.80]*
    - leukemia NEC C95.9 ☑ *[M36.1]*
    - malignant histiocytosis C96.A *[M36.1]*
    - metabolic disease NOS E88.9 *[M14.8-]*
    - multiple myeloma C90.0 ☑ *[M36.1]*

- **Arthropathy** — *continued*
  - in — *continued*
    - neoplastic disease NOS (see also Neoplasm) D49.9 *[M36.1]*
    - nutritional deficiency (*see also* subcategory M14.8-)E63.9
    - psoriasis NOS L40.50
    - sarcoidosis D86.86
    - syphilis (late) A52.77
      - congenital A50.55 *[M12.80]*
    - thyrotoxicosis (*see also* subcategory M14.8-) E05.90
    - ulcerative colitis K51.90 *[M07.60]*
    - viral hepatitis (postinfectious) NEC B19.9 *[M12.80]*
    - Whipple's disease (*see also* subcategory M14.8-) K90.81
  - Jaccoud — *see* Arthropathy, postrheumatic, chronic
  - juvenile — *see* Arthritis, juvenile
    - psoriatic L40.54
  - mutilans (psoriatic) L40.52
  - neuropathic (Charcot) M14.60
    - ankle M14.67 ☑
    - diabetic — *see* Diabetes, arthropathy, neuropathic
    - elbow M14.62 ☑
    - foot joint M14.67 ☑
    - hand joint M14.64 ☑
    - hip M14.65 ☑
    - knee M14.66 ☑
    - multiple site M14.69
    - nonsyphilitic NEC G98.0
    - shoulder M14.61 ☑
    - syringomyelic G95.0
    - vertebra M14.68
    - wrist M14.63 ☑
  - osteopulmonary — *see* Osteoarthropathy, hypertrophic, specified NEC
  - postdysenteric M02.10
    - ankle M02.17 ☑
    - elbow M02.12 ☑
    - foot joint M02.17 ☑
    - hand joint M02.14 ☑
    - hip M02.15 ☑
    - knee M02.16 ☑
    - multiple site M02.19
    - shoulder M02.11 ☑
    - vertebra M02.18
    - wrist M02.13 ☑
  - postimmunization M02.20
    - ankle M02.27 ☑
    - elbow M02.22 ☑
    - foot joint M02.27 ☑
    - hand joint M02.24 ☑
    - hip M02.25 ☑
    - knee M02.26 ☑
    - multiple site M02.29
    - shoulder M02.21 ☑
    - vertebra M02.28
    - wrist M02.23 ☑
  - postinfectious NEC B99 ☑ *[M12.80]*
    - in (due to)
      - enteritis due to Yersinia enterocolitica A04.6 *[M12.80]*
      - syphilis A52.77
      - viral hepatitis NEC B19.9 *[M12.80]*
  - postrheumatic, chronic (Jaccoud) M12.00
    - ankle M12.07 ☑
    - elbow M12.02 ☑
    - foot joint M12.07 ☑
    - hand joint M12.04 ☑
    - hip M12.05 ☑
    - knee M12.06 ☑
    - multiple site M12.09
    - shoulder M12.01 ☑
    - specified joint NEC M12.08
    - vertebrae M12.08
    - wrist M12.03 ☑
  - psoriatic NEC L40.59
    - interphalangeal, distal L40.51
  - reactive M02.9
    - in (due to)
      - infective endocarditis I33.0 *[M02.9]*
    - specified type NEC M02.80
      - ankle M02.87 ☑
      - elbow M02.82 ☑
      - foot joint M02.87 ☑
      - hand joint M02.84 ☑
      - hip M02.85 ☑
      - knee M02.86 ☑
      - multiple site M02.89

- **Arthropathy** — *continued*
  - reactive — *continued*
      - shoulder M02.81 ☑
      - vertebra M02.88
      - wrist M02.83 ☑
  - specified form NEC M12.80
    - ankle M12.87 ☑
    - elbow M12.82 ☑
    - foot joint M12.87 ☑
    - hand joint M12.84 ☑
    - hip M12.85 ☑
    - knee M12.86 ☑
    - multiple site M12.89
    - shoulder M12.81 ☑
    - specified joint NEC M12.88
    - vertebrae M12.88
    - wrist M12.83 ☑
  - syringomyelic G95.0
  - tabes dorsalis A52.16
  - tabetic A52.16
  - transient — *see* Arthropathy, specified form NEC
  - traumatic M12.50
    - ankle M12.57 ☑
    - elbow M12.52 ☑
    - foot joint M12.57 ☑
    - hand joint M12.54 ☑
    - hip M12.55 ☑
    - knee M12.56 ☑
    - multiple site M12.59
    - shoulder M12.51 ☑
    - specified joint NEC M12.58
    - vertebrae M12.58
    - wrist M12.53 ☑
- **Arthropyosis** — *see* Arthritis, pyogenic or pyemic
- **Arthrosis** (deformans) (degenerative) (localized) (*see also* Osteoarthritis)M19.90
  - spine — *see* Spondylosis
- **Arthus'** phenomenon or reaction T78.41 ☑
  - due to
    - drug — *see* Table of Drugs and Chemicals, by drug
- **Articular** — *see* condition
- **Articulation,** reverse (teeth) M26.24
- **Artificial**
  - insemination complication — *see* Complications, artificial, fertilization
  - opening status (functioning) (without complication) Z93.9
    - anus (colostomy) Z93.3
    - colostomy Z93.3
    - cystostomy Z93.50
      - appendico-vesicostomy Z93.52
      - cutaneous Z93.51
      - specified NEC Z93.59
    - enterostomy Z93.4
    - gastrostomy Z93.1
    - ileostomy Z93.2
    - intestinal tract NEC Z93.4
    - jejunostomy Z93.4
    - nephrostomy Z93.6
    - specified site NEC Z93.8
    - tracheostomy Z93.0
    - ureterostomy Z93.6
    - urethrostomy Z93.6
    - urinary tract NEC Z93.6
    - vagina Z93.8
  - vagina status Z93.8
- **Arytenoid** — *see* condition
- **Asbestosis** (occupational) J61
- **ASC-H** (atypical squamous cells cannot exclude high grade squamous intraepithelial lesion on cytologic smear)
  - anus R85.611
  - cervix R87.611
  - vagina R87.621
- **ASC-US** (atypical squamous cells of undetermined significance on cytologic smear)
  - anus R85.610
  - cervix R87.610
  - vagina R87.620
- **Ascariasis** B77.9
  - with
    - complications NEC B77.89
    - intestinal complications B77.0
    - pneumonia, pneumonitis B77.81
- **Ascaridosis,** ascaridiasis — *see* Ascariasis
- **Ascaris** (infection) (infestation) (lumbricoides) — *see* Ascariasis
- **Ascending** — *see* condition
- **Aschoff's** bodies — *see* Myocarditis, rheumatic
- **Ascites** (abdominal) R18.8
  - cardiac I50.9

- **Ascites** — *continued*
  - chylous (nonfilarial) I89.8
    - filarial — *see* Infestation, filarial
  - due to
    - cirrhosis, alcoholic K70.31
    - hepatitis
      - alcoholic K70.11
      - chronic active K71.51
    - S. japonicum B65.2
  - heart I50.9
  - malignant R18.0
  - pseudochylous R18.8
  - syphilitic A52.74
  - tuberculous A18.31
- **Aseptic** — *see* condition
- **Asherman's** syndrome N85.6
- **Asialia** K11.7
- **Asiatic** cholera — *see* Cholera
- **Asimultagnosia** (simultanagnosia) R48.3
- **Askin's** tumor — *see* Neoplasm, connective tissue, malignant
- **Asocial** personality F60.2
- **Asomatognosia** R41.4
- **Aspartylglucosaminuria** E77.1
- **Asperger's** disease or syndrome F84.5
- **Aspergilloma** — *see* Aspergillosis
- **Aspergillosis** (with pneumonia) B44.9
  - bronchopulmonary, allergic B44.81
  - disseminated B44.7
  - generalized B44.7
  - pulmonary NEC B44.1
    - allergic B44.81
    - invasive B44.0
  - specified NEC B44.89
  - tonsillar B44.2
- **Aspergillus** (flavus) (fumigatus) (infection) (terreus) — *see* Aspergillosis
- **Aspermatogenesis** — *see* Azoospermia
- **Aspermia** (testis) — *see* Azoospermia
- **Asphyxia,** asphyxiation (by) R09.01
  - antenatal P84
  - birth P84
  - bunny bag — *see* Asphyxia, due to, mechanical threat to breathing, trapped in bed clothes
  - crushing S28.0 ☑
  - drowning T75.1 ☑
  - gas, fumes, or vapor — *see* Table of Drugs and Chemicals
  - inhalation — *see* Inhalation
  - intrauterine P84
  - local I73.00
    - with gangrene I73.01
  - mucus (*see also* Foreign body, respiratory tract, causing asphyxia)
  - newborn P84
  - pathological R09.01
  - postnatal P84
    - mechanical — *see* Asphyxia, due to, mechanical threat to breathing
  - prenatal P84
  - reticularis R23.1
  - strangulation — *see* Asphyxia, due to, mechanical threat to breathing
  - submersion T75.1 ☑
  - traumatic T71.9 ☑
    - due to
      - crushed chest S28.0 ☑
      - foreign body (in) — *see* Foreign body, respiratory tract, causing asphyxia
      - low oxygen content of ambient air T71.20 ☑
        - due to
          - being trapped in
            - low oxygen environment T71.29 ☑
              - in car trunk T71.221 ☑
                - circumstances undetermined T71.224 ☑
                - done with intent to harm by
                  - another person T71.223 ☑
                  - self T71.222 ☑
              - in refrigerator T71.231 ☑
                - circumstances undetermined T71.234 ☑
                - done with intent to harm by
                  - another person T71.233 ☑
                  - self T71.232 ☑
          - cave-in T71.21 ☑
      - mechanical threat to breathing (accidental) T71.191 ☑
        - circumstances undetermined T71.194 ☑
        - done with intent to harm by
          - another person T71.193 ☑
          - self T71.192 ☑

- **Asphyxia** — *continued*
  - traumatic — *continued*
      - hanging T71.161 ☑
        - circumstances undetermined T71.164 ☑
        - done with intent to harm by
          - another person T71.163 ☑
          - self T71.162 ☑
      - plastic bag T71.121 ☑
        - circumstances undetermined T71.124 ☑
        - done with intent to harm by
          - another person T71.123 ☑
          - self T71.122 ☑
      - smothering
        - in furniture T71.151 ☑
          - circumstances undetermined T71.154 ☑
          - done with intent to harm by
            - another person T71.153 ☑
            - self T71.152 ☑
        - under
          - another person's body T71.141 ☑
            - circumstances undetermined T71.144 ☑
            - done with intent to harm T71.143 ☑
          - pillow T71.111 ☑
            - circumstances undetermined T71.114 ☑
            - done with intent to harm by
              - another person T71.113 ☑
              - self T71.112 ☑
      - trapped in bed clothes T71.131 ☑
        - circumstances undetermined T71.134 ☑
        - done with intent to harm by
          - another person T71.133 ☑
          - self T71.132 ☑
  - vomiting, vomitus — *see* Foreign body, respiratory tract, causing asphyxia
- **Aspiration**
  - amniotic (clear) fluid (newborn) P24.10
    - with
      - pneumonia (pneumonitis) P24.11
      - respiratory symptoms P24.11
  - blood
    - newborn (without respiratory symptoms) P24.20
      - with
        - pneumonia (pneumonitis) P24.21
        - respiratory symptoms P24.21
    - specified age NEC — *see* Foreign body, respiratory tract
  - bronchitis J69.0
  - food or foreign body (with asphyxiation) — *see* Asphyxia, food
  - liquor (amnii) (newborn) P24.10
    - with
      - pneumonia (pneumonitis) P24.11
      - respiratory symptoms P24.11
  - meconium (newborn) (without respiratory symptoms) P24.00
    - with
      - pneumonitis (pneumonitis) P24.01
      - respiratory symptoms P24.01
  - milk (newborn) (without respiratory symptoms) P24.30
    - with
      - pneumonia (pneumonitis) P24.31
      - respiratory symptoms P24.31
    - specified age NEC — *see* Foreign body, respiratory tract
  - mucus (*see also* Foreign body, by site, causing asphyxia)
    - newborn P24.10
      - with
        - pneumonia (pneumonitis) P24.11
        - respiratory symptoms P24.11
  - neonatal P24.9
    - specific NEC (without respiratory symptoms) P24.80
      - with
        - pneumonia (pneumonitis) P24.81
        - respiratory symptoms P24.81
  - newborn P24.9
    - specific NEC (without respiratory symptoms) P24.80
      - with
        - pneumonia (pneumonitis) P24.81
        - respiratory symptoms P24.81
  - pneumonia J69.0
  - pneumonitis J69.0
  - syndrome of newborn — *see* Aspiration, by substance, with pneumonia

- **Aspiration** — *continued*
  - vernix caseosa (newborn) P24.80
    - with
      - pneumonia (pneumonitis) P24.81
      - respiratory symptoms P24.81
  - vomitus (*see also* Foreign body, respiratory tract)
    - newborn (without respiratory symptoms) P24.30
      - with
        - pneumonia (pneumonitis) P24.31
        - respiratory symptoms P24.31
- **Asplenia** (congenital) Q89.01
  - postsurgical Z90.81
- **Assam** fever B55.0
- **Assault,** sexual — *see* Maltreatment
- **Assmann's** focus NEC A15.0
- **Astasia** (-abasia) (hysterical) F44.4
- **Asteatosis** cutis L85.3
- **Astereognosia,** astereognosis R48.1
- **Asterixis** R27.8
  - in liver disease K71.3
- **Asteroid** hyalitis — *see* Deposit, crystalline
- **Asthenia,** asthenic R53.1
  - cardiac (*see also* Failure, heart)I50.9
    - psychogenic F45.8
  - cardiovascular (*see also* Failure, heart)I50.9
    - psychogenic F45.8
  - heart (*see also* Failure, heart)I50.9
    - psychogenic F45.8
  - hysterical F44.4
  - myocardial (*see also* Failure, heart)I50.9
    - psychogenic F45.8
  - nervous F48.8
  - neurocirculatory F45.8
  - neurotic F48.8
  - psychogenic F48.8
  - psychoneurotic F48.8
  - psychophysiologic F48.8
  - reaction (psychophysiologic) F48.8
  - senile R54
- **Asthenopia** (*see also* Discomfort, visual)
  - hysterical F44.6
  - psychogenic F44.6
- **Asthenospermia** — *see* Abnormal, specimen, male genital organs
- **Asthma,** asthmatic (bronchial) (catarrh) (spasmodic) J45.909
  - with
    - chronic obstructive bronchitis J44.9
      - with
        - acute lower respiratory infection J44.0
        - exacerbation (acute) J44.1
    - chronic obstructive pulmonary disease J44.9
      - with
        - acute lower respiratory infection J44.0
        - exacerbation (acute) J44.1
    - exacerbation (acute) J45.901
    - hay fever — *see* Asthma, allergic extrinsic
    - rhinitis, allergic — *see* Asthma, allergic extrinsic
    - status asthmaticus J45.902
  - allergic extrinsic J45.909
    - with
      - exacerbation (acute) J45.901
      - status asthmaticus J45.902
  - atopic — *see* Asthma, allergic extrinsic
  - cardiac — *see* Failure, ventricular, left
  - cardiobronchial I50.1
  - childhood J45.909
    - with
      - exacerbation (acute) J45.901
      - status asthmaticus J45.902
  - chronic obstructive J44.9
    - with
      - acute lower respiratory infection J44.0
      - exacerbation (acute) J44.1
  - collier's J60
  - cough variant J45.991
  - detergent J69.8
  - due to
    - detergent J69.8
    - inhalation of fumes J68.3
  - eosinophilic J82
  - extrinsic, allergic — *see* Asthma, allergic extrinsic
  - grinder's J62.8
  - hay — *see* Asthma, allergic extrinsic
  - heart I50.1
  - idiosyncratic — *see* Asthma, nonallergic
  - intermittent (mild) J45.20
    - with
      - exacerbation (acute) J45.21
      - status asthmaticus J45.22
  - intrinsic, nonallergic — *see* Asthma, nonallergic

- **Asthma** — *continued*
  - Kopp's E32.8
  - late-onset J45.909
    - with
      - exacerbation (acute) J45.901
      - status asthmaticus J45.902
  - mild intermittent J45.20
    - with
      - exacerbation (acute) J45.21
      - status asthmaticus J45.22
  - mild persistent J45.30
    - with
      - exacerbation (acute) J45.31
      - status asthmaticus J45.32
  - Millar's (laryngismus stridulus) J38.5
  - miner's J60
  - mixed J45.909
    - with
      - exacerbation (acute) J45.901
      - status asthmaticus J45.902
  - moderate persistent J45.40
    - with
      - exacerbation (acute) J45.41
      - status asthmaticus J45.42
  - nervous — *see* Asthma, nonallergic
  - nonallergic (intrinsic) J45.909
    - with
      - exacerbation (acute) J45.901
      - status asthmaticus J45.902
  - persistent
    - mild J45.30
      - with
        - exacerbation (acute) J45.31
        - status asthmaticus J45.32
    - moderate J45.40
      - with
        - exacerbation (acute) J45.41
        - status asthmaticus J45.42
    - severe J45.50
      - with
        - exacerbation (acute) J45.51
        - status asthmaticus J45.52
  - platinum J45.998
  - pneumoconiotic NEC J64
  - potter's J62.8
  - predominantly allergic J45.909
  - psychogenic F54
  - pulmonary eosinophilic J82
  - red cedar J67.8
  - Rostan's I50.1
  - sandblaster's J62.8
  - sequoiosis J67.8
  - severe persistent J45.50
    - with
      - exacerbation (acute) J45.51
      - status asthmaticus J45.52
  - specified NEC J45.998
  - stonemason's J62.8
  - thymic E32.8
  - tuberculous — *see* Tuberculosis, pulmonary
  - Wichmann's (laryngismus stridulus) J38.5
  - wood J67.8
- **Astigmatism** (compound) (congenital) H52.20 ☑
  - irregular H52.21 ☑
  - regular H52.22 ☑
- **Astraphobia** F40.220
- **Astroblastoma**
  - specified site — *see* Neoplasm, malignant, by site
  - unspecified site C71.9
- **Astrocytoma** (cystic)
  - anaplastic
    - specified site — *see* Neoplasm, malignant, by site
    - unspecified site C71.9
  - fibrillary
    - specified site — *see* Neoplasm, malignant, by site
    - unspecified site C71.9
  - fibrous
    - specified site — *see* Neoplasm, malignant, by site
    - unspecified site C71.9
  - gemistocytic
    - specified site — *see* Neoplasm, malignant, by site
    - unspecified site C71.9
  - juvenile
    - specified site — *see* Neoplasm, malignant, by site
    - unspecified site C71.9
  - pilocytic
    - specified site — *see* Neoplasm, malignant, by site
    - unspecified site C71.9
- **Astrocytoma** — *continued*
  - piloid
    - specified site — *see* Neoplasm, malignant, by site
    - unspecified site C71.9
  - protoplasmic
    - specified site — *see* Neoplasm, malignant, by site
    - unspecified site C71.9
  - specified site NEC — *see* Neoplasm, malignant, by site
  - subependymal D43.2
    - giant cell
      - specified site — *see* Neoplasm, uncertain behavior, by site
      - unspecified site D43.2
    - specified site — *see* Neoplasm, uncertain behavior, by site
    - unspecified site D43.2
  - unspecified site C71.9
- **Astroglioma**
  - specified site — *see* Neoplasm, malignant, by site
  - unspecified site C71.9
- **Asymbolia** R48.8
- **Asymmetry** (*see also* Distortion)
  - between native and reconstructed breast N65.1
  - face Q67.0
  - jaw (lower) — *see* Anomaly, dentofacial, jaw-cranial base relationship, asymmetry
- **Asynergia,** asynergy R27.8
  - ventricular I51.89
- **Asystole** (heart) — *see* Arrest, cardiac
- **At risk**
  - for falling Z91.81
- **Ataxia,** ataxy, ataxic R27.0
  - acute R27.8
  - brain (hereditary) G11.9
  - cerebellar (hereditary) G11.9
    - with defective DNA repair G11.3
    - alcoholic G31.2
    - early-onset G11.1
    - in
      - alcoholism G31.2
      - myxedema E03.9 *[G13.2]*
      - neoplastic disease (*see also* Neoplasm)D49.9 *[G32.81]*
      - specified disease NEC G32.81
    - late-onset (Marie's) G11.2
  - cerebral (hereditary) G11.9
  - congenital nonprogressive G11.0
  - family, familial — *see* Ataxia, hereditary
  - following
    - cerebrovascular disease I69.993
      - cerebral infarction I69.393
      - intracerebral hemorrhage I69.193
      - nontraumatic intracranial hemorrhage NEC I69.293
      - specified disease NEC I69.893
      - subarachnoid hemorrhage I69.093
  - Friedreich's (heredofamilial) (cerebellar) (spinal) G11.1
  - gait R26.0
    - hysterical F44.4
  - general R27.8
  - gluten M35.9 *[G32.81]*
    - with celiac disease K90.0 *[G32.81]*
  - hereditary G11.9
    - with neuropathy G60.2
    - cerebellar — *see* Ataxia, cerebellar
    - spastic G11.4
    - specified NEC G11.8
    - spinal (Friedreich's) G11.1
  - heredofamilial — *see* Ataxia, hereditary
  - Hunt's G11.1
  - hysterical F44.4
  - locomotor (progressive) (syphilitic) (partial) (spastic) A52.11
    - diabetic — *see* Diabetes, ataxia
  - Marie's (cerebellar) (heredofamilial) (late- onset) G11.2
  - nonorganic origin F44.4
  - nonprogressive, congenital G11.0
  - psychogenic F44.4
  - Roussy-Lévy G60.0
  - Sanger-Brown's (hereditary) G11.2
  - spastic hereditary G11.4
  - spinal
    - hereditary (Friedreich's) G11.1
    - progressive (syphilitic) A52.11
  - spinocerebellar, X-linked recessive G11.1
  - telangiectasia (Louis-Bar) G11.3
- **Ataxia-telangiectasia** (Louis-Bar) G11.3
- **Atelectasis** (massive) (partial) (pressure) (pulmonary) J98.11
  - newborn P28.10
    - due to resorption P28.11
    - partial P28.19
    - primary P28.0
    - secondary P28.19
  - primary (newborn) P28.0
  - tuberculous — *see* Tuberculosis, pulmonary
- **Atelocardia** Q24.9
- **Atelomyelia** Q06.1
- **Atheroembolism**
  - of
    - extremities
      - lower I75.02 ☑
      - upper I75.01 ☑
    - kidney I75.81
    - specified NEC I75.89
- **Atheroma,** atheromatous (*see also* Arteriosclerosis)I70.90
  - aorta, aortic I70.0
    - valve (*see also* Endocarditis, aortic)I35.8
  - aorto-iliac I70.0
  - artery — *see* Arteriosclerosis
  - basilar (artery) I67.2
  - carotid (artery) (common) (internal) I67.2
  - cerebral (arteries) I67.2
  - coronary (artery) I25.10
    - with angina pectoris — *see* Arteriosclerosis, coronary (artery),
  - degeneration — *see* Arteriosclerosis
  - heart, cardiac — *see* Disease, heart, ischemic, atherosclerotic
  - mitral (valve) I34.8
  - myocardium, myocardial — *see* Disease, heart, ischemic, atherosclerotic
  - pulmonary valve (heart) (*see also* Endocarditis, pulmonary)I37.8
  - tricuspid (heart) (valve) I36.8
  - valve, valvular — *see* Endocarditis
  - vertebral (artery) I67.2
- **Atheromatosis** — *see* Arteriosclerosis
- **Atherosclerosis** (*see also* Arteriosclerosis)
  - coronary
    - artery I25.10
      - with angina pectoris — *see* Arteriosclerosis, coronary (artery),
      - due to
        - calcified coronary lesion (severely) I25.84
        - lipid rich plaque I25.83
    - transplanted heart I25.811
      - bypass graft I25.812
        - with angina pectoris — *see* Arteriosclerosis, coronary (artery),
      - native coronary artery I25.811
        - with angina pectoris — *see* Arteriosclerosis, coronary (artery),
- **Athetosis** (acquired) R25.8
  - bilateral (congenital) G80.3
  - congenital (bilateral) (double) G80.3
  - double (congenital) G80.3
  - unilateral R25.8
- **Athlete's**
  - foot B35.3
  - heart I51.7
- **Athrepsia** E41
- **Athyrea** (acquired) (*see also* Hypothyroidism)
  - congenital E03.1
- **Atonia,** atony, atonic
  - bladder (sphincter) (neurogenic) N31.2
  - capillary I78.8
  - cecum K59.8
    - psychogenic F45.8
  - colon — *see* Atony, intestine
  - congenital P94.2
  - esophagus K22.8
  - intestine K59.8
    - psychogenic F45.8
  - stomach K31.89
    - neurotic or psychogenic F45.8
  - uterus (during labor) O62.2
    - with hemorrhage (postpartum) O72.1
    - postpartum (with hemorrhage) O72.1
      - without hemorrhage O75.89
- **Atopy** — *see* History, allergy
- **Atransferrinemia,** congenital E88.09
- **Atresia,** atretic
  - alimentary organ or tract NEC Q45.8
    - upper Q40.8
  - ani, anus, anal (canal) Q42.3
    - with fistula Q42.2
  - aorta (ring) Q25.29

Atresia - Atrophy

- **Atresia** — *continued*
  - aortic (orifice) (valve) Q23.0
    - arch Q25.21
    - congenital with hypoplasia of ascending aorta and defective development of left ventricle (with mitral stenosis) Q23.4
    - in hypoplastic left heart syndrome Q23.4
  - aqueduct of Sylvius Q03.0
    - with spina bifida — *see* Spina bifida, with hydrocephalus
  - artery NEC Q27.8
    - cerebral Q28.3
    - coronary Q24.5
    - digestive system Q27.8
    - eye Q15.8
    - lower limb Q27.8
    - pulmonary Q25.5
    - specified site NEC Q27.8
    - umbilical Q27.0
    - upper limb Q27.8
  - auditory canal (external) Q16.1
  - bile duct (common) (congenital) (hepatic) Q44.2
    - acquired — *see* Obstruction, bile duct
  - bladder (neck) Q64.39
    - obstruction Q64.31
  - bronchus Q32.4
  - cecum Q42.8
  - cervix (acquired) N88.2
    - congenital Q51.828
    - in pregnancy or childbirth — *see* Anomaly, cervix, in pregnancy or childbirth
      - causing obstructed labor O65.5
  - choana Q30.0
  - colon Q42.9
    - specified NEC Q42.8
  - common duct Q44.2
  - cricoid cartilage Q31.8
  - cystic duct Q44.2
    - acquired K82.8
      - with obstruction K82.0
  - digestive organs NEC Q45.8
  - duodenum Q41.0
  - ear canal Q16.1
  - ejaculatory duct Q55.4
  - epiglottis Q31.8
  - esophagus Q39.0
    - with tracheoesophageal fistula Q39.1
  - eustachian tube Q17.8
  - fallopian tube (congenital) Q50.6
    - acquired N97.1
  - follicular cyst N83.0 ☑
  - foramen of
    - Luschka Q03.1
      - with spina bifida — *see* Spina bifida, with hydrocephalus
    - Magendie Q03.1
      - with spina bifida — *see* Spina bifida, with hydrocephalus
  - gallbladder Q44.1
  - genital organ
    - external
      - female Q52.79
      - male Q55.8
    - internal
      - female Q52.8
      - male Q55.8
  - glottis Q31.8
  - gullet Q39.0
    - with tracheoesophageal fistula Q39.1
  - heart valve NEC Q24.8
    - pulmonary Q22.0
    - tricuspid Q22.4
  - hymen Q52.3
    - acquired (postinfective) N89.6
  - ileum Q41.2
  - intestine (small) Q41.9
    - large Q42.9
      - specified NEC Q42.8
  - iris, filtration angle Q15.0
  - jejunum Q41.1
  - lacrimal apparatus Q10.4
  - larynx Q31.8
  - meatus urinarius Q64.33
  - mitral valve Q23.2
    - in hypoplastic left heart syndrome Q23.4
  - nares (anterior) (posterior) Q30.0
  - nasopharynx Q34.8
  - nose, nostril Q30.0
    - acquired J34.89
  - organ or site NEC Q89.8
  - osseous meatus (ear) Q16.1
  - oviduct (congenital) Q50.6
    - acquired N97.1
  - parotid duct Q38.4
    - acquired K11.8
  - pulmonary (artery) Q25.5
    - valve Q22.0
  - pulmonic Q22.0
  - pupil Q13.2
  - rectum Q42.1
    - with fistula Q42.0
  - salivary duct Q38.4
    - acquired K11.8
  - sublingual duct Q38.4
    - acquired K11.8
  - submandibular duct Q38.4
    - acquired K11.8
  - submaxillary duct Q38.4
    - acquired K11.8
  - thyroid cartilage Q31.8
  - trachea Q32.1
  - tricuspid valve Q22.4
  - ureter Q62.10
    - pelvic junction Q62.11
    - vesical orifice Q62.12
  - ureteropelvic junction Q62.11
  - ureterovesical orifice Q62.12
  - urethra (valvular) Q64.39
    - stricture Q64.32
  - urinary tract NEC Q64.8
  - uterus Q51.818
    - acquired N85.8
  - vagina (congenital) Q52.4
    - acquired (postinfectional) (senile) N89.5
  - vas deferens Q55.3
  - vascular NEC Q27.8
    - cerebral Q28.3
    - digestive system Q27.8
    - lower limb Q27.8
    - specified site NEC Q27.8
    - upper limb Q27.8
  - vein NEC Q27.8
    - digestive system Q27.8
    - great Q26.8
    - lower limb Q27.8
    - portal Q26.5
    - pulmonary Q26.3
    - specified site NEC Q27.8
    - upper limb Q27.8
  - vena cava (inferior) (superior) Q26.8
  - vesicourethral orifice Q64.31
  - vulva Q52.79
    - acquired N90.5
- **Atrichia**, atrichosis — *see* Alopecia
- **Atrophia** (*see also* Atrophy)
  - cutis senilis L90.8
    - due to radiation L57.8
  - gyrata of choroid and retina H31.23
  - senilis R54
    - dermatological L90.8
      - due to radiation (nonionizing) (solar) L57.8
  - unguium L60.3
    - congenita Q84.6
- **Atrophie** blanche (en plaque) (de Milian) L95.0
- **Atrophoderma**, atrophodermia (of) L90.9
  - diffusum (idiopathic) L90.4
  - maculatum L90.8
    - et striatum L90.8
      - due to syphilis A52.79
    - syphilitic A51.39
  - neuriticum L90.8
  - Pasini and Pierini L90.3
  - pigmentosum Q82.1
  - reticulatum symmetricum faciei L66.4
  - senile L90.8
    - due to radiation (nonionizing) (solar) L57.8
  - vermiculata (cheeks) L66.4
- **Atrophy**, atrophic (of)
  - adrenal (capsule) (gland) E27.49
    - primary (autoimmune) E27.1
  - alveolar process or ridge (edentulous) K08.20
  - anal sphincter (disuse) N81.84
  - appendix K38.8
  - arteriosclerotic — *see* Arteriosclerosis
  - bile duct (common) (hepatic) K83.8
  - bladder N32.89
    - neurogenic N31.8
  - blanche (en plaque) (of Milian) L95.0
  - bone (senile) NEC (*see also* Disorder, bone, specified type NEC)
    - due to
      - tabes dorsalis (neurogenic) A52.11
  - brain (cortex) (progressive) G31.9
    - frontotemporal circumscribed G31.01 *[F02.80]*
      - with behavioral disturbance G31.01 *[F02.81]*
    - senile NEC G31.1
  - breast N64.2
    - obstetric — *see* Disorder, breast, specified type NEC
  - buccal cavity K13.79
  - cardiac — *see* Degeneration, myocardial
  - cartilage (infectional) (joint) — *see* Disorder, cartilage, specified NEC
  - cerebellar — *see* Atrophy, brain
  - cerebral — *see* Atrophy, brain
  - cervix (mucosa) (senile) (uteri) N88.8
    - menopausal N95.8
  - Charcot-Marie-Tooth G60.0
  - choroid (central) (macular) (myopic) (retina) H31.10 ☑
    - diffuse secondary H31.12 ☑
    - gyrate H31.23
    - senile H31.11 ☑
  - ciliary body — *see* Atrophy, iris
  - conjunctiva (senile) H11.89
  - corpus cavernosum N48.89
  - cortical — *see* Atrophy, brain
  - cystic duct K82.8
  - Déjérine-Thomas G23.8
  - disuse NEC — *see* Atrophy, muscle
  - Duchenne-Aran G12.21
  - ear H93.8 ☑
  - edentulous alveolar ridge K08.20
  - endometrium (senile) N85.8
    - cervix N88.8
  - enteric K63.89
  - epididymis N50.89
  - eyeball — *see* Disorder, globe, degenerated condition, atrophy
  - eyelid (senile) — *see* Disorder, eyelid, degenerative
  - facial (skin) L90.9
  - fallopian tube (senile) N83.32 ☑
    - with ovary N83.33 ☑
  - fascioscapulohumeral (Landouzy- Déjérine) G71.0
  - fatty, thymus (gland) E32.8
  - gallbladder K82.8
  - gastric K29.40
    - with bleeding K29.41
  - gastrointestinal K63.89
  - glandular I89.8
  - globe H44.52 ☑
  - gum (*see also* Recession, gingival)K06.0
  - hair L67.8
  - heart (brown) — *see* Degeneration, myocardial
  - hemifacial Q67.4
    - Romberg G51.8
  - infantile E41
    - paralysis, acute — *see* Poliomyelitis, paralytic
  - intestine K63.89
  - iris (essential) (progressive) H21.26 ☑
    - specified NEC H21.29
  - kidney (senile) (terminal) (*see also* Sclerosis, renal)N26.1
    - congenital or infantile Q60.5
      - bilateral Q60.4
      - unilateral Q60.3
    - hydronephrotic — *see* Hydronephrosis
  - lacrimal gland (primary) H04.14 ☑
    - secondary H04.15 ☑
  - Landouzy-Déjérine G71.0
  - laryngitis, infective J37.0
  - larynx J38.7
  - Leber's optic (hereditary) H47.22
  - lip K13.0
  - liver (yellow) K72.90
    - with coma K72.91
    - acute, subacute K72.00
      - with coma K72.01
    - chronic K72.10
      - with coma K72.11
  - lung (senile) J98.4
  - macular (dermatological) L90.8
    - syphilitic, skin A51.39
      - striated A52.79
  - mandible (edentulous) K08.20
    - minimal K08.21
    - moderate K08.22
    - severe K08.23
  - maxilla K08.20
    - minimal K08.24
    - moderate K08.25
    - severe K08.26

Atrophy — *continued*
- muscle, muscular (diffuse) (general) (idiopathic) (primary) M62.50
  - ankle M62.57 ☑
  - Duchenne-Aran G12.21
  - foot M62.57 ☑
  - forearm M62.53 ☑
  - hand M62.54 ☑
  - infantile spinal G12.0
  - lower leg M62.56 ☑
  - multiple sites M62.59
  - myelopathic — *see* Atrophy, muscle, spinal
  - myotonic G71.11
  - neuritic G58.9
  - neuropathic (peroneal) (progressive) G60.0
  - pelvic (disuse) N81.84
  - peroneal G60.0
  - progressive (bulbar) G12.21
    - adult G12.1
    - infantile (spinal) G12.0
    - spinal G12.9
      - adult G12.1
      - infantile G12.0
  - pseudohypertrophic G71.0
  - shoulder region M62.51 ☑
  - specified site NEC M62.58
  - spinal G12.9
    - adult form G12.1
    - Aran-Duchenne G12.21
    - childhood form, type II G12.1
    - distal G12.1
    - hereditary NEC G12.1
    - infantile, type I (Werdnig-Hoffmann) G12.0
    - juvenile form, type III (Kugelberg- Welander) G12.1
    - progressive G12.21
    - scapuloperoneal form G12.1
    - specified NEC G12.8
  - syphilitic A52.78
  - thigh M62.55 ☑
  - upper arm M62.52 ☑
- myocardium — *see* Degeneration, myocardial
- myometrium (senile) N85.8
  - cervix N88.8
- myopathic NEC — *see* Atrophy, muscle
- myotonia G71.11
- nail L60.3
- nasopharynx J31.1
- nerve (*see also* Disorder, nerve)
  - abducens — *see* Strabismus, paralytic, sixth nerve
  - accessory G52.8
  - acoustic or auditory — *see* subcategory H93.3
  - cranial G52.9
    - eighth (auditory) — *see* subcategory H93.3
    - eleventh (accessory) G52.8
    - fifth (trigeminal) G50.8
    - first (olfactory) G52.0
    - fourth (trochlear) — *see* Strabismus, paralytic, fourth nerve
    - second (optic) H47.20
    - sixth (abducens) — *see* Strabismus, paralytic, sixth nerve
    - tenth (pneumogastric) (vagus) G52.2
    - third (oculomotor) — *see* Strabismus, paralytic, third nerve
    - twelfth (hypoglossal) G52.3
  - hypoglossal G52.3
  - oculomotor — *see* Strabismus, paralytic, third nerve
  - olfactory G52.0
  - optic (papillomacular bundle)
    - syphilitic (late) A52.15
      - congenital A50.44
  - pneumogastric G52.2
  - trigeminal G50.8
  - trochlear — *see* Strabismus, paralytic, fourth nerve
  - vagus (pneumogastric) G52.2
- neurogenic, bone, tabetic A52.11
- nutritional E41
- old age R54
- olivopontocerebellar G23.8
- optic (nerve) H47.20
  - glaucomatous H47.23 ☑
  - hereditary H47.22
  - primary H47.21 ☑
  - specified type NEC H47.29 ☑
  - syphilitic (late) A52.15
    - congenital A50.44
- orbit H05.31 ☑
- ovary (senile) N83.31 ☑
  - with fallopian tube N83.33 ☑

Atrophy — *continued*
- oviduct (senile) — *see* Atrophy, fallopian tube
- palsy, diffuse (progressive) G12.22
- pancreas (duct) (senile) K86.89
- parotid gland K11.0
- pelvic muscle N81.84
- penis N48.89
- pharynx J39.2
- pluriglandular E31.8
  - autoimmune E31.0
- polyarthritis M15.9
- prostate N42.89
- pseudohypertrophic (muscle) G71.0
- renal (*see also* Sclerosis, renal)N26.1
- retina, retinal (postinfectional) H35.89
- rhinitis J31.0
- salivary gland K11.0
- scar L90.5
- sclerosis, lobar (of brain) G31.09 *[F02.80]*
  - with behavioral disturbance G31.09 *[F02.81]*
- scrotum N50.89
- seminal vesicle N50.89
- senile R54
  - due to radiation (nonionizing) (solar) L57.8
- skin (patches) (spots) L90.9
  - degenerative (senile) L90.8
  - due to radiation (nonionizing) (solar) L57.8
  - senile L90.8
- spermatic cord N50.89
- spinal (acute) (cord) G95.89
  - muscular — *see* Atrophy, muscle, spinal
  - paralysis G12.20
    - acute — *see* Poliomyelitis, paralytic
    - meaning progressive muscular atrophy G12.21
- spine (column) — *see* Spondylopathy, specified NEC
- spleen (senile) D73.0
- stomach K29.40
  - with bleeding K29.41
- striate (skin) L90.6
  - syphilitic A52.79
- subcutaneous L90.9
- sublingual gland K11.0
- submandibular gland K11.0
- submaxillary gland K11.0
- Sudeck's — *see* Algoneurodystrophy
- suprarenal (capsule) (gland) E27.49
  - primary E27.1
- systemic affecting central nervous system
  - in
    - myxedema E03.9 *[G13.2]*
    - neoplastic disease (*see also* Neoplasm)D49.9 *[G13.1]*
    - specified disease NEC G13.8
- tarso-orbital fascia, congenital Q10.3
- testis N50.0
- thenar, partial — *see* Syndrome, carpal tunnel
- thymus (fatty) E32.8
- thyroid (gland) (acquired) E03.4
  - with cretinism E03.1
  - congenital (with myxedema) E03.1
- tongue (senile) K14.8
  - papillae K14.4
- trachea J39.8
- tunica vaginalis N50.89
- turbinate J34.89
- tympanic membrane (nonflaccid) H73.82 ☑
  - flaccid H73.81 ☑
- upper respiratory tract J39.8
- uterus, uterine (senile) N85.8
  - cervix N88.8
  - due to radiation (intended effect) N85.8
    - adverse effect or misadventure N99.89
- vagina (senile) N95.2
- vas deferens N50.89
- vascular I99.8
- vertebra (senile) — *see* Spondylopathy, specified NEC
- vulva (senile) N90.5
- Werdnig-Hoffmann G12.0
- yellow — *see* Failure, hepatic

Attack, attacks
- with alteration of consciousness (with automatisms) — *see* Epilepsy, localization-related, symptomatic, with complex partial seizures
- Adams-Stokes I45.9
- akinetic — *see* Epilepsy, generalized, specified NEC
- angina — *see* Angina
- atonic — *see* Epilepsy, generalized, specified NEC

Attack — *continued*
- benign shuddering G25.83
- cataleptic — *see* Catalepsy
- coronary — *see* Infarct, myocardium
- cyanotic, newborn P28.2
- drop NEC R55
- epileptic — *see* Epilepsy
- heart — *see* infarct, myocardium
- hysterical F44.9
- jacksonian — *see* Epilepsy, localization-related, symptomatic, with simple partial seizures
- myocardium, myocardial — *see* Infarct, myocardium
- myoclonic — *see* Epilepsy, generalized, specified NEC
- panic F41.0
- psychomotor — *see* Epilepsy, localization-related, symptomatic, with complex partial seizures
- salaam — *see* Epilepsy, spasms
- schizophreniform, brief F23
- shuddering, benign G25.83
- Stokes-Adams I45.9
- syncope R55
- transient ischemic (TIA) G45.9
  - specified NEC G45.8
- unconsciousness R55
  - hysterical F44.89
- vasomotor R55
- vasovagal (paroxysmal) (idiopathic) R55
- without alteration of consciousness — *see* Epilepsy, localization-related, symptomatic, with simple partial seizures

Attention (to)
- artificial
  - opening (of) Z43.9
    - digestive tract NEC Z43.4
      - colon Z43.3
      - ilium Z43.2
      - stomach Z43.1
    - specified NEC Z43.8
    - trachea Z43.0
    - urinary tract NEC Z43.6
      - cystostomy Z43.5
      - nephrostomy Z43.6
      - ureterostomy Z43.6
      - urethrostomy Z43.6
  - vagina Z43.7
- colostomy Z43.3
- cystostomy Z43.5
- deficit disorder or syndrome F98.8
  - with hyperactivity — *see* Disorder, attention-deficit hyperactivity
- gastrostomy Z43.1
- ileostomy Z43.2
- jejunostomy Z43.4
- nephrostomy Z43.6
- surgical dressings Z48.01
- sutures Z48.02
- tracheostomy Z43.0
- ureterostomy Z43.6
- urethrostomy Z43.6

Attrition
- gum (*see also* Recession, gingival)K06.0
- tooth, teeth (excessive) (hard tissues) K03.0

Atypical, atypism (*see also* condition)
- cells (on cytological smear) (endocervical) (endometrial) (glandular)
  - cervix R87.619
  - vagina R87.629
- cervical N87.9
- endometrium N85.9
  - hyperplasia N85.00
- parenting situation Z62.9

Auditory — *see* condition

Aujeszky's disease B33.8

Aurantiasis, cutis E67.1

Auricle, auricular (*see also* condition)
- cervical Q18.2

Auriculotemporal syndrome G50.8

Austin Flint murmur (aortic insufficiency) I35.1

Australian
- Q fever A78
- X disease A83.4

Autism, autistic (childhood) (infantile) F84.0
- atypical F84.9
- spectrum disorder F84.0

Autodigestion R68.89

Autoerythrocyte sensitization (syndrome) D69.2

Autographism L50.3

Autoimmune
- disease (systemic) M35.9
- inhibitors to clotting factors D68.311

- **Autoimmune** — *continued*
  - lymphoproliferative syndrome [ALPS] D89.82
  - thyroiditis E06.3
- **Autointoxication** R68.89
- **Automatism** G93.89
  - with temporal sclerosis G93.81
  - epileptic — *see* Epilepsy, localization-related, symptomatic, with complex partial seizures
  - paroxysmal, idiopathic — *see* Epilepsy, localization-related, symptomatic, with complex partial seizures
- **Autonomic,** autonomous
  - bladder (neurogenic) N31.2
  - hysteria seizure F44.5
- **Autosensitivity,** erythrocyte D69.2
- **Autosensitization,** cutaneous L30.2
- **Autosome** — *see* condition by chromosome involved
- **Autotopagnosia** R48.1
- **Autotoxemia** R68.89
- **Autumn** — *see* condition
- **Avellis'** syndrome G46.8
- **Aversion**
  - oral R63.3
    - newborn P92. ☑
    - nonorganic origin F98.2 ☑
  - sexual F52.1
- **Aviator's**
  - disease or sickness — *see* Effect, adverse, high altitude
  - ear T70.0 ☑
- **Avitaminosis** (multiple) (*see also* Deficiency, vitamin)E56.9
  - B E53.9
    - with
      - beriberi E51.11
      - pellagra E52
  - B2 E53.0
  - B6 E53.1
  - B12 E53.8
  - D E55.9
    - with rickets E55.0
  - G E53.0
  - K E56.1
  - nicotinic acid E52
- **AVNRT** (atrioventricular nodal re-entrant tachycardia) I47.1
- **AVRT** (atrioventricular nodal re-entrant tachycardia) I47.1
- **Avulsion** (traumatic)
  - blood vessel — *see* Injury, blood vessel
  - bone — *see* Fracture, by site
  - cartilage (*see also* Dislocation, by site)
    - symphyseal (inner), complicating delivery O71.6
  - external site other than limb — *see* Wound, open, by site
  - eye S05.7 ☑
  - head (intracranial)
    - external site NEC S08.89 ☑
    - scalp S08.0 ☑
  - internal organ or site — *see* Injury, by site
  - joint (*see also* Dislocation, by site)
    - capsule — *see* Sprain, by site
  - kidney S37.06 ☑
  - ligament — *see* Sprain, by site
  - limb (*see also* Amputation, traumatic, by site)
    - skin and subcutaneous tissue — *see* Wound, open, by site
  - muscle — *see* Injury, muscle
  - nerve (root) — *see* Injury, nerve
  - scalp S08.0 ☑
  - skin and subcutaneous tissue — *see* Wound, open, by site
  - spleen S36.032 ☑
  - symphyseal cartilage (inner), complicating delivery O71.6
  - tendon — *see* Injury, muscle
  - tooth S03.2 ☑
- **Awareness** of heart beat R00.2
- **Axenfeld's**
  - anomaly or syndrome Q15.0
  - degeneration (calcareous) Q13.4
- **Axilla,** axillary (*see also* condition)
  - breast Q83.1
- **Axonotmesis** — *see* Injury, nerve
- **Ayerza's** disease or syndrome (pulmonary artery sclerosis with pulmonary hypertension) I27.0
- **Azoospermia** (organic) N46.01
  - due to
    - drug therapy N46.021
    - efferent duct obstruction N46.023
- **Azoospermia** — *continued*
  - due to — *continued*
    - infection N46.022
    - radiation N46.024
    - specified cause NEC N46.029
    - systemic disease N46.025
- **Azotemia** R79.89
  - meaning uremia N19
- **Aztec** ear Q17.3
- **Azygos**
  - continuation inferior vena cava Q26.8
  - lobe (lung) Q33.1

B

- **Baastrup's** disease — *see* Kissing spine
- **Babesiosis** B60.0
- **Babington's** disease (familial hemorrhagic telangiectasia) I78.0
- **Babinski's** syndrome A52.79
- **Baby**
  - crying constantly R68.11
  - floppy (syndrome) P94.2
- **Bacillary** — *see* condition
- **Bacilluria** R82.71
- **Bacillus** (*see also* Infection, bacillus)
  - abortus infection A23.1
  - anthracis infection A22.9
  - coli infection (*see also* Escherichia coli)B96.20
  - Flexner's A03.1
  - mallei infection A24.0
  - Shiga's A03.0
  - suipestifer infection — *see* Infection, salmonella
- **Back** — *see* condition
- **Backache** (postural) M54.9
  - sacroiliac M53.3
  - specified NEC M54.89
- **Backflow** — *see* Reflux
- **Backward** reading (dyslexia) F81.0
- **Bacteremia** R78.81
  - with sepsis — *see* Sepsis
- **Bactericholia** — *see* Cholecystitis, acute
- **Bacterid,** bacteride (pustular) L40.3
- **Bacterium,** bacteria, bacterial
  - agent NEC, as cause of disease classified elsewhere B96.89
  - in blood — *see* Bacteremia
  - in urine — *see* Bacteriuria
- **Bacteriuria,** bacteruria R82.71
  - asymptomatic R82.71
- **Bacteroides**
  - fragilis, as cause of disease classified elsewhere B96.6
- **Bad**
  - heart — *see* Disease, heart
  - trip
    - due to drug abuse — *see* Abuse, drug, hallucinogen
    - due to drug dependence — *see* Dependence, drug, hallucinogen
- **Baelz's** disease (cheilitis glandularis apostematosa) K13.0
- **Baerensprung's** disease (eczema marginatum) B35.6
- **Bagasse** disease or pneumonitis J67.1
- **Bagassosis** J67.1
- **Baker's** cyst — *see* Cyst, Baker's
- **Bakwin-Krida** syndrome (metaphyseal dysplasia) Q78.5
- **Balancing** side interference M26.56
- **Balanitis** (circinata) (erosiva) (gangrenosa) (phagedenic) (vulgaris) N48.1
  - amebic A06.82
  - candidal B37.42
  - due to Haemophilus ducreyi A57
  - gonococcal (acute) (chronic) A54.09
  - xerotica obliterans N48.0
- **Balanoposthitis** N47.6
  - gonococcal (acute) (chronic) A54.09
  - ulcerative (specific) A63.8
- **Balanorrhagia** — *see* Balanitis
- **Balantidiasis,** balantidiosis A07.0
- **Bald** tongue K14.4
- **Baldness** (*see also* Alopecia)
  - male-pattern — *see* Alopecia, androgenic
- **Balkan** grippe A78
- **Balloon** disease — *see* Effect, adverse, high altitude
- **Balo's** disease (concentric sclerosis) G37.5
- **Bamberger-Marie** disease — *see* Osteoarthropathy, hypertrophic, specified type NEC
- **Bancroft's** filariasis B74.0
- **Band** (s)
  - adhesive — *see* Adhesions, peritoneum
  - anomalous or congenital (*see also* Anomaly, by site)
    - heart (atrial) (ventricular) Q24.8
    - intestine Q43.3
    - omentum Q43.3
  - cervix N88.1
  - constricting, congenital Q79.8
  - gallbladder (congenital) Q44.1
  - intestinal (adhesive) — *see* Adhesions, peritoneum
  - obstructive
    - intestine K56.5
    - peritoneum K56.5
  - periappendiceal, congenital Q43.3
  - peritoneal (adhesive) — *see* Adhesions, peritoneum
  - uterus N73.6
    - internal N85.6
  - vagina N89.5
- **Bandemia** D72.825
- **Bandl's** ring (contraction), complicating delivery O62.4
- **Bangkok** hemorrhagic fever A91
- **Bang's** disease (brucella abortus) A23.1
- **Bankruptcy,** anxiety concerning Z59.8
- **Bannister's** disease T78.3 ☑
  - hereditary D84.1
- **Banti's** disease or syndrome (with cirrhosis) (with portal hypertension) K76.6
- **Bar,** median, prostate — *see* Enlargement, enlarged, prostate
- **Barcoo** disease or rot — *see* Ulcer, skin
- **Barlow's** disease E54
- **Barodontalgia** T70.29 ☑
- **Baron** Münchausen syndrome — *see* Disorder, factitious
- **Barosinusitis** T70.1 ☑
- **Barotitis** T70.0 ☑
- **Barotrauma** T70.29 ☑
  - odontalgia T70.29 ☑
  - otitic T70.0 ☑
  - sinus T70.1 ☑
- **Barraquer** (-Simons) disease or syndrome (progressive lipodystrophy) E88.1
- **Barré-Guillain** disease or syndrome G61.0
- **Barré-Liéou** syndrome (posterior cervical sympathetic) M53.0
- **Barrel** chest M95.4
- **Barrett's**
  - disease — *see* Barrett's, esophagus
  - esophagus K22.70
    - with dysplasia K22.719
      - high grade K22.711
      - low grade K22.710
    - without dysplasia K22.70
  - syndrome — *see* Barrett's, esophagus
  - ulcer K22.10
    - with bleeding K22.11
    - without bleeding K22.10
- **Bársony** (-Polgár) (-Teschendorf) syndrome (corkscrew esophagus) K22.4
- **Bartholinitis** (suppurating) N75.8
  - gonococcal (acute) (chronic) (with abscess) A54.1
- **Barth** syndrome E78.71
- **Bartonellosis** A44.9
  - cutaneous A44.1
  - mucocutaneous A44.1
  - specified NEC A44.8
  - systemic A44.0
- **Barton's** fracture S52.56 ☑
- **Bartter's** syndrome E26.81
- **Basal** — *see* condition
- **Basan's** (hidrotic) ectodermal dysplasia Q82.4
- **Baseball** finger — *see* Dislocation, finger
- **Basedow's** disease (exophthalmic goiter) — *see* Hyperthyroidism, with, goiter
- **Basic** — *see* condition
- **Basilar** — *see* condition
- **Bason's** (hidrotic) ectodermal dysplasia Q82.4
- **Basopenia** — *see* Agranulocytosis
- **Basophilia** D72.824
- **Basophilism** (cortico-adrenal) (Cushing's) (pituitary) E24.0
- **Bassen-Kornzweig** disease or syndrome E78.6
- **Bat** ear Q17.5
- **Bateman's**
  - disease B08.1
  - purpura (senile) D69.2
- **Bathing** cramp T75.1 ☑
- **Bathophobia** F40.248

Batten (-Mayou) disease E75.4
- retina E75.4 *[H36]*

Batten-Steinert syndrome G71.11
Battered — *see* Maltreatment
Battey Mycobacterium infection A31.0
Battle exhaustion F43.0
Battledore placenta O43.19 ☑
Baumgarten-Cruveilhier cirrhosis, disease or syndrome K74.69
Bauxite fibrosis (of lung) J63.1
Bayle's disease (general paresis) A52.17
Bazin's disease (primary) (tuberculous) A18.4
Beach ear — *see* Swimmer's, ear
Beaded hair (congenital) Q84.1
Béal conjunctivitis or syndrome B30.2
Beard's disease (neurasthenia) F48.8
Beat (s)
- atrial, premature I49.1
- ectopic I49.49
- elbow — *see* Bursitis, elbow
- escaped, heart I49.49
- hand — *see* Bursitis, hand
- knee — *see* Bursitis, knee
- premature I49.40
  - atrial I49.1
  - auricular I49.1
  - supraventricular I49.1

Beau's
- disease or syndrome — *see* Degeneration, myocardial
- lines (transverse furrows on fingernails) L60.4

Bechterev's syndrome — *see* Spondylitis, ankylosing
Beck's syndrome (anterior spinal artery occlusion) I65.8
Becker's
- cardiomyopathy I42.8
- disease
  - idiopathic mural endomyocardial disease I42.3
  - myotonia congenita, recessive form G71.12
- dystrophy G71.0
- pigmented hairy nevus D22.5

Beckwith-Wiedemann syndrome Q87.3
Bed confinement status Z74.01
Bed sore — *see* Ulcer, pressure, by site
Bedbug bite (s) — *see* Bite (s), by site, superficial, insect
Bedclothes, asphyxiation or suffocation by — *see* Asphyxia, traumatic, due to, mechanical, trapped
Bednar's
- aphthae K12.0
- tumor — *see* Neoplasm, malignant, by site

Bedridden Z74.01
Bedsore — *see* Ulcer, pressure, by site
Bedwetting — *see* Enuresis
Bee sting (with allergic or anaphylactic shock) — *see* Toxicity, venom, arthropod, bee
Beer drinker's heart (disease) I42.6
Begbie's disease (exophthalmic goiter) — *see* Hyperthyroidism, with, goiter
Behavior
- antisocial
  - adult Z72.811
  - child or adolescent Z72.810
- disorder, disturbance — *see* Disorder, conduct
- disruptive — *see* Disorder, conduct
- drug seeking Z76.5
- inexplicable R46.2
- marked evasiveness R46.5
- obsessive-compulsive R46.81
- overactivity R46.3
- poor responsiveness R46.4
- self-damaging (life-style) Z72.89
- sleep-incompatible Z72.821
- slowness R46.4
- specified NEC R46.89
- strange (and inexplicable) R46.2
- suspiciousness R46.5
- type A pattern Z73.1
- undue concern or preoccupation with stressful events R46.6
- verbosity and circumstantial detail obscuring reason for contact R46.7

Behçet's disease or syndrome M35.2
Behr's disease — *see* Degeneration, macula
Beigel's disease or morbus (white piedra) B36.2
Bejel A65
Bekhterev's syndrome — *see* Spondylitis, ankylosing
Belching — *see* Eructation
Bell's
- mania F30.8
- palsy, paralysis G51.0
  - infant or newborn P11.3
- spasm G51.3

Bence Jones albuminuria or proteinuria NEC R80.3
Bends T70.3 ☑
Benedikt's paralysis or syndrome G46.3
Benign (*see also* condition)
- prostatic hyperplasia — *see* Hyperplasia, prostate

Bennett's fracture (displaced) S62.21 ☑
Benson's disease — *see* Deposit, crystalline
Bent
- back (hysterical) F44.4
- nose M95.0
  - congenital Q67.4

Bereavement (uncomplicated) Z63.4
Bergeron's disease (hysterical chorea) F44.4
Berger's disease — *see* Nephropathy, IgA
Beriberi (dry) E51.11
- heart (disease) E51.12
- polyneuropathy E51.11
- wet E51.12
  - involving circulatory system E51.11

Berlin's disease or edema (traumatic) S05.8X ☑
Berlock (berloque) dermatitis L56.2
Bernard-Horner syndrome G90.2
Bernard-Soulier disease or thrombopathia D69.1
Bernhardt (-Roth) disease — *see* Mononeuropathy, lower limb, meralgia paresthetica
Bernheim's syndrome — *see* Failure, heart, congestive
Bertielliasis B71.8
Berylliosis (lung) J63.2
Besnier-Boeck (-Schaumann) disease — *see* Sarcoidosis
Besnier's
- lupus pernio D86.3
- prurigo L20.0

Bestiality F65.89
Best's disease H35.50
Beta-mercaptolactate-cysteine disulfiduria E72.09
Betalipoproteinemia, broad or floating E78.2
Betting and gambling Z72.6
- pathological (compulsive) F63.0

Bezoar T18.9 ☑
- intestine T18.3 ☑
- stomach T18.2 ☑

Bezold's abscess — *see* Mastoiditis, acute
Bianchi's syndrome R48.8
Bicornate or bicornis uterus Q51.3
- in pregnancy or childbirth O34.0 ☑
  - causing obstructed labor O65.5

Bicuspid aortic valve Q23.1
Biedl-Bardet syndrome Q87.89
Bielschowsky (-Jansky) disease E75.4
Biermer's (pernicious) anemia or disease D51.0
Biett's disease L93.0
Bifid (congenital)
- apex, heart Q24.8
- clitoris Q52.6
- kidney Q63.8
- nose Q30.2
- patella Q74.1
- scrotum Q55.29
- toe NEC Q74.2
- tongue Q38.3
- ureter Q62.8
- uterus Q51.3
- uvula Q35.7

Biforis uterus (suprasimplex) Q51.3
Bifurcation (congenital)
- gallbladder Q44.1
- kidney pelvis Q63.8
- renal pelvis Q63.8
- rib Q76.6
- tongue, congenital Q38.3
- trachea Q32.1
- ureter Q62.8
- urethra Q64.74
- vertebra Q76.49

Big spleen syndrome D73.1
Bigeminal pulse R00.8
Bilateral — *see* condition
Bile
- duct — *see* condition
- pigments in urine R82.2

Bilharziasis (*see also* Schistosomiasis)
- chyluria B65.0
- cutaneous B65.3
- galacturia B65.0
- hematochyluria B65.0
- intestinal B65.1
- lipemia B65.9
- lipuria B65.0
- oriental B65.2
- piarhemia B65.9
- pulmonary NOS B65.9 *[J99]*
  - pneumonia B65.9 *[J17]*
- tropical hematuria B65.0
- vesical B65.0

Biliary — *see* condition
Bilirubin metabolism disorder E80.7
- specified NEC E80.6

Bilirubinemia, familial nonhemolytic E80.4
Bilirubinuria R82.2
Biliuria R82.2
Bilocular stomach K31.2
Binswanger's disease I67.3
Biparta, bipartite
- carpal scaphoid Q74.0
- patella Q74.1
- vagina Q52.10

Bird
- face Q75.8
- fancier's disease or lung J67.2

Birt-Hogg-Dube syndrome Q87.89
Birth
- complications in mother — *see* Delivery, complicated
- compression during NOS P15.9
- defect — *see* Anomaly
- immature (less than 37 completed weeks) — *see* Preterm, newborn
  - extremely (less than 28 completed weeks) — *see* Immaturity, extreme
- inattention, at or after — *see* Maltreatment, child, neglect
- injury NOS P15.9
  - basal ganglia P11.1
  - brachial plexus NEC P14.3
  - brain (compression) (pressure) P11.2
  - central nervous system NOS P11.9
  - cerebellum P11.1
  - cerebral hemorrhage P10.1
  - external genitalia P15.5
  - eye P15.3
  - face P15.4
  - fracture
    - bone P13.9
      - specified NEC P13.8
    - clavicle P13.4
    - femur P13.2
    - humerus P13.3
    - long bone, except femur P13.3
    - radius and ulna P13.3
    - skull P13.0
    - spine P11.5
    - tibia and fibula P13.3
  - intracranial P11.2
    - laceration or hemorrhage P10.9
      - specified NEC P10.8
  - intraventricular hemorrhage P10.2
  - laceration
    - brain P10.1
    - by scalpel P15.8
    - peripheral nerve P14.9
  - liver P15.0
  - meninges
    - brain P11.1
    - spinal cord P11.5
  - nerve
    - brachial plexus P14.3
    - cranial NEC (except facial) P11.4
    - facial P11.3
    - peripheral P14.9
    - phrenic (paralysis) P14.2
  - paralysis
    - facial nerve P11.3
    - spinal P11.5
  - penis P15.5
  - rupture
    - spinal cord P11.5
  - scalp P12.9
  - scalpel wound P15.8
  - scrotum P15.5
  - skull NEC P13.1
    - fracture P13.0
  - specified type NEC P15.8
  - spinal cord P11.5
  - spine P11.5
  - spleen P15.1
  - sternomastoid (hematoma) P15.2
  - subarachnoid hemorrhage P10.3
  - subcutaneous fat necrosis P15.6
  - subdural hemorrhage P10.0
  - tentorial tear P10.4
  - testes P15.5

- **Birth** — *continued*
  - injury NOS — *continued*
    - vulva P15.5
  - lack of care, at or after — *see* Maltreatment, child, neglect
  - neglect, at or after — *see* Maltreatment, child, neglect
  - palsy or paralysis, newborn, NOS (birth injury) P14.9
  - premature (infant) — *see* Preterm, newborn
  - shock, newborn P96.89
  - trauma — *see* Birth, injury
  - weight
    - low (2499 grams or less) — *see* Low, birthweight
      - extremely (999 grams or less) — *see* Low, birthweight, extreme
    - 4000 grams to 4499 grams P08.1
    - 4500 grams or more P08.0
- **Birthmark** Q82.5
- **Bisalbuminemia** E88.09
- **Biskra's** button B55.1
- **Bite** (s) (animal) (human)
  - abdomen, abdominal
    - wall S31.159 ☑
      - with penetration into peritoneal cavity S31.659 ☑
      - epigastric region S31.152 ☑
        - with penetration into peritoneal cavity S31.652 ☑
      - left
        - lower quadrant S31.154 ☑
          - with penetration into peritoneal cavity S31.654 ☑
        - upper quadrant S31.151 ☑
          - with penetration into peritoneal cavity S31.651 ☑
      - periumbilic region S31.155 ☑
        - with penetration into peritoneal cavity S31.655 ☑
      - right
        - lower quadrant S31.153 ☑
          - with penetration into peritoneal cavity S31.653 ☑
        - upper quadrant S31.150 ☑
          - with penetration into peritoneal cavity S31.650 ☑
      - superficial NEC S30.871 ☑
        - insect S30.861 ☑
  - alveolar (process) — *see* Bite, oral cavity
  - amphibian (venomous) — *see* Venom, bite, amphibian
  - animal (*see also* Bite, by site)
    - venomous — *see* Venom
  - ankle S91.05 ☑
    - superficial NEC S90.57 ☑
      - insect S90.56 ☑
  - antecubital space — *see* Bite, elbow
  - anus S31.835 ☑
    - superficial NEC S30.877 ☑
      - insect S30.867 ☑
  - arm (upper) S41.15 ☑
    - lower — *see* Bite, forearm
    - superficial NEC S40.87 ☑
      - insect S40.86 ☑
  - arthropod NEC — *see* Venom, bite, arthropod
  - auditory canal (external) (meatus) — *see* Bite, ear
  - auricle, ear — *see* Bite, ear
  - axilla — *see* Bite, arm
  - back (*see also* Bite, thorax, back)
    - lower S31.050 ☑
      - with penetration into retroperitoneal space S31.051 ☑
      - superficial NEC S30.870 ☑
        - insect S30.860 ☑
  - bedbug — *see* Bite (s), by site, superficial, insect
  - breast S21.05 ☑
    - superficial NEC S20.17 ☑
      - insect S20.16 ☑
  - brow — *see* Bite, head, specified site NEC
  - buttock S31.805 ☑
    - left S31.825 ☑
    - right S31.815 ☑
    - superficial NEC S30.870 ☑
      - insect S30.860 ☑
  - calf — *see* Bite, leg
  - canaliculus lacrimalis — *see* Bite, eyelid
  - canthus, eye — *see* Bite, eyelid
  - centipede — *see* Toxicity, venom, arthropod, centipede
  - cheek (external) S01.45 ☑
    - superficial NEC S00.87 ☑

- **Bite** — *continued*
  - cheek — *continued*
      - insect S00.86 ☑
    - internal — *see* Bite, oral cavity
  - chest wall — *see* Bite, thorax
  - chigger B88.0
  - chin — *see* Bite, head, specified site NEC
  - clitoris — *see* Bite, vulva
  - costal region — *see* Bite, thorax
  - digit (s)
    - hand — *see* Bite, finger
    - toe — *see* Bite, toe
  - ear (canal) (external) S01.35 ☑
    - superficial NEC S00.47 ☑
      - insect S00.46 ☑
  - elbow S51.05 ☑
    - superficial NEC S50.37 ☑
      - insect S50.36 ☑
  - epididymis — *see* Bite, testis
  - epigastric region — *see* Bite, abdomen
  - epiglottis — *see* Bite, neck, specified site NEC
  - esophagus, cervical S11.25 ☑
    - superficial NEC S10.17 ☑
      - insect S10.16 ☑
  - eyebrow — *see* Bite, eyelid
  - eyelid S01.15 ☑
    - superficial NEC S00.27 ☑
      - insect S00.26 ☑
  - face NEC — *see* Bite, head, specified site NEC
  - finger (s) S61.259 ☑
    - with
      - damage to nail S61.359 ☑
    - index S61.258 ☑
      - with
        - damage to nail S61.358 ☑
      - left S61.251 ☑
        - with
          - damage to nail S61.351 ☑
      - right S61.250 ☑
        - with
          - damage to nail S61.350 ☑
      - superficial NEC S60.478 ☑
        - insect S60.46 ☑
    - little S61.25 ☑
      - with
        - damage to nail S61.35 ☑
      - superficial NEC S60.47 ☑
        - insect S60.46 ☑
    - middle S61.25 ☑
      - with
        - damage to nail S61.35 ☑
      - superficial NEC S60.47 ☑
        - insect S60.46 ☑
    - ring S61.25 ☑
      - with
        - damage to nail S61.35 ☑
      - superficial NEC S60.47 ☑
        - insect S60.46 ☑
    - superficial NEC S60.479 ☑
      - insect S60.469 ☑
    - thumb — *see* Bite, thumb
  - flank — *see* Bite, abdomen, wall
  - flea — *see* Bite, by site, superficial, insect
  - foot (except toe (s) alone) S91.35 ☑
    - superficial NEC S90.87 ☑
      - insect S90.86 ☑
    - toe — *see* Bite, toe
  - forearm S51.85 ☑
    - elbow only — *see* Bite, elbow
    - superficial NEC S50.87 ☑
      - insect S50.86 ☑
  - forehead — *see* Bite, head, specified site NEC
  - genital organs, external
    - female S31.552 ☑
      - superficial NEC S30.876 ☑
        - insect S30.866 ☑
      - vagina and vulva — *see* Bite, vulva
    - male S31.551 ☑
      - penis — *see* Bite, penis
      - scrotum — *see* Bite, scrotum
      - superficial NEC S30.875 ☑
        - insect S30.865 ☑
      - testes — *see* Bite, testis
  - groin — *see* Bite, abdomen, wall
  - gum — *see* Bite, oral cavity
  - hand S61.45 ☑
    - finger — *see* Bite, finger
    - superficial NEC S60.57 ☑
      - insect S60.56 ☑
    - thumb — *see* Bite, thumb
  - head S01.95 ☑
    - cheek — *see* Bite, cheek

- **Bite** — *continued*
  - head — *continued*
    - ear — *see* Bite, ear
    - eyelid — *see* Bite, eyelid
    - lip — *see* Bite, lip
    - nose — *see* Bite, nose
    - oral cavity — *see* Bite, oral cavity
    - scalp — *see* Bite, scalp
    - specified site NEC S01.85 ☑
      - superficial NEC S00.87 ☑
        - insect S00.86 ☑
    - superficial NEC S00.97 ☑
      - insect S00.96 ☑
    - temporomandibular area — *see* Bite, cheek
  - heel — *see* Bite, foot
  - hip S71.05 ☑
    - superficial NEC S70.27 ☑
      - insect S70.26 ☑
  - hymen S31.45 ☑
  - hypochondrium — *see* Bite, abdomen, wall
  - hypogastric region — *see* Bite, abdomen, wall
  - inguinal region — *see* Bite, abdomen, wall
  - insect — *see* Bite, by site, superficial, insect
  - instep — *see* Bite, foot
  - interscapular region — *see* Bite, thorax, back
  - jaw — *see* Bite, head, specified site NEC
  - knee S81.05 ☑
    - superficial NEC S80.27 ☑
      - insect S80.26 ☑
  - labium (majus) (minus) — *see* Bite, vulva
  - lacrimal duct — *see* Bite, eyelid
  - larynx S11.015 ☑
    - superficial NEC S10.17 ☑
      - insect S10.16 ☑
  - leg (lower) S81.85 ☑
    - ankle — *see* Bite, ankle
    - foot — *see* Bite, foot
    - knee — *see* Bite, knee
    - superficial NEC S80.87 ☑
      - insect S80.86 ☑
    - toe — *see* Bite, toe
    - upper — *see* Bite, thigh
  - lip S01.551 ☑
    - superficial NEC S00.571 ☑
      - insect S00.561 ☑
  - lizard (venomous) — *see* Venom, bite, reptile
  - loin — *see* Bite, abdomen, wall
  - lower back — *see* Bite, back, lower
  - lumbar region — *see* Bite, back, lower
  - malar region — *see* Bite, head, specified site NEC
  - mammary — *see* Bite, breast
  - marine animals (venomous) — *see* Toxicity, venom, marine animal
  - mastoid region — *see* Bite, head, specified site NEC
  - mouth — *see* Bite, oral cavity
  - nail
    - finger — *see* Bite, finger
    - toe — *see* Bite, toe
  - nape — *see* Bite, neck, specified site NEC
  - nasal (septum) (sinus) — *see* Bite, nose
  - nasopharynx — *see* Bite, head, specified site NEC
  - neck S11.95 ☑
    - involving
      - cervical esophagus — *see* Bite, esophagus, cervical
      - larynx — *see* Bite, larynx
      - pharynx — *see* Bite, pharynx
      - thyroid gland S11.15 ☑
      - trachea — *see* Bite, trachea
    - specified site NEC S11.85 ☑
      - superficial NEC S10.87 ☑
        - insect S10.86 ☑
    - superficial NEC S10.97 ☑
      - insect S10.96 ☑
    - throat S11.85 ☑
      - superficial NEC S10.17 ☑
        - insect S10.16 ☑
  - nose (septum) (sinus) S01.25 ☑
    - superficial NEC S00.37 ☑
      - insect S00.36 ☑
  - occipital region — *see* Bite, scalp
  - oral cavity S01.552 ☑
    - superficial NEC S00.572 ☑
      - insect S00.562 ☑
  - orbital region — *see* Bite, eyelid
  - palate — *see* Bite, oral cavity
  - palm — *see* Bite, hand
  - parietal region — *see* Bite, scalp
  - pelvis S31.050 ☑
    - with penetration into retroperitoneal space S31.051 ☑

- **Bite** — *continued*
  - pelvis — *continued*
    - superficial NEC S30.870 ☑
      - insect S30.860 ☑
  - penis S31.25 ☑
    - superficial NEC S30.872 ☑
      - insect S30.862 ☑
  - perineum
    - female — *see* Bite, vulva
    - male — *see* Bite, pelvis
  - periocular area (with or without lacrimal passages) — *see* Bite, eyelid
  - phalanges
    - finger — *see* Bite, finger
    - toe — *see* Bite, toe
  - pharynx S11.25 ☑
    - superficial NEC S10.17 ☑
      - insect S10.16 ☑
  - pinna — *see* Bite, ear
  - poisonous — *see* Venom
  - popliteal space — *see* Bite, knee
  - prepuce — *see* Bite, penis
  - pubic region — *see* Bite, abdomen, wall
  - rectovaginal septum — *see* Bite, vulva
  - red bug B88.0
  - reptile NEC (*see also* Venom, bite, reptile)
    - nonvenomous — *see* Bite, by site
    - snake — *see* Venom, bite, snake
  - sacral region — *see* Bite, back, lower
  - sacroiliac region — *see* Bite, back, lower
  - salivary gland — *see* Bite, oral cavity
  - scalp S01.05 ☑
    - superficial NEC S00.07 ☑
      - insect S00.06 ☑
  - scapular region — *see* Bite, shoulder
  - scrotum S31.35 ☑
    - superficial NEC S30.873 ☑
      - insect S30.863 ☑
  - sea-snake (venomous) — *see* Toxicity, venom, snake, sea snake
  - shin — *see* Bite, leg
  - shoulder S41.05 ☑
    - superficial NEC S40.27 ☑
      - insect S40.26 ☑
  - snake (*see also* Venom, bite, snake)
    - nonvenomous — *see* Bite, by site
  - spermatic cord — *see* Bite, testis
  - spider (venomous) — *see* Toxicity, venom, spider
    - nonvenomous — *see* Bite, by site, superficial, insect
  - sternal region — *see* Bite, thorax, front
  - submaxillary region — *see* Bite, head, specified site NEC
  - submental region — *see* Bite, head, specified site NEC
  - subungual
    - finger (s) — *see* Bite, finger
    - toe — *see* Bite, toe
  - superficial — *see* Bite, by site, superficial
  - supraclavicular fossa S11.85 ☑
  - supraorbital — *see* Bite, head, specified site NEC
  - temple, temporal region — *see* Bite, head, specified site NEC
  - temporomandibular area — *see* Bite, cheek
  - testis S31.35 ☑
    - superficial NEC S30.873 ☑
      - insect S30.863 ☑
  - thigh S71.15 ☑
    - superficial NEC S70.37 ☑
      - insect S70.36 ☑
  - thorax, thoracic (wall) S21.95 ☑
    - back S21.25 ☑
      - with penetration into thoracic cavity S21.45 ☑
    - breast — *see* Bite, breast
    - front S21.15 ☑
      - with penetration into thoracic cavity S21.35 ☑
    - superficial NEC S20.97 ☑
      - back S20.47 ☑
      - front S20.37 ☑
      - insect S20.96 ☑
        - back S20.46 ☑
        - front S20.36 ☑
  - throat — *see* Bite, neck, throat
  - thumb S61.05 ☑
    - with
      - damage to nail S61.15 ☑
    - superficial NEC S60.37 ☑
      - insect S60.36 ☑
  - thyroid S11.15 ☑
    - superficial NEC S10.87 ☑
      - insect S10.86 ☑

- **Bite** — *continued*
  - toe (s) S91.15 ☑
    - with
      - damage to nail S91.25 ☑
    - great S91.15 ☑
      - with
        - damage to nail S91.25 ☑
    - lesser S91.15 ☑
      - with
        - damage to nail S91.25 ☑
    - superficial NEC S90.47 ☑
      - great S90.47 ☑
      - insect S90.46 ☑
        - great S90.46 ☑
  - tongue S01.552 ☑
  - trachea S11.025 ☑
    - superficial NEC S10.17 ☑
      - insect S10.16 ☑
  - tunica vaginalis — *see* Bite, testis
  - tympanum, tympanic membrane — *see* Bite, ear
  - umbilical region S31.155 ☑
  - uvula — *see* Bite, oral cavity
  - vagina — *see* Bite, vulva
  - venomous — *see* Venom
  - vocal cords S11.035 ☑
    - superficial NEC S10.17 ☑
      - insect S10.16 ☑
  - vulva S31.45 ☑
    - superficial NEC S30.874 ☑
      - insect S30.864 ☑
  - wrist S61.55 ☑
    - superficial NEC S60.87 ☑
      - insect S60.86 ☑
- **Biting,** cheek or lip K13.1
- **Biventricular** failure (heart) I50.9
- **Björck** (-Thorson) syndrome (malignant carcinoid) E34.0
- **Black**
  - death A20.9
  - eye S00.1 ☑
  - hairy tongue K14.3
  - heel (foot) S90.3 ☑
  - lung (disease) J60
  - palm (hand) S60.22 ☑
- **Blackfan-Diamond** anemia or syndrome (congenital hypoplastic anemia) D61.01
- **Blackhead** L70.0
- **Blackout** R55
- **Bladder** — *see* condition
- **Blast** (air) (hydraulic) (immersion) (underwater)
  - blindness S05.8X ☑
  - injury
    - abdomen or thorax — *see* Injury, by site
    - ear (acoustic nerve trauma) — *see* Injury, nerve, acoustic, specified type NEC
    - syndrome NEC T70.8 ☑
- **Blastoma** — *see* Neoplasm, malignant, by site
  - pulmonary — *see* Neoplasm, lung, malignant
- **Blastomycosis,** blastomycotic B40.9
  - Brazilian — *see* Paracoccidioidomycosis
  - cutaneous B40.3
  - disseminated B40.7
  - European — *see* Cryptococcosis
  - generalized B40.7
  - keloidal B48.0
  - North American B40.9
  - primary pulmonary B40.0
  - pulmonary B40.2
    - acute B40.0
    - chronic B40.1
  - skin B40.3
  - South American — *see* Paracoccidioidomycosis
  - specified NEC B40.89
- **Bleb** (s) R23.8
  - emphysematous (lung) (solitary) J43.9
  - endophthalmitis H59.43
  - filtering (vitreous), after glaucoma surgery Z98.83
  - inflamed (infected), postprocedural H59.40
    - stage 1 H59.41
    - stage 2 H59.42
    - stage 3 H59.43
  - lung (ruptured) J43.9
    - congenital — *see* Atelectasis
    - newborn P25.8
  - subpleural (emphysematous) J43.9
- **Blebitis,** postprocedural H59.40
  - stage 1 H59.41
  - stage 2 H59.42
  - stage 3 H59.43
- **Bleeder** (familial) (hereditary) — *see* Hemophilia

- **Bleeding** (*see also* Hemorrhage)
  - anal K62.5
  - anovulatory N97.0
  - atonic, following delivery O72.1
  - capillary I78.8
    - puerperal O72.2
  - contact (postcoital) N93.0
  - due to uterine subinvolution N85.3
  - ear — *see* Otorrhagia
  - excessive, associated with menopausal onset N92.4
  - familial — *see* Defect, coagulation
  - following intercourse N93.0
  - gastrointestinal K92.2
  - hemorrhoids — *see* Hemorrhoids
  - intermenstrual (regular) N92.3
    - irregular N92.1
  - intraoperative — *see* Complication, intraoperative, hemorrhage
  - irregular N92.6
  - menopausal N92.4
  - newborn, intraventricular — *see* Newborn, affected by, hemorrhage, intraventricular
  - nipple N64.59
  - nose R04.0
  - ovulation N92.3
  - postclimacteric N95.0
  - postcoital N93.0
  - postmenopausal N95.0
  - postoperative — *see* Complication, postprocedural, hemorrhage
  - preclimacteric N92.4
  - pre-pubertal vaginal N93.1
  - puberty (excessive, with onset of menstrual periods) N92.2
  - rectum, rectal K62.5
    - newborn P54.2
  - tendencies — *see* Defect, coagulation
  - throat R04.1
  - tooth socket (post-extraction) K91.840
  - umbilical stump P51.9
  - uterus, uterine NEC N93.9
    - climacteric N92.4
    - dysfunctional of functional N93.8
    - menopausal N92.4
    - preclimacteric or premenopausal N92.4
    - unrelated to menstrual cycle N93.9
  - vagina, vaginal (abnormal) N93.9
    - dysfunctional or functional N93.8
    - newborn P54.6
    - pre-pubertal N93.1
  - vicarious N94.89
- **Blennorrhagia,** blennorrhagic — *see* Gonorrhea
- **Blennorrhea** (acute) (chronic) (*see also* Gonorrhea)
  - inclusion (neonatal) (newborn) P39.1
  - lower genitourinary tract (gonococcal) A54.00
  - neonatorum (gonococcal ophthalmia) A54.31
- **Blepharelosis** — *see* Entropion
- **Blepharitis** (angularis) (ciliaris) (eyelid) (marginal) (nonulcerative) H01.009
  - herpes zoster B02.39
  - left H01.006
    - lower H01.005
    - upper H01.004
  - right H01.003
    - lower H01.002
    - upper H01.001
  - squamous H01.029
    - left H01.026
      - lower H01.025
      - upper H01.024
    - right H01.023
      - lower H01.022
      - upper H01.021
  - ulcerative H01.019
    - left H01.016
      - lower H01.015
      - upper H01.014
    - right H01.013
      - lower H01.012
      - upper H01.011
- **Blepharochalasis** H02.30
  - congenital Q10.0
  - left H02.36
    - lower H02.35
    - upper H02.34
  - right H02.33
    - lower H02.32
    - upper H02.31
- **Blepharoclonus** H02.59
- **Blepharoconjunctivitis** H10.50 ☑
  - angular H10.52 ☑

Blepharoconjunctivitis — *continued*
- contact H10.53 ☑
- ligneous H10.51 ☑

Blepharophimosis (eyelid) H02.529
- congenital Q10.3
- left H02.526
  - lower H02.525
  - upper H02.524
- right H02.523
  - lower H02.522
  - upper H02.521

Blepharoptosis H02.40 ☑
- congenital Q10.0
- mechanical H02.41 ☑
- myogenic H02.42 ☑
- neurogenic H02.43 ☑
- paralytic H02.43 ☑

Blepharopyorrhea, gonococcal A54.39

Blepharospasm G24.5
- drug induced G24.01

Blighted ovum O02.0

Blind (*see also* Blindness)
- bronchus (congenital) Q32.4
- loop syndrome K90.2
  - congenital Q43.8
- sac, fallopian tube (congenital) Q50.6
- spot, enlarged — *see* Defect, visual field, localized, scotoma, blind spot area
- tract or tube, congenital NEC — *see* Atresia, by site

Blindness (acquired) (congenital) (both eyes) H54.0
- blast S05.8X ☑
- color — *see* Deficiency, color vision
- concussion S05.8X ☑
- cortical H47.619
  - left brain H47.612
  - right brain H47.611
- day H53.11
- due to injury (current episode) S05.9 ☑
  - sequelae -- code to injury with seventh character S
- eclipse (total) — *see* Retinopathy, solar
- emotional (hysterical) F44.6
- face H53.16
- hysterical F44.6
- legal (both eyes) (USA definition) H54.8
- mind R48.8
- night H53.60
  - abnormal dark adaptation curve H53.61
  - acquired H53.62
  - congenital H53.63
  - specified type NEC H53.69
  - vitamin A deficiency E50.5
- one eye (other eye normal) H54.40
  - left (normal vision on right) H54.42
    - low vision on right H54.12
  - low vision, other eye H54.10
  - right (normal vision on left) H54.41
    - low vision on left H54.11
- psychic R48.8
- river B73.01
- snow — *see* Photokeratitis
- sun, solar — *see* Retinopathy, solar
- transient — *see* Disturbance, vision, subjective, loss, transient
- traumatic (current episode) S05.9 ☑
- word (developmental) F81.0
  - acquired R48.0
  - secondary to organic lesion R48.0

Blister (nonthermal)
- abdominal wall S30.821 ☑
- alveolar process S00.522 ☑
- ankle S90.52 ☑
- antecubital space — *see* Blister, elbow
- anus S30.827 ☑
- arm (upper) S40.82 ☑
- auditory canal — *see* Blister, ear
- auricle — *see* Blister, ear
- axilla — *see* Blister, arm
- back, lower S30.820 ☑
- beetle dermatitis L24.89
- breast S20.12 ☑
- brow S00.82 ☑
- calf — *see* Blister, leg
- canthus — *see* Blister, eyelid
- cheek S00.82 ☑
  - internal S00.522 ☑
- chest wall — *see* Blister, thorax
- chin S00.82 ☑
- costal region — *see* Blister, thorax
- digit (s)
  - foot — *see* Blister, toe
  - hand — *see* Blister, finger

Blister — *continued*
- due to burn — *see* Burn, by site, second degree
- ear S00.42 ☑
- elbow S50.32 ☑
- epiglottis S10.12 ☑
- esophagus, cervical S10.12 ☑
- eyebrow — *see* Blister, eyelid
- eyelid S00.22 ☑
- face S00.82 ☑
- fever B00.1
- finger (s) S60.429 ☑
  - index S60.42 ☑
  - little S60.42 ☑
  - middle S60.42 ☑
  - ring S60.42 ☑
- foot (except toe (s) alone) S90.82 ☑
  - toe — *see* Blister, toe
- forearm S50.82 ☑
  - elbow only — *see* Blister, elbow
- forehead S00.82 ☑
- fracture - omit code
- genital organ
  - female S30.826 ☑
  - male S30.825 ☑
- gum S00.522 ☑
- hand S60.52 ☑
- head S00.92 ☑
  - ear — *see* Blister, ear
  - eyelid — *see* Blister, eyelid
  - lip S00.521 ☑
  - nose S00.32 ☑
  - oral cavity S00.522 ☑
  - scalp S00.02 ☑
  - specified site NEC S00.82 ☑
- heel — *see* Blister, foot
- hip S70.22 ☑
- interscapular region S20.429 ☑
- jaw S00.82 ☑
- knee S80.22 ☑
- larynx S10.12 ☑
- leg (lower) S80.82 ☑
  - knee — *see* Blister, knee
  - upper — *see* Blister, thigh
- lip S00.521 ☑
- malar region S00.82 ☑
- mammary — *see* Blister, breast
- mastoid region S00.82 ☑
- mouth S00.522 ☑
- multiple, skin, nontraumatic R23.8
- nail
  - finger — *see* Blister, finger
  - toe — *see* Blister, toe
- nasal S00.32 ☑
- neck S10.92 ☑
  - specified site NEC S10.82 ☑
  - throat S10.12 ☑
- nose S00.32 ☑
- occipital region S00.02 ☑
- oral cavity S00.522 ☑
- orbital region — *see* Blister, eyelid
- palate S00.522 ☑
- palm — *see* Blister, hand
- parietal region S00.02 ☑
- pelvis S30.820 ☑
- penis S30.822 ☑
- periocular area — *see* Blister, eyelid
- phalanges
  - finger — *see* Blister, finger
  - toe — *see* Blister, toe
- pharynx S10.12 ☑
- pinna — *see* Blister, ear
- popliteal space — *see* Blister, knee
- scalp S00.02 ☑
- scapular region — *see* Blister, shoulder
- scrotum S30.823 ☑
- shin — *see* Blister, leg
- shoulder S40.22 ☑
- sternal region S20.329 ☑
- submaxillary region S00.82 ☑
- submental region S00.82 ☑
- subungual
  - finger (s) — *see* Blister, finger
  - toe (s) — *see* Blister, toe
- supraclavicular fossa S10.82 ☑
- supraorbital S00.82 ☑
- temple S00.82 ☑
- temporal region S00.82 ☑
- testis S30.823 ☑
- thermal — *see* Burn, second degree, by site
- thigh S70.32 ☑
- thorax, thoracic (wall) S20.92 ☑
  - back S20.42 ☑
  - front S20.32 ☑

Blister — *continued*
- throat S10.12 ☑
- thumb S60.32 ☑
- toe (s) S90.42 ☑
  - great S90.42 ☑
- tongue S00.522 ☑
- trachea S10.12 ☑
- tympanum, tympanic membrane — *see* Blister, ear
- upper arm — *see* Blister, arm (upper)
- uvula S00.522 ☑
- vagina S30.824 ☑
- vocal cords S10.12 ☑
- vulva S30.824 ☑
- wrist S60.82 ☑

Bloating R14.0

Bloch-Sulzberger disease or syndrome Q82.3

Block, blocked
- alveolocapillary J84.10
- arborization (heart) I45.5
- arrhythmic I45.9
- atrioventricular (incomplete) (partial) I44.30
  - with atrioventricular dissociation I44.2
  - complete I44.2
    - congenital Q24.6
  - congenital Q24.6
  - first degree I44.0
  - second degree (types I and II) I44.1
  - specified NEC I44.39
  - third degree I44.2
  - types I and II I44.1
- auriculoventricular — *see* Block, atrioventricular
- bifascicular (cardiac) I45.2
- bundle-branch (complete) (false) (incomplete) I45.4
  - bilateral I45.2
  - left I44.7
    - with right bundle branch block I45.2
    - hemiblock I44.60
      - anterior I44.4
      - posterior I44.5
    - incomplete I44.7
      - with right bundle branch block I45.2
  - right I45.10
    - with
      - left bundle branch block I45.2
      - left fascicular block I45.2
    - specified NEC I45.19
  - Wilson's type I45.19
- cardiac I45.9
- conduction I45.9
  - complete I44.2
- fascicular (left) I44.60
  - anterior I44.4
  - posterior I44.5
  - right I45.0
  - specified NEC I44.69
- foramen Magendie (acquired) G91.1
  - congenital Q03.1
    - with spina bifida — *see* Spina bifida, by site, with hydrocephalus
- heart I45.9
  - bundle branch I45.4
    - bilateral I45.2
  - complete (atrioventricular) I44.2
  - congenital Q24.6
  - first degree (atrioventricular) I44.0
  - second degree (atrioventricular) I44.1
  - specified type NEC I45.5
  - third degree (atrioventricular) I44.2
- hepatic vein I82.0
- intraventricular (nonspecific) I45.4
  - bundle branch
    - bilateral I45.2
- kidney N28.9
  - postcystoscopic or postprocedural N99.0
- Mobitz (types I and II) I44.1
- myocardial — *see* Block, heart
- nodal I45.5
- organ or site, congenital NEC — *see* Atresia, by site
- portal (vein) I81
- second degree (types I and II) I44.1
- sinoatrial I45.5
- sinoauricular I45.5
- third degree I44.2
- trifascicular I45.3
- tubal N97.1
- vein NOS I82.90
- Wenckebach (types I and II) I44.1

Blockage — *see* Obstruction

Blocq's disease F44.4

- **Blood**
  - constituents, abnormal R78.9
  - disease D75.9
  - donor — *see* Donor, blood
  - dyscrasia D75.9
    - with
      - abortion — *see* Abortion, by type, complicated by, hemorrhage
      - ectopic pregnancy O08.1
      - molar pregnancy O08.1
    - following ectopic or molar pregnancy O08.1
    - newborn P61.9
    - puerperal, postpartum O72.3
  - flukes NEC — *see* Schistosomiasis
  - in
    - feces K92.1
      - occult R19.5
    - urine — *see* Hematuria
  - mole O02.0
  - occult in feces R19.5
  - pressure
    - decreased, due to shock following injury T79.4 ☑
    - examination only Z01.30
    - fluctuating I99.8
    - high — *see* Hypertension
      - borderline R03.0
      - incidental reading, without diagnosis of hypertension R03.0
    - low (*see also* Hypotension)
      - incidental reading, without diagnosis of hypotension R03.1
  - spitting — *see* Hemoptysis
  - staining cornea — *see* Pigmentation, cornea, stromal
  - transfusion
    - reaction or complication — *see* Complications, transfusion
  - type
    - A (Rh positive) Z67.10
      - Rh negative Z67.11
    - AB (Rh positive) Z67.30
      - Rh negative Z67.31
    - B (Rh positive) Z67.20
      - Rh negative Z67.21
    - O (Rh positive) Z67.40
      - Rh negative Z67.41
    - Rh (positive) Z67.90
      - negative Z67.91
  - vessel rupture — *see* Hemorrhage
  - vomiting — *see* Hematemesis
- **Blood-forming** organs, disease D75.9
- **Bloodgood's** disease — *see* Mastopathy, cystic
- **Bloom** (-Machacek) (-Torre) syndrome Q82.8
- **Blount's** disease or osteochondrosis — *see* Osteochondrosis, juvenile, tibia
- **Blue**
  - baby Q24.9
  - diaper syndrome E72.09
  - dome cyst (breast) — *see* Cyst, breast
  - dot cataract Q12.0
  - nevus D22.9
  - sclera Q13.5
    - with fragility of bone and deafness Q78.0
  - toe syndrome I75.02 ☑
- **Blueness** — *see* Cyanosis
- **Blues,** postpartal O90.6
  - baby O90.6
- **Blurring,** visual H53.8
- **Blushing** (abnormal) (excessive) R23.2
- **BMI** — *see* Body, mass index
- **Boarder,** hospital NEC Z76.4
  - accompanying sick person Z76.3
  - healthy infant or child Z76.2
    - foundling Z76.1
- **Bockhart's** impetigo L01.02
- **Bodechtel-Guttman** disease (subacute sclerosing panencephalitis) A81.1
- **Boder-Sedgwick** syndrome (ataxia-telangiectasia) G11.3
- **Body,** bodies
  - Aschoff's — *see* Myocarditis, rheumatic
  - asteroid, vitreous — *see* Deposit, crystalline
  - cytoid (retina) — *see* Occlusion, artery, retina
  - drusen (degenerative) (macula) (retinal) (*see also* Degeneration, macula, drusen)
    - optic disc — *see* Drusen, optic disc
  - foreign — *see* Foreign body
  - loose
    - joint, except knee — *see* Loose, body, joint
      - knee M23.4 ☑

- **Body** — *continued*
  - loose — *continued*
    - sheath, tendon — *see* Disorder, tendon, specified type NEC
  - mass index (BMI)
    - adult
      - 19 or less Z68.1
      - 20.0-20.9 Z68.20
      - 21.0-21.9 Z68.21
      - 22.0-22.9 Z68.22
      - 23.0-23.9 Z68.23
      - 24.0-24.9 Z68.24
      - 25.0-25.9 Z68.25
      - 26.0-26.9 Z68.26
      - 27.0-27.9 Z68.27
      - 28.0-28.9 Z68.28
      - 29.0-29.9 Z68.29
      - 30.0-30.9 Z68.30
      - 31.0-31.9 Z68.31
      - 32.0-32.9 Z68.32
      - 33.0-33.9 Z68.33
      - 34.0-34.9 Z68.34
      - 35.0-35.9 Z68.35
      - 36.0-36.9 Z68.36
      - 37.0-37.9 Z68.37
      - 38.0-38.9 Z68.38
      - 39.0-39.9 Z68.39
      - 40.0-44.9 Z68.41
      - 45.0-49.9 Z68.42
      - 50.0-59.9 Z68.43
      - 60.0-69.9 Z68.44
      - 70 and over Z68.45
    - pediatric
      - 5th percentile to less than 85th percentile for age Z68.52
      - 85th percentile to less than 95th percentile for age Z68.53
      - greater than or equal to ninety-fifth percentile for age Z68.54
      - less than fifth percentile for age Z68.51
  - Mooser's A75.2
  - rice (*see also* Loose, body, joint)
    - knee M23.4 ☑
  - rocking F98.4
- **Boeck's**
  - disease or sarcoid — *see* Sarcoidosis
  - lupoid (miliary) D86.3
- **Boerhaave's** syndrome (spontaneous esophageal rupture) K22.3
- **Boggy**
  - cervix N88.8
  - uterus N85.8
- **Boil** (*see also* Furuncle, by site)
  - Aleppo B55.1
  - Baghdad B55.1
  - Delhi B55.1
  - lacrimal
    - gland — *see* Dacryoadenitis
    - passages (duct) (sac) — *see* Inflammation, lacrimal, passages, acute
  - Natal B55.1
  - orbit, orbital — *see* Abscess, orbit
  - tropical B55.1
- **Bold** hives — *see* Urticaria
- **Bombé,** iris — *see* Membrane, pupillary
- **Bone** — *see* condition
- **Bonnevie-Ullrich** syndrome (*see also* Turner's syndrome)Q87.1
- **Bonnier's** syndrome — *see* subcategory H81.8
- **Bonvale** dam fever T73.3 ☑
- **Bony** block of joint — *see* Ankylosis
- **BOOP** (bronchiolitis obliterans organized pneumonia) J84.89
- **Borderline**
  - diabetes mellitus R73.03
  - hypertension R03.0
  - osteopenia M85.8 ☑
  - pelvis, with obstruction during labor O65.1
  - personality F60.3
- **Borna** disease A83.9
- **Bornholm** disease B33.0
- **Boston** exanthem A88.0
- **Botalli,** ductus (patent) (persistent) Q25.0
- **Bothriocephalus** latus infestation B70.0
- **Botulism** (food-borne intoxication) A05.1
  - infant A48.51
  - non-food-borne A48.52
  - wound A48.52
- **Bouba** — *see* Yaws
- **Bouchard's** nodes (with arthropathy) M15.2
- **Bouffée** délirante F23

- **Bouillaud's** disease or syndrome (rheumatic heart disease) I01.9
- **Bourneville's** disease Q85.1
- **Boutonniere** deformity (finger) — *see* Deformity, finger, boutonniere
- **Bouveret** (-Hoffmann) syndrome (paroxysmal tachycardia) I47.9
- **Bovine** heart — *see* Hypertrophy, cardiac
- **Bowel** — *see* condition
- **Bowen's**
  - dermatosis (precancerous) — *see* Neoplasm, skin, in situ
  - disease — *see* Neoplasm, skin, in situ
  - epithelioma — *see* Neoplasm, skin, in situ
  - type
    - epidermoid carcinoma-in-situ — *see* Neoplasm, skin, in situ
    - intraepidermal squamous cell carcinoma — *see* Neoplasm, skin, in situ
- **Bowing**
  - femur (*see also* Deformity, limb, specified type NEC, thigh)
    - congenital Q68.3
  - fibula (*see also* Deformity, limb, specified type NEC, lower leg)
    - congenital Q68.4
  - forearm — *see* Deformity, limb, specified type NEC, forearm
  - leg (s), long bones, congenital Q68.5
  - radius — *see* Deformity, limb, specified type NEC, forearm
  - tibia (*see also* Deformity, limb, specified type NEC, lower leg)
    - congenital Q68.4
- **Bowleg** (s) (acquired) M21.16 ☑
  - congenital Q68.5
  - rachitic E64.3
- **Boyd's** dysentery A03.2
- **Brachial** — *see* condition
- **Brachycardia** R00.1
- **Brachycephaly** Q75.0
- **Bradley's** disease A08.19
- **Bradyarrhythmia,** cardiac I49.8
- **Bradycardia** (sinoatrial) (sinus) (vagal) R00.1
  - neonatal P29.12
  - reflex G90.09
  - tachycardia syndrome I49.5
- **Bradykinesia** R25.8
- **Bradypnea** R06.89
- **Bradytachycardia** I49.5
- **Brailsford's** disease or osteochondrosis — *see* Osteochondrosis, juvenile, radius
- **Brain** (*see also* condition)
  - death G93.82
  - syndrome — *see* Syndrome, brain
- **Branched-chain** amino-acid disorder E71.2
- **Branchial** — *see* condition
  - cartilage, congenital Q18.2
- **Branchiogenic** remnant (in neck) Q18.0
- **Brandt's** syndrome (acrodermatitis enteropathica) E83.2
- **Brash** (water) R12
- **Bravais-Jacksonian** epilepsy — *see* Epilepsy, localization-related, symptomatic, with simple partial seizures
- **Braxton** Hicks contractions — *see* False, labor
- **Brazilian** leishmaniasis B55.2
- **BRBPR** K62.5
- **Break,** retina (without detachment) H33.30 ☑
  - with retinal detachment — *see* Detachment, retina
  - horseshoe tear H33.31 ☑
  - multiple H33.33 ☑
  - round hole H33.32 ☑
- **Breakdown**
  - device, graft or implant (*see also* Complications, by site and type, mechanical)T85.618 ☑
    - arterial graft NEC — *see* Complication, cardiovascular device, mechanical, vascular
    - breast (implant) T85.41 ☑
    - catheter NEC T85.618 ☑
      - cystostomy T83.010 ☑
      - Hopkins T83.018 ☑
      - ileostomy T83.018 ☑
      - dialysis (renal) T82.41 ☑
        - intraperitoneal T85.611 ☑
      - infusion NEC T82.514 ☑
        - cranial T85.610 ☑
        - epidural T85.610 ☑
        - intrathecal T85.610 ☑
        - spinal T85.610 ☑
        - subarachnoid T85.610 ☑

Breakdown - Bronchitis

- **Breakdown** — *continued*
  - device, graft or implant — *continued*
        - subdural T85.610 ☑
      - nephrostomy T83.012 ☑
      - urethral indwelling T83.011 ☑
      - urinary NEC T83.018 ☑
      - urostomy T83.018 ☑
    - electronic (electrode) (pulse generator) (stimulator)
      - bone T84.310 ☑
      - cardiac T82.119 ☑
        - electrode T82.110 ☑
        - pulse generator T82.111 ☑
        - specified type NEC T82.118 ☑
      - nervous system — *see* Complication, prosthetic device, mechanical, electronic nervous system stimulator
      - urinary — *see* Complication, genitourinary, device, urinary, mechanical
    - fixation, internal (orthopedic) NEC — *see* Complication, fixation device, mechanical
    - gastrointestinal — *see* Complications, prosthetic device, mechanical, gastrointestinal device
    - genital NEC T83.418 ☑
      - intrauterine contraceptive device T83.31 ☑
      - penile prosthesis (cylinder) (implanted) (pump) (reservoir) T83.410 ☑
      - testicular prosthesis T83.411 ☑
    - heart NEC — *see* Complication, cardiovascular device, mechanical
    - intrathecal infusion pump T85.615 ☑
    - joint prosthesis — *see* Complications..., joint prosthesis, internal, mechanical, by site
    - nervous system, specified device NEC T85.615 ☑
    - ocular NEC — *see* Complications, prosthetic device, mechanical, ocular device
    - orthopedic NEC — *see* Complication, orthopedic, device, mechanical
    - specified NEC T85.618 ☑
    - subcutaneous device pocket
      - nervous system prosthetic device, implant, or graft T85.890 ☑
      - other internal prosthetic device, implant, or graft T85.898 ☑
    - sutures, permanent T85.612 ☑
      - used in bone repair — *see* Complications, fixation device, internal (orthopedic), mechanical
    - urinary NEC T83.118 ☑
      - graft T83.21 ☑
      - sphincter, implanted T83.111 ☑
      - stent (ileal conduit) (nephroureteral) T83.113 ☑
        - ureteral indwelling T83.112 ☑
    - vascular NEC — *see* Complication, cardiovascular device, mechanical
    - ventricular intracranial shunt T85.01 ☑
  - nervous F48.8
  - perineum O90.1
  - respirator J95.850
    - specified NEC J95.859
  - ventilator J95.850
    - specified NEC J95.859
- **Breast** (*see also* condition)
  - buds E30.1
    - in newborn P96.89
  - dense R92.2
  - nodule N63
- **Breath**
  - foul R19.6
  - holder, child R06.89
  - holding spell R06.89
  - shortness R06.02
- **Breathing**
  - labored — *see* Hyperventilation
  - mouth R06.5
    - causing malocclusion M26.5 ☑
  - periodic R06.3
    - high altitude G47.32
- **Breathlessness** R06.81
- **Breda's** disease — *see* Yaws
- **Breech** presentation (mother) O32.1 ☑
  - causing obstructed labor O64.1 ☑
  - footling O32.8 ☑
    - causing obstructed labor O64.8 ☑
  - incomplete O32.8 ☑
    - causing obstructed labor O64.8 ☑
- **Breisky's** disease N90.4
- **Brennemann's** syndrome I88.0
- **Brenner**
  - tumor (benign) D27.9
    - borderline malignancy D39.1 ☑
    - malignant C56 ☑
    - proliferating D39.1 ☑
- **Bretonneau's** disease or angina A36.0
- **Breus'** mole O02.0
- **Brevicollis** Q76.49
- **Brickmakers'** anemia B76.9 *[D63.8]*
- **Bridge,** myocardial Q24.5
- **Bright** red blood per rectum (BRBPR) K62.5
- **Bright's** disease (*see also* Nephritis)
  - arteriosclerotic — *see* Hypertension, kidney
- **Brill** (-Zinsser) disease (recrudescent typhus) A75.1
  - flea-borne A75.2
  - louse-borne A75.1
- **Brill-Symmers'** disease C82.90
- **Brion-Kayser** disease — *see* Fever, parathyroid
- **Briquet's** disorder or syndrome F45.0
- **Brissaud's**
  - infantilism or dwarfism E23.0
  - motor-verbal tic F95.2
- **Brittle**
  - bones disease Q78.0
  - nails L60.3
    - congenital Q84.6
- **Broad** (*see also* condition)
  - beta disease E78.2
  - ligament laceration syndrome N83.8
- **Broad-** or floating-betalipoproteinemia E78.2
- **Brock's** syndrome (atelectasis due to enlarged lymph nodes) J98.19
- **Brocq-Duhring** disease (dermatitis herpetiformis) L13.0
- **Brodie's** abscess or disease M86.8X ☑
- **Broken**
  - arches (*see also* Deformity, limb, flat foot)
  - arm (meaning upper limb) — *see* Fracture, arm
  - back — *see* Fracture, vertebra
  - bone — *see* Fracture
  - implant or internal device — *see* Complications, by site and type, mechanical
  - leg (meaning lower limb) — *see* Fracture, leg
  - nose S02.2 ☑
  - tooth, teeth — *see* Fracture, tooth
- **Bromhidrosis,** bromidrosis L75.0
- **Bromidism,** bromism G92
  - due to
    - correct substance properly administered — *see* Table of Drugs and Chemicals, by drug, adverse effect
    - overdose or wrong substance given or taken — *see* Table of Drugs and Chemicals, by drug, poisoning
  - chronic (dependence) F13.20
- **Bromidrosiphobia** F40.298
- **Bronchi,** bronchial — *see* condition
- **Bronchiectasis** (cylindrical) (diffuse) (fusiform) (localized) (saccular) J47.9
  - with
    - acute
      - bronchitis J47.0
      - lower respiratory infection J47.0
    - exacerbation (acute) J47.1
  - congenital Q33.4
  - tuberculous NEC — *see* Tuberculosis, pulmonary
- **Bronchiolectasis** — *see* Bronchiectasis
- **Bronchiolitis** (acute) (infective) (subacute) J21.9
  - with
    - bronchospasm or obstruction J21.9
    - influenza, flu or grippe — *see* Influenza, with, respiratory manifestations NEC
  - chemical (chronic) J68.4
    - acute J68.0
  - chronic (fibrosing) (obliterative) J44.9
  - due to
    - external agent — *see* Bronchitis, acute, due to
    - human metapneumovirus J21.1
    - respiratory syncytial virus J21.0
    - specified organism NEC J21.8
  - fibrosa obliterans J44.9
  - influenzal — *see* Influenza, with, respiratory manifestations NEC
  - obliterans J42
    - with organizing pneumonia (BOOP) J84.89
  - obliterative (chronic) (subacute) J44.9
    - due to fumes or vapors J68.4
    - due to chemicals, gases, fumes or vapors (inhalation) J68.4
  - respiratory, interstitial lung disease J84.115
- **Bronchitis** (diffuse) (fibrinous) (hypostatic) (infective) (membranous) J40
- **Bronchitis** — *continued*
  - with
    - influenza, flu or grippe — *see* Influenza, with, respiratory manifestations NEC
    - obstruction (airway) (lung) J44.9
    - tracheitis (15 years of age and above) J40
      - acute or subacute J20.9
      - chronic J42
      - under 15 years of age J20.9
  - acute or subacute (with bronchospasm or obstruction) J20.9
    - with
      - bronchiectasis J47.0
      - chronic obstructive pulmonary disease J44.0
    - chemical (due to gases, fumes or vapors) J68.0
    - due to
      - fumes or vapors J68.0
      - Haemophilus influenzae J20.1
      - Mycoplasma pneumoniae J20.0
      - radiation J70.0
      - specified organism NEC J20.8
      - Streptococcus J20.2
      - virus
        - coxsackie J20.3
        - echovirus J20.7
        - parainfluenzae J20.4
        - respiratory syncytial J20.5
        - rhinovirus J20.6
    - viral NEC J20.8
  - allergic (acute) J45.909
    - with
      - exacerbation (acute) J45.901
      - status asthmaticus J45.902
  - arachidic T17.528 ☑
  - aspiration (due to fumes or vapors) J68.0
  - asthmatic J45.9 ☑
    - chronic J44.9
      - with
        - acute lower respiratory infection J44.0
        - exacerbation (acute) J44.1
  - capillary — *see* Pneumonia, broncho
  - caseous (tuberculous) A15.5
  - Castellani's A69.8
  - catarrhal (15 years of age and above) J40
    - acute — *see* Bronchitis, acute
    - chronic J41.0
    - under 15 years of age J20.9
  - chemical (acute) (subacute) J68.0
    - chronic J68.4
    - due to fumes or vapors J68.0
      - chronic J68.4
  - chronic J42
    - with
      - airways obstruction J44.9
      - tracheitis (chronic) J42
    - asthmatic (obstructive) J44.9
    - catarrhal J41.0
    - chemical (due to fumes or vapors) J68.4
    - due to
      - chemicals, gases, fumes or vapors (inhalation) J68.4
      - radiation J70.1
      - tobacco smoking J41.0
    - emphysematous J44.9
    - mucopurulent J41.1
    - non-obstructive J41.0
    - obliterans J44.9
    - obstructive J44.9
    - purulent J41.1
    - simple J41.0
  - croupous — *see* Bronchitis, acute
  - due to gases, fumes or vapors (chemical) J68.0
  - emphysematous (obstructive) J44.9
  - exudative — *see* Bronchitis, acute
  - fetid J41.1
  - grippal — *see* Influenza, with, respiratory manifestations NEC
  - in those under 15 years age — *see* Bronchitis, acute
    - chronic — *see* Bronchitis, chronic
  - influenzal — *see* Influenza, with, respiratory manifestations NEC
  - mixed simple and mucopurulent J41.8
  - moulder's J62.8
  - mucopurulent (chronic) (recurrent) J41.1
    - acute or subacute J20.9
    - simple (mixed) J41.8
  - obliterans (chronic) J44.9
  - obstructive (chronic) (diffuse) J44.9
  - pituitous J41.1
  - pneumococcal, acute or subacute J20.2

- **Bronchitis** — *continued*
  - pseudomembranous, acute or subacute — *see* Bronchitis, acute
  - purulent (chronic) (recurrent) J41.1
    - acute or subacute — *see* Bronchitis, acute
  - putrid J41.1
  - senile (chronic) J42
  - simple and mucopurulent (mixed) J41.8
  - smokers' J41.0
  - spirochetal NEC A69.8
  - subacute — *see* Bronchitis, acute
  - suppurative (chronic) J41.1
    - acute or subacute — *see* Bronchitis, acute
  - tuberculous A15.5
  - under I5 years of age — *see* Bronchitis, acute
    - chronic — *see* Bronchitis, chronic
  - viral NEC, acute or subacute (*see also* Bronchitis, acute)J20.8
- **Bronchoalveolitis** J18.0
- **Bronchoaspergillosis** B44.1
- **Bronchocele** meaning goiter E04.0
- **Broncholithiasis** J98.09
  - tuberculous NEC A15.5
- **Bronchomalacia** J98.09
  - congenital Q32.2
- **Bronchomycosis** NOS B49 *[J99]*
  - candidal B37.1
- **Bronchopleuropneumonia** — *see* Pneumonia, broncho
- **Bronchopneumonia** — *see* Pneumonia, broncho
- **Bronchopneumonitis** — *see* Pneumonia, broncho
- **Bronchopulmonary** — *see* condition
- **Bronchopulmonitis** — *see* Pneumonia, broncho
- **Bronchorrhagia** (see Hemoptysis)
- **Bronchorrhea** J98.09
  - acute J20.9
  - chronic (infective) (purulent) J42
- **Bronchospasm** (acute) J98.01
  - with
    - bronchiolitis, acute J21.9
    - bronchitis, acute (conditions in J20) — *see* Bronchitis, acute
  - due to external agent — *see* condition, respiratory, acute, due to
  - exercise induced J45.990
- **Bronchospirochetosis** A69.8
  - Castellani A69.8
- **Bronchostenosis** J98.09
- **Bronchus** — *see* condition
- **Brontophobia** F40.220
- **Bronze** baby syndrome P83.8
- **Brooke's** tumor — *see* Neoplasm, skin, benign
- **Brown** enamel of teeth (hereditary) K00.5
- **Brown's** sheath syndrome H50.61 ☑
- **Brown-Séquard** disease, paralysis or syndrome G83.81
- **Bruce** sepsis A23.0
- **Brucellosis** (infection) A23.9
  - abortus A23.1
  - canis A23.3
  - dermatitis A23.9
  - melitensis A23.0
  - mixed A23.8
  - sepsis A23.9
    - melitensis A23.0
    - specified NEC A23.8
  - suis A23.2
- **Bruck-de** Lange disease Q87.1
- **Bruck's** disease — *see* Deformity, limb
- **Brugsch's** syndrome Q82.8
- **Bruise** (skin surface intact) (*see also* Contusion)
  - with
    - open wound — *see* Wound, open
  - internal organ — *see* Injury, by site
  - newborn P54.5
  - scalp, due to birth injury, newborn P12.3
  - umbilical cord O69.5 ☑
- **Bruit** (arterial) R09.89
  - cardiac R01.1
- **Brush** burn — *see* Abrasion, by site
- **Bruton's** X-linked agammaglobulinemia D80.0
- **Bruxism**
  - psychogenic F45.8
  - sleep related G47.63
- **Bubbly** lung syndrome P27.0
- **Bubo** I88.8
  - blennorrhagic (gonococcal) A54.89
  - chancroidal A57
  - climatic A55
  - due to Haemophilus ducreyi A57
  - gonococcal A54.89
  - indolent (nonspecific) I88.8
- **Bubo** — *continued*
  - inguinal (nonspecific) I88.8
    - chancroidal A57
    - climatic A55
    - due to H. ducreyi A57
    - infective I88.8
  - scrofulous (tuberculous) A18.2
  - soft chancre A57
  - suppurating — *see* Lymphadenitis, acute
  - syphilitic (primary) A51.0
    - congenital A50.07
  - tropical A55
  - virulent (chancroidal) A57
- **Bubonic** plague A20.0
- **Bubonocele** — *see* Hernia, inguinal
- **Buccal** — *see* condition
- **Buchanan's** disease or osteochondrosis M91.0
- **Buchem's** syndrome (hyperostosis corticalis) M85.2
- **Bucket-handle** fracture or tear (semilunar cartilage) — *see* Tear, meniscus
- **Budd-Chiari** syndrome (hepatic vein thrombosis) I82.0
- **Budgerigar** fancier's disease or lung J67.2
- **Buds**
  - breast E30.1
    - in newborn P96.89
- **Buerger's** disease (thromboangiitis obliterans) I73.1
- **Bulbar** — *see* condition
- **Bulbus** cordis (left ventricle) (persistent) Q21.8
- **Bulimia** (nervosa) F50.2
  - atypical F50.9
  - normal weight F50.9
- **Bulky**
  - stools R19.5
  - uterus N85.2
- **Bulla** (e) R23.8
  - lung (emphysematous) (solitary) J43.9
    - newborn P25.8
- **Bullet** wound (*see also* Wound, open)
  - fracture - code as Fracture, by site
  - internal organ — *see* Injury, by site
- **Bundle**
  - branch block (complete) (false) (incomplete) — *see* Block, bundle-branch
  - of His — *see* condition
- **Bunion** M21.61 ☑
  - tailor's M21.62 ☑
- **Bunionette** M21.62 ☑
- **Buphthalmia**, buphthalmos (congenital) Q15.0
- **Burdwan** fever B55.0
- **Bürger-Grütz** disease or syndrome E78.3
- **Buried**
  - penis (congenital) Q55.64
    - acquired N48.83
  - roots K08.3
- **Burke's** syndrome K86.89
- **Burkitt**
  - cell leukemia C91.0 ☑
  - lymphoma (malignant) C83.7 ☑
    - small noncleaved, diffuse C83.7 ☑
    - spleen C83.77
    - undifferentiated C83.7 ☑
  - tumor C83.7 ☑
  - type
    - acute lymphoblastic leukemia C91.0 ☑
    - undifferentiated C83.7 ☑
- **Burn** (electricity) (flame) (hot gas, liquid or hot object) (radiation) (steam) (thermal) T30.0
  - abdomen, abdominal (muscle) (wall) T21.02 ☑
    - first degree T21.12 ☑
    - second degree T21.22 ☑
    - third degree T21.32 ☑
  - above elbow T22.039 ☑
    - first degree T22.139 ☑
    - left T22.032 ☑
      - first degree T22.132 ☑
      - second degree T22.232 ☑
      - third degree T22.332 ☑
    - right T22.031 ☑
      - first degree T22.131 ☑
      - second degree T22.231 ☑
      - third degree T22.331 ☑
    - second degree T22.239 ☑
    - third degree T22.339 ☑
  - acid (caustic) (external) (internal) — *see* Corrosion, by site
  - alimentary tract NEC T28.2 ☑
    - esophagus T28.1 ☑
    - mouth T28.0 ☑
    - pharynx T28.0 ☑
  - alkaline (caustic) (external) (internal) — *see* Corrosion, by site
- **Burn** — *continued*
  - ankle T25.019 ☑
    - first degree T25.119 ☑
    - left T25.012 ☑
      - first degree T25.112 ☑
      - second degree T25.212 ☑
      - third degree T25.312 ☑
    - multiple with foot — *see* Burn, lower, limb, multiple, ankle and foot
    - right T25.011 ☑
      - first degree T25.111 ☑
      - second degree T25.211 ☑
      - third degree T25.311 ☑
    - second degree T25.219 ☑
    - third degree T25.319 ☑
  - anus — *see* Burn, buttock
  - arm (lower) (upper) — *see* Burn, upper, limb
  - axilla T22.049 ☑
    - first degree T22.149 ☑
    - left T22.042 ☑
      - first degree T22.142 ☑
      - second degree T22.242 ☑
      - third degree T22.342 ☑
    - right T22.041 ☑
      - first degree T22.141 ☑
      - second degree T22.241 ☑
      - third degree T22.341 ☑
    - second degree T22.249 ☑
    - third degree T22.349 ☑
  - back (lower) T21.04 ☑
    - first degree T21.14 ☑
    - second degree T21.24 ☑
    - third degree T21.34 ☑
    - upper T21.03 ☑
      - first degree T21.13 ☑
      - second degree T21.23 ☑
      - third degree T21.33 ☑
  - blisters - code as Burn, second degree, by site
  - breast (s) — *see* Burn, chest wall
  - buttock (s) T21.05 ☑
    - first degree T21.15 ☑
    - second degree T21.25 ☑
    - third degree T21.35 ☑
  - calf T24.039 ☑
    - first degree T24.139 ☑
    - left T24.032 ☑
      - first degree T24.132 ☑
      - second degree T24.232 ☑
      - third degree T24.332 ☑
    - right T24.031 ☑
      - first degree T24.131 ☑
      - second degree T24.231 ☑
      - third degree T24.331 ☑
    - second degree T24.239 ☑
    - third degree T24.339 ☑
  - canthus (eye) — *see* Burn, eyelid
  - caustic acid or alkaline — *see* Corrosion, by site
  - cervix T28.3 ☑
  - cheek T20.06 ☑
    - first degree T20.16 ☑
    - second degree T20.26 ☑
    - third degree T20.36 ☑
  - chemical (acids) (alkalines) (caustics) (external) (internal) — *see* Corrosion, by site
  - chest wall T21.01 ☑
    - first degree T21.11 ☑
    - second degree T21.21 ☑
    - third degree T21.31 ☑
  - chin T20.03 ☑
    - first degree T20.13 ☑
    - second degree T20.23 ☑
    - third degree T20.33 ☑
  - colon T28.2 ☑
  - conjunctiva (and cornea) — *see* Burn, cornea
  - cornea (and conjunctiva) T26.1 ☑
    - chemical — *see* Corrosion, cornea
  - corrosion (external) (internal) — *see* Corrosion, by site
  - deep necrosis of underlying tissue - code as Burn, third degree, by site
  - dorsum of hand T23.069 ☑
    - first degree T23.169 ☑
    - left T23.062 ☑
      - first degree T23.162 ☑
      - second degree T23.262 ☑
      - third degree T23.362 ☑
    - right T23.061 ☑
      - first degree T23.161 ☑
      - second degree T23.261 ☑
      - third degree T23.361 ☑
    - second degree T23.269 ☑
    - third degree T23.369 ☑

Burn — *continued*
- due to ingested chemical agent — *see* Corrosion, by site
- ear (auricle) (external) (canal) T20.01 ☑
  - first degree T20.11 ☑
  - second degree T20.21 ☑
  - third degree T20.31 ☑
- elbow T22.029 ☑
  - first degree T22.129 ☑
  - left T22.022 ☑
    - first degree T22.122 ☑
    - second degree T22.222 ☑
    - third degree T22.322 ☑
  - right T22.021 ☑
    - first degree T22.121 ☑
    - second degree T22.221 ☑
    - third degree T22.321 ☑
  - second degree T22.229 ☑
  - third degree T22.329 ☑
- epidermal loss - code as Burn, second degree, by site
- erythema, erythematous - code as Burn, first degree, by site
- esophagus T28.1 ☑
- extent (percentage of body surface)
  - less than 10 percent T31.0
  - 10-19 percent T31.10
    - with 0-9 percent third degree burns T31.10
    - with 10-19 percent third degree burns T31.11
  - 20-29 percent T31.20
    - with 0-9 percent third degree burns T31.20
    - with 10-19 percent third degree burns T31.21
    - with 20-29 percent third degree burns T31.22
  - 30-39 percent T31.30
    - with 0-9 percent third degree burns T31.30
    - with 10-19 percent third degree burns T31.31
    - with 20-29 percent third degree burns T31.32
    - with 30-39 percent third degree burns T31.33
  - 40-49 percent T31.40
    - with 0-9 percent third degree burns T31.40
    - with 10-19 percent third degree burns T31.41
    - with 20-29 percent third degree burns T31.42
    - with 30-39 percent third degree burns T31.43
    - with 40-49 percent third degree burns T31.44
  - 50-59 percent T31.50
    - with 0-9 percent third degree burns T31.50
    - with 10-19 percent third degree burns T31.51
    - with 20-29 percent third degree burns T31.52
    - with 30-39 percent third degree burns T31.53
    - with 40-49 percent third degree burns T31.54
    - with 50-59 percent third degree burns T31.55
  - 60-69 percent T31.60
    - with 0-9 percent third degree burns T31.60
    - with 10-19 percent third degree burns T31.61
    - with 20-29 percent third degree burns T31.62
    - with 30-39 percent third degree burns T31.63
    - with 40-49 percent third degree burns T31.64
    - with 50-59 percent third degree burns T31.65
    - with 60-69 percent third degree burns T31.66
  - 70-79 percent T31.70
    - with 0-9 percent third degree burns T31.70
    - with 10-19 percent third degree burns T31.71
    - with 20-29 percent third degree burns T31.72
    - with 30-39 percent third degree burns T31.73
    - with 40-49 percent third degree burns T31.74
    - with 50-59 percent third degree burns T31.75
    - with 60-69 percent third degree burns T31.76
    - with 70-79 percent third degree burns T31.77
  - 80-89 percent T31.80
    - with 0-9 percent third degree burns T31.80
    - with 10-19 percent third degree burns T31.81
    - with 20-29 percent third degree burns T31.82
    - with 30-39 percent third degree burns T31.83
    - with 40-49 percent third degree burns T31.84
    - with 50-59 percent third degree burns T31.85
    - with 60-69 percent third degree burns T31.86
    - with 70-79 percent third degree burns T31.87
    - with 80-89 percent third degree burns T31.88
  - 90 percent or more T31.90
    - with 0-9 percent third degree burns T31.90
    - with 10-19 percent third degree burns T31.91
    - with 20-29 percent third degree burns T31.92
    - with 30-39 percent third degree burns T31.93
    - with 40-49 percent third degree burns T31.94
    - with 50-59 percent third degree burns T31.95
    - with 60-69 percent third degree burns T31.96
    - with 70-79 percent third degree burns T31.97
    - with 80-89 percent third degree burns T31.98
    - with 90 percent or more third degree burns T31.99
- extremity — *see* Burn, limb

Burn — *continued*
- eye (s) and adnexa T26.4 ☑
  - with resulting rupture and destruction of eyeball T26.2 ☑
  - conjunctival sac — *see* Burn, cornea
  - cornea — *see* Burn, cornea
  - lid — *see* Burn, eyelid
  - periocular area — *see* Burn, eyelid
  - specified site NEC T26.3 ☑
- eyeball — *see* Burn, eye
- eyelid (s) T26.0 ☑
  - chemical — *see* Corrosion, eyelid
- face — *see* Burn, head
- finger T23.029 ☑
  - first degree T23.129 ☑
  - left T23.022 ☑
    - first degree T23.122 ☑
    - second degree T23.222 ☑
    - third degree T23.322 ☑
  - multiple sites (without thumb) T23.039 ☑
    - with thumb T23.049 ☑
      - first degree T23.149 ☑
      - left T23.042 ☑
        - first degree T23.142 ☑
        - second degree T23.242 ☑
        - third degree T23.342 ☑
      - right T23.041 ☑
        - first degree T23.141 ☑
        - second degree T23.241 ☑
        - third degree T23.341 ☑
      - second degree T23.249 ☑
      - third degree T23.349 ☑
    - first degree T23.139 ☑
    - left T23.032 ☑
      - first degree T23.132 ☑
      - second degree T23.232 ☑
      - third degree T23.332 ☑
    - right T23.031 ☑
      - first degree T23.131 ☑
      - second degree T23.231 ☑
      - third degree T23.331 ☑
    - second degree T23.239 ☑
    - third degree T23.339 ☑
  - right T23.021 ☑
    - first degree T23.121 ☑
    - second degree T23.221 ☑
    - third degree T23.321 ☑
  - second degree T23.229 ☑
  - third degree T23.329 ☑
- flank — *see* Burn, abdominal wall
- foot T25.029 ☑
  - first degree T25.129 ☑
  - left T25.022 ☑
    - first degree T25.122 ☑
    - second degree T25.222 ☑
    - third degree T25.322 ☑
  - multiple with ankle — *see* Burn, lower, limb, multiple, ankle and foot
  - right T25.021 ☑
    - first degree T25.121 ☑
    - second degree T25.221 ☑
    - third degree T25.321 ☑
  - second degree T25.229 ☑
  - third degree T25.329 ☑
- forearm T22.019 ☑
  - first degree T22.119 ☑
  - left T22.012 ☑
    - first degree T22.112 ☑
    - second degree T22.212 ☑
    - third degree T22.312 ☑
  - right T22.011 ☑
    - first degree T22.111 ☑
    - second degree T22.211 ☑
    - third degree T22.311 ☑
  - second degree T22.219 ☑
  - third degree T22.319 ☑
- forehead T20.06 ☑
  - first degree T20.16 ☑
  - second degree T20.26 ☑
  - third degree T20.36 ☑
- fourth degree - code as Burn, third degree, by site
- friction — *see* Burn, by site
- from swallowing caustic or corrosive substance NEC — *see* Corrosion, by site
- full thickness skin loss - code as Burn, third degree, by site
- gastrointestinal tract NEC T28.2 ☑
  - from swallowing caustic or corrosive substance T28.7 ☑
- genital organs
  - external
    - female T21.07 ☑

Burn — *continued*
- genital organs — *continued*
      - first degree T21.17 ☑
      - second degree T21.27 ☑
      - third degree T21.37 ☑
    - male T21.06 ☑
      - first degree T21.16 ☑
      - second degree T21.26 ☑
      - third degree T21.36 ☑
  - internal T28.3 ☑
    - from caustic or corrosive substance T28.8 ☑
- groin — *see* Burn, abdominal wall
- hand (s) T23.009 ☑
  - back — *see* Burn, dorsum of hand
  - finger — *see* Burn, finger
  - first degree T23.109 ☑
  - left T23.002 ☑
    - first degree T23.102 ☑
    - second degree T23.202 ☑
    - third degree T23.302 ☑
  - multiple sites with wrist T23.099 ☑
    - first degree T23.199 ☑
    - left T23.092 ☑
      - first degree T23.192 ☑
      - second degree T23.292 ☑
      - third degree T23.392 ☑
    - right T23.091 ☑
      - first degree T23.191 ☑
      - second degree T23.291 ☑
      - third degree T23.391 ☑
    - second degree T23.299 ☑
    - third degree T23.399 ☑
  - palm — *see* Burn, palm
  - right T23.001 ☑
    - first degree T23.101 ☑
    - second degree T23.201 ☑
    - third degree T23.301 ☑
  - second degree T23.209 ☑
  - third degree T23.309 ☑
  - thumb — *see* Burn, thumb
- head (and face) (and neck) T20.00 ☑
  - cheek — *see* Burn, cheek
  - chin — *see* Burn, chin
  - ear — *see* Burn, ear
  - eye (s) only — *see* Burn, eye
  - first degree T20.10 ☑
  - forehead — *see* Burn, forehead
  - lip — *see* Burn, lip
  - multiple sites T20.09 ☑
    - first degree T20.19 ☑
    - second degree T20.29 ☑
    - third degree T20.39 ☑
  - neck — *see* Burn, neck
  - nose — *see* Burn, nose
  - scalp — *see* Burn, scalp
  - second degree T20.20 ☑
  - third degree T20.30 ☑
- hip (s) — *see* Burn, thigh
- inhalation — *see* Burn, respiratory tract
  - caustic or corrosive substance (fumes) — *see* Corrosion, respiratory tract
- internal organ (s) T28.40 ☑
  - alimentary tract T28.2 ☑
    - esophagus T28.1 ☑
  - eardrum T28.41 ☑
  - esophagus T28.1 ☑
  - from caustic or corrosive substance (swallowing) NEC — *see* Corrosion, by site
  - genitourinary T28.3 ☑
  - mouth T28.0 ☑
  - pharynx T28.0 ☑
  - respiratory tract — *see* Burn, respiratory tract
  - specified organ NEC T28.49 ☑
- interscapular region — *see* Burn, back, upper
- intestine (large) (small) T28.2 ☑
- knee T24.029 ☑
  - first degree T24.129 ☑
  - left T24.022 ☑
    - first degree T24.122 ☑
    - second degree T24.222 ☑
    - third degree T24.322 ☑
  - right T24.021 ☑
    - first degree T24.121 ☑
    - second degree T24.221 ☑
    - third degree T24.321 ☑
  - second degree T24.229 ☑
  - third degree T24.329 ☑
- labium (majus) (minus) — *see* Burn, genital organs, external, female
- lacrimal apparatus, duct, gland or sac — *see* Burn, eye, specified site NEC
- larynx T27.0 ☑
  - with lung T27.1 ☑

Burn — *continued*
- leg (s) (lower) (upper) — *see* Burn, lower, limb
- lightning — *see* Burn, by site
- limb (s)
  - lower (except ankle or foot alone) — *see* Burn, lower, limb
  - upper — *see* Burn, upper limb
- lip (s) T20.02 ☑
  - first degree T20.12 ☑
  - second degree T20.22 ☑
  - third degree T20.32 ☑
- lower
  - back — *see* Burn, back
  - limb T24.009 ☑
    - ankle — *see* Burn, ankle
    - calf — *see* Burn, calf
    - first degree T24.109 ☑
    - foot — *see* Burn, foot
    - hip — *see* Burn, thigh
    - knee — *see* Burn, knee
    - left T24.002 ☑
      - first degree T24.102 ☑
      - second degree T24.202 ☑
      - third degree T24.302 ☑
    - multiple sites, except ankle and foot T24.099 ☑
      - ankle and foot T25.099 ☑
        - first degree T25.199 ☑
        - left T25.092 ☑
          - first degree T25.192 ☑
          - second degree T25.292 ☑
          - third degree T25.392 ☑
        - right T25.091 ☑
          - first degree T25.191 ☑
          - second degree T25.291 ☑
          - third degree T25.391 ☑
        - second degree T25.299 ☑
        - third degree T25.399 ☑
      - first degree T24.199 ☑
      - left T24.092 ☑
        - first degree T24.192 ☑
        - second degree T24.292 ☑
        - third degree T24.392 ☑
      - right T24.091 ☑
        - first degree T24.191 ☑
        - second degree T24.291 ☑
        - third degree T24.391 ☑
      - second degree T24.299 ☑
      - third degree T24.399 ☑
    - right T24.001 ☑
      - first degree T24.101 ☑
      - second degree T24.201 ☑
      - third degree T24.301 ☑
    - second degree T24.209 ☑
    - thigh — *see* Burn, thigh
    - third degree T24.309 ☑
    - toe — *see* Burn, toe
- lung (with larynx and trachea) T27.1 ☑
- mouth T28.0 ☑
- neck T20.07 ☑
  - first degree T20.17 ☑
  - second degree T20.27 ☑
  - third degree T20.37 ☑
- nose (septum) T20.04 ☑
  - first degree T20.14 ☑
  - second degree T20.24 ☑
  - third degree T20.34 ☑
- ocular adnexa — *see* Burn, eye
- orbit region — *see* Burn, eyelid
- palm T23.059 ☑
  - first degree T23.159 ☑
  - left T23.052 ☑
    - first degree T23.152 ☑
    - second degree T23.252 ☑
    - third degree T23.352 ☑
  - right T23.051 ☑
    - first degree T23.151 ☑
    - second degree T23.251 ☑
    - third degree T23.351 ☑
  - second degree T23.259 ☑
  - third degree T23.359 ☑
- partial thickness - code as Burn, unspecified degree, by site
- pelvis — *see* Burn, trunk
- penis — *see* Burn, genital organs, external, male
- perineum
  - female — *see* Burn, genital organs, external, female
  - male — *see* Burn, genital organs, external, male
- periocular area — *see* Burn, eyelid
- pharynx T28.0 ☑
- rectum T28.2 ☑

Burn — *continued*
- respiratory tract T27.3 ☑
  - larynx — *see* Burn, larynx
  - specified part NEC T27.2 ☑
  - trachea — *see* Burn, trachea
- sac, lacrimal — *see* Burn, eye, specified site NEC
- scalp T20.05 ☑
  - first degree T20.15 ☑
  - second degree T20.25 ☑
  - third degree T20.35 ☑
- scapular region T22.069 ☑
  - first degree T22.169 ☑
  - left T22.062 ☑
    - first degree T22.162 ☑
    - second degree T22.262 ☑
    - third degree T22.362 ☑
  - right T22.061 ☑
    - first degree T22.161 ☑
    - second degree T22.261 ☑
    - third degree T22.361 ☑
  - second degree T22.269 ☑
  - third degree T22.369 ☑
- sclera — *see* Burn, eye, specified site NEC
- scrotum — *see* Burn, genital organs, external, male
- shoulder T22.059 ☑
  - first degree T22.159 ☑
  - left T22.052 ☑
    - first degree T22.152 ☑
    - second degree T22.252 ☑
    - third degree T22.352 ☑
  - right T22.051 ☑
    - first degree T22.151 ☑
    - second degree T22.251 ☑
    - third degree T22.351 ☑
  - second degree T22.259 ☑
  - third degree T22.359 ☑
- stomach T28.2 ☑
- temple — *see* Burn, head
- testis — *see* Burn, genital organs, external, male
- thigh T24.019 ☑
  - first degree T24.119 ☑
  - left T24.012 ☑
    - first degree T24.112 ☑
    - second degree T24.212 ☑
    - third degree T24.312 ☑
  - right T24.011 ☑
    - first degree T24.111 ☑
    - second degree T24.211 ☑
    - third degree T24.311 ☑
  - second degree T24.219 ☑
  - third degree T24.319 ☑
- thorax (external) — *see* Burn, trunk
- throat (meaning pharynx) T28.0 ☑
- thumb (s) T23.019 ☑
  - first degree T23.119 ☑
  - left T23.012 ☑
    - first degree T23.112 ☑
    - second degree T23.212 ☑
    - third degree T23.312 ☑
  - multiple sites with fingers T23.049 ☑
    - first degree T23.149 ☑
    - left T23.042 ☑
      - first degree T23.142 ☑
      - second degree T23.242 ☑
      - third degree T23.342 ☑
    - right T23.041 ☑
      - first degree T23.141 ☑
      - second degree T23.241 ☑
      - third degree T23.341 ☑
    - second degree T23.249 ☑
    - third degree T23.349 ☑
  - right T23.011 ☑
    - first degree T23.111 ☑
    - second degree T23.211 ☑
    - third degree T23.311 ☑
  - second degree T23.219 ☑
  - third degree T23.319 ☑
- toe T25.039 ☑
  - first degree T25.139 ☑
  - left T25.032 ☑
    - first degree T25.132 ☑
    - second degree T25.232 ☑
    - third degree T25.332 ☑
  - right T25.031 ☑
    - first degree T25.131 ☑
    - second degree T25.231 ☑
    - third degree T25.331 ☑
  - second degree T25.239 ☑
  - third degree T25.339 ☑
- tongue T28.0 ☑
- tonsil (s) T28.0 ☑

Burn — *continued*
- trachea T27.0 ☑
  - with lung T27.1 ☑
- trunk T21.00 ☑
  - abdominal wall — *see* Burn, abdominal wall
  - anus — *see* Burn, buttock
  - axilla — *see* Burn, upper limb
  - back — *see* Burn, back
  - breast — *see* Burn, chest wall
  - buttock — *see* Burn, buttock
  - chest wall — *see* Burn, chest wall
  - first degree T21.10 ☑
  - flank — *see* Burn, abdominal wall
  - genital
    - female — *see* Burn, genital organs, external, female
    - male — *see* Burn, genital organs, external, male
  - groin — *see* Burn, abdominal wall
  - interscapular region — *see* Burn, back, upper
  - labia — *see* Burn, genital organs, external, female
  - lower back — *see* Burn, back
  - penis — *see* Burn, genital organs, external, male
  - perineum
    - female — *see* Burn, genital organs, external, female
    - male — *see* Burn, genital organs, external, male
  - scapula region — *see* Burn, scapular region
  - scrotum — *see* Burn, genital organs, external, male
  - second degree T21.20 ☑
  - specified site NEC T21.09 ☑
    - first degree T21.19 ☑
    - second degree T21.29 ☑
    - third degree T21.39 ☑
  - testes — *see* Burn, genital organs, external, male
  - third degree T21.30 ☑
  - upper back — *see* Burn, back, upper
  - vulva — *see* Burn, genital organs, external, female
- unspecified site with extent of body surface involved specified
  - less than 10 per cent T31.0
  - 10-19 per cent (0-9 percent third degree) T31.10
    - with 10-19 percent third degree T31.11
  - 20-29 per cent (0-9 percent third degree) T31.20
    - with
      - 10-19 percent third degree T31.21
      - 20-29 percent third degree T31.22
  - 30-39 per cent (0-9 percent third degree) T31.30
    - with
      - 10-19 percent third degree T31.31
      - 20-29 percent third degree T31.32
      - 30-39 percent third degree T31.33
  - 40-49 per cent (0-9 percent third degree) T31.40
    - with
      - 10-19 percent third degree T31.41
      - 20-29 percent third degree T31.42
      - 30-39 percent third degree T31.43
      - 40-49 percent third degree T31.44
  - 50-59 per cent (0-9 percent third degree) T31.50
    - with
      - 10-19 percent third degree T31.51
      - 20-29 percent third degree T31.52
      - 30-39 percent third degree T31.53
      - 40-49 percent third degree T31.54
      - 50-59 percent third degree T31.55
  - 60-69 per cent (0-9 percent third degree) T31.60
    - with
      - 10-19 percent third degree T31.61
      - 20-29 percent third degree T31.62
      - 30-39 percent third degree T31.63
      - 40-49 percent third degree T31.64
      - 50-59 percent third degree T31.65
      - 60-69 percent third degree T31.66
  - 70-79 per cent (0-9 percent third degree) T31.70
    - with
      - 10-19 percent third degree T31.71
      - 20-29 percent third degree T31.72
      - 30-39 percent third degree T31.73
      - 40-49 percent third degree T31.74

Burn — *continued*
- unspecified site — *continued*
        - 50-59 percent third degree T31.75
        - 60-69 percent third degree T31.76
        - 70-79 percent third degree T31.77
    - 80-89 per cent (0-9 percent third degree) T31.80
        - with
            - 10-19 percent third degree T31.81
            - 20-29 percent third degree T31.82
            - 30-39 percent third degree T31.83
            - 40-49 percent third degree T31.84
            - 50-59 percent third degree T31.85
            - 60-69 percent third degree T31.86
            - 70-79 percent third degree T31.87
            - 80-89 percent third degree T31.88
    - 90 per cent or more (0-9 percent third degree) T31.90
        - with
            - 10-19 percent third degree T31.91
            - 20-29 percent third degree T31.92
            - 30-39 percent third degree T31.93
            - 40-49 percent third degree T31.94
            - 50-59 percent third degree T31.95
            - 60-69 percent third degree T31.96
            - 70-79 percent third degree T31.97
            - 80-89 percent third degree T31.98
            - 90-99 percent third degree T31.99
- upper limb T22.00 ☑
    - above elbow — *see* Burn, above elbow
    - axilla — *see* Burn, axilla
    - elbow — *see* Burn, elbow
    - first degree T22.10 ☑
    - forearm — *see* Burn, forearm
    - hand — *see* Burn, hand
    - interscapular region — *see* Burn, back, upper
    - multiple sites T22.099 ☑
        - first degree T22.199 ☑
        - left T22.092 ☑
            - first degree T22.192 ☑
            - second degree T22.292 ☑
            - third degree T22.392 ☑
        - right T22.091 ☑
            - first degree T22.191 ☑
            - second degree T22.291 ☑
            - third degree T22.391 ☑
        - second degree T22.299 ☑
        - third degree T22.399 ☑
    - scapular region — *see* Burn, scapular region
    - second degree T22.20 ☑
    - shoulder — *see* Burn, shoulder
    - third degree T22.30 ☑
    - wrist — *see* Burn, wrist
- uterus T28.3 ☑
- vagina T28.3 ☑
- vulva — *see* Burn, genital organs, external, female
- wrist T23.079 ☑
    - first degree T23.179 ☑
    - left T23.072 ☑
        - first degree T23.172 ☑
        - second degree T23.272 ☑
        - third degree T23.372 ☑
    - multiple sites with hand T23.099 ☑
        - first degree T23.199 ☑
        - left T23.092 ☑
            - first degree T23.192 ☑
            - second degree T23.292 ☑
            - third degree T23.392 ☑
        - right T23.091 ☑
            - first degree T23.191 ☑
            - second degree T23.291 ☑
            - third degree T23.391 ☑
        - second degree T23.299 ☑
        - third degree T23.399 ☑
    - right T23.071 ☑
        - first degree T23.171 ☑
        - second degree T23.271 ☑
        - third degree T23.371 ☑
    - second degree T23.279 ☑
    - third degree T23.379 ☑

Burnett's syndrome E83.52

Burning
- feet syndrome E53.9
- sensation R20.8
- tongue K14.6

Burn-out (state) Z73.0

Burns' disease or osteochondrosis — *see* Osteochondrosis, juvenile, ulna

Bursa — *see* condition

Bursitis M71.9
- Achilles — *see* Tendinitis, Achilles
- adhesive — *see* Bursitis, specified NEC

Bursitis — *continued*
- ankle — *see* Enthesopathy, lower limb, ankle, specified type NEC
- calcaneal — *see* Enthesopathy, foot, specified type NEC
- collateral ligament, tibial — *see* Bursitis, tibial collateral
- due to use, overuse, pressure (*see also* Disorder, soft tissue, due to use, specified type NEC)
    - specified NEC — *see* Disorder, soft tissue, due to use, specified NEC
- Duplay's M75.0 ☑
- elbow NEC M70.3 ☑
    - olecranon M70.2 ☑
- finger — *see* Disorder, soft tissue, due to use, specified type NEC, hand
- foot — *see* Enthesopathy, foot, specified type NEC
- gonococcal A54.49
- gouty — *see* Gout
- hand M70.1 ☑
- hip NEC M70.7 ☑
    - trochanteric M70.6 ☑
- infective NEC M71.10
    - abscess — *see* Abscess, bursa
    - ankle M71.17 ☑
    - elbow M71.12 ☑
    - foot M71.17 ☑
    - hand M71.14 ☑
    - hip M71.15 ☑
    - knee M71.16 ☑
    - multiple sites M71.19
    - shoulder M71.11 ☑
    - specified site NEC M71.18
    - wrist M71.13 ☑
- ischial — *see* Bursitis, hip
- knee NEC M70.5 ☑
    - prepatellar M70.4 ☑
- occupational NEC (*see also* Disorder, soft tissue, due to, use)
- olecranon — *see* Bursitis, elbow, olecranon
- pharyngeal J39.1
- popliteal — *see* Bursitis, knee
- prepatellar M70.4 ☑
- radiohumeral M77.8
- rheumatoid M06.20
    - ankle M06.27 ☑
    - elbow M06.22 ☑
    - foot joint M06.27 ☑
    - hand joint M06.24 ☑
    - hip M06.25 ☑
    - knee M06.26 ☑
    - multiple site M06.29
    - shoulder M06.21 ☑
    - vertebra M06.28
    - wrist M06.23 ☑
- scapulohumeral — *see* Bursitis, shoulder
- semimembranous muscle (knee) — *see* Bursitis, knee
- shoulder M75.5 ☑
    - adhesive — *see* Capsulitis, adhesive
- specified NEC M71.50
    - ankle M71.57 ☑
    - due to use, overuse or pressure — *see* Disorder, soft tissue, due to, use
    - elbow M71.52 ☑
    - foot M71.57 ☑
    - hand M71.54 ☑
    - hip M71.55 ☑
    - knee M71.56 ☑
    - shoulder — *see* Bursitis, shoulder
    - specified site NEC M71.58
    - tibial collateral M76.4 ☑
    - wrist M71.53 ☑
- subacromial — *see* Bursitis, shoulder
- subcoracoid — *see* Bursitis, shoulder
- subdeltoid — *see* Bursitis, shoulder
- syphilitic A52.78
- Thornwaldt, Tornwaldt J39.2
- tibial collateral M76.4 ☑
- toe — *see* Enthesopathy, foot, specified type NEC
- trochanteric (area) — *see* Bursitis, hip, trochanteric
- wrist — *see* Bursitis, hand

Bursopathy M71.9
- specified type NEC M71.80
    - ankle M71.87 ☑
    - elbow M71.82 ☑
    - foot M71.87 ☑
    - hand M71.84 ☑
    - hip M71.85 ☑
    - knee M71.86 ☑
    - multiple sites M71.89

Bursopathy — *continued*
- specified type NEC — *continued*
    - shoulder M71.81 ☑
    - specified site NEC M71.88
    - wrist M71.83 ☑

Burst stitches or sutures (complication of surgery) T81.31 ☑
- external operation wound T81.31 ☑
- internal operation wound T81.32 ☑

Buruli ulcer A31.1

Bury's disease L95.1

Buschke's
- disease B45.3
- scleredema — *see* Sclerosis, systemic

Busse-Buschke disease B45.3

Buttock — *see* condition

Button
- Biskra B55.1
- Delhi B55.1
- oriental B55.1

Buttonhole deformity (finger) — *see* Deformity, finger, boutonniere

Bwamba fever A92.8

Byssinosis J66.0

Bywaters' syndrome T79.5 ☑

C

Cachexia R64
- cancerous R64
- cardiac — *see* Disease, heart
- dehydration E86.0
- due to malnutrition R64
- exophthalmic — *see* Hyperthyroidism
- heart — *see* Disease, heart
- hypophyseal E23.0
- hypopituitary E23.0
- lead — *see* Poisoning, lead
- malignant R64
- marsh — *see* Malaria
- nervous F48.8
- old age R54
- paludal — *see* Malaria
- pituitary E23.0
- renal N28.9
- saturnine — *see* Poisoning, lead
- senile R54
- Simmonds' E23.0
- splenica D73.0
- strumipriva E03.4
- tuberculous NEC — *see* Tuberculosis

Café, au lait spots L81.3

Caffeine-induced
- anxiety disorder F15.980
- sleep disorder F15.982

Caffey's syndrome Q78.8

Caisson disease T70.3 ☑

Cake kidney Q63.1

Caked breast (puerperal, postpartum) O92.79

Calabar swelling B74.3

Calcaneal spur — *see* Spur, bone, calcaneal

Calcaneo-apophysitis M92.8

Calcareous — *see* condition

Calcicosis J62.8

Calciferol (vitamin D) deficiency E55.9
- with rickets E55.0

Calcification
- adrenal (capsule) (gland) E27.49
    - tuberculous E35 *[B90.8]*
- aorta I70.0
- artery (annular) — *see* Arteriosclerosis
- auricle (ear) — *see* Disorder, pinna, specified type NEC
- basal ganglia G23.8
- bladder N32.89
    - due to Schistosoma hematobium B65.0
- brain (cortex) — *see* Calcification, cerebral
- bronchus J98.09
- bursa M71.40
    - ankle M71.47 ☑
    - elbow M71.42 ☑
    - foot M71.47 ☑
    - hand M71.44 ☑
    - hip M71.45 ☑
    - knee M71.46 ☑
    - multiple sites M71.49
    - shoulder M75.3 ☑
    - specified site NEC M71.48
    - wrist M71.43 ☑
- cardiac — *see* Degeneration, myocardial

Calcification — *continued*
- cerebral (cortex) G93.89
  - artery I67.2
- cervix (uteri) N88.8
- choroid plexus G93.89
- conjunctiva — *see* Concretion, conjunctiva
- corpora cavernosa (penis) N48.89
- cortex (brain) — *see* Calcification, cerebral
- dental pulp (nodular) K04.2
- dentinal papilla K00.4
- fallopian tube N83.8
- falx cerebri G96.19
- gallbladder K82.8
- general E83.59
- heart (*see also* Degeneration, myocardial)
  - valve — *see* Endocarditis
- idiopathic infantile arterial (IIAC) Q28.8
- intervertebral cartilage or disc (postinfective) — *see* Disorder, disc, specified NEC
- intracranial — *see* Calcification, cerebral
- joint — *see* Disorder, joint, specified type NEC
- kidney N28.89
  - tuberculous N29 *[B90.1]*
- larynx (senile) J38.7
- lens — *see* Cataract, specified NEC
- lung (active) (postinfectional) J98.4
  - tuberculous B90.9
- lymph gland or node (postinfectional) I89.8
  - tuberculous (*see also* Tuberculosis, lymph gland)B90.8
- mammographic R92.1
- massive (paraplegic) — *see* Myositis, ossificans, in, quadriplegia
- medial — *see* Arteriosclerosis, extremities
- meninges (cerebral) (spinal) G96.19
- metastatic E83.59
- Mönckeberg's — *see* Arteriosclerosis, extremities
- muscle M61.9
  - due to burns — *see* Myositis, ossificans, in, burns
  - paralytic — *see* Myositis, ossificans, in, quadriplegia
  - specified type NEC M61.40
    - ankle M61.47 ☑
    - foot M61.47 ☑
    - forearm M61.43 ☑
    - hand M61.44 ☑
    - lower leg M61.46 ☑
    - multiple sites M61.49
    - pelvic region M61.45 ☑
    - shoulder region M61.41 ☑
    - specified site NEC M61.48
    - thigh M61.45 ☑
    - upper arm M61.42 ☑
- myocardium, myocardial — *see* Degeneration, myocardial
- ovary N83.8
- pancreas K86.89
- penis N48.89
- periarticular — *see* Disorder, joint, specified type NEC
- pericardium (*see also* Pericarditis)I31.1
- pineal gland E34.8
- pleura J94.8
  - postinfectional J94.8
  - tuberculous NEC B90.9
- pulpal (dental) (nodular) K04.2
- sclera H15.89
- spleen D73.89
- subcutaneous L94.2
- suprarenal (capsule) (gland) E27.49
- tendon (sheath) (*see also* Tenosynovitis, specified type NEC)
  - with bursitis, synovitis or tenosynovitis — *see* Tendinitis, calcific
- trachea J39.8
- ureter N28.89
- uterus N85.8
- vitreous — *see* Deposit, crystalline

Calcified — *see* Calcification

Calcinosis (interstitial) (tumoral) (universalis) E83.59
- with Raynaud's phenomenon, esophageal dysfunction, sclerodactyly, telangiectasia (CREST syndrome) M34.1
- circumscripta (skin) L94.2
- cutis L94.2

Calciphylaxis (*see also* Calcification, by site)E83.59

Calcium
- deposits — *see* Calcification, by site
- metabolism disorder E83.50
- salts or soaps in vitreous — *see* Deposit, crystalline

Calciuria R82.99

Calculi — *see* Calculus

Calculosis, intrahepatic — *see* Calculus, bile duct

Calculus, calculi, calculous
- ampulla of Vater — *see* Calculus, bile duct
- anuria (impacted) (recurrent) (*see also* Calculus, urinary)N20.9
- appendix K38.1
- bile duct (common) (hepatic) K80.50
  - with
    - calculus of gallbladder — *see* Calculus, gallbladder and bile duct
    - cholangitis K80.30
      - with
        - cholecystitis — *see* Calculus, bile duct, with cholecystitis
        - obstruction K80.31
      - acute K80.32
        - with
          - chronic cholangitis K80.36
            - with obstruction K80.37
          - obstruction K80.33
      - chronic K80.34
        - with
          - acute cholangitis K80.36
            - with obstruction K80.37
          - obstruction K80.35
    - cholecystitis (with cholangitis) K80.40
      - with obstruction K80.41
      - acute K80.42
        - with
          - chronic cholecystitis K80.46
            - with obstruction K80.47
          - obstruction K80.43
      - chronic K80.44
        - with
          - acute cholecystitis K80.46
            - with obstruction K80.47
          - obstruction K80.45
    - obstruction K80.51
- biliary (*see also* Calculus, gallbladder)
  - specified NEC K80.80
    - with obstruction K80.81
- bilirubin, multiple — *see* Calculus, gallbladder
- bladder (encysted) (impacted) (urinary) (diverticulum) N21.0
- bronchus J98.09
- calyx (kidney) (renal) — *see* Calculus, kidney
- cholesterol (pure) (solitary) — *see* Calculus, gallbladder
- common duct (bile) — *see* Calculus, bile duct
- conjunctiva — *see* Concretion, conjunctiva
- cystic N21.0
  - duct — *see* Calculus, gallbladder
- dental (subgingival) (supragingival) K03.6
- diverticulum
  - bladder N21.0
  - kidney N20.0
- epididymis N50.89
- gallbladder K80.20
  - with
    - bile duct calculus — *see* Calculus, gallbladder and bile duct
    - cholecystitis K80.10
      - with obstruction K80.11
      - acute K80.00
        - with
          - chronic cholecystitis K80.12
            - with obstruction K80.13
          - obstruction K80.01
      - chronic K80.10
        - with
          - acute cholecystitis K80.12
            - with obstruction K80.13
          - obstruction K80.11
      - specified NEC K80.18
        - with obstruction K80.19
    - obstruction K80.21
- gallbladder and bile duct K80.70
  - with
    - cholecystitis K80.60
      - with obstruction K80.61
      - acute K80.62
        - with
          - chronic cholecystitis K80.66
            - with obstruction K80.67
          - obstruction K80.63
      - chronic K80.64
        - with
          - acute cholecystitis K80.66
            - with obstruction K80.67
          - obstruction K80.65
    - obstruction K80.71

Calculus — *continued*
- hepatic (duct) — *see* Calculus, bile duct
- hepatobiliary K80.80
  - with obstruction K80.81
- ileal conduit N21.8
- intestinal (impaction) (obstruction) K56.49
- kidney (impacted) (multiple) (pelvis) (recurrent) (staghorn) N20.0
  - with calculus, ureter N20.2
  - congenital Q63.8
- lacrimal passages — *see* Dacryolith
- liver (impacted) — *see* Calculus, bile duct
- lung J98.4
- mammographic R92.1
- nephritic (impacted) (recurrent) — *see* Calculus, kidney
- nose J34.89
- pancreas (duct) K86.89
- parotid duct or gland K11.5
- pelvis, encysted — *see* Calculus, kidney
- prostate N42.0
- pulmonary J98.4
- pyelitis (impacted) (recurrent) N20.0
  - with hydronephrosis N13.2
- pyelonephritis (impacted) (recurrent) N20
  - with hydronephrosis N13.2
- renal (impacted) (recurrent) — *see* Calculus, kidney
- salivary (duct) (gland) K11.5
- seminal vesicle N50.89
- staghorn — *see* Calculus, kidney
- Stensen's duct K11.5
- stomach K31.89
- sublingual duct or gland K11.5
  - congenital Q38.4
- submandibular duct, gland or region K11.5
- submaxillary duct, gland or region K11.5
- suburethral N21.8
- tonsil J35.8
- tooth, teeth (subgingival) (supragingival) K03.6
- tunica vaginalis N50.89
- ureter (impacted) (recurrent) N20.1
  - with calculus, kidney N20.2
    - with hydronephrosis N13.2
      - with infection N13.6
- urethra (impacted) N21.1
- urinary (duct) (impacted) (passage) (tract) N20.9
  - with hydronephrosis N13.2
    - with infection N13.6
  - in (due to)
  - lower N21.9
    - specified NEC N21.8
- vagina N89.8
- vesical (impacted) N21.0
- Wharton's duct K11.5
- xanthine E79.8 *[N22]*

Calicectasis N28.89

Caliectasis N28.89

California
- disease B38.9
- encephalitis A83.5

Caligo cornea — *see* Opacity, cornea, central

Callositas, callosity (infected) L84

Callus (infected) L84
- bone — *see* Osteophyte
  - excessive, following fracture - code as Sequelae of fracture

CALME (childhood asymmetric labium majus enlargement) N90.61

Calorie deficiency or malnutrition (*see also* Malnutrition)E46

Calvé-Perthes disease — *see* Legg-Calvé-Perthes disease

Calvé's disease — *see* Osteochondrosis, juvenile, spine

Calvities — *see* Alopecia, androgenic

Cameroon fever — *see* Malaria

Camptocormia (hysterical) F44.4

Camurati-Engelmann syndrome Q78.3

Canal (*see also* condition)
- atrioventricular common Q21.2

Canaliculitis (lacrimal) (acute) (subacute) H04.33 ☑
- Actinomyces A42.89
- chronic H04.42 ☑

Canavan's disease E75.29

Canceled procedure (surgical) Z53.9
- because of
  - contraindication Z53.09
    - smoking Z53.01
  - left against medical advice (AMA) Z53.21
  - patient's decision Z53.20
    - for reasons of belief or group pressure Z53.1

- **Canceled** procedure — *continued*
  - because of — *continued*
    - specified reason NEC Z53.29
  - specified reason NEC Z53.8
- **Cancer** (*see also* Neoplasm, by site, malignant)
  - bile duct type liver C22.1
  - blood — *see* Leukemia
  - breast (*see also* Neoplasm, breast, malignant)C50.91 ☑
  - hepatocellular C22.0
  - lung (*see also* Neoplasm, lung, malignant)C34.90
  - ovarian (*see also* Neoplasm ovary, malignant)C56.9
  - unspecified site (primary) C80.1
- **Cancer** (o)phobia F45.29
- **Cancerous** — *see* Neoplasm, malignant, by site
- **Cancrum** oris A69.0
- **Candidiasis,** candidal B37.9
  - balanitis B37.42
  - bronchitis B37.1
  - cheilitis B37.83
  - congenital P37.5
  - cystitis B37.41
  - disseminated B37.7
  - endocarditis B37.6
  - enteritis B37.82
  - esophagitis B37.81
  - intertrigo B37.2
  - lung B37.1
  - meningitis B37.5
  - mouth B37.0
  - nails B37.2
  - neonatal P37.5
  - onychia B37.2
  - oral B37.0
  - osteomyelitis B37.89
  - otitis externa B37.84
  - paronychia B37.2
  - perionyxis B37.2
  - pneumonia B37.1
  - proctitis B37.82
  - pulmonary B37.1
  - pyelonephritis B37.49
  - sepsis B37.7
  - skin B37.2
  - specified site NEC B37.89
  - stomatitis B37.0
  - systemic B37.7
  - urethritis B37.41
  - urogenital site NEC B37.49
  - vagina B37.3
  - vulva B37.3
  - vulvovaginitis B37.3
- **Candidid** L30.2
- **Candidosis** — *see* Candidiasis
- **Candiru** infection or infestation B88.8
- **Canities** (premature) L67.1
  - congenital Q84.2
- **Canker** (mouth) (sore) K12.0
  - rash A38.9
- **Cannabinosis** J66.2
- **Cannabis** induced
  - anxiety disorder F12.980
  - psychotic disorder F12.959
  - sleep disorder F12.988
- **Canton** fever A75.9
- **Cantrell**'s syndrome Q87.89
- **Capillariasis** (intestinal) B81.1
  - hepatic B83.8
- **Capillary** — *see* condition
- **Caplan's** syndrome — *see* Rheumatoid, lung
- **Capsule** — *see* condition
- **Capsulitis** (joint) (*see also* Enthesopathy)
  - adhesive (shoulder) M75.0 ☑
  - hepatic K65.8
  - labyrinthine — *see* Otosclerosis, specified NEC
  - thyroid E06.9
- **Caput**
  - crepitus Q75.8
  - medusae I86.8
  - succedaneum P12.81
- **Car** sickness T75.3 ☑
- **Carapata** (disease) A68.0
- **Carate** — *see* Pinta
- **Carbon** lung J60
- **Carbuncle** L02.93
  - abdominal wall L02.231
  - anus K61.0
  - auditory canal, external — *see* Abscess, ear, external
  - auricle ear — *see* Abscess, ear, external
  - axilla L02.43 ☑
- **Carbuncle** — *continued*
  - back (any part) L02.232
  - breast N61.1
  - buttock L02.33
  - cheek (external) L02.03
  - chest wall L02.233
  - chin L02.03
  - corpus cavernosum N48.21
  - ear (any part) (external) (middle) — *see* Abscess, ear, external
  - external auditory canal — *see* Abscess, ear, external
  - eyelid — *see* Abscess, eyelid
  - face NEC L02.03
  - femoral (region) — *see* Carbuncle, lower limb
  - finger — *see* Carbuncle, hand
  - flank L02.231
  - foot L02.63 ☑
  - forehead L02.03
  - genital — *see* Abscess, genital
  - gluteal (region) L02.33
  - groin L02.234
  - hand L02.53 ☑
  - head NEC L02.831
  - heel — *see* Carbuncle, foot
  - hip — *see* Carbuncle, lower limb
  - kidney — *see* Abscess, kidney
  - knee — *see* Carbuncle, lower limb
  - labium (majus) (minus) N76.4
  - lacrimal
    - gland — *see* Dacryoadenitis
    - passages (duct) (sac) — *see* Inflammation, lacrimal, passages, acute
  - leg — *see* Carbuncle, lower limb
  - lower limb L02.43 ☑
  - malignant A22.0
  - navel L02.236
  - neck L02.13
  - nose (external) (septum) J34.0
  - orbit, orbital — *see* Abscess, orbit
  - palmar (space) — *see* Carbuncle, hand
  - partes posteriores L02.33
  - pectoral region L02.233
  - penis N48.21
  - perineum L02.235
  - pinna — *see* Abscess, ear, external
  - popliteal — *see* Carbuncle, lower limb
  - scalp L02.831
  - seminal vesicle N49.0
  - shoulder — *see* Carbuncle, upper limb
  - specified site NEC L02.838
  - temple (region) L02.03
  - thumb — *see* Carbuncle, hand
  - toe — *see* Carbuncle, foot
  - trunk L02.239
    - abdominal wall L02.231
    - back L02.232
    - chest wall L02.233
    - groin L02.234
    - perineum L02.235
    - umbilicus L02.236
  - umbilicus L02.236
  - upper limb L02.43 ☑
  - urethra N34.0
  - vulva N76.4
- **Carbunculus** — *see* Carbuncle
- **Carcinoid** (tumor) — *see* Tumor, carcinoid
- **Carcinoidosis** E34.0
- **Carcinoma** (malignant) (*see also* Neoplasm, by site, malignant)
  - acidophil
    - specified site — *see* Neoplasm, malignant, by site
    - unspecified site C75.1
  - acidophil-basophil, mixed
    - specified site — *see* Neoplasm, malignant, by site
    - unspecified site C75.1
  - adnexal (skin) — *see* Neoplasm, skin, malignant
  - adrenal cortical C74.0 ☑
  - alveolar — *see* Neoplasm, lung, malignant
    - cell — *see* Neoplasm, lung, malignant
  - ameloblastic C41.1
    - upper jaw (bone) C41.0
  - apocrine
    - breast — *see* Neoplasm, breast, malignant
    - specified site NEC — *see* Neoplasm, skin, malignant
    - unspecified site C44.99
  - basal cell (pigmented) (see also Neoplasm, skin, malignant) C44.91
- **Carcinoma** — *continued*
  - basal cell — *continued*
    - fibro-epithelial — *see* Neoplasm, skin, malignant
    - morphea — *see* Neoplasm, skin, malignant
    - multicentric — *see* Neoplasm, skin, malignant
  - basaloid
  - basal-squamous cell, mixed — *see* Neoplasm, skin, malignant
  - basophil
    - specified site — *see* Neoplasm, malignant, by site
    - unspecified site C75.1
  - basophil-acidophil, mixed
    - specified site — *see* Neoplasm, malignant, by site
    - unspecified site C75.1
  - basosquamous — *see* Neoplasm, skin, malignant
  - bile duct
    - with hepatocellular, mixed C22.0
    - liver C22.1
    - specified site NEC — *see* Neoplasm, malignant, by site
    - unspecified site C22.1
  - branchial or branchiogenic C10.4
  - bronchial or bronchogenic — *see* Neoplasm, lung, malignant
  - bronchiolar — *see* Neoplasm, lung, malignant
  - bronchioloalveolar — *see* Neoplasm, lung, malignant
  - C cell
    - specified site — *see* Neoplasm, malignant, by site
    - unspecified site C73
  - ceruminous C44.29 ☑
  - cervix uteri
    - in situ D06.9
      - endocervix D06.0
      - exocervix D06.1
      - specified site NEC D06.7
  - chorionic
    - specified site — *see* Neoplasm, malignant, by site
    - unspecified site
      - female C58
      - male C62.90
  - chromophobe
    - specified site — *see* Neoplasm, malignant, by site
    - unspecified site C75.1
  - cloacogenic
    - specified site — *see* Neoplasm, malignant, by site
    - unspecified site C21.2
  - diffuse type
    - specified site — *see* Neoplasm, malignant, by site
    - unspecified site C16.9
  - duct (cell)
    - with Paget's disease — *see* Neoplasm, breast, malignant
    - infiltrating
      - with lobular carcinoma (in situ)
        - specified site — *see* Neoplasm, malignant, by site
        - unspecified site (female) C50.91 ☑
          - male C50.92 ☑
      - specified site — *see* Neoplasm, malignant, by site
        - unspecified site (female) C50.91 ☑
          - male C50.92 ☑
  - ductal
    - with lobular
      - specified site — *see* Neoplasm, malignant, by site
      - unspecified site (female) C50.91 ☑
        - male C50.92 ☑
  - ductular, infiltrating
    - specified site — *see* Neoplasm, malignant, by site
    - unspecified site (female) C50.91 ☑
      - male C50.92 ☑
  - embryonal
    - liver C22.7
  - endometrioid
    - specified site — *see* Neoplasm, malignant, by site
    - unspecified site
      - female C56.9
      - male C61
  - eosinophil

Carcinoma — *continued*
- eosinophil — *continued*
  - specified site — *see* Neoplasm, malignant, by site
  - unspecified site C75.1
- epidermoid (*see also* Neoplasm, skin malignant)
  - in situ, Bowen's type — *see* Neoplasm, skin, in situ
- fibroepithelial, basal cell — *see* Neoplasm, skin, malignant
- follicular
  - with papillary (mixed) C73
  - moderately differentiated C73
  - pure follicle C73
  - specified site — *see* Neoplasm, malignant, by site
  - trabecular C73
  - unspecified site C73
  - well differentiated C73
- generalized, with unspecified primary site C80.0
- glycogen-rich — *see* Neoplasm, breast, malignant
- granulosa cell C56 ☑
- hepatic cell C22.0
- hepatocellular C22.0
  - with bile duct, mixed C22.0
  - fibrolamellar C22.0
- hepatocholangiolitic C22.0
- Hurthle cell C73
- in
  - adenomatous
    - polyposis coli C18.9
  - pleomorphic adenoma — *see* Neoplasm, salivary glands, malignant
  - situ — *see* Carcinoma-in-situ
- infiltrating
  - duct
    - with lobular
      - specified site — *see* Neoplasm, malignant, by site
      - unspecified site (female) C50.91 ☑
        - male C50.92 ☑
    - with Paget's disease — *see* Neoplasm, breast, malignant
    - specified site — *see* Neoplasm, malignant
    - unspecified site (female) C50.91 ☑
      - male C50.92 ☑
  - ductular
    - specified site — *see* Neoplasm, malignant
    - unspecified site (female) C50.91 ☑
      - male C50.92 ☑
  - lobular
    - specified site — *see* Neoplasm, malignant
    - unspecified site (female) C50.91 ☑
      - male C50.92 ☑
- inflammatory
  - specified site — *see* Neoplasm, malignant
  - unspecified site (female) C50.91 ☑
    - male C50.92 ☑
- intestinal type
  - specified site — *see* Neoplasm, malignant, by site
  - unspecified site C16.9
- intracystic
  - noninfiltrating — *see* Neoplasm, in situ, by site
- intraductal (noninfiltrating)
  - with Paget's disease — *see* Neoplasm, breast, malignant
  - breast D05.1 ☑
  - papillary
    - with invasion
      - specified site — *see* Neoplasm, malignant, by site
      - unspecified site (female) C50.91 ☑
        - male C50.92 ☑
    - breast D05.1 ☑
    - specified site NEC — *see* Neoplasm, in situ, by site
    - unspecified site (female) D05.1 ☑
  - specified site NEC — *see* Neoplasm, in situ, by site
  - unspecified site (female) D05.1 ☑
- intraepidermal — *see* Neoplasm, in situ
  - squamous cell, Bowen's type — *see* Neoplasm, skin, in situ
- intraepithelial — *see* Neoplasm, in situ, by site
  - squamous cell — *see* Neoplasm, in situ, by site
- intraosseous C41.1
  - upper jaw (bone) C41.0
- islet cell
  - with exocrine, mixed
    - specified site — *see* Neoplasm, malignant, by site

Carcinoma — *continued*
- islet cell — *continued*
    - unspecified site C25.9
  - pancreas C25.4
  - specified site NEC — *see* Neoplasm, malignant, by site
  - unspecified site C25.4
- juvenile, breast — *see* Neoplasm, breast, malignant
- large cell
  - small cell
    - specified site — *see* Neoplasm, malignant, by site
    - unspecified site C34.90
- Leydig cell (testis)
  - specified site — *see* Neoplasm, malignant, by site
  - unspecified site
    - female C56.9
    - male C62.90
- lipid-rich (female) C50.91 ☑
  - male C50.92 ☑
- liver cell C22.0
- liver NEC C22.7
- lobular (infiltrating)
  - with intraductal
    - specified site — *see* Neoplasm, malignant, by site
    - unspecified site (female) C50.91 ☑
      - male C50.92 ☑
  - noninfiltrating
    - breast D05.0 ☑
    - specified site NEC — *see* Neoplasm, in situ, by site
    - unspecified site D05.0 ☑
  - specified site — *see* Neoplasm, malignant, by site
  - unspecified site (female) C50.91 ☑
    - male C50.92 ☑
- medullary
  - with
    - amyloid stroma
      - specified site — *see* Neoplasm, malignant, by site
      - unspecified site C73
    - lymphoid stroma
      - specified site — *see* Neoplasm, malignant, by site
      - unspecified site (female) C50.91 ☑
        - male C50.92 ☑
- Merkel cell C4A.9
  - anal margin C4A.51
  - anal skin C4A.51
  - canthus C4A.1 ☑
  - ear and external auricular canal C4A.2 ☑
  - external auricular canal C4A.2 ☑
  - eyelid, including canthus C4A.1 ☑
  - face C4A.30
    - specified NEC C4A.39
  - hip C4A.7 ☑
  - lip C4A.0
  - lower limb, including hip C4A.7 ☑
  - neck C4A.4
  - nodal presentation C7B.1
  - nose C4A.31
  - overlapping sites C4A.8
  - perianal skin C4A.51
  - scalp C4A.4
  - secondary C7B.1
  - shoulder C4A.6 ☑
  - skin of breast C4A.52
  - trunk NEC C4A.59
  - upper limb, including shoulder C4A.6 ☑
  - visceral metastatic C7B.1
- metastatic — *see* Neoplasm, secondary, by site
- metatypical — *see* Neoplasm, skin, malignant
- morphea, basal cell — *see* Neoplasm, skin, malignant
- mucoid
  - cell
    - specified site — *see* Neoplasm, malignant, by site
    - unspecified site C75.1
- neuroendocrine (*see also* Tumor, neuroendocrine)
  - high grade, any site C7A.1
  - poorly differentiated, any site C7A.1
- nonencapsulated sclerosing C73
- noninfiltrating
  - intracystic — *see* Neoplasm, in situ, by site
  - intraductal
    - breast D05.1 ☑
    - papillary

Carcinoma — *continued*
- noninfiltrating — *continued*
      - breast D05.1 ☑
      - specified site NEC — *see* Neoplasm, in situ, by site
      - unspecified site D05.1 ☑
    - specified site — *see* Neoplasm, in situ, by site
    - unspecified site D05.1 ☑
  - lobular
    - breast D05.0 ☑
    - specified site NEC — *see* Neoplasm, in situ, by site
    - unspecified site (female) D05.0 ☑
- oat cell
  - specified site — *see* Neoplasm, malignant, by site
  - unspecified site C34.90
- odontogenic C41.1
  - upper jaw (bone) C41.0
- papillary
  - with follicular (mixed) C73
  - follicular variant C73
  - intraductal (noninfiltrating)
    - with invasion
      - specified site — *see* Neoplasm, malignant, by site
      - unspecified site (female) C50.91 ☑
        - male C50.92 ☑
    - breast D05.1 ☑
    - specified site NEC — *see* Neoplasm, in situ, by site
    - unspecified site D05.1 ☑
  - serous
    - specified site — *see* Neoplasm, malignant, by site
    - surface
      - specified site — *see* Neoplasm, malignant, by site
      - unspecified site C56.9
    - unspecified site C56.9
- papillocystic
  - specified site — *see* Neoplasm, malignant, by site
  - unspecified site C56.9
- parafollicular cell
  - specified site — *see* Neoplasm, malignant, by site
  - unspecified site C73
- pilomatrix — *see* Neoplasm, skin, malignant
- pseudomucinous
  - specified site — *see* Neoplasm, malignant, by site
  - unspecified site C56.9
- renal cell C64 ☑
- Schmincke — *see* Neoplasm, nasopharynx, malignant
- Schneiderian
  - specified site — *see* Neoplasm, malignant, by site
  - unspecified site C30.0
- sebaceous — *see* Neoplasm, skin, malignant
- secondary (*see also* Neoplasm, secondary, by site)
  - Merkel cell C7B.1
- secretory, breast — *see* Neoplasm, breast, malignant
- serous
  - papillary
    - specified site — *see* Neoplasm, malignant, by site
    - unspecified site C56.9
  - surface, papillary
    - specified site — *see* Neoplasm, malignant, by site
    - unspecified site C56.9
- Sertoli cell
  - specified site — *see* Neoplasm, malignant, by site
  - unspecified site C62.90
    - female C56.9
    - male C62.90
- skin appendage — *see* Neoplasm, skin, malignant
- small cell
  - fusiform cell
    - specified site — *see* Neoplasm, malignant, by site
    - unspecified site C34.90
  - intermediate cell
    - specified site — *see* Neoplasm, malignant, by site
    - unspecified site C34.90
  - large cell

- **Carcinoma** — *continued*
  - small cell — *continued*
    - specified site — *see* Neoplasm, malignant, by site
    - unspecified site C34.90
  - solid
    - with amyloid stroma
      - specified site — *see* Neoplasm, malignant, by site
      - unspecified site C73
    - microinvasive
      - specified site — *see* Neoplasm, malignant, by site
      - unspecified site C53.9
  - sweat gland — *see* Neoplasm, skin, malignant
  - theca cell C56. ☑
  - thymic C37
  - unspecified site (primary) C80.1
  - water-clear cell C75.0
- **Carcinoma-in-situ** (*see also* Neoplasm, in situ, by site)
  - breast NOS D05.9 ☑
    - specified type NEC D05.8 ☑
  - epidermoid (*see also* Neoplasm, in situ, by site)
    - with questionable stromal invasion
      - cervix D06.9
      - specified site NEC — *see* Neoplasm, in situ, by site
      - unspecified site D06.9
    - Bowen's type — *see* Neoplasm, skin, in situ
  - intraductal
    - breast D05.1 ☑
    - specified site NEC — *see* Neoplasm, in situ, by site
    - unspecified site D05.1 ☑
  - lobular
    - with
      - infiltrating duct
        - breast (female) C50.91 ☑
          - male C50.92 ☑
        - specified site NEC — *see* Neoplasm, malignant
        - unspecified site (female) C50.91 ☑
          - male C50.92 ☑
      - intraductal
        - breast D05.8 ☑
        - specified site NEC — *see* Neoplasm, in situ, by site
        - unspecified site (female) D05.8 ☑
    - breast D05.0 ☑
    - specified site NEC — *see* Neoplasm, in situ, by site
    - unspecified site D05.0 ☑
  - squamous cell (*see also* Neoplasm, in situ, by site)
    - with questionable stromal invasion
      - cervix D06.9
      - specified site NEC — *see* Neoplasm, in situ, by site
      - unspecified site D06.9
- **Carcinomaphobia** F45.29
- **Carcinomatosis** C80.0
  - peritonei C78.6
  - unspecified site (primary) (secondary) C80.0
- **Carcinosarcoma** — *see* Neoplasm, malignant, by site
  - embryonal — *see* Neoplasm, malignant, by site
- **Cardia,** cardial — *see* condition
- **Cardiac** (*see also* condition)
  - death, sudden — *see* Arrest, cardiac
  - pacemaker
    - in situ Z95.0
    - management or adjustment Z45.018
  - tamponade I31.4
- **Cardialgia** — *see* Pain, precordial
- **Cardiectasis** — *see* Hypertrophy, cardiac
- **Cardiochalasia** K21.9
- **Cardiomalacia** I51.5
- **Cardiomegalia** glycogenica diffusa E74.02 *[I43]*
- **Cardiomegaly** (*see also* Hypertrophy, cardiac)
  - congenital Q24.8
  - glycogen E74.02 *[I43]*
  - idiopathic I51.7
- **Cardiomyoliposis** I51.5
- **Cardiomyopathy** (familial) (idiopathic) I42.9
  - alcoholic I42.6
  - amyloid E85.4 *[I43]*
  - arteriosclerotic — *see* Disease, heart, ischemic, atherosclerotic
  - beriberi E51.12
  - cobalt-beer I42.6
  - congenital I42.4
  - congestive I42.0
  - constrictive NOS I42.5
  - dilated I42.0
- **Cardiomyopathy** — *continued*
  - due to
    - alcohol I42.6
    - beriberi E51.12
    - cardiac glycogenosis E74.02 *[I43]*
    - drugs I42.7
    - external agents NEC I42.7
    - Friedreich's ataxia G11.1
    - myotonia atrophica G71.11 *[I43]*
    - progressive muscular dystrophy G71.0
  - glycogen storage E74.02 *[I43]*
  - hypertensive — *see* Hypertension, heart
  - hypertrophic (nonobstructive) I42.2
    - obstructive I42.1
      - congenital Q24.8
  - in
    - Chagas' disease (chronic) B57.2
      - acute B57.0
    - sarcoidosis D86.85
  - ischemic I25.5
  - metabolic E88.9 *[I43]*
    - thyrotoxic E05.90 *[I43]*
      - with thyroid storm E05.91 *[I43]*
  - newborn I42.8
    - congenital I42.4
  - nutritional E63.9 *[I43]*
    - beriberi E51.12
  - obscure of Africa I42.8
  - peripartum O90.3
  - postpartum O90.3
  - restrictive NEC I42.5
  - rheumatic I09.0
  - secondary I42.9
  - stress induced I51.81
  - takotsubo I51.81
  - thyrotoxic E05.90 *[I43]*
    - with thyroid storm E05.91 *[I43]*
  - toxic NEC I42.7
  - tuberculous A18.84
  - viral B33.24
- **Cardionephritis** — *see* Hypertension, cardiorenal
- **Cardionephropathy** — *see* Hypertension, cardiorenal
- **Cardionephrosis** — *see* Hypertension, cardiorenal
- **Cardiopathia** nigra I27.0
- **Cardiopathy** (*see also* Disease, heart)I51.9
  - idiopathic I42.9
  - mucopolysaccharidosis E76.3 *[I52]*
- **Cardiopericarditis** — *see* Pericarditis
- **Cardiophobia** F45.29
- **Cardiorenal** — *see* condition
- **Cardiorrhexis** — *see* Infarct, myocardium
- **Cardiosclerosis** — *see* Disease, heart, ischemic, atherosclerotic
- **Cardiosis** — *see* Disease, heart
- **Cardiospasm** (esophagus) (reflex) (stomach) K22.0
  - congenital Q39.5
    - with megaesophagus Q39.5
- **Cardiostenosis** — *see* Disease, heart
- **Cardiosymphysis** I31.0
- **Cardiovascular** — *see* condition
- **Carditis** (acute) (bacterial) (chronic) (subacute) I51.89
  - meningococcal A39.50
  - rheumatic — *see* Disease, heart, rheumatic
  - rheumatoid — *see* Rheumatoid, carditis
  - viral B33.20
- **Care** (of) (for) (following)
  - child (routine) Z76.2
  - family member (handicapped) (sick)
    - creating problem for family Z63.6
    - provided away from home for holiday relief Z75.5
    - unavailable, due to
      - absence (person rendering care) (sufferer) Z74.2
      - inability (any reason) of person rendering care Z74.2
  - foundling Z76.1
  - holiday relief Z75.5
  - improper — *see* Maltreatment
  - lack of (at or after birth) (infant) — *see* Maltreatment, child, neglect
  - lactating mother Z39.1
  - palliative Z51.5
  - postpartum
    - immediately after delivery Z39.0
    - routine follow-up Z39.2
  - respite Z75.5
  - unavailable, due to
    - absence of person rendering care Z74.2
    - inability (any reason) of person rendering care Z74.2
  - well-baby Z76.2
- **Caries**
  - bone NEC A18.03
  - dental (dentino enamel junction) (early childhood) (of dentine) (pre-eruptive) (recurrent) (to the pulp) K02.9
    - arrested (coronal) (root) K02.3
    - chewing surface
      - limited to enamel K02.51
      - penetrating into dentin K02.52
      - penetrating into pulp K02.53
    - coronal surface
      - chewing surface
        - limited to enamel K02.51
        - penetrating into dentin K02.52
        - penetrating into pulp K02.53
      - pit and fissure surface
        - limited to enamel K02.51
        - penetrating into dentin K02.52
        - penetrating into pulp K02.53
      - smooth surface
        - limited to enamel K02.61
        - penetrating into dentin K02.62
        - penetrating into pulp K02.63
    - pit and fissure surface
      - limited to enamel K02.51
      - penetrating into dentin K02.52
      - penetrating into pulp K02.53
    - primary, cervical origin K02.52
    - root K02.7
    - smooth surface
      - limited to enamel K02.61
      - penetrating into dentin K02.62
      - penetrating into pulp K02.63
  - external meatus — *see* Disorder, ear, external, specified type NEC
  - hip (tuberculous) A18.02
  - initial (tooth)
    - chewing surface K02.51
    - pit and fissure surface K02.51
    - smooth surface K02.61
  - knee (tuberculous) A18.02
  - labyrinth — *see* subcategory H83.8
  - limb NEC (tuberculous) A18.03
  - mastoid process (chronic) — *see* Mastoiditis, chronic
    - tuberculous A18.03
  - middle ear — *see* subcategory H74.8
  - nose (tuberculous) A18.03
  - orbit (tuberculous) A18.03
  - ossicles, ear — *see* Abnormal, ear ossicles
  - petrous bone — *see* Petrositis
  - root (dental) (tooth) K02.7
  - sacrum (tuberculous) A18.01
  - spine, spinal (column) (tuberculous) A18.01
  - syphilitic A52.77
    - congenital (early) A50.02 *[M90.80]*
  - tooth, teeth — *see* Caries, dental
  - tuberculous A18.03
  - vertebra (column) (tuberculous) A18.01
- **Carious** teeth — *see* Caries, dental
- **Carneous** mole O02.0
- **Carnitine** insufficiency E71.40
- **Carotid** body or sinus syndrome G90.01
- **Carotidynia** G90.01
- **Carotinemia** (dietary) E67.1
- **Carotinosis** (cutis) (skin) E67.1
- **Carpal** tunnel syndrome — *see* Syndrome, carpal tunnel
- **Carpenter's** syndrome Q87.0
- **Carpopedal** spasm — *see* Tetany
- **Carr-Barr-Plunkett** syndrome Q97.1
- **Carrier** (suspected) of
  - amebiasis Z22.1
  - bacterial disease NEC Z22.39
    - diphtheria Z22.2
    - intestinal infectious NEC Z22.1
      - typhoid Z22.0
    - meningococcal Z22.31
    - sexually transmitted Z22.4
    - specified NEC Z22.39
    - staphylococcal (Methicillin susceptible) Z22.321
      - Methicillin resistant Z22.322
    - streptococcal Z22.338
      - group B Z22.330
        - complicating pregnancy or delivery O99.82 ☑
    - typhoid Z22.0
  - cholera Z22.1
  - diphtheria Z22.2
  - gastrointestinal pathogens NEC Z22.1

- **Carrier** — *continued*
  - genetic Z14.8
    - cystic fibrosis Z14.1
    - hemophilia A (asymptomatic) Z14.01
      - symptomatic Z14.02
  - gestational, pregnant Z33.1
  - gonorrhea Z22.4
  - HAA (hepatitis Australian-antigen) B18.8
  - HB (c) (s)-AG B18.1
  - hepatitis (viral) B18.9
    - Australia-antigen (HAA) B18.8
    - B surface antigen (HBsAg) B18.1
      - with acute delta- (super)infection B17.0
    - C B18.2
    - specified NEC B18.8
  - human T-cell lymphotropic virus type-1 (HTLV-1) infection Z22.6
  - infectious organism Z22.9
    - specified NEC Z22.8
  - meningococci Z22.31
  - Salmonella typhosa Z22.0
  - serum hepatitis — *see* Carrier, hepatitis
  - staphylococci (Methicillin susceptible) Z22.321
    - Methicillin resistant Z22.322
  - streptococci Z22.338
    - group B Z22.330
      - complicating pregnancy or delivery O99.82 ☑
  - syphilis Z22.4
  - typhoid Z22.0
  - venereal disease NEC Z22.4
- **Carrion's** disease A44.0
- **Carter's** relapsing fever (Asiatic) A68.1
- **Cartilage** — *see* condition
- **Caruncle** (inflamed)
  - conjunctiva (acute) — *see* Conjunctivitis, acute
  - labium (majus) (minus) N90.89
  - lacrimal — *see* Inflammation, lacrimal, passages
  - myrtiform N89.8
  - urethral (benign) N36.2
- **Cascade** stomach K31.2
- **Caseation** lymphatic gland (tuberculous) A18.2
- **Cassidy** (-Scholte) syndrome (malignant carcinoid) E34.0
- **Castellani's** disease A69.8
- **Castration,** traumatic, male S38.231 ☑
- **Casts** in urine R82.99
- **Cat**
  - cry syndrome Q93.4
  - ear Q17.3
  - eye syndrome Q92.8
- **Catabolism,** senile R54
- **Catalepsy** (hysterical) F44.2
  - schizophrenic F20.2
- **Cataplexy** (idiopathic) — *see* - Narcolepsy
- **Cataract** (cortical) (immature) (incipient) H26.9
  - with
    - neovascularization — *see* Cataract, complicated
  - age-related — *see* Cataract, senile
  - anterior
    - and posterior axial embryonal Q12.0
    - pyramidal Q12.0
  - associated with
    - galactosemia E74.21 *[H28]*
    - myotonic disorders G71.19 *[H28]*
  - blue Q12.0
  - central Q12.0
  - cerulean Q12.0
  - complicated H26.20
    - with
      - neovascularization H26.21 ☑
      - ocular disorder H26.22 ☑
    - glaucomatous flecks H26.23 ☑
  - congenital Q12.0
  - coraliform Q12.0
  - coronary Q12.0
  - crystalline Q12.0
  - diabetic — *see* Diabetes, cataract
  - drug-induced H26.3 ☑
  - due to
    - ocular disorder — *see* Cataract, complicated
    - radiation H26.8
  - electric H26.8
  - extraction status Z98.4 ☑
  - glass-blower's H26.8
  - heat ray H26.8
  - heterochromic — *see* Cataract, complicated
  - hypermature — *see* Cataract, senile, morgagnian type
  - in (due to)
    - chronic iridocyclitis — *see* Cataract, complicated
- **Cataract** — *continued*
  - in — *continued*
    - diabetes — *see* Diabetes, cataract
    - endocrine disease E34.9 *[H28]*
    - eye disease — *see* Cataract, complicated
    - hypoparathyroidism E20.9 *[H28]*
    - malnutrition-dehydration E46 *[H28]*
    - metabolic disease E88.9 *[H28]*
    - myotonic disorders G71.19 *[H28]*
    - nutritional disease E63.9 *[H28]*
  - infantile — *see* Cataract, presenile
  - irradiational — *see* Cataract, specified NEC
  - juvenile — *see* Cataract, presenile
  - malnutrition-dehydration E46 *[H28]*
  - morgagnian — *see* Cataract, senile, morgagnian type
  - myotonic G71.19 *[H28]*
  - myxedema E03.9 *[H28]*
  - nuclear
    - embryonal Q12.0
    - sclerosis — *see* Cataract, senile, nuclear
  - presenile H26.00 ☑
    - combined forms H26.06 ☑
    - cortical H26.01 ☑
    - lamellar — *see* Cataract, presenile, cortical
    - nuclear H26.03 ☑
    - specified NEC H26.09
    - subcapsular polar (anterior) H26.04 ☑
      - posterior H26.05 ☑
    - zonular — *see* Cataract, presenile, cortical
  - secondary H26.40
    - Soemmering's ring H26.41 ☑
    - specified NEC H26.49 ☑
    - to eye disease — *see* Cataract, complicated
  - senile H25.9
    - brunescens — *see* Cataract, senile, nuclear
    - combined forms H25.81 ☑
    - coronary — *see* Cataract, senile, incipient
    - cortical H25.01 ☑
    - hypermature — *see* Cataract, senile, morgagnian type
    - incipient (mature) (total) H25.09 ☑
      - cortical — *see* Cataract, senile, cortical
      - subcapsular — *see* Cataract, senile, subcapsular
    - morgagnian type (hypermature) H25.2 ☑
    - nuclear (sclerosis) H25.1 ☑
    - polar subcapsular (anterior) (posterior) — *see* Cataract, senile, incipient
    - punctate — *see* Cataract, senile, incipient
    - specified NEC H25.89
    - subcapsular polar (anterior) H25.03 ☑
      - posterior H25.04 ☑
  - snowflake — *see* Diabetes, cataract
  - specified NEC H26.8
  - toxic — *see* Cataract, drug-induced
  - traumatic H26.10 ☑
    - localized H26.11 ☑
    - partially resolved H26.12 ☑
    - total H26.13 ☑
  - zonular (perinuclear) Q12.0
- **Cataracta** (*see also* Cataract)
  - brunescens — *see* Cataract, senile, nuclear
  - centralis pulverulenta Q12.0
  - cerulea Q12.0
  - complicata — *see* Cataract, complicated
  - congenita Q12.0
  - coralliformis Q12.0
  - coronaria Q12.0
  - diabetic — *see* Diabetes, cataract
  - membranacea
    - accreta — *see* Cataract, secondary
    - congenita Q12.0
  - nigra — *see* Cataract, senile, nuclear
  - sunflower — *see* Cataract, complicated
- **Catarrh,** catarrhal (acute) (febrile) (infectious) (inflammation) (*see also* condition) J00
  - bronchial — *see* Bronchitis
  - chest — *see* Bronchitis
  - chronic J31.0
  - due to congenital syphilis A50.03
  - enteric — *see* Enteritis
  - eustachian H68.009
  - fauces — *see* Pharyngitis
  - gastrointestinal — *see* Enteritis
  - gingivitis K05.00
    - nonplaque induced K05.01
    - plaque induced K05.00
  - hay — *see* Fever, hay
  - intestinal — *see* Enteritis
  - larynx, chronic J37.0
  - liver B15.9
    - with hepatic coma B15.0
- **Catarrh** — *continued*
  - lung — *see* Bronchitis
  - middle ear, chronic — *see* Otitis, media, nonsuppurative, chronic, serous
  - mouth K12.1
  - nasal (chronic) — *see* Rhinitis
  - nasobronchial J31.1
  - nasopharyngeal (chronic) J31.1
    - acute J00
  - pulmonary — *see* Bronchitis
  - spring (eye) (vernal) — *see* Conjunctivitis, acute, atopic
  - summer (hay) — *see* Fever, hay
  - throat J31.2
  - tubotympanal (*see also* Otitis, media, nonsuppurative)
    - chronic — *see* Otitis, media, nonsuppurative, chronic, serous
- **Catatonia** (schizophrenic) F20.2
- **Catatonic**
  - disorder due to known physiologic condition F06.1
  - schizophrenia F20.2
  - stupor R40.1
- **Cat-scratch** (*see also* Abrasion)
  - disease or fever A28.1
- **Cauda** equina — *see* condition
- **Cauliflower** ear M95.1 ☑
- **Causalgia** (upper limb) G56.4 ☑
  - lower limb G57.7 ☑
- **Cause**
  - external, general effects T75.89 ☑
- **Caustic** burn — *see* Corrosion, by site
- **Cavare's** disease (familial periodic paralysis) G72.3
- **Cave-in,** injury
  - crushing (severe) — *see* Crush
  - suffocation — *see* Asphyxia, traumatic, due to low oxygen, due to cave-in
- **Cavernitis** (penis) N48.29
- **Cavernositis** N48.29
- **Cavernous** — *see* condition
- **Cavitation** of lung (*see also* Tuberculosis, pulmonary)
  - nontuberculous J98.4
- **Cavities,** dental — *see* Caries, dental
- **Cavity**
  - lung — *see* Cavitation of lung
  - optic papilla Q14.2
  - pulmonary — *see* Cavitation of lung
- **Cavovarus** foot, congenital Q66.1
- **Cavus** foot (congenital) Q66.7
  - acquired — *see* Deformity, limb, foot, specified NEC
- **Cazenave's** disease L10.2
- **Cecitis** K52.9
  - with perforation, peritonitis, or rupture K65.8
- **Cecum** — *see* condition
- **Celiac**
  - artery compression syndrome I77.4
  - disease (with steatorrhea) K90.0
  - infantilism K90.0
- **Cell** (s), cellular (*see also* condition)
  - in urine R82.99
- **Cellulitis** (diffuse) (phlegmonous) (septic) (suppurative) L03.90
  - abdominal wall L03.311
  - anaerobic A48.0
  - ankle — *see* Cellulitis, lower limb
  - anus K61.0
  - arm — *see* Cellulitis, upper limb
  - auricle (ear) — *see* Cellulitis, ear
  - axilla L03.11 ☑
  - back (any part) L03.312
  - breast (acute) (nonpuerperal) (subacute) N61.0
    - nipple N61.0
  - broad ligament
    - acute N73.0
  - buttock L03.317
  - cervical (meaning neck) L03.221
  - cervix (uteri) — *see* Cervicitis
  - cheek (external) L03.211
    - internal K12.2
  - chest wall L03.313
  - chronic L03.90
  - clostridial A48.0
  - corpus cavernosum N48.22
  - digit
    - finger — *see* Cellulitis, finger
    - toe — *see* Cellulitis, toe
  - Douglas' cul-de-sac or pouch
    - acute N73.0
  - drainage site (following operation) T81.48
  - ear (external) H60.1 ☑

Cellulitis — *continued*
- eosinophilic (granulomatous) L98.3
- erysipelatous — *see* Erysipelas
- external auditory canal — *see* Cellulitis, ear
- eyelid — *see* Abscess, eyelid
- face NEC L03.211
- finger (intrathecal) (periosteal) (subcutaneous) (subcuticular) L03.01 ☑
- foot — *see* Cellulitis, lower limb
- gangrenous — *see* Gangrene
- genital organ NEC
  - female (external) N76.4
  - male N49.9
    - multiple sites N49.8
    - specified NEC N49.8
- gluteal (region) L03.317
- gonococcal A54.89
- groin L03.314
- hand — *see* Cellulitis, upper limb
- head NEC L03.811
  - face (any part, except ear, eye and nose) L03.211
- heel — *see* Cellulitis, lower limb
- hip — *see* Cellulitis, lower limb
- jaw (region) L03.211
- knee — *see* Cellulitis, lower limb
- labium (majus) (minus) — *see* Vulvitis
- lacrimal passages — *see* Inflammation, lacrimal, passages
- larynx J38.7
- leg — *see* Cellulitis, lower limb
- lip K13.0
- lower limb L03.11 ☑
  - toe — *see* Cellulitis, toe
- mouth (floor) K12.2
- multiple sites, so stated L03.90
- nasopharynx J39.1
- navel L03.316
  - newborn P38.9
    - with mild hemorrhage P38.1
    - without hemorrhage P38.9
- neck (region) L03.221
- nipple (acute) (nonpuerperal) (subacute) N61.0
- nose (septum) (external) J34.0
- orbit, orbital H05.01 ☑
- palate (soft) K12.2
- pectoral (region) L03.313
- pelvis, pelvic (chronic)
  - female (*see also* Disease, pelvis, inflammatory)N73.2
    - acute N73.0
  - following ectopic or molar pregnancy O08.0
  - male K65.0
- penis N48.22
- perineal, perineum L03.315
- periorbital L03.213
- perirectal K61.1
- peritonsillar J36
- periurethral N34.0
- periuterine (*see also* Disease, pelvis, inflammatory)N73.2
  - acute N73.0
- pharynx J39.1
- preseptal L03.213
- rectum K61.1
- retroperitoneal K68.9
- round ligament
  - acute N73.0
- scalp (any part) L03.811
- scrotum N49.2
- seminal vesicle N49.0
- shoulder — *see* Cellulitis, upper limb
- specified site NEC L03.818
- submandibular (region) (space) (triangle) K12.2
  - gland K11.3
- submaxillary (region) K12.2
  - gland K11.3
- thigh — *see* Cellulitis, lower limb
- thumb (intrathecal) (periosteal) (subcutaneous) (subcuticular) — *see* Cellulitis, finger
- toe (intrathecal) (periosteal) (subcutaneous) (subcuticular) L03.03 ☑
- tonsil J36
- trunk L03.319
  - abdominal wall L03.311
  - back (any part) L03.312
  - buttock L03.317
  - chest wall L03.313
  - groin L03.314
  - perineal, perineum L03.315
  - umbilicus L03.316
- tuberculous (primary) A18.4

Cellulitis — *continued*
- umbilicus L03.316
- upper limb L03.11 ☑
  - axilla — *see* Cellulitis, axilla
  - finger — *see* Cellulitis, finger
  - thumb — *see* Cellulitis, finger
- vaccinal T88.0 ☑
- vocal cord J38.3
- vulva — *see* Vulvitis
- wrist — *see* Cellulitis, upper limb

Cementoblastoma, benign — *see* Cyst, calcifying odontogenic
Cementoma — *see* Cyst, calcifying odontogenic
Cementoperiostitis — *see* Periodontitis
Cementosis K03.4
Central auditory processing disorder H93.25
Central pain syndrome G89.0
Cephalematocele, cephal (o)hematocele
- newborn P52.8
  - birth injury P10.8
- traumatic — *see* Hematoma, brain

Cephalematoma, cephalhematoma (calcified)
- newborn (birth injury) P12.0
- traumatic — *see* Hematoma, brain

Cephalgia, cephalalgia (*see also* Headache)
- histamine G44.009
  - intractable G44.001
  - not intractable G44.009
- trigeminal autonomic (TAC) NEC G44.099
  - intractable G44.091
  - not intractable G44.099

Cephalic — *see* condition
Cephalitis — *see* Encephalitis
Cephalocele — *see* Encephalocele
Cephalomenia N94.89
Cephalopelvic — *see* condition
Cerclage (with cervical incompetence) in pregnancy — *see* Incompetence, cervix, in pregnancy
Cerebellitis — *see* Encephalitis
Cerebellum, cerebellar — *see* condition
Cerebral — *see* condition
Cerebritis — *see* Encephalitis
Cerebro-hepato-renal syndrome Q87.89
Cerebromalacia — *see* Softening, brain
- sequelae of cerebrovascular disease I69.398

Cerebroside lipidosis E75.22
Cerebrospasticity (congenital) G80.1
Cerebrospinal — *see* condition
Cerebrum — *see* condition
Ceroid-lipofuscinosis, neuronal E75.4
Cerumen (accumulation) (impacted) H61.2 ☑
Cervical (*see also* condition)
- auricle Q18.2
- dysplasia in pregnancy — *see* Abnormal, cervix, in pregnancy or childbirth
- erosion in pregnancy — *see* Abnormal, cervix, in pregnancy or childbirth
- fibrosis in pregnancy — *see* Abnormal, cervix, in pregnancy or childbirth
- fusion syndrome Q76.1
- rib Q76.5
- shortening (complicating pregnancy) O26.87 ☑

Cervicalgia M54.2
Cervicitis (acute) (chronic) (nonvenereal) (senile (atrophic)) (subacute) (with ulceration) N72
- with
  - abortion — *see* Abortion, by type complicated by genital tract and pelvic infection
  - ectopic pregnancy O08.0
  - molar pregnancy O08.0
- chlamydial A56.09
- gonococcal A54.03
- herpesviral A60.03
- puerperal (postpartum) O86.11
- syphilitic A52.76
- trichomonal A59.09
- tuberculous A18.16

Cervicocolpitis (emphysematosa) (see also Cervicitis) N72
Cervix — *see* condition
Cesarean delivery, previous, affecting management of pregnancy O34.219
- classical (vertical) scar O34.212
- low transverse scar O34.211

Céstan (-Chenais) paralysis or syndrome G46.3
Céstan-Raymond syndrome I65.8
Cestode infestation B71.9
- specified type NEC B71.8

Cestodiasis B71.9
Chabert's disease A22.9
Chacaleh E53.8
Chafing L30.4
Chagas' (-Mazza) disease (chronic) B57.2
- with
  - cardiovascular involvement NEC B57.2
  - digestive system involvement B57.30
    - megacolon B57.32
    - megaesophagus B57.31
    - other specified B57.39
  - megacolon B57.32
  - megaesophagus B57.31
  - myocarditis B57.2
  - nervous system involvement B57.40
    - meningitis B57.41
    - meningoencephalitis B57.42
    - other specified B57.49
  - specified organ involvement NEC B57.5
- acute (with) B57.1
  - cardiovascular NEC B57.0
  - myocarditis B57.0

Chagres fever B50.9
Chair-ridden Z74.09
Chalasia (cardiac sphincter) K21.9
Chalazion H00.19
- left H00.16
  - lower H00.15
  - upper H00.14
- right H00.13
  - lower H00.12
  - upper H00.11

Chalcosis (*see also* Disorder, globe, degenerative, chalcosis)
- cornea — *see* Deposit, cornea
- crystalline lens — *see* Cataract, complicated
- retina H35.89

Chalicosis (pulmonum) J62.8
Chancre (any genital site) (hard) (hunterian) (mixed) (primary) (seronegative) (seropositive) (syphilitic) A51.0
- congenital A50.07
- conjunctiva NEC A51.2
- Ducrey's A57
- extragenital A51.2
- eyelid A51.2
- lip A51.2
- nipple A51.2
- Nisbet's A57
- of
  - carate A67.0
  - pinta A67.0
  - yaws A66.0
- palate, soft A51.2
- phagedenic A57
- simple A57
- soft A57
  - bubo A57
  - palate A51.2
- urethra A51.0
- yaws A66.0

Chancroid (anus) (genital) (penis) (perineum) (rectum) (urethra) (vulva) A57
Chandler's disease (osteochondritis dissecans, hip) — *see* Osteochondritis, dissecans, hip
Change (s) (in) (of) (*see also* Removal)
- arteriosclerotic — *see* Arteriosclerosis
- bone (*see also* Disorder, bone)
  - diabetic — *see* Diabetes, bone change
- bowel habit R19.4
- cardiorenal (vascular) — *see* Hypertension, cardiorenal
- cardiovascular — *see* Disease, cardiovascular
- circulatory I99.9
- cognitive (mild) (organic) R41.89
- color, tooth, teeth
  - during formation K00.8
  - posteruptive K03.7
- contraceptive device Z30.433
- corneal membrane H18.30
  - Bowman's membrane fold or rupture H18.31 ☑
  - Descemet's membrane
    - fold H18.32 ☑
    - rupture H18.33 ☑
- coronary — *see* Disease, heart, ischemic
- degenerative, spine or vertebra — *see* Spondylosis
- dental pulp, regressive K04.2
- dressing (nonsurgical) Z48.00
  - surgical Z48.01
- heart — *see* Disease, heart
- hip joint — *see* Derangement, joint, hip
- hyperplastic larynx J38.7
- hypertrophic
  - nasal sinus J34.89
  - turbinate, nasal J34.3
  - upper respiratory tract J39.8

Cholesteatoma - Cicatrix

Cholesteatoma — *continued*
- external ear (canal) H60.4 ☑
- mastoid H71.2 ☑
- postmastoidectomy cavity (recurrent) — *see* Complications, postmastoidectomy, recurrent cholesteatoma
- recurrent (postmastoidectomy) — *see* Complications, postmastoidectomy, recurrent cholesteatoma
- tympanum H71.1 ☑

Cholesteatosis, diffuse H71.3 ☑
Cholesteremia E78.00
Cholesterin in vitreous — *see* Deposit, crystalline
Cholesterol
- deposit
  - retina H35.89
  - vitreous — *see* Deposit, crystalline
- elevated (high) E78.00
  - with elevated (high) triglycerides E78.2
  - screening for Z13.220
- imbibition of gallbladder K82.4

Cholesterolemia (essential) (pure) E78.00
- familial E78.01
- hereditary E78.01

Cholesterolosis, cholesterosis (gallbladder) K82.4
- cerebrotendinous E75.5

Cholocolic fistula K82.3
Choluria R82.2
Chondritis M94.8X9
- aurical H61.03 ☑
- costal (Tietze's) M94.0
- external ear H61.03 ☑
- patella, posttraumatic — *see* Chondromalacia, patella
- pinna H61.03 ☑
- purulent M94.8X ☑
- tuberculous NEC A18.02
  - intervertebral A18.01

Chondroblastoma (*see also* Neoplasm, bone, benign)
- malignant — *see* Neoplasm, bone, malignant

Chondrocalcinosis M11.20
- ankle M11.27 ☑
- elbow M11.22 ☑
- familial M11.10
  - ankle M11.17 ☑
  - elbow M11.12 ☑
  - foot joint M11.17 ☑
  - hand joint M11.14 ☑
  - hip M11.15 ☑
  - knee M11.16 ☑
  - multiple site M11.19
  - shoulder M11.11 ☑
  - vertebrae M11.18
  - wrist M11.13 ☑
- foot joint M11.27 ☑
- hand joint M11.24 ☑
- hip M11.25 ☑
- knee M11.26 ☑
- multiple site M11.29
- shoulder M11.21 ☑
- vertebrae M11.28
- specified type NEC M11.20
  - ankle M11.27 ☑
  - elbow M11.22 ☑
  - foot joint M11.27 ☑
  - hand joint M11.24 ☑
  - hip M11.25 ☑
  - knee M11.26 ☑
  - multiple site M11.29
  - shoulder M11.21 ☑
  - vertebrae M11.28
  - wrist M11.23 ☑
- wrist M11.23 ☑

Chondrodermatitis nodularis helicis or anthelicis — *see* Perichondritis, ear
Chondrodysplasia Q78.9
- with hemangioma Q78.4
- calcificans congenita Q77.3
- fetalis Q77.4
- metaphyseal (Jansen's) (McKusick's) (Schmid's) Q78.8
- punctata Q77.3

Chondrodystrophy, chondrodystrophia (familial) (fetalis) (hypoplastic) Q78.9
- calcificans congenita Q77.3
- myotonic (congenital) G71.13
- punctata Q77.3

Chondroectodermal dysplasia Q77.6
Chondrogenesis imperfecta Q77.4
Chondrolysis M94.35 ☑
Chondroma (*see also* Neoplasm, cartilage, benign)
- juxtacortical — *see* Neoplasm, bone, benign
- periosteal — *see* Neoplasm, bone, benign

Chondromalacia (systemic) M94.20
- acromioclavicular joint M94.21 ☑
- ankle M94.27 ☑
- elbow M94.22 ☑
- foot joint M94.27 ☑
- glenohumeral joint M94.21 ☑
- hand joint M94.24 ☑
- hip M94.25 ☑
- knee M94.26 ☑
  - patella M22.4 ☑
- multiple sites M94.29
- patella M22.4 ☑
- rib M94.28
- sacroiliac joint M94.259
- shoulder M94.21 ☑
- sternoclavicular joint M94.21 ☑
- vertebral joint M94.28
- wrist M94.23 ☑

Chondromatosis (*see also* Neoplasm, cartilage, uncertain behavior)
- internal Q78.4

Chondromyxosarcoma — *see* Neoplasm, cartilage, malignant
Chondro-osteodysplasia (Morquio-Brailsford type) E76.219
Chondro-osteodystrophy E76.29
Chondro-osteoma — *see* Neoplasm, bone, benign
Chondropathia tuberosa M94.0
Chondrosarcoma — *see* Neoplasm, cartilage, malignant
- juxtacortical — *see* Neoplasm, bone, malignant
- mesenchymal — *see* Neoplasm, connective tissue, malignant
- myxoid — *see* Neoplasm, cartilage, malignant

Chordee (nonvenereal) N48.89
- congenital Q54.4
- gonococcal A54.09

Chorditis (fibrinous) (nodosa) (tuberosa) J38.2
Chordoma — *see* Neoplasm, vertebral (column), malignant
Chorea (chronic) (gravis) (posthemiplegic) (senile) (spasmodic) G25.5
- with
  - heart involvement I02.0
    - active or acute (conditions in I01-) I02.0
    - rheumatic I02.9
      - with valvular disorder I02.0
  - rheumatic heart disease (chronic) (inactive) (quiescent) - code to rheumatic heart condition involved
- drug-induced G25.4
- habit F95.8
- hereditary G10
- Huntington's G10
- hysterical F44.4
- minor I02.9
  - with heart involvement I02.0
- progressive G25.5
  - hereditary G10
- rheumatic (chronic) I02.9
  - with heart involvement I02.0
- Sydenham's I02.9
  - with heart involvement — *see* Chorea, with rheumatic heart disease
  - nonrheumatic G25.5

Choreoathetosis (paroxysmal) G25.5
Chorioadenoma (destruens) D39.2
Chorioamnionitis O41.12 ☑
Chorioangioma D26.7
Choriocarcinoma — *see* Neoplasm, malignant, by site
- combined with
  - embryonal carcinoma — *see* Neoplasm, malignant, by site
  - other germ cell elements — *see* Neoplasm, malignant, by site
  - teratoma — *see* Neoplasm, malignant, by site
- specified site — *see* Neoplasm, malignant, by site
- unspecified site
  - female C58
  - male C62.90

Chorioencephalitis (acute) (lymphocytic) (serous) A87.2
Chorioepithelioma — *see* Choriocarcinoma
Choriomeningitis (acute) (lymphocytic) (serous) A87.2
Chorionepithelioma — *see* Choriocarcinoma
Chorioretinitis (*see also* Inflammation, chorioretinal)
Chorioretinitis — *continued*
- disseminated (*see also* Inflammation, chorioretinal, disseminated)
  - in neurosyphilis A52.19
- Egyptian B76.9 *[D63.8]*
- focal (*see also* Inflammation, chorioretinal, focal)
- histoplasmic B39.9 *[H32]*
- in (due to)
  - histoplasmosis B39.9 *[H32]*
  - syphilis (secondary) A51.43
    - late A52.71
  - toxoplasmosis (acquired) B58.01
    - congenital (active) P37.1 *[H32]*
  - tuberculosis A18.53
- juxtapapillary, juxtapapillaris — *see* Inflammation, chorioretinal, focal, juxtapapillary
- leprous A30.9 *[H32]*
- miner's B76.9 *[D63.8]*
- progressive myopia (degeneration) H44.2 ☑
- syphilitic (secondary) A51.43
  - congenital (early) A50.01 *[H32]*
    - late A50.32
  - late A52.71
- tuberculous A18.53

Chorioretinopathy, central serous H35.71 ☑
Choroid — *see* condition
Choroideremia H31.21
Choroiditis — *see* Chorioretinitis
Choroidopathy — *see* Disorder, choroid
Choroidoretinitis — *see* Chorioretinitis
Choroidoretinopathy, central serous — *see* Chorioretinopathy, central serous
Christian-Weber disease M35.6
Christmas disease D67
Chromaffinoma (*see also* Neoplasm, benign, by site)
- malignant — *see* Neoplasm, malignant, by site

Chromatopsia — *see* Deficiency, color vision
Chromhidrosis, chromidrosis L75.1
Chromoblastomycosis — *see* Chromomycosis
Chromoconversion R82.91
Chromomycosis B43.9
- brain abscess B43.1
- cerebral B43.1
- cutaneous B43.0
- skin B43.0
- specified NEC B43.8
- subcutaneous abscess or cyst B43.2

Chromophytosis B36.0
Chromosome — *see* condition by chromosome involved
- D (1) — *see* condition, chromosome 13
- E (3) — *see* condition, chromosome 18
- G — *see* condition, chromosome 21

Chromotrichomycosis B36.8
Chronic — *see* condition
- fracture — *see* Fracture, pathological

Churg-Strauss syndrome M30.1
Chyle cyst, mesentery I89.8
Chylocele (nonfilarial) I89.8
- filarial (*see also* Infestation, filarial)B74.9 *[N51]*
- tunica vaginalis N50.89
  - filarial (*see also* Infestation, filarial)B74.9 *[N51]*

Chylomicronemia (fasting) (with hyperprebetalipoproteinemia) E78.3
Chylopericardium I31.3
- acute I30.9

Chylothorax (nonfilarial) I89.8
- filarial (*see also* Infestation, filarial)B74.9 *[J91.8]*

Chylous — *see* condition
Chyluria (nonfilarial) R82.0
- due to
  - bilharziasis B65.0
  - Brugia (malayi) B74.1
    - timori B74.2
  - schistosomiasis (bilharziasis) B65.0
  - Wuchereria (bancrofti) B74.0
- filarial — *see* Infestation, filarial

Cicatricial (deformity) — *see* Cicatrix
Cicatrix (adherent) (contracted) (painful) (vicious) (*see also* Scar)L90.5
- adenoid (and tonsil) J35.8
- alveolar process M26.79
- anus K62.89
- auricle — *see* Disorder, pinna, specified type NEC
- bile duct (common) (hepatic) K83.8
- bladder N32.89
- bone — *see* Disorder, bone, specified type NEC
- brain G93.89
- cervix (postoperative) (postpartal) N88.1
- common duct K83.8
- cornea H17.9
  - tuberculous A18.59

- **Cicatrix** — *continued*
  - duodenum (bulb), obstructive K31.5
  - esophagus K22.2
  - eyelid — *see* Disorder, eyelid function
  - hypopharynx J39.2
  - lacrimal passages — *see* Obstruction, lacrimal
  - larynx J38.7
  - lung J98.4
  - middle ear — *see* subcategory H74.8
  - mouth K13.79
  - muscle M62.89
    - with contracture — *see* Contraction, muscle NEC
  - nasopharynx J39.2
  - palate (soft) K13.79
  - penis N48.89
  - pharynx J39.2
  - prostate N42.89
  - rectum K62.89
  - retina — *see* Scar, chorioretinal
  - semilunar cartilage — *see* Derangement, meniscus
  - seminal vesicle N50.89
  - skin L90.5
    - infected L08.89
    - postinfective L90.5
    - tuberculous B90.8
  - specified site NEC L90.5
  - throat J39.2
  - tongue K14.8
  - tonsil (and adenoid) J35.8
  - trachea J39.8
  - tuberculous NEC B90.9
  - urethra N36.8
  - uterus N85.8
  - vagina N89.8
    - postoperative N99.2
  - vocal cord J38.3
  - wrist, constricting (annular) L90.5
- **CIDP** (chronic inflammatory demyelinating polyneuropathy) G61.81
- **CIN** — *see* Neoplasia, intraepithelial, cervix
- **CINCA** (chronic infantile neurological, cutaneous and articular syndrome) M04.2
- **Cinchonism** — *see* Deafness, ototoxic
  - correct substance properly administered — *see* Table of Drugs and Chemicals, by drug, adverse effect
  - overdose or wrong substance given or taken — *see* Table of Drugs and Chemicals, by drug, poisoning
- **Circle** of Willis — *see* condition
- **Circular** — *see* condition
- **Circulating** anticoagulants (*see also* - Disorder, hemorrhagic)D68.318
  - due to drugs (*see also* - Disorder, hemorrhagic)D68.32
  - following childbirth O72.3
- **Circulation**
  - collateral, any site I99.8
  - defective (lower extremity) I99.8
    - congenital Q28.9
  - embryonic Q28.9
  - failure (peripheral) R57.9
    - newborn P29.89
  - fetal, persistent P29.3
  - heart, incomplete Q28.9
- **Circulatory** system — *see* condition
- **Circulus** senilis (cornea) — *see* Degeneration, cornea, senile
- **Circumcision** (in absence of medical indication) (ritual) (routine) Z41.2
- **Circumscribed** — *see* condition
- **Circumvallate** placenta O43.11 ☑
- **Cirrhosis**, cirrhotic (hepatic) (liver) K74.60
  - alcoholic K70.30
    - with ascites K70.31
  - atrophic — *see* Cirrhosis, liver
  - Baumgarten-Cruveilhier K74.69
  - biliary (cholangiolitic) (cholangitic) (hypertrophic) (obstructive) (pericholangiolitic) K74.5
    - due to
      - Clonorchiasis B66.1
      - flukes B66.3
    - primary K74.3
    - secondary K74.4
  - cardiac (of liver) K76.1
  - Charcot's K74.3
  - cholangiolitic, cholangitic, cholostatic (primary) K74.3
  - congestive K76.1
  - Cruveilhier-Baumgarten K74.69
- **Cirrhosis** — *continued*
  - cryptogenic (liver) K74.69
  - due to
    - hepatolenticular degeneration E83.01
    - Wilson's disease E83.01
    - xanthomatosis E78.2
  - fatty K76.0
    - alcoholic K70.0
  - Hanot's (hypertrophic) K74.3
  - hepatic — *see* Cirrhosis, liver
  - hypertrophic K74.3
  - Indian childhood K74.69
  - kidney — *see* Sclerosis, renal
  - Laennec's K70.30
    - with ascites K70.31
    - alcoholic K70.30
      - with ascites K70.31
    - nonalcoholic K74.69
  - liver K74.60
    - alcoholic K70.30
      - with ascites K70.31
      - fatty K70.0
    - congenital P78.81
    - syphilitic A52.74
  - lung (chronic) J84.10
  - macronodular K74.69
    - alcoholic K70.30
      - with ascites K70.31
  - micronodular K74.69
    - alcoholic K70.30
      - with ascites K70.31
  - mixed type K74.69
  - monolobular K74.3
  - nephritis — *see* Sclerosis, renal
  - nutritional K74.69
    - alcoholic K70.30
      - with ascites K70.31
  - obstructive — *see* Cirrhosis, biliary
  - ovarian N83.8
  - pancreas (duct) K86.89
  - pigmentary E83.110
  - portal K74.69
    - alcoholic K70.30
      - with ascites K70.31
  - postnecrotic K74.69
    - alcoholic K70.30
      - with ascites K70.31
  - pulmonary J84.10
  - renal — *see* Sclerosis, renal
  - spleen D73.2
  - stasis K76.1
  - Todd's K74.3
  - unilobar K74.3
  - xanthomatous (biliary) K74.5
    - due to xanthomatosis (familial) (metabolic) (primary) E78.2
- **Cistern**, subarachnoid R93.0
- **Citrullinemia** E72.23
- **Citrullinuria** E72.23
- **Civatte's** disease or poikiloderma L57.3
- **Clam** digger's itch B65.3
- **Clammy** skin R23.1
- **Clap** — *see* Gonorrhea
- **Clarke-Hadfield** syndrome (pancreatic infantilism) K86.89
- **Clark's** paralysis G80.9
- **Clastothrix** L67.8
- **Claude** Bernard-Horner syndrome G90.2
  - traumatic — *see* Injury, nerve, cervical sympathetic
- **Claude's** disease or syndrome G46.3
- **Claudication** (intermittent) I73.9
  - cerebral (artery) G45.9
  - spinal cord (arteriosclerotic) G95.19
    - syphilitic A52.09
  - venous (axillary) I87.8
- **Claudicatio** venosa intermittens I87.8
- **Claustrophobia** F40.240
- **Clavus** (infected) L84
- **Clawfoot** (congenital) Q66.89
  - acquired — *see* Deformity, limb, clawfoot
- **Clawhand** (acquired) (*see also* Deformity, limb, clawhand)
  - congenital Q68.1
- **Clawtoe** (congenital) Q66.89
  - acquired — *see* Deformity, toe, specified NEC
- **Clay** eating — *see* Pica
- **Cleansing** of artificial opening — *see* Attention to, artificial, opening
- **Cleft** (congenital) (*see also* Imperfect, closure)
  - alveolar process M26.79
  - branchial (cyst) (persistent) Q18.2
- **Cleft** — *continued*
  - cricoid cartilage, posterior Q31.8
  - foot Q72.7 ☑
  - hand Q71.6 ☑
  - lip (unilateral) Q36.9
    - with cleft palate Q37.9
      - hard Q37.1
        - with soft Q37.5
      - soft Q37.3
        - with hard Q37.5
    - bilateral Q36.0
      - with cleft palate Q37.8
        - hard Q37.0
          - with soft Q37.4
        - soft Q37.2
          - with hard Q37.4
    - median Q36.1
  - nose Q30.2
  - palate Q35.9
    - with cleft lip (unilateral) Q37.9
      - bilateral Q37.8
    - hard Q35.1
      - with
        - cleft lip (unilateral) Q37.1
          - bilateral Q37.0
        - soft Q35.5
          - with cleft lip (unilateral) Q37.5
            - bilateral Q37.4
    - medial Q35.5
    - soft Q35.3
      - with
        - cleft lip (unilateral) Q37.3
          - bilateral Q37.2
        - hard Q35.5
          - with cleft lip (unilateral) Q37.5
            - bilateral Q37.4
  - penis Q55.69
  - scrotum Q55.29
  - thyroid cartilage Q31.8
  - uvula Q35.7
- **Cleidocranial** dysostosis Q74.0
- **Cleptomania** F63.2
- **Clicking** hip (newborn) R29.4
- **Climacteric** (female) (*see also* Menopause)
  - arthritis (any site) NEC — *see* Arthritis, specified form NEC
  - depression (single episode) F32.89
    - recurrent episode F33.8
  - melancholia (single episode) F32.89
    - recurrent episode F33.8
  - male (symptoms) (syndrome) NEC N50.89
  - paranoid state F22
  - polyarthritis NEC — *see* Arthritis, specified form NEC
  - symptoms (female) N95.1
- **Clinical** research investigation (clinical trial) (control subject) (normal comparison) (participant) Z00.6
- **Clitoris** — *see* condition
- **Cloaca** (persistent) Q43.7
- **Clonorchiasis**, clonorchis infection (liver) B66.1
- **Clonus** R25.8
- **Closed** bite M26.29
- **Clostridium** (C.) perfringens, as cause of disease classified elsewhere B96.7
- **Closure**
  - congenital, nose Q30.0
  - cranial sutures, premature Q75.0
  - defective or imperfect NEC — *see* Imperfect, closure
  - fistula, delayed — *see* Fistula
  - foramen ovale, imperfect Q21.1
  - hymen N89.6
  - interauricular septum, defective Q21.1
  - interventricular septum, defective Q21.0
  - lacrimal duct (*see also* Stenosis, lacrimal, duct)
    - congenital Q10.5
  - nose (congenital) Q30.0
    - acquired M95.0
  - of artificial opening — *see* Attention to, artificial, opening
  - primary angle, without glaucoma damage H40.06 ☑
  - vagina N89.5
  - valve — *see* Endocarditis
  - vulva N90.5
- **Clot** (blood) (*see also* Embolism)
  - artery (obstruction) (occlusion) — *see* Embolism
  - bladder N32.89
  - brain (intradural or extradural) — *see* Occlusion, artery, cerebral
  - circulation I74.9
  - heart (*see also* Infarct, myocardium)
    - not resulting in infarction I51.3
  - vein — *see* Thrombosis

Clouded - Collapse

- **Clouded** state R40.1
  - epileptic — *see* Epilepsy, specified NEC
  - paroxysmal — *see* Epilepsy, specified NEC
- **Cloudy** antrum, antra J32.0
- **Clouston's** (hidrotic) ectodermal dysplasia Q82.4
- **Clubbed** nail pachydermoperiostosis M89.40 *[L62]*
- **Clubbing** of finger (s) (nails) R68.3
- **Clubfinger** R68.3
  - congenital Q68.1
- **Clubfoot** (congenital) Q66.89
  - acquired — *see* Deformity, limb, clubfoot
  - equinovarus Q66.0
  - paralytic — *see* Deformity, limb, clubfoot
- **Clubhand** (congenital) (radial) Q71.4 ☑
  - acquired — *see* Deformity, limb, clubhand
- **Clubnail** R68.3
  - congenital Q84.6
- **Clump,** kidney Q63.1
- **Clumsiness,** clumsy child syndrome F82
- **Cluttering** F80.81
- **Clutton's** joints A50.51 *[M12.80]*
- **Coagulation,** intravascular (diffuse) (disseminated) (*see also* Defibrination syndrome)
  - complicating abortion — *see* Abortion, by type, complicated by, intravascular coagulation
  - following ectopic or molar pregnancy O08.1
- **Coagulopathy** (*see also* Defect, coagulation)
  - consumption D65
  - intravascular D65
    - newborn P60
- **Coalition**
  - calcaneo-scaphoid Q66.89
  - tarsal Q66.89
- **Coalminer's**
  - elbow — *see* Bursitis, elbow, olecranon
  - lung or pneumoconiosis J60
- **Coalworker's** lung or pneumoconiosis J60
- **Coarctation**
  - aorta (preductal) (postductal) Q25.1
  - pulmonary artery Q25.71
- **Coated** tongue K14.3
- **Coats'** disease (exudative retinopathy) — *see* Retinopathy, exudative
- **Cocaine-induced**
  - anxiety disorder F14.980
  - bipolar and related disorder F14.94
  - depressive disorder F14.94
  - obsessive-compulsive and related disorder F14.988
  - psychotic disorder F14.959
  - sleep disorder F14.982
  - sexual dysfunction F14.981
- **Cocainism** — *see* Disorder, cocaine use
- **Coccidioidomycosis** B38.9
  - cutaneous B38.3
  - disseminated B38.7
  - generalized B38.7
  - meninges B38.4
  - prostate B38.81
  - pulmonary B38.2
    - acute B38.0
    - chronic B38.1
  - skin B38.3
  - specified NEC B38.89
- **Coccidioidosis** — *see* Coccidioidomycosis
- **Coccidiosis** (intestinal) A07.3
- **Coccydynia,** coccygodynia M53.3
- **Coccyx** — *see* condition
- **Cochin-China** diarrhea K90.1
- **Cockayne's** syndrome Q87.1
- **Cocked** up toe — *see* Deformity, toe, specified NEC
- **Cock's** peculiar tumor L72.3
- **Codman's** tumor — *see* Neoplasm, bone, benign
- **Coenurosis** B71.8
- **Coffee-worker's** lung J67.8
- **Cogan's** syndrome H16.32 ☑
  - oculomotor apraxia H51.8
- **Coitus,** painful (female) N94.10
  - male N53.12
  - psychogenic F52.6
- **Cold** J00
  - with influenza, flu, or grippe — *see* Influenza, with, respiratory manifestations NEC
  - agglutinin disease or hemoglobinuria (chronic) D59.1
  - bronchial — *see* Bronchitis
  - chest — *see* Bronchitis
  - common (head) J00
  - effects of T69.9 ☑
    - specified effect NEC T69.8 ☑
  - excessive, effects of T69.9 ☑
    - specified effect NEC T69.8 ☑

Cold — *continued*

  - exhaustion from T69.8 ☑
  - exposure to T69.9 ☑
    - specified effect NEC T69.8 ☑
  - head J00
  - injury syndrome (newborn) P80.0
  - on lung — *see* Bronchitis
  - rose J30.1
  - sensitivity, auto-immune D59.1
  - virus J00
- **Coldsore** B00.1
- **Colibacillosis** A49.8
  - as the cause of other disease (*see also* Escherichia coli)B96.20
  - generalized A41.50
- **Colic** (bilious) (infantile) (intestinal) (recurrent) (spasmodic) R10.83
  - abdomen R10.83
    - psychogenic F45.8
  - appendix, appendicular K38.8
  - bile duct — *see* Calculus, bile duct
  - biliary — *see* Calculus, bile duct
  - common duct — *see* Calculus, bile duct
  - cystic duct — *see* Calculus, gallbladder
  - Devonshire NEC — *see* Poisoning, lead
  - gallbladder — *see* Calculus, gallbladder
  - gallstone — *see* Calculus, gallbladder
    - gallbladder or cystic duct — *see* Calculus, gallbladder
  - hepatic (duct) — *see* Calculus, bile duct
  - hysterical F45.8
  - kidney N23
  - lead NEC — *see* Poisoning, lead
  - mucous K58.9
    - with diarrhea K58.0
    - psychogenic F54
  - nephritic N23
  - painter's NEC — *see* Poisoning, lead
  - pancreas K86.89
  - psychogenic F45.8
  - renal N23
  - saturnine NEC — *see* Poisoning, lead
  - ureter N23
  - urethral N36.8
    - due to calculus N21.1
  - uterus NEC N94.89
    - menstrual — *see* Dysmenorrhea
  - worm NOS B83.9
- **Colicystitis** — *see* Cystitis
- **Colitis** (acute) (catarrhal) (chronic) (noninfective) (hemorrhagic) (*see also* Enteritis)K52.9
  - allergic K52.29
    - with
      - food protein-induced enterocolitis syndrome K52.21
      - proctocolitis K52.82
  - amebic (acute) (*see also* Amebiasis)A06.0
    - nondysenteric A06.2
  - anthrax A22.2
  - bacillary — *see* Infection, Shigella
  - balantidial A07.0
  - Clostridium difficile A04.7
  - coccidial A07.3
  - collagenous K52.831
  - cystica superficialis K52.89
  - dietary counseling and surveillance (for) Z71.3
  - dietetic (*see also* Colitis, allergic)K52.29
  - drug-induced K52.1
  - due to radiation K52.0
  - eosinophilic K52.82
  - food hypersensitivity (*see also* Colitis, allergic)K52.29
  - giardial A07.1
  - granulomatous — *see* Enteritis, regional, large intestine
  - indeterminate, so stated K52.3
  - infectious — *see* Enteritis, infectious
  - ischemic K55.9
    - acute (subacute) (*see also* Ischemia, intestine, acute)K55.039
    - chronic K55.1
    - due to mesenteric artery insufficiency K55.1
    - fulminant (acute) (*see also* Ischemia, intestine, acute)K55.039
  - left sided K51.50
    - with
      - abscess K51.514
      - complication K51.519
        - specified NEC K51.518
      - fistula K51.513
      - obstruction K51.512
      - rectal bleeding K51.511

Colitis — *continued*

  - lymphocytic K52.832
  - membranous
    - psychogenic F54
  - microscopic K52.839
    - specified NEC K52.838
  - mucous — *see* Syndrome, irritable, bowel
    - psychogenic F54
  - noninfective K52.9
    - specified NEC K52.89
  - polyposa — *see* Polyp, colon, inflammatory
  - protozoal A07.9
  - pseudomembranous A04.7
  - pseudomucinous — *see* Syndrome, irritable, bowel
  - regional — *see* Enteritis, regional, large intestine
  - segmental — *see* Enteritis, regional, large intestine
  - septic — *see* Enteritis, infectious
  - spastic K58.9
    - with diarrhea K58.0
    - psychogenic F54
  - staphylococcal A04.8
    - food-borne A05.0
  - subacute ischemic (*see also* Ischemia, intestine, acute)K55.039
  - thromboulcerative (*see also* Ischemia, intestine, acute)K55.039
  - toxic NEC K52.1
    - due to Clostridium difficile A04.7
  - transmural — *see* Enteritis, regional, large intestine
  - trichomonal A07.8
  - tuberculous (ulcerative) A18.32
  - ulcerative (chronic) K51.90
    - with
      - complication K51.919
        - abscess K51.914
        - fistula K51.913
        - obstruction K51.912
        - rectal bleeding K51.911
        - specified complication NEC K51.918
    - enterocolitis — *see* Enterocolitis, ulcerative
    - ileocolitis — *see* Ileocolitis, ulcerative
    - mucosal proctocolitis — *see* Proctocolitis, mucosal
    - proctitis — *see* Proctitis, ulcerative
    - pseudopolyposis — *see* Polyp, colon, inflammatory
    - psychogenic F54
    - rectosigmoiditis — *see* Rectosigmoiditis, ulcerative
    - specified type NEC K51.80
      - with
        - complication K51.819
          - abscess K51.814
          - fistula K51.813
          - obstruction K51.812
          - rectal bleeding K51.811
          - specified complication NEC K51.818
- **Collagenosis,** collagen disease (nonvascular) (vascular) M35.9
  - cardiovascular I42.8
  - reactive perforating L87.1
  - specified NEC M35.8
- **Collapse** R55
  - adrenal E27.2
  - cardiorespiratory R57.0
  - cardiovascular R57.0
    - newborn P29.89
  - circulatory (peripheral) R57.9
    - during or after labor and delivery O75.1
    - following ectopic or molar pregnancy O08.3
    - newborn P29.89
  - during or
    - after labor and delivery O75.1
    - resulting from a procedure, not elsewhere classified T81.10 ☑
  - external ear canal — *see* Stenosis, external ear canal
  - general R55
  - heart — *see* Disease, heart
  - heat T67.1 ☑
  - hysterical F44.89
  - labyrinth, membranous (congenital) Q16.5
  - lung (massive) (*see also* Atelectasis)J98.19
    - pressure due to anesthesia (general) (local) or other sedation T88.2 ☑
      - during labor and delivery O74.1
      - in pregnancy O29.02 ☑
      - postpartum, puerperal O89.09
  - myocardial — *see* Disease, heart

Collapse — *continued*
- nervous F48.8
- neurocirculatory F45.8
- nose M95.0
- postoperative T81.10 ☑
- pulmonary (*see also* Atelectasis)J98.19
  - newborn — *see* Atelectasis
- trachea J39.8
- tracheobronchial J98.09
- valvular — *see* Endocarditis
- vascular (peripheral) R57.9
  - during or after labor and delivery O75.1
  - following ectopic or molar pregnancy O08.3
  - newborn P29.89
- vertebra M48.50 ☑
  - cervical region M48.52 ☑
  - cervicothoracic region M48.53 ☑
  - in (due to)
    - metastasis — *see* Collapse, vertebra, in, specified disease NEC
    - osteoporosis (*see also* Osteoporosis)M80.88 ☑
      - cervical region M80.88 ☑
      - cervicothoracic region M80.88 ☑
      - lumbar region M80.88 ☑
      - lumbosacral region M80.88 ☑
      - multiple sites M80.88 ☑
      - occipito-atlanto-axial region M80.88 ☑
      - sacrococcygeal region M80.88 ☑
      - thoracic region M80.88 ☑
      - thoracolumbar region M80.88 ☑
    - specified disease NEC M48.50 ☑
      - cervical region M48.52 ☑
      - cervicothoracic region M48.53 ☑
      - lumbar region M48.56 ☑
      - lumbosacral region M48.57 ☑
      - occipito-atlanto-axial region M48.51 ☑
      - sacrococcygeal region M48.58 ☑
      - thoracic region M48.54 ☑
      - thoracolumbar region M48.55 ☑
  - lumbar region M48.56 ☑
  - lumbosacral region M48.57 ☑
  - occipito-atlanto-axial region M48.51 ☑
  - sacrococcygeal region M48.58 ☑
  - thoracic region M48.54 ☑
  - thoracolumbar region M48.55 ☑

Collateral (*see also* condition)
- circulation (venous) I87.8
- dilation, veins I87.8

Colles' fracture S52.53 ☑

Collet (-Sicard) syndrome G52.7

Collier's asthma or lung J60

Collodion baby Q80.2

Colloid nodule (of thyroid) (cystic) E04.1

Coloboma (iris) Q13.0
- eyelid Q10.3
- fundus Q14.8
- lens Q12.2
- optic disc (congenital) Q14.2
  - acquired H47.31 ☑

Coloenteritis — *see* Enteritis

Colon — *see* condition

Colonization
- MRSA (Methicillin resistant Staphylococcus aureus) Z22.322
- MSSA (Methicillin susceptible Staphylococcus aureus) Z22.321
- status — *see* Carrier (suspected) of

Coloptosis K63.4

Color blindness — *see* Deficiency, color vision

Colostomy
- attention to Z43.3
- fitting or adjustment Z46.89
- malfunctioning K94.03
- status Z93.3

Colpitis (acute) — *see* Vaginitis

Colpocele N81.5

Colpocystitis — *see* Vaginitis

Colpospasm N94.2

Column, spinal, vertebral — *see* condition

Coma R40.20
- with
  - motor response (none) R40.231 ☑
    - abnormal R40.233 ☑
    - extension R40.232 ☑
    - flexion withdrawal R40.234 ☑
    - localizes pain R40.235 ☑
    - obeys commands R40.236 ☑
  - opening of eyes (never) R40.211 ☑
    - in response to
      - pain R40.212 ☑
      - sound R40.213 ☑

Coma — *continued*
- with — *continued*
  - opening of eyes — *continued*
    - spontaneous R40.214 ☑
  - verbal response (none) R40.221 ☑
    - confused conversation R40.224 ☑
    - inappropriate words R40.223 ☑
    - incomprehensible words R40.222 ☑
    - oriented R40.225 ☑
- eclamptic — *see* Eclampsia
- epileptic — *see* Epilepsy
- Glasgow, scale score — *see* Glasgow coma scale
- hepatic — *see* Failure, hepatic, by type, with coma
- hyperglycemic (diabetic) — *see* Diabetes, by type, with hyperosmolarity, with coma
- hyperosmolar (diabetic) — *see* Diabetes, by type, with hyperosmolarity, with coma
- hypoglycemic (diabetic) — *see* Diabetes, by type, with hypoglycemia, with coma
  - nondiabetic E15
- in diabetes — *see* Diabetes, coma
- insulin-induced — *see* Coma, hypoglycemic
- myxedematous E03.5
- newborn P91.5
- persistent vegetative state R40.3
- specified NEC, without documented Glasgow coma scale score, or with partial Glasgow coma scale score reported R40.244 ☑

Comatose — *see* Coma

Combat fatigue F43.0

Combined — *see* condition

Comedo, comedones (giant) L70.0

Comedocarcinoma (*see also* Neoplasm, breast, malignant)
- noninfiltrating
  - breast D05.8 ☑
  - specified site — *see* Neoplasm, in situ, by site
  - unspecified site D05.8 ☑

Comedomastitis — *see* Ectasia, mammary duct

Comminuted fracture - code as Fracture, closed

Common
- arterial trunk Q20.0
- atrioventricular canal Q21.2
- atrium Q21.1
- cold (head) J00
- truncus (arteriosus) Q20.0
- variable immunodeficiency — *see* Immunodeficiency, common variable
- ventricle Q20.4

Commotio, commotion (current)
- brain — *see* Injury, intracranial, concussion
- cerebri — *see* Injury, intracranial, concussion
- retinae S05.8X ☑
- spinal cord — *see* Injury, spinal cord, by region
- spinalis — *see* Injury, spinal cord, by region

Communication
- between
  - base of aorta and pulmonary artery Q21.4
  - left ventricle and right atrium Q20.5
  - pericardial sac and pleural sac Q34.8
  - pulmonary artery and pulmonary vein, congenital Q25.72
- congenital between uterus and digestive or urinary tract Q51.7

Compartment syndrome (deep) (posterior) (traumatic) T79.A0 ☑
- abdomen T79.A3 ☑
- lower extremity (hip, buttock, thigh, leg, foot, toes) T79.A2 ☑
- nontraumatic
  - abdomen M79.A3
  - lower extremity (hip, buttock, thigh, leg, foot, toes) M79.A2 ☑
  - specified site NEC M79.A9
  - upper extremity (shoulder, arm, forearm, wrist, hand, fingers) M79.A1 ☑
- specified site NEC T79.A9 ☑
- upper extremity (shoulder, arm, forearm, wrist, hand, fingers) T79.A1 ☑

Compensation
- failure — *see* Disease, heart
- neurosis, psychoneurosis — *see* Disorder, factitious

Complaint (*see also* Disease)
- bowel, functional K59.9
  - psychogenic F45.8
- intestine, functional K59.9
  - psychogenic F45.8
- kidney — *see* Disease, renal
- miners' J60

Complete — *see* condition

Complex
- Addison-Schilder E71.528

Complex — *continued*
- cardiorenal — *see* Hypertension, cardiorenal
- Costen's M26.69
- disseminated mycobacterium avium-intracellulare (DMAC) A31.2
- Eisenmenger's (ventricular septal defect) I27.89
- hypersexual F52.8
- jumped process, spine — *see* Dislocation, vertebra
- primary, tuberculous A15.7
- Schilder-Addison E71.528
- subluxation (vertebral) M99.19
  - abdomen M99.19
  - acromioclavicular M99.17
  - cervical region M99.11
  - cervicothoracic M99.11
  - costochondral M99.18
  - costovertebral M99.18
  - head region M99.10
  - hip M99.15
  - lower extremity M99.16
  - lumbar region M99.13
  - lumbosacral M99.13
  - occipitocervical M99.10
  - pelvic region M99.15
  - pubic M99.15
  - rib cage M99.18
  - sacral region M99.14
  - sacrococcygeal M99.14
  - sacroiliac M99.14
  - specified NEC M99.19
  - sternochondral M99.18
  - sternoclavicular M99.17
  - thoracic region M99.12
  - thoracolumbar M99.12
  - upper extremity M99.17
- Taussig-Bing (transposition, aorta and overriding pulmonary artery) Q20.1

Complication (s) (from) (of)
- accidental puncture or laceration during a procedure (of) — *see* Complications, intraoperative (intraprocedural), puncture or laceration
- amputation stump (surgical) (late) NEC T87.9
  - dehiscence T87.81
  - infection or inflammation T87.40
    - lower limb T87.4 ☑
    - upper limb T87.4 ☑
  - necrosis T87.50
    - lower limb T87.5 ☑
    - upper limb T87.5 ☑
  - neuroma T87.30
    - lower limb T87.3 ☑
    - upper limb T87.3 ☑
  - specified type NEC T87.89
- anastomosis (and bypass) (*see also* Complications, prosthetic device or implant)
  - intestinal (internal) NEC K91.89
    - involving urinary tract N99.89
  - urinary tract (involving intestinal tract) N99.89
  - vascular — *see* Complications, cardiovascular device or implant
- anesthesia, anesthetic (*see also* Anesthesia, complication)T88.59 ☑
  - brain, postpartum, puerperal O89.2
  - cardiac
    - in
      - labor and delivery O74.2
      - pregnancy O29.19 ☑
    - postpartum, puerperal O89.1
  - central nervous system
    - in
      - labor and delivery O74.3
      - pregnancy O29.29 ☑
    - postpartum, puerperal O89.2
  - difficult or failed intubation T88.4 ☑
    - in pregnancy O29.6 ☑
  - failed sedation (conscious) (moderate) during procedure T88.52 ☑
  - general, unintended awareness during procedure T88.53 ☑
  - hyperthermia, malignant T88.3 ☑
  - hypothermia T88.51 ☑
  - intubation failure T88.4 ☑
  - malignant hyperthermia T88.3 ☑
  - pulmonary
    - in
      - labor and delivery O74.1
      - pregnancy NEC O29.09 ☑
    - postpartum, puerperal O89.09
  - shock T88.2 ☑
  - spinal and epidural

Complication — *continued*
- anesthesia, anesthetic — *continued*
  - in
    - labor and delivery NEC O74.6
      - headache O74.5
    - pregnancy NEC O29.5X ☑
    - postpartum, puerperal NEC O89.5
      - headache O89.4
  - unintended awareness under general anesthesia during procedure T88.53 ☑
- anti-reflux device — *see* Complications, esophageal anti-reflux device
- aortic (bifurcation) graft — *see* Complications, graft, vascular
- aortocoronary (bypass) graft — *see* Complications, coronary artery (bypass) graft
- aortofemoral (bypass) graft — *see* Complications, extremity artery (bypass) graft
- arteriovenous
  - fistula, surgically created T82.9 ☑
    - embolism T82.818 ☑
    - fibrosis T82.828 ☑
    - hemorrhage T82.838 ☑
    - infection or inflammation T82.7 ☑
    - mechanical
      - breakdown T82.510 ☑
      - displacement T82.520 ☑
      - leakage T82.530 ☑
      - malposition T82.520 ☑
      - obstruction T82.590 ☑
      - perforation T82.590 ☑
      - protrusion T82.590 ☑
    - pain T82.848 ☑
    - specified type NEC T82.898 ☑
    - stenosis T82.858 ☑
    - thrombosis T82.868 ☑
  - shunt, surgically created T82.9 ☑
    - embolism T82.818 ☑
    - fibrosis T82.828 ☑
    - hemorrhage T82.838 ☑
    - infection or inflammation T82.7 ☑
    - mechanical
      - breakdown T82.511 ☑
      - displacement T82.521 ☑
      - leakage T82.531 ☑
      - malposition T82.521 ☑
      - obstruction T82.591 ☑
      - perforation T82.591 ☑
      - protrusion T82.591 ☑
    - pain T82.848 ☑
    - specified type NEC T82.898 ☑
    - stenosis T82.858 ☑
    - thrombosis T82.868 ☑
- arthroplasty — *see* Complications, joint prosthesis
- artificial
  - fertilization or insemination N98.9
    - attempted introduction (of)
      - embryo in embryo transfer N98.3
      - ovum following in vitro fertilization N98.2
    - hyperstimulation of ovaries N98.1
    - infection N98.0
    - specified NEC N98.8
  - heart T82.9 ☑
    - embolism T82.817 ☑
    - fibrosis T82.827 ☑
    - hemorrhage T82.837 ☑
    - infection or inflammation T82.7 ☑
    - mechanical
      - breakdown T82.512 ☑
      - displacement T82.522 ☑
      - leakage T82.532 ☑
      - malposition T82.522 ☑
      - obstruction T82.592 ☑
      - perforation T82.592 ☑
      - protrusion T82.592 ☑
    - pain T82.847 ☑
    - specified type NEC T82.897 ☑
    - stenosis T82.857 ☑
    - thrombosis T82.867 ☑
  - opening
    - cecostomy — *see* Complications, colostomy
    - colostomy — *see* Complications, colostomy
    - cystostomy — *see* Complications, cystostomy
    - enterostomy — *see* Complications, enterostomy
    - gastrostomy — *see* Complications, gastrostomy
    - ileostomy — *see* Complications, enterostomy
    - jejunostomy — *see* Complications, enterostomy

Complication — *continued*
- artificial — *continued*
    - nephrostomy — *see* Complications, stoma, urinary tract
    - tracheostomy — *see* Complications, tracheostomy
    - ureterostomy — *see* Complications, stoma, urinary tract
    - urethrostomy — *see* Complications, stoma, urinary tract
- balloon implant or device
  - gastrointestinal T85.9 ☑
    - embolism T85.818 ☑
    - fibrosis T85.828 ☑
    - hemorrhage T85.838 ☑
    - infection and inflammation T85.79 ☑
    - pain T85.848 ☑
    - specified type NEC T85.898 ☑
    - stenosis T85.858 ☑
    - thrombosis T85.868 ☑
  - vascular (counterpulsation) T82.9 ☑
    - embolism T82.818 ☑
    - fibrosis T82.828 ☑
    - hemorrhage T82.838 ☑
    - infection or inflammation T82.7 ☑
    - mechanical
      - breakdown T82.513 ☑
      - displacement T82.523 ☑
      - leakage T82.533 ☑
      - malposition T82.523 ☑
      - obstruction T82.593 ☑
      - perforation T82.593 ☑
      - protrusion T82.593 ☑
    - pain T82.848 ☑
    - specified type NEC T82.898 ☑
    - stenosis T82.858 ☑
    - thrombosis T82.868 ☑
- bariatric procedure
  - gastric band procedure K95.09
    - infection K95.01
  - specified procedure NEC K95.89
    - infection K95.81
- bile duct implant (prosthetic) T85.9 ☑
  - embolism T85.818 ☑
  - fibrosis T85.828 ☑
  - hemorrhage T85.838 ☑
  - infection and inflammation T85.79 ☑
  - mechanical
    - breakdown T85.510 ☑
    - displacement T85.520 ☑
    - malfunction T85.510 ☑
    - malposition T85.520 ☑
    - obstruction T85.590 ☑
    - perforation T85.590 ☑
    - protrusion T85.590 ☑
    - specified NEC T85.590 ☑
  - pain T85.848 ☑
  - specified type NEC T85.898 ☑
  - stenosis T85.858 ☑
  - thrombosis T85.868 ☑
- bladder device (auxiliary) — *see* Complications, genitourinary, device or implant, urinary system
- bleeding (postoperative) — *see* Complication, postoperative, hemorrhage
  - intraoperative — *see* Complication, intraoperative, hemorrhage
- blood vessel graft — *see* Complications, graft, vascular
- bone
  - device NEC T84.9 ☑
    - embolism T84.81 ☑
    - fibrosis T84.82 ☑
    - hemorrhage T84.83 ☑
    - infection or inflammation T84.7 ☑
    - mechanical
      - breakdown T84.318 ☑
      - displacement T84.328 ☑
      - malposition T84.328 ☑
      - obstruction T84.398 ☑
      - perforation T84.398 ☑
      - protrusion T84.398 ☑
    - pain T84.84 ☑
    - specified type NEC T84.89 ☑
    - stenosis T84.85 ☑
    - thrombosis T84.86 ☑
  - graft — *see* Complications, graft, bone
  - growth stimulator (electrode) — *see* Complications, electronic stimulator device, bone
  - marrow transplant — *see* Complications, transplant, bone, marrow

Complication — *continued*
- brain neurostimulator (electrode) — *see* Complications, electronic stimulator device, brain
- breast implant (prosthetic) T85.9 ☑
  - capsular contracture T85.44 ☑
  - embolism T85.818 ☑
  - fibrosis T85.828 ☑
  - hemorrhage T85.838 ☑
  - infection and inflammation T85.79 ☑
  - mechanical
    - breakdown T85.41 ☑
    - displacement T85.42 ☑
    - leakage T85.43 ☑
    - malposition T85.42 ☑
    - obstruction T85.49 ☑
    - perforation T85.49 ☑
    - protrusion T85.49 ☑
    - specified NEC T85.49 ☑
  - pain T85.848 ☑
  - specified type NEC T85.898 ☑
  - stenosis T85.858 ☑
  - thrombosis T85.868 ☑
- bypass (*see also* Complications, prosthetic device or implant)
  - aortocoronary — *see* Complications, coronary artery (bypass) graft
  - arterial (*see also* Complications, graft, vascular)
    - extremity — *see* Complications, extremity artery (bypass) graft
- cardiac (*see also* Disease, heart)
  - device, implant or graft T82.9 ☑
    - embolism T82.817 ☑
    - fibrosis T82.827 ☑
    - hemorrhage T82.837 ☑
    - infection or inflammation T82.7 ☑
      - valve prosthesis T82.6 ☑
    - mechanical
      - breakdown T82.519 ☑
        - specified device NEC T82.518 ☑
      - displacement T82.529 ☑
        - specified device NEC T82.528 ☑
      - leakage T82.539 ☑
        - specified device NEC T82.538 ☑
      - malposition T82.529 ☑
        - specified device NEC T82.528 ☑
      - obstruction T82.599 ☑
        - specified device NEC T82.598 ☑
      - perforation T82.599 ☑
        - specified device NEC T82.598 ☑
      - protrusion T82.599 ☑
        - specified device NEC T82.598 ☑
    - pain T82.847 ☑
    - specified type NEC T82.897 ☑
    - stenosis T82.857 ☑
    - thrombosis T82.867 ☑
- cardiovascular device, graft or implant T82.9 ☑
  - aortic graft — *see* Complications, graft, vascular
  - arteriovenous
    - fistula, artificial — *see* Complication, arteriovenous, fistula, surgically created
    - shunt — *see* Complication, arteriovenous, shunt, surgically created
  - artificial heart — *see* Complication, artificial, heart
  - balloon (counterpulsation) device — *see* Complication, balloon implant, vascular
  - carotid artery graft — *see* Complications, graft, vascular
  - coronary bypass graft — *see* Complication, coronary artery (bypass) graft
  - dialysis catheter (vascular) — *see* Complication, catheter, dialysis
  - electronic T82.9 ☑
    - electrode T82.9 ☑
      - embolism T82.817 ☑
      - fibrosis T82.827 ☑
      - hemorrhage T82.837 ☑
      - infection T82.7 ☑
      - mechanical
        - breakdown T82.110 ☑
        - displacement T82.120 ☑
        - leakage T82.190 ☑
        - obstruction T82.190 ☑
        - perforation T82.190 ☑
        - protrusion T82.190 ☑
        - specified type NEC T82.190 ☑
      - pain T82.847 ☑
      - specified NEC T82.897 ☑
      - stenosis T82.857 ☑
      - thrombosis T82.867 ☑
    - embolism T82.817 ☑

Complication — *continued*
- cardiovascular device — *continued*
  - fibrosis T82.827 ☑
  - hemorrhage T82.837 ☑
  - infection T82.7 ☑
  - mechanical
    - breakdown T82.119 ☑
    - displacement T82.129 ☑
    - leakage T82.199 ☑
    - obstruction T82.199 ☑
    - perforation T82.199 ☑
    - protrusion T82.199 ☑
    - specified type NEC T82.199 ☑
  - pain T82.847 ☑
  - pulse generator T82.9 ☑
    - embolism T82.817 ☑
    - fibrosis T82.827 ☑
    - hemorrhage T82.837 ☑
    - infection T82.7 ☑
    - mechanical
      - breakdown T82.111 ☑
      - displacement T82.121 ☑
      - leakage T82.191 ☑
      - obstruction T82.191 ☑
      - perforation T82.191 ☑
      - protrusion T82.191 ☑
      - specified type NEC T82.191 ☑
    - pain T82.847 ☑
    - specified NEC T82.897 ☑
    - stenosis T82.857 ☑
    - thrombosis T82.867 ☑
  - specified condition NEC T82.897 ☑
  - specified device NEC T82.9 ☑
    - embolism T82.817 ☑
    - fibrosis T82.827 ☑
    - hemorrhage T82.837 ☑
    - infection T82.7 ☑
    - mechanical
      - breakdown T82.118 ☑
      - displacement T82.128 ☑
      - leakage T82.198 ☑
      - obstruction T82.198 ☑
      - perforation T82.198 ☑
      - protrusion T82.198 ☑
      - specified type NEC T82.198 ☑
    - pain T82.847 ☑
    - specified NEC T82.897 ☑
    - stenosis T82.857 ☑
    - thrombosis T82.867 ☑
  - stenosis T82.857 ☑
  - thrombosis T82.867 ☑
  - extremity artery graft — *see* Complication, extremity artery (bypass) graft
  - femoral artery graft — *see* Complication, extremity artery (bypass) graft
  - heart-lung transplant — *see* Complication, transplant, heart, with lung
  - heart
    - transplant — *see* Complication, transplant, heart
    - valve — *see* Complication, prosthetic device, heart valve
      - graft — *see* Complication, heart, valve, graft
  - infection or inflammation T82.7 ☑
  - umbrella device — *see* Complication, umbrella device, vascular
  - vascular graft (or anastomosis) — *see* Complication, graft, vascular
- carotid artery (bypass) graft — *see* Complications, graft, vascular
- catheter (device) NEC (*see also* Complications, prosthetic device or implant)
  - cranial infusion
    - infection and inflammation T85.735 ☑
    - mechanical
      - breakdown T85.610 ☑
      - displacement T85.620 ☑
      - leakage T85.630 ☑
      - malfunction T85.690 ☑
      - malposition T85.620 ☑
      - obstruction T85.690 ☑
      - perforation T85.690 ☑
      - protrusion T85.690 ☑
      - specified NEC T85.690 ☑
  - cystostomy T83.9 ☑
    - embolism T83.81 ☑
    - fibrosis T83.82 ☑
    - hemorrhage T83.83 ☑
    - infection and inflammation T83.510 ☑
    - mechanical
      - breakdown T83.010 ☑

Complication — *continued*
- catheter — *continued*
      - displacement T83.020 ☑
      - leakage T83.030 ☑
      - malposition T83.020 ☑
      - obstruction T83.090 ☑
      - perforation T83.090 ☑
      - protrusion T83.090 ☑
      - specified NEC T83.090 ☑
    - pain T83.84 ☑
    - specified type NEC T83.89 ☑
    - stenosis T83.85 ☑
    - thrombosis T83.86 ☑
  - dialysis (vascular) T82.9 ☑
    - embolism T82.818 ☑
    - fibrosis T82.828 ☑
    - hemorrhage T82.838 ☑
    - infection and inflammation T82.7 ☑
    - intraperitoneal — *see* Complications, catheter, intraperitoneal
    - mechanical
      - breakdown T82.41 ☑
      - displacement T82.42 ☑
      - leakage T82.43 ☑
      - malposition T82.42 ☑
      - obstruction T82.49 ☑
      - perforation T82.49 ☑
      - protrusion T82.49 ☑
    - pain T82.848 ☑
    - specified type NEC T82.898 ☑
    - stenosis T82.858 ☑
    - thrombosis T82.868 ☑
  - epidural infusion T85.9 ☑
    - embolism T85.810 ☑
    - fibrosis T85.820 ☑
    - hemorrhage T85.830 ☑
    - infection and inflammation T85.735 ☑
    - mechanical
      - breakdown T85.610 ☑
      - displacement T85.620 ☑
      - leakage T85.630 ☑
      - malfunction T85.610 ☑
      - malposition T85.620 ☑
      - obstruction T85.690 ☑
      - perforation T85.690 ☑
      - protrusion T85.690 ☑
      - specified NEC T85.690 ☑
    - pain T85.840 ☑
    - specified type NEC T85.890 ☑
    - stenosis T85.850 ☑
    - thrombosis T85.860 ☑
  - intraperitoneal dialysis T85.9 ☑
    - embolism T85.818 ☑
    - fibrosis T85.828 ☑
    - hemorrhage T85.838 ☑
    - infection and inflammation T85.71 ☑
    - mechanical
      - breakdown T85.611 ☑
      - displacement T85.621 ☑
      - leakage T85.631 ☑
      - malfunction T85.611 ☑
      - malposition T85.621 ☑
      - obstruction T85.691 ☑
      - perforation T85.691 ☑
      - protrusion T85.691 ☑
      - specified NEC T85.691 ☑
    - pain T85.848 ☑
    - specified type NEC T85.898 ☑
    - stenosis T85.858 ☑
    - thrombosis T85.868 ☑
  - intrathecal infusion
    - infection and inflammation T85.735 ☑
    - mechanical
      - breakdown T85.610 ☑
      - displacement T85.620 ☑
      - leakage T85.630 ☑
      - malfunction T85.690 ☑
      - malposition T85.620 ☑
      - obstruction T85.690 ☑
      - perforation T85.690 ☑
      - protrusion T85.690 ☑
      - specified NEC T85.690 ☑
  - intravenous infusion T82.9 ☑
    - embolism T82.818 ☑
    - fibrosis T82.828 ☑
    - hemorrhage T82.838 ☑
    - infection or inflammation T82.7 ☑
    - mechanical
      - breakdown T82.514 ☑
      - displacement T82.524 ☑
      - leakage T82.534 ☑
      - malposition T82.524 ☑

Complication — *continued*
- catheter — *continued*
      - obstruction T82.594 ☑
      - perforation T82.594 ☑
      - protrusion T82.594 ☑
    - pain T82.848 ☑
    - specified type NEC T82.898 ☑
    - stenosis T82.858 ☑
    - thrombosis T82.868 ☑
  - spinal infusion
    - infection and inflammation T85.735 ☑
    - mechanical
      - breakdown T85.610 ☑
      - displacement T85.620 ☑
      - leakage T85.630 ☑
      - malfunction T85.690 ☑
      - malposition T85.620 ☑
      - obstruction T85.690 ☑
      - perforation T85.690 ☑
      - protrusion T85.690 ☑
      - specified NEC T85.690 ☑
  - subarachnoid infusion
    - infection and inflammation T85.735 ☑
    - mechanical
      - breakdown T85.610 ☑
      - displacement T85.620 ☑
      - leakage T85.630 ☑
      - malfunction T85.690 ☑
      - malposition T85.620 ☑
      - obstruction T85.690 ☑
      - perforation T85.690 ☑
      - protrusion T85.690 ☑
      - specified NEC T85.690 ☑
  - subdural infusion T85.9 ☑
    - embolism T85.810 ☑
    - fibrosis T85.820 ☑
    - hemorrhage T85.830 ☑
    - infection and inflammation T85.735 ☑
    - mechanical
      - breakdown T85.610 ☑
      - displacement T85.620 ☑
      - leakage T85.630 ☑
      - malfunction T85.610 ☑
      - malposition T85.620 ☑
      - obstruction T85.690 ☑
      - perforation T85.690 ☑
      - protrusion T85.690 ☑
      - specified NEC T85.690 ☑
    - pain T85.840 ☑
    - specified type NEC T85.890 ☑
    - stenosis T85.850 ☑
    - thrombosis T85.860 ☑
  - urethral T83.9 ☑
    - displacement T83.028 ☑
    - embolism T83.81 ☑
    - fibrosis T83.82 ☑
    - hemorrhage T83.83 ☑
    - indwelling
      - breakdown T83.011 ☑
      - displacement T83.021 ☑
      - infection and inflammation T83.511 ☑
      - leakage T83.031 ☑
      - specified complication NEC T83.091 ☑
    - infection and inflammation T83.511 ☑
    - leakage T83.038 ☑
    - malposition T83.028 ☑
    - mechanical
      - breakdown T83.011 ☑
    - obstruction (mechanical) T83.091 ☑
    - pain T83.84 ☑
    - perforation T83.091 ☑
    - protrusion T83.091 ☑
    - specified type NEC T83.091 ☑
    - stenosis T83.85 ☑
    - thrombosis T83.86 ☑
  - urinary NEC
    - breakdown T83.018 ☑
    - displacement T83.028 ☑
    - infection and inflammation T83.518 ☑
    - leakage T83.038 ☑
    - specified complication NEC T83.098 ☑
- cecostomy (stoma) — *see* Complications, colostomy
- cesarean delivery wound NEC O90.89
  - disruption O90.0
  - hematoma O90.2
  - infection (following delivery) O86.0
- chemotherapy (antineoplastic) NEC T88.7 ☑
- chin implant (prosthetic) — *see* Complication, prosthetic device or implant, specified NEC
- circulatory system I99.8
  - intraoperative I97.88

- **Complication** — *continued*
  - circulatory system — *continued*
    - postprocedural I97.89
      - following cardiac surgery I97.19 ☑
        - postcardiotomy syndrome I97.0
      - hypertension I97.3
      - lymphedema after mastectomy I97.2
      - postcardiotomy syndrome I97.0
      - specified NEC I97.89
  - colostomy (stoma) K94.00
    - hemorrhage K94.01
    - infection K94.02
    - malfunction K94.03
    - mechanical K94.03
    - specified complication NEC K94.09
  - contraceptive device, intrauterine — *see* Complications, intrauterine, contraceptive device
  - cord (umbilical) — *see* Complications, umbilical cord
  - corneal graft — *see* Complications, graft, cornea
  - coronary artery (bypass) graft T82.9 ☑
    - atherosclerosis — *see* Arteriosclerosis, coronary (artery),
    - embolism T82.818 ☑
    - fibrosis T82.828 ☑
    - hemorrhage T82.838 ☑
    - infection and inflammation T82.7 ☑
    - mechanical
      - breakdown T82.211 ☑
      - displacement T82.212 ☑
      - leakage T82.213 ☑
      - malposition T82.212 ☑
      - obstruction T82.218 ☑
      - perforation T82.218 ☑
      - protrusion T82.218 ☑
      - specified NEC T82.218 ☑
    - pain T82.848 ☑
    - specified type NEC T82.898 ☑
    - stenosis T82.858 ☑
    - thrombosis T82.868 ☑
  - counterpulsation device (balloon), intra- aortic — *see* Complications, balloon implant, vascular
  - cystostomy (stoma) N99.518
    - catheter — *see* Complications, catheter, cystostomy
    - hemorrhage N99.510
    - infection N99.511
    - malfunction N99.512
    - specified type NEC N99.518
  - delivery (*see also* Complications, obstetric)O75.9
    - procedure (instrumental) (manual) (surgical) O75.4
    - specified NEC O75.89
  - dialysis (peritoneal) (renal) (*see also* Complications, infusion)
    - catheter (vascular) — *see* Complication, catheter, dialysis
      - peritoneal, intraperitoneal — *see* Complications, catheter, intraperitoneal
  - dorsal column (spinal) neurostimulator — *see* Complications, electronic stimulator device, spinal cord
  - drug NEC T88.7 ☑
  - ear procedure (*see also* Disorder, ear)
    - intraoperative H95.88
      - hematoma — *see* Complications, intraoperative, hemorrhage (hematoma) (of), ear
      - hemorrhage — *see* Complications, intraoperative, hemorrhage (hematoma) (of), ear
      - laceration — *see* Complications, intraoperative, puncture or laceration..., ear
      - specified NEC H95.88
    - postoperative H95.89
      - external ear canal stenosis H95.81 ☑
      - hematoma — *see* Complications, postprocedural, hematoma (of), ear
      - hemorrhage — *see* Complications, postprocedural, hemorrhage (of), ear
      - postmastoidectomy — *see* Complications, postmastoidectomy
      - seroma — *see* Complications, postprocedural, seroma (of), mastoid process
      - specified NEC H95.89
  - ectopic pregnancy O08.9
    - damage to pelvic organs O08.6
    - embolism O08.2
    - genital infection O08.0
    - hemorrhage (delayed) (excessive) O08.1

- **Complication** — *continued*
  - ectopic pregnancy — *continued*
    - metabolic disorder O08.5
    - renal failure O08.4
    - shock O08.3
    - specified type NEC O08.0
    - venous complication NEC O08.7
  - electronic stimulator device
    - bladder (urinary) — *see* Complications, electronic stimulator device, urinary
    - bone T84.9 ☑
      - breakdown T84.310 ☑
      - displacement T84.320 ☑
      - embolism T84.81 ☑
      - fibrosis T84.82 ☑
      - hemorrhage T84.83 ☑
      - infection or inflammation T84.7 ☑
      - malfunction T84.310 ☑
      - malposition T84.320 ☑
      - mechanical NEC T84.390 ☑
      - obstruction T84.390 ☑
      - pain T84.84 ☑
      - perforation T84.390 ☑
      - protrusion T84.390 ☑
      - specified type NEC T84.89 ☑
      - stenosis T84.85 ☑
      - thrombosis T84.86 ☑
    - brain T85.9 ☑
      - embolism T85.810 ☑
      - fibrosis T85.820 ☑
      - hemorrhage T85.830 ☑
      - infection and inflammation T85.731 ☑
      - mechanical
        - breakdown T85.110 ☑
        - displacement T85.120 ☑
        - leakage T85.190 ☑
        - malposition T85.120 ☑
        - obstruction T85.190 ☑
        - perforation T85.190 ☑
        - protrusion T85.190 ☑
        - specified NEC T85.190 ☑
      - pain T85.840 ☑
      - specified type NEC T85.890 ☑
      - stenosis T85.850 ☑
      - thrombosis T85.860 ☑
    - cardiac (defibrillator) (pacemaker) — *see* Complications, cardiovascular device or implant, electronic
    - generator (brain) (gastric) (peripheral) (sacral) (spinal)
      - breakdown T85.113 ☑
      - displacement T85.123 ☑
      - leakage T85.193 ☑
      - malposition T85.123 ☑
      - obstruction T85.193 ☑
      - perforation T85.193 ☑
      - protrusion T85.193 ☑
      - specified type NEC T85.193 ☑
    - muscle T84.9 ☑
      - breakdown T84.418 ☑
      - displacement T84.428 ☑
      - embolism T84.81 ☑
      - fibrosis T84.82 ☑
      - hemorrhage T84.83 ☑
      - infection or inflammation T84.7 ☑
      - mechanical NEC T84.498 ☑
      - pain T84.84 ☑
      - specified type NEC T84.89 ☑
      - stenosis T84.85 ☑
      - thrombosis T84.86 ☑
    - nervous system T85.9 ☑
      - brain — *see* Complications, electronic stimulator device, brain
      - cranial nerve — *see* Complications, electronic stimulator device, peripheral nerve
      - embolism T85.810 ☑
      - fibrosis T85.820 ☑
      - gastric nerve — *see* Complications, electronic stimulator device, peripheral nerve
      - hemorrhage T85.830 ☑
      - infection and inflammation T85.738 ☑
      - mechanical
        - breakdown T85.118 ☑
        - displacement T85.128 ☑
        - leakage T85.199 ☑
        - malposition T85.128 ☑
        - obstruction T85.199 ☑
        - perforation T85.199 ☑
        - protrusion T85.199 ☑
        - specified NEC T85.199 ☑
      - pain T85.840 ☑

- **Complication** — *continued*
  - electronic stimulator device — *continued*
      - peripheral nerve — *see* Complications, electronic stimulator device, peripheral nerve
      - sacral nerve — *see* Complications, electronic stimulator device, peripheral nerve
      - specified type NEC T85.890 ☑
      - spinal cord — *see* Complications, electronic stimulator device, spinal cord
      - stenosis T85.850 ☑
      - thrombosis T85.860 ☑
      - vagal nerve — *see* Complications, electronic stimulator device, peripheral nerve
    - peripheral nerve T85.9 ☑
      - embolism T85.810 ☑
      - fibrosis T85.820 ☑
      - hemorrhage T85.830 ☑
      - infection and inflammation T85.732 ☑
      - mechanical
        - breakdown T85.111 ☑
        - displacement T85.121 ☑
        - leakage T85.191 ☑
        - malposition T85.121 ☑
        - obstruction T85.191 ☑
        - perforation T85.191 ☑
        - protrusion T85.191 ☑
        - specified NEC T85.191 ☑
      - pain T85.840 ☑
      - specified type NEC T85.890 ☑
      - stenosis T85.850 ☑
      - thrombosis T85.860 ☑
    - spinal cord T85.9 ☑
      - embolism T85.810 ☑
      - fibrosis T85.820 ☑
      - hemorrhage T85.830 ☑
      - infection and inflammation T85.733 ☑
      - mechanical
        - breakdown T85.112 ☑
        - displacement T85.122 ☑
        - leakage T85.192 ☑
        - malposition T85.122 ☑
        - obstruction T85.192 ☑
        - perforation T85.192 ☑
        - protrusion T85.192 ☑
        - specified NEC T85.192 ☑
      - pain T85.840 ☑
      - specified type NEC T85.890 ☑
      - stenosis T85.850 ☑
      - thrombosis T85.860 ☑
    - urinary T83.9 ☑
      - embolism T83.81 ☑
      - fibrosis T83.82 ☑
      - hemorrhage T83.83 ☑
      - infection and inflammation T83.598 ☑
      - mechanical
        - breakdown T83.110 ☑
        - displacement T83.120 ☑
        - malposition T83.120 ☑
        - perforation T83.190 ☑
        - protrusion T83.190 ☑
        - specified NEC T83.190 ☑
      - pain T83.84 ☑
      - specified type NEC T83.89 ☑
      - stenosis T83.85 ☑
      - thrombosis T83.86 ☑
  - electroshock therapy T88.9 ☑
    - specified NEC T88.8 ☑
  - endocrine E34.9
    - postprocedural
      - adrenal hypofunction E89.6
      - hypoinsulinemia E89.1
      - hypoparathyroidism E89.2
      - hypopituitarism E89.3
      - hypothyroidism E89.0
      - ovarian failure E89.40
        - asymptomatic E89.40
        - symptomatic E89.41
      - specified NEC E89.89
      - testicular hypofunction E89.5
  - endodontic treatment NEC M27.59
  - enterostomy (stoma) K94.10
    - hemorrhage K94.11
    - infection K94.12
    - malfunction K94.13
    - mechanical K94.13
    - specified complication NEC K94.19
  - episiotomy, disruption O90.1
  - esophageal anti-reflux device T85.9 ☑
    - embolism T85.818 ☑
    - fibrosis T85.828 ☑
    - hemorrhage T85.838 ☑

- **Complication** — *continued*
  - esophageal anti-reflux device — *continued*
    - infection and inflammation T85.79 ☑
    - mechanical
      - breakdown T85.511 ☑
      - displacement T85.521 ☑
      - malfunction T85.511 ☑
      - malposition T85.521 ☑
      - obstruction T85.591 ☑
      - perforation T85.591 ☑
      - protrusion T85.591 ☑
      - specified NEC T85.591 ☑
    - pain T85.848 ☑
    - specified type NEC T85.898 ☑
    - stenosis T85.858 ☑
    - thrombosis T85.868 ☑
  - esophagostomy K94.30
    - hemorrhage K94.31
    - infection K94.32
    - malfunction K94.33
    - mechanical K94.33
    - specified complication NEC K94.39
  - extracorporeal circulation T80.90 ☑
  - extremity artery (bypass) graft T82.9 ☑
    - arteriosclerosis — *see* Arteriosclerosis, extremities, bypass graft
    - embolism T82.818 ☑
    - fibrosis T82.828 ☑
    - hemorrhage T82.838 ☑
    - infection and inflammation T82.7 ☑
    - mechanical
      - breakdown T82.318 ☑
        - femoral artery T82.312 ☑
      - displacement T82.328 ☑
        - femoral artery T82.322 ☑
      - leakage T82.338 ☑
        - femoral artery T82.332 ☑
      - malposition T82.328 ☑
        - femoral artery T82.322 ☑
      - obstruction T82.398 ☑
        - femoral artery T82.392 ☑
      - perforation T82.398 ☑
        - femoral artery T82.392 ☑
      - protrusion T82.398 ☑
        - femoral artery T82.392 ☑
    - pain T82.848 ☑
    - specified type NEC T82.898 ☑
    - stenosis T82.858 ☑
    - thrombosis T82.868 ☑
  - eye H57.9
    - corneal graft — *see* Complications, graft, cornea
    - implant (prosthetic) T85.9 ☑
      - embolism T85.818 ☑
      - fibrosis T85.828 ☑
      - hemorrhage T85.838 ☑
      - infection and inflammation T85.79 ☑
      - mechanical
        - breakdown T85.318 ☑
        - displacement T85.328 ☑
        - leakage T85.398 ☑
        - malposition T85.328 ☑
        - obstruction T85.398 ☑
        - perforation T85.398 ☑
        - protrusion T85.398 ☑
        - specified NEC T85.398 ☑
      - pain T85.848 ☑
      - specified type NEC T85.898 ☑
      - stenosis T85.858 ☑
      - thrombosis T85.868 ☑
    - intraocular lens — *see* Complications, intraocular lens
    - orbital prosthesis — *see* Complications, orbital prosthesis
  - female genital N94.9
    - device, implant or graft NEC — *see* Complications, genitourinary, device or implant, genital tract
  - femoral artery (bypass) graft — *see* Complication, extremity artery (bypass) graft
  - fixation device, internal (orthopedic) T84.9 ☑
    - infection and inflammation T84.60 ☑
      - arm T84.61 ☑
        - humerus T84.61 ☑
        - radius T84.61 ☑
        - ulna T84.61 ☑
      - leg T84.629 ☑
        - femur T84.62 ☑
        - fibula T84.62 ☑
        - tibia T84.62 ☑
      - specified site NEC T84.69 ☑
      - spine T84.63 ☑

- **Complication** — *continued*
  - fixation device, internal — *continued*
    - mechanical
      - breakdown
        - limb T84.119 ☑
          - carpal T84.210 ☑
          - femur T84.11 ☑
          - fibula T84.11 ☑
          - humerus T84.11 ☑
          - metacarpal T84.210 ☑
          - metatarsal T84.213 ☑
          - phalanx
            - foot T84.213 ☑
            - hand T84.210 ☑
          - radius T84.11 ☑
          - tarsal T84.213 ☑
          - tibia T84.11 ☑
          - ulna T84.11 ☑
        - specified bone NEC T84.218 ☑
        - spine T84.216 ☑
      - displacement
        - limb T84.129 ☑
          - carpal T84.220 ☑
          - femur T84.12 ☑
          - fibula T84.12 ☑
          - humerus T84.12 ☑
          - metacarpal T84.220 ☑
          - metatarsal T84.223 ☑
          - phalanx
            - foot T84.223 ☑
            - hand T84.220 ☑
          - radius T84.12 ☑
          - tarsal T84.223 ☑
          - tibia T84.12 ☑
          - ulna T84.12 ☑
        - specified bone NEC T84.228 ☑
        - spine T84.226 ☑
      - malposition — *see* Complications, fixation device, internal, mechanical, displacement
      - obstruction — *see* Complications, fixation device, internal, mechanical, specified type NEC
      - perforation — *see* Complications, fixation device, internal, mechanical, specified type NEC
      - protrusion — *see* Complications, fixation device, internal, mechanical, specified type NEC
      - specified type NEC
        - limb T84.199 ☑
          - carpal T84.290 ☑
          - femur T84.19 ☑
          - fibula T84.19 ☑
          - humerus T84.19 ☑
          - metacarpal T84.290 ☑
          - metatarsal T84.293 ☑
          - phalanx
            - foot T84.293 ☑
            - hand T84.290 ☑
          - radius T84.19 ☑
          - tarsal T84.293 ☑
          - tibia T84.19 ☑
          - ulna T84.19 ☑
        - specified bone NEC T84.298 ☑
        - vertebra T84.296 ☑
    - specified type NEC T84.89 ☑
      - embolism T84.81 ☑
      - fibrosis T84.82 ☑
      - hemorrhage T84.83 ☑
      - pain T84.84 ☑
      - specified complication NEC T84.89 ☑
      - stenosis T84.85 ☑
      - thrombosis T84.86 ☑
  - following
    - acute myocardial infarction NEC I23.8
      - aneurysm (false) (of cardiac wall) (of heart wall) (ruptured) I23.3
      - angina I23.7
      - atrial
        - septal defect I23.1
        - thrombosis I23.6
      - cardiac wall rupture I23.3
      - chordae tendinae rupture I23.4
      - defect
        - septal
          - atrial (heart) I23.1
          - ventricular (heart) I23.2
      - hemopericardium I23.0
      - papillary muscle rupture I23.5
      - rupture
        - cardiac wall I23.3

- **Complication** — *continued*
  - following — *continued*
          - with hemopericardium I23.0
        - chordae tendineae I23.4
        - papillary muscle I23.5
      - specified NEC I23.8
      - thrombosis
        - atrium I23.6
        - auricular appendage I23.6
        - ventricle (heart) I23.6
      - ventricular
        - septal defect I23.2
        - thrombosis I23.6
    - ectopic or molar pregnancy O08.9
      - cardiac arrest O08.81
      - sepsis O08.82
      - specified type NEC O08.89
      - urinary tract infection O08.83
    - termination of pregnancy — *see* Abortion
  - gastrointestinal K92.9
    - bile duct prosthesis — *see* Complications, bile duct implant
    - esophageal anti-reflux device — *see* Complications, esophageal anti-reflux device
    - postoperative
      - colostomy — *see* Complications, colostomy
      - dumping syndrome K91.1
      - enterostomy — *see* Complications, enterostomy
      - gastrostomy — *see* Complications, gastrostomy
      - malabsorption NEC K91.2
      - obstruction K91.3
      - postcholecystectomy syndrome K91.5
      - specified NEC K91.89
      - vomiting after GI surgery K91.0
    - prosthetic device or implant
      - bile duct prosthesis — *see* Complications, bile duct implant
      - esophageal anti-reflux device — *see* Complications, esophageal anti-reflux device
      - specified type NEC
        - embolism T85.818 ☑
        - fibrosis T85.828 ☑
        - hemorrhage T85.838 ☑
        - mechanical
          - breakdown T85.518 ☑
          - displacement T85.528 ☑
          - malfunction T85.518 ☑
          - malposition T85.528 ☑
          - obstruction T85.598 ☑
          - perforation T85.598 ☑
          - protrusion T85.598 ☑
          - specified NEC T85.598 ☑
        - pain T85.848 ☑
        - specified complication NEC T85.898 ☑
        - stenosis T85.858 ☑
        - thrombosis T85.868 ☑
  - gastrostomy (stoma) K94.20
    - hemorrhage K94.21
    - infection K94.22
    - malfunction K94.23
    - mechanical K94.23
    - specified complication NEC K94.29
  - genitourinary
    - device or implant T83.9 ☑
      - genital tract T83.9 ☑
        - infection or inflammation T83.69 ☑
        - intrauterine contraceptive device — *see* Complications, intrauterine, contraceptive device
        - mechanical — *see* Complications, by device, mechanical
        - mesh — *see* Complications, mesh
        - penile prosthesis — *see* Complications, prosthetic device, penile
        - specified type NEC T83.89 ☑
          - embolism T83.81 ☑
          - fibrosis T83.82 ☑
          - hemorrhage T83.83 ☑
          - pain T83.84 ☑
          - specified complication NEC T83.89 ☑
          - stenosis T83.85 ☑
          - thrombosis T83.86 ☑
        - vaginal mesh — *see* Complications, mesh
      - urinary system T83.9 ☑
        - cystostomy catheter — *see* Complication, catheter, cystostomy
        - electronic stimulator — *see* Complications, electronic stimulator device, urinary

Complication — *continued*
- insulin pump
  - infection and inflammation T85.72 ☑
  - mechanical
    - breakdown T85.614 ☑
    - displacement T85.624 ☑
    - leakage T85.633 ☑
    - malposition T85.624 ☑
    - obstruction T85.694 ☑
    - perforation T85.694 ☑
    - protrusion T85.694 ☑
    - specified NEC T85.694 ☑
- intestinal pouch NEC K91.858
- intraocular lens (prosthetic) T85.9 ☑
  - embolism T85.818 ☑
  - fibrosis T85.828 ☑
  - hemorrhage T85.838 ☑
  - infection and inflammation T85.79 ☑
  - mechanical
    - breakdown T85.21 ☑
    - displacement T85.22 ☑
    - malposition T85.22 ☑
    - obstruction T85.29 ☑
    - perforation T85.29 ☑
    - protrusion T85.29 ☑
    - specified NEC T85.29 ☑
  - pain T85.848 ☑
  - specified type NEC T85.898 ☑
  - stenosis T85.858 ☑
  - thrombosis T85.868 ☑
- intraoperative (intraprocedural)
  - cardiac arrest
    - during cardiac surgery I97.710
    - during other surgery I97.711
  - cardiac functional disturbance NEC
    - during cardiac surgery I97.790
    - during other surgery I97.791
  - hemorrhage (hematoma) (of)
    - circulatory system organ or structure
      - during cardiac bypass I97.411
      - during cardiac catheterization I97.410
      - during other circulatory system procedure I97.418
      - during other procedure I97.42
    - digestive system organ
      - during procedure on digestive system K91.61
      - during procedure on other organ K91.62
    - ear
      - during procedure on ear and mastoid process H95.21
      - during procedure on other organ H95.22
    - endocrine system organ or structure
      - during procedure on endocrine system organ or structure E36.01
      - during procedure on other organ E36.02
    - eye and adnexa
      - during ophthalmic procedure H59.11 ☑
      - during other procedure H59.12 ☑
    - genitourinary organ or structure
      - during procedure on genitourinary organ or structure N99.61
      - during procedure on other organ N99.62
    - mastoid process
      - during procedure on ear and mastoid process H95.21
      - during procedure on other organ H95.22
    - musculoskeletal structure
      - during musculoskeletal surgery M96.810
      - during non-orthopedic surgery M96.811
      - during orthopedic surgery M96.810
    - nervous system
      - during a nervous system procedure G97.31
      - during other procedure G97.32
    - respiratory system
      - during other procedure J95.62
      - during procedure on respiratory system organ or structure J95.61
    - skin and subcutaneous tissue
      - during a dermatologic procedure L76.01
      - during a procedure on other organ L76.02
    - spleen
      - during a procedure on other organ D78.02
      - during a procedure on the spleen D78.01
  - puncture or laceration (accidental) (unintentional) (of)
    - brain
      - during a nervous system procedure G97.48
      - during other procedure G97.49
    - circulatory system organ or structure
      - during circulatory system procedure I97.51
      - during other procedure I97.52

Complication — *continued*
- intraoperative — *continued*
  - puncture or laceration — (continued)
    - digestive system
      - during procedure on digestive system K91.71
      - during procedure on other organ K91.72
    - ear
      - during procedure on ear and mastoid process H95.31
      - during procedure on other organ H95.32
    - endocrine system organ or structure
      - during procedure on endocrine system organ or structure E36.11
      - during procedure on other organ E36.12
    - eye and adnexa
      - during ophthalmic procedure H59.21 ☑
      - during other procedure H59.22 ☑
    - genitourinary organ or structure
      - during procedure on genitourinary organ or structure N99.71
      - during procedure on other organ N99.72
    - mastoid process
      - during procedure on ear and mastoid process H95.31
      - during procedure on other organ H95.32
    - musculoskeletal structure
      - during musculoskeletal surgery M96.820
      - during non-orthopedic surgery M96.821
      - during orthopedic surgery M96.820
    - nervous system
      - during a nervous system procedure G97.48
      - during other procedure G97.49
    - respiratory system
      - during other procedure J95.72
      - during procedure on respiratory system organ or structure J95.71
    - skin and subcutaneous tissue
      - during a dermatologic procedure L76.11
      - during a procedure on other organ L76.12
    - spleen
      - during a procedure on other organ D78.12
      - during a procedure on the spleen D78.11
  - specified NEC
    - circulatory system I97.88
    - digestive system K91.81
    - ear H95.88
    - endocrine system E36.8
    - eye and adnexa H59.88
    - genitourinary system N99.81
    - mastoid process H95.88
    - musculoskeletal structure M96.89
    - nervous system G97.81
    - respiratory system J95.88
    - skin and subcutaneous tissue L76.81
    - spleen D78.81
- intraperitoneal catheter (dialysis) (infusion) — *see* Complications, catheter, intraperitoneal
- intrathecal infusion pump
  - infection and inflammation T85.738 ☑
  - mechanical
    - breakdown T85.615 ☑
    - displacement T85.625 ☑
    - leakage T85.635 ☑
    - malfunction T85.695 ☑
    - malposition T85.625 ☑
    - obstruction T85.695 ☑
    - perforation T85.695 ☑
    - protrusion T85.695 ☑
    - specified NEC T85.695 ☑
- intrauterine
  - contraceptive device
    - embolism T83.81 ☑
    - fibrosis T83.82 ☑
    - hemorrhage T83.83 ☑
    - infection and inflammation T83.69 ☑
    - mechanical
      - breakdown T83.31 ☑
      - displacement T83.32 ☑
      - malposition T83.32 ☑
      - obstruction T83.39 ☑
      - perforation T83.39 ☑
      - protrusion T83.39 ☑
      - specified NEC T83.39 ☑
    - pain T83.84 ☑
    - specified type NEC T83.89 ☑
    - stenosis T83.85 ☑
    - thrombosis T83.86 ☑
  - procedure (fetal), to newborn P96.5
- jejunostomy (stoma) — *see* Complications, enterostomy
- joint prosthesis, internal T84.9 ☑
  - breakage (fracture) T84.01 ☑

Complication — *continued*
- joint prosthesis, internal — *continued*
  - dislocation T84.02 ☑
  - fracture T84.01 ☑
  - infection or inflammation T84.50 ☑
    - hip T84.5 ☑
    - knee T84.5 ☑
    - specified joint NEC T84.59 ☑
  - instability T84.02 ☑
  - malposition — *see* Complications, joint prosthesis, mechanical, displacement
  - mechanical
    - breakage, broken T84.01 ☑
    - dislocation T84.02 ☑
    - fracture T84.01 ☑
    - instability T84.02 ☑
    - leakage — *see* Complications, joint prosthesis, mechanical, specified NEC
    - loosening T84.039 ☑
      - hip T84.03 ☑
      - knee T84.03 ☑
      - specified joint NEC T84.038 ☑
    - obstruction — *see* Complications, joint prosthesis, mechanical, specified NEC
    - perforation — *see* Complications, joint prosthesis, mechanical, specified NEC
    - osteolysis T84.059 ☑
      - hip T84.05 ☑
      - knee T84.05 ☑
      - other specified joint T84.058 ☑
    - protrusion — *see* Complications, joint prosthesis, mechanical, specified NEC
    - specified complication NEC T84.099 ☑
      - hip T84.09 ☑
      - knee T84.09 ☑
      - other specified joint T84.098 ☑
    - subluxation T84.02 ☑
    - wear of articular bearing surface T84.069 ☑
      - hip T84.06 ☑
      - knee T84.06 ☑
      - other specified joint T84.068 ☑
  - specified joint NEC T84.89 ☑
    - embolism T84.81 ☑
    - fibrosis T84.82 ☑
    - hemorrhage T84.83 ☑
    - pain T84.84 ☑
    - specified complication NEC T84.89 ☑
    - stenosis T84.85 ☑
    - thrombosis T84.86 ☑
  - subluxation T84.02 ☑
- kidney transplant — *see* Complications, transplant, kidney
- labor O75.9
  - specified NEC O75.89
- liver transplant (immune or nonimmune) — *see* Complications, transplant, liver
- lumbar puncture G97.1
  - cerebrospinal fluid leak G97.0
  - headache or reaction G97.1
- lung transplant — *see* Complications, transplant, lung
  - and heart — *see* Complications, transplant, lung, with heart
- male genital N50.9
  - device, implant or graft — *see* Complications, genitourinary, device or implant, genital tract
  - postprocedural or postoperative — *see* Complications, genitourinary, postprocedural
    - specified NEC N99.89
- mastoid (process) procedure
  - intraoperative H95.88
    - hematoma — *see* Complications, intraoperative, hemorrhage (hematoma) (of), mastoid process
    - hemorrhage — *see* Complications, intraoperative, hemorrhage (hematoma) (of), mastoid process
    - laceration — *see* Complications, intraoperative, puncture or laceration..., mastoid process
    - specified NEC H95.88
  - postmastoidectomy — *see* Complications, postmastoidectomy
  - postoperative H95.89
    - external ear canal stenosis H95.81 ☑
    - hematoma — *see* Complications..., postprocedural, hematoma (of), mastoid process

- **Complication** — *continued*
  - mastoid procedure — *continued*
    - hemorrhage — *see* Complications..., postprocedural, hemorrhage (of), mastoid process
    - postmastoidectomy — *see* Complications, postmastoidectomy
    - seroma — *see* Complications, postprocedural, seroma (of), mastoid process
    - specified NEC H95.89
  - mastoidectomy cavity — *see* Complications, postmastoidectomy
  - mechanical — *see* Complications, by site and type, mechanical
  - medical procedures (*see also* Complication (s), intraoperative)T88.9 ☑
  - metabolic E88.9
    - postoperative E89.89
      - specified NEC E89.89
  - molar pregnancy NOS O08.9
    - damage to pelvic organs O08.6
    - embolism O08.2
    - genital infection O08.0
    - hemorrhage (delayed) (excessive) O08.1
    - metabolic disorder O08.5
    - renal failure O08.4
    - shock O08.3
    - specified type NEC O08.0
    - venous complication NEC O08.7
  - musculoskeletal system (*see also* Complication, intraoperative (intraprocedural), by site)
    - device, implant or graft NEC — *see* Complications, orthopedic, device or implant
    - internal fixation (nail) (plate) (rod) — *see* Complications, fixation device, internal
    - joint prosthesis — *see* Complications, joint prosthesis
    - postoperative (postprocedural) M96.89
      - with osteoporosis — *see* Osteoporosis
      - fracture following insertion of device — *see* Fracture, following insertion of orthopedic implant, joint prosthesis or bone plate
      - joint instability after prosthesis removal M96.89
      - lordosis M96.4
      - postlaminectomy syndrome NEC M96.1
        - kyphosis M96.3
      - pseudarthrosis M96.0
      - specified complication NEC M96.89
    - post radiation M96.89
      - kyphosis M96.2
      - scoliosis M96.5
      - specified complication NEC M96.89
  - nephrostomy (stoma) — *see* Complications, stoma, urinary tract, external NEC
  - nervous system G98.8
    - central G96.9
    - device, implant or graft (*see also* Complication, prosthetic device or implant, specified NEC)
      - electronic stimulator (electrode (s)) — *see* Complications, electronic stimulator device
      - specified NEC
        - infection and inflammation T85.738 ☑
        - mechanical T85.695 ☑
          - breakdown T85.615 ☑
          - displacement T85.625 ☑
          - leakage T85.635 ☑
          - malfunction T85.695 ☑
          - malposition T85.625 ☑
          - obstruction T85.695 ☑
          - perforation T85.695 ☑
          - protrusion T85.695 ☑
          - specified NEC T85.695 ☑
      - ventricular shunt — *see* Complications, ventricular shunt
    - electronic stimulator (electrode (s)) — *see* Complications, electronic stimulator device
    - postprocedural G97.82
      - intracranial hypotension G97.2
      - specified NEC G97.82
      - spinal fluid leak G97.0
  - newborn, due to intrauterine (fetal) procedure P96.5
  - nonabsorbable (permanent) sutures — *see* Complication, sutures, permanent
  - obstetric O75.9
    - procedure (instrumental) (manual) (surgical)
      - specified NEC O75.4

- **Complication** — *continued*
  - obstetric — *continued*
    - specified NEC O75.89
    - surgical wound NEC O90.89
      - hematoma O90.2
      - infection O86.0
  - ocular lens implant — *see* Complications, intraocular lens
  - ophthalmologic
    - postprocedural bleb — *see* Blebitis
  - orbital prosthesis T85.9 ☑
    - embolism T85.818 ☑
    - fibrosis T85.828 ☑
    - hemorrhage T85.838 ☑
    - infection and inflammation T85.79 ☑
    - mechanical
      - breakdown T85.31 ☑
      - displacement T85.32 ☑
      - malposition T85.32 ☑
      - obstruction T85.39 ☑
      - perforation T85.39 ☑
      - protrusion T85.39 ☑
      - specified NEC T85.39 ☑
    - pain T85.848 ☑
    - specified type NEC T85.898 ☑
    - stenosis T85.858 ☑
    - thrombosis T85.868 ☑
  - organ or tissue transplant (partial) (total) — *see* Complications, transplant
  - orthopedic (*see also* Disorder, soft tissue)
    - device or implant T84.9 ☑
      - bone
        - device or implant — *see* Complication, bone, device NEC
        - graft — *see* Complication, graft, bone
      - breakdown T84.418 ☑
      - displacement T84.428 ☑
      - electronic bone stimulator — *see* Complications, electronic stimulator device, bone
      - embolism T84.81 ☑
      - fibrosis T84.82 ☑
      - fixation device — *see* Complication, fixation device, internal
      - hemorrhage T84.83 ☑
      - infection or inflammation T84.7 ☑
      - joint prosthesis — *see* Complication, joint prosthesis, internal
      - malfunction T84.418 ☑
      - malposition T84.428 ☑
      - mechanical NEC T84.498 ☑
      - muscle graft — *see* Complications, graft, muscle
      - obstruction T84.498 ☑
      - pain T84.84 ☑
      - perforation T84.498 ☑
      - protrusion T84.498 ☑
      - specified complication NEC T84.89 ☑
      - stenosis T84.85 ☑
      - tendon graft — *see* Complications, graft, tendon
      - thrombosis T84.86 ☑
    - fracture (following insertion of device) — *see* Fracture, following insertion of orthopedic implant, joint prosthesis or bone plate
    - postprocedural M96.89
      - fracture — *see* Fracture, following insertion of orthopedic implant, joint prosthesis or bone plate
      - postlaminectomy syndrome NEC M96.1
        - kyphosis M96.3
        - lordosis M96.4
      - postradiation
        - kyphosis M96.2
        - scoliosis M96.5
      - pseudarthrosis post-fusion M96.0
      - specified type NEC M96.89
  - pacemaker (cardiac) — *see* Complications, cardiovascular device or implant, electronic
  - pancreas transplant — *see* Complications, transplant, pancreas
  - penile prosthesis (implant) — *see* Complications, prosthetic device, penile
  - perfusion NEC T80.90 ☑
  - perineal repair (obstetrical) NEC O90.89
    - disruption O90.1
    - hematoma O90.2
    - infection (following delivery) O86.0
  - phototherapy T88.9 ☑
    - specified NEC T88.8 ☑
  - postmastoidectomy NEC H95.19 ☑
    - cyst, mucosal H95.13 ☑

- **Complication** — *continued*
  - postmastoidectomy NEC — *continued*
    - granulation H95.12 ☑
    - inflammation, chronic H95.11 ☑
    - recurrent cholesteatoma H95.0 ☑
  - postoperative — *see* Complications, postprocedural
    - circulatory — *see* Complications, circulatory system
    - ear — *see* Complications, ear
    - endocrine — *see* Complications, endocrine
    - eye — *see* Complications, eye
    - lumbar puncture G97.1
      - cerebrospinal fluid leak G97.0
    - nervous system (central) (peripheral) — *see* Complications, nervous system
    - respiratory system — *see* Complications, respiratory system
  - postprocedural (*see also* Complications, surgical procedure)
    - cardiac arrest
      - following cardiac surgery I97.120
      - following other surgery I97.121
    - cardiac functional disturbance NEC
      - following cardiac surgery I97.190
      - following other surgery I97.191
    - cardiac insufficiency
      - following cardiac surgery I97.110
      - following other surgery I97.111
    - chorioretinal scars following retinal surgery H59.81 ☑
    - following cataract surgery
      - cataract (lens) fragments H59.02 ☑
      - cystoid macular edema H59.03 ☑
      - specified NEC H59.09 ☑
      - vitreous (touch) syndrome H59.01 ☑
    - heart failure
      - following cardiac surgery I97.130
      - following other surgery I97.131
    - hematoma (of)
      - circulatory system organ or structure
        - following cardiac bypass I97.631
        - following cardiac catheterization I97.630
        - following other circulatory system procedure I97.638
        - following other procedure I97.621
      - digestive system
        - following procedure on digestive system K91.870
        - following procedure on other organ K91.871
      - ear
        - following other procedure H95.52
        - following procedure on ear and mastoid process H95.51
      - endocrine system
        - following endocrine system procedure E89.820
        - following other procedure E89.821
      - eye and adnexa
        - following ophthalmic procedure H59.33 ☑
        - following other procedure H59.34 ☑
      - genitourinary organ or structure
        - following procedure on genitourinary organ or structure N99.840
        - following procedure on other organ N99.841
      - mastoid process
        - following other procedure H95.52
        - following procedure on ear and mastoid process H95.51
      - musculoskeletal structure
        - following musculoskeletal surgery M96.840
        - following non-orthopedic surgery M96.841
        - following orthopedic surgery M96.840
      - nervous system
        - following nervous system procedure G97.61
        - following other procedure G97.62
      - respiratory system
        - following other procedure J95.861
        - following procedure on respiratory system organ or structure J95.860
      - skin and subcutaneous tissue
        - following dermatologic procedure L76.31
        - following procedure on other organ L76.32
      - spleen
        - following procedure on other organ D78.32
        - following procedure on the spleen D78.31
    - hemorrhage (of)
      - circulatory system organ or structure

- **Complication** — *continued*
  - postprocedural — *continued*
    - seroma (of) — *continued*
      - circulatory system organ or structure — *continued*
        - following cardiac bypass I97.611
        - following cardiac catheterization I97.610
        - following other circulatory system procedure I97.618
        - following other procedure I97.620
      - digestive system
        - following procedure on digestive system K91.840
        - following procedure on other organ K91.841
      - ear
        - following other procedure H95.42
        - following procedure on ear and mastoid process H95.41
      - endocrine system
        - following endocrine system procedure E89.810
        - following other procedure E89.811
      - eye and adnexa
        - following ophthalmic procedure H59.31 ☑
        - following other procedure H59.32 ☑
      - genitourinary organ or structure
        - following procedure on genitourinary organ or structure N99.820
        - following procedure on other organ N99.821
      - mastoid process
        - following other procedure H95.42
        - following procedure on ear and mastoid process H95.41
      - musculoskeletal structure
        - following musculoskeletal surgery M96.830
        - following non-orthopedic surgery M96.831
        - following orthopedic surgery M96.830
      - nervous system
        - following nervous system procedure G97.51
        - following other procedure G97.52
      - respiratory system
        - following other procedure J95.831
        - following procedure on respiratory system organ or structure J95.830
      - skin and subcutaneous tissue
        - following dermatologic procedure L76.21
        - following a procedure on other organ L76.22
      - spleen
        - following procedure on other organ D78.22
        - following procedure on the spleen D78.21
    - seroma (of)
      - circulatory system organ or structure
        - following cardiac bypass I97.641
        - following cardiac catheterization I97.640
        - following other circulatory system procedure I97.648
        - following other procedure I97.622
      - digestive system
        - following procedure on digestive system K91.872
        - following procedure on other organ K91.873
      - ear
        - following other procedure H95.54
        - following procedure on ear and mastoid process H95.53
      - endocrine system
        - following endocrine system procedure E89.822
        - following other procedure E89.823
      - eye and adnexa
        - following ophthalmic procedure H59.35 ☑
        - following other procedure H59.36 ☑
      - genitourinary organ or structure
        - following procedure on genitourinary organ or structure N99.842
        - following procedure on other organ N99.843
      - mastoid process
        - following other procedure H95.54
        - following procedure on ear and mastoid process H95.53
      - musculoskeletal structure
        - following musculoskeletal surgery M96.842
        - following non-orthopedic surgery M96.843
        - following orthopedic surgery M96.842
      - nervous system
        - following nervous system procedure G97.63
        - following other procedure G97.64

- **Complication** — *continued*
  - postprocedural — *continued*
    - seroma (of) — *continued*
      - respiratory system
        - following other procedure J95.863
        - following procedure on respiratory system organ or structure J95.862
      - skin and subcutaneous tissue
        - following dermatologic procedure L76.33
        - following procedure on other organ L76.34
      - spleen
        - following procedure on other organ D78.34
        - following procedure on the spleen D78.33
    - specified NEC
      - circulatory system I97.89
      - digestive K91.89
      - ear H95.89
      - endocrine E89.89
      - eye and adnexa H59.89
      - genitourinary N99.89
      - mastoid process H95.89
      - metabolic E89.89
      - musculoskeletal structure M96.89
      - nervous system G97.82
      - respiratory system J95.89
      - skin and subcutaneous tissue L76.82
      - spleen D78.89
  - pregnancy NEC — *see* Pregnancy, complicated by
  - prosthetic device or implant T85.9 ☑
    - bile duct — *see* Complications, bile duct implant
    - breast — *see* Complications, breast implant
    - bulking agent
      - ureteral
        - erosion T83.714 ☑
        - exposure T83.724 ☑
      - urethral
        - erosion T83.713 ☑
        - exposure T83.723 ☑
    - cardiac and vascular NEC — *see* Complications, cardiovascular device or implant
    - corneal transplant — *see* Complications, graft, cornea
    - electronic nervous system stimulator — *see* Complications, electronic stimulator device
    - epidural infusion catheter — *see* Complications, catheter, epidural
    - esophageal anti-reflux device — *see* Complications, esophageal anti-reflux device
    - genital organ or tract — *see* Complications, genitourinary, device or implant, genital tract
      - specified NEC T83.79 ☑
    - heart valve — *see* Complications, heart, valve, prosthesis
    - infection or inflammation T85.79 ☑
      - intestine transplant T86.892
      - liver transplant T86.43
      - lung transplant T86.812
      - pancreas transplant T86.892
      - skin graft T86.822
    - intraocular lens — *see* Complications, intraocular lens
    - intraperitoneal (dialysis) catheter — *see* Complications, catheter, intraperitoneal
    - joint — *see* Complications, joint prosthesis, internal
    - mechanical NEC T85.698 ☑
      - dialysis catheter (vascular) (*see also* Complication, catheter, dialysis, mechanical)
        - peritoneal — *see* Complication, catheter, intraperitoneal, mechanical
      - gastrointestinal device T85.598 ☑
      - ocular device T85.398 ☑
      - subdural (infusion) catheter T85.690 ☑
      - suture, permanent T85.692 ☑
        - that for bone repair — *see* Complications, fixation device, internal (orthopedic), mechanical
      - ventricular shunt
        - breakdown T85.01 ☑
        - displacement T85.02 ☑
        - leakage T85.03 ☑
        - malposition T85.02 ☑
        - obstruction T85.09 ☑
        - perforation T85.09 ☑
        - protrusion T85.09 ☑
        - specified NEC T85.09 ☑
    - mesh

- **Complication** — *continued*
  - prosthetic device or implant — *continued*
    - mesh — *continued*
      - erosion (to surrounding organ or tissue) T83.717
        - urethral (into pelvic floor muscles) T83.712 ☑
        - vaginal (into pelvic floor muscles) T83.711 ☑
      - exposure (into surrounding organ or tissue) T83.727
        - urethral (through urethral wall) T83.722 ☑
        - vaginal (into vagina) (through vaginal wall) T83.721 ☑
    - orbital — *see* Complications, orbital prosthesis
    - penile T83.9 ☑
      - embolism T83.81 ☑
      - fibrosis T83.82 ☑
      - hemorrhage T83.83 ☑
      - infection and inflammation T83.61 ☑
      - mechanical
        - breakdown T83.410 ☑
        - displacement T83.420 ☑
        - leakage T83.490 ☑
        - malposition T83.420 ☑
        - obstruction T83.490 ☑
        - perforation T83.490 ☑
        - protrusion T83.490 ☑
        - specified NEC T83.490 ☑
      - pain T83.84 ☑
      - specified type NEC T83.89 ☑
      - stenosis T83.85 ☑
      - thrombosis T83.86 ☑
    - prosthetic materials NEC
      - erosion (to surrounding organ or tissue) T83.718 ☑
      - exposure (into surrounding organ or tissue) T83.728 ☑
    - skin graft T86.829
      - artificial skin or decellularized allodermis
        - embolism T85.818 ☑
        - fibrosis T85.828 ☑
        - hemorrhage T85.838 ☑
        - infection and inflammation T85.79 ☑
        - mechanical
          - breakdown T85.613 ☑
          - displacement T85.623 ☑
          - malfunction T85.613 ☑
          - malposition T85.623 ☑
          - obstruction T85.693 ☑
          - perforation T85.693 ☑
          - protrusion T85.693 ☑
          - specified NEC T85.693 ☑
        - pain T85.848 ☑
        - specified type NEC T85.898 ☑
        - stenosis T85.858 ☑
        - thrombosis T85.868 ☑
      - failure T86.821
      - infection T86.822
      - rejection T86.820
      - specified NEC T86.828
    - sling
      - urethral (female) (male)
        - erosion T83.712 ☑
        - exposure T83.722 ☑
    - specified NEC T85.9 ☑
      - embolism T85.818 ☑
      - fibrosis T85.828 ☑
      - hemorrhage T85.838 ☑
      - infection and inflammation T85.79 ☑
      - mechanical
        - breakdown T85.618 ☑
        - displacement T85.628 ☑
        - leakage T85.638 ☑
        - malfunction T85.618 ☑
        - malposition T85.628 ☑
        - obstruction T85.698 ☑
        - perforation T85.698 ☑
        - protrusion T85.698 ☑
        - specified NEC T85.698 ☑
      - pain T85.848 ☑
      - specified type NEC T85.898 ☑
      - stenosis T85.858 ☑
      - thrombosis T85.868 ☑
    - subdural infusion catheter — *see* Complications, catheter, subdural
    - sutures — *see* Complications, sutures
    - urinary organ or tract NEC — *see* Complications, genitourinary, device or implant, urinary system
    - vascular — *see* Complications, cardiovascular device or implant

Complication — *continued*
- prosthetic device or implant — *continued*
  - ventricular shunt — *see* Complications, ventricular shunt (device)
- puerperium — *see* Puerperal
- puncture, spinal G97.1
  - cerebrospinal fluid leak G97.0
  - headache or reaction G97.1
- pyelogram N99.89
- radiation
  - kyphosis M96.2
  - scoliosis M96.5
- reattached
  - extremity (infection) (rejection)
    - lower T87.1X ☑
    - upper T87.0X ☑
  - specified body part NEC T87.2
- reconstructed breast
  - asymmetry between native and reconstructed breast N65.1
  - deformity N65.0
  - disproportion between native and reconstructed breast N65.1
  - excess tissue N65.0
  - misshapen N65.0
- reimplant NEC (*see also* Complications, prosthetic device or implant)
  - limb (infection) (rejection) — *see* Complications, reattached, extremity
  - organ (partial) (total) — *see* Complications, transplant
  - prosthetic device NEC — *see* Complications, prosthetic device
- renal N28.9
  - allograft — *see* Complications, transplant, kidney
  - dialysis — *see* Complications, dialysis
- respirator
  - mechancial J95.850
  - specified NEC J95.859
- respiratory system J98.9
  - device, implant or graft — *see* Complication, prosthetic device or implant, specified NEC
  - lung transplant — *see* Complications, prosthetic device or implant, lung transplant
  - postoperative J95.89
    - air leak J95.812
    - Mendelson's syndrome (chemical pneumonitis) J95.4
    - pneumothorax J95.811
    - pulmonary insufficiency (acute) (after nonthoracic surgery) J95.2
      - chronic J95.3
      - following thoracic surgery J95.1
    - respiratory failure (acute) J95.821
      - acute and chronic J95.822
    - specified NEC J95.89
    - subglottic stenosis J95.5
    - tracheostomy complication — *see* Complications, tracheostomy
  - therapy T81.89 ☑
- sedation during labor and delivery O74.9
  - cardiac O74.2
  - central nervous system O74.3
  - pulmonary NEC O74.1
- shunt (*see also* Complications, prosthetic device or implant)
  - arteriovenous — *see* Complications, arteriovenous, shunt
  - ventricular (communicating) — *see* Complications, ventricular shunt
- skin
  - graft T86.829
    - failure T86.821
    - infection T86.822
    - rejection T86.820
    - specified type NEC T86.828
- spinal
  - anesthesia — *see* Complications, anesthesia, spinal
  - catheter (epidural) (subdural) — *see* Complications, catheter
  - puncture or tap G97.1
    - cerebrospinal fluid leak G97.0
    - headache or reaction G97.1
- stent
  - bile duct — *see* Complications, bile duct prosthesis
  - ureteral indwelling
    - breakdown T83.112 ☑
    - displacement T83.122 ☑

Complication — *continued*
- stent — *continued*
    - leakage T83.192 ☑
    - malposition T83.122 ☑
    - obstruction T83.192 ☑
    - perforation T83.192 ☑
    - protrusion T83.192 ☑
    - specified NEC T83.192 ☑
  - urinary NEC (ileal conduit) (nephroureteral) T83.193 ☑
    - embolism T83.81 ☑
    - fibrosis T83.82 ☑
    - hemorrhage T83.83 ☑
    - infection and inflammation T83.593 ☑
    - mechanical
      - breakdown T83.113 ☑
      - displacement T83.123 ☑
      - leakage T83.193 ☑
      - malposition T83.123 ☑
      - obstruction T83.193 ☑
      - perforation T83.193 ☑
      - protrusion T83.193 ☑
      - specified NEC T83.193 ☑
    - pain T83.84 ☑
    - specified type NEC T83.89 ☑
    - stenosis T83.85 ☑
    - thrombosis T83.86 ☑
  - vascular
    - end stent stenosis — *see* Restenosis, stent
    - in stent stenosis — *see* Restenosis, stent
- stoma
  - digestive tract
    - colostomy — *see* Complications, colostomy
    - enterostomy — *see* Complications, enterostomy
    - esophagostomy — *see* Complications, esophagostomy
    - gastrostomy — *see* Complications, gastrostomy
  - urinary tract N99.528
    - continent N99.538
      - hemorrhage N99.530
      - herniation N99.533
      - infection N99.531
      - malfunction N99.532
      - specified type NEC N99.538
      - stenosis N99.534
    - cystostomy — *see* Complications, cystostomy
    - external NOS N99.528
    - hemorrhage N99.520
    - herniation N99.523
    - incontinent N99.528
      - hemorrhage N99.520
      - herniation N99.523
      - infection N99.521
      - malfunction N99.522
      - specified type NEC N99.528
      - stenosis N99.524
    - infection N99.521
    - malfunction N99.522
    - specified type NEC N99.528
    - stenosis N99.524
- stomach banding — *see* Complication (s), bariatric procedure
- stomach stapling — *see* Complication (s), bariatric procedure
- surgical material, nonabsorbable — *see* Complication, suture, permanent
- surgical procedure (on) T81.9 ☑
  - amputation stump (late) — *see* Complications, amputation stump
  - cardiac — *see* Complications, circulatory system
  - cholesteatoma, recurrent — *see* Complications, postmastoidectomy, recurrent cholesteatoma
  - circulatory (early) — *see* Complications, circulatory system
  - digestive system — *see* Complications, gastrointestinal
  - dumping syndrome (postgastrectomy) K91.1
  - ear — *see* Complications, ear
  - elephantiasis or lymphedema I97.89
    - postmastectomy I97.2
  - emphysema (surgical) T81.82 ☑
  - endocrine — *see* Complications, endocrine
  - eye — *see* Complications, eye
  - fistula (persistent postoperative) T81.83 ☑
  - foreign body inadvertently left in wound (sponge) (suture) (swab) — *see* Foreign body, accidentally left during a procedure

Complication — *continued*
- surgical procedure — *continued*
  - gastrointestinal — *see* Complications, gastrointestinal
  - genitourinary NEC N99.89
  - hematoma
    - intraoperative — *see* Complication, intraoperative, hemorrhage
    - postprocedural — *see* Complication, postprocedural, hematoma
  - hemorrhage
    - intraoperative — *see* Complication, intraoperative, hemorrhage
    - postprocedural — *see* Complication, postprocedural, hemorrhage
  - hepatic failure K91.82
  - hyperglycemia (postpancreatectomy) E89.1
  - hypoinsulinemia (postpancreatectomy) E89.1
  - hypoparathyroidism (postparathyroidectomy) E89.2
  - hypopituitarism (posthypophysectomy) E89.3
  - hypothyroidism (post-thyroidectomy) E89.0
  - intestinal obstruction K91.3
  - intracranial hypotension following ventricular shunting (ventriculostomy) G97.2
  - lymphedema I97.89
    - postmastectomy I97.2
  - malabsorption (postsurgical) NEC K91.2
    - osteoporosis — *see* Osteoporosis, postsurgical malabsorption
  - mastoidectomy cavity NEC — *see* Complications, postmastoidectomy
  - metabolic E89.89
    - specified NEC E89.89
  - musculoskeletal — *see* Complications, musculoskeletal system
  - nervous system (central) (peripheral) — *see* Complications, nervous system
  - ovarian failure E89.40
    - asymptomatic E89.40
    - symptomatic E89.41
  - peripheral vascular — *see* Complications, surgical procedure, vascular
  - postcardiotomy syndrome I97.0
  - postcholecystectomy syndrome K91.5
  - postcommissurotomy syndrome I97.0
  - postgastrectomy dumping syndrome K91.1
  - postlaminectomy syndrome NEC M96.1
    - kyphosis M96.3
  - postmastectomy lymphedema syndrome I97.2
  - postmastoidectomy cholesteatoma — *see* Complications, postmastoidectomy, recurrent cholesteatoma
  - postvagotomy syndrome K91.1
  - postvalvulotomy syndrome I97.0
  - pulmonary insufficiency (acute) J95.2
    - chronic J95.3
    - following thoracic surgery J95.1
  - reattached body part — *see* Complications, reattached
  - respiratory — *see* Complications, respiratory system
  - shock (hypovolemic) T81.19 ☑
  - spleen (postoperative) D78.89
    - intraoperative D78.81
  - stitch abscess T81.48
  - subglottic stenosis (postsurgical) J95.5
  - testicular hypofunction E89.5
  - transplant — *see* Complications, organ or tissue transplant
  - urinary NEC N99.89
  - vaginal vault prolapse (posthysterectomy) N99.3
  - vascular (peripheral)
    - artery T81.719 ☑
      - mesenteric T81.710 ☑
      - renal T81.711 ☑
      - specified NEC T81.718 ☑
    - vein T81.72 ☑
  - wound infection T81.40
- suture, permanent (wire) NEC T85.9 ☑
  - with repair of bone — *see* Complications, fixation device, internal
  - embolism T85.818 ☑
  - fibrosis T85.828 ☑
  - hemorrhage T85.838 ☑
  - infection and inflammation T85.79 ☑
  - mechanical
    - breakdown T85.612 ☑
    - displacement T85.622 ☑
    - malfunction T85.612 ☑
    - malposition T85.622 ☑

Complication — *continued*
- suture, permanent — *continued*
      - obstruction T85.692 ☑
      - perforation T85.692 ☑
      - protrusion T85.692 ☑
      - specified NEC T85.692 ☑
  - pain T85.848 ☑
  - specified type NEC T85.898 ☑
  - stenosis T85.858 ☑
  - thrombosis T85.868 ☑
- tracheostomy J95.00
  - granuloma J95.09
  - hemorrhage J95.01
  - infection J95.02
  - malfunction J95.03
  - mechanical J95.03
  - obstruction J95.03
  - specified type NEC J95.09
  - tracheo-esophageal fistula J95.04
- transfusion (blood) (lymphocytes) (plasma) T80.92 ☑
  - air emblism T80.0 ☑
  - circulatory overload E87.71
  - febrile nonhemolytic transfusion reaction R50.84
  - hemolysis T80.89 ☑
  - hemochromatosis E83.111
  - hemolytic reaction (antigen unspecified) T80.919 ☑
  - incompatibility reaction (antigen unspecified) T80.919 ☑
    - ABO T80.30 ☑
      - delayed serologic (DSTR) T80.39 ☑
      - hemolytic transfusion reaction (HTR) (unspecified time after transfusion) T80.319 ☑
        - acute (AHTR) (less than 24 hours after transfusion) T80.310 ☑
        - delayed (DHTR) (24 hours or more after transfusion) T80.311 ☑
      - specified NEC T80.39 ☑
    - acute (antigen unspecified) T80.910 ☑
    - delayed (antigen unspecified) T80.911 ☑
    - delayed serologic (DSTR) T80.89 ☑
    - Non-ABO (minor antigens (Duffy) (Kell) (Kidd) (Lewis) (M) (N) (P) (S)) T80.A0 ☑
      - delayed serologic (DSTR) T80.A9 ☑
      - hemolytic transfusion reaction (HTR) (unspecified time after transfusion) T80.A19 ☑
        - acute (AHTR) (less than 24 hours after transfusion) T80.A10 ☑
        - delayed (DHTR) (24 hours or more after transfusion) T80.A11 ☑
      - specified NEC T80.A9 ☑
    - Rh (antigens (C) (c) (D) (E) (e)) (factor) T80.40 ☑
      - delayed serologic (DSTR) T80.49 ☑
      - hemolytic transfusion reaction (HTR) (unspecified time after transfusion) T80.419 ☑
        - acute (AHTR) (less than 24 hours after transfusion) T80.410 ☑
        - delayed (DHTR) (24 hours or more after transfusion) T80.411 ☑
      - specified NEC T80.49 ☑
  - infection T80.29 ☑
    - acute T80.22 ☑
  - reaction NEC T80.89 ☑
  - sepsis T80.29 ☑
  - shock T80.89 ☑
- transplant T86.90
  - bone T86.839
    - failure T86.831
    - infection T86.832
    - rejection T86.830
    - specified type NEC T86.838
  - bone marrow T86.00
    - failure T86.02
    - infection T86.03
    - rejection T86.01
    - specified type NEC T86.09
  - cornea T86.849
    - failure T86.841
    - infection T86.842
    - rejection T86.840
    - specified type NEC T86.848
  - failure T86.92
  - heart T86.20
    - with lung T86.30
    - cardiac allograft vasculopathy T86.290
      - failure T86.32

Complication — *continued*
- transplant — *continued*
      - infection T86.33
      - rejection T86.31
      - specified type NEC T86.39
    - failure T86.22
    - infection T86.23
    - rejection T86.21
    - specified type NEC T86.298
  - infection T86.93
  - intestine T86.859
    - failure T86.851
    - infection T86.852
    - rejection T86.850
    - specified type NEC T86.858
  - kidney T86.10
    - failure T86.12
    - infection T86.13
    - rejection T86.11
    - specified type NEC T86.19
  - liver T86.40
    - failure T86.42
    - infection T86.43
    - rejection T86.41
    - specified type NEC T86.49
  - lung T86.819
    - with heart T86.30
      - failure T86.32
      - infection T86.33
      - rejection T86.31
      - specified type NEC T86.39
    - failure T86.811
    - infection T86.812
    - rejection T86.810
    - specified type NEC T86.818
  - malignant neoplasm C80.2
  - pancreas T86.899
    - failure T86.891
    - infection T86.892
    - rejection T86.890
    - specified type NEC T86.898
  - peripheral blood stem cells T86.5
  - post-transplant lymphoproliferative disorder (PTLD) D47.Z1
  - rejection T86.91
  - skin T86.829
    - failure T86.821
    - infection T86.822
    - rejection T86.820
    - specified type NEC T86.828
  - specified
    - tissue T86.899
      - failure T86.891
      - infection T86.892
      - rejection T86.890
      - specified type NEC T86.898
    - type NEC T86.99
  - stem cell (from peripheral blood) (from umbilical cord) T86.5
  - umbilical cord stem cells T86.5
- trauma (early) T79.9 ☑
  - specified NEC T79.8 ☑
- ultrasound therapy NEC T88.9 ☑
- umbilical cord NEC
  - complicating delivery O69.9 ☑
    - specified NEC O69.89 ☑
- umbrella device, vascular T82.9 ☑
  - embolism T82.818 ☑
  - fibrosis T82.828 ☑
  - hemorrhage T82.838 ☑
  - infection or inflammation T82.7 ☑
  - mechanical
    - breakdown T82.515 ☑
    - displacement T82.525 ☑
    - leakage T82.535 ☑
    - malposition T82.525 ☑
    - obstruction T82.595 ☑
    - perforation T82.595 ☑
    - protrusion T82.595 ☑
  - pain T82.848 ☑
  - specified type NEC T82.898 ☑
  - stenosis T82.858 ☑
  - thrombosis T82.868 ☑
- urethral catheter — *see* Complications, catheter, urethral, indwelling
- vaccination T88.1 ☑
  - anaphylaxis NEC T80.52 ☑
  - arthropathy — *see* Arthropathy, postimmunization
  - cellulitis T88.0 ☑
  - encephalitis or encephalomyelitis G04.02
  - infection (general) (local) NEC T88.0 ☑

Complication — *continued*
- vaccination — *continued*
  - meningitis G03.8
  - myelitis G04.02
  - protein sickness T80.62 ☑
  - rash T88.1 ☑
  - reaction (allergic) T88.1 ☑
    - serum T80.62 ☑
  - sepsis T88.0 ☑
  - serum intoxication, sickness, rash, or other serum reaction NEC T80.62 ☑
    - anaphylactic shock T80.52 ☑
  - shock (allergic) (anaphylactic) T80.52 ☑
  - vaccinia (generalized) (localized) T88.1 ☑
- vas deferens device or implant — *see* Complications, genitourinary, device or implant, genital tract
- vascular I99.9
  - device or implant T82.9 ☑
    - embolism T82.818 ☑
    - fibrosis T82.828 ☑
    - hemorrhage T82.838 ☑
    - infection or inflammation T82.7 ☑
    - mechanical
      - breakdown T82.519 ☑
        - specified device NEC T82.518 ☑
      - displacement T82.529 ☑
        - specified device NEC T82.528 ☑
      - leakage T82.539 ☑
        - specified device NEC T82.538 ☑
      - malposition T82.529 ☑
        - specified device NEC T82.528 ☑
      - obstruction T82.599 ☑
        - specified device NEC T82.598 ☑
      - perforation T82.599 ☑
        - specified device NEC T82.598 ☑
      - protrusion T82.599 ☑
        - specified device NEC T82.598 ☑
    - pain T82.848 ☑
    - specified type NEC T82.898 ☑
    - stenosis T82.858 ☑
    - thrombosis T82.868 ☑
  - dialysis catheter — *see* Complication, catheter, dialysis
  - following infusion, therapeutic injection or transfusion T80.1 ☑
  - graft T82.9 ☑
    - embolism T82.818 ☑
    - fibrosis T82.828 ☑
    - hemorrhage T82.838 ☑
    - mechanical
      - breakdown T82.319 ☑
        - aorta (bifurcation) T82.310 ☑
        - carotid artery T82.311 ☑
        - specified vessel NEC T82.318 ☑
      - displacement T82.329 ☑
        - aorta (bifurcation) T82.320 ☑
        - carotid artery T82.321 ☑
        - specified vessel NEC T82.328 ☑
      - leakage T82.339 ☑
        - aorta (bifurcation) T82.330 ☑
        - carotid artery T82.331 ☑
        - specified vessel NEC T82.338 ☑
      - malposition T82.329 ☑
        - aorta (bifurcation) T82.320 ☑
        - carotid artery T82.321 ☑
        - specified vessel NEC T82.328 ☑
      - obstruction T82.399 ☑
        - aorta (bifurcation) T82.390 ☑
        - carotid artery T82.391 ☑
        - specified vessel NEC T82.398 ☑
      - perforation T82.399 ☑
        - aorta (bifurcation) T82.390 ☑
        - carotid artery T82.391 ☑
        - specified vessel NEC T82.398 ☑
      - protrusion T82.399 ☑
        - aorta (bifurcation) T82.390 ☑
        - carotid artery T82.391 ☑
        - specified vessel NEC T82.398 ☑
    - pain T82.848 ☑
    - specified complication NEC T82.898 ☑
    - stenosis T82.858 ☑
    - thrombosis T82.868 ☑
  - postoperative — *see* Complications, postoperative, circulatory
- vena cava device (filter) (sieve) (umbrella) — *see* Complications, umbrella device, vascular
- ventilation therapy NEC T81.81 ☑
- ventilator
  - mechanical J95.850
    - specified NEC J95.859

- **Complication** — *continued*
  - ventricular (communicating) shunt (device) T85.9 ☑
    - embolism T85.810 ☑
    - fibrosis T85.820 ☑
    - hemorrhage T85.830 ☑
    - infection and inflammation T85.730 ☑
    - mechanical
      - breakdown T85.01 ☑
      - displacement T85.02 ☑
      - leakage T85.03 ☑
      - malposition T85.02 ☑
      - obstruction T85.09 ☑
      - perforation T85.09 ☑
      - protrusion T85.09 ☑
      - specified NEC T85.09 ☑
    - pain T85.840 ☑
    - specified type NEC T85.890 ☑
    - stenosis T85.850 ☑
    - thrombosis T85.860 ☑
  - wire suture, permanent (implanted) — *see* Complications, suture, permanent
- **Compressed** air disease T70.3 ☑
- **Compression**
  - with injury - code by Nature of injury
  - artery I77.1
    - celiac, syndrome I77.4
  - brachial plexus G54.0
  - brain (stem) G93.5
    - due to
      - contusion (diffuse) — *see* Injury, intracranial, diffuse
        - focal — *see* Injury, intracranial, focal
      - injury NEC — *see* Injury, intracranial, diffuse
    - traumatic — *see* Injury, intracranial, diffuse
  - bronchus J98.09
  - cauda equina G83.4
  - celiac (artery) (axis) I77.4
  - cerebral — *see* Compression, brain
  - cervical plexus G54.2
  - cord
    - spinal — *see* Compression, spinal
    - umbilical — *see* Compression, umbilical cord
  - cranial nerve G52.9
    - eighth — *see* subcategory H93.3
    - eleventh G52.8
    - fifth G50.8
    - first G52.0
    - fourth — *see* Strabismus, paralytic, fourth nerve
    - ninth G52.1
    - second — *see* Disorder, nerve, optic
    - seventh G52.8
    - sixth — *see* Strabismus, paralytic, sixth nerve
    - tenth G52.2
    - third — *see* Strabismus, paralytic, third nerve
    - twelfth G52.3
  - diver's squeeze T70.3 ☑
  - during birth (newborn) P15.9
  - esophagus K22.2
  - eustachian tube — *see* Obstruction, eustachian tube, cartilaginous
  - facies Q67.1
  - fracture
    - nontraumatic NOS — *see* Collapse, vertebra
    - pathological — *see* Fracture, pathological
    - traumatic — *see* Fracture, traumatic
  - heart — *see* Disease, heart
  - intestine — *see* Obstruction, intestine
  - laryngeal nerve, recurrent G52.2
    - with paralysis of vocal cords and larynx J38.00
      - bilateral J38.02
      - unilateral J38.01
  - lumbosacral plexus G54.1
  - lung J98.4
  - lymphatic vessel I89.0
  - medulla — *see* Compression, brain
  - nerve (*see also* Disorder, nerve)G58.9
    - arm NEC — *see* Mononeuropathy, upper limb
    - axillary G54.0
    - cranial — *see* Compression, cranial nerve
    - leg NEC — *see* Mononeuropathy, lower limb
    - median (in carpal tunnel) — *see* Syndrome, carpal tunnel
    - optic — *see* Disorder, nerve, optic
    - plantar — *see* Lesion, nerve, plantar
    - posterior tibial (in tarsal tunnel) — *see* Syndrome, tarsal tunnel
    - root or plexus NOS (in) G54.9
      - intervertebral disc disorder NEC — *see* Disorder, disc, with, radiculopathy
        - with myelopathy — *see* Disorder, disc, with, myelopathy

- **Compression** — *continued*
  - nerve — *continued*
      - neoplastic disease (*see also* Neoplasm)D49.9 *[G55]*
      - spondylosis — *see* Spondylosis, with radiculopathy
    - sciatic (acute) — *see* Lesion, nerve, sciatic
    - sympathetic G90.8
    - traumatic — *see* Injury, nerve
    - ulnar — *see* Lesion, nerve, ulnar
    - upper extremity NEC — *see* Mononeuropathy, upper limb
  - spinal (cord) G95.20
    - by displacement of intervertebral disc NEC (*see also* Disorder, disc, with, myelopathy)
    - nerve root NOS G54.9
      - due to displacement of intervertebral disc NEC — *see* Disorder, disc, with, radiculopathy
        - with myelopathy — *see* Disorder, disc, with, myelopathy
    - specified NEC G95.29
    - spondylogenic (cervical) (lumbar, lumbosacral) (thoracic) — *see* Spondylosis, with myelopathy NEC
      - anterior — *see* Syndrome, anterior, spinal artery, compression
    - traumatic — *see* Injury, spinal cord, by region
  - subcostal nerve (syndrome) — *see* Mononeuropathy, upper limb, specified NEC
  - sympathetic nerve NEC G90.8
  - syndrome T79.5 ☑
  - trachea J39.8
  - ulnar nerve (by scar tissue) — *see* Lesion, nerve, ulnar
  - umbilical cord
    - complicating delivery O69.2 ☑
      - cord around neck O69.1 ☑
      - prolapse O69.0 ☑
      - specified NEC O69.2 ☑
  - ureter N13.5
  - vein I87.1
  - vena cava (inferior) (superior) I87.1
- **Compulsion, compulsive**
  - gambling F63.0
  - neurosis F42.8
  - personality F60.5
  - states F42.8
  - swearing F42.8
    - in Gilles de la Tourette's syndrome F95.2
  - tics and spasms F95.9
- **Concato's** disease (pericardial polyserositis) A19.9
  - nontubercular I31.1
  - pleural — *see* Pleurisy, with effusion
- **Concavity** chest wall M95.4
- **Concealed** penis Q55.69
- **Concern** (normal) about sick person in family Z63.6
- **Concrescence** (teeth) K00.2
- **Concretio** cordis I31.1
  - rheumatic I09.2
- **Concretion** (*see also* Calculus)
  - appendicular K38.1
  - canaliculus — *see* Dacryolith
  - clitoris N90.89
  - conjunctiva H11.12 ☑
  - eyelid — *see* Disorder, eyelid, specified type NEC
  - lacrimal passages — *see* Dacryolith
  - prepuce (male) N47.8
  - salivary gland (any) K11.5
  - seminal vesicle N50.89
  - tonsil J35.8
- **Concussion** (brain) (cerebral) (current) S06.0X9 ☑
  - with
    - loss of consciousness of 30 minutes or less S06.0X1 ☑
    - loss of consciousness of unspecified durationS06.0X9
  - blast (air) (hydraulic) (immersion) (underwater)
    - abdomen or thorax — *see* Injury, blast, by site
    - ear with acoustic nerve injury — *see* Injury, nerve, acoustic, specified type NEC
  - cauda equina S34.3 ☑
  - conus medullaris S34.02 ☑
  - ocular S05.8X ☑
  - spinal (cord)
    - cervical S14.0 ☑
    - lumbar S34.01 ☑
    - sacral S34.02 ☑
    - thoracic S24.0 ☑
  - syndrome F07.81
- **without** loss of consciousness S06.0X0 ☑
- **Condition** — *see* Disease

- **Conditions** arising in the perinatal period — *see* Newborn, affected by
- **Conduct** disorder — *see* Disorder, conduct
- **Condyloma** A63.0
  - acuminatum A63.0
  - gonorrheal A54.09
  - latum A51.31
  - syphilitic A51.31
    - congenital A50.07
  - venereal, syphilitic A51.31
- **Conflagration** (*see also* Burn)
  - asphyxia (by inhalation of gases, fumes or vapors) (*see also* Table of Drugs and Chemicals)T59.9 ☑
- **Conflict** (with) (*see also* Discord)
  - family Z73.9
  - marital Z63.0
    - involving divorce or estrangement Z63.5
  - parent-child Z62.820
    - parent-adopted child Z62.821
    - parent-biological child Z62.820
    - parent-foster child Z62.822
  - social role NEC Z73.5
- **Confluent** — *see* condition
- **Confusion,** confused R41.0
  - epileptic F05
  - mental state (psychogenic) F44.89
  - psychogenic F44.89
  - reactive (from emotional stress, psychological trauma) F44.89
- **Confusional** arousals G47.51
- **Congelation** T69.9 ☑
- **Congenital** (*see also* condition)
  - aortic septum Q25.49
  - intrinsic factor deficiency D51.0
  - malformation — *see* Anomaly
- **Congestion,** congestive
  - bladder N32.89
  - bowel K63.89
  - brain G93.89
  - breast N64.59
  - bronchial J98.09
  - catarrhal J31.0
  - chest R09.89
  - chill, malarial — *see* Malaria
  - circulatory NEC I99.8
  - duodenum K31.89
  - eye — *see* Hyperemia, conjunctiva
  - facial, due to birth injury P15.4
  - general R68.89
  - glottis J37.0
  - heart — *see* Failure, heart, congestive
  - hepatic K76.1
  - hypostatic (lung) — *see* Edema, lung
  - intestine K63.89
  - kidney N28.89
  - labyrinth — *see* subcategory H83.8
  - larynx J37.0
  - liver K76.1
  - lung R09.89
    - active or acute — *see* Pneumonia
  - malaria, malarial — *see* Malaria
  - nasal R09.81
  - nose R09.81
  - orbit, orbital (*see also* Exophthalmos)
    - inflammatory (chronic) — *see* Inflammation, orbit
  - ovary N83.8
  - pancreas K86.89
  - pelvic, female N94.89
  - pleural J94.8
  - prostate (active) N42.1
  - pulmonary — *see* Congestion, lung
  - renal N28.89
  - retina H35.81
  - seminal vesicle N50.1
  - spinal cord G95.19
  - spleen (chronic) D73.2
  - stomach K31.89
  - trachea — *see* Tracheitis
  - urethra N36.8
  - uterus N85.8
    - with subinvolution N85.3
  - venous (passive) I87.8
  - viscera R68.89
- **Congestive** — *see* Congestion
- **Conical**
  - cervix (hypertrophic elongation) N88.4
  - cornea — *see* Keratoconus
  - teeth K00.2
- **Conjoined** twins Q89.4
- **Conjugal** maladjustment Z63.0
  - involving divorce or estrangement Z63.5

- **Conjunctiva** — *see* condition
- **Conjunctivitis** (staphylococcal) (streptococcal) NOS H10.9
  - Acanthamoeba B60.12
  - acute H10.3 ☑
    - atopic H10.1 ☑
    - mucopurulent H10.02 ☑
      - follicular H10.01 ☑
    - chemical (*see also* Corrosion, cornea)H10.21 ☑
    - pseudomembranous H10.22 ☑
    - serous except viral H10.23 ☑
      - viral — *see* Conjunctivitis, viral
    - toxic H10.21 ☑
  - adenoviral (acute) (follicular) B30.1
  - allergic (acute) — *see* Conjunctivitis, acute, atopic
    - chronic H10.45
      - vernal H10.44
  - anaphylactic — *see* Conjunctivitis, acute, atopic
  - Apollo B30.3
  - atopic (acute) — *see* Conjunctivitis, acute, atopic
  - Béal's B30.2
  - blennorrhagic (gonococcal) (neonatorum) A54.31
  - chemical (acute) (*see also* Corrosion, cornea)H10.21 ☑
  - chlamydial A74.0
    - due to trachoma A71.1
    - neonatal P39.1
  - chronic (nodosa) (petrificans) (phlyctenular) H10.40 ☑
    - allergic H10.45
      - vernal H10.44
    - follicular H10.43 ☑
    - giant papillary H10.41 ☑
    - simple H10.42 ☑
    - vernal H10.44
  - coxsackievirus 24 B30.3
  - diphtheritic A36.86
  - due to
    - dust — *see* Conjunctivitis, acute, atopic
    - filariasis B74.9
    - mucocutaneous leishmaniasis B55.2
  - enterovirus type 70 (hemorrhagic) B30.3
  - epidemic (viral) B30.9
    - hemorrhagic B30.3
  - gonococcal (neonatorum) A54.31
  - granular (trachomatous) A71.1
    - sequelae (late effect) B94.0
  - hemorrhagic (acute) (epidemic) B30.3
  - herpes zoster B02.31
  - in (due to)
    - Acanthamoeba B60.12
    - adenovirus (acute) (follicular) B30.1
    - Chlamydia A74.0
    - coxsackievirus 24 B30.3
    - diphtheria A36.86
    - enterovirus type 70 (hemorrhagic) B30.3
    - filariasis B74.9
    - gonococci A54.31
    - herpes (simplex) virus B00.53
      - zoster B02.31
    - infectious disease NEC B99 ☑
    - meningococci A39.89
    - mucocutaneous leishmaniasis B55.2
    - rosacea L71.9
    - syphilis (late) A52.71
    - zoster B02.31
  - inclusion A74.0
  - infantile P39.1
    - gonococcal A54.31
  - Koch-Weeks' — *see* Conjunctivitis, acute, mucopurulent
  - light — *see* Conjunctivitis, acute, atopic
  - ligneous — *see* Blepharoconjunctivitis, ligneous
  - meningococcal A39.89
  - mucopurulent — *see* Conjunctivitis, acute, mucopurulent
  - neonatal P39.1
    - gonococcal A54.31
  - Newcastle B30.8
  - of Béal B30.2
  - parasitic
    - filariasis B74.9
    - mucocutaneous leishmaniasis B55.2
  - Parinaud's H10.89
  - petrificans H10.89
  - rosacea L71.9
  - specified NEC H10.89
  - swimming-pool B30.1
  - trachomatous A71.1
    - acute A71.0
    - sequelae (late effect) B94.0
  - traumatic NEC H10.89

- **Conjunctivitis** — *continued*
  - tuberculous A18.59
  - tularemic A21.1
  - tularensis A21.1
  - viral B30.9
    - due to
      - adenovirus B30.1
      - enterovirus B30.3
    - specified NEC B30.8
- **Conjunctivochalasis** H11.82 ☑
- **Connective** tissue — *see* condition
- **Conn's** syndrome E26.01
- **Conradi** (-Hunermann) disease Q77.3
- **Consanguinity** Z84.3
  - counseling Z71.89
- **Conscious** simulation (of illness) Z76.5
- **Consecutive** — *see* condition
- **Consolidation** lung (base) — *see* Pneumonia, lobar
- **Constipation** (atonic) (neurogenic) (simple) (spastic) K59.00
  - chronic K59.09
    - idiopathic K59.04
  - drug-induced K59.03
  - functional K59.04
  - outlet dysfunction K59.02
  - psychogenic F45.8
  - slow transit K59.01
  - specified NEC K59.09
- **Constitutional** (*see also* condition)
  - substandard F60.7
- **Constitutionally** substandard F60.7
- **Constriction** (*see also* Stricture)
  - auditory canal — *see* Stenosis, external ear canal
  - bronchial J98.09
  - duodenum K31.5
  - esophagus K22.2
  - external
    - abdomen, abdominal (wall) S30.841 ☑
    - alveolar process S00.542 ☑
    - ankle S90.54 ☑
    - antecubital space — *see* Constriction, external, forearm
    - arm (upper) S40.84 ☑
    - auricle — *see* Constriction, external, ear
    - axilla — *see* Constriction, external, arm
    - back, lower S30.840 ☑
    - breast S20.14 ☑
    - brow S00.84 ☑
    - buttock S30.840 ☑
    - calf — *see* Constriction, external, leg
    - canthus — *see* Constriction, external, eyelid
    - cheek S00.84 ☑
      - internal S00.542 ☑
    - chest wall — *see* Constriction, external, thorax
    - chin S00.84 ☑
    - clitoris S30.844 ☑
    - costal region — *see* Constriction, external, thorax
    - digit (s)
      - foot — *see* Constriction, external, toe
      - hand — *see* Constriction, external, finger
    - ear S00.44 ☑
    - elbow S50.34 ☑
    - epididymis S30.843 ☑
    - epigastric region S30.841 ☑
    - esophagus, cervical S10.14 ☑
    - eyebrow — *see* Constriction, external, eyelid
    - eyelid S00.24 ☑
    - face S00.84 ☑
    - finger (s) S60.44 ☑
      - index S60.44 ☑
      - little S60.44 ☑
      - middle S60.44 ☑
      - ring S60.44 ☑
    - flank S30.841 ☑
    - foot (except toe (s) alone) S90.84 ☑
      - toe — *see* Constriction, external, toe
    - forearm S50.84 ☑
      - elbow only — *see* Constriction, external, elbow
    - forehead S00.84 ☑
    - genital organs, external
      - female S30.846 ☑
      - male S30.845 ☑
    - groin S30.841 ☑
    - gum S00.542 ☑
    - hand S60.54 ☑
    - head S00.94 ☑
      - ear — *see* Constriction, external, ear
      - eyelid — *see* Constriction, external, eyelid
      - lip S00.541 ☑
      - nose S00.34 ☑

- **Constriction** — *continued*
  - external — *continued*
      - oral cavity S00.542 ☑
      - scalp S00.04 ☑
      - specified site NEC S00.84 ☑
    - heel — *see* Constriction, external, foot
    - hip S70.24 ☑
    - inguinal region S30.841 ☑
    - interscapular region S20.449 ☑
    - jaw S00.84 ☑
    - knee S80.24 ☑
    - labium (majus) (minus) S30.844 ☑
    - larynx S10.14 ☑
    - leg (lower) S80.84 ☑
      - knee — *see* Constriction, external, knee
      - upper — *see* Constriction, external, thigh
    - lip S00.541 ☑
    - lower back S30.840 ☑
    - lumbar region S30.840 ☑
    - malar region S00.84 ☑
    - mammary — *see* Constriction, external, breast
    - mastoid region S00.84 ☑
    - mouth S00.542 ☑
    - nail
      - finger — *see* Constriction, external, finger
      - toe — *see* Constriction, external, toe
    - nasal S00.34 ☑
    - neck S10.94 ☑
      - specified site NEC S10.84 ☑
      - throat S10.14 ☑
    - nose S00.34 ☑
    - occipital region S00.04 ☑
    - oral cavity S00.542 ☑
    - orbital region — *see* Constriction, external, eyelid
    - palate S00.542 ☑
    - palm — *see* Constriction, external, hand
    - parietal region S00.04 ☑
    - pelvis S30.840 ☑
    - penis S30.842 ☑
    - perineum
      - female S30.844 ☑
      - male S30.840 ☑
    - periocular area — *see* Constriction, external, eyelid
    - phalanges
      - finger — *see* Constriction, external, finger
      - toe — *see* Constriction, external, toe
    - pharynx S10.14 ☑
    - pinna — *see* Constriction, external, ear
    - popliteal space — *see* Constriction, external, knee
    - prepuce S30.842 ☑
    - pubic region S30.840 ☑
    - pudendum
      - female S30.846 ☑
      - male S30.845 ☑
    - sacral region S30.840 ☑
    - scalp S00.04 ☑
    - scapular region — *see* Constriction, external, shoulder
    - scrotum S30.843 ☑
    - shin — *see* Constriction, external, leg
    - shoulder S40.24 ☑
    - sternal region S20.349 ☑
    - submaxillary region S00.84 ☑
    - submental region S00.84 ☑
    - subungual
      - finger (s) — *see* Constriction, external, finger
      - toe (s) — *see* Constriction, external, toe
    - supraclavicular fossa S10.84 ☑
    - supraorbital S00.84 ☑
    - temple S00.84 ☑
    - temporal region S00.84 ☑
    - testis S30.843 ☑
    - thigh S70.34 ☑
    - thorax, thoracic (wall) S20.94 ☑
      - back S20.44 ☑
      - front S20.34 ☑
    - throat S10.14 ☑
    - thumb S60.34 ☑
    - toe (s) (lesser) S90.44 ☑
      - great S90.44 ☑
    - tongue S00.542 ☑
    - trachea S10.14 ☑
    - tunica vaginalis S30.843 ☑
    - uvula S00.542 ☑
    - vagina S30.844 ☑
    - vulva S30.844 ☑
    - wrist S60.84 ☑
  - gallbladder — *see* Obstruction, gallbladder
  - intestine — *see* Obstruction, intestine

- **Constriction** — *continued*
  - larynx J38.6
    - congenital Q31.8
      - specified NEC Q31.8
      - subglottic Q31.1
  - organ or site, congenital NEC — *see* Atresia, by site
  - prepuce (acquired) (congenital) N47.1
  - pylorus (adult hypertrophic) K31.1
    - congenital or infantile Q40.0
    - newborn Q40.0
  - ring dystocia (uterus) O62.4
  - spastic (*see also* Spasm)
    - ureter N13.5
  - ureter N13.5
    - with infection N13.6
  - urethra — *see* Stricture, urethra
  - visual field (peripheral) (functional) — *see* Defect, visual field
- **Constrictive** — *see* condition
- **Consultation**
  - medical — *see* Counseling, medical
  - religious Z71.81
  - specified reason NEC Z71.89
  - spiritual Z71.81
  - without complaint or sickness Z71.9
    - feared complaint unfounded Z71.1
    - specified reason NEC Z71.89
- **Consumption** — *see* Tuberculosis
- **Contact** (with) (*see also* Exposure (to))
  - acariasis Z20.7
  - AIDS virus Z20.6
  - air pollution Z77.110
  - algae and algae toxins Z77.121
  - algae bloom Z77.121
  - anthrax Z20.810
  - aromatic amines Z77.020
  - aromatic (hazardous) compounds NEC Z77.028
  - aromatic dyes NOS Z77.028
  - arsenic Z77.010
  - asbestos Z77.090
  - bacterial disease NEC Z20.818
  - benzene Z77.021
  - blue-green algae bloom Z77.121
  - body fluids (potentially hazardous) Z77.21
  - brown tide Z77.121
  - chemicals (chiefly nonmedicinal) (hazardous) NEC Z77.098
  - cholera Z20.09
  - chromium compounds Z77.018
  - communicable disease Z20.9
    - bacterial NEC Z20.818
    - specified NEC Z20.89
    - viral NEC Z20.828
  - cyanobacteria bloom Z77.121
  - dyes Z77.098
  - Escherichia coli (E. coli) Z20.01
  - fiberglass — *see* Table of Drugs and Chemicals, fiberglass
  - German measles Z20.4
  - gonorrhea Z20.2
  - hazardous metals NEC Z77.018
  - hazardous substances NEC Z77.29
  - hazards in the physical environment NEC Z77.128
  - hazards to health NEC Z77.9
  - HIV Z20.6
  - HTLV-III/LAV Z20.6
  - human immunodeficiency virus (HIV) Z20.6
  - infection Z20.9
    - specified NEC Z20.89
  - infestation (parasitic) NEC Z20.7
  - intestinal infectious disease NEC Z20.09
    - Escherichia coli (E. coli) Z20.01
  - lead Z77.011
  - meningococcus Z20.811
  - mold (toxic) Z77.120
  - nickel dust Z77.018
  - noise Z77.122
  - parasitic disease Z20.7
  - pediculosis Z20.7
  - pfiesteria piscicida Z77.121
  - poliomyelitis Z20.89
  - pollution
    - air Z77.110
    - environmental NEC Z77.118
    - soil Z77.112
    - water Z77.111
  - polycyclic aromatic hydrocarbons Z77.028
  - rabies Z20.3
  - radiation, naturally occurring NEC Z77.123
  - radon Z77.123
  - red tide (Florida) Z77.121
- **Contact** — *continued*
  - rubella Z20.4
  - sexually-transmitted disease Z20.2
  - smallpox (laboratory) Z20.89
  - syphilis Z20.2
  - tuberculosis Z20.1
  - uranium Z77.012
  - varicella Z20.820
  - venereal disease Z20.2
  - viral disease NEC Z20.828
  - viral hepatitis Z20.5
  - water pollution Z77.111
- **Contamination,** food — *see* Intoxication, food-borne
- **Contraception,** contraceptive
  - advice Z30.09
  - counseling Z30.09
  - device (intrauterine) (in situ) Z97.5
    - causing menorrhagia T83.83 ☑
    - checking Z30.431
    - complications — *see* Complications, intrauterine, contraceptive device
    - in place Z97.5
    - initial prescription Z30.014
    - reinsertion Z30.433
    - removal Z30.432
    - replacement Z30.433
  - emergency (postcoital) Z30.012
  - initial prescription Z30.019
    - barrier Z30.018
    - diaphragm Z30.018
    - injectable Z30.013
    - intrauterine device Z30.014
    - pills Z30.011
    - postcoital (emergency) Z30.012
    - specified type NEC Z30.018
    - subdermal implantable Z30.017
    - transdermal patch hormonal Z30.016
    - vaginal ring hormonal Z30.015
  - maintenance Z30.40
    - barrier Z30.49
    - diaphragm Z30.49
    - examination Z30.8
    - injectable Z30.42
    - intrauterine device Z30.431
    - pills Z30.41
    - specified type NEC Z30.49
    - subdermal implantable Z30.46
    - transdermal patch hormonal Z30.45
    - vaginal ring hormonal Z30.44
  - management Z30.9
    - specified NEC Z30.8
  - postcoital (emergency) Z30.012
  - prescription Z30.019
    - repeat Z30.40
  - sterilization Z30.2
  - surveillance (drug) — *see* Contraception, maintenance
- **Contraction** (s), contracture, contracted
  - Achilles tendon (*see also* Short, tendon, Achilles)
    - congenital Q66.89
  - amputation stump (surgical) (flexion) (late) (next proximal joint) T87.89
  - anus K59.8
  - bile duct (common) (hepatic) K83.8
  - bladder N32.89
    - neck or sphincter N32.0
  - bowel, cecum, colon or intestine, any part — *see* Obstruction, intestine
  - Braxton Hicks — *see* False, labor
  - breast implant, capsular T85.44 ☑
  - bronchial J98.09
  - burn (old) — *see* Cicatrix
  - cervix — *see* Stricture, cervix
  - cicatricial — *see* Cicatrix
  - conjunctiva, trachomatous, active A71.1
    - sequelae (late effect) B94.0
  - Dupuytren's M72.0
  - eyelid — *see* Disorder, eyelid function
  - fascia (lata) (postural) M72.8
    - Dupuytren's M72.0
    - palmar M72.0
    - plantar M72.2
  - finger NEC (*see also* Deformity, finger)
    - congenital Q68.1
    - joint — *see* Contraction, joint, hand
  - flaccid — *see* Contraction, paralytic
  - gallbladder K82.0
  - heart valve — *see* Endocarditis
  - hip — *see* Contraction, joint, hip
  - hourglass
    - bladder N32.89
      - congenital Q64.79
- **Contraction** — *continued*
  - hourglass — *continued*
    - gallbladder K82.0
      - congenital Q44.1
    - stomach K31.89
      - congenital Q40.2
      - psychogenic F45.8
    - uterus (complicating delivery) O62.4
  - hysterical F44.4
  - internal os — *see* Stricture, cervix
  - joint (abduction) (acquired) (adduction) (flexion) (rotation) M24.50
    - ankle M24.57 ☑
    - congenital NEC Q68.8
      - hip Q65.89
    - elbow M24.52 ☑
    - foot joint M24.57 ☑
    - hand joint M24.54 ☑
    - hip M24.55 ☑
      - congenital Q65.89
    - hysterical F44.4
    - knee M24.56 ☑
    - shoulder M24.51 ☑
    - wrist M24.53 ☑
  - kidney (granular) (secondary) N26.9
    - congenital Q63.8
    - hydronephritic — *see* Hydronephrosis
    - Page N26.2
    - pyelonephritic — *see* Pyelitis, chronic
    - tuberculous A18.11
  - ligament (*see also* Disorder, ligament)
    - congenital Q79.8
  - muscle (postinfective) (postural) NEC M62.40
    - with contracture of joint — *see* Contraction, joint
    - ankle M62.47 ☑
    - congenital Q79.8
      - sternocleidomastoid Q68.0
    - extraocular — *see* Strabismus
    - eye (extrinsic) — *see* Strabismus
    - foot M62.47 ☑
    - forearm M62.43 ☑
    - hand M62.44 ☑
    - hysterical F44.4
    - ischemic (Volkmann's) T79.6 ☑
    - lower leg M62.46 ☑
    - multiple sites M62.49
    - pelvic region M62.45 ☑
    - posttraumatic — *see* Strabismus, paralytic
    - psychogenic F45.8
      - conversion reaction F44.4
    - shoulder region M62.41 ☑
    - specified site NEC M62.48
    - thigh M62.45 ☑
    - upper arm M62.42 ☑
  - neck — *see* Torticollis
  - ocular muscle — *see* Strabismus
  - organ or site, congenital NEC — *see* Atresia, by site
  - outlet (pelvis) — *see* Contraction, pelvis
  - palmar fascia M72.0
  - paralytic
    - joint — *see* Contraction, joint
    - muscle (*see also* Contraction, muscle NEC)
      - ocular — *see* Strabismus, paralytic
  - pelvis (acquired) (general) M95.5
    - with disproportion (fetopelvic) O33.1
      - causing obstructed labor O65.1
      - inlet O33.2
      - mid-cavity O33.3 ☑
      - outlet O33.3 ☑
  - plantar fascia M72.2
  - premature
    - atrium I49.1
    - auriculoventricular I49.49
    - heart I49.49
    - junctional I49.2
    - supraventricular I49.1
    - ventricular I49.3
  - prostate N42.89
  - pylorus NEC (*see also* Pylorospasm)
    - psychogenic F45.8
  - rectum, rectal (sphincter) K59.8
  - ring (Bandl's) (complicating delivery) O62.4
  - scar — *see* Cicatrix
  - spine — *see* Dorsopathy, deforming
  - sternocleidomastoid (muscle), congenital Q68.0
  - stomach K31.89
    - hourglass K31.89
      - congenital Q40.2
      - psychogenic F45.8
    - psychogenic F45.8

Contraction — *continued*
- tendon (sheath) M62.40
  - with contracture of joint — *see* Contraction, joint
  - Achilles — *see* Short, tendon, Achilles
  - ankle M62.47 ☑
    - Achilles — *see* Short, tendon, Achilles
  - foot M62.47 ☑
  - forearm M62.43 ☑
  - hand M62.44 ☑
  - lower leg M62.46 ☑
  - multiple sites M62.49
  - neck M62.48
  - pelvic region M62.45 ☑
  - shoulder region M62.41 ☑
  - specified site NEC M62.48
  - thigh M62.45 ☑
  - thorax M62.48
  - trunk M62.48
  - upper arm M62.42 ☑
- toe — *see* Deformity, toe, specified NEC
- ureterovesical orifice (postinfectional) N13.5
  - with infection N13.6
- urethra (*see also* Stricture, urethra)
  - orifice N32.0
- uterus N85.8
  - abnormal NEC O62.9
  - clonic (complicating delivery) O62.4
  - dyscoordinate (complicating delivery) O62.4
  - hourglass (complicating delivery) O62.4
  - hypertonic O62.4
  - hypotonic NEC O62.2
  - inadequate
    - primary O62.0
    - secondary O62.1
  - incoordinate (complicating delivery) O62.4
  - poor O62.2
  - tetanic (complicating delivery) O62.4
- vagina (outlet) N89.5
- vesical N32.89
  - neck or urethral orifice N32.0
- visual field — *see* Defect, visual field, generalized
- Volkmann's (ischemic) T79.6 ☑

Contusion (skin surface intact) T14.8
- abdomen, abdominal (muscle) (wall) S30.1 ☑
- adnexa, eye NEC S05.8X ☑
- adrenal gland S37.812 ☑
- alveolar process S00.532 ☑
- ankle S90.0 ☑
- antecubital space — *see* Contusion, forearm
- anus S30.3 ☑
- arm (upper) S40.02 ☑
  - lower (with elbow) — *see* Contusion, forearm
- auditory canal — *see* Contusion, ear
- auricle — *see* Contusion, ear
- axilla — *see* Contusion, arm, upper
- back (*see also* Contusion, thorax, back)
  - lower S30.0 ☑
- bile duct S36.13 ☑
- bladder S37.22 ☑
- bone NEC T14.8
- brain (diffuse) — *see* Injury, intracranial, diffuse
  - focal — *see* Injury, intracranial, focal
- brainstem S06.38 ☑
- breast S20.0 ☑
- broad ligament S37.892 ☑
- brow S00.83 ☑
- buttock S30.0 ☑
- canthus, eye S00.1 ☑
- cauda equina S34.3 ☑
- cerebellar, traumatic S06.37 ☑
- cerebral S06.33 ☑
  - left side S06.32 ☑
  - right side S06.31 ☑
- cheek S00.83 ☑
  - internal S00.532 ☑
- chest (wall) — *see* Contusion, thorax
- chin S00.83 ☑
- clitoris S30.23 ☑
- colon — *see* Injury, intestine, large, contusion
- common bile duct S36.13 ☑
- conjunctiva S05.1 ☑
  - with foreign body (in conjunctival sac) — *see* Foreign body, conjunctival sac
- conus medullaris (spine) S34.139 ☑
- cornea — *see* Contusion, eyeball
  - with foreign body — *see* Foreign body, cornea
- corpus cavernosum S30.21 ☑
- cortex (brain) (cerebral) — *see* Injury, intracranial, diffuse
  - focal — *see* Injury, intracranial, focal
- costal region — *see* Contusion, thorax

Contusion — *continued*
- cystic duct S36.13 ☑
- diaphragm S27.802 ☑
- duodenum S36.420 ☑
- ear S00.43 ☑
- elbow S50.0 ☑
  - with forearm — *see* Contusion, forearm
- epididymis S30.22 ☑
- epigastric region S30.1 ☑
- epiglottis S10.0 ☑
- esophagus (thoracic) S27.812 ☑
  - cervical S10.0 ☑
- eyeball S05.1 ☑
- eyebrow S00.1 ☑
- eyelid (and periocular area) S00.1 ☑
- face NEC S00.83 ☑
- fallopian tube S37.529 ☑
  - bilateral S37.522 ☑
  - unilateral S37.521 ☑
- femoral triangle S30.1 ☑
- finger (s) S60.00 ☑
  - with damage to nail (matrix) S60.10 ☑
  - index S60.02 ☑
    - with damage to nail S60.12 ☑
  - little S60.05 ☑
    - with damage to nail S60.15 ☑
  - middle S60.03 ☑
    - with damage to nail S60.13 ☑
  - ring S60.04 ☑
    - with damage to nail S60.14 ☑
  - thumb — *see* Contusion, thumb
- flank S30.1 ☑
- foot (except toe (s) alone) S90.3 ☑
  - toe — *see* Contusion, toe
- forearm S50.1 ☑
  - elbow only — *see* Contusion, elbow
- forehead S00.83 ☑
- gallbladder S36.122 ☑
- genital organs, external
  - female S30.202 ☑
  - male S30.201 ☑
- globe (eye) — *see* Contusion, eyeball
- groin S30.1 ☑
- gum S00.532 ☑
- hand S60.22 ☑
  - finger (s) — *see* Contusion, finger
  - wrist — *see* Contusion, wrist
- head S00.93 ☑
  - ear — *see* Contusion, ear
  - eyelid — *see* Contusion, eyelid
  - lip S00.531 ☑
  - nose S00.33 ☑
  - oral cavity S00.532 ☑
  - scalp S00.03 ☑
  - specified part NEC S00.83 ☑
- heart (*see also* Injury, heart)S26.91 ☑
- heel — *see* Contusion, foot
- hepatic duct S36.13 ☑
- hip S70.0 ☑
- ileum S36.428 ☑
- iliac region S30.1 ☑
- inguinal region S30.1 ☑
- interscapular region S20.229 ☑
- intra-abdominal organ S36.92 ☑
  - colon — *see* Injury, intestine, large, contusion
  - liver S36.112 ☑
  - pancreas — *see* Contusion, pancreas
  - rectum S36.62 ☑
  - small intestine — *see* Injury, intestine, small, contusion
  - specified organ NEC S36.892 ☑
  - spleen — *see* Contusion, spleen
  - stomach S36.32 ☑
- iris (eye) — *see* Contusion, eyeball
- jaw S00.83 ☑
- jejunum S36.428 ☑
- kidney S37.01 ☑
  - major (greater than 2 cm) S37.02 ☑
  - minor (less than 2 cm) S37.01 ☑
- knee S80.0 ☑
- labium (majus) (minus) S30.23 ☑
- lacrimal apparatus, gland or sac S05.8X ☑
- larynx S10.0 ☑
- leg (lower) S80.1 ☑
  - knee — *see* Contusion, knee
- lens — *see* Contusion, eyeball
- lip S00.531 ☑
- liver S36.112 ☑
- lower back S30.0 ☑
- lumbar region S30.0 ☑
- lung S27.329 ☑
  - bilateral S27.322 ☑
  - unilateral S27.321 ☑

Contusion — *continued*
- malar region S00.83 ☑
- mastoid region S00.83 ☑
- membrane, brain — *see* Injury, intracranial, diffuse
  - focal — *see* Injury, intracranial, focal
- mesentery S36.892 ☑
- mesosalpinx S37.892 ☑
- mouth S00.532 ☑
- muscle — *see* Contusion, by site
- nail
  - finger — *see* Contusion, finger, with damage to nail
  - toe — *see* Contusion, toe, with damage to nail
- nasal S00.33 ☑
- neck S10.93 ☑
  - specified site NEC S10.83 ☑
  - throat S10.0 ☑
- nerve — *see* Injury, nerve
- newborn P54.5
- nose S00.33 ☑
- occipital
  - lobe (brain) — *see* Injury, intracranial, diffuse
    - focal — *see* Injury, intracranial, focal
  - region (scalp) S00.03 ☑
- orbit (region) (tissues) S05.1 ☑
- ovary S37.429 ☑
  - bilateral S37.422 ☑
  - unilateral S37.421 ☑
- palate S00.532 ☑
- pancreas S36.229 ☑
  - body S36.221 ☑
  - head S36.220 ☑
  - tail S36.222 ☑
- parietal
  - lobe (brain) — *see* Injury, intracranial, diffuse
    - focal — *see* Injury, intracranial, focal
  - region (scalp) S00.03 ☑
- pelvic organ S37.92 ☑
  - adrenal gland S37.812 ☑
  - bladder S37.22 ☑
  - fallopian tube — *see* Contusion, fallopian tube
  - kidney — *see* Contusion, kidney
  - ovary — *see* Contusion, ovary
  - prostate S37.822 ☑
  - specified organ NEC S37.892 ☑
  - ureter S37.12 ☑
  - urethra S37.32 ☑
  - uterus S37.62 ☑
- pelvis S30.0 ☑
- penis S30.21 ☑
- perineum
  - female S30.23 ☑
  - male S30.0 ☑
- periocular area S00.1 ☑
- peritoneum S36.81 ☑
- periurethral tissue — *see* Contusion, urethra
- pharynx S10.0 ☑
- pinna — *see* Contusion, ear
- popliteal space — *see* Contusion, knee
- prepuce S30.21 ☑
- prostate S37.822 ☑
- pubic region S30.1 ☑
- pudendum
  - female S30.202 ☑
  - male S30.201 ☑
- quadriceps femoris — *see* Contusion, thigh
- rectum S36.62 ☑
- retroperitoneum S36.892 ☑
- round ligament S37.892 ☑
- sacral region S30.0 ☑
- scalp S00.03 ☑
  - due to birth injury P12.3
- scapular region — *see* Contusion, shoulder
- sclera — *see* Contusion, eyeball
- scrotum S30.22 ☑
- seminal vesicle S37.892 ☑
- shoulder S40.01 ☑
- skin NEC T14.8
- small intestine — *see* Injury, intestine, small, contusion
- spermatic cord S30.22 ☑
- spinal cord — *see* Injury, spinal cord, by region
  - cauda equina S34.3 ☑
  - conus medullaris S34.139 ☑
- spleen S36.029 ☑
  - major S36.021 ☑
  - minor S36.020 ☑
- sternal region S20.219 ☑
- stomach S36.32 ☑
- subconjunctival S05.1 ☑
- subcutaneous NEC T14.8

Contusion - Corrosion

- **Contusion** — *continued*
  - submaxillary region S00.83 ☑
  - submental region S00.83 ☑
  - subperiosteal NEC T14.8
  - subungual
    - finger — *see* Contusion, finger, with damage to nail
    - toe — *see* Contusion, toe, with damage to nail
  - supraclavicular fossa S10.83 ☑
  - supraorbital S00.83 ☑
  - suprarenal gland S37.812 ☑
  - temple (region) S00.83 ☑
  - temporal
    - lobe (brain) — *see* Injury, intracranial, diffuse
      - focal — *see* Injury, intracranial, focal
    - region S00.83 ☑
  - testis S30.22 ☑
  - thigh S70.1 ☑
  - thorax (wall) S20.20 ☑
    - back S20.22 ☑
    - front S20.21 ☑
  - throat S10.0 ☑
  - thumb S60.01 ☑
    - with damage to nail S60.11 ☑
  - toe (s) (lesser) S90.12 ☑
    - with damage to nail S90.22 ☑
    - great S90.11 ☑
      - with damage to nail S90.21 ☑
      - specified type NEC S90.221 ☑
  - tongue S00.532 ☑
  - trachea (cervical) S10.0 ☑
    - thoracic S27.52 ☑
  - tunica vaginalis S30.22 ☑
  - tympanum, tympanic membrane — *see* Contusion, ear
  - ureter S37.12 ☑
  - urethra S37.32 ☑
  - urinary organ NEC S37.892 ☑
  - uterus S37.62 ☑
  - uvula S00.532 ☑
  - vagina S30.23 ☑
  - vas deferens S37.892 ☑
  - vesical S37.22 ☑
  - vocal cord (s) S10.0 ☑
  - vulva S30.23 ☑
  - wrist S60.21 ☑
- **Conus** (congenital) (any type) Q14.8
  - cornea — *see* Keratoconus
  - medullaris syndrome G95.81
- **Conversion** hysteria, neurosis or reaction F44.9
- **Converter,** tuberculosis (test reaction) R76.11
- **Conviction** (legal), anxiety concerning Z65.0
  - with imprisonment Z65.1
- **Convulsions** (idiopathic) (*see also* Seizure (s))R56.9
  - apoplectiform (cerebral ischemia) I67.82
  - dissociative F44.5
  - epileptic — *see* Epilepsy
  - epileptiform, epileptoid — *see* Seizure, epileptiform
  - ether (anesthetic) — *see* Table of Drugs and Chemicals, by drug
  - febrile R56.00
    - with status epilepticus G40.901
    - complex R56.01
      - with status epilepticus G40.901
    - simple R56.00
  - hysterical F44.5
  - infantile P90
    - epilepsy — *see* Epilepsy
  - jacksonian — *see* Epilepsy, localization-related, symptomatic, with simple partial seizures
  - myoclonic G25.3
  - newborn P90
  - obstetrical (nephritic) (uremic) — *see* Eclampsia
  - paretic A52.17
  - post traumatic R56.1
  - psychomotor — *see* Epilepsy, localization-related, symptomatic, with complex partial seizures
  - recurrent R56.9
  - reflex R25.8
  - scarlatinal A38.8
  - tetanus, tetanic — *see* Tetanus
  - thymic E32.8
- **Convulsive** (*see also* Convulsions)
- **Cooley's** anemia D56.1
- **Coolie** itch B76.9
- **Cooper's**
  - disease — *see* Mastopathy, cystic
  - hernia — *see* Hernia, abdomen, specified site NEC
- **Copra** itch B88.0
- **Coprophagy** F50.89
- **Coprophobia** F40.298
- **Coproporphyria,** hereditary E80.29
- **Cor**
  - biloculare Q20.8
  - bovis, bovinum — *see* Hypertrophy, cardiac
  - pulmonale (chronic) I27.81
    - acute I26.09
  - triatriatum, triatrium Q24.2
  - triloculare Q20.8
    - biatrium Q20.4
    - biventriculare Q21.1
- **Corbus'** disease (gangrenous balanitis) N48.1
- **Cord** (*see also* condition)
  - around neck (tightly) (with compression)
    - complicating delivery O69.1 ☑
  - bladder G95.89
    - tabetic A52.19
- **Cordis** ectopia Q24.8
- **Corditis** (spermatic) N49.1
- **Corectopia** Q13.2
- **Cori's** disease (glycogen storage) E74.03
- **Corkhandler's** disease or lung J67.3
- **Corkscrew** esophagus K22.4
- **Corkworker's** disease or lung J67.3
- **Corn** (infected) L84
- **Cornea** (*see also* condition)
  - donor Z52.5
  - plana Q13.4
- **Cornelia** de Lange syndrome Q87.1
- **Cornu** cutaneum L85.8
- **Cornual** gestation or pregnancy O00.80
  - with intrauterine pregnancy O00.81
- **Coronary** (artery) — *see* condition
- **Coronavirus,** as cause of disease classified elsewhere B97.29
  - SARS-associated B97.21
- **Corpora** (*see also* condition)
  - amylacea, prostate N42.89
  - cavernosa — *see* condition
- **Corpulence** — *see* Obesity
- **Corpus** — *see* condition
- **Corrected** transposition Q20.5
- **Corrosion** (injury) (acid) (caustic) (chemical) (lime) (external) (internal) T30.4
  - abdomen, abdominal (muscle) (wall) T21.42 ☑
    - first degree T21.52 ☑
    - second degree T21.62 ☑
    - third degree T21.72 ☑
  - above elbow T22.439 ☑
    - first degree T22.539 ☑
    - left T22.432 ☑
      - first degree T22.532 ☑
      - second degree T22.632 ☑
      - third degree T22.732 ☑
    - right T22.431 ☑
      - first degree T22.531 ☑
      - second degree T22.631 ☑
      - third degree T22.731 ☑
    - second degree T22.639 ☑
    - third degree T22.739 ☑
  - alimentary tract NEC T28.7 ☑
  - ankle T25.419 ☑
    - first degree T25.519 ☑
    - left T25.412 ☑
      - first degree T25.512 ☑
      - second degree T25.612 ☑
      - third degree T25.712 ☑
    - multiple with foot — *see* Corrosion, lower, limb, multiple, ankle and foot
    - right T25.411 ☑
      - first degree T25.511 ☑
      - second degree T25.611 ☑
      - third degree T25.711 ☑
    - second degree T25.619 ☑
    - third degree T25.719 ☑
  - anus — *see* Corrosion, buttock
  - arm (s) (meaning upper limb (s)) — *see* Corrosion, upper limb
  - axilla T22.449 ☑
    - first degree T22.549 ☑
    - left T22.442 ☑
      - first degree T22.542 ☑
      - second degree T22.642 ☑
      - third degree T22.742 ☑
    - right T22.441 ☑
      - first degree T22.541 ☑
      - second degree T22.641 ☑
      - third degree T22.741 ☑
    - second degree T22.649 ☑
    - third degree T22.749 ☑
  - back (lower) T21.44 ☑
    - first degree T21.54 ☑
    - second degree T21.64 ☑
- **Corrosion** — *continued*
  - back — *continued*
    - third degree T21.74 ☑
    - upper T21.43 ☑
      - first degree T21.53 ☑
      - second degree T21.63 ☑
      - third degree T21.73 ☑
  - blisters - code as Corrosion, second degree, by site
  - breast (s) — *see* Corrosion, chest wall
  - buttock (s) T21.45 ☑
    - first degree T21.55 ☑
    - second degree T21.65 ☑
    - third degree T21.75 ☑
  - calf T24.439 ☑
    - first degree T24.539 ☑
    - left T24.432 ☑
      - first degree T24.532 ☑
      - second degree T24.632 ☑
      - third degree T24.732 ☑
    - right T24.431 ☑
      - first degree T24.531 ☑
      - second degree T24.631 ☑
      - third degree T24.731 ☑
    - second degree T24.639 ☑
    - third degree T24.739 ☑
  - canthus (eye) — *see* Corrosion, eyelid
  - cervix T28.8 ☑
  - cheek T20.46 ☑
    - first degree T20.56 ☑
    - second degree T20.66 ☑
    - third degree T20.76 ☑
  - chest wall T21.41 ☑
    - first degree T21.51 ☑
    - second degree T21.61 ☑
    - third degree T21.71 ☑
  - chin T20.43 ☑
    - first degree T20.53 ☑
    - second degree T20.63 ☑
    - third degree T20.73 ☑
  - colon T28.7 ☑
  - conjunctiva (and cornea) — *see* Corrosion, cornea
  - cornea (and conjunctiva) T26.6 ☑
  - deep necrosis of underlying tissue - code as Corrosion, third degree, by site
  - dorsum of hand T23.469 ☑
    - first degree T23.569 ☑
    - left T23.462 ☑
      - first degree T23.562 ☑
      - second degree T23.662 ☑
      - third degree T23.762 ☑
    - right T23.461 ☑
      - first degree T23.561 ☑
      - second degree T23.661 ☑
      - third degree T23.761 ☑
    - second degree T23.669 ☑
    - third degree T23.769 ☑
  - ear (auricle) (external) (canal) T20.41 ☑
    - drum T28.91 ☑
    - first degree T20.51 ☑
    - second degree T20.61 ☑
    - third degree T20.71 ☑
  - elbow T22.429 ☑
    - first degree T22.529 ☑
    - left T22.422 ☑
      - first degree T22.522 ☑
      - second degree T22.622 ☑
      - third degree T22.722 ☑
    - right T22.421 ☑
      - first degree T22.521 ☑
      - second degree T22.621 ☑
      - third degree T22.721 ☑
    - second degree T22.629 ☑
    - third degree T22.729 ☑
  - entire body — *see* Corrosion, multiple body regions
  - epidermal loss - code as Corrosion, second degree, by site
  - epiglottis T27.4 ☑
  - erythema, erythematous - code as Corrosion, first degree, by site
  - esophagus T28.6 ☑
  - extent (percentage of body surface)
    - less than 10 per cent T32.0
    - 10-19 per cent (0-9 percent third degree) T32.10
      - with 10-19 percent third degree T32.11
    - 20-29 per cent (0-9 percent third degree) T32.20
      - with
        - 10-19 percent third degree T32.21
        - 20-29 percent third degree T32.22

- **Corrosion** — *continued*
  - extent — *continued*
    - 30-39 per cent (0-9 percent third degree) T32.30
      - with
        - 10-19 percent third degree T32.31
        - 20-29 percent third degree T32.32
        - 30-39 percent third degree T32.33
    - 40-49 per cent (0-9 percent third degree) T32.40
      - with
        - 10-19 percent third degree T32.41
        - 20-29 percent third degree T32.42
        - 30-39 percent third degree T32.43
        - 40-49 percent third degree T32.44
    - 50-59 per cent (0-9 percent third degree) T32.50
      - with
        - 10-19 percent third degree T32.51
        - 20-29 percent third degree T32.52
        - 30-39 percent third degree T32.53
        - 40-49 percent third degree T32.54
        - 50-59 percent third degree T32.55
    - 60-69 per cent (0-9 percent third degree) T32.60
      - with
        - 10-19 percent third degree T32.61
        - 20-29 percent third degree T32.62
        - 30-39 percent third degree T32.63
        - 40-49 percent third degree T32.64
        - 50-59 percent third degree T32.65
        - 60-69 percent third degree T32.66
    - 70-79 per cent (0-9 percent third degree) T32.70
      - with
        - 10-19 percent third degree T32.71
        - 20-29 percent third degree T32.72
        - 30-39 percent third degree T32.73
        - 40-49 percent third degree T32.74
        - 50-59 percent third degree T32.75
        - 60-69 percent third degree T32.76
        - 70-79 percent third degree T32.77
    - 80-89 per cent (0-9 percent third degree) T32.80
      - with
        - 10-19 percent third degree T32.81
        - 20-29 percent third degree T32.82
        - 30-39 percent third degree T32.83
        - 40-49 percent third degree T32.84
        - 50-59 percent third degree T32.85
        - 60-69 percent third degree T32.86
        - 70-79 percent third degree T32.87
        - 80-89 percent third degree T32.88
    - 90 per cent or more (0-9 percent third degree) T32.90
      - with
        - 10-19 percent third degree T32.91
        - 20-29 percent third degree T32.92
        - 30-39 percent third degree T32.93
        - 40-49 percent third degree T32.94
        - 50-59 percent third degree T32.95
        - 60-69 percent third degree T32.96
        - 70-79 percent third degree T32.97
        - 80-89 percent third degree T32.98
        - 90-99 percent third degree T32.99
  - extremity — *see* Corrosion, limb
  - eye (s) and adnexa T26.9 ☑
    - with resulting rupture and destruction of eyeball T26.7 ☑
    - conjunctival sac — *see* Corrosion, cornea
    - cornea — *see* Corrosion, cornea
    - lid — *see* Corrosion, eyelid
    - periocular area — *see* Corrosion eyelid
    - specified site NEC T26.8 ☑
  - eyeball — *see* Corrosion, eye
  - eyelid (s) T26.5 ☑
  - face — *see* Corrosion, head
  - finger T23.429 ☑
    - first degree T23.529 ☑
    - left T23.422 ☑
      - first degree T23.522 ☑
      - second degree T23.622 ☑
      - third degree T23.722 ☑
    - multiple sites (without thumb) T23.439 ☑
      - with thumb T23.449 ☑
        - first degree T23.549 ☑
        - left T23.442 ☑
          - first degree T23.542 ☑
          - second degree T23.642 ☑
          - third degree T23.742 ☑
        - right T23.441 ☑
          - first degree T23.541 ☑

- **Corrosion** — *continued*
  - finger — *continued*
          - second degree T23.641 ☑
          - third degree T23.741 ☑
        - second degree T23.649 ☑
        - third degree T23.749 ☑
      - first degree T23.539 ☑
      - left T23.432 ☑
        - first degree T23.532 ☑
        - second degree T23.632 ☑
        - third degree T23.732 ☑
      - right T23.431 ☑
        - first degree T23.531 ☑
        - second degree T23.631 ☑
        - third degree T23.731 ☑
      - second degree T23.639 ☑
      - third degree T23.739 ☑
    - right T23.421 ☑
      - first degree T23.521 ☑
      - second degree T23.621 ☑
      - third degree T23.721 ☑
    - second degree T23.629 ☑
    - third degree T23.729 ☑
  - flank — *see* Corrosion, abdomen
  - foot T25.429 ☑
    - first degree T25.529 ☑
    - left T25.422 ☑
      - first degree T25.522 ☑
      - second degree T25.622 ☑
      - third degree T25.722 ☑
    - multiple with ankle — *see* Corrosion, lower, limb, multiple, ankle and foot
    - right T25.421 ☑
      - first degree T25.521 ☑
      - second degree T25.621 ☑
      - third degree T25.721 ☑
    - second degree T25.629 ☑
    - third degree T25.729 ☑
  - forearm T22.419 ☑
    - first degree T22.519 ☑
    - left T22.412 ☑
      - first degree T22.512 ☑
      - second degree T22.612 ☑
      - third degree T22.712 ☑
    - right T22.411 ☑
      - first degree T22.511 ☑
      - second degree T22.611 ☑
      - third degree T22.711 ☑
    - second degree T22.619 ☑
    - third degree T22.719 ☑
  - forehead T20.46 ☑
    - first degree T20.56 ☑
    - second degree T20.66 ☑
    - third degree T20.76 ☑
  - fourth degree - code as Corrosion, third degree, by site
  - full thickness skin loss - code as Corrosion, third degree, by site
  - gastrointestinal tract NEC T28.7 ☑
  - genital organs
    - external
      - female T21.47 ☑
        - first degree T21.57 ☑
        - second degree T21.67 ☑
        - third degree T21.77 ☑
      - male T21.46 ☑
        - first degree T21.56 ☑
        - second degree T21.66 ☑
        - third degree T21.76 ☑
    - internal T28.8 ☑
  - groin — *see* Corrosion, abdominal wall
  - hand (s) T23.409 ☑
    - back — *see* Corrosion, dorsum of hand
    - finger — *see* Corrosion, finger
    - first degree T23.509 ☑
    - left T23.402 ☑
      - first degree T23.502 ☑
      - second degree T23.602 ☑
      - third degree T23.702 ☑
    - multiple sites with wrist T23.499 ☑
      - first degree T23.599 ☑
      - left T23.492 ☑
        - first degree T23.592 ☑
        - second degree T23.692 ☑
        - third degree T23.792 ☑
      - right T23.491 ☑
        - first degree T23.591 ☑
        - second degree T23.691 ☑
        - third degree T23.791 ☑
      - second degree T23.699 ☑
      - third degree T23.799 ☑
    - palm — *see* Corrosion, palm

- **Corrosion** — *continued*
  - hand — *continued*
    - right T23.401 ☑
      - first degree T23.501 ☑
      - second degree T23.601 ☑
      - third degree T23.701 ☑
    - second degree T23.609 ☑
    - third degree T23.709 ☑
    - thumb — *see* Corrosion, thumb
  - head (and face) (and neck) T20.40 ☑
    - cheek — *see* Corrosion, cheek
    - chin — *see* Corrosion, chin
    - ear — *see* Corrosion, ear
    - eye (s) only — *see* Corrosion, eye
    - first degree T20.50 ☑
    - forehead — *see* Corrosion, forehead
    - lip — *see* Corrosion, lip
    - multiple sites T20.49 ☑
      - first degree T20.59 ☑
      - second degree T20.69 ☑
      - third degree T20.79 ☑
    - neck — *see* Corrosion, neck
    - nose — *see* Corrosion, nose
    - scalp — *see* Corrosion, scalp
    - second degree T20.60 ☑
    - third degree T20.70 ☑
  - hip (s) — *see* Corrosion, lower, limb
  - inhalation — *see* Corrosion, respiratory tract
  - internal organ (s) (*see also* Corrosion, by site)T28.90 ☑
    - alimentary tract T28.7 ☑
      - esophagus T28.6 ☑
    - esophagus T28.6 ☑
    - genitourinary T28.8 ☑
    - mouth T28.5 ☑
    - pharynx T28.5 ☑
    - specified organ NEC T28.99 ☑
  - interscapular region — *see* Corrosion, back, upper
  - intestine (large) (small) T28.7 ☑
  - knee T24.429 ☑
    - first degree T24.529 ☑
    - left T24.422 ☑
      - first degree T24.522 ☑
      - second degree T24.622 ☑
      - third degree T24.722 ☑
    - right T24.421 ☑
      - first degree T24.521 ☑
      - second degree T24.621 ☑
      - third degree T24.721 ☑
    - second degree T24.629 ☑
    - third degree T24.729 ☑
  - labium (majus) (minus) — *see* Corrosion, genital organs, external, female
  - lacrimal apparatus, duct, gland or sac — *see* Corrosion, eye, specified site NEC
  - larynx T27.4 ☑
    - with lung T27.5 ☑
  - leg (s) (meaning lower limb (s)) — *see* Corrosion, lower limb
  - limb (s)
    - lower — *see* Corrosion, lower, limb
    - upper — *see* Corrosion, upper limb
  - lip (s) T20.42 ☑
    - first degree T20.52 ☑
    - second degree T20.62 ☑
    - third degree T20.72 ☑
  - lower
    - back — *see* Corrosion, back
    - limb T24.409 ☑
      - ankle — *see* Corrosion, ankle
      - calf — *see* Corrosion, calf
      - first degree T24.509 ☑
      - foot — *see* Corrosion, foot
      - knee — *see* Corrosion, knee
      - left T24.402 ☑
        - first degree T24.502 ☑
        - second degree T24.602 ☑
        - third degree T24.702 ☑
      - multiple sites, except ankle and foot T24.499 ☑
        - ankle and foot T25.499 ☑
          - first degree T25.599 ☑
          - left T25.492 ☑
            - first degree T25.592 ☑
            - second degree T25.692 ☑
            - third degree T25.792 ☑
          - right T25.491 ☑
            - first degree T25.591 ☑
            - second degree T25.691 ☑
            - third degree T25.791 ☑
          - second degree T25.699 ☑
          - third degree T25.799 ☑

Corrosion — *continued*
- upper limb (axilla) (scapular region) T22.40 ☑
  - above elbow — *see* Corrosion, above elbow
  - axilla — *see* Corrosion, axilla
  - elbow — *see* Corrosion, elbow
  - first degree T22.50 ☑
  - forearm — *see* Corrosion, forearm
  - hand — *see* Corrosion, hand
  - interscapular region — *see* Corrosion, back, upper
  - multiple sites T22.499 ☑
    - first degree T22.599 ☑
    - left T22.492 ☑
      - first degree T22.592 ☑
      - second degree T22.692 ☑
      - third degree T22.792 ☑
    - right T22.491 ☑
      - first degree T22.591 ☑
      - second degree T22.691 ☑
      - third degree T22.791 ☑
    - second degree T22.699 ☑
    - third degree T22.799 ☑
  - scapular region — *see* Corrosion, scapular region
  - second degree T22.60 ☑
  - shoulder — *see* Corrosion, shoulder
  - third degree T22.70 ☑
  - wrist — *see* Corrosion, hand
- uterus T28.8 ☑
- vagina T28.8 ☑
- vulva — *see* Corrosion, genital organs, external, female
- wrist T23.479 ☑
  - first degree T23.579 ☑
  - left T23.472 ☑
    - first degree T23.572 ☑
    - second degree T23.672 ☑
    - third degree T23.772 ☑
  - multiple sites with hand T23.499 ☑
    - first degree T23.599 ☑
    - left T23.492 ☑
      - first degree T23.592 ☑
      - second degree T23.692 ☑
      - third degree T23.792 ☑
    - right T23.491 ☑
      - first degree T23.591 ☑
      - second degree T23.691 ☑
      - third degree T23.791 ☑
    - second degree T23.699 ☑
    - third degree T23.799 ☑
  - right T23.471 ☑
    - first degree T23.571 ☑
    - second degree T23.671 ☑
    - third degree T23.771 ☑
  - second degree T23.679 ☑
  - third degree T23.779 ☑

Corrosive burn — *see* Corrosion

Corsican fever — *see* Malaria

Cortical — *see* condition

Cortico-adrenal — *see* condition

Coryza (acute) J00
- with grippe or influenza — *see* Influenza, with, respiratory manifestations NEC
- syphilitic
  - congenital (chronic) A50.05

Costen's syndrome or complex M26.69

Costiveness — *see* Constipation

Costochondritis M94.0

Cotard's syndrome F22

Cot death R99

Cotia virus B08.8

Cotton wool spots (retinal) H35.81

Cotungo's disease — *see* Sciatica

Cough (affected) (chronic) (epidemic) (nervous) R05
- with hemorrhage — *see* Hemoptysis
- bronchial R05
  - with grippe or influenza — *see* Influenza, with, respiratory manifestations NEC
- functional F45.8
- hysterical F45.8
- laryngeal, spasmodic R05
- psychogenic F45.8
- smokers' J41.0
- tea taster's B49

Counseling (for) Z71.9
- abuse NEC
  - perpetrator Z69.82
  - victim Z69.81
- alcohol abuser Z71.41
  - family Z71.42
- child abuse
  - nonparental
    - perpetrator Z69.021
    - victim Z69.020
  - parental
    - perpetrator Z69.011
    - victim Z69.010
- consanguinity Z71.89
- contraceptive Z30.09
- dietary Z71.3
- drug abuser Z71.51
  - family member Z71.52
- family Z71.89
- fertility preservation (prior to cancer therapy) (prior to removal of gonads) Z31.62
- for non-attending third party Z71.0
  - related to sexual behavior or orientation Z70.2
- genetic NEC Z31.5
- gestational carrier Z31.7
- health (advice) (education) (instruction) — *see* Counseling, medical
- human immunodeficiency virus (HIV) Z71.7
- impotence Z70.1
- insulin pump use Z46.81
- medical (for) Z71.9
  - boarding school resident Z59.3
  - consanguinity Z71.89
  - feared complaint and no disease found Z71.1
  - human immunodeficiency virus (HIV) Z71.7
  - institutional resident Z59.3
  - on behalf of another Z71.0
    - related to sexual behavior or orientation Z70.2
  - person living alone Z60.2
  - specified reason NEC Z71.89
- natural family planning
  - procreative Z31.61
  - to avoid pregnancy Z30.02
- perpetrator (of)
  - abuse NEC Z69.82
  - child abuse
    - non-parental Z69.021
    - parental Z69.011
  - rape NEC Z69.82
  - spousal abuse Z69.12
- procreative NEC Z31.69
  - fertility preservation (prior to cancer therapy) (prior to removal of gonads) Z31.62
  - using natural family planning Z31.61
- promiscuity Z70.1
- rape victim Z69.81
- religious Z71.81
- sex, sexual (related to) Z70.9
  - attitude (s) Z70.0
  - behavior or orientation Z70.1
  - combined concerns Z70.3
  - non-responsiveness Z70.1
  - on behalf of third party Z70.2
  - specified reason NEC Z70.8
- specified reason NEC Z71.89
- spiritual Z71.81
- spousal abuse (perpetrator) Z69.12
  - victim Z69.11
- substance abuse Z71.89
  - alcohol Z71.41
  - drug Z71.51
  - tobacco Z71.6
- tobacco use Z71.6
- use (of)
  - insulin pump Z46.81
- victim (of)
  - abuse Z69.81
  - child abuse
    - by parent Z69.010
    - non-parental Z69.020
  - rape NEC Z69.81

Coupled rhythm R00.8

Couvelaire syndrome or uterus (complicating delivery) O45.8X ☑

Cowperitis — *see* Urethritis

Cowper's gland — *see* condition

Cowpox B08.010
- due to vaccination T88.1 ☑

Coxa
- magna M91.4 ☑
- plana M91.2 ☑
- valga (acquired) (*see also* Deformity, limb, specified type NEC, thigh)
  - congenital Q65.81
  - sequelae (late effect) of rickets E64.3
- vara (acquired) (*see also* Deformity, limb, specified type NEC, thigh)

Coxa — *continued*
- vara — *continued*
  - congenital Q65.82
  - sequelae (late effect) of rickets E64.3

Coxalgia, coxalgic (nontuberculous) (*see also* Pain, joint, hip)
- tuberculous A18.02

Coxitis — *see* Monoarthritis, hip

Coxsackie (virus) (infection) B34.1
- as cause of disease classified elsewhere B97.11
- carditis B33.20
- central nervous system NEC A88.8
- endocarditis B33.21
- enteritis A08.39
- meningitis (aseptic) A87.0
- myocarditis B33.22
- pericarditis B33.23
- pharyngitis B08.5
- pleurodynia B33.0
- specific disease NEC B33.8

Crabs, meaning pubic lice B85.3

Crack baby P04.41

Cracked nipple N64.0
- associated with
  - lactation O92.13
  - pregnancy O92.11 ☑
  - puerperium O92.12

Cracked tooth K03.81

Cradle cap L21.0

Craft neurosis F48.8

Cramp (s) R25.2
- abdominal — *see* Pain, abdominal
- bathing T75.1 ☑
- colic R10.83
  - psychogenic F45.8
- due to immersion T75.1 ☑
- fireman T67.2 ☑
- heat T67.2 ☑
- immersion T75.1 ☑
- intestinal — *see* Pain, abdominal
  - psychogenic F45.8
- leg, sleep related G47.62
- limb (lower) (upper) NEC R25.2
  - sleep related G47.62
- linotypist's F48.8
  - organic G25.89
- muscle (limb) (general) R25.2
  - due to immersion T75.1 ☑
  - psychogenic F45.8
- occupational (hand) F48.8
  - organic G25.89
- salt-depletion E87.1
- sleep related, leg G47.62
- stoker's T67.2 ☑
- swimmer's T75.1 ☑
- telegrapher's F48.8
  - organic G25.89
- typist's F48.8
  - organic G25.89
- uterus N94.89
  - menstrual — *see* Dysmenorrhea
- writer's F48.8
  - organic G25.89

Cranial — *see* condition

Craniocleidodysostosis Q74.0

Craniofenestria (skull) Q75.8

Craniolacunia (skull) Q75.8

Craniopagus Q89.4

Craniopathy, metabolic M85.2

Craniopharyngeal — *see* condition

Craniopharyngioma D44.4

Craniorachischisis (totalis) Q00.1

Cranioschisis Q75.8

Craniostenosis Q75.0

Craniosynostosis Q75.0

Craniotabes (cause unknown) M83.8
- neonatal P96.3
- rachitic E64.3
- syphilitic A50.56

Cranium — *see* condition

Craw-craw — *see* Onchocerciasis

Creaking joint — *see* Derangement, joint, specified type NEC

Creeping
- eruption B76.9
- palsy or paralysis G12.22

Crenated tongue K14.8

Creotoxism A05.9

Crepitus
- caput Q75.8
- joint — *see* Derangement, joint, specified type NEC

- **Crescent** or conus choroid, congenital Q14.3
- **CREST** syndrome M34.1
- **Cretin,** cretinism (congenital) (endemic) (nongoitrous) (sporadic) E00.9
  - pelvis
    - with disproportion (fetopelvic) O33.0
      - causing obstructed labor O65.0
  - type
    - hypothyroid E00.1
    - mixed E00.2
    - myxedematous E00.1
    - neurological E00.0
- **Creutzfeldt-Jakob** disease or syndrome (with dementia) A81.00
  - familial A81.09
  - iatrogenic A81.09
  - specified NEC A81.09
  - sporadic A81.09
  - variant (vCJD) A81.01
- **Crib** death R99
- **Cribriform** hymen Q52.3
- **Cri-du-chat** syndrome Q93.4
- **Crigler-Najjar** disease or syndrome E80.5
- **Crime,** victim of Z65.4
- **Crimean** hemorrhagic fever A98.0
- **Criminalism** F60.2
- **Crisis**
  - abdomen R10.0
  - acute reaction F43.0
  - addisonian E27.2
  - adrenal (cortical) E27.2
  - celiac K90.0
  - Dietl's N13.8
  - emotional (*see also* Disorder, adjustment)
    - acute reaction to stress F43.0
    - specific to childhood and adolescence F93.8
  - glaucomatocyclitic — *see* Glaucoma, secondary, inflammation
  - heart — *see* Failure, heart
  - nitritoid I95.2
    - correct substance properly administered — *see* Table of Drugs and Chemicals, by drug, adverse effect
    - overdose or wrong substance given or taken — *see* Table of Drugs and Chemicals, by drug, poisoning
  - oculogyric H51.8
    - psychogenic F45.8
  - Pel's (tabetic) A52.11
  - psychosexual identity F64.2
  - renal N28.0
  - sickle-cell D57.00
    - with
      - acute chest syndrome D57.01
      - splenic sequestration D57.02
  - state (acute reaction) F43.0
  - tabetic A52.11
  - thyroid — *see* Thyrotoxicosis with thyroid storm
  - thyrotoxic — *see* Thyrotoxicosis with thyroid storm
- **Crocq's** disease (acrocyanosis) I73.89
- **Crohn's** disease — *see* Enteritis, regional
- **Crooked** septum, nasal J34.2
- **Cross** syndrome E70.328
- **Crossbite** (anterior) (posterior) M26.24
- **Cross-eye** — *see* Strabismus, convergent concomitant
- **Croup,** croupous (catarrhal) (infectious) (inflammatory) (nondiphtheritic) J05.0
  - bronchial J20.9
  - diphtheritic A36.2
  - false J38.5
  - spasmodic J38.5
    - diphtheritic A36.2
  - stridulous J38.5
    - diphtheritic A36.2
- **Crouzon's** disease Q75.1
- **Crowding,** tooth, teeth, fully erupted M26.31
- **CRST** syndrome M34.1
- **Cruchet's** disease A85.8
- **Cruelty** in children (*see also* Disorder, conduct)
- **Crural** ulcer — *see* Ulcer, lower limb
- **Crush,** crushed, crushing T14.8
  - abdomen S38.1 ☑
  - ankle S97.0 ☑
  - arm (upper) (and shoulder) S47. ☑
  - axilla — *see* Crush, arm
  - back, lower S38.1 ☑
  - buttock S38.1 ☑
  - cheek S07.0 ☑
  - chest S28.0 ☑
  - cranium S07.1 ☑

Crush — *continued*

  - ear S07.0 ☑
  - elbow S57.0 ☑
  - extremity
    - lower
      - ankle — *see* Crush, ankle
      - below knee — *see* Crush, leg
      - foot — *see* Crush, foot
      - hip — *see* Crush, hip
      - knee — *see* Crush, knee
      - thigh — *see* Crush, thigh
      - toe — *see* Crush, toe
    - upper
      - below elbow S67.9 ☑
      - elbow — *see* Crush, elbow
      - finger — *see* Crush, finger
      - forearm — *see* Crush, forearm
      - hand — *see* Crush, hand
      - thumb — *see* Crush, thumb
      - upper arm — *see* Crush, arm
      - wrist — *see* Crush, wrist
  - face S07.0 ☑
  - finger (s) S67.1 ☑
    - with hand (and wrist) — *see* Crush, hand, specified site NEC
    - index S67.19 ☑
    - little S67.19 ☑
    - middle S67.19 ☑
    - ring S67.19 ☑
    - thumb — *see* Crush, thumb
  - foot S97.8 ☑
    - toe — *see* Crush, toe
  - forearm S57.8 ☑
  - genitalia, external
    - female S38.002 ☑
      - vagina S38.03 ☑
      - vulva S38.03 ☑
    - male S38.001 ☑
      - penis S38.01 ☑
      - scrotum S38.02 ☑
      - testis S38.02 ☑
  - hand (except fingers alone) S67.2 ☑
    - with wrist S67.4 ☑
  - head S07.9 ☑
    - specified NEC S07.8 ☑
  - heel — *see* Crush, foot
  - hip S77.0 ☑
    - with thigh S77.2 ☑
  - internal organ (abdomen, chest, or pelvis) NEC T14.8
  - knee S87.0 ☑
  - labium (majus) (minus) S38.03 ☑
  - larynx S17.0 ☑
  - leg (lower) S87.8 ☑
    - knee — *see* Crush, knee
  - lip S07.0 ☑
  - lower
    - back S38.1 ☑
    - leg — *see* Crush, leg
  - neck S17.9 ☑
  - nerve — *see* Injury, nerve
  - nose S07.0 ☑
  - pelvis S38.1 ☑
  - penis S38.01 ☑
  - scalp S07.8 ☑
  - scapular region — *see* Crush, arm
  - scrotum S38.02 ☑
  - severe, unspecified site T14.8
  - shoulder (and upper arm) — *see* Crush, arm
  - skull S07.1 ☑
  - syndrome (complication of trauma) T79.5 ☑
  - testis S38.02 ☑
  - thigh S77.1 ☑
    - with hip S77.2 ☑
  - throat S17.8 ☑
  - thumb S67.0 ☑
    - with hand (and wrist) — *see* Crush, hand, specified site NEC
  - toe (s) S97.10 ☑
    - great S97.11 ☑
    - lesser S97.12 ☑
  - trachea S17.0 ☑
  - vagina S38.03 ☑
  - vulva S38.03 ☑
  - wrist S67.3 ☑
    - with hand S67.4 ☑
- **Crusta** lactea L21.0
- **Crusts** R23.4
- **Crutch** paralysis — *see* Injury, brachial plexus
- **Cruveilhier-Baumgarten** cirrhosis, disease or syndrome K74.69
- **Cruveilhier's** atrophy or disease G12.8
- **Crying** (constant) (continuous) (excessive)
  - child, adolescent, or adult R45.83
  - infant (baby) (newborn) R68.11
- **Cryofibrinogenemia** D89.2
- **Cryoglobulinemia** (essential) (idiopathic) (mixed) (primary) (purpura) (secondary) (vasculitis) D89.1
  - with lung involvement D89.1 *[J99]*
- **Cryptitis** (anal) (rectal) K62.89
- **Cryptococcosis,** cryptococcus (infection) (neoformans) B45.9
  - bone B45.3
  - cerebral B45.1
  - cutaneous B45.2
  - disseminated B45.7
  - generalized B45.7
  - meningitis B45.1
  - meningocerebralis B45.1
  - osseous B45.3
  - pulmonary B45.0
  - skin B45.2
  - specified NEC B45.8
- **Cryptopapillitis** (anus) K62.89
- **Cryptophthalmos** Q11.2
  - syndrome Q87.0
- **Cryptorchid,** cryptorchism, cryptorchidism Q53.9
  - bilateral Q53.20
    - abdominal Q53.21
    - perineal Q53.22
  - unilateral Q53.10
    - abdominal Q53.11
    - perineal Q53.12
- **Cryptosporidiosis** A07.2
  - hepatobiliary B88.8
  - respiratory B88.8
- **Cryptostromosis** J67.6
- **Crystalluria** R82.99
- **Cubitus**
  - congenital Q68.8
  - valgus (acquired) M21.0 ☑
    - congenital Q68.8
    - sequelae (late effect) of rickets E64.3
  - varus (acquired) M21.1 ☑
    - congenital Q68.8
    - sequelae (late effect) of rickets E64.3
- **Cultural** deprivation or shock Z60.3
- **Curling** esophagus K22.4
- **Curling's** ulcer — *see* Ulcer, peptic, acute
- **Curschmann** (-Batten) (-Steinert) disease or syndrome G71.11
- **Curse,** Ondine's — *see* Apnea, sleep
- **Curvature**
  - organ or site, congenital NEC — *see* Distortion
  - penis (lateral) Q55.61
  - Pott's (spinal) A18.01
  - radius, idiopathic, progressive (congenital) Q74.0
  - spine (acquired) (angular) (idiopathic) (incorrect) (postural) — *see* Dorsopathy, deforming
    - congenital Q67.5
    - due to or associated with
      - Charcot-Marie-Tooth disease (*see also* subcategory M49.8)G60.0
      - osteitis
        - deformans M88.88
        - fibrosa cystica (*see also* subcategory M49.8)E21.0
      - tuberculosis (Pott's curvature) A18.01
    - sequelae (late effect) of rickets E64.3
    - tuberculous A18.01
- **Cushingoid** due to steroid therapy E24.2
  - correct substance properly administered — *see* Table of Drugs and Chemicals, by drug, adverse effect
  - overdose or wrong substance given or taken — *see* Table of Drugs and Chemicals, by drug, poisoning
- **Cushing's**
  - syndrome or disease E24.9
    - drug-induced E24.2
    - iatrogenic E24.2
    - pituitary-dependent E24.0
    - specified NEC E24.8
  - ulcer — *see* Ulcer, peptic, acute
- **Cusp,** Carabelli - omit code
- **Cut** (external) (*see also* Laceration)
  - muscle — *see* Injury, muscle
- **Cutaneous** (*see also* condition)
  - hemorrhage R23.3
  - larva migrans B76.9
- **Cutis** (*see also* condition)
  - hyperelastica Q82.8
    - acquired L57.4
  - laxa (hyperelastica) — *see* Dermatolysis

Cutis — *continued*
- marmorata R23.8
- osteosis L94.2
- pendula — *see* Dermatolysis
- rhomboidalis nuchae L57.2
- verticis gyrata Q82.8
  - acquired L91.8

Cyanosis R23.0
- due to
  - patent foramen botalli Q21.1
  - persistent foramen ovale Q21.1
- enterogenous D74.8
- paroxysmal digital — *see* Raynaud's disease
  - with gangrene I73.01
- retina, retinal H35.89

Cyanotic heart disease I24.9
- congenital Q24.9

Cycle
- anovulatory N97.0
- menstrual, irregular N92.6

Cyclencephaly Q04.9

Cyclical vomiting (*see also* Vomiting, cyclical)G43.A0
- psychogenic F50.89

Cyclitis (*see also* Iridocyclitis)H20.9
- chronic — *see* Iridocyclitis, chronic
- Fuchs' heterochromic H20.81 ☑
- granulomatous — *see* Iridocyclitis, chronic
- lens-induced — *see* Iridocyclitis, lens-induced
- posterior H30.2 ☑

Cycloid personality F34.0

Cyclophoria H50.54

Cyclopia, cyclops Q87.0

Cyclopism Q87.0

Cyclosporiasis A07.4

Cyclothymia F34.0

Cyclothymic personality F34.0

Cyclotropia H50.41 ☑

Cylindroma (*see also* Neoplasm, malignant, by site)
- eccrine dermal — *see* Neoplasm, skin, benign
- skin — *see* Neoplasm, skin, benign

Cylindruria R82.99

Cynanche
- diphtheritic A36.2
- tonsillaris J36

Cynophobia F40.218

Cynorexia R63.2

Cyphosis — *see* Kyphosis

Cyprus fever — *see* Brucellosis

Cyst (colloid) (mucous) (simple) (retention)
- adenoid (infected) J35.8
- adrenal gland E27.8
  - congenital Q89.1
- air, lung J98.4
- allantoic Q64.4
- alveolar process (jaw bone) M27.40
- amnion, amniotic O41.8X ☑
- aneurysmal M27.49
- anterior
  - chamber (eye) — *see* Cyst, iris
  - nasopalatine K09.1
- antrum J34.1
- anus K62.89
- apical (tooth) (periodontal) K04.8
- appendix K38.8
- arachnoid, brain (acquired) G93.0
  - congenital Q04.6
- arytenoid J38.7
- Baker's M71.2 ☑
  - ruptured M66.0
  - tuberculous A18.02
- Bartholin's gland N75.0
- bile duct (common) (hepatic) K83.5
- bladder (multiple) (trigone) N32.89
- blue dome (breast) — *see* Cyst, breast
- bone (local) NEC M85.60
  - aneurysmal M85.50
    - ankle M85.57 ☑
    - foot M85.57 ☑
    - forearm M85.53 ☑
    - hand M85.54 ☑
    - jaw M27.49
    - lower leg M85.56 ☑
    - multiple site M85.59
    - neck M85.58
    - rib M85.58
    - shoulder M85.51 ☑
    - skull M85.58
    - specified site NEC M85.58
    - thigh M85.55 ☑
    - toe M85.57 ☑
    - upper arm M85.52 ☑
    - vertebra M85.58

Cyst — *continued*
- bone — *continued*
  - solitary M85.40
    - ankle M85.47 ☑
    - fibula M85.46 ☑
    - foot M85.47 ☑
    - hand M85.44 ☑
    - humerus M85.42 ☑
    - jaw M27.49
    - neck M85.48
    - pelvis M85.45 ☑
    - radius M85.43 ☑
    - rib M85.48
    - shoulder M85.41 ☑
    - skull M85.48
    - specified site NEC M85.48
    - tibia M85.46 ☑
    - toe M85.47 ☑
    - ulna M85.43 ☑
    - vertebra M85.48
  - specified type NEC M85.60
    - ankle M85.67 ☑
    - foot M85.67 ☑
    - forearm M85.63 ☑
    - hand M85.64 ☑
    - jaw M27.40
      - developmental (nonodontogenic) K09.1
        - odontogenic K09.0
      - latent M27.0
    - lower leg M85.66 ☑
    - multiple site M85.69
    - neck M85.68
    - rib M85.68
    - shoulder M85.61 ☑
    - skull M85.68
    - specified site NEC M85.68
    - thigh M85.65 ☑
    - toe M85.67 ☑
    - upper arm M85.62 ☑
    - vertebra M85.68
- brain (acquired) G93.0
  - congenital Q04.6
  - hydatid B67.99 *[G94]*
  - third ventricle (colloid), congenital Q04.6
- branchial (cleft) Q18.0
- branchiogenic Q18.0
- breast (benign) (blue dome) (pedunculated) (solitary) N60.0 ☑
  - involution — *see* Dysplasia, mammary, specified type NEC
  - sebaceous — *see* Dysplasia, mammary, specified type NEC
- broad ligament (benign) N83.8
- bronchogenic (mediastinal) (sequestration) J98.4
  - congenital Q33.0
- buccal K09.8
- bulbourethral gland N36.8
- bursa, bursal NEC M71.30
  - with rupture — *see* Rupture, synovium
  - ankle M71.37 ☑
  - elbow M71.32 ☑
  - foot M71.37 ☑
  - hand M71.34 ☑
  - hip M71.35 ☑
  - multiple sites M71.39
  - pharyngeal J39.2
  - popliteal space — *see* Cyst, Baker's
  - shoulder M71.31 ☑
  - specified site NEC M71.38
  - wrist M71.33 ☑
- calcifying odontogenic D16.5
  - upper jaw (bone) (maxilla) D16.4
- canal of Nuck (female) N94.89
  - congenital Q52.4
- canthus — *see* Cyst, conjunctiva
- carcinomatous — *see* Neoplasm, malignant, by site
- cauda equina G95.89
- cavum septi pellucidi — *see* Cyst, brain
- celomic (pericardium) Q24.8
- cerebellopontine (angle) — *see* Cyst, brain
- cerebellum — *see* Cyst, brain
- cerebral — *see* Cyst, brain
- cervical lateral Q18.0
- cervix NEC N88.8
  - embryonic Q51.6
  - nabothian N88.8
- chiasmal optic NEC — *see* Disorder, optic, chiasm
- chocolate (ovary) N80.1
- choledochus, congenital Q44.4
- chorion O41.8X ☑
- choroid plexus G93.0

Cyst — *continued*
- ciliary body — *see* Cyst, iris
- clitoris N90.7
- colon K63.89
- common (bile) duct K83.5
- congenital NEC Q89.8
  - adrenal gland Q89.1
  - epiglottis Q31.8
  - esophagus Q39.8
  - fallopian tube Q50.4
  - kidney Q61.00
    - more than one (multiple) Q61.02
      - specified as polycystic Q61.3
        - adult type Q61.2
        - infantile type NEC Q61.19
          - collecting duct dilation Q61.11
    - solitary Q61.01
  - larynx Q31.8
  - liver Q44.6
  - lung Q33.0
  - mediastinum Q34.1
  - ovary Q50.1
  - oviduct Q50.4
  - periurethral (tissue) Q64.79
  - prepuce Q55.69
  - salivary gland (any) Q38.4
  - sublingual Q38.6
  - submaxillary gland Q38.6
  - thymus (gland) Q89.2
  - tongue Q38.3
  - ureterovesical orifice Q62.8
  - vulva Q52.79
- conjunctiva H11.44 ☑
- cornea H18.89 ☑
- corpora quadrigemina G93.0
- corpus
  - albicans N83.29 ☑
  - luteum (hemorrhagic) (ruptured) N83.1 ☑
- Cowper's gland (benign) (infected) N36.8
- cranial meninges G93.0
- craniobuccal pouch E23.6
- craniopharyngeal pouch E23.6
- cystic duct K82.8
- Cysticercus — *see* Cysticercosis
- Dandy-Walker Q03.1
  - with spina bifida — *see* Spina bifida
- dental (root) K04.8
  - developmental K09.0
  - eruption K09.0
  - primordial K09.0
- dentigerous (mandible) (maxilla) K09.0
- dermoid — *see* Neoplasm, benign, by site
  - with malignant transformation C56. ☑
  - implantation
    - external area or site (skin) NEC L72.0
    - iris — *see* Cyst, iris, implantation
    - vagina N89.8
    - vulva N90.7
  - mouth K09.8
  - oral soft tissue K09.8
  - sacrococcygeal — *see* Cyst, pilonidal
- developmental K09.1
  - odontogenic K09.0
  - oral region (nonodontogenic) K09.1
  - ovary, ovarian Q50.1
- dura (cerebral) G93.0
  - spinal G96.19
- ear (external) Q18.1
- echinococcal — *see* Echinococcus
- embryonic
  - cervix uteri Q51.6
  - fallopian tube Q50.4
  - vagina Q51.6
- endometrium, endometrial (uterus) N85.8
  - ectopic — *see* Endometriosis
- enterogenous Q43.8
- epidermal, epidermoid (inclusion) (see also Cyst, skin) L72.0
  - mouth K09.8
  - oral soft tissue K09.8
- epididymis N50.3
- epiglottis J38.7
- epiphysis cerebri E34.8
- epithelial (inclusion) L72.0
- epoophoron Q50.5
- eruption K09.0
- esophagus K22.8
- ethmoid sinus J34.1
- external female genital organs NEC N90.7
- eye NEC H57.8
  - congenital Q15.8
- eyelid (sebaceous) H02.829

Cyst

- **Cyst** — *continued*
  - eyelid — *continued*
    - infected — *see* Hordeolum
    - left H02.826
      - lower H02.825
      - upper H02.824
    - right H02.823
      - lower H02.822
      - upper H02.821
  - fallopian tube N83.8
    - congenital Q50.4
  - fimbrial (twisted) Q50.4
  - fissural (oral region) K09.1
  - follicle (graafian) (hemorrhagic) N83.0 ☑
    - nabothian N88.8
  - follicular (atretic) (hemorrhagic) (ovarian) N83.0 ☑
    - dentigerous K09.0
    - odontogenic K09.0
    - skin L72.9
      - specified NEC L72.8
  - frontal sinus J34.1
  - gallbladder K82.8
  - ganglion — *see* Ganglion
  - Gartner's duct Q52.4
  - gingiva K09.0
  - gland of Moll — *see* Cyst, eyelid
  - globulomaxillary K09.1
  - graafian follicle (hemorrhagic) N83.0 ☑
  - granulosal lutein (hemorrhagic) N83.1 ☑
  - hemangiomatous D18.00
    - intra-abdominal D18.03
    - intracranial D18.02
    - skin D18.01
    - specified site NEC D18.09
  - hemorrhagic M27.49
  - hydatid (*see also* Echinococcus)B67.90
    - brain B67.99 *[G94]*
    - liver (*see also* Cyst, liver, hydatid)B67.8
    - lung NEC B67.99 *[J99]*
    - Morgagni
      - female Q50.5
      - male (epididymal) Q55.4
        - testicular Q55.29
    - specified site NEC B67.99
  - hymen N89.8
    - embryonic Q52.4
  - hypopharynx J39.2
  - hypophysis, hypophyseal (duct) (recurrent) E23.6
    - cerebri E23.6
  - implantation (dermoid)
    - external area or site (skin) NEC L72.0
    - iris — *see* Cyst, iris, implantation
    - vagina N89.8
    - vulva N90.7
  - incisive canal K09.1
  - inclusion (epidermal) (epithelial) (epidermoid) (squamous) L72.0
    - not of skin - code under Cyst, by site
  - intestine (large) (small) K63.89
  - intracranial — *see* Cyst, brain
  - intraligamentous (*see also* Disorder, ligament)
    - knee — *see* Derangement, knee
  - intrasellar E23.6
  - iris H21.309
    - exudative H21.31 ☑
    - idiopathic H21.30 ☑
    - implantation H21.32 ☑
    - parasitic H21.33 ☑
    - pars plana (primary) H21.34 ☑
      - exudative H21.35 ☑
  - jaw (bone) M27.40
    - aneurysmal M27.49
    - hemorrhagic M27.49
    - traumatic M27.49
    - developmental (odontogenic) K09.0
    - fissural K09.1
  - joint NEC — *see* Disorder, joint, specified type NEC
  - kidney (acquired) N28.1
    - calyceal — *see* Hydronephrosis
    - congenital Q61.00
    - more than one (multiple) Q61.02
      - specified as polycystic Q61.3
        - adult type (autosomal dominant) Q61.2
        - infantile type (autosomal recessive) NEC Q61.19
          - collecting duct dilation Q61.11
    - pyelogenic — *see* Hydronephrosis
    - simple N28.1
    - solitary (single) Q61.01
      - acquired N28.1

- **Cyst** — *continued*
  - labium (majus) (minus) N90.7
    - sebaceous N90.7
  - lacrimal (*see also* Disorder, lacrimal system, specified NEC)
    - gland H04.13 ☑
    - passages or sac — *see* Disorder, lacrimal system, specified NEC
  - larynx J38.7
  - lateral periodontal K09.0
  - lens H27.8
    - congenital Q12.8
  - lip (gland) K13.0
  - liver (idiopathic) (simple) K76.89
    - congenital Q44.6
    - hydatid B67.8
      - granulosus B67.0
      - multilocularis B67.5
  - lung J98.4
    - congenital Q33.0
    - giant bullous J43.9
  - lutein N83.1 ☑
  - lymphangiomatous D18.1
  - lymphoepithelial, oral soft tissue K09.8
  - macula — *see* Degeneration, macula, hole
  - malignant — *see* Neoplasm, malignant, by site
  - mammary gland — *see* Cyst, breast
  - mandible M27.40
    - dentigerous K09.0
    - radicular K04.8
  - maxilla M27.40
    - dentigerous K09.0
    - radicular K04.8
  - medial, face and neck Q18.8
  - median
    - anterior maxillary K09.1
    - palatal K09.1
  - mediastinum, congenital Q34.1
  - meibomian (gland) — *see* Chalazion
    - infected — *see* Hordeolum
  - membrane, brain G93.0
  - meninges (cerebral) G93.0
    - spinal G96.19
  - meniscus, knee — *see* Derangement, knee, meniscus, cystic
  - mesentery, mesenteric K66.8
    - chyle I89.8
  - mesonephric duct
    - female Q50.5
    - male Q55.4
  - milk N64.89
  - Morgagni (hydatid)
    - female Q50.5
    - male (epididymal) Q55.4
      - testicular Q55.29
  - mouth K09.8
  - Müllerian duct Q50.4
    - appendix testis Q55.29
    - cervix Q51.6
    - fallopian tube Q50.4
    - female Q50.4
    - male Q55.29
    - prostatic utricle Q55.4
    - vagina (embryonal) Q52.4
  - multilocular (ovary) D39.10
    - benign — *see* Neoplasm, benign, by site
  - myometrium N85.8
  - nabothian (follicle) (ruptured) N88.8
  - nasoalveolar K09.1
  - nasolabial K09.1
  - nasopalatine (anterior) (duct) K09.1
  - nasopharynx J39.2
  - neoplastic — *see* Neoplasm, uncertain behavior, by site
    - benign — *see* Neoplasm, benign, by site
  - nervous system NEC G96.8
  - neuroenteric (congenital) Q06.8
  - nipple — *see* Cyst, breast
  - nose (turbinates) J34.1
    - sinus J34.1
  - odontogenic, developmental K09.0
  - omentum (lesser) K66.8
    - congenital Q45.8
  - ora serrata — *see* Cyst, retina, ora serrata
  - oral
    - region K09.9
      - developmental (nonodontogenic) K09.1
      - specified NEC K09.8
    - soft tissue K09.9
      - specified NEC K09.8
  - orbit H05.81 ☑

- **Cyst** — *continued*
  - ovary, ovarian (twisted) N83.20 ☑
    - adherent N83.20 ☑
    - chocolate N80.1
    - corpus
      - albicans N83.29 ☑
      - luteum (hemorrhagic) N83.1 ☑
    - dermoid D27.9
    - developmental Q50.1
    - due to failure of involution NEC N83.20 ☑
    - endometrial N80.1
    - follicular (graafian) (hemorrhagic) N83.0 ☑
    - hemorrhagic N83.20 ☑
    - in pregnancy or childbirth O34.8 ☑
      - with obstructed labor O65.5
    - multilocular D39.10
    - pseudomucinous D27.9
    - retention N83.29 ☑
    - serous N83.20 ☑
    - specified NEC N83.29 ☑
    - theca lutein (hemorrhagic) N83.1 ☑
    - tuberculous A18.18
  - oviduct N83.8
  - palate (median) (fissural) K09.1
  - palatine papilla (jaw) K09.1
  - pancreas, pancreatic (hemorrhagic) (true) K86.2
    - congenital Q45.2
    - false K86.3
  - paralabral
    - hip M24.85 ☑
    - shoulder S43.43 ☑
  - paramesonephric duct Q50.4
    - female Q50.4
    - male Q55.29
  - paranephric N28.1
  - paraphysis, cerebri, congenital Q04.6
  - parasitic B89
  - parathyroid (gland) E21.4
  - paratubal N83.8
  - paraurethral duct N36.8
  - paroophoron Q50.5
  - parotid gland K11.6
  - parovarian Q50.5
  - pelvis, female N94.89
    - in pregnancy or childbirth O34.8 ☑
      - causing obstructed labor O65.5
  - penis (sebaceous) N48.89
  - periapical K04.8
  - pericardial (congenital) Q24.8
    - acquired (secondary) I31.8
  - pericoronal K09.0
  - periodontal K04.8
    - lateral K09.0
  - peripelvic (lymphatic) N28.1
  - peritoneum K66.8
    - chylous I89.8
  - periventricular, acquired, newborn P91.1
  - pharynx (wall) J39.2
  - pilar L72.11
  - pilonidal (infected) (rectum) L05.91
    - with abscess L05.01
    - malignant C44.59 ☑
  - pituitary (duct) (gland) E23.6
  - placenta O43.19 ☑
  - pleura J94.8
  - popliteal — *see* Cyst, Baker's
  - porencephalic Q04.6
    - acquired G93.0
  - postanal (infected) — *see* Cyst, pilonidal
  - postmastoidectomy cavity (mucosal) — *see* Complications, postmastoidectomy, cyst
  - preauricular Q18.1
  - prepuce N47.4
    - congenital Q55.69
  - primordial (jaw) K09.0
  - prostate N42.83
  - pseudomucinous (ovary) D27.9
  - pupillary, miotic H21.27 ☑
  - radicular (residual) K04.8
  - radiculodental K04.8
  - ranular K11.8
  - Rathke's pouch E23.6
  - rectum (epithelium) (mucous) K62.89
  - renal — *see* Cyst, kidney
  - residual (radicular) K04.8
  - retention (ovary) N83.29 ☑
    - salivary gland K11.6
  - retina H33.19 ☑
    - ora serrata H33.11 ☑
    - parasitic H33.12 ☑
  - retroperitoneal K68.9
  - sacrococcygeal (dermoid) — *see* Cyst, pilonidal

- **Cyst** — *continued*
  - salivary gland or duct (mucous extravasation or retention) K11.6
  - Sampson's N80.1
  - sclera H15.89
  - scrotum L72.9
    - sebaceous L72.3
  - sebaceous (duct) (gland) L72.3
    - breast — *see* Dysplasia, mammary, specified type NEC
    - eyelid — *see* Cyst, eyelid
    - genital organ NEC
      - female N94.89
      - male N50.89
    - scrotum L72.3
  - semilunar cartilage (knee) (multiple) — *see* Derangement, knee, meniscus, cystic
  - seminal vesicle N50.89
  - serous (ovary) N83.20 ☑
  - sinus (accessory) (nasal) J34.1
  - Skene's gland N36.8
  - skin L72.9
    - breast — *see* Dysplasia, mammary, specified type NEC
    - epidermal, epidermoid L72.0
    - epithelial L72.0
    - eyelid — *see* Cyst, eyelid
    - genital organ NEC
      - female N90.7
      - male N50.89
    - inclusion L72.0
    - scrotum L72.9
    - sebaceous L72.3
    - sweat gland or duct L74.8
  - solitary
    - bone — *see* Cyst, bone, solitary
    - jaw M27.40
    - kidney N28.1
  - spermatic cord N50.89
  - sphenoid sinus J34.1
  - spinal meninges G96.19
  - spleen NEC D73.4
    - congenital Q89.09
    - hydatid (*see also* Echinococcus)B67.99 *[D77]*
  - Stafne's M27.0
  - subarachnoid intrasellar R93.0
  - subcutaneous, pheomycotic (chromomycotic) B43.2
  - subdural (cerebral) G93.0
    - spinal cord G96.19
  - sublingual gland K11.6
  - submandibular gland K11.6
  - submaxillary gland K11.6
  - suburethral N36.8
  - suprarenal gland E27.8
  - suprasellar — *see* Cyst, brain
  - sweat gland or duct L74.8
  - synovial (*see also* Cyst, bursa)
    - ruptured — *see* Rupture, synovium
  - tarsal — *see* Chalazion
  - tendon (sheath) — *see* Disorder, tendon, specified type NEC
  - testis N44.2
    - tunica albuginea N44.1
  - theca lutein (ovary) N83.1 ☑
  - Thornwaldt's J39.2
  - thymus (gland) E32.8
  - thyroglossal duct (infected) (persistent) Q89.2
  - thyrolingual duct (infected) (persistent) Q89.2
  - thyroid (gland) E04.1
  - tongue K14.8
  - tonsil J35.8
  - tooth — *see* Cyst, dental
  - Tornwaldt's J39.2
  - trichilemmal (proliferating) L72.12
  - trichodermal L72.12
  - tubal (fallopian) N83.8
    - inflammatory — *see* Salpingitis, chronic
  - tubo-ovarian N83.8
    - inflammatory N70.13
  - tunica
    - albuginea testis N44.1
    - vaginalis N50.89
  - turbinate (nose) J34.1
  - Tyson's gland N48.89
  - urachus, congenital Q64.4
  - ureter N28.89
  - ureterovesical orifice N28.89
  - urethra, urethral (gland) N36.8
  - uterine ligament N83.8
  - uterus (body) (corpus) (recurrent) N85.8
    - embryonic Q51.818
      - cervix Q51.6
- **Cyst** — *continued*
  - vagina, vaginal (implantation) (inclusion) (squamous cell) (wall) N89.8
    - embryonic Q52.4
  - vallecula, vallecular (epiglottis) J38.7
  - vesical (orifice) N32.89
  - vitreous body H43.89
  - vulva (implantation) (inclusion) N90.7
    - congenital Q52.79
    - sebaceous gland N90.7
  - vulvovaginal gland N90.7
  - wolffian
    - female Q50.5
    - male Q55.4
- **Cystadenocarcinoma** — *see* Neoplasm, malignant, by site
  - bile duct C22.1
  - endometrioid — *see* Neoplasm, malignant, by site
    - specified site — *see* Neoplasm, malignant, by site
    - unspecified site
      - female C56.9
      - male C61
  - mucinous
    - papillary
      - specified site — *see* Neoplasm, malignant, by site
      - unspecified site C56.9
    - specified site — *see* Neoplasm, malignant, by site
    - unspecified site C56.9
  - papillary
    - mucinous
      - specified site — *see* Neoplasm, malignant, by site
      - unspecified site C56.9
    - pseudomucinous
      - specified site — *see* Neoplasm, malignant, by site
      - unspecified site C56.9
    - serous
      - specified site — *see* Neoplasm, malignant, by site
      - unspecified site C56.9
    - specified site — *see* Neoplasm, malignant, by site
    - unspecified site C56.9
  - pseudomucinous
    - papillary
      - specified site — *see* Neoplasm, malignant, by site
      - unspecified site C56.9
    - specified site — *see* Neoplasm, malignant, by site
    - unspecified site C56.9
  - serous
    - papillary
      - specified site — *see* Neoplasm, malignant, by site
      - unspecified site C56.9
    - specified site — *see* Neoplasm, malignant, by site
    - unspecified site C56.9
- **Cystadenofibroma**
  - clear cell — *see* Neoplasm, benign, by site
  - endometrioid D27.9
    - borderline malignancy D39.1 ☑
    - malignant C56. ☑
  - mucinous
    - specified site — *see* Neoplasm, benign, by site
    - unspecified site D27.9
  - serous
    - specified site — *see* Neoplasm, benign, by site
    - unspecified site D27.9
  - specified site — *see* Neoplasm, benign, by site
  - unspecified site D27.9
- **Cystadenoma** (*see also* Neoplasm, benign, by site)
  - bile duct D13.4
  - endometrioid — *see* Neoplasm, benign, by site
    - borderline malignancy — *see* Neoplasm, uncertain behavior, by site
  - malignant — *see* Neoplasm, malignant, by site
  - mucinous
    - borderline malignancy
      - ovary C56. ☑
      - specified site NEC — *see* Neoplasm, uncertain behavior, by site
      - unspecified site C56.9
    - papillary
      - borderline malignancy
        - ovary C56. ☑
- **Cystadenoma** — *continued*
  - mucinous — *continued*
    - papillary
      - borderline malignancy
        - specified site NEC — *see* Neoplasm, uncertain behavior, by site
        - unspecified site C56.9
      - specified site — *see* Neoplasm, benign, by site
      - unspecified site D27.9
    - specified site — *see* Neoplasm, benign, by site
    - unspecified site D27.9
  - papillary
    - borderline malignancy
      - ovary C56. ☑
      - specified site NEC — *see* Neoplasm, uncertain behavior, by site
      - unspecified site C56.9
    - lymphomatosum
      - specified site — *see* Neoplasm, benign, by site
      - unspecified site D11.9
    - mucinous
      - borderline malignancy
        - ovary C56. ☑
        - specified site NEC — *see* Neoplasm, uncertain behavior, by site
        - unspecified site C56.9
      - specified site — *see* Neoplasm, benign, by site
      - unspecified site D27.9
    - pseudomucinous
      - borderline malignancy
        - ovary C56. ☑
        - specified site NEC — *see* Neoplasm, uncertain behavior, by site
        - unspecified site C56.9
      - specified site — *see* Neoplasm, benign, by site
      - unspecified site D27.9
    - serous
      - borderline malignancy
        - ovary C56. ☑
        - specified site NEC — *see* Neoplasm, uncertain behavior, by site
        - unspecified site C56.9
      - specified site — *see* Neoplasm, benign, by site
      - unspecified site D27.9
    - specified site — *see* Neoplasm, benign, by site
    - unspecified site D27.9
  - pseudomucinous
    - borderline malignancy
      - ovary C56. ☑
      - specified site NEC — *see* Neoplasm, uncertain behavior, by site
      - unspecified site C56.9
    - papillary
      - borderline malignancy
        - ovary C56. ☑
        - specified site NEC — *see* Neoplasm, uncertain behavior, by site
        - unspecified site C56.9
      - specified site — *see* Neoplasm, benign, by site
      - unspecified site D27.9
    - specified site — *see* Neoplasm, benign, by site
    - unspecified site D27.9
  - serous
    - borderline malignancy
      - ovary C56. ☑
      - specified site NEC — *see* Neoplasm, uncertain behavior, by site
      - unspecified site C56.9
    - papillary
      - borderline malignancy
        - ovary C56. ☑
        - specified site NEC — *see* Neoplasm, uncertain behavior, by site
        - unspecified site C56.9
      - specified site — *see* Neoplasm, benign, by site
      - unspecified site D27.9
    - specified site — *see* Neoplasm, benign, by site
    - unspecified site D27.9
- **Cystathionine** synthase deficiency E72.11
- **Cystathioninemia** E72.19
- **Cystathioninuria** E72.19
- **Cystic** (*see also* condition)
  - breast (chronic) — *see* Mastopathy, cystic
  - corpora lutea (hemorrhagic) N83.1 ☑
  - duct — *see* condition
  - eyeball (congenital) Q11.0
  - fibrosis — *see* Fibrosis, cystic

- **Cystic** — *continued*
  - kidney (congenital) Q61.9
    - adult type Q61.2
    - infantile type NEC Q61.19
      - collecting duct dilatation Q61.11
    - medullary Q61.5
  - liver, congenital Q44.6
  - lung disease J98.4
    - congenital Q33.0
  - mastitis, chronic — *see* Mastopathy, cystic
  - medullary, kidney Q61.5
  - meniscus — *see* Derangement, knee, meniscus, cystic
  - ovary N83.20 ☑
- **Cysticercosis,** cysticerciasis B69.9
  - with
    - epileptiform fits B69.0
    - myositis B69.81
  - brain B69.0
  - central nervous system B69.0
  - cerebral B69.0
  - ocular B69.1
  - specified NEC B69.89
- **Cysticercus** cellulose infestation — *see* Cysticercosis
- **Cystinosis** (malignant) E72.04
- **Cystinuria** E72.01
- **Cystitis** (exudative) (hemorrhagic) (septic) (suppurative) N30.90
  - with
    - fibrosis — *see* Cystitis, chronic, interstitial
    - hematuria N30.91
    - leukoplakia — *see* Cystitis, chronic, interstitial
    - malakoplakia — *see* Cystitis, chronic, interstitial
    - metaplasia — *see* Cystitis, chronic, interstitial
    - prostatitis N41.3
  - acute N30.00
    - with hematuria N30.01
    - of trigone N30.30
      - with hematuria N30.31
  - allergic — *see* Cystitis, specified type NEC
  - amebic A06.81
  - bilharzial B65.9 *[N33]*
  - blennorrhagic (gonococcal) A54.01
  - bullous — *see* Cystitis, specified type NEC
  - calculous N21.0
  - chlamydial A56.01
  - chronic N30.20
    - with hematuria N30.21
    - interstitial N30.10
      - with hematuria N30.11
    - of trigone N30.30
      - with hematuria N30.31
    - specified NEC N30.20
      - with hematuria N30.21
  - cystic (a) — *see* Cystitis, specified type NEC
  - diphtheritic A36.85
  - echinococcal
    - granulosus B67.39
    - multilocularis B67.69
  - emphysematous — *see* Cystitis, specified type NEC
  - encysted — *see* Cystitis, specified type NEC
  - eosinophilic — *see* Cystitis, specified type NEC
  - follicular — *see* Cystitis, of trigone
  - gangrenous — *see* Cystitis, specified type NEC
  - glandularis — *see* Cystitis, specified type NEC
  - gonococcal A54.01
  - incrusted — *see* Cystitis, specified type NEC
  - interstitial (chronic) — *see* Cystitis, chronic, interstitial
  - irradiation N30.40
    - with hematuria N30.41
  - irritation — *see* Cystitis, specified type NEC
  - malignant — *see* Cystitis, specified type NEC
  - of trigone N30.30
    - with hematuria N30.31
  - panmural — *see* Cystitis, chronic, interstitial
  - polyposa — *see* Cystitis, specified type NEC
  - prostatic N41.3
  - puerperal (postpartum) O86.22
  - radiation — *see* Cystitis, irradiation
  - specified type NEC N30.80
    - with hematuria N30.81
  - subacute — *see* Cystitis, chronic
  - submucous — *see* Cystitis, chronic, interstitial
  - syphilitic (late) A52.76
  - trichomonal A59.03
  - tuberculous A18.12
  - ulcerative — *see* Cystitis, chronic, interstitial
- **Cystocele** (-urethrocele)
  - female N81.10
    - with prolapse of uterus — *see* Prolapse, uterus
- **Cystocele** — *continued*
  - female — *continued*
    - lateral N81.12
    - midline N81.11
    - paravaginal N81.12
  - in pregnancy or childbirth O34.8 ☑
    - causing obstructed labor O65.5
  - male N32.89
- **Cystolithiasis** N21.0
- **Cystoma** (*see also* Neoplasm, benign, by site)
  - endometrial, ovary N80.1
  - mucinous
    - specified site — *see* Neoplasm, benign, by site
    - unspecified site D27.9
  - serous
    - specified site — *see* Neoplasm, benign, by site
    - unspecified site D27.9
  - simple (ovary) N83.29 ☑
- **Cystoplegia** N31.2
- **Cystoptosis** N32.89
- **Cystopyelitis** — *see* Pyelonephritis
- **Cystorrhagia** N32.89
- **Cystosarcoma** phyllodes D48.6 ☑
  - benign D24 ☑
  - malignant — *see* Neoplasm, breast, malignant
- **Cystostomy**
  - attention to Z43.5
  - complication — *see* Complications, cystostomy
  - status Z93.50
    - appendico-vesicostomy Z93.52
    - cutaneous Z93.51
    - specified NEC Z93.59
- **Cystourethritis** — *see* Urethritis
- **Cystourethrocele** (*see also* Cystocele)
  - female N81.10
    - with uterine prolapse — *see* Prolapse, uterus
    - lateral N81.12
    - midline N81.11
    - paravaginal N81.12
  - male N32.89
- **Cytomegalic** inclusion disease
  - congenital P35.1
- **Cytomegalovirus** infection B25.9
- **Cytomycosis** (reticuloendothelial) B39.4
- **Cytopenia** D75.9
  - refractory
    - with multilineage dysplasia D46.A
      - and ring sideroblasts (RCMD RS) D46.B
- **Czerny's** disease (periodic hydrarthrosis of the knee) — *see* Effusion, joint, knee

D

- **Daae** (-Finsen) disease (epidemic pleurodynia) B33.0
- **Da** Costa's syndrome F45.8
- **Dabney's** grip B33.0
- **Dacryoadenitis,** dacryadenitis H04.00 ☑
  - acute H04.01 ☑
  - chronic H04.02 ☑
- **Dacryocystitis** H04.30 ☑
  - acute H04.32 ☑
  - chronic H04.41 ☑
  - neonatal P39.1
  - phlegmonous H04.31 ☑
  - syphilitic A52.71
    - congenital (early) A50.01
  - trachomatous, active A71.1
    - sequelae (late effect) B94.0
- **Dacryocystoblenorrhea** — *see* Inflammation, lacrimal, passages, chronic
- **Dacryocystocele** — *see* Disorder, lacrimal system, changes
- **Dacryolith,** dacryolithiasis H04.51 ☑
- **Dacryoma** — *see* Disorder, lacrimal system, changes
- **Dacryopericystitis** — *see* Dacryocystitis
- **Dacryops** H04.11 ☑
- **Dacryostenosis** (*see also* Stenosis, lacrimal)
  - congenital Q10.5
- **Dactylitis**
  - bone — *see* Osteomyelitis
  - sickle-cell D57.00
    - Hb C D57.219
    - Hb SS D57.00
    - specified NEC D57.819
  - skin L08.9
  - syphilitic A52.77
  - tuberculous A18.03
- **Dactylolysis** spontanea (ainhum) L94.6
- **Dactylosymphysis** Q70.9
  - fingers — *see* Syndactylism, complex, fingers
  - toes — *see* Syndactylism, complex, toes
- **Damage**
  - arteriosclerotic — *see* Arteriosclerosis
  - brain (nontraumatic) G93.9
    - anoxic, hypoxic G93.1
      - resulting from a procedure G97.82
    - child NEC G80.9
    - due to birth injury P11.2
  - cardiorenal (vascular) — *see* Hypertension, cardiorenal
  - cerebral NEC — *see* Damage, brain
  - coccyx, complicating delivery O71.6
  - coronary — *see* Disease, heart, ischemic
  - eye, birth injury P15.3
  - liver (nontraumatic) K76.9
    - alcoholic K70.9
    - due to drugs — *see* Disease, liver, toxic
    - toxic — *see* Disease, liver, toxic
  - medication T88.7 ☑
  - pelvic
    - joint or ligament, during delivery O71.6
    - organ NEC
      - during delivery O71.5
      - following ectopic or molar pregnancy O08.6
  - renal — *see* Disease, renal
  - subendocardium, subendocardial — *see* Degeneration, myocardial
  - vascular I99.9
- **Dana-Putnam** syndrome (subacute combined sclerosis with pernicious anemia) — *see* Degeneration, combined
- **Danbolt** (-Cross) syndrome (acrodermatitis enteropathica) E83.2
- **Dandruff** L21.0
- **Dandy-Walker** syndrome Q03.1
  - with spina bifida — *see* Spina bifida
- **Danlos'** syndrome Q79.6
- **Darier** (-White) disease (congenital) Q82.8
  - meaning erythema annulare centrifugum L53.1
- **Darier-Roussy** sarcoid D86.3
- **Darling's** disease or histoplasmosis B39.4
- **Darwin's** tubercle Q17.8
- **Dawson's** (inclusion body) encephalitis A81.1
- **De** Beurmann (-Gougerot) disease B42.1
- **De** la Tourette's syndrome F95.2
- **De** Lange's syndrome Q87.1
- **De** Morgan's spots (senile angiomas) I78.1
- **De** Quervain's
  - disease (tendon sheath) M65.4
  - syndrome E34.51
  - thyroiditis (subacute granulomatous thyroiditis) E06.1
- **De** Toni-Fanconi (-Debré) syndrome E72.09
  - with cystinosis E72.04
- **Dead**
  - fetus, retained (mother) O36.4 ☑
    - early pregnancy O02.1
  - labyrinth — *see* subcategory H83.2
  - ovum, retained O02.0
- **Deaf** nonspeaking NEC H91.3
- **Deaf mutism** (acquired) (congenital) NEC H91.3
  - hysterical F44.6
  - syphilitic, congenital (*see also* subcategory H94.8)A50.09
- **Deafness** (acquired) (complete) (hereditary) (partial) H91.9 ☑
  - with blue sclera and fragility of bone Q78.0
  - auditory fatigue — *see* Deafness, specified type NEC
  - aviation T70.0 ☑
    - nerve injury — *see* Injury, nerve, acoustic, specified type NEC
  - boilermaker's — *see* subcategory H83.3
  - central — *see* Deafness, sensorineural
  - conductive H90.2
    - and sensorineural
      - mixed H90.8
        - bilateral H90.6
    - bilateral H90.0
    - unilateral H90.1 ☑
      - with restricted hearing on the contralateral side H90.A ☑
  - congenital H90.5
    - with blue sclera and fragility of bone Q78.0
  - due to toxic agents — *see* Deafness, ototoxic
  - emotional (hysterical) F44.6
  - functional (hysterical) F44.6
  - high frequency H91.9 ☑
  - hysterical F44.6
  - low frequency H91.9 ☑
  - mental R48.8
  - mixed conductive and sensorineural H90.8
    - bilateral H90.6
    - unilateral H90.7 ☑

Deafness — *continued*
- nerve — *see* Deafness, sensorineural
- neural — *see* Deafness, sensorineural
- noise-induced (*see also* subcategory)H83.3 ☑
  - nerve injury — *see* Injury, nerve, acoustic, specified type NEC
- nonspeaking H91.3
- ototoxic — *see* subcategory H91.0
- perceptive — *see* Deafness, sensorineural
- psychogenic (hysterical) F44.6
- sensorineural H90.5
  - and conductive
    - mixed H90.8
      - bilateral H90.6
  - bilateral H90.3
  - unilateral H90.4 ☑
    - with restricted hearing on the contralateral side H90.A ☑
- sensory — *see* Deafness, sensorineural
- specified type NEC — *see* subcategory H91.8
- sudden (idiopathic) H91.2 ☑
- syphilitic A52.15
- transient ischemic H93.01 ☑
- traumatic — *see* Injury, nerve, acoustic, specified type NEC
- word (developmental) H93.25

Death (cause unknown) (of) (unexplained) (unspecified cause) R99
- brain G93.82
- cardiac (sudden) (with successful resuscitation) - code to underlying disease
  - family history of Z82.41
  - personal history of Z86.74
- family member (assumed) Z63.4

Debility (chronic) (general) (nervous) R53.81
- congenital or neonatal NOS P96.9
- nervous R53.81
- old age R54
- senile R54

Débove's disease (splenomegaly) R16.1

Decalcification
- bone — *see* Osteoporosis
- teeth K03.89

Decapsulation, kidney N28.89

Decay
- dental — *see* Caries, dental
- senile R54
- tooth, teeth — *see* Caries, dental

Deciduitis (acute)
- following ectopic or molar pregnancy O08.0

Decline (general) — *see* Debility
- cognitive, age-associated R41.81

Decompensation
- cardiac (acute) (chronic) — *see* Disease, heart
- cardiovascular — *see* Disease, cardiovascular
- heart — *see* Disease, heart
- hepatic — *see* Failure, hepatic
- myocardial (acute) (chronic) — *see* Disease, heart
- respiratory J98.8

Decompression sickness T70.3 ☑

Decrease (d)
- absolute neutrophil count — *see* Neutropenia
- blood
  - platelets — *see* Thrombocytopenia
  - pressure R03.1
    - due to shock following
      - injury T79.4 ☑
      - operation T81.19 ☑
- estrogen E28.39
  - postablative E89.40
    - asymptomatic E89.40
    - symptomatic E89.41
- fragility of erythrocytes D58.8
- function
  - lipase (pancreatic) K90.3
  - ovary in hypopituitarism E23.0
  - parenchyma of pancreas K86.89
  - pituitary (gland) (anterior) (lobe) E23.0
    - posterior (lobe) E23.0
- functional activity R68.89
- glucose R73.09
- hematocrit R71.0
- hemoglobin R71.0
- leukocytes D72.819
  - specified NEC D72.818
- libido R68.82
- lymphocytes D72.810
- platelets D69.6
- respiration, due to shock following injury T79.4 ☑
- sexual desire R68.82
- tear secretion NEC — *see* Syndrome, dry eye

Decrease — *continued*
- tolerance
  - fat K90.49
  - glucose R73.09
  - pancreatic K90.3
  - salt and water E87.8
- vision NEC H54.7
- white blood cell count D72.819
  - specified NEC D72.818

Decubitus (ulcer) — *see* Ulcer, pressure, by site
- cervix N86

Deepening acetabulum — *see* Derangement, joint, specified type NEC, hip

Defect, defective Q89.9
- 3-beta-hydroxysteroid dehydrogenase E25.0
- 11-hydroxylase E25.0
- 21-hydroxylase E25.0
- abdominal wall, congenital Q79.59
- antibody immunodeficiency D80.9
- aorticopulmonary septum Q21.4
- atrial septal (ostium secundum type) Q21.1
  - following acute myocardial infarction (current complication) I23.1
  - ostium primum type Q21.2
- atrioventricular
  - canal Q21.2
  - septum Q21.2
- auricular septal Q21.1
- bilirubin excretion NEC E80.6
- biosynthesis, androgen (testicular) E29.1
- bulbar septum Q21.0
- catalase E80.3
- cell membrane receptor complex (CR3) D71
- circulation I99.9
  - congenital Q28.9
  - newborn Q28.9
- coagulation (factor) (*see also* Deficiency, factor)D68.9
  - with
    - ectopic pregnancy O08.1
    - molar pregnancy O08.1
  - acquired D68.4
  - antepartum with hemorrhage — *see* Hemorrhage, antepartum, with coagulation defect
  - due to
    - liver disease D68.4
    - vitamin K deficiency D68.4
  - hereditary NEC D68.2
  - intrapartum O67.0
  - newborn, transient P61.6
  - postpartum O72.3
  - specified type NEC D68.8
- complement system D84.1
- conduction (heart) I45.9
  - bone — *see* Deafness, conductive
- congenital, organ or site not listed — *see* Anomaly, by site
- coronary sinus Q21.1
- cushion, endocardial Q21.2
- degradation, glycoprotein E77.1
- dental bridge, crown, fillings — *see* Defect, dental restoration
- dental restoration K08.50
  - specified NEC K08.59
- dentin (hereditary) K00.5
- Descemet's membrane, congenital Q13.89
- developmental (*see also* Anomaly)
  - cauda equina Q06.3
- diaphragm
  - with elevation, eventration or hernia — *see* Hernia, diaphragm
  - congenital Q79.1
    - with hernia Q79.0
    - gross (with hernia) Q79.0
- ectodermal, congenital Q82.9
- Eisenmenger's Q21.8
- enzyme
  - catalase E80.3
  - peroxidase E80.3
- esophagus, congenital Q39.9
- extensor retinaculum M62.89
- fibrin polymerization D68.2
- filling
  - bladder R93.41
  - kidney R93.42 ☑
  - renal pelvis R93.41
  - stomach R93.3
  - ureter R93.41
  - urinary organs, specified NEC R93.49
- Gerbode Q21.0
- glycoprotein degradation E77.1

Defect — *continued*
- Hageman (factor) D68.2
- hearing — *see* Deafness
- high grade F70
- interatrial septal Q21.1
- interauricular septal Q21.1
- interventricular septal Q21.0
  - with dextroposition of aorta, pulmonary stenosis and hypertrophy of right ventricle Q21.3
  - in tetralogy of Fallot Q21.3
- learning (specific) — *see* Disorder, learning
- lymphocyte function antigen-1 (LFA-1) D84.0
- lysosomal enzyme, post-translational modification E77.0
- major osseous M89.70
  - ankle M89.77 ☑
  - carpus M89.74 ☑
  - clavicle M89.71 ☑
  - femur M89.75 ☑
  - fibula M89.76 ☑
  - fingers M89.74 ☑
  - foot M89.77 ☑
  - forearm M89.73 ☑
  - hand M89.74 ☑
  - humerus M89.72 ☑
  - lower leg M89.76 ☑
  - metacarpus M89.74 ☑
  - metatarsus M89.77 ☑
  - multiple sites M89.79
  - pelvic region M89.75 ☑
  - pelvis M89.75 ☑
  - radius M89.73 ☑
  - scapula M89.71 ☑
  - shoulder region M89.71 ☑
  - specified NEC M89.78
  - tarsus M89.77 ☑
  - thigh M89.75 ☑
  - tibia M89.76 ☑
  - toes M89.77 ☑
  - ulna M89.73 ☑
- mental — *see* Disability, intellectual
- modification, lysosomal enzymes, post-translational E77.0
- obstructive, congenital
  - renal pelvis Q62.39
  - ureter Q62.39
    - atresia — *see* Atresia, ureter
    - cecoureterocele Q62.32
    - megaureter Q62.2
    - orthotopic ureterocele Q62.31
- osseous, major M89.70
  - ankle M89.77 ☑
  - carpus M89.74 ☑
  - clavicle M89.71 ☑
  - femur M89.75 ☑
  - fibula M89.76 ☑
  - fingers M89.74 ☑
  - foot M89.77 ☑
  - forearm M89.73 ☑
  - hand M89.74 ☑
  - humerus M89.72 ☑
  - lower leg M89.76 ☑
  - metacarpus M89.74 ☑
  - metatarsus M89.77 ☑
  - multiple sites M89.9
  - pelvic region M89.75 ☑
  - pelvis M89.75 ☑
  - radius M89.73 ☑
  - scapula M89.71 ☑
  - shoulder region M89.71 ☑
  - specified NEC M89.78
  - tarsus M89.77 ☑
  - thigh M89.75 ☑
  - tibia M89.76 ☑
  - toes M89.77 ☑
  - ulna M89.73 ☑
- osteochondral NEC (*see also* Deformity)M95.8
- ostium
  - primum Q21.2
  - secundum Q21.1
- peroxidase E80.3
- placental blood supply — *see* Insufficiency, placental
- platelets, qualitative D69.1
  - constitutional D68.0
- postural NEC, spine — *see* Dorsopathy, deforming
- reduction
  - limb Q73.8
    - lower Q72.9 ☑
      - absence — *see* Agenesis, leg
        - foot — *see* Agenesis, foot

Defect — *continued*
- reduction — *continued*
  - longitudinal
    - femur Q72.4 ☑
    - fibula Q72.6 ☑
    - tibia Q72.5 ☑
  - specified type NEC Q72.89 ☑
  - split foot Q72.7 ☑
  - specified type NEC Q73.8
  - upper Q71.9 ☑
    - absence — *see* Agenesis, arm
      - forearm — *see* Agenesis, forearm
      - hand — *see* Agenesis, hand
    - lobster-claw hand Q71.6 ☑
    - longitudinal
      - radius Q71.4 ☑
      - ulna Q71.5 ☑
    - specified type NEC Q71.89 ☑
- renal pelvis Q63.8
  - obstructive Q62.39
- respiratory system, congenital Q34.9
- restoration, dental K08.50
  - specified NEC K08.59
- retinal nerve bundle fibers H35.89
- septal (heart) NOS Q21.9
  - acquired (atrial) (auricular) (ventricular) (old) I51.0
  - atrial Q21.1
    - concurrent with acute myocardial infarction — *see* Infarct, myocardium
    - following acute myocardial infarction (current complication) I23.1
  - ventricular (*see also* Defect, ventricular septal)Q21.0
- sinus venosus Q21.1
- speech R47.9
  - developmental F80.9
  - specified NEC R47.89
- Taussig-Bing (aortic transposition and overriding pulmonary artery) Q20.1
- teeth, wedge K03.1
- vascular (local) I99.9
  - congenital Q27.9
- ventricular septal Q21.0
  - concurrent with acute myocardial infarction — *see* Infarct, myocardium
  - following acute myocardial infarction (current complication) I23.2
  - in tetralogy of Fallot Q21.3
- vision NEC H54.7
- visual field H53.40
  - bilateral
    - heteronymous H53.47
    - homonymous H53.46 ☑
  - generalized contraction H53.48 ☑
  - localized
    - arcuate H53.43 ☑
    - scotoma (central area) H53.41 ☑
      - blind spot area H53.42 ☑
    - sector H53.43 ☑
    - specified type NEC H53.45 ☑
- voice R49.9
  - specified NEC R49.8
- wedge, tooth, teeth (abrasion) K03.1

Deferentitis N49.1
- gonorrheal (acute) (chronic) A54.23

Defibrination (syndrome) D65
- antepartum — *see* Hemorrhage, antepartum, with coagulation defect, disseminated intravascular coagulation
- following ectopic or molar pregnancy O08.1
- intrapartum O67.0
- newborn P60
- postpartum O72.3

Deficiency, deficient
- 3-beta hydroxysteroid dehydrogenase E25.0
- 5-alpha reductase (with male pseudohermaphroditism) E29.1
- 11-hydroxylase E25.0
- 21-hydroxylase E25.0
- abdominal muscle syndrome Q79.4
- accelerator globulin (Ac G) (blood) D68.2
- AC globulin (congenital) (hereditary) D68.2
  - acquired D68.4
- acid phosphatase E83.39
- activating factor (blood) D68.2
- adenosine deaminase (ADA) D81.3
- aldolase (hereditary) E74.19
- alpha-1-antitrypsin E88.01
- amino-acids E72.9
- anemia — *see* Anemia
- aneurin E51.9

Deficiency — *continued*
- antibody with
  - hyperimmunoglobulinemia D80.6
  - near-normal immunoglobins D80.6
- antidiuretic hormone E23.2
- anti-hemophilic
  - factor (A) D66
    - B D67
    - C D68.1
  - globulin (AHG) NEC D66
- antithrombin (antithrombin III) D68.59
- ascorbic acid E54
- attention (disorder) (syndrome) F98.8
  - with hyperactivity — *see* Disorder, attention-deficit hyperactivity
- autoprothrombin
  - I D68.2
  - II D67
  - C D68.2
- beta-glucuronidase E76.29
- biotin E53.8
- biotin-dependent carboxylase D81.819
- biotinidase D81.810
- brancher enzyme (amylopectinosis) E74.03
- calciferol E55.9
  - with
    - adult osteomalacia M83.8
    - rickets — *see* Rickets
- calcium (dietary) E58
- calorie, severe E43
  - with marasmus E41
    - and kwashiorkor E42
- cardiac — *see* Insufficiency, myocardial
- carnitine E71.40
  - due to
    - hemodialysis E71.43
    - inborn errors of metabolism E71.42
    - Valproic acid therapy E71.43
  - iatrogenic E71.43
  - muscle palmityltransferase E71.314
  - primary E71.41
  - secondary E71.448
- carotene E50.9
- central nervous system G96.8
- ceruloplasmin (Wilson) E83.01
- choline E53.8
- Christmas factor D67
- chromium E61.4
- clotting (blood) (*see also* Deficiency, coagulation factor)D68.9
- clotting factor NEC (hereditary) (*see also* Deficiency, factor)D68.2
- coagulation NOS D68.9
  - with
    - ectopic pregnancy O08.1
    - molar pregnancy O08.1
  - acquired (any) D68.4
  - antepartum hemorrhage — *see* Hemorrhage, antepartum, with coagulation defect
  - clotting factor NEC (*see also* Deficiency, factor)D68.2
  - due to
    - hyperprothrombinemia D68.4
    - liver disease D68.4
    - vitamin K deficiency D68.4
  - newborn, transient P61.6
  - postpartum O72.3
  - specified NEC D68.8
- cognitive F09
- color vision H53.50
  - achromatopsia H53.51
  - acquired H53.52
  - deuteranomaly H53.53
  - protanomaly H53.54
  - specified type NEC H53.59
  - tritanomaly H53.55
- combined glucocorticoid and mineralocorticoid E27.49
- contact factor D68.2
- copper (nutritional) E61.0
- corticoadrenal E27.40
  - primary E27.1
- craniofacial axis Q75.0
- cyanocobalamin E53.8
- C1 esterase inhibitor (C1-INH) D84.1
- debrancher enzyme (limit dextrinosis) E74.03
- dehydrogenase
  - long chain/very long chain acyl CoA E71.310
  - medium chain acyl CoA E71.311
  - short chain acyl CoA E71.312
- diet E63.9
- dihydropyrimidine dehydrogenase (DPD) E88.89

Deficiency — *continued*
- disaccharidase E73.9
- edema — *see* Malnutrition, severe
- endocrine E34.9
- energy-supply — *see* Malnutrition
- enzymes, circulating NEC E88.09
- ergosterol E55.9
  - with
    - adult osteomalacia M83.8
    - rickets — *see* Rickets
- essential fatty acid (EFA) E63.0
- factor (*see also* Deficiency, coagulation)
  - Hageman D68.2
  - I (congenital) (hereditary) D68.2
  - II (congenital) (hereditary) D68.2
  - IX (congenital) (functional) (hereditary) (with functional defect) D67
  - multiple (congenital) D68.8
    - acquired D68.4
  - V (congenital) (hereditary) D68.2
  - VII (congenital) (hereditary) D68.2
  - VIII (congenital) (functional) (hereditary) (with functional defect) D66
    - with vascular defect D68.0
  - X (congenital) (hereditary) D68.2
  - XI (congenital) (hereditary) D68.1
  - XII (congenital) (hereditary) D68.2
  - XIII (congenital) (hereditary) D68.2
- femoral, proximal focal (congenital) — *see* Defect, reduction, lower limb, longitudinal, femur
- fibrin-stabilizing factor (congenital) (hereditary) D68.2
  - acquired D68.4
- fibrinase D68.2
- fibrinogen (congenital) (hereditary) D68.2
  - acquired D65
- folate E53.8
- folic acid E53.8
- foreskin N47.3
- fructokinase E74.11
- fructose 1,6-diphosphatase E74.19
- fructose-1-phosphate aldolase E74.19
- galactokinase E74.29
- galactose-1-phosphate uridyl transferase E74.29
- gamma globulin in blood D80.1
  - hereditary D80.0
- glass factor D68.2
- glucocorticoid E27.49
  - mineralocorticoid E27.49
- glucose-6-phosphatase E74.01
- glucose-6-phosphate dehydrogenase anemia D55.0
- glucuronyl transferase E80.5
- glycogen synthetase E74.09
- gonadotropin (isolated) E23.0
- growth hormone (idiopathic) (isolated) E23.0
- Hageman factor D68.2
- hemoglobin D64.9
- hepatophosphorylase E74.09
- homogentisate 1,2-dioxygenase E70.29
- hormone
  - anterior pituitary (partial) NEC E23.0
    - growth E23.0
  - growth (isolated) E23.0
  - pituitary E23.0
  - testicular E29.1
- hypoxanthine- (guanine)-phosphoribosyltransferase (HG- PRT) (total H-PRT) E79.1
- immunity D84.9
  - cell-mediated D84.8
    - with thrombocytopenia and eczema D82.0
  - combined D81.9
  - humoral D80.9
  - IgA (secretory) D80.2
  - IgG D80.3
  - IgM D80.4
- immuno — *see* Immunodeficiency
- immunoglobulin, selective
  - A (IgA) D80.2
  - G (IgG) (subclasses) D80.3
  - M (IgM) D80.4
- inositol (B complex) E53.8
- intrinsic
  - factor (congenital) D51.0
  - sphincter N36.42
    - with urethral hypermobility N36.43
- iodine E61.8
  - congenital syndrome — *see* Syndrome, iodine-deficiency, congenital
- iron E61.1
  - anemia D50.9

Deficiency — *continued*
- kalium E87.6
- kappa-light chain D80.8
- labile factor (congenital) (hereditary) D68.2
  - acquired D68.4
- lacrimal fluid (acquired) (*see also* Syndrome, dry eye)
  - congenital Q10.6
- lactase
  - congenital E73.0
  - secondary E73.1
- Laki-Lorand factor D68.2
- lecithin cholesterol acyltransferase E78.6
- lipocaic K86.89
- lipoprotein (familial) (high density) E78.6
- liver phosphorylase E74.09
- lysosomal alpha-1, 4 glucosidase E74.02
- magnesium E61.2
- major histocompatibility complex
  - class I D81.6
  - class II D81.7
- manganese E61.3
- menadione (vitamin K) E56.1
  - newborn P53
- mental (familial) (hereditary) — *see* Disability, intellectual
- methylenetetrahydrofolate reductase (MTHFR) E72.12
- mevalonate kinase M04.1
- mineral NEC E61.8
- mineralocorticoid E27.49
  - with glucocorticoid E27.49
- molybdenum (nutritional) E61.5
- moral F60.2
- multiple nutrient elements E61.7
- muscle
  - carnitine (palmityltransferase) E71.314
  - phosphofructokinase E74.09
- myoadenylate deaminase E79.2
- myocardial — *see* Insufficiency, myocardial
- myophosphorylase E74.04
- NADH diaphorase or reductase (congenital) D74.0
- NADH-methemoglobin reductase (congenital) D74.0
- natrium E87.1
- niacin (amide) (-tryptophan) E52
- nicotinamide E52
- nicotinic acid E52
- number of teeth — *see* Anodontia
- nutrient element E61.9
  - multiple E61.7
  - specified NEC E61.8
- nutrition, nutritional E63.9
  - sequelae — *see* Sequelae, nutritional deficiency
  - specified NEC E63.8
- of interleukin 1 receptor antagonist [DIRA] M04.8
- ornithine transcarbamylase E72.4
- ovarian E28.39
- oxygen — *see* Anoxia
- pantothenic acid E53.8
- parathyroid (gland) E20.9
- perineum (female) N81.89
- phenylalanine hydroxylase E70.1
- phosphoenolpyruvate carboxykinase E74.4
- phosphofructokinase E74.19
- phosphomannomutuse E74.8
- phosphomannose isomerase E74.8
- phosphomannosyl mutase E74.8
- phosphorylase kinase, liver E74.09
- pituitary hormone (isolated) E23.0
- plasma thromboplastin
  - antecedent (PTA) D68.1
  - component (PTC) D67
- platelet NEC D69.1
  - constitutional D68.0
- polyglandular E31.8
  - autoimmune E31.0
- potassium (K) E87.6
- prepuce N47.3
- proaccelerin (congenital) (hereditary) D68.2
  - acquired D68.4
- proconvertin factor (congenital) (hereditary) D68.2
  - acquired D68.4
- protein (*see also* Malnutrition)E46
  - anemia D53.0
  - C D68.59
  - S D68.59
- prothrombin (congenital) (hereditary) D68.2
  - acquired D68.4
- Prower factor D68.2

Deficiency — *continued*
- pseudocholinesterase E88.09
- PTA (plasma thromboplastin antecedent) D68.1
- PTC (plasma thromboplastin component) D67
- purine nucleoside phosphorylase (PNP) D81.5
- pyracin (alpha) (beta) E53.1
- pyridoxal E53.1
- pyridoxamine E53.1
- pyridoxine (derivatives) E53.1
- pyruvate
  - carboxylase E74.4
  - dehydrogenase E74.4
- riboflavin (vitamin B2) E53.0
- salt E87.1
- secretion
  - ovary E28.39
  - salivary gland (any) K11.7
  - urine R34
- selenium (dietary) E59
- serum antitrypsin, familial E88.01
- short stature homeobox gene (SHOX)
  - with
    - dyschondrosteosis Q78.8
    - short stature (idiopathic) E34.3
    - Turner's syndrome Q96.9
- sodium (Na) E87.1
- SPCA (factor VII) D68.2
- sphincter, intrinsic N36.42
  - with urethral hypermobility N36.43
- stable factor (congenital) (hereditary) D68.2
  - acquired D68.4
- Stuart-Prower (factor X) D68.2
- sucrase E74.39
- sulfatase E75.29
- sulfite oxidase E72.19
- thiamin, thiaminic (chloride) E51.9
  - beriberi (dry) E51.11
    - wet E51.12
- thrombokinase D68.2
  - newborn P53
- thyroid (gland) — *see* Hypothyroidism
- tocopherol E56.0
- tooth bud K00.0
- transcobalamine II (anemia) D51.2
- vanadium E61.6
- vascular I99.9
- vasopressin E23.2
- vertical ridge K06.8
- viosterol — *see* Deficiency, calciferol
- vitamin (multiple) NOS E56.9
  - A E50.9
    - with
      - Bitot's spot (corneal) E50.1
      - follicular keratosis E50.8
      - keratomalacia E50.4
      - manifestations NEC E50.8
      - night blindness E50.5
      - scar of cornea, xerophthalmic E50.6
      - xeroderma E50.8
      - xerophthalmia E50.7
      - xerosis
        - conjunctival E50.0
          - and Bitot's spot E50.1
        - cornea E50.2
          - and ulceration E50.3
    - sequelae E64.1
  - B (complex) NOS E53.9
    - with
      - beriberi (dry) E51.11
        - wet E51.12
      - pellagra E52
  - B1 NOS E51.9
    - beriberi (dry) E51.11
      - with circulatory system manifestations E51.11
      - wet E51.12
  - B12 E53.8
  - B2 (riboflavin) E53.0
  - B6 E53.1
  - C E54
    - sequelae E64.2
  - D E55.9
    - with
      - adult osteomalacia M83.8
      - rickets — *see* Rickets
    - 25-hydroxylase E83.32
  - E E56.0
  - folic acid E53.8
  - G E53.0
  - group B E53.9
    - specified NEC E53.8
  - H (biotin) E53.8

Deficiency — *continued*
- vitamin — *continued*
  - K E56.1
    - of newborn P53
  - nicotinic E52
  - P E56.8
  - PP (pellagra-preventing) E52
  - specified NEC E56.8
  - thiamin E51.9
    - beriberi — *see* Beriberi
- zinc, dietary E60

Deficit (*see also* Deficiency)
- attention and concentration R41.840
  - following
    - cerebral infarction I69.310
    - cerebrovascular disease I69.910
      - specified disease NEC I69.810
    - nontraumatic
      - intracerebral hemorrhage I69.110
      - specified intracranial hemorrhage NEC I69.210
      - subarachnoid hemorrhage I69.010
  - disorder — *see* Attention, deficit
- cognitive
  - communication R41.841
  - emotional
    - following
      - cerebral infarction I69.315
      - cerebrovascular disease I69.915
        - specified disease NEC I69.815
      - nontraumatic
        - intracerebral hemorrhage I69.115
        - specified intracranial hemorrhage NEC I69.215
        - subarachnoid hemorrhage I69.015
  - following
    - cerebral infarction I69.319
    - cerebrovascular disease I69.919
      - specified disease NEC I69.819
    - nontraumatic
      - intracerebral hemorrhage I69.119
      - specified intracranial hemorrhage NEC I69.219
      - subarachnoid hemorrhage I69.019
  - social
    - following
      - cerebral infarction I69.315
      - cerebrovascular disease I69.915
        - specified disease NEC I69.815
      - nontraumatic
        - intracerebral hemorrhage I69.115
        - specified intracranial hemorrhage NEC I69.215
        - subarachnoid hemorrhage I69.015
- cognitive NEC R41.89
  - following
    - cerebral infarction I69.318
    - cerebrovascular disease I69.918
      - specified disease NEC I69.818
    - nontraumatic
      - intracerebral hemorrhage I69.118
      - specified intracranial hemorrhage NEC I69.218
      - subarachnoid hemorrhage I69.018
- concentration R41.840
- executive function R41.844
  - following
    - cerebral infarction I69.314
    - cerebrovascular disease I69.914
      - specified disease NEC I69.814
    - nontraumatic
      - intracerebral hemorrhage I69.114
      - specified intracranial hemorrhage NEC I69.214
      - subarachnoid hemorrhage I69.014
- frontal lobe R41.844
  - following
    - cerebral infarction I69.314
    - cerebrovascular disease I69.914
      - specified disease NEC I69.814
    - nontraumatic
      - intracerebral hemorrhage I69.114
      - specified intracranial hemorrhage NEC I69.214
      - subarachnoid hemorrhage I69.014
- memory
  - following
    - cerebral infarction I69.311
    - cerebrovascular disease I69.911
      - specified disease NEC I69.811
    - nontraumatic
      - intracerebral hemorrhage I69.111

Deficit - Deformity

- **Deficit** — *continued*
  - memory — *continued*
      - specified intracranial hemorrhage NEC I69.211
      - subarachnoid hemorrhage I69.011
  - neurologic NEC R29.818
    - ischemic
      - reversible (RIND) I63.9
        - prolonged (PRIND) I63.9
  - oxygen R09.02
  - prolonged reversible ischemic neurologic (PRIND) I63.9
  - psychomotor R41.843
    - following
      - cerebral infarction I69.313
      - cerebrovascular disease I69.913
        - specified disease NEC I69.813
      - nontraumatic
        - intracerebral hemorrhage I69.113
        - specified intracranial hemorrhage NEC I69.213
        - subarachnoid hemorrhage I69.013
  - visuospatial R41.842
    - following
      - cerebral infarction I69.312
      - cerebrovascular disease I69.912
        - specified disease NEC I69.812
      - nontraumatic
        - intracerebral hemorrhage I69.112
        - specified intracranial hemorrhage NEC I69.212
        - subarachnoid hemorrhage I69.012
- **Deflection**
  - radius — *see* Deformity, limb, specified type NEC, forearm
  - septum (acquired) (nasal) (nose) J34.2
  - spine — *see* Curvature, spine
  - turbinate (nose) J34.2
- **Defluvium**
  - capillorum — *see* Alopecia
  - ciliorum — *see* Madarosis
  - unguium L60.8
- **Deformity** Q89.9
  - abdomen, congenital Q89.9
  - abdominal wall
    - acquired M95.8
    - congenital Q79.59
  - acquired (unspecified site) M95.9
  - adrenal gland Q89.1
  - alimentary tract, congenital Q45.9
    - upper Q40.9
  - ankle (joint) (acquired) (*see also* Deformity, limb, lower leg)
    - abduction — *see* Contraction, joint, ankle
    - congenital Q68.8
    - contraction — *see* Contraction, joint, ankle
    - specified type NEC — *see* Deformity, limb, foot, specified NEC
  - anus (acquired) K62.89
    - congenital Q43.9
  - aorta (arch) (congenital) Q25.40
    - acquired I77.89
  - aortic
    - arch, acquired I77.89
    - cusp or valve (congenital) Q23.8
      - acquired (*see also* Endocarditis, aortic)I35.8
  - arm (acquired) (upper) (*see also* Deformity, limb, upper arm)
    - congenital Q68.8
    - forearm — *see* Deformity, limb, forearm
  - artery (congenital) (peripheral) NOS Q27.9
    - acquired I77.89
    - coronary (acquired) I25.9
      - congenital Q24.5
    - umbilical Q27.0
  - atrial septal Q21.1
  - auditory canal (external) (congenital) (*see also* Malformation, ear, external)
    - acquired — *see* Disorder, ear, external, specified type NEC
  - auricle
    - ear (congenital) (*see also* Malformation, ear, external)
      - acquired — *see* Disorder, pinna, deformity
  - back — *see* Dorsopathy, deforming
  - bile duct (common) (congenital) (hepatic) Q44.5
    - acquired K83.8
  - biliary duct or passage (congenital) Q44.5
    - acquired K83.8
  - bladder (neck) (trigone) (sphincter) (acquired) N32.89
    - congenital Q64.79

- **Deformity** — *continued*
  - bone (acquired) NOS M95.9
    - congenital Q79.9
    - turbinate M95.0
  - brain (congenital) Q04.9
    - acquired G93.89
    - reduction Q04.3
  - breast (acquired) N64.89
    - congenital Q83.9
    - reconstructed N65.0
  - bronchus (congenital) Q32.4
    - acquired NEC J98.09
  - bursa, congenital Q79.9
  - canaliculi (lacrimalis) (acquired) (*see also* Disorder, lacrimal system, changes)
    - congenital Q10.6
  - canthus, acquired — *see* Disorder, eyelid, specified type NEC
  - capillary (acquired) I78.8
  - cardiovascular system, congenital Q28.9
  - caruncle, lacrimal (acquired) (*see also* Disorder, lacrimal system, changes)
    - congenital Q10.6
  - cascade, stomach K31.2
  - cecum (congenital) Q43.9
    - acquired K63.89
  - cerebral, acquired G93.89
    - congenital Q04.9
  - cervix (uterus) (acquired) NEC N88.8
    - congenital Q51.9
  - cheek (acquired) M95.2
    - congenital Q18.9
  - chest (acquired) (wall) M95.4
    - congenital Q67.8
    - sequelae (late effect) of rickets E64.3
  - chin (acquired) M95.2
    - congenital Q18.9
  - choroid (congenital) Q14.3
    - acquired H31.8
    - plexus Q07.8
      - acquired G96.19
  - cicatricial — *see* Cicatrix
  - cilia, acquired — *see* Disorder, eyelid, specified type NEC
  - clavicle (acquired) M95.8
    - congenital Q68.8
  - clitoris (congenital) Q52.6
    - acquired N90.89
  - clubfoot — *see* Clubfoot
  - coccyx (acquired) — *see* subcategory M43.8
  - colon (congenital) Q43.9
    - acquired K63.89
  - concha (ear), congenital (*see also* Malformation, ear, external)
    - acquired — *see* Disorder, pinna, deformity
  - cornea (acquired) H18.70
    - congenital Q13.4
    - descemetocele — *see* Descemetocele
    - ectasia — *see* Ectasia, cornea
    - specified NEC H18.79 ☑
    - staphyloma — *see* Staphyloma, cornea
  - coronary artery (acquired) I25.9
    - congenital Q24.5
  - cranium (acquired) — *see* Deformity, skull
  - cricoid cartilage (congenital) Q31.8
    - acquired J38.7
  - cystic duct (congenital) Q44.5
    - acquired K82.8
  - Dandy-Walker Q03.1
    - with spina bifida — *see* Spina bifida
  - diaphragm (congenital) Q79.1
    - acquired J98.6
  - digestive organ NOS Q45.9
  - ductus arteriosus Q25.0
  - duodenal bulb K31.89
  - duodenum (congenital) Q43.9
    - acquired K31.89
  - dura — *see* Deformity, meninges
  - ear (acquired) (*see also* Disorder, pinna, deformity)
    - congenital (external) Q17.9
      - internal Q16.5
      - middle Q16.4
        - ossicles Q16.3
      - ossicles Q16.3
  - ectodermal (congenital) NEC Q84.9
  - ejaculatory duct (congenital) Q55.4
    - acquired N50.89
  - elbow (joint) (acquired) (*see also* Deformity, limb, upper arm)
    - congenital Q68.8
    - contraction — *see* Contraction, joint, elbow

- **Deformity** — *continued*
  - endocrine gland NEC Q89.2
  - epididymis (congenital) Q55.4
    - acquired N50.89
  - epiglottis (congenital) Q31.8
    - acquired J38.7
  - esophagus (congenital) Q39.9
    - acquired K22.8
  - eustachian tube (congenital) NEC Q17.8
  - eye, congenital Q15.9
  - eyebrow (congenital) Q18.8
  - eyelid (acquired) (*see also* Disorder, eyelid, specified type NEC)
    - congenital Q10.3
  - face (acquired) M95.2
    - congenital Q18.9
  - fallopian tube, acquired N83.8
  - femur (acquired) — *see* Deformity, limb, specified type NEC, thigh
  - fetal
    - with fetopelvic disproportion O33.7 ☑
    - causing obstructed labor O66.3
  - finger (acquired) M20.00 ☑
    - boutonniere M20.02 ☑
    - congenital Q68.1
    - flexion contracture — *see* Contraction, joint, hand
    - mallet finger M20.01 ☑
    - specified NEC M20.09 ☑
    - swan-neck M20.03 ☑
  - flexion (joint) (acquired) (*see also* Deformity, limb, flexion)M21.20
    - congenital NOS Q74.9
      - hip Q65.89
  - foot (acquired) (*see also* Deformity, limb, lower leg)
    - cavovarus (congenital) Q66.1
    - congenital NOS Q66.9
      - specified type NEC Q66.89
    - specified type NEC — *see* Deformity, limb, foot, specified NEC
    - valgus (congenital) Q66.6
      - acquired — *see* Deformity, valgus, ankle
    - varus (congenital) NEC Q66.3
      - acquired — *see* Deformity, varus, ankle
  - forearm (acquired) (*see also* Deformity, limb, forearm)
    - congenital Q68.8
  - forehead (acquired) M95.2
    - congenital Q75.8
  - frontal bone (acquired) M95.2
    - congenital Q75.8
  - gallbladder (congenital) Q44.1
    - acquired K82.8
  - gastrointestinal tract (congenital) NOS Q45.9
    - acquired K63.89
  - genitalia, genital organ (s) or system NEC
    - female (congenital) Q52.9
      - acquired N94.89
      - external Q52.70
    - male (congenital) Q55.9
      - acquired N50.89
  - globe (eye) (congenital) Q15.8
    - acquired H44.89
  - gum, acquired NEC K06.8
  - hand (acquired) — *see* Deformity, limb, hand
    - congenital Q68.1
  - head (acquired) M95.2
    - congenital Q75.8
  - heart (congenital) Q24.9
    - septum Q21.9
      - auricular Q21.1
      - ventricular Q21.0
    - valve (congenital) NEC Q24.8
      - acquired — *see* Endocarditis
  - heel (acquired) — *see* Deformity, foot
  - hepatic duct (congenital) Q44.5
    - acquired K83.8
  - hip (joint) (acquired) (*see also* Deformity, limb, thigh)
    - congenital Q65.9
    - due to (previous) juvenile osteochondrosis — *see* Coxa, plana
    - flexion — *see* Contraction, joint, hip
  - hourglass — *see* Contraction, hourglass
  - humerus (acquired) M21.82 ☑
    - congenital Q74.0
  - hypophyseal (congenital) Q89.2
  - ileocecal (coil) (valve) (acquired) K63.89
    - congenital Q43.9
  - ileum (congenital) Q43.9
    - acquired K63.89

Deformity - Degeneration

Deformity — *continued*
- Sprengel's (congenital) Q74.0
- sternocleidomastoid (muscle), congenital Q68.0
- sternum (acquired) M95.4
  - congenital NEC Q76.7
- stomach (congenital) Q40.3
  - acquired K31.89
- submandibular gland (congenital) Q38.4
- submaxillary gland (congenital) Q38.4
  - acquired K11.8
- talipes — *see* Talipes
- testis (congenital) (*see also* Malformation, testis and scrotum)
  - acquired N44.8
    - torsion — *see* Torsion, testis
- thigh (acquired) (*see also* Deformity, limb, thigh)
  - congenital NEC Q68.8
- thorax (acquired) (wall) M95.4
  - congenital Q67.8
  - sequelae of rickets E64.3
- thumb (acquired) (*see also* Deformity, finger)
  - congenital NEC Q68.1
- thymus (tissue) (congenital) Q89.2
- thyroid (gland) (congenital) Q89.2
  - cartilage Q31.8
    - acquired J38.7
- tibia (acquired) (*see also* Deformity, limb, specified type NEC, lower leg)
  - congenital NEC Q68.8
  - saber (syphilitic) A50.56
- toe (acquired) M20.6 ☑
  - congenital Q66.9
  - hallux rigidus M20.2 ☑
  - hallux valgus M20.1 ☑
  - hallux varus M20.3 ☑
  - hammer toe M20.4 ☑
  - specified NEC M20.5X ☑
- tongue (congenital) Q38.3
  - acquired K14.8
- tooth, teeth K00.2
- trachea (rings) (congenital) Q32.1
  - acquired J39.8
- transverse aortic arch (congenital) Q25.49
- tricuspid (leaflets) (valve) I07.8
  - atresia or stenosis Q22.4
  - Ebstein's Q22.5
- trunk (acquired) M95.8
  - congenital Q89.9
- ulna (acquired) (*see also* Deformity, limb, forearm)
  - congenital NEC Q68.8
- urachus, congenital Q64.4
- ureter (opening) (congenital) Q62.8
  - acquired N28.89
- urethra (congenital) Q64.79
  - acquired N36.8
- urinary tract (congenital) Q64.9
  - urachus Q64.4
- uterus (congenital) Q51.9
  - acquired N85.8
- uvula (congenital) Q38.5
- vagina (acquired) N89.8
  - congenital Q52.4
- valgus NEC M21.00
  - ankle M21.07 ☑
  - elbow M21.02 ☑
  - hip M21.05 ☑
  - knee M21.06 ☑
- valve, valvular (congenital) (heart) Q24.8
  - acquired — *see* Endocarditis
- varus NEC M21.10
  - ankle M21.17 ☑
  - elbow M21.12 ☑
  - hip M21.15 ☑
  - knee M21.16 ☑
  - tibia — *see* Osteochondrosis, juvenile, tibia
- vas deferens (congenital) Q55.4
  - acquired N50.89
- vein (congenital) Q27.9
  - great Q26.9
- vertebra — *see* Dorsopathy, deforming
- vertical talus (congenital) Q66.80
  - left foot Q66.82
  - right foot Q66.81
- vesicourethral orifice (acquired) N32.89
  - congenital NEC Q64.79
- vessels of optic papilla (congenital) Q14.2
- visual field (contraction) — *see* Defect, visual field
- vitreous body, acquired H43.89
- vulva (congenital) Q52.79
  - acquired N90.89
- wrist (joint) (acquired) (*see also* Deformity, limb, forearm)
  - congenital Q68.8
  - contraction — *see* Contraction, joint, wrist

Degeneration, degenerative
- adrenal (capsule) (fatty) (gland) (hyaline) (infectional) E27.8
- amyloid (*see also* Amyloidosis)E85.9
- anterior cornua, spinal cord G12.29
- anterior labral S43.49 ☑
- aorta, aortic I70.0
  - fatty I77.89
- aortic valve (heart) — *see* Endocarditis, aortic
- arteriovascular — *see* Arteriosclerosis
- artery, arterial (atheromatous) (calcareous) (*see also* Arteriosclerosis)
  - cerebral, amyloid E85.4 *[I68.0]*
  - medial — *see* Arteriosclerosis, extremities
- articular cartilage NEC — *see* Derangement, joint, articular cartilage, by site
- atheromatous — *see* Arteriosclerosis
- basal nuclei or ganglia G23.9
  - specified NEC G23.8
- bone NEC — *see* Disorder, bone, specified type NEC
- brachial plexus G54.0
- brain (cortical) (progressive) G31.9
  - alcoholic G31.2
  - arteriosclerotic I67.2
  - childhood G31.9
    - specified NEC G31.89
  - cystic G31.89
    - congenital Q04.6
  - in
    - alcoholism G31.2
    - beriberi E51.2
    - cerebrovascular disease I67.9
    - congenital hydrocephalus Q03.9
      - with spina bifida (*see also* Spina bifida)
    - Fabry-Anderson disease E75.21
    - Gaucher's disease E75.22
    - Hunter's syndrome E76.1
    - lipidosis
      - cerebral E75.4
      - generalized E75.6
    - mucopolysaccharidosis — *see* Mucopolysaccharidosis
    - myxedema E03.9 *[G32.89]*
    - neoplastic disease (*see also* Neoplasm)D49.6 *[G32.89]*
    - Niemann-Pick disease E75.249 *[G32.89]*
    - sphingolipidosis E75.3 *[G32.89]*
    - vitamin B12 deficiency E53.8 *[G32.89]*
  - senile NEC G31.1
- breast N64.89
- Bruch's membrane — *see* Degeneration, choroid
- capillaries (fatty) I78.8
  - amyloid E85.8 *[I79.8]*
- cardiac (*see also* Degeneration, myocardial)
  - valve, valvular — *see* Endocarditis
- cardiorenal — *see* Hypertension, cardiorenal
- cardiovascular (*see also* Disease, cardiovascular)
  - renal — *see* Hypertension, cardiorenal
- cerebellar NOS G31.9
  - alcoholic G31.2
  - primary (hereditary) (sporadic) G11.9
- cerebral — *see* Degeneration, brain
- cerebrovascular I67.9
  - due to hypertension I67.4
- cervical plexus G54.2
- cervix N88.8
  - due to radiation (intended effect) N88.8
    - adverse effect or misadventure N99.89
- chamber angle H21.21 ☑
- changes, spine or vertebra — *see* Spondylosis
- chorioretinal (*see also* Degeneration, choroid)
  - hereditary H31.20
- choroid (colloid) (drusen) H31.10 ☑
  - atrophy — *see* Atrophy, choroidal
  - hereditary — *see* Dystrophy, choroidal, hereditary
- ciliary body H21.22 ☑
- cochlear — *see* subcategory H83.8
- combined (spinal cord) (subacute) E53.8 *[G32.0]*
  - with anemia (pernicious) D51.0 *[G32.0]*
    - due to dietary vitamin B12 deficiency D51.3 *[G32.0]*
  - in (due to)
    - vitamin B12 deficiency E53.8 *[G32.0]*
      - anemia D51.9 *[G32.0]*
- conjunctiva H11.10
  - concretions — *see* Concretion, conjunctiva

Degeneration — *continued*
- conjunctiva — *continued*
  - deposits — *see* Deposit, conjunctiva
  - pigmentations — *see* Pigmentation, conjunctiva
  - pinguecula — *see* Pinguecula
  - xerosis — *see* Xerosis, conjunctiva
- cornea H18.40
  - calcerous H18.43
    - band keratopathy H18.42 ☑
  - familial, hereditary — *see* Dystrophy, cornea
  - hyaline (of old scars) H18.49
  - keratomalacia — *see* Keratomalacia
  - nodular H18.45 ☑
  - peripheral H18.46 ☑
  - senile H18.41 ☑
  - specified type NEC H18.49
- cortical (cerebellar) (parenchymatous) G31.89
  - alcoholic G31.2
  - diffuse, due to arteriopathy I67.2
- corticobasal G31.85
- cutis L98.8
  - amyloid E85.4 *[L99]*
- dental pulp K04.2
- disc disease — *see* Degeneration, intervertebral disc NEC
- dorsolateral (spinal cord) — *see* Degeneration, combined
- extrapyramidal G25.9
- eye, macular (*see also* Degeneration, macula)
  - congenital or hereditary — *see* Dystrophy, retina
- facet joints — *see* Spondylosis
- fatty
  - liver NEC K76.0
    - alcoholic K70.0
- grey matter (brain) (Alpers') G31.81
- heart (*see also* Degeneration, myocardial)
  - amyloid E85.4 *[I43]*
  - atheromatous — *see* Disease, heart, ischemic, atherosclerotic
  - ischemic — *see* Disease, heart, ischemic
- hepatolenticular (Wilson's) E83.01
- hepatorenal K76.7
- hyaline (diffuse) (generalized)
  - localized — *see* Degeneration, by site
- infrapatellar fat pad M79.4
- intervertebral disc NOS
  - with
    - myelopathy — *see* Disorder, disc, with, myelopathy
    - radiculitis or radiculopathy — *see* Disorder, disc, with, radiculopathy
  - cervical, cervicothoracic — *see* Disorder, disc, cervical, degeneration
    - with
      - myelopathy — *see* Disorder, disc, cervical, with myelopathy
      - neuritis, radiculitis or radiculopathy — *see* Disorder, disc, cervical, with neuritis
  - lumbar region M51.36
    - with
      - myelopathy M51.06
      - neuritis, radiculitis, radiculopathy or sciatica M51.16
  - lumbosacral region M51.37
    - with
      - neuritis, radiculitis, radiculopathy or sciatica M51.17
  - sacrococcygeal region M53.3
  - thoracic region M51.34
    - with
      - myelopathy M51.04
      - neuritis, radiculitis, radiculopathy M51.14
  - thoracolumbar region M51.35
    - with
      - myelopathy M51.05
      - neuritis, radiculitis, radiculopathy M51.15
- intestine, amyloid E85.4
- iris (pigmentary) H21.23 ☑
- ischemic — *see* Ischemia
- joint disease — *see* Osteoarthritis
- kidney N28.89
  - amyloid E85.4 *[N29]*
  - cystic, congenital Q61.9
  - fatty N28.89
  - polycystic Q61.3
    - adult type (autosomal dominant) Q61.2
    - infantile type (autosomal recessive) NEC Q61.19
      - collecting duct dilatation Q61.11

Degeneration — *continued*
- Kuhnt-Junius (*see also* Degeneration, macula)H35.32 ☑
- lens — *see* Cataract
- lenticular (familial) (progressive) (Wilson's) (with cirrhosis of liver) E83.01
- liver (diffuse) NEC K76.89
  - amyloid E85.4 *[K77]*
  - cystic K76.89
    - congenital Q44.6
  - fatty NEC K76.0
    - alcoholic K70.0
  - hypertrophic K76.89
  - parenchymatous, acute or subacute K72.00
    - with coma K72.01
  - pigmentary K76.89
  - toxic (acute) K71.9
- lung J98.4
- lymph gland I89.8
  - hyaline I89.8
- macula, macular (acquired) (age-related) (senile) H35.30 ☑
  - angioid streaks H35.33
  - atrophic age-related H35.31 ☑
  - congenital or hereditary — *see* Dystrophy, retina
  - cystoid H35.35 ☑
  - drusen H35.36 ☑
  - dry age-related H35.31 ☑
  - exudative H35.32 ☑
  - hole H35.34 ☑
  - nonexudative H35.31 ☑
  - puckering H35.37 ☑
  - toxic H35.38 ☑
  - wet age-related H35.32 ☑
- membranous labyrinth, congenital (causing impairment of hearing) Q16.5
- meniscus — *see* Derangement, meniscus
- mitral — *see* Insufficiency, mitral
- Mönckeberg's — *see* Arteriosclerosis, extremities
- motor centers, senile G31.1
- multi-system G90.3
- mural — *see* Degeneration, myocardial
- muscle (fatty) (fibrous) (hyaline) (progressive) M62.89
  - heart — *see* Degeneration, myocardial
- myelin, central nervous system G37.9
- myocardial, myocardium (fatty) (hyaline) (senile) I51.5
  - with rheumatic fever (conditions in I00) I09.0
    - active, acute or subacute I01.2
      - with chorea I02.0
    - inactive or quiescent (with chorea) I09.0
  - hypertensive — *see* Hypertension, heart
  - rheumatic — *see* Degeneration, myocardial, with rheumatic fever
  - syphilitic A52.06
- nasal sinus (mucosa) J32.9
  - frontal J32.1
  - maxillary J32.0
- nerve — *see* Disorder, nerve
- nervous system G31.9
  - alcoholic G31.2
  - amyloid E85.4 *[G99.8]*
  - autonomic G90.9
  - fatty G31.89
  - specified NEC G31.89
- nipple N64.89
- olivopontocerebellar (hereditary) (familial) G23.8
- osseous labyrinth — *see* subcategory H83.8
- ovary N83.8
  - cystic N83.20 ☑
  - microcystic N83.20 ☑
- pallidal pigmentary (progressive) G23.0
- pancreas K86.89
  - tuberculous A18.83
- penis N48.89
- pigmentary (diffuse) (general)
  - localized — *see* Degeneration, by site
  - pallidal (progressive) G23.0
- pineal gland E34.8
- pituitary (gland) E23.6
- popliteal fat pad M79.4
- posterolateral (spinal cord) — *see* Degeneration, combined
- pulmonary valve (heart) I37.8
- pulp (tooth) K04.2
- pupillary margin H21.24 ☑
- renal — *see* Degeneration, kidney
- retina H35.9

Degeneration — *continued*
- retina — *continued*
  - hereditary (cerebroretinal) (congenital) (juvenile) (macula) (peripheral) (pigmentary) — *see* Dystrophy, retina
  - Kuhnt-Junius (*see also* Degeneration, macula)H35.32 ☑
  - macula (cystic) (exudative) (hole) (nonexudative) (pseudohole) (senile) (toxic) — *see* Degeneration, macula
  - peripheral H35.40
    - lattice H35.41 ☑
    - microcystoid H35.42 ☑
    - paving stone H35.43 ☑
    - secondary
      - pigmentary H35.45 ☑
      - vitreoretinal H35.46 ☑
    - senile reticular H35.44 ☑
  - pigmentary (primary) (*see also* Dystrophy, retina)
    - secondary — *see* Degeneration, retina, peripheral, secondary
  - posterior pole — *see* Degeneration, macula
- saccule, congenital (causing impairment of hearing) Q16.5
- senile R54
  - brain G31.1
  - cardiac, heart or myocardium — *see* Degeneration, myocardial
  - motor centers G31.1
  - vascular — *see* Arteriosclerosis
- sinus (cystic) (*see also* Sinusitis)
  - polypoid J33.1
- skin L98.8
  - amyloid E85.4 *[L99]*
  - colloid L98.8
- spinal (cord) G31.89
  - amyloid E85.4 *[G32.89]*
  - combined (subacute) — *see* Degeneration, combined
  - dorsolateral — *see* Degeneration, combined
  - familial NEC G31.89
  - fatty G31.89
  - funicular — *see* Degeneration, combined
  - posterolateral — *see* Degeneration, combined
  - subacute combined — *see* Degeneration, combined
  - tuberculous A17.81
- spleen D73.0
  - amyloid E85.4 *[D77]*
- stomach K31.89
- striatonigral G23.2
- suprarenal (capsule) (gland) E27.8
- synovial membrane (pulpy) — *see* Disorder, synovium, specified type NEC
- tapetoretinal — *see* Dystrophy, retina
- thymus (gland) E32.8
  - fatty E32.8
- thyroid (gland) E07.89
- tricuspid (heart) (valve) I07.9
- tuberculous NEC — *see* Tuberculosis
- turbinate J34.89
- uterus (cystic) N85.8
- vascular (senile) — *see* Arteriosclerosis
  - hypertensive — *see* Hypertension
- vitreoretinal, secondary — *see* Degeneration, retina, peripheral, secondary, vitreoretinal
- vitreous (body) H43.81 ☑
- Wallerian — *see* Disorder, nerve
- Wilson's hepatolenticular E83.01

Deglutition
- paralysis R13.0
  - hysterical F44.4
- pneumonia J69.0

Degos' disease I77.89

Dehiscence (of)
- amputation stump T87.81
- cesarean wound O90.0
- closure of
  - cornea T81.31 ☑
  - craniotomy T81.32 ☑
  - fascia (muscular) (superficial) T81.32 ☑
  - internal organ or tissue T81.32 ☑
  - laceration (external) (internal) T81.33 ☑
  - ligament T81.32 ☑
  - mucosa T81.31 ☑
  - muscle or muscle flap T81.32 ☑
  - ribs or rib cage T81.32 ☑
  - skin and subcutaneous tissue (full-thickness) (superficial) T81.31 ☑
  - skull T81.32 ☑
  - sternum (sternotomy) T81.32 ☑

Dehiscence — *continued*
- closure of — *continued*
  - tendon T81.32 ☑
  - traumatic laceration (external) (internal) T81.33 ☑
- episiotomy O90.1
- operation wound NEC T81.31 ☑
  - external operation wound (superficial) T81.31 ☑
  - internal operation wound (deep) T81.32 ☑
- perineal wound (postpartum) O90.1
- traumatic injury wound repair T81.33 ☑
- wound T81.30 ☑
  - traumatic repair T81.33 ☑

Dehydration E86.0
- newborn P74.1

Déjérine-Roussy syndrome G89.0

Déjérine-Sottas disease or neuropathy (hypertrophic) G60.0

Déjérine-Thomas atrophy G23.8

Delay, delayed
- any plane in pelvis
  - complicating delivery O66.9
- birth or delivery NOS O63.9
- closure, ductus arteriosus (Botalli) P29.3
- coagulation — *see* Defect, coagulation
- conduction (cardiac) (ventricular) I45.9
- delivery, second twin, triplet, etc O63.2
- development R62.50
  - global F88
  - intellectual (specific) F81.9
  - language F80.9
    - due to hearing loss F80.4
  - learning F81.9
  - pervasive F84.9
  - physiological R62.50
    - specified stage NEC R62.0
  - reading F81.0
  - sexual E30.0
  - speech F80.9
    - due to hearing loss F80.4
  - spelling F81.81
- ejaculation F52.32
- gastric emptying K30
- menarche E30.0
- menstruation (cause unknown) N91.0
- milestone R62.0
- passage of meconium (newborn) P76.0
- primary respiration P28.9
- puberty (constitutional) E30.0
- separation of umbilical cord P96.82
- sexual maturation, female E30.0
- sleep phase syndrome G47.21
- union, fracture — *see* Fracture, by site
- vaccination Z28.9

Deletion (s)
- autosome Q93.9
  - identified by fluorescence in situ hybridization (FISH) Q93.89
  - identified by in situ hybridization (ISH) Q93.89
- chromosome
  - with complex rearrangements NEC Q93.7
  - part of NEC Q93.5
  - seen only at prometaphase Q93.89
  - short arm
    - 4 Q93.3
    - 5p Q93.4
    - 22q11.2 Q93.81
  - specified NEC Q93.89
- long arm chromosome 18 or 21 Q93.89
  - with complex rearrangements NEC Q93.7
- microdeletions NEC Q93.88

Delhi boil or button B55.1

Delinquency (juvenile) (neurotic) F91.8
- group Z72.810

Delinquent immunization status Z28.3

Delirium, delirious (acute or subacute) (not alcohol- or drug-induced) (with dementia) R41.0
- alcoholic (acute) (tremens) (withdrawal) F10.921
  - with intoxication F10.921
    - in
      - abuse F10.121
      - dependence F10.221
- due to (secondary to)
  - alcohol
    - intoxication F10.921
      - in
        - abuse F10.121
        - dependence F10.221
    - withdrawal F10.231
  - amphetamine intoxication F15.921
    - in

- **Delirium** — *continued*
  - due to — *continued*
        - abuse F15.121
        - dependence F15.221
    - anxiolytic
      - intoxication F13.921
        - in
          - abuse F13.121
          - dependence F13.221
      - withdrawal F13.231
    - cannabis intoxication (acute) F12.921
      - in
        - abuse F12.121
        - dependence F12.221
    - cocaine intoxication (acute) F14.921
      - in
        - abuse F14.121
        - dependence F14.221
    - general medical condition F05
    - hallucinogen intoxication F16.921
      - in
        - abuse F16.121
        - dependence F16.221
    - hypnotic
      - intoxication F13.921
        - in
          - abuse F13.121
          - dependence F13.221
      - withdrawal F13.231
    - inhalant intoxication (acute) F18.921
      - in
        - abuse F18.121
        - dependence F18.221
    - multiple etiologies F05
    - opioid intoxication (acute) F11.921
      - in
        - abuse F11.121
        - dependence F11.221
    - other (or unknown) substance F19.921
    - phencyclidine intoxication (acute) F16.921
      - in
        - abuse F16.121
        - dependence F16.221
    - psychoactive substance NEC intoxication (acute) F19.921
      - in
        - abuse F19.121
        - dependence F19.221
    - sedative
      - intoxication F13.921
        - in
          - abuse F13.121
          - dependence F13.221
      - withdrawal F13.231
    - unknown etiology F05
  - exhaustion F43.0
  - hysterical F44.89
  - postprocedural (postoperative) F05
  - puerperal F05
  - thyroid — *see* Thyrotoxicosis with thyroid storm
  - traumatic — *see* Injury, intracranial
  - tremens (alcohol-induced) F10.231
    - sedative-induced F13.231
- **Delivery** (childbirth) (labor)
  - arrested active phase O62.1
  - cesarean (for)
    - abnormal
      - pelvis (bony) (deformity) (major) NEC with disproportion (fetopelvic) O33.0
        - with obstructed labor O65.0
      - presentation or position O32.9 ☑
    - abruptio placentae (*see also* Abruptio placentae)O45.9 ☑
    - acromion presentation O32.2 ☑
    - atony, uterus O62.2
    - breech presentation O32.1 ☑
      - incomplete O32.8 ☑
    - brow presentation O32.3 ☑
    - cephalopelvic disproportion O33.9
    - cerclage O34.3 ☑
    - chin presentation O32.3 ☑
    - cicatrix of cervix O34.4 ☑
    - contracted pelvis (general)
      - inlet O33.2
      - outlet O33.3 ☑
    - cord presentation or prolapse O69.0 ☑
    - cystocele O34.8 ☑
    - deformity (acquired) (congenital)
      - pelvic organs or tissues NEC O34.8 ☑
      - pelvis (bony) NEC O33.0
    - disproportion NOS O33.9
    - eclampsia — *see* Eclampsia

- **Delivery** — *continued*
  - cesarean — *continued*
    - face presentation O32.3 ☑
    - failed
      - forceps O66.5
      - induction of labor O61.9
        - instrumental O61.1
        - mechanical O61.1
        - medical O61.0
        - specified NEC O61.8
        - surgical O61.1
      - trial of labor NOS O66.40
        - following previous cesarean delivery O66.41
      - vacuum extraction O66.5
      - ventouse O66.5
    - fetal-maternal hemorrhage O43.01 ☑
    - hemorrhage (intrapartum) O67.9
      - with coagulation defect O67.0
      - specified cause NEC O67.8
    - high head at term O32.4 ☑
    - hydrocephalic fetus O33.6 ☑
    - incarceration of uterus O34.51 ☑
    - incoordinate uterine action O62.4
    - increased size, fetus O33.5 ☑
    - inertia, uterus O62.2
      - primary O62.0
      - secondary O62.1
    - lateroversion, uterus O34.59 ☑
    - mal lie O32.9 ☑
    - malposition
      - fetus O32.9 ☑
      - pelvic organs or tissues NEC O34.8 ☑
      - uterus NEC O34.59 ☑
    - malpresentation NOS O32.9 ☑
    - oblique presentation O32.2 ☑
    - occurring after 37 completed weeks of gestation but before 39 completed weeks gestation due to (spontaneous) onset of labor O75.82
    - oversize fetus O33.5 ☑
    - pelvic tumor NEC O34.8 ☑
    - placenta previa O44.0 ☑
      - complete O44.0 ☑
        - with hemorrhage O44.1 ☑
    - placental insufficiency O36.51 ☑
    - planned, occurring after 37 completed weeks of gestation but before 39 completed weeks gestation due to (spontaneous) onset of labor O75.82
    - polyp, cervix O34.4 ☑
      - causing obstructed labor O65.5
    - poor dilatation, cervix O62.0
    - pre-eclampsia O14.94
      - mild O14.04
      - moderate O14.04
      - severe O14.14
        - with hemolysis, elevated liver enzymes and low platelet count (HELLP) O14.24
    - previous
      - cesarean delivery O34.219
        - classical (vertical) scar O34.212
        - low transverse scar O34.211
      - surgery (to)
        - cervix O34.4 ☑
        - gynecological NEC O34.8 ☑
        - rectum O34.7 ☑
        - uterus O34.29
        - vagina O34.6 ☑
    - prolapse
      - arm or hand O32.2 ☑
      - uterus O34.52 ☑
    - prolonged labor NOS O63.9
    - rectocele O34.8 ☑
    - retroversion
      - uterus O34.53 ☑
    - rigid
      - cervix O34.4 ☑
      - pelvic floor O34.8 ☑
      - perineum O34.7 ☑
      - vagina O34.6 ☑
      - vulva O34.7 ☑
    - sacculation, pregnant uterus O34.59 ☑
    - scar (s)
      - cervix O34.4 ☑
      - cesarean delivery O34.219
        - classical (vertical) O34.212
        - low transverse O34.211
      - transmural uterine O34.29
      - uterus O34.29
    - Shirodkar suture in situ O34.3 ☑
    - shoulder presentation O32.2 ☑

- **Delivery** — *continued*
  - cesarean — *continued*
    - stenosis or stricture, cervix O34.4 ☑
    - streptococcus group B (GBS) carrier state O99.824
    - transmural uterine scar O34.29
    - transverse presentation or lie O32.2 ☑
    - tumor, pelvic organs or tissues NEC O34.8 ☑
      - cervix O34.4 ☑
    - umbilical cord presentation or prolapse O69.0 ☑
    - without indication O82
  - completely normal case O80
  - complicated O75.9
    - by
      - abnormal, abnormality (of)
        - forces of labor O62.9
          - specified type NEC O62.8
        - glucose O99.814
        - uterine contractions NOS O62.9
      - abruptio placentae (*see also* Abruptio placentae)O45.9 ☑
      - abuse
        - physical O9A.32
        - psychological O9A.52
        - sexual O9A.42
      - adherent placenta O72.0
        - without hemorrhage O73.0
      - alcohol use O99.314
      - anemia (pre-existing) O99.02
      - anesthetic death O74.8
      - annular detachment of cervix O71.3
      - atony, uterus O62.2
      - attempted vacuum extraction and forceps O66.5
      - Bandl's ring O62.4
      - bariatric surgery status O99.844
      - biliary tract disorder O26.62
      - bleeding — *see* Delivery, complicated by, hemorrhage
      - blood disorder NEC O99.12
      - cervical dystocia (hypotonic) O62.2
        - primary O62.0
        - secondary O62.1
      - circulatory system disorder O99.42
      - compression of cord (umbilical) NEC O69.2 ☑
      - condition NEC O99.89
      - contraction, contracted ring O62.4
      - cord (umbilical)
        - around neck
          - with compression O69.1 ☑
          - without compression O69.81 ☑
        - bruising O69.5 ☑
        - complication O69.9 ☑
          - specified NEC O69.89 ☑
        - compression NEC O69.2 ☑
        - entanglement O69.2 ☑
          - without compression O69.82 ☑
        - hematoma O69.5 ☑
        - presentation O69.0 ☑
        - prolapse O69.0 ☑
        - short O69.3 ☑
        - thrombosis (vessels) O69.5 ☑
        - vascular lesion O69.5 ☑
      - Couvelaire uterus O45.8X ☑
      - damage to (injury to) NEC
        - perineum O71.82
        - periurethral tissue O71.82
        - vulva O71.82
      - delay following rupture of membranes (spontaneous) — *see* Pregnancy, complicated by, premature rupture of membranes
      - depressed fetal heart tones O76
      - diabetes O24.92
        - gestational O24.429
          - diet controlled O24.420
          - insulin controlled O24.424
          - oral drug controlled (antidiabetic) (hypoglycemic) O24.425
        - pre-existing O24.32
          - specified NEC O24.82
          - type 1 O24.02
          - type 2 O24.12
      - diastasis recti (abdominis) O71.89
      - dilatation
        - bladder O66.8
        - cervix incomplete, poor or slow O62.0
      - disease NEC O99.89
      - disruptio uteri — *see* Delivery, complicated by, rupture, uterus
      - drug use O99.324

- **Delivery** — *continued*
  - complicated — *continued*
    - dysfunction, uterus NOS O62.9
      - hypertonic O62.4
      - hypotonic O62.2
        - primary O62.0
        - secondary O62.1
      - incoordinate O62.4
    - eclampsia O15.1
    - embolism (pulmonary) — *see* Embolism, obstetric
    - endocrine, nutritional or metabolic disease NEC O99.284
    - failed
      - attempted vaginal birth after previous cesarean delivery O66.41
      - induction of labor O61.9
        - instrumental O61.1
        - mechanical O61.1
        - medical O61.0
        - specified NEC O61.8
        - surgical O61.1
      - trial of labor O66.40
    - female genital mutilation O65.5
    - fetal
      - abnormal acid-base balance O68
      - acidemia O68
      - acidosis O68
      - alkalosis O68
      - death, early O02.1
      - deformity O66.3
      - heart rate or rhythm (abnormal) (non-reassuring) O76
      - hypoxia O77.8
      - stress O77.9
        - due to drug administration O77.1
        - electrocardiographic evidence of O77.8
        - specified NEC O77.8
        - ultrasound evidence of O77.8
    - fever during labor O75.2
    - gastric banding status O99.844
    - gastric bypass status O99.844
    - gastrointestinal disease NEC O99.62
    - gestational
      - diabetes O24.429
        - diet controlled O24.420
        - insulin (and diet) controlled O24.424
        - oral drug controlled (antidiabetic) (hypoglycemic) O24.425
      - edema O12.04
        - with proteinuria O12.24
      - proteinuria O12.14
    - gonorrhea O98.22
    - hematoma O71.7
      - ischial spine O71.7
      - pelvic O71.7
      - vagina O71.7
      - vulva or perineum O71.7
    - hemorrhage (uterine) O67.9
      - associated with
        - afibrinogenemia O67.0
        - coagulation defect O67.0
        - hyperfibrinolysis O67.0
        - hypofibrinogenemia O67.0
      - due to
        - low implantation of placenta O44.5 ☑
        - low lying placenta O44.5 ☑
        - placenta previa O44.1 ☑
          - marginal O44.3 ☑
          - partial O44.3 ☑
        - premature separation of placenta (normally implanted) (*see also* Abruptio placentae)O45.9 ☑
        - retained placenta O72.0
        - uterine leiomyoma O67.8
      - placenta NEC O67.8
      - postpartum NEC (atonic) (immediate) O72.1
        - with retained or trapped placenta O72.0
        - delayed O72.2
        - secondary O72.2
        - third stage O72.0
    - hourglass contraction, uterus O62.4
    - hypertension, hypertensive (pre-existing) — *see* Hypertension, complicated by, childbirth (labor)
    - hypotension O26.5 ☑
    - incomplete dilatation (cervix) O62.0
    - incoordinate uterus contractions O62.4
    - inertia, uterus O62.2
      - during latent phase of labor O62.0
      - primary O62.0
      - secondary O62.1
    - infection (maternal) O98.92
      - carrier state NEC O99.834
      - gonorrhea O98.22
      - human immunodeficiency virus (HIV) O98.72
      - sexually transmitted NEC O98.32
      - specified NEC O98.82
      - syphilis O98.12
      - tuberculosis O98.02
      - viral hepatitis O98.42
      - viral NEC O98.52
    - injury (to mother) (*see also* Delivery, complicated, by, damage to)O71.9
      - nonobstetric O9A.22
        - caused by abuse — *see* Delivery, complicated by, abuse
    - intrauterine fetal death, early O02.1
    - inversion, uterus O71.2
    - laceration (perineal) O70.9
      - anus (sphincter) O70.4
        - with third degree laceration (*see also* Delivery, complicated, by, laceration, perineum, third degree)O70.20
          - with mucosa O70.3
        - without third degree laceration O70.4
      - bladder (urinary) O71.5
      - bowel O71.5
      - cervix (uteri) O71.3
      - fourchette O70.0
      - hymen O70.0
      - labia O70.0
      - pelvic
        - floor O70.1
        - organ NEC O71.5
      - perineum, perineal O70.9
        - first degree O70.0
        - fourth degree O70.3
        - muscles O70.1
        - second degree O70.1
        - skin O70.0
        - slight O70.0
        - third degree O70.20
          - with
            - both external anal sphincter (EAS) and internal anal sphincter (IAS) torn (IIIc) O70.23
            - less than 50% of external anal sphincter (EAS) thickness torn (IIIa) O70.21
            - more than 50% external anal sphincter (EAS) thickness torn (IIIb) O70.22
          - IIIa O70.21
          - IIIb O70.22
          - IIIc O70.23
      - peritoneum (pelvic) O71.5
      - rectovaginal (septum) (without perineal laceration) O71.4
        - with perineum (*see also* Delivery, complicated, by, laceration, perineum, third degree)O70.20
          - with anal or rectal mucosa O70.3
      - specified NEC O71.89
      - sphincter ani — *see* Delivery, complicated, by, laceration, anus (sphincter)
      - urethra O71.5
      - uterus O71.81
        - before labor O71.81
      - vagina, vaginal (deep) (high) (without perineal laceration) O71.4
        - with perineum O70.0
        - muscles, with perineum O70.1
      - vulva O70.0
    - liver disorder O26.62
    - malignancy O9A.12
    - malnutrition O25.2
    - malposition, malpresentation
      - placenta O44.0 ☑
        - with hemorrhage O44.1 ☑
      - uterus or cervix O65.5
      - without obstruction (*see also* Delivery, complicated by, obstruction)O32.9 ☑
        - breech O32.1 ☑
        - compound O32.6 ☑
        - face (brow) (chin) O32.3 ☑
        - footling O32.8 ☑
        - high head O32.4 ☑
        - oblique O32.2 ☑
        - specified NEC O32.8 ☑
        - transverse O32.2 ☑
        - unstable lie O32.0 ☑
    - meconium in amniotic fluid O77.0
    - mental disorder NEC O99.344
    - metrorrhexis — *see* Delivery, complicated by, rupture, uterus
    - nervous system disorder O99.354
    - obesity (pre-existing) O99.214
    - obesity surgery status O99.844
    - obstetric trauma O71.9
      - specified NEC O71.89
    - obstructed labor
      - due to
        - breech (complete) (frank) presentation O64.1 ☑
          - incomplete O64.8 ☑
        - brow presentation O64.3 ☑
        - buttock presentation O64.1 ☑
        - chin presentation O64.2 ☑
        - compound presentation O64.5 ☑
        - contracted pelvis O65.1
        - deep transverse arrest O64.0 ☑
        - deformed pelvis O65.0
        - dystocia (fetal) O66.9
          - due to
            - conjoined twins O66.3
            - fetal
              - abnormality NEC O66.3
              - ascites O66.3
              - hydrops O66.3
              - meningomyelocele O66.3
              - sacral teratoma O66.3
              - tumor O66.3
            - hydrocephalic fetus O66.3
          - shoulder O66.0
        - face presentation O64.2 ☑
        - fetopelvic disproportion O65.4
        - footling presentation O64.8 ☑
        - impacted shoulders O66.0
        - incomplete rotation of fetal head O64.0 ☑
        - large fetus O66.2
        - locked twins O66.1
        - malposition O64.9 ☑
          - specified NEC O64.8 ☑
        - malpresentation O64.9 ☑
          - specified NEC O64.8 ☑
        - multiple fetuses NEC O66.6
        - pelvic
          - abnormality (maternal) O65.9
            - organ O65.5
            - specified NEC O65.8
          - contraction
            - inlet O65.2
            - mid-cavity O65.3
            - outlet O65.3
        - persistent (position)
          - occipitoiliac O64.0 ☑
          - occipitoposterior O64.0 ☑
          - occipitosacral O64.0 ☑
          - occipitotransverse O64.0 ☑
        - prolapsed arm O64.4 ☑
        - shoulder presentation O64.4 ☑
      - specified NEC O66.8
    - pathological retraction ring, uterus O62.4
    - penetration, pregnant uterus by instrument O71.1
    - perforation — *see* Delivery, complicated by, laceration
    - placenta, placental
      - ablatio (*see also* Abruptio placentae)O45.9 ☑
      - abnormality O43.9 ☑
        - specified NEC O43.89 ☑
      - abruptio (*see also* Abruptio placentae)O45.9 ☑
      - accreta O43.21 ☑
      - adherent (with hemorrhage) O72.0
        - without hemorrhage O73.0
      - detachment (premature) (*see also* Abruptio placentae)O45.9 ☑
      - disorder O43.9 ☑
        - specified NEC O43.89 ☑
      - hemorrhage NEC O67.8
      - increta O43.22 ☑
      - low (implantation) (lying) O44.4 ☑
        - with hemorrhage O44.5 ☑
      - malformation O43.10 ☑
      - malposition O44.0 ☑
        - without hemorrhage O44.1 ☑

Delivery - Dependence

- **Delivery** — *continued*
  - complicated — *continued*
      - percreta O43.23 ☑
      - previa (central) (complete) (lateral) (total) O44.0 ☑
        - with hemorrhage O44.1 ☑
        - marginal O44.2 ☑
          - with hemorrhage O44.3 ☑
        - partial O44.2 ☑
          - with hemorrhage O44.3 ☑
      - retained (with hemorrhage) O72.0
        - without hemorrhage O73.0
      - separation (premature) O45.9 ☑
        - specified NEC O45.8X ☑
      - vicious insertion O44.1 ☑
    - precipitate labor O62.3
    - premature rupture, membranes (*see also* Pregnancy, complicated by, premature rupture of membranes)O42.90
    - prolapse
      - arm or hand O32.2 ☑
      - cord (umbilical) O69.0 ☑
      - foot or leg O32.8 ☑
      - uterus O34.52 ☑
    - prolonged labor O63.9
      - first stage O63.0
      - second stage O63.1
    - protozoal disease (maternal) O98.62
    - respiratory disease NEC O99.52
    - retained membranes or portions of placenta O72.2
      - without hemorrhage O73.1
    - retarded birth O63.9
    - retention of secundines (with hemorrhage) O72.0
      - without hemorrhage O73.0
      - partial O72.2
        - without hemorrhage O73.1
    - rupture
      - bladder (urinary) O71.5
      - cervix O71.3
      - pelvic organ NEC O71.5
      - urethra O71.5
      - uterus (during or after labor) O71.1
        - before labor O71.0 ☑
    - separation, pubic bone (symphysis pubis) O71.6
    - shock O75.1
    - shoulder presentation O64.4 ☑
    - skin disorder NEC O99.72
    - spasm, cervix O62.4
    - stenosis or stricture, cervix O65.5
    - streptococcus group B (GBS) carrier state O99.824
    - subluxation of symphysis (pubis) O26.72
    - syphilis (maternal) O98.12
    - tear — *see* Delivery, complicated by, laceration
    - tetanic uterus O62.4
    - trauma (obstetrical) (*see also* Delivery, complicated, by, damage to)O71.9
      - non-obstetric O9A.22
      - periurethral O71.82
      - specified NEC O71.89
    - tuberculosis (maternal) O98.02
    - tumor, pelvic organs or tissues NEC O65.5
    - umbilical cord around neck
      - with compression O69.1 ☑
      - without compression O69.81 ☑
    - uterine inertia O62.2
      - during latent phase of labor O62.0
      - primary O62.0
      - secondary O62.1
    - vasa previa O69.4 ☑
    - velamentous insertion of cord O43.12 ☑
    - specified complication NEC O75.89
  - delayed NOS O63.9
    - following rupture of membranes
      - artificial O75.5
    - second twin, triplet, etc. O63.2
  - forceps, low following failed vacuum extraction O66.5
  - missed (at or near term) O36.4 ☑
  - normal O80
  - obstructed — *see* Delivery, complicated by, obstruction
  - precipitate O62.3
  - preterm (*see also* Pregnancy, complicated by, preterm labor)O60.10 ☑
  - spontaneous O80
  - term pregnancy NOS O80
  - uncomplicated O80

- **Delivery** — *continued*
  - vaginal, following previous cesarean delivery O34.219
    - classical (vertical) scar O34.212
    - low transverse scar O34.211
- **Delusions** (paranoid) — *see* Disorder, delusional
- **Dementia** (degenerative (primary)) (old age) (persisting) F03.90
  - with
    - aggressive behavior F03.91
    - behavioral disturbance F03.91
    - combative behavior F03.91
    - Lewy bodies G31.83 *[F02.80]*
      - with behavioral disturbance G31.83 *[F02.81]*
    - Parkinsonism G31.83 *[F02.80]*
      - with behavioral disturbance G31.83 *[F02.81]*
    - Parkinson's disease G20 *[F02.80]*
      - with behavioral disturbance G20 *[F02.81]*
    - violent behavior F03.91
  - alcoholic F10.97
    - with dependence F10.27
  - Alzheimer's type — *see* Disease, Alzheimer's
  - arteriosclerotic — *see* Dementia, vascular
  - atypical, Alzheimer's type — *see* Disease, Alzheimer's, specified NEC
  - congenital — *see* Disability, intellectual
  - frontal (lobe) G31.09 *[F02.80]*
    - with behavioral disturbance G31.09 *[F02.81]*
  - frontotemporal G31.09 *[F02.80]*
    - with behavioral disturbance G31.09 *[F02.81]*
    - specified NEC G31.09 *[F02.80]*
      - with behavioral disturbance G31.09 *[F02.81]*
  - in (due to)
    - alcohol F10.97
      - with dependence F10.27
    - Alzheimer's disease — *see* Disease, Alzheimer's
    - arteriosclerotic brain disease — *see* Dementia, vascular
    - cerebral lipidoses E75. ☑ *[F02.80]*
      - with behavioral disturbance E75. ☑ *[F02.81]*
    - Creutzfeldt-Jakob disease (*see also* Creutzfeldt-Jakob disease or syndrome (with dementia))A81.00
    - epilepsy G40. ☑ *[F02.80]*
      - with behavioral disturbance G40. ☑ *[F02.81]*
    - hepatolenticular degeneration E83.01 *[F02.80]*
      - with behavioral disturbance E83.01 *[F02.81]*
    - human immunodeficiency virus (HIV) disease B20 *[F02.80]*
      - with behavioral disturbance B20 *[F02.81]*
    - Huntington's disease or chorea G10
    - hypercalcemia E83.52 *[F02.80]*
      - with behavioral disturbance E83.52 *[F02.81]*
    - hypothyroidism, acquired E03.9 *[F02.80]*
      - with behavioral disturbance E03.9 *[F02.81]*
      - due to iodine deficiency E01.8 *[F02.80]*
        - with behavioral disturbance E01.8 *[F02.81]*
    - inhalants F18.97
      - with dependence F18.27
    - multiple
      - etiologies F03 ☑
      - sclerosis G35 *[F02.80]*
        - with behavioral disturbance G35 *[F02.81]*
    - neurosyphilis A52.17 *[F02.80]*
      - with behavioral disturbance A52.17 *[F02.81]*
      - juvenile A50.49 *[F02.80]*
        - with behavioral disturbance A50.49 *[F02.81]*
    - niacin deficiency E52 *[F02.80]*
      - with behavioral disturbance E52 *[F02.81]*
    - paralysis agitans G20 *[F02.80]*
      - with behavioral disturbance G20 *[F02.81]*
    - Parkinson's disease G20 *[F02.80]*
    - pellagra E52 *[F02.80]*
      - with behavioral disturbance E52 *[F02.81]*
    - Pick's G31.01 *[F02.80]*
      - with behavioral disturbance G31.01 *[F02.81]*
    - polyarteritis nodosa M30.0 *[F02.80]*
      - with behavioral disturbance M30.0 *[F02.81]*
    - psychoactive drug F19.97
      - with dependence F19.27
      - inhalants F18.97
        - with dependence F18.27
      - sedatives, hypnotics or anxiolytics F13.97
        - with dependence F13.27
    - sedatives, hypnotics or anxiolytics F13.97
      - with dependence F13.27
    - systemic lupus erythematosus M32. ☑ *[F02.80]*
      - with behavioral disturbance M32. ☑ *[F02.81]*
    - trypanosomiasis
      - African B56.9 *[F02.80]*
        - with behavioral disturbance B56.9 *[F02.81]*

- **Dementia** — *continued*
  - in — *continued*
    - unknown etiology F03 ☑
    - vitamin B12 deficiency E53.8 *[F02.80]*
      - with behavioral disturbance E53.8 *[F02.81]*
    - volatile solvents F18.97
      - with dependence F18.27
    - with behavioral disturbance G31.83 *[F02.81]*
  - infantile, infantilis F84.3
  - Lewy body G31.83 *[F02.80]*
    - with behavioral disturbance G31.83 *[F02.81]*
  - multi-infarct — *see* Dementia, vascular
  - paralytica, paralytic (syphilitic) A52.17 *[F02.80]*
    - with behavioral disturbance A52.17 *[F02.81]*
    - juvenilis A50.45
  - paretic A52.17
  - praecox — *see* Schizophrenia
  - presenile F03 ☑
    - Alzheimer's type — *see* Disease, Alzheimer's, early onset
  - primary degenerative F03 ☑
  - progressive, syphilitic A52.17
  - senile F03 ☑
    - with acute confusional state F05
    - Alzheimer's type — *see* Disease, Alzheimer's, late onset
    - depressed or paranoid type F03 ☑
  - vascular (acute onset) (mixed) (multi-infarct) (subcortical) F01.50
    - with behavioral disturbance F01.51
- **Demineralization,** bone — *see* Osteoporosis
- **Demodex** folliculorum (infestation) B88.0
- **Demophobia** F40.248
- **Demoralization** R45.3
- **Demyelination,** demyelinization
  - central nervous system G37.9
    - specified NEC G37.8
  - corpus callosum (central) G37.1
  - disseminated, acute G36.9
    - specified NEC G36.8
  - global G35
  - in optic neuritis G36.0
- **Dengue** (classical) (fever) A90
  - hemorrhagic A91
  - sandfly A93.1
- **Dennie-Marfan** syphilitic syndrome A50.45
- **Dens** evaginatus, in dente or invaginatus K00.2
- **Dense** breasts R92.2
- **Density**
  - increased, bone (disseminated) (generalized) (spotted) — *see* Disorder, bone, density and structure, specified type NEC
  - lung (nodular) J98.4
- **Dental** (*see also* condition)
  - examination Z01.20
    - with abnormal findings Z01.21
  - restoration
    - aesthetically inadequate or displeasing K08.56
    - defective K08.50
      - specified NEC K08.59
    - failure of marginal integrity K08.51
    - failure of periodontal anatomical integrity K08.54
- **Dentia** praecox K00.6
- **Denticles** (pulp) K04.2
- **Dentigerous** cyst K09.0
- **Dentin**
  - irregular (in pulp) K04.3
  - opalescent K00.5
  - secondary (in pulp) K04.3
  - sensitive K03.89
- **Dentinogenesis** imperfecta K00.5
- **Dentinoma** — *see* Cyst, calcifying odontogenic
- **Dentition** (syndrome) K00.7
  - delayed K00.6
  - difficult K00.7
  - precocious K00.6
  - premature K00.6
  - retarded K00.6
- **Dependence** (on) (syndrome) F19.20
  - with remission F19.21
  - alcohol (ethyl) (methyl) (without remission) F10.20
    - with
      - amnestic disorder, persisting F10.26
      - anxiety disorder F10.280
      - dementia, persisting F10.27
      - intoxication F10.229
        - with delirium F10.221
        - uncomplicated F10.220
      - mood disorder F10.24
      - psychotic disorder F10.259

- **Dependence** — *continued*
  - alcohol — *continued*
        - with
          - delusions F10.250
          - hallucinations F10.251
      - remission F10.21
      - sexual dysfunction F10.281
      - sleep disorder F10.282
      - specified disorder NEC F10.288
      - withdrawal F10.239
        - with
          - delirium F10.231
          - perceptual disturbance F10.232
        - uncomplicated F10.230
    - counseling and surveillance Z71.41
  - amobarbital — *see* Dependence, drug, sedative
  - amphetamine (s) (type) — *see* Dependence, drug, stimulant NEC
  - amytal (sodium) — *see* Dependence, drug, sedative
  - analgesic NEC F55.8
  - anesthetic (agent) (gas) (general) (local) NEC — *see* Dependence, drug, psychoactive NEC
  - anxiolytic NEC — *see* Dependence, drug, sedative
  - barbital (s) — *see* Dependence, drug, sedative
  - barbiturate (s) (compounds) (drugs classifiable to T42) — *see* Dependence, drug, sedative
  - benzedrine — *see* Dependence, drug, stimulant NEC
  - bhang — *see* Dependence, drug, cannabis
  - bromide (s) NEC — *see* Dependence, drug, sedative
  - caffeine — *see* Dependence, drug, stimulant NEC
  - cannabis (sativa) (indica) (resin) (derivatives) (type) — *see* Dependence, drug, cannabis
  - chloral (betaine) (hydrate) — *see* Dependence, drug, sedative
  - chlordiazepoxide — *see* Dependence, drug, sedative
  - coca (leaf) (derivatives) — *see* Dependence, drug, cocaine
  - cocaine — *see* Dependence, drug, cocaine
  - codeine — *see* Dependence, drug, opioid
  - combinations of drugs F19.20
  - dagga — *see* Dependence, drug, cannabis
  - Demerol® — *see* Dependence, drug, opioid
  - dexamphetamine — *see* Dependence, drug, stimulant NEC
  - dexedrine — *see* Dependence, drug, stimulant NEC
  - dextromethorphan — *see* Dependence, drug, opioid
  - dextromoramide — *see* Dependence, drug, opioid
  - dextro-nor-pseudo-ephedrine — *see* Dependence, drug, stimulant NEC
  - dextrorphan — *see* Dependence, drug, opioid
  - diazepam — *see* Dependence, drug, sedative
  - dilaudid — *see* Dependence, drug, opioid
  - D-lysergic acid diethylamide — *see* Dependence, drug, hallucinogen
  - drug NEC F19.20
    - with sleep disorder F19.282
    - cannabis F12.20
      - with
        - anxiety disorder F12.280
        - intoxication F12.229
          - with
            - delirium F12.221
            - perceptual disturbance F12.222
          - uncomplicated F12.220
        - other specified disorder F12.288
        - psychosis F12.259
          - delusions F12.250
          - hallucinations F12.251
        - unspecified disorder F12.29
      - in remission F12.21
    - cocaine F14.20
      - with
        - anxiety disorder F14.280
        - intoxication F14.229
          - with
            - delirium F14.221
            - perceptual disturbance F14.222
          - uncomplicated F14.220
        - mood disorder F14.24
        - other specified disorder F14.288
        - psychosis F14.259
          - delusions F14.250
          - hallucinations F14.251
        - sexual dysfunction F14.281
        - sleep disorder F14.282

- **Dependence** — *continued*
  - drug NEC — *continued*
        - unspecified disorder F14.29
        - withdrawal F14.23
      - in remission F14.21
      - withdrawal symptoms in newborn P96.1
    - counseling and surveillance Z71.51
    - hallucinogen F16.20
      - with
        - anxiety disorder F16.280
        - flashbacks F16.283
        - intoxication F16.229
          - with delirium F16.221
          - uncomplicated F16.220
        - mood disorder F16.24
        - other specified disorder F16.288
        - perception disorder, persisting F16.283
        - psychosis F16.259
          - delusions F16.250
          - hallucinations F16.251
        - unspecified disorder F16.29
      - in remission F16.21
    - in remission F19.21
    - inhalant F18.20
      - with
        - anxiety disorder F18.280
        - dementia, persisting F18.27
        - intoxication F18.229
          - with delirium F18.221
          - uncomplicated F18.220
        - mood disorder F18.24
        - other specified disorder F18.288
        - psychosis F18.259
          - delusions F18.250
          - hallucinations F18.251
        - unspecified disorder F18.29
      - in remission F18.21
    - nicotine F17.200
      - with disorder F17.209
        - remission F17.201
        - specified disorder NEC F17.208
        - withdrawal F17.203
      - chewing tobacco F17.220
        - with disorder F17.229
          - remission F17.221
          - specified disorder NEC F17.228
          - withdrawal F17.223
      - cigarettes F17.210
        - with disorder F17.219
          - remission F17.211
          - specified disorder NEC F17.218
          - withdrawal F17.213
      - specified product NEC F17.290
        - with disorder F17.299
          - remission F17.291
          - specified disorder NEC F17.298
          - withdrawal F17.293
    - opioid F11.20
      - with
        - intoxication F11.229
          - with
            - delirium F11.221
            - perceptual disturbance F11.222
          - uncomplicated F11.220
        - mood disorder F11.24
        - other specified disorder F11.288
        - psychosis F11.259
          - delusions F11.250
          - hallucinations F11.251
        - sexual dysfunction F11.281
        - sleep disorder F11.282
        - unspecified disorder F11.29
        - withdrawal F11.23
      - in remission F11.21
    - psychoactive NEC F19.20
      - with
        - amnestic disorder F19.26
        - anxiety disorder F19.280
        - dementia F19.27
        - intoxication F19.229
          - with
            - delirium F19.221
            - perceptual disturbance F19.222
          - uncomplicated F19.220
        - mood disorder F19.24
        - other specified disorder F19.288
        - psychosis F19.259
          - delusions F19.250
          - hallucinations F19.251
        - sexual dysfunction F19.281
        - sleep disorder F19.282
        - unspecified disorder F19.29

- **Dependence** — *continued*
  - drug NEC — *continued*
        - withdrawal F19.239
          - with
            - delirium F19.231
            - perceptual disturbance F19.232
          - uncomplicated F19.230
    - sedative, hypnotic or anxiolytic F13.20
      - with
        - amnestic disorder F13.26
        - anxiety disorder F13.280
        - dementia, persisting F13.27
        - intoxication F13.229
          - with delirium F13.221
          - uncomplicated F13.220
        - mood disorder F13.24
        - other specified disorder F13.288
        - psychosis F13.259
          - delusions F13.250
          - hallucinations F13.251
        - sexual dysfunction F13.281
        - sleep disorder F13.282
        - unspecified disorder F13.29
        - withdrawal F13.239
          - with
            - delirium F13.231
            - perceptual disturbance F13.232
          - uncomplicated F13.230
      - in remission F13.21
    - stimulant NEC F15.20
      - with
        - anxiety disorder F15.280
        - intoxication F15.229
          - with
            - delirium F15.221
            - perceptual disturbance F15.222
          - uncomplicated F15.220
        - mood disorder F15.24
        - other specified disorder F15.288
        - psychosis F15.259
          - delusions F15.250
          - hallucinations F15.251
        - sexual dysfunction F15.281
        - sleep disorder F15.282
        - unspecified disorder F15.29
        - withdrawal F15.23
      - in remission F15.21
  - ethyl
    - alcohol (without remission) F10.20
      - with remission F10.21
    - bromide — *see* Dependence, drug, sedative
    - carbamate F19.20
    - chloride F19.20
    - morphine — *see* Dependence, drug, opioid
  - ganja — *see* Dependence, drug, cannabis
  - glue (airplane) (sniffing) — *see* Dependence, drug, inhalant
  - glutethimide — *see* Dependence, drug, sedative
  - hallucinogenics — *see* Dependence, drug, hallucinogen
  - hashish — *see* Dependence, drug, cannabis
  - hemp — *see* Dependence, drug, cannabis
  - heroin (salt) (any) — *see* Dependence, drug, opioid
  - hypnotic NEC — *see* Dependence, drug, sedative
  - Indian hemp — *see* Dependence, drug, cannabis
  - inhalants — *see* Dependence, drug, inhalant
  - khat — *see* Dependence, drug, stimulant NEC
  - laudanum — *see* Dependence, drug, opioid
  - LSD (-25) (derivatives) — *see* Dependence, drug, hallucinogen
  - luminal — *see* Dependence, drug, sedative
  - lysergic acid — *see* Dependence, drug, hallucinogen
  - maconha — *see* Dependence, drug, cannabis
  - marihuana — *see* Dependence, drug, cannabis
  - meprobamate — *see* Dependence, drug, sedative
  - mescaline — *see* Dependence, drug, hallucinogen
  - methadone — *see* Dependence, drug, opioid
  - methamphetamine (s) — *see* Dependence, drug, stimulant NEC
  - methaqualone — *see* Dependence, drug, sedative
  - methyl
    - alcohol (without remission) F10.20
      - with remission F10.21
    - bromide — *see* Dependence, drug, sedative
    - morphine — *see* Dependence, drug, opioid
    - phenidate — *see* Dependence, drug, stimulant NEC
    - sulfonal — *see* Dependence, drug, sedative

Dependence - Derangement

Dependence — *continued*
- morphine (sulfate) (sulfite) (type) — *see* Dependence, drug, opioid
- narcotic (drug) NEC — *see* Dependence, drug, opioid
- nembutal — *see* Dependence, drug, sedative
- neraval — *see* Dependence, drug, sedative
- neravan — *see* Dependence, drug, sedative
- neurobarb — *see* Dependence, drug, sedative
- nicotine — *see* Dependence, drug, nicotine
- nitrous oxide F19.20
- nonbarbiturate sedatives and tranquilizers with similar effect — *see* Dependence, drug, sedative
- on
  - artificial heart (fully implantable) (mechanical) Z95.812
  - aspirator Z99.0
  - care provider (because of) Z74.9
    - impaired mobility Z74.09
    - need for
      - assistance with personal care Z74.1
      - continuous supervision Z74.3
    - no other household member able to render care Z74.2
    - specified reason NEC Z74.8
  - machine Z99.89
    - enabling NEC Z99.89
    - specified type NEC Z99.89
  - renal dialysis (hemodialysis) (peritoneal) Z99.2
  - respirator Z99.11
  - ventilator Z99.11
  - wheelchair Z99.3
- opiate — *see* Dependence, drug, opioid
- opioids — *see* Dependence, drug, opioid
- opium (alkaloids) (derivatives) (tincture) — *see* Dependence, drug, opioid
- oxygen (long-term) (supplemental) Z99.81
- paraldehyde — *see* Dependence, drug, sedative
- paregoric — *see* Dependence, drug, opioid
- PCP (phencyclidine) (or related substance) — *see* Dependence, drug, hallucinogen
- pentobarbital — *see* Dependence, drug, sedative
- pentobarbitone (sodium) — *see* Dependence, drug, sedative
- pentothal — *see* Dependence, drug, sedative
- peyote — *see* Dependence, drug, hallucinogen
- phencyclidine (PCP) (or related substance) — *see* Dependence, drug, hallucinogen
- phenmetrazine — *see* Dependence, drug, stimulant NEC
- phenobarbital — *see* Dependence, drug, sedative
- polysubstance F19.20
- psilocibin, psilocin, psilocyn, psilocyline — *see* Dependence, drug, hallucinogen
- psychostimulant NEC — *see* Dependence, drug, stimulant NEC
- secobarbital — *see* Dependence, drug, sedative
- seconal — *see* Dependence, drug, sedative
- sedative NEC — *see* Dependence, drug, sedative
- specified drug NEC — *see* Dependence, drug
- stimulant NEC — *see* Dependence, drug, stimulant NEC
- substance NEC — *see* Dependence, drug
- supplemental oxygen Z99.81
- tobacco — *see* Dependence, drug, nicotine
  - counseling and surveillance Z71.6
- tranquilizer NEC — *see* Dependence, drug, sedative
- vitamin B6 E53.1
- volatile solvents — *see* Dependence, drug, inhalant

Dependency
- care-provider Z74.9
- passive F60.7
- reactions (persistent) F60.7

Depersonalization (in neurotic state) (neurotic) (syndrome) F48.1

Depletion
- extracellular fluid E86.9
- plasma E86.1
- potassium E87.6
  - nephropathy N25.89
- salt or sodium E87.1
  - causing heat exhaustion or prostration T67.4 ☑
  - nephropathy N28.9
- volume NOS E86.9

Deployment (current) (military) status Z56.82
- in theater or in support of military war, peacekeeping and humanitarian operations Z56.82

Deployment — *continued*
- personal history of Z91.82
  - military war, peacekeeping and humanitarian deployment (current or past conflict) Z91.82
- returned from Z91.82

Depolarization, premature I49.40
- atrial I49.1
- junctional I49.2
- specified NEC I49.49
- ventricular I49.3

Deposit
- bone in Boeck's sarcoid D86.89
- calcareous, calcium — *see* Calcification
- cholesterol
  - retina H35.89
  - vitreous (body) (humor) — *see* Deposit, crystalline
- conjunctiva H11.11 ☑
- cornea H18.00 ☑
  - argentous H18.02 ☑
  - due to metabolic disorder H18.03 ☑
  - Kayser-Fleischer ring H18.04 ☑
  - pigmentation — *see* Pigmentation, cornea
- crystalline, vitreous (body) (humor) H43.2 ☑
- hemosiderin in old scars of cornea — *see* Pigmentation, cornea, stromal
- metallic in lens — *see* Cataract, specified NEC
- skin R23.8
- tooth, teeth (betel) (black) (green) (materia alba) (orange) (tobacco) K03.6
- urate, kidney — *see* Calculus, kidney

Depraved appetite — *see* Pica

Depressed
- HDL cholesterol E78.6

Depression (acute) (mental) F32.9
- agitated (single episode) F32.2
- anaclitic — *see* Disorder, adjustment
- anxiety F41.8
  - persistent F34.1
- arches (*see also* Deformity, limb, flat foot)
- atypical (single episode) F32.89
  - recurrent episode F33.8
- basal metabolic rate R94.8
- bone marrow D75.89
- central nervous system R09.2
- cerebral R29.818
  - newborn P91.4
- cerebrovascular I67.9
- chest wall M95.4
- climacteric (single episode) F32.89
  - recurrent episode F33.8
- endogenous (without psychotic symptoms) F33.2
  - with psychotic symptoms F33.3
- functional activity R68.89
- hysterical F44.89
- involutional (single episode) F32.89
  - recurrent episode F33.8
- major F32.9
  - with psychotic symptoms F32.3
  - recurrent — *see* Disorder, depressive, recurrent
- manic-depressive — *see* Disorder, depressive, recurrent
- masked (single episode) F32.89
- medullary G93.89
- menopausal (single episode) F32.89
  - recurrent episode F33.8
- metatarsus — *see* Depression, arches
- monopolar F33.9
- nervous F34.1
- neurotic F34.1
- nose M95.0
- postnatal F53
- postpartum F53
- post-psychotic of schizophrenia F32.89
- post-schizophrenic F32.89
- psychogenic (reactive) (single episode) F32.9
- psychoneurotic F34.1
- psychotic (single episode) F32.3
  - recurrent F33.3
- reactive (psychogenic) (single episode) F32.9
  - psychotic (single episode) F32.3
- recurrent — *see* Disorder, depressive, recurrent
- respiratory center G93.89
- seasonal — *see* Disorder, depressive, recurrent
- senile F03 ☑
- severe, single episode F32.2
- situational F43.21
- skull Q67.4
- specified NEC (single episode) F32.89
- sternum M95.4
- visual field — *see* Defect, visual field

Depression — *continued*
- vital (recurrent) (without psychotic symptoms) F33.2
  - with psychotic symptoms F33.3
  - single episode F32.2

Deprivation
- cultural Z60.3
- effects NOS T73.9 ☑
  - specified NEC T73.8 ☑
- emotional NEC Z65.8
  - affecting infant or child — *see* Maltreatment, child, psychological
- food T73.0 ☑
- protein — *see* Malnutrition
- sleep Z72.820
- social Z60.4
  - affecting infant or child — *see* Maltreatment, child, psychological
- specified NEC T73.8 ☑
- vitamins — *see* Deficiency, vitamin
- water T73.1 ☑

Derangement
- ankle (internal) — *see* Derangement, joint, ankle
- cartilage (articular) NEC — *see* Derangement, joint, articular cartilage, by site
  - recurrent — *see* Dislocation, recurrent
- cruciate ligament, anterior, current injury — *see* Sprain, knee, cruciate, anterior
- elbow (internal) — *see* Derangement, joint, elbow
- hip (joint) (internal) (old) — *see* Derangement, joint, hip
- joint (internal) M24.9
  - ankylosis — *see* Ankylosis
  - articular cartilage M24.10
    - ankle M24.17 ☑
    - elbow M24.12 ☑
    - foot M24.17 ☑
    - hand M24.14 ☑
    - hip M24.15 ☑
    - knee NEC M23.9 ☑
    - loose body — *see* Loose, body
    - shoulder M24.11 ☑
    - wrist M24.13 ☑
  - contracture — *see* Contraction, joint
  - current injury (*see also* Dislocation)
    - knee, meniscus or cartilage — *see* Tear, meniscus
  - dislocation
    - pathological — *see* Dislocation, pathological
    - recurrent — *see* Dislocation, recurrent
  - knee — *see* Derangement, knee
  - ligament — *see* Disorder, ligament
  - loose body — *see* Loose, body
  - recurrent — *see* Dislocation, recurrent
  - specified type NEC M24.80
    - ankle M24.87 ☑
    - elbow M24.82 ☑
    - foot joint M24.87 ☑
    - hand joint M24.84 ☑
    - hip M24.85 ☑
    - shoulder M24.81 ☑
    - wrist M24.83 ☑
  - temporomandibular M26.69
- knee (recurrent) M23.9 ☑
  - ligament disruption, spontaneous M23.60 ☑
    - anterior cruciate M23.61 ☑
    - capsular M23.67 ☑
    - instability, chronic M23.5 ☑
    - lateral collateral M23.64 ☑
    - medial collateral M23.63 ☑
    - posterior cruciate M23.62 ☑
  - loose body M23.4 ☑
  - meniscus M23.30 ☑
    - cystic M23.00 ☑
      - lateral M23.002
        - anterior horn M23.04 ☑
        - posterior horn M23.05 ☑
        - specified NEC M23.06 ☑
      - medial M23.005
        - anterior horn M23.01 ☑
        - posterior horn M23.02 ☑
        - specified NEC M23.03 ☑
    - degenerate — *see* Derangement, knee, meniscus, specified NEC
    - detached — *see* Derangement, knee, meniscus, specified NEC
    - due to old tear or injury M23.20 ☑
      - lateral M23.20 ☑
        - anterior horn M23.24 ☑
        - posterior horn M23.25 ☑
        - specified NEC M23.26 ☑
      - medial M23.20 ☑

Dermatitis - Development

- **Dermatitis** — *continued*
  - flexural NEC L20.82
  - friction L30.4
  - fungus B36.9
    - specified type NEC B36.8
  - gangrenosa, gangrenous infantum L08.0
  - harvest mite B88.0
  - heat L59.0
  - herpesviral, vesicular (ear) (lip) B00.1
  - herpetiformis (bullous) (erythematous) (pustular) (vesicular) L13.0
    - juvenile L12.2
    - senile L12.0
  - hiemalis L30.8
  - hypostatic, hypostatica — *see* Varix, leg, with, inflammation
  - infectious eczematoid L30.3
  - infective L30.3
  - irritant — *see* Dermatitis, contact, irritant
  - Jacquet's (diaper dermatitis) L22
  - Leptus B88.0
  - lichenified NEC L28.0
  - medicamentosa (generalized) (internal use) — *see* Dermatitis, due to drugs
  - mite B88.0
  - multiformis L13.0
    - juvenile L12.2
  - napkin L22
  - neurotica L13.0
  - nummular L30.0
  - papillaris capillitii L73.0
  - pellagrous E52
  - perioral L71.0
  - photocontact L56.2
  - polymorpha dolorosa L13.0
  - pruriginosa L13.0
  - pruritic NEC L30.8
  - psychogenic F54
  - purulent L08.0
  - pustular
    - contagious B08.02
    - subcorneal L13.1
  - pyococcal L08.0
  - pyogenica L08.0
  - repens L40.2
  - Ritter's (exfoliativa) L00
  - Schamberg's L81.7
  - schistosome B65.3
  - seasonal bullous L30.8
  - seborrheic L21.9
    - infantile L21.1
    - specified NEC L21.8
  - sensitization NOS L23.9
  - septic L08.0
  - solare L57.8
  - specified NEC L30.8
  - stasis I87.2
    - with
      - varicose ulcer — *see* Varix, leg, with ulcer, with inflammation
      - varicose veins — *see* Varix, leg, with, inflammation
    - due to postthrombotic syndrome — *see* Syndrome, postthrombotic
  - suppurative L08.0
  - traumatic NEC L30.4
  - trophoneurotica L13.0
  - ultraviolet (sun) (chronic exposure) L57.8
    - acute L56.8
  - varicose — *see* Varix, leg, with, inflammation
  - vegetans L10.1
  - verrucosa B43.0
  - vesicular, herpesviral B00.1
- **Dermatoarthritis,** lipoid E78.81
- **Dermatochalasis,** eyelid H02.839
  - left H02.836
    - lower H02.835
    - upper H02.834
  - right H02.833
    - lower H02.832
    - upper H02.831
- **Dermatofibroma** (lenticulare) — *see* Neoplasm, skin, benign
  - protuberans — *see* Neoplasm, skin, uncertain behavior
- **Dermatofibrosarcoma** (pigmented) (protuberans) — *see* Neoplasm, skin, malignant
- **Dermatographia** L50.3
- **Dermatolysis** (exfoliativa) (congenital) Q82.8
  - acquired L57.4
  - eyelids — *see* Blepharochalasis
  - palpebrarum — *see* Blepharochalasis
  - senile L57.4
- **Dermatomegaly** NEC Q82.8
- **Dermatomucosomyositis** M33.10
  - with
    - myopathy M33.12
    - respiratory involvement M33.11
    - specified organ involvement NEC M33.19
- **Dermatomycosis** B36.9
  - furfuracea B36.0
  - specified type NEC B36.8
- **Dermatomyositis** (acute) (chronic) — *see also* Dermatopolymyositis
  - in (due to) neoplastic disease (*see also* Neoplasm)D49.9 *[M36.0]*
- **Dermatoneuritis** of children — *see* Poisoning, mercury
- **Dermatophilosis** A48.8
- **Dermatophytid** L30.2
- **Dermatophytide** — *see* Dermatophytosis
- **Dermatophytosis** (epidermophyton) (infection) (Microsporum) (tinea) (Trichophyton) B35.9
  - beard B35.0
  - body B35.4
  - capitis B35.0
  - corporis B35.4
  - deep-seated B35.8
  - disseminated B35.8
  - foot B35.3
  - granulomatous B35.8
  - groin B35.6
  - hand B35.2
  - nail B35.1
  - perianal (area) B35.6
  - scalp B35.0
  - specified NEC B35.8
- **Dermatopolymyositis** M33.90
  - with
    - myopathy M33.92
    - respiratory involvement M33.91
    - specified organ involvement NEC M33.99
  - in neoplastic disease (*see also* Neoplasm)D49.9 *[M36.0]*
  - juvenile M33.00
    - with
      - myopathy M33.02
      - respiratory involvement M33.01
      - specified organ involvement NEC M33.09
  - specified NEC M33.10
    - myopathy M33.12
    - respiratory involvement M33.11
    - specified organ involvement NEC M33.19
- **Dermatopolyneuritis** — *see* Poisoning, mercury
- **Dermatorrhexis** Q79.6
  - acquired L57.4
- **Dermatosclerosis** (*see also* Scleroderma)
  - localized L94.0
- **Dermatosis** L98.9
  - Andrews' L08.89
  - Bowen's — *see* Neoplasm, skin, in situ
  - bullous L13.9
    - specified NEC L13.8
  - exfoliativa L26
  - eyelid (noninfectious)
    - dermatitis — *see* Dermatitis, eyelid
    - discoid lupus erythematosus — *see* Lupus, erythematosus, eyelid
    - xeroderma — *see* Xeroderma, acquired, eyelid
  - factitial L98.1
  - febrile neutrophilic L98.2
  - gonococcal A54.89
  - herpetiformis L13.0
    - juvenile L12.2
  - linear IgA L13.8
  - menstrual NEC L98.8
  - neutrophilic, febrile L98.2
  - occupational — *see* Dermatitis, contact
  - papulosa nigra L82.1
  - pigmentary L81.9
    - progressive L81.7
    - Schamberg's L81.7
  - psychogenic F54
  - purpuric, pigmented L81.7
  - pustular, subcorneal L13.1
  - transient acantholytic L11.1
- **Dermographia,** dermographism L50.3
- **Dermoid** (cyst) (*see also* Neoplasm, benign, by site)
  - with malignant transformation C56 ☑
  - due to radiation (nonionizing) L57.8
- **Dermopathy**
  - infiltrative with thyrotoxicosis — *see* Thyrotoxicosis
  - nephrogenic fibrosing L90.8
- **Dermophytosis** — *see* Dermatophytosis
- **Descemetocele** H18.73 ☑
- **Descemet's** membrane — *see* condition
- **Descending** — *see* condition
- **Descensus** uteri — *see* Prolapse, uterus
- **Desert**
  - rheumatism B38.0
  - sore — *see* Ulcer, skin
- **Desertion** (newborn) — *see* Maltreatment
- **Desmoid** (extra-abdominal) (tumor) — *see* Neoplasm, connective tissue, uncertain behavior
  - abdominal D48.1
- **Despondency** F32.9
- **Desquamation,** skin R23.4
- **Destruction,** destructive (*see also* Damage)
  - articular facet (*see also* Derangement, joint, specified type NEC)
    - knee M23.8X ☑
    - vertebra — *see* Spondylosis
  - bone (*see also* Disorder, bone, specified type NEC)
    - syphilitic A52.77
  - joint (*see also* Derangement, joint, specified type NEC)
    - sacroiliac M53.3
  - rectal sphincter K62.89
  - septum (nasal) J34.89
  - tuberculous NEC — *see* Tuberculosis
  - tympanum, tympanic membrane (nontraumatic) — *see* Disorder, tympanic membrane, specified NEC
  - vertebral disc — *see* Degeneration, intervertebral disc
- **Destructiveness** (*see also* Disorder, conduct)
  - adjustment reaction — *see* Disorder, adjustment
- **Desultory** labor O62.2
- **Detachment**
  - cartilage — *see* Sprain
  - cervix, annular N88.8
    - complicating delivery O71.3
  - choroid (old) (postinfectional) (simple) (spontaneous) H31.40 ☑
    - hemorrhagic H31.41 ☑
    - serous H31.42 ☑
  - ligament — *see* Sprain
  - meniscus (knee) (*see also* Derangement, knee, meniscus, specified NEC)
    - current injury — *see* Tear, meniscus
    - due to old tear or injury — *see* Derangement, knee, meniscus, due to old tear
  - retina (without retinal break) (serous) H33.2 ☑
    - with retinal:
      - break H33.00 ☑
        - giant H33.03 ☑
        - multiple H33.02 ☑
        - single H33.01 ☑
      - dialysis H33.04 ☑
    - pigment epithelium — *see* Degeneration, retina, separation of layers, pigment epithelium detachment
    - rhegmatogenous — *see* Detachment, retina, with retinal, break
    - specified NEC H33.8
    - total H33.05 ☑
    - traction H33.4 ☑
  - vitreous (body) H43.81 ☑
- **Detergent** asthma J69.8
- **Deterioration**
  - epileptic F06.8
  - general physical R53.81
  - heart, cardiac — *see* Degeneration, myocardial
  - mental — *see* Psychosis
  - myocardial, myocardium — *see* Degeneration, myocardial
  - senile (simple) R54
- **Deuteranomaly** (anomalous trichromat) H53.53
- **Deuteranopia** (complete) (incomplete) H53.53
- **Development**
  - abnormal, bone Q79.9
  - arrested R62.50
    - bone — *see* Arrest, development or growth, bone
    - child R62.50
    - due to malnutrition E45
  - defective, congenital (*see also* Anomaly, by site)
    - cauda equina Q06.3
    - left ventricle Q24.8
      - in hypoplastic left heart syndrome Q23.4
    - valve Q24.8
      - pulmonary Q22.3
  - delayed (*see also* Delay, development)R62.50
    - arithmetical skills F81.2
    - language (skills) (expressive) F80.1
    - learning skill F81.9

Dermatitis - Development

- **Development** — *continued*
  - delayed — *continued*
    - mixed skills F88
    - motor coordination F82
    - reading F81.0
    - specified learning skill NEC F81.89
    - speech F80.9
    - spelling F81.81
    - written expression F81.81
  - imperfect, congenital (*see also* Anomaly, by site)
    - heart Q24.9
    - lungs Q33.6
  - incomplete
    - bronchial tree Q32.4
    - organ or site not listed — *see* Hypoplasia, by site
    - respiratory system Q34.9
  - sexual, precocious NEC E30.1
  - tardy, mental (*see also* Disability, intellectual)F79
- **Developmental** — *see* condition
  - testing, infant or child — *see* Examination, child
- **Devergie's** disease (pityriasis rubra pilaris) L44.0
- **Deviation** (in)
  - conjugate palsy (eye) (spastic) H51.0
  - esophagus (acquired) K22.8
  - eye, skew H51.8
  - midline (jaw) (teeth) (dental arch) M26.29
    - specified site NEC — *see* Malposition
  - nasal septum J34.2
    - congenital Q67.4
  - opening and closing of the mandible M26.53
  - organ or site, congenital NEC — *see* Malposition, congenital
  - septum (nasal) (acquired) J34.2
    - congenital Q67.4
  - sexual F65.9
    - bestiality F65.89
    - erotomania F52.8
    - exhibitionism F65.2
    - fetishism, fetishistic F65.0
      - transvestism F65.1
    - frotteurism F65.81
    - masochism F65.51
    - multiple F65.89
    - necrophilia F65.89
    - nymphomania F52.8
    - pederosis F65.4
    - pedophilia F65.4
    - sadism, sadomasochism F65.52
    - satyriasis F52.8
    - specified type NEC F65.89
    - transvestism F64.1
    - voyeurism F65.3
  - teeth, midline M26.29
  - trachea J39.8
  - ureter, congenital Q62.61
- **Device**
  - cerebral ventricle (communicating) in situ Z98.2
  - contraceptive — *see* Contraceptive, device
  - drainage, cerebrospinal fluid, in situ Z98.2
- **Devic's** disease G36.0
- **Devil's**
  - grip B33.0
  - pinches (purpura simplex) D69.2
- **Devitalized** tooth K04.99
- **Devonshire** colic — *see* Poisoning, lead
- **Dextraposition,** aorta Q20.3
  - in tetralogy of Fallot Q21.3
- **Dextrinosis,** limit (debrancher enzyme deficiency) E74.03
- **Dextrocardia** (true) Q24.0
  - with
    - complete transposition of viscera Q89.3
    - situs inversus Q89.3
- **Dextrotransposition,** aorta Q20.3
- **d-glycericacidemia** E72.59
- **Dhat** syndrome F48.8
- **Dhobi** itch B35.6
- **Di** George's syndrome D82.1
- **Di** Guglielmo's disease C94.0 ☑
- **Diabetes,** diabetic (mellitus) (sugar) E11.9
  - with
    - amyotrophy E11.44
    - arthropathy NEC E11.618
    - autonomic (poly)neuropathy E11.43
    - cataract E11.36
    - Charcot's joints E11.610
    - chronic kidney disease E11.22
    - circulatory complication NEC E11.59
    - complication E11.8
      - specified NEC E11.69
    - dermatitis E11.620

- **Diabetes** — *continued*
  - with — *continued*
    - foot ulcer E11.621
    - gangrene E11.52
    - gastroparalysis E11.43
    - gastroparesis E11.43
    - glomerulonephrosis, intracapillary E11.21
    - glomerulosclerosis, intercapillary E11.21
    - hyperglycemia E11.65
    - hyperosmolarity E11.00
      - with coma E11.01
    - hypoglycemia E11.649
      - with coma E11.641
    - kidney complications NEC E11.29
    - Kimmelstiel-Wilson disease E11.21
    - loss of protective sensation (LOPS) — *see* Diabetes, by type, with neuropathy
    - mononeuropathy E11.41
    - myasthenia E11.44
    - necrobiosis lipoidica E11.620
    - nephropathy E11.21
    - neuralgia E11.42
    - neurologic complication NEC E11.49
    - neuropathic arthropathy E11.610
    - neuropathy E11.40
    - ophthalmic complication NEC E11.39
    - oral complication NEC E11.638
    - osteomyelitis E11.69
    - periodontal disease E11.630
    - peripheral angiopathy E11.51
      - with gangrene E11.52
    - polyneuropathy E11.42
    - renal complication NEC E11.29
    - renal tubular degeneration E11.29
    - retinopathy E11.319
      - with macular edema E11.311
        - resolved following treatment E11.37 ☑
      - nonproliferative E11.329 ☑
        - with macular edema E11.321 ☑
        - mild E11.329 ☑
          - with macular edema E11.321 ☑
        - moderate E11.339 ☑
          - with macular edema E11.331 ☑
        - severe E11.349 ☑
          - with macular edema E11.341 ☑
      - proliferative E11.359 ☑
        - with
          - combined traction retinal detachment and rhegmatogenous retinal detachment E11.354 ☑
          - macular edema E11.351 ☑
          - stable proliferative diabetic retinopathy E11.355 ☑
          - traction retinal detachment involving the macula E11.352 ☑
          - traction retinal detachment not involving the macula E11.353 ☑
    - skin complication NEC E11.628
    - skin ulcer NEC E11.622
  - brittle — *see* Diabetes, type 1
  - bronzed E83.110
  - complicating pregnancy — *see* Pregnancy, complicated by, diabetes
  - dietary counseling and surveillance Z71.3
  - due to
    - autoimmune process — *see* Diabetes, type 1
    - immune mediated pancreatic islet beta-cell destruction — *see* Diabetes, type 1
  - due to drug or chemical E09.9
    - with
      - amyotrophy E09.44
      - arthropathy NEC E09.618
      - autonomic (poly)neuropathy E09.43
      - cataract E09.36 ☑
      - Charcot's joints E09.610
      - chronic kidney disease E09.22
      - circulatory complication NEC E09.59
      - complication E09.8
        - specified NEC E09.69
      - dermatitis E09.620
      - foot ulcer E09.621
      - gangrene E09.52
      - gastroparalysis E09.43
      - gastroparesis E09.43
      - glomerulonephrosis, intracapillary E09.21
      - glomerulosclerosis, intercapillary E09.21
      - hyperglycemia E09.65
      - hyperosmolarity E09.00
        - with coma E09.01
      - hypoglycemia E09.649
        - with coma E09.641
      - ketoacidosis E09.10

- **Diabetes** — *continued*
  - due to drug or chemical — *continued*
        - with coma E09.11
      - kidney complications NEC E09.29
      - Kimmelstiel-Wilson disease E09.21
      - mononeuropathy E09.41
      - myasthenia E09.44
      - necrobiosis lipoidica E09.620
      - nephropathy E09.21
      - neuralgia E09.42
      - neurologic complication NEC E09.49
      - neuropathic arthropathy E09.610
      - neuropathy E09.40
      - ophthalmic complication NEC E09.39
      - oral complication NEC E09.638
      - periodontal disease E09.630
      - peripheral angiopathy E09.51
        - with gangrene E09.52
      - polyneuropathy E09.42
      - renal complication NEC E09.29
      - renal tubular degeneration E09.29
      - retinopathy E09.319
        - with macular edema E09.311
        - resolved following treatment E09.37 ☑
        - nonproliferative E09.329 ☑
          - with macular edema E09.321 ☑
          - mild E09.329 ☑
            - with macular edema E09.321 ☑
          - moderate E09.339 ☑
            - with macular edema E09.331 ☑
          - severe E09.349 ☑
            - with macular edema E09.341 ☑
        - proliferative E09.359 ☑
        - with
          - combined traction retinal detachment and rhegmatogenous retinal detachment E09.354 ☑
          - macular edema E09.351 ☑
          - stable proliferative diabetic retinopathy E09.355 ☑
          - traction retinal detachment involving the macula E09.352 ☑
          - traction retinal detachment not involving the macula E09.353 ☑
      - skin complication NEC E09.628
      - skin ulcer NEC E09.622
  - due to underlying condition E08.9
    - with
      - amyotrophy E08.44
      - arthropathy NEC E08.618
      - autonomic (poly)neuropathy E08.43
      - cataract E08.36
      - Charcot's joints E08.610
      - chronic kidney disease E08.22
      - circulatory complication NEC E08.59
      - complication E08.8
        - specified NEC E08.69
      - dermatitis E08.620
      - foot ulcer E08.621
      - gangrene E08.52
      - gastroparalysis E08.43
      - gastroparesis E08.43
      - glomerulonephrosis, intracapillary E08.21
      - glomerulosclerosis, intercapillary E08.21
      - hyperglycemia E08.65
      - hyperosmolarity E08.00
        - with coma E08.01
      - hypoglycemia E08.649
        - with coma E08.641
      - ketoacidosis E08.10
        - with coma E08.11
      - kidney complications NEC E08.29
      - Kimmelstiel-Wilson disease E08.21
      - mononeuropathy E08.41
      - myasthenia E08.44
      - necrobiosis lipoidica E08.620
      - nephropathy E08.21
      - neuralgia E08.42
      - neurologic complication NEC E08.49
      - neuropathic arthropathy E08.610
      - neuropathy E08.40
      - ophthalmic complication NEC E08.39
      - oral complication NEC E08.638
      - periodontal disease E08.630
      - peripheral angiopathy E08.51
        - with gangrene E08.52
      - polyneuropathy E08.42
      - renal complication NEC E08.29
      - renal tubular degeneration E08.29
      - retinopathy E08.319
        - with macular edema E08.311
        - resolved following treatment E08.37 ☑

- **Diabetes** — *continued*
  - due to underlying condition — *continued*
        - nonproliferative E08.329 ☑
          - with macular edema E08.321 ☑
          - mild E08.329 ☑
            - with macular edema E08.321 ☑
          - moderate E08.339 ☑
            - with macular edema E08.331 ☑
          - severe E08.349 ☑
            - with macular edema E08.341 ☑
        - proliferative E08.359 ☑
          - with
            - combined traction retinal detachment and rhegmatogenous retinal detachment E08.354 ☑
            - macular edema E08.351 ☑
            - stable proliferative diabetic retinopathy E08.355 ☑
            - traction retinal detachment involving the macula E08.352 ☑
            - traction retinal detachment not involving the macula E08.353 ☑
      - skin complication NEC E08.628
      - skin ulcer NEC E08.622
  - gestational (in pregnancy) O24.419
    - affecting newborn P70.0
    - diet controlled O24.410
    - in childbirth O24.429
      - diet controlled O24.420
      - insulin (and diet) controlled O24.424
      - oral drug controlled (antidiabetic) (hypoglycemic) O24.425
    - insulin (and diet) controlled O24.414
    - oral drug controlled (antidiabetic) (hypoglycemic) O24.415
    - puerperal O24.439
      - diet controlled O24.430
      - insulin (and diet) controlled O24.434
      - oral drug controlled (antidiabetic) (hypoglycemic) O24.435
  - hepatogenous E13.9
  - idiopathic — *see* Diabetes, type 1
  - inadequately controlled - code to Diabetes, by type, with hyperglycemia
  - insipidus E23.2
    - nephrogenic N25.1
    - pituitary E23.2
    - vasopressin resistant N25.1
  - insulin dependent - code to type of diabetes
  - juvenile-onset — *see* Diabetes, type 1
  - ketosis-prone — *see* Diabetes, type 1
  - latent R73.03
  - neonatal (transient) P70.2
  - non-insulin dependent - code to type of diabetes
  - out of control - code to Diabetes, by type, with hyperglycemia
  - phosphate E83.39
  - poorly controlled - code to Diabetes, by type, with hyperglycemia
  - postpancreatectomy — *see* Diabetes, specified type NEC
  - postprocedural — *see* Diabetes, specified type NEC
  - secondary diabetes mellitus NEC — *see* Diabetes, specified type NEC
  - specified type NEC E13.9
    - with
      - amyotrophy E13.44
      - arthropathy NEC E13.618
      - autonomic (poly)neuropathy E13.43
      - cataract E13.36
      - Charcot's joints E13.610
      - chronic kidney disease E13.22
      - circulatory complication NEC E13.59
      - complication E13.8
        - specified NEC E13.69
      - dermatitis E13.620
      - foot ulcer E13.621
      - gangrene E13.52
      - gastroparalysis E13.43
      - gastroparesis E13.43
      - glomerulonephrosis, intracapillary E13.21
      - glomerulosclerosis, intercapillary E13.21
      - hyperglycemia E13.65
      - hyperosmolarity E13.00
        - with coma E13.01
      - hypoglycemia E13.649
        - with coma E13.641
      - ketoacidosis E13.10
        - with coma E13.11
      - kidney complications NEC E13.29
      - Kimmelstiel-Wilson disease E13.21

- **Diabetes** — *continued*
  - specified type NEC — *continued*
      - mononeuropathy E13.41
      - myasthenia E13.44
      - necrobiosis lipoidica E13.620
      - nephropathy E13.21
      - neuralgia E13.42
      - neurologic complication NEC E13.49
      - neuropathic arthropathy E13.610
      - neuropathy E13.40
      - ophthalmic complication NEC E13.39
      - oral complication NEC E13.638
      - periodontal disease E13.630
      - peripheral angiopathy E13.51
        - with gangrene E13.52
      - polyneuropathy E13.42
      - renal complication NEC E13.29
      - renal tubular degeneration E13.29
      - retinopathy E13.319
        - with macular edema E13.311
        - resolved following treatment E13.37 ☑
        - nonproliferative E13.329 ☑
          - with macular edema E13.321 ☑
          - mild E13.329 ☑
            - with macular edema E13.321 ☑
          - moderate E13.339 ☑
            - with macular edema E13.331 ☑
          - severe E13.349 ☑
            - with macular edema E13.341 ☑
        - proliferative E13.359 ☑
          - with
            - combined traction retinal detachment and rhegmatogenous retinal detachment E13.354 ☑
            - macular edema E13.351 ☑
            - stable proliferative diabetic retinopathy E13.355 ☑
            - traction retinal detachment involving the macula E13.352 ☑
            - traction retinal detachment not involving the macula E13.353 ☑
      - skin complication NEC E13.628
      - skin ulcer NEC E13.622
  - steroid-induced — *see* Diabetes, due to, drug or chemical
  - type 1 E10.9
    - with
      - amyotrophy E10.44
      - arthropathy NEC E10.618
      - autonomic (poly)neuropathy E10.43
      - cataract E10.36
      - Charcot's joints E10.610
      - chronic kidney disease E10.22
      - circulatory complication NEC E10.59
      - complication E10.8
        - specified NEC E10.69
      - dermatitis E10.620
      - foot ulcer E10.621
      - gangrene E10.52
      - gastroparalysis E10.43
      - gastroparesis E10.43
      - glomerulonephrosis, intracapillary E10.21
      - glomerulosclerosis, intercapillary E10.21
      - hyperglycemia E10.65
      - hypoglycemia E10.649
        - with coma E10.641
      - ketoacidosis E10.10
        - with coma E10.11
      - kidney complications NEC E10.29
      - Kimmelstiel-Wilson disease E10.21
      - mononeuropathy E10.41
      - myasthenia E10.44
      - necrobiosis lipoidica E10.620
      - nephropathy E10.21
      - neuralgia E10.42
      - neurologic complication NEC E10.49
      - neuropathic arthropathy E10.610
      - neuropathy E10.40
      - ophthalmic complication NEC E10.39
      - oral complication NEC E10.638
      - periodontal disease E10.630
      - peripheral angiopathy E10.51
        - with gangrene E10.52
      - polyneuropathy E10.42
      - renal complication NEC E10.29
      - renal tubular degeneration E10.29
      - retinopathy E10.319
        - with macular edema E10.311
        - resolved following treatment E10.37 ☑
        - nonproliferative E10.329 ☑
          - with macular edema E10.321 ☑
          - mild E10.329 ☑

- **Diabetes** — *continued*
  - type 1 — *continued*
            - with macular edema E10.321 ☑
          - moderate E10.339 ☑
            - with macular edema E10.331 ☑
          - severe E10.349 ☑
            - with macular edema E10.341 ☑
        - proliferative E10.359 ☑
          - with
            - combined traction retinal detachment and rhegmatogenous retinal detachment E10.354 ☑
            - macular edema E10.351 ☑
            - stable proliferative diabetic retinopathy E10.355 ☑
            - traction retinal detachment involving the macula E10.352 ☑
            - traction retinal detachment not involving the macula E10.353 ☑
      - skin complication NEC E10.628
      - skin ulcer NEC E10.622
  - type 2 E11.9
    - with
      - amyotrophy E11.44
      - arthropathy NEC E11.618
      - autonomic (poly)neuropathy E11.43
      - cataract E11.36
      - Charcot's joints E11.610
      - chronic kidney disease E11.22
      - circulatory complication NEC E11.59
      - complication E11.8
        - specified NEC E11.69
      - dermatitis E11.620
      - foot ulcer E11.621
      - gangrene E11.52
      - gastroparalysis E11.43
      - gastroparesis E11.43
      - glomerulonephrosis, intracapillary E11.21
      - glomerulosclerosis, intercapillary E11.21
      - hyperglycemia E11.65
      - hyperosmolarity E11.00
        - with coma E11.01
      - hypoglycemia E11.649
        - with coma E11.641
      - kidney complications NEC E11.29
      - Kimmelstiel-Wilson disease E11.21
      - mononeuropathy E11.41
      - myasthenia E11.44
      - necrobiosis lipoidica E11.620
      - nephropathy E11.21
      - neuralgia E11.42
      - neurologic complication NEC E11.49
      - neuropathic arthropathy E11.610
      - neuropathy E11.40
      - ophthalmic complication NEC E11.39
      - oral complication NEC E11.638
      - periodontal disease E11.630
      - peripheral angiopathy E11.51
        - with gangrene E11.52
      - polyneuropathy E11.42
      - renal complication NEC E11.29
      - renal tubular degeneration E11.29
      - retinopathy E11.319
        - with macular edema E11.311
        - resolved following treatment E11.37 ☑
        - nonproliferative E11.329 ☑
          - with macular edema E11.321 ☑
          - mild E11.329 ☑
            - with macular edema E11.321 ☑
          - moderate E11.339 ☑
            - with macular edema E11.331 ☑
          - severe E11.349 ☑
            - with macular edema E11.341 ☑
        - proliferative E11.359 ☑
          - with
            - combined traction retinal detachment and rhegmatogenous retinal detachment E11.354 ☑
            - macular edema E11.351 ☑
            - stable proliferative diabetic retinopathy E11.355 ☑
            - traction retinal detachment involving the macula E11.352 ☑
            - traction retinal detachment not involving the macula E11.353 ☑
      - skin complication NEC E11.628
      - skin ulcer NEC E11.622
  - uncontrolled
    - meaning
      - hyperglycemia — *see* Diabetes, by type, with, hyperglycemia
      - hypoglycemia — *see* Diabetes, by type, with, hypoglycemia

- **Diacyclothrombopathia** D69.1
- **Diagnosis** deferred R69
- **Dialysis** (intermittent) (treatment)
  - noncompliance (with) Z91.15
  - renal (hemodialysis) (peritoneal), status Z99.2
  - retina, retinal — *see* Detachment, retina, with retinal, dialysis
- **Diamond-Blackfan** anemia (congenital hypoplastic) D61.01
- **Diamond-Gardener** syndrome (autoerythrocyte sensitization) D69.2
- **Diaper** rash L22
- **Diaphoresis** (excessive) R61
- **Diaphragm** — *see* condition
- **Diaphragmalgia** R07.1
- **Diaphragmatitis,** diaphragmitis J98.6
- **Diaphysial** aclasis Q78.6
- **Diaphysitis** — *see* Osteomyelitis, specified type NEC
- **Diarrhea,** diarrheal (disease) (infantile) (inflammatory) R19.7
  - achlorhydric K31.83
  - allergic K52.29
    - due to
      - colitis — *see* Colitis, allergic
      - enteritis — *see* Enteritis, allergic
  - amebic (*see also* Amebiasis)A06.0
    - with abscess — *see* Abscess, amebic
    - acute A06.0
    - chronic A06.1
    - nondysenteric A06.2
  - bacillary — *see* Dysentery, bacillary
  - balantidial A07.0
  - cachectic NEC K52.89
  - Chilomastix A07.8
  - choleriformis A00.1
  - chronic (noninfectious) K52.9
  - coccidial A07.3
  - Cochin-China K90.1
    - strongyloidiasis B78.0
  - Dientamoeba A07.8
  - dietetic (*see also* Diarrhea, allergic)K52.29
  - drug-induced K52.1
  - due to
    - bacteria A04.9
      - specified NEC A04.8
    - Campylobacter A04.5
    - Capillaria philippinensis B81.1
    - Clostridium difficile A04.7
    - Clostridium perfringens (C) (F) A04.8
    - Cryptosporidium A07.2
    - drugs K52.1
    - Escherichia coli A04.4
      - enteroaggregative A04.4
      - enterohemorrhagic A04.3
      - enteroinvasive A04.2
      - enteropathogenic A04.0
      - enterotoxigenic A04.1
      - specified NEC A04.4
    - food hypersensitivity (*see also* Diarrhea, allergic)K52.29
    - Necator americanus B76.1
    - S. japonicum B65.2
    - specified organism NEC A08.8
      - bacterial A04.8
      - viral A08.39
    - Staphylococcus A04.8
    - Trichuris trichiuria B79
    - virus — *see* Enteritis, viral
    - Yersinia enterocolitica A04.6
  - dysenteric A09
  - endemic A09
  - epidemic A09
  - flagellate A07.9
  - Flexner's (ulcerative) A03.1
  - functional K59.1
    - following gastrointestinal surgery K91.89
    - psychogenic F45.8
  - Giardia lamblia A07.1
  - giardial A07.1
  - hill K90.1
  - infectious A09
  - malarial — *see* Malaria
  - mite B88.0
  - mycotic NEC B49
  - neonatal (noninfectious) P78.3
  - nervous F45.8
  - neurogenic K59.1
  - noninfectious K52.9
  - postgastrectomy K91.1
  - postvagotomy K91.1
  - protozoal A07.9
    - specified NEC A07.8

Diarrhea — *continued*

  - psychogenic F45.8
  - specified
    - bacterium NEC A04.8
    - virus NEC A08.39
  - strongyloidiasis B78.0
  - toxic K52.1
  - trichomonal A07.8
  - tropical K90.1
  - tuberculous A18.32
  - viral — *see* Enteritis, viral
- **Diastasis**
  - cranial bones M84.88
    - congenital NEC Q75.8
  - joint (traumatic) — *see* Dislocation
  - muscle M62.00
    - ankle M62.07 ☑
    - congenital Q79.8
    - foot M62.07 ☑
    - forearm M62.03 ☑
    - hand M62.04 ☑
    - lower leg M62.06 ☑
    - pelvic region M62.05 ☑
    - shoulder region M62.01 ☑
    - specified site NEC M62.08
    - thigh M62.05 ☑
    - upper arm M62.02 ☑
  - recti (abdomen)
    - complicating delivery O71.89
    - congenital Q79.59
- **Diastema,** tooth, teeth, fully erupted M26.32
- **Diastematomyelia** Q06.2
- **Diataxia,** cerebral G80.4
- **Diathesis**
  - allergic — *see* History, allergy
  - bleeding (familial) D69.9
  - cystine (familial) E72.00
  - gouty — *see* Gout
  - hemorrhagic (familial) D69.9
    - newborn NEC P53
  - spasmophilic R29.0
- **Diaz's** disease or osteochondrosis (juvenile) (talus) — *see* Osteochondrosis, juvenile, tarsus
- **Dibothriocephalus,** dibothriocephaliasis (latus) (infection) (infestation) B70.0
  - larval B70.1
- **Dicephalus,** dicephaly Q89.4
- **Dichotomy,** teeth K00.2
- **Dichromat,** dichromatopsia (congenital) — *see* Deficiency, color vision
- **Dichuchwa** A65
- **Dicroceliasis** B66.2
- **Didelphia,** didelphys — *see* Double uterus
- **Didymytis** N45.1
  - with orchitis N45.3
- **Dietary**
  - inadequacy or deficiency E63.9
  - surveillance and counseling Z71.3
- **Dietl's** crisis N13.8
- **Dieulafoy** lesion (hemorrhagic)
  - duodenum K31.82
  - esophagus K22.8
  - intestine (colon) K63.81
  - stomach K31.82
- **Difficult,** difficulty (in)
  - acculturation Z60.3
  - feeding R63.3
    - newborn P92.9
      - breast P92.5
      - specified NEC P92.8
    - nonorganic (infant or child) F98.29
  - intubation, in anesthesia T88.4 ☑
  - mechanical, gastroduodenal stoma K91.89
    - causing obstruction K91.3
  - micturition
    - need to immediately re-void R39.191
    - position dependent R39.192
    - specified NEC R39.198
  - reading (developmental) F81.0
    - secondary to emotional disorders F93.9
  - spelling (specific) F81.81
    - with reading disorder F81.89
    - due to inadequate teaching Z55.8
  - swallowing — *see* Dysphagia
  - walking R26.2
  - work
    - conditions NEC Z56.5
    - schedule Z56.3
- **Diffuse** — *see* condition
- **DiGeorge's** syndrome (thymic hypoplasia) D82.1
- **Digestive** — *see* condition
- **Dihydropyrimidine** dehydrogenase disease (DPD) E88.89
- **Diktyoma** — *see* Neoplasm, malignant, by site
- **Dilaceration,** tooth K00.4
- **Dilatation**
  - anus K59.8
    - venule — *see* Hemorrhoids
  - aorta (focal) (general) — *see* Ectasia, aorta
    - with aneurysm — *see* Aneurysm, aorta
    - congenital Q25.44
  - artery — *see* Aneurysm
  - bladder (sphincter) N32.89
    - congenital Q64.79
  - blood vessel I99.8
  - bronchial J47.9
    - with
      - exacerbation (acute) J47.1
      - lower respiratory infection J47.0
  - calyx (due to obstruction) — *see* Hydronephrosis
  - capillaries I78.8
  - cardiac (acute) (chronic) (*see also* Hypertrophy, cardiac)
    - congenital Q24.8
      - valve NEC Q24.8
        - pulmonary Q22.3
    - valve — *see* Endocarditis
  - cavum septi pellucidi Q06.8
  - cervix (uteri) (*see also* Incompetency, cervix)
    - incomplete, poor, slow complicating delivery O62.0
  - colon K59.39
    - congenital Q43.1
    - psychogenic F45.8
    - toxic K59.31
  - common duct (acquired) K83.8
    - congenital Q44.5
  - cystic duct (acquired) K82.8
    - congenital Q44.5
  - duct, mammary — *see* Ectasia, mammary duct
  - duodenum K59.8
  - esophagus K22.8
    - congenital Q39.5
    - due to achalasia K22.0
  - eustachian tube, congenital Q17.8
  - gallbladder K82.8
  - gastric — *see* Dilatation, stomach
  - heart (acute) (chronic) (*see also* Hypertrophy, cardiac)
    - congenital Q24.8
    - valve — *see* Endocarditis
  - ileum K59.8
    - psychogenic F45.8
  - jejunum K59.8
    - psychogenic F45.8
  - kidney (calyx) (collecting structures) (cystic) (parenchyma) (pelvis) (idiopathic) N28.89
  - lacrimal passages or duct — *see* Disorder, lacrimal system, changes
  - lymphatic vessel I89.0
  - mammary duct — *see* Ectasia, mammary duct
  - Meckel's diverticulum (congenital) Q43.0
    - malignant — *see* Table of Neoplasms, small intestine, malignant
  - myocardium (acute) (chronic) — *see* Hypertrophy, cardiac
  - organ or site, congenital NEC — *see* Distortion
  - pancreatic duct K86.89
  - pericardium — *see* Pericarditis
  - pharynx J39.2
  - prostate N42.89
  - pulmonary
    - artery (idiopathic) I28.8
    - valve, congenital Q22.3
  - pupil H57.04
  - rectum K59.39
  - saccule, congenital Q16.5
  - salivary gland (duct) K11.8
  - sphincter ani K62.89
  - stomach K31.89
    - acute K31.0
    - psychogenic F45.8
  - submaxillary duct K11.8
  - trachea, congenital Q32.1
  - ureter (idiopathic) N28.82
    - congenital Q62.2
    - due to obstruction N13.4
  - urethra (acquired) N36.8
  - vasomotor I73.9
  - vein I86.8
  - ventricular, ventricle (acute) (chronic) (*see also* Hypertrophy, cardiac)
    - cerebral, congenital Q04.8

- **Dilatation** — *continued*
  - venule NEC I86.8
  - vesical orifice N32.89
- **Dilated,** dilation — *see* Dilatation
- **Diminished,** diminution
  - hearing (acuity) — *see* Deafness
  - sense or sensation (cold) (heat) (tactile) (vibratory) R20.8
  - vision NEC H54.7
  - vital capacity R94.2
- **Diminuta** taenia B71.0
- **Dimitri-Sturge-Weber** disease Q85.8
- **Dimple**
  - congenital sacral Q82.6
  - parasacral Q82.6
  - pilonidal or postanal — *see* Cyst, pilonidal
- **Dioctophyme** renalis (infection) (infestation) B83.8
- **Dipetalonemiasis** B74.4
- **Diphallus** Q55.69
- **Diphtheria,** diphtheritic (gangrenous) (hemorrhagic) A36.9
  - carrier (suspected) Z22.2
  - cutaneous A36.3
  - faucial A36.0
  - infection of wound A36.3
  - laryngeal A36.2
  - myocarditis A36.81
  - nasal, anterior A36.89
  - nasopharyngeal A36.1
  - neurological complication A36.89
  - pharyngeal A36.0
  - specified site NEC A36.89
  - tonsillar A36.0
- **Diphyllobothriasis** (intestine) B70.0
  - larval B70.1
- **Diplacusis** H93.22 ☑
- **Diplegia** (upper limbs) G83.0
  - congenital (cerebral) G80.8
  - facial G51.0
  - lower limbs G82.20
  - spastic G80.1
- **Diplococcus,** diplococcal — *see* condition
- **Diplopia** H53.2
- **Dipsomania** F10.20
  - with
    - psychosis — *see* Psychosis, alcoholic
    - remission F10.21
- **Dipylidiasis** B71.1
- **DIRA** (deficiency of interleukin 1 receptor antagonist) M04.8
- **Direction,** teeth, abnormal, fully erupted M26.30
- **Dirofilariasis** B74.8
- **Dirt-eating** child F98.3
- **Disability,** disabilities
  - heart — *see* Disease, heart
  - intellectual F79
    - with
      - autistic features F84.9
    - mild (I.Q.50-69) F70
    - moderate (I.Q.35-49) F71
    - profound (I.Q. under 20) F73
    - severe (I.Q.20-34) F72
    - specified level NEC F78
  - knowledge acquisition F81.9
  - learning F81.9
  - limiting activities Z73.6
  - spelling, specific F81.81
- **Disappearance** of family member Z63.4
- **Disarticulation** — *see* Amputation
  - meaning traumatic amputation — *see* Amputation, traumatic
- **Discharge** (from)
  - abnormal finding in — *see* Abnormal, specimen
  - breast (female) (male) N64.52
  - diencephalic autonomic idiopathic — *see* Epilepsy, specified NEC
  - ear (*see also* Otorrhea)
    - blood — *see* Otorrhagia
  - excessive urine R35.8
  - nipple N64.52
  - penile R36.9
  - postnasal R09.82
  - prison, anxiety concerning Z65.2
  - urethral R36.9
    - without blood R36.0
    - hematospermia R36.1
  - vaginal N89.8
- **Discitis,** diskitis M46.40
  - cervical region M46.42
  - cervicothoracic region M46.43
  - lumbar region M46.46
  - lumbosacral region M46.47
- **Discitis** — *continued*
  - multiple sites M46.49
  - occipito-atlanto-axial region M46.41
  - pyogenic — *see* Infection, intervertebral disc, pyogenic
  - sacrococcygeal region M46.48
  - thoracic region M46.44
  - thoracolumbar region M46.45
- **Discoid**
  - meniscus (congenital) Q68.6
  - semilunar cartilage (congenital) — *see* Derangement, knee, meniscus, specified NEC
- **Discoloration**
  - nails L60.8
  - teeth (posteruptive) K03.7
    - during formation K00.8
- **Discomfort**
  - chest R07.89
  - visual H53.14 ☑
- **Discontinuity,** ossicles, ear H74.2 ☑
- **Discord** (with)
  - boss Z56.4
  - classmates Z55.4
  - counselor Z64.4
  - employer Z56.4
  - family Z63.8
  - fellow employees Z56.4
  - in-laws Z63.1
  - landlord Z59.2
  - lodgers Z59.2
  - neighbors Z59.2
  - probation officer Z64.4
  - social worker Z64.4
  - teachers Z55.4
  - workmates Z56.4
- **Discordant** connection
  - atrioventricular (congenital) Q20.5
  - ventriculoarterial Q20.3
- **Discrepancy**
  - centric occlusion maximum intercuspation M26.55
  - leg length (acquired) — *see* Deformity, limb, unequal length
    - congenital — *see* Defect, reduction, lower limb
  - uterine size date O26.84 ☑
- **Discrimination**
  - ethnic Z60.5
  - political Z60.5
  - racial Z60.5
  - religious Z60.5
  - sex Z60.5
- **Disease,** diseased (*see also* Syndrome)
  - absorbent system I87.8
  - acid-peptic K30
  - Acosta's T70.29 ☑
  - Adams-Stokes (-Morgagni) (syncope with heart block) I45.9
  - Addison's anemia (pernicious) D51.0
  - adenoids (and tonsils) J35.9
  - adrenal (capsule) (cortex) (gland) (medullary) E27.9
    - hyperfunction E27.0
    - specified NEC E27.8
  - ainhum L94.6
  - airway
    - obstructive, chronic J44.9
      - due to
        - cotton dust J66.0
        - specific organic dusts NEC J66.8
    - reactive — *see* Asthma
  - akamushi (scrub typhus) A75.3
  - Albers-Schönberg (marble bones) Q78.2
  - Albert's — *see* Tendinitis, Achilles
  - alimentary canal K63.9
  - alligator-skin Q80.9
    - acquired L85.0
  - alpha heavy chain C88.3
  - alpine T70.29 ☑
  - altitude T70.20 ☑
  - alveolar ridge
    - edentulous K06.9
      - specified NEC K06.8
  - alveoli, teeth K08.9
  - Alzheimer's G30.9 *[F02.80]*
    - with behavioral disturbance G30.9 *[F02.81]*
    - early onset G30.0 *[F02.80]*
      - with behavioral disturbance G30.0 *[F02.81]*
    - late onset G30.1 *[F02.80]*
      - with behavioral disturbance G30.1 *[F02.81]*
    - specified NEC G30.8 *[F02.80]*
      - with behavioral disturbance G30.8 *[F02.81]*
  - amyloid — *see* Amyloidosis
- **Disease** — *continued*
  - Andersen's (glycogenosis IV) E74.09
  - Andes T70.29 ☑
  - Andrews' (bacterid) L08.89
  - angiospastic I73.9
    - cerebral G45.9
    - vein I87.8
  - anterior
    - chamber H21.9
    - horn cell G12.29
  - antiglomerular basement membrane (anti- GBM) antibody M31.0
    - tubulo-interstitial nephritis N12
  - antral — *see* Sinusitis, maxillary
  - anus K62.9
    - specified NEC K62.89
  - aorta (nonsyphilitic) I77.9
    - syphilitic NEC A52.02
  - aortic (heart) (valve) I35.9
    - rheumatic I06.9
  - Apollo B30.3
  - aponeuroses — *see* Enthesopathy
  - appendix K38.9
    - specified NEC K38.8
  - aqueous (chamber) H21.9
  - Arnold-Chiari — *see* Arnold-Chiari disease
  - arterial I77.9
    - occlusive — *see* Occlusion, by site
      - due to stricture or stenosis I77.1
  - arteriocardiorenal — *see* Hypertension, cardiorenal
  - arteriolar (generalized) (obliterative) I77.9
  - arteriorenal — *see* Hypertension, kidney
  - arteriosclerotic (*see also* Arteriosclerosis)
    - cardiovascular — *see* Disease, heart, ischemic, atherosclerotic
    - coronary (artery) — *see* Disease, heart, ischemic, atherosclerotic
    - heart — *see* Disease, heart, ischemic, atherosclerotic
  - artery I77.9
    - cerebral I67.9
    - coronary I25.10
      - with angina pectoris — *see* Arteriosclerosis, coronary (artery),
  - arthropod-borne NOS (viral) A94
    - specified type NEC A93.8
  - atticoantral, chronic H66.20
    - left H66.22
      - with right H66.23
    - right H66.21
      - with left H66.23
  - auditory canal — *see* Disorder, ear, external
  - auricle, ear NEC — *see* Disorder, pinna
  - Australian X A83.4
  - autoimmune (systemic) NOS M35.9
    - hemolytic (cold type) (warm type) D59.1
      - drug-induced D59.0
    - thyroid E06.3
  - aviator's — *see* Effect, adverse, high altitude
  - Ayerza's (pulmonary artery sclerosis with pulmonary hypertension) I27.0
  - Babington's (familial hemorrhagic telangiectasia) I78.0
  - bacterial A49.9
    - specified NEC A48.8
    - zoonotic A28.9
      - specified type NEC A28.8
  - Baelz's (cheilitis glandularis apostematosa) K13.0
  - bagasse J67.1
  - balloon — *see* Effect, adverse, high altitude
  - Bang's (brucella abortus) A23.1
  - Bannister's T78.3 ☑
  - barometer makers' — *see* Poisoning, mercury
  - Barraquer (-Simons') (progressive lipodystrophy) E88.1
  - Barrett's — *see* Barrett's, esophagus
  - Bartholin's gland N75.9
  - basal ganglia G25.9
    - degenerative G23.9
      - specified NEC G23.8
    - specified NEC G25.89
  - Basedow's (exophthalmic goiter) — *see* Hyperthyroidism, with, goiter (diffuse)
  - Bateman's B08.1
  - Batten-Steinert G71.11
  - Battey A31.0
  - Beard's (neurasthenia) F48.8
  - Becker
    - idiopathic mural endomyocardial I42.3
    - myotonia congenita G71.12

Disease — *continued*
- Begbie's (exophthalmic goiter) — *see* Hyperthyroidism, with, goiter (diffuse)
- behavioral, organic F07.9
- Beigel's (white piedra) B36.2
- Benson's — *see* Deposit, crystalline
- Bernard-Soulier (thrombopathy) D69.1
- Bernhardt (-Roth) — *see* Mononeuropathy, lower limb, meralgia paresthetica
- Biermer's (pernicious anemia) D51.0
- bile duct (common) (hepatic) K83.9
  - with calculus, stones — *see* Calculus, bile duct
  - specified NEC K83.8
- biliary (tract) K83.9
  - specified NEC K83.8
- Billroth's — *see* Spina bifida
- bird fancier's J67.2
- black lung J60
- bladder N32.9
  - in (due to)
    - schistosomiasis (bilharziasis) B65.0 *[N33]*
  - specified NEC N32.89
- bleeder's D66
- blood D75.9
  - forming organs D75.9
  - vessel I99.9
- Bloodgood's — *see* Mastopathy, cystic
- Bodechtel-Guttmann (subacute sclerosing panencephalitis) A81.1
- bone (*see also* Disorder, bone)
  - aluminum M83.4
  - fibrocystic NEC
    - jaw M27.49
- bone-marrow D75.9
- Borna A83.9
- Bornholm (epidemic pleurodynia) B33.0
- Bouchard's (myopathic dilatation of the stomach) K31.0
- Bouillaud's (rheumatic heart disease) I01.9
- Bourneville (-Brissaud) (tuberous sclerosis) Q85.1
- Bouveret (-Hoffmann) (paroxysmal tachycardia) I47.9
- bowel K63.9
  - functional K59.9
    - psychogenic F45.8
- brain G93.9
  - arterial, artery I67.9
  - arteriosclerotic I67.2
  - congenital Q04.9
  - degenerative — *see* Degeneration, brain
  - inflammatory — *see* Encephalitis
  - organic G93.9
    - arteriosclerotic I67.2
  - parasitic NEC B71.9 *[G94]*
  - senile NEC G31.1
  - specified NEC G93.89
- breast (*see also* Disorder, breast)N64.9
  - cystic (chronic) — *see* Mastopathy, cystic
  - fibrocystic — *see* Mastopathy, cystic
  - Paget's
    - female, unspecified side C50.91 ☑
    - male, unspecified side C50.92 ☑
  - specified NEC N64.89
- Breda's — *see* Yaws
- Bretonneau's (diphtheritic malignant angina) A36.0
- Bright's — *see* Nephritis
  - arteriosclerotic — *see* Hypertension, kidney
- Brill's (recrudescent typhus) A75.1
- Brill-Zinsser (recrudescent typhus) A75.1
- Brion-Kayser — *see* Fever, paratyphoid
- broad
  - beta E78.2
  - ligament (noninflammatory) N83.9
    - inflammatory — *see* Disease, pelvis, inflammatory
    - specified NEC N83.8
- Brocq-Duhring (dermatitis herpetiformis) L13.0
- Brocq's
  - meaning
    - dermatitis herpetiformis L13.0
    - prurigo L28.2
- bronchopulmonary J98.4
- bronchus NEC J98.09
- bronze Addison's E27.1
  - tuberculous A18.7
- budgerigar fancier's J67.2
- bullous L13.9
  - chronic of childhood L12.2
  - specified NEC L13.8
- Buerger's (thromboangiitis obliterans) I73.1
- Bürger-Grütz (essential familial hyperlipemia) E78.3
- bursa — *see* Bursopathy
- caisson T70.3 ☑
- California — *see* Coccidioidomycosis
- capillaries I78.9
  - specified NEC I78.8
- Carapata A68.0
- cardiac — *see* Disease, heart
- cardiopulmonary, chronic I27.9
- cardiorenal (hepatic) (hypertensive) (vascular) — *see* Hypertension, cardiorenal
- cardiovascular (atherosclerotic) I25.10
  - with angina pectoris — *see* Arteriosclerosis, coronary (artery),
  - congenital Q28.9
  - newborn P29.9
    - specified NEC P29.89
  - hypertensive — *see* Hypertension, heart
  - renal (hypertensive) — *see* Hypertension, cardiorenal
  - syphilitic (asymptomatic) A52.00
- cartilage — *see* Disorder, cartilage
- Castellani's A69.8
- Castleman (unicentric) (multicentric) D47.Z2
  - HHV-8-associated (*see also* Herpesvirus, human, 8)D47.Z2
- cat-scratch A28.1
- Cavare's (familial periodic paralysis) G72.3
- cecum K63.9
- celiac (adult) (infantile) (with steatorrhea) K90.0
- cellular tissue L98.9
- central core G71.2
- cerebellar, cerebellum — *see* Disease, brain
- cerebral (*see also* Disease, brain)
  - degenerative — *see* Degeneration, brain
- cerebrospinal G96.9
- cerebrovascular I67.9
  - acute I67.89
    - embolic I63.4 ☑
    - thrombotic I63.3 ☑
  - arteriosclerotic I67.2
  - specified NEC I67.89
- cervix (uteri) (noninflammatory) N88.9
  - inflammatory — *see* Cervicitis
  - specified NEC N88.8
- Chabert's A22.9
- Chandler's (osteochondritis dissecans, hip) — *see* Osteochondritis, dissecans, hip
- Charlouis — *see* Yaws
- Chédiak-Steinbrinck (-Higashi) (congenital gigantism of peroxidase granules) E70.330
- chest J98.9
- Chiari's (hepatic vein thrombosis) I82.0
- Chicago B40.9
- Chignon B36.8
- chigo, chigoe B88.1
- childhood granulomatous D71
- Chinese liver fluke B66.1
- chlamydial A74.9
  - specified NEC A74.89
- cholecystic K82.9
- choroid H31.9
  - specified NEC H31.8
- Christmas D67
- chronic bullous of childhood L12.2
- chylomicron retention E78.3
- ciliary body H21.9
  - specified NEC H21.89
- circulatory (system) NEC I99.8
  - newborn P29.9
  - syphilitic A52.00
    - congenital A50.54
- coagulation factor deficiency (congenital) — *see* Defect, coagulation
- coccidioidal — *see* Coccidioidomycosis
- cold
  - agglutinin or hemoglobinuria D59.1
    - paroxysmal D59.6
  - hemagglutinin (chronic) D59.1
- collagen NOS (nonvascular) (vascular) M35.9
  - specified NEC M35.8
- colon K63.9
  - functional K59.9
    - congenital Q43.2
  - ischemic (*see also* Ischemia, intestine, acute)K55.039
- colonic inflammatory bowel, unclassified (IBDU) K52.3
- combined system — *see* Degeneration, combined
- compressed air T70.3 ☑
- Concato's (pericardial polyserositis) A19.9
  - nontubercular I31.1
  - pleural — *see* Pleurisy, with effusion
- conjunctiva H11.9
  - chlamydial A74.0
  - specified NEC H11.89
  - viral B30.9
    - specified NEC B30.8
- connective tissue, systemic (diffuse) M35.9
  - in (due to)
    - hypogamma globulinemia D80.1 *[M36.8]*
    - ochronosis E70.29 *[M36.8]*
  - specified NEC M35.8
- Conor and Bruch's (boutonneuse fever) A77.1
- Cooper's — *see* Mastopathy, cystic
- Cori's (glycogenosis III) E74.03
- corkhandler's or corkworker's J67.3
- cornea H18.9
  - specified NEC H18.89 ☑
- coronary (artery) — *see* Disease, heart, ischemic, atherosclerotic
  - congenital Q24.5
  - ostial, syphilitic (aortic) (mitral) (pulmonary) A52.03
- corpus cavernosum N48.9
  - specified NEC N48.89
- Cotugno's — *see* Sciatica
- coxsackie (virus) NEC B34.1
- cranial nerve NOS G52.9
- Creutzfeldt-Jakob — *see* Creutzfeldt-Jakob disease or syndrome
- Crocq's (acrocyanosis) I73.89
- Crohn's — *see* Enteritis, regional
- Curschmann G71.11
- cystic
  - breast (chronic) — *see* Mastopathy, cystic
  - kidney, congenital Q61.9
  - liver, congenital Q44.6
  - lung J98.4
    - congenital Q33.0
- cytomegalic inclusion (generalized) B25.9
  - with pneumonia B25.0
  - congenital P35.1
- cytomegaloviral B25.9
  - specified NEC B25.8
- Czerny's (periodic hydrarthrosis of the knee) — *see* Effusion, joint, knee
- Daae (-Finsen) (epidemic pleurodynia) B33.0
- Darling's — *see* Histoplasmosis capsulati
- Débove's (splenomegaly) R16.1
- deer fly — *see* Tularemia
- Degos' I77.89
- demyelinating, demyelinizating (nervous system) G37.9
  - multiple sclerosis G35
  - specified NEC G37.8
- dense deposit (*see also* N00-N07 with fourth character .6)N05.6
- deposition, hydroxyapatite — *see* Disease, hydroxyapatite deposition
- de Quervain's (tendon sheath) M65.4
  - thyroid (subacute granulomatous thyroiditis) E06.1
- Devergie's (pityriasis rubra pilaris) L44.0
- Devic's G36.0
- diaphorase deficiency D74.0
- diaphragm J98.6
- diarrheal, infectious NEC A09
- digestive system K92.9
  - specified NEC K92.89
- disc, degenerative — *see* Degeneration, intervertebral disc
- discogenic (*see also* Displacement, intervertebral disc NEC)
  - with myelopathy — *see* Disorder, disc, with, myelopathy
- diverticular — *see* Diverticula
- Dubois (thymus) A50.59 *[E35]*
- Duchenne-Griesinger G71.0
- Duchenne's
  - muscular dystrophy G71.0
  - pseudohypertrophy, muscles G71.0
- ductless glands E34.9
- Duhring's (dermatitis herpetiformis) L13.0
- duodenum K31.9
  - specified NEC K31.89
- Dupré's (meningism) R29.1
- Dupuytren's (muscle contracture) M72.0
- Durand-Nicholas-Favre (climatic bubo) A55
- Duroziez's (congenital mitral stenosis) Q23.2

Disease

Disease — *continued*
- ear — *see* Disorder, ear
- Eberth's — *see* Fever, typhoid
- Ebola (virus) A98.4
- Ebstein's heart Q22.5
- Echinococcus — *see* Echinococcus
- echovirus NEC B34.1
- Eddowes' (brittle bones and blue sclera) Q78.0
- edentulous (alveolar) ridge K06.9
  - specified NEC K06.8
- Edsall's T67.2 ☑
- Eichstedt's (pityriasis versicolor) B36.0
- Ellis-van Creveld (chondroectodermal dysplasia) Q77.6
- end stage renal (ESRD) N18.6
  - due to hypertension I12.0
- endocrine glands or system NEC E34.9
- endomyocardial (eosinophilic) I42.3
- English (rickets) E55.0
- enteroviral, enterovirus NEC B34.1
  - central nervous system NEC A88.8
- epidemic B99.9
  - specified NEC B99.8
- epididymis N50.9
- Erb (-Landouzy) G71.0
- Erdheim-Chester (ECD) E88.89
- esophagus K22.9
  - functional K22.4
  - psychogenic F45.8
  - specified NEC K22.8
- Eulenburg's (congenital paramyotonia) G71.19
- eustachian tube — *see* Disorder, eustachian tube
- external
  - auditory canal — *see* Disorder, ear, external
  - ear — *see* Disorder, ear, external
- extrapyramidal G25.9
  - specified NEC G25.89
- eye H57.9
  - anterior chamber H21.9
  - inflammatory NEC H57.8
  - muscle (external) — *see* Strabismus
  - specified NEC H57.8
  - syphilitic — *see* Oculopathy, syphilitic
- eyeball H44.9
  - specified NEC H44.89
- eyelid — *see* Disorder, eyelid
  - specified NEC — *see* Disorder, eyelid, specified type NEC
- eyeworm of Africa B74.3
- facial nerve (seventh) G51.9
  - newborn (birth injury) P11.3
- Fahr (of brain) G23.8
- Fahr Volhard (of kidney) I12. ☑
- fallopian tube (noninflammatory) N83.9
  - inflammatory — *see* Salpingo-oophoritis
  - specified NEC N83.8
- familial periodic paralysis G72.3
- Fanconi's (congenital pancytopenia) D61.09
- fascia NEC (*see also* Disorder, muscle)
  - inflammatory — *see* Myositis
  - specified NEC M62.89
- Fauchard's (periodontitis) — *see* Periodontitis
- Favre-Durand-Nicolas (climatic bubo) A55
- Fede's K14.0
- Feer's — *see* Poisoning, mercury
- female pelvic inflammatory (*see also* Disease, pelvis, inflammatory)N73.9
  - syphilitic (secondary) A51.42
  - tuberculous A18.17
- Fernels' (aortic aneurysm) I71.9
- fibrocaseous of lung — *see* Tuberculosis, pulmonary
- fibrocystic — *see* Fibrocystic disease
- Fiedler's (leptospiral jaundice) A27.0
- fifth B08.3
- file-cutter's — *see* Poisoning, lead
- fish-skin Q80.9
  - acquired L85.0
- Flajani (-Basedow) (exophthalmic goiter) — *see* Hyperthyroidism, with, goiter (diffuse)
- flax-dresser's J66.1
- fluke — *see* Infestation, fluke
- foot and mouth B08.8
- foot process N04.9
- Forbes' (glycogenosis III) E74.03
- Fordyce-Fox (apocrine miliaria) L75.2
- Fordyce's (ectopic sebaceous glands) (mouth) Q38.6
- Forestier's (rhizomelic pseudopolyarthritis) M35.3
  - meaning ankylosing hyperostosis — *see* Hyperostosis, ankylosing
- Fothergill's
  - neuralgia — *see* Neuralgia, trigeminal
  - scarlatina anginosa A38.9

Disease — *continued*
- Fournier (gangrene) N49.3
  - female N76.89
- fourth B08.8
- Fox (-Fordyce) (apocrine miliaria) L75.2
- Francis' — *see* Tularemia
- Franklin C88.2
- Frei's (climatic bubo) A55
- Friedreich's
  - combined systemic or ataxia G11.1
  - myoclonia G25.3
- frontal sinus — *see* Sinusitis, frontal
- fungus NEC B49
- Gaisböck's (polycythemia hypertonica) D75.1
- gallbladder K82.9
  - calculus — *see* Calculus, gallbladder
  - cholecystitis — *see* Cholecystitis
  - cholesterolosis K82.4
  - fistula — *see* Fistula, gallbladder
  - hydrops K82.1
  - obstruction — *see* Obstruction, gallbladder
  - perforation K82.2
  - specified NEC K82.8
- gamma heavy chain C88.2
- Gamna's (siderotic splenomegaly) D73.2
- Gamstorp's (adynamia episodica hereditaria) G72.3
- Gandy-Nanta (siderotic splenomegaly) D73.2
- ganister J62.8
- gastric — *see* Disease, stomach
- gastroesophageal reflux (GERD) K21.9
  - with esophagitis K21.0
- gastrointestinal (tract) K92.9
  - amyloid E85.4
  - functional K59.9
    - psychogenic F45.8
  - specified NEC K92.89
- Gee (-Herter) (-Heubner) (-Thaysen) (nontropical sprue) K90.0
- genital organs
  - female N94.9
  - male N50.9
- Gerhardt's (erythromelalgia) I73.81
- Gibert's (pityriasis rosea) L42
- Gierke's (glycogenosis I) E74.01
- Gilles de la Tourette's (motor-verbal tic) F95.2
- gingiva K06.9
  - plaque induced K05.00
  - specified NEC K06.8
- gland (lymph) I89.9
- Glanzmann's (hereditary hemorrhagic thrombasthenia) D69.1
- glass-blower's (cataract) — *see* Cataract, specified NEC
  - salivary gland hypertrophy K11.1
- Glisson's — *see* Rickets
- globe H44.9
  - specified NEC H44.89
- glomerular (*see also* Glomerulonephritis)
  - with edema — *see* Nephrosis
  - acute — *see* Nephritis, acute
  - chronic — *see* Nephritis, chronic
  - minimal change N05.0
  - rapidly progressive N01.9
- glycogen storage E74.00
  - Andersen's E74.09
  - Cori's E74.03
  - Forbes' E74.03
  - generalized E74.00
  - glucose-6-phosphatase deficiency E74.01
  - heart E74.02 *[I43]*
  - hepatorenal E74.09
  - Hers' E74.09
  - liver and kidney E74.09
  - McArdle's E74.04
  - muscle phosphofructokinase E74.09
  - myocardium E74.02 *[I43]*
  - Pompe's E74.02
  - Tauri's E74.09
  - type 0 E74.09
  - type I E74.01
  - type II E74.02
  - type III E74.03
  - type IV E74.09
  - type V E74.04
  - type VI-XI E74.09
  - Von Gierke's E74.01
- Goldstein's (familial hemorrhagic telangiectasia) I78.0
- gonococcal NOS A54.9
- graft-versus-host (GVH) D89.813
  - acute D89.810
  - acute on chronic D89.812
  - chronic D89.811

Disease — *continued*
- grainhandler's J67.8
- granulomatous (childhood) (chronic) D71
- Graves' (exophthalmic goiter) — *see* Hyperthyroidism, with, goiter (diffuse)
- Griesinger's — *see* Ancylostomiasis
- Grisel's M43.6
- Gruby's (tinea tonsurans) B35.0
- Guillain-Barré G61.0
- Guinon's (motor-verbal tic) F95.2
- gum K06.9
- gynecological N94.9
- H (Hartnup's) E72.02
- Haff — *see* Poisoning, mercury
- Hageman (congenital factor XII deficiency) D68.2
- hair (color) (shaft) L67.9
  - follicles L73.9
    - specified NEC L73.8
- Hamman's (spontaneous mediastinal emphysema) J98.2
- hand, foot and mouth B08.4
- Hansen's — *see* Leprosy
- Hantavirus, with pulmonary manifestations B33.4
  - with renal manifestations A98.5
- Harada's H30.81 ☑
- Hartnup (pellagra-cerebellar ataxia-renal aminoaciduria) E72.02
- Hart's (pellagra-cerebellar ataxia-renal aminoaciduria) E72.02
- Hashimoto's (struma lymphomatosa) E06.3
- Hb — *see* Disease, hemoglobin
- heart (organic) I51.9
  - with
    - pulmonary edema (acute) (*see also* Failure, ventricular, left)I50.1
    - rheumatic fever (conditions in I00)
      - active I01.9
        - with chorea I02.0
        - specified NEC I01.8
      - inactive or quiescent (with chorea) I09.9
        - specified NEC I09.89
  - amyloid E85.4 *[I43]*
  - aortic (valve) I35.9
  - arteriosclerotic or sclerotic (senile) — *see* Disease, heart, ischemic, atherosclerotic
  - artery, arterial — *see* Disease, heart, ischemic, atherosclerotic
  - beer drinkers' I42.6
  - beriberi (wet) E51.12
  - black I27.0
  - congenital Q24.9
    - cyanotic Q24.9
    - specified NEC Q24.8
  - coronary — *see* Disease, heart, ischemic
  - cryptogenic I51.9
  - fibroid — *see* Myocarditis
  - functional I51.89
    - psychogenic F45.8
  - glycogen storage E74.02 *[I43]*
  - gonococcal A54.83
  - hypertensive — *see* Hypertension, heart
  - hyperthyroid (*see also* Hyperthyroidism)E05.90 *[I43]*
    - with thyroid storm E05.91 *[I43]*
  - ischemic (chronic or with a stated duration of over 4 weeks) I25.9
    - atherosclerotic (of) I25.10
      - with angina pectoris — *see* Arteriosclerosis, coronary (artery)
      - coronary artery bypass graft — *see* Arteriosclerosis, coronary (artery),
    - cardiomyopathy I25.5
    - diagnosed on ECG or other special investigation, but currently presenting no symptoms I25.6
    - silent I25.6
    - specified form NEC I25.89
  - kyphoscoliotic I27.1
  - meningococcal A39.50
    - endocarditis A39.51
    - myocarditis A39.52
    - pericarditis A39.53
  - mitral I05.9
    - specified NEC I05.8
  - muscular — *see* Degeneration, myocardial
  - psychogenic (functional) F45.8
  - pulmonary (chronic) I27.9
    - in schistosomiasis B65.9 *[I52]*
    - specified NEC I27.89
  - rheumatic (chronic) (inactive) (old) (quiescent) (with chorea) I09.9
    - active or acute I01.9

- **Disease** — *continued*
  - heart — *continued*
        - with chorea (acute) (rheumatic) (Sydenham's) I02.0
      - specified NEC I09.89
    - senile — *see* Myocarditis
    - syphilitic A52.06
      - aortic A52.03
        - aneurysm A52.01
      - congenital A50.54 *[I52]*
    - thyrotoxic (*see also* Thyrotoxicosis)E05.90 *[I43]*
      - with thyroid storm E05.91 *[I43]*
    - valve, valvular (obstructive) (regurgitant) (*see also* Endocarditis)
      - congenital NEC Q24.8
        - pulmonary Q22.3
    - vascular — *see* Disease, cardiovascular
  - heavy chain NEC C88.2
    - alpha C88.3
    - gamma C88.2
    - mu C88.2
  - Hebra's
    - pityriasis
      - maculata et circinata L42
      - rubra pilaris L44.0
    - prurigo L28.2
  - hematopoietic organs D75.9
  - hemoglobin or Hb
    - abnormal (mixed) NEC D58.2
      - with thalassemia D56.9
    - AS genotype D57.3
    - Bart's D56.0
    - C (Hb-C) D58.2
      - with other abnormal hemoglobin NEC D58.2
      - elliptocytosis D58.1
      - Hb-S D57.2 ☑
      - sickle-cell D57.2 ☑
      - thalassemia D56.8
    - Constant Spring D58.2
    - D (Hb-D) D58.2
    - E (Hb-E) D58.2
    - E-beta thalassemia D56.5
    - elliptocytosis D58.1
    - H (Hb-H) (thalassemia) D56.0
      - with other abnormal hemoglobin NEC D56.9
      - Constant Spring D56.0
    - I thalassemia D56.9
    - M D74.0
    - S or SS D57.1
    - SC D57.2 ☑
    - SD D57.8 ☑
    - SE D57.8 ☑
    - spherocytosis D58.0
    - unstable, hemolytic D58.2
  - hemolytic (newborn) P55.9
    - autoimmune (cold type) (warm type) D59.1
    - drug-induced D59.0
    - due to or with
      - incompatibility
        - ABO (blood group) P55.1
        - blood (group) (Duffy) (K (ell)) (Kidd) (Lewis) (M) (S) NEC P55.8
        - Rh (blood group) (factor) P55.0
      - Rh negative mother P55.0
    - specified type NEC P55.8
    - unstable hemoglobin D58.2
  - hemorrhagic D69.9
    - newborn P53
  - Henoch (-Schönlein) (purpura nervosa) D69.0
  - hepatic — *see* Disease, liver
  - hepatobiliary K83.9
    - toxic K71.9
  - hepatolenticular E83.01
  - heredodegenerative NEC
    - spinal cord G95.89
  - herpesviral, disseminated B00.7
  - Hers' (glycogenosis VI) E74.09
  - Herter (-Gee) (-Heubner) (nontropical sprue) K90.0
  - Heubner-Herter (nontropical sprue) K90.0
  - high fetal gene or hemoglobin thalassemia D56.9
  - Hildenbrand's — *see* Typhus
  - hip (joint) M25.9
    - congenital Q65.89
    - suppurative M00.9
    - tuberculous A18.02
  - His (-Werner) (trench fever) A79.0
  - Hodgson's I71.2
    - ruptured I71.1
  - Holla — *see* Spherocytosis
  - hookworm B76.9
    - specified NEC B76.8

- **Disease** — *continued*
  - host-versus-graft D89.813
    - acute D89.810
    - acute on chronic D89.812
    - chronic D89.811
  - human immunodeficiency virus (HIV) B20
  - Huntington's G10
  - Hutchinson's (cheiropompholyx) — *see* Hutchinson's disease
  - hyaline (diffuse) (generalized)
    - membrane (lung) (newborn) P22.0
      - adult J80
  - hydatid — *see* Echinococcus
  - hydroxyapatite deposition M11.00
    - ankle M11.07 ☑
    - elbow M11.02 ☑
    - foot joint M11.07 ☑
    - hand joint M11.04 ☑
    - hip M11.05 ☑
    - knee M11.06 ☑
    - multiple site M11.09
    - shoulder M11.01 ☑
    - vertebra M11.08
    - wrist M11.03 ☑
  - hyperkinetic — *see* Hyperkinesia
  - hypertensive — *see* Hypertension
  - hypophysis E23.7
  - Iceland G93.3
  - I-cell E77.0
  - immune D89.9
  - immunoproliferative (malignant) C88.9
    - small intestinal C88.3
    - specified NEC C88.8
  - inclusion B25.9
    - salivary gland B25.9
  - infectious, infective B99.9
    - congenital P37.9
      - specified NEC P37.8
      - viral P35.9
        - specified type NEC P35.8
    - specified NEC B99.8
  - inflammatory
    - penis N48.29
      - abscess N48.21
      - cellulitis N48.22
    - prepuce N47.7
      - balanoposthitis N47.6
    - tubo-ovarian — *see* Salpingo-oophoritis
  - intervertebral disc (*see also* Disorder, disc)
    - with myelopathy — *see* Disorder, disc, with, myelopathy
    - cervical, cervicothoracic — *see* Disorder, disc, cervical
      - with
        - myelopathy — *see* Disorder, disc, cervical, with myelopathy
        - neuritis, radiculitis or radiculopathy — *see* Disorder, disc, cervical, with neuritis
        - specified NEC — *see* Disorder, disc, cervical, specified type NEC
    - lumbar (with)
      - myelopathy M51.06
      - neuritis, radiculitis, radiculopathy or sciatica M51.16
      - specified NEC M51.86
    - lumbosacral (with)
      - neuritis, radiculitis, radiculopathy or sciatica M51.17
      - specified NEC M51.87
    - specified NEC — *see* Disorder, disc, specified NEC
    - thoracic (with)
      - myelopathy M51.04
      - neuritis, radiculitis or radiculopathy M51.14
      - specified NEC M51.84
    - thoracolumbar (with)
      - myelopathy M51.05
      - neuritis, radiculitis or radiculopathy M51.15
      - specified NEC M51.85
  - intestine K63.9
    - functional K59.9
      - psychogenic F45.8
      - specified NEC K59.8
    - organic K63.9
    - protozoal A07.9
    - specified NEC K63.89
  - iris H21.9
    - specified NEC H21.89
  - iron metabolism or storage E83.10
  - island (scrub typhus) A75.3
  - itai-itai — *see* Poisoning, cadmium

- **Disease** — *continued*
  - Jakob-Creutzfeldt — *see* Creutzfeldt-Jakob disease or syndrome
  - jaw M27.9
    - fibrocystic M27.49
    - specified NEC M27.8
  - jigger B88.1
  - joint (*see also* Disorder, joint)
    - Charcot's — *see* Arthropathy, neuropathic (Charcot)
    - degenerative — *see* Osteoarthritis
      - multiple M15.9
      - spine — *see* Spondylosis
    - hypertrophic — *see* Osteoarthritis
    - sacroiliac M53.3
    - specified NEC — *see* Disorder, joint, specified type NEC
    - spine NEC — *see* Dorsopathy
    - suppurative — *see* Arthritis, pyogenic or pyemic
  - Jourdain's (acute gingivitis) K05.00
    - nonplaque induced K05.01
    - plaque induced K05.00
  - Kaschin-Beck (endemic polyarthritis) M12.10
    - ankle M12.17 ☑
    - elbow M12.12 ☑
    - foot joint M12.17 ☑
    - hand joint M12.14 ☑
    - hip M12.15 ☑
    - knee M12.16 ☑
    - multiple site M12.19
    - shoulder M12.11 ☑
    - vertebra M12.18
    - wrist M12.13 ☑
  - Katayama B65.2
  - Kedani (scrub typhus) A75.3
  - Keshan E59
  - kidney (functional) (pelvis) N28.9
    - chronic N18.9
      - hypertensive — *see* Hypertension, kidney
      - stage 1 N18.1
      - stage 2 (mild) N18.2
      - stage 3 (moderate) N18.3
      - stage 4 (severe) N18.4
      - stage 5 N18.5
    - complicating pregnancy — *see* Pregnancy, complicated by, renal disease
    - cystic (congenital) Q61.9
    - diabetic — *see* E08-E13 with .22
    - fibrocystic (congenital) Q61.8
    - hypertensive — *see* Hypertension, kidney
    - in (due to)
      - schistosomiasis (bilharziasis) B65.9 *[N29]*
    - multicystic Q61.4
    - polycystic Q61.3
      - adult type Q61.2
      - childhood type NEC Q61.19
        - collecting duct dilatation Q61.11
  - Kimmelstiel (-Wilson) (intercapillary polycystic (congenital) glomerulosclerosis) — *see* E08-E13 with .21
  - Kimura D21.9
    - specified site (see Neoplasm, connective tissue benign)
  - Kinnier Wilson's (hepatolenticular degeneration) E83.01
  - kissing — *see* Mononucleosis, infectious
  - Klebs' (*see also* Glomerulonephritis)N05. ☑
  - Klippel-Feil (brevicollis) Q76.1
  - Köhler-Pellegrini-Stieda (calcification, knee joint) — *see* Bursitis, tibial collateral
  - Kok Q89.8
  - König's (osteochondritis dissecans) — *see* Osteochondritis, dissecans
  - Korsakoff's (nonalcoholic) F04
    - alcoholic F10.96
      - with dependence F10.26
  - Kostmann's (infantile genetic agranulocytosis) D70.0
  - kuru A81.81
  - Kyasanur Forest A98.2
  - labyrinth, ear — *see* Disorder, ear, inner
  - lacrimal system — *see* Disorder, lacrimal system
  - Lafora's — *see* Epilepsy, generalized, idiopathic
  - Lancereaux-Mathieu (leptospiral jaundice) A27.0
  - Landry's G61.0
  - Larrey-Weil (leptospiral jaundice) A27.0
  - larynx J38.7
  - legionnaires' A48.1
    - nonpneumonic A48.2
  - Lenegre's I44.2
  - lens H27.9
    - specified NEC H27.8

Disease — *continued*
- Lev's (acquired complete heart block) I44.2
- Lewy body (dementia) G31.83 *[F02.80]*
  - with behavioral disturbance G31.83 *[F02.81]*
- Lichtheim's (subacute combined sclerosis with pernicious anemia) D51.0
- Lightwood's (renal tubular acidosis) N25.89
- Lignac's (cystinosis) E72.04
- lip K13.0
- lipid-storage E75.6
  - specified NEC E75.5
- Lipschütz's N76.6
- liver (chronic) (organic) K76.9
  - alcoholic (chronic) K70.9
    - acute — *see* Disease, liver, alcoholic, hepatitis
    - cirrhosis K70.30
      - with ascites K70.31
    - failure K70.40
      - with coma K70.41
    - fatty liver K70.0
    - fibrosis K70.2
    - hepatitis K70.10
      - with ascites K70.11
    - sclerosis K70.2
  - cystic, congenital Q44.6
  - drug-induced (idiosyncratic) (toxic) (predictable) (unpredictable) — *see* Disease, liver, toxic
  - end stage K72.90
    - due to hepatitis — *see* Hepatitis
  - fatty, nonalcoholic (NAFLD) K76.0
    - alcoholic K70.0
  - fibrocystic (congenital) Q44.6
  - fluke
    - Chinese B66.1
    - oriental B66.1
    - sheep B66.3
  - glycogen storage E74.09 *[K77]*
  - in (due to)
    - schistosomiasis (bilharziasis) B65.9 *[K77]*
  - inflammatory K75.9
    - alcoholic K70.1 ☑
    - specified NEC K75.89
  - polycystic (congenital) Q44.6
  - toxic K71.9
    - with
      - cholestasis K71.0
      - cirrhosis (liver) K71.7
      - fibrosis (liver) K71.7
      - focal nodular hyperplasia K71.8
      - hepatic granuloma K71.8
      - hepatic necrosis K71.10
        - with coma K71.11
      - hepatitis NEC K71.6
        - acute K71.2
        - chronic
          - active K71.50
            - with ascites K71.51
          - lobular K71.4
          - persistent K71.3
        - lupoid K71.50
          - with ascites K71.51
      - peliosis hepatis K71.8
      - veno-occlusive disease (VOD) of liver K71.8
  - veno-occlusive K76.5
- Lobo's (keloid blastomycosis) B48.0
- Lobstein's (brittle bones and blue sclera) Q78.0
- Ludwig's (submaxillary cellulitis) K12.2
- lumbosacral region M53.87
- lung J98.4
  - black J60
  - congenital Q33.9
  - cystic J98.4
    - congenital Q33.0
  - fibroid (chronic) — *see* Fibrosis, lung
  - fluke B66.4
    - oriental B66.4
  - in
    - amyloidosis E85.4 *[J99]*
    - sarcoidosis D86.0
    - Sjögren's syndrome M35.02
    - systemic
      - lupus erythematosus M32.13
      - sclerosis M34.81
  - interstitial J84.9
    - of childhood, specified NEC J84.848
    - respiratory bronchiolitis J84.115
    - specified NEC J84.89
  - obstructive (chronic) J44.9
    - with
      - acute
        - bronchitis J44.0

Disease — *continued*
- lung — *continued*
  - obstructive (chronic) — *continued*
    - with — *continued*
      - acute — *continued*
        - exacerbation NEC J44.1
        - lower respiratory infection J44.0
      - alveolitis, allergic J67.9
      - asthma J44.9
      - bronchiectasis J47.9
        - with
          - exacerbation (acute) J47.1
          - lower respiratory infection J47.0
      - bronchitis J44.9
        - with
          - exacerbation (acute) J44.1
          - lower respiratory infection J44.0
      - emphysema J44.9
      - hypersensitivity pneumonitis J67.9
    - decompensated J44.1
      - with
        - exacerbation (acute) J44.1
  - polycystic J98.4
    - congenital Q33.0
  - rheumatoid (diffuse) (interstitial) — *see* Rheumatoid, lung
- Lutembacher's (atrial septal defect with mitral stenosis) Q21.1
- Lyme A69.20
- lymphatic (gland) (system) (channel) (vessel) I89.9
- lymphoproliferative D47.9
  - specified NEC D47.Z9
  - T-gamma D47.Z9
  - X-linked D82.3
- Magitot's M27.2
- malarial — *see* Malaria
- malignant (*see also* Neoplasm, malignant, by site)
- Manson's B65.1
- maple bark J67.6
- maple-syrup-urine E71.0
- Marburg (virus) A98.3
- Marion's (bladder neck obstruction) N32.0
- Marsh's (exophthalmic goiter) — *see* Hyperthyroidism, with, goiter (diffuse)
- mastoid (process) — *see* Disorder, ear, middle
- Mathieu's (leptospiral jaundice) A27.0
- Maxcy's A75.2
- McArdle (-Schmid-Pearson) (glycogenosis V) E74.04
- mediastinum J98.59
- medullary center (idiopathic) (respiratory) G93.89
- Meige's (chronic hereditary edema) Q82.0
- meningococcal — *see* Infection, meningococcal
- mental F99
  - organic F09
- mesenchymal M35.9
- mesenteric embolic (*see also* Ischemia, intestine, acute)K55.039
- metabolic, metabolism E88.9
  - bilirubin E80.7
- metal-polisher's J62.8
- metastatic (*see also* Neoplasm, secondary, by site)C79.9
- microvascular - code to condition
- microvillus
  - atrophy Q43.8
  - inclusion (MVD) Q43.8
- middle ear — *see* Disorder, ear, middle
- Mikulicz' (dryness of mouth, absent or decreased lacrimation) K11.8
- Milroy's (chronic hereditary edema) Q82.0
- Minamata — *see* Poisoning, mercury
- minicore G71.2
- Minor's G95.19
- Minot's (hemorrhagic disease, newborn) P53
- Minot-von Willebrand-Jürgens (angiohemophilia) D68.0
- Mitchell's (erythromelalgia) I73.81
- mitral (valve) I05.9
  - nonrheumatic I34.9
- mixed connective tissue M35.1
- moldy hay J67.0
- Monge's T70.29 ☑
- Morgagni-Adams-Stokes (syncope with heart block) I45.9
- Morgagni's (syndrome) (hyperostosis frontalis interna) M85.2
- Morton's (with metatarsalgia) — *see* Lesion, nerve, plantar
- Morvan's G60.8
- motor neuron (bulbar) (familial) (mixed type) (spinal) G12.20
  - amyotrophic lateral sclerosis G12.21
  - progressive bulbar palsy G12.22
  - specified NEC G12.29

Disease — *continued*
- moyamoya I67.5
- mu heavy chain disease C88.2
- multicore G71.2
- muscle (*see also* Disorder, muscle)
  - inflammatory — *see* Myositis
  - ocular (external) — *see* Strabismus
- musculoskeletal system, soft tissue — *see* also Disorder, soft tissue
  - specified NEC — *see* Disorder, soft tissue, specified type NEC
- mushroom workers' J67.5
- mycotic B49
- myelodysplastic, not classified C94.6
- myeloproliferative, not classified C94.6
  - chronic D47.1
- myocardium, myocardial (*see also* Degeneration, myocardial)I51.5
  - primary (idiopathic) I42.9
- myoneural G70.9
- Naegeli's D69.1
- nails L60.9
  - specified NEC L60.8
- Nairobi (sheep virus) A93.8
- nasal J34.9
- nemaline body G71.2
- nerve — *see* Disorder, nerve
- nervous system G98.8
  - autonomic G90.9
  - central G96.9
    - specified NEC G96.8
  - congenital Q07.9
  - parasympathetic G90.9
  - specified NEC G98.8
  - sympathetic G90.9
  - vegetative G90.9
- neuromuscular system G70.9
- Newcastle B30.8
- Nicolas (-Durand)-Favre (climatic bubo) A55
- nipple N64.9
  - Paget's C50.01 ☑
    - female C50.01 ☑
    - male C50.02 ☑
- Nishimoto (-Takeuchi) I67.5
- nonarthropod-borne NOS (viral) B34.9
  - enterovirus NEC B34.1
- nonautoimmune hemolytic D59.4
  - drug-induced D59.2
- Nonne-Milroy-Meige (chronic hereditary edema) Q82.0
- nose J34.9
- nucleus pulposus — *see* Disorder, disc
- nutritional E63.9
- oast-house-urine E72.19
  - ocular
    - herpesviral B00.50
    - zoster B02.30
- obliterative vascular I77.1
- Ohara's — *see* Tularemia
- Opitz's (congestive splenomegaly) D73.2
- Oppenheim-Urbach (necrobiosis lipoidica diabeticorum) — *see* E08-E13 with .620
- optic nerve NEC — *see* Disorder, nerve, optic
- orbit — *see* Disorder, orbit
- Oriental liver fluke B66.1
- Oriental lung fluke B66.4
- Ormond's N13.5
- Oropouche virus A93.0
- Osler-Rendu (familial hemorrhagic telangiectasia) I78.0
- osteofibrocystic E21.0
- Otto's M24.7
- outer ear — *see* Disorder, ear, external
- ovary (noninflammatory) N83.9
  - cystic N83.20 ☑
  - inflammatory — *see* Salpingo-oophoritis
  - polycystic E28.2
  - specified NEC N83.8
- Owren's (congenital) — *see* Defect, coagulation
- pancreas K86.9
  - cystic K86.2
  - fibrocystic E84.9
  - specified NEC K86.89
- panvalvular I08.9
  - specified NEC I08.8
- parametrium (noninflammatory) N83.9
- parasitic B89
  - cerebral NEC B71.9 *[G94]*
  - intestinal NOS B82.9
  - mouth B37.0
  - skin NOS B88.9
  - specified type — *see* Infestation
  - tongue B37.0

Disease — *continued*
- parathyroid (gland) E21.5
  - specified NEC E21.4
- Parkinson's G20
- parodontal K05.6
- Parrot's (syphilitic osteochondritis) A50.02
- Parry's (exophthalmic goiter) — *see* Hyperthyroidism, with, goiter (diffuse)
- Parson's (exophthalmic goiter) — *see* Hyperthyroidism, with, goiter (diffuse)
- Paxton's (white piedra) B36.2
- pearl-worker's — *see* Osteomyelitis, specified type NEC
- Pellegrini-Stieda (calcification, knee joint) — *see* Bursitis, tibial collateral
- pelvis, pelvic
  - female NOS N94.9
    - specified NEC N94.89
  - gonococcal (acute) (chronic) A54.24
  - inflammatory (female) N73.9
    - acute N73.0
    - chlamydial A56.11
    - chronic N73.1
    - specified NEC N73.8
    - syphilitic (secondary) A51.42
      - late A52.76
    - tuberculous A18.17
  - organ, female N94.9
  - peritoneum, female NEC N94.89
- penis N48.9
  - inflammatory N48.29
    - abscess N48.21
    - cellulitis N48.22
  - specified NEC N48.89
- periapical tissues NOS K04.90
- periodontal K05.6
  - specified NEC K05.5
- periosteum — *see* Disorder, bone, specified type NEC
- peripheral
  - arterial I73.9
  - autonomic nervous system G90.9
  - nerves — *see* Polyneuropathy
  - vascular NOS I73.9
- peritoneum K66.9
  - pelvic, female NEC N94.89
  - specified NEC K66.8
- persistent mucosal (middle ear) H66.20
  - left H66.22
    - with right H66.23
  - right H66.21
    - with left H66.23
- Petit's — *see* Hernia, abdomen, specified site NEC
- pharynx J39.2
  - specified NEC J39.2
- Phocas' — *see* Mastopathy, cystic
- photochromogenic (acid-fast bacilli) (pulmonary) A31.0
  - nonpulmonary A31.9
- Pick's G31.01 *[F02.80]*
  - with behavioral disturbance G31.01 *[F02.81]*
  - brain G31.01 *[F02.80]*
    - with behavioral disturbance G31.01 *[F02.81]*
  - of pericardium (pericardial pseudocirrhosis of liver) I31.1
- pigeon fancier's J67.2
- pineal gland E34.8
- pink — *see* Poisoning, mercury
- Pinkus' (lichen nitidus) L44.1
- pinworm B80
- Piry virus A93.8
- pituitary (gland) E23.7
- pituitary-snuff-taker's J67.8
- pleura (cavity) J94.9
  - specified NEC J94.8
- pneumatic drill (hammer) T75.21 ☑
- Pollitzer's (hidradenitis suppurativa) L73.2
- polycystic
  - kidney or renal Q61.3
    - adult type Q61.2
    - childhood type NEC Q61.19
      - collecting duct dilatation Q61.11
  - liver or hepatic Q44.6
  - lung or pulmonary J98.4
    - congenital Q33.0
  - ovary, ovaries E28.2
  - spleen Q89.09
- polyethylene T84.05 ☑
- Pompe's (glycogenosis II) E74.02
- Posadas-Wernicke B38.9
- Potain's (pulmonary edema) — *see* Edema, lung

Disease — *continued*
- prepuce N47.8
  - inflammatory N47.7
    - balanoposthitis N47.6
- Pringle's (tuberous sclerosis) Q85.1
- prion, central nervous system A81.9
  - specified NEC A81.89
- prostate N42.9
  - specified NEC N42.89
- protozoal B64
  - acanthamebiasis — *see* Acanthamebiasis
  - African trypanosomiasis — *see* African trypanosomiasis
  - babesiosis B60.0
  - Chagas disease — *see* Chagas disease
  - intestine, intestinal A07.9
  - leishmaniasis — *see* Leishmaniasis
  - malaria — *see* Malaria
  - naegleriasis B60.2
  - pneumocystosis B59
  - specified organism NEC B60.8
  - toxoplasmosis — *see* Toxoplasmosis
- pseudo-Hurler's E77.0
- psychiatric F99
- psychotic — *see* Psychosis
- Puente's (simple glandular cheilitis) K13.0
- puerperal (*see also* Puerperal)O90.89
- pulmonary (*see also* Disease, lung)
  - artery I28.9
  - chronic obstructive J44.9
    - with
      - acute bronchitis J44.0
      - exacerbation (acute) J44.1
      - lower respiratory infection (acute) J44.0
    - decompensated J44.1
      - with
        - exacerbation (acute) J44.1
  - heart I27.9
    - specified NEC I27.89
  - hypertensive (vascular) I27.0
  - valve I37.9
    - rheumatic I09.89
- pulp (dental) NOS K04.90
- pulseless M31.4
- Putnam's (subacute combined sclerosis with pernicious anemia) D51.0
- Pyle (-Cohn) (metaphyseal dysplasia) Q78.5
- ragpicker's or ragsorter's A22.1
- Raynaud's — *see* Raynaud's disease
- reactive airway — *see* Asthma
- Reclus' (cystic) — *see* Mastopathy, cystic
- rectum K62.9
  - specified NEC K62.89
- Refsum's (heredopathia atactica polyneuritiformis) G60.1
- renal (functional) (pelvis) (*see also* Disease, kidney)N28.9
  - with
    - edema — *see* Nephrosis
    - glomerular lesion — *see* Glomerulonephritis
      - with edema — *see* Nephrosis
    - interstitial nephritis N12
  - acute N28.9
  - chronic (*see also* Disease, kidney, chronic)N18.9
  - cystic, congenital Q61.9
  - diabetic — *see* E08-E13 with .22
  - end-stage (failure) N18.6
    - due to hypertension I12.0
  - fibrocystic (congenital) Q61.8
  - hypertensive — *see* Hypertension, kidney
  - lupus M32.14
  - phosphate-losing (tubular) N25.0
  - polycystic (congenital) Q61.3
    - adult type Q61.2
    - childhood type NEC Q61.19
      - collecting duct dilatation Q61.11
  - rapidly progressive N01.9
  - subacute N01.9
- Rendu-Osler-Weber (familial hemorrhagic telangiectasia) I78.0
- renovascular (arteriosclerotic) — *see* Hypertension, kidney
- respiratory (tract) J98.9
  - acute or subacute NOS J06.9
    - due to
      - chemicals, gases, fumes or vapors (inhalation) J68.3
      - external agent J70.9
        - specified NEC J70.8
      - radiation J70.0
      - smoke inhalation J70.5
    - noninfectious J39.8

Disease — *continued*
- respiratory — *continued*
  - chronic NOS J98.9
    - due to
      - chemicals, gases, fumes or vapors J68.4
      - external agent J70.9
        - specified NEC J70.8
      - radiation J70.1
    - newborn P27.9
      - specified NEC P27.8
  - due to
    - chemicals, gases, fumes or vapors J68.9
      - acute or subacute NEC J68.3
      - chronic J68.4
    - external agent J70.9
      - specified NEC J70.8
  - newborn P28.9
    - specified type NEC P28.89
  - upper J39.9
    - acute or subacute J06.9
    - noninfectious NEC J39.8
    - specified NEC J39.8
    - streptococcal J06.9
- retina, retinal H35.9
  - Batten's or Batten-Mayou E75.4 *[H36]*
  - specified NEC H35.89
- rheumatoid — *see* Arthritis, rheumatoid
- rickettsial NOS A79.9
  - specified type NEC A79.89
- Riga (-Fede) (cachectic aphthae) K14.0
- Riggs' (compound periodontitis) — *see* Periodontitis
- Ritter's L00
- Rivalta's (cervicofacial actinomycosis) A42.2
- Robles' (onchocerciasis) B73.01
- Roger's (congenital interventricular septal defect) Q21.0
- Rosenthal's (factor XI deficiency) D68.1
- Rossbach's (hyperchlorhydria) K30
- Ross River B33.1
- Rotes Quérol — *see* Hyperostosis, ankylosing
- Roth (-Bernhardt) — *see* Mononeuropathy, lower limb, meralgia paresthetica
- Runeberg's (progressive pernicious anemia) D51.0
- sacroiliac NEC M53.3
- salivary gland or duct K11.9
  - inclusion B25.9
  - specified NEC K11.8
  - virus B25.9
- sandworm B76.9
- Schimmelbusch's — *see* Mastopathy, cystic
- Schmorl's — *see* Schmorl's disease or nodes
- Schönlein (-Henoch) (purpura rheumatica) D69.0
- Schottmüller's — *see* Fever, paratyphoid
- Schultz's (agranulocytosis) — *see* Agranulocytosis
- Schwalbe-Ziehen-Oppenheim G24.1
- Schwartz-Jampel G71.13
- sclera H15.9
  - specified NEC H15.89
- scrofulous (tuberculous) A18.2
- scrotum N50.9
- sebaceous glands L73.9
- semilunar cartilage, cystic (*see also* Derangement, knee, meniscus, cystic)
- seminal vesicle N50.9
- serum NEC (*see also* Reaction, serum)T80.69 ☑
- sexually transmitted A64
  - anogenital
    - herpesviral infection — *see* Herpes, anogenital
    - warts A63.0
  - chancroid A57
  - chlamydial infection — *see* Chlamydia
  - gonorrhea — *see* Gonorrhea
  - granuloma inguinale A58
  - specified organism NEC A63.8
  - syphilis — *see* Syphilis
  - trichomoniasis — *see* Trichomoniasis
- Sézary C84.1 ☑
- shimamushi (scrub typhus) A75.3
- shipyard B30.0
- sickle-cell D57.1
  - with crisis (vasoocclusive pain) D57.00
    - with
      - acute chest syndrome D57.01
      - splenic sequestration D57.02
  - elliptocytosis D57.8 ☑
  - Hb-C D57.20
    - with crisis (vasoocclusive pain) D57.219
      - with
        - acute chest syndrome D57.211

Disease

- Disease — *continued*
  - sickle-cell — *continued*
          - splenic sequestration D57.212
      - without crisis D57.20
    - Hb-SD D57.80
      - with crisis D57.819
        - with
          - acute chest syndrome D57.811
          - splenic sequestration D57.812
    - Hb-SE D57.80
      - with crisis D57.819
        - with
          - acute chest syndrome D57.811
          - splenic sequestration D57.812
    - specified NEC D57.80
      - with crisis D57.819
        - with
          - acute chest syndrome D57.811
          - splenic sequestration D57.812
    - spherocytosis D57.80
      - with crisis D57.819
        - with
          - acute chest syndrome D57.811
          - splenic sequestration D57.812
    - thalassemia D57.40
      - with crisis (vasoocclusive pain) D57.419
        - with
          - acute chest syndrome D57.411
          - splenic sequestration D57.412
      - without crisis D57.40
  - silo-filler's J68.8
    - bronchitis J68.0
    - pneumonitis J68.0
    - pulmonary edema J68.1
  - simian B B00.4
  - Simons' (progressive lipodystrophy) E88.1
  - sin nombre virus B33.4
  - sinus — *see* Sinusitis
  - Sirkari's B55.0
  - sixth B08.20
    - due to human herpesvirus 6 B08.21
    - due to human herpesvirus 7 B08.22
  - skin L98.9
    - due to metabolic disorder NEC E88.9 *[L99]*
    - specified NEC L98.8
  - slim (HIV) B20
  - small vessel I73.9
  - Sneddon-Wilkinson (subcorneal pustular dermatosis) L13.1
  - South African creeping B88.0
  - spinal (cord) G95.9
    - congenital Q06.9
    - specified NEC G95.89
  - spine (*see also* Spondylopathy)
    - joint — *see* Dorsopathy
    - tuberculous A18.01
  - spinocerebellar (hereditary) G11.9
    - specified NEC G11.8
  - spleen D73.9
    - amyloid E85.4 *[D77]*
    - organic D73.9
    - polycystic Q89.09
    - postinfectional D73.89
  - sponge-diver's — *see* Toxicity, venom, marine animal, sea anemone
  - Startle Q89.8
  - Steinert's G71.11
  - Sticker's (erythema infectiosum) B08.3
  - Stieda's (calcification, knee joint) — *see* Bursitis, tibial collateral
  - Stokes' (exophthalmic goiter) — *see* Hyperthyroidism, with, goiter (diffuse)
  - Stokes-Adams (syncope with heart block) I45.9
  - stomach K31.9
    - functional, psychogenic F45.8
    - specified NEC K31.89
  - stonemason's J62.8
  - storage
    - glycogen — *see* Disease, glycogen storage
    - mucopolysaccharide — *see* Mucopolysaccharidosis
  - striatopallidal system NEC G25.89
  - Stuart-Prower (congenital factor X deficiency) D68.2
  - Stuart's (congenital factor X deficiency) D68.2
  - subcutaneous tissue — *see* Disease, skin
  - supporting structures of teeth K08.9
    - specified NEC K08.89
  - suprarenal (capsule) (gland) E27.9
    - hyperfunction E27.0
    - specified NEC E27.8
  - sweat glands L74.9
    - specified NEC L74.8

- Disease — *continued*
  - Sweeley-Klionsky E75.21
  - Swift (-Feer) — *see* Poisoning, mercury
  - swimming-pool granuloma A31.1
  - Sylvest's (epidemic pleurodynia) B33.0
  - sympathetic nervous system G90.9
  - synovium — *see* Disorder, synovium
  - syphilitic — *see* Syphilis
  - systemic tissue mast cell C96.2
  - tanapox (virus) B08.71
  - Tangier E78.6
  - Tarral-Besnier (pityriasis rubra pilaris) L44.0
  - Tauri's E74.09
  - tear duct — *see* Disorder, lacrimal system
  - tendon, tendinous (*see also* Disorder, tendon)
    - nodular — *see* Trigger finger
  - terminal vessel I73.9
  - testis N50.9
  - thalassemia Hb-S — *see* Disease, sickle-cell, thalassemia
  - Thaysen-Gee (nontropical sprue) K90.0
  - Thomsen G71.12
  - throat J39.2
    - septic J02.0
  - thromboembolic — *see* Embolism
  - thymus (gland) E32.9
    - specified NEC E32.8
  - thyroid (gland) E07.9
    - heart (*see also* Hyperthyroidism)E05.90 *[I43]*
      - with thyroid storm E05.91 *[I43]*
    - specified NEC E07.89
  - Tietze's M94.0
  - tongue K14.9
    - specified NEC K14.8
  - tonsils, tonsillar (and adenoids) J35.9
  - tooth, teeth K08.9
    - hard tissues K03.9
      - specified NEC K03.89
    - pulp NEC K04.99
    - specified NEC K08.89
  - Tourette's F95.2
  - trachea NEC J39.8
  - tricuspid I07.9
    - nonrheumatic I36.9
  - triglyceride-storage E75.5
  - trophoblastic — *see* Mole, hydatidiform
  - tsutsugamushi A75.3
  - tube (fallopian) (noninflammatory) N83.9
    - inflammatory — *see* Salpingitis
    - specified NEC N83.8
  - tuberculous NEC — *see* Tuberculosis
  - tubo-ovarian (noninflammatory) N83.9
    - inflammatory — *see* Salpingo-oophoritis
    - specified NEC N83.8
  - tubotympanic, chronic — *see* Otitis, media, suppurative, chronic, tubotympanic
  - tubulo-interstitial N15.9
    - specified NEC N15.8
  - tympanum — *see* Disorder, tympanic membrane
  - Uhl's Q24.8
  - Underwood's (sclerema neonatorum) P83.0
  - Unverricht (-Lundborg) — *see* Epilepsy, generalized, idiopathic
  - Urbach-Oppenheim (necrobiosis lipoidica diabeticorum) — *see* E08-E13 with .620
  - ureter N28.9
    - in (due to)
      - schistosomiasis (bilharziasis) B65.0 *[N29]*
  - urethra N36.9
    - specified NEC N36.8
  - urinary (tract) N39.9
    - bladder N32.9
      - specified NEC N32.89
    - specified NEC N39.8
  - uterus (noninflammatory) N85.9
    - infective — *see* Endometritis
    - inflammatory — *see* Endometritis
    - specified NEC N85.8
  - uveal tract (anterior) H21.9
    - posterior H31.9
  - vagabond's B85.1
  - vagina, vaginal (noninflammatory) N89.9
    - inflammatory NEC N76.89
    - specified NEC N89.8
  - valve, valvular I38
    - multiple I08.9
      - specified NEC I08.8
  - van Creveld-von Gierke (glycogenosis I) E74.01
  - vas deferens N50.9
  - vascular I99.9
    - arteriosclerotic — *see* Arteriosclerosis
    - ciliary body NEC — *see* Disorder, iris, vascular

- Disease — *continued*
  - vascular — *continued*
    - hypertensive — *see* Hypertension
    - iris NEC — *see* Disorder, iris, vascular
    - obliterative I77.1
      - peripheral I73.9
    - occlusive I99.8
    - peripheral (occlusive) I73.9
      - in diabetes mellitus — *see* E08-E13 with .51
  - vasomotor I73.9
  - vasospastic I73.9
  - vein I87.9
  - venereal (*see also* Disease, sexually transmitted)A64
    - chlamydial NEC A56.8
      - anus A56.3
      - genitourinary NOS A56.2
      - pharynx A56.4
      - rectum A56.3
    - fifth A55
    - sixth A55
    - specified nature or type NEC A63.8
  - vertebra, vertebral (*see also* Spondylopathy)
    - disc — *see* Disorder, disc
  - vibration — *see* Vibration, adverse effects
  - viral, virus (*see also* Disease, by type of virus)B34.9
    - arbovirus NOS A94
    - arthropod-borne NOS A94
    - congenital P35.9
      - specified NEC P35.8
    - Hanta (with renal manifestations) (Dobrava) (Puumala) (Seoul) A98.5
      - with pulmonary manifestations (Andes) (Bayou) (Bermejo) (Black Creek Canal) (Choclo) (Juquitiba) (Laguna negra) (Lechiguanas) (New York) (Oran) (Sin nombre) B33.4
    - Hantaan (Korean hemorrhagic fever) A98.5
    - human immunodeficiency (HIV) B20
    - Kunjin A83.4
    - nonarthropod-borne NOS B34.9
    - Powassan A84.8
    - Rocio (encephalitis) A83.6
    - Sin nombre (Hantavirus) (cardio)-pulmonary syndrome) B33.4
    - Tahyna B33.8
    - vesicular stomatitis A93.8
  - vitreous H43.9
    - specified NEC H43.89
  - vocal cord J38.3
  - Volkmann's, acquired T79.6 ☑
  - von Eulenburg's (congenital paramyotonia) G71.19
  - von Gierke's (glycogenosis I) E74.01
  - von Graefe's — *see* Strabismus, paralytic, ophthalmoplegia, progressive
  - von Willebrand (-Jürgens) (angiohemophilia) D68.0
  - Vrolik's (osteogenesis imperfecta) Q78.0
  - vulva (noninflammatory) N90.9
    - inflammatory NEC N76.89
    - specified NEC N90.89
  - Wallgren's (obstruction of splenic vein with collateral circulation) I87.8
  - Wassilieff's (leptospiral jaundice) A27.0
  - wasting NEC R64
    - due to malnutrition E41
  - Waterhouse-Friderichsen A39.1
  - Wegner's (syphilitic osteochondritis) A50.02
  - Weil's (leptospiral jaundice of lung) A27.0
  - Weir Mitchell's (erythromelalgia) I73.81
  - Werdnig-Hoffmann G12.0
  - Wermer's E31.21
  - Werner-His (trench fever) A79.0
  - Werner-Schultz (neutropenic splenomegaly) D73.81
  - Wernicke-Posadas B38.9
  - whipworm B79
  - white blood cells D72.9
    - specified NEC D72.89
  - white matter R90.82
  - white-spot, meaning lichen sclerosus et atrophicus L90.0
    - penis N48.0
    - vulva N90.4
  - Wilkie's K55.1
  - Wilkinson-Sneddon (subcorneal pustular dermatosis) L13.1
  - Willis' — *see* Diabetes
  - Wilson's (hepatolenticular degeneration) E83.01
  - woolsorter's A22.1
  - yaba monkey tumor B08.72

- **Disease** — *continued*
  - yaba pox (virus) B08.72
  - Zika virus A92.5
  - zoonotic, bacterial A28.9
    - specified type NEC A28.8
- **Disfigurement** (due to scar) L90.5
- **Disgerminoma** — *see* Dysgerminoma
- **DISH** (diffuse idiopathic skeletal hyperostosis) — *see* Hyperostosis, ankylosing
- **Disinsertion,** retina — *see* Detachment, retina
- **Dislocatable** hip, congenital Q65.6
- **Dislocation** (articular)
  - with fracture — *see* Fracture
  - acromioclavicular (joint) S43.10 ☑
    - with displacement
      - 100%-200% S43.12 ☑
      - more than 200% S43.13 ☑
    - inferior S43.14 ☑
    - posterior S43.15 ☑
  - ankle S93.0 ☑
  - astragalus — *see* Dislocation, ankle
  - atlantoaxial S13.121 ☑
  - atlantooccipital S13.111 ☑
  - atloidooccipital S13.111 ☑
  - breast bone S23.29 ☑
  - capsule, joint - code by site under Dislocation
  - carpal (bone) — *see* Dislocation, wrist
  - carpometacarpal (joint) NEC S63.05 ☑
    - thumb S63.04 ☑
  - cartilage (joint) - code by site under Dislocation
  - cervical spine (vertebra) — *see* Dislocation, vertebra, cervical
  - chronic — *see* Dislocation, recurrent
  - clavicle — *see* Dislocation, acromioclavicular joint
  - coccyx S33.2 ☑
  - congenital NEC Q68.8
  - coracoid — *see* Dislocation, shoulder
  - costal cartilage S23.29 ☑
  - costochondral S23.29 ☑
  - cricoarytenoid articulation S13.29 ☑
  - cricothyroid articulation S13.29 ☑
  - dorsal vertebra — *see* Dislocation, vertebra, thoracic
  - ear ossicle — *see* Discontinuity, ossicles, ear
  - elbow S53.10 ☑
    - congenital Q68.8
    - pathological — *see* Dislocation, pathological NEC, elbow
    - radial head alone — *see* Dislocation, radial head
    - recurrent — *see* Dislocation, recurrent, elbow
    - traumatic S53.10 ☑
      - anterior S53.11 ☑
      - lateral S53.14 ☑
      - medial S53.13 ☑
      - posterior S53.12 ☑
      - specified type NEC S53.19 ☑
  - eye, nontraumatic — *see* Luxation, globe
  - eyeball, nontraumatic — *see* Luxation, globe
  - femur
    - distal end — *see* Dislocation, knee
    - proximal end — *see* Dislocation, hip
  - fibula
    - distal end — *see* Dislocation, ankle
    - proximal end — *see* Dislocation, knee
  - finger S63.25 ☑
    - index S63.25 ☑
    - interphalangeal S63.27 ☑
      - distal S63.29 ☑
        - index S63.29 ☑
        - little S63.29 ☑
        - middle S63.29 ☑
        - ring S63.29 ☑
      - index S63.27 ☑
      - little S63.27 ☑
      - middle S63.27 ☑
      - proximal S63.28 ☑
        - index S63.28 ☑
        - little S63.28 ☑
        - middle S63.28 ☑
        - ring S63.28 ☑
      - ring S63.27 ☑
    - little S63.25 ☑
    - metacarpophalangeal S63.26 ☑
      - index S63.26 ☑
      - little S63.26 ☑
      - middle S63.26 ☑
      - ring S63.26 ☑
    - middle S63.25 ☑
    - recurrent — *see* Dislocation, recurrent, finger
    - ring S63.25 ☑
    - thumb — *see* Dislocation, thumb

- **Dislocation** — *continued*
  - foot S93.30 ☑
    - recurrent — *see* Dislocation, recurrent, foot
    - specified site NEC S93.33 ☑
    - tarsal joint S93.31 ☑
    - tarsometatarsal joint S93.32 ☑
    - toe — *see* Dislocation, toe
  - fracture — *see* Fracture
  - glenohumeral (joint) — *see* Dislocation, shoulder
  - glenoid — *see* Dislocation, shoulder
  - habitual — *see* Dislocation, recurrent
  - hip S73.00 ☑
    - anterior S73.03 ☑
      - obturator S73.02 ☑
    - central S73.04 ☑
    - congenital (total) Q65.2
      - bilateral Q65.1
      - partial Q65.5
        - bilateral Q65.4
        - unilateral Q65.3 ☑
      - unilateral Q65.0 ☑
    - developmental M24.85 ☑
    - pathological — *see* Dislocation, pathological NEC, hip
    - posterior S73.01 ☑
    - recurrent — *see* Dislocation, recurrent, hip
  - humerus, proximal end — *see* Dislocation, shoulder
  - incomplete — *see* Subluxation, by site
  - incus — *see* Discontinuity, ossicles, ear
  - infracoracoid — *see* Dislocation, shoulder
  - innominate (pubic junction) (sacral junction) S33.39 ☑
    - acetabulum — *see* Dislocation, hip
  - interphalangeal (joint (s))
    - finger S63.279 ☑
      - distal S63.29 ☑
        - index S63.29 ☑
        - little S63.29 ☑
        - middle S63.29 ☑
        - ring S63.29 ☑
      - index S63.27 ☑
      - little S63.27 ☑
      - middle S63.27 ☑
      - proximal S63.28 ☑
        - index S63.28 ☑
        - little S63.28 ☑
        - middle S63.28 ☑
        - ring S63.28 ☑
      - ring S63.27 ☑
    - foot or toe — *see* Dislocation, toe
    - thumb S63.12 ☑
      - distal joint S63.14 ☑
      - proximal joint S63.13 ☑
  - jaw (cartilage) (meniscus) S03.0 ☑
  - joint prosthesis — *see* Complications, joint prosthesis, mechanical, displacement, by site
  - knee S83.106 ☑
    - cap — *see* Dislocation, patella
    - congenital Q68.2
    - old M23.8X ☑
    - patella — *see* Dislocation, patella
    - pathological — *see* Dislocation, pathological NEC, knee
    - proximal tibia
      - anteriorly S83.11 ☑
      - laterally S83.14 ☑
      - medially S83.13 ☑
      - posteriorly S83.12 ☑
    - recurrent (*see also* Derangement, knee, specified NEC)
    - specified type NEC S83.19 ☑
  - lacrimal gland H04.16 ☑
  - lens (complete) H27.10
    - anterior H27.12 ☑
    - congenital Q12.1
    - ocular implant — *see* Complications, intraocular lens
    - partial H27.11 ☑
    - posterior H27.13 ☑
    - traumatic S05.8X ☑
  - ligament - code by site under Dislocation
  - lumbar (vertebra) — *see* Dislocation, vertebra, lumbar
  - lumbosacral (vertebra) (*see also* Dislocation, vertebra, lumbar)
    - congenital Q76.49
  - mandible S03.0 ☑
  - meniscus (knee) — *see* Tear, meniscus
    - other sites - code by site under Dislocation
  - metacarpal (bone)
    - distal end — *see* Dislocation, finger
    - proximal end S63.06 ☑

- **Dislocation** — *continued*
  - metacarpophalangeal (joint)
    - finger S63.26 ☑
      - index S63.26 ☑
      - little S63.26 ☑
      - middle S63.26 ☑
      - ring S63.26 ☑
    - thumb S63.11 ☑
  - metatarsal (bone) — *see* Dislocation, foot
  - metatarsophalangeal (joint (s)) — *see* Dislocation, toe
  - midcarpal (joint) S63.03 ☑
  - midtarsal (joint) — *see* Dislocation, foot
  - neck S13.20 ☑
    - specified site NEC S13.29 ☑
    - vertebra — *see* Dislocation, vertebra, cervical
  - nose (septal cartilage) S03.1 ☑
  - occipitoatloid S13.111 ☑
  - old — *see* Derangement, joint, specified type NEC
  - ossicles, ear — *see* Discontinuity, ossicles, ear
  - partial — *see* Subluxation, by site
  - patella S83.006 ☑
    - congenital Q74.1
    - lateral S83.01 ☑
    - recurrent (nontraumatic) M22.0 ☑
      - incomplete M22.1 ☑
    - specified type NEC S83.09 ☑
  - pathological NEC M24.30
    - ankle M24.37 ☑
    - elbow M24.32 ☑
    - foot joint M24.37 ☑
    - hand joint M24.34 ☑
    - hip M24.35 ☑
    - knee M24.36 ☑
    - lumbosacral joint — *see* subcategory M53.2
    - pelvic region — *see* Dislocation, pathological, hip
    - sacroiliac — *see* subcategory M53.2
    - shoulder M24.31 ☑
    - wrist M24.33 ☑
  - pelvis NEC S33.30 ☑
    - specified NEC S33.39 ☑
  - phalanx
    - finger or hand — *see* Dislocation, finger
    - foot or toe — *see* Dislocation, toe
  - prosthesis, internal — *see* Complications, prosthetic device, by site, mechanical
  - radial head S53.006 ☑
    - anterior S53.01 ☑
    - posterior S53.02 ☑
    - specified type NEC S53.09 ☑
  - radiocarpal (joint) S63.02 ☑
  - radiohumeral (joint) — *see* Dislocation, radial head
  - radioulnar (joint)
    - distal S63.01 ☑
    - proximal — *see* Dislocation, elbow
  - radius
    - distal end — *see* Dislocation, wrist
    - proximal end — *see* Dislocation, radial head
  - recurrent M24.40
    - ankle M24.47 ☑
    - elbow M24.42 ☑
    - finger M24.44 ☑
    - foot joint M24.47 ☑
    - hand joint M24.44 ☑
    - hip M24.45 ☑
    - knee M24.46 ☑
      - patella — *see* Dislocation, patella, recurrent
    - patella — *see* Dislocation, patella, recurrent
    - sacroiliac — *see* subcategory M53.2
    - shoulder M24.41 ☑
    - toe M24.47 ☑
    - vertebra (*see also* subcategory)M43.5 ☑
      - atlantoaxial M43.4
        - with myelopathy M43.3
    - wrist M24.43 ☑
  - rib (cartilage) S23.29 ☑
  - sacrococcygeal S33.2 ☑
  - sacroiliac (joint) (ligament) S33.2 ☑
    - congenital Q74.2
    - recurrent — *see* subcategory M53.2
  - sacrum S33.2 ☑
  - scaphoid (bone) (hand) (wrist) — *see* Dislocation, wrist
    - foot — *see* Dislocation, foot
  - scapula — *see* Dislocation, shoulder, girdle, scapula
  - semilunar cartilage, knee — *see* Tear, meniscus
  - septal cartilage (nose) S03.1 ☑
  - septum (nasal) (old) J34.2
  - sesamoid bone - code by site under Dislocation

- **Dislocation** — *continued*
  - shoulder (blade) (ligament) (joint) (traumatic) S43.006 ☑
    - acromioclavicular — *see* Dislocation, acromioclavicular
    - chronic — *see* Dislocation, recurrent, shoulder
    - congenital Q68.8
    - girdle S43.30 ☑
      - scapula S43.31 ☑
      - specified site NEC S43.39 ☑
    - humerus S43.00 ☑
      - anterior S43.01 ☑
      - inferior S43.03 ☑
      - posterior S43.02 ☑
    - pathological — *see* Dislocation, pathological NEC, shoulder
    - recurrent — *see* Dislocation, recurrent, shoulder
    - specified type NEC S43.08 ☑
  - spine
    - cervical — *see* Dislocation, vertebra, cervical
    - congenital Q76.49
    - due to birth trauma P11.5
    - lumbar — *see* Dislocation, vertebra, lumbar
    - thoracic — *see* Dislocation, vertebra, thoracic
  - spontaneous — *see* Dislocation, pathological
  - sternoclavicular (joint) S43.206 ☑
    - anterior S43.21 ☑
    - posterior S43.22 ☑
  - sternum S23.29 ☑
  - subglenoid — *see* Dislocation, shoulder
  - symphysis pubis S33.4 ☑
  - talus — *see* Dislocation, ankle
  - tarsal (bone (s)) (joint (s)) — *see* Dislocation, foot
  - tarsometatarsal (joint (s)) — *see* Dislocation, foot
  - temporomandibular (joint) S03.0 ☑
  - thigh, proximal end — *see* Dislocation, hip
  - thorax S23.20 ☑
    - specified site NEC S23.29 ☑
    - vertebra — *see* Dislocation, vertebra
  - thumb S63.10 ☑
    - interphalangeal joint — *see* Dislocation, interphalangeal (joint), thumb
    - metacarpophalangeal joint — *see* Dislocation, metacarpophalangeal (joint), thumb
  - thyroid cartilage S13.29 ☑
  - tibia
    - distal end — *see* Dislocation, ankle
    - proximal end — *see* Dislocation, knee
  - tibiofibular (joint)
    - distal — *see* Dislocation, ankle
    - superior — *see* Dislocation, knee
  - toe (s) S93.106 ☑
    - great S93.10 ☑
      - interphalangeal joint S93.11 ☑
      - metatarsophalangeal joint S93.12 ☑
    - interphalangeal joint S93.119 ☑
    - lesser S93.106 ☑
      - interphalangeal joint S93.11 ☑
      - metatarsophalangeal joint S93.12 ☑
    - metatarsophalangeal joint S93.12 ☑
  - tooth S03.2 ☑
  - trachea S23.29 ☑
  - ulna
    - distal end S63.07 ☑
    - proximal end — *see* Dislocation, elbow
  - ulnohumeral (joint) — *see* Dislocation, elbow
  - vertebra (articular process) (body) (traumatic)
    - cervical S13.101 ☑
      - atlantoaxial joint S13.121 ☑
      - atlantooccipital joint S13.111 ☑
      - atloidooccipital joint S13.111 ☑
      - joint between
        - C0 and C1 S13.111 ☑
        - C1 and C2 S13.121 ☑
        - C2 and C3 S13.131 ☑
        - C3 and C4 S13.141 ☑
        - C4 and C5 S13.151 ☑
        - C5and C6 S13.161 ☑
        - C6and C7 S13.171 ☑
        - C7and T1 S13.181 ☑
      - occipitoatloid joint S13.111 ☑
    - congenital Q76.49
    - lumbar S33.101 ☑
      - joint between
        - L1and L2 S33.111 ☑
        - L2and L3 S33.121 ☑
        - L3 and L4 S33.131 ☑
        - L4and L5 S33.141 ☑
    - nontraumatic — *see* Displacement, intervertebral disc
    - partial — *see* Subluxation, by site
    - recurrent NEC — *see* subcategory M43.5

- **Dislocation** — *continued*
  - vertebra — *continued*
    - thoracic S23.101 ☑
      - joint between
        - T1 and T2 S23.111 ☑
        - T2 and T3 S23.121 ☑
        - T3 and T4 S23.123 ☑
        - T4 and T5 S23.131 ☑
        - T5 and T6 S23.133 ☑
        - T6 and T7 S23.141 ☑
        - T7 and T8 S23.143 ☑
        - T8 and T9 S23.151 ☑
        - T9 and T10 S23.153 ☑
        - T10 and T11 S23.161 ☑
        - T11 and T12 S23.163 ☑
        - T12 and L1 S23.171 ☑
  - wrist (carpal bone) S63.006 ☑
    - carpometacarpal joint — *see* Dislocation, carpometacarpal (joint)
    - distal radioulnar joint — *see* Dislocation, radioulnar (joint), distal
    - metacarpal bone, proximal — *see* Dislocation, metacarpal (bone), proximal end
    - midcarpal — *see* Dislocation, midcarpal (joint)
    - radiocarpal joint — *see* Dislocation, radiocarpal (joint)
    - recurrent — *see* Dislocation, recurrent, wrist
    - specified site NEC S63.09 ☑
    - ulna — *see* Dislocation, ulna, distal end
  - xiphoid cartilage S23.29 ☑
- **Disorder** (of) (*see also* Disease)
  - acantholytic L11.9
    - specified NEC L11.8
  - acute
    - psychotic — *see* Psychosis, acute
    - stress F43.0
  - adjustment (grief) F43.20
    - with
      - anxiety F43.22
        - with depressed mood F43.23
      - conduct disturbance F43.24
        - with emotional disturbance F43.25
      - depressed mood F43.21
        - with anxiety F43.23
      - other specified symptom F43.29
  - adrenal (capsule) (gland) (medullary) E27.9
    - specified NEC E27.8
  - adrenogenital E25.9
    - drug-induced E25.8
    - iatrogenic E25.8
    - idiopathic E25.8
  - adult personality (and behavior) F69
    - specified NEC F68.8
  - affective (mood) — *see* Disorder, mood
  - aggressive, unsocialized F91.1
  - alcohol-related F10.99
    - with
      - amnestic disorder, persisting F10.96
      - anxiety disorder F10.980
      - dementia, persisting F10.97
      - intoxication F10.929
        - with delirium F10.921
        - uncomplicated F10.920
      - mood disorder F10.94
      - other specified F10.988
      - psychotic disorder F10.959
        - with
          - delusions F10.950
          - hallucinations F10.951
      - sexual dysfunction F10.981
      - sleep disorder F10.982
  - alcohol use
    - mild F10.10
      - with
        - alcohol-induced
          - anxiety disorder F10.180
          - bipolar and related disorder F10.14
          - depressive disorder F10.14
          - psychotic disorder F10.159
          - sexual dysfunction F10.181
          - sleep disorder F10.182
        - alcohol intoxication F10.129
          - delirium F10.121
    - moderate or severe F10.20
      - with
        - alcohol-induced
          - anxiety disorder F10.280
          - bipolar and related disorder F10.24
          - depressive disorder F10.24
          - major neurocognitive disorder, amnestic-confabulatory type F10.26

- **Disorder** — *continued*
  - alcohol use — *continued*
          - major neurocognitive disorder, nonamnestic-confabulatory type F10.27
          - mild neurocognitive disorder F10.288
          - psychotic disorder F10.259
          - sexual dysfunction F10.281
          - sleep disorder F10.282
        - alcohol intoxication F10.229
          - delirium F10.221
  - allergic — *see* Allergy
  - alveolar NEC J84.09
  - amino-acid
    - cystathioninuria E72.19
    - cystinosis E72.04
    - cystinuria E72.01
    - glycinuria E72.09
    - homocystinuria E72.11
    - metabolism — *see* Disturbance, metabolism, amino-acid
      - specified NEC E72.8
    - neonatal, transitory P74.8
    - renal transport NEC E72.09
    - transport NEC E72.09
  - amnesic, amnestic
    - alcohol-induced F10.96
      - with dependence F10.26
    - due to (secondary to) general medical condition F04
    - psychoactive NEC-induced F19.96
      - with
        - abuse F19.16
        - dependence F19.26
    - sedative, hypnotic or anxiolytic-induced F13.96
      - with dependence F13.26
  - amphetamine-type substance use
    - mild F15.10
    - moderate F15.20
    - severe F15.20
  - amphetamine (or other stimulant) use
    - mild
      - with
        - amphetamine (or other stimulant)-induced
          - anxiety disorder F15.180
          - bipolar and related disorder F15.14
          - depressive disorder F15.14
          - obsessive-compulsive and related disorder F15.188
          - psychotic disorder F15.159
          - sexual dysfunction F15.181
        - amphetamine, cocaine, or other stimulant intoxication
          - with perceptual disturbances F15.122
          - without perceptual disturbances F15.129
        - intoxication delirium F15.121
    - moderate or severe
      - with
        - amphetamine (or other stimulant)-induced
          - anxiety disorder F15.280
          - obsessive-compulsive and related disorder F15.288
          - sexual dysfunction F15.281
          - bipolar and related disorder F15.24
          - depressive disorder F15.24
          - psychotic disorder F15.259
        - amphetamine, cocaine, or other stimulant intoxication
          - with perceptual disturbances F15.222
          - without perceptual disturbances F15.229
        - intoxication delirium F15.221
  - anaerobic glycolysis with anemia D55.2
  - anxiety F41.9
    - due to (secondary to)
      - alcohol F10.980
      - amphetamine F15.980
        - in
          - abuse F15.180
          - dependence F15.280
      - anxiolytic F13.980
        - in
          - abuse F13.180
          - dependence F13.280
      - caffeine F15.980
        - in
          - abuse F15.180
          - dependence F15.280
      - cannabis F12.980
        - in
          - abuse F12.180
          - dependence F12.280
      - cocaine F14.980

- **Disorder** — *continued*
  - anxiety — *continued*
        - in
          - abuse F14.180
          - dependence F14.180
      - general medical condition F06.4
      - hallucinogen F16.980
        - in
          - abuse F16.180
          - dependence F16.280
      - hypnotic F13.980
        - in
          - abuse F13.180
          - dependence F13.280
      - inhalant F18.980
        - in
          - abuse F18.180
          - dependence F18.280
      - phencyclidine F16.980
        - in
          - abuse F16.180
          - dependence F16.280
      - psychoactive substance NEC F19.980
        - in
          - abuse F19.180
          - dependence F19.280
      - sedative F13.980
        - in
          - abuse F13.180
          - dependence F13.280
      - volatile solvents F18.980
        - in
          - abuse F18.180
          - dependence F18.280
    - generalized F41.1
    - illness F45.21
    - mixed
      - with depression (mild) F41.8
      - specified NEC F41.3
    - organic F06.4
    - phobic F40.9
      - of childhood F40.8
    - specified NEC F41.8
  - aortic valve — *see* Endocarditis, aortic
  - aromatic amino-acid metabolism E70.9
    - specified NEC E70.8
  - arteriole NEC I77.89
  - artery NEC I77.89
  - articulation — *see* Disorder, joint
  - attachment (childhood)
    - disinhibited F94.2
    - reactive F94.1
  - attention-deficit hyperactivity (adolescent) (adult) (child) F90.9
    - combined type F90.2
    - hyperactive type F90.1
    - inattentive type F90.0
    - specified type NEC F90.8
  - attention-deficit without hyperactivity (adolescent) (adult) (child) F98.8
  - auditory processing (central) H93.25
  - autistic F84.0
  - autism spectrum F84.0
  - autonomic nervous system G90.9
    - specified NEC G90.8
  - avoidant
    - child or adolescent F40.10
    - restrictive food intake F50.89
  - balance
    - acid-base E87.8
      - mixed E87.4
    - electrolyte E87.8
    - fluid NEC E87.8
  - behavioral (disruptive) — *see* Disorder, conduct
  - beta-amino-acid metabolism E72.8
  - bile acid and cholesterol metabolism E78.70
    - Barth syndrome E78.71
    - other specified E78.79
    - Smith-Lemli-Opitz syndrome E78.72
  - bilirubin excretion E80.6
  - binge eating F50.81
  - binocular
    - movement H51.9
      - convergence
        - excess H51.12
        - insufficiency H51.11
      - internuclear ophthalmoplegia — *see* Ophthalmoplegia, internuclear
      - palsy of conjugate gaze H51.0
      - specified type NEC H51.8
    - vision NEC — *see* Disorder, vision, binocular

- **Disorder** — *continued*
  - bipolar (I) F31.9
    - current episode
      - depressed F31.9
        - with psychotic features F31.5
        - without psychotic features F31.30
          - mild F31.31
          - moderate F31.32
          - severe (without psychotic features) F31.4
            - with psychotic features F31.5
      - hypomanic F31.0
      - manic F31.9
        - with psychotic features F31.2
        - without psychotic features F31.10
          - mild F31.11
          - moderate F31.12
          - severe (without psychotic features) F31.13
            - with psychotic features F31.2
      - mixed F31.60
        - mild F31.61
        - moderate F31.62
        - severe (without psychotic features) F31.63
          - with psychotic features F31.64
      - severe depression (without psychotic features) F31.4
        - with psychotic features F31.5
    - in remission (currently) F31.70
      - in full remission
        - most recent episode
          - depressed F31.76
          - hypomanic F31.72
          - manic F31.74
          - mixed F31.78
      - in partial remission
        - most recent episode
          - depressed F31.75
          - hypomanic F31.71
          - manic F31.73
          - mixed F31.77
    - specified NEC F31.89
    - II F31.81
    - organic F06.30
    - single manic episode F30.9
      - mild F30.11
      - moderate F30.12
      - severe (without psychotic symptoms) F30.13
        - with psychotic symptoms F30.2
  - bladder N32.9
    - functional NEC N31.9
    - in schistosomiasis B65.0 *[N33]*
    - specified NEC N32.89
  - bleeding D68.9
  - blood D75.9
    - in congenital early syphilis A50.09 *[D77]*
  - body dysmorphic F45.22
  - bone M89.9
    - continuity M84.9
      - specified type NEC M84.80
        - ankle M84.87 ☑
        - fibula M84.86 ☑
        - foot M84.87 ☑
        - hand M84.84 ☑
        - humerus M84.82 ☑
        - neck M84.88
        - pelvis M84.859
        - radius M84.83 ☑
        - rib M84.88
        - shoulder M84.81 ☑
        - skull M84.88
        - thigh M84.85 ☑
        - tibia M84.86 ☑
        - ulna M84.83 ☑
        - vertebra M84.88
    - density and structure M85.9
      - cyst (*see also* Cyst, bone, specified type NEC)
        - aneurysmal — *see* Cyst, bone, aneurysmal
        - solitary — *see* Cyst, bone, solitary
      - diffuse idiopathic skeletal hyperostosis — *see* Hyperostosis, ankylosing
      - fibrous dysplasia (monostotic) — *see* Dysplasia, fibrous, bone
      - fluorosis — *see* Fluorosis, skeletal
      - hyperostosis of skull M85.2
      - osteitis condensans — *see* Osteitis, condensans
      - specified type NEC M85.8 ☑
        - ankle M85.87 ☑
        - foot M85.87 ☑
        - forearm M85.83 ☑
        - hand M85.84 ☑
        - lower leg M85.86 ☑

- **Disorder** — *continued*
  - bone — *continued*
        - multiple sites M85.89
        - neck M85.88
        - rib M85.88
        - shoulder M85.81 ☑
        - skull M85.88
        - thigh M85.85 ☑
        - upper arm M85.82 ☑
        - vertebra M85.88
    - development and growth NEC M89.20
      - carpus M89.24 ☑
      - clavicle M89.21 ☑
      - femur M89.25 ☑
      - fibula M89.26 ☑
      - finger M89.24 ☑
      - humerus M89.22 ☑
      - ilium M89.259
      - ischium M89.259
      - metacarpus M89.24 ☑
      - metatarsus M89.27 ☑
      - multiple sites M89.29
      - neck M89.28
      - radius M89.23 ☑
      - rib M89.28
      - scapula M89.21 ☑
      - skull M89.28
      - tarsus M89.27 ☑
      - tibia M89.26 ☑
      - toe M89.27 ☑
      - ulna M89.23 ☑
      - vertebra M89.28
    - specified type NEC M89.8X ☑
  - brachial plexus G54.0
  - branched-chain amino-acid metabolism E71.2
    - specified NEC E71.19
  - breast N64.9
    - agalactia — *see* Agalactia
    - associated with
      - lactation O92.70
        - specified NEC O92.79
      - pregnancy O92.20
        - specified NEC O92.29
      - puerperium O92.20
        - specified NEC O92.29
    - cracked nipple — *see* Cracked nipple
    - galactorrhea — *see* Galactorrhea
    - hypogalactia O92.4
    - lactation disorder NEC O92.79
    - mastitis — *see* Mastitis
    - nipple infection — *see* Infection, nipple
    - retracted nipple — *see* Retraction, nipple
    - specified type NEC N64.89
  - Briquet's F45.0
  - bullous, in diseases classified elsewhere L14
  - caffeine use
    - mild
      - with
        - caffeine-induced
          - anxiety disorder F15.180
          - sleep disorder F15.182
    - moderate or severe
      - with
        - caffeine-induced
          - anxiety disorder F15.280
          - sleep disorder F15.282
  - cannabis use
    - mild F12.10
      - with
        - cannabis-induced
          - anxiety disorder F12.180
          - psychotic disorder F12.159
          - sleep disorder F12.188
        - cannabis intoxication delirium F12.121
          - with perceptual disturbances F12.122
          - without perceptual disturbances F12.129
    - moderate or severe F12.20
      - with
        - cannabis-induced
          - anxiety disorder F12.280
          - psychotic disorder F12.259
          - sleep disorder F12.288
        - cannabis intoxication
          - with perceptual disturbances F12.222
          - without perceptual disturbances F12.229
        - delirium F12.221
  - carbohydrate
    - absorption, intestinal NEC E74.39
    - metabolism (congenital) E74.9
      - specified NEC E74.8
  - cardiac, functional I51.89
  - carnitine metabolism E71.40

Disorder — *continued*
- cartilage M94.9
  - articular NEC — *see* Derangement, joint, articular cartilage
    - chondrocalcinosis — *see* Chondrocalcinosis
  - specified type NEC M94.8X ☑
    - articular — *see* Derangement, joint, articular cartilage
    - multiple sites M94.8X0
- catatonia (due to known physiological condition) (with another mental disorder) F06.1
- catatonic
  - due to (secondary to) known physiological condition F06.1
  - organic F06.1
- central auditory processing H93.25
- cervical
  - region NEC M53.82
  - root (nerve) NEC G54.2
- character NOS F60.9
- childhood disintegrative NEC F84.3
- cholesterol and bile acid metabolism E78.70
  - Barth syndrome E78.71
  - other specified E78.79
  - Smith-Lemli-Opitz syndrome E78.72
- choroid H31.9
  - atrophy — *see* Atrophy, choroid
  - degeneration — *see* Degeneration, choroid
  - detachment — *see* Detachment, choroid
  - dystrophy — *see* Dystrophy, choroid
  - hemorrhage — *see* Hemorrhage, choroid
  - rupture — *see* Rupture, choroid
  - scar — *see* Scar, chorioretinal
  - solar retinopathy — *see* Retinopathy, solar
  - specified type NEC H31.8
- ciliary body — *see* Disorder, iris
  - degeneration — *see* Degeneration, ciliary body
- coagulation (factor) (*see also* Defect, coagulation)D68.9
  - newborn, transient P61.6
- cocaine use
  - mild F14.10
    - with
      - amphetamine, cocaine, or other stimulant intoxication
        - with perceptual disturbances F14.122
        - without perceptual disturbances F14.129
      - cocaine-induced
        - anxiety disorder F14.180
        - bipolar and related disorder F14.14
        - depressive disorder F14.14
        - obsessive-compulsive and related disorder F14.188
        - psychotic disorder F14.159
        - sexual dysfunction F14.181
        - sleep disorder F14.182
      - cocaine intoxication delirium F14.121
  - moderate or severe F14.20
    - with
      - amphetamine, cocaine, or other stimulant intoxication
        - with perceptual disturbances F14.222
        - without perceptual disturbances F14.229
      - cocaine-induced
        - anxiety disorder F14.280
        - bipolar and related disorder F14.24
        - depressive disorder F14.24
        - obsessive-compulsive and related disorder F14.288
        - psychotic disorder F14.259
        - sexual dysfunction F14.281
        - sleep disorder F14.282
      - cocaine intoxication delirium F14.221
- coccyx NEC M53.3
- cognitive F09
  - due to (secondary to) general medical condition F09
  - persisting R41.89
    - due to
      - alcohol F10.97
        - with dependence F10.27
      - anxiolytics F13.97
        - with dependence F13.27
      - hypnotics F13.97
        - with dependence F13.27
      - sedatives F13.97
        - with dependence F13.27
      - specified substance NEC F19.97
        - with
          - abuse F19.17
          - dependence F19.27

Disorder — *continued*
- communication F80.9
  - social pragmatic F80.82
- conduct (childhood) F91.9
  - adjustment reaction — *see* Disorder, adjustment
  - adolescent onset type F91.2
  - childhood onset type F91.1
  - compulsive F63.9
  - confined to family context F91.0
  - depressive F91.8
  - group type F91.2
  - hyperkinetic — *see* Disorder, attention-deficit hyperactivity
  - oppositional defiance F91.3
  - socialized F91.2
  - solitary aggressive type F91.1
  - specified NEC F91.8
  - unsocialized (aggressive) F91.1
- conduction, heart I45.9
- congenital glycosylation (CDG) E74.8
- conjunctiva H11.9
  - infection — *see* Conjunctivitis
- connective tissue, localized L94.9
  - specified NEC L94.8
- conversion (functional neurological symptom disorder)
  - with
    - abnormal movement F44.4
    - anesthesia or sensory loss F44.6
    - attacks or seizures F44.5
    - mixed symptoms F44.7
    - special sensory symptoms F44.6
    - speech symptoms F44.4
    - swallowing symptoms F44.4
    - weakness or paralysis F44.4
- convulsive (secondary) — *see* Convulsions
- cornea H18.9
  - deformity — *see* Deformity, cornea
  - degeneration — *see* Degeneration, cornea
  - deposits — *see* Deposit, cornea
  - due to contact lens H18.82 ☑
    - specified as edema — *see* Edema, cornea
  - edema — *see* Edema, cornea
  - keratitis — *see* Keratitis
  - keratoconjunctivitis — *see* Keratoconjunctivitis
  - membrane change — *see* Change, corneal membrane
  - neovascularization — *see* Neovascularization, cornea
  - scar — *see* Opacity, cornea
  - specified type NEC H18.89 ☑
  - ulcer — *see* Ulcer, cornea
- corpus cavernosum N48.9
- cranial nerve — *see* Disorder, nerve, cranial
- cyclothymic F34.0
- defiant oppositional F91.3
- delusional (persistent) (systematized) F22
  - induced F24
- depersonalization F48.1
- depressive F32.9
  - major F32.9
    - with psychotic symptoms F32.3
    - in remission (full) F32.5
      - partial F32.4
    - recurrent F33.9
    - single episode F32.9
      - mild F32.0
      - moderate F32.1
      - severe (without psychotic symptoms) F32.2
        - with psychotic symptoms F32.3
  - organic F06.31
  - persistent F34.1
  - recurrent F33.9
    - current episode
      - mild F33.0
      - moderate F33.1
      - severe (without psychotic symptoms) F33.2
        - with psychotic symptoms F33.3
    - in remission F33.40
      - full F33.42
      - partial F33.41
    - specified NEC F33.8
  - single episode — *see* Episode, depressive
  - specified NEC F32.89
- developmental F89
  - arithmetical skills F81.2
  - coordination (motor) F82
  - expressive writing F81.81
  - language F80.9
    - expressive F80.1
    - mixed receptive and expressive F80.2

Disorder — *continued*
- developmental — *continued*
    - receptive type F80.2
    - specified NEC F80.89
  - learning F81.9
    - arithmetical F81.2
    - reading F81.0
  - mixed F88
  - motor coordination or function F82
  - pervasive F84.9
    - specified NEC F84.8
  - phonological F80.0
  - reading F81.0
  - scholastic skills (*see also* Disorder, learning)
    - mixed F81.89
  - specified NEC F88
  - speech F80.9
    - articulation F80.0
    - specified NEC F80.89
  - written expression F81.81
- diaphragm J98.6
- digestive (system) K92.9
  - newborn P78.9
    - specified NEC P78.89
  - postprocedural — *see* Complication, gastrointestinal
  - psychogenic F45.8
- disc (intervertebral) M51.9
  - with
    - myelopathy
      - cervical region M50.00
      - cervicothoracic region M50.03
      - high cervical region M50.01
      - lumbar region M51.06
      - mid-cervical region M50.020
      - sacrococcygeal region M53.3
      - thoracic region M51.04
      - thoracolumbar region M51.05
    - radiculopathy
      - cervical region M50.10
      - cervicothoracic region M50.13
      - high cervical region M50.11
      - lumbar region M51.16
      - lumbosacral region M51.17
      - mid-cervical region M50.120
      - sacrococcygeal region M53.3
      - thoracic region M51.14
      - thoracolumbar region M51.15
  - cervical M50.90
    - with
      - myelopathy M50.00
        - C2-C3 M50.01
        - C3-C4 M50.01
        - C4-C5 M50.021
        - C5-C6 M50.022
        - C6-C7 M50.023
        - C7-T1 M50.03
        - cervicothoracic region M50.03
        - high cervical region M50.01
        - mid-cervical region M50.020
      - neuritis, radiculitis or radiculopathy M50.10
        - C2-C3 M50.11
        - C3-C4 M50.11
        - C4-C5 M50.121
        - C5-C6 M50.122
        - C6-C7 M50.123
        - C7-T1 M50.13
        - cervicothoracic region M50.13
        - high cervical region M50.11
        - mid-cervical region M50.120
    - C2-C3 M50.91
    - C3-C4 M50.91
    - C4-C5 M50.921
    - C5-C6 M50.922
    - C6-C7 M50.923
    - C7-T1 M50.93
    - cervicothoracic region M50.93
    - degeneration M50.30
      - C2-C3 M50.31
      - C3-C4 M50.31
      - C4-C5 M50.321
      - C5-C6 M50.322
      - C6-C7 M50.323
      - C7-T1 M50.33
      - cervicothoracic region M50.33
      - high cervical region M50.31
      - mid-cervical region M50.320
    - displacement M50.20
      - C2-C3 M50.21
      - C3-C4 M50.21
      - C4-C5 M50.221
      - C5-C6 M50.222

Disorder — *continued*
digestive — *continued*
C6-C7 M50.223
C7-T1 M50.23
cervicothoracic region M50.23
high cervical region M50.21
mid-cervical region M50.220
high cervical region M50.91
mid-cervical region M50.920
specified type NEC M50.80
C2-C3 M50.81
C3-C4 M50.81
C4-C5 M50.821
C5-C6 M50.822
C6-C7 M50.823
C7-T1 M50.83
cervicothoracic region M50.83
high cervical region M50.81
mid-cervical region M50.820
specified NEC
lumbar region M51.86
lumbosacral region M51.87
sacrococcygeal region M53.3
thoracic region M51.84
thoracolumbar region M51.85
disinhibited attachment (childhood) F94.2
disintegrative, childhood NEC F84.3
disruptive F91.9
mood dysregulation F34.81
specified NEC F91.8
disruptive behavior F91.9
dissocial personality F60.2
dissociative F44.9
affecting
motor function F44.4
and sensation F44.7
sensation F44.6
and motor function F44.7
brief reactive F43.0
due to (secondary to) general medical condition F06.8
mixed F44.7
organic F06.8
other specified NEC F44.89
double heterozygous sickling — *see* Disease, sickle-cell
dream anxiety F51.5
drug induced hemorrhagic D68.32
drug related F19.99
abuse — *see* Abuse, drug
dependence — *see* Dependence, drug
dysmorphic body F45.22
dysthymic F34.1
ear H93.9 ☑
bleeding — *see* Otorrhagia
deafness — *see* Deafness
degenerative H93.09 ☑
discharge — *see* Otorrhea
external H61.9 ☑
auditory canal stenosis — *see* Stenosis, external ear canal
exostosis — *see* Exostosis, external ear canal
impacted cerumen — *see* Impaction, cerumen
otitis — *see* Otitis, externa
perichondritis — *see* Perichondritis, ear
pinna — *see* Disorder, pinna
specified type NEC H61.89 ☑
in diseases classified elsewhere H62.8X ☑
inner H83.9 ☑
vestibular dysfunction — *see* Disorder, vestibular function
middle H74.9 ☑
adhesive H74.1 ☑
ossicle — *see* Abnormal, ear ossicles
polyp — *see* Polyp, ear (middle)
specified NEC, in diseases classified elsewhere H75.8 ☑
postprocedural — *see* Complications, ear, procedure
specified NEC, in diseases classified elsewhere H94.8 ☑
eating (adult) (psychogenic) F50.9
anorexia — *see* Anorexia
binge F50.81
bulimia F50.2
child F98.29
pica F98.3
rumination disorder F98.21
pica F50.89
childhood F98.3

Disorder — *continued*
electrolyte (balance) NEC E87.8
with
abortion — *see* Abortion by type complicated by specified condition NEC
ectopic pregnancy O08.5
molar pregnancy O08.5
acidosis (metabolic) (respiratory) E87.2
alkalosis (metabolic) (respiratory) E87.3
elimination, transepidermal L87.9
specified NEC L87.8
emotional (persistent) F34.9
of childhood F93.9
specified NEC F93.8
endocrine E34.9
postprocedural E89.89
specified NEC E89.89
erectile (male) (organic) (*see also* Dysfunction, sexual, male, erectile)N52.9
nonorganic F52.21
erythematous — *see* Erythema
esophagus K22.9
functional K22.4
psychogenic F45.8
eustachian tube H69.9 ☑
infection — *see* Salpingitis, eustachian
obstruction — *see* Obstruction, eustachian tube
patulous — *see* Patulous, eustachian tube
specified NEC H69.8 ☑
extrapyramidal G25.9
in diseases classified elsewhere G26
specified type NEC G25.89
eye H57.9
postprocedural — *see* Complication, postprocedural, eye
eyelid H02.9
cyst — *see* Cyst, eyelid
degenerative H02.70
chloasma — *see* Chloasma, eyelid
madarosis — *see* Madarosis
specified type NEC H02.79
vitiligo — *see* Vitiligo, eyelid
xanthelasma — *see* Xanthelasma
dermatochalasis — *see* Dermatochalasis
edema — *see* Edema, eyelid
elephantiasis — *see* Elephantiasis, eyelid
foreign body, retained — *see* Foreign body, retained, eyelid
function H02.59
abnormal innervation syndrome — *see* Syndrome, abnormal innervation
blepharochalasis — *see* Blepharochalasis
blepharoclonus — *see* Blepharoclonus
blepharophimosis — *see* Blepharophimosis
blepharoptosis — *see* Blepharoptosis
lagophthalmos — *see* Lagophthalmos
lid retraction — *see* Retraction, lid
hypertrichosis — *see* Hypertrichosis, eyelid
specified type NEC H02.89
vascular H02.879
left H02.876
lower H02.875
upper H02.874
right H02.873
lower H02.872
upper H02.871
factitious F68.10
with predominantly
psychological symptoms F68.11
with physical symptoms F68.13
physical symptoms F68.12
with psychological symptoms F68.13
factor, coagulation — *see* Defect, coagulation
fatty acid
metabolism E71.30
specified NEC E71.39
oxidation
LCAD E71.310
MCAD E71.311
SCAD E71.312
specified deficiency NEC E71.318
feeding (infant or child) (*see also* Disorder, eating)R63.3
feigned (with obvious motivation) Z76.5
without obvious motivation — *see* Disorder, factitious
female
hypoactive sexual desire F52.0
orgasmic F52.31
sexual arousal F52.22

Disorder — *continued*
fibroblastic M72.9
specified NEC M72.8
fluency
adult onset F98.5
childhood onset F80.81
following
cerebral infarction I69.323
cerebrovascular disease I69.923
specified disease NEC I69.823
intracerebral hemorrhage I69.123
nontraumatic intracranial hemorrhage NEC I69.223
subarachnoid hemorrhage I69.023
in conditions classified elsewhere R47.82
fluid balance E87.8
follicular (skin) L73.9
specified NEC L73.8
fructose metabolism E74.10
essential fructosuria E74.11
fructokinase deficiency E74.11
fructose-1, 6-diphosphatase deficiency E74.19
hereditary fructose intolerance E74.12
other specified E74.19
functional polymorphonuclear neutrophils D71
gallbladder, biliary tract and pancreas in diseases classified elsewhere K87
gamma-glutamyl cycle E72.8
gastric (functional) K31.9
motility K30
psychogenic F45.8
secretion K30
gastrointestinal (functional) NOS K92.9
newborn P78.9
psychogenic F45.8
gender-identity or -role F64.9
childhood F64.2
effect on relationship F66
of adolescence or adulthood F64.0
nontranssexual F64.8
specified NEC F64.8
uncertainty F66
genito-pelvic pain penetration F52.6
genitourinary system
female N94.9
male N50.9
psychogenic F45.8
globe H44.9
degenerated condition H44.50
absolute glaucoma H44.51 ☑
atrophy H44.52 ☑
leucocoria H44.53 ☑
degenerative H44.30
chalcosis H44.31 ☑
myopia H44.2 ☑
siderosis H44.32 ☑
specified type NEC H44.39 ☑
endophthalmitis — *see* Endophthalmitis
foreign body, retained — *see* Foreign body, intraocular, old, retained
hemophthalmos — *see* Hemophthalmos
hypotony H44.40
due to
ocular fistula H44.42 ☑
specified disorder NEC H44.43 ☑
flat anterior chamber H44.41 ☑
primary H44.44 ☑
luxation — *see* Luxation, globe
specified type NEC H44.89
glomerular (in) N05.9
amyloidosis E85.4 *[N08]*
cryoglobulinemia D89.1 *[N08]*
disseminated intravascular coagulation D65 *[N08]*
Fabry's disease E75.21 *[N08]*
familial lecithin cholesterol acyltransferase deficiency E78.6 *[N08]*
Goodpasture's syndrome M31.0
hemolytic-uremic syndrome D59.3
Henoch (-Schönlein) purpura D69.0 *[N08]*
malariae malaria B52.0
microscopic polyangiitis M31.7 *[N08]*
multiple myeloma C90.0 ☑ *[N08]*
mumps B26.83
schistosomiasis B65.9 *[N08]*
sepsis NEC A41. ☑ *[N08]*
streptococcal A40. ☑ *[N08]*
sickle-cell disorders D57. ☑ *[N08]*
strongyloidiasis B78.9 *[N08]*
subacute bacterial endocarditis I33.0 *[N08]*
syphilis A52.75
systemic lupus erythematosus M32.14

Disorder — *continued*
- glomerular — *continued*
  - thrombotic thrombocytopenic purpura M31.1 *[N08]*
  - Waldenström macroglobulinemia C88.0 *[N08]*
  - Wegener's granulomatosis M31.31
- gluconeogenesis E74.4
- glucosaminoglycan metabolism — *see* Disorder, metabolism, glucosaminoglycan
- glycine metabolism E72.50
  - d-glycericacidemia E72.59
  - hyperhydroxyprolinemia E72.59
  - hyperoxaluria E72.53
  - hyperprolinemia E72.59
  - non-ketotic hyperglycinemia E72.51
  - oxalosis E72.53
  - oxaluria E72.53
  - sarcosinemia E72.59
  - trimethylaminuria E72.52
- glycoprotein metabolism E77.9
  - specified NEC E77.8
- habit (and impulse) F63.9
  - involving sexual behavior NEC F65.9
  - specified NEC F63.89
- hallucinogen use
  - mild F16.10
    - with
      - hallucinogen-induced
        - anxiety disorder F16.180
        - bipolar and related disorder F16.14
        - depressive disorder F16.14
        - psychotic disorder F16.159
      - hallucinogen intoxication delirium F16.121
      - other hallucinogen intoxication F16.129
  - moderate or severe F16.20
    - with
      - hallucinogen-induced
        - anxiety disorder F16.280
        - bipolar and related disorder F16.24
        - depressive disorder F16.24
        - psychotic disorder F16.259
      - hallucinogen intoxication delirium F16.221
      - other hallucinogen intoxication F16.229
- heart action I49.9
- hematological D75.9
  - newborn (transient) P61.9
    - specified NEC P61.8
- hematopoietic organs D75.9
- hemorrhagic NEC D69.9
  - drug-induced D68.32
  - due to
    - extrinsic circulating anticoagulants D68.32
    - increase in
      - anti-IIa D68.32
      - anti-Xa D68.32
    - intrinsic
      - circulating anticoagulants D68.318
      - increase in
        - antithrombin D68.318
        - anti-VIIIa D68.318
        - anti-IXa D68.318
        - anti-XIa D68.318
  - following childbirth O72.3
- hemostasis — *see* Defect, coagulation
- histidine metabolism E70.40
  - histidinemia E70.41
  - other specified E70.49
- hoarding F42.3
- hyperkinetic — *see* Disorder, attention-deficit hyperactivity
- hyperleucine-isoleucinemia E71.19
- hypervalinemia E71.19
- hypoactive sexual desire F52.0
- hypochondriacal F45.20
  - body dysmorphic F45.22
  - neurosis F45.21
  - other specified F45.29
- identity
  - dissociative F44.81
  - of childhood F93.8
  - illness anxiety F45.21
- immune mechanism (immunity) D89.9
  - specified type NEC D89.89
- impaired renal tubular function N25.9
  - specified NEC N25.89
- impulse (control) F63.9
- inflammatory
  - pelvic, in diseases classified elsewhere N74
  - penis N48.29
    - abscess N48.21
    - cellulitis N48.22

Disorder — *continued*
- inhalant use
  - mild F18.10
    - with
      - inhalant-induced
        - anxiety disorder F18.180
        - depressive disorder F18.14
        - major neurocognitive disorder F18.17
        - mild neurocognitive disorder F18.188
        - psychotic disorder F18.159
      - inhalant intoxication F18.129
      - inhalant intoxication delirium F18.121
  - moderate or severe F18.20
    - with
      - inhalant-induced
        - anxiety disorder F18.280
        - depressive disorder F18.24
        - major neurocognitive disorder F18.27
        - mild neurocognitive disorder F18.288
        - psychotic disorder F18.259
      - inhalant intoxication F18.229
      - inhalant intoxication delirium F18.221
- integument, newborn P83.9
  - specified NEC P83.8
- intermittent explosive F63.81
- internal secretion pancreas — *see* Increased, secretion, pancreas, endocrine
- intestine, intestinal
  - carbohydrate absorption NEC E74.39
    - postoperative K91.2
  - functional NEC K59.9
    - postoperative K91.89
  - psychogenic F45.8
  - vascular K55.9
    - chronic K55.1
    - specified NEC K55.8
- intraoperative (intraprocedural) — *see* Complications, intraoperative
- involuntary emotional expression (IEED) F48.2
- iris H21.9
  - adhesions — *see* Adhesions, iris
  - atrophy — *see* Atrophy, iris
  - chamber angle recession — *see* Recession, chamber angle
  - cyst — *see* Cyst, iris
  - degeneration — *see* Degeneration, iris
  - in diseases classified elsewhere H22
  - iridodialysis — *see* Iridodialysis
  - iridoschisis — *see* Iridoschisis
  - miotic pupillary cyst — *see* Cyst, pupillary
  - pupillary
    - abnormality — *see* Abnormality, pupillary
    - membrane — *see* Membrane, pupillary
  - specified type NEC H21.89
  - vascular NEC H21.1X ☑
- iron metabolism E83.10
  - specified NEC E83.19
- isovaleric acidemia E71.110
- jaw, developmental M27.0
  - temporomandibular (*see also* Anomaly, dentofacial, temporomandibular joint)M26.60 ☑
- joint M25.9
  - derangement — *see* Derangement, joint
  - effusion — *see* Effusion, joint
  - fistula — *see* Fistula, joint
  - hemarthrosis — *see* Hemarthrosis
  - instability — *see* Instability, joint
  - osteophyte — *see* Osteophyte
  - pain — *see* Pain, joint
  - psychogenic F45.8
  - specified type NEC M25.80
    - ankle M25.87 ☑
    - elbow M25.82 ☑
    - foot joint M25.87 ☑
    - hand joint M25.84 ☑
    - hip M25.85 ☑
    - knee M25.86 ☑
    - shoulder M25.81 ☑
    - wrist M25.83 ☑
  - stiffness — *see* Stiffness, joint
- ketone metabolism E71.32
- kidney N28.9
  - functional (tubular) N25.9
  - in
    - schistosomiasis B65.9 *[N29]*
  - tubular function N25.9
    - specified NEC N25.89
- lacrimal system H04.9
  - changes H04.69
    - fistula — *see* Fistula, lacrimal
  - gland H04.19

Disorder — *continued*
- lacrimal system — *continued*
    - atrophy — *see* Atrophy, lacrimal gland
    - cyst — *see* Cyst, lacrimal, gland
    - dacryops — *see* Dacryops
    - dislocation — *see* Dislocation, lacrimal gland
    - dry eye syndrome — *see* Syndrome, dry eye
    - infection — *see* Dacryoadenitis
  - granuloma — *see* Granuloma, lacrimal
  - inflammation — *see* Inflammation, lacrimal
  - obstruction — *see* Obstruction, lacrimal
  - specified NEC H04.89
- lactation NEC O92.79
- language (developmental) F80.9
  - expressive F80.1
  - mixed receptive and expressive F80.2
  - receptive F80.2
- late luteal phase dysphoric N94.89
- learning (specific) F81.9
  - acalculia R48.8
  - alexia R48.0
  - mathematics F81.2
  - reading F81.0
  - specified NEC F81.89
  - spelling F81.81
  - written expression F81.81
- lens H27.9
  - aphakia — *see* Aphakia
  - cataract — *see* Cataract
  - dislocation — *see* Dislocation, lens
  - specified type NEC H27.8
- ligament M24.20
  - ankle M24.27 ☑
  - attachment, spine — *see* Enthesopathy, spinal
  - elbow M24.22 ☑
  - foot joint M24.27 ☑
  - hand joint M24.24 ☑
  - hip M24.25 ☑
  - knee — *see* Derangement, knee, specified NEC
  - shoulder M24.21 ☑
  - vertebra M24.28
  - wrist M24.23 ☑
- ligamentous attachments (*see also* Enthesopathy)
  - spine — *see* Enthesopathy, spinal
- lipid
  - metabolism, congenital E78.9
  - storage E75.6
    - specified NEC E75.5
- lipoprotein
  - deficiency (familial) E78.6
  - metabolism E78.9
    - specified NEC E78.89
- liver K76.9
  - malarial B54 *[K77]*
- low back (*see also* Dorsopathy, specified NEC)
- lumbosacral
  - plexus G54.1
  - root (nerve) NEC G54.4
- lung, interstitial, drug-induced J70.4
  - acute J70.2
  - chronic J70.3
- lymphoproliferative, post-transplant (PTLD) D47.Z1
- lysine and hydroxylysine metabolism E72.3
- major neurocognitive — *see* Dementia, in (due to)
- male
  - erectile (organic) (*see also* Dysfunction, sexual, male, erectile)N52.9
    - nonorganic F52.21
  - hypoactive sexual desire F52.0
  - orgasmic F52.32
- manic F30.9
  - organic F06.33
- mast cell activation — *see* Activation, mast cell
- mastoid (*see also* Disorder, ear, middle)
  - postprocedural — *see* Complications, ear, procedure
- meniscus — *see* Derangement, knee, meniscus
- menopausal N95.9
  - specified NEC N95.8
- menstrual N92.6
  - psychogenic F45.8
  - specified NEC N92.5
- mental (or behavioral) (nonpsychotic) F99
  - due to (secondary to)
    - amphetamine
      - due to drug abuse — *see* Abuse, drug, stimulant
      - due to drug dependence — *see* Dependence, drug, stimulant
    - brain disease, damage and dysfunction F09

- **Disorder** — *continued*
  - mental — *continued*
    - caffeine use
      - due to drug abuse — *see* Abuse, drug, stimulant
      - due to drug dependence — *see* Dependence, drug, stimulant
    - cannabis use
      - due to drug abuse — *see* Abuse, drug, cannabis
      - due to drug dependence — *see* Dependence, drug, cannabis
    - general medical condition F09
    - sedative or hypnotic use
      - due to drug abuse — *see* Abuse, drug, sedative
      - due to drug dependence — *see* Dependence, drug, sedative
    - tobacco (nicotine) use — *see* Dependence, drug, nicotine
  - following organic brain damage F07.9
    - frontal lobe syndrome F07.0
    - personality change F07.0
    - postconcussional syndrome F07.81
    - specified NEC F07.89
  - infancy, childhood or adolescence F98.9
  - neurotic — *see* Neurosis
  - organic or symptomatic F09
  - presenile, psychotic F03 ☑
  - problem NEC
  - psychoneurotic — *see* Neurosis
  - psychotic — *see* Psychosis
  - puerperal F53
  - senile, psychotic NEC F03 ☑
  - metabolic, amino acid, transitory, newborn P74.8
  - metabolism NOS E88.9
    - amino-acid E72.9
      - aromatic E70.9
        - albinism — *see* Albinism
        - histidine E70.40
          - histidinemia E70.41
          - other specified E70.49
        - hyperphenylalaninemia E70.1
          - classical phenylketonuria E70.0
        - other specified E70.8
        - tryptophan E70.5
        - tyrosine E70.20
          - hypertyrosinemia E70.21
          - other specified E70.29
      - branched chain E71.2
        - 3-methylglutaconic aciduria E71.111
        - hyperleucine-isoleucinemia E71.19
        - hypervalinemia E71.19
        - isovaleric acidemia E71.110
        - maple syrup urine disease E71.0
        - methylmalonic acidemia E71.120
        - organic aciduria NEC E71.118
        - other specified E71.19
        - proprionate NEC E71.128
        - proprionic acidemia E71.121
      - glycine E72.50
        - d-glycericacidemia E72.59
        - hyperhydroxyprolinemia E72.59
        - hyperoxaluria E72.53
        - hyperprolinemia E72.59
        - non-ketotic hyperglycinemia E72.51
        - other specified E72.59
        - sarcosinemia E72.59
        - trimethylaminuria E72.52
      - hydroxylysine E72.3
      - lysine E72.3
      - ornithine E72.4
      - other specified E72.8
        - beta-amino acid E72.8
        - gamma-glutamyl cycle E72.8
      - straight-chain E72.8
      - sulfur-bearing E72.10
        - homocystinuria E72.11
        - methylenetetrahydrofolate reductase deficiency E72.12
        - other specified E72.19
    - bile acid and cholesterol metabolism E78.70
    - bilirubin E80.7
      - specified NEC E80.6
    - calcium E83.50
      - hypercalcemia E83.52
      - hypocalcemia E83.51
      - other specified E83.59
    - carbohydrate E74.9
      - specified NEC E74.8
    - cholesterol and bile acid metabolism E78.70
    - congenital E88.9

- **Disorder** — *continued*
  - metabolism — *continued*
    - copper E83.00
      - Wilson's disease E83.01
      - specified type NEC E83.09
    - cystinuria E72.01
    - fructose E74.10
    - galactose E74.20
    - glucosaminoglycan E76.9
      - mucopolysaccharidosis — *see* Mucopolysaccharidosis
      - specified NEC E76.8
    - glutamine E72.8
    - glycine E72.50
    - glycogen storage (hepatorenal) E74.09
    - glycoprotein E77.9
      - specified NEC E77.8
    - glycosaminoglycan E76.9
      - specified NEC E76.8
    - in labor and delivery O75.89
    - iron E83.10
    - isoleucine E71.19
    - leucine E71.19
    - lipoid E78.9
    - lipoprotein E78.9
      - specified NEC E78.89
    - magnesium E83.40
      - hypermagnesemia E83.41
      - hypomagnesemia E83.42
      - other specified E83.49
    - mineral E83.9
      - specified NEC E83.89
    - mitochondrial E88.40
      - MELAS syndrome E88.41
      - MERRF syndrome (myoclonic epilepsy associated with ragged-red fibers) E88.42
      - other specified E88.49
    - ornithine E72.4
    - phosphatases E83.30
    - phosphorus E83.30
      - acid phosphatase deficiency E83.39
      - hypophosphatasia E83.39
      - hypophosphatemia E83.39
        - familial E83.31
      - other specified E83.39
      - pseudovitamin D deficiency E83.32
    - plasma protein NEC E88.09
    - porphyrin — *see* Porphyria
    - postprocedural E89.89
      - specified NEC E89.89
    - purine E79.9
      - specified NEC E79.8
    - pyrimidine E79.9
      - specified NEC E79.8
    - pyruvate E74.4
    - serine E72.8
    - sodium E87.8
    - specified NEC E88.89
    - threonine E72.8
    - valine E71.19
    - zinc E83.2
  - methylmalonic acidemia E71.120
  - micturition NEC (*see also* Difficulty, micturition)R39.198
    - feeling of incomplete emptying R39.14
    - hesitancy R39.11
    - poor stream R39.12
    - psychogenic F45.8
    - split stream R39.13
    - straining R39.16
    - urgency R39.15
  - mild neurocognitive G31.84
  - mitochondrial metabolism E88.40
  - mitral (valve) — *see* Endocarditis, mitral
  - mixed
    - anxiety and depressive F41.8
    - of scholastic skills (developmental) F81.89
    - receptive expressive language F80.2
  - mood F39
    - bipolar — *see* Disorder, bipolar
    - depressive — *see* Disorder, depressive
    - due to (secondary to)
      - alcohol F10.94
      - amphetamine F15.94
        - in
          - abuse F15.14
          - dependence F15.24
      - anxiolytic F13.94
        - in
          - abuse F13.14
          - dependence F13.24
      - cocaine F14.94

- **Disorder** — *continued*
  - mood — *continued*
        - in
          - abuse F14.14
          - dependence F14.24
      - general medical condition F06.30
      - hallucinogen F16.94
        - in
          - abuse F16.14
          - dependence F16.24
      - hypnotic F13.94
        - in
          - abuse F13.14
          - dependence F13.24
      - inhalant F18.94
        - in
          - abuse F18.14
          - dependence F18.24
      - opioid F11.94
        - in
          - abuse F11.14
          - dependence F11.24
      - phencyclidine (PCP) F16.94
        - in
          - abuse F16.14
          - dependence F16.24
      - physiological condition F06.30
        - with
          - depressive features F06.31
          - major depressive-like episode F06.32
          - manic features F06.33
          - mixed features F06.34
      - psychoactive substance NEC F19.94
        - in
          - abuse F19.14
          - dependence F19.24
      - sedative F13.94
        - in
          - abuse F13.14
          - dependence F13.24
      - volatile solvents F18.94
        - in
          - abuse F18.14
          - dependence F18.24
    - manic episode F30.9
      - with psychotic symptoms F30.2
      - in remission (full) F30.4
        - partial F30.3
      - specified type NEC F30.8
      - without psychotic symptoms F30.10
        - mild F30.11
        - moderate F30.12
        - severe F30.13
    - organic F06.30
      - right hemisphere F07.89
    - persistent F34.9
      - cyclothymia F34.0
      - dysthymia F34.1
      - specified type NEC F34.89
    - recurrent F39
    - right hemisphere organic F07.89
  - movement G25.9
    - drug-induced G25.70
      - akathisia G25.71
      - specified NEC G25.79
    - hysterical F44.4
    - in diseases classified elsewhere G26
    - periodic limb G47.61
      - sleep related G47.61
    - specified NEC G25.89
    - sleep related NEC G47.69
    - stereotyped F98.4
    - treatment-induced G25.9
  - multiple personality F44.81
  - muscle M62.9
    - attachment, spine — *see* Enthesopathy, spinal
    - in trichinellosis — *see* Trichinellosis, with muscle disorder
    - psychogenic F45.8
    - specified type NEC M62.89
    - tone, newborn P94.9
      - specified NEC P94.8
  - muscular
    - attachments (*see also* Enthesopathy)
      - spine — *see* Enthesopathy, spinal
    - urethra N36.44
  - musculoskeletal system, soft tissue — *see* Disorder, soft tissue
    - postprocedural M96.89
    - psychogenic F45.8
  - myoneural G70.9
    - due to lead G70.1

Disorder — *continued*
- myoneural — *continued*
  - specified NEC G70.89
  - toxic G70.1
- myotonic NEC G71.19
- nail, in diseases classified elsewhere L62
- neck region NEC — *see* Dorsopathy, specified NEC
- neonatal onset multisystemic inflammatory (NOMID) M04.2
- nerve G58.9
  - abducent NEC — *see* Strabismus, paralytic, sixth nerve
  - accessory G52.8
  - acoustic — *see* subcategory H93.3
  - auditory — *see* subcategory H93.3
  - auriculotemporal G50.8
  - axillary G54.0
  - cerebral — *see* Disorder, nerve, cranial
  - cranial G52.9
    - eighth — *see* subcategory H93.3
    - eleventh G52.8
    - fifth G50.9
    - first G52.0
    - fourth NEC — *see* Strabismus, paralytic, fourth nerve
    - multiple G52.7
    - ninth G52.1
    - second NEC — *see* Disorder, nerve, optic
    - seventh NEC G51.8
    - sixth NEC — *see* Strabismus, paralytic, sixth nerve
    - specified NEC G52.8
    - tenth G52.2
    - third NEC — *see* Strabismus, paralytic, third nerve
    - twelfth G52.3
  - entrapment — *see* Neuropathy, entrapment
  - facial G51.9
    - specified NEC G51.8
  - femoral — *see* Lesion, nerve, femoral
  - glossopharyngeal NEC G52.1
  - hypoglossal G52.3
  - intercostal G58.0
  - lateral
    - cutaneous of thigh — *see* Mononeuropathy, lower limb, meralgia paresthetica
    - popliteal — *see* Lesion, nerve, popliteal
  - lower limb — *see* Mononeuropathy, lower limb
  - medial popliteal — *see* Lesion, nerve, popliteal, medial
  - median NEC — *see* Lesion, nerve, median
  - multiple G58.7
  - oculomotor NEC — *see* Strabismus, paralytic, third nerve
  - olfactory G52.0
  - optic NEC H47.09 ☑
    - hemorrhage into sheath — *see* Hemorrhage, optic nerve
    - ischemic H47.01 ☑
  - peroneal — *see* Lesion, nerve, popliteal
  - phrenic G58.8
  - plantar — *see* Lesion, nerve, plantar
  - pneumogastric G52.2
  - posterior tibial — *see* Syndrome, tarsal tunnel
  - radial — *see* Lesion, nerve, radial
  - recurrent laryngeal G52.2
  - root G54.9
    - cervical G54.2
    - lumbosacral G54.1
    - specified NEC G54.8
    - thoracic G54.3
  - sciatic NEC — *see* Lesion, nerve, sciatic
  - specified NEC G58.8
    - lower limb — *see* Mononeuropathy, lower limb, specified NEC
    - upper limb — *see* Mononeuropathy, upper limb, specified NEC
  - sympathetic G90.9
  - tibial — *see* Lesion, nerve, popliteal, medial
  - trigeminal G50.9
    - specified NEC G50.8
  - trochlear NEC — *see* Strabismus, paralytic, fourth nerve
  - ulnar — *see* Lesion, nerve, ulnar
  - upper limb — *see* Mononeuropathy, upper limb
  - vagus G52.2
- nervous system G98.8
  - autonomic (peripheral) G90.9
    - specified NEC G90.8
  - central G96.9

Disorder — *continued*
- nervous system — *continued*
    - specified NEC G96.8
  - parasympathetic G90.9
  - specified NEC G98.8
  - sympathetic G90.9
  - vegetative G90.9
- neurocognitive
  - major
    - with
      - aggressive behavior F01.51
      - combative behavior F01.51
      - violent behavior F01.51
    - due to vascular disease, with behavioral disturbance F01.51
    - in (due to) (other diseases classified elsewhere) (*see also* Dementia, in (due to))F02.80
      - with
        - aggressive behavior F02.81
        - combative behavior F02.81
        - violent behavior F02.81
    - without behavioral disturbance F01.50
  - mild G31.84
- neurodevelopmental F89
  - specified NEC F88
- neurohypophysis NEC E23.3
- neurological NEC R29.818
- neuromuscular G70.9
  - hereditary NEC G71.9
  - specified NEC G70.89
  - toxic G70.1
- neurotic F48.9
  - specified NEC F48.8
- neutrophil, polymorphonuclear D71
- nicotine use — *see* Dependence, drug, nicotine
- nightmare F51.5
- nose J34.9
  - specified NEC J34.89
- obsessive-compulsive F42.9
- odontogenesis NOS K00.9
- opioid use
  - with
    - opioid-induced psychotic disorder F11.959
      - with
        - delusions F11.950
        - hallucinations F11.951
  - due to drug abuse — *see* Abuse, drug, opioid
  - due to drug dependence — *see* Dependence, drug, opioid
  - mild F11.10
    - with
      - opioid-induced
        - anxiety disorder F11.188
        - depressive disorder F11.14
        - sexual dysfunction F11.181
      - opioid intoxication
        - with perceptual disturbances F11.122
        - delirium F11.121
        - without perceptual disturbances F11.129
  - moderate or severe F11.20
    - with
      - opioid-induced
        - anxiety disorder F11.288
        - anxiety disorder F11.988
        - depressive disorder F11.24
        - depressive disorder F11.94
        - sexual dysfunction F11.281
        - sexual dysfunction F11.981
      - opioid intoxication
        - with perceptual disturbances F11.222
        - delirium F11.221
        - without perceptual disturbances F11.229
- oppositional defiant F91.3
- optic
  - chiasm H47.49
    - due to
      - inflammatory disorder H47.41
      - neoplasm H47.42
      - vascular disorder H47.43
  - disc H47.39 ☑
    - coloboma — *see* Coloboma, optic disc
    - drusen — *see* Drusen, optic disc
    - pseudopapilledema — *see* Pseudopapilledema
  - radiations — *see* Disorder, visual, pathway
  - tracts — *see* Disorder, visual, pathway
- orbit H05.9
  - cyst — *see* Cyst, orbit
  - deformity — *see* Deformity, orbit
  - edema — *see* Edema, orbit
  - enophthalmos — *see* Enophthalmos

Disorder — *continued*
- orbit — *continued*
  - exophthalmos — *see* Exophthalmos
  - hemorrhage — *see* Hemorrhage, orbit
  - inflammation — *see* Inflammation, orbit
  - myopathy — *see* Myopathy, extraocular muscles
  - retained foreign body — *see* Foreign body, orbit, old
  - specified type NEC H05.89
- organic
  - anxiety F06.4
  - catatonic F06.1
  - delusional F06.2
  - dissociative F06.8
  - emotionally labile (asthenic) F06.8
  - mood (affective) F06.30
  - schizophrenia-like F06.2
- orgasmic (female) F52.31
  - male F52.32
- ornithine metabolism E72.4
- overanxious F41.1
  - of childhood F93.8
- pain
  - with related psychological factors F45.42
  - exclusively related to psychological factors F45.41
  - genito-pelvic penetration disorder F52.6
- pancreatic internal secretion E16.9
  - specified NEC E16.8
- panic F41.0
  - with agoraphobia F40.01
- papulosquamous L44.9
  - in diseases classified elsewhere L45
  - specified NEC L44.8
- paranoid F22
  - induced F24
  - shared F24
- parathyroid (gland) E21.5
  - specified NEC E21.4
- parietoalveolar NEC J84.09
- paroxysmal, mixed R56.9
- patella M22.9 ☑
  - chondromalacia — *see* Chondromalacia, patella
  - derangement NEC M22.3X ☑
  - recurrent
    - dislocation — *see* Dislocation, patella, recurrent
    - subluxation — *see* Dislocation, patella, recurrent, incomplete
  - specified NEC M22.8X ☑
- patellofemoral M22.2X ☑
- pentose phosphate pathway with anemia D55.1
- perception, due to hallucinogens F16.983
  - in
    - abuse F16.183
    - dependence F16.283
- peripheral nervous system NEC G64
- peroxisomal E71.50
  - biogenesis
    - neonatal adrenoleukodystrophy E71.511
    - specified disorder NEC E71.518
    - Zellweger syndrome E71.510
  - rhizomelic chondrodysplasia punctata E71.540
  - specified form NEC E71.548
    - group 1 E71.518
    - group 2 E71.53
    - group 3 E71.542
  - X-linked adrenoleukodystrophy E71.529
    - adolescent E71.521
    - adrenomyeloneuropathy E71.522
    - childhood E71.520
    - specified form NEC E71.528
  - Zellweger-like syndrome E71.541
- persistent
  - (somatoform) pain F45.41
  - affective (mood) F34.9
- personality (*see also* Personality)F60.9
  - affective F34.0
  - aggressive F60.3
  - amoral F60.2
  - anankastic F60.5
  - antisocial F60.2
  - anxious F60.6
  - asocial F60.2
  - asthenic F60.7
  - avoidant F60.6
  - borderline F60.3
  - change (secondary) due to general medical condition F07.0
  - compulsive F60.5
  - cyclothymic F34.0

- **Disorder** — *continued*
  - personality — *continued*
    - dependent (passive) F60.7
    - depressive F34.1
    - dissocial F60.2
    - emotional instability F60.3
    - expansive paranoid F60.0
    - explosive F60.3
    - following organic brain damage F07.9
    - histrionic F60.4
    - hyperthymic F34.0
    - hypothymic F34.1
    - hysterical F60.4
    - immature F60.89
    - inadequate F60.7
    - labile F60.3
    - mixed (nonspecific) F60.89
    - moral deficiency F60.2
    - narcissistic F60.81
    - negativistic F60.89
    - obsessional F60.5
    - obsessive (-compulsive) F60.5
    - organic F07.9
    - overconscientious F60.5
    - paranoid F60.0
    - passive (-dependent) F60.7
    - passive-aggressive F60.89
    - pathological NEC F60.9
    - pseudosocial F60.2
    - psychopathic F60.2
    - schizoid F60.1
    - schizotypal F21
    - self-defeating F60.7
    - specified NEC F60.89
    - type A F60.5
    - unstable (emotional) F60.3
  - pervasive, developmental F84.9
  - phencyclidine use
    - mild F16.10
      - with
        - phencyclidine-induced
          - anxiety disorder F16.180
          - bipolar and related disorder F16.14
          - depressive disorder F16.14
          - psychotic disorder F16.159
        - phencyclidine intoxication F16.129
        - phencyclidine intoxication delirium F16.121
    - moderate or severe F16.20
      - with
        - phencyclidine-induced
          - anxiety disorder F16.280
          - bipolar and related disorder F16.24
          - depressive disorder F16.24
          - psychotic disorder F16.259
        - phencyclidine intoxication F16.229
        - phencyclidine intoxication delirium F16.221
  - phobic anxiety, childhood F40.8
  - phosphate-losing tubular N25.0
  - pigmentation L81.9
    - choroid, congenital Q14.3
    - diminished melanin formation L81.6
    - iron L81.8
    - specified NEC L81.8
  - pinna (noninfective) H61.10 ☑
    - deformity, acquired H61.11 ☑
    - hematoma H61.12 ☑
    - perichondritis — *see* Perichondritis, ear
    - specified type NEC H61.19 ☑
  - pituitary gland E23.7
    - iatrogenic (postprocedural) E89.3
    - specified NEC E23.6
  - platelets D69.1
  - plexus G54.9
    - specified NEC G54.8
  - polymorphonuclear neutrophils D71
  - porphyrin metabolism — *see* Porphyria
  - postconcussional F07.81
  - posthallucinogen perception F16.983
    - in
      - abuse F16.183
      - dependence F16.283
  - postmenopausal N95.9
    - specified NEC N95.8
  - postprocedural (postoperative) — *see* Complications, postprocedural
  - post-transplant lymphoproliferative D47.Z1
  - post-traumatic stress (PTSD) F43.10
    - acute F43.11
    - chronic F43.12
  - premenstrual dysphoric (PMDD) F32.81

- **Disorder** — *continued*
  - prepuce N47.8
  - propionic acidemia E71.121
  - prostate N42.9
    - specified NEC N42.89
  - psychogenic NOS (*see also* condition)F45.9
    - anxiety F41.8
    - appetite F50.9
    - asthenic F48.8
    - cardiovascular (system) F45.8
    - compulsive F42.8
    - cutaneous F54
    - depressive F32.9
    - digestive (system) F45.8
    - dysmenorrheic F45.8
    - dyspneic F45.8
    - endocrine (system) F54
    - eye NEC F45.8
    - feeding — *see* Disorder, eating
    - functional NEC F45.8
    - gastric F45.8
    - gastrointestinal (system) F45.8
    - genitourinary (system) F45.8
    - heart (function) (rhythm) F45.8
    - hyperventilatory F45.8
    - hypochondriacal — *see* Disorder, hypochondriacal
    - intestinal F45.8
    - joint F45.8
    - learning F81.9
    - limb F45.8
    - lymphatic (system) F45.8
    - menstrual F45.8
    - micturition F45.8
    - monoplegic NEC F44.4
    - motor F44.4
    - muscle F45.8
    - musculoskeletal F45.8
    - neurocirculatory F45.8
    - obsessive F42.8
    - occupational F48.8
    - organ or part of body NEC F45.8
    - paralytic NEC F44.4
    - phobic F40.9
    - physical NEC F45.8
    - rectal F45.8
    - respiratory (system) F45.8
    - rheumatic F45.8
    - sexual (function) F52.9
    - skin (allergic) (eczematous) F54
    - sleep F51.9
    - specified part of body NEC F45.8
    - stomach F45.8
  - psychological F99
    - associated with
      - disease classified elsewhere F54
      - sexual
        - development F66
        - relationship F66
      - uncertainty about gender identity F64.9
  - psychomotor NEC F44.4
    - hysterical F44.4
  - psychoneurotic (*see also* Neurosis)
    - mixed NEC F48.8
  - psychophysiologic — *see* Disorder, somatoform
  - psychosexual F65.9
    - development F66
    - identity of childhood F64.2
  - psychosomatic NOS — *see* Disorder, somatoform
    - multiple F45.0
    - undifferentiated F45.1
  - psychotic — *see* Psychosis
    - transient (acute) F23
  - puberty E30.9
    - specified NEC E30.8
  - pulmonary (valve) — *see* Endocarditis, pulmonary
  - purine metabolism E79.9
  - pyrimidine metabolism E79.9
  - pyruvate metabolism E74.4
  - reactive attachment (childhood) F94.1
  - reading R48.0
    - developmental (specific) F81.0
  - receptive language F80.2
  - receptor, hormonal, peripheral (*see also* Syndrome, androgen insensitivity)E34.50
  - recurrent brief depressive F33.8
  - reflex R29.2
  - refraction H52.7
    - aniseikonia H52.32
    - anisometropia H52.31
    - astigmatism — *see* Astigmatism
    - hypermetropia — *see* Hypermetropia

- **Disorder** — *continued*
  - refraction — *continued*
    - myopia — *see* Myopia
    - presbyopia H52.4
    - specified NEC H52.6
  - relationship F68.8
    - due to sexual orientation F66
  - REM sleep behavior G47.52
  - renal function, impaired (tubular) N25.9
  - resonance R49.9
    - specified NEC R49.8
  - respiratory function, impaired (*see also* Failure, respiration)
    - postprocedural — *see* Complication, postoperative, respiratory system
    - psychogenic F45.8
  - retina H35.9
    - angioid streaks H35.33
    - changes in vascular appearance H35.01 ☑
    - degeneration — *see* Degeneration, retina
    - dystrophy (hereditary) — *see* Dystrophy, retina
    - edema H35.81
    - hemorrhage — *see* Hemorrhage, retina
    - ischemia H35.82
    - macular degeneration — *see* Degeneration, macula
    - microaneurysms H35.04 ☑
    - microvascular abnormality NEC H35.09
    - neovascularization — *see* Neovascularization, retina
    - retinopathy — *see* Retinopathy
    - separation of layers H35.70
      - central serous chorioretinopathy H35.71 ☑
      - pigment epithelium detachment (serous) H35.72 ☑
        - hemorrhagic H35.73 ☑
    - specified type NEC H35.89
    - telangiectasis — *see* Telangiectasis, retina
    - vasculitis — *see* Vasculitis, retina
  - retroperitoneal K68.9
  - right hemisphere organic affective F07.89
  - rumination (infant or child) F98.21
  - sacrum, sacrococcygeal NEC M53.3
  - schizoaffective F25.9
    - bipolar type F25.0
    - depressive type F25.1
    - manic type F25.0
    - mixed type F25.0
    - specified NEC F25.8
  - schizoid of childhood F84.5
  - schizophreniform F20.81
    - brief F23
  - schizotypal (personality) F21
  - secretion, thyrocalcitonin E07.0
  - sedative, hypnotic, or anxiolytic use
    - mild F13.10
      - with
        - sedative, hypnotic, or anxiolytic-induced
          - anxiety disorder F13.180
          - bipolar and related disorder F13.14
          - depressive disorder F13.14
          - psychotic disorder F13.159
          - sexual dysfunction F13.181
        - sedative, hypnotic, or anxiolytic intoxication F13.129
        - sedative, hypnotic, or anxiolytic intoxication delirium F13.121
    - moderate or severe F13.20
      - with
        - sedative, hypnotic, or anxiolytic-induced
          - anxiety disorder F13.280
          - bipolar and related disorder F13.24
          - depressive disorder F13.24
          - major neurocognitive disorder F13.27
          - mild neurocognitive disorder F13.288
          - psychotic disorder F13.259
          - sexual dysfunction F13.281
        - sedative, hypnotic, or anxiolytic intoxication F13.229
        - sedative, hypnotic, or anxiolytic intoxication delirium F13.221
  - seizure (*see also* Epilepsy)G40.909
    - intractable G40.919
      - with status epilepticus G40.911
  - semantic pragmatic F80.89
    - with autism F84.0
  - sense of smell R43.1
    - psychogenic F45.8
  - separation anxiety, of childhood F93.0
  - sexual
    - arousal, female F52.22
    - aversion F52.1

- **Disorder** — *continued*
  - sexual — *continued*
    - function, psychogenic F52.9
    - maturation F66
    - nonorganic F52.9
    - preference (*see also* Deviation, sexual) F65.9
      - fetishistic transvestism F65.1
    - relationship F66
  - shyness, of childhood and adolescence F40.10
  - sibling rivalry F93.8
  - sickle-cell (sickling) (homozygous) — *see* Disease, sickle-cell
    - heterozygous D57.3
    - specified type NEC D57.8 ☑
    - trait D57.3
  - sinus (nasal) J34.9
    - specified NEC J34.89
  - skin L98.9
    - atrophic L90.9
      - specified NEC L90.8
    - granulomatous L92.9
      - specified NEC L92.8
    - hypertrophic L91.9
      - specified NEC L91.8
    - infiltrative NEC L98.6
    - newborn P83.9
      - specified NEC P83.8
    - picking F42.4
    - psychogenic (allergic) (eczematous) F54
  - sleep G47.9
    - breathing-related — *see* Apnea, sleep
    - circadian rhythm G47.20
      - advance sleep phase type G47.22
      - delayed sleep phase type G47.21
      - due to
        - alcohol
          - abuse F10.182
          - dependence F10.282
          - use F10.982
        - amphetamines
          - abuse F15.182
          - dependence F15.282
          - use F15.982
        - caffeine
          - abuse F15.182
          - dependence F15.282
          - use F15.982
        - cocaine
          - abuse F14.182
          - dependence F14.282
          - use F14.982
        - drug NEC
          - abuse F19.182
          - dependence F19.282
          - use F19.982
        - opioid
          - abuse F11.182
          - dependence F11.282
          - use F11.982
        - psychoactive substance NEC
          - abuse F19.182
          - dependence F19.282
          - use F19.982
        - sedative, hypnotic, or anxiolytic
          - abuse F13.182
          - dependence F13.282
          - use F13.982
        - stimulant NEC
          - abuse F15.182
          - dependence F15.282
          - use F15.982
      - free running type G47.24
      - in conditions classified elsewhere G47.27
      - irregular sleep wake type G47.23
      - jet lag type G47.25
      - shift work type G47.26
      - specified NEC G47.29
    - due to
      - alcohol
        - abuse F10.182
        - dependence F10.282
        - use F10.982
      - amphetamine
        - abuse F15.182
        - dependence F15.282
        - use F15.982
      - anxiolytic
        - abuse F13.182
        - dependence F13.282
        - use F13.982
      - caffeine
        - abuse F15.182

- **Disorder** — *continued*
  - sleep — *continued*
        - dependence F15.282
        - use F15.982
      - cocaine
        - abuse F14.182
        - dependence F14.282
        - use F14.982
      - drug NEC
        - abuse F19.182
        - dependence F19.282
        - use F19.982
      - hypnotic
        - abuse F13.182
        - dependence F13.282
        - use F13.982
      - opioid
        - abuse F11.182
        - dependence F11.282
        - use F11.982
      - psychoactive substance NEC
        - abuse F19.182
        - dependence F19.282
        - use F19.982
      - sedative
        - abuse F13.182
        - dependence F13.282
        - use F13.982
      - stimulant NEC
        - abuse F15.182
        - dependence F15.282
        - use F15.982
    - emotional F51.9
    - excessive somnolence — *see* Hypersomnia
    - hypersomnia type — *see* Hypersomnia
    - initiating or maintaining — *see* Insomnia
    - nightmares F51.5
    - nonorganic F51.9
      - specified NEC F51.8
    - parasomnia type G47.50
    - specified NEC G47.8
    - terrors F51.4
    - walking F51.3
  - sleep-wake pattern or schedule — *see* Disorder, sleep, circadian rhythm
  - social
    - anxiety of childhood F40.10
    - functioning in childhood F94.9
      - specified NEC F94.8
    - pragmatic F80.82
  - soft tissue M79.9
    - ankle M79.9
    - due to use, overuse and pressure M70.90
      - ankle M70.97 ☑
      - bursitis — *see* Bursitis
      - foot M70.97 ☑
      - forearm M70.93 ☑
      - hand M70.94 ☑
      - lower leg M70.96 ☑
      - multiple sites M70.99
      - pelvic region M70.95 ☑
      - shoulder region M70.91 ☑
      - specified site NEC M70.98
      - specified type NEC M70.80
        - ankle M70.87 ☑
        - foot M70.87 ☑
        - forearm M70.83 ☑
        - hand M70.84 ☑
        - lower leg M70.86 ☑
        - multiple sites M70.89
        - pelvic region M70.85 ☑
        - shoulder region M70.81 ☑
        - specified site NEC M70.88
        - thigh M70.85 ☑
        - upper arm M70.82 ☑
      - thigh M70.95 ☑
      - upper arm M70.92 ☑
    - foot M79.9
    - forearm M79.9
    - hand M79.9
    - lower leg M79.9
    - multiple sites M79.9
    - occupational — *see* Disorder, soft tissue, due to use, overuse and pressure
    - pelvic region M79.9
    - shoulder region M79.9
    - specified type NEC M79.89
    - thigh M79.9
    - upper arm M79.9
  - somatic symptom F45.1
  - somatization F45.0

- **Disorder** — *continued*
  - somatoform F45.9
    - pain (persistent) F45.41
    - somatization (multiple) (long-lasting) F45.0
    - specified NEC F45.8
    - undifferentiated F45.1
  - somnolence, excessive — *see* Hypersomnia
  - specific
    - arithmetical F81.2
    - developmental, of motor F82
    - reading F81.0
    - speech and language F80.9
    - spelling F81.81
    - written expression F81.81
  - speech R47.9
    - articulation (functional) (specific) F80.0
    - developmental F80.9
    - specified NEC R47.89
  - speech-sound F80.0
  - spelling (specific) F81.81
  - spine (*see also* Dorsopathy)
    - ligamentous or muscular attachments, peripheral — *see* Enthesopathy, spinal
    - specified NEC — *see* Dorsopathy, specified NEC
  - stereotyped, habit or movement F98.4
  - stimulant use (other) (unspecified)
    - mild F15.10
    - moderate or severe F15.20
  - stomach (functional) — *see* Disorder, gastric
  - stress F43.9
    - acute F43.0
    - post-traumatic F43.10
      - acute F43.11
      - chronic F43.12
  - substance use (other) (unknown)
    - mild F19.10
      - with substance-induced
        - anxiety disorder F19.180
        - bipolar and related disorder F19.14
        - depressive disorder F19.14
        - major neurocognitive disorder F19.17
        - mild neurocognitive disorder F19.188
        - obsessive-compulsive and related disorder F19.188
        - sexual dysfunction F19.181
      - substance intoxication F19.129
      - substance intoxication delirium F19.121
    - moderate or severe F19.20
      - with substance-induced
        - anxiety disorder F19.280
        - bipolar and related disorder F19.24
        - depressive disorder F19.24
        - major neurocognitive disorder F19.27
        - mild neurocognitive disorder F19.288
        - obsessive-compulsive and related disorder F19.288
        - sexual dysfunction F19.281
      - substance intoxication F19.229
      - substance intoxication delirium F19.221
  - sulfur-bearing amino-acid metabolism E72.10
  - sweat gland (eccrine) L74.9
    - apocrine L75.9
      - specified NEC L75.8
    - specified NEC L74.8
  - synovium M67.90
    - acromioclavicular M67.91 ☑
    - ankle M67.97 ☑
    - elbow M67.92 ☑
    - foot M67.97 ☑
    - forearm M67.93 ☑
    - hand M67.94 ☑
    - hip M67.95 ☑
    - knee M67.96 ☑
    - multiple sites M67.99
    - rupture — *see* Rupture, synovium
    - shoulder M67.91 ☑
    - specified type NEC M67.80
      - acromioclavicular M67.81 ☑
      - ankle M67.87 ☑
      - elbow M67.82 ☑
      - foot M67.87 ☑
      - hand M67.84 ☑
      - hip M67.85 ☑
      - knee M67.86 ☑
      - multiple sites M67.89
      - wrist M67.83 ☑
    - synovitis — *see* Synovitis
    - upper arm M67.92 ☑
    - wrist M67.93 ☑
  - temperature regulation, newborn P81.9
    - specified NEC P81.8
  - temporomandibular joint M26.60 ☑

- **Disorder** — *continued*
  - tendon M67.90
    - acromioclavicular M67.91 ☑
    - ankle M67.97 ☑
    - contracture — *see* Contracture, tendon
    - elbow M67.92 ☑
    - foot M67.97 ☑
    - forearm M67.93 ☑
    - hand M67.94 ☑
    - hip M67.95 ☑
    - knee M67.96 ☑
    - multiple sites M67.99
    - rupture — *see* Rupture, tendon
    - shoulder M67.91 ☑
    - specified type NEC M67.80
      - acromioclavicular M67.81 ☑
      - ankle M67.87 ☑
      - elbow M67.82 ☑
      - foot M67.87 ☑
      - hand M67.84 ☑
      - hip M67.85 ☑
      - knee M67.86 ☑
      - multiple sites M67.89
      - trunk M67.88
      - wrist M67.83 ☑
    - synovitis — *see* Synovitis
    - tendinitis — *see* Tendinitis
    - tenosynovitis — *see* Tenosynovitis
    - trunk M67.98
    - upper arm M67.92 ☑
    - wrist M67.93 ☑
  - thoracic root (nerve) NEC G54.3
  - thyrocalcitonin hypersecretion E07.0
  - thyroid (gland) E07.9
    - function NEC, neonatal, transitory P72.2
    - iodine-deficiency related E01.8
    - specified NEC E07.89
  - tic — *see* Tic
  - tobacco use
    - mild Z72.0
    - moderate F17.200
    - severe F17.200
  - tooth K08.9
    - development K00.9
      - specified NEC K00.8
    - eruption K00.6
  - Tourette's F95.2
  - trance and possession F44.89
  - trauma and stressor-related F43.9
    - other specified F43.8
  - tricuspid (valve) — *see* Endocarditis, tricuspid
  - tryptophan metabolism E70.5
  - tubular, phosphate-losing N25.0
  - tubulo-interstitial (in)
    - brucellosis A23.9 *[N16]*
    - cystinosis E72.04
    - diphtheria A36.84
    - glycogen storage disease E74.00 *[N16]*
    - leukemia NEC C95.9 ☑ *[N16]*
    - lymphoma NEC C85.9 ☑ *[N16]*
    - mixed cryoglobulinemia D89.1 *[N16]*
    - multiple myeloma C90.0 ☑ *[N16]*
    - Salmonella infection A02.25
    - sarcoidosis D86.84
    - sepsis A41.9 *[N16]*
      - streptococcal A40.9 *[N16]*
    - systemic lupus erythematosus M32.15
    - toxoplasmosis B58.83
    - transplant rejection T86.91 *[N16]*
    - Wilson's disease E83.01 *[N16]*
  - tubulo-renal function, impaired N25.9
    - specified NEC N25.89
  - tympanic membrane H73.9 ☑
    - atrophy — *see* Atrophy, tympanic membrane
    - infection — *see* Myringitis
    - perforation — *see* Perforation, tympanum
    - specified NEC H73.89 ☑
  - unsocialized aggressive F91.1
  - urea cycle metabolism E72.20
    - argininemia E72.21
    - arginosuccinic aciduria E72.22
    - citrullinemia E72.23
    - ornithine transcarbamylase deficiency E72.4
    - other specified E72.29
  - ureter (in) N28.9
    - schistosomiasis B65.0 *[N29]*
    - tuberculosis A18.11
  - urethra N36.9
    - specified NEC N36.8
  - urinary system N39.9
    - specified NEC N39.8
- **Disorder** — *continued*
  - valve, heart
    - aortic — *see* Endocarditis, aortic
    - mitral — *see* Endocarditis, mitral
    - pulmonary — *see* Endocarditis, pulmonary
    - rheumatic
      - aortic — *see* Endocarditis, aortic, rheumatic
      - mitral — *see* Endocarditis, mitral
      - pulmonary — *see* Endocarditis, pulmonary, rheumatic
      - tricuspid — *see* Endocarditis, tricuspid
    - tricuspid — *see* Endocarditis, tricuspid
  - vestibular function H81.9 ☑
    - specified NEC — *see* subcategory H81.8
      - in diseases classified elsewhere H82. ☑
    - vertigo — *see* Vertigo
  - vision, binocular H53.30
    - abnormal retinal correspondence H53.31
    - diplopia H53.2
    - fusion with defective stereopsis H53.32
    - simultaneous perception H53.33
    - suppression H53.34
  - visual
    - cortex
      - blindness H47.619
        - left brain H47.612
        - right brain H47.611
      - due to
        - inflammatory disorder H47.629
          - left brain H47.622
          - right brain H47.621
        - neoplasm H47.639
          - left brain H47.632
          - right brain H47.631
        - vascular disorder H47.649
          - left brain H47.642
          - right brain H47.641
    - pathway H47.9
      - due to
        - inflammatory disorder H47.51 ☑
        - neoplasm H47.52 ☑
        - vascular disorder H47.53 ☑
      - optic chiasm — *see* Disorder, optic, chiasm
  - vitreous body H43.9
    - crystalline deposits — *see* Deposit, crystalline
    - degeneration — *see* Degeneration, vitreous
    - hemorrhage — *see* Hemorrhage, vitreous
    - opacities — *see* Opacity, vitreous
    - prolapse — *see* Prolapse, vitreous
    - specified type NEC H43.89
  - voice R49.9
    - specified type NEC R49.8
  - volatile solvent use
    - due to drug abuse — *see* Abuse, drug, inhalant
    - due to drug dependence — *see* Dependence, drug, inhalant
  - white blood cells D72.9
    - specified NEC D72.89
  - withdrawing, child or adolescent F40.10
- **Disorientation** R41.0
- **Displacement,** displaced
  - acquired traumatic of bone, cartilage, joint, tendon NEC — *see* Dislocation
  - adrenal gland (congenital) Q89.1
  - appendix, retrocecal (congenital) Q43.8
  - auricle (congenital) Q17.4
  - bladder (acquired) N32.89
    - congenital Q64.19
  - brachial plexus (congenital) Q07.8
  - brain stem, caudal (congenital) Q04.8
  - canaliculus (lacrimalis), congenital Q10.6
  - cardia through esophageal hiatus (congenital) Q40.1
  - cerebellum, caudal (congenital) Q04.8
  - cervix — *see* Malposition, uterus
  - colon (congenital) Q43.3
  - device, implant or graft (*see also* Complications, by site and type, mechanical)T85.628 ☑
    - arterial graft NEC — *see* Complication, cardiovascular device, mechanical, vascular
    - breast (implant) T85.42 ☑
    - catheter NEC T85.628 ☑
      - dialysis (renal) T82.42 ☑
        - intraperitoneal T85.621 ☑
      - infusion NEC T82.524 ☑
        - spinal (epidural) (subdural) T85.620 ☑
      - urinary
        - cystostomy T83.020 ☑
        - Hopkins T83.028 ☑
        - ileostomy T83.028 ☑
        - indwelling T83.021 ☑
        - nephrostomy T83.022 ☑
- **Displacement** — *continued*
  - device, implant or graft — *continued*
        - specified NEC T83.028 ☑
        - urostomy T83.028 ☑
    - electronic (electrode) (pulse generator) (stimulator) — *see* Complication, electronic stimulator
    - fixation, internal (orthopedic) NEC — *see* Complication, fixation device, mechanical
    - gastrointestinal — *see* Complications, prosthetic device, mechanical, gastrointestinal device
    - genital NEC T83.428 ☑
      - intrauterine contraceptive device (string) T83.32 ☑
      - penile prosthesis (cylinder) (implanted) (pump) (reservoir) T83.420 ☑
      - testicular prosthesis T83.421 ☑
    - heart NEC — *see* Complication, cardiovascular device, mechanical
    - joint prosthesis — *see* Complications, joint prosthesis, mechanical
    - ocular — *see* Complications, prosthetic device, mechanical, ocular device
    - orthopedic NEC — *see* Complication, orthopedic, device or graft, mechanical
    - specified NEC T85.628 ☑
    - urinary NEC T83.128 ☑
      - graft T83.22 ☑
      - sphincter, implanted T83.121 ☑
      - stent (ileal conduit) (nephroureteral) T83.123 ☑
        - ureteral indwelling T83.122 ☑
    - vascular NEC — *see* Complication, cardiovascular device, mechanical
    - ventricular intracranial shunt T85.02 ☑
  - electronic stimulator
    - bone T84.320 ☑
    - cardiac — *see* Complications, cardiac device, electronic
    - nervous system — *see* Complication, prosthetic device, mechanical, electronic nervous system stimulator
    - urinary — *see* Complications, electronic stimulator, urinary
  - esophageal mucosa into cardia of stomach, congenital Q39.8
  - esophagus (acquired) K22.8
    - congenital Q39.8
  - eyeball (acquired) (lateral) (old) — *see* Displacement, globe
    - congenital Q15.8
    - current — *see* Avulsion, eye
  - fallopian tube (acquired) N83.4 ☑
    - congenital Q50.6
    - opening (congenital) Q50.6
  - gallbladder (congenital) Q44.1
  - gastric mucosa (congenital) Q40.2
  - globe (acquired) (old) (lateral) H05.21 ☑
    - current — *see* Avulsion, eye
  - heart (congenital) Q24.8
    - acquired I51.89
  - hymen (upward) (congenital) Q52.4
  - intervertebral disc NEC
    - with myelopathy — *see* Disorder, disc, with, myelopathy
    - cervical, cervicothoracic (with) M50.20
      - myelopathy — *see* Disorder, disc, cervical, with myelopathy
      - neuritis, radiculitis or radiculopathy — *see* Disorder, disc, cervical, with neuritis
    - due to trauma — *see* Dislocation, vertebra
    - lumbar region M51.26
      - with
        - myelopathy M51.06
        - neuritis, radiculitis, radiculopathy or sciatica M51.16
    - lumbosacral region M51.27
      - with
        - neuritis, radiculitis, radiculopathy or sciatica M51.17
    - sacrococcygeal region M53.3
    - thoracic region M51.24
      - with
        - myelopathy M51.04
        - neuritis, radiculitis, radiculopathy M51.14
    - thoracolumbar region M51.25
      - with
        - myelopathy M51.05
        - neuritis, radiculitis, radiculopathy M51.15
  - intrauterine device (string) T83.32 ☑
  - kidney (acquired) N28.83
    - congenital Q63.2

Displacement — *continued*
- lachrymal, lacrimal apparatus or duct (congenital) Q10.6
- lens, congenital Q12.1
- macula (congenital) Q14.1
- Meckel's diverticulum Q43.0
  - malignant — *see* Table of Neoplasms, small intestine, malignant
- nail (congenital) Q84.6
  - acquired L60.8
- opening of Wharton's duct in mouth Q38.4
- organ or site, congenital NEC — *see* Malposition, congenital
- ovary (acquired) N83.4 ☑
  - congenital Q50.39
  - free in peritoneal cavity (congenital) Q50.39
  - into hernial sac N83.4 ☑
- oviduct (acquired) N83.4 ☑
  - congenital Q50.6
- parathyroid (gland) E21.4
- parotid gland (congenital) Q38.4
- punctum lacrimale (congenital) Q10.6
- sacro-iliac (joint) (congenital) Q74.2
  - current injury S33.2 ☑
  - old — *see* subcategory M53.2
- salivary gland (any) (congenital) Q38.4
- spleen (congenital) Q89.09
- stomach, congenital Q40.2
- sublingual duct Q38.4
- tongue (downward) (congenital) Q38.3
- tooth, teeth, fully erupted M26.30
  - horizontal M26.33
  - vertical M26.34
- trachea (congenital) Q32.1
- ureter or ureteric opening or orifice (congenital) Q62.62
- uterine opening of oviducts or fallopian tubes Q50.6
- uterus, uterine — *see* Malposition, uterus
- ventricular septum Q21.0
  - with rudimentary ventricle Q20.4

Disproportion
- between native and reconstructed breast N65.1
- fiber-type G71.2

Disruptio uteri — *see* Rupture, uterus

Disruption (of)
- ciliary body NEC H21.89
- closure of
  - cornea T81.31 ☑
  - craniotomy T81.32 ☑
  - fascia (muscular) (superficial) T81.32 ☑
  - internal organ or tissue T81.32 ☑
  - laceration (external) (internal) T81.33 ☑
  - ligament T81.32 ☑
  - mucosa T81.31 ☑
  - muscle or muscle flap T81.32 ☑
  - ribs or rib cage T81.32 ☑
  - skin and subcutaneous tissue (full-thickness) (superficial) T81.31 ☑
  - skull T81.32 ☑
  - sternum (sternotomy) T81.32 ☑
  - tendon T81.32 ☑
  - traumatic laceration (external) (internal) T81.33 ☑
- family Z63.8
  - due to
    - absence of family member due to military deployment Z63.31
    - absence of family member NEC Z63.32
    - alcoholism and drug addiction in family Z63.72
    - bereavement Z63.4
    - death (assumed) or disappearance of family member Z63.4
    - divorce or separation Z63.5
    - drug addiction in family Z63.72
    - return of family member from military deployment (current or past conflict) Z63.71
    - stressful life events NEC Z63.79
- iris NEC H21.89
- ligament (s) (*see also* Sprain)
  - knee
    - current injury — *see* Dislocation, knee
    - old (chronic) — *see* Derangement, knee, ligament, instability, chronic
    - spontaneous NEC — *see* Derangement, knee, disruption ligament
- ossicular chain — *see* Discontinuity, ossicles, ear
- pelvic ring (stable) S32.810 ☑
  - unstable S32.811 ☑

Disruption — *continued*
- wound T81.30 ☑
  - episiotomy O90.1
  - operation T81.31 ☑
    - cesarean O90.0
    - external operation wound (superficial) T81.31 ☑
    - internal operation wound (deep) T81.32 ☑
  - perineal (obstetric) O90.1
  - traumatic injury repair T81.33 ☑
- traumatic injury wound repair T81.33 ☑

Dissatisfaction with
- employment Z56.9
- school environment Z55.4

Dissecting — *see* condition

Dissection
- aorta I71.00
  - abdominal I71.02
  - thoracic I71.01
  - thoracoabdominal I71.03
- artery I77.70
  - basilar (trunk) I77.75
  - carotid I77.71
  - cerebral (nonruptured) I67.0
    - ruptured — *see* Hemorrhage, intracranial, subarachnoid
  - coronary I25.42
  - extremity
    - lower I77.77
    - upper I77.76
  - iliac I77.72
  - precerebral
    - congenital (nonruptured) Q28.1
    - specified site NEC I77.75
  - renal I77.73
  - specified NEC I77.79
  - vertebral I77.74
- traumatic — *see* Wound, open, by site
- vascular I99.8
- wound — *see* Wound, open

Disseminated — *see* condition

Dissociation
- auriculoventricular or atrioventricular (AV) (any degree) (isorhythmic) I45.89
  - with heart block I44.2
- interference I45.89

Dissociative reaction, state F44.9

Dissolution, vertebra — *see* Osteoporosis

Distension, distention
- abdomen R14.0
- bladder N32.89
- cecum K63.89
- colon K63.89
- gallbladder K82.8
- intestine K63.89
- kidney N28.89
- liver K76.89
- seminal vesicle N50.89
- stomach K31.89
  - acute K31.0
  - psychogenic F45.8
- ureter — *see* Dilatation, ureter
- uterus N85.8

Distoma hepaticum infestation B66.3

Distomiasis B66.9
- bile passages B66.3
- hemic B65.9
- hepatic B66.3
  - due to Clonorchis sinensis B66.1
- intestinal B66.5
- liver B66.3
  - due to Clonorchis sinensis B66.1
- lung B66.4
- pulmonary B66.4

Distomolar (fourth molar) K00.1

Disto-occlusion (Division I) (Division II) M26.212

Distortion (s) (congenital)
- adrenal (gland) Q89.1
- arm NEC Q68.8
- bile duct or passage Q44.5
- bladder Q64.79
- brain Q04.9
- cervix (uteri) Q51.9
- chest (wall) Q67.8
  - bones Q76.8
- clavicle Q74.0
- clitoris Q52.6
- coccyx Q76.49
- common duct Q44.5
- coronary Q24.5
- cystic duct Q44.5

Distortion — *continued*
- ear (auricle) (external) Q17.3
  - inner Q16.5
  - middle Q16.4
    - ossicles Q16.3
- endocrine NEC Q89.2
- eustachian tube Q17.8
- eye (adnexa) Q15.8
- face bone (s) NEC Q75.8
- fallopian tube Q50.6
- femur NEC Q68.8
- fibula NEC Q68.8
- finger (s) Q68.1
- foot Q66.9
- genitalia, genital organ (s)
  - female Q52.8
    - external Q52.79
    - internal NEC Q52.8
- gyri Q04.8
- hand bone (s) Q68.1
- heart (auricle) (ventricle) Q24.8
  - valve (cusp) Q24.8
- hepatic duct Q44.5
- humerus NEC Q68.8
- hymen Q52.4
- intrafamilial communications Z63.8
- jaw NEC M26.89
- labium (majus) (minus) Q52.79
- leg NEC Q68.8
- lens Q12.8
- liver Q44.7
- lumbar spine Q76.49
  - with disproportion O33.8
    - causing obstructed labor O65.0
- lumbosacral (joint) (region) Q76.49
  - kyphosis — *see* Kyphosis, congenital
  - lordosis — *see* Lordosis, congenital
- nerve Q07.8
- nose Q30.8
- organ
  - of Corti Q16.5
  - or site not listed — *see* Anomaly, by site
- ossicles, ear Q16.3
- oviduct Q50.6
- pancreas Q45.3
- parathyroid (gland) Q89.2
- pituitary (gland) Q89.2
- radius NEC Q68.8
- sacroiliac joint Q74.2
- sacrum Q76.49
- scapula Q74.0
- shoulder girdle Q74.0
- skull bone (s) NEC Q75.8
  - with
    - anencephalus Q00.0
    - encephalocele — *see* Encephalocele
    - hydrocephalus Q03.9
      - with spina bifida — *see* Spina bifida, with hydrocephalus
    - microcephaly Q02
- spinal cord Q06.8
- spine Q76.49
  - kyphosis — *see* Kyphosis, congenital
  - lordosis — *see* Lordosis, congenital
- spleen Q89.09
- sternum NEC Q76.7
- thorax (wall) Q67.8
  - bony Q76.8
- thymus (gland) Q89.2
- thyroid (gland) Q89.2
- tibia NEC Q68.8
- toe (s) Q66.9
- tongue Q38.3
- trachea (cartilage) Q32.1
- ulna NEC Q68.8
- ureter Q62.8
- urethra Q64.79
  - causing obstruction Q64.39
- uterus Q51.9
- vagina Q52.4
- vertebra Q76.49
  - kyphosis — *see* Kyphosis, congenital
  - lordosis — *see* Lordosis, congenital
- visual (*see also* Disturbance, vision)
  - shape and size H53.15
- vulva Q52.79
- wrist (bones) (joint) Q68.8

Distress
- abdomen — *see* Pain, abdominal
- acute respiratory R06.00
  - syndrome (adult) (child) J80
- epigastric R10.13

Distress — *continued*
- fetal P84
  - complicating pregnancy — *see* Stress, fetal
- gastrointestinal (functional) K30
  - psychogenic F45.8
- intestinal (functional) NOS K59.9
  - psychogenic F45.8
- maternal, during labor and delivery O75.0
- respiratory (adult) (child) R06.00
  - newborn P22.9
    - specified NEC P22.8
  - orthopnea R06.01
  - psychogenic F45.8
  - shortness of breath R06.02
  - specified type NEC R06.09

Distribution vessel, atypical Q27.9
- coronary artery Q24.5
- precerebral Q28.1

Districhiasis L68.8

Disturbance (s) (*see also* Disease)
- absorption K90.9
  - calcium E58
  - carbohydrate K90.49
  - fat K90.49
    - pancreatic K90.3
  - protein K90.49
  - starch K90.49
  - vitamin — *see* Deficiency, vitamin
- acid-base equilibrium E87.8
  - mixed E87.4
- activity and attention (with hyperkinesis) — *see* Disorder, attention-deficit hyperactivity
- amino acid transport E72.00
- assimilation, food K90.9
- auditory nerve, except deafness — *see* subcategory H93.3
- behavior — *see* Disorder, conduct
- blood clotting (mechanism) (*see also* Defect, coagulation)D68.9
- cerebral
  - nerve — *see* Disorder, nerve, cranial
  - status, newborn P91.9
    - specified NEC P91.8
- circulatory I99.9
- conduct (*see also* Disorder, conduct)F91.9
  - adjustment reaction — *see* Disorder, adjustment
  - compulsive F63.9
  - disruptive F91.9
  - hyperkinetic — *see* Disorder, attention-deficit hyperactivity
  - socialized F91.2
  - specified NEC F91.8
  - unsocialized F91.1
- coordination R27.8
- cranial nerve — *see* Disorder, nerve, cranial
- deep sensibility — *see* Disturbance, sensation
- digestive K30
  - psychogenic F45.8
- electrolyte (*see also* Imbalance, electrolyte)
  - newborn, transitory P74.4
    - hyperammonemia P74.6
    - potassium balance P74.3
    - sodium balance P74.2
    - specified type NEC P74.4
- emotions specific to childhood and adolescence F93.9
  - with
    - anxiety and fearfulness NEC F93.8
    - elective mutism F94.0
    - oppositional disorder F91.3
    - sensitivity (withdrawal) F40.10
    - shyness F40.10
    - social withdrawal F40.10
  - involving relationship problems F93.8
  - mixed F93.8
  - specified NEC F93.8
- endocrine (gland) E34.9
  - neonatal, transitory P72.9
    - specified NEC P72.8
- equilibrium R42
- fructose metabolism E74.10
- gait — *see* Gait
  - hysterical F44.4
  - psychogenic F44.4
- gastrointestinal (functional) K30
  - psychogenic F45.8
- habit, child F98.9
- hearing, except deafness and tinnitus — *see* Abnormal, auditory perception
- heart, functional (conditions in I44-I50)

Disturbance — *continued*
- heart, functional — *continued*
  - due to presence of (cardiac) prosthesis I97.19 ☑
  - postoperative I97.89
    - cardiac surgery I97.19 ☑
- hormones E34.9
- innervation uterus (parasympathetic) (sympathetic) N85.8
- keratinization NEC
  - gingiva K05.10
    - nonplaque induced K05.11
    - plaque induced K05.10
  - lip K13.0
  - oral (mucosa) (soft tissue) K13.29
  - tongue K13.29
- learning (specific) — *see* Disorder, learning
- memory — *see* Amnesia
  - mild, following organic brain damage F06.8
- mental F99
  - associated with diseases classified elsewhere F54
- metabolism E88.9
  - with
    - abortion — *see* Abortion, by type with other specified complication
    - ectopic pregnancy O08.5
    - molar pregnancy O08.5
  - amino-acid E72.9
    - aromatic E70.9
    - branched-chain E71.2
    - straight-chain E72.8
    - sulfur-bearing E72.10
  - ammonia E72.20
  - arginine E72.21
  - arginosuccinic acid E72.22
  - carbohydrate E74.9
  - cholesterol E78.9
  - citrulline E72.23
  - cystathionine E72.19
  - general E88.9
  - glutamine E72.8
  - histidine E70.40
  - homocystine E72.19
  - hydroxylysine E72.3
  - in labor or delivery O75.89
  - iron E83.10
  - lipoid E78.9
  - lysine E72.3
  - methionine E72.19
  - neonatal, transitory P74.9
    - calcium and magnesium P71.9
      - specified type NEC P71.8
    - carbohydrate metabolism P70.9
      - specified type NEC P70.8
    - specified NEC P74.8
  - ornithine E72.4
  - phosphate E83.39
  - sodium NEC E87.8
  - threonine E72.8
  - tryptophan E70.5
  - tyrosine E70.20
  - urea cycle E72.20
- motor R29.2
- nervous, functional R45.0
- neuromuscular mechanism (eye), due to syphilis A52.15
- nutritional E63.9
  - nail L60.3
- ocular motion H51.9
  - psychogenic F45.8
- oculogyric H51.8
  - psychogenic F45.8
- oculomotor H51.9
  - psychogenic F45.8
- olfactory nerve R43.1
- optic nerve NEC — *see* Disorder, nerve, optic
- oral epithelium, including tongue NEC K13.29
- perceptual due to
  - alcohol withdrawal F10.232
  - amphetamine intoxication F15.922
    - in
      - abuse F15.122
      - dependence F15.222
  - anxiolytic withdrawal F13.232
  - cannabis intoxication (acute) F12.922
    - in
      - abuse F12.122
      - dependence F12.222
  - cocaine intoxication (acute) F14.922
    - in
      - abuse F14.122

Disturbance — *continued*
- perceptual due to — *continued*
  - cocaine intoxication (acute) F14.922
    - in
      - dependence F14.222
  - hypnotic withdrawal F13.232
  - opioid intoxication (acute) F11.922
    - in
      - abuse F11.122
      - dependence F11.222
  - phencyclidine intoxication (acute) F16.122
  - sedative withdrawal F13.232
- personality (pattern) (trait) (*see also* Disorder, personality)F60.9
  - following organic brain damage F07.9
- polyglandular E31.9
  - specified NEC E31.8
- potassium balance, newborn P74.3
- psychogenic F45.9
- psychomotor F44.4
- psychophysical visual H53.16
- pupillary — *see* Anomaly, pupil, function
- reflex R29.2
- rhythm, heart I49.9
- salivary secretion K11.7
- sensation (cold) (heat) (localization) (tactile discrimination) (texture) (vibratory) NEC R20.9
  - hysterical F44.6
  - skin R20.9
    - anesthesia R20.0
    - hyperesthesia R20.3
    - hypoesthesia R20.1
    - paresthesia R20.2
    - specified type NEC R20.8
  - smell R43.9
    - and taste (mixed) R43.8
    - anosmia R43.0
    - parosmia R43.1
    - specified NEC R43.8
  - taste R43.9
    - and smell (mixed) R43.8
    - parageusia R43.2
    - specified NEC R43.8
- sensory — *see* Disturbance, sensation
- situational (transient) (*see also* Disorder, adjustment)
  - acute F43.0
- sleep G47.9
  - nonorganic origin F51.9
- smell — *see* Disturbance, sensation, smell
- sociopathic F60.2
- sodium balance, newborn P74.2
- speech R47.9
  - developmental F80.9
  - specified NEC R47.89
- stomach (functional) K31.9
- sympathetic (nerve) G90.9
- taste — *see* Disturbance, sensation, taste
- temperature
  - regulation, newborn P81.9
    - specified NEC P81.8
  - sense R20.8
    - hysterical F44.6
- tooth
  - eruption K00.6
  - formation K00.4
  - structure, hereditary NEC K00.5
- touch — *see* Disturbance, sensation
- vascular I99.9
  - arteriosclerotic — *see* Arteriosclerosis
- vasomotor I73.9
- vasospastic I73.9
- vision, visual H53.9
  - following
    - cerebral infarction I69.398
    - cerebrovascular disease I69.998
      - specified NEC I69.898
    - intracerebral hemorrhage I69.198
    - nontraumatic intracranial hemorrhage NEC I69.298
    - specified disease NEC I69.898
    - subarachnoid hemorrhage I69.098
  - psychophysical H53.16
  - specified NEC H53.8
  - subjective H53.10
    - day blindness H53.11
    - discomfort H53.14 ☑
    - distortions of shape and size H53.15
    - loss
      - sudden H53.13 ☑
      - transient H53.12 ☑
    - specified type NEC H53.19

- **Disturbance** — *continued*
  - voice R49.9
    - psychogenic F44.4
    - specified NEC R49.8
- **Diuresis** R35.8
- **Diver's** palsy, paralysis or squeeze T70.3 ☑
- **Diverticulitis** (acute) K57.92
  - bladder — *see* Cystitis
  - ileum — *see* Diverticulitis, intestine, small
  - intestine K57.92
    - with
      - abscess, perforation or peritonitis K57.80
        - with bleeding K57.81
      - bleeding K57.93
    - congenital Q43.8
    - large K57.32
      - with
        - abscess, perforation or peritonitis K57.20
          - with bleeding K57.21
        - bleeding K57.33
        - small intestine K57.52
          - with
            - abscess, perforation or peritonitis K57.40
              - with bleeding K57.41
            - bleeding K57.53
    - small K57.12
      - with
        - abscess, perforation or peritonitis K57.00
          - with bleeding K57.01
        - bleeding K57.13
        - large intestine K57.52
          - with
            - abscess, perforation or peritonitis K57.40
              - with bleeding K57.41
            - bleeding K57.53
- **Diverticulosis** K57.90
  - with bleeding K57.91
  - large intestine K57.30
    - with
      - bleeding K57.31
      - small intestine K57.50
        - with bleeding K57.51
  - small intestine K57.10
    - with
      - bleeding K57.11
      - large intestine K57.50
        - with bleeding K57.51
- **Diverticulum,** diverticula (multiple) K57.90
  - appendix (noninflammatory) K38.2
  - bladder (sphincter) N32.3
    - congenital Q64.6
  - bronchus (congenital) Q32.4
    - acquired J98.09
  - calyx, calyceal (kidney) N28.89
  - cardia (stomach) K31.4
  - cecum — *see* Diverticulosis, intestine, large
    - congenital Q43.8
  - colon — *see* Diverticulosis, intestine, large
    - congenital Q43.8
  - duodenum — *see* Diverticulosis, intestine, small
    - congenital Q43.8
  - epiphrenic (esophagus) K22.5
  - esophagus (congenital) Q39.6
    - acquired (epiphrenic) (pulsion) (traction) K22.5
  - eustachian tube — *see* Disorder, eustachian tube, specified NEC
  - fallopian tube N83.8
  - gastric K31.4
  - heart (congenital) Q24.8
  - ileum — *see* Diverticulosis, intestine, small
  - jejunum — *see* Diverticulosis, intestine, small
  - kidney (pelvis) (calyces) N28.89
    - with calculus — *see* Calculus, kidney
  - Meckel's (displaced) (hypertrophic) Q43.0
    - malignant — *see* Table of Neoplasms, small intestine, malignant
  - midthoracic K22.5
  - organ or site, congenital NEC — *see* Distortion
  - pericardium (congenital) (cyst) Q24.8
    - acquired I31.8
  - pharyngoesophageal (congenital) Q39.6
    - acquired K22.5
  - pharynx (congenital) Q38.7
  - rectosigmoid — *see* Diverticulosis, intestine, large
    - congenital Q43.8
  - rectum — *see* Diverticulosis, intestine, large
  - Rokitansky's K22.5
  - seminal vesicle N50.89
  - sigmoid — *see* Diverticulosis, intestine, large
    - congenital Q43.8
- **Diverticulum** — *continued*
  - stomach (acquired) K31.4
    - congenital Q40.2
  - trachea (acquired) J39.8
  - ureter (acquired) N28.89
    - congenital Q62.8
  - ureterovesical orifice N28.89
  - urethra (acquired) N36.1
    - congenital Q64.79
  - ventricle, left (congenital) Q24.8
  - vesical N32.3
    - congenital Q64.6
  - Zenker's (esophagus) K22.5
- **Division**
  - cervix uteri (acquired) N88.8
  - glans penis Q55.69
  - labia minora (congenital) Q52.79
  - ligament (partial or complete) (current) (*see also* Sprain)
    - with open wound — *see* Wound, open
  - muscle (partial or complete) (current) (*see also* Injury, muscle)
    - with open wound — *see* Wound, open
  - nerve (traumatic) — *see* Injury, nerve
  - spinal cord — *see* Injury, spinal cord, by region
  - vein I87.8
- **Divorce,** causing family disruption Z63.5
- **Dix-Hallpike** neurolabyrinthitis — *see* Neuronitis, vestibular
- **Dizziness** R42
  - hysterical F44.89
  - psychogenic F45.8
- **DMAC** (disseminated mycobacterium avium-intracellulare complex) A31.2
- **DNR** (do not resuscitate) Z66
- **Doan-Wiseman** syndrome (primary splenic neutropenia) — *see* Agranulocytosis
- **Doehle-Heller** aortitis A52.02
- **Dog** bite — *see* Bite
- **Dohle** body panmyelopathic syndrome D72.0
- **Dolichocephaly** Q67.2
- **Dolichocolon** Q43.8
- **Dolichostenomelia** — *see* Syndrome, Marfan's
- **Donohue's** syndrome E34.8
- **Donor** (organ or tissue) Z52.9
  - blood (whole) Z52.000
    - autologous Z52.010
    - specified component (lymphocytes) (platelets) NEC Z52.008
      - autologous Z52.018
      - specified donor NEC Z52.098
    - specified donor NEC Z52.090
    - stem cells Z52.001
      - autologous Z52.011
      - specified donor NEC Z52.091
  - bone Z52.20
    - autologous Z52.21
    - marrow Z52.3
    - specified type NEC Z52.29
  - cornea Z52.5
  - egg (Oocyte) Z52.819
    - age 35 and over Z52.812
      - anonymous recipient Z52.812
      - designated recipient Z52.813
    - under age 35 Z52.810
      - anonymous recipient Z52.810
      - designated recipient Z52.811
  - kidney Z52.4
  - liver Z52.6
  - lung Z52.89
  - lymphocyte — *see* Donor, blood, specified components NEC
  - Oocyte — *see* Donor, egg
  - platelets Z52.008
  - potential, examination of Z00.5
  - semen Z52.89
  - skin Z52.10
    - autologous Z52.11
    - specified type NEC Z52.19
  - specified organ or tissue NEC Z52.89
  - sperm Z52.89
- **Donovanosis** A58
- **Dorsalgia** M54.9
  - psychogenic F45.41
  - specified NEC M54.89
- **Dorsopathy** M53.9
  - deforming M43.9
    - specified NEC — *see* subcategory M43.8
  - specified NEC M53.80
    - cervical region M53.82
    - cervicothoracic region M53.83
    - lumbar region M53.86
- **Dorsopathy** — *continued*
  - specified NEC — *continued*
    - lumbosacral region M53.87
    - occipito-atlanto-axial region M53.81
    - sacrococcygeal region M53.88
    - thoracic region M53.84
    - thoracolumbar region M53.85
- **Double**
  - albumin E88.09
  - aortic arch Q25.45
  - auditory canal Q17.8
  - auricle (heart) Q20.8
  - bladder Q64.79
  - cervix Q51.820
    - with doubling of uterus (and vagina) Q51.10
      - with obstruction Q51.11
  - inlet ventricle Q20.4
  - kidney with double pelvis (renal) Q63.0
  - meatus urinarius Q64.75
  - monster Q89.4
  - outlet
    - left ventricle Q20.2
    - right ventricle Q20.1
  - pelvis (renal) with double ureter Q62.5
  - tongue Q38.3
  - ureter (one or both sides) Q62.5
    - with double pelvis (renal) Q62.5
  - urethra Q64.74
  - urinary meatus Q64.75
  - uterus Q51.2
    - with
      - doubling of cervix (and vagina) Q51.10
        - with obstruction Q51.11
    - in pregnancy or childbirth O34.59 ☑
      - causing obstructed labor O65.5
  - vagina Q52.10
    - with doubling of uterus (and cervix) Q51.10
      - with obstruction Q51.11
  - vision H53.2
  - vulva Q52.79
- **Douglas'** pouch, cul-de-sac — *see* condition
- **Down** syndrome Q90.9
  - meiotic nondisjunction Q90.0
  - mitotic nondisjunction Q90.1
  - mosaicism Q90.1
  - translocation Q90.2
- **DPD** (dihydropyrimidine dehydrogenase deficiency) E88.89
- **Dracontiasis** B72
- **Dracunculiasis,** dracunculosis B72
- **Dream** state, hysterical F44.89
- **Dreschlera** (hawaiiensis) (infection) B43.8
- **Drepanocytic** anemia — *see* Disease, sickle-cell
- **Dresbach's** syndrome (elliptocytosis) D58.1
- **Dressler's** syndrome I24.1
- **Drift,** ulnar — *see* Deformity, limb, specified type NEC, forearm
- **Drinking** (alcohol)
  - excessive, to excess NEC (without dependence) F10.10
    - habitual (continual) (without remission) F10.20
      - with remission F10.21
- **Drip,** postnasal (chronic) R09.82
  - due to
    - allergic rhinitis — *see* Rhinitis, allergic
    - common cold J00
    - gastroesophageal reflux — *see* Reflux, gastroesophageal
    - nasopharyngitis — *see* Nasopharyngitis
    - other know condition - code to condition
    - sinusitis — *see* Sinusitis
- **Droop**
  - facial R29.810
    - cerebrovascular disease I69.992
      - cerebral infarction I69.392
      - intracerebral hemorrhage I69.192
      - nontraumatic intracranial hemorrhage NEC I69.292
      - specified disease NEC I69.892
      - subarachnoid hemorrhage I69.092
- **Drop** (in)
  - attack NEC R55
  - finger — *see* Deformity, finger
  - foot — *see* Deformity, limb, foot, drop
  - hematocrit (precipitous) R71.0
  - hemoglobin R71.0
  - toe — *see* Deformity, toe, specified NEC
  - wrist — *see* Deformity, limb, wrist drop
- **Dropped** heart beats I45.9
- **Dropsy,** dropsical (*see also* Hydrops)
  - abdomen R18.8
  - brain — *see* Hydrocephalus

Dropsy — *continued*
- cardiac, heart — *see* Failure, heart, congestive
- gangrenous — *see* Gangrene
- heart — *see* Failure, heart, congestive
- kidney — *see* Nephrosis
- lung — *see* Edema, lung
- newborn due to isoimmunization P56.0
- pericardium — *see* Pericarditis

Drowned, drowning (near) T75.1 ☑
Drowsiness R40.0
Drug
- abuse counseling and surveillance Z71.51
- addiction — *see* Dependence
- dependence — *see* Dependence
- habit — *see* Dependence
- harmful use — *see* Abuse, drug
- induced fever R50.2
- overdose — *see* Table of Drugs and Chemicals, by drug, poisoning
- poisoning — *see* Table of Drugs and Chemicals, by drug, poisoning
- resistant organism infection (*see also* Resistant, organism, to, drug)Z16.30
- therapy
  - long term (current) (prophylactic) — *see* Therapy, drug long-term (current) (prophylactic)
  - short term - omit code
- wrong substance given or taken in error — *see* Table of Drugs and Chemicals, by drug, poisoning

Drunkenness (without dependence) F10.129
- acute in alcoholism F10.229
- chronic (without remission) F10.20
  - with remission F10.21
- pathological (without dependence) F10.129
  - with dependence F10.229
- sleep F51.9

Drusen
- macula (degenerative) (retina) — *see* Degeneration, macula, drusen
- optic disc H47.32 ☑

Dry, dryness (*see also* condition)
- larynx J38.7
- mouth R68.2
  - due to dehydration E86.0
- nose J34.89
- socket (teeth) M27.3
- throat J39.2

DSAP L56.5
Duane's syndrome H50.81 ☑
Dubin-Johnson disease or syndrome E80.6
Dubois' disease (thymus gland) A50.59 *[E35]*
Dubowitz' syndrome Q87.1
Duchenne-Aran muscular atrophy G12.21
Duchenne-Griesinger disease G71.0
Duchenne's
- disease or syndrome
  - motor neuron disease G12.22
  - muscular dystrophy G71.0
- locomotor ataxia (syphilitic) A52.11
- paralysis
  - birth injury P14.0
  - due to or associated with
    - motor neuron disease G12.22
    - muscular dystrophy G71.0

Ducrey's chancre A57
Duct, ductus — *see* condition
Duhring's disease (dermatitis herpetiformis) L13.0
Dullness, cardiac (decreased) (increased) R01.2
Dumb ague — *see* Malaria
Dumbness — *see* Aphasia
Dumdum fever B55.0
Dumping syndrome (postgastrectomy) K91.1
Duodenitis (nonspecific) (peptic) K29.80
- with bleeding K29.81

Duodenocholangitis — *see* Cholangitis
Duodenum, duodenal — *see* condition
Duplay's bursitis or periarthritis — *see* Tendinitis, calcific, shoulder
Duplication, duplex (*see also* Accessory)
- alimentary tract Q45.8
- anus Q43.4
- appendix (and cecum) Q43.4
- biliary duct (any) Q44.5
- bladder Q64.79
- cecum (and appendix) Q43.4
- cervix Q51.820
- chromosome NEC
  - with complex rearrangements NEC Q92.5
  - seen only at prometaphase Q92.8
- cystic duct Q44.5

Duplication — *continued*
- digestive organs Q45.8
- esophagus Q39.8
- frontonasal process Q75.8
- intestine (large) (small) Q43.4
- kidney Q63.0
- liver Q44.7
- pancreas Q45.3
- penis Q55.69
- respiratory organs NEC Q34.8
- salivary duct Q38.4
- spinal cord (incomplete) Q06.2
- stomach Q40.2

Dupré's disease (meningism) R29.1
Dupuytren's contraction or disease M72.0
Durand-Nicolas-Favre disease A55
Durotomy (inadvertent) (incidental) G97.41
Duroziez's disease (congenital mitral stenosis) Q23.2
Dutton's relapsing fever (West African) A68.1
Dwarfism E34.3
- achondroplastic Q77.4
- congenital E34.3
- constitutional E34.3
- hypochondroplastic Q77.4
- hypophyseal E23.0
- infantile E34.3
- Laron-type E34.3
- Lorain (-Levi) type E23.0
- metatropic Q77.8
- nephrotic-glycosuric (with hypophosphatemic rickets) E72.09
- nutritional E45
- pancreatic K86.89
- pituitary E23.0
- renal N25.0
- thanatophoric Q77.1

Dyke-Young anemia (secondary) (symptomatic) D59.1
Dysacusis — *see* Abnormal, auditory perception
Dysadrenocortism E27.9
- hyperfunction E27.0

Dysarthria R47.1
- following
  - cerebral infarction I69.322
  - cerebrovascular disease I69.922
    - specified disease NEC I69.822
  - intracerebral hemorrhage I69.122
  - nontraumatic intracranial hemorrhage NEC I69.222
  - subarachnoid hemorrhage I69.022

Dysautonomia (familial) G90.1
Dysbarism T70.3 ☑
Dysbasia R26.2
- angiosclerotica intermittens I73.9
- hysterical F44.4
- lordotica (progressiva) G24.1
- nonorganic origin F44.4
- psychogenic F44.4

Dysbetalipoproteinemia (familial) E78.2
Dyscalculia R48.8
- developmental F81.2

Dyschezia K59.00
Dyschondroplasia (with hemangiomata) Q78.4
Dyschromia (skin) L81.9
Dyscollagenosis M35.9
Dyscranio-pygo-phalangy Q87.0
Dyscrasia
- blood (with) D75.9
  - antepartum hemorrhage — *see* Hemorrhage, antepartum, with coagulation defect
  - newborn P61.9
    - specified type NEC P61.8
  - intrapartum hemorrhage O67.0
  - puerperal, postpartum O72.3
- polyglandular, pluriglandular E31.9

Dysendocrinism E34.9
Dysentery, dysenteric (catarrhal) (diarrhea) (epidemic) (hemorrhagic) (infectious) (sporadic) (tropical) A09
- abscess, liver A06.4
- amebic (*see also* Amebiasis)A06.0
  - with abscess — *see* Abscess, amebic
  - acute A06.0
  - chronic A06.1
- arthritis (*see also* category M01)A09
  - bacillary (*see also* category M01)A03.9
- bacillary A03.9
  - arthritis (*see also* category M01)A03.9
  - Boyd A03.2
  - Flexner A03.1
  - Schmitz (-Stutzer) A03.0
  - Shiga (-Kruse) A03.0

Dysentery — *continued*
- bacillary — *continued*
  - Shigella A03.9
    - boydii A03.2
    - dysenteriae A03.0
    - flexneri A03.1
    - group A A03.0
    - group B A03.1
    - group C A03.2
    - group D A03.3
    - sonnei A03.3
    - specified type NEC A03.8
  - Sonne A03.3
  - specified type NEC A03.8
- balantidial A07.0
- Balantidium coli A07.0
- Boyd's A03.2
- candidal B37.82
- Chilomastix A07.8
- Chinese A03.9
- coccidial A07.3
- Dientamoeba (fragilis) A07.8
- Embadomonas A07.8
- Entamoeba, entamebic — *see* Dysentery, amebic
- Flexner-Boyd A03.2
- Flexner's A03.1
- Giardia lamblia A07.1
- Hiss-Russell A03.1
- Lamblia A07.1
- leishmanial B55.0
- malarial — *see* Malaria
- metazoal B82.0
- monilial B37.82
- protozoal A07.9
- Salmonella A02.0
- schistosomal B65.1
- Schmitz (-Stutzer) A03.0
- Shiga (-Kruse) A03.0
- Shigella NOS — *see* Dysentery, bacillary
- Sonne A03.3
- strongyloidiasis B78.0
- trichomonal A07.8
- viral (*see also* Enteritis, viral)A08.4

Dysequilibrium R42
Dysesthesia R20.8
- hysterical F44.6

Dysfibrinogenemia (congenital) D68.2
Dysfunction
- adrenal E27.9
  - hyperfunction E27.0
- autonomic
  - due to alcohol G31.2
  - somatoform F45.8
- bladder N31.9
  - neurogenic NOS — *see* Dysfunction, bladder, neuromuscular
  - neuromuscular NOS N31.9
    - atonic (motor) (sensory) N31.2
    - autonomous N31.2
    - flaccid N31.2
    - nonreflex N31.2
    - reflex N31.1
    - specified NEC N31.8
    - uninhibited N31.0
- bleeding, uterus N93.8
- cerebral G93.89
- colon K59.9
  - psychogenic F45.8
- colostomy K94.03
- cystic duct K82.8
- cystostomy (stoma) — *see* Complications, cystostomy
- ejaculatory N53.19
  - anejaculatory orgasm N53.13
  - painful N53.12
  - premature F52.4
  - retarded N53.11
- endocrine NOS E34.9
- endometrium N85.8
- enterostomy K94.13
- erectile — *see* Dysfunction, sexual, male, erectile
- gallbladder K82.8
- gastrostomy (stoma) K94.23
- gland, glandular NOS E34.9
- heart I51.89
- hemoglobin D75.89
- hepatic K76.89
- hypophysis E23.7
- hypothalamic NEC E23.3
- ileostomy (stoma) K94.13
- jejunostomy (stoma) K94.13
- kidney — *see* Disease, renal

Dysfunction - Dyspepsia

- **Dysfunction** — *continued*
  - labyrinthine — *see* subcategory H83.2
  - left ventricular, following sudden emotional stress I51.81
  - liver K76.89
  - male — *see* Dysfunction, sexual, male
  - orgasmic (female) F52.31
    - male F52.32
  - ovary E28.9
    - specified NEC E28.8
  - papillary muscle I51.89
  - parathyroid E21.4
  - physiological NEC R68.89
    - psychogenic F59
  - pineal gland E34.8
  - pituitary (gland) E23.3
  - platelets D69.1
  - polyglandular E31.9
    - specified NEC E31.8
  - psychophysiologic F59
  - psychosexual F52.9
    - with
      - dyspareunia F52.6
      - premature ejaculation F52.4
      - vaginismus F52.5
  - pylorus K31.9
  - rectum K59.9
    - psychogenic F45.8
  - reflex (sympathetic) — *see* Syndrome, pain, complex regional I
  - segmental — *see* Dysfunction, somatic
  - senile R54
  - sexual (due to) R37
    - alcohol F10.981
    - amphetamine F15.981
      - in
        - abuse F15.181
        - dependence F15.281
    - anxiolytic F13.981
      - in
        - abuse F13.181
        - dependence F13.281
    - cocaine F14.981
      - in
        - abuse F14.181
        - dependence F14.281
    - excessive sexual drive F52.8
    - failure of genital response (male) F52.21
      - female F52.22
    - female N94.9
      - aversion F52.1
      - dyspareunia N94.10
        - psychogenic F52.6
      - frigidity F52.22
      - nymphomania F52.8
      - orgasmic F52.31
      - psychogenic F52.9
        - aversion F52.1
        - dyspareunia F52.6
        - frigidity F52.22
        - nymphomania F52.8
        - orgasmic F52.31
        - vaginismus F52.5
      - vaginismus N94.2
        - psychogenic F52.5
    - hypnotic F13.981
      - in
        - abuse F13.181
        - dependence F13.281
    - inhibited orgasm (female) F52.31
      - male F52.32
    - lack
      - of sexual enjoyment F52.1
      - or loss of sexual desire F52.0
    - male N53.9
      - anejaculatory orgasm N53.13
      - ejaculatory N53.19
        - painful N53.12
        - premature F52.4
        - retarded N53.11
      - erectile N52.9
        - drug induced N52.2
        - due to
          - disease classified elsewhere N52.1
          - drug N52.2
        - postoperative (postprocedural) N52.39
          - following
            - cryotherapy N52.37
            - interstitial seed therapy N52.36
            - prostate ablative therapy N52.37
            - prostatectomy N52.34
              - radical N52.31

- **Dysfunction** — *continued*
  - sexual — *continued*
            - radiation therapy N52.35
            - radical cystectomy N52.32
            - ultrasound ablative therapy N52.37
            - urethral surgery N52.33
        - psychogenic F52.21
        - specified cause NEC N52.8
        - vasculogenic
          - arterial insufficiency N52.01
            - with corporo-venous occlusive N52.03
          - corporo-venous occlusive N52.02
            - with arterial insufficiency N52.03
      - impotence — *see* Dysfunction, sexual, male, erectile
      - psychogenic F52.9
        - aversion F52.1
        - erectile F52.21
        - orgasmic F52.32
        - premature ejaculation F52.4
        - satyriasis F52.8
        - specified type NEC F52.8
      - specified type NEC N53.8
    - nonorganic F52.9
      - specified NEC F52.8
    - opioid F11.981
      - in
        - abuse F11.181
        - dependence F11.281
    - orgasmic dysfunction (female) F52.31
      - male F52.32
    - premature ejaculation F52.4
    - psychoactive substances NEC F19.981
      - in
        - abuse F19.181
        - dependence F19.281
    - psychogenic F52.9
    - sedative F13.981
      - in
        - abuse F13.181
        - dependence F13.281
    - sexual aversion F52.1
    - vaginismus (nonorganic) (psychogenic) F52.5
  - sinoatrial node I49.5
  - somatic M99.09
    - abdomen M99.09
    - acromioclavicular M99.07
    - cervical region M99.01
    - cervicothoracic M99.01
    - costochondral M99.08
    - costovertebral M99.08
    - head region M99.00
    - hip M99.05
    - lower extremity M99.06
    - lumbar region M99.03
    - lumbosacral M99.03
    - occipitocervical M99.00
    - pelvic region M99.05
    - pubic M99.05
    - rib cage M99.08
    - sacral region M99.04
    - sacrococcygeal M99.04
    - sacroiliac M99.04
    - specified NEC M99.09
    - sternochondral M99.08
    - sternoclavicular M99.07
    - thoracic region M99.02
    - thoracolumbar M99.02
    - upper extremity M99.07
  - somatoform autonomic F45.8
  - stomach K31.89
    - psychogenic F45.8
  - suprarenal E27.9
    - hyperfunction E27.0
  - symbolic R48.9
    - specified type NEC R48.8
  - temporomandibular (joint) M26.69
    - joint-pain syndrome M26.62 ☑
  - testicular (endocrine) E29.9
    - specified NEC E29.8
  - thymus E32.9
  - thyroid E07.9
  - ureterostomy (stoma) — *see* Complications, stoma, urinary tract
  - urethrostomy (stoma) — *see* Complications, stoma, urinary tract
  - uterus, complicating delivery O62.9
    - hypertonic O62.4
    - hypotonic O62.2
      - primary O62.0
      - secondary O62.1

- **Dysfunction** — *continued*
  - ventricular I51.9
    - with congestive heart failure I50.9- - left, reversible, following sudden emotional stress I51.81
- **Dysgenesis**
  - gonadal (due to chromosomal anomaly) Q96.9
    - pure Q99.1
  - renal Q60.5
    - bilateral Q60.4
    - unilateral Q60.3
  - reticular D72.0
  - tidal platelet D69.3
- **Dysgerminoma**
  - specified site — *see* Neoplasm, malignant, by site
  - unspecified site
    - female C56.9
    - male C62.90
- **Dysgeusia** R43.2
- **Dysgraphia** R27.8
- **Dyshidrosis,** dysidrosis L30.1
- **Dyskaryotic** cervical smear R87.619
- **Dyskeratosis** L85.8
  - cervix — *see* Dysplasia, cervix
  - congenital Q82.8
  - uterus NEC N85.8
- **Dyskinesia** G24.9
  - biliary (cystic duct or gallbladder) K82.8
  - drug induced
    - orofacial G24.01
  - esophagus K22.4
  - hysterical F44.4
  - intestinal K59.8
  - nonorganic origin F44.4
  - orofacial (idiopathic) G24.4
    - drug induced G24.01
  - psychogenic F44.4
  - subacute, drug induced G24.01
  - tardive G24.01
    - neuroleptic induced G24.01
  - trachea J39.8
  - tracheobronchial J98.09
- **Dyslalia** (developmental) F80.0
- **Dyslexia** R48.0
  - developmental F81.0
- **Dyslipidemia** E78.5
  - depressed HDL cholesterol E78.6
  - elevated fasting triglycerides E78.1
- **Dysmaturity** (*see also* Light for dates)
  - pulmonary (newborn) (Wilson-Mikity) P27.0
- **Dysmenorrhea** (essential) (exfoliative) N94.6
  - congestive (syndrome) N94.6
  - primary N94.4
  - psychogenic F45.8
  - secondary N94.5
- **Dysmetabolic** syndrome X E88.81
- **Dysmetria** R27.8
- **Dysmorphism** (due to)
  - alcohol Q86.0
  - exogenous cause NEC Q86.8
  - hydantoin Q86.1
  - warfarin Q86.2
- **Dysmorphophobia** (nondelusional) F45.22
  - delusional F22
- **Dysnomia** R47.01
- **Dysorexia** R63.0
  - psychogenic F50.89
- **Dysostosis**
  - cleidocranial, cleidocranialis Q74.0
  - craniofacial Q75.1
  - Fairbank's (idiopathic familial generalized osteophytosis) Q78.9
  - mandibulofacial (incomplete) Q75.4
  - multiplex E76.01
  - oculomandibular Q75.5
- **Dyspareunia** (female) N94.10
  - deep N94.12
  - male N53.12
  - nonorganic F52.6
  - psychogenic F52.6
  - secondary N94.19
  - specified NEC N94.19
  - superficial (introital) N94.11
- **Dyspepsia** R10.13
  - atonic K30
  - functional (allergic) (congenital) (gastrointestinal) (occupational) (reflex) K30
  - intestinal K59.8
  - nervous F45.8
  - neurotic F45.8
  - psychogenic F45.8

- **Dysphagia** R13.10
  - cervical R13.19
  - following
    - cerebral infarction I69.391
    - cerebrovascular disease I69.991
      - specified NEC I69.891
    - intracerebral hemorrhage I69.191
    - nontraumatic intracranial hemorrhage NEC I69.291
    - specified disease NEC I69.891
    - subarachnoid hemorrhage I69.091
  - functional (hysterical) F45.8
  - hysterical F45.8
  - nervous (hysterical) F45.8
  - neurogenic R13.19
  - oral phase R13.11
  - oropharyngeal phase R13.12
  - pharyngeal phase R13.13
  - pharyngoesophageal phase R13.14
  - psychogenic F45.8
  - sideropenic D50.1
  - spastica K22.4
  - specified NEC R13.19
- **Dysphagocytosis,** congenital D71
- **Dysphasia** R47.02
  - developmental
    - expressive type F80.1
    - receptive type F80.2
  - following
    - cerebrovascular disease I69.921
      - cerebral infarction I69.321
      - intracerebral hemorrhage I69.121
      - nontraumatic intracranial hemorrhage NEC I69.221
      - specified disease NEC I69.821
      - subarachnoid hemorrhage I69.021
- **Dysphonia** R49.0
  - functional F44.4
  - hysterical F44.4
  - psychogenic F44.4
  - spastica J38.3
- **Dysphoria**
  - gender
    - in
      - adolescence and adulthood F64.0
      - children F64.2
  - postpartal O90.6
- **Dyspituitarism** E23.3
- **Dysplasia** (*see also* Anomaly)
  - acetabular, congenital Q65.89
  - alveolar capillary, with vein misalignment J84.843
  - anus (histologically confirmed) (mild) (moderate) K62.82
    - severe D01.3
  - arrhythmogenic right ventricular I42.8
  - arterial, fibromuscular I77.3
  - asphyxiating thoracic (congenital) Q77.2
  - brain Q07.9
  - bronchopulmonary, perinatal P27.1
  - cervix (uteri) N87.9
    - mild N87.0
    - moderate N87.1
    - severe D06.9
  - chondroectodermal Q77.6
  - colon D12.6
  - craniometaphyseal Q78.8
  - dentinal K00.5
  - diaphyseal, progressive Q78.3
  - dystrophic Q77.5
  - ectodermal (anhidrotic) (congenital) (hereditary) Q82.4
    - hydrotic Q82.8
  - epithelial, uterine cervix — *see* Dysplasia, cervix
  - eye (congenital) Q11.2
  - fibrous
    - bone NEC (monostotic) M85.00
      - ankle M85.07 ☑
      - foot M85.07 ☑
      - forearm M85.03 ☑
      - hand M85.04 ☑
      - lower leg M85.06 ☑
      - multiple site M85.09
      - neck M85.08
      - rib M85.08
      - shoulder M85.01 ☑
      - skull M85.08
      - specified site NEC M85.08
      - thigh M85.05 ☑
      - toe M85.07 ☑
      - upper arm M85.02 ☑
      - vertebra M85.08
    - diaphyseal, progressive Q78.3

- **Dysplasia** — *continued*
  - fibrous — *continued*
    - jaw M27.8
    - polyostotic Q78.1
  - florid osseous (*see also* Cyst, calcifying odontogenic)
  - high grade, focal D12.6
  - hip, congenital Q65.89
  - joint, congenital Q74.8
  - kidney Q61.4
    - multicystic Q61.4
  - leg Q74.2
  - lung, congenital (not associated with short gestation) Q33.6
  - mammary (gland) (benign) N60.9 ☑
    - cyst (solitary) — *see* Cyst, breast
    - cystic — *see* Mastopathy, cystic
    - duct ectasia — *see* Ectasia, mammary duct
    - fibroadenosis — *see* Fibroadenosis, breast
    - fibrosclerosis — *see* Fibrosclerosis, breast
    - specified type NEC N60.8 ☑
  - metaphyseal Q78.5
  - muscle Q79.8
  - oculodentodigital Q87.0
  - periapical (cemental) (cemento-osseous) — *see* Cyst, calcifying odontogenic
  - periosteum — *see* Disorder, bone, specified type NEC
  - polyostotic fibrous Q78.1
  - prostate (*see also* Neoplasia, intraepithelial, prostate)N42.30
    - severe D07.5
    - specified NEC N42.39
  - renal Q61.4
    - multicystic Q61.4
  - retinal, congenital Q14.1
  - right ventricular, arrhythmogenic I42.8
  - septo-optic Q04.4
  - skin L98.8
  - spinal cord Q06.1
  - spondyloepiphyseal Q77.7
  - thymic, with immunodeficiency D82.1
  - vagina N89.3
    - mild N89.0
    - moderate N89.1
    - severe NEC D07.2
  - vulva N90.3
    - mild N90.0
    - moderate N90.1
    - severe NEC D07.1
- **Dyspnea** (nocturnal) (paroxysmal) R06.00
  - asthmatic (bronchial) J45.909
    - with
      - exacerbation (acute) J45.901
      - bronchitis J45.909
        - with
          - exacerbation (acute) J45.901
          - status asthmaticus J45.902
        - chronic J44.9
      - status asthmaticus J45.902
    - cardiac — *see* Failure, ventricular, left
  - cardiac — *see* Failure, ventricular, left
  - functional F45.8
  - hyperventilation R06.4
  - hysterical F45.8
  - newborn P28.89
  - orthopnea R06.01
  - psychogenic F45.8
  - shortness of breath R06.02
  - specified type NEC R06.09
- **Dyspraxia** R27.8
  - developmental (syndrome) F82
- **Dysproteinemia** E88.09
- **Dysreflexia,** autonomic G90.4
- **Dysrhythmia**
  - cardiac I49.9
    - newborn
      - bradycardia P29.12
      - occurring before birth P03.819
        - before onset of labor P03.810
        - during labor P03.811
      - tachycardia P29.11
    - postoperative I97.89
  - cerebral or cortical — *see* Epilepsy
- **Dyssomnia** — *see* Disorder, sleep
- **Dyssynergia**
  - biliary K83.8
  - bladder sphincter N36.44
  - cerebellaris myoclonica (Hunt's ataxia) G11.1
- **Dysthymia** F34.1
- **Dysthyroidism** E07.9

- **Dystocia** O66.9
  - affecting newborn P03.1
  - cervical (hypotonic) O62.2
    - affecting newborn P03.6
    - primary O62.0
    - secondary O62.1
  - contraction ring O62.4
  - fetal O66.9
    - abnormality NEC O66.3
    - conjoined twins O66.3
    - oversize O66.2
  - maternal O66.9
  - positional O64.9 ☑
  - shoulder (girdle) O66.0
    - causing obstructed labor O66.0
  - uterine NEC O62.4
- **Dystonia** G24.9
  - deformans progressiva G24.1
  - drug induced NEC G24.09
    - acute G24.02
    - specified NEC G24.09
  - familial G24.1
  - idiopathic G24.1
    - familial G24.1
    - nonfamilial G24.2
    - orofacial G24.4
  - lenticularis G24.8
  - musculorum deformans G24.1
  - neuroleptic induced (acute) G24.02
  - orofacial (idiopathic) G24.4
  - oromandibular G24.4
    - due to drug G24.01
  - specified NEC G24.8
  - torsion (familial) (idiopathic) G24.1
    - acquired G24.8
    - genetic G24.1
    - symptomatic (nonfamilial) G24.2
- **Dystonic** movements R25.8
- **Dystrophy,** dystrophia
  - adiposogenital E23.6
  - Becker's type G71.0
  - cervical sympathetic G90.2
  - choroid (hereditary) H31.20
    - central areolar H31.22
    - choroideremia H31.21
    - gyrate atrophy H31.23
    - specified type NEC H31.29
  - cornea (hereditary) H18.50
    - endothelial H18.51
    - epithelial H18.52
    - granular H18.53
    - lattice H18.54
    - macular H18.55
    - specified type NEC H18.59
  - Duchenne's type G71.0
  - due to malnutrition E45
  - Erb's G71.0
  - Fuchs' H18.51
  - Gower's muscular G71.0
  - hair L67.8
  - infantile neuraxonal G31.89
  - Landouzy-Déjérine G71.0
  - Leyden-Möbius G71.0
  - muscular G71.0
    - benign (Becker type) G71.0
    - congenital (hereditary) (progressive) (with specific morphological abnormalities of the muscle fiber) G71.0
      - myotonic G71.11
    - distal G71.0
    - Duchenne type G71.0
    - Emery-Dreifuss G71.0
    - Erb type G71.0
    - facioscapulohumeral G71.0
    - Gower's G71.0
    - hereditary (progressive) G71.0
    - Landouzy-Déjérine type G71.0
    - limb-girdle G71.0
    - myotonic G71.11
    - progressive (hereditary) G71.0
      - Charcot-Marie (-Tooth) type G60.0
    - pseudohypertrophic (infantile) G71.0
    - severe (Duchenne type) G71.0
  - myocardium, myocardial — *see* Degeneration, myocardial
  - myotonic, myotonica G71.11
  - nail L60.3
    - congenital Q84.6
  - nutritional E45
  - ocular G71.0
  - oculocerebrorenal E72.03
  - oculopharyngeal G71.0

Dystrophy - Edema

- **Dystrophy** — *continued*
  - ovarian N83.8
  - polyglandular E31.8
  - reflex (neuromuscular) (sympathetic) — *see* Syndrome, pain, complex regional I
  - retinal (hereditary) H35.50
    - in
      - lipid storage disorders E75.6 *[H36]*
      - systemic lipidoses E75.6 *[H36]*
    - involving
      - pigment epithelium H35.54
      - sensory area H35.53
    - pigmentary H35.52
    - vitreoretinal H35.51
  - Salzmann's nodular — *see* Degeneration, cornea, nodular
  - scapuloperoneal G71.0
  - skin NEC L98.8
  - sympathetic (reflex) — *see* Syndrome, pain, complex regional I
    - cervical G90.2
  - tapetoretinal H35.54
  - thoracic, asphyxiating Q77.2
  - unguium L60.3
    - congenital Q84.6
  - vitreoretinal H35.51
  - vulva N90.4
  - yellow (liver) — *see* Failure, hepatic
- **Dysuria** R30.0
  - psychogenic F45.8

E

- **Eales'** disease H35.06 ☑
- **Ear** (*see also* condition)
  - piercing Z41.3
  - tropical NEC B36.9 *[H62.40]*
    - in
      - aspergillosis B44.89
      - candidiasis B37.84
      - moniliasis B37.84
  - wax (impacted) H61.20
    - left H61.22
      - with right H61.23
    - right H61.21
      - with left H61.23
- **Earache** — *see* subcategory H92.0
- **Early** satiety R68.81
- **Eaton-Lambert** syndrome — *see* Syndrome, Lambert-Eaton
- **Eberth's** disease (typhoid fever) A01.00
- **Ebola** virus disease A98.4
- **Ebstein's** anomaly or syndrome (heart) Q22.5
- **Eccentro-osteochondrodysplasia** E76.29
- **Ecchondroma** — *see* Neoplasm, bone, benign
- **Ecchondrosis** D48.0
- **Ecchymosis** R58
  - conjunctiva — *see* Hemorrhage, conjunctiva
  - eye (traumatic) — *see* Contusion, eyeball
  - eyelid (traumatic) — *see* Contusion, eyelid
  - newborn P54.5
  - spontaneous R23.3
  - traumatic — *see* Contusion
- **Echinococciasis** — *see* Echinococcus
- **Echinococcosis** — *see* Echinococcus
- **Echinococcus** (infection) B67.90
  - granulosus B67.4
    - bone B67.2
    - liver B67.0
    - lung B67.1
    - multiple sites B67.32
    - specified site NEC B67.39
    - thyroid B67.31
  - liver NOS B67.8
    - granulosus B67.0
    - multilocularis B67.5
  - lung NEC B67.99
    - granulosus B67.1
    - multilocularis B67.69
  - multilocularis B67.7
    - liver B67.5
    - multiple sites B67.61
    - specified site NEC B67.69
  - specified site NEC B67.99
    - granulosus B67.39
    - multilocularis B67.69
  - thyroid NEC B67.99
    - granulosus B67.31
    - multilocularis B67.69 *[E35]*
- **Echinorhynchiasis** B83.8
- **Echinostomiasis** B66.8
- **Echolalia** R48.8
- **Echovirus,** as cause of disease classified elsewhere B97.12
- **Eclampsia,** eclamptic (coma) (convulsions) (delirium) (with hypertension) NEC O15.9
  - complicating
    - labor and delivery O15.1
    - postpartum O15.2
    - pregnancy O15.0 ☑
    - puerperium O15.2
- **Economic** circumstances affecting care Z59.9
- **Economo's** disease A85.8
- **Ectasia,** ectasis
  - annuloaortic I35.8
  - aorta I77.819
    - with aneurysm — *see* Aneurysm, aorta
    - abdominal I77.811
    - thoracic I77.810
    - thoracoabdominal I77.812
  - breast — *see* Ectasia, mammary duct
  - capillary I78.8
  - cornea H18.71 ☑
  - gastric antral vascular (GAVE) K31.819
    - with hemorrhage K31.811
    - without hemorrhage K31.819
  - mammary duct N60.4 ☑
  - salivary gland (duct) K11.8
  - sclera — *see* Sclerectasia
- **Ecthyma** L08.0
  - contagiosum B08.02
  - gangrenosum L08.0
  - infectiosum B08.02
- **Ectocardia** Q24.8
- **Ectodermal** dysplasia (anhidrotic) Q82.4
- **Ectodermosis** erosiva pluriorificialis L51.1
- **Ectopic,** ectopia (congenital)
  - abdominal viscera Q45.8
    - due to defect in anterior abdominal wall Q79.59
  - ACTH syndrome E24.3
  - adrenal gland Q89.1
  - anus Q43.5
  - atrial beats I49.1
  - beats I49.49
    - atrial I49.1
    - ventricular I49.3
  - bladder Q64.10
  - bone and cartilage in lung Q33.5
  - brain Q04.8
  - breast tissue Q83.8
  - cardiac Q24.8
  - cerebral Q04.8
  - cordis Q24.8
  - endometrium — *see* Endometriosis
  - gastric mucosa Q40.2
  - gestation — *see* Pregnancy, by site
  - heart Q24.8
  - hormone secretion NEC E34.2
  - kidney (crossed) (pelvis) Q63.2
  - lens, lentis Q12.1
  - mole — *see* Pregnancy, by site
  - organ or site NEC — *see* Malposition, congenital
  - pancreas Q45.3
  - pregnancy — *see* Pregnancy, ectopic
  - pupil — *see* Abnormality, pupillary
  - renal Q63.2
  - sebaceous glands of mouth Q38.6
  - spleen Q89.09
  - testis Q53.00
    - bilateral Q53.02
    - unilateral Q53.01
  - thyroid Q89.2
  - tissue in lung Q33.5
  - ureter Q62.63
  - ventricular beats I49.3
  - vesicae Q64.10
- **Ectromelia** Q73.8
  - lower limb — *see* Defect, reduction, limb, lower, specified type NEC
  - upper limb — *see* Defect, reduction, limb, upper, specified type NEC
- **Ectropion** H02.109
  - cervix N86
    - with cervicitis N72
  - congenital Q10.1
  - eyelid (paralytic) H02.109
    - cicatricial H02.119
      - left H02.116
        - lower H02.115
        - upper H02.114
      - right H02.113
- **Ectropion** — *continued*
  - eyelid — *continued*
        - lower H02.112
        - upper H02.111
    - congenital Q10.1
    - left H02.106
      - lower H02.105
      - upper H02.104
    - mechanical H02.129
      - left H02.126
        - lower H02.125
        - upper H02.124
      - right H02.123
        - lower H02.122
        - upper H02.121
    - right H02.103
      - lower H02.102
      - upper H02.101
    - senile H02.139
      - left H02.136
        - lower H02.135
        - upper H02.134
      - right H02.133
        - lower H02.132
        - upper H02.131
    - spastic H02.149
      - left H02.146
        - lower H02.145
        - upper H02.144
      - right H02.143
        - lower H02.142
        - upper H02.141
  - iris H21.89
  - lip (acquired) K13.0
    - congenital Q38.0
  - urethra N36.8
  - uvea H21.89
- **Eczema** (acute) (chronic) (erythematous) (fissum) (rubrum) (squamous) (*see also* Dermatitis)L30.9
  - contact — *see* Dermatitis, contact
  - dyshydrotic L30.1
  - external ear — *see* Otitis, externa, acute, eczematoid
  - flexural L20.82
  - herpeticum B00.0
  - hypertrophicum L28.0
  - hypostatic — *see* Varix, leg, with, inflammation
  - impetiginous L01.1
  - infantile (due to any substance) L20.83
    - intertriginous L21.1
    - seborrheic L21.1
  - intertriginous NEC L30.4
    - infantile L21.1
  - intrinsic (allergic) L20.84
  - lichenified NEC L28.0
  - marginatum (hebrae) B35.6
  - pustular L30.3
  - stasis I87.2
    - with varicose veins — *see* Varix, leg, with, inflammation
  - vaccination, vaccinatum T88.1 ☑
  - varicose — *see* Varix, leg, with, inflammation
- **Eczematid** L30.2
- **Eddowes** (-Spurway) syndrome Q78.0
- **Edema,** edematous (infectious) (pitting) (toxic) R60.9
  - with nephritis — *see* Nephrosis
  - allergic T78.3 ☑
  - amputation stump (surgical) (sequelae (late effect)) T87.89
  - angioneurotic (allergic) (any site) (with urticaria) T78.3 ☑
    - hereditary D84.1
  - angiospastic I73.9
  - Berlin's (traumatic) S05.8X ☑
  - brain (cytotoxic) (vasogenic) G93.6
    - due to birth injury P11.0
    - newborn (anoxia or hypoxia) P52.4
      - birth injury P11.0
    - traumatic — *see* Injury, intracranial, cerebral edema
  - cardiac — *see* Failure, heart, congestive
  - cardiovascular — *see* Failure, heart, congestive
  - cerebral — *see* Edema, brain
  - cerebrospinal — *see* Edema, brain
  - cervix (uteri) (acute) N88.8
    - puerperal, postpartum O90.89
  - chronic hereditary Q82.0
  - circumscribed, acute T78.3 ☑
    - hereditary D84.1
  - conjunctiva H11.42 ☑
  - cornea H18.2 ☑
    - idiopathic H18.22 ☑

- **Edema** — *continued*
  - cornea — *continued*
    - secondary H18.23 ☑
      - due to contact lens H18.21 ☑
  - due to
    - lymphatic obstruction I89.0
    - salt retention E87.0
  - epiglottis — *see* Edema, glottis
  - essential, acute T78.3 ☑
    - hereditary D84.1
  - extremities, lower — *see* Edema, legs
  - eyelid NEC H02.849
    - left H02.846
      - lower H02.845
      - upper H02.844
    - right H02.843
      - lower H02.842
      - upper H02.841
  - familial, hereditary Q82.0
  - famine — *see* Malnutrition, severe
  - generalized R60.1
  - glottis, glottic, glottidis (obstructive) (passive) J38.4
    - allergic T78.3 ☑
      - hereditary D84.1
  - heart — *see* Failure, heart, congestive
  - heat T67.7 ☑
  - hereditary Q82.0
  - inanition — *see* Malnutrition, severe
  - intracranial G93.6
  - iris H21.89
  - joint — *see* Effusion, joint
  - larynx — *see* Edema, glottis
  - legs R60.0
    - due to venous obstruction I87.1
    - hereditary Q82.0
  - localized R60.0
    - due to venous obstruction I87.1
  - lower limbs — *see* Edema, legs
  - lung J81.1
    - with heart condition or failure — *see* Failure, ventricular, left
    - acute J81.0
    - chemical (acute) J68.1
      - chronic J68.1
    - chronic J81.1
      - due to
        - chemicals, gases, fumes or vapors (inhalation) J68.1
        - external agent J70.9
          - specified NEC J70.8
        - radiation J70.1
    - due to
      - chemicals, fumes or vapors (inhalation) J68.1
      - external agent J70.9
        - specified NEC J70.8
      - high altitude T70.29 ☑
      - near drowning T75.1 ☑
      - radiation J70.0
    - meaning failure, left ventricle I50.1
  - lymphatic I89.0
    - due to mastectomy I97.2
  - macula H35.81
    - cystoid, following cataract surgery — *see* Complications, postprocedural, following cataract surgery
    - diabetic — *see* Diabetes, by type, with, retinopathy, with macular edema
  - malignant — *see* Gangrene, gas
  - Milroy's Q82.0
  - nasopharynx J39.2
  - newborn P83.30
    - hydrops fetalis — *see* Hydrops, fetalis
    - specified NEC P83.39
  - nutritional (*see also* Malnutrition, severe)
    - with dyspigmentation, skin and hair E40
  - optic disc or nerve — *see* Papilledema
  - orbit H05.22 ☑
  - pancreas K86.89
  - papilla, optic — *see* Papilledema
  - penis N48.89
  - periodic T78.3 ☑
    - hereditary D84.1
  - pharynx J39.2
  - pulmonary — *see* Edema, lung
  - Quincke's T78.3 ☑
    - hereditary D84.1
  - renal — *see* Nephrosis
  - retina H35.81
    - diabetic — *see* Diabetes, by type, with, retinopathy, with macular edema
  - salt E87.0
- **Edema** — *continued*
  - scrotum N50.89
  - seminal vesicle N50.89
  - spermatic cord N50.89
  - spinal (cord) (vascular) (nontraumatic) G95.19
  - starvation — *see* Malnutrition, severe
  - stasis — *see* Hypertension, venous, (chronic)
  - subglottic — *see* Edema, glottis
  - supraglottic — *see* Edema, glottis
  - testis N44.8
  - tunica vaginalis N50.89
  - vas deferens N50.89
  - vulva (acute) N90.89
- **Edentulism** — *see* Absence, teeth, acquired
- **Edsall's** disease T67.2 ☑
- **Educational** handicap Z55.9
  - specified NEC Z55.8
- **Edward's** syndrome — *see* Trisomy, 18
- **Effect, adverse**
  - abnormal gravitational (G) forces or states T75.81 ☑
  - abuse — *see* Maltreatment
  - air pressure T70.9 ☑
    - specified NEC T70.8 ☑
  - altitude (high) — *see* Effect, adverse, high altitude
  - anesthesia (*see also* Anesthesia)T88.59 ☑
    - in labor and delivery O74.9
    - local, toxic
      - in labor and delivery O74.4
      - in pregnancy NEC O29.3 ☑
      - postpartum, puerperal O89.3
    - postpartum, puerperal O89.9
    - specified NEC T88.59 ☑
      - in labor and delivery O74.8
      - postpartum, puerperal O89.8
    - spinal and epidural T88.59 ☑
      - headache T88.59 ☑
        - in labor and delivery O74.5
        - postpartum, puerperal O89.4
      - specified NEC
        - in labor and delivery O74.6
        - postpartum, puerperal O89.5
  - antitoxin — *see* Complications, vaccination
  - atmospheric pressure T70.9 ☑
    - due to explosion T70.8 ☑
    - high T70.3 ☑
    - low — *see* Effect, adverse, high altitude
    - specified effect NEC T70.8 ☑
  - biological, correct substance properly administered — *see* Effect, adverse, drug
  - blood (derivatives) (serum) (transfusion) — *see* Complications, transfusion
  - chemical substance — *see* Table of Drugs and Chemicals
  - cold (temperature) (weather) T69.9 ☑
    - chilblains T69.1 ☑
    - frostbite — *see* Frostbite
    - specified effect NEC T69.8 ☑
  - drugs and medicaments T88.7 ☑
    - specified drug — *see* Table of Drugs and Chemicals, by drug, adverse effect
    - specified effect - code to condition
  - electric current, electricity (shock) T75.4 ☑
    - burn — *see* Burn
  - exertion (excessive) T73.3 ☑
  - exposure — *see* Exposure
  - external cause NEC T75.89 ☑
  - foodstuffs T78.1 ☑
    - allergic reaction — *see* Allergy, food
      - causing anaphylaxis — *see* Shock, anaphylactic, due to food
    - noxious — *see* Poisoning, food, noxious
  - gases, fumes, or vapors T59.9 ☑
    - specified agent — *see* Table of Drugs and Chemicals
  - glue (airplane) sniffing
    - due to drug abuse — *see* Abuse, drug, inhalant
    - due to drug dependence — *see* Dependence, drug, inhalant
  - heat — *see* Heat
  - high altitude NEC T70.29 ☑
    - anoxia T70.29 ☑
    - on
      - ears T70.0 ☑
      - sinuses T70.1 ☑
    - polycythemia D75.1
  - high pressure fluids T70.4 ☑
  - hot weather — *see* Heat
  - hunger T73.0 ☑
  - immersion, foot — *see* Immersion
  - immunization — *see* Complications, vaccination
- **Effect** — *continued*
  - immunological agents — *see* Complications, vaccination
  - infrared (radiation) (rays) NOS T66 ☑
    - dermatitis or eczema L59.8
  - infusion — *see* Complications, infusion
  - lack of care of infants — *see* Maltreatment, child
  - lightning — *see* Lightning
  - medical care T88.9 ☑
    - specified NEC T88.8 ☑
  - medicinal substance, correct, properly administered — *see* Effect, adverse, drug
  - motion T75.3 ☑
  - noise, on inner ear — *see* subcategory H83.3
  - overheated places — *see* Heat
  - psychosocial, of work environment Z56.5
  - radiation (diagnostic) (infrared) (natural source) (therapeutic) (ultraviolet) (X-ray) NOS T66 ☑
    - dermatitis or eczema — *see* Dermatitis, due to, radiation
    - fibrosis of lung J70.1
    - pneumonitis J70.0
    - pulmonary manifestations
      - acute J70.0
      - chronic J70.1
    - skin L59.9
  - radioactive substance NOS
    - dermatitis or eczema — *see* Radiodermatitis
  - reduced temperature T69.9 ☑
    - immersion foot or hand — *see* Immersion
    - specified effect NEC T69.8 ☑
  - serum NEC (*see also* Reaction, serum)T80.69 ☑
  - specified NEC T78.8 ☑
    - external cause NEC T75.89 ☑
  - strangulation — *see* Asphyxia, traumatic
  - submersion T75.1 ☑
  - thirst T73.1 ☑
  - toxic — *see* Toxicity
  - transfusion — *see* Complications, transfusion
  - ultraviolet (radiation) (rays) NOS T66 ☑
    - burn — *see* Burn
    - dermatitis or eczema — *see* Dermatitis, due to, ultraviolet rays
      - acute L56.8
  - vaccine (any) — *see* Complications, vaccination
  - vibration — *see* Vibration, adverse effects
  - water pressure NEC T70.9 ☑
    - specified NEC T70.8 ☑
  - weightlessness T75.82 ☑
  - whole blood — *see* Complications, transfusion
  - work environment Z56.5
- **Effect** (s) (of) (from) — *see* Effect, adverse NEC
- **Effects,** late — *see* Sequelae
- **Effluvium**
  - anagen L65.1
  - telogen L65.0
- **Effort** syndrome (psychogenic) F45.8
- **Effusion**
  - amniotic fluid — *see* Pregnancy, complicated by, premature rupture of membranes
  - brain (serous) G93.6
  - bronchial — *see* Bronchitis
  - cerebral G93.6
  - cerebrospinal (*see also* Meningitis)
    - vessel G93.6
  - chest — *see* Effusion, pleura
  - chylous, chyliform (pleura) J94.0
  - intracranial G93.6
  - joint M25.40
    - ankle M25.47 ☑
    - elbow M25.42 ☑
    - foot joint M25.47 ☑
    - hand joint M25.44 ☑
    - hip M25.45 ☑
    - knee M25.46 ☑
    - shoulder M25.41 ☑
    - specified joint NEC M25.48
    - wrist M25.43 ☑
  - malignant pleural J91.0
  - meninges — *see* Meningitis
  - pericardium, pericardial (noninflammatory) I31.3
    - acute — *see* Pericarditis, acute
  - peritoneal (chronic) R18.8
  - pleura, pleurisy, pleuritic, pleuropericardial J90
    - chylous, chyliform J94.0
    - due to systemic lupus erythematosis M32.13
    - influenzal — *see* Influenza, with, respiratory manifestations NEC
    - malignant J91.0
    - newborn P28.89
    - tuberculous NEC A15.6
      - primary (progressive) A15.7

- **Effusion** — *continued*
  - spinal — *see* Meningitis
  - thorax, thoracic — *see* Effusion, pleura
- **Egg** shell nails L60.3
  - congenital Q84.6
- **Egyptian** splenomegaly B65.1
- **Ehrlichiosis** A77.40
  - due to
    - E. chafeensis A77.41
    - E. sennetsu A79.81
    - specified organism NEC A77.49
- **Ehlers-Danlos** syndrome Q79.6
- **Eichstedt's** disease B36.0
- **Eisenmenger's**
  - complex or syndrome I27.89
  - defect Q21.8
- **Ejaculation**
  - delayed F52.32
  - painful N53.12
  - premature F52.4
  - retarded N53.11
  - retrograde N53.14
  - semen, painful N53.12
    - psychogenic F52.6
- **Ekbom's** syndrome (restless legs) G25.81
- **Ekman's** syndrome (brittle bones and blue sclera) Q78.0
- **Elastic** skin Q82.8
  - acquired L57.4
- **Elastofibroma** — *see* Neoplasm, connective tissue, benign
- **Elastoma** (juvenile) Q82.8
  - Miescher's L87.2
- **Elastomyofibrosis** I42.4
- **Elastosis**
  - actinic, solar L57.8
  - atrophicans (senile) L57.4
  - perforans serpiginosa L87.2
  - senilis L57.4
- **Elbow** — *see* condition
- **Electric** current, electricity, effects (concussion) (fatal) (nonfatal) (shock) T75.4 ☑
  - burn — *see* Burn
- **Electric** feet syndrome E53.8
- **Electrocution** T75.4 ☑
  - from electroshock gun (taser) T75.4 ☑
- **Electrolyte** imbalance E87.8
  - with
    - abortion — *see* Abortion by type, complicated by, electrolyte imbalance
    - ectopic pregnancy O08.5
    - molar pregnancy O08.5
- **Elephantiasis** (nonfilarial) I89.0
  - arabicum — *see* Infestation, filarial
  - bancroftian B74.0
  - congenital (any site) (hereditary) Q82.0
  - due to
    - Brugia (malayi) B74.1
      - timori B74.2
    - mastectomy I97.2
    - Wuchereria (bancrofti) B74.0
  - eyelid H02.859
    - left H02.856
      - lower H02.855
      - upper H02.854
    - right H02.853
      - lower H02.852
      - upper H02.851
  - filarial, filariensis — *see* Infestation, filarial
  - glandular I89.0
  - graecorum A30.9
  - lymphangiectatic I89.0
  - lymphatic vessel I89.0
    - due to mastectomy I97.2
  - scrotum (nonfilarial) I89.0
  - streptococcal I89.0
  - surgical I97.89
    - postmastectomy I97.2
  - telangiectodes I89.0
  - vulva (nonfilarial) N90.89
- **Elevated**, elevation
  - antibody titer R76.0
  - basal metabolic rate R94.8
  - blood pressure (*see also* Hypertension)
    - reading (incidental) (isolated) (nonspecific), no diagnosis of hypertension R03.0
  - blood sugar R73.9
  - body temperature (of unknown origin) R50.9
  - C-reactive protein (CRP) R79.82
  - cancer antigen 125 [CA 125] R97.1
  - carcinoembryonic antigen [CEA] R97.0
  - cholesterol E78.00
    - with high triglycerides E78.2
- **Elevated** — *continued*
  - conjugate, eye H51.0
  - diaphragm, congenital Q79.1
  - erythrocyte sedimentation rate R70.0
  - fasting glucose R73.01
  - fasting triglycerides E78.1
  - finding on laboratory examination — *see* Findings, abnormal, inconclusive, without diagnosis, by type of exam
  - GFR (glomerular filtration rate) — *see* Findings, abnormal, inconclusive, without diagnosis, by type of exam
  - glucose tolerance (oral) R73.02
  - immunoglobulin level R76.8
  - indoleacetic acid R82.5
  - lactic acid dehydrogenase (LDH) level R74.0
  - leukocytes D72.829
  - lipoprotein a level E78.8 ☑
  - liver function
    - study R94.5
    - test R79.89
      - alkaline phosphatase R74.8
      - aminotransferase R74.0
      - bilirubin R17
      - hepatic enzyme R74.8
      - lactate dehydrogenase R74.0
  - lymphocytes D72.820
  - prostate specific antigen [PSA] R97.20
  - Rh titer — *see* Complication (s), transfusion, incompatibility reaction, Rh (factor)
  - scapula, congenital Q74.0
  - sedimentation rate R70.0
  - SGOT R74.0
  - SGPT R74.0
  - transaminase level R74.0
  - triglycerides E78.1
    - with high cholesterol E78.2
  - tumor associated antigens [TAA] NEC R97.8
  - tumor specific antigens [TSA] NEC R97.8
  - urine level of
    - catecholamine R82.5
    - indoleacetic acid R82.5
    - 17-ketosteroids R82.5
    - steroids R82.5
    - vanillylmandelic acid (VMA) R82.5
  - venous pressure I87.8
  - white blood cell count D72.829
    - specified NEC D72.828
- **Elliptocytosis** (congenital) (hereditary) D58.1
  - Hb C (disease) D58.1
  - hemoglobin disease D58.1
  - sickle-cell (disease) D57.8 ☑
    - trait D57.3
- **Ellison-Zollinger** syndrome E16.4
- **Ellis-van** Creveld syndrome (chondroectodermal dysplasia) Q77.6
- **Elongated,** elongation (congenital) (*see also* Distortion)
  - bone Q79.9
  - cervix (uteri) Q51.828
    - acquired N88.4
    - hypertrophic N88.4
  - colon Q43.8
  - common bile duct Q44.5
  - cystic duct Q44.5
  - frenulum, penis Q55.69
  - labia minora (acquired) N90.69
  - ligamentum patellae Q74.1
  - petiolus (epiglottidis) Q31.8
  - tooth, teeth K00.2
  - uvula Q38.6
- **El Tor** cholera A00.1
- **Emaciation** (due to malnutrition) E41
- **Embadomoniasis** A07.8
- **Embedded** tooth, teeth K01.0
  - root only K08.3
- **Embolic** — *see* condition
- **Embolism** (multiple) (paradoxical) I74.9
  - air (any site) (traumatic) T79.0 ☑
    - following
      - abortion — *see* Abortion by type complicated by embolism
      - ectopic pregnancy O08.2
      - infusion, therapeutic injection or transfusion T80.0 ☑
      - molar pregnancy O08.2
      - procedure NEC
        - artery T81.719 ☑
          - mesenteric T81.710 ☑
          - renal T81.711 ☑
          - specified NEC T81.718 ☑
        - vein T81.72 ☑
- **Embolism** — *continued*
  - air — *continued*
    - in pregnancy, childbirth or puerperium — *see* Embolism, obstetric
  - amniotic fluid (pulmonary) (*see also* Embolism, obstetric)
    - following
      - abortion — *see* Abortion by type complicated by embolism
      - ectopic pregnancy O08.2
      - molar pregnancy O08.2
  - aorta, aortic I74.10
    - abdominal I74.09
      - saddle I74.01
    - bifurcation I74.09
    - saddle I74.01
    - thoracic I74.11
  - artery I74.9
    - auditory, internal I65.8
    - basilar — *see* Occlusion, artery, basilar
    - carotid (common) (internal) — *see* Occlusion, artery, carotid
    - cerebellar (anterior inferior) (posterior inferior) (superior) I66.3
    - cerebral — *see* Occlusion, artery, cerebral
    - choroidal (anterior) I66.8
    - communicating posterior I66.8
    - coronary (*see also* Infarct, myocardium)
      - not resulting in infarction I24.0
    - extremity I74.4
      - lower I74.3
      - upper I74.2
    - hypophyseal I66.8
    - iliac I74.5
    - limb I74.4
      - lower I74.3
      - upper I74.2
    - mesenteric (with gangrene) (*see also* Ischemia, intestine, acute)K55.059
    - ophthalmic — *see* Occlusion, artery, retina
    - peripheral I74.4
    - pontine I66.8
    - precerebral — *see* Occlusion, artery, precerebral
    - pulmonary — *see* Embolism, pulmonary
    - renal N28.0
    - retinal — *see* Occlusion, artery, retina
    - septic I76
    - specified NEC I74.8
    - vertebral — *see* Occlusion, artery, vertebral
  - basilar (artery) I65.1
  - blood clot
    - following
      - abortion — *see* Abortion by type complicated by embolism
      - ectopic or molar pregnancy O08.2
    - in pregnancy, childbirth or puerperium — *see* Embolism, obstetric
  - brain (*see also* Occlusion, artery, cerebral)
    - following
      - abortion — *see* Abortion by type complicated by embolism
      - ectopic or molar pregnancy O08.2
    - puerperal, postpartum, childbirth — *see* Embolism, obstetric
  - capillary I78.8
  - cardiac (*see also* Infarct, myocardium)
    - not resulting in infarction I51.3
  - carotid (artery) (common) (internal) — *see* Occlusion, artery, carotid
  - cavernous sinus (venous) — *see* Embolism, intracranial venous sinus
  - cerebral — *see* Occlusion, artery, cerebral
  - cholesterol — *see* Atheroembolism
  - coronary (artery or vein) (systemic) — *see* Occlusion, coronary
  - due to device, implant or graft (*see also* Complications, by site and type, specified NEC)
    - arterial graft NEC T82.818 ☑
    - breast (implant) T85.818 ☑
    - catheter NEC T85.818 ☑
      - dialysis (renal) T82.818 ☑
        - intraperitoneal T85.818 ☑
      - infusion NEC T82.818 ☑
        - spinal (epidural) (subdural) T85.810 ☑
      - urinary (indwelling) T83.81 ☑
    - electronic (electrode) (pulse generator) (stimulator)
      - bone T84.81 ☑
      - cardiac T82.817 ☑
      - nervous system (brain) (peripheral nerve) (spinal) T85.810 ☑

- **Embolism** — *continued*
  - due to device — *continued*
    - urinary T83.81 ☑
    - fixation, internal (orthopedic) NEC T84.81 ☑
    - gastrointestinal (bile duct) (esophagus) T85.818 ☑
    - genital NEC T83.81 ☑
    - heart (graft) (valve) T82.817 ☑
    - joint prosthesis T84.81 ☑
    - ocular (corneal graft) (orbital implant) T85.818 ☑
    - orthopedic (bone graft) NEC T86.838
    - specified NEC T85.818 ☑
    - urinary (graft) NEC T83.81 ☑
    - vascular NEC T82.818 ☑
    - ventricular intracranial shunt T85.810 ☑
  - extremities
    - lower — *see* Embolism, vein, lower extremity
      - arterial I74.3
    - upper I74.2
  - eye H34.9
  - fat (cerebral) (pulmonary) (systemic) T79.1 ☑
    - following
      - abortion — *see* Abortion by type complicated by embolism
      - ectopic or molar pregnancy O08.2
    - complicating delivery — *see* Embolism, obstetric
  - following
    - abortion — *see* Abortion by type complicated by embolism
    - ectopic or molar pregnancy O08.2
    - infusion, therapeutic injection or transfusion
      - air T80.0 ☑
  - heart (fatty) (*see also* Infarct, myocardium)
    - not resulting in infarction I51.3
  - hepatic (vein) I82.0
  - in pregnancy, childbirth or puerperium — *see* Embolism, obstetric
  - intestine (artery) (vein) (with gangrene) (*see also* Ischemia, intestine, acute)K55.039
  - intracranial (*see also* Occlusion, artery, cerebral)
    - venous sinus (any) G08
      - nonpyogenic I67.6
  - intraspinal venous sinuses or veins G08
    - nonpyogenic G95.19
  - kidney (artery) N28.0
  - lateral sinus (venous) — *see* Embolism, intracranial, venous sinus
  - leg — *see* Embolism, vein, lower extremity
    - arterial I74.3
  - longitudinal sinus (venous) — *see* Embolism, intracranial, venous sinus
  - lung (massive) — *see* Embolism, pulmonary
  - meninges I66.8
  - mesenteric (artery) (vein) (with gangrene) (*see also* Ischemia, intestine, acute)K55.059
  - obstetric (in) (pulmonary)
    - childbirth O88.22
      - air O88.02
      - amniotic fluid O88.12
      - blood clot O88.22
      - fat O88.82
      - pyemic O88.32
      - septic O88.32
      - specified type NEC O88.82
    - pregnancy O88.21 ☑
      - air O88.01 ☑
      - amniotic fluid O88.11 ☑
      - blood clot O88.21 ☑
      - fat O88.81 ☑
      - pyemic O88.31 ☑
      - septic O88.31 ☑
      - specified type NEC O88.81 ☑
    - puerperal O88.23
      - air O88.03
      - amniotic fluid O88.13
      - blood clot O88.23
      - fat O88.83
      - pyemic O88.33
      - septic O88.33
      - specified type NEC O88.83
  - ophthalmic — *see* Occlusion, artery, retina
  - penis N48.81
  - peripheral artery NOS I74.4
  - pituitary E23.6
  - popliteal (artery) I74.3
  - portal (vein) I81
  - postoperative, postprocedural
    - artery T81.719 ☑
      - mesenteric T81.710 ☑
      - renal T81.711 ☑

- **Embolism** — *continued*
  - postoperative — *continued*
    - specified NEC T81.718 ☑
    - vein T81.72 ☑
  - precerebral artery — *see* Occlusion, artery, precerebral
  - puerperal — *see* Embolism, obstetric
  - pulmonary (acute) (artery) (vein) I26.99
    - with acute cor pulmonale I26.09
    - chronic I27.82
    - following
      - abortion — *see* Abortion by type complicated by embolism
      - ectopic or molar pregnancy O08.2
    - healed or old Z86.711
    - in pregnancy, childbirth or puerperium — *see* Embolism, obstetric
    - personal history of Z86.711
    - saddle I26.92
      - with acute cor pulmonale I26.02
    - septic I26.90
      - with acute cor pulmonale I26.01
  - pyemic (multiple) I76
    - following
      - abortion — *see* Abortion by type complicated by embolism
      - ectopic or molar pregnancy O08.2
    - Hemophilus influenzae A41.3
    - pneumococcal A40.3
      - with pneumonia J13
    - puerperal, postpartum, childbirth (any organism) — *see* Embolism, obstetric
    - specified organism NEC A41.89
    - staphylococcal A41.2
    - streptococcal A40.9
  - renal (artery) N28.0
    - vein I82.3
  - retina, retinal — *see* Occlusion, artery, retina
  - saddle
    - abdominal aorta I74.01
    - pulmonary artery I26.92
      - with acute cor pulmonale I26.02
  - septic (arterial) I76
    - complicating abortion — *see* Abortion, by type, complicated by, embolism
  - sinus — *see* Embolism, intracranial, venous sinus
  - soap complicating abortion — *see* Abortion, by type, complicated by, embolism
  - spinal cord G95.19
    - pyogenic origin G06.1
  - spleen, splenic (artery) I74.8
  - upper extremity I74.2
  - vein (acute) I82.90
    - antecubital I82.61 ☑
      - chronic I82.71 ☑
    - axillary I82.A1 ☑
      - chronic I82.A2 ☑
    - basilic I82.61 ☑
      - chronic I82.71 ☑
    - brachial I82.62 ☑
      - chronic I82.72 ☑
    - brachiocephalic (innominate) I82.290
      - chronic I82.291
    - cephalic I82.61 ☑
      - chronic I82.71 ☑
    - chronic I82.91
    - deep (DVT) I82.40 ☑
      - calf I82.4Z ☑
        - chronic I82.5Z ☑
      - lower leg I82.4Z ☑
        - chronic I82.5Z ☑
      - thigh I82.4Y ☑
        - chronic I82.5Y ☑
      - upper leg I82.4Y ☑
        - chronic I82.5y ☑
    - femoral I82.41 ☑
      - chronic I82.51 ☑
    - iliac (iliofemoral) I82.42 ☑
      - chronic I82.52 ☑
    - innominate I82.290
      - chronic I82.291
    - internal jugular I82.C1 ☑
      - chronic I82.C2 ☑
    - lower extremity
      - deep I82.40 ☑
        - chronic I82.50 ☑
        - specified NEC I82.49 ☑
          - chronic NEC I82.59 ☑
      - distal
        - deep I82.4Z ☑
      - proximal
        - deep I82.4Y ☑

- **Embolism** — *continued*
  - vein — *continued*
        - chronic I82.5Y ☑
      - superficial I82.81 ☑
    - popliteal I82.43 ☑
      - chronic I82.53 ☑
    - radial I82.62 ☑
      - chronic I82.72 ☑
    - renal I82.3
    - saphenous (greater) (lesser) I82.81 ☑
    - specified NEC I82.890
      - chronic NEC I82.891
    - subclavian I82.B1 ☑
      - chronic I82.B2 ☑
    - thoracic NEC I82.290
      - chronic I82.291
    - tibial I82.44 ☑
      - chronic I82.54 ☑
    - ulnar I82.62 ☑
      - chronic I82.72 ☑
    - upper extremity I82.60 ☑
      - chronic I82.70 ☑
      - deep I82.62 ☑
        - chronic I82.72 ☑
      - superficial I82.61 ☑
        - chronic I82.71 ☑
  - vena cava
    - inferior (acute) I82.220
      - chronic I82.221
    - superior (acute) I82.210
      - chronic I82.211
  - venous sinus G08
  - vessels of brain — *see* Occlusion, artery, cerebral
- **Embolus** — *see* Embolism
- **Embryoma** (*see also* Neoplasm, uncertain behavior, by site)
  - benign — *see* Neoplasm, benign, by site
  - kidney C64. ☑
  - liver C22.0
  - malignant (*see also* Neoplasm, malignant, by site)
    - kidney C64. ☑
    - liver C22.0
    - testis C62.9 ☑
      - descended (scrotal) C62.1 ☑
      - undescended C62.0 ☑
  - testis C62.9 ☑
    - descended (scrotal) C62.1 ☑
    - undescended C62.0 ☑
- **Embryonic**
  - circulation Q28.9
  - heart Q28.9
  - vas deferens Q55.4
- **Embryopathia** NOS Q89.9
- **Embryotoxon** Q13.4
- **Emesis** — *see* Vomiting
- **Emotional** lability R45.86
- **Emotionality,** pathological F60.3
- **Emotogenic** disease — *see* Disorder, psychogenic
- **Emphysema** (atrophic) (bullous) (chronic) (interlobular) (lung) (obstructive) (pulmonary) (senile) (vesicular) J43.9
  - cellular tissue (traumatic) T79.7 ☑
    - surgical T81.82 ☑
  - centrilobular J43.2
  - compensatory J98.3
  - congenital (interstitial) P25.0
  - conjunctiva H11.89
  - connective tissue (traumatic) T79.7 ☑
    - surgical T81.82 ☑
  - due to chemicals, gases, fumes or vapors J68.4
  - eyelid (s) — *see* Disorder, eyelid, specified type NEC
    - surgical T81.82 ☑
    - traumatic T79.7 ☑
  - interstitial J98.2
    - congenital P25.0
    - perinatal period P25.0
  - laminated tissue T79.7 ☑
    - surgical T81.82 ☑
  - mediastinal J98.2
    - newborn P25.2
  - orbit, orbital — *see* Disorder, orbit, specified type NEC
  - panacinar J43.1
  - panlobular J43.1
  - specified NEC J43.8
  - subcutaneous (traumatic) T79.7 ☑
    - nontraumatic J98.2
    - postprocedural T81.82 ☑
    - surgical T81.82 ☑
  - surgical T81.82 ☑
  - thymus (gland) (congenital) E32.8

Emphysema - Encephalopathy

- **Emphysema** — *continued*
  - traumatic (subcutaneous) T79.7 ☑
  - unilateral J43.0
- **Empty** nest syndrome Z60.0
- **Empyema** (acute) (chest) (double) (pleura) (supradiaphragmatic) (thorax) J86.9
  - with fistula J86.0
  - accessory sinus (chronic) — *see* Sinusitis
  - antrum (chronic) — *see* Sinusitis, maxillary
  - brain (any part) — *see* Abscess, brain
  - ethmoidal (chronic) (sinus) — *see* Sinusitis, ethmoidal
  - extradural — *see* Abscess, extradural
  - frontal (chronic) (sinus) — *see* Sinusitis, frontal
  - gallbladder K81.0
  - mastoid (process) (acute) — *see* Mastoiditis, acute
  - maxilla, maxillary M27.2
    - sinus (chronic) — *see* Sinusitis, maxillary
  - nasal sinus (chronic) — *see* Sinusitis
  - sinus (accessory) (chronic) (nasal) — *see* Sinusitis
  - sphenoidal (sinus) (chronic) — *see* Sinusitis, sphenoidal
  - subarachnoid — *see* Abscess, extradural
  - subdural — *see* Abscess, subdural
  - tuberculous A15.6
  - ureter — *see* Ureteritis
  - ventricular — *see* Abscess, brain
- **En coup** de sabre lesion L94.1
- **Enamel** pearls K00.2
- **Enameloma** K00.2
- **Enanthema**, viral B09
- **Encephalitis** (chronic) (hemorrhagic) (idiopathic) (nonepidemic) (spurious) (subacute) G04.90
  - acute (*see also* Encephalitis, viral)A86
    - disseminated G04.00
      - infectious G04.01
      - noninfectious G04.81
      - postimmunization (postvaccination) G04.02
      - postinfectious G04.01
    - inclusion body A85.8
    - necrotizing hemorrhagic G04.30
      - postimmunization G04.32
      - postinfectious G04.31
      - specified NEC G04.39
  - arboviral, arbovirus NEC A85.2
  - arthropod-borne NEC (viral) A85.2
  - Australian A83.4
  - California (virus) A83.5
  - Central European (tick-borne) A84.1
  - Czechoslovakian A84.1
  - Dawson's (inclusion body) A81.1
  - diffuse sclerosing A81.1
  - disseminated, acute G04.00
  - due to
    - cat scratch disease A28.1
    - human immunodeficiency virus (HIV) disease B20 *[G05.3]*
    - malaria — *see* Malaria
    - rickettsiosis — *see* Rickettsiosis
    - smallpox inoculation G04.02
    - typhus — *see* Typhus
  - Eastern equine A83.2
  - endemic (viral) A86
  - epidemic NEC (viral) A86
  - equine (acute) (infectious) (viral) A83.9
    - Eastern A83.2
    - Venezuelan A92.2
    - Western A83.1
  - Far Eastern (tick-borne) A84.0
  - following vaccination or other immunization procedure G04.02
  - herpes zoster B02.0
  - herpesviral B00.4
    - due to herpesvirus 6 B10.01
    - due to herpesvirus 7 B10.09
    - specified NEC B10.09
  - Ilheus (virus) A83.8
  - inclusion body A81.1
  - in (due to)
    - actinomycosis A42.82
    - adenovirus A85.1
    - African trypanosomiasis B56.9 *[G05.3]*
    - Chagas' disease (chronic) B57.42
    - cytomegalovirus B25.8
    - enterovirus A85.0
    - herpes (simplex) virus B00.4
      - due to herpesvirus 6 B10.01
      - due to herpesvirus 7 B10.09
      - specified NEC B10.09
    - infectious disease NEC B99 ☑ *[G05.3]*
    - influenza — *see* Influenza, with, encephalopathy

- **Encephalitis** — *continued*
  - in — *continued*
    - listeriosis A32.12
    - measles B05.0
    - mumps B26.2
    - naegleriasis B60.2
    - parasitic disease NEC B89 *[G05.3]*
    - poliovirus A80.9 *[G05.3]*
    - rubella B06.01
    - syphilis
      - congenital A50.42
      - late A52.14
    - systemic lupus erythematosus M32.19
    - toxoplasmosis (acquired) B58.2
      - congenital P37.1
    - tuberculosis A17.82
    - zoster B02.0
  - infectious (acute) (virus) NEC A86
  - Japanese (B type) A83.0
  - La Crosse A83.5
  - lead — *see* Poisoning, lead
  - lethargica (acute) (infectious) A85.8
  - louping ill A84.8
  - lupus erythematosus, systemic M32.19
  - lymphatica A87.2
  - Mengo A85.8
  - meningococcal A39.81
  - Murray Valley A83.4
  - otitic NEC H66.40 *[G05.3]*
  - parasitic NOS B71.9
  - periaxial G37.0
  - periaxialis (concentrica) (diffuse) G37.5
  - postchickenpox B01.11
  - postexanthematous NEC B09
  - postimmunization G04.02
  - postinfectious NEC G04.01
  - postmeasles B05.0
  - postvaccinal G04.02
  - postvaricella B01.11
  - postviral NEC A86
  - Powassan A84.8
  - Rasmussen G04.81
  - Rio Bravo A85.8
  - Russian
    - autumnal A83.0
    - spring-summer (taiga) A84.0
  - saturnine — *see* Poisoning, lead
  - specified NEC G04.81
  - St. Louis A83.3
  - subacute sclerosing A81.1
  - summer A83.0
  - suppurative G04.81
  - tick-borne A84.9
  - Torula, torular (cryptococcal) B45.1
  - toxic NEC G92
  - trichinosis B75 *[G05.3]*
  - type
    - B A83.0
    - C A83.3
  - van Bogaert's A81.1
  - Venezuelan equine A92.2
  - Vienna A85.8
  - viral, virus A86
    - arthropod-borne NEC A85.2
      - mosquito-borne A83.9
        - Australian X disease A83.4
        - California virus A83.5
        - Eastern equine A83.2
        - Japanese (B type) A83.0
        - Murray Valley A83.4
        - specified NEC A83.8
        - St. Louis A83.3
        - type B A83.0
        - type C A83.3
        - Western equine A83.1
      - tick-borne A84.9
        - biundulant A84.1
        - central European A84.1
        - Czechoslovakian A84.1
        - diphasic meningoencephalitis A84.1
        - Far Eastern A84.0
        - Russian spring-summer (taiga) A84.0
        - specified NEC A84.8
    - specified type NEC A85.8
  - Western equine A83.1
- **Encephalocele** Q01.9
  - frontal Q01.0
  - nasofrontal Q01.1
  - occipital Q01.2
  - specified NEC Q01.8
- **Encephalocystocele** — *see* Encephalocele

- **Encephaloduroarteriomyosynangiosis** (EDAMS) I67.5
- **Encephalomalacia** (brain) (cerebellar) (cerebral) — *see* Softening, brain
- **Encephalomeningitis** — *see* Meningoencephalitis
- **Encephalomeningocele** — *see* Encephalocele
- **Encephalomeningomyelitis** — *see* Meningoencephalitis
- **Encephalomyelitis** (*see also* Encephalitis)G04.90
  - acute disseminated G04.00
    - infectious G04.01
    - noninfectious G04.81
    - postimmunization G04.02
    - postinfectious G04.01
  - acute necrotizing hemorrhagic G04.30
    - postimmunization G04.32
    - postinfectious G04.31
    - specified NEC G04.39
  - benign myalgic G93.3
  - equine A83.9
    - Eastern A83.2
    - Venezuelan A92.2
    - Western A83.1
  - in diseases classified elsewhere G05.3
  - myalgic, benign G93.3
  - postchickenpox B01.11
  - postinfectious NEC G04.01
  - postmeasles B05.0
  - postvaccinal G04.02
  - postvaricella B01.11
  - rubella B06.01
  - specified NEC G04.81
  - Venezuelan equine A92.2
- **Encephalomyelocele** — *see* Encephalocele
- **Encephalomyelomeningitis** — *see* Meningoencephalitis
- **Encephalomyelopathy** G96.9
- **Encephalomyeloradiculitis** (acute) G61.0
- **Encephalomyeloradiculoneuritis** (acute) (Guillain-Barré) G61.0
- **Encephalomyeloradiculopathy** G96.9
- **Encephalopathia** hyperbilirubinemica, newborn P57.9
  - due to isoimmunization (conditions in P55) P57.0
- **Encephalopathy** (acute) G93.40
  - acute necrotizing hemorrhagic G04.30
    - postimmunization G04.32
    - postinfectious G04.31
    - specified NEC G04.39
  - alcoholic G31.2
  - anoxic — *see* Damage, brain, anoxic
  - arteriosclerotic I67.2
  - centrolobar progressive (Schilder) G37.0
  - congenital Q07.9
  - degenerative, in specified disease NEC G32.89
  - demyelinating callosal G37.1
  - due to
    - drugs - (*see also* Table of Drugs and Chemicals)G92
  - hepatic — *see* Failure, hepatic
  - hyperbilirubinemic, newborn P57.9
    - due to isoimmunization (conditions in P55) P57.0
  - hypertensive I67.4
  - hypoglycemic E16.2
  - hypoxic — *see* Damage, brain, anoxic
  - hypoxic ischemic P91.60
    - mild P91.61
    - moderate P91.62
    - severe P91.63
  - in (due to) (with)
    - birth injury P11.1
    - hyperinsulinism E16.1 *[G94]*
    - influenza — *see* Influenza, with, encephalopathy
    - lack of vitamin (*see also* Deficiency, vitamin)E56.9 *[G32.89]*
    - neoplastic disease (see also Neoplasm) D49.9 *[G13.1]*
    - serum (*see also* Reaction, serum)T80.69 ☑
    - syphilis A52.17
    - trauma (postconcussional) F07.81
      - current injury — *see* Injury, intracranial
    - vaccination G04.02
  - lead — *see* Poisoning, lead
  - metabolic G93.41
    - drug induced G92
    - toxic G92
  - myoclonic, early, symptomatic — *see* Epilepsy, generalized, specified NEC
  - necrotizing, subacute (Leigh) G31.82
  - pellagrous E52 *[G32.89]*

Encephalopathy — *continued*
- portosystemic — *see* Failure, hepatic
- postcontusional F07.81
  - current injury — *see* Injury, intracranial, diffuse
- posthypoglycemic (coma) E16.1 *[G94]*
- postradiation G93.89
- saturnine — *see* Poisoning, lead
- septic G93.41
- specified NEC G93.49
- spongiform, subacute (viral) A81.09
- toxic G92
  - metabolic G92
- traumatic (postconcussional) F07.81
  - current injury — *see* Injury, intracranial
- vitamin B deficiency NEC E53.9 *[G32.89]*
  - vitamin B1 E51.2
- Wernicke's E51.2

Encephalorrhagia — *see* Hemorrhage, intracranial, intracerebral

Encephalosis, posttraumatic F07.81

Enchondroma (*see also* Neoplasm, bone, benign)

Enchondromatosis (cartilaginous) (multiple) Q78.4

Encopresis R15.9
- functional F98.1
- nonorganic origin F98.1
- psychogenic F98.1

Encounter (with health service) (for) Z76.89
- adjustment and management (of)
  - breast implant Z45.81 ☑
  - implanted device NEC Z45.89
  - myringotomy device (stent) (tube) Z45.82
- administrative purpose only Z02.9
  - examination for
    - adoption Z02.82
    - armed forces Z02.3
    - disability determination Z02.71
    - driving license Z02.4
    - employment Z02.1
    - insurance Z02.6
    - medical certificate NEC Z02.79
    - paternity testing Z02.81
    - residential institution admission Z02.2
    - school admission Z02.0
    - sports Z02.5
  - specified reason NEC Z02.89
- aftercare — *see* Aftercare
- antenatal screening Z36
- assisted reproductive fertility procedure cycle Z31.83
- blood typing Z01.83
  - Rh typing Z01.83
- breast augmentation or reduction Z41.1
- breast implant exchange (different material) (different size) Z45.81 ☑
- breast reconstruction following mastectomy Z42.1
- check-up — *see* Examination
- chemotherapy for neoplasm Z51.11
- colonoscopy, screening Z12.11
- counseling — *see* Counseling
- delivery, full-term, uncomplicated O80
  - cesarean, without indication O82
- desensitization to allergens Z51.6
- ear piercing Z41.3
- examination — *see* Examination
- expectant parent (s) (adoptive) pre-birth pediatrician visit Z76.81
- fertility preservation procedure (prior to cancer therapy) (prior to removal of gonads) Z31.84
- fitting (of) — *see* Fitting (and adjustment) (of)
- genetic
  - counseling Z31.5
  - testing — *see* Test, genetic
- hearing conservation and treatment Z01.12
- immunotherapy for neoplasm Z51.12
- in vitro fertilization cycle Z31.83
- instruction (in)
  - childbirth Z32.2
  - child care (postpartal) (prenatal) Z32.3
  - natural family planning
    - procreative Z31.61
    - to avoid pregnancy Z30.02
- insulin pump titration Z46.81
- joint prosthesis insertion following prior explantation of joint prosthesis (staged procedure)
  - hip Z47.32
  - knee Z47.33
  - shoulder Z47.31
- laboratory (as part of a general medical examination) Z00.00
  - with abnormal findings Z00.01

Encounter — *continued*
- mental health services (for)
  - abuse NEC
    - perpetrator Z69.82
    - victim Z69.81
  - child abuse
    - nonparental
      - perpetrator Z69.021
      - victim Z69.020
    - parental
      - perpetrator Z69.011
      - victim Z69.010
  - spousal or partner abuse
    - perpetrator Z69.12
    - victim Z69.11
- observation (for) (ruled out)
  - exposure to (suspected)
    - anthrax Z03.810
    - biological agent NEC Z03.818
- pediatrician visit, by expectant parent (s) (adoptive) Z76.81
- plastic and reconstructive surgery following medical procedure or healed injury NEC Z42.8
- pregnancy
  - supervision of — *see* Pregnancy, supervision of
  - test Z32.00
    - result negative Z32.02
    - result positive Z32.01
- procreative management and counseling for gestational carrier Z31.7
- prophylactic measures Z29.9
  - antivenin Z29.12
  - fluoride administration Z29.3
  - immunotherapy for respiratory syncytial virus (RSV) Z29.11
  - rabies immune globin Z29.14
  - Rho (D) immune globulin Z29.13
  - specified NEC Z29.8
- radiation therapy (antineoplastic) Z51.0
- radiological (as part of a general medical examination) Z00.00
  - with abnormal findings Z00.01
- reconstructive surgery following medical procedure or healed injury NEC Z42.8
- removal (of) (*see also* Removal)
  - artificial
    - arm Z44.00 ☑
      - complete Z44.01 ☑
      - partial Z44.02 ☑
    - eye Z44.2 ☑
    - leg Z44.10 ☑
      - complete Z44.11 ☑
      - partial Z44.12 ☑
  - breast implant Z45.81 ☑
    - tissue expander (without synchronous insertion of permanent implant) Z45.81 ☑
  - device Z46.9
    - specified NEC Z46.89
  - external
    - fixation device - code to fracture with seventh character D
    - prosthesis, prosthetic device Z44.9
      - breast Z44.3 ☑
      - specified NEC Z44.8
  - implanted device NEC Z45.89
  - insulin pump Z46.81
  - internal fixation device Z47.2
  - myringotomy device (stent) (tube) Z45.82
  - nervous system device NEC Z46.2
    - brain neuropacemaker Z46.2
    - visual substitution device Z46.2
      - implanted Z45.31
  - non-vascular catheter Z46.82
  - orthodontic device Z46.4
  - stent
    - ureteral Z46.6
  - urinary device Z46.6
- repeat cervical smear to confirm findings of recent normal smear following initial abnormal smear Z01.42
- respirator [ventilator] use during power failure Z99.12
- Rh typing Z01.83
- screening — *see* Screening
- specified NEC Z76.89
- sterilization Z30.2
- suspected condition, ruled out
  - amniotic cavity and membrane Z03.71
  - cervical shortening Z03.75
  - fetal anomaly Z03.73

Encounter — *continued*
- suspected condition — *continued*
  - fetal growth Z03.74
  - maternal and fetal conditions NEC Z03.79
  - oligohydramnios Z03.71
  - placental problem Z03.72
  - polyhydramnios Z03.71
- suspected exposure (to), ruled out
  - anthrax Z03.810
  - biological agents NEC Z03.818
- termination of pregnancy, elective Z33.2
- testing — *see* Test
- therapeutic drug level monitoring Z51.81
- titration, insulin pump Z46.81
- to determine fetal viability of pregnancy O36.80 ☑
- training
  - insulin pump Z46.81
- X-ray of chest (as part of a general medical examination) Z00.00
  - with abnormal findings Z00.01

Encystment — *see* Cyst

Endarteritis (bacterial, subacute) (infective) I77.6
- brain I67.7
- cerebral or cerebrospinal I67.7
- deformans — *see* Arteriosclerosis
- embolic — *see* Embolism
- obliterans (*see also* Arteriosclerosis)
  - pulmonary I28.8
- pulmonary I28.8
- retina — *see* Vasculitis, retina
- senile — *see* Arteriosclerosis
- syphilitic A52.09
  - brain or cerebral A52.04
  - congenital A50.54 *[I79.8]*
- tuberculous A18.89

Endemic — *see* condition

Endocarditis (chronic) (marantic) (nonbacterial) (thrombotic) (valvular) I38
- with rheumatic fever (conditions in I00)
  - active — *see* Endocarditis, acute, rheumatic
  - inactive or quiescent (with chorea) I09.1
- acute or subacute I33.9
  - infective I33.0
  - rheumatic (aortic) (mitral) (pulmonary) (tricuspid) I01.1
    - with chorea (acute) (rheumatic) (Sydenham's) I02.0
- aortic (heart) (nonrheumatic) (valve) I35.8
  - with
    - mitral disease I08.0
      - with tricuspid (valve) disease I08.3
      - active or acute I01.1
        - with chorea (acute) (rheumatic) (Sydenham's) I02.0
    - rheumatic fever (conditions in I00)
      - active — *see* Endocarditis, acute, rheumatic
      - inactive or quiescent (with chorea) I06.9
    - tricuspid (valve) disease I08.2
      - with mitral (valve) disease I08.3
  - acute or subacute I33.9
  - arteriosclerotic I35.8
  - rheumatic I06.9
    - with mitral disease I08.0
      - with tricuspid (valve) disease I08.3
      - active or acute I01.1
        - with chorea (acute) (rheumatic) (Sydenham's) I02.0
    - active or acute I01.1
      - with chorea (acute) (rheumatic) (Sydenham's) I02.0
    - specified NEC I06.8
  - specified cause NEC I35.8
  - syphilitic A52.03
- arteriosclerotic I38
- atypical verrucous (Libman-Sacks) M32.11
- bacterial (acute) (any valve) (subacute) I33.0
- candidal B37.6
- congenital Q24.8
- constrictive I33.0
- Coxiella burnetii A78 *[I39]*
- Coxsackie B33.21
- due to
  - prosthetic cardiac valve T82.6 ☑
  - Q fever A78 *[I39]*
  - Serratia marcescens I33.0
  - typhoid (fever) A01.02
- gonococcal A54.83
- infectious or infective (acute) (any valve) (subacute) I33.0
- lenta (acute) (any valve) (subacute) I33.0
- Libman-Sacks M32.11
- listerial A32.82

Endocarditis - Enteritis

Endocarditis — *continued*
- Löffler's I42.3
- malignant (acute) (any valve) (subacute) I33.0
- meningococcal A39.51
- mitral (chronic) (double) (fibroid) (heart) (inactive) (valve) (with chorea) I05.9
  - with
    - aortic (valve) disease I08.0
      - with tricuspid (valve) disease I08.3
      - active or acute I01.1
        - with chorea (acute) (rheumatic) (Sydenham's) I02.0
    - rheumatic fever (conditions in I00)
      - active — *see* Endocarditis, acute, rheumatic
      - inactive or quiescent (with chorea) I05.9
    - tricuspid (valve) disease I08.1
      - with aortic (valve) disease I08.3
  - active or acute I01.1
    - with chorea (acute) (rheumatic) (Sydenham's) I02.0
    - bacterial I33.0
  - arteriosclerotic I34.8
  - nonrheumatic I34.8
    - acute or subacute I33.9
  - specified NEC I05.8
- monilial B37.6
- multiple valves I08.9
  - specified disorders I08.8
- mycotic (acute) (any valve) (subacute) I33.0
- pneumococcal (acute) (any valve) (subacute) I33.0
- pulmonary (chronic) (heart) (valve) I37.8
  - with rheumatic fever (conditions in I00)
    - active — *see* Endocarditis, acute, rheumatic
    - inactive or quiescent (with chorea) I09.89
      - with aortic, mitral or tricuspid disease I08.8
  - acute or subacute I33.9
    - rheumatic I01.1
      - with chorea (acute) (rheumatic) (Sydenham's) I02.0
  - arteriosclerotic I37.8
  - congenital Q22.2
  - rheumatic (chronic) (inactive) (with chorea) I09.89
    - active or acute I01.1
      - with chorea (acute) (rheumatic) (Sydenham's) I02.0
  - syphilitic A52.03
- purulent (acute) (any valve) (subacute) I33.0
- Q fever A78 *[I39]*
- rheumatic (chronic) (inactive) (with chorea) I09.1
  - active or acute (aortic) (mitral) (pulmonary) (tricuspid) I01.1
    - with chorea (acute) (rheumatic) (Sydenham's) I02.0
- rheumatoid — *see* Rheumatoid, carditis
- septic (acute) (any valve) (subacute) I33.0
- streptococcal (acute) (any valve) (subacute) I33.0
- subacute — *see* Endocarditis, acute
- suppurative (acute) (any valve) (subacute) I33.0
- syphilitic A52.03
- toxic I33.9
- tricuspid (chronic) (heart) (inactive) (rheumatic) (valve) (with chorea) I07.9
  - with
    - aortic (valve) disease I08.2
      - mitral (valve) disease I08.3
    - mitral (valve) disease I08.1
      - aortic (valve) disease I08.3
    - rheumatic fever (conditions in I00)
      - active — *see* Endocarditis, acute, rheumatic
      - inactive or quiescent (with chorea) I07.8
  - active or acute I01.1
    - with chorea (acute) (rheumatic) (Sydenham's) I02.0
  - arteriosclerotic I36.8
  - nonrheumatic I36.8
    - acute or subacute I33.9
  - specified cause, except rheumatic I36.8
- tuberculous — *see* Tuberculosis, endocarditis
- typhoid A01.02
- ulcerative (acute) (any valve) (subacute) I33.0
- vegetative (acute) (any valve) (subacute) I33.0
- verrucous (atypical) (nonbacterial) (nonrheumatic) M32.11

Endocardium, endocardial (*see also* condition)
- cushion defect Q21.2

Endocervicitis (*see also* Cervicitis)
- due to intrauterine (contraceptive) device T83.69 ☑
- hyperplastic N72

Endocrine — *see* condition

Endocrinopathy, pluriglandular E31.9

Endodontic
- overfill M27.52
- underfill M27.53

Endodontitis K04.01
- irreversible K04.02
- reversible K04.01

Endomastoiditis — *see* Mastoiditis

Endometrioma N80.9

Endometriosis N80.9
- appendix N80.5
- bladder N80.8
- bowel N80.5
- broad ligament N80.3
- cervix N80.0
- colon N80.5
- cul-de-sac (Douglas') N80.3
- exocervix N80.0
- fallopian tube N80.2
- female genital organ NEC N80.8
- gallbladder N80.8
- in scar of skin N80.6
- internal N80.0
- intestine N80.5
- lung N80.8
- myometrium N80.0
- ovary N80.1
- parametrium N80.3
- pelvic peritoneum N80.3
- peritoneal (pelvic) N80.3
- rectovaginal septum N80.4
- rectum N80.5
- round ligament N80.3
- skin (scar) N80.6
- specified site NEC N80.8
- stromal D39.0
- umbilicus N80.8
- uterus (internal) N80.0
- vagina N80.4
- vulva N80.8

Endometritis (decidual) (nonspecific) (purulent) (senile) (atrophic) (suppurative) N71.9
- with ectopic pregnancy O08.0
- acute N71.0
- blenorrhagic (gonococcal) (acute) (chronic) A54.24
- cervix, cervical (with erosion or ectropion) (*see also* Cervicitis)
  - hyperplastic N72
- chlamydial A56.11
- chronic N71.1
- following
  - abortion — *see* Abortion by type complicated by genital infection
  - ectopic or molar pregnancy O08.0
- gonococcal, gonorrheal (acute) (chronic) A54.24
- hyperplastic (*see also* Hyperplasia, endometrial)N85.00
  - cervix N72
- puerperal, postpartum, childbirth O86.12
- subacute N71.0
- tuberculous A18.17

Endometrium — *see* condition

Endomyocardiopathy, South African I42.3

Endomyocarditis — *see* Endocarditis

Endomyofibrosis I42.3

Endomyometritis — *see* Endometritis

Endopericarditis — *see* Endocarditis

Endoperineuritis — *see* Disorder, nerve

Endophlebitis — *see* Phlebitis

Endophthalmia — *see* Endophthalmitis, purulent

Endophthalmitis (acute) (infective) (metastatic) (subacute) H44.009
- bleb associated H59.4 — *see* also Bleb, inflamed (infected), postprocedural
- gonorrheal A54.39
- in (due to)
  - cysticercosis B69.1
  - onchocerciasis B73.01
  - toxocariasis B83.0
- panuveitis — *see* Panuveitis
- parasitic H44.12 ☑
- purulent H44.00 ☑
  - panophthalmitis — *see* Panophthalmitis
  - vitreous abscess H44.02 ☑
- specified NEC H44.19
- sympathetic — *see* Uveitis, sympathetic

Endosalpingioma D28.2

Endosalpingiosis N94.89

Endosteitis — *see* Osteomyelitis

Endothelioma, bone — *see* Neoplasm, bone, malignant

Endotheliosis (hemorrhagic infectional) D69.8

Endotoxemia - code to condition

Endotrachelitis — *see* Cervicitis

Engelmann (-Camurati) syndrome Q78.3

English disease — *see* Rickets

Engman's disease L30.3

Engorgement
- breast N64.59
  - newborn P83.4
  - puerperal, postpartum O92.79
- lung (passive) — *see* Edema, lung
- pulmonary (passive) — *see* Edema, lung
- stomach K31.89
- venous, retina — *see* Occlusion, retina, vein, engorgement

Enlargement, enlarged (*see also* Hypertrophy)
- adenoids J35.2
  - with tonsils J35.3
- alveolar ridge K08.89
  - congenital — *see* Anomaly, alveolar
- apertures of diaphragm (congenital) Q79.1
- gingival K06.1
- heart, cardiac — *see* Hypertrophy, cardiac
- labium majus, childhood asymmetric (CALME) N90.61
- lacrimal gland, chronic H04.03 ☑
- liver — *see* Hypertrophy, liver
- lymph gland or node R59.9
  - generalized R59.1
  - localized R59.0
- orbit H05.34 ☑
- organ or site, congenital NEC — *see* Anomaly, by site
- parathyroid (gland) E21.0
- pituitary fossa R93.0
- prostate N40.0
  - with lower urinary tract symptoms (LUTS) N40.1
  - without lower urinary tract symptoms (LUTS) N40.0
- sella turcica R93.0
- spleen — *see* Splenomegaly
- thymus (gland) (congenital) E32.0
- thyroid (gland) — *see* Goiter
- tongue K14.8
- tonsils J35.1
  - with adenoids J35.3
- uterus N85.2

Enophthalmos H05.40 ☑
- due to
  - orbital tissue atrophy H05.41 ☑
  - trauma or surgery H05.42 ☑

Enostosis M27.8

Entamebic, entamebiasis — *see* Amebiasis

Entanglement
- umbilical cord (s) O69.2 ☑
  - with compression O69.2 ☑
    - without compression O69.82 ☑
  - around neck (with compression) O69.1 ☑
    - without compression O69.81 ☑
  - of twins in monoamniotic sac O69.2 ☑

Enteralgia — *see* Pain, abdominal

Enteric — *see* condition

Enteritis (acute) (diarrheal) (hemorrhagic) (noninfective) K52.9
- adenovirus A08.2
- aertrycke infection A02.0
- allergic K52.29
  - with
    - eosinophilic gastritis or gastroenteritis K52.81
    - food protein-induced enterocolitis syndrome K52.21
    - food protein-induced enteropathy K52.22
- amebic (acute) A06.0
  - with abscess — *see* Abscess, amebic
  - chronic A06.1
    - with abscess — *see* Abscess, amebic
    - nondysenteric A06.2
  - nondysenteric A06.2
- astrovirus A08.32
- bacillary NOS A03.9
- bacterial A04.9
  - specified NEC A04.8
- calicivirus A08.31
- candidal B37.82
- Chilomastix A07.8
- choleriformis A00.1
- chronic (noninfectious) K52.9
  - ulcerative — *see* Colitis, ulcerative
- cicatrizing (chronic) — *see* Enteritis, regional, small intestine

☑ Additional character required

Enthesopathy - Epilepsy

- **Enthesopathy** — *continued*
  - multiple sites M77.9
  - patellar tendinitis — *see* Tendinitis, patellar
  - pelvis M77.9
  - periarthritis of wrist — *see* Periarthritis, wrist
  - peroneal tendinitis — *see* Tendinitis, peroneal
  - posterior tibial syndrome M76.82 ☑
  - psoas tendinitis — *see* Tendinitis, psoas
  - shoulder region — *see* Lesion, shoulder
  - specified site NEC M77.9
  - specified type NEC M77.8
  - spinal M46.00
    - cervical region M46.02
    - cervicothoracic region M46.03
    - lumbar region M46.06
    - lumbosacral region M46.07
    - multiple sites M46.09
    - occipito-atlanto-axial region M46.01
    - sacrococcygeal region M46.08
    - thoracic region M46.04
    - thoracolumbar region M46.05
  - tibial collateral bursitis — *see* Bursitis, tibial collateral
  - upper arm M77.9
  - wrist and carpus NEC M77.8
    - calcaneal spur — *see* Spur, bone, calcaneal
    - periarthritis of wrist — *see* Periarthritis, wrist
- **Entomophobia** F40.218
- **Entomophthoromycosis** B46.8
- **Entrance,** air into vein — *see* Embolism, air
- **Entrapment,** nerve — *see* Neuropathy, entrapment
- **Entropion** (eyelid) (paralytic) H02.009
  - cicatricial H02.019
    - left H02.016
      - lower H02.015
      - upper H02.014
    - right H02.013
      - lower H02.012
      - upper H02.011
  - congenital Q10.2
  - left H02.006
    - lower H02.005
    - upper H02.004
  - mechanical H02.029
    - left H02.026
      - lower H02.025
      - upper H02.024
    - right H02.023
      - lower H02.022
      - upper H02.021
  - right H02.003
    - lower H02.002
    - upper H02.001
  - senile H02.039
    - left H02.036
      - lower H02.035
      - upper H02.034
    - right H02.033
      - lower H02.032
      - upper H02.031
  - spastic H02.049
    - left H02.046
      - lower H02.045
      - upper H02.044
    - right H02.043
      - lower H02.042
      - upper H02.041
- **Enucleated** eye (traumatic, current) S05.7 ☑
- **Enuresis** R32
  - functional F98.0
  - habit disturbance F98.0
  - nocturnal N39.44
    - psychogenic F98.0
  - nonorganic origin F98.0
  - psychogenic F98.0
- **Eosinopenia** — *see* Agranulocytosis
- **Eosinophilia** (allergic) (hereditary) (idiopathic) (secondary) D72.1
  - with
    - angiolymphoid hyperplasia (ALHE) D18.01
  - infiltrative J82
  - Löffler's J82
  - peritoneal — *see* Peritonitis, eosinophilic
  - pulmonary NEC J82
  - tropical (pulmonary) J82
- **Eosinophilia-myalgia** syndrome M35.8
- **Ependymitis** (acute) (cerebral) (chronic) (granular) — *see* Encephalomyelitis
- **Ependymoblastoma**
  - specified site — *see* Neoplasm, malignant, by site
  - unspecified site C71.9
- **Ependymoma** (epithelial) (malignant)
  - anaplastic
    - specified site — *see* Neoplasm, malignant, by site
    - unspecified site C71.9
  - benign
    - specified site — *see* Neoplasm, benign, by site
    - unspecified site D33.2
  - myxopapillary D43.2
    - specified site — *see* Neoplasm, uncertain behavior, by site
    - unspecified site D43.2
  - papillary D43.2
    - specified site — *see* Neoplasm, uncertain behavior, by site
    - unspecified site D43.2
  - specified site — *see* Neoplasm, malignant, by site
  - unspecified site C71.9
- **Ependymopathy** G93.89
- **Ephelis,** ephelides L81.2
- **Epiblepharon** (congenital) Q10.3
- **Epicanthus,** epicanthic fold (eyelid) (congenital) Q10.3
- **Epicondylitis** (elbow)
  - lateral M77.1 ☑
  - medial M77.0 ☑
- **Epicystitis** — *see* Cystitis
- **Epidemic** — *see* condition
- **Epidermidalization,** cervix — *see* Dysplasia, cervix
- **Epidermis,** epidermal — *see* condition
- **Epidermodysplasia** verruciformis B07.8
- **Epidermolysis**
  - bullosa (congenital) Q81.9
    - acquired L12.30
      - drug-induced L12.31
      - specified cause NEC L12.35
    - dystrophica Q81.2
    - letalis Q81.1
    - simplex Q81.0
    - specified NEC Q81.8
  - necroticans combustiformis L51.2
    - due to drug — *see* Table of Drugs and Chemicals, by drug
- **Epidermophytid** — *see* Dermatophytosis
- **Epidermophytosis** (infected) — *see* Dermatophytosis
- **Epididymis** — *see* condition
- **Epididymitis** (acute) (nonvenereal) (recurrent) (residual) N45.1
  - with orchitis N45.3
  - blennorrhagic (gonococcal) A54.23
  - caseous (tuberculous) A18.15
  - chlamydial A56.19
  - filarial (*see also* Infestation, filarial)B74.9 *[N51]*
  - gonococcal A54.23
  - syphilitic A52.76
  - tuberculous A18.15
- **Epididymo-orchitis** (*see also* Epididymitis)N45.3
- **Epidural** — *see* condition
- **Epigastrium,** epigastric — *see* condition
- **Epigastrocele** — *see* Hernia, ventral
- **Epiglottis** — *see* condition
- **Epiglottitis,** epiglottiditis (acute) J05.10
  - with obstruction J05.11
  - chronic J37.0
- **Epignathus** Q89.4
- **Epilepsia** partialis continua (*see also* Kozhevnikof's epilepsy)G40.1 ☑
- **Epilepsy,** epileptic, epilepsia (attack) (cerebral) (convulsion) (fit) (seizure) G40.909
  - Note: the following terms are to be considered equivalent to intractable: pharmacoresistant (pharmacologically resistant), treatment resistant, refractory (medically) and poorly controlled
  - with
    - complex partial seizures — *see* Epilepsy, localization-related, symptomatic, with complex partial seizures
    - grand mal seizures on awakening — *see* Epilepsy, generalized, specified NEC
    - myoclonic absences — *see* Epilepsy, generalized, specified NEC
    - myoclonic-astatic seizures — *see* Epilepsy, generalized, specified NEC
    - simple partial seizures — *see* Epilepsy, localization-related, symptomatic, with simple partial seizures
  - akinetic — *see* Epilepsy, generalized, specified NEC
- **Epilepsy** — *continued*
  - benign childhood with centrotemporal EEG spikes — *see* Epilepsy, localization-related, idiopathic
  - benign myoclonic in infancy G40.80 ☑
  - Bravais-jacksonian — *see* Epilepsy, localization-related, symptomatic, with simple partial seizures
  - childhood
    - with occipital EEG paroxysms — *see* Epilepsy, localization-related, idiopathic
    - absence G40.A09
      - intractable G40.A19
        - with status epilepticus G40.A11
        - without status epilepticus G40.A19
      - not intractable G40.A09
        - with status epilepticus G40.A01
        - without status epilepticus G40.A09
  - climacteric — *see* Epilepsy, specified NEC
  - cysticercosis B69.0
  - deterioration (mental) F06.8
  - due to syphilis A52.19
  - focal — *see* Epilepsy, localization-related, symptomatic, with simple partial seizures
  - generalized
    - idiopathic G40.309
      - intractable G40.319
        - with status epilepticus G40.311
        - without status epilepticus G40.319
      - not intractable G40.309
        - with status epilepticus G40.301
        - without status epilepticus G40.309
    - specified NEC G40.409
      - intractable G40.419
        - with status epilepticus G40.411
        - without status epilepticus G40.419
      - not intractable G40.409
        - with status epilepticus G40.401
        - without status epilepticus G40.409
  - impulsive petit mal — *see* Epilepsy, juvenile myoclonic
  - intractable G40.919
    - with status epilepticus G40.911
    - without status epilepticus G40.919
  - juvenile absence G40.A09
    - intractable G40.A19
      - with status epilepticus G40.A11
      - without status epilepticus G40.A19
    - not intractable G40.A09
      - with status epilepticus G40.A01
      - without status epilepticus G40.A09
  - juvenile myoclonic G40.B09
    - intractable G40.B19
      - with status epilepticus G40.B11
      - without status epilepticus G40.B19
    - not intractable G40.B09
      - with status epilepticus G40.B01
      - without status epilepticus G40.B09
  - localization-related (focal) (partial)
    - idiopathic G40.009
      - with seizures of localized onset G40.009
        - intractable G40.019
          - with status epilepticus G40.011
          - without status epilepticus G40.019
        - not intractable G40.009
          - with status epilepticus G40.001
          - without status epilepticus G40.009
    - symptomatic
      - with complex partial seizures G40.209
        - intractable G40.219
          - with status epilepticus G40.211
          - without status epilepticus G40.219
        - not intractable G40.209
          - with status epilepticus G40.201
          - without status epilepticus G40.209
      - with simple partial seizures G40.109
        - intractable G40.119
          - with status epilepticus G40.111
          - without status epilepticus G40.119
        - not intractable G40.109
          - with status epilepticus G40.101
          - without status epilepticus G40.109
  - myoclonus, myoclonic — *see* Epilepsy, generalized, specified NEC
    - progressive — *see* Epilepsy, generalized, idiopathic
  - not intractable G40.909
    - with status epilepticus G40.901
    - without status epilepticus G40.909
  - on awakening — *see* Epilepsy, generalized, specified NEC
  - parasitic NOS B71.9 *[G94]*

Epilepsy — *continued*
- partialis continua (*see also* Kozhevnikof's epilepsy)G40.1 ☑
- peripheral — *see* Epilepsy, specified NEC
- procursiva — *see* Epilepsy, localization-related, symptomatic, with simple partial seizures
- progressive (familial) myoclonic — *see* Epilepsy, generalized, idiopathic
- reflex — *see* Epilepsy, specified NEC
- related to
  - alcohol G40.509
    - not intractable G40.509
      - with status epilepticus G40.501
      - without status epliepticus G40.509
  - drugs G40.509
    - not intractable G40.509
      - with status epilepticus G40.501
      - without status epliepticus G40.509
  - external causes G40.509
    - not intractable G40.509
      - with status epilepticus G40.501
      - without status epilepticus G40.509
  - hormonal changes G40.509
    - not intractable G40.509
      - with status epilepticus G40.501
      - without status epilepticus G40.509
  - sleep deprivation G40.509
    - not intractable G40.509
      - with status epilepticus G40.501
      - without status epliepticus G40.509
  - stress G40.509
    - not intractable G40.509
      - with status epilepticus G40.501
      - without status epliepticus G40.509
- somatomotor — *see* Epilepsy, localization-related, symptomatic, with simple partial seizures
- somatosensory — *see* Epilepsy, localization-related, symptomatic, with simple partial seizures
- spasms G40.822
  - intractable G40.824
    - with status epilepticus G40.823
    - without status epilepticus G40.824
  - not intractable G40.822
    - with status epilepticus G40.821
    - without status epilepticus G40.822
- specified NEC G40.802
  - intractable G40.804
    - with status epilepticus G40.803
    - without status epilepticus G40.804
  - not intractable G40.802
    - with status epilepticus G40.801
    - without status epilepticus G40.802
- syndromes
  - generalized
    - idiopathic G40.309
      - intractable G40.319
        - with status epilepticus G40.311
        - without status epilepticus G40.319
      - not intractable G40.309
        - with status epilepticus G40.301
        - without status epilepticus G40.309
    - specified NEC G40.409
      - intractable G40.419
        - with status epilepticus G40.411
        - without status epilepticus G40.419
      - not intractable G40.409
        - with status epilepticus G40.401
        - without status epilepticus G40.409
  - localization-related (focal) (partial)
    - idiopathic G40.009
      - with seizures of localized onset G40.009
        - intractable G40.019
          - with status epilepticus G40.011
          - without status epilepticus G40.019
        - not intractable G40.009
          - with status epilepticus G40.001
          - without status epilepticus G40.009
    - symptomatic
      - with complex partial seizures G40.209
        - intractable G40.219
          - with status epilepticus G40.211
          - without status epilepticus G40.219
        - not intractable G40.209
          - with status epilepticus G40.201
          - without status epilepticus G40.209
      - with simple partial seizures G40.109
        - intractable G40.119
          - with status epilepticus G40.111
          - without status epilepticus G40.119
        - not intractable G40.109
          - with status epilepticus G40.101

Epilepsy — *continued*
- syndromes — *continued*
  - without status epilepticus G40.109
  - specified NEC G40.802
    - intractable G40.804
      - with status epilepticus G40.803
      - without status epilepticus G40.804
    - not intractable G40.802
      - with status epilepticus G40.801
      - without status epilepticus G40.802
- tonic (-clonic) — *see* Epilepsy, generalized, specified NEC
- twilight F05
- uncinate (gyrus) — *see* Epilepsy, localization-related, symptomatic, with complex partial seizures
- Unverricht (-Lundborg) (familial myoclonic) — *see* Epilepsy, generalized, idiopathic
- visceral — *see* Epilepsy, specified NEC
- visual — *see* Epilepsy, specified NEC

Epiloia Q85.1

Epimenorrhea N92.0

Epipharyngitis — *see* Nasopharyngitis

Epiphora H04.20 ☑
- due to
  - excess lacrimation H04.21 ☑
  - insufficient drainage H04.22 ☑

Epiphyseal arrest — *see* Arrest, epiphyseal

Epiphyseolysis, epiphysiolysis — *see* Osteochondropathy

Epiphysitis (*see also* Osteochondropathy)
- juvenile M92.9
- syphilitic (congenital) A50.02

Epiplocele — *see* Hernia, abdomen

Epiploitis — *see* Peritonitis

Epiplosarcomphalocele — *see* Hernia, umbilicus

Episcleritis (suppurative) H15.10 ☑
- in (due to)
  - syphilis A52.71
  - tuberculosis A18.51
- nodular H15.12 ☑
- periodica fugax H15.11 ☑
  - angioneurotic — *see* Edema, angioneurotic
- syphilitic (late) A52.71
- tuberculous A18.51

Episode
- affective, mixed F39
- depersonalization (in neurotic state) F48.1
- depressive F32.9
  - major F32.9
    - mild F32.0
    - moderate F32.1
    - severe (without psychotic symptoms) F32.2
      - with psychotic symptoms F32.3
  - recurrent F33.9
    - brief F33.8
  - specified NEC F32.89
- hypomanic F30.8
- manic F30.9
  - with
    - psychotic symptoms F30.2
    - remission (full) F30.4
      - partial F30.3
  - other specified F30.8
  - recurrent F31.89
  - without psychotic symptoms F30.10
    - mild F30.11
    - moderate F30.12
    - severe (without psychotic symptoms) F30.13
      - with psychotic symptoms F30.2
- psychotic F23
  - organic F06.8
- schizophrenic (acute) NEC, brief F23

Epispadias (female) (male) Q64.0

Episplenitis D73.89

Epistaxis (multiple) R04.0
- hereditary I78.0
- vicarious menstruation N94.89

Epithelioma (malignant) — *see* also Neoplasm, malignant, by site
- adenoides cysticum — *see* Neoplasm, skin, benign
- basal cell — *see* Neoplasm, skin, malignant
- benign — *see* Neoplasm, benign, by site
- Bowen's — *see* Neoplasm, skin, in situ
- calcifying, of Malherbe — *see* Neoplasm, skin, benign
- external site — *see* Neoplasm, skin, malignant
- intraepidermal, Jadassohn — *see* Neoplasm, skin, benign
- squamous cell — *see* Neoplasm, malignant, by site

Epitheliomatosis pigmented Q82.1

Epitheliopathy, multifocal placoid pigment H30.14 ☑

Epithelium, epithelial — *see* condition

Epituberculosis (with atelectasis) (allergic) A15.7

Eponychia Q84.6

Epstein's
- nephrosis or syndrome — *see* Nephrosis
- pearl K09.8

Epulis (gingiva) (fibrous) (giant cell) K06.8

Equinia A24.0

Equinovarus (congenital) (talipes) Q66.0
- acquired — *see* Deformity, limb, clubfoot

Equivalent
- convulsive (abdominal) — *see* Epilepsy, specified NEC
- epileptic (psychic) — *see* Epilepsy, localization-related, symptomatic, with complex partial seizures

Erb (-Duchenne) paralysis (birth injury) (newborn) P14.0

Erb-Goldflam disease or syndrome G70.00
- with exacerbation (acute) G70.01
- in crisis G70.01

Erb's
- disease G71.0
- palsy, paralysis (brachial) (birth) (newborn) P14.0
  - spinal (spastic) syphilitic A52.17
- pseudohypertrophic muscular dystrophy G71.0

Erdheim's syndrome (acromegalic macrospondylitis) E22.0

Erection, painful (persistent) — *see* Priapism

Ergosterol deficiency (vitamin D) E55.9
- with
  - adult osteomalacia M83.8
  - rickets — *see* Rickets

Ergotism (*see also* Poisoning, food, noxious, plant)
- from ergot used as drug (migraine therapy) — *see* Table of Drugs and Chemicals

Erosio interdigitalis blastomycetica B37.2

Erosion
- artery I77.2
  - without rupture I77.89
- bone — *see* Disorder, bone, density and structure, specified NEC
- bronchus J98.09
- cartilage (joint) — *see* Disorder, cartilage, specified type NEC
- cervix (uteri) (acquired) (chronic) (congenital) N86
  - with cervicitis N72
- cornea (nontraumatic) — *see* Ulcer, cornea
  - recurrent H18.83 ☑
  - traumatic — *see* Abrasion, cornea
- dental (idiopathic) (occupational) (due to diet, drugs or vomiting) K03.2
- duodenum, postpyloric — *see* Ulcer, duodenum
- esophagus K22.10
  - with bleeding K22.11
- gastric — *see* Ulcer, stomach
- gastrojejunal — *see* Ulcer, gastrojejunal
- implanted mesh — *see* Complications, mesh
- intestine K63.3
- lymphatic vessel I89.8
- pylorus, pyloric (ulcer) — *see* Ulcer, stomach
- spine, aneurysmal A52.09
- stomach — *see* Ulcer, stomach
- subcutaneous device pocket
  - nervous system prosthetic device, implant, or graft T85.890 ☑
  - other internal prosthetic device, implant, or graft T85.898 ☑
- teeth (idiopathic) (occupational) (due to diet, drugs or vomiting) K03.2
- urethra N36.8
- uterus N85.8

Erotomania F52.8

Error
- metabolism, inborn -- se Disorder, metabolism
- refractive — *see* Disorder, refraction

Eructation R14.2
- nervous or psychogenic F45.8

Eruption
- creeping B76.9
- drug (generalized) (taken internally) L27.0
  - fixed L27.1
  - in contact with skin — *see* Dermatitis, due to drugs
  - localized L27.1
- Hutchinson, summer L56.4
- Kaposi's varicelliform B00.0
- napkin L22

- **Eruption** — *continued*
  - polymorphous light (sun) L56.4
  - recalcitrant pustular L13.8
  - ringed R23.8
  - skin (nonspecific) R21
    - creeping (meaning hookworm) B76.9
    - due to inoculation/vaccination (generalized) (*see also* Dermatitis, due to, vaccine)L27.0
      - localized L27.1
    - erysipeloid A26.0
    - feigned L98.1
    - Kaposi's varicelliform B00.0
    - lichenoid L28.0
    - meaning dermatitis — *see* Dermatitis
    - toxic NEC L53.0
  - tooth, teeth, abnormal (incomplete) (late) (premature) (sequence) K00.6
  - vesicular R23.8
- **Erysipelas** (gangrenous) (infantile) (newborn) (phlegmonous) (suppurative) A46
  - external ear A46 *[H62.40]*
  - puerperal, postpartum O86.89
- **Erysipeloid** A26.9
  - cutaneous (Rosenbach's) A26.0
  - disseminated A26.8
  - sepsis A26.7
  - specified NEC A26.8
- **Erythema,** erythematous (infectional) (inflammation) L53.9
  - ab igne L59.0
  - annulare (centrifugum) (rheumaticum) L53.1
  - arthriticum epidemicum A25.1
  - brucellum — *see* Brucellosis
  - chronic figurate NEC L53.3
  - chronicum migrans (Borrelia burgdorferi) A69.20
  - diaper L22
  - due to
    - chemical NEC L53.0
      - in contact with skin L24.5
    - drug (internal use) — *see* Dermatitis, due to, drugs
  - elevatum diutinum L95.1
  - endemic E52
  - epidemic, arthritic A25.1
  - figuratum perstans L53.3
  - gluteal L22
  - heat - code by site under Burn, first degree
  - ichthyosiforme congenitum bullous Q80.3
  - in diseases classified elsewhere L54
  - induratum (nontuberculous) L52
    - tuberculous A18.4
  - infectiosum B08.3
  - intertrigo L30.4
  - iris L51.9
  - marginatum L53.2
    - in (due to) acute rheumatic fever I00
  - medicamentosum — *see* Dermatitis, due to, drugs
  - migrans A26.0
    - chronicum A69.20
    - tongue K14.1
  - multiforme (major) (minor) L51.9
    - bullous, bullosum L51.1
    - conjunctiva L51.1
    - nonbullous L51.0
    - pemphigoides L12.0
    - specified NEC L51.8
  - napkin L22
  - neonatorum P83.8
    - toxic P83.1
  - nodosum L52
    - tuberculous A18.4
  - palmar L53.8
  - pernio T69.1 ☑
  - rash, newborn P83.8
  - scarlatiniform (recurrent) (exfoliative) L53.8
  - solare L55.0
  - specified NEC L53.8
  - toxic, toxicum NEC L53.0
    - newborn P83.1
  - tuberculous (primary) A18.4
- **Erythematous,** erythematosus — *see* condition
- **Erythermalgia** (primary) I73.81
- **Erythralgia** I73.81
- **Erythrasma** L08.1
- **Erythredema** (polyneuropathy) — *see* Poisoning, mercury
- **Erythremia** (acute) C94.0 ☑
  - chronic D45
  - secondary D75.1
- **Erythroblastopenia** (*see also* Aplasia, red cell)D60.9
  - congenital D61.01
- **Erythroblastophthisis** D61.09
- **Erythroblastosis** (fetalis) (newborn) P55.9
  - due to
    - ABO (antibodies) (incompatibility) (isoimmunization) P55.1
    - Rh (antibodies) (incompatibility) (isoimmunization) P55.0
- **Erythrocyanosis** (crurum) I73.89
- **Erythrocythemia** — *see* Erythremia
- **Erythrocytosis** (megalosplenic) (secondary) D75.1
  - familial D75.0
  - oval, hereditary — *see* Elliptocytosis
  - secondary D75.1
  - stress D75.1
- **Erythroderma** (secondary) (*see also* Erythema)L53.9
  - bullous ichthyosiform, congenital Q80.3
  - desquamativum L21.1
  - ichthyosiform, congenital (bullous) Q80.3
  - neonatorum P83.8
  - psoriaticum L40.8
- **Erythrodysesthesia,** palmar plantar (PPE) L27.1
- **Erythrogenesis** imperfecta D61.09
- **Erythroleukemia** C94.0 ☑
- **Erythromelalgia** I73.81
- **Erythrophagocytosis** D75.89
- **Erythrophobia** F40.298
- **Erythroplakia,** oral epithelium, and tongue K13.29
- **Erythroplasia** (Queyrat) D07.4
  - specified site — *see* Neoplasm, skin, in situ
  - unspecified site D07.4
- **Escherichia** coli (E. coli), as cause of disease classified elsewhere B96.20
  - non-O157 Shiga toxin-producing (with known O group) B96.22
  - non-Shiga toxin-producing B96.29
  - O157 with confirmation of Shiga toxin when H antigen is unknown, or is not H7 B96.21
  - O157:H- (nonmotile) with confirmation of Shiga toxin B96.21
  - O157:H7 with or without confirmation of Shiga toxin-production B96.21
  - Shiga toxin-producing (with unspecified O group) (STEC) B96.23
    - O157 B96.21
    - O157:H7 with or without confirmation of Shiga toxin-production B96.21
    - specified NEC B96.22
  - specified NEC B96.29
- **Esophagismus** K22.4
- **Esophagitis** (acute) (alkaline) (chemical) (chronic) (infectional) (necrotic) (peptic) (postoperative) K20.9
  - candidal B37.81
  - due to gastrointestinal reflux disease K21.0
  - eosinophilic K20.0
  - reflux K21.0
  - specified NEC K20.8
  - tuberculous A18.83
  - ulcerative K22.10
    - with bleeding K22.11
- **Esophagocele** K22.5
- **Esophagomalacia** K22.8
- **Esophagospasm** K22.4
- **Esophagostenosis** K22.2
- **Esophagostomiasis** B81.8
- **Esophagotracheal** — *see* condition
- **Esophagus** — *see* condition
- **Esophoria** H50.51
  - convergence, excess H51.12
  - divergence, insufficiency H51.8
- **Esotropia** — *see* Strabismus, convergent concomitant
- **Espundia** B55.2
- **Essential** — *see* condition
- **Esthesioneuroblastoma** C30.0
- **Esthesioneurocytoma** C30.0
- **Esthesioneuroepithelioma** C30.0
- **Esthiomene** A55
- **Estivo-autumnal** malaria (fever) B50.9
- **Estrangement** (marital) Z63.5
  - parent-child NEC Z62.890
- **Estriasis** — *see* Myiasis
- **Ethanolism** — *see* Alcoholism
- **Etherism** — *see* Dependence, drug, inhalant
- **Ethmoid,** ethmoidal — *see* condition
- **Ethmoiditis** (chronic) (nonpurulent) (purulent) (*see also* Sinusitis, ethmoidal)
  - influenzal — *see* Influenza, with, respiratory manifestations NEC
  - Woakes' J33.1
- **Ethylism** — *see* Alcoholism
- **Eulenburg's** disease (congenital paramyotonia) G71.19
- **Eumycetoma** B47.0
- **Eunuchoidism** E29.1
  - hypogonadotropic E23.0
- **European** blastomycosis — *see* Cryptococcosis
- **Eustachian** — *see* condition
- **Evaluation** (for) (of)
  - development state
    - adolescent Z00.3
    - period of
      - delayed growth in childhood Z00.70
        - with abnormal findings Z00.71
      - rapid growth in childhood Z00.2
    - puberty Z00.3
  - growth and developmental state (period of rapid growth) Z00.2
    - delayed growth Z00.70
      - with abnormal findings Z00.71
  - mental health (status) Z00.8
    - requested by authority Z04.6
  - period of
    - delayed growth in childhood Z00.70
      - with abnormal findings Z00.71
    - rapid growth in childhood Z00.2
  - suspected condition — *see* Observation
- **Evans** syndrome D69.41
- **Event,** apparent life threatening in newborn and infant (ALTE) R68.13
- **Eventration** (*see also* Hernia, ventral)
  - colon into chest — *see* Hernia, diaphragm
  - diaphragm (congenital) Q79.1
- **Eversion**
  - bladder N32.89
  - cervix (uteri) N86
    - with cervicitis N72
  - foot NEC (*see also* Deformity, valgus, ankle)
    - congenital Q66.6
  - punctum lacrimale (postinfectional) (senile) H04.52 ☑
  - ureter (meatus) N28.89
  - urethra (meatus) N36.8
  - uterus N81.4
- **Evidence**
  - cytologic
    - of malignancy on anal smear R85.614
    - of malignancy on cervical smear R87.614
    - of malignancy on vaginal smear R87.624
- **Evisceration**
  - birth injury P15.8
  - traumatic NEC
    - eye — *see* Enucleated eye
- **Evulsion** — *see* Avulsion
- **Ewing's** sarcoma or tumor - — *see* Neoplasm, bone, malignant
- **Examination** (for) (following) (general) (of) (routine) Z00.00
  - with abnormal findings Z00.01
  - abuse, physical (alleged), ruled out
    - adult Z04.71
    - child Z04.72
  - adolescent (development state) Z00.3
  - alleged rape or sexual assault (victim), ruled out
    - adult Z04.41
    - child Z04.42
  - allergy Z01.82
  - annual (adult) (periodic) (physical) Z00.00
    - with abnormal findings Z00.01
    - gynecological Z01.419
      - with abnormal findings Z01.411
  - antibody response Z01.84
  - blood — *see* Examination, laboratory
  - blood pressure Z01.30
    - with abnormal findings Z01.31
  - cancer staging — *see* Neoplasm, malignant, by site
  - cervical Papanicolaou smear Z12.4
    - as part of routine gynecological examination Z01.419
      - with abnormal findings Z01.411
  - child (over 28 days old) Z00.129
    - with abnormal findings Z00.121
    - under 28 days old — *see* Newborn, examination
  - clinical research control or normal comparison (control) (participant) Z00.6
  - contraceptive (drug) maintenance (routine) Z30.8
    - device (intrauterine) Z30.431
  - dental Z01.20
    - with abnormal findings Z01.21
  - developmental — *see* Examination, child
  - donor (potential) Z00.5

Examination — *continued*
- ear Z01.10
  - with abnormal findings NEC Z01.118
- eye Z01.00
  - with abnormal findings Z01.01
- following
  - accident NEC Z04.3
    - transport Z04.1
    - work Z04.2
  - assault, alleged, ruled out
    - adult Z04.71
    - child Z04.72
  - motor vehicle accident Z04.1
  - treatment (for) Z09
    - combined NEC Z09
      - fracture Z09
      - malignant neoplasm Z08
    - malignant neoplasm Z08
    - mental disorder Z09
    - specified condition NEC Z09
- follow-up (routine) (following) Z09
  - chemotherapy NEC Z09
    - malignant neoplasm Z08
  - fracture Z09
  - malignant neoplasm Z08
  - postpartum Z39.2
  - psychotherapy Z09
  - radiotherapy NEC Z09
    - malignant neoplasm Z08
  - surgery NEC Z09
    - malignant neoplasm Z08
- gynecological Z01.419
  - with abnormal findings Z01.411
  - for contraceptive maintenance Z30.8
- health — *see* Examination, medical
- hearing Z01.10
  - with abnormal findings NEC Z01.118
  - following failed hearing screening Z01.110
- immunity status testing Z01.84
- laboratory (as part of a general medical examination) Z00.00
  - with abnormal findings Z00.01
  - preprocedural Z01.812
- lactating mother Z39.1
- medical (adult) (for) (of) Z00.00
  - with abnormal findings Z00.01
  - administrative purpose only Z02.9
    - specified NEC Z02.89
  - admission to
    - armed forces Z02.3
    - old age home Z02.2
    - prison Z02.89
    - residential institution Z02.2
    - school Z02.0
      - following illness or medical treatment Z02.0
    - summer camp Z02.89
  - adoption Z02.82
  - blood alcohol or drug level Z02.83
  - camp (summer) Z02.89
  - clinical research, normal subject (control) (participant) Z00.6
  - control subject in clinical research (normal comparison) (participant) Z00.6
  - donor (potential) Z00.5
  - driving license Z02.4
  - general (adult) Z00.00
    - with abnormal findings Z00.01
  - immigration Z02.89
  - insurance purposes Z02.6
  - marriage Z02.89
  - medicolegal reasons NEC Z04.8
  - naturalization Z02.89
  - participation in sport Z02.5
  - paternity testing Z02.81
  - population survey Z00.8
  - pre-employment Z02.1
  - pre-operative — *see* Examination, pre-procedural
  - pre-procedural
    - cardiovascular Z01.810
    - respiratory Z01.811
    - specified NEC Z01.818
  - preschool children
    - for admission to school Z02.0
  - prisoners
    - for entrance into prison Z02.89
  - recruitment for armed forces Z02.3
  - specified NEC Z00.8
  - sport competition Z02.5
- medicolegal reason NEC Z04.8
- newborn — *see* Newborn, examination

Examination — *continued*
- pelvic (annual) (periodic) Z01.419
  - with abnormal findings Z01.411
- period of rapid growth in childhood Z00.2
- periodic (adult) (annual) (routine) Z00.00
  - with abnormal findings Z00.01
- physical (adult) (*see also* Examination, medical Z00.00)
  - sports Z02.5
- postpartum
  - immediately after delivery Z39.0
  - routine follow-up Z39.2
- prenatal (normal pregnancy) (*see also* Pregnancy, normal)Z34.9 ☑
- pre-chemotherapy (antineoplastic) Z01.818
- pre-procedural (pre-operative)
  - cardiovascular Z01.810
  - laboratory Z01.812
  - respiratory Z01.811
  - specified NEC Z01.818
- prior to chemotherapy (antineoplastic) Z01.818
- psychiatric NEC Z00.8
  - follow-up not needing further care Z09
  - requested by authority Z04.6
- radiological (as part of a general medical examination) Z00.00
  - with abnormal findings Z00.01
- repeat cervical smear to confirm findings of recent normal smear following initial abnormal smear Z01.42
- skin (hypersensitivity) Z01.82
- special (*see also* Examination, by type)Z01.89
  - specified type NEC Z01.89
- specified type or reason NEC Z04.8
- teeth Z01.20
  - with abnormal findings Z01.21
- urine — *see* Examination, laboratory
- vision Z01.00
  - with abnormal findings Z01.01

Exanthem, exanthema (*see also* Rash)
- with enteroviral vesicular stomatitis B08.4
- Boston A88.0
- epidemic with meningitis A88.0 *[G02]*
- subitum B08.20
  - due to human herpesvirus 6 B08.21
  - due to human herpesvirus 7 B08.22
- viral, virus B09
  - specified type NEC B08.8

Excess, excessive, excessively
- alcohol level in blood R78.0
- androgen (ovarian) E28.1
- attrition, tooth, teeth K03.0
- carotene, carotin (dietary) E67.1
- cold, effects of T69.9 ☑
  - specified effect NEC T69.8 ☑
- convergence H51.12
- crying
  - in child, adolescent, or adult R45.83
  - in infant R68.11
- development, breast N62
- divergence H51.8
- drinking (alcohol) NEC (without dependence) F10.10
  - habitual (continual) (without remission) F10.20
- eating R63.2
- estrogen E28.0
- fat (*see also* Obesity)
  - in heart — *see* Degeneration, myocardial
  - localized E65
- foreskin N47.8
- gas R14.0
- glucagon E16.3
- heat — *see* Heat
- intermaxillary vertical dimension of fully erupted teeth M26.37
- interocclusal distance of fully erupted teeth M26.37
- kalium E87.5
- large
  - colon K59.39
    - congenital Q43.8
  - infant P08.0
  - organ or site, congenital NEC — *see* Anomaly, by site
- long
  - organ or site, congenital NEC — *see* Anomaly, by site
- menstruation (with regular cycle) N92.0
  - with irregular cycle N92.1
- napping Z72.821
- natrium E87.0
- number of teeth K00.1

Excess — *continued*
- nutrient (dietary) NEC R63.2
- potassium (K) E87.5
- salivation K11.7
- secretion (*see also* Hypersecretion)
  - milk O92.6
  - sputum R09.3
  - sweat R61
- sexual drive F52.8
- short
  - organ or site, congenital NEC — *see* Anomaly, by site
  - umbilical cord in labor or delivery O69.3 ☑
- skin L98.7
  - and subcutaneous tissue L98.7
  - eyelid (acquired) — *see* Blepharochalasis
    - congenital Q10.3
- sodium (Na) E87.0
- spacing of fully erupted teeth M26.32
- sputum R09.3
- sweating R61
- thirst R63.1
  - due to deprivation of water T73.1 ☑
- tuberosity of jaw M26.07
- vitamin
  - A (dietary) E67.0
    - administered as drug (prolonged intake) — *see* Table of Drugs and Chemicals, vitamins, adverse effect
    - overdose or wrong substance given or taken — *see* Table of Drugs and Chemicals, vitamins, poisoning
  - D (dietary) E67.3
    - administered as drug (prolonged intake) — *see* Table of Drugs and Chemicals, vitamins, adverse effect
    - overdose or wrong substance given or taken — *see* Table of Drugs and Chemicals, vitamins, poisoning
- weight
  - gain R63.5
  - loss R63.4

Excitability, abnormal, under minor stress (personality disorder) F60.3

Excitation
- anomalous atrioventricular I45.6
- psychogenic F30.8
- reactive (from emotional stress, psychological trauma) F30.8

Excitement
- hypomanic F30.8
- manic F30.9
- mental, reactive (from emotional stress, psychological trauma) F30.8
- state, reactive (from emotional stress, psychological trauma) F30.8

Excoriation (traumatic) (*see also* Abrasion)
- neurotic L98.1
- skin picking disorder F42.4

Exfoliation
- due to erythematous conditions according to extent of body surface involved L49.0
  - 10-19 percent of body surface L49.1
  - 20-29 percent of body surface L49.2
  - 30-39 percent of body surface L49.3
  - 40-49 percent of body surface L49.4
  - 50-59 percent of body surface L49.5
  - 60-69 percent of body surface L49.6
  - 70-79 percent of body surface L49.7
  - 80-89 percent of body surface L49.8
  - 90-99 percent of body surface L49.9
  - less than 10 percent of body surface L49.0
- teeth, due to systemic causes K08.0

Exfoliative — *see* condition

Exhaustion, exhaustive (physical NEC) R53.83
- battle F43.0
- cardiac — *see* Failure, heart
- delirium F43.0
- due to
  - cold T69.8 ☑
  - excessive exertion T73.3 ☑
  - exposure T73.2 ☑
  - neurasthenia F48.8
- heart — *see* Failure, heart
- heat (*see also* Heat, exhaustion)T67.5 ☑
  - due to
    - salt depletion T67.4 ☑
    - water depletion T67.3 ☑
- maternal, complicating delivery O75.81
- mental F48.8
- myocardium, myocardial — *see* Failure, heart
- nervous F48.8

Exhaustion - Failure

Exhaustion — *continued*
- old age R54
- psychogenic F48.8
- psychosis F43.0
- senile R54
- vital NEC Z73.0

Exhibitionism F65.2
Exocervicitis — *see* Cervicitis
Exomphalos Q79.2
- meaning hernia — *see* Hernia, umbilicus

Exophoria H50.52
- convergence, insufficiency H51.11
- divergence, excess H51.8

Exophthalmos H05.2 ☑
- congenital Q15.8
- constant NEC H05.24 ☑
- displacement, globe — *see* Displacement, globe
- due to thyrotoxicosis (hyperthyroidism) — *see* Hyperthyroidism, with, goiter (diffuse)
- dysthyroid — *see* Hyperthyroidism, with, goiter (diffuse)
- goiter — *see* Hyperthyroidism, with, goiter (diffuse)
- intermittent NEC H05.25 ☑
- malignant — *see* Hyperthyroidism, with, goiter (diffuse)
- orbital
  - edema — *see* Edema, orbit
  - hemorrhage — *see* Hemorrhage, orbit
- pulsating NEC H05.26 ☑
- thyrotoxic, thyrotropic — *see* Hyperthyroidism, with, goiter (diffuse)

Exostosis (*see also* Disorder, bone)
- cartilaginous — *see* Neoplasm, bone, benign
- congenital (multiple) Q78.6
- external ear canal H61.81 ☑
- gonococcal A54.49
- jaw (bone) M27.8
- multiple, congenital Q78.6
- orbit H05.35 ☑
- osteocartilaginous — *see* Neoplasm, bone, benign
- syphilitic A52.77

Exotropia — *see* Strabismus, divergent concomitant
Explanation of
- investigation finding Z71.2
- medication Z71.89

Exposure (to) (*see also* Contact, with)T75.89 ☑
- acariasis Z20.7
- AIDS virus Z20.6
- air pollution Z77.110
- algae and algae toxins Z77.121
- algae bloom Z77.121
- anthrax Z20.810
- aromatic amines Z77.020
- aromatic (hazardous) compounds NEC Z77.028
- aromatic dyes NOS Z77.028
- arsenic Z77.010
- asbestos Z77.090
- bacterial disease NEC Z20.818
- benzene Z77.021
- blue-green algae bloom Z77.121
- body fluids (potentially hazardous) Z77.21
- brown tide Z77.121
- chemicals (chiefly nonmedicinal) (hazardous) NEC Z77.098
- cholera Z20.09
- chromium compounds Z77.018
- cold, effects of T69.9 ☑
  - specified effect NEC T69.8 ☑
- communicable disease Z20.9
  - bacterial NEC Z20.818
  - specified NEC Z20.89
  - viral NEC Z20.828
- cyanobacteria bloom Z77.121
- disaster Z65.5
- discrimination Z60.5
- dyes Z77.098
- effects of T73.9 ☑
- environmental tobacco smoke (acute) (chronic) Z77.22
- Escherichia coli (E. coli) Z20.01
- exhaustion due to T73.2 ☑
- fiberglass — *see* Table of Drugs and Chemicals, fiberglass
- German measles Z20.4
- gonorrhea Z20.2
- hazardous metals NEC Z77.018
- hazardous substances NEC Z77.29
- hazards in the physical environment NEC Z77.128
- hazards to health NEC Z77.9
- human immunodeficiency virus (HIV) Z20.6

Exposure — *continued*
- human T-lymphotropic virus type-1 (HTLV-1) Z20.89
- implanted
  - mesh — *see* Complications, mesh
  - prosthetic materials NEC — *see* Complications, prosthetic materials NEC
- infestation (parasitic) NEC Z20.7
- intestinal infectious disease NEC Z20.09
  - Escherichia coli (E. coli) Z20.01
- lead Z77.011
- meningococcus Z20.811
- mold (toxic) Z77.120
- nickel dust Z77.018
- noise Z77.122
- occupational
  - air contaminants NEC Z57.39
  - dust Z57.2
  - environmental tobacco smoke Z57.31
  - extreme temperature Z57.6
  - noise Z57.0
  - radiation Z57.1
  - risk factors Z57.9
    - specified NEC Z57.8
  - toxic agents (gases) (liquids) (solids) (vapors) in agriculture Z57.4
  - toxic agents (gases) (liquids) (solids) (vapors) in industry NEC Z57.5
  - vibration Z57.7
- parasitic disease NEC Z20.7
- pediculosis Z20.7
- persecution Z60.5
- pfiesteria piscicida Z77.121
- poliomyelitis Z20.89
- polycyclic aromatic hydrocarbons Z77.028
- pollution
  - air Z77.110
  - environmental NEC Z77.118
  - soil Z77.112
  - water Z77.111
- prenatal (drugs) (toxic chemicals) — *see* Newborn, affected by, noxious substances transmitted via placenta or breast milk
- rabies Z20.3
- radiation, naturally occurring NEC Z77.123
- radon Z77.123
- red tide (Florida) Z77.121
- rubella Z20.4
- second hand tobacco smoke (acute) (chronic) Z77.22
  - in the perinatal period P96.81
- sexually-transmitted disease Z20.2
- smallpox (laboratory) Z20.89
- syphilis Z20.2
- terrorism Z65.4
- torture Z65.4
- tuberculosis Z20.1
- uranium Z77.012
- varicella Z20.820
- venereal disease Z20.2
- viral disease NEC Z20.828
- war Z65.5
- water pollution Z77.111

Exsanguination — *see* Hemorrhage
Exstrophy
- abdominal contents Q45.8
- bladder Q64.10
  - cloacal Q64.12
  - specified type NEC Q64.19
  - supravesical fissure Q64.11

Extensive — *see* condition
Extra (*see also* Accessory)
- marker chromosomes (normal individual) Q92.61
  - in abnormal individual Q92.62
- rib Q76.6
  - cervical Q76.5

Extrasystoles (supraventricular) I49.49
- atrial I49.1
- auricular I49.1
- junctional I49.2
- ventricular I49.3

Extrauterine gestation or pregnancy - — *see* Pregnancy, by site
Extravasation
- blood R58
- chyle into mesentery I89.8
- pelvicalyceal N13.8
- pyelosinus N13.8
- urine (from ureter) R39.0
- vesicant agent
  - antineoplastic chemotherapy T80.810 ☑
  - other agent NEC T80.818 ☑

Extremity — *see* condition, limb
Extrophy — *see* Exstrophy
Extroversion
- bladder Q64.19
- uterus N81.4
  - complicating delivery O71.2
  - postpartal (old) N81.4

Extruded tooth (teeth) M26.34
Extrusion
- breast implant (prosthetic) T85.42 ☑
- eye implant (globe) (ball) T85.328 ☑
- intervertebral disc — *see* Displacement, intervertebral disc
- ocular lens implant (prosthetic) — *see* Complications, intraocular lens
- vitreous — *see* Prolapse, vitreous

Exudate
- pleural — *see* Effusion, pleura
- retina H35.89

Exudative — *see* condition
Eye, eyeball, eyelid — *see* condition
Eyestrain — *see* Disturbance, vision, subjective
Eyeworm disease of Africa B74.3

F

Faber's syndrome (achlorhydric anemia) D50.9
Fabry (-Anderson) disease E75.21
Faciocephalalgia, autonomic (*see also* Neuropathy, peripheral, autonomic)G90.09
Factor (s)
- psychic, associated with diseases classified elsewhere F54
- psychological
  - affecting physical conditions F54
  - or behavioral
    - affecting general medical condition F54
    - associated with disorders or diseases classified elsewhere F54

Fahr disease (of brain) G23.8
Fahr Volhard disease (of kidney) I12. ☑
Failure, failed
- abortion — *see* Abortion, attempted
- aortic (valve) I35.8
  - rheumatic I06.8
- attempted abortion — *see* Abortion, attempted
- biventricular I50.9
- bone marrow — *see* Anemia, aplastic
- cardiac — *see* Failure, heart
- cardiorenal (chronic) I50.9
  - hypertensive I13.2
- cardiorespiratory (*see also* Failure, heart)R09.2
- cardiovascular (chronic) — *see* Failure, heart
- cerebrovascular I67.9
- cervical dilatation in labor O62.0
- circulation, circulatory (peripheral) R57.9
  - newborn P29.89
- compensation — *see* Disease, heart
- compliance with medical treatment or regimen — *see* Noncompliance
- congestive — *see* Failure, heart, congestive
- dental implant (endosseous) M27.69
  - due to
    - failure of dental prosthesis M27.63
    - lack of attached gingiva M27.62
    - occlusal trauma (poor prosthetic design) M27.62
    - parafunctional habits M27.62
    - periodontal infection (peri-implantitis) M27.62
    - poor oral hygiene M27.62
  - osseointegration M27.61
    - due to
      - complications of systemic disease M27.61
      - poor bone quality M27.61
    - iatrogenic M27.61
  - post-osseointegration
    - biological M27.62
    - due to complications of systemic disease M27.62
    - iatrogenic M27.62
    - mechanical M27.63
  - pre-integration M27.61
  - pre-osseointegration M27.61
  - specified NEC M27.69
- descent of head (at term) of pregnancy (mother) O32.4 ☑
- endosseous dental implant — *see* Failure, dental implant

Failure — *continued*
- engagement of head (term of pregnancy) (mother) O32.4 ☑
- erection (penile) (*see also* Dysfunction, sexual, male, erectile)N52.9
  - nonorganic F52.21
- examination (s), anxiety concerning Z55.2
- expansion terminal respiratory units (newborn) (primary) P28.0
- forceps NOS (with subsequent cesarean delivery) O66.5
- gain weight (child over 28 days old) R62.51
  - adult R62.7
  - newborn P92.6
- genital response (male) F52.21
  - female F52.22
- heart (acute) (senile) (sudden) I50.9
  - with
    - acute pulmonary edema — *see* Failure, ventricular, left
    - decompensation — *see* Failure, heart, congestive
    - dilatation — *see* Disease, heart
  - arteriosclerotic I70.90
  - biventricular I50.9
  - combined left-right sided I50.9
  - compensated I50.9
  - complicating
    - anesthesia (general) (local) or other sedation
      - in labor and delivery O74.2
      - in pregnancy O29.12 ☑
      - postpartum, puerperal O89.1
    - delivery (cesarean) (instrumental) O75.4
  - congestive (compensated) (decompensated) I50.9
    - with rheumatic fever (conditions in I00)
      - active I01.8
      - inactive or quiescent (with chorea) I09.81
    - newborn P29.0
    - rheumatic (chronic) (inactive) (with chorea) I09.81
      - active or acute I01.8
        - with chorea I02.0
  - decompensated I50.9
  - degenerative — *see* Degeneration, myocardial
  - diastolic (congestive) I50.30
    - acute (congestive) I50.31
      - and (on) chronic (congestive) I50.33
    - chronic (congestive) I50.32
      - and (on) acute (congestive) I50.33
    - combined with systolic (congestive) I50.40
      - acute (congestive) I50.41
        - and (on) chronic (congestive) I50.43
      - chronic (congestive) I50.42
        - and (on) acute (congestive) I50.43
  - due to presence of cardiac prosthesis I97.13 ☑
  - following cardiac surgery I97.13 ☑
  - high output NOS I50.9
  - hypertensive — *see* Hypertension, heart
  - left (ventricular) — *see* Failure, ventricular, left
  - low output (syndrome) NOS I50.9
  - newborn P29.0
  - organic — *see* Disease, heart
  - peripartum O90.3
  - postprocedural I97.13 ☑
  - rheumatic (chronic) (inactive) I09.9
  - right (ventricular) (secondary to left heart failure) — *see* Failure, heart, congestive
  - systolic (congestive) I50.20
    - acute (congestive) I50.21
      - and (on) chronic (congestive) I50.23
    - chronic (congestive) I50.22
      - and (on) acute (congestive) I50.23
    - combined with diastolic (congestive) I50.40
      - acute (congestive) I50.41
        - and (on) chronic (congestive) I50.43
      - chronic (congestive) I50.42
        - and (on) acute (congestive) I50.43
  - thyrotoxic (*see also* Thyrotoxicosis)E05.90 *[I43]*
    - with thyroid storm E05.91 *[I43]*
  - valvular — *see* Endocarditis
- hepatic K72.90
  - with coma K72.91
  - acute or subacute K72.00
    - with coma K72.01
    - due to drugs K71.10
      - with coma K71.11
  - alcoholic (acute) (chronic) (subacute) K70.40
    - with coma K70.41
  - chronic K72.10
    - with coma K72.11

Failure — *continued*
- hepatic — *continued*
    - due to drugs (acute) (subacute) (chronic) K71.10
      - with coma K71.11
  - due to drugs (acute) (subacute) (chronic) K71.10
    - with coma K71.11
  - postprocedural K91.82
- hepatorenal K76.7
- induction (of labor) O61.9
  - abortion — *see* Abortion, attempted
  - by
    - oxytocic drugs O61.0
    - prostaglandins O61.0
  - instrumental O61.1
  - mechanical O61.1
  - medical O61.0
  - specified NEC O61.8
  - surgical O61.1
- intubation during anesthesia T88.4 ☑
  - in pregnancy O29.6 ☑
  - labor and delivery O74.7
  - postpartum, puerperal O89.6
- involution, thymus (gland) E32.0
- kidney (*see also* Disease, kidney, chronic)N19
  - acute (*see also* Failure, renal, acute)N17.9
  - diabetic — *see* E08-E13 with .22
- lactation (complete) O92.3
  - partial O92.4
- Leydig's cell, adult E29.1
- liver — *see* Failure, hepatic
- menstruation at puberty N91.0
- mitral I05.8
- myocardial, myocardium (*see also* Failure, heart)I50.9
  - chronic (*see also* Failure, heart, congestive)I50.9
  - congestive (*see also* Failure, heart, congestive)I50.9
- orgasm (female) (psychogenic) F52.31
  - male F52.32
- ovarian (primary) E28.39
  - iatrogenic E89.40
    - asymptomatic E89.40
    - symptomatic E89.41
  - postprocedural (postablative) (postirradiation) (postsurgical) E89.40
    - asymptomatic E89.40
    - symptomatic E89.41
- ovulation causing infertility N97.0
- polyglandular, autoimmune E31.0
- prosthetic joint implant — *see* Complications, joint prosthesis, mechanical, breakdown, by site
- renal N19
  - with
    - tubular necrosis (acute) N17.0
  - acute N17.9
    - with
      - cortical necrosis N17.1
      - medullary necrosis N17.2
      - tubular necrosis N17.0
    - specified NEC N17.8
  - chronic N18.9
    - hypertensive — *see* Hypertension, kidney
  - congenital P96.0
  - end stage (chronic) N18.6
    - due to hypertension I12.0
  - following
    - abortion — *see* Abortion by type complicated by specified condition NEC
    - crushing T79.5 ☑
    - ectopic or molar pregnancy O08.4
    - labor and delivery (acute) O90.4
  - hypertensive — *see* Hypertension, kidney
  - postprocedural N99.0
- respiration, respiratory J96.90
  - with
    - hypercapnia J96.92
    - hypoxia J96.91
  - acute J96.00
    - with
      - hypercapnia J96.02
      - hypoxia J96.01
  - center G93.89
  - acute and (on) chronic J96.20
    - with
      - hypercapnia J96.22
      - hypoxia J96.21
  - chronic J96.10
    - with
      - hypercapnia J96.12

Failure — *continued*
- respiration, respiratory — *continued*
      - hypoxia J96.11
  - newborn P28.5
  - postprocedural (acute) J95.821
    - acute and chronic J95.822
- rotation
  - cecum Q43.3
  - colon Q43.3
  - intestine Q43.3
  - kidney Q63.2
- sedation (conscious) (moderate) during procedure T88.52 ☑
  - history of Z92.83
- segmentation (*see also* Fusion)
  - fingers — *see* Syndactylism, complex, fingers
  - vertebra Q76.49
    - with scoliosis Q76.3
- seminiferous tubule, adult E29.1
- senile (general) R54
- sexual arousal (male) F52.21
  - female F52.22
- testicular endocrine function E29.1
- to thrive (child over 28 days old) R62.51
  - adult R62.7
  - newborn P92.6
- transplant T86.92
  - bone T86.831
    - marrow T86.02
  - cornea T86.841
  - heart T86.22
    - with lung (s) T86.32
  - intestine T86.851
  - kidney T86.12
  - liver T86.42
  - lung (s) T86.811
    - with heart T86.32
  - pancreas T86.891
  - skin (allograft) (autograft) T86.821
  - specified organ or tissue NEC T86.891
  - stem cell (peripheral blood) (umbilical cord) T86.5
- trial of labor (with subsequent cesarean delivery) O66.40
  - following previous cesarean delivery O66.41
- tubal ligation N99.89
- urinary — *see* Disease, kidney, chronic
- vacuum extraction NOS (with subsequent cesarean delivery) O66.5
- vasectomy N99.89
- ventouse NOS (with subsequent cesarean delivery) O66.5
- ventricular (*see also* Failure, heart)I50.9
  - left I50.1
    - with rheumatic fever (conditions in I00)
      - active I01.8
        - with chorea I02.0
      - inactive or quiescent (with chorea) I09.81
    - rheumatic (chronic) (inactive) (with chorea) I09.81
      - active or acute I01.8
        - with chorea I02.0
  - right (*see also* Failure, heart, congestive)I50.9
- vital centers, newborn P91.8

Fainting (fit) R55

Fallen arches — *see* Deformity, limb, flat foot

Falling, falls (repeated) R29.6
- any organ or part — *see* Prolapse

Fallopian
- insufflation Z31.41
- tube — *see* condition

Fallot's
- pentalogy Q21.8
- tetrad or tetralogy Q21.3
- triad or trilogy Q22.3

False (*see also* condition)
- croup J38.5
- joint — *see* Nonunion, fracture
- labor (pains) O47.9
  - at or after 37 completed weeks of gestation O47.1
  - before 37 completed weeks of gestation O47.0 ☑
- passage, urethra (prostatic) N36.5
- pregnancy F45.8

Family, familial (*see also* condition)
- disruption Z63.8
  - involving divorce or separation Z63.5
- Li-Fraumeni (syndrome) Z15.01
- planning advice Z30.09
- problem Z63.9
  - specified NEC Z63.8
- retinoblastoma C69.2 ☑

- **Famine** (effects of) T73.0 ☑
  - edema — *see* Malnutrition, severe
- **Fanconi** (-de Toni) (-Debré) syndrome E72.09
  - with cystinosis E72.04
- **Fanconi's** anemia (congenital pancytopenia) D61.09
- **Farber's** disease or syndrome E75.29
- **Farcy** A24.0
- **Farmer's**
  - lung J67.0
  - skin L57.8
- **Farsightedness** — *see* Hypermetropia
- **Fascia** — *see* condition
- **Fasciculation** R25.3
- **Fasciitis** M72.9
  - diffuse (eosinophilic) M35.4
  - infective M72.8
    - necrotizing M72.6
  - necrotizing M72.6
  - nodular M72.4
  - perirenal (with ureteral obstruction) N13.5
    - with infection N13.6
  - plantar M72.2
  - specified NEC M72.8
  - traumatic (old) M72.8
    - current - code by site under Sprain
- **Fascioliasis** B66.3
- **Fasciolopsis,** fasciolopsiasis (intestinal) B66.5
- **Fascioscapulohumeral** myopathy G71.0
- **Fast** pulse R00.0
- **Fat**
  - embolism — *see* Embolism, fat
  - excessive (*see also* Obesity)
    - in heart — *see* Degeneration, myocardial
  - in stool R19.5
  - localized (pad) E65
    - heart — *see* Degeneration, myocardial
    - knee M79.4
    - retropatellar M79.4
  - necrosis
    - breast N64.1
    - mesentery K65.4
    - omentum K65.4
  - pad E65
    - knee M79.4
- **Fatigue** R53.83
  - auditory deafness — *see* Deafness
  - chronic R53.82
  - combat F43.0
  - general R53.83
    - psychogenic F48.8
  - heat (transient) T67.6 ☑
  - muscle M62.89
  - myocardium — *see* Failure, heart
  - neoplasm-related R53.0
  - nervous, neurosis F48.8
  - operational F48.8
  - psychogenic (general) F48.8
  - senile R54
  - voice R49.8
- **Fatness** — *see* Obesity
- **Fatty** (*see also* condition)
  - apron E65
  - degeneration — *see* Degeneration, fatty
  - heart (enlarged) — *see* Degeneration, myocardial
  - liver NEC K76.0
    - alcoholic K70.0
    - nonalcoholic K76.0
  - necrosis — *see* Degeneration, fatty
- **Fauces** — *see* condition
- **Fauchard's** disease (periodontitis) — *see* Periodontitis
- **Faucitis** J02.9
- **Favism** (anemia) D55.0
- **Favus** — *see* Dermatophytosis
- **Fazio-Londe** disease or syndrome G12.1
- **Fear** complex or reaction F40.9
- **Fear** of — *see* Phobia
- **Feared** complaint unfounded Z71.1
- **Febris,** febrile (*see also* Fever)
  - flava (*see also* Fever, yellow)A95.9
  - melitensis A23.0
  - pestis — *see* Plague
  - recurrens — *see* Fever, relapsing
  - rubra A38.9
- **Fecal**
  - incontinence R15.9
  - smearing R15.1
  - soiling R15.1
  - urgency R15.2
- **Fecalith** (impaction) K56.41
  - appendix K38.1
  - congenital P76.8
- **Fede's** disease K14.0
- **Feeble** rapid pulse due to shock following injury T79.4 ☑
- **Feeble-minded** F70
- **Feeding**
  - difficulties R63.3
  - problem R63.3
    - newborn P92.9
      - specified NEC P92.8
    - nonorganic (adult) — *see* Disorder, eating
- **Feeling** (of)
  - foreign body in throat R09.89
- **Feer's** disease — *see* Poisoning, mercury
- **Feet** — *see* condition
- **Feigned** illness Z76.5
- **Feil-Klippel** syndrome (brevicollis) Q76.1
- **Feinmesser's** (hidrotic) ectodermal dysplasia Q82.4
- **Felinophobia** F40.218
- **Felon** (*see also* Cellulitis, digit)
  - with lymphangitis — *see* Lymphangitis, acute, digit
- **Felty's** syndrome M05.00
  - ankle M05.07 ☑
  - elbow M05.02 ☑
  - foot joint M05.07 ☑
  - hand joint M05.04 ☑
  - hip M05.05 ☑
  - knee M05.06 ☑
  - multiple site M05.09
  - shoulder M05.01 ☑
  - vertebra — *see* Spondylitis, ankylosing
  - wrist M05.03 ☑
- **Female** genital cutting status — *see* Female genital mutilation status (FGM)
- **Female** genital mutilation status (FGM) N90.810
  - specified NEC N90.818
  - type I (clitorectomy status) N90.811
  - type II (clitorectomy with excision of labia minora status) N90.812
  - type III (infibulation status) N90.813
  - type IV N90.818
- **Femur,** femoral — *see* condition
- **Fenestration,** fenestrated (*see also* Imperfect, closure)
  - aortico-pulmonary Q21.4
  - cusps, heart valve NEC Q24.8
    - pulmonary Q22.3
  - pulmonic cusps Q22.3
- **Fernell's** disease (aortic aneurysm) I71.9
- **Fertile** eunuch syndrome E23.0
- **Fetid**
  - breath R19.6
  - sweat L75.0
- **Fetishism** F65.0
  - transvestic F65.1
- **Fetus,** fetal (*see also* condition)
  - alcohol syndrome (dysmorphic) Q86.0
  - compressus O31.0 ☑
  - hydantoin syndrome Q86.1
  - lung tissue P28.0
  - papyraceous O31.0 ☑
- **Fever** (inanition) (of unknown origin) (persistent) (with chills) (with rigor) R50.9
  - abortus A23.1
  - Aden (dengue) A90
  - African tick-borne A68.1
  - American
    - mountain (tick) A93.2
    - spotted A77.0
  - aphthous B08.8
  - arbovirus, arboviral A94
    - hemorrhagic A94
    - specified NEC A93.8
  - Argentinian hemorrhagic A96.0
  - Assam B55.0
  - Australian Q A78
  - Bangkok hemorrhagic A91
  - Barmah forest A92.8
  - Bartonella A44.0
  - bilious, hemoglobinuric B50.8
  - blackwater B50.8
  - blister B00.1
  - Bolivian hemorrhagic A96.1
  - Bonvale dam T73.3 ☑
  - boutonneuse A77.1
  - brain — *see* Encephalitis
  - Brazilian purpuric A48.4
  - breakbone A90
  - Bullis A77.0
  - Bunyamwera A92.8
  - Burdwan B55.0
  - Bwamba A92.8

Fever — *continued*

  - Cameroon — *see* Malaria
  - Canton A75.9
  - catarrhal (acute) J00
    - chronic J31.0
  - cat-scratch A28.1
  - Central Asian hemorrhagic A98.0
  - cerebral — *see* Encephalitis
  - cerebrospinal meningococcal A39.0
  - Chagres B50.9
  - Chandipura A92.8
  - Changuinola A93.1
  - Charcot's (biliary) (hepatic) (intermittent) - — *see* Calculus, bile duct
  - Chikungunya (viral) (hemorrhagic) A92.0
  - Chitral A93.1
  - Colombo — *see* Fever, paratyphoid
  - Colorado tick (virus) A93.2
  - congestive (remittent) — *see* Malaria
  - Congo virus A98.0
  - continued malarial B50.9
  - Corsican — *see* Malaria
  - Crimean-Congo hemorrhagic A98.0
  - Cyprus — *see* Brucellosis
  - dandy A90
  - deer fly — *see* Tularemia
  - dengue (virus) A90
    - hemorrhagic A91
    - sandfly A93.1
  - desert B38.0
  - drug induced R50.2
  - due to
    - conditions classified elsewhere R50.81
    - heat T67.0 ☑
  - enteric A01.00
  - enteroviral exanthematous (Boston exanthem) A88.0
  - ephemeral (of unknown origin) R50.9
  - epidemic hemorrhagic A98.5
  - erysipelatous — *see* Erysipelas
  - estivo-autumnal (malarial) B50.9
  - famine A75.0
  - five day A79.0
  - following delivery O86.4
  - Fort Bragg A27.89
  - gastroenteric A01.00
  - gastromalarial — *see* Malaria
  - Gibraltar — *see* Brucellosis
  - glandular — *see* Mononucleosis, infectious
  - Guama (viral) A92.8
  - Haverhill A25.1
  - hay (allergic) J30.1
    - with asthma (bronchial) J45.909
      - with
        - exacerbation (acute) J45.901
        - status asthmaticus J45.902
    - due to
      - allergen other than pollen J30.89
      - pollen, any plant or tree J30.1
  - heat (effects) T67.0 ☑
  - hematuric, bilious B50.8
  - hemoglobinuric (malarial) (bilious) B50.8
  - hemorrhagic (arthropod-borne) NOS A94
    - with renal syndrome A98.5
    - arenaviral A96.9
      - specified NEC A96.8
    - Argentinian A96.0
    - Bangkok A91
    - Bolivian A96.1
    - Central Asian A98.0
    - Chikungunya A92.0
    - Crimean-Congo A98.0
    - dengue (virus) A91
    - epidemic A98.5
    - Junin (virus) A96.0
    - Korean A98.5
    - Kyasanur forest A98.2
    - Machupo (virus) A96.1
    - mite-borne A93.8
    - mosquito-borne A92.8
    - Omsk A98.1
    - Philippine A91
    - Russian A98.5
    - Singapore A91
    - Southeast Asia A91
    - Thailand A91
    - tick-borne NEC A93.8
    - viral A99
      - specified NEC A98.8
  - hepatic — *see* Cholecystitis
  - herpetic — *see* Herpes
  - icterohemorrhagic A27.0

Fever — *continued*
- Indiana A93.8
- infective B99.9
  - specified NEC B99.8
- intermittent (bilious) (*see also* Malaria)
  - of unknown origin R50.9
  - pernicious B50.9
- iodide R50.2
- Japanese river A75.3
- jungle (*see also* Malaria)
  - yellow A95.0
- Junin (virus) hemorrhagic A96.0
- Katayama B65.2
- kedani A75.3
- Kenya (tick) A77.1
- Kew Garden A79.1
- Korean hemorrhagic A98.5
- Lassa A96.2
- Lone Star A77.0
- Machupo (virus) hemorrhagic A96.1
- malaria, malarial — *see* Malaria
- Malta A23.9
- Marseilles A77.1
- marsh — *see* Malaria
- Mayaro (viral) A92.8
- Mediterranean (*see also* Brucellosis)A23.9
  - familial M04.1
  - tick A77.1
- meningeal — *see* Meningitis
- Meuse A79.0
- Mexican A75.2
- mianeh A68.1
- miasmatic — *see* Malaria
- mosquito-borne (viral) A92.9
  - hemorrhagic A92.8
- mountain (*see also* Brucellosis)
  - meaning Rocky Mountain spotted fever A77.0
  - tick (American) (Colorado) (viral) A93.2
- Mucambo (viral) A92.8
- mud A27.9
- Neapolitan — *see* Brucellosis
- neutropenic D70.9
- newborn P81.9
  - environmental P81.0
- Nine-Mile A78
- non-exanthematous tick A93.2
- North Asian tick-borne A77.2
- Omsk hemorrhagic A98.1
- O'nyong-nyong (viral) A92.1
- Oropouche (viral) A93.0
- Oroya A44.0
- paludal — *see* Malaria
- Panama (malarial) B50.9
- Pappataci A93.1
- paratyphoid A01.4
  - A A01.1
  - B A01.2
  - C A01.3
- parrot A70
- periodic (Mediterranean) M04.1
- persistent (of unknown origin) R50.9
- petechial A39.0
- pharyngoconjunctival B30.2
- Philippine hemorrhagic A91
- phlebotomus A93.1
- Piry (virus) A93.8
- Pixuna (viral) A92.8
- Plasmodium ovale B53.0
- polioviral (nonparalytic) A80.4
- Pontiac A48.2
- postimmunization R50.83
- postoperative R50.82
  - due to infection T81.40
- posttransfusion R50.84
- postvaccination R50.83
- presenting with conditions classified elsewhere R50.81
- pretibial A27.89
- puerperal O86.4
- Q A78
- quadrilateral A78
- quartan (malaria) B52.9
- Queensland (coastal) (tick) A77.3
- quintan A79.0
- rabbit — *see* Tularemia
- rat-bite A25.9
  - due to
    - Spirillum A25.0
    - Streptobacillus moniliformis A25.1
- recurrent — *see* Fever, relapsing
- relapsing (Borrelia) A68.9
  - Carter's (Asiatic) A68.1

Fever — *continued*
- relapsing — *continued*
  - Dutton's (West African) A68.1
  - Koch's A68.9
  - louse-borne A68.0
  - Novy's
    - louse-borne A68.0
    - tick-borne A68.1
  - Obermeyer's (European) A68.0
  - tick-borne A68.1
- remittent (bilious) (congestive) (gastric) — *see* Malaria
- rheumatic (active) (acute) (chronic) (subacute) I00
  - with central nervous system involvement I02.9
  - active with heart involvement — *see* categoryI01 ☑
  - inactive or quiescent with
    - cardiac hypertrophy I09.89
    - carditis I09.9
    - endocarditis I09.1
      - aortic (valve) I06.9
        - with mitral (valve) disease I08.0
      - mitral (valve) I05.9
        - with aortic (valve) disease I08.0
      - pulmonary (valve) I09.89
      - tricuspid (valve) I07.8
    - heart disease NEC I09.89
    - heart failure (congestive) (conditions in I50.9) I09.81
    - left ventricular failure (conditions in I50.1) I09.81
    - myocarditis, myocardial degeneration (conditions in I51.4) I09.0
    - pancarditis I09.9
    - pericarditis I09.2
- Rift Valley (viral) A92.4
- Rocky Mountain spotted A77.0
- rose J30.1
- Ross River B33.1
- Russian hemorrhagic A98.5
- San Joaquin (Valley) B38.0
- sandfly A93.1
- Sao Paulo A77.0
- scarlet A38.9
- seven day (leptospirosis) (autumnal) (Japanese) A27.89
  - dengue A90
- shin-bone A79.0
- Singapore hemorrhagic A91
- solar A90
- Songo A98.5
- sore B00.1
- South African tick-bite A68.1
- Southeast Asia hemorrhagic A91
- spinal — *see* Meningitis
- spirillary A25.0
- splenic — *see* Anthrax
- spotted A77.9
  - American A77.0
  - Brazilian A77.0
  - cerebrospinal meningitis A39.0
  - Colombian A77.0
  - due to Rickettsia
    - australis A77.3
    - conorii A77.1
    - rickettsii A77.0
    - sibirica A77.2
    - specified type NEC A77.8
  - Ehrlichiosis A77.40
    - due to
      - E. chafeensis A77.41
      - specified organism NEC A77.49
  - Rocky Mountain A77.0
- steroid R50.2
- streptobacillary A25.1
- subtertian B50.9
- Sumatran mite A75.3
- sun A90
- swamp A27.9
- swine A02.8
- sylvatic, yellow A95.0
- Tahyna B33.8
- tertian — *see* Malaria, tertian
- Thailand hemorrhagic A91
- thermic T67.0 ☑
- three-day A93.1
- tick
  - American mountain A93.2
  - Colorado A93.2
  - Kemerovo A93.8
  - Mediterranean A77.1
  - mountain A93.2

Fever — *continued*
- tick — *continued*
  - nonexanthematous A93.2
  - Quaranfil A93.8
- tick-bite NEC A93.8
- tick-borne (hemorrhagic) NEC A93.8
- trench A79.0
- tsutsugamushi A75.3
- typhogastric A01.00
- typhoid (abortive) (hemorrhagic) (intermittent) (malignant) A01.00
  - complicated by
    - arthritis A01.04
    - heart involvement A01.02
    - meningitis A01.01
    - osteomyelitis A01.05
    - pneumonia A01.03
    - specified NEC A01.09
- typhomalarial — *see* Malaria
- typhus — *see* Typhus (fever)
- undulant — *see* Brucellosis
- unknown origin R50.9
- uveoparotid D86.89
- valley B38.0
- Venezuelan equine A92.2
- vesicular stomatitis A93.8
- viral hemorrhagic — *see* Fever, hemorrhagic, by type of virus
- Volhynian A79.0
- Wesselsbron (viral) A92.8
- West
  - African B50.8
  - Nile (viral) A92.30
    - with
      - complications NEC A92.39
      - cranial nerve disorders A92.32
      - encephalitis A92.31
      - encephalomyelitis A92.31
      - neurologic manifestation NEC A92.32
      - optic neuritis A92.32
      - polyradiculitis A92.32
- Whitmore's — *see* Melioidosis
- Wolhynian A79.0
- worm B83.9
- yellow A95.9
  - jungle A95.0
  - sylvatic A95.0
  - urban A95.1
- Zika virus A92.5

Fibrillation
- atrial or auricular (established) I48.91
  - chronic I48.2
  - paroxysmal I48.0
  - permanent I48.2
  - persistent I48.1
- cardiac I49.8
- heart I49.8
- muscular M62.89
- ventricular I49.01

Fibrin
- ball or bodies, pleural (sac) J94.1
- chamber, anterior (eye) (gelatinous exudate) — *see* Iridocyclitis, acute

Fibrinogenolysis — *see* Fibrinolysis

Fibrinogenopenia D68.8
- acquired D65
- congenital D68.2

Fibrinolysis (hemorrhagic) (acquired) D65
- antepartum hemorrhage — *see* Hemorrhage, antepartum, with coagulation defect
- following
  - abortion — *see* Abortion by type complicated by hemorrhage
  - ectopic or molar pregnancy O08.1
- intrapartum O67.0
- newborn, transient P60
- postpartum O72.3

Fibrinopenia (hereditary) D68.2
- acquired D68.4

Fibrinopurulent — *see* condition

Fibrinous — *see* condition

Fibroadenoma
- cellular intracanalicular D24 ☑
- giant D24 ☑
- intracanalicular
  - cellular D24 ☑
  - giant D24 ☑
  - specified site — *see* Neoplasm, benign, by site
  - unspecified site D24 ☑
- juvenile D24 ☑
- pericanalicular
  - specified site — *see* Neoplasm, benign, by site
  - unspecified site D24 ☑

Fibroadenoma - Fibroxanthosarcoma

- **Fibroadenoma** — *continued*
  - phyllodes D24 ☑
  - prostate D29.1
  - specified site NEC — *see* Neoplasm, benign, by site
  - unspecified site D24 ☑
- **Fibroadenosis,** breast (chronic) (cystic) (diffuse) (periodic) (segmental) N60.2 ☑
- **Fibroangioma** (*see also* Neoplasm, benign, by site)
  - juvenile
    - specified site — *see* Neoplasm, benign, by site
    - unspecified site D10.6
- **Fibrochondrosarcoma** — *see* Neoplasm, cartilage, malignant
- **Fibrocystic**
  - disease (*see also* Fibrosis, cystic)
    - breast — *see* Mastopathy, cystic
    - jaw M27.49
    - kidney (congenital) Q61.8
    - liver Q44.6
    - pancreas E84.9
  - kidney (congenital) Q61.8
- **Fibrodysplasia** ossificans progressiva - — *see* Myositis, ossificans, progressiva
- **Fibroelastosis** (cordis) (endocardial) (endomyocardial) I42.4
- **Fibroid** (tumor) (*see also* Neoplasm, connective tissue, benign)
  - disease, lung (chronic) — *see* Fibrosis, lung
  - heart (disease) — *see* Myocarditis
  - in pregnancy or childbirth O34.1 ☑
    - causing obstructed labor O65.5
  - induration, lung (chronic) — *see* Fibrosis, lung
  - lung — *see* Fibrosis, lung
  - pneumonia (chronic) — *see* Fibrosis, lung
  - uterus D25.9
- **Fibrolipoma** — *see* Lipoma
- **Fibroliposarcoma** — *see* Neoplasm, connective tissue, malignant
- **Fibroma** (*see also* Neoplasm, connective tissue, benign)
  - ameloblastic — *see* Cyst, calcifying odontogenic
  - bone (nonossifying) — *see* Disorder, bone, specified type NEC
    - ossifying — *see* Neoplasm, bone, benign
  - cementifying — *see* Neoplasm, bone, benign
  - chondromyxoid — *see* Neoplasm, bone, benign
  - desmoplastic — *see* Neoplasm, connective tissue, uncertain behavior
  - durum — *see* Neoplasm, connective tissue, benign
  - fascial — *see* Neoplasm, connective tissue, benign
  - invasive — *see* Neoplasm, connective tissue, uncertain behavior
  - molle — *see* Lipoma
  - myxoid — *see* Neoplasm, connective tissue, benign
  - nasopharynx, nasopharyngeal (juvenile) D10.6
  - nonosteogenic (nonossifying) — *see* Dysplasia, fibrous
  - odontogenic (central) — *see* Cyst, calcifying odontogenic
  - ossifying — *see* Neoplasm, bone, benign
  - periosteal — *see* Neoplasm, bone, benign
  - soft — *see* Lipoma
- **Fibromatosis** M72.9
  - abdominal — *see* Neoplasm, connective tissue, uncertain behavior
  - aggressive — *see* Neoplasm, connective tissue, uncertain behavior
  - congenital generalized — *see* Neoplasm, connective tissue, uncertain behavior
  - Dupuytren's M72.0
  - gingival K06.1
  - palmar (fascial) M72.0
  - plantar (fascial) M72.2
  - pseudosarcomatous (proliferative) (subcutaneous) M72.4
  - retroperitoneal D48.3
  - specified NEC M72.8
- **Fibromyalgia** M79.7
- **Fibromyoma** (*see also* Neoplasm, connective tissue, benign)
  - uterus (corpus) (*see also* Leiomyoma, uterus)
    - in pregnancy or childbirth — *see* Fibroid, in pregnancy or childbirth
      - causing obstructed labor O65.5
- **Fibromyositis** M79.7
- **Fibromyxolipoma** D17.9
- **Fibromyxoma** — *see* Neoplasm, connective tissue, benign
- **Fibromyxosarcoma** — *see* Neoplasm, connective tissue, malignant
- **Fibro-odontoma,** ameloblastic — *see* Cyst, calcifying odontogenic
- **Fibro-osteoma** — *see* Neoplasm, bone, benign
- **Fibroplasia,** retrolental H35.17 ☑
- **Fibropurulent** — *see* condition
- **Fibrosarcoma** (*see also* Neoplasm, connective tissue, malignant)
  - ameloblastic C41.1
    - upper jaw (bone) C41.0
  - congenital — *see* Neoplasm, connective tissue, malignant
  - fascial — *see* Neoplasm, connective tissue, malignant
  - infantile — *see* Neoplasm, connective tissue, malignant
  - odontogenic C41.1
    - upper jaw (bone) C41.0
  - periosteal — *see* Neoplasm, bone, malignant
- **Fibrosclerosis**
  - breast N60.3 ☑
  - multifocal M35.5
  - penis (corpora cavernosa) N48.6
- **Fibrosis,** fibrotic
  - adrenal (gland) E27.8
  - amnion O41.8X ☑
  - anal papillae K62.89
  - arteriocapillary — *see* Arteriosclerosis
  - bladder N32.89
    - interstitial — *see* Cystitis, chronic, interstitial
    - localized submucosal — *see* Cystitis, chronic, interstitial
    - panmural — *see* Cystitis, chronic, interstitial
  - breast — *see* Fibrosclerosis, breast
  - capillary (*see also* Arteriosclerosis)I70.90
    - lung (chronic) — *see* Fibrosis, lung
  - cardiac — *see* Myocarditis
  - cervix N88.8
  - chorion O41.8X ☑
  - corpus cavernosum (sclerosing) N48.6
  - cystic (of pancreas) E84.9
    - with
      - distal intestinal obstruction syndrome E84.19
      - fecal impaction E84.19
      - intestinal manifestations NEC E84.19
      - pulmonary manifestations E84.0
      - specified manifestations NEC E84.8
  - due to device, implant or graft (*see also* Complications, by site and type, specified NEC)T85.828 ☑
    - arterial graft NEC T82.828 ☑
    - breast (implant) T85.828 ☑
    - catheter NEC T85.828 ☑
      - dialysis (renal) T82.828 ☑
        - intraperitoneal T85.828 ☑
      - infusion NEC T82.828 ☑
        - spinal (epidural) (subdural) T85.820 ☑
      - urinary (indwelling) T83.82 ☑
    - electronic (electrode) (pulse generator) (stimulator)
      - bone T84.82 ☑
      - cardiac T82.827 ☑
      - nervous system (brain) (peripheral nerve) (spinal) T85.820 ☑
      - urinary T83.82 ☑
    - fixation, internal (orthopedic) NEC T84.82 ☑
    - gastrointestinal (bile duct) (esophagus) T85.828 ☑
    - genital NEC T83.82 ☑
    - heart NEC T82.827 ☑
    - joint prosthesis T84.82 ☑
    - ocular (corneal graft) (orbital implant) NEC T85.828 ☑
    - orthopedic NEC T84.82 ☑
    - specified NEC T85.828 ☑
    - urinary NEC T83.82 ☑
    - vascular NEC T82.828 ☑
    - ventricular intracranial shunt T85.820 ☑
  - ejaculatory duct N50.89
  - endocardium — *see* Endocarditis
  - endomyocardial (tropical) I42.3
  - epididymis N50.89
  - eye muscle — *see* Strabismus, mechanical
  - heart — *see* Myocarditis
  - hepatic — *see* Fibrosis, liver
  - hepatolienal (portal hypertension) K76.6
  - hepatosplenic (portal hypertension) K76.6
  - infrapatellar fat pad M79.4
  - intrascrotal N50.89
  - kidney N26.9
  - liver K74.0
- **Fibrosis** — *continued*
  - liver — *continued*
    - with sclerosis K74.2
    - alcoholic K70.2
  - lung (atrophic) (chronic) (confluent) (massive) (perialveolar) (peribronchial) J84.10
    - with
      - anthracosilicosis J60
      - anthracosis J60
      - asbestosis J61
      - bagassosis J67.1
      - bauxite J63.1
      - berylliosis J63.2
      - byssinosis J66.0
      - calcicosis J62.8
      - chalicosis J62.8
      - dust reticulation J64
      - farmer's lung J67.0
      - ganister disease J62.8
      - graphite J63.3
      - pneumoconiosis NOS J64
      - siderosis J63.4
      - silicosis J62.8
    - capillary J84.10
    - congenital P27.8
    - diffuse (idiopathic) J84.10
      - chemicals, gases, fumes or vapors (inhalation) J68.4
      - interstitial J84.10
        - acute J84.114
      - talc J62.0
    - following radiation J70.1
    - idiopathic J84.112
    - postinflammatory J84.10
    - silicotic J62.8
    - tuberculous — *see* Tuberculosis, pulmonary
  - lymphatic gland I89.8
  - median bar — *see* Hyperplasia, prostate
  - mediastinum (idiopathic) J98.59
  - meninges G96.19
  - myocardium, myocardial — *see* Myocarditis
  - ovary N83.8
  - oviduct N83.8
  - pancreas K86.89
  - penis NEC N48.6
  - pericardium I31.0
  - perineum, in pregnancy or childbirth O34.7 ☑
    - causing obstructed labor O65.5
  - pleura J94.1
  - popliteal fat pad M79.4
  - prostate (chronic) — *see* Hyperplasia, prostate
  - pulmonary (*see also* Fibrosis, lung)J84.10
    - congenital P27.8
    - idiopathic J84.112
  - rectal sphincter K62.89
  - retroperitoneal, idiopathic (with ureteral obstruction) N13.5
    - with infection N13.6
  - sclerosing mesenteric (idiopathic) K65.4
  - scrotum N50.89
  - seminal vesicle N50.89
  - senile R54
  - skin L90.5
  - spermatic cord N50.89
  - spleen D73.89
    - in schistosomiasis (bilharziasis) B65.9 *[D77]*
  - subepidermal nodular — *see* Neoplasm, skin, benign
  - submucous (oral) (tongue) K13.5
  - testis N44.8
    - chronic, due to syphilis A52.76
  - thymus (gland) E32.8
  - tongue, submucous K13.5
  - tunica vaginalis N50.89
  - uterus (non-neoplastic) N85.8
  - vagina N89.8
  - valve, heart — *see* Endocarditis
  - vas deferens N50.89
  - vein I87.8
- **Fibrositis** (periarticular) M79.7
  - nodular, chronic (Jaccoud's) (rheumatoid) — *see* Arthropathy, postrheumatic, chronic
- **Fibrothorax** J94.1
- **Fibrotic** — *see* Fibrosis
- **Fibrous** — *see* condition
- **Fibroxanthoma** (*see also* Neoplasm, connective tissue, benign)
  - atypical — *see* Neoplasm, connective tissue, uncertain behavior
  - malignant — *see* Neoplasm, connective tissue, malignant
- **Fibroxanthosarcoma** — *see* Neoplasm, connective tissue, malignant

Fibroadenoma - Fibroxanthosarcoma

- **Fiedler's**
  - disease (icterohemorrhagic leptospirosis) A27.0
  - myocarditis (acute) I40.1
- **Fifth disease** B08.3
  - venereal A55
- **Filaria,** filarial, filariasis — *see* Infestation, filarial
- **Filatov's** disease — *see* Mononucleosis, infectious
- **File-cutter's** disease — *see* Poisoning, lead
- **Filling** defect
  - biliary tract R93.2
  - bladder R93.41
  - duodenum R93.3
  - gallbladder R93.2
  - gastrointestinal tract R93.3
  - intestine R93.3
  - kidney R93.42 ☑
  - stomach R93.3
  - ureter R93.41
  - urinary organs, specified NEC R93.49
- **Fimbrial** cyst Q50.4
- **Financial** problem affecting care NOS Z59.9
  - bankruptcy Z59.8
  - foreclosure on loan Z59.8
- **Findings,** abnormal, inconclusive, without diagnosis (*see also* Abnormal)
  - 17-ketosteroids, elevated R82.5
  - acetonuria R82.4
  - alcohol in blood R78.0
  - anisocytosis R71.8
  - antenatal screening of mother O28.9
    - biochemical O28.1
    - chromosomal O28.5
    - cytological O28.2
    - genetic O28.5
    - hematological O28.0
    - radiological O28.4
    - specified NEC O28.8
    - ultrasonic O28.3
  - antibody titer, elevated R76.0
  - anticardiolipin antibody R76.0
  - antiphosphatidylglycerol antibody R76.0
  - antiphosphatidylinositol antibody R76.0
  - antiphosphatidylserine antibody R76.0
  - antiphospholipid antibody R76.0
  - bacteriuria R82.71
  - bicarbonate E87.8
  - bile in urine R82.2
  - blood sugar R73.09
    - high R73.9
    - low (transient) E16.2
  - body fluid or substance, specified NEC R88.8
  - casts, urine R82.99
  - catecholamines R82.5
  - cells, urine R82.99
  - chloride E87.8
  - cholesterol E78.9
    - high E78.00
      - with high triglycerides E78.2
  - chyluria R82.0
  - cloudy
    - dialysis effluent R88.0
    - urine R82.90
  - creatinine clearance R94.4
  - crystals, urine R82.99
  - culture
    - blood R78.81
    - positive — *see* Positive, culture
  - echocardiogram R93.1
  - electrolyte level, urinary R82.99
  - function study NEC R94.8
    - bladder R94.8
    - endocrine NEC R94.7
      - thyroid R94.6
    - kidney R94.4
    - liver R94.5
    - pancreas R94.8
    - placenta R94.8
    - pulmonary R94.2
    - spleen R94.8
  - gallbladder, nonvisualization R93.2
  - glucose (tolerance test) (non-fasting) R73.09
  - glycosuria R81
  - heart
    - shadow R93.1
    - sounds R01.2
  - hematinuria R82.3
  - hematocrit drop (precipitous) R71.0
  - hemoglobinuria R82.3
  - human papillomavirus (HPV) DNA test positive
    - cervix
      - high risk R87.810
      - low risk R87.820

- **Findings** abnormal — *continued*
  - human papillomavirus — *continued*
    - vagina
      - high risk R87.811
      - low risk R87.821
  - in blood (of substance not normally found in blood) R78.9
    - addictive drug NEC R78.4
    - alcohol (excessive level) R78.0
    - cocaine R78.2
    - hallucinogen R78.3
    - heavy metals (abnormal level) R78.79
    - lead R78.71
    - lithium (abnormal level) R78.89
    - opiate drug R78.1
    - psychotropic drug R78.5
    - specified substance NEC R78.89
    - steroid agent R78.6
  - indoleacetic acid, elevated R82.5
  - ketonuria R82.4
  - lactic acid dehydrogenase (LDH) R74.0
  - liver function test R79.89
  - mammogram NEC R92.8
    - calcification (calculus) R92.1
    - inconclusive result (due to dense breasts) R92.2
    - microcalcification R92.0
  - mediastinal shift R93.8
  - melanin, urine R82.99
  - myoglobinuria R82.1
  - neonatal screening P09
  - nonvisualization of gallbladder R93.2
  - odor of urine NOS R82.90
  - Papanicolaou cervix R87.619
    - non-atypical endometrial cells R87.618
  - pneumoencephalogram R93.0
  - poikilocytosis R71.8
  - potassium (deficiency) E87.6
    - excess E87.5
  - PPD R76.11
  - radiologic (X-ray) R93.8
    - abdomen R93.5
    - biliary tract R93.2
    - breast R92.8
    - gastrointestinal tract R93.3
    - genitourinary organs R93.8
    - head R93.0
    - inconclusive due to excess body fat of patient R93.9
    - intrathoracic organs NEC R93.1
    - placenta R93.8
    - retroperitoneum R93.5
    - skin R93.8
    - skull R93.0
    - subcutaneous tissue R93.8
  - red blood cell (count) (morphology) (sickling) (volume) R71.8
  - scan NEC R94.8
    - bladder R94.8
    - bone R94.8
    - kidney R94.4
    - liver R93.2
    - lung R94.2
    - pancreas R94.8
    - placental R94.8
    - spleen R94.8
    - thyroid R94.6
  - sedimentation rate, elevated R70.0
  - SGOT R74.0
  - SGPT R74.0
  - sodium (deficiency) E87.1
    - excess E87.0
  - specified body fluid NEC R88.8
  - stress test R94.39
  - thyroid (function) (metabolic rate) (scan) (uptake) R94.6
  - transaminase (level) R74.0
  - triglycerides E78.9
    - high E78.1
      - with high cholesterol E78.2
  - tuberculin skin test (without active tuberculosis) R76.11
  - urine R82.90
    - acetone R82.4
    - bacteria R82.71
    - bile R82.2
    - casts or cells R82.99
    - chyle R82.0
    - culture positive R82.79
    - glucose R81
    - hemoglobin R82.3
    - ketone R82.4
    - sugar R81

- **Findings** abnormal — *continued*
  - vanillylmandelic acid (VMA), elevated R82.5
  - vectorcardiogram (VCG) R94.39
  - ventriculogram R93.0
  - white blood cell (count) (differential) (morphology) D72.9
  - xerography R92.8
- **Finger** — *see* condition
- **Fire,** Saint Anthony's — *see* Erysipelas
- **Fire-setting**
  - pathological (compulsive) F63.1
- **Fish hook** stomach K31.89
- **Fishmeal-worker's** lung J67.8
- **Fissure,** fissured
  - anus, anal K60.2
    - acute K60.0
    - chronic K60.1
    - congenital Q43.8
  - ear, lobule, congenital Q17.8
  - epiglottis (congenital) Q31.8
  - larynx J38.7
    - congenital Q31.8
  - lip K13.0
    - congenital — *see* Cleft, lip
  - nipple N64.0
    - associated with
      - lactation O92.13
      - pregnancy O92.11 ☑
      - puerperium O92.12
  - nose Q30.2
  - palate (congenital) — *see* Cleft, palate
  - skin R23.4
  - spine (congenital) (*see also* Spina bifida)
    - with hydrocephalus — *see* Spina bifida, by site, with hydrocephalus
  - tongue (acquired) K14.5
    - congenital Q38.3
- **Fistula** (cutaneous) L98.8
  - abdomen (wall) K63.2
    - bladder N32.2
    - intestine NEC K63.2
    - ureter N28.89
    - uterus N82.5
  - abdominorectal K63.2
  - abdominosigmoidal K63.2
  - abdominothoracic J86.0
  - abdominouterine N82.5
    - congenital Q51.7
  - abdominovesical N32.2
  - accessory sinuses — *see* Sinusitis
  - actinomycotic — *see* Actinomycosis
  - alveolar antrum — *see* Sinusitis, maxillary
  - alveolar process K04.6
  - anorectal K60.5
  - antrobuccal — *see* Sinusitis, maxillary
  - antrum — *see* Sinusitis, maxillary
  - anus, anal (recurrent) (infectional) K60.3
    - congenital Q43.6
      - with absence, atresia and stenosis Q42.2
    - tuberculous A18.32
  - aorta-duodenal I77.2
  - appendix, appendicular K38.3
  - arteriovenous (acquired) (nonruptured) I77.0
    - brain I67.1
      - congenital Q28.2
        - ruptured I60.8
      - ruptured I60.8
    - cerebral — *see* Fistula, arteriovenous, brain
    - congenital (peripheral) (*see also* Malformation, arteriovenous)
      - brain Q28.2
        - ruptured I60.8
      - coronary Q24.5
      - pulmonary Q25.72
    - coronary I25.41
      - congenital Q24.5
    - pulmonary I28.0
      - congenital Q25.72
    - surgically created (for dialysis) Z99.2
      - complication — *see* Complication, arteriovenous, fistula, surgically created
    - traumatic — *see* Injury, blood vessel
  - artery I77.2
  - aural (mastoid) — *see* Mastoiditis, chronic
  - auricle (*see also* Disorder, pinna, specified type NEC)
    - congenital Q18.1
  - Bartholin's gland N82.8
  - bile duct (common) (hepatic) K83.3
    - with calculus, stones — *see* Calculus, bile duct
  - biliary (tract) — *see* Fistula, bile duct

- **Fistula** — *continued*
  - bladder (sphincter) NEC (*see also* Fistula, vesico-) N32.2
    - into seminal vesicle N32.2
  - bone (*see also* Disorder, bone, specified type NEC)
    - with osteomyelitis, chronic — *see* Osteomyelitis, chronic, with draining sinus
  - brain G93.89
    - arteriovenous (acquired) I67.1
      - congenital Q28.2
  - branchial (cleft) Q18.0
  - branchiogenous Q18.0
  - breast N61.0
    - puerperal, postpartum or gestational, due to mastitis (purulent) — *see* Mastitis, obstetric, purulent
  - bronchial J86.0
  - bronchocutaneous, bronchomediastinal, bronchopleural, bronchopleuromediastinal (infective) J86.0
    - tuberculous NEC A15.5
  - bronchoesophageal J86.0
    - congenital Q39.2
      - with atresia of esophagus Q39.1
  - bronchovisceral J86.0
  - buccal cavity (infective) K12.2
  - cecosigmoidal K63.2
  - cecum K63.2
  - cerebrospinal (fluid) G96.0
  - cervical, lateral Q18.1
  - cervicoaural Q18.1
  - cervicosigmoidal N82.4
  - cervicovesical N82.1
  - cervix N82.8
  - chest (wall) J86.0
  - cholecystenteric — *see* Fistula, gallbladder
  - cholecystocolic — *see* Fistula, gallbladder
  - cholecystocolonic — *see* Fistula, gallbladder
  - cholecystoduodenal — *see* Fistula, gallbladder
  - cholecystogastric — *see* Fistula, gallbladder
  - cholecystointestinal — *see* Fistula, gallbladder
  - choledochoduodenal — *see* Fistula, bile duct
  - cholocolic K82.3
  - coccyx — *see* Sinus, pilonidal
  - colon K63.2
  - colostomy K94.09
  - common duct — *see* Fistula, bile duct
  - congenital, site not listed — *see* Anomaly, by site
  - coronary, arteriovenous I25.41
    - congenital Q24.5
  - costal region J86.0
  - cul-de-sac, Douglas' N82.8
  - cystic duct (*see also* Fistula, gallbladder)
    - congenital Q44.5
  - dental K04.6
  - diaphragm J86.0
  - duodenum K31.6
  - ear (external) (canal) — *see* Disorder, ear, external, specified type NEC
  - enterocolic K63.2
  - enterocutaneous K63.2
  - enterouterine N82.4
    - congenital Q51.7
  - enterovaginal N82.4
    - congenital Q52.2
    - large intestine N82.3
    - small intestine N82.2
  - enterovesical N32.1
  - epididymis N50.89
    - tuberculous A18.15
  - esophagobronchial J86.0
    - congenital Q39.2
      - with atresia of esophagus Q39.1
  - esophagocutaneous K22.8
  - esophagopleural-cutaneous J86.0
  - esophagotracheal J86.0
    - congenital Q39.2
      - with atresia of esophagus Q39.1
  - esophagus K22.8
    - congenital Q39.2
      - with atresia of esophagus Q39.1
  - ethmoid — *see* Sinusitis, ethmoidal
  - eyeball (cornea) (sclera) — *see* Disorder, globe, hypotony
  - eyelid H01.8
  - fallopian tube, external N82.5
  - fecal K63.2
    - congenital Q43.6
  - from periapical abscess K04.6
  - frontal sinus — *see* Sinusitis, frontal
  - gallbladder K82.3

- **Fistula** — *continued*
  - gallbladder — *continued*
    - with calculus, cholelithiasis, stones — *see* Calculus, gallbladder
  - gastric K31.6
  - gastrocolic K31.6
    - congenital Q40.2
    - tuberculous A18.32
  - gastroenterocolic K31.6
  - gastroesophageal K31.6
  - gastrojejunal K31.6
  - gastrojejunocolic K31.6
  - genital tract (female) N82.9
    - specified NEC N82.8
    - to intestine NEC N82.4
    - to skin N82.5
  - hepatic artery-portal vein, congenital Q26.6
  - hepatopleural J86.0
  - hepatopulmonary J86.0
  - ileorectal or ileosigmoidal K63.2
  - ileovaginal N82.2
  - ileovesical N32.1
  - ileum K63.2
  - in ano K60.3
    - tuberculous A18.32
  - inner ear (labyrinth) — *see* subcategory H83.1
  - intestine NEC K63.2
  - intestinocolonic (abdominal) K63.2
  - intestinoureteral N28.89
  - intestinouterine N82.4
  - intestinovaginal N82.4
    - large intestine N82.3
    - small intestine N82.2
  - intestinovesical N32.1
  - ischiorectal (fossa) K61.3
  - jejunum K63.2
  - joint M25.10
    - ankle M25.17 ☑
    - elbow M25.12 ☑
    - foot joint M25.17 ☑
    - hand joint M25.14 ☑
    - hip M25.15 ☑
    - knee M25.16 ☑
    - shoulder M25.11 ☑
    - specified joint NEC M25.18
    - tuberculous — *see* Tuberculosis, joint
    - vertebrae M25.18
    - wrist M25.13 ☑
  - kidney N28.89
  - labium (majus) (minus) N82.8
  - labyrinth — *see* subcategory H83.1
  - lacrimal (gland) (sac) H04.61 ☑
  - lacrimonasal duct — *see* Fistula, lacrimal
  - laryngotracheal, congenital Q34.8
  - larynx J38.7
  - lip K13.0
    - congenital Q38.0
  - lumbar, tuberculous A18.01
  - lung J86.0
  - lymphatic I89.8
  - mammary (gland) N61.0
  - mastoid (process) (region) — *see* Mastoiditis, chronic
  - maxillary J32.0
  - medial, face and neck Q18.8
  - mediastinal J86.0
  - mediastinobronchial J86.0
  - mediastinocutaneous J86.0
  - middle ear — *see* subcategory H74.8
  - mouth K12.2
  - nasal J34.89
    - sinus — *see* Sinusitis
  - nasopharynx J39.2
  - nipple N64.0
  - nose J34.89
  - oral (cutaneous) K12.2
    - maxillary J32.0
    - nasal (with cleft palate) — *see* Cleft, palate
  - orbit, orbital — *see* Disorder, orbit, specified type NEC
  - oroantral J32.0
  - oviduct, external N82.5
  - palate (hard) M27.8
  - pancreatic K86.89
  - pancreaticoduodenal K86.89
  - parotid (gland) K11.4
    - region K12.2
  - penis N48.89
  - perianal K60.3
  - pericardium (pleura) (sac) — *see* Pericarditis
  - pericecal K63.2
  - perineorectal K60.4

- **Fistula** — *continued*
  - perineosigmoidal K63.2
  - perineum, perineal (with urethral involvement) NEC N36.0
    - tuberculous A18.13
    - ureter N28.89
  - perirectal K60.4
    - tuberculous A18.32
  - peritoneum K65.9
  - pharyngoesophageal J39.2
  - pharynx J39.2
    - branchial cleft (congenital) Q18.0
  - pilonidal (infected) (rectum) — *see* Sinus, pilonidal
  - pleura, pleural, pleurocutaneous, pleuroperitoneal J86.0
    - tuberculous NEC A15.6
  - pleuropericardial I31.8
  - portal vein-hepatic artery, congenital Q26.6
  - postauricular H70.81 ☑
  - postoperative, persistent T81.83 ☑
    - specified site — *see* Fistula, by site
  - preauricular (congenital) Q18.1
  - prostate N42.89
  - pulmonary J86.0
    - arteriovenous I28.0
      - congenital Q25.72
    - tuberculous — *see* Tuberculosis, pulmonary
  - pulmonoperitoneal J86.0
  - rectolabial N82.4
  - rectosigmoid (intercommunicating) K63.2
  - rectoureteral N28.89
  - rectourethral N36.0
    - congenital Q64.73
  - rectouterine N82.4
    - congenital Q51.7
  - rectovaginal N82.3
    - congenital Q52.2
    - tuberculous A18.18
  - rectovesical N32.1
    - congenital Q64.79
  - rectovesicovaginal N82.3
  - rectovulval N82.4
    - congenital Q52.79
  - rectum (to skin) K60.4
    - congenital Q43.6
      - with absence, atresia and stenosis Q42.0
    - tuberculous A18.32
  - renal N28.89
  - retroauricular — *see* Fistula, postauricular
  - salivary duct or gland (any) K11.4
    - congenital Q38.4
  - scrotum (urinary) N50.89
    - tuberculous A18.15
  - semicircular canals — *see* subcategory H83.1
  - sigmoid K63.2
    - to bladder N32.1
  - sinus — *see* Sinusitis
  - skin L98.8
    - to genital tract (female) N82.5
  - splenocolic D73.89
  - stercoral K63.2
  - stomach K31.6
  - sublingual gland K11.4
  - submandibular gland K11.4
  - submaxillary (gland) K11.4
    - region K12.2
  - thoracic J86.0
    - duct I89.8
  - thoracoabdominal J86.0
  - thoracogastric J86.0
  - thoracointestinal J86.0
  - thorax J86.0
  - thyroglossal duct Q89.2
  - thyroid E07.89
  - trachea, congenital (external) (internal) Q32.1
  - tracheoesophageal J86.0
    - congenital Q39.2
      - with atresia of esophagus Q39.1
    - following tracheostomy J95.04
  - traumatic arteriovenous — *see* Injury, blood vessel, by site
  - tuberculous - code by site under Tuberculosis
  - typhoid A01.09
  - umbilicourinary Q64.8
  - urachus, congenital Q64.4
  - ureter (persistent) N28.89
  - ureteroabdominal N28.89
  - ureterorectal N28.89
  - ureterosigmoido-abdominal N28.89
  - ureterovaginal N82.1
  - ureterovesical N32.2

- **Fistula** — *continued*
  - urethra N36.0
    - congenital Q64.79
    - tuberculous A18.13
  - urethroperineal N36.0
  - urethroperineovesical N32.2
  - urethrorectal N36.0
    - congenital Q64.73
  - urethroscrotal N50.89
  - urethrovaginal N82.1
  - urethrovesical N32.2
  - urinary (tract) (persistent) (recurrent) N36.0
  - uteroabdominal N82.5
    - congenital Q51.7
  - uteroenteric, uterointestinal N82.4
    - congenital Q51.7
  - uterorectal N82.4
    - congenital Q51.7
  - uteroureteric N82.1
  - uterourethral Q51.7
  - uterovaginal N82.8
  - uterovesical N82.1
    - congenital Q51.7
  - uterus N82.8
  - vagina (postpartal) (wall) N82.8
  - vaginocutaneous (postpartal) N82.5
  - vaginointestinal NEC N82.4
    - large intestine N82.3
    - small intestine N82.2
  - vaginoperineal N82.5
  - vasocutaneous, congenital Q55.7
  - vesical NEC N32.2
  - vesicoabdominal N32.2
  - vesicocervicovaginal N82.1
  - vesicocolic N32.1
  - vesicocutaneous N32.2
  - vesicoenteric N32.1
  - vesicointestinal N32.1
  - vesicometrorectal N82.4
  - vesicoperineal N32.2
  - vesicorectal N32.1
    - congenital Q64.79
  - vesicosigmoidal N32.1
  - vesicosigmoidovaginal N82.3
  - vesicoureteral N32.2
  - vesicoureterovaginal N82.1
  - vesicourethral N32.2
  - vesicourethrorectal N32.1
  - vesicouterine N82.1
    - congenital Q51.7
  - vesicovaginal N82.0
  - vulvorectal N82.4
    - congenital Q52.79
- **Fit** R56.9
  - epileptic — *see* Epilepsy
  - fainting R55
  - hysterical F44.5
  - newborn P90
- **Fitting** (and adjustment) (of)
  - artificial
    - arm — *see* Admission, adjustment, artificial, arm
    - breast Z44.3 ☑
    - eye Z44.2 ☑
    - leg — *see* Admission, adjustment, artificial, leg
  - automatic implantable cardiac defibrillator (with synchronous cardiac pacemaker) Z45.02
  - brain neuropacemaker Z46.2
    - implanted Z45.42
  - cardiac defibrillator — *see* Fitting (and adjustment) (of), automatic implantable cardiac defibrillator
  - catheter, non-vascular Z46.82
  - colostomy belt Z46.89
  - contact lenses Z46.0
  - CRT-D (resynchronization therapy defibrillator) Z45.02
  - CRT-P (cardiac resynchronization therapy pacemaker) Z45.018
    - pulse generator Z45.010
  - cystostomy device Z46.6
  - defibrillator, cardiac — *see* Fitting (and adjustment) (of), automatic implantable cardiac defibrillator
  - dentures Z46.3
  - device NOS Z46.9
    - abdominal Z46.89
    - gastrointestinal NEC Z46.59
    - implanted NEC Z45.89
    - nervous system Z46.2
      - implanted — *see* Admission, adjustment, device, implanted, nervous system

- **Fitting** — *continued*
  - device NOS — *continued*
    - orthodontic Z46.4
    - orthoptic Z46.0
    - orthotic Z46.89
    - prosthetic (external) Z44.9
      - breast Z44.3 ☑
      - dental Z46.3
      - eye Z44.2 ☑
      - specified NEC Z44.8
    - specified NEC Z46.89
    - substitution
      - auditory Z46.2
        - implanted — *see* Admission, adjustment, device, implanted, hearing device
      - nervous system Z46.2
        - implanted — *see* Admission, adjustment, device, implanted, nervous system
      - visual Z46.2
        - implanted Z45.31
    - urinary Z46.6
  - gastric lap band Z46.51
  - gastrointestinal appliance NEC Z46.59
  - glasses (reading) Z46.0
  - hearing aid Z46.1
  - ileostomy device Z46.89
  - insulin pump Z46.81
  - intestinal appliance NEC Z46.89
  - myringotomy device (stent) (tube) Z45.82
  - neuropacemaker Z46.2
    - implanted Z45.42
  - non-vascular catheter Z46.82
  - orthodontic device Z46.4
  - orthopedic device (brace) (cast) (corset) (shoes) Z46.89
  - pacemaker (cardiac) (cardiac resynchronization therapy (CRT-P)) Z45.018
    - nervous system (brain) (peripheral nerve) (spinal cord) Z46.2
      - implanted Z45.42
    - pulse generator Z45.010
  - portacath (Port-a-Cath®) Z45.2
  - prosthesis (external) Z44.9
    - arm — *see* Admission, adjustment, artificial, arm
    - breast Z44.3 ☑
    - dental Z46.3
    - eye Z44.2 ☑
    - leg — *see* Admission, adjustment, artificial, leg
    - specified NEC Z44.8
  - spectacles Z46.0
  - wheelchair Z46.89
- **Fitzhugh-Curtis** syndrome
  - due to
    - Chlamydia trachomatis A74.81
    - Neisseria gonorrhoeae (gonococcal peritonitis) A54.85
- **Fitz's** syndrome (acute hemorrhagic pancreatitis) (*see also* Pancreatitis, acute)K85.80
- **Fixation**
  - joint — *see* Ankylosis
  - larynx J38.7
  - stapes — *see* Ankylosis, ear ossicles
    - deafness — *see* Deafness, conductive
  - uterus (acquired) — *see* Malposition, uterus
  - vocal cord J38.3
- **Flabby** ridge K06.8
- **Flaccid** (*see also* condition)
  - palate, congenital Q38.5
- **Flail**
  - chest S22.5 ☑
    - newborn (birth injury) P13.8
  - joint (paralytic) M25.20
    - ankle M25.27 ☑
    - elbow M25.22 ☑
    - foot joint M25.27 ☑
    - hand joint M25.24 ☑
    - hip M25.25 ☑
    - knee M25.26 ☑
    - shoulder M25.21 ☑
    - specified joint NEC M25.28
    - wrist M25.23 ☑
- **Flajani's** disease — *see* Hyperthyroidism, with, goiter (diffuse)
- **Flap**, liver K71.3
- **Flashbacks** (residual to hallucinogen use) F16.283
- **Flat**
  - chamber (eye) — *see* Disorder, globe, hypotony, flat anterior chamber
  - chest, congenital Q67.8
  - foot (acquired) (fixed type) (painful) (postural) (*see also* Deformity, limb, flat foot)

- **Flat** — *continued*
  - foot — *continued*
    - congenital (rigid) (spastic (everted)) Q66.5 ☑
    - rachitic sequelae (late effect) E64.3
  - organ or site, congenital NEC — *see* Anomaly, by site
  - pelvis M95.5
    - with disproportion (fetopelvic) O33.0
      - causing obstructed labor O65.0
    - congenital Q74.2
- **Flatau-Schilder** disease G37.0
- **Flatback** syndrome M40.30
  - lumbar region M40.36
  - lumbosacral region M40.37
  - thoracolumbar region M40.35
- **Flattening**
  - head, femur M89.8X5
  - hip — *see* Coxa, plana
  - lip (congenital) Q18.8
  - nose (congenital) Q67.4
    - acquired M95.0
- **Flatulence** R14.3
  - psychogenic F45.8
- **Flatus** R14.3
  - vaginalis N89.8
- **Flax-dresser's** disease J66.1
- **Flea** bite — *see* Injury, bite, by site, superficial, insect
- **Flecks,** glaucomatous (subcapsular) — *see* Cataract, complicated
- **Fleischer** (-Kayser) ring (cornea) H18.04 ☑
- **Fleshy** mole O02.0
- **Flexibilitas** cerea — *see* Catalepsy
- **Flexion**
  - amputation stump (surgical) T87.89
  - cervix — *see* Malposition, uterus
  - contracture, joint — *see* Contraction, joint
  - deformity, joint (*see also* Deformity, limb, flexion)M21.20
    - hip, congenital Q65.89
  - uterus (*see also* Malposition, uterus)
    - lateral — *see* Lateroversion, uterus
- **Flexner-Boyd** dysentery A03.2
- **Flexner's** dysentery A03.1
- **Flexure** — *see* Flexion
- **Flint** murmur (aortic insufficiency) I35.1
- **Floater,** vitreous — *see* Opacity, vitreous
- **Floating**
  - cartilage (joint) (*see also* Loose, body, joint)
    - knee — *see* Derangement, knee, loose body
  - gallbladder, congenital Q44.1
  - kidney N28.89
    - congenital Q63.8
  - spleen D73.89
- **Flooding** N92.0
- **Floor** — *see* condition
- **Floppy**
  - baby syndrome (nonspecific) P94.2
  - iris syndrome (intraoperative) (IFIS) H21.81
  - nonrheumatic mitral valve syndrome I34.1
- **Flu** (*see also* Influenza)
  - avian (*see also* Influenza, due to, identified novel influenza A virus)J09.X2
  - bird (*see also* Influenza, due to, identified novel influenza A virus)J09.X2
  - intestinal NEC A08.4
  - swine (viruses that normally cause infections in pigs) (*see also* Influenza, due to, identified novel influenza A virus)J09.X2
- **Fluctuating** blood pressure I99.8
- **Fluid**
  - abdomen R18.8
  - chest J94.8
  - heart — *see* Failure, heart, congestive
  - joint — *see* Effusion, joint
  - loss (acute) E86.9
  - lung — *see* Edema, lung
  - overload E87.70
    - specified NEC E87.79
  - peritoneal cavity R18.8
  - pleural cavity J94.8
  - retention R60.9
- **Flukes** NEC (*see also* Infestation, fluke)
  - blood NEC — *see* Schistosomiasis
  - liver B66.3
- **Fluor** (vaginalis) N89.8
  - trichomonal or due to Trichomonas (vaginalis) A59.00
- **Fluorosis**
  - dental K00.3
  - skeletal M85.10
    - ankle M85.17 ☑
    - foot M85.17 ☑

- **Fluorosis** — *continued*
  - skeletal — *continued*
    - forearm M85.13 ☑
    - hand M85.14 ☑
    - lower leg M85.16 ☑
    - multiple site M85.19
    - neck M85.18
    - rib M85.18
    - shoulder M85.11 ☑
    - skull M85.18
    - specified site NEC M85.18
    - thigh M85.15 ☑
    - toe M85.17 ☑
    - upper arm M85.12 ☑
    - vertebra M85.18
- **Flush** syndrome E34.0
- **Flushing** R23.2
  - menopausal N95.1
- **Flutter**
  - atrial or auricular I48.92
    - atypical I48.4
    - type I I48.3
    - type II I48.4
    - typical I48.3
  - heart I49.8
    - atrial or auricular I48.92
      - atypical I48.4
      - type I I48.3
      - type II I48.4
      - typical I48.3
    - ventricular I49.02
  - ventricular I49.02
- **FNHTR** (febrile nonhemolytic transfusion reaction) R50.84
- **Fochier's** abscess - code by site under Abscess
- **Focus,** Assmann's — *see* Tuberculosis, pulmonary
- **Fogo** selvagem L10.3
- **Foix-Alajouanine** syndrome G95.19
- **Fold,** folds (anomalous) (*see also* Anomaly, by site)
  - Descemet's membrane — *see* Change, corneal membrane, Descemet's, fold
  - epicanthic Q10.3
  - heart Q24.8
- **Folie** à deux F24
- **Follicle**
  - cervix (nabothian) (ruptured) N88.8
  - graafian, ruptured, with hemorrhage N83.0 ☑
  - nabothian N88.8
- **Follicular** — *see* condition
- **Folliculitis** (superficial) L73.9
  - abscedens et suffodiens L66.3
  - cyst N83.0 ☑
  - decalvans L66.2
  - deep — *see* Furuncle, by site
  - gonococcal (acute) (chronic) A54.01
  - keloid, keloidalis L73.0
  - pustular L01.02
  - ulerythematosa reticulata L66.4
- **Folliculome** lipidique
  - specified site — *see* Neoplasm, benign, by site
  - unspecified site
    - female D27.9
    - male D29.20
- **Følling's** disease E70.0
- **Follow-up** — *see* Examination, follow-up
- **Fong's** syndrome (hereditary osteo-onychodysplasia) Q87.2
- **Food**
  - allergy L27.2
  - asphyxia (from aspiration or inhalation) — *see* Foreign body, by site
  - choked on — *see* Foreign body, by site
  - deprivation T73.0 ☑
    - specified kind of food NEC E63.8
  - intoxication — *see* Poisoning, food
  - lack of T73.0 ☑
  - poisoning — *see* Poisoning, food
  - rejection NEC — *see* Disorder, eating
  - strangulation or suffocation — *see* Foreign body, by site
  - toxemia — *see* Poisoning, food
- **Foot** — *see* condition
- **Foramen** ovale (nonclosure) (patent) (persistent) Q21.1
- **Forbes'** glycogen storage disease E74.03
- **Fordyce-Fox** disease L75.2
- **Fordyce's** disease (mouth) Q38.6
- **Forearm** — *see* condition
- **Foreign** body
  - with
    - laceration — *see* Laceration, by site, with foreign body

- **Foreign** body — *continued*
  - with — *continued*
    - puncture wound — *see* Puncture, by site, with foreign body
  - accidentally left following a procedure T81.509 ☑
    - aspiration T81.506 ☑
      - resulting in
        - adhesions T81.516 ☑
        - obstruction T81.526 ☑
        - perforation T81.536 ☑
        - specified complication NEC T81.596 ☑
    - cardiac catheterization T81.505 ☑
      - resulting in
        - acute reaction T81.60 ☑
          - aseptic peritonitis T81.61 ☑
          - specified NEC T81.69 ☑
        - adhesions T81.515 ☑
        - obstruction T81.525 ☑
        - perforation T81.535 ☑
        - specified complication NEC T81.595 ☑
    - causing
      - acute reaction T81.60 ☑
        - aseptic peritonitis T81.61 ☑
        - specified complication NEC T81.69 ☑
      - adhesions T81.519 ☑
      - aseptic peritonitis T81.61 ☑
      - obstruction T81.529 ☑
      - perforation T81.539 ☑
      - specified complication NEC T81.599 ☑
    - endoscopy T81.504 ☑
      - resulting in
        - adhesions T81.514 ☑
        - obstruction T81.524 ☑
        - perforation T81.534 ☑
        - specified complication NEC T81.594 ☑
    - immunization T81.503 ☑
      - resulting in
        - adhesions T81.513 ☑
        - obstruction T81.523 ☑
        - perforation T81.533 ☑
        - specified complication NEC T81.593 ☑
    - infusion T81.501 ☑
      - resulting in
        - adhesions T81.511 ☑
        - obstruction T81.521 ☑
        - perforation T81.531 ☑
        - specified complication NEC T81.591 ☑
    - injection T81.503 ☑
      - resulting in
        - adhesions T81.513 ☑
        - obstruction T81.523 ☑
        - perforation T81.533 ☑
        - specified complication NEC T81.593 ☑
    - kidney dialysis T81.502 ☑
      - resulting in
        - adhesions T81.512 ☑
        - obstruction T81.522 ☑
        - perforation T81.532 ☑
        - specified complication NEC T81.592 ☑
    - packing removal T81.507 ☑
      - resulting in
        - acute reaction T81.60 ☑
          - aseptic peritonitis T81.61 ☑
          - specified NEC T81.69 ☑
        - adhesions T81.517 ☑
        - obstruction T81.527 ☑
        - perforation T81.537 ☑
        - specified complication NEC T81.597 ☑
    - puncture T81.506 ☑
      - resulting in
        - adhesions T81.516 ☑
        - obstruction T81.526 ☑
        - perforation T81.536 ☑
        - specified complication NEC T81.596 ☑
    - specified procedure NEC T81.508 ☑
      - resulting in
        - acute reaction T81.60 ☑
          - aseptic peritonitis T81.61 ☑
          - specified NEC T81.69 ☑
        - adhesions T81.518 ☑
        - obstruction T81.528 ☑
        - perforation T81.538 ☑
        - specified complication NEC T81.598 ☑
    - surgical operation T81.500 ☑
      - resulting in
        - acute reaction T81.60 ☑
          - aseptic peritonitis T81.61 ☑
          - specified NEC T81.69 ☑
        - adhesions T81.510 ☑
        - obstruction T81.520 ☑
        - perforation T81.530 ☑
        - specified complication NEC T81.590 ☑

- **Foreign** body — *continued*
  - accidentally left following a procedure — *continued*
    - transfusion T81.501 ☑
      - resulting in
        - adhesions T81.511 ☑
        - obstruction T81.521 ☑
        - perforation T81.531 ☑
        - specified complication NEC T81.591 ☑
  - alimentary tract T18.9 ☑
    - anus T18.5 ☑
    - colon T18.4 ☑
    - esophagus — *see* Foreign body, esophagus
    - mouth T18.0 ☑
    - multiple sites T18.8 ☑
    - rectosigmoid (junction) T18.5 ☑
    - rectum T18.5 ☑
    - small intestine T18.3 ☑
    - specified site NEC T18.8 ☑
    - stomach T18.2 ☑
  - anterior chamber (eye) S05.5 ☑
  - auditory canal — *see* Foreign body, entering through orifice, ear
  - bronchus T17.508 ☑
    - causing
      - asphyxiation T17.500 ☑
        - food (bone) (seed) T17.520 ☑
        - gastric contents (vomitus) T17.510 ☑
        - specified type NEC T17.590 ☑
      - injury NEC T17.508 ☑
        - food (bone) (seed) T17.528 ☑
        - gastric contents (vomitus) T17.518 ☑
        - specified type NEC T17.598 ☑
  - canthus — *see* Foreign body, conjunctival sac
  - ciliary body (eye) S05.5 ☑
  - conjunctival sac T15.1 ☑
  - cornea T15.0 ☑
  - entering through orifice
    - accessory sinus T17.0 ☑
    - alimentary canal T18.9 ☑
      - multiple parts T18.8 ☑
      - specified part NEC T18.8 ☑
    - alveolar process T18.0 ☑
    - antrum (Highmore's) T17.0 ☑
    - anus T18.5 ☑
    - appendix T18.4 ☑
    - auditory canal — *see* Foreign body, entering through orifice, ear
    - auricle — *see* Foreign body, entering through orifice, ear
    - bladder T19.1 ☑
    - bronchioles — *see* Foreign body, respiratory tract, specified site NEC
    - bronchus (main) — *see* Foreign body, bronchus
    - buccal cavity T18.0 ☑
    - canthus (inner) — *see* Foreign body, conjunctival sac
    - cecum T18.4 ☑
    - cervix (canal) (uteri) T19.3 ☑
    - colon T18.4 ☑
    - conjunctival sac — *see* Foreign body, conjunctival sac
    - cornea — *see* Foreign body, cornea
    - digestive organ or tract NOS T18.9 ☑
      - multiple parts T18.8 ☑
      - specified part NEC T18.8 ☑
    - duodenum T18.3 ☑
    - ear (external) T16. ☑
    - esophagus — *see* Foreign body, esophagus
    - eye (external) NOS T15.9 ☑
      - conjunctival sac — *see* Foreign body, conjunctival sac
      - cornea — *see* Foreign body, cornea
      - specified part NEC T15.8 ☑
    - eyeball (*see also* Foreign body, entering through orifice, eye, specified part NEC)
      - with penetrating wound — *see* Puncture, eyeball
    - eyelid (*see also* Foreign body, conjunctival sac)
      - with
        - laceration — *see* Laceration, eyelid, with foreign body
        - puncture — *see* Puncture, eyelid, with foreign body
        - superficial injury — *see* Foreign body, superficial, eyelid
    - gastrointestinal tract T18.9 ☑
      - multiple parts T18.8 ☑
      - specified part NEC T18.8 ☑
    - genitourinary tract T19.9 ☑
      - multiple parts T19.8 ☑
      - specified part NEC T19.8 ☑

- **Foreign** body — *continued*
  - entering through orifice — *continued*
    - globe — *see* Foreign body, entering through orifice, eyeball
    - gum T18.0 ☑
    - Highmore's antrum T17.0 ☑
    - hypopharynx — *see* Foreign body, pharynx
    - ileum T18.3 ☑
    - intestine (small) T18.3 ☑
      - large T18.4 ☑
    - lacrimal apparatus (punctum) — *see* Foreign body, entering through orifice, eye, specified part NEC
    - large intestine T18.4 ☑
    - larynx — *see* Foreign body, larynx
    - lung — *see* Foreign body, respiratory tract, specified site NEC
    - maxillary sinus T17.0 ☑
    - mouth T18.0 ☑
    - nasal sinus T17.0 ☑
    - nasopharynx — *see* Foreign body, pharynx
    - nose (passage) T17.1 ☑
    - nostril T17.1 ☑
    - oral cavity T18.0 ☑
    - palate T18.0 ☑
    - penis T19.4 ☑
    - pharynx — *see* Foreign body, pharynx
    - piriform sinus — *see* Foreign body, pharynx
    - rectosigmoid (junction) T18.5 ☑
    - rectum T18.5 ☑
    - respiratory tract — *see* Foreign body, respiratory tract
    - sinus (accessory) (frontal) (maxillary) (nasal) T17.0 ☑
      - piriform — *see* Foreign body, pharynx
    - small intestine T18.3 ☑
    - stomach T18.2 ☑
    - suffocation by — *see* Foreign body, by site
    - tear ducts or glands — *see* Foreign body, entering through orifice, eye, specified part NEC
    - throat — *see* Foreign body, pharynx
    - tongue T18.0 ☑
    - tonsil, tonsillar (fossa) — *see* Foreign body, pharynx
    - trachea — *see* Foreign body, trachea
    - ureter T19.8 ☑
    - urethra T19.0 ☑
    - uterus (any part) T19.3 ☑
    - vagina T19.2 ☑
    - vulva T19.2 ☑
  - esophagus T18.108 ☑
    - causing
      - injury NEC T18.108 ☑
        - food (bone) (seed) T18.128 ☑
        - gastric contents (vomitus) T18.118 ☑
        - specified type NEC T18.198 ☑
      - tracheal compression T18.100 ☑
        - food (bone) (seed) T18.120 ☑
        - gastric contents (vomitus) T18.110 ☑
        - specified type NEC T18.190 ☑
  - feeling of, in throat R09.89
  - fragment — *see* Retained, foreign body fragments (type of)
  - genitourinary tract T19.9 ☑
    - bladder T19.1 ☑
    - multiple parts T19.8 ☑
    - penis T19.4 ☑
    - specified site NEC T19.8 ☑
    - urethra T19.0 ☑
    - uterus T19.3 ☑
      - IUD Z97.5
    - vagina T19.2 ☑
      - contraceptive device Z97.5
    - vulva T19.2 ☑
  - granuloma (old) (soft tissue) (*see also* Granuloma, foreign body)
    - skin L92.3
  - in
    - laceration — *see* Laceration, by site, with foreign body
    - puncture wound — *see* Puncture, by site, with foreign body
    - soft tissue (residual) M79.5
  - inadvertently left in operation wound — *see* Foreign body, accidentally left during a procedure
  - ingestion, ingested NOS T18.9 ☑
  - inhalation or inspiration — *see* Foreign body, by site

- **Foreign** body — *continued*
  - internal organ, not entering through a natural orifice - code as specific injury with foreign body
  - intraocular S05.5 ☑
    - old, retained (nonmagnetic) H44.70 ☑
      - anterior chamber H44.71 ☑
      - ciliary body H44.72 ☑
      - iris H44.72 ☑
      - lens H44.73 ☑
      - magnetic H44.60 ☑
        - anterior chamber H44.61 ☑
        - ciliary body H44.62 ☑
        - iris H44.62 ☑
        - lens H44.63 ☑
        - posterior wall H44.64 ☑
        - specified site NEC H44.69 ☑
        - vitreous body H44.65 ☑
      - posterior wall H44.74 ☑
      - specified site NEC H44.79 ☑
      - vitreous body H44.75 ☑
  - iris — *see* Foreign body, intraocular
  - lacrimal punctum — *see* Foreign body, entering through orifice, eye, specified part NEC
  - larynx T17.308 ☑
    - causing
      - asphyxiation T17.300 ☑
        - food (bone) (seed) T17.320 ☑
        - gastric contents (vomitus) T17.310 ☑
        - specified type NEC T17.390 ☑
      - injury NEC T17.308 ☑
        - food (bone) (seed) T17.328 ☑
        - gastric contents (vomitus) T17.318 ☑
        - specified type NEC T17.398 ☑
  - lens — *see* Foreign body, intraocular
  - ocular muscle S05.4 ☑
    - old, retained — *see* Foreign body, orbit, old
  - old or residual
    - soft tissue (residual) M79.5
  - operation wound, left accidentally — *see* Foreign body, accidentally left during a procedure
  - orbit S05.4 ☑
    - old, retained H05.5 ☑
  - pharynx T17.208 ☑
    - causing
      - asphyxiation T17.200 ☑
        - food (bone) (seed) T17.220 ☑
        - gastric contents (vomitus) T17.210 ☑
        - specified type NEC T17.290 ☑
      - injury NEC T17.208 ☑
        - food (bone) (seed) T17.228 ☑
        - gastric contents (vomitus) T17.218 ☑
        - specified type NEC T17.298 ☑
  - respiratory tract T17.908 ☑
    - bronchioles — *see* Foreign body, respiratory tract, specified site NEC
    - bronchus — *see* Foreign body, bronchus
    - causing
      - asphyxiation T17.900 ☑
        - food (bone) (seed) T17.920 ☑
        - gastric contents (vomitus) T17.910 ☑
        - specified type NEC T17.990 ☑
      - injury NEC T17.908 ☑
        - food (bone) (seed) T17.928 ☑
        - gastric contents (vomitus) T17.918 ☑
        - specified type NEC T17.998 ☑
    - larynx — *see* Foreign body, larynx
    - lung — *see* Foreign body, respiratory tract, specified site NEC
    - multiple parts — *see* Foreign body, respiratory tract, specified site NEC
    - nasal sinus T17.0 ☑
    - nasopharynx — *see* Foreign body, pharynx
    - nose T17.1 ☑
    - nostril T17.1 ☑
    - pharynx — *see* Foreign body, pharynx
    - specified site NEC T17.808 ☑
      - causing
        - asphyxiation T17.800 ☑
          - food (bone) (seed) T17.820 ☑
          - gastric contents (vomitus) T17.810 ☑
          - specified type NEC T17.890 ☑
        - injury NEC T17.808 ☑
          - food (bone) (seed) T17.828 ☑
          - gastric contents (vomitus) T17.818 ☑
          - specified type NEC T17.898 ☑
    - throat — *see* Foreign body, pharynx
    - trachea — *see* Foreign body, trachea
  - retained (old) (nonmagnetic) (in)
    - anterior chamber (eye) — *see* Foreign body, intraocular, old, retained, anterior chamber

- **Foreign** body — *continued*
  - retained — *continued*
      - magnetic — *see* Foreign body, intraocular, old, retained, magnetic, anterior chamber
    - ciliary body — *see* Foreign body, intraocular, old, retained, ciliary body
      - magnetic — *see* Foreign body, intraocular, old, retained, magnetic, ciliary body
    - eyelid H02.819
      - left H02.816
        - lower H02.815
        - upper H02.814
      - right H02.813
        - lower H02.812
        - upper H02.811
    - fragments — *see* Retained, foreign body fragments (type of)
    - globe — *see* Foreign body, intraocular, old, retained
      - magnetic — *see* Foreign body, intraocular, old, retained, magnetic
    - intraocular — *see* Foreign body, intraocular, old, retained
      - magnetic — *see* Foreign body, intraocular, old, retained, magnetic
    - iris — *see* Foreign body, intraocular, old, retained, iris
      - magnetic — *see* Foreign body, intraocular, old, retained, magnetic, iris
    - lens — *see* Foreign body, intraocular, old, retained, lens
      - magnetic — *see* Foreign body, intraocular, old, retained, magnetic, lens
    - muscle — *see* Foreign body, retained, soft tissue
    - orbit — *see* Foreign body, orbit, old
    - posterior wall of globe — *see* Foreign body, intraocular, old, retained, posterior wall
      - magnetic — *see* Foreign body, intraocular, old, retained, magnetic, posterior wall
    - retrobulbar — *see* Foreign body, orbit, old, retrobulbar
    - soft tissue M79.5
    - vitreous — *see* Foreign body, intraocular, old, retained, vitreous body
      - magnetic — *see* Foreign body, intraocular, old, retained, magnetic, vitreous body
  - retina S05.5 ☑
  - superficial, without open wound
    - abdomen, abdominal (wall) S30.851 ☑
    - alveolar process S00.552 ☑
    - ankle S90.55 ☑
    - antecubital space — *see* Foreign body, superficial, forearm
    - anus S30.857 ☑
    - arm (upper) S40.85 ☑
    - auditory canal — *see* Foreign body, superficial, ear
    - auricle — *see* Foreign body, superficial, ear
    - axilla — *see* Foreign body, superficial, arm
    - back, lower S30.850 ☑
    - breast S20.15 ☑
    - brow S00.85 ☑
    - buttock S30.850 ☑
    - calf — *see* Foreign body, superficial, leg
    - canthus — *see* Foreign body, superficial, eyelid
    - cheek S00.85 ☑
      - internal S00.552 ☑
    - chest wall — *see* Foreign body, superficial, thorax
    - chin S00.85 ☑
    - clitoris S30.854 ☑
    - costal region — *see* Foreign body, superficial, thorax
    - digit (s)
      - hand — *see* Foreign body, superficial, finger
      - foot — *see* Foreign body, superficial, toe
    - ear S00.45 ☑
    - elbow S50.35 ☑
    - epididymis S30.853 ☑
    - epigastric region S30.851 ☑
    - epiglottis S10.15 ☑
    - esophagus, cervical S10.15 ☑
    - eyebrow — *see* Foreign body, superficial, eyelid
    - eyelid S00.25 ☑
    - face S00.85 ☑
    - finger (s) S60.459 ☑
      - index S60.45 ☑
      - little S60.45 ☑
      - middle S60.45 ☑
      - ring S60.45 ☑

Foreign body — *continued*
  superficial, without open wound — *continued*
    flank S30.851 ☑
    foot (except toe (s) alone) S90.85 ☑
      toe — *see* Foreign body, superficial, toe
    forearm S50.85 ☑
      elbow only — *see* Foreign body, superficial, elbow
    forehead S00.85 ☑
    genital organs, external
      female S30.856 ☑
      male S30.855 ☑
    groin S30.851 ☑
    gum S00.552 ☑
    hand S60.55 ☑
    head S00.95 ☑
      ear — *see* Foreign body, superficial, ear
      eyelid — *see* Foreign body, superficial, eyelid
      lip S00.551 ☑
      nose S00.35 ☑
      oral cavity S00.552 ☑
      scalp S00.05 ☑
      specified site NEC S00.85 ☑
    heel — *see* Foreign body, superficial, foot
    hip S70.25 ☑
    inguinal region S30.851 ☑
    interscapular region S20.459 ☑
    jaw S00.85 ☑
    knee S80.25 ☑
    labium (majus) (minus) S30.854 ☑
    larynx S10.15 ☑
    leg (lower) S80.85 ☑
      knee — *see* Foreign body, superficial, knee
      upper — *see* Foreign body, superficial, thigh
    lip S00.551 ☑
    lower back S30.850 ☑
    lumbar region S30.850 ☑
    malar region S00.85 ☑
    mammary — *see* Foreign body, superficial, breast
    mastoid region S00.85 ☑
    mouth S00.552 ☑
    nail
      finger — *see* Foreign body, superficial, finger
      toe — *see* Foreign body, superficial, toe
    nape S10.85 ☑
    nasal S00.35 ☑
    neck S10.95 ☑
      specified site NEC S10.85 ☑
      throat S10.15 ☑
    nose S00.35 ☑
    occipital region S00.05 ☑
    oral cavity S00.552 ☑
    orbital region — *see* Foreign body, superficial, eyelid
    palate S00.552 ☑
    palm — *see* Foreign body, superficial, hand
    parietal region S00.05 ☑
    pelvis S30.850 ☑
    penis S30.852 ☑
    perineum
      female S30.854 ☑
      male S30.850 ☑
    periocular area — *see* Foreign body, superficial, eyelid
    phalanges
      finger — *see* Foreign body, superficial, finger
      toe — *see* Foreign body, superficial, toe
    pharynx S10.15 ☑
    pinna — *see* Foreign body, superficial, ear
    popliteal space — *see* Foreign body, superficial, knee
    prepuce S30.852 ☑
    pubic region S30.850 ☑
    pudendum
      female S30.856 ☑
      male S30.855 ☑
    sacral region S30.850 ☑
    scalp S00.05 ☑
    scapular region — *see* Foreign body, superficial, shoulder
    scrotum S30.853 ☑
    shin — *see* Foreign body, superficial, leg
    shoulder S40.25 ☑
    sternal region S20.359 ☑
    submaxillary region S00.85 ☑
    submental region S00.85 ☑
    subungual
      finger (s) — *see* Foreign body, superficial, finger
      toe (s) — *see* Foreign body, superficial, toe
    supraclavicular fossa S10.85 ☑

Foreign body — *continued*
  superficial, without open wound — *continued*
    supraorbital S00.85 ☑
    temple S00.85 ☑
    temporal region S00.85 ☑
    testis S30.853 ☑
    thigh S70.35 ☑
    thorax, thoracic (wall) S20.95 ☑
      back S20.45 ☑
      front S20.35 ☑
    throat S10.15 ☑
    thumb S60.35 ☑
    toe (s) (lesser) S90.456 ☑
      great S90.45 ☑
    tongue S00.552 ☑
    trachea S10.15 ☑
    tunica vaginalis S30.853 ☑
    tympanum, tympanic membrane — *see* Foreign body, superficial, ear
    uvula S00.552 ☑
    vagina S30.854 ☑
    vocal cords S10.15 ☑
    vulva S30.854 ☑
    wrist S60.85 ☑
  swallowed T18.9 ☑
  trachea T17.408 ☑
    causing
      asphyxiation T17.400 ☑
        food (bone) (seed) T17.420 ☑
        gastric contents (vomitus) T17.410 ☑
        specified type NEC T17.490 ☑
      injury NEC T17.408 ☑
        food (bone) (seed) T17.428 ☑
        gastric contents (vomitus) T17.418 ☑
        specified type NEC T17.498 ☑
  type of fragment — *see* Retained, foreign body fragments (type of)
  vitreous (humor) S05.5 ☑
Forestier's disease (rhizomelic pseudopolyarthritis) M35.3
  meaning ankylosing hyperostosis — *see* Hyperostosis, ankylosing
Formation
  hyalin in cornea — *see* Degeneration, cornea
  sequestrum in bone (due to infection) — *see* Osteomyelitis, chronic
  valve
    colon, congenital Q43.8
    ureter (congenital) Q62.39
Formication R20.2
Fort Bragg fever A27.89
Fossa (*see also* condition)
  pyriform — *see* condition
Foster-Kennedy syndrome H47.14 ☑
Fothergill's
  disease (trigeminal neuralgia) (*see also* Neuralgia, trigeminal)
  scarlatina anginosa A38.9
Foul breath R19.6
Foundling Z76.1
Fournier disease or gangrene N49.3
  female N76.89
Fourth
  cranial nerve — *see* condition
  molar K00.1
Foville's (peduncular) disease or syndrome G46.3
Fox (-Fordyce) disease (apocrine miliaria) L75.2
Fracture, burst — *see* Fracture, traumatic, by site
Fracture, chronic — *see* Fracture, pathological
Fracture, insufficiency — *see* Fracture, pathologic, by site
Fracture, nontraumatic, NEC
  atypical
    femur M84.750 ☑
      complete
        oblique M84.759 ☑
          left side M84.758 ☑
          right side M84.757 ☑
        transverse M84.756 ☑
          left side M84.755 ☑
          right side M84.754 ☑
      incomplete M84.753 ☑
        left side M84.752 ☑
        right side M84.751 ☑
Fracture, pathological (pathologic) (*see also* Fracture, traumatic M84.40)
  ankle M84.47 ☑
  carpus M84.44 ☑
  clavicle M84.41 ☑
  compression (not due to trauma) (*see also* Collapse, vertebra)M48.50 ☑
  dental implant M27.63

Fracture, pathological — *continued*
  dental restorative material K08.539
    with loss of material K08.531
    without loss of material K08.530
  due to
    neoplastic disease NEC (*see also* Neoplasm)M84.50 ☑
      ankle M84.57 ☑
      carpus M84.54 ☑
      clavicle M84.51 ☑
      femur M84.55 ☑
      fibula M84.56 ☑
      finger M84.54 ☑
      hip M84.559 ☑
      humerus M84.52 ☑
      ilium M84.550 ☑
      ischium M84.550 ☑
      metacarpus M84.54 ☑
      metatarsus M84.57 ☑
      neck M84.58 ☑
      pelvis M84.550 ☑
      radius M84.53 ☑
      rib M84.58 ☑
      scapula M84.51 ☑
      skull M84.58 ☑
      specified site NEC M84.58 ☑
      tarsus M84.57 ☑
      tibia M84.56 ☑
      toe M84.57 ☑
      ulna M84.53 ☑
      vertebra M84.58 ☑
    osteoporosis M80.00 ☑
      disuse — *see* Osteoporosis, specified type NEC, with pathological fracture
      drug-induced — *see* Osteoporosis, drug induced, with pathological fracture
      idiopathic — *see* Osteoporosis, specified type NEC, with pathological fracture
      postmenopausal — *see* Osteoporosis, postmenopausal, with pathological fracture
      postoophorectomy — *see* Osteoporosis, postoophorectomy, with pathological fracture
      postsurgical malabsorption — *see* Osteoporosis, specified type NEC, with pathological fracture
      specified cause NEC — *see* Osteoporosis, specified type NEC, with pathological fracture
    specified disease NEC M84.60 ☑
      ankle M84.67 ☑
      carpus M84.64 ☑
      clavicle M84.61 ☑
      femur M84.65 ☑
      fibula M84.66 ☑
      finger M84.64 ☑
      hip M84.65 ☑
      humerus M84.62 ☑
      ilium M84.650 ☑
      ischium M84.650 ☑
      metacarpus M84.64 ☑
      metatarsus M84.67 ☑
      neck M84.68 ☑
      radius M84.63 ☑
      rib M84.68 ☑
      scapula M84.61 ☑
      skull M84.68 ☑
      tarsus M84.67 ☑
      tibia M84.66 ☑
      toe M84.67 ☑
      ulna M84.63 ☑
      vertebra M84.68 ☑
  femur M84.45 ☑
  fibula M84.46 ☑
  finger M84.44 ☑
  hip M84.459 ☑
  humerus M84.42 ☑
  ilium M84.454 ☑
  ischium M84.454 ☑
  joint prosthesis — *see* Complications, joint prosthesis, mechanical, breakdown, by site
    periprosthetic — *see* Fracture, pathological, periprosthetic
  metacarpus M84.44 ☑
  metatarsus M84.47 ☑
  neck M84.48 ☑
  pelvis M84.454 ☑
  periprosthetic M97.9 ☑
    ankle M97.2 ☑
    elbow M97.4 ☑
    finger M97.8 ☑

- **Fracture**, pathological — *continued*
  - periprosthetic — *continued*
    - hip M97.0 ☑
    - knee M97.1 ☑
    - other specified joint M97.8 ☑
    - shoulder M97.3 ☑
    - spinal joint M97.8 ☑
    - toe joint M97.8 ☑
    - wrist joint M97.8 ☑
  - radius M84.43 ☑
  - restorative material (dental) K08.539
    - with loss of material K08.531
    - without loss of material K08.530
  - rib M84.48 ☑
  - scapula M84.41 ☑
  - skull M84.48 ☑
  - tarsus M84.47 ☑
  - tibia M84.46 ☑
  - toe M84.47 ☑
  - ulna M84.43 ☑
  - vertebra M84.48 ☑
- **Fracture**, traumatic (abduction) (adduction) (separation) (*see also* Fracture, pathological)T14.8
  - acetabulum S32.40 ☑
    - column
      - anterior (displaced) (iliopubic) S32.43 ☑
        - nondisplaced S32.436 ☑
      - posterior (displaced) (ilioischial) S32.443 ☑
        - nondisplaced S32.44 ☑
    - dome (displaced) S32.48 ☑
      - nondisplaced S32.48 ☑
    - specified NEC S32.49 ☑
    - transverse (displaced) S32.45 ☑
      - with associated posterior wall fracture (displaced) S32.46 ☑
        - nondisplaced S32.46 ☑
      - nondisplaced S32.45 ☑
    - wall
      - anterior (displaced) S32.41 ☑
        - nondisplaced S32.41 ☑
      - medial (displaced) S32.47 ☑
        - nondisplaced S32.47 ☑
      - posterior (displaced) S32.42 ☑
        - with associated transverse fracture (displaced) S32.46 ☑
          - nondisplaced S32.46 ☑
        - nondisplaced S32.42 ☑
  - acromion — *see* Fracture, scapula, acromial process
  - ankle S82.899 ☑
    - bimalleolar (displaced) S82.84 ☑
      - nondisplaced S82.84 ☑
    - lateral malleolus only (displaced) S82.6 ☑
      - nondisplaced S82.6 ☑
    - medial malleolus (displaced) S82.5 ☑
      - associated with Maisonneuve's fracture — *see* Fracture, Maisonneuve's
      - nondisplaced S82.5 ☑
    - talus — *see* Fracture, tarsal, talus
    - trimalleolar (displaced) S82.85 ☑
      - nondisplaced S82.85 ☑
  - arm (upper) (*see also* Fracture, humerus, shaft)
    - humerus — *see* Fracture, humerus
    - radius — *see* Fracture, radius
    - ulna — *see* Fracture, ulna
  - astragalus — *see* Fracture, tarsal, talus
  - atlas — *see* Fracture, neck, cervical vertebra, first
  - axis — *see* Fracture, neck, cervical vertebra, second
  - back — *see* Fracture, vertebra
  - Barton's — *see* Barton's fracture
  - base of skull — *see* Fracture, skull, base
  - basicervical (basal) (femoral) S72.0 ☑
  - Bennett's — *see* Bennett's fracture
  - bimalleolar — *see* Fracture, ankle, bimalleolar
  - blow-out S02.3 ☑
  - bone NEC T14.8
    - birth injury P13.9
    - following insertion of orthopedic implant, joint prosthesis or bone plate — *see* Fracture, following insertion of orthopedic implant, joint prosthesis or bone plate
    - in (due to) neoplastic disease NEC — *see* Fracture, pathological, due to, neoplastic disease
    - pathological (cause unknown) — *see* Fracture, pathological
  - breast bone — *see* Fracture, sternum
  - bucket handle (semilunar cartilage) — *see* Tear, meniscus
  - burst — *see* Fracture, traumatic, by site
  - calcaneus — *see* Fracture, tarsal, calcaneus

- **Fracture**, traumatic — *continued*
  - carpal bone (s) S62.10 ☑
    - capitate (displaced) S62.13 ☑
      - nondisplaced S62.13 ☑
    - cuneiform — *see* Fracture, carpal bone, triquetrum
    - hamate (body) (displaced) S62.143 ☑
      - hook process (displaced) S62.15 ☑
        - nondisplaced S62.15 ☑
      - nondisplaced S62.14 ☑
    - larger multangular — *see* Fracture, carpal bones, trapezium
    - lunate (displaced) S62.12 ☑
      - nondisplaced S62.12 ☑
    - navicular S62.00 ☑
      - distal pole (displaced) S62.01 ☑
        - nondisplaced S62.01 ☑
      - middle third (displaced) S62.02 ☑
        - nondisplaced S62.02 ☑
      - proximal third (displaced) S62.03 ☑
        - nondisplaced S62.03 ☑
      - volar tuberosity — *see* Fracture, carpal bones, navicular, distal pole
    - os magnum — *see* Fracture, carpal bones, capitate
    - pisiform (displaced) S62.16 ☑
      - nondisplaced S62.16 ☑
    - semilunar — *see* Fracture, carpal bones, lunate
    - smaller multangular — *see* Fracture, carpal bones, trapezoid
    - trapezium (displaced) S62.17 ☑
      - nondisplaced S62.17 ☑
    - trapezoid (displaced) S62.18 ☑
      - nondisplaced S62.18 ☑
    - triquetrum (displaced) S62.11 ☑
      - nondisplaced S62.11 ☑
    - unciform — *see* Fracture, carpal bones, hamate
  - cervical — *see* Fracture, vertebra, cervical
  - clavicle S42.00 ☑
    - acromial end (displaced) S42.03 ☑
      - nondisplaced S42.03 ☑
    - birth injury P13.4
    - lateral end — *see* Fracture, clavicle, acromial end
    - shaft (displaced) S42.02 ☑
      - nondisplaced S42.02 ☑
    - sternal end (anterior) (displaced) S42.01 ☑
      - nondisplaced S42.01 ☑
      - posterior S42.01 ☑
  - coccyx S32.2 ☑
  - collapsed — *see* Collapse, vertebra
  - collar bone — *see* Fracture, clavicle
  - Colles' — *see* Colles' fracture
  - coronoid process — *see* Fracture, ulna, upper end, coronoid process
  - corpus cavernosum penis S39.840 ☑
  - costochondral cartilage S23.41 ☑
  - costochondral, costosternal junction — *see* Fracture, rib
  - cranium — *see* Fracture, skull
  - cricoid cartilage S12.8 ☑
  - cuboid (ankle) — *see* Fracture, tarsal, cuboid
  - cuneiform
    - foot — *see* Fracture, tarsal, cuneiform
    - wrist — *see* Fracture, carpal, triquetrum
  - delayed union — *see* Delay, union, fracture
  - dental restorative material K08.539
    - with loss of material K08.531
    - without loss of material K08.530
  - due to
    - birth injury — *see* Birth, injury, fracture
    - osteoporosis — *see* Osteoporosis, with fracture
  - Dupuytren's — *see* Fracture, ankle, lateral malleolus
  - elbow S42.40 ☑
  - ethmoid (bone) (sinus) — *see* Fracture, skull, base
  - face bone S02.92 ☑
  - fatigue (*see also* Fracture, stress)
    - vertebra M48.40 ☑
      - cervical region M48.42 ☑
      - cervicothoracic region M48.43 ☑
      - lumbar region M48.46 ☑
      - lumbosacral region M48.47 ☑
      - occipito-atlanto-axial region M48.41 ☑
      - sacrococcygeal region M48.48 ☑
      - thoracic region M48.44 ☑
      - thoracolumbar region M48.45 ☑
  - femur, femoral S72.9 ☑
    - basicervical (basal) S72.0 ☑
    - birth injury P13.2
    - capital epiphyseal S79.01 ☑

- **Fracture**, traumatic — *continued*
  - femur, femoral — *continued*
    - condyles, epicondyles — *see* Fracture, femur, lower end
    - distal end — *see* Fracture, femur, lower end
    - epiphysis
      - head — *see* Fracture, femur, upper end, epiphysis
      - lower — *see* Fracture, femur, lower end, epiphysis
      - upper — *see* Fracture, femur, upper end, epiphysis
    - following insertion of implant, prosthesis or plate M96.66 ☑
    - head — *see* Fracture, femur, upper end, head
    - intertrochanteric — *see* Fracture, femur, trochanteric
    - intratrochanteric — *see* Fracture, femur, trochanteric
    - lower end S72.40 ☑
      - condyle (displaced) S72.41 ☑
        - lateral (displaced) S72.42 ☑
          - nondisplaced S72.42 ☑
        - medial (displaced) S72.43 ☑
          - nondisplaced S72.43 ☑
        - nondisplaced S72.41 ☑
      - epiphysis (displaced) S72.44 ☑
        - nondisplaced S72.44 ☑
      - physeal S79.10 ☑
        - Salter-Harris
          - Type I S79.11 ☑
          - Type II S79.12 ☑
          - Type III S79.13 ☑
          - Type IV S79.14 ☑
        - specified NEC S79.19 ☑
      - specified NEC S72.49 ☑
      - supracondylar (displaced) S72.45 ☑
        - with intracondylar extension (displaced) S72.46 ☑
          - nondisplaced S72.46 ☑
        - nondisplaced S72.45 ☑
      - torus S72.47 ☑
    - neck — *see* Fracture, femur, upper end, neck
    - pertrochanteric — *see* Fracture, femur, trochanteric
    - shaft (lower third) (middle third) (upper third) S72.30 ☑
      - comminuted (displaced) S72.35 ☑
        - nondisplaced S72.35 ☑
      - oblique (displaced) S72.33 ☑
        - nondisplaced S72.33 ☑
      - segmental (displaced) S72.36 ☑
        - nondisplaced S72.36 ☑
      - specified NEC S72.39 ☑
      - spiral (displaced) S72.34 ☑
        - nondisplaced S72.34 ☑
      - transverse (displaced) S72.32 ☑
        - nondisplaced S72.32 ☑
    - specified site NEC — *see* subcategory S72.8
    - subcapital (displaced) S72.01 ☑
    - subtrochanteric (region) (section) (displaced) S72.2 ☑
      - nondisplaced S72.2 ☑
    - transcervical — *see* Fracture, femur, upper end, neck
    - transtrochanteric — *see* Fracture, femur, trochanteric
    - trochanteric S72.10 ☑
      - apophyseal (displaced) S72.13 ☑
        - nondisplaced S72.13 ☑
      - greater trochanter (displaced) S72.11 ☑
        - nondisplaced S72.11 ☑
      - intertrochanteric (displaced) S72.14 ☑
        - nondisplaced S72.14 ☑
      - lesser trochanter (displaced) S72.12 ☑
        - nondisplaced S72.12 ☑
    - upper end S72.00 ☑
      - apophyseal (displaced) S72.13 ☑
        - nondisplaced S72.13 ☑
      - cervicotrochanteric — *see* Fracture, femur, upper end, neck, base
      - epiphysis (displaced) S72.02 ☑
        - nondisplaced S72.02 ☑
      - head S72.05 ☑
        - articular (displaced) S72.06 ☑
          - nondisplaced S72.06 ☑
        - specified NEC S72.09 ☑
      - intertrochanteric (displaced) S72.14 ☑
        - nondisplaced S72.14 ☑
      - intracapsular S72.01 ☑
      - midcervical (displaced) S72.03 ☑
        - nondisplaced S72.03 ☑

Fracture, traumatic — *continued*
- femur, femoral — *continued*
  - neck S72.00 ☑
    - base (displaced) S72.04 ☑
      - nondisplaced S72.04 ☑
    - specified NEC S72.09 ☑
  - pertrochanteric — *see* Fracture, femur, upper end, trochanteric
  - physeal S79.00 ☑
    - Salter-Harris type I S79.01 ☑
    - specified NEC S79.09 ☑
  - subcapital (displaced) S72.01 ☑
  - subtrochanteric (displaced) S72.2 ☑
    - nondisplaced S72.2 ☑
  - transcervical — *see* Fracture, femur, upper end, midcervical
  - trochanteric S72.10 ☑
    - greater (displaced) S72.11 ☑
      - nondisplaced S72.11 ☑
    - lesser (displaced) S72.12 ☑
      - nondisplaced S72.12 ☑
- fibula (shaft) (styloid) S82.40 ☑
  - comminuted (displaced) S82.45 ☑
    - nondisplaced S82.45 ☑
  - following insertion of implant, prosthesis or plate M96.67 ☑
  - involving ankle or malleolus — *see* Fracture, fibula, lateral malleolus
  - lateral malleolus (displaced) S82.6 ☑
    - nondisplaced S82.6 ☑
  - lower end
    - physeal S89.30 ☑
      - Salter-Harris
        - Type I S89.31 ☑
        - Type II S89.32 ☑
      - specified NEC S89.39 ☑
    - specified NEC S82.83 ☑
    - torus S82.82 ☑
  - oblique (displaced) S82.43 ☑
    - nondisplaced S82.43 ☑
  - segmental (displaced) S82.46 ☑
    - nondisplaced S82.46 ☑
  - specified NEC S82.49 ☑
  - spiral (displaced) S82.44 ☑
    - nondisplaced S82.44 ☑
  - transverse (displaced) S82.42 ☑
    - nondisplaced S82.42 ☑
  - upper end
    - physeal S89.20 ☑
      - Salter-Harris
        - Type I S89.21 ☑
        - Type II S89.22 ☑
      - specified NEC S89.29 ☑
    - specified NEC S82.83 ☑
    - torus S82.81 ☑
- finger (except thumb) S62.60 ☑
  - distal phalanx (displaced) S62.63 ☑
    - nondisplaced S62.66 ☑
  - index S62.60 ☑
    - distal phalanx (displaced) S62.63 ☑
      - nondisplaced S62.66 ☑
    - medial phalanx (displaced) S62.62 ☑
      - nondisplaced S62.65 ☑
    - proximal phalanx (displaced) S62.61 ☑
      - nondisplaced S62.64 ☑
  - little S62.60 ☑
    - distal phalanx (displaced) S62.63 ☑
      - nondisplaced S62.66 ☑
    - medial phalanx (displaced) S62.62 ☑
      - nondisplaced S62.65 ☑
    - proximal phalanx (displaced) S62.61 ☑
      - nondisplaced S62.64 ☑
  - medial phalanx (displaced) S62.62 ☑
    - nondisplaced S62.65 ☑
  - middle S62.60 ☑
    - distal phalanx (displaced) S62.63 ☑
      - nondisplaced S62.66 ☑
    - medial phalanx (displaced) S62.62 ☑
      - nondisplaced S62.65 ☑
    - proximal phalanx (displaced) S62.61 ☑
      - nondisplaced S62.64 ☑
  - proximal phalanx (displaced) S62.61 ☑
    - nondisplaced S62.64 ☑
  - ring S62.60 ☑
    - distal phalanx (displaced) S62.63 ☑
      - nondisplaced S62.66 ☑
    - medial phalanx (displaced) S62.62 ☑
      - nondisplaced S62.65 ☑
    - proximal phalanx (displaced) S62.61 ☑
      - nondisplaced S62.64 ☑
  - thumb — *see* Fracture, thumb

Fracture, traumatic — *continued*
- following insertion (intraoperative) (postoperative) of orthopedic implant, joint prosthesis or bone plate M96.69
  - femur M96.66 ☑
  - fibula M96.67 ☑
  - humerus M96.62 ☑
  - pelvis M96.65
  - radius M96.63 ☑
  - specified bone NEC M96.69
  - tibia M96.67 ☑
  - ulna M96.63 ☑
- foot S92.90 ☑
  - astragalus — *see* Fracture, tarsal, talus
  - calcaneus — *see* Fracture, tarsal, calcaneus
  - cuboid — *see* Fracture, tarsal, cuboid
  - cuneiform — *see* Fracture, tarsal, cuneiform
  - metatarsal — *see* Fracture, metatarsal
  - navicular — *see* Fracture, tarsal, navicular
  - sesamoid S92.81 ☑
  - specified NEC S92.81 ☑
  - talus — *see* Fracture, tarsal, talus
  - tarsal — *see* Fracture, tarsal
  - toe — *see* Fracture, toe
- forearm S52.9 ☑
  - radius — *see* Fracture, radius
  - ulna — *see* Fracture, ulna
- fossa (anterior) (middle) (posterior) S02.19 ☑
- frontal (bone) (skull) S02.0 ☑
  - sinus S02.19 ☑
- glenoid (cavity) (scapula) — *see* Fracture, scapula, glenoid cavity
- greenstick — *see* Fracture, by site
- hallux — *see* Fracture, toe, great
- hand S62.9 ☑
  - carpal — *see* Fracture, carpal bone
  - finger (except thumb) — *see* Fracture, finger
  - metacarpal — *see* Fracture, metacarpal
  - navicular (scaphoid) (hand) — *see* Fracture, carpal bone, navicular
  - thumb — *see* Fracture, thumb
- healed or old
  - with complications - code by Nature of the complication
- heel bone — *see* Fracture, tarsal, calcaneus
- Hill-Sachs S42.29 ☑
- hip — *see* Fracture, femur, neck
- humerus S42.30 ☑
  - anatomical neck — *see* Fracture, humerus, upper end
  - articular process — *see* Fracture, humerus, lower end
  - capitellum — *see* Fracture, humerus, lower end, condyle, lateral
  - distal end — *see* Fracture, humerus, lower end
  - epiphysis
    - lower — *see* Fracture, humerus, lower end, physeal
    - upper — *see* Fracture, humerus, upper end, physeal
  - external condyle — *see* Fracture, humerus, lower end, condyle, lateral
  - following insertion of implant, prosthesis or plate M96.62 ☑
  - great tuberosity — *see* Fracture, humerus, upper end, greater tuberosity
  - intercondylar — *see* Fracture, humerus, lower end
  - internal epicondyle — *see* Fracture, humerus, lower end, epicondyle, medial
  - lesser tuberosity — *see* Fracture, humerus, upper end, lesser tuberosity
  - lower end S42.40 ☑
    - condyle
      - lateral (displaced) S42.45 ☑
        - nondisplaced S42.45 ☑
      - medial (displaced) S42.46 ☑
        - nondisplaced S42.46 ☑
    - epicondyle
      - lateral (displaced) S42.43 ☑
        - nondisplaced S42.43 ☑
      - medial (displaced) S42.44 ☑
        - incarcerated S42.44 ☑
        - nondisplaced S42.44 ☑
    - physeal S49.10 ☑
      - Salter-Harris
        - Type I S49.11 ☑
        - Type II S49.12 ☑
        - Type III S49.13 ☑
        - Type IV S49.14 ☑
      - specified NEC S49.19 ☑

Fracture, traumatic — *continued*
- humerus — *continued*
    - specified NEC (displaced) S42.49 ☑
      - nondisplaced S42.49 ☑
    - supracondylar (simple) (displaced) S42.41 ☑
      - with intercondylar fracture — *see* Fracture, humerus, lower end
      - comminuted (displaced) S42.42 ☑
        - nondisplaced S42.42 ☑
      - nondisplaced S42.41 ☑
    - torus S42.48 ☑
    - transcondylar (displaced) S42.47 ☑
      - nondisplaced S42.47 ☑
  - proximal end — *see* Fracture, humerus, upper end
  - shaft S42.30 ☑
    - comminuted (displaced) S42.35 ☑
      - nondisplaced S42.35 ☑
    - greenstick S42.31 ☑
    - oblique (displaced) S42.33 ☑
      - nondisplaced S42.33 ☑
    - segmental (displaced) S42.36 ☑
      - nondisplaced S42.36 ☑
    - specified NEC S42.39 ☑
    - spiral (displaced) S42.34 ☑
      - nondisplaced S42.34 ☑
    - transverse (displaced) S42.32 ☑
      - nondisplaced S42.32 ☑
  - supracondylar — *see* Fracture, humerus, lower end
  - surgical neck — *see* Fracture, humerus, upper end, surgical neck
  - trochlea — *see* Fracture, humerus, lower end, condyle, medial
  - tuberosity — *see* Fracture, humerus, upper end
  - upper end S42.20 ☑
    - anatomical neck — *see* Fracture, humerus, upper end, specified NEC
    - articular head — *see* Fracture, humerus, upper end, specified NEC
    - epiphysis — *see* Fracture, humerus, upper end, physeal
    - greater tuberosity (displaced) S42.25 ☑
      - nondisplaced S42.25 ☑
    - lesser tuberosity (displaced) S42.26 ☑
      - nondisplaced S42.26 ☑
    - physeal S49.00 ☑
      - Salter-Harris
        - Type I S49.01 ☑
        - Type II S49.02 ☑
        - Type III S49.03 ☑
        - Type IV S49.04 ☑
      - specified NEC S49.09 ☑
    - specified NEC (displaced) S42.29 ☑
      - nondisplaced S42.29 ☑
    - surgical neck (displaced) S42.21 ☑
      - four-part S42.24 ☑
      - nondisplaced S42.21 ☑
      - three-part S42.23 ☑
      - two-part (displaced) S42.22 ☑
        - nondisplaced S42.22 ☑
    - torus S42.27 ☑
    - transepiphyseal — *see* Fracture, humerus, upper end, physeal
- hyoid bone S12.8 ☑
- ilium S32.30 ☑
  - with disruption of pelvic ring — *see* Disruption, pelvic ring
  - avulsion (displaced) S32.31 ☑
    - nondisplaced S32.31 ☑
  - specified NEC S32.39 ☑
- impaction, impacted - code as Fracture, by site
- innominate bone — *see* Fracture, ilium
- instep — *see* Fracture, foot
- ischium S32.60 ☑
  - with disruption of pelvic ring — *see* Disruption, pelvic ring
  - avulsion (displaced) S32.61 ☑
    - nondisplaced S32.61 ☑
  - specified NEC S32.69 ☑
- jaw (bone) (lower) — *see* Fracture, mandible
  - upper — *see* Fracture, maxilla
- joint prosthesis — *see* Complications, joint prosthesis, mechanical, breakdown, by site
  - periprosthetic — *see* Fracture, traumatic, periprosthetic
- knee cap — *see* Fracture, patella
- larynx S12.8 ☑
- late effects — *see* Sequelae, fracture
- leg (lower) S82.9 ☑
  - ankle — *see* Fracture, ankle
  - femur — *see* Fracture, femur

- **Fracture,** traumatic — *continued*
  - leg — *continued*
    - fibula — *see* Fracture, fibula
    - malleolus — *see* Fracture, ankle
    - patella — *see* Fracture, patella
    - specified site NEC S82.89 ☑
    - tibia — *see* Fracture, tibia
  - lumbar spine — *see* Fracture, vertebra, lumbar
  - lumbosacral spine S32.9 ☑
  - Maisonneuve's (displaced) S82.86 ☑
    - nondisplaced S82.86 ☑
  - malar bone (*see also* Fracture, maxilla)S02.400 ☑
    - left side S02.40B ☑
    - right side S02.40A ☑
  - malleolus — *see* Fracture, ankle
  - malunion — *see* Fracture, by site
  - mandible (lower jaw (bone)) S02.609 ☑
    - alveolus S02.67 ☑
    - angle (of jaw) S02.65 ☑
    - body, unspecified S02.600 ☑
      - left side S02.602 ☑
      - right side S02.601 ☑
    - condylar process S02.61 ☑
    - coronoid process S02.63 ☑
    - ramus, unspecified S02.64 ☑
    - specified site NEC S02.69 ☑
    - subcondylar process S02.62 ☑
    - symphysis S02.66 ☑
  - manubrium (sterni) S22.21 ☑
    - dissociation from sternum S22.23 ☑
  - march — *see* Fracture, traumatic, stress, by site
  - maxilla, maxillary (bone) (sinus) (superior) (upper jaw) S02.401 ☑
    - alveolus S02.42 ☑
    - inferior — *see* Fracture, mandible
    - LeFort I S02.411 ☑
    - LeFort II S02.412 ☑
    - LeFort III S02.413 ☑
    - left side S02.40D ☑
    - right side S02.40C ☑
  - metacarpal S62.309 ☑
    - base (displaced) S62.319 ☑
      - nondisplaced S62.349 ☑
    - fifth S62.30 ☑
      - base (displaced) S62.31 ☑
        - nondisplaced S62.34 ☑
      - neck (displaced) S62.33 ☑
        - nondisplaced S62.36 ☑
      - shaft (displaced) S62.32 ☑
        - nondisplaced S62.35 ☑
      - specified NEC S62.398 ☑
    - first S62.20 ☑
      - base NEC (displaced) S62.23 ☑
        - nondisplaced S62.23 ☑
      - Bennett's — *see* Bennett's fracture
      - neck (displaced) S62.25 ☑
        - nondisplaced S62.25 ☑
      - shaft (displaced) S62.24 ☑
        - nondisplaced S62.24 ☑
      - specified NEC S62.29 ☑
    - fourth S62.30 ☑
      - base (displaced) S62.31 ☑
        - nondisplaced S62.34 ☑
      - neck (displaced) S62.33 ☑
        - nondisplaced S62.36 ☑
      - shaft (displaced) S62.32 ☑
        - nondisplaced S62.35 ☑
      - specified NEC S62.39 ☑
    - neck (displaced) S62.33 ☑
      - nondisplaced S62.36 ☑
    - Rolando's — *see* Rolando's fracture
    - second S62.30 ☑
      - base (displaced) S62.31 ☑
        - nondisplaced S62.34 ☑
      - neck (displaced) S62.33 ☑
        - nondisplaced S62.36 ☑
      - shaft (displaced) S62.32 ☑
        - nondisplaced S62.35 ☑
      - specified NEC S62.39 ☑
    - shaft (displaced) S62.32 ☑
      - nondisplaced S62.35 ☑
    - third S62.30 ☑
      - base (displaced) S62.31 ☑
        - nondisplaced S62.34 ☑
      - neck (displaced) S62.33 ☑
        - nondisplaced S62.36 ☑
      - shaft (displaced) S62.32 ☑
        - nondisplaced S62.35 ☑
      - specified NEC S62.39 ☑
    - specified NEC S62.399 ☑
  - metastatic — *see* Fracture, pathological, due to, neoplastic disease (*see also* Neoplasm)

- **Fracture,** traumatic — *continued*
  - metatarsal bone S92.30 ☑
    - fifth (displaced) S92.35 ☑
      - nondisplaced S92.35 ☑
    - first (displaced) S92.31 ☑
      - nondisplaced S92.31 ☑
    - fourth (displaced) S92.34 ☑
      - nondisplaced S92.34 ☑
    - physeal S99.10 ☑
      - Salter-Harris
        - Type I S99.11 ☑
        - Type II S99.12 ☑
        - Type III S99.13 ☑
        - Type IV S99.14 ☑
      - specified NEC S99.19 ☑
    - second (displaced) S92.32 ☑
      - nondisplaced S92.32 ☑
    - third (displaced) S92.33 ☑
      - nondisplaced S92.33 ☑
  - Monteggia's — *see* Monteggia's fracture
  - multiple
    - hand (and wrist) NEC — *see* Fracture, by site
    - ribs — *see* Fracture, rib, multiple
  - nasal (bone (s)) S02.2 ☑
  - navicular (scaphoid) (foot) (*see also* Fracture, tarsal, navicular)
    - hand — *see* Fracture, carpal, navicular
  - neck S12.9 ☑
    - cervical vertebra S12.9 ☑
      - fifth (displaced) S12.400 ☑
        - nondisplaced S12.401 ☑
        - specified type NEC (displaced) S12.490 ☑
          - nondisplaced S12.491 ☑
      - first (displaced) S12.000 ☑
        - burst (stable) S12.01 ☑
          - unstable S12.02 ☑
        - lateral mass (displaced) S12.040 ☑
          - nondisplaced S12.041 ☑
        - nondisplaced S12.001 ☑
        - posterior arch (displaced) S12.030 ☑
          - nondisplaced S12.031 ☑
        - specified type NEC (displaced) S12.090 ☑
          - nondisplaced S12.091 ☑
      - fourth (displaced) S12.300 ☑
        - nondisplaced S12.301 ☑
        - specified type NEC (displaced) S12.390 ☑
          - nondisplaced S12.391 ☑
      - second (displaced) S12.100 ☑
        - nondisplaced S12.101 ☑
        - dens (anterior) (displaced) (type II) S12.110 ☑
          - nondisplaced S12.112 ☑
          - posterior S12.111 ☑
          - specified type NEC (displaced) S12.120 ☑
            - nondisplaced S12.121 ☑
        - specified type NEC (displaced) S12.190 ☑
          - nondisplaced S12.191 ☑
      - seventh (displaced) S12.600 ☑
        - nondisplaced S12.601 ☑
        - specified type NEC (displaced) S12.690 ☑
          - nondisplaced S12.691 ☑
      - sixth (displaced) S12.500 ☑
        - nondisplaced S12.501 ☑
        - specified type NEC (displaced) S12.590 ☑
          - nondisplaced S12.591 ☑
      - third (displaced) S12.200 ☑
        - nondisplaced S12.201 ☑
        - specified type NEC (displaced) S12.290 ☑
          - nondisplaced S12.291 ☑
    - hyoid bone S12.8 ☑
    - larynx S12.8 ☑
    - specified site NEC S12.8 ☑
    - thyroid cartilage S12.8 ☑
    - trachea S12.8 ☑
  - neoplastic NEC — *see* Fracture, pathological, due to, neoplastic disease
  - neural arch — *see* Fracture, vertebra
  - newborn — *see* Birth, injury, fracture
  - nontraumatic — *see* Fracture, pathological
  - nonunion — *see* Nonunion, fracture
  - nose, nasal (bone) (septum) S02.2 ☑
  - occiput — *see* Fracture, skull, base, occiput
  - odontoid process — *see* Fracture, neck, cervical vertebra, second
  - olecranon (process) (ulna) — *see* Fracture, ulna, upper end, olecranon process
  - orbit, orbital (bone) (region) S02.8 ☑
    - floor (blow-out) S02.3 ☑
    - roof S02.19 ☑
  - os
    - calcis — *see* Fracture, tarsal, calcaneus
    - magnum — *see* Fracture, carpal, capitate
    - pubis — *see* Fracture, pubis

- **Fracture,** traumatic — *continued*
  - palate S02.8 ☑
  - parietal bone (skull) S02.0 ☑
  - patella S82.00 ☑
    - comminuted (displaced) S82.04 ☑
      - nondisplaced S82.04 ☑
    - longitudinal (displaced) S82.02 ☑
      - nondisplaced S82.02 ☑
    - osteochondral (displaced) S82.01 ☑
      - nondisplaced S82.01 ☑
    - specified NEC S82.09 ☑
    - transverse (displaced) S82.03 ☑
      - nondisplaced S82.03 ☑
  - pedicle (of vertebral arch) — *see* Fracture, vertebra
  - pelvis, pelvic (bone) S32.9 ☑
    - acetabulum — *see* Fracture, acetabulum
    - circle — *see* Disruption, pelvic ring
    - following insertion of implant, prosthesis or plate M96.65
    - ilium — *see* Fracture, ilium
    - ischium — *see* Fracture, ischium
    - multiple
      - with disruption of pelvic ring (circle) — *see* Disruption, pelvic ring
      - without disruption of pelvic ring (circle) S32.82 ☑
    - pubis — *see* Fracture, pubis
    - specified site NEC S32.89 ☑
    - sacrum — *see* Fracture, sacrum
  - periprosthetic, around internal prosthetic joint M97.9 ☑
    - ankle M97.2 ☑
    - elbow M97.4 ☑
    - finger M97.8 ☑
    - hip M97.0 ☑
    - knee M97.1--
    - shoulder M97.3 ☑
    - specified joint NEC M97.8 ☑
    - spine M97.8 ☑
    - toe M97.8 ☑
    - wrist M97.8 ☑
  - phalanx
    - foot — *see* Fracture, toe
    - hand — *see* Fracture, finger
  - pisiform — *see* Fracture, carpal, pisiform
  - pond — *see* Fracture, skull
  - prosthetic device, internal — *see* Complications, prosthetic device, by site, mechanical
  - pubis S32.50 ☑
    - with disruption of pelvic ring — *see* Disruption, pelvic ring
    - specified site NEC S32.59 ☑
    - superior rim S32.51 ☑
  - radius S52.9 ☑
    - distal end — *see* Fracture, radius, lower end
    - following insertion of implant, prosthesis or plate M96.63 ☑
    - head — *see* Fracture, radius, upper end, head
    - lower end S52.50 ☑
      - Barton's — *see* Barton's fracture
      - Colles' — *see* Colles' fracture
      - extraarticular NEC S52.55 ☑
      - intraarticular NEC S52.57 ☑
      - physeal S59.20 ☑
        - Salter-Harris
          - Type I S59.21 ☑
          - Type II S59.22 ☑
          - Type III S59.23 ☑
          - Type IV S59.24 ☑
        - specified NEC S59.29 ☑
      - Smith's — *see* Smith's fracture
      - specified NEC S52.59 ☑
      - styloid process (displaced) S52.51 ☑
        - nondisplaced S52.51 ☑
      - torus S52.52 ☑
    - neck — *see* Fracture, radius, upper end
    - proximal end — *see* Fracture, radius, upper end
    - shaft S52.30 ☑
      - bent bone S52.38 ☑
      - comminuted (displaced) S52.35 ☑
        - nondisplaced S52.35 ☑
      - Galeazzi's — *see* Galeazzi's fracture
      - greenstick S52.31 ☑
      - oblique (displaced) S52.33 ☑
        - nondisplaced S52.33 ☑
      - segmental (displaced) S52.36 ☑
        - nondisplaced S52.36 ☑
      - specified NEC S52.39 ☑
      - spiral (displaced) S52.34 ☑
        - nondisplaced S52.34 ☑
      - transverse (displaced) S52.32 ☑

- **Fracture,** traumatic — *continued*
  - radius — *continued*
        - nondisplaced S52.32 ☑
    - upper end S52.10 ☑
      - head (displaced) S52.12 ☑
        - nondisplaced S52.12 ☑
      - neck (displaced) S52.13 ☑
        - nondisplaced S52.13 ☑
      - specified NEC S52.18 ☑
      - physeal S59.10 ☑
        - Salter-Harris
          - Type I S59.11 ☑
          - Type II S59.12 ☑
          - Type III S59.13 ☑
          - Type IV S59.14 ☑
        - specified NEC S59.19 ☑
      - torus S52.11 ☑
  - ramus
    - inferior or superior, pubis — *see* Fracture, pubis
    - mandible — *see* Fracture, mandible
  - restorative material (dental) K08.539
    - with loss of material K08.531
    - without loss of material K08.530
  - rib S22.3 ☑
    - with flail chest — *see* Flail, chest
    - multiple S22.4 ☑
      - with flail chest — *see* Flail, chest
  - root, tooth — *see* Fracture, tooth
  - sacrum S32.10 ☑
    - specified NEC S32.19 ☑
    - Type
      - 1 S32.14 ☑
      - 2 S32.15 ☑
      - 3 S32.16 ☑
      - 4 S32.17 ☑
    - Zone
      - I S32.119 ☑
        - displaced (minimally) S32.111 ☑
          - severely S32.112 ☑
        - nondisplaced S32.110 ☑
      - II S32.129 ☑
        - displaced (minimally) S32.121 ☑
          - severely S32.122 ☑
        - nondisplaced S32.120 ☑
      - III S32.139 ☑
        - displaced (minimally) S32.131 ☑
          - severely S32.132 ☑
        - nondisplaced S32.130 ☑
  - scaphoid (hand) (*see also* Fracture, carpal, navicular)
    - foot — *see* Fracture, tarsal, navicular
  - scapula S42.10 ☑
    - acromial process (displaced) S42.12 ☑
      - nondisplaced S42.12 ☑
    - body (displaced) S42.11 ☑
      - nondisplaced S42.11 ☑
    - coracoid process (displaced) S42.13 ☑
      - nondisplaced S42.13 ☑
    - glenoid cavity (displaced) S42.14 ☑
      - nondisplaced S42.14 ☑
    - neck (displaced) S42.15 ☑
      - nondisplaced S42.15 ☑
    - specified NEC S42.19 ☑
  - semilunar bone, wrist — *see* Fracture, carpal, lunate
  - sequelae — *see* Sequelae, fracture
  - sesamoid bone
    - foot S92.81 ☑
    - hand — *see* Fracture, carpal
    - other — *see* Fracture, traumatic, by site
  - shepherd's — *see* Fracture, tarsal, talus
  - shoulder (girdle) S42.9 ☑
    - blade — *see* Fracture, scapula
  - sinus (ethmoid) (frontal) S02.19 ☑
  - skull S02.91 ☑
    - base S02.10 ☑
      - occiput S02.119 ☑
        - condyle S02.113 ☑
          - type I S02.110 ☑
            - left side S02.11B ☑
            - right side S02.11A ☑
          - type II S02.111 ☑
            - left side S02.11D ☑
            - right side S02.11C ☑
          - type III S02.112 ☑
            - left side S02.11F ☑
            - right side S02.11E ☑
          - specified NEC S02.118 ☑
            - left side S02.11H ☑
            - right side S02.11G ☑
      - specified NEC S02.19 ☑
    - birth injury P13.0

- **Fracture,** traumatic — *continued*
  - skull — *continued*
    - frontal bone S02.0 ☑
    - parietal bone S02.0 ☑
    - specified site NEC S02.8 ☑
    - temporal bone S02.19 ☑
    - vault S02.0 ☑
  - Smith's — *see* Smith's fracture
  - sphenoid (bone) (sinus) S02.19 ☑
  - spine — *see* Fracture, vertebra
  - spinous process — *see* Fracture, vertebra
  - spontaneous (cause unknown) — *see* Fracture, pathological
  - stave (of thumb) — *see* Fracture, metacarpal, first
  - sternum S22.20 ☑
    - with flail chest — *see* Flail, chest
    - body S22.22 ☑
    - manubrium S22.21 ☑
    - xiphoid (process) S22.24 ☑
  - stress M84.30 ☑
    - ankle M84.37 ☑
    - carpus M84.34 ☑
    - clavicle M84.31 ☑
    - femoral neck M84.359 ☑
    - femur M84.35 ☑
    - fibula M84.36 ☑
    - finger M84.34 ☑
    - hip M84.359 ☑
    - humerus M84.32 ☑
    - ilium M84.350 ☑
    - ischium M84.350 ☑
    - metacarpus M84.34 ☑
    - metatarsus M84.37 ☑
    - neck — *see* Fracture, fatigue, vertebra
    - pelvis M84.350 ☑
    - radius M84.33 ☑
    - rib M84.38 ☑
    - scapula M84.31 ☑
    - skull M84.38 ☑
    - tarsus M84.37 ☑
    - tibia M84.36 ☑
    - toe M84.37 ☑
    - ulna M84.33 ☑
    - vertebra — *see* Fracture, fatigue, vertebra
  - supracondylar, elbow — *see* Fracture, humerus, lower end, supracondylar
  - symphysis pubis — *see* Fracture, pubis
  - talus (ankle bone) — *see* Fracture, tarsal, talus
  - tarsal bone (s) S92.20 ☑
    - astragalus — *see* Fracture, tarsal, talus
    - calcaneus S92.00 ☑
      - anterior process (displaced) S92.02 ☑
        - nondisplaced S92.02 ☑
      - body (displaced) S92.01 ☑
        - nondisplaced S92.01 ☑
      - extraarticular NEC (displaced) S92.05 ☑
        - nondisplaced S92.05 ☑
      - intraarticular (displaced) S92.06 ☑
        - nondisplaced S92.06 ☑
      - physeal S99.00 ☑
        - Salter-Harris
          - Type I S99.01 ☑
          - Type II S99.02 ☑
          - Type III S99.03 ☑
          - Type IV S99.04 ☑
        - specified NEC S99.09 ☑
      - tuberosity (displaced) S92.04 ☑
        - avulsion (displaced) S92.03 ☑
          - nondisplaced S92.03 ☑
        - nondisplaced S92.04 ☑
    - cuboid (displaced) S92.21 ☑
      - nondisplaced S92.21 ☑
    - cuneiform
      - intermediate (displaced) S92.23 ☑
        - nondisplaced S92.23 ☑
      - lateral (displaced) S92.22 ☑
        - nondisplaced S92.22 ☑
      - medial (displaced) S92.24 ☑
        - nondisplaced S92.24 ☑
    - navicular (displaced) S92.25 ☑
      - nondisplaced S92.25 ☑
    - scaphoid — *see* Fracture, tarsal, navicular
    - talus S92.10 ☑
      - avulsion (displaced) S92.15 ☑
        - nondisplaced S92.15 ☑
      - body (displaced) S92.12 ☑
        - nondisplaced S92.12 ☑
      - dome (displaced) S92.14 ☑
        - nondisplaced S92.14 ☑
      - head (displaced) S92.12 ☑
        - nondisplaced S92.12 ☑
      - lateral process (displaced) S92.14 ☑

- **Fracture,** traumatic — *continued*
  - tarsal bone (s) — *continued*
        - nondisplaced S92.14 ☑
      - neck (displaced) S92.11 ☑
        - nondisplaced S92.11 ☑
      - posterior process (displaced) S92.13 ☑
        - nondisplaced S92.13 ☑
      - specified NEC S92.19 ☑
  - temporal bone (styloid) S02.19 ☑
  - thorax (bony) S22.9 ☑
    - with flail chest — *see* Flail, chest
    - rib S22.3 ☑
      - multiple S22.4 ☑
        - with flail chest — *see* Flail, chest
    - sternum S22.20 ☑
      - body S22.22 ☑
      - manubrium S22.21 ☑
      - xiphoid process S22.24 ☑
    - vertebra (displaced) S22.009 ☑
      - burst (stable) S22.001 ☑
        - unstable S22.002 ☑
      - eighth S22.069 ☑
        - burst (stable) S22.061 ☑
          - unstable S22.062 ☑
        - specified type NEC S22.068 ☑
        - wedge compression S22.060 ☑
      - eleventh S22.089 ☑
        - burst (stable) S22.081 ☑
          - unstable S22.082 ☑
        - specified type NEC S22.088 ☑
        - wedge compression S22.080 ☑
      - fifth S22.059 ☑
        - burst (stable) S22.051 ☑
          - unstable S22.052 ☑
        - specified type NEC S22.058 ☑
        - wedge compression S22.050 ☑
      - first S22.019 ☑
        - burst (stable) S22.011 ☑
          - unstable S22.012 ☑
        - specified type NEC S22.018 ☑
        - wedge compression S22.010 ☑
      - fourth S22.049 ☑
        - burst (stable) S22.041 ☑
          - unstable S22.042 ☑
        - specified type NEC S22.048 ☑
        - wedge compression S22.040 ☑
      - ninth S22.079 ☑
        - burst (stable) S22.071 ☑
          - unstable S22.072 ☑
        - specified type NEC S22.078 ☑
        - wedge compression S22.070 ☑
      - nondisplaced S22.001 ☑
      - second S22.029 ☑
        - burst (stable) S22.021 ☑
          - unstable S22.022 ☑
        - specified type NEC S22.028 ☑
        - wedge compression S22.020 ☑
      - seventh S22.069 ☑
        - burst (stable) S22.061 ☑
          - unstable S22.062 ☑
        - specified type NEC S22.068 ☑
        - wedge compression S22.060 ☑
      - sixth S22.059 ☑
        - burst (stable) S22.051 ☑
          - unstable S22.052 ☑
        - specified type NEC S22.058 ☑
        - wedge compression S22.050 ☑
      - specified type NEC S22.008 ☑
      - tenth S22.079 ☑
        - burst (stable) S22.071 ☑
          - unstable S22.072 ☑
        - specified type NEC S22.078 ☑
        - wedge compression S22.070 ☑
      - third S22.039 ☑
        - burst (stable) S22.031 ☑
          - unstable S22.032 ☑
        - specified type NEC S22.038 ☑
        - wedge compression S22.030 ☑
      - twelfth S22.089 ☑
        - burst (stable) S22.081 ☑
          - unstable S22.082 ☑
        - specified type NEC S22.088 ☑
        - wedge compression S22.080 ☑
      - wedge compression S22.000 ☑
  - thumb S62.50 ☑
    - distal phalanx (displaced) S62.52 ☑
      - nondisplaced S62.52 ☑
    - proximal phalanx (displaced) S62.51 ☑
      - nondisplaced S62.51 ☑
  - thyroid cartilage S12.8 ☑
  - tibia (shaft) S82.20 ☑
    - comminuted (displaced) S82.25 ☑

Fracture, traumatic — *continued*
- tibia — *continued*
      - nondisplaced S82.25 ☑
    - condyles — *see* Fracture, tibia, upper end
    - distal end — *see* Fracture, tibia, lower end
    - epiphysis
        - lower — *see* Fracture, tibia, lower end
        - upper — *see* Fracture, tibia, upper end
    - following insertion of implant, prosthesis or plate M96.67 ☑
    - head (involving knee joint) — *see* Fracture, tibia, upper end
    - intercondyloid eminence — *see* Fracture, tibia, upper end
    - involving ankle or malleolus — *see* Fracture, ankle, medial malleolus
    - lower end S82.30 ☑
        - physeal S89.10 ☑
            - Salter-Harris
                - Type I S89.11 ☑
                - Type II S89.12 ☑
                - Type III S89.13 ☑
                - Type IV S89.14 ☑
            - specified NEC S89.19 ☑
        - pilon (displaced) S82.87 ☑
            - nondisplaced S82.87 ☑
        - specified NEC S82.39 ☑
        - torus S82.31 ☑
    - malleolus — *see* Fracture, ankle, medial malleolus
    - oblique (displaced) S82.23 ☑
        - nondisplaced S82.23 ☑
    - pilon — *see* Fracture, tibia, lower end, pilon
    - proximal end — *see* Fracture, tibia, upper end
    - segmental (displaced) S82.26 ☑
        - nondisplaced S82.26 ☑
    - specified NEC S82.29 ☑
    - spine — *see* Fracture, upper end, spine
    - spiral (displaced) S82.24 ☑
        - nondisplaced S82.24 ☑
    - transverse (displaced) S82.22 ☑
        - nondisplaced S82.22 ☑
    - tuberosity — *see* Fracture, tibia, upper end, tuberosity
    - upper end S82.10 ☑
        - bicondylar (displaced) S82.14 ☑
            - nondisplaced S82.14 ☑
        - lateral condyle (displaced) S82.12 ☑
            - nondisplaced S82.12 ☑
        - medial condyle (displaced) S82.13 ☑
            - nondisplaced S82.13 ☑
        - physeal S89.00 ☑
            - Salter-Harris
                - Type I S89.01 ☑
                - Type II S89.02 ☑
                - Type III S89.03 ☑
                - Type IV S89.04 ☑
            - specified NEC S89.09 ☑
        - plateau — *see* Fracture, tibia, upper end, bicondylar
        - spine (displaced) S82.11 ☑
            - nondisplaced S82.11 ☑
        - torus S82.16 ☑
        - specified NEC S82.19 ☑
        - tuberosity (displaced) S82.15 ☑
            - nondisplaced S82.15 ☑
- toe S92.91 ☑
    - great (displaced) S92.40 ☑
        - distal phalanx (displaced) S92.42 ☑
            - nondisplaced S92.42 ☑
        - nondisplaced S92.40 ☑
        - proximal phalanx (displaced) S92.41 ☑
            - nondisplaced S92.41 ☑
        - specified NEC S92.49 ☑
    - lesser (displaced) S92.50 ☑
        - distal phalanx (displaced) S92.53 ☑
            - nondisplaced S92.53 ☑
        - medial phalanx (displaced) S92.52 ☑
            - nondisplaced S92.52 ☑
        - nondisplaced S92.50 ☑
        - proximal phalanx (displaced) S92.51 ☑
            - nondisplaced S92.51 ☑
        - specified NEC S92.59 ☑
    - physeal
        - phalanx S99.20 ☑
            - Salter-Harris
                - Type I S99.21 ☑
                - Type II S99.22 ☑
                - Type III S99.23 ☑
                - Type IV S99.24 ☑
            - specified NEC S99.29 ☑
- tooth (root) S02.5 ☑

Fracture, traumatic — *continued*
- trachea (cartilage) S12.8 ☑
- transverse process — *see* Fracture, vertebra
- trapezium or trapezoid bone — *see* Fracture, carpal
- trimalleolar — *see* Fracture, ankle, trimalleolar
- triquetrum (cuneiform of carpus) — *see* Fracture, carpal, triquetrum
- trochanter — *see* Fracture, femur, trochanteric
- tuberosity (external) — *see* Fracture, traumatic, by site
- ulna (shaft) S52.20 ☑
    - bent bone S52.28 ☑
    - coronoid process — *see* Fracture, ulna, upper end, coronoid process
    - distal end — *see* Fracture, ulna, lower end
    - following insertion of implant, prosthesis or plate M96.63 ☑
    - head S52.00 ☑
    - lower end S52.60 ☑
        - physeal S59.00 ☑
            - Salter-Harris
                - Type I S59.01 ☑
                - Type II S59.02 ☑
                - Type III S59.03 ☑
                - Type IV S59.04 ☑
            - specified NEC S59.09 ☑
        - specified NEC S52.69 ☑
        - styloid process (displaced) S52.61 ☑
            - nondisplaced S52.61 ☑
        - torus S52.62 ☑
    - proximal end — *see* Fracture, ulna, upper end
    - shaft S52.20 ☑
        - comminuted (displaced) S52.25 ☑
            - nondisplaced S52.25 ☑
        - greenstick S52.21 ☑
        - Monteggia's — *see* Monteggia's fracture
        - oblique (displaced) S52.23 ☑
            - nondisplaced S52.23 ☑
        - segmental (displaced) S52.26 ☑
            - nondisplaced S52.26 ☑
        - specified NEC S52.29 ☑
        - spiral (displaced) S52.24 ☑
            - nondisplaced S52.24 ☑
        - transverse (displaced) S52.22 ☑
            - nondisplaced S52.22 ☑
    - upper end S52.00 ☑
        - coronoid process (displaced) S52.04 ☑
            - nondisplaced S52.04 ☑
        - olecranon process (displaced) S52.02 ☑
            - with intraarticular extension S52.03 ☑
            - nondisplaced S52.02 ☑
                - with intraarticular extension S52.03 ☑
        - specified NEC S52.09 ☑
        - torus S52.01 ☑
- unciform — *see* Fracture, carpal, hamate
- vault of skull S02.0 ☑
- vertebra, vertebral (arch) (body) (column) (neural arch) (pedicle) (spinous process) (transverse process)
    - atlas — *see* Fracture, neck, cervical vertebra, first
    - axis — *see* Fracture, neck, cervical vertebra, second
    - cervical (teardrop) S12.9 ☑
        - axis — *see* Fracture, neck, cervical vertebra, second
        - first (atlas) — *see* Fracture, neck, cervical vertebra, first
        - second (axis) — *see* Fracture, neck, cervical vertebra, second
    - chronic M84.48 ☑
    - coccyx S32.2 ☑
    - dorsal — *see* Fracture, thorax, vertebra
    - lumbar S32.009 ☑
        - burst (stable) S32.001 ☑
            - unstable S32.002 ☑
        - fifth S32.059 ☑
            - burst (stable) S32.051 ☑
                - unstable S32.052 ☑
            - specified type NEC S32.058 ☑
            - wedge compression S32.050 ☑
        - first S32.019 ☑
            - burst (stable) S32.011 ☑
                - unstable S32.012 ☑
            - specified type NEC S32.018 ☑
            - wedge compression S32.010 ☑
        - fourth S32.049 ☑
            - burst (stable) S32.041 ☑
                - unstable S32.042 ☑
            - specified type NEC S32.048 ☑
            - wedge compression S32.040 ☑

Fracture, traumatic — *continued*
- vertebra, vertebral — *continued*
        - second S32.029 ☑
            - burst (stable) S32.021 ☑
                - unstable S32.022 ☑
            - specified type NEC S32.028 ☑
            - wedge compression S32.020 ☑
        - specified type NEC S32.008 ☑
        - third S32.039 ☑
            - burst (stable) S32.031 ☑
                - unstable S32.032 ☑
            - specified type NEC S32.038 ☑
            - wedge compression S32.030 ☑
        - wedge compression S32.000 ☑
    - metastatic — *see* Collapse, vertebra, in, specified disease NEC (*see also* Neoplasm)
    - newborn (birth injury) P11.5
    - sacrum S32.10 ☑
        - specified NEC S32.19 ☑
        - Type
            - 1 S32.14 ☑
            - 2 S32.15 ☑
            - 3 S32.16 ☑
            - 4 S32.17 ☑
        - Zone
            - I S32.119 ☑
                - displaced (minimally) S32.111 ☑
                    - severely S32.112 ☑
                - nondisplaced S32.110 ☑
            - II S32.129 ☑
                - displaced (minimally) S32.121 ☑
                    - severely S32.122 ☑
                - nondisplaced S32.120 ☑
            - III S32.139 ☑
                - displaced (minimally) S32.131 ☑
                    - severely S32.132 ☑
                - nondisplaced S32.130 ☑
    - thoracic — *see* Fracture, thorax, vertebra
- vertex S02.0 ☑
- vomer (bone) S02.2 ☑
- wrist S62.10 ☑
    - carpal — *see* Fracture, carpal bone
    - navicular (scaphoid) (hand) — *see* Fracture, carpal, navicular
- xiphisternum, xiphoid (process) S22.24 ☑
- zygoma S02.402 ☑
    - left side S02.40F ☑
    - right side S02.40E ☑

Fragile, fragility
- autosomal site Q95.5
- bone, congenital (with blue sclera) Q78.0
- capillary (hereditary) D69.8
- hair L67.8
- nails L60.3
- non-sex chromosome site Q95.5
- X chromosome Q99.2

Fragilitas
- crinium L67.8
- ossium (with blue sclerae) (hereditary) Q78.0
- unguium L60.3
    - congenital Q84.6

Fragments, cataract (lens), following cataract surgery H59.02 ☑
- retained foreign body — *see* Retained, foreign body fragments (type of)

Frailty (frail) R54
- mental R41.81

Frambesia, frambesial (tropica) (*see also* Yaws)
- initial lesion or ulcer A66.0
- primary A66.0

Frambeside
- gummatous A66.4
- of early yaws A66.2

Frambesioma A66.1

Franceschetti-Klein (-Wildervanck) disease or syndrome Q75.4

Francis' disease — *see* Tularemia

Franklin disease C88.2

Frank's essential thrombocytopenia D69.3

Fraser's syndrome Q87.0

Freckle(s) L81.2
- malignant melanoma in — *see* Melanoma
- melanotic (Hutchinson's) — *see* Melanoma, in situ
- retinal D49.81

Frederickson's hyperlipoproteinemia, type
- I and V E78.3
- IIA E78.00
- IIB and III E78.2
- IV E78.1

Freeman Sheldon syndrome Q87.0

Freezing (*see also* Effect, adverse, cold)T69.9 ☑

- **Freiberg's** disease (infraction of metatarsal head or osteochondrosis) — *see* Osteochondrosis, juvenile, metatarsus
- **Frei's** disease A55
- **Fremitus,** friction, cardiac R01.2
- **Frenum,** frenulum
  - external os Q51.828
  - tongue (shortening) (congenital) Q38.1
- **Frequency** micturition (nocturnal) R35.0
  - psychogenic F45.8
- **Frey's** syndrome
  - auriculotemporal G50.8
  - hyperhidrosis L74.52
- **Friction**
  - burn — *see* Burn, by site
  - fremitus, cardiac R01.2
  - precordial R01.2
  - sounds, chest R09.89
- **Friderichsen-Waterhouse** syndrome or disease A39.1
- **Friedländer's** B (bacillus) NEC (*see also* condition)A49.8
- **Friedreich's**
  - ataxia G11.1
  - combined systemic disease G11.1
  - facial hemihypertrophy Q67.4
  - sclerosis (cerebellum) (spinal cord) G11.1
- **Frigidity** F52.22
- **Fröhlich's** syndrome E23.6
- **Frontal** (*see also* condition)
  - lobe syndrome F07.0
- **Frostbite** (superficial) T33.90 ☑
  - with
    - partial thickness skin loss — *see* Frostbite (superficial), by site
    - tissue necrosis T34.90 ☑
  - abdominal wall T33.3 ☑
    - with tissue necrosis T34.3 ☑
  - ankle T33.81 ☑
    - with tissue necrosis T34.81 ☑
  - arm T33.4 ☑
    - with tissue necrosis T34.4 ☑
    - finger (s) — *see* Frostbite, finger
    - hand — *see* Frostbite, hand
    - wrist — *see* Frostbite, wrist
  - ear T33.01 ☑
    - with tissue necrosis T34.01 ☑
  - face T33.09 ☑
    - with tissue necrosis T34.09 ☑
  - finger T33.53 ☑
    - with tissue necrosis T34.53 ☑
  - foot T33.82 ☑
    - with tissue necrosis T34.82 ☑
  - hand T33.52 ☑
    - with tissue necrosis T34.52 ☑
  - head T33.09 ☑
    - with tissue necrosis T34.09 ☑
    - ear — *see* Frostbite, ear
    - nose — *see* Frostbite, nose
  - hip (and thigh) T33.6 ☑
    - with tissue necrosis T34.6 ☑
  - knee T33.7 ☑
    - with tissue necrosis T34.7 ☑
  - leg T33.9 ☑
    - with tissue necrosis T34.9 ☑
    - ankle — *see* Frostbite, ankle
    - foot — *see* Frostbite, foot
    - knee — *see* Frostbite, knee
    - lower T33.7 ☑
      - with tissue necrosis T34.7 ☑
    - thigh — *see* Frostbite, hip
    - toe — *see* Frostbite, toe
  - limb
    - lower T33.99 ☑
      - with tissue necrosis T34.99 ☑
    - upper — *see* Frostbite, arm
  - neck T33.1 ☑
    - with tissue necrosis T34.1 ☑
  - nose T33.02 ☑
    - with tissue necrosis T34.02 ☑
  - pelvis T33.3 ☑
    - with tissue necrosis T34.3 ☑
  - specified site NEC T33.99 ☑
    - with tissue necrosis T34.99 ☑
  - thigh — *see* Frostbite, hip
  - thorax T33.2 ☑
    - with tissue necrosis T34.2 ☑
  - toes T33.83 ☑
    - with tissue necrosis T34.83 ☑
  - trunk T33.99 ☑
    - with tissue necrosis T34.99 ☑

Frostbite — *continued*

  - wrist T33.51 ☑
    - with tissue necrosis T34.51 ☑
- **Frotteurism** F65.81
- **Frozen** (*see also* Effect, adverse, cold)T69.9 ☑
  - pelvis (female) N94.89
    - male K66.8
  - shoulder — *see* Capsulitis, adhesive
- **Fructokinase** deficiency E74.11
- **Fructose** 1,6 diphosphatase deficiency E74.19
- **Fructosemia** (benign) (essential) E74.12
- **Fructosuria** (benign) (essential) E74.11
- **Fuchs'**
  - black spot (myopic) H44.2 ☑
  - dystrophy (corneal endothelium) H18.51
  - heterochromic cyclitis — *see* Cyclitis, Fuchs' heterochromic
- **Fucosidosis** E77.1
- **Fugue** R68.89
  - dissociative F44.1
  - hysterical (dissociative) F44.1
  - postictal in epilepsy — *see* Epilepsy
  - reaction to exceptional stress (transient) F43.0
- **Fulminant,** fulminating — *see* condition
- **Functional** (*see also* condition)
  - bleeding (uterus) N93.8
- **Functioning,** intellectual, borderline R41.83
- **Fundus** — *see* condition
- **Fungemia** NOS B49
- **Fungus,** fungous
  - cerebral G93.89
  - disease NOS B49
  - infection — *see* Infection, fungus
- **Funiculitis** (acute) (chronic) (endemic) N49.1
  - gonococcal (acute) (chronic) A54.23
  - tuberculous A18.15
- **Funnel**
  - breast (acquired) M95.4
    - congenital Q67.6
    - sequelae (late effect) of rickets E64.3
  - chest (acquired) M95.4
    - congenital Q67.6
    - sequelae (late effect) of rickets E64.3
  - pelvis (acquired) M95.5
    - with disproportion (fetopelvic) O33.3 ☑
      - causing obstructed labor O65.3
    - congenital Q74.2
- **FUO** (fever of unknown origin) R50.9
- **Furfur** L21.0
  - microsporon B36.0
- **Furrier's** lung J67.8
- **Furrowed** K14.5
  - nail (s) (transverse) L60.4
    - congenital Q84.6
  - tongue K14.5
    - congenital Q38.3
- **Furuncle** L02.92
  - abdominal wall L02.221
  - ankle — *see* Furuncle, lower limb
  - anus K61.0
  - antecubital space — *see* Furuncle, upper limb
  - arm — *see* Furuncle, upper limb
  - auditory canal, external — *see* Abscess, ear, external
  - auricle (ear) — *see* Abscess, ear, external
  - axilla (region) L02.42 ☑
  - back (any part) L02.222
  - breast N61.1
  - buttock L02.32
  - cheek (external) L02.02
  - chest wall L02.223
  - chin L02.02
  - corpus cavernosum N48.21
  - ear, external — *see* Abscess, ear, external
  - external auditory canal — *see* Abscess, ear, external
  - eyelid — *see* Abscess, eyelid
  - face L02.02
  - femoral (region) — *see* Furuncle, lower limb
  - finger — *see* Furuncle, hand
  - flank L02.221
  - foot L02.62 ☑
  - forehead L02.02
  - gluteal (region) L02.32
  - groin L02.224
  - hand L02.52 ☑
  - head L02.821
    - face L02.02
  - hip — *see* Furuncle, lower limb
  - kidney — *see* Abscess, kidney
  - knee — *see* Furuncle, lower limb
  - labium (majus) (minus) N76.4

Furuncle — *continued*

  - lacrimal
    - gland — *see* Dacryoadenitis
    - passages (duct) (sac) — *see* Inflammation, lacrimal, passages, acute
  - leg (any part) — *see* Furuncle, lower limb
  - lower limb L02.42 ☑
  - malignant A22.0
  - mouth K12.2
  - navel L02.226
  - neck L02.12
  - nose J34.0
  - orbit, orbital — *see* Abscess, orbit
  - palmar (space) — *see* Furuncle, hand
  - partes posteriores L02.32
  - pectoral region L02.223
  - penis N48.21
  - perineum L02.225
  - pinna — *see* Abscess, ear, external
  - popliteal — *see* Furuncle, lower limb
  - prepatellar — *see* Furuncle, lower limb
  - scalp L02.821
  - seminal vesicle N49.0
  - shoulder — *see* Furuncle, upper limb
  - specified site NEC L02.828
  - submandibular K12.2
  - temple (region) L02.02
  - thumb — *see* Furuncle, hand
  - toe — *see* Furuncle, foot
  - trunk L02.229
    - abdominal wall L02.221
    - back L02.222
    - chest wall L02.223
    - groin L02.224
    - perineum L02.225
    - umbilicus L02.226
  - umbilicus L02.226
  - upper limb L02.42 ☑
  - vulva N76.4
- **Furunculosis** — *see* Furuncle
- **Fused** — *see* Fusion, fused
- **Fusion,** fused (congenital)
  - astragaloscaphoid Q74.2
  - atria Q21.1
  - auditory canal Q16.1
  - auricles, heart Q21.1
  - binocular with defective stereopsis H53.32
  - bone Q79.8
  - cervical spine M43.22
  - choanal Q30.0
  - commissure, mitral valve Q23.2
  - cusps, heart valve NEC Q24.8
    - mitral Q23.2
    - pulmonary Q22.1
    - tricuspid Q22.4
  - ear ossicles Q16.3
  - fingers Q70.0 ☑
  - hymen Q52.3
  - joint (acquired) (*see also* Ankylosis)
    - congenital Q74.8
  - kidneys (incomplete) Q63.1
  - labium (majus) (minus) Q52.5
  - larynx and trachea Q34.8
  - limb, congenital Q74.8
    - lower Q74.2
    - upper Q74.0
  - lobes, lung Q33.8
  - lumbosacral (acquired) M43.27
    - arthrodesis status Z98.1
    - congenital Q76.49
    - postprocedural status Z98.1
  - nares, nose, nasal, nostril (s) Q30.0
  - organ or site not listed — *see* Anomaly, by site
  - ossicles Q79.9
    - auditory Q16.3
  - pulmonic cusps Q22.1
  - ribs Q76.6
  - sacroiliac (joint) (acquired) M43.28
    - arthrodesis status Z98.1
    - congenital Q74.2
    - postprocedural status Z98.1
  - spine (acquired) NEC M43.20
    - arthrodesis status Z98.1
    - cervical region M43.22
    - cervicothoracic region M43.23
    - congenital Q76.49
    - lumbar M43.26
    - lumbosacral region M43.27
    - occipito-atlanto-axial region M43.21
    - postoperative status Z98.1
    - sacrococcygeal region M43.28
    - thoracic region M43.24
    - thoracolumbar region M43.25

- **Fusion** — *continued*
  - sublingual duct with submaxillary duct at opening in mouth Q38.4
  - testes Q55.1
  - toes Q70.2 ☑
  - tooth, teeth K00.2
  - trachea and esophagus Q39.8
  - twins Q89.4
  - vagina Q52.4
  - ventricles, heart Q21.0
  - vertebra (arch) — *see* Fusion, spine
  - vulva Q52.5
- **Fusospirillosis** (mouth) (tongue) (tonsil) A69.1
- **Fussy** baby R68.12

G

- **Gain** in weight (abnormal) (excessive) (*see also* Weight, gain)
- **Gaisböck's** disease (polycythemia hypertonica) D75.1
- **Gait** abnormality R26.9
  - ataxic R26.0
  - falling R29.6
  - hysterical (ataxic) (staggering) F44.4
  - paralytic R26.1
  - spastic R26.1
  - specified type NEC R26.89
  - staggering R26.0
  - unsteadiness R26.81
  - walking difficulty NEC R26.2
- **Galactocele** (breast) N64.89
  - puerperal, postpartum O92.79
- **Galactokinase** deficiency E74.29
- **Galactophoritis** N61.0
  - gestational, puerperal, postpartum O91.2 ☑
- **Galactorrhea** O92.6
  - not associated with childbirth N64.3
- **Galactosemia** (classic) (congenital) E74.21
- **Galactosuria** E74.29
- **Galacturia** R82.0
  - schistosomiasis (bilharziasis) B65.0
- **Galeazzi's** fracture S52.37 ☑
- **Galen's** vein — *see* condition
- **Galeophobia** F40.218
- **Gall** duct — *see* condition
- **Gallbladder** (*see also* condition)
  - acute K81.0
- **Gallop** rhythm R00.8
- **Gallstone** (colic) (cystic duct) (gallbladder) (impacted) (multiple) (*see also* Calculus, gallbladder)
  - with
    - cholecystitis — *see* Calculus, gallbladder, with cholecystitis
    - bile duct (common) (hepatic) — *see* Calculus, bile duct
    - causing intestinal obstruction K56.3
    - specified NEC K80.80
      - with obstruction K80.81
- **Gambling** Z72.6
  - pathological (compulsive) F63.0
- **Gammopathy** (of undetermined significance [MGUS]) D47.2
  - associated with lymphoplasmacytic dyscrasia D47.2
  - monoclonal D47.2
  - polyclonal D89.0
- **Gamna's** disease (siderotic splenomegaly) D73.1
- **Gamophobia** F40.298
- **Gampsodactylia** (congenital) Q66.7
- **Gamstorp's** disease (adynamia episodica hereditaria) G72.3
- **Gandy-Nanta** disease (siderotic splenomegaly) D73.1
- **Gang**
  - membership offenses Z72.810
- **Gangliocytoma** D36.10
- **Ganglioglioma** — *see* Neoplasm, uncertain behavior, by site
- **Ganglion** (compound) (diffuse) (joint) (tendon (sheath)) M67.40
  - ankle M67.47 ☑
  - foot M67.47 ☑
  - forearm M67.43 ☑
  - hand M67.44 ☑
  - lower leg M67.46 ☑
  - multiple sites M67.49
  - of yaws (early) (late) A66.6
  - pelvic region M67.45 ☑
- **Ganglion** — *continued*
  - periosteal — *see* Periostitis
  - shoulder region M67.41 ☑
  - specified site NEC M67.48
  - thigh region M67.45 ☑
  - tuberculous A18.09
  - upper arm M67.42 ☑
  - wrist M67.43 ☑
- **Ganglioneuroblastoma** — *see* Neoplasm, nerve, malignant
- **Ganglioneuroma** D36.10
  - malignant — *see* Neoplasm, nerve, malignant
- **Ganglioneuromatosis** D36.10
- **Ganglionitis**
  - fifth nerve — *see* Neuralgia, trigeminal
  - gasserian (postherpetic) (postzoster) B02.21
  - geniculate G51.1
    - newborn (birth injury) P11.3
    - postherpetic, postzoster B02.21
  - herpes zoster B02.21
  - postherpetic geniculate B02.21
- **Gangliosidosis** E75.10
  - GM1 E75.19
  - GM2 E75.00
    - other specified E75.09
    - Sandhoff disease E75.01
    - Tay-Sachs disease E75.02
  - GM3 E75.19
  - mucolipidosis IV E75.11
- **Gangosa** A66.5
- **Gangrene**, gangrenous (connective tissue) (dropsical) (dry) (moist) (skin) (ulcer) (*see also* Necrosis)I96
  - with diabetes (mellitus) — *see* Diabetes, gangrene
  - abdomen (wall) I96
  - alveolar M27.3
  - appendix K35.80
    - with
      - perforation or rupture K35.2
      - peritoneal abscess K35.3
      - peritonitis NEC K35.3
        - generalized (with perforation or rupture) K35.2
        - localized (with perforation or rupture) K35.3
  - arteriosclerotic (general) (senile) — *see* Arteriosclerosis, extremities, with, gangrene
  - auricle I96
  - Bacillus welchii A48.0
  - bladder (infectious) — *see* Cystitis, specified type NEC
  - bowel, cecum, or colon — *see* Gangrene, intestine
  - Clostridium perfringens or welchii A48.0
  - cornea H18.89 ☑
  - corpora cavernosa N48.29
    - noninfective N48.89
  - cutaneous, spreading I96
  - decubital — *see* Ulcer, pressure, by site
  - diabetic (any site) — *see* Diabetes, gangrene
  - epidemic — *see* Poisoning, food, noxious, plant
  - epididymis (infectional) N45.1
  - erysipelas — *see* Erysipelas
  - emphysematous — *see* Gangrene, gas
  - extremity (lower) (upper) I96
  - Fournier N49.3
    - female N76.89
  - fusospirochetal A69.0
  - gallbladder — *see* Cholecystitis, acute
  - gas (bacillus) A48.0
    - following
      - abortion — *see* Abortion by type complicated by infection
      - ectopic or molar pregnancy O08.0
  - glossitis K14.0
  - hernia — *see* Hernia, by site, with gangrene
  - intestine, intestinal (hemorrhagic) (massive) (*see also* Infarct, intestine)K55.069
    - with
      - mesenteric embolism (*see also* Infarct, intestine)K55.069
      - obstruction — *see* Obstruction, intestine
  - laryngitis J04.0
  - limb (lower) (upper) I96
  - lung J85.0
    - spirochetal A69.8
  - lymphangitis I89.1
  - Meleney's (synergistic) — *see* Ulcer, skin
  - mesentery (*see also* Infarct, intestine)K55.069
    - with
      - embolism (*see also* Infarct, intestine)K55.069
      - intestinal obstruction — *see* Obstruction, intestine
- **Gangrene** — *continued*
  - mouth A69.0
  - ovary — *see* Oophoritis
  - pancreas — *see* Pancreatitis, acute
  - penis N48.29
    - noninfective N48.89
  - perineum I96
  - pharynx (*see also* Pharyngitis)
    - Vincent's A69.1
  - presenile I73.1
  - progressive synergistic — *see* Ulcer, skin
  - pulmonary J85.0
  - pulpal (dental) K04.1
  - quinsy J36
  - Raynaud's (symmetric gangrene) I73.01
  - retropharyngeal J39.2
  - scrotum N49.3
    - noninfective N50.89
  - senile (atherosclerotic) — *see* Arteriosclerosis, extremities, with, gangrene
  - spermatic cord N49.1
    - noninfective N50.89
  - spine I96
  - spirochetal NEC A69.8
  - spreading cutaneous I96
  - stomatitis A69.0
  - symmetrical I73.01
  - testis (infectional) N45.2
    - noninfective N44.8
  - throat (*see also* Pharyngitis)
    - diphtheritic A36.0
    - Vincent's A69.1
  - thyroid (gland) E07.89
  - tooth (pulp) K04.1
  - tuberculous NEC — *see* Tuberculosis
  - tunica vaginalis N49.1
    - noninfective N50.89
  - umbilicus I96
  - uterus — *see* Endometritis
  - uvulitis K12.2
  - vas deferens N49.1
    - noninfective N50.89
  - vulva N76.89
- **Ganister** disease J62.8
- **Ganser's** syndrome (hysterical) F44.89
- **Gardner-Diamond** syndrome (autoerythrocyte sensitization) D69.2
- **Gargoylism** E76.01
- **Garré's** disease, osteitis (sclerosing), osteomyelitis — *see* Osteomyelitis, specified type NEC
- **Garrod's** pad, knuckle M72.1
- **Gartner's** duct
  - cyst Q52.4
  - persistent Q50.6
- **Gas** R14.3
  - asphyxiation, inhalation, poisoning, suffocation NEC — *see* Table of Drugs and Chemicals
  - excessive R14.0
  - gangrene A48.0
    - following
      - abortion — *see* Abortion by type complicated by infection
      - ectopic or molar pregnancy O08.0
  - on stomach R14.0
  - pains R14.1
- **Gastralgia** (*see also* Pain, abdominal)
- **Gastrectasis** K31.0
  - psychogenic F45.8
- **Gastric** — *see* condition
- **Gastrinoma**
  - malignant
    - pancreas C25.4
    - specified site NEC — *see* Neoplasm, malignant, by site
    - unspecified site C25.4
  - specified site — *see* Neoplasm, uncertain behavior
  - unspecified site D37.9
- **Gastritis** (simple) K29.70
  - with bleeding K29.71
  - acute (erosive) K29.00
    - with bleeding K29.01
  - alcoholic K29.20
    - with bleeding K29.21
  - allergic K29.60
    - with bleeding K29.61
  - atrophic (chronic) K29.40
    - with bleeding K29.41
  - chronic (antral) (fundal) K29.50
    - with bleeding K29.51
    - atrophic K29.40
      - with bleeding K29.41

Gastritis - Glaucoma

- **Gastritis** — *continued*
  - chronic — *continued*
    - superficial K29.30
      - with bleeding K29.31
  - dietary counseling and surveillance Z71.3
  - due to diet deficiency E63.9
  - eosinophilic K52.81
  - giant hypertrophic K29.60
    - with bleeding K29.61
  - granulomatous K29.60
    - with bleeding K29.61
  - hypertrophic (mucosa) K29.60
    - with bleeding K29.61
  - nervous F54
  - spastic K29.60
    - with bleeding K29.61
  - specified NEC K29.60
    - with bleeding K29.61
  - superficial chronic K29.30
    - with bleeding K29.31
  - tuberculous A18.83
  - viral NEC A08.4
- **Gastrocarcinoma** — *see* Neoplasm, malignant, stomach
- **Gastrocolic** — *see* condition
- **Gastrodisciasis,** gastrodiscoidiasis B66.8
- **Gastroduodenitis** K29.90
  - with bleeding K29.91
  - virus, viral A08.4
    - specified type NEC A08.39
- **Gastrodynia** — *see* Pain, abdominal
- **Gastroenteritis** (acute) (chronic) (noninfectious) (*see also* Enteritis)K52.9
  - allergic K52.29
    - with
      - eosinophilic gastritis or gastroenteritis K52.81
      - food protein-induced enterocolitis syndrome K52.21
      - food protein-induced enteropathy K52.22
  - dietetic (*see also* Gastroenteritis, allergic)K52.29
  - drug-induced K52.1
  - due to
    - Cryptosporidium A07.2
    - drugs K52.1
    - food poisoning — *see* Intoxication, food-borne
    - radiation K52.0
  - eosinophilic K52.81
  - epidemic (infectious) A09
  - food hypersensitivity (*see also* Gastroenteritis, allergic)K52.29
  - infectious — *see* Enteritis, infectious
  - influenzal — *see* Influenza, with gastroenteritis
  - noninfectious K52.9
    - specified NEC K52.89
  - rotaviral A08.0
  - Salmonella A02.0
  - toxic K52.1
  - viral NEC A08.4
    - acute infectious A08.39
      - type Norwalk A08.11
    - infantile (acute) A08.39
    - Norwalk agent A08.11
    - rotaviral A08.0
    - severe of infants A08.39
    - specified type NEC A08.39
- **Gastroenteropathy** (*see also* Gastroenteritis)K52.9
  - acute, due to Norwalk agent A08.11
  - acute, due to Norovirus A08.11
  - infectious A09
- **Gastroenteroptosis** K63.4
- **Gastroesophageal** laceration- hemorrhage syndrome K22.6
- **Gastrointestinal** — *see* condition
- **Gastrojejunal** — *see* condition
- **Gastrojejunitis** (*see also* Enteritis)K52.9
- **Gastrojejunocolic** — *see* condition
- **Gastroliths** K31.89
- **Gastromalacia** K31.89
- **Gastroparalysis** K31.84
  - diabetic — *see* Diabetes, gastroparalysis
- **Gastroparesis** K31.84
  - diabetic — *see* Diabetes, by type, with gastroparesis
- **Gastropathy** K31.9
  - congestive portal K31.89
  - erythematous K29.70
  - exudative K90.89
  - portal hypertensive K31.89
- **Gastroptosis** K31.89
- **Gastrorrhagia** K92.2
  - psychogenic F45.8
- **Gastroschisis** (congenital) Q79.3
- **Gastrospasm** (neurogenic) (reflex) K31.89
  - neurotic F45.8
  - psychogenic F45.8
- **Gastrostaxis** — *see* Gastritis, with bleeding
- **Gastrostenosis** K31.89
- **Gastrostomy**
  - attention to Z43.1
  - status Z93.1
- **Gastrosuccorrhea** (continuous) (intermittent) K31.89
  - neurotic F45.8
  - psychogenic F45.8
- **Gatophobia** F40.218
- **Gaucher's** disease or splenomegaly (adult) (infantile) E75.22
- **Gee** (-Herter) (-Thaysen) disease (nontropical sprue) K90.0
- **Gélineau's** syndrome G47.419
  - with cataplexy G47.411
- **Gemination,** tooth, teeth K00.2
- **Gemistocytoma**
  - specified site — *see* Neoplasm, malignant, by site
  - unspecified site C71.9
- **General,** generalized — *see* condition
- **Genetic**
  - carrier (status)
    - cystic fibrosis Z14.1
    - hemophilia A (asymptomatic) Z14.01
      - symptomatic Z14.02
    - specified NEC Z14.8
  - susceptibility to disease NEC Z15.89
    - malignant neoplasm Z15.09
      - breast Z15.01
      - endometrium Z15.04
      - ovary Z15.02
      - prostate Z15.03
      - specified NEC Z15.09
    - multiple endocrine neoplasia Z15.81
- **Genital** — *see* condition
- **Genito-anorectal** syndrome A55
- **Genitourinary** system — *see* condition
- **Genu**
  - congenital Q74.1
  - extrorsum (acquired) (*see also* Deformity, varus, knee)
    - congenital Q74.1
    - sequelae (late effect) of rickets E64.3
  - introrsum (acquired) (*see also* Deformity, valgus, knee)
    - congenital Q74.1
    - sequelae (late effect) of rickets E64.3
  - rachitic (old) E64.3
  - recurvatum (acquired) (*see also* Deformity, limb, specified type NEC, lower leg)
    - congenital Q68.2
    - sequelae (late effect) of rickets E64.3
  - valgum (acquired) (knock-knee) M21.06 ☑
    - congenital Q74.1
    - sequelae (late effect) of rickets E64.3
  - varum (acquired) (bowleg) M21.16 ☑
    - congenital Q74.1
    - sequelae (late effect) of rickets E64.3
- **Geographic** tongue K14.1
- **Geophagia** — *see* Pica
- **Geotrichosis** B48.3
  - stomatitis B48.3
- **Gephyrophobia** F40.242
- **Gerbode** defect Q21.0
- **GERD** (gastroesophageal reflux disease) K21.9
- **Gerhardt's**
  - disease (erythromelalgia) I73.81
  - syndrome (vocal cord paralysis) J38.00
    - bilateral J38.02
    - unilateral J38.01
- **German** measles (*see also* Rubella)
  - exposure to Z20.4
- **Germinoblastoma** (diffuse) C85.9 ☑
  - follicular C82.9 ☑
- **Germinoma** — *see* Neoplasm, malignant, by site
- **Gerontoxon** — *see* Degeneration, cornea, senile
- **Gerstmann-Sträussler-Scheinker** syndrome (GSS) A81.82
- **Gerstmann's** syndrome R48.8
  - developmental F81.2
- **Gestation** (period) (*see also* Pregnancy)
  - ectopic — *see* Pregnancy, by site
  - multiple O30.9 ☑
    - greater than quadruplets — *see* Pregnancy, multiple (gestation), specified NEC
    - specified NEC — *see* Pregnancy, multiple (gestation), specified NEC
- **Gestational**
  - mammary abscess O91.11 ☑
  - purulent mastitis O91.11 ☑
  - subareolar abscess O91.11 ☑
- **Ghon** tubercle, primary infection A15.7
- **Ghost**
  - teeth K00.4
  - vessels (cornea) H16.41 ☑
- **Ghoul** hand A66.3
- **Gianotti-Crosti** disease L44.4
- **Giant**
  - cell
    - epulis K06.8
    - peripheral granuloma K06.8
  - esophagus, congenital Q39.5
  - kidney, congenital Q63.3
  - urticaria T78.3 ☑
    - hereditary D84.1
- **Giardiasis** A07.1
- **Gibert's** disease or pityriasis L42
- **Giddiness** R42
  - hysterical F44.89
  - psychogenic F45.8
- **Gierke's** disease (glycogenosis I) E74.01
- **Gigantism** (cerebral) (hypophyseal) (pituitary) E22.0
  - constitutional E34.4
- **Gilbert's** disease or syndrome E80.4
- **Gilchrist's** disease B40.9
- **Gilford-Hutchinson** disease E34.8
- **Gilles** de la Tourette's disease or syndrome (motor-verbal tic) F95.2
- **Gingivitis** K05.10
  - acute (catarrhal) K05.00
    - necrotizing A69.1
    - nonplaque induced K05.01
    - plaque induced K05.00
  - chronic (desquamative) (hyperplastic) (simple marginal) (pregnancy associated) (ulcerative) K05.10
    - nonplaque induced K05.11
    - plaque induced K05.10
  - expulsiva — *see* Periodontitis
  - necrotizing ulcerative (acute) A69.1
  - pellagrous E52
    - acute necrotizing A69.1
  - Vincent's A69.1
- **Gingivoglossitis** K14.0
- **Gingivopericementitis** — *see* Periodontitis
- **Gingivosis** — *see* Gingivitis, chronic
- **Gingivostomatitis** K05.10
  - herpesviral B00.2
  - necrotizing ulcerative (acute) A69.1
- **Gland,** glandular — *see* condition
- **Glanders** A24.0
- **Glanzmann** (-Naegeli) disease or thrombasthenia D69.1
- **Glasgow** coma scale
  - total score
    - 3-8 R40.243 ☑
    - 9-12 R40.242 ☑
    - 13-15 R40.241 ☑
- **Glass-blower's** disease (cataract) — *see* Cataract, specified NEC
- **Glaucoma** H40.9
  - with
    - increased episcleral venous pressure H40.81 ☑
    - pseudoexfoliation of lens — *see* Glaucoma, open angle, primary, capsular
  - absolute H44.51 ☑
  - angle-closure (primary) H40.20 ☑
    - acute (attack) (crisis) H40.21 ☑
    - chronic H40.22 ☑
    - intermittent H40.23 ☑
    - residual stage H40.24 ☑
  - borderline H40.00 ☑
  - capsular (with pseudoexfoliation of lens) — *see* Glaucoma, open angle, primary, capsular
  - childhood Q15.0
  - closed angle — *see* Glaucoma, angle-closure
  - congenital Q15.0
  - corticosteroid-induced — *see* Glaucoma, secondary, drugs
  - hypersecretion H40.82 ☑
  - in (due to)
    - amyloidosis E85.4 *[H42]*
    - aniridia Q13.1 *[H42]*
    - concussion of globe — *see* Glaucoma, secondary, trauma
    - dislocation of lens — *see* Glaucoma, secondary
    - disorder of lens NEC — *see* Glaucoma, secondary
    - drugs — *see* Glaucoma, secondary, drugs

- **Glaucoma** — *continued*
  - in — *continued*
    - endocrine disease NOS E34.9 *[H42]*
    - eye
      - inflammation — *see* Glaucoma, secondary, inflammation
      - trauma — *see* Glaucoma, secondary, trauma
    - hypermature cataract — *see* Glaucoma, secondary
    - iridocyclitis — *see* Glaucoma, secondary, inflammation
    - lens disorder — *see* Glaucoma, secondary,
    - Lowe's syndrome E72.03 *[H42]*
    - metabolic disease NOS E88.9 *[H42]*
    - ocular disorders NEC — *see* Glaucoma, secondary
    - onchocerciasis B73.02
    - pupillary block — *see* Glaucoma, secondary
    - retinal vein occlusion — *see* Glaucoma, secondary
    - Rieger's anomaly Q13.81 *[H42]*
    - rubeosis of iris — *see* Glaucoma, secondary
    - tumor of globe — *see* Glaucoma, secondary
  - infantile Q15.0
  - low tension — *see* Glaucoma, open angle, primary, low-tension
  - malignant H40.83 ☑
  - narrow angle — *see* Glaucoma, angle-closure
  - newborn Q15.0
  - noncongestive (chronic) — *see* Glaucoma, open angle
  - nonobstructive — *see* Glaucoma, open angle
  - obstructive (*see also* Glaucoma, angle-closure)
    - due to lens changes — *see* Glaucoma, secondary
  - open angle H40.10 ☑
    - primary H40.11 ☑
      - capsular (with pseudoexfoliation of lens) H40.14 ☑
      - low-tension H40.12 ☑
      - pigmentary H40.13 ☑
      - residual stage H40.15 ☑
  - phacolytic — *see* Glaucoma, secondary
  - pigmentary — *see* Glaucoma, open angle, primary, pigmentary
  - postinfectious — *see* Glaucoma, secondary, inflammation
  - secondary (to) H40.5 ☑
    - drugs H40.6 ☑
    - inflammation H40.4 ☑
    - trauma H40.3 ☑
  - simple (chronic) H40.11 ☑
  - simplex H40.11 ☑
  - specified type NEC H40.89
  - suspect H40.00 ☑
  - syphilitic A52.71
  - traumatic (*see also* Glaucoma, secondary, trauma)
    - newborn (birth injury) P15.3
  - tuberculous A18.59
- **Glaucomatous** flecks (subcapsular) — *see* Cataract, complicated
- **Glazed** tongue K14.4
- **Gleet** (gonococcal) A54.01
- **Glénard's** disease K63.4
- **Glioblastoma** (multiforme)
  - with sarcomatous component
    - specified site — *see* Neoplasm, malignant, by site
    - unspecified site C71.9
  - giant cell
    - specified site — *see* Neoplasm, malignant, by site
    - unspecified site C71.9
  - specified site — *see* Neoplasm, malignant, by site
  - unspecified site C71.9
- **Glioma** (malignant)
  - astrocytic
    - specified site — *see* Neoplasm, malignant, by site
    - unspecified site C71.9
  - mixed
    - specified site — *see* Neoplasm, malignant, by site
    - unspecified site C71.9
  - nose Q30.8
  - specified site NEC — *see* Neoplasm, malignant, by site
  - subependymal D43.2
    - specified site — *see* Neoplasm, uncertain behavior, by site
    - unspecified site D43.2
  - unspecified site C71.9
- **Gliomatosis** cerebri C71.0
- **Glioneuroma** — *see* Neoplasm, uncertain behavior, by site
- **Gliosarcoma**
  - specified site — *see* Neoplasm, malignant, by site
  - unspecified site C71.9
- **Gliosis** (cerebral) G93.89
  - spinal G95.89
- **Glisson's** disease — *see* Rickets
- **Globinuria** R82.3
- **Globus** (hystericus) F45.8
- **Glomangioma** D18.00
  - intra-abdominal D18.03
  - intracranial D18.02
  - skin D18.01
  - specified site NEC D18.09
- **Glomangiomyoma** D18.00
  - intra-abdominal D18.03
  - intracranial D18.02
  - skin D18.01
  - specified site NEC D18.09
- **Glomangiosarcoma** — *see* Neoplasm, connective tissue, malignant
- **Glomerular**
  - disease in syphilis A52.75
  - nephritis — *see* Glomerulonephritis
- **Glomerulitis** — *see* Glomerulonephritis
- **Glomerulonephritis** (*see also* Nephritis)N05.9
  - with
    - edema — *see* Nephrosis
    - minimal change N05.0
    - minor glomerular abnormality N05.0
  - acute N00.9
  - chronic N03.9
  - crescentic (diffuse) NEC (*see also* N00-N07 with fourth character .7)N05.7
  - dense deposit (*see also* N00-N07 with fourth character .6)N05.6
  - diffuse
    - crescentic (*see also* N00-N07 with fourth character .7)N05.7
    - endocapillary proliferative (*see also* N00-N07 with fourth character .4)N05.4
    - membranous (*see also* N00-N07 with fourth character .2)N05.2
    - mesangial proliferative (*see also* N00-N07 with fourth character .3)N05.3
    - mesangiocapillary (*see also* N00-N07 with fourth character .5)N05.5
    - sclerosing N05.8
  - endocapillary proliferative (diffuse) NEC (*see also* N00-N07 with fourth character .4)N05.4
  - extracapillary NEC (*see also* N00-N07 with fourth character .7)N05.7
  - focal (and segmental) (*see also* N00-N07 with fourth character .1)N05.1
  - hypocomplementemic — *see* Glomerulonephritis, membranoproliferative
  - IgA — *see* Nephropathy, IgA
  - immune complex (circulating) NEC N05.8
  - in (due to)
    - amyloidosis E85.4 *[N08]*
    - bilharziasis B65.9 *[N08]*
    - cryoglobulinemia D89.1 *[N08]*
    - defibrination syndrome D65 *[N08]*
    - diabetes mellitus — *see* Diabetes, glomerulosclerosis
    - disseminated intravascular coagulation D65 *[N08]*
    - Fabry (-Anderson) disease E75.21 *[N08]*
    - Goodpasture's syndrome M31.0
    - hemolytic-uremic syndrome D59.3
    - Henoch (-Schönlein) purpura D69.0 *[N08]*
    - lecithin cholesterol acyltransferase deficiency E78.6 *[N08]*
    - microscopic polyangiitis M31.7 *[N08]*
    - multiple myeloma C90.0 ☑ *[N08]*
    - Plasmodium malariae B52.0
    - schistosomiasis B65.9 *[N08]*
    - sepsis A41.9 *[N08]*
      - streptococcal A40 ☑ *[N08]*
    - sickle-cell disorders D57. ☑ *[N08]*
    - strongyloidiasis B78.9 *[N08]*
    - subacute bacterial endocarditis I33.0 *[N08]*
    - syphilis (late) congenital A50.59 *[N08]*
    - systemic lupus erythematosus M32.14
    - thrombotic thrombocytopenic purpura M31.1 *[N08]*
    - typhoid fever A01.09
    - Waldenström macroglobulinemia C88.0 *[N08]*
    - Wegener's granulomatosis M31.31
  - latent or quiescent N03.9
- **Glomerulonephritis** — *continued*
  - lobular, lobulonodular — *see* Glomerulonephritis, membranoproliferative
  - membranoproliferative (diffuse) (type 1 or 3) (*see also* N00-N07 with fourth character .5)N05.5
    - dense deposit (type 2) NEC (*see also* N00-N07 with fourth character .6)N05.6
  - membranous (diffuse) NEC (*see also* N00-N07 with fourth character .2)N05.2
  - mesangial
    - IgA/IgG — *see* Nephropathy, IgA
    - proliferative (diffuse) NEC (*see also* N00-N07 with fourth character .3)N05.3
  - mesangiocapillary (diffuse) NEC (*see also* N00-N07 with fourth character .5)N05.5
  - necrotic, necrotizing NEC (*see also* N00-N07 with fourth character .8)N05.8
  - nodular — *see* Glomerulonephritis, membranoproliferative
  - poststreptococcal NEC N05.9
    - acute N00.9
    - chronic N03.9
    - rapidly progressive N01.9
  - proliferative NEC (*see also* N00-N07 with fourth character .8)N05.8
    - diffuse (lupus) M32.14
  - rapidly progressive N01.9
  - sclerosing, diffuse N05.8
  - specified pathology NEC (*see also* N00-N07 with fourth character .8)N05.8
  - subacute N01.9
- **Glomerulopathy** — *see* Glomerulonephritis
- **Glomerulosclerosis** (*see also* Sclerosis, renal)
  - intercapillary (nodular) (with diabetes) — *see* Diabetes, glomerulosclerosis
  - intracapillary — *see* Diabetes, glomerulosclerosis
- **Glossagra** K14.6
- **Glossalgia** K14.6
- **Glossitis** (chronic superficial) (gangrenous) (Moeller's) K14.0
  - areata exfoliativa K14.1
  - atrophic K14.4
  - benign migratory K14.1
  - cortical superficial, sclerotic K14.0
  - Hunter's D51.0
  - interstitial, sclerous K14.0
  - median rhomboid K14.2
  - pellagrous E52
  - superficial, chronic K14.0
- **Glossocele** K14.8
- **Glossodynia** K14.6
  - exfoliativa K14.4
- **Glossoncus** K14.8
- **Glossopathy** K14.9
- **Glossophytia** K14.3
- **Glossoplegia** K14.8
- **Glossoptosis** K14.8
- **Glossopyrosis** K14.6
- **Glossotrichia** K14.3
- **Glossy** skin L90.8
- **Glottis** — *see* condition
- **Glottitis** (*see also* Laryngitis)J04.0
- **Glucagonoma**
  - pancreas
    - benign D13.7
    - malignant C25.4
    - uncertain behavior D37.8
  - specified site NEC
    - benign — *see* Neoplasm, benign, by site
    - malignant — *see* Neoplasm, malignant, by site
    - uncertain behavior — *see* Neoplasm, uncertain behavior, by site
  - unspecified site
    - benign D13.7
    - malignant C25.4
    - uncertain behavior D37.8
- **Glucoglycinuria** E72.51
- **Glucose-galactose** malabsorption E74.39
- **Glue**
  - ear — *see* Otitis, media, nonsuppurative, chronic, mucoid
  - sniffing (airplane) — *see* Abuse, drug, inhalant
    - dependence — *see* Dependence, drug, inhalant
- **Glutaric** aciduria E72.3
- **Glycinemia** E72.51
- **Glycinuria** (renal) (with ketosis) E72.09
- **Glycogen**
  - infiltration — *see* Disease, glycogen storage
  - storage disease — *see* Disease, glycogen storage
- **Glycogenosis** (diffuse) (generalized) (*see also* Disease, glycogen storage)
  - cardiac E74.02 *[I43]*

- **Glycogenosis** — *continued*
  - diabetic, secondary — *see* Diabetes, glycogenosis, secondary
  - pulmonary interstitial J84.842
- **Glycopenia** E16.2
- **Glycosuria** R81
  - renal E74.8
- **Gnathostoma** spinigerum (infection) (infestation), gnathostomiasis (wandering swelling) B83.1
- **Goiter** (plunging) (substernal) E04.9
  - with
    - hyperthyroidism (recurrent) — *see* Hyperthyroidism, with, goiter
    - thyrotoxicosis — *see* Hyperthyroidism, with, goiter
  - adenomatous — *see* Goiter, nodular
  - cancerous C73
  - congenital (nontoxic) E03.0
    - diffuse E03.0
    - parenchymatous E03.0
    - transitory, with normal functioning P72.0
  - cystic E04.2
    - due to iodine-deficiency E01.1
  - due to
    - enzyme defect in synthesis of thyroid hormone E07.1
    - iodine-deficiency (endemic) E01.2
  - dyshormonogenetic (familial) E07.1
  - endemic (iodine-deficiency) E01.2
    - diffuse E01.0
    - multinodular E01.1
  - exophthalmic — *see* Hyperthyroidism, with, goiter
  - iodine-deficiency (endemic) E01.2
    - diffuse E01.0
    - multinodular E01.1
    - nodular E01.1
  - lingual Q89.2
  - lymphadenoid E06.3
  - malignant C73
  - multinodular (cystic) (nontoxic) E04.2
    - toxic or with hyperthyroidism E05.20
      - with thyroid storm E05.21
  - neonatal NEC P72.0
  - nodular (nontoxic) (due to) E04.9
    - with
      - hyperthyroidism E05.20
        - with thyroid storm E05.21
      - thyrotoxicosis E05.20
        - with thyroid storm E05.21
    - endemic E01.1
    - iodine-deficiency E01.1
    - sporadic E04.9
    - toxic E05.20
      - with thyroid storm E05.21
  - nontoxic E04.9
    - diffuse (colloid) E04.0
    - multinodular E04.2
    - simple E04.0
    - specified NEC E04.8
    - uninodular E04.1
  - simple E04.0
  - toxic — *see* Hyperthyroidism, with, goiter
  - uninodular (nontoxic) E04.1
    - toxic or with hyperthyroidism E05.10
      - with thyroid storm E05.11
- **Goiter-deafness** syndrome E07.1
- **Goldberg** syndrome Q89.8
- **Goldberg-Maxwell** syndrome E34.51
- **Goldblatt's** hypertension or kidney I70.1
- **Goldenhar** (-Gorlin) syndrome Q87.0
- **Goldflam-Erb** disease or syndrome G70.00
  - with exacerbation (acute) G70.01
  - in crisis G70.01
- **Goldscheider's** disease Q81.8
- **Goldstein's** disease (familial hemorrhagic telangiectasia) I78.0
- **Golfer's** elbow — *see* Epicondylitis, medial
- **Gonadoblastoma**
  - specified site — *see* Neoplasm, uncertain behavior, by site
  - unspecified site
    - female D39.10
    - male D40.10
- **Gonecystitis** — *see* Vesiculitis
- **Gongylonemiasis** B83.8
- **Goniosynechiae** — *see* Adhesions, iris, goniosynechiae
- **Gonococcemia** A54.86
- **Gonococcus**, gonococcal (disease) (infection) (*see also* condition)A54.9
  - anus A54.6
- **Gonococcus** — *continued*
  - bursa, bursitis A54.49
  - conjunctiva, conjunctivitis (neonatorum) A54.31
  - endocardium A54.83
  - eye A54.30
    - conjunctivitis A54.31
    - iridocyclitis A54.32
    - keratitis A54.33
    - newborn A54.31
    - other specified A54.39
  - fallopian tubes (acute) (chronic) A54.24
  - genitourinary (organ) (system) (tract) (acute)
    - lower A54.00
      - with abscess (accessory gland) (periurethral) A54.1
    - upper (*see also* condition)A54.29
  - heart A54.83
  - iridocyclitis A54.32
  - joint A54.42
  - lymphatic (gland) (node) A54.89
  - meninges, meningitis A54.81
  - musculoskeletal A54.40
    - arthritis A54.42
    - osteomyelitis A54.43
    - other specified A54.49
    - spondylopathy A54.41
  - pelviperitonitis A54.24
  - pelvis (acute) (chronic) A54.24
  - pharynx A54.5
  - proctitis A54.6
  - pyosalpinx (acute) (chronic) A54.24
  - rectum A54.6
  - skin A54.89
  - specified site NEC A54.89
  - tendon sheath A54.49
  - throat A54.5
  - urethra (acute) (chronic) A54.01
    - with abscess (accessory gland) (periurethral) A54.1
  - vulva (acute) (chronic) A54.02
- **Gonocytoma**
  - specified site — *see* Neoplasm, uncertain behavior, by site
  - unspecified site
    - female D39.10
    - male D40.10
- **Gonorrhea** (acute) (chronic) A54.9
  - Bartholin's gland (acute) (chronic) (purulent) A54.02
    - with abscess (accessory gland) (periurethral) A54.1
  - bladder A54.01
  - cervix A54.03
  - conjunctiva, conjunctivitis (neonatorum) A54.31
  - contact Z20.2
  - Cowper's gland (with abscess) A54.1
  - exposure to Z20.2
  - fallopian tube (acute) (chronic) A54.24
  - kidney (acute) (chronic) A54.21
  - lower genitourinary tract A54.00
    - with abscess (accessory gland) (periurethral) A54.1
  - ovary (acute) (chronic) A54.24
  - pelvis (acute) (chronic) A54.24
    - female pelvic inflammatory disease A54.24
  - penis A54.09
  - prostate (acute) (chronic) A54.22
  - seminal vesicle (acute) (chronic) A54.23
  - specified site not listed (*see also* Gonococcus)A54.89
  - spermatic cord (acute) (chronic) A54.23
  - urethra A54.01
    - with abscess (accessory gland) (periurethral) A54.1
  - vagina A54.02
  - vas deferens (acute) (chronic) A54.23
  - vulva A54.02
- **Goodall's** disease A08.19
- **Goodpasture's** syndrome M31.0
- **Gopalan's** syndrome (burning feet) E53.0
- **Gorlin-Chaudry-Moss** syndrome Q87.0
- **Gottron's** papules L94.4
- **Gougerot's** syndrome (trisymptomatic) L81.7
- **Gougerot-Blum** syndrome (pigmented purpuric lichenoid dermatitis) L81.7
- **Gougerot-Carteaud** disease or syndrome (confluent reticulate papillomatosis) L83
- **Gouley's** syndrome (constrictive pericarditis) I31.1
- **Goundou** A66.6
- **Gout**, gouty (acute) (attack) (flare) (*see also* Gout, chronic)M10.9
  - drug-induced M10.20
    - ankle M10.27 ☑
- **Gout** — *continued*
  - drug-induced — *continued*
    - elbow M10.22 ☑
    - foot joint M10.27 ☑
    - hand joint M10.24 ☑
    - hip M10.25 ☑
    - knee M10.26 ☑
    - multiple site M10.29
    - shoulder M10.21 ☑
    - vertebrae M10.28
    - wrist M10.23 ☑
  - idiopathic M10.00
    - ankle M10.07 ☑
    - elbow M10.02 ☑
    - foot joint M10.07 ☑
    - hand joint M10.04 ☑
    - hip M10.05 ☑
    - knee M10.06 ☑
    - multiple site M10.09
    - shoulder M10.01 ☑
    - vertebrae M10.08
    - wrist M10.03 ☑
  - in (due to) renal impairment M10.30
    - ankle M10.37 ☑
    - elbow M10.32 ☑
    - foot joint M10.37 ☑
    - hand joint M10.34 ☑
    - hip M10.35 ☑
    - knee M10.36 ☑
    - multiple site M10.39
    - shoulder M10.31 ☑
    - vertebrae M10.38
    - wrist M10.33 ☑
  - lead-induced M10.10
    - ankle M10.17 ☑
    - elbow M10.12 ☑
    - foot joint M10.17 ☑
    - hand joint M10.14 ☑
    - hip M10.15 ☑
    - knee M10.16 ☑
    - multiple site M10.19
    - shoulder M10.11 ☑
    - vertebrae M10.18
    - wrist M10.13 ☑
  - primary — *see* Gout, idiopathic
  - saturnine — *see* Gout, lead-induced
  - secondary NEC M10.40
    - ankle M10.47 ☑
    - elbow M10.42 ☑
    - foot joint M10.47 ☑
    - hand joint M10.44 ☑
    - hip M10.45 ☑
    - knee M10.46 ☑
    - multiple site M10.49
    - shoulder M10.41 ☑
    - vertebrae M10.48
    - wrist M10.43 ☑
  - syphilitic (*see also* subcategory M14.8-)A52.77
  - tophi — *see* Gout, chronic
- **Gout**, chronic (*see also* Gout, gouty)M1A.9 ☑
  - drug-induced M1A.20 ☑
    - ankle M1A.27 ☑
    - elbow M1A.22 ☑
    - foot joint M1A.27 ☑
    - hand joint M1A.24 ☑
    - hip M1A.25 ☑
    - knee M1A.26 ☑
    - multiple site M1A.29 ☑
    - shoulder M1A.21 ☑
    - vertebrae M1A.28 ☑
    - wrist M1A.23 ☑
  - idiopathic M1A.00 ☑
    - ankle M1A.07 ☑
    - elbow M1A.02 ☑
    - foot joint M1A.07 ☑
    - hand joint M1A.04 ☑
    - hip M1A.05 ☑
    - knee M1A.06 ☑
    - multiple site M1A.09 ☑
    - shoulder M1A.01 ☑
    - vertebrae M1A.08 ☑
    - wrist M1A.03 ☑
  - in (due to) renal impairment M1A.30 ☑
    - ankle M1A.37 ☑
    - elbow M1A.32 ☑
    - foot joint M1A.37 ☑
    - hand joint M1A.34 ☑
    - hip M1A.35 ☑
    - knee M1A.36 ☑
    - multiple site M1A.39 ☑
    - shoulder M1A.31 ☑
    - vertebrae M1A.38 ☑
    - wrist M1A.33 ☑

- **Gout**, chronic — *continued*
  - lead-induced M1A.10 ☑
    - ankle M1A.17 ☑
    - elbow M1A.12 ☑
    - foot joint M1A.17 ☑
    - hand joint M1A.14 ☑
    - hip M1A.15 ☑
    - knee M1A.16 ☑
    - multiple site M1A.19 ☑
    - shoulder M1A.11 ☑
    - vertebrae M1A.18 ☑
    - wrist M1A.13 ☑
  - primary — *see* Gout, chronic, idiopathic
  - saturnine — *see* Gout, chronic, lead-induced
  - secondary NEC M1A.40 ☑
    - ankle M1A.47 ☑
    - elbow M1A.42 ☑
    - foot joint M1A.47 ☑
    - hand joint M1A.44 ☑
    - hip M1A.45 ☑
    - knee M1A.46 ☑
    - multiple site M1A.49 ☑
    - shoulder M1A.41 ☑
    - vertebrae M1A.48 ☑
    - wrist M1A.43 ☑
  - syphilitic (*see also* subcategory M14.8-)A52.77
  - tophi M1A.9 ☑
- **Gower's**
  - muscular dystrophy G71.0
  - syndrome (vasovagal attack) R55
- **Gradenigo's** syndrome — *see* Otitis, media, suppurative, acute
- **Graefe's** disease — *see* Strabismus, paralytic, ophthalmoplegia, progressive
- **Graft-versus-host** disease D89.813
  - acute D89.810
  - acute on chronic D89.812
  - chronic D89.811
- **Grainhandler's** disease or lung J67.8
- **Grain** mite (itch) B88.0
- **Grand** mal — *see* Epilepsy, generalized, specified NEC
- **Grand** multipara status only (not pregnant) Z64.1
  - pregnant — *see* Pregnancy, complicated by, grand multiparity
- **Granite** worker's lung J62.8
- **Granular** (*see also* condition)
  - inflammation, pharynx J31.2
  - kidney (contracting) — *see* Sclerosis, renal
  - liver K74.69
- **Granulation** tissue (abnormal) (excessive) L92.9
  - postmastoidectomy cavity — *see* Complications, postmastoidectomy, granulation
- **Granulocytopenia** (primary) (malignant) — *see* Agranulocytosis
- **Granuloma** L92.9
  - abdomen K66.8
    - from residual foreign body L92.3
    - pyogenicum L98.0
  - actinic L57.5
  - annulare (perforating) L92.0
  - apical K04.5
  - aural — *see* Otitis, externa, specified NEC
  - beryllium (skin) L92.3
  - bone
    - eosinophilic C96.6
    - from residual foreign body — *see* Osteomyelitis, specified type NEC
    - lung C96.6
  - brain (any site) G06.0
    - schistosomiasis B65.9 *[G07]*
  - canaliculus lacrimalis — *see* Granuloma, lacrimal
  - candidal (cutaneous) B37.2
  - cerebral (any site) G06.0
  - coccidioidal (primary) (progressive) B38.7
    - lung B38.1
    - meninges B38.4
  - colon K63.89
  - conjunctiva H11.22 ☑
  - dental K04.5
  - ear, middle — *see* Cholesteatoma
  - eosinophilic C96.6
    - bone C96.6
    - lung C96.6
    - oral mucosa K13.4
    - skin L92.2
  - eyelid H01.8
  - facial (e) L92.2
  - foreign body (in soft tissue) NEC M60.20
    - ankle M60.27 ☑
    - foot M60.27 ☑
    - forearm M60.23 ☑
- **Granuloma** — *continued*
  - foreign body — *continued*
    - hand M60.24 ☑
    - in operation wound — *see* Foreign body, accidentally left during a procedure
    - lower leg M60.26 ☑
    - pelvic region M60.25 ☑
    - shoulder region M60.21 ☑
    - skin L92.3
    - specified site NEC M60.28
    - subcutaneous tissue L92.3
    - thigh M60.25 ☑
    - upper arm M60.22 ☑
  - gangraenescens M31.2
  - genito-inguinale A58
  - giant cell (central) (reparative) (jaw) M27.1
    - gingiva (peripheral) K06.8
  - gland (lymph) I88.8
  - hepatic NEC K75.3
    - in (due to)
      - berylliosis J63.2 *[K77]*
      - sarcoidosis D86.89
  - Hodgkin C81.9 ☑
  - ileum K63.89
  - infectious B99.9
    - specified NEC B99.8
  - inguinale (Donovan) (venereal) A58
  - intestine NEC K63.89
  - intracranial (any site) G06.0
  - intraspinal (any part) G06.1
  - iridocyclitis — *see* Iridocyclitis, chronic
  - jaw (bone) (central) M27.1
    - reparative giant cell M27.1
  - kidney (*see also* Infection, kidney)N15.8
  - lacrimal H04.81 ☑
  - larynx J38.7
  - lethal midline (faciale (e)) M31.2
  - liver NEC — *see* Granuloma, hepatic
  - lung (infectious) (*see also* Fibrosis, lung)
    - coccidioidal B38.1
    - eosinophilic C96.6
  - Majocchi's B35.8
  - malignant (facial (e)) M31.2
  - mandible (central) M27.1
  - midline (lethal) M31.2
  - monilial (cutaneous) B37.2
  - nasal sinus — *see* Sinusitis
  - operation wound T81.89 ☑
    - foreign body — *see* Foreign body, accidentally left during a procedure
    - stitch T81.89 ☑
    - talc — *see* Foreign body, accidentally left during a procedure
  - oral mucosa K13.4
  - orbit, orbital H05.11 ☑
  - paracoccidioidal B41.8
  - penis, venereal A58
  - periapical K04.5
  - peritoneum K66.8
    - due to ova of helminths NOS (*see also* Helminthiasis)B83.9 *[K67]*
  - postmastoidectomy cavity — *see* Complications, postmastoidectomy, recurrent cholesteatoma
  - prostate N42.89
  - pudendi (ulcerating) A58
  - pulp, internal (tooth) K03.3
  - pyogenic, pyogenicum (of) (skin) L98.0
    - gingiva K06.8
    - maxillary alveolar ridge K04.5
    - oral mucosa K13.4
  - rectum K62.89
  - reticulohistiocytic D76.3
  - rubrum nasi L74.8
  - Schistosoma — *see* Schistosomiasis
  - septic (skin) L98.0
  - silica (skin) L92.3
  - sinus (accessory) (infective) (nasal) — *see* Sinusitis
  - skin L92.9
    - from residual foreign body L92.3
    - pyogenicum L98.0
  - spine
    - syphilitic (epidural) A52.19
    - tuberculous A18.01
  - stitch (postoperative) T81.89 ☑
  - suppurative (skin) L98.0
  - swimming pool A31.1
  - talc (*see also* Granuloma, foreign body)
    - in operation wound — *see* Foreign body, accidentally left during a procedure
  - telangiectaticum (skin) L98.0
  - tracheostomy J95.09
- **Granuloma** — *continued*
  - trichophyticum B35.8
  - tropicum A66.4
  - umbilicus L92.9
  - urethra N36.8
  - uveitis — *see* Iridocyclitis, chronic
  - vagina A58
  - venereum A58
  - vocal cord J38.3
- **Granulomatosis** L92.9
  - lymphoid C83.8 ☑
  - miliary (listerial) A32.89
  - necrotizing, respiratory M31.30
  - progressive septic D71
  - specified NEC L92.8
  - Wegener's M31.30
    - with renal involvement M31.31
- **Granulomatous** tissue (abnormal) (excessive) L92.9
- **Granulosis** rubra nasi L74.8
- **Graphite** fibrosis (of lung) J63.3
- **Graphospasm** F48.8
  - organic G25.89
- **Grating** scapula M89.8X1
- **Gravel** (urinary) — *see* Calculus, urinary
- **Graves'** disease — *see* Hyperthyroidism, with, goiter
- **Gravis** — *see* condition
- **Grawitz** tumor C64. ☑
- **Gray** syndrome (newborn) P93.0
- **Grayness**, hair (premature) L67.1
  - congenital Q84.2
- **Green** sickness D50.8
- **Greenfield's** disease
  - meaning
    - concentric sclerosis (encephalitis periaxialis concentrica) G37.5
    - metachromatic leukodystrophy E75.25
- **Greenstick** fracture - code as Fracture, by site
- **Grey** syndrome (newborn) P93.0
- **Grief** F43.21
  - prolonged F43.29
  - reaction (*see also* Disorder, adjustment)F43.20
- **Griesinger's** disease B76.9
- **Grinder's** lung or pneumoconiosis J62.8
- **Grinding**, teeth
  - psychogenic F45.8
  - sleep related G47.63
- **Grip**
  - Dabney's B33.0
  - devil's B33.0
- **Grippe**, grippal (*see also* Influenza)
  - Balkan A78
  - summer, of Italy A93.1
- **Grisel's** disease M43.6
- **Groin** — *see* condition
- **Grooved** tongue K14.5
- **Ground** itch B76.9
- **Grover's** disease or syndrome L11.1
- **Growing** pains, children R29.898
- **Growth** (fungoid) (neoplastic) (new) (*see also* Neoplasm)
  - adenoid (vegetative) J35.8
  - benign — *see* Neoplasm, benign, by site
  - malignant — *see* Neoplasm, malignant, by site
  - rapid, childhood Z00.2
  - secondary — *see* Neoplasm, secondary, by site
- **Gruby's** disease B35.0
- **Gubler-Millard** paralysis or syndrome G46.3
- **Guerin-Stern** syndrome Q74.3
- **Guidance**, insufficient anterior (occlusal) M26.54
- **Guillain-Barré** disease or syndrome G61.0
  - sequelae G65.0
- **Guinea** worms (infection) (infestation) B72
- **Guinon's** disease (motor-verbal tic) F95.2
- **Gull's** disease E03.4
- **Gum** — *see* condition
- **Gumboil** K04.7
  - with sinus K04.6
- **Gumma** (syphilitic) A52.79
  - artery A52.09
    - cerebral A52.04
  - bone A52.77
    - of yaws (late) A66.6
  - brain A52.19
  - cauda equina A52.19
  - central nervous system A52.3
  - ciliary body A52.71
  - congenital A50.59
  - eyelid A52.71
  - heart A52.06
  - intracranial A52.19
  - iris A52.71
  - kidney A52.75

Gumma — *continued*
- larynx A52.73
- leptomeninges A52.19
- liver A52.74
- meninges A52.19
- myocardium A52.06
- nasopharynx A52.73
- neurosyphilitic A52.3
- nose A52.73
- orbit A52.71
- palate (soft) A52.79
- penis A52.76
- pericardium A52.06
- pharynx A52.73
- pituitary A52.79
- scrofulous (tuberculous) A18.4
- skin A52.79
- specified site NEC A52.79
- spinal cord A52.19
- tongue A52.79
- tonsil A52.73
- trachea A52.73
- tuberculous A18.4
- ulcerative due to yaws A66.4
- ureter A52.75
- yaws A66.4
  - bone A66.6

Gunn's syndrome Q07.8
Gunshot wound (*see also* Wound, open)
- fracture - code as Fracture, by site
- internal organs — *see* Injury, by site

Gynandrism Q56.0
Gynandroblastoma
- specified site — *see* Neoplasm, uncertain behavior, by site
- unspecified site
  - female D39.10
  - male D40.10

Gynecological examination (periodic) (routine) Z01.419
- with abnormal findings Z01.411

Gynecomastia N62
Gynephobia F40.291
Gyrate scalp Q82.8

H

H (Hartnup's) disease E72.02
Haas' disease or osteochondrosis (juvenile) (head of humerus) — *see* Osteochondrosis, juvenile, humerus
Habit, habituation
- bad sleep Z72.821
- chorea F95.8
- disturbance, child F98.9
- drug — *see* Dependence, drug
- irregular sleep Z72.821
- laxative F55.2
- spasm — *see* Tic
- tic — *see* Tic

Haemophilus (H.) influenzae, as cause of disease classified elsewhere B96.3
Haff disease — *see* Poisoning, mercury
Hageman's factor defect, deficiency or disease D68.2
Haglund's disease or osteochondrosis (juvenile) (os tibiale externum) — *see* Osteochondrosis, juvenile, tarsus
Hailey-Hailey disease Q82.8
Hair (*see also* condition)
- plucking F63.3
  - in stereotyped movement disorder F98.4
- tourniquet syndrome (*see also* Constriction, external, by site)
  - finger S60.44 ☑
  - penis S30.842 ☑
  - thumb S60.34 ☑
  - toe S90.44 ☑

Hairball in stomach T18.2 ☑
Hair-pulling, pathological (compulsive) F63.3
Hairy black tongue K14.3
Half vertebra Q76.49
Halitosis R19.6
Hallerman-Streiff syndrome Q87.0
Hallervorden-Spatz disease G23.0
Hallopeau's acrodermatitis or disease L40.2
Hallucination R44.3
- auditory R44.0
- gustatory R44.2
- olfactory R44.2
- specified NEC R44.2
- tactile R44.2
- visual R44.1

Hallucinosis (chronic) F28
- alcoholic (acute) F10.951
  - in
    - abuse F10.151
    - dependence F10.251
- drug-induced F19.951
  - cannabis F12.951
  - cocaine F14.951
  - hallucinogen F16.151
  - in
    - abuse F19.151
      - cannabis F12.151
      - cocaine F14.151
      - hallucinogen F16.151
      - inhalant F18.151
      - opioid F11.151
      - sedative, anxiolytic or hypnotic F13.151
      - stimulant NEC F15.151
    - dependence F19.251
      - cannabis F12.251
      - cocaine F14.251
      - hallucinogen F16.251
      - inhalant F18.251
      - opioid F11.251
      - sedative, anxiolytic or hypnotic F13.251
      - stimulant NEC F15.251
  - inhalant F18.951
  - opioid F11.951
  - sedative, anxiolytic or hypnotic F13.951
  - stimulant NEC F15.951
- organic F06.0

Hallux
- deformity (acquired) NEC M20.5X ☑
- limitus M20.5X ☑
- malleus (acquired) NEC M20.3 ☑
- rigidus (acquired) M20.2 ☑
  - congenital Q74.2
  - sequelae (late effect) of rickets E64.3
- valgus (acquired) M20.1 ☑
  - congenital Q66.6
- varus (acquired) M20.3 ☑
  - congenital Q66.3

Halo, visual H53.19
Hamartoma, hamartoblastoma Q85.9
- epithelial (gingival), odontogenic, central or peripheral — *see* Cyst, calcifying odontogenic

Hamartosis Q85.9
Hamman-Rich syndrome J84.114
Hammer toe (acquired) NEC (*see also* Deformity, toe, hammer toe)
- congenital Q66.89
- sequelae (late effect) of rickets E64.3

Hand — *see* condition
Hand-foot syndrome L27.1
Handicap, handicapped
- educational Z55.9
  - specified NEC Z55.8

Hand-Schüller-Christian disease or syndrome C96.5
Hanging (asphyxia) (strangulation) (suffocation) — *see* Asphyxia, traumatic, due to mechanical threat
Hangnail (*see also* Cellulitis, digit)
- with lymphangitis — *see* Lymphangitis, acute, digit

Hangover (alcohol) F10.129
Hanhart's syndrome Q87.0
Hanot-Chauffard (-Troisier) syndrome E83.19
Hanot's cirrhosis or disease K74.3
Hansen's disease — *see* Leprosy
Hantaan virus disease (Korean hemorrhagic fever) A98.5
Hantavirus disease (with renal manifestations) (Dobrava) (Puumala) (Seoul) A98.5
- with pulmonary manifestations (Andes) (Bayou) (Bermejo) (Black Creek Canal) (Choclo) (Juquitiba) (Laguna negra) (Lechiguanas) (New York) (Oran) (Sin nombre) B33.4

Happy puppet syndrome Q93.5
Harada's disease or syndrome H30.81 ☑
Hardening
- artery — *see* Arteriosclerosis
- brain G93.89

Harelip (complete) (incomplete) — *see* Cleft, lip
Harlequin (newborn) Q80.4
Harley's disease D59.6
Harmful use (of)
- alcohol F10.10
- anxiolytics — *see* Abuse, drug, sedative
- cannabinoids — *see* Abuse, drug, cannabis
- cocaine — *see* Abuse, drug, cocaine
- drug — *see* Abuse, drug
- hallucinogens — *see* Abuse, drug, hallucinogen
- hypnotics — *see* Abuse, drug, sedative
- opioids — *see* Abuse, drug, opioid
- PCP (phencyclidine) — *see* Abuse, drug, hallucinogen
- sedatives — *see* Abuse, drug, sedative
- stimulants NEC — *see* Abuse, drug, stimulant

Harris' lines — *see* Arrest, epiphyseal
Hartnup's disease E72.02
Harvester's lung J67.0
Harvesting ovum for in vitro fertilization Z31.83
Hashimoto's disease or thyroiditis E06.3
Hashitoxicosis (transient) E06.3
Hassal-Henle bodies or warts (cornea) H18.49
Haut mal — *see* Epilepsy, generalized, specified NEC
Haverhill fever A25.1
Hay fever (*see also* Fever, hay)J30.1
Hayem-Widal syndrome D59.8
Haygarth's nodes M15.8
Haymaker's lung J67.0
Hb (abnormal)
- Bart's disease D56.0
- disease — *see* Disease, hemoglobin
- trait — *see* Trait

Head — *see* condition
Headache R51
- allergic NEC G44.89
- associated with sexual activity G44.82
- chronic daily R51
- cluster G44.009
  - chronic G44.029
    - intractable G44.021
    - not intractable G44.029
  - episodic G44.019
    - intractable G44.011
    - not intractable G44.019
  - intractable G44.001
  - not intractable G44.009
- cough (primary) G44.83
- daily chronic R51
- drug-induced NEC G44.40
  - intractable G44.41
  - not intractable G44.40
- exertional (primary) G44.84
- histamine G44.009
  - intractable G44.001
  - not intractable G44.009
- hypnic G44.81
- lumbar puncture G97.1
- medication overuse G44.40
  - intractable G44.41
  - not intractable G44.40
- menstrual — *see* Migraine, menstrual
- migraine (type) (*see also* Migraine)G43.909
- nasal septum R51
- neuralgiform, short lasting unilateral, with conjunctival injection and tearing (SUNCT) G44.059
  - intractable G44.051
  - not intractable G44.059
- new daily persistent (NDPH) G44.52
- orgasmic G44.82
- periodic syndromes in adults and children G43.C0
  - with refractory migraine G43.C1
  - intractable G43.C1
  - not intractable G43.C0
  - without refractory migraine G43.C0
- postspinal puncture G97.1
- post-traumatic G44.309
  - acute G44.319
    - intractable G44.311
    - not intractable G44.319
  - chronic G44.329
    - intractable G44.321
    - not intractable G44.329
  - intractable G44.301
  - not intractable G44.309
- pre-menstrual — *see* Migraine, menstrual
- preorgasmic G44.82
- primary
  - cough G44.83
  - exertional G44.84
  - stabbing G44.85
  - thunderclap G44.53
- rebound G44.40
  - intractable G44.41
  - not intractable G44.40

- **Headache** — *continued*
  - short lasting unilateral neuralgiform, with conjunctival injection and tearing (SUNCT) G44.059
    - intractable G44.051
    - not intractable G44.059
  - specified syndrome NEC G44.89
  - spinal and epidural anesthesia - induced T88.59 ☑
    - in labor and delivery O74.5
    - in pregnancy O29.4 ☑
    - postpartum, puerperal O89.4
  - spinal fluid loss (from puncture) G97.1
  - stabbing (primary) G44.85
  - tension (-type) G44.209
    - chronic G44.229
      - intractable G44.221
      - not intractable G44.229
    - episodic G44.219
      - intractable G44.211
      - not intractable G44.219
    - intractable G44.201
    - not intractable G44.209
  - thunderclap (primary) G44.53
  - vascular NEC G44.1
- **Healthy**
  - infant
    - accompanying sick mother Z76.3
    - receiving care Z76.2
  - person accompanying sick person Z76.3
- **Hearing** examination Z01.10
  - with abnormal findings NEC Z01.118
  - following failed hearing screening Z01.110
  - for hearing conservation and treatment Z01.12
- **Heart** — *see* condition
- **Heart** beat
  - abnormality R00.9
    - specified NEC R00.8
  - awareness R00.2
  - rapid R00.0
  - slow R00.1
- **Heartburn** R12
  - psychogenic F45.8
- **Heat** (effects) T67.9 ☑
  - apoplexy T67.0 ☑
  - burn (*see also* Burn)L55.9
  - collapse T67.1 ☑
  - cramps T67.2 ☑
  - dermatitis or eczema L59.0
  - edema T67.7 ☑
  - erythema - code by site under Burn, first degree
  - excessive T67.9 ☑
    - specified effect NEC T67.8 ☑
  - exhaustion T67.5 ☑
    - anhydrotic T67.3 ☑
    - due to
      - salt (and water) depletion T67.4 ☑
      - water depletion T67.3 ☑
        - with salt depletion T67.4 ☑
  - fatigue (transient) T67.6 ☑
  - fever T67.0 ☑
  - hyperpyrexia T67.0 ☑
  - prickly L74.0
  - prostration — *see* Heat, exhaustion
  - pyrexia T67.0 ☑
  - rash L74.0
  - specified effect NEC T67.8 ☑
  - stroke T67.0 ☑
  - sunburn — *see* Sunburn
  - syncope T67.1 ☑
- **Heavy-for-dates** NEC (infant) (4000g to 4499g) P08.1
  - exceptionally (4500g or more) P08.0
- **Hebephrenia,** hebephrenic (schizophrenia) F20.1
- **Heberden's** disease or nodes (with arthropathy) M15.1
- **Hebra's**
  - pityriasis L26
  - prurigo L28.2
- **Heel** — *see* condition
- **Heerfordt's** disease D86.89
- **Hegglin's** anomaly or syndrome D72.0
- **Heilmeyer-Schoner** disease D45
- **Heine-Medin** disease A80.9
- **Heinz** body anemia, congenital D58.2
- **Heliophobia** F40.228
- **Heller's** disease or syndrome F84.3
- **HELLP** syndrome (hemolysis, elevated liver enzymes and low platelet count) O14.2 ☑
  - complicating
    - childbirth O14.24
    - puerperium O14.25
- **Helminthiasis** (*see also* Infestation, helminth)
  - Ancylostoma B76.0
  - intestinal B82.0
    - mixed types (types classifiable to more than one of the titles B65.0-B81.3 and B81.8) B81.4
    - specified type NEC B81.8
  - mixed types (intestinal) (types classifiable to more than one of the titles B65.0-B81.3 and B81.8) B81.4
  - Necator (americanus) B76.1
  - specified type NEC B83.8
- **Heloma** L84
- **Hemangioblastoma** — *see* Neoplasm, connective tissue, uncertain behavior
  - malignant — *see* Neoplasm, connective tissue, malignant
- **Hemangioendothelioma** (*see also* Neoplasm, uncertain behavior, by site)
  - benign D18.00
    - intra-abdominal D18.03
    - intracranial D18.02
    - skin D18.01
    - specified site NEC D18.09
  - bone (diffuse) — *see* Neoplasm, bone, malignant
  - epithelioid (*see also* Neoplasm, uncertain behavior, by site)
    - malignant — *see* Neoplasm, malignant, by site
  - malignant — *see* Neoplasm, connective tissue, malignant
- **Hemangiofibroma** — *see* Neoplasm, benign, by site
- **Hemangiolipoma** — *see* Lipoma
- **Hemangioma** D18.00
  - arteriovenous D18.00
    - intra-abdominal D18.03
    - intracranial D18.02
    - skin D18.01
    - specified site NEC D18.09
  - capillary D18.00
    - intra-abdominal D18.03
    - intracranial D18.02
    - skin D18.01
    - specified site NEC D18.09
  - cavernous D18.00
    - intra-abdominal D18.03
    - intracranial D18.02
    - skin D18.01
    - specified site NEC D18.09
  - epithelioid D18.00
    - intra-abdominal D18.03
    - intracranial D18.02
    - skin D18.01
    - specified site NEC D18.09
  - histiocytoid D18.00
    - intra-abdominal D18.03
    - intracranial D18.02
    - skin D18.01
    - specified site NEC D18.09
  - infantile D18.00
    - intra-abdominal D18.03
    - intracranial D18.02
    - skin D18.01
    - specified site NEC D18.09
  - intra-abdominal D18.03
  - intracranial D18.02
  - intramuscular D18.00
    - intra-abdominal D18.03
    - intracranial D18.02
    - skin D18.01
    - specified site NEC D18.09
  - intrathoracic structures D18.09
  - juvenile D18.00
  - malignant — *see* Neoplasm,connective tissue, malignant
  - plexiform D18.00
    - intra-abdominal D18.03
    - intracranial D18.02
    - skin D18.01
    - specified site NEC D18.09
  - racemose D18.00
    - intra-abdominal D18.03
    - intracranial D18.02
    - skin D18.01
    - specified site NEC D18.09
  - sclerosing — *see* Neoplasm,skin, benign
  - simplex D18.00
    - intra-abdominal D18.03
    - intracranial D18.02
    - skin D18.01
    - specified site NEC D18.09
  - skin D18.01
  - specified site NEC D18.09
- **Hemangioma** — *continued*
  - venous D18.00
    - intra-abdominal D18.03
    - intracranial D18.02
    - skin D18.01
    - specified site NEC D18.09
  - verrucous keratotic D18.00
    - intra-abdominal D18.03
    - intracranial D18.02
    - skin D18.01
    - specified site NEC D18.09
- **Hemangiomatosis** (systemic) I78.8
  - involving single site — *see* Hemangioma
- **Hemangiopericytoma** (*see also* Neoplasm, connective tissue, uncertain behavior)
  - benign — *see* Neoplasm, connective tissue, benign
  - malignant — *see* Neoplasm, connective tissue, malignant
- **Hemangiosarcoma** — *see* Neoplasm, connective tissue, malignant
- **Hemarthrosis** (nontraumatic) M25.00
  - ankle M25.07 ☑
  - elbow M25.02 ☑
  - foot joint M25.07 ☑
  - hand joint M25.04 ☑
  - hip M25.05 ☑
  - in hemophilic arthropathy — *see* Arthropathy, hemophilic
  - knee M25.06 ☑
  - shoulder M25.01 ☑
  - specified joint NEC M25.08
  - traumatic — *see* Sprain, by site
  - vertebrae M25.08
  - wrist M25.03 ☑
- **Hematemesis** K92.0
  - with ulcer - code by site under Ulcer, with hemorrhage K27.4
  - newborn, neonatal P54.0
    - due to swallowed maternal blood P78.2
- **Hematidrosis** L74.8
- **Hematinuria** (*see also* Hemoglobinuria)
  - malarial B50.8
- **Hematobilia** K83.8
- **Hematocele**
  - female NEC N94.89
    - with ectopic pregnancy O00.90
      - with intrauterine pregnancy O00.91
    - ovary N83.8
  - male N50.1
- **Hematochezia** (*see also* Melena)K92.1
- **Hematochyluria** (*see also* Infestation, filarial)
  - schistosomiasis (bilharziasis) B65.0
- **Hematocolpos** (with hematometra or hematosalpinx) N89.7
- **Hematocornea** — *see* Pigmentation, cornea, stromal
- **Hematogenous** — *see* condition
- **Hematoma** (traumatic) (skin surface intact) (*see also* Contusion)
  - with
    - injury of internal organs — *see* Injury, by site
    - open wound — *see* Wound, open
  - amputation stump (surgical) (late) T87.89
  - aorta, dissecting I71.00
    - abdominal I71.02
    - thoracic I71.01
    - thoracoabdominal I71.03
  - aortic intramural — *see* Dissection, aorta
  - arterial (complicating trauma) — *see* Injury, blood vessel, by site
  - auricle — *see* Contusion, ear
    - nontraumatic — *see* Disorder, pinna, hematoma
  - birth injury NEC P15.8
  - brain (traumatic)
    - with
      - cerebral laceration or contusion (diffuse) — *see* Injury, intracranial, diffuse
        - focal — *see* Injury, intracranial, focal
    - cerebellar, traumatic S06.37 ☑
    - newborn NEC P52.4
      - birth injury P10.1
    - intracerebral, traumatic — *see* Injury, intracranial, intracerebral hemorrhage
    - nontraumatic — *see* Hemorrhage, intracranial
    - subarachnoid, arachnoid, traumatic — *see* Injury, intracranial, subarachnoid hemorrhage
    - subdural, traumatic — *see* Injury, intracranial, subdural hemorrhage
  - breast (nontraumatic) N64.89
  - broad ligament (nontraumatic) N83.7
    - traumatic S37.892 ☑

Hematoma - Hemoglobinuria

Hematoma — *continued*
- cerebellar, traumatic S06.37 ☑
- cerebral — *see* Hematoma, brain
- cerebrum S06.36 ☑
  - left S06.35 ☑
  - right S06.34 ☑
- cesarean delivery wound O90.2
- complicating delivery (perineal) (pelvic) (vagina) (vulva) O71.7
- corpus cavernosum (nontraumatic) N48.89
- epididymis (nontraumatic) N50.1
- epidural (traumatic) — *see* Injury, intracranial, epidural hemorrhage
  - spinal — *see* Injury, spinal cord, by region
- episiotomy O90.2
- face, birth injury P15.4
- genital organ NEC (nontraumatic)
  - female (nonobstetric) N94.89
    - traumatic S30.202 ☑
  - male N50.1
    - traumatic S30.201 ☑
- internal organs — *see* Injury, by site
- intracerebral, traumatic — *see* Injury, intracranial, intracerebral hemorrhage
- intraoperative — *see* Complications, intraoperative, hemorrhage
- labia (nontraumatic) (nonobstetric) N90.89
- liver (subcapsular) (nontraumatic) K76.89
  - birth injury P15.0
- mediastinum — *see* Injury, intrathoracic
- mesosalpinx (nontraumatic) N83.7
  - traumatic S37.898 ☑
- muscle - code by site under Contusion
- nontraumatic
  - muscle M79.81
  - soft tissue M79.81
- obstetrical surgical wound O90.2
- orbit, orbital (nontraumatic) (*see also* Hemorrhage, orbit)
  - traumatic — *see* Contusion, orbit
- pelvis (female) (nontraumatic) (nonobstetric) N94.89
  - obstetric O71.7
  - traumatic — *see* Injury, by site
- penis (nontraumatic) N48.89
  - birth injury P15.5
- perianal (nontraumatic) K64.5
- perineal S30.23 ☑
  - complicating delivery O71.7
- perirenal — *see* Injury, kidney
- pinna — *see* Contusion, ear
  - nontraumatic — *see* Disorder, pinna, hematoma
- placenta O43.89 ☑
- postoperative (postprocedural) — *see* Complication, postprocedural, hematoma
- retroperitoneal (nontraumatic) K66.1
  - traumatic S36.892 ☑
- scrotum, superficial S30.22 ☑
  - birth injury P15.5
- seminal vesicle (nontraumatic) N50.1
  - traumatic S37.892 ☑
- spermatic cord (traumatic) S37.892 ☑
  - nontraumatic N50.1
- spinal (cord) (meninges) (*see also* Injury, spinal cord, by region)
  - newborn (birth injury) P11.5
- spleen D73.5
  - intraoperative — *see* Complications, intraoperative, hemorrhage, spleen
  - postprocedural (postoperative) — *see* Complications, postprocedural, hemorrhage, spleen
- sternocleidomastoid, birth injury P15.2
- sternomastoid, birth injury P15.2
- subarachnoid (traumatic) — *see* Injury, intracranial, subarachnoid hemorrhage
  - newborn (nontraumatic) P52.5
    - due to birth injury P10.3
  - nontraumatic — *see* Hemorrhage, intracranial, subarachnoid
- subdural (traumatic) — *see* Injury, intracranial, subdural hemorrhage
  - newborn (localized) P52.8
    - birth injury P10.0
  - nontraumatic — *see* Hemorrhage, intracranial, subdural
- superficial, newborn P54.5
- testis (nontraumatic) N50.1
  - birth injury P15.5
- tunica vaginalis (nontraumatic) N50.1
- umbilical cord, complicating delivery O69.5 ☑

Hematoma — *continued*
- uterine ligament (broad) (nontraumatic) N83.7
  - traumatic S37.892 ☑
- vagina (ruptured) (nontraumatic) N89.8
  - complicating delivery O71.7
- vas deferens (nontraumatic) N50.1
  - traumatic S37.892 ☑
- vitreous — *see* Hemorrhage, vitreous
- vulva (nontraumatic) (nonobstetric) N90.89
  - complicating delivery O71.7
  - newborn (birth injury) P15.5

Hematometra N85.7
- with hematocolpos N89.7

Hematomyelia (central) G95.19
- newborn (birth injury) P11.5
- traumatic T14.8

Hematomyelitis G04.90

Hematoperitoneum — *see* Hemoperitoneum

Hematophobia F40.230

Hematopneumothorax (see Hemothorax)

Hematopoiesis, cyclic D70.4

Hematoporphyria — *see* Porphyria

Hematorachis, hematorrhachis G95.19
- newborn (birth injury) P11.5

Hematosalpinx N83.6
- with
  - hematocolpos N89.7
  - hematometra N85.7
    - with hematocolpos N89.7
- infectional — *see* Salpingitis

Hematospermia R36.1

Hematothorax (see Hemothorax)

Hematuria R31.9
- due to sulphonamide, sulfonamide — *see* Table of Drugs and Chemicals, by drug
- benign (familial) (of childhood) (*see also* Hematuria, idiopathic)
  - essential microscopic R31.1
- endemic (*see also* Schistosomiasis)B65.0
- gross R31.0
- idiopathic N02.9
  - with glomerular lesion
    - crescentic (diffuse) glomerulonephritis N02.7
    - dense deposit disease N02.6
    - endocapillary proliferative glomerulonephritis N02.4
    - focal and segmental hyalinosis or sclerosis N02.1
    - membranoproliferative (diffuse) N02.5
    - membranous (diffuse) N02.2
    - mesangial proliferative (diffuse) N02.3
    - mesangiocapillary (diffuse) N02.5
    - minor abnormality N02.0
    - proliferative NEC N02.8
    - specified pathology NEC N02.8
- intermittent — *see* Hematuria, idiopathic
- malarial B50.8
- microscopic NEC (with symptoms) R31.29
  - asymptomatic R31.21
  - benign essential R31.1
- paroxysmal (*see also* Hematuria, idiopathic)
  - nocturnal D59.5
- persistent — *see* Hematuria, idiopathic
- recurrent — *see* Hematuria, idiopathic
- tropical (*see also* Schistosomiasis)B65.0
- tuberculous A18.13

Hemeralopia (day blindness) H53.11
- vitamin A deficiency E50.5

Hemi-akinesia R41.4

Hemianalgesia R20.0

Hemianencephaly Q00.0

Hemianesthesia R20.0

Hemianopia, hemianopsia (heteronymous) H53.47
- homonymous H53.46 ☑
- syphilitic A52.71

Hemiathetosis R25.8

Hemiatrophy R68.89
- cerebellar G31.9
- face, facial, progressive (Romberg) G51.8
- tongue K14.8

Hemiballism (us) G25.5

Hemicardia Q24.8

Hemicephalus, hemicephaly Q00.0

Hemichorea G25.5

Hemicolitis, left — *see* Colitis, left sided

Hemicrania
- congenital malformation Q00.0
- continua G44.51
- meaning migraine (*see also* Migraine)G43.909
- paroxysmal G44.039
  - chronic G44.049
    - intractable G44.041

Hemicrania — *continued*
- paroxysmal — *continued*
    - not intractable G44.049
  - episodic G44.039
    - intractable G44.031
    - not intractable G44.039
  - intractable G44.031
  - not intractable G44.039

Hemidystrophy — *see* Hemiatrophy

Hemiectromelia Q73.8

Hemihypalgesia R20.8

Hemihypesthesia R20.1

Hemi-inattention R41.4

Hemimelia Q73.8
- lower limb — *see* Defect, reduction, lower limb, specified type NEC
- upper limb — *see* Defect, reduction, upper limb, specified type NEC

Hemiparalysis — *see* Hemiplegia

Hemiparesis — *see* Hemiplegia

Hemiparesthesia R20.2

Hemiparkinsonism G20

Hemiplegia G81.9 ☑
- alternans facialis G83.89
- ascending NEC G81.90
  - spinal G95.89
- congenital (cerebral) G80.8
  - spastic G80.2
- embolic (current episode) I63.4 ☑
- flaccid G81.0 ☑
- following
  - cerebrovascular disease I69.959
    - cerebral infarction I69.35 ☑
    - intracerebral hemorrhage I69.15 ☑
    - nontraumatic intracranial hemorrhage NEC I69.25 ☑
    - specified disease NEC I69.85 ☑
    - stroke NOS I69.35 ☑
    - subarachnoid hemorrhage I69.05 ☑
- hysterical F44.4
- newborn NEC P91.8
  - birth injury P11.9
- spastic G81.1 ☑
  - congenital G80.2
- thrombotic (current episode) I63.3 ☑

Hemisection, spinal cord — *see* Injury, spinal cord, by region

Hemispasm (facial) R25.2

Hemisporosis B48.8

Hemitremor R25.1

Hemivertebra Q76.49
- failure of segmentation with scoliosis Q76.3
- fusion with scoliosis Q76.3

Hemochromatosis E83.119
- with refractory anemia D46.1
- due to repeated red blood cell transfusion E83.111
- hereditary (primary) E83.110
- primary E83.110
- specified NEC E83.118

Hemoglobin (*see also* condition)
- abnormal (disease) — *see* Disease, hemoglobin
- AS genotype D57.3
- Constant Spring D58.2
- E-beta thalassemia D56.5
- fetal, hereditary persistence (HPFH) D56.4
- H Constant Spring D56.0
- low NOS D64.9
- S (Hb S), heterozygous D57.3

Hemoglobinemia D59.9
- due to blood transfusion T80.89 ☑
- paroxysmal D59.6
  - nocturnal D59.5

Hemoglobinopathy (mixed) D58.2
- with thalassemia D56.8
- sickle-cell D57.1
  - with thalassemia D57.40
    - with crisis (vasoocclusive pain) D57.419
      - with
        - acute chest syndrome D57.411
        - splenic sequestration D57.412
    - without crisis D57.40

Hemoglobinuria R82.3
- with anemia, hemolytic, acquired (chronic) NEC D59.6
- cold (agglutinin) (paroxysmal) (with Raynaud's syndrome) D59.6
- due to exertion or hemolysis NEC D59.6
- intermittent D59.6
- malarial B50.8
- march D59.6
- nocturnal (paroxysmal) D59.5

- **Hemoglobinuria** — *continued*
  - paroxysmal (cold) D59.6
    - nocturnal D59.5
- **Hemolymphangioma** D18.1
- **Hemolysis**
  - intravascular
    - with
      - abortion — *see* Abortion, by type, complicated by, hemorrhage
      - ectopic or molar pregnancy O08.1
      - hemorrhage
        - antepartum — *see* Hemorrhage, antepartum, with coagulation defect
        - intrapartum (*see also* Hemorrhage, complicating, delivery)O67.0
    - postpartum O72.3
  - neonatal (excessive) P58.9
    - specified NEC P58.8
- **Hemolytic** — *see* condition
- **Hemopericardium** I31.2
  - following acute myocardial infarction (current complication) I23.0
  - newborn P54.8
  - traumatic — *see* Injury, heart, with hemopericardium
- **Hemoperitoneum** K66.1
  - infectional K65.9
  - traumatic S36.899 ☑
    - with open wound — *see* Wound, open, with penetration into peritoneal cavity
- **Hemophilia** (classical) (familial) (hereditary) D66
  - A D66
  - B D67
  - C D68.1
  - acquired D68.311
  - autoimmune D68.311
  - calcipriva (*see also* Defect, coagulation)D68.4
  - nonfamilial (*see also* Defect, coagulation)D68.4
  - secondary D68.311
  - vascular D68.0
- **Hemophthalmos** H44.81 ☑
- **Hemopneumothorax** (*see also* Hemothorax)
  - traumatic S27.2 ☑
- **Hemoptysis** R04.2
  - newborn P26.9
  - tuberculous — *see* Tuberculosis, pulmonary
- **Hemorrhage,** hemorrhagic (concealed) R58
  - abdomen R58
  - accidental antepartum — *see* Hemorrhage, antepartum
  - acute idiopathic pulmonary, in infants R04.81
  - adenoid J35.8
  - adrenal (capsule) (gland) E27.49
    - medulla E27.8
    - newborn P54.4
  - after delivery — *see* Hemorrhage, postpartum
  - alveolar
    - lung, newborn P26.8
    - process K08.89
  - alveolus K08.89
  - amputation stump (surgical) T87.89
  - anemia (chronic) D50.0
    - acute D62
  - antepartum (with) O46.90
    - with coagulation defect O46.00 ☑
      - afibrinogenemia O46.01 ☑
      - disseminated intravascular coagulation O46.02 ☑
      - hypofibrinogenemia O46.01 ☑
      - specified defect NEC O46.09 ☑
    - before 20 weeks gestation O20.9
      - specified type NEC O20.8
      - threatened abortion O20.0
    - due to
      - abruptio placenta (*see also* Abruptio placentae)O45.9 ☑
      - leiomyoma, uterus — *see* Hemorrhage, antepartum, specified cause NEC
      - placenta previa O44.1 ☑
    - specified cause NEC — *see* subcategory O46.8X-
  - anus (sphincter) K62.5
  - apoplexy (stroke) — *see* Hemorrhage, intracranial, intracerebral
  - arachnoid — *see* Hemorrhage, intracranial, subarachnoid
  - artery R58
    - brain — *see* Hemorrhage, intracranial, intracerebral
  - basilar (ganglion) I61.0
  - bladder N32.89
  - bowel K92.2
    - newborn P54.3

- **Hemorrhage** — *continued*
  - brain (miliary) (nontraumatic) — *see* Hemorrhage, intracranial, intracerebral
    - due to
      - birth injury P10.1
      - syphilis A52.05
    - epidural or extradural (traumatic) — *see* Injury, intracranial, epidural hemorrhage
    - newborn P52.4
      - birth injury P10.1
    - subarachnoid — *see* Hemorrhage, intracranial, subarachnoid
    - subdural — *see* Hemorrhage, intracranial, subdural
  - brainstem (nontraumatic) I61.3
    - traumatic S06.38 ☑
  - breast N64.59
  - bronchial tube — *see* Hemorrhage, lung
  - bronchopulmonary — *see* Hemorrhage, lung
  - bronchus — *see* Hemorrhage, lung
  - bulbar I61.5
  - capillary I78.8
    - primary D69.8
  - cecum K92.2
  - cerebellar, cerebellum (nontraumatic) I61.4
    - newborn P52.6
    - traumatic S06.37 ☑
  - cerebral, cerebrum (*see also* Hemorrhage, intracranial, intracerebral)
    - newborn (anoxic) P52.4
      - birth injury P10.1
    - lobe I61.1
  - cerebromeningeal I61.8
  - cerebrospinal — *see* Hemorrhage, intracranial, intracerebral
  - cervix (uteri) (stump) NEC N88.8
  - chamber, anterior (eye) — *see* Hyphema
  - childbirth — *see* Hemorrhage, complicating, delivery
  - choroid H31.30 ☑
    - expulsive H31.31 ☑
  - ciliary body — *see* Hyphema
  - cochlea — *see* subcategory H83.8
  - colon K92.2
  - complicating
    - abortion — *see* Abortion, by type, complicated by, hemorrhage
    - delivery O67.9
      - associated with coagulation defect (afibrinogenemia) (DIC) (hyperfibrinolysis) O67.0
      - specified cause NEC O67.8
    - surgical procedure — *see* Hemorrhage, intraoperative
  - conjunctiva H11.3 ☑
    - newborn P54.8
  - cord, newborn (stump) P51.9
  - corpus luteum (ruptured) cyst N83.1 ☑
  - cortical (brain) I61.1
  - cranial — *see* Hemorrhage, intracranial
  - cutaneous R23.3
    - due to autosensitivity, erythrocyte D69.2
    - newborn P54.5
  - delayed
    - following ectopic or molar pregnancy O08.1
    - postpartum O72.2
  - diathesis (familial) D69.9
  - disease D69.9
    - newborn P53
    - specified type NEC D69.8
  - due to or associated with
    - afibrinogenemia or other coagulation defect (conditions in categories D65-D69)
      - antepartum — *see* Hemorrhage, antepartum, with coagulation defect
      - intrapartum O67.0
    - dental implant M27.61
    - device, implant or graft (*see also* Complications, by site and type, specified NEC)T85.838 ☑
      - arterial graft NEC T82.838 ☑
      - breast T85.838 ☑
      - catheter NEC T85.838 ☑
        - dialysis (renal) T82.838 ☑
          - intraperitoneal T85.838 ☑
        - infusion NEC T82.838 ☑
          - spinal (epidural) (subdural) T85.830 ☑
        - urinary (indwelling) T83.83 ☑
      - electronic (electrode) (pulse generator) (stimulator)
        - bone T84.83 ☑
        - cardiac T82.837 ☑

- **Hemorrhage** — *continued*
  - due to — *continued*
        - nervous system (brain) (peripheral nerve) (spinal) T85.830 ☑
        - urinary T83.83 ☑
      - fixation, internal (orthopedic) NEC T84.83 ☑
      - gastrointestinal (bile duct) (esophagus) T85.838 ☑
      - genital NEC T83.83 ☑
      - heart NEC T82.837 ☑
      - joint prosthesis T84.83 ☑
      - ocular (corneal graft) (orbital implant) NEC T85.838 ☑
      - orthopedic NEC T84.83 ☑
        - bone graft T86.838
      - specified NEC T85.838 ☑
      - urinary NEC T83.83 ☑
      - vascular NEC T82.838 ☑
      - ventricular intracranial shunt T85.830 ☑
  - duodenum, duodenal K92.2
    - ulcer — *see* Ulcer, duodenum, with hemorrhage
  - dura mater — *see* Hemorrhage, intracranial, subdural
  - endotracheal — *see* Hemorrhage, lung
  - epicranial subaponeurotic (massive), birth injury P12.2
  - epidural (traumatic) (*see also* Injury, intracranial, epidural hemorrhage)
    - nontraumatic I62.1
  - esophagus K22.8
    - varix I85.01
      - secondary I85.11
  - excessive, following ectopic gestation (subsequent episode) O08.1
  - extradural (traumatic) — *see* Injury, intracranial, epidural hemorrhage
    - birth injury P10.8
    - newborn (anoxic) (nontraumatic) P52.8
    - nontraumatic I62.1
  - eye NEC H57.8
    - fundus — *see* Hemorrhage, retina
    - lid — *see* Disorder, eyelid, specified type NEC
  - fallopian tube N83.6
  - fibrinogenolysis — *see* Fibrinolysis
  - fibrinolytic (acquired) — *see* Fibrinolysis
  - from
    - ear (nontraumatic) — *see* Otorrhagia
    - tracheostomy stoma J95.01
  - fundus, eye — *see* Hemorrhage, retina
  - funis — *see* Hemorrhage, umbilicus, cord
  - gastric — *see* Hemorrhage, stomach
  - gastroenteric K92.2
    - newborn P54.3
  - gastrointestinal (tract) K92.2
    - newborn P54.3
  - genital organ, male N50.1
  - genitourinary (tract) NOS R31.9
  - gingiva K06.8
  - globe (eye) — *see* Hemophthalmos
  - graafian follicle cyst (ruptured) N83.0 ☑
  - gum K06.8
  - heart I51.89
  - hypopharyngeal (throat) R04.1
  - intermenstrual (regular) N92.3
    - irregular N92.1
  - internal (organs) NEC R58
    - capsule I61.0
    - ear — *see* subcategory H83.8
    - newborn P54.8
  - intestine K92.2
    - newborn P54.3
  - intra-abdominal R58
  - intra-alveolar (lung), newborn P26.8
  - intracerebral (nontraumatic) — *see* Hemorrhage, intracranial, intracerebral
  - intracranial (nontraumatic) I62.9
    - birth injury P10.9
    - epidural, nontraumatic I62.1
    - extradural, nontraumatic I62.1
    - newborn P52.9
      - specified NEC P52.8
    - intracerebral (nontraumatic) (in) I61.9
      - brain stem I61.3
      - cerebellum I61.4
      - newborn P52.4
        - birth injury P10.1
      - hemisphere I61.2
        - cortical (superficial) I61.1
        - subcortical (deep) I61.0
      - intraoperative
        - during a nervous system procedure G97.31

- **Hemorrhage** — *continued*
  - intracranial — *continued*
        - during other procedure G97.32
      - intraventricular I61.5
      - multiple localized I61.6
      - postprocedural
        - following a nervous system procedure G97.51
        - following other procedure G97.52
      - specified NEC I61.8
      - superficial I61.1
      - traumatic (diffuse) — *see* Injury, intracranial, diffuse
        - focal — *see* Injury, intracranial, focal
    - subarachnoid (nontraumatic) (from) I60.9
      - newborn P52.5
        - birth injury P10.3
      - intracranial (cerebral) artery I60.7
        - anterior communicating I60.2 ☑
        - basilar I60.4
        - carotid siphon and bifurcation I60.0 ☑
        - communicating I60.7
          - anterior I60.2 ☑
          - posterior I60.3 ☑
        - middle cerebral I60.1 ☑
        - posterior communicating I60.3 ☑
        - specified artery NEC I60.6
        - vertebral I60.5 ☑
      - specified NEC I60.8
      - traumatic S06.6X ☑
    - subdural (nontraumatic) I62.00
      - acute I62.01
      - birth injury P10.0
      - chronic I62.03
      - newborn (anoxic) (hypoxic) P52.8
        - birth injury P10.0
      - spinal G95.19
      - subacute I62.02
      - traumatic — *see* Injury, intracranial, subdural hemorrhage
    - traumatic — *see* Injury, intracranial, focal brain injury
  - intramedullary NEC G95.19
  - intraocular — *see* Hemophthalmos
  - intraoperative, intraprocedural — *see* Complication, hemorrhage (hematoma), intraoperative (intraprocedural), by site
  - intrapartum — *see* Hemorrhage, complicating, delivery
  - intrapelvic
    - female N94.89
    - male K66.1
  - intraperitoneal K66.1
  - intrapontine I61.3
  - intraprocedural — *see* Complication, hemorrhage (hematoma), intraoperative (intraprocedural), by site
  - intrauterine N85.7
    - complicating delivery (*see also* Hemorrhage, complicating, delivery)O67.9
    - postpartum — *see* Hemorrhage, postpartum
  - intraventricular I61.5
    - newborn (nontraumatic) (*see also* Newborn, affected by, hemorrhage)P52.3
      - due to birth injury P10.2
      - grade
        - 1 P52.0
        - 2 P52.1
        - 3 P52.21
        - 4 P52.22
  - intravesical N32.89
  - iris (postinfectional) (postinflammatory) (toxic) — *see* Hyphema
  - joint (nontraumatic) — *see* Hemarthrosis
  - kidney N28.89
  - knee (joint) (nontraumatic) — *see* Hemarthrosis, knee
  - labyrinth — *see* subcategory H83.8
  - lenticular striate artery I61.0
  - ligature, vessel — *see* Hemorrhage, postoperative
  - liver K76.89
  - lung R04.89
    - newborn P26.9
      - massive P26.1
      - specified NEC P26.8
    - tuberculous — *see* Tuberculosis, pulmonary
  - massive umbilical, newborn P51.0
  - mediastinum — *see* Hemorrhage, lung
  - medulla I61.3
  - membrane (brain) I60.8
    - spinal cord — *see* Hemorrhage, spinal cord
  - meninges, meningeal (brain) (middle) I60.8
    - spinal cord — *see* Hemorrhage, spinal cord

- **Hemorrhage** — *continued*
  - mesentery K66.1
  - metritis — *see* Endometritis
  - mouth K13.79
  - mucous membrane NEC R58
    - newborn P54.8
  - muscle M62.89
  - nail (subungual) L60.8
  - nasal turbinate R04.0
    - newborn P54.8
  - navel, newborn P51.9
  - newborn P54.9
    - specified NEC P54.8
  - nipple N64.59
  - nose R04.0
    - newborn P54.8
  - omentum K66.1
  - optic nerve (sheath) H47.02 ☑
  - orbit, orbital H05.23 ☑
  - ovary NEC N83.8
  - oviduct N83.6
  - pancreas K86.89
  - parathyroid (gland) (spontaneous) E21.4
  - parturition — *see* Hemorrhage, complicating, delivery
  - penis N48.89
  - pericardium, pericarditis I31.2
  - peritoneum, peritoneal K66.1
  - peritonsillar tissue J35.8
    - due to infection J36
  - petechial R23.3
    - due to autosensitivity, erythrocyte D69.2
  - pituitary (gland) E23.6
  - pleura — *see* Hemorrhage, lung
  - polioencephalitis, superior E51.2
  - polymyositis — *see* Polymyositis
  - pons, pontine I61.3
  - posterior fossa (nontraumatic) I61.8
    - newborn P52.6
  - postmenopausal N95.0
  - postnasal R04.0
  - postoperative — *see* Complications, postprocedural, hemorrhage, by site
  - postpartum NEC (following delivery of placenta) O72.1
    - delayed or secondary O72.2
    - retained placenta O72.0
    - third stage O72.0
  - pregnancy — *see* Hemorrhage, antepartum
  - preretinal — *see* Hemorrhage, retina
  - prostate N42.1
  - puerperal — *see* Hemorrhage, postpartum
    - delayed or secondary O72.2
  - pulmonary R04.89
    - newborn P26.9
      - massive P26.1
      - specified NEC P26.8
    - tuberculous — *see* Tuberculosis, pulmonary
  - purpura (primary) D69.3
  - rectum (sphincter) K62.5
    - newborn P54.2
  - recurring, following initial hemorrhage at time of injury T79.2 ☑
  - renal N28.89
  - respiratory passage or tract R04.9
    - specified NEC R04.89
  - retina, retinal (vessels) H35.6 ☑
    - diabetic — *see* Diabetes, retinal, hemorrhage
  - retroperitoneal R58
  - scalp R58
  - scrotum N50.1
  - secondary (nontraumatic) R58
    - following initial hemorrhage at time of injury T79.2 ☑
  - seminal vesicle N50.1
  - skin R23.3
    - newborn P54.5
  - slipped umbilical ligature P51.8
  - spermatic cord N50.1
  - spinal (cord) G95.19
    - newborn (birth injury) P11.5
  - spleen D73.5
    - intraoperative — *see* Complications, intraoperative, hemorrhage, spleen
    - postprocedural — *see* Complications, postprocedural, hemorrhage, spleen
  - stomach K92.2
    - newborn P54.3
    - ulcer — *see* Ulcer, stomach, with hemorrhage
  - subarachnoid (nontraumatic) — *see* Hemorrhage, intracranial, subarachnoid

- **Hemorrhage** — *continued*
  - subconjunctival (*see also* Hemorrhage, conjunctiva)
    - birth injury P15.3
  - subcortical (brain) I61.0
  - subcutaneous R23.3
  - subdiaphragmatic R58
  - subdural (acute) (nontraumatic) — *see* Hemorrhage, intracranial, subdural
  - subependymal
    - newborn P52.0
      - with intraventricular extension P52.1
        - and intracerebral extension P52.22
  - subgaleal P12.2
  - subhyaloid — *see* Hemorrhage, retina
  - subperiosteal — *see* Disorder, bone, specified type NEC
  - subretinal — *see* Hemorrhage, retina
  - subtentorial — *see* Hemorrhage, intracranial, subdural
  - subungual L60.8
  - suprarenal (capsule) (gland) E27.49
    - newborn P54.4
  - tentorium (traumatic) NEC — *see* Hemorrhage, brain
    - newborn (birth injury) P10.4
  - testis N50.1
  - third stage (postpartum) O72.0
  - thorax — *see* Hemorrhage, lung
  - throat R04.1
  - thymus (gland) E32.8
  - thyroid (cyst) (gland) E07.89
  - tongue K14.8
  - tonsil J35.8
  - trachea — *see* Hemorrhage, lung
  - tracheobronchial R04.89
    - newborn P26.0
  - traumatic - code to specific injury
    - cerebellar — *see* Hemorrhage, brain
    - intracranial — *see* Hemorrhage, brain
    - recurring or secondary (following initial hemorrhage at time of injury) T79.2 ☑
  - tuberculous NEC (*see also* Tuberculosis, pulmonary)A15.0
  - tunica vaginalis N50.1
  - ulcer - code by site under Ulcer, with hemorrhage K27.4
  - umbilicus, umbilical
    - cord
      - after birth, newborn P51.9
      - complicating delivery O69.5 ☑
    - newborn P51.9
      - massive P51.0
      - slipped ligature P51.8
    - stump P51.9
  - urethra (idiopathic) N36.8
  - uterus, uterine (abnormal) N93.9
    - climacteric N92.4
    - complicating delivery — *see* Hemorrhage, complicating, delivery
    - dysfunctional or functional N93.8
    - intermenstrual (regular) N92.3
      - irregular N92.1
    - postmenopausal N95.0
    - postpartum — *see* Hemorrhage, postpartum
    - preclimacteric or premenopausal N92.4
    - prepubertal N93.8
    - pubertal N92.2
  - vagina (abnormal) N93.9
    - newborn P54.6
  - vas deferens N50.1
  - vasa previa O69.4 ☑
  - ventricular I61.5
  - vesical N32.89
  - viscera NEC R58
    - newborn P54.8
  - vitreous (humor) (intraocular) H43.1 ☑
  - vulva N90.89
- **Hemorrhoids** (bleeding) (without mention of degree) K64.9
  - 1st degree (grade/stage I) (without prolapse outside of anal canal) K64.0
  - 2nd degree (grade/stage II) (that prolapse with straining but retract spontaneously) K64.1
  - 3rd degree (grade/stage III) (that prolapse with straining and require manual replacement back inside anal canal) K64.2
  - 4th degree (grade/stage IV) (with prolapsed tissue that cannot be manually replaced) K64.3
  - complicating
    - pregnancy O22.4 ☑
    - puerperium O87.2

- **Hemorrhoids** — *continued*
  - external K64.4
    - with
      - thrombosis K64.5
  - internal (without mention of degree) K64.8
  - prolapsed K64.8
  - skin tags
    - anus K64.4
    - residual K64.4
  - specified NEC K64.8
  - strangulated (*see also* Hemorrhoids, by degree)K64.8
  - thrombosed (*see also* Hemorrhoids, by degree)K64.5
  - ulcerated (*see also* Hemorrhoids, by degree)K64.8
- **Hemosalpinx** N83.6
  - with
    - hematocolpos N89.7
    - hematometra N85.7
      - with hematocolpos N89.7
- **Hemosiderosis** (dietary) E83.19
  - pulmonary, idiopathic E83.1 ☑ *[J84.03]*
  - transfusion T80.89 ☑
- **Hemothorax** (bacterial) (nontuberculous) J94.2
  - newborn P54.8
  - traumatic S27.1 ☑
    - with pneumothorax S27.2 ☑
  - tuberculous NEC A15.6
- **Henoch** (-Schönlein) disease or syndrome (purpura) D69.0
- **Henpue**, henpuye A66.6
- **Hepar** lobatum (syphilitic) A52.74
- **Hepatalgia** K76.89
- **Hepatitis** K75.9
  - acute B17.9
    - with coma K72.01
    - with hepatic failure — *see* Failure, hepatic
    - alcoholic — *see* Hepatitis, alcoholic
    - infectious B17.9
    - non-viral K72.0 ☑
    - viral B17.9
  - alcoholic (acute) (chronic) K70.10
    - with ascites K70.11
  - amebic — *see* Abscess, liver, amebic
  - anicteric, (viral) — *see* Hepatitis, viral
  - antigen-associated (HAA) — *see* Hepatitis, B
  - Australia-antigen (positive) — *see* Hepatitis, B
  - autoimmune K75.4
  - B B19.10
    - with hepatic coma B19.11
    - acute B16.9
      - with
        - delta-agent (coinfection) (without hepatic coma) B16.1
          - with hepatic coma B16.0
        - hepatic coma (without delta-agent coinfection) B16.2
    - chronic B18.1
      - with delta-agent B18.0
  - bacterial NEC K75.89
  - C (viral) B19.20
    - with hepatic coma B19.21
    - acute B17.10
      - with hepatic coma B17.11
    - chronic B18.2
  - catarrhal (acute) B15.9
    - with hepatic coma B15.0
  - cholangiolitic K75.89
  - cholestatic K75.89
  - chronic K73.9
    - active NEC K73.2
    - lobular NEC K73.1
    - persistent NEC K73.0
    - specified NEC K73.8
  - cytomegaloviral B25.1
  - due to ethanol (acute) (chronic) — *see* Hepatitis, alcoholic
  - epidemic B15.9
    - with hepatic coma B15.0
  - fulminant NEC (viral) — *see* Hepatitis, viral
  - neonatal giant cell P59.29
  - granulomatous NEC K75.3
  - herpesviral B00.81
  - history of
    - B Z86.19
    - C Z86.19
  - homologous serum — *see* Hepatitis, viral, type B
  - in (due to)
    - mumps B26.81
    - toxoplasmosis (acquired) B58.1
      - congenital (active) P37.1 *[K77]*
  - infectious, infective B15.9

- **Hepatitis** — *continued*
  - infectious, infective — *continued*
    - acute (subacute) B17.9
    - chronic B18.9
  - inoculation — *see* Hepatitis, viral, type B
  - interstitial (chronic) K74.69
  - lupoid NEC K75.4
  - malignant NEC (with hepatic failure) K72.90
    - with coma K72.91
  - neonatal (idiopathic) (toxic) P59.29
  - newborn P59.29
  - postimmunization — *see* Hepatitis, viral, type B
  - post-transfusion — *see* Hepatitis, viral, type B
  - reactive, nonspecific K75.2
  - serum — *see* Hepatitis, viral, type B
  - specified type NEC
    - with hepatic failure — *see* Failure, hepatic
  - syphilitic (late) A52.74
    - congenital (early) A50.08 *[K77]*
      - late A50.59 *[K77]*
    - secondary A51.45
  - toxic (*see also* Disease, liver, toxic)K71.6
  - tuberculous A18.83
  - viral, virus B19.9
    - with hepatic coma B19.0
    - acute B17.9
    - chronic B18.9
      - specified NEC B18.8
      - type
        - B B18.1
          - with delta-agent B18.0
        - C B18.2
    - congenital P35.3
    - coxsackie B33.8 *[K77]*
    - cytomegalic inclusion B25.1
    - in remission, any type - code to Hepatitis, chronic, by type
    - non-A, non-B B17.8
    - specified type NEC (with or without coma) B17.8
    - type
      - A B15.9
        - with hepatic coma B15.0
      - B B19.10
        - with hepatic coma B19.11
        - acute B16.9
          - with
            - delta-agent (coinfection) (without hepatic coma) B16.1
              - with hepatic coma B16.0
            - hepatic coma (without delta-agent coinfection) B16.2
        - chronic B18.1
          - with delta-agent B18.0
      - C B19.20
        - with hepatic coma B19.21
        - acute B17.10
          - with hepatic coma B17.11
        - chronic B18.2
      - E B17.2
      - non-A, non-B B17.8
- **Hepatization** lung (acute) — *see* Pneumonia, lobar
- **Hepatoblastoma** C22.2
- **Hepatocarcinoma** C22.0
- **Hepatocholangiocarcinoma** C22.0
- **Hepatocholangioma,** benign D13.4
- **Hepatocholangitis** K75.89
- **Hepatolenticular** degeneration E83.01
- **Hepatoma** (malignant) C22.0
  - benign D13.4
  - embryonal C22.0
- **Hepatomegaly** (*see also* Hypertrophy, liver)
  - with splenomegaly R16.2
  - congenital Q44.7
  - in mononucleosis
    - gammaherpesviral B27.09
    - infectious specified NEC B27.89
- **Hepatoptosis** K76.89
- **Hepatorenal** syndrome following labor and delivery O90.4
- **Hepatosis** K76.89
- **Hepatosplenomegaly** R16.2
  - hyperlipemic (Bürger-Grütz type) E78.3 *[K77]*
- **Hereditary** — *see* condition
- **Heredodegeneration,** macular — *see* Dystrophy, retina
- **Heredopathia** atactica polyneuritiformis G60.1
- **Heredosyphilis** — *see* Syphilis, congenital
- **Herlitz'** syndrome Q81.1
- **Hermansky-Pudlak** syndrome E70.331
- **Hermaphrodite,** hermaphroditism (true) Q56.0
  - 46,XX with streak gonads Q99.1

- **Hermaphrodite** — *continued*
  - 46,XX/46,XY Q99.0
  - 46,XY with streak gonads Q99.1
  - chimera 46,XX/46,XY Q99.0
- **Hernia,** hernial (acquired) (recurrent) K46.9
  - with
    - gangrene — *see* Hernia, by site, with, gangrene
    - incarceration — *see* Hernia, by site, with, obstruction
    - irreducible — *see* Hernia, by site, with, obstruction
    - obstruction — *see* Hernia, by site, with, obstruction
    - strangulation — *see* Hernia, by site, with, obstruction
  - abdomen, abdominal K46.9
    - with
      - gangrene (and obstruction) K46.1
      - obstruction K46.0
    - femoral — *see* Hernia, femoral
    - incisional — *see* Hernia, incisional
    - inguinal — *see* Hernia, inguinal
    - specified site NEC K45.8
      - with
        - gangrene (and obstruction) K45.1
        - obstruction K45.0
    - umbilical — *see* Hernia, umbilical
    - wall — *see* Hernia, ventral
  - appendix — *see* Hernia, abdomen
  - bladder (mucosa) (sphincter)
    - congenital (female) (male) Q79.51
    - female — *see* Cystocele
    - male N32.89
  - brain, congenital — *see* Encephalocele
  - cartilage, vertebra — *see* Displacement, intervertebral disc
  - cerebral, congenital (*see also* Encephalocele)
    - endaural Q01.8
  - ciliary body (traumatic) S05.2 ☑
  - colon — *see* Hernia, abdomen
  - Cooper's — *see* Hernia, abdomen, specified site NEC
  - crural — *see* Hernia, femoral
  - diaphragm, diaphragmatic K44.9
    - with
      - gangrene (and obstruction) K44.1
      - obstruction K44.0
    - congenital Q79.0
  - direct (inguinal) — *see* Hernia, inguinal
  - diverticulum, intestine — *see* Hernia, abdomen
  - double (inguinal) — *see* Hernia, inguinal, bilateral
  - due to adhesions (with obstruction) K56.5
  - epigastric (*see also* Hernia, ventral)K43.9
  - esophageal hiatus — *see* Hernia, hiatal
  - external (inguinal) — *see* Hernia, inguinal
  - fallopian tube N83.4 ☑
  - fascia M62.89
  - femoral K41.90
    - with
      - gangrene (and obstruction) K41.40
        - not specified as recurrent K41.40
        - recurrent K41.41
      - obstruction K41.30
        - not specified as recurrent K41.30
        - recurrent K41.31
    - bilateral K41.20
      - with
        - gangrene (and obstruction) K41.10
          - not specified as recurrent K41.10
          - recurrent K41.11
        - obstruction K41.00
          - not specified as recurrent K41.00
          - recurrent K41.01
      - not specified as recurrent K41.20
      - recurrent K41.21
    - unilateral K41.90
      - with
        - gangrene (and obstruction) K41.40
          - not specified as recurrent K41.40
          - recurrent K41.41
        - obstruction K41.30
          - not specified as recurrent K41.30
          - recurrent K41.31
      - not specified as recurrent K41.90
      - recurrent K41.91
    - not specified as recurrent K41.90
    - recurrent K41.91
  - foramen magnum G93.5
    - congenital Q01.8
  - funicular (umbilical) (*see also* Hernia, umbilicus)
    - spermatic (cord) — *see* Hernia, inguinal
  - gastrointestinal tract — *see* Hernia, abdomen

Hernia - Herpesvirus

- **Hernia** — *continued*
  - Hesselbach's — *see* Hernia, femoral, specified site NEC
  - hiatal (esophageal) (sliding) K44.9
    - with
      - gangrene (and obstruction) K44.1
      - obstruction K44.0
    - congenital Q40.1
  - hypogastric — *see* Hernia, ventral
  - incarcerated (*see also* Hernia, by site, with obstruction)
    - with gangrene — *see* Hernia, by site, with gangrene
  - incisional K43.2
    - with
      - gangrene (and obstruction) K43.1
      - obstruction K43.0
  - indirect (inguinal) — *see* Hernia, inguinal
  - inguinal (direct) (external) (funicular) (indirect) (internal) (oblique) (scrotal) (sliding) K40.90
    - with
      - gangrene (and obstruction) K40.40
        - not specified as recurrent K40.40
        - recurrent K40.41
      - obstruction K40.30
        - not specified as recurrent K40.30
        - recurrent K40.31
    - not specified as recurrent K40.90
    - recurrent K40.91
    - bilateral K40.20
      - with
        - gangrene (and obstruction) K40.10
          - not specified as recurrent K40.10
          - recurrent K40.11
        - obstruction K40.00
          - not specified as recurrent K40.00
          - recurrent K40.01
      - not specified as recurrent K40.20
      - recurrent K40.21
    - unilateral K40.90
      - with
        - gangrene (and obstruction) K40.40
          - not specified as recurrent K40.40
          - recurrent K40.41
        - obstruction K40.30
          - not specified as recurrent K40.30
          - recurrent K40.31
      - not specified as recurrent K40.90
      - recurrent K40.91
  - internal (*see also* Hernia, abdomen)
    - inguinal — *see* Hernia, inguinal
  - interstitial — *see* Hernia, abdomen
  - intervertebral cartilage or disc — *see* Displacement, intervertebral disc
  - intestine, intestinal — *see* Hernia, by site
  - intra-abdominal — *see* Hernia, abdomen
  - iris (traumatic) S05.2 ☑
  - irreducible (*see also* Hernia, by site, with obstruction)
    - with gangrene — *see* Hernia, by site, with gangrene
  - ischiatic — *see* Hernia, abdomen, specified site NEC
  - ischiorectal — *see* Hernia, abdomen, specified site NEC
  - lens (traumatic) S05.2 ☑
  - linea (alba) (semilunaris) — *see* Hernia, ventral
  - Littre's — *see* Hernia, abdomen
  - lumbar — *see* Hernia, abdomen, specified site NEC
  - lung (subcutaneous) J98.4
  - mediastinum J98.59
  - mesenteric (internal) — *see* Hernia, abdomen
  - midline — *see* Hernia, ventral
  - muscle (sheath) M62.89
  - nucleus pulposus — *see* Displacement, intervertebral disc
  - oblique (inguinal) — *see* Hernia, inguinal
  - obstructive (*see also* Hernia, by site, with obstruction)
    - with gangrene — *see* Hernia, by site, with gangrene
  - obturator — *see* Hernia, abdomen, specified site NEC
  - omental — *see* Hernia, abdomen
  - ovary N83.4 ☑
  - oviduct N83.4 ☑
  - paraesophageal (*see also* Hernia, diaphragm)
    - congenital Q40.1
  - parastomal K43.5
    - with
      - gangrene (and obstruction) K43.4
      - obstruction K43.3

- **Hernia** — *continued*
  - paraumbilical — *see* Hernia, umbilicus
  - perineal — *see* Hernia, abdomen, specified site NEC
  - Petit's — *see* Hernia, abdomen, specified site NEC
  - postoperative — *see* Hernia, incisional
  - pregnant uterus — *see* Abnormal, uterus in pregnancy or childbirth
  - prevesical N32.89
  - properitoneal — *see* Hernia, abdomen, specified site NEC
  - pudendal — *see* Hernia, abdomen, specified site NEC
  - rectovaginal N81.6
  - retroperitoneal — *see* Hernia, abdomen, specified site NEC
  - Richter's — *see* Hernia, abdomen, with obstruction
  - Rieux's, Riex's — *see* Hernia, abdomen, specified site NEC
  - sac condition (adhesion) (dropsy) (inflammation) (laceration) (suppuration) - code by site under Hernia
  - sciatic — *see* Hernia, abdomen, specified site NEC
  - scrotum, scrotal — *see* Hernia, inguinal
  - sliding (inguinal) (*see also* Hernia, inguinal)
    - hiatus — *see* Hernia, hiatal
  - spigelian — *see* Hernia, ventral
  - spinal — *see* Spina bifida
  - strangulated (*see also* Hernia, by site, with obstruction)
    - with gangrene — *see* Hernia, by site, with gangrene
  - subxiphoid — *see* Hernia, ventral
  - supra-umbilicus — *see* Hernia, ventral
  - tendon — *see* Disorder, tendon, specified type NEC
  - Treitz's (fossa) — *see* Hernia, abdomen, specified site NEC
  - tunica vaginalis Q55.29
  - umbilicus, umbilical K42.9
    - with
      - gangrene (and obstruction) K42.1
      - obstruction K42.0
  - ureter N28.89
  - urethra, congenital Q64.79
  - urinary meatus, congenital Q64.79
  - uterus N81.4
    - pregnant — *see* Abnormal, uterus in pregnancy or childbirth
  - vaginal (anterior) (wall) — *see* Cystocele
  - Velpeau's — *see* Hernia, femoral
  - ventral K43.9
    - with
      - gangrene (and obstruction) K43.7
      - obstruction K43.6
    - recurrent — *see* Hernia, incisional
    - incisional K43.2
      - with
        - gangrene (and obstruction) K43.1
        - obstruction K43.0
    - specified NEC K43.9
      - with
        - gangrene (and obstruction) K43.7
        - obstruction K43.6
  - vesical
    - congenital (female) (male) Q79.51
    - female — *see* Cystocele
    - male N32.89
  - vitreous (into wound) S05.2 ☑
    - into anterior chamber — *see* Prolapse, vitreous
- **Herniation** (*see also* Hernia)
  - brain (stem) G93.5
  - cerebral G93.5
  - mediastinum J98.59
  - nucleus pulposus — *see* Displacement, intervertebral disc
- **Herpangina** B08.5
- **Herpes,** herpesvirus, herpetic B00.9
  - anogenital A60.9
    - perianal skin A60.1
    - rectum A60.1
    - urogenital tract A60.00
      - cervix A60.03
      - male genital organ NEC A60.02
      - penis A60.01
      - specified site NEC A60.09
      - vagina A60.04
      - vulva A60.04
  - blepharitis (zoster) B02.39
    - simplex B00.59
  - circinatus B35.4
    - bullosus L12.0

- **Herpes** — *continued*
  - conjunctivitis (simplex) B00.53
    - zoster B02.31
  - cornea B02.33
  - encephalitis B00.4
    - due to herpesvirus 6 B10.01
    - due to herpesvirus 7 B10.09
    - specified NEC B10.09
  - eye (zoster) B02.30
    - simplex B00.50
  - eyelid (zoster) B02.39
    - simplex B00.59
  - facialis B00.1
  - febrilis B00.1
  - geniculate ganglionitis B02.21
  - genital, genitalis A60.00
    - female A60.09
    - male A60.02
  - gestational, gestationis O26.4 ☑
  - gingivostomatitis B00.2
  - human B00.9
    - 1 — *see* Herpes, simplex
    - 2 — *see* Herpes, simplex
    - 3 — *see* Varicella
    - 4 — *see* Mononucleosis, Epstein-Barr (virus)
    - 5 — *see* Disease, cytomegalic inclusion (generalized)
    - 6
      - encephalitis B10.01
      - specified NEC B10.81
    - 7
      - encephalitis B10.09
      - specified NEC B10.82
    - 8 B10.89
  - infection NEC B10.89
    - Kaposi's sarcoma associated B10.89
  - iridocyclitis (simplex) B00.51
    - zoster B02.32
  - iris (vesicular erythema multiforme) L51.9
  - iritis (simplex) B00.51
  - Kaposi's sarcoma associated B10.89
  - keratitis (simplex) (dendritic) (disciform) (interstitial) B00.52
    - zoster (interstitial) B02.33
  - keratoconjunctivitis (simplex) B00.52
    - zoster B02.33
  - labialis B00.1
  - lip B00.1
  - meningitis (simplex) B00.3
    - zoster B02.1
  - ophthalmicus (zoster) NEC B02.30
    - simplex B00.50
  - penis A60.01
  - perianal skin A60.1
  - pharyngitis, pharyngotonsillitis B00.2
  - rectum A60.1
  - scrotum A60.02
  - sepsis B00.7
  - simplex B00.9
    - complicated NEC B00.89
    - congenital P35.2
    - conjunctivitis B00.53
    - external ear B00.1
    - eyelid B00.59
    - hepatitis B00.81
    - keratitis (interstitial) B00.52
    - myleitis B00.82
    - specified complication NEC B00.89
    - visceral B00.89
  - stomatitis B00.2
  - tonsurans B35.0
  - visceral B00.89
  - vulva A60.04
  - whitlow B00.89
  - zoster (*see also* condition)B02.9
    - auricularis B02.21
    - complicated NEC B02.8
    - conjunctivitis B02.31
    - disseminated B02.7
    - encephalitis B02.0
    - eye (lid) B02.39
    - geniculate ganglionitis B02.21
    - keratitis (interstitial) B02.33
    - meningitis B02.1
    - myelitis B02.24
    - neuritis, neuralgia B02.29
    - ophthalmicus NEC B02.30
    - oticus B02.21
    - polyneuropathy B02.23
    - specified complication NEC B02.8
    - trigeminal neuralgia B02.22
- **Herpesvirus** (human) — *see* Herpes

- **Herpetophobia** F40.218
- **Herrick's** anemia — *see* Disease, sickle-cell
- **Hers'** disease E74.09
- **Herter-Gee** syndrome K90.0
- **Herxheimer's** reaction R68.89
- **Hesitancy**
  - of micturition R39.11
  - urinary R39.11
- **Hesselbach's** hernia — *see* Hernia, femoral, specified site NEC
- **Heterochromia** (congenital) Q13.2
  - cataract — *see* Cataract, complicated
  - cyclitis (Fuchs) — *see* Cyclitis, Fuchs' heterochromic
  - hair L67.1
  - iritis — *see* Cyclitis, Fuchs' heterochromic
  - retained metallic foreign body (nonmagnetic) — *see* Foreign body, intraocular, old, retained
    - magnetic — *see* Foreign body, intraocular, old, retained, magnetic
  - uveitis — *see* Cyclitis, Fuchs' heterochromic
- **Heterophoria** — *see* Strabismus, heterophoria
- **Heterophyes,** heterophyiasis (small intestine) B66.8
- **Heterotopia,** heterotopic (*see also* Malposition, congenital)
  - cerebralis Q04.8
- **Heterotropia** — *see* Strabismus
- **Heubner-Herter** disease K90.0
- **Hexadactylism** Q69.9
- **HGSIL** (cytology finding) (high grade squamous intraepithelial lesion on cytologic smear) (Pap smear finding)
  - anus R85.613
  - cervix R87.613
    - biopsy (histology) finding — *see* Neoplasia, intraepithelial, cervix, grade II or grade III
  - vagina R87.623
    - biopsy (histology) finding — *see* Neoplasia, intraepithelial, vagina, grade II or grade III
- **Hibernoma** — *see* Lipoma
- **Hiccup,** hiccough R06.6
  - epidemic B33.0
  - psychogenic F45.8
- **Hidden** penis (congenital) Q55.64
  - acquired N48.83
- **Hidradenitis** (axillaris) (suppurative) L73.2
- **Hidradenoma** (nodular) (*see also* Neoplasm, skin, benign)
  - clear cell — *see* Neoplasm, skin, benign
  - papillary — *see* Neoplasm, skin, benign
- **Hidrocystoma** — *see* Neoplasm, skin, benign
- **High**
  - altitude effects T70.20 ☑
    - anoxia T70.29 ☑
    - on
      - ears T70.0 ☑
      - sinuses T70.1 ☑
    - polycythemia D75.1
  - arch
    - foot Q66.7
    - palate, congenital Q38.5
  - arterial tension — *see* Hypertension
  - basal metabolic rate R94.8
  - blood pressure (*see also* Hypertension)
    - borderline R03.0
    - reading (incidental) (isolated) (nonspecific), without diagnosis of hypertension R03.0
  - cholesterol E78.00
    - with high triglycerides E78.2
  - diaphragm (congenital) Q79.1
  - expressed emotional level within family Z63.8
  - head at term O32.4 ☑
  - palate, congenital Q38.5
  - risk
    - infant NEC Z76.2
    - sexual behavior (heterosexual) Z72.51
      - bisexual Z72.53
      - homosexual Z72.52
  - temperature (of unknown origin) R50.9
  - thoracic rib Q76.6
  - triglycerides E78.1
    - with high cholesterol E78.2
- **Hildenbrand's** disease A75.0
- **Hilum** — *see* condition
- **Hip** — *see* condition
- **Hippel's** disease Q85.8
- **Hippophobia** F40.218
- **Hippus** H57.09
- **Hirschsprung's** disease or megacolon Q43.1
- **Hirsutism,** hirsuties L68.0
- **Hirudiniasis**
  - external B88.3
  - internal B83.4
- **Hiss-Russell** dysentery A03.1
- **Histidinemia,** histidinuria E70.41
- **Histiocytoma** (*see also* Neoplasm, skin, benign)
  - fibrous (*see also* Neoplasm, skin, benign)
    - atypical — *see* Neoplasm, connective tissue, uncertain behavior
    - malignant — *see* Neoplasm, connective tissue, malignant
- **Histiocytosis** D76.3
  - acute differentiated progressive C96.0
  - Langerhans' cell NEC C96.6
    - multifocal X
      - multisystemic (disseminated) C96.0
      - unisystemic C96.5
    - pulmonary, adult (adult PLCH) J84.82
    - unifocal (X) C96.6
  - lipid, lipoid D76.3
    - essential E75.29
  - malignant C96.A
  - mononuclear phagocytes NEC D76.1
    - Langerhans' cells C96.6
  - non-Langerhans cell D76.3
  - polyostotic sclerosing D76.3
  - sinus, with massive lymphadenopathy D76.3
  - syndrome NEC D76.3
  - X NEC C96.6
    - acute (progressive) C96.0
    - chronic C96.6
    - multifocal C96.5
    - multisystemic C96.0
    - unifocal C96.6
- **Histoplasmosis** B39.9
  - with pneumonia NEC B39.2
  - African B39.5
  - American — *see* Histoplasmosis, capsulati
  - capsulati B39.4
    - disseminated B39.3
    - generalized B39.3
    - pulmonary B39.2
      - acute B39.0
      - chronic B39.1
  - Darling's B39.4
  - duboisii B39.5
  - lung NEC B39.2
- **History**
  - family (of) (*see also* History, personal (of))
    - alcohol abuse Z81.1
    - allergy NEC Z84.89
    - anemia Z83.2
    - arthritis Z82.61
    - asthma Z82.5
    - blindness Z82.1
    - cardiac death (sudden) Z82.41
    - carrier of genetic disease Z84.81
    - chromosomal anomaly Z82.79
    - chronic
      - disabling disease NEC Z82.8
      - lower respiratory disease Z82.5
    - colonic polyps Z83.71
    - congenital malformations and deformations Z82.79
      - polycystic kidney Z82.71
    - consanguinity Z84.3
    - deafness Z82.2
    - diabetes mellitus Z83.3
    - disability NEC Z82.8
    - disease or disorder (of)
      - allergic NEC Z84.89
      - behavioral NEC Z81.8
      - blood and blood-forming organs Z83.2
      - cardiovascular NEC Z82.49
      - chronic disabling NEC Z82.8
      - digestive Z83.79
      - ear NEC Z83.52
      - endocrine NEC Z83.49
      - eye NEC Z83.518
        - glaucoma Z83.511
      - familial hypercholesterolemia Z83.42
      - genitourinary NEC Z84.2
      - glaucoma Z83.511
      - hematological Z83.2
      - immune mechanism Z83.2
      - infectious NEC Z83.1
      - ischemic heart Z82.49
      - kidney Z84.1
      - mental NEC Z81.8
      - metabolic Z83.49
      - musculoskeletal NEC Z82.69
      - neurological NEC Z82.0
      - nutritional Z83.49
      - parasitic NEC Z83.1
      - psychiatric NEC Z81.8

History — *continued*

  - family — *continued*
      - respiratory NEC Z83.6
      - skin and subcutaneous tissue NEC Z84.0
      - specified NEC Z84.89
    - drug abuse NEC Z81.3
    - epilepsy Z82.0
    - familial hypercholesterolemia Z83.42
    - genetic disease carrier Z84.81
    - glaucoma Z83.511
    - hearing loss Z82.2
    - human immunodeficiency virus (HIV) infection Z83.0
    - Huntington's chorea Z82.0
    - intellectual disability Z81.0
    - leukemia Z80.6
    - malignant neoplasm (of) NOS Z80.9
      - bladder Z80.52
      - breast Z80.3
      - bronchus Z80.1
      - digestive organ Z80.0
      - gastrointestinal tract Z80.0
      - genital organ Z80.49
        - ovary Z80.41
        - prostate Z80.42
        - specified organ NEC Z80.49
        - testis Z80.43
      - hematopoietic NEC Z80.7
      - intrathoracic organ NEC Z80.2
      - kidney Z80.51
      - lung Z80.1
      - lymphatic NEC Z80.7
      - ovary Z80.41
      - prostate Z80.42
      - respiratory organ NEC Z80.2
      - specified site NEC Z80.8
      - testis Z80.43
      - trachea Z80.1
      - urinary organ or tract Z80.59
        - bladder Z80.52
        - kidney Z80.51
    - mental
      - disorder NEC Z81.8
    - multiple endocrine neoplasia (MEN) syndrome Z83.41
    - osteoporosis Z82.62
    - polycystic kidney Z82.71
    - polyps (colon) Z83.71
    - psychiatric disorder Z81.8
    - psychoactive substance abuse NEC Z81.3
    - respiratory condition NEC Z83.6
      - asthma and other lower respiratory conditions Z82.5
    - self-harmful behavior Z81.8
    - SIDS (sudden infant death syndrome) Z84.82
    - skin condition Z84.0
    - specified condition NEC Z84.89
    - stroke (cerebrovascular) Z82.3
    - substance abuse NEC Z81.4
      - alcohol Z81.1
      - drug NEC Z81.3
      - psychoactive NEC Z81.3
      - tobacco Z81.2
    - sudden
      - cardiac death Z82.41
      - infant death syndrome (SIDS) Z84.82
    - tobacco abuse Z81.2
    - violence, violent behavior Z81.8
    - visual loss Z82.1
  - personal (of) (*see also* History, family (of))
    - abuse
      - childhood Z62.819
        - physical Z62.810
        - psychological Z62.811
        - sexual Z62.810
      - adult Z91.419
        - physical and sexual Z91.410
        - psychological Z91.411
    - alcohol dependence F10.21
    - allergy (to) Z88.9
      - analgesic agent NEC Z88.6
      - anesthetic Z88.4
      - antibiotic agent NEC Z88.1
      - anti-infective agent NEC Z88.3
      - contrast media Z91.041
      - drugs, medicaments and biological substances Z88.9
        - specified NEC Z88.8
      - food Z91.018
        - additives Z91.02
        - eggs Z91.012
        - milk products Z91.011

- **History** — *continued*
  - personal — *continued*
        - peanuts Z91.010
        - seafood Z91.013
        - specified food NEC Z91.018
      - insect Z91.038
        - bee Z91.030
      - latex Z91.040
      - medicinal agents Z88.9
        - specified NEC Z88.8
      - narcotic agent NEC Z88.5
      - nonmedicinal agents Z91.048
      - penicillin Z88.0
      - serum Z88.7
      - specified NEC Z91.09
      - sulfonamides Z88.2
      - vaccine Z88.7
    - anaphylactic shock Z87.892
    - anaphylaxis Z87.892
    - behavioral disorders Z86.59
    - benign carcinoid tumor Z86.012
    - benign neoplasm Z86.018
      - carcinoid Z86.012
      - brain Z86.011
      - colonic polyps Z86.010
    - brain injury (traumatic) Z87.820
    - breast implant removal Z98.86
    - calculi, renal Z87.442
    - cancer — *see* History, personal (of), malignant neoplasm (of)
    - cardiac arrest (death), successfully resuscitated Z86.74
    - cerebral infarction without residual deficit Z86.73
    - cervical dysplasia Z87.410
    - chemotherapy for neoplastic condition Z92.21
    - childhood abuse — *see* History, personal (of), abuse
    - cleft lip (corrected) Z87.730
    - cleft palate (corrected) Z87.730
    - collapsed vertebra (healed) Z87.311
      - due to osteoporosis Z87.310
    - combat and operational stress reaction Z86.51
    - congenital malformation (corrected) Z87.798
      - circulatory system (corrected) Z87.74
      - digestive system (corrected) NEC Z87.738
      - ear (corrected) Z87.720
      - eye (corrected) Z87.721
      - face and neck (corrected) Z87.790
      - genitourinary system (corrected) NEC Z87.718
      - heart (corrected) Z87.74
      - integument (corrected) Z87.76
      - limb (s) (corrected) Z87.76
      - musculoskeletal system (corrected) Z87.76
      - neck (corrected) Z87.790
      - nervous system (corrected) NEC Z87.728
      - respiratory system (corrected) Z87.75
      - sense organs (corrected) NEC Z87.728
      - specified NEC Z87.798
    - contraception Z92.0
    - deployment (military) Z91.82
    - diabetic foot ulcer Z86.31
    - disease or disorder (of) Z87.898
      - blood and blood-forming organs Z86.2
      - circulatory system Z86.79
        - specified condition NEC Z86.79
      - connective tissue NEC Z87.39
      - digestive system Z87.19
        - colonic polyp Z86.010
        - peptic ulcer disease Z87.11
        - specified condition NEC Z87.19
      - ear Z86.69
      - endocrine Z86.39
        - diabetic foot ulcer Z86.31
        - gestational diabetes Z86.32
        - specified type NEC Z86.39
      - eye Z86.69
      - genital (track) system NEC
        - female Z87.42
        - male Z87.438
      - hematological Z86.2
      - Hodgkin Z85.71
      - immune mechanism Z86.2
      - infectious Z86.19
        - malaria Z86.13
        - Methicillin resistant Staphylococcus aureus (MRSA) Z86.14
        - poliomyelitis Z86.12
        - specified NEC Z86.19
        - tuberculosis Z86.11
      - mental NEC Z86.59

- **History** — *continued*
  - personal — *continued*
      - metabolic Z86.39
        - diabetic foot ulcer Z86.31
        - gestational diabetes Z86.32
        - specified type NEC Z86.39
      - musculoskeletal NEC Z87.39
      - nervous system Z86.69
      - nutritional Z86.39
      - parasitic Z86.19
      - respiratory system NEC Z87.09
      - sense organs Z86.69
      - skin Z87.2
      - specified site or type NEC Z87.898
      - subcutaneous tissue Z87.2
      - trophoblastic Z87.59
      - urinary system NEC Z87.448
    - drug dependence — *see* Dependence, drug, by type, in remission
    - drug therapy
      - antineoplastic chemotherapy Z92.21
      - estrogen Z92.23
      - immunosuppression Z92.25
      - inhaled steroids Z92.240
      - monoclonal drug Z92.22
      - specified NEC Z92.29
      - steroid Z92.241
      - systemic steroids Z92.241
    - dysplasia
      - cervical (mild) (moderate) Z87.410
        - severe (grade III) Z86.001
      - prostatic Z87.430
      - vaginal (mild) (moderate) Z87.411
        - severe (grade III) Z86.008
      - vulvar (mild) (moderate) Z87.412
        - severe (grade III) Z86.008
    - embolism (venous) Z86.718
      - pulmonary Z86.711
    - encephalitis Z86.61
    - estrogen therapy Z92.23
    - extracorporeal membrane oxygenation (ECMO) Z92.81
    - failed moderate sedation Z92.83
    - failed conscious sedation Z92.83
    - fall, falling Z91.81
    - fracture (healed)
      - fatigue Z87.312
      - fragility Z87.310
      - osteoporosis Z87.310
      - pathological NEC Z87.311
      - stress Z87.312
      - traumatic Z87.81
    - gestational diabetes Z86.32
    - hepatitis
      - B Z86.19
      - C Z86.19
    - Hodgkin disease Z85.71
    - hyperthermia, malignant Z88.4
    - hypospadias (corrected) Z87.710
    - hysterectomy Z90.710
    - immunosuppression therapy Z92.25
    - in situ neoplasm
      - breast Z86.000
      - cervix uteri Z86.001
      - specified NEC Z86.008
    - infection NEC Z86.19
      - central nervous system Z86.61
      - Methicillin resistant Staphylococcus aureus (MRSA) Z86.14
      - urinary (recurrent) (tract) Z87.440
    - injury NEC Z87.828
    - in utero procedure during pregnancy Z98.870
    - in utero procedure while a fetus Z98.871
    - irradiation Z92.3
    - kidney stones Z87.442
    - leukemia Z85.6
    - lymphoma (non-Hodgkin) Z85.72
    - malignant melanoma (skin) Z85.820
    - malignant neoplasm (of) Z85.9
      - accessory sinuses Z85.22
      - anus NEC Z85.048
        - carcinoid Z85.040
      - bladder Z85.51
      - bone Z85.830
      - brain Z85.841
      - breast Z85.3
      - bronchus NEC Z85.118
        - carcinoid Z85.110
      - carcinoid — *see* History, personal (of), malignant neoplasm, by site, carciniold
      - cervix Z85.41
      - colon NEC Z85.038

- **History** — *continued*
  - personal — *continued*
        - carcinoid Z85.030
      - digestive organ Z85.00
        - specified NEC Z85.09
      - endocrine gland NEC Z85.858
      - epididymis Z85.48
      - esophagus Z85.01
      - eye Z85.840
      - gastrointestinal tract — *see* History, malignant neoplasm, digestive organ
      - genital organ
        - female Z85.40
          - specified NEC Z85.44
        - male Z85.45
          - specified NEC Z85.49
      - hematopoietic NEC Z85.79
      - intrathoracic organ Z85.20
      - kidney NEC Z85.528
        - carcinoid Z85.520
      - large intestine NEC Z85.038
        - carcinoid Z85.030
      - larynx Z85.21
      - liver Z85.05
      - lung NEC Z85.118
        - carcinoid Z85.110
      - mediastinum Z85.29
      - Merkel cell Z85.821
      - middle ear Z85.22
      - nasal cavities Z85.22
      - nervous system NEC Z85.848
      - oral cavity Z85.819
        - specified site NEC Z85.818
      - ovary Z85.43
      - pancreas Z85.07
      - pharynx Z85.819
        - specified site NEC Z85.818
      - pelvis Z85.53
      - pleura Z85.29
      - prostate Z85.46
      - rectosigmoid junction NEC Z85.048
        - carcinoid Z85.040
      - rectum NEC Z85.048
        - carcinoid Z85.040
      - respiratory organ Z85.20
      - sinuses, accessory Z85.22
      - skin NEC Z85.828
        - melanoma Z85.820
        - Merkel cell Z85.821
      - small intestine NEC Z85.068
        - carcinoid Z85.060
      - soft tissue Z85.831
      - specified site NEC Z85.89
      - stomach NEC Z85.028
        - carcinoid Z85.020
      - testis Z85.47
      - thymus NEC Z85.238
        - carcinoid Z85.230
      - thyroid Z85.850
      - tongue Z85.810
      - trachea Z85.12
      - ureter Z85.54
      - urinary organ or tract Z85.50
        - specified NEC Z85.59
      - uterus Z85.42
    - maltreatment Z91.89
    - medical treatment NEC Z92.89
    - melanoma (malignant) (skin) Z85.820
    - meningitis Z86.61
    - mental disorder Z86.59
    - Merkel cell carcinoma (skin) Z85.821
    - Methicillin resistant Staphylococcus aureus (MRSA) Z86.14
    - military deployment Z91.82
    - military war, peacekeeping and humanitarian deployment (current or past conflict) Z91.82
    - myocardial infarction (old) I25.2
    - neglect (in)
      - adult Z91.412
      - childhood Z62.812
    - neoplasm
      - benign Z86.018
        - brain Z86.011
        - colon polyp Z86.010
      - in situ
        - breast Z86.000
        - cervix uteri Z86.001
        - specified NEC Z86.008
      - malignant — *see* History of, malignant neoplasm
      - uncertain behavior Z86.03

- **Hydrarthrosis** — *continued*
  - of yaws (early) (late) (*see also* subcategory M14.8-) A66.6
  - syphilitic (late) A52.77
    - congenital A50.55 *[M12.80]*
- **Hydremia** D64.89
- **Hydrencephalocele** (congenital) — *see* Encephalocele
- **Hydrencephalomeningocele** (congenital) — *see* Encephalocele
- **Hydroa** R23.8
  - aestivale L56.4
  - vacciniforme L56.4
- **Hydroadenitis** (axillaris) (suppurative) L73.2
- **Hydrocalycosis** — *see* Hydronephrosis
- **Hydrocele** (spermatic cord) (testis) (tunica vaginalis) N43.3
  - canal of Nuck N94.89
  - communicating N43.2
    - congenital P83.5
  - congenital P83.5
  - encysted N43.0
  - female NEC N94.89
  - infected N43.1
  - newborn P83.5
  - round ligament N94.89
  - specified NEC N43.2
  - spinalis — *see* Spina bifida
  - vulva N90.89
- **Hydrocephalus** (acquired) (external) (internal) (malignant) (recurrent) G91.9
  - aqueduct Sylvius stricture Q03.0
  - causing disproportion O33.6 ☑
    - with obstructed labor O66.3
  - communicating G91.0
  - congenital (external) (internal) Q03.9
    - with spina bifida Q05.4
      - cervical Q05.0
      - dorsal Q05.1
      - lumbar Q05.2
      - lumbosacral Q05.2
      - sacral Q05.3
      - thoracic Q05.1
      - thoracolumbar Q05.1
    - specified NEC Q03.8
  - due to toxoplasmosis (congenital) P37.1
  - foramen Magendie block (acquired) G91.1
    - congenital (*see also* Hydrocephalus, congenital)Q03.1
  - in (due to)
    - infectious disease NEC B89 *[G91.4]*
    - neoplastic disease NEC (see also Neoplasm) G91.4
    - parasitic disease B89 *[G91.4]*
  - newborn Q03.9
    - with spina bifida — *see* Spina bifida, with hydrocephalus
  - noncommunicating G91.1
  - normal pressure G91.2
    - secondary G91.0
  - obstructive G91.1
  - otitic G93.2
  - post-traumatic NEC G91.3
  - secondary G91.4
    - post-traumatic G91.3
  - specified NEC G91.8
  - syphilitic, congenital A50.49
- **Hydrocolpos** (congenital) N89.8
- **Hydrocystoma** — *see* Neoplasm, skin, benign
- **Hydroencephalocele** (congenital) — *see* Encephalocele
- **Hydroencephalomeningocele** (congenital) — *see* Encephalocele
- **Hydrohematopneumothorax** — *see* Hemothorax
- **Hydromeningitis** — *see* Meningitis
- **Hydromeningocele** (spinal) (*see also* Spina bifida)
  - cranial — *see* Encephalocele
- **Hydrometra** N85.8
- **Hydrometrocolpos** N89.8
- **Hydromicrocephaly** Q02
- **Hydromphalos** (since birth) Q45.8
- **Hydromyelia** Q06.4
- **Hydromyelocele** — *see* Spina bifida
- **Hydronephrosis** (atrophic) (early) (functionless) (intermittent) (primary) (secondary) NEC N13.30
  - with
    - infection N13.6
    - obstruction (by) (of)
      - renal calculus N13.2
        - with infection N13.6
      - ureteral NEC N13.1
        - with infection N13.6
- **Hydronephrosis** — *continued*
  - with — *continued*
      - calculus N13.2
        - with infection N13.6
      - ureteropelvic junction (congenital) Q62.0
        - acquired N13.0
          - with infection N13.6
    - ureteral stricture NEC N13.1
      - with infection N13.6
  - congenital Q62.0
    - due to acquired occlusion of ureteropelvic junction N13.0
  - specified type NEC N13.39
  - tuberculous A18.11
- **Hydropericarditis** — *see* Pericarditis
- **Hydropericardium** — *see* Pericarditis
- **Hydroperitoneum** R18.8
- **Hydrophobia** — *see* Rabies
- **Hydrophthalmos** Q15.0
- **Hydropneumohemothorax** — *see* Hemothorax
- **Hydropneumopericarditis** — *see* Pericarditis
- **Hydropneumopericardium** — *see* Pericarditis
- **Hydropneumothorax** J94.8
  - traumatic — *see* Injury, intrathoracic, lung
  - tuberculous NEC A15.6
- **Hydrops** R60.9
  - abdominis R18.8
  - articulorum intermittens — *see* Hydrarthrosis, intermittent
  - cardiac — *see* Failure, heart, congestive
  - causing obstructed labor (mother) O66.3
  - endolymphatic H81.0 ☑
  - fetal — *see* Pregnancy, complicated by, hydrops, fetalis
  - fetalis P83.2
    - due to
      - ABO isoimmunization P56.0
      - alpha thalassemia D56.0
      - hemolytic disease P56.90
        - specified NEC P56.99
      - isoimmunization (ABO) (Rh) P56.0
      - other specified nonhemolytic disease NEC P83.2
      - Rh incompatibility P56.0
    - during pregnancy — *see* Pregnancy, complicated by, hydrops, fetalis
  - gallbladder K82.1
  - joint — *see* Effusion, joint
  - labyrinth H81.0 ☑
  - newborn (idiopathic) P83.2
    - due to
      - ABO isoimmunization P56.0
      - alpha thalassemia D56.0
      - hemolytic disease P56.90
        - specified NEC P56.99
      - isoimmunization (ABO) (Rh) P56.0
      - Rh incompatibility P56.0
  - nutritional — *see* Malnutrition, severe
  - pericardium — *see* Pericarditis
  - pleura — *see* Hydrothorax
  - spermatic cord — *see* Hydrocele
- **Hydropyonephrosis** N13.6
- **Hydrorachis** Q06.4
- **Hydrorrhea** (nasal) J34.89
  - pregnancy — *see* Rupture, membranes, premature
- **Hydrosadenitis** (axillaris) (suppurative) L73.2
- **Hydrosalpinx** (fallopian tube) (follicularis) N70.11
- **Hydrothorax** (double) (pleura) J94.8
  - chylous (nonfilarial) I89.8
    - filarial (*see also* Infestation, filarial)B74.9 *[J91.8]*
  - traumatic — *see* Injury, intrathoracic
  - tuberculous NEC (non primary) A15.6
- **Hydroureter** (*see also* Hydronephrosis)N13.4
  - with infection N13.6
  - congenital Q62.39
- **Hydroureteronephrosis** — *see* Hydronephrosis
- **Hydrourethra** N36.8
- **Hydroxykynureninuria** E70.8
- **Hydroxylysinemia** E72.3
- **Hydroxyprolinemia** E72.59
- **Hygiene,** sleep
  - abuse Z72.821
  - inadequate Z72.821
  - poor Z72.821
- **Hygroma** (congenital) (cystic) D18.1
  - praepatellare, prepatellar — *see* Bursitis, prepatellar
- **Hymen** — *see* condition
- **Hymenolepis,** hymenolepiasis (diminuta) (infection) (infestation) (nana) B71.0
- **Hypalgesia** R20.8
- **Hyperacidity** (gastric) K31.89
  - psychogenic F45.8
- **Hyperactive,** hyperactivity F90.9
  - basal cell, uterine cervix — *see* Dysplasia, cervix
  - bowel sounds R19.12
  - cervix epithelial (basal) — *see* Dysplasia, cervix
  - child F90.9
    - attention deficit — *see* Disorder, attention-deficit hyperactivity
  - detrusor muscle N32.81
  - gastrointestinal K31.89
    - psychogenic F45.8
  - nasal mucous membrane J34.3
  - stomach K31.89
  - thyroid (gland) — *see* Hyperthyroidism
- **Hyperacusis** H93.23 ☑
- **Hyperadrenalism** E27.5
- **Hyperadrenocorticism** E24.9
  - congenital E25.0
  - iatrogenic E24.2
    - correct substance properly administered — *see* Table of Drugs and Chemicals, by drug, adverse effect
    - overdose or wrong substance given or taken — *see* Table of Drugs and Chemicals, by drug, poisoning
  - not associated with Cushing's syndrome E27.0
  - pituitary-dependent E24.0
- **Hyperaldosteronism** E26.9
  - familial (type I) E26.02
  - glucocorticoid-remediable E26.02
  - primary (due to (bilateral) adrenal hyperplasia) E26.09
  - primary NEC E26.09
  - secondary E26.1
  - specified NEC E26.89
- **Hyperalgesia** R20.8
- **Hyperalimentation** R63.2
  - carotene, carotin E67.1
  - specified NEC E67.8
  - vitamin
    - A E67.0
    - D E67.3
- **Hyperaminoaciduria**
  - arginine E72.21
  - cystine E72.01
  - lysine E72.3
  - ornithine E72.4
- **Hyperammonemia** (congenital) E72.20
- **Hyperazotemia** — *see* Uremia
- **Hyperbetalipoproteinemia** (familial) E78.00
  - with prebetalipoproteinemia E78.2
- **Hyperbilirubinemia**
  - constitutional E80.6
  - familial conjugated E80.6
  - neonatal (transient) — *see* Jaundice, newborn
- **Hypercalcemia,** hypocalciuric, familial E83.52
- **Hypercalciuria,** idiopathic E83.52
- **Hypercapnia** R06.89
  - newborn P84
- **Hypercarotenemia,** hypercarotinemia (dietary) E67.1
- **Hypercementosis** K03.4
- **Hyperchloremia** E87.8
- **Hyperchlorhydria** K31.89
  - neurotic F45.8
  - psychogenic F45.8
- **Hypercholesterinemia** — *see* Hypercholesterolemia
- **Hypercholesterolemia** (essential) (primary) (pure) E78.00
  - with hyperglyceridemia, endogenous E78.2
  - dietary counseling and surveillance Z71.3
  - familial E78.01
  - hereditary E78.01
- **Hyperchylia** gastrica, psychogenic F45.8
- **Hyperchylomicronemia** (familial) (primary) E78.3
  - with hyperbetalipoproteinemia E78.3
- **Hypercoagulable** (state) D68.59
  - activated protein C resistance D68.51
  - antithrombin (III) deficiency D68.59
  - factor V Leiden mutation D68.51
  - primary NEC D68.59
  - protein C deficiency D68.59
  - protein S deficiency D68.59
  - prothrombin gene mutation D68.52
  - secondary D68.69
  - specified NEC D68.69
- **Hypercoagulation** (state) D68.59
- **Hypercorticalism,** pituitary-dependent E24.0
- **Hypercorticosolism** — *see* Cushing's, syndrome
- **Hypercorticosteronism** E24.2

Hypercorticosteronism — *continued*
- correct substance properly administered — *see* Table of Drugs and Chemicals, by drug, adverse effect
- overdose or wrong substance given or taken — *see* Table of Drugs and Chemicals, by drug, poisoning

Hypercortisonism E24.2
- correct substance properly administered — *see* Table of Drugs and Chemicals, by drug, adverse effect
- overdose or wrong substance given or taken — *see* Table of Drugs and Chemicals, by drug, poisoning

Hyperekplexia Q89.8

Hyperelectrolytemia E87.8

Hyperemesis R11.10
- with nausea R11.2
- gravidarum (mild) O21.0
  - with
    - carbohydrate depletion O21.1
    - dehydration O21.1
    - electrolyte imbalance O21.1
    - metabolic disturbance O21.1
  - severe (with metabolic disturbance) O21.1
- projectile R11.12
- psychogenic F45.8

Hyperemia (acute) (passive) R68.89
- anal mucosa K62.89
- bladder N32.89
- cerebral I67.89
- conjunctiva H11.43 ☑
- ear internal, acute — *see* subcategory H83.0
- enteric K59.8
- eye — *see* Hyperemia, conjunctiva
- eyelid (active) (passive) — *see* Disorder, eyelid, specified type NEC
- intestine K59.8
- iris — *see* Disorder, iris, vascular
- kidney N28.89
- labyrinth — *see* subcategory H83.0
- liver (active) K76.89
- lung (passive) — *see* Edema, lung
- pulmonary (passive) — *see* Edema, lung
- renal N28.89
- retina H35.89
- stomach K31.89

Hyperesthesia (body surface) R20.3
- larynx (reflex) J38.7
  - hysterical F44.89
- pharynx (reflex) J39.2
  - hysterical F44.89

Hyperestrogenism (drug-induced) (iatrogenic) E28.0

Hyperexplexia Q89.8

Hyperfibrinolysis — *see* Fibrinolysis

Hyperfructosemia E74.19

Hyperfunction
- adrenal cortex, not associated with Cushing's syndrome E27.0
  - medulla E27.5
    - adrenomedullary E27.5
  - virilism E25.9
    - congenital E25.0
- ovarian E28.8
- pancreas K86.89
- parathyroid (gland) E21.3
- pituitary (gland) (anterior) E22.9
  - specified NEC E22.8
- polyglandular E31.1
- testicular E29.0

Hypergammaglobulinemia D89.2
- polyclonal D89.0
- Waldenström D89.0

Hypergastrinemia E16.4

Hyperglobulinemia R77.1

Hyperglycemia, hyperglycemic (transient) R73.9
- coma — *see* Diabetes, by type, with coma
- postpancreatectomy E89.1

Hyperglyceridemia (endogenous) (essential) (familial) (hereditary) (pure) E78.1
- mixed E78.3

Hyperglycinemia (non-ketotic) E72.51

Hypergonadism
- ovarian E28.8
- testicular (primary) (infantile) E29.0

Hyperheparinemia D68.32

Hyperhidrosis, hyperidrosis R61
- focal
  - primary L74.519
    - axilla L74.510
    - face L74.511
    - palms L74.512

Hyperhidrosis — *continued*
- focal — *continued*
    - soles L74.513
  - secondary L74.52
- generalized R61
- localized
  - primary L74.519
    - axilla L74.510
    - face L74.511
    - palms L74.512
    - soles L74.513
  - secondary L74.52
- psychogenic F45.8
- secondary R61
  - focal L74.52

Hyperhistidinemia E70.41

Hyperhomocysteinemia E72.11

Hyperhydroxyprolinemia E72.59

Hyperinsulinism (functional) E16.1
- with
  - coma (hypoglycemic) E15
  - encephalopathy E16.1 *[G94]*
- ectopic E16.1
- therapeutic misadventure (from administration of insulin) — *see* subcategory T38.3

Hyperkalemia E87.5

Hyperkeratosis (*see also* Keratosis)L85.9
- cervix N88.0
- due to yaws (early) (late) (palmar or plantar) A66.3
- follicularis Q82.8
  - penetrans (in cutem) L87.0
- palmoplantaris climacterica L85.1
- pinta A67.1
- senile (with pruritus) L57.0
- universalis congenita Q80.8
- vocal cord J38.3
- vulva N90.4

Hyperkinesia, hyperkinetic (disease) (reaction) (syndrome) (childhood) (adolescence) (*see also* Disorder, attention-deficit hyperactivity)
- heart I51.89

Hyperleucine-isoleucinemia E71.19

Hyperlipemia, hyperlipidemia E78.5
- combined E78.2
  - familial E78.4
- group
  - A E78.00
  - B E78.1
  - C E78.2
  - D E78.3
- mixed E78.2
- specified NEC E78.4

Hyperlipidosis E75.6
- hereditary NEC E75.5

Hyperlipoproteinemia E78.5
- Fredrickson's type
  - I E78.3
  - IIa E78.00
  - IIb E78.2
  - III E78.2
  - IV E78.1
  - V E78.3
- low-density-lipoprotein-type (LDL) E78.00
- very-low-density-lipoprotein-type (VLDL) E78.1

Hyperlucent lung, unilateral J43.0

Hyperlysinemia E72.3

Hypermagnesemia E83.41
- neonatal P71.8

Hypermenorrhea N92.0

Hypermethioninemia E72.19

Hypermetropia (congenital) H52.0 ☑

Hypermobility, hypermotility
- cecum — *see* Syndrome, irritable bowel
- coccyx — *see* subcategory M53.2
- colon — *see* Syndrome, irritable bowel
  - psychogenic F45.8
- ileum K58.9
- intestine (*see also* Syndrome, irritable bowel)K58.9
  - psychogenic F45.8
- meniscus (knee) — *see* Derangement, knee, meniscus
- scapula — *see* Instability, joint, shoulder
- stomach K31.89
  - psychogenic F45.8
- syndrome M35.7
- urethra N36.41
  - with intrinsic sphincter deficiency N36.43

Hypernasality R49.21

Hypernatremia E87.0

Hypernephroma C64. ☑

Hyperopia — *see* Hypermetropia

Hyperorexia nervosa F50.2

Hyperornithinemia E72.4

Hyperosmia R43.1

Hyperosmolality E87.0

Hyperostosis (monomelic) (*see also* Disorder, bone, density and structure, specified NEC)
- ankylosing (spine) M48.10
  - cervical region M48.12
  - cervicothoracic region M48.13
  - lumbar region M48.16
  - lumbosacral region M48.17
  - multiple sites M48.19
  - occipito-atlanto-axial region M48.11
  - sacrococcygeal region M48.18
  - thoracic region M48.14
  - thoracolumbar region M48.15
- cortical (skull) M85.2
  - infantile M89.8X ☑
- frontal, internal of skull M85.2
- interna frontalis M85.2
- skeletal, diffuse idiopathic — *see* Hyperostosis, ankylosing
- skull M85.2
  - congenital Q75.8
- vertebral, ankylosing — *see* Hyperostosis, ankylosing

Hyperovarism E28.8

Hyperoxaluria (primary) E72.53

Hyperparathyroidism E21.3
- primary E21.0
- secondary (renal) N25.81
  - non-renal E21.1
- specified NEC E21.2
- tertiary E21.2

Hyperpathia R20.8

Hyperperistalsis R19.2
- psychogenic F45.8

Hyperpermeability, capillary I78.8

Hyperphagia R63.2

Hyperphenylalaninemia NEC E70.1

Hyperphoria (alternating) H50.53

Hyperphosphatemia E83.39

Hyperpiesis, hyperpiesia — *see* Hypertension

Hyperpigmentation (*see also* Pigmentation)
- melanin NEC L81.4
- postinflammatory L81.0

Hyperpinealism E34.8

Hyperpituitarism E22.9

Hyperplasia, hyperplastic
- adenoids J35.2
- adrenal (capsule) (cortex) (gland) E27.8
  - with
    - sexual precocity (male) E25.9
      - congenital E25.0
    - virilism, adrenal E25.9
      - congenital E25.0
    - virilization (female) E25.9
      - congenital E25.0
  - congenital E25.0
    - salt-losing E25.0
- adrenomedullary E27.5
- angiolymphoid, eosinophilia (ALHE) D18.01
- appendix (lymphoid) K38.0
- artery, fibromuscular I77.3
- bone (*see also* Hypertrophy, bone)
  - marrow D75.89
- breast (*see also* Hypertrophy, breast)
  - ductal (atypical) N60.9 ☑
- C-cell, thyroid E07.0
- cementation (tooth) (teeth) K03.4
- cervical gland R59.0
- cervix (uteri) (basal cell) (endometrium) (polypoid) (*see also* Dysplasia, cervix)
  - congenital Q51.828
- clitoris, congenital Q52.6
- denture K06.2
- endocervicitis N72
- endometrium, endometrial (adenomatous) (benign) (cystic) (glandular) (glandular-cystic) (polypoid) N85.00
  - with atypia N85.02
  - cervix — *see* Dysplasia, cervix
  - complex (without atypia) N85.01
  - simple (without atypia) N85.01
- epithelial L85.9
  - focal, oral, including tongue K13.29
  - nipple N62
  - skin L85.9
  - tongue K13.29
  - vaginal wall N89.3
- erythroid D75.89

Hyperplasia - Hypertension

- **Hyperplasia** — *continued*
  - fibromuscular of artery (carotid) (renal) I77.3
  - genital
    - female NEC N94.89
    - male N50.89
  - gingiva K06.1
  - glandularis cystica uteri (interstitialis) (*see also* Hyperplasia, endometrial)N85.00
  - gum K06.1
  - hymen, congenital Q52.4
  - irritative, edentulous (alveolar) K06.2
  - jaw M26.09
    - alveolar M26.79
    - lower M26.03
      - alveolar M26.72
    - upper M26.01
      - alveolar M26.71
  - kidney (congenital) Q63.3
  - labia N90.69
    - epithelial N90.3
  - liver (congenital) Q44.7
    - nodular, focal K76.89
  - lymph gland or node R59.9
  - mandible, mandibular M26.03
    - alveolar M26.72
    - unilateral condylar M27.8
  - maxilla, maxillary M26.01
    - alveolar M26.71
  - myometrium, myometrial N85.2
  - neuroendocrine cell, of infancy J84.841
  - nose
    - lymphoid J34.89
    - polypoid J33.9
  - oral mucosa (irritative) K13.6
  - organ or site, congenital NEC — *see* Anomaly, by site
  - ovary N83.8
  - palate, papillary (irritative) K13.6
  - pancreatic islet cells E16.9
    - alpha E16.8
      - with excess
        - gastrin E16.4
        - glucagon E16.3
    - beta E16.1
  - parathyroid (gland) E21.0
  - pharynx (lymphoid) J39.2
  - prostate (adenofibromatous) (nodular) N40.0
    - with lower urinary tract symptoms (LUTS) N40.1
    - without lower urinary tract symptoms (LUTS) N40.0
  - renal artery I77.89
  - reticulo-endothelial (cell) D75.89
  - salivary gland (any) K11.1
  - Schimmelbusch's — *see* Mastopathy, cystic
  - suprarenal capsule (gland) E27.8
  - thymus (gland) (persistent) E32.0
  - thyroid (gland) — *see* Goiter
  - tonsils (faucial) (infective) (lingual) (lymphoid) J35.1
    - with adenoids J35.3
  - unilateral condylar M27.8
  - uterus, uterine N85.2
    - endometrium (glandular) (*see also* Hyperplasia, endometrial)N85.00
  - vulva N90.69
    - epithelial N90.3
- **Hyperpnea** — *see* Hyperventilation
- **Hyperpotassemia** E87.5
- **Hyperprebetalipoproteinemia** (familial) E78.1
- **Hyperprolactinemia** E22.1
- **Hyperprolinemia** (type I) (type II) E72.59
- **Hyperproteinemia** E88.09
- **Hyperprothrombinemia,** causing coagulation factor deficiency D68.4
- **Hyperpyrexia** R50.9
  - heat (effects) T67.0 ☑
  - malignant, due to anesthetic T88.3 ☑
  - rheumatic — *see* Fever, rheumatic
  - unknown origin R50.9
- **Hyper-reflexia** R29.2
- **Hypersalivation** K11.7
- **Hypersecretion**
  - ACTH (not associated with Cushing's syndrome) E27.0
    - pituitary E24.0
  - adrenaline E27.5
  - adrenomedullary E27.5
  - androgen (testicular) E29.0
    - ovarian (drug-induced) (iatrogenic) E28.1
  - calcitonin E07.0
  - catecholamine E27.5
- **Hypersecretion** — *continued*
  - corticoadrenal E24.9
  - cortisol E24.9
  - epinephrine E27.5
  - estrogen E28.0
  - gastric K31.89
    - psychogenic F45.8
  - gastrin E16.4
  - glucagon E16.3
  - hormone (s)
    - ACTH (not associated with Cushing's syndrome) E27.0
      - pituitary E24.0
    - antidiuretic E22.2
    - growth E22.0
    - intestinal NEC E34.1
    - ovarian androgen E28.1
    - pituitary E22.9
    - testicular E29.0
    - thyroid stimulating E05.80
      - with thyroid storm E05.81
  - insulin — *see* Hyperinsulinism
  - lacrimal glands — *see* Epiphora
  - medulloadrenal E27.5
  - milk O92.6
  - ovarian androgens E28.1
  - salivary gland (any) K11.7
  - thyrocalcitonin E07.0
  - upper respiratory J39.8
- **Hypersegmentation,** leukocytic, hereditary D72.0
- **Hypersensitive,** hypersensitiveness, hypersensitivity (*see also* Allergy)
  - carotid sinus G90.01
  - colon — *see* Irritable, colon
  - drug T88.7 ☑
  - gastrointestinal K52.29
    - immediate K52.29
    - psychogenic F45.8
  - labyrinth — *see* subcategory H83.2
  - pain R20.8
  - pneumonitis — *see* Pneumonitis, allergic
  - reaction T78.40 ☑
    - upper respiratory tract NEC J39.3
- **Hypersomnia** (organic) G47.10
  - due to
    - alcohol
      - abuse F10.182
      - dependence F10.282
      - use F10.982
    - amphetamines
      - abuse F15.182
      - dependence F15.282
      - use F15.982
    - caffeine
      - abuse F15.182
      - dependence F15.282
      - use F15.982
    - cocaine
      - abuse F14.182
      - dependence F14.282
      - use F14.982
    - drug NEC
      - abuse F19.182
      - dependence F19.282
      - use F19.982
    - medical condition G47.14
    - mental disorder F51.13
    - opioid
      - abuse F11.182
      - dependence F11.282
      - use F11.982
    - psychoactive substance NEC
      - abuse F19.182
      - dependence F19.282
      - use F19.982
    - sedative, hypnotic, or anxiolytic
      - abuse F13.182
      - dependence F13.282
      - use F13.982
    - stimulant NEC
      - abuse F15.182
      - dependence F15.282
      - use F15.982
  - idiopathic G47.11
    - with long sleep time G47.11
    - without long sleep time G47.12
  - menstrual related G47.13
  - nonorganic origin F51.11
    - specified NEC F51.19
  - not due to a substance or known physiological condition F51.11
    - specified NEC F51.19
- **Hypersomnia** — *continued*
  - primary F51.11
  - recurrent G47.13
  - specified NEC G47.19
- **Hypersplenia,** hypersplenism D73.1
- **Hyperstimulation,** ovaries (associated with induced ovulation) N98.1
- **Hypersusceptibility** — *see* Allergy
- **Hypertelorism** (ocular) (orbital) Q75.2
- **Hypertension,** hypertensive (accelerated) (benign) (essential) (idiopathic) (malignant) (systemic) I10
  - with
    - heart involvement (conditions in I51.4- I51.9 due to hypertension) — *see* Hypertension, heart
    - kidney involvement — *see* Hypertension, kidney
  - benign, intracranial G93.2
  - borderline R03.0
  - cardiorenal (disease) I13.10
    - with heart failure I13.0
      - with stage 1 through stage 4 chronic kidney disease I13.0
      - with stage 5 or end stage renal disease I13.2
    - without heart failure I13.10
      - with stage 1 through stage 4 chronic kidney disease I13.10
      - with stage 5 or end stage renal disease I13.11
  - cardiovascular
    - disease (arteriosclerotic) (sclerotic) — *see* Hypertension, heart
    - renal (disease) — *see* Hypertension, cardiorenal
  - chronic venous — *see* Hypertension, venous (chronic)
  - complicating
    - childbirth (labor) O16.4
      - pre-existing O10.92
        - with
          - heart disease O10.12
            - with renal disease O10.32
          - pre-eclampsia O11.4
          - renal disease O10.22
            - with heart disease O10.32
        - essential O10.02
      - secondary O10.42
    - pregnancy O16. ☑
      - with edema (*see also* Pre-eclampsia)O14.9 ☑
      - gestational (pregnancy induced) (without proteinuria) O13. ☑
        - with proteinuria O14.9 ☑
          - mild pre-eclampsia O14.0 ☑
          - moderate pre-eclampsia O14.0 ☑
          - severe pre-eclampsia O14.1 ☑
            - with hemolysis, elevated liver enzymes and low platelet count (HELLP) O14.2 ☑
      - pre-existing O10.91 ☑
        - with
          - heart disease O10.11 ☑
            - with renal disease O10.31 ☑
          - pre-eclampsia O11
          - renal disease O10.21 ☑
            - with heart disease O10.31 ☑
        - essential O10.01 ☑
        - secondary O10.41 ☑
      - transient O13. ☑
    - puerperium, pre-existing O16.5
      - pre-existing
        - with
          - heart disease O10.13
            - with renal disease O10.33
          - pre-eclampsia O11.5
          - renal disease O10.23
            - with heart disease O10.33
        - essential O10.03
      - pregnancy-induced O13.9
      - secondary O10.43
  - crisis I16.9
  - due to
    - endocrine disorders I15.2
    - pheochromocytoma I15.2
    - renal disorders NEC I15.1
      - arterial I15.0
    - renovascular disorders I15.0
    - specified disease NEC I15.8
  - emergency I16.2
  - encephalopathy I67.4
  - gestational (without significant proteinuria) (pregnancy-induced) (transient) O13. ☑
    - with significant proteinuria — *see* Pre-eclampsia
    - complicating
      - delivery O13.4
      - puerperium O13.5

Hypertension — *continued*
- Goldblatt's I70.1
- heart (disease) (conditions in I51.4-I51.9 due to hypertension) I11.9
  - with
    - heart failure (congestive) I11.0
    - kidney disease (chronic) — *see* Hypertension, cardiorenal
- intracranial (benign) G93.2
- kidney I12.9
  - with
    - heart disease — *see* Hypertension, cardiorenal
    - stage 5 chronic kidney disease (CKD) or end stage renal disease (ESRD) I12.0
    - stage 1 through stage 4 chronic kidney disease I12.9
- lesser circulation I27.0
- maternal O16. ☑
- newborn P29.2
  - pulmonary (persistent) P29.3
- ocular H40.05 ☑
- pancreatic duct - code to underlying condition
  - with chronic pancreatitis K86.1
- portal (due to chronic liver disease) (idiopathic) K76.6
  - gastropathy K31.89
  - in (due to) schistosomiasis (bilharziasis) B65.9 *[K77]*
- postoperative I97.3
- psychogenic F45.8
- pulmonary (artery) (secondary) NEC I27.2
  - with
    - cor pulmonale (chronic) I27.2
      - acute I26.09
    - right heart ventricular strain/failure I27.2
      - acute I26.09
  - of newborn (persistent) P29.3
  - primary (idiopathic) I27.0
- renal — *see* Hypertension, kidney
- renovascular I15.0
- secondary NEC I15.9
  - due to
    - endocrine disorders I15.2
    - pheochromocytoma I15.2
    - renal disorders NEC I15.1
      - arterial I15.0
    - renovascular disorders I15.0
  - specified NEC I15.8
- transient, of pregnancy O13. ☑
- urgency I16.0
- venous (chronic)
  - due to
    - deep vein thrombosis — *see* Syndrome, postthrombotic
  - idiopathic I87.309
    - with
      - inflammation I87.32 ☑
        - with ulcer I87.33 ☑
      - specified complication NEC I87.39 ☑
      - ulcer I87.31 ☑
        - with inflammation I87.33 ☑
    - asymptomatic I87.30 ☑

Hypertensive urgency — *see* Hypertension

Hyperthecosis ovary E28.8

Hyperthermia (of unknown origin) (*see also* Hyperpyrexia)
- malignant, due to anesthesia T88.3 ☑
- newborn P81.9
  - environmental P81.0

Hyperthyroid (recurrent) — *see* Hyperthyroidism

Hyperthyroidism (latent) (pre-adult) (recurrent) E05.90
- with
  - goiter (diffuse) E05.00
    - with thyroid storm E05.01
    - nodular (multinodular) E05.20
      - with thyroid storm E05.21
      - uninodular E05.10
        - with thyroid storm E05.11
  - storm E05.91
- due to ectopic thyroid tissue E05.30
  - with thyroid storm E05.31
- neonatal, transitory P72.1
- specified NEC E05.80
  - with thyroid storm E05.81

Hypertony, hypertonia, hypertonicity
- bladder N31.8
- congenital P94.1
- stomach K31.89
  - psychogenic F45.8

Hypertony — *continued*
- uterus, uterine (contractions) (complicating delivery) O62.4

Hypertrichosis L68.9
- congenital Q84.2
- eyelid H02.869
  - left H02.866
    - lower H02.865
    - upper H02.864
  - right H02.863
    - lower H02.862
    - upper H02.861
- lanuginosa Q84.2
  - acquired L68.1
- localized L68.2
- specified NEC L68.8

Hypertriglyceridemia, essential E78.1

Hypertrophy, hypertrophic
- adenofibromatous, prostate — *see* Enlargement, enlarged, prostate
- adenoids (infective) J35.2
  - with tonsils J35.3
- adrenal cortex E27.8
- alveolar process or ridge — *see* Anomaly, alveolar
- anal papillae K62.89
- artery I77.89
  - congenital NEC Q27.8
    - digestive system Q27.8
    - lower limb Q27.8
    - specified site NEC Q27.8
    - upper limb Q27.8
- auricular — *see* Hypertrophy, cardiac
- Bartholin's gland N75.8
- bile duct (common) (hepatic) K83.8
- bladder (sphincter) (trigone) N32.89
- bone M89.30
  - carpus M89.34 ☑
  - clavicle M89.31 ☑
  - femur M89.35 ☑
  - fibula M89.36 ☑
  - finger M89.34 ☑
  - humerus M89.32 ☑
  - ilium M89.359
  - ischium M89.359
  - metacarpus M89.34 ☑
  - metatarsus M89.37 ☑
  - multiple sites M89.39
  - neck M89.38
  - radius M89.33 ☑
  - rib M89.38
  - scapula M89.31 ☑
  - skull M89.38
  - tarsus M89.37 ☑
  - tibia M89.36 ☑
  - toe M89.37 ☑
  - ulna M89.33 ☑
  - vertebra M89.38
- brain G93.89
- breast N62
  - cystic — *see* Mastopathy, cystic
  - newborn P83.4
  - pubertal, massive N62
  - puerperal, postpartum — *see* Disorder, breast, specified type NEC
  - senile (parenchymatous) N62
- cardiac (chronic) (idiopathic) I51.7
  - with rheumatic fever (conditions in I00)
    - active I01.8
    - inactive or quiescent (with chorea) I09.89
  - congenital NEC Q24.8
  - fatty — *see* Degeneration, myocardial
  - hypertensive — *see* Hypertension, heart
  - rheumatic (with chorea) I09.89
    - active or acute I01.8
      - with chorea I02.0
  - valve — *see* Endocarditis
- cartilage — *see* Disorder, cartilage, specified type NEC
- cecum — *see* Megacolon
- cervix (uteri) N88.8
  - congenital Q51.828
  - elongation N88.4
- clitoris (cirrhotic) N90.89
  - congenital Q52.6
- colon (*see also* Megacolon)
  - congenital Q43.2
- conjunctiva, lymphoid H11.89
- corpora cavernosa N48.89
- cystic duct K82.8
- duodenum K31.89
- endometrium (glandular) (*see also* Hyperplasia, endometrial)N85.00
  - cervix N88.8

Hypertrophy — *continued*
- epididymis N50.89
- esophageal hiatus (congenital) Q79.1
  - with hernia — *see* Hernia, hiatal
- eyelid — *see* Disorder, eyelid, specified type NEC
- fat pad E65
  - knee (infrapatellar) (popliteal) (prepatellar) (retropatellar) M79.4
- foot (congenital) Q74.2
- frenulum, frenum (tongue) K14.8
  - lip K13.0
- gallbladder K82.8
- gastric mucosa K29.60
  - with bleeding K29.61
- gland, glandular R59.9
  - generalized R59.1
  - localized R59.0
- gum (mucous membrane) K06.1
- heart (idiopathic) (*see also* Hypertrophy, cardiac)
  - valve (*see also* Endocarditis)I38
- hemifacial Q67.4
- hepatic — *see* Hypertrophy, liver
- hiatus (esophageal) Q79.1
- hilus gland R59.0
- hymen, congenital Q52.4
- ileum K63.89
- intestine NEC K63.89
- jejunum K63.89
- kidney (compensatory) N28.81
  - congenital Q63.3
- labium (majus) (minus) N90.60
- ligament — *see* Disorder, ligament
- lingual tonsil (infective) J35.1
  - with adenoids J35.3
- lip K13.0
  - congenital Q18.6
- liver R16.0
  - acute K76.89
  - congenital Q44.7
  - cirrhotic — *see* Cirrhosis, liver
  - fatty — *see* Fatty, liver
- lymph, lymphatic gland R59.9
  - generalized R59.1
  - localized R59.0
  - tuberculous — *see* Tuberculosis, lymph gland
- mammary gland — *see* Hypertrophy, breast
- Meckel's diverticulum (congenital) Q43.0
  - malignant — *see* Table of Neoplasms, small intestine, malignant
- median bar — *see* Hyperplasia, prostate
- meibomian gland — *see* Chalazion
- meniscus, knee, congenital Q74.1
- metatarsal head — *see* Hypertrophy, bone, metatarsus
- metatarsus — *see* Hypertrophy, bone, metatarsus
- mucous membrane
  - alveolar ridge K06.2
  - gum K06.1
  - nose (turbinate) J34.3
- muscle M62.89
- muscular coat, artery I77.89
- myocardium (*see also* Hypertrophy, cardiac)
  - idiopathic I42.2
- myometrium N85.2
- nail L60.2
  - congenital Q84.5
- nasal J34.89
  - alae J34.89
  - bone J34.89
  - cartilage J34.89
  - mucous membrane (septum) J34.3
  - sinus J34.89
  - turbinate J34.3
- nasopharynx, lymphoid (infectional) (tissue) (wall) J35.2
- nipple N62
- organ or site, congenital NEC — *see* Anomaly, by site
- ovary N83.8
- palate (hard) M27.8
  - soft K13.79
- pancreas, congenital Q45.3
- parathyroid (gland) E21.0
- parotid gland K11.1
- penis N48.89
- pharyngeal tonsil J35.2
- pharynx J39.2
  - lymphoid (infectional) (tissue) (wall) J35.2
- pituitary (anterior) (fossa) (gland) E23.6
- prepuce (congenital) N47.8
  - female N90.89
- prostate — *see* Enlargement, enlarged, prostate
  - congenital Q55.4

Hypertrophy — *continued*
- pseudomuscular G71.0
- pylorus (adult) (muscle) (sphincter) K31.1
  - congenital or infantile Q40.0
- rectal, rectum (sphincter) K62.89
- rhinitis (turbinate) J31.0
- salivary gland (any) K11.1
  - congenital Q38.4
- scaphoid (tarsal) — *see* Hypertrophy, bone, tarsus
- scar L91.0
- scrotum N50.89
- seminal vesicle N50.89
- sigmoid — *see* Megacolon
- skin L91.9
  - specified NEC L91.8
- spermatic cord N50.89
- spleen — *see* Splenomegaly
- spondylitis — *see* Spondylosis
- stomach K31.89
- sublingual gland K11.1
- submandibular gland K11.1
- suprarenal cortex (gland) E27.8
- synovial NEC M67.20
  - acromioclavicular M67.21 ☑
  - ankle M67.27 ☑
  - elbow M67.22 ☑
  - foot M67.27 ☑
  - hand M67.24 ☑
  - hip M67.25 ☑
  - knee M67.26 ☑
  - multiple sites M67.29
  - specified site NEC M67.28
  - wrist M67.23 ☑
- tendon — *see* Disorder, tendon, specified type NEC
- testis N44.8
  - congenital Q55.29
- thymic, thymus (gland) (congenital) E32.0
- thyroid (gland) — *see* Goiter
- toe (congenital) Q74.2
  - acquired (*see also* Deformity, toe, specified NEC)
- tongue K14.8
  - congenital Q38.2
  - papillae (foliate) K14.3
- tonsils (faucial) (infective) (lingual) (lymphoid) J35.1
  - with adenoids J35.3
- tunica vaginalis N50.89
- ureter N28.89
- urethra N36.8
- uterus N85.2
  - neck (with elongation) N88.4
  - puerperal O90.89
- uvula K13.79
- vagina N89.8
- vas deferens N50.89
- vein I87.8
- ventricle, ventricular (heart) (*see also* Hypertrophy, cardiac)
  - congenital Q24.8
  - in tetralogy of Fallot Q21.3
- verumontanum N36.8
- vocal cord J38.3
- vulva N90.60
  - stasis (nonfilarial) N90.69

Hypertropia H50.2 ☑
Hypertyrosinemia E70.21
Hyperuricemia (asymptomatic) E79.0
Hypervalinemia E71.19
Hyperventilation (tetany) R06.4
- hysterical F45.8
- psychogenic F45.8
- syndrome F45.8

Hypervitaminosis (dietary) NEC E67.8
- A E67.0
  - administered as drug (prolonged intake) — *see* Table of Drugs and Chemicals, vitamins, adverse effect
  - overdose or wrong substance given or taken — *see* Table of Drugs and Chemicals, vitamins, poisoning
- B6 E67.2
- D E67.3
  - administered as drug (prolonged intake) — *see* Table of Drugs and Chemicals, vitamins, adverse effect
  - overdose or wrong substance given or taken — *see* Table of Drugs and Chemicals, vitamins, poisoning
- K E67.8

Hypervitaminosis — *continued*
- K — *continued*
  - administered as drug (prolonged intake) — *see* Table of Drugs and Chemicals, vitamins, adverse effect
  - overdose or wrong substance given or taken — *see* Table of Drugs and Chemicals, vitamins, poisoning

Hypervolemia E87.70
- specified NEC E87.79

Hypesthesia R20.1
- cornea — *see* Anesthesia, cornea

Hyphema H21.0 ☑
- traumatic S05.1 ☑

Hypoacidity, gastric K31.89
- psychogenic F45.8

Hypoadrenalism, hypoadrenia E27.40
- primary E27.1
- tuberculous A18.7

Hypoadrenocorticism E27.40
- pituitary E23.0
- primary E27.1

Hypoalbuminemia E88.09
Hypoaldosteronism E27.40
Hypoalphalipoproteinemia E78.6
Hypobarism T70.29 ☑
Hypobaropathy T70.29 ☑
Hypobetalipoproteinemia (familial) E78.6
Hypocalcemia E83.51
- dietary E58
- neonatal P71.1
  - due to cow's milk P71.0
- phosphate-loading (newborn) P71.1

Hypochloremia E87.8
Hypochlorhydria K31.89
- neurotic F45.8
- psychogenic F45.8

Hypochondria, hypochondriac, hypochondriasis (reaction) F45.21
- sleep F51.03

Hypochondrogenesis Q77.0
Hypochondroplasia Q77.4
Hypochromasia, blood cells D50.8
Hypodontia — *see* Anodontia
Hypoeosinophilia D72.89
Hypoesthesia R20.1
Hypofibrinogenemia D68.8
- acquired D65
- congenital (hereditary) D68.2

Hypofunction
- adrenocortical E27.40
  - drug-induced E27.3
  - postprocedural E89.6
  - primary E27.1
- adrenomedullary, postprocedural E89.6
- cerebral R29.818
- corticoadrenal NEC E27.40
- intestinal K59.8
- labyrinth — *see* subcategory H83.2
- ovary E28.39
- pituitary (gland) (anterior) E23.0
- testicular E29.1
  - postprocedural (postsurgical) (postirradiation) (iatrogenic) E89.5

Hypogalactia O92.4
Hypogammaglobulinemia (*see also* Agammaglobulinemia)D80.1
- hereditary D80.0
- nonfamilial D80.1
- transient, of infancy D80.7

Hypogenitalism (congenital) — *see* Hypogonadism
Hypoglossia Q38.3
Hypoglycemia (spontaneous) E16.2
- coma E15
  - diabetic — *see* Diabetes, coma
- diabetic — *see* Diabetes, hypoglycemia
- dietary counseling and surveillance Z71.3
- drug-induced E16.0
  - with coma (nondiabetic) E15
- due to insulin E16.0
  - with coma (nondiabetic) E15
  - therapeutic misadventure — *see* subcategory T38.3
- functional, nonhyperinsulinemic E16.1
- iatrogenic E16.0
  - with coma (nondiabetic) E15
- in infant of diabetic mother P70.1
  - gestational diabetes P70.0
- infantile E16.1
- leucine-induced E71.19
- neonatal (transitory) P70.4
  - iatrogenic P70.3

Hypoglycemia — *continued*
- reactive (not drug-induced) E16.1
- transitory neonatal P70.4

Hypogonadism
- female E28.39
- hypogonadotropic E23.0
- male E29.1
- ovarian (primary) E28.39
- pituitary E23.0
- testicular (primary) E29.1

Hypohidrosis, hypoidrosis L74.4
Hypoinsulinemia, postprocedural E89.1
Hypokalemia E87.6
Hypoleukocytosis — *see* Agranulocytosis
Hypolipoproteinemia (alpha) (beta) E78.6
Hypomagnesemia E83.42
- neonatal P71.2

Hypomania, hypomanic reaction F30.8
Hypomenorrhea — *see* Oligomenorrhea
Hypometabolism R63.8
Hypomotility
- gastrointestinal (tract) K31.89
  - psychogenic F45.8
- intestine K59.8
  - psychogenic F45.8
- stomach K31.89
  - psychogenic F45.8

Hyponasality R49.22
Hyponatremia E87.1
Hypo-osmolality E87.1
Hypo-ovarianism, hypo-ovarism E28.39
Hypoparathyroidism E20.9
- familial E20.8
- idiopathic E20.0
- neonatal, transitory P71.4
- postprocedural E89.2
- specified NEC E20.8

Hypoperfusion (in)
- newborn P96.89

Hypopharyngitis — *see* Laryngopharyngitis
Hypophoria H50.53
Hypophosphatemia, hypophosphatasia (acquired) (congenital) (renal) E83.39
- familial E83.31

Hypophyseal, hypophysis (*see also* condition)
- dwarfism E23.0
- gigantism E22.0

Hypopiesis — *see* Hypotension
Hypopinealism E34.8
Hypopituitarism (juvenile) E23.0
- drug-induced E23.1
- due to
  - hypophysectomy E89.3
  - radiotherapy E89.3
- iatrogenic NEC E23.1
- postirradiation E89.3
- postpartum O99.285
- postprocedural E89.3

Hypoplasia, hypoplastic
- adrenal (gland), congenital Q89.1
- alimentary tract, congenital Q45.8
  - upper Q40.8
- anus, anal (canal) Q42.3
  - with fistula Q42.2
- aorta, aortic Q25.42
  - ascending, in hypoplastic left heart syndrome Q23.4
  - valve Q23.1
    - in hypoplastic left heart syndrome Q23.4
- areola, congenital Q83.8
- arm (congenital) — *see* Defect, reduction, upper limb
- artery (peripheral) Q27.8
  - brain (congenital) Q28.3
  - coronary Q24.5
  - digestive system Q27.8
  - lower limb Q27.8
  - pulmonary Q25.79
    - functional, unilateral J43.0
  - retinal (congenital) Q14.1
  - specified site NEC Q27.8
  - umbilical Q27.0
  - upper limb Q27.8
- auditory canal Q17.8
  - causing impairment of hearing Q16.9
- biliary duct or passage Q44.5
- bone NOS Q79.9
  - face Q75.8
  - marrow D61.9
    - megakaryocytic D69.49
  - skull — *see* Hypoplasia, skull

- **Hypoplasia** — *continued*
  - brain Q02
    - gyri Q04.3
    - part of Q04.3
  - breast (areola) N64.82
  - bronchus Q32.4
  - cardiac Q24.8
  - carpus — *see* Defect, reduction, upper limb, specified type NEC
  - cartilage hair Q78.8
  - cecum Q42.8
  - cementum K00.4
  - cephalic Q02
  - cerebellum Q04.3
  - cervix (uteri), congenital Q51.821
  - clavicle (congenital) Q74.0
  - coccyx Q76.49
  - colon Q42.9
    - specified NEC Q42.8
  - corpus callosum Q04.0
  - cricoid cartilage Q31.2
  - digestive organ (s) or tract NEC Q45.8
    - upper (congenital) Q40.8
  - ear (auricle) (lobe) Q17.2
    - middle Q16.4
  - enamel of teeth (neonatal) (postnatal) (prenatal) K00.4
  - endocrine (gland) NEC Q89.2
  - endometrium N85.8
  - epididymis (congenital) Q55.4
  - epiglottis Q31.2
  - erythroid, congenital D61.01
  - esophagus (congenital) Q39.8
  - eustachian tube Q17.8
  - eye Q11.2
  - eyelid (congenital) Q10.3
  - face Q18.8
    - bone (s) Q75.8
  - femur (congenital) — *see* Defect, reduction, lower limb, specified type NEC
  - fibula (congenital) — *see* Defect, reduction, lower limb, specified type NEC
  - finger (congenital) — *see* Defect, reduction, upper limb, specified type NEC
  - focal dermal Q82.8
  - foot — *see* Defect, reduction, lower limb, specified type NEC
  - gallbladder Q44.0
  - genitalia, genital organ (s)
    - female, congenital Q52.8
      - external Q52.79
      - internal NEC Q52.8
    - in adiposogenital dystrophy E23.6
  - glottis Q31.2
  - hair Q84.2
  - hand (congenital) — *see* Defect, reduction, upper limb, specified type NEC
  - heart Q24.8
  - humerus (congenital) — *see* Defect, reduction, upper limb, specified type NEC
  - intestine (small) Q41.9
    - large Q42.9
      - specified NEC Q42.8
  - jaw M26.09
    - alveolar M26.79
    - lower M26.04
      - alveolar M26.74
    - upper M26.02
      - alveolar M26.73
  - kidney (s) Q60.5
    - bilateral Q60.4
    - unilateral Q60.3
  - labium (majus) (minus), congenital Q52.79
  - larynx Q31.2
  - left heart syndrome Q23.4
  - leg (congenital) — *see* Defect, reduction, lower limb
  - limb Q73.8
    - lower (congenital) — *see* Defect, reduction, lower limb
    - upper (congenital) — *see* Defect, reduction, upper limb
  - liver Q44.7
  - lung (lobe) (not associated with short gestation) Q33.6
    - associated with immaturity, low birth weight, prematurity, or short gestation P28.0
  - mammary (areola), congenital Q83.8
  - mandible, mandibular M26.04
    - alveolar M26.74
    - unilateral condylar M27.8
  - maxillary M26.02
    - alveolar M26.73
- **Hypoplasia** — *continued*
  - medullary D61.9
  - megakaryocytic D69.49
  - metacarpus — *see* Defect, reduction, upper limb, specified type NEC
  - metatarsus — *see* Defect, reduction, lower limb, specified type NEC
  - muscle Q79.8
  - nail (s) Q84.6
  - nose, nasal Q30.1
  - optic nerve H47.03 ☑
  - osseous meatus (ear) Q17.8
  - ovary, congenital Q50.39
  - pancreas Q45.0
  - parathyroid (gland) Q89.2
  - parotid gland Q38.4
  - patella Q74.1
  - pelvis, pelvic girdle Q74.2
  - penis (congenital) Q55.62
  - peripheral vascular system Q27.8
    - digestive system Q27.8
    - lower limb Q27.8
    - specified site NEC Q27.8
    - upper limb Q27.8
  - pituitary (gland) (congenital) Q89.2
  - pulmonary (not associated with short gestation) Q33.6
    - artery, functional J43.0
    - associated with short gestation P28.0
  - radioulnar — *see* Defect, reduction, upper limb, specified type NEC
  - radius — *see* Defect, reduction, upper limb
  - rectum Q42.1
    - with fistula Q42.0
  - respiratory system NEC Q34.8
  - rib Q76.6
  - right heart syndrome Q22.6
  - sacrum Q76.49
  - scapula Q74.0
  - scrotum Q55.1
  - shoulder girdle Q74.0
  - skin Q82.8
  - skull (bone) Q75.8
    - with
      - anencephaly Q00.0
      - encephalocele — *see* Encephalocele
      - hydrocephalus Q03.9
        - with spina bifida — *see* Spina bifida, by site, with hydrocephalus
      - microcephaly Q02
  - spinal (cord) (ventral horn cell) Q06.1
  - spine Q76.49
  - sternum Q76.7
  - tarsus — *see* Defect, reduction, lower limb, specified type NEC
  - testis Q55.1
  - thymic, with immunodeficiency D82.1
  - thymus (gland) Q89.2
    - with immunodeficiency D82.1
  - thyroid (gland) E03.1
    - cartilage Q31.2
  - tibiofibular (congenital) — *see* Defect, reduction, lower limb, specified type NEC
  - toe — *see* Defect, reduction, lower limb, specified type NEC
  - tongue Q38.3
  - Turner's K00.4
  - ulna (congenital) — *see* Defect, reduction, upper limb
  - umbilical artery Q27.0
  - unilateral condylar M27.8
  - ureter Q62.8
  - uterus, congenital Q51.811
  - vagina Q52.4
  - vascular NEC peripheral Q27.8
    - brain Q28.3
    - digestive system Q27.8
    - lower limb Q27.8
    - specified site NEC Q27.8
    - upper limb Q27.8
  - vein (s) (peripheral) Q27.8
    - brain Q28.3
    - digestive system Q27.8
    - great Q26.8
    - lower limb Q27.8
    - specified site NEC Q27.8
    - upper limb Q27.8
  - vena cava (inferior) (superior) Q26.8
  - vertebra Q76.49
  - vulva, congenital Q52.79
  - zonule (ciliary) Q12.8
- **Hypopotassemia** E87.6
- **Hypoproconvertinemia,** congenital (hereditary) D68.2
- **Hypoproteinemia** E77.8
- **Hypoprothrombinemia** (congenital) (hereditary) (idiopathic) D68.2
  - acquired D68.4
  - newborn, transient P61.6
- **Hypoptyalism** K11.7
- **Hypopyon** (eye) (anterior chamber) — *see* Iridocyclitis, acute, hypopyon
- **Hypopyrexia** R68.0
- **Hyporeflexia** R29.2
- **Hyposecretion**
  - ACTH E23.0
  - antidiuretic hormone E23.2
  - ovary E28.39
  - salivary gland (any) K11.7
  - vasopressin E23.2
- **Hyposegmentation,** leukocytic, hereditary D72.0
- **Hyposiderinemia** D50.9
- **Hypospadias** Q54.9
  - balanic Q54.0
  - coronal Q54.0
  - glandular Q54.0
  - penile Q54.1
  - penoscrotal Q54.2
  - perineal Q54.3
  - specified NEC Q54.8
- **Hypospermatogenesis** — *see* Oligospermia
- **Hyposplenism** D73.0
- **Hypostasis** pulmonary, passive — *see* Edema, lung
- **Hypostatic** — *see* condition
- **Hyposthenuria** N28.89
- **Hypotension** (arterial) (constitutional) I95.9
  - chronic I95.89
  - due to (of) hemodialysis I95.3
  - drug-induced I95.2
  - iatrogenic I95.89
  - idiopathic (permanent) I95.0
  - intracranial, following ventricular shunting (ventriculostomy) G97.2
  - intra-dialytic I95.3
  - maternal, syndrome (following labor and delivery) O26.5 ☑
  - neurogenic, orthostatic G90.3
  - orthostatic (chronic) I95.1
    - due to drugs I95.2
    - neurogenic G90.3
  - postoperative I95.81
  - postural I95.1
  - specified NEC I95.89
- **Hypothermia** (accidental) T68 ☑
  - due to anesthesia, anesthetic T88.51 ☑
  - low environmental temperature T68 ☑
  - neonatal P80.9
    - environmental (mild) NEC P80.8
    - mild P80.8
    - severe (chronic) (cold injury syndrome) P80.0
    - specified NEC P80.8
  - not associated with low environmental temperature R68.0
- **Hypothyroidism** (acquired) E03.9
  - congenital (without goiter) E03.1
    - with goiter (diffuse) E03.0
  - due to
    - exogenous substance NEC E03.2
    - iodine-deficiency, acquired E01.8
      - subclinical E02
    - irradiation therapy E89.0
    - medicament NEC E03.2
    - P-aminosalicylic acid (PAS) E03.2
    - phenylbutazone E03.2
    - resorcinol E03.2
    - sulfonamide E03.2
    - surgery E89.0
    - thiourea group drugs E03.2
  - iatrogenic NEC E03.2
  - iodine-deficiency (acquired) E01.8
    - congenital — *see* Syndrome, iodine- deficiency, congenital
    - subclinical E02
  - neonatal, transitory P72.2
  - postinfectious E03.3
  - postirradiation E89.0
  - postprocedural E89.0
  - postsurgical E89.0
  - specified NEC E03.8
  - subclinical, iodine-deficiency related E02
- **Hypotonia,** hypotonicity, hypotony
  - bladder N31.2
  - congenital (benign) P94.2
  - eye — *see* Disorder, globe, hypotony

Hypotrichosis - Immunodeficiency

Hypotrichosis — *see* Alopecia
Hypotropia H50.2 ☑
Hypoventilation R06.89
- congenital central alveolar G47.35
- sleep related
  - idiopathic nonobstructive alveolar G47.34
  - in conditions classified elsewhere G47.36

Hypovitaminosis — *see* Deficiency, vitamin
Hypovolemia E86.1
- surgical shock T81.19 ☑
- traumatic (shock) T79.4 ☑

Hypoxemia R09.02
- newborn P84
- sleep related, in conditions classified elsewhere G47.36

Hypoxia (*see also* Anoxia)R09.02
- cerebral, during a procedure NEC G97.81
  - postprocedural NEC G97.82
- intrauterine P84
- myocardial — *see* Insufficiency, coronary
- newborn P84
- sleep-related G47.34

Hypsarhythmia — *see* Epilepsy, generalized, specified NEC
Hysteralgia, pregnant uterus O26.89 ☑
Hysteria, hysterical (conversion) (dissociative state) F44.9
- anxiety F41.8
- convulsions F44.5
- psychosis, acute F44.9

Hysteroepilepsy F44.5

I

IBDU (colonic inflammatory bowel disease unclassified) K52.3
Ichthyoparasitism due to Vandellia cirrhosa B88.8
Ichthyosis (congenital) Q80.9
- acquired L85.0
- fetalis Q80.4
- hystrix Q80.8
- lamellar Q80.2
- lingual K13.29
- palmaris and plantaris Q82.8
- simplex Q80.0
- vera Q80.8
- vulgaris Q80.0
- X-linked Q80.1

Ichthyotoxism — *see* Poisoning, fish
- bacterial — *see* Intoxication, food-borne

Icteroanemia, hemolytic (acquired) D59.9
- congenital — *see* Spherocytosis

Icterus (*see also* Jaundice)
- conjunctiva R17
- newborn P59.9
- gravis, newborn P55.0
- hematogenous (acquired) D59.9
- hemolytic (acquired) D59.9
  - congenital — *see* Spherocytosis
- hemorrhagic (acute) (leptospiral) (spirochetal) A27.0
  - newborn P53
- infectious B15.9
  - with hepatic coma B15.0
  - leptospiral A27.0
  - spirochetal A27.0
- neonatorum — *see* Jaundice, newborn
- spirochetal A27.0

Ictus solaris, solis T67.0 ☑
Ideation
- homicidal R45.850
- suicidal R45.851

Identity disorder (child) F64.9
- gender role F64.2
- psychosexual F64.2

Id reaction (due to bacteria) L30.2
Idioglossia F80.0
Idiopathic — *see* condition
Idiot, idiocy (congenital) F73
- amaurotic (Bielschowsky (-Jansky)) (family) (infantile (late)) (juvenile (late)) (Vogt-Spielmeyer) E75.4
- microcephalic Q02

IgE asthma J45.909
IIAC (idiopathic infantile arterial calcification) Q28.8
Ileitis (chronic) (noninfectious) (*see also* Enteritis)K52.9
- backwash — *see* Pancolitis, ulcerative (chronic)
- infectious A09

Ileitis — *continued*
- regional (ulcerative) — *see* Enteritis, regional, small intestine
- segmental — *see* Enteritis, regional
- terminal (ulcerative) — *see* Enteritis, regional, small intestine

Ileocolitis (*see also* Enteritis)K52.9
- regional — *see* Enteritis, regional
- infectious A09

Ileostomy
- attention to Z43.2
- malfunctioning K94.13
- status Z93.2
  - with complication — *see* Complications, enterostomy

Ileotyphus — *see* Typhoid
Ileum — *see* condition
Ileus (bowel) (colon) (inhibitory) (intestine) K56.7
- adynamic K56.0
- due to gallstone (in intestine) K56.3
- duodenal (chronic) K31.5
- gallstone K56.3
- mechanical NEC K56.69
- meconium P76.0
  - in cystic fibrosis E84.11
  - meaning meconium plug (without cystic fibrosis) P76.0
- myxedema K59.8
- neurogenic K56.0
  - Hirschsprung's disease or megacolon Q43.1
- newborn
  - due to meconium P76.0
    - in cystic fibrosis E84.11
    - meaning meconium plug (without cystic fibrosis) P76.0
  - transitory P76.1
- obstructive K56.69
- paralytic K56.0

Iliac — *see* condition
Iliotibial band syndrome M76.3 ☑
Illiteracy Z55.0
Illness (*see also* Disease)R69
- manic-depressive — *see* Disorder, bipolar

Imbalance R26.89
- autonomic G90.8
- constituents of food intake E63.1
- electrolyte E87.8
  - with
    - abortion — *see* Abortion by type, complicated by, electrolyte imbalance
    - molar pregnancy O08.5
  - due to hyperemesis gravidarum O21.1
  - following ectopic or molar pregnancy O08.5
  - neonatal, transitory NEC P74.4
    - potassium P74.3
    - sodium P74.2
- endocrine E34.9
- eye muscle NOS H50.9
- hormone E34.9
- hysterical F44.4
- labyrinth — *see* subcategory H83.2
- posture R29.3
- protein-energy — *see* Malnutrition
- sympathetic G90.8

Imbecile, imbecility (I.Q.35-49) F71
Imbedding, intrauterine device T83.39 ☑
Imbibition, cholesterol (gallbladder) K82.4
Imbrication, teeth,, fully erupted M26.30
Imerslund (-Gräsbeck) syndrome D51.1
Immature (*see also* Immaturity)
- birth (less than 37 completed weeks) — *see* Preterm, newborn
  - extremely (less than 28 completed weeks) — *see* Immaturity, extreme
- personality F60.89

Immaturity (less than 37 completed weeks) (*see also* Preterm, newborn)
- extreme of newborn (less than 28 completed weeks of gestation) (less than 196 completed days of gestation) (unspecified weeks of gestation) P07.20
  - gestational age
    - 23 completed weeks (23 weeks, 0 days through 23 weeks, 6 days) P07.22
    - 24 completed weeks (24 weeks, 0 days through 24 weeks, 6 days) P07.23
    - 25 completed weeks (25 weeks, 0 days through 25 weeks, 6 days) P07.24
    - 26 completed weeks (26 weeks, 0 days through 26 weeks, 6 days) P07.25
    - 27 completed weeks (27 weeks, 0 days through 27 weeks, 6 days) P07.26

Immaturity — *continued*
- extreme of newborn — *continued*
    - less than 23 completed weeks P07.21
- fetus or infant light-for-dates — *see* Light-for-dates
- lung, newborn P28.0
- organ or site NEC — *see* Hypoplasia
- pulmonary, newborn P28.0
- reaction F60.89
- sexual (female) (male), after puberty E30.0

Immersion T75.1 ☑
- hand T69.01 ☑
- foot T69.02 ☑

Immobile, immobility
- complete, due to severe physical disability or frailty R53.2
- intestine K59.8
- syndrome (paraplegic) M62.3

Immune reconstitution (inflammatory) syndrome [IRIS] D89.3
Immunization (*see also* Vaccination)
- ABO — *see* Incompatibility, ABO
  - in newborn P55.1
- complication — *see* Complications, vaccination
- encounter for Z23
- not done (not carried out) Z28.9
  - because (of)
    - acute illness of patient Z28.01
    - allergy to vaccine (or component) Z28.04
    - caregiver refusal Z28.82
    - chronic illness of patient Z28.02
    - contraindication NEC Z28.09
    - group pressure Z28.1
    - guardian refusal Z28.82
    - immune compromised state of patient Z28.03
    - parent refusal Z28.82
    - patient's belief Z28.1
    - patient had disease being vaccinated against Z28.81
    - patient refusal Z28.21
    - religious beliefs of patient Z28.1
    - specified reason NEC Z28.89
      - of patient Z28.29
    - unspecified patient reason Z28.20
- Rh factor
  - affecting management of pregnancy NEC O36.09 ☑
    - anti-D antibody O36.01 ☑
  - from transfusion — *see* Complication (s), transfusion, incompatibility reaction, Rh (factor)

Immunocytoma C83.0 ☑
Immunodeficiency D84.9
- with
  - adenosine-deaminase deficiency D81.3
  - antibody defects D80.9
    - specified type NEC D80.8
  - hyperimmunoglobulinemia D80.6
  - increased immunoglobulin M (IgM) D80.5
  - major defect D82.9
    - specified type NEC D82.8
  - partial albinism D82.8
  - short-limbed stature D82.2
  - thrombocytopenia and eczema D82.0
- antibody with
  - hyperimmunoglobulinemia D80.6
  - near-normal immunoglobulins D80.6
- autosomal recessive, Swiss type D80.0
- combined D81.9
  - biotin-dependent carboxylase D81.819
    - biotinidase D81.810
    - holocarboxylase synthetase D81.818
    - specified type NEC D81.818
  - severe (SCID) D81.9
    - with
      - low or normal B-cell numbers D81.2
      - low T- and B-cell numbers D81.1
      - reticular dysgenesis D81.0
  - specified type NEC D81.89
- common variable D83.9
  - with
    - abnormalities of B-cell numbers and function D83.0
    - autoantibodies to B- or T-cells D83.2
    - immunoregulatory T-cell disorders D83.1
  - specified type NEC D83.8
- following hereditary defective response to Epstein-Barr virus (EBV) D82.3
- selective, immunoglobulin
  - A (IgA) D80.2
  - G (IgG) (subclasses) D80.3
  - M (IgM) D80.4

- **Immunodeficiency** — *continued*
  - severe combined (SCID) D81.9
  - specified type NEC D84.8
  - X-linked, with increased IgM D80.5
- **Immunotherapy** (encounter for)
  - antineoplastic Z51.12
- **Impaction,** impacted
  - bowel, colon, rectum (*see also* Impaction, fecal)K56.49
    - by gallstone K56.3
  - calculus — *see* Calculus
  - cerumen (ear) (external) H61.2 ☑
  - cuspid — *see* Impaction, tooth
  - dental (same or adjacent tooth) K01.1
  - fecal, feces K56.41
  - fracture — *see* Fracture, by site
  - gallbladder — *see* Calculus, gallbladder
  - gallstone (s) — *see* Calculus, gallbladder
    - bile duct (common) (hepatic) — *see* Calculus, bile duct
    - cystic duct — *see* Calculus, gallbladder
    - in intestine, with obstruction (any part) K56.3
  - intestine (calculous) NEC (*see also* Impaction, fecal)K56.49
    - gallstone, with ileus K56.3
  - intrauterine device (IUD) T83.39 ☑
  - molar — *see* Impaction, tooth
  - shoulder, causing obstructed labor O66.0
  - tooth, teeth K01.1
  - turbinate J34.89
- **Impaired,** impairment (function)
  - auditory discrimination — *see* Abnormal, auditory perception
  - cognitive, mild, so stated G31.84
  - dual sensory Z73.82
  - fasting glucose R73.01
  - glucose tolerance (oral) R73.02
  - hearing — *see* Deafness
  - heart — *see* Disease, heart
  - kidney N28.9
    - disorder resulting from N25.9
      - specified NEC N25.89
  - liver K72.90
    - with coma K72.91
  - mastication K08.89
  - mild cognitive, so stated G31.84
  - mobility
    - ear ossicles — *see* Ankylosis, ear ossicles
    - requiring care provider Z74.09
  - myocardium, myocardial — *see* Insufficiency, myocardial
  - rectal sphincter R19.8
  - renal (acute) (chronic) N28.9
    - disorder resulting from N25.9
      - specified NEC N25.89
  - vision NEC H54.7
    - both eyes H54.3
- **Impediment,** speech R47.9
  - psychogenic (childhood) F98.8
  - slurring R47.81
  - specified NEC R47.89
- **Impending**
  - coronary syndrome I20.0
  - delirium tremens F10.239
  - myocardial infarction I20.0
- **Imperception** auditory (acquired) (*see also* Deafness)
  - congenital H93.25
- **Imperfect**
  - aeration, lung (newborn) NEC — *see* Atelectasis
  - closure (congenital)
    - alimentary tract NEC Q45.8
      - lower Q43.8
      - upper Q40.8
    - atrioventricular ostium Q21.2
    - atrium (secundum) Q21.1
    - branchial cleft or sinus Q18.0
    - choroid Q14.3
    - cricoid cartilage Q31.8
    - cusps, heart valve NEC Q24.8
      - pulmonary Q22.3
    - ductus
      - arteriosus Q25.0
      - Botalli Q25.0
    - ear drum (causing impairment of hearing) Q16.4
    - esophagus with communication to bronchus or trachea Q39.1
    - eyelid Q10.3
    - foramen
      - botalli Q21.1
      - ovale Q21.1
    - genitalia, genital organ (s) or system

- **Imperfect** — *continued*
  - closure — *continued*
      - female Q52.8
        - external Q52.79
        - internal NEC Q52.8
      - male Q55.8
    - glottis Q31.8
    - interatrial ostium or septum Q21.1
    - interauricular ostium or septum Q21.1
    - interventricular ostium or septum Q21.0
    - larynx Q31.8
    - lip — *see* Cleft, lip
    - nasal septum Q30.3
    - nose Q30.2
    - omphalomesenteric duct Q43.0
    - optic nerve entry Q14.2
    - organ or site not listed — *see* Anomaly, by site
    - ostium
      - interatrial Q21.1
      - interauricular Q21.1
      - interventricular Q21.0
    - palate — *see* Cleft, palate
    - preauricular sinus Q18.1
    - retina Q14.1
    - roof of orbit Q75.8
    - sclera Q13.5
    - septum
      - aorticopulmonary Q21.4
      - atrial (secundum) Q21.1
      - between aorta and pulmonary artery Q21.4
      - heart Q21.9
      - interatrial (secundum) Q21.1
      - interauricular (secundum) Q21.1
      - interventricular Q21.0
        - in tetralogy of Fallot Q21.3
      - nasal Q30.3
      - ventricular Q21.0
        - with pulmonary stenosis or atresia, dextraposition of aorta, and hypertrophy of right ventricle Q21.3
        - in tetralogy of Fallot Q21.3
    - skull Q75.0
      - with
        - anencephaly Q00.0
        - encephalocele — *see* Encephalocele
        - hydrocephalus Q03.9
          - with spina bifida — *see* Spina bifida, by site, with hydrocephalus
        - microcephaly Q02
    - spine (with meningocele) — *see* Spina bifida
    - trachea Q32.1
    - tympanic membrane (causing impairment of hearing) Q16.4
    - uterus Q51.818
    - vitelline duct Q43.0
  - erection — *see* Dysfunction, sexual, male, erectile
  - fusion — *see* Imperfect, closure
  - inflation, lung (newborn) — *see* Atelectasis
  - posture R29.3
  - rotation, intestine Q43.3
  - septum, ventricular Q21.0
- **Imperfectly** descended testis — *see* Cryptorchid
- **Imperforate** (congenital) (*see also* Atresia)
  - anus Q42.3
    - with fistula Q42.2
  - cervix (uteri) Q51.828
  - esophagus Q39.0
    - with tracheoesophageal fistula Q39.1
  - hymen Q52.3
  - jejunum Q41.1
  - pharynx Q38.8
  - rectum Q42.1
    - with fistula Q42.0
  - urethra Q64.39
  - vagina Q52.4
- **Impervious** (congenital) (*see also* Atresia)
  - anus Q42.3
    - with fistula Q42.2
  - bile duct Q44.2
  - esophagus Q39.0
    - with tracheoesophageal fistula Q39.1
  - intestine (small) Q41.9
    - large Q42.9
      - specified NEC Q42.8
  - rectum Q42.1
    - with fistula Q42.0
  - ureter — *see* Atresia, ureter
  - urethra Q64.39
- **Impetiginization** of dermatoses L01.1
- **Impetigo** (any organism) (any site) (circinate) (contagiosa) (simplex) (vulgaris) L01.00
  - Bockhart's L01.02

- **Impetigo** — *continued*
  - bullous, bullosa L01.03
  - external ear L01.00 *[H62.40]*
  - follicularis L01.02
  - furfuracea L30.5
  - herpetiformis L40.1
    - nonobstetrical L40.1
  - neonatorum L01.03
  - nonbullous L01.01
  - specified type NEC L01.09
  - ulcerative L01.09
- **Impingement** (on teeth)
  - soft tissue
    - anterior M26.81
    - posterior M26.82
- **Implant,** endometrial N80.9
- **Implantation**
  - anomalous — *see* Anomaly, by site
    - ureter Q62.63
  - cyst
    - external area or site (skin) NEC L72.0
    - iris — *see* Cyst, iris, implantation
    - vagina N89.8
    - vulva N90.7
  - dermoid (cyst) — *see* Implantation, cyst
- **Impotence** (sexual) N52.9
  - counseling Z70.1
  - organic origin (*see also* Dysfunction, sexual, male, erectile)N52.9
  - psychogenic F52.21
- **Impression,** basilar Q75.8
- **Imprisonment,** anxiety concerning Z65.1
- **Improper** care (child) (newborn) — *see* Maltreatment
- **Improperly** tied umbilical cord (causing hemorrhage) P51.8
- **Impulsiveness** (impulsive) R45.87
- **Inability** to swallow — *see* Aphagia
- **Inaccessible,** inaccessibility
  - health care NEC Z75.3
    - due to
      - waiting period Z75.2
        - for admission to facility elsewhere Z75.1
  - other helping agencies Z75.4
- **Inactive** — *see* condition
- **Inadequate,** inadequacy
  - aesthetics of dental restoration K08.56
  - biologic, constitutional, functional, or social F60.7
  - development
    - child R62.50
    - genitalia
      - after puberty NEC E30.0
      - congenital
        - female Q52.8
          - external Q52.79
          - internal Q52.8
        - male Q55.8
    - lungs Q33.6
      - associated with short gestation P28.0
    - organ or site not listed — *see* Anomaly, by site
  - diet (causing nutritional deficiency) E63.9
  - eating habits Z72.4
  - environment, household Z59.1
  - family support Z63.8
  - food (supply) NEC Z59.4
    - hunger effects T73.0 ☑
  - functional F60.7
  - household care, due to
    - family member
      - handicapped or ill Z74.2
      - on vacation Z75.5
      - temporarily away from home Z74.2
    - technical defects in home Z59.1
    - temporary absence from home of person rendering care Z74.2
  - housing (heating) (space) Z59.1
  - income (financial) Z59.6
  - intrafamilial communication Z63.8
  - material resources Z59.9
  - mental — *see* Disability, intellectual
  - parental supervision or control of child Z62.0
  - personality F60.7
  - pulmonary
    - function R06.89
      - newborn P28.5
    - ventilation, newborn P28.5
  - sample of cytologic smear
    - anus R85.615
    - cervix R87.615
    - vagina R87.625
  - social F60.7
    - insurance Z59.7
    - skills NEC Z73.4

Inadequate - Infant

Inadequate — *continued*
- supervision of child by parent Z62.0
- teaching affecting education Z55.8
- welfare support Z59.7

Inanition R64
- with edema — *see* Malnutrition, severe
- due to
  - deprivation of food T73.0 ☑
  - malnutrition — *see* Malnutrition
- fever R50.9

Inappropriate
- change in quantitative human chorionic gonadotropin (hCG) in early pregnancy O02.81
- diet or eating habits Z72.4
- level of quantitative human chorionic gonadotropin (hCG) for gestational age in early pregnancy O02.81
- secretion
  - antidiuretic hormone (ADH) (excessive) E22.2
    - deficiency E23.2
  - pituitary (posterior) E22.2

Inattention at or after birth — *see* Neglect

Incarceration, incarcerated
- enterocele K46.0
  - gangrenous K46.1
- epiplocele K46.0
  - gangrenous K46.1
- exomphalos K42.0
  - gangrenous K42.1
- hernia (*see also* Hernia, by site, with obstruction)
  - with gangrene — *see* Hernia, by site, with gangrene
- iris, in wound — *see* Injury, eye, laceration, with prolapse
- lens, in wound — *see* Injury, eye, laceration, with prolapse
- omphalocele K42.0
- prison, anxiety concerning Z65.1
- rupture — *see* Hernia, by site
- sarcoepiplocele K46.0
  - gangrenous K46.1
- sarcoepiplomphalocele K42.0
  - with gangrene K42.1
- uterus N85.8
  - gravid O34.51 ☑
    - causing obstructed labor O65.5

Incised wound
- external — *see* Laceration
- internal organs — *see* Injury, by site

Incision, incisional
- hernia K43.2
  - with
    - gangrene (and obstruction) K43.1
    - obstruction K43.0
- surgical, complication — *see* Complications, surgical procedure
- traumatic
  - external — *see* Laceration
  - internal organs — *see* Injury, by site

Inclusion
- azurophilic leukocytic D72.0
- blennorrhea (neonatal) (newborn) P39.1
- gallbladder in liver (congenital) Q44.1

Incompatibility
- ABO
  - affecting management of pregnancy O36.11 ☑
    - anti-A sensitization O36.11 ☑
    - anti-B sensitization O36.19 ☑
    - specified NEC O36.19 ☑
  - infusion or transfusion reaction — *see* Complication (s), transfusion, incompatibility reaction, ABO
  - newborn P55.1
- blood (group) (Duffy) (K (ell)) (Kidd) (Lewis) (M) (S) NEC
  - affecting management of pregnancy O36.11 ☑
    - anti-A sensitization O36.11 ☑
    - anti-B sensitization O36.19 ☑
  - infusion or transfusion reaction T80.89 ☑
  - newborn P55.8
- divorce or estrangement Z63.5
- Rh (blood group) (factor) Z31.82
  - affecting management of pregnancy NEC O36.09 ☑
    - anti-D antibody O36.01 ☑
  - infusion or transfusion reaction — *see* Complication (s), transfusion, incompatibility reaction, Rh (factor)
  - newborn P55.0
- rhesus — *see* Incompatibility, Rh

Incompetency, incompetent, incompetence
- annular
  - aortic (valve) — *see* Insufficiency, aortic
  - mitral (valve) I34.0
  - pulmonary valve (heart) I37.1
- aortic (valve) — *see* Insufficiency, aortic
- cardiac valve — *see* Endocarditis
- cervix, cervical (os) N88.3
  - in pregnancy O34.3 ☑
- chronotropic I45.89
  - with
    - autonomic dysfunction G90.8
    - ischemic heart disease I25.89
    - left ventricular dysfunction I51.89
    - sinus node dysfunction I49.8
- esophagogastric (junction) (sphincter) K22.0
- mitral (valve) — *see* Insufficiency, mitral
- pelvic fundus N81.89
- pubocervical tissue N81.82
- pulmonary valve (heart) I37.1
  - congenital Q22.3
- rectovaginal tissue N81.83
- tricuspid (annular) (valve) — *see* Insufficiency, tricuspid
- valvular — *see* Endocarditis
  - congenital Q24.8
- vein, venous (saphenous) (varicose) — *see* Varix, leg

Incomplete (*see also* condition)
- bladder, emptying R33.9
- defecation R15.0
- expansion lungs (newborn) NEC — *see* Atelectasis
- rotation, intestine Q43.3

Inconclusive
- diagnostic imaging due to excess body fat of patient R93.9
- findings on diagnostic imaging of breast NEC R92.8
- mammogram (due to dense breasts) R92.2

Incontinence R32
- anal sphincter R15.9
- coital N39.491
- feces R15.9
  - nonorganic origin F98.1
- insensible (urinary) N39.42
- overflow N39.490
- postural (urinary) N39.492
- psychogenic F45.8
- rectal R15.9
- reflex N39.498
- stress (female) (male) N39.3
  - and urge N39.46
- urethral sphincter R32
- urge N39.41
  - and stress (female) (male) N39.46
- urine (urinary) R32
  - continuous N39.45
  - due to cognitive impairment, or severe physical disability or immobility R39.81
  - functional R39.81
  - insensible N39.42
  - mixed (stress and urge) N39.46
  - nocturnal N39.44
  - nonorganic origin F98.0
  - overflow N39.490
  - post dribbling N39.43
  - postural N39.492
  - reflex N39.498
  - specified NEC N39.498
  - stress (female) (male) N39.3
    - and urge N39.46
  - total N39.498
  - unaware N39.42
  - urge N39.41
    - and stress (female) (male) N39.46

Incontinentia pigmenti Q82.3

Incoordinate, incoordination
- esophageal-pharyngeal (newborn) — *see* Dysphagia
- muscular R27.8
- uterus (action) (contractions) (complicating delivery) O62.4

Increase, increased
- abnormal, in development R63.8
- androgens (ovarian) E28.1
- anticoagulants (antithrombin) (anti-VIIIa) (anti-IXa) (anti-Xa) (anti-XIa) — *see* Circulating anticoagulants
- cold sense R20.8
- estrogen E28.0

Increase — *continued*
- function
  - adrenal
    - cortex — *see* Cushing's, syndrome
    - medulla E27.5
  - pituitary (gland) (anterior) (lobe) E22.9
    - posterior E22.2
- heat sense R20.8
- intracranial pressure (benign) G93.2
- permeability, capillaries I78.8
- pressure, intracranial G93.2
- secretion
  - gastrin E16.4
  - glucagon E16.3
  - pancreas, endocrine E16.9
    - growth hormone-releasing hormone E16.8
    - pancreatic polypeptide E16.8
    - somatostatin E16.8
    - vasoactive-intestinal polypeptide E16.8
- sphericity, lens Q12.4
- splenic activity D73.1
- venous pressure I87.8
  - portal K76.6

Increta placenta O43.22 ☑

Incrustation, cornea, foreign body (lead) (zinc) — *see* Foreign body, cornea

Incyclophoria H50.54

Incyclotropia — *see* Cyclotropia

Indeterminate sex Q56.4

India rubber skin Q82.8

Indigestion (acid) (bilious) (functional) K30
- catarrhal K31.89
- due to decomposed food NOS A05.9
- nervous F45.8
- psychogenic F45.8

Indirect — *see* condition

Induratio penis plastica N48.6

Induration, indurated
- brain G93.89
- breast (fibrous) N64.51
  - puerperal, postpartum O92.29
- broad ligament N83.8
- chancre
  - anus A51.1
  - congenital A50.07
  - extragenital NEC A51.2
- corpora cavernosa (penis) (plastic) N48.6
- liver (chronic) K76.89
- lung (black) (chronic) (fibroid) (*see also* Fibrosis, lung)J84.10
  - essential brown J84.03
- penile (plastic) N48.6
- phlebitic — *see* Phlebitis
- skin R23.4

Inebriety (without dependence) — *see* Alcohol, intoxication

Inefficiency, kidney N28.9

Inelasticity, skin R23.4

Inequality, leg (length) (acquired) (*see also* Deformity, limb, unequal length)
- congenital — *see* Defect, reduction, lower limb
- lower leg — *see* Deformity, limb, unequal length

Inertia
- bladder (neurogenic) N31.2
- stomach K31.89
  - psychogenic F45.8
- uterus, uterine during labor O62.2
  - during latent phase of labor O62.0
  - primary O62.0
  - secondary O62.1
- vesical (neurogenic) N31.2

Infancy, infantile, infantilism (*see also* condition)
- celiac K90.0
- genitalia, genitals (after puberty) E30.0
- Herter's (nontropical sprue) K90.0
- intestinal K90.0
- Lorain E23.0
- pancreatic K86.89
- pelvis M95.5
  - with disproportion (fetopelvic) O33.1
    - causing obstructed labor O65.1
- pituitary E23.0
- renal N25.0
- uterus — *see* Infantile, genitalia

Infant (s) (*see also* Infancy)
- excessive crying R68.11
- irritable child R68.12
- lack of care — *see* Neglect
- liveborn (singleton) Z38.2
  - born in hospital Z38.00
    - by cesarean Z38.01
  - born outside hospital Z38.1

- **Infant** — *continued*
  - liveborn — *continued*
    - multiple NEC Z38.8
      - born in hospital Z38.68
        - by cesarean Z38.69
      - born outside hospital Z38.7
    - quadruplet Z38.8
      - born in hospital Z38.63
        - by cesarean Z38.64
      - born outside hospital Z38.7
    - quintuplet Z38.8
      - born in hospital Z38.65
        - by cesarean Z38.66
      - born outside hospital Z38.7
    - triplet Z38.8
      - born in hospital Z38.61
        - by cesarean Z38.62
      - born outside hospital Z38.7
    - twin Z38.5
      - born in hospital Z38.30
        - by cesarean Z38.31
      - born outside hospital Z38.4
  - of diabetic mother (syndrome of) P70.1
    - gestational diabetes P70.0
- **Infantile** (*see also* condition)
  - genitalia, genitals E30.0
  - os, uterine E30.0
  - penis E30.0
  - testis E29.1
  - uterus E30.0
- **Infantilism** — *see* Infancy
- **Infarct,** infarction
  - adrenal (capsule) (gland) E27.49
  - appendices epiploicae (*see also* Infarct, intestine)K55.069
  - bowel (*see also* Infarct, intestine)K55.069
  - brain (stem) — *see* Infarct, cerebral
  - breast N64.89
  - brewer's (kidney) N28.0
  - cardiac — *see* Infarct, myocardium
  - cerebellar — *see* Infarct, cerebral
  - cerebral (*see also* Occlusion, artery cerebral or precerebral, with infarction)I63.9
    - aborted I63.9
    - cortical I63.9
    - due to
      - cerebral venous thrombosis, nonpyogenic I63.6
      - embolism
        - cerebral arteries I63.4 ☑
        - precerebral arteries I63.1 ☑
      - occlusion NEC
        - cerebral arteries I63.5 ☑
        - precerebral arteries I63.2 ☑
      - stenosis NEC
        - cerebral arteries I63.5 ☑
        - precerebral arteries I63.2 ☑
      - thrombosis
        - cerebral artery I63.3 ☑
        - precerebral artery I63.0 ☑
    - intraoperative
      - during cardiac surgery I97.810
      - during other surgery I97.811
    - postprocedural
      - following cardiac surgery I97.820
      - following other surgery I97.821
    - specified NEC I63.8
  - colon (acute) (agnogenic) (embolic) (hemorrhagic) (nonocclusive) (nonthrombotic) (occlusive) (segmental) (thrombotic) (with gangrene) (*see also* Infarct, intestine)K55.049
  - coronary artery — *see* Infarct, myocardium
  - embolic — *see* Embolism
  - fallopian tube N83.8
  - gallbladder K82.8
  - heart — *see* Infarct, myocardium
  - hepatic K76.3
  - hypophysis (anterior lobe) E23.6
  - impending (myocardium) I20.0
  - intestine (acute) (agnogenic) (embolic) (hemorrhagic) (nonocclusive) (nonthrombotic) (occlusive) (thrombotic) (with gangrene) K55.069
    - diffuse K55.062
    - focal K55.061
    - large K55.049
      - diffuse K55.042
      - focal K55.041
    - small K55.029
      - diffuse K55.022
      - focal K55.021
- **Infarct,** infarction — *continued*
  - kidney N28.0
  - liver K76.3
  - lung (embolic) (thrombotic) — *see* Embolism, pulmonary
  - lymph node I89.8
  - mesentery, mesenteric (embolic) (thrombotic) (with gangrene) (*see also* Infarct, intestine)K55.069
  - muscle (ischemic) M62.20
    - ankle M62.27 ☑
    - foot M62.27 ☑
    - forearm M62.23 ☑
    - hand M62.24 ☑
    - lower leg M62.26 ☑
    - pelvic region M62.25 ☑
    - shoulder region M62.21 ☑
    - specified site NEC M62.28
    - thigh M62.25 ☑
    - upper arm M62.22 ☑
  - myocardium, myocardial (acute) (with stated duration of 4 weeks or less) I21.3
    - diagnosed on ECG, but presenting no symptoms I25.2
    - healed or old I25.2
    - intraoperative
      - during cardiac surgery I97.790
      - during other surgery I97.791
    - non-Q wave I21.4
    - non-ST elevation (NSTEMI) I21.4
      - subsequent I22.2
    - nontransmural I21.4
    - past (diagnosed on ECG or other investigation, but currently presenting no symptoms) I25.2
    - postprocedural
      - following cardiac surgery I97.190
      - following other surgery I97.191
    - Q wave (see also, Infarct, myocardium, by site) I21.3
    - ST elevation (STEMI) I21.3
      - anterior (anteroapical) (anterolateral) (anteroseptal) (Q wave) (wall) I21.09
        - subsequent I22.0
      - inferior (diaphragmatic) (inferolateral) (inferoposterior) (wall) NEC I21.19
        - subsequent I22.1
      - inferoposterior transmural (Q wave) I21.11
      - involving
        - coronary artery of anterior wall NEC I21.09
        - coronary artery of inferior wall NEC I21.19
        - diagonal coronary artery I21.02
        - left anterior descending coronary artery I21.02
        - left circumflex coronary artery I21.21
        - left main coronary artery I21.01
        - oblique marginal coronary artery I21.21
        - right coronary artery I21.11
      - lateral (apical-lateral) (basal-lateral) (high) I21.29
        - subsequent I22.8
      - posterior (posterobasal) (posterolateral) (posteroseptal) (true) I21.29
        - subsequent I22.8
      - septal I21.29
        - subsequent I22.8
      - specified NEC I21.29
        - subsequent I22.8
      - subsequent I22.9
    - subsequent (recurrent) (reinfarction) I22.9
      - anterior (anteroapical) (anterolateral) (anteroseptal) (wall) I22.0
      - diaphragmatic (wall) I22.1
      - inferior (diaphragmatic) (inferolateral) (inferoposterior) (wall) I22.1
      - lateral (apical-lateral) (basal-lateral) (high) I22.8
      - non-ST elevation (NSTEMI) I22.2
      - posterior (posterobasal) (posterolateral) (posteroseptal) (true) I22.8
      - septal I22.8
      - specified NEC I22.8
      - ST elevation I22.9
        - anterior (anteroapical) (anterolateral) (anteroseptal) (wall) I22.0
        - inferior (diaphragmatic) (inferolateral) (inferoposterior) (wall) I22.1
        - specified NEC I22.8
      - subendocardial I22.2
      - transmural I22.9
- **Infarct,** infarction — *continued*
  - myocardium, myocardial — *continued*
      - anterior (anteroapical) (anterolateral) (anteroseptal) (wall) I22.0
      - diaphragmatic (wall) I22.1
      - inferior (diaphragmatic) (inferolateral) (inferoposterior) (wall) I22.1
      - lateral (apical-lateral) (basal-lateral) (high) I22.8
      - posterior (posterobasal) (posterolateral) (posteroseptal) (true) I22.8
      - specified NEC I22.8
    - syphilitic A52.06
    - transmural I21.3
      - anterior (anteroapical) (anterolateral) (anteroseptal) (Q wave) (wall) NEC I21.09
      - inferior (diaphragmatic) (inferolateral) (inferoposterior) (Q wave) (wall) NEC I21.19
      - inferoposterior (Q wave) I21.11
      - lateral (apical-lateral) (basal-lateral) (high) NEC I21.29
      - posterior (posterobasal) (posterolateral) (posteroseptal) (true) NEC I21.29
      - septal NEC I21.29
      - specified NEC I21.29
  - nontransmural I21.4
  - omentum (*see also* Infarct, intestine)K55.069
  - ovary N83.8
  - pancreas K86.89
  - papillary muscle — *see* Infarct, myocardium
  - parathyroid gland E21.4
  - pituitary (gland) E23.6
  - placenta O43.81 ☑
  - prostate N42.89
  - pulmonary (artery) (vein) (hemorrhagic) — *see* Embolism, pulmonary
  - renal (embolic) (thrombotic) N28.0
  - retina, retinal (artery) — *see* Occlusion, artery, retina
  - spinal (cord) (acute) (embolic) (nonembolic) G95.11
  - spleen D73.5
    - embolic or thrombotic I74.8
  - subendocardial (acute) (nontransmural) I21.4
  - suprarenal (capsule) (gland) E27.49
  - testis N50.1
  - thrombotic (*see also* Thrombosis)
    - artery, arterial — *see* Embolism
  - thyroid (gland) E07.89
  - ventricle (heart) — *see* Infarct, myocardium
- **Infecting** — *see* condition
- **Infection,** infected, infective (opportunistic) B99.9
  - with
    - drug resistant organism — *see* Resistance (to), drug (*see also* specific organism)
    - lymphangitis — *see* Lymphangitis
    - organ dysfunction (acute) R65.20
      - with septic shock R65.21
  - abscess (skin) - code by site under Abscess
  - Absidia — *see* Mucormycosis
  - Acanthamoeba — *see* Acanthamebiasis
  - Acanthocheilonema (perstans) (streptocerca) B74.4
  - accessory sinus (chronic) — *see* Sinusitis
  - achorion — *see* Dermatophytosis
  - Acremonium falciforme B47.0
  - acromioclavicular M00.9
  - Actinobacillus (actinomycetem-comitans) A28.8
    - mallei A24.0
    - muris A25.1
  - Actinomadura B47.1
  - Actinomyces (israelii) (*see also* Actinomycosis)A42.9
  - Actinomycetales — *see* Actinomycosis
  - actinomycotic NOS — *see* Actinomycosis
  - adenoid (and tonsil) J03.90
    - chronic J35.02
  - adenovirus NEC
    - as cause of disease classified elsewhere B97.0
    - unspecified nature or site B34.0
  - aerogenes capsulatus A48.0
  - aertrycke — *see* Infection, salmonella
  - alimentary canal NOS — *see* Enteritis, infectious
  - Allescheria boydii B48.2
  - Alternaria B48.8
  - alveolus, alveolar (process) K04.7
  - Ameba, amebic (histolytica) — *see* Amebiasis
  - amniotic fluid, sac or cavity O41.10 ☑
    - chorioamnionitis O41.12 ☑
    - placentitis O41.14 ☑

Infection — *continued*
- amputation stump (surgical) — *see* Complication, amputation stump, infection
- Ancylostoma (duodenalis) B76.0
- Anisakiasis, Anisakis larvae B81.0
- anthrax — *see* Anthrax
- antrum (chronic) — *see* Sinusitis, maxillary
- anus, anal (papillae) (sphincter) K62.89
- arbovirus (arbor virus) A94
  - specified type NEC A93.8
- artificial insemination N98.0
- Ascaris lumbricoides — *see* Ascariasis
- Ascomycetes B47.0
- Aspergillus (flavus) (fumigatus) (terreus) — *see* Aspergillosis
- atypical
  - acid-fast (bacilli) — *see* Mycobacterium, atypical
  - mycobacteria — *see* Mycobacterium, atypical
  - virus A81.9
    - specified type NEC A81.89
- auditory meatus (external) — *see* Otitis, externa, infective
- auricle (ear) — *see* Otitis, externa, infective
- axillary gland (lymph) L04.2
- Bacillus A49.9
  - abortus A23.1
  - anthracis — *see* Anthrax
  - Ducrey's (any location) A57
  - Flexner's A03.1
  - Friedländer's NEC A49.8
  - gas (gangrene) A48.0
  - mallei A24.0
  - melitensis A23.0
  - paratyphoid, paratyphosus A01.4
    - A A01.1
    - B A01.2
    - C A01.3
  - Shiga (-Kruse) A03.0
  - suipestifer — *see* Infection, salmonella
  - swimming pool A31.1
  - typhosa A01.00
  - welchii — *see* Gangrene, gas
- bacterial NOS A49.9
  - as cause of disease classified elsewhere B96.89
    - Clostridium perfringens [C. perfringens] B96.7
    - Bacteroides fragilis [B. fragilis] B96.6
    - Enterobacter sakazakii B96.89
    - Enterococcus B95.2
    - Escherichia coli [E. coli] (*see also* Escherichia coli)B96.20
    - Helicobacter pylori [H. pylori] B96.81
    - Hemophilus influenzae [H. influenzae] B96.3
    - Klebsiella pneumoniae [K. pneumoniae] B96.1
    - Mycoplasma pneumoniae [M. pneumoniae] B96.0
    - Proteus (mirabilis) (morganii) B96.4
    - Pseudomonas (aeruginosa) (mallei) (pseudomallei) B96.5
    - Staphylococcus B95.8
      - aureus (methicillin susceptible) (MSSA) B95.61
        - methicillin resistant (MRSA) B95.62
      - specified NEC B95.7
    - Streptococcus B95.5
      - group A B95.0
      - group B B95.1
      - pneumoniae B95.3
      - specified NEC B95.4
    - Vibrio vulnificus B96.82
  - specified NEC A48.8
- Bacterium
  - paratyphosum A01.4
    - A A01.1
    - B A01.2
    - C A01.3
  - typhosum A01.00
- Bacteroides NEC A49.8
  - fragilis, as cause of disease classified elsewhere B96.6
- Balantidium coli A07.0
- Bartholin's gland N75.8
- Basidiobolus B46.8
- bile duct (common) (hepatic) — *see* Cholangitis
- bladder — *see* Cystitis
- Blastomyces, blastomycotic (*see also* Blastomycosis)
  - brasiliensis — *see* Paracoccidioidomycosis
  - dermatitidis — *see* Blastomycosis
  - European — *see* Cryptococcosis

Infection — *continued*
- Blastomyces, blastomycotic — *continued*
  - Loboi B48.0
  - North American B40.9
  - South American — *see* Paracoccidioidomycosis
- bleb, postprocedure — *see* Blebitis
- bone — *see* Osteomyelitis
- Bordetella — *see* Whooping cough
- Borrelia bergdorfi A69.20
- brain (*see also* Encephalitis)G04.90
  - membranes — *see* Meningitis
  - septic G06.0
    - meninges — *see* Meningitis, bacterial
- branchial cyst Q18.0
- breast — *see* Mastitis
- bronchus — *see* Bronchitis
- Brucella A23.9
  - abortus A23.1
  - canis A23.3
  - melitensis A23.0
  - mixed A23.8
  - specified NEC A23.8
  - suis A23.2
- Brugia (malayi) B74.1
  - timori B74.2
- bursa — *see* Bursitis, infective
- buttocks (skin) L08.9
- Campylobacter, intestinal A04.5
  - as cause of disease classified elsewhere B96.81
- Candida (albicans) (tropicalis) — *see* Candidiasis
- candiru B88.8
- Capillaria (intestinal) B81.1
  - hepatica B83.8
  - philippinensis B81.1
- cartilage — *see* Disorder, cartilage, specified type NEC
- catheter-related bloodstream (CRBSI) T80.211 ☑
- cat liver fluke B66.0
- cellulitis - code by site under Cellulitis
- central line-associated T80.219 ☑
  - bloodstream (CLABSI) T80.211 ☑
  - specified NEC T80.218 ☑
- Cephalosporium falciforme B47.0
- cerebrospinal — *see* Meningitis
- cervical gland (lymph) L04.0
- cervix — *see* Cervicitis
- cesarean delivery wound (puerperal) O86.0
- cestodes — *see* Infestation, cestodes
- chest J22
- Chilomastix (intestinal) A07.8
- Chlamydia, chlamydial A74.9
  - anus A56.3
  - genitourinary tract A56.2
    - lower A56.00
    - specified NEC A56.19
  - lymphogranuloma A55
  - pharynx A56.4
  - psittaci A70
  - rectum A56.3
  - sexually transmitted NEC A56.8
- cholera — *see* Cholera
- Cladosporium
  - bantianum (brain abscess) B43.1
  - carrionii B43.0
  - castellanii B36.1
  - trichoides (brain abscess) B43.1
  - werneckii B36.1
- Clonorchis (sinensis) (liver) B66.1
- Clostridium NEC
  - bifermentans A48.0
  - botulinum (food poisoning) A05.1
    - infant A48.51
    - wound A48.52
  - difficile
    - as cause of disease classified elsewhere B96.89
    - food-borne (disease) A04.7
    - gas gangrene A48.0
    - necrotizing enterocolitis A04.7
    - sepsis A41.4
  - gas-forming NEC A48.0
  - histolyticum A48.0
  - novyi, causing gas gangrene A48.0
  - oedematiens A48.0
  - perfringens
    - as cause of disease classified elsewhere B96.7
    - due to food A05.2
    - food-borne (disease) A05.2
    - gas gangrene A48.0
    - sepsis A41.4
  - septicum, causing gas gangrene A48.0
  - sordellii, causing gas gangrene A48.0

Infection — *continued*
- Clostridium NEC — *continued*
  - welchii
    - as cause of disease classified elsewhere B96.7
    - food-borne (disease) A05.2
    - gas gangrene A48.0
    - necrotizing enteritis A05.2
    - sepsis A41.4
- Coccidioides (immitis) — *see* Coccidioidomycosis
- colon — *see* Enteritis, infectious
- colostomy K94.02
- common duct — *see* Cholangitis
- congenital P39.9
  - Candida (albicans) P37.5
  - cytomegalovirus P35.1
  - hepatitis, viral P35.3
  - herpes simplex P35.2
  - infectious or parasitic disease P37.9
    - specified NEC P37.8
  - listeriosis (disseminated) P37.2
  - malaria NEC P37.4
    - falciparum P37.3
  - Plasmodium falciparum P37.3
  - poliomyelitis P35.8
  - rubella P35.0
  - skin P39.4
  - toxoplasmosis (acute) (subacute) (chronic) P37.1
  - tuberculosis P37.0
  - urinary (tract) P39.3
  - vaccinia P35.8
  - virus P35.9
    - specified type NEC P35.8
- Conidiobolus B46.8
- coronavirus NEC B34.2
  - as cause of disease classified elsewhere B97.29
  - severe acute respiratory syndrome (SARS associated) B97.21
- corpus luteum — *see* Salpingo-oophoritis
- Corynebacterium diphtheriae — *see* Diphtheria
- cotia virus B08.8
- Coxiella burnetii A78
- coxsackie — *see* Coxsackie
- Cryptococcus neoformans — *see* Cryptococcosis
- Cryptosporidium A07.2
- Cunninghamella — *see* Mucormycosis
- cyst — *see* Cyst
- cystic duct (*see also* Cholecystitis)K81.9
- Cysticercus cellulosae — *see* Cysticercosis
- cytomegalovirus, cytomegaloviral B25.9
  - congenital P35.1
  - maternal, maternal care for (suspected) damage to fetus O35.3 ☑
  - mononucleosis B27.10
    - with
      - complication NEC B27.19
      - meningitis B27.12
      - polyneuropathy B27.11
- delta-agent (acute), in hepatitis B carrier B17.0
- dental (pulpal origin) K04.7
- Deuteromycetes B47.0
- Dicrocoelium dendriticum B66.2
- Dipetalonema (perstans) (streptocerca) B74.4
- diphtherial — *see* Diphtheria
- Diphyllobothrium (adult) (latum) (pacificum) B70.0
  - larval B70.1
- Diplogonoporus (grandis) B71.8
- Dipylidium caninum B67.4
- Dirofilaria B74.8
- Dracunculus medinensis B72
- Drechslera (hawaiiensis) B43.8
- Ducrey Haemophilus (any location) A57
- due to or resulting from
  - artificial insemination N98.0
  - central venous catheter T80.219 ☑
    - bloodstream T80.211 ☑
    - exit or insertion site T80.212 ☑
    - localized T80.212 ☑
    - port or reservoir T80.212 ☑
    - specified NEC T80.218 ☑
    - tunnel T80.212 ☑
  - device, implant or graft (*see also* Complications, by site and type, infection or inflammation)T85.79 ☑
    - arterial graft NEC T82.7 ☑
    - breast (implant) T85.79 ☑
    - catheter NEC T85.79 ☑
      - dialysis (renal) T82.7 ☑
        - intraperitoneal T85.71 ☑
      - infusion NEC T82.7 ☑
        - cranial T85.735 ☑

- **Infection** — *continued*
  - due to or resulting from — *continued*
    - (continued)
      - (continued)
        - intrathecal T85.735 ☑
          - spinal (epidural) (subdural) T85.735 ☑
          - subarachnoid T85.735 ☑
        - urinary T83.518 ☑
          - cystostomy T83.510 ☑
          - Hopkins T83.518 ☑
          - ileostomy T83.518 ☑
          - nephrostomy T83.512 ☑
          - specified NEC T83.518 ☑
          - urethral indwelling T83.511 ☑
          - urostomy T83.518 ☑
      - electronic (electrode) (pulse generator) (stimulator)
        - bone T84.7 ☑
        - cardiac T82.7 ☑
        - nervous system T85.738 ☑
          - brain T85.731 ☑
          - cranial nerve T85.732 ☑
          - gastric nerve T85.732 ☑
          - generator pocket T85.734 ☑
          - neurostimulator generator T85.734 ☑
          - peripheral nerve T85.732 ☑
          - sacral nerve T85.732 ☑
          - spinal cord T85.733 ☑
          - vagal nerve T85.732 ☑
        - urinary T83.590 ☑
      - fixation, internal (orthopedic) NEC — *see* Complication, fixation device, infection
      - gastrointestinal (bile duct) (esophagus) T85.79 ☑
        - neurostimulator electrode (lead) T85.732 ☑
      - genital NEC T83.69 ☑
      - heart NEC T82.7 ☑
        - valve (prosthesis) T82.6 ☑
          - graft T82.7 ☑
      - joint prosthesis — *see* Complication, joint prosthesis, infection
      - ocular (corneal graft) (orbital implant) NEC T85.79 ☑
      - orthopedic NEC T84.7 ☑
      - penile (cylinder) (pump) (reservoir) T83.61 ☑
      - specified NEC T85.79 ☑
      - testicular T83.62 ☑
      - urinary NEC T83.598 ☑
        - ileal conduit stent T83.593 ☑
        - implanted neurostimulation T83.590 ☑
        - implanted sphincter T83.591 ☑
        - indwelling ureteral stent T83.592 ☑
        - nephroureteral stent T83.593 ☑
        - specified stent NEC T83.593 ☑
      - vascular NEC T82.7 ☑
      - ventricular intracranial (communicating) shunt T85.730 ☑
    - Hickman catheter T80.219 ☑
      - bloodstream T80.211 ☑
      - localized T80.212 ☑
      - specified NEC T80.218 ☑
    - immunization or vaccination T88.0 ☑
    - infusion, injection or transfusion NEC T80.29 ☑
      - acute T80.22 ☑
    - injury NEC - code by site under Wound, open
    - peripherally inserted central catheter (PICC) T80.219 ☑
      - bloodstream T80.211 ☑
      - localized T80.212 ☑
      - specified NEC T80.218 ☑
    - portacath (Port-a-Cath®) T80.219 ☑
      - bloodstream T80.211 ☑
      - localized T80.212 ☑
      - specified NEC T80.218 ☑
    - pulmonary artery catheter — *see* Infection, due to or resulting from, central venous catheter
    - surgery T81.40
    - Swan Ganz catheter — *see* Infection, due to or resulting from, central venous catheter
    - triple lumen catheter T80.219 ☑
      - bloodstream T80.211 ☑
      - localized T80.212 ☑
      - specified NEC T80.218 ☑
    - umbilical venous catheter T80.219 ☑
      - bloodstream T80.211 ☑
      - localized T80.212 ☑
      - specified NEC T80.218 ☑
  - during labor NEC O75.3
  - ear (middle) (*see also* Otitis media)
    - external — *see* Otitis, externa, infective
    - inner — *see* subcategory H83.0
  - Eberthella typhosa A01.00
  - Echinococcus — *see* Echinococcus

- **Infection** — *continued*
  - echovirus
    - as cause of disease classified elsewhere B97.12
    - unspecified nature or site B34.1
  - endocardium I33.0
  - endocervix — *see* Cervicitis
  - Entamoeba — *see* Amebiasis
  - enteric — *see* Enteritis, infectious
  - Enterobacter sakazakii B96.89
  - Enterobius vermicularis B80
  - enterostomy K94.12
  - enterovirus B34.1
    - as cause of disease classified elsewhere B97.10
      - coxsackievirus B97.11
      - echovirus B97.12
      - specified NEC B97.19
  - Entomophthora B46.8
  - Epidermophyton — *see* Dermatophytosis
  - epididymis — *see* Epididymitis
  - episiotomy (puerperal) O86.0
  - Erysipelothrix (insidiosa) (rhusiopathiae) — *see* Erysipeloid
  - erythema infectiosum B08.3
  - Escherichia (E.) coli NEC A49.8
    - as cause of disease classified elsewhere (*see also* Escherichia coli)B96.20
    - congenital P39.8
      - sepsis P36.4
    - generalized A41.51
    - intestinal — *see* Enteritis, infectious, due to, Escherichia coli
  - ethmoidal (chronic) (sinus) — *see* Sinusitis, ethmoidal
  - eustachian tube (ear) — *see* Salpingitis, eustachian
  - external auditory canal (meatus) NEC — *see* Otitis, externa, infective
  - eye (purulent) — *see* Endophthalmitis, purulent
  - eyelid — *see* Inflammation, eyelid
  - fallopian tube — *see* Salpingo-oophoritis
  - Fasciola (gigantica) (hepatica) (indica) B66.3
  - Fasciolopsis (buski) B66.5
  - filarial — *see* Infestation, filarial
  - finger (skin) L08.9
    - nail L03.01 ☑
      - fungus B35.1
  - fish tapeworm B70.0
    - larval B70.1
  - flagellate, intestinal A07.9
  - fluke — *see* Infestation, fluke
  - focal
    - teeth (pulpal origin) K04.7
    - tonsils J35.01
  - Fonsecaea (compactum) (pedrosoi) B43.0
  - food — *see* Intoxication, food-borne
  - foot (skin) L08.9
    - dermatophytic fungus B35.3
  - Francisella tularensis — *see* Tularemia
  - frontal (sinus) (chronic) — *see* Sinusitis, frontal
  - fungus NOS B49
    - beard B35.0
    - dermatophytic — *see* Dermatophytosis
    - foot B35.3
    - groin B35.6
    - hand B35.2
    - nail B35.1
    - pathogenic to compromised host only B48.8
    - perianal (area) B35.6
    - scalp B35.0
    - skin B36.9
      - foot B35.3
      - hand B35.2
      - toenails B35.1
  - Fusarium B48.8
  - gallbladder — *see* Cholecystitis
  - gas bacillus — *see* Gangrene, gas
  - gastrointestinal — *see* Enteritis, infectious
  - generalized NEC — *see* Sepsis
  - generator pocket, implanted electronic
    - neurostimulator T85.734 ☑
  - genital organ or tract
    - female — *see* Disease, pelvis, inflammatory
    - male N49.9
      - multiple sites N49.8
      - specified NEC N49.8
  - Ghon tubercle, primary A15.7
  - Giardia lamblia A07.1
  - gingiva (chronic) K05.10
    - acute K05.00
      - nonplaque induced K05.01
      - plaque induced K05.00
    - nonplaque induced K05.11
    - plaque induced K05.10

- **Infection** — *continued*
  - glanders A24.0
  - glenosporopsis B48.0
  - Gnathostoma (spinigerum) B83.1
  - Gongylonema B83.8
  - gonococcal — *see* Gonococcus
  - gram-negative bacilli NOS A49.9
  - guinea worm B72
  - gum (chronic) K05.10
    - acute K05.00
      - nonplaque induced K05.01
      - plaque induced K05.00
    - nonplaque induced K05.11
    - plaque induced K05.10
  - Haemophilus — *see* Infection, Hemophilus
  - heart — *see* Carditis
  - Helicobacter pylori A04.8
    - as cause of disease classified elsewhere B96.81
  - helminths B83.9
    - intestinal B82.0
      - mixed (types classifiable to more than one of the titles B65.0-B81.3 and B81.8) B81.4
      - specified type NEC B81.8
    - specified type NEC B83.8
  - Hemophilus
    - aegyptius, systemic A48.4
    - ducrey (any location) A57
    - influenzae NEC A49.2
      - as cause of disease classified elsewhere B96.3
    - generalized A41.3
  - herpes (simplex) (*see also* Herpes)
    - congenital P35.2
    - disseminated B00.7
    - zoster B02.9
  - herpesvirus, herpesviral — *see* Herpes
  - hip (joint) NEC M00.9
    - due to internal joint prosthesis
      - left T84.52 ☑
      - right T84.51 ☑
    - skin NEC L08.9
  - Heterophyes (heterophyes) B66.8
  - Histoplasma — *see* Histoplasmosis
    - American B39.4
    - capsulatum B39.4
  - hookworm B76.9
  - human
    - papilloma virus A63.0
    - T-cell lymphotropic virus type-1 (HTLV-1) B33.3
  - hydrocele N43.0
  - Hymenolepis B71.0
  - hypopharynx — *see* Pharyngitis
  - inguinal (lymph) glands L04.1
    - due to soft chancre A57
  - intervertebral disc, pyogenic M46.30
    - cervical region M46.32
    - cervicothoracic region M46.33
    - lumbar region M46.36
    - lumbosacral region M46.37
    - multiple sites M46.39
    - occipito-atlanto-axial region M46.31
    - sacrococcygeal region M46.38
    - thoracic region M46.34
    - thoracolumbar region M46.35
  - intestine, intestinal — *see* Enteritis, infectious
    - specified NEC A08.8
  - intra-amniotic affecting newborn NEC P39.2
  - Isospora belli or hominis A07.3
  - Japanese B encephalitis A83.0
  - jaw (bone) (lower) (upper) M27.2
  - joint NEC M00.9
    - due to internal joint prosthesis T84.50 ☑
  - kidney (cortex) (hematogenous) N15.9
    - with calculus N20.0
      - with hydronephrosis N13.6
    - following ectopic gestation O08.83
    - pelvis and ureter (cystic) N28.85
    - puerperal (postpartum) O86.21
    - specified NEC N15.8
  - Klebsiella (K.) pneumoniae NEC A49.8
    - as cause of disease classified elsewhere B96.1
  - knee (joint) NEC M00.9
    - joint M00.9
    - due to internal joint prosthesis
      - left T84.54 ☑
      - right T84.53 ☑
    - skin L08.9
  - Koch's — *see* Tuberculosis
  - labia (majora) (minora) (acute) — *see* Vulvitis
  - lacrimal
    - gland — *see* Dacryoadenitis
    - passages (duct) (sac) — *see* Inflammation, lacrimal, passages

Infection

- **Infection** — *continued*
  - lancet fluke B66.2
  - larynx NEC J38.7
  - leg (skin) NOS L08.9
  - Legionella pneumophila A48.1
    - nonpneumonic A48.2
  - Leishmania (*see also* Leishmaniasis)
    - aethiopica B55.1
    - braziliensis B55.2
    - chagasi B55.0
    - donovani B55.0
    - infantum B55.0
    - major B55.1
    - mexicana B55.1
    - tropica B55.1
  - lentivirus, as cause of disease classified elsewhere B97.31
  - Leptosphaeria senegalensis B47.0
  - Leptospira interrogans A27.9
    - autumnalis A27.89
    - canicola A27.89
    - hebdomadis A27.89
    - icterohaemorrhagiae A27.0
    - pomona A27.89
    - specified type NEC A27.89
  - leptospirochetal NEC — *see* Leptospirosis
  - Listeria monocytogenes (*see also* Listeriosis)
    - congenital P37.2
  - Loa loa B74.3
    - with conjunctival infestation B74.3
    - eyelid B74.3
  - Loboa loboi B48.0
  - local, skin (staphylococcal) (streptococcal) L08.9
    - abscess - code by site under Abscess
    - cellulitis - code by site under Cellulitis
    - specified NEC L08.89
    - ulcer — *see* Ulcer, skin
  - Loefflerella mallei A24.0
  - lung (*see also* Pneumonia)J18.9
    - atypical Mycobacterium A31.0
    - spirochetal A69.8
    - tuberculous — *see* Tuberculosis, pulmonary
    - virus — *see* Pneumonia, viral
  - lymph gland (*see also* Lymphadenitis, acute)
    - mesenteric I88.0
  - lymphoid tissue, base of tongue or posterior pharynx, NEC (chronic) J35.03
  - Madurella (grisea) (mycetomii) B47.0
  - major
    - following ectopic or molar pregnancy O08.0
    - puerperal, postpartum, childbirth O85
  - Malassezia furfur B36.0
  - Malleomyces
    - mallei A24.0
    - pseudomallei (whitmori) — *see* Melioidosis
  - mammary gland N61.0
  - Mansonella (ozzardi) (perstans) (streptocerca) B74.4
  - mastoid — *see* Mastoiditis
  - maxilla, maxillary M27.2
    - sinus (chronic) — *see* Sinusitis, maxillary
  - mediastinum J98.51
  - Medina (worm) B72
  - meibomian cyst or gland — *see* Hordeolum
  - meninges — *see* Meningitis, bacterial
  - meningococcal (*see also* condition)A39.9
    - adrenals A39.1
    - brain A39.81
    - cerebrospinal A39.0
    - conjunctiva A39.89
    - endocardium A39.51
    - heart A39.50
      - endocardium A39.51
      - myocardium A39.52
      - pericardium A39.53
    - joint A39.83
    - meninges A39.0
    - meningococcemia A39.4
      - acute A39.2
      - chronic A39.3
    - myocardium A39.52
    - pericardium A39.53
    - retrobulbar neuritis A39.82
    - specified site NEC A39.89
  - mesenteric lymph nodes or glands NEC I88.0
  - Metagonimus B66.8
  - metatarsophalangeal M00.9
  - methicillin
    - resistant Staphylococcus aureus (MRSA) A49.02
    - susceptible Staphylococcus aureus (MSSA) A49.01

- **Infection** — *continued*
  - Microsporum, microsporic — *see* Dermatophytosis
  - mixed flora (bacterial) NEC A49.8
  - Monilia — *see* Candidiasis
  - Monosporium apiospermum B48.2
  - mouth, parasitic B37.0
  - Mucor — *see* Mucormycosis
  - muscle NEC — *see* Myositis, infective
  - mycelium NOS B49
  - mycetoma B47.9
    - actinomycotic NEC B47.1
    - mycotic NEC B47.0
  - Mycobacterium, mycobacterial — *see* Mycobacterium
  - Mycoplasma NEC A49.3
    - pneumoniae, as cause of disease classified elsewhere B96.0
  - mycotic NOS B49
    - pathogenic to compromised host only B48.8
    - skin NOS B36.9
  - myocardium NEC I40.0
  - nail (chronic)
    - with lymphangitis — *see* Lymphangitis, acute, digit
    - finger L03.01 ☑
      - fungus B35.1
    - ingrowing L60.0
    - toe L03.03 ☑
      - fungus B35.1
  - nasal sinus (chronic) — *see* Sinusitis
  - nasopharynx — *see* Nasopharyngitis
  - navel L08.82
  - Necator americanus B76.1
  - Neisseria — *see* Gonococcus
  - Neotestudina rosatii B47.0
  - newborn P39.9
    - intra-amniotic NEC P39.2
    - skin P39.4
    - specified type NEC P39.8
  - nipple N61.0
    - associated with
      - lactation O91.03
      - pregnancy O91.01 ☑
      - puerperium O91.02
  - Nocardia — *see* Nocardiosis
  - obstetrical surgical wound (puerperal) O86.0
  - Oesophagostomum (apiostomum) B81.8
  - Oestrus ovis — *see* Myiasis
  - Oidium albicans B37.9
  - Onchocerca (volvulus) — *see* Onchocerciasis
  - oncovirus, as cause of disease classified elsewhere B97.32
  - operation wound T81.40
  - Opisthorchis (felineus) (viverrini) B66.0
  - orbit, orbital — *see* Inflammation, orbit
  - orthopoxvirus NEC B08.09
  - ovary — *see* Salpingo-oophoritis
  - Oxyuris vermicularis B80
  - pancreas (acute) — *see* Pancreatitis, acute
    - abscess — *see* Pancreatitis, acute
    - specified NEC (*see also* Pancreatitis, acute)K85.80
  - papillomavirus, as cause of disease classified elsewhere B97.7
  - papovavirus NEC B34.4
  - Paracoccidioides brasiliensis — *see* Paracoccidioidomycosis
  - Paragonimus (westermani) B66.4
  - parainfluenza virus B34.8
  - parameningococcus NOS A39.9
  - parapoxvirus B08.60
    - specified NEC B08.69
  - parasitic B89
  - Parastrongylus
    - cantonensis B83.2
    - costaricensis B81.3
    - paratyphoid A01.4
      - Type A A01.1
      - Type B A01.2
      - Type C A01.3
  - paraurethral ducts N34.2
  - parotid gland — *see* Sialoadenitis
  - parvovirus NEC B34.3
    - as cause of disease classified elsewhere B97.6
  - Pasteurella NEC A28.0
    - multocida A28.0
    - pestis — *see* Plague
    - pseudotuberculosis A28.0
    - septica (cat bite) (dog bite) A28.0
    - tularensis — *see* Tularemia
  - pelvic, female — *see* Disease, pelvis, inflammatory

- **Infection** — *continued*
  - Penicillium (marneffei) B48.4
  - penis (glans) (retention) NEC N48.29
  - periapical K04.5
  - peridental, periodontal K05.20
    - generalized — *see* Periodontitis, aggressive, generalized
    - localized — *see* Periodontitis, aggressive, localized
  - perinatal period P39.9
    - specified type NEC P39.8
  - perineal repair (puerperal) O86.0
  - periorbital — *see* Inflammation, orbit
  - perirectal K62.89
  - perirenal — *see* Infection, kidney
  - peritoneal — *see* Peritonitis
  - periureteral N28.89
  - Petriellidium boydii B48.2
  - pharynx (*see also* Pharyngitis)
    - coxsackievirus B08.5
    - posterior, lymphoid (chronic) J35.03
  - Phialophora
    - gougerotii (subcutaneous abscess or cyst) B43.2
    - jeanselmei (subcutaneous abscess or cyst) B43.2
    - verrucosa (skin) B43.0
  - Piedraia hortae B36.3
  - pinta A67.9
    - intermediate A67.1
    - late A67.2
    - mixed A67.3
    - primary A67.0
  - pinworm B80
  - pityrosporum furfur B36.0
  - pleuro-pneumonia-like organism (PPLO) NEC A49.3
    - as cause of disease classified elsewhere B96.0
  - pneumococcus, pneumococcal NEC A49.1
    - as cause of disease classified elsewhere B95.3
    - generalized (purulent) A40.3
      - with pneumonia J13
  - Pneumocystis carinii (pneumonia) B59
  - Pneumocystis jiroveci (pneumonia) B59
  - port or reservoir T80.212 ☑
  - postoperative T81.40
  - postoperative wound T81.40
  - postprocedural T81.40
    - deep incisional surgical site T81.42
    - organ and space surgical site T81.43
    - sepsis T81.49
    - specified surgical site NEC T81.48
    - superficial incisional surgical site T81.41
  - postvaccinal T88.0 ☑
  - prepuce NEC N47.7
    - with penile inflammation N47.6
  - prion — *see* Disease, prion, central nervous system
  - prostate (capsule) — *see* Prostatitis
  - Proteus (mirabilis) (morganii) (vulgaris) NEC A49.8
    - as cause of disease classified elsewhere B96.4
  - protozoal NEC B64
    - intestinal A07.9
      - specified NEC A07.8
    - specified NEC B60.8
  - Pseudoallescheria boydii B48.2
  - Pseudomonas NEC A49.8
    - as cause of disease classified elsewhere B96.5
    - mallei A24.0
    - pneumonia J15.1
    - pseudomallei — *see* Melioidosis
  - puerperal O86.4
    - genitourinary tract NEC O86.89
    - major or generalized O85
    - minor O86.4
    - specified NEC O86.89
  - pulmonary — *see* Infection, lung
  - purulent — *see* Abscess
  - Pyrenochaeta romeroi B47.0
  - Q fever A78
  - rectum (sphincter) K62.89
  - renal (*see also* Infection, kidney)
    - pelvis and ureter (cystic) N28.85
  - reovirus, as cause of disease classified elsewhere B97.5
  - respiratory (tract) NEC J98.8
    - acute J22
    - chronic J98.8
    - influenzal (upper) (acute) — *see* Influenza, with, respiratory manifestations NEC
    - lower (acute) J22
      - chronic — *see* Bronchitis, chronic

- **Infection** — *continued*
  - respiratory — *continued*
    - rhinovirus J00
    - syncytial virus, as cause of disease classified elsewhere B97.4
    - upper (acute) NOS J06.9
      - chronic J39.8
      - streptococcal J06.9
      - viral NOS J06.9
  - resulting from
    - presence of internal prosthesis, implant, graft — *see* Complications, by site and type, infection
  - retortamoniasis A07.8
  - retroperitoneal NEC K68.9
  - retrovirus B33.3
    - as cause of disease classified elsewhere B97.30
      - human
        - immunodeficiency, type 2 (HIV 2) B97.35
        - T-cell lymphotropic
          - type I (HTLV-I) B97.33
          - type II (HTLV-II) B97.34
      - lentivirus B97.31
      - oncovirus B97.32
      - specified NEC B97.39
  - Rhinosporidium (seeberi) B48.1
  - rhinovirus
    - as cause of disease classified elsewhere B97.89
    - unspecified nature or site B34.8
  - Rhizopus — *see* Mucormycosis
  - rickettsial NOS A79.9
  - roundworm (large) NEC B82.0
    - Ascariasis (*see also* Ascariasis)B77.9
  - rubella — *see* Rubella
  - Saccharomyces — *see* Candidiasis
  - salivary duct or gland (any) — *see* Sialoadenitis
  - Salmonella (aertrycke) (arizonae) (callinarum) (cholerae-suis) (enteritidis) (suipestifer) (typhimurium) A02.9
    - with
      - (gastro)enteritis A02.0
      - sepsis A02.1
      - specified manifestation NEC A02.8
    - due to food (poisoning) A02.9
    - hirschfeldii A01.3
    - localized A02.20
      - arthritis A02.23
      - meningitis A02.21
      - osteomyelitis A02.24
      - pneumonia A02.22
      - pyelonephritis A02.25
      - specified NEC A02.29
    - paratyphi A01.4
      - A A01.1
      - B A01.2
      - C A01.3
    - schottmuelleri A01.2
    - typhi, typhosa — *see* Typhoid
  - Sarcocystis A07.8
  - scabies B86
  - Schistosoma — *see* Infestation, Schistosoma
  - scrotum (acute) NEC N49.2
  - seminal vesicle — *see* Vesiculitis
  - septic
    - localized, skin — *see* Abscess
  - sheep liver fluke B66.3
  - Shigella A03.9
    - boydii A03.2
    - dysenteriae A03.0
    - flexneri A03.1
    - group
      - A A03.0
      - B A03.1
      - C A03.2
      - D A03.3
    - Schmitz (-Stutzer) A03.0
    - schmitzii A03.0
    - shigae A03.0
    - sonnei A03.3
    - specified NEC A03.8
  - shoulder (joint) NEC M00.9
    - due to internal joint prosthesis T84.59 ☑
    - skin NEC L08.9
  - sinus (accessory) (chronic) (nasal) (*see also* Sinusitis)
    - pilonidal — *see* Sinus, pilonidal
    - skin NEC L08.89
  - Skene's duct or gland — *see* Urethritis
  - skin (local) (staphylococcal) (streptococcal) L08.9
    - abscess - code by site under Abscess
    - cellulitis - code by site under Cellulitis
    - due to fungus B36.9

- **Infection** — *continued*
  - skin — *continued*
    - due to fungus — *continued*
      - specified type NEC B36.8
    - mycotic B36.9
      - specified type NEC B36.8
    - newborn P39.4
    - ulcer — *see* Ulcer, skin
  - slow virus A81.9
    - specified NEC A81.89
  - Sparganum (mansoni) (proliferum) (baxteri) B70.1
  - specific (*see also* Syphilis)
    - to perinatal period — *see* Infection, congenital
  - specified NEC B99.8
  - spermatic cord NEC N49.1
  - sphenoidal (sinus) — *see* Sinusitis, sphenoidal
  - spinal cord NOS (*see also* Myelitis)G04.91
    - abscess G06.1
    - meninges — *see* Meningitis
    - streptococcal G04.89
  - Spirillum A25.0
  - spirochetal NOS A69.9
    - lung A69.8
    - specified NEC A69.8
  - Spirometra larvae B70.1
  - spleen D73.89
  - Sporotrichum, Sporothrix (schenckii) — *see* Sporotrichosis
  - staphylococcal, unspecified site
    - aureus (methicillin susceptible) (MSSA) A49.01
      - methicillin resistant (MRSA) A49.02
    - as cause of disease classified elsewhere B95.8
      - aureus (methicillin susceptible) (MSSA) B95.61
        - methicillin resistant (MRSA) B95.62
      - specified NEC B95.7
    - food poisoning A05.0
    - generalized (purulent) A41.2
    - pneumonia — *see* Pneumonia, staphylococcal
  - Stellantchasmus falcatus B66.8
  - streptobacillus moniliformis A25.1
  - streptococcal NEC A49.1
    - as cause of disease classified elsewhere B95.5
    - B genitourinary complicating
      - childbirth O98.82
      - pregnancy O98.81 ☑
      - puerperium O98.83
    - congenital
      - sepsis P36.10
        - group B P36.0
        - specified NEC P36.19
    - generalized (purulent) A40.9
  - Streptomyces B47.1
  - Strongyloides (stercoralis) — *see* Strongyloidiasis
  - stump (amputation) (surgical) — *see* Complication, amputation stump, infection
  - subcutaneous tissue, local L08.9
  - suipestifer — *see* Infection, salmonella
  - swimming pool bacillus A31.1
  - Taenia — *see* Infestation, Taenia
  - Taeniarhynchus saginatus B68.1
  - tapeworm — *see* Infestation, tapeworm
  - tendon (sheath) — *see* Tenosynovitis, infective NEC
  - Ternidens diminutus B81.8
  - testis — *see* Orchitis
  - threadworm B80
  - throat — *see* Pharyngitis
  - thyroglossal duct K14.8
  - toe (skin) L08.9
    - cellulitis L03.03 ☑
      - fungus B35.1
    - nail L03.03 ☑
      - fungus B35.1
  - tongue NEC K14.0
    - parasitic B37.0
  - tonsil (and adenoid) (faucial) (lingual) (pharyngeal) — *see* Tonsillitis
  - tooth, teeth K04.7
    - periapical K04.7
    - peridental, periodontal K05.20
      - generalized — *see* Periodontitis, aggressive, generalized
      - localized — *see* Periodontitis, aggressive, localized
    - pulp K04.01
    - irreversible K04.02
    - reversible K04.01
    - socket M27.3
  - TORCH — *see* Infection, congenital
    - without active infection P00.2
  - Torula histolytica — *see* Cryptococcosis
  - Toxocara (canis) (cati) (felis) B83.0

- **Infection** — *continued*
  - Toxoplasma gondii — *see* Toxoplasma
  - trachea, chronic J42
  - trematode NEC — *see* Infestation, fluke
  - trench fever A79.0
  - Treponema pallidum — *see* Syphilis
  - Trichinella (spiralis) B75
  - Trichomonas A59.9
    - cervix A59.09
    - intestine A07.8
    - prostate A59.02
    - specified site NEC A59.8
    - urethra A59.03
    - urogenitalis A59.00
    - vagina A59.01
    - vulva A59.01
  - Trichophyton, trichophytic — *see* Dermatophytosis
  - Trichosporon (beigelii) cutaneum B36.2
  - Trichostrongylus B81.2
  - Trichuris (trichiura) B79
  - Trombicula (irritans) B88.0
  - Trypanosoma
    - brucei
      - gambiense B56.0
      - rhodesiense B56.1
    - cruzi — *see* Chagas' disease
  - tubal — *see* Salpingo-oophoritis
  - tuberculous NEC — *see* Tuberculosis
  - tubo-ovarian — *see* Salpingo-oophoritis
  - tunnel T80.212 ☑
  - tunica vaginalis N49.1
  - tympanic membrane NEC — *see* Myringitis
  - typhoid (abortive) (ambulant) (bacillus) — *see* Typhoid
  - typhus A75.9
    - flea-borne A75.2
    - mite-borne A75.3
    - recrudescent A75.1
    - tick-borne A77.9
      - African A77.1
      - North Asian A77.2
  - umbilicus L08.82
  - ureter N28.86
  - urethra — *see* Urethritis
  - urinary (tract) N39.0
    - bladder — *see* Cystitis
    - complicating
      - pregnancy O23.4 ☑
        - specified type NEC O23.3 ☑
    - kidney — *see* Infection, kidney
    - newborn P39.3
    - puerperal (postpartum) O86.20
    - tuberculous A18.13
    - urethra — *see* Urethritis
  - uterus, uterine — *see* Endometritis
  - vaccination T88.0 ☑
  - vaccinia not from vaccination B08.011
  - vagina (acute) — *see* Vaginitis
  - varicella B01.9
  - varicose veins — *see* Varix
  - vas deferens NEC N49.1
  - vesical — *see* Cystitis
  - Vibrio
    - cholerae A00.0
      - El Tor A00.1
    - parahaemolyticus (food poisoning) A05.3
    - vulnificus
      - as cause of disease classified elsewhere B96.82
      - food-borne intoxication A05.5
  - Vincent's (gum) (mouth) (tonsil) A69.1
  - virus, viral NOS B34.9
    - adenovirus
      - as cause of disease classified elsewhere B97.0
      - unspecified nature or site B34.0
    - arborvirus, arbovirus arthropod-borne A94
    - as cause of disease classified elsewhere B97.89
      - adenovirus B97.0
      - coronavirus B97.29
        - SARS-associated B97.21
      - coxsackievirus B97.11
      - echovirus B97.12
      - enterovirus B97.10
        - coxsackievirus B97.11
        - echovirus B97.12
        - specified NEC B97.19
      - human
        - immunodeficiency, type 2 (HIV 2) B97.35
        - T-cell lymphotropic,
          - type I (HTLV-I) B97.33
          - type II (HTLV-II) B97.34

Infection - Infestation

Infection — *continued*
- virus, viral NOS — *continued*
      - metapneumovirus B97.81
    - papillomavirus B97.7
    - parvovirus B97.6
    - reovirus B97.5
    - respiratory syncytial B97.4
    - retrovirus B97.30
        - human
            - immunodeficiency, type 2 (HIV 2) B97.35
            - T-cell lymphotropic,
                - type I (HTLV-I) B97.33
                - type II (HTLV-II) B97.34
        - lentivirus B97.31
        - oncovirus B97.32
        - specified NEC B97.39
    - specified NEC B97.89
  - central nervous system A89
    - atypical A81.9
        - specified NEC A81.89
    - enterovirus NEC A88.8
        - meningitis A87.0
    - slow virus A81.9
        - specified NEC A81.89
    - specified NEC A88.8
  - chest J98.8
  - cotia B08.8
  - coxsackie (*see also* Infection, coxsackie)B34.1
    - as cause of disease classified elsewhere B97.11
  - ECHO
    - as cause of disease classified elsewhere B97.12
    - unspecified nature or site B34.1
  - encephalitis, tick-borne A84.9
  - enterovirus, as cause of disease classified elsewhere B97.10
    - coxsackievirus B97.11
    - echovirus B97.12
    - specified NEC B97.19
  - exanthem NOS B09
  - human papilloma as cause of disease classified elsewhere B97.7
  - human metapneumovirus as cause of disease classified elsewhere B97.81
  - intestine — *see* Enteritis, viral
  - respiratory syncytial
    - as cause of disease classified elsewhere B97.4
    - bronchopneumonia J12.1
    - common cold syndrome J00
    - nasopharyngitis (acute) J00
  - rhinovirus
    - as cause of disease classified elsewhere B97.89
    - unspecified nature or site B34.8
  - slow A81.9
    - specified NEC A81.89
  - specified type NEC B33.8
    - as cause of disease classified elsewhere B97.89
    - unspecified nature or site B34.8
  - unspecified nature or site B34.9
  - West Nile — *see* Virus, West Nile
- vulva (acute) — *see* Vulvitis
- West Nile — *see* Virus, West Nile
- whipworm B79
- worms B83.9
  - specified type NEC B83.8
- Wuchereria (bancrofti) B74.0
  - malayi B74.1
- yatapoxvirus B08.70
  - specified NEC B08.79
- yeast (*see also* Candidiasis)B37.9
- yellow fever — *see* Fever, yellow
- Yersinia
  - enterocolitica (intestinal) A04.6
  - pestis — *see* Plague
  - pseudotuberculosis A28.2
- Zeis' gland — *see* Hordeolum
- Zika virus A92.5
- zoonotic bacterial NOS A28.9
- Zopfia senegalensis B47.0

Infective, infectious — *see* condition

Infertility
- female N97.9
  - age-related N97.8
  - associated with
    - anovulation N97.0
    - cervical (mucus) disease or anomaly N88.3
    - congenital anomaly
        - cervix N88.3
        - fallopian tube N97.1
        - uterus N97.2
        - vagina N97.8
    - dysmucorrhea N88.3
    - fallopian tube disease or anomaly N97.1
    - pituitary-hypothalamic origin E23.0
    - specified origin NEC N97.8
    - Stein-Leventhal syndrome E28.2
    - uterine disease or anomaly N97.2
    - vaginal disease or anomaly N97.8
  - due to
    - cervical anomaly N88.3
    - fallopian tube anomaly N97.1
    - ovarian failure E28.39
    - Stein-Leventhal syndrome E28.2
    - uterine anomaly N97.2
    - vaginal anomaly N97.8
  - nonimplantation N97.2
  - origin
    - cervical N88.3
    - tubal (block) (occlusion) (stenosis) N97.1
    - uterine N97.2
    - vaginal N97.8
- male N46.9
  - azoospermia N46.01
    - extratesticular cause N46.029
        - drug therapy N46.021
        - efferent duct obstruction N46.023
        - infection N46.022
        - radiation N46.024
        - specified cause NEC N46.029
        - systemic disease N46.025
  - oligospermia N46.11
    - extratesticular cause N46.129
        - drug therapy N46.121
        - efferent duct obstruction N46.123
        - infection N46.122
        - radiation N46.124
        - specified cause NEC N46.129
        - systemic disease N46.125
  - specified type NEC N46.8

Infestation B88.9
- Acanthocheilonema (perstans) (streptocerca) B74.4
- Acariasis B88.0
  - demodex folliculorum B88.0
  - sarcoptes scabiei B86
  - trombiculae B88.0
- Agamofilaria streptocerca B74.4
- Ancylostoma, ankylostoma (braziliense) (caninum) (ceylanicum) (duodenale) B76.0
  - americanum B76.1
  - new world B76.1
- Anisakis larvae, anisakiasis B81.0
- arthropod NEC B88.2
- Ascaris lumbricoides — *see* Ascariasis
- Balantidium coli A07.0
- beef tapeworm B68.1
- Bothriocephalus (latus) B70.0
  - larval B70.1
- broad tapeworm B70.0
  - larval B70.1
- Brugia (malayi) B74.1
  - timori B74.2
- candiru B88.8
- Capillaria
  - hepatica B83.8
  - philippinensis B81.1
- cat liver fluke B66.0
- cestodes B71.9
  - diphyllobothrium — *see* Infestation, diphyllobothrium
  - dipylidiasis B71.1
  - hymenolepiasis B71.0
  - specified type NEC B71.8
- chigger B88.0
- chigo, chigoe B88.1
- Clonorchis (sinensis) (liver) B66.1
- coccidial A07.3
- crab-lice B85.3
- Cysticercus cellulosae — *see* Cysticercosis
- Demodex (folliculorum) B88.0
- Dermanyssus gallinae B88.0
- Dermatobia (hominis) — *see* Myiasis
- Dibothriocephalus (latus) B70.0
  - larval B70.1
- Dicrocoelium dendriticum B66.2
- Diphyllobothrium (adult) (latum) (intestinal) (pacificum) B70.0
  - larval B70.1
- Diplogonoporus (grandis) B71.8

Infestation — *continued*
- Dipylidium caninum B67.4
- Distoma hepaticum B66.3
- dog tapeworm B67.4
- Dracunculus medinensis B72
- dragon worm B72
- dwarf tapeworm B71.0
- Echinococcus — *see* Echinococcus
- Echinostomum ilocanum B66.8
- Entamoeba (histolytica) — *see* Infection, Ameba
- Enterobius vermicularis B80
- eyelid
  - in (due to)
    - leishmaniasis B55.1
    - loiasis B74.3
    - onchocerciasis B73.09
    - phthiriasis B85.3
  - parasitic NOS B89
- eyeworm B74.3
- Fasciola (gigantica) (hepatica) (indica) B66.3
- Fasciolopsis (buski) (intestine) B66.5
- filarial B74.9
  - bancroftian B74.0
  - conjunctiva B74.9
  - due to
    - Acanthocheilonema (perstans) (streptocerca) B74.4
    - Brugia (malayi) B74.1
        - timori B74.2
    - Dracunculus medinensis B72
    - guinea worm B72
    - loa loa B74.3
    - Mansonella (ozzardi) (perstans) (streptocerca) B74.4
    - Onchocerca volvulus B73.00
        - eye B73.00
        - eyelid B73.09
    - Wuchereria (bancrofti) B74.0
  - Malayan B74.1
  - ozzardi B74.4
  - specified type NEC B74.8
- fish tapeworm B70.0
  - larval B70.1
- fluke B66.9
  - blood NOS — *see* Schistosomiasis
  - cat liver B66.0
  - intestinal B66.5
  - liver (sheep) B66.3
    - cat B66.0
    - Chinese B66.1
    - due to clonorchiasis B66.1
    - oriental B66.1
  - lancet B66.2
  - lung (oriental) B66.4
  - sheep liver B66.3
  - specified type NEC B66.8
- fly larvae — *see* Myiasis
- Gasterophilus (intestinalis) — *see* Myiasis
- Gastrodiscoides hominis B66.8
- Giardia lamblia A07.1
- Gnathostoma (spinigerum) B83.1
- Gongylonema B83.8
- guinea worm B72
- helminth B83.9
  - angiostrongyliasis B83.2
    - intestinal B81.3
  - gnathostomiasis B83.1
  - hirudiniasis, internal B83.4
  - intestinal B82.0
    - angiostrongyliasis B81.3
    - anisakiasis B81.0
    - ascariasis — *see* Ascariasis
    - capillariasis B81.1
    - cysticercosis — *see* Cysticercosis
    - diphyllobothriasis — *see* Infestation, diphyllobothriasis
    - dracunculiasis B72
    - echinococcus — *see* Echinococcosis
    - enterobiasis B80
    - filariasis - — *see* Infestation, filarial
    - fluke — *see* Infestation, fluke
    - hookworm — *see* Infestation, hookworm
    - mixed (types classifiable to more than one of the titles B65.0-B81.3 and B81.8) B81.4
    - onchocerciasis — *see* Onchocerciasis
    - schistosomiasis — *see* Infestation, schistosoma
    - specified
        - cestode NEC — *see* Infestation, cestode
        - type NEC B81.8
    - strongyloidiasis — *see* Strongyloidiasis
    - taenia — *see* Infestation, taenia

- **Infestation** — *continued*
  - helminth — *continued*
      - trichinellosis B75
      - trichostrongyliasis B81.2
      - trichuriasis B79
    - specified type NEC B83.8
    - syngamiasis B83.3
    - visceral larva migrans B83.0
  - Heterophyes (heterophyes) B66.8
  - hookworm B76.9
    - ancylostomiasis B76.0
    - necatoriasis B76.1
    - specified type NEC B76.8
  - Hymenolepis (diminuta) (nana) B71.0
  - intestinal NEC B82.9
  - leeches (aquatic) (land) — *see* Hirudiniasis
  - Leishmania — *see* Leishmaniasis
  - lice, louse — *see* Infestation, Pediculus
  - Linguatula B88.8
  - Liponyssoides sanguineus B88.0
  - Loa loa B74.3
    - conjunctival B74.3
    - eyelid B74.3
  - louse — *see* Infestation, Pediculus
  - maggots — *see* Myiasis
  - Mansonella (ozzardi) (perstans) (streptocerca) B74.4
  - Medina (worm) B72
  - Metagonimus (yokogawai) B66.8
  - microfilaria streptocerca — *see* Onchocerciasis
    - eye B73.00
    - eyelid B73.09
  - mites B88.9
    - scabic B86
  - Monilia (albicans) — *see* Candidiasis
  - mouth B37.0
  - Necator americanus B76.1
  - nematode NEC (intestinal) B82.0
    - Ancylostoma B76.0
    - conjunctiva NEC B83.9
    - Enterobius vermicularis B80
    - Gnathostoma spinigerum B83.1
    - physaloptera B80
    - specified NEC B81.8
    - trichostrongylus B81.2
    - trichuris (trichuria) B79
  - Oesophagostomum (apiostomum) B81.8
  - Oestrus ovis (*see also* Myiasis)B87.9
  - Onchocerca (volvulus) — *see* Onchocerciasis
  - Opisthorchis (felineus) (viverrini) B66.0
  - orbit, parasitic NOS B89
  - Oxyuris vermicularis B80
  - Paragonimus (westermani) B66.4
  - parasite, parasitic B89
    - eyelid B89
    - intestinal NOS B82.9
    - mouth B37.0
    - skin B88.9
    - tongue B37.0
  - Parastrongylus
    - cantonensis B83.2
    - costaricensis B81.3
  - Pediculus B85.2
    - body B85.1
    - capitis (humanus) (any site) B85.0
    - corporis (humanus) (any site) B85.1
    - head B85.0
    - mixed (classifiable to more than one of the titles B85.0-B85.3) B85.4
    - pubis (any site) B85.3
  - Pentastoma B88.8
  - Phthirus (pubis) (any site) B85.3
    - with any infestation classifiable to B85.0-B85.2 B85.4
  - pinworm B80
  - pork tapeworm (adult) B68.0
  - protozoal NEC B64
    - intestinal A07.9
      - specified NEC A07.8
    - specified NEC B60.8
  - pubic, louse B85.3
  - rat tapeworm B71.0
  - red bug B88.0
  - roundworm (large) NEC B82.0
    - Ascariasis (*see also* Ascariasis)B77.9
  - sandflea B88.1
  - Sarcoptes scabiei B86
  - scabies B86
  - Schistosoma B65.9
    - bovis B65.8
    - cercariae B65.3
    - haematobium B65.0
- **Infestation** — *continued*
  - Schistosoma — *continued*
    - intercalatum B65.8
    - japonicum B65.2
    - mansoni B65.1
    - mattheei B65.8
    - mekongi B65.8
    - specified type NEC B65.8
    - spindale B65.8
  - screw worms — *see* Myiasis
  - skin NOS B88.9
  - Sparganum (mansoni) (proliferum) (baxteri) B70.1
    - larval B70.1
  - specified type NEC B88.8
  - Spirometra larvae B70.1
  - Stellantchasmus falcatus B66.8
  - Strongyloides stercoralis — *see* Strongyloidiasis
  - Taenia B68.9
    - diminuta B71.0
    - echinococcus — *see* Echinococcus
    - mediocanellata B68.1
    - nana B71.0
    - saginata B68.1
    - solium (intestinal form) B68.0
      - larval form — *see* Cysticercosis
  - Taeniarhynchus saginatus B68.1
  - tapeworm B71.9
    - beef B68.1
    - broad B70.0
      - larval B70.1
    - dog B67.4
    - dwarf B71.0
    - fish B70.0
      - larval B70.1
    - pork B68.0
    - rat B71.0
  - Ternidens diminutus B81.8
  - Tetranychus molestissimus B88.0
  - threadworm B80
  - tongue B37.0
  - Toxocara (canis) (cati) (felis) B83.0
  - trematode (s) NEC — *see* Infestation, fluke
  - Trichinella (spiralis) B75
  - Trichocephalus B79
  - Trichomonas — *see* Trichomoniasis
  - Trichostrongylus B81.2
  - Trichuris (trichiura) B79
  - Trombicula (irritans) B88.0
  - Tunga penetrans B88.1
  - Uncinaria americana B76.1
  - Vandellia cirrhosa B88.8
  - whipworm B79
  - worms B83.9
    - intestinal B82.0
  - Wuchereria (bancrofti) B74.0
- **Infiltrate,** infiltration
  - amyloid (generalized) (localized) — *see* Amyloidosis
  - calcareous NEC R89.7
    - localized — *see* Degeneration, by site
  - calcium salt R89.7
  - cardiac
    - fatty — *see* Degeneration, myocardial
    - glycogenic E74.02 *[I43]*
  - corneal — *see* Edema, cornea
  - eyelid — *see* Inflammation, eyelid
  - glycogen, glycogenic — *see* Disease, glycogen storage
  - heart, cardiac
    - fatty — *see* Degeneration, myocardial
    - glycogenic E74.02 *[I43]*
  - inflammatory in vitreous H43.89
  - kidney N28.89
  - leukemic — *see* Leukemia
  - liver K76.89
    - fatty — *see* Fatty, liver NEC
    - glycogen (*see also* Disease, glycogen storage)E74.03 *[K77]*
  - lung R91.8
    - eosinophilic J82
  - lymphatic (*see also* Leukemia, lymphatic)C91.9 ☑
    - gland I88.9
  - muscle, fatty M62.89
  - myocardium, myocardial
    - fatty — *see* Degeneration, myocardial
    - glycogenic E74.02 *[I43]*
  - on chest x-ray R91.8
  - pulmonary R91.8
    - with eosinophilia J82
  - skin (lymphocytic) L98.6
  - thymus (gland) (fatty) E32.8
  - urine R39.0
- **Infiltrate** — *continued*
  - vesicant agent
    - antineoplastic chemotherapy T80.810 ☑
    - other agent NEC T80.818 ☑
  - vitreous body H43.89
- **Infirmity** R68.89
  - senile R54
- **Inflammation,** inflamed, inflammatory (with exudation)
  - abducent (nerve) — *see* Strabismus, paralytic, sixth nerve
  - accessory sinus (chronic) — *see* Sinusitis
  - adrenal (gland) E27.8
  - alveoli, teeth M27.3
    - scorbutic E54
  - anal canal, anus K62.89
  - antrum (chronic) — *see* Sinusitis, maxillary
  - appendix — *see* Appendicitis
  - arachnoid — *see* Meningitis
  - areola N61.0
    - puerperal, postpartum or gestational — *see* Infection, nipple
  - areolar tissue NOS L08.9
  - artery — *see* Arteritis
  - auditory meatus (external) — *see* Otitis, externa
  - Bartholin's gland N75.8
  - bile duct (common) (hepatic) or passage — *see* Cholangitis
  - bladder — *see* Cystitis
  - bone — *see* Osteomyelitis
  - brain (*see also* Encephalitis)
    - membrane — *see* Meningitis
  - breast N61.0
    - puerperal, postpartum, gestational — *see* Mastitis, obstetric
  - broad ligament — *see* Disease, pelvis, inflammatory
  - bronchi — *see* Bronchitis
  - catarrhal J00
  - cecum — *see* Appendicitis
  - cerebral (*see also* Encephalitis)
    - membrane — *see* Meningitis
  - cerebrospinal
    - meningococcal A39.0
  - cervix (uteri) — *see* Cervicitis
  - chest J98.8
  - chorioretinal H30.9 ☑
    - cyclitis — *see* Cyclitis
    - disseminated H30.10 ☑
      - generalized H30.13 ☑
      - peripheral H30.12 ☑
      - posterior pole H30.11 ☑
    - epitheliopathy — *see* Epitheliopathy
    - focal H30.00 ☑
      - juxtapapillary H30.01 ☑
      - macular H30.04 ☑
      - paramacular — *see* Inflammation, chorioretinal, focal, macular
      - peripheral H30.03 ☑
      - posterior pole H30.02 ☑
    - specified type NEC H30.89 ☑
  - choroid — *see* Inflammation, chorioretinal
  - chronic, postmastoidectomy cavity — *see* Complications, postmastoidectomy, inflammation
  - colon — *see* Enteritis
  - connective tissue (diffuse) NEC — *see* Disorder, soft tissue, specified type NEC
  - cornea — *see* Keratitis
  - corpora cavernosa N48.29
  - cranial nerve — *see* Disorder, nerve, cranial
  - Douglas' cul-de-sac or pouch (chronic) N73.0
  - due to device, implant or graft (*see also* Complications, by site and type, infection or inflammation)
    - arterial graft T82.7 ☑
    - breast (implant) T85.79 ☑
    - catheter T85.79 ☑
      - dialysis (renal) T82.7 ☑
        - intraperitoneal T85.71 ☑
      - infusion T82.7 ☑
        - cranial T85.735 ☑
        - intrathecal T85.735 ☑
        - spinal (epidural) (subdural) T85.735 ☑
        - subarachnoid T85.735 ☑
      - urinary T83.518 ☑
        - cystostomy T83.510 ☑
        - Hopkins T83.518 ☑
        - ileostomy T83.518 ☑
        - nephrostomy T83.512 ☑
        - specified NEC T83.518 ☑
        - urethral indwelling T83.511 ☑

Inflammation - Influenza

- **Inflammation** — *continued*
  - due to device, implant or graft — *continued*
        - urostomy T83.518 ☑
    - electronic (electrode) (pulse generator) (stimulator)
      - bone T84.7 ☑
      - cardiac T82.7 ☑
      - nervous system T85.738 ☑
        - brain T85.731 ☑
        - cranial nerve T85.732 ☑
        - gastric nerve T85.732 ☑
        - neurostimulator generator T85.734 ☑
        - peripheral nerve T85.732 ☑
        - sacral nerve T85.732 ☑
        - spinal cord T85.733 ☑
        - vagal nerve T85.732 ☑
      - urinary T83.590 ☑
    - fixation, internal (orthopedic) NEC — *see* Complication, fixation device, infection
    - gastrointestinal (bile duct) (esophagus) T85.79 ☑
      - neurostimulator electrode (lead) T85.732 ☑
    - genital NEC T83.69 ☑
    - heart NEC T82.7 ☑
      - valve (prosthesis) T82.6 ☑
        - graft T82.7 ☑
    - joint prosthesis — *see* Complication, joint prosthesis, infection
    - ocular (corneal graft) (orbital implant) NEC T85.79 ☑
    - orthopedic NEC T84.7 ☑
    - penile (cylinder) (pump) (reservoir) T83.61 ☑
    - specified NEC T85.79 ☑
    - testicular T83.62 ☑
    - urinary NEC T83.598 ☑
      - ileal conduit stent T83.593 ☑
      - implanted neurostimulation T83.590 ☑
      - implanted sphincter T83.591 ☑
      - indwelling ureteral stent T83.592 ☑
      - nephroureteral stent T83.593 ☑
      - specified stent NEC T83.593 ☑
    - vascular NEC T82.7 ☑
    - ventricular intracranial (communicating) shunt T85.730 ☑
  - duodenum K29.80
    - with bleeding K29.81
  - dura mater — *see* Meningitis
  - ear (middle) (*see also* Otitis, media)
    - external — *see* Otitis, externa
    - inner — *see* subcategory H83.0
  - epididymis — *see* Epididymitis
  - esophagus K20.9
  - ethmoidal (sinus) (chronic) — *see* Sinusitis, ethmoidal
  - eustachian tube (catarrhal) — *see* Salpingitis, eustachian
  - eyelid H01.9
    - abscess — *see* Abscess, eyelid
    - blepharitis — *see* Blepharitis
    - chalazion — *see* Chalazion
    - dermatosis (noninfectious) — *see* Dermatosis, eyelid
    - hordeolum — *see* Hordeolum
    - specified NEC H01.8
  - fallopian tube — *see* Salpingo-oophoritis
  - fascia — *see* Myositis
  - follicular, pharynx J31.2
  - frontal (sinus) (chronic) — *see* Sinusitis, frontal
  - gallbladder — *see* Cholecystitis
  - gastric — *see* Gastritis
  - gastrointestinal — *see* Enteritis
  - genital organ (internal) (diffuse)
    - female — *see* Disease, pelvis, inflammatory
    - male N49.9
      - multiple sites N49.8
      - specified NEC N49.8
  - gland (lymph) — *see* Lymphadenitis
  - glottis — *see* Laryngitis
  - granular, pharynx J31.2
  - gum K05.10
    - nonplaque induced K05.11
    - plaque induced K05.10
  - heart — *see* Carditis
  - hepatic duct — *see* Cholangitis
  - ileoanal (internal) pouch K91.850
  - ileum (*see also* Enteritis)
    - regional or terminal — *see* Enteritis, regional
  - intestine (any part) — *see* Enteritis
  - intestinal pouch K91.850
  - jaw (acute) (bone) (chronic) (lower) (suppurative) (upper) M27.2
  - joint NEC — *see* Arthritis
    - sacroiliac M46.1
- **Inflammation** — *continued*
  - kidney — *see* Nephritis
  - knee (joint) M13.169
    - tuberculous A18.02
  - labium (majus) (minus) — *see* Vulvitis
  - lacrimal
    - gland — *see* Dacryoadenitis
    - passages (duct) (sac) (*see also* Dacryocystitis)
      - canaliculitis — *see* Canaliculitis, lacrimal
  - larynx — *see* Laryngitis
  - leg NOS L08.9
  - lip K13.0
  - liver (capsule) (*see also* Hepatitis)
    - chronic K73.9
    - suppurative K75.0
  - lung (acute) (*see also* Pneumonia)
    - chronic J98.4
  - lymph gland or node — *see* Lymphadenitis
  - lymphatic vessel — *see* Lymphangitis
  - maxilla, maxillary M27.2
    - sinus (chronic) — *see* Sinusitis, maxillary
  - membranes of brain or spinal cord — *see* Meningitis
  - meninges — *see* Meningitis
  - mouth K12.1
  - muscle — *see* Myositis
  - myocardium — *see* Myocarditis
  - nasal sinus (chronic) — *see* Sinusitis
  - nasopharynx — *see* Nasopharyngitis
  - navel L08.82
  - nerve NEC — *see* Neuralgia
  - nipple N61.0
    - puerperal, postpartum or gestational — *see* Infection, nipple
  - nose — *see* Rhinitis
  - oculomotor (nerve) — *see* Strabismus, paralytic, third nerve
  - optic nerve — *see* Neuritis, optic
  - orbit (chronic) H05.10
    - acute H05.00
      - abscess — *see* Abscess, orbit
      - cellulitis — *see* Cellulitis, orbit
      - osteomyelitis — *see* Osteomyelitis, orbit
      - periostitis — *see* Periostitis, orbital
      - tenonitis — *see* Tenonitis, eye
    - granuloma — *see* Granuloma, orbit
    - myositis — *see* Myositis, orbital
  - ovary — *see* Salpingo-oophoritis
  - oviduct — *see* Salpingo-oophoritis
  - pancreas (acute) — *see* Pancreatitis
  - parametrium N73.0
  - parotid region L08.9
  - pelvis, female — *see* Disease, pelvis, inflammatory
  - penis (corpora cavernosa) N48.29
  - perianal K62.89
  - pericardium — *see* Pericarditis
  - perineum (female) (male) L08.9
  - perirectal K62.89
  - peritoneum — *see* Peritonitis
  - periuterine — *see* Disease, pelvis, inflammatory
  - perivesical — *see* Cystitis
  - petrous bone (acute) (chronic) — *see* Petrositis
  - pharynx (acute) — *see* Pharyngitis
  - pia mater — *see* Meningitis
  - pleura — *see* Pleurisy
  - polyp, colon (*see also* Polyp, colon, inflammatory)K51.40
  - prostate (*see also* Prostatitis)
    - specified type NEC N41.8
  - rectosigmoid — *see* Rectosigmoiditis
  - rectum (*see also* Proctitis)K62.89
  - respiratory, upper (*see also* Infection, respiratory, upper)J06.9
    - acute, due to radiation J70.0
    - chronic, due to external agent — *see* condition, respiratory, chronic, due to
    - due to
      - chemicals, gases, fumes or vapors (inhalation) J68.2
      - radiation J70.1
  - retina — *see* Chorioretinitis
  - retrocecal — *see* Appendicitis
  - retroperitoneal — *see* Peritonitis
  - salivary duct or gland (any) (suppurative) — *see* Sialoadenitis
  - scorbutic, alveoli, teeth E54
  - scrotum N49.2
  - seminal vesicle — *see* Vesiculitis
  - sigmoid — *see* Enteritis
  - sinus — *see* Sinusitis
  - Skene's duct or gland — *see* Urethritis
  - skin L08.9
- **Inflammation** — *continued*
  - spermatic cord N49.1
  - sphenoidal (sinus) — *see* Sinusitis, sphenoidal
  - spinal
    - cord — *see* Encephalitis
    - membrane — *see* Meningitis
    - nerve — *see* Disorder, nerve
  - spine — *see* Spondylopathy, inflammatory
  - spleen (capsule) D73.89
  - stomach — *see* Gastritis
  - subcutaneous tissue L08.9
  - suprarenal (gland) E27.8
  - synovial — *see* Tenosynovitis
  - tendon (sheath) NEC — *see* Tenosynovitis
  - testis — *see* Orchitis
  - throat (acute) — *see* Pharyngitis
  - thymus (gland) E32.8
  - thyroid (gland) — *see* Thyroiditis
  - tongue K14.0
  - tonsil — *see* Tonsillitis
  - trachea — *see* Tracheitis
  - trochlear (nerve) — *see* Strabismus, paralytic, fourth nerve
  - tubal — *see* Salpingo-oophoritis
  - tuberculous NEC — *see* Tuberculosis
  - tubo-ovarian — *see* Salpingo-oophoritis
  - tunica vaginalis N49.1
  - tympanic membrane — *see* Tympanitis
  - umbilicus, umbilical L08.82
  - uterine ligament — *see* Disease, pelvis, inflammatory
  - uterus (catarrhal) — *see* Endometritis
  - uveal tract (anterior) NOS (*see also* Iridocyclitis)
    - posterior — *see* Chorioretinitis
  - vagina — *see* Vaginitis
  - vas deferens N49.1
  - vein (*see also* Phlebitis)
    - intracranial or intraspinal (septic) G08
    - thrombotic I80.9
      - leg — *see* Phlebitis, leg
      - lower extremity — *see* Phlebitis, leg
  - vocal cord J38.3
  - vulva — *see* Vulvitis
  - Wharton's duct (suppurative) — *see* Sialoadenitis
- **Inflation**, lung, imperfect (newborn) — *see* Atelectasis
- **Influenza** (bronchial) (epidemic) (respiratory (upper)) (unidentified influenza virus) J11.1
  - with
    - digestive manifestations J11.2
    - encephalopathy J11.81
    - enteritis J11.2
    - gastroenteritis J11.2
    - gastrointestinal manifestations J11.2
    - laryngitis J11.1
    - myocarditis J11.82
    - otitis media J11.83
    - pharyngitis J11.1
    - pneumonia J11.00
      - specified type J11.08
    - respiratory manifestations NEC J11.1
    - specified manifestation NEC J11.89
  - A/H5N1 (*see also* Influenza, due to, identified novel influenza A virus)J09.X2
  - avian (*see also* Influenza, due to, identified novel influenza A virus)J09.X2
  - bird (*see also* Influenza, due to, identified novel influenza A virus)J09.X2
  - novel (2009) H1N1 influenza (*see also* Influenza, due to, identified influenza virus NEC)J10.1
  - novel influenza A/H1N1 (*see also* Influenza, due to, identified influenza virus NEC)J10.1
  - due to
    - avian (*see also* Influenza, due to, identified novel influenza A virus)J09.X2
    - identified influenza virus NEC J10.1
      - with
        - digestive manifestations J10.2
        - encephalopathy J10.81
        - enteritis J10.2
        - gastroenteritis J10.2
        - gastrointestinal manifestations J10.2
        - laryngitis J10.1
        - myocarditis J10.82
        - otitis media J10.83
        - pharyngitis J10.1
        - pneumonia (unspecified type) J10.00
          - with same identified influenza virus J10.01
          - specified type NEC J10.08
        - respiratory manifestations NEC J10.1
        - specified manifestation NEC J10.89

- **Influenza** — *continued*
  - due to — *continued*
    - identified novel influenza A virus J09.X2
      - with
        - digestive manifestations J09.X3
        - encephalopathy J09.X9
        - enteritis J09.X3
        - gastroenteritis J09.X3
        - gastrointestinal manifestations J09.X3
        - laryngitis J09.X2
        - myocarditis J09.X9
        - otitis media J09.X9
        - pharyngitis J09.X2
        - pneumonia J09.X1
        - respiratory manifestations NEC J09.X2
        - specified manifestation NEC J09.X9
        - upper respiratory symptoms J09.X2
    - of other animal origin, not bird or swine (*see also* Influenza, due to, identified novel influenza A virus)J09.X2
    - swine (viruses that normally cause infections in pigs) (*see also* Influenza, due to, identified novel influenza A virus)J09.X2
- **Influenza-like** disease — *see* Influenza
- **Influenzal** — *see* Influenza
- **Infraction,** Freiberg's (metatarsal head) — *see* Osteochondrosis, juvenile, metatarsus
- **Infraeruption** of tooth (teeth) M26.34
- **Infusion** complication, misadventure, or reaction — *see* Complications, infusion
- **Ingestion**
  - chemical — *see* Table of Drugs and Chemicals, by substance, poisoning
  - drug or medicament
    - correct substance properly administered — *see* Table of Drugs and Chemicals, by drug, adverse effect
    - overdose or wrong substance given or taken — *see* Table of Drugs and Chemicals, by drug, poisoning
  - foreign body — *see* Foreign body, alimentary tract
  - tularemia A21.3
- **Ingrowing**
  - hair (beard) L73.1
  - nail (finger) (toe) L60.0
- **Inguinal** (*see also* condition)
  - testicle Q53.9
    - bilateral Q53.21
    - unilateral Q53.11
- **Inhalant-induced**
  - anxiety disorder F18.980
  - depressive disorder F18.94
  - major neurocognitive disorder F18.97
  - mild neurocognitive disorder F18.988
  - psychotic disorder F18.959
- **Inhalation**
  - anthrax A22.1
  - flame T27.3 ☑
  - food or foreign body — *see* Foreign body, by site
  - gases, fumes, or vapors NEC T59.9 ☑
    - specified agent — *see* Table of Drugs and Chemicals, by substance
  - liquid or vomitus — *see* Asphyxia
  - meconium (newborn) P24.00
    - with
      - pneumonia (pneumonitis) P24.01
      - with respiratory symptoms P24.01
  - mucus — *see* Asphyxia, mucus
  - oil or gasoline (causing suffocation) — *see* Foreign body, by site
  - smoke J70.5
    - due to chemicals, gases, fumes and vapors J68.9
  - steam — *see* Toxicity, vapors
  - stomach contents or secretions — *see* Foreign body, by site
    - due to anesthesia (general) (local) or other sedation T88.59 ☑
      - in labor and delivery O74.0
      - in pregnancy O29.01 ☑
      - postpartum, puerperal O89.01
- **Inhibition,** orgasm
  - female F52.31
  - male F52.32
- **Inhibitor,** systemic lupus erythematosus (presence of) D68.62
- **Iniencephalus,** iniencephaly Q00.2
- **Injection,** traumatic jet (air) (industrial) (water) (paint or dye) T70.4 ☑
- **Injury** (*see also* specified injury type)T14.90
  - abdomen, abdominal S39.91 ☑
    - blood vessel — *see* Injury, blood vessel, abdomen
    - cavity — *see* Injury, intra-abdominal
    - contusion S30.1 ☑
    - internal — *see* Injury, intra-abdominal
    - intra-abdominal organ — *see* Injury, intra-abdominal
    - nerve — *see* Injury, nerve, abdomen
    - open — *see* Wound, open, abdomen
    - specified NEC S39.81 ☑
    - superficial — *see* Injury, superficial, abdomen
  - Achilles tendon S86.00 ☑
    - laceration S86.02 ☑
    - specified type NEC S86.09 ☑
    - strain S86.01 ☑
  - acoustic, resulting in deafness — *see* Injury, nerve, acoustic
  - adrenal (gland) S37.819 ☑
    - contusion S37.812 ☑
    - laceration S37.813 ☑
    - specified type NEC S37.818 ☑
  - alveolar (process) S09.93 ☑
  - ankle S99.91 ☑
    - contusion — *see* Contusion, ankle
    - dislocation — *see* Dislocation, ankle
    - fracture — *see* Fracture, ankle
    - nerve — *see* Injury, nerve, ankle
    - open — *see* Wound, open, ankle
    - specified type NEC S99.81 ☑
    - sprain — *see* Sprain, ankle
    - superficial — *see* Injury, superficial, ankle
  - anterior chamber, eye — *see* Injury, eye, specified site NEC
  - anus — *see* Injury, abdomen
  - aorta (thoracic) S25.00 ☑
    - abdominal S35.00 ☑
      - laceration (minor) (superficial) S35.01 ☑
        - major S35.02 ☑
      - specified type NEC S35.09 ☑
    - laceration (minor) (superficial) S25.01 ☑
      - major S25.02 ☑
    - specified type NEC S25.09 ☑
  - arm (upper) S49.9 ☑
    - blood vessel — *see* Injury, blood vessel, arm
    - contusion — *see* Contusion, arm, upper
    - fracture — *see* Fracture, humerus
    - lower — *see* Injury, forearm
    - muscle — *see* Injury, muscle, shoulder
    - nerve — *see* Injury, nerve, arm
    - open — *see* Wound, open, arm
    - specified type NEC S49.8 ☑
    - superficial — *see* Injury, superficial, arm
  - artery (complicating trauma) (*see also* Injury, blood vessel, by site)
    - cerebral or meningeal — *see* Injury, intracranial
  - auditory canal (external) (meatus) S09.91 ☑
  - auricle, auris, ear S09.91 ☑
  - axilla — *see* Injury, shoulder
  - back — *see* Injury, back, lower
  - bile duct S36.13 ☑
  - birth (*see also* Birth, injury)P15.9
  - bladder (sphincter) S37.20 ☑
    - at delivery O71.5
    - contusion S37.22 ☑
    - laceration S37.23 ☑
    - obstetrical trauma O71.5
    - specified type NEC S37.29 ☑
  - blast (air) (hydraulic) (immersion) (underwater) NEC T14.8
    - acoustic nerve trauma — *see* Injury, nerve, acoustic
    - bladder — *see* Injury, bladder
    - brain — *see* Concussion
    - colon — *see* Injury, intestine, large, blast injury
    - ear (primary) S09.31 ☑
      - secondary S09.39 ☑
    - generalized T70.8 ☑
    - lung — *see* Injury, intrathoracic, lung, blast injury
    - multiple body organs T70.8 ☑
    - peritoneum S36.81 ☑
    - rectum S36.61 ☑
    - retroperitoneum S36.898 ☑
    - small intestine S36.419 ☑
      - duodenum S36.410 ☑
      - specified site NEC S36.418 ☑
    - specified
      - intra-abdominal organ NEC S36.898 ☑
      - pelvic organ NEC S37.899 ☑
- **Injury** — *continued*
  - blood vessel NEC T14.8
    - abdomen S35.9 ☑
      - aorta — *see* Injury, aorta, abdominal
      - celiac artery — *see* Injury, blood vessel, celiac artery
      - iliac vessel — *see* Injury, blood vessel, iliac
      - laceration S35.91 ☑
      - mesenteric vessel — *see* Injury, mesenteric
      - portal vein — *see* Injury, blood vessel, portal vein
      - renal vessel — *see* Injury, blood vessel, renal
      - specified vessel NEC S35.8X ☑
      - splenic vessel — *see* Injury, blood vessel, splenic
      - vena cava — *see* Injury, vena cava, inferior
    - ankle — *see* Injury, blood vessel, foot
    - aorta (abdominal) (thoracic) — *see* Injury, aorta
    - arm (upper) NEC S45.90 ☑
      - forearm — *see* Injury, blood vessel, forearm
      - laceration S45.91 ☑
      - specified
        - site NEC S45.80 ☑
          - laceration S45.81 ☑
          - specified type NEC S45.89 ☑
        - type NEC S45.99 ☑
      - superficial vein S45.30 ☑
        - laceration S45.31 ☑
        - specified type NEC S45.39 ☑
    - axillary
      - artery S45.00 ☑
        - laceration S45.01 ☑
        - specified type NEC S45.09 ☑
      - vein S45.20 ☑
        - laceration S45.21 ☑
        - specified type NEC S45.29 ☑
    - azygos vein — *see* Injury, blood vessel, thoracic, specified site NEC
    - brachial
      - artery S45.10 ☑
        - laceration S45.11 ☑
        - specified type NEC S45.19 ☑
      - vein S45.20 ☑
        - laceration S45.219 ☑
        - specified type NEC S45.29 ☑
    - carotid artery (common) (external) (internal, extracranial) S15.00 ☑
      - internal, intracranial S06.8 ☑
      - laceration (minor) (superficial) S15.01 ☑
        - major S15.02 ☑
      - specified type NEC S15.09 ☑
    - celiac artery S35.219 ☑
      - branch S35.299 ☑
        - laceration (minor) (superficial) S35.291 ☑
          - major S35.292 ☑
        - specified NEC S35.298 ☑
      - laceration (minor) (superficial) S35.211 ☑
        - major S35.212 ☑
      - specified type NEC S35.218 ☑
    - cerebral — *see* Injury, intracranial
    - deep plantar — *see* Injury, blood vessel, plantar artery
    - digital (hand) — *see* Injury, blood vessel, finger
    - dorsal
      - artery (foot) S95.00 ☑
        - laceration S95.01 ☑
        - specified type NEC S95.09 ☑
      - vein (foot) S95.20 ☑
        - laceration S95.21 ☑
        - specified type NEC S95.29 ☑
    - due to accidental laceration during procedure — *see* Laceration, accidental complicating surgery
    - extremity — *see* Injury, blood vessel, limb
    - femoral
      - artery (common) (superficial) S75.00 ☑
        - laceration (minor) (superficial) S75.01 ☑
          - major S75.02 ☑
        - specified type NEC S75.09 ☑
      - vein (hip level) (thigh level) S75.10 ☑
        - laceration (minor) (superficial) S75.11 ☑
          - major S75.12 ☑
        - specified type NEC S75.19 ☑
    - finger S65.50 ☑
      - index S65.50 ☑
        - laceration S65.51 ☑
        - specified type NEC S65.59 ☑
      - laceration S65.51 ☑
      - little S65.50 ☑
        - laceration S65.51 ☑
        - specified type NEC S65.59 ☑
      - middle S65.50 ☑

- **Injury** — *continued*
  - blood vessel NEC — *continued*
        - laceration S65.51 ☑
        - specified type NEC S65.59 ☑
      - specified type NEC S65.59 ☑
      - thumb — *see* Injury, blood vessel, thumb
    - foot S95.90 ☑
      - dorsal
        - artery — *see* Injury, blood vessel, dorsal, artery
        - vein — *see* Injury, blood vessel, dorsal, vein
      - laceration S95.91 ☑
      - plantar artery — *see* Injury, blood vessel, plantar artery
      - specified
        - site NEC S95.80 ☑
          - laceration S95.81 ☑
          - specified type NEC S95.89 ☑
        - specified type NEC S95.99 ☑
    - forearm S55.90 ☑
      - laceration S55.91 ☑
      - radial artery — *see* Injury, blood vessel, radial artery
      - specified
        - site NEC S55.80 ☑
          - laceration S55.81 ☑
          - specified type NEC S55.89 ☑
        - type NEC S55.99 ☑
      - ulnar artery — *see* Injury, blood vessel, ulnar artery
      - vein S55.20 ☑
        - laceration S55.21 ☑
        - specified type NEC S55.29 ☑
    - gastric
      - artery — *see* Injury, mesenteric, artery, branch
      - vein — *see* Injury, blood vessel, abdomen
    - gastroduodenal artery — *see* Injury, mesenteric, artery, branch
    - greater saphenous vein (lower leg level) S85.30 ☑
      - hip (and thigh) level S75.20 ☑
        - laceration (minor) (superficial) S75.21 ☑
          - major S75.22 ☑
        - specified type NEC S75.29 ☑
      - laceration S85.31 ☑
      - specified type NEC S85.39 ☑
    - hand (level) S65.90 ☑
      - finger — *see* Injury, blood vessel, finger
      - laceration S65.91 ☑
      - palmar arch — *see* Injury, blood vessel, palmar arch
      - radial artery — *see* Injury, blood vessel, radial artery, hand
      - specified
        - site NEC S65.80 ☑
          - laceration S65.81 ☑
          - specified type NEC S65.89 ☑
        - type NEC S65.99 ☑
      - thumb — *see* Injury, blood vessel, thumb
      - ulnar artery — *see* Injury, blood vessel, ulnar artery, hand
    - head S09.0 ☑
      - intracranial — *see* Injury, intracranial
      - multiple S09.0 ☑
    - hepatic
      - artery — *see* Injury, mesenteric, artery
      - vein — *see* Injury, vena cava, inferior
    - hip S75.90 ☑
      - femoral artery — *see* Injury, blood vessel, femoral, artery
      - femoral vein — *see* Injury, blood vessel, femoral, vein
      - greater saphenous vein — *see* Injury, blood vessel, greater saphenous, hip level
      - laceration S75.91 ☑
      - specified
        - site NEC S75.80 ☑
          - laceration S75.81 ☑
          - specified type NEC S75.89 ☑
        - type NEC S75.99 ☑
    - hypogastric (artery) (vein) — *see* Injury, blood vessel, iliac
    - iliac S35.5 ☑
      - artery S35.51 ☑
      - specified vessel NEC S35.5 ☑
      - uterine vessel — *see* Injury, blood vessel, uterine
      - vein S35.51 ☑
    - innominate — *see* Injury, blood vessel, thoracic, innominate

- **Injury** — *continued*
  - blood vessel NEC — *continued*
    - intercostal (artery) (vein) — *see* Injury, blood vessel, thoracic, intercostal
    - jugular vein (external) S15.20 ☑
      - internal S15.30 ☑
        - laceration (minor) (superficial) S15.31 ☑
          - major S15.32 ☑
        - specified type NEC S15.39 ☑
      - laceration (minor) (superficial) S15.21 ☑
        - major S15.22 ☑
      - specified type NEC S15.29 ☑
    - leg (level) (lower) S85.90 ☑
      - greater saphenous — *see* Injury, blood vessel, greater saphenous
      - laceration S85.91 ☑
      - lesser saphenous — *see* Injury, blood vessel, lesser saphenous
      - peroneal artery — *see* Injury, blood vessel, peroneal artery
      - popliteal
        - artery — *see* Injury, blood vessel, popliteal, artery
        - vein — *see* Injury, blood vessel, popliteal, vein
      - specified
        - site NEC S85.80 ☑
          - laceration S85.81 ☑
          - specified type NEC S85.89 ☑
        - type NEC S85.99 ☑
      - thigh — *see* Injury, blood vessel, hip
      - tibial artery — *see* Injury, blood vessel, tibial artery
    - lesser saphenous vein (lower leg level) S85.40 ☑
      - laceration S85.41 ☑
      - specified type NEC S85.49 ☑
    - limb
      - lower — *see* Injury, blood vessel, leg
      - upper — *see* Injury, blood vessel, arm
    - lower back — *see* Injury, blood vessel, abdomen
      - specified NEC — *see* Injury, blood vessel, abdomen, specified, site NEC
    - mammary (artery) (vein) — *see* Injury, blood vessel, thoracic, specified site NEC
    - mesenteric (inferior) (superior)
      - artery — *see* Injury, mesenteric, artery
      - vein — *see* Injury, mesenteric, vein
    - neck S15.9 ☑
      - specified site NEC S15.8 ☑
    - ovarian (artery) (vein) — *see* subcategory S35.8
    - palmar arch (superficial) S65.20 ☑
      - deep S65.30 ☑
        - laceration S65.31 ☑
        - specified type NEC S65.39 ☑
      - laceration S65.21 ☑
      - specified type NEC S65.29 ☑
    - pelvis — *see* Injury, blood vessel, abdomen
      - specified NEC — *see* Injury, blood vessel, abdomen, specified, site NEC
    - peroneal artery S85.20 ☑
      - laceration S85.21 ☑
      - specified type NEC S85.29 ☑
    - plantar artery (deep) (foot) S95.10 ☑
      - laceration S95.11 ☑
      - specified type NEC S95.19 ☑
    - popliteal
      - artery S85.00 ☑
        - laceration S85.01 ☑
        - specified type NEC S85.09 ☑
      - vein S85.50 ☑
        - laceration S85.51 ☑
        - specified type NEC S85.59 ☑
    - portal vein S35.319 ☑
      - laceration S35.311 ☑
      - specified type NEC S35.318 ☑
    - precerebral — *see* Injury, blood vessel, neck
    - pulmonary (artery) (vein) — *see* Injury, blood vessel, thoracic, pulmonary
    - radial artery (forearm level) S55.10 ☑
      - hand and wrist (level) S65.10 ☑
        - laceration S65.11 ☑
        - specified type NEC S65.19 ☑
      - laceration S55.11 ☑
      - specified type NEC S55.19 ☑
    - renal
      - artery S35.40 ☑
        - laceration S35.41 ☑
        - specified NEC S35.49 ☑
      - vein S35.40 ☑
        - laceration S35.41 ☑

- **Injury** — *continued*
  - blood vessel NEC — *continued*
        - specified NEC S35.49 ☑
    - saphenous vein (greater) (lower leg level) — *see* Injury, blood vessel, greater saphenous
      - hip and thigh level — *see* Injury, blood vessel, greater saphenous, hip level
      - lesser — *see* Injury, blood vessel, lesser saphenous
    - shoulder
      - specified NEC — *see* Injury, blood vessel, arm, specified site NEC
      - superficial vein — *see* Injury, blood vessel, arm, superficial vein
    - specified NEC T14.8
    - splenic
      - artery — *see* Injury, blood vessel, celiac artery, branch
      - vein S35.329 ☑
        - laceration S35.321 ☑
        - specified NEC S35.328 ☑
    - subclavian — *see* Injury, blood vessel, thoracic, innominate
    - thigh — *see* Injury, blood vessel, hip
    - thoracic S25.90 ☑
      - aorta S25.00 ☑
        - laceration (minor) (superficial) S25.01 ☑
          - major S25.02 ☑
        - specified type NEC S25.09 ☑
      - azygos vein — *see* Injury, blood vessel, thoracic, specified, site NEC
      - innominate
        - artery S25.10 ☑
          - laceration (minor) (superficial) S25.11 ☑
            - major S25.12 ☑
          - specified type NEC S25.19 ☑
        - vein S25.30 ☑
          - laceration (minor) (superficial) S25.31 ☑
            - major S25.32 ☑
          - specified type NEC S25.39 ☑
      - intercostal S25.50 ☑
        - laceration S25.51 ☑
        - specified type NEC S25.59 ☑
      - laceration S25.91 ☑
      - mammary vessel — *see* Injury, blood vessel, thoracic, specified, site NEC
      - pulmonary S25.40 ☑
        - laceration (minor) (superficial) S25.41 ☑
          - major S25.42 ☑
        - specified type NEC S25.49 ☑
      - specified
        - site NEC S25.80 ☑
          - laceration S25.81 ☑
          - specified type NEC S25.89 ☑
        - type NEC S25.99 ☑
      - subclavian — *see* Injury, blood vessel, thoracic, innominate
      - vena cava (superior) S25.20 ☑
        - laceration (minor) (superficial) S25.21 ☑
          - major S25.22 ☑
        - specified type NEC S25.29 ☑
    - thumb S65.40 ☑
      - laceration S65.41 ☑
      - specified type NEC S65.49 ☑
    - tibial artery S85.10 ☑
      - anterior S85.13 ☑
        - laceration S85.14 ☑
        - specified injury NEC S85.15 ☑
      - laceration S85.11 ☑
      - posterior S85.16 ☑
        - laceration S85.17 ☑
        - specified injury NEC S85.18 ☑
      - specified injury NEC S85.12 ☑
    - ulnar artery (forearm level) S55.00 ☑
      - hand and wrist (level) S65.00 ☑
        - laceration S65.01 ☑
        - specified type NEC S65.09 ☑
      - laceration S55.01 ☑
      - specified type NEC S55.09 ☑
    - upper arm (level) — *see* Injury, blood vessel, arm
      - superficial vein — *see* Injury, blood vessel, arm, superficial vein
    - uterine S35.5 ☑
      - artery S35.53 ☑
      - vein S35.53 ☑
    - vena cava — *see* Injury, vena cava
    - vertebral artery S15.10 ☑
      - laceration (minor) (superficial) S15.11 ☑
        - major S15.12 ☑
      - specified type NEC S15.19 ☑
    - wrist (level) — *see* Injury, blood vessel, hand

Injury — *continued*
- brachial plexus S14.3 ☑
  - newborn P14.3
- brain (traumatic) S06.9 ☑
  - diffuse (axonal) S06.2X ☑
  - focal S06.30 ☑
- brainstem S06.38 ☑
- breast NOS S29.9 ☑
- broad ligament — *see* Injury, pelvic organ, specified site NEC
- bronchus, bronchi — *see* Injury, intrathoracic, bronchus
- brow S09.90 ☑
- buttock S39.92 ☑
- canthus, eye S05.90 ☑
- cardiac plexus — *see* Injury, nerve, thorax, sympathetic
- cauda equina S34.3 ☑
- cavernous sinus — *see* Injury, intracranial
- cecum — *see* Injury, colon
- celiac ganglion or plexus — *see* Injury, nerve, lumbosacral, sympathetic
- cerebellum — *see* Injury, intracranial
- cerebral — *see* Injury, intracranial
- cervix (uteri) — *see* Injury, uterus
- cheek (wall) S09.93 ☑
- chest — *see* Injury, thorax
- childbirth (newborn) (*see also* Birth, injury)
  - maternal NEC O71.9
- chin S09.93 ☑
- choroid (eye) — *see* Injury, eye, specified site NEC
- clitoris S39.94 ☑
- coccyx (*see also* Injury, back, lower)
  - complicating delivery O71.6
- colon — *see* Injury, intestine, large
- common bile duct — *see* Injury, liver
- conjunctiva (superficial) — *see* Injury, eye, conjunctiva
- conus medullaris — *see* Injury, spinal, sacral
- cord
  - spermatic (pelvic region) S37.898 ☑
    - scrotal region S39.848 ☑
  - spinal — *see* Injury, spinal cord, by region
- cornea — *see* Injury, eye, specified site NEC
  - abrasion — *see* Injury, eye, cornea, abrasion
- cortex (cerebral) (*see also* Injury, intracranial)
  - visual — *see* Injury, nerve, optic
- costal region NEC S29.9 ☑
- costochondral NEC S29.9 ☑
- cranial
  - cavity — *see* Injury, intracranial
  - nerve — *see* Injury, nerve, cranial
- crushing — *see* Crush
- cutaneous sensory nerve
- cystic duct — *see* Injury, liver
- deep tissue — *see* Contusion, by site
  - meaning pressure ulcer — *see* Ulcer, pressure, unstageable, by site
- delivery (newborn) P15.9
  - maternal NEC O71.9
- Descemet's membrane — *see* Injury, eyeball, penetrating
- diaphragm — *see* Injury, intrathoracic, diaphragm
- duodenum — *see* Injury, intestine, small, duodenum
- ear (auricle) (external) (canal) S09.91 ☑
  - abrasion — *see* Abrasion, ear
  - bite — *see* Bite, ear
  - blister — *see* Blister, ear
  - bruise — *see* Contusion, ear
  - contusion — *see* Contusion, ear
  - external constriction — *see* Constriction, external, ear
  - hematoma — *see* Hematoma, ear
  - inner — *see* Injury, ear, middle
  - laceration — *see* Laceration, ear
  - middle S09.30 ☑
    - blast — *see* Injury, blast, ear
    - specified NEC S09.39 ☑
  - puncture — *see* Puncture, ear
  - superficial — *see* Injury, superficial, ear
- eighth cranial nerve (acoustic or auditory) — *see* Injury, nerve, acoustic
- elbow S59.90 ☑
  - contusion — *see* Contusion, elbow
  - dislocation — *see* Dislocation, elbow
  - fracture — *see* Fracture, ulna, upper end
  - open — *see* Wound, open, elbow
  - specified NEC S59.80 ☑
  - sprain — *see* Sprain, elbow
  - superficial — *see* Injury, superficial, elbow

Injury — *continued*
- eleventh cranial nerve (accessory) — *see* Injury, nerve, accessory
- epididymis S39.94 ☑
- epigastric region S39.91 ☑
- epiglottis NEC S19.89 ☑
- esophageal plexus — *see* Injury, nerve, thorax, sympathetic
- esophagus (thoracic part) (*see also* Injury, intrathoracic, esophagus)
  - cervical NEC S19.85 ☑
- eustachian tube S09.30 ☑
- eye S05.9 ☑
  - avulsion S05.7 ☑
  - ball — *see* Injury, eyeball
  - conjunctiva S05.0 ☑
  - cornea
    - abrasion S05.0 ☑
  - laceration S05.3 ☑
    - with prolapse S05.2 ☑
  - lacrimal apparatus S05.8X ☑
  - orbit penetration S05.4 ☑
  - specified site NEC S05.8X ☑
- eyeball S05.8X ☑
  - contusion S05.1 ☑
  - penetrating S05.6 ☑
    - with
      - foreign body S05.5 ☑
      - prolapse or loss of intraocular tissue S05.2 ☑
    - without prolapse or loss of intraocular tissue S05.3 ☑
  - specified type NEC S05.8 ☑
- eyebrow S09.93 ☑
- eyelid S09.93 ☑
  - abrasion — *see* Abrasion, eyelid
  - contusion — *see* Contusion, eyelid
  - open — *see* Wound, open, eyelid
- face S09.93 ☑
- fallopian tube S37.509 ☑
  - bilateral S37.502 ☑
    - blast injury S37.512 ☑
    - contusion S37.522 ☑
    - laceration S37.532 ☑
    - specified type NEC S37.592 ☑
  - blast injury (primary) S37.519 ☑
    - bilateral S37.512 ☑
    - secondary — *see* Injury, fallopian tube, specified type NEC
    - unilateral S37.511 ☑
  - contusion S37.529 ☑
    - bilateral S37.522 ☑
    - unilateral S37.521 ☑
  - laceration S37.539 ☑
    - bilateral S37.532 ☑
    - unilateral S37.531 ☑
  - specified type NEC S37.599 ☑
    - bilateral S37.592 ☑
    - unilateral S37.591 ☑
  - unilateral S37.501 ☑
    - blast injury S37.511 ☑
    - contusion S37.521 ☑
    - laceration S37.531 ☑
    - specified type NEC S37.591 ☑
- fascia — *see* Injury, muscle
- fifth cranial nerve (trigeminal) — *see* Injury, nerve, trigeminal
- finger (nail) S69.9 ☑
  - blood vessel — *see* Injury, blood vessel, finger
  - contusion — *see* Contusion, finger
  - dislocation — *see* Dislocation, finger
  - fracture — *see* Fracture, finger
  - muscle — *see* Injury, muscle, finger
  - nerve — *see* Injury, nerve, digital, finger
  - open — *see* Wound, open, finger
  - specified NEC S69.8 ☑
  - sprain — *see* Sprain, finger
  - superficial — *see* Injury, superficial, finger
- first cranial nerve (olfactory) — *see* Injury, nerve, olfactory
- flank — *see* Injury, abdomen
- foot S99.92 ☑
  - blood vessel — *see* Injury, blood vessel, foot
  - contusion — *see* Contusion, foot
  - dislocation — *see* Dislocation, foot
  - fracture — *see* Fracture, foot
  - muscle — *see* Injury, muscle, foot
  - open — *see* Wound, open, foot
  - specified type NEC S99.82 ☑
  - sprain — *see* Sprain, foot
  - superficial — *see* Injury, superficial, foot
- forceps NOS P15.9

Injury — *continued*
- forearm S59.91 ☑
  - blood vessel — *see* Injury, blood vessel, forearm
  - contusion — *see* Contusion, forearm
  - fracture — *see* Fracture, forearm
  - muscle — *see* Injury, muscle, forearm
  - nerve — *see* Injury, nerve, forearm
  - open — *see* Wound, open, forearm
  - specified NEC S59.81 ☑
  - superficial — *see* Injury, superficial, forearm
- forehead S09.90 ☑
- fourth cranial nerve (trochlear) — *see* Injury, nerve, trochlear
- gallbladder S36.129 ☑
  - contusion S36.122 ☑
  - laceration S36.123 ☑
  - specified NEC S36.128 ☑
- ganglion
  - celiac, coeliac — *see* Injury, nerve, lumbosacral, sympathetic
  - gasserian — *see* Injury, nerve, trigeminal
  - stellate — *see* Injury, nerve, thorax, sympathetic
  - thoracic sympathetic — *see* Injury, nerve, thorax, sympathetic
- gasserian ganglion — *see* Injury, nerve, trigeminal
- gastric artery — *see* Injury, blood vessel, celiac artery, branch
- gastroduodenal artery — *see* Injury, blood vessel, celiac artery, branch
- gastrointestinal tract — *see* Injury, intra-abdominal
  - with open wound into abdominal cavity — *see* Wound, open, with penetration into peritoneal cavity
  - colon — *see* Injury, intestine, large
  - rectum — *see* Injury, intestine, large, rectum
    - with open wound into abdominal cavity S36.61 ☑
  - specified site NEC — *see* Injury, intra-abdominal, specified, site NEC
  - stomach — *see* Injury, stomach
  - small intestine — *see* Injury, intestine, small
- genital organ (s)
  - external S39.94 ☑
    - specified NEC S39.848 ☑
  - internal S37.90 ☑
    - fallopian tube — *see* Injury, fallopian tube
    - ovary — *see* Injury, ovary
    - prostate — *see* Injury, prostate
    - seminal vesicle — *see* Injury, pelvis, organ, specified site NEC
    - uterus — *see* Injury, uterus
    - vas deferens — *see* Injury, pelvis, organ, specified site NEC
  - obstetrical trauma O71.9
- gland
  - lacrimal laceration — *see* Injury, eye, specified site NEC
  - salivary S09.93 ☑
  - thyroid NEC S19.84 ☑
- globe (eye) S05.90 ☑
  - specified NEC S05.8X ☑
- groin — *see* Injury, abdomen
- gum S09.90 ☑
- hand S69.9 ☑
  - blood vessel — *see* Injury, blood vessel, hand
  - contusion — *see* Contusion, hand
  - fracture — *see* Fracture, hand
  - muscle — *see* Injury, muscle, hand
  - nerve — *see* Injury, nerve, hand
  - open — *see* Wound, open, hand
  - specified NEC S69.8 ☑
  - sprain — *see* Sprain, hand
  - superficial — *see* Injury, superficial, hand
- head S09.90 ☑
  - with loss of consciousness S06.9 ☑
  - specified NEC S09.8 ☑
- heart S26.90 ☑
  - with hemopericardium S26.00 ☑
    - contusion S26.01 ☑
    - laceration (mild) S26.020 ☑
      - moderate S26.021 ☑
      - major S26.022 ☑
    - specified type NEC S26.09 ☑
  - contusion S26.91 ☑
  - laceration S26.92 ☑
  - specified type NEC S26.99 ☑
  - without hemopericardium S26.10 ☑
    - contusion S26.11 ☑
    - laceration S26.12 ☑
    - specified type NEC S26.19 ☑
- heel — *see* Injury, foot

- **Injury** — *continued*
  - intrathoracic — *continued*
      - contusion S27.892 ☑
      - laceration S27.893 ☑
      - specified type NEC S27.898 ☑
    - thoracic duct — *see* Injury, intrathoracic, specified organ NEC
    - thymus gland — *see* Injury, intrathoracic, specified organ NEC
    - trachea, thoracic S27.50 ☑
      - blast (primary) S27.51 ☑
      - contusion S27.52 ☑
      - laceration S27.53 ☑
      - specified type NEC S27.59 ☑
  - iris — *see* Injury, eye, specified site NEC
    - penetrating — *see* Injury, eyeball, penetrating
  - jaw S09.93 ☑
  - jejunum — *see* Injury, intestine, small
  - joint NOS T14.8
    - old or residual — *see* Disorder, joint, specified type NEC
  - kidney S37.00 ☑
    - acute (nontraumatic) N17.9
    - contusion — *see* Contusion, kidney
    - laceration — *see* Laceration, kidney
    - specified NEC S37.09 ☑
  - knee S89.9 ☑
    - contusion — *see* Contusion, knee
    - dislocation — *see* Dislocation, knee
    - meniscus (lateral) (medial) — *see* Sprain, knee, specified site NEC
      - old injury or tear — *see* Derangement, knee, meniscus, due to old injury
    - open — *see* Wound, open, knee
    - specified NEC S89.8 ☑
    - sprain — *see* Sprain, knee
    - superficial — *see* Injury, superficial, knee
  - labium (majus) (minus) S39.94 ☑
  - labyrinth, ear S09.30 ☑
  - lacrimal apparatus, duct, gland, or sac — *see* Injury, eye, specified site NEC
  - larynx NEC S19.81 ☑
  - leg (lower) S89.9 ☑
    - blood vessel — *see* Injury, blood vessel, leg
    - contusion — *see* Contusion, leg
    - fracture — *see* Fracture, leg
    - muscle — *see* Injury, muscle, leg
    - nerve — *see* Injury, nerve, leg
    - open — *see* Wound, open, leg
    - specified NEC S89.8 ☑
    - superficial — *see* Injury, superficial, leg
  - lens, eye — *see* Injury, eye, specified site NEC
    - penetrating — *see* Injury, eyeball, penetrating
  - limb NEC T14.8
  - lip S09.93 ☑
  - liver S36.119 ☑
    - contusion S36.112 ☑
    - laceration S36.113 ☑
      - major (stellate) S36.116 ☑
      - minor S36.114 ☑
      - moderate S36.115 ☑
    - specified NEC S36.118 ☑
  - lower back S39.92 ☑
    - specified NEC S39.82 ☑
  - lumbar, lumbosacral (region) S39.92 ☑
    - plexus — *see* Injury, lumbosacral plexus
  - lumbosacral plexus S34.4 ☑
  - lung (*see also* Injury, intrathoracic, lung)
    - aspiration J69.0
    - transfusion-related (TRALI) J95.84
  - lymphatic thoracic duct — *see* Injury, intrathoracic, specified organ NEC
  - malar region S09.93 ☑
  - mastoid region S09.90 ☑
  - maxilla S09.93 ☑
  - mediastinum — *see* Injury, intrathoracic, specified organ NEC
  - membrane, brain — *see* Injury, intracranial
  - meningeal artery — *see* Injury, intracranial, subdural hemorrhage
  - meninges (cerebral) — *see* Injury, intracranial
  - mesenteric
    - artery
      - branch S35.299 ☑
        - laceration (minor) (superficial) S35.291 ☑
          - major S35.292 ☑
        - specified NEC S35.298 ☑
      - inferior S35.239 ☑
        - laceration (minor) (superficial) S35.231 ☑
          - major S35.232 ☑
        - specified NEC S35.238 ☑
      - superior S35.229 ☑

- **Injury** — *continued*
  - mesenteric — *continued*
        - laceration (minor) (superficial) S35.221 ☑
          - major S35.222 ☑
        - specified NEC S35.228 ☑
    - plexus (inferior) (superior) — *see* Injury, nerve, lumbosacral, sympathetic
    - vein
      - inferior S35.349 ☑
        - laceration S35.341 ☑
        - specified NEC S35.348 ☑
      - superior S35.339 ☑
        - laceration S35.331 ☑
        - specified NEC S35.338 ☑
  - mesentery — *see* Injury, intra-abdominal, specified site NEC
  - mesosalpinx — *see* Injury, pelvic organ, specified site NEC
  - middle ear S09.30 ☑
  - midthoracic region NOS S29.9 ☑
  - mouth S09.93 ☑
  - multiple NOS T07
  - muscle (and fascia) (and tendon)
    - abdomen S39.001 ☑
      - laceration S39.021 ☑
      - specified type NEC S39.091 ☑
      - strain S39.011 ☑
    - abductor
      - thumb, forearm level — *see* Injury, muscle, thumb, abductor
    - adductor
      - thigh S76.20 ☑
        - laceration S76.22 ☑
        - specified type NEC S76.29 ☑
        - strain S76.21 ☑
    - ankle — *see* Injury, muscle, foot
    - anterior muscle group, at leg level (lower) S86.20 ☑
      - laceration S86.22 ☑
      - specified type NEC S86.29 ☑
      - strain S86.21 ☑
    - arm (upper) — *see* Injury, muscle, shoulder
    - biceps (parts NEC) S46.20 ☑
      - laceration S46.22 ☑
      - long head S46.10 ☑
        - laceration S46.12 ☑
        - strain S46.11 ☑
        - specified type NEC S46.19 ☑
      - specified type NEC S46.29 ☑
      - strain S46.21 ☑
    - extensor
      - finger (s) (other than thumb) — *see* Injury, muscle, finger by site, extensor
      - forearm level, specified NEC — *see* Injury, muscle, forearm, extensor
      - thumb — *see* Injury, muscle, thumb, extensor
      - toe (large) (ankle level) (foot level) — *see* Injury, muscle, toe, extensor
    - finger
      - extensor (forearm level) S56.40 ☑
        - hand level S66.309 ☑
          - laceration S66.329 ☑
          - specified type NEC S66.399 ☑
          - strain S66.319 ☑
        - laceration S56.429 ☑
        - specified type NEC S56.499 ☑
        - strain S56.419 ☑
      - flexor (forearm level) S56.10 ☑
        - hand level S66.109 ☑
          - laceration S66.129 ☑
          - specified type NEC S66.199 ☑
          - strain S66.119 ☑
        - laceration S56.129 ☑
        - specified type NEC S56.199 ☑
        - strain S56.119 ☑
      - intrinsic S66.509 ☑
        - laceration S66.529 ☑
        - specified type NEC S66.599 ☑
        - strain S66.519 ☑
      - index
        - extensor (forearm level)
          - hand level S66.308 ☑
            - laceration S66.32 ☑
            - specified type NEC S66.39 ☑
            - strain S66.31 ☑
          - specified type NEC S56.492 ☑
        - flexor (forearm level)
          - hand level S66.108 ☑
            - laceration S66.12 ☑
            - specified type NEC S66.19 ☑
            - strain S66.11 ☑
          - specified type NEC S56.19 ☑

- **Injury** — *continued*
  - muscle — *continued*
          - strain S56.11 ☑
        - intrinsic S66.50 ☑
          - laceration S66.52 ☑
          - specified type NEC S66.59 ☑
          - strain S66.51 ☑
      - little
        - extensor (forearm level)
          - hand level S66.30 ☑
            - laceration S66.32 ☑
            - specified type NEC S66.39 ☑
            - strain S66.31 ☑
          - laceration S56.42 ☑
          - specified type NEC S56.49 ☑
          - strain S56.41 ☑
        - flexor (forearm level)
          - hand level S66.10 ☑
            - laceration S66.12 ☑
            - specified type NEC S66.19 ☑
            - strain S66.11 ☑
          - laceration S56.12 ☑
          - specified type NEC S56.19 ☑
          - strain S56.11 ☑
        - intrinsic S66.50 ☑
          - laceration S66.52 ☑
          - specified type NEC S66.59 ☑
          - strain S66.51 ☑
      - middle
        - extensor (forearm level)
          - hand level S66.30 ☑
            - laceration S66.32 ☑
            - specified type NEC S66.39 ☑
            - strain S66.31 ☑
          - laceration S56.42 ☑
          - specified type NEC S56.49 ☑
          - strain S56.41 ☑
        - flexor (forearm level)
          - hand level S66.10 ☑
            - laceration S66.12 ☑
            - specified type NEC S66.19 ☑
            - strain S66.11 ☑
          - laceration S56.12 ☑
          - specified type NEC S56.19 ☑
          - strain S56.11 ☑
        - intrinsic S66.50 ☑
          - laceration S66.52 ☑
          - specified type NEC S66.59 ☑
          - strain S66.51 ☑
      - ring
        - extensor (forearm level)
          - hand level S66.30 ☑
            - laceration S66.32 ☑
            - specified type NEC S66.39 ☑
            - strain S66.31 ☑
          - laceration S56.42 ☑
          - specified type NEC S56.49 ☑
          - strain S56.41 ☑
        - flexor (forearm level)
          - hand level S66.10 ☑
            - laceration S66.12 ☑
            - specified type NEC S66.19 ☑
            - strain S66.11 ☑
          - laceration S56.12 ☑
          - specified type NEC S56.19 ☑
          - strain S56.11 ☑
        - intrinsic S66.50 ☑
          - laceration S66.52 ☑
          - specified type NEC S66.59 ☑
          - strain S66.51 ☑
    - flexor
      - finger (s) (other than thumb) — *see* Injury, muscle, finger
      - forearm level, specified NEC — *see* Injury, muscle, forearm, flexor
      - thumb — *see* Injury, muscle, thumb, flexor
      - toe (long) (ankle level) (foot level) — *see* Injury, muscle, toe, flexor
    - foot S96.90 ☑
      - intrinsic S96.20 ☑
        - laceration S96.22 ☑
        - specified type NEC S96.29 ☑
        - strain S96.21 ☑
      - laceration S96.92 ☑
      - long extensor, toe — *see* Injury, muscle, toe, extensor
      - long flexor, toe — *see* Injury, muscle, toe, flexor
      - specified
        - site NEC S96.80 ☑
          - laceration S96.82 ☑
          - specified type NEC S96.89 ☑

- **Injury** — *continued*
  - muscle — *continued*
        - strain S96.81 ☑
      - type NEC S96.99 ☑
    - strain S96.91 ☑
    - forearm (level) S56.90 ☑
      - extensor S56.50 ☑
        - laceration S56.52 ☑
        - specified type NEC S56.59 ☑
        - strain S56.51 ☑
      - flexor S56.20 ☑
        - laceration S56.22 ☑
        - specified type NEC S56.29 ☑
        - strain S56.21 ☑
      - laceration S56.92 ☑
      - specified S56.99 ☑
        - site NEC S56.80 ☑
          - laceration S56.82 ☑
          - strain S56.81 ☑
          - type NEC S56.89 ☑
      - strain S56.91 ☑
    - hand (level) S66.90 ☑
      - laceration S66.92 ☑
      - specified
        - site NEC S66.80 ☑
          - laceration S66.82 ☑
          - specified type NEC S66.89 ☑
          - strain S66.81 ☑
        - type NEC S66.99 ☑
      - strain S66.91 ☑
    - head S09.10 ☑
      - laceration S09.12 ☑
      - specified type NEC S09.19 ☑
      - strain S09.11 ☑
    - hip NEC S76.00 ☑
      - laceration S76.02 ☑
      - specified type NEC S76.09 ☑
      - strain S76.01 ☑
    - intrinsic
      - ankle and foot level — *see* Injury, muscle, foot, intrinsic
      - finger (other than thumb) — *see* Injury, muscle, finger by site, intrinsic
      - foot (level) — *see* Injury, muscle, foot, intrinsic
      - thumb — *see* Injury, muscle, thumb, intrinsic
    - leg (level) (lower) S86.90 ☑
      - Achilles tendon — *see* Injury, Achilles tendon
      - anterior muscle group — *see* Injury, muscle, anterior muscle group
      - laceration S86.92 ☑
      - peroneal muscle group — *see* Injury, muscle, peroneal muscle group
      - posterior muscle group — *see* Injury, muscle, posterior muscle group, leg level
      - specified
        - site NEC S86.80 ☑
          - laceration S86.82 ☑
          - specified type NEC S86.89 ☑
          - strain S86.81 ☑
        - type NEC S86.99 ☑
      - strain S86.91 ☑
    - long
      - extensor toe, at ankle and foot level — *see* Injury, muscle, toe, extensor
      - flexor, toe, at ankle and foot level — *see* Injury, muscle, toe, flexor
      - head, biceps — *see* Injury, muscle, biceps, long head
    - lower back S39.002 ☑
      - laceration S39.022 ☑
      - specified type NEC S39.092 ☑
      - strain S39.012 ☑
    - neck (level) S16.9 ☑
      - laceration S16.2 ☑
      - specified type NEC S16.8 ☑
      - strain S16.1 ☑
    - pelvis S39.003 ☑
      - laceration S39.023 ☑
      - specified type NEC S39.093 ☑
      - strain S39.013 ☑
    - peroneal muscle group, at leg level (lower) S86.30 ☑
      - laceration S86.32 ☑
      - specified type NEC S86.39 ☑
      - strain S86.31 ☑
    - posterior muscle (group)
      - leg level (lower) S86.10 ☑
        - laceration S86.12 ☑
        - specified type NEC S86.19 ☑
        - strain S86.11 ☑
      - thigh level S76.30 ☑

- **Injury** — *continued*
  - muscle — *continued*
        - laceration S76.32 ☑
        - specified type NEC S76.39 ☑
        - strain S76.31 ☑
    - quadriceps (thigh) S76.10 ☑
      - laceration S76.12 ☑
      - specified type NEC S76.19 ☑
      - strain S76.11 ☑
    - shoulder S46.90 ☑
      - laceration S46.92 ☑
      - rotator cuff — *see* Injury, rotator cuff
      - specified site NEC S46.80 ☑
        - laceration S46.82 ☑
        - strain S46.81 ☑
        - specified type NEC S46.89 ☑
      - strain S46.91 ☑
      - specified type NEC S46.99 ☑
    - thigh NEC (level) S76.90 ☑
      - adductor — *see* Injury, muscle, adductor, thigh
      - laceration S76.92 ☑
      - posterior muscle (group) — *see* Injury, muscle, posterior muscle, thigh level
      - quadriceps — *see* Injury, muscle, quadriceps
      - specified
        - site NEC S76.80 ☑
          - laceration S76.82 ☑
          - specified type NEC S76.89 ☑
          - strain S76.81 ☑
        - type NEC S76.99 ☑
      - strain S76.91 ☑
    - thorax (level) S29.009 ☑
      - back wall S29.002 ☑
      - front wall S29.001 ☑
      - laceration S29.029 ☑
        - back wall S29.022 ☑
        - front wall S29.021 ☑
      - specified type NEC S29.099 ☑
        - back wall S29.092 ☑
        - front wall S29.091 ☑
      - strain S29.019 ☑
        - back wall S29.012 ☑
        - front wall S29.011 ☑
    - thumb
      - abductor (forearm level) S56.30 ☑
        - laceration S56.32 ☑
        - specified type NEC S56.39 ☑
        - strain S56.31 ☑
      - extensor (forearm level) S56.30 ☑
        - hand level S66.20 ☑
          - laceration S66.22 ☑
          - specified type NEC S66.29 ☑
          - strain S66.21 ☑
        - laceration S56.32 ☑
        - specified type NEC S56.39 ☑
        - strain S56.31 ☑
      - flexor (forearm level) S56.00 ☑
        - hand level S66.00 ☑
          - laceration S66.02 ☑
          - specified type NEC S66.09 ☑
          - strain S66.01 ☑
        - laceration S56.02 ☑
        - specified type NEC S56.09 ☑
        - strain S56.01 ☑
        - wrist level — *see* Injury, muscle, thumb, flexor, hand level
      - intrinsic S66.40 ☑
        - laceration S66.42 ☑
        - specified type NEC S66.49 ☑
        - strain S66.41 ☑
    - toe (*see also* Injury, muscle, foot)
      - extensor, long S96.10 ☑
        - laceration S96.12 ☑
        - specified type NEC S96.19 ☑
        - strain S96.11 ☑
      - flexor, long S96.00 ☑
        - laceration S96.02 ☑
        - specified type NEC S96.09 ☑
        - strain S96.01 ☑
    - triceps S46.30 ☑
      - laceration S46.32 ☑
      - specified type NEC S46.39 ☑
      - strain S46.31 ☑
    - wrist (and hand) level — *see* Injury, muscle, hand
  - musculocutaneous nerve — *see* Injury, nerve, musculocutaneous
  - myocardium — *see* Injury, heart
  - nape — *see* Injury, neck
  - nasal (septum) (sinus) S09.92 ☑
  - nasopharynx S09.92 ☑

- **Injury** — *continued*
  - neck S19.9 ☑
    - specified NEC S19.80 ☑
      - specified site NEC S19.89 ☑
  - nerve NEC T14.8
    - abdomen S34.9 ☑
      - peripheral S34.6 ☑
      - specified site NEC S34.8 ☑
    - abducens S04.4 ☑
      - contusion S04.4 ☑
      - laceration S04.4 ☑
      - specified type NEC S04.4 ☑
    - abducent — *see* Injury, nerve, abducens
    - accessory S04.7 ☑
      - contusion S04.7 ☑
      - laceration S04.7 ☑
      - specified type NEC S04.7 ☑
    - acoustic S04.6 ☑
      - contusion S04.6 ☑
      - laceration S04.6 ☑
      - specified type NEC S04.6 ☑
    - ankle S94.9 ☑
      - cutaneous sensory S94.3 ☑
      - specified site NEC — *see* subcategory S94.8
    - anterior crural, femoral — *see* Injury, nerve, femoral
    - arm (upper) S44.9 ☑
      - axillary — *see* Injury, nerve, axillary
      - cutaneous — *see* Injury, nerve, cutaneous, arm
      - median — *see* Injury, nerve, median, upper arm
      - musculocutaneous — *see* Injury, nerve, musculocutaneous
      - radial — *see* Injury, nerve, radial, upper arm
      - specified site NEC — *see* subcategory S44.8
      - ulnar — *see* Injury, nerve, ulnar, arm
    - auditory — *see* Injury, nerve, acoustic
    - axillary S44.3 ☑
    - brachial plexus — *see* Injury, brachial plexus
    - cervical sympathetic S14.5 ☑
    - cranial S04.9 ☑
      - contusion S04.9 ☑
      - eighth (acoustic or auditory) — *see* Injury, nerve, acoustic
      - eleventh (accessory) — *see* Injury, nerve, accessory
      - fifth (trigeminal) — *see* Injury, nerve, trigeminal
      - first (olfactory) — *see* Injury, nerve, olfactory
      - fourth (trochlear) — *see* Injury, nerve, trochlear
      - laceration S04.9 ☑
      - ninth (glossopharyngeal) — *see* Injury, nerve, glossopharyngeal
      - second (optic) — *see* Injury, nerve, optic
      - seventh (facial) — *see* Injury, nerve, facial
      - sixth (abducent) — *see* Injury, nerve, abducens
      - specified
        - nerve NEC S04.89 ☑
          - contusion S04.89 ☑
          - laceration S04.89 ☑
          - specified type NEC S04.89 ☑
        - type NEC S04.9 ☑
      - tenth (pneumogastric or vagus) — *see* Injury, nerve, vagus
      - third (oculomotor) — *see* Injury, nerve, oculomotor
      - twelfth (hypoglossal) — *see* Injury, nerve, hypoglossal
    - cutaneous sensory
      - ankle (level) S94.3 ☑
      - arm (upper) (level) S44.5 ☑
      - foot (level) — *see* Injury, nerve, cutaneous sensory, ankle
      - forearm (level) S54.3 ☑
      - hip (level) S74.2 ☑
      - leg (lower level) S84.2 ☑
      - shoulder (level) — *see* Injury, nerve, cutaneous sensory, arm
      - thigh (level) — *see* Injury, nerve, cutaneous sensory, hip
    - deep peroneal — *see* Injury, nerve, peroneal, foot
    - digital
      - finger S64.4 ☑
        - index S64.49 ☑
        - little S64.49 ☑
        - middle S64.49 ☑
        - ring S64.49 ☑
      - thumb S64.3 ☑

- **Injury** — *continued*
  - nerve NEC — *continued*
    - toe — *see* Injury, nerve, ankle, specified site NEC
    - eighth cranial (acoustic or auditory) — *see* Injury, nerve, acoustic
    - eleventh cranial (accessory) — *see* Injury, nerve, accessory
    - facial S04.5 ☑
      - contusion S04.5 ☑
      - laceration S04.5 ☑
      - newborn P11.3
      - specified type NEC S04.5 ☑
    - femoral (hip level) (thigh level) S74.1 ☑
    - fifth cranial (trigeminal) — *see* Injury, nerve, trigeminal
    - finger (digital) — *see* Injury, nerve, digital, finger
    - first cranial (olfactory) — *see* Injury, nerve, olfactory
    - foot S94.9 ☑
      - cutaneous sensory S94.3 ☑
      - deep peroneal S94.2 ☑
      - lateral plantar S94.0 ☑
      - medial plantar S94.1 ☑
      - specified site NEC — *see* subcategory S94.8
    - forearm (level) S54.9 ☑
      - cutaneous sensory — *see* Injury, nerve, cutaneous sensory, forearm
      - median — *see* Injury, nerve, median
      - radial — *see* Injury, nerve, radial
      - specified site NEC — *see* subcategory S54.8
      - ulnar — *see* Injury, nerve, ulnar
    - fourth cranial (trochlear) — *see* Injury, nerve, trochlear
    - glossopharyngeal S04.89 ☑
      - specified type NEC S04.89 ☑
    - hand S64.9 ☑
      - median — *see* Injury, nerve, median, hand
      - radial — *see* Injury, nerve, radial, hand
      - specified NEC — *see* subcategory S64.8
      - ulnar — *see* Injury, nerve, ulnar, hand
    - hip (level) S74.9 ☑
      - cutaneous sensory — *see* Injury, nerve, cutaneous sensory, hip
      - femoral — *see* Injury, nerve, femoral
      - sciatic — *see* Injury, nerve, sciatic
      - specified site NEC — *see* subcategory S74.8
    - hypoglossal S04.89 ☑
      - specified type NEC S04.89 ☑
    - lateral plantar S94.0 ☑
    - leg (lower) S84.9 ☑
      - cutaneous sensory — *see* Injury, nerve, cutaneous sensory, leg
      - peroneal — *see* Injury, nerve, peroneal
      - specified site NEC — *see* subcategory S84.8
      - tibial — *see* Injury, nerve, tibial
      - upper — *see* Injury, nerve, thigh
    - lower
      - back — *see* Injury, nerve, abdomen, specified site NEC
        - peripheral — *see* Injury, nerve, abdomen, peripheral
      - limb — *see* Injury, nerve, leg
    - lumbar spinal — *see* Injury, nerve, spinal, lumbar
    - lumbar plexus — *see* Injury, nerve, lumbosacral, sympathetic
    - lumbosacral
      - plexus — *see* Injury, nerve, lumbosacral, sympathetic
      - sympathetic S34.5 ☑
    - medial plantar S94.1 ☑
    - median (forearm level) S54.1 ☑
      - hand (level) S64.1 ☑
      - upper arm (level) S44.1 ☑
      - wrist (level) — *see* Injury, nerve, median, hand
    - musculocutaneous S44.4 ☑
    - musculospiral (upper arm level) — *see* Injury, nerve, radial, upper arm
    - neck S14.9 ☑
      - peripheral S14.4 ☑
      - specified site NEC S14.8 ☑
      - sympathetic S14.5 ☑
    - ninth cranial (glossopharyngeal) — *see* Injury, nerve, glossopharyngeal
    - oculomotor S04.1 ☑
      - contusion S04.1 ☑
      - laceration S04.1 ☑
      - specified type NEC S04.1 ☑
    - olfactory S04.81 ☑

- **Injury** — *continued*
  - nerve NEC — *continued*
      - specified type NEC S04.81 ☑
    - optic S04.01 ☑
      - contusion S04.01 ☑
      - laceration S04.01 ☑
      - specified type NEC S04.01 ☑
    - pelvic girdle — *see* Injury, nerve, hip
    - pelvis — *see* Injury, nerve, abdomen, specified site NEC
      - peripheral — *see* Injury, nerve, abdomen, peripheral
    - peripheral NEC T14.8
      - abdomen — *see* Injury, nerve, abdomen, peripheral
      - lower back — *see* Injury, nerve, abdomen, peripheral
      - neck — *see* Injury, nerve, neck, peripheral
      - pelvis — *see* Injury, nerve, abdomen, peripheral
      - specified NEC T14.8
    - peroneal (lower leg level) S84.1 ☑
      - foot S94.2 ☑
    - plexus
      - brachial — *see* Injury, brachial plexus
      - celiac, coeliac — *see* Injury, nerve, lumbosacral, sympathetic
      - mesenteric, inferior — *see* Injury, nerve, lumbosacral, sympathetic
      - sacral — *see* Injury, lumbosacral plexus
      - spinal
        - brachial — *see* Injury, brachial plexus
        - lumbosacral — *see* Injury, lumbosacral plexus
    - pneumogastric — *see* Injury, nerve, vagus
    - radial (forearm level) S54.2 ☑
      - hand (level) S64.2 ☑
      - upper arm (level) S44.2 ☑
      - wrist (level) — *see* Injury, nerve, radial, hand
    - root — *see* Injury, nerve, spinal, root
    - sacral plexus — *see* Injury, lumbosacral plexus
    - sacral spinal — *see* Injury, nerve, spinal, sacral
    - sciatic (hip level) (thigh level) S74.0 ☑
    - second cranial (optic) — *see* Injury, nerve, optic
    - seventh cranial (facial) — *see* Injury, nerve, facial
    - shoulder — *see* Injury, nerve, arm
    - sixth cranial (abducent) — *see* Injury, nerve, abducens
    - spinal
      - plexus — *see* Injury, nerve, plexus, spinal
      - root
        - cervical S14.2 ☑
        - dorsal S24.2 ☑
        - lumbar S34.21 ☑
        - sacral S34.22 ☑
        - thoracic — *see* Injury, nerve, spinal, root, dorsal
    - splanchnic — *see* Injury, nerve, lumbosacral, sympathetic
    - sympathetic NEC — *see* Injury, nerve, lumbosacral, sympathetic
      - cervical — *see* Injury, nerve, cervical sympathetic
    - tenth cranial (pneumogastric or vagus) — *see* Injury, nerve, vagus
    - thigh (level) — *see* Injury, nerve, hip
      - cutaneous sensory — *see* Injury, nerve, cutaneous sensory, hip
      - femoral — *see* Injury, nerve, femoral
      - sciatic — *see* Injury, nerve, sciatic
      - specified NEC — *see* Injury, nerve, hip
    - third cranial (oculomotor) — *see* Injury, nerve, oculomotor
    - thorax S24.9 ☑
      - peripheral S24.3 ☑
      - specified site NEC S24.8 ☑
      - sympathetic S24.4 ☑
    - thumb, digital — *see* Injury, nerve, digital, thumb
    - tibial (lower leg level) (posterior) S84.0 ☑
    - toe — *see* Injury, nerve, ankle
    - trigeminal S04.3 ☑
      - contusion S04.3 ☑
      - laceration S04.3 ☑
      - specified type NEC S04.3 ☑
    - trochlear S04.2 ☑
      - contusion S04.2 ☑
      - laceration S04.2 ☑
      - specified type NEC S04.2 ☑
    - twelfth cranial (hypoglossal) — *see* Injury, nerve, hypoglossal

- **Injury** — *continued*
  - nerve NEC — *continued*
    - ulnar (forearm level) S54.0 ☑
      - arm (upper) (level) S44.0 ☑
      - hand (level) S64.0 ☑
      - wrist (level) — *see* Injury, nerve, ulnar, hand
    - vagus S04.89 ☑
      - specified type NEC S04.89 ☑
    - wrist (level) — *see* Injury, nerve, hand
  - ninth cranial nerve (glossopharyngeal) — *see* Injury, nerve, glossopharyngeal
  - nose (septum) S09.92 ☑
  - obstetrical O71.9
    - specified NEC O71.89
  - occipital (region) (scalp) S09.90 ☑
    - lobe — *see* Injury, intracranial
  - optic chiasm S04.02 ☑
  - optic radiation S04.03 ☑
  - optic tract and pathways S04.03 ☑
  - orbit, orbital (region) — *see* Injury, eye
    - penetrating (with foreign body) — *see* Injury, eye, orbit, penetrating
    - specified NEC — *see* Injury, eye, specified site NEC
  - ovary, ovarian S37.409 ☑
    - bilateral S37.402 ☑
      - contusion S37.422 ☑
      - laceration S37.432 ☑
      - specified type NEC S37.492 ☑
    - blood vessel — *see* Injury, blood vessel, ovarian
    - contusion S37.429 ☑
      - bilateral S37.422 ☑
      - unilateral S37.421 ☑
    - laceration S37.439 ☑
      - bilateral S37.432 ☑
      - unilateral S37.431 ☑
    - specified type NEC S37.499 ☑
      - bilateral S37.492 ☑
      - unilateral S37.491 ☑
    - unilateral S37.401 ☑
      - contusion S37.421 ☑
      - laceration S37.431 ☑
      - specified type NEC S37.491 ☑
  - palate (hard) (soft) S09.93 ☑
  - pancreas S36.209 ☑
    - body S36.201 ☑
      - contusion S36.221 ☑
      - laceration S36.231 ☑
        - major S36.261 ☑
        - minor S36.241 ☑
        - moderate S36.251 ☑
      - specified type NEC S36.291 ☑
    - contusion S36.229 ☑
    - head S36.200 ☑
      - contusion S36.220 ☑
      - laceration S36.230 ☑
        - major S36.260 ☑
        - minor S36.240 ☑
        - moderate S36.250 ☑
      - specified type NEC S36.290 ☑
    - laceration S36.239 ☑
      - major S36.269 ☑
      - minor S36.249 ☑
      - moderate S36.259 ☑
    - specified type NEC S36.299 ☑
    - tail S36.202 ☑
      - contusion S36.222 ☑
      - laceration S36.232 ☑
        - major S36.262 ☑
        - minor S36.242 ☑
        - moderate S36.252 ☑
      - specified type NEC S36.292 ☑
  - parietal (region) (scalp) S09.90 ☑
    - lobe — *see* Injury, intracranial
  - patellar ligament (tendon) S76.10 ☑
    - laceration S76.12 ☑
    - specified NEC S76.19 ☑
    - strain S76.11 ☑
  - pelvis, pelvic (floor) S39.93 ☑
    - complicating delivery O70.1
    - joint or ligament, complicating delivery O71.6
    - organ S37.90 ☑
      - with ectopic or molar pregnancy O08.6
      - complication of abortion — *see* Abortion
      - contusion S37.92 ☑
      - following ectopic or molar pregnancy O08.6
      - laceration S37.93 ☑
      - obstetrical trauma NEC O71.5
      - specified
        - site NEC S37.899 ☑
          - contusion S37.892 ☑
          - laceration S37.893 ☑

- **Injury** — *continued*
  - pelvis, pelvic — *continued*
        - specified type NEC S37.898 ☑
      - type NEC S37.99 ☑
    - specified NEC S39.83 ☑
  - penis S39.94 ☑
  - perineum S39.94 ☑
  - peritoneum S36.81 ☑
    - laceration S36.893 ☑
  - periurethral tissue — *see* Injury, urethra
    - complicating delivery O71.82
  - phalanges
    - foot — *see* Injury, foot
    - hand — *see* Injury, hand
  - pharynx NEC S19.85 ☑
  - pleura — *see* Injury, intrathoracic, pleura
  - plexus
    - brachial — *see* Injury, brachial plexus
    - cardiac — *see* Injury, nerve, thorax, sympathetic
    - celiac, coeliac — *see* Injury, nerve, lumbosacral, sympathetic
    - esophageal — *see* Injury, nerve, thorax, sympathetic
    - hypogastric — *see* Injury, nerve, lumbosacral, sympathetic
    - lumbar, lumbosacral — *see* Injury, lumbosacral plexus
    - mesenteric — *see* Injury, nerve, lumbosacral, sympathetic
    - pulmonary — *see* Injury, nerve, thorax, sympathetic
  - postcardiac surgery (syndrome) I97.0
  - prepuce S39.94 ☑
  - prostate S37.829 ☑
    - contusion S37.822 ☑
    - laceration S37.823 ☑
    - specified type NEC S37.828 ☑
  - pubic region S39.94 ☑
  - pudendum S39.94 ☑
  - pulmonary plexus — *see* Injury, nerve, thorax, sympathetic
  - rectovaginal septum NEC S39.83 ☑
  - rectum — *see* Injury, intestine, large, rectum
  - retina — *see* Injury, eye, specified site NEC
    - penetrating — *see* Injury, eyeball, penetrating
  - retroperitoneal — *see* Injury, intra-abdominal, specified site NEC
  - rotator cuff (muscle (s)) (tendon (s)) S46.00 ☑
    - laceration S46.02 ☑
    - specified type NEC S46.09 ☑
    - strain S46.01 ☑
  - round ligament — *see* Injury, pelvic organ, specified site NEC
  - sacral plexus — *see* Injury, lumbosacral plexus
  - salivary duct or gland S09.93 ☑
  - scalp S09.90 ☑
    - newborn (birth injury) P12.9
      - due to monitoring (electrode) (sampling incision) P12.4
      - specified NEC P12.89
        - caput succedaneum P12.81
  - scapular region — *see* Injury, shoulder
  - sclera — *see* Injury, eye, specified site NEC
    - penetrating — *see* Injury, eyeball, penetrating
  - scrotum S39.94 ☑
  - second cranial nerve (optic) — *see* Injury, nerve, optic
  - seminal vesicle — *see* Injury, pelvic organ, specified site NEC
  - seventh cranial nerve (facial) — *see* Injury, nerve, facial
  - shoulder S49.9 ☑
    - blood vessel — *see* Injury, blood vessel, arm
    - contusion — *see* Contusion, shoulder
    - dislocation — *see* Dislocation, shoulder
    - fracture — *see* Fracture, shoulder
    - muscle — *see* Injury, muscle, shoulder
    - nerve — *see* Injury, nerve, shoulder
    - open — *see* Wound, open, shoulder
    - specified type NEC S49.8 ☑
    - sprain — *see* Sprain, shoulder girdle
    - superficial — *see* Injury, superficial, shoulder
  - sinus
    - cavernous — *see* Injury, intracranial
    - nasal S09.92 ☑
  - sixth cranial nerve (abducent) — *see* Injury, nerve, abducens
  - skeleton, birth injury P13.9
    - specified part NEC P13.8
  - skin NEC T14.8
    - surface intact — *see* Injury, superficial
  - skull NEC S09.90 ☑

- **Injury** — *continued*
  - specified NEC T14.8
  - spermatic cord (pelvic region) S37.898 ☑
    - scrotal region S39.848 ☑
  - spinal (cord)
    - cervical (neck) S14.109 ☑
      - anterior cord syndrome S14.139 ☑
        - C1 level S14.131 ☑
        - C2 level S14.132 ☑
        - C3 level S14.133 ☑
        - C4 level S14.134 ☑
        - C5 level S14.135 ☑
        - C6 level S14.136 ☑
        - C7 level S14.137 ☑
        - C8 level S14.138 ☑
      - Brown-Séquard syndrome S14.149 ☑
        - C1 level S14.141 ☑
        - C2 level S14.142 ☑
        - C3 level S14.143 ☑
        - C4 level S14.144 ☑
        - C5 level S14.145 ☑
        - C6 level S14.146 ☑
        - C7 level S14.147 ☑
        - C8 level S14.148 ☑
      - C1 level S14.101 ☑
      - C2 level S14.102 ☑
      - C3 level S14.103 ☑
      - C4 level S14.104 ☑
      - C5 level S14.105 ☑
      - C6 level S14.106 ☑
      - C7 level S14.107 ☑
      - C8 level S14.108 ☑
      - central cord syndrome S14.129 ☑
        - C1 level S14.121 ☑
        - C2 level S14.122 ☑
        - C3 level S14.123 ☑
        - C4 level S14.124 ☑
        - C5 level S14.125 ☑
        - C6 level S14.126 ☑
        - C7 level S14.127 ☑
        - C8 level S14.128 ☑
      - complete lesion S14.119 ☑
        - C1 level S14.111 ☑
        - C2 level S14.112 ☑
        - C3 level S14.113 ☑
        - C4 level S14.114 ☑
        - C5 level S14.115 ☑
        - C6 level S14.116 ☑
        - C7 level S14.117 ☑
        - C8 level S14.118 ☑
      - concussion S14.0 ☑
      - edema S14.0 ☑
      - incomplete lesion specified NEC S14.159 ☑
        - C1 level S14.151 ☑
        - C2 level S14.152 ☑
        - C3 level S14.153 ☑
        - C4 level S14.154 ☑
        - C5 level S14.155 ☑
        - C6 level S14.156 ☑
        - C7 level S14.157 ☑
        - C8 level S14.158 ☑
      - posterior cord syndrome S14.159 ☑
        - C1 level S14.151 ☑
        - C2 level S14.152 ☑
        - C3 level S14.153 ☑
        - C4 level S14.154 ☑
        - C5 level S14.155 ☑
        - C6 level S14.156 ☑
        - C7 level S14.157 ☑
        - C8 level S14.158 ☑
    - dorsal — *see* Injury, spinal, thoracic
    - lumbar S34.109 ☑
      - complete lesion S34.119 ☑
        - L1 level S34.111 ☑
        - L2 level S34.112 ☑
        - L3 level S34.113 ☑
        - L4 level S34.114 ☑
        - L5 level S34.115 ☑
      - concussion S34.01 ☑
      - edema S34.01 ☑
      - incomplete lesion S34.129 ☑
        - L1 level S34.121 ☑
        - L2 level S34.122 ☑
        - L3 level S34.123 ☑
        - L4 level S34.124 ☑
        - L5 level S34.125 ☑
      - L1 level S34.101 ☑
      - L2 level S34.102 ☑
      - L3 level S34.103 ☑
      - L4 level S34.104 ☑
      - L5 level S34.105 ☑
    - nerve root NEC

- **Injury** — *continued*
  - spinal — *continued*
      - cervical — *see* Injury, nerve, spinal, root, cervical
      - dorsal — *see* Injury, nerve, spinal, root, dorsal
      - lumbar S34.21 ☑
      - sacral S34.22 ☑
      - thoracic — *see* Injury, nerve, spinal, root, dorsal
    - plexus
      - brachial — *see* Injury, brachial plexus
      - lumbosacral — *see* Injury, lumbosacral plexus
    - sacral S34.139 ☑
      - complete lesion S34.131 ☑
      - incomplete lesion S34.132 ☑
    - thoracic S24.109 ☑
      - anterior cord syndrome S24.139 ☑
        - T1 level S24.131 ☑
        - T2-T6 level S24.132 ☑
        - T7-T10 level S24.133 ☑
        - T11-T12 level S24.134 ☑
      - Brown-Séquard syndrome S24.149 ☑
        - T1 level S24.141 ☑
        - T2-T6 level S24.142 ☑
        - T7-T10 level S24.143 ☑
        - T11-T12 level S24.144 ☑
      - complete lesion S24.119 ☑
        - T1 level S24.111 ☑
        - T2-T6 level S24.112 ☑
        - T7-T10 level S24.113 ☑
        - T11-T12 level S24.114 ☑
      - concussion S24.0 ☑
      - edema S24.0 ☑
      - incomplete lesion specified NEC S24.159 ☑
        - T1 level S24.151 ☑
        - T2-T6 level S24.152 ☑
        - T7-T10 level S24.153 ☑
        - T11-T12 level S24.154 ☑
      - posterior cord syndrome S24.159 ☑
        - T1 level S24.151 ☑
        - T2-T6 level S24.152 ☑
        - T7-T10 level S24.153 ☑
        - T11-T12 level S24.154 ☑
      - T1 level S24.101 ☑
      - T2-T6 level S24.102 ☑
      - T7-T10 level S24.103 ☑
      - T11-T12 level S24.104 ☑
  - splanchnic nerve — *see* Injury, nerve, lumbosacral, sympathetic
  - spleen S36.00 ☑
    - contusion S36.029 ☑
      - major S36.021 ☑
      - minor S36.020 ☑
    - laceration S36.039 ☑
      - major (massive) (stellate) S36.032 ☑
      - moderate S36.031 ☑
      - superficial (capsular) (minor) S36.030 ☑
    - specified type NEC S36.09 ☑
  - splenic artery — *see* Injury, blood vessel, celiac artery, branch
  - stellate ganglion — *see* Injury, nerve, thorax, sympathetic
  - sternal region S29.9 ☑
  - stomach S36.30 ☑
    - contusion S36.32 ☑
    - laceration S36.33 ☑
    - specified type NEC S36.39 ☑
  - subconjunctival — *see* Injury, eye, conjunctiva
  - subcutaneous NEC T14.8
  - submaxillary region S09.93 ☑
  - submental region S09.93 ☑
  - subungual
    - fingers — *see* Injury, hand
    - toes — *see* Injury, foot
  - superficial NEC T14.8
    - abdomen, abdominal (wall) S30.92 ☑
      - abrasion S30.811 ☑
      - bite S30.871 ☑
        - insect S30.861 ☑
      - contusion S30.1 ☑
      - external constriction S30.841 ☑
      - foreign body S30.851 ☑
    - abrasion — *see* Abrasion, by site
    - adnexa, eye NEC — *see* Injury, eye, specified site NEC
    - alveolar process — *see* Injury, superficial, oral cavity
    - ankle S90.91 ☑
      - abrasion — *see* Abrasion, ankle
      - blister — *see* Blister, ankle
      - bite — *see* Bite, ankle
      - contusion — *see* Contusion, ankle

- **Injury** — *continued*
  - superficial NEC — *continued*
      - external constriction — *see* Constriction, external, ankle
      - foreign body — *see* Foreign body, superficial, ankle
    - anus S30.98 ☑
    - arm (upper) S40.92 ☑
      - abrasion — *see* Abrasion, arm
      - bite — *see* Bite, superficial, arm
      - blister — *see* Blister, arm (upper)
      - contusion — *see* Contusion, arm
      - external constriction — *see* Constriction, external, arm
      - foreign body — *see* Foreign body, superficial, arm
    - auditory canal (external) (meatus) — *see* Injury, superficial, ear
    - auricle — *see* Injury, superficial, ear
    - axilla — *see* Injury, superficial, arm
    - back (*see also* Injury, superficial, thorax, back)
      - lower S30.91 ☑
        - abrasion S30.810 ☑
        - contusion S30.0 ☑
        - external constriction S30.840 ☑
        - superficial
          - bite NEC S30.870 ☑
            - insect S30.860 ☑
          - foreign body S30.850 ☑
    - bite NEC — *see* Bite, superficial NEC, by site
    - blister — *see* Blister, by site
    - breast S20.10 ☑
      - abrasion — *see* Abrasion, breast
      - bite — *see* Bite, superficial, breast
      - contusion — *see* Contusion, breast
      - external constriction — *see* Constriction, external, breast
      - foreign body — *see* Foreign body, superficial, breast
    - brow — *see* Injury, superficial, head, specified NEC
    - buttock S30.91 ☑
    - calf — *see* Injury, superficial, leg
    - canthus, eye — *see* Injury, superficial, periocular area
    - cheek (external) — *see* Injury, superficial, head, specified NEC
      - internal — *see* Injury, superficial, oral cavity
    - chest wall — *see* Injury, superficial, thorax
    - chin — *see* Injury, superficial, head NEC
    - clitoris S30.95 ☑
    - conjunctiva — *see* Injury, eye, conjunctiva
      - with foreign body (in conjunctival sac) — *see* Foreign body, conjunctival sac
    - contusion — *see* Contusion, by site
    - costal region — *see* Injury, superficial, thorax
    - digit (s)
      - hand — *see* Injury, superficial, finger
    - ear (auricle) (canal) (external) S00.40 ☑
      - abrasion — *see* Abrasion, ear
      - bite — *see* Bite, superficial, ear
      - contusion — *see* Contusion, ear
      - external constriction — *see* Constriction, external, ear
      - foreign body — *see* Foreign body, superficial, ear
    - elbow S50.90 ☑
      - abrasion — *see* Abrasion, elbow
      - bite — *see* Bite, superficial, elbow
      - blister — *see* Blister, elbow
      - contusion — *see* Contusion, elbow
      - external constriction — *see* Constriction, external, elbow
      - foreign body — *see* Foreign body, superficial, elbow
    - epididymis S30.94 ☑
    - epigastric region S30.92 ☑
    - epiglottis — *see* Injury, superficial, throat
    - esophagus
      - cervical — *see* Injury, superficial, throat
    - external constriction — *see* Constriction, external, by site
    - extremity NEC T14.8
    - eyeball NEC — *see* Injury, eye, specified site NEC
    - eyebrow — *see* Injury, superficial, periocular area
    - eyelid S00.20 ☑
      - abrasion — *see* Abrasion, eyelid
      - bite — *see* Bite, superficial, eyelid
      - contusion — *see* Contusion, eyelid
      - external constriction — *see* Constriction, external, eyelid
      - foreign body — *see* Foreign body, superficial, eyelid
    - face NEC — *see* Injury, superficial, head, specified NEC
    - finger (s) S60.949 ☑
      - abrasion — *see* Abrasion, finger
      - bite — *see* Bite, superficial, finger
      - blister — *see* Blister, finger
      - contusion — *see* Contusion, finger
      - external constriction — *see* Constriction, external, finger
      - foreign body — *see* Foreign body, superficial, finger
      - insect bite — *see* Bite, by site, superficial, insect
      - index S60.94 ☑
      - little S60.94 ☑
      - middle S60.94 ☑
      - ring S60.94 ☑
    - flank S30.92 ☑
    - foot S90.92 ☑
      - abrasion — *see* Abrasion, foot
      - bite — *see* Bite, foot
      - blister — *see* Blister, foot
      - contusion — *see* Contusion, foot
      - external constriction — *see* Constriction, external, foot
      - foreign body — *see* Foreign body, superficial, foot
    - forearm S50.91 ☑
      - abrasion — *see* Abrasion, forearm
      - bite — *see* Bite, forearm, superficial
      - blister — *see* Blister, forearm
      - contusion — *see* Contusion, forearm
      - elbow only — *see* Injury, superficial, elbow
      - external constriction — *see* Constriction, external, forearm
      - foreign body — *see* Foreign body, superficial, forearm
    - forehead — *see* Injury, superficial, head NEC
    - foreign body — *see* Foreign body, superficial
    - genital organs, external
      - female S30.97 ☑
      - male S30.96 ☑
    - globe (eye) — *see* Injury, eye, specified site NEC
    - groin S30.92 ☑
    - gum — *see* Injury, superficial, oral cavity
    - hand S60.92 ☑
      - abrasion — *see* Abrasion, hand
      - bite — *see* Bite, superficial, hand
      - contusion — *see* Contusion, hand
      - external constriction — *see* Constriction, external, hand
      - foreign body — *see* Foreign body, superficial, hand
    - head S00.90 ☑
      - ear — *see* Injury, superficial, ear
      - eyelid — *see* Injury, superficial, eyelid
      - nose S00.30 ☑
      - oral cavity S00.502 ☑
      - scalp S00.00 ☑
      - specified site NEC S00.80 ☑
    - heel — *see* Injury, superficial, foot
    - hip S70.91 ☑
      - abrasion — *see* Abrasion, hip
      - bite — *see* Bite, superficial, hip
      - blister — *see* Blister, hip
      - contusion — *see* Contusion, hip
      - external constriction — *see* Constriction, external, hip
      - foreign body — *see* Foreign body, superficial, hip
    - iliac region — *see* Injury, superficial, abdomen
    - inguinal region — *see* Injury, superficial, abdomen
    - insect bite — *see* Bite, by site, superficial, insect
    - interscapular region — *see* Injury, superficial, thorax, back
    - jaw — *see* Injury, superficial, head, specified NEC
    - knee S80.91 ☑
      - abrasion — *see* Abrasion, knee
      - bite — *see* Bite, superficial, knee
      - blister — *see* Blister, knee
      - contusion — *see* Contusion, knee
      - external constriction — *see* Constriction, external, knee
      - foreign body — *see* Foreign body, superficial, knee
    - labium (majus) (minus) S30.95 ☑
    - lacrimal (apparatus) (gland) (sac) — *see* Injury, eye, specified site NEC
    - larynx — *see* Injury, superficial, throat
    - leg (lower) S80.92 ☑
      - abrasion — *see* Abrasion, leg
      - bite — *see* Bite, superficial, leg
      - contusion — *see* Contusion, leg
      - external constriction — *see* Constriction, external, leg
      - foreign body — *see* Foreign body, superficial, leg
      - knee — *see* Injury, superficial, knee
    - limb NEC T14.8
    - lip S00.501 ☑
    - lower back S30.91 ☑
    - lumbar region S30.91 ☑
    - malar region — *see* Injury, superficial, head, specified NEC
    - mammary — *see* Injury, superficial, breast
    - mastoid region — *see* Injury, superficial, head, specified NEC
    - mouth — *see* Injury, superficial, oral cavity
    - muscle NEC T14.8
    - nail NEC T14.8
      - finger — *see* Injury, superficial, finger
      - toe — *see* Injury, superficial, toe
    - nasal (septum) — *see* Injury, superficial, nose
    - neck S10.90 ☑
      - specified site NEC S10.80 ☑
    - nose (septum) S00.30 ☑
    - occipital region — *see* Injury, superficial, scalp
    - oral cavity S00.502 ☑
    - orbital region — *see* Injury, superficial, periocular area
    - palate — *see* Injury, superficial, oral cavity
    - palm — *see* Injury, superficial, hand
    - parietal region — *see* Injury, superficial, scalp
    - pelvis S30.91 ☑
      - girdle — *see* Injury, superficial, hip
    - penis S30.93 ☑
    - perineum
      - female S30.95 ☑
      - male S30.91 ☑
    - periocular area S00.20 ☑
      - abrasion — *see* Abrasion, eyelid
      - bite — *see* Bite, superficial, eyelid
      - contusion — *see* Contusion, eyelid
      - external constriction — *see* Constriction, external, eyelid
      - foreign body — *see* Foreign body, superficial, eyelid
    - phalanges
      - finger — *see* Injury, superficial, finger
      - toe — *see* Injury, superficial, toe
    - pharynx — *see* Injury, superficial, throat
    - pinna — *see* Injury, superficial, ear
    - popliteal space — *see* Injury, superficial, knee
    - prepuce S30.93 ☑
    - pubic region S30.91 ☑
    - pudendum
      - female S30.97 ☑
      - male S30.96 ☑
    - sacral region S30.91 ☑
    - scalp S00.00 ☑
    - scapular region — *see* Injury, superficial, shoulder
    - sclera — *see* Injury, eye, specified site NEC
    - scrotum S30.94 ☑
    - shin — *see* Injury, superficial, leg
    - shoulder S40.91 ☑
      - abrasion — *see* Abrasion, shoulder
      - bite — *see* Bite, superficial, shoulder
      - blister — *see* Blister, shoulder
      - contusion — *see* Contusion, shoulder
      - external constriction — *see* Constriction, external, shoulder
      - foreign body — *see* Foreign body, superficial, shoulder
    - skin NEC T14.8
    - sternal region — *see* Injury, superficial, thorax, front
    - subconjunctival — *see* Injury, eye, specified site NEC
    - subcutaneous NEC T14.8
    - submaxillary region — *see* Injury, superficial, head, specified NEC

- **Injury** — *continued*
  - superficial NEC — *continued*
    - submental region — *see* Injury, superficial, head, specified NEC
    - subungual
      - finger (s) — *see* Injury, superficial, finger
      - toe (s) — *see* Injury, superficial, toe
    - supraclavicular fossa — *see* Injury, superficial, neck
    - supraorbital — *see* Injury, superficial, head, specified NEC
    - temple — *see* Injury, superficial, head, specified NEC
    - temporal region — *see* Injury, superficial, head, specified NEC
    - testis S30.94 ☑
    - thigh S70.92 ☑
      - abrasion — *see* Abrasion, thigh
      - bite — *see* Bite, superficial, thigh
      - blister — *see* Blister, thigh
      - contusion — *see* Contusion, thigh
      - external constriction — *see* Constriction, external, thigh
      - foreign body — *see* Foreign body, superficial, thigh
    - thorax, thoracic (wall) S20.90 ☑
      - abrasion — *see* Abrasion, thorax
      - back S20.40 ☑
      - bite — *see* Bite, thorax, superficial
      - blister — *see* Blister, thorax
      - contusion — *see* Contusion, thorax
      - external constriction — *see* Constriction, external, thorax
      - foreign body — *see* Foreign body, superficial, thorax
      - front S20.30 ☑
    - throat S10.10 ☑
      - abrasion S10.11 ☑
      - bite S10.17 ☑
        - insect S10.16 ☑
      - blister S10.12 ☑
      - contusion S10.0 ☑
      - external constriction S10.14 ☑
      - foreign body S10.15 ☑
    - thumb S60.93 ☑
      - abrasion — *see* Abrasion, thumb
      - bite — *see* Bite, superficial, thumb
      - blister — *see* Blister, thumb
      - contusion — *see* Contusion, thumb
      - external constriction — *see* Constriction, external, thumb
      - foreign body — *see* Foreign body, superficial, thumb
      - insect bite — *see* Bite, by site, superficial, insect
      - specified type NEC S60.39 ☑
    - toe (s) S90.93 ☑
      - abrasion — *see* Abrasion, toe
      - bite — *see* Bite, toe
      - blister — *see* Blister, toe
      - contusion — *see* Contusion, toe
      - external constriction — *see* Constriction, external, toe
      - foreign body — *see* Foreign body, superficial, toe
      - great S90.93 ☑
    - tongue — *see* Injury, superficial, oral cavity
    - tooth, teeth — *see* Injury, superficial, oral cavity
    - trachea S10.10 ☑
    - tunica vaginalis S30.94 ☑
    - tympanum, tympanic membrane — *see* Injury, superficial, ear
    - uvula — *see* Injury, superficial, oral cavity
    - vagina S30.95 ☑
    - vocal cords — *see* Injury, superficial, throat
    - vulva S30.95 ☑
    - wrist S60.91 ☑
  - supraclavicular region — *see* Injury, neck
  - supraorbital S09.93 ☑
  - suprarenal gland (multiple) — *see* Injury, adrenal
  - surgical complication (external or internal site) — *see* Laceration, accidental complicating surgery
  - temple S09.90 ☑
  - temporal region S09.90 ☑
  - tendon (*see also* Injury, muscle, by site)
    - abdomen — *see* Injury, muscle, abdomen
    - Achilles — *see* Injury, Achilles tendon
    - lower back — *see* Injury, muscle, lower back
    - pelvic organs — *see* Injury, muscle, pelvis
  - tenth cranial nerve (pneumogastric or vagus) — *see* Injury, nerve, vagus
  - testis S39.94 ☑
  - thigh S79.92 ☑
    - blood vessel — *see* Injury, blood vessel, hip
    - contusion — *see* Contusion, thigh
    - fracture — *see* Fracture, femur
    - muscle — *see* Injury, muscle, thigh
    - nerve — *see* Injury, nerve, thigh
    - open — *see* Wound, open, thigh
    - specified NEC S79.82 ☑
    - superficial — *see* Injury, superficial, thigh
  - third cranial nerve (oculomotor) — *see* Injury, nerve, oculomotor
  - thorax, thoracic S29.9 ☑
    - blood vessel — *see* Injury, blood vessel, thorax
    - cavity — *see* Injury, intrathoracic
    - dislocation — *see* Dislocation, thorax
    - external (wall) S29.9 ☑
      - contusion — *see* Contusion, thorax
      - nerve — *see* Injury, nerve, thorax
      - open — *see* Wound, open, thorax
      - specified NEC S29.8 ☑
      - sprain — *see* Sprain, thorax
      - superficial — *see* Injury, superficial, thorax
    - fracture — *see* Fracture, thorax
    - internal — *see* Injury, intrathoracic
    - intrathoracic organ — *see* Injury, intrathoracic
    - sympathetic ganglion — *see* Injury, nerve, thorax, sympathetic
  - throat (*see also* Injury, neck)S19.9 ☑
  - thumb S69.9 ☑
    - blood vessel — *see* Injury, blood vessel, thumb
    - contusion — *see* Contusion, thumb
    - dislocation — *see* Dislocation, thumb
    - fracture — *see* Fracture, thumb
    - muscle — *see* Injury, muscle, thumb
    - nerve — *see* Injury, nerve, digital, thumb
    - open — *see* Wound, open, thumb
    - specified NEC S69.8 ☑
    - sprain — *see* Sprain, thumb
    - superficial — *see* Injury, superficial, thumb
  - thymus (gland) — *see* Injury, intrathoracic, specified organ NEC
  - thyroid (gland) NEC S19.84 ☑
  - toe S99.92 ☑
    - contusion — *see* Contusion, toe
    - dislocation — *see* Dislocation, toe
    - fracture — *see* Fracture, toe
    - muscle — *see* Injury, muscle, toe
    - open — *see* Wound, open, toe
    - specified type NEC S99.82 ☑
    - sprain — *see* Sprain, toe
    - superficial — *see* Injury, superficial, toe
  - tongue S09.93 ☑
  - tonsil S09.93 ☑
  - tooth S09.93 ☑
  - trachea (cervical) NEC S19.82 ☑
    - thoracic — *see* Injury, intrathoracic, trachea, thoracic
  - transfusion-related acute lung (TRALI) J95.84
  - tunica vaginalis S39.94 ☑
  - twelfth cranial nerve (hypoglossal) — *see* Injury, nerve, hypoglossal
  - ureter S37.10 ☑
    - contusion S37.12 ☑
    - laceration S37.13 ☑
    - specified type NEC S37.19 ☑
  - urethra (sphincter) S37.30 ☑
    - at delivery O71.5
    - contusion S37.32 ☑
    - laceration S37.33 ☑
    - specified type NEC S37.39 ☑
  - urinary organ S37.90 ☑
    - contusion S37.92 ☑
    - laceration S37.93 ☑
    - specified
      - site NEC S37.899 ☑
        - contusion S37.892 ☑
        - laceration S37.893 ☑
        - specified type NEC S37.898 ☑
      - type NEC S37.99 ☑
  - uterus, uterine S37.60 ☑
    - with ectopic or molar pregnancy O08.6
    - blood vessel — *see* Injury, blood vessel, iliac
    - contusion S37.62 ☑
    - laceration S37.63 ☑
      - cervix at delivery O71.3
    - rupture associated with obstetrics — *see* Rupture, uterus
    - specified type NEC S37.69 ☑
  - uvula S09.93 ☑
  - vagina S39.93 ☑
    - abrasion S30.814 ☑
    - bite S31.45 ☑
      - insect S30.864 ☑
      - superficial NEC S30.874 ☑
    - contusion S30.23 ☑
    - crush S38.03 ☑
    - during delivery — *see* Laceration, vagina, during delivery
    - external constriction S30.844 ☑
    - insect bite S30.864 ☑
    - laceration S31.41 ☑
      - with foreign body S31.42 ☑
    - open wound S31.40 ☑
    - puncture S31.43 ☑
      - with foreign body S31.44 ☑
    - superficial S30.95 ☑
      - foreign body S30.854 ☑
  - vas deferens — *see* Injury, pelvic organ, specified site NEC
  - vascular NEC T14.8
  - vein — *see* Injury, blood vessel
  - vena cava (superior) S25.20 ☑
    - inferior S35.10 ☑
      - laceration (minor) (superficial) S35.11 ☑
        - major S35.12 ☑
      - specified type NEC S35.19 ☑
    - laceration (minor) (superficial) S25.21 ☑
      - major S25.22 ☑
    - specified type NEC S25.29 ☑
  - vesical (sphincter) — *see* Injury, bladder
  - visual cortex S04.04 ☑
  - vitreous (humor) S05.90 ☑
    - specified NEC S05.8X ☑
  - vocal cord NEC S19.83 ☑
  - vulva S39.94 ☑
    - abrasion S30.814 ☑
    - bite S31.45 ☑
      - insect S30.864 ☑
      - superficial NEC S30.874 ☑
    - contusion S30.23 ☑
    - crush S38.03 ☑
    - during delivery — *see* Laceration, perineum, female, during delivery
    - external constriction S30.844 ☑
    - insect bite S30.864 ☑
    - laceration S31.41 ☑
      - with foreign body S31.42 ☑
    - open wound S31.40 ☑
    - puncture S31.43 ☑
      - with foreign body S31.44 ☑
    - superficial S30.95 ☑
      - foreign body S30.854 ☑
  - whiplash (cervical spine) S13.4 ☑
  - wrist S69.9 ☑
    - blood vessel — *see* Injury, blood vessel, hand
    - contusion — *see* Contusion, wrist
    - dislocation — *see* Dislocation, wrist
    - fracture — *see* Fracture, wrist
    - muscle — *see* Injury, muscle, hand
    - nerve — *see* Injury, nerve, hand
    - open — *see* Wound, open, wrist
    - specified NEC S69.8 ☑
    - sprain — *see* Sprain, wrist
    - superficial — *see* Injury, superficial, wrist
- **Inoculation** (*see also* Vaccination)
  - complication or reaction — *see* Complications, vaccination
- **Insanity**, insane (*see also* Psychosis)
  - adolescent — *see* Schizophrenia
  - confusional F28
    - acute or subacute F05
  - delusional F22
  - senile F03 ☑
- **Insect**
  - bite — *see* Bite, by site, superficial, insect
  - venomous, poisoning NEC (by) — *see* Venom, arthropod
- **Insensitivity**
  - adrenocorticotropin hormone (ACTH) E27.49
  - androgen E34.50
    - complete E34.51
    - partial E34.52
- **Insertion**
  - cord (umbilical) lateral or velamentous O43.12 ☑
  - intrauterine contraceptive device (encounter for) — *see* Intrauterine contraceptive device
- **Insolation** (sunstroke) T67.0 ☑
- **Insomnia** (organic) G47.00
  - adjustment F51.02
  - adjustment disorder F51.02

- **Insomnia** — *continued*
  - behavioral, of childhood Z73.819
    - combined type Z73.812
    - limit setting type Z73.811
    - sleep-onset association type Z73.810
  - childhood Z73.819
  - chronic F51.04
    - somatized tension F51.04
  - conditioned F51.04
  - due to
    - alcohol
      - abuse F10.182
      - dependence F10.282
      - use F10.982
    - amphetamines
      - abuse F15.182
      - dependence F15.282
      - use F15.982
    - anxiety disorder F51.05
    - caffeine
      - abuse F15.182
      - dependence F15.282
      - use F15.982
    - cocaine
      - abuse F14.182
      - dependence F14.282
      - use F14.982
    - depression F51.05
    - drug NEC
      - abuse F19.182
      - dependence F19.282
      - use F19.982
    - medical condition G47.01
    - mental disorder NEC F51.05
    - opioid
      - abuse F11.182
      - dependence F11.282
      - use F11.982
    - psychoactive substance NEC
      - abuse F19.182
      - dependence F19.282
      - use F19.982
    - sedative, hypnotic, or anxiolytic
      - abuse F13.182
      - dependence F13.282
      - use F13.982
    - stimulant NEC
      - abuse F15.182
      - dependence F15.282
      - use F15.982
  - fatal familial (FFI) A81.83
  - idiopathic F51.01
  - learned F51.3
  - nonorganic origin F51.01
  - not due to a substance or known physiological condition F51.01
    - specified NEC F51.09
  - paradoxical F51.03
  - primary F51.01
  - psychiatric F51.05
  - psychophysiologic F51.04
  - related to psychopathology F51.05
  - short-term F51.02
  - specified NEC G47.09
  - stress-related F51.02
  - transient F51.02
  - without objective findings F51.02
- **Inspiration**
  - food or foreign body — *see* Foreign body, by site
  - mucus — *see* Asphyxia, mucus
- **Inspissated** bile syndrome (newborn) P59.1
- **Instability**
  - emotional (excessive) F60.3
  - joint (post-traumatic) M25.30
    - ankle M25.37 ☑
    - due to old ligament injury — *see* Disorder, ligament
    - elbow M25.32 ☑
    - flail — *see* Flail, joint
    - foot M25.37 ☑
    - hand M25.34 ☑
    - hip M25.35 ☑
    - knee M25.36 ☑
    - lumbosacral — *see* subcategory M53.2
    - prosthesis — *see* Complications, joint prosthesis, mechanical, displacement, by site
    - sacroiliac — *see* subcategory M53.2
    - secondary to
      - old ligament injury — *see* Disorder, ligament
      - removal of joint prosthesis M96.89
    - shoulder (region) M25.31 ☑
- **Instability** — *continued*
  - joint — *continued*
    - spine — *see* subcategory M53.2
    - wrist M25.33 ☑
  - knee (chronic) M23.5 ☑
  - lumbosacral — *see* subcategory M53.2
  - nervous F48.8
  - personality (emotional) F60.3
  - spine — *see* Instability, joint, spine
  - vasomotor R55
- **Institutional** syndrome (childhood) F94.2
- **Institutionalization,** affecting child Z62.22
  - disinhibited attachment F94.2
- **Insufficiency,** insufficient
  - accommodation, old age H52.4
  - adrenal (gland) E27.40
    - primary E27.1
  - adrenocortical E27.40
    - drug-induced E27.3
    - iatrogenic E27.3
    - primary E27.1
  - anatomic crown height K08.89
  - anterior (occlusal) guidance M26.54
  - anus K62.89
  - aortic (valve) I35.1
    - with
      - mitral (valve) disease I08.0
        - with tricuspid (valve) disease I08.3
      - stenosis I35.2
      - tricuspid (valve) disease I08.2
        - with mitral (valve) disease I08.3
    - congenital Q23.1
    - rheumatic I06.1
      - with
        - mitral (valve) disease I08.0
          - with tricuspid (valve) disease I08.3
        - stenosis I06.2
          - with mitral (valve) disease I08.0
            - with tricuspid (valve) disease I08.3
        - tricuspid (valve) disease I08.2
          - with mitral (valve) disease I08.3
    - specified cause NEC I35.1
    - syphilitic A52.03
  - arterial I77.1
    - basilar G45.0
    - carotid (hemispheric) G45.1
    - cerebral I67.81
    - coronary (acute or subacute) I24.8
    - mesenteric K55.1
    - peripheral I73.9
    - precerebral (multiple) (bilateral) G45.2
    - vertebral G45.0
  - arteriovenous I99.8
  - biliary K83.8
  - cardiac (*see also* Insufficiency, myocardial)
    - due to presence of (cardiac) prosthesis I97.11 ☑
    - postprocedural I97.11 ☑
  - cardiorenal, hypertensive I13.2
  - cardiovascular — *see* Disease, cardiovascular
  - cerebrovascular (acute) I67.81
    - with transient focal neurological signs and symptoms G45.8
  - circulatory NEC I99.8
    - newborn P29.89
  - clinical crown length K08.89
  - convergence H51.11
  - coronary (acute or subacute) I24.8
    - chronic or with a stated duration of over 4 weeks I25.89
  - corticoadrenal E27.40
    - primary E27.1
  - dietary E63.9
  - divergence H51.8
  - food T73.0 ☑
  - gastroesophageal K22.8
  - gonadal
    - ovary E28.39
    - testis E29.1
  - heart (*see also* Insufficiency, myocardial)
    - newborn P29.0
    - valve — *see* Endocarditis
  - hepatic — *see* Failure, hepatic
  - idiopathic autonomic G90.09
  - interocclusal distance of fully erupted teeth (ridge) M26.36
  - kidney N28.9
    - acute N28.9
    - chronic N18.9
  - lacrimal (secretion) H04.12 ☑
    - passages — *see* Stenosis, lacrimal
  - liver — *see* Failure, hepatic
- **Insufficiency** — *continued*
  - lung — *see* Insufficiency, pulmonary
  - mental (congenital) — *see* Disability, intellectual
  - mesenteric K55.1
  - mitral (valve) I34.0
    - with
      - aortic valve disease I08.0
        - with tricuspid (valve) disease I08.3
      - obstruction or stenosis I05.2
        - with aortic valve disease I08.0
      - tricuspid (valve) disease I08.1
        - with aortic (valve) disease I08.3
    - congenital Q23.3
    - rheumatic I05.1
      - with
        - aortic valve disease I08.0
          - with tricuspid (valve) disease I08.3
        - obstruction or stenosis I05.2
          - with aortic valve disease I08.0
            - with tricuspid (valve) disease I08.3
        - tricuspid (valve) disease I08.1
          - with aortic (valve) disease I08.3
      - active or acute I01.1
        - with chorea, rheumatic (Sydenham's) I02.0
    - specified cause, except rheumatic I34.0
  - muscle (*see also* Disease, muscle)
    - heart — *see* Insufficiency, myocardial
    - ocular NEC H50.9
  - myocardial, myocardium (with arteriosclerosis) I50.9
    - with
      - rheumatic fever (conditions in I00) I09.0
        - active, acute or subacute I01.2
          - with chorea I02.0
        - inactive or quiescent (with chorea) I09.0
    - congenital Q24.8
    - hypertensive — *see* Hypertension, heart
    - newborn P29.0
    - rheumatic I09.0
      - active, acute, or subacute I01.2
    - syphilitic A52.06
  - nourishment T73.0 ☑
  - pancreatic K86.89
    - exocrine K86.81
  - parathyroid (gland) E20.9
  - peripheral vascular (arterial) I73.9
  - pituitary E23.0
  - placental (mother) O36.51 ☑
  - platelets D69.6
  - prenatal care affecting management of pregnancy O09.3 ☑
  - progressive pluriglandular E31.0
  - pulmonary J98.4
    - acute, following surgery (nonthoracic) J95.2
      - thoracic J95.1
    - chronic, following surgery J95.3
    - following
      - shock J98.4
      - trauma J98.4
    - newborn P28.5
    - valve I37.1
      - with stenosis I37.2
      - congenital Q22.2
      - rheumatic I09.89
        - with aortic, mitral or tricuspid (valve) disease I08.8
  - pyloric K31.89
  - renal (acute) N28.9
    - chronic N18.9
  - respiratory R06.89
    - newborn P28.5
  - rotation — *see* Malrotation
  - sleep syndrome F51.12
  - social insurance Z59.7
  - suprarenal E27.40
    - primary E27.1
  - tarso-orbital fascia, congenital Q10.3
  - testis E29.1
  - thyroid (gland) (acquired) E03.9
    - congenital E03.1
  - tricuspid (valve) (rheumatic) I07.1
    - with
      - aortic (valve) disease I08.2
        - with mitral (valve) disease I08.3
      - mitral (valve) disease I08.1
        - with aortic (valve) disease I08.3
      - obstruction or stenosis I07.2
        - with aortic (valve) disease I08.2
          - with mitral (valve) disease I08.3
    - congenital Q22.8
    - nonrheumatic I36.1
      - with stenosis I36.2

Insomnia - Insufficiency

ICD-10-CM INDEX TO DISEASES AND INJURIES

- **Insufficiency** — *continued*
  - urethral sphincter R32
  - valve, valvular (heart) — *see* Endocarditis
    - congenital Q24.8
  - vascular I99.8
    - intestine K55.9
      - acute (*see also* Ischemia, intestine, acute)K55.059
    - mesenteric K55.1
    - peripheral I73.9
    - renal — *see* Hypertension, kidney
  - velopharyngeal
    - acquired K13.79
    - congenital Q38.8
  - venous (chronic) (peripheral) I87.2
  - ventricular — *see* Insufficiency, myocardial
  - welfare support Z59.7
- **Insufflation,** fallopian Z31.41
- **Insular** — *see* condition
- **Insulinoma**
  - pancreas
    - benign D13.7
    - malignant C25.4
    - uncertain behavior D37.8
  - specified site
    - benign — *see* Neoplasm, by site, benign
    - malignant — *see* Neoplasm, by site, malignant
    - uncertain behavior — *see* Neoplasm, by site, uncertain behavior
  - unspecified site
    - benign D13.7
    - malignant C25.4
    - uncertain behavior D37.8
- **Insuloma** — *see* Insulinoma
- **Interference**
  - balancing side M26.56
  - non-working side M26.56
- **Intermenstrual** — *see* condition
- **Intermittent** — *see* condition
- **Internal** — *see* condition
- **Interrogation**
  - cardiac defibrillator (automatic) (implantable) Z45.02
  - cardiac pacemaker Z45.018
  - cardiac (event) (loop) recorder Z45.09
  - infusion pump (implanted) (intrathecal) Z45.1
  - neurostimulator Z46.2
- **Interruption**
  - aortic arch Q25.21
  - bundle of His I44.30
  - phase-shift, sleep cycle — *see* Disorder, sleep, circadian rhythm
  - sleep phase-shift, or 24 hour sleep-wake cycle — *see* Disorder, sleep, circadian rhythm
- **Interstitial** — *see* condition
- **Intertrigo** L30.4
  - labialis K13.0
- **Intervertebral** disc — *see* condition
- **Intestine,** intestinal — *see* condition
- **Intolerance**
  - carbohydrate K90.49
  - disaccharide, hereditary E73.0
  - fat NEC K90.49
    - pancreatic K90.3
  - food K90.49
    - dietary counseling and surveillance Z71.3
  - fructose E74.10
    - hereditary E74.12
  - glucose (-galactose) E74.39
  - gluten K90.41
  - lactose E73.9
    - specified NEC E73.8
  - lysine E72.3
  - milk NEC K90.49
    - lactose E73.9
  - protein K90.49
  - starch NEC K90.49
  - sucrose (-isomaltose) E74.31
- **Intoxicated** NEC (without dependence) — *see* Alcohol, intoxication
- **Intoxication**
  - acid E87.2
  - alcoholic (acute) (without dependence) — *see* Alcohol, intoxication
  - alimentary canal K52.1
  - amphetamine (without dependence) — *see* Abuse, drug, stimulant, with intoxication
    - with dependence — *see* Dependence, drug, stimulant, with intoxication
  - anxiolytic (acute) (without dependence) — *see* Abuse, drug, sedative, with intoxication
- **Intoxication** — *continued*
  - anxiolytic — *continued*
    - with dependence — *see* Dependence, drug, sedative, with intoxication
  - caffeine F15.929
    - with dependence — *see* Dependence, drug, stimulant, with intoxication
  - cannabinoids (acute) (without dependence) — *see* Use, cannabis, with intoxication
    - with
      - abuse — *see* Abuse, drug, cannabis, with intoxication
      - dependence — *see* Dependence, drug, cannabis, with intoxication
  - chemical — *see* Table of Drugs and Chemicals
    - via placenta or breast milk — *see* - Absorption, chemical, through placenta
  - cocaine (acute) (without dependence) — *see* Abuse, drug, cocaine, with intoxication
    - with dependence — *see* Dependence, drug, cocaine, with intoxication
  - drug
    - acute (without dependence) — *see* Abuse, drug, by type with intoxication
      - with dependence — *see* Dependence, drug, by type with intoxication
    - addictive
      - via placenta or breast milk — *see* Absorption, drug, addictive, through placenta
    - newborn P93.8
      - gray baby syndrome P93.0
    - overdose or wrong substance given or taken — *see* Table of Drugs and Chemicals, by drug, poisoning
  - enteric K52.1
  - food-borne A05.9
    - bacterial A05.9
    - classical (Clostridium botulinum) A05.1
    - due to
      - Bacillus cereus A05.4
      - bacterium A05.9
        - specified NEC A05.8
      - Clostridium
        - botulinum A05.1
        - perfringens A05.2
        - welchii A05.2
      - Salmonella A02.9
        - with
          - (gastro)enteritis A02.0
          - localized infection (s) A02.20
            - arthritis A02.23
            - meningitis A02.21
            - osteomyelitis A02.24
            - pneumonia A02.22
            - pyelonephritis A02.25
            - specified NEC A02.29
          - sepsis A02.1
          - specified manifestation NEC A02.8
      - Staphylococcus A05.0
      - Vibrio
        - parahaemolyticus A05.3
        - vulnificus A05.5
    - enterotoxin, staphylococcal A05.0
    - noxious — *see* Poisoning, food, noxious
  - gastrointestinal K52.1
  - hallucinogenic (without dependence) — *see* Abuse, drug, hallucinogen, with intoxication
    - with dependence — *see* Dependence, drug, hallucinogen, with intoxication
  - hypnotic (acute) (without dependence) — *see* Abuse, drug, sedative, with intoxication
    - with dependence — *see* Dependence, drug, sedative, with intoxication
  - inhalant (acute) (without dependence) — *see* Abuse, drug, inhalant, with intoxication
    - with dependence — *see* Dependence, drug, inhalant, with intoxication
  - meaning
    - inebriation F10
    - poisoning — *see* Table of Drugs and Chemicals
  - methyl alcohol (acute) (without dependence) — *see* Alcohol, intoxication
  - opioid (acute) (without dependence) — *see* Abuse, drug, opioid, with intoxication
    - with dependence — *see* Dependence, drug, opioid, with intoxication
  - pathologic NEC (without dependence) — *see* Alcohol, intoxication
  - phencyclidine (without dependence) — *see* Abuse, drug, hallucinogen, with intoxication
    - with dependence - — *see* Dependence, drug, hallucinogen, with intoxication
- **Intoxication** — *continued*
  - potassium (K) E87.5
  - psychoactive substance NEC (without dependence) — *see* Abuse, drug, psychoactive NEC, with intoxication
    - with dependence — *see* Dependence, drug, psychoactive NEC, with intoxication
  - sedative (acute) (without dependence) — *see* Abuse, drug, sedative, with intoxication
    - with dependence — *see* Dependence, drug, sedative, with intoxication
  - serum (*see also* Reaction, serum)T80.69 ☑
  - uremic — *see* Uremia
  - volatile solvents (acute) (without dependence) — *see* Abuse, drug, inhalant, with intoxication
    - with dependence — *see* Dependence, drug, inhalant, with intoxication
  - water E87.79
- **Intracranial** — *see* condition
- **Intrahepatic** gallbladder Q44.1
- **Intraligamentous** — *see* condition
- **Intrathoracic** (*see also* condition)
  - kidney Q63.2
- **Intrauterine** contraceptive device
  - checking Z30.431
  - insertion Z30.430
    - immediately following removal Z30.433
  - in situ Z97.5
  - management Z30.431
  - reinsertion Z30.433
  - removal Z30.432
  - replacement Z30.433
  - retention in pregnancy O26.3 ☑
- **Intraventricular** — *see* condition
- **Intrinsic** deformity — *see* Deformity
- **Intubation,** difficult or failed T88.4 ☑
- **Intumescence,** lens (eye) (cataract) — *see* Cataract
- **Intussusception** (bowel) (colon) (enteric) (ileocecal) (ileocolic) (intestine) (rectum) K56.1
  - appendix K38.8
  - congenital Q43.8
  - ureter (with obstruction) N13.5
- **Invagination** (bowel, colon, intestine or rectum) K56.1
- **Inversion**
  - albumin-globulin (A-G) ratio E88.09
  - bladder N32.89
  - cecum — *see* Intussusception
  - cervix N88.8
  - chromosome in normal individual Q95.1
  - circadian rhythm — *see* Disorder, sleep, circadian rhythm
  - nipple N64.59
    - congenital Q83.8
    - gestational — *see* Retraction, nipple
    - puerperal, postpartum — *see* Retraction, nipple
  - nyctohemeral rhythm — *see* Disorder, sleep, circadian rhythm
  - optic papilla Q14.2
  - organ or site, congenital NEC — *see* Anomaly, by site
  - sleep rhythm — *see* Disorder, sleep, circadian rhythm
  - testis (congenital) Q55.29
  - uterus (chronic) (postinfectional) (postpartal, old) N85.5
    - postpartum O71.2
  - vagina (posthysterectomy) N99.3
  - ventricular Q20.5
- **Investigation** (*see also* Examination)Z04.9
  - clinical research subject (control) (normal comparison) (participant) Z00.6
- **Involuntary** movement, abnormal R25.9
- **Involution,** involutional (*see also* condition)
  - breast, cystic — *see* Dysplasia, mammary, specified type NEC
  - depression (single episode) F32.89
    - recurrent episode F33.9
  - melancholia (single episode) F32.89
    - recurrent episode F33.8
  - ovary, senile — *see* Atrophy, ovary
  - thymus failure E32.8
- **I.Q.**
  - under 20 F73
  - 20-34 F72
  - 35-49 F71
  - 50-69 F70
- **IRDS** (type I) P22.0
  - type II P22.1
- **Irideremia** Q13.1
- **Iridis** rubeosis — *see* Disorder, iris, vascular
- **Iridochoroiditis** (panuveitis) — *see* Panuveitis

- **Iridocyclitis** H20.9
  - acute H20.0 ☑
    - hypopyon H20.05 ☑
    - primary H20.01 ☑
    - recurrent H20.02 ☑
    - secondary (noninfectious) H20.04 ☑
      - infectious H20.03 ☑
  - chronic H20.1 ☑
  - due to allergy — *see* Iridocyclitis, acute, secondary
  - endogenous — *see* Iridocyclitis, acute, primary
  - Fuchs' — *see* Cyclitis, Fuchs' heterochromic
  - gonococcal A54.32
  - granulomatous — *see* Iridocyclitis, chronic
  - herpes, herpetic (simplex) B00.51
    - zoster B02.32
  - hypopyon — *see* Iridocyclitis, acute, hypopyon
  - in (due to)
    - ankylosing spondylitis M45.9
    - gonococcal infection A54.32
    - herpes (simplex) virus B00.51
      - zoster B02.32
    - infectious disease NOS B99 ☑
    - parasitic disease NOS B89 *[H22]*
    - sarcoidosis D86.83
    - syphilis A51.43
    - tuberculosis A18.54
    - zoster B02.32
  - lens-induced H20.2 ☑
  - nongranulomatous — *see* Iridocyclitis, acute
  - recurrent — *see* Iridocyclitis, acute, recurrent
  - rheumatic — *see* Iridocyclitis, chronic
  - subacute — *see* Iridocyclitis, acute
  - sympathetic — *see* Uveitis, sympathetic
  - syphilitic (secondary) A51.43
  - tuberculous (chronic) A18.54
  - Vogt-Koyanagi H20.82 ☑
- **Iridocyclochoroiditis** (panuveitis) — *see* Panuveitis
- **Iridodialysis** H21.53 ☑
- **Iridodonesis** H21.89
- **Iridoplegia** (complete) (partial) (reflex) H57.09
- **Iridoschisis** H21.25 ☑
- **Iris** (*see also* condition)
  - bombé — *see* Membrane, pupillary
- **Iritis** (*see also* Iridocyclitis)
  - chronic — *see* Iridocyclitis, chronic
  - diabetic — *see* E08-E13 with .39
  - due to
    - herpes simplex B00.51
    - leprosy A30.9 *[H22]*
  - gonococcal A54.32
  - gouty (*see also* Gout, by type)M10.9 *[H22]*
  - granulomatous — *see* Iridocyclitis, chronic
  - lens induced — *see* Iridocyclitis, lens-induced
  - papulosa (syphilitic) A52.71
  - rheumatic — *see* Iridocyclitis, chronic
  - syphilitic (secondary) A51.43
    - congenital (early) A50.01
    - late A52.71
  - tuberculous A18.54
- **Iron** — *see* condition
- **Iron-miner's** lung J63.4
- **Irradiated** enamel (tooth, teeth) K03.89
- **Irradiation** effects, adverse T66 ☑
- **Irreducible**, irreducibility — *see* condition
- **Irregular**, irregularity
  - action, heart I49.9
  - alveolar process K08.89
  - bleeding N92.6
  - breathing R06.89
  - contour of cornea (acquired) — *see* Deformity, cornea
    - congenital Q13.4
  - contour, reconstructed breast N65.0
  - dentin (in pulp) K04.3
  - eye movements H55.89
    - nystagmus — *see* Nystagmus
    - saccadic H55.81
  - labor O62.2
  - menstruation (cause unknown) N92.6
  - periods N92.6
  - prostate N42.9
  - pupil — *see* Abnormality, pupillary
  - reconstructed breast N65.0
  - respiratory R06.89
  - septum (nasal) J34.2
  - shape, organ or site, congenital NEC — *see* Distortion
  - sleep-wake pattern (rhythm) G47.23
- **Irritable**, irritability R45.4
  - bladder N32.89
  - bowel (syndrome) K58.9
- **Irritable**, irritability — *continued*
  - bowel — *continued*
    - with
      - constipation K58.1
      - diarrhea K58.0
    - mixed K58.2
    - psychogenic F45.8
    - specified NEC K58.8
  - bronchial — *see* Bronchitis
  - cerebral, in newborn P91.3
  - colon (*see also* Irritable, bowel)K58.9
    - with diarrhea K58.0
    - psychogenic F45.8
  - duodenum K59.8
  - heart (psychogenic) F45.8
  - hip — *see* Derangement, joint, specified type NEC, hip
  - ileum K59.8
  - infant R68.12
  - jejunum K59.8
  - rectum K59.8
  - stomach K31.89
    - psychogenic F45.8
  - sympathetic G90.8
  - urethra N36.8
- **Irritation**
  - anus K62.89
  - axillary nerve G54.0
  - bladder N32.89
  - brachial plexus G54.0
  - bronchial — *see* Bronchitis
  - cervical plexus G54.2
  - cervix — *see* Cervicitis
  - choroid, sympathetic — *see* Endophthalmitis
  - cranial nerve — *see* Disorder, nerve, cranial
  - gastric K31.89
    - psychogenic F45.8
  - globe, sympathetic — *see* Uveitis, sympathetic
  - labyrinth — *see* subcategory H83.2
  - lumbosacral plexus G54.1
  - meninges (traumatic) — *see* Injury, intracranial
    - nontraumatic — *see* Meningismus
  - nerve — *see* Disorder, nerve
  - nervous R45.0
  - penis N48.89
  - perineum NEC L29.3
  - peripheral autonomic nervous system G90.8
  - peritoneum — *see* Peritonitis
  - pharynx J39.2
  - plantar nerve — *see* Lesion, nerve, plantar
  - spinal (cord) (traumatic) (*see also* Injury, spinal cord, by region)
    - nerve G58.9
      - root NEC — *see* Radiculopathy
    - nontraumatic — *see* Myelopathy
  - stomach K31.89
    - psychogenic F45.8
  - sympathetic nerve NEC G90.8
  - ulnar nerve — *see* Lesion, nerve, ulnar
  - vagina N89.8
- **Ischemia**, ischemic I99.8
  - brain — *see* Ischemia, cerebral
  - bowel (transient)
    - acute (*see also* Ischemia, intestine, acute)K55.059
    - chronic K55.1
    - due to mesenteric artery insufficiency K55.1
  - cardiac (see Disease, heart, ischemic)
  - cardiomyopathy I25.5
  - cerebral (chronic) (generalized) I67.82
    - arteriosclerotic I67.2
    - intermittent G45.9
    - newborn P91.0
    - recurrent focal G45.8
    - transient G45.9
  - colon chronic (due to mesenteric artery insufficiency) K55.1
  - coronary — *see* Disease, heart, ischemic
  - demand (coronary) (*see also* Angina)I24.8
  - heart (chronic or with a stated duration of over 4 weeks) I25.9
    - acute or with a stated duration of 4 weeks or less I24.9
    - subacute I24.9
  - infarction, muscle — *see* Infarct, muscle
  - intestine (large) (small) (transient) K55.9
    - acute K55.059
      - diffuse K55.052
      - focal K55.051
      - large K55.039
        - diffuse K55.032
        - focal K55.031
- **Ischemia** — *continued*
  - intestine — *continued*
      - small K55.019
        - diffuse K55.012
        - focal K55.011
    - chronic K55.1
    - due to mesenteric artery insufficiency K55.1
  - kidney N28.0
  - mesenteric, acute (*see also* Ischemia, intestine, acute)K55.059
  - muscle, traumatic T79.6 ☑
  - myocardium, myocardial (chronic or with a stated duration of over 4 weeks) I25.9
    - acute, without myocardial infarction I51.3
    - silent (asymptomatic) I25.6
    - transient of newborn P29.4
  - renal N28.0
  - retina, retinal — *see* Occlusion, artery, retina
  - small bowel
    - acute K55.019
      - diffuse K55.012
      - focal K55.011
    - chronic K55.1
    - due to mesenteric artery insufficiency K55.1
  - spinal cord G95.11
  - subendocardial — *see* Insufficiency, coronary
  - supply (coronary) (*see also* Angina)I25.9
    - due to vasospasm I20.1
- **Ischial** spine — *see* condition
- **Ischialgia** — *see* Sciatica
- **Ischiopagus** Q89.4
- **Ischium**, ischial — *see* condition
- **Ischuria** R34
- **Iselin's** disease or osteochondrosis — *see* Osteochondrosis, juvenile, metatarsus
- **Islands** of
  - parotid tissue in
    - lymph nodes Q38.6
    - neck structures Q38.6
  - submaxillary glands in
    - fascia Q38.6
    - lymph nodes Q38.6
    - neck muscles Q38.6
- **Islet** cell tumor, pancreas D13.7
- **Isoimmunization** NEC (*see also* Incompatibility)
  - affecting management of pregnancy (ABO) (with hydrops fetalis) O36.11 ☑
    - anti-A sensitization O36.11 ☑
    - anti-B sensitization O36.19 ☑
    - anti-c sensitization O36.09 ☑
    - anti-C sensitization O36.09 ☑
    - anti-e sensitization O36.09 ☑
    - anti-E sensitization O36.09 ☑
    - Rh NEC O36.09 ☑
      - anti-D antibody O36.01 ☑
    - specified NEC O36.19 ☑
  - newborn P55.9
    - with
      - hydrops fetalis P56.0
      - kernicterus P57.0
    - ABO (blood groups) P55.1
    - Rhesus (Rh) factor P55.0
    - specified type NEC P55.8
- **Isolation**, isolated
  - dwelling Z59.8
  - family Z63.79
  - social Z60.4
- **Isoleucinosis** E71.19
- **Isomerism** atrial appendages (with asplenia or polysplenia) Q20.6
- **Isosporiasis**, isosporosis A07.3
- **Isovaleric** acidemia E71.110
- **Issue** of
  - medical certificate Z02.79
    - for disability determination Z02.71
  - repeat prescription (appliance) (glasses) (medicinal substance, medicament, medicine) Z76.0
    - contraception — *see* Contraception
- **Itch**, itching (*see also* Pruritus)
  - baker's L23.6
  - barber's B35.0
  - bricklayer's L24.5
  - cheese B88.0
  - clam digger's B65.3
  - coolie B76.9
  - copra B88.0
  - dew B76.9
  - dhobi B35.6
  - filarial — *see* Infestation, filarial
  - grain B88.0
  - grocer's B88.0

- **Itch,** itching — *continued*
  - ground B76.9
  - harvest B88.0
  - jock B35.6
  - Malabar B35.5
    - beard B35.0
    - foot B35.3
    - scalp B35.0
  - meaning scabies B86
  - Norwegian B86
  - perianal L29.0
  - poultrymen's B88.0
  - sarcoptic B86
  - scabies B86
  - scrub B88.0
  - straw B88.0
  - swimmer's B65.3
  - water B76.9
  - winter L29.8
- **Ivemark's** syndrome (asplenia with congenital heart disease) Q89.01
- **Ivory** bones Q78.2
- **Ixodiasis** NEC B88.8

J

- **Jaccoud's** syndrome — *see* Arthropathy, postrheumatic, chronic
- **Jackson's**
  - membrane Q43.3
  - paralysis or syndrome G83.89
  - veil Q43.3
- **Jacquet's** dermatitis (diaper dermatitis) L22
- **Jadassohn-Pellizari's** disease or anetoderma L90.2
- **Jadassohn's**
  - blue nevus — *see* Nevus
  - intraepidermal epithelioma — *see* Neoplasm, skin, benign
- **Jaffe-Lichtenstein** (-Uehlinger) syndrome — *see* Dysplasia, fibrous, bone NEC
- **Jakob-Creutzfeldt** disease or syndrome — *see* Creutzfeldt-Jakob disease or syndrome
- **Jaksch-Luzet** disease D64.89
- **Jamaican**
  - neuropathy G92
  - paraplegic tropical ataxic-spastic syndrome G92
- **Janet's** disease F48.8
- **Janiceps** Q89.4
- **Jansky-Bielschowsky** amaurotic idiocy E75.4
- **Japanese**
  - B-type encephalitis A83.0
  - river fever A75.3
- **Jaundice** (yellow) R17
  - acholuric (familial) (splenomegalic) (*see also* Spherocytosis)
    - acquired D59.8
  - breast-milk (inhibitor) P59.3
  - catarrhal (acute) B15.9
    - with hepatic coma B15.0
  - cholestatic (benign) R17
  - due to or associated with
    - delayed conjugation P59.8
      - associated with (due to) preterm delivery P59.0
    - preterm delivery P59.0
  - epidemic (catarrhal) B15.9
    - with hepatic coma B15.0
    - leptospiral A27.0
    - spirochetal A27.0
  - familial nonhemolytic (congenital) (Gilbert) E80.4
    - Crigler-Najjar E80.5
  - febrile (acute) B15.9
    - with hepatic coma B15.0
    - leptospiral A27.0
    - spirochetal A27.0
  - hematogenous D59.9
  - hemolytic (acquired) D59.9
    - congenital — *see* Spherocytosis
  - hemorrhagic (acute) (leptospiral) (spirochetal) A27.0
  - infectious (acute) (subacute) B15.9
    - with hepatic coma B15.0
    - leptospiral A27.0
    - spirochetal A27.0
  - leptospiral (hemorrhagic) A27.0
  - malignant (without coma) K72.90
    - with coma K72.91
  - newborn P59.9
    - due to or associated with
      - ABO

- **Jaundice** — *continued*
  - newborn — *continued*
      - antibodies P55.1
      - incompatibility, maternal/fetal P55.1
      - isoimmunization P55.1
    - absence or deficiency of enzyme system for bilirubin conjugation (congenital) P59.8
    - bleeding P58.1
    - breast milk inhibitors to conjugation P59.3
      - associated with preterm delivery P59.0
    - bruising P58.0
    - Crigler-Najjar syndrome E80.5
    - delayed conjugation P59.8
      - associated with preterm delivery P59.0
    - drugs or toxins
      - given to newborn P58.42
      - transmitted from mother P58.41
    - excessive hemolysis P58.9
      - due to
        - bleeding P58.1
        - bruising P58.0
        - drugs or toxins
          - given to newborn P58.42
          - transmitted from mother P58.41
        - infection P58.2
        - polycythemia P58.3
        - swallowed maternal blood P58.5
      - specified type NEC P58.8
    - galactosemia E74.21
    - Gilbert syndrome E80.4
    - hemolytic disease P55.9
      - ABO isoimmunization P55.1
      - Rh isoimmunization P55.0
      - specified NEC P55.8
    - hepatocellular damage P59.20
      - specified NEC P59.29
    - hereditary hemolytic anemia P58.8
    - hypothyroidism, congenital E03.1
    - incompatibility, maternal/fetal NOS P55.9
    - infection P58.2
    - inspissated bile syndrome P59.1
    - isoimmunization NOS P55.9
    - mucoviscidosis E84.9
    - polycythemia P58.3
    - preterm delivery P59.0
    - Rh
      - antibodies P55.0
      - incompatibility, maternal/fetal P55.0
      - isoimmunization P55.0
    - specified cause NEC P59.8
    - swallowed maternal blood P58.5
    - spherocytosis (congenital) D58.0
  - neonatal — *see* Jaundice, newborn
  - nonhemolytic congenital familial (Gilbert) E80.4
  - nuclear, newborn (*see also* Kernicterus of newborn)P57.9
  - obstructive (*see also* Obstruction, bile duct)K83.1
  - post-immunization — *see* Hepatitis, viral, type, B
  - post-transfusion — *see* Hepatitis, viral, type, B
  - regurgitation (*see also* Obstruction, bile duct)K83.1
  - serum (homologous) (prophylactic) (therapeutic) — *see* Hepatitis, viral, type, B
  - spirochetal (hemorrhagic) A27.0
  - symptomatic R17
    - newborn P59.9
- **Jaw** — *see* condition
- **Jaw-winking** phenomenon or syndrome Q07.8
- **Jealousy**
  - alcoholic F10.988
  - childhood F93.8
  - sibling F93.8
- **Jejunitis** — *see* Enteritis
- **Jejunostomy** status Z93.4
- **Jejunum,** jejunal — *see* condition
- **Jensen's** disease — *see* Inflammation, chorioretinal, focal, juxtapapillary
- **Jerks,** myoclonic G25.3
- **Jervell-Lange-Nielsen** syndrome I45.81
- **Jeune's** disease Q77.2
- **Jigger** disease B88.1
- **Job's** syndrome (chronic granulomatous disease) D71
- **Joint** (*see also* condition)
  - mice — *see* Loose, body, joint
    - knee M23.4 ☑
- **Jordan's** anomaly or syndrome D72.0
- **Joseph-Diamond-Blackfan** anemia (congenital hypoplastic) D61.01
- **Jungle** yellow fever A95.0
- **Jüngling's** disease — *see* Sarcoidosis
- **Juvenile** — *see* condition

K

- **Kahler's** disease C90.0 ☑
- **Kakke** E51.11
- **Kala-azar** B55.0
- **Kallmann's** syndrome E23.0
- **Kanner's** syndrome (autism) — *see* Psychosis, childhood
- **Kaposi's**
  - dermatosis (xeroderma pigmentosum) Q82.1
  - lichen ruber L44.0
    - acuminatus L44.0
  - sarcoma
    - colon C46.4
    - connective tissue C46.1
    - gastrointestinal organ C46.4
    - lung C46.5 ☑
    - lymph node (multiple) C46.3
    - palate (hard) (soft) C46.2
    - rectum C46.4
    - skin (multiple sites) C46.0
    - specified site NEC C46.7
    - stomach C46.4
    - unspecified site C46.9
  - varicelliform eruption B00.0
    - vaccinia T88.1 ☑
- **Kartagener's** syndrome or triad (sinusitis, bronchiectasis, situs inversus) Q89.3
- **Karyotype**
  - with abnormality except iso (Xq) Q96.2
  - 45,X Q96.0
  - 46,X
    - iso (Xq) Q96.1
  - 46,XX Q98.3
    - with streak gonads Q50.32
    - hermaphrodite (true) Q99.1
    - male Q98.3
  - 46,XY
    - with streak gonads Q56.1
    - female Q97.3
    - hermaphrodite (true) Q99.1
  - 47,XXX Q97.0
  - 47,XXY Q98.0
  - 47,XYY Q98.5
- **Kaschin-Beck** disease — *see* Disease, Kaschin-Beck
- **Katayama's** disease or fever B65.2
- **Kawasaki's** syndrome M30.3
- **Kayser-Fleischer** ring (cornea) (pseudosclerosis) H18.04 ☑
- **Kaznelson's** syndrome (congenital hypoplastic anemia) D61.01
- **Kearns-Sayre** syndrome H49.81 ☑
- **Kedani** fever A75.3
- **Kelis** L91.0
- **Kelly** (-Patterson) syndrome (sideropenic dysphagia) D50.1
- **Keloid,** cheloid L91.0
  - acne L73.0
  - Addison's L94.0
  - cornea — *see* Opacity, cornea
  - Hawkin's L91.0
  - scar L91.0
- **Keloma** L91.0
- **Kenya** fever A77.1
- **Keratectasia** (*see also* Ectasia, cornea)
  - congenital Q13.4
- **Keratinization** of alveolar ridge mucosa
  - excessive K13.23
  - minimal K13.22
- **Keratinized** residual ridge mucosa
  - excessive K13.23
  - minimal K13.22
- **Keratitis** (nodular) (nonulcerative) (simple) (zonular) H16.9
  - with ulceration (central) (marginal) (perforated) (ring) — *see* Ulcer, cornea
  - actinic — *see* Photokeratitis
  - arborescens (herpes simplex) B00.52
  - areolar H16.11 ☑
  - bullosa H16.8
  - deep H16.309
    - specified type NEC H16.399
  - dendritic (a) (herpes simplex) B00.52
  - disciform (is) (herpes simplex) B00.52
    - varicella B01.81
  - filamentary H16.12 ☑
  - gonococcal (congenital or prenatal) A54.33
  - herpes, herpetic (simplex) B00.52
    - zoster B02.33
  - in (due to)
    - acanthamebiasis B60.13

- **Keratitis** — *continued*
  - In — *continued*
    - adenovirus B30.0
    - exanthema (*see also* Exanthem)B09
    - herpes (simplex) virus B00.52
    - measles B05.81
    - syphilis A50.31
    - tuberculosis A18.52
    - zoster B02.33
  - interstitial (nonsyphilitic) H16.30 ☑
    - diffuse H16.32 ☑
    - herpes, herpetic (simplex) B00.52
      - zoster B02.33
    - sclerosing H16.33 ☑
    - specified type NEC H16.39 ☑
    - syphilitic (congenital) (late) A50.31
    - tuberculous A18.52
  - macular H16.11 ☑
  - nummular H16.11 ☑
  - oyster shuckers' H16.8
  - parenchymatous — *see* Keratitis, interstitial
  - petrificans H16.8
  - postmeasles B05.81
  - punctata
    - leprosa A30.9 *[H16.14-]*
    - syphilitic (profunda) A50.31
  - punctate H16.14 ☑
  - purulent H16.8
  - rosacea L71.8
  - sclerosing H16.33 ☑
  - specified type NEC H16.8
  - stellate H16.11 ☑
  - striate H16.11 ☑
  - superficial H16.10 ☑
    - with conjunctivitis — *see* Keratoconjunctivitis
    - due to light — *see* Photokeratitis
  - suppurative H16.8
  - syphilitic (congenital) (prenatal) A50.31
  - trachomatous A71.1
    - sequelae B94.0
  - tuberculous A18.52
  - vesicular H16.8
  - xerotic (*see also* Keratomalacia)H16.8
    - vitamin A deficiency E50.4
- **Keratoacanthoma** L85.8
- **Keratocele** — *see* Descemetocele
- **Keratoconjunctivitis** H16.20 ☑
  - Acanthamoeba B60.13
  - adenoviral B30.0
  - epidemic B30.0
  - exposure H16.21 ☑
  - herpes, herpetic (simplex) B00.52
    - zoster B02.33
  - in exanthema (*see also* Exanthem)B09
  - infectious B30.0
  - lagophthalmic — *see* Keratoconjunctivitis, specified type NEC
  - neurotrophic H16.23 ☑
  - phlyctenular H16.25 ☑
  - postmeasles B05.81
  - shipyard B30.0
  - sicca (Sjogren's) M35.0 ☑
    - not Sjogren's H16.22 ☑
  - specified type NEC H16.29 ☑
  - tuberculous (phlyctenular) A18.52
  - vernal H16.26 ☑
- **Keratoconus** H18.60 ☑
  - congenital Q13.4
  - stable H18.61 ☑
  - unstable H18.62 ☑
- **Keratocyst** (dental) (odontogenic) — *see* Cyst, calcifying odontogenic
- **Keratoderma,** keratodermia (congenital) (palmaris et plantaris) (symmetrical) Q82.8
  - acquired L85.1
    - in diseases classified elsewhere L86
  - climactericum L85.1
  - gonococcal A54.89
  - gonorrheal A54.89
  - punctata L85.2
  - Reiter's — *see* Reiter's disease
- **Keratodermatocele** — *see* Descemetocele
- **Keratoglobus** H18.79 ☑
  - congenital Q15.8
    - with glaucoma Q15.0
- **Keratohemia** — *see* Pigmentation, cornea, stromal
- **Keratoiritis** (*see also* Iridocyclitis)
  - syphilitic A50.39
  - tuberculous A18.54
- **Keratoma** L57.0
  - palmaris and plantaris hereditarium Q82.8
  - senile L57.0
- **Keratomalacia** H18.44 ☑
  - vitamin A deficiency E50.4
- **Keratomegaly** Q13.4
- **Keratomycosis** B49
  - nigrans, nigricans (palmaris) B36.1
- **Keratopathy** H18.9
  - band H18.42 ☑
  - bullous H18.1 ☑
  - bullous (aphakic), following cataract surgery H59.01 ☑
- **Keratoscleritis,** tuberculous A18.52
- **Keratosis** L57.0
  - actinic L57.0
  - arsenical L85.8
  - congenital, specified NEC Q80.8
  - female genital NEC N94.89
  - follicularis Q82.8
    - acquired L11.0
    - congenita Q82.8
    - et parafollicularis in cutem penetrans L87.0
    - spinulosa (decalvans) Q82.8
    - vitamin A deficiency E50.8
  - gonococcal A54.89
  - male genital (external) N50.89
  - nigricans L83
  - obturans, external ear (canal) — *see* Cholesteatoma, external ear
  - palmaris et plantaris (inherited) (symmetrical) Q82.8
    - acquired L85.1
  - penile N48.89
  - pharynx J39.2
  - pilaris, acquired L85.8
  - punctata (palmaris et plantaris) L85.2
  - scrotal N50.89
  - seborrheic L82.1
    - inflamed L82.0
  - senile L57.0
  - solar L57.0
  - tonsillaris J35.8
  - vagina N89.4
  - vegetans Q82.8
  - vitamin A deficiency E50.8
  - vocal cord J38.3
- **Kerato-uveitis** — *see* Iridocyclitis
- **Kerunoparalysis** T75.09 ☑
- **Kerion** (celsi) B35.0
- **Kernicterus** of newborn (not due to isoimmunization) P57.9
  - due to isoimmunization (conditions in P55.0-P55.9) P57.0
  - specified type NEC P57.8
- **Keshan** disease E59
- **Ketoacidosis** E87.2
  - diabetic — *see* Diabetes, by type, with ketoacidosis
- **Ketonuria** R82.4
- **Ketosis** NEC E88.89
  - diabetic — *see* Diabetes, by type, with ketoacidosis
- **Kew** Garden fever A79.1
- **Kidney** — *see* condition
- **Kienböck's** disease (*see also* Osteochondrosis, juvenile, hand, carpal lunate)
  - adult M93.1
- **Kimmelstiel** (-Wilson) disease — *see* Diabetes, Kimmelstiel (-Wilson) disease
- **Kimura** disease D21.9
  - specified site (see Neoplasm, connective tissue benign)
- **Kink,** kinking
  - artery I77.1
  - hair (acquired) L67.8
  - ileum or intestine — *see* Obstruction, intestine
  - Lane's — *see* Obstruction, intestine
  - organ or site, congenital NEC — *see* Anomaly, by site
  - ureter (pelvic junction) N13.5
    - with
      - hydronephrosis N13.1
        - with infection N13.6
      - pyelonephritis (chronic) N11.1
    - congenital Q62.39
  - vein(s) I87.8
    - caval I87.1
    - peripheral I87.1
- **Kinnier** Wilson's disease (hepatolenticular degeneration) E83.01
- **Kissing** spine M48.20
  - cervical region M48.22
  - cervicothoracic region M48.23
  - lumbar region M48.26
- **Kissing** spine — *continued*
  - lumbosacral region M48.27
  - occipito-atlanto-axial region M48.21
  - thoracic region M48.24
  - thoracolumbar region M48.25
- **Klatskin's** tumor C24.0
- **Klauder's** disease A26.8
- **Klebs'** disease (*see also* Glomerulonephritis)N05. ☑
- **Klebsiella** (K.) pneumoniae, as cause of disease classified elsewhere B96.1
- **Klein** (e)-Levin syndrome G47.13
- **Kleptomania** F63.2
- **Klinefelter's** syndrome Q98.4
  - karyotype 47,XXY Q98.0
  - male with more than two X chromosomes Q98.1
- **Klippel-Feil** deficiency, disease, or syndrome (brevicollis) Q76.1
- **Klippel's** disease I67.2
- **Klippel-Trenaunay** (-Weber) syndrome Q87.2
- **Klumpke** (-Déjerine) palsy, paralysis (birth) (newborn) P14.1
- **Knee** — *see* condition
- **Knock** knee (acquired) M21.06 ☑
  - congenital Q74.1
- **Knot** (s)
  - intestinal, syndrome (volvulus) K56.2
  - surfer S89.8 ☑
  - umbilical cord (true) O69.2 ☑
- **Knotting** (of)
  - hair L67.8
  - intestine K56.2
- **Knuckle** pad (Garrod's) M72.1
- **Koch's**
  - infection — *see* Tuberculosis
  - relapsing fever A68.9
- **Koch-Weeks'** conjunctivitis — *see* Conjunctivitis, acute, mucopurulent
- **Köebner's** syndrome Q81.8
- **Köenig's** disease (osteochondritis dissecans) — *see* Osteochondritis, dissecans
- **Köhler-Pellegrini-Steida** disease or syndrome (calcification, knee joint) — *see* Bursitis, tibial collateral
- **Köhler's** disease
  - patellar — *see* Osteochondrosis, juvenile, patella
  - tarsal navicular — *see* Osteochondrosis, juvenile, tarsus
- **Koilonychia** L60.3
  - congenital Q84.6
- **Kojevnikov's,** epilepsy — *see* Kozhevnikof's epilepsy
- **Koplik's** spots B05.9
- **Kopp's** asthma E32.8
- **Korsakoff's** (Wernicke) disease, psychosis or syndrome (alcoholic) F10.96
  - with dependence F10.26
  - drug-induced
    - due to drug abuse — *see* Abuse, drug, by type, with amnestic disorder
    - due to drug dependence — *see* Dependence, drug, by type, with amnestic disorder
  - nonalcoholic F04
- **Korsakov's** disease, psychosis or syndrome — *see* Korsakoff's disease
- **Korsakow's** disease, psychosis or syndrome — *see* Korsakoff's disease
- **Kostmann's** disease or syndrome (infantile genetic agranulocytosis) — *see* Agranulocytosis
- **Kozhevnikof's** epilepsy G40.109
  - intractable G40.119
    - with status epilepticus G40.111
    - without status epilepticus G40.119
  - not intractable G40.109
    - with status epilepticus G40.101
    - without status epilepticus G40.109
- **Krabbe's**
  - disease E75.23
  - syndrome, congenital muscle hypoplasia Q79.8
- **Kraepelin-Morel** disease — *see* Schizophrenia
- **Kraft-Weber-Dimitri** disease Q85.8
- **Kraurosis**
  - ani K62.89
  - penis N48.0
  - vagina N89.8
  - vulva N90.4
- **Kreotoxism** A05.9
- **Krukenberg's**
  - spindle — *see* Pigmentation, cornea, posterior
  - tumor C79.6 ☑
- **Kufs'** disease E75.4
- **Kugelberg-Welander** disease G12.1
- **Kuhnt-Junius** degeneration (*see also* Degeneration, macula)H35.32 ☑

- **Kümmell's** disease or spondylitis — *see* Spondylopathy, traumatic
- **Kupffer** cell sarcoma C22.3
- **Kuru** A81.81
- **Kussmaul's**
  - disease M30.0
  - respiration E87.2
    - in diabetic acidosis — *see* Diabetes, by type, with ketoacidosis
- **Kwashiorkor** E40
  - marasmic, marasmus type E42
- **Kyasanur** Forest disease A98.2
- **Kyphoscoliosis,** kyphoscoliotic (acquired) (*see also* Scoliosis)M41.9
  - congenital Q67.5
  - heart (disease) I27.1
  - sequelae of rickets E64.3
  - tuberculous A18.01
- **Kyphosis,** kyphotic (acquired) M40.209
  - cervical region M40.202
  - cervicothoracic region M40.203
  - congenital Q76.419
    - cervical region Q76.412
    - cervicothoracic region Q76.413
    - occipito-atlanto-axial region Q76.411
    - thoracic region Q76.414
    - thoracolumbar region Q76.415
  - Morquio-Brailsford type (spinal) (*see also* subcategory M49.8)E76.219
  - postlaminectomy M96.3
  - postradiation therapy M96.2
  - postural (adolescent) M40.00
    - cervicothoracic region M40.03
    - thoracic region M40.04
    - thoracolumbar region M40.05
  - secondary NEC M40.10
    - cervical region M40.12
    - cervicothoracic region M40.13
    - thoracic region M40.14
    - thoracolumbar region M40.15
  - sequelae of rickets E64.3
  - specified type NEC M40.299
    - cervical region M40.292
    - cervicothoracic region M40.293
    - thoracic region M40.294
    - thoracolumbar region M40.295
  - syphilitic, congenital A50.56
  - thoracic region M40.204
  - thoracolumbar region M40.205
  - tuberculous A18.01
- **Kyrle** disease L87.0

L

- **Labia,** labium — *see* condition
- **Labile**
  - blood pressure R09.89
  - vasomotor system I73.9
- **Labioglossal** paralysis G12.29
- **Labium** leporinum — *see* Cleft, lip
- **Labor** — *see* Delivery
- **Labored** breathing — *see* Hyperventilation
- **Labyrinthitis** (circumscribed) (destructive) (diffuse) (inner ear) (latent) (purulent) (suppurative) (*see also* subcategory)H83.0 ☑
  - syphilitic A52.79
- **Laceration**
  - with abortion — *see* Abortion, by type, complicated by laceration of pelvic organs
  - abdomen, abdominal
    - wall S31.119 ☑
      - with
        - foreign body S31.129 ☑
        - penetration into peritoneal cavity S31.619 ☑
          - with foreign body S31.629 ☑
      - epigastric region S31.112 ☑
        - with
          - foreign body S31.122 ☑
          - penetration into peritoneal cavity S31.612 ☑
            - with foreign body S31.622 ☑
      - left
        - lower quadrant S31.114 ☑
          - with
            - foreign body S31.124 ☑
            - penetration into peritoneal cavity S31.614 ☑
              - with foreign body S31.624 ☑
        - upper quadrant S31.111 ☑

Laceration — *continued*

abdomen, abdominal — *continued*

- with
  - foreign body S31.121 ☑
  - penetration into peritoneal cavity S31.611 ☑
    - with foreign body S31.621 ☑
- periumbilic region S31.115 ☑
  - with
    - foreign body S31.125 ☑
    - penetration into peritoneal cavity S31.615 ☑
      - with foreign body S31.625 ☑
- right
  - lower quadrant S31.113 ☑
    - with
      - foreign body S31.123 ☑
      - penetration into peritoneal cavity S31.613 ☑
        - with foreign body S31.623 ☑
  - upper quadrant S31.110 ☑
    - with
      - foreign body S31.120 ☑
      - penetration into peritoneal cavity S31.610 ☑
        - with foreign body S31.620 ☑

- accidental, complicating surgery — *see* Complications, surgical, accidental puncture or laceration
- Achilles tendon S86.02 ☑
- adrenal gland S37.813 ☑
- alveolar (process) — *see* Laceration, oral cavity
- ankle S91.01 ☑
  - with
    - foreign body S91.02 ☑
- antecubital space — *see* Laceration, elbow
- anus (sphincter) S31.831 ☑
  - with
    - ectopic or molar pregnancy O08.6
    - foreign body S31.832 ☑
  - complicating delivery — *see* Delivery, complicated, by, laceration, anus (sphincter)
  - following ectopic or molar pregnancy O08.6
  - nontraumatic, nonpuerperal — *see* Fissure, anus
- arm (upper) S41.11 ☑
  - with foreign body S41.12 ☑
  - lower — *see* Laceration, forearm
- auditory canal (external) (meatus) — *see* Laceration, ear
- auricle, ear — *see* Laceration, ear
- axilla — *see* Laceration, arm
- back (*see also* Laceration, thorax, back)
  - lower S31.010 ☑
    - with
      - foreign body S31.020 ☑
        - with penetration into retroperitoneal space S31.021 ☑
      - penetration into retroperitoneal space S31.011 ☑
- bile duct S36.13 ☑
- bladder S37.23 ☑
  - with ectopic or molar pregnancy O08.6
  - following ectopic or molar pregnancy O08.6
  - obstetrical trauma O71.5
- blood vessel — *see* Injury, blood vessel
- bowel (*see also* Laceration, intestine)
  - with ectopic or molar pregnancy O08.6
  - complicating abortion — *see* Abortion, by type, complicated by, specified condition NEC
  - following ectopic or molar pregnancy O08.6
  - obstetrical trauma O71.5
- brain (any part) (cortex) (diffuse) (membrane) (*see also* Injury, intracranial, diffuse)
  - during birth P10.8
    - with hemorrhage P10.1
  - focal — *see* Injury, intracranial, focal brain injury
- brainstem S06.38 ☑
- breast S21.01 ☑
  - with foreign body S21.02 ☑
- broad ligament S37.893 ☑
  - with ectopic or molar pregnancy O08.6
  - following ectopic or molar pregnancy O08.6
  - laceration syndrome N83.8
  - obstetrical trauma O71.6
  - syndrome (laceration) N83.8
- buttock S31.801 ☑
  - with foreign body S31.802 ☑
  - left S31.821 ☑
    - with foreign body S31.822 ☑
  - right S31.811 ☑
    - with foreign body S31.812 ☑

Laceration — *continued*

- calf — *see* Laceration, leg
- canaliculus lacrimalis — *see* Laceration, eyelid
- canthus, eye — *see* Laceration, eyelid
- capsule, joint — *see* Sprain
- causing eversion of cervix uteri (old) N86
- central (perineal), complicating delivery O70.9
- cerebellum, traumatic S06.37 ☑
- cerebral S06.33 ☑
  - left side S06.32 ☑
  - during birth P10.8
    - with hemorrhage P10.1
  - right side S06.31 ☑
- cervix (uteri)
  - with ectopic or molar pregnancy O08.6
  - following ectopic or molar pregnancy O08.6
  - nonpuerperal, nontraumatic N88.1
  - obstetrical trauma (current) O71.3
  - old (postpartal) N88.1
  - traumatic S37.63 ☑
- cheek (external) S01.41 ☑
  - with foreign body S01.42 ☑
  - internal — *see* Laceration, oral cavity
- chest wall — *see* Laceration, thorax
- chin — *see* Laceration, head, specified site NEC
- chordae tendinae NEC I51.1
  - concurrent with acute myocardial infarction — *see* Infarct, myocardium
  - following acute myocardial infarction (current complication) I23.4
- clitoris — *see* Laceration, vulva
- colon — *see* Laceration, intestine, large, colon
- common bile duct S36.13 ☑
- cortex (cerebral) — *see* Injury, intracranial, diffuse
- costal region — *see* Laceration, thorax
- cystic duct S36.13 ☑
- diaphragm S27.803 ☑
- digit (s)
  - hand — *see* Laceration, finger
  - foot — *see* Laceration, toe
- duodenum S36.430 ☑
- ear (canal) (external) S01.31 ☑
  - with foreign body S01.32 ☑
  - drum S09.2 ☑
- elbow S51.01 ☑
  - with
    - foreign body S51.02 ☑
- epididymis — *see* Laceration, testis
- epigastric region — *see* Laceration, abdomen, wall, epigastric region
- esophagus K22.8
  - traumatic
    - cervical S11.21 ☑
      - with foreign body S11.22 ☑
    - thoracic S27.813 ☑
- eye (ball) S05.3 ☑
  - with prolapse or loss of intraocular tissue S05.2 ☑
  - penetrating S05.6 ☑
- eyebrow — *see* Laceration, eyelid
- eyelid S01.11 ☑
  - with foreign body S01.12 ☑
- face NEC — *see* Laceration, head, specified site NEC
- fallopian tube S37.539 ☑
  - bilateral S37.532 ☑
  - unilateral S37.531 ☑
- finger (s) S61.219 ☑
  - with
    - damage to nail S61.319 ☑
      - with
        - foreign body S61.329 ☑
    - foreign body S61.229 ☑
  - index S61.218 ☑
    - with
      - damage to nail S61.318 ☑
        - with
          - foreign body S61.328 ☑
      - foreign body S61.228 ☑
    - left S61.211 ☑
      - with
        - damage to nail S61.311 ☑
          - with
            - foreign body S61.321 ☑
        - foreign body S61.221 ☑
    - right S61.210 ☑
      - with
        - damage to nail S61.310 ☑
          - with
            - foreign body S61.320 ☑
        - foreign body S61.220 ☑
  - little S61.218 ☑

- **Laceration** — *continued*
  - finger (s) — *continued*
      - with
        - damage to nail S61.318 ☑
          - with
            - foreign body S61.328 ☑
        - foreign body S61.228 ☑
      - left S61.217 ☑
        - with
          - damage to nail S61.317 ☑
            - with
              - foreign body S61.327 ☑
          - foreign body S61.227 ☑
      - right S61.216 ☑
        - with
          - damage to nail S61.316 ☑
            - with
              - foreign body S61.326 ☑
          - foreign body S61.226 ☑
    - middle S61.218 ☑
      - with
        - damage to nail S61.318 ☑
          - with
            - foreign body S61.328 ☑
        - foreign body S61.228 ☑
      - left S61.213 ☑
        - with
          - damage to nail S61.313 ☑
            - with
              - foreign body S61.323 ☑
          - foreign body S61.223 ☑
      - right S61.212 ☑
        - with
          - damage to nail S61.312 ☑
            - with
              - foreign body S61.322 ☑
          - foreign body S61.222 ☑
    - ring S61.218 ☑
      - with
        - damage to nail S61.318 ☑
          - with
            - foreign body S61.328 ☑
        - foreign body S61.228 ☑
      - left S61.215 ☑
        - with
          - damage to nail S61.315 ☑
            - with
              - foreign body S61.325 ☑
          - foreign body S61.225 ☑
      - right S61.214 ☑
        - with
          - damage to nail S61.314 ☑
            - with
              - foreign body S61.324 ☑
          - foreign body S61.224 ☑
  - flank S31.119 ☑
    - with foreign body S31.129 ☑
  - foot (except toe (s) alone) S91.319 ☑
    - with foreign body S91.329 ☑
    - left S91.312 ☑
      - with foreign body S91.322 ☑
    - right S91.311 ☑
      - with foreign body S91.321 ☑
    - toe — *see* Laceration, toe
  - forearm S51.819 ☑
    - with
      - foreign body S51.829 ☑
    - elbow only — *see* Laceration, elbow
    - left S51.812 ☑
      - with
        - foreign body S51.822 ☑
    - right S51.811 ☑
      - with
        - foreign body S51.821 ☑
  - forehead S01.81 ☑
    - with foreign body S01.82 ☑
  - fourchette O70.0
    - with ectopic or molar pregnancy O08.6
    - complicating delivery O70.0
    - following ectopic or molar pregnancy O08.6
  - gallbladder S36.123 ☑
  - genital organs, external
    - female S31.512 ☑
      - with foreign body S31.522 ☑
      - vagina — *see* Laceration, vagina
      - vulva — *see* Laceration, vulva
    - male S31.511 ☑
      - with foreign body S31.521 ☑
      - penis — *see* Laceration, penis
      - scrotum — *see* Laceration, scrotum
      - testis — *see* Laceration, testis

- **Laceration** — *continued*
  - groin — *see* Laceration, abdomen, wall
  - gum — *see* Laceration, oral cavity
  - hand S61.419 ☑
    - with
      - foreign body S61.429 ☑
    - finger — *see* Laceration, finger
    - left S61.412 ☑
      - with
        - foreign body S61.422 ☑
    - right S61.411 ☑
      - with
        - foreign body S61.421 ☑
    - thumb — *see* Laceration, thumb
  - head S01.91 ☑
    - with foreign body S01.92 ☑
    - cheek — *see* Laceration, cheek
    - ear — *see* Laceration, ear
    - eyelid — *see* Laceration, eyelid
    - lip — *see* Laceration, lip
    - nose — *see* Laceration, nose
    - oral cavity — *see* Laceration, oral cavity
    - scalp S01.01 ☑
      - with foreign body S01.02 ☑
    - specified site NEC S01.81 ☑
      - with foreign body S01.82 ☑
    - temporomandibular area — *see* Laceration, cheek
  - heart — *see* Injury, heart, laceration
  - heel — *see* Laceration, foot
  - hepatic duct S36.13 ☑
  - hip S71.019 ☑
    - with foreign body S71.029 ☑
    - left S71.012 ☑
      - with foreign body S71.022 ☑
    - right S71.011 ☑
      - with foreign body S71.021 ☑
  - hymen — *see* Laceration, vagina
  - hypochondrium — *see* Laceration, abdomen, wall
  - hypogastric region — *see* Laceration, abdomen, wall
  - ileum S36.438 ☑
  - inguinal region — *see* Laceration, abdomen, wall
  - instep — *see* Laceration, foot
  - internal organ — *see* Injury, by site
  - interscapular region — *see* Laceration, thorax, back
  - intestine
    - large
      - colon S36.539 ☑
        - ascending S36.530 ☑
        - descending S36.532 ☑
        - sigmoid S36.533 ☑
        - specified site NEC S36.538 ☑
      - rectum S36.63 ☑
        - transverse S36.531 ☑
    - small S36.439 ☑
      - duodenum S36.430 ☑
      - specified site NEC S36.438 ☑
  - intra-abdominal organ S36.93 ☑
    - intestine — *see* Laceration, intestine
    - liver — *see* Laceration, liver
    - pancreas — *see* Laceration, pancreas
    - peritoneum S36.81 ☑
    - specified site NEC S36.893 ☑
    - spleen — *see* Laceration, spleen
    - stomach — *see* Laceration, stomach
  - intracranial NEC (*see also* Injury, intracranial, diffuse)
    - birth injury P10.9
  - jaw — *see* Laceration, head, specified site NEC
  - jejunum S36.438 ☑
  - joint capsule — *see* Sprain, by site
  - kidney S37.03 ☑
    - major (greater than 3 cm) (massive) (stellate) S37.06 ☑
    - minor (less than 1 cm) S37.04 ☑
    - moderate (1 to 3 cm) S37.05 ☑
      - multiple S37.06 ☑
  - knee S81.01 ☑
    - with foreign body S81.02 ☑
  - labium (majus) (minus) — *see* Laceration, vulva
  - lacrimal duct — *see* Laceration, eyelid
  - large intestine — *see* Laceration, intestine, large
  - larynx S11.011 ☑
    - with foreign body S11.012 ☑
  - leg (lower) S81.819 ☑
    - with foreign body S81.829 ☑
    - foot — *see* Laceration, foot
    - knee — *see* Laceration, knee
    - left S81.812 ☑
      - with foreign body S81.822 ☑

- **Laceration** — *continued*
  - leg — *continued*
    - right S81.811 ☑
      - with foreign body S81.821 ☑
    - upper — *see* Laceration, thigh
  - ligament — *see* Sprain
  - lip S01.511 ☑
    - with foreign body S01.521 ☑
  - liver S36.113 ☑
    - major (stellate) S36.116 ☑
    - minor S36.114 ☑
    - moderate S36.115 ☑
  - loin — *see* Laceration, abdomen, wall
  - lower back — *see* Laceration, back, lower
  - lumbar region — *see* Laceration, back, lower
  - lung S27.339 ☑
    - bilateral S27.332 ☑
    - unilateral S27.331 ☑
  - malar region — *see* Laceration, head, specified site NEC
  - mammary — *see* Laceration, breast
  - mastoid region — *see* Laceration, head, specified site NEC
  - meninges — *see* Injury, intracranial, diffuse
  - meniscus — *see* Tear, meniscus
  - mesentery S36.893 ☑
  - mesosalpinx S37.893 ☑
  - mouth — *see* Laceration, oral cavity
  - muscle — *see* Injury, muscle, by site, laceration
  - nail
    - finger — *see* Laceration, finger, with damage to nail
    - toe — *see* Laceration, toe, with damage to nail
  - nasal (septum) (sinus) — *see* Laceration, nose
  - nasopharynx — *see* Laceration, head, specified site NEC
  - neck S11.91 ☑
    - with foreign body S11.92 ☑
    - involving
      - cervical esophagus S11.21 ☑
        - with foreign body S11.22 ☑
      - larynx — *see* Laceration, larynx
      - pharynx — *see* Laceration, pharynx
      - thyroid gland — *see* Laceration, thyroid gland
      - trachea — *see* Laceration, trachea
    - specified site NEC S11.81 ☑
      - with foreign body S11.82 ☑
  - nerve — *see* Injury, nerve
  - nose (septum) (sinus) S01.21 ☑
    - with foreign body S01.22 ☑
  - ocular NOS S05.3 ☑
    - adnexa NOS S01.11 ☑
  - oral cavity S01.512 ☑
    - with foreign body S01.522 ☑
  - orbit (eye) — *see* Wound, open, ocular, orbit
  - ovary S37.439 ☑
    - bilateral S37.432 ☑
    - unilateral S37.431 ☑
  - palate — *see* Laceration, oral cavity
  - palm — *see* Laceration, hand
  - pancreas S36.239 ☑
    - body S36.231 ☑
      - major S36.261 ☑
      - minor S36.241 ☑
      - moderate S36.251 ☑
    - head S36.230 ☑
      - major S36.260 ☑
      - minor S36.240 ☑
      - moderate S36.250 ☑
    - major S36.269 ☑
    - minor S36.249 ☑
    - moderate S36.259 ☑
    - tail S36.232 ☑
      - major S36.262 ☑
      - minor S36.242 ☑
      - moderate S36.252 ☑
  - pelvic S31.010 ☑
    - with
      - foreign body S31.020 ☑
        - penetration into retroperitoneal cavity S31.021 ☑
      - penetration into retroperitoneal cavity S31.011 ☑
    - floor (*see also* Laceration, back, lower)
      - with ectopic or molar pregnancy O08.6
      - complicating delivery O70.1
      - following ectopic or molar pregnancy O08.6
      - old (postpartal) N81.89
    - organ S37.93 ☑
      - with ectopic or molar pregnancy O08.6
      - adrenal gland S37.813 ☑
      - bladder S37.23 ☑

Laceration - Lack

Laceration — *continued*
- pelvic — *continued*
  - fallopian tube — *see* Laceration, fallopian tube
  - following ectopic or molar pregnancy O08.6
  - kidney — *see* Laceration, kidney
  - obstetrical trauma O71.5
  - ovary — *see* Laceration, ovary
  - prostate S37.823 ☑
  - specified site NEC S37.893 ☑
  - ureter S37.13 ☑
  - urethra S37.33 ☑
  - uterus S37.63 ☑
- penis S31.21 ☑
  - with foreign body S31.22 ☑
- perineum
  - female S31.41 ☑
    - with
      - ectopic or molar pregnancy O08.6
      - foreign body S31.42 ☑
    - during delivery O70.9
      - first degree O70.0
      - fourth degree O70.3
      - second degree O70.1
      - third degree (*see also* Delivery, complicated, by, laceration, perineum, third degree)O70.20
    - old (postpartal) N81.89
    - postpartal N81.89
    - secondary (postpartal) O90.1
  - male S31.119 ☑
    - with foreign body S31.129 ☑
- periocular area (with or without lacrimal passages) — *see* Laceration, eyelid
- peritoneum S36.893 ☑
- periumbilic region — *see* Laceration, abdomen, wall, periumbilic
- periurethral tissue — *see* Laceration, urethra
- phalanges
  - finger — *see* Laceration, finger
  - toe — *see* Laceration, toe
- pharynx S11.21 ☑
  - with foreign body S11.22 ☑
- pinna — *see* Laceration, ear
- popliteal space — *see* Laceration, knee
- prepuce — *see* Laceration, penis
- prostate S37.823 ☑
- pubic region S31.119 ☑
  - with foreign body S31.129 ☑
- pudendum — *see* Laceration, genital organs, external
- rectovaginal septum — *see* Laceration, vagina
- rectum S36.63 ☑
- retroperitoneum S36.893 ☑
- round ligament S37.893 ☑
- sacral region — *see* Laceration, back, lower
- sacroiliac region — *see* Laceration, back, lower
- salivary gland — *see* Laceration, oral cavity
- scalp S01.01 ☑
  - with foreign body S01.02 ☑
- scapular region — *see* Laceration, shoulder
- scrotum S31.31 ☑
  - with foreign body S31.32 ☑
- seminal vesicle S37.893 ☑
- shin — *see* Laceration, leg
- shoulder S41.019 ☑
  - with foreign body S41.029 ☑
  - left S41.012 ☑
    - with foreign body S41.022 ☑
  - right S41.011 ☑
    - with foreign body S41.021 ☑
- small intestine — *see* Laceration, intestine, small
- spermatic cord — *see* Laceration, testis
- spinal cord (meninges) (*see also* Injury, spinal cord, by region)
  - due to injury at birth P11.5
  - newborn (birth injury) P11.5
- spleen S36.039 ☑
  - major (massive) (stellate) S36.032 ☑
  - moderate S36.031 ☑
  - superficial (minor) S36.030 ☑
- sternal region — *see* Laceration, thorax, front
- stomach S36.33 ☑
- submaxillary region — *see* Laceration, head, specified site NEC
- submental region — *see* Laceration, head, specified site NEC
- subungual
  - finger (s) — *see* Laceration, finger, with damage to nail
  - toe (s) — *see* Laceration, toe, with damage to nail
- suprarenal gland — *see* Laceration, adrenal gland
- temple, temporal region — *see* Laceration, head, specified site NEC
- temporomandibular area — *see* Laceration, cheek
- tendon — *see* Injury, muscle, by site, laceration
  - Achilles S86.02 ☑
- tentorium cerebelli — *see* Injury, intracranial, diffuse
- testis S31.31 ☑
  - with foreign body S31.32 ☑
- thigh S71.11 ☑
  - with foreign body S71.12 ☑
- thorax, thoracic (wall) S21.91 ☑
  - with foreign body S21.92 ☑
    - back S21.22 ☑
      - with penetration into thoracic cavity S21.42 ☑
    - front S21.12 ☑
      - with penetration into thoracic cavity S21.32 ☑
  - back S21.21 ☑
    - with
      - foreign body S21.22 ☑
        - with penetration into thoracic cavity S21.42 ☑
      - penetration into thoracic cavity S21.41 ☑
  - breast — *see* Laceration, breast
  - front S21.11 ☑
    - with
      - foreign body S21.12 ☑
        - with penetration into thoracic cavity S21.32 ☑
      - penetration into thoracic cavity S21.31 ☑
- thumb S61.019 ☑
  - with
    - damage to nail S61.119 ☑
      - with
        - foreign body S61.129 ☑
    - foreign body S61.029 ☑
  - left S61.012 ☑
    - with
      - damage to nail S61.112 ☑
        - with
          - foreign body S61.122 ☑
      - foreign body S61.022 ☑
  - right S61.011 ☑
    - with
      - damage to nail S61.111 ☑
        - with
          - foreign body S61.121 ☑
      - foreign body S61.021 ☑
- thyroid gland S11.11 ☑
  - with foreign body S11.12 ☑
- toe (s) S91.119 ☑
  - with
    - damage to nail S91.219 ☑
      - with
        - foreign body S91.229 ☑
    - foreign body S91.129 ☑
  - great S91.113 ☑
    - with
      - damage to nail S91.213 ☑
        - with
          - foreign body S91.223 ☑
      - foreign body S91.123 ☑
    - left S91.112 ☑
      - with
        - damage to nail S91.212 ☑
          - with
            - foreign body S91.222 ☑
        - foreign body S91.122 ☑
    - right S91.111 ☑
      - with
        - damage to nail S91.211 ☑
          - with
            - foreign body S91.221 ☑
        - foreign body S91.121 ☑
  - lesser S91.116 ☑
    - with
      - damage to nail S91.216 ☑
        - with
          - foreign body S91.226 ☑
      - foreign body S91.126 ☑
    - left S91.115 ☑
      - with
        - damage to nail S91.215 ☑
          - with
            - foreign body S91.225 ☑
        - foreign body S91.125 ☑
    - right S91.114 ☑
      - with

Laceration — *continued*
- toe (s) — *continued*
        - damage to nail S91.214 ☑
          - with
            - foreign body S91.224 ☑
        - foreign body S91.124 ☑
- tongue — *see* Laceration, oral cavity
- trachea S11.021 ☑
  - with foreign body S11.022 ☑
- tunica vaginalis — *see* Laceration, testis
- tympanum, tympanic membrane — *see* Laceration, ear, drum
- umbilical region S31.115 ☑
  - with foreign body S31.125 ☑
- ureter S37.13 ☑
- urethra S37.33 ☑
  - with or following ectopic or molar pregnancy O08.6
  - obstetrical trauma O71.5
- urinary organ NEC S37.893 ☑
- uterus S37.63 ☑
  - with ectopic or molar pregnancy O08.6
  - following ectopic or molar pregnancy O08.6
  - nonpuerperal, nontraumatic N85.8
  - obstetrical trauma NEC O71.81
  - old (postpartal) N85.8
- uvula — *see* Laceration, oral cavity
- vagina S31.41 ☑
  - with
    - ectopic or molar pregnancy O08.6
    - foreign body S31.42 ☑
  - during delivery O71.4
    - with perineal laceration — *see* Laceration, perineum, female, during delivery
  - following ectopic or molar pregnancy O08.6
  - nonpuerperal, nontraumatic N89.8
  - old (postpartal) N89.8
- vas deferens S37.893 ☑
- vesical — *see* Laceration, bladder
- vocal cords S11.031 ☑
  - with foreign body S11.032 ☑
- vulva S31.41 ☑
  - with
    - ectopic or molar pregnancy O08.6
    - foreign body S31.42 ☑
  - complicating delivery O70.0
  - following ectopic or molar pregnancy O08.6
  - nonpuerperal, nontraumatic N90.89
  - old (postpartal) N90.89
- wrist S61.519 ☑
  - with
    - foreign body S61.529 ☑
  - left S61.512 ☑
    - with
      - foreign body S61.522 ☑
  - right S61.511 ☑
    - with
      - foreign body S61.521 ☑

Lack of
- achievement in school Z55.3
- adequate
  - food Z59.4
  - intermaxillary vertical dimension of fully erupted teeth M26.36
  - sleep Z72.820
- appetite (see Anorexia) R63.0
- awareness R41.9
- care
  - in home Z74.2
  - of infant (at or after birth) T76.02 ☑
    - confirmed T74.02 ☑
- cognitive functions R41.9
- coordination R27.9
  - ataxia R27.0
  - specified type NEC R27.8
- development (physiological) R62.50
  - failure to thrive (child over 28 days old) R62.51
    - adult R62.7
    - newborn P92.6
  - short stature R62.52
  - specified type NEC R62.59
- energy R53.83
- financial resources Z59.6
- food T73.0 ☑
- growth R62.52
- heating Z59.1
- housing (permanent) (temporary) Z59.0
  - adequate Z59.1
- learning experiences in childhood Z62.898
- leisure time (affecting life-style) Z73.2
- material resources Z59.9

- **Lack** of — *continued*
  - memory (*see also* Amnesia)
    - mild, following organic brain damage F06.8
  - ovulation N97.0
  - parental supervision or control of child Z62.0
  - person able to render necessary care Z74.2
  - physical exercise Z72.3
  - play experience in childhood Z62.898
  - posterior occlusal support M26.57
  - relaxation (affecting life-style) Z73.2
  - sexual
    - desire F52.0
    - enjoyment F52.1
  - shelter Z59.0
  - sleep (adequate) Z72.820
  - supervision of child by parent Z62.0
  - support, posterior occlusal M26.57
  - water T73.1 ☑
- **Lacrimal** — *see* condition
- **Lacrimation,** abnormal — *see* Epiphora
- **Lacrimonasal** duct — *see* condition
- **Lactation,** lactating (breast) (puerperal, postpartum)
  - associated
    - cracked nipple O92.13
    - retracted nipple O92.03
  - defective O92.4
  - disorder NEC O92.79
  - excessive O92.6
  - failed (complete) O92.3
    - partial O92.4
  - mastitis NEC — *see* Mastitis, obstetric
  - mother (care and/or examination) Z39.1
  - nonpuerperal N64.3
- **Lacticemia,** excessive E87.2
- **Lacunar** skull Q75.8
- **Laennec's** cirrhosis K70.30
  - with ascites K70.31
  - nonalcoholic K74.69
- **Lafora's** disease — *see* Epilepsy, generalized, idiopathic
- **Lag,** lid (nervous) — *see* Retraction, lid
- **Lagophthalmos** (eyelid) (nervous) H02.209
  - cicatricial H02.219
    - left H02.216
      - lower H02.215
      - upper H02.214
    - right H02.213
      - lower H02.212
      - upper H02.211
  - keratoconjunctivitis — *see* Keratoconjunctivitis
  - left H02.206
    - lower H02.205
    - upper H02.204
  - mechanical H02.229
    - left H02.226
      - lower H02.225
      - upper H02.224
    - right H02.223
      - lower H02.222
      - upper H02.221
  - paralytic H02.239
    - left H02.236
      - lower H02.235
      - upper H02.234
    - right H02.233
      - lower H02.232
      - upper H02.231
  - right H02.203
    - lower H02.202
    - upper H02.201
- **Laki-Lorand** factor deficiency — *see* Defect, coagulation, specified type NEC
- **Lalling** F80.0
- **Lambert-Eaton** syndrome — *see* Syndrome, Lambert-Eaton
- **Lambliasis,** lambliosis A07.1
- **Landau-Kleffner** syndrome — *see* Epilepsy, specified NEC
- **Landouzy-Déjérine** dystrophy or facioscapulohumeral atrophy G71.0
- **Landouzy's** disease (icterohemorrhagic leptospirosis) A27.0
- **Landry-Guillain-Barré,** syndrome or paralysis G61.0
- **Landry's** disease or paralysis G61.0
- **Lane's**
  - band Q43.3
  - kink — *see* Obstruction, intestine
  - syndrome K90.2
- **Langdon** Down syndrome — *see* Trisomy, 21
- **Lapsed** immunization schedule status Z28.3
- **Large**
  - baby (regardless of gestational age) (4000g to 4499g) P08.1
- **Large** — *continued*
  - ear, congenital Q17.1
  - physiological cup Q14.2
  - stature R68.89
- **Large-for-dates** NEC (infant) (4000g to 4499g) P08.1
  - affecting management of pregnancy O36.6 ☑
  - exceptionally (4500g or more) P08.0
- **Larsen-Johansson** disease orosteochondrosis — *see* Osteochondrosis, juvenile, patella
- **Larsen's** syndrome (flattened facies and multiple congenital dislocations) Q74.8
- **Larva** migrans
  - cutaneous B76.9
    - Ancylostoma B76.0
  - visceral B83.0
- **Laryngeal** — *see* condition
- **Laryngismus** (stridulus) J38.5
  - congenital P28.89
  - diphtheritic A36.2
- **Laryngitis** (acute) (edematous) (fibrinous) (infective) (infiltrative) (malignant) (membranous) (phlegmonous) (pneumococcal) (pseudomembranous) (septic) (subglottic) (suppurative) (ulcerative) J04.0
  - with
    - influenza, flu, or grippe — *see* Influenza, with, laryngitis
    - tracheitis (acute) — *see* Laryngotracheitis
  - atrophic J37.0
  - catarrhal J37.0
  - chronic J37.0
    - with tracheitis (chronic) J37.1
  - diphtheritic A36.2
  - due to external agent — *see* Inflammation, respiratory, upper, due to
  - Hemophilus influenzae J04.0
  - H. influenzae J04.0
  - hypertrophic J37.0
  - influenzal — *see* Influenza, with, respiratory manifestations NEC
  - obstructive J05.0
  - sicca J37.0
  - spasmodic J05.0
    - acute J04.0
  - streptococcal J04.0
  - stridulous J05.0
  - syphilitic (late) A52.73
    - congenital A50.59 *[J99]*
      - early A50.03 *[J99]*
  - tuberculous A15.5
  - Vincent's A69.1
- **Laryngocele** (congenital) (ventricular) Q31.3
- **Laryngofissure** J38.7
  - congenital Q31.8
- **Laryngomalacia** (congenital) Q31.5
- **Laryngopharyngitis** (acute) J06.0
  - chronic J37.0
  - due to external agent — *see* Inflammation, respiratory, upper, due to
- **Laryngoplegia** J38.00
  - bilateral J38.02
  - unilateral J38.01
- **Laryngoptosis** J38.7
- **Laryngospasm** J38.5
- **Laryngostenosis** J38.6
- **Laryngotracheitis** (acute) (Infectional) (infective) (viral) J04.2
  - atrophic J37.1
  - catarrhal J37.1
  - chronic J37.1
  - diphtheritic A36.2
  - due to external agent — *see* Inflammation, respiratory, upper, due to
  - Hemophilus influenzae J04.2
  - hypertrophic J37.1
  - influenzal — *see* Influenza, with, respiratory manifestations NEC
  - pachydermic J38.7
  - sicca J37.1
  - spasmodic J38.5
    - acute J05.0
  - streptococcal J04.2
  - stridulous J38.5
  - syphilitic (late) A52.73
    - congenital A50.59 *[J99]*
      - early A50.03 *[J99]*
  - tuberculous A15.5
  - Vincent's A69.1
- **Laryngotracheobronchitis** — *see* Bronchitis
- **Larynx,** laryngeal — *see* condition
- **Lassa** fever A96.2
- **Lassitude** — *see* Weakness
- **Late**
  - talker R62.0
  - walker R62.0
- **Late** effect (s) — *see* Sequelae
- **Latent** — *see* condition
- **Laterocession** — *see* Lateroversion
- **Lateroflexion** — *see* Lateroversion
- **Lateroversion**
  - cervix — *see* Lateroversion, uterus
  - uterus, uterine (cervix) (postinfectional) (postpartal, old) N85.4
    - congenital Q51.818
    - in pregnancy or childbirth O34.59 ☑
- **Lathyrism** — *see* Poisoning, food, noxious, plant
- **Launois'** syndrome (pituitary gigantism) E22.0
- **Launois-Bensaude** adenolipomatosis E88.89
- **Laurence-Moon** (-Bardet)-Biedl syndrome Q87.89
- **Lax,** laxity (*see also* Relaxation)
  - ligament (ous) (*see also* Disorder, ligament)
    - familial M35.7
    - knee — *see* Derangement, knee
  - skin (acquired) L57.4
    - congenital Q82.8
- **Laxative** habit F55.2
- **Lazy** leukocyte syndrome D70.8
- **Lead** miner's lung J63.6
- **Leak,** leakage
  - air NEC J93.82
    - postprocedural J95.812
  - amniotic fluid — *see* Rupture, membranes, premature
  - blood (microscopic), fetal, into maternal circulation affecting management of pregnancy — *see* Pregnancy, complicated by
  - cerebrospinal fluid G96.0
    - from spinal (lumbar) puncture G97.0
  - device, implant or graft (*see also* Complications, by site and type, mechanical)
    - arterial graft NEC — *see* Complication, cardiovascular device, mechanical, vascular
    - breast (implant) T85.43 ☑
    - catheter NEC T85.638 ☑
      - urinary T83.038 ☑
        - cystostomy T83.030 ☑
        - Hopkins T83.038 ☑
        - ileostomy T83.038 ☑
        - indwelling T83.031 ☑
        - nephrostomy T83.032 ☑
        - specified NEC T83.038 ☑
        - urostomy T83.038 ☑
      - dialysis (renal) T82.43 ☑
        - intraperitoneal T85.631 ☑
      - infusion NEC T82.534 ☑
        - spinal (epidural) (subdural) T85.630 ☑
    - gastrointestinal — *see* Complications, prosthetic device, mechanical, gastrointestinal device
    - genital NEC T83.498 ☑
      - penile prosthesis (cylinder) (implanted) (pump) (reservoir) T83.490 ☑
      - testicular prosthesis T83.491 ☑
    - heart NEC — *see* Complication, cardiovascular device, mechanical
    - joint prosthesis — *see* Complications, joint prosthesis, mechanical, specified NEC, by site
    - ocular NEC — *see* Complications, prosthetic device, mechanical, ocular device
    - orthopedic NEC — *see* Complication, orthopedic, device, mechanical
    - persistent air J93.82
    - specified NEC T85.638 ☑
    - urinary NEC (*see also* Complication, genitourinary, device, urinary, mechanical)
      - graft T83.23 ☑
    - vascular NEC — *see* Complication, cardiovascular device, mechanical
    - ventricular intracranial shunt T85.03 ☑
  - urine — *see* Incontinence
- **Leaky** heart — *see* Endocarditis
- **Learning** defect (specific) F81.9
- **Leather** bottle stomach C16.9
- **Leber's**
  - congenital amaurosis H35.50
  - optic atrophy (hereditary) H47.22
- **Lederer's** anemia D59.1
- **Leeches** (external) — *see* Hirudiniasis
- **Leg** — *see* condition
- **Legg** (-Calvé)-Perthes disease, syndrome or osteochondrosis M91.1 ☑
- **Legionellosis** A48.1
  - nonpneumonic A48.2

Legionnaires - Lesion

- **Legionnaires'**
  - disease A48.1
    - nonpneumonic A48.2
  - pneumonia A48.1
- **Leigh's** disease G31.82
- **Leiner's** disease L21.1
- **Leiofibromyoma** — *see* Leiomyoma
- **Leiomyoblastoma** — *see* Neoplasm, connective tissue, benign
- **Leiomyofibroma** (*see also* Neoplasm, connective tissue, benign)
  - uterus (cervix) (corpus) D25.9
- **Leiomyoma** (*see also* Neoplasm, connective tissue, benign)
  - bizarre — *see* Neoplasm, connective tissue, benign
  - cellular — *see* Neoplasm, connective tissue, benign
  - epithelioid — *see* Neoplasm, connective tissue, benign
  - uterus (cervix) (corpus) D25.9
    - intramural D25.1
    - submucous D25.0
    - subserosal D25.2
  - vascular — *see* Neoplasm, connective tissue, benign
- **Leiomyoma,** leiomyomatosis (intravascular) — *see* Neoplasm, connective tissue, uncertain behavior
- **Leiomyosarcoma** (*see also* Neoplasm, connective tissue, malignant)
  - epithelioid — *see* Neoplasm, connective tissue, malignant
  - myxoid — *see* Neoplasm, connective tissue, malignant
- **Leishmaniasis** B55.9
  - American (mucocutaneous) B55.2
    - cutaneous B55.1
  - Asian Desert B55.1
  - Brazilian B55.2
  - cutaneous (any type) B55.1
  - dermal (*see also* Leishmaniasis, cutaneous)
    - post-kala-azar B55.0
  - eyelid B55.1
  - infantile B55.0
  - Mediterranean B55.0
  - mucocutaneous (American) (New World) B55.2
  - naso-oral B55.2
  - nasopharyngeal B55.2
  - old world B55.1
  - tegumentaria diffusa B55.1
  - visceral B55.0
- **Leishmanoid,** dermal (*see also* Leishmaniasis, cutaneous)
  - post-kala-azar B55.0
- **Lenegre's** disease I44.2
- **Lengthening,** leg — *see* Deformity, limb, unequal length
- **Lennert's** lymphoma — *see* Lymphoma, Lennert's
- **Lennox-Gastaut** syndrome G40.812
  - intractable G40.814
    - with status epilepticus G40.813
    - without status epilepticus G40.814
  - not intractable G40.812
    - with status epilepticus G40.811
    - without status epilepticus G40.812
- **Lens** — *see* condition
- **Lenticonus** (anterior) (posterior) (congenital) Q12.8
- **Lenticular** degeneration, progressive E83.01
- **Lentiglobus** (posterior) (congenital) Q12.8
- **Lentigo** (congenital) L81.4
  - maligna (*see also* Melanoma, in situ)
    - melanoma — *see* Melanoma
- **Lentivirus,** as cause of disease classified elsewhere B97.31
- **Leontiasis**
  - ossium M85.2
  - syphilitic (late) A52.78
    - congenital A50.59
- **Lepothrix** A48.8
- **Lepra** — *see* Leprosy
- **Leprechaunism** E34.8
- **Leprosy** A30. ☑
  - with muscle disorder A30.9 *[M63.80]*
    - ankle A30.9 *[M63.87-]*
    - foot A30.9 *[M63.87-]*
    - forearm A30.9 *[M63.83-]*
    - hand A30.9 *[M63.84-]*
    - lower leg A30.9 *[M63.86-]*
    - multiple sites A30.9 *[M63.89]*
    - pelvic region A30.9 *[M63.85-]*
    - shoulder region A30.9 *[M63.81-]*
    - specified site NEC A30.9 *[M63.88]*

- **Leprosy** — *continued*
  - with muscle disorder — *continued*
    - thigh A30.9 *[M63.85-]*
    - upper arm A30.9 *[M63.82-]*
  - anesthetic A30.9
  - BB A30.3
  - BL A30.4
  - borderline (infiltrated) (neuritic) A30.3
    - lepromatous A30.4
    - tuberculoid A30.2
  - BT A30.2
  - dimorphous (infiltrated) (neuritic) A30.3
  - I A30.0
  - indeterminate (macular) (neuritic) A30.0
  - lepromatous (diffuse) (infiltrated) (macular) (neuritic) (nodular) A30.5
  - LL A30.5
  - macular (early) (neuritic) (simple) A30.9
  - maculoanesthetic A30.9
  - mixed A30.3
  - neural A30.9
  - nodular A30.5
  - primary neuritic A30.3
  - specified type NEC A30.8
  - TT A30.1
  - tuberculoid (major) (minor) A30.1
- **Leptocytosis,** hereditary D56.9
- **Leptomeningitis** (chronic) (circumscribed) (hemorrhagic) (nonsuppurative) — *see* Meningitis
- **Leptomeningopathy** G96.19
- **Leptospiral** — *see* condition
- **Leptospirochetal** — *see* condition
- **Leptospirosis** A27.9
  - canicola A27.89
  - due to Leptospira interrogans serovar icterohaemorrhagiae A27.0
  - icterohemorrhagica A27.0
  - pomona A27.89
  - Weil's disease A27.0
- **Leptus** dermatitis B88.0
- **Leriche's** syndrome (aortic bifurcation occlusion) I74.09
- **Leri's** pleonosteosis Q78.8
- **Leri-Weill** syndrome Q77.8
- **Lermoyez'** syndrome — *see* Vertigo, peripheral NEC
- **Lesch-Nyhan** syndrome E79.1
- **Leser-Trélat** disease L82.1
  - inflamed L82.0
- **Lesion** (s) (nontraumatic)
  - abducens nerve — *see* Strabismus, paralytic, sixth nerve
  - alveolar process K08.9
  - angiocentric immunoproliferative D47.Z9
  - anorectal K62.9
  - aortic (valve) I35.9
  - auditory nerve — *see* subcategory H93.3
  - basal ganglion G25.9
  - bile duct — *see* Disease, bile duct
  - biomechanical M99.9
    - specified type NEC M99.89
      - abdomen M99.89
      - acromioclavicular M99.87
      - cervical region M99.81
      - cervicothoracic M99.81
      - costochondral M99.88
      - costovertebral M99.88
      - head region M99.80
      - hip M99.85
      - lower extremity M99.86
      - lumbar region M99.83
      - lumbosacral M99.83
      - occipitocervical M99.80
      - pelvic region M99.85
      - pubic M99.85
      - rib cage M99.88
      - sacral region M99.84
      - sacrococcygeal M99.84
      - sacroiliac M99.84
      - specified NEC M99.89
      - sternochondral M99.88
      - sternoclavicular M99.87
      - thoracic region M99.82
      - thoracolumbar M99.82
      - upper extremity M99.87
  - bladder N32.9
  - bone — *see* Disorder, bone
  - brachial plexus G54.0
  - brain G93.9
    - congenital Q04.9
    - vascular I67.9
      - degenerative I67.9
      - hypertensive I67.4

- **Lesion** (s) — *continued*
  - buccal cavity K13.79
  - calcified — *see* Calcification
  - canthus — *see* Disorder, eyelid
  - carate — *see* Pinta, lesions
  - cardia K31.9
  - cardiac (*see also* Disease, heart)I51.9
    - congenital Q24.9
    - valvular — *see* Endocarditis
  - cauda equina G83.4
  - cecum K63.9
  - cerebral — *see* Lesion, brain
  - cerebrovascular I67.9
    - degenerative I67.9
    - hypertensive I67.4
  - cervical (nerve) root NEC G54.2
  - chiasmal — *see* Disorder, optic, chiasm
  - chorda tympani G51.8
  - coin, lung R91.1
  - colon K63.9
  - combined periodontic - endodontic K05.5
  - congenital — *see* Anomaly, by site
  - conjunctiva H11.9
  - conus medullaris — *see* Injury, conus medullaris
  - coronary artery — *see* Ischemia, heart
  - cranial nerve G52.9
    - eighth — *see* Disorder, ear
    - eleventh G52.9
    - fifth G50.9
    - first G52.0
    - fourth — *see* Strabismus, paralytic, fourth nerve
    - seventh G51.9
    - sixth — *see* Strabismus, paralytic, sixth nerve
    - tenth G52.2
    - twelfth G52.3
  - cystic — *see* Cyst
  - degenerative — *see* Degeneration
  - duodenum K31.9
  - edentulous (alveolar) ridge, associated with trauma, due to traumatic occlusion K06.2
  - en coup de sabre L94.1
  - eyelid — *see* Disorder, eyelid
  - gasserian ganglion G50.8
  - gastric K31.9
  - gastroduodenal K31.9
  - gastrointestinal K63.9
  - gingiva, associated with trauma K06.2
  - glomerular
    - focal and segmental (*see also* N00-N07 with fourth character .1)N05.1
    - minimal change (*see also* N00-N07 with fourth character .0)N05.0
  - heart (organic) — *see* Disease, heart
  - hyperchromic, due to pinta (carate) A67.1
  - hyperkeratotic — *see* Hyperkeratosis
  - hypothalamic E23.7
  - ileocecal K63.9
  - ileum K63.9
  - iliohypogastric nerve G57.8 ☑
  - inflammatory — *see* Inflammation
  - intestine K63.9
  - intracerebral — *see* Lesion, brain
  - intrachiasmal (optic) — *see* Disorder, optic, chiasm
  - intracranial, space-occupying R90.0
  - joint — *see* Disorder, joint
    - sacroiliac (old) M53.3
  - keratotic — *see* Keratosis
  - kidney — *see* Disease, renal
  - laryngeal nerve (recurrent) G52.2
  - lip K13.0
  - liver K76.9
  - lumbosacral
    - plexus G54.1
    - root (nerve) NEC G54.4
  - lung (coin) R91.1
  - maxillary sinus J32.0
  - mitral I05.9
  - Morel-Lavallée — *see* Hematoma, by site
  - motor cortex NEC G93.89
  - mouth K13.79
  - nerve G58.9
    - femoral G57.2 ☑
    - median G56.1 ☑
      - carpal tunnel syndrome — *see* Syndrome, carpal tunnel
    - plantar G57.6 ☑
    - popliteal (lateral) G57.3 ☑
      - medial G57.4 ☑
    - radial G56.3 ☑
    - sciatic G57.0 ☑
    - spinal — *see* Injury, nerve, spinal
    - ulnar G56.2 ☑

- **Lesion** (s) — *continued*
  - nervous system, congenital Q07.9
  - nonallopathic — *see* Lesion, biomechanical
  - nose (internal) J34.89
  - obstructive — *see* Obstruction
  - obturator nerve G57.8 ☑
  - oral mucosa K13.70
  - organ or site NEC — *see* Disease, by site
  - osteolytic — *see* Osteolysis
  - peptic K27.9
  - periodontal, due to traumatic occlusion K05.5
  - pharynx J39.2
  - pigment, pigmented (skin) L81.9
  - pinta — *see* Pinta, lesions
  - polypoid — *see* Polyp
  - prechiasmal (optic) — *see* Disorder, optic, chiasm
  - primary (*see also* Syphilis, primary)A51.0
    - carate A67.0
    - pinta A67.0
    - yaws A66.0
  - pulmonary J98.4
    - valve I37.9
  - pylorus K31.9
  - rectosigmoid K63.9
  - retina, retinal H35.9
  - sacroiliac (joint) (old) M53.3
  - salivary gland K11.9
    - benign lymphoepithelial K11.8
  - saphenous nerve G57.8 ☑
  - sciatic nerve G57.0 ☑
  - secondary — *see* Syphilis, secondary
  - shoulder (region) M75.9 ☑
    - specified NEC M75.8 ☑
  - sigmoid K63.9
  - sinus (accessory) (nasal) J34.89
  - skin L98.9
    - suppurative L08.0
  - SLAP S43.43 ☑
  - spinal cord G95.9
    - congenital Q06.9
  - spleen D73.89
  - stomach K31.9
  - superior glenoid labrum S43.43 ☑
  - syphilitic — *see* Syphilis
  - tertiary — *see* Syphilis, tertiary
  - thoracic root (nerve) NEC G54.3
  - tonsillar fossa J35.9
  - tooth, teeth K08.9
    - white spot
      - chewing surface K02.51
      - pit and fissure surface K02.51
      - smooth surface K02.61
  - traumatic — *see* specific type of injury by site
  - tricuspid (valve) I07.9
    - nonrheumatic I36.9
  - trigeminal nerve G50.9
  - ulcerated or ulcerative — *see* Ulcer, skin
  - uterus N85.9
  - vagus nerve G52.2
  - valvular — *see* Endocarditis
  - vascular I99.9
    - affecting central nervous system I67.9
    - following trauma NEC T14.8
    - umbilical cord, complicating delivery O69.5 ☑
  - warty — *see* Verruca
  - white spot (tooth)
    - chewing surface K02.51
    - pit and fissure surface K02.51
    - smooth surface K02.61
- **Lethargic** — *see* condition
- **Lethargy** R53.83
- **Letterer-Siwe's** disease C96.0
- **Leukemia,** leukemic C95.9 ☑
  - acute basophilic C94.8 ☑
  - acute bilineal C95.0 ☑
  - acute erythroid C94.0 ☑
  - acute lymphoblastic C91.0 ☑
  - acute megakaryoblastic C94.2 ☑
  - acute megakaryocytic C94.2 ☑
  - acute mixed lineage C95.0 ☑
  - acute monoblastic (monoblastic/monocytic) C93.0 ☑
  - acute monocytic (monoblastic/monocytic) C93.0 ☑
  - acute myeloblastic (minimal differentiation) (with maturation) C92.0 ☑
  - acute myeloid
    - with
      - 11q23-abnormality C92.6 ☑
      - dysplasia of remaining hematopoiesis and/ or myelodysplastic disease in its history C92.A ☑
- **Leukemia** — *continued*
  - acute myeloid — *continued*
      - multilineage dysplasia C92.A ☑
      - variation of MLL-gene C92.6 ☑
    - M6 (a) (b) C94.0 ☑
    - M7 C94.2 ☑
  - acute myelomonocytic C92.5 ☑
  - acute promyelocytic C92.4 ☑
  - adult T-cell (HTLV-1-associated) (acute variant) (chronic variant) (lymphomatoid variant) (smouldering variant) C91.5 ☑
  - aggressive NK-cell C94.8 ☑
  - AML (1/ETO) (M0) (M1) (M2) (without a FAB classification) C92.0 ☑
  - AML M3 C92.4 ☑
  - AML M4 (Eo with inv (16) or t (16;16)) C92.5 ☑
  - AML M5 C93.0 ☑
  - AML M5a C93.0 ☑
  - AML M5b C93.0 ☑
  - AML Me with t (15;17) and variants C92.4 ☑
  - atypical chronic myeloid, BCR/ABL-negative C92.2 ☑
  - biphenotypic acute C95.0 ☑
  - blast cell C95.0 ☑
  - Burkitt-type, mature B-cell C91.A ☑
  - chronic lymphocytic, of B-cell type C91.1 ☑
  - chronic monocytic C93.1 ☑
  - chronic myelogenous (Philadelphia chromosome (Ph1) positive) (t (9;22)) (q34;q11) (with crisis of blast cells) C92.1 ☑
  - chronic myeloid, BCR/ABL-positive C92.1 ☑
    - atypical, BCR/ABL-negative C92.2 ☑
  - chronic myelomonocytic C93.1 ☑
  - chronic neutrophilic D47.1
  - CMML (-1) (-2) (with eosinophilia) C93.1 ☑
  - granulocytic (*see also* Category C92)C92.9 ☑
  - hairy cell C91.4 ☑
  - juvenile myelomonocytic C93.3 ☑
  - lymphoid C91.9 ☑
    - specified NEC C91.Z ☑
  - mast cell C94.3 ☑
  - mature B-cell, Burkitt-type C91.A ☑
  - monocytic (subacute) C93.9 ☑
    - specified NEC C93.Z ☑
  - myelogenous (*see also* Category C92)C92.9 ☑
  - myeloid C92.9 ☑
    - specified NEC C92.Z ☑
  - plasma cell C90.1 ☑
  - plasmacytic C90.1 ☑
  - prolymphocytic
    - of B-cell type C91.3 ☑
    - of T-cell type C91.6 ☑
  - specified NEC C94.8 ☑
  - stem cell, of unclear lineage C95.0 ☑
  - subacute lymphocytic C91.9 ☑
  - T-cell large granular lymphocytic C91.Z ☑
  - unspecified cell type C95.9 ☑
    - acute C95.0 ☑
    - chronic C95.1 ☑
- **Leukemoid** reaction (*see also* Reaction, leukemoid)D72.823
- **Leukoaraiosis** (hypertensive) I67.81
- **Leukoariosis** — *see* Leukoaraiosis
- **Leukocoria** — *see* Disorder, globe, degenerated condition, leucocoria
- **Leukocytopenia** D72.819
- **Leukocytosis** D72.829
  - eosinophilic D72.1
- **Leukoderma,** leukodermia NEC L81.5
  - syphilitic A51.39
    - late A52.79
- **Leukodystrophy** E75.29
- **Leukoedema,** oral epithelium K13.29
- **Leukoencephalitis** G04.81
  - acute (subacute) hemorrhagic G36.1
    - postimmunization or postvaccinal G04.02
  - postinfectious G04.01
  - subacute sclerosing A81.1
  - van Bogaert's (sclerosing) A81.1
- **Leukoencephalopathy** (*see also* Encephalopathy)G93.49
  - Binswanger's I67.3
  - heroin vapor G92
  - metachromatic E75.25
  - multifocal (progressive) A81.2
  - postimmunization and postvaccinal G04.02
  - progressive multifocal A81.2
  - reversible, posterior G93.6
  - van Bogaert's (sclerosing) A81.1
  - vascular, progressive I67.3
- **Leukoerythroblastosis** D75.9
- **Leukokeratosis** (*see also* Leukoplakia)
  - mouth K13.21
  - nicotina palati K13.24
  - oral mucosa K13.21
  - tongue K13.21
  - vocal cord J38.3
- **Leukokraurosis** vulva (e) N90.4
- **Leukoma** (cornea) (*see also* Opacity, cornea)
  - adherent H17.0 ☑
  - interfering with central vision — *see* Opacity, cornea, central
- **Leukomalacia,** cerebral, newborn P91.2
  - periventricular P91.2
- **Leukomelanopathy,** hereditary D72.0
- **Leukonychia** (punctata) (striata) L60.8
  - congenital Q84.4
- **Leukopathia** unguium L60.8
  - congenital Q84.4
- **Leukopenia** D72.819
  - basophilic D72.818
  - chemotherapy (cancer) induced D70.1
  - congenital D70.0
  - cyclic D70.0
  - drug induced NEC D70.2
    - due to cytoreductive cancer chemotherapy D70.1
  - eosinophilic D72.818
  - familial D70.0
  - infantile genetic D70.0
  - malignant D70.9
  - periodic D70.0
  - transitory neonatal P61.5
- **Leukopenic** — *see* condition
- **Leukoplakia**
  - anus K62.89
  - bladder (postinfectional) N32.89
  - buccal K13.21
  - cervix (uteri) N88.0
  - esophagus K22.8
  - gingiva K13.21
  - hairy (oral mucosa) (tongue) K13.3
  - kidney (pelvis) N28.89
  - larynx J38.7
  - lip K13.21
  - mouth K13.21
  - oral epithelium, including tongue (mucosa) K13.21
  - palate K13.21
  - pelvis (kidney) N28.89
  - penis (infectional) N48.0
  - rectum K62.89
  - syphilitic (late) A52.79
  - tongue K13.21
  - ureter (postinfectional) N28.89
  - urethra (postinfectional) N36.8
  - uterus N85.8
  - vagina N89.4
  - vocal cord J38.3
  - vulva N90.4
- **Leukorrhea** N89.8
  - due to Trichomonas (vaginalis) A59.00
  - trichomonal A59.00
- **Leukosarcoma** C85.9 ☑
- **Levocardia** (isolated) Q24.1
  - with situs inversus Q89.3
- **Levotransposition** Q20.5
- **Lev's** disease or syndrome (acquired complete heart block) I44.2
- **Levulosuria** — *see* Fructosuria
- **Levurid** L30.2
- **Lewy** body (ies) (dementia) (disease) G31.83
- **Leyden-Moebius** dystrophy G71.0
- **Leydig** cell
  - carcinoma
    - specified site — *see* Neoplasm, malignant, by site
    - unspecified site
      - female C56.9
      - male C62.9 ☑
  - tumor
    - benign
      - specified site — *see* Neoplasm, benign, by site
      - unspecified site
        - female D27. ☑
        - male D29.2 ☑
    - malignant
      - specified site — *see* Neoplasm, malignant, by site
      - unspecified site
        - female C56. ☑
        - male C62.9 ☑

- **Leydig** cell — *continued*
  - tumor — *continued*
    - specified site — *see* Neoplasm, uncertain behavior, by site
    - unspecified site
      - female D39.1 ☑
      - male D40.1 ☑
- **Leydig-Sertoli** cell tumor
  - specified site — *see* Neoplasm, benign, by site
  - unspecified site
    - female D27. ☑
    - male D29.2 ☑
- **LGSIL** (Low grade squamous intraepithelial lesion on cytologic smear of)
  - anus R85.612
  - cervix R87.612
  - vagina R87.622
- **Liar**, pathologic F60.2
- **Libido**
  - decreased R68.82
- **Libman-Sacks** disease M32.11
- **Lice** (infestation) B85.2
  - body (Pediculus corporis) B85.1
  - crab B85.3
  - head (Pediculus capitis) B85.0
  - mixed (classifiable to more than one of the titles B85.0-B85.3) B85.4
  - pubic (Phthirus pubis) B85.3
- **Lichen** L28.0
  - albus L90.0
    - penis N48.0
    - vulva N90.4
  - amyloidosis E85.4 *[L99]*
  - atrophicus L90.0
    - penis N48.0
    - vulva N90.4
  - congenital Q82.8
  - myxedematosus L98.5
  - nitidus L44.1
  - pilaris Q82.8
    - acquired L85.8
  - planopilaris L66.1
  - planus (chronicus) L43.9
    - annularis L43.8
    - bullous L43.1
    - follicular L66.1
    - hypertrophic L43.0
    - moniliformis L44.3
    - of Wilson L43.9
    - specified NEC L43.8
    - subacute (active) L43.3
    - tropicus L43.3
  - ruber
    - acuminatus L44.0
    - moniliformis L44.3
    - planus L43.9
  - sclerosus (et atrophicus) L90.0
    - penis N48.0
    - vulva N90.4
  - scrofulosus (primary) (tuberculous) A18.4
  - simplex (chronicus) (circumscriptus) L28.0
  - striatus L44.2
  - urticatus L28.2
- **Lichenification** L28.0
- **Lichenoides** tuberculosis (primary) A18.4
- **Lichtheim's** disease or syndrome — *see* Degeneration, combined
- **Lien** migrans D73.89
- **Ligament** — *see* condition
- **Light**
  - for gestational age — *see* Light for dates
  - headedness R42
- **Light-for-dates** (infant) P05.00
  - with weight of
    - 499 grams or less P05.01
    - 500-749 grams P05.02
    - 750-999 grams P05.03
    - 1000-1249 grams P05.04
    - 1250-1499 grams P05.05
    - 1500-1749 grams P05.06
    - 1750-1999 grams P05.07
    - 2000-2499 grams P05.08
    - 2500 grams and over P05.09
  - specified NEC P05.09
  - and small-for-dates — *see* Small for dates
  - affecting management of pregnancy O36.59 ☑
- **Lightning** (effects) (stroke) (struck by) T75.00 ☑
  - burn — *see* Burn
  - foot E53.8
  - shock T75.01 ☑
  - specified effect NEC T75.09 ☑
- **Lightwood-Albright** syndrome N25.89
- **Lightwood's** disease or syndrome (renal tubular acidosis) N25.89
- **Lignac** (-de Toni) (-Fanconi) (-Debré) disease or syndrome E72.09
  - with cystinosis E72.04
- **Ligneous** thyroiditis E06.5
- **Likoff's** syndrome I20.8
- **Limb** — *see* condition
- **Limbic** epilepsy personality syndrome F07.0
- **Limitation,** limited
  - activities due to disability Z73.6
  - cardiac reserve — *see* Disease, heart
  - eye muscle duction, traumatic — *see* Strabismus, mechanical
  - mandibular range of motion M26.52
- **Lindau** (-von Hippel) disease Q85.8
- **Line** (s)
  - Beau's L60.4
  - Harris' — *see* Arrest, epiphyseal
  - Hudson's (cornea) — *see* Pigmentation, cornea, anterior
  - Stähli's (cornea) — *see* Pigmentation, cornea, anterior
- **Linea** corneae senilis — *see* Change, cornea, senile
- **Lingua**
  - geographica K14.1
  - nigra (villosa) K14.3
  - plicata K14.5
  - tylosis K13.29
- **Lingual** — *see* condition
- **Linguatulosis** B88.8
- **Linitis** (gastric) plasticaC16.9
- **Lip** — *see* condition
- **Lipedema** — *see* Edema
- **Lipemia** (*see also* Hyperlipidemia)
  - retina, retinalis E78.3
- **Lipidosis** E75.6
  - cerebral (infantile) (juvenile) (late) E75.4
  - cerebroretinal E75.4
  - cerebroside E75.22
  - cholesterol (cerebral) E75.5
  - glycolipid E75.21
  - hepatosplenomegalic E78.3
  - sphingomyelin — *see* Niemann-Pick disease or syndrome
  - sulfatide E75.29
- **Lipoadenoma** — *see* Neoplasm, benign, by site
- **Lipoblastoma** — *see* Lipoma
- **Lipoblastomatosis** — *see* Lipoma
- **Lipochondrodystrophy** E76.01
- **Lipodermatosclerosis** — *see* Varix, leg, with, inflammation
  - ulcerated — *see* Varix, leg, with, ulcer, with inflammation by site
- **Lipochrome** histiocytosis (familial) D71
- **Lipodystrophia** progressiva E88.1
- **Lipodystrophy** (progressive) E88.1
  - insulin E88.1
  - intestinal K90.81
  - mesenteric K65.4
- **Lipofibroma** — *see* Lipoma
- **Lipofuscinosis,** neuronal (with ceroidosis) E75.4
- **Lipogranuloma,** sclerosing L92.8
- **Lipogranulomatosis** E78.89
- **Lipoid** (*see also* condition)
  - histiocytosis D76.3
    - essential E75.29
  - nephrosis N04.9
  - proteinosis of Urbach E78.89
- **Lipoidemia** — *see* Hyperlipidemia
- **Lipoidosis** — *see* Lipidosis
- **Lipoma** D17.9
  - fetal D17.9
    - fat cell D17.9
  - infiltrating D17.9
  - intramuscular D17.9
  - pleomorphic D17.9
  - site classification
    - arms (skin) (subcutaneous) D17.2 ☑
    - connective tissue D17.30
      - intra-abdominal D17.5
      - intrathoracic D17.4
      - peritoneum D17.79
      - retroperitoneum D17.79
      - specified site NEC D17.39
      - spermatic cord D17.6
    - face (skin) (subcutaneous) D17.0
    - genitourinary organ NEC D17.72
    - head (skin) (subcutaneous) D17.0
    - intra-abdominal D17.5
    - intrathoracic D17.4
    - kidney D17.71
- **Lipoma** — *continued*
  - site classification — *continued*
    - legs (skin) (subcutaneous) D17.2 ☑
    - neck (skin) (subcutaneous) D17.0
    - peritoneum D17.79
    - retroperitoneum D17.79
    - skin D17.30
      - specified site NEC D17.39
    - specified site NEC D17.79
    - spermatic cord D17.6
    - subcutaneous D17.30
      - specified site NEC D17.39
    - trunk (skin) (subcutaneous) D17.1
    - unspecified D17.9
  - spindle cell D17.9
- **Lipomatosis** E88.2
  - dolorosa (Dercum) E88.2
  - fetal — *see* Lipoma
  - Launois-Bensaude E88.89
- **Lipomyoma** — *see* Lipoma
- **Lipomyxoma** — *see* Lipoma
- **Lipomyxosarcoma** — *see* Neoplasm, connective tissue, malignant
- **Lipoprotein** metabolism disorder E78.9
- **Lipoproteinemia** E78.5
  - broad-beta E78.2
  - floating-beta E78.2
  - hyper-pre-beta E78.1
- **Liposarcoma** (*see also* Neoplasm, connective tissue, malignant)
  - dedifferentiated — *see* Neoplasm, connective tissue, malignant
  - differentiated type — *see* Neoplasm, connective tissue, malignant
  - embryonal — *see* Neoplasm, connective tissue, malignant
  - mixed type — *see* Neoplasm, connective tissue, malignant
  - myxoid — *see* Neoplasm, connective tissue, malignant
  - pleomorphic — *see* Neoplasm, connective tissue, malignant
  - round cell — *see* Neoplasm, connective tissue, malignant
  - well differentiated type — *see* Neoplasm, connective tissue, malignant
- **Liposynovitis** prepatellaris E88.89
- **Lipping,** cervix N86
- **Lipschütz** disease or ulcer N76.6
- **Lipuria** R82.0
  - schistosomiasis (bilharziasis) B65.0
- **Lisping** F80.0
- **Lissauer's** paralysis A52.17
- **Lissencephalia,** lissencephaly Q04.3
- **Listeriosis,** listerellosis A32.9
  - congenital (disseminated) P37.2
  - cutaneous A32.0
  - neonatal, newborn (disseminated) P37.2
  - oculoglandular A32.81
  - specified NEC A32.89
- **Lithemia** E79.0
- **Lithiasis** — *see* Calculus
- **Lithosis** J62.8
- **Lithuria** R82.99
- **Litigation,** anxiety concerning Z65.3
- **Little** leaguer's elbow — *see* Epicondylitis, medial
- **Little's** disease G80.9
- **Littre's**
  - gland — *see* condition
  - hernia — *see* Hernia, abdomen
- **Littritis** — *see* Urethritis
- **Livedo** (annularis) (racemosa) (reticularis) R23.1
- **Liver** — *see* condition
- **Living** alone (problems with) Z60.2
  - with handicapped person Z74.2
- **Lloyd's** syndrome — *see* Adenomatosis, endocrine
- **Loa** loa, loaiasis, loasis B74.3
- **Lobar** — *see* condition
- **Lobomycosis** B48.0
- **Lobo's** disease B48.0
- **Lobotomy** syndrome F07.0
- **Lobstein** (-Ekman) disease or syndrome Q78.0
- **Lobster-claw** hand Q71.6 ☑
- **Lobulation** (congenital) (*see also* Anomaly, by site)
  - kidney, Q63.1
  - liver, abnormal Q44.7
  - spleen Q89.09
- **Lobule,** lobular — *see* condition
- **Local,** localized — *see* condition
- **Locked-in** state G83.5
- **Locked** twins causing obstructed labor O66.1

Lumbago - Lymphocytic

- **Lumbago** — *continued*
  - due to displacement, intervertebral disc M51.27
    - with sciatica M51.17
- **Lumbar** — *see* condition
- **Lumbarization,** vertebra, congenital Q76.49
- **Lumbermen's** itch B88.0
- **Lump** — *see* Mass
- **Lunacy** — *see* Psychosis
- **Lung** — *see* condition
- **Lupoid** (miliary) of Boeck D86.3
- **Lupus**
  - anticoagulant D68.62
    - with
      - hemorrhagic disorder D68.312
      - hypercoagulable state D68.62
    - finding without diagnosis R76.0
  - discoid (local) L93.0
  - erythematosus (discoid) (local) L93.0
    - disseminated — *see* Lupus, erythematosus, systemic
    - eyelid H01.129
      - left H01.126
        - lower H01.125
        - upper H01.124
      - right H01.123
        - lower H01.122
        - upper H01.121
    - profundus L93.2
    - specified NEC L93.2
    - subacute cutaneous L93.1
    - systemic M32.9
      - with organ or system involvement M32.10
        - endocarditis M32.11
        - lung M32.13
        - pericarditis M32.12
        - renal (glomerular) M32.14
          - tubulo-interstitial M32.15
        - specified organ or system NEC M32.19
      - drug-induced M32.0
      - inhibitor (presence of) D68.62
        - with
          - hemorrhagic disorder D68.312
          - hypercoagulable state D68.62
        - finding without diagnosis R76.0
      - specified NEC M32.8
  - exedens A18.4
  - hydralazine M32.0
    - correct substance properly administered — *see* Table of Drugs and Chemicals, by drug, adverse effect
    - overdose or wrong substance given or taken — *see* Table of Drugs and Chemicals, by drug, poisoning
  - nephritis (chronic) M32.14
  - nontuberculous, not disseminated L93.0
  - panniculitis L93.2
  - pernio (Besnier) D86.3
  - systemic — *see* Lupus, erythematosus, systemic
  - tuberculous A18.4
    - eyelid A18.4
  - vulgaris A18.4
    - eyelid A18.4
- **Luteinoma** D27.☑
- **Lutembacher's** disease or syndrome (atrial septal defect with mitral stenosis) Q21.1
- **Luteoma** D27.☑
- **Lutz** (-Splendore-de Almeida) disease — *see* Paracoccidioidomycosis
- **Luxation** (*see also* Dislocation)
  - eyeball (nontraumatic) — *see* Luxation, globe
    - birth injury P15.3
  - globe, nontraumatic H44.82☑
  - lacrimal gland — *see* Dislocation, lacrimal gland
  - lens (old) (partial) (spontaneous)
    - congenital Q12.1
      - syphilitic A50.39
- **Lycanthropy** F22
- **Lyell's** syndrome L51.2
  - due to drug L51.2
    - correct substance properly administered — *see* Table of Drugs and Chemicals, by drug, adverse effect
    - overdose or wrong substance given or taken — *see* Table of Drugs and Chemicals, by drug, poisoning
- **Lyme** disease A69.20
- **Lymph**
  - gland or node — *see* condition
  - scrotum — *see* Infestation, filarial
- **Lymphadenitis** I88.9
  - with ectopic or molar pregnancy O08.0
  - acute L04.9
- **Lymphadenitis** — *continued*
  - acute — *continued*
    - axilla L04.2
    - face L04.0
    - head L04.0
    - hip L04.3
    - limb
      - lower L04.3
      - upper L04.2
    - neck L04.0
    - shoulder L04.2
    - specified site NEC L04.8
    - trunk L04.1
  - anthracosis (occupational) J60
  - any site, except mesenteric I88.9
    - chronic I88.1
    - subacute I88.1
  - breast
    - gestational — *see* Mastitis, obstetric
    - puerperal, postpartum (nonpurulent) O91.22
  - chancroidal (congenital) A57
  - chronic I88.1
    - mesenteric I88.0
  - due to
    - Brugia (malayi) B74.1
      - timori B74.2
    - chlamydial lymphogranuloma A55
    - diphtheria (toxin) A36.89
    - lymphogranuloma venereum A55
    - Wuchereria bancrofti B74.0
  - following ectopic or molar pregnancy O08.0
  - gonorrheal A54.89
  - infective — *see* Lymphadenitis, acute
  - mesenteric (acute) (chronic) (nonspecific) (subacute) I88.0
    - due to Salmonella typhi A01.09
    - tuberculous A18.39
  - mycobacterial A31.8
  - purulent — *see* Lymphadenitis, acute
  - pyogenic — *see* Lymphadenitis, acute
  - regional, nonbacterial I88.8
  - septic — *see* Lymphadenitis, acute
  - subacute, unspecified site I88.1
  - suppurative — *see* Lymphadenitis, acute
  - syphilitic (early) (secondary) A51.49
    - late A52.79
  - tuberculous — *see* Tuberculosis, lymph gland
  - venereal (chlamydial) A55
- **Lymphadenoid** goiter E06.3
- **Lymphadenopathy** (generalized) R59.1
  - angioimmunoblastic, with dysproteinemia (AILD) C86.5
  - due to toxoplasmosis (acquired) B58.89
    - congenital (acute) (subacute) (chronic) P37.1
  - localized R59.0
  - syphilitic (early) (secondary) A51.49
- **Lymphadenosis** R59.1
- **Lymphangiectasis** I89.0
  - conjunctiva H11.89
  - postinfectional I89.0
  - scrotum I89.0
- **Lymphangiectatic** elephantiasis, nonfilarial I89.0
- **Lymphangioendothelioma** D18.1
  - malignant — *see* Neoplasm, connective tissue, malignant
- **Lymphangioleiomyomatosis** J84.81
- **Lymphangioma** D18.1
  - capillary D18.1
  - cavernous D18.1
  - cystic D18.1
  - malignant — *see* Neoplasm, connective tissue, malignant
- **Lymphangiomyoma** D18.1
- **Lymphangiomyomatosis** J84.81
- **Lymphangiosarcoma** — *see* Neoplasm, connective tissue, malignant
- **Lymphangitis** I89.1
  - with
    - abscess - code by site under Abscess
    - cellulitis - code by site under Cellulitis
    - ectopic or molar pregnancy O08.0
  - acute L03.91
    - abdominal wall L03.321
    - ankle — *see* Lymphangitis, acute, lower limb
    - arm — *see* Lymphangitis, acute, upper limb
    - auricle (ear) — *see* Lymphangitis, acute, ear
    - axilla L03.12☑
    - back (any part) L03.322
    - buttock L03.327
    - cervical (meaning neck) L03.222
    - cheek (external) L03.212
    - chest wall L03.323
- **Lymphangitis** — *continued*
  - acute — *continued*
    - digit
      - finger — *see* Lymphangitis, acute, finger
      - toe — *see* Lymphangitis, acute, toe
    - ear (external) H60.1☑
    - external auditory canal — *see* Lymphangitis, acute, ear
    - eyelid — *see* Abscess, eyelid
    - face NEC L03.212
    - finger (intrathecal) (periosteal) (subcutaneous) (subcuticular) L03.02☑
    - foot — *see* Lymphangitis, acute, lower limb
    - gluteal (region) L03.327
    - groin L03.324
    - hand — *see* Lymphangitis, acute, upper limb
    - head NEC L03.891
      - face (any part, except ear, eye and nose) L03.212
    - heel — *see* Lymphangitis, acute, lower limb
    - hip — *see* Lymphangitis, acute, lower limb
    - jaw (region) L03.212
    - knee — *see* Lymphangitis, acute, lower limb
    - leg — *see* Lymphangitis, acute, lower limb
    - lower limb L03.12☑
      - toe — *see* Lymphangitis, acute, toe
    - navel L03.326
    - neck (region) L03.222
    - orbit, orbital — *see* Cellulitis, orbit
    - pectoral (region) L03.323
    - perineal, perineum L03.325
    - scalp (any part) L03.891
    - shoulder — *see* Lymphangitis, acute, upper limb
    - specified site NEC L03.898
    - thigh — *see* Lymphangitis, acute, lower limb
    - thumb (intrathecal) (periosteal) (subcutaneous) (subcuticular) — *see* Lymphangitis, acute, finger
    - toe (intrathecal) (periosteal) (subcutaneous) (subcuticular) L03.04☑
    - trunk L03.329
      - abdominal wall L03.321
      - back (any part) L03.322
      - buttock L03.327
      - chest wall L03.323
      - groin L03.324
      - perineal, perineum L03.325
      - umbilicus L03.326
    - umbilicus L03.326
    - upper limb L03.12☑
      - axilla — *see* Lymphangitis, acute, axilla
      - finger — *see* Lymphangitis, acute, finger
      - thumb — *see* Lymphangitis, acute, finger
    - wrist — *see* Lymphangitis, acute, upper limb
  - breast
    - gestational — *see* Mastitis, obstetric
  - chancroidal A57
  - chronic (any site) I89.1
  - due to
    - Brugia (malayi) B74.1
      - timori B74.2
    - Wuchereria bancrofti B74.0
  - following ectopic or molar pregnancy O08.89
  - penis
    - acute N48.29
    - gonococcal (acute) (chronic) A54.09
  - puerperal, postpartum, childbirth O86.89
  - strumous, tuberculous A18.2
  - subacute (any site) I89.1
  - tuberculous — *see* Tuberculosis, lymph gland
- **Lymphatic** (vessel) — *see* condition
- **Lymphatism** E32.8
- **Lymphectasia** I89.0
- **Lymphedema** (acquired) (*see also* Elephantiasis)
  - congenital Q82.0
  - hereditary (chronic) (idiopathic) Q82.0
  - postmastectomy I97.2
  - praecox I89.0
  - secondary I89.0
  - surgical NEC I97.89
    - postmastectomy (syndrome) I97.2
- **Lymphoblastic** — *see* condition
- **Lymphoblastoma** (diffuse) — *see* Lymphoma, lymphoblastic (diffuse)
  - giant follicular — *see* Lymphoma, lymphoblastic (diffuse)
  - macrofollicular — *see* Lymphoma, lymphoblastic (diffuse)
- **Lymphocele** I89.8
- **Lymphocytic**
  - chorioencephalitis (acute) (serous) A87.2

Lymphocytic — *continued*
- choriomeningitis (acute) (serous) A87.2
- meningoencephalitis A87.2

Lymphocytoma, benign cutis L98.8
Lymphocytopenia D72.810
Lymphocytosis (symptomatic) D72.820
- infectious (acute) B33.8

Lymphoepithelioma — *see* Neoplasm, malignant, by site
Lymphogranuloma (malignant) (*see also* Lymphoma, Hodgkin)
- chlamydial A55
- inguinale A55
- venereum (any site) (chlamydial) (with stricture of rectum) A55

Lymphogranulomatosis (malignant) (*see also* Lymphoma, Hodgkin)
- benign (Boeck's sarcoid) (Schaumann's) D86.1

Lymphohistiocytosis, hemophagocytic (familial) D76.1
Lymphoid — *see* condition
Lymphoma (of) (malignant) C85.90
- adult T-cell (HTLV-1-associated) (acute variant) (chronic variant) (lymphomatoid variant) (smouldering variant) C91.5 ☑
- anaplastic large cell
  - ALK-negative C84.7 ☑
  - ALK-positive C84.6 ☑
  - CD30-positive C84.6 ☑
  - primary cutaneous C86.6
- angioimmunoblastic T-cell C86.5
- BALT C88.4
- B-cell C85.1 ☑
- B-precursor C83.5 ☑
- blastic NK-cell C86.4
- bronchial-associated lymphoid tissue [BALT-lymphoma] C88.4
- Burkitt (atypical) C83.7 ☑
- Burkitt-like C83.7 ☑
- centrocytic C83.1 ☑
- cutaneous follicle center C82.6 ☑
- cutaneous T-cell C84.A ☑
- diffuse follicle center C82.5 ☑
- diffuse large cell C83.3 ☑
  - anaplastic C83.3 ☑
  - B-cell C83.3 ☑
  - CD30-positive C83.3 ☑
  - centroblastic C83.3 ☑
  - immunoblastic C83.3 ☑
  - plasmablastic C83.3 ☑
  - subtype not specified C83.3 ☑
  - T-cell rich C83.3 ☑
- enteropathy-type (associated) (intestinal) T-cell C86.2
- extranodal NK/T-cell, nasal type C86.0
- extranodal marginal zone B-cell lymphoma of mucosa-associated lymphoid tissue [MALT-lymphoma] C88.4
- follicular C82.9 ☑
  - grade
    - I C82.0 ☑
    - II C82.1 ☑
    - III C82.2 ☑
    - IIIa C82.3 ☑
    - IIIb C82.4 ☑
  - specified NEC C82.8 ☑
- hepatosplenic T-cell (alpha-beta) (gamma-delta) C86.1
- histiocytic C85.9 ☑
  - true C96.A
- Hodgkin C81.9 ☑
  - lymphocyte-rich (classical) C81.4 ☑
  - lymphocyte depleted (classical) C81.3 ☑
  - mixed cellularity (classical) C81.2 ☑
  - nodular sclerosis (classical) C81.1 ☑
  - specified NEC (classical) C81.7 ☑
  - lymphocyte-rich classical C81.4 ☑
  - lymphocyte depleted classical C81.3 ☑
  - mixed cellularity classical C81.2 ☑
  - nodular
    - lymphocyte predominant C81.0 ☑
    - sclerosis (classical) C81.1 ☑
- intravascular large B-cell C83.8 ☑
- Lennert's C84.4 ☑
- lymphoblastic B-cell C83.5 ☑
- lymphoblastic (diffuse) C83.5 ☑
- lymphoblastic T-cell C83.5 ☑
- lymphoepithelioid C84.4 ☑
- lymphoplasmacytic C83.0 ☑
  - with IgM-production C88.0
- MALT C88.4
- mantle cell C83.1 ☑
- mature T-cell NEC C84.4 ☑
- mature T/NK-cell C84.9 ☑
  - specified NEC C84.Z ☑
- mediastinal (thymic) large B-cell C85.2 ☑
- Mediterranean C88.3
- mucosa-associated lymphoid tissue [MALT-lymphoma] C88.4
- NK/T cell C84.9 ☑
- nodal marginal zone C83.0 ☑
- non-follicular (diffuse) C83.9 ☑
  - specified NEC C83.8 ☑
- non-Hodgkin (*see also* Lymphoma, by type)C85.9 ☑
  - specified NEC C85.8 ☑
- non-leukemic variant of B-CLL C83.0 ☑
- peripheral T-cell, not classified C84.4 ☑
- primary cutaneous
  - anaplastic large cell C86.6
  - CD30-positive large T-cell C86.6
- primary effusion B-cell C83.8 ☑
- SALT C88.4
- skin-associated lymphoid tissue [SALT-lymphoma] C88.4
- small cell B-cell C83.0 ☑
- splenic marginal zone C83.0 ☑
- subcutaneous panniculitis-like T-cell C86.3
- T-precursor C83.5 ☑
- true histiocytic C96.A

Lymphomatosis — *see* Lymphoma
Lymphopathia venereum, veneris A55
Lymphopenia D72.810
Lymphoplasmacytic leukemia — *see* Leukemia, chronic lymphocytic, B-cell type
Lymphoproliferation, X-linked disease D82.3
Lymphoreticulosis, benign (of inoculation) A28.1
Lymphorrhea I89.8
Lymphosarcoma (diffuse) (*see also* Lymphoma)C85.9 ☑
Lymphostasis I89.8
Lypemania — *see* Melancholia
Lysine and hydroxylysine metabolism disorder E72.3
Lyssa — *see* Rabies

M

Macacus ear Q17.3
Maceration, wet feet, tropical (syndrome) T69.02 ☑
MacLeod's syndrome J43.0
Macrocephalia, macrocephaly Q75.3
Macrocheilia, macrochilia (congenital) Q18.6
Macrocolon (*see also* Megacolon)Q43.1
Macrocornea Q15.8
- with glaucoma Q15.0

Macrocytic — *see* condition
Macrocytosis D75.89
Macrodactylia, macrodactylism (fingers) (thumbs) Q74.0
- toes Q74.2

Macrodontia K00.2
Macrogenia M26.05
Macrogenitosomia (adrenal) (male) (praecox) E25.9
- congenital E25.0

Macroglobulinemia (idiopathic) (primary) C88.0
- monoclonal (essential) D47.2
- Waldenström C88.0

Macroglossia (congenital) Q38.2
- acquired K14.8

Macrognathia, macrognathism (congenital) (mandibular) (maxillary) M26.09
Macrogyria (congenital) Q04.8
Macrohydrocephalus — *see* Hydrocephalus
Macromastia — *see* Hypertrophy, breast
Macrophthalmos Q11.3
- in congenital glaucoma Q15.0

Macropsia H53.15
Macrosigmoid K59.39
- congenital Q43.2

Macrospondylitis , acromegalic E22.0
Macrostomia (congenital) Q18.4
Macrotia (external ear) (congenital) Q17.1
Macula
- cornea, corneal — *see* Opacity, cornea
- degeneration (atrophic) (exudative) (senile) (*see also* Degeneration, macula)
  - hereditary — *see* Dystrophy, retina

Maculae ceruleae -- B85.1
Maculopathy, toxic — *see* Degeneration, macula, toxic
Madarosis (eyelid) H02.729
- left H02.726
  - lower H02.725
  - upper H02.724
- right H02.723
  - lower H02.722
  - upper H02.721

Madelung's
- deformity (radius) Q74.0
- disease
  - radial deformity Q74.0
  - symmetrical lipomas, neck E88.89

Madness — *see* Psychosis
Madura
- foot B47.9
  - actinomycotic B47.1
  - mycotic B47.0

Maduromycosis B47.0
Maffucci's syndrome Q78.4
Magnesium metabolism disorder — *see* Disorder, metabolism, magnesium
Main en griffe (acquired) (*see also* Deformity, limb, clawhand)
- congenital Q74.0

Maintenance (encounter for)
- antineoplastic chemotherapy Z51.11
- antineoplastic radiation therapy Z51.0
- methadone F11.20

Majocchi's
- disease L81.7
- granuloma B35.8

Major — *see* condition
Malabar itch (any site) B35.5
Malabsorption K90.9
- calcium K90.89
- carbohydrate K90.49
- disaccharide E73.9
- fat K90.49
- galactose E74.20
- glucose (-galactose) E74.39
- intestinal K90.9
  - specified NEC K90.89
- isomaltose E74.31
- lactose E73.9
- methionine E72.19
- monosaccharide E74.39
- postgastrectomy K91.2
- postsurgical K91.2
- protein K90.49
- starch K90.49
- sucrose E74.39
- syndrome K90.9
  - postsurgical K91.2

Malacia, bone (adult) M83.9
- juvenile — *see* Rickets

Malacoplakia
- bladder N32.89
- pelvis (kidney) N28.89
- ureter N28.89
- urethra N36.8

Malacosteon, juvenile — *see* Rickets
Maladaptation — *see* Maladjustment
Maladie de Roger Q21.0
Maladjustment
- conjugal Z63.0
  - involving divorce or estrangement Z63.5
- educational Z55.4
- family Z63.9
- marital Z63.0
  - involving divorce or estrangement Z63.5
- occupational NEC Z56.89
- simple, adult — *see* Disorder, adjustment
- situational — *see* Disorder, adjustment
- social Z60.9
  - due to
    - acculturation difficulty Z60.3
    - discrimination and persecution (perceived) Z60.5
    - exclusion and isolation Z60.4
    - life-cycle (phase of life) transition Z60.0
    - rejection Z60.4
    - specified reason NEC Z60.8

Malaise R53.81
Malakoplakia — *see* Malacoplakia
Malaria, malarial (fever) B54
- with
  - blackwater fever B50.8
    - hemoglobinuric (bilious) B50.8
  - hemoglobinuria B50.8
- accidentally induced (therapeutically) - code by type under Malaria
- algid B50.9

- **Malaria** — *continued*
  - cerebral B50.0 *[G94]*
  - clinically diagnosed (without parasitological confirmation) B54
  - congenital NEC P37.4
    - falciparum P37.3
  - congestion, congestive B54
  - continued (fever) B50.9
  - estivo-autumnal B50.9
  - falciparum B50.9
    - with complications NEC B50.8
      - cerebral B50.0 *[G94]*
    - severe B50.8
  - hemorrhagic B54
  - malariae B52.9
    - with
      - complications NEC B52.8
      - glomerular disorder B52.0
  - malignant (tertian) — *see* Malaria, falciparum
  - mixed infections - code to first listed type in B50-B53
  - ovale B53.0
  - parasitologically confirmed NEC B53.8
  - pernicious, acute — *see* Malaria, falciparum
  - Plasmodium (P.)
    - falciparum NEC — *see* Malaria, falciparum
    - malariae NEC B52.9
      - with Plasmodium
        - falciparum (and or vivax) — *see* Malaria, falciparum
        - vivax (*see also* Malaria, vivax)
          - and falciparum — *see* Malaria, falciparum
    - ovale B53.0
      - with Plasmodium malariae (*see also* Malaria, malariae)
        - and vivax (*see also* Malaria, vivax)
          - and falciparum — *see* Malaria, falciparum
    - simian B53.1
      - with Plasmodium malariae (*see also* Malaria, malariae)
        - and vivax (*see also* Malaria, vivax)
          - and falciparum — *see* Malaria, falciparum
    - vivax NEC B51.9
      - with Plasmodium falciparum — *see* Malaria, falciparum
  - quartan — *see* Malaria, malariae
  - quotidian — *see* Malaria, falciparum
  - recurrent B54
  - remittent B54
  - specified type NEC (parasitologically confirmed) B53.8
  - spleen B54
  - subtertian (fever) — *see* Malaria, falciparum
  - tertian (benign) (*see also* Malaria, vivax)
    - malignant B50.9
  - tropical B50.9
  - typhoid B54
  - vivax B51.9
    - with
      - complications NEC B51.8
      - ruptured spleen B51.0
- **Malassimilation** K90.9
- **Malassez's** disease (cystic) N50.89
- **Mal** de los pintos — *see* Pinta
- **Mal** de mer T75.3 ☑
- **Maldescent,** testis Q53.9
  - bilateral Q53.20
    - abdominal Q53.21
    - perineal Q53.22
  - unilateral Q53.10
    - abdominal Q53.11
    - perineal Q53.12
- **Maldevelopment** (*see also* Anomaly)
  - brain Q07.9
  - colon Q43.9
  - hip Q74.2
    - congenital dislocation Q65.2
      - bilateral Q65.1
      - unilateral Q65.0 ☑
  - mastoid process Q75.8
  - middle ear Q16.4
    - except ossicles Q16.4
    - ossicles Q16.3
  - ossicles Q16.3
  - spine Q76.49
  - toe Q74.2
- **Male** type pelvis Q74.2
  - with disproportion (fetopelvic) O33.3 ☑
    - causing obstructed labor O65.3
- **Malformation** (congenital) (*see also* Anomaly)
  - adrenal gland Q89.1

- **Malformation** — *continued*
  - affecting multiple systems with skeletal changes NEC Q87.5
  - alimentary tract Q45.9
    - specified type NEC Q45.8
    - upper Q40.9
      - specified type NEC Q40.8
  - aorta Q25.40
    - absence Q25.41
    - aneurysm, congenital Q25.43
    - aplasia Q25.41
    - atresia Q25.29
      - aortic arch Q25.21
    - coarctation (preductal) (postductal) Q25.1
    - dilatation, congenital Q25.44
    - hypoplasia Q25.42
    - patent ductus arteriosus Q25.0
    - specified type NEC Q25.49
    - stenosis Q25.1
      - supravalvular Q25.3
  - aortic valve Q23.9
    - specified NEC Q23.8
  - arteriovenous, aneurysmatic (congenital) Q27.30
    - brain Q28.2
    - cerebral Q28.2
    - peripheral Q27.30
      - digestive system Q27.33
      - lower limb Q27.32
      - other specified site Q27.39
      - renal vessel Q27.34
      - upper limb Q27.31
    - precerebral vessels (nonruptured) Q28.0
  - auricle
    - ear (congenital) Q17.3
      - acquired H61.119
        - left H61.112
          - with right H61.113
        - right H61.111
          - with left H61.113
  - bile duct Q44.5
  - bladder Q64.79
    - aplasia Q64.5
    - diverticulum Q64.6
    - exstrophy — *see* Exstrophy, bladder
    - neck obstruction Q64.31
  - bone Q79.9
    - face Q75.9
      - specified type NEC Q75.8
    - skull Q75.9
      - specified type NEC Q75.8
  - brain (multiple) Q04.9
    - arteriovenous Q28.2
    - specified type NEC Q04.8
  - branchial cleft Q18.2
  - breast Q83.9
    - specified type NEC Q83.8
  - broad ligament Q50.6
  - bronchus Q32.4
  - bursa Q79.9
  - cardiac
    - chambers Q20.9
      - specified type NEC Q20.8
    - septum Q21.9
      - specified type NEC Q21.8
  - cerebral Q04.9
    - vessels Q28.3
  - cervix uteri Q51.9
    - specified type NEC Q51.828
  - Chiari
    - Type I G93.5
    - Type II Q07.01
  - choroid (congenital) Q14.3
    - plexus Q07.8
  - circulatory system Q28.9
  - cochlea Q16.5
  - cornea Q13.4
  - coronary vessels Q24.5
  - corpus callosum (congenital) Q04.0
  - diaphragm Q79.1
  - digestive system NEC, specified type NEC Q45.8
  - dura Q07.9
    - brain Q04.9
    - spinal Q06.9
  - ear Q17.9
    - causing impairment of hearing Q16.9
    - external Q17.9
      - accessory auricle Q17.0
      - causing impairment of hearing Q16.9
      - absence of
        - auditory canal Q16.1
        - auricle Q16.0
      - macrotia Q17.1

- **Malformation** — *continued*
  - ear — *continued*
      - microtia Q17.2
      - misplacement Q17.4
      - misshapen NEC Q17.3
      - prominence Q17.5
      - specified type NEC Q17.8
    - inner Q16.5
    - middle Q16.4
      - absence of eustachian tube Q16.2
      - ossicles (fusion) Q16.3
    - ossicles Q16.3
    - specified type NEC Q17.8
  - epididymis Q55.4
  - esophagus Q39.9
    - specified type NEC Q39.8
  - eye Q15.9
    - lid Q10.3
    - specified NEC Q15.8
  - fallopian tube Q50.6
  - genital organ — *see* Anomaly, genitalia
  - great
    - artery Q25.9
      - aorta — *see* Malformation, aorta
      - pulmonary artery — *see* Malformation, pulmonary, artery
      - specified type NEC Q25.8
    - vein Q26.9
      - anomalous
        - portal venous connection Q26.5
        - pulmonary venous connection Q26.4
          - partial Q26.3
          - total Q26.2
      - persistent left superior vena cava Q26.1
      - portal vein-hepatic artery fistula Q26.6
      - specified type NEC Q26.8
      - vena cava stenosis, congenital Q26.0
  - gum Q38.6
  - hair Q84.2
  - heart Q24.9
    - specified type NEC Q24.8
  - integument Q84.9
    - specified type NEC Q84.8
  - internal ear Q16.5
  - intestine Q43.9
    - specified type NEC Q43.8
  - iris Q13.2
  - joint Q74.9
    - ankle Q74.2
    - lumbosacral Q76.49
    - sacroiliac Q74.2
    - specified type NEC Q74.8
  - kidney Q63.9
    - accessory Q63.0
    - giant Q63.3
    - horseshoe Q63.1
    - hydronephrosis Q62.0
    - malposition Q63.2
    - specified type NEC Q63.8
  - lacrimal apparatus Q10.6
  - lip Q38.0
  - lingual Q38.3
  - liver Q44.7
  - lung Q33.9
  - meninges or membrane (congenital) Q07.9
    - cerebral Q04.8
    - spinal (cord) Q06.9
  - middle ear Q16.4
    - ossicles Q16.3
  - mitral valve Q23.9
    - specified NEC Q23.8
  - Mondini's (congenital) (malformation, cochlea) Q16.5
  - mouth (congenital) Q38.6
  - multiple types NEC Q89.7
  - musculoskeletal system Q79.9
  - myocardium Q24.8
  - nail Q84.6
  - nervous system (central) Q07.9
  - nose Q30.9
    - specified type NEC Q30.8
  - optic disc Q14.2
  - orbit Q10.7
  - ovary Q50.39
  - palate Q38.5
  - parathyroid gland Q89.2
  - pelvic organs or tissues NEC
    - in pregnancy or childbirth O34.8 ☑
      - causing obstructed labor O65.5
  - penis Q55.69
    - aplasia Q55.5
    - curvature (lateral) Q55.61
    - hypoplasia Q55.62

Malformation — *continued*
- pericardium Q24.8
- peripheral vascular system Q27.9
  - specified type NEC Q27.8
- pharynx Q38.8
- precerebral vessels Q28.1
- prostate Q55.4
- pulmonary
  - arteriovenous Q25.72
  - artery Q25.9
    - atresia Q25.5
    - specified type NEC Q25.79
    - stenosis Q25.6
  - valve Q22.3
- renal artery Q27.2
- respiratory system Q34.9
- retina Q14.1
- scrotum — *see* Malformation, testis and scrotum
- seminal vesicles Q55.4
- sense organs NEC Q07.9
- skin Q82.9
- specified NEC Q89.8
- spinal
  - cord Q06.9
  - nerve root Q07.8
- spine Q76.49
  - kyphosis — *see* Kyphosis, congenital
  - lordosis — *see* Lordosis, congenital
- spleen Q89.09
- stomach Q40.3
  - specified type NEC Q40.2
- teeth, tooth K00.9
- tendon Q79.9
- testis and scrotum Q55.20
  - aplasia Q55.0
  - hypoplasia Q55.1
  - polyorchism Q55.21
  - retractile testis Q55.22
  - scrotal transposition Q55.23
  - specified NEC Q55.29
- throat Q38.8
- thorax, bony Q76.9
- thyroid gland Q89.2
- tongue (congenital) Q38.3
  - hypertrophy Q38.2
  - tie Q38.1
- trachea Q32.1
- tricuspid valve Q22.9
  - specified type NEC Q22.8
- umbilical cord NEC (complicating delivery) O69.89 ☑
- umbilicus Q89.9
- ureter Q62.8
  - agenesis Q62.4
  - duplication Q62.5
  - malposition — *see* Malposition, congenital, ureter
  - obstructive defect — *see* Defect, obstructive, ureter
  - vesico-uretero-renal reflux Q62.7
- urethra Q64.79
  - aplasia Q64.5
  - duplication Q64.74
  - posterior valves Q64.2
  - prolapse Q64.71
  - stricture Q64.32
- urinary system Q64.9
- uterus Q51.9
  - specified type NEC Q51.818
- vagina Q52.4
- vascular system, peripheral Q27.9
- vas deferens Q55.4
  - atresia Q55.3
- venous — *see* Anomaly, vein (s)
- vulva Q52.70

Malfunction (*see also* Dysfunction)
- cardiac electronic device T82.119 ☑
  - electrode T82.110 ☑
  - pulse generator T82.111 ☑
  - specified type NEC T82.118 ☑
- catheter device NEC T85.618 ☑
  - cystostomy T83.010 ☑
  - dialysis (renal) (vascular) T82.41 ☑
    - intraperitoneal T85.611 ☑
  - infusion NEC T82.514 ☑
    - cranial T85.610 ☑
    - epidural T85.610 ☑
    - intrathecal T85.610 ☑
    - spinal T85.610 ☑
    - subarachnoid T85.610 ☑
    - subdural T85.610 ☑

Malfunction — *continued*
- catheter device NEC — *continued*
  - urinary (*see also* Breakdown, device, catheter)T83.018 ☑
- colostomy K94.03
  - valve K94.03
- cystostomy (stoma) N99.512
  - catheter T83.010 ☑
- enteric stoma K94.13
- enterostomy K94.13
- esophagostomy K94.33
- gastroenteric K31.89
- gastrostomy K94.23
- ileostomy K94.13
  - valve K94.13
- intrathecal infusion pump T85.615 ☑
- jejunostomy K94.13
- nervous system device, implant or graft, specified NEC T85.615 ☑
- pacemaker — *see* Malfunction, cardiac electronic device
- prosthetic device, internal — *see* Complications, prosthetic device, by site, mechanical
- tracheostomy J95.03
- urinary device NEC — *see* Complication, genitourinary, device, urinary, mechanical
- valve
  - colostomy K94.03
  - heart T82.09 ☑
  - ileostomy K94.13
- vascular graft or shunt NEC — *see* Complication, cardiovascular device, mechanical, vascular
- ventricular (communicating shunt) T85.01 ☑

Malherbe's tumor — *see* Neoplasm, skin, benign

Malibu disease L98.8

Malignancy (*see also* Neoplasm, malignant, by site)
- unspecified site (primary) C80.1

Malignant — *see* condition

Malingerer, malingering Z76.5

Mallet finger (acquired) — *see* Deformity, finger, mallet finger
- congenital Q74.0
- sequelae of rickets E64.3

Malleus A24.0

Mallory's bodies R89.7

Mallory-Weiss syndrome K22.6

Malnutrition E46
- degree
  - first E44.1
  - mild (protein) E44.1
  - moderate (protein) E44.0
  - second E44.0
  - severe (protein-energy) E43
    - intermediate form E42
      - with
        - kwashiorkor (and marasmus) E42
        - marasmus E41
  - third E43
- following gastrointestinal surgery K91.2
- intrauterine
  - light-for-dates — *see* Light for dates
  - small-for-dates — *see* Small for dates
- lack of care, or neglect (child) (infant) T76.02 ☑
  - confirmed T74.02 ☑
- malignant E40
- protein E46
  - calorie E46
    - mild E44.1
    - moderate E44.0
    - severe E43
      - intermediate form E42
        - with
          - kwashiorkor (and marasmus) E42
          - marasmus E41
  - energy E46
    - mild E44.1
    - moderate E44.0
    - severe E43
      - intermediate form E42
        - with
          - kwashiorkor (and marasmus) E42
          - marasmus E41
- severe (protein-energy) E43
  - with
    - kwashiorkor (and marasmus) E42
    - marasmus E41

Malocclusion (teeth) M26.4
- Angle's M26.219
  - class I M26.211
  - class II M26.212
  - class III M26.213

Malocclusion — *continued*
- due to
  - abnormal swallowing M26.59
  - mouth breathing M26.59
  - tongue, lip or finger habits M26.59
- temporomandibular (joint) M26.69

Malposition
- cervix — *see* Malposition, uterus
- congenital
  - adrenal (gland) Q89.1
  - alimentary tract Q45.8
    - lower Q43.8
    - upper Q40.8
  - aorta Q25.49
  - appendix Q43.8
  - arterial trunk Q20.0
  - artery (peripheral) Q27.8
    - coronary Q24.5
    - digestive system Q27.8
    - lower limb Q27.8
    - pulmonary Q25.79
    - specified site NEC Q27.8
    - upper limb Q27.8
  - auditory canal Q17.8
    - causing impairment of hearing Q16.9
  - auricle (ear) Q17.4
    - causing impairment of hearing Q16.9
    - cervical Q18.2
  - biliary duct or passage Q44.5
  - bladder (mucosa) — *see* Exstrophy, bladder
  - brachial plexus Q07.8
  - brain tissue Q04.8
  - breast Q83.8
  - bronchus Q32.4
  - cecum Q43.8
  - clavicle Q74.0
  - colon Q43.8
  - digestive organ or tract NEC Q45.8
    - lower Q43.8
    - upper Q40.8
  - ear (auricle) (external) Q17.4
    - ossicles Q16.3
  - endocrine (gland) NEC Q89.2
  - epiglottis Q31.8
  - eustachian tube Q17.8
  - eye Q15.8
  - facial features Q18.8
  - fallopian tube Q50.6
  - finger (s) Q68.1
    - supernumerary Q69.0
  - foot Q66.9
  - gallbladder Q44.1
  - gastrointestinal tract Q45.8
  - genitalia, genital organ (s) or tract
    - female Q52.8
      - external Q52.79
      - internal NEC Q52.8
    - male Q55.8
  - glottis Q31.8
  - hand Q68.1
  - heart Q24.8
    - dextrocardia Q24.0
      - with complete transposition of viscera Q89.3
  - hepatic duct Q44.5
  - hip (joint) Q65.89
  - intestine (large) (small) Q43.8
    - with anomalous adhesions, fixation or malrotation Q43.3
  - joint NEC Q68.8
  - kidney Q63.2
  - larynx Q31.8
  - limb Q68.8
    - lower Q68.8
    - upper Q68.8
  - liver Q44.7
  - lung (lobe) Q33.8
  - nail (s) Q84.6
  - nerve Q07.8
  - nervous system NEC Q07.8
  - nose, nasal (septum) Q30.8
  - organ or site not listed — *see* Anomaly, by site
  - ovary Q50.39
  - pancreas Q45.3
  - parathyroid (gland) Q89.2
  - patella Q74.1
  - peripheral vascular system Q27.8
  - pituitary (gland) Q89.2
  - respiratory organ or system NEC Q34.8
  - rib (cage) Q76.6
    - supernumerary in cervical region Q76.5
  - scapula Q74.0

Malposition - Mass

Malposition — *continued*
- congenital — *continued*
  - shoulder Q74.0
  - spinal cord Q06.8
  - spleen Q89.09
  - sternum NEC Q76.7
  - stomach Q40.2
  - symphysis pubis Q74.2
  - thymus (gland) Q89.2
  - thyroid (gland) (tissue) Q89.2
    - cartilage Q31.8
  - toe (s) Q66.9
    - supernumerary Q69.2
  - tongue Q38.3
  - trachea Q32.1
  - ureter Q62.60
    - deviation Q62.61
    - displacement Q62.62
    - ectopia Q62.63
    - specified type NEC Q62.69
  - uterus Q51.818
  - vein (s) (peripheral) Q27.8
    - great Q26.8
  - vena cava (inferior) (superior) Q26.8
- device, implant or graft (*see also* Complications, by site and type, mechanical)T85.628 ☑
  - arterial graft NEC — *see* Complication, cardiovascular device, mechanical, vascular
  - breast (implant) T85.42 ☑
  - catheter NEC T85.628 ☑
    - cystostomy T83.020 ☑
    - dialysis (renal) T82.42 ☑
      - intraperitoneal T85.621 ☑
    - infusion NEC T82.524 ☑
      - spinal (epidural) (subdural) T85.620 ☑
    - urinary (*see also* Displacement, device, catheter, urinary)T83.028 ☑
  - electronic (electrode) (pulse generator) (stimulator)
    - bone T84.320 ☑
    - cardiac T82.129 ☑
      - electrode T82.120 ☑
      - pulse generator T82.121 ☑
      - specified type NEC T82.128 ☑
    - nervous system — *see* Complication, prosthetic device, mechanical, electronic nervous system stimulator
    - urinary — *see* Complication, genitourinary, device, urinary, mechanical
  - fixation, internal (orthopedic) NEC — *see* Complication, fixation device, mechanical
  - gastrointestinal — *see* Complications, prosthetic device, mechanical, gastrointestinal device
  - genital NEC T83.428 ☑
    - intrauterine contraceptive device (string) T83.32 ☑
    - penile prosthesis (cylinder) (implanted) (pump) (reservoir) T83.420 ☑
    - testicular prosthesis T83.421 ☑
  - heart NEC — *see* Complication, cardiovascular device, mechanical
  - joint prosthesis — *see* Complication, joint prosthesis, mechanical
  - ocular NEC — *see* Complications, prosthetic device, mechanical, ocular device
  - orthopedic NEC — *see* Complication, orthopedic, device, mechanical
  - specified NEC T85.628 ☑
  - urinary NEC (*see also* Complication, genitourinary, device, urinary, mechanical)
    - graft T83.22 ☑
  - vascular NEC — *see* Complication, cardiovascular device, mechanical
  - ventricular intracranial shunt T85.02 ☑
- fetus — *see* Pregnancy, complicated by (management affected by), presentation, fetal
- gallbladder K82.8
- gastrointestinal tract, congenital Q45.8
- heart, congenital NEC Q24.8
- joint prosthesis — *see* Complications, joint prosthesis, mechanical, displacement, by site
- stomach K31.89
  - congenital Q40.2
- tooth, teeth, fully erupted M26.30
- uterus (acute) (acquired) (adherent) (asymptomatic) (postinfectional) (postpartal, old) N85.4
  - anteflexion or anteversion N85.4
    - congenital Q51.818
  - flexion N85.4

Malposition — *continued*
- uterus — *continued*
  - flexion
    - lateral — *see* Lateroversion, uterus
  - inversion N85.5
  - lateral (flexion) (version) — *see* Lateroversion, uterus
    - in pregnancy or childbirth — *see* subcategory O34.5
  - retroflexion or retroversion — *see* Retroversion, uterus

Malposture R29.3

Malrotation
- cecum Q43.3
- colon Q43.3
- intestine Q43.3
- kidney Q63.2

Maltreatment
- adult
  - abandonment
    - confirmed T74.01 ☑
    - suspected T76.01 ☑
  - confirmed T74.91 ☑
  - history of Z91.419
  - neglect
    - confirmed T74.01 ☑
    - suspected T76.01 ☑
  - physical abuse
    - confirmed T74.11 ☑
    - suspected T76.11 ☑
  - psychological abuse
    - confirmed T74.31 ☑
    - suspected T76.31 ☑
    - history of Z91.411
  - sexual abuse
    - confirmed T74.21 ☑
    - suspected T76.21 ☑
  - suspected T76.91 ☑
- child
  - abandonment
    - confirmed T74.02 ☑
    - suspected T76.02 ☑
  - confirmed T74.92 ☑
  - history of — *see* History, personal (of), abuse
  - neglect
    - confirmed T74.02 ☑
    - history of — *see* History, personal (of), abuse
    - suspected T76.02 ☑
  - physical abuse
    - confirmed T74.12 ☑
    - history of — *see* History, personal (of), abuse
    - suspected T76.12 ☑
  - psychological abuse
    - confirmed T74.32 ☑
    - history of — *see* History, personal (of), abuse
    - suspected T76.32 ☑
  - sexual abuse
    - confirmed T74.22 ☑
    - history of — *see* History, personal (of), abuse
    - suspected T76.22 ☑
  - suspected T76.92 ☑
- personal history of Z91.89

Malta fever — *see* Brucellosis

Maltworker's lung J67.4

Malunion, fracture — *see* Fracture, by site

Mammillitis N61.0
- puerperal, postpartum O91.02

Mammitis — *see* Mastitis

Mammogram (examination) Z12.39
- routine Z12.31

Mammoplasia N62

Management (of)
- bone conduction hearing device (implanted) Z45.320
- cardiac pacemaker NEC Z45.018
- cerebrospinal fluid drainage device Z45.41
- cochlear device (implanted) Z45.321
- contraceptive Z30.9
  - specified NEC Z30.8
- implanted device Z45.9
  - specified NEC Z45.89
- infusion pump Z45.1
- procreative Z31.9
  - male factor infertility in female Z31.81
  - specified NEC Z31.89
- prosthesis (external) (*see also* Fitting)Z44.9
  - implanted Z45.9
    - specified NEC Z45.89
- renal dialysis catheter Z49.01
- vascular access device Z45.2

Mangled — *see* specified injury by site

Mania (monopolar) (*see also* Disorder, mood, manic episode)

Mania — *continued*
- with psychotic symptoms F30.2
- without psychotic symptoms F30.10
  - mild F30.11
  - moderate F30.12
  - severe F30.13
- Bell's F30.8
- chronic (recurrent) F31.89
- hysterical F44.89
- puerperal F30.8
- recurrent F31.89

Manic-depressive insanity, psychosis, or syndrome — *see* Disorder, bipolar

Mannosidosis E77.1

Mansonelliasis, mansonellosis B74.4

Manson's
- disease B65.1
- schistosomiasis B65.1

Manual — *see* condition

Maple-bark-stripper's lung (disease) J67.6

Maple-syrup-urine disease E71.0

Marable's syndrome (celiac artery compression) I77.4

Marasmus E41
- due to malnutrition E41
- intestinal E41
- nutritional E41
- senile R54
- tuberculous NEC — *see* Tuberculosis

Marble
- bones Q78.2
- skin R23.8

Marburg virus disease A98.3

March
- fracture — *see* Fracture, traumatic, stress, by site
- hemoglobinuria D59.6

Marchesani (-Weill) syndrome Q87.0

Marchiafava (-Bignami) syndrome or disease G37.1

Marchiafava-Micheli syndrome D59.5

Marcus Gunn's syndrome Q07.8

Marfan's syndrome — *see* Syndrome, Marfan's

Marie-Bamberger disease — *see* Osteoarthropathy, hypertrophic, specified NEC

Marie-Charcot-Tooth neuropathic muscular atrophy G60.0

Marie's
- cerebellar ataxia (late-onset) G11.2
- disease or syndrome (acromegaly) E22.0

Marie-Strümpell arthritis, disease or spondylitis — *see* Spondylitis, ankylosing

Marion's disease (bladder neck obstruction) N32.0

Marital conflict Z63.0

Mark
- port wine Q82.5
- raspberry Q82.5
- strawberry Q82.5
- stretch L90.6
- tattoo L81.8

Marker heterochromatin — *see* Extra, marker chromosomes

Maroteaux-Lamy syndrome (mild) (severe) E76.29

Marrow (bone)
- arrest D61.9
- poor function D75.89

Marseilles fever A77.1

Marsh fever — *see* Malaria

Marshall's (hidrotic) ectodermal dysplasia Q82.4

Marsh's disease (exophthalmic goiter) E05.00
- with storm E05.01

Masculinization (female) with adrenal hyperplasia E25.9
- congenital E25.0

Masculinovoblastoma D27. ☑

Masochism (sexual) F65.51

Mason's lung J62.8

Mass
- abdominal R19.00
  - epigastric R19.06
  - generalized R19.07
  - left lower quadrant R19.04
  - left upper quadrant R19.02
  - periumbilic R19.05
  - right lower quadrant R19.03
  - right upper quadrant R19.01
  - specified site NEC R19.09
- breast N63
- chest R22.2
- cystic — *see* Cyst
- ear H93.8 ☑
- head R22.0
- intra-abdominal (diffuse) (generalized) — *see* Mass, abdominal

- **Mass** — *continued*
  - kidney N28.89
  - liver R16.0
  - localized (skin) R22.9
    - chest R22.2
    - head R22.0
    - limb
      - lower R22.4 ☑
      - upper R22.3 ☑
    - neck R22.1
    - trunk R22.2
  - lung R91.8
  - malignant — *see* Neoplasm, malignant, by site
  - neck R22.1
  - pelvic (diffuse) (generalized) — *see* Mass, abdominal
  - specified organ NEC — *see* Disease, by site
  - splenic R16.1
  - substernal thyroid — *see* Goiter
  - superficial (localized) R22.9
  - umbilical (diffuse) (generalized) R19.09
- **Massive** — *see* condition
- **Mast cell**
  - disease, systemic tissue D47.0
  - leukemia C94.3 ☑
  - sarcoma C96.2
  - tumor D47.0
    - malignant C96.2
- **Mastalgia** N64.4
- **Masters-Allen** syndrome N83.8
- **Mastitis** (acute) (diffuse) (nonpuerperal) (subacute) N61.0
  - with abscess N61.1
  - chronic (cystic) — *see* Mastopathy, cystic
  - cystic (Schimmelbusch's type) — *see* Mastopathy, cystic
  - fibrocystic — *see* Mastopathy, cystic
  - infective N61.0
    - newborn P39.0
  - interstitial, gestational or puerperal — *see* Mastitis, obstetric
  - neonatal (noninfective) P83.4
    - infective P39.0
  - obstetric (interstitial) (nonpurulent)
    - associated with
      - lactation O91.23
      - pregnancy O91.21 ☑
      - puerperium O91.22
    - purulent
      - associated with
        - lactation O91.13
        - pregnancy O91.11 ☑
        - puerperium O91.12
  - periductal — *see* Ectasia, mammary duct
  - phlegmonous — *see* Mastopathy, cystic
  - plasma cell — *see* Ectasia, mammary duct
  - without abscess N61.0
- **Mastocytoma** D47.0
  - malignant C96.2
- **Mastocytosis** Q82.2
  - aggressive systemic C96.2
  - indolent systemic D47.0
  - malignant C96.2
  - systemic, associated with clonal hematopoietic non-mast-cell disease (SM-AHNMD) D47.0
- **Mastodynia** N64.4
- **Mastoid** — *see* condition
- **Mastoidalgia** — *see* subcategory H92.0
- **Mastoiditis** (coalescent) (hemorrhagic) (suppurative) H70.9 ☑
  - acute, subacute H70.00 ☑
    - complicated NEC H70.09 ☑
    - subperiosteal H70.01 ☑
  - chronic (necrotic) (recurrent) H70.1 ☑
  - in (due to)
    - infectious disease NEC B99 ☑ *[H75.0-]*
    - parasitic disease NEC B89 *[H75.0-]*
    - tuberculosis A18.03
  - petrositis — *see* Petrositis
  - postauricular fistula — *see* Fistula, postauricular
  - specified NEC H70.89 ☑
  - tuberculous A18.03
- **Mastopathy,** mastopathia N64.9
  - chronica cystica — *see* Mastopathy, cystic
  - cystic (chronic) (diffuse) N60.1 ☑
    - with epithelial proliferation N60.3 ☑
  - diffuse cystic — *see* Mastopathy, cystic
  - estrogenic, oestrogenica N64.89
  - ovarian origin N64.89
- **Mastoplasia,** mastoplastia N62
- **Masturbation** (excessive) F98.8
- **Maternal** care (for) — *see* Pregnancy (complicated by) (management affected by)
- **Matheiu's** disease (leptospiral jaundice) A27.0
- **Mauclaire's** disease or osteochondrosis — *see* Osteochondrosis, juvenile, hand, metacarpal
- **Maxcy's** disease A75.2
- **Maxilla,** maxillary — *see* condition
- **May** (-Hegglin) anomaly or syndrome D72.0
- **McArdle** (-Schmid) (-Pearson) disease (glycogen storage) E74.04
- **McCune-Albright** syndrome Q78.1
- **McQuarrie's** syndrome (idiopathic familial hypoglycemia) E16.2
- **Meadow's** syndrome Q86.1
- **Measles** (black) (hemorrhagic) (suppressed) B05.9
  - with
    - complications NEC B05.89
    - encephalitis B05.0
    - intestinal complications B05.4
    - keratitis (keratoconjunctivitis) B05.81
    - meningitis B05.1
    - otitis media B05.3
    - pneumonia B05.2
  - French — *see* Rubella
  - German — *see* Rubella
  - Liberty — *see* Rubella
- **Meatitis,** urethral — *see* Urethritis
- **Meatus,** meatal — *see* condition
- **Meat-wrappers'** asthma J68.9
- **Meckel-Gruber** syndrome Q61.9
- **Meckel's** diverticulitis, diverticulum (displaced) (hypertrophic) Q43.0
  - malignant — *see* Table of Neoplasms, small intestine, malignant
- **Meconium**
  - ileus, newborn P76.0
    - in cystic fibrosis E84.11
    - meaning meconium plug (without cystic fibrosis) P76.0
  - obstruction, newborn P76.0
    - due to fecaliths P76.0
    - in mucoviscidosis E84.11
  - peritonitis P78.0
  - plug syndrome (newborn) NEC P76.0
- **Median** (*see also* condition)
  - arcuate ligament syndrome I77.4
  - bar (prostate) (vesical orifice) — *see* Hyperplasia, prostate
  - rhomboid glossitis K14.2
- **Mediastinal** shift R93.8
- **Mediastinitis** (acute) (chronic) J98.51
  - syphilitic A52.73
  - tuberculous A15.8
- **Mediastinopericarditis** (*see also* Pericarditis)
  - acute I30.9
  - adhesive I31.0
  - chronic I31.8
    - rheumatic I09.2
- **Mediastinum,** mediastinal — *see* condition
- **Medicine** poisoning — *see* Table of Drugs and Chemicals, by drug, poisoning
- **Mediterranean**
  - fever — *see* Brucellosis
    - familial M04.1
    - tick A77.1
  - kala-azar B55.0
  - leishmaniasis B55.0
  - tick fever A77.1
- **Medulla** — *see* condition
- **Medullary** cystic kidney Q61.5
- **Medullated** fibers
  - optic (nerve) Q14.8
  - retina Q14.1
- **Medulloblastoma**
  - desmoplastic C71.6
  - specified site — *see* Neoplasm, malignant, by site
  - unspecified site C71.6
- **Medulloepithelioma** (*see also* Neoplasm, malignant, by site)
  - teratoid — *see* Neoplasm, malignant, by site
- **Medullomyoblastoma**
  - specified site — *see* Neoplasm, malignant, by site
  - unspecified site C71.6
- **Meekeren-Ehlers-Danlos** syndrome Q79.6
- **Megacolon** (acquired) (functional) (not Hirschsprung's disease) (in) K59.39
  - Chagas' disease B57.32
  - congenital, congenitum (aganglionic) Q43.1
  - Hirschsprung's (disease) Q43.1
  - toxic NEC K59.31
    - due to Clostridium difficile A04.7
- **Megaesophagus** (functional) K22.0
  - congenital Q39.5
  - in (due to) Chagas' disease B57.31
- **Megalencephaly** Q04.5
- **Megalerythema** (epidemic) B08.3
- **Megaloappendix** Q43.8
- **Megalocephalus,** megalocephaly NEC Q75.3
- **Megalocornea** Q15.8
  - with glaucoma Q15.0
- **Megalocytic** anemia D53.1
- **Megalodactylia** (fingers) (thumbs) (congenital) Q74.0
  - toes Q74.2
- **Megaloduodenum** Q43.8
- **Megaloesophagus** (functional) K22.0
  - congenital Q39.5
- **Megalogastria** (acquired) K31.89
  - congenital Q40.2
- **Megalophthalmos** Q11.3
- **Megalopsia** H53.15
- **Megalosplenia** — *see* Splenomegaly
- **Megaloureter** N28.82
  - congenital Q62.2
- **Megarectum** K62.89
- **Megasigmoid** K59.39
  - congenital Q43.2
- **Megaureter** N28.82
  - congenital Q62.2
- **Megavitamin-B6** syndrome E67.2
- **Megrim** — *see* Migraine
- **Meibomian**
  - cyst, infected — *see* Hordeolum
  - gland — *see* condition
  - sty, stye — *see* Hordeolum
- **Meibomitis** — *see* Hordeolum
- **Meige-Milroy** disease (chronic hereditary edema) Q82.0
- **Meige's** syndrome Q82.0
- **Melalgia,** nutritional E53.8
- **Melancholia** F32.9
  - climacteric (single episode) F32.89
    - recurrent episode F33.8
  - hypochondriac F45.29
  - intermittent (single episode) F32.89
    - recurrent episode F33.8
  - involutional (single episode) F32.89
    - recurrent episode F33.8
  - menopausal (single episode) F32.89
    - recurrent episode F33.8
  - puerperal F32.89
  - reactive (emotional stress or trauma) F32.3
  - recurrent F33.9
  - senile F03 ☑
  - stuporous (single episode) F32.89
    - recurrent episode F33.8
- **Melanemia** R79.89
- **Melanoameloblastoma** — *see* Neoplasm, bone, benign
- **Melanoblastoma** — *see* Melanoma
- **Melanocarcinoma** — *see* Melanoma
- **Melanocytoma,** eyeball D31.9 ☑
- **Melanocytosis,** neurocutaneous Q82.8
- **Melanoderma,** melanodermia L81.4
- **Melanodontia,** infantile K03.89
- **Melanodontoclasia** K03.89
- **Melanoepithelioma** — *see* Melanoma
- **Melanoma** (malignant) C43.9
  - acral lentiginous, malignant — *see* Melanoma, skin, by site
  - amelanotic — *see* Melanoma, skin, by site
  - balloon cell — *see* Melanoma, skin, by site
  - benign — *see* Nevus
  - desmoplastic, malignant — *see* Melanoma, skin, by site
  - epithelioid cell — *see* Melanoma, skin, by site
    - with spindle cell, mixed — *see* Melanoma, skin, by site
  - in
    - giant pigmented nevus — *see* Melanoma, skin, by site
    - Hutchinson's melanotic freckle — *see* Melanoma, skin, by site
    - junctional nevus — *see* Melanoma, skin, by site
    - precancerous melanosis — *see* Melanoma, skin, by site
  - in situ D03.9
    - abdominal wall D03.59
    - ala nasi D03.39
    - ankle D03.7 ☑
    - anus, anal (margin) (skin) D03.51
    - arm D03.6 ☑
    - auditory canal D03.2 ☑
    - auricle (ear) D03.2 ☑
    - auricular canal (external) D03.2 ☑
    - axilla, axillary fold D03.59

Melanoma - Meningioma

- **Melanoma** — *continued*
  - in situ — *continued*
    - back D03.59
    - breast D03.52
    - brow D03.39
    - buttock D03.59
    - canthus (eye) D03.1 ☑
    - cheek (external) D03.39
    - chest wall D03.59
    - chin D03.39
    - choroid D03.8
    - conjunctiva D03.8
    - ear (external) D03.2 ☑
    - external meatus (ear) D03.2 ☑
    - eye D03.8
    - eyebrow D03.39
    - eyelid (lower) (upper) D03.1 ☑
    - face D03.30
      - specified NEC D03.39
    - female genital organ (external) NEC D03.8
    - finger D03.6 ☑
    - flank D03.59
    - foot D03.7 ☑
    - forearm D03.6 ☑
    - forehead D03.39
    - foreskin D03.8
    - gluteal region D03.59
    - groin D03.59
    - hand D03.6 ☑
    - heel D03.7 ☑
    - helix D03.2 ☑
    - hip D03.7 ☑
    - interscapular region D03.59
    - iris D03.8
    - jaw D03.39
    - knee D03.7 ☑
    - labium (majus) (minus) D03.8
    - lacrimal gland D03.8
    - leg D03.7 ☑
    - lip (lower) (upper) D03.0
    - lower limb NEC D03.7 ☑
    - male genital organ (external) NEC D03.8
    - nail D03.9
      - finger D03.6 ☑
      - toe D03.7 ☑
    - neck D03.4
    - nose (external) D03.39
    - orbit D03.8
    - penis D03.8
    - perianal skin D03.51
    - perineum D03.51
    - pinna D03.2 ☑
    - popliteal fossa or space D03.7 ☑
    - prepuce D03.8
    - pudendum D03.8
    - retina D03.8
    - retrobulbar D03.8
    - scalp D03.4
    - scrotum D03.8
    - shoulder D03.6 ☑
    - specified site NEC D03.8
    - submammary fold D03.52
    - temple D03.39
    - thigh D03.7 ☑
    - toe D03.7 ☑
    - trunk NEC D03.59
    - umbilicus D03.59
    - upper limb NEC D03.6 ☑
    - vulva D03.8
  - juvenile — *see* Nevus
  - malignant, of soft parts except skin — *see* Neoplasm, connective tissue, malignant
  - metastatic
    - breast C79.81
    - genital organ C79.82
    - specified site NEC C79.89
  - neurotropic, malignant — *see* Melanoma, skin, by site
  - nodular — *see* Melanoma, skin, by site
  - regressing, malignant — *see* Melanoma, skin, by site
  - skin C43.9
    - abdominal wall C43.59
    - ala nasi C43.31
    - ankle C43.7 ☑
    - anus, anal (skin) C43.51
    - arm C43.6 ☑
    - auditory canal (external) C43.2 ☑
    - auricle (ear) C43.2 ☑
    - auricular canal (external) C43.2 ☑
    - axilla, axillary fold C43.59
    - back C43.59
- **Melanoma** — *continued*
  - skin — *continued*
    - breast (female) (male) C43.52
    - brow C43.39
    - buttock C43.59
    - canthus (eye) C43.1 ☑
    - cheek (external) C43.39
    - chest wall C43.59
    - chin C43.39
    - ear (external) C43.2 ☑
    - elbow C43.6 ☑
    - external meatus (ear) C43.2 ☑
    - eyebrow C43.39
    - eyelid (lower) (upper) C43.1 ☑
    - face C43.30
      - specified NEC C43.39
    - female genital organ (external) NEC C51.9
    - finger C43.6 ☑
    - flank C43.59
    - foot C43.7 ☑
    - forearm C43.6 ☑
    - forehead C43.39
    - foreskin C60.0
    - glabella C43.39
    - gluteal region C43.59
    - groin C43.59
    - hand C43.6 ☑
    - heel C43.7 ☑
    - helix C43.2 ☑
    - hip C43.7 ☑
    - interscapular region C43.59
    - jaw (external) C43.39
    - knee C43.7 ☑
    - labium C51.9
      - majus C51.0
      - minus C51.1
    - leg C43.7 ☑
    - lip (lower) (upper) C43.0
    - lower limb NEC C43.7 ☑
    - male genital organ (external) NEC C63.9
    - nail
      - finger C43.6 ☑
      - toe C43.7 ☑
    - nasolabial groove C43.39
    - nates C43.59
    - neck C43.4
    - nose (external) C43.31
    - overlapping site C43.8
    - palpbrae C43.1 ☑
    - penis C60.9
    - perianal skin C43.51
    - perineum C43.51
    - pinna C43.2 ☑
    - popliteal fossa or space C43.7 ☑
    - prepuce C60.0
    - pudendum C51.9
    - scalp C43.4
    - scrotum C63.2
    - shoulder C43.6 ☑
    - skin NEC C43.9
    - submammary fold C43.52
    - temple C43.39
    - thigh C43.7 ☑
    - toe C43.7 ☑
    - trunk NEC C43.59
    - umbilicus C43.59
    - upper limb NEC C43.6 ☑
    - vulva C51.9
      - overlapping sites C51.8
  - spindle cell
    - with epithelioid, mixed — *see* Melanoma, skin, by site
    - type A C69.4 ☑
    - type B C69.4 ☑
  - superficial spreading — *see* Melanoma, skin, by site
- **Melanosarcoma** (*see also* Melanoma)
  - epithelioid cell — *see* Melanoma
- **Melanosis** L81.4
  - addisonian E27.1
    - tuberculous A18.7
  - adrenal E27.1
  - colon K63.89
  - conjunctiva — *see* Pigmentation, conjunctiva
    - congenital Q13.89
  - cornea (presenile) (senile) (*see also* Pigmentation, cornea)
    - congenital Q13.4
  - eye NEC H57.8
    - congenital Q15.8
  - lenticularis progressiva Q82.1
  - liver K76.89
- **Melanosis** — *continued*
  - precancerous (*see also* Melanoma, in situ)
    - malignant melanoma in — *see* Melanoma
  - Riehl's L81.4
  - sclera H15.89
    - congenital Q13.89
  - suprarenal E27.1
  - tar L81.4
  - toxic L81.4
- **Melanuria** R82.99
- **MELAS** syndrome E88.41
- **Melasma** L81.1
  - adrenal (gland) E27.1
  - suprarenal (gland) E27.1
- **Melena** K92.1
  - with ulcer - code by site under Ulcer, with hemorrhage K27.4
  - due to swallowed maternal blood P78.2
  - newborn, neonatal P54.1
    - due to swallowed maternal blood P78.2
- **Meleney's**
  - gangrene (cutaneous) — *see* Ulcer, skin
  - ulcer (chronic undermining) — *see* Ulcer, skin
- **Melioidosis** A24.9
  - acute A24.1
  - chronic A24.2
  - fulminating A24.1
  - pneumonia A24.1
  - pulmonary (chronic) A24.2
    - acute A24.1
    - subacute A24.2
  - sepsis A24.1
  - specified NEC A24.3
  - subacute A24.2
- **Melitensis,** febris A23.0
- **Melkersson** (-Rosenthal) syndrome G51.2
- **Mellitus,** diabetes — *see* Diabetes
- **Melorheostosis** (bone) — *see* Disorder, bone, density and structure, specified NEC
- **Meloschisis** Q18.4
- **Melotia** Q17.4
- **Membrana**
  - capsularis lentis posterior Q13.89
  - epipapillaris Q14.2
- **Membranacea** placenta O43.19 ☑
- **Membranaceous** uterus N85.8
- **Membrane** (s), membranous (*see also* condition)
  - cyclitic — *see* Membrane, pupillary
  - folds, congenital — *see* Web
  - Jackson's Q43.3
  - over face of newborn P28.9
  - premature rupture — *see* Rupture, membranes, premature
  - pupillary H21.4 ☑
    - persistent Q13.89
  - retained (with hemorrhage) (complicating delivery) O72.2
    - without hemorrhage O73.1
  - secondary cataract — *see* Cataract, secondary
  - unruptured (causing asphyxia) — *see* Asphyxia, newborn
  - vitreous — *see* Opacity, vitreous, membranes and strands
- **Membranitis** — *see* Chorioamnionitis
- **Memory** disturbance, lack or loss (*see also* Amnesia)
  - mild, following organic brain damage F06.8
- **Menadione** deficiency E56.1
- **Menarche**
  - delayed E30.0
  - precocious E30.1
- **Mendacity,** pathologic F60.2
- **Mendelson's** syndrome (due to anesthesia) J95.4
  - in labor and delivery O74.0
  - in pregnancy O29.01 ☑
  - obstetric O74.0
  - postpartum, puerperal O89.01
- **Ménétrier's** disease or syndrome K29.60
  - with bleeding K29.61
- **Ménière's** disease, syndrome or vertigo H81.0 ☑
- **Meninges,** meningeal — *see* condition
- **Meningioma** (*see also* Neoplasm, meninges, benign)
  - angioblastic — *see* Neoplasm, meninges, benign
  - angiomatous — *see* Neoplasm, meninges, benign
  - endotheliomatous — *see* Neoplasm, meninges, benign
  - fibroblastic — *see* Neoplasm, meninges, benign
  - fibrous — *see* Neoplasm, meninges, benign
  - hemangioblastic — *see* Neoplasm, meninges, benign
  - hemangiopericytic — *see* Neoplasm, meninges, benign
  - malignant — *see* Neoplasm, meninges, malignant

Meningioma — *continued*
- meningiothelial — *see* Neoplasm, meninges, benign
- meningotheliomatous — *see* Neoplasm, meninges, benign
- mixed — *see* Neoplasm, meninges, benign
- multiple — *see* Neoplasm, meninges, uncertain behavior
- papillary — *see* Neoplasm, meninges, uncertain behavior
- psammomatous — *see* Neoplasm, meninges, benign
- syncytial — *see* Neoplasm, meninges, benign
- transitional — *see* Neoplasm, meninges, benign

Meningiomatosis (diffuse) — *see* Neoplasm, meninges, uncertain behavior

Meningism — *see* Meningismus

Meningismus (infectional) (pneumococcal) R29.1
- due to serum or vaccine R29.1
- influenzal — *see* Influenza, with, manifestations NEC

Meningitis (basal) (basic) (brain) (cerebral) (cervical) (congestive) (diffuse) (hemorrhagic) (infantile) (membranous) (metastatic) (nonspecific) (pontine) (progressive) (simple) (spinal) (subacute) (sympathetic) (toxic) G03.9
- abacterial G03.0
- actinomycotic A42.81
- adenoviral A87.1
- arbovirus A87.8
- aseptic (acute) G03.0
- bacterial G00.9
  - Escherichia coli (E. coli) G00.8
  - Friedländer (bacillus) G00.8
  - gram-negative G00.9
  - H. influenzae G00.0
  - Klebsiella G00.8
  - pneumococcal G00.1
  - specified organism NEC G00.8
  - staphylococcal G00.3
  - streptococcal (acute) G00.2
- benign recurrent (Mollaret) G03.2
- candidal B37.5
- caseous (tuberculous) A17.0
- cerebrospinal A39.0
- chronic NEC G03.1
- clear cerebrospinal fluid NEC G03.0
- coxsackievirus A87.0
- cryptococcal B45.1
- diplococcal (gram positive) A39.0
- echovirus A87.0
- enteroviral A87.0
- eosinophilic B83.2
- epidemic NEC A39.0
- Escherichia coli (E. coli) G00.8
- fibrinopurulent G00.9
  - specified organism NEC G00.8
- Friedländer (bacillus) G00.8
- gonococcal A54.81
- gram-negative cocci G00.9
- gram-positive cocci G00.9
- Haemophilus (influenzae) G00.0
- H. influenzae G00.0
- in (due to)
  - adenovirus A87.1
  - African trypanosomiasis B56.9 *[G02]*
  - anthrax A22.8
  - bacterial disease NEC A48.8 *[G01]*
  - Chagas' disease (chronic) B57.41
  - chickenpox B01.0
  - coccidioidomycosis B38.4
  - Diplococcus pneumoniae G00.1
  - enterovirus A87.0
  - herpes (simplex) virus B00.3
    - zoster B02.1
  - infectious mononucleosis B27.92
  - leptospirosis A27.81
  - Listeria monocytogenes A32.11
  - Lyme disease A69.21
  - measles B05.1
  - mumps (virus) B26.1
  - neurosyphilis (late) A52.13
  - parasitic disease NEC B89 *[G02]*
  - poliovirus A80.9 *[G02]*
  - preventive immunization, inoculation or vaccination G03.8
  - rubella B06.02
  - Salmonella infection A02.21
  - specified cause NEC G03.8
  - Streptococcal pneumoniae G00.1
  - typhoid fever A01.01
  - varicella B01.0

Meningitis — *continued*
- in — *continued*
  - viral disease NEC A87.8
  - whooping cough A37.90
  - zoster B02.1
- infectious G00.9
- influenzal (H. influenzae) G00.0
- Klebsiella G00.8
- leptospiral (aseptic) A27.81
- lymphocytic (acute) (benign) (serous) A87.2
- meningococcal A39.0
- Mima polymorpha G00.8
- Mollaret (benign recurrent) G03.2
- monilial B37.5
- mycotic NEC B49 *[G02]*
- Neisseria A39.0
- nonbacterial G03.0
- nonpyogenic NEC G03.0
- ossificans G96.19
- pneumococcal streptococcus pneumoniae G00.1
- poliovirus A80.9 *[G02]*
- postmeasles B05.1
- purulent G00.9
  - specified organism NEC G00.8
- pyogenic G00.9
  - specified organism NEC G00.8
- Salmonella (arizonae) (Cholerae-Suis) (enteritidis) (typhimurium) A02.21
- septic G00.9
  - specified organism NEC G00.8
- serosa circumscripta NEC G03.0
- serous NEC G93.2
- specified organism NEC G00.8
- sporotrichosis B42.81
- staphylococcal G00.3
- sterile G03.0
- Streptococcal (acute) G00.2
  - pneumoniae G00.1
- suppurative G00.9
  - specified organism NEC G00.8
- syphilitic (late) (tertiary) A52.13
  - acute A51.41
  - congenital A50.41
  - secondary A51.41
- Torula histolytica (cryptococcal) B45.1
- traumatic (complication of injury) T79.8 ☑
- tuberculous A17.0
- typhoid A01.01
- viral NEC A87.9
- Yersinia pestis A20.3

Meningocele (spinal) (*see also* Spina bifida)
- with hydrocephalus — *see* Spina bifida, by site, with hydrocephalus
- acquired (traumatic) G96.19
- cerebral — *see* Encephalocele

Meningocerebritis — *see* Meningoencephalitis

Meningococcemia A39.4
- acute A39.2
- chronic A39.3

Meningococcus, meningococcal (*see also* condition)A39.9
- adrenalitis, hemorrhagic A39.1
- carrier (suspected) of Z22.31
- meningitis (cerebrospinal) A39.0

Meningoencephalitis (*see also* Encephalitis)G04.90
- acute NEC (*see also* Encephalitis, viral)A86
- bacterial NEC G04.2
- California A83.5
- diphasic A84.1
- eosinophilic B83.2
- epidemic A39.81
- herpesviral, herpetic B00.4
  - due to herpesvirus 6 B10.01
  - due to herpesvirus 7 B10.09
  - specified NEC B10.09
- in (due to)
  - blastomycosis NEC B40.81
  - diseases classified elsewhere G05.3
  - free-living amoebae B60.2
  - Hemophilus influenzae (H .influenzae) G00.0
  - herpes B00.4
    - due to herpesvirus 6 B10.01
    - due to herpesvirus 7 B10.09
    - specified NEC B10.09
  - H. influenzae G00.0
  - Lyme disease A69.22
  - mercury — *see* subcategory T56.1
  - mumps B26.2
  - Naegleria (amoebae) (organisms) (fowleri) B60.2
  - Parastrongylus cantonensis B83.2
  - toxoplasmosis (acquired) B58.2
    - congenital P37.1

Meningoencephalitis — *continued*
- infectious (acute) (viral) A86
- influenzal (H. influenzae) G00.0
- Listeria monocytogenes A32.12
- lymphocytic (serous) A87.2
- mumps B26.2
- parasitic NEC B89 *[G05.3]*
- pneumococcal G04.2
- primary amebic B60.2
- specific (syphilitic) A52.14
- specified organism NEC G04.81
- staphylococcal G04.2
- streptococcal G04.2
- syphilitic A52.14
- toxic NEC G92
  - due to mercury — *see* subcategory T56.1
- tuberculous A17.82
- virus NEC A86

Meningoencephalocele (*see also* Encephalocele)
- syphilitic A52.19
  - congenital A50.49

Meningoencephalomyelitis (*see also* Meningoencephalitis)
- acute NEC (viral) A86
  - disseminated G04.00
    - postimmunization or postvaccination G04.02
    - postinfectious G04.01
- due to
  - actinomycosis A42.82
  - Torula B45.1
  - Toxoplasma or toxoplasmosis (acquired) B58.2
    - congenital P37.1
- postimmunization or postvaccination G04.02

Meningoencephalomyelopathy G96.9

Meningoencephalopathy G96.9

Meningomyelitis (*see also* Meningoencephalitis)
- bacterial NEC G04.2
- blastomycotic NEC B40.81
- cryptococcal B45.1
- in diseases classified elsewhere G05.4
- meningococcal A39.81
- syphilitic A52.14
- tuberculous A17.82

Meningomyelocele (*see also* Spina bifida)
- syphilitic A52.19

Meningomyeloneuritis — *see* Meningoencephalitis

Meningoradiculitis — *see* Meningitis

Meningovascular — *see* condition

Menkes' disease or syndrome E83.09
- meaning maple-syrup-urine disease E71.0

Menometrorrhagia N92.1

Menopause, menopausal (asymptomatic) (state) Z78.0
- arthritis (any site) NEC — *see* Arthritis, specified form NEC
- bleeding N92.4
- depression (single episode) F32.89
  - agitated (single episode) F32.2
    - recurrent episode F33.9
  - psychotic (single episode) F32.89
    - recurrent episode F33.9
  - recurrent episode F33.8
- melancholia (single episode) F32.89
  - recurrent episode F33.8
- paranoid state F22
- premature E28.319
  - asymptomatic E28.319
    - postirradiation E89.40
    - postsurgical E89.40
  - symptomatic E28.310
    - postirradiation E89.41
    - postsurgical E89.41
- psychosis NEC F28
- symptomatic N95.1
- toxic polyarthritis NEC — *see* Arthritis, specified form NEC

Menorrhagia (primary) N92.0
- climacteric N92.4
  - menopausal N92.4
- menopausal N92.4
- postclimacteric N95.0
- postmenopausal N95.0
- preclimacteric or premenopausal N92.4
- pubertal (menses retained) N92.2

Menostaxis N92.0

Menses, retention N94.89

Menstrual — *see* Menstruation

Menstruation
- absent — *see* Amenorrhea
- anovulatory N97.0
- cycle, irregular N92.6
- delayed N91.0

- **Mohr's** syndrome (Types I and II) Q87.0
- **Mola** destruens D39.2
- **Molar** pregnancy O02.0
- **Molarization** of premolars K00.2
- **Molding,** head (during birth) - omit code
- **Mole** (pigmented) (*see also* Nevus)
  - blood O02.0
  - Breus' O02.0
  - cancerous — *see* Melanoma
  - carneous O02.0
  - destructive D39.2
  - fleshy O02.0
  - hydatid, hydatidiform (benign) (complicating pregnancy) (delivered) (undelivered) O01.9
    - classical O01.0
    - complete O01.0
    - incomplete O01.1
    - invasive D39.2
    - malignant D39.2
    - partial O01.1
  - intrauterine O02.0
  - invasive (hydatidiform) D39.2
  - malignant
    - meaning
      - malignant hydatidiform mole D39.2
      - melanoma — *see* Melanoma
  - nonhydatidiform O02.0
  - nonpigmented — *see* Nevus
  - pregnancy NEC O02.0
  - skin — *see* Nevus
  - tubal O00.10
    - with intrauterine pregnancy O00.11
  - vesicular — *see* Mole, hydatidiform
- **Molimen,** molimina (menstrual) N94.3
- **Molluscum** contagiosum (epitheliale) B08.1
- **Mönckeberg's** arteriosclerosis, disease, or sclerosis — *see* Arteriosclerosis, extremities
- **Mondini's** malformation (cochlea) Q16.5
- **Mondor's** disease I80.8
- **Monge's** disease T70.29 ☑
- **Monilethrix** (congenital) Q84.1
- **Moniliasis** (*see also* Candidiasis)B37.9
  - neonatal P37.5
- **Monitoring** (encounter for)
  - therapeutic drug level Z51.81
- **Monkey** malaria B53.1
- **Monkeypox** B04
- **Monoarthritis** M13.10
  - ankle M13.17 ☑
  - elbow M13.12 ☑
  - foot joint M13.17 ☑
  - hand joint M13.14 ☑
  - hip M13.15 ☑
  - knee M13.16 ☑
  - shoulder M13.11 ☑
  - wrist M13.13 ☑
- **Monoblastic** — *see* condition
- **Monochromat** (ism), monochromatopsia (acquired) (congenital) H53.51
- **Monocytic** — *see* condition
- **Monocytopenia** D72.818
- **Monocytosis** (symptomatic) D72.821
- **Monomania** — *see* Psychosis
- **Mononeuritis** G58.9
  - cranial nerve — *see* Disorder, nerve, cranial
  - femoral nerve G57.2 ☑
  - lateral
    - cutaneous nerve of thigh G57.1 ☑
    - popliteal nerve G57.3 ☑
  - lower limb G57.9 ☑
    - specified nerve NEC G57.8 ☑
  - medial popliteal nerve G57.4 ☑
  - median nerve G56.1 ☑
  - multiplex G58.7
  - plantar nerve G57.6 ☑
  - posterior tibial nerve G57.5 ☑
  - radial nerve G56.3 ☑
  - sciatic nerve G57.0 ☑
  - specified NEC G58.8
  - tibial nerve G57.4 ☑
  - ulnar nerve G56.2 ☑
  - upper limb G56.9 ☑
    - specified nerve NEC G56.8 ☑
  - vestibular — *see* subcategory H93.3
- **Mononeuropathy** G58.9
  - carpal tunnel syndrome — *see* Syndrome, carpal tunnel
  - diabetic NEC — *see* E08-E13 with .41
  - femoral nerve — *see* Lesion, nerve, femoral
  - ilioinguinal nerve G57.8 ☑
  - in diseases classified elsewhere G59
- **Mononeuropathy** — *continued*
  - intercostal G58.0
  - lower limb G57.9 ☑
    - causalgia — *see* Causalgia, lower limb
    - femoral nerve — *see* Lesion, nerve, femoral
    - meralgia paresthetica G57.1 ☑
    - plantar nerve — *see* Lesion, nerve, plantar
    - popliteal nerve — *see* Lesion, nerve, popliteal
    - sciatic nerve — *see* Lesion, nerve, sciatic
    - specified NEC G57.8 ☑
    - tarsal tunnel syndrome — *see* Syndrome, tarsal tunnel
  - median nerve — *see* Lesion, nerve, median
  - multiplex G58.7
  - obturator nerve G57.8 ☑
  - popliteal nerve — *see* Lesion, nerve, popliteal
  - radial nerve — *see* Lesion, nerve, radial
  - saphenous nerve G57.8 ☑
  - specified NEC G58.8
  - tarsal tunnel syndrome — *see* Syndrome, tarsal tunnel
  - tuberculous A17.83
  - ulnar nerve — *see* Lesion, nerve, ulnar
  - upper limb G56.9 ☑
    - carpal tunnel syndrome — *see* Syndrome, carpal tunnel
    - causalgia — *see* Causalgia
    - median nerve — *see* Lesion, nerve, median
    - radial nerve — *see* Lesion, nerve, radial
    - specified site NEC G56.8 ☑
    - ulnar nerve — *see* Lesion, nerve, ulnar
- **Mononucleosis,** infectious B27.90
  - with
    - complication NEC B27.99
    - meningitis B27.92
    - polyneuropathy B27.91
  - cytomegaloviral B27.10
    - with
      - complication NEC B27.19
      - meningitis B27.12
      - polyneuropathy B27.11
  - Epstein-Barr (virus) B27.00
    - with
      - complication NEC B27.09
      - meningitis B27.02
      - polyneuropathy B27.01
  - gammaherpesviral B27.00
    - with
      - complication NEC B27.09
      - meningitis B27.02
      - polyneuropathy B27.01
  - specified NEC B27.80
    - with
      - complication NEC B27.89
      - meningitis B27.82
      - polyneuropathy B27.81
- **Monoplegia** G83.3 ☑
  - congenital (cerebral) G80.8
    - spastic G80.1
  - embolic (current episode) I63.4 ☑
  - following
    - cerebrovascular disease
      - cerebral infarction
        - lower limb I69.34 ☑
        - upper limb I69.33 ☑
      - intracerebral hemorrhage
        - lower limb I69.14 ☑
        - upper limb I69.13 ☑
      - lower limb I69.94 ☑
      - nontraumatic intracranial hemorrhage NEC
        - lower limb I69.24 ☑
        - upper limb I69.23 ☑
      - specified disease NEC
        - lower limb I69.84 ☑
        - upper limb I69.83 ☑
      - stroke NOS
        - lower limb I69.34 ☑
        - upper limb I69.33 ☑
      - subarachnoid hemorrhage
        - lower limb I69.04 ☑
        - upper limb I69.03 ☑
      - upper limb I69.93 ☑
  - hysterical (transient) F44.4
  - lower limb G83.1 ☑
  - psychogenic (conversion reaction) F44.4
  - thrombotic (current episode) I63.3 ☑
  - transient R29.818
  - upper limb G83.2 ☑
- **Monorchism,** monorchidism Q55.0
- **Monosomy** (*see also* Deletion, chromosome)Q93.9
  - specified NEC Q93.89
  - whole chromosome
- **Monosomy** — *continued*
  - whole chromosome — *continued*
    - meiotic nondisjunction Q93.0
    - mitotic nondisjunction Q93.1
    - mosaicism Q93.1
  - X Q96.9
- **Monster,** monstrosity (single) Q89.7
  - acephalic Q00.0
  - twin Q89.4
- **Monteggia's** fracture (-dislocation) S52.27 ☑
- **Mooren's** ulcer (cornea) — *see* Ulcer, cornea, Mooren's
- **Moore's** syndrome — *see* Epilepsy, specified NEC
- **Mooser-Neill** reaction A75.2
- **Mooser's** bodies A75.2
- **Morbidity** not stated or unknown R69
- **Morbilli** — *see* Measles
- **Morbus** (*see also* Disease)
  - angelicus, anglorum E55.0
  - Beigel B36.2
  - caducus — *see* Epilepsy
  - celiacus K90.0
  - comitialis — *see* Epilepsy
  - cordis (*see also* Disease, heart)I51.9
    - valvulorum — *see* Endocarditis
  - coxae senilis M16.9
    - tuberculous A18.02
  - hemorrhagicus neonatorum P53
  - maculosus neonatorum P54.5
- **Morel** (-Stewart) (-Morgagni) syndrome M85.2
- **Morel-Kraepelin** disease — *see* Schizophrenia
- **Morel-Moore** syndrome M85.2
- **Morgagni's**
  - cyst, organ, hydatid, or appendage
    - female Q50.5
    - male (epididymal) Q55.4
      - testicular Q55.29
  - syndrome M85.2
- **Morgagni-Stokes-Adams** syndrome I45.9
- **Morgagni-Stewart-Morel** syndrome M85.2
- **Morgagni-Turner** (-Albright) syndrome Q96.9
- **Moria** F07.0
- **Moron** (I.Q.50-69) F70
- **Morphea** L94.0
- **Morphinism** (without remission) F11.20
  - with remission F11.21
- **Morphinomania** (without remission) F11.20
  - with remission F11.21
- **Morquio** (-Ullrich) (-Brailsford) disease or syndrome — *see* Mucopolysaccharidosis
- **Mortification** (dry) (moist) — *see* Gangrene
- **Morton's** metatarsalgia (neuralgia) (neuroma) (syndrome) G57.6 ☑
- **Morvan's** disease or syndrome G60.8
- **Mosaicism,** mosaic (autosomal) (chromosomal)
  - 45,X/other cell lines NEC with abnormal sex chromosome Q96.4
  - 45,X/46,XX Q96.3
  - sex chromosome
    - female Q97.8
    - lines with various numbers of X chromosomes Q97.2
    - male Q98.7
  - XY Q96.3
- **Moschowitz'** disease M31.1
- **Mother** yaw A66.0
- **Motion** sickness (from travel, any vehicle) (from roundabouts or swings) T75.3 ☑
- **Mottled,** mottling, teeth (enamel) (endemic) (nonendemic) K00.3
- **Mounier-Kuhn** syndrome Q32.4
  - with bronchiectasis J47.9
    - exacerbation (acute) J47.1
    - lower respiratory infection J47.0
  - acquired J98.09
    - with bronchiectasis J47.9
      - with
        - exacerbation (acute) J47.1
        - lower respiratory infection J47.0
- **Mountain**
  - sickness T70.29 ☑
    - with polycythemia , acquired (acute) D75.1
  - tick fever A93.2
- **Mouse,** joint — *see* Loose, body, joint
  - knee M23.4 ☑
- **Mouth** — *see* condition
- **Movable**
  - coccyx — *see* subcategory M53.2
  - kidney N28.89
    - congenital Q63.8
  - spleen D73.89
- **Movements,** dystonic R25.8

Myeloblastoma - Myopathy

Myeloblastoma — *continued*
- granular cell — *continued*
  - malignant — *see* Neoplasm, connective tissue, malignant
  - tongue D10.1

Myelocele — *see* Spina bifida
Myelocystocele — *see* Spina bifida
Myelocytic — *see* condition
Myelodysplasia D46.9
- specified NEC D46.Z
- spinal cord (congenital) Q06.1

Myelodysplastic syndrome D46.9
- with
  - 5q deletion D46.C
  - isolated del (5q) chromosomal abnormality D46.C
- specified NEC D46.Z

Myeloencephalitis — *see* Encephalitis
Myelofibrosis D75.81
- with myeloid metaplasia D47.4
- acute C94.4 ☑
- idiopathic (chronic) D47.4
- primary D47.1
- secondary D75.81
  - in myeloproliferative disease D47.4

Myelogenous — *see* condition
Myeloid — *see* condition
Myelokathexis D70.9
Myeloleukodystrophy E75.29
Myelolipoma — *see* Lipoma
Myeloma (multiple) C90.0 ☑
- monostotic C90.3 ☑
  - plasma cell C90.0 ☑
- plasma cell C90.0 ☑
- solitary (*see also* Plasmacytoma, solitary)C90.3 ☑

Myelomalacia G95.89
Myelomatosis C90.0 ☑
Myelomeningitis — *see* Meningoencephalitis
Myelomeningocele (spinal cord) — *see* Spina bifida
Myelo-osteo-musculodysplasia hereditaria Q79.8
Myelopathic
- anemia D64.89
- muscle atrophy — *see* Atrophy, muscle, spinal
- pain syndrome G89.0

Myelopathy (spinal cord) G95.9
- drug-induced G95.89
- in (due to)
  - degeneration or displacement, intervertebral disc NEC — *see* Disorder, disc, with, myelopathy
  - infection — *see* Encephalitis
  - intervertebral disc disorder (*see also* Disorder, disc, with, myelopathy)
  - mercury — *see* subcategory T56.1
  - neoplastic disease (*see also* Neoplasm)D49.9 *[G99.2]*
  - pernicious anemia D51.0 *[G99.2]*
  - spondylosis — *see* Spondylosis, with myelopathy NEC
- necrotic (subacute) (vascular) G95.19
- radiation-induced G95.89
- spondylogenic NEC — *see* Spondylosis, with myelopathy NEC
- toxic G95.89
- transverse, acute G37.3
- vascular G95.19
- vitamin B12 E53.8 *[G32.0]*

Myelophthisis D61.82
Myeloradiculitis G04.91
Myeloradiculodysplasia (spinal) Q06.1
Myelosarcoma C92.3 ☑
Myelosclerosis D75.89
- with myeloid metaplasia D47.4
- disseminated, of nervous system G35
- megakaryocytic D47.4
  - with myeloid metaplasia D47.4

Myelosis
- acute C92.0 ☑
- aleukemic C92.9 ☑
- chronic D47.1
- erythremic (acute) C94.0 ☑
- megakaryocytic C94.2 ☑
- nonleukemic D72.828
- subacute C92.9 ☑

Myiasis (cavernous) B87.9
- aural B87.4
- creeping B87.0
- cutaneous B87.0
- dermal B87.0
- ear (external) (middle) B87.4
- eye B87.2
- genitourinary B87.81

Myiasis — *continued*
- intestinal B87.82
- laryngeal B87.3
- nasopharyngeal B87.3
- ocular B87.2
- orbit B87.2
- skin B87.0
- specified site NEC B87.89
- traumatic B87.1
- wound B87.1

Myoadenoma, prostate — *see* Hyperplasia, prostate
Myoblastoma
- granular cell (*see also* Neoplasm, connective tissue, benign)
  - malignant — *see* Neoplasm, connective tissue, malignant
- tongue D10.1

Myocardial — *see* condition
Myocardiopathy (congestive) (constrictive) (familial) (hypertrophic nonobstructive) (idiopathic) (infiltrative) (obstructive) (primary) (restrictive) (sporadic) (*see also* Cardiomyopathy)I42.9
- alcoholic I42.6
- cobalt-beer I42.6
- glycogen storage E74.02 *[I43]*
- hypertrophic obstructive I42.1
- in (due to)
  - beriberi E51.12
  - cardiac glycogenosis E74.02 *[I43]*
  - Friedreich's ataxia G11.1 *[I43]*
  - myotonia atrophica G71.11 *[I43]*
  - progressive muscular dystrophy G71.0 *[I43]*
- obscure (African) I42.8
- secondary I42.9
- thyrotoxic E05.90 *[I43]*
  - with storm E05.91 *[I43]*
- toxic NEC I42.7

Myocarditis (with arteriosclerosis) (chronic) (fibroid) (interstitial) (old) (progressive) (senile) I51.4
- with
  - rheumatic fever (conditions in I00) I09.0
    - active — *see* Myocarditis, acute, rheumatic
    - inactive or quiescent (with chorea) I09.0
- active I40.9
  - rheumatic I01.2
    - with chorea (acute) (rheumatic) (Sydenham's) I02.0
- acute or subacute (interstitial) I40.9
  - due to
    - streptococcus (beta-hemolytic) I01.2
  - idiopathic I40.1
  - rheumatic I01.2
    - with chorea (acute) (rheumatic) (Sydenham's) I02.0
  - specified NEC I40.8
- aseptic of newborn B33.22
- bacterial (acute) I40.0
- Coxsackie (virus) B33.22
- diphtheritic A36.81
- eosinophilic I40.1
- epidemic of newborn (Coxsackie) B33.22
- Fiedler's (acute) (isolated) I40.1
- giant cell (acute) (subacute) I40.1
- gonococcal A54.83
- granulomatous (idiopathic) (isolated) (nonspecific) I40.1
- hypertensive — *see* Hypertension, heart
- idiopathic (granulomatous) I40.1
- in (due to)
  - diphtheria A36.81
  - epidemic louse-borne typhus A75.0 *[I41]*
  - Lyme disease A69.29
  - sarcoidosis D86.85
  - scarlet fever A38.1
  - toxoplasmosis (acquired) B58.81
  - typhoid A01.02
  - typhus NEC A75.9 *[I41]*
- infective I40.0
- influenzal — *see* Influenza, with, myocarditis
- isolated (acute) I40.1
- meningococcal A39.52
- mumps B26.82
- nonrheumatic, active I40.9
- parenchymatous I40.9
- pneumococcal I40.0
- rheumatic (chronic) (inactive) (with chorea) I09.0
  - active or acute I01.2
    - with chorea (acute) (rheumatic) (Sydenham's) I02.0
- rheumatoid — *see* Rheumatoid, carditis
- septic I40.0
- staphylococcal I40.0

Myocarditis — *continued*
- suppurative I40.0
- syphilitic (chronic) A52.06
- toxic I40.8
  - rheumatic — *see* Myocarditis, acute, rheumatic
- tuberculous A18.84
- typhoid A01.02
- valvular — *see* Endocarditis
- virus, viral I40.0
  - of newborn (Coxsackie) B33.22

Myocardium, myocardial — *see* condition
Myocardosis — *see* Cardiomyopathy
Myoclonus, myoclonic, myoclonia (familial) (essential) (multifocal) (simplex) G25.3
- drug-induced G25.3
- epilepsy (*see also* Epilepsy, generalized, specified NEC)G40.4 ☑
  - familial (progressive) G25.3
- epileptica G40.409
  - with status epilepticus G40.401
- facial G51.3
- familial progressive G25.3
- Friedreich's G25.3
- jerks G25.3
- massive G25.3
- palatal G25.3
- pharyngeal G25.3

Myocytolysis I51.5
Myodiastasis — *see* Diastasis, muscle
Myoendocarditis — *see* Endocarditis
Myoepithelioma — *see* Neoplasm, benign, by site
Myofasciitis (acute) — *see* Myositis
Myofibroma (*see also* Neoplasm, connective tissue, benign)
- uterus (cervix) (corpus) — *see* Leiomyoma

Myofibromatosis D48.1
- infantile Q89.8

Myofibrosis M62.89
- heart — *see* Myocarditis
- scapulohumeral — *see* Lesion, shoulder, specified NEC

Myofibrositis M79.7
- scapulohumeral — *see* Lesion, shoulder, specified NEC

Myoglobulinuria, myoglobinuria (primary) R82.1
Myokymia, facial G51.4
Myolipoma — *see* Lipoma
Myoma (*see also* Neoplasm, connective tissue, benign)
- malignant — *see* Neoplasm, connective tissue, malignant
- prostate D29.1
- uterus (cervix) (corpus) — *see* Leiomyoma

Myomalacia M62.89
Myometritis — *see* Endometritis
Myometrium — *see* condition
Myonecrosis, clostridial A48.0
Myopathy G72.9
- acute
  - necrotizing G72.81
  - quadriplegic G72.81
- alcoholic G72.1
- benign congenital G71.2
- central core G71.2
- centronuclear G71.2
- congenital (benign) G71.2
- critical illness G72.81
- distal G71.0
- drug-induced G72.0
- endocrine NEC E34.9 *[G73.7]*
- extraocular muscles H05.82 ☑
- facioscapulohumeral G71.0
- hereditary G71.9
  - specified NEC G71.8
- immune NEC G72.49
- in (due to)
  - Addison's disease E27.1 *[G73.7]*
  - alcohol G72.1
  - amyloidosis E85.0 *[G73.7]*
  - cretinism E00.9 *[G73.7]*
  - Cushing's syndrome E24.9 *[G73.7]*
  - drugs G72.0
  - endocrine disease NEC E34.9 *[G73.7]*
  - giant cell arteritis M31.6 *[G73.7]*
  - glycogen storage disease E74.00 *[G73.7]*
  - hyperadrenocorticism E24.9 *[G73.7]*
  - hyperparathyroidism NEC E21.3 *[G73.7]*
  - hypoparathyroidism E20.9 *[G73.7]*
  - hypopituitarism E23.0 *[G73.7]*
  - hypothyroidism E03.9 *[G73.7]*
  - infectious disease NEC B99 ☑ *[G73.7]*
  - lipid storage disease E75.6 *[G73.7]*

Myopathy — *continued*
- in — *continued*
  - metabolic disease NEC E88.9 *[G73.7]*
  - myxedema E03.9 *[G73.7]*
  - parasitic disease NEC B89 *[G73.7]*
  - polyarteritis nodosa M30.0 *[G73.7]*
  - rheumatoid arthritis — *see* Rheumatoid, myopathy
  - sarcoidosis D86.87
  - scleroderma M34.82
  - sicca syndrome M35.03
  - Sjögren's syndrome M35.03
  - systemic lupus erythematosus M32.19
  - thyrotoxicosis (hyperthyroidism) E05.90 *[G73.7]*
    - with thyroid storm E05.91 *[G73.7]*
  - toxic agent NEC G72.2
- inflammatory NEC G72.49
- intensive care (ICU) G72.81
- limb-girdle G71.0
- mitochondrial NEC G71.3
- myotonic, proximal (PROMM) G71.11
- myotubular G71.2
- nemaline G71.2
- ocular G71.0
- oculopharyngeal G71.0
- of critical illness G72.81
- primary G71.9
  - specified NEC G71.8
- progressive NEC G72.89
- proximal myotonic (PROMM) G71.11
- rod G71.2
- scapulohumeral G71.0
- specified NEC G72.89
- toxic G72.2

Myopericarditis (*see also* Pericarditis)
- chronic rheumatic I09.2

Myopia (axial) (congenital) H52.1 ☑
- degenerative (malignant) H44.2 ☑
- malignant H44.2 ☑
- pernicious H44.2 ☑
- progressive high (degenerative) H44.2 ☑

Myosarcoma — *see* Neoplasm, connective tissue, malignant

Myosis (pupil) H57.03
- stromal (endolymphatic) D39.0

Myositis M60.9
- clostridial A48.0
- due to posture — *see* Myositis, specified type NEC
- epidemic B33.0
- fibrosa or fibrous (chronic), Volkmann's T79.6 ☑
- foreign body granuloma — *see* Granuloma, foreign body
- in (due to)
  - bilharziasis B65.9 *[M63.8-]*
  - cysticercosis B69.81
  - leprosy A30.9 *[M63.8-]*
  - mycosis B49 *[M63.8-]*
  - sarcoidosis D86.87
  - schistosomiasis B65.9 *[M63.8-]*
  - syphilis
    - late A52.78
    - secondary A51.49
  - toxoplasmosis (acquired) B58.82
  - trichinellosis B75 *[M63.8-]*
  - tuberculosis A18.09
- inclusion body [IBM] G72.41
- infective M60.009
  - arm M60.002
    - left M60.001
    - right M60.000
  - leg M60.005
    - left M60.004
    - right M60.003
  - lower limb M60.005
    - ankle M60.07 ☑
    - foot M60.07 ☑
    - lower leg M60.06 ☑
    - thigh M60.05 ☑
    - toe M60.07 ☑
  - multiple sites M60.09
  - specified site NEC M60.08
  - upper limb M60.002
    - finger M60.04 ☑
    - forearm M60.03 ☑
    - hand M60.04 ☑
    - shoulder region M60.01 ☑
    - upper arm M60.02 ☑
- interstitial M60.10
  - ankle M60.17 ☑
  - foot M60.17 ☑
  - forearm M60.13 ☑
  - hand M60.14 ☑

Myositis — *continued*
- interstitial — *continued*
  - lower leg M60.16 ☑
  - multiple sites M60.19
  - shoulder region M60.11 ☑
  - specified site NEC M60.18
  - thigh M60.15 ☑
  - upper arm M60.12 ☑
- mycotic B49 *[M63.8-]*
- orbital, chronic H05.12 ☑
- ossificans or ossifying (circumscripta) (*see also* Ossification, muscle, specified NEC)
  - in (due to)
    - burns M61.30
      - ankle M61.37 ☑
      - foot M61.37 ☑
      - forearm M61.33 ☑
      - hand M61.34 ☑
      - lower leg M61.36 ☑
      - multiple sites M61.39
      - pelvic region M61.35 ☑
      - shoulder region M61.31 ☑
      - specified site NEC M61.38
      - thigh M61.35 ☑
      - upper arm M61.32 ☑
    - quadriplegia or paraplegia M61.20
      - ankle M61.27 ☑
      - foot M61.27 ☑
      - forearm M61.23 ☑
      - hand M61.24 ☑
      - lower leg M61.26 ☑
      - multiple sites M61.29
      - pelvic region M61.25 ☑
      - shoulder region M61.21 ☑
      - specified site NEC M61.28
      - thigh M61.25 ☑
      - upper arm M61.22 ☑
  - progressiva M61.10
    - ankle M61.17 ☑
    - finger M61.14 ☑
    - foot M61.17 ☑
    - forearm M61.13 ☑
    - hand M61.14 ☑
    - lower leg M61.16 ☑
    - multiple sites M61.19
    - pelvic region M61.15 ☑
    - shoulder region M61.11 ☑
    - specified site NEC M61.18
    - thigh M61.15 ☑
    - toe M61.17 ☑
    - upper arm M61.12 ☑
  - traumatica M61.00
    - ankle M61.07 ☑
    - foot M61.07 ☑
    - forearm M61.03 ☑
    - hand M61.04 ☑
    - lower leg M61.06 ☑
    - multiple sites M61.09
    - pelvic region M61.05 ☑
    - shoulder region M61.01 ☑
    - specified site NEC M61.08
    - thigh M61.05 ☑
    - upper arm M61.02 ☑
- purulent — *see* Myositis, infective
- specified type NEC M60.80
  - ankle M60.87 ☑
  - foot M60.87 ☑
  - forearm M60.83 ☑
  - hand M60.84 ☑
  - lower leg M60.86 ☑
  - multiple sites M60.89
  - pelvic region M60.85 ☑
  - shoulder region M60.81 ☑
  - specified site NEC M60.88
  - thigh M60.85 ☑
  - upper arm M60.82 ☑
- suppurative — *see* Myositis, infective
- traumatic (old) — *see* Myositis, specified type NEC

Myospasia impulsiva F95.2

Myotonia (acquisita) (intermittens) M62.89
- atrophica G71.11
- chondrodystrophic G71.13
- congenita (acetazolamide responsive) (dominant) (recessive) G71.12
- drug-induced G71.14
- dystrophica G71.11
- fluctuans G71.19
- levior G71.12
- permanens G71.19
- symptomatic G71.19

Myotonic pupil — *see* Anomaly, pupil, function, tonic pupil

Myriapodiasis B88.2

Myringitis H73.2 ☑
- with otitis media — *see* Otitis, media
- acute H73.00 ☑
  - bullous H73.01 ☑
  - specified NEC H73.09 ☑
- bullous — *see* Myringitis, acute, bullous
- chronic H73.1 ☑

Mysophobia F40.228

Mytilotoxism — *see* Poisoning, fish

Myxadenitis labialis K13.0

Myxedema (adult) (idiocy) (infantile) (juvenile) (*see also* Hypothyroidism)E03.9
- circumscribed E05.90
  - with storm E05.91
- coma E03.5
- congenital E00.1
- cutis L98.5
- localized (pretibial) E05.90
  - with storm E05.91
- papular L98.5

Myxochondrosarcoma — *see* Neoplasm, cartilage, malignant

Myxofibroma — *see* Neoplasm, connective tissue, benign
- odontogenic — *see* Cyst, calcifying odontogenic

Myxofibrosarcoma — *see* Neoplasm, connective tissue, malignant

Myxolipoma D17.9

Myxoliposarcoma — *see* Neoplasm, connective tissue, malignant

Myxoma (*see also* Neoplasm, connective tissue, benign)
- nerve sheath — *see* Neoplasm, nerve, benign
- odontogenic — *see* Cyst, calcifying odontogenic

Myxosarcoma — *see* Neoplasm, connective tissue, malignant

N

Naegeli's
- disease Q82.8
- leukemia, monocytic C93.1 ☑

Naegleriasis (with meningoencephalitis) B60.2

Naffziger's syndrome G54.0

Naga sore — *see* Ulcer, skin

Nägele's pelvis M95.5
- with disproportion (fetopelvic) O33.0
  - causing obstructed labor O65.0

Nail (*see also* condition)
- biting F98.8
- patella syndrome Q87.2

Nanism, nanosomia — *see* Dwarfism

Nanophyetiasis B66.8

Nanukayami A27.89

Napkin rash L22

Narcolepsy G47.419
- with cataplexy G47.411
- in conditions classified elsewhere G47.429
  - with cataplexy G47.421

Narcosis R06.89

Narcotism — *see* Dependence

NARP (Neuropathy, Ataxia and Retinitis pigmentosa) syndrome E88.49

Narrow
- anterior chamber angle H40.03 ☑
- gingival width (of periodontal soft tissue) K05.5
- pelvis — *see* Contraction, pelvis

Narrowing (*see also* Stenosis)
- artery I77.1
  - auditory, internal I65.8
  - basilar — *see* Occlusion, artery, basilar
  - carotid — *see* Occlusion, artery, carotid
  - cerebellar — *see* Occlusion, artery, cerebellar
  - cerebral — *see* Occlusion artery, cerebral
  - choroidal — *see* Occlusion, artery, cerebral, specified NEC
  - communicating posterior — *see* Occlusion, artery, cerebral, specified NEC
  - coronary (*see also* Disease, heart, ischemic, atherosclerotic)
    - congenital Q24.5
      - syphilitic A50.54 *[I52]*
    - due to syphilis NEC A52.06
  - hypophyseal — *see* Occlusion, artery, cerebral, specified NEC
  - pontine — *see* Occlusion, artery, cerebral, specified NEC
  - precerebral — *see* Occlusion, artery, precerebral
  - vertebral — *see* Occlusion, artery, vertebral

Narrowing - Nephritis

Narrowing — *continued*
- auditory canal (external) — *see* Stenosis, external ear canal
- eustachian tube — *see* Obstruction, eustachian tube
- eyelid — *see* Disorder, eyelid function
- larynx J38.6
- mesenteric artery (*see also* Ischemia, intestine, acute)K55.059
- palate M26.89
- palpebral fissure — *see* Disorder, eyelid function
- ureter N13.5
  - with infection N13.6
- urethra — *see* Stricture, urethra

Narrowness, abnormal, eyelid Q10.3
Nasal — *see* condition
Nasolachrymal, nasolacrimal — *see* condition
Nasopharyngeal (*see also* condition)
- pituitary gland Q89.2
- torticollis M43.6

Nasopharyngitis (acute) (infective) (streptococcal) (subacute) J00
- chronic (suppurative) (ulcerative) J31.1

Nasopharynx, nasopharyngeal — *see* condition
Natal tooth, teeth K00.6
Nausea (without vomiting) R11.0
- with vomiting R11.2
- gravidarum — *see* Hyperemesis, gravidarum
- marina T75.3 ☑
- navalis T75.3 ☑

Navel — *see* condition
Neapolitan fever — *see* Brucellosis
Near drowning T75.1 ☑
Nearsightedness — *see* Myopia
Near-syncope R55
Nebula, cornea — *see* Opacity, cornea
Necator americanus infestation B76.1
Necatoriasis B76.1
Neck — *see* condition
Necrobiosis R68.89
- lipoidica NEC L92.1
  - with diabetes — *see* E08-E13 with .620

Necrolysis, toxic epidermal L51.2
- due to drug
  - correct substance properly administered — *see* Table of Drugs and Chemicals, by drug, adverse effect
  - overdose or wrong substance given or taken — *see* Table of Drugs and Chemicals, by drug, poisoning

Necrophilia F65.89
Necrosis, necrotic (ischemic) (*see also* Gangrene)
- adrenal (capsule) (gland) E27.49
- amputation stump (surgical) (late) T87.50
  - arm T87.5 ☑
  - leg T87.5 ☑
- antrum J32.0
- aorta (hyaline) (*see also* Aneurysm, aorta)
  - cystic medial — *see* Dissection, aorta
- artery I77.5
- bladder (aseptic) (sphincter) N32.89
- bone (*see also* Osteonecrosis)M87.9
  - aseptic or avascular — *see* Osteonecrosis
    - idiopathic M87.00
  - ethmoid J32.2
  - jaw M27.2
  - tuberculous — *see* Tuberculosis, bone
- brain I67.89
- breast (aseptic) (fat) (segmental) N64.1
- bronchus J98.09
- central nervous system NEC I67.89
- cerebellar I67.89
- cerebral I67.89
- colon (*see also* Infarct, intestine)K55.049
- cornea H18.89 ☑
- cortical (acute) (renal) N17.1
- cystic medial (aorta) — *see* Dissection, aorta
- dental pulp K04.1
- esophagus K22.8
- ethmoid (bone) J32.2
- eyelid — *see* Disorder, eyelid, degenerative
- fat, fatty (generalized) (*see also* Disorder, soft tissue, specified type NEC)
  - abdominal wall K65.4
  - breast (aseptic) (segmental) N64.1
  - localized — *see* Degeneration, by site, fatty
  - mesentery K65.4
  - omentum K65.4
  - pancreas K86.89
  - peritoneum K65.4
  - skin (subcutaneous), newborn P83.0
  - subcutaneous, due to birth injury P15.6

Necrosis — *continued*
- gallbladder — *see* Cholecystitis, acute
- heart — *see* Infarct, myocardium
- hip, aseptic or avascular — *see* Osteonecrosis, by type, femur
- intestine (acute) (hemorrhagic) (massive) (*see also* Infarct, intestine)K55.069
- jaw M27.2
- kidney (bilateral) N28.0
  - acute N17.9
  - cortical (acute) (bilateral) N17.1
    - with ectopic or molar pregnancy O08.4
  - medullary (bilateral) (in acute renal failure) (papillary) N17.2
  - papillary (bilateral) (in acute renal failure) N17.2
  - tubular N17.0
    - with ectopic or molar pregnancy O08.4
    - complicating
      - abortion — *see* Abortion, by type, complicated by, tubular necrosis
      - ectopic or molar pregnancy O08.4
      - pregnancy — *see* Pregnancy, complicated by, diseases of, specified type or system NEC
    - following ectopic or molar pregnancy O08.4
    - traumatic T79.5 ☑
- larynx J38.7
- liver (with hepatic failure) (cell) — *see* Failure, hepatic
  - hemorrhagic, central K76.2
- lung J85.0
- lymphatic gland — *see* Lymphadenitis, acute
- mammary gland (fat) (segmental) N64.1
- mastoid (chronic) — *see* Mastoiditis, chronic
- medullary (acute) (renal) N17.2
- mesentery (*see also* Infarct, intestine)K55.069
  - fat K65.4
- mitral valve — *see* Insufficiency, mitral
- myocardium, myocardial — *see* Infarct, myocardium
- nose J34.0
- omentum (with mesenteric infarction) (*see also* Infarct, intestine)K55.069
  - fat K65.4
- orbit, orbital — *see* Osteomyelitis, orbit
- ossicles, ear — *see* Abnormal, ear ossicles
- ovary N70.92
- pancreas (aseptic) (duct) (fat) K86.89
  - acute (infective) — *see* Pancreatitis, acute
  - infective — *see* Pancreatitis, acute
- papillary (acute) (renal) N17.2
- perineum N90.89
- peritoneum (with mesenteric infarction) (*see also* Infarct, intestine)K55.069
  - fat K65.4
- pharynx J02.9
  - in granulocytopenia — *see* Neutropenia
  - Vincent's A69.1
- phosphorus — *see* subcategory T54.2
- pituitary (gland) E23.0
  - postpartum O99.285
  - Sheehan O99.285
- pressure — *see* Ulcer, pressure, by site
- pulmonary J85.0
- pulp (dental) K04.1
- radiation — *see* Necrosis, by site
- radium — *see* Necrosis, by site
- renal — *see* Necrosis, kidney
- sclera H15.89
- scrotum N50.89
- skin or subcutaneous tissue NEC I96
- spine, spinal (column) (*see also* Osteonecrosis, by type, vertebra)
  - cord G95.19
- spleen D73.5
- stomach K31.89
- stomatitis (ulcerative) A69.0
- subcutaneous fat, newborn P83.8
- subendocardial (acute) I21.4
  - chronic I25.89
- suprarenal (capsule) (gland) E27.49
- testis N50.89
- thymus (gland) E32.8
- tonsil J35.8
- trachea J39.8
- tuberculous NEC — *see* Tuberculosis
- tubular (acute) (anoxic) (renal) (toxic) N17.0
  - postprocedural N99.0
- vagina N89.8
- vertebra (*see also* Osteonecrosis, by type, vertebra)
  - tuberculous A18.01

Necrosis — *continued*
- vulva N90.89
- X-ray — *see* Necrosis, by site

Necrospermia — *see* Infertility, male
Need (for)
- care provider because (of)
  - assistance with personal care Z74.1
  - continuous supervision required Z74.3
  - impaired mobility Z74.09
  - no other household member able to render care Z74.2
  - specified reason NEC Z74.8
- immunization — *see* Vaccination
- vaccination — *see* Vaccination

Neglect
- adult
  - confirmed T74.01 ☑
  - history of Z91.412
  - suspected T76.01 ☑
- child (childhood)
  - confirmed T74.02 ☑
  - history of Z62.812
  - suspected T76.02 ☑
- emotional, in childhood Z62.898
- hemispatial R41.4
- left-sided R41.4
- sensory R41.4
- visuospatial R41.4

Neisserian infection NEC — *see* Gonococcus
Nelaton's syndrome G60.8
Nelson's syndrome E24.1
Nematodiasis (intestinal) B82.0
- Ancylostoma B76.0

Neonatal (*see also* Newborn)
- acne L70.4
- bradycardia P29.12
- tachycardia P29.11
- screening, abnormal findings on P09
- tooth, teeth K00.6

Neonatorum — *see* condition
Neoplasia
- endocrine, multiple (MEN) E31.20
  - type I E31.21
  - type IIA E31.22
  - type IIB E31.23
- intraepithelial (histologically confirmed)
  - anal (AIN) (histologically confirmed) K62.82
    - grade I K62.82
    - grade II K62.82
    - severe D01.3
  - cervical glandular (histologically confirmed) D06.9
  - cervix (uteri) (CIN) (histologically confirmed) N87.9
    - glandular D06.9
    - grade I N87.0
    - grade II N87.1
    - grade III (severe dysplasia) (*see also* Carcinoma, cervix uteri, in situ)D06.9
  - prostate (histologically confirmed) (PIN) N42.31
    - grade I N42.31
    - grade II N42.31
    - grade III (severe dysplasia) D07.5
  - vagina (histologically confirmed) (VAIN) N89.3
    - grade I N89.0
    - grade II N89.1
    - grade III (severe dysplasia) D07.2
  - vulva (histologically confirmed) (VIN) N90.3
    - grade I N90.0
    - grade II N90.1
    - grade III (severe dysplasia) D07.1

Neoplasm, neoplastic (*see also* Table of Neoplasms)
- lipomatous, benign — *see* Lipoma

Neovascularization
- ciliary body — *see* Disorder, iris, vascular
- cornea H16.40 ☑
  - deep H16.44 ☑
  - ghost vessels — *see* Ghost, vessels
  - localized H16.43 ☑
  - pannus — *see* Pannus
- iris — *see* Disorder, iris, vascular
- retina H35.05 ☑

Nephralgia N23
Nephritis, nephritic (albuminuric) (azotemic) (congenital) (disseminated) (epithelial) (familial) (focal) (granulomatous) (hemorrhagic) (infantile) (nonsuppurative, excretory) (uremic) N05.9
- with
  - dense deposit disease N05.6
  - diffuse
    - crescentic glomerulonephritis N05.7

- **Nephritis** — *continued*
  - with — *continued*
      - endocapillary proliferative glomerulonephritis N05.4
      - membranous glomerulonephritis N05.2
      - mesangial proliferative glomerulonephritis N05.3
      - mesangiocapillary glomerulonephritis N05.5
    - edema — *see* Nephrosis
    - focal and segmental glomerular lesions N05.1
    - foot process disease N04.9
    - glomerular lesion
      - diffuse sclerosing N05.8
      - hypocomplementemic — *see* Nephritis, membranoproliferative
      - IgA — *see* Nephropathy, IgA
      - lobular, lobulonodular — *see* Nephritis, membranoproliferative
      - nodular — *see* Nephritis, membranoproliferative
    - lesion of
      - glomerulonephritis, proliferative N05.8
      - renal necrosis N05.9
    - minor glomerular abnormality N05.0
    - specified morphological changes NEC N05.8
  - acute N00.9
    - with
      - dense deposit disease N00.6
      - diffuse
        - crescentic glomerulonephritis N00.7
        - endocapillary proliferative glomerulonephritis N00.4
        - membranous glomerulonephritis N00.2
        - mesangial proliferative glomerulonephritis N00.3
        - mesangiocapillary glomerulonephritis N00.5
      - focal and segmental glomerular lesions N00.1
      - minor glomerular abnormality N00.0
      - specified morphological changes NEC N00.8
  - amyloid E85.4 *[N08]*
  - antiglomerular basement membrane (anti-GBM) antibody NEC
    - in Goodpasture's syndrome M31.0
  - antitubular basement membrane (tubulo-interstitial) NEC N12
    - toxic — *see* Nephropathy, toxic
  - arteriolar — *see* Hypertension, kidney
  - arteriosclerotic — *see* Hypertension, kidney
  - ascending — *see* Nephritis, tubulo-interstitial
  - atrophic N03.9
  - Balkan (endemic) N15.0
  - calculous, calculus — *see* Calculus, kidney
  - cardiac — *see* Hypertension, kidney
  - cardiovascular — *see* Hypertension, kidney
  - chronic N03.9
    - with
      - dense deposit disease N03.6
      - diffuse
        - crescentic glomerulonephritis N03.7
        - endocapillary proliferative glomerulonephritis N03.4
        - membranous glomerulonephritis N03.2
        - mesangial proliferative glomerulonephritis N03.3
        - mesangiocapillary glomerulonephritis N03.5
      - focal and segmental glomerular lesions N03.1
      - minor glomerular abnormality N03.0
      - specified morphological changes NEC N03.8
    - arteriosclerotic — *see* Hypertension, kidney
  - cirrhotic N26.9
  - complicating pregnancy O26.83 ☑
  - croupous N00.9
  - degenerative — *see* Nephrosis
  - diffuse sclerosing N05.8
  - due to
    - diabetes mellitus — *see* E08-E13 with .21
    - subacute bacterial endocarditis I33.0
    - systemic lupus erythematosus (chronic) M32.14
    - typhoid fever A01.09
  - gonococcal (acute) (chronic) A54.21
  - hypocomplementemic — *see* Nephritis, membranoproliferative
  - IgA — *see* Nephropathy, IgA
  - immune complex (circulating) NEC N05.8
  - infective — *see* Nephritis, tubulo-interstitial
  - interstitial — *see* Nephritis, tubulo-interstitial
  - lead N14.3

- **Nephritis** — *continued*
  - membranoproliferative (diffuse) (type 1 or 3) (*see also* N00-N07 with fourth character .5)N05.5
    - type 2 (*see also* N00-N07 with fourth character .6)N05.6
  - minimal change N05.0
  - necrotic, necrotizing NEC (*see also* N00-N07 with fourth character .8)N05.8
  - nephrotic — *see* Nephrosis
  - nodular — *see* Nephritis, membranoproliferative
  - polycystic Q61.3
    - adult type Q61.2
    - autosomal
      - dominant Q61.2
      - recessive NEC Q61.19
    - childhood type NEC Q61.19
    - infantile type NEC Q61.19
  - poststreptococcal N05.9
    - acute N00.9
    - chronic N03.9
    - rapidly progressive N01.9
  - proliferative NEC (*see also* N00-N07 with fourth character .8)N05.8
  - purulent — *see* Nephritis, tubulo-interstitial
  - rapidly progressive N01.9
    - with
      - dense deposit disease N01.6
      - diffuse
        - crescentic glomerulonephritis N01.7
        - endocapillary proliferative glomerulonephritis N01.4
        - membranous glomerulonephritis N01.2
        - mesangial proliferative glomerulonephritis N01.3
        - mesangiocapillary glomerulonephritis N01.5
      - focal and segmental glomerular lesions N01.1
      - minor glomerular abnormality N01.0
      - specified morphological changes NEC N01.8
  - salt losing or wasting NEC N28.89
  - saturnine N14.3
  - sclerosing, diffuse N05.8
  - septic — *see* Nephritis, tubulo-interstitial
  - specified pathology NEC (*see also* N00-N07 with fourth character .8)N05.8
  - subacute N01.9
  - suppurative — *see* Nephritis, tubulo-interstitial
  - syphilitic (late) A52.75
    - congenital A50.59 *[N08]*
    - early (secondary) A51.44
  - toxic — *see* Nephropathy, toxic
  - tubal, tubular — *see* Nephritis, tubulo-interstitial
  - tuberculous A18.11
  - tubulo-interstitial (in) N12
    - acute (infectious) N10
    - chronic (infectious) N11.9
      - nonobstructive N11.8
        - reflux-associated N11.0
      - obstructive N11.1
      - specified NEC N11.8
    - due to
      - brucellosis A23.9 *[N16]*
      - cryoglobulinemia D89.1 *[N16]*
      - glycogen storage disease E74.00 *[N16]*
    - Sjögren's syndrome M35.04
  - vascular — *see* Hypertension, kidney
  - war N00.9
- **Nephroblastoma** (epithelial) (mesenchymal) C64 ☑
- **Nephrocalcinosis** E83.59 *[N29]*
- **Nephrocystitis,** pustular — *see* Nephritis, tubulo-interstitial
- **Nephrolithiasis** (congenital) (pelvis) (recurrent) (*see also* Calculus, kidney)
- **Nephroma** C64 ☑
  - mesoblastic D41.0 ☑
- **Nephronephritis** — *see* Nephrosis
- **Nephronophthisis** Q61.5
- **Nephropathia** epidemica A98.5
- **Nephropathy** (*see also* Nephritis)N28.9
  - with
    - edema — *see* Nephrosis
    - glomerular lesion — *see* Glomerulonephritis
  - amyloid, hereditary E85.0
  - analgesic N14.0
    - with medullary necrosis, acute N17.2
  - Balkan (endemic) N15.0
  - chemical — *see* Nephropathy, toxic
  - diabetic — *see* E08-E13 with .21
  - drug-induced N14.2
    - specified NEC N14.1
  - focal and segmental hyalinosis or sclerosis N02.1

- **Nephropathy** — *continued*
  - heavy metal-induced N14.3
  - hereditary NEC N07.9
    - with
      - dense deposit disease N07.6
      - diffuse
        - crescentic glomerulonephritis N07.7
        - endocapillary proliferative glomerulonephritis N07.4
        - membranous glomerulonephritis N07.2
        - mesangial proliferative glomerulonephritis N07.3
        - mesangiocapillary glomerulonephritis N07.5
      - focal and segmental glomerular lesions N07.1
      - minor glomerular abnormality N07.0
      - specified morphological changes NEC N07.8
  - hypercalcemic N25.89
  - hypertensive — *see* Hypertension, kidney
  - hypokalemic (vacuolar) N25.89
  - IgA N02.8
    - with glomerular lesion N02.9
      - focal and segmental hyalinosis or sclerosis N02.1
      - membranoproliferative (diffuse) N02.5
      - membranous (diffuse) N02.2
      - mesangial proliferative (diffuse) N02.3
      - mesangiocapillary (diffuse) N02.5
      - proliferative NEC N02.8
      - specified pathology NEC N02.8
  - lead N14.3
  - membranoproliferative (diffuse) N02.5
  - membranous (diffuse) N02.2
  - mesangial (IgA/IgG) — *see* Nephropathy, IgA
    - proliferative (diffuse) N02.3
  - mesangiocapillary (diffuse) N02.5
  - obstructive N13.8
  - phenacetin N17.2
  - phosphate-losing N25.0
  - potassium depletion N25.89
  - pregnancy-related O26.83 ☑
  - proliferative NEC (*see also* N00-N07 with fourth character .8)N05.8
  - protein-losing N25.89
  - saturnine N14.3
  - sickle-cell D57.☑ *[N08]*
  - toxic NEC N14.4
    - due to
      - drugs N14.2
        - analgesic N14.0
        - specified NEC N14.1
      - heavy metals N14.3
  - vasomotor N17.0
  - water-losing N25.89
- **Nephroptosis** N28.83
- **Nephropyosis** — *see* Abscess, kidney
- **Nephrorrhagia** N28.89
- **Nephrosclerosis** (arteriolar) (arteriosclerotic) (chronic) (hyaline) (*see also* Hypertension, kidney)
  - hyperplastic — *see* Hypertension, kidney
  - senile N26.9
- **Nephrosis,** nephrotic (Epstein's) (syndrome) (congenital) N04.9
  - with
    - foot process disease N04.9
    - glomerular lesion N04.1
      - hypocomplementemic N04.5
  - acute N04.9
  - anoxic — *see* Nephrosis, tubular
  - chemical — *see* Nephrosis, tubular
  - cholemic K76.7
  - diabetic — *see* E08-E13 with .21
  - Finnish type (congenital) Q89.8
  - hemoglobin N10
  - hemoglobinuric — *see* Nephrosis, tubular
  - in
    - amyloidosis E85.4 *[N08]*
    - diabetes mellitus — *see* E08-E13 with .21
    - epidemic hemorrhagic fever A98.5
    - malaria (malariae) B52.0
  - ischemic — *see* Nephrosis, tubular
  - lipoid N04.9
  - lower nephron — *see* Nephrosis, tubular
  - malarial (malariae) B52.0
  - minimal change N04.0
  - myoglobin N10
  - necrotizing — *see* Nephrosis, tubular
  - osmotic (sucrose) N25.89
  - radiation N04.9
  - syphilitic (late) A52.75
  - toxic — *see* Nephrosis, tubular

Nephrosis - Neuropathy

- **Nephrosis** — *continued*
  - tubular (acute) N17.0
    - postprocedural N99.0
    - radiation N04.9
- **Nephrosonephritis,** hemorrhagic (endemic) A98.5
- **Nephrostomy**
  - attention to Z43.6
  - status Z93.6
- **Nerve** (*see also* condition)
  - injury — *see* Injury, nerve, by body site
- **Nerves** R45.0
- **Nervous** (*see also* condition)R45.0
  - heart F45.8
  - stomach F45.8
  - tension R45.0
- **Nervousness** R45.0
- **Nesidioblastoma**
  - pancreas D13.7
  - specified site NEC — *see* Neoplasm, benign, by site
  - unspecified site D13.7
- **Nettleship's** syndrome Q82.2
- **Neumann's** disease or syndrome L10.1
- **Neuralgia,** neuralgic (acute) M79.2
  - accessory (nerve) G52.8
  - acoustic (nerve) — *see* subcategory H93.3
  - auditory (nerve) — *see* subcategory H93.3
  - ciliary G44.009
    - intractable G44.001
    - not intractable G44.009
  - cranial
    - nerve (*see also* Disorder, nerve, cranial)
      - fifth or trigeminal — *see* Neuralgia, trigeminal
    - postherpetic, postzoster B02.29
  - ear — *see* subcategory H92.0
  - facialis vera G51.1
  - Fothergill's — *see* Neuralgia, trigeminal
  - glossopharyngeal (nerve) G52.1
  - Horton's G44.099
    - intractable G44.091
    - not intractable G44.099
  - Hunt's B02.21
  - hypoglossal (nerve) G52.3
  - infraorbital — *see* Neuralgia, trigeminal
  - malarial — *see* Malaria
  - migrainous G44.009
    - intractable G44.001
    - not intractable G44.009
  - Morton's G57.6 ☑
  - nerve, cranial — *see* Disorder, nerve, cranial
  - nose G52.0
  - occipital M54.81
  - olfactory G52.0
  - penis N48.9
  - perineum R10.2
  - postherpetic NEC B02.29
    - trigeminal B02.22
  - pubic region R10.2
  - scrotum R10.2
  - Sluder's G44.89
  - specified nerve NEC G58.8
  - spermatic cord R10.2
  - sphenopalatine (ganglion) G90.09
  - trifacial — *see* Neuralgia, trigeminal
  - trigeminal G50.0
    - postherpetic, postzoster B02.22
  - vagus (nerve) G52.2
  - writer's F48.8
    - organic G25.89
- **Neurapraxia** — *see* Injury, nerve
- **Neurasthenia** F48.8
  - cardiac F45.8
  - gastric F45.8
  - heart F45.8
- **Neurilemmoma** (*see also* Neoplasm, nerve, benign)
  - acoustic (nerve) D33.3
  - malignant (*see also* Neoplasm, nerve, malignant)
    - acoustic (nerve) C72.4 ☑
- **Neurilemmosarcoma** — *see* Neoplasm, nerve, malignant
- **Neurinoma** — *see* Neoplasm, nerve, benign
- **Neurinomatosis** — *see* Neoplasm, nerve, uncertain behavior
- **Neuritis** (rheumatoid) M79.2
  - abducens (nerve) — *see* Strabismus, paralytic, sixth nerve
  - accessory (nerve) G52.8
  - acoustic (nerve) (*see also* subcategory)H93.3 ☑
    - in (due to)
      - infectious disease NEC B99 ☑ *[H94.0-]*
      - parasitic disease NEC B89 *[H94.0-]*
    - syphilitic A52.15
- **Neuritis** — *continued*
  - alcoholic G62.1
    - with psychosis — *see* Psychosis, alcoholic
  - amyloid, any site E85.4 *[G63]*
  - auditory (nerve) — *see* subcategory H93.3
  - brachial — *see* Radiculopathy
    - due to displacement, intervertebral disc — *see* Disorder, disc, cervical, with neuritis
  - cranial nerve
    - due to Lyme disease A69.22
    - eighth or acoustic or auditory — *see* subcategory H93.3
    - eleventh or accessory G52.8
    - fifth or trigeminal G51.0
    - first or olfactory G52.0
    - fourth or trochlear — *see* Strabismus, paralytic, fourth nerve
    - second or optic — *see* Neuritis, optic
    - seventh or facial G51.8
      - newborn (birth injury) P11.3
    - sixth or abducent — *see* Strabismus, paralytic, sixth nerve
    - tenth or vagus G52.2
    - third or oculomotor — *see* Strabismus, paralytic, third nerve
    - twelfth or hypoglossal G52.3
  - Déjérine-Sottas G60.0
  - diabetic (mononeuropathy) — *see* E08-E13 with .41
    - polyneuropathy — *see* E08-E13 with .42
  - due to
    - beriberi E51.11
    - displacement, prolapse or rupture, intervertebral disc — *see* Disorder, disc, with, radiculopathy
    - herniation, nucleus pulposus M51.9 *[G55]*
  - endemic E51.11
  - facial G51.8
    - newborn (birth injury) P11.3
  - general — *see* Polyneuropathy
  - geniculate ganglion G51.1
    - due to herpes (zoster) B02.21
  - gouty (*see also* Gout, by type)M10.9 *[G63]*
  - hypoglossal (nerve) G52.3
  - ilioinguinal (nerve) G57.9 ☑
  - infectious (multiple) NEC G61.0
  - interstitial hypertrophic progressive G60.0
  - lumbar M54.16
  - lumbosacral M54.17
  - multiple (*see also* Polyneuropathy)
    - endemic E51.11
    - infective, acute G61.0
  - multiplex endemica E51.11
  - nerve root — *see* Radiculopathy
  - oculomotor (nerve) — *see* Strabismus, paralytic, third nerve
  - olfactory nerve G52.0
  - optic (nerve) (hereditary) (sympathetic) H46.9
    - with demyelination G36.0
    - in myelitis G36.0
    - nutritional H46.2
    - papillitis — *see* Papillitis, optic
    - retrobulbar H46.1 ☑
    - specified type NEC H46.8
    - toxic H46.3
  - peripheral (nerve) G62.9
    - multiple — *see* Polyneuropathy
    - single — *see* Mononeuritis
  - pneumogastric (nerve) G52.2
  - postherpetic, postzoster B02.29
  - progressive hypertrophic interstitial G60.0
  - retrobulbar (*see also* Neuritis, optic, retrobulbar)
    - in (due to)
      - late syphilis A52.15
      - meningococcal infection A39.82
    - meningococcal A39.82
    - syphilitic A52.15
  - sciatic (nerve) (*see also* Sciatica)
    - due to displacement of intervertebral disc — *see* Disorder, disc, with, radiculopathy
  - serum (*see also* Reaction, serum)T80.69 ☑
  - shoulder-girdle G54.5
  - specified nerve NEC G58.8
  - spinal (nerve) root — *see* Radiculopathy
  - syphilitic A52.15
  - thenar (median) G56.1 ☑
  - thoracic M54.14
  - toxic NEC G62.2
  - trochlear (nerve) — *see* Strabismus, paralytic, fourth nerve
  - vagus (nerve) G52.2
- **Neuroastrocytoma** — *see* Neoplasm, uncertain behavior, by site
- **Neuroavitaminosis** E56.9 *[G99.8]*
- **Neuroblastoma**
  - olfactory C30.0
  - specified site — *see* Neoplasm, malignant, by site
  - unspecified site C74.90
- **Neurochorioretinitis** — *see* Chorioretinitis
- **Neurocirculatory** asthenia F45.8
- **Neurocysticercosis** B69.0
- **Neurocytoma** — *see* Neoplasm, benign, by site
- **Neurodermatitis** (circumscribed) (circumscripta) (local) L28.0
  - atopic L20.81
  - diffuse (Brocq) L20.81
  - disseminated L20.81
- **Neuroencephalomyelopathy,** optic G36.0
- **Neuroepithelioma** (*see also* Neoplasm, malignant, by site)
  - olfactory C30.0
- **Neurofibroma** (*see also* Neoplasm, nerve, benign)
  - melanotic — *see* Neoplasm, nerve, benign
  - multiple — *see* Neurofibromatosis
  - plexiform — *see* Neoplasm, nerve, benign
- **Neurofibromatosis** (multiple) (nonmalignant) Q85.00
  - acoustic Q85.02
  - malignant — *see* Neoplasm, nerve, malignant
  - specified NEC Q85.09
  - type 1 (von Recklinghausen) Q85.01
  - type 2 Q85.02
- **Neurofibrosarcoma** — *see* Neoplasm, nerve, malignant
- **Neurogenic** (*see also* condition)
  - bladder (*see also* Dysfunction, bladder, neuromuscular)N31.9
    - cauda equina syndrome G83.4
  - bowel NEC K59.2
  - heart F45.8
- **Neuroglioma** — *see* Neoplasm, uncertain behavior, by site
- **Neurolabyrinthitis** (of Dix and Hallpike) — *see* Neuronitis, vestibular
- **Neurolathyrism** — *see* Poisoning, food, noxious, plant
- **Neuroleprosy** A30.9
- **Neuroma** (*see also* Neoplasm, nerve, benign)
  - acoustic (nerve) D33.3
  - amputation (stump) (traumatic) (surgical complication) (late) T87.3 ☑
    - arm T87.3 ☑
    - leg T87.3 ☑
  - digital (toe) G57.6 ☑
  - interdigital G58.8
    - lower limb (toe) G57.8 ☑
    - upper limb G56.8 ☑
  - intermetatarsal G57.8 ☑
  - Morton's G57.6 ☑
  - nonneoplastic
    - arm G56.9 ☑
    - leg G57.9 ☑
    - lower extremity G57.9 ☑
    - upper extremity G56.9 ☑
  - optic (nerve) D33.3
  - plantar G57.6 ☑
  - plexiform — *see* Neoplasm, nerve, benign
  - surgical (nonneoplastic)
    - arm G56.9 ☑
    - leg G57.9 ☑
    - lower extremity G57.9 ☑
    - upper extremity G56.9 ☑
- **Neuromyalgia** — *see* Neuralgia
- **Neuromyasthenia** (epidemic) (postinfectious) G93.3
- **Neuromyelitis** G36.9
  - ascending G61.0
  - optica G36.0
- **Neuromyopathy** G70.9
  - paraneoplastic D49.9 *[G13.0]*
- **Neuromyotonia** (Isaacs) G71.19
- **Neuronevus** — *see* Nevus
- **Neuronitis** G58.9
  - ascending (acute) G57.2 ☑
  - vestibular H81.2 ☑
- **Neuroparalytic** — *see* condition
- **Neuropathy,** neuropathic G62.9
  - acute motor G62.81
  - alcoholic G62.1
    - with psychosis — *see* Psychosis, alcoholic
  - arm G56.9 ☑
  - autonomic, peripheral — *see* Neuropathy, peripheral, autonomic
  - axillary G56.9 ☑

- **Neuropathy** — *continued*
  - bladder N31.9
    - atonic (motor) (sensory) N31.2
    - autonomous N31.2
    - flaccid N31.2
    - nonreflex N31.2
    - reflex N31.1
    - uninhibited N31.0
  - brachial plexus G54.0
  - cervical plexus G54.2
  - chronic
    - progressive segmentally demyelinating G62.89
    - relapsing demyelinating G62.89
  - Déjérine-Sottas G60.0
  - diabetic — *see* E08-E13 with .40
    - mononeuropathy — *see* E08-E13 with .41
    - polyneuropathy — *see* E08-E13 with .42
  - entrapment G58.9
    - iliohypogastric nerve G57.8 ☑
    - ilioinguinal nerve G57.8 ☑
    - lateral cutaneous nerve of thigh G57.1 ☑
    - median nerve G56.0 ☑
    - obturator nerve G57.8 ☑
    - peroneal nerve G57.3 ☑
    - posterior tibial nerve G57.5 ☑
    - saphenous nerve G57.8 ☑
    - ulnar nerve G56.2 ☑
  - facial nerve G51.9
  - hereditary G60.9
    - motor and sensory (types I-IV) G60.0
    - sensory G60.8
    - specified NEC G60.8
  - hypertrophic G60.0
    - Charcot-Marie-Tooth G60.0
    - Déjérine-Sottas G60.0
    - interstitial progressive G60.0
    - of infancy G60.0
    - Refsum G60.1
  - idiopathic G60.9
    - progressive G60.3
    - specified NEC G60.8
  - in association with hereditary ataxia G60.2
  - intercostal G58.0
  - ischemic — *see* Disorder, nerve
  - Jamaica (ginger) G62.2
  - leg NEC G57.9 ☑
  - lower extremity G57.9 ☑
  - lumbar plexus G54.1
  - median nerve G56.1 ☑
  - motor and sensory (*see also* Polyneuropathy)
    - hereditary (types I-IV) G60.0
  - multifocal motor (MMN) G61.82
  - multiple (acute) (chronic) — *see* Polyneuropathy
  - optic (nerve) (*see also* Neuritis, optic)
    - ischemic H47.01 ☑
  - paraneoplastic (sensorial) (Denny Brown) D49.9 *[G13.0]*
  - peripheral (nerve) (*see also* Polyneuropathy)G62.9
    - autonomic G90.9
      - idiopathic G90.09
      - in (due to)
        - amyloidosis E85.4 *[G99.0]*
        - diabetes mellitus — *see* E08-E13 with .43
        - endocrine disease NEC E34.9 *[G99.0]*
        - gout M10.00 *[G99.0]*
        - hyperthyroidism E05.90 *[G99.0]*
          - with thyroid storm E05.91 *[G99.0]*
        - metabolic disease NEC E88.9 *[G99.0]*
    - idiopathic G60.9
      - progressive G60.3
    - in (due to)
      - antitetanus serum G62.0
      - arsenic G62.2
      - drugs NEC G62.0
      - lead G62.2
      - organophosphate compounds G62.2
      - toxic agent NEC G62.2
  - plantar nerves G57.6 ☑
  - progressive
    - hypertrophic interstitial G60.0
    - inflammatory G62.81
  - radicular NEC — *see* Radiculopathy
  - sacral plexus G54.1
  - sciatic G57.0 ☑
  - serum G61.1
  - toxic NEC G62.2
  - trigeminal sensory G50.8
  - ulnar nerve G56.2 ☑
  - uremic N18.9 *[G63]*
  - vitamin B12 E53.8 *[G63]*
    - with anemia (pernicious) D51.0 *[G63]*
      - due to dietary deficiency D51.3 *[G63]*
- **Neurophthisis** (*see also* Disorder, nerve)
  - peripheral, diabetic — *see* E08-E13 with .42
- **Neuroretinitis** — *see* Chorioretinitis
- **Neuroretinopathy,** hereditary optic H47.22
- **Neurosarcoma** — *see* Neoplasm, nerve, malignant
- **Neurosclerosis** — *see* Disorder, nerve
- **Neurosis,** neurotic F48.9
  - anankastic F42.8
  - anxiety (state) F41.1
    - panic type F41.0
  - asthenic F48.8
  - bladder F45.8
  - cardiac (reflex) F45.8
  - cardiovascular F45.8
  - character F60.9
  - colon F45.8
  - compensation F68.1 ☑
  - compulsive, compulsion F42.8
  - conversion F44.9
  - craft F48.8
  - cutaneous F45.8
  - depersonalization F48.1
  - depressive (reaction) (type) F34.1
  - environmental F48.8
  - excoriation L98.1
  - fatigue F48.8
  - functional — *see* Disorder, somatoform
  - gastric F45.8
  - gastrointestinal F45.8
  - heart F45.8
  - hypochondriacal F45.21
  - hysterical F44.9
  - incoordination F45.8
    - larynx F45.8
    - vocal cord F45.8
  - intestine F45.8
  - larynx (sensory) F45.8
    - hysterical F44.4
  - mixed NEC F48.8
  - musculoskeletal F45.8
  - obsessional F42.8
  - obsessive-compulsive F42.8
  - occupational F48.8
  - ocular NEC F45.8
  - organ — *see* Disorder, somatoform
  - pharynx F45.8
  - phobic F40.9
  - posttraumatic (situational) F43.10
    - acute F43.11
    - chronic F43.12
  - psychasthenic (type) F48.8
  - railroad F48.8
  - rectum F45.8
  - respiratory F45.8
  - rumination F45.8
  - sexual F65.9
  - situational F48.8
  - social F40.10
    - generalized F40.11
  - specified type NEC F48.8
  - state F48.9
    - with depersonalization episode F48.1
  - stomach F45.8
  - traumatic F43.10
    - acute F43.11
    - chronic F43.12
  - vasomotor F45.8
  - visceral F45.8
  - war F48.8
- **Neurospongioblastosis** diffusa Q85.1
- **Neurosyphilis** (arrested) (early) (gumma) (late) (latent) (recurrent) (relapse) A52.3
  - with ataxia (cerebellar) (locomotor) (spastic) (spinal) A52.19
  - aneurysm (cerebral) A52.05
  - arachnoid (adhesive) A52.13
  - arteritis (any artery) (cerebral) A52.04
  - asymptomatic A52.2
  - congenital A50.40
  - dura (mater) A52.13
  - general paresis A52.17
  - hemorrhagic A52.05
  - juvenile (asymptomatic) (meningeal) A50.40
  - leptomeninges (aseptic) A52.13
  - meningeal, meninges (adhesive) A52.13
  - meningitis A52.13
  - meningovascular (diffuse) A52.13
  - optic atrophy A52.15
  - parenchymatous (degenerative) A52.19
  - paresis, paretic A52.17
    - juvenile A50.45
  - remission in (sustained) A52.3
- **Neurosyphilis** — *continued*
  - serological (without symptoms) A52.2
  - specified nature or site NEC A52.19
  - tabes, tabetic (dorsalis) A52.11
    - juvenile A50.45
  - taboparesis A52.17
    - juvenile A50.45
  - thrombosis (cerebral) A52.05
  - vascular (cerebral) NEC A52.05
- **Neurothekeoma** — *see* Neoplasm, nerve, benign
- **Neurotic** — *see* Neurosis
- **Neurotoxemia** — *see* Toxemia
- **Neutroclusion** M26.211
- **Neutropenia,** neutropenic (chronic) (genetic) (idiopathic) (immune) (infantile) (malignant) (pernicious) (splenic) D70.9
  - congenital (primary) D70.0
  - cyclic D70.4
  - cytoreductive cancer chemotherapy sequela D70.1
  - drug-induced D70.2
    - due to cytoreductive cancer chemotherapy D70.1
  - due to infection D70.3
  - fever D70.9
  - neonatal, transitory (isoimmune) (maternal transfer) P61.5
  - periodic D70.4
  - secondary (cyclic) (periodic) (splenic) D70.4
    - drug-induced D70.2
      - due to cytoreductive cancer chemotherapy D70.1
  - toxic D70.8
- **Neutrophilia,** hereditary giant D72.0
- **Nevocarcinoma** — *see* Melanoma
- **Nevus** D22.9
  - achromic — *see* Neoplasm, skin, benign
  - amelanotic — *see* Neoplasm, skin, benign
  - angiomatousD18.00
    - intra-abdominal D18.03
    - intracranial D18.02
    - skin D18.01
    - specified site NEC D18.09
  - araneus I78.1
  - balloon cell — *see* Neoplasm, skin, benign
  - bathing trunk D48.5
  - blue — *see* Neoplasm, skin, benign
    - cellular — *see* Neoplasm, skin, benign
    - giant — *see* Neoplasm, skin, benign
    - Jadassohn's — *see* Neoplasm, skin, benign
    - malignant — *see* Melanoma
  - capillary D18.00
    - intra-abdominal D18.03
    - intracranial D18.02
    - skin D18.01
    - specified site NEC D18.09
  - cavernous D18.00
    - intra-abdominal D18.03
    - intracranial D18.02
    - skin D18.01
    - specified site NEC D18.09
  - cellular — *see* Neoplasm, skin, benign
    - blue — *see* Neoplasm, skin, benign
  - choroid D31.3 ☑
  - comedonicus Q82.5
  - conjunctiva D31.0 ☑
  - dermal — *see* Neoplasm, skin, benign
    - with epidermal nevus — *see* Neoplasm, skin, benign
  - dysplastic — *see* Neoplasm, skin, benign
  - eye D31.9 ☑
  - flammeus Q82.5
  - hemangiomatous D18.00
    - intra-abdominal D18.03
    - intracranial D18.02
    - skin D18.01
    - specified site NEC D18.09
  - iris D31.4 ☑
  - lacrimal gland D31.5 ☑
  - lymphatic D18.1
  - magnocellular
    - specified site — *see* Neoplasm, benign, by site
    - unspecified site D31.40
  - malignant — *see* Melanoma
  - meaning hemangioma D18.00
    - intra-abdominal D18.03
    - intracranial D18.02
    - skin D18.01
    - specified site NEC D18.09
  - mouth (mucosa) D10.30
    - specified site NEC D10.39
    - white sponge Q38.6

- **Nevus** — *continued*
  - multiplex Q85.1
  - non-neoplastic I78.1
  - oral mucosa D10.30
    - specified site NEC D10.39
    - white sponge Q38.6
  - orbit D31.6 ☑
  - pigmented
    - giant (*see also* Neoplasm, skin, uncertain behavior) D48.5
      - malignant melanoma in — *see* Melanoma
  - portwine Q82.5
  - retina D31.2 ☑
  - retrobulbar D31.6 ☑
  - sanguineous Q82.5
  - senile I78.1
  - skin D22.9
    - abdominal wall D22.5
    - ala nasi D22.39
    - ankle D22.7 ☑
    - anus, anal D22.5
    - arm D22.6 ☑
    - auditory canal (external) D22.2 ☑
    - auricle (ear) D22.2 ☑
    - auricular canal (external) D22.2 ☑
    - axilla, axillary fold D22.5
    - back D22.5
    - breast D22.5
    - brow D22.39
    - buttock D22.5
    - canthus (eye) D22.1 ☑
    - cheek (external) D22.39
    - chest wall D22.5
    - chin D22.39
    - ear (external) D22.2 ☑
    - external meatus (ear) D22.2 ☑
    - eyebrow D22.39
    - eyelid (lower) (upper) D22.1 ☑
    - face D22.30
      - specified NEC D22.39
    - female genital organ (external) NEC D28.0
    - finger D22.6 ☑
    - flank D22.5
    - foot D22.7 ☑
    - forearm D22.6 ☑
    - forehead D22.39
    - foreskin D29.0
    - genital organ (external) NEC
      - female D28.0
      - male D29.9
    - gluteal region D22.5
    - groin D22.5
    - hand D22.6 ☑
    - heel D22.7 ☑
    - helix D22.2 ☑
    - hip D22.7 ☑
    - interscapular region D22.5
    - jaw D22.39
    - knee D22.7 ☑
    - labium (majus) (minus) D28.0
    - leg D22.7 ☑
    - lip (lower) (upper) D22.0
    - lower limb D22.7 ☑
    - male genital organ (external) D29.9
    - nail D22.9
      - finger D22.6 ☑
      - toe D22.7 ☑
    - nasolabial groove D22.39
    - nates D22.5
    - neck D22.4
    - nose (external) D22.39
    - palpbrae D22.1 ☑
    - penis D29.0
    - perianal skin D22.5
    - perineum D22.5
    - pinna D22.2 ☑
    - popliteal fossa or space D22.7 ☑
    - prepuce D29.0
    - pudendum D28.0
    - scalp D22.4
    - scrotum D29.4
    - shoulder D22.6 ☑
    - submammary fold D22.5
    - temple D22.39
    - thigh D22.7 ☑
    - toe D22.7 ☑
    - trunk NEC D22.5
    - umbilicus D22.5
    - upper limb D22.6 ☑
    - vulva D28.0
  - specified site NEC — *see* Neoplasm, by site, benign

- **Nevus** — *continued*
  - spider I78.1
  - stellar I78.1
  - strawberry Q82.5
  - Sutton's — *see* Neoplasm, skin, benign
  - unius lateris Q82.5
  - Unna's Q82.5
  - vascular Q82.5
  - verrucous Q82.5
- **Newborn** (infant) (liveborn) (singleton) Z38.2
  - acne L70.4
  - abstinence syndrome P96.1
  - affected by
    - abnormalities of membranes P02.9
      - specified NEC P02.8
    - abruptio placenta P02.1
    - amino-acid metabolic disorder, transitory P74.8
    - amniocentesis (while in utero) P00.6
    - amnionitis P02.7
    - apparent life threatening event (ALTE) R68.13
    - bleeding (into)
      - cerebral cortex P52.22
      - germinal matrix P52.0
      - ventricles P52.1
    - breech delivery P03.0
    - cardiac arrest P29.81
    - cardiomyopathy I42.8
      - congenital I42.4
    - cerebral ischemia P91.0
    - Cesarean delivery P03.4
    - chemotherapy agents P04.1
    - chorioamnionitis P02.7
    - cocaine (crack) P04.41
    - complications of labor and delivery P03.9
      - specified NEC P03.89
    - compression of umbilical cord NEC P02.5
    - contracted pelvis P03.1
    - delivery P03.9
      - Cesarean P03.4
      - forceps P03.2
      - vacuum extractor P03.3
    - environmental chemicals P04.6
    - entanglement (knot) in umbilical cord P02.5
    - fetal (intrauterine)
      - growth retardation P05.9
      - malnutrition not light or small for gestational age P05.2
    - forceps delivery P03.2
    - heart rate abnormalities
      - bradycardia P29.12
      - intrauterine P03.819
        - before onset of labor P03.810
        - during labor P03.811
      - tachycardia P29.11
    - hemorrhage (antepartum) P02.1
      - cerebellar (nontraumatic) P52.6
      - intracerebral (nontraumatic) P52.4
      - intracranial (nontraumatic) P52.9
        - specified NEC P52.8
      - intraventricular (nontraumatic) P52.3
        - grade 1 P52.0
        - grade 2 P52.1
        - grade 3 P52.21
        - grade 4 P52.22
      - posterior fossa (nontraumatic) P52.6
      - subarachnoid (nontraumatic) P52.5
      - subependymal P52.0
        - with intracerebral extension P52.22
        - with intraventricular extension P52.1
          - with enlargement of ventricles P52.21
        - without intraventricular extension P52.0
    - hypoxic ischemic encephalopathy [HIE] P91.60
      - mild P91.61
      - moderate P91.62
      - severe P91.63
    - induction of labor P03.89
    - intestinal perforation P78.0
    - intrauterine (fetal) blood loss P50.9
      - due to (from)
        - cut end of co-twin cord P50.5
        - hemorrhage into
          - co-twin P50.3
          - maternal circulation P50.4
        - placenta P50.2
        - ruptured cord blood P50.1
        - vasa previa P50.0
      - specified NEC P50.8
    - intrauterine (fetal) hemorrhage P50.9
    - intrauterine (in utero) procedure P96.5
    - malpresentation (malposition) NEC P03.1
    - maternal (complication of) (use of)
      - alcohol P04.3

- **Newborn** — *continued*
  - affected by — *continued*
      - analgesia (maternal) P04.0
      - anesthesia (maternal) P04.0
      - blood loss P02.1
      - circulatory disease P00.3
      - condition P00.9
        - specified NEC P00.89
      - delivery P03.9
        - Cesarean P03.4
        - forceps P03.2
        - vacuum extractor P03.3
      - diabetes mellitus (pre-existing) P70.1
      - disorder P00.9
        - specified NEC P00.89
      - drugs (addictive) (illegal) NEC P04.49
      - ectopic pregnancy P01.4
      - gestational diabetes P70.0
      - hemorrhage P02.1
      - hypertensive disorder P00.0
      - incompetent cervix P01.0
      - infectious disease P00.2
      - injury P00.5
      - labor and delivery P03.9
      - malpresentation before labor P01.7
      - maternal death P01.6
      - medical procedure P00.7
      - medication P04.1
      - multiple pregnancy P01.5
      - nutritional disorder P00.4
      - oligohydramnios P01.2
      - parasitic disease P00.2
      - periodontal disease P00.81
      - placenta previa P02.0
      - polyhydramnios P01.3
      - precipitate delivery P03.5
      - pregnancy P01.9
        - specified P01.8
      - premature rupture of membranes P01.1
      - renal disease P00.1
      - respiratory disease P00.3
      - surgical procedure P00.6
      - urinary tract disease P00.1
      - uterine contraction (abnormal) P03.6
    - meconium peritonitis P78.0
    - medication (legal) (maternal use) (prescribed) P04.1
    - membrane abnormalities P02.9
      - specified NEC P02.8
    - membranitis P02.7
    - methamphetamine (s) P04.49
    - mixed metabolic and respiratory acidosis P84
    - neonatal abstinence syndrome P96.1
    - noxious substances transmitted via placenta or breast milk P04.9
      - specified NEC P04.8
    - nutritional supplements P04.5
    - placenta previa P02.0
    - placental
      - abnormality (functional) (morphological) P02.20
        - specified NEC P02.29
      - dysfunction P02.29
      - infarction P02.29
      - insufficiency P02.29
      - separation NEC P02.1
      - transfusion syndromes P02.3
    - placentitis P02.7
    - precipitate delivery P03.5
    - prolapsed cord P02.4
    - respiratory arrest P28.81
    - slow intrauterine growth P05.9
    - tobacco P04.2
    - twin to twin transplacental transfusion P02.3
    - umbilical cord (tightly) around neck P02.5
    - umbilical cord condition P02.60
      - short cord P02.69
      - specified NEC P02.69
    - uterine contractions (abnormal) P03.6
    - vasa previa P02.69
      - from intrauterine blood loss P50.0
  - apnea P28.4
    - primary P28.3
    - obstructive P28.4
    - sleep (central) (obstructive) (primary) P28.3
  - born in hospital Z38.00
    - by cesarean Z38.01
  - born outside hospital Z38.1
  - breast buds P96.89
  - breast engorgement P83.4
  - check-up — *see* Newborn, examination
  - convulsion P90

- **Newborn** — *continued*
  - dehydration P74.1
  - examination
    - 8 to 28 days old Z00.111
    - under 8 days old Z00.110
  - fever P81.9
    - environmentally-induced P81.0
  - hyperbilirubinemia P59.9
    - of prematurity P59.0
  - hypernatremia P74.2
  - hyponatremia P74.2
  - infection P39.9
    - candidal P37.5
    - specified NEC P39.8
    - urinary tract P39.3
  - jaundice P59.9
    - due to
      - breast milk inhibitor P59.3
      - hepatocellular damage P59.20
        - specified NEC P59.29
      - preterm delivery P59.0
    - of prematurity P59.0
    - specified NEC P59.8
  - late metabolic acidosis P74.0
  - mastitis P39.0
    - infective P39.0
    - noninfective P83.4
  - multiple born NEC Z38.8
    - born in hospital Z38.68
      - by cesarean Z38.69
    - born outside hospital Z38.7
  - omphalitis P38.9
    - with mild hemorrhage P38.1
    - without hemorrhage P38.9
  - post-term P08.21
  - prolonged gestation (over 42 completed weeks) P08.22
  - quadruplet Z38.8
    - born in hospital Z38.63
      - by cesarean Z38.64
    - born outside hospital Z38.7
  - quintuplet Z38.8
    - born in hospital Z38.65
      - by cesarean Z38.66
    - born outside hospital Z38.7
  - seizure P90
  - sepsis (congenital) P36.9
    - due to
      - anaerobes NEC P36.5
      - Escherichia coli P36.4
      - Staphylococcus P36.30
        - aureus P36.2
        - specified NEC P36.39
      - Streptococcus P36.10
        - group B P36.0
        - specified NEC P36.19
    - specified NEC P36.8
  - triplet Z38.8
    - born in hospital Z38.61
      - by cesarean Z38.62
    - born outside hospital Z38.7
  - twin Z38.5
    - born in hospital Z38.30
      - by cesarean Z38.31
    - born outside hospital Z38.4
  - vomiting P92.09
    - bilious P92.01
  - weight check Z00.111
- **Newcastle** conjunctivitis or disease B30.8
- **Nezelof's** syndrome (pure alymphocytosis) D81.4
- **Niacin** (amide) deficiency E52
- **Nicolas** (-Durand)-Favre disease A55
- **Nicotine** — *see* Tobacco
- **Nicotinic** acid deficiency E52
- **Niemann-Pick** disease or syndrome E75.249
  - specified NEC E75.248
  - type
    - A E75.240
    - B E75.241
    - C E75.242
    - D E75.243
- **Night**
  - blindness — *see* Blindness, night
  - sweats R61
  - terrors (child) F51.4
- **Nightmares** (REM sleep type) F51.5
- **NIHSS** (National Institutes of Health Stroke Scale) score R29.7 ☑
- **Nipple** — *see* condition
- **Nisbet's** chancre A57
- **Nishimoto** (-Takeuchi) disease I67.5
- **Nitritoid** crisis or reaction — *see* Crisis, nitritoid
- **Nitrosohemoglobinemia** D74.8
- **Njovera** A65
- **Nocardiosis,** nocardiasis A43.9
  - cutaneous A43.1
  - lung A43.0
  - pneumonia A43.0
  - pulmonary A43.0
  - specified site NEC A43.8
- **Nocturia** R35.1
  - psychogenic F45.8
- **Nocturnal** — *see* condition
- **Nodal** rhythm I49.8
- **Node** (s) (*see also* Nodule)
  - Bouchard's (with arthropathy) M15.2
  - Haygarth's M15.8
  - Heberden's (with arthropathy) M15.1
  - larynx J38.7
  - lymph — *see* condition
  - milker's B08.03
  - Osler's I33.0
  - Schmorl's — *see* Schmorl's disease
  - singer's J38.2
  - teacher's J38.2
  - tuberculous — *see* Tuberculosis, lymph gland
  - vocal cord J38.2
- **Nodule** (s), nodular
  - actinomycotic — *see* Actinomycosis
  - breast NEC N63
  - colloid (cystic), thyroid E04.1
  - cutaneous — *see* Swelling, localized
  - endometrial (stromal) D26.1
  - Haygarth's M15.8
  - inflammatory — *see* Inflammation
  - juxta-articular
    - syphilitic A52.77
    - yaws A66.7
  - larynx J38.7
  - lung, solitary (subsegmental branch of the bronchial tree) R91.1
    - multiple R91.8
  - milker's B08.03
  - prostate N40.2
    - with lower urinary tract symptoms (LUTS) N40.3
    - without lower urinary tract symptoms (LUTS) N40.2
  - pulmonary, solitary (subsegmental branch of the bronchial tree) R91.1
  - retrocardiac R09.89
  - rheumatoid M06.30
    - ankle M06.37 ☑
    - elbow M06.32 ☑
    - foot joint M06.37 ☑
    - hand joint M06.34 ☑
    - hip M06.35 ☑
    - knee M06.36 ☑
    - multiple site M06.39
    - shoulder M06.31 ☑
    - vertebra M06.38
    - wrist M06.33 ☑
  - scrotum (inflammatory) N49.2
  - singer's J38.2
  - solitary, lung (subsegmental branch of the bronchial tree) R91.1
    - multiple R91.8
  - subcutaneous — *see* Swelling, localized
  - teacher's J38.2
  - thyroid (cold) (gland) (nontoxic) E04.1
    - with thyrotoxicosis E05.20
      - with thyroid storm E05.21
    - toxic or with hyperthyroidism E05.20
      - with thyroid storm E05.21
  - vocal cord J38.2
- **Noma** (gangrenous) (hospital) (infective) A69.0
  - auricle I96
  - mouth A69.0
  - pudendi N76.89
  - vulvae N76.89
- **Nomad,** nomadism Z59.0
- **NOMID** (neonatal onset multisystemic inflammatory disorder) M04.2
- **Nonautoimmune** hemolytic anemia D59.4
  - drug-induced D59.2
- **Nonclosure** (*see also* Imperfect, closure)
  - ductus arteriosus (Botallo's) Q25.0
  - foramen
    - botalli Q21.1
    - ovale Q21.1
- **Noncompliance** Z91.19
  - with
    - dietary regimen Z91.11
    - dialysis Z91.15
- **Noncompliance** — *continued*
  - with — *continued*
    - medical treatment Z91.19
    - medication regimen NEC Z91.14
      - underdosing (*see also* Table of Drugs and Chemicals, categories T36-T50, with final character 6)Z91.14
        - intentional NEC Z91.128
          - due to financial hardship of patient Z91.120
        - unintentional NEC Z91.138
          - due to patient's age related debility Z91.130
    - renal dialysis Z91.15
- **Nondescent** (congenital) (*see also* Malposition, congenital)
  - cecum Q43.3
  - colon Q43.3
  - testicle Q53.9
    - bilateral Q53.20
      - abdominal Q53.21
      - perineal Q53.22
    - unilateral Q53.10
      - abdominal Q53.11
      - perineal Q53.12
- **Nondevelopment**
  - brain Q02
    - part of Q04.3
  - heart Q24.8
  - organ or site, congenital NEC — *see* Hypoplasia
- **Nonengagement**
  - head NEC O32.4 ☑
    - in labor, causing obstructed labor O64.8 ☑
- **Nonexanthematous** tick fever A93.2
- **Nonexpansion,** lung (newborn) P28.0
- **Nonfunctioning**
  - cystic duct (*see also* Disease, gallbladder)K82.8
  - gallbladder (*see also* Disease, gallbladder)K82.8
  - kidney N28.9
  - labyrinth — *see* subcategory H83.2
- **Non-Hodgkin** lymphoma NEC — *see* Lymphoma, non-Hodgkin
- **Non-working** side interference M26.56
- **Nonimplantation,** ovum N97.2
- **Noninsufflation,** fallopian tube N97.1
- **Non-ketotic** hyperglycinemia E72.51
- **Nonne-Milroy** syndrome Q82.0
- **Nonovulation** N97.0
- **Nonpatent** fallopian tube N97.1
- **Nonpneumatization,** lung NEC P28.0
- **Nonrotation** — *see* Malrotation
- **Nonsecretion,** urine — *see* Anuria
- **Nonunion**
  - fracture — *see* Fracture, by site
  - joint, following fusion or arthrodesis M96.0
  - organ or site, congenital NEC — *see* Imperfect, closure
  - symphysis pubis, congenital Q74.2
- **Nonvisualization,** gallbladder R93.2
- **Nonvital,** nonvitalized tooth K04.99
- **Noonan's** syndrome Q87.1
- **Normocytic** anemia (infectional) due to blood loss (chronic) D50.0
  - acute D62
- **Norrie's** disease (congenital) Q15.8
- **North** American blastomycosis B40.9
- **Norwegian** itch B86
- **Nose,** nasal — *see* condition
- **Nosebleed** R04.0
- **Nose-picking** F98.8
- **Nosomania** F45.21
- **Nosophobia** F45.22
- **Nostalgia** F43.20
- **Notch** of iris Q13.2
- **Notching** nose, congenital (tip) Q30.2
- **Nothnagel's**
  - syndrome — *see* Strabismus, paralytic, third nerve
  - vasomotor acroparesthesia I73.89
- **Novy's** relapsing fever A68.9
  - louse-borne A68.0
  - tick-borne A68.1
- **Noxious**
  - foodstuffs, poisoning by — *see* Poisoning, food, noxious, plant
  - substances transmitted through placenta or breast milk P04.9
- **Nucleus** pulposus — *see* condition
- **Numbness** R20.0
- **Nuns'** knee — *see* Bursitis, prepatellar
- **Nursemaid's** elbow S53.03 ☑
- **Nutcracker** esophagus K22.4

- **Nutmeg** liver K76.1
- **Nutrient** element deficiency E61.9
  - specified NEC E61.8
- **Nutrition** deficient or insufficient (*see also* Malnutrition)E46
  - due to
    - insufficient food T73.0 ☑
    - lack of
      - care (child) T76.02 ☑
        - adult T76.01 ☑
      - food T73.0 ☑
- **Nutritional** stunting E45
- **Nyctalopia** (night blindness) — *see* Blindness, night
- **Nycturia** R35.1
  - psychogenic F45.8
- **Nymphomania** F52.8
- **Nystagmus** H55.00
  - benign paroxysmal — *see* Vertigo, benign paroxysmal
  - central positional H81.4 ☑
  - congenital H55.01
  - dissociated H55.04
  - latent H55.02
  - miners' H55.09
  - positional
    - benign paroxysmal H81.4 ☑
    - central H81.4 ☑
  - specified form NEC H55.09
  - visual deprivation H55.03

O

- **Obermeyer's** relapsing fever (European) A68.0
- **Obesity** E66.9
  - with alveolar hypoventilation E66.2
  - adrenal E27.8
  - complicating
    - childbirth O99.214
    - pregnancy O99.21 ☑
    - puerperium O99.215
  - constitutional E66.8
  - dietary counseling and surveillance Z71.3
  - drug-induced E66.1
  - due to
    - drug E66.1
    - excess calories E66.09
      - morbid E66.01
      - severe E66.01
  - endocrine E66.8
  - endogenous E66.8
  - exogenous E66.09
  - familial E66.8
  - glandular E66.8
  - hypothyroid — *see* Hypothyroidism
  - hypoventilation syndrome (OHS) E66.2
  - morbid E66.01
    - with
      - alveolar hypoventilation E66.2
      - obesity hypoventilation syndrome (OHS) E66.2
    - due to excess calories E66.01
  - nutritional E66.09
  - pituitary E23.6
  - severe E66.01
  - specified type NEC E66.8
- **Oblique** — *see* condition
- **Obliteration**
  - appendix (lumen) K38.8
  - artery I77.1
  - bile duct (noncalculous) K83.1
  - common duct (noncalculous) K83.1
  - cystic duct — *see* Obstruction, gallbladder
  - disease, arteriolar I77.1
  - endometrium N85.8
  - eye, anterior chamber — *see* Disorder, globe, hypotony
  - fallopian tube N97.1
  - lymphatic vessel I89.0
    - due to mastectomy I97.2
  - organ or site, congenital NEC — *see* Atresia, by site
  - ureter N13.5
    - with infection N13.6
  - urethra — *see* Stricture, urethra
  - vein I87.8
  - vestibule (oral) K08.89
- **Observation** (following) (for) (without need for further medical care) Z04.9
  - accident NEC Z04.3
    - at work Z04.2
    - transport Z04.1

Observation — *continued*

  - adverse effect of drug Z03.6
  - alleged rape or sexual assault (victim), ruled out
    - adult Z04.41
    - child Z04.42
  - criminal assault Z04.8
  - development state
    - adolescent Z00.3
    - period of rapid growth in childhood Z00.2
    - puberty Z00.3
  - disease, specified NEC Z03.89
  - following work accident Z04.2
  - growth and development state — *see* Observation, development state
  - injuries (accidental) NEC (*see also* Observation, accident)
  - newborn (for)
    - suspected condition, related to exposure from the mother or birth process — *see* - Newborn, affected by, maternal
      - ruled out Z05.9
        - cardiac Z05.0
        - connective tissue Z05.73
        - gastrointestinal Z05.5
        - genetic Z05.41
        - genitourinary Z05.6
        - immunologic Z05.43
        - infectious Z05.1
        - metabolic Z05.42
        - musculoskeletal Z05.72
        - neurological Z05.2
        - respiratory Z05.3
        - skin and subcutaneous tissue Z05.71
        - specified condition NEC Z05.8
  - postpartum
    - immediately after delivery Z39.0
    - routine follow-up Z39.2
  - pregnancy (normal) (without complication) Z34.9 ☑
    - high risk O09.9 ☑
  - suicide attempt, alleged NEC Z03.89
    - self-poisoning Z03.6
  - suspected, ruled out (*see also* Suspected condition, ruled out)
    - abuse, physical
      - adult Z04.71
      - child Z04.72
    - accident at work Z04.2
    - adult battering victim Z04.71
    - child battering victim Z04.72
    - condition NEC Z03.89
      - newborn (*see also* Observation, newborn (for), suspected condition, ruled out)Z05.9
    - drug poisoning or adverse effect Z03.6
    - exposure (to)
      - anthrax Z03.810
      - biological agent NEC Z03.818
    - inflicted injury NEC Z04.8
    - suicide attempt, alleged Z03.89
      - self-poisoning Z03.6
    - toxic effects from ingested substance (drug) (poison) Z03.6
  - toxic effects from ingested substance (drug) (poison) Z03.6
- **Obsession,** obsessional state F42.8
  - mixed thoughts and acts F42.2
- **Obsessive-compulsive** neurosis or reaction F42.8
- **Obstetric** embolism, septic — *see* Embolism, obstetric, septic
- **Obstetrical** trauma (complicating delivery) O71.9
  - with or following ectopic or molar pregnancy O08.6
  - specified type NEC O71.89
- **Obstipation** — *see* Constipation
- **Obstruction,** obstructed, obstructive
  - airway J98.8
    - with
      - allergic alveolitis J67.9
      - asthma J45.909
        - with
          - exacerbation (acute) J45.901
          - status asthmaticus J45.902
      - bronchiectasis J47.9
        - with
          - exacerbation (acute) J47.1
          - lower respiratory infection J47.0
      - bronchitis (chronic) J44.9
      - emphysema J43.9
    - chronic J44.9
      - with

Obstruction — *continued*

  - airway — *continued*
        - allergic alveolitis — *see* Pneumonitis, hypersensitivity
        - bronchiectasis J47.9
          - with
            - exacerbation (acute) J47.1
            - lower respiratory infection J47.0
    - due to
      - foreign body — *see* Foreign body, by site, causing asphyxia
      - inhalation of fumes or vapors J68.9
      - laryngospasm J38.5
  - ampulla of Vater K83.1
  - aortic (heart) (valve) — *see* Stenosis, aortic
  - aortoiliac I74.09
  - aqueduct of Sylvius G91.1
    - congenital Q03.0
      - with spina bifida — *see* Spina bifida, by site, with hydrocephalus
  - Arnold-Chiari — *see* Arnold-Chiari disease
  - artery (*see also* Embolism, artery)I74.9
    - stent — *see* Restenosis, stent
    - basilar (complete) (partial) — *see* Occlusion, artery, basilar
    - carotid (complete) (partial) — *see* Occlusion, artery, carotid
    - cerebellar — *see* Occlusion, artery, cerebellar
    - cerebral (anterior) (middle) (posterior) — *see* Occlusion, artery, cerebral
    - precerebral — *see* Occlusion, artery, precerebral
    - renal N28.0
    - retinal NEC — *see* Occlusion, artery, retina
    - vertebral (complete) (partial) — *see* Occlusion, artery, vertebral
  - band (intestinal) K56.69
  - bile duct or passage (common) (hepatic) (noncalculous) K83.1
    - with calculus K80.51
    - congenital (causing jaundice) Q44.3
  - biliary (duct) (tract) K83.1
    - gallbladder K82.0
  - bladder-neck (acquired) N32.0
    - congenital Q64.31
    - due to hyperplasia (hypertrophy) of prostate — *see* Hyperplasia, prostate
  - bowel — *see* Obstruction, intestine
  - bronchus J98.09
  - canal, ear — *see* Stenosis, external ear canal
  - cardia K22.2
  - caval veins (inferior) (superior) I87.1
  - cecum — *see* Obstruction, intestine
  - circulatory I99.8
  - colon — *see* Obstruction, intestine
  - common duct (noncalculous) K83.1
  - coronary (artery) — *see* Occlusion, coronary
  - cystic duct (*see also* Obstruction, gallbladder)
    - with calculus K80.21
  - device, implant or graft (*see also* Complications, by site and type, mechanical)T85.698 ☑
    - arterial graft NEC — *see* Complication, cardiovascular device, mechanical, vascular
    - catheter NEC T85.628 ☑
      - cystostomy T83.090 ☑
      - dialysis (renal) T82.49 ☑
        - intraperitoneal T85.691 ☑
      - Hopkins T83.098 ☑
      - ileostomy T83.098 ☑
      - infusion NEC T82.594 ☑
        - spinal (epidural) (subdural) T85.690 ☑
      - nephrostomy T83.092 ☑
      - urethral indwelling T83.091 ☑
      - urinary T83.098 ☑
      - urostomy T83.098 ☑
    - due to infection T85.79 ☑
    - gastrointestinal — *see* Complications, prosthetic device, mechanical, gastrointestinal device
    - genital NEC T83.498 ☑
      - intrauterine contraceptive device T83.39 ☑
      - penile prosthesis (cylinder) (implanted) (pump) (reservoir) T83.490 ☑
      - testicular prosthesis T83.491 ☑
    - heart NEC — *see* Complication, cardiovascular device, mechanical
    - joint prosthesis — *see* Complications, joint prosthesis, mechanical, specified NEC, by site
    - orthopedic NEC — *see* Complication, orthopedic, device, mechanical
    - specified NEC T85.628 ☑

- **Obstruction** — *continued*
  - device, implant or graft — *continued*
    - urinary NEC (*see also* Complication, genitourinary, device, urinary, mechanical)
      - graft T83.29 ☑
    - vascular NEC — *see* Complication, cardiovascular device, mechanical
    - ventricular intracranial shunt T85.09 ☑
  - due to foreign body accidentally left in operative wound T81.529 ☑
  - duodenum K31.5
  - ejaculatory duct N50.89
  - esophagus K22.2
  - eustachian tube (complete) (partial) H68.10 ☑
    - cartilagenous (extrinsic) H68.13 ☑
      - intrinsic H68.12 ☑
    - osseous H68.11 ☑
  - fallopian tube (bilateral) N97.1
  - fecal K56.41
    - with hernia — *see* Hernia, by site, with obstruction
  - foramen of Monro (congenital) Q03.8
    - with spina bifida — *see* Spina bifida, by site, with hydrocephalus
  - foreign body — *see* Foreign body
  - gallbladder K82.0
    - with calculus, stones K80.21
    - congenital Q44.1
  - gastric outlet K31.1
  - gastrointestinal — *see* Obstruction, intestine
  - hepatic K76.89
    - duct (noncalculous) K83.1
  - hepatobiliary K83.1
  - ileum — *see* Obstruction, intestine
  - iliofemoral (artery) I74.5
  - intestine K56.60
    - with
      - adhesions (intestinal) (peritoneal) K56.5
    - adynamic K56.0
    - by gallstone K56.3
    - congenital (small) Q41.9
      - large Q42.9
        - specified part NEC Q42.8
    - neurogenic K56.0
      - Hirschsprung's disease or megacolon Q43.1
    - newborn P76.9
      - due to
        - fecaliths P76.8
        - inspissated milk P76.2
        - meconium (plug) P76.0
          - in mucoviscidosis E84.11
      - specified NEC P76.8
    - postoperative K91.3
    - reflex K56.0
    - specified NEC K56.69
    - volvulus K56.2
  - intracardiac ball valve prosthesis T82.09 ☑
  - jejunum — *see* Obstruction, intestine
  - joint prosthesis — *see* Complications, joint prosthesis, mechanical, specified NEC, by site
  - kidney (calices) N28.89
  - labor — *see* Delivery
  - lacrimal (passages) (duct)
    - by
      - dacryolith — *see* Dacryolith
      - stenosis — *see* Stenosis, lacrimal
    - congenital Q10.5
    - neonatal H04.53 ☑
  - lacrimonasal duct — *see* Obstruction, lacrimal
  - lacteal, with steatorrhea K90.2
  - laryngitis — *see* Laryngitis
  - larynx NEC J38.6
    - congenital Q31.8
  - lung J98.4
    - disease, chronic J44.9
  - lymphatic I89.0
  - meconium (plug)
    - newborn P76.0
      - due to fecaliths P76.0
      - in mucoviscidosis E84.11
  - mitral — *see* Stenosis, mitral
  - nasal J34.89
  - nasolacrimal duct (*see also* Obstruction, lacrimal)
    - congenital Q10.5
  - nasopharynx J39.2
  - nose J34.89
  - organ or site, congenital NEC — *see* Atresia, by site
  - pancreatic duct K86.89
  - parotid duct or gland K11.8
  - pelviureteral junction N13.5
    - with hydronephrosis N13.0
    - congenital Q62.39

- **Obstruction** — *continued*
  - pharynx J39.2
  - portal (circulation) (vein) I81
  - prostate (*see also* Hyperplasia, prostate)
    - valve (urinary) N32.0
  - pulmonary valve (heart) I37.0
  - pyelonephritis (chronic) N11.1
  - pylorus
    - adult K31.1
    - congenital or infantile Q40.0
  - rectosigmoid — *see* Obstruction, intestine
  - rectum K62.4
  - renal N28.89
    - outflow N13.8
    - pelvis, congenital Q62.39
  - respiratory J98.8
    - chronic J44.9
  - retinal (vessels) H34.9
  - salivary duct (any) K11.8
    - with calculus K11.5
  - sigmoid — *see* Obstruction, intestine
  - sinus (accessory) (nasal) J34.89
  - Stensen's duct K11.8
  - stomach NEC K31.89
    - acute K31.0
    - congenital Q40.2
    - due to pylorospasm K31.3
  - submandibular duct K11.8
  - submaxillary gland K11.8
    - with calculus K11.5
  - thoracic duct I89.0
  - thrombotic — *see* Thrombosis
  - trachea J39.8
  - tracheostomy airway J95.03
  - tricuspid (valve) — *see* Stenosis, tricuspid
  - upper respiratory, congenital Q34.8
  - ureter (functional) (pelvic junction) NEC N13.5
    - with
      - hydronephrosis N13.1
        - with infection N13.6
      - pyelonephritis (chronic) N11.1
    - congenital Q62.39
    - due to calculus — *see* Calculus, ureter
  - urethra NEC N36.8
    - congenital Q64.39
  - urinary (moderate) N13.9
    - due to hyperplasia (hypertrophy) of prostate — *see* Hyperplasia, prostate
    - organ or tract (lower) N13.9
    - prostatic valve N32.0
    - specified NEC N13.8
  - uropathy N13.9
  - uterus N85.8
  - vagina N89.5
  - valvular — *see* Endocarditis
  - vein, venous I87.1
    - caval (inferior) (superior) I87.1
    - thrombotic — *see* Thrombosis
  - vena cava (inferior) (superior) I87.1
  - vesical NEC N32.0
  - vesicourethral orifice N32.0
    - congenital Q64.31
  - vessel NEC I99.8
    - stent — *see* Restenosis, stent
- **Obturator** — *see* condition
- **Occlusal** wear, teeth K03.0
- **Occlusio** pupillae — *see* Membrane, pupillary
- **Occlusion,** occluded
  - anus K62.4
    - congenital Q42.3
      - with fistula Q42.2
  - aortoiliac (chronic) I74.09
  - aqueduct of Sylvius G91.1
    - congenital Q03.0
      - with spina bifida — *see* Spina bifida, by site, with hydrocephalus
  - artery (*see also* Embolism, artery)I74.9
    - auditory, internal I65.8
    - basilar I65.1
      - with
        - infarction I63.22
          - due to
            - embolism I63.12
            - thrombosis I63.02
    - brain or cerebral I66.9
      - with infarction (due to) I63.5 ☑
        - embolism I63.4 ☑
        - thrombosis I63.3 ☑
    - carotid I65.2 ☑
      - with
        - infarction I63.23 ☑
          - due to

- **Occlusion** — *continued*
  - artery — *continued*
            - embolism I63.13 ☑
            - thrombosis I63.03 ☑
    - cerebellar (anterior inferior) (posterior inferior) (superior) I66.3
      - with infarction I63.54 ☑
        - due to
          - embolism I63.44 ☑
          - thrombosis I63.34 ☑
    - cerebral I66.9
      - with infarction I63.50
        - due to
          - embolism I63.40
            - specified NEC I63.49
          - thrombosis I63.30
            - specified NEC I63.39
      - anterior I66.1 ☑
        - with infarction I63.52 ☑
          - due to
            - embolism I63.42 ☑
            - thrombosis I63.32 ☑
      - middle I66.0 ☑
        - with infarction I63.51 ☑
          - due to
            - embolism I63.41 ☑
            - thrombosis I63.31 ☑
      - posterior I66.2 ☑
        - with infarction I63.53 ☑
          - due to
            - embolism I63.43 ☑
            - thrombosis I63.33 ☑
      - specified NEC I66.8
        - with infarction I63.59
          - due to
            - embolism I63.4 ☑
            - thrombosis I63.3 ☑
    - choroidal (anterior) — *see* Occlusion, artery, precerebral, specified NEC
    - communicating posterior — *see* Occlusion, artery, cerebral, specified NEC
    - complete
      - coronary I25.82
      - extremities I70.92
    - coronary (acute) (thrombotic) (without myocardial infarction) I24.0
      - with myocardial infarction — *see* Infarction, myocardium
      - chronic total I25.82
      - complete I25.82
      - healed or old I25.2
      - total (chronic) I25.82
    - hypophyseal — *see* Occlusion, artery, precerebral, specified NEC
    - iliac I74.5
    - lower extremities due to stenosis or stricture I77.1
    - mesenteric (embolic) (thrombotic) (*see also* Infarct, intestine)K55.069
    - perforating — *see* Occlusion, artery, cerebral, specified NEC
    - peripheral I77.9
      - thrombotic or embolic I74.4
    - pontine — *see* Occlusion, artery, cerebral, specified NEC
    - precerebral I65.9
      - with infarction I63.20
        - specified NEC I63.29
        - due to
          - embolism I63.10
            - specified NEC I63.19
          - thrombosis I63.00
            - specified NEC I63.09
      - basilar — *see* Occlusion, artery, basilar
      - carotid — *see* Occlusion, artery, carotid
      - puerperal O88.23
      - specified NEC I65.8
        - with infarction I63.29
          - due to
            - embolism I63.19
            - thrombosis I63.00
      - vertebral — *see* Occlusion, artery, vertebral
    - renal N28.0
    - retinal
      - central H34.1 ☑
      - partial H34.21 ☑
      - branch H34.23 ☑
      - transient H34.0 ☑
    - spinal — *see* Occlusion, artery, precerebral, vertebral
    - total (chronic)
      - coronary I25.82

Occlusion - Opacity

Occlusion — *continued*
- artery — *continued*
  - extremities I70.92
  - vertebral I65.0 ☑
    - with
      - infarction I63.21 ☑
        - due to
          - embolism I63.11 ☑
          - thrombosis I63.01 ☑
- basilar artery — *see* Occlusion, artery, basilar
- bile duct (common) (hepatic) (noncalculous) K83.1
- bowel — *see* Obstruction, intestine
- carotid (artery) (common) (internal) — *see* Occlusion, artery, carotid
- centric (of teeth) M26.59
  - maximum intercuspation discrepancy M26.55
- cerebellar (artery) — *see* Occlusion, artery, cerebellar
- cerebral (artery) — *see* Occlusion, artery, cerebral
- cerebrovascular (*see also* Occlusion, artery, cerebral)
  - with infarction I63.5 ☑
- cervical canal — *see* Stricture, cervix
- cervix (uteri) — *see* Stricture, cervix
- choanal Q30.0
- choroidal (artery) — *see* Occlusion, artery, precerebral, specified NEC
- colon — *see* Obstruction, intestine
- communicating posterior artery — *see* Occlusion, artery, precerebral, specified NEC
- coronary (artery) (vein) (thrombotic) (*see also* Infarct, myocardium)
  - chronic total I25.82
  - healed or old I25.2
  - not resulting in infarction I24.0
  - total (chronic) I25.82
- cystic duct — *see* Obstruction, gallbladder
- embolic — *see* Embolism
- fallopian tube N97.1
  - congenital Q50.6
- gallbladder (*see also* Obstruction, gallbladder)
  - congenital (causing jaundice) Q44.1
- gingiva, traumatic K06.2
- hymen N89.6
  - congenital Q52.3
- hypophyseal (artery) — *see* Occlusion, artery, precerebral, specified NEC
- iliac artery I74.5
- intestine — *see* Obstruction, intestine
- lacrimal passages — *see* Obstruction, lacrimal
- lung J98.4
- lymph or lymphatic channel I89.0
- mammary duct N64.89
- mesenteric artery (embolic) (thrombotic) (*see also* Infarct, intestine)K55.069
- nose J34.89
  - congenital Q30.0
- organ or site, congenital NEC — *see* Atresia, by site
- oviduct N97.1
  - congenital Q50.6
- peripheral arteries
  - due to stricture or stenosis I77.1
  - upper extremity I74.2
- pontine (artery) — *see* Occlusion, artery, precerebral, specified NEC
- posterior lingual, of mandibular teeth M26.29
- precerebral artery — *see* Occlusion, artery, precerebral
- punctum lacrimale — *see* Obstruction, lacrimal
- pupil — *see* Membrane, pupillary
- pylorus, adult (*see also* Stricture, pylorus)K31.1
- renal artery N28.0
- retina, retinal
  - artery — *see* Occlusion, artery, retinal
  - vein (central) H34.81 ☑
    - engorgement H34.82 ☑
    - tributary H34.83 ☑
  - vessels H34.9
- spinal artery — *see* Occlusion, artery, precerebral, vertebral
- teeth (mandibular) (posterior lingual) M26.29
- thoracic duct I89.0
- thrombotic — *see* Thrombosis, artery
- traumatic
  - edentulous (alveolar) ridge K06.2
  - gingiva K06.2
  - periodontal K05.5
- tubal N97.1
- ureter (complete) (partial) N13.5
  - congenital Q62.10
- ureteropelvic junction N13.5
  - congenital Q62.11
- ureterovesical orifice N13.5
  - congenital Q62.12
- urethra — *see* Stricture, urethra
- uterus N85.8
- vagina N89.5
- vascular NEC I99.8
- vein — *see* Thrombosis
  - retinal — *see* Occlusion, retinal, vein
- vena cava (inferior) (superior) — *see* Embolism, vena cava
- ventricle (brain) NEC G91.1
- vertebral (artery) — *see* Occlusion, artery, vertebral
- vessel (blood) I99.8
- vulva N90.5

Occult
- blood in feces (stools) R19.5

Occupational
- problems NEC Z56.89

Ochlophobia — *see* Agoraphobia

Ochronosis (endogenous) E70.29

Ocular muscle — *see* condition

Oculogyric crisis or disturbance H51.8
- psychogenic F45.8

Oculomotor syndrome H51.9

Oculopathy
- syphilitic NEC A52.71
  - congenital
    - early A50.01
    - late A50.30
  - early (secondary) A51.43
  - late A52.71

Oddi's sphincter spasm K83.4

Odontalgia K08.89

Odontoameloblastoma — *see* Cyst, calcifying odontogenic

Odontoclasia K03.89

Odontodysplasia, regional K00.4

Odontogenesis imperfecta K00.5

Odontoma (ameloblastic) (complex) (compound) (fibroameloblastic) — *see* Cyst, calcifying odontogenic

Odontomyelitis (closed) (open) K04.01
- irreversible K04.02
- reversible K04.01

Odontorrhagia K08.89

Odontosarcoma, ameloblastic C41.1
- upper jaw (bone) C41.0

Oestriasis — *see* Myiasis

Oguchi's disease H53.63

Ohara's disease — *see* Tularemia

OHS (obesity hypoventilation syndrome) E66.2

Oidiomycosis — *see* Candidiasis

Oidium albicans infection — *see* Candidiasis

Old age (without mention of debility) R54
- dementia F03 ☑

Old (previous) myocardial infarction I25.2

Olfactory — *see* condition

Oligemia — *see* Anemia

Oligoastrocytoma
- specified site — *see* Neoplasm, malignant, by site
- unspecified site C71.9

Oligocythemia D64.9

Oligodendroblastoma
- specified site — *see* Neoplasm, malignant
- unspecified site C71.9

Oligodendroglioma
- anaplastic type
  - specified site — *see* Neoplasm, malignant, by site
  - unspecified site C71.9
- specified site — *see* Neoplasm, malignant, by site
- unspecified site C71.9

Oligodontia — *see* Anodontia

Oligoencephalon Q02

Oligohidrosis L74.4

Oligohydramnios O41.0 ☑

Oligohydrosis L74.4

Oligomenorrhea N91.5
- primary N91.3
- secondary N91.4

Oligophrenia (*see also* Disability, intellectual)
- phenylpyruvic E70.0

Oligospermia N46.11
- due to
  - drug therapy N46.121
  - efferent duct obstruction N46.123
  - infection N46.122
  - radiation N46.124

Oligospermia — *continued*
- due to — *continued*
  - specified cause NEC N46.129
  - systemic disease N46.125

Oligotrichia — *see* Alopecia

Oliguria R34
- with, complicating or following ectopic or molar pregnancy O08.4
- postprocedural N99.0

Ollier's disease Q78.4

Omentitis — *see* Peritonitis

Omenotocele — *see* Hernia, abdomen, specified site NEC

Omentum, omental — *see* condition

Omphalitis (congenital) (newborn) P38.9
- with mild hemorrhage P38.1
- without hemorrhage P38.9
- not of newborn L08.82
- tetanus A33

Omphalocele Q79.2

Omphalomesenteric duct, persistent Q43.0

Omphalorrhagia, newborn P51.9

Omsk hemorrhagic fever A98.1

Onanism (excessive) F98.8

Onchocerciasis, onchocercosis B73.1
- with
  - eye disease B73.00
    - endophthalmitis B73.01
    - eyelid B73.09
    - glaucoma B73.02
    - specified NEC B73.09
- eye NEC B73.00
- eyelid B73.09

Oncocytoma — *see* Neoplasm, benign, by site

Oncovirus, as cause of disease classified elsewhere B97.32

Ondine's curse — *see* Apnea, sleep

Oneirophrenia F23

Onychauxis L60.2
- congenital Q84.5

Onychia (*see also* Cellulitis, digit)
- with lymphangitis — *see* Lymphangitis, acute, digit
- candidal B37.2
- dermatophytic B35.1

Onychitis (*see also* Cellulitis, digit)
- with lymphangitis — *see* Lymphangitis, acute, digit

Onychocryptosis L60.0

Onychodystrophy L60.3
- congenital Q84.6

Onychogryphosis, onychogryposis L60.2

Onycholysis L60.1

Onychomadesis L60.8

Onychomalacia L60.3

Onychomycosis (finger) (toe) B35.1

Onycho-osteodysplasia Q87.2

Onychophagia F98.8

Onychophosis L60.8

Onychoptosis L60.8

Onychorrhexis L60.3
- congenital Q84.6

Onychoschizia L60.3

Onyxis (finger) (toe) L60.0

Onyxitis (*see also* Cellulitis, digit)
- with lymphangitis — *see* Lymphangitis, acute, digit

Oophoritis (cystic) (infectional) (interstitial) N70.92
- with salpingitis N70.93
- acute N70.02
  - with salpingitis N70.03
- chronic N70.12
  - with salpingitis N70.13
- complicating abortion — *see* Abortion, by type, complicated by, oophoritis

Oophorocele N83.4 ☑

Opacity, opacities
- cornea H17. ☑
  - central H17.1 ☑
  - congenital Q13.3
  - degenerative — *see* Degeneration, cornea
  - hereditary — *see* Dystrophy, cornea
  - inflammatory — *see* Keratitis
  - minor H17.81 ☑
  - peripheral H17.82 ☑
  - sequelae of trachoma (healed) B94.0
  - specified NEC H17.89
- enamel (teeth) (fluoride) (nonfluoride) K00.3
- lens — *see* Cataract
- snowball — *see* Deposit, crystalline
- vitreous (humor) NEC H43.39 ☑
  - congenital Q14.0
  - membranes and strands H43.31 ☑

- **Opalescent** dentin (hereditary) K00.5
- **Open,** opening
  - abnormal, organ or site, congenital — *see* Imperfect, closure
  - angle with
    - borderline
      - findings
        - high risk H40.02 ☑
        - low risk H40.01 ☑
      - intraocular pressure H40.00 ☑
    - cupping of discs H40.01 ☑
    - glaucoma (primary) — *see* Glaucoma, open angle
  - bite
    - anterior M26.220
    - posterior M26.221
  - false — *see* Imperfect, closure
  - margin on tooth restoration K08.51
  - restoration margins of tooth K08.51
  - wound — *see* Wound, open
- **Operational** fatigue F48.8
- **Operative** — *see* condition
- **Operculitis** — *see* Periodontitis
- **Operculum** — *see* Break, retina
- **Ophiasis** L63.2
- **Ophthalmia** (*see also* Conjunctivitis)H10.9
  - actinic rays — *see* Photokeratitis
  - allergic (acute) — *see* Conjunctivitis, acute, atopic
  - blennorrhagic (gonococcal) (neonatorum) A54.31
  - diphtheritic A36.86
  - Egyptian A71.1
  - electrica — *see* Photokeratitis
  - gonococcal (neonatorum) A54.31
  - metastatic — *see* Endophthalmitis, purulent
  - migraine — *see* Migraine, ophthalmoplegic
  - neonatorum, newborn P39.1
    - gonococcal A54.31
  - nodosa H16.24 ☑
  - purulent — *see* Conjunctivitis, acute, mucopurulent
  - spring — *see* Conjunctivitis, acute, atopic
  - sympathetic — *see* Uveitis, sympathetic
- **Ophthalmitis** — *see* Ophthalmia
- **Ophthalmocele** (congenital) Q15.8
- **Ophthalmoneuromyelitis** G36.0
- **Ophthalmoplegia** (*see also* Strabismus, paralytic)
  - anterior internuclear — *see* Ophthalmoplegia, internuclear
  - ataxia-areflexia G61.0
  - diabetic — *see* E08-E13 with .39
  - exophthalmic E05.00
    - with thyroid storm E05.01
  - external H49.88 ☑
    - progressive H49.4 ☑
      - with pigmentary retinopathy — *see* Kearns-Sayre syndrome
    - total H49.3 ☑
  - internal (complete) (total) H52.51 ☑
  - internuclear H51.2 ☑
  - migraine — *see* Migraine, ophthalmoplegic
  - Parinaud's H49.88 ☑
  - progressive external — *see* Ophthalmoplegia, external, progressive
  - supranuclear, progressive G23.1
  - total (external) — *see* Ophthalmoplegia, external, total
- **Opioid** (s)
  - abuse — *see* Abuse, drug, opioids
  - dependence — *see* Dependence, drug, opioids
  - induced, without use disorder
    - anxiety disorder F11.988
    - delirium F11.921
    - depressive disorder F11.94
    - sexual dysfunction F11.981
    - sleep disorder F11.982
- **Opisthognathism** M26.09
- **Opisthorchiasis** (felineus) (viverrini) B66.0
- **Opitz'** disease D73.2
- **Opiumism** — *see* Dependence, drug, opioid
- **Oppenheim's** disease G70.2
- **Oppenheim-Urbach** disease (necrobiosis lipoidica diabeticorum) — *see* E08-E13 with .620
- **Optic** nerve — *see* condition
- **Orbit** — *see* condition
- **Orchioblastoma** C62.9 ☑
- **Orchitis** (gangrenous) (nonspecific) (septic) (suppurative) N45.2
  - blennorrhagic (gonococcal) (acute) (chronic) A54.23
  - chlamydial A56.19
  - filarial (*see also* Infestation, filarial)B74.9 *[N51]*
  - gonococcal (acute) (chronic) A54.23
- **Orchitis** — *continued*
  - mumps B26.0
  - syphilitic A52.76
  - tuberculous A18.15
- **Orf** (virus disease) B08.02
- **Organic** (*see also* condition)
  - brain syndrome F09
  - heart — *see* Disease, heart
  - mental disorder F09
  - psychosis F09
- **Orgasm**
  - anejaculatory N53.13
- **Oriental**
  - bilharziasis B65.2
  - schistosomiasis B65.2
- **Orifice** — *see* condition
- **Origin** of both great vessels from right ventricle Q20.1
- **Ormond's** disease (with ureteral obstruction) N13.5
  - with infection N13.6
- **Ornithine** metabolism disorder E72.4
- **Ornithinemia** (Type I) (Type II) E72.4
- **Ornithosis** A70
- **Orotaciduria,** oroticaciduria (congenital) (hereditary) (pyrimidine deficiency) E79.8
  - anemia D53.0
- **Orthodontics**
  - adjustment Z46.4
  - fitting Z46.4
- **Orthopnea** R06.01
- **Orthopoxvirus** B08.09
  - specified NEC B08.09
- **Os,** uterus — *see* condition
- **Osgood-Schlatter** disease or osteochondrosis — *see* Osteochondrosis, juvenile, tibia
- **Osler** (-Weber)-Rendu disease I78.0
- **Osler's** nodes I33.0
- **Osmidrosis** L75.0
- **Osseous** — *see* condition
- **Ossification**
  - artery — *see* Arteriosclerosis
  - auricle (ear) — *see* Disorder, pinna, specified type NEC
  - bronchial J98.09
  - cardiac — *see* Degeneration, myocardial
  - cartilage (senile) — *see* Disorder, cartilage, specified type NEC
  - coronary (artery) — *see* Disease, heart, ischemic, atherosclerotic
  - diaphragm J98.6
  - ear, middle — *see* Otosclerosis
  - falx cerebri G96.19
  - fontanel, premature Q75.0
  - heart (*see also* Degeneration, myocardial)
    - valve — *see* Endocarditis
  - larynx J38.7
  - ligament — *see* Disorder, tendon, specified type NEC
    - posterior longitudinal — *see* Spondylopathy, specified NEC
  - meninges (cerebral) (spinal) G96.19
  - multiple, eccentric centers — *see* Disorder, bone, development or growth
  - muscle (*see also* Calcification, muscle)
    - due to burns — *see* Myositis, ossificans, in, burns
    - paralytic — *see* Myositis, ossificans, in, quadriplegia
    - progressive — *see* Myositis, ossificans, progressiva
    - specified NEC M61.50
      - ankle M61.57 ☑
      - foot M61.57 ☑
      - forearm M61.53 ☑
      - hand M61.54 ☑
      - lower leg M61.56 ☑
      - multiple sites M61.59
      - pelvic region M61.55 ☑
      - shoulder region M61.51 ☑
      - specified site NEC M61.58
      - thigh M61.55 ☑
      - upper arm M61.52 ☑
    - traumatic — *see* Myositis, ossificans, traumatica
  - myocardium, myocardial — *see* Degeneration, myocardial
  - penis N48.89
  - periarticular — *see* Disorder, joint, specified type NEC
  - pinna — *see* Disorder, pinna, specified type NEC
  - rider's bone — *see* Ossification, muscle, specified NEC
  - sclera H15.89
- **Ossification** — *continued*
  - subperiosteal, post-traumatic M89.8X ☑
  - tendon — *see* Disorder, tendon, specified type NEC
  - trachea J39.8
  - tympanic membrane — *see* Disorder, tympanic membrane, specified NEC
  - vitreous (humor) — *see* Deposit, crystalline
- **Osteitis** (*see also* Osteomyelitis)
  - alveolar M27.3
  - condensans M85.30
    - ankle M85.37 ☑
    - foot M85.37 ☑
    - forearm M85.33 ☑
    - hand M85.34 ☑
    - lower leg M85.36 ☑
    - multiple site M85.39
    - neck M85.38
    - rib M85.38
    - shoulder M85.31 ☑
    - skull M85.38
    - specified site NEC M85.38
    - thigh M85.35 ☑
    - toe M85.37 ☑
    - upper arm M85.32 ☑
    - vertebra M85.38
  - deformans M88.9
    - in (due to)
      - malignant neoplasm of bone C41.9 *[M90.60]*
      - neoplastic disease (*see also* Neoplasm)D49.9 *[M90.60]*
        - carpus D49.9 *[M90.64-]*
        - clavicle D49.9 *[M90.61-]*
        - femur D49.9 *[M90.65-]*
        - fibula D49.9 *[M90.66-]*
        - finger D49.9 *[M90.64-]*
        - humerus D49.9 *[M90.62-]*
        - ilium D49.9 *[M90.65-]*
        - ischium D49.9 *[M90.65-]*
        - metacarpus D49.9 *[M90.64-]*
        - metatarsus D49.9 *[M90.67-]*
        - multiple sites D49.9 *[M90.69]*
        - neck D49.9 *[M90.68]*
        - radius D49.9 *[M90.63-]*
        - rib D49.9 *[M90.68]*
        - scapula D49.9 *[M90.61-]*
        - skull D49.9 *[M90.68]*
        - tarsus D49.9 *[M90.67-]*
        - tibia D49.9 *[M90.66-]*
        - toe D49.9 *[M90.67-]*
        - ulna D49.9 *[M90.63-]*
        - vertebra D49.9 *[M90.68]*
    - skull M88.0
    - specified NEC — *see* Paget's disease, bone, by site
    - vertebra M88.1
  - due to yaws A66.6
  - fibrosa NEC — *see* Cyst, bone, by site
    - circumscripta — *see* Dysplasia, fibrous, bone NEC
    - cystica (generalisata) E21.0
    - disseminata Q78.1
    - osteoplastica E21.0
  - fragilitans Q78.0
  - Garr's (sclerosing) — *see* Osteomyelitis, specified type NEC
  - jaw (acute) (chronic) (lower) (suppurative) (upper) M27.2
  - parathyroid E21.0
  - petrous bone (acute) (chronic) — *see* Petrositis
  - sclerotic, nonsuppurative — *see* Osteomyelitis, specified type NEC
  - tuberculosa A18.09
    - cystica D86.89
    - multiplex cystoides D86.89
- **Osteoarthritis** M19.90
  - ankle M19.07 ☑
  - elbow M19.02 ☑
  - foot joint M19.07 ☑
  - generalized M15.9
    - erosive M15.4
    - primary M15.0
    - specified NEC M15.8
  - hand joint M19.04 ☑
    - first carpometacarpal joint M18.9
  - hip M16.1 ☑
    - bilateral M16.0
    - due to hip dysplasia (unilateral) M16.3 ☑
      - bilateral M16.2
  - interphalangeal
    - distal (Heberden) M15.1
    - proximal (Bouchard) M15.2

- **Osteoarthritis** — *continued*
  - knee M17.9
    - bilateral M17.0
  - shoulder M19.01 ☑
  - spine — *see* Spondylosis
  - wrist M19.03 ☑
  - post-traumatic NEC M19.92
    - ankle M19.17 ☑
    - elbow M19.12 ☑
    - foot joint M19.17 ☑
    - hand joint M19.14 ☑
      - first carpometacarpal joint M18.3 ☑
        - bilateral M18.2
    - hip M16.5 ☑
      - bilateral M16.4
    - knee M17.3 ☑
      - bilateral M17.2
    - shoulder M19.11 ☑
    - wrist M19.13 ☑
  - primary M19.91
    - ankle M19.07 ☑
    - elbow M19.02 ☑
    - foot joint M19.07 ☑
    - hand joint M19.04 ☑
      - first carpometacarpal joint M18.1 ☑
        - bilateral M18.0
    - hip M16.1 ☑
      - bilateral M16.0
    - knee M17.1 ☑
      - bilateral M17.0
    - shoulder M19.01 ☑
    - spine — *see* Spondylosis
    - wrist M19.03 ☑
  - secondary M19.93
    - ankle M19.27 ☑
    - elbow M19.22 ☑
    - foot joint M19.27 ☑
    - hand joint M19.24 ☑
      - first carpometacarpal joint M18.5 ☑
        - bilateral M18.4
    - hip M16.7
      - bilateral M16.6
    - knee M17.5
      - bilateral M17.4
    - multiple M15.3
    - shoulder M19.21 ☑
    - spine — *see* Spondylosis
    - wrist M19.23 ☑
- **Osteoarthropathy** (hypertrophic) M19.90
  - ankle — *see* Osteoarthritis, primary, ankle
  - elbow — *see* Osteoarthritis, primary, elbow
  - foot joint — *see* Osteoarthritis, primary, foot
  - hand joint — *see* Osteoarthritis, primary, hand joint
  - knee joint — *see* Osteoarthritis, primary, knee
  - multiple site — *see* Osteoarthritis, primary, multiple joint
  - pulmonary (*see also* Osteoarthropathy, specified type NEC)
    - hypertrophic — *see* Osteoarthropathy, hypertrophic, specified type NEC
  - secondary hypertrophic — *see* Osteoarthropathy, specified type NEC
  - shoulder — *see* Osteoarthritis, primary, shoulder
  - specified joint NEC — *see* Osteoarthritis, primary, specified joint NEC
  - specified type NEC M89.40
    - carpus M89.44 ☑
    - clavicle M89.41 ☑
    - femur M89.45 ☑
    - fibula M89.46 ☑
    - finger M89.44 ☑
    - humerus M89.42 ☑
    - ilium M89.459
    - ischium M89.459
    - metacarpus M89.44 ☑
    - metatarsus M89.47 ☑
    - multiple sites M89.49
    - neck M89.48
    - radius M89.43 ☑
    - rib M89.48
    - scapula M89.41 ☑
    - skull M89.48
    - tarsus M89.47 ☑
    - tibia M89.46 ☑
    - toe M89.47 ☑
    - ulna M89.43 ☑
    - vertebra M89.48
  - secondary — *see* Osteoarthropathy, specified type NEC
  - spine — *see* Spondylosis
  - wrist — *see* Osteoarthritis, primary, wrist
- **Osteoarthropathy** (degenerative) (hypertrophic) (joint) (*see also* Osteoarthritis)
  - deformans alkaptonurica E70.29 *[M36.8]*
  - erosive M15.4
  - generalized M15.9
    - primary M15.0
  - polyarticular M15.9
  - spine — *see* Spondylosis
- **Osteoblastoma** — *see* Neoplasm, bone, benign
  - aggressive — *see* Neoplasm, bone, uncertain behavior
- **Osteochondroarthrosis** deformans endemica — *see* Disease, Kaschin-Beck
- **Osteochondritis** (*see also* Osteochondropathy, by site)
  - Brailsford's — *see* Osteochondrosis, juvenile, radius
  - dissecans M93.20
    - ankle M93.27 ☑
    - elbow M93.22 ☑
    - foot M93.27 ☑
    - hand M93.24 ☑
    - hip M93.25 ☑
    - knee M93.26 ☑
    - multiple sites M93.29
    - shoulder joint M93.21 ☑
    - specified site NEC M93.28
    - wrist M93.23 ☑
  - juvenile M92.9
    - patellar — *see* Osteochondrosis, juvenile, patella
  - syphilitic (congenital) (early) A50.02 *[M90.80]*
    - ankle A50.02 *[M90.87-]*
    - elbow A50.02 *[M90.82-]*
    - foot A50.02 *[M90.87-]*
    - forearm A50.02 *[M90.83-]*
    - hand A50.02 *[M90.84-]*
    - hip A50.02 *[M90.85-]*
    - knee A50.02 *[M90.86-]*
    - multiple sites A50.02 *[M90.89]*
    - shoulder joint A50.02 *[M90.81-]*
    - specified site NEC A50.02 *[M90.88]*
- **Osteochondrodysplasia** Q78.9
  - with defects of growth of tubular bones and spine Q77.9
    - specified NEC Q77.8
  - specified NEC Q78.8
- **Osteochondrodystrophy** E78.9
- **Osteochondrolysis** — *see* Osteochondritis, dissecans
- **Osteochondroma** — *see* Neoplasm, bone, benign
- **Osteochondromatosis** D48.0
  - syndrome Q78.4
- **Osteochondromyxosarcoma** — *see* Neoplasm, bone, malignant
- **Osteochondropathy** M93.90
  - ankle M93.97 ☑
  - elbow M93.92 ☑
  - foot M93.97 ☑
  - hand M93.94 ☑
  - hip M93.95 ☑
  - Kienböck's disease of adults M93.1
  - knee M93.96 ☑
  - multiple joints M93.99
  - osteochondritis dissecans — *see* Osteochondritis, dissecans
  - osteochondrosis — *see* Osteochondrosis
  - shoulder region M93.91 ☑
  - slipped upper femoral epiphysis — *see* Slipped, epiphysis, upper femoral
  - specified joint NEC M93.98
  - specified type NEC M93.80
    - ankle M93.87 ☑
    - elbow M93.82 ☑
    - foot M93.87 ☑
    - hand M93.84 ☑
    - hip M93.85 ☑
    - knee M93.86 ☑
    - multiple joints M93.89
    - shoulder region M93.81 ☑
    - specified joint NEC M93.88
    - wrist M93.83 ☑
  - syphilitic, congenital
    - early A50.02 *[M90.80]*
    - late A50.56 *[M90.80]*
  - wrist M93.93 ☑
- **Osteochondrosarcoma** — *see* Neoplasm, bone, malignant
- **Osteochondrosis** (*see also* Osteochondropathy, by site)
  - acetabulum (juvenile) M91.0
  - adult — *see* Osteochondropathy, specified type NEC, by site
- **Osteochondrosis** — *continued*
  - astragalus (juvenile) — *see* Osteochondrosis, juvenile, tarsus
  - Blount's — *see* Osteochondrosis, juvenile, tibia
  - Buchanan's M91.0
  - Burns' — *see* Osteochondrosis, juvenile, ulna
  - calcaneus (juvenile) — *see* Osteochondrosis, juvenile, tarsus
  - capitular epiphysis (femur) (juvenile) — *see* Legg-Calvé-Perthes disease
  - carpal (juvenile) (lunate) (scaphoid) — *see* Osteochondrosis, juvenile, hand, carpal lunate
    - adult M93.1
  - coxae juvenilis — *see* Legg-Calvé-Perthes disease
  - deformans juvenilis, coxae — *see* Legg-Calvé-Perthes disease
  - Diaz's — *see* Osteochondrosis, juvenile, tarsus
  - dissecans (knee) (shoulder) — *see* Osteochondritis, dissecans
  - femoral capital epiphysis (juvenile) — *see* Legg-Calvé-Perthes disease
  - femur (head), juvenile — *see* Legg-Calvé-Perthes disease
  - fibula (juvenile) — *see* Osteochondrosis, juvenile, fibula
  - foot NEC (juvenile) M92.8
  - Freiberg's — *see* Osteochondrosis, juvenile, metatarsus
  - Haas' (juvenile) — *see* Osteochondrosis, juvenile, humerus
  - Haglund's — *see* Osteochondrosis, juvenile, tarsus
  - hip (juvenile) — *see* Legg-Calvé-Perthes disease
  - humerus (capitulum) (head) (juvenile) — *see* Osteochondrosis, juvenile, humerus
  - ilium, iliac crest (juvenile) M91.0
  - ischiopubic synchondrosis M91.0
  - Iselin's — *see* Osteochondrosis, juvenile, metatarsus
  - juvenile, juvenilis M92.9
    - after congenital dislocation of hip reduction — *see* Osteochondrosis, juvenile, hip, specified NEC
    - arm — *see* Osteochondrosis, juvenile, upper limb NEC
    - capitular epiphysis (femur) — *see* Legg-Calvé-Perthes disease
    - clavicle, sternal epiphysis — *see* Osteochondrosis, juvenile, upper limb NEC
    - coxae — *see* Legg-Calvé-Perthes disease
    - deformans M92.9
    - fibula M92.5 ☑
    - foot NEC M92.8
    - hand M92.20 ☑
      - carpal lunate M92.21 ☑
      - metacarpal head M92.22 ☑
      - specified site NEC M92.29 ☑
    - head of femur — *see* Legg-Calvé-Perthes disease
    - hip and pelvis M91.9 ☑
      - coxa plana — *see* Coxa, plana
      - femoral head — *see* Legg-Calvé-Perthes disease
      - pelvis M91.0
      - pseudocoxalgia — *see* Pseudocoxalgia
      - specified NEC M91.8 ☑
    - humerus M92.0 ☑
    - limb
      - lower NEC M92.8
      - upper NEC — *see* Osteochondrosis, juvenile, upper limb NEC
    - medial cuneiform bone — *see* Osteochondrosis, juvenile, tarsus
    - metatarsus M92.7 ☑
    - patella M92.4 ☑
    - radius M92.1 ☑
    - specified site NEC M92.8
    - spine M42.00
      - cervical region M42.02
      - cervicothoracic region M42.03
      - lumbar region M42.06
      - lumbosacral region M42.07
      - multiple sites M42.09
      - occipito-atlanto-axial region M42.01
      - sacrococcygeal region M42.08
      - thoracic region M42.04
      - thoracolumbar region M42.05
    - tarsus M92.6 ☑
    - tibia M92.5 ☑
    - ulna M92.1 ☑
    - upper limb NEC M92.3 ☑

- **Osteochondrosis** — *continued*
  - juvenile, juvenilis — *continued*
    - vertebra (body) (epiphyseal plates) (Calvé's) (Scheuermann's) — *see* Osteochondrosis, juvenile, spine
  - Kienböck's — *see* Osteochondrosis, juvenile, hand, carpal lunate
    - adult M93.1
  - Köhler's
    - patellar — *see* Osteochondrosis, juvenile, patella
    - tarsal navicular — *see* Osteochondrosis, juvenile, tarsus
  - Legg-Perthes (-Calvé) (-Waldenström) — *see* Legg-Calvé-Perthes disease
  - limb
    - lower NEC (juvenile) M92.8
    - upper NEC (juvenile) — *see* Osteochondrosis, juvenile, upper limb NEC
  - lunate bone (carpal) (juvenile) (*see also* Osteochondrosis, juvenile, hand, carpal lunate)
    - adult M93.1
  - Mauclaire's — *see* Osteochondrosis, juvenile, hand, metacarpal
  - metacarpal (head) (juvenile) — *see* Osteochondrosis, juvenile, hand, metacarpal
  - metatarsus (fifth) (head) (juvenile) (second) — *see* Osteochondrosis, juvenile, metatarsus
  - navicular (juvenile) — *see* Osteochondrosis, juvenile, tarsus
  - os
    - calcis (juvenile) — *see* Osteochondrosis, juvenile, tarsus
    - tibiale externum (juvenile) — *see* Osteochondrosis, juvenile, tarsus
  - Osgood-Schlatter — *see* Osteochondrosis, juvenile, tibia
  - Panner's — *see* Osteochondrosis, juvenile, humerus
  - patellar center (juvenile) (primary) (secondary) — *see* Osteochondrosis, juvenile, patella
  - pelvis (juvenile) M91.0
  - Pierson's M91.0
  - radius (head) (juvenile) — *see* Osteochondrosis, juvenile, radius
  - Scheuermann's — *see* Osteochondrosis, juvenile, spine
  - Sever's — *see* Osteochondrosis, juvenile, tarsus
  - Sinding-Larsen — *see* Osteochondrosis, juvenile, patella
  - spine M42.9
    - adult M42.10
      - cervical region M42.12
      - cervicothoracic region M42.13
      - lumbar region M42.16
      - lumbosacral region M42.17
      - multiple sites M42.19
      - occipito-atlanto-axial region M42.11
      - sacrococcygeal region M42.18
      - thoracic region M42.14
      - thoracolumbar region M42.15
    - juvenile — *see* Osteochondrosis, juvenile, spine
  - symphysis pubis (juvenile) M91.0
  - syphilitic (congenital) A50.02
  - talus (juvenile) — *see* Osteochondrosis, juvenile, tarsus
  - tarsus (navicular) (juvenile) — *see* Osteochondrosis, juvenile, tarsus
  - tibia (proximal) (tubercle) (juvenile) — *see* Osteochondrosis, juvenile, tibia
  - tuberculous — *see* Tuberculosis, bone
  - ulna (lower) (juvenile) — *see* Osteochondrosis, juvenile, ulna
  - van Neck's M91.0
  - vertebral — *see* Osteochondrosis, spine
- **Osteoclastoma** D48.0
  - malignant — *see* Neoplasm, bone, malignant
- **Osteodynia** — *see* Disorder, bone, specified type NEC
- **Osteodystrophy** Q78.9
  - azotemic N25.0
  - congenital Q78.9
  - parathyroid, secondary E21.1
  - renal N25.0
- **Osteofibroma** — *see* Neoplasm, bone, benign
- **Osteofibrosarcoma** — *see* Neoplasm, bone, malignant
- **Osteogenesis** imperfecta Q78.0
- **Osteogenic** — *see* condition
- **Osteolysis** M89.50
  - carpus M89.54 ☑
- **Osteolysis** — *continued*
  - clavicle M89.51 ☑
  - femur M89.55 ☑
  - fibula M89.56 ☑
  - finger M89.54 ☑
  - humerus M89.52 ☑
  - ilium M89.559
  - ischium M89.559
  - joint prosthesis (periprosthetic) — *see* Complications, joint prosthesis, mechanical, periprosthetic, osteolysis, by site
  - metacarpus M89.54 ☑
  - metatarsus M89.57 ☑
  - multiple sites M89.59
  - neck M89.58
  - periprosthetic — *see* Complications, joint prosthesis, mechanical, periprosthetic, osteolysis, by site
  - radius M89.53 ☑
  - rib M89.58
  - scapula M89.51 ☑
  - skull M89.58
  - tarsus M89.57 ☑
  - tibia M89.56 ☑
  - toe M89.57 ☑
  - ulna M89.53 ☑
  - vertebra M89.58
- **Osteoma** (*see also* Neoplasm, bone, benign)
  - osteoid (*see also* Neoplasm, bone, benign)
    - giant — *see* Neoplasm, bone, benign
- **Osteomalacia** M83.9
  - adult M83.9
    - drug-induced NEC M83.5
    - due to
      - malabsorption (postsurgical) M83.2
      - malnutrition M83.3
    - specified NEC M83.8
  - aluminium-induced M83.4
  - infantile — *see* Rickets
  - juvenile — *see* Rickets
  - oncogenic E83.89
  - pelvis M83.8
  - puerperal M83.0
  - senile M83.1
  - vitamin-D-resistant in adults E83.31 *[M90.8-]*
    - carpus E83.31 *[M90.84-]*
    - clavicle E83.31 *[M90.81-]*
    - femur E83.31 *[M90.85-]*
    - fibula E83.31 *[M90.86-]*
    - finger E83.31 *[M90.84-]*
    - humerus E83.31 *[M90.82-]*
    - ilium E83.31 *[M90.859]*
    - ischium E83.31 *[M90.859]*
    - metacarpus E83.31 *[M90.84-]*
    - metatarsus E83.31 *[M90.87-]*
    - multiple sites E83.31 *[M90.89]*
    - neck E83.31 *[M90.88]*
    - radius E83.31 *[M90.83-]*
    - rib E83.31 *[M90.88]*
    - scapula E83.31 *[M90.819]*
    - skull E83.31 *[M90.88]*
    - tarsus E83.31 *[M90.879]*
    - tibia E83.31 *[M90.869]*
    - toe E83.31 *[M90.879]*
    - ulna E83.31 *[M90.839]*
    - vertebra E83.31 *[M90.88]*
- **Osteomyelitis** (general) (infective) (localized) (neonatal) (purulent) (septic) (staphylococcal) (streptococcal) (suppurative) (with periostitis) M86.9
  - acute M86.10
    - carpus M86.14 ☑
    - clavicle M86.11 ☑
    - femur M86.15 ☑
    - fibula M86.16 ☑
    - finger M86.14 ☑
    - hematogenous M86.00
      - carpus M86.04 ☑
      - clavicle M86.01 ☑
      - femur M86.05 ☑
      - fibula M86.06 ☑
      - finger M86.04 ☑
      - humerus M86.02 ☑
      - ilium M86.059
      - ischium M86.059
      - mandible M27.2
      - metacarpus M86.04 ☑
      - metatarsus M86.07 ☑
      - multiple sites M86.09
      - neck M86.08
      - orbit H05.02 ☑
      - petrous bone — *see* Petrositis
- **Osteomyelitis** — *continued*
  - acute — *continued*
      - radius M86.03 ☑
      - rib M86.08
      - scapula M86.01 ☑
      - skull M86.08
      - tarsus M86.07 ☑
      - tibia M86.06 ☑
      - toe M86.07 ☑
      - ulna M86.03 ☑
      - vertebra — *see* Osteomyelitis, vertebra
    - humerus M86.12 ☑
    - ilium M86.159
    - ischium M86.159
    - mandible M27.2
    - metacarpus M86.14 ☑
    - metatarsus M86.17 ☑
    - multiple sites M86.19
    - neck M86.18
    - orbit H05.02 ☑
    - petrous bone — *see* Petrositis
    - radius M86.13 ☑
    - rib M86.18
    - scapula M86.11 ☑
    - skull M86.18
    - tarsus M86.17 ☑
    - tibia M86.16 ☑
    - toe M86.17 ☑
    - ulna M86.13 ☑
    - vertebra — *see* Osteomyelitis, vertebra
  - chronic (or old) M86.60
    - with draining sinus M86.40
      - carpus M86.44 ☑
      - clavicle M86.41 ☑
      - femur M86.45 ☑
      - fibula M86.46 ☑
      - finger M86.44 ☑
      - humerus M86.42 ☑
      - ilium M86.459
      - ischium M86.459
      - mandible M27.2
      - metacarpus M86.44 ☑
      - metatarsus M86.47 ☑
      - multiple sites M86.49
      - neck M86.48
      - orbit H05.02 ☑
      - petrous bone — *see* Petrositis
      - radius M86.43 ☑
      - rib M86.48
      - scapula M86.41 ☑
      - skull M86.48
      - tarsus M86.47 ☑
      - tibia M86.46 ☑
      - toe M86.47 ☑
      - ulna M86.43 ☑
      - vertebra — *see* Osteomyelitis, vertebra
    - carpus M86.64 ☑
    - clavicle M86.61 ☑
    - femur M86.65 ☑
    - fibula M86.66 ☑
    - finger M86.64 ☑
    - hematogenous NEC M86.50
      - carpus M86.54 ☑
      - clavicle M86.51 ☑
      - femur M86.55 ☑
      - fibula M86.56 ☑
      - finger M86.54 ☑
      - humerus M86.52 ☑
      - ilium M86.559
      - ischium M86.559
      - mandible M27.2
      - metacarpus M86.54 ☑
      - metatarsus M86.57 ☑
      - multifocal M86.30
        - carpus M86.34 ☑
        - clavicle M86.31 ☑
        - femur M86.35 ☑
        - fibula M86.36 ☑
        - finger M86.34 ☑
        - humerus M86.32 ☑
        - ilium M86.359
        - ischium M86.359
        - metacarpus M86.34 ☑
        - metatarsus M86.37 ☑
        - multiple sites M86.39
        - neck M86.38
        - radius M86.33 ☑
        - rib M86.38
        - scapula M86.31 ☑
        - skull M86.38
        - tarsus M86.37 ☑
        - tibia M86.36 ☑

- **Osteomyelitis** — *continued*
  - chronic — *continued*
        - toe M86.37 ☑
        - ulna M86.33 ☑
        - vertebra — *see* Osteomyelitis, vertebra
      - multiple sites M86.59
      - neck M86.58
      - orbit H05.02 ☑
      - petrous bone — *see* Petrositis
      - radius M86.53 ☑
      - rib M86.58
      - scapula M86.51 ☑
      - skull M86.58
      - tarsus M86.57 ☑
      - tibia M86.56 ☑
      - toe M86.57 ☑
      - ulna M86.53 ☑
      - vertebra — *see* Osteomyelitis, vertebra
    - humerus M86.62 ☑
    - ilium M86.659
    - ischium M86.659
    - mandible M27.2
    - metacarpus M86.64 ☑
    - metatarsus M86.67 ☑
    - multifocal — *see* Osteomyelitis, chronic, hematogenous, multifocal
    - multiple sites M86.69
    - neck M86.68
    - orbit H05.02 ☑
    - petrous bone — *see* Petrositis
    - radius M86.63 ☑
    - rib M86.68
    - scapula M86.61 ☑
    - skull M86.68
    - tarsus M86.67 ☑
    - tibia M86.66 ☑
    - toe M86.67 ☑
    - ulna M86.63 ☑
    - vertebra — *see* Osteomyelitis, vertebra
  - echinococcal B67.2
  - Garr's — *see* Osteomyelitis, specified type NEC
  - in diabetes mellitus — *see* E08-E13 with .69
  - jaw (acute) (chronic) (lower) (neonatal) (suppurative) (upper) M27.2
  - nonsuppurating — *see* Osteomyelitis, specified type NEC
  - orbit H05.02 ☑
  - petrous bone — *see* Petrositis
  - Salmonella (arizonae) (cholerae-suis) (enteritidis) (typhimurium) A02.24
  - sclerosing, nonsuppurative — *see* Osteomyelitis, specified type NEC
  - specified type NEC (*see also* subcategory)M86.8X ☑
    - mandible M27.2
    - orbit H05.02 ☑
    - petrous bone — *see* Petrositis
    - vertebra — *see* Osteomyelitis, vertebra
  - subacute M86.20
    - carpus M86.24 ☑
    - clavicle M86.21 ☑
    - femur M86.25 ☑
    - fibula M86.26 ☑
    - finger M86.24 ☑
    - humerus M86.22 ☑
    - mandible M27.2
    - metacarpus M86.24 ☑
    - metatarsus M86.27 ☑
    - multiple sites M86.29
    - neck M86.28
    - orbit H05.02 ☑
    - petrous bone — *see* Petrositis
    - radius M86.23 ☑
    - rib M86.28
    - scapula M86.21 ☑
    - skull M86.28
    - tarsus M86.27 ☑
    - tibia M86.26 ☑
    - toe M86.27 ☑
    - ulna M86.23 ☑
    - vertebra — *see* Osteomyelitis, vertebra
  - syphilitic A52.77
    - congenital (early) A50.02 *[M90.80]*
  - tuberculous — *see* Tuberculosis, bone
  - typhoid A01.05
  - vertebra M46.20
    - cervical region M46.22
    - cervicothoracic region M46.23
    - lumbar region M46.26
    - lumbosacral region M46.27
    - occipito-atlanto-axial region M46.21
    - sacrococcygeal region M46.28

- **Osteomyelitis** — *continued*
  - vertebra — *continued*
    - thoracic region M46.24
    - thoracolumbar region M46.25
- **Osteomyelofibrosis** D47.4
- **Osteomyelosclerosis** D75.89
- **Osteonecrosis** M87.9
  - due to
    - drugs — *see* Osteonecrosis, secondary, due to, drugs
    - trauma — *see* Osteonecrosis, secondary, due to, trauma
  - idiopathic aseptic M87.00
    - ankle M87.07 ☑
    - carpus M87.03 ☑
    - clavicle M87.01 ☑
    - femur M87.05 ☑
    - fibula M87.06 ☑
    - finger M87.04 ☑
    - humerus M87.02 ☑
    - ilium M87.050
    - ischium M87.050
    - metacarpus M87.04 ☑
    - metatarsus M87.07 ☑
    - multiple sites M87.09
    - neck M87.08
    - pelvis M87.050
    - radius M87.03 ☑
    - rib M87.08
    - scapula M87.01 ☑
    - skull M87.08
    - tarsus M87.07 ☑
    - tibia M87.06 ☑
    - toe M87.07 ☑
    - ulna M87.03 ☑
    - vertebra M87.08
  - secondary NEC M87.30
    - carpus M87.33 ☑
    - clavicle M87.31 ☑
    - due to
      - drugs M87.10
        - carpus M87.13 ☑
        - clavicle M87.11 ☑
        - femur M87.15 ☑
        - fibula M87.16 ☑
        - finger M87.14 ☑
        - humerus M87.12 ☑
        - ilium M87.159
        - ischium M87.159
        - jaw M87.180
        - metacarpus M87.14 ☑
        - metatarsus M87.17 ☑
        - multiple sites M87.19
        - neck M87.18 ☑
        - radius M87.13 ☑
        - rib M87.18 ☑
        - scapula M87.11 ☑
        - skull M87.18 ☑
        - tarsus M87.17 ☑
        - tibia M87.16 ☑
        - toe M87.17 ☑
        - ulna M87.13 ☑
        - vertebra M87.18 ☑
      - hemoglobinopathy NEC D58.2 *[M90.50]*
        - carpus D58.2 *[M90.54-]*
        - clavicle D58.2 *[M90.51-]*
        - femur D58.2 *[M90.55-]*
        - fibula D58.2 *[M90.56-]*
        - finger D58.2 *[M90.54-]*
        - humerus D58.2 *[M90.52-]*
        - ilium D58.2 *[M90.55-]*
        - ischium D58.2 *[M90.55-]*
        - metacarpus D58.2 *[M90.54-]*
        - metatarsus D58.2 *[M90.57-]*
        - multiple sites D58.2 *[M90.58]*
        - neck D58.2 *[M90.58]*
        - radius D58.2 *[M90.53-]*
        - rib D58.2 *[M90.58]*
        - scapula D58.2 *[M90.51-]*
        - skull D58.2 *[M90.58]*
        - tarsus D58.2 *[M90.57-]*
        - tibia D58.2 *[M90.56-]*
        - toe D58.2 *[M90.57-]*
        - ulna D58.2 *[M90.53-]*
        - vertebra D58.2 *[M90.58]*
      - trauma (previous) M87.20
        - carpus M87.23 ☑
        - clavicle M87.21 ☑
        - femur M87.25 ☑
        - fibula M87.26 ☑
        - finger M87.24 ☑
        - humerus M87.22 ☑

- **Osteonecrosis** — *continued*
  - secondary NEC — *continued*
        - ilium M87.25 ☑
        - ischium M87.25 ☑
        - metacarpus M87.24 ☑
        - metatarsus M87.27 ☑
        - multiple sites M87.29
        - neck M87.28
        - radius M87.23 ☑
        - rib M87.28
        - scapula M87.21 ☑
        - skull M87.28
        - tarsus M87.27 ☑
        - tibia M87.26 ☑
        - toe M87.27 ☑
        - ulna M87.23 ☑
        - vertebra M87.28
    - femur M87.35 ☑
    - fibula M87.36 ☑
    - finger M87.34 ☑
    - humerus M87.32 ☑
    - ilium M87.350
    - in
      - caisson disease T70.3 ☑ *[M90.50]*
        - carpus T70.3 ☑ *[M90.54-]*
        - clavicle T70.3 ☑ *[M90.51-]*
        - femur T70.3 ☑ *[M90.55-]*
        - fibula T70.3 ☑ *[M90.56-]*
        - finger T70.3 ☑ *[M90.54-]*
        - humerus T70.3 ☑ *[M90.52-]*
        - ilium T70.3 ☑ *[M90.55-]*
        - ischium T70.3 ☑ *[M90.55-]*
        - metacarpus T70.3 ☑ *[M90.54-]*
        - metatarsus T70.3 ☑ *[M90.57-]*
        - multiple sites T70.3 ☑ *[M90.59]*
        - neck T70.3 ☑ *[M90.58]*
        - radius T70.3 ☑ *[M90.53-]*
        - rib T70.3 ☑ *[M90.58]*
        - scapula T70.3 ☑ *[M90.51-]*
        - skull T70.3 ☑ *[M90.58]*
        - tarsus T70.3 ☑ *[M90.57-]*
        - tibia T70.3 ☑ *[M90.56-]*
        - toe T70.3 ☑ *[M90.57-]*
        - ulna T70.3 ☑ *[M90.53-]*
        - vertebra T70.3 ☑ *[M90.58]*
    - ischium M87.350
    - metacarpus M87.34 ☑
    - metatarsus M87.37 ☑
    - multiple site M87.39
    - neck M87.38
    - radius M87.33 ☑
    - rib M87.38
    - scapula M87.319
    - skull M87.38
    - tarsus M87.379
    - tibia M87.366
    - toe M87.379
    - ulna M87.33 ☑
    - vertebra M87.38
  - specified type NEC M87.80
    - carpus M87.83 ☑
    - clavicle M87.81 ☑
    - femur M87.85 ☑
    - fibula M87.86 ☑
    - finger M87.84 ☑
    - humerus M87.82 ☑
    - ilium M87.85 ☑
    - ischium M87.85 ☑
    - metacarpus M87.84 ☑
    - metatarsus M87.87 ☑
    - multiple sites M87.89
    - neck M87.88
    - radius M87.83 ☑
    - rib M87.88
    - scapula M87.81 ☑
    - skull M87.88
    - tarsus M87.87 ☑
    - tibia M87.86 ☑
    - toe M87.87 ☑
    - ulna M87.83 ☑
    - vertebra M87.88
- **Osteo-onycho-arthro-dysplasia** Q87.2
- **Osteo-onychodysplasia,** hereditary Q87.2
- **Osteopathia** condensans disseminata Q78.8
- **Osteopathy** (*see also* Osteomyelitis, Osteonecrosis, Osteoporosis)
  - after poliomyelitis M89.60
    - carpus M89.64 ☑
    - clavicle M89.61 ☑
    - femur M89.65 ☑
    - fibula M89.66 ☑
    - finger M89.64 ☑

- **Otitis** — *continued*
  - media — *continued*
    - transudative — *see* Otitis, media, nonsuppurative, chronic, mucoid
    - exudative — *see* Otitis, media, suppurative
    - in (due to) (with)
      - influenza — *see* Influenza, with, otitis media
      - measles B05.3
      - scarlet fever A38.0
      - tuberculosis A18.6
      - viral disease NEC B34. ☑ *[H67.☑]*
    - mucoid — *see* Otitis, media, nonsuppurative
    - nonsuppurative H65.9 ☑
      - acute or subacute NEC H65.19 ☑
        - allergic H65.11 ☑
          - recurrent H65.11 ☑
        - recurrent H65.19 ☑
        - secretory — *see* Otitis, media, nonsuppurative, serous
        - serous H65.0 ☑
          - recurrent H65.0 ☑
      - chronic H65.49 ☑
        - allergic H65.41 ☑
        - mucoid H65.3 ☑
        - serous H65.2 ☑
    - postmeasles B05.3
    - purulent — *see* Otitis, media, suppurative
    - secretory — *see* Otitis, media, nonsuppurative
    - seromucinous — *see* Otitis, media, nonsuppurative
    - serous — *see* Otitis, media, nonsuppurative
    - suppurative H66.4 ☑
      - acute H66.00 ☑
        - with rupture of ear drum H66.01 ☑
        - recurrent H66.00 ☑
          - with rupture of ear drum H66.01 ☑
      - chronic (*see also* subcategory)H66.3 ☑
        - atticoantral H66.2 ☑
        - benign — *see* Otitis, media, suppurative, chronic, tubotympanic
        - tubotympanic H66.1 ☑
    - transudative — *see* Otitis, media, nonsuppurative
    - tuberculous A18.6
- **Otocephaly** Q18.2
- **Otolith** syndrome — *see* subcategory H81.8
- **Otomycosis** (diffuse) NEC B36.9 *[H62.40]*
  - in
    - aspergillosis B44.89
    - candidiasis B37.84
    - moniliasis B37.84
- **Otoporosis** — *see* Otosclerosis
- **Otorrhagia** (nontraumatic) H92.2 ☑
  - traumatic - code by Type of injury
- **Otorrhea** H92.1 ☑
  - cerebrospinal G96.0
- **Otosclerosis** (general) H80.9 ☑
  - cochlear (endosteal) H80.2 ☑
  - involving
    - otic capsule — *see* Otosclerosis, cochlear
    - oval window
      - nonobliterative H80.0 ☑
      - obliterative H80.1 ☑
    - round window — *see* Otosclerosis, cochlear
  - nonobliterative — *see* Otosclerosis, involving, oval window, nonobliterative
  - obliterative — *see* Otosclerosis, involving, oval window, obliterative
  - specified NEC H80.8 ☑
- **Otospongiosis** — *see* Otosclerosis
- **Otto's** disease or pelvis M24.7
- **Outcome** of delivery Z37.9
  - multiple births Z37.9
    - all liveborn Z37.50
      - quadruplets Z37.52
      - quintuplets Z37.53
      - sextuplets Z37.54
      - specified number NEC Z37.59
      - triplets Z37.51
    - all stillborn Z37.7
    - some liveborn Z37.60
      - quadruplets Z37.62
      - quintuplets Z37.63
      - sextuplets Z37.64
      - specified number NEC Z37.69
      - triplets Z37.61
  - single NEC Z37.9
    - liveborn Z37.0
    - stillborn Z37.1
  - twins NEC Z37.9
    - both liveborn Z37.2
    - both stillborn Z37.4
    - one liveborn, one stillborn Z37.3
- **Outlet** — *see* condition
- **Ovalocytosis** (congenital) (hereditary) — *see* Elliptocytosis
- **Ovarian** — *see* Condition
- **Ovariocele** N83.4 ☑
- **Ovaritis** (cystic) — *see* Oophoritis
- **Ovary,** ovarian (*see also* condition)
  - resistant syndrome E28.39
  - vein syndrome N13.8
- **Overactive** (*see also* Hyperfunction)
  - adrenal cortex NEC E27.0
  - bladder N32.81
  - hypothalamus E23.3
  - thyroid — *see* Hyperthyroidism
- **Overactivity** R46.3
  - child — *see* Disorder, attention-deficit hyperactivity
- **Overbite** (deep) (excessive) (horizontal) (vertical) M26.29
- **Overbreathing** — *see* Hyperventilation
- **Overconscientious** personality F60.5
- **Overdevelopment** — *see* Hypertrophy
- **Overdistension** — *see* Distension
- **Overdose,** overdosage (drug) — *see* Table of Drugs and Chemicals, by drug, poisoning
- **Overeating** R63.2
  - nonorganic origin F50.89
  - psychogenic F50.89
- **Overexertion** (effects) (exhaustion) T73.3 ☑
- **Overexposure** (effects) T73.9 ☑
  - exhaustion T73.2 ☑
- **Overfeeding** — *see* Overeating
  - newborn P92.4
- **Overfill,** endodontic M27.52
- **Overgrowth,** bone — *see* Hypertrophy, bone
- **Overhanging** of dental restorative material (unrepairable) K08.52
- **Overheated** (places) (effects) — *see* Heat
- **Overjet** (excessive horizontal) M26.23
- **Overlaid,** overlying (suffocation) — *see* Asphyxia, traumatic, due to mechanical threat
- **Overlap,** excessive horizontal (teeth) M26.23
- **Overlapping** toe (acquired) (*see also* Deformity, toe, specified NEC)
  - congenital (fifth toe) Q66.89
- **Overload**
  - circulatory, due to transfusion (blood) (blood components) (TACO) E87.71
  - fluid E87.70
    - due to transfusion (blood) (blood components) E87.71
    - specified NEC E87.79
  - iron, due to repeated red blood cell transfusions E83.111
  - potassium (K) E87.5
  - sodium (Na) E87.0
- **Overnutrition** — *see* Hyperalimentation
- **Overproduction** (*see also* Hypersecretion)
  - ACTH E27.0
  - catecholamine E27.5
  - growth hormone E22.0
- **Overprotection,** child by parent Z62.1
- **Overriding**
  - aorta Q25.49
  - finger (acquired) — *see* Deformity, finger
    - congenital Q68.1
  - toe (acquired) (*see also* Deformity, toe, specified NEC)
    - congenital Q66.89
- **Overstrained** R53.83
  - heart — *see* Hypertrophy, cardiac
- **Overuse,** muscle NEC M70.8 ☑
- **Overweight** E66.3
- **Overworked** R53.83
- **Oviduct** — *see* condition
- **Ovotestis** Q56.0
- **Ovulation** (cycle)
  - failure or lack of N97.0
  - pain N94.0
- **Ovum** — *see* condition
- **Owren's** disease or syndrome (parahemophilia) D68.2
- **Ox heart** — *see* Hypertrophy, cardiac
- **Oxalosis** E72.53
- **Oxaluria** E72.53
- **Oxycephaly,** oxycephalic Q75.0
  - syphilitic, congenital A50.02
- **Oxyuriasis** B80
- **Oxyuris** vermicularis (infestation) B80
- **Ozena** J31.0

P

- **Pachyderma,** pachydermia L85.9
  - larynx (verrucosa) J38.7
- **Pachydermatocele** (congenital) Q82.8
- **Pachydermoperiostosis** (*see also* Osteoarthropathy, hypertrophic, specified type NEC)
  - clubbed nail M89.40 *[L62]*
- **Pachygyria** Q04.3
- **Pachymeningitis** (adhesive) (basal) (brain) (cervical) (chronic) (circumscribed) (external) (fibrous) (hemorrhagic) (hypertrophic) (internal) (purulent) (spinal) (suppurative) — *see* Meningitis
- **Pachyonychia** (congenital) Q84.5
- **Pacinian** tumor — *see* Neoplasm, skin, benign
- **Pad,** knuckle or Garrod's M72.1
- **Paget-Schroetter** syndrome I82.890
- **Paget's** disease
  - with infiltrating duct carcinoma — *see* Neoplasm, breast, malignant
  - bone M88.9
    - carpus M88.84 ☑
    - clavicle M88.81 ☑
    - femur M88.85 ☑
    - fibula M88.86 ☑
    - finger M88.84 ☑
    - humerus M88.82 ☑
    - ilium M88.85 ☑
    - in neoplastic disease — *see* Osteitis, deformans, in neoplastic disease
    - ischium M88.85 ☑
    - metacarpus M88.84 ☑
    - metatarsus M88.87 ☑
    - multiple sites M88.89
    - neck M88.88
    - radius M88.83 ☑
    - rib M88.88
    - scapula M88.81 ☑
    - skull M88.0
    - tarsus M88.87 ☑
    - tibia M88.86 ☑
    - toe M88.87 ☑
    - ulna M88.83 ☑
    - vertebra M88.88
  - breast (female) C50.01 ☑
    - male C50.02 ☑
  - extramammary (*see also* Neoplasm, skin, malignant)
    - anus C21.0
      - margin C44.590
      - skin C44.590
  - intraductal carcinoma — *see* Neoplasm, breast, malignant
  - malignant — *see* Neoplasm, skin, malignant
    - breast (female) C50.01 ☑
      - male C50.02 ☑
    - unspecified site (female) C50.01 ☑
      - male C50.02 ☑
  - mammary — *see* Paget's disease, breast
  - nipple — *see* Paget's disease, breast
  - osteitis deformans — *see* Paget's disease, bone
- **Pain** (s) (*see also* Painful)R52
  - abdominal R10.9
    - colic R10.83
    - generalized R10.84
      - with acute abdomen R10.0
    - lower R10.30
      - left quadrant R10.32
      - pelvic or perineal R10.2
      - periumbilical R10.33
      - right quadrant R10.31
    - rebound — *see* Tenderness, abdominal, rebound
    - severe with abdominal rigidity R10.0
    - tenderness — *see* Tenderness, abdominal
    - upper R10.10
      - epigastric R10.13
      - left quadrant R10.12
      - right quadrant R10.11
  - acute R52
    - due to trauma G89.11
    - neoplasm related G89.3
    - postprocedural NEC G89.18
    - post-thoracotomy G89.12
    - specified by site - code to Pain, by site
  - adnexa (uteri) R10.2
  - anginoid — *see* Pain, precordial
  - anus K62.89
  - arm — *see* Pain, limb, upper
  - axillary (axilla) M79.62 ☑
  - back (postural) M54.9

Pain — *continued*
- bladder R39.89
  - associated with micturition — *see* Micturition, painful
  - chronic R39.82
- bone — *see* Disorder, bone, specified type NEC
- breast N64.4
- broad ligament R10.2
- cancer associated (acute) (chronic) G89.3
- cecum — *see* Pain, abdominal
- cervicobrachial M53.1
- chest (central) R07.9
  - anterior wall R07.89
  - atypical R07.89
  - ischemic I20.9
  - musculoskeletal R07.89
  - non-cardiac R07.89
  - on breathing R07.1
  - pleurodynia R07.81
  - precordial R07.2
  - wall (anterior) R07.89
- chronic G89.29
  - associated with significant psychosocial dysfunction G89.4
  - due to trauma G89.21
  - neoplasm related G89.3
  - postoperative NEC G89.28
  - postprocedural NEC G89.28
  - post-thoracotomy G89.22
  - specified NEC G89.29
- coccyx M53.3
- colon — *see* Pain, abdominal
- coronary — *see* Angina
- costochondral R07.1
- diaphragm R07.1
- due to cancer G89.3
- due to device, implant or graft (*see also* Complications, by site and type, specified NEC)T85.848 ☑
  - arterial graft NEC T82.848 ☑
  - breast (implant) T85.848 ☑
  - catheter NEC T85.848 ☑
    - dialysis (renal) T82.848 ☑
      - intraperitoneal T85.848 ☑
    - infusion NEC T82.848 ☑
      - spinal (epidural) (subdural) T85.840 ☑
    - urinary (indwelling) T83.84 ☑
  - electronic (electrode) (pulse generator) (stimulator)
    - bone T84.84 ☑
    - cardiac T82.847 ☑
    - nervous system (brain) (peripheral nerve) (spinal) T85.840 ☑
    - urinary T83.84 ☑
  - fixation, internal (orthopedic) NEC T84.84 ☑
  - gastrointestinal (bile duct) (esophagus) T85.848 ☑
  - genital NEC T83.84 ☑
  - heart NEC T82.847 ☑
  - infusion NEC T85.848 ☑
  - joint prosthesis T84.84 ☑
  - ocular (corneal graft) (orbital implant) NEC T85.848 ☑
  - orthopedic NEC T84.84 ☑
  - specified NEC T85.848 ☑
  - urinary NEC T83.84 ☑
  - vascular NEC T82.848 ☑
  - ventricular intracranial shunt T85.840 ☑
- due to malignancy (primary) (secondary) G89.3
- ear — *see* subcategory H92.0
- epigastric, epigastrium R10.13
- eye — *see* Pain, ocular
- face, facial R51
  - atypical G50.1
- female genital organs NEC N94.89
- finger — *see* Pain, limb, upper
- flank — *see* Pain, abdominal
- foot — *see* Pain, limb, lower
- gallbladder K82.9
- gas (intestinal) R14.1
- gastric — *see* Pain, abdominal
- generalized NOS R52
- genital organ
  - female N94.89
  - male N50.89
- groin — *see* Pain, abdominal, lower
- hand — *see* Pain, limb, upper
- head — *see* Headache
- heart — *see* Pain, precordial
- infra-orbital — *see* Neuralgia, trigeminal
- intercostal R07.82
- intermenstrual N94.0

Pain — *continued*
- jaw R68.84
- joint M25.50
  - ankle M25.57 ☑
  - elbow M25.52 ☑
  - finger M25.54 ☑
  - foot M25.57 ☑
  - hand M25.54 ☑
  - hip M25.55 ☑
  - knee M25.56 ☑
  - shoulder M25.51 ☑
  - toe M25.57 ☑
  - wrist M25.53 ☑
- kidney N23
- laryngeal R07.0
- leg — *see* Pain, limb, lower
- limb M79.609
  - lower M79.60 ☑
    - foot M79.67 ☑
    - lower leg M79.66 ☑
    - thigh M79.65 ☑
    - toe M79.67 ☑
  - upper M79.60 ☑
    - axilla M79.62 ☑
    - finger M79.64 ☑
    - forearm M79.63 ☑
    - hand M79.64 ☑
    - upper arm M79.62 ☑
- loin M54.5
- low back M54.5
- lumbar region M54.5
- mandibular R68.84
- mastoid — *see* subcategory H92.0
- maxilla R68.84
- menstrual (*see also* Dysmenorrhea)N94.6
- metacarpophalangeal (joint) — *see* Pain, joint, hand
- metatarsophalangeal (joint) — *see* Pain, joint, foot
- mouth K13.79
- muscle — *see* Myalgia
- musculoskeletal (*see also* Pain, by site)M79.1
- myofascial M79.1
- nasal J34.89
- nasopharynx J39.2
- neck NEC M54.2
- nerve NEC — *see* Neuralgia
- neuromuscular — *see* Neuralgia
- nose J34.89
- ocular H57.1 ☑
- ophthalmic — *see* Pain, ocular
- orbital region — *see* Pain, ocular
- ovary N94.89
- over heart — *see* Pain, precordial
- ovulation N94.0
- pelvic (female) R10.2
- penis N48.89
- pericardial — *see* Pain, precordial
- perineal, perineum R10.2
- pharynx J39.2
- pleura, pleural, pleuritic R07.81
- postoperative NOS G89.18
- postprocedural NOS G89.18
- post-thoracotomy G89.12
- precordial (region) R07.2
- premenstrual N94.3
- psychogenic (persistent) (any site) F45.41
- radicular (spinal) — *see* Radiculopathy
- rectum K62.89
- respiration R07.1
- retrosternal R07.2
- rheumatoid, muscular — *see* Myalgia
- rib R07.81
- root (spinal) — *see* Radiculopathy
- round ligament (stretch) R10.2
- sacroiliac M53.3
- sciatic — *see* Sciatica
- scrotum N50.82
- seminal vesicle N50.89
- shoulder M25.51 ☑
- spermatic cord N50.89
- spinal root — *see* Radiculopathy
- spine M54.9
  - cervical M54.2
  - low back M54.5
    - with sciatica M54.4 ☑
  - thoracic M54.6
- stomach — *see* Pain, abdominal
- substernal R07.2
- temporomandibular (joint) M26.62 ☑
- testis N50.81 ☑
- thoracic spine M54.6
  - with radicular and visceral pain M54.14

Pain — *continued*
- throat R07.0
- tibia — *see* Pain, limb, lower
- toe — *see* Pain, limb, lower
- tongue K14.6
- tooth K08.89
- trigeminal — *see* Neuralgia, trigeminal
- tumor associated G89.3
- ureter N23
- urinary (organ) (system) N23
- uterus NEC N94.89
- vagina R10.2
- vertebrogenic (syndrome) M54.89
- vesical R39.89
  - associated with micturition — *see* Micturition, painful
- vulva R10.2

Painful (*see also* Pain)
- coitus
  - female N94.10
  - male N53.12
  - psychogenic F52.6
- ejaculation (semen) N53.12
  - psychogenic F52.6
- erection — *see* Priapism
- feet syndrome E53.8
- joint replacement (hip) (knee) T84.84 ☑
- menstruation — *see* Dysmenorrhea
  - psychogenic F45.8
- micturition — *see* Micturition, painful
- respiration R07.1
- scar NEC L90.5
- wire sutures T81.89 ☑

Painter's colic — *see* subcategory T56.0

Palate — *see* condition

Palatoplegia K13.79

Palatoschisis — *see* Cleft, palate

Palilalia R48.8

Palliative care Z51.5

Pallor R23.1
- optic disc, temporal — *see* Atrophy, optic

Palmar (*see also* condition)
- fascia — *see* condition

Palpable
- cecum K63.89
- kidney N28.89
- ovary N83.8
- prostate N42.9
- spleen — *see* Splenomegaly

Palpitations (heart) R00.2
- psychogenic F45.8

Palsy (*see also* Paralysis)G83.9
- atrophic diffuse (progressive) G12.22
- Bell's (*see also* Palsy, facial)
  - newborn P11.3
- brachial plexus NEC G54.0
  - newborn (birth injury) P14.3
- brain — *see* Palsy, cerebral
- bulbar (progressive) (chronic) G12.22
  - of childhood (Fazio-Londe) G12.1
  - pseudo NEC G12.29
  - supranuclear (progressive) G23.1
- cerebral (congenital) G80.9
  - ataxic G80.4
  - athetoid G80.3
  - choreathetoid G80.3
  - diplegic G80.8
    - spastic G80.1
  - dyskinetic G80.3
    - athetoid G80.3
    - choreathetoid G80.3
    - distonic G80.3
  - dystonic G80.3
  - hemiplegic G80.8
    - spastic G80.2
  - mixed G80.8
  - monoplegic G80.8
    - spastic G80.1
  - paraplegic G80.8
    - spastic G80.1
  - quadriplegic G80.8
    - spastic G80.0
  - spastic G80.1
    - diplegic G80.1
    - hemiplegic G80.2
    - monoplegic G80.1
    - quadriplegic G80.0
    - specified NEC G80.1
    - tetrapelgic G80.0
  - specified NEC G80.8
  - syphilitic A52.12
    - congenital A50.49

Palsy - Paraganglioma

- **Palsy** — *continued*
  - cerebral — *continued*
    - tetraplegic G80.8
      - spastic G80.0
  - cranial nerve (*see also* Disorder, nerve, cranial)
    - multiple G52.7
      - in
        - infectious disease B99 ☑ *[G53]*
        - neoplastic disease (*see also* Neoplasm)D49.9 *[G53]*
        - parasitic disease B89 *[G53]*
        - sarcoidosis D86.82
  - creeping G12.22
  - diver's T70.3 ☑
  - Erb's P14.0
  - facial G51.0
    - newborn (birth injury) P11.3
  - glossopharyngeal G52.1
  - Klumpke (-Déjérine) P14.1
  - lead — *see* subcategory T56.0
  - median nerve (tardy) G56.1 ☑
  - nerve G58.9
    - specified NEC G58.8
  - peroneal nerve (acute) (tardy) G57.3 ☑
  - progressive supranuclear G23.1
  - pseudobulbar NEC G12.29
  - radial nerve (acute) G56.3 ☑
  - seventh nerve (*see also* Palsy, facial)
    - newborn P11.3
  - shaking — *see* Parkinsonism
  - spastic (cerebral) (spinal) G80.1
  - ulnar nerve (tardy) G56.2 ☑
  - wasting G12.29
- **Paludism** — *see* Malaria
- **Panangiitis** M30.0
- **Panaris,** panaritium (*see also* Cellulitis, digit)
  - with lymphangitis — *see* Lymphangitis, acute, digit
- **Panarteritis** nodosa M30.0
  - brain or cerebral I67.7
- **Pancake** heart R93.1
  - with cor pulmonale (chronic) I27.81
- **Pancarditis** (acute) (chronic) I51.89
  - rheumatic I09.89
    - active or acute I01.8
- **Pancoast's** syndrome or tumor C34.1 ☑
- **Pancolitis,** ulcerative (chronic) K51.00
  - with
    - complication K51.019
    - abscess K51.014
    - fistula K51.013
    - obstruction K51.012
    - rectal bleeding K51.011
    - specified complication NEC K51.018
- **Pancreas,** pancreatic — *see* condition
- **Pancreatitis** (annular) (apoplectic) (calcareous) (edematous) (hemorrhagic) (malignant) (recurrent) (subacute) (suppurative) K85.90
  - with necrosis (uninfected) K85.91
    - infected K85.92
  - acute (without necrosis or infection) K85.90
    - with necrosis (uninfected) K85.91
      - infected K85.92
    - alcohol induced (without necrosis or infection) K85.20
      - with necrosis (uninfected) K85.21
        - infected K85.22
    - biliary (without necrosis or infection) K85.10
      - with necrosis (uninfected) K85.11
        - infected K85.12
    - drug induced (without necrosis or infection) K85.30
      - with necrosis (uninfected) K85.31
        - infected K85.32
    - gallstone (without necrosis or infection) K85.10
      - with necrosis (uninfected) K85.11
        - infected K85.12
    - idiopathic (without necrosis or infection) K85.00
      - with necrosis (uninfected) K85.01
        - infected K85.02
    - specified NEC (without necrosis or infection) K85.80
      - with necrosis (uninfected) K85.81
        - infected K85.82
  - chronic (infectious) K86.1
    - alcohol-induced K86.0
    - recurrent K86.1
    - relapsing K86.1
  - cystic (chronic) K86.1
  - cytomegaloviral B25.2
  - fibrous (chronic) K86.1
- **Pancreatitis** — *continued*
  - gangrenous — *see* Pancreatitis, acute
  - gallstone (without necrosis or infection) K85.10
    - with necrosis (uninfected) K85.11
      - infected K85.12
  - interstitial (chronic) K86.1
    - acute (*see also* Pancreatitis, acute)K85.80
  - mumps B26.3
  - recurrent (chronic) K86.1
  - relapsing, chronic K86.1
  - syphilitic A52.74
- **Pancreatoblastoma** — *see* Neoplasm, pancreas, malignant
- **Pancreolithiasis** K86.89
- **Pancytolysis** D75.89
- **Pancytopenia** (acquired) D61.818
  - with
    - malformations D61.09
    - myelodysplastic syndrome — *see* Syndrome, myelodysplastic
  - antineoplastic chemotherapy induced D61.810
  - congenital D61.09
  - drug-induced NEC D61.811
- **Panencephalitis,** subacute, sclerosing A81.1
- **Panhematopenia** D61.9
  - congenital D61.09
  - constitutional D61.09
  - splenic, primary D73.1
- **Panhemocytopenia** D61.9
  - congenital D61.09
  - constitutional D61.09
- **Panhypogonadism** E29.1
- **Panhypopituitarism** E23.0
  - prepubertal E23.0
- **Panic** (attack) (state) F41.0
  - reaction to exceptional stress (transient) F43.0
- **Panmyelopathy,** familial, constitutional D61.09
- **Panmyelophthisis** D61.82
  - congenital D61.09
- **Panmyelosis** (acute) (with myelofibrosis) C94.4 ☑
- **Panner's** disease — *see* Osteochondrosis, juvenile, humerus
- **Panneuritis** endemica E51.11
- **Panniculitis** (nodular) (nonsuppurative) M79.3
  - back M54.00
    - cervical region M54.02
    - cervicothoracic region M54.03
    - lumbar region M54.06
    - lumbosacral region M54.07
    - multiple sites M54.09
    - occipito-atlanto-axial region M54.01
    - sacrococcygeal region M54.08
    - thoracic region M54.04
    - thoracolumbar region M54.05
  - lupus L93.2
  - mesenteric K65.4
  - neck M54.02
    - cervicothoracic region M54.03
    - occipito-atlanto-axial region M54.01
  - relapsing M35.6
- **Panniculus** adiposus (abdominal) E65
- **Pannus** (allergic) (cornea) (degenerativus) (keratic) H16.42 ☑
  - abdominal (symptomatic) E65
  - trachomatosus, trachomatous (active) A71.1
- **Panophthalmitis** H44.01 ☑
- **Pansinusitis** (chronic) (hyperplastic) (nonpurulent) (purulent) J32.4
  - acute J01.40
    - recurrent J01.41
  - tuberculous A15.8
- **Panuveitis** (sympathetic) H44.11 ☑
- **Panvalvular** disease I08.9
  - specified NEC I08.8
- **PAPA** (pyogenic arthritis, pyoderma gangrenosum, and acne syndrome) M04.8
- **Papanicolaou** smear, cervix Z12.4
  - as part of routine gynecological examination Z01.419
    - with abnormal findings Z01.411
  - for suspected neoplasm Z12.4
  - nonspecific abnormal finding R87.619
  - routine Z01.419
    - with abnormal findings Z01.411
- **Papilledema** (choked disc) H47.10
  - associated with
    - decreased ocular pressure H47.12
    - increased intracranial pressure H47.11
    - retinal disorder H47.13
  - Foster-Kennedy syndrome H47.14 ☑
- **Papillitis** H46.00
  - anus K62.89
- **Papillitis** — *continued*
  - chronic lingual K14.4
  - necrotizing, kidney N17.2
  - optic H46.0 ☑
  - rectum K62.89
  - renal, necrotizing N17.2
  - tongue K14.0
- **Papilloma** (*see also* Neoplasm, benign, by site)
  - acuminatum (female) (male) (anogenital) A63.0
  - basal cell L82.1
    - inflamed L82.0
  - benign pinta (primary) A67.0
  - bladder (urinary) (transitional cell) D41.4
  - choroid plexus (lateral ventricle) (third ventricle) D33.0
    - anaplastic C71.5
    - fourth ventricle D33.1
    - malignant C71.5
  - renal pelvis (transitional cell) D41.1 ☑
    - benign D30.1 ☑
  - Schneiderian
    - specified site — *see* Neoplasm, benign, by site
    - unspecified site D14.0
  - serous surface
    - borderline malignancy
      - specified site — *see* Neoplasm, uncertain behavior, by site
      - unspecified site D39.10
    - specified site — *see* Neoplasm, benign, by site
    - unspecified site D27.9
  - transitional (cell)
    - bladder (urinary) D41.4
    - inverted type — *see* Neoplasm, uncertain behavior, by site
    - renal pelvis D41.1 ☑
    - ureter D41.2 ☑
  - ureter (transitional cell) D41.2 ☑
    - benign D30.2 ☑
  - urothelial — *see* Neoplasm, uncertain behavior, by site
  - villous — *see* Neoplasm, uncertain behavior, by site
    - adenocarcinoma in — *see* Neoplasm, malignant, by site
    - in situ — *see* Neoplasm, in situ
  - yaws, plantar or palmar A66.1
- **Papillomata,** multiple, of yaws A66.1
- **Papillomatosis** (*see also* Neoplasm, benign, by site)
  - confluent and reticulated L83
  - cystic, breast — *see* Mastopathy, cystic
  - ductal, breast — *see* Mastopathy, cystic
  - intraductal (diffuse) — *see* Neoplasm, benign, by site
  - subareolar duct D24 ☑
- **Papillomavirus,** as cause of disease classified elsewhere B97.7
- **Papillon-Léage** and Psaume syndrome Q87.0
- **Papule** (s) R23.8
  - carate (primary) A67.0
  - fibrous, of nose D22.39
  - Gottron's L94.4
  - pinta (primary) A67.0
- **Papulosis**
  - lymphomatoid C86.6
  - malignant I77.89
- **Papyraceous** fetus O31.0 ☑
- **Para-albuminemia** E88.09
- **Paracephalus** Q89.7
- **Parachute** mitral valve Q23.2
- **Paracoccidioidomycosis** B41.9
  - disseminated B41.7
  - generalized B41.7
  - mucocutaneous-lymphangitic B41.8
  - pulmonary B41.0
  - specified NEC B41.8
  - visceral B41.8
- **Paradentosis** K05.4
- **Paraffinoma** T88.8 ☑
- **Paraganglioma** D44.7
  - adrenal D35.0 ☑
    - malignant C74.1 ☑
  - aortic body D44.7
    - malignant C75.5
  - carotid body D44.6
    - malignant C75.4
  - chromaffin (*see also* Neoplasm, benign, by site)
    - malignant — *see* Neoplasm, malignant, by site
  - extra-adrenal D44.7
    - malignant C75.5
      - specified site — *see* Neoplasm, malignant, by site
      - unspecified site C75.5

☑ **Additional character required**

- **Paraganglioma** — *continued*
  - extra-adrenal — *continued*
    - specified site — *see* Neoplasm, uncertain behavior, by site
    - unspecified site D44.7
  - gangliocytic D13.2
    - specified site — *see* Neoplasm, benign, by site
    - unspecified site D13.2
  - glomus jugulare D44.7
    - malignant C75.5
  - jugular D44.7
  - malignant C75.5
    - specified site — *see* Neoplasm, malignant, by site
    - unspecified site C75.5
  - nonchromaffin D44.7
    - malignant C75.5
      - specified site — *see* Neoplasm, malignant, by site
      - unspecified site C75.5
    - specified site — *see* Neoplasm, uncertain behavior, by site
    - unspecified site D44.7
  - parasympathetic D44.7
    - specified site — *see* Neoplasm, uncertain behavior, by site
    - unspecified site D44.7
  - specified site — *see* Neoplasm, uncertain behavior, by site
  - sympathetic D44.7
    - specified site — *see* Neoplasm, uncertain behavior, by site
    - unspecified site D44.7
  - unspecified site D44.7
- **Parageusia** R43.2
  - psychogenic F45.8
- **Paragonimiasis** B66.4
- **Paragranuloma,** Hodgkin — *see* Lymphoma, Hodgkin, classical, specified NEC
- **Parahemophilia** (*see also* Defect, coagulation)D68.2
- **Parakeratosis** R23.4
  - variegata L41.0
- **Paralysis,** paralytic (complete) (incomplete) G83.9
  - with
    - syphilis A52.17
  - abducens, abducent (nerve) — *see* Strabismus, paralytic, sixth nerve
  - abductor, lower extremity G57.9 ☑
  - accessory nerve G52.8
  - accommodation (*see also* Paresis, of accommodation)
    - hysterical F44.89
  - acoustic nerve (except Deafness) — *see* subcategory H93.3
  - agitans (*see also* Parkinsonism)G20
    - arteriosclerotic G21.4
  - alternating (oculomotor) G83.89
  - amyotrophic G12.21
  - ankle G57.9 ☑
  - anus (sphincter) K62.89
  - arm — *see* Monoplegia, upper limb
  - ascending (spinal), acute G61.0
  - association G12.29
  - asthenic bulbar G70.00
    - with exacerbation (acute) G70.01
    - in crisis G70.01
  - ataxic (hereditary) G11.9
    - general (syphilitic) A52.17
  - atrophic G58.9
    - infantile, acute — *see* Poliomyelitis, paralytic
    - progressive G12.22
    - spinal (acute) — *see* Poliomyelitis, paralytic
  - axillary G54.0
  - Babinski-Nageotte's G83.89
  - Bell's G51.0
    - newborn P11.3
  - Benedikt's G46.3
  - birth injury P14.9
    - spinal cord P11.5
  - bladder (neurogenic) (sphincter) N31.2
  - bowel, colon or intestine K56.0
  - brachial plexus G54.0
    - birth injury P14.3
    - newborn (birth injury) P14.3
  - brain G83.9
    - diplegia G83.0
    - triplegia G83.89
  - bronchial J98.09
  - Brown-Séquard G83.81
  - bulbar (chronic) (progressive) G12.22
    - infantile — *see* Poliomyelitis, paralytic
    - poliomyelitic — *see* Poliomyelitis, paralytic
    - pseudo G12.29

- **Paralysis** — *continued*
  - bulbospinal G70.00
    - with exacerbation (acute) G70.01
    - in crisis G70.01
  - cardiac (*see also* Failure, heart)I50.9
  - cerebrocerebellar, diplegic G80.1
  - cervical
    - plexus G54.2
    - sympathetic G90.09
  - Céstan-Chenais G46.3
  - Charcot-Marie-Tooth type G60.0
  - Clark's G80.9
  - colon K56.0
  - compressed air T70.3 ☑
  - compression
    - arm G56.9 ☑
    - leg G57.9 ☑
    - lower extremity G57.9 ☑
    - upper extremity G56.9 ☑
  - congenital (cerebral) — *see* Palsy, cerebral
  - conjugate movement (gaze) (of eye) H51.0
    - cortical (nuclear) (supranuclear) H51.0
  - cordis — *see* Failure, heart
  - cranial or cerebral nerve G52.9
  - creeping G12.22
  - crossed leg G83.89
  - crutch — *see* Injury, brachial plexus
  - deglutition R13.0
    - hysterical F44.4
  - dementia A52.17
  - descending (spinal) NEC G12.29
  - diaphragm (flaccid) J98.6
    - due to accidental dissection of phrenic nerve during procedure — *see* Puncture, accidental complicating surgery
  - digestive organs NEC K59.8
  - diplegic — *see* Diplegia
  - divergence (nuclear) H51.8
  - diver's T70.3 ☑
  - Duchenne's
    - birth injury P14.0
    - due to or associated with
      - motor neuron disease G12.22
      - muscular dystrophy G71.0
  - due to intracranial or spinal birth injury — *see* Palsy, cerebral
  - embolic (current episode) I63.4 ☑
  - Erb (-Duchenne) (birth) (newborn) P14.0
  - Erb's syphilitic spastic spinal A52.17
  - esophagus K22.8
  - eye muscle (extrinsic) H49.9
    - intrinsic (*see also* Paresis, of accommodation)
  - facial (nerve) G51.0
    - birth injury P11.3
    - congenital P11.3
    - following operation NEC — *see* Puncture, accidental complicating surgery
    - newborn (birth injury) P11.3
  - familial (recurrent) (periodic) G72.3
    - spastic G11.4
  - fauces J39.2
  - finger G56.9 ☑
  - gait R26.1
  - gastric nerve (nondiabetic) G52.2
  - gaze, conjugate H51.0
  - general (progressive) (syphilitic) A52.17
    - juvenile A50.45
  - glottis J38.00
    - bilateral J38.02
    - unilateral J38.01
  - gluteal G54.1
  - Gubler (-Millard) G46.3
  - hand — *see* Monoplegia, upper limb
  - heart — *see* Arrest, cardiac
  - hemiplegic — *see* Hemiplegia
  - hyperkalemic periodic (familial) G72.3
  - hypoglossal (nerve) G52.3
  - hypokalemic periodic G72.3
  - hysterical F44.4
  - ileus K56.0
  - infantile (*see also* Poliomyelitis, paralytic)A80.30
    - bulbar — *see* Poliomyelitis, paralytic
    - cerebral — *see* Palsy, cerebral
    - spastic — *see* Palsy, cerebral, spastic
  - infective — *see* Poliomyelitis, paralytic
  - inferior nuclear G83.9
  - internuclear — *see* Ophthalmoplegia, internuclear
  - intestine K56.0
  - iris H57.09
    - due to diphtheria (toxin) A36.89

- **Paralysis** — *continued*
  - ischemic, Volkmann's (complicating trauma) T79.6 ☑
  - Jackson's G83.89
  - jake — *see* Poisoning, food, noxious, plant
  - Jamaica ginger (jake) G62.2
  - juvenile general A50.45
  - Klumpke (-Déjérine) (birth) (newborn) P14.1
  - labioglossal (laryngeal) (pharyngeal) G12.29
  - Landry's G61.0
  - laryngeal nerve (recurrent) (superior) (unilateral) J38.00
    - bilateral J38.02
    - unilateral J38.01
  - larynx J38.00
    - bilateral J38.02
    - due to diphtheria (toxin) A36.2
    - unilateral J38.01
  - lateral G12.21
  - lead — *see* subcategory T56.0
  - left side — *see* Hemiplegia
  - leg G83.1 ☑
    - both — *see* Paraplegia
    - crossed G83.89
    - hysterical F44.4
    - psychogenic F44.4
    - transient or transitory R29.818
      - traumatic NEC — *see* Injury, nerve, leg
  - levator palpebrae superioris — *see* Blepharoptosis, paralytic
  - limb — *see* Monoplegia
  - lip K13.0
  - Lissauer's A52.17
  - lower limb — *see* Monoplegia, lower limb
    - both — *see* Paraplegia
  - lung J98.4
  - median nerve G56.1 ☑
  - medullary (tegmental) G83.89
  - mesencephalic NEC G83.89
    - tegmental G83.89
  - middle alternating G83.89
  - Millard-Gubler-Foville G46.3
  - monoplegic — *see* Monoplegia
  - motor G83.9
  - muscle, muscular NEC G72.89
    - due to nerve lesion G58.9
    - eye (extrinsic) H49.9
      - intrinsic — *see* Paresis, of accommodation
      - oblique — *see* Strabismus, paralytic, fourth nerve
    - iris sphincter H21.9
    - ischemic (Volkmann's) (complicating trauma) T79.6 ☑
    - progressive G12.21
    - pseudohypertrophic G71.0
  - musculocutaneous nerve G56.9 ☑
  - musculospiral G56.9 ☑
  - nerve (*see also* Disorder, nerve)
    - abducent — *see* Strabismus, paralytic, sixth nerve
    - accessory G52.8
    - auditory (except Deafness) — *see* subcategory H93.3
    - birth injury P14.9
    - cranial or cerebral G52.9
    - facial G51.0
      - birth injury P11.3
      - congenital P11.3
      - newborn (birth injury) P11.3
    - fourth or trochlear — *see* Strabismus, paralytic, fourth nerve
    - newborn (birth injury) P14.9
    - oculomotor — *see* Strabismus, paralytic, third nerve
    - phrenic (birth injury) P14.2
    - radial G56.3 ☑
    - seventh or facial G51.0
      - newborn (birth injury) P11.3
    - sixth or abducent — *see* Strabismus, paralytic, sixth nerve
    - syphilitic A52.15
    - third or oculomotor — *see* Strabismus, paralytic, third nerve
    - trigeminal G50.9
    - trochlear — *see* Strabismus, paralytic, fourth nerve
    - ulnar G56.2 ☑
  - normokalemic periodic G72.3
  - ocular H49.9
    - alternating G83.89
  - oculofacial, congenital (Moebius) Q87.0

☑ **Additional character required**

Paralysis — *continued*
- oculomotor (external bilateral) (nerve) — *see* Strabismus, paralytic, third nerve
- palate (soft) K13.79
- paratrigeminal G50.9
- periodic (familial) (hyperkalemic) (hypokalemic) (myotonic) (normokalemic) (potassium sensitive) (secondary) G72.3
- peripheral autonomic nervous system — *see* Neuropathy, peripheral, autonomic
- peroneal (nerve) G57.3 ☑
- pharynx J39.2
- phrenic nerve G56.8 ☑
- plantar nerve (s) G57.6 ☑
- pneumogastric nerve G52.2
- poliomyelitis (current) — *see* Poliomyelitis, paralytic
- popliteal nerve G57.3 ☑
- postepileptic transitory G83.84
- progressive (atrophic) (bulbar) (spinal) G12.22
  - general A52.17
  - infantile acute — *see* Poliomyelitis, paralytic
  - supranuclear G23.1
- pseudobulbar G12.29
- pseudohypertrophic (muscle) G71.0
- psychogenic F44.4
- quadriceps G57.9 ☑
- quadriplegic — *see* Tetraplegia
- radial nerve G56.3 ☑
- rectus muscle (eye) H49.9
- recurrent isolated sleep G47.53
- respiratory (muscle) (system) (tract) R06.81
  - center NEC G93.89
  - congenital P28.89
  - newborn P28.89
- right side — *see* Hemiplegia
- saturnine — *see* subcategory T56.0
- sciatic nerve G57.0 ☑
- senile G83.9
- shaking — *see* Parkinsonism
- shoulder G56.9 ☑
- sleep, recurrent isolated G47.53
- spastic G83.9
  - cerebral — *see* Palsy, cerebral, spastic
  - congenital (cerebral) — *see* Palsy, cerebral, spastic
  - familial G11.4
  - hereditary G11.4
  - quadriplegic G80.0
  - syphilitic (spinal) A52.17
- sphincter, bladder — *see* Paralysis, bladder
- spinal (cord) G83.9
  - accessory nerve G52.8
  - acute — *see* Poliomyelitis, paralytic
  - ascending acute G61.0
  - atrophic (acute) (*see also* Poliomyelitis, paralytic)
    - spastic, syphilitic A52.17
  - congenital NEC — *see* Palsy, cerebral
  - infantile — *see* Poliomyelitis, paralytic
  - hereditary G95.89
  - progressive G12.21
  - sequelae NEC G83.89
- sternomastoid G52.8
- stomach K31.84
  - diabetic — *see* Diabetes, by type, with gastroparesis
  - nerve G52.2
    - diabetic — *see* Diabetes, by type, with gastroparesis
- stroke — *see* Infarct, brain
- subcapsularis G56.8 ☑
- supranuclear (progressive) G23.1
- sympathetic G90.8
  - cervical G90.09
  - nervous system — *see* Neuropathy, peripheral, autonomic
- syndrome G83.9
  - specified NEC G83.89
- syphilitic spastic spinal (Erb's) A52.17
- thigh G57.9 ☑
- throat J39.2
  - diphtheritic A36.0
  - muscle J39.2
- thrombotic (current episode) I63.3 ☑
- thumb G56.9 ☑
- tick — *see* Toxicity, venom, arthropod, specified NEC
- Todd's (postepileptic transitory paralysis) G83.84
- toe G57.6 ☑
- tongue K14.8
- transient R29.5

Paralysis — *continued*
- transient — *continued*
  - arm or leg NEC R29.818
  - traumatic NEC — *see* Injury, nerve
- trapezius G52.8
- traumatic, transient NEC — *see* Injury, nerve
- trembling — *see* Parkinsonism
- triceps brachii G56.9 ☑
- trigeminal nerve G50.9
- trochlear (nerve) — *see* Strabismus, paralytic, fourth nerve
- ulnar nerve G56.2 ☑
- upper limb — *see* Monoplegia, upper limb
- uremic N18.9 *[G99.8]*
- uveoparotitic D86.89
- uvula K13.79
  - postdiphtheritic A36.0
- vagus nerve G52.2
- vasomotor NEC G90.8
- velum palati K13.79
- vesical — *see* Paralysis, bladder
- vestibular nerve (except Vertigo) — *see* subcategory H93.3
- vocal cords J38.00
  - bilateral J38.02
  - unilateral J38.01
- Volkmann's (complicating trauma) T79.6 ☑
- wasting G12.29
- Weber's G46.3
- wrist G56.9 ☑

Paramedial urethrovesical orifice Q64.79

Paramenia N92.6

Parametritis (*see also* Disease, pelvis, inflammatory)N73.2
- acute N73.0
- complicating abortion — *see* Abortion, by type, complicated by, parametritis

Parametrium, parametric — *see* condition

Paramnesia — *see* Amnesia

Paramolar K00.1

Paramyloidosis E85.8

Paramyoclonus multiplex G25.3

Paramyotonia (congenita) G71.19

Parangi — *see* Yaws

Paranoia (querulans) F22
- senile F03 ☑

Paranoid
- dementia (senile) F03 ☑
  - praecox — *see* Schizophrenia
- personality F60.0
- psychosis (climacteric) (involutional) (menopausal) F22
  - psychogenic (acute) F23
  - senile F03 ☑
- reaction (acute) F23
  - chronic F22
- schizophrenia F20.0
- state (climacteric) (involutional) (menopausal) (simple) F22
  - senile F03 ☑
- tendencies F60.0
- traits F60.0
- trends F60.0
- type, psychopathic personality F60.0

Paraparesis — *see* Paraplegia

Paraphasia R47.02

Paraphilia F65.9

Paraphimosis (congenital) N47.2
- chancroidal A57

Paraphrenia, paraphrenic (late) F22
- schizophrenia F20.0

Paraplegia (lower) G82.20
- ataxic — *see* Degeneration, combined, spinal cord
- complete G82.21
- congenital (cerebral) G80.8
  - spastic G80.1
- familial spastic G11.4
- functional (hysterical) F44.4
- hereditary, spastic G11.4
- hysterical F44.4
- incomplete G82.22
- Pott's A18.01
- psychogenic F44.4
- spastic
  - Erb's spinal, syphilitic A52.17
  - hereditary G11.4
  - tropical G04.1
- syphilitic (spastic) A52.17
- tropical spastic G04.1

Parapoxvirus B08.60
- specified NEC B08.69

Paraproteinemia D89.2
- benign (familial) D89.2
- monoclonal D47.2
- secondary to malignant disease D47.2

Parapsoriasis L41.9
- en plaques L41.4
- guttata L41.1
- large plaque L41.4
- retiform, retiformis L41.5
- small plaque L41.3
- specified NEC L41.8
- varioliformis (acuta) L41.0

Parasitic (*see also* condition)
- disease NEC B89
- stomatitis B37.0
- sycosis (beard) (scalp) B35.0
- twin Q89.4

Parasitism B89
- intestinal B82.9
- skin B88.9
- specified — *see* Infestation

Parasitophobia F40.218

Parasomnia G47.50
- due to
  - alcohol
    - abuse F10.182
    - dependence F10.282
    - use F10.982
  - amphetamines
    - abuse F15.182
    - dependence F15.282
    - use F15.982
  - caffeine
    - abuse F15.182
    - dependence F15.282
    - use F15.982
  - cocaine
    - abuse F14.182
    - dependence F14.282
    - use F14.982
  - drug NEC
    - abuse F19.182
    - dependence F19.282
    - use F19.982
  - opioid
    - abuse F11.182
    - dependence F11.282
    - use F11.982
  - psychoactive substance NEC
    - abuse F19.182
    - dependence F19.282
    - use F19.982
  - sedative, hypnotic, or anxiolytic
    - abuse F13.182
    - dependence F13.282
    - use F13.982
  - stimulant NEC
    - abuse F15.182
    - dependence F15.282
    - use F15.982
- in conditions classified elsewhere G47.54
- nonorganic origin F51.8
- organic G47.50
- specified NEC G47.59

Paraspadias Q54.9

Paraspasmus facialis G51.8

Parasuicide (attempt)
- history of (personal) Z91.5
  - in family Z81.8

Parathyroid gland — *see* condition

Parathyroid tetany E20.9

Paratrachoma A74.0

Paratyphilitis — *see* Appendicitis

Paratyphoid (fever) — *see* Fever, paratyphoid

Paratyphus — *see* Fever, paratyphoid

Paraurethral duct Q64.79
- nonorganic origin F51.5

Paraurethritis (*see also* Urethritis)
- gonococcal (acute) (chronic) (with abscess) A54.1

Paravaccinia NEC B08.04

Paravaginitis — *see* Vaginitis

Parencephalitis (*see also* Encephalitis)
- sequelae G09

Parent-child conflict — *see* Conflict, parent-child
- estrangement NEC Z62.890

Paresis (*see also* Paralysis)
- accommodation — *see* Paresis, of accommodation
- Bernhardt's G57.1 ☑
- bladder (sphincter) (*see also* Paralysis, bladder)
  - tabetic A52.17
- bowel, colon or intestine K56.0

- **Paresis** — *continued*
  - extrinsic muscle, eye H49.9
  - general (progressive) (syphilitic) A52.17
    - juvenile A50.45
  - heart — *see* Failure, heart
  - insane (syphilitic) A52.17
  - juvenile (general) A50.45
  - of accommodation H52.52 ☑
  - peripheral progressive (idiopathic) G60.3
  - pseudohypertrophic G71.0
  - senile G83.9
  - syphilitic (general) A52.17
    - congenital A50.45
  - vesical NEC N31.2
- **Paresthesia** (*see also* Disturbance, sensation)
  - Bernhardt G57.1 ☑
- **Paretic** — *see* condition
- **Parinaud's**
  - conjunctivitis H10.89
  - oculoglandular syndrome H10.89
  - ophthalmoplegia H49.88 ☑
- **Parkinsonism** (idiopathic) (primary) G20
  - with neurogenic orthostatic hypotension (symptomatic) G90.3
  - arteriosclerotic G21.4
  - dementia G31.83 *[F02.80]*
    - with behavioral disturbance G31.83 *[F02.81]*
  - due to
    - drugs NEC G21.19
      - neuroleptic G21.11
  - neuroleptic induced G21.11
  - postencephalitic G21.3
  - secondary G21.9
    - due to
      - arteriosclerosis G21.4
      - drugs NEC G21.19
        - neuroleptic G21.11
      - encephalitis G21.3
      - external agents NEC G21.2
      - syphilis A52.19
    - specified NEC G21.8
  - syphilitic A52.19
  - treatment-induced NEC G21.19
  - vascular G21.4
- **Parkinson's** disease, syndrome or tremor — *see* Parkinsonism
- **Parodontitis** — *see* Periodontitis
- **Parodontosis** K05.4
- **Paronychia** (*see also* Cellulitis, digit)
  - with lymphangitis — *see* Lymphangitis, acute, digit
  - candidal (chronic) B37.2
  - tuberculous (primary) A18.4
- **Parorexia** (psychogenic) F50.89
- **Parosmia** R43.1
  - psychogenic F45.8
- **Parotid** gland — *see* condition
- **Parotitis**, parotiditis (allergic) (nonspecific toxic) (purulent) (septic) (suppurative) (*see also* Sialoadenitis)
  - epidemic — *see* Mumps
  - infectious — *see* Mumps
  - postoperative K91.89
  - surgical K91.89
- **Parrot** fever A70
- **Parrot's** disease (early congenital syphilitic pseudoparalysis) A50.02
- **Parry-Romberg** syndrome G51.8
- **Parry's** disease or syndrome E05.00
  - with thyroid storm E05.01
- **Pars** planitis — *see* Cyclitis
- **Parsonage** (-Aldren)-Turner syndrome G54.5
- **Parson's** disease (exophthalmic goiter) E05.00
  - with thyroid storm E05.01
- **Particolored** infant Q82.8
- **Parturition** — *see* Delivery
- **Parulis** K04.7
  - with sinus K04.6
- **Parvovirus**, as cause of disease classified elsewhere B97.6
- **Pasini** and Pierini's atrophoderma L90.3
- **Passage**
  - false, urethra N36.5
  - meconium (newborn) during delivery P03.82
  - of sounds or bougies — *see* Attention to, artificial, opening
- **Passive** — *see* condition
  - smoking Z77.22
- **Pasteurella** septica A28.0
- **Pasteurellosis** — *see* Infection, Pasteurella
- **PAT** (paroxysmal atrial tachycardia) I47.1
- **Patau's** syndrome — *see* Trisomy, 13
- **Patches**
  - mucous (syphilitic) A51.39
    - congenital A50.07
  - smokers' (mouth) K13.24
- **Patellar** — *see* condition
- **Patent** (*see also* Imperfect, closure)
  - canal of Nuck Q52.4
  - cervix N88.3
  - ductus arteriosus or Botallo's Q25.0
  - foramen
    - botalli Q21.1
    - ovale Q21.1
  - interauricular septum Q21.1
  - interventricular septum Q21.0
  - omphalomesenteric duct Q43.0
  - os (uteri) — *see* Patent, cervix
  - ostium secundum Q21.1
  - urachus Q64.4
  - vitelline duct Q43.0
- **Paterson** (-Brown) (-Kelly) syndrome or web D50.1
- **Pathologic**, pathological (*see also* condition)
  - asphyxia R09.01
  - fire-setting F63.1
  - gambling F63.0
  - ovum O02.0
  - resorption, tooth K03.3
  - stealing F63.2
- **Pathology** (of) — *see* Disease
  - periradicular, associated with previous endodontic treatment NEC M27.59
- **Pattern**, sleep-wake, irregular G47.23
- **Patulous** (*see also* Imperfect, closure (congenital))
  - alimentary tract Q45.8
    - lower Q43.8
    - upper Q40.8
  - eustachian tube H69.0 ☑
- **Pause**, sinoatrial I49.5
- **Paxton's** disease B36.2
- **Pearl** (s)
  - enamel K00.2
  - Epstein's K09.8
- **Pearl-worker's** disease — *see* Osteomyelitis, specified type NEC
- **Pectenosis** K62.4
- **Pectoral** — *see* condition
- **Pectus**
  - carinatum (congenital) Q67.7
    - acquired M95.4
    - rachitic sequelae (late effect) E64.3
  - excavatum (congenital) Q67.6
    - acquired M95.4
    - rachitic sequelae (late effect) E64.3
  - recurvatum (congenital) Q67.6
- **Pedatrophia** E41
- **Pederosis** F65.4
- **Pediculosis** (infestation) B85.2
  - capitis (head-louse) (any site) B85.0
  - corporis (body-louse) (any site) B85.1
  - eyelid B85.0
  - mixed (classifiable to more than one of the titles B85.0-B85.3) B85.4
  - pubis (pubic louse) (any site) B85.3
  - vestimenti B85.1
  - vulvae B85.3
- **Pediculus** (infestation) — *see* Pediculosis
- **Pedophilia** F65.4
- **Peg-shaped** teeth K00.2
- **Pelade** — *see* Alopecia, areata
- **Pelger-Huët** anomaly or syndrome D72.0
- **Peliosis** (rheumatica) D69.0
  - hepatis K76.4
    - with toxic liver disease K71.8
- **Pelizaeus-Merzbacher** disease E75.29
- **Pellagra** (alcoholic) (with polyneuropathy) E52
- **Pellagra-cerebellar-ataxia-renal** aminoaciduria syndrome E72.02
- **Pellegrini** (-Stieda) disease or syndrome — *see* Bursitis, tibial collateral
- **Pellizzi's** syndrome E34.8
- **Pel's** crisis A52.11
- **Pelvic** (*see also* condition)
  - examination (periodic) (routine) Z01.419
    - with abnormal findings Z01.411
  - kidney, congenital Q63.2
- **Pelviolithiasis** — *see* Calculus, kidney
- **Pelviperitonitis** (*see also* Peritonitis, pelvic)
  - gonococcal A54.24
  - puerperal O85
- **Pelvis** — *see* condition or type
- **Pemphigoid** L12.9
  - benign, mucous membrane L12.1
  - bullous L12.0
- **Pemphigoid** — *continued*
  - cicatricial L12.1
  - juvenile L12.2
  - ocular L12.1
  - specified NEC L12.8
- **Pemphigus** L10.9
  - benign familial (chronic) Q82.8
  - Brazilian L10.3
  - circinatus L13.0
  - conjunctiva L12.1
  - drug-induced L10.5
  - erythematosus L10.4
  - foliaceous L10.2
  - gangrenous — *see* Gangrene
  - neonatorum L01.03
  - ocular L12.1
  - paraneoplastic L10.81
  - specified NEC L10.89
  - syphilitic (congenital) A50.06
  - vegetans L10.1
  - vulgaris L10.0
  - wildfire L10.3
- **Pendred's** syndrome E07.1
- **Pendulous**
  - abdomen, in pregnancy — *see* Pregnancy, complicated by, abnormal, pelvic organs or tissues NEC
  - breast N64.89
- **Penetrating** wound (*see also* Puncture)
  - with internal injury — *see* Injury, by site
  - eyeball — *see* Puncture, eyeball
  - orbit (with or without foreign body) — *see* Puncture, orbit
  - uterus by instrument with or following ectopic or molar pregnancy O08.6
- **Penicillosis** B48.4
- **Penis** — *see* condition
- **Penitis** N48.29
- **Pentalogy** of Fallot Q21.8
- **Pentasomy** X syndrome Q97.1
- **Pentosuria** (essential) E74.8
- **Percreta** placenta O43.23 ☑
- **Peregrinating** patient — *see* Disorder, factitious
- **Perforation**, perforated (nontraumatic) (of)
  - accidental during procedure (blood vessel) (nerve) (organ) — *see* Complication, accidental puncture or laceration
  - antrum — *see* Sinusitis, maxillary
  - appendix K35.2
    - with localized peritonitis K35.3
  - atrial septum, multiple Q21.1
  - attic, ear — *see* Perforation, tympanum, attic
  - bile duct (common) (hepatic) K83.2
    - cystic K82.2
  - bladder (urinary)
    - with or following ectopic or molar pregnancy O08.6
    - obstetrical trauma O71.5
    - traumatic S37.29 ☑
      - at delivery O71.5
  - bowel K63.1
    - with or following ectopic or molar pregnancy O08.6
    - newborn P78.0
    - obstetrical trauma O71.5
    - traumatic — *see* Laceration, intestine
  - broad ligament N83.8
    - with or following ectopic or molar pregnancy O08.6
    - obstetrical trauma O71.6
  - by
    - device, implant or graft (*see also* Complications, by site and type, mechanical)T85.628 ☑
      - arterial graft NEC — *see* Complication, cardiovascular device, mechanical, vascular
      - breast (implant) T85.49 ☑
      - catheter NEC T85.698 ☑
        - cystostomy T83.090 ☑
        - dialysis (renal) T82.49 ☑
          - intraperitoneal T85.691 ☑
        - infusion NEC T82.594 ☑
          - spinal (epidural) (subdural) T85.690 ☑
        - urinary (*see also* Complications, catheter, urinary)T83.098 ☑
      - electronic (electrode) (pulse generator) (stimulator)
        - bone T84.390 ☑
        - cardiac T82.199 ☑
          - electrode T82.190 ☑
          - pulse generator T82.191 ☑
          - specified type NEC T82.198 ☑

Perforation — *continued*
- by — *continued*
      - nervous system — *see* Complication, prosthetic device, mechanical, electronic nervous system stimulator
      - urinary — *see* Complication, genitourinary, device, urinary, mechanical
    - fixation, internal (orthopedic) NEC — *see* Complication, fixation device, mechanical
    - gastrointestinal — *see* Complications, prosthetic device, mechanical, gastrointestinal device
    - genital NEC T83.498 ☑
      - intrauterine contraceptive device T83.39 ☑
      - penile prosthesis T83.490 ☑
    - heart NEC — *see* Complication, cardiovascular device, mechanical
    - joint prosthesis — *see* Complications, joint prosthesis, mechanical, specified NEC, by site
    - ocular NEC — *see* Complications, prosthetic device, mechanical, ocular device
    - orthopedic NEC — *see* Complication, orthopedic, device, mechanical
    - specified NEC T85.628 ☑
    - urinary NEC (*see also* Complication, genitourinary, device, urinary, mechanical)
      - graft T83.29 ☑
    - vascular NEC — *see* Complication, cardiovascular device, mechanical
    - ventricular intracranial shunt T85.09 ☑
  - foreign body left accidentally in operative wound T81.539 ☑
  - instrument (any) during a procedure, accidental — *see* Puncture, accidental complicating surgery
- cecum K35.2
  - with localized peritonitis K35.3
- cervix (uteri) N88.8
  - with or following ectopic or molar pregnancy O08.6
  - obstetrical trauma O71.3
- colon K63.1
  - newborn P78.0
  - obstetrical trauma O71.5
  - traumatic — *see* Laceration, intestine, large
- common duct (bile) K83.2
- cornea (due to ulceration) — *see* Ulcer, cornea, perforated
- cystic duct K82.2
- diverticulum (intestine) K57.80
  - with bleeding K57.81
  - large intestine K57.20
    - with
      - bleeding K57.21
      - small intestine K57.40
        - with bleeding K57.41
  - small intestine K57.00
    - with
      - bleeding K57.01
      - large intestine K57.40
        - with bleeding K57.41
- ear drum — *see* Perforation, tympanum
- esophagus K22.3
- ethmoidal sinus — *see* Sinusitis, ethmoidal
- frontal sinus — *see* Sinusitis, frontal
- gallbladder K82.2
- heart valve — *see* Endocarditis
- ileum K63.1
  - newborn P78.0
  - obstetrical trauma O71.5
  - traumatic — *see* Laceration, intestine, small
- instrumental, surgical (accidental) (blood vessel) (nerve) (organ) — *see* Puncture, accidental complicating surgery
- intestine NEC K63.1
  - with ectopic or molar pregnancy O08.6
  - newborn P78.0
  - obstetrical trauma O71.5
  - traumatic — *see* Laceration, intestine
  - ulcerative NEC K63.1
    - newborn P78.0
- jejunum, jejunal K63.1
  - obstetrical trauma O71.5
  - traumatic — *see* Laceration, intestine, small
  - ulcer — *see* Ulcer, gastrojejunal, with perforation
- joint prosthesis — *see* Complications, joint prosthesis, mechanical, specified NEC, by site

Perforation — *continued*
- mastoid (antrum) (cell) — *see* Disorder, mastoid, specified NEC
- maxillary sinus — *see* Sinusitis, maxillary
- membrana tympani — *see* Perforation, tympanum
- nasal
  - septum J34.89
    - congenital Q30.3
    - syphilitic A52.73
  - sinus J34.89
    - congenital Q30.8
    - due to sinusitis — *see* Sinusitis
- palate (*see also* Cleft, palate)Q35.9
  - syphilitic A52.79
- palatine vault (*see also* Cleft, palate, hard)Q35.1
  - syphilitic A52.79
    - congenital A50.59
- pars flaccida (ear drum) — *see* Perforation, tympanum, attic
- pelvic
  - floor S31.030 ☑
    - with
      - ectopic or molar pregnancy O08.6
      - penetration into retroperitoneal space S31.031 ☑
      - retained foreign body S31.040 ☑
        - with penetration into retroperitoneal space S31.041 ☑
    - following ectopic or molar pregnancy O08.6
    - obstetrical trauma O70.1
  - organ S37.99 ☑
    - adrenal gland S37.818 ☑
    - bladder — *see* Perforation, bladder
    - fallopian tube S37.599 ☑
      - bilateral S37.592 ☑
      - unilateral S37.591 ☑
    - kidney S37.09 ☑
    - obstetrical trauma O71.5
    - ovary S37.499 ☑
      - bilateral S37.492 ☑
      - unilateral S37.491 ☑
    - prostate S37.828 ☑
    - specified organ NEC S37.898 ☑
    - ureter — *see* Perforation, ureter
    - urethra — *see* Perforation, urethra
    - uterus — *see* Perforation, uterus
- perineum — *see* Laceration, perineum
- pharynx J39.2
- rectum K63.1
  - newborn P78.0
  - obstetrical trauma O71.5
  - traumatic S36.63 ☑
- root canal space due to endodontic treatment M27.51
- sigmoid K63.1
  - newborn P78.0
  - obstetrical trauma O71.5
  - traumatic S36.533 ☑
- sinus (accessory) (chronic) (nasal) J34.89
- sphenoidal sinus — *see* Sinusitis, sphenoidal
- surgical (accidental) (by instrument) (blood vessel) (nerve) (organ) — *see* Puncture, accidental complicating surgery
- traumatic
  - external — *see* Puncture
  - eye — *see* Puncture, eyeball
  - internal organ — *see* Injury, by site
- tympanum, tympanic (membrane) (persistent post-traumatic) (postinflammatory) H72.9 ☑
  - attic H72.1 ☑
    - multiple — *see* Perforation, tympanum, multiple
    - total — *see* Perforation, tympanum, total
  - central H72.0 ☑
    - multiple — *see* Perforation, tympanum, multiple
    - total — *see* Perforation, tympanum, total
  - marginal NEC — *see* subcategory H72.2
  - multiple H72.81 ☑
  - pars flaccida — *see* Perforation, tympanum, attic
  - total H72.82 ☑
  - traumatic, current episode S09.2 ☑
- typhoid, gastrointestinal — *see* Typhoid
- ulcer — *see* Ulcer, by site, with perforation
- ureter N28.89
  - traumatic S37.19 ☑
- urethra N36.8
  - with ectopic or molar pregnancy O08.6
  - following ectopic or molar pregnancy O08.6
  - obstetrical trauma O71.5

Perforation — *continued*
- urethra — *continued*
  - traumatic S37.39 ☑
    - at delivery O71.5
- uterus
  - with ectopic or molar pregnancy O08.6
  - by intrauterine contraceptive device T83.39 ☑
  - following ectopic or molar pregnancy O08.6
  - obstetrical trauma O71.1
  - traumatic S37.69 ☑
    - obstetric O71.1
- uvula K13.79
  - syphilitic A52.79
- vagina
  - obstetrical trauma O71.4
  - other trauma — *see* Puncture, vagina

Periadenitis mucosa necrotica recurrens K12.0

Periappendicitis (acute) — *see* Appendicitis

Periarteritis nodosa (disseminated) (infectious) (necrotizing) M30.0

Periarthritis (joint) (*see also* Enthesopathy)
- Duplay's M75.0 ☑
- gonococcal A54.42
- humeroscapularis — *see* Capsulitis, adhesive
- scapulohumeral — *see* Capsulitis, adhesive
- shoulder — *see* Capsulitis, adhesive
- wrist M77.2 ☑

Periarthrosis (angioneural) — *see* Enthesopathy

Pericapsulitis, adhesive (shoulder) — *see* Capsulitis, adhesive

Pericarditis (with decompensation) (with effusion) I31.9
- with rheumatic fever (conditions in I00)
  - active — *see* Pericarditis, rheumatic
  - inactive or quiescent I09.2
- acute (hemorrhagic) (nonrheumatic) (Sicca) I30.9
  - with chorea (acute) (rheumatic) (Sydenham's) I02.0
  - benign I30.8
  - nonspecific I30.0
  - rheumatic I01.0
    - with chorea (acute) (Sydenham's) I02.0
- adhesive or adherent (chronic) (external) (internal) I31.0
  - acute — *see* Pericarditis, acute
  - rheumatic I09.2
- bacterial (acute) (subacute) (with serous or seropurulent effusion) I30.1
- calcareous I31.1
- cholesterol (chronic) I31.8
  - acute I30.9
- chronic (nonrheumatic) I31.9
  - rheumatic I09.2
- constrictive (chronic) I31.1
- coxsackie B33.23
- fibrinocaseous (tuberculous) A18.84
- fibrinopurulent I30.1
- fibrinous I30.8
- fibrous I31.0
- gonococcal A54.83
- idiopathic I30.0
- in systemic lupus erythematosus M32.12
- infective I30.1
- meningococcal A39.53
- neoplastic (chronic) I31.8
  - acute I30.9
- obliterans, obliterating I31.0
- plastic I31.0
- pneumococcal I30.1
- postinfarction I24.1
- purulent I30.1
- rheumatic (active) (acute) (with effusion) (with pneumonia) I01.0
  - with chorea (acute) (rheumatic) (Sydenham's) I02.0
  - chronic or inactive (with chorea) I09.2
- rheumatoid — *see* Rheumatoid, carditis
- septic I30.1
- serofibrinous I30.8
- staphylococcal I30.1
- streptococcal I30.1
- suppurative I30.1
- syphilitic A52.06
- tuberculous A18.84
- uremic N18.9 *[I32]*
- viral I30.1

Pericardium, pericardial — *see* condition

Pericellulitis — *see* Cellulitis

Pericementitis (chronic) (suppurative) (*see also* Periodontitis)
- acute K05.20

Persistence, persistent — *continued*
- right aortic arch Q25.47
- rhesus (Rh) titer — *see* Complication (s), transfusion, incompatibility reaction, Rh (factor)
- sinus
  - urogenitalis
    - female Q52.8
    - male Q55.8
  - venosus with imperfect incorporation in right auricle Q26.8
- thymus (gland) (hyperplasia) E32.0
- thyroglossal duct Q89.2
- thyrolingual duct Q89.2
- truncus arteriosus or communis Q20.0
- tunica vasculosa lentis Q12.2
- umbilical sinus Q64.4
- urachus Q64.4
- vitelline duct Q43.0

Person (with)
- admitted for clinical research, as a control subject (normal comparison) (participant) Z00.6
- awaiting admission to adequate facility elsewhere Z75.1
- concern (normal) about sick person in family Z63.6
- consulting on behalf of another Z71.0
- feigning illness Z76.5
- living (in)
  - alone Z60.2
  - boarding school Z59.3
  - residential institution Z59.3
  - without
    - adequate housing (heating) (space) Z59.1
    - housing (permanent) (temporary) Z59.0
    - person able to render necessary care Z74.2
    - shelter Z59.0
- on waiting list Z75.1
- sick or handicapped in family Z63.6

Personality (disorder) F60.9
- accentuation of traits (type A pattern) Z73.1
- affective F34.0
- aggressive F60.3
- amoral F60.2
- anacastic, anankastic F60.5
- antisocial F60.2
- anxious F60.6
- asocial F60.2
- asthenic F60.7
- avoidant F60.6
- borderline F60.3
- change due to organic condition (enduring) F07.0
- compulsive F60.5
- cycloid F34.0
- cyclothymic F34.0
- dependent F60.7
- depressive F34.1
- dissocial F60.2
- dual F44.81
- eccentric F60.89
- emotionally unstable F60.3
- expansive paranoid F60.0
- explosive F60.3
- fanatic F60.0
- haltlose type F60.89
- histrionic F60.4
- hyperthymic F34.0
- hypothymic F34.1
- hysterical F60.4
- immature F60.89
- inadequate F60.7
- labile (emotional) F60.3
- mixed (nonspecific) F60.89
- morally defective F60.2
- multiple F44.81
- narcissistic F60.81
- obsessional F60.5
- obsessive (-compulsive) F60.5
- organic F07.0
- overconscientious F60.5
- paranoid F60.0
- passive (-dependent) F60.7
- passive-aggressive F60.89
- pathologic F60.9
- pattern defect or disturbance F60.9
- pseudopsychopathic (organic) F07.0
- pseudoretarded (organic) F07.0
- psychoinfantile F60.4
- psychoneurotic NEC F60.89
- psychopathic F60.2
- querulant F60.0

Personality — *continued*
- sadistic F60.89
- schizoid F60.1
- self-defeating F60.7
- sensitive paranoid F60.0
- sociopathic (amoral) (antisocial) (asocial) (dissocial) F60.2
- specified NEC F60.89
- type A Z73.1
- unstable (emotional) F60.3

Perthes' disease — *see* Legg-Calvé-Perthes disease
Pertussis (*see also* Whooping cough)A37.90
Perversion, perverted
- appetite F50.89
  - psychogenic F50.89
- function
  - pituitary gland E23.2
    - posterior lobe E22.2
- sense of smell and taste R43.8
  - psychogenic F45.8
- sexual — *see* Deviation, sexual

Pervious, congenital (*see also* Imperfect, closure)
- ductus arteriosus Q25.0

Pes (congenital) (*see also* Talipes)
- acquired (*see also* Deformity, limb, foot, specified NEC)
  - planus — *see* Deformity, limb, flat foot
- adductus Q66.89
- cavus Q66.7
- deformity NEC, acquired — *see* Deformity, limb, foot, specified NEC
- planus (acquired) (any degree) (*see also* Deformity, limb, flat foot)
  - rachitic sequelae (late effect) E64.3
- valgus Q66.6

Pest, pestis — *see* Plague
Petechia, petechiae R23.3
- newborn P54.5

Petechial typhus A75.9
Peter's anomaly Q13.4
Petit mal seizure — *see* Epilepsy, generalized, specified NEC
Petit's hernia — *see* Hernia, abdomen, specified site NEC
Petrellidosis B48.2
Petrositis H70.20 ☑
- acute H70.21 ☑
- chronic H70.22 ☑

Peutz-Jeghers disease or syndrome Q85.8
Peyronie's disease N48.6
PFAPA (periodic fever, aphthous stomatitis, pharyngitis, and adenopathy syndrome) M04.8
Pfeiffer's disease — *see* Mononucleosis, infectious
Phagedena (dry) (moist) (sloughing) (*see also* Gangrene)
- geometric L88
- penis N48.29
- tropical — *see* Ulcer, skin
- vulva N76.6

Phagedenic — *see* condition
Phakoma H35.89
Phakomatosis (*see also* specific eponymous syndromes)Q85.9
- Bourneville's Q85.1
- specified NEC Q85.8

Phantom limb syndrome (without pain) G54.7
- with pain G54.6

Pharyngeal pouch syndrome D82.1
Pharyngitis (acute) (catarrhal) (gangrenous) (infective) (malignant) (membranous) (phlegmonous) (pseudomembranous) (simple) (subacute) (suppurative) (ulcerative) (viral) J02.9
- with influenza, flu, or grippe — *see* Influenza, with, pharyngitis
- aphthous B08.5
- atrophic J31.2
- chlamydial A56.4
- chronic (atrophic) (granular) (hypertrophic) J31.2
- coxsackievirus B08.5
- diphtheritic A36.0
- enteroviral vesicular B08.5
- follicular (chronic) J31.2
- fusospirochetal A69.1
- gonococcal A54.5
- granular (chronic) J31.2
- herpesviral B00.2
- hypertrophic J31.2
- infectional, chronic J31.2
- influenzal — *see* Influenza, with, respiratory manifestations NEC
- lymphonodular, acute (enteroviral) B08.8
- pneumococcal J02.8

Pharyngitis — *continued*
- purulent J02.9
- putrid J02.9
- septic J02.0
- sicca J31.2
- specified organism NEC J02.8
- staphylococcal J02.8
- streptococcal J02.0
- syphilitic, congenital (early) A50.03
- tuberculous A15.8
- vesicular, enteroviral B08.5
- viral NEC J02.8

Pharyngoconjunctivitis, viral B30.2
Pharyngolaryngitis (acute) J06.0
- chronic J37.0

Pharyngoplegia J39.2
Pharyngotonsillitis, herpesviral B00.2
Pharyngotracheitis, chronic J42
Pharynx, pharyngeal — *see* condition
Phencyclidine-induced
- anxiety disorder F16.980
- bipolar and related disorder F16.94
- depressive disorder F16.94
- psychotic disorder F16.959

Phenomenon
- Arthus' — *see* Arthus' phenomenon
- jaw-winking Q07.8
- lupus erythematosus (LE) cell M32.9
- Raynaud's (secondary) I73.00
  - with gangrene I73.01
- vasomotor R55
- vasospastic I73.9
- vasovagal R55
- Wenckebach's I44.1

Phenylketonuria E70.1
- classical E70.0
- maternal E70.1

Pheochromoblastoma
- specified site — *see* Neoplasm, malignant, by site
- unspecified site C74.10

Pheochromocytoma
- malignant
  - specified site — *see* Neoplasm, malignant, by site
  - unspecified site C74.10
- specified site — *see* Neoplasm, benign, by site
- unspecified site D35.00

Pheohyphomycosis — *see* Chromomycosis
Pheomycosis — *see* Chromomycosis
Phimosis (congenital) (due to infection) N47.1
- chancroidal A57

Phlebectasia (*see also* Varix)
- congenital Q27.4

Phlebitis (infective) (pyemic) (septic) (suppurative) I80.9
- antepartum — *see* Thrombophlebitis, antepartum
- blue — *see* Phlebitis, leg, deep
- breast, superficial I80.8
- cavernous (venous) sinus — *see* Phlebitis, intracranial (venous) sinus
- cerebral (venous) sinus — *see* Phlebitis, intracranial (venous) sinus
- chest wall, superficial I80.8
- cranial (venous) sinus — *see* Phlebitis, intracranial (venous) sinus
- deep (vessels) — *see* Phlebitis, leg, deep
- due to implanted device — *see* Complications, by site and type, specified NEC
- during or resulting from a procedure T81.72 ☑
- femoral vein (superficial) I80.1 ☑
- femoropopliteal vein I80.0 ☑
- gestational — *see* Phlebopathy, gestational
- hepatic veins I80.8
- iliofemoral — *see* Phlebitis, femoral vein
- intracranial (venous) sinus (any) G08
  - nonpyogenic I67.6
- intraspinal venous sinuses and veins G08
  - nonpyogenic G95.19
- lateral (venous) sinus — *see* Phlebitis, intracranial (venous) sinus
- leg I80.3
  - antepartum — *see* Thrombophlebitis, antepartum
  - deep (vessels) NEC I80.20 ☑
    - iliac I80.21 ☑
    - popliteal vein I80.22 ☑
    - specified vessel NEC I80.29 ☑
    - tibial vein I80.23 ☑
  - femoral vein (superficial) I80.1 ☑
  - superficial (vessels) I80.0 ☑

Phlebitis — *continued*
- longitudinal sinus — *see* Phlebitis, intracranial (venous) sinus
- lower limb — *see* Phlebitis, leg
- migrans, migrating (superficial) I82.1
- pelvic
  - with ectopic or molar pregnancy O08.0
  - following ectopic or molar pregnancy O08.0
  - puerperal, postpartum O87.1
- popliteal vein — *see* Phlebitis, leg, deep, popliteal
- portal (vein) K75.1
- postoperative T81.72 ☑
- pregnancy — *see* Thrombophlebitis, antepartum
- puerperal, postpartum, childbirth O87.0
  - deep O87.1
  - pelvic O87.1
  - superficial O87.0
- retina — *see* Vasculitis, retina
- saphenous (accessory) (great) (long) (small) — *see* Phlebitis, leg, superficial
- sinus (meninges) — *see* Phlebitis, intracranial (venous) sinus
- specified site NEC I80.8
- syphilitic A52.09
- tibial vein — *see* Phlebitis, leg, deep, tibial
- ulcerative I80.9
  - leg — *see* Phlebitis, leg
- umbilicus I80.8
- uterus (septic) — *see* Endometritis
- varicose (leg) (lower limb) — *see* Varix, leg, with, inflammation

Phlebofibrosis I87.8
Phleboliths I87.8
Phlebopathy,
- gestational O22.9 ☑
- puerperal O87.9

Phlebosclerosis I87.8
Phlebothrombosis (*see also* Thrombosis)
- antepartum — *see* Thrombophlebitis, antepartum
- pregnancy — *see* Thrombophlebitis, antepartum
- puerperal — *see* Thrombophlebitis, puerperal

Phlebotomus fever A93.1
Phlegmasia
- alba dolens O87.1
  - nonpuerperal — *see* Phlebitis, femoral vein
- cerulea dolens — *see* Phlebitis, leg, deep

Phlegmon — *see* Abscess
Phlegmonous — *see* condition
Phlyctenulosis (allergic) (keratoconjunctivitis) (nontuberculous) (*see also* Keratoconjunctivitis)
- cornea — *see* Keratoconjunctivitis
- tuberculous A18.52

Phobia, phobic F40.9
- animal F40.218
  - spiders F40.210
- examination F40.298
- reaction F40.9
- simple F40.298
- social F40.10
  - generalized F40.11
- specific (isolated) F40.298
  - animal F40.218
    - spiders F40.210
  - blood F40.230
  - injection F40.231
  - injury F40.233
  - men F40.290
  - natural environment F40.228
    - thunderstorms F40.220
  - situational F40.248
    - bridges F40.242
    - closed in spaces F40.240
    - flying F40.243
    - heights F40.241
  - specified focus NEC F40.298
  - transfusion F40.231
  - women F40.291
- specified NEC F40.8
  - medical care NEC F40.232
- state F40.9

Phocas' disease — *see* Mastopathy, cystic
Phocomelia Q73.1
- lower limb — *see* Agenesis, leg, with foot present
- upper limb — *see* Agenesis, arm, with hand present

Phoria H50.50
Phosphate-losing tubular disorder N25.0
Phosphatemia E83.39
Phosphaturia E83.39
Photodermatitis (sun) L56.8
- chronic L57.8

Photodermatitis — *continued*
- due to drug L56.8
- light other than sun L59.8

Photokeratitis H16.13 ☑
Photophobia H53.14 ☑
Photophthalmia — *see* Photokeratitis
Photopsia H53.19
Photoretinitis — *see* Retinopathy, solar
Photosensitivity, photosensitization (sun) skin L56.8
- light other than sun L59.8

Phrenitis — *see* Encephalitis
Phrynoderma (vitamin A deficiency) E50.8
Phthiriasis (pubis) B85.3
- with any infestation classifiable to B85.0-B85.2 B85.4

Phthirus infestation — *see* Phthiriasis
Phthisis (*see also* Tuberculosis)
- bulbi (infectional) — *see* Disorder, globe, degenerated condition, atrophy
- eyeball (due to infection) — *see* Disorder, globe, degenerated condition, atrophy

Phycomycosis — *see* Zygomycosis
Physalopteriasis B81.8
Physical restraint status Z78.1
Phytobezoar T18.9 ☑
- intestine T18.3 ☑
- stomach T18.2 ☑

Pian — *see* Yaws
Pianoma A66.1
Pica F50.89
- in adults F50.89
- infant or child F98.3

Picking, nose F98.8
Pick-Niemann disease — *see* Niemann-Pick disease or syndrome
Pick's
- cerebral atrophy G31.01 *[F02.80]*
  - with behavioral disturbance G31.01 *[F02.81]*
- disease or syndrome (brain) G31.01 *[F02.80]*
  - with behavioral disturbance G31.01 *[F02.81]*
  - brain G31.01 *[F02.80]*
    - with behavioral disturbance G31.01 *[F02.81]*
  - pericardium (pericardial pseudocirrhosis of liver) I31.1
- syndrome
  - brain G31.01 *[F02.80]*
    - with behavioral disturbance G31.01 *[F02.81]*
  - of heart (pericardial pseudocirrhosis of liver) I31.1

Pickwickian syndrome E66.2
Piebaldism E70.39
Piedra (beard) (scalp) B36.8
- black B36.3
- white B36.2

Pierre Robin deformity or syndrome Q87.0
Pierson's disease or osteochondrosis M91.0
Pig-bel A05.2
Pigeon
- breast or chest (acquired) M95.4
  - congenital Q67.7
  - rachitic sequelae (late effect) E64.3
- breeder's disease or lung J67.2
- fancier's disease or lung J67.2
- toe — *see* Deformity, toe, specified NEC

Pigmentation (abnormal) (anomaly) L81.9
- conjunctiva H11.13 ☑
- cornea (anterior) H18.01 ☑
  - posterior H18.05 ☑
  - stromal H18.06 ☑
- diminished melanin formation NEC L81.6
- iron L81.8
- lids, congenital Q82.8
- limbus corneae — *see* Pigmentation, cornea
- metals L81.8
- optic papilla, congenital Q14.2
- retina, congenital (grouped) (nevoid) Q14.1
- scrotum, congenital Q82.8
- tattoo L81.8

Piles (*see also* Hemorrhoids)K64.9
Pili
- annulati or torti (congenital) Q84.1
- incarnati L73.1

Pill roller hand (intrinsic) — *see* Parkinsonism
Pilomatrixoma — *see* Neoplasm, skin, benign
- malignant — *see* Neoplasm, skin, malignant

Pilonidal — *see* condition
Pimple R23.8
PIN — *see* Neoplasia, intraepithelial, prostate
Pinched nerve — *see* Neuropathy, entrapment
Pindborg tumor — *see* Cyst, calcifying odontogenic
Pineal body or gland — *see* condition
Pinealoblastoma C75.3
Pinealoma D44.5
- malignant C75.3

Pineoblastoma C75.3
Pineocytoma D44.5
Pinguecula H11.15 ☑
Pingueculitis H10.81 ☑
Pinhole meatus (*see also* Stricture, urethra)N35.9
Pink
- disease — *see* subcategory T56.1
- eye — *see* Conjunctivitis, acute, mucopurulent

Pinkus' disease (lichen nitidus) L44.1
Pinpoint
- meatus — *see* Stricture, urethra
- os (uteri) — *see* Stricture, cervix

Pins and needles R20.2
Pinta A67.9
- cardiovascular lesions A67.2
- chancre (primary) A67.0
- erythematous plaques A67.1
- hyperchromic lesions A67.1
- hyperkeratosis A67.1
- lesions A67.9
  - cardiovascular A67.2
  - hyperchromic A67.1
  - intermediate A67.1
  - late A67.2
  - mixed A67.3
  - primary A67.0
  - skin (achromic) (cicatricial) (dyschromic) A67.2
    - hyperchromic A67.1
    - mixed (achromic and hyperchromic) A67.3
- papule (primary) A67.0
- skin lesions (achromic) (cicatricial) (dyschromic) A67.2
  - hyperchromic A67.1
  - mixed (achromic and hyperchromic) A67.3
- vitiligo A67.2

Pintids A67.1
Pinworm (disease) (infection) (infestation) B80
Piroplasmosis B60.0
Pistol wound — *see* Gunshot wound
Pitchers' elbow — *see* Derangement, joint, specified type NEC, elbow
Pithecoid pelvis Q74.2
- with disproportion (fetopelvic) O33.0
  - causing obstructed labor O65.0

Pithiatism F48.8
Pitted — *see* Pitting
Pitting (*see also* Edema)R60.9
- lip R60.0
- nail L60.8
- teeth K00.4

Pituitary gland — *see* condition
Pituitary-snuff-taker's disease J67.8
Pityriasis (capitis) L21.0
- alba L30.5
- circinata (et maculata) L42
- furfuracea L21.0
- Hebra's L26
- lichenoides L41.0
  - chronica L41.1
  - et varioliformis (acuta) L41.0
- maculata (et circinata) L30.5
- nigra B36.1
- pilaris, Hebra's L44.0
- rosea L42
- rotunda L44.8
- rubra (Hebra) pilaris L44.0
- simplex L30.5
- specified type NEC L30.5
- streptogenes L30.5
- versicolor (scrotal) B36.0

Placenta, placental — *see* Pregnancy, complicated by (care of) (management affected by), specified condition
Placentitis O41.14 ☑
Plagiocephaly Q67.3
Plague A20.9
- abortive A20.8
- ambulatory A20.8
- asymptomatic A20.8
- bubonic A20.0
- cellulocutaneous A20.1
- cutaneobubonic A20.1
- lymphatic gland A20.0
- meningitis A20.3
- pharyngeal A20.8
- pneumonic (primary) (secondary) A20.2
- pulmonary, pulmonic A20.2
- septicemic A20.7
- tonsillar A20.8
  - septicemic A20.7

Planning, family
- contraception Z30.9
- procreation Z31.69

Plaque (s)
- artery, arterial — *see* Arteriosclerosis
- calcareous — *see* Calcification
- coronary, lipid rich I25.83
- epicardial I31.8
- erythematous, of pinta A67.1
- Hollenhorst's — *see* Occlusion, artery, retina
- lipid rich, coronary I25.83
- pleural (without asbestos) J92.9
  - with asbestos J92.0
- tongue K13.29

Plasmacytoma C90.3 ☑
- extramedullary C90.2 ☑
- medullary C90.0 ☑
- solitary C90.3 ☑

Plasmacytopenia D72.818

Plasmacytosis D72.822

Plaster ulcer — *see* Ulcer, pressure, by site

Plateau iris syndrome (post-iridectomy) (postprocedural) (without glaucoma) H21.82
- with glaucoma H40.22 ☑

Platybasia Q75.8

Platyonychia (congenital) Q84.6
- acquired L60.8

Platypelloid pelvis M95.5
- with disproportion (fetopelvic) O33.0
  - causing obstructed labor O65.0
- congenital Q74.2

Platyspondylisis Q76.49

Plaut (-Vincent) disease (*see also* Vincent's)A69.1

Plethora R23.2
- newborn P61.1

Pleura, pleural — *see* condition

Pleuralgia R07.81

Pleurisy (acute) (adhesive) (chronic) (costal) (diaphragmatic) (double) (dry) (fibrinous) (fibrous) (interlobar) (latent) (plastic) (primary) (residual) (sicca) (sterile) (subacute) (unresolved) R09.1
- with
  - adherent pleura J86.0
  - effusion J90
    - chylous, chyliform J94.0
    - tuberculous (non primary) A15.6
      - primary (progressive) A15.7
  - tuberculosis — *see* Pleurisy, tuberculous (non primary)
- encysted — *see* Pleurisy, with effusion
- exudative — *see* Pleurisy, with effusion
- fibrinopurulent, fibropurulent — *see* Pyothorax
- hemorrhagic — *see* Hemothorax
- pneumococcal J90
- purulent — *see* Pyothorax
- septic — *see* Pyothorax
- serofibrinous — *see* Pleurisy, with effusion
- seropurulent — *see* Pyothorax
- serous — *see* Pleurisy, with effusion
- staphylococcal J86.9
- streptococcal J90
- suppurative — *see* Pyothorax
- traumatic (post) (current) — *see* Injury, intrathoracic, pleura
- tuberculous (with effusion) (non primary) A15.6
  - primary (progressive) A15.7

Pleuritis sicca — *see* Pleurisy

Pleurobronchopneumonia — *see* Pneumonia, broncho-

Pleurodynia R07.81
- epidemic B33.0
- viral B33.0

Pleuropericarditis (*see also* Pericarditis)
- acute I30.9

Pleuropneumonia (acute) (bilateral) (double) (septic) (*see also* Pneumonia)J18.8
- chronic — *see* Fibrosis, lung

Pleuro-pneumonia-like-organism (PPLO), as cause of disease classified elsewhere B96.0

Pleurorrhea — *see* Pleurisy, with effusion

Plexitis, brachial G54.0

Plica
- polonica B85.0
- syndrome, knee M67.5 ☑
- tonsil J35.8

Plicated tongue K14.5

Plug
- bronchus NEC J98.09
- meconium (newborn) NEC syndrome P76.0
- mucus — *see* Asphyxia, mucus

Plumbism — *see* subcategory T56.0

Plummer's disease E05.20
- with thyroid storm E05.21

Plummer-Vinson syndrome D50.1

Pluricarential syndrome of infancy E40

Plus (and minus) hand (intrinsic) — *see* Deformity, limb, specified type NEC, forearm

Pneumathemia — *see* Air, embolism

Pneumatic hammer (drill) syndrome T75.21 ☑

Pneumatocele (lung) J98.4
- intracranial G93.89
- tension J44.9

Pneumatosis
- cystoides intestinalis K63.89
- intestinalis K63.89
- peritonei K66.8

Pneumaturia R39.89

Pneumoblastoma — *see* Neoplasm, lung, malignant

Pneumocephalus G93.89

Pneumococcemia A40.3

Pneumococcus, pneumococcal — *see* condition

Pneumoconiosis (due to) (inhalation of) J64
- with tuberculosis (any type in A15) J65
- aluminum J63.0
- asbestos J61
- bagasse, bagassosis J67.1
- bauxite J63.1
- beryllium J63.2
- coal miners' (simple) J60
- coalworkers' (simple) J60
- collier's J60
- cotton dust J66.0
- diatomite (diatomaceous earth) J62.8
- dust
  - inorganic NEC J63.6
  - lime J62.8
  - marble J62.8
  - organic NEC J66.8
- fumes or vapors (from silo) J68.9
- graphite J63.3
- grinder's J62.8
- kaolin J62.8
- mica J62.8
- millstone maker's J62.8
- mineral fibers NEC J61
- miner's J60
- moldy hay J67.0
- potter's J62.8
- rheumatoid — *see* Rheumatoid, lung
- sandblaster's J62.8
- silica, silicate NEC J62.8
  - with carbon J60
- stonemason's J62.8
- talc (dust) J62.0

Pneumocystis carinii pneumonia B59

Pneumocystis jiroveci (pneumonia) B59

Pneumocystosis (with pneumonia) B59

Pneumohemopericardium I31.2

Pneumohemothorax J94.2
- traumatic S27.2 ☑

Pneumohydropericardium — *see* Pericarditis

Pneumohydrothorax — *see* Hydrothorax

Pneumomediastinum J98.2
- congenital or perinatal P25.2

Pneumomycosis B49 *[J99]*

Pneumonia (acute) (double) (migratory) (purulent) (septic) (unresolved) J18.9
- with
  - lung abscess J85.1
    - due to specified organism — *see* Pneumonia, in (due to)
  - influenza — *see* Influenza, with, pneumonia
- adenoviral J12.0
- adynamic J18.2
- alba A50.04
- allergic (eosinophilic) J82
- alveolar — *see* Pneumonia, lobar
- anaerobes J15.8
- anthrax A22.1
- apex, apical — *see* Pneumonia, lobar
- Ascaris B77.81
- aspiration J69.0
  - due to
    - aspiration of microorganisms
      - bacterial J15.9
      - viral J12.9
    - food (regurgitated) J69.0
    - gastric secretions J69.0
    - milk (regurgitated) J69.0
    - oils, essences J69.1
    - solids, liquids NEC J69.8
    - vomitus J69.0
  - newborn P24.81

Pneumonia — *continued*
- aspiration — *continued*
    - amniotic fluid (clear) P24.11
    - blood P24.21
    - liquor (amnii) P24.11
    - meconium P24.01
    - milk P24.31
    - mucus P24.11
    - food (regurgitated) P24.31
    - specified NEC P24.81
    - stomach contents P24.31
  - postprocedural J95.4
- atypical NEC J18.9
- bacillus J15.9
  - specified NEC J15.8
- bacterial J15.9
  - specified NEC J15.8
- Bacteroides (fragilis) (oralis) (melaninogenicus) J15.8
- basal, basic, basilar — *see* Pneumonia, by type
- bronchiolitis obliterans organized (BOOP) J84.89
- broncho-, bronchial (confluent) (croupous) (diffuse) (disseminated) (hemorrhagic) (involving lobes) (lobar) (terminal) J18.0
  - allergic (eosinophilic) J82
  - aspiration — *see* Pneumonia, aspiration
  - bacterial J15.9
    - specified NEC J15.8
  - chronic — *see* Fibrosis, lung
  - diplococcal J13
  - Eaton's agent J15.7
  - Escherichia coli (E. coli) J15.5
  - Friedländer's bacillus J15.0
  - Hemophilus influenzae J14
  - hypostatic J18.2
  - inhalation (*see also* Pneumonia, aspiration)
    - due to fumes or vapors (chemical) J68.0
    - of oils or essences J69.1
  - Klebsiella (pneumoniae) J15.0
  - lipid, lipoid J69.1
    - endogenous J84.89
  - Mycoplasma (pneumoniae) J15.7
  - pleuro-pneumonia-like-organisms (PPLO) J15.7
  - pneumococcal J13
  - Proteus J15.6
  - Pseudomonas J15.1
  - Serratia marcescens J15.6
  - specified organism NEC J16.8
  - staphylococcal — *see* Pneumonia, staphylococcal
  - streptococcal NEC J15.4
    - group B J15.3
    - pneumoniae J13
  - viral, virus — *see* Pneumonia, viral
- Butyrivibrio (fibriosolvens) J15.8
- Candida B37.1
- caseous — *see* Tuberculosis, pulmonary
- catarrhal — *see* Pneumonia, broncho
- chlamydial J16.0
  - congenital P23.1
- cholesterol J84.89
- cirrhotic (chronic) — *see* Fibrosis, lung
- Clostridium (haemolyticum) (novyi) J15.8
- confluent — *see* Pneumonia, broncho
- congenital (infective) P23.9
  - due to
    - bacterium NEC P23.6
    - Chlamydia P23.1
    - Escherichia coli P23.4
    - Haemophilus influenzae P23.6
    - infective organism NEC P23.8
    - Klebsiella pneumoniae P23.6
    - Mycoplasma P23.6
    - Pseudomonas P23.5
    - Staphylococcus P23.2
    - Streptococcus (except group B) P23.6
      - group B P23.3
    - viral agent P23.0
  - specified NEC P23.8
- croupous — *see* Pneumonia, lobar
- cryptogenic organizing J84.116
- cytomegalic inclusion B25.0
- cytomegaloviral B25.0
- deglutition — *see* Pneumonia, aspiration
- desquamative interstitial J84.117
- diffuse — *see* Pneumonia, broncho
- diplococcal, diplococcus (broncho-) (lobar) J13
- disseminated (focal) — *see* Pneumonia, broncho
- Eaton's agent J15.7
- embolic, embolism — *see* Embolism, pulmonary
- Enterobacter J15.6
- eosinophilic J82

Pneumonia — *continued*
- Escherichia coli (E. coli) J15.5
- Eubacterium J15.8
- fibrinous — *see* Pneumonia, lobar
- fibroid, fibrous (chronic) — *see* Fibrosis, lung
- Friedländer's bacillus J15.0
- Fusobacterium (nucleatum) J15.8
- gangrenous J85.0
- giant cell (measles) B05.2
- gonococcal A54.84
- gram-negative bacteria NEC J15.6
  - anaerobic J15.8
- Hemophilus influenzae (broncho) (lobar) J14
- human metapneumovirus J12.3
- hypostatic (broncho) (lobar) J18.2
- in (due to)
  - actinomycosis A42.0
  - adenovirus J12.0
  - anthrax A22.1
  - ascariasis B77.81
  - aspergillosis B44.9
  - Bacillus anthracis A22.1
  - Bacterium anitratum J15.6
  - candidiasis B37.1
  - chickenpox B01.2
  - Chlamydia J16.0
    - neonatal P23.1
  - coccidioidomycosis B38.2
    - acute B38.0
    - chronic B38.1
  - cytomegalovirus disease B25.0
  - Diplococcus (pneumoniae) J13
  - Eaton's agent J15.7
  - Enterobacter J15.6
  - Escherichia coli (E. coli) J15.5
  - Friedländer's bacillus J15.0
  - fumes and vapors (chemical) (inhalation) J68.0
  - gonorrhea A54.84
  - Hemophilus influenzae (H. influenzae) J14
  - Herellea J15.6
  - histoplasmosis B39.2
    - acute B39.0
    - chronic B39.1
  - human metapneumovirus J12.3
  - Klebsiella (pneumoniae) J15.0
  - measles B05.2
  - Mycoplasma (pneumoniae) J15.7
  - nocardiosis, nocardiasis A43.0
  - ornithosis A70
  - parainfluenza virus J12.2
  - pleuro-pneumonia-like-organism (PPLO) J15.7
  - pneumococcus J13
  - pneumocystosis (Pneumocystis carinii) (Pneumocystis jiroveci) B59
  - Proteus J15.6
  - Pseudomonas NEC J15.1
    - pseudomallei A24.1
  - psittacosis A70
  - Q fever A78
  - respiratory syncytial virus J12.1
  - rheumatic fever I00 *[J17]*
  - rubella B06.81
  - Salmonella (infection) A02.22
    - typhi A01.03
  - schistosomiasis B65.9 *[J17]*
  - Serratia marcescens J15.6
  - specified
    - bacterium NEC J15.8
    - organism NEC J16.8
  - spirochetal NEC A69.8
  - Staphylococcus J15.20
    - aureus (methicillin susceptible) (MSSA) J15.211
      - methicillin resistant (MRSA) J15.212
    - specified NEC J15.29
  - Streptococcus J15.4
    - group B J15.3
    - pneumoniae J13
    - specified NEC J15.4
  - toxoplasmosis B58.3
  - tularemia A21.2
  - typhoid (fever) A01.03
  - varicella B01.2
  - virus — *see* Pneumonia, viral
  - whooping cough A37.91
    - due to
      - Bordetella parapertussis A37.11
      - Bordetella pertussis A37.01
      - specified NEC A37.81
  - Yersinia pestis A20.2
- inhalation of food or vomit — *see* Pneumonia, aspiration

Pneumonia — *continued*
- interstitial J84.9
  - chronic J84.111
  - desquamative J84.117
  - due to
    - collagen vascular disease J84.17
    - known underlying cause J84.17
  - idiopathic NOS J84.111
  - in disease classified elsewhere J84.17
  - lymphocytic (due to collagen vascular disease) (in diseases classified elsewhere) J84.17
  - lymphoid J84.2
  - non-specific J84.89
    - due to
      - collagen vascular disease J84.17
      - known underlying cause J84.17
    - idiopathic J84.113
    - in diseases classified elsewhere J84.17
  - plasma cell B59
  - pseudomonas J15.1
  - usual J84.112
    - due to collagen vascular disease J84.17
    - idiopathic J84.112
    - in diseases classified elsewhere J84.17
- Klebsiella (pneumoniae) J15.0
- lipid, lipoid (exogenous) J69.1
  - endogenous J84.89
- lobar (disseminated) (double) (interstitial) J18.1
  - bacterial J15.9
    - specified NEC J15.8
  - chronic — *see* Fibrosis, lung
  - Escherichia coli (E. coli) J15.5
  - Friedländer's bacillus J15.0
  - Hemophilus influenzae J14
  - hypostatic J18.2
  - Klebsiella (pneumoniae) J15.0
  - pneumococcal J13
  - Proteus J15.6
  - Pseudomonas J15.1
  - specified organism NEC J16.8
  - staphylococcal — *see* Pneumonia, staphylococcal
  - streptococcal NEC J15.4
  - Streptococcus pneumoniae J13
  - viral, virus — *see* Pneumonia, viral
- lobular — *see* Pneumonia, broncho
- Löffler's J82
- lymphoid interstitial J84.2
- massive — *see* Pneumonia, lobar
- meconium P24.01
- MRSA (Methicillin resistant Staphylococcus aureus) J15.212
- MSSA (methicillin susceptible Staphylococcus aureus) J15.211
- multilobar — *see* Pneumonia, by type
- Mycoplasma (pneumoniae) J15.7
- necrotic J85.0
- neonatal P23.9
  - aspiration — *see* Aspiration, by substance, with pneumonia
- nitrogen dioxide J68.0
- organizing J84.89
  - due to
    - collagen vascular disease J84.17
    - known underlying cause J84.17
  - in diseases classified elsewhere J84.17
- orthostatic J18.2
- parainfluenza virus J12.2
- parenchymatous — *see* Fibrosis, lung
- passive J18.2
- patchy — *see* Pneumonia, broncho
- Peptococcus J15.8
- Peptostreptococcus J15.8
- plasma cell (of infants) B59
- pleurolobar — *see* Pneumonia, lobar
- pleuro-pneumonia-like organism (PPLO) J15.7
- pneumococcal (broncho) (lobar) J13
- Pneumocystis (carinii) (jiroveci) B59
- postinfectional NEC B99 ☑ *[J17]*
- postmeasles B05.2
- Proteus J15.6
- Pseudomonas J15.1
- psittacosis A70
- radiation J70.0
- respiratory syncytial virus J12.1
- resulting from a procedure J95.89
- rheumatic I00 *[J17]*
- Salmonella (arizonae) (cholerae-suis) (enteritidis) (typhimurium) A02.22
  - typhi A01.03
  - typhoid fever A01.03
- SARS-associated coronavirus J12.81

Pneumonia — *continued*
- segmented, segmental — *see* Pneumonia, broncho-
- Serratia marcescens J15.6
- specified NEC J18.8
  - bacterium NEC J15.8
  - organism NEC J16.8
  - virus NEC J12.89
- spirochetal NEC A69.8
- staphylococcal (broncho) (lobar) J15.20
  - aureus (methicillin susceptible) (MSSA) J15.211
    - methicillin resistant (MRSA) J15.212
  - specified NEC J15.29
- static, stasis J18.2
- streptococcal NEC (broncho) (lobar) J15.4
  - group
    - A J15.4
    - B J15.3
    - specified NEC J15.4
- Streptococcus pneumoniae J13
- syphilitic, congenital (early) A50.04
- traumatic (complication) (early) (secondary) T79.8 ☑
- tuberculous (any) — *see* Tuberculosis, pulmonary
- tularemic A21.2
- varicella B01.2
- Veillonella J15.8
- ventilator associated J95.851
- viral, virus (broncho) (interstitial) (lobar) J12.9
  - adenoviral J12.0
  - congenital P23.0
  - human metapneumovirus J12.3
  - parainfluenza J12.2
  - respiratory syncytial J12.1
  - SARS-associated coronavirus J12.81
  - specified NEC J12.89
- white (congenital) A50.04

Pneumonic — *see* condition

Pneumonitis (acute) (primary) (*see also* Pneumonia)
- air-conditioner J67.7
- allergic (due to) J67.9
  - organic dust NEC J67.8
  - red cedar dust J67.8
  - sequoiosis J67.8
  - wood dust J67.8
- aspiration J69.0
  - due to
    - anesthesia J95.4
      - during
        - labor and delivery O74.0
        - pregnancy O29.01 ☑
        - puerperium O89.01
    - fumes or gases J68.0
  - obstetric O74.0
- chemical (due to gases, fumes or vapors) (inhalation) J68.0
  - due to anesthesia J95.4
- cholesterol J84.89
- crack (cocaine) J68.0
- chronic — *see* Fibrosis, lung
- congenital rubella P35.0
- due to
  - beryllium J68.0
  - cadmium J68.0
  - crack (cocaine) J68.0
  - detergent J69.8
  - fluorocarbon-polymer J68.0
  - food, vomit (aspiration) J69.0
  - fumes or vapors J68.0
  - gases, fumes or vapors (inhalation) J68.0
  - inhalation
    - blood J69.8
    - essences J69.1
    - food (regurgitated), milk, vomit J69.0
    - oils, essences J69.1
    - saliva J69.0
    - solids, liquids NEC J69.8
  - manganese J68.0
  - nitrogen dioxide J68.0
  - oils, essences J69.1
  - solids, liquids NEC J69.8
  - toxoplasmosis (acquired) B58.3
    - congenital P37.1
  - vanadium J68.0
  - ventilator J95.851
- eosinophilic J82
- hypersensitivity J67.9
  - air conditioner lung J67.7
  - bagassosis J67.1
  - bird fancier's lung J67.2
  - farmer's lung J67.0
  - maltworker's lung J67.4

Pneumonitis - Polycythemia

Pneumonitis — *continued*
- hypersensitivity — *continued*
  - maple bark-stripper's lung J67.6
  - mushroom worker's lung J67.5
  - specified organic dust NEC J67.8
  - suberosis J67.3
- interstitial (chronic) J84.89
  - acute J84.114
  - lymphoid J84.2
  - non-specific J84.89
    - idiopathic J84.113
- lymphoid, interstitial J84.2
- meconium P24.01
- postanesthetic J95.4
  - correct substance properly administered — *see* Table of Drugs and Chemicals, by drug, adverse effect
  - in labor and delivery O74.0
  - in pregnancy O29.01 ☑
  - obstetric O74.0
  - overdose or wrong substance given or taken (by accident) — *see* Table of Drugs and Chemicals, by drug, poisoning
  - postpartum, puerperal O89.01
- postoperative J95.4
  - obstetric O74.0
- radiation J70.0
- rubella, congenital P35.0
- ventilation (air-conditioning) J67.7
- ventilator associated J95.851
- wood-dust J67.8

Pneumonoconiosis — *see* Pneumoconiosis

Pneumoparotid K11.8

Pneumopathy NEC J98.4
- alveolar J84.09
- due to organic dust NEC J66.8
- parietoalveolar J84.09

Pneumopericarditis (*see also* Pericarditis)
- acute I30.9

Pneumopericardium (*see also* Pericarditis)
- congenital P25.3
- newborn P25.3
- traumatic (post) — *see* Injury, heart

Pneumophagia (psychogenic) F45.8

Pneumopleurisy, pneumopleuritis (*see also* Pneumonia)J18.8

Pneumopyopericardium I30.1

Pneumopyothorax — *see* Pyopneumothorax
- with fistula J86.0

Pneumorrhagia (*see also* Hemorrhage, lung)
- tuberculous — *see* Tuberculosis, pulmonary

Pneumothorax NOS J93.9
- acute J93.83
- chronic J93.81
- congenital P25.1
- perinatal period P25.1
- postprocedural J95.811
- specified NEC J93.83
- spontaneous NOS J93.83
  - newborn P25.1
  - primary J93.11
  - secondary J93.12
  - tension J93.0
- tense valvular, infectional J93.0
- tension (spontaneous) J93.0
- traumatic S27.0 ☑
  - with hemothorax S27.2 ☑
- tuberculous — *see* Tuberculosis, pulmonary

Podagra (*see also* Gout)M10.9

Podencephalus Q01.9

Poikilocytosis R71.8

Poikiloderma L81.6
- Civatte's L57.3
- congenital Q82.8
- vasculare atrophicans L94.5

Poikilodermatomyositis M33.10
- with
  - myopathy M33.12
  - respiratory involvement M33.11
  - specified organ involvement NEC M33.19

Pointed ear (congenital) Q17.3

Poison ivy, oak, sumac or other plant dermatitis (allergic) (contact) L23.7

Poisoning (acute) (*see also* Table of Drugs and Chemicals)
- algae and toxins T65.82 ☑
- Bacillus B (aertrycke) (cholerae (suis)) (paratyphosus) (suipestifer) A02.9
  - botulinus A05.1
- bacterial toxins A05.9
- berries, noxious — *see* Poisoning, food, noxious, berries

Poisoning — *continued*
- botulism A05.1
- ciguatera fish T61.0 ☑
- Clostridium botulinum A05.1
- death-cap (Amanita phalloides) (Amanita verna) — *see* Poisoning, food, noxious, mushrooms
- drug — *see* Table of Drugs and Chemicals, by drug, poisoning
- epidemic, fish (noxious) — *see* Poisoning, seafood
  - bacterial A05.9
- fava bean D55.0
- fish (noxious) T61.9 ☑
  - bacterial — *see* Intoxication, food-borne, by agent
  - ciguatera fish — *see* Poisoning, ciguatera fish
  - scombroid fish — *see* Poisoning, scombroid fish
  - specified type NEC T61.77 ☑
- food (acute) (diseased) (infected) (noxious) NEC T62.9 ☑
  - bacterial — *see* Intoxication, food-borne, by agent
  - due to
    - Bacillus (aertrycke) (choleraesuis) (paratyphosus) (suipestifer) A02.9
      - botulinus A05.1
    - Clostridium (perfringens) (Welchii) A05.2
    - salmonella (aertrycke) (callinarum) (choleraesuis) (enteritidis) (paratyphi) (suipestifer) A02.9
      - with
        - gastroenteritis A02.0
        - sepsis A02.1
    - staphylococcus A05.0
    - Vibrio
      - parahaemolyticus A05.3
      - vulnificus A05.5
  - noxious or naturally toxic T62.9 ☑
    - berries — *see* subcategory T62.1-
    - fish — *see* Poisoning, seafood
    - mushrooms — *see* subcategory T62.0X-
    - plants NEC — *see* subcategory T62.2X-
    - seafood — *see* Poisoning, seafood
    - specified NEC — *see* subcategory T62.8X-
- ichthyotoxism — *see* Poisoning, seafood
- kreotoxism, food A05.9
- latex T65.81 ☑
- lead T56.0 ☑
- mushroom — *see* Poisoning, food, noxious, mushroom
- mussels (*see also* Poisoning, shellfish)
  - bacterial — *see* Intoxication, food-borne, by agent
- nicotine (tobacco) T65.2 ☑
- noxious foodstuffs — *see* Poisoning, food, noxious
- plants, noxious — *see* Poisoning, food, noxious, plants NEC
- ptomaine — *see* Poisoning, food
- radiation J70.0
- Salmonella (arizonae) (cholerae-suis) (enteritidis) (typhimurium) A02.9
- scombroid fish T61.1 ☑
- seafood (noxious) T61.9 ☑
  - bacterial — *see* Intoxication, food-borne, by agent
  - fish — *see* Poisoning, fish
  - shellfish — *see* Poisoning, shellfish
  - specified NEC — *see* subcategory T61.8X-
- shellfish (amnesic) (azaspiracid) (diarrheic) (neurotoxic) (noxious) (paralytic) T61.78 ☑
  - bacterial — *see* Intoxication, food-borne, by agent
  - ciguatera mollusk — *see* Poisoning, ciguatera fish
- specified substance NEC T65.891 ☑
- Staphylococcus, food A05.0
- tobacco (nicotine) T65.2 ☑
- water E87.79

Poker spine — *see* Spondylitis, ankylosing

Poland syndrome Q79.8

Polioencephalitis (acute) (bulbar) A80.9
- inferior G12.22
- influenzal — *see* Influenza, with, encephalopathy
- superior hemorrhagic (acute) (Wernicke's) E51.2
- Wernicke's E51.2

Polioencephalomyelitis (acute) (anterior) A80.9
- with beriberi E51.2

Polioencephalopathy, superior hemorrhagic E51.2
- with
  - beriberi E51.11
  - pellagra E52

Poliomeningoencephalitis — *see* Meningoencephalitis

Poliomyelitis (acute) (anterior) (epidemic) A80.9
- with paralysis (bulbar) — *see* Poliomyelitis, paralytic
- abortive A80.4
- ascending (progressive) — *see* Poliomyelitis, paralytic
- bulbar (paralytic) — *see* Poliomyelitis, paralytic
- congenital P35.8
- nonepidemic A80.9
- nonparalytic A80.4
- paralytic A80.30
  - specified NEC A80.39
  - vaccine-associated A80.0
  - wild virus
    - imported A80.1
    - indigenous A80.2
- spinal, acute A80.9

Poliosis (eyebrow) (eyelashes) L67.1
- circumscripta, acquired L67.1

Pollakiuria R35.0
- psychogenic F45.8

Pollinosis J30.1

Pollitzer's disease L73.2

Polyadenitis (*see also* Lymphadenitis)
- malignant A20.0

Polyalgia M79.89

Polyangiitis M30.0
- microscopic M31.7
- overlap syndrome M30.8

Polyarteritis
- microscopic M31.7
- nodosa M30.0
  - with lung involvement M30.1
  - juvenile M30.2
  - related condition NEC M30.8

Polyarthralgia — *see* Pain, joint

Polyarthritis, polyarthropathy (*see also* Arthritis)M13.0
- due to or associated with other specified conditions — *see* Arthritis
- epidemic (Australian) (with exanthema) B33.1
- infective — *see* Arthritis, pyogenic or pyemic
- inflammatory M06.4
- juvenile (chronic) (seronegative) M08.3
- migratory — *see* Fever, rheumatic
- rheumatic, acute — *see* Fever, rheumatic

Polyarthrosis M15.9
- post-traumatic M15.3
- primary M15.0
- specified NEC M15.8

Polycarential syndrome of infancy E40

Polychondritis (atrophic) (chronic) (*see also* Disorder, cartilage, specified type NEC)
- relapsing M94.1

Polycoria Q13.2

Polycystic (disease)
- degeneration, kidney Q61.3
  - autosomal dominant (adult type) Q61.2
  - autosomal recessive (infantile type) NEC Q61.19
- kidney Q61.3
  - autosomal
    - dominant Q61.2
    - recessive NEC Q61.19
  - autosomal dominant (adult type) Q61.2
  - autosomal recessive (childhood type) NEC Q61.19
  - infantile type NEC Q61.19
- liver Q44.6
- lung J98.4
  - congenital Q33.0
- ovary, ovaries E28.2
- spleen Q89.09

Polycythemia (secondary) D75.1
- acquired D75.1
- benign (familial) D75.0
- due to
  - donor twin P61.1
  - erythropoietin D75.1
  - fall in plasma volume D75.1
  - high altitude D75.1
  - maternal-fetal transfusion P61.1
  - stress D75.1
- emotional D75.1
- erythropoietin D75.1
- familial (benign) D75.0
- Gaisböck's (hypertonica) D75.1
- high altitude D75.1
- hypertonica D75.1
- hypoxemic D75.1

☑ **Additional character required**

Polyposis - Pregnancy

Polyposis — *continued*
- familial D12.6
  - adenocarcinoma in situ in — *see* Neoplasm, in situ, by site
- intestinal (adenomatous) D12.6
- malignant lymphomatous C83.1 ☑
- multiple, adenomatous (*see also* Neoplasm, benign)D36.9

Polyradiculitis — *see* Polyneuropathy
Polyradiculoneuropathy (acute) (postinfective) (segmentally demyelinating) G61.0
Polyserositis
- due to pericarditis I31.1
- pericardial I31.1
- periodic, familial E85.0
- tuberculous A19.9
  - acute A19.1
  - chronic A19.8

Polysplenia syndrome Q89.09
Polysyndactyly (*see also* Syndactylism, syndactyly)Q70.4
Polytrichia L68.3
Polyunguia Q84.6
Polyuria R35.8
- nocturnal R35.1
- psychogenic F45.8

Pompe's disease (glycogen storage) E74.02
Pompholyx L30.1
Poncet's disease (tuberculous rheumatism) A18.09
Pond fracture — *see* Fracture, skull
Ponos B55.0
Pons, pontine — *see* condition
Poor
- aesthetic of existing restoration of tooth K08.56
- contractions, labor O62.2
- gingival margin to tooth restoration K08.51
- personal hygiene R46.0
- prenatal care, affecting management of pregnancy — *see* Pregnancy, complicated by, insufficient, prenatal care
- sucking reflex (newborn) R29.2
- urinary stream R39.12
- vision NEC H54.7

Poradenitis, nostras inguinalis or venereal A55
Porencephaly (congenital) (developmental) (true) Q04.6
- acquired G93.0
- nondevelopmental G93.0
- traumatic (post) F07.89

Porocephaliasis B88.8
Porokeratosis Q82.8
Poroma, eccrine — *see* Neoplasm, skin, benign
Porphyria (South African) E80.20
- acquired E80.20
- acute intermittent (hepatic) (Swedish) E80.21
- cutanea tarda (hereditary) (symptomatic) E80.1
- due to drugs E80.20
  - correct substance properly administered — *see* Table of Drugs and Chemicals, by drug, adverse effect
  - overdose or wrong substance given or taken — *see* Table of Drugs and Chemicals, by drug, poisoning
- erythropoietic (congenital) (hereditary) E80.0
- hepatocutaneous type E80.1
- secondary E80.20
- toxic NEC E80.20
- variegata E80.20

Porphyrinuria — *see* Porphyria
Porphyruria — *see* Porphyria
Portal — *see* condition
Port wine nevus, mark, or stain Q82.5
Posadas-Wernicke disease B38.9
Positive
- culture (nonspecific)
  - blood R78.81
  - bronchial washings R84.5
  - cerebrospinal fluid R83.5
  - cervix uteri R87.5
  - nasal secretions R84.5
  - nipple discharge R89.5
  - nose R84.5
    - staphylococcus (Methicillin susceptible) Z22.321
      - Methicillin resistant Z22.322
  - peritoneal fluid R85.5
  - pleural fluid R84.5
  - prostatic secretions R86.5
  - saliva R85.5
  - seminal fluid R86.5
  - sputum R84.5
  - synovial fluid R89.5

Positive — *continued*
- culture — *continued*
  - throat scrapings R84.5
  - urine R82.79
  - vagina R87.5
  - vulva R87.5
  - wound secretions R89.5
- PPD (skin test) R76.11
- serology for syphilis A53.0
  - false R76.8
  - with signs or symptoms - code as Syphilis, by site and stage
- skin test, tuberculin (without active tuberculosis) R76.11
- test, human immunodeficiency virus (HIV) R75
- VDRL A53.0
  - with signs or symptoms - code by site and stage under Syphilis A53.9
- Wassermann reaction A53.0

Postcardiotomy syndrome I97.0
Postcaval ureter Q62.62
Postcholecystectomy syndrome K91.5
Postclimacteric bleeding N95.0
Postcommissurotomy syndrome I97.0
Postconcussional syndrome F07.81
Postcontusional syndrome F07.81
Postcricoid region — *see* condition
Post-dates (40-42 weeks) (pregnancy) (mother) O48.0
- more than 42 weeks gestation O48.1

Postencephalitic syndrome F07.89
Posterior — *see* condition
Posterolateral sclerosis (spinal cord) — *see* Degeneration, combined
Postexanthematous — *see* condition
Postfebrile — *see* condition
Postgastrectomy dumping syndrome K91.1
Posthemiplegic chorea — *see* Monoplegia
Posthemorrhagic anemia (chronic) D50.0
- acute D62
- newborn P61.3

Postherpetic neuralgia (zoster) B02.29
- trigeminal B02.22

Posthitis N47.7
Postimmunization complication or reaction — *see* Complications, vaccination
Postinfectious — *see* condition
Postlaminectomy syndrome NEC M96.1
Postleukotomy syndrome F07.0
Postmastectomy lymphedema (syndrome) I97.2
Postmaturity, postmature (over 42 weeks)
- maternal (over 42 weeks gestation) O48.1
- newborn P08.22

Postmeasles complication NEC (*see also* condition)B05.89
Postmenopausal
- endometrium (atrophic) N95.8
  - suppurative (*see also* Endometritis)N71.9
- osteoporosis — *see* Osteoporosis, postmenopausal

Postnasal drip R09.82
- due to
  - allergic rhinitis — *see* Rhinitis, allergic
  - common cold J00
  - gastroesophageal reflux — *see* Reflux, gastroesophageal
  - nasopharyngitis — *see* Nasopharyngitis
  - other know condition - code to condition
  - sinusitis — *see* Sinusitis

Postnatal — *see* condition
Postoperative (postprocedural) — *see* Complication, postoperative
- pneumothorax, therapeutic Z98.3
- state NEC Z98.890

Postpancreatectomy hyperglycemia E89.1
Postpartum — *see* Puerperal
Postphlebitic syndrome — *see* Syndrome, postthrombotic
Postpoliomyelitic (*see also* condition)
- osteopathy — *see* Osteopathy, after poliomyelitis

Postpolio (myelitic) syndrome G14
Postprocedural (*see also* Postoperative)
- hypoinsulinemia E89.1

Postschizophrenic depression F32.89
Postsurgery status (*see also* Status (post))
- pneumothorax, therapeutic Z98.3

Post-term (40-42 weeks) (pregnancy) (mother) O48.0
- infant P08.21
- more than 42 weeks gestation (mother) O48.1

Post-traumatic brain syndrome, nonpsychotic F07.81
Post-typhoid abscess A01.09

Postures, hysterical F44.2
Postvaccinal reaction or complication — *see* Complications, vaccination
Postvalvulotomy syndrome I97.0
Potain's
- disease (pulmonary edema) — *see* Edema, lung
- syndrome (gastrectasis with dyspepsia) K31.0

Potter's
- asthma J62.8
- facies Q60.6
- lung J62.8
- syndrome (with renal agenesis) Q60.6

Pott's
- curvature (spinal) A18.01
- disease or paraplegia A18.01
- spinal curvature A18.01
- tumor, puffy — *see* Osteomyelitis, specified type NEC

Pouch
- bronchus Q32.4
- Douglas' — *see* condition
- esophagus, esophageal, congenital Q39.6
  - acquired K22.5
- gastric K31.4
- Hartmann's K82.8
- pharynx, pharyngeal (congenital) Q38.7

Pouchitis K91.850
Poultrymen's itch B88.0
Poverty NEC Z59.6
- extreme Z59.5

Poxvirus NEC B08.8
Prader-Willi syndrome Q87.1
Preauricular appendage or tag Q17.0
Prebetalipoproteinemia (acquired) (essential) (familial) (hereditary) (primary) (secondary) E78.1
- with chylomicronemia E78.3

Precipitate labor or delivery O62.3
Preclimacteric bleeding (menorrhagia) N92.4
Precocious
- adrenarche E30.1
- menarche E30.1
- menstruation E30.1
- pubarche E30.1
- puberty E30.1
  - central E22.8
- sexual development NEC E30.1
- thelarche E30.8

Precocity, sexual (constitutional) (cryptogenic) (female) (idiopathic) (male) E30.1
- with adrenal hyperplasia E25.9
  - congenital E25.0

Precordial pain R07.2
Predeciduous teeth K00.2
Prediabetes, prediabetic R73.03
- complicating
  - pregnancy — *see* Pregnancy, complicated by, diseases of, specified type or system NEC
  - puerperium O99.89

Predislocation status of hip at birth Q65.6
Pre-eclampsia O14.9 ☑
- with pre-existing hypertension — *see* Hypertension, complicating pregnancy, pre-existing, with, pre-eclampsia
- complicating
  - childbirth O14.94
  - puerperium O14.95
- mild O14.0 ☑
  - complicating
    - childbirth O14.04
    - puerperium O14.05
- moderate O14.0 ☑
  - complicating
    - childbirth O14.04
    - puerperium O14.05
- severe O14.1 ☑
  - with hemolysis, elevated liver enzymes and low platelet count (HELLP) O14.2 ☑
    - complicating
      - childbirth O14.24
      - puerperium O14.25
  - complicating
    - childbirth O14.14
    - puerperium O14.15

Pre-eruptive color change, teeth, tooth K00.8
Pre-excitation atrioventricular conduction I45.6
Preglaucoma H40.00 ☑
Pregnancy (single) (uterine) (*see also* Delivery and Puerperal)
- Note: The Tabular must be reviewed for assignment of the appropriate character indicating the trimester of the pregnancy

Pregnancy — *continued*

Note: The Tabular must be reviewed for assignment of appropriate seventh character for multiple gestation codes in Chapter 15

- abdominal (ectopic) O00.00
  - with intrauterine pregnancy O00.01
  - with viable fetus O36.7 ☑
- ampullar O00.10
  - with intrauterine pregnancy O00.11
- biochemical O02.81
- broad ligament O00.80
  - with intrauterine pregnancy O00.81
- cervical O00.80
  - with intrauterine pregnancy O00.81
- chemical O02.81
- complicated NOS O26.9 ☑
- complicated by (care of) (management affected by)
  - abnormal, abnormality
    - cervix O34.4 ☑
      - causing obstructed labor O65.5
    - cord (umbilical) O69.9 ☑
    - findings on antenatal screening of mother O28.9
      - biochemical O28.1
      - cytological O28.2
      - chromosomal O28.5
      - genetic O28.5
      - hematological O28.0
      - radiological O28.4
      - specified NEC O28.8
      - ultrasonic O28.3
    - glucose (tolerance) NEC O99.810
    - pelvic organs O34.9 ☑
      - specified NEC O34.8 ☑
        - causing obstructed labor O65.5
    - pelvis (bony) (major) NEC O33.0
    - perineum O34.7 ☑
    - position
      - placenta O44.0 ☑
        - with hemorrhage O44.1 ☑
      - uterus O34.59 ☑
    - uterus O34.59 ☑
      - causing obstructed labor O65.5
      - congenital O34.0 ☑
    - vagina O34.6 ☑
      - causing obstructed labor O65.5
    - vulva O34.7 ☑
      - causing obstructed labor O65.5
  - abruptio placentae — *see* Abruptio placentae
  - abscess or cellulitis
    - bladder O23.1 ☑
    - breast O91.11 ☑
    - genital organ or tract O23.9 ☑
  - abuse
    - physical O9A.31 ☑
    - psychological O9A.51 ☑
    - sexual O9A.41 ☑
  - adverse effect anesthesia O29.9 ☑
    - aspiration pneumonitis O29.01 ☑
    - cardiac arrest O29.11 ☑
    - cardiac complication NEC O29.19 ☑
    - cardiac failure O29.12 ☑
    - central nervous system complication NEC O29.29 ☑
    - cerebral anoxia O29.21 ☑
    - failed or difficult intubation O29.6 ☑
    - inhalation of stomach contents or secretions NOS O29.01 ☑
    - local, toxic reaction O29.3X ☑
    - Mendelson's syndrome O29.01 ☑
    - pressure collapse of lung O29.02 ☑
    - pulmonary complications NEC O29.09 ☑
    - specified NEC O29.8X ☑
    - spinal and epidural type NEC O29.5X ☑
      - induced headache O29.4 ☑
  - albuminuria (*see also* Proteinuria, gestational)O12.1 ☑
  - alcohol use O99.31 ☑
  - amnionitis O41.12 ☑
  - anaphylactoid syndrome of pregnancy O88.01 ☑
  - anemia (conditions in D50-D64) (pre-existing) O99.01 ☑
    - complicating the puerperium O99.03
  - antepartum hemorrhage O46.9 ☑
    - with coagulation defect — *see* Hemorrhage, antepartum, with coagulation defect
    - specified NEC O46.8X ☑
  - appendicitis O99.61 ☑
  - atrophy (yellow) (acute) liver (subacute) O26.61 ☑

Pregnancy — *continued*

- complicated by — *continued*
  - bariatric surgery status O99.84 ☑
  - bicornis or bicornuate uterus O34.0 ☑
  - biliary tract problems O26.61 ☑
  - breech presentation O32.1 ☑
  - cardiovascular diseases (conditions in I00-I09, I20-I52, I70-I99) O99.41 ☑
  - cerebrovascular disorders (conditions in I60-I69) O99.41 ☑
  - cervical shortening O26.87 ☑
  - cervicitis O23.51 ☑
  - chloasma (gravidarum) O26.89 ☑
  - cholestasis (intrahepatic) O26.61 ☑
  - cholecystitis O99.61 ☑
  - chorioamnionitis O41.12 ☑
  - circulatory system disorder (conditions in I00-I09, I20-I99, O99.41-)
  - compound presentation O32.6 ☑
  - conjoined twins O30.02 ☑
  - connective system disorders (conditions in M00-M99) O99.89
  - contracted pelvis (general) O33.1
    - inlet O33.2
    - outlet O33.3 ☑
  - convulsions (eclamptic) (uremic) (*see also* Eclampsia)O15.9
  - cracked nipple O92.11 ☑
  - cystitis O23.1 ☑
  - cystocele O34.8 ☑
  - death of fetus (near term) O36.4 ☑
    - early pregnancy O02.1
    - of one fetus or more in multiple gestation O31.2 ☑
  - deciduitis O41.14 ☑
  - decreased fetal movement O36.81 ☑
  - dental problems O99.61 ☑
  - diabetes (mellitus) O24.91 ☑
    - gestational (pregnancy induced) — *see* - Diabetes, gestational
    - pre-existing O24.31 ☑
      - specified NEC O24.81 ☑
      - type 1 O24.01 ☑
      - type 2 O24.11 ☑
  - digestive system disorders (conditions in K00-K93) O99.61 ☑
  - diseases of — *see* Pregnancy, complicated by, specified body system disease
    - biliary tract O26.61 ☑
    - blood NEC (conditions in D65-D77) O99.11 ☑
    - liver O26.61 ☑
    - specified NEC O99.89
  - disorders of — *see* Pregnancy, complicated by, specified body system disorder
    - amniotic fluid and membranes O41.9 ☑
      - specified NEC O41.8X ☑
    - biliary tract O26.61 ☑
    - ear and mastoid process (conditions in H60-H95) O99.89
    - eye and adnexa (conditions in H00-H59) O99.89
    - liver O26.61 ☑
    - skin (conditions in L00-L99) O99.71 ☑
    - specified NEC O99.89
  - displacement, uterus NEC O34.59 ☑
    - causing obstructed labor O65.5
  - disproportion (due to) O33.9
    - fetal (ascites) (hydrops) (meningomyelocele) (sacral teratoma) (tumor) deformities NEC O33.7 ☑
    - generally contracted pelvis O33.1
    - hydrocephalic fetus O33.6 ☑
    - inlet contraction of pelvis O33.2
    - mixed maternal and fetal origin O33.4 ☑
    - specified NEC O33.8
  - double uterus O34.0 ☑
    - causing obstructed labor O65.5
  - drug use (conditions in F11-F19) O99.32 ☑
  - eclampsia, eclamptic (coma) (convulsions) (delirium) (nephritis) (uremia) (*see also* Eclampsia) O15. ☑
  - ectopic pregnancy — *see* Pregnancy, ectopic
  - edema O12.0 ☑
    - with
      - gestational hypertension, mild (*see also* Pre-eclampsia)O14.0 ☑
      - proteinuria O12.2 ☑
  - effusion, amniotic fluid — *see* Pregnancy, complicated by, premature rupture of membranes
  - elderly
    - multigravida O09.52 ☑

Pregnancy — *continued*

- complicated by — *continued*
    - primigravida O09.51 ☑
  - embolism (*see also* Embolism, obstetric, pregnancy) O88. ☑
  - endocrine diseases NEC O99.28 ☑
  - endometritis O86.12
  - excessive weight gain O26.0 ☑
  - exhaustion O26.81 ☑
    - during labor and delivery O75.81
  - face presentation O32.3 ☑
  - failed induction of labor O61.9
    - instrumental O61.1
    - mechanical O61.1
    - medical O61.0
    - specified NEC O61.8
    - surgical O61.1
  - failed or difficult intubation for anesthesia O29.6 ☑
  - false labor (pains) O47.9
    - at or after 37 completed weeks of pregnancy O47.1
    - before 37 completed weeks of pregnancy O47.0 ☑
  - fatigue O26.81 ☑
    - during labor and delivery O75.81
  - fatty metamorphosis of liver O26.61 ☑
  - female genital mutilation O34.8 ☑ *[N90.81-]*
  - fetal (maternal care for)
    - abnormality or damage O35.9 ☑
      - acid-base balance O68
      - specified type NEC O35.8 ☑
    - acidemia O68
    - acidosis O68
    - alkalosis O68
    - anemia and thrombocytopenia O36.82 ☑
    - anencephaly O35.0 ☑
    - chromosomal abnormality (conditions in Q90-Q99) O35.1 ☑
    - conjoined twins O30.02 ☑
    - damage from
      - amniocentesis O35.7 ☑
      - biopsy procedures O35.7 ☑
      - drug addiction O35.5 ☑
      - hematological investigation O35.7 ☑
      - intrauterine contraceptive device O35.7 ☑
      - maternal
        - alcohol addiction O35.4 ☑
        - cytomegalovirus infection O35.3 ☑
        - disease NEC O35.8 ☑
        - drug addiction O35.5 ☑
        - listeriosis O35.8 ☑
        - rubella O35.3 ☑
        - toxoplasmosis O35.8 ☑
        - viral infection O35.3 ☑
      - medical procedure NEC O35.7 ☑
      - radiation O35.6 ☑
    - death (near term) O36.4 ☑
      - early pregnancy O02.1
    - decreased movement O36.81 ☑
    - disproportion due to deformity (fetal) O33.7 ☑
    - excessive growth (large for dates) O36.6 ☑
    - growth retardation O36.59 ☑
      - light for dates O36.59 ☑
      - small for dates O36.59 ☑
    - heart rate irregularity (bradycardia) (decelerations) (tachycardia) O76
    - hereditary disease O35.2 ☑
    - hydrocephalus O35.0 ☑
    - intrauterine death O36.4 ☑
    - poor growth O36.59 ☑
      - light for dates O36.59 ☑
      - small for dates O36.59 ☑
    - problem O36.9 ☑
      - specified NEC O36.89 ☑
    - reduction (elective) O31.3 ☑
    - selective termination O31.3 ☑
    - spina bifida O35.0 ☑
    - thrombocytopenia O36.82 ☑
  - fibroid (tumor) (uterus) O34.1 ☑
  - fissure of nipple O92.11 ☑
  - gallstones O99.61 ☑
  - gastric banding status O99.84 ☑
  - gastric bypass status O99.84 ☑
  - genital herpes (asymptomatic) (history of) (inactive) O98.51 ☑
  - genital tract infection O23.9 ☑
  - glomerular diseases (conditions in N00-N07) O26.83 ☑

- **Pregnancy** — *continued*
  - complicated by — *continued*
    - with hypertension, pre-existing — *see* Hypertension, complicating, pregnancy, pre-existing, with, renal disease
    - gonorrhea O98.21 ☑
    - grand multiparity O09.4 ☑
    - habitual aborter — *see* Pregnancy, complicated by, recurrent pregnancy loss
    - HELLP syndrome (hemolysis, elevated liver enzymes and low platelet count) O14.2 ☑
    - hemorrhage
      - antepartum — *see* Hemorrhage, antepartum
      - before 20 completed weeks gestation O20.9
        - specified NEC O20.8
      - due to premature separation, placenta (*see also* Abruptio placentae)O45.9 ☑
      - early O20.9
        - specified NEC O20.8
      - threatened abortion O20.0
    - hemorrhoids O22.4 ☑
    - hepatitis (viral) O98.41 ☑
    - herniation of uterus O34.59 ☑
    - high
      - head at term O32.4 ☑
      - risk — *see* Supervision (of) (for), high-risk
    - history of in utero procedure during previous pregnancy O09.82 ☑
    - HIV O98.71 ☑
    - human immunodeficiency virus (HIV) disease O98.71 ☑
    - hydatidiform mole (*see also* Mole, hydatidiform)O01.9
    - hydramnios O40. ☑
    - hydrocephalic fetus (disproportion) O33.6 ☑
    - hydrops
      - amnii O40. ☑
      - fetalis O36.2 ☑
        - associated with isoimmunization (*see also* Pregnancy, complicated by, isoimmunization)O36.11 ☑
    - hydrorrhea O42.90
    - hyperemesis (gravidarum) (mild) (*see also* Hyperemesis, gravidarum)O21.0
    - hypertension — *see* Hypertension, complicating pregnancy
    - hypertensive
      - heart and renal disease, pre-existing — *see* Hypertension, complicating, pregnancy, pre-existing, with, heart disease, with renal disease
      - heart disease, pre-existing — *see* Hypertension, complicating, pregnancy, pre-existing, with, heart disease
      - renal disease, pre-existing — *see* Hypertension, complicating, pregnancy, pre-existing, with, renal disease
    - hypotension O26.5 ☑
    - immune disorders NEC (conditions in D80-D89) O99.11 ☑
    - incarceration, uterus O34.51 ☑
    - incompetent cervix O34.3 ☑
    - inconclusive fetal viability O36.80 ☑
    - infection (s) O98.91 ☑
      - amniotic fluid or sac O41.10 ☑
      - bladder O23.1 ☑
      - carrier state NEC O99.830
        - streptococcus B O99.820
      - genital organ or tract O23.9 ☑
        - specified NEC O23.59 ☑
      - genitourinary tract O23.9 ☑
      - gonorrhea O98.21 ☑
      - hepatitis (viral) O98.41 ☑
      - HIV O98.71 ☑
      - human immunodeficiency virus (HIV) O98.71 ☑
      - kidney O23.0 ☑
      - nipple O91.01 ☑
      - parasitic disease O98.91 ☑
        - specified NEC O98.81 ☑
      - protozoal disease O98.61 ☑
      - sexually transmitted NEC O98.31 ☑
      - specified type NEC O98.81 ☑
      - syphilis O98.11 ☑
      - tuberculosis O98.01 ☑
      - urethra O23.2 ☑
      - urinary (tract) O23.4 ☑
        - specified NEC O23.3 ☑
      - viral disease O98.51 ☑
    - injury or poisoning (conditions in S00-T88) O9A.21 ☑
      - due to abuse
        - physical O9A.31 ☑
        - psychological O9A.51 ☑
        - sexual O9A.41 ☑
    - insufficient
      - prenatal care O09.3 ☑
      - weight gain O26.1 ☑
    - insulin resistance O26.89 ☑
    - intrauterine fetal death (near term) O36.4 ☑
      - early pregnancy O02.1
      - multiple gestation (one fetus or more) O31.2 ☑
    - isoimmunization O36.11 ☑
      - anti-A sensitization O36.11 ☑
      - anti-B sensitization O36.19 ☑
      - Rh O36.09 ☑
        - anti-D antibody O36.01 ☑
      - specified NEC O36.19 ☑
    - laceration of uterus NEC O71.81
    - malformation
      - placenta, placental (vessel) O43.10 ☑
        - specified NEC O43.19 ☑
      - uterus (congenital) O34.0 ☑
    - malnutrition (conditions in E40-E46) O25.1 ☑
    - maternal hypotension syndrome O26.5 ☑
    - mental disorders (conditions in F01-F09, F20-F99) O99.34 ☑
      - alcohol use O99.31 ☑
      - drug use O99.32 ☑
      - smoking O99.33 ☑
    - mentum presentation O32.3 ☑
    - metabolic disorders O99.28 ☑
    - missed
      - abortion O02.1
      - delivery O36.4 ☑
    - multiple gestations O30.9 ☑
      - conjoined twins O30.02 ☑
      - specified number of multiples NEC — *see* Pregnancy, multiple (gestation), specified NEC
      - quadruplet — *see* Pregnancy, quadruplet
      - specified complication NEC O31.8X ☑
      - triplet — *see* Pregnancy, triplet
      - twin — *see* Pregnancy, twin
    - musculoskeletal condition (conditions is M00-M99) O99.89
    - necrosis, liver (conditions in K72) O26.61 ☑
    - neoplasm
      - benign
        - cervix O34.4 ☑
        - corpus uteri O34.1 ☑
        - uterus O34.1 ☑
      - malignant O9A.11 ☑
    - nephropathy NEC O26.83 ☑
    - nervous system condition (conditions in G00-G99) O99.35 ☑
    - nutritional diseases NEC O99.28 ☑
    - obesity (pre-existing) O99.21 ☑
    - obesity surgery status O99.84 ☑
    - oblique lie or presentation O32.2 ☑
    - older mother — *see* Pregnancy, complicated by, elderly
    - oligohydramnios O41.0 ☑
      - with premature rupture of membranes (*see also* Pregnancy, complicated by, premature rupture of membranes) O42. ☑
    - onset (spontaneous) of labor after 37 completed weeks of gestation but before 39 completed weeks gestation, with delivery by (planned) cesarean section O75.82
    - oophoritis O23.52 ☑
    - overdose, drug (*see also* Table of Drugs and Chemicals, by drug, poisoning)O9A.21 ☑
    - oversize fetus O33.5 ☑
    - papyraceous fetus O31.0 ☑
    - pelvic inflammatory disease O99.89
    - periodontal disease O99.61 ☑
    - peripheral neuritis O26.82 ☑
    - peritoneal (pelvic) adhesions O99.89
    - phlebitis O22.9 ☑
    - phlebopathy O22.9 ☑
    - phlebothrombosis (superficial) O22.2 ☑
      - deep O22.3 ☑
    - placenta accreta O43.21 ☑
    - placenta increta O43.22 ☑
    - placenta percreta O43.23 ☑
    - placenta previa O44.0 ☑
      - complete O44.0 ☑
        - with hemorrhage O44.1 ☑
      - marginal O44.2 ☑
        - with hemorrhage O44.3 ☑
      - partial O44.2 ☑
        - with hemorrhage O44.3 ☑
    - placental disorder O43.9 ☑
      - specified NEC O43.89 ☑
    - placental dysfunction O43.89 ☑
    - placental infarction O43.81 ☑
    - placental insufficiency O36.51 ☑
    - placental transfusion syndromes
      - fetomaternal O43.01 ☑
      - fetus to fetus O43.02 ☑
      - maternofetal O43.01 ☑
    - placentitis O41.14 ☑
    - pneumonia O99.51 ☑
    - poisoning (*see also* Table of Drugs and Chemicals)O9A.21 ☑
    - polyhydramnios O40 ☑
    - polymorphic eruption of pregnancy O26.86
    - poor obstetric history NEC O09.29 ☑
    - postmaturity (post-term) (40 to 42 weeks) O48.0
      - more than 42 completed weeks gestation (prolonged) O48.1
    - pre-eclampsia O14.9 ☑
      - mild O14.0 ☑
      - moderate O14.0 ☑
      - severe O14.1 ☑
        - with hemolysis, elevated liver enzymes and low platelet count (HELLP) O14.2 ☑
    - premature labor — *see* Pregnancy, complicated by, preterm labor
    - premature rupture of membranes O42.90
      - full-term, unspecified as to length of time between rupture and onset of labor O42.92
      - with onset of labor
        - within 24 hours O42.00
          - at or after 37 weeks gestation, onset of labor within 24 hours of rupture O42.02
          - pre-term (before 37 completed weeks of gestation) O42.01 ☑
        - after 24 hours O42.10
          - at or after 37 weeks gestation, onset of labor more than 24 hours following rupture O42.12
          - pre-term (before 37 completed weeks of gestation) O42.11 ☑
      - at or after 37 weeks gestation, unspecified as to length of time between rupture and onset of labor O42.92
      - pre-term (before 37 completed weeks of gestation) O42.91 ☑
    - premature separation of placenta (*see also* Abruptio placentae)O45.9 ☑
    - presentation, fetal - — *see* Delivery, complicated by, malposition
    - preterm delivery O60.10 ☑
    - preterm labor
      - with delivery O60.10 ☑
        - preterm O60.10 ☑
        - term O60.20 ☑
      - second trimester
        - with term delivery O60.22 ☑
        - without delivery O60.02
        - with preterm delivery
          - second trimester O60.12 ☑
          - third trimester O60.13 ☑
      - third trimester
        - with term delivery O60.23 ☑
        - without delivery O60.03
        - with third trimester preterm delivery O60.14 ☑
      - without delivery O60.00
        - second trimester O60.02
        - third trimester O60.03
    - previous history of — *see* Pregnancy, supervision of, high-risk
    - prolapse, uterus O34.52 ☑
    - proteinuria (gestational) (*see also* Proteinuria, gestational)O12.1 ☑
      - with edema O12.2 ☑
    - pruritic urticarial papules and plaques of pregnancy (PUPPP) O26.86
    - pruritus (neurogenic) O26.89 ☑
    - psychosis or psychoneurosis (puerperal) F53
    - ptyalism O26.89 ☑
    - PUPPP (pruritic urticarial papules and plaques of pregnancy) O26.86
    - pyelitis O23.0 ☑

- **Presence** — *continued*
  - implanted device (artificial) (functional) (prosthetic) Z96.9
    - automatic cardiac defibrillator (with synchronous cardiac pacemaker) Z95.810
    - cardiac pacemaker Z95.0
    - cochlear Z96.21
    - dental Z96.5
    - heart Z95.812
    - heart valve Z95.2
      - prosthetic Z95.2
      - specified NEC Z95.4
      - xenogenic Z95.3
    - insulin pump Z96.41
    - intraocular lens Z96.1
    - joint Z96.60
      - ankle Z96.66 ☑
      - elbow Z96.62 ☑
      - finger Z96.69 ☑
      - hip Z96.64 ☑
      - knee Z96.65 ☑
      - shoulder Z96.61 ☑
      - specified NEC Z96.698
      - wrist Z96.63 ☑
    - larynx Z96.3
    - myringotomy tube Z96.22
    - otological Z96.20
      - cochlear Z96.21
      - eustachian stent Z96.29
      - myringotomy Z96.22
      - specified NEC Z96.29
      - stapes Z96.29
    - skin Z96.81
    - skull plate Z96.7
    - specified NEC Z96.89
    - urogenital Z96.0
  - insulin pump (functional) Z96.41
  - intestinal bypass or anastomosis Z98.0
  - intraocular lens (functional) Z96.1
  - intrauterine contraceptive device (IUD) Z97.5
  - intravascular implant (functional) (prosthetic) NEC Z95.9
    - coronary artery Z95.5
    - defibrillator (with synchronous cardiac pacemaker) Z95.810
    - peripheral vessel (with angioplasty) Z95.820
  - joint implant (prosthetic) (any) Z96.60
    - ankle — *see* Presence, ankle joint implant
    - elbow — *see* Presence, elbow joint implant
    - finger — *see* Presence, finger joint implant
    - hip — *see* Presence, hip joint implant
    - knee — *see* Presence, knee joint implant
    - shoulder — *see* Presence, shoulder joint implant
    - specified joint NEC Z96.698
    - wrist — *see* Presence, wrist joint implant
  - knee-joint implant (functional) (prosthesis) Z96.65 ☑
  - laryngeal implant (functional) Z96.3
  - mandibular implant (dental) Z96.5
  - myringotomy tube (s) Z96.22
  - orthopedic-joint implant (prosthetic) (any) — *see* Presence, joint implant
  - otological implant (functional) Z96.29
  - shoulder-joint implant (functional) (prosthesis) Z96.61 ☑
  - skull-plate implant Z96.7
  - spectacles Z97.3
  - stapes implant (functional) Z96.29
  - systemic lupus erythematosus [SLE] inhibitor D68.62
  - tendon implant (functional) (graft) Z96.7
  - tooth root (s) implant Z96.5
  - ureteral stent Z96.0
  - urethral stent Z96.0
  - urogenital implant (functional) Z96.0
  - vascular implant or device Z95.9
    - access port device Z95.828
    - specified type NEC Z95.828
  - wrist-joint implant (functional) (prosthesis) Z96.63 ☑
- **Presenile** (*see also* condition)
  - dementia F03 ☑
  - premature aging E34.8
- **Presentation,** fetal — *see* Delivery , complicated by, malposition
- **Prespondylolisthesis** (congenital) Q76.2
- **Pressure**
  - area, skin — *see* Ulcer, pressure, by site
  - brachial plexus G54.0
  - brain G93.5
    - injury at birth NEC P11.1
- **Pressure** — *continued*
  - cerebral — *see* Pressure, brain
  - chest R07.89
  - cone, tentorial G93.5
  - hyposystolic (*see also* Hypotension)
    - incidental reading, without diagnosis of hypotension R03.1
  - increased
    - intracranial (benign) G93.2
      - injury at birth P11.0
    - intraocular H40.05 ☑
  - lumbosacral plexus G54.1
  - mediastinum J98.59
  - necrosis (chronic) — *see* Ulcer, pressure, by site
  - parental, inappropriate (excessive) Z62.6
  - sore (chronic) — *see* Ulcer, pressure, by site
  - spinal cord G95.20
  - ulcer (chronic) — *see* Ulcer, pressure, by site
  - venous, increased I87.8
- **Pre-syncope** R55
- **Preterm**
  - delivery (*see also* Pregnancy, complicated by, preterm labor)O60.10 ☑
  - labor — *see* Pregnancy, complicated by, preterm labor
  - newborn (infant) P07.30
    - gestational age
      - 28 completed weeks (28 weeks, 0 days through 28 weeks, 6 days) P07.31
      - 29 completed weeks (29 weeks, 0 days through 29 weeks, 6 days) P07.32
      - 30 completed weeks (30 weeks, 0 days through 30 weeks, 6 days) P07.33
      - 31 completed weeks (31 weeks, 0 days through 31 weeks, 6 days) P07.34
      - 32 completed weeks (32 weeks, 0 days through 32 weeks, 6 days) P07.35
      - 33 completed weeks (33 weeks, 0 days through 33 weeks, 6 days) P07.36
      - 34 completed weeks (34 weeks, 0 days through 34 weeks, 6 days) P07.37
      - 35 completed weeks (35 weeks, 0 days through 35 weeks, 6 days) P07.38
      - 36 completed weeks (36 weeks, 0 days through 36 weeks, 6 days) P07.39
- **Previa**
  - placenta (total) (without hemorrhage) O44.0 ☑
    - with hemorrhage O44.1 ☑
    - complete O44.0 ☑
      - with hemorrhage O44.1 ☑
    - low (*see also* Delivery, complicated, by, placenta, low)O44.4 ☑
      - with hemorrhage O44.5 ☑
    - marginal O44.2 ☑
      - with hemorrhage O44.3 ☑
    - partial O44.2 ☑
      - with hemorrhage O44.3 ☑
  - vasa O69.4 ☑
- **Priapism** N48.30
  - due to
    - disease classified elsewhere N48.32
    - drug N48.33
    - specified cause NEC N48.39
    - trauma N48.31
- **Prickling** sensation (skin) R20.2
- **Prickly** heat L74.0
- **Primary** — *see* condition
- **Primigravida**
  - elderly, affecting management of pregnancy, labor and delivery (supervision only) — *see* Pregnancy, complicated by, elderly, primigravida
  - older, affecting management of pregnancy, labor and delivery (supervision only) — *see* Pregnancy, complicated by, elderly, primigravida
  - very young, affecting management of pregnancy, labor and delivery (supervision only) — *see* Pregnancy, complicated by, young mother, primigravida
- **Primipara**
  - elderly, affecting management of pregnancy, labor and delivery (supervision only) — *see* Pregnancy, complicated by, elderly, primigravida
  - older, affecting management of pregnancy, labor and delivery (supervision only) — *see* Pregnancy, complicated by, elderly, primigravida
  - very young, affecting management of pregnancy, labor and delivery (supervision only) — *see* Pregnancy, complicated by, young mother, primigravida
- **Primus** varus (bilateral) Q66.2 ☑
- **PRIND** (Prolonged reversible ischemic neurologic deficit) I63.9
- **Pringle's** disease (tuberous sclerosis) Q85.1
- **Prinzmetal** angina I20.1
- **Prizefighter** ear — *see* Cauliflower ear
- **Problem** (with) (related to)
  - academic Z55.8
  - acculturation Z60.3
  - adjustment (to)
    - change of job Z56.1
    - life-cycle transition Z60.0
    - pension Z60.0
    - retirement Z60.0
  - adopted child Z62.821
  - alcoholism in family Z63.72
  - atypical parenting situation Z62.9
  - bankruptcy Z59.8
  - behavioral (adult) F69
    - drug seeking Z76.5
  - birth of sibling affecting child Z62.898
  - care (of)
    - provider dependency Z74.9
      - specified NEC Z74.8
    - sick or handicapped person in family or household Z63.6
  - child
    - abuse (affecting the child) — *see* Maltreatment, child
    - custody or support proceedings Z65.3
    - in welfare custody Z62.21
    - in care of non-parental family member Z62.21
    - in foster care Z62.21
    - living in orphanage or group home Z62.22
  - child-rearing Z62.9
    - specified NEC Z62.898
  - communication (developmental) F80.9
  - conflict or discord (with)
    - boss Z56.4
    - classmates Z55.4
    - counselor Z64.4
    - employer Z56.4
    - family Z63.9
      - specified NEC Z63.8
    - probation officer Z64.4
    - social worker Z64.4
    - teachers Z55.4
    - workmates Z56.4
  - conviction in legal proceedings Z65.0
    - with imprisonment Z65.1
  - counselor Z64.4
  - creditors Z59.8
  - digestive K92.9
  - drug addict in family Z63.72
  - ear — *see* Disorder, ear
  - economic Z59.9
    - affecting care Z59.9
    - specified NEC Z59.8
  - education Z55.9
    - specified NEC Z55.8
  - employment Z56.9
    - change of job Z56.1
    - discord Z56.4
    - environment Z56.5
    - sexual harassment Z56.81
    - specified NEC Z56.89
    - stress NEC Z56.6
    - stressful schedule Z56.3
    - threat of job loss Z56.2
    - unemployment Z56.0
  - enuresis, child F98.0
  - eye H57.9
  - failed examinations (school) Z55.2
  - falling Z91.81
  - family (*see also* Disruption, family)Z63.9
    - specified NEC Z63.8
  - feeding (elderly) (infant) R63.3
    - newborn P92.9
      - breast P92.5
      - overfeeding P92.4
      - slow P92.2
      - specified NEC P92.8
      - underfeeding P92.3
    - nonorganic F50.89
  - finance Z59.9
    - specified NEC Z59.8
  - foreclosure on loan Z59.8
  - foster child Z62.822
  - frightening experience (s) in childhood Z62.898
  - genital NEC
    - female N94.9
    - male N50.9

- **Problem** — *continued*
  - health care Z75.9
    - specified NEC Z75.8
  - hearing — *see* Deafness
  - homelessness Z59.0
  - housing Z59.9
    - inadequate Z59.1
    - isolated Z59.8
    - specified NEC Z59.8
  - identity (of childhood) F93.8
  - illegitimate pregnancy (unwanted) Z64.0
  - illiteracy Z55.0
  - impaired mobility Z74.09
  - imprisonment or incarceration Z65.1
  - inadequate teaching affecting education Z55.8
  - inappropriate (excessive) parental pressure Z62.6
  - influencing health status NEC Z78.9
  - in-law Z63.1
  - institutionalization, affecting child Z62.22
  - intrafamilial communication Z63.8
  - jealousy, child F93.8
  - landlord Z59.2
  - language (developmental) F80.9
  - learning (developmental) F81.9
  - legal Z65.3
    - conviction without imprisonment Z65.0
    - imprisonment Z65.1
    - release from prison Z65.2
  - life-management Z73.9
    - specified NEC Z73.89
  - life-style Z72.9
    - gambling Z72.6
    - high-risk sexual behavior (heterosexual) Z72.51
      - bisexual Z72.53
      - homosexual Z72.52
    - inappropriate eating habits Z72.4
    - self-damaging behavior NEC Z72.89
    - specified NEC Z72.89
    - tobacco use Z72.0
  - literacy Z55.9
    - low level Z55.0
    - specified NEC Z55.8
  - living alone Z60.2
  - lodgers Z59.2
  - loss of love relationship in childhood Z62.898
  - marital Z63.0
    - involving
      - divorce Z63.5
      - estrangement Z63.5
      - gender identity F66
  - mastication K08.89
  - medical
    - care, within family Z63.6
    - facilities Z75.9
      - specified NEC Z75.8
  - mental F48.9
  - multiparity Z64.1
  - negative life events in childhood Z62.9
    - altered pattern of family relationships Z62.898
    - frightening experience Z62.898
    - loss of
      - love relationship Z62.898
      - self-esteem Z62.898
    - physical abuse (alleged) — *see* Maltreatment, child
    - removal from home Z62.29
    - specified event NEC Z62.898
  - neighbor Z59.2
  - neurological NEC R29.818
  - new step-parent affecting child Z62.898
  - none (feared complaint unfounded) Z71.1
  - occupational NEC Z56.89
  - parent-child — *see* Conflict, parent-child
  - personal hygiene Z91.89
  - personality F69
  - phase-of-life transition, adjustment Z60.0
  - presence of sick or disabled person in family or household Z63.79
    - needing care Z63.6
  - primary support group (family) Z63.9
    - specified NEC Z63.8
  - probation officer Z64.4
  - psychiatric F99
  - psychosexual (development) F66
  - psychosocial Z65.9
    - specified NEC Z65.8
  - relationship Z63.9
    - childhood F93.8
  - release from prison Z65.2
  - removal from home affecting child Z62.29
  - seeking and accepting known hazardous and harmful

- **Problem** — *continued*
  - seeking and accepting known hazardous and harmful — *continued*
    - behavioral or psychological interventions Z65.8
    - chemical, nutritional or physical interventions Z65.8
  - sexual function (nonorganic) F52.9
  - sight H54.7
  - sleep disorder, child F51.9
  - smell — *see* Disturbance, sensation, smell
  - social
    - environment Z60.9
      - specified NEC Z60.8
    - exclusion and rejection Z60.4
    - worker Z64.4
  - speech R47.9
    - developmental F80.9
    - specified NEC R47.89
  - swallowing — *see* Dysphagia
  - taste — *see* Disturbance, sensation, taste
  - tic, child F95.0
  - underachievement in school Z55.3
  - unemployment Z56.0
    - threatened Z56.2
  - unwanted pregnancy Z64.0
  - upbringing Z62.9
    - specified NEC Z62.898
  - urinary N39.9
  - voice production R47.89
  - work schedule (stressful) Z56.3
- **Procedure** (surgical)
  - converted
    - arthroscopic to open Z53.33
    - laparoscopic to open Z53.31
    - specified procedure NEC to open Z53.39
    - thoracoscopic to open Z53.32
  - for purpose other than remedying health state Z41.9
    - specified NEC Z41.8
  - not done Z53.9
    - because of
      - administrative reasons Z53.8
      - contraindication Z53.09
        - smoking Z53.01
      - patient's decision Z53.20
        - for reasons of belief or group pressure Z53.1
        - left against medical advice (AMA) Z53.21
        - specified reason NEC Z53.29
      - specified reason NEC Z53.8
- **Procidentia** (uteri) N81.3
- **Proctalgia** K62.89
  - fugax K59.4
  - spasmodic K59.4
- **Proctitis** K62.89
  - amebic (acute) A06.0
  - chlamydial A56.3
  - gonococcal A54.6
  - granulomatous — *see* Enteritis, regional, large intestine
  - herpetic A60.1
  - radiation K62.7
  - tuberculous A18.32
  - ulcerative (chronic) K51.20
    - with
      - complication K51.219
        - abscess K51.214
        - fistula K51.213
        - obstruction K51.212
        - rectal bleeding K51.211
        - specified NEC K51.218
- **Proctocele**
  - female (without uterine prolapse) N81.6
    - with uterine prolapse N81.2
      - complete N81.3
  - male K62.3
- **Proctocolitis**
  - food-induced eosinophilic K52.82
  - food protein-induced K52.82
  - milk protein-induced K52.82
  - mucosal — *see* Rectosigmoiditis, ulcerative
- **Proctoptosis** K62.3
- **Proctorrhagia** K62.5
- **Proctosigmoiditis** K63.89
  - ulcerative (chronic) — *see* Rectosigmoiditis, ulcerative
- **Proctospasm** K59.4
  - psychogenic F45.8
- **Profichet's** disease — *see* Disorder, soft tissue, specified type NEC
- **Progeria** E34.8
- **Prognathism** (mandibular) (maxillary) M26.19

- **Progonoma** (melanotic) — *see* Neoplasm, benign, by site
- **Progressive** — *see* condition
- **Prolactinoma**
  - specified site — *see* Neoplasm, benign, by site
  - unspecified site D35.2
- **Prolapse,** prolapsed
  - anus, anal (canal) (sphincter) K62.2
  - arm or hand O32.2 ☑
    - causing obstructed labor O64.4 ☑
  - bladder (mucosa) (sphincter) (acquired)
    - congenital Q79.4
    - female — *see* Cystocele
    - male N32.89
  - breast implant (prosthetic) T85.49 ☑
  - cecostomy K94.09
  - cecum K63.4
  - cervix, cervical (hypertrophied) N81.2
    - anterior lip, obstructing labor O65.5
    - congenital Q51.828
    - postpartal, old N81.2
    - stump N81.85
  - ciliary body (traumatic) — *see* Laceration, eye (ball), with prolapse or loss of interocular tissue
  - colon (pedunculated) K63.4
  - colostomy K94.09
  - disc (intervertebral) — *see* Displacement, intervertebral disc
  - eye implant (orbital) T85.398 ☑
    - lens (ocular) — *see* Complications, intraocular lens
  - fallopian tube N83.4 ☑
  - gastric (mucosa) K31.89
  - genital, female N81.9
    - specified NEC N81.89
  - globe, nontraumatic — *see* Luxation, globe
  - ileostomy bud K94.19
  - intervertebral disc — *see* Displacement, intervertebral disc
  - intestine (small) K63.4
  - iris (traumatic) — *see* Laceration, eye (ball), with prolapse or loss of interocular tissue
    - nontraumatic H21.89
  - kidney N28.83
    - congenital Q63.2
  - laryngeal muscles or ventricle J38.7
  - liver K76.89
  - meatus urinarius N36.8
  - mitral (valve) I34.1
  - ocular lens implant — *see* Complications, intraocular lens
  - organ or site, congenital NEC — *see* Malposition, congenital
  - ovary N83.4 ☑
  - pelvic floor, female N81.89
  - perineum, female N81.89
  - rectum (mucosa) (sphincter) K62.3
    - due to trichuris trichuria B79
  - spleen D73.89
  - stomach K31.89
  - umbilical cord
    - complicating delivery O69.0 ☑
  - urachus, congenital Q64.4
  - ureter N28.89
    - with obstruction N13.5
      - with infection N13.6
  - ureterovesical orifice N28.89
  - urethra (acquired) (infected) (mucosa) N36.8
    - congenital Q64.71
  - urinary meatus N36.8
    - congenital Q64.72
  - uterovaginal N81.4
    - complete N81.3
    - incomplete N81.2
  - uterus (with prolapse of vagina) N81.4
    - complete N81.3
    - congenital Q51.818
    - first degree N81.2
    - in pregnancy or childbirth — *see* Pregnancy, complicated by, abnormal, uterus
    - incomplete N81.2
    - postpartal (old) N81.4
    - second degree N81.2
    - third degree N81.3
  - uveal (traumatic) — *see* Laceration, eye (ball), with prolapse or loss of interocular tissue
  - vagina (anterior) (wall) — *see* Cystocele
    - with prolapse of uterus N81.4
      - complete N81.3
      - incomplete N81.2
    - posterior wall N81.6
    - posthysterectomy N99.3

Prolapse — *continued*
- vitreous (humor) H43.0 ☑
  - in wound — *see* Laceration, eye (ball), with prolapse or loss of interocular tissue
- womb — *see* Prolapse, uterus

Prolapsus, female N81.9
- specified NEC N81.89

Proliferation (s)
- prostate, atypical small acinar N42.32
- primary cutaneous CD30-positive large T-cell C86.6

Proliferative — *see* condition

Prolonged, prolongation (of)
- bleeding (time) (idiopathic) R79.1
- coagulation (time) R79.1
- gestation (over 42 completed weeks)
  - mother O48.1
  - newborn P08.22
- interval I44.0
- labor O63.9
  - first stage O63.0
  - second stage O63.1
- partial thromboplastin time (PTT) R79.1
- pregnancy (more than 42 weeks gestation) O48.1
- prothrombin time R79.1
- QT interval I45.81
- uterine contractions in labor O62.4

Prominence, prominent
- auricle (congenital) (ear) Q17.5
- ischial spine or sacral promontory
- with disproportion (fetopelvic) O33.0
  - causing obstructed labor O65.0
- nose (congenital) acquired M95.0

Promiscuity — *see* High, risk, sexual behavior

Pronation
- ankle — *see* Deformity, limb, foot, specified NEC
- foot (*see also* Deformity, limb, foot, specified NEC)
  - congenital Q74.2

Prophylactic
- administration of
  - antibiotics, long-term Z79.2
    - short-term use - omit code
  - drug (*see also* Long-term (current) drug therapy (use of)) Z79.899
- medication Z79.899
- organ removal (for neoplasia management) Z40.00
  - breast Z40.01
  - ovary Z40.02
  - specified site NEC Z40.09
- surgery Z40.9
  - for risk factors related to malignant neoplasm — *see* Prophylactic, organ removal
  - specified NEC Z40.8
- vaccination Z23

Propionic acidemia E71.121

Proptosis (ocular) (*see also* Exophthalmos)
- thyroid — *see* Hyperthyroidism, with goiter

Prosecution, anxiety concerning Z65.3

Prosopagnosia R48.3

Prostadynia N42.81

Prostate, prostatic — *see* condition

Prostatism — *see* Hyperplasia, prostate

Prostatitis (congestive) (suppurative) (with cystitis) N41.9
- acute N41.0
- cavitary N41.8
- chronic N41.1
- diverticular N41.8
- due to Trichomonas (vaginalis) A59.02
- fibrous N41.1
- gonococcal (acute) (chronic) A54.22
- granulomatous N41.4
- hypertrophic N41.1
- subacute N41.1
- trichomonal A59.02
- tuberculous A18.14

Prostatocystitis N41.3

Prostatorrhea N42.89

Prostatosis N42.82

Prostration R53.83
- heat (*see also* Heat, exhaustion)
  - anhydrotic T67.3 ☑
  - due to
    - salt (and water) depletion T67.4 ☑
    - water depletion T67.3 ☑
- nervous F48.8
- senile R54

Protanomaly (anomalous trichromat) H53.54

Protanopia (complete) (incomplete) H53.54

Protection (against) (from) — *see* Prophylactic

Protein
- deficiency NEC — *see* Malnutrition
- malnutrition — *see* Malnutrition
- sickness (*see also* Reaction, serum) T80.69 ☑

Proteinemia R77.9

Proteinosis
- alveolar (pulmonary) J84.01
- lipid or lipoid (of Urbach) E78.89

Proteinuria R80.9
- Bence Jones R80.3
- complicating pregnancy — *see* Proteinuria, gestational
- gestational
  - complicating
    - childbirth O12.14
    - pregnancy O12.1 ☑
      - with edema O12.2 ☑
    - puerperium O12.15
- idiopathic R80.0
- isolated R80.0
  - with glomerular lesion N06.9
    - dense deposit disease N06.6
    - diffuse
      - crescentic glomerulonephritis N06.7
      - endocapillary proliferative glomerulonephritis N06.4
      - mesangiocapillary glomerulonephritis N06.5
    - focal and segmental hyalinosis or sclerosis N06.1
    - membranous (diffuse) N06.2
    - mesangial proliferative (diffuse) N06.3
    - minimal change N06.0
    - specified pathology NEC N06.8
- orthostatic R80.2
  - with glomerular lesion — *see* Proteinuria, isolated, with glomerular lesion
- persistent R80.1
  - with glomerular lesion — *see* Proteinuria, isolated, with glomerular lesion
- postural R80.2
  - with glomerular lesion — *see* Proteinuria, isolated, with glomerular lesion
- pre-eclamptic — *see* Pre-eclampsia
- puerperal O12.15
- specified type NEC R80.8

Proteolysis, pathologic D65

Proteus (mirabilis) (morganii), as cause of disease classified elsewhere B96.4

Prothrombin gene mutation D68.52

Protoporphyria, erythropoietic E80.0

Protozoal (*see also* condition)
- disease B64
  - specified NEC B60.8

Protrusion, protrusio
- acetabuli M24.7
- acetabulum (into pelvis) M24.7
- device, implant or graft (*see also* Complications, by site and type, mechanical) T85.698 ☑
  - arterial graft NEC — *see* Complication, cardiovascular device, mechanical, vascular
  - breast (implant) T85.49 ☑
  - catheter NEC T85.698 ☑
    - cystostomy T83.090 ☑
    - dialysis (renal) T82.49 ☑
      - intraperitoneal T85.691 ☑
    - infusion NEC T82.594 ☑
      - spinal (epidural) (subdural) T85.690 ☑
    - urinary (*see also* Complications, catheter, urinary) T83.098 ☑
  - electronic (electrode) (pulse generator) (stimulator)
    - bone T84.390 ☑
    - nervous system — *see* Complication, prosthetic device, mechanical, electronic nervous system stimulator
  - fixation, internal (orthopedic) NEC — *see* Complication, fixation device, mechanical
  - gastrointestinal — *see* Complications, prosthetic device, mechanical, gastrointestinal device
  - genital NEC T83.498 ☑
    - intrauterine contraceptive device T83.39 ☑
    - penile prosthesis (cylinder) (implanted) (pump) (reservoir) T83.490 ☑
    - testicular prosthesis T83.491 ☑
  - heart NEC — *see* Complication, cardiovascular device, mechanical
  - joint prosthesis — *see* Complications, joint prosthesis, mechanical, specified NEC, by site

Protrusion — *continued*
- device, implant or graft — *continued*
  - ocular NEC — *see* Complications, prosthetic device, mechanical, ocular device
  - orthopedic NEC — *see* Complication, orthopedic, device, mechanical
  - specified NEC T85.628 ☑
  - urinary NEC (*see also* Complication, genitourinary, device, urinary, mechanical)
    - graft T83.29 ☑
  - vascular NEC — *see* Complication, cardiovascular device, mechanical
  - ventricular intracranial shunt T85.09 ☑
- intervertebral disc — *see* Displacement, intervertebral disc
- joint prosthesis — *see* Complications, joint prosthesis, mechanical, specified NEC, by site
- nucleus pulposus — *see* Displacement, intervertebral disc

Prune belly (syndrome) Q79.4

Prurigo (ferox) (gravis) (Hebrae) (Hebra's) (mitis) (simplex) L28.2
- Besnier's L20.0
- estivalis L56.4
- nodularis L28.1
- psychogenic F45.8

Pruritus, pruritic (essential) L29.9
- ani, anus L29.0
  - psychogenic F45.8
- anogenital L29.3
  - psychogenic F45.8
- due to onchocerca volvulus B73.1
- gravidarum — *see* Pregnancy, complicated by, specified pregnancy-related condition NEC
- hiemalis L29.8
- neurogenic (any site) F45.8
- perianal L29.0
- psychogenic (any site) F45.8
- scroti, scrotum L29.1
  - psychogenic F45.8
- senile, senilis L29.8
- specified NEC L29.8
  - psychogenic F45.8
- Trichomonas A59.9
- vulva, vulvae L29.2
  - psychogenic F45.8

Pseudarthrosis, pseudoarthrosis (bone) — *see* Nonunion, fracture
- clavicle, congenital Q74.0
- joint, following fusion or arthrodesis M96.0

Pseudoaneurysm — *see* Aneurysm

Pseudoangioma I81

Pseudoangina (pectoris) — *see* Angina

Pseudoarteriosus Q28.8

Pseudoarthrosis — *see* Pseudarthrosis

Pseudobulbar affect (PBA) F48.2

Pseudochromhidrosis L67.8

Pseudocirrhosis, liver, pericardial I31.1

Pseudocowpox B08.03

Pseudocoxalgia M91.3 ☑

Pseudocroup J38.5

Pseudo-Cushing's syndrome, alcohol-induced E24.4

Pseudocyesis F45.8

Pseudocyst
- lung J98.4
- pancreas K86.3
- retina — *see* Cyst, retina

Pseudoelephantiasis neuroarthritica Q82.0

Pseudoexfoliation, capsule (lens) — *see* Cataract, specified NEC

Pseudofolliculitis barbae L73.1

Pseudoglioma H44.89

Pseudohemophilia (Bernuth's) (hereditary) (type B) D68.0
- Type A D69.8
- vascular D69.8

Pseudohermaphroditism Q56.3
- adrenal E25.8
- female Q56.2
  - with adrenocortical disorder E25.8
  - without adrenocortical disorder Q56.2
  - adrenal (congenital) E25.0
- male Q56.1
  - with
    - adrenocortical disorder E25.8
    - androgen resistance E34.51
    - cleft scrotum Q56.1
    - feminizing testis E34.51
    - 5-alpha-reductase deficiency E29.1
  - without gonadal disorder Q56.1
  - adrenal E25.8

Pseudo-Hurler's polydystrophy E77.0

Pseudohydrocephalus - Psychosis

- **Pseudohydrocephalus** G93.2
- **Pseudohypertrophic** muscular dystrophy (Erb's) G71.0
- **Pseudohypertrophy,** muscle G71.0
- **Pseudohypoparathyroidism** E20.1
- **Pseudoinsomnia** F51.03
- **Pseudoleukemia,** infantile D64.89
- **Pseudomembranous** — *see* condition
- **Pseudomenses** (newborn) P54.6
- **Pseudomenstruation** (newborn) P54.6
- **Pseudomeningocele** (cerebral) (infective) (post-traumatic) G96.19
  - postprocedural (spinal) G97.82
- **Pseudomonas**
  - aeruginosa, as cause of disease classified elsewhere B96.5
  - mallei infection A24.0
    - as cause of disease classified elsewhere B96.5
  - pseudomallei, as cause of disease classified elsewhere B96.5
- **Pseudomyotonia** G71.19
- **Pseudomyxoma** peritonei C78.6
- **Pseudoneuritis,** optic (nerve) (disc) (papilla), congenital Q14.2
- **Pseudo-obstruction** intestine (acute) (chronic) (idiopathic) (intermittent secondary) (primary) K59.8
- **Pseudopapilledema** H47.33 ☑
  - congenital Q14.2
- **Pseudoparalysis**
  - arm or leg R29.818
  - atonic, congenital P94.2
- **Pseudopelade** L66.0
- **Pseudophakia** Z96.1
- **Pseudopolyarthritis,** rhizomelic M35.3
- **Pseudopolycythemia** D75.1
- **Pseudopseudohypoparathyroidism** E20.1
- **Pseudopterygium** H11.81 ☑
- **Pseudoptosis** (eyelid) — *see* Blepharochalasis
- **Pseudopuberty,** precocious
  - female heterosexual E25.8
  - male isosexual E25.8
- **Pseudorickets** (renal) N25.0
- **Pseudorubella** B08.20
- **Pseudosclerema,** newborn P83.8
- **Pseudosclerosis** (brain)
  - of Westphal (Strümpell) E83.01
  - Jakob's — *see* Creutzfeldt-Jakob disease or syndrome
  - spastic — *see* Creutzfeldt-Jakob disease or syndrome
- **Pseudotetanus** — *see* Convulsions
- **Pseudotetany** R29.0
  - hysterical F44.5
- **Pseudotruncus** arteriosus Q25.49
- **Pseudotuberculosis** A28.2
  - enterocolitis A04.8
  - pasteurella (infection) A28.0
- **Pseudotumor**
  - cerebri G93.2
  - orbital H05.11 ☑
- **Pseudoxanthoma** elasticum Q82.8
- **Psilosis** (sprue) (tropical) K90.1
  - nontropical K90.0
- **Psittacosis** A70
- **Psoitis** M60.88
- **Psoriasis** L40.9
  - arthropathic L40.50
    - arthritis mutilans L40.52
    - distal interphalangeal L40.51
    - juvenile L40.54
    - other specified L40.59
    - spondylitis L40.53
  - buccal K13.29
  - flexural L40.8
  - guttate L40.4
  - mouth K13.29
  - nummular L40.0
  - plaque L40.0
  - psychogenic F54
  - pustular (generalized) L40.1
    - palmaris et plantaris L40.3
  - specified NEC L40.8
  - vulgaris L40.0
- **Psychasthenia** F48.8
- **Psychiatric** disorder or problem F99
- **Psychogenic** (*see also* condition)
  - factors associated with physical conditions F54
- **Psychological** and behavioral factors affecting medical condition F59
- **Psychoneurosis,** psychoneurotic (*see also* Neurosis)
  - anxiety (state) F41.1
- **Psychoneurosis** — *continued*
  - depersonalization F48.1
  - hypochondriacal F45.21
  - hysteria F44.9
  - neurasthenic F48.8
  - personality NEC F60.89
- **Psychopathy,** psychopathic
  - affectionless F94.2
  - autistic F84.5
  - constitution, post-traumatic F07.81
  - personality — *see* Disorder, personality
  - sexual — *see* Deviation, sexual
  - state F60.2
- **Psychosexual** identity disorder of childhood F64.2
- **Psychosis,** psychotic F29
  - acute (transient) F23
    - hysterical F44.9
  - affective — *see* Disorder, mood
  - alcoholic F10.959
    - with
      - abuse F10.159
      - anxiety disorder F10.980
        - with
          - abuse F10.180
          - dependence F10.280
      - delirium tremens F10.231
      - delusions F10.950
        - with
          - abuse F10.150
          - dependence F10.250
      - dementia F10.97
        - with dependence F10.27
      - dependence F10.259
      - hallucinosis F10.951
        - with
          - abuse F10.151
          - dependence F10.251
      - mood disorder F10.94
        - with
          - abuse F10.14
          - dependence F10.24
      - paranoia F10.950
        - with
          - abuse F10.150
          - dependence F10.250
      - persisting amnesia F10.96
        - with dependence F10.26
    - amnestic confabulatory F10.96
      - with dependence F10.26
    - delirium tremens F10.231
    - Korsakoff's, Korsakov's, Korsakow's F10.26
    - paranoid type F10.950
      - with
        - abuse F10.150
        - dependence F10.250
  - anergastic — *see* Psychosis, organic
  - arteriosclerotic (simple type) (uncomplicated) F01.50
    - with behavioral disturbance F01.51
  - childhood F84.0
    - atypical F84.8
  - climacteric — *see* Psychosis, involutional
  - confusional F29
    - acute or subacute F05
    - reactive F23
  - cycloid F23
  - depressive — *see* Disorder, depressive
  - disintegrative (childhood) F84.3
  - drug-induced — *see* F11-F19 with .x59
    - paranoid and hallucinatory states — *see* F11-F19 with .x50 or .x51
  - due to or associated with
    - addiction, drug — *see* F11-F19 with .x59
    - dependence
      - alcohol F10.259
      - drug — *see* F11-F19 with .x59
    - epilepsy F06.8
    - Huntington's chorea F06.8
    - ischemia, cerebrovascular (generalized) F06.8
    - multiple sclerosis F06.8
    - physical disease F06.8
    - presenile dementia F03 ☑
    - senile dementia F03 ☑
    - vascular disease (arteriosclerotic) (cerebral) F01.50
      - with behavioral disturbance F01.51
  - epileptic F06.8
  - episode F23
    - due to or associated with physical condition F06.8
  - exhaustive F43.0
  - hallucinatory, chronic F28
- **Psychosis** — *continued*
  - hypomanic F30.8
  - hysterical (acute) F44.9
  - induced F24
  - infantile F84.0
    - atypical F84.8
  - infective (acute) (subacute) F05
  - involutional F28
    - depressive — *see* Disorder, depressive
    - melancholic — *see* Disorder, depressive
    - paranoid (state) F22
  - Korsakoff's, Korsakov's, Korsakow's (nonalcoholic) F04
    - alcoholic F10.96
      - in dependence F10.26
    - induced by other psychoactive substance — *see* categories F11-F19 with .x5x
  - mania, manic (single episode) F30.2
    - recurrent type F31.89
  - manic-depressive — *see* Disorder, bipolar
  - menopausal — *see* Psychosis, involutional
  - mixed schizophrenic and affective F25.8
  - multi-infarct (cerebrovascular) F01.50
    - with behavioral disturbance F01.51
  - nonorganic F29
    - specified NEC F28
  - organic F09
    - due to or associated with
      - arteriosclerosis (cerebral) — *see* Psychosis, arteriosclerotic
      - cerebrovascular disease, arteriosclerotic — *see* Psychosis, arteriosclerotic
      - childbirth — *see* Psychosis, puerperal
      - Creutzfeldt-Jakob disease or syndrome — *see* Creutzfeldt-Jakob disease or syndrome
      - dependence, alcohol F10.259
      - disease
        - alcoholic liver F10.259
        - brain, arteriosclerotic — *see* Psychosis, arteriosclerotic
        - cerebrovascular F01.50
          - with behavioral disturbance F01.51
        - Creutzfeldt-Jakob — *see* Creutzfeldt-Jakob disease or syndrome
        - endocrine or metabolic F06.8
          - acute or subacute F05
        - liver, alcoholic F10.259
      - epilepsy transient (acute) F05
      - infection
        - brain (intracranial) F06.8
          - acute or subacute F05
      - intoxication
        - alcoholic (acute) F10.259
        - drug F19 with .x59 F11 ☑
      - ischemia, cerebrovascular (generalized) — *see* Psychosis, arteriosclerotic
      - puerperium — *see* Psychosis, puerperal
      - trauma, brain (birth) (from electric current) (surgical) F06.8
        - acute or subacute F05
    - infective F06.8
      - acute or subacute F05
    - post-traumatic F06.8
      - acute or subacute F05
  - paranoiac F22
  - paranoid (climacteric) (involutional) (menopausal) F22
    - psychogenic (acute) F23
    - schizophrenic F20.0
    - senile F03 ☑
  - postpartum F53
  - presbyophrenic (type) F03 ☑
  - presenile F03 ☑
  - psychogenic (paranoid) F23
    - depressive F32.3
  - puerperal F53
    - specified type — *see* Psychosis, by type
  - reactive (brief) (transient) (emotional stress) (psychological trauma) F23
    - depressive F32.3
      - recurrent F33.3
    - excitative type F30.8
  - schizoaffective F25.9
    - depressive type F25.1
    - manic type F25.0
  - schizophrenia, schizophrenic — *see* Schizophrenia
  - schizophrenia-like, in epilepsy F06.2
  - schizophreniform F20.81
    - affective type F25.9
    - brief F23
    - confusional type F23

Psychosis — *continued*
- schizophreniform — *continued*
  - depressive type F25.1
  - manic type F25.0
  - mixed type F25.0
- senile NEC F03 ☑
  - depressed or paranoid type F03 ☑
  - simple deterioration F03 ☑
  - specified type - code to condition
- shared F24
- situational (reactive) F23
- symbiotic (childhood) F84.3
- symptomatic F09

Psychosomatic — *see* Disorder, psychosomatic
Psychosyndrome, organic F07.9
Psychotic episode due to or associated with physical condition F06.8
Pterygium (eye) H11.00 ☑
- amyloid H11.01 ☑
- central H11.02 ☑
- colli Q18.3
- double H11.03 ☑
- peripheral
  - progressive H11.05 ☑
  - stationary H11.04 ☑
- recurrent H11.06 ☑

Ptilosis (eyelid) — *see* Madarosis
Ptomaine (poisoning) — *see* Poisoning, food
Ptosis (*see also* Blepharoptosis)
- adiposa (false) — *see* Blepharoptosis
- breast N64.81
- cecum K63.4
- colon K63.4
- congenital (eyelid) Q10.0
  - specified site NEC — *see* Anomaly, by site
- eyelid — *see* Blepharoptosis
  - congenital Q10.0
- gastric K31.89
- intestine K63.4
- kidney N28.83
- liver K76.89
- renal N28.83
- splanchnic K63.4
- spleen D73.89
- stomach K31.89
- viscera K63.4

PTP D69.51
Ptyalism (periodic) K11.7
- hysterical F45.8
- pregnancy — *see* Pregnancy, complicated by, specified pregnancy-related condition NEC
- psychogenic F45.8

Ptyalolithiasis K11.5
Pubarche, precocious E30.1
Pubertas praecox E30.1
Puberty (development state) Z00.3
- bleeding (excessive) N92.2
- delayed E30.0
- precocious (constitutional) (cryptogenic) (idiopathic) E30.1
  - central E22.8
  - due to
    - ovarian hyperfunction E28.1
      - estrogen E28.0
    - testicular hyperfunction E29.0
- premature E30.1
  - due to
    - adrenal cortical hyperfunction E25.8
    - pineal tumor E34.8
    - pituitary (anterior) hyperfunction E22.8

Puckering, macula — *see* Degeneration, macula, puckering
Pudenda, pudendum — *see* condition
Puente's disease (simple glandular cheilitis) K13.0
Puerperal, puerperium (complicated by, complications)
- abnormal glucose (tolerance test) O99.815
- abscess
  - areola O91.02
    - associated with lactation O91.03
  - Bartholin's gland O86.19
  - breast O91.12
    - associated with lactation O91.13
  - cervix (uteri) O86.11
  - genital organ NEC O86.19
  - kidney O86.21
  - mammary O91.12
    - associated with lactation O91.13
  - nipple O91.02
    - associated with lactation O91.03
  - peritoneum O85
  - subareolar O91.12

Puerperal — *continued*
- abscess — *continued*
    - associated with lactation O91.13
  - urinary tract — *see* Puerperal, infection, urinary
  - uterus O86.12
  - vagina (wall) O86.13
  - vaginorectal O86.13
  - vulvovaginal gland O86.13
- adnexitis O86.19
- afibrinogenemia, or other coagulation defect O72.3
- albuminuria (acute) (subacute) — *see* Proteinuria, gestational
- alcohol use O99.315
- anemia O90.81
  - pre-existing (pre-pregnancy) O99.03
- anesthetic death O89.8
- apoplexy O99.43
- bariatric surgery status O99.845
- blood disorder NEC O99.13
- blood dyscrasia O72.3
- cardiomyopathy O90.3
- cerebrovascular disorder (conditions in I60-I69) O99.43
- cervicitis O86.11
- circulatory system disorder O99.43
- coagulopathy (any) O72.3
- complications O90.9
  - specified NEC O90.89
- convulsions — *see* Eclampsia
- cystitis O86.22
- cystopyelitis O86.29
- delirium NEC F05
- diabetes O24.93
  - gestational — *see* Puerperal, gestational diabetes
  - pre-existing O24.33
    - specified NEC O24.83
    - type 1 O24.03
    - type 2 O24.13
- digestive system disorder O99.63
- disease O90.9
  - breast NEC O92.29
  - cerebrovascular (acute) O99.43
  - nonobstetric NEC O99.89
  - tubo-ovarian O86.19
  - Valsuani's O99.03
- disorder O90.9
  - biliary tract O26.63
  - lactation O92.70
  - liver O26.63
  - nonobstetric NEC O99.89
- disruption
  - cesarean wound O90.0
  - episiotomy wound O90.1
  - perineal laceration wound O90.1
- drug use O99.325
- eclampsia (with pre-existing hypertension) O15.2
- embolism (pulmonary) (blood clot) — *see* Embolism, obstetric, puerperal
- endocrine, nutritional or metabolic disease NEC O99.285
- endophlebitis — *see* Puerperal, phlebitis
- endotrachelitis O86.11
- failure
  - lactation (complete) O92.3
    - partial O92.4
  - renal, acute O90.4
- fever (of unknown origin) O86.4
  - septic O85
- fissure, nipple O92.12
  - associated with lactation O92.13
- fistula
  - breast (due to mastitis) O91.12
    - associated with lactation O91.13
  - nipple O91.02
    - associated with lactation O91.03
- galactophoritis O91.22
  - associated with lactation O91.23
- galactorrhea O92.6
- gastric banding status O99.845
- gastric bypass status O99.845
- gastrointestinal disease NEC O99.63
- gestational
  - diabetes O24.439
    - diet controlled O24.430
    - insulin (and diet) controlled O24.434
    - oral drug controlled (antidiabetic) (hypoglycemic) O24.435
  - edema O12.05
    - with proteinuria O12.25
  - proteinuria O12.15

Puerperal — *continued*
- gonorrhea O98.23
- hematoma, subdural O99.43
- hemiplegia, cerebral O99.355
  - due to cerebrovascular disorder O99.43
- hemorrhage O72.1
  - brain O99.43
  - bulbar O99.43
  - cerebellar O99.43
  - cerebral O99.43
  - cortical O99.43
  - delayed or secondary O72.2
  - extradural O99.43
  - internal capsule O99.43
  - intracranial O99.43
  - intrapontine O99.43
  - meningeal O99.43
  - pontine O99.43
  - retained placenta O72.0
  - subarachnoid O99.43
  - subcortical O99.43
  - subdural O99.43
  - third stage O72.0
  - uterine, delayed O72.2
  - ventricular O99.43
- hemorrhoids O87.2
- hepatorenal syndrome O90.4
- hypertension — *see* Hypertension, complicating, puerperium
- hypertrophy, breast O92.29
- induration breast (fibrous) O92.29
- infection O86.4
  - cervix O86.11
  - generalized O85
  - genital tract NEC O86.19
    - obstetric surgical wound O86.0
  - kidney (bacillus coli) O86.21
  - maternal O98.93
    - carrier state NEC O99.835
    - gonorrhea O98.23
    - human immunodeficiency virus (HIV) O98.73
    - protozoal O98.63
    - sexually transmitted NEC O98.33
    - specified NEC O98.83
    - streptococcus group B (GBS) carrier state O99.825
    - syphilis O98.13
    - tuberculosis O98.03
    - viral hepatitis O98.43
    - viral NEC O98.53
  - nipple O91.02
    - associated with lactation O91.03
  - peritoneum O85
  - renal O86.21
  - specified NEC O86.89
  - urinary (asymptomatic) (tract) NEC O86.20
    - bladder O86.22
    - kidney O86.21
    - specified site NEC O86.29
    - urethra O86.22
  - vagina O86.13
  - vein — *see* Puerperal, phlebitis
- ischemia, cerebral O99.43
- lymphangitis O86.89
  - breast O91.22
    - associated with lactation O91.23
- malignancy O9A.13
- malnutrition O25.3
- mammillitis O91.02
  - associated with lactation O91.03
- mammitis O91.22
  - associated with lactation O91.23
- mania F30.8
- mastitis O91.22
  - associated with lactation O91.23
  - purulent O91.12
    - associated with lactation O91.13
- melancholia — *see* Disorder, depressive
- mental disorder NEC O99.345
- metroperitonitis O85
- metrorrhagia — *see* Hemorrhage, postpartum
- metrosalpingitis O86.19
- metrovaginitis O86.13
- milk leg O87.1
- monoplegia, cerebral O99.43
- mood disturbance O90.6
- necrosis, liver (acute) (subacute) (conditions in subcategory K72.0) O26.63
  - with renal failure O90.4
- nervous system disorder O99.355
- neuritis O90.89
- obesity (pre-existing prior to pregnancy) O99.215

Puerperal — *continued*
- obesity surgery status O99.845
- occlusion, precerebral artery O99.43
- paralysis
  - bladder (sphincter) O90.89
  - cerebral O99.43
- paralytic stroke O99.43
- parametritis O85
- paravaginitis O86.13
- pelviperitonitis O85
- perimetritis O86.12
- perimetrosalpingitis O86.19
- perinephritis O86.21
- periphlebitis — *see* Puerperal phlebitis
- peritoneal infection O85
- peritonitis (pelvic) O85
- perivaginitis O86.13
- phlebitis O87.0
  - deep O87.1
  - pelvic O87.1
  - superficial O87.0
- phlebothrombosis, deep O87.1
- phlegmasia alba dolens O87.1
- placental polyp O90.89
- pneumonia, embolic — *see* Embolism, obstetric, puerperal
- pre-eclampsia — *see* Pre-eclampsia
- psychosis F53
- pyelitis O86.21
- pyelocystitis O86.29
- pyelonephritis O86.21
- pyelonephrosis O86.21
- pyemia O85
- pyocystitis O86.29
- pyohemia O85
- pyometra O86.12
- pyonephritis O86.21
- pyosalpingitis O86.19
- pyrexia (of unknown origin) O86.4
- renal
  - disease NEC O90.89
  - failure O90.4
- respiratory disease NEC O99.53
- retention
  - decidua — *see* Retention, decidua
  - placenta O72.0
  - secundines — *see* Retention, secundines
- retracted nipple O92.02
- salpingo-ovaritis O86.19
- salpingoperitonitis O85
- secondary perineal tear O90.1
- sepsis (pelvic) O85
- sepsis O85
- septic thrombophlebitis O86.81
- skin disorder NEC O99.73
- specified condition NEC O99.89
- stroke O99.43
- subinvolution (uterus) O90.89
- subluxation of symphysis (pubis) O26.73
- suppuration — *see* Puerperal, abscess
- tetanus A34
- thelitis O91.02
  - associated with lactation O91.03
- thrombocytopenia O72.3
- thrombophlebitis (superficial) O87.0
  - deep O87.1
  - pelvic O87.1
  - septic O86.81
- thrombosis (venous) — *see* Thrombosis, puerperal
- thyroiditis O90.5
- toxemia (eclamptic) (pre-eclamptic) (with convulsions) O15.2
- trauma, non-obstetric O9A.23
  - caused by abuse (physical) (suspected) O9A.33
    - confirmed O9A.33
    - psychological (suspected) O9A.53
      - confirmed O9A.53
    - sexual (suspected) O9A.43
      - confirmed O9A.43
- uremia (due to renal failure) O90.4
- urethritis O86.22
- vaginitis O86.13
- varicose veins (legs) O87.4
  - vulva or perineum O87.8
- venous O87.9
- vulvitis O86.19
- vulvovaginitis O86.13
- white leg O87.1

Puerperium — *see* Puerperal

Pulmolithiasis J98.4

Pulmonary — *see* condition

Pulpitis (acute) (anachoretic) (chronic) (hyperplastic) (putrescent) (suppurative) (ulcerative) K04.01
- irreversible K04.02
- reversible K04.01

Pulpless tooth K04.99

Pulse
- alternating R00.8
- bigeminal R00.8
- fast R00.0
- feeble, rapid due to shock following injury T79.4 ☑
- rapid R00.0
- weak R09.89

Pulsus alternans or trigeminus R00.8

Punch drunk F07.81

Punctum lacrimale occlusion — *see* Obstruction, lacrimal

Puncture
- abdomen, abdominal
  - wall S31.139 ☑
    - with
      - foreign body S31.149 ☑
      - penetration into peritoneal cavity S31.639 ☑
        - with foreign body S31.649 ☑
    - epigastric region S31.132 ☑
      - with
        - foreign body S31.142 ☑
        - penetration into peritoneal cavity S31.632 ☑
          - with foreign body S31.642 ☑
    - left
      - lower quadrant S31.134 ☑
        - with
          - foreign body S31.144 ☑
          - penetration into peritoneal cavity S31.634 ☑
            - with foreign body S31.644 ☑
      - upper quadrant S31.131 ☑
        - with
          - foreign body S31.141 ☑
          - penetration into peritoneal cavity S31.631 ☑
            - with foreign body S31.641 ☑
    - periumbilic region S31.135 ☑
      - with
        - foreign body S31.145 ☑
        - penetration into peritoneal cavity S31.635 ☑
          - with foreign body S31.645 ☑
    - right
      - lower quadrant S31.133 ☑
        - with
          - foreign body S31.143 ☑
          - penetration into peritoneal cavity S31.633 ☑
            - with foreign body S31.643 ☑
      - upper quadrant S31.130 ☑
        - with
          - foreign body S31.140 ☑
          - penetration into peritoneal cavity S31.630 ☑
            - with foreign body S31.640 ☑
- accidental, complicating surgery — *see* Complication, accidental puncture or laceration
- alveolar (process) — *see* Puncture, oral cavity
- ankle S91.039 ☑
  - with
    - foreign body S91.049 ☑
  - left S91.032 ☑
    - with
      - foreign body S91.042 ☑
  - right S91.031 ☑
    - with
      - foreign body S91.041 ☑
- anus S31.833 ☑
  - with foreign body S31.834 ☑
- arm (upper) S41.139 ☑
  - with foreign body S41.149 ☑
  - left S41.132 ☑
    - with foreign body S41.142 ☑
  - lower — *see* Puncture, forearm
  - right S41.131 ☑
    - with foreign body S41.141 ☑
- auditory canal (external) (meatus) — *see* Puncture, ear
- auricle, ear — *see* Puncture, ear
- axilla — *see* Puncture, arm
- back (*see also* Puncture, thorax, back)
  - lower S31.030 ☑
    - with

Puncture — *continued*
- back — *continued*
      - foreign body S31.040 ☑
        - with penetration into retroperitoneal space S31.041 ☑
      - penetration into retroperitoneal space S31.031 ☑
- bladder (traumatic) S37.29 ☑
  - nontraumatic N32.89
- breast S21.039 ☑
  - with foreign body S21.049 ☑
  - left S21.032 ☑
    - with foreign body S21.042 ☑
  - right S21.031 ☑
    - with foreign body S21.041 ☑
- buttock S31.803 ☑
  - with foreign body S31.804 ☑
  - left S31.823 ☑
    - with foreign body S31.824 ☑
  - right S31.813 ☑
    - with foreign body S31.814 ☑
- by
  - device, implant or graft — *see* Complications, by site and type, mechanical
  - foreign body left accidentally in operative wound T81.539 ☑
  - instrument (any) during a procedure, accidental — *see* Puncture, accidental complicating surgery
- calf — *see* Puncture, leg
- canaliculus lacrimalis — *see* Puncture, eyelid
- canthus, eye — *see* Puncture, eyelid
- cervical esophagus S11.23 ☑
  - with foreign body S11.24 ☑
- cheek (external) S01.439 ☑
  - with foreign body S01.449 ☑
  - left S01.432 ☑
    - with foreign body S01.442 ☑
  - right S01.431 ☑
    - with foreign body S01.441 ☑
  - internal — *see* Puncture, oral cavity
- chest wall — *see* Puncture, thorax
- chin — *see* Puncture, head, specified site NEC
- clitoris — *see* Puncture, vulva
- costal region — *see* Puncture, thorax
- digit (s)
  - hand — *see* Puncture, finger
  - foot — *see* Puncture, toe
- ear (canal) (external) S01.339 ☑
  - with foreign body S01.349 ☑
  - left S01.332 ☑
    - with foreign body S01.342 ☑
  - right S01.331 ☑
    - with foreign body S01.341 ☑
  - drum S09.2 ☑
- elbow S51.039 ☑
  - with
    - foreign body S51.049 ☑
  - left S51.032 ☑
    - with
      - foreign body S51.042 ☑
  - right S51.031 ☑
    - with
      - foreign body S51.041 ☑
- epididymis — *see* Puncture, testis
- epigastric region — *see* Puncture, abdomen, wall, epigastric
- epiglottis S11.83 ☑
  - with foreign body S11.84 ☑
- esophagus
  - cervical S11.23 ☑
    - with foreign body S11.24 ☑
  - thoracic S27.818 ☑
- eyeball S05.6 ☑
  - with foreign body S05.5 ☑
- eyebrow — *see* Puncture, eyelid
- eyelid S01.13 ☑
  - with foreign body S01.14 ☑
  - left S01.132 ☑
    - with foreign body S01.142 ☑
  - right S01.131 ☑
    - with foreign body S01.141 ☑
- face NEC — *see* Puncture, head, specified site NEC
- finger (s) S61.239 ☑
  - with
    - damage to nail S61.339 ☑
      - with
        - foreign body S61.349 ☑
    - foreign body S61.249 ☑
  - index S61.238 ☑
    - with
      - damage to nail S61.338 ☑

- **Puncture** — *continued*
  - finger (s) — *continued*
          - with
            - foreign body S61.348 ☑
        - foreign body S61.248 ☑
      - left S61.231 ☑
        - with
          - damage to nail S61.331 ☑
            - with
              - foreign body S61.341 ☑
          - foreign body S61.241 ☑
      - right S61.230 ☑
        - with
          - damage to nail S61.330 ☑
            - with
              - foreign body S61.340 ☑
          - foreign body S61.240 ☑
    - little S61.238 ☑
      - with
        - damage to nail S61.338 ☑
          - with
            - foreign body S61.348 ☑
        - foreign body S61.248 ☑
      - left S61.237 ☑
        - with
          - damage to nail S61.337 ☑
            - with
              - foreign body S61.347 ☑
          - foreign body S61.247 ☑
      - right S61.236 ☑
        - with
          - damage to nail S61.336 ☑
            - with
              - foreign body S61.346 ☑
          - foreign body S61.246 ☑
    - middle S61.238 ☑
      - with
        - damage to nail S61.338 ☑
          - with
            - foreign body S61.348 ☑
        - foreign body S61.248 ☑
      - left S61.233 ☑
        - with
          - damage to nail S61.333 ☑
            - with
              - foreign body S61.343 ☑
          - foreign body S61.243 ☑
      - right S61.232 ☑
        - with
          - damage to nail S61.332 ☑
            - with
              - foreign body S61.342 ☑
          - foreign body S61.242 ☑
    - ring S61.238 ☑
      - with
        - damage to nail S61.338 ☑
          - with
            - foreign body S61.348 ☑
        - foreign body S61.248 ☑
      - left S61.235 ☑
        - with
          - damage to nail S61.335 ☑
            - with
              - foreign body S61.345 ☑
          - foreign body S61.245 ☑
      - right S61.234 ☑
        - with
          - damage to nail S61.334 ☑
            - with
              - foreign body S61.344 ☑
          - foreign body S61.244 ☑
  - flank S31.139 ☑
    - with foreign body S31.149 ☑
  - foot (except toe (s) alone) S91.339 ☑
    - with foreign body S91.349 ☑
    - left S91.332 ☑
      - with foreign body S91.342 ☑
    - right S91.331 ☑
      - with foreign body S91.341 ☑
    - toe — *see* Puncture, toe
  - forearm S51.839 ☑
    - with
      - foreign body S51.849 ☑
    - elbow only — *see* Puncture, elbow
    - left S51.832 ☑
      - with
        - foreign body S51.842 ☑
    - right S51.831 ☑
      - with
        - foreign body S51.841 ☑
  - forehead — *see* Puncture, head, specified site NEC

- **Puncture** — *continued*
  - genital organs, external
    - female S31.532 ☑
      - with foreign body S31.542 ☑
      - vagina — *see* Puncture, vagina
      - vulva — *see* Puncture, vulva
    - male S31.531 ☑
      - with foreign body S31.541 ☑
      - penis — *see* Puncture, penis
      - scrotum — *see* Puncture, scrotum
      - testis — *see* Puncture, testis
  - groin — *see* Puncture, abdomen, wall
  - gum — *see* Puncture, oral cavity
  - hand S61.439 ☑
    - with
      - foreign body S61.449 ☑
    - finger — *see* Puncture, finger
    - left S61.432 ☑
      - with
        - foreign body S61.442 ☑
    - right S61.431 ☑
      - with
        - foreign body S61.441 ☑
    - thumb — *see* Puncture, thumb
  - head S01.93 ☑
    - with foreign body S01.94 ☑
    - cheek — *see* Puncture, cheek
    - ear — *see* Puncture, ear
    - eyelid — *see* Puncture, eyelid
    - lip — *see* Puncture, oral cavity
    - nose — *see* Puncture, nose
    - oral cavity — *see* Puncture, oral cavity
    - scalp S01.03 ☑
      - with foreign body S01.04 ☑
    - specified site NEC S01.83 ☑
      - with foreign body S01.84 ☑
    - temporomandibular area — *see* Puncture, cheek
  - heart S26.99 ☑
    - with hemopericardium S26.09 ☑
    - without hemopericardium S26.19 ☑
  - heel — *see* Puncture, foot
  - hip S71.039 ☑
    - with foreign body S71.049 ☑
    - left S71.032 ☑
      - with foreign body S71.042 ☑
    - right S71.031 ☑
      - with foreign body S71.041 ☑
  - hymen — *see* Puncture, vagina
  - hypochondrium — *see* Puncture, abdomen, wall
  - hypogastric region — *see* Puncture, abdomen, wall
  - inguinal region — *see* Puncture, abdomen, wall
  - instep — *see* Puncture, foot
  - internal organs — *see* Injury, by site
  - interscapular region — *see* Puncture, thorax, back
  - intestine
    - large
      - colon S36.599 ☑
        - ascending S36.590 ☑
        - descending S36.592 ☑
        - sigmoid S36.593 ☑
        - specified site NEC S36.598 ☑
        - transverse S36.591 ☑
      - rectum S36.69 ☑
    - small S36.499 ☑
      - duodenum S36.490 ☑
      - specified site NEC S36.498 ☑
  - intra-abdominal organ S36.99 ☑
    - gallbladder S36.128 ☑
    - intestine — *see* Puncture, intestine
    - liver S36.118 ☑
    - pancreas — *see* Puncture, pancreas
    - peritoneum S36.81 ☑
    - specified site NEC S36.898 ☑
    - spleen S36.09 ☑
    - stomach S36.39 ☑
  - jaw — *see* Puncture, head, specified site NEC
  - knee S81.039 ☑
    - with foreign body S81.049 ☑
    - left S81.032 ☑
      - with foreign body S81.042 ☑
    - right S81.031 ☑
      - with foreign body S81.041 ☑
  - labium (majus) (minus) — *see* Puncture, vulva
  - lacrimal duct — *see* Puncture, eyelid
  - larynx S11.013 ☑
    - with foreign body S11.014 ☑
  - leg (lower) S81.839 ☑
    - with foreign body S81.849 ☑
    - foot — *see* Puncture, foot
    - knee — *see* Puncture, knee

- **Puncture** — *continued*
  - leg — *continued*
    - left S81.832 ☑
      - with foreign body S81.842 ☑
    - right S81.831 ☑
      - with foreign body S81.841 ☑
    - upper — *see* Puncture, thigh
  - lip S01.531 ☑
    - with foreign body S01.541 ☑
  - loin — *see* Puncture, abdomen, wall
  - lower back — *see* Puncture, back, lower
  - lumbar region — *see* Puncture, back, lower
  - malar region — *see* Puncture, head, specified site NEC
  - mammary — *see* Puncture, breast
  - mastoid region — *see* Puncture, head, specified site NEC
  - mouth — *see* Puncture, oral cavity
  - nail
    - finger — *see* Puncture, finger, with damage to nail
    - toe — *see* Puncture, toe, with damage to nail
  - nasal (septum) (sinus) — *see* Puncture, nose
  - nasopharynx — *see* Puncture, head, specified site NEC
  - neck S11.93 ☑
    - with foreign body S11.94 ☑
    - involving
      - cervical esophagus — *see* Puncture, cervical esophagus
      - larynx — *see* Puncture, larynx
      - pharynx — *see* Puncture, pharynx
      - thyroid gland — *see* Puncture, thyroid gland
      - trachea — *see* Puncture, trachea
    - specified site NEC S11.83 ☑
      - with foreign body S11.84 ☑
  - nose (septum) (sinus) S01.23 ☑
    - with foreign body S01.24 ☑
  - ocular — *see* Puncture, eyeball
  - oral cavity S01.532 ☑
    - with foreign body S01.542 ☑
  - orbit S05.4 ☑
  - palate — *see* Puncture, oral cavity
  - palm — *see* Puncture, hand
  - pancreas S36.299 ☑
    - body S36.291 ☑
    - head S36.290 ☑
    - tail S36.292 ☑
  - pelvis — *see* Puncture, back, lower
  - penis S31.23 ☑
    - with foreign body S31.24 ☑
  - perineum
    - female S31.43 ☑
      - with foreign body S31.44 ☑
    - male S31.139 ☑
      - with foreign body S31.149 ☑
  - periocular area (with or without lacrimal passages) — *see* Puncture, eyelid
  - phalanges
    - finger — *see* Puncture, finger
    - toe — *see* Puncture, toe
  - pharynx S11.23 ☑
    - with foreign body S11.24 ☑
  - pinna — *see* Puncture, ear
  - popliteal space — *see* Puncture, knee
  - prepuce — *see* Puncture, penis
  - pubic region S31.139 ☑
    - with foreign body S31.149 ☑
  - pudendum — *see* Puncture, genital organs, external
  - rectovaginal septum — *see* Puncture, vagina
  - sacral region — *see* Puncture, back, lower
  - sacroiliac region — *see* Puncture, back, lower
  - salivary gland — *see* Puncture, oral cavity
  - scalp S01.03 ☑
    - with foreign body S01.04 ☑
  - scapular region — *see* Puncture, shoulder
  - scrotum S31.33 ☑
    - with foreign body S31.34 ☑
  - shin — *see* Puncture, leg
  - shoulder S41.039 ☑
    - with foreign body S41.049 ☑
    - left S41.032 ☑
      - with foreign body S41.042 ☑
    - right S41.031 ☑
      - with foreign body S41.041 ☑
  - spermatic cord — *see* Puncture, testis
  - sternal region — *see* Puncture, thorax, front
  - submaxillary region — *see* Puncture, head, specified site NEC
  - submental region — *see* Puncture, head, specified site NEC

- **Puncture** — *continued*
  - subungual
    - finger (s) — *see* Puncture, finger, with damage to nail
    - toe — *see* Puncture, toe, with damage to nail
  - supraclavicular fossa — *see* Puncture, neck, specified site NEC
  - temple, temporal region — *see* Puncture, head, specified site NEC
  - temporomandibular area — *see* Puncture, cheek
  - testis S31.33 ☑
    - with foreign body S31.34 ☑
  - thigh S71.139 ☑
    - with foreign body S71.149 ☑
    - left S71.132 ☑
      - with foreign body S71.142 ☑
    - right S71.131 ☑
      - with foreign body S71.141 ☑
  - thorax, thoracic (wall) S21.93 ☑
    - with foreign body S21.94 ☑
    - back S21.23 ☑
      - with
        - foreign body S21.24 ☑
          - with penetration S21.44 ☑
        - penetration S21.43 ☑
    - breast — *see* Puncture, breast
    - front S21.13 ☑
      - with
        - foreign body S21.14 ☑
          - with penetration S21.34 ☑
        - penetration S21.33 ☑
  - throat — *see* Puncture, neck
  - thumb S61.039 ☑
    - with
      - damage to nail S61.139 ☑
        - with
          - foreign body S61.149 ☑
      - foreign body S61.049 ☑
    - left S61.032 ☑
      - with
        - damage to nail S61.132 ☑
          - with
            - foreign body S61.142 ☑
        - foreign body S61.042 ☑
    - right S61.031 ☑
      - with
        - damage to nail S61.131 ☑
          - with
            - foreign body S61.141 ☑
        - foreign body S61.041 ☑
  - thyroid gland S11.13 ☑
    - with foreign body S11.14 ☑
  - toe (s) S91.139 ☑
    - with
      - damage to nail S91.239 ☑
        - with
          - foreign body S91.249 ☑
      - foreign body S91.149 ☑
    - great S91.133 ☑
      - with
        - damage to nail S91.233 ☑
          - with
            - foreign body S91.243 ☑
        - foreign body S91.143 ☑
      - left S91.132 ☑
        - with
          - damage to nail S91.232 ☑
            - with
              - foreign body S91.242 ☑
          - foreign body S91.142 ☑
      - right S91.131 ☑
        - with
          - damage to nail S91.231 ☑
            - with
              - foreign body S91.241 ☑
          - foreign body S91.141 ☑
    - lesser S91.136 ☑
      - with
        - damage to nail S91.236 ☑
          - with
            - foreign body S91.246 ☑
        - foreign body S91.146 ☑
      - left S91.135 ☑
        - with
          - damage to nail S91.235 ☑
            - with
              - foreign body S91.245 ☑
          - foreign body S91.145 ☑
      - right S91.134 ☑
        - with
          - damage to nail S91.234 ☑
            - with

- **Puncture** — *continued*
  - toe (s) — *continued*
              - foreign body S91.244 ☑
          - foreign body S91.144 ☑
  - tongue — *see* Puncture, oral cavity
  - trachea S11.023 ☑
    - with foreign body S11.024 ☑
  - tunica vaginalis — *see* Puncture, testis
  - tympanum, tympanic membrane S09.2 ☑
  - umbilical region S31.135 ☑
    - with foreign body S31.145 ☑
  - uvula — *see* Puncture, oral cavity
  - vagina S31.43 ☑
    - with foreign body S31.44 ☑
  - vocal cords S11.033 ☑
    - with foreign body S11.034 ☑
  - vulva S31.43 ☑
    - with foreign body S31.44 ☑
  - wrist S61.539 ☑
    - with
      - foreign body S61.549 ☑
    - left S61.532 ☑
      - with
        - foreign body S61.542 ☑
    - right S61.531 ☑
      - with
        - foreign body S61.541 ☑
- **PUO** (pyrexia of unknown origin) R50.9
- **Pupillary** membrane (persistent) Q13.89
- **Pupillotonia** — *see* Anomaly, pupil, function, tonic pupil
- **Purpura** D69.2
  - abdominal D69.0
  - allergic D69.0
  - anaphylactoid D69.0
  - annularis telangiectodes L81.7
  - arthritic D69.0
  - autoerythrocyte sensitization D69.2
  - autoimmune D69.0
  - bacterial D69.0
  - Bateman's (senile) D69.2
  - capillary fragility (hereditary) (idiopathic) D69.8
  - cryoglobulinemic D89.1
  - Devil's pinches D69.2
  - fibrinolytic — *see* Fibrinolysis
  - fulminans, fulminous D65
  - gangrenous D65
  - hemorrhagic, hemorrhagica D69.3
    - not due to thrombocytopenia D69.0
  - Henoch (-Schönlein) (allergic) D69.0
  - hypergammaglobulinemic (benign) (Waldenström) D89.0
  - idiopathic (thrombocytopenic) D69.3
    - nonthrombocytopenic D69.0
  - immune thrombocytopenic D69.3
  - infectious D69.0
  - malignant D69.0
  - neonatorum P54.5
  - nervosa D69.0
  - newborn P54.5
  - nonthrombocytopenic D69.2
    - hemorrhagic D69.0
    - idiopathic D69.0
  - nonthrombopenic D69.2
  - peliosis rheumatica D69.0
  - posttransfusion (post-transfusion) (from (fresh) whole blood or blood products) D69.51
  - primary D69.49
  - red cell membrane sensitivity D69.2
  - rheumatica D69.0
  - Schönlein (-Henoch) (allergic) D69.0
  - scorbutic E54 *[D77]*
  - senile D69.2
  - simplex D69.2
  - symptomatica D69.0
  - telangiectasia annularis L81.7
  - thrombocytopenic D69.49
    - congenital D69.42
    - hemorrhagic D69.3
    - hereditary D69.42
    - idiopathic D69.3
    - immune D69.3
    - neonatal, transitory P61.0
    - thrombotic M31.1
  - thrombohemolytic — *see* Fibrinolysis
  - thrombolytic — *see* Fibrinolysis
  - thrombopenic D69.49
  - thrombotic, thrombocytopenic M31.1
  - toxic D69.0
  - vascular D69.0
  - visceral symptoms D69.0
- **Purpuric** spots R23.3

- **Purulent** — *see* condition
- **Pus**
  - in
    - stool R19.5
    - urine N39.0
  - tube (rupture) — *see* Salpingo-oophoritis
- **Pustular** rash L08.0
- **Pustule** (nonmalignant) L08.9
  - malignant A22.0
- **Pustulosis** palmaris et plantaris L40.3
- **Putnam** (-Dana) disease or syndrome — *see* Degeneration, combined
- **Putrescent** pulp (dental) K04.1
- **Pyarthritis,** pyarthrosis — *see* Arthritis, pyogenic or pyemic
  - tuberculous — *see* Tuberculosis, joint
- **Pyelectasis** — *see* Hydronephrosis
- **Pyelitis** (congenital) (uremic) (*see also* Pyelonephritis)
  - with
    - calculus N20
      - with hydronephrosis N13.2
    - contracted kidney N11.9
  - acute N10
  - chronic N11.9
    - with calculus N20
      - with hydronephrosis N13.2
  - cystica N28.84
  - puerperal (postpartum) O86.21
  - tuberculous A18.11
- **Pyelocystitis** — *see* Pyelonephritis
- **Pyelonephritis** (*see also* Nephritis, tubulo-interstitial)
  - with
    - calculus N20
      - with hydronephrosis N13.2
    - contracted kidney N11.9
  - acute N10
  - calculous N20
    - with hydronephrosis N13.2
  - chronic N11.9
    - with calculus N20
      - with hydronephrosis N13.2
    - associated with ureteral obstruction or stricture N11.1
    - nonobstructive N11.8
      - with reflux (vesicoureteral) N11.0
    - obstructive N11.1
    - specified NEC N11.8
  - in (due to)
    - brucellosis A23.9 *[N16]*
    - cryoglobulinemia (mixed) D89.1 *[N16]*
    - cystinosis E72.04
    - diphtheria A36.84
    - glycogen storage disease E74.09 *[N16]*
    - leukemia NEC C95.9 ☑ *[N16]*
    - lymphoma NEC C85.90 *[N16]*
    - multiple myeloma C90.0 ☑ *[N16]*
    - obstruction N11.1
    - Salmonella infection A02.25
    - sarcoidosis D86.84
    - sepsis A41.9 *[N16]*
    - Sjögren's disease M35.04
    - toxoplasmosis B58.83
    - transplant rejection T86.91 *[N16]*
    - Wilson's disease E83.01 *[N16]*
  - nonobstructive N12
    - with reflux (vesicoureteral) N11.0
    - chronic N11.8
  - syphilitic A52.75
- **Pyelonephrosis** (obstructive) N11.1
  - chronic N11.9
- **Pyelophlebitis** I80.8
- **Pyeloureteritis** cystica N28.85
- **Pyemia,** pyemic (fever) (infection) (purulent) (*see also* Sepsis)
  - joint — *see* Arthritis, pyogenic or pyemic
  - liver K75.1
  - pneumococcal A40.3
  - portal K75.1
  - postvaccinal T88.0 ☑
  - puerperal, postpartum, childbirth O85
  - specified organism NEC A41.89
  - tuberculous — *see* Tuberculosis, miliary
- **Pygopagus** Q89.4
- **Pyknoepilepsy** (idiopathic) — *see* Pyknolepsy
- **Pyknolepsy** G40.A09
  - intractable G40.A19
    - with status epilepticus G40.A11
    - without status epilepticus G40.A19
  - not intractable G40.A09
    - with status epilepticus G40.A01
    - without status epilepticus G40.A09
- **Pylephlebitis** K75.1

☑ **Additional character required**

- **Pyle's** syndrome Q78.5
- **Pylethrombophlebitis** K75.1
- **Pylethrombosis** K75.1
- **Pyloritis** K29.90
  - with bleeding K29.91
- **Pylorospasm** (reflex) NEC K31.3
  - congenital or infantile Q40.0
  - newborn Q40.0
  - neurotic F45.8
  - psychogenic F45.8
- **Pylorus,** pyloric — *see* condition
- **Pyoarthrosis** — *see* Arthritis, pyogenic or pyemic
- **Pyocele**
  - mastoid — *see* Mastoiditis, acute
  - sinus (accessory) — *see* Sinusitis
  - turbinate (bone) J32.9
  - urethra (*see also* Urethritis)N34.0
- **Pyocolpos** — *see* Vaginitis
- **Pyocystitis** N30.80
  - with hematuria N30.81
- **Pyoderma,** pyodermia L08.0
  - gangrenosum L88
  - newborn P39.4
  - phagedenic L88
  - vegetans L08.81
- **Pyodermatitis** L08.0
  - vegetans L08.81
- **Pyogenic** — *see* condition
- **Pyohydronephrosis** N13.6
- **Pyometra,** pyometrium, pyometritis — *see* Endometritis
- **Pyomyositis** (tropical) — *see* Myositis, infective
- **Pyonephritis** N12
- **Pyonephrosis** N13.6
  - tuberculous A18.11
- **Pyo-oophoritis** — *see* Salpingo-oophoritis
- **Pyo-ovarium** — *see* Salpingo-oophoritis
- **Pyopericarditis,** pyopericardium I30.1
- **Pyophlebitis** — *see* Phlebitis
- **Pyopneumopericardium** I30.1
- **Pyopneumothorax** (infective) J86.9
  - with fistula J86.0
  - tuberculous NEC A15.6
- **Pyosalpinx,** pyosalpingitis (*see also* Salpingo-oophoritis)
- **Pyothorax** J86.9
  - with fistula J86.0
  - tuberculous NEC A15.6
- **Pyoureter** N28.89
  - tuberculous A18.11
- **Pyramidopallidonigral** syndrome G20
- **Pyrexia** (of unknown origin) R50.9
  - atmospheric T67.0 ☑
  - during labor NEC O75.2
  - heat T67.0 ☑
  - newborn P81.9
    - environmentally-induced P81.0
  - persistent R50.9
  - puerperal O86.4
- **Pyroglobulinemia** NEC E88.09
- **Pyromania** F63.1
- **Pyrosis** R12
- **Pyuria** (bacterial) N39.0

Q

- **Q fever** A78
  - with pneumonia A78
- **Quadricuspid** aortic valve Q23.8
- **Quadrilateral** fever A78
- **Quadriparesis** — *see* Quadriplegia
  - meaning muscle weakness M62.81
- **Quadriplegia** G82.50
  - complete
    - C1-C4 level G82.51
    - C5-C7 level G82.53
  - congenital (cerebral) (spinal) G80.8
    - spastic G80.0
  - embolic (current episode) I63.4 ☑
  - functional R53.2
  - incomplete
    - C1-C4 level G82.52
    - C5-C7 level G82.54
  - thrombotic (current episode) I63.3 ☑
  - traumatic -- code to injury with seventh character S
    - current episode — *see* Injury, spinal (cord), cervical
- **Quadruplet,** pregnancy — *see* Pregnancy, quadruplet
- **Quarrelsomeness** F60.3
- **Queensland** fever A77.3
- **Quervain's** disease M65.4
  - thyroid E06.1
- **Queyrat's** erythroplasia D07.4
  - penis D07.4
  - specified site — *see* Neoplasm, skin, in situ
  - unspecified site D07.4
- **Quincke's** disease or edema T78.3 ☑
  - hereditary D84.1
- **Quinsy** (gangrenous) J36
- **Quintan** fever A79.0
- **Quintuplet,** pregnancy — *see* Pregnancy, quintuplet

R

- **Rabbit** fever — *see* Tularemia
- **Rabies** A82.9
  - contact Z20.3
  - exposure to Z20.3
  - inoculation reaction — *see* Complications, vaccination
  - sylvatic A82.0
  - urban A82.1
- **Rachischisis** — *see* Spina bifida
- **Rachitic** (*see also* condition)
  - deformities of spine (late effect) (sequelae) E64.3
  - pelvis (late effect) (sequelae) E64.3
    - with disproportion (fetopelvic) O33.0
      - causing obstructed labor O65.0
- **Rachitis,** rachitism (acute) (tarda) (*see also* Rickets)
  - renalis N25.0
  - sequelae E64.3
- **Radial** nerve — *see* condition
- **Radiation**
  - burn — *see* Burn
  - effects NOS T66 ☑
  - sickness NOS T66 ☑
  - therapy, encounter for Z51.0
- **Radiculitis** (pressure) (vertebrogenic) — *see* Radiculopathy
- **Radiculomyelitis** (*see also* Encephalitis)
  - toxic, due to
    - Clostridium tetani A35
    - Corynebacterium diphtheriae A36.82
- **Radiculopathy** M54.10
  - cervical region M54.12
  - cervicothoracic region M54.13
  - due to
    - disc disorder
      - C3 M50.11
      - C4 M50.11
      - C5 M50.121
      - C6 M50.122
      - C7 M50.123
      - C8 M50.13
    - displacement of intervertebral disc — *see* Disorder, disc, with, radiculopathy
  - leg M54.1 ☑
  - lumbar region M54.16
  - lumbosacral region M54.17
  - occipito-atlanto-axial region M54.11
  - postherpetic B02.29
  - sacrococcygeal region M54.18
  - syphilitic A52.11
  - thoracic region (with visceral pain) M54.14
  - thoracolumbar region M54.15
- **Radiodermal** burns (acute, chronic, or occupational) — *see* Burn
- **Radiodermatitis** L58.9
  - acute L58.0
  - chronic L58.1
- **Radiotherapy** session Z51.0
- **RAEB** (refractory anemia with excess blasts) D46.2 ☑
- **Rage,** meaning rabies — *see* Rabies
- **Ragpicker's** disease A22.1
- **Ragsorter's** disease A22.1
- **Raillietiniasis** B71.8
- **Railroad** neurosis F48.8
- **Railway** spine F48.8
- **Raised** (*see also* Elevated)
  - antibody titer R76.0
- **Rake** teeth, tooth M26.39
- **Rales** R09.89
- **Ramifying** renal pelvis Q63.8
- **Ramsay-Hunt** disease or syndrome (*see also* Hunt's disease)B02.21
  - meaning dyssynergia cerebellaris myoclonica G11.1
- **Ranula** K11.6
  - congenital Q38.4
- **Rape**
  - adult
    - confirmed T74.21 ☑
    - suspected T76.21 ☑
  - alleged, observation or examination, ruled out
    - adult Z04.41
    - child Z04.42
  - child
    - confirmed T74.22 ☑
    - suspected T76.22 ☑
- **Rapid**
  - feeble pulse, due to shock, following injury T79.4 ☑
  - heart (beat) R00.0
    - psychogenic F45.8
  - second stage (delivery) O62.3
  - time-zone change syndrome — *see* Disorder, sleep, circadian rhythm, psychogenic
- **Rarefaction,** bone — *see* Disorder, bone, density and structure, specified NEC
- **Rash** (toxic) R21
  - canker A38.9
  - diaper L22
  - drug (internal use) L27.0
    - contact (*see also* Dermatitis, due to, drugs, external)L25.1
  - following immunization T88.1 ☑
  - food — *see* Dermatitis, due to, food
  - heat L74.0
  - napkin (psoriasiform) L22
  - nettle — *see* Urticaria
  - pustular L08.0
  - rose R21
    - epidemic B06.9
  - scarlet A38.9
  - serum (*see also* Reaction, serum)T80.69 ☑
  - wandering tongue K14.1
- **Rasmussen** aneurysm — *see* Tuberculosis, pulmonary
- **Rasmussen** encephalitis G04.81
- **Rat-bite** fever A25.9
  - due to Streptobacillus moniliformis A25.1
  - spirochetal (morsus muris) A25.0
- **Rathke's** pouch tumor D44.3
- **Raymond** (-Céstan) syndrome I65.8
- **Raynaud's** disease, phenomenon or syndrome (secondary) I73.00
  - with gangrene (symmetric) I73.01
- **RDS** (newborn) (type I) P22.0
  - type II P22.1
- **Reaction** (*see also* Disorder)
  - adaptation — *see* Disorder, adjustment
  - adjustment (anxiety) (conduct disorder) (depressiveness) (distress) — *see* Disorder, adjustment
    - with
      - mutism, elective (child) (adolescent) F94.0
  - adverse
    - food (any) (ingested) NEC T78.1 ☑
      - anaphylactic — *see* Shock, anaphylactic, due to food
  - affective — *see* Disorder, mood
  - allergic — *see* Allergy
  - anaphylactic — *see* Shock, anaphylactic
  - anaphylactoid — *see* Shock, anaphylactic
  - anesthesia — *see* Anesthesia, complication
  - antitoxin (prophylactic) (therapeutic) — *see* Complications, vaccination
  - anxiety F41.1
  - Arthus — *see* Arthus' phenomenon
  - asthenic F48.8
  - combat and operational stress F43.0
  - compulsive F42.8
  - conversion F44.9
  - crisis, acute F43.0
  - deoxyribonuclease (DNA) (DNase) hypersensitivity D69.2
  - depressive (single episode) F32.9
    - affective (single episode) F31.4
      - recurrent episode F33.9
    - neurotic F34.1
    - psychoneurotic F34.1
    - psychotic F32.3
    - recurrent — *see* Disorder, depressive, recurrent
  - dissociative F44.9
  - drug NEC T88.7 ☑
    - addictive — *see* Dependence, drug
      - transmitted via placenta or breast milk — *see* Absorption, drug, addictive, through placenta
    - allergic — *see* Allergy, drug
    - lichenoid L43.2

Reaction - Regurgitation

- **Reaction** — *continued*
  - drug NEC — *continued*
    - newborn P93.8
      - gray baby syndrome P93.0
    - overdose or poisoning (by accident) — *see* Table of Drugs and Chemicals, by drug, poisoning
    - photoallergic L56.1
    - phototoxic L56.0
    - withdrawal — *see* Dependence, by drug, with, withdrawal
      - infant of dependent mother P96.1
      - newborn P96.1
    - wrong substance given or taken (by accident) — *see* Table of Drugs and Chemicals, by drug, poisoning
  - fear F40.9
    - child (abnormal) F93.8
  - febrile nonhemolytic transfusion (FNHTR) R50.84
  - fluid loss, cerebrospinal G97.1
  - foreign
    - body NEC — *see* Granuloma, foreign body
      - in operative wound (inadvertently left) — *see* Foreign body, accidentally left during a procedure
    - substance accidentally left during a procedure (chemical) (powder) (talc) T81.60 ☑
      - aseptic peritonitis T81.61 ☑
      - body or object (instrument) (sponge) (swab) — *see* Foreign body, accidentally left during a procedure
      - specified reaction NEC T81.69 ☑
  - grief — *see* Disorder, adjustment
  - Herxheimer's R68.89
  - hyperkinetic — *see* Hyperkinesia
  - hypochondriacal F45.20
  - hypoglycemic, due to insulin E16.0
    - with coma (diabetic) — *see* Diabetes, coma
      - nondiabetic E15
    - therapeutic misadventure — *see* subcategory T38.3
  - hypomanic F30.8
  - hysterical F44.9
  - immunization — *see* Complications, vaccination
  - incompatibility
    - ABO blood group (infusion) (transfusion) — *see* Complication (s), transfusion, incompatibility reaction, ABO
      - delayed serologic T80.39 ☑
    - minor blood group (Duffy) (E) (K (ell)) (Kidd) (Lewis) (M) (N) (P) (S) T80.89 ☑
    - Rh (factor) (infusion) (transfusion) — *see* Complication (s), transfusion, incompatibility reaction, Rh (factor)
  - inflammatory — *see* Infection
  - infusion — *see* Complications, infusion
  - inoculation (immune serum) — *see* Complications, vaccination
  - insulin T38.3 ☑
  - involutional psychotic — *see* Disorder, depressive
  - leukemoid D72.823
    - basophilic D72.823
    - lymphocytic D72.823
    - monocytic D72.823
    - myelocytic D72.823
    - neutrophilic D72.823
  - LSD (acute)
    - due to drug abuse — *see* Abuse, drug, hallucinogen
    - due to drug dependence — *see* Dependence, drug, hallucinogen
  - lumbar puncture G97.1
  - manic-depressive — *see* Disorder, bipolar
  - neurasthenic F48.8
  - neurogenic — *see* Neurosis
  - neurotic F48.9
  - neurotic-depressive F34.1
  - nitritoid — *see* Crisis, nitritoid
  - nonspecific
    - to
      - cell mediated immunity measurement of gamma interferon antigen response without active tuberculosis R76.12
      - QuantiFERON-TB test (QFT) without active tuberculosis R76.12
      - tuberculin test (*see also* Reaction, tuberculin skin test)R76.11
  - obsessive-compulsive F42.8
  - organic, acute or subacute — *see* Delirium
  - paranoid (acute) F23
    - chronic F22
    - senile F03 ☑
- **Reaction** — *continued*
  - passive dependency F60.7
  - phobic F40.9
  - post-traumatic stress, uncomplicated Z73.3
  - psychogenic F99
  - psychoneurotic (*see also* Neurosis)
    - compulsive F42.8
    - depersonalization F48.1
    - depressive F34.1
    - hypochondriacal F45.20
    - neurasthenic F48.8
    - obsessive F42.8
  - psychophysiologic — *see* Disorder, somatoform
  - psychosomatic — *see* Disorder, somatoform
  - psychotic — *see* Psychosis
  - scarlet fever toxin — *see* Complications, vaccination
  - schizophrenic F23
    - acute (brief) (undifferentiated) F23
    - latent F21
    - undifferentiated (acute) (brief) F23
  - serological for syphilis — *see* Serology for syphilis
  - serum T80.69 ☑
    - anaphylactic (immediate) (*see also* Shock, anaphylactic)T80.59 ☑
    - specified reaction NEC
      - due to
        - administration of blood and blood products T80.61 ☑
        - immunization T80.62 ☑
        - serum specified NEC T80.69 ☑
        - vaccination T80.62 ☑
  - situational — *see* Disorder, adjustment
  - somatization — *see* Disorder, somatoform
  - spinal puncture G97.1
  - stress (severe) F43.9
    - acute (agitation) ("daze") (disorientation) (disturbance of consciousness) (flight reaction) (fugue) F43.0
    - specified NEC F43.8
  - surgical procedure — *see* Complications, surgical procedure
  - tetanus antitoxin — *see* Complications, vaccination
  - toxic, to local anesthesia T88.59 ☑
    - in labor and delivery O74.4
    - in pregnancy O29.3X ☑
    - postpartum, puerperal O89.3
  - toxin-antitoxin — *see* Complications, vaccination
  - transfusion (blood) (bone marrow) (lymphocytes) (allergic) — *see* Complications, transfusion
  - tuberculin skin test, abnormal R76.11
  - vaccination (any) — *see* Complications, vaccination
  - withdrawing, child or adolescent F93.8
- **Reactive** airway disease — *see* Asthma
- **Reactive** depression — *see* Reaction, depressive
- **Rearrangement**
  - chromosomal
    - balanced (in) Q95.9
      - abnormal individual (autosomal) Q95.2
        - non-sex (autosomal) chromosomes Q95.2
        - sex/non-sex chromosomes Q95.3
      - specified NEC Q95.8
- **Recalcitrant** patient — *see* Noncompliance
- **Recanalization,** thrombus — *see* Thrombosis
- **Recession,** receding
  - chamber angle (eye) H21.55 ☑
  - chin M26.09
  - gingival (generalized) (localized) (postinfective) (postoperative) K06.00
    - Miller Class I K06.01
    - Miller Class II K06.02
    - Miller Class III K06.03
    - Miller Class IV K06.04
- **Recklinghausen** disease Q85.01
  - bones E21.0
- **Reclus'** disease (cystic) — *see* Mastopathy, cystic
- **Recrudescent** typhus (fever) A75.1
- **Recruitment,** auditory H93.21 ☑
- **Rectalgia** K62.89
- **Rectitis** K62.89
- **Rectocele**
  - female (without uterine prolapse) N81.6
    - with uterine prolapse N81.4
      - incomplete N81.2
  - in pregnancy — *see* Pregnancy, complicated by, abnormal, pelvic organs or tissues NEC
  - male K62.3
- **Rectosigmoid** junction — *see* condition
- **Rectosigmoiditis** K63.89
  - ulcerative (chronic) K51.30
    - with
      - complication K51.319
        - abscess K51.314
        - fistula K51.313
        - obstruction K51.312
        - rectal bleeding K51.311
        - specified NEC K51.318
- **Rectourethral** — *see* condition
- **Rectovaginal** — *see* condition
- **Rectovesical** — *see* condition
- **Rectum,** rectal — *see* condition
- **Recurrent** — *see* condition
  - pregnancy loss — *see* Loss (of), pregnancy, recurrent
- **Red** bugs B88.0
- **Red-cedar** lung or pneumonitis J67.8
- **Red** tide (*see also* Table of Drugs and Chemicals)T65.82 ☑
- **Reduced**
  - mobility Z74.09
  - ventilatory or vital capacity R94.2
- **Redundant,** redundancy
  - anus (congenital) Q43.8
  - clitoris N90.89
  - colon (congenital) Q43.8
  - foreskin (congenital) N47.8
  - intestine (congenital) Q43.8
  - labia N90.69
  - organ or site, congenital NEC — *see* Accessory
  - panniculus (abdominal) E65
  - prepuce (congenital) N47.8
  - pylorus K31.89
  - rectum (congenital) Q43.8
  - scrotum N50.89
  - sigmoid (congenital) Q43.8
  - skin L98.7
    - and subcutaneous tissue L98.7
    - of face L57.4
      - eyelids — *see* Blepharochalasis
  - stomach K31.89
- **Reduplication** — *see* Duplication
- **Reflex** R29.2
  - hyperactive gag J39.2
  - pupillary, abnormal — *see* Anomaly, pupil, function
  - vasoconstriction I73.9
  - vasovagal R55
- **Reflux** K21.9
  - acid K21.9
  - esophageal K21.9
    - with esophagitis K21.0
    - newborn P78.83
  - gastroesophageal K21.9
    - with esophagitis K21.0
  - mitral — *see* Insufficiency, mitral
  - ureteral — *see* Reflux, vesicoureteral
  - vesicoureteral (with scarring) N13.70
    - with
      - nephropathy N13.729
        - with hydroureter N13.739
          - bilateral N13.732
          - unilateral N13.731
        - bilateral N13.722
        - unilateral N13.721
        - without hydroureter N13.729
          - bilateral N13.722
          - unilateral N13.721
      - pyelonephritis (chronic) N11.0
    - congenital Q62.7
    - without nephropathy N13.71
- **Reforming,** artificial openings — *see* Attention to, artificial, opening
- **Refractive** error — *see* Disorder, refraction
- **Refsum's** disease or syndrome G60.1
- **Refusal** of
  - food, psychogenic F50.89
  - treatment (because of) Z53.20
    - left against medical advice (AMA) Z53.21
    - patient's decision NEC Z53.29
    - reasons of belief or group pressure Z53.1
- **Regional** — *see* condition
- **Regurgitation** R11.10
  - aortic (valve) — *see* Insufficiency, aortic
  - food (*see also* Vomiting)
    - with reswallowing — *see* Rumination
    - newborn P92.1
  - gastric contents — *see* Vomiting
  - heart — *see* Endocarditis
  - mitral (valve) — *see* Insufficiency, mitral
    - congenital Q23.3

Restless - Retrognathia

- **Restless** legs (syndrome) G25.81
- **Restlessness** R45.1
- **Restriction** of housing space Z59.1
- **Restoration** (of)
  - dental
    - aesthetically inadequate or displeasing K08.56
    - defective K08.50
      - specified NEC K08.59
    - failure of marginal integrity K08.51
    - failure of periodontal anatomical integrity K08.54
  - organ continuity from previous sterilization (tuboplasty) (vasoplasty) Z31.0
    - aftercare Z31.42
  - tooth (existing)
    - contours biologically incompatible with oral health K08.54
    - open margins K08.51
    - overhanging K08.52
    - poor aesthetic K08.56
    - poor gingival margins K08.51
  - unsatisfactory, of tooth K08.50
    - specified NEC K08.59
- **Restorative** material (dental)
  - allergy to K08.55
  - fractured K08.539
    - with loss of material K08.531
    - without loss of material K08.530
  - unrepairable overhanging of K08.52
- **Rests,** ovarian, in fallopian tube Q50.6
- **Restzustand** (schizophrenic) F20.5
- **Retained** (*see also* Retention)
  - cholelithiasis following cholecystectomy K91.86
  - foreign body fragments (type of) Z18.9
    - acrylics Z18.2
    - animal quill (s) or spines Z18.31
    - cement Z18.83
    - concrete Z18.83
    - crystalline Z18.83
    - depleted isotope Z18.09
    - depleted uranium Z18.01
    - diethylhexylphthalates Z18.2
    - glass Z18.81
    - isocyanate Z18.2
    - magnetic metal Z18.11
    - metal Z18.10
    - nonmagnetic metal Z18.12
    - nontherapeutic radioactive Z18.09
    - organic NEC Z18.39
    - plastic Z18.2
    - quill (s) (animal) Z18.31
    - radioactive (nontherapeutic) NEC Z18.09
    - specified NEC Z18.89
    - spine (s) (animal) Z18.31
    - stone Z18.83
    - tooth (teeth) Z18.32
    - wood Z18.33
  - fragments (type of) Z18.9
    - acrylics Z18.2
    - animal quill (s) or spines Z18.31
    - cement Z18.83
    - concrete Z18.83
    - crystalline Z18.83
    - depleted isotope Z18.09
    - depleted uranium Z18.01
    - diethylhexylphthalates Z18.2
    - glass Z18.81
    - isocyanate Z18.2
    - magnetic metal Z18.11
    - metal Z18.10
    - nonmagnetic metal Z18.12
    - nontherapeutic radioactive Z18.09
    - organic NEC Z18.39
    - plastic Z18.2
    - quill (s) (animal) Z18.31
    - radioactive (nontherapeutic) NEC Z18.09
    - specified NEC Z18.89
    - spine (s) (animal) Z18.31
    - stone Z18.83
    - tooth (teeth) Z18.32
    - wood Z18.33
  - gallstones, following cholecystectomy K91.86
- **Retardation**
  - development, developmental, specific — *see* Disorder, developmental
  - endochondral bone growth — *see* Disorder, bone, development or growth
  - growth R62.50
    - due to malnutrition E45
  - mental — *see* Disability, intellectual
  - motor function, specific F82
  - physical (child) R62.52
    - due to malnutrition E45

Retardation — *continued*

  - reading (specific) F81.0
  - spelling (specific) (without reading disorder) F81.81
- **Retching** — *see* Vomiting
- **Retention** (*see also* Retained)
  - bladder — *see* Retention, urine
  - carbon dioxide E87.2
  - cholelithiasis following cholecystectomy K91.86
  - cyst — *see* Cyst
  - dead
    - fetus (at or near term) (mother) O36.4 ☑
      - early fetal death O02.1
    - ovum O02.0
  - decidua (fragments) (following delivery) (with hemorrhage) O72.2
    - without hemorrhage O73.1
  - deciduous tooth K00.6
  - dental root K08.3
  - fecal — *see* Constipation
  - fetus
    - dead O36.4 ☑
      - early O02.1
  - fluid R60.9
  - foreign body (*see also* Foreign body, retained)
    - current trauma - code as Foreign body, by site or type
  - gallstones, following cholecystectomy K91.86
  - gastric K31.89
  - intrauterine contraceptive device, in pregnancy — *see* Pregnancy, complicated by, retention, intrauterine device
  - membranes (complicating delivery) (with hemorrhage) O72.2
    - with abortion — *see* Abortion, by type
    - without hemorrhage O73.1
  - meniscus — *see* Derangement, meniscus
  - menses N94.89
  - milk (puerperal, postpartum) O92.79
  - nitrogen, extrarenal R39.2
  - ovary syndrome N99.83
  - placenta (total) (with hemorrhage) O72.0
    - without hemorrhage O73.0
    - portions or fragments (with hemorrhage) O72.2
      - without hemorrhage O73.1
  - products of conception
    - early pregnancy (dead fetus) O02.1
    - following
      - delivery (with hemorrhage) O72.2
        - without hemorrhage O73.1
  - secundines (following delivery) (with hemorrhage) O72.0
    - without hemorrhage O73.0
    - complicating puerperium (delayed hemorrhage) O72.2
    - partial O72.2
      - without hemorrhage O73.1
  - smegma, clitoris N90.89
  - urine R33.9
    - due to hyperplasia (hypertrophy) of prostate — *see* Hyperplasia, prostate
    - drug-induced R33.0
    - organic R33.8
      - drug-induced R33.0
    - psychogenic F45.8
    - specified NEC R33.8
  - water (in tissues) — *see* Edema
- **Reticular** erythematous mucinosis L98.5
- **Reticulation,** dust — *see* Pneumoconiosis
- **Reticulocytosis** R70.1
- **Reticuloendotheliosis**
  - acute infantile C96.0
  - leukemic C91.4 ☑
  - nonlipid C96.0
- **Reticulohistiocytoma** (giant-cell) D76.3
- **Reticuloid,** actinic L57.1
- **Reticulosis** (skin)
  - acute of infancy C96.0
  - hemophagocytic, familial D76.1
  - histiocytic medullary C96.A
  - lipomelanotic I89.8
  - malignant (midline) C86.0
  - polymorphic C86.0
  - Sézary — *see* Sézary disease
- **Retina,** retinal (*see also* condition)
  - dark area D49.81
- **Retinitis** (*see also* Inflammation, chorioretinal)
  - albuminurica N18.9 *[H32]*
  - diabetic — *see* Diabetes, retinitis
  - disciformis — *see* Degeneration, macula
  - focal — *see* Inflammation, chorioretinal, focal

Retinitis — *continued*

  - gravidarum — *see* Pregnancy, complicated by, specified pregnancy-related condition NEC
  - juxtapapillaris — *see* Inflammation, chorioretinal, focal, juxtapapillary
  - luetic — *see* Retinitis, syphilitic
  - pigmentosa H35.52
  - proliferans — *see* Disorder, globe, degenerative, specified type NEC
  - proliferating — *see* Disorder, globe, degenerative, specified type NEC
  - renal N18.9 *[H32]*
  - syphilitic (early) (secondary) A51.43
    - central, recurrent A52.71
    - congenital (early) A50.01 *[H32]*
    - late A52.71
  - tuberculous A18.53
- **Retinoblastoma** C69.2 ☑
  - differentiated C69.2 ☑
  - undifferentiated C69.2 ☑
- **Retinochoroiditis** (*see also* Inflammation, chorioretinal)
  - disseminated — *see* Inflammation, chorioretinal, disseminated
    - syphilitic A52.71
  - focal — *see* Inflammation, chorioretinal
  - juxtapapillaris — *see* Inflammation, chorioretinal, focal, juxtapapillary
- **Retinopathy** (background) H35.00
  - arteriosclerotic I70.8 *[H35.0-]*
  - atherosclerotic I70.8 *[H35.0-]*
  - central serous — *see* Chorioretinopathy, central serous
  - Coats H35.02 ☑
  - diabetic — *see* Diabetes, retinopathy
  - exudative H35.02 ☑
  - hypertensive H35.03 ☑
  - in (due to)
    - diabetes — *see* Diabetes, retinopathy
    - sickle-cell disorders D57. ☑ *[H36]*
  - of prematurity H35.10 ☑
    - stage 0 H35.11 ☑
    - stage 1 H35.12 ☑
    - stage 2 H35.13 ☑
    - stage 3 H35.14 ☑
    - stage 4 H35.15 ☑
    - stage 5 H35.16 ☑
  - pigmentary, congenital — *see* Dystrophy, retina
  - proliferative NEC H35.2 ☑
    - diabetic — *see* Diabetes, retinopathy, proliferative
    - sickle-cell D57. ☑ *[H36]*
  - solar H31.02 ☑
- **Retinoschisis** H33.10 ☑
  - congenital Q14.1
  - specified type NEC H33.19 ☑
- **Retortamoniasis** A07.8
- **Retractile** testis Q55.22
- **Retraction**
  - cervix — *see* Retroversion, uterus
  - drum (membrane) — *see* Disorder, tympanic membrane, specified NEC
  - finger — *see* Deformity, finger
  - lid H02.539
    - left H02.536
      - lower H02.535
      - upper H02.534
    - right H02.533
      - lower H02.532
      - upper H02.531
  - lung J98.4
  - mediastinum J98.59
  - nipple N64.53
    - associated with
      - lactation O92.03
      - pregnancy O92.01 ☑
      - puerperium O92.02
    - congenital Q83.8
  - palmar fascia M72.0
  - pleura — *see* Pleurisy
  - ring, uterus (Bandl's) (pathological) O62.4
  - sternum (congenital) Q76.7
    - acquired M95.4
  - uterus — *see* Retroversion, uterus
  - valve (heart) — *see* Endocarditis
- **Retrobulbar** — *see* condition
- **Retrocecal** — *see* condition
- **Retrocession** — *see* Retroversion
- **Retrodisplacement** — *see* Retroversion
- **Retroflection,** retroflexion — *see* Retroversion
- **Retrognathia,** retrognathism (mandibular) (maxillary) M26.19

Retrograde menstruation N92.5
Retroperineal — *see* condition
Retroperitoneal — *see* condition
Retroperitonitis K68.9
Retropharyngeal — *see* condition
Retroplacental — *see* condition
Retroposition — *see* Retroversion
Retroprosthetic membrane T85.398 ☑
Retrosternal thyroid (congenital) Q89.2
Retroversion, retroverted
- cervix — *see* Retroversion, uterus
- female NEC — *see* Retroversion, uterus
- iris H21.89
- testis (congenital) Q55.29
- uterus (acquired) (acute) (any degree) (asymptomatic) (cervix) (postinfectional) (postpartal, old) N85.4
  - congenital Q51.818
  - in pregnancy O34.53 ☑

Retrovirus, as cause of disease classified elsewhere B97.30
- human
  - immunodeficiency, type 2 (HIV 2) B97.35
  - T-cell lymphotropic
    - type I (HTLV-I) B97.33
    - type II (HTLV-II) B97.34
- lentivirus B97.31
- oncovirus B97.32
- specified NEC B97.39

Retrusion, premaxilla (developmental) M26.09
Rett's disease or syndrome F84.2
Reverse peristalsis R19.2
Reye's syndrome G93.7
Rh (factor)
- hemolytic disease (newborn) P55.0
- incompatibility, immunization or sensitization
  - affecting management of pregnancy NEC O36.09 ☑
    - anti-D antibody O36.01 ☑
  - newborn P55.0
  - transfusion reaction — *see* Complication (s), transfusion, incompatibility reaction, Rh (factor)
- negative mother affecting newborn P55.0
- titer elevated — *see* Complication (s), transfusion, incompatibility reaction, Rh (factor)
- transfusion reaction — *see* Complication (s), transfusion, incompatibility reaction, Rh (factor)

Rhabdomyolysis (idiopathic) NEC M62.82
- traumatic T79.6 ☑

Rhabdomyoma (*see also* Neoplasm, connective tissue, benign)
- adult — *see* Neoplasm, connective tissue, benign
- fetal — *see* Neoplasm, connective tissue, benign
- glycogenic — *see* Neoplasm, connective tissue, benign

Rhabdomyosarcoma (any type) — *see* Neoplasm, connective tissue, malignant
Rhabdosarcoma — *see* Rhabdomyosarcoma
Rhesus (factor) incompatibility — *see* Rh, incompatibility
Rheumatic (acute) (subacute) (chronic)
- adherent pericardium I09.2
- coronary arteritis I01.9
- degeneration, myocardium I09.0
- fever (acute) — *see* Fever, rheumatic
- heart — *see* Disease, heart, rheumatic
- myocardial degeneration — *see* Degeneration, myocardium
- myocarditis (chronic) (inactive) (with chorea) I09.0
  - active or acute I01.2
  - with chorea (acute) (rheumatic) (Sydenham's) I02.0
- pancarditis, acute I01.8
  - with chorea (acute (rheumatic) Sydenham's) I02.0
- pericarditis (active) (acute) (with effusion) (with pneumonia) I01.0
  - with chorea (acute) (rheumatic) (Sydenham's) I02.0
  - chronic or inactive I09.2
- pneumonia I00 *[J17]*
- torticollis M43.6
- typhoid fever A01.09

Rheumatism (articular) (neuralgic) (nonarticular) M79.0
- gout — *see* Arthritis, rheumatoid
- intercostal, meaning Tietze's disease M94.0
- palindromic (any site) M12.30
  - ankle M12.37 ☑

Rheumatism — *continued*
- palindromic — *continued*
  - elbow M12.32 ☑
  - foot joint M12.37 ☑
  - hand joint M12.34 ☑
  - hip M12.35 ☑
  - knee M12.36 ☑
  - multiple site M12.39
  - shoulder M12.31 ☑
  - specified joint NEC M12.38
  - vertebrae M12.38
  - wrist M12.33 ☑
- sciatic M54.4 ☑

Rheumatoid (*see also* condition)
- arthritis (*see also* Arthritis, rheumatoid)
  - with involvement of organs NEC M05.60
    - ankle M05.67 ☑
    - elbow M05.62 ☑
    - foot joint M05.67 ☑
    - hand joint M05.64 ☑
    - hip M05.65 ☑
    - knee M05.66 ☑
    - multiple site M05.69
    - shoulder M05.61 ☑
    - vertebra — *see* Spondylitis, ankylosing
    - wrist M05.63 ☑
  - seronegative — *see* Arthritis, rheumatoid, seronegative
  - seropositive — *see* Arthritis, rheumatoid, seropositive
- carditis M05.30
  - ankle M05.37 ☑
  - elbow M05.32 ☑
  - foot joint M05.37 ☑
  - hand joint M05.34 ☑
  - hip M05.35 ☑
  - knee M05.36 ☑
  - multiple site M05.39
  - shoulder M05.31 ☑
  - vertebra — *see* Spondylitis, ankylosing
  - wrist M05.33 ☑
- endocarditis — *see* Rheumatoid, carditis
- lung (disease) M05.10
  - ankle M05.17 ☑
  - elbow M05.12 ☑
  - foot joint M05.17 ☑
  - hand joint M05.14 ☑
  - hip M05.15 ☑
  - knee M05.16 ☑
  - multiple site M05.19
  - shoulder M05.11 ☑
  - vertebra — *see* Spondylitis, ankylosing
  - wrist M05.13 ☑
- myocarditis — *see* Rheumatoid, carditis
- myopathy M05.40
  - ankle M05.47 ☑
  - elbow M05.42 ☑
  - foot joint M05.47 ☑
  - hand joint M05.44 ☑
  - hip M05.45 ☑
  - knee M05.46 ☑
  - multiple site M05.49
  - shoulder M05.41 ☑
  - vertebra — *see* Spondylitis, ankylosing
  - wrist M05.43 ☑
- pericarditis — *see* Rheumatoid, carditis
- polyarthritis — *see* Arthritis, rheumatoid
- polyneuropathy M05.50
  - ankle M05.57 ☑
  - elbow M05.52 ☑
  - foot joint M05.57 ☑
  - hand joint M05.54 ☑
  - hip M05.55 ☑
  - knee M05.56 ☑
  - multiple site M05.59
  - shoulder M05.51 ☑
  - vertebra — *see* Spondylitis, ankylosing
  - wrist M05.53 ☑
- vasculitis M05.20
  - ankle M05.27 ☑
  - elbow M05.22 ☑
  - foot joint M05.27 ☑
  - hand joint M05.24 ☑
  - hip M05.25 ☑
  - knee M05.26 ☑
  - multiple site M05.29
  - shoulder M05.21 ☑
  - vertebra — *see* Spondylitis, ankylosing
  - wrist M05.23 ☑

Rhinitis (atrophic) (catarrhal) (chronic) (croupous) (fibrinous) (granulomatous) (hyperplastic)

Rhinitis — *continued*
(hypertrophic) (membranous) (obstructive) (purulent) (suppurative) (ulcerative) J31.0
- with
  - sore throat — *see* Nasopharyngitis
- acute J00
- allergic J30.9
  - with asthma J45.909
    - with
      - exacerbation (acute) J45.901
      - status asthmaticus J45.902
  - due to
    - food J30.5
    - pollen J30.1
  - nonseasonal J30.89
  - perennial J30.89
  - seasonal NEC J30.2
  - specified NEC J30.89
- infective J00
- pneumococcal J00
- syphilitic A52.73
  - congenital A50.05 *[J99]*
- tuberculous A15.8
- vasomotor J30.0

Rhinoantritis (chronic) — *see* Sinusitis, maxillary
Rhinodacryolith — *see* Dacryolith
Rhinolith (nasal sinus) J34.89
Rhinomegaly J34.89
Rhinopharyngitis (acute) (subacute) (*see also* Nasopharyngitis)
- chronic J31.1
- destructive ulcerating A66.5
- mutilans A66.5

Rhinophyma L71.1
Rhinorrhea J34.89
- cerebrospinal (fluid) G96.0
- paroxysmal — *see* Rhinitis, allergic
- spasmodic — *see* Rhinitis, allergic

Rhinosalpingitis — *see* Salpingitis, eustachian
Rhinoscleroma A48.8
Rhinosporidiosis B48.1
Rhinovirus infection NEC B34.8
Rhizomelic chondrodysplasia punctata E71.540
Rhythm
- atrioventricular nodal I49.8
- disorder I49.9
  - coronary sinus I49.8
  - ectopic I49.8
  - nodal I49.8
- escape I49.9
- heart, abnormal I49.9
- idioventricular I44.2
- nodal I49.8
- sleep, inversion G47.2 ☑
  - nonorganic origin — *see* Disorder, sleep, circadian rhythm, psychogenic

Rhytidosis facialis L98.8
Rib (*see also* condition)
- cervical Q76.5

Riboflavin deficiency E53.0
Rice bodies (*see also* Loose, body, joint)
- knee M23.4 ☑

Richter syndrome — *see* Leukemia, chronic lymphocytic, B-cell type
Richter's hernia — *see* Hernia, abdomen, with obstruction
Ricinism — *see* Poisoning, food, noxious, plant
Rickets (active) (acute) (adolescent) (chest wall) (congenital) (current) (infantile) (intestinal) E55.0
- adult — *see* Osteomalacia
- celiac K90.0
- hypophosphatemic with nephrotic-glycosuric dwarfism E72.09
- inactive E64.3
- kidney N25.0
- renal N25.0
- sequelae, any E64.3
- vitamin-D-resistant E83.31 *[M90.80]*

Rickettsial disease A79.9
- specified type NEC A79.89

Rickettsialpox (Rickettsia akari) A79.1
Rickettsiosis A79.9
- due to
  - Ehrlichia sennetsu A79.81
  - Rickettsia akari (rickettsialpox) A79.1
- specified type NEC A79.89
- tick-borne A77.9
- vesicular A79.1

Rider's bone — *see* Ossification, muscle, specified NEC
Ridge, alveolus (*see also* condition)
- flabby K06.8

Ridged ear, congenital Q17.3
Riedel's
- lobe, liver Q44.7
- struma, thyroiditis or disease E06.5

Rieger's anomaly or syndrome Q13.81
Riehl's melanosis L81.4
Rietti-Greppi-Micheli anemia D56.9
Rieux's hernia — *see* Hernia, abdomen, specified site NEC
Riga (-Fede) disease K14.0
Riggs' disease — *see* Periodontitis
Right aortic arch Q25.47
Right middle lobe syndrome J98.11
Rigid, rigidity (*see also* condition)
- abdominal R19.30
  - with severe abdominal pain R10.0
  - epigastric R19.36
  - generalized R19.37
  - left lower quadrant R19.34
  - left upper quadrant R19.32
  - periumbilic R19.35
  - right lower quadrant R19.33
  - right upper quadrant R19.31
- articular, multiple, congenital Q68.8
- cervix (uteri) in pregnancy — *see* Pregnancy, complicated by, abnormal, cervix
- hymen (acquired) (congenital) N89.6
- nuchal R29.1
- pelvic floor in pregnancy — *see* Pregnancy, complicated by, abnormal, pelvic organs or tissues NEC
- perineum or vulva in pregnancy — *see* Pregnancy, complicated by, abnormal, vulva
- spine — *see* Dorsopathy, specified NEC
- vagina in pregnancy — *see* Pregnancy, complicated by, abnormal, vagina

Rigors R68.89
- with fever R50.9

Riley-Day syndrome G90.1
RIND (reversible ischemic neurologic deficit) I63.9
Ring (s)
- aorta (vascular) Q25.45
- Bandl's O62.4
- contraction, complicating delivery O62.4
- esophageal, lower (muscular) K22.2
- Fleischer's (cornea) H18.04 ☑
- hymenal, tight (acquired) (congenital) N89.6
- Kayser-Fleischer (cornea) H18.04 ☑
- retraction, uterus, pathological O62.4
- Schatzki's (esophagus) (lower) K22.2
  - congenital Q39.3
- Soemmerring's — *see* Cataract, secondary
- vascular (congenital) Q25.8
  - aorta Q25.45

Ringed hair (congenital) Q84.1
Ringworm B35.9
- beard B35.0
- black dot B35.0
- body B35.4
- Burmese B35.5
- corporeal B35.4
- foot B35.3
- groin B35.6
- hand B35.2
- honeycomb B35.0
- nails B35.1
- perianal (area) B35.6
- scalp B35.0
- specified NEC B35.8
- Tokelau B35.5

Rise, venous pressure I87.8
Rising, PSA following treatment for malignant neoplasm of prostate R97.21
Risk, suicidal
- meaning personal history of attempted suicide Z91.5
- meaning suicidal ideation — *see* Ideation, suicidal

Ritter's disease L00
Rivalry, sibling Z62.891
Rivalta's disease A42.2
River blindness B73.01
Robert's pelvis Q74.2
- with disproportion (fetopelvic) O33.0
  - causing obstructed labor O65.0

Robin (-Pierre) syndrome Q87.0
Robinow-Silvermann-Smith syndrome Q87.1
Robinson's (hidrotic) ectodermal dysplasia or syndrome Q82.4
Robles' disease B73.01
Rocky Mountain (spotted) fever A77.0
Roetheln — *see* Rubella
Roger's disease Q21.0
Rokitansky-Aschoff sinuses (gallbladder) K82.8
Rolando's fracture (displaced) S62.22 ☑
- nondisplaced S62.22 ☑

Romano-Ward (prolonged QT interval) syndrome I45.81
Romberg's disease or syndrome G51.8
Roof, mouth — *see* condition
Rosacea L71.9
- acne L71.9
- keratitis L71.8
- specified NEC L71.8

Rosary, rachitic E55.0
Rose
- cold J30.1
- fever J30.1
- rash R21
  - epidemic B06.9

Rosenbach's erysipeloid A26.0
Rosenthal's disease or syndrome D68.1
Roseola B09
- infantum B08.20
  - due to human herpesvirus 6 B08.21
  - due to human herpesvirus 7 B08.22

Rossbach's disease K31.89
- psychogenic F45.8

Ross River disease or fever B33.1
Rostan's asthma (cardiac) — *see* Failure, ventricular, left
Rotation
- anomalous, incomplete or insufficient, intestine Q43.3
- cecum (congenital) Q43.3
- colon (congenital) Q43.3
- spine, incomplete or insufficient — *see* Dorsopathy, deforming, specified NEC
- tooth, teeth, fully erupted M26.35
- vertebra, incomplete or insufficient — *see* Dorsopathy, deforming, specified NEC

Rotes Quérol disease or syndrome — *see* Hyperostosis, ankylosing
Roth (-Bernhardt) disease or syndrome — *see* Meralgia paraesthetica
Rothmund (-Thomson) syndrome Q82.8
Rotor's disease or syndrome E80.6
Round
- back (with wedging of vertebrae) — *see* Kyphosis
  - sequelae (late effect) of rickets E64.3
- worms (large) (infestation) NEC B82.0
  - Ascariasis (*see also* Ascariasis)B77.9

Roussy-Lévy syndrome G60.0
Rubella (German measles) B06.9
- complication NEC B06.09
  - neurological B06.00
- congenital P35.0
- contact Z20.4
- exposure to Z20.4
- maternal
  - manifest rubella in infant P35.0
  - care for (suspected) damage to fetus O35.3 ☑
  - suspected damage to fetus affecting management of pregnancy O35.3 ☑
- specified complications NEC B06.89

Rubeola (meaning measles) — *see* Measles
- meaning rubella — *see* Rubella

Rubeosis, iris — *see* Disorder, iris, vascular
Rubinstein-Taybi syndrome Q87.2
Rudimentary (congenital) (*see also* Agenesis)
- arm — *see* Defect, reduction, upper limb
- bone Q79.9
- cervix uteri Q51.828
- eye Q11.2
- lobule of ear Q17.3
- patella Q74.1
- respiratory organs in thoracopagus Q89.4
- tracheal bronchus Q32.4
- uterus Q51.818
  - in male Q56.1
- vagina Q52.0

Ruled out condition — *see* Observation, suspected
Rumination R11.10
- with nausea R11.2
- disorder of infancy F98.21
- neurotic F42.8
- newborn P92.1
- obsessional F42.8
- psychogenic F42.8

Runeberg's disease D51.0
Runny nose R09.89
Rupia (syphilitic) A51.39
- congenital A50.06
- tertiary A52.79

Rupture, ruptured
- abscess (spontaneous) - code by site under Abscess
- aneurysm — *see* Aneurysm
- anus (sphincter) — *see* Laceration, anus
- aorta, aortic I71.8
  - abdominal I71.3
  - arch I71.1
  - ascending I71.1
  - descending I71.8
    - abdominal I71.3
    - thoracic I71.1
  - syphilitic A52.01
  - thoracoabdominal I71.5
  - thorax, thoracic I71.1
  - transverse I71.1
  - traumatic — *see* Injury, aorta, laceration, major
  - valve or cusp (*see also* Endocarditis, aortic)I35.8
- appendix (with peritonitis) K35.2
  - with localized peritonitis K35.3
- arteriovenous fistula, brain I60.8
- artery I77.2
  - brain — *see* Hemorrhage, intracranial, intracerebral
  - coronary — *see* Infarct, myocardium
  - heart — *see* Infarct, myocardium
  - pulmonary I28.8
  - traumatic (complication) — *see* Injury, blood vessel
- bile duct (common) (hepatic) K83.2
  - cystic K82.2
- bladder (sphincter) (nontraumatic) (spontaneous) N32.89
  - following ectopic or molar pregnancy O08.6
  - obstetrical trauma O71.5
  - traumatic S37.29 ☑
- blood vessel (*see also* Hemorrhage)
  - brain — *see* Hemorrhage, intracranial, intracerebral
  - heart — *see* Infarct, myocardium
  - traumatic (complication) — *see* Injury, blood vessel, laceration, major, by site
- bone — *see* Fracture
- bowel (nontraumatic) K63.1
- brain
  - aneurysm (congenital) (*see also* Hemorrhage, intracranial, subarachnoid)
    - syphilitic A52.05
  - hemorrhagic — *see* Hemorrhage, intracranial, intracerebral
- capillaries I78.8
- cardiac (auricle) (ventricle) (wall) I23.3
  - with hemopericardium I23.0
  - infectional I40.9
  - traumatic — *see* Injury, heart
- cartilage (articular) (current) (*see also* Sprain)
  - knee S83.3 ☑
  - semilunar — *see* Tear, meniscus
- cecum (with peritonitis) K65.0
  - with peritoneal abscess K35.3
  - traumatic S36.598 ☑
- celiac artery, traumatic — *see* Injury, blood vessel, celiac artery, laceration, major
- cerebral aneurysm (congenital) (see Hemorrhage, intracranial, subarachnoid)
- cervix (uteri)
  - with ectopic or molar pregnancy O08.6
  - following ectopic or molar pregnancy O08.6
  - obstetrical trauma O71.3
  - traumatic S37.69 ☑
- chordae tendineae NEC I51.1
  - concurrent with acute myocardial infarction — *see* Infarct, myocardium
  - following acute myocardial infarction (current complication) I23.4
- choroid (direct) (indirect) (traumatic) H31.32 ☑
- circle of Willis I60.6
- colon (nontraumatic) K63.1
  - traumatic — *see* Injury, intestine, large
- cornea (traumatic) — *see* Injury, eye, laceration
- coronary (artery) (thrombotic) — *see* Infarct, myocardium
- corpus luteum (infected) (ovary) N83.1 ☑
- cyst — *see* Cyst
- cystic duct K82.2
- Descemet's membrane — *see* Change, corneal membrane, Descemet's, rupture
  - traumatic — *see* Injury, eye, laceration
- diaphragm, traumatic — *see* Injury, intrathoracic, diaphragm
- disc — *see* Rupture, intervertebral disc

☑ **Additional character required**

Rupture — *continued*
- diverticulum (intestine) K57.80
  - with bleeding K57.81
  - bladder N32.3
  - large intestine K57.20
    - with
      - bleeding K57.21
      - small intestine K57.40
        - with bleeding K57.41
  - small intestine K57.00
    - with
      - bleeding K57.01
      - large intestine K57.40
        - with bleeding K57.41
- duodenal stump K31.89
- ear drum (nontraumatic) (*see also* Perforation, tympanum)
  - traumatic S09.2 ☑
    - due to blast injury — *see* Injury, blast, ear
- esophagus K22.3
- eye (without prolapse or loss of intraocular tissue) — *see* Injury, eye, laceration
- fallopian tube NEC (nonobstetric) (nontraumatic) N83.8
  - due to pregnancy O00.10
    - with intrauterine pregnancy O00.11
- fontanel P13.1
- gallbladder K82.2
  - traumatic S36.128 ☑
- gastric (*see also* Rupture, stomach)
  - vessel K92.2
- globe (eye) (traumatic) — *see* Injury, eye, laceration
- graafian follicle (hematoma) N83.0 ☑
- heart — *see* Rupture, cardiac
- hymen (nontraumatic) (nonintentional) N89.8
- internal organ, traumatic — *see* Injury, by site
- intervertebral disc — *see* Displacement, intervertebral disc
  - traumatic — *see* Rupture, traumatic, intervertebral disc
- intestine NEC (nontraumatic) K63.1
  - traumatic — *see* Injury, intestine
- iris (*see also* Abnormality, pupillary)
  - traumatic — *see* Injury, eye, laceration
- joint capsule, traumatic — *see* Sprain
- kidney (traumatic) S37.06 ☑
  - birth injury P15.8
  - nontraumatic N28.89
- lacrimal duct (traumatic) — *see* Injury, eye, specified site NEC
- lens (cataract) (traumatic) — *see* Cataract, traumatic
- ligament, traumatic — *see* Rupture, traumatic, ligament, by site
- liver S36.116 ☑
  - birth injury P15.0
- lymphatic vessel I89.8
- marginal sinus (placental) (with hemorrhage) — *see* Hemorrhage, antepartum, specified cause NEC
- membrana tympani (nontraumatic) — *see* Perforation, tympanum
- membranes (spontaneous)
  - artificial
    - delayed delivery following O75.5
  - delayed delivery following — *see* Pregnancy, complicated by, premature rupture of membranes
- meningeal artery I60.8
- meniscus (knee) (*see also* Tear, meniscus)
  - old — *see* Derangement, meniscus
  - site other than knee - code as Sprain
- mesenteric artery, traumatic — *see* Injury, mesenteric, artery, laceration, major
- mesentery (nontraumatic) K66.8
  - traumatic — *see* Injury, intra-abdominal, specified, site NEC
- mitral (valve) I34.8
- muscle (traumatic) (*see also* Strain)
  - diastasis — *see* Diastasis, muscle
  - nontraumatic M62.10
    - ankle M62.17 ☑
    - foot M62.17 ☑
    - forearm M62.13 ☑
    - hand M62.14 ☑
    - lower leg M62.16 ☑
    - pelvic region M62.15 ☑
    - shoulder region M62.11 ☑
    - specified site NEC M62.18
    - thigh M62.15 ☑
    - upper arm M62.12 ☑
  - traumatic — *see* Strain, by site

Rupture — *continued*
- musculotendinous junction NEC, nontraumatic — *see* Rupture, tendon, spontaneous
- mycotic aneurysm causing cerebral hemorrhage — *see* Hemorrhage, intracranial, subarachnoid
- myocardium, myocardial — *see* Rupture, cardiac
  - traumatic — *see* Injury, heart
- nontraumatic, meaning hernia — *see* Hernia
- obstructed — *see* Hernia, by site, obstructed
- operation wound — *see* Disruption, wound, operation
- ovary, ovarian N83.8
  - corpus luteum cyst N83.1 ☑
  - follicle (graafian) N83.0 ☑
- oviduct (nonobstetric) (nontraumatic) N83.8
  - due to pregnancy O00.10
    - with intrauterine pregnancy O00.11
- pancreas (nontraumatic) K86.89
  - traumatic S36.299 ☑
- papillary muscle NEC I51.2
  - following acute myocardial infarction (current complication) I23.5
- pelvic
  - floor, complicating delivery O70.1
  - organ NEC, obstetrical trauma O71.5
- perineum (nonobstetric) (nontraumatic) N90.89
  - complicating delivery — *see* Delivery, complicated, by, laceration, anus (sphincter)
- postoperative wound — *see* Disruption, wound, operation
- prostate (traumatic) S37.828 ☑
- pulmonary
  - artery I28.8
  - valve (heart) I37.8
  - vein I28.8
  - vessel I28.8
- pus tube — *see* Salpingitis
- pyosalpinx — *see* Salpingitis
- rectum (nontraumatic) K63.1
  - traumatic S36.69 ☑
- retina, retinal (traumatic) (without detachment) (*see also* Break, retina)
  - with detachment — *see* Detachment, retina, with retinal, break
- rotator cuff (nontraumatic) M75.10 ☑
  - complete M75.12 ☑
  - incomplete M75.11 ☑
- sclera — *see* Injury, eye, laceration
- sigmoid (nontraumatic) K63.1
  - traumatic S36.593 ☑
- spinal cord (*see also* Injury, spinal cord, by region)
  - due to injury at birth P11.5
  - newborn (birth injury) P11.5
- spleen (traumatic) S36.09 ☑
  - birth injury P15.1
  - congenital (birth injury) P15.1
  - due to P. vivax malaria B51.0
  - nontraumatic D73.5
  - spontaneous D73.5
- splenic vein R58
  - traumatic — *see* Injury, blood vessel, splenic vein
- stomach (nontraumatic) (spontaneous) K31.89
  - traumatic S36.39 ☑
- supraspinatus (complete) (incomplete) (nontraumatic) — *see* Tear, rotator cuff
- symphysis pubis
  - obstetric O71.6
  - traumatic S33.4 ☑
- synovium (cyst) M66.10
  - ankle M66.17 ☑
  - elbow M66.12 ☑
  - finger M66.14 ☑
  - foot M66.17 ☑
  - forearm M66.13 ☑
  - hand M66.14 ☑
  - pelvic region M66.15 ☑
  - shoulder region M66.11 ☑
  - specified site NEC M66.18
  - thigh M66.15 ☑
  - toe M66.17 ☑
  - upper arm M66.12 ☑
  - wrist M66.13 ☑
- tendon (traumatic) — *see* Strain
  - nontraumatic (spontaneous) M66.9
    - ankle M66.87 ☑
    - extensor M66.20
      - ankle M66.27 ☑
      - foot M66.27 ☑
      - forearm M66.23 ☑

Rupture — *continued*
- tendon — *continued*
      - hand M66.24 ☑
      - lower leg M66.26 ☑
      - multiple sites M66.29
      - pelvic region M66.25 ☑
      - shoulder region M66.21 ☑
      - specified site NEC M66.28
      - thigh M66.25 ☑
      - upper arm M66.22 ☑
    - flexor M66.30
      - ankle M66.37 ☑
      - foot M66.37 ☑
      - forearm M66.33 ☑
      - hand M66.34 ☑
      - lower leg M66.36 ☑
      - multiple sites M66.39
      - pelvic region M66.35 ☑
      - shoulder region M66.31 ☑
      - specified site NEC M66.38
      - thigh M66.35 ☑
      - upper arm M66.32 ☑
    - foot M66.87 ☑
    - forearm M66.83 ☑
    - hand M66.84 ☑
    - lower leg M66.86 ☑
    - multiple sites M66.89
    - pelvic region M66.85 ☑
    - shoulder region M66.81 ☑
    - specified
      - site NEC M66.88
      - tendon M66.80
    - thigh M66.85 ☑
    - upper arm M66.82 ☑
- thoracic duct I89.8
- tonsil J35.8
- traumatic
  - aorta — *see* Injury, aorta, laceration, major
  - diaphragm — *see* Injury, intrathoracic, diaphragm
  - external site — *see* Wound, open, by site
  - eye — *see* Injury, eye, laceration
  - internal organ — *see* Injury, by site
  - intervertebral disc
    - cervical S13.0 ☑
    - lumbar S33.0 ☑
    - thoracic S23.0 ☑
  - kidney S37.06 ☑
  - ligament (*see also* Sprain)
    - ankle — *see* Sprain, ankle
    - carpus — *see* Rupture, traumatic, ligament, wrist
    - collateral (hand) — *see* Rupture, traumatic, ligament, finger, collateral
    - finger (metacarpophalangeal) (interphalangeal) S63.40 ☑
      - collateral S63.41 ☑
        - index S63.41 ☑
        - little S63.41 ☑
        - middle S63.41 ☑
        - ring S63.41 ☑
      - index S63.40 ☑
      - little S63.40 ☑
      - middle S63.40 ☑
      - palmar S63.42 ☑
        - index S63.42 ☑
        - little S63.42 ☑
        - middle S63.42 ☑
        - ring S63.42 ☑
      - ring S63.40 ☑
      - specified site NEC S63.499 ☑
        - index S63.49 ☑
        - little S63.49 ☑
        - middle S63.49 ☑
        - ring S63.49 ☑
      - volar plate S63.43 ☑
        - index S63.43 ☑
        - little S63.43 ☑
        - middle S63.43 ☑
        - ring S63.43 ☑
    - foot — *see* Sprain, foot
    - radial collateral S53.2 ☑
    - radiocarpal — *see* Rupture, traumatic, ligament, wrist, radiocarpal
    - ulnar collateral S53.3 ☑
    - ulnocarpal — *see* Rupture, traumatic, ligament, wrist, ulnocarpal
    - wrist S63.30 ☑
      - collateral S63.31 ☑
      - radiocarpal S63.32 ☑
      - specified site NEC S63.39 ☑
      - ulnocarpal (palmar) S63.33 ☑

- **Rupture** — *continued*
  - traumatic — *continued*
    - liver S36.116 ☑
    - membrana tympani — *see* Rupture, ear drum, traumatic
    - muscle or tendon — *see* Strain
    - myocardium — *see* Injury, heart
    - pancreas S36.299 ☑
    - rectum S36.69 ☑
    - sigmoid S36.593 ☑
    - spleen S36.09 ☑
    - stomach S36.39 ☑
    - symphysis pubis S33.4 ☑
    - tympanum, tympanic (membrane) — *see* Rupture, ear drum, traumatic
    - ureter S37.19 ☑
    - uterus S37.69 ☑
    - vagina — *see* Injury, vagina
    - vena cava — *see* Injury, vena cava, laceration, major
  - tricuspid (heart) (valve) I07.8
  - tube, tubal (nonobstetric) (nontraumatic) N83.8
    - abscess — *see* Salpingitis
    - due to pregnancy O00.10
      - with intrauterine pregnancy O00.11
  - tympanum, tympanic (membrane) (nontraumatic) (*see also* Perforation, tympanic membrane)H72.9 ☑
    - traumatic — *see* Rupture, ear drum, traumatic
  - umbilical cord, complicating delivery O69.89 ☑
  - ureter (traumatic) S37.19 ☑
    - nontraumatic N28.89
  - urethra (nontraumatic) N36.8
    - with ectopic or molar pregnancy O08.6
    - following ectopic or molar pregnancy O08.6
    - obstetrical trauma O71.5
    - traumatic S37.39 ☑
  - uterosacral ligament (nonobstetric) (nontraumatic) N83.8
  - uterus (traumatic) S37.69 ☑
    - before labor O71.0 ☑
    - during or after labor O71.1
    - nonpuerperal, nontraumatic N85.8
    - pregnant (during labor) O71.1
      - before labor O71.0 ☑
  - vagina — *see* Injury, vagina
  - valve, valvular (heart) — *see* Endocarditis
  - varicose vein — *see* Varix
  - varix — *see* Varix
  - vena cava R58
    - traumatic — *see* Injury, vena cava, laceration, major
  - vesical (urinary) N32.89
  - vessel (blood) R58
    - pulmonary I28.8
    - traumatic — *see* Injury, blood vessel
  - viscus R19.8
  - vulva complicating delivery O70.0
- **Russell-Silver** syndrome Q87.1
- **Russian** spring-summer type encephalitis A84.0
- **Rust's** disease (tuberculous cervical spondylitis) A18.01
- **Ruvalcaba-Myhre-Smith** syndrome E71.440
- **Rytand-Lipsitch** syndrome I44.2

S

- **Saber,** sabre shin or tibia (syphilitic) A50.56 *[M90.8-]*
- **Sac** lacrimal — *see* condition
- **Saccharomyces** infection B37.9
- **Saccharopinuria** E72.3
- **Saccular** — *see* condition
- **Sacculation**
  - aorta (nonsyphilitic) — *see* Aneurysm, aorta
  - bladder N32.3
  - intralaryngeal (congenital) (ventricular) Q31.3
  - larynx (congenital) (ventricular) Q31.3
  - organ or site, congenital — *see* Distortion
  - pregnant uterus — *see* Pregnancy, complicated by, abnormal, uterus
  - ureter N28.89
  - urethra N36.1
  - vesical N32.3
- **Sachs'** amaurotic familial idiocy or disease E75.02
- **Sachs-Tay** disease E75.02
- **Sacks-Libman** disease M32.11
- **Sacralgia** M53.3
- **Sacralization** Q76.49
- **Sacrodynia** M53.3
- **Sacroiliac** joint — *see* condition
- **Sacroiliitis** NEC M46.1
- **Sacrum** — *see* condition
- **Saddle**
  - back — *see* Lordosis
  - embolus
    - abdominal aorta I74.01
    - pulmonary artery I26.92
      - with acute cor pulmonale I26.02
  - injury - code to condition
  - nose M95.0
    - due to syphilis A50.57
- **Sadism** (sexual) F65.52
- **Sadness,** postpartal O90.6
- **Sadomasochism** F65.50
- **Saemisch's** ulcer (cornea) — *see* Ulcer, cornea, central
- **Sagging**
  - skin and subcutaneous tissue (following bariatric surgery weight loss) (following dietary weight loss) L98.7
- **Sahib** disease B55.0
- **Sailors'** skin L57.8
- **Saint**
  - Anthony's fire — *see* Erysipelas
  - triad — *see* Hernia, diaphragm
  - Vitus' dance — *see* Chorea, Sydenham's
- **Salaam**
  - attack (s) — *see* Epilepsy, spasms
  - tic R25.8
- **Salicylism**
  - abuse F55.8
  - overdose or wrong substance given — *see* Table of Drugs and Chemicals, by drug, poisoning
- **Salivary** duct or gland — *see* condition
- **Salivation,** excessive K11.7
- **Salmonella** — *see* Infection, Salmonella
- **Salmonellosis** A02.0
- **Salpingitis** (catarrhal) (fallopian tube) (nodular) (pseudofollicular) (purulent) (septic) N70.91
  - with oophoritis N70.93
  - acute N70.01
    - with oophoritis N70.03
  - chlamydial A56.11
  - chronic N70.11
    - with oophoritis N70.13
  - complicating abortion — *see* Abortion, by type, complicated by, salpingitis
  - ear — *see* Salpingitis, eustachian
  - eustachian (tube) H68.00 ☑
    - acute H68.01 ☑
    - chronic H68.02 ☑
  - follicularis N70.11
    - with oophoritis N70.13
  - gonococcal (acute) (chronic) A54.24
  - interstitial, chronic N70.11
    - with oophoritis N70.13
  - isthmica nodosa N70.11
    - with oophoritis N70.13
  - specific (gonococcal) (acute) (chronic) A54.24
  - tuberculous (acute) (chronic) A18.17
  - venereal (gonococcal) (acute) (chronic) A54.24
- **Salpingocele** N83.4 ☑
- **Salpingo-oophoritis** (catarrhal) (purulent) (ruptured) (septic) (suppurative) N70.93
  - acute N70.03
    - with ectopic or molar pregnancy O08.0
    - following ectopic or molar pregnancy O08.0
    - gonococcal A54.24
  - chronic N70.13
  - following ectopic or molar pregnancy O08.0
  - gonococcal (acute) (chronic) A54.24
  - puerperal O86.19
  - specific (gonococcal) (acute) (chronic) A54.24
  - subacute N70.03
  - tuberculous (acute) (chronic) A18.17
  - venereal (gonococcal) (acute) (chronic) A54.24
- **Salpingo-ovaritis** — *see* Salpingo-oophoritis
- **Salpingoperitonitis** — *see* Salpingo-oophoritis
- **Salzmann's** nodular dystrophy — *see* Degeneration, cornea, nodular
- **Sampson's** cyst or tumor N80.1
- **San** Joaquin (Valley) fever B38.0
- **Sandblaster's** asthma, lung or pneumoconiosis J62.8
- **Sander's** disease (paranoia) F22
- **Sandfly** fever A93.1
- **Sandhoff's** disease E75.01
- **Sanfilippo** (Type B) (Type C) (Type D) syndrome E76.22
- **Sanger-Brown** ataxia G11.2
- **Sao** Paulo fever or typhus A77.0
- **Saponification,** mesenteric K65.8
- **Sarcocele** (benign)
  - syphilitic A52.76
    - congenital A50.59
- **Sarcocystosis** A07.8
- **Sarcoepiplocele** — *see* Hernia
- **Sarcoepiplomphalocele** Q79.2
- **Sarcoid** (*see also* Sarcoidosis)
  - arthropathy D86.86
  - Boeck's D86.9
  - Darier-Roussy D86.3
  - iridocyclitis D86.83
  - meningitis D86.81
  - myocarditis D86.85
  - myositis D86.87
  - pyelonephritis D86.84
  - Spiegler-Fendt L08.89
- **Sarcoidosis** D86.9
  - with
    - cranial nerve palsies D86.82
    - hepatic granuloma D86.89
    - polyarthritis D86.86
    - tubulo-interstitial nephropathy D86.84
  - combined sites NEC D86.89
  - lung D86.0
    - and lymph nodes D86.2
  - lymph nodes D86.1
    - and lung D86.2
  - meninges D86.81
  - skin D86.3
  - specified type NEC D86.89
- **Sarcoma** (of) (*see also* Neoplasm, connective tissue, malignant)
  - alveolar soft part — *see* Neoplasm, connective tissue, malignant
  - ameloblastic C41.1
    - upper jaw (bone) C41.0
  - botryoid — *see* Neoplasm, connective tissue, malignant
  - botryoides — *see* Neoplasm, connective tissue, malignant
  - cerebellar C71.6
    - circumscribed (arachnoidal) C71.6
  - circumscribed (arachnoidal) cerebellar C71.6
  - clear cell (*see also* Neoplasm, connective tissue, malignant)
    - kidney C64. ☑
  - dendritic cells (accessory cells) C96.4
  - embryonal — *see* Neoplasm, connective tissue, malignant
  - endometrial (stromal) C54.1
    - isthmus C54.0
  - epithelioid (cell) — *see* Neoplasm, connective tissue, malignant
  - Ewing's — *see* Neoplasm, bone, malignant
  - follicular dendritic cell C96.4
  - germinoblastic (diffuse) — *see* Lymphoma, diffuse large cell
    - follicular — *see* Lymphoma, follicular, specified NEC
  - giant cell (except of bone) (*see also* Neoplasm, connective tissue, malignant)
    - bone — *see* Neoplasm, bone, malignant
  - glomoid — *see* Neoplasm, connective tissue, malignant
  - granulocytic C92.3 ☑
  - hemangioendothelial — *see* Neoplasm, connective tissue, malignant
  - hemorrhagic, multiple — *see* Sarcoma, Kaposi's
  - histiocytic C96.A
  - Hodgkin — *see* Lymphoma, Hodgkin
  - immunoblastic (diffuse) — *see* Lymphoma, diffuse large cell
  - interdigitating dendritic cell C96.4
  - Kaposi's
    - colon C46.4
    - connective tissue C46.1
    - gastrointestinal organ C46.4
    - lung C46.5 ☑
    - lymph node (s) C46.3
    - palate (hard) (soft) C46.2
    - rectum C46.4
    - skin C46.0
    - specified site NEC C46.7
    - stomach C46.4
    - unspecified site C46.9
  - Kupffer cell C22.3
  - Langerhans cell C96.4
  - leptomeningeal — *see* Neoplasm, meninges, malignant
  - liver NEC C22.4
  - lymphangioendothelial — *see* Neoplasm, connective tissue, malignant

Sarcoma — *continued*
- lymphoblastic — *see* Lymphoma, lymphoblastic (diffuse)
- lymphocytic — *see* Lymphoma, small cell B-cell
- mast cell C96.2
- melanotic — *see* Melanoma
- meningeal — *see* Neoplasm, meninges, malignant
- meningothelial — *see* Neoplasm, meninges, malignant
- mesenchymal (*see also* Neoplasm, connective tissue, malignant)
  - mixed — *see* Neoplasm, connective tissue, malignant
- mesothelial — *see* Mesothelioma
- monstrocellular
  - specified site — *see* Neoplasm, malignant, by site
  - unspecified site C71.9
- myeloid C92.3 ☑
- neurogenic — *see* Neoplasm, nerve, malignant
- odontogenic C41.1
  - upper jaw (bone) C41.0
- osteoblastic — *see* Neoplasm, bone, malignant
- osteogenic (*see also* Neoplasm, bone, malignant)
  - juxtacortical — *see* Neoplasm, bone, malignant
  - periosteal — *see* Neoplasm, bone, malignant
- periosteal (*see also* Neoplasm, bone, malignant)
  - osteogenic — *see* Neoplasm, bone, malignant
- pleomorphic cell — *see* Neoplasm, connective tissue, malignant
- reticulum cell (diffuse) — *see* Lymphoma, diffuse large cell
  - nodular — *see* Lymphoma, follicular
  - pleomorphic cell type — *see* Lymphoma, diffuse large cell
- rhabdoid — *see* Neoplasm, malignant, by site
- round cell — *see* Neoplasm, connective tissue, malignant
- small cell — *see* Neoplasm, connective tissue, malignant
- soft tissue — *see* Neoplasm, connective tissue, malignant
- spindle cell — *see* Neoplasm, connective tissue, malignant
- stromal (endometrial) C54.1
  - isthmus C54.0
- synovial (*see also* Neoplasm, connective tissue, malignant)
  - biphasic — *see* Neoplasm, connective tissue, malignant
  - epithelioid cell — *see* Neoplasm, connective tissue, malignant
  - spindle cell — *see* Neoplasm, connective tissue, malignant

Sarcomatosis
- meningeal — *see* Neoplasm, meninges, malignant
- specified site NEC — *see* Neoplasm, connective tissue, malignant
- unspecified site C80.1

Sarcopenia (age-related) M62.84
Sarcosinemia E72.59
Sarcosporidiosis (intestinal) A07.8
Satiety, early R68.81
Saturnine — *see* condition
Saturnism
- overdose or wrong substance given or taken — *see* Table of Drugs and Chemicals, by drug, poisoning

Satyriasis F52.8
Sauriasis — *see* Ichthyosis
SBE (subacute bacterial endocarditis) I33.0
Scabs R23.4
Scabies (any site) B86
Scaglietti-Dagnini syndrome E22.0
Scald — *see* Burn
Scalenus anticus (anterior) syndrome G54.0
Scales R23.4
Scaling, skin R23.4
Scalp — *see* condition
Scapegoating affecting child Z62.3
Scaphocephaly Q75.0
Scapulalgia M89.8X1
Scapulohumeral myopathy G71.0
Scar, scarring (*see also* Cicatrix)L90.5
- adherent L90.5
- atrophic L90.5
- cervix
  - in pregnancy or childbirth — *see* Pregnancy, complicated by, abnormal cervix
- cheloid L91.0
- chorioretinal H31.00 ☑
  - posterior pole macula H31.01 ☑
  - postsurgical H59.81 ☑
  - solar retinopathy H31.02 ☑
  - specified type NEC H31.09 ☑
- choroid — *see* Scar, chorioretinal
- conjunctiva H11.24 ☑
- cornea H17.9
  - xerophthalmic (*see also* Opacity, cornea)
    - vitamin A deficiency E50.6
- duodenum, obstructive K31.5
- hypertrophic L91.0
- keloid L91.0
- labia N90.89
- lung (base) J98.4
- macula — *see* Scar, chorioretinal, posterior pole
- muscle M62.89
- myocardium, myocardial I25.2
- painful L90.5
- posterior pole (eye) — *see* Scar, chorioretinal, posterior pole
- retina — *see* Scar, chorioretinal
- trachea J39.8
- transmural uterine, in pregnancy O34.29
- uterus N85.8
  - in pregnancy O34.29
- vagina N89.8
  - postoperative N99.2
- vulva N90.89

Scarabiasis B88.2
Scarlatina (anginosa) (maligna) (ulcerosa) A38.9
- myocarditis (acute) A38.1
  - old — *see* Myocarditis
- otitis media A38.0

Scarlet fever (albuminuria) (angina) A38.9
Schamberg's disease (progressive pigmentary dermatosis) L81.7
Schatzki's ring (acquired) (esophagus) (lower) K22.2
- congenital Q39.3

Schaufenster krankheit I20.8
Schaumann's
- benign lymphogranulomatosis D86.1
- disease or syndrome — *see* Sarcoidosis

Scheie's syndrome E76.03
Schenck's disease B42.1
Scheuermann's disease or osteochondrosis — *see* Osteochondrosis, juvenile, spine
Schilder (-Flatau) disease G37.0
Schilling-type monocytic leukemia C93.0 ☑
Schimmelbusch's disease, cystic mastitis, or hyperplasia — *see* Mastopathy, cystic
Schistosoma infestation — *see* Infestation, Schistosoma
Schistosomiasis B65.9
- with muscle disorder B65.9 *[M63.80]*
  - ankle B65.9 *[M63.87-]*
  - foot B65.9 *[M63.87-]*
  - forearm B65.9 *[M63.83-]*
  - hand B65.9 *[M63.84-]*
  - lower leg B65.9 *[M63.86-]*
  - multiple sites B65.9 *[M63.89]*
  - pelvic region B65.9 *[M63.85-]*
  - shoulder region B65.9 *[M63.81-]*
  - specified site NEC B65.9 *[M63.88]*
  - thigh B65.9 *[M63.85-]*
  - upper arm B65.9 *[M63.82-]*
- Asiatic B65.2
- bladder B65.0
- chestermani B65.8
- colon B65.1
- cutaneous B65.3
- due to
  - S. haematobium B65.0
  - S. japonicum B65.2
  - S. mansoni B65.1
  - S. mattheii B65.8
- Eastern B65.2
- genitourinary tract B65.0
- intestinal B65.1
- lung NEC B65.9 *[J99]*
  - pneumonia B65.9 *[J17]*
- Manson's (intestinal) B65.1
- oriental B65.2
- pulmonary NEC B65.9 *[J99]*
  - pneumonia B65.9
- Schistosoma
  - haematobium B65.0
  - japonicum B65.2
  - mansoni B65.1
- specified type NEC B65.8
- urinary B65.0
- vesical B65.0

Schizencephaly Q04.6
Schizoaffective psychosis F25.9
Schizodontia K00.2
Schizoid personality F60.1
Schizophrenia, schizophrenic F20.9
- acute (brief) (undifferentiated) F23
- atypical (form) F20.3
- borderline F21
- catalepsy F20.2
- catatonic (type) (excited) (withdrawn) F20.2
- cenesthopathic, cenesthesiopathic F20.89
- childhood type F84.5
- chronic undifferentiated F20.5
- cyclic F25.0
- disorganized (type) F20.1
- flexibilitas cerea F20.2
- hebephrenic (type) F20.1
- incipient F21
- latent F21
- negative type F20.5
- paranoid (type) F20.0
- paraphrenic F20.0
- post-psychotic depression F32.89
- prepsychotic F21
- prodromal F21
- pseudoneurotic F21
- pseudopsychopathic F21
- reaction F23
- residual (state) (type) F20.5
- restzustand F20.5
- schizoaffective (type) — *see* Psychosis, schizoaffective
- simple (type) F20.89
- simplex F20.89
- specified type NEC F20.89
- stupor F20.2
- syndrome of childhood F84.5
- undifferentiated (type) F20.3
  - chronic F20.5

Schizothymia (persistent) F60.1
Schlatter-Osgood disease or osteochondrosis — *see* Osteochondrosis, juvenile, tibia
Schlatter's tibia — *see* Osteochondrosis, juvenile, tibia
Schmidt's syndrome (polyglandular, autoimmune) E31.0
Schmincke's carcinoma or tumor — *see* Neoplasm, nasopharynx, malignant
Schmitz (-Stutzer) dysentery A03.0
Schmorl's disease or nodes
- lumbar region M51.46
- lumbosacral region M51.47
- sacrococcygeal region M53.3
- thoracic region M51.44
- thoracolumbar region M51.45

Schneiderian
- papilloma — *see* Neoplasm, nasopharynx, benign
  - specified site — *see* Neoplasm, benign, by site
  - unspecified site D14.0
- specified site — *see* Neoplasm, malignant, by site
  - unspecified site C30.0

Scholte's syndrome (malignant carcinoid) E34.0
Scholz (-Bielchowsky-Henneberg) disease or syndrome E75.25
Schönlein (-Henoch) disease or purpura (primary) (rheumatic) D69.0
Schottmuller's disease A01.4
Schroeder's syndrome (endocrine hypertensive) E27.0
Schüller-Christian disease or syndrome C96.5
Schultze's type acroparesthesia, simple I73.89
Schultz's disease or syndrome — *see* Agranulocytosis
Schwalbe-Ziehen-Oppenheim disease G24.1
Schwannoma (*see also* Neoplasm, nerve, benign)
- malignant (*see also* Neoplasm, nerve, malignant)
  - with rhabdomyoblastic differentiation — *see* Neoplasm, nerve, malignant
- melanocytic — *see* Neoplasm, nerve, benign
- pigmented — *see* Neoplasm, nerve, benign

Schwannomatosis Q85.03
Schwartz (-Jampel) syndrome G71.13
Schwartz-Bartter syndrome E22.2
Schweniger-Buzzi anetoderma L90.1
Sciatic — *see* condition
Sciatica (infective)
- with lumbago M54.4 ☑
  - due to intervertebral disc disorder — *see* Disorder, disc, with, radiculopathy
- due to displacement of intervertebral disc (with lumbago) — *see* Disorder, disc, with, radiculopathy
- wallet M54.3 ☑

Scimitar - Scratchy

- **Scimitar** syndrome Q26.8
- **Sclera** — *see* condition
- **Sclerectasia** H15.84 ☑
- **Scleredema**
  - adultorum — *see* Sclerosis, systemic
  - Buschke's — *see* Sclerosis, systemic
  - newborn P83.0
- **Sclerema** (adiposum) (edematosum) (neonatorum) (newborn) P83.0
  - adultorum — *see* Sclerosis, systemic
- **Scleriasis** — *see* Scleroderma
- **Scleritis** H15.00 ☑
  - with corneal involvement H15.04 ☑
  - anterior H15.01 ☑
  - brawny H15.02 ☑
  - in (due to) zoster B02.34
  - posterior H15.03 ☑
  - specified type NEC H15.09 ☑
  - syphilitic A52.71
  - tuberculous (nodular) A18.51
- **Sclerochoroiditis** H31.8
- **Scleroconjunctivitis** — *see* Scleritis
- **Sclerocystic** ovary syndrome E28.2
- **Sclerodactyly,** sclerodactylia L94.3
- **Scleroderma,** sclerodermia (acrosclerotic) (diffuse) (generalized) (progressive) (pulmonary) (*see also* Sclerosis, systemic)M34.9
  - circumscribed L94.0
  - linear L94.1
  - localized L94.0
  - newborn P83.8
  - systemic M34.9
- **Sclerokeratitis** H16.8
  - tuberculous A18.52
- **Scleroma** nasi A48.8
- **Scleromalacia** (perforans) H15.05 ☑
- **Scleromyxedema** L98.5
- **Sclérose** en plaques G35
- **Sclerosis,** sclerotic
  - adrenal (gland) E27.8
  - Alzheimer's — *see* Disease, Alzheimer's
  - amyotrophic (lateral) G12.21
  - aorta, aortic I70.0
    - valve — *see* Endocarditis, aortic
  - artery, arterial, arteriolar, arteriovascular — *see* Arteriosclerosis
  - ascending multiple G35
  - brain (generalized) (lobular) G37.9
    - artery, arterial I67.2
    - diffuse G37.0
    - disseminated G35
    - insular G35
    - Krabbe's E75.23
    - miliary G35
    - multiple G35
    - presenile (Alzheimer's) — *see* Disease, Alzheimer's, early onset
    - senile (arteriosclerotic) I67.2
    - stem, multiple G35
    - tuberous Q85.1
  - bulbar, multiple G35
  - bundle of His I44.39
  - cardiac — *see* Disease, heart, ischemic, atherosclerotic
  - cardiorenal — *see* Hypertension, cardiorenal
  - cardiovascular (*see also* Disease, cardiovascular)
    - renal — *see* Hypertension, cardiorenal
  - cerebellar — *see* Sclerosis, brain
  - cerebral — *see* Sclerosis, brain
  - cerebrospinal (disseminated) (multiple) G35
  - cerebrovascular I67.2
  - choroid — *see* Degeneration, choroid
  - combined (spinal cord) (*see also* Degeneration, combined)
    - multiple G35
  - concentric (Balo) G37.5
  - cornea — *see* Opacity, cornea
  - coronary (artery) I25.10
    - with angina pectoris — *see* Arteriosclerosis, coronary (artery),
  - corpus cavernosum
    - female N90.89
    - male N48.6
  - diffuse (brain) (spinal cord) G37.0
  - disseminated G35
  - dorsal G35
  - dorsolateral (spinal cord) — *see* Degeneration, combined
  - endometrium N85.5
  - extrapyramidal G25.9
  - eye, nuclear (senile) — *see* Cataract, senile, nuclear

Sclerosis — *continued*

  - focal and segmental (glomerular) (*see also* N00-N07 with fourth character .1)N05.1
  - Friedreich's (spinal cord) G11.1
  - funicular (spermatic cord) N50.89
  - general (vascular) — *see* Arteriosclerosis
  - gland (lymphatic) I89.8
  - hepatic K74.1
    - alcoholic K70.2
  - hereditary
    - cerebellar G11.9
    - spinal (Friedreich's ataxia) G11.1
  - hippocampal G93.81
  - insular G35
  - kidney — *see* Sclerosis, renal
  - larynx J38.7
  - lateral (amyotrophic) (descending) (primary) (spinal) G12.21
  - lens, senile nuclear — *see* Cataract, senile, nuclear
  - liver K74.1
    - with fibrosis K74.2
      - alcoholic K70.2
    - alcoholic K70.2
    - cardiac K76.1
  - lung — *see* Fibrosis, lung
  - mastoid — *see* Mastoiditis, chronic
  - mesial temporal G93.81
  - mitral I05.8
  - Mönckeberg's (medial) — *see* Arteriosclerosis, extremities
  - multiple (brain stem) (cerebral) (generalized) (spinal cord) G35
  - myocardium, myocardial — *see* Disease, heart, ischemic, atherosclerotic
  - nuclear (senile), eye — *see* Cataract, senile, nuclear
  - ovary N83.8
  - pancreas K86.89
  - penis N48.6
  - peripheral arteries — *see* Arteriosclerosis, extremities
  - plaques G35
  - pluriglandular E31.8
  - polyglandular E31.8
  - posterolateral (spinal cord) — *see* Degeneration, combined
  - presenile (Alzheimer's) — *see* Disease, Alzheimer's, early onset
  - primary, lateral G12.29
  - progressive, systemic M34.0
  - pulmonary — *see* Fibrosis, lung
    - artery I27.0
    - valve (heart) — *see* Endocarditis, pulmonary
  - renal N26.9
    - with
      - cystine storage disease E72.09
      - hypertensive heart disease (conditions in I11) — *see* Hypertension, cardiorenal
    - arteriolar (hyaline) (hyperplastic) — *see* Hypertension, kidney
  - retina (senile) (vascular) H35.00
  - senile (vascular) — *see* Arteriosclerosis
  - spinal (cord) (progressive) G95.89
    - ascending G61.0
    - combined (*see also* Degeneration, combined)
      - multiple G35
      - syphilitic A52.11
    - disseminated G35
    - dorsolateral — *see* Degeneration, combined
    - hereditary (Friedreich's) (mixed form) G11.1
    - lateral (amyotrophic) G12.21
    - multiple G35
    - posterior (syphilitic) A52.11
  - stomach K31.89
  - subendocardial, congenital I42.4
  - systemic M34.9
    - with
      - lung involvement M34.81
      - myopathy M34.82
      - polyneuropathy M34.83
    - drug-induced M34.2
    - due to chemicals NEC M34.2
    - progressive M34.0
    - specified NEC M34.89
  - temporal (mesial) G93.81
  - tricuspid (heart) (valve) I07.8
  - tuberous (brain) Q85.1
  - tympanic membrane — *see* Disorder, tympanic membrane, specified NEC
  - valve, valvular (heart) — *see* Endocarditis
  - vascular — *see* Arteriosclerosis
  - vein I87.8

- **Scoliosis** (acquired) (postural) M41.9
  - adolescent (idiopathic) — *see* Scoliosis, idiopathic, adolescent
  - congenital Q67.5
    - due to bony malformation Q76.3
    - failure of segmentation (hemivertebra) Q76.3
    - hemivertebra fusion Q76.3
    - postural Q67.5
  - idiopathic M41.20
    - adolescent M41.129
      - cervical region M41.122
      - cervicothoracic region M41.123
      - lumbar region M41.126
      - lumbosacral region M41.127
      - thoracic region M41.124
      - thoracolumbar region M41.125
    - cervical region M41.22
    - cervicothoracic region M41.23
    - infantile M41.00
      - cervical region M41.02
      - cervicothoracic region M41.03
      - lumbar region M41.06
      - lumbosacral region M41.07
      - sacrococcygeal region M41.08
      - thoracic region M41.04
      - thoracolumbar region M41.05
    - juvenile M41.119
      - cervical region M41.112
      - cervicothoracic region M41.113
      - lumbar region M41.116
      - lumbosacral region M41.117
      - thoracic region M41.114
      - thoracolumbar region M41.115
    - lumbar region M41.26
    - lumbosacral region M41.27
    - thoracic region M41.24
    - thoracolumbar region M41.25
  - infantile — *see* Scoliosis, idiopathic, infantile
  - neuromuscular M41.40
    - cervical region M41.42
    - cervicothoracic region M41.43
    - lumbar region M41.46
    - lumbosacral region M41.47
    - occipito-atlanto-axial region M41.41
    - thoracic region M41.44
    - thoracolumbar region M41.45
  - paralytic — *see* Scoliosis, neuromuscular
  - postradiation therapy M96.5
  - rachitic (late effect or sequelae) E64.3 *[M49.80]*
    - cervical region E64.3 *[M49.82]*
    - cervicothoracic region E64.3 *[M49.83]*
    - lumbar region E64.3 *[M49.86]*
    - lumbosacral region E64.3 *[M49.87]*
    - multiple sites E64.3 *[M49.89]*
    - occipito-atlanto-axial region E64.3 *[M49.81]*
    - sacrococcygeal region E64.3 *[M49.88]*
    - thoracic region E64.3 *[M49.84]*
    - thoracolumbar region E64.3 *[M49.85]*
  - sciatic M54.4 ☑
  - secondary (to) NEC M41.50
    - cerebral palsy, Friedreich's ataxia, poliomyelitis, neuromuscular disorders — *see* Scoliosis, neuromuscular
    - cervical region M41.52
    - cervicothoracic region M41.53
    - lumbar region M41.56
    - lumbosacral region M41.57
    - thoracic region M41.54
    - thoracolumbar region M41.55
  - specified form NEC M41.80
    - cervical region M41.82
    - cervicothoracic region M41.83
    - lumbar region M41.86
    - lumbosacral region M41.87
    - thoracic region M41.84
    - thoracolumbar region M41.85
  - thoracogenic M41.30
    - thoracic region M41.34
    - thoracolumbar region M41.35
  - tuberculous A18.01
- **Scoliotic** pelvis
  - with disproportion (fetopelvic) O33.0
    - causing obstructed labor O65.0
- **Scorbutus,** scorbutic (*see also* Scurvy)
  - anemia D53.2
- **Score,** NIHSS (National Institutes of Health Stroke Scale) R29.7 ☑
- **Scotoma** (arcuate) (Bjerrum) (central) (ring) (*see also* Defect, visual field, localized, scotoma)
  - scintillating H53.19
- **Scratch** — *see* Abrasion
- **Scratchy** throat R09.89

- **Screening** (for) Z13.9
  - alcoholism Z13.89
  - anemia Z13.0
  - anomaly, congenital Z13.89
  - antenatal, of mother Z36
  - arterial hypertension Z13.6
  - arthropod-borne viral disease NEC Z11.59
  - bacteriuria, asymptomatic Z13.89
  - behavioral disorder Z13.89
  - brain injury, traumatic Z13.850
  - bronchitis, chronic Z13.83
  - brucellosis Z11.2
  - cardiovascular disorder Z13.6
  - cataract Z13.5
  - chlamydial diseases Z11.8
  - cholera Z11.0
  - chromosomal abnormalities (nonprocreative) NEC Z13.79
  - colonoscopy Z12.11
  - congenital
    - dislocation of hip Z13.89
    - eye disorder Z13.5
    - malformation or deformation Z13.89
  - contamination NEC Z13.88
  - cystic fibrosis Z13.228
  - dengue fever Z11.59
  - dental disorder Z13.84
  - depression Z13.89
  - developmental handicap Z13.42
    - in early childhood Z13.42
    - infant Z13.41
  - diabetes mellitus Z13.1
  - diphtheria Z11.2
  - disability, intellectual Z13.42
    - infant Z13.41
  - disease or disorder Z13.9
    - bacterial NEC Z11.2
      - intestinal infectious Z11.0
      - respiratory tuberculosis Z11.1
    - blood or blood-forming organ Z13.0
    - cardiovascular Z13.6
    - Chagas' Z11.6
    - chlamydial Z11.8
    - dental Z13.89
    - developmental Z13.42
      - in child Z13.42
      - infant Z13.41
    - digestive tract NEC Z13.818
      - lower GI Z13.811
      - upper GI Z13.810
    - ear Z13.5
    - endocrine Z13.29
    - eye Z13.5
    - genitourinary Z13.89
    - heart Z13.6
    - human immunodeficiency virus (HIV) infection Z11.4
    - immunity Z13.0
    - infection
      - intestinal Z11.0
        - specified NEC Z11.6
    - infectious Z11.9
    - mental Z13.89
    - metabolic Z13.228
    - neurological Z13.89
    - nutritional Z13.21
      - metabolic Z13.228
        - lipoid disorders Z13.220
    - protozoal Z11.6
      - intestinal Z11.0
    - respiratory Z13.83
    - rheumatic Z13.828
    - rickettsial Z11.8
    - sexually-transmitted NEC Z11.3
      - human immunodeficiency virus (HIV) Z11.4
    - sickle-cell (trait) Z13.0
    - skin Z13.89
    - specified NEC Z13.89
    - spirochetal Z11.8
    - thyroid Z13.29
    - vascular Z13.6
    - venereal Z11.3
    - viral NEC Z11.59
      - human immunodeficiency virus (HIV) Z11.4
      - intestinal Z11.0
  - elevated titer Z13.89
  - emphysema Z13.83
  - encephalitis, viral (mosquito- or tick-borne) Z11.59
  - exposure to contaminants (toxic) Z13.88
  - fever
    - dengue Z11.59

- **Screening** — *continued*
  - fever — *continued*
    - hemorrhagic Z11.59
    - yellow Z11.59
  - filariasis Z11.6
  - galactosemia Z13.228
  - gastrointestinal condition Z13.818
  - genetic (nonprocreative) - for procreative management — *see* Testing, genetic, for procreative management
    - disease carrier status (nonprocreative) Z13.71
    - specified NEC (nonprocreative) Z13.79
  - genitourinary condition Z13.89
  - glaucoma Z13.5
  - gonorrhea Z11.3
  - gout Z13.89
  - helminthiasis (intestinal) Z11.6
  - hematopoietic malignancy Z12.89
  - hemoglobinopathies NEC Z13.0
  - hemorrhagic fever Z11.59
  - Hodgkin disease Z12.89
  - human immunodeficiency virus (HIV) Z11.4
  - human papillomavirus Z11.51
  - hypertension Z13.6
  - immunity disorders Z13.0
  - infection
    - mycotic Z11.8
    - parasitic Z11.8
  - ingestion of radioactive substance Z13.88
  - intellectual disability Z13.42
    - infant Z13.41
  - intestinal
    - helminthiasis Z11.6
    - infectious disease Z11.0
  - leishmaniasis Z11.6
  - leprosy Z11.2
  - leptospirosis Z11.8
  - leukemia Z12.89
  - lymphoma Z12.89
  - malaria Z11.6
  - malnutrition Z13.29
    - metabolic Z13.228
    - nutritional Z13.21
  - measles Z11.59
  - mental disorder Z13.89
  - metabolic errors, inborn Z13.228
  - multiphasic Z13.89
  - musculoskeletal disorder Z13.828
    - osteoporosis Z13.820
  - mycoses Z11.8
  - myocardial infarction (acute) Z13.6
  - neoplasm (malignant) (of) Z12.9
    - bladder Z12.6
    - blood Z12.89
    - breast Z12.39
      - routine mammogram Z12.31
    - cervix Z12.4
    - colon Z12.11
    - genitourinary organs NEC Z12.79
      - bladder Z12.6
      - cervix Z12.4
      - ovary Z12.73
      - prostate Z12.5
      - testis Z12.71
      - vagina Z12.72
    - hematopoietic system Z12.89
    - intestinal tract Z12.10
      - colon Z12.11
      - rectum Z12.12
      - small intestine Z12.13
    - lung Z12.2
    - lymph (glands) Z12.89
    - nervous system Z12.82
    - oral cavity Z12.81
    - prostate Z12.5
    - rectum Z12.12
    - respiratory organs Z12.2
    - skin Z12.83
    - small intestine Z12.13
    - specified site NEC Z12.89
    - stomach Z12.0
  - nephropathy Z13.89
  - nervous system disorders NEC Z13.858
  - neurological condition Z13.89
  - osteoporosis Z13.820
  - parasitic infestation Z11.9
    - specified NEC Z11.8
  - phenylketonuria Z13.228
  - plague Z11.2
  - poisoning (chemical) (heavy metal) Z13.88
  - poliomyelitis Z11.59
  - postnatal, chromosomal abnormalities Z13.89

- **Screening** — *continued*
  - prenatal, of mother Z36
  - protozoal disease Z11.6
    - intestinal Z11.0
  - pulmonary tuberculosis Z11.1
  - radiation exposure Z13.88
  - respiratory condition Z13.83
  - respiratory tuberculosis Z11.1
  - rheumatoid arthritis Z13.828
  - rubella Z11.59
  - schistosomiasis Z11.6
  - sexually-transmitted disease NEC Z11.3
    - human immunodeficiency virus (HIV) Z11.4
  - sickle-cell disease or trait Z13.0
  - skin condition Z13.89
  - sleeping sickness Z11.6
  - special Z13.9
    - specified NEC Z13.89
  - syphilis Z11.3
  - tetanus Z11.2
  - trachoma Z11.8
  - traumatic brain injury Z13.850
  - trypanosomiasis Z11.6
  - tuberculosis, respiratory Z11.1
  - venereal disease Z11.3
  - viral encephalitis (mosquito- or tick-borne) Z11.59
  - whooping cough Z11.2
  - worms, intestinal Z11.6
  - yaws Z11.8
  - yellow fever Z11.59
- **Scrofula,** scrofulosis (tuberculosis of cervical lymph glands) A18.2
- **Scrofulide** (primary) (tuberculous) A18.4
- **Scrofuloderma,** scrofulodermia (any site) (primary) A18.4
- **Scrofulosus** lichen (primary) (tuberculous) A18.4
- **Scrofulous** — *see* condition
- **Scrotal** tongue K14.5
- **Scrotum** — *see* condition
- **Scurvy,** scorbutic E54
  - anemia D53.2
  - gum E54
  - infantile E54
  - rickets E55.0 *[M90.80]*
- **Sealpox** B08.62
- **Seasickness** T75.3 ☑
- **Seatworm** (infection) (infestation) B80
- **Sebaceous** (*see also* condition)
  - cyst — *see* Cyst, sebaceous
- **Seborrhea,** seborrheic L21.9
  - capillitii R23.8
  - capitis L21.0
  - dermatitis L21.9
    - infantile L21.1
  - eczema L21.9
    - infantile L21.1
  - sicca L21.0
- **Seckel's** syndrome Q87.1
- **Seclusion,** pupil — *see* Membrane, pupillary
- **Second** hand tobacco smoke exposure (acute) (chronic) Z77.22
  - in the perinatal period P96.81
- **Secondary**
  - dentin (in pulp) K04.3
  - neoplasm, secondaries — *see* Table of Neoplasms, secondary
- **Secretion**
  - antidiuretic hormone, inappropriate E22.2
  - catecholamine, by pheochromocytoma E27.5
  - hormone
    - antidiuretic, inappropriate (syndrome) E22.2
    - by
      - carcinoid tumor E34.0
      - pheochromocytoma E27.5
    - ectopic NEC E34.2
  - urinary
    - excessive R35.8
    - suppression R34
- **Section**
  - nerve, traumatic — *see* Injury, nerve
- **Sedative,** hypnotic, or anxiolytic-induced
  - anxiety disorder F13.980
  - bipolar and related disorder F13.94
  - delirium F13.921
  - depressive disorder F13.94
  - major neurocognitive disorder F13.97
  - mild neurocognitive disorder F13.988
  - psychotic disorder F13.959
  - sexual dysfunction F13.981
  - sleep disorder F13.982

Segmentation - Sepsis

- **Sepsis** — *continued*
  - tracheostomy stoma J95.02
  - tularemic A21.7
  - umbilical, umbilical cord (newborn) — *see* Sepsis, newborn
  - Yersinia pestis A20.7
- **Septate** — *see* Septum
- **Septic** — *see* condition
  - arm — *see* Cellulitis, upper limb
    - with lymphangitis — *see* Lymphangitis, acute, upper limb
  - embolus — *see* Embolism
  - finger — *see* Cellulitis, digit
    - with lymphangitis — *see* Lymphangitis, acute, digit
  - foot — *see* Cellulitis, lower limb
    - with lymphangitis — *see* Lymphangitis, acute, lower limb
  - gallbladder (acute) K81.0
  - hand — *see* Cellulitis, upper limb
    - with lymphangitis — *see* Lymphangitis, acute, upper limb
  - joint — *see* Arthritis, pyogenic or pyemic
  - leg — *see* Cellulitis, lower limb
    - with lymphangitis — *see* Lymphangitis, acute, lower limb
  - nail (*see also* Cellulitis, digit)
    - with lymphangitis — *see* Lymphangitis, acute, digit
  - sore (*see also* Abscess)
    - throat J02.0
      - streptococcal J02.0
  - spleen (acute) D73.89
  - teeth, tooth (pulpal origin) K04.4
  - throat — *see* Pharyngitis
  - thrombus — *see* Thrombosis
  - toe — *see* Cellulitis, digit
    - with lymphangitis — *see* Lymphangitis, acute, digit
  - tonsils, chronic J35.01
    - with adenoiditis J35.03
  - uterus — *see* Endometritis
- **Septicemia** A41.9
  - meaning sepsis — *see* Sepsis
- **Septum**, septate (congenital) (*see also* Anomaly, by site)
  - anal Q42.3
    - with fistula Q42.2
  - aqueduct of Sylvius Q03.0
    - with spina bifida — *see* Spina bifida, by site, with hydrocephalus
  - uterus (complete) (partial) Q51.2
  - vagina Q52.10
    - in pregnancy — *see* Pregnancy, complicated by, abnormal vagina
      - causing obstructed labor O65.5
    - longitudinal Q52.129
      - microperforate
        - left side Q52.124
        - right side Q52.123
      - nonobstruction Q52.120
      - obstructing Q52.129
        - left side Q52.122
        - right side Q52.121
    - transverse Q52.11
- **Sequelae** (of) (*see also* condition)
  - abscess, intracranial or intraspinal (conditions in G06) G09
  - amputation -- code to injury with seventh character S
  - burn and corrosion -- code to injury with seventh character S
  - calcium deficiency E64.8
  - cerebrovascular disease — *see* Sequelae, disease, cerebrovascular
  - childbirth O94
  - contusion -- code to injury with seventh character S
  - corrosion — *see* Sequelae, burn and corrosion
  - crushing injury -- code to injury with seventh character S
  - disease
    - cerebrovascular I69.90
      - alteration of sensation I69.998
      - aphasia I69.920
      - apraxia I69.990
      - ataxia I69.993
      - cognitive deficits I69.91 ☑
      - disturbance of vision I69.998
      - dysarthria I69.922
      - dysphagia I69.991
      - dysphasia I69.921

- **Sequelae** — *continued*
  - disease — *continued*
      - facial droop I69.992
      - facial weakness I69.992
      - fluency disorder I69.923
      - hemiplegia I69.95 ☑
      - hemorrhage
        - intracerebral — *see* Sequelae, hemorrhage, intracerebral
        - intracranial, nontraumatic NEC — *see* Sequelae, hemorrhage, intracranial, nontraumatic
        - subarachnoid — *see* Sequelae, hemorrhage, subarachnoid
      - language deficit I69.928
      - monoplegia
        - lower limb I69.84 ☑
        - upper limb I69.93 ☑
      - paralytic syndrome I69.96 ☑
      - specified effect NEC I69.998
      - specified type NEC I69.80
        - alteration of sensation I69.898
        - aphasia I69.820
        - apraxia I69.890
        - ataxia I69.893
        - cognitive deficits I69.81 ☑
        - disturbance of vision I69.898
        - dysarthria I69.822
        - dysphagia I69.891
        - dysphasia I69.821
        - facial droop I69.892
        - facial weakness I69.892
        - fluency disorder I69.823
        - hemiplegia I69.85 ☑
        - language deficit I69.828
        - monoplegia
          - lower limb I69.84 ☑
          - upper limb I69.83 ☑
        - paralytic syndrome I69.86 ☑
        - specified effect NEC I69.898
      - speech deficit I69.928
        - speech deficit I69.828
      - stroke NOS — *see* Sequelae, stroke NOS
  - dislocation -- code to injury with seventh character S
  - encephalitis or encephalomyelitis (conditions in G04) G09
    - in infectious disease NEC B94.8
    - viral B94.1
  - external cause -- code to injury with seventh character S
  - foreign body entering natural orifice -- code to injury with seventh character S
  - fracture -- code to injury with seventh character S
  - frostbite -- code to injury with seventh character S
  - Hansen's disease B92
  - hemorrhage
    - intracerebral I69.10
      - alteration of sensation I69.198
      - aphasia I69.120
      - apraxia I69.190
      - ataxia I69.193
      - cognitive deficits I69.11 ☑
      - disturbance of vision I69.198
      - dysarthria I69.122
      - dysphagia I69.191
      - dysphasia I69.121
      - facial droop I69.192
      - facial weakness I69.192
      - fluency disorder I69.123
      - hemiplegia I69.15 ☑
      - language deficit NEC I69.128
      - monoplegia
        - lower limb I69.14 ☑
        - upper limb I69.13 ☑
      - paralytic syndrome I69.16 ☑
      - specified effect NEC I69.198
      - speech deficit NEC I69.128
    - intracranial, nontraumatic NEC I69.20
      - alteration of sensation I69.298
      - aphasia I69.220
      - apraxia I69.290
      - ataxia I69.293
      - cognitive deficits I69.21 ☑
      - disturbance of vision I69.298
      - dysarthria I69.222
      - dysphagia I69.291
      - dysphasia I69.221
      - facial droop I69.292
      - facial weakness I69.292
      - fluency disorder I69.223

- **Sequelae** — *continued*
  - hemorrhage — *continued*
      - hemiplegia I69.25 ☑
      - language deficit NEC I69.228
      - monoplegia
        - lower limb I69.24 ☑
        - upper limb I69.23 ☑
      - paralytic syndrome I69.26 ☑
      - specified effect NEC I69.298
      - speech deficit NEC I69.228
    - subarachnoid I69.00
      - alteration of sensation I69.098
      - aphasia I69.020
      - apraxia I69.090
      - ataxia I69.093
      - cognitive deficits — *see* subcategory I69.01-
      - disturbance of vision I69.098
      - dysarthria I69.022
      - dysphagia I69.091
      - dysphasia I69.021
      - facial droop I69.092
      - facial weakness I69.092
      - fluency disorder I69.023
      - hemiplegia I69.05 ☑
      - language deficit NEC I69.028
      - monoplegia
        - lower limb I69.04 ☑
        - upper limb I69.03 ☑
      - paralytic syndrome I69.06 ☑
      - specified effect NEC I69.098
      - speech deficit NEC I69.028
  - hepatitis, viral B94.2
  - hyperalimentation E68
  - infarction
    - cerebral I69.30
      - alteration of sensation I69.398
      - aphasia I69.320
      - apraxia I69.390
      - ataxia I69.393
      - cognitive deficits I69.31 ☑
      - disturbance of vision I69.398
      - dysarthria I69.322
      - dysphagia I69.391
      - dysphasia I69.321
      - facial droop I69.392
      - facial weakness I69.392
      - fluency disorder I69.323
      - hemiplegia I69.35 ☑
      - language deficit NEC I69.328
      - monoplegia
        - lower limb I69.34 ☑
        - upper limb I69.33 ☑
      - paralytic syndrome I69.36 ☑
      - specified effect NEC I69.398
      - speech deficit NEC I69.328
  - infection, pyogenic, intracranial or intraspinal G09
  - infectious disease B94.9
    - specified NEC B94.8
  - injury -- code to injury with seventh character S
  - leprosy B92
  - meningitis
    - bacterial (conditions in G00) G09
    - other or unspecified cause (conditions in G03) G09
  - muscle (and tendon) injury -- code to injury with seventh character S
  - myelitis — *see* Sequelae, encephalitis
  - niacin deficiency E64.8
  - nutritional deficiency E64.9
    - specified NEC E64.8
  - obstetrical condition O94
  - parasitic disease B94.9
  - phlebitis or thrombophlebitis of intracranial or intraspinal venous sinuses and veins (conditions in G08) G09
  - poisoning -- code to poisoning with seventh character S
    - nonmedicinal substance — *see* Sequelae, toxic effect, nonmedicinal substance
  - poliomyelitis (acute) B91
  - pregnancy O94
  - protein-energy malnutrition E64.0
  - puerperium O94
  - rickets E64.3
  - selenium deficiency E64.8
  - sprain and strain -- code to injury with seventh character S
  - stroke NOS I69.30
    - alteration in sensation I69.398
    - aphasia I69.320
    - apraxia I69.390

- **Sequelae** — *continued*
  - stroke NOS — *continued*
    - ataxia I69.393
    - cognitive deficits I69.31 ☑
    - disturbance of vision I69.398
    - dysarthria I69.322
    - dysphagia I69.391
    - dysphasia I69.321
    - facial droop I69.392
    - facial weakness I69.392
    - hemiplegia I69.35 ☑
    - language deficit NEC I69.328
    - monoplegia
      - lower limb I69.34 ☑
      - upper limb I69.33 ☑
    - paralytic syndrome I69.36 ☑
    - specified effect NEC I69.398
    - speech deficit NEC I69.328
  - tendon and muscle injury -- code to injury with seventh character S
  - thiamine deficiency E64.8
  - trachoma B94.0
  - tuberculosis B90.9
    - bones and joints B90.2
    - central nervous system B90.0
    - genitourinary B90.1
    - pulmonary (respiratory) B90.9
    - specified organs NEC B90.8
  - viral
    - encephalitis B94.1
    - hepatitis B94.2
  - vitamin deficiency NEC E64.8
    - A E64.1
    - B E64.8
    - C E64.2
  - wound, open -- code to injury with seventh character S
- **Sequestration** (*see also* Sequestrum)
  - disk — *see* Displacement, intervertebral disk
  - lung, congenital Q33.2
- **Sequestrum**
  - bone — *see* Osteomyelitis, chronic
  - dental M27.2
  - jaw bone M27.2
  - orbit — *see* Osteomyelitis, orbit
  - sinus (accessory) (nasal) — *see* Sinusitis
- **Sequoiosis** lung or pneumonitis J67.8
- **Serology** for syphilis
  - doubtful
    - with signs or symptoms - code by site and stage under Syphilis
    - follow-up of latent syphilis — *see* Syphilis, latent
  - negative, with signs or symptoms - code by site and stage under Syphilis
  - positive A53.0
    - with signs or symptoms - code by site and stage under Syphilis
  - reactivated A53.0
- **Seroma** (*see also* Hematoma)
  - postprocedural — *see* Complication, postprocedural, seroma
  - traumatic, secondary and recurrent T79.2 ☑
- **Seropurulent** — *see* condition
- **Serositis**, multiple K65.8
  - pericardial I31.1
  - peritoneal K65.8
- **Serous** — *see* condition
- **Sertoli** cell
  - adenoma
    - specified site — *see* Neoplasm, benign, by site
    - unspecified site
      - female D27.9
      - male D29.20
  - carcinoma
    - specified site — *see* Neoplasm, malignant, by site
    - unspecified site (male) C62.9 ☑
      - female C56.9
  - tumor
    - with lipid storage
      - specified site — *see* Neoplasm, benign, by site
      - unspecified site
        - female D27.9
        - male D29.20
    - specified site — *see* Neoplasm, benign, by site
    - unspecified site
      - female D27.9
      - male D29.20
- **Sertoli-Leydig** cell tumor — *see* Neoplasm, benign, by site
- **Sertoli-Leydig** cell tumor — *continued*
  - specified site — *see* Neoplasm, benign, by site
  - unspecified site
    - female D27.9
    - male D29.20
- **Serum**
  - allergy, allergic reaction (*see also* Reaction, serum)T80.69 ☑
    - shock (*see also* Shock, anaphylactic)T80.59 ☑
  - arthritis (*see also* Reaction, serum)T80.69 ☑
  - complication or reaction NEC (*see also* Reaction, serum)T80.69 ☑
  - disease NEC (*see also* Reaction, serum)T80.69 ☑
  - hepatitis (*see also* Hepatitis, viral, type B)
    - carrier (suspected) of B18.1
  - intoxication (*see also* Reaction, serum)T80.69 ☑
  - neuritis (*see also* Reaction, serum)T80.69 ☑
  - neuropathy G61.1
  - poisoning NEC (*see also* Reaction, serum)T80.69 ☑
  - rash NEC (*see also* Reaction, serum)T80.69 ☑
  - reaction NEC (*see also* Reaction, serum)T80.69 ☑
  - sickness NEC (*see also* Reaction, serum)T80.69 ☑
  - urticaria (*see also* Reaction, serum)T80.69 ☑
- **Sesamoiditis** M25.8 ☑
- **Sever's** disease or osteochondrosis — *see* Osteochondrosis, juvenile, tarsus
- **Severe** sepsis R65.20
  - with septic shock R65.21
- **Sex**
  - chromosome mosaics Q97.8
    - lines with various numbers of X chromosomes Q97.2
  - education Z70.8
  - reassignment surgery status Z87.890
- **Sextuplet** pregnancy — *see* Pregnancy, sextuplet
- **Sexual**
  - function, disorder of (psychogenic) F52.9
  - immaturity (female) (male) E30.0
  - impotence (psychogenic) organic origin NEC — *see* Dysfunction, sexual, male
  - precocity (constitutional) (cryptogenic) (female) (idiopathic) (male) E30.1
- **Sexuality**, pathologic — *see* Deviation, sexual
- **Sézary** disease C84.1 ☑
- **Shadow**, lung R91.8
- **Shaking** palsy or paralysis — *see* Parkinsonism
- **Shallowness**, acetabulum — *see* Derangement, joint, specified type NEC, hip
- **Shaver's** disease J63.1
- **Sheath** (tendon) — *see* condition
- **Sheathing**, retinal vessels H35.01 ☑
- **Shedding**
  - nail L60.8
  - premature, primary (deciduous) teeth K00.6
- **Sheehan's** disease or syndrome E23.0
- **Shelf**, rectal K62.89
- **Shell** teeth K00.5
- **Shellshock** (current) F43.0
  - lasting state — *see* Disorder, post-traumatic stress
- **Shield** kidney Q63.1
- **Shift**
  - auditory threshold (temporary) H93.24 ☑
  - mediastinal R93.8
- **Shifting** sleep-work schedule (affecting sleep) G47.26
- **Shiga** (-Kruse) dysentery A03.0
- **Shiga's** bacillus A03.0
- **Shigella** (dysentery) — *see* Dysentery, bacillary
- **Shigellosis** A03.9
  - Group A A03.0
  - Group B A03.1
  - Group C A03.2
  - Group D A03.3
- **Shin** splints S86.89 ☑
- **Shingles** — *see* Herpes, zoster
- **Shipyard** disease or eye B30.0
- **Shirodkar** suture, in pregnancy — *see* Pregnancy, complicated by, incompetent cervix
- **Shock** R57.9
  - with ectopic or molar pregnancy O08.3
  - adrenal (cortical) (Addisonian) E27.2
  - adverse food reaction (anaphylactic) — *see* Shock, anaphylactic, due to food
  - allergic — *see* Shock, anaphylactic
  - anaphylactic T78.2 ☑
    - chemical — *see* Table of Drugs and Chemicals
    - due to drug or medicinal substance
      - correct substance properly administered T88.6 ☑
- **Shock** — *continued*
  - anaphylactic — *continued*
      - overdose or wrong substance given or taken (by accident) — *see* Table of Drugs and Chemicals, by drug, poisoning
    - due to food (nonpoisonous) T78.00 ☑
      - additives T78.06 ☑
      - dairy products T78.07 ☑
      - eggs T78.08 ☑
      - fish T78.03 ☑
        - shellfish T78.02 ☑
      - fruit T78.04 ☑
      - milk T78.07 ☑
      - nuts T78.05 ☑
        - multiple types T78.05 ☑
        - peanuts T78.01 ☑
      - peanuts T78.01 ☑
      - seeds T78.05 ☑
      - specified type NEC T78.09 ☑
      - vegetable T78.04 ☑
    - following sting (s) — *see* Venom
    - immunization T80.52 ☑
    - serum T80.59 ☑
      - blood and blood products T80.51 ☑
      - immunization T80.52 ☑
      - specified NEC T80.59 ☑
      - vaccination T80.52 ☑
  - anaphylactoid — *see* Shock, anaphylactic
  - anesthetic
    - correct substance properly administered T88.2 ☑
    - overdose or wrong substance given or taken — *see* Table of Drugs and Chemicals, by drug, poisoning
      - specified anesthetic — *see* Table of Drugs and Chemicals, by drug, poisoning
  - cardiogenic R57.0
  - chemical substance — *see* Table of Drugs and Chemicals
  - complicating ectopic or molar pregnancy O08.3
  - culture — *see* Disorder, adjustment
  - drug
    - due to correct substance properly administered T88.6 ☑
    - overdose or wrong substance given or taken (by accident) — *see* Table of Drugs and Chemicals, by drug, poisoning
  - during or after labor and delivery O75.1
  - electric T75.4 ☑
    - (taser) T75.4 ☑
  - endotoxic R65.21
    - postprocedural (resulting from a procedure, not elsewhere classified) T81.12 ☑
  - following
    - ectopic or molar pregnancy O08.3
    - injury (immediate) (delayed) T79.4 ☑
    - labor and delivery O75.1
  - food (anaphylactic) — *see* Shock, anaphylactic, due to food
  - from electroshock gun (taser) T75.4 ☑
  - gram-negative R65.21
    - postprocedural (resulting from a procedure, not elsewhere classified) T81.12 ☑
  - hematologic R57.8
  - hemorrhagic
    - surgery (intraoperative) (postoperative) T81.19 ☑
    - trauma T79.4 ☑
  - hypovolemic R57.1
    - surgical T81.19 ☑
    - traumatic T79.4 ☑
  - insulin E15
    - therapeutic misadventure — *see* subcategory T38.3
  - kidney N17.0
    - traumatic (following crushing) T79.5 ☑
  - liver K72.00
  - lightning T75.01 ☑
  - lung J80
  - obstetric O75.1
    - with ectopic or molar pregnancy O08.3
    - following ectopic or molar pregnancy O08.3
  - pleural (surgical) T81.19 ☑
    - due to trauma T79.4 ☑
  - postprocedural (postoperative) T81.10 ☑
    - with ectopic or molar pregnancy O08.3
    - cardiogenic T81.11 ☑
    - endotoxic T81.12 ☑
    - following ectopic or molar pregnancy O08.3
    - gram-negative T81.12 ☑
    - hypovolemic T81.19 ☑
    - septic T81.12 ☑
    - specified type NEC T81.19 ☑

- **Sinusitis** — *continued*
  - sphenoidal J32.3
    - acute J01.30
      - recurrent J01.31
  - tuberculous, any sinus A15.8
- **Sinusitis-bronchiectasis-situs** inversus (syndrome) (triad) Q89.3
- **Sipple's** syndrome E31.22
- **Sirenomelia** (syndrome) Q87.2
- **Siriasis** T67.0 ☑
- **Sirkari's** disease B55.0
- **Siti** A65
- **Situation**, psychiatric F99
- **Situational**
  - disturbance (transient) — *see* Disorder, adjustment
    - acute F43.0
  - maladjustment — *see* Disorder, adjustment
  - reaction — *see* Disorder, adjustment
    - acute F43.0
- **Situs** inversus or transversus (abdominalis) (thoracis) Q89.3
- **Sixth** disease B08.20
  - due to human herpesvirus 6 B08.21
  - due to human herpesvirus 7 B08.22
- **Sjögren-Larsson** syndrome Q87.1
- **Sjögren's** syndrome or disease — *see* Sicca syndrome
- **Skeletal** — *see* condition
- **Skene's** gland — *see* condition
- **Skenitis** — *see* Urethritis
- **Skerljevo** A65
- **Skevas-Zerfus** disease — *see* Toxicity, venom, marine animal, sea anemone
- **Skin** (*see also* condition)
  - clammy R23.1
  - donor — *see* Donor, skin
  - hidebound M35.9
- **Slate-dressers'** or slate-miners' lung J62.8
- **Sleep**
  - apnea — *see* Apnea, sleep
  - deprivation Z72.820
  - disorder or disturbance G47.9
    - child F51.9
    - nonorganic origin F51.9
    - specified NEC G47.8
  - disturbance G47.9
    - nonorganic origin F51.9
  - drunkenness F51.9
  - rhythm inversion G47.2 ☑
  - terrors F51.4
  - walking F51.3
    - hysterical F44.89
- **Sleep hygiene**
  - abuse Z72.821
  - inadequate Z72.821
  - poor Z72.821
- **Sleeping** sickness — *see* Sickness, sleeping
- **Sleeplessness** — *see* Insomnia
  - menopausal N95.1
- **Sleep-wake** schedule disorder G47.20
- **Slim** disease (in HIV infection) B20
- **Slipped**, slipping
  - epiphysis (traumatic) (*see also* Osteochondropathy, specified type NEC)
    - capital femoral (traumatic)
      - acute (on chronic) S79.01 ☑
    - current traumatic - code as Fracture, by site
    - upper femoral (nontraumatic) M93.00 ☑
      - acute M93.01 ☑
        - on chronic M93.03 ☑
      - chronic M93.02 ☑
  - intervertebral disc — *see* Displacement, intervertebral disc
  - ligature, umbilical P51.8
  - patella — *see* Disorder, patella, derangement NEC
  - rib M89.8X8
  - sacroiliac joint — *see* subcategory M53.2
  - tendon — *see* Disorder, tendon
  - ulnar nerve, nontraumatic — *see* Lesion, nerve, ulnar
  - vertebra NEC — *see* Spondylolisthesis
- **Slocumb's** syndrome E27.0
- **Sloughing** (multiple) (phagedena) (skin) (*see also* Gangrene)
  - abscess — *see* Abscess
  - appendix K38.8
  - fascia — *see* Disorder, soft tissue, specified type NEC
  - scrotum N50.89
  - tendon — *see* Disorder, tendon
  - transplanted organ — *see* Rejection, transplant
  - ulcer — *see* Ulcer, skin
- **Slow**
  - feeding, newborn P92.2
  - flow syndrome, coronary I20.8
  - heart (beat) R00.1
- **Slowing**, urinary stream R39.198
- **Sluder's** neuralgia (syndrome) G44.89
- **Slurred**, slurring speech R47.81
- **Small** (ness)
  - for gestational age — *see* Small for dates
  - introitus, vagina N89.6
  - kidney (unknown cause) N27.9
    - bilateral N27.1
    - unilateral N27.0
  - ovary (congenital) Q50.39
  - pelvis
    - with disproportion (fetopelvic) O33.1
      - causing obstructed labor O65.1
  - uterus N85.8
  - white kidney N03.9
- **Small-and-light-for-dates** — *see* Small for dates
- **Small-for-dates** (infant) P05.10
  - with weight of
    - 499 grams or less P05.11
    - 500-749 grams P05.12
    - 750-999 grams P05.13
    - 1000-1249 grams P05.14
    - 1250-1499 grams P05.15
    - 1500-1749 grams P05.16
    - 1750-1999 grams P05.17
    - 2000-2499 grams P05.18
    - 2500 grams and over P05.19
  - specified NEC P05.19
- **Smallpox** B03
- **Smearing**, fecal R15.1
- **Smith-Lemli-Opitz** syndrome E78.72
- **Smith's** fracture S52.54 ☑
- **Smoker** — *see* Dependence, drug, nicotine
- **Smoker's**
  - bronchitis J41.0
  - cough J41.0
  - palate K13.24
  - throat J31.2
  - tongue K13.24
- **Smoking**
  - passive Z77.22
- **Smothering** spells R06.81
- **Snaggle** teeth, tooth M26.39
- **Snapping**
  - finger — *see* Trigger finger
  - hip — *see* Derangement, joint, specified type NEC, hip
    - involving the iliotibial band M76.3 ☑
  - knee — *see* Derangement, knee
    - involving the iliotibial band M76.3 ☑
- **Sneddon-Wilkinson** disease or syndrome (subcorneal pustular dermatosis) L13.1
- **Sneezing** (intractable) R06.7
- **Sniffing**
  - cocaine
    - abuse — *see* Abuse, drug, cocaine
    - dependence — *see* Dependence, drug, cocaine
  - gasoline
    - abuse — *see* Abuse, drug, inhalant
    - dependence — *see* Dependence, drug, inhalant
  - glue (airplane)
    - abuse — *see* Abuse, drug, inhalant
    - drug dependence — *see* Dependence, drug, inhalant
- **Sniffles**
  - newborn P28.89
- **Snoring** R06.83
- **Snow** blindness — *see* Photokeratitis
- **Snuffles** (non-syphilitic) R06.5
  - newborn P28.89
  - syphilitic (infant) A50.05 *[J99]*
- **Social**
  - exclusion Z60.4
    - due to discrimination or persecution (perceived) Z60.5
  - migrant Z59.0
    - acculturation difficulty Z60.3
  - rejection Z60.4
    - due to discrimination or persecution Z60.5
  - role conflict NEC Z73.5
  - skills inadequacy NEC Z73.4
  - transplantation Z60.3
- **Sodoku** A25.0
- **Soemmerring's** ring — *see* Cataract, secondary
- **Soft** (*see also* condition)
  - nails L60.3
- **Softening**
  - bone — *see* Osteomalacia
- **Softening** — *continued*
  - brain (necrotic) (progressive) G93.89
    - congenital Q04.8
    - embolic I63.4 ☑
    - hemorrhagic — *see* Hemorrhage, intracranial, intracerebral
    - occlusive I63.5 ☑
    - thrombotic I63.3 ☑
  - cartilage M94.2 ☑
    - patella M22.4 ☑
  - cerebellar — *see* Softening, brain
  - cerebral — *see* Softening, brain
  - cerebrospinal — *see* Softening, brain
  - myocardial, heart — *see* Degeneration, myocardial
  - spinal cord G95.89
  - stomach K31.89
- **Soldier's**
  - heart F45.8
  - patches I31.0
- **Solitary**
  - cyst, kidney N28.1
  - kidney, congenital Q60.0
- **Solvent** abuse — *see* Abuse, drug, inhalant
  - dependence — *see* Dependence, drug, inhalant
- **Somatization** reaction, somatic reaction — *see* Disorder, somatoform
- **Somnambulism** F51.3
  - hysterical F44.89
- **Somnolence** R40.0
  - nonorganic origin F51.11
- **Sonne** dysentery A03.3
- **Soor** B37.0
- **Sore**
  - bed — *see* Ulcer, pressure, by site
  - chiclero B55.1
  - Delhi B55.1
  - desert — *see* Ulcer, skin
  - eye H57.1 ☑
  - Lahore B55.1
  - mouth K13.79
    - canker K12.0
  - muscle M79.1
  - Naga — *see* Ulcer, skin
  - of skin — *see* Ulcer, skin
  - oriental B55.1
  - pressure — *see* Ulcer, pressure, by site
  - skin L98.9
  - soft A57
  - throat (acute) (*see also* Pharyngitis)
    - with influenza, flu, or grippe — *see* Influenza, with, respiratory manifestations NEC
    - chronic J31.2
    - coxsackie (virus) B08.5
    - diphtheritic A36.0
    - herpesviral B00.2
    - influenzal — *see* Influenza, with, respiratory manifestations NEC
    - septic J02.0
    - streptococcal (ulcerative) J02.0
    - viral NEC J02.8
      - coxsackie B08.5
  - tropical — *see* Ulcer, skin
  - veldt — *see* Ulcer, skin
- **Soto's** syndrome (cerebral gigantism) Q87.3
- **South** African cardiomyopathy syndrome I42.8
- **Southeast** Asian hemorrhagic fever A91
- **Spacing**
  - abnormal, tooth, teeth, fully erupted M26.30
  - excessive, tooth, fully erupted M26.32
- **Spade-like** hand (congenital) Q68.1
- **Spading** nail L60.8
  - congenital Q84.6
- **Spanish** collar N47.1
- **Sparganosis** B70.1
- **Spasm** (s), spastic, spasticity (*see also* condition) R25.2
  - accommodation — *see* Spasm, of accommodation
  - ampulla of Vater K83.4
  - anus, ani (sphincter) (reflex) K59.4
    - psychogenic F45.8
  - artery I73.9
    - cerebral G45.9
  - Bell's G51.3
  - bladder (sphincter, external or internal) N32.89
    - psychogenic F45.8
  - bronchus, bronchiole J98.01
  - cardia K22.0
  - cardiac I20.1
  - carpopedal — *see* Tetany
  - cerebral (arteries) (vascular) G45.9
  - cervix, complicating delivery O62.4

Spasm — *continued*
- ciliary body (of accommodation) — *see* Spasm, of accommodation
- colon (*see also* Irritable, bowel)K58.9
  - with diarrhea K58.0
  - psychogenic F45.8
- common duct K83.8
- compulsive — *see* Tic
- conjugate H51.8
- coronary (artery) I20.1
- diaphragm (reflex) R06.6
  - epidemic B33.0
  - psychogenic F45.8
- duodenum K59.8
- epidemic diaphragmatic (transient) B33.0
- esophagus (diffuse) K22.4
  - psychogenic F45.8
- facial G51.3
- fallopian tube N83.8
- gastrointestinal (tract) K31.89
  - psychogenic F45.8
- glottis J38.5
  - hysterical F44.4
  - psychogenic F45.8
    - conversion reaction F44.4
  - reflex through recurrent laryngeal nerve J38.5
- habit — *see* Tic
- heart I20.1
- hemifacial (clonic) G51.3
- hourglass — *see* Contraction, hourglass
- hysterical F44.4
- infantile — *see* Epilepsy, spasms
- inferior oblique, eye H51.8
- intestinal (*see also* Syndrome, irritable bowel)K58.9
  - psychogenic F45.8
- larynx, laryngeal J38.5
  - hysterical F44.4
  - psychogenic F45.8
    - conversion reaction F44.4
- levator palpebrae superioris — *see* Disorder, eyelid function
- muscle NEC M62.838
  - back M62.830
- nerve, trigeminal G51.0
- nervous F45.8
- nodding F98.4
- occupational F48.8
- oculogyric H51.8
  - psychogenic F45.8
- of accommodation H52.53 ☑
- ophthalmic artery — *see* Occlusion, artery, retina
- perineal, female N94.89
- peroneo-extensor (*see also* Deformity, limb, flat foot)
- pharynx (reflex) J39.2
  - hysterical F45.8
  - psychogenic F45.8
- psychogenic F45.8
- pylorus NEC K31.3
  - adult hypertrophic K31.89
  - congenital or infantile Q40.0
  - psychogenic F45.8
- rectum (sphincter) K59.4
  - psychogenic F45.8
- retinal (artery) — *see* Occlusion, artery, retina
- sigmoid (*see also* Syndrome, irritable bowel)K58.9
  - psychogenic F45.8
- sphincter of Oddi K83.4
- stomach K31.89
  - neurotic F45.8
- throat J39.2
  - hysterical F45.8
  - psychogenic F45.8
- tic F95.9
  - chronic F95.1
  - transient of childhood F95.0
- tongue K14.8
- torsion (progressive) G24.1
- trigeminal nerve — *see* Neuralgia, trigeminal
- ureter N13.5
- urethra (sphincter) N35.9
- uterus N85.8
  - complicating labor O62.4
- vagina N94.2
  - psychogenic F52.5
- vascular I73.9
- vasomotor I73.9
- vein NEC I87.8
- viscera — *see* Pain, abdominal

Spasmodic — *see* condition
Spasmophilia — *see* Tetany
Spasmus nutans F98.4
Spastic, spasticity (*see also* Spasm)
- child (cerebral) (congenital) (paralysis) G80.1

Speaker's throat R49.8
Specific, specified — *see* condition
Speech
- defect, disorder, disturbance, impediment R47.9
  - psychogenic, in childhood and adolescence F98.8
  - slurring R47.81
  - specified NEC R47.89

Spencer's disease A08.19
Spens' syndrome (syncope with heart block) I45.9
Sperm counts (fertility testing) Z31.41
- postvasectomy Z30.8
  - reversal Z31.42

Spermatic cord — *see* condition
Spermatocele N43.40
- congenital Q55.4
- multiple N43.42
- single N43.41

Spermatocystitis N49.0
Spermatocytoma C62.9 ☑
- specified site — *see* Neoplasm, malignant, by site

Spermatorrhea N50.89
Sphacelus — *see* Gangrene
Sphenoidal — *see* condition
Sphenoiditis (chronic) — *see* Sinusitis, sphenoidal
Sphenopalatine ganglion neuralgia G90.09
Sphericity, increased, lens (congenital) Q12.4
Spherocytosis (congenital) (familial) (hereditary) D58.0
- hemoglobin disease D58.0
- sickle-cell (disease) D57.8 ☑

Spherophakia Q12.4
Sphincter — *see* condition
Sphincteritis, sphincter of Oddi — *see* Cholangitis
Sphingolipidosis E75.3
- specified NEC E75.29

Sphingomyelinosis E75.3
Spicule tooth K00.2
Spider
- bite — *see* Toxicity, venom, spider
- fingers — *see* Syndrome, Marfan's
- nevus I78.1
- toes — *see* Syndrome, Marfan's
- vascular I78.1

Spiegler-Fendt
- benign lymphocytoma L98.8
- sarcoid L08.89

Spielmeyer-Vogt disease E75.4
Spina bifida (aperta) Q05.9
- with hydrocephalus NEC Q05.4
- cervical Q05.5
  - with hydrocephalus Q05.0
- dorsal Q05.6
  - with hydrocephalus Q05.1
- lumbar Q05.7
  - with hydrocephalus Q05.2
- lumbosacral Q05.7
  - with hydrocephalus Q05.2
- occulta Q76.0
- sacral Q05.8
  - with hydrocephalus Q05.3
- thoracic Q05.6
  - with hydrocephalus Q05.1
- thoracolumbar Q05.6
  - with hydrocephalus Q05.1

Spindle, Krukenberg's — *see* Pigmentation, cornea, posterior
Spine, spinal — *see* condition
Spiradenoma (eccrine) — *see* Neoplasm, skin, benign
Spirillosis A25.0
Spirillum
- minus A25.0
- obermeieri infection A68.0

Spirochetal — *see* condition
Spirochetosis A69.9
- arthritic, arthritica A69.9
- bronchopulmonary A69.8
- icterohemorrhagic A27.0
- lung A69.8

Spirometrosis B70.1
Spitting blood — *see* Hemoptysis
Splanchnoptosis K63.4
Spleen, splenic — *see* condition
Splenectasis — *see* Splenomegaly
Splenitis (interstitial) (malignant) (nonspecific) D73.89
- malarial (*see also* Malaria)B54 *[D77]*
- tuberculous A18.85

Splenocele D73.89
Splenomegaly, splenomegalia (Bengal) (cryptogenic) (idiopathic) (tropical) R16.1
- with hepatomegaly R16.2
- cirrhotic D73.2
- congenital Q89.09
- congestive, chronic D73.2
- Egyptian B65.1
- Gaucher's E75.22
- malarial (*see also* Malaria)B54 *[D77]*
- neutropenic D73.81
- Niemann-Pick — *see* Niemann-Pick disease or syndrome
- siderotic D73.2
- syphilitic A52.79
  - congenital (early) A50.08 *[D77]*

Splenopathy D73.9
Splenoptosis D73.89
Splenosis D73.89
Splinter — *see* Foreign body, superficial, by site
Split, splitting
- foot Q72.7 ☑
- hand Q71.6 ☑
- heart sounds R01.2
- lip, congenital — *see* Cleft, lip
- nails L60.3
- urinary stream R39.13

Spondylarthrosis — *see* Spondylosis
Spondylitis (chronic) (*see also* Spondylopathy, inflammatory)
- ankylopoietica — *see* Spondylitis, ankylosing
- ankylosing (chronic) M45.9
  - with lung involvement M45.9 *[J99]*
  - cervical region M45.2
  - cervicothoracic region M45.3
  - juvenile M08.1
  - lumbar region M45.6
  - lumbosacral region M45.7
  - multiple sites M45.0
  - occipito-atlanto-axial region M45.1
  - sacrococcygeal region M45.8
  - thoracic region M45.4
  - thoracolumbar region M45.5
- atrophic (ligamentous) — *see* Spondylitis, ankylosing
- deformans (chronic) — *see* Spondylosis
- gonococcal A54.41
- gouty (*see also* Gout, by type, vertebrae)M10.08
- in (due to)
  - brucellosis A23.9 *[M49.80]*
    - cervical region A23.9 *[M49.82]*
    - cervicothoracic region A23.9 *[M49.83]*
    - lumbar region A23.9 *[M49.86]*
    - lumbosacral region A23.9 *[M49.87]*
    - multiple sites A23.9 *[M49.89]*
    - occipito-atlanto-axial region A23.9 *[M49.81]*
    - sacrococcygeal region A23.9 *[M49.88]*
    - thoracic region A23.9 *[M49.84]*
    - thoracolumbar region A23.9 *[M49.85]*
  - enterobacteria (*see also* subcategory M49.8)A04.9
  - tuberculosis A18.01
- infectious NEC — *see* Spondylopathy, infective
- juvenile ankylosing (chronic) M08.1
- Kümmell's — *see* Spondylopathy, traumatic
- Marie-Strümpell — *see* Spondylitis, ankylosing
- muscularis — *see* Spondylopathy, specified NEC
- psoriatic L40.53
- rheumatoid — *see* Spondylitis, ankylosing
- rhizomelica — *see* Spondylitis, ankylosing
- sacroiliac NEC M46.1
- senescent, senile — *see* Spondylosis
- traumatic (chronic) or post-traumatic — *see* Spondylopathy, traumatic
- tuberculous A18.01
- typhosa A01.05

Spondylolisthesis (acquired) (degenerative) M43.10
- with disproportion (fetopelvic) O33.0
  - causing obstructed labor O65.0
- cervical region M43.12
- cervicothoracic region M43.13
- congenital Q76.2
- lumbar region M43.16
- lumbosacral region M43.17
- multiple sites M43.19
- occipito-atlanto-axial region M43.11
- sacrococcygeal region M43.18
- thoracic region M43.14
- thoracolumbar region M43.15
- traumatic (old) M43.10
  - acute
    - fifth cervical (displaced) S12.430 ☑

Spondylolisthesis - Sprain

Spondylolisthesis — *continued*
- traumatic — *continued*
    - nondisplaced S12.431 ☑
    - specified type NEC (displaced) S12.450 ☑
        - nondisplaced S12.451 ☑
    - type III S12.44 ☑
  - fourth cervical (displaced) S12.330 ☑
    - nondisplaced S12.331 ☑
    - specified type NEC (displaced) S12.350 ☑
        - nondisplaced S12.351 ☑
    - type III S12.34 ☑
  - second cervical (displaced) S12.130 ☑
    - nondisplaced S12.131 ☑
    - specified type NEC (displaced) S12.150 ☑
        - nondisplaced S12.151 ☑
    - type III S12.14 ☑
  - seventh cervical (displaced) S12.630 ☑
    - nondisplaced S12.631 ☑
    - specified type NEC (displaced) S12.650 ☑
        - nondisplaced S12.651 ☑
    - type III S12.64 ☑
  - sixth cervical (displaced) S12.530 ☑
    - nondisplaced S12.531 ☑
    - specified type NEC (displaced) S12.550 ☑
        - nondisplaced S12.551 ☑
    - type III S12.54 ☑
  - third cervical (displaced) S12.230 ☑
    - nondisplaced S12.231 ☑
    - specified type NEC (displaced) S12.250 ☑
        - nondisplaced S12.251 ☑
    - type III S12.24 ☑

Spondylolysis (acquired) M43.00
- cervical region M43.02
- cervicothoracic region M43.03
- congenital Q76.2
- lumbar region M43.06
- lumbosacral region M43.07
  - with disproportion (fetopelvic) O33.0
    - causing obstructed labor O65.8
- multiple sites M43.09
- occipito-atlanto-axial region M43.01
- sacrococcygeal region M43.08
- thoracic region M43.04
- thoracolumbar region M43.05

Spondylopathy M48.9
- infective NEC M46.50
  - cervical region M46.52
  - cervicothoracic region M46.53
  - lumbar region M46.56
  - lumbosacral region M46.57
  - multiple sites M46.59
  - occipito-atlanto-axial region M46.51
  - sacrococcygeal region M46.58
  - thoracic region M46.54
  - thoracolumbar region M46.55
- inflammatory M46.90
  - cervical region M46.92
  - cervicothoracic region M46.93
  - lumbar region M46.96
  - lumbosacral region M46.97
  - multiple sites M46.99
  - occipito-atlanto-axial region M46.91
  - sacrococcygeal region M46.98
  - specified type NEC M46.80
    - cervical region M46.82
    - cervicothoracic region M46.83
    - lumbar region M46.86
    - lumbosacral region M46.87
    - multiple sites M46.89
    - occipito-atlanto-axial region M46.81
    - sacrococcygeal region M46.88
    - thoracic region M46.84
    - thoracolumbar region M46.85
  - thoracic region M46.94
  - thoracolumbar region M46.95
- neuropathic, in
  - syringomyelia and syringobulbia G95.0
  - tabes dorsalis A52.11
- specified NEC — *see* subcategory M48.8
- traumatic M48.30
  - cervical region M48.32
  - cervicothoracic region M48.33
  - lumbar region M48.36
  - lumbosacral region M48.37
  - occipito-atlanto-axial region M48.31
  - sacrococcygeal region M48.38
  - thoracic region M48.34
  - thoracolumbar region M48.35

Spondylosis M47.9
- with
  - disproportion (fetopelvic) O33.0
    - causing obstructed labor O65.0

Spondylosis — *continued*
- with — *continued*
  - myelopathy NEC M47.10
    - cervical region M47.12
    - cervicothoracic region M47.13
    - lumbar region M47.16
    - occipito-atlanto-axial region M47.11
    - thoracic region M47.14
    - thoracolumbar region M47.15
  - radiculopathy M47.20
    - cervical region M47.22
    - cervicothoracic region M47.23
    - lumbar region M47.26
    - lumbosacral region M47.27
    - occipito-atlanto-axial region M47.21
    - sacrococcygeal region M47.28
    - thoracic region M47.24
    - thoracolumbar region M47.25
- specified NEC M47.899
  - cervical region M47.892
  - cervicothoracic region M47.893
  - lumbar region M47.896
  - lumbosacral region M47.897
  - occipito-atlanto-axial region M47.891
  - sacrococcygeal region M47.898
  - thoracic region M47.894
  - thoracolumbar region M47.895
- traumatic — *see* Spondylopathy, traumatic
- without myelopathy or radiculopathy M47.819
  - cervical region M47.812
  - cervicothoracic region M47.813
  - lumbar region M47.816
  - lumbosacral region M47.817
  - occipito-atlanto-axial region M47.811
  - sacrococcygeal region M47.818
  - thoracic region M47.814
  - thoracolumbar region M47.815

Sponge
- inadvertently left in operation wound — *see* Foreign body, accidentally left during a procedure
- kidney (medullary) Q61.5

Sponge-diver's disease — *see* Toxicity, venom, marine animal, sea anemone

Spongioblastoma (any type) — *see* Neoplasm, malignant, by site
- specified site — *see* Neoplasm, malignant, by site
- unspecified site C71.9

Spongioneuroblastoma — *see* Neoplasm, malignant, by site

Spontaneous (*see also* condition)
- fracture (cause unknown) — *see* Fracture, pathological

Spoon nail L60.3
- congenital Q84.6

Sporadic — *see* condition

Sporothrix schenckii infection — *see* Sporotrichosis

Sporotrichosis B42.9
- arthritis B42.82
- disseminated B42.7
- generalized B42.7
- lymphocutaneous (fixed) (progressive) B42.1
- pulmonary B42.0
- specified NEC B42.89

Spots, spotting (in) (of)
- Bitot's (*see also* Pigmentation, conjunctiva)
  - in the young child E50.1
  - vitamin A deficiency E50.1
- café au lait L81.3
- Cayenne pepper I78.1
- cotton wool, retina — *see* Occlusion, artery, retina
- de Morgan's (senile angiomas) I78.1
- Fuchs' black (myopic) H44.2 ☑
- intermenstrual (regular) N92.0
  - irregular N92.1
- Koplik's B05.9
- liver L81.4
- pregnancy O26.85 ☑
- purpuric R23.3
- ruby I78.1

Spotted fever — *see* Fever, spottedN92.3

Sprain (joint) (ligament)
- acromioclavicular joint or ligament S43.5 ☑
- ankle S93.40 ☑
  - calcaneofibular ligament S93.41 ☑
  - deltoid ligament S93.42 ☑
  - internal collateral ligament — *see* Sprain, ankle, specified ligament NEC
  - specified ligament NEC S93.49 ☑
  - talofibular ligament — *see* Sprain, ankle, specified ligament NEC
  - tibiofibular ligament S93.43 ☑

Sprain — *continued*
- anterior longitudinal, cervical S13.4 ☑
- atlas, atlanto-axial, atlanto-occipital S13.4 ☑
- breast bone — *see* Sprain, sternum
- calcaneofibular — *see* Sprain, ankle
- carpal — *see* Sprain, wrist
- carpometacarpal — *see* Sprain, hand, specified site NEC
- cartilage
  - costal S23.41 ☑
  - semilunar (knee) — *see* Sprain, knee, specified site NEC
    - with current tear — *see* Tear, meniscus
  - thyroid region S13.5 ☑
  - xiphoid — *see* Sprain, sternum
- cervical, cervicodorsal, cervicothoracic S13.4 ☑
- chondrosternal S23.421 ☑
- coracoclavicular S43.8 ☑
- coracohumeral S43.41 ☑
- coronary, knee — *see* Sprain, knee, specified site NEC
- costal cartilage S23.41 ☑
- cricoarytenoid articulation or ligament S13.5 ☑
- cricothyroid articulation S13.5 ☑
- cruciate, knee — *see* Sprain, knee, cruciate
- deltoid, ankle — *see* Sprain, ankle
- dorsal (spine) S23.3 ☑
- elbow S53.40 ☑
  - radial collateral ligament S53.43 ☑
  - radiohumeral S53.41 ☑
  - rupture
    - radial collateral ligament — *see* Rupture, traumatic, ligament, radial collateral
    - ulnar collateral ligament — *see* Rupture, traumatic, ligament, ulnar collateral
  - specified type NEC S53.49 ☑
  - ulnar collateral ligament S53.44 ☑
  - ulnohumeral S53.42 ☑
- femur, head — *see* Sprain, hip
- fibular collateral, knee — *see* Sprain, knee, collateral
- fibulocalcaneal — *see* Sprain, ankle
- finger (s) S63.61 ☑
  - index S63.61 ☑
  - interphalangeal (joint) S63.63 ☑
    - index S63.63 ☑
    - little S63.63 ☑
    - middle S63.63 ☑
    - ring S63.63 ☑
  - little S63.61 ☑
  - middle S63.61 ☑
  - ring S63.61 ☑
  - metacarpophalangeal (joint) S63.65 ☑
  - specified site NEC S63.69 ☑
    - index S63.69 ☑
    - little S63.69 ☑
    - middle S63.69 ☑
    - ring S63.69 ☑
- foot S93.60 ☑
  - specified ligament NEC S93.69 ☑
  - tarsal ligament S93.61 ☑
  - tarsometatarsal ligament S93.62 ☑
  - toe — *see* Sprain, toe
- hand S63.9 ☑
  - finger — *see* Sprain, finger
  - specified site NEC — *see* subcategory S63.8
  - thumb — *see* Sprain, thumb
- head S03.9 ☑
- hip S73.10 ☑
  - iliofemoral ligament S73.11 ☑
  - ischiocapsular (ligament) S73.12 ☑
  - specified NEC S73.19 ☑
- iliofemoral — *see* Sprain, hip
- innominate
  - acetabulum — *see* Sprain, hip
  - sacral junction S33.6 ☑
- internal
  - collateral, ankle — *see* Sprain, ankle
  - semilunar cartilage — *see* Sprain, knee, specified site NEC
- interphalangeal
  - finger — *see* Sprain, finger, interphalangeal (joint)
  - toe — *see* Sprain, toe, interphalangeal joint
- ischiocapsular — *see* Sprain, hip
- ischiofemoral — *see* Sprain, hip
- jaw (articular disc) (cartilage) (meniscus) S03.4 ☑
  - old M26.69
- knee S83.9 ☑
  - collateral ligament S83.40 ☑
    - lateral (fibular) S83.42 ☑
    - medial (tibial) S83.41 ☑

- **Sprain** — *continued*
  - knee — *continued*
    - cruciate ligament S83.50 ☑
      - anterior S83.51 ☑
      - posterior S83.52 ☑
    - lateral (fibular) collateral ligament S83.42 ☑
    - medial (tibial) collateral ligament S83.41 ☑
    - patellar ligament S76.11 ☑
    - specified site NEC S83.8X ☑
    - superior tibiofibular joint (ligament) S83.6 ☑
  - lateral collateral, knee — *see* Sprain, knee, collateral
  - lumbar (spine) S33.5 ☑
  - lumbosacral S33.9 ☑
  - mandible (articular disc) S03.4 ☑
    - old M26.69
  - medial collateral, knee — *see* Sprain, knee, collateral
  - meniscus
    - jaw S03.4 ☑
      - old M26.69
    - knee — *see* Sprain, knee, specified site NEC
      - with current tear — *see* Tear, meniscus
        - old — *see* Derangement, knee, meniscus, due to old tear
    - mandible S03.4 ☑
      - old M26.69
  - metacarpal (distal) (proximal) — *see* Sprain, hand, specified site NEC
  - metacarpophalangeal — *see* Sprain, finger, metacarpophalangeal (joint)
  - metatarsophalangeal — *see* Sprain, toe, metatarsophalangeal joint
  - midcarpal — *see* Sprain, hand, specified site NEC
  - midtarsal — *see* Sprain, foot, specified site NEC
  - neck S13.9 ☑
    - anterior longitudinal cervical ligament S13.4 ☑
    - atlanto-axial joint S13.4 ☑
    - atlanto-occipital joint S13.4 ☑
    - cervical spine S13.4 ☑
    - cricoarytenoid ligament S13.5 ☑
    - cricothyroid ligament S13.5 ☑
    - specified site NEC S13.8 ☑
    - thyroid region (cartilage) S13.5 ☑
  - nose S03.8 ☑
  - orbicular, hip — *see* Sprain, hip
  - patella — *see* Sprain, knee, specified site NEC
  - patellar ligament S76.11 ☑
  - pelvis NEC S33.8 ☑
  - phalanx
    - finger — *see* Sprain, finger
    - toe — *see* Sprain, toe
  - pubofemoral — *see* Sprain, hip
  - radiocarpal — *see* Sprain, wrist
  - radiohumeral — *see* Sprain, elbow
  - radius, collateral — *see* Rupture, traumatic, ligament, radial collateral
  - rib (cage) S23.41 ☑
  - rotator cuff (capsule) S43.42 ☑
  - sacroiliac (region)
    - chronic or old — *see* subcategory M53.2
    - joint S33.6 ☑
  - scaphoid (hand) — *see* Sprain, hand, specified site NEC
  - scapula (r) — *see* Sprain, shoulder girdle, specified site NEC
  - semilunar cartilage (knee) — *see* Sprain, knee, specified site NEC
    - with current tear — *see* Tear, meniscus
      - old — *see* Derangement, knee, meniscus, due to old tear
  - shoulder joint S43.40 ☑
    - acromioclavicular joint (ligament) — *see* Sprain, acromioclavicular joint
    - blade — *see* Sprain, shoulder, girdle, specified site NEC
    - coracoclavicular joint (ligament) — *see* Sprain, coracoclavicular joint
    - coracohumeral ligament — *see* Sprain, coracohumeral joint
    - girdle S43.9 ☑
      - specified site NEC S43.8 ☑
    - rotator cuff — *see* Sprain, rotator cuff
    - specified site NEC S43.49 ☑
    - sternoclavicular joint (ligament) — *see* Sprain, sternoclavicular joint
  - spine
    - cervical S13.4 ☑
    - lumbar S33.5 ☑
    - thoracic S23.3 ☑
  - sternoclavicular joint S43.6 ☑
- **Sprain** — *continued*
  - sternum S23.429 ☑
    - chondrosternal joint S23.421 ☑
    - specified site NEC S23.428 ☑
    - sternoclavicular (joint) (ligament) S23.420 ☑
  - symphysis
    - jaw S03.4 ☑
      - old M26.69
    - mandibular S03.4 ☑
      - old M26.69
  - talofibular — *see* Sprain, ankle
  - tarsal — *see* Sprain, foot, specified site NEC
  - tarsometatarsal — *see* Sprain, foot, specified site NEC
  - temporomandibular S03.4 ☑
    - old M26.69
  - thorax S23.9 ☑
    - ribs S23.41 ☑
    - specified site NEC S23.8 ☑
    - spine S23.3 ☑
    - sternum — *see* Sprain, sternum
  - thumb S63.60 ☑
    - interphalangeal (joint) S63.62 ☑
    - metacarpophalangeal (joint) S63.64 ☑
    - specified site NEC S63.68 ☑
  - thyroid cartilage or region S13.5 ☑
  - tibia (proximal end) — *see* Sprain, knee, specified site NEC
  - tibial collateral, knee — *see* Sprain, knee, collateral
  - tibiofibular
    - distal — *see* Sprain, ankle
    - superior — *see* Sprain, knee, specified site NEC
  - toe (s) S93.50 ☑
    - great S93.50 ☑
    - interphalangeal joint S93.51 ☑
      - great S93.51 ☑
      - lesser S93.51 ☑
    - lesser S93.50 ☑
    - metatarsophalangeal joint S93.52 ☑
      - great S93.52 ☑
      - lesser S93.52 ☑
  - ulna, collateral — *see* Rupture, traumatic, ligament, ulnar collateral
  - ulnohumeral — *see* Sprain, elbow
  - wrist S63.50 ☑
    - carpal S63.51 ☑
    - radiocarpal S63.52 ☑
    - specified site NEC S63.59 ☑
  - xiphoid cartilage — *see* Sprain, sternum
- **Sprengel's** deformity (congenital) Q74.0
- **Sprue** (tropical) K90.1
  - celiac K90.0
  - idiopathic K90.49
  - meaning thrush B37.0
  - nontropical K90.0
- **Spur,** bone (*see also* Enthesopathy)
  - calcaneal M77.3 ☑
  - iliac crest M76.2 ☑
  - nose (septum) J34.89
- **Spurway's** syndrome Q78.0
- **Sputum**
  - abnormal (amount) (color) (odor) (purulent) R09.3
  - blood-stained R04.2
  - excessive (cause unknown) R09.3
- **Squamous** (*see also* condition)
  - epithelium in
    - cervical canal (congenital) Q51.828
    - uterine mucosa (congenital) Q51.818
- **Squashed** nose M95.0
  - congenital Q67.4
- **Squeeze,** diver's T70.3 ☑
- **Squint** (*see also* Strabismus)
  - accommodative — *see* Strabismus, convergent concomitant
- **St. Hubert's** disease A82.9
- **Stab** (*see also* Laceration)
  - internal organs — *see* Injury, by site
- **Stafne's** cyst or cavity M27.0
- **Staggering** gait R26.0
  - hysterical F44.4
- **Staghorn** calculus — *see* Calculus, kidney
- **Stähli's** line (cornea) (pigment) — *see* Pigmentation, cornea, anterior
- **Stain,** staining
  - meconium (newborn) P96.83
  - port wine Q82.5
  - tooth, teeth (hard tissues) (extrinsic) K03.6
    - due to
      - accretions K03.6
- **Stain,** staining — *continued*
  - tooth, teeth — *continued*
      - deposits (betel) (black) (green) (materia alba) (orange) (soft) (tobacco) K03.6
      - metals (copper) (silver) K03.7
      - nicotine K03.6
      - pulpal bleeding K03.7
      - tobacco K03.6
    - intrinsic K00.8
- **Stammering** (*see also* Disorder, fluency)F80.81
- **Standstill**
  - auricular I45.5
  - cardiac — *see* Arrest, cardiac
  - sinoatrial I45.5
  - ventricular — *see* Arrest, cardiac
- **Stannosis** J63.5
- **Stanton's** disease — *see* Melioidosis
- **Staphylitis** (acute) (catarrhal) (chronic) (gangrenous) (membranous) (suppurative) (ulcerative) K12.2
- **Staphylococcal** scalded skin syndrome L00
- **Staphylococcemia** A41.2
- **Staphylococcus,** staphylococcal (*see also* condition)
  - as cause of disease classified elsewhere B95.8
    - aureus (methicillin susceptible) (MSSA) B95.61
      - methicillin resistant (MRSA) B95.62
  - specified NEC, as cause of disease classified elsewhere B95.7
- **Staphyloma** (sclera)
  - cornea H18.72 ☑
  - equatorial H15.81 ☑
  - localized (anterior) H15.82 ☑
  - posticum H15.83 ☑
  - ring H15.85 ☑
- **Stargardt's** disease — *see* Dystrophy, retina
- **Starvation** (inanition) (due to lack of food) T73.0 ☑
  - edema — *see* Malnutrition, severe
- **Stasis**
  - bile (noncalculous) K83.1
  - bronchus J98.09
    - with infection — *see* Bronchitis
  - cardiac — *see* Failure, heart, congestive
  - cecum K59.8
  - colon K59.8
  - dermatitis I87.2
    - with
      - varicose ulcer — *see* Varix, leg, with ulcer, with inflammation
      - varicose veins — *see* Varix, leg, with, inflammation
    - due to postthrombotic syndrome — *see* Syndrome, postthrombotic
  - duodenal K31.5
  - eczema — *see* Varix, leg, with, inflammation
  - edema — *see* Hypertension, venous (chronic), idiopathic
  - foot T69.0 ☑
  - ileocecal coil K59.8
  - ileum K59.8
  - intestinal K59.8
  - jejunum K59.8
  - kidney N19
  - liver (cirrhotic) K76.1
  - lymphatic I89.8
  - pneumonia J18.2
  - pulmonary — *see* Edema, lung
  - rectal K59.8
  - renal N19
    - tubular N17.0
  - ulcer — *see* Varix, leg, with, ulcer
    - without varicose veins I87.2
  - urine — *see* Retention, urine
  - venous I87.8
- **State** (of)
  - affective and paranoid, mixed, organic psychotic F06.8
  - agitated R45.1
    - acute reaction to stress F43.0
  - anxiety (neurotic) F41.1
  - apprehension F41.1
  - burn-out Z73.0
  - climacteric, female Z78.0
    - symptomatic N95.1
  - compulsive F42.8
    - mixed with obsessional thoughts F42.2
  - confusional (psychogenic) F44.89
    - acute (*see also* Delirium)
      - with
        - arteriosclerotic dementia F01.50
          - with behavioral disturbance F01.51
        - senility or dementia F05
      - alcoholic F10.231
    - epileptic F05

- **State** — *continued*
  - confusional — *continued*
    - reactive (from emotional stress, psychological trauma) F44.89
    - subacute — *see* Delirium
  - convulsive — *see* Convulsions
  - crisis F43.0
  - depressive F32.9
    - neurotic F34.1
  - dissociative F44.9
  - emotional shock (stress) R45.7
  - hypercoagulation — *see* Hypercoagulable
  - locked-in G83.5
  - menopausal Z78.0
    - symptomatic N95.1
  - neurotic F48.9
    - with depersonalization F48.1
  - obsessional F42.8
  - oneiroid (schizophrenia-like) F23
  - organic
    - hallucinatory (nonalcoholic) F06.0
    - paranoid (-hallucinatory) F06.2
  - panic F41.0
  - paranoid F22
    - climacteric F22
    - involutional F22
    - menopausal F22
    - organic F06.2
    - senile F03 ☑
    - simple F22
  - persistent vegetative R40.3
  - phobic F40.9
  - postleukotomy F07.0
  - pregnant
    - gestational carrier Z33.3
    - incidental Z33.1
  - psychogenic, twilight F44.89
  - psychopathic (constitutional) F60.2
  - psychotic, organic (*see also* Psychosis, organic)
    - mixed paranoid and affective F06.8
    - senile or presenile F03 ☑
    - transient NEC F06.8
      - with
        - hallucinations F06.0
        - depression F06.31
  - residual schizophrenic F20.5
  - restlessness R45.1
  - stress (emotional) R45.7
  - tension (mental) F48.9
    - specified NEC F48.8
  - transient organic psychotic NEC F06.8
    - depressive type F06.31
    - hallucinatory type F06.0
  - twilight
    - epileptic F05
    - psychogenic F44.89
  - vegetative, persistent R40.3
  - vital exhaustion Z73.0
  - withdrawal, — *see* Withdrawal, state
- **Status** (post) (*see also* Presence (of))
  - absence, epileptic — *see* Epilepsy, by type, with status epilepticus
  - administration of tPA (rtPA) in a different facility within the last 24 hours prior to admission to current facility Z92.82
  - adrenalectomy (unilateral) (bilateral) E89.6
  - anastomosis Z98.0
  - angioplasty (peripheral) Z98.62
    - with implant Z95.820
    - coronary artery Z98.61
      - with implant Z95.5
  - anginosus I20.9
  - aortocoronary bypass Z95.1
  - arthrodesis Z98.1
  - artificial opening (of) Z93.9
    - gastrointestinal tract Z93.4
    - specified NEC Z93.8
    - urinary tract Z93.6
    - vagina Z93.8
  - asthmaticus — *see* Asthma, by type, with status asthmaticus
  - awaiting organ transplant Z76.82
  - bariatric surgery Z98.84
  - bed confinement Z74.01
  - bleb, filtering (vitreous), after glaucoma surgery Z98.83
  - breast implant Z98.82
    - removal Z98.86
  - cataract extraction Z98.4 ☑
  - cholecystectomy Z90.49
  - clitorectomy N90.811
    - with excision of labia minora N90.812
  - colectomy (complete) (partial) Z90.49
  - colonization — *see* Carrier (suspected) of
  - colostomy Z93.3
  - convulsivus idiopathicus — *see* Epilepsy, by type, with status epilepticus
  - coronary artery angioplasty — *see* Status, angioplasty, coronary artery
  - cystectomy (urinary bladder) Z90.6
  - cystostomy Z93.50
    - appendico-vesicostomy Z93.52
    - cutaneous Z93.51
    - specified NEC Z93.59
  - delinquent immunization Z28.3
  - dental Z98.818
    - crown Z98.811
    - fillings Z98.811
    - restoration Z98.811
    - sealant Z98.810
    - specified NEC Z98.818
  - deployment (current) (military) Z56.82
  - dialysis (hemodialysis) (peritoneal) Z99.2
  - do not resuscitate (DNR) Z66
  - donor — *see* Donor
  - embedded fragments — *see* Retained, foreign body fragments (type of)
  - embedded splinter — *see* Retained, foreign body fragments (type of)
  - enterostomy Z93.4
  - epileptic, epilepticus (*see also* Epilepsy, by type, with status epilepticus)G40.901
  - estrogen receptor
    - negative Z17.1
    - positive Z17.0
  - female genital cutting — *see* Female genital mutilation status
  - female genital mutilation — *see* Female genital mutilation status
  - filtering (vitreous) bleb after glaucoma surgery Z98.83
  - gastrectomy (complete) (partial) Z90.3
  - gastric banding Z98.84
  - gastric bypass for obesity Z98.84
  - gastrostomy Z93.1
  - human immunodeficiency virus (HIV) infection, asymptomatic Z21
  - hysterectomy (complete) (total) Z90.710
    - partial (with remaining cervical stump) Z90.711
  - ileostomy Z93.2
  - implant
    - breast Z98.82
  - infibulation N90.813
  - intestinal bypass Z98.0
  - jejunostomy Z93.4
  - laryngectomy Z90.02
  - lapsed immunization schedule Z28.3
  - lymphaticus E32.8
  - malignancy
    - castrate resistant prostate Z19.2
    - hormone resistant Z19.2
    - hormone sensitive Z19.1
  - marmoratus G80.3
  - mastectomy (unilateral) (bilateral) Z90.1 ☑
  - military deployment status (current) Z56.82
    - in theater or in support of military war, peacekeeping and humanitarian operations Z56.82
  - nephrectomy (unilateral) (bilateral) Z90.5
  - nephrostomy Z93.6
  - obesity surgery Z98.84
  - oophorectomy
    - bilateral Z90.722
    - unilateral Z90.721
  - organ replacement
    - by artificial or mechanical device or prosthesis of
      - artery Z95.828
      - bladder Z96.0
      - blood vessel Z95.828
      - breast Z97.8
      - eye globe Z97.0
      - heart Z95.812
        - valve Z95.2
      - intestine Z97.8
      - joint Z96.60
        - hip — *see* Presence, hip joint implant
        - knee — *see* Presence, knee joint implant
        - specified site NEC Z96.698
      - kidney Z97.8
      - larynx Z96.3
      - lens Z96.1
      - limbs — *see* Presence, artificial, limb
      - liver Z97.8
      - lung Z97.8
      - pancreas Z97.8
    - by organ transplant (heterologous) (homologous) — *see* Transplant
  - pacemaker
    - brain Z96.89
    - cardiac Z95.0
    - specified NEC Z96.89
  - pancreatectomy Z90.410
    - complete Z90.410
    - partial Z90.411
    - total Z90.410
  - physical restraint Z78.1
  - pneumonectomy (complete) (partial) Z90.2
  - pneumothorax, therapeutic Z98.3
  - postcommotio cerebri F07.81
  - postoperative (postprocedural) NEC Z98.890
    - breast implant Z98.82
    - dental Z98.818
      - crown Z98.811
      - fillings Z98.811
      - restoration Z98.811
      - sealant Z98.810
      - specified NEC Z98.818
    - uterine scar Z98.891
    - pneumothorax, therapeutic Z98.3
  - postpartum (routine follow-up) Z39.2
    - care immediately after delivery Z39.0
  - postsurgical (postprocedural) NEC Z98.890
    - pneumothorax, therapeutic Z98.3
  - pregnancy, incidental Z33.1
  - prosthesis coronary angioplasty Z95.5
  - pseudophakia Z96.1
  - renal dialysis (hemodialysis) (peritoneal) Z99.2
  - retained foreign body — *see* Retained, foreign body fragments (type of)
  - reversed jejunal transposition (for bypass) Z98.0
  - salpingo-oophorectomy
    - bilateral Z90.722
    - unilateral Z90.721
  - sex reassignment surgery status Z87.890
  - shunt
    - arteriovenous (for dialysis) Z99.2
    - cerebrospinal fluid Z98.2
    - ventricular (communicating) (for drainage) Z98.2
  - splenectomy Z90.81
  - thymicolymphaticus E32.8
  - thymicus E32.8
  - thymolymphaticus E32.8
  - thyroidectomy (hypothyroidism) E89.0
  - tooth (teeth) extraction (*see also* Absence, teeth, acquired)K08.409
  - tPA (rtPA) administration in a different facility within the last 24 hours prior to admission to current facility Z92.82
  - tracheostomy Z93.0
  - transplant — *see* Transplant
    - organ removed Z98.85
  - tubal ligation Z98.51
  - underimmunization Z28.3
  - ureterostomy Z93.6
  - urethrostomy Z93.6
  - vagina, artificial Z93.8
  - vasectomy Z98.52
  - wheelchair confinement Z99.3
- **Stealing**
  - child problem F91.8
    - in company with others Z72.810
  - pathological (compulsive) F63.2
- **Steam** burn — *see* Burn
- **Steatocystoma** multiplex L72.2
- **Steatohepatitis** (nonalcoholic) (NASH) K75.81
- **Steatoma** L72.3
  - eyelid (cystic) — *see* Dermatosis, eyelid
    - infected — *see* Hordeolum
- **Steatorrhea** (chronic) K90.9
  - with lacteal obstruction K90.2
  - idiopathic (adult) (infantile) K90.9
  - pancreatic K90.3
  - primary K90.0
  - tropical K90.1
- **Steatosis** E88.89
  - heart — *see* Degeneration, myocardial
  - kidney N28.89
  - liver NEC K76.0
- **Steele-Richardson-Olszewski** disease or syndrome G23.1
- **Steinbrocker's** syndrome G90.8

- **Stenosis** — *continued*
  - neural canal — *continued*
      - sacroiliac M99.34
      - specified NEC M99.39
      - thoracic region M99.32
      - thoracolumbar M99.32
      - upper extremity M99.37
    - subluxation M99.29
      - cervical region M99.21
      - cervicothoracic M99.21
      - head region M99.20
      - lower extremity M99.26
      - lumbar region M99.23
      - lumbosacral M99.23
      - occipitocervical M99.20
      - pelvic M99.25
      - rib cage M99.28
      - sacral region M99.24
      - sacrococcygeal M99.24
      - sacroiliac M99.24
      - specified NEC M99.29
      - thoracic region M99.22
      - thoracolumbar M99.22
      - upper extremity M99.27
  - organ or site, congenital NEC — *see* Atresia, by site
  - papilla of Vater K83.1
  - pulmonary (artery) (congenital) Q25.6
    - with ventricular septal defect, transposition of aorta, and hypertrophy of right ventricle Q21.3
    - acquired I28.8
    - in tetralogy of Fallot Q21.3
    - infundibular Q24.3
    - subvalvular Q24.3
    - supravalvular Q25.6
    - valve I37.0
      - with insufficiency I37.2
      - congenital Q22.1
      - rheumatic I09.89
        - with aortic, mitral or tricuspid (valve) disease I08.8
    - vein, acquired I28.8
    - vessel NEC I28.8
  - pulmonic (congenital) Q22.1
    - infundibular Q24.3
    - subvalvular Q24.3
  - pylorus (hypertrophic) (acquired) K31.1
    - adult K31.1
    - congenital Q40.0
    - infantile Q40.0
  - rectum (sphincter) — *see* Stricture, rectum
  - renal artery I70.1
    - congenital Q27.1
  - salivary duct (any) K11.8
  - sphincter of Oddi K83.1
  - spinal M48.00
    - cervical region M48.02
    - cervicothoracic region M48.03
    - lumbar region M48.06
    - lumbosacral region M48.07
    - occipito-atlanto-axial region M48.01
    - sacrococcygeal region M48.08
    - thoracic region M48.04
    - thoracolumbar region M48.05
  - stent
    - vascular
      - end stent
        - adjacent to stent — *see* Arteriosclerosis
        - within the stent
          - coronary T82.855 ☑
          - peripheral T82.856 ☑
      - in stent
        - coronary vessel T82.855 ☑
        - peripheral vessel T82.856 ☑
  - stomach, hourglass K31.2
  - subaortic (congenital) Q24.4
    - hypertrophic (idiopathic) I42.1
  - subglottic J38.6
    - congenital Q31.1
    - postprocedural J95.5
  - trachea J39.8
    - congenital Q32.1
    - syphilitic A52.73
    - tuberculous NEC A15.5
  - tracheostomy J95.03
  - tricuspid (valve) I07.0
    - with
      - aortic (valve) disease I08.2
      - incompetency, insufficiency or regurgitation I07.2
        - with aortic (valve) disease I08.2

- **Stenosis** — *continued*
  - tricuspid — *continued*
        - with mitral (valve) disease I08.3
      - mitral (valve) disease I08.1
        - with aortic (valve) disease I08.3
    - congenital Q22.4
    - nonrheumatic I36.0
      - with insufficiency I36.2
  - tubal N97.1
  - ureter — *see* Atresia, ureter
  - ureteropelvic junction, congenital Q62.11
  - ureterovesical orifice, congenital Q62.12
  - urethra (valve) (*see also* Stricture, urethra)
    - congenital Q64.32
  - urinary meatus, congenital Q64.33
  - vagina N89.5
    - congenital Q52.4
    - in pregnancy — *see* Pregnancy, complicated by, abnormal vagina
      - causing obstructed labor O65.5
  - valve (cardiac) (heart) (*see also* Endocarditis)I38
    - congenital Q24.8
      - aortic Q23.0
      - mitral Q23.2
      - pulmonary Q22.1
      - tricuspid Q22.4
  - vena cava (inferior) (superior) I87.1
    - congenital Q26.0
  - vesicourethral orifice Q64.31
  - vulva N90.5
- **Stent** jail T82.897 ☑
- **Stercolith** (impaction) K56.41
  - appendix K38.1
- **Stercoraceous,** stercoral ulcer K63.3
  - anus or rectum K62.6
- **Stereotypies** NEC F98.4
- **Sterility** — *see* Infertility
- **Sterilization** — *see* Encounter (for), sterilization
- **Sternalgia** — *see* Angina
- **Sternopagus** Q89.4
- **Sternum** bifidum Q76.7
- **Steroid**
  - effects (adverse) (adrenocortical) (iatrogenic)
    - cushingoid E24.2
      - correct substance properly administered — *see* Table of Drugs and Chemicals, by drug, adverse effect
      - overdose or wrong substance given or taken — *see* Table of Drugs and Chemicals, by drug, poisoning
    - diabetes E09
      - correct substance properly administered — *see* Table of Drugs and Chemicals, by drug, adverse effect
      - overdose or wrong substance given or taken — *see* Table of Drugs and Chemicals, by drug, poisoning
    - fever R50.2
    - insufficiency E27.3
      - correct substance properly administered — *see* Table of Drugs and Chemicals, by drug, adverse effect
      - overdose or wrong substance given or taken — *see* Table of Drugs and Chemicals, by drug, poisoning
  - responder H40.04 ☑
- **Stevens-Johnson** disease or syndrome L51.1
  - toxic epidermal necrolysis overlap L51.3
- **Stewart-Morel** syndrome M85.2
- **Sticker's** disease B08.3
- **Sticky** eye — *see* Conjunctivitis, acute, mucopurulent
- **Stieda's** disease — *see* Bursitis, tibial collateral
- **Stiff** neck — *see* Torticollis
- **Stiff-man** syndrome G25.82
- **Stiffness,** joint NEC M25.60
  - ankle M25.67 ☑
  - ankylosis — *see* Ankylosis, joint
  - contracture — *see* Contraction, joint
  - elbow M25.62 ☑
  - foot M25.67 ☑
  - hand M25.64 ☑
  - hip M25.65 ☑
  - knee M25.66 ☑
  - shoulder M25.61 ☑
  - wrist M25.63 ☑
- **Stigmata** congenital syphilis A50.59
- **Stillbirth** P95
- **Still-Felty** syndrome — *see* Felty's syndrome
- **Still's** disease or syndrome (juvenile) M08.20
  - adult-onset M06.1
  - ankle M08.27 ☑
  - elbow M08.22 ☑

- **Still's** disease or syndrome — *continued*
  - foot joint M08.27 ☑
  - hand joint M08.24 ☑
  - hip M08.25 ☑
  - knee M08.26 ☑
  - multiple site M08.29
  - shoulder M08.21 ☑
  - vertebra M08.28
  - wrist M08.23 ☑
- **Stimulation,** ovary E28.1
- **Sting** (venomous) (with allergic or anaphylactic shock) — *see* Table of Drugs and Chemicals, by animal or substance, poisoning
- **Stippled** epiphyses Q78.8
- **Stitch**
  - abscess T81.48
  - burst (in operation wound) — *see* Disruption, wound, operation
- **Stokes-Adams** disease or syndrome I45.9
- **Stokes'** disease E05.00
  - with thyroid storm E05.01
- **Stokvis** (-Talma) disease D74.8
- **Stoma** malfunction
  - colostomy K94.03
  - enterostomy K94.13
  - gastrostomy K94.23
  - ileostomy K94.13
  - tracheostomy J95.03
- **Stomach** — *see* condition
- **Stomatitis** (denture) (ulcerative) K12.1
  - angular K13.0
    - due to dietary or vitamin deficiency E53.0
  - aphthous K12.0
  - bovine B08.61
  - candidal B37.0
  - catarrhal K12.1
  - diphtheritic A36.89
  - due to
    - dietary deficiency E53.0
    - thrush B37.0
    - vitamin deficiency
      - B group NEC E53.9
      - B2 (riboflavin) E53.0
  - epidemic B08.8
  - epizootic B08.8
  - follicular K12.1
  - gangrenous A69.0
  - Geotrichum B48.3
  - herpesviral, herpetic B00.2
  - herpetiformis K12.0
  - malignant K12.1
  - membranous acute K12.1
  - monilial B37.0
  - mycotic B37.0
  - necrotizing ulcerative A69.0
  - parasitic B37.0
  - septic K12.1
  - spirochetal A69.1
  - suppurative (acute) K12.2
  - ulceromembranous A69.1
  - vesicular K12.1
    - with exanthem (enteroviral) B08.4
    - virus disease A93.8
  - Vincent's A69.1
- **Stomatocytosis** D58.8
- **Stomatomycosis** B37.0
- **Stomatorrhagia** K13.79
- **Stone** (s) (*see also* Calculus)
  - bladder (diverticulum) N21.0
  - cystine E72.09
  - heart syndrome I50.1
  - kidney N20.0
  - prostate N42.0
  - pulpal (dental) K04.2
  - renal N20.0
  - salivary gland or duct (any) K11.5
  - urethra (impacted) N21.1
  - urinary (duct) (impacted) (passage) N20.9
    - bladder (diverticulum) N21.0
    - lower tract N21.9
    - specified NEC N21.8
  - xanthine E79.8 *[N22]*
- **Stonecutter's** lung J62.8
- **Stonemason's** asthma, disease, lung or pneumoconiosis J62.8
- **Stoppage**
  - heart — *see* Arrest, cardiac
  - urine — *see* Retention, urine
- **Storm,** thyroid — *see* Thyrotoxicosis
- **Strabismus** (congenital) (nonparalytic) H50.9
  - concomitant H50.40

- **Strabismus** — *continued*
  - concomitant — *continued*
    - convergent — *see* Strabismus, convergent concomitant
    - divergent — *see* Strabismus, divergent concomitant
  - convergent concomitant H50.00
    - accommodative component H50.43
    - alternating H50.05
      - with
        - A pattern H50.06
        - specified nonconcomitances NEC H50.08
        - V pattern H50.07
    - monocular H50.01 ☑
      - with
        - A pattern H50.02 ☑
        - specified nonconcomitances NEC H50.04 ☑
        - V pattern H50.03 ☑
      - intermittent H50.31 ☑
        - alternating H50.32
  - cyclotropia H50.41 ☑
  - divergent concomitant H50.10
    - alternating H50.15
      - with
        - A pattern H50.16
        - specified noncomitances NEC H50.18
        - V pattern H50.17
    - monocular H50.11 ☑
      - with
        - A pattern H50.12 ☑
        - specified noncomitances NEC H50.14 ☑
        - V pattern H50.13 ☑
      - intermittent H50.33 ☑
        - alternating H50.34
  - Duane's syndrome H50.81 ☑
  - due to adhesions, scars H50.69
  - heterophoria H50.50
    - alternating H50.55
    - cyclophoria H50.54
    - esophoria H50.51
    - exophoria H50.52
    - vertical H50.53
  - heterotropia H50.40
    - intermittent H50.30
  - hypertropia H50.2 ☑
  - hypotropia — *see* Hypertropia
  - latent H50.50
  - mechanical H50.60
    - Brown's sheath syndrome H50.61 ☑
    - specified type NEC H50.69
  - monofixation syndrome H50.42
  - paralytic H49.9
    - abducens nerve H49.2 ☑
    - fourth nerve H49.1 ☑
    - Kearns-Sayre syndrome H49.81 ☑
    - ophthalmoplegia (external)
      - progressive H49.4 ☑
        - with pigmentary retinopathy H49.81 ☑
      - total H49.3 ☑
    - sixth nerve H49.2 ☑
    - specified type NEC H49.88 ☑
    - third nerve H49.0 ☑
    - trochlear nerve H49.1 ☑
  - specified type NEC H50.89
  - vertical H50.2 ☑
- **Strain**
  - back S39.012 ☑
  - cervical S16.1 ☑
  - eye NEC — *see* Disturbance, vision, subjective
  - heart — *see* Disease, heart
  - low back S39.012 ☑
  - mental NOS Z73.3
    - work-related Z56.6
  - muscle (tendon) — *see* Injury, muscle, by site, strain
  - neck S16.1 ☑
  - postural (*see also* Disorder, soft tissue, due to use)
  - physical NOS Z73.3
    - work-related Z56.6
  - psychological NEC Z73.3
  - tendon — *see* Injury, muscle, by site, strain
- **Straining,** on urination R39.16
- **Strand,** vitreous — *see* Opacity, vitreous, membranes and strands
- **Strangulation,** strangulated (*see also* Asphyxia, traumatic)
  - appendix K38.8
  - bladder-neck N32.0
  - bowel or colon K56.2
  - food or foreign body — *see* Foreign body, by site
- **Strangulation** — *continued*
  - hemorrhoids — *see* Hemorrhoids, with complication
  - hernia (*see also* Hernia, by site, with obstruction)
    - with gangrene — *see* Hernia, by site, with gangrene
  - intestine (large) (small) K56.2
    - with hernia (*see also* Hernia, by site, with obstruction)
      - with gangrene — *see* Hernia, by site, with gangrene
  - mesentery K56.2
  - mucus — *see* Asphyxia, mucus
  - omentum K56.2
  - organ or site, congenital NEC — *see* Atresia, by site
  - ovary — *see* Torsion, ovary
  - penis N48.89
    - foreign body T19.4 ☑
  - rupture — *see* Hernia, by site, with obstruction
  - stomach due to hernia (*see also* Hernia, by site, with obstruction)
    - with gangrene — *see* Hernia, by site, with gangrene
  - vesicourethral orifice N32.0
- **Strangury** R30.0
- **Straw** itch B88.0
- **Strawberry**
  - gallbladder K82.4
  - mark Q82.5
  - tongue (red) (white) K14.3
- **Streak** (s)
  - macula, angioid H35.33
  - ovarian Q50.32
- **Strephosymbolia** F81.0
  - secondary to organic lesion R48.8
- **Streptobacillary** fever A25.1
- **Streptobacillosis** A25.1
- **Streptobacillus** moniliformis A25.1
- **Streptococcus,** streptococcal (*see also* condition)
  - as cause of disease classified elsewhere B95.5
  - group
    - A, as cause of disease classified elsewhere B95.0
    - B, as cause of disease classified elsewhere B95.1
    - D, as cause of disease classified elsewhere B95.2
  - pneumoniae, as cause of disease classified elsewhere B95.3
  - specified NEC, as cause of disease classified elsewhere B95.4
- **Streptomycosis** B47.1
- **Streptotrichosis** A48.8
- **Stress** F43.9
  - family — *see* Disruption, family
  - fetal P84
    - complicating pregnancy O77.9
      - due to drug administration O77.1
  - mental NEC Z73.3
    - work-related Z56.6
  - physical NEC Z73.3
    - work-related Z56.6
  - polycythemia D75.1
  - reaction (*see also* Reaction, stress)F43.9
  - work schedule Z56.3
- **Stretching,** nerve — *see* Injury, nerve
- **Striae** albicantes, atrophicae or distensae (cutis) L90.6
- **Stricture** (*see also* Stenosis)
  - ampulla of Vater K83.1
  - anus (sphincter) K62.4
    - congenital Q42.3
      - with fistula Q42.2
    - infantile Q42.3
      - with fistula Q42.2
  - aorta (ascending) (congenital) Q25.1
    - arteriosclerotic I70.0
    - calcified I70.0
    - supravalvular, congenital Q25.3
  - aortic (valve) — *see* Stenosis, aortic
  - aqueduct of Sylvius (congenital) Q03.0
    - with spina bifida — *see* Spina bifida, by site, with hydrocephalus
    - acquired G91.1
  - artery I77.1
    - basilar — *see* Occlusion, artery, basilar
    - carotid — *see* Occlusion, artery, carotid
    - celiac I77.4
    - congenital (peripheral) Q27.8
      - cerebral Q28.3
      - coronary Q24.5
      - digestive system Q27.8
- **Stricture** — *continued*
  - artery — *continued*
      - lower limb Q27.8
      - retinal Q14.1
      - specified site NEC Q27.8
      - umbilical Q27.0
      - upper limb Q27.8
    - coronary — *see* Disease, heart, ischemic, atherosclerotic
      - congenital Q24.5
    - precerebral — *see* Occlusion, artery, precerebral
    - pulmonary (congenital) Q25.6
      - acquired I28.8
    - renal I70.1
    - vertebral — *see* Occlusion, artery, vertebral
  - auditory canal (external) (congenital)
    - acquired — *see* Stenosis, external ear canal
  - bile duct (common) (hepatic) K83.1
    - congenital Q44.3
    - postoperative K91.89
  - bladder N32.89
    - neck N32.0
  - bowel — *see* Obstruction, intestine
  - brain G93.89
  - bronchus J98.09
    - congenital Q32.3
    - syphilitic A52.72
  - cardia (stomach) K22.2
    - congenital Q39.3
  - cardiac (*see also* Disease, heart)
    - orifice (stomach) K22.2
  - cecum — *see* Obstruction, intestine
  - cervix, cervical (canal) N88.2
    - congenital Q51.828
    - in pregnancy — *see* Pregnancy, complicated by, abnormal cervix
      - causing obstructed labor O65.5
  - colon (*see also* Obstruction, intestine)
    - congenital Q42.9
      - specified NEC Q42.8
  - colostomy K94.03
  - common (bile) duct K83.1
  - coronary (artery) — *see* Disease, heart, ischemic, atherosclerotic
  - cystic duct — *see* Obstruction, gallbladder
  - digestive organs NEC, congenital Q45.8
  - duodenum K31.5
    - congenital Q41.0
  - ear canal (external) (congenital) Q16.1
    - acquired — *see* Stricture, auditory canal, acquired
  - ejaculatory duct N50.89
  - enterostomy K94.13
  - esophagus K22.2
    - congenital Q39.3
    - syphilitic A52.79
      - congenital A50.59 *[K23]*
  - eustachian tube (*see also* Obstruction, eustachian tube)
    - congenital Q17.8
  - fallopian tube N97.1
    - gonococcal A54.24
    - tuberculous A18.17
  - gallbladder — *see* Obstruction, gallbladder
  - glottis J38.6
  - heart (*see also* Disease, heart)
    - valve (*see also* Endocarditis)I38
      - aortic Q23.0
      - mitral Q23.4
      - pulmonary Q22.1
      - tricuspid Q22.4
  - hepatic duct K83.1
  - hourglass, of stomach K31.2
  - hymen N89.6
  - hypopharynx J39.2
  - ileum K56.69
    - congenital Q41.2
  - intestine (*see also* Obstruction, intestine)
    - congenital (small) Q41.9
      - large Q42.9
        - specified NEC Q42.8
      - specified NEC Q41.8
    - ischemic K55.1
  - jejunum K56.69
    - congenital Q41.1
  - lacrimal passages (*see also* Stenosis, lacrimal)
    - congenital Q10.5
  - larynx J38.6
    - congenital NEC Q31.8
      - subglottic Q31.1
    - syphilitic A52.73
      - congenital A50.59 *[J99]*

Strabismus - Stricture

ICD-10-CM INDEX TO DISEASES AND INJURIES

- **Stricture** — *continued*
  - meatus
    - ear (congenital) Q16.1
      - acquired — *see* Stricture, auditory canal, acquired
    - osseous (ear) (congenital) Q16.1
      - acquired — *see* Stricture, auditory canal, acquired
    - urinarius (*see also* Stricture, urethra)
      - congenital Q64.33
  - mitral (valve) — *see* Stenosis, mitral
  - myocardium, myocardial I51.5
    - hypertrophic subaortic (idiopathic) I42.1
  - nares (anterior) (posterior) J34.89
    - congenital Q30.0
  - nasal duct (*see also* Stenosis, lacrimal, duct)
    - congenital Q10.5
  - nasolacrimal duct (*see also* Stenosis, lacrimal, duct)
    - congenital Q10.5
  - nasopharynx J39.2
    - syphilitic A52.73
  - nose J34.89
    - congenital Q30.0
  - nostril (anterior) (posterior) J34.89
    - congenital Q30.0
    - syphilitic A52.73
      - congenital A50.59 *[J99]*
  - organ or site, congenital NEC — *see* Atresia, by site
  - os uteri — *see* Stricture, cervix
  - osseous meatus (ear) (congenital) Q16.1
    - acquired — *see* Stricture, auditory canal, acquired
  - oviduct — *see* Stricture, fallopian tube
  - pelviureteric junction (congenital) Q62.11
    - acquired, with hydronephrosis N13.0
  - penis, by foreign body T19.4 ☑
  - pharynx J39.2
  - prostate N42.89
  - pulmonary, pulmonic
    - artery (congenital) Q25.6
      - acquired I28.8
      - noncongenital I28.8
    - infundibulum (congenital) Q24.3
    - valve I37.0
      - congenital Q22.1
    - vein, acquired I28.8
    - vessel NEC I28.8
  - punctum lacrimale (*see also* Stenosis, lacrimal, punctum)
    - congenital Q10.5
  - pylorus (hypertrophic) K31.1
    - adult K31.1
    - congenital Q40.0
    - infantile Q40.0
  - rectosigmoid K56.69
  - rectum (sphincter) K62.4
    - congenital Q42.1
      - with fistula Q42.0
    - due to
      - chlamydial lymphogranuloma A55
      - irradiation K91.89
      - lymphogranuloma venereum A55
    - gonococcal A54.6
    - inflammatory (chlamydial) A55
    - syphilitic A52.74
    - tuberculous A18.32
  - renal artery I70.1
    - congenital Q27.1
  - salivary duct or gland (any) K11.8
  - sigmoid (flexure) — *see* Obstruction, intestine
  - spermatic cord N50.89
  - stoma (following) (of)
    - colostomy K94.03
    - enterostomy K94.13
    - gastrostomy K94.23
    - ileostomy K94.13
    - tracheostomy J95.03
  - stomach K31.89
    - congenital Q40.2
    - hourglass K31.2
  - subaortic Q24.4
    - hypertrophic (acquired) (idiopathic) I42.1
  - subglottic J38.6
  - syphilitic NEC A52.79
  - trachea J39.8
    - congenital Q32.1
    - syphilitic A52.73
    - tuberculous NEC A15.5
  - tracheostomy J95.03
  - tricuspid (valve) — *see* Stenosis, tricuspid

- **Stricture** — *continued*
  - tunica vaginalis N50.89
  - ureter (postoperative) N13.5
    - with
      - hydronephrosis N13.1
        - with infection N13.6
      - pyelonephritis (chronic) N11.1
    - congenital — *see* Atresia, ureter
    - tuberculous A18.11
  - ureteropelvic junction (congenital) Q62.11
    - acquired, with hydronephrosis N13.0
  - ureterovesical orifice N13.5
    - with infection N13.6
  - urethra (organic) (spasmodic) N35.9
    - associated with schistosomiasis B65.0 *[N37]*
    - congenital Q64.39
      - valvular (posterior) Q64.2
    - due to
      - infection — *see* Stricture, urethra, postinfective
      - trauma — *see* Stricture, urethra, post-traumatic
    - gonococcal, gonorrheal A54.01
    - infective NEC — *see* Stricture, urethra, postinfective
    - late effect (sequelae) of injury — *see* Stricture, urethra, post-traumatic
    - postcatheterization — *see* Stricture, urethra, postprocedural
    - postinfective NEC
      - female N35.12
      - male N35.119
        - anterior urethra N35.114
        - bulbous urethra N35.112
        - meatal N35.111
        - membranous urethra N35.113
    - postobstetric N35.021
    - postoperative — *see* Stricture, urethra, postprocedural
    - postprocedural
      - female N99.12
      - male N99.114
        - anterior bulbous urethra N99.113
        - bulbous urethra N99.111
        - fossa navicularis N99.115
        - meatal N99.110
        - membranous urethra N99.112
    - post-traumatic
      - female N35.028
        - due to childbirth N35.021
      - male N35.014
        - anterior urethra N35.013
        - bulbous urethra N35.011
        - meatal N35.010
        - membranous urethra N35.012
    - sequela (late effect) of
      - childbirth N35.021
      - injury — *see* Stricture, urethra, post-traumatic
    - specified cause NEC N35.8
    - syphilitic A52.76
    - traumatic — *see* Stricture, urethra, post-traumatic
    - valvular (posterior), congenital Q64.2
  - urinary meatus — *see* Stricture, urethra
  - uterus, uterine (synechiae) N85.6
    - os (external) (internal) — *see* Stricture, cervix
  - vagina (outlet) — *see* Stenosis, vagina
  - valve (cardiac) (heart) (*see also* Endocarditis)
    - congenital
      - aortic Q23.0
      - mitral Q23.2
      - pulmonary Q22.1
      - tricuspid Q22.4
  - vas deferens N50.89
    - congenital Q55.4
  - vein I87.1
  - vena cava (inferior) (superior) NEC I87.1
    - congenital Q26.0
  - vesicourethral orifice N32.0
    - congenital Q64.31
  - vulva (acquired) N90.5
- **Stridor** R06.1
  - congenital (larynx) P28.89
- **Stridulous** — *see* condition
- **Stroke** (apoplectic) (brain) (embolic) (ischemic) (paralytic) (thrombotic) I63.9
  - epileptic — *see* Epilepsy
  - heat T67.0 ☑
  - in evolution I63.9
  - intraoperative
    - during cardiac surgery I97.810
    - during other surgery I97.811

- **Stroke** — *continued*
  - lightning — *see* Lightning
  - meaning
    - cerebral hemorrhage - code to Hemorrhage, intracranial
    - cerebral infarction - code to Infarction, cerebral
  - postprocedural
    - following cardiac surgery I97.820
    - following other surgery I97.821
  - unspecified (NOS) I63.9
- **Stromatosis,** endometrial D39.0
- **Strongyloidiasis,** strongyloidosis B78.9
  - cutaneous B78.1
  - disseminated B78.7
  - intestinal B78.0
- **Strophulus** pruriginosus L28.2
- **Struck** by lightning — *see* Lightning
- **Struma** (*see also* Goiter)
  - Hashimoto E06.3
  - lymphomatosa E06.3
  - nodosa (simplex) E04.9
    - endemic E01.2
      - multinodular E01.1
    - multinodular E04.2
      - iodine-deficiency related E01.1
    - toxic or with hyperthyroidism E05.20
      - with thyroid storm E05.21
      - multinodular E05.20
        - with thyroid storm E05.21
      - uninodular E05.10
        - with thyroid storm E05.11
    - toxicosa E05.20
      - with thyroid storm E05.21
      - multinodular E05.20
        - with thyroid storm E05.21
      - uninodular E05.10
        - with thyroid storm E05.11
    - uninodular E04.1
  - ovarii D27. ☑
  - Riedel's E06.5
- **Strumipriva** cachexia E03.4
- **Strümpell-Marie** spine — *see* Spondylitis, ankylosing
- **Strümpell-Westphal** pseudosclerosis E83.01
- **Stuart** deficiency disease (factor X) D68.2
- **Stuart-Prower** factor deficiency (factor X) D68.2
- **Student's** elbow — *see* Bursitis, elbow, olecranon
- **Stump** — *see* Amputation
- **Stunting,** nutritional E45
- **Stupor** (catatonic) R40.1
  - depressive (single episode) F32.89
    - recurrent episode F33.8
  - dissociative F44.2
  - manic F30.2
  - manic-depressive F31.89
  - psychogenic (anergic) F44.2
  - reaction to exceptional stress (transient) F43.0
- **Sturge** (-Weber) (-Dimitri) (-Kalischer) disease or syndrome Q85.8
- **Stuttering** F80.81
  - adult onset F98.5
  - childhood onset F80.81
  - following cerebrovascular disease — *see* Disorder, fluency. following cerebrovascular disease
  - in conditions classified elsewhere R47.82
- **Sty,** stye (external) (internal) (meibomian) (zeisian) — *see* Hordeolum
- **Subacidity,** gastric K31.89
  - psychogenic F45.8
- **Subacute** — *see* condition
- **Subarachnoid** — *see* condition
- **Subcortical** — *see* condition
- **Subcostal** syndrome, nerve compression — *see* Mononeuropathy, upper limb, specified site NEC
- **Subcutaneous,** subcuticular — *see* condition
- **Subdural** — *see* condition
- **Subendocardium** — *see* condition
- **Subependymoma**
  - specified site — *see* Neoplasm, uncertain behavior, by site
  - unspecified site D43.2
- **Suberosis** J67.3
- **Subglossitis** — *see* Glossitis
- **Subhemophilia** D66
- **Subinvolution**
  - breast (postlactational) (postpuerperal) N64.89
  - puerperal O90.89
  - uterus (chronic) (nonpuerperal) N85.3
    - puerperal O90.89
- **Sublingual** — *see* condition
- **Sublinguitis** — *see* Sialoadenitis
- **Subluxatable** hip Q65.6

- **Subluxation** (*see also* Dislocation)
  - acromioclavicular S43.11 ☑
  - ankle S93.0 ☑
  - atlantoaxial, recurrent M43.4
    - with myelopathy M43.3
  - carpometacarpal (joint) NEC S63.05 ☑
    - thumb S63.04 ☑
  - complex, vertebral — *see* Complex, subluxation
  - congenital (*see also* Malposition, congenital)
    - hip — *see* Dislocation, hip, congenital, partial
    - joint (excluding hip)
      - lower limb Q68.8
      - shoulder Q68.8
      - upper limb Q68.8
  - elbow (traumatic) S53.10 ☑
    - anterior S53.11 ☑
    - lateral S53.14 ☑
    - medial S53.13 ☑
    - posterior S53.12 ☑
    - specified type NEC S53.19 ☑
  - finger S63.20 ☑
    - index S63.20 ☑
    - interphalangeal S63.22 ☑
      - distal S63.24 ☑
        - index S63.24 ☑
        - little S63.24 ☑
        - middle S63.24 ☑
        - ring S63.24 ☑
      - index S63.22 ☑
      - little S63.22 ☑
      - middle S63.22 ☑
      - proximal S63.23 ☑
        - index S63.23 ☑
        - little S63.23 ☑
        - middle S63.23 ☑
        - ring S63.23 ☑
      - ring S63.22 ☑
    - little S63.20 ☑
    - metacarpophalangeal S63.21 ☑
      - index S63.21 ☑
      - little S63.21 ☑
      - middle S63.21 ☑
      - ring S63.21 ☑
    - middle S63.20 ☑
    - ring S63.20 ☑
  - foot S93.30 ☑
    - specified site NEC S93.33 ☑
    - tarsal joint S93.31 ☑
    - tarsometatarsal joint S93.32 ☑
    - toe — *see* Subluxation, toe
  - hip S73.00 ☑
    - anterior S73.03 ☑
      - obturator S73.02 ☑
    - central S73.04 ☑
    - posterior S73.01 ☑
  - interphalangeal (joint)
    - finger S63.22 ☑
      - distal joint S63.24 ☑
        - index S63.24 ☑
        - little S63.24 ☑
        - middle S63.24 ☑
        - ring S63.24 ☑
      - index S63.22 ☑
      - little S63.22 ☑
      - middle S63.22 ☑
      - proximal joint S63.23 ☑
        - index S63.23 ☑
        - little S63.23 ☑
        - middle S63.23 ☑
        - ring S63.23 ☑
      - ring S63.22 ☑
    - thumb S63.12 ☑
      - distal joint S63.14 ☑
      - proximal joint S63.13 ☑
    - toe S93.13 ☑
      - great S93.13 ☑
      - lesser S93.13 ☑
  - joint prosthesis — *see* Complications, joint prosthesis, mechanical, displacement, by site
  - knee S83.10 ☑
    - cap — *see* Subluxation, patella
    - patella — *see* Subluxation, patella
    - proximal tibia
      - anteriorly S83.11 ☑
      - laterally S83.14 ☑
      - medially S83.13 ☑
      - posteriorly S83.12 ☑
    - specified type NEC S83.19 ☑
  - lens — *see* Dislocation, lens, partial
  - ligament, traumatic — *see* Sprain, by site
  - metacarpal (bone)
    - proximal end S63.06 ☑

- **Subluxation** — *continued*
  - metacarpophalangeal (joint)
    - finger S63.21 ☑
      - index S63.21 ☑
      - little S63.21 ☑
      - middle S63.21 ☑
      - ring S63.21 ☑
    - thumb S63.11 ☑
  - metatarsophalangeal joint S93.14 ☑
    - great toe S93.14 ☑
    - lesser toe S93.14 ☑
  - midcarpal (joint) S63.03 ☑
  - patella S83.00 ☑
    - lateral S83.01 ☑
    - recurrent (nontraumatic) — *see* Dislocation, patella, recurrent, incomplete
    - specified type NEC S83.09 ☑
  - pathological — *see* Dislocation, pathological
  - radial head S53.00 ☑
    - anterior S53.01 ☑
    - nursemaid's elbow S53.03 ☑
    - posterior S53.02 ☑
    - specified type NEC S53.09 ☑
  - radiocarpal (joint) S63.02 ☑
  - radioulnar (joint)
    - distal S63.01 ☑
    - proximal — *see* Subluxation, elbow
  - shoulder
    - congenital Q68.8
    - girdle S43.30 ☑
      - scapula S43.31 ☑
      - specified site NEC S43.39 ☑
    - traumatic S43.00 ☑
      - anterior S43.01 ☑
      - inferior S43.03 ☑
      - posterior S43.02 ☑
      - specified type NEC S43.08 ☑
  - sternoclavicular (joint) S43.20 ☑
    - anterior S43.21 ☑
    - posterior S43.22 ☑
  - symphysis (pubis)
  - thumb S63.103 ☑
    - interphalangeal joint — *see* Subluxation, interphalangeal (joint), thumb
    - metacarpophalangeal joint — *see* Subluxation, metacarpophalangeal (joint), thumb
  - toe (s) S93.10 ☑
    - great S93.10 ☑
      - interphalangeal joint S93.13 ☑
      - metatarsophalangeal joint S93.14 ☑
    - interphalangeal joint S93.13 ☑
    - lesser S93.10 ☑
      - interphalangeal joint S93.13 ☑
      - metatarsophalangeal joint S93.14 ☑
    - metatarsophalangeal joint S93.149 ☑
  - ulnohumeral joint — *see* Subluxation, elbow
  - vertebral
    - recurrent NEC — *see* subcategory M43.5
    - traumatic
      - cervical S13.100 ☑
        - atlantoaxial joint S13.120 ☑
        - atlantooccipital joint S13.110 ☑
        - atloidooccipital joint S13.110 ☑
        - joint between
          - C0 and C1 S13.110 ☑
          - C1 and C2 S13.120 ☑
          - C2 and C3 S13.130 ☑
          - C3 and C4 S13.140 ☑
          - C4 and C5 S13.150 ☑
          - C5and C6 S13.160 ☑
          - C6and C7 S13.170 ☑
          - C7and T1 S13.180 ☑
        - occipitoatloid joint S13.110 ☑
      - lumbar S33.100 ☑
        - joint between
          - L1and L2 S33.110 ☑
          - L2and L3 S33.120 ☑
          - L3 and L4 S33.130 ☑
          - L4and L5 S33.140 ☑
      - thoracic S23.100 ☑
        - joint between
          - T1and T2 S23.110 ☑
          - T2and T3 S23.120 ☑
          - T3 and T4 S23.122 ☑
          - T4 and T5 S23.130 ☑
          - T5 and T6 S23.132 ☑
          - T6 and T7 S23.140 ☑
          - T7 and T8 S23.142 ☑
          - T8 and T9 S23.150 ☑
          - T9 and T10 S23.152 ☑
          - T10 and T11 S23.160 ☑
          - T11 and T12 S23.162 ☑
          - T12 and L1 S23.170 ☑

- **Subluxation** — *continued*
  - ulna
    - distal end S63.07 ☑
    - proximal end — *see* Subluxation, elbow
  - wrist (carpal bone) S63.00 ☑
    - carpometacarpal joint — *see* Subluxation, carpometacarpal (joint)
    - distal radioulnar joint — *see* Subluxation, radioulnar (joint), distal
    - metacarpal bone, proximal — *see* Subluxation, metacarpal (bone), proximal end
    - midcarpal — *see* Subluxation, midcarpal (joint)
    - radiocarpal joint — *see* Subluxation, radiocarpal (joint)
    - recurrent — *see* Dislocation, recurrent, wrist
    - specified site NEC S63.09 ☑
    - ulna — *see* Subluxation, ulna, distal end
- **Submaxillary** — *see* condition
- **Submersion** (fatal) (nonfatal) T75.1 ☑
- **Submucous** — *see* condition
- **Subnormal,** subnormality
  - accommodation (old age) H52.4
  - mental — *see* Disability, intellectual
  - temperature (accidental) T68 ☑
- **Subphrenic** — *see* condition
- **Subscapular** nerve — *see* condition
- **Subseptus** uterus Q51.2
- **Subsiding** appendicitis K36
- **Substance** (other psychoactive)-induced
  - anxiety disorder F19.980
  - bipolar and related disorder F19.94
  - delirium F19.921
  - depressive disorder F19.94
  - major neurocognitive disorder F19.97
  - mild neurocognitive disorder F19.988
  - obsessive-compulsive and related disorder F19.988
  - psychotic disorder F19.959
  - sexual dysfunction F19.981
  - sleep disorder F19.982
- **Substernal** thyroid E04.9
  - congenital Q89.2
- **Substitution** disorder F44.9
- **Subtentorial** — *see* condition
- **Subthyroidism** (acquired) (*see also* Hypothyroidism)
  - congenital E03.1
- **Succenturiate** placenta O43.19 ☑
- **Sucking** thumb, child (excessive) F98.8
- **Sudamen,** sudamina L74.1
- **Sudanese** kala-azar B55.0
- **Sudden**
  - heart failure — *see* Failure, heart
  - hearing loss — *see* Deafness, sudden
- **Sudeck's** atrophy, disease, or syndrome — *see* Algoneurodystrophy
- **Suffocation** — *see* Asphyxia, traumatic
- **Sugar**
  - blood
    - high (transient) R73.9
    - low (transient) E16.2
  - in urine R81
- **Suicide,** suicidal (attempted) T14.91
  - by poisoning — *see* Table of Drugs and Chemicals
  - history of (personal) Z91.5
    - in family Z81.8
  - ideation — *see* Ideation, suicidal
  - risk
    - meaning personal history of attempted suicide Z91.5
    - meaning suicidal ideation — *see* Ideation, suicidal
  - tendencies
    - meaning personal history of attempted suicide Z91.5
    - meaning suicidal ideation — *see* Ideation, suicidal
  - trauma — *see* nature of injury by site
- **Suipestifer** infection — *see* Infection, salmonella
- **Sulfhemoglobinemia,** sulphemoglobinemia (acquired) (with methemoglobinemia) D74.8
- **Sumatran** mite fever A75.3
- **Summer** — *see* condition
- **Sunburn** L55.9
  - due to
    - tanning bed (acute) L56.8
      - chronic L57.8
    - ultraviolet radiation (acute) L56.8
      - chronic L57.8
  - first degree L55.0
  - second degree L55.1
  - third degree L55.2

- **SUNCT** (short lasting unilateral neuralgiform headache with conjunctival injection and tearing) G44.059
  - intractable G44.051
  - not intractable G44.059
- **Sunken** acetabulum — *see* Derangement, joint, specified type NEC, hip
- **Sunstroke** T67.0 ☑
- **Superfecundation** — *see* Pregnancy, multiple
- **Superfetation** — *see* Pregnancy, multiple
- **Superinvolution** (uterus) N85.8
- **Supernumerary** (congenital)
  - aortic cusps Q23.8
  - auditory ossicles Q16.3
  - bone Q79.8
  - breast Q83.1
  - carpal bones Q74.0
  - cusps, heart valve NEC Q24.8
    - aortic Q23.8
    - mitral Q23.2
    - pulmonary Q22.3
  - digit (s) Q69.9
  - ear (lobule) Q17.0
  - fallopian tube Q50.6
  - finger Q69.0
  - hymen Q52.4
  - kidney Q63.0
  - lacrimonasal duct Q10.6
  - lobule (ear) Q17.0
  - mitral cusps Q23.2
  - muscle Q79.8
  - nipple (s) Q83.3
  - organ or site not listed — *see* Accessory
  - ossicles, auditory Q16.3
  - ovary Q50.31
  - oviduct Q50.6
  - pulmonary, pulmonic cusps Q22.3
  - rib Q76.6
    - cervical or first (syndrome) Q76.5
  - roots (of teeth) K00.2
  - spleen Q89.09
  - tarsal bones Q74.2
  - teeth K00.1
  - testis Q55.29
  - thumb Q69.1
  - toe Q69.2
  - uterus Q51.2
  - vagina Q52.1 ☑
  - vertebra Q76.49
- **Supervision** (of)
  - contraceptive — *see* Prescription, contraceptives
  - dietary (for) Z71.3
    - allergy (food) Z71.3
    - colitis Z71.3
    - diabetes mellitus Z71.3
    - food allergy or intolerance Z71.3
    - gastritis Z71.3
    - hypercholesterolemia Z71.3
    - hypoglycemia Z71.3
    - intolerance (food) Z71.3
    - obesity Z71.3
    - specified NEC Z71.3
  - healthy infant or child Z76.2
    - foundling Z76.1
  - high-risk pregnancy — *see* Pregnancy, complicated by, high, risk
  - lactation Z39.1
  - pregnancy — *see* Pregnancy, supervision of
- **Supplemental** teeth K00.1
- **Suppression**
  - binocular vision H53.34
  - lactation O92.5
  - menstruation N94.89
  - ovarian secretion E28.39
  - renal N28.9
  - urine, urinary secretion R34
- **Suppuration,** suppurative (*see also* condition)
  - accessory sinus (chronic) — *see* Sinusitis
  - adrenal gland
  - antrum (chronic) — *see* Sinusitis, maxillary
  - bladder — *see* Cystitis
  - brain G06.0
    - sequelae G09
  - breast N61.1
    - puerperal, postpartum or gestational — *see* Mastitis, obstetric, purulent
  - dental periosteum M27.3
  - ear (middle) (*see also* Otitis, media)
    - external NEC — *see* Otitis, externa, infective
    - internal — *see* subcategory H83.0
  - ethmoidal (chronic) (sinus) — *see* Sinusitis, ethmoidal

Suppuration — *continued*

  - fallopian tube — *see* Salpingo-oophoritis
  - frontal (chronic) (sinus) — *see* Sinusitis, frontal
  - gallbladder (acute) K81.0
  - gum K05.20
    - generalized — *see* Periodontitis, aggressive, generalized
    - localized — *see* Periodontitis, aggressive, localized
  - intracranial G06.0
  - joint — *see* Arthritis, pyogenic or pyemic
  - labyrinthine — *see* subcategory H83.0
  - lung — *see* Abscess, lung
  - mammary gland N61.1
    - puerperal, postpartum O91.12
      - associated with lactation O91.13
  - maxilla, maxillary M27.2
    - sinus (chronic) — *see* Sinusitis, maxillary
  - muscle — *see* Myositis, infective
  - nasal sinus (chronic) — *see* Sinusitis
  - pancreas, acute (*see also* Pancreatitis, acute)K85.80
  - parotid gland — *see* Sialoadenitis
  - pelvis, pelvic
    - female — *see* Disease, pelvis, inflammatory
    - male K65.0
  - pericranial — *see* Osteomyelitis
  - salivary duct or gland (any) — *see* Sialoadenitis
  - sinus (accessory) (chronic) (nasal) — *see* Sinusitis
  - sphenoidal sinus (chronic) — *see* Sinusitis, sphenoidal
  - thymus (gland) E32.1
  - thyroid (gland) E06.0
  - tonsil — *see* Tonsillitis
  - uterus — *see* Endometritis
- **Supraeruption** of tooth (teeth) M26.34
- **Supraglottitis** J04.30
  - with obstruction J04.31
- **Suprarenal** (gland) — *see* condition
- **Suprascapular** nerve — *see* condition
- **Suprasellar** — *see* condition
- **Surfer's** knots or nodules S89.8 ☑
- **Surgical**
  - emphysema T81.82 ☑
  - procedures, complication or misadventure — *see* Complications, surgical procedures
  - shock T81.10 ☑
- **Surveillance** (of) (for) (*see also* Observation)
  - alcohol abuse Z71.41
  - contraceptive — *see* Prescription, contraceptives
  - dietary Z71.3
  - drug abuse Z71.51
- **Susceptibility** to disease, genetic Z15.89
  - malignant neoplasm Z15.09
    - breast Z15.01
    - endometrium Z15.04
    - ovary Z15.02
    - prostate Z15.03
    - specified NEC Z15.09
  - multiple endocrine neoplasia Z15.81
- **Suspected** condition, ruled out (*see also* Observation, suspected)
  - amniotic cavity and membrane Z03.71
  - cervical shortening Z03.75
  - fetal anomaly Z03.73
  - fetal growth Z03.74
  - maternal and fetal conditions NEC Z03.79
  - newborn (*see also* Observation, newborn, suspected condition ruled out)Z05.9
  - oligohydramnios Z03.71
  - placental problem Z03.72
  - polyhydramnios Z03.71
- **Suspended** uterus
  - in pregnancy or childbirth — *see* Pregnancy, complicated by, abnormal uterus
- **Sutton's** nevus D22.9
- **Suture**
  - burst (in operation wound) T81.31 ☑
    - external operation wound T81.31 ☑
    - internal operation wound T81.32 ☑
  - inadvertently left in operation wound — *see* Foreign body, accidentally left during a procedure
  - removal Z48.02
- **Swab** inadvertently left in operation wound — *see* Foreign body, accidentally left during a procedure
- **Swallowed,** swallowing
  - difficulty — *see* Dysphagia
  - foreign body — *see* Foreign body, alimentary tract
- **Swan-neck** deformity (finger) — *see* Deformity, finger, swan-neck
- **Swearing,** compulsive F42.8
  - in Gilles de la Tourette's syndrome F95.2
- **Sweat,** sweats
  - fetid L75.0
  - night R61
- **Sweating,** excessive R61
- **Sweeley-Klionsky** disease E75.21
- **Sweet's** disease or dermatosis L98.2
- **Swelling** (of) R60.9
  - abdomen, abdominal (not referable to any particular organ) — *see* Mass, abdominal
  - ankle — *see* Effusion, joint, ankle
  - arm M79.89
    - forearm M79.89
  - breast N63
  - Calabar B74.3
  - cervical gland R59.0
  - chest, localized R22.2
  - ear H93.8 ☑
  - extremity (lower) (upper) — *see* Disorder, soft tissue, specified type NEC
  - finger M79.89
  - foot M79.89
  - glands R59.9
    - generalized R59.1
    - localized R59.0
  - hand M79.89
  - head (localized) R22.0
  - inflammatory — *see* Inflammation
  - intra-abdominal — *see* Mass, abdominal
  - joint — *see* Effusion, joint
  - leg M79.89
    - lower M79.89
  - limb — *see* Disorder, soft tissue, specified type NEC
  - localized (skin) R22.9
    - chest R22.2
    - head R22.0
    - limb
      - lower — *see* Mass, localized, limb, lower
      - upper — *see* Mass, localized, limb, upper
    - neck R22.1
    - trunk R22.2
  - neck (localized) R22.1
  - pelvic — *see* Mass, abdominal
  - scrotum N50.89
  - splenic — *see* Splenomegaly
  - testis N50.89
  - toe M79.89
  - umbilical R19.09
  - wandering, due to Gnathostoma (spinigerum) B83.1
  - white — *see* Tuberculosis, arthritis
- **Swift** (-Feer) disease
  - overdose or wrong substance given or taken — *see* Table of Drugs and Chemicals, by drug, poisoning
- **Swimmer's**
  - cramp T75.1 ☑
  - ear H60.33 ☑
  - itch B65.3
- **Swimming** in the head R42
- **Swollen** — *see* Swelling
- **Swyer** syndrome Q99.1
- **Sycosis** L73.8
  - barbae (not parasitic) L73.8
  - contagiosa (mycotic) B35.0
  - lupoides L73.8
  - mycotic B35.0
  - parasitic B35.0
  - vulgaris L73.8
- **Sydenham's** chorea — *see* Chorea, Sydenham's
- **Sylvatic** yellow fever A95.0
- **Sylvest's** disease B33.0
- **Symblepharon** H11.23 ☑
  - congenital Q10.3
- **Symond's** syndrome G93.2
- **Sympathetic** — *see* condition
- **Sympatheticotonia** G90.8
- **Sympathicoblastoma**
  - specified site — *see* Neoplasm, malignant, by site
  - unspecified site C74.90
- **Sympathogonioma** — *see* Sympathicoblastoma
- **Symphalangy** (fingers) (toes) Q70.9
- **Symptoms** NEC R68.89
  - breast NEC N64.59
  - development NEC R63.8
  - factitious, self-induced — *see* Disorder, factitious
  - genital organs, female R10.2
  - involving
    - abdomen NEC R19.8
    - appearance NEC R46.89

- **Symptoms** — *continued*
  - involving — *continued*
    - awareness R41.9
      - altered mental status R41.82
      - amnesia — *see* Amnesia
      - borderline intellectual functioning R41.83
      - coma — *see* Coma
      - disorientation R41.0
      - neurologic neglect syndrome R41.4
      - senile cognitive decline R41.81
      - specified symptom NEC R41.89
    - behavior NEC R46.89
    - cardiovascular system NEC R09.89
    - chest NEC R09.89
    - circulatory system NEC R09.89
    - cognitive functions R41.9
      - altered mental status R41.82
      - amnesia — *see* Amnesia
      - borderline intellectual functioning R41.83
      - coma — *see* Coma
      - disorientation R41.0
      - neurologic neglect syndrome R41.4
      - senile cognitive decline R41.81
      - specified symptom NEC R41.89
    - development NEC R62.50
    - digestive system NEC R19.8
    - emotional state NEC R45.89
      - emotional lability R45.86
    - food and fluid intake R63.8
    - general perceptions and sensations R44.9
      - specified NEC R44.8
    - musculoskeletal system R29.91
      - specified NEC R29.898
    - nervous system R29.90
      - specified NEC R29.818
    - pelvis NEC R19.8
    - respiratory system NEC R09.89
    - skin and integument R23.9
    - urinary system R39.9
  - menopausal N95.1
  - metabolism NEC R63.8
  - neurotic F48.8
  - of infancy R68.19
  - pelvis NEC, female R10.2
  - skin and integument NEC R23.9
  - subcutaneous tissue NEC R23.9
- **Sympus** Q74.2
- **Syncephalus** Q89.4
- **Synchondrosis**
  - abnormal (congenital) Q78.8
  - ischiopubic M91.0
- **Synchysis** (scintillans) (senile) (vitreous body) H43.89
- **Syncope** (near) (pre-) R55
  - anginosa I20.8
  - bradycardia R00.1
  - cardiac R55
  - carotid sinus G90.01
  - due to spinal (lumbar) puncture G97.1
  - heart R55
  - heat T67.1 ☑
  - laryngeal R05
  - psychogenic F48.8
  - tussive R05
  - vasoconstriction R55
  - vasodepressor R55
  - vasomotor R55
  - vasovagal R55
- **Syndactylism,** syndactyly Q70.9
  - complex (with synostosis)
    - fingers Q70.0 ☑
    - toes Q70.2 ☑
  - simple (without synostosis)
    - fingers Q70.1 ☑
    - toes Q70.3 ☑
- **Syndrome** (*see also* Disease)
  - 5q minus NOS D46.C
  - 48,XXXX Q97.1
  - 49,XXXXX Q97.1
  - abdominal
    - acute R10.0
    - muscle deficiency Q79.4
  - abnormal innervation H02.519
    - left H02.516
      - lower H02.515
      - upper H02.514
    - right H02.513
      - lower H02.512
      - upper H02.511
  - abstinence, neonatal P96.1
  - acid pulmonary aspiration, obstetric O74.0
  - acquired immunodeficiency — *see* Human, immunodeficiency virus (HIV) disease

- **Syndrome** — *continued*
  - acute abdominal R10.0
  - acute respiratory distress (adult) (child) J80
    - idiopathic J84.114
  - Adair-Dighton Q78.0
  - Adams-Stokes (-Morgagni) I45.9
  - adiposogenital E23.6
  - adrenal
    - hemorrhage (meningococcal) A39.1
    - meningococcic A39.1
  - adrenocortical — *see* Cushing's, syndrome
  - adrenogenital E25.9
    - congenital, associated with enzyme deficiency E25.0
  - afferent loop NEC K91.89
  - Alagille's Q44.7
  - alcohol withdrawal (without convulsions) — *see* Dependence, alcohol, with, withdrawal
  - Alder's D72.0
  - Aldrich (-Wiskott) D82.0
  - alien hand R41.4
  - Alport Q87.81
  - alveolar hypoventilation E66.2
  - alveolocapillary block J84.10
  - amnesic, amnestic (confabulatory) (due to) — *see* Disorder, amnesic
  - amyostatic (Wilson's disease) E83.01
  - androgen insensitivity E34.50
    - complete E34.51
    - partial E34.52
  - androgen resistance (*see also* Syndrome, androgen insensitivity)E34.50
  - Angelman Q93.5
  - anginal — *see* Angina
  - ankyloglossia superior Q38.1
  - anterior
    - chest wall R07.89
    - cord G83.82
    - spinal artery G95.19
      - compression M47.019
        - cervical region M47.012
        - cervicothoracic region M47.013
        - lumbar region M47.016
        - occipito-atlanto-axial region M47.011
        - thoracic region M47.014
        - thoracolumbar region M47.015
    - tibial M76.81 ☑
  - antibody deficiency D80.9
    - agammaglobulinemic D80.1
      - hereditary D80.0
    - congenital D80.0
    - hypogammaglobulinemic D80.1
      - hereditary D80.0
  - anticardiolipin (-antibody) D68.61
  - antiphospholipid (-antibody) D68.61
  - aortic
    - arch M31.4
    - bifurcation I74.09
  - aortomesenteric duodenum occlusion K31.5
  - apical ballooning (transient left ventricular) I51.81
  - arcuate ligament I77.4
  - argentaffin, argintaffinoma E34.0
  - Arnold-Chiari — *see* Arnold-Chiari disease
  - Arrillaga-Ayerza I27.0
  - arterial tortuosity Q87.82
  - arteriovenous steal T82.898 ☑
  - Asherman's N85.6
  - aspiration, of newborn — *see* Aspiration, by substance, with pneumonia
    - meconium P24.01
  - ataxia-telangiectasia G11.3
  - auriculotemporal G50.8
  - autoerythrocyte sensitization (Gardner-Diamond) D69.2
  - autoimmune polyglandular E31.0
  - autoimmune lymphoproliferative [ALPS] D89.82
  - autoinflammatory M04.9
    - specified type NEC M04.8
  - autosomal — *see* Abnormal, autosomes
  - Avellis' G46.8
  - Ayerza (-Arrillaga) I27.0
  - Babinski-Nageotte G83.89
  - Bakwin-Krida Q78.5
  - bare lymphocyte D81.6
  - Barré-Guillain G61.0
  - Barré-Liéou M53.0
  - Barrett's — *see* Barrett's, esophagus
  - Barsony-Polgar K22.4
  - Barsony-Teschendorf K22.4
  - Barth E78.71
  - Bartter's E26.81

- **Syndrome** — *continued*
  - basal cell nevus Q87.89
  - Basedow's E05.00
    - with thyroid storm E05.01
  - basilar artery G45.0
  - Batten-Steinert G71.11
  - battered
    - baby or child — *see* Maltreatment, child, physical abuse
    - spouse — *see* Maltreatment, adult, physical abuse
  - Beals Q87.40
  - Beau's I51.5
  - Beck's I65.8
  - Benedikt's G46.3
  - Béquez César (-Steinbrinck-Chédiak-Higashi) E70.330
  - Bernhardt-Roth — *see* Meralgia paresthetica
  - Bernheim's I50.9
  - big spleen D73.1
  - bilateral polycystic ovarian E28.2
  - Bing-Horton's — *see* Horton's headache
  - Birt-Hogg-Dube syndrome Q87.89
  - Björck (-Thorsen) E34.0
  - black
    - lung J60
    - widow spider bite — *see* Toxicity, venom, spider, black widow
  - Blackfan-Diamond D61.01
  - Blau M04.8
  - blind loop K90.2
    - congenital Q43.8
    - postsurgical K91.2
  - blue sclera Q78.0
  - blue toe I75.02 ☑
  - Boder-Sedgewick G11.3
  - Boerhaave's K22.3
  - Borjeson Forssman Lehmann Q89.8
  - Bouillaud's I01.9
  - Bourneville (-Pringle) Q85.1
  - Bouveret (-Hoffman) I47.9
  - brachial plexus G54.0
  - bradycardia-tachycardia I49.5
  - brain (nonpsychotic) F09
    - with psychosis, psychotic reaction F09
    - acute or subacute — *see* Delirium
    - congenital — *see* Disability, intellectual
    - organic F09
      - post-traumatic (nonpsychotic) F07.81
        - psychotic F09
    - personality change F07.0
    - postcontusional F07.81
    - post-traumatic, nonpsychotic F07.81
    - psycho-organic F09
    - psychotic F06.8
  - brain stem stroke G46.3
  - Brandt's (acrodermatitis enteropathica) E83.2
  - broad ligament laceration N83.8
  - Brock's J98.11
  - bronze baby P83.8
  - Brown-Sequard G83.81
  - bubbly lung P27.0
  - Buchem's M85.2
  - Budd-Chiari I82.0
  - bulbar (progressive) G12.22
  - Bürger-Grütz E78.3
  - Burke's K86.89
  - Burnett's (milk-alkali) E83.52
  - burning feet E53.9
  - Bywaters' T79.5 ☑
  - Call-Fleming I67.841
  - carbohydrate-deficient glycoprotein (CDGS) E77.8
  - carcinogenic thrombophlebitis I82.1
  - carcinoid E34.0
  - cardiac asthma I50.1
  - cardiacos negros I27.0
  - cardiofaciocutaneous Q87.89
  - cardiopulmonary-obesity E66.2
  - cardiorenal — *see* Hypertension, cardiorenal
  - cardiorespiratory distress (idiopathic), newborn P22.0
  - cardiovascular renal — *see* Hypertension, cardiorenal
  - carotid
    - artery (hemispheric) (internal) G45.1
    - body G90.01
    - sinus G90.01
  - carpal tunnel G56.0 ☑
  - Cassidy (-Scholte) E34.0
  - cat cry Q93.4
  - cat eye Q92.8

Syndrome

Syndrome — *continued*
- fragile X Q99.2
- Franceschetti Q75.4
- Frey's
  - auriculotemporal G50.8
  - hyperhidrosis L74.52
- Friderichsen-Waterhouse A39.1
- Froin's G95.89
- frontal lobe F07.0
- Fukuhara E88.49
- functional
  - bowel K59.9
  - prepubertal castrate E29.1
- Gaisböck's D75.1
- ganglion (basal ganglia brain) G25.9
  - geniculi G51.1
- Gardner-Diamond D69.2
- gastroesophageal
  - junction K22.0
  - laceration-hemorrhage K22.6
- gastrojejunal loop obstruction K91.89
- Gee-Herter-Heubner K90.0
- Gelineau's G47.419
  - with cataplexy G47.411
- genito-anorectal A55
- Gerstmann-Sträussler-Scheinker (GSS) A81.82
- Gianotti-Crosti L44.4
- giant platelet (Bernard-Soulier) D69.1
- Gilles de la Tourette's F95.2
- goiter-deafness E07.1
- Goldberg Q89.8
- Goldberg-Maxwell E34.51
- Good's D83.8
- Gopalan' (burning feet) E53.8
- Gorlin's Q87.89
- Gougerot-Blum L81.7
- Gouley's I31.1
- Gower's R55
- gray or grey (newborn) P93.0
  - platelet D69.1
- Gubler-Millard G46.3
- Guillain-Barré (-Strohl) G61.0
- gustatory sweating G50.8
- Hadfield-Clarke K86.89
- hair tourniquet — *see* Constriction, external, by site
- Hamman's J98.19
- hand-foot L27.1
- hand-shoulder G90.8
- hantavirus (cardio)-pulmonary (HPS) (HCPS) B33.4
- happy puppet Q93.5
- Harada's H30.81 ☑
- Hayem-Faber D50.9
- headache NEC G44.89
  - complicated NEC G44.59
- Heberden's I20.8
- Hedinger's E34.0
- Hegglin's D72.0
- HELLP (hemolysis, elevated liver enzymes and low platelet count) O14.2 ☑
  - complicating
    - childbirth O14.24
    - puerperium O14.25
- hemolytic-uremic D59.3
- hemophagocytic, infection-associated D76.2
- Henoch-Schönlein D69.0
- hepatic flexure K59.8
- hepatopulmonary K76.81
- hepatorenal K76.7
  - following delivery O90.4
  - postoperative or postprocedural K91.83
  - postpartum, puerperal O90.4
- hepatourologic K76.7
- Herter (-Gee) (nontropical sprue) K90.0
- Heubner-Herter K90.0
- Heyd's K76.7
- Hilger's G90.09
- histamine-like (fish poisoning) — *see* Poisoning, fish
- histiocytic D76.3
- histiocytosis NEC D76.3
- HIV infection, acute B20
- Hoffmann-Werdnig G12.0
- Hollander-Simons E88.1
- Hoppe-Goldflam G70.00
  - with exacerbation (acute) G70.01
  - in crisis G70.01
- Horner's G90.2
- hungry bone E83.81
- hunterian glossitis D51.0
- Hutchinson's triad A50.53

Syndrome — *continued*
- hyperabduction G54.0
- hyperammonemia-hyperornithinemia-homocitrullinemia E72.4
- hypereosinophilic (idiopathic) D72.1
- hyperimmunoglobulin D M04.1
- hyperimmunoglobulin E (IgE) D82.4
- hyperkalemic E87.5
- hyperkinetic — *see* Hyperkinesia
- hypermobility M35.7
- hypernatremia E87.0
- hyperosmolarity E87.0
- hyperperfusion G97.82
- hypersplenic D73.1
- hypertransfusion, newborn P61.1
- hyperventilation F45.8
- hyperviscosity (of serum)
  - polycythemic D75.1
  - sclerothymic D58.8
- hypoglycemic (familial) (neonatal) E16.2
- hypokalemic E87.6
- hyponatremic E87.1
- hypopituitarism E23.0
- hypoplastic left-heart Q23.4
- hypopotassemia E87.6
- hyposmolality E87.1
- hypotension, maternal O26.5 ☑
- hypothenar hammer I73.89
- hypoventilation, obesity (OHS) E66.2
- ICF (intravascular coagulation-fibrinolysis) D65
- idiopathic
  - cardiorespiratory distress, newborn P22.0
  - nephrotic (infantile) N04.9
- iliotibial band M76.3 ☑
- immobility, immobilization (paraplegic) M62.3
- immune reconstitution D89.3
- immune reconstitution inflammatory [IRIS] D89.3
- immunity deficiency, combined D81.9
- immunodeficiency
  - acquired — *see* Human, immunodeficiency virus (HIV) disease
  - combined D81.9
- impending coronary I20.0
- impingement, shoulder M75.4 ☑
- inappropriate secretion of antidiuretic hormone E22.2
- infant
  - of diabetic mother P70.1
  - gestational diabetes P70.0
- infantilism (pituitary) E23.0
- inferior vena cava I87.1
- inspissated bile (newborn) P59.1
- institutional (childhood) F94.2
- insufficient sleep F51.12
- intermediate coronary (artery) I20.0
- interspinous ligament — *see* Spondylopathy, specified NEC
- intestinal
  - carcinoid E34.0
  - knot K56.2
- intravascular coagulation-fibrinolysis (ICF) D65
- iodine-deficiency, congenital E00.9
  - type
    - mixed E00.2
    - myxedematous E00.1
    - neurological E00.0
- IRDS (idiopathic respiratory distress, newborn) P22.0
- irritable
  - bowel K58.9
    - with
      - constipation K58.1
      - diarrhea K58.0
    - mixed K58.2
    - psychogenic F45.8
    - specified NEC K58.8
  - heart (psychogenic) F45.8
  - weakness F48.8
- ischemic
  - bowel (transient) K55.9
    - chronic K55.1
    - due to mesenteric artery insufficiency K55.1
  - steal T82.898 ☑
- IVC (intravascular coagulopathy) D65
- Ivemark's Q89.01
- Jaccoud's — *see* Arthropathy, postrheumatic, chronic
- Jackson's G83.89
- Jakob-Creutzfeldt — *see* Creutzfeldt-Jakob disease or syndrome
- jaw-winking Q07.8
- Jervell-Lange-Nielsen I45.81

Syndrome — *continued*
- jet lag G47.25
- Job's D71
- Joseph-Diamond-Blackfan D61.01
- jugular foramen G52.7
- Kabuki Q89.8
- Kanner's (autism) F84.0
- Kartagener's Q89.3
- Kelly's D50.1
- Kimmelstiel-Wilson — *see* Diabetes, specified type, with Kimmelstiel-Wilson disease
- Klein (e)-Levine G47.13
- Klippel-Feil (brevicollis) Q76.1
- Köhler-Pellegrini-Steida — *see* Bursitis, tibial collateral
- König's K59.8
- Korsakoff (-Wernicke) (nonalcoholic) F04
  - alcoholic F10.26
- Kostmann's D70.0
- Krabbe's congenital muscle hypoplasia Q79.8
- labyrinthine — *see* subcategory H83.2
- lacunar NEC G46.7
- Lambert-Eaton G70.80
  - in
    - neoplastic disease G73.1
    - specified disease NEC G70.81
- Landau-Kleffner — *see* Epilepsy, specified NEC
- Larsen's Q74.8
- lateral
  - cutaneous nerve of thigh G57.1 ☑
  - medullary G46.4
- Launois' E22.0
- lazy
  - leukocyte D70.8
  - posture M62.3
- Lemiere I80.8
- Lennox-Gastaut G40.812
  - intractable G40.814
    - with status epilepticus G40.813
    - without status epilepticus G40.814
  - not intractable G40.812
    - with status epilepticus G40.811
    - without status epilepticus G40.812
- lenticular, progressive E83.01
- Leopold-Levi's E05.90
- Lev's I44.2
- Li-Fraumeni Z15.01
- Lichtheim's D51.0
- Lightwood's N25.89
- Lignac (de Toni) (-Fanconi) (-Debré) E72.09
  - with cystinosis E72.04
- Likoff's I20.8
- limbic epilepsy personality F07.0
- liver-kidney K76.7
- lobotomy F07.0
- Loffler's J82
- long arm 18 or 21 deletion Q93.89
- long QT I45.81
- Louis-Barré G11.3
- low
  - atmospheric pressure T70.29 ☑
  - back M54.5
  - output (cardiac) I50.9
- lower radicular, newborn (birth injury) P14.8
- Luetscher's (dehydration) E86.0
- Lupus anticoagulant D68.62
- Lutembacher's Q21.1
- macrophage activation D76.1
  - due to infection D76.2
- magnesium-deficiency R29.0
- Majeed M04.8
- Mal de Debarquement R42
- malabsorption K90.9
  - postsurgical K91.2
- malformation, congenital, due to
  - alcohol Q86.0
  - exogenous cause NEC Q86.8
  - hydantoin Q86.1
  - warfarin Q86.2
- malignant
  - carcinoid E34.0
  - neuroleptic G21.0
- Mallory-Weiss K22.6
- mandibulofacial dysostosis Q75.4
- manic-depressive — *see* Disorder, bipolar
- maple-syrup-urine E71.0
- Marable's I77.4
- Marfan's Q87.40
  - with
    - cardiovascular manifestations Q87.418
      - aortic dilation Q87.410
    - ocular manifestations Q87.42
    - skeletal manifestations Q87.43

☑ **Additional character required**

Syndrome — *continued*
- Marie's (acromegaly) E22.0
- mast cell activation — *see* Activation, mast cell
- maternal hypotension — *see* Syndrome, hypotension, maternal
- May (-Hegglin) D72.0
- McArdle (-Schmidt) (-Pearson) E74.04
- McQuarrie's E16.2
- meconium plug (newborn) P76.0
- median arcuate ligament I77.4
- Meekeren-Ehlers-Danlos Q79.6
- megavitamin-B6 E67.2
- Meige G24.4
- MELAS E88.41
- Mendelson's O74.0
- MERRF (myoclonic epilepsy associated with ragged-red fibers) E88.42
- mesenteric
  - artery (superior) K55.1
  - vascular insufficiency K55.1
- metabolic E88.81
- metastatic carcinoid E34.0
- micrognathia-glossoptosis Q87.0
- midbrain NEC G93.89
- middle lobe (lung) J98.19
- middle radicular G54.0
- migraine (*see also* Migraine)G43.909
- Mikulicz' K11.8
- milk-alkali E83.52
- Millard-Gubler G46.3
- Miller-Dieker Q93.88
- Miller-Fisher G61.0
- Minkowski-Chauffard D58.0
- Mirizzi's K83.1
- MNGIE (Mitochondrial Neurogastrointestinal Encephalopathy) E88.49
- Möbius, ophthalmoplegic migraine — *see* Migraine, ophthalmoplegic
- monofixation H50.42
- Morel-Moore M85.2
- Morel-Morgagni M85.2
- Morgagni (-Morel) (-Stewart) M85.2
- Morgagni-Adams-Stokes I45.9
- Muckle-Wells M04.2
- mucocutaneous lymph node (acute febrile) (MCLS) M30.3
- multiple endocrine neoplasia (MEN) — *see* Neoplasia, endocrine, multiple (MEN)
- multiple operations — *see* Disorder, factitious
- Mounier-Kuhn Q32.4
  - with bronchiectasis J47.9
    - with
      - exacerbation (acute) J47.1
      - lower respiratory infection J47.0
  - acquired J98.09
    - with bronchiectasis J47.9
      - with
        - exacerbation (acute) J47.1
        - lower respiratory infection J47.0
- myasthenic G70.9
  - in
    - diabetes mellitus — *see* Diabetes, amyotrophy
    - endocrine disease NEC E34.9 *[G73.3]*
    - neoplastic disease (*see also* Neoplasm)D49.9 *[G73.3]*
    - thyrotoxicosis (hyperthyroidism) E05.90 *[G73.3]*
      - with thyroid storm E05.91 *[G73.3]*
- myelodysplastic D46.9
  - with
    - 5q deletion D46.C
    - isolated del (5q) chromosomal abnormality D46.C
  - lesions, low grade D46.20
  - specified NEC D46.Z
- myelopathic pain G89.0
- myeloproliferative (chronic) D47.1
- myofascial pain M79.1
- Naffziger's G54.0
- nail patella Q87.2
- NARP (Neuropathy, Ataxia and Retinitis pigmentosa) E88.49
- neonatal abstinence P96.1
- nephritic (*see also* Nephritis)
  - with edema — *see* Nephrosis
  - acute N00.9
  - chronic N03.9
  - rapidly progressive N01.9
- nephrotic (congenital) (*see also* Nephrosis)N04.9
  - with
    - dense deposit disease N04.6

Syndrome — *continued*
- nephrotic — *continued*
    - diffuse
      - crescentic glomerulonephritis N04.7
      - endocapillary proliferative glomerulonephritis N04.4
      - membranous glomerulonephritis N04.2
      - mesangial proliferative glomerulonephritis N04.3
      - mesangiocapillary glomerulonephritis N04.5
    - focal and segmental glomerular lesions N04.1
    - minor glomerular abnormality N04.0
    - specified morphological changes NEC N04.8
  - diabetic — *see* Diabetes, nephrosis
- neurologic neglect R41.4
- Nezelof's D81.4
- Nonne-Milroy-Meige Q82.0
- Nothnagel's vasomotor acroparesthesia I73.89
- obesity hypoventilation (OHS) E66.2
- oculomotor H51.9
- ophthalmoplegia-cerebellar ataxia — *see* Strabismus, paralytic, third nerve
- oral allergy T78.1 ☑
- oral-facial-digital Q87.0
- organic
  - affective F06.30
  - amnesic (not alcohol- or drug-induced) F04
  - brain F09
  - depressive F06.31
  - hallucinosis F06.0
  - personality F07.0
- Ormond's N13.5
- oro-facial-digital Q87.0
- os trigonum Q68.8
- Osler-Weber-Rendu I78.0
- osteoporosis-osteomalacia M83.8
- Osterreicher-Turner Q87.2
- otolith — *see* subcategory H81.8
- oto-palatal-digital Q87.0
- outlet (thoracic) G54.0
- ovary
  - polycystic E28.2
  - resistant E28.39
  - sclerocystic E28.2
- Owren's D68.2
- Paget-Schroetter I82.890
- pain (*see also* Pain)
  - complex regional I G90.50
    - lower limb G90.52 ☑
    - specified site NEC G90.59
    - upper limb G90.51 ☑
  - complex regional II — *see* Causalgia
- painful
  - bruising D69.2
  - feet E53.8
  - prostate N42.81
- paralysis agitans — *see* Parkinsonism
- paralytic G83.9
  - specified NEC G83.89
- Parinaud's H51.0
- parkinsonian — *see* Parkinsonism
- Parkinson's — *see* Parkinsonism
- paroxysmal facial pain G50.0
- Parry's E05.00
  - with thyroid storm E05.01
- Parsonage (-Aldren)-Turner G54.5
- patella clunk M25.86 ☑
- Paterson (-Brown) (-Kelly) D50.1
- pectoral girdle I77.89
- pectoralis minor I77.89
- Pelger-Huet D72.0
- pellagra-cerebellar ataxia-renal aminoaciduria E72.02
- pellagroid E52
- Pellegrini-Stieda — *see* Bursitis, tibial collateral
- pelvic congestion-fibrosis, female N94.89
- penta X Q97.1
- peptic ulcer — *see* Ulcer, peptic
- perabduction I77.89
- periodic fever M04.1
- periodic fever, aphthous stomatitis, pharyngitis, and adenopathy [PFAPA] M04.8
- periodic headache, in adults and children — *see* Headache, periodic syndromes in adults and children
- periurethral fibrosis N13.5
- phantom limb (without pain) G54.7
  - with pain G54.6
- pharyngeal pouch D82.1
- Pick's — *see* Disease, Pick's

Syndrome — *continued*
- Pickwickian E66.2
- PIE (pulmonary infiltration with eosinophilia) J82
- pigmentary pallidal degeneration (progressive) G23.0
- pineal E34.8
- pituitary E22.0
- plantar fascia M72.2
- placental transfusion — *see* Pregnancy, complicated by, placental transfusion syndromes
- plateau iris (post-iridectomy) (postprocedural) H21.82
- Plummer-Vinson D50.1
- pluricarential of infancy E40
- pluricdeficiency E40
- pluriglandular (compensatory) E31.8
  - autoimmune E31.0
- pneumatic hammer T75.21 ☑
- polyangiitis overlap M30.8
- polycarential of infancy E40
- polyglandular E31.8
  - autoimmune E31.0
- polysplenia Q89.09
- pontine NEC G93.89
- popliteal
  - artery entrapment I77.89
  - web Q87.89
- postcardiac injury
  - postcardiotomy I97.0
  - postmyocardial infarction I24.1
- postcardiotomy I97.0
- post chemoembolization - code to associated conditions
- postcholecystectomy K91.5
- postcommissurotomy I97.0
- postconcussional F07.81
- postcontusional F07.81
- postencephalitic F07.89
- posterior
  - cervical sympathetic M53.0
  - cord G83.83
  - fossa compression G93.5
  - reversible encephalopathy (PRES) I67.83
- postgastrectomy (dumping) K91.1
- postgastric surgery K91.1
- postinfarction I24.1
- postlaminectomy NEC M96.1
- postleukotomy F07.0
- postmastectomy lymphedema I97.2
- postmyocardial infarction I24.1
- postoperative NEC T81.9 ☑
  - blind loop K90.2
- postpartum panhypopituitary (Sheehan) E23.0
- postpolio (myelitic) G14
- postthrombotic I87.009
  - with
    - inflammation I87.02 ☑
      - with ulcer I87.03 ☑
    - specified complication NEC I87.09 ☑
    - ulcer I87.01 ☑
      - with inflammation I87.03 ☑
  - asymptomatic I87.00 ☑
- postvagotomy K91.1
- postvalvulotomy I97.0
- postviral NEC G93.3
  - fatigue G93.3
- Potain's K31.0
- potassium intoxication E87.5
- precerebral artery (multiple) (bilateral) G45.2
- preinfarction I20.0
- preleukemic D46.9
- premature senility E34.8
- premenstrual dysphoric F32.89
- premenstrual tension N94.3
- Prinzmetal-Massumi R07.1
- prune belly Q79.4
- pseudocarpal tunnel (sublimis) — *see* Syndrome, carpal tunnel
- pseudoparalytica G70.00
  - with exacerbation (acute) G70.01
  - in crisis G70.01
- pseudo -Turner's Q87.1
- psycho-organic (nonpsychotic severity) F07.9
  - acute or subacute F05
  - depressive type F06.31
  - hallucinatory type F06.0
  - nonpsychotic severity F07.0
  - specified NEC F07.89
- pulmonary
  - arteriosclerosis I27.0
  - dysmaturity (Wilson-Mikity) P27.0
  - hypoperfusion (idiopathic) P22.0

- **Syndrome** — *continued*
  - pulmonary — *continued*
    - renal (hemorrhagic) (Goodpasture's) M31.0
  - pure
    - motor lacunar G46.5
    - sensory lacunar G46.6
  - Putnam-Dana D51.0
  - pyogenic arthritis, pyoderma gangrenosum, and acne [PAPA] M04.8
  - pyramidopallidonigral G20
  - pyriformis — *see* Lesion, nerve, sciatic
  - QT interval prolongation I45.81
  - radicular NEC — *see* Radiculopathy
    - upper limbs, newborn (birth injury) P14.3
  - rapid time-zone change G47.25
  - Rasmussen G04.81
  - Raymond (-Céstan) I65.8
  - Raynaud's I73.00
    - with gangrene I73.01
  - RDS (respiratory distress syndrome, newborn) P22.0
  - reactive airways dysfunction J68.3
  - Refsum's G60.1
  - Reifenstein E34.52
  - renal glomerulohyalinosis-diabetic — *see* Diabetes, nephrosis
  - Rendu-Osler-Weber I78.0
  - residual ovary N99.83
  - resistant ovary E28.39
  - respiratory
    - distress
      - acute J80
        - adult J80
        - child J80
        - idiopathic J84.114
      - newborn (idiopathic) (type I) P22.0
        - type II P22.1
  - restless legs G25.81
  - retinoblastoma (familial) C69.2 ☑
  - retroperitoneal fibrosis N13.5
  - retroviral seroconversion (acute) Z21
  - Reye's G93.7
  - Richter — *see* Leukemia, chronic lymphocytic, B-cell type
  - Ridley's I50.1
  - right
    - heart, hypoplastic Q22.6
    - ventricular obstruction — *see* Failure, heart, congestive
  - Romano-Ward (prolonged QT interval) I45.81
  - rotator cuff, shoulder (*see also* Tear, rotator cuff)M75.10 ☑
  - Rotes Quérol — *see* Hyperostosis, ankylosing
  - Roth — *see* Meralgia paresthetica
  - rubella (congenital) P35.0
  - Ruvalcaba-Myhre-Smith E71.440
  - Rytand-Lipsitch I44.2
  - salt
    - depletion E87.1
      - due to heat NEC T67.8 ☑
        - causing heat exhaustion or prostration T67.4 ☑
    - low E87.1
  - salt-losing N28.89
  - Scaglietti-Dagnini E22.0
  - scalenus anticus (anterior) G54.0
  - scapulocostal — *see* Mononeuropathy, upper limb, specified site NEC
  - scapuloperoneal G71.0
  - schizophrenic, of childhood NEC F84.5
  - Schnitzler D47.2
  - Scholte's E34.0
  - Schroeder's E27.0
  - Schüller-Christian C96.5
  - Schwachman's — *see* Syndrome, Shwachman's
  - Schwartz (-Jampel) G71.13
  - Schwartz-Bartter E22.2
  - scimitar Q26.8
  - sclerocystic ovary E28.2
  - Seitelberger's G31.89
  - septicemic adrenal hemorrhage A39.1
  - seroconversion, retroviral (acute) Z21
  - serous meningitis G93.2
  - severe acute respiratory (SARS) J12.81
  - shaken infant T74.4 ☑
  - shock (traumatic) T79.4 ☑
    - kidney N17.0
      - following crush injury T79.5 ☑
    - toxic A48.3
  - shock-lung J80
  - Shone's - code to specific anomalies
  - short
    - bowel K91.2
    - rib Q77.2
  - shoulder-hand — *see* Algoneurodystrophy
  - Shwachman's D70.4
  - sicca — *see* Sicca syndrome
  - sick
    - cell E87.1
    - sinus I49.5
  - sick-euthyroid E07.81
  - sideropenic D50.1
  - Siemens' ectodermal dysplasia Q82.4
  - Silfverskköld's Q78.9
  - Simons' E88.1
  - sinus tarsi M25.57 ☑
  - sinusitis-bronchiectasis-situs inversus Q89.3
  - Sipple's E31.22
  - sirenomelia Q87.2
  - Slocumb's E27.0
  - slow flow, coronary I20.8
  - Sluder's G44.89
  - Smith-Magenis Q93.88
  - Sneddon-Wilkinson L13.1
  - Soto's Q87.3
  - South African cardiomyopathy I42.8
  - spasmodic
    - upward movement, eyes H51.8
    - winking F95.8
  - Spen's I45.9
  - splenic
    - agenesis Q89.01
    - flexure K59.8
    - neutropenia D73.81
  - Spurway's Q78.0
  - staphylococcal scalded skin L00
  - steal
    - arteriovenous T82.898 ☑
    - ischemic T82.898 ☑
    - subclavian G45.8
  - Stein-Leventhal E28.2
  - Stein's E28.2
  - Stevens-Johnson syndrome L51.1
    - toxic epidermal necrolysis overlap L51.3
  - Stewart-Morel M85.2
  - Stickler Q89.8
  - stiff baby Q89.8
  - stiff man G25.82
  - Still-Felty — *see* Felty's syndrome
  - Stokes (-Adams) I45.9
  - stone heart I50.1
  - straight back, congenital Q76.49
  - subclavian steal G45.8
  - subcoracoid-pectoralis minor G54.0
  - subcostal nerve compression I77.89
  - subphrenic interposition Q43.3
  - superior
    - cerebellar artery I63.8
    - mesenteric artery K55.1
    - semi-circular canal dehiscence H83.8X ☑
    - vena cava I87.1
  - supine hypotensive (maternal) — *see* Syndrome, hypotension, maternal
  - suprarenal cortical E27.0
  - supraspinatus (*see also* Tear, rotator cuff)M75.10 ☑
  - Susac G93.49
  - swallowed blood P78.2
  - sweat retention L74.0
  - Swyer Q99.1
  - Symond's G93.2
  - sympathetic
    - cervical paralysis G90.2
    - pelvic, female N94.89
  - systemic inflammatory response (SIRS), of non-infectious origin (without organ dysfunction) R65.10
    - with acute organ dysfunction R65.11
  - tachycardia-bradycardia I49.5
  - takotsubo I51.81
  - TAR (thrombocytopenia with absent radius) Q87.2
  - tarsal tunnel G57.5 ☑
  - teething K00.7
  - tegmental G93.89
  - telangiectasic-pigmentation-cataract Q82.8
  - temporal pyramidal apex — *see* Otitis, media, suppurative, acute
  - temporomandibular joint-pain-dysfunction M26.62 ☑
  - Terry's H44.2 ☑
  - testicular feminization (*see also* Syndrome, androgen insensitivity)E34.51
  - thalamic pain (hyperesthetic) G89.0
  - thoracic outlet (compression) G54.0
  - Thorson-Björck E34.0
  - thrombocytopenia with absent radius (TAR) Q87.2
  - thyroid-adrenocortical insufficiency E31.0
  - tibial
    - anterior M76.81 ☑
    - posterior M76.82 ☑
  - Tietze's M94.0
  - time-zone (rapid) G47.25
  - Toni-Fanconi E72.09
    - with cystinosis E72.04
  - Touraine's Q79.8
  - tourniquet — *see* Constriction, external, by site
  - toxic shock A48.3
  - transient left ventricular apical ballooning I51.81
  - traumatic vasospastic T75.22 ☑
  - Treacher Collins Q75.4
  - triple X, female Q97.0
  - trisomy Q92.9
    - 13 Q91.7
      - meiotic nondisjunction Q91.4
      - mitotic nondisjunction Q91.5
      - mosaicism Q91.5
      - translocation Q91.6
    - 18 Q91.3
      - meiotic nondisjunction Q91.0
      - mitotic nondisjunction Q91.1
      - mosaicism Q91.1
      - translocation Q91.2
    - 20 (q) (p) Q92.8
    - 21 Q90.9
      - meiotic nondisjunction Q90.0
      - mitotic nondisjunction Q90.1
      - mosaicism Q90.1
      - translocation Q90.2
    - 22 Q92.8
  - tropical wet feet T69.0 ☑
  - Trousseau's I82.1
  - tumor lysis (following antineoplastic chemotherapy) (spontaneous) NEC E88.3
  - tumor necrosis factor receptor associated periodic (TRAPS) M04.1
  - Twiddler's (due to)
    - automatic implantable defibrillator T82.198 ☑
    - cardiac pacemaker T82.198 ☑
  - Unverricht (-Lundborg) — *see* Epilepsy, generalized, idiopathic
  - upward gaze H51.8
  - uremia, chronic (*see also* Disease, kidney, chronic)N18.9
  - urethral N34.3
  - urethro-oculo-articular — *see* Reiter's disease
  - urohepatic K76.7
  - vago-hypoglossal G52.7
  - vascular NEC in cerebrovascular disease G46.8
  - vasoconstriction, reversible cerebrovascular I67.841
  - vasomotor I73.9
  - vasospastic (traumatic) T75.22 ☑
  - vasovagal R55
  - van Buchem's M85.2
  - van der Hoeve's Q78.0
  - VATER Q87.2
  - velo-cardio-facial Q93.81
  - vena cava (inferior) (superior) (obstruction) I87.1
  - vertebral
    - artery G45.0
      - compression — *see* Syndrome, anterior, spinal artery, compression
    - steal G45.0
  - vertebro-basilar artery G45.0
  - vertebrogenic (pain) M54.89
  - vertiginous — *see* Disorder, vestibular function
  - Vinson-Plummer D50.1
  - virus B34.9
  - visceral larva migrans B83.0
  - visual disorientation H53.8
  - vitamin B6 deficiency E53.1
  - vitreal corneal H59.01 ☑
  - vitreous (touch) H59.01 ☑
  - Vogt-Koyanagi H20.82 ☑
  - Volkmann's T79.6 ☑
  - von Schroetter's I82.890
  - von Willebrand (-Jürgen) D68.0
  - Waldenström-Kjellberg D50.1
  - Wallenberg's G46.3
  - water retention E87.79

- **Syndrome** — *continued*
  - Waterhouse (-Friderichsen) A39.1
  - Weber-Gubler G46.3
  - Weber-Leyden G46.3
  - Weber's G46.3
  - Wegener's M31.30
    - with
      - kidney involvement M31.31
      - lung involvement M31.30
        - with kidney involvement M31.31
  - Weingarten's (tropical eosinophilia) J82
  - Weiss-Baker G90.09
  - Werdnig-Hoffman G12.0
  - Wermer's E31.21
  - Werner's E34.8
  - Wernicke-Korsakoff (nonalcoholic) F04
    - alcoholic F10.26
  - West's — *see* Epilepsy, spasms
  - Westphal-Strümpell E83.01
  - wet
    - feet (maceration) (tropical) T69.0 ☑
    - lung, newborn P22.1
  - whiplash S13.4 ☑
  - whistling face Q87.0
  - Wilkie's K55.1
  - Wilkinson-Sneddon L13.1
  - Willebrand (-Jürgens) D68.0
  - Wilson's (hepatolenticular degeneration) E83.01
  - Wiskott-Aldrich D82.0
  - withdrawal — *see* Withdrawal, state
    - drug
      - infant of dependent mother P96.1
      - therapeutic use, newborn P96.2
  - Woakes' (ethmoiditis) J33.1
  - Wright's (hyperabduction) I77.89
  - X I20.9
  - XXXX Q97.1
  - XXXXX Q97.1
  - XXXXY Q98.1
  - XXY Q98.0
  - yellow nail L60.5
  - Zahorsky's B08.5
  - Zellweger syndrome E71.510
  - Zellweger-like syndrome E71.541
- **Synechia** (anterior) (iris) (posterior) (pupil) (*see also* Adhesions, iris)
  - intra-uterine (traumatic) N85.6
- **Synesthesia** R20.8
- **Syngamiasis,** syngamosis B83.3
- **Synodontia** K00.2
- **Synorchidism,** synorchism Q55.1
- **Synostosis** (congenital) Q78.8
  - astragalo-scaphoid Q74.2
  - radioulnar Q74.0
- **Synovial** sarcoma — *see* Neoplasm, connective tissue, malignant
- **Synovioma** (malignant) (*see also* Neoplasm, connective tissue, malignant)
  - benign — *see* Neoplasm, connective tissue, benign
- **Synoviosarcoma** — *see* Neoplasm, connective tissue, malignant
- **Synovitis** (*see also* Tenosynovitis)M65.9
  - crepitant
    - hand M70.0 ☑
    - wrist M70.03 ☑
  - gonococcal A54.49
  - gouty — *see* Gout
  - in (due to)
    - crystals M65.8 ☑
    - gonorrhea A54.49
    - syphilis (late) A52.78
    - use, overuse, pressure — *see* Disorder, soft tissue, due to use
  - infective NEC — *see* Tenosynovitis, infective NEC
  - specified NEC — *see* Tenosynovitis, specified type NEC
  - syphilitic A52.78
    - congenital (early) A50.02
  - toxic — *see* Synovitis, transient
  - transient M67.3 ☑
    - ankle M67.37 ☑
    - elbow M67.32 ☑
    - foot joint M67.37 ☑
    - hand joint M67.34 ☑
    - hip M67.35 ☑
    - knee M67.36 ☑
    - multiple site M67.39
    - pelvic region M67.35 ☑
    - shoulder M67.31 ☑
    - specified joint NEC M67.38
    - wrist M67.33 ☑

- **Synovitis** — *continued*
  - traumatic, current — *see* Sprain
  - tuberculous — *see* Tuberculosis, synovitis
  - villonodular (pigmented) M12.2 ☑
    - ankle M12.27 ☑
    - elbow M12.22 ☑
    - foot joint M12.27 ☑
    - hand joint M12.24 ☑
    - hip M12.25 ☑
    - knee M12.26 ☑
    - multiple site M12.29
    - pelvic region M12.25 ☑
    - shoulder M12.21 ☑
    - specified joint NEC M12.28
    - vertebrae M12.28
    - wrist M12.23 ☑
- **Syphilid** A51.39
  - congenital A50.06
  - newborn A50.06
  - tubercular (late) A52.79
- **Syphilis,** syphilitic (acquired) A53.9
  - abdomen (late) A52.79
  - acoustic nerve A52.15
  - adenopathy (secondary) A51.49
  - adrenal (gland) (with cortical hypofunction) A52.79
  - age under 2 years NOS (*see also* Syphilis, congenital, early)
    - acquired A51.9
  - alopecia (secondary) A51.32
  - anemia (late) A52.79 *[D63.8]*
  - aneurysm (aorta) (ruptured) A52.01
    - central nervous system A52.05
    - congenital A50.54 *[I79.0]*
  - anus (late) A52.74
    - primary A51.1
    - secondary A51.39
  - aorta (arch) (abdominal) (thoracic) A52.02
    - aneurysm A52.01
  - aortic (insufficiency) (regurgitation) (stenosis) A52.03
    - aneurysm A52.01
  - arachnoid (adhesive) (cerebral) (spinal) A52.13
  - asymptomatic — *see* Syphilis, latent
  - ataxia (locomotor) A52.11
  - atrophoderma maculatum A51.39
  - auricular fibrillation A52.06
  - bladder (late) A52.76
  - bone A52.77
    - secondary A51.46
  - brain A52.17
  - breast (late) A52.79
  - bronchus (late) A52.72
  - bubo (primary) A51.0
  - bulbar palsy A52.19
  - bursa (late) A52.78
  - cardiac decompensation A52.06
  - cardiovascular A52.00
  - central nervous system (late) (recurrent) (relapse) (tertiary) A52.3
    - with
      - ataxia A52.11
      - general paralysis A52.17
        - juvenile A50.45
      - paresis (general) A52.17
        - juvenile A50.45
      - tabes (dorsalis) A52.11
        - juvenile A50.45
      - taboparesis A52.17
        - juvenile A50.45
    - aneurysm A52.05
    - congenital A50.40
    - juvenile A50.40
    - remission in (sustained) A52.3
    - serology doubtful, negative, or positive A52.3
    - specified nature or site NEC A52.19
    - vascular A52.05
  - cerebral A52.17
    - meningovascular A52.13
    - nerves (multiple palsies) A52.15
    - sclerosis A52.17
    - thrombosis A52.05
  - cerebrospinal (tabetic type) A52.12
  - cerebrovascular A52.05
  - cervix (late) A52.76
  - chancre (multiple) A51.0
    - extragenital A51.2
    - Rollet's A51.0
  - Charcot's joint A52.16
  - chorioretinitis A51.43
    - congenital A50.01
    - late A52.71
    - prenatal A50.01

- **Syphilis,** syphilitic — *continued*
  - choroiditis — *see* Syphilitic chorioretinitis
  - choroidoretinitis — *see* Syphilitic chorioretinitis
  - ciliary body (secondary) A51.43
    - late A52.71
  - colon (late) A52.74
  - combined spinal sclerosis A52.11
  - condyloma (latum) A51.31
  - congenital A50.9
    - with
      - paresis (general) A50.45
      - tabes (dorsalis) A50.45
      - taboparesis A50.45
    - chorioretinitis, choroiditis A50.01 *[H32]*
    - early, or less than 2 years after birth NEC A50.2
      - with manifestations — *see* Syphilis, congenital, early, symptomatic
      - latent (without manifestations) A50.1
        - negative spinal fluid test A50.1
        - serology positive A50.1
      - symptomatic A50.09
        - cutaneous A50.06
        - mucocutaneous A50.07
        - oculopathy A50.01
        - osteochondropathy A50.02
        - pharyngitis A50.03
        - pneumonia A50.04
        - rhinitis A50.05
        - visceral A50.08
    - interstitial keratitis A50.31
    - juvenile neurosyphilis A50.45
    - late, or 2 years or more after birth NEC A50.7
      - chorioretinitis, choroiditis A50.32
      - interstitial keratitis A50.31
      - juvenile neurosyphilis A50.45
      - latent (without manifestations) A50.6
        - negative spinal fluid test A50.6
        - serology positive A50.6
      - symptomatic or with manifestations NEC A50.59
        - arthropathy A50.55
        - cardiovascular A50.54
        - Clutton's joints A50.51
        - Hutchinson's teeth A50.52
        - Hutchinson's triad A50.53
        - osteochondropathy A50.56
        - saddle nose A50.57
  - conjugal A53.9
    - tabes A52.11
  - conjunctiva (late) A52.71
  - contact Z20.2
  - cord bladder A52.19
  - cornea, late A52.71
  - coronary (artery) (sclerosis) A52.06
  - coryza, congenital A50.05
  - cranial nerve A52.15
    - multiple palsies A52.15
  - cutaneous — *see* Syphilis, skin
  - dacryocystitis (late) A52.71
  - degeneration, spinal cord A52.12
  - dementia paralytica A52.17
    - juvenilis A50.45
  - destruction of bone A52.77
  - dilatation, aorta A52.01
  - due to blood transfusion A53.9
  - dura mater A52.13
  - ear A52.79
    - inner A52.79
      - nerve (eighth) A52.15
      - neurorecurrence A52.15
  - early A51.9
    - cardiovascular A52.00
    - central nervous system A52.3
    - latent (without manifestations) (less than 2 years after infection) A51.5
      - negative spinal fluid test A51.5
      - serological relapse after treatment A51.5
      - serology positive A51.5
    - relapse (treated, untreated) A51.9
    - skin A51.39
    - symptomatic A51.9
      - extragenital chancre A51.2
      - primary, except extragenital chancre A51.0
      - secondary (*see also* Syphilis, secondary)A51.39
        - relapse (treated, untreated) A51.49
    - ulcer A51.39
  - eighth nerve (neuritis) A52.15
  - endemic A65
  - endocarditis A52.03
    - aortic A52.03
    - pulmonary A52.03

Syphilis — *continued*
- uveal tract (secondary) A51.43
  - late A52.71
- uveitis (secondary) A51.43
  - late A52.71
- uvula (late) (perforated) A52.79
- vagina A51.0
  - late A52.76
- valvulitis NEC A52.03
- vascular A52.00
  - brain (cerebral) A52.05
- ventriculi A52.74
- vesicae urinariae (late) A52.76
- viscera (abdominal) (late) A52.74
  - secondary A51.49
- vitreous (opacities) (late) A52.71
  - hemorrhage A52.71
- vulva A51.0
  - late A52.76
  - secondary A51.39

Syphiloma A52.79
- cardiovascular system A52.00
- central nervous system A52.3
- circulatory system A52.00
- congenital A50.59

Syphilophobia F45.29

Syringadenoma (*see also* Neoplasm, skin, benign)
- papillary — *see* Neoplasm, skin, benign

Syringobulbia G95.0

Syringocystadenoma — *see* Neoplasm, skin, benign
- papillary — *see* Neoplasm, skin, benign

Syringoma (*see also* Neoplasm, skin, benign)
- chondroid — *see* Neoplasm, skin, benign

Syringomyelia G95.0

Syringomyelitis — *see* Encephalitis

Syringomyelocele — *see* Spina bifida

Syringopontia G95.0

System, systemic (*see also* condition)
- disease, combined — *see* Degeneration, combined
- inflammatory response syndrome (SIRS) of non-infectious origin (without organ dysfunction) R65.10
  - with acute organ dysfunction R65.11
- lupus erythematosus M32.9
  - inhibitor present D68.62

T

Tabacism, tabacosis, tabagism (*see also* Poisoning, tobacco)
- meaning dependence (without remission) F17.200
  - with
    - disorder F17.299
      - remission F17.211
      - specified disorder NEC F17.298
      - withdrawal F17.203

Tabardillo A75.9
- flea-borne A75.2
- louse-borne A75.0

Tabes, tabetic A52.10
- with
  - central nervous system syphilis A52.10
  - Charcot's joint A52.16
  - cord bladder A52.19
  - crisis, viscera (any) A52.19
  - paralysis, general A52.17
  - paresis (general) A52.17
  - perforating ulcer (foot) A52.19
- arthropathy (Charcot) A52.16
- bladder A52.19
- bone A52.11
- cerebrospinal A52.12
- congenital A50.45
- conjugal A52.10
- dorsalis A52.11
  - juvenile A50.49
- juvenile A50.49
- latent A52.19
- mesenterica A18.39
- paralysis, insane, general A52.17
- spasmodic A52.17
- syphilis (cerebrospinal) A52.12

Taboparalysis A52.17

Taboparesis (remission) A52.17
- juvenile A50.45

TAC (trigeminal autonomic cephalgia) NEC G44.099
- intractable G44.091
- not intractable G44.099

Tache noir S60.22 ☑

Tachyalimentation K91.2

Tachyarrhythmia, tachyrhythmia — *see* Tachycardia

Tachycardia R00.0
- atrial (paroxysmal) I47.1
- auricular I47.1
- AV nodal re-entry (re-entrant) I47.1
- junctional (paroxysmal) I47.1
- newborn P29.11
- nodal (paroxysmal) I47.1
- non-paroxysmal AV nodal I45.89
- paroxysmal (sustained) (nonsustained) I47.9
  - with sinus bradycardia I49.5
  - atrial (PAT) I47.1
  - atrioventricular (AV) (re-entrant) I47.1
    - psychogenic F54
  - junctional I47.1
    - ectopic I47.1
  - nodal I47.1
  - psychogenic (atrial) (supraventricular) (ventricular) F54
  - supraventricular (sustained) I47.1
    - psychogenic F54
  - ventricular I47.2
    - psychogenic F54
- psychogenic F45.8
- sick sinus I49.5
- sinoauricular NOS R00.0
  - paroxysmal I47.1
- sinus [sinusal] NOS R00.0
  - paroxysmal I47.1
- supraventricular I47.1
- ventricular (paroxysmal) (sustained) I47.2
  - psychogenic F54

Tachygastria K31.89

Tachypnea R06.82
- hysterical F45.8
- newborn (idiopathic) (transitory) P22.1
- psychogenic F45.8
- transitory, of newborn P22.1

Taenia (infection) (infestation) B68.9
- diminuta B71.0
- echinococcal infestation B67.90
- mediocanellata B68.1
- nana B71.0
- saginata B68.1
- solium (intestinal form) B68.0
  - larval form — *see* Cysticercosis

Taeniasis (intestine) — *see* Taenia

TACO (transfusion associated circulatory overload) E87.71

Tag (hypertrophied skin) (infected) L91.8
- adenoid J35.8
- anus K64.4
- hemorrhoidal K64.4
- hymen N89.8
- perineal N90.89
- preauricular Q17.0
- sentinel K64.4
- skin L91.8
  - accessory (congenital) Q82.8
  - anus K64.4
  - congenital Q82.8
  - preauricular Q17.0
- tonsil J35.8
- urethra, urethral N36.8
- vulva N90.89

Tahyna fever B33.8

Takahara's disease E80.3

Takayasu's disease or syndrome M31.4

Talcosis (pulmonary) J62.0

Talipes (congenital) Q66.89
- acquired, planus — *see* Deformity, limb, flat foot
- asymmetric Q66.89
- calcaneovalgus Q66.4
- calcaneovarus Q66.1
- calcaneus Q66.89
- cavus Q66.7
- equinovalgus Q66.6
- equinovarus Q66.0
- equinus Q66.89
- percavus Q66.7
- planovalgus Q66.6
- planus (acquired) (any degree) (*see also* Deformity, limb, flat foot)
  - congenital Q66.5 ☑
  - due to rickets (sequelae) E64.3
- valgus Q66.6
- varus Q66.3

Tall stature, constitutional E34.4

Talma's disease M62.89

Talon noir S90.3 ☑
- hand S60.22 ☑
- heel S90.3 ☑
- toe S90.1 ☑

Tamponade, heart I31.4

Tanapox (virus disease) B08.71

Tangier disease E78.6

Tantrum, child problem F91.8

Tapeworm (infection) (infestation) — *see* Infestation, tapeworm

Tapia's syndrome G52.7

TAR (thrombocytopenia with absent radius) syndrome Q87.2

Tarral-Besnier disease L44.0

Tarsal tunnel syndrome — *see* Syndrome, tarsal tunnel

Tarsalgia — *see* Pain, limb, lower

Tarsitis (eyelid) H01.8
- syphilitic A52.71
- tuberculous A18.4

Tartar (teeth) (dental calculus) K03.6

Tattoo (mark) L81.8

Tauri's disease E74.09

Taurodontism K00.2

Taussig-Bing syndrome Q20.1

Taybi's syndrome Q87.2

Tay-Sachs amaurotic familial idiocy or disease E75.02

TBI (traumatic brain injury) S06.9 ☑

Teacher's node or nodule J38.2

Tear, torn (traumatic) (*see also* Laceration)
- with abortion — *see* Abortion
- annular fibrosis M51.35
- anus, anal (sphincter) S31.831 ☑
  - complicating delivery
    - with third degree perineal laceration (*see also* Delivery, complicated, by, laceration, perineum, third degree)O70.20
      - with mucosa O70.3
    - without third degree perineal laceration O70.4
  - nontraumatic (healed) (old) K62.81
- articular cartilage, old — *see* Derangement, joint, articular cartilage, by site
- bladder
  - with ectopic or molar pregnancy O08.6
  - following ectopic or molar pregnancy O08.6
  - obstetrical O71.5
  - traumatic — *see* Injury, bladder
- bowel
  - with ectopic or molar pregnancy O08.6
  - following ectopic or molar pregnancy O08.6
  - obstetrical trauma O71.5
- broad ligament
  - with ectopic or molar pregnancy O08.6
  - following ectopic or molar pregnancy O08.6
  - obstetrical trauma O71.6
- bucket handle (knee) (meniscus) — *see* Tear, meniscus
- capsule, joint — *see* Sprain
- cartilage (*see also* Sprain)
  - articular, old — *see* Derangement, joint, articular cartilage, by site
- cervix
  - with ectopic or molar pregnancy O08.6
  - following ectopic or molar pregnancy O08.6
  - obstetrical trauma (current) O71.3
  - old N88.1
  - traumatic — *see* Injury, uterus
- dural G97.41
  - nontraumatic G96.11
- internal organ — *see* Injury, by site
- knee cartilage
  - articular (current) S83.3 ☑
  - old — *see* Derangement, knee, meniscus, due to old tear
- ligament — *see* Sprain
- meniscus (knee) (current injury) S83.209 ☑
  - bucket-handle S83.20 ☑
  - lateral
    - bucket-handle S83.25 ☑
    - complex S83.27 ☑
    - peripheral S83.26 ☑
    - specified type NEC S83.28 ☑
  - medial
    - bucket-handle S83.21 ☑
    - complex S83.23 ☑
    - peripheral S83.22 ☑
    - specified type NEC S83.24 ☑
  - old — *see* Derangement, knee, meniscus, due to old tear
  - site other than knee - code as Sprain
  - specified type NEC S83.20 ☑

Tear — *continued*
- muscle — *see* Strain
- pelvic
  - floor, complicating delivery O70.1
  - organ NEC, obstetrical trauma O71.5
    - with ectopic or molar pregnancy O08.6
    - following ectopic or molar pregnancy O08.6
- perineal, secondary O90.1
- periurethral tissue, obstetrical trauma O71.82
  - with ectopic or molar pregnancy O08.6
  - following ectopic or molar pregnancy O08.6
- rectovaginal septum — *see* Laceration, vagina
- retina, retinal (without detachment) (horseshoe) (*see also* Break, retina, horseshoe)
  - with detachment — *see* Detachment, retina, with retinal, break
- rotator cuff (nontraumatic) M75.10 ☑
  - complete M75.12 ☑
  - incomplete M75.11 ☑
  - traumatic S46.01 ☑
    - capsule S43.42 ☑
- semilunar cartilage, knee — *see* Tear, meniscus
- supraspinatus (complete) (incomplete) (nontraumatic) (*see also* Tear, rotator cuff)M75.10 ☑
- tendon — *see* Strain
- tentorial, at birth P10.4
- umbilical cord
  - complicating delivery O69.89 ☑
- urethra
  - with ectopic or molar pregnancy O08.6
  - following ectopic or molar pregnancy O08.6
  - obstetrical trauma O71.5
- uterus — *see* Injury, uterus
- vagina — *see* Laceration, vagina
- vessel, from catheter — *see* Puncture, accidental complicating surgery
- vulva, complicating delivery O70.0

Tear-stone — *see* Dacryolith

Teeth (*see also* condition)
- grinding
  - psychogenic F45.8
  - sleep related G47.63

Teething (syndrome) K00.7

Telangiectasia, telangiectasis (verrucous) I78.1
- ataxic (cerebellar) (Louis-Bar) G11.3
- familial I78.0
- hemorrhagic, hereditary (congenital) (senile) I78.0
- hereditary, hemorrhagic (congenital) (senile) I78.0
- juxtafoveal H35.07 ☑
- macular H35.07 ☑
- parafoveal H35.07 ☑
- retinal (idiopathic) (juxtafoveal) (macular) (parafoveal) H35.07 ☑
- spider I78.1

Telephone scatologia F65.89

Telescoped bowel or intestine K56.1
- congenital Q43.8

Temperature
- body, high (of unknown origin) R50.9
- cold, trauma from T69.9 ☑
  - newborn P80.0
  - specified effect NEC T69.8 ☑

Temple — *see* condition

Temporal — *see* condition

Temporomandibular joint pain-dysfunction syndrome M26.62 ☑

Temporosphenoidal — *see* condition

Tendency
- bleeding — *see* Defect, coagulation
- suicide
  - meaning personal history of attempted suicide Z91.5
  - meaning suicidal ideation — *see* Ideation, suicidal
- to fall R29.6

Tenderness, abdominal R10.819
- epigastric R10.816
- generalized R10.817
- left lower quadrant R10.814
- left upper quadrant R10.812
- periumbilic R10.815
- right lower quadrant R10.813
- right upper quadrant R10.811
- rebound R10.829
  - epigastric R10.826
  - generalized R10.827
  - left lower quadrant R10.824
  - left upper quadrant R10.822
  - periumbilic R10.825

Tenderness — *continued*
- rebound — *continued*
  - right lower quadrant R10.823
  - right upper quadrant R10.821

Tendinitis, tendonitis (*see also* Enthesopathy)
- Achilles M76.6 ☑
- adhesive — *see* Tenosynovitis, specified type NEC
  - shoulder — *see* Capsulitis, adhesive
- bicipital M75.2 ☑
- calcific M65.2 ☑
  - ankle M65.27 ☑
  - foot M65.27 ☑
  - forearm M65.23 ☑
  - hand M65.24 ☑
  - lower leg M65.26 ☑
  - multiple sites M65.29
  - pelvic region M65.25 ☑
  - shoulder M75.3 ☑
  - specified site NEC M65.28
  - thigh M65.25 ☑
  - upper arm M65.22 ☑
- due to use, overuse, pressure (*see also* Disorder, soft tissue, due to use)
  - specified NEC — *see* Disorder, soft tissue, due to use, specified NEC
- gluteal M76.0 ☑
- patellar M76.5 ☑
- peroneal M76.7 ☑
- psoas M76.1 ☑
- tibial (posterior) M76.82 ☑
  - anterior M76.81 ☑
- trochanteric — *see* Bursitis, hip, trochanteric

Tendon — *see* condition

Tendosynovitis — *see* Tenosynovitis

Tenesmus (rectal) R19.8
- vesical R30.1

Tennis elbow — *see* Epicondylitis, lateral

Tenonitis (*see also* Tenosynovitis)
- eye (capsule) H05.04 ☑

Tenontosynovitis — *see* Tenosynovitis

Tenontothecitis — *see* Tenosynovitis

Tenophyte — *see* Disorder, synovium, specified type NEC

Tenosynovitis (*see also* Synovitis)M65.9
- adhesive — *see* Tenosynovitis, specified type NEC
  - shoulder — *see* Capsulitis, adhesive
- bicipital (calcifying) — *see* Tendinitis, bicipital
- gonococcal A54.49
- in (due to)
  - crystals M65.8 ☑
  - gonorrhea A54.49
  - syphilis (late) A52.78
  - use, overuse, pressure (*see also* Disorder, soft tissue, due to use)
    - specified NEC — *see* Disorder, soft tissue, due to use, specified NEC
- infective NEC M65.1 ☑
  - ankle M65.17 ☑
  - foot M65.17 ☑
  - forearm M65.13 ☑
  - hand M65.14 ☑
  - lower leg M65.16 ☑
  - multiple sites M65.19
  - pelvic region M65.15 ☑
  - shoulder region M65.11 ☑
  - specified site NEC M65.18
  - thigh M65.15 ☑
  - upper arm M65.12 ☑
- radial styloid M65.4
- shoulder region M65.81 ☑
  - adhesive — *see* Capsulitis, adhesive
- specified type NEC M65.88
  - ankle M65.87 ☑
  - foot M65.87 ☑
  - forearm M65.83 ☑
  - hand M65.84 ☑
  - lower leg M65.86 ☑
  - multiple sites M65.89
  - pelvic region M65.85 ☑
  - shoulder region M65.81 ☑
  - specified site NEC M65.88
  - thigh M65.85 ☑
  - upper arm M65.82 ☑
- tuberculous — *see* Tuberculosis, tenosynovitis

Tenovaginitis — *see* Tenosynovitis

Tension
- arterial, high (*see also* Hypertension)
  - without diagnosis of hypertension R03.0
- headache G44.209
  - intractable G44.201
  - not intractable G44.209

Tension — *continued*
- nervous R45.0
- pneumothorax J93.0
- premenstrual N94.3
- state (mental) F48.9

Tentorium — *see* condition

Teratencephalus Q89.8

Teratism Q89.7

Teratoblastoma (malignant) — *see* Neoplasm, malignant, by site

Teratocarcinoma (*see also* Neoplasm, malignant, by site)
- liver C22.7

Teratoma (solid) (*see also* Neoplasm, uncertain behavior, by site)
- with embryonal carcinoma, mixed — *see* Neoplasm, malignant, by site
- with malignant transformation — *see* Neoplasm, malignant, by site
- adult (cystic) — *see* Neoplasm, benign, by site
- benign — *see* Neoplasm, benign, by site
- combined with choriocarcinoma — *see* Neoplasm, malignant, by site
- cystic (adult) — *see* Neoplasm, benign, by site
- differentiated — *see* Neoplasm, benign, by site
- embryonal (*see also* Neoplasm, malignant, by site)
  - liver C22.7
- immature — *see* Neoplasm, malignant, by site
- liver C22.7
  - adult, benign, cystic, differentiated type or mature D13.4
- malignant (*see also* Neoplasm, malignant, by site)
  - anaplastic — *see* Neoplasm, malignant, by site
  - intermediate — *see* Neoplasm, malignant, by site
  - specified site — *see* Neoplasm, malignant, by site
  - unspecified site C62.90
  - undifferentiated — *see* Neoplasm, malignant, by site
- mature — *see* Neoplasm, uncertain behavior, by site
  - malignant — *see* Neoplasm, by site, malignant, by site
- ovary D27. ☑
  - embryonal, immature or malignant C56 ☑
- solid — *see* Neoplasm, uncertain behavior, by site
- testis C62.9 ☑
  - adult, benign, cystic, differentiated type or mature D29.2 ☑
  - scrotal C62.1 ☑
  - undescended C62.0 ☑

Termination
- anomalous (*see also* Malposition, congenital)
  - right pulmonary vein Q26.3
- pregnancy, elective Z33.2

Ternidens diminutus infestation B81.8

Ternidensiasis B81.8

Terror (s) night (child) F51.4

Terrorism, victim of Z65.4

Terry's syndrome H44.2 ☑

Tertiary — *see* condition

Test, tests, testing (for)
- adequacy (for dialysis)
  - hemodialysis Z49.31
  - peritoneal Z49.32
- blood pressure Z01.30
  - abnormal reading — *see* Blood, pressure
- blood-alcohol Z04.8
  - positive — *see* Findings, abnormal, in blood
- blood-drug Z04.8
  - positive — *see* Findings, abnormal, in blood
- blood typing Z01.83
  - Rh typing Z01.83
- cardiac pulse generator (battery) Z45.010
- fertility Z31.41
- genetic
  - disease carrier status for procreative management
    - female Z31.430
    - male Z31.440
  - male partner of patient with recurrent pregnancy loss Z31.441
  - procreative management NEC
    - female Z31.438
    - male Z31.448
- hearing Z01.10
  - with abnormal findings NEC Z01.118
- HIV (human immunodeficiency virus)
  - nonconclusive (in infants) R75
  - positive Z21
  - seropositive Z21

Test - Thrombophlebitis

- **Test,** tests, testing — *continued*
  - immunity status Z01.84
  - intelligence NEC Z01.89
  - laboratory (as part of a general medical examination) Z00.00
    - with abnormal finding Z00.01
    - for medicolegal reason NEC Z04.8
  - male partner of patient with recurrent pregnancy loss Z31.441
  - Mantoux (for tuberculosis) Z11.1
    - abnormal result R76.11
  - pregnancy, positive first pregnancy — *see* Pregnancy, normal, first
  - procreative Z31.49
    - fertility Z31.41
  - skin, diagnostic
    - allergy Z01.82
      - special screening examination — *see* Screening, by name of disease
    - Mantoux Z11.1
    - tuberculin Z11.1
  - specified NEC Z01.89
  - tuberculin Z11.1
    - abnormal result R76.11
  - vision Z01.00
    - with abnormal findings Z01.01
  - Wassermann Z11.3
    - positive — *see* Serology for syphilis, positive
- **Testicle,** testicular, testis (*see also* condition)
  - feminization syndrome (*see also* Syndrome, androgen insensitivity)E34.51
  - migrans Q55.29
- **Tetanus,** tetanic (cephalic) (convulsions) A35
  - with
    - abortion A34
    - ectopic or molar pregnancy O08.0
  - following ectopic or molar pregnancy O08.0
  - inoculation reaction (due to serum) — *see* Complications, vaccination
  - neonatorum A33
  - obstetrical A34
  - puerperal, postpartum, childbirth A34
- **Tetany** (due to) R29.0
  - alkalosis E87.3
  - associated with rickets E55.0
  - convulsions R29.0
    - hysterical F44.5
  - functional (hysterical) F44.5
  - hyperkinetic R29.0
    - hysterical F44.5
  - hyperpnea R06.4
    - hysterical F44.5
    - psychogenic F45.8
  - hyperventilation (*see also* Hyperventilation)R06.4
    - hysterical F44.5
  - neonatal (without calcium or magnesium deficiency) P71.3
  - parathyroid (gland) E20.9
  - parathyroprival E89.2
  - post- (para)thyroidectomy E89.2
  - postoperative E89.2
  - pseudotetany R29.0
  - psychogenic (conversion reaction) F44.5
- **Tetralogy** of Fallot Q21.3
- **Tetraplegia** (chronic) (*see also* Quadriplegia)G82.50
- **Thailand** hemorrhagic fever A91
- **Thalassanemia** — *see* Thalassemia
- **Thalassemia** (anemia) (disease) D56.9
  - with other hemoglobinopathy D56.8
  - alpha (major) (severe) (triple gene defect) D56.0
    - minor D56.3
    - silent carrier D56.3
    - trait D56.3
  - beta (severe) D56.1
    - homozygous D56.1
    - major D56.1
    - minor D56.3
    - trait D56.3
  - delta-beta (homozygous) D56.2
    - minor D56.3
    - trait D56.3
  - dominant D56.8
  - hemoglobin
    - C D56.8
    - E-beta D56.5
  - intermedia D56.1
  - major D56.1
  - minor D56.3
  - mixed D56.8
  - sickle-cell — *see* Disease, sickle-cell, thalassemia
  - specified type NEC D56.8
  - trait D56.3
  - variants D56.8
- **Thanatophoric** dwarfism or short stature Q77.1
- **Thaysen-Gee** disease (nontropical sprue) K90.0
- **Thaysen's** disease K90.0
- **Thecoma** D27 ☑
  - luteinized D27 ☑
  - malignant C56 ☑
- **Thelarche,** premature E30.8
- **Thelaziasis** B83.8
- **Thelitis** N61.0
  - puerperal, postpartum or gestational — *see* Infection, nipple
- **Therapeutic** — *see* condition
- **Therapy**
  - drug, long-term (current) (prophylactic)
    - agents affecting estrogen receptors and estrogen levels NEC Z79.818
    - anastrozole (Arimidex) Z79.811
    - antibiotics Z79.2
      - short-term use - omit code
    - anticoagulants Z79.01
    - anti-inflammatory Z79.1
    - antiplatelet Z79.02
    - antithrombotics Z79.02
    - aromatase inhibitors Z79.811
    - aspirin Z79.82
    - birth control pill or patch Z79.3
    - bisphosphonates Z79.83
    - contraceptive, oral Z79.3
    - drug, specified NEC Z79.899
    - estrogen receptor downregulators Z79.818
    - Evista Z79.810
    - exemestane (Aromasin) Z79.811
    - Fareston Z79.810
    - fulvestrant (Faslodex) Z79.818
    - gonadotropin-releasing hormone (GnRH) agonist Z79.818
    - goserelin acetate (Zoladex) Z79.818
    - hormone replacement (postmenopausal) Z79.890
    - insulin Z79.4
    - letrozole (Femara) Z79.811
    - leuprolide acetate (leuprorelin) (Lupron) Z79.818
    - megestrol acetate (Megace) Z79.818
    - methadone
      - for pain management Z79.891
      - maintenance therapy F11.20
    - Nolvadex Z79.810
    - opiate analgesic Z79.891
    - oral contraceptive Z79.3
    - raloxifene (Evista) Z79.810
    - selective estrogen receptor modulators (SERMs) Z79.810
    - short term - omit code
    - steroids
      - inhaled Z79.51
      - systemic Z79.52
    - tamoxifen (Nolvadex) Z79.810
    - toremifene (Fareston) Z79.810
- **Thermic** — *see* condition
- **Thermography** (abnormal) (*see also* Abnormal, diagnostic imaging)R93.8
  - breast R92.8
- **Thermoplegia** T67.0 ☑
- **Thesaurismosis,** glycogen — *see* Disease, glycogen storage
- **Thiamin** deficiency E51.9
  - specified NEC E51.8
- **Thiaminic** deficiency with beriberi E51.11
- **Thibierge-Weissenbach** syndrome — *see* Sclerosis, systemic
- **Thickening**
  - bone — *see* Hypertrophy, bone
  - breast N64.59
  - endometrium R93.8
  - epidermal L85.9
    - specified NEC L85.8
  - hymen N89.6
  - larynx J38.7
  - nail L60.2
    - congenital Q84.5
  - periosteal — *see* Hypertrophy, bone
  - pleura J92.9
    - with asbestos J92.0
  - skin R23.4
  - subepiglottic J38.7
  - tongue K14.8
  - valve, heart — *see* Endocarditis
- **Thigh** — *see* condition
- **Thinning** vertebra — *see* Spondylopathy, specified NEC
- **Thirst,** excessive R63.1
  - due to deprivation of water T73.1 ☑
- **Thomsen** disease G71.12
- **Thoracic** (*see also* condition)
  - kidney Q63.2
  - outlet syndrome G54.0
- **Thoracogastroschisis** (congenital) Q79.8
- **Thoracopagus** Q89.4
- **Thorax** — *see* condition
- **Thorn's** syndrome N28.89
- **Thorson-Björck** syndrome E34.0
- **Threadworm** (infection) (infestation) B80
- **Threatened**
  - abortion O20.0
    - with subsequent abortion O03.9
  - job loss, anxiety concerning Z56.2
  - labor (without delivery) O47.9
    - at or after 37 completed weeks of gestation O47.1
    - before 37 completed weeks of gestation O47.0 ☑
  - loss of job, anxiety concerning Z56.2
  - miscarriage O20.0
  - unemployment, anxiety concerning Z56.2
- **Three-day** fever A93.1
- **Threshers'** lung J67.0
- **Thrix** annulata (congenital) Q84.1
- **Throat** — *see* condition
- **Thrombasthenia** (Glanzmann) (hemorrhagic) (hereditary) D69.1
- **Thromboangiitis** I73.1
  - obliterans (general) I73.1
    - cerebral I67.89
    - vessels
      - brain I67.89
      - spinal cord I67.89
- **Thromboarteritis** — *see* Arteritis
- **Thromboasthenia** (Glanzmann) (hemorrhagic) (hereditary) D69.1
- **Thrombocytasthenia** (Glanzmann) D69.1
- **Thrombocythemia** (essential) (hemorrhagic) (idiopathic) (primary) D47.3
- **Thrombocytopathy** (dystrophic) (granulopenic) D69.1
- **Thrombocytopenia,** thrombocytopenic D69.6
  - with absent radius (TAR) Q87.2
  - congenital D69.42
  - dilutional D69.59
  - due to
    - drugs D69.59
    - extracorporeal circulation of blood D69.59
    - (massive) blood transfusion D69.59
    - platelet alloimmunization D69.59
  - essential D69.3
  - heparin induced (HIT) D75.82
  - hereditary D69.42
  - idiopathic D69.3
  - neonatal, transitory P61.0
    - due to
      - exchange transfusion P61.0
      - idiopathic maternal thrombocytopenia P61.0
      - isoimmunization P61.0
  - primary NEC D69.49
    - idiopathic D69.3
  - puerperal, postpartum O72.3
  - secondary D69.59
  - transient neonatal P61.0
- **Thrombocytosis,** essential D47.3
  - primary D47.3
- **Thromboembolism** — *see* Embolism
- **Thrombopathy** (Bernard-Soulier) D69.1
  - constitutional D68.0
  - Willebrand-Jurgens D68.0
- **Thrombopenia** — *see* Thrombocytopenia
- **Thrombophilia** D68.59
  - primary NEC D68.59
  - secondary NEC D68.69
  - specified NEC D68.69
- **Thrombophlebitis** I80.9
  - antepartum O22.2 ☑
    - deep O22.3 ☑
    - superficial O22.2 ☑
  - cavernous (venous) sinus G08
    - complicating pregnancy O22.5 ☑
    - nonpyogenic I67.6
  - cerebral (sinus) (vein) G08
    - nonpyogenic I67.6
    - sequelae G09
  - due to implanted device — *see* Complications, by site and type, specified NEC
  - during or resulting from a procedure NEC T81.72 ☑

Thrombosis - Tocopherol

- **Thrombosis** — *continued*
  - vein — *continued*
      - calf I82.4Z ☑
        - chronic I82.5Z ☑
      - lower leg I82.4Z ☑
        - chronic I82.5Z ☑
      - thigh I82.4Y ☑
        - chronic I82.5Y ☑
      - upper leg I82.4Y ☑
        - chronic I82.5y ☑
    - femoral I82.41 ☑
      - chronic I82.51 ☑
    - iliac (iliofemoral) I82.42 ☑
      - chronic I82.52 ☑
    - innominate I82.290
      - chronic I82.291
    - internal jugular I82.C1 ☑
      - chronic I82.C2 ☑
    - lower extremity
      - deep I82.40 ☑
        - chronic I82.50 ☑
        - specified NEC I82.49 ☑
          - chronic NEC I82.59 ☑
      - distal
        - deep I82.4Z ☑
      - proximal
        - deep I82.4Y ☑
          - chronic I82.5Y ☑
      - superficial I82.81 ☑
    - perianal K64.5
    - popliteal I82.43 ☑
      - chronic I82.53 ☑
    - radial I82.62 ☑
      - chronic I82.72 ☑
    - renal I82.3
    - saphenous (greater) (lesser) I82.81 ☑
    - specified NEC I82.890
      - chronic NEC I82.891
    - subclavian I82.B1 ☑
      - chronic I82.B2 ☑
    - thoracic NEC I82.290
      - chronic I82.291
    - tibial I82.44 ☑
      - chronic I82.54 ☑
    - ulnar I82.62 ☑
      - chronic I82.72 ☑
    - upper extremity I82.60 ☑
      - chronic I82.70 ☑
      - deep I82.62 ☑
        - chronic I82.72 ☑
      - superficial I82.61 ☑
        - chronic I82.71 ☑
  - vena cava
    - inferior I82.220
      - chronic I82.221
    - superior I82.210
      - chronic I82.211
  - venous, perianal K64.5
  - ventricle (*see also* Infarct, myocardium)
    - following acute myocardial infarction (current complication) I23.6
    - not resulting in infarction I24.0
- **Thrombus** — *see* Thrombosis
- **Thrush** (*see also* Candidiasis)
  - oral B37.0
  - newborn P37.5
  - vaginal B37.3
- **Thumb** (*see also* condition)
  - sucking (child problem) F98.8
- **Thymitis** E32.8
- **Thymoma** (benign) D15.0
  - malignant C37
- **Thymus**, thymic (gland) — *see* condition
- **Thyrocele** — *see* Goiter
- **Thyroglossal** (*see also* condition)
  - cyst Q89.2
  - duct, persistent Q89.2
- **Thyroid** (gland) (body) (*see also* condition)
  - hormone resistance E07.89
  - lingual Q89.2
  - nodule (cystic) (nontoxic) (single) E04.1
- **Thyroiditis** E06.9
  - acute (nonsuppurative) (pyogenic) (suppurative) E06.0
  - autoimmune E06.3
  - chronic (nonspecific) (sclerosing) E06.5
    - with thyrotoxicosis, transient E06.2
    - fibrous E06.5
    - lymphadenoid E06.3
    - lymphocytic E06.3
    - lymphoid E06.3
  - de Quervain's E06.1
- **Thyroiditis** — *continued*
  - drug-induced E06.4
  - fibrous (chronic) E06.5
  - giant-cell (follicular) E06.1
  - granulomatous (de Quervain) (subacute) E06.1
  - Hashimoto's (struma lymphomatosa) E06.3
  - iatrogenic E06.4
  - ligneous E06.5
  - lymphocytic (chronic) E06.3
  - lymphoid E06.3
  - lymphomatous E06.3
  - nonsuppurative E06.1
  - postpartum, puerperal O90.5
  - pseudotuberculous E06.1
  - pyogenic E06.0
  - radiation E06.4
  - Riedel's E06.5
  - subacute (granulomatous) E06.1
  - suppurative E06.0
  - tuberculous A18.81
  - viral E06.1
  - woody E06.5
- **Thyrolingual** duct, persistent Q89.2
- **Thyromegaly** E01.0
- **Thyrotoxic**
  - crisis — *see* Thyrotoxicosis
  - heart disease or failure (*see also* Thyrotoxicosis)E05.90 *[I43]*
    - with thyroid storm E05.91 *[I43]*
  - storm — *see* Thyrotoxicosis
- **Thyrotoxicosis** (recurrent) E05.90
  - with
    - goiter (diffuse) E05.00
      - with thyroid storm E05.01
      - adenomatous uninodular E05.10
        - with thyroid storm E05.11
      - multinodular E05.20
        - with thyroid storm E05.21
      - nodular E05.20
        - with thyroid storm E05.21
      - uninodular E05.10
        - with thyroid storm E05.11
    - infiltrative
      - dermopathy E05.00
        - with thyroid storm E05.01
      - ophthalmopathy E05.00
        - with thyroid storm E05.01
    - single thyroid nodule E05.10
      - with thyroid storm E05.11
    - thyroid storm E05.91
  - due to
    - ectopic thyroid nodule or tissue E05.30
      - with thyroid storm E05.31
    - ingestion of (excessive) thyroid material E05.40
      - with thyroid storm E05.41
    - overproduction of thyroid-stimulating hormone E05.80
      - with thyroid storm E05.81
    - specified cause NEC E05.80
      - with thyroid storm E05.81
  - factitia E05.40
    - with thyroid storm E05.41
  - heart E05.90 *[I43]*
    - with thyroid storm E05.91 *[I43]*
    - failure E05.90 *[I43]*
  - neonatal (transient) P72.1
  - transient with chronic thyroiditis E06.2
- **Tibia vara** — *see* Osteochondrosis, juvenile, tibia
- **Tic** (disorder) F95.9
  - breathing F95.8
  - child problem F95.0
  - compulsive F95.1
  - de la Tourette F95.2
  - degenerative (generalized) (localized) G25.69
    - facial G25.69
  - disorder
    - chronic
      - motor F95.1
      - vocal F95.1
    - combined vocal and multiple motor F95.2
    - transient F95.0
  - douloureux G50.0
    - atypical G50.1
    - postherpetic, postzoster B02.22
  - drug-induced G25.61
  - eyelid F95.8
  - habit F95.9
    - chronic F95.1
    - transient of childhood F95.0
  - lid, transient of childhood F95.0
  - motor-verbal F95.2
  - occupational F48.8
- **Tic** — *continued*
  - orbicularis F95.8
    - transient of childhood F95.0
  - organic origin G25.69
  - provisional F95.0
  - postchoreic G25.69
  - psychogenic, compulsive F95.1
  - salaam R25.8
  - spasm (motor or vocal) F95.9
    - chronic F95.1
    - transient of childhood F95.0
  - specified NEC F95.8
- **Tick-borne** — *see* condition
- **Tietze's** disease or syndrome M94.0
- **Tight**, tightness
  - anus K62.89
  - chest R07.89
  - fascia (lata) M62.89
  - foreskin (congenital) N47.1
  - hymen, hymenal ring N89.6
  - introitus (acquired) (congenital) N89.6
  - rectal sphincter K62.89
  - tendon — *see* Short, tendon
  - urethral sphincter N35.9
- **Tilting** vertebra — *see* Dorsopathy, deforming, specified NEC
- **Timidity**, child F93.8
- **Tin-miner's** lung J63.5
- **Tinea** (intersecta) (tarsi) B35.9
  - amiantacea L44.8
  - asbestina B35.0
  - barbae B35.0
  - beard B35.0
  - black dot B35.0
  - blanca B36.2
  - capitis B35.0
  - corporis B35.4
  - cruris B35.6
  - flava B36.0
  - foot B35.3
  - furfuracea B36.0
  - imbricata (Tokelau) B35.5
  - kerion B35.0
  - manuum B35.2
  - microsporic — *see* Dermatophytosis
  - nigra B36.1
  - nodosa — *see* Piedra
  - pedis B35.3
  - scalp B35.0
  - specified site NEC B35.8
  - sycosis B35.0
  - tonsurans B35.0
  - trichophytic — *see* Dermatophytosis
  - unguium B35.1
  - versicolor B36.0
- **Tingling** sensation (skin) R20.2
- **Tinnitus** NOS H93.1 ☑
  - audible H93.1 ☑
  - aurium H93.1 ☑
  - pulsatile H93.A ☑
  - subjective H93.1 ☑
- **Tipped** tooth (teeth) M26.33
- **Tipping**
  - pelvis M95.5
    - with disproportion (fetopelvic) O33.0
      - causing obstructed labor O65.0
  - tooth (teeth), fully erupted M26.33
- **Tiredness** R53.83
- **Tissue** — *see* condition
- **Tobacco** (nicotine)
  - abuse — *see* Tobacco, use
  - dependence — *see* Dependence, drug, nicotine
  - harmful use Z72.0
  - heart — *see* Tobacco, toxic effect
  - maternal use, affecting newborn P04.2
  - toxic effect — *see* Table of Drugs and Chemicals, by substance, poisoning
    - chewing tobacco — *see* Table of Drugs and Chemicals, by substance, poisoning
    - cigarettes — *see* Table of Drugs and Chemicals, by substance, poisoning
  - use Z72.0
    - complicating
      - childbirth O99.334
      - pregnancy O99.33 ☑
      - puerperium O99.335
    - counseling and surveillance Z71.6
    - history Z87.891
  - withdrawal state (*see also* Dependence, drug, nicotine)F17.203
- **Tocopherol** deficiency E56.0

Todd's
- cirrhosis K74.3
- paralysis (postepileptic) (transitory) G83.84

Toe — *see* condition

Toilet, artificial opening — *see* Attention to, artificial, opening

Tokelau (ringworm) B35.5

Tollwut — *see* Rabies

Tommaselli's disease R31.9
- correct substance properly administered — *see* Table of Drugs and Chemicals, by drug, adverse effect
- overdose or wrong substance given or taken — *see* Table of Drugs and Chemicals, by drug, poisoning

Tongue (*see also* condition)
- tie Q38.1

Tonic pupil — *see* Anomaly, pupil, function, tonic pupil

Toni-Fanconi syndrome (cystinosis) E72.09
- with cystinosis E72.04

Tonsil — *see* condition

Tonsillitis (acute) (catarrhal) (croupous) (follicular) (gangrenous) (infective) (lacunar) (lingual) (malignant) (membranous) (parenchymatous) (phlegmonous) (pseudomembranous) (purulent) (septic) (subacute) (suppurative) (toxic) (ulcerative) (vesicular) (viral) J03.90
- chronic J35.01
  - with adenoiditis J35.03
- diphtheritic A36.0
- hypertrophic J35.01
  - with adenoiditis J35.03
- recurrent J03.91
- specified organism NEC J03.80
  - recurrent J03.81
- staphylococcal J03.80
  - recurrent J03.81
- streptococcal J03.00
  - recurrent J03.01
- tuberculous A15.8
- Vincent's A69.1

Tooth, teeth — *see* condition

Toothache K08.89

Topagnosis R20.8

Tophi — *see* Gout, chronic

TORCH infection — *see* Infection, congenital
- without active infection P00.2

Torn — *see* Tear

Tornwaldt's cyst or disease J39.2

Torsion
- accessory tube — *see* Torsion, fallopian tube
- adnexa (female) — *see* Torsion, fallopian tube
- aorta, acquired I77.1
- appendix epididymis N44.04
- appendix testis N44.03
- bile duct (common) (hepatic) K83.8
  - congenital Q44.5
- bowel, colon or intestine K56.2
- cervix — *see* Malposition, uterus
- cystic duct K82.8
- dystonia — *see* Dystonia, torsion
- epididymis (appendix) N44.04
- fallopian tube N83.52 ☑
  - with ovary N83.53
- gallbladder K82.8
  - congenital Q44.1
- hydatid of Morgagni
  - female N83.52 ☑
  - male N44.03
- kidney (pedicle) (leading to infarction) N28.0
- Meckel's diverticulum (congenital) Q43.0
  - malignant — *see* Table of Neoplasms, small intestine, malignant
- mesentery K56.2
- omentum K56.2
- organ or site, congenital NEC — *see* Anomaly, by site
- ovary (pedicle) N83.51 ☑
  - with fallopian tube N83.53
  - congenital Q50.2
- oviduct — *see* Torsion, fallopian tube
- penis (acquired) N48.82
  - congenital Q55.63
- spasm — *see* Dystonia, torsion
- spermatic cord N44.02
  - extravaginal N44.01
  - intravaginal N44.02
- spleen D73.5
- testis, testicle N44.00
  - appendix N44.03

Torsion — *continued*
- tibia — *see* Deformity, limb, specified type NEC, lower leg
- uterus — *see* Malposition, uterus

Torticollis (intermittent) (spastic) M43.6
- congenital (sternomastoid) Q68.0
- due to birth injury P15.8
- hysterical F44.4
- ocular R29.891
- psychogenic F45.8
  - conversion reaction F44.4
- rheumatic M43.6
- rheumatoid M06.88
- spasmodic G24.3
- traumatic, current S13.4 ☑

Tortipelvis G24.1

Tortuous
- aortic arch Q25.46
- artery I77.1
- organ or site, congenital NEC — *see* Distortion
- retinal vessel, congenital Q14.1
- ureter N13.8
- urethra N36.8
- vein — *see* Varix

Torture, victim of Z65.4

Torula, torular (histolytica) (infection) — *see* Cryptococcosis

Torulosis — *see* Cryptococcosis

Torus (mandibularis) (palatinus) M27.0
- fracture — *see* Fracture, by site, torus

Touraine's syndrome Q79.8

Tourette's syndrome F95.2

Tourniquet syndrome — *see* Constriction, external, by site

Tower skull Q75.0
- with exophthalmos Q87.0

Toxemia R68.89
- bacterial — *see* Sepsis
- burn — *see* Burn
- eclamptic (with pre-existing hypertension) — *see* Eclampsia
- erysipelatous — *see* Erysipelas
- fatigue R68.89
- food — *see* Poisoning, food
- gastrointestinal K52.1
- intestinal K52.1
- kidney — *see* Uremia
- malarial — *see* Malaria
- myocardial — *see* Myocarditis, toxic
- of pregnancy — *see* Pre-eclampsia
- pre-eclamptic — *see* Pre-eclampsia
- small intestine K52.1
- staphylococcal, due to food A05.0
- stasis R68.89
- uremic — *see* Uremia
- urinary — *see* Uremia

Toxemica cerebropathia psychica (nonalcoholic) F04
- alcoholic — *see* Alcohol, amnestic disorder

Toxic (poisoning) (*see also* condition)T65.91 ☑
- effect — *see* Table of Drugs and Chemicals, by substance, poisoning
- shock syndrome A48.3
- thyroid (gland) — *see* Thyrotoxicosis

Toxicemia — *see* Toxemia

Toxicity — *see* Table of Drugs and Chemicals, by substance, poisoning
- fava bean D55.0
- food, noxious — *see* Poisoning, food
- from drug or nonmedicinal substance — *see* Table of Drugs and Chemicals, by drug

Toxicosis (*see also* Toxemia)
- capillary, hemorrhagic D69.0

Toxinfection, gastrointestinal K52.1

Toxocariasis B83.0

Toxoplasma, toxoplasmosis (acquired) B58.9
- with
  - hepatitis B58.1
  - meningoencephalitis B58.2
  - ocular involvement B58.00
  - other organ involvement B58.89
  - pneumonia, pneumonitis B58.3
- congenital (acute) (subacute) (chronic) P37.1
- maternal, manifest toxoplasmosis in infant (acute) (subacute) (chronic) P37.1

tPA (rtPA) administration in a different facility within the last 24 hours prior to admission to current facility Z92.82

Trabeculation, bladder N32.89

Trachea — *see* condition

Tracheitis (catarrhal) (infantile) (membranous) (plastic) (septal) (suppurative) (viral) J04.10
- with
  - bronchitis (15 years of age and above) J40
    - acute or subacute — *see* Bronchitis, acute
    - chronic J42
    - tuberculous NEC A15.5
    - under 15 years of age J20.9
  - laryngitis (acute) J04.2
    - chronic J37.1
    - tuberculous NEC A15.5
- acute J04.10
  - with obstruction J04.11
- chronic J42
  - with
    - bronchitis (chronic) J42
    - laryngitis (chronic) J37.1
- diphtheritic (membranous) A36.89
- due to external agent — *see* Inflammation, respiratory, upper, due to
- syphilitic A52.73
- tuberculous A15.5

Trachelitis (nonvenereal) — *see* Cervicitis

Tracheobronchial — *see* condition

Tracheobronchitis (15 years of age and above) (*see also* Bronchitis)
- due to
  - Bordetella bronchiseptica A37.80
    - with pneumonia A37.81
  - Francisella tularensis A21.8

Tracheobronchomegaly Q32.4
- with bronchiectasis J47.9
  - with
    - exacerbation (acute) J47.1
    - lower respiratory infection J47.0
- acquired J98.09
  - with bronchiectasis J47.9
    - with
      - exacerbation (acute) J47.1
      - lower respiratory infection J47.0

Tracheobronchopneumonitis — *see* Pneumonia, broncho-

Tracheocele (external) (internal) J39.8
- congenital Q32.1

Tracheomalacia J39.8
- congenital Q32.0

Tracheopharyngitis (acute) J06.9
- chronic J42
- due to external agent — *see* Inflammation, respiratory, upper, due to

Tracheostenosis J39.8

Tracheostomy
- complication — *see* Complication, tracheostomy
- status Z93.0
  - attention to Z43.0
  - malfunctioning J95.03

Trachoma, trachomatous A71.9
- active (stage) A71.1
- contraction of conjunctiva A71.1
- dubium A71.0
- initial (stage) A71.0
- healed or sequelae B94.0
- pannus A71.1
- Türck's J37.0

Traction, vitreomacular H43.82 ☑

Train sickness T75.3 ☑

Trait (s)
- Hb-S D57.3
- hemoglobin
  - abnormal NEC D58.2
    - with thalassemia D56.3
  - C — *see* Disease, hemoglobin C
  - S (Hb-S) D57.3
- Lepore D56.3
- personality, accentuated Z73.1
- sickle-cell D57.3
  - with elliptocytosis or spherocytosis D57.3
- type A personality Z73.1

Tramp Z59.0

Trance R41.89
- hysterical F44.89

Transection
- abdomen (partial) S38.3 ☑
- aorta (incomplete) (*see also* Injury, aorta)
  - complete — *see* Injury, aorta, laceration, major
- carotid artery (incomplete) (*see also* Injury, blood vessel, carotid, laceration)
  - complete — *see* Injury, blood vessel, carotid, laceration, major
- celiac artery (incomplete) S35.211 ☑
  - branch (incomplete) S35.291 ☑
    - complete S35.292 ☑
  - complete S35.212 ☑

Transection — *continued*
- innominate
  - artery (incomplete) (*see also* Injury, blood vessel, thoracic, innominate, artery, laceration)
    - complete — *see* Injury, blood vessel, thoracic, innominate, artery, laceration, major
  - vein (incomplete) (*see also* Injury, blood vessel, thoracic, innominate, vein, laceration)
    - complete — *see* Injury, blood vessel, thoracic, innominate, vein, laceration, major
- jugular vein (external) (incomplete) (*see also* Injury, blood vessel, jugular vein, laceration)
  - complete — *see* Injury, blood vessel, jugular vein, laceration, major
  - internal (incomplete) (*see also* Injury, blood vessel, jugular vein, internal, laceration)
    - complete — *see* Injury, blood vessel, jugular vein, internal, laceration, major
- mesenteric artery (incomplete) (*see also* Injury, mesenteric, artery, laceration)
  - complete — *see* Injury, mesenteric artery, laceration, major
- pulmonary vessel (incomplete) (*see also* Injury, blood vessel, thoracic, pulmonary, laceration)
  - complete — *see* Injury, blood vessel, thoracic, pulmonary, laceration, major
- subclavian — *see* Transection, innominate
- vena cava (incomplete) (*see also* Injury, vena cava)
  - complete — *see* Injury, vena cava, laceration, major
- vertebral artery (incomplete) (*see also* Injury, blood vessel, vertebral, laceration)
  - complete — *see* Injury, blood vessel, vertebral, laceration, major

Transaminasemia R74.0

Transfusion
- associated (red blood cell) hemochromatosis E83.111
- blood
  - ABO incompatible — *see* Complication (s), transfusion, incompatibility reaction, ABO
  - minor blood group (Duffy) (E) (K (ell)) (Kidd) (Lewis) (M) (N) (P) (S) T80.89 ☑
  - reaction or complication — *see* Complications, transfusion
- fetomaternal (mother) — *see* Pregnancy, complicated by, placenta, transfusion syndrome
- maternofetal (mother) — *see* Pregnancy, complicated by, placenta, transfusion syndrome
- placental (syndrome) (mother) — *see* Pregnancy, complicated by, placenta, transfusion syndrome
- reaction (adverse) — *see* Complications, transfusion
- related acute lung injury (TRALI) J95.84
- twin-to-twin — *see* Pregnancy, complicated by, placenta, transfusion syndrome, fetus to fetus

Transient (meaning homeless) (*see also* condition)Z59.0

Translocation
- balanced autosomal Q95.9
  - in normal individual Q95.0
- chromosomes NEC Q99.8
  - balanced and insertion in normal individual Q95.0
- Down syndrome Q90.2
- trisomy
  - 13 Q91.6
  - 18 Q91.2
  - 21 Q90.2

Translucency, iris — *see* Degeneration, iris

Transmission of chemical substances through the placenta — *see* Absorption, chemical, through placenta

Transparency, lung, unilateral J43.0

Transplant (ed) (status) Z94.9
- awaiting organ Z76.82
- bone Z94.6
  - marrow Z94.81
- candidate Z76.82
- complication — *see* Complication, transplant
- cornea Z94.7
- heart Z94.1
  - and lung (s) Z94.3
  - valve Z95.2
    - prosthetic Z95.2
    - specified NEC Z95.4
    - xenogenic Z95.3

Transplant — *continued*
- intestine Z94.82
- kidney Z94.0
- liver Z94.4
- lung (s) Z94.2
  - and heart Z94.3
- organ (failure) (infection) (rejection) Z94.9
  - removal status Z98.85
- pancreas Z94.83
- skin Z94.5
- social Z60.3
- specified organ or tissue NEC Z94.89
- stem cells Z94.84
- tissue Z94.9

Transplants, ovarian, endometrial N80.1

Transposed — *see* Transposition

Transposition (congenital) (*see also* Malposition, congenital)
- abdominal viscera Q89.3
- aorta (dextra) Q20.3
- appendix Q43.8
- colon Q43.8
- corrected Q20.5
- great vessels (complete) (partial) Q20.3
- heart Q24.0
  - with complete transposition of viscera Q89.3
- intestine (large) (small) Q43.8
- reversed jejunal (for bypass) (status) Z98.0
- scrotum Q55.23
- stomach Q40.2
  - with general transposition of viscera Q89.3
- tooth, teeth, fully erupted M26.30
- vessels, great (complete) (partial) Q20.3
- viscera (abdominal) (thoracic) Q89.3

Transsexualism F64.0

Transverse (*see also* condition)
- arrest (deep), in labor O64.0 ☑
- lie (mother) O32.2 ☑
  - causing obstructed labor O64.8 ☑

Transvestism, transvestitism (dual-role) F64.1
- fetishistic F65.1

Trapped placenta (with hemorrhage) O72.0
- without hemorrhage O73.0

TRAPS (tumor necrosis factor receptor associated periodic syndrome) M04.1

Trauma, traumatism (*see also* Injury)
- acoustic — *see* subcategory H83.3
- birth — *see* Birth, injury
- complicating ectopic or molar pregnancy O08.6
- during delivery O71.9
- following ectopic or molar pregnancy O08.6
- obstetric O71.9
  - specified NEC O71.89
- occlusal
  - primary K08.81
  - secondary K08.82

Traumatic (*see also* condition)
- brain injury S06.9 ☑

Treacher Collins syndrome Q75.4

Treitz's hernia — *see* Hernia, abdomen, specified site NEC

Trematode infestation — *see* Infestation, fluke

Trematodiasis — *see* Infestation, fluke

Trembling paralysis — *see* Parkinsonism

Tremor (s) R25.1
- drug induced G25.1
- essential (benign) G25.0
- familial G25.0
- hereditary G25.0
- hysterical F44.4
- intention G25.2
- medication induced postural G25.1
- mercurial — *see* subcategory T56.1
- Parkinson's — *see* Parkinsonism
- psychogenic (conversion reaction) F44.4
- senilis R54
- specified type NEC G25.2

Trench
- fever A79.0
- foot — *see* Immersion, foot
- mouth A69.1

Treponema pallidum infection — *see* Syphilis

Treponematosis
- due to
  - T. pallidum — *see* Syphilis
  - T. pertenue — *see* Yaws

Triad
- Hutchinson's (congenital syphilis) A50.53
- Kartagener's Q89.3
- Saint's — *see* Hernia, diaphragm

Trichiasis (eyelid) H02.059
- with entropion — *see* Entropion

Trichiasis — *continued*
- left H02.056
  - lower H02.055
  - upper H02.054
- right H02.053
  - lower H02.052
  - upper H02.051

Trichinella spiralis (infection) (infestation) B75

Trichinellosis, trichiniasis, trichinelliasis, trichinosis B75
- with muscle disorder B75 *[M63.80]*
  - ankle B75 *[M63.87-]*
  - foot B75 *[M63.87-]*
  - forearm B75 *[M63.83-]*
  - hand B75 *[M63.84-]*
  - lower leg B75 *[M63.86-]*
  - multiple sites B75 *[M63.89]*
  - pelvic region B75 *[M63.85-]*
  - shoulder region B75 *[M63.81-]*
  - specified site NEC B75 *[M63.88]*
  - thigh B75 *[M63.85-]*
  - upper arm B75 *[M63.82-]*

Trichobezoar T18.9 ☑
- intestine T18.3 ☑
- stomach T18.2 ☑

Trichocephaliasis, trichocephalosis B79

Trichocephalus infestation B79

Trichoclasis L67.8

Trichoepithelioma (*see also* Neoplasm, skin, benign)
- malignant — *see* Neoplasm, skin, malignant

Trichofolliculoma — *see* Neoplasm, skin, benign

Tricholemmoma — *see* Neoplasm, skin, benign

Trichomoniasis A59.9
- bladder A59.03
- cervix A59.09
- intestinal A07.8
- prostate A59.02
- seminal vesicles A59.09
- specified site NEC A59.8
- urethra A59.03
- urogenitalis A59.00
- vagina A59.01
- vulva A59.01

Trichomycosis
- axillaris A48.8
- nodosa, nodularis B36.8

Trichonodosis L67.8

Trichophytid, trichophyton infection — *see* Dermatophytosis

Trichophytobezoar T18.9 ☑
- intestine T18.3 ☑
- stomach T18.2 ☑

Trichophytosis — *see* Dermatophytosis

Trichoptilosis L67.8

Trichorrhexis (nodosa) (invaginata) L67.0

Trichosis axillaris A48.8

Trichosporosis nodosa B36.2

Trichostasis spinulosa (congenital) Q84.1

Trichostrongyliasis, trichostrongylosis (small intestine) B81.2

Trichostrongylus infection B81.2

Trichotillomania F63.3

Trichromat, trichromatopsia, anomalous (congenital) H53.55

Trichuriasis B79

Trichuris trichiura (infection) (infestation) (any site) B79

Tricuspid (valve) — *see* condition

Trifid (*see also* Accessory)
- kidney (pelvis) Q63.8
- tongue Q38.3

Trigeminal neuralgia — *see* Neuralgia, trigeminal

Trigeminy R00.8

Trigger finger (acquired) M65.30
- congenital Q74.0
- index finger M65.32 ☑
- little finger M65.35 ☑
- middle finger M65.33 ☑
- ring finger M65.34 ☑
- thumb M65.31 ☑

Trigonitis (bladder) (chronic) (pseudomembranous) N30.30
- with hematuria N30.31

Trigonocephaly Q75.0

Trilocular heart — *see* Cor triloculare

Trimethylaminuria E72.52

Tripartite placenta O43.19 ☑

Triphalangeal thumb Q74.0

Triple (*see also* Accessory)
- kidneys Q63.0
- uteri Q51.818
- X, female Q97.0

- **Triplegia** G83.89
  - congenital G80.8
- **Triplet** (newborn) (*see also* Newborn, triplet)
  - complicating pregnancy — *see* Pregnancy, triplet
- **Triplication** — *see* Accessory
- **Triploidy** Q92.7
- **Trismus** R25.2
  - neonatorum A33
  - newborn A33
- **Trisomy** (syndrome) Q92.9
  - autosomes Q92.9
  - chromosome specified NEC Q92.8
    - partial Q92.2
      - due to unbalanced translocation Q92.5
    - whole (nonsex chromosome)
      - meiotic nondisjunction Q92.0
      - mitotic nondisjunction Q92.1
      - mosaicism Q92.1
    - specified NEC Q92.8
  - due to
    - dicentrics — *see* Extra, marker chromosomes
    - extra rings — *see* Extra, marker chromosomes
    - isochromosomes — *see* Extra, marker chromosomes
  - specified NEC Q92.8
  - whole chromosome Q92.9
    - meiotic nondisjunction Q92.0
    - mitotic nondisjunction Q92.1
    - mosaicism Q92.1
    - partial Q92.9
    - specified NEC Q92.8
  - 13 (partial) Q91.7
    - meiotic nondisjunction Q91.4
    - mitotic nondisjunction Q91.5
    - mosaicism Q91.5
    - translocation Q91.6
  - 18 (partial) Q91.3
    - meiotic nondisjunction Q91.0
    - mitotic nondisjunction Q91.1
    - mosaicism Q91.1
    - translocation Q91.2
  - 20 Q92.8
  - 21 (partial) Q90.9
    - meiotic nondisjunction Q90.0
    - mitotic nondisjunction Q90.1
    - mosaicism Q90.1
    - translocation Q90.2
  - 22 Q92.8
- **Tritanomaly,** tritanopia H53.55
- **Trombiculosis,** trombiculiasis, trombidiosis B88.0
- **Trophedema** (congenital) (hereditary) Q82.0
- **Trophoblastic** disease (*see also* Mole, hydatidiform)O01.9
- **Tropholymphedema** Q82.0
- **Trophoneurosis** NEC G96.8
  - disseminated M34.9
- **Tropical** — *see* condition
- **Trouble** (*see also* Disease)
  - heart — *see* Disease, heart
  - kidney — *see* Disease, renal
  - nervous R45.0
  - sinus — *see* Sinusitis
- **Trousseau's** syndrome (thrombophlebitis migrans) I82.1
- **Truancy,** childhood
  - from school Z72.810
- **Truncus**
  - arteriosus (persistent) Q20.0
  - communis Q20.0
- **Trunk** — *see* condition
- **Trypanosomiasis**
  - African B56.9
    - by Trypanosoma brucei
      - gambiense B56.0
      - rhodesiense B56.1
  - American — *see* Chagas' disease
  - Brazilian — *see* Chagas' disease
  - by Trypanosoma
    - brucei gambiense B56.0
    - brucei rhodesiense B56.1
    - cruzi — *see* Chagas' disease
  - gambiensis, Gambian B56.0
  - rhodesiensis, Rhodesian B56.1
  - South American — *see* Chagas' disease
  - where
    - African trypanosomiasis is prevalent B56.9
    - Chagas' disease is prevalent B57.2
- **T-shaped** incisors K00.2
- **Tsutsugamushi** (disease) (fever) A75.3
- **Tube,** tubal, tubular — *see* condition
- **Tubercle** (*see also* Tuberculosis)
  - brain, solitary A17.81
  - Darwin's Q17.8
  - Ghon, primary infection A15.7
- **Tuberculid,** tuberculide (indurating, subcutaneous) (lichenoid) (miliary) (papulonecrotic) (primary) (skin) A18.4
- **Tuberculoma** (*see also* Tuberculosis)
  - brain A17.81
  - meninges (cerebral) (spinal) A17.1
  - spinal cord A17.81
- **Tuberculosis,** tubercular, tuberculous (calcification) (calcified) (caseous) (chromogenic acid-fast bacilli) (degeneration) (fibrocaseous) (fistula) (interstitial) (isolated circumscribed lesions) (necrosis) (parenchymatous) (ulcerative) A15.9
  - with pneumoconiosis (any condition in J60-J64) J65
  - abdomen (lymph gland) A18.39
  - abscess (respiratory) A15.9
    - bone A18.03
      - hip A18.02
      - knee A18.02
      - sacrum A18.01
      - specified site NEC A18.03
      - spinal A18.01
      - vertebra A18.01
    - brain A17.81
    - breast A18.89
    - Cowper's gland A18.15
    - dura (mater) (cerebral) (spinal) A17.81
    - epidural (cerebral) (spinal) A17.81
    - female pelvis A18.17
    - frontal sinus A15.8
    - genital organs NEC A18.10
    - genitourinary A18.10
    - gland (lymphatic) — *see* Tuberculosis, lymph gland
    - hip A18.02
    - intestine A18.32
    - ischiorectal A18.32
    - joint NEC A18.02
      - hip A18.02
      - knee A18.02
      - specified NEC A18.02
      - vertebral A18.01
    - kidney A18.11
    - knee A18.02
    - latent R76.11
    - lumbar (spine) A18.01
    - lung — *see* Tuberculosis, pulmonary
    - meninges (cerebral) (spinal) A17.0
    - muscle A18.09
    - perianal (fistula) A18.32
    - perinephritic A18.11
    - perirectal A18.32
    - rectum A18.32
    - retropharyngeal A15.8
    - sacrum A18.01
    - scrofulous A18.2
    - scrotum A18.15
    - skin (primary) A18.4
    - spinal cord A17.81
    - spine or vertebra (column) A18.01
    - subdiaphragmatic A18.31
    - testis A18.15
    - urinary A18.13
    - uterus A18.17
  - accessory sinus — *see* Tuberculosis, sinus
  - Addison's disease A18.7
  - adenitis — *see* Tuberculosis, lymph gland
  - adenoids A15.8
  - adenopathy — *see* Tuberculosis, lymph gland
  - adherent pericardium A18.84
  - adnexa (uteri) A18.17
  - adrenal (capsule) (gland) A18.7
  - alimentary canal A18.32
  - anemia A18.89
  - ankle (joint) (bone) A18.02
  - anus A18.32
  - apex, apical — *see* Tuberculosis, pulmonary
  - appendicitis, appendix A18.32
  - arachnoid A17.0
  - artery, arteritis A18.89
    - cerebral A18.89
  - arthritis (chronic) (synovial) A18.02
    - spine or vertebra (column) A18.01
  - articular — *see* Tuberculosis, joint
  - ascites A18.31
  - asthma — *see* Tuberculosis, pulmonary
  - axilla, axillary (gland) A18.2
  - bladder A18.12

Tuberculosis, tubercular, tuberculous — *continued*

  - bone A18.03
    - hip A18.02
    - knee A18.02
    - limb NEC A18.03
    - sacrum A18.01
    - spine or vertebral column A18.01
  - bowel (miliary) A18.32
  - brain A17.81
  - breast A18.89
  - broad ligament A18.17
  - bronchi, bronchial, bronchus A15.5
    - ectasia, ectasis (bronchiectasis) — *see* Tuberculosis, pulmonary
    - fistula A15.5
      - primary (progressive) A15.7
    - gland or node A15.4
      - primary (progressive) A15.7
    - lymph gland or node A15.4
      - primary (progressive) A15.7
  - bronchiectasis — *see* Tuberculosis, pulmonary
  - bronchitis A15.5
  - bronchopleural A15.6
  - bronchopneumonia, bronchopneumonic — *see* Tuberculosis, pulmonary
  - bronchorrhagia A15.5
  - bronchotracheal A15.5
  - bronze disease A18.7
  - buccal cavity A18.83
  - bulbourethral gland A18.15
  - bursa A18.09
  - cachexia A15.9
  - cardiomyopathy A18.84
  - caries — *see* Tuberculosis, bone
  - cartilage A18.02
    - intervertebral A18.01
  - catarrhal — *see* Tuberculosis, respiratory
  - cecum A18.32
  - cellulitis (primary) A18.4
  - cerebellum A17.81
  - cerebral, cerebrum A17.81
  - cerebrospinal A17.81
    - meninges A17.0
  - cervical (lymph gland or node) A18.2
  - cervicitis, cervix (uteri) A18.16
  - chest — *see* Tuberculosis, respiratory
  - chorioretinitis A18.53
  - choroid, choroiditis A18.53
  - ciliary body A18.54
  - colitis A18.32
  - collier's J65
  - colliquativa (primary) A18.4
  - colon A18.32
  - complex, primary A15.7
  - congenital P37.0
  - conjunctiva A18.59
  - connective tissue (systemic) A18.89
  - contact Z20.1
  - cornea (ulcer) A18.52
  - Cowper's gland A18.15
  - coxae A18.02
  - coxalgia A18.02
  - cul-de-sac of Douglas A18.17
  - curvature, spine A18.01
  - cutis (colliquativa) (primary) A18.4
  - cyst, ovary A18.18
  - cystitis A18.12
  - dactylitis A18.03
  - diarrhea A18.32
  - diffuse — *see* Tuberculosis, miliary
  - digestive tract A18.32
  - disseminated — *see* Tuberculosis, miliary
  - duodenum A18.32
  - dura (mater) (cerebral) (spinal) A17.0
    - abscess (cerebral) (spinal) A17.81
  - dysentery A18.32
  - ear (inner) (middle) A18.6
    - bone A18.03
    - external (primary) A18.4
    - skin (primary) A18.4
  - elbow A18.02
  - emphysema — *see* Tuberculosis, pulmonary
  - empyema A15.6
  - encephalitis A17.82
  - endarteritis A18.89
  - endocarditis A18.84
    - aortic A18.84
    - mitral A18.84
    - pulmonary A18.84
    - tricuspid A18.84
  - endocrine glands NEC A18.82
  - endometrium A18.17

Tuberculosis, tubercular, tuberculous — *continued*
- tonsil, tonsillitis A15.8
- trachea, tracheal A15.5
  - lymph gland or node A15.4
    - primary (progressive) A15.7
- tracheobronchial A15.5
  - lymph gland or node A15.4
    - primary (progressive) A15.7
- tubal (acute) (chronic) A18.17
- tunica vaginalis A18.15
- ulcer (skin) (primary) A18.4
  - bowel or intestine A18.32
  - specified NEC - code under Tuberculosis, by site
- unspecified site A15.9
- ureter A18.11
- urethra, urethral (gland) A18.13
- urinary organ or tract A18.13
- uterus A18.17
- uveal tract A18.54
- uvula A18.83
- vagina A18.18
- vas deferens A18.15
- verruca, verrucosa (cutis) (primary) A18.4
- vertebra (column) A18.01
- vesiculitis A18.15
- vulva A18.18
- wrist (joint) A18.02

Tuberculum
- Carabelli — *see* Note atK00.2
- occlusal — *see* Note atK00.2
- paramolare K00.2

Tuberosity, entire maxillary M26.07

Tuberous sclerosis (brain) Q85.1

Tubo-ovarian — *see* condition

Tuboplasty, after previous sterilization Z31.0
- aftercare Z31.42

Tubotympanitis, catarrhal (chronic) — *see* Otitis, media, nonsuppurative, chronic, serous

Tularemia A21.9
- with
  - conjunctivitis A21.1
  - pneumonia A21.2
- abdominal A21.3
- bronchopneumonic A21.2
- conjunctivitis A21.1
- cryptogenic A21.3
- enteric A21.3
- gastrointestinal A21.3
- generalized A21.7
- ingestion A21.3
- intestinal A21.3
- oculoglandular A21.1
- ophthalmic A21.1
- pneumonia (any), pneumonic A21.2
- pulmonary A21.2
- sepsis A21.7
- specified NEC A21.8
- typhoidal A21.7
- ulceroglandular A21.0

Tularensis conjunctivitis A21.1

Tumefaction (*see also* Swelling)
- liver — *see* Hypertrophy, liver

Tumor (*see also* Neoplasm, unspecified behavior, by site)
- acinar cell — *see* Neoplasm, uncertain behavior, by site
- acinic cell — *see* Neoplasm, uncertain behavior, by site
- adenocarcinoid — *see* Neoplasm, malignant, by site
- adenomatoid (*see also* Neoplasm, benign, by site)
  - odontogenic — *see* Cyst, calcifying odontogenic
- adnexal (skin) — *see* Neoplasm, skin, benign, by site
- adrenal
  - cortical (benign) D35.0 ☑
    - malignant C74.0 ☑
  - rest — *see* Neoplasm, benign, by site
- alpha-cell
  - malignant
    - pancreas C25.4
    - specified site NEC — *see* Neoplasm, malignant, by site
    - unspecified site C25.4
  - pancreas D13.7
  - specified site NEC — *see* Neoplasm, benign, by site
  - unspecified site D13.7
- aneurysmal — *see* Aneurysm
- aortic body D44.7
  - malignant C75.5

Tumor — *continued*
- Askin's — *see* Neoplasm, connective tissue, malignant
- basal cell (*see also* Neoplasm, skin, uncertain behavior)D48.5
- Bednar — *see* Neoplasm, skin, malignant
- benign (unclassified) — *see* Neoplasm, benign, by site
- beta-cell
  - malignant
    - pancreas C25.4
    - specified site NEC — *see* Neoplasm, malignant, by site
    - unspecified site C25.4
  - pancreas D13.7
  - specified site NEC — *see* Neoplasm, benign, by site
  - unspecified site D13.7
- Brenner D27.9
  - borderline malignancy D39.1 ☑
  - malignant C56 ☑
  - proliferating D39.1 ☑
- bronchial alveolar, intravascular D38.1
- Brooke's — *see* Neoplasm, skin, benign
- brown fat — *see* Lipoma
- Burkitt — *see* Lymphoma, Burkitt
- calcifying epithelial odontogenic — *see* Cyst, calcifying odontogenic
- carcinoid
  - benign D3A.00
    - appendix D3A.020
    - ascending colon D3A.022
    - bronchus (lung) D3A.090
    - cecum D3A.021
    - colon D3A.029
    - descending colon D3A.024
    - duodenum D3A.010
    - foregut NOS D3A.094
    - hindgut NOS D3A.096
    - ileum D3A.012
    - jejunum D3A.011
    - kidney D3A.093
    - large intestine D3A.029
    - lung (bronchus) D3A.090
    - midgut NOS D3A.095
    - rectum D3A.026
    - sigmoid colon D3A.025
    - small intestine D3A.019
    - specified NEC D3A.098
    - stomach D3A.092
    - thymus D3A.091
    - transverse colon D3A.023
  - malignant C7A.00
    - appendix C7A.020
    - ascending colon C7A.022
    - bronchus (lung) C7A.090
    - cecum C7A.021
    - colon C7A.029
    - descending colon C7A.024
    - duodenum C7A.010
    - foregut NOS C7A.094
    - hindgut NOS C7A.096
    - ileum C7A.012
    - jejunum C7A.011
    - kidney C7A.093
    - large intestine C7A.029
    - lung (bronchus) C7A.090
    - midgut NOS C7A.095
    - rectum C7A.026
    - sigmoid colon C7A.025
    - small intestine C7A.019
    - specified NEC C7A.098
    - stomach C7A.092
    - thymus C7A.091
    - transverse colon C7A.023
  - mesentery metastasis C7B.04
  - secondary C7B.00
    - bone C7B.03
    - distant lymph nodes C7B.01
    - liver C7B.02
    - peritoneum C7B.04
    - specified NEC C7B.09
- carotid body D44.6
  - malignant C75.4
- cells (*see also* Neoplasm, unspecified behavior, by site)
  - benign — *see* Neoplasm, benign, by site
  - malignant — *see* Neoplasm, malignant, by site
  - uncertain whether benign or malignant — *see* Neoplasm, uncertain behavior, by site
- cervix, in pregnancy or childbirth — *see* Pregnancy, complicated by, tumor, cervix

Tumor — *continued*
- chondromatous giant cell — *see* Neoplasm, bone, benign
- chromaffin (*see also* Neoplasm, benign, by site)
  - malignant — *see* Neoplasm, malignant, by site
- Cock's peculiar L72.3
- Codman's — *see* Neoplasm, bone, benign
- dentigerous, mixed — *see* Cyst, calcifying odontogenic
- dermoid — *see* Neoplasm, benign, by site
  - with malignant transformation C56 ☑
- desmoid (extra-abdominal) (*see also* Neoplasm, connective tissue, uncertain behavior)
  - abdominal — *see* Neoplasm, connective tissue, uncertain behavior
- embolus — *see* Neoplasm, secondary, by site
- embryonal (mixed) (*see also* Neoplasm, uncertain behavior, by site)
  - liver C22.7
- endodermal sinus
  - specified site — *see* Neoplasm, malignant, by site
  - unspecified site
    - female C56. ☑
    - male C62.90
- epithelial
  - benign — *see* Neoplasm, benign, by site
  - malignant — *see* Neoplasm, malignant, by site
- Ewing's — *see* Neoplasm, bone, malignant, by site
- fatty — *see* Lipoma
- fibroid — *see* Leiomyoma
- G cell
  - malignant
    - pancreas C25.4
    - specified site NEC — *see* Neoplasm, malignant, by site
    - unspecified site C25.4
  - specified site — *see* Neoplasm, uncertain behavior, by site
  - unspecified site D37.8
- germ cell (*see also* Neoplasm, malignant, by site)
  - mixed — *see* Neoplasm, malignant, by site
- ghost cell, odontogenic — *see* Cyst, calcifying odontogenic
- giant cell (*see also* Neoplasm, uncertain behavior, by site)
  - bone D48.0
    - malignant — *see* Neoplasm, bone, malignant
  - chondromatous — *see* Neoplasm, bone, benign
  - malignant — *see* Neoplasm, malignant, by site
  - soft parts — *see* Neoplasm, connective tissue, uncertain behavior
    - malignant — *see* Neoplasm, connective tissue, malignant
- glomus D18.00
  - intra-abdominal D18.03
  - intracranial D18.02
  - jugulare D44.7
    - malignant C75.5
  - skin D18.01
  - specified site NEC D18.09
- gonadal stromal — *see* Neoplasm, uncertain behavior, by site
- granular cell (*see also* Neoplasm, connective tissue, benign)
  - malignant — *see* Neoplasm, connective tissue, malignant
- granulosa cell D39.1 ☑
  - juvenile D39.1 ☑
  - malignant C56 ☑
- granulosa cell-theca cell D39.1 ☑
  - malignant C56 ☑
- Grawitz's C64 ☑
- hemorrhoidal — *see* Hemorrhoids
- hilar cell D27 ☑
- hilus cell D27 ☑
- Hurthle cell (benign) D34
  - malignant C73
- hydatid — *see* Echinococcus
- hypernephroid (*see also* Neoplasm, uncertain behavior, by site)
- interstitial cell (*see also* Neoplasm, uncertain behavior, by site)
  - benign — *see* Neoplasm, benign, by site
  - malignant — *see* Neoplasm, malignant, by site
- intravascular bronchial alveolar D38.1
- islet cell — *see* Neoplasm, benign, by site
  - malignant — *see* Neoplasm, malignant, by site
    - pancreas C25.4
    - specified site NEC — *see* Neoplasm, malignant, by site
    - unspecified site C25.4

- **Tumor** — *continued*
  - islet cell — *continued*
    - pancreas D13.7
    - specified site NEC — *see* Neoplasm, benign, by site
    - unspecified site D13.7
  - juxtaglomerular D41.0 ☑
  - Klatskin's C24.0
  - Krukenberg's C79.6 ☑
  - Leydig cell — *see* Neoplasm, uncertain behavior, by site
    - benign — *see* Neoplasm, benign, by site
      - specified site — *see* Neoplasm, benign, by site
      - unspecified site
        - female D27.9
        - male D29.20
    - malignant — *see* Neoplasm, malignant, by site
      - specified site — *see* Neoplasm, malignant, by site
      - unspecified site
        - female C56.9
        - male C62.90
    - specified site — *see* Neoplasm, uncertain behavior, by site
    - unspecified site
      - female D39.10
      - male D40.10
  - lipid cell, ovary D27 ☑
  - lipoid cell, ovary D27 ☑
  - malignant (*see also* Neoplasm, malignant, by site)C80.1
    - fusiform cell (type) C80.1
    - giant cell (type) C80.1
    - localized, plasma cell — *see* Plasmacytoma, solitary
    - mixed NEC C80.1
    - small cell (type) C80.1
    - spindle cell (type) C80.1
    - unclassified C80.1
  - mast cell D47.0
    - malignant C96.2
  - melanotic, neuroectodermal — *see* Neoplasm, benign, by site
  - Merkel cell — *see* Carcinoma, Merkel cell
  - mesenchymal
    - malignant — *see* Neoplasm, connective tissue, malignant
    - mixed — *see* Neoplasm, connective tissue, uncertain behavior
  - mesodermal, mixed (*see also* Neoplasm, malignant, by site)
    - liver C22.4
  - mesonephric (*see also* Neoplasm, uncertain behavior, by site)
    - malignant — *see* Neoplasm, malignant, by site
  - metastatic
    - from specified site — *see* Neoplasm, malignant, by site
    - of specified site — *see* Neoplasm, malignant, by site
    - to specified site — *see* Neoplasm, secondary, by site
  - mixed NEC (*see also* Neoplasm, benign, by site)
    - malignant — *see* Neoplasm, malignant, by site
  - mucinous of low malignant potential
    - specified site — *see* Neoplasm, malignant, by site
    - unspecified site C56.9
  - mucocarcinoid
    - specified site — *see* Neoplasm, malignant, by site
    - unspecified site C18.1
  - mucoepidermoid — *see* Neoplasm, uncertain behavior, by site
  - Müllerian, mixed
    - specified site — *see* Neoplasm, malignant, by site
    - unspecified site C54.9
  - myoepithelial — *see* Neoplasm, benign, by site
  - neuroectodermal (peripheral) — *see* Neoplasm, malignant, by site
    - primitive
      - specified site — *see* Neoplasm, malignant, by site
      - unspecified site C71.9
  - neuroendocrine D3A.8
    - malignant poorly differentiated C7A.1
    - secondary NEC C7B.8
    - specified NEC C7A.8
  - neurogenic olfactory C30.0
  - nonencapsulated sclerosing C73

- **Tumor** — *continued*
  - odontogenic (adenomatoid) (benign) (calcifying epithelial) (keratocystic) (squamous) — *see* Cyst, calcifying odontogenic
    - malignant C41.1
      - upper jaw (bone) C41.0
  - ovarian stromal D39.1 ☑
  - ovary, in pregnancy — *see* Pregnancy, complicated by
  - pacinian — *see* Neoplasm, skin, benign
  - Pancoast's — *see* Pancoast's syndrome
  - papillary (*see also* Papilloma)
    - cystic D37.9
      - mucinous of low malignant potential C56 ☑
        - specified site — *see* Neoplasm, malignant, by site
        - unspecified site C56.9
      - serous of low malignant potential
        - specified site — *see* Neoplasm, malignant, by site
        - unspecified site C56.9
  - pelvic, in pregnancy or childbirth — *see* Pregnancy, complicated by
  - phantom F45.8
  - phyllodes D48.6 ☑
    - benign D24 ☑
    - malignant — *see* Neoplasm, breast, malignant
  - Pindborg — *see* Cyst, calcifying odontogenic
  - placental site trophoblastic D39.2
  - plasma cell (malignant) (localized) — *see* Plasmacytoma, solitary
  - polyvesicular vitelline
    - specified site — *see* Neoplasm, malignant, by site
    - unspecified site
      - female C56.9
      - male C62.90
  - Pott's puffy — *see* Osteomyelitis, specified NEC
  - Rathke's pouch D44.3
  - retinal anlage — *see* Neoplasm, benign, by site
  - salivary gland type, mixed — *see* Neoplasm, salivary gland, benign
    - malignant — *see* Neoplasm, salivary gland, malignant
  - Sampson's N80.1
  - Schmincke's — *see* Neoplasm, nasopharynx, malignant
  - sclerosing stromal D27 ☑
  - sebaceous — *see* Cyst, sebaceous
  - secondary — *see* Neoplasm, secondary, by site
    - carcinoid C7B.00
      - bone C7B.03
      - distant lymph nodes C7B.01
      - liver C7B.02
      - peritoneum C7B.04
      - specified NEC C7B.09
    - neuroendocrine NEC C7B.8
  - serous of low malignant potential
    - specified site — *see* Neoplasm, malignant, by site
    - unspecified site C56.9
  - Sertoli cell — *see* Neoplasm, benign, by site
    - with lipid storage
      - specified site — *see* Neoplasm, benign, by site
      - unspecified site
        - female D27.9
        - male D29.20
    - specified site — *see* Neoplasm, benign, by site
    - unspecified site
      - female D27.9
      - male D29.20
  - Sertoli-Leydig cell — *see* Neoplasm, benign, by site
    - specified site — *see* Neoplasm, benign, by site
    - unspecified site
      - female D27.9
      - male D29.20
  - sex cord (-stromal) — *see* Neoplasm, uncertain behavior, by site
    - with annular tubules D39.1 ☑
  - skin appendage — *see* Neoplasm, skin, benign
  - smooth muscle — *see* Neoplasm, connective tissue, uncertain behavior
  - soft tissue
    - benign — *see* Neoplasm, connective tissue, benign
    - malignant — *see* Neoplasm, connective tissue, malignant
  - sternomastoid (congenital) Q68.0
  - stromal
    - endometrial D39.0

- **Tumor** — *continued*
  - stromal — *continued*
    - gastric D48.1
      - benign D21.4
      - malignant C16.9
      - uncertain behavior D48.1
    - gastrointestinal C49.A ☑
      - benign D21.4
      - esophagus C49.A1
      - large intestine C49.A4
      - malignant C49.A0
        - colon C49.A4
        - duodenum C49.A3
        - esophagus C49.A1
        - ileum C49.A3
        - jejunum C49.A3
        - Meckel diverticulum C49.A3
        - large intestine C49.A4
        - omentum C49.A9
        - peritoneum C49.A9
        - rectum C49.A5
        - small intestine C49.A3
        - specified site NEC C49.A9
        - stomach C49.A2
      - large intestine C49.A4
      - rectum C49.A5
      - small intestine C49.A3
      - specified site NEC C49.A9
      - stomach C49.A2
      - uncertain behavior D48.1
    - intestine
      - benign D21.4
      - malignant
        - large C49.A4
        - small C49.A3
      - uncertain behavior D48.1
    - ovarian D39.1 ☑
    - stomach C49.A2
      - benign D21.4
      - malignant C49.A2
      - uncertain behavior D48.1
  - testicular D40.10
  - sweat gland (*see also* Neoplasm, skin, uncertain behavior)
    - benign — *see* Neoplasm, skin, benign
    - malignant — *see* Neoplasm, skin, malignant
  - syphilitic, brain A52.17
  - testicular stromal D40.1 ☑
  - theca cell D27. ☑
  - theca cell-granulosa cell D39.1 ☑
  - Triton, malignant — *see* Neoplasm, nerve, malignant
  - trophoblastic, placental site D39.2
  - turban D23.4
  - uterus (body), in pregnancy or childbirth — *see* Pregnancy, complicated by, tumor, uterus
  - vagina, in pregnancy or childbirth — *see* Pregnancy, complicated by
  - varicose — *see* Varix
  - von Recklinghausen's — *see* Neurofibromatosis
  - vulva or perineum, in pregnancy or childbirth — *see* Pregnancy, complicated by
    - causing obstructed labor O65.5
  - Warthin's — *see* Neoplasm, salivary gland, benign
  - Wilms' C64 ☑
  - yolk sac — *see* Neoplasm, malignant, by site
    - specified site — *see* Neoplasm, malignant, by site
    - unspecified site
      - female C56.9
      - male C62.90
- **Tumor** lysis syndrome (following antineoplastic chemotherapy) (spontaneous) NEC E88.3
- **Tumorlet** — *see* Neoplasm, uncertain behavior, by site
- **Tungiasis** B88.1
- **Tunica** vasculosa lentis Q12.2
- **Turban** tumor D23.4
- **Türck's** trachoma J37.0
- **Turner-Kieser** syndrome Q87.2
- **Turner-like** syndrome Q87.1
- **Turner's**
  - hypoplasia (tooth) K00.4
  - syndrome Q96.9
    - specified NEC Q96.8
  - tooth K00.4
- **Turner-Ullrich** syndrome Q96.9
- **Tussis** convulsiva — *see* Whooping cough
- **Twiddler's** syndrome (due to)
  - automatic implantable defibrillator T82.198 ☑
  - cardiac pacemaker T82.198 ☑

- **Twilight** state
  - epileptic F05
  - psychogenic F44.89
- **Twin** (newborn) (*see also* Newborn, twin)
  - conjoined Q89.4
  - pregnancy — *see* Pregnancy, twin, conjoined
- **Twinning**, teeth K00.2
- **Twist, twisted**
  - bowel, colon or intestine K56.2
  - hair (congenital) Q84.1
  - mesentery K56.2
  - omentum K56.2
  - organ or site, congenital NEC — *see* Anomaly, by site
  - ovarian pedicle — *see* Torsion, ovary
- **Twitching** R25.3
- **Tylosis** (acquired) L84
  - buccalis K13.29
  - linguae K13.29
  - palmaris et plantaris (congenital) (inherited) Q82.8
    - acquired L85.1
- **Tympanism** R14.0
- **Tympanites** (abdominal) (intestinal) R14.0
- **Tympanitis** — *see* Myringitis
- **Tympanosclerosis** — *see* subcategory H74.0
- **Tympanum** — *see* condition
- **Tympany**
  - abdomen R14.0
  - chest R09.89
- **Type** A behavior pattern Z73.1
- **Typhlitis** — *see* Appendicitis
- **Typhoenteritis** — *see* Typhoid
- **Typhoid** (abortive) (ambulant) (any site) (clinical) (fever) (hemorrhagic) (infection) (intermittent) (malignant) (rheumatic) (Widal negative) A01.00
  - with pneumonia A01.03
  - abdominal A01.09
  - arthritis A01.04
  - carrier (suspected) of Z22.0
  - cholecystitis (current) A01.09
  - endocarditis A01.02
  - heart involvement A01.02
  - inoculation reaction — *see* Complications, vaccination
  - meningitis A01.01
  - mesenteric lymph nodes A01.09
  - myocarditis A01.02
  - osteomyelitis A01.05
  - perichondritis, larynx A01.09
  - pneumonia A01.03
  - spine A01.05
  - specified NEC A01.09
  - ulcer (perforating) A01.09
- **Typhomalaria** (fever) — *see* Malaria
- **Typhomania** A01.00
- **Typhoperitonitis** A01.09
- **Typhus** (fever) A75.9
  - abdominal, abdominalis — *see* Typhoid
  - African tick A77.1
  - amarillic A95.9
  - brain A75.9 *[G94]*
  - cerebral A75.9 *[G94]*
  - classical A75.0
  - due to Rickettsia
    - prowazekii A75.0
      - recrudescent A75.1
    - tsutsugamushi A75.3
    - typhi A75.2
  - endemic (flea-borne) A75.2
  - epidemic (louse-borne) A75.0
  - exanthematic NEC A75.0
  - exanthematicus SAI A75.0
    - brillii SAI A75.1
    - mexicanus SAI A75.2
    - typhus murinus A75.2
  - flea-borne A75.2
  - India tick A77.1
  - Kenya (tick) A77.1
  - louse-borne A75.0
  - Mexican A75.2
  - mite-borne A75.3
  - murine A75.2
  - North Asian tick-borne A77.2
  - petechial A75.9
  - Queensland tick A77.3
  - rat A75.2
  - recrudescent A75.1
  - recurrens — *see* Fever, relapsing
  - Sao Paulo A77.0
  - scrub (China) (India) (Malaysia) (New Guinea) A75.3

- **Typhus** — *continued*
  - shop (of Malaysia) A75.2
  - Siberian tick A77.2
  - tick-borne A77.9
  - tropical (mite-borne) A75.3
- **Tyrosinemia** E70.21
  - newborn, transitory P74.5
- **Tyrosinosis** E70.21
- **Tyrosinuria** E70.29

U

- **Uhl's** anomaly or disease Q24.8
- **Ulcer,** ulcerated, ulcerating, ulceration, ulcerative
  - alveolar process M27.3
  - amebic (intestine) A06.1
    - skin A06.7
  - anastomotic — *see* Ulcer, gastrojejunal
  - anorectal K62.6
  - antral — *see* Ulcer, stomach
  - anus (sphincter) (solitary) K62.6
  - aorta — *see* Aneurysm
  - aphthous (oral) (recurrent) K12.0
    - genital organ (s)
      - female N76.6
      - male N50.89
  - artery I77.2
  - atrophic — *see* Ulcer, skin
    - decubitus — *see* Ulcer, pressure, by site
  - back L98.429
    - with
      - bone necrosis L98.424
      - exposed fat layer L98.422
      - muscle necrosis L98.423
      - skin breakdown only L98.421
  - Barrett's (esophagus) K22.10
    - with bleeding K22.11
  - bile duct (common) (hepatic) K83.8
  - bladder (solitary) (sphincter) NEC N32.89
    - bilharzial B65.9 *[N33]*
    - in schistosomiasis (bilharzial) B65.9 *[N33]*
    - submucosal — *see* Cystitis, interstitial
    - tuberculous A18.12
  - bleeding K27.4
  - bone — *see* Osteomyelitis, specified type NEC
  - bowel — *see* Ulcer, intestine
  - breast N61.1
  - bronchus J98.09
  - buccal (cavity) (traumatic) K12.1
  - Buruli A31.1
  - buttock L98.419
    - with
      - bone necrosis L98.414
      - exposed fat layer L98.412
      - muscle necrosis L98.413
      - skin breakdown only L98.411
  - cancerous — *see* Neoplasm, malignant, by site
  - cardia K22.10
    - with bleeding K22.11
  - cardioesophageal (peptic) K22.10
    - with bleeding K22.11
  - cecum — *see* Ulcer, intestine
  - cervix (uteri) (decubitus) (trophic) N86
    - with cervicitis N72
  - chancroidal A57
  - chiclero B55.1
  - chronic (cause unknown) — *see* Ulcer, skin
  - Cochin-China B55.1
  - colon — *see* Ulcer, intestine
  - conjunctiva H10.89
  - cornea H16.00 ☑
    - with hypopyon H16.03 ☑
    - central H16.01 ☑
    - dendritic (herpes simplex) B00.52
    - marginal H16.04 ☑
    - Mooren's H16.05 ☑
    - mycotic H16.06 ☑
    - perforated H16.07 ☑
    - ring H16.02 ☑
    - tuberculous (phlyctenular) A18.52
  - corpus cavernosum (chronic) N48.5
  - crural — *see* Ulcer, lower limb
  - Curling's — *see* Ulcer, peptic, acute
  - Cushing's — *see* Ulcer, peptic, acute
  - cystic duct K82.8
  - cystitis (interstitial) — *see* Cystitis, interstitial
  - decubitus — *see* Ulcer, pressure, by site
  - dendritic, cornea (herpes simplex) B00.52
  - diabetes, diabetic — *see* Diabetes, ulcer
  - Dieulafoy's K25.0

- **Ulcer,** ulcerated, ulcerating, ulceration, ulcerative — *continued*
  - due to
    - infection NEC — *see* Ulcer, skin
    - radiation NEC L59.8
    - trophic disturbance (any region) — *see* Ulcer, skin
    - X-ray L58.1
  - duodenum, duodenal (eroded) (peptic) K26.9
    - with
      - hemorrhage K26.4
        - and perforation K26.6
      - perforation K26.5
    - acute K26.3
      - with
        - hemorrhage K26.0
          - and perforation K26.2
        - perforation K26.1
    - chronic K26.7
      - with
        - hemorrhage K26.4
          - and perforation K26.6
        - perforation K26.5
  - dysenteric A09
  - elusive — *see* Cystitis, interstitial
  - endocarditis (acute) (chronic) (subacute) I28.8
  - epiglottis J38.7
  - esophagus (peptic) K22.10
    - with bleeding K22.11
    - due to
      - aspirin K22.10
        - with bleeding K22.11
      - gastrointestinal reflux disease K21.0
      - ingestion of chemical or medicament K22.10
        - with bleeding K22.11
    - fungal K22.10
      - with bleeding K22.11
    - infective K22.10
      - with bleeding K22.11
    - varicose — *see* Varix, esophagus
  - eyelid (region) H01.8
  - fauces J39.2
  - Fenwick (-Hunner) (solitary) — *see* Cystitis, interstitial
  - fistulous — *see* Ulcer, skin
  - foot (indolent) (trophic) — *see* Ulcer, lower limb
  - frambesial, initial A66.0
  - frenum (tongue) K14.0
  - gallbladder or duct K82.8
  - gangrenous — *see* Gangrene
  - gastric — *see* Ulcer, stomach
  - gastrocolic — *see* Ulcer, gastrojejunal
  - gastroduodenal — *see* Ulcer, peptic
  - gastroesophageal — *see* Ulcer, stomach
  - gastrointestinal — *see* Ulcer, gastrojejunal
  - gastrojejunal (peptic) K28.9
    - with
      - hemorrhage K28.4
        - and perforation K28.6
      - perforation K28.5
    - acute K28.3
      - with
        - hemorrhage K28.0
          - and perforation K28.2
        - perforation K28.1
    - chronic K28.7
      - with
        - hemorrhage K28.4
          - and perforation K28.6
        - perforation K28.5
  - gastrojejunocolic — *see* Ulcer, gastrojejunal
  - gingiva K06.8
  - gingivitis K05.10
    - nonplaque induced K05.11
    - plaque induced K05.10
  - glottis J38.7
  - granuloma of pudenda A58
  - gum K06.8
  - gumma, due to yaws A66.4
  - heel — *see* Ulcer, lower limb
  - hemorrhoid (*see also* Hemorrhoids, by degree)K64.8
  - Hunner's — *see* Cystitis, interstitial
  - hypopharynx J39.2
  - hypopyon (chronic) (subacute) — *see* Ulcer, cornea, with hypopyon
  - hypostaticum — *see* Ulcer, varicose
  - ileum — *see* Ulcer, intestine
  - intestine, intestinal K63.3
    - with perforation K63.1
    - amebic A06.1
    - duodenal — *see* Ulcer, duodenum

- **Ulcer,** ulcerated, ulcerating, ulceration, ulcerative — *continued*
  - intestine, intestinal — *continued*
    - granulocytopenic (with hemorrhage) — *see* Neutropenia
    - marginal — *see* Ulcer, gastrojejunal
    - perforating K63.1
      - newborn P78.0
    - primary, small intestine K63.3
    - rectum K62.6
    - stercoraceous, stercoral K63.3
    - tuberculous A18.32
    - typhoid (fever) — *see* Typhoid
    - varicose I86.8
  - jejunum, jejunal — *see* Ulcer, gastrojejunal
  - keratitis — *see* Ulcer, cornea
  - knee — *see* Ulcer, lower limb
  - labium (majus) (minus) N76.6
  - laryngitis — *see* Laryngitis
  - larynx (aphthous) (contact) J38.7
    - diphtheritic A36.2
  - leg — *see* Ulcer, lower limb
  - lip K13.0
  - Lipschütz's N76.6
  - lower limb (atrophic) (chronic) (neurogenic) (perforating) (pyogenic) (trophic) (tropical) L97.909
    - with
      - bone necrosis L97.904
      - exposed fat layer L97.902
      - muscle necrosis L97.903
      - skin breakdown only L97.901
    - ankle L97.309
      - with
        - bone necrosis L97.304
        - exposed fat layer L97.302
        - muscle necrosis L97.303
        - skin breakdown only L97.301
      - left L97.329
        - with
          - bone necrosis L97.324
          - exposed fat layer L97.322
          - muscle necrosis L97.323
          - skin breakdown only L97.321
      - right L97.319
        - with
          - bone necrosis L97.314
          - exposed fat layer L97.312
          - muscle necrosis L97.313
          - skin breakdown only L97.311
    - calf L97.209
      - with
        - bone necrosis L97.204
        - exposed fat layer L97.202
        - muscle necrosis L97.203
        - skin breakdown only L97.201
      - left L97.229
        - with
          - bone necrosis L97.224
          - exposed fat layer L97.222
          - muscle necrosis L97.223
          - skin breakdown only L97.221
      - right L97.219
        - with
          - bone necrosis L97.214
          - exposed fat layer L97.212
          - muscle necrosis L97.213
          - skin breakdown only L97.211
    - decubitus — *see* Ulcer, pressure, by site
    - foot specified NEC L97.509
      - with
        - bone necrosis L97.504
        - exposed fat layer L97.502
        - muscle necrosis L97.503
        - skin breakdown only L97.501
      - left L97.529
        - with
          - bone necrosis L97.524
          - exposed fat layer L97.522
          - muscle necrosis L97.523
          - skin breakdown only L97.521
      - right L97.519
        - with
          - bone necrosis L97.514
          - exposed fat layer L97.512
          - muscle necrosis L97.513
          - skin breakdown only L97.511
    - heel L97.409
      - with
        - bone necrosis L97.404
        - exposed fat layer L97.402
        - muscle necrosis L97.403
        - skin breakdown only L97.401

- **Ulcer,** ulcerated, ulcerating, ulceration, ulcerative — *continued*
  - lower limb — *continued*
      - left L97.429
        - with
          - bone necrosis L97.424
          - exposed fat layer L97.422
          - muscle necrosis L97.423
          - skin breakdown only L97.421
      - right L97.419
        - with
          - bone necrosis L97.414
          - exposed fat layer L97.412
          - muscle necrosis L97.413
          - skin breakdown only L97.411
    - left L97.929
      - with
        - bone necrosis L97.924
        - exposed fat layer L97.922
        - muscle necrosis L97.923
        - skin breakdown only L97.921
    - lower leg NOS L97.909
      - with
        - bone necrosis L97.904
        - exposed fat layer L97.902
        - muscle necrosis L97.903
        - skin breakdown only L97.901
      - left L97.929
        - with
          - bone necrosis L97.924
          - exposed fat layer L97.922
          - muscle necrosis L97.923
          - skin breakdown only L97.921
      - right L97.919
        - with
          - bone necrosis L97.914
          - exposed fat layer L97.912
          - muscle necrosis L97.913
          - skin breakdown only L97.911
      - specified site NEC L97.809
        - with
          - bone necrosis L97.804
          - exposed fat layer L97.802
          - muscle necrosis L97.803
          - skin breakdown only L97.801
        - left L97.829
          - with
            - bone necrosis L97.824
            - exposed fat layer L97.822
            - muscle necrosis L97.823
            - skin breakdown only L97.821
        - right L97.819
          - with
            - bone necrosis L97.814
            - exposed fat layer L97.812
            - muscle necrosis L97.813
            - skin breakdown only L97.811
    - midfoot L97.409
      - with
        - bone necrosis L97.404
        - exposed fat layer L97.402
        - muscle necrosis L97.403
        - skin breakdown only L97.401
      - left L97.429
        - with
          - bone necrosis L97.424
          - exposed fat layer L97.422
          - muscle necrosis L97.423
          - skin breakdown only L97.421
      - right L97.419
        - with
          - bone necrosis L97.414
          - exposed fat layer L97.412
          - muscle necrosis L97.413
          - skin breakdown only L97.411
    - right L97.919
      - with
        - bone necrosis L97.914
        - exposed fat layer L97.912
        - muscle necrosis L97.913
        - skin breakdown only L97.911
    - thigh L97.109
      - with
        - bone necrosis L97.104
        - exposed fat layer L97.102
        - muscle necrosis L97.103
        - skin breakdown only L97.101
      - left L97.129
        - with
          - bone necrosis L97.124
          - exposed fat layer L97.122
          - muscle necrosis L97.123
          - skin breakdown only L97.121

- **Ulcer,** ulcerated, ulcerating, ulceration, ulcerative — *continued*
  - lower limb — *continued*
      - right L97.119
        - with
          - bone necrosis L97.114
          - exposed fat layer L97.112
          - muscle necrosis L97.113
          - skin breakdown only L97.111
    - toe L97.509
      - with
        - bone necrosis L97.504
        - exposed fat layer L97.502
        - muscle necrosis L97.503
        - skin breakdown only L97.501
      - left L97.529
        - with
          - bone necrosis L97.524
          - exposed fat layer L97.522
          - muscle necrosis L97.523
          - skin breakdown only L97.521
      - right L97.519
        - with
          - bone necrosis L97.514
          - exposed fat layer L97.512
          - muscle necrosis L97.513
          - skin breakdown only L97.511
    - leprous A30.1
    - syphilitic A52.19
    - varicose — *see* Varix, leg, with, ulcer
  - luetic — *see* Ulcer, syphilitic
  - lung J98.4
    - tuberculous — *see* Tuberculosis, pulmonary
  - malignant — *see* Neoplasm, malignant, by site
  - marginal NEC — *see* Ulcer, gastrojejunal
  - meatus (urinarius) N34.2
  - Meckel's diverticulum Q43.0
    - malignant — *see* Table of Neoplasms, small intestine, malignant
  - Meleney's (chronic undermining) — *see* Ulcer, skin
  - Mooren's (cornea) — *see* Ulcer, cornea, Mooren's
  - mycobacterial (skin) A31.1
  - nasopharynx J39.2
  - neck, uterus N86
  - neurogenic NEC — *see* Ulcer, skin
  - nose, nasal (passage) (infective) (septum) J34.0
    - skin — *see* Ulcer, skin
    - spirochetal A69.8
    - varicose (bleeding) I86.8
  - oral mucosa (traumatic) K12.1
  - palate (soft) K12.1
  - penis (chronic) N48.5
  - peptic (site unspecified) K27.9
    - with
      - hemorrhage K27.4
        - and perforation K27.6
      - perforation K27.5
    - acute K27.3
      - with
        - hemorrhage K27.0
          - and perforation K27.2
        - perforation K27.1
    - chronic K27.7
      - with
        - hemorrhage K27.4
          - and perforation K27.6
        - perforation K27.5
    - esophagus K22.10
      - with bleeding K22.11
    - newborn P78.82
  - perforating K27.5
    - skin — *see* Ulcer, skin
  - peritonsillar J35.8
  - phagedenic (tropical) — *see* Ulcer, skin
  - pharynx J39.2
  - phlebitis — *see* Phlebitis
  - plaster — *see* Ulcer, pressure, by site
  - popliteal space — *see* Ulcer, lower limb
  - postpyloric — *see* Ulcer, duodenum
  - prepuce N47.7
  - prepyloric — *see* Ulcer, stomach
  - pressure (pressure area) L89.9 ☑
    - ankle L89.5 ☑
    - back L89.1 ☑
    - buttock L89.3 ☑
    - coccyx L89.15 ☑
    - contiguous site of back, buttock, hip L89.4 ☑
    - elbow L89.0 ☑
    - face L89.81 ☑
    - head L89.81 ☑
    - heel L89.6 ☑
    - hip L89.2 ☑

Ulcer, ulcerated, ulcerating, ulceration, ulcerative — *continued* — *continued*
- pressure — *continued*
  - sacral region (tailbone) L89.15 ☑
  - specified site NEC L89.89 ☑
  - stage 1 (healing) (pre-ulcer skin changes limited to persistent focal edema)
    - ankle L89.5 ☑
    - back L89.1 ☑
    - buttock L89.3 ☑
    - coccyx L89.15 ☑
    - contiguous site of back, buttock, hip L89.4 ☑
    - elbow L89.0 ☑
    - face L89.81 ☑
    - head L89.81 ☑
    - heel L89.6 ☑
    - hip L89.2 ☑
    - sacral region (tailbone) L89.15 ☑
    - specified site NEC L89.89 ☑
  - stage 2 (healing) (abrasion, blister, partial thickness skin loss involving epidermis and/or dermis)
    - ankle L89.5 ☑
    - back L89.1 ☑
    - buttock L89.3 ☑
    - coccyx L89.15 ☑
    - contiguous site of back, buttock, hip L89.4 ☑
    - elbow L89.0 ☑
    - face L89.81 ☑
    - head L89.81 ☑
    - heel L89.6 ☑
    - hip L89.2 ☑
    - sacral region (tailbone) L89.15 ☑
    - specified site NEC L89.89 ☑
  - stage 3 (healing) (full thickness skin loss involving damage or necrosis of subcutaneous tissue)
    - ankle L89.5 ☑
    - back L89.1 ☑
    - buttock L89.3 ☑
    - coccyx L89.15 ☑
    - contiguous site of back, buttock, hip L89.4 ☑
    - elbow L89.0 ☑
    - face L89.81 ☑
    - head L89.81 ☑
    - heel L89.6 ☑
    - hip L89.2 ☑
    - sacral region (tailbone) L89.15 ☑
    - specified site NEC L89.89 ☑
  - stage 4 (healing) (necrosis of soft tissues through to underlying muscle, tendon, or bone)
    - ankle L89.5 ☑
    - back L89.1 ☑
    - buttock L89.3 ☑
    - coccyx L89.15 ☑
    - contiguous site of back, buttock, hip L89.4 ☑
    - elbow L89.0 ☑
    - face L89.81 ☑
    - head L89.81 ☑
    - heel L89.6 ☑
    - hip L89.2 ☑
    - sacral region (tailbone) L89.15 ☑
    - specified site NEC L89.89 ☑
  - unspecified stage
    - ankle L89.5 ☑
    - back L89.1 ☑
    - buttock L89.3 ☑
    - coccyx L89.15 ☑
    - contiguous site of back, buttock, hip L89.4 ☑
    - elbow L89.0 ☑
    - face L89.81 ☑
    - head L89.81 ☑
    - heel L89.6 ☑
    - hip L89.2 ☑
    - sacral region (tailbone) L89.15 ☑
    - specified site NEC L89.89 ☑
  - unstageable
    - ankle L89.5 ☑
    - back L89.1 ☑
    - buttock L89.3 ☑
    - coccyx L89.15 ☑
    - contiguous site of back, buttock, hip L89.4 ☑
    - elbow L89.0 ☑
    - face L89.81 ☑
    - head L89.81 ☑
    - heel L89.6 ☑
    - hip L89.2 ☑
    - sacral region (tailbone) L89.15 ☑
    - specified site NEC L89.89 ☑
- primary of intestine K63.3
  - with perforation K63.1

Ulcer — *continued*
- prostate N41.9
- pyloric — *see* Ulcer, stomach
- rectosigmoid K63.3
  - with perforation K63.1
- rectum (sphincter) (solitary) K62.6
  - stercoraceous, stercoral K62.6
- retina — *see* Inflammation, chorioretinal
- rodent (*see also* Neoplasm, skin, malignant)
- sclera — *see* Scleritis
- scrofulous (tuberculous) A18.2
- scrotum N50.89
  - tuberculous A18.15
  - varicose I86.1
- seminal vesicle N50.89
- sigmoid — *see* Ulcer, intestine
- skin (atrophic) (chronic) (neurogenic) (non-healing) (perforating) (pyogenic) (trophic) (tropical) L98.499
  - with gangrene — *see* Gangrene
  - amebic A06.7
  - back — *see* Ulcer, back
  - buttock — *see* Ulcer, buttock
  - decubitus — *see* Ulcer, pressure
  - lower limb — *see* Ulcer, lower limb
  - mycobacterial A31.1
  - specified site NEC L98.499
    - with
      - bone necrosis L98.494
      - exposed fat layer L98.492
      - muscle necrosis L98.493
      - skin breakdown only L98.491
  - tuberculous (primary) A18.4
  - varicose — *see* Ulcer, varicose
- sloughing — *see* Ulcer, skin
- solitary, anus or rectum (sphincter) K62.6
- sore throat J02.9
  - streptococcal J02.0
- spermatic cord N50.89
- spine (tuberculous) A18.01
- stasis (venous) — *see* Varix, leg, with, ulcer
  - without varicose veins I87.2
- stercoraceous, stercoral K63.3
  - with perforation K63.1
  - anus or rectum K62.6
- stoma, stomal — *see* Ulcer, gastrojejunal
- stomach (eroded) (peptic) (round) K25.9
  - with
    - hemorrhage K25.4
      - and perforation K25.6
    - perforation K25.5
  - acute K25.3
    - with
      - hemorrhage K25.0
        - and perforation K25.2
      - perforation K25.1
  - chronic K25.7
    - with
      - hemorrhage K25.4
        - and perforation K25.6
      - perforation K25.5
- stomal — *see* Ulcer, gastrojejunal
- stomatitis K12.1
- stress — *see* Ulcer, peptic
- strumous (tuberculous) A18.2
- submucosal, bladder — *see* Cystitis, interstitial
- syphilitic (any site) (early) (secondary) A51.39
  - late A52.79
  - perforating A52.79
    - foot A52.11
- testis N50.89
- thigh — *see* Ulcer, lower limb
- throat J39.2
  - diphtheritic A36.0
- toe — *see* Ulcer, lower limb
- tongue (traumatic) K14.0
- tonsil J35.8
  - diphtheritic A36.0
- trachea J39.8
- trophic — *see* Ulcer, skin
- tropical — *see* Ulcer, skin
- tuberculous — *see* Tuberculosis, ulcer
- tunica vaginalis N50.89
- turbinate J34.89
- typhoid (perforating) — *see* Typhoid
- unspecified site — *see* Ulcer, skin
- urethra (meatus) — *see* Urethritis
- uterus N85.8
  - cervix N86
    - with cervicitis N72
  - neck N86
    - with cervicitis N72

Ulcer — *continued*
- vagina N76.5
  - in Behçet's disease M35.2 *[N77.0]*
  - pessary N89.8
- valve, heart I33.0
- varicose (lower limb, any part) (*see also* Varix, leg, with, ulcer)
  - broad ligament I86.2
  - esophagus — *see* Varix, esophagus
  - inflamed or infected — *see* Varix, leg, with ulcer, with inflammation
  - nasal septum I86.8
  - perineum I86.3
  - scrotum I86.1
  - specified site NEC I86.8
  - sublingual I86.0
  - vulva I86.3
- vas deferens N50.89
- vulva (acute) (infectional) N76.6
  - in (due to)
    - Behçet's disease M35.2 *[N77.0]*
    - herpesviral (herpes simplex) infection A60.04
    - tuberculosis A18.18
- vulvobuccal, recurring N76.6
- X-ray L58.1
- yaws A66.4

Ulcerosa scarlatina A38.8
Ulcus (*see also* Ulcer)
- cutis tuberculosum A18.4
- duodeni — *see* Ulcer, duodenum
- durum (syphilitic) A51.0
  - extragenital A51.2
- gastrojejunale — *see* Ulcer, gastrojejunal
- hypostaticum — *see* Ulcer, varicose
- molle (cutis) (skin) A57
- serpens corneae — *see* Ulcer, cornea, central
- ventriculi — *see* Ulcer, stomach

Ulegyria Q04.8
Ulerythema
- ophryogenes, congenital Q84.2
- sycosiforme L73.8

Ullrich (-Bonnevie) (-Turner) syndrome (*see also* Turner's syndrome)Q87.1
Ullrich-Feichtiger syndrome Q87.0
Ulnar — *see* condition
Ulorrhagia, ulorrhea K06.8
Umbilicus, umbilical — *see* condition
Unacceptable
- contours of tooth K08.54
- morphology of tooth K08.54

Unavailability (of)
- bed at medical facility Z75.1
- health service-related agencies Z75.4
- medical facilities (at) Z75.3
  - due to
    - investigation by social service agency Z75.2
    - lack of services at home Z75.0
    - remoteness from facility Z75.3
    - waiting list Z75.1
  - home Z75.0
  - outpatient clinic Z75.3
- schooling Z55.1
- social service agencies Z75.4

Uncinaria americana infestation B76.1
Uncinariasis B76.9
Uncongenial work Z56.5
Unconscious (ness) — *see* Coma
Under observation — *see* Observation
Underachievement in school Z55.3
Underdevelopment (*see also* Undeveloped)
- nose Q30.1
- sexual E30.0

Underdosing (*see also* Table of Drugs and Chemicals, categories T36-T50, with final character 6)Z91.14
- intentional NEC Z91.128
  - due to financial hardship of patient Z91.120
- unintentional NEC Z91.138
  - due to patient's age related debility Z91.130

Underfeeding, newborn P92.3
Underfill, endodontic M27.53
Underimmunization status Z28.3
Undernourishment — *see* Malnutrition
Undernutrition — *see* Malnutrition
Underweight R63.6
- for gestational age — *see* Light for dates

Underwood's disease P83.0
Undescended (*see also* Malposition, congenital)
- cecum Q43.3
- colon Q43.3
- testicle — *see* Cryptorchid

Undeveloped, undevelopment (*see also* Hypoplasia)
- brain (congenital) Q02

- **Undeveloped** — *continued*
  - cerebral (congenital) Q02
  - heart Q24.8
  - lung Q33.6
  - testis E29.1
  - uterus E30.0
- **Undiagnosed** (disease) R69
- **Undulant** fever — *see* Brucellosis
- **Unemployment,** anxiety concerning Z56.0
  - threatened Z56.2
- **Unequal** length (acquired) (limb) (*see also* Deformity, limb, unequal length)
  - leg (*see also* Deformity, limb, unequal length)
    - congenital Q72.9 ☑
- **Unextracted** dental root K08.3
- **Unguis** incarnatus L60.0
- **Unhappiness** R45.2
- **Unicornate** uterus Q51.4
- **Unilateral** (*see also* condition)
  - development, breast N64.89
  - organ or site, congenital NEC — *see* Agenesis, by site
- **Unilocular** heart Q20.8
- **Union,** abnormal (*see also* Fusion)
  - larynx and trachea Q34.8
- **Universal** mesentery Q43.3
- **Unrepairable** overhanging of dental restorative materials K08.52
- **Unsatisfactory**
  - restoration of tooth K08.50
    - specified NEC K08.59
  - sample of cytologic smear
    - anus R85.615
    - cervix R87.615
    - vagina R87.625
  - surroundings Z59.1
    - work Z56.5
- **Unsoundness** of mind — *see* Psychosis
- **Unstable**
  - back NEC — *see* Instability, joint, spine
  - hip (congenital) Q65.6
    - acquired — *see* Derangement, joint, specified type NEC, hip
  - joint — *see* Instability, joint
    - secondary to removal of joint prosthesis M96.89
  - lie (mother) O32.0 ☑
  - lumbosacral joint (congenital)
    - acquired — *see* subcategory M53.2
  - sacroiliac — *see* subcategory M53.2
  - spine NEC — *see* Instability, joint, spine
- **Unsteadiness** on feet R26.81
- **Untruthfulness,** child problem F91.8
- **Unverricht** (-Lundborg) disease or epilepsy — *see* Epilepsy, generalized, idiopathic
- **Unwanted** pregnancy Z64.0
- **Upbringing,** institutional Z62.22
  - away from parents NEC Z62.29
  - in care of non-parental family member Z62.21
  - in foster care Z62.21
  - in orphanage or group home Z62.22
  - in welfare custody Z62.21
- **Upper** respiratory — *see* condition
- **Upset**
  - gastric K30
  - gastrointestinal K30
    - psychogenic F45.8
  - intestinal (large) (small) K59.9
    - psychogenic F45.8
  - menstruation N93.9
  - mental F48.9
  - stomach K30
    - psychogenic F45.8
- **Urachus** (*see also* condition)
  - patent or persistent Q64.4
- **Urbach-Oppenheim** disease (necrobiosis lipoidica diabeticorum) — *see* E08-E13 with .620
- **Urbach's** lipoid proteinosis E78.89
- **Urbach-Wiethe** disease E78.89
- **Urban** yellow fever A95.1
- **Urea**
  - blood, high — *see* Uremia
  - cycle metabolism disorder — *see* Disorder, urea cycle metabolism
- **Uremia,** uremic N19
  - with
    - ectopic or molar pregnancy O08.4
    - polyneuropathy N18.9 *[G63]*
  - chronic (*see also* Disease, kidney, chronic)N18.9
    - due to hypertension — *see* Hypertensive, kidney
  - complicating
    - ectopic or molar pregnancy O08.4
- **Uremia** — *continued*
  - congenital P96.0
  - extrarenal R39.2
  - following ectopic or molar pregnancy O08.4
  - newborn P96.0
  - prerenal R39.2
- **Ureter,** ureteral — *see* condition
- **Ureteralgia** N23
- **Ureterectasis** — *see* Hydroureter
- **Ureteritis** N28.89
  - cystica N28.86
  - due to calculus N20.1
    - with calculus, kidney N20.2
      - with hydronephrosis N13.2
  - gonococcal (acute) (chronic) A54.21
  - nonspecific N28.89
- **Ureterocele** N28.89
  - congenital (orthotopic) Q62.31
    - ectopic Q62.32
- **Ureterolith,** ureterolithiasis — *see* Calculus, ureter
- **Ureterostomy**
  - attention to Z43.6
  - status Z93.6
- **Urethra,** urethral — *see* condition
- **Urethralgia** R39.89
- **Urethritis** (anterior) (posterior) N34.2
  - calculous N21.1
  - candidal B37.41
  - chlamydial A56.01
  - diplococcal (gonococcal) A54.01
    - with abscess (accessory gland) (periurethral) A54.1
  - gonococcal A54.01
    - with abscess (accessory gland) (periurethral) A54.1
  - nongonococcal N34.1
    - Reiter's — *see* Reiter's disease
  - nonspecific N34.1
  - nonvenereal N34.1
  - postmenopausal N34.2
  - puerperal O86.22
  - Reiter's — *see* Reiter's disease
  - specified NEC N34.2
  - trichomonal or due to Trichomonas (vaginalis) A59.03
- **Urethrocele** N81.0
  - with
    - cystocele — *see* Cystocele
    - prolapse of uterus — *see* Prolapse, uterus
- **Urethrolithiasis** (with colic or infection) N21.1
- **Urethrorectal** — *see* condition
- **Urethrorrhagia** N36.8
- **Urethrorrhea** R36.9
- **Urethrostomy**
  - attention to Z43.6
  - status Z93.6
- **Urethrotrigonitis** — *see* Trigonitis
- **Urethrovaginal** — *see* condition
- **Urgency**
  - fecal R15.2
  - hypertensive — *see* Hypertension
  - urinary R39.15
- **Urhidrosis,** uridrosis L74.8
- **Uric** acid in blood (increased) E79.0
- **Uricacidemia** (asymptomatic) E79.0
- **Uricemia** (asymptomatic) E79.0
- **Uricosuria** R82.99
- **Urinary** — *see* condition
- **Urination**
  - frequent R35.0
  - painful R30.9
- **Urine**
  - blood in — *see* Hematuria
  - discharge, excessive R35.8
  - enuresis, nonorganic origin F98.0
  - extravasation R39.0
  - frequency R35.0
  - incontinence R32
    - nonorganic origin F98.0
  - intermittent stream R39.198
  - pus in N39.0
  - retention or stasis R33.9
    - organic R33.8
      - drug-induced R33.0
    - psychogenic F45.8
  - secretion
    - deficient R34
    - excessive R35.8
    - frequency R35.0
  - stream
    - intermittent R39.198
    - slowing R39.198
- **Urine** — *continued*
  - stream — *continued*
    - splitting R39.13
    - weak R39.12
- **Urinemia** — *see* Uremia
- **Urinoma,** urethra N36.8
- **Uroarthritis,** infectious (Reiter's) — *see* Reiter's disease
- **Urodialysis** R34
- **Urolithiasis** — *see* Calculus, urinary
- **Uronephrosis** — *see* Hydronephrosis
- **Uropathy** N39.9
  - obstructive N13.9
    - specified NEC N13.8
  - reflux N13.9
    - specified NEC N13.8
  - vesicoureteral reflux-associated — *see* Reflux, vesicoureteral
- **Urosepsis** - code to condition
- **Urticaria** L50.9
  - with angioneurotic edema T78.3 ☑
    - hereditary D84.1
  - allergic L50.0
  - cholinergic L50.5
  - chronic L50.8
  - cold, familial L50.2
  - contact L50.6
  - dermatographic L50.3
  - due to
    - cold or heat L50.2
    - drugs L50.0
    - food L50.0
    - inhalants L50.0
    - plants L50.6
    - serum (*see also* Reaction, serum)T80.69 ☑
  - factitial L50.3
  - familial cold M04.2
  - giant T78.3 ☑
    - hereditary D84.1
  - gigantea T78.3 ☑
  - idiopathic L50.1
  - larynx T78.3 ☑
    - hereditary D84.1
  - neonatorum P83.8
  - nonallergic L50.1
  - papulosa (Hebra) L28.2
  - pigmentosa Q82.2
  - recurrent periodic L50.8
  - serum (*see also* Reaction, serum)T80.69 ☑
  - solar L56.3
  - specified type NEC L50.8
  - thermal (cold) (heat) L50.2
  - vibratory L50.4
  - xanthelasmoidea Q82.2
- **Use** (of)
  - alcohol Z72.89
    - with
      - intoxication F10.929
      - sleep disorder F10.982
    - harmful — *see* Abuse, alcohol
  - amphetamines — *see* Use, stimulant NEC
  - caffeine — *see* Use, stimulant NEC
  - cannabis F12.90
    - with
      - anxiety disorder F12.980
      - intoxication F12.929
        - with
          - delirium F12.921
          - perceptual disturbance F12.922
        - uncomplicated F12.920
      - other specified disorder F12.988
      - psychosis F12.959
        - delusions F12.950
        - hallucinations F12.951
      - unspecified disorder F12.99
  - cocaine F14.90
    - with
      - anxiety disorder F14.980
      - intoxication F14.929
        - with
          - delirium F14.921
          - perceptual disturbance F14.922
        - uncomplicated F14.920
      - other specified disorder F14.988
      - psychosis F14.959
        - delusions F14.950
        - hallucinations F14.951
      - sexual dysfunction F14.981
      - sleep disorder F14.982
      - unspecified disorder F14.99
    - harmful — *see* Abuse, drug, cocaine

- **Use** — *continued*
  - drug (s) NEC F19.90
    - with sleep disorder F19.982
    - harmful — *see* Abuse, drug, by type
  - hallucinogen NEC F16.90
    - with
      - anxiety disorder F16.980
      - intoxication F16.929
        - with
          - delirium F16.921
        - uncomplicated F16.920
      - mood disorder F16.94
      - other specified disorder F16.988
      - perception disorder (flashbacks) F16.983
      - psychosis F16.959
        - delusions F16.950
        - hallucinations F16.951
      - unspecified disorder F16.99
    - harmful — *see* Abuse, drug, hallucinogen NEC
  - inhalants F18.90
    - with
      - anxiety disorder F18.980
      - intoxication F18.929
        - with delirium F18.921
        - uncomplicated F18.920
      - mood disorder F18.94
      - other specified disorder F18.988
      - persisting dementia F18.97
      - psychosis F18.959
        - delusions F18.950
        - hallucinations F18.951
      - unspecified disorder F18.99
    - harmful — *see* Abuse, drug, inhalant
  - methadone — *see* Use, opioid
  - nonprescribed drugs F19.90
    - harmful — *see* Abuse, non-psychoactive substance
  - opioid F11.90
    - with
      - disorder F11.99
        - mood F11.94
        - sleep F11.982
        - specified type NEC F11.988
      - intoxication F11.929
        - with
          - delirium F11.921
          - perceptual disturbance F11.922
        - uncomplicated F11.920
      - withdrawal F11.93
    - harmful — *see* Abuse, drug, opioid
  - patent medicines F19.90
    - harmful — *see* Abuse, non-psychoactive substance
  - psychoactive drug NEC F19.90
    - with
      - anxiety disorder F19.980
      - intoxication F19.929
        - with
          - delirium F19.921
          - perceptual disturbance F19.922
        - uncomplicated F19.920
      - mood disorder F19.94
      - other specified disorder F19.988
      - persisting
        - amnestic disorder F19.96
        - dementia F19.97
      - psychosis F19.959
        - delusions F19.950
        - hallucinations F19.951
      - sexual dysfunction F19.981
      - sleep disorder F19.982
      - unspecified disorder F19.99
      - withdrawal F19.939
        - with
          - delirium F19.931
          - perceptual disturbance F19.932
        - uncomplicated F19.930
    - harmful — *see* Abuse, drug NEC, psychoactive NEC
  - sedative, hypnotic, or anxiolytic F13.90
    - with
      - anxiety disorder F13.980
      - intoxication F13.929
        - with
          - delirium F13.921
        - uncomplicated F13.920
      - other specified disorder F13.988
      - persisting
        - amnestic disorder F13.96
        - dementia F13.97
      - psychosis F13.959
        - delusions F13.950
- **Use** — *continued*
  - sedative, hypnotic, or anxiolytic — *continued*
        - hallucinations F13.951
      - sexual dysfunction F13.981
      - sleep disorder F13.982
      - unspecified disorder F13.99
    - harmful — *see* Abuse, drug, sedative, hypnotic, or anxiolytic
  - stimulant NEC F15.90
    - with
      - anxiety disorder F15.980
      - intoxication F15.929
        - with
          - delirium F15.921
          - perceptual disturbance F15.922
        - uncomplicated F15.920
      - mood disorder F15.94
      - other specified disorder F15.988
      - psychosis F15.959
        - delusions F15.950
        - hallucinations F15.951
      - sexual dysfunction F15.981
      - sleep disorder F15.982
      - unspecified disorder F15.99
      - withdrawal F15.93
    - harmful — *see* Abuse, drug, stimulant NEC
  - tobacco Z72.0
    - with dependence — *see* Dependence, drug, nicotine
  - volatile solvents (*see also* Use, inhalant)F18.90
    - harmful — *see* Abuse, drug, inhalant
- **Usher-Senear** disease or syndrome L10.4
- **Uta** B55.1
- **Uteromegaly** N85.2
- **Uterovaginal** — *see* condition
- **Uterovesical** — *see* condition
- **Uveal** — *see* condition
- **Uveitis** (anterior) (*see also* Iridocyclitis)
  - acute — *see* Iridocyclitis, acute
  - chronic — *see* Iridocyclitis, chronic
  - due to toxoplasmosis (acquired) B58.09
    - congenital P37.1
  - granulomatous — *see* Iridocyclitis, chronic
  - heterochromic — *see* Cyclitis, Fuchs' heterochromic
  - lens-induced — *see* Iridocyclitis, lens-induced
  - posterior — *see* Chorioretinitis
  - sympathetic H44.13 ☑
  - syphilitic (secondary) A51.43
    - congenital (early) A50.01
    - late A52.71
  - tuberculous A18.54
- **Uveoencephalitis** — *see* Inflammation, chorioretinal
- **Uveokeratitis** — *see* Iridocyclitis
- **Uveoparotitis** D86.89
- **Uvula** — *see* condition
- **Uvulitis** (acute) (catarrhal) (chronic) (membranous) (suppurative) (ulcerative) K12.2

V

- **Vaccination** (prophylactic)
  - complication or reaction — *see* Complications, vaccination
  - delayed Z28.9
  - encounter for Z23
  - not done — *see* Immunization, not done, because (of)
- **Vaccinia** (generalized) (localized) T88.1 ☑
  - congenital P35.8
  - without vaccination B08.011
- **Vacuum**, in sinus (accessory) (nasal) J34.89
- **Vagabond**, vagabondage Z59.0
- **Vagabond's** disease B85.1
- **Vagina**, vaginal — *see* condition
- **Vaginalitis** (tunica) (testis) N49.1
- **Vaginismus** (reflex) N94.2
  - functional F52.5
  - nonorganic F52.5
  - psychogenic F52.5
  - secondary N94.2
- **Vaginitis** (acute) (circumscribed) (diffuse) (emphysematous) (nonvenereal) (ulcerative) N76.0
  - with ectopic or molar pregnancy O08.0
  - amebic A06.82
  - atrophic, postmenopausal N95.2
  - bacterial N76.0
  - blennorrhagic (gonococcal) A54.02
  - candidal B37.3
  - chlamydial A56.02
- **Vaginitis** — *continued*
  - chronic N76.1
  - due to Trichomonas (vaginalis) A59.01
  - following ectopic or molar pregnancy O08.0
  - gonococcal A54.02
    - with abscess (accessory gland) (periurethral) A54.1
  - granuloma A58
  - in (due to)
    - candidiasis B37.3
    - herpesviral (herpes simplex) infection A60.04
    - pinworm infection B80 *[N77.1]*
  - monilial B37.3
  - mycotic (candidal) B37.3
  - postmenopausal atrophic N95.2
  - puerperal (postpartum) O86.13
  - senile (atrophic) N95.2
  - subacute or chronic N76.1
  - syphilitic (early) A51.0
    - late A52.76
  - trichomonal A59.01
  - tuberculous A18.18
- **Vaginosis** — *see* Vaginitis
- **Vagotonia** G52.2
- **Vagrancy** Z59.0
- **VAIN** — *see* Neoplasia, intraepithelial, vagina
- **Vallecula** — *see* condition
- **Valley** fever B38.0
- **Valsuani's** disease — *see* Anemia, obstetric
- **Valve**, valvular (formation) (*see also* condition)
  - cerebral ventricle (communicating) in situ Z98.2
  - cervix, internal os Q51.828
  - congenital NEC — *see* Atresia, by site
  - ureter (pelvic junction) (vesical orifice) Q62.39
  - urethra (congenital) (posterior) Q64.2
- **Valvulitis** (chronic) — *see* Endocarditis
- **Valvulopathy** — *see* Endocarditis
- **Van** Bogaert's leukoencephalopathy (sclerosing) (subacute) A81.1
- **Van** Bogaert-Scherer-Epstein disease or syndrome E75.5
- **Van** Buchem's syndrome M85.2
- **Van** Creveld-von Gierke disease E74.01
- **Van** der Hoeve (-de Kleyn) syndrome Q78.0
- **Van** der Woude's syndrome Q38.0
- **Van** Neck's disease or osteochondrosis M91.0
- **Vanishing** lung J44.9
- **Vapor** asphyxia or suffocation T59.9 ☑
  - specified agent — *see* Table of Drugs and Chemicals
- **Variance**, lethal ball, prosthetic heart valve T82.09 ☑
- **Variants**, thalassemic D56.8
- **Variations** in hair color L67.1
- **Varicella** B01.9
  - with
    - complications NEC B01.89
    - encephalitis B01.11
    - encephalomyelitis B01.11
    - meningitis B01.0
    - myelitis B01.12
    - pneumonia B01.2
  - congenital P35.8
- **Varices** — *see* Varix
- **Varicocele** (scrotum) (thrombosed) I86.1
  - ovary I86.2
  - perineum I86.3
  - spermatic cord (ulcerated) I86.1
- **Varicose**
  - aneurysm (ruptured) I77.0
  - dermatitis — *see* Varix, leg, with, inflammation
  - eczema — *see* Varix, leg, with, inflammation
  - phlebitis — *see* Varix, with, inflammation
  - tumor — *see* Varix
  - ulcer (lower limb, any part) (*see also* Varix, leg, with, ulcer)
    - anus (*see also* Hemorrhoids)K64.8
    - esophagus — *see* Varix, esophagus
    - inflamed or infected — *see* Varix, leg, with ulcer, with inflammation
    - nasal septum I86.8
    - perineum I86.3
    - scrotum I86.1
    - specified site NEC I86.8
  - vein — *see* Varix
  - vessel — *see* Varix, leg
- **Varicosis**, varicosities, varicosity — *see* Varix
- **Variola** (major) (minor) B03
- **Varioloid** B03
- **Varix** (lower limb) (ruptured) I83.90
  - with
    - edema I83.899
    - inflammation I83.10

W

Wasting - Wound

- **Wasting** — *continued*
  - extreme (due to malnutrition) E41
  - muscle NEC — *see* Atrophy, muscle
- **Water**
  - clefts (senile cataract) — *see* Cataract, senile, incipient
  - deprivation of T73.1 ☑
  - intoxication E87.79
  - itch B76.9
  - lack of T73.1 ☑
  - loading E87.70
  - on
    - brain — *see* Hydrocephalus
    - chest J94.8
  - poisoning E87.79
- **Waterbrash** R12
- **Waterhouse** (-Friderichsen) syndrome or disease (meningococcal) A39.1
- **Water-losing** nephritis N25.89
- **Watermelon** stomach K31.819
  - with hemorrhage K31.811
  - without hemorrhage K31.819
- **Watsoniasis** B66.8
- **Wax** in ear — *see* Impaction, cerumen
- **Weak, weakening, weakness** (generalized) R53.1
  - arches (acquired) (*see also* Deformity, limb, flat foot)
  - bladder (sphincter) R32
  - facial R29.810
    - following
      - cerebrovascular disease I69.992
        - cerebral infarction I69.392
        - intracerebral hemorrhage I69.192
        - nontraumatic intracranial hemorrhage NEC I69.292
        - specified disease NEC I69.892
        - stroke I69.392
        - subarachnoid hemorrhage I69.092
  - foot (double) — *see* Weak, arches
  - heart, cardiac — *see* Failure, heart
  - mind F70
  - muscle M62.81
  - myocardium — *see* Failure, heart
  - newborn P96.89
  - pelvic fundus N81.89
  - pubocervical tissue N81.82
  - senile R54
  - rectovaginal tissue N81.83
  - urinary stream R39.12
  - valvular — *see* Endocarditis
- **Wear, worn** (with normal or routine use)
  - articular bearing surface of internal joint prosthesis — *see* Complications, joint prosthesis, mechanical, wear of articular bearing surfaces, by site
  - device, implant or graft — *see* Complications, by site, mechanical complication
  - tooth, teeth (approximal) (hard tissues) (interproximal) (occlusal) K03.0
- **Weather, weathered**
  - effects of
    - cold T69.9 ☑
      - specified effect NEC T69.8 ☑
    - hot — *see* Heat
  - skin L57.8
- **Weaver's** syndrome Q87.3
- **Web, webbed** (congenital)
  - duodenal Q43.8
  - esophagus Q39.4
  - fingers Q70.1 ☑
  - larynx (glottic) (subglottic) Q31.0
  - neck (pterygium colli) Q18.3
  - Paterson-Kelly D50.1
  - popliteal syndrome Q87.89
  - toes Q70.3 ☑
- **Weber-Christian** disease M35.6
- **Weber-Cockayne** syndrome (epidermolysis bullosa) Q81.8
- **Weber-Gubler** syndrome G46.3
- **Weber-Leyden** syndrome G46.3
- **Weber-Osler** syndrome I78.0
- **Weber's** paralysis or syndrome G46.3
- **Wedge-shaped** or wedging vertebra — *see* Collapse, vertebra NEC
- **Wegener's** granulomatosis or syndrome M31.30
  - with
    - kidney involvement M31.31
    - lung involvement M31.30
      - with kidney involvement M31.31
- **Wegner's** disease A50.02
- **Weight**
  - 1000-2499 grams at birth (low) — *see* Low, birthweight
  - 999 grams or less at birth (extremely low) — *see* Low, birthweight, extreme
  - and length below 10th percentile for gestational age P05.1 ☑
  - below but length above 10th percentile for gestational age P05.0 ☑
  - gain (abnormal) (excessive) R63.5
    - in pregnancy — *see* Pregnancy, complicated by, excessive weight gain
      - low — *see* Pregnancy, complicated by, insufficient, weight gain
  - loss (abnormal) (cause unknown) R63.4
- **Weightlessness** (effect of) T75.82 ☑
- **Weil** (l)-Marchesani syndrome Q87.1
- **Weil's** disease A27.0
- **Weingarten's** syndrome J82
- **Weir** Mitchell's disease I73.81
- **Weiss-Baker** syndrome G90.09
- **Wells'** disease L98.3
- **Wen** — *see* Cyst, sebaceous
- **Wenckebach's** block or phenomenon I44.1
- **Werdnig-Hoffmann** syndrome (muscular atrophy) G12.0
- **Werlhof's** disease D69.3
- **Wermer's** disease or syndrome E31.21
- **Werner-His** disease A79.0
- **Werner's** disease or syndrome E34.8
- **Wernicke-Korsakoff's** syndrome or psychosis (alcoholic) F10.96
  - with dependence F10.26
  - drug-induced
    - due to drug abuse — *see* Abuse, drug, by type, with amnestic disorder
    - due to drug dependence — *see* Dependence, drug, by type, with amnestic disorder
  - nonalcoholic F04
- **Wernicke-Posadas** disease B38.9
- **Wernicke's**
  - developmental aphasia F80.2
  - disease or syndrome E51.2
  - encephalopathy E51.2
  - polioencephalitis, superior E51.2
- **West** African fever B50.8
- **Westphal-Strümpell** syndrome E83.01
- **West's** syndrome — *see* Epilepsy, spasms
- **Wet**
  - feet, tropical (maceration) (syndrome) — *see* Immersion, foot
  - lung (syndrome), newborn P22.1
- **Wharton's** duct — *see* condition
- **Wheal** — *see* Urticaria
- **Wheezing** R06.2
- **Whiplash** injury S13.4 ☑
- **Whipple's** disease (*see also* subcategory M14.8-) K90.81
- **Whipworm** (disease) (infection) (infestation) B79
- **Whistling** face Q87.0
- **White** (*see also* condition)
  - kidney, small N03.9
  - leg, puerperal, postpartum, childbirth O87.1
  - mouth B37.0
  - patches of mouth K13.29
  - spot lesions, teeth
    - chewing surface K02.51
    - pit and fissure surface K02.51
    - smooth surface K02.61
- **Whitehead** L70.0
- **Whitlow** (*see also* Cellulitis, digit)
  - with lymphangitis — *see* Lymphangitis, acute, digit
  - herpesviral B00.89
- **Whitmore's** disease or fever — *see* Melioidosis
- **Whooping** cough A37.90
  - with pneumonia A37.91
    - due to Bordetella
      - bronchiseptica A37.81
      - parapertussis A37.11
      - pertussis A37.01
    - specified organism NEC A37.81
  - due to
    - Bordetella
      - bronchiseptica A37.80
        - with pneumonia A37.81
      - parapertussis A37.10
        - with pneumonia A37.11
      - pertussis A37.00
        - with pneumonia A37.01
      - specified NEC A37.80
        - with pneumonia A37.81
- **Wichman's** asthma J38.5
- **Wide** cranial sutures, newborn P96.3
- **Widening** aorta — *see* Ectasia, aorta
  - with aneurysm — *see* Aneurysm, aorta
- **Wilkie's** disease or syndrome K55.1
- **Wilkinson-Sneddon** disease or syndrome L13.1
- **Willebrand** (-Jürgens) thrombopathy D68.0
- **Willige-Hunt** disease or syndrome G23.1
- **Wilms'** tumor C64 ☑
- **Wilson-Mikity** syndrome P27.0
- **Wilson's**
  - disease or syndrome E83.01
  - hepatolenticular degeneration E83.01
  - lichen ruber L43.9
- **Window** (*see also* Imperfect, closure)
  - aorticopulmonary Q21.4
- **Winter** — *see* condition
- **Wiskott-Aldrich** syndrome D82.0
- **Withdrawal** state (*see also* Dependence, drug by type, with withdrawal)
  - alcohol
    - with perceptual disturbances F10.232
    - without perceptual disturbances F10.239
  - caffeine F15.93
  - cannabis F12.288
  - newborn
    - correct therapeutic substance properly administered P96.2
    - infant of dependent mother P96.1
  - therapeutic substance, neonatal P96.2
- **Witts'** anemia D50.8
- **Witzelsucht** F07.0
- **Woakes'** ethmoiditis or syndrome J33.1
- **Wolff-Hirschorn** syndrome Q93.3
- **Wolff-Parkinson-White** syndrome I45.6
- **Wolhynian** fever A79.0
- **Wolman's** disease E75.5
- **Wood** lung or pneumonitis J67.8
- **Woolly,** wooly hair (congenital) (nevus) Q84.1
- **Woolsorter's** disease A22.1
- **Word**
  - blindness (congenital) (developmental) F81.0
  - deafness (congenital) (developmental) H93.25
- **Worm** (s) (infection) (infestation) (*see also* Infestation, helminth)
  - guinea B72
  - in intestine NEC B82.0
- **Worm-eaten** soles A66.3
- **Worn** out — *see* Exhaustion
  - cardiac
    - defibrillator (with synchronous cardiac pacemaker) Z45.02
    - pacemaker
      - battery Z45.010
      - lead Z45.018
  - device, implant or graft — *see* Complications, by site, mechanical
- **Worried** well Z71.1
- **Worries** R45.82
- **Wound,** open
  - abdomen, abdominal
    - wall S31.109 ☑
      - with penetration into peritoneal cavity S31.609 ☑
      - bite — *see* Bite, abdomen, wall
      - epigastric region S31.102 ☑
        - with penetration into peritoneal cavity S31.602 ☑
        - bite — *see* Bite, abdomen, wall, epigastric region
        - laceration — *see* Laceration, abdomen, wall, epigastric region
        - puncture — *see* Puncture, abdomen, wall, epigastric region
      - laceration — *see* Laceration, abdomen, wall
      - left
        - lower quadrant S31.104 ☑
          - with penetration into peritoneal cavity S31.604 ☑
          - bite — *see* Bite, abdomen, wall, left, lower quadrant
          - laceration — *see* Laceration, abdomen, wall, left, lower quadrant
          - puncture — *see* Puncture, abdomen, wall, left, lower quadrant
        - upper quadrant S31.101 ☑
          - with penetration into peritoneal cavity S31.601 ☑
          - bite — *see* Bite, abdomen, wall, left, upper quadrant
          - laceration — *see* Laceration, abdomen, wall, left, upper quadrant

Wound, open — *continued*
- abdomen, abdominal — *continued*
          - puncture — *see* Puncture, abdomen, wall, left, upper quadrant
      - periumbilic region S31.105 ☑
        - with penetration into peritoneal cavity S31.605 ☑
        - bite — *see* Bite, abdomen, wall, periumbilic region
        - laceration — *see* Laceration, abdomen, wall, periumbilic region
        - puncture — *see* Puncture, abdomen, wall, periumbilic region
      - puncture — *see* Puncture, abdomen, wall
      - right
        - lower quadrant S31.103 ☑
          - with penetration into peritoneal cavity S31.603 ☑
          - bite — *see* Bite, abdomen, wall, right, lower quadrant
          - laceration — *see* Laceration, abdomen, wall, right, lower quadrant
          - puncture — *see* Puncture, abdomen, wall, right, lower quadrant
        - upper quadrant S31.100 ☑
          - with penetration into peritoneal cavity S31.600 ☑
          - bite — *see* Bite, abdomen, wall, right, upper quadrant
          - laceration — *see* Laceration, abdomen, wall, right, upper quadrant
          - puncture — *see* Puncture, abdomen, wall, right, upper quadrant
- alveolar (process) — *see* Wound, open, oral cavity
- ankle S91.00 ☑
  - bite — *see* Bite, ankle
  - laceration — *see* Laceration, ankle
  - puncture — *see* Puncture, ankle
- antecubital space — *see* Wound, open, elbow
- anterior chamber, eye — *see* Wound, open, ocular
- anus S31.839 ☑
  - bite S31.835 ☑
  - laceration — *see* Laceration, anus
  - puncture — *see* Puncture, anus
- arm (upper) S41.10 ☑
  - with amputation — *see* Amputation, traumatic, arm
  - bite — *see* Bite, arm
  - forearm — *see* Wound, open, forearm
  - laceration — *see* Laceration, arm
  - puncture — *see* Puncture, arm
- auditory canal (external) (meatus) — *see* Wound, open, ear
- auricle, ear — *see* Wound, open, ear
- axilla — *see* Wound, open, arm
- back (*see also* Wound, open, thorax, back)
  - lower S31.000 ☑
    - with penetration into retroperitoneal space S31.001 ☑
    - bite — *see* Bite, back, lower
    - laceration — *see* Laceration, back, lower
    - puncture — *see* Puncture, back, lower
- bite — *see* Bite
- blood vessel — *see* Injury, blood vessel
- breast S21.00 ☑
  - with amputation — *see* Amputation, traumatic, breast
  - bite — *see* Bite, breast
  - laceration — *see* Laceration, breast
  - puncture — *see* Puncture, breast
- buttock S31.809 ☑
  - bite — *see* Bite, buttock
  - laceration — *see* Laceration, buttock
  - left S31.829 ☑
  - puncture — *see* Puncture, buttock
  - right S31.819 ☑
- calf — *see* Wound, open, leg
- canaliculus lacrimalis — *see* Wound, open, eyelid
- canthus, eye — *see* Wound, open, eyelid
- cervical esophagus S11.20 ☑
  - bite S11.25 ☑
  - laceration — *see* Laceration, esophagus, traumatic, cervical
  - puncture — *see* Puncture, cervical esophagus
- cheek (external) S01.40 ☑
  - bite — *see* Bite, cheek
  - laceration — *see* Laceration, cheek
  - puncture — *see* Puncture, cheek
  - internal — *see* Wound, open, oral cavity
- chest wall — *see* Wound, open, thorax
- chin — *see* Wound, open, head, specified site NEC
- choroid — *see* Wound, open, ocular

Wound, open — *continued*
- ciliary body (eye) — *see* Wound, open, ocular
- clitoris S31.40 ☑
  - with amputation — *see* Amputation, traumatic, clitoris
  - bite S31.45 ☑
  - laceration — *see* Laceration, vulva
  - puncture — *see* Puncture, vulva
- conjunctiva — *see* Wound, open, ocular
- cornea — *see* Wound, open, ocular
- costal region — *see* Wound, open, thorax
- Descemet's membrane — *see* Wound, open, ocular
- digit (s)
  - foot — *see* Wound, open, toe
  - hand — *see* Wound, open, finger
- ear (canal) (external) S01.30 ☑
  - with amputation — *see* Amputation, traumatic, ear
  - bite — *see* Bite, ear
  - laceration — *see* Laceration, ear
  - puncture — *see* Puncture, ear
  - drum S09.2 ☑
- elbow S51.00 ☑
  - bite — *see* Bite, elbow
  - laceration — *see* Laceration, elbow
  - puncture — *see* Puncture, elbow
- epididymis — *see* Wound, open, testis
- epigastric region S31.102 ☑
  - with penetration into peritoneal cavity S31.602 ☑
  - bite — *see* Bite, abdomen, wall, epigastric region
  - laceration — *see* Laceration, abdomen, wall, epigastric region
  - puncture — *see* Puncture, abdomen, wall, epigastric region
- epiglottis — *see* Wound, open, neck, specified site NEC
- esophagus (thoracic) S27.819 ☑
  - cervical — *see* Wound, open, cervical esophagus
  - laceration S27.813 ☑
  - specified type NEC S27.818 ☑
- eye — *see* Wound, open, ocular
- eyeball — *see* Wound, open, ocular
- eyebrow — *see* Wound, open, eyelid
- eyelid S01.10 ☑
  - bite — *see* Bite, eyelid
  - laceration — *see* Laceration, eyelid
  - puncture — *see* Puncture, eyelid
- face NEC — *see* Wound, open, head, specified site NEC
- finger (s) S61.209 ☑
  - with
    - amputation — *see* Amputation, traumatic, finger
    - damage to nail S61.309 ☑
  - bite — *see* Bite, finger
  - index S61.208 ☑
    - with
      - damage to nail S61.308 ☑
    - left S61.201 ☑
      - with
        - damage to nail S61.301 ☑
    - right S61.200 ☑
      - with
        - damage to nail S61.300 ☑
  - laceration — *see* Laceration, finger
  - little S61.208 ☑
    - with
      - damage to nail S61.308 ☑
    - left S61.207 ☑
      - with damage to nail S61.307 ☑
    - right S61.206 ☑
      - with damage to nail S61.306 ☑
  - middle S61.208 ☑
    - with
      - damage to nail S61.308 ☑
    - left S61.203 ☑
      - with damage to nail S61.303 ☑
    - right S61.202 ☑
      - with damage to nail S61.302 ☑
  - puncture — *see* Puncture, finger
  - ring S61.208 ☑
    - with
      - damage to nail S61.308 ☑
    - left S61.205 ☑
      - with damage to nail S61.305 ☑
    - right S61.204 ☑
      - with damage to nail S61.304 ☑
- flank — *see* Wound, open, abdomen, wall

Wound, open — *continued*
- foot (except toe (s) alone) S91.30 ☑
  - with amputation — *see* Amputation, traumatic, foot
  - bite — *see* Bite, foot
  - laceration — *see* Laceration, foot
  - puncture — *see* Puncture, foot
  - toe — *see* Wound, open, toe
- forearm S51.80 ☑
  - with
    - amputation — *see* Amputation, traumatic, forearm
  - bite — *see* Bite, forearm
  - elbow only — *see* Wound, open, elbow
  - laceration — *see* Laceration, forearm
  - puncture — *see* Puncture, forearm
- forehead — *see* Wound, open, head, specified site NEC
- genital organs, external
  - with amputation — *see* Amputation, traumatic, genital organs
  - bite — *see* Bite, genital organ
  - female S31.502 ☑
    - vagina S31.40 ☑
    - vulva S31.40 ☑
  - laceration — *see* Laceration, genital organ
  - male S31.501 ☑
    - penis S31.20 ☑
    - scrotum S31.30 ☑
    - testes S31.30 ☑
  - puncture — *see* Puncture, genital organ
- globe (eye) — *see* Wound, open, ocular
- groin — *see* Wound, open, abdomen, wall
- gum — *see* Wound, open, oral cavity
- hand S61.40 ☑
  - with
    - amputation — *see* Amputation, traumatic, hand
  - bite — *see* Bite, hand
  - finger (s) — *see* Wound, open, finger
  - laceration — *see* Laceration, hand
  - puncture — *see* Puncture, hand
  - thumb — *see* Wound, open, thumb
- head S01.90 ☑
  - bite — *see* Bite, head
  - cheek — *see* Wound, open, cheek
  - ear — *see* Wound, open, ear
  - eyelid — *see* Wound, open, eyelid
  - laceration — *see* Laceration, head
  - lip — *see* Wound, open, lip
  - nose S01.20 ☑
  - oral cavity — *see* Wound, open, oral cavity
  - puncture — *see* Puncture, head
  - scalp — *see* Wound, open, scalp
  - specified site NEC S01.80 ☑
  - temporomandibular area — *see* Wound, open, cheek
- heel — *see* Wound, open, foot
- hip S71.00 ☑
  - with amputation — *see* Amputation, traumatic, hip
  - bite — *see* Bite, hip
  - laceration — *see* Laceration, hip
  - puncture — *see* Puncture, hip
- hymen S31.40 ☑
  - bite — *see* Bite, vulva
  - laceration — *see* Laceration, vagina
  - puncture — *see* Puncture, vagina
- hypochondrium S31.109 ☑
  - bite — *see* Bite, hypochondrium
  - laceration — *see* Laceration, hypochondrium
  - puncture — *see* Puncture, hypochondrium
- hypogastric region S31.109 ☑
  - bite — *see* Bite, hypogastric region
  - laceration — *see* Laceration, hypogastric region
  - puncture — *see* Puncture, hypogastric region
- iliac (region) — *see* Wound, open, inguinal region
- inguinal region S31.109 ☑
  - bite — *see* Bite, abdomen, wall, lower quadrant
  - laceration — *see* Laceration, inguinal region
  - puncture — *see* Puncture, inguinal region
- instep — *see* Wound, open, foot
- interscapular region — *see* Wound, open, thorax, back
- intraocular — *see* Wound, open, ocular
- iris — *see* Wound, open, ocular
- jaw — *see* Wound, open, head, specified site NEC
- knee S81.00 ☑
  - bite — *see* Bite, knee
  - laceration — *see* Laceration, knee
  - puncture — *see* Puncture, knee

- **Wound,** open — *continued*
  - labium (majus) (minus) — *see* Wound, open, vulva
  - laceration — *see* Laceration, by site
  - lacrimal duct — *see* Wound, open, eyelid
  - larynx S11.019 ☑
    - bite — *see* Bite, larynx
    - laceration — *see* Laceration, larynx
    - puncture — *see* Puncture, larynx
  - left
    - lower quadrant S31.104 ☑
      - with penetration into peritoneal cavity S31.604 ☑
      - bite — *see* Bite, abdomen, wall, left, lower quadrant
      - laceration — *see* Laceration, abdomen, wall, left, lower quadrant
      - puncture — *see* Puncture, abdomen, wall, left, lower quadrant
    - upper quadrant S31.101 ☑
      - with penetration into peritoneal cavity S31.601 ☑
      - bite — *see* Bite, abdomen, wall, left, upper quadrant
      - laceration — *see* Laceration, abdomen, wall, left, upper quadrant
      - puncture — *see* Puncture, abdomen, wall, left, upper quadrant
  - leg (lower) S81.80 ☑
    - with amputation — *see* Amputation, traumatic, leg
    - ankle — *see* Wound, open, ankle
    - bite — *see* Bite, leg
    - foot — *see* Wound, open, foot
    - knee — *see* Wound, open, knee
    - laceration — *see* Laceration, leg
    - puncture — *see* Puncture, leg
    - toe — *see* Wound, open, toe
    - upper — *see* Wound, open, thigh
  - lip S01.501 ☑
    - bite — *see* Bite, lip
    - laceration — *see* Laceration, lip
    - puncture — *see* Puncture, lip
  - loin S31.109 ☑
    - bite — *see* Bite, abdomen, wall
    - laceration — *see* Laceration, loin
    - puncture — *see* Puncture, loin
  - lower back — *see* Wound, open, back, lower
  - lumbar region — *see* Wound, open, back, lower
  - malar region — *see* Wound, open, head, specified site NEC
  - mammary — *see* Wound, open, breast
  - mastoid region — *see* Wound, open, head, specified site NEC
  - mouth — *see* Wound, open, oral cavity
  - nail
    - finger — *see* Wound, open, finger, with damage to nail
    - toe — *see* Wound, open, toe, with damage to nail
  - nape (neck) — *see* Wound, open, neck
  - nasal (septum) (sinus) — *see* Wound, open, nose
  - nasopharynx — *see* Wound, open, head, specified site NEC
  - neck S11.90 ☑
    - bite — *see* Bite, neck
    - involving
      - cervical esophagus S11.20 ☑
      - larynx — *see* Wound, open, larynx
      - pharynx S11.20 ☑
      - thyroid S11.10 ☑
      - trachea (cervical) S11.029 ☑
        - bite — *see* Bite, trachea
        - laceration S11.021 ☑
          - with foreign body S11.022 ☑
        - puncture S11.023 ☑
          - with foreign body S11.024 ☑
    - laceration — *see* Laceration, neck
    - puncture — *see* Puncture, neck
    - specified site NEC S11.80 ☑
      - specified type NEC S11.89 ☑
  - nose (septum) (sinus) S01.20 ☑
    - with amputation — *see* Amputation, traumatic, nose
    - bite — *see* Bite, nose
    - laceration — *see* Laceration, nose
    - puncture — *see* Puncture, nose
  - ocular S05.90 ☑
    - avulsion (traumatic enucleation) S05.7 ☑
    - eyeball S05.6 ☑
      - with foreign body S05.5 ☑
    - eyelid — *see* Wound, open, eyelid

- **Wound,** open — *continued*
  - ocular — *continued*
    - laceration and rupture S05.3 ☑
      - with prolapse or loss of intraocular tissue S05.2 ☑
    - orbit (penetrating) (with or without foreign body) S05.4 ☑
    - periocular area — *see* Wound, open, eyelid
    - specified NEC S05.8X ☑
  - oral cavity S01.502 ☑
    - bite S01.552 ☑
    - laceration — *see* Laceration, oral cavity
    - puncture — *see* Puncture, oral cavity
  - orbit — *see* Wound, open, ocular, orbit
  - palate — *see* Wound, open, oral cavity
  - palm — *see* Wound, open, hand
  - pelvis, pelvic (*see also* Wound, open, back, lower)
    - girdle — *see* Wound, open, hip
  - penetrating — *see* Puncture, by site
  - penis S31.20 ☑
    - with amputation — *see* Amputation, traumatic, penis
    - bite S31.25 ☑
    - laceration — *see* Laceration, penis
    - puncture — *see* Puncture, penis
  - perineum
    - bite — *see* Bite, perineum
    - female S31.502 ☑
    - laceration — *see* Laceration, perineum
    - male S31.501 ☑
    - puncture — *see* Puncture, perineum
  - periocular area (with or without lacrimal passages) — *see* Wound, open, eyelid
  - periumbilic region S31.105 ☑
    - with penetration into peritoneal cavity S31.605 ☑
    - bite — *see* Bite, abdomen, wall, periumbilic region
    - laceration — *see* Laceration, abdomen, wall, periumbilic region
    - puncture — *see* Puncture, abdomen, wall, periumbilic region
  - phalanges
    - finger — *see* Wound, open, finger
    - toe — *see* Wound, open, toe
  - pharynx S11.20 ☑
  - pinna — *see* Wound, open, ear
  - popliteal space — *see* Wound, open, knee
  - prepuce — *see* Wound, open, penis
  - pubic region — *see* Wound, open, back, lower
  - pudendum — *see* Wound, open, genital organs, external
  - puncture wound — *see* Puncture
  - rectovaginal septum — *see* Wound, open, vagina
  - right
    - lower quadrant S31.103 ☑
      - with penetration into peritoneal cavity S31.603 ☑
      - bite — *see* Bite, abdomen, wall, right, lower quadrant
      - laceration — *see* Laceration, abdomen, wall, right, lower quadrant
      - puncture — *see* Puncture, abdomen, wall, right, lower quadrant
    - upper quadrant S31.100 ☑
      - with penetration into peritoneal cavity S31.600 ☑
      - bite — *see* Bite, abdomen, wall, right, upper quadrant
      - laceration — *see* Laceration, abdomen, wall, right, upper quadrant
      - puncture — *see* Puncture, abdomen, wall, right, upper quadrant
  - sacral region — *see* Wound, open, back, lower
  - sacroiliac region — *see* Wound, open, back, lower
  - salivary gland — *see* Wound, open, oral cavity
  - scalp S01.00 ☑
    - bite S01.05 ☑
    - laceration — *see* Laceration, scalp
    - puncture — *see* Puncture, scalp
  - scalpel, newborn (birth injury) P15.8
  - scapular region — *see* Wound, open, shoulder
  - sclera — *see* Wound, open, ocular
  - scrotum S31.30 ☑
    - with amputation — *see* Amputation, traumatic, scrotum
    - bite S31.35 ☑
    - laceration — *see* Laceration, scrotum
    - puncture — *see* Puncture, scrotum
  - shin — *see* Wound, open, leg
  - shoulder S41.00 ☑

- **Wound,** open — *continued*
  - shoulder — *continued*
    - with amputation — *see* Amputation, traumatic, arm
    - bite — *see* Bite, shoulder
    - laceration — *see* Laceration, shoulder
    - puncture — *see* Puncture, shoulder
  - skin NOS T14.8
  - spermatic cord — *see* Wound, open, testis
  - sternal region — *see* Wound, open, thorax, front wall
  - submaxillary region — *see* Wound, open, head, specified site NEC
  - submental region — *see* Wound, open, head, specified site NEC
  - subungual
    - finger (s) — *see* Wound, open, finger
    - toe (s) — *see* Wound, open, toe
  - supraclavicular region — *see* Wound, open, neck, specified site NEC
  - temple, temporal region — *see* Wound, open, head, specified site NEC
  - temporomandibular area — *see* Wound, open, cheek
  - testis S31.30 ☑
    - with amputation — *see* Amputation, traumatic, testes
    - bite S31.35 ☑
    - laceration — *see* Laceration, testis
    - puncture — *see* Puncture, testis
  - thigh S71.10 ☑
    - with amputation — *see* Amputation, traumatic, hip
    - bite — *see* Bite, thigh
    - laceration — *see* Laceration, thigh
    - puncture — *see* Puncture, thigh
  - thorax, thoracic (wall) S21.90 ☑
    - back S21.20 ☑
      - with penetration S21.40 ☑
    - bite — *see* Bite, thorax
    - breast — *see* Wound, open, breast
    - front S21.10 ☑
      - with penetration S21.30 ☑
    - laceration — *see* Laceration, thorax
    - puncture — *see* Puncture, thorax
  - throat — *see* Wound, open, neck
  - thumb S61.009 ☑
    - with
      - amputation — *see* Amputation, traumatic, thumb
      - damage to nail S61.109 ☑
    - bite — *see* Bite, thumb
    - laceration — *see* Laceration, thumb
    - left S61.002 ☑
      - with
        - damage to nail S61.102 ☑
    - puncture — *see* Puncture, thumb
    - right S61.001 ☑
      - with
        - damage to nail S61.101 ☑
  - thyroid (gland) — *see* Wound, open, neck, thyroid
  - toe (s) S91.109 ☑
    - with
      - amputation — *see* Amputation, traumatic, toe
      - damage to nail S91.209 ☑
    - bite — *see* Bite, toe
    - great S91.103 ☑
      - with
        - damage to nail S91.203 ☑
      - left S91.102 ☑
        - with
          - damage to nail S91.202 ☑
      - right S91.101 ☑
        - with
          - damage to nail S91.201 ☑
    - laceration — *see* Laceration, toe
    - lesser S91.106 ☑
      - with
        - damage to nail S91.206 ☑
      - left S91.105 ☑
        - with
          - damage to nail S91.205 ☑
      - right S91.104 ☑
        - with
          - damage to nail S91.204 ☑
    - puncture — *see* Puncture, toe
  - tongue — *see* Wound, open, oral cavity
  - trachea (cervical region) — *see* Wound, open, neck, trachea

X

Y

Z

This page intentionally left blank

ICD-10-CM Table of Neoplasms

The list below gives the code numbers for neoplasms by anatomical site. For each site, there are six possible code numbers according to whether the neoplasm in question is malignant, benign, in situ, of uncertain behavior, or of unspecified nature. The description of the neoplasm will often indicate which of the six columns is appropriate; e.g., malignant melanoma of skin, benign fibroadenoma of breast, carcinoma in situ of cervix uteri.

Where such descriptors are not present, the remainder of the Index to Diseases and Injuries should be consulted where guidance is given to the appropriate column for each morphological (histological) variety listed; e.g., Mesonephroma—*see* Neoplasm, malignant; Embryoma— *see also* Neoplasm, uncertain behavior; Disease, Bowen's—*see* Neoplasm, skin, in situ. However, the guidance in the Index to Diseases and Injuries can be overridden if one of the descriptors mentioned above is present; e.g., malignant adenoma of colon is coded to C18.9 and not to D12.6 as the adjective "malignant" overrides the Index entry "Adenoma—*see also* Neoplasm, benign."

Codes listed with a dash -, following the code have a required additional character for laterality. The tabular must be reviewed for the complete code.

Neoplasm	Malignant Primary	Malignant Secondary	Ca in situ	Benign	Uncertain Behavior	Unspecified Behavior
Neoplasm, neoplastic	C80.1	C79.9	D09.9	D36.9	D48.9	D49.9
abdomen, abdominal	C76.2	C79.8-	D09.8	D36.7	D48.7	D49.89
cavity	C76.2	C79.8-	D09.8	D36.7	D48.7	D49.89
organ	C76.2	C79.8-	D09.8	D36.7	D48.7	D49.89
viscera	C76.2	C79.8-	D09.8	D36.7	D48.7	D49.89
wall (*see also* Neoplasm, abdomen, wall, skin)	C44.509	C79.2-	D04.5	D23.5	D48.5	D49.2
connective tissue	C49.4	C79.8-	-	D21.4	D48.1	D49.2
skin	C44.509					
basal cell carcinoma	C44.519	-	-	-	-	-
specified type NEC	C44.599	-	-	-	-	-
squamous cell carcinoma	C44.529	-	-	-	-	-
abdominopelvic	C76.8	C79.8-	-	D36.7	D48.7	D49.89
accessory sinus — *see* Neoplasm, sinus						
acoustic nerve	C72.4-	C79.49	-	D33.3	D43.3	D49.7
adenoid (pharynx) (tissue)	C11.1	C79.89	D00.08	D10.6	D37.05	D49.0
adipose tissue (*see also* Neoplasm, connective tissue)	C49.4	C79.89	-	D21.9	D48.1	D49.2
adnexa (uterine)	C57.4	C79.89	D07.39	D28.7	D39.8	D49.59
adrenal	C74.9-	C79.7-	D09.3	D35.0-	D44.1-	D49.7
capsule	C74.9-	C79.7-	D09.3	D35.0-	D44.1-	D49.7
cortex	C74.0-	C79.7-	D09.3	D35.0-	D44.1-	D49.7
gland	C74.9-	C79.7-	D09.3	D35.0-	D44.1-	D49.7
medulla	C74.1-	C79.7-	D09.3	D35.0-	D44.1-	D49.7
ala nasi (external) (*see also* Neoplasm, skin, nose)	C44.301	C79.2	D04.39	D23.39	D48.5	D49.2
alimentary canal or tract NEC	C26.9	C78.80	D01.9	D13.9	D37.9	D49.0
alveolar	C03.9	C79.89	D00.03	D10.39	D37.09	D49.0
mucosa	C03.9	C79.89	D00.03	D10.39	D37.09	D49.0
lower	C03.1	C79.89	D00.03	D10.39	D37.09	D49.0
upper	C03.0	C79.89	D00.03	D10.39	D37.09	D49.0
ridge or process	C41.1	C79.51	-	D16.5-	D48.0	D49.2
carcinoma	C03.9	C79.8-	-	-	-	-
lower	C03.1	C79.8-	-	-	-	-
upper	C03.0	C79.8-	-	-	-	-
lower	C41.1	C79.51	-	D16.5-	D48.0	D49.2
mucosa	C03.9	C79.89	D00.03	D10.39	D37.09	D49.0
lower	C03.1	C79.89	D00.03	D10.39	D37.09	D49.0
upper	C03.0	C79.89	D00.03	D10.39	D37.09	D49.0
upper	C41.0	C79.51	-	D16.4-	D48.0	D49.2
sulcus	C06.1	C79.89	D00.02	D10.39	D37.09	D49.0
alveolus	C03.9	C79.89	D00.03	D10.39	D37.09	D49.0
lower	C03.1	C79.89	D00.03	D10.39	D37.09	D49.0
upper	C03.0	C79.89	D00.03	D10.39	D37.09	D49.0
ampulla of Vater	C24.1	C78.89	D01.5	D13.5	D37.6	D49.0
ankle NEC	C76.5-	C79.89	D04.7-	D36.7	D48.7	D49.89
anorectum, anorectal (junction)	C21.8	C78.5	D01.3	D12.9	D37.8	D49.0
antecubital fossa or space	C76.4-	C79.89	D04.6-	D36.7	D48.7	D49.89
antrum (Highmore) (maxillary)	C31.0	C78.39	D02.3	D14.0	D38.5	D49.1
pyloric	C16.3	C78.89	D00.2	D13.1	D37.1	D49.0
tympanicum	C30.1	C78.39	D02.3	D14.0	D38.5	D49.1
anus, anal	C21.0	C78.5	D01.3	D12.9	D37.8	D49.0
canal	C21.1	C78.5	D01.3	D12.9	D37.8	D49.0
cloacogenic zone	C21.2	C78.5	D01.3	D12.9	D37.8	D49.0
margin (*see also* Neoplasm, anus, skin)	C44.500	C79.2	D04.5	D23.5	D48.5	D49.2
overlapping lesion with rectosigmoid junction or rectum	C21.8	-	-	-	-	-
skin						
basal cell carcinoma						
specified type NEC	C44.590	-	-	-	-	-
squamous cell carcinoma	C44.520	-	-	-	-	-
sphincter	C21.1	C78.5	D01.3	D12.9	D37.8	D49.0
aorta (thoracic)	C49.3	C79.89	-	D21.3	D48.1	D49.2
abdominal	C49.4	C79.89	-	D21.4	D48.1	D49.2
aortic body	C75.5	C79.89	-	D35.6	D44.7	D49.7
aponeurosis	C49.9	C79.89	-	D21.9	D48.1	D49.2
palmar	C49.1-	C79.89	-	D21.1-	D48.1	D49.2
plantar	C49.2-	C79.89	-	D21.2-	D48.1	D49.2
appendix	C18.1	C78.5	D01.0	D12.1	D37.3	D49.0
arachnoid	C70.9	C79.49	-	D32.9	D42.9	D49.7
cerebral	C70.0	C79.32	-	D32.0	D42.0	D49.7
spinal	C70.1	C79.49	-	D32.1	D42.1	D49.7
areola	C50.0-	C79.81	D05.-	D24.-	D48.6-	D49.3
arm NEC	C76.4-	C79.89	D04.6-	D36.7	D48.7	D49.89
artery — *see* Neoplasm, connective tissue						
aryepiglottic fold	C13.1	C79.89	D00.08	D10.7	D37.05	D49.0
hypopharyngeal aspect	C13.1	C79.89	D00.08	D10.7	D37.05	D49.0
laryngeal aspect	C32.1	C78.39	D02.0	D14.1	D38.0	D49.1
marginal zone	C13.1	C79.89	D00.08	D10.7	D37.05	D49.0
arytenoid (cartilage)	C32.3	C78.39	D02.0	D14.1	D38.0	D49.1
fold — *see* Neoplasm, aryepiglottic						
associated with transplanted organ	C80.2	-	-	-	-	-
atlas	C41.2	C79.51	-	D16.6	D48.0	D49.2
atrium, cardiac	C38.0	C79.89	-	D15.1	D48.7	D49.89
auditory						
canal (external) (skin)	C44.20-	C79.2	D04.2-	D23.2-	D48.5	D49.2
internal	C30.1	C78.39	D02.3	D14.0	D38.5	D49.1
nerve	C72.4-	C79.49	-	D33.3	D43.3	D49.7
tube	C30.1	C78.39	D02.3	D14.0	D38.5	D49.1
opening	C11.2	C79.89	D00.08	D10.6	D37.05	D49.0
auricle, ear (*see also* Neoplasm, skin, ear)	C44.20-	C79.2	D04.2-	D23.2-	D48.5	D49.2
auricular canal (external) (*see also* Neoplasm, skin, ear)	C44.20-	C79.2	D04.2-	D23.2-	D48.5	D49.2
internal	C30.1	C78.39	D02.3	D14.0	D38.5	D49.2
autonomic nerve or nervous system NEC (*see* Neoplasm, nerve, peripheral)						
axilla, axillary	C76.1	C79.89	D09.8	D36.7	D48.7	D49.89
fold (*see also* Neoplasm, skin, trunk)	C44.509	C79.2	D04.5	D23.5	D48.5	D49.2
back NEC	C76.8	C79.89	D04.5	D36.7	D48.7	D49.89
Bartholin's gland	C51.0	C79.82	D07.1	D28.0	D39.8	D49.59
basal ganglia	C71.0	C79.31	-	D33.0	D43.0	D49.6
basis pedunculi	C71.7	C79.31	-	D33.1	D43.1	D49.6
bile or biliary (tract)	C24.9	C78.89	D01.5	D13.5	D37.6	D49.0
canaliculi (biliferi) (intrahepatic)	C22.1	C78.7	D01.5	D13.4	D37.6	D49.0
canals, interlobular	C22.1	C78.89	D01.5	D13.4	D37.6	D49.0
duct or passage (common) (cystic) (extrahepatic)	C24.0	C78.89	D01.5	D13.5	D37.6	D49.0
interlobular	C22.1	C78.89	D01.5	D13.4	D37.6	D49.0
intrahepatic	C22.1	C78.7	D01.5	D13.4	D37.6	D49.0
and extrahepatic	C24.8	C78.89	D01.5	D13.5	D37.6	D49.0
bladder (urinary)	C67.9	C79.11	D09.0	D30.3	D41.4	D49.4
dome	C67.1	C79.11	D09.0	D30.3	D41.4	D49.4
neck	C67.5	C79.11	D09.0	D30.3	D41.4	D49.4
orifice	C67.9	C79.11	D09.0	D30.3	D41.4	D49.4
ureteric	C67.6	C79.11	D09.0	D30.3	D41.4	D49.4
urethral	C67.5	C79.11	D09.0	D30.3	D41.4	D49.4
overlapping lesion	C67.8	-	-	-	-	-
sphincter	C67.8	C79.11	D09.0	D30.3	D41.4	D49.4
trigone	C67.0	C79.11	D09.0	D30.3	D41.4	D49.4
urachus	C67.7	C79.11	D09.0	D30.3	D41.4	D49.4
wall	C67.9	C79.11	D09.0	D30.3	D41.4	D49.4
anterior	C67.3	C79.11	D09.0	D30.3	D41.4	D49.4
lateral	C67.2	C79.11	D09.0	D30.3	D41.4	D49.4
posterior	C67.4	C79.11	D09.0	D30.3	D41.4	D49.4
blood vessel — *see* Neoplasm, connective tissue						
bone (periosteum)	C41.9	C79.51	-	D16.9-	D48.0	D49.2
acetabulum	C41.4	C79.51	-	D16.8-	D48.0	D49.2
ankle	C40.3-	C79.51	-	D16.3-	-	-
arm NEC	C40.0-	C79.51	-	D16.0-	-	-
astragalus	C40.3-	C79.51	-	D16.3-	-	-
atlas	C41.2	C79.51	-	D16.6-	D48.0	D49.2
axis	C41.2	C79.51	-	D16.6-	D48.0	D49.2
back NEC	C41.2	C79.51	-	D16.6-	D48.0	D49.2
calcaneus	C40.3-	C79.51	-	D16.3-	-	-
calvarium	C41.0	C79.51	-	D16.4-	D48.0	D49.2
carpus (any)	C40.1-	C79.51	-	D16.1-	-	-
cartilage NEC	C41.9	C79.51	-	D16.9-	D48.0	D49.2
clavicle	C41.3	C79.51	-	D16.7-	D48.0	D49.2
clivus	C41.0	C79.51	-	D16.4-	D48.0	D49.2
coccygeal vertebra	C41.4	C79.51	-	D16.8-	D48.0	D49.2
coccyx	C41.4	C79.51	-	D16.8-	D48.0	D49.2
costal cartilage	C41.3	C79.51	-	D16.7-	D48.0	D49.2
costovertebral joint	C41.3	C79.51	-	D16.7-	D48.0	D49.2
cranial	C41.0	C79.51	-	D16.4-	D48.0	D49.2
cuboid	C40.3-	C79.51	-	D16.3-	-	-
cuneiform	C41.9	C79.51	-	D16.9-	D48.0	D49.2
elbow	C40.0-	C79.51	-	D16.0-	-	-

Neoplasm	Malignant Primary	Malignant Secondary	Ca in situ	Benign	Uncertain Behavior	Unspecified Behavior
bone — *continued*						
ethmoid (labyrinth)	C41.0	C79.51	-	D16.4-	D48.0	D49.2
face	C41.0	C79.51	-	D16.4-	D48.0	D49.2
femur (any part)	C40.2-	C79.51	-	D16.2-	-	-
fibula (any part)	C40.2-	C79.51	-	D16.2-	-	-
finger (any)	C40.1-	C79.51	-	D16.1-	-	-
foot	C40.3-	C79.51	-	D16.3-	-	-
forearm	C40.0-	C79.51	-	D16.0-	-	-
frontal	C41.0	C79.51	-	D16.4-	D48.0	D49.2
hand	C40.1-	C79.51	-	D16.1-	-	-
heel	C40.3-	C79.51	-	D16.3-	-	-
hip	C41.4	C79.51	-	D16.8-	D48.0	D49.2
humerus (any part)	C40.0-	C79.51	-	D16.0-	-	-
hyoid	C41.0	C79.51	-	D16.4-	D48.0	D49.2
ilium	C41.4	C79.51	-	D16.8-	D48.0	D49.2
innominate	C41.4	C79.51	-	D16.8-	D48.0	D49.2
intervertebral cartilage or disc	C41.2	C79.51	-	D16.6-	D48.0	D49.2
ischium	C41.4	C79.51	-	D16.8-	D48.0	D49.2
jaw (lower)	C41.1	C79.51	-	D16.5-	D48.0	D49.2
knee	C40.2-	C79.51	-	D16.2-	-	-
leg NEC	C40.2-	C79.51	-	D16.2-	-	-
limb NEC	C40.9-	C79.51	-	D16.9-	-	-
lower (long bones)	C40.2-	C79.51	-	D16.2-	-	-
short bones	C40.3-	C79.51	-	D16.3-	-	-
upper (long bones)	C40.0-	C79.51	-	D16.0-	-	-
short bones	C40.1-	C79.51	-	D16.1-	-	-
malar	C41.0	C79.51	-	D16.4-	D48.0	D49.2
mandible	C41.1	C79.51	-	D16.5-	D48.0	D49.2
marrow NEC (any bone)	C96.9	C79.52	-	-	D47.9	D49.89
mastoid	C41.0	C79.51	-	D16.4-	D48.0	D49.2
maxilla, maxillary (superior)	C41.0	C79.51	-	D16.4-	D48.0	D49.2
inferior	C41.1	C79.51	-	D16.5-	D48.0	D49.2
metacarpus (any)	C40.1-	C79.51	-	D16.1-	-	-
metatarsus (any)	C40.3-	C79.51	-	D16.3-	-	-
overlapping sites	C40.8-	-	-	-	-	-
navicular						
ankle	C40.3-	C79.51	-	-	-	-
hand	C40.1-	C79.51	-	-	-	-
nose, nasal	C41.0	C79.51	-	D16.4-	D48.0	D49.2
occipital	C41.0	C79.51	-	D16.4-	D48.0	D49.2
orbit	C41.0	C79.51	-	D16.4-	D48.0	D49.2
parietal	C41.0	C79.51	-	D16.4-	D48.0	D49.2
patella	C40.2-	C79.51	-	-	-	-
pelvic	C41.4	C79.51	-	D16.8	D48.0	D49.2
phalanges						
foot	C40.3-	C79.51	-	-	-	-
hand	C40.1-	C79.51	-	-	-	-
pubic	C41.4	C79.51	-	D16.8	D48.0	D49.2
radius (any part)	C40.0-	C79.51	-	D16.0-	-	-
rib	C41.3	C79.51	-	D16.7	D48.0	D49.2
sacral vertebra	C41.4	C79.51	-	D16.8	D48.0	D49.2
sacrum	C41.4	C79.51	-	D16.8	D48.0	D49.2
scaphoid	-	-				
of ankle	C40.3-	C79.51	-	-	-	-
of hand	C40.1-	C79.51	-	-	-	-
scapula (any part)	C40.0-	C79.51	-	D16.0-	-	-
sella turcica	C41.0	C79.51	-	D16.4-	D48.0	D49.2
shoulder	C40.0-	C79.51	-	D16.0-	-	-
skull	C41.0	C79.51	-	D16.4-	D48.0	D49.2
sphenoid	C41.0	C79.51	-	D16.4-	D48.0	D49.2
spine, spinal (column)	C41.2	C79.51	-	D16.6	D48.0	D49.2
coccyx	C41.4	C79.51	-	D16.8	D48.0	D49.2
sacrum	C41.4	C79.51	-	D16.8	D48.0	D49.2
sternum	C41.3	C79.51	-	D16.7	D48.0	D49.2
tarsus (any)	C40.3-	C79.51	-	-	-	-
temporal	C41.0	C79.51	-	D16.4-	D48.0	D49.2
thumb	C40.1-	C79.51	-	-	-	-
tibia (any part)	C40.2-	C79.51	-	-	-	-
toe (any)	C40.3-	C79.51	-	-	-	-
trapezium	C40.1-	C79.51	-	-	-	-
trapezoid	C40.1-	C79.51	-	-	-	-
turbinate	C41.0	C79.51	-	D16.4-	D48.0	D49.2
ulna (any part)	C40.0-	C79.51	-	D16.0-	-	-
unciform	C40.1-	C79.51	-	-	-	-
vertebra (column)	C41.2	C79.51	-	D16.6	D48.0	D49.2
coccyx	C41.4	C79.51	-	D16.8	D48.0	D49.2
sacrum	C41.4	C79.51	-	D16.8	D48.0	D49.2
vomer	C41.0	C79.51	-	D16.4-	D48.0	D49.2
wrist	C40.1-	C79.51	-	-	-	-
xiphoid process	C41.3	C79.51	-	D16.7	D48.0	D49.2
zygomatic	C41.0	C79.51	-	D16.4-	D48.0	D49.2
book-leaf (mouth) – *ventral surface of tongue and floor of mouth*	C06.89	C79.89	D00.00	D10.39	D37.09	D49.0
bowel — *see* Neoplasm, intestine						
brachial plexus	C47.1-	C79.89	-	D36.12	D48.2	D49.2
brain NEC	C71.9	C79.31	-	D33.2	D43.2	D49.6
basal ganglia	C71.0	C79.31	-	D33.0	D43.0	D49.6
brain NEC — *continued*						
cerebellopontine angle	C71.6	C79.31	-	D33.1	D43.1	D49.6
cerebellum NOS	C71.6	C79.31	-	D33.1	D43.1	D49.6
cerebrum	C71.0	C79.31	-	D33.0	D43.0	D49.6
choroid plexus	C71.7	C79.31	-	D33.1	D43.1	D49.6
corpus callosum	C71.8	C79.31	-	D33.2	D43.2	D49.6
corpus striatum	C71.0	C79.31	-	D33.0	D43.0	D49.6
cortex (cerebral)	C71.0	C79.31	-	D33.0	D43.0	D49.6
frontal lobe	C71.1	C79.31	-	D33.0	D43.0	D49.6
globus pallidus	C71.0	C79.31	-	D33.0	D43.0	D49.6
hippocampus	C71.2	C79.31	-	D33.0	D43.0	D49.6
hypothalamus	C71.0	C79.31	-	D33.0	D43.0	D49.6
internal capsule	C71.0	C79.31	-	D33.0	D43.0	D49.6
medulla oblongata	C71.7	C79.31	-	D33.1	D43.1	D49.6
meninges	C70.0	C79.32	-	D32.0	D42.0	D49.7
midbrain	C71.7	C79.31	-	D33.1	D43.1	D49.6
occipital lobe	C71.4	C79.31	-	D33.0	D43.0	D49.6
overlapping lesion	C71.8	C79.31	-	-	-	-
parietal lobe	C71.3	C79.31	-	D33.0	D43.0	D49.6
peduncle	C71.7	C79.31	-	D33.1	D43.1	D49.6
pons	C71.7	C79.31	-	D33.1	D43.1	D49.6
stem	C71.7	C79.31	-	D33.1	D43.1	D49.6
tapetum	C71.8	C79.31	-	D33.2	D43.2	D49.6
temporal lobe	C71.2	C79.31	-	D33.0	D43.0	D49.6
thalamus	C71.0	C79.31	-	D33.0	D43.0	D49.6
uncus	C71.2	C79.31	-	D33.0	D43.0	D49.6
ventricle (floor)	C71.5	C79.31	-	D33.0	D43.0	D49.6
fourth	C71.7	C79.31	-	D33.1	D43.1	D49.6
branchial (cleft) (cyst) (vestiges)	C10.4	C79.89	D00.08	D10.5	D37.05	D49.0
breast (connective tissue) (glandular tissue) (soft parts)	C50.9-	C79.81	D05.-	D24.-	D48.6-	D49.3
areola	C50.0-	C79.81	D05.-	D24.-	D48.6-	D49.3
axillary tail	C50.6-	C79.81	D05.-	D24.-	D48.6-	D49.3
central portion	C50.1-	C79.81	D05.-	D24.-	D48.6-	D49.3
inner	C50.8-	C79.81	D05.-	D24.-	D48.6-	D49.3
lower	C50.8-	C79.81	D05.-	D24.-	D48.6-	D49.3
lower-inner quadrant	C50.3-	C79.81	D05.-	D24.-	D48.6-	D49.3
lower-outer quadrant	C50.5-	C79.81	D05.-	D24.-	D48.6-	D49.3
mastectomy site (skin) (*see also* Neoplasm, breast, skin)	C44.501	C79.2	-	-	-	-
specified as breast tissue	C50.8-	C79.81	-	-	-	-
midline	C50.8-	C79.81	D05.-	D24.-	D48.6-	D49.3
nipple	C50.0-	C79.81	D05.-	D24.-	D48.6-	D49.3
outer	C50.8-	C79.81	D05.-	D24.-	D48.6-	D49.3
overlapping lesion	C50.8-	-	-	-	-	-
skin	C44.501	C79.2	D04.5	D23.5	D48.5	D49.2
basal cell carcinoma	C44.511	-	-	-	-	-
specified type NEC	C44.591	-	-	-	-	-
squamous cell carcinoma	C44.521	-	-	-	-	-
tail (axillary)	C50.6-	C79.81	D05.-	D24.-	D48.6-	D49.3
upper	C50.8-	C79.81	D05.-	D24.-	D48.6-	D49.3
upper-inner quadrant	C50.2-	C79.81	D05.-	D24.-	D48.6-	D49.3
upper-outer quadrant	C50.4-	C79.81	D05.-	D24.-	D48.6-	D49.3
broad ligament	C57.1	C79.82	D07.39	D28.2	D39.8	D49.59
bronchiogenic, bronchogenic (lung)	C34.9-	C78.0-	D02.2-	D14.3-	D38.1	D49.1
bronchiole	C34.9-	C78.0-	D02.2-	D14.3-	D38.1	D49.1
bronchus	C34.9-	C78.0-	D02.2-	D14.3-	D38.1	D49.1
carina	C34.0-	C78.0-	D02.2-	D14.3-	D38.1	D49.1
lower lobe of lung	C34.3-	C78.0-	D02.2-	D14.3-	D38.1	D49.1
main	C34.0-	C78.0-	D02.2-	D14.3-	D38.1	D49.1
middle lobe of lung	C34.2	C78.0-	D02.21	D14.31	D38.1	D49.1
overlapping lesion	C34.8-	-	-	-	-	-
upper lobe of lung	C34.1-	C78.0-	D02.2-	D14.3-	D38.1	D49.1
brow	C44.309	C79.2	D04.39	D23.39	D48.5	D49.2
basal cell carcinoma	C44.319	-	-	-	-	-
specified type NEC	C44.399	-	-	-	-	-
squamous cell carcinoma	C44.329	-	-	-	-	-
buccal (cavity)	C06.9	C79.89	D00.00	D10.39	D37.09	D49.0
commissure	C06.0	C79.89	D00.02	D10.39	D37.09	D49.0
groove (lower) (upper)	C06.1	C79.89	D00.02	D10.39	D37.09	D49.0
mucosa	C06.0	C79.89	D00.02	D10.39	D37.09	D49.0
sulcus (lower) (upper)	C06.1	C79.89	D00.02	D10.39	D37.09	D49.0
bulbourethral gland	C68.0	C79.19	D09.19	D30.4	D41.3	D49.59
bursa — *see* Neoplasm, connective tissue						
buttock NEC	C76.3	C79.89	D04.5	D36.7	D48.7	D49.89
calf	C76.5-	C79.89	D04.7-	D36.7	D48.7	D49.89
calvarium	C41.0	C79.51	-	D16.4-	D48.0	D49.2
calyx, renal	C65.-	C79.0-	D09.19	D30.1-	D41.1-	D49.51-
canal						
anal	C21.1	C78.5	D01.3	D12.9	D37.8	D49.0
auditory (external) (*see also* Neoplasm, skin, ear)	C44.20-	C79.2	D04.2-	D23.2-	D48.5	D49.2
auricular (external) (*see also* Neoplasm, skin, ear)	C44.20-	C79.2	D04.2-	D23.2-	D48.5	D49.2
canaliculi, biliary (biliferi) (intrahepatic)	C22.1	C78.7	D01.5	D13.4	D37.6	D49.0
canthus (eye) (inner) (outer)	C44.10-	C79.2	D04.1-	D23.1-	D48.5	D49.2
basal cell carcinoma	C44.11-	-	-	-	-	-
specified type NEC	C44.19-	-	-	-	-	-
squamous cell carcinoma	C44.12-	-	-	-	-	-

Neoplasm	Malignant Primary	Malignant Secondary	Ca in situ	Benign	Uncertain Behavior	Unspecified Behavior
capillary — *see* Neoplasm, connective tissue						
caput coli	C18.0	C78.5	D01.0	D12.0	D37.4	D49.0
carcinoid — *see* Tumor, carcinoid						
cardia (gastric)	C16.0	C78.89	D00.2	D13.1	D37.1	D49.0
cardiac orifice (stomach)	C16.0	C78.89	D00.2	D13.1	D37.1	D49.0
cardio-esophageal junction	C16.0	C78.89	D00.2	D13.1	D37.1	D49.0
cardio-esophagus	C16.0	C78.89	D00.2	D13.1	D37.1	D49.0
carina (bronchus)	C34.0-	C78.0-	D02.2-	D14.3-	D38.1	D49.1
carotid (artery)	C49.0	C79.89	-	D21.0	D48.1	D49.2
body	C75.4	C79.89	-	D35.5	D44.6	D49.7
carpus (any bone)	C40.1-	C79.51	-	D16.1-	-	-
cartilage (articular) (joint) NEC (*see also* Neoplasm, bone)	C41.9	C79.51	-	D16.9-	D48.0	D49.2
arytenoid	C32.3	C78.39	D02.0	D14.1	D38.0	D49.1
auricular	C49.0	C79.89	-	D21.0	D48.1	D49.2
bronchi	C34.0-	C78.39	-	D14.3-	D38.1	D49.1
costal	C41.3	C79.51	-	D16.7	D48.0	D49.2
cricoid	C32.3	C78.39	D02.0	D14.1	D38.0	D49.1
cuneiform	C32.3	C78.39	D02.0	D14.1	D38.0	D49.1
ear (external)	C49.0	C79.89	-	D21.0	D48.1	D49.2
ensiform	C41.3	C79.51	-	D16.7	D48.0	D49.2
epiglottis	C32.1	C78.39	D02.0	D14.1	D38.0	D49.1
anterior surface	C10.1	C79.89	D00.08	D10.5	D37.05	D49.0
eyelid	C49.0	C79.89	-	D21.0	D48.1	D49.2
intervertebral	C41.2	C79.51	-	D16.6	D48.0	D49.2
larynx, laryngeal	C32.3	C78.39	D02.0	D14.1	D38.0	D49.1
nose, nasal	C30.0	C78.39	D02.3	D14.0	D38.5	D49.1
pinna	C49.0	C79.89	-	D21.0	D48.1	D49.2
rib	C41.3	C79.51	-	D16.7	D48.0	D49.2
semilunar (knee)	C40.2-	C79.51	-	D16.2-	D48.0	D49.2
thyroid	C32.3	C78.39	D02.0	D14.1	D38.0	D49.1
trachea	C33	C78.39	D02.1	D14.2	D38.1	D49.1
cauda equina	C72.1	C79.49	-	D33.4	D43.4	D49.7
cavity						
buccal	C06.9	C79.89	D00.00	D10.30	D37.09	D49.0
nasal	C30.0	C78.39	D02.3	D14.0	D38.5	D49.1
oral	C06.9	C79.89	D00.00	D10.30	D37.09	D49.0
peritoneal	C48.2	C78.6	-	D20.1	D48.4	D49.0
tympanic	C30.1	C78.39	D02.3	D14.0	D38.5	D49.1
cecum	C18.0	C78.5	D01.0	D12.0	D37.4	D49.0
central nervous system	C72.9	C79.40	-	-	-	-
cerebellopontine (angle)	C71.6	C79.31	-	D33.1	D43.1	D49.6
cerebellum, cerebellar	C71.6	C79.31	-	D33.1	D43.1	D49.6
cerebrum, cerebral (cortex) (hemisphere) (white matter)	C71.0	C79.31	-	D33.0	D43.0	D49.6
meninges	C70.0	C79.32	-	D32.0	D42.0	D49.7
peduncle	C71.7	C79.31	-	D33.1	D43.1	D49.6
ventricle	C71.5	C79.31	-	D33.0	D43.0	D49.6
fourth	C71.7	C79.31	-	D33.1	D43.1	D49.6
cervical region	C76.0	C79.89	D09.8	D36.7	D48.7	D49.89
cervix (cervical) (uteri) (uterus)	C53.9	C79.82	D06.9	D26.0	D39.0	D49.59
canal	C53.0	C79.82	D06.0	D26.0	D39.0	D49.59
endocervix (canal) (gland)	C53.0	C79.82	D06.0	D26.0	D39.0	D49.59
exocervix	C53.1	C79.82	D06.1	D26.0	D39.0	D49.59
external os	C53.1	C79.82	D06.1	D26.0	D39.0	D49.59
internal os	C53.0	C79.82	D06.0	D26.0	D39.0	D49.59
nabothian gland	C53.0	C79.82	D06.0	D26.0	D39.0	D49.59
overlapping lesion	C53.8	-	-	-	-	-
squamocolumnar junction	C53.8	C79.82	D06.7	D26.0	D39.0	D49.59
stump	C53.8	C79.82	D06.7	D26.0	D39.0	D49.59
cheek	C76.0	C79.89	D09.8	D36.7	D48.7	D49.89
external	C44.309	C79.2	D04.39	D23.39	D48.5	D49.2
basal cell carcinoma	C44.319	-	-	-	-	-
specified type NEC	C44.399	-	-	-	-	-
squamous cell carcinoma	C44.329	-	-	-	-	-
inner aspect	C06.0	C79.89	D00.02	D10.39	D37.09	D49.0
internal	C06.0	C79.89	D00.02	D10.39	D37.09	D49.0
mucosa	C06.0	C79.89	D00.02	D10.39	D37.09	D49.0
chest (wall) NEC	C76.1	C79.89	D09.8	D36.7	D48.7	D49.89
chiasma opticum	C72.3-	C79.49	-	D33.3	D43.3	D49.7
chin	C44.309	C79.2	D04.39	D23.39	D48.5	D49.2
basal cell carcinoma	C44.319	-	-	-	-	-
specified type NEC	C44.399	-	-	-	-	-
squamous cell carcinoma	C44.329	-	-	-	-	-
choana	C11.3	C79.89	D00.08	D10.6	D37.05	D49.0
cholangiole	C22.1	C78.89	D01.5	D13.4	D37.6	D49.0
choledochal duct	C24.0	C78.89	D01.5	D13.5	D37.6	D49.0
choroid	C69.3-	C79.49	D09.2-	D31.3-	D48.7	D49.81
plexus	C71.5	C79.31	-	D33.0	D43.0	D49.6
ciliary body	C69.4-	C79.49	D09.2-	D31.4-	D48.7	D49.89
clavicle	C41.3	C79.51	-	D16.7	D48.0	D49.2
clitoris	C51.2	C79.82	D07.1	D28.0	D39.8	D49.59
clivus	C41.0	C79.51	-	D16.4-	D48.0	D49.2
cloacogenic zone	C21.2	C78.5	D01.3	D12.9	D37.8	D49.0
coccygeal						
body or glomus	C49.5	C79.89	-	D21.5	D48.1	D49.2
vertebra	C41.4	C79.51	-	D16.8	D48.0	D49.2

Neoplasm	Malignant Primary	Malignant Secondary	Ca in situ	Benign	Uncertain Behavior	Unspecified Behavior
coccyx	C41.4	C79.51	-	D16.8	D48.0	D49.2
colon (*see also* Neoplasm, intestine, large)	C18.9	C78.5	-	-	-	-
with rectum	C19	C78.5	D01.1	D12.7	D37.5	D49.0
column, spinal — *see* Neoplasm, spine						
columnella (*see also* Neoplasm, skin, face)	C44.390	C79.2	D04.39	D23.39	D48.5	D49.2
commissure						
labial, lip	C00.6	C79.89	D00.01	D10.39	D37.01	D49.0
laryngeal	C32.0	C78.39	D02.0	D14.1	D38.0	D49.1
common (bile) duct	C24.0	C78.89	D01.5	D13.5	D37.6	D49.0
concha (*see also* Neoplasm, skin, ear)	C44.20-	C79.2	D04.2-	D23.2-	D48.5	D49.2
nose	C30.0	C78.39	D02.3	D14.0	D38.5	D49.1
conjunctiva	C69.0-	C79.49	D09.2-	D31.0-	D48.7	D49.89
connective tissue NEC	C49.9	C79.89	-	D21.9	D48.1	D49.2

Note: For neoplasms of connective tissue (blood vessel, bursa, fascia, ligament, muscle, peripheral nerves, sympathetic and parasympathetic nerves and ganglia, synovia, tendon, etc.) or of morphological types that indicate connective tissue, code according to the list under "Neoplasm, connective tissue". For sites that do not appear in this list, code to neoplasm of that site; e.g., fibrosarcoma, pancreas (C25.9)

Note: Morphological types that indicate connective tissue appear in their proper place in the alphabetic index with the instruction "*see* Neoplasm, connective tissue ...."

Neoplasm	Malignant Primary	Malignant Secondary	Ca in situ	Benign	Uncertain Behavior	Unspecified Behavior
abdomen	C49.4	C79.89	-	D21.4	D48.1	D49.2
abdominal wall	C49.4	C79.89	-	D21.4	D48.1	D49.2
ankle	C49.2-	C79.89	-	D21.2-	D48.1	D49.2
antecubital fossa or space	C49.1-	C79.89	-	D21.1-	D48.1	D49.2
arm	C49.1-	C79.89	-	D21.1-	D48.1	D49.2
auricle (ear)	C49.0	C79.89	-	D21.0	D48.1	D49.2
axilla	C49.3	C79.89	-	D21.3	D48.1	D49.2
back	C49.6	C79.89	-	D21.6	D48.1	D49.2
breast — *see* Neoplasm, breast						
buttock	C49.5	C79.89	-	D21.5	D48.1	D49.2
calf	C49.2-	C79.89	-	D21.2-	D48.1	D49.2
cervical region	C49.0	C79.89	-	D21.0	D48.1	D49.2
cheek	C49.0	C79.89	-	D21.0	D48.1	D49.2
chest (wall)	C49.3	C79.89	-	D21.3	D48.1	D49.2
chin	C49.0	C79.89	-	D21.0	D48.1	D49.2
diaphragm	C49.3	C79.89	-	D21.3	D48.1	D49.2
ear (external)	C49.0	C79.89	-	D21.0	D48.1	D49.2
elbow	C49.1-	C79.89	-	D21.1-	D48.1	D49.2
extrarectal	C49.5	C79.89	-	D21.5	D48.1	D49.2
extremity	C49.9	C79.89	-	D21.9	D48.1	D49.2
lower	C49.2-	C79.89	-	D21.2-	D48.1	D49.2
upper	C49.1-	C79.89	-	D21.1-	D48.1	D49.2
eyelid	C49.0	C79.89	-	D21.0	D48.1	D49.2
face	C49.0	C79.89	-	D21.0	D48.1	D49.2
finger	C49.1-	C79.89	-	D21.1-	D48.1	D49.2
flank	C49.6	C79.89	-	D21.6	D48.1	D49.2
foot	C49.2-	C79.89	-	D21.2-	D48.1	D49.2
forearm	C49.1-	C79.89	-	D21.1-	D48.1	D49.2
forehead	C49.0	C79.89	-	D21.0	D48.1	D49.2
gastric	C49.4	C79.89	-	D21.4	D48.1	D49.2
gastrointestinal	C49.4	C79.89	-	D21.4	D48.1	D49.2
gluteal region	C49.5	C79.89	-	D21.5	D48.1	D49.2
great vessels NEC	C49.3	C79.89	-	D21.3	D48.1	D49.2
groin	C49.5	C79.89	-	D21.5	D48.1	D49.2
hand	C49.1-	C79.89	-	D21.1-	D48.1	D49.2
head	C49.0	C79.89	-	D21.0	D48.1	D49.2
heel	C49.2-	C79.89	-	D21.2-	D48.1	D49.2
hip	C49.2-	C79.89	-	D21.2-	D48.1	D49.2
hypochondrium	C49.4	C79.89	-	D21.4	D48.1	D49.2
iliopsoas muscle	C49.5	C79.89	-	D21.5	D48.1	D49.2
infraclavicular region	C49.3	C79.89	-	D21.3	D48.1	D49.2
inguinal (canal) (region)	C49.5	C79.89	-	D21.5	D48.1	D49.2
intestinal	C49.4	C79.89	-	D21.4	D48.1	D49.2
intrathoracic	C49.3	C79.89	-	D21.3	D48.1	D49.2
ischiorectal fossa	C49.5	C79.89	-	D21.5	D48.1	D49.2
jaw	C03.9	C79.89	D00.03	D10.39	D48.1	D49.0
knee	C49.2-	C79.89	-	D21.2-	D48.1	D49.2
leg	C49.2-	C79.89	-	D21.2-	D48.1	D49.2
limb NEC	C49.9	C79.89	-	D21.9	D48.1	D49.2
lower	C49.2-	C79.89	-	D21.2-	D48.1	D49.2
upper	C49.1-	C79.89	-	D21.1-	D48.1	D49.2
nates	C49.5	C79.89	-	D21.5	D48.1	D49.2
neck	C49.0	C79.89	-	D21.0	D48.1	D49.2
orbit	C69.6-	C79.49	D09.2-	D31.6-	D48.1	D49.89
overlapping lesion	C49.8	-	-	-	-	-
pararectal	C49.5	C79.89	-	D21.5	D48.1	D49.2
para-urethral	C49.5	C79.89	-	D21.5	D48.1	D49.2
paravaginal	C49.5	C79.89	-	D21.5	D48.1	D49.2
pelvis (floor)	C49.5	C79.89	-	D21.5	D48.1	D49.2
pelvo-abdominal	C49.8	C79.89	-	D21.6	D48.1	D49.2
perineum	C49.5	C79.89	-	D21.5	D48.1	D49.2
perirectal (tissue)	C49.5	C79.89	-	D21.5	D48.1	D49.2
periurethral (tissue)	C49.5	C79.89	-	D21.5	D48.1	D49.2
popliteal fossa or space	C49.2-	C79.89	-	D21.2-	D48.1	D49.2
presacral	C49.5	C79.89	-	D21.5	D48.1	D49.2

Neoplasm	Malignant Primary	Malignant Secondary	Ca in situ	Benign	Uncertain Behavior	Unspecified Behavior
connective tissue NEC — *continued*						
psoas muscle	C49.4	C79.89	-	D21.4	D48.1	D49.2
pterygoid fossa	C49.0	C79.89	-	D21.0	D48.1	D49.2
rectovaginal septum or wall	C49.5	C79.89	-	D21.5	D48.1	D49.2
rectovesical	C49.5	C79.89	-	D21.5	D48.1	D49.2
retroperitoneum	C48.0	C78.6	-	D20.0	D48.3	D49.0
sacrococcygeal region	C49.5	C79.89	-	D21.5	D48.1	D49.2
scalp	C49.0	C79.89	-	D21.0	D48.1	D49.2
scapular region	C49.3	C79.89	-	D21.3	D48.1	D49.2
shoulder	C49.1-	C79.89	-	D21.1-	D48.1	D49.2
skin (dermis) NEC (*see also* Neoplasm, skin, by site)	C44.90	C79.2	D04.9	D23.9	D48.5	D49.2
stomach	C49.4	C79.89	-	D21.4	D48.1	D49.2
submental	C49.0	C79.89	-	D21.0	D48.1	D49.2
supraclavicular region	C49.0	C79.89	-	D21.0	D48.1	D49.2
temple	C49.0	C79.89	-	D21.0	D48.1	D49.2
temporal region	C49.0	C79.89	-	D21.0	D48.1	D49.2
thigh	C49.2-	C79.89	-	D21.2-	D48.1	D49.2
thoracic (duct) (wall)	C49.3	C79.89	-	D21.3	D48.1	D49.2
thorax	C49.3	C79.89	-	D21.3	D48.1	D49.2
thumb	C49.1-	C79.89	-	D21.1-	D48.1	D49.2
toe	C49.2-	C79.89	-	D21.2-	D48.1	D49.2
trunk	C49.6	C79.89	-	D21.6	D48.1	D49.2
umbilicus	C49.4	C79.89	-	D21.4	D48.1	D49.2
vesicorectal	C49.5	C79.89	-	D21.5	D48.1	D49.2
wrist	C49.1-	C79.89	-	D21.1-	D48.1	D49.2
conus medullaris	C72.0	C79.49	-	D33.4	D43.4	D49.7
cord (true) (vocal)	C32.0	C78.39	D02.0	D14.1	D38.0	D49.1
false	C32.1	C78.39	D02.0	D14.1	D38.0	D49.1
spermatic	C63.1-	C79.82	D07.69	D29.8	D40.8	D49.59
spinal (cervical) (lumbar) (thoracic)	C72.0	C79.49	-	D33.4	D43.4	D49.7
cornea (limbus)	C69.1-	C79.49	D09.2-	D31.1-	D48.7	D49.89
corpus						
albicans	C56.-	C79.6-	D07.39	D27.-	D39.1-	D49.59
callosum, brain	C71.0	C79.31	-	D33.2	D43.2	D49.6
cavernosum	C60.2	C79.82	D07.4	D29.0	D40.8	D49.59
gastric	C16.2	C78.89	D00.2	D13.1	D37.1	D49.0
overlapping sites	C54.8	-	-	-	-	-
penis	C60.2	C79.82	D07.4	D29.0	D40.8	D49.59
striatum, cerebrum	C71.0	C79.31	-	D33.0	D43.0	D49.6
uteri	C54.9	C79.82	D07.0	D26.1	D39.0	D49.59
isthmus	C54.0	C79.82	D07.0	D26.1	D39.0	D49.59
cortex						
adrenal	C74.0-	C79.7-	D09.3	D35.0-	D44.1-	D49.7
cerebral	C71.0	C79.31	-	D33.0	D43.0	D49.6
costal cartilage	C41.3	C79.51	-	D16.7	D48.0	D49.2
costovertebral joint	C41.3	C79.51	-	D16.7	D48.0	D49.2
Cowper's gland	C68.0	C79.19	D09.19	D30.4	D41.3	D49.59
cranial (fossa, any)	C71.9	C79.31	-	D33.2	D43.2	D49.6
meninges	C70.0	C79.32	-	D32.0	D42.0	D49.7
nerve	C72.50	C79.49	-	D33.3	D43.3	D49.7
specified NEC	C72.59	C79.49	-	D33.3	D43.3	D49.7
craniobuccal pouch	C75.2	C79.89	D09.3	D35.2	D44.3	D49.7
craniopharyngeal (duct) (pouch)	C75.2	C79.89	D09.3	D35.3	D44.4	D49.7
cricoid	C13.0	C79.89	D00.08	D10.7	D37.05	D49.0
cartilage	C32.3	C78.39	D02.0	D14.1	D38.0	D49.1
cricopharynx	C13.0	C79.89	D00.08	D10.7	D37.05	D49.0
crypt of Morgagni	C21.8	C78.5	D01.3	D12.9	D37.8	D49.0
crystalline lens	C69.4-	C79.49	D09.2-	D31.4-	D48.7	D49.89
cul-de-sac (Douglas')	C48.1	C78.6	-	D20.1	D48.4	D49.0
cuneiform cartilage	C32.3	C78.39	D02.0	D14.1	D38.0	D49.1
cutaneous — *see* Neoplasm, skin						
cutis — *see* Neoplasm, skin						
cystic (bile) duct (common)	C24.0	C78.89	D01.5	D13.5	D37.6	D49.0
dermis — *see* Neoplasm, skin						
diaphragm	C49.3	C79.89	-	D21.3	D48.1	D49.2
digestive organs, system, tube, or tract NEC	C26.9	C78.89	D01.9	D13.9	D37.9	D49.0
disc, intervertebral	C41.2	C79.51	-	D16.6	D48.0	D49.2
disease, generalized	C80.0	-	-	-	-	-
disseminated	C80.0	-	-	-	-	-
Douglas' cul-de-sac or pouch	C48.1	C78.6	-	D20.1	D48.4	D49.0
duodenojejunal junction	C17.8	C78.4	D01.49	D13.39	D37.2	D49.0
duodenum	C17.0	C78.4	D01.49	D13.2	D37.2	D49.0
dura (cranial) (mater)	C70.9	C79.49	-	D32.9	D42.9	D49.7
cerebral	C70.0	C79.32	-	D32.0	D42.0	D49.7
spinal	C70.1	C79.49	-	D32.1	D42.1	D49.7
ear (external) (*see also* Neoplasm, skin, ear)	C44.20-	C79.2	D04.2-	D23.2-	D48.5	D49.2
auricle or auris (*see also* Neoplasm, skin, ear)	C44.20-	C79.2	D04.2-	D23.2-	D48.5	D49.2
canal, external (*see also* Neoplasm, skin, ear)	C44.20-	C79.2	D04.2-	D23.2-	D48.5	D49.2
cartilage	C49.0	C79.89	-	D21.0	D48.1	D49.2
external meatus (*see also* Neoplasm, skin, ear)	C44.20-	C79.2	D04.2-	D23.2-	D48.5	D49.2
inner	C30.1	C78.39	D02.3	D14.0	D38.5	D49.1
lobule (*see also* Neoplasm, skin, ear)	C44.20-	C79.2	D04.2-	D23.2-	D48.5	D49.2

Neoplasm	Malignant Primary	Malignant Secondary	Ca in situ	Benign	Uncertain Behavior	Unspecified Behavior
ear — *continued*						
middle	C30.1	C78.39	D02.3	D14.0	D38.5	D49.1
overlapping lesion with accessory sinuses	C31.8	-	-	-	-	-
skin	C44.20-	C79.2	D04.2-	D23.2-	D48.5	D49.2
basal cell carcinoma	C44.21-	-	-	-	-	-
specified type NEC	C44.29-	-	-	-	-	-
squamous cell carcinoma	C44.22-	-	-	-	-	-
earlobe	C44.20-	C79.2	D04.2-	D23.2-	D48.5	D49.2
basal cell carcinoma	C44.21-	-	-	-	-	-
specified type NEC	C44.29-	-	-	-	-	-
squamous cell carcinoma	C44.22-	-	-	-	-	-
ejaculatory duct	C63.7	C79.82	D07.69	D29.8	D40.8	D49.59
elbow NEC	C76.4-	C79.89	D04.6-	D36.7	D48.7	D49.89
endocardium	C38.0	C79.89	-	D15.1	D48.7	D49.89
endocervix (canal) (gland)	C53.0	C79.82	D06.0	D26.0	D39.0	D49.59
endocrine gland NEC	C75.9	C79.89	D09.3	D35.9	D44.9	D49.7
pluriglandular	C75.8	C79.89	D09.3	D35.7	D44.9	D49.7
endometrium (gland) (stroma)	C54.1	C79.82	D07.0	D26.1	D39.0	D49.59
ensiform cartilage	C41.3	C79.51	-	D16.7	D48.0	D49.2
enteric — *see* Neoplasm, intestine						
ependyma (brain)	C71.5	C79.31	-	D33.0	D43.0	D49.6
fourth ventricle	C71.7	C79.31	-	D33.1	D43.1	D49.6
epicardium	C38.0	C79.89	-	D15.1	D48.7	D49.89
epididymis	C63.0-	C79.82	D07.69	D29.3-	D40.8	D49.59
epidural	C72.9	C79.49	-	D33.9	D43.9	D49.7
epiglottis	C32.1	C78.39	D02.0	D14.1	D38.0	D49.1
anterior aspect or surface	C10.1	C79.89	D00.08	D10.5	D37.05	D49.0
cartilage	C32.3	C78.39	D02.0	D14.1	D38.0	D49.1
free border (margin)	C10.1	C79.89	D00.08	D10.5	D37.05	D49.0
junctional region	C10.8	C79.89	D00.08	D10.5	D37.05	D49.0
posterior (laryngeal) surface	C32.1	C78.39	D02.0	D14.1	D38.0	D49.1
suprahyoid portion	C32.1	C78.39	D02.0	D14.1	D38.0	D49.1
esophagogastric junction	C16.0	C78.89	D00.2	D13.1	D37.1	D49.0
esophagus	C15.9	C78.89	D00.1	D13.0	D37.8	D49.0
abdominal	C15.5	C78.89	D00.1	D13.0	D37.8	D49.0
cervical	C15.3	C78.89	D00.1	D13.0	D37.8	D49.0
distal (third)	C15.5	C78.89	D00.1	D13.0	D37.8	D49.0
lower (third)	C15.5	C78.89	D00.1	D13.0	D37.8	D49.0
middle (third)	C15.4	C78.89	D00.1	D13.0	D37.8	D49.0
overlapping lesion	C15.8	-	-	-	-	-
proximal (third)	C15.3	C78.89	D00.1	D13.0	D37.8	D49.0
thoracic	C15.4	C78.89	D00.1	D13.0	D37.8	D49.0
upper (third)	C15.3	C78.89	D00.1	D13.0	D37.8	D49.0
ethmoid (sinus)	C31.1	C78.39	D02.3	D14.0	D38.5	D49.1
bone or labyrinth	C41.0	C79.51	-	D16.4-	D48.0	D49.2
eustachian tube	C30.1	C78.39	D02.3	D14.0	D38.5	D49.1
exocervix	C53.1	C79.82	D06.1	D26.0	D39.0	D49.59
external						
meatus (ear) (*see also* Neoplasm, skin, ear)	C44.20-	C79.2	D04.2-	D23.2-	D48.5	D49.2
os, cervix uteri	C53.1	C79.82	D06.1	D26.0	D39.0	D49.59
extradural	C72.9	C79.49	-	D33.9	D43.9	D49.7
extrahepatic (bile) duct	C24.0	C78.89	D01.5	D13.5	D37.6	D49.0
overlapping lesion with gallbladder	C24.8	-	-	-	-	-
extraocular muscle	C69.6-	C79.49	D09.2-	D31.6-	D48.7	D49.89
extrarectal	C76.3	C79.89	D09.8	D36.7	D48.7	D49.89
extremity	C76.8	C79.89	D04.8	D36.7	D48.7	D49.89
lower	C76.5-	C79.89	D04.7-	D36.7	D48.7	D49.89
upper	C76.4-	C79.89	D04.6-	D36.7	D48.7	D49.89
eye NEC	C69.9-	C79.49	D09.2	D31.9	D48.7	D49.89
overlapping sites	C69.8	-	-	-	-	-
eyeball	C69.9-	C79.49	D09.2-	D31.9-	D48.7	D49.89
eyebrow	C44.309	C79.2	D04.39	D23.39	D48.5	D49.2
basal cell carcinoma	C44.319	-	-	-	-	-
specified type NEC	C44.399	-	-	-	-	-
squamous cell carcinoma	C44.329	-	-	-	-	-
eyelid (lower) (skin) (upper)	C44.10-	-	-	-	-	-
basal cell carcinoma	C44.11-	-	-	-	-	-
specified type NEC	C44.19-	-	-	-	-	-
squamous cell carcinoma	C44.12-	-	-	-	-	-
cartilage	C49.0	C79.89	-	D21.0	D48.1	D49.2
face NEC	C76.0	C79.89	D04.39	D36.7	D48.7	D49.89
fallopian tube (accessory)	C57.0-	C79.82	D07.39	D28.2	D39.8	D49.59
falx (cerebella) (cerebri)	C70.0	C79.32	-	D32.0	D42.0	D49.7
fascia (*see also* Neoplasm, connective tissue)						
palmar	C49.1-	C79.89	-	D21.1-	D48.1	D49.2
plantar	C49.2-	C79.89	-	D21.2-	D48.1	D49.2
fatty tissue — *see* Neoplasm, connective tissue						
fauces, faucial NEC	C10.9	C79.89	D00.08	D10.5	D37.05	D49.0
pillars	C09.1	C79.89	D00.08	D10.5	D37.05	D49.0
tonsil	C09.9	C79.89	D00.08	D10.4	D37.05	D49.0
femur (any part)	C40.2-	-	-	D16.2-	-	-
fetal membrane	C58	C79.82	D07.0	D26.7	D39.2	D49.59
fibrous tissue — *see* Neoplasm, connective tissue						
fibula (any part)	C40.2-	C79.51	-	D16.2-	-	-

Neoplasm	Malignant Primary	Malignant Secondary	Ca in situ	Benign	Uncertain Behavior	Unspecified Behavior
filum terminale	C72.0	C79.49	-	D33.4	D43.4	D49.7
finger NEC	C76.4-	C79.89	D04.6-	D36.7	D48.7	D49.89
flank NEC	C76.8	C79.89	D04.5	D36.7	D48.7	D49.89
follicle, nabothian	C53.0	C79.82	D06.0	D26.0	D39.0	D49.59
foot NEC	C76.5-	C79.89	D04.7-	D36.7	D48.7	D49.89
forearm NEC	C76.4-	C79.89	D04.6-	D36.7	D48.7	D49.89
forehead (skin)	C44.309	C79.2	D04.39	D23.39	D48.5	D49.2
basal cell carcinoma	C44.319	-	-	-	-	-
specified type NEC	C44.399	-	-	-	-	-
squamous cell carcinoma	C44.329	-	-	-	-	-
foreskin	C60.0	C79.82	D07.4	D29.0	D40.8	D49.59
fornix						
pharyngeal	C11.3	C79.89	D00.08	D10.6	D37.05	D49.0
vagina	C52	C79.82	D07.2	D28.1	D39.8	D49.59
fossa (of)						
anterior (cranial)	C71.9	C79.31	-	D33.2	D43.2	D49.6
cranial	C71.9	C79.31	-	D33.2	D43.2	D49.6
ischiorectal	C76.3	C79.89	D09.8	D36.7	D48.7	D49.89
middle (cranial)	C71.9	C79.31	-	D33.2	D43.2	D49.6
piriform	C12	C79.89	D00.08	D10.7	D37.05	D49.0
pituitary	C75.1	C79.89	D09.3	D35.2	D44.3	D49.7
posterior (cranial)	C71.9	C79.31	-	D33.2	D43.2	D49.6
pterygoid	C49.0	C79.89	-	D21.0	D48.1	D49.2
pyriform	C12	C79.89	D00.08	D10.7	D37.05	D49.0
Rosenmuller	C11.2	C79.89	D00.08	D10.6	D37.05	D49.0
tonsillar	C09.0	C79.89	D00.08	D10.5	D37.05	D49.0
fourchette	C51.9	C79.82	D07.1	D28.0	D39.8	D49.59
frenulum						
labii — *see* Neoplasm, lip, internal						
linguae	C02.2	C79.89	D00.07	D10.1	D37.02	D49.0
frontal						
bone	C41.0	C79.51	-	D16.4-	D48.0	D49.2
lobe, brain	C71.1	C79.31	-	D33.0	D43.0	D49.6
pole	C71.1	C79.31	-	D33.0	D43.0	D49.6
sinus	C31.2	C78.39	D02.3	D14.0	D38.5	D49.1
fundus						
stomach	C16.1	C78.89	D00.2	D13.1	D37.1	D49.0
uterus	C54.3	C79.82	D07.0	D26.1	D39.0	D49.59
gall duct (extrahepatic)	C24.0	C78.89	D01.5	D13.5	D37.6	D49.0
intrahepatic	C22.1	C78.7	D01.5	D13.4	D37.6	D49.0
gallbladder	C23	C78.89	D01.5	D13.5	D37.6	D49.0
overlapping lesion with extrahepatic bile ducts	C24.8	-	-	-	-	-
ganglia (*see also* Neoplasm, nerve, peripheral)	C47.9	C79.89	-	D36.10	D48.2	D49.2
basal	C71.0	C79.31	-	D33.0	D43.0	D49.6
cranial nerve	C72.50	C79.49	-	D33.3	D43.3	D49.7
Gartner's duct	C52	C79.82	D07.2	D28.1	D39.8	D49.59
gastric — *see* Neoplasm, stomach						
gastrocolic	C26.9	C78.89	D01.9	D13.9	D37.9	D49.0
gastroesophageal junction	C16.0	C78.89	D00.2	D13.1	D37.1	D49.0
gastrointestinal (tract) NEC	C26.9	C78.89	D01.9	D13.9	D37.9	D49.0
generalized	C80.0	-	-	-	-	-
genital organ or tract						
female NEC	C57.9	C79.82	D07.30	D28.9	D39.9	D49.59
overlapping lesion	C57.8	-	-	-	-	-
specified site NEC	C57.7	C79.82	D07.39	D28.7	D39.8	D49.59
male NEC	C63.9	C79.82	D07.60	D29.9	D40.9	D49.59
overlapping lesion	C63.8	-	-	-	-	-
specified site NEC	C63.7	C79.82	D07.69	D29.8	D40.8	D49.59
genitourinary tract						
female	C57.9	C79.82	D07.30	D28.9	D39.9	D49.59
male	C63.9	C79.82	D07.60	D29.9	D40.9	D49.59
gingiva (alveolar) (marginal)	C03.9	C79.89	D00.03	D10.39	D37.09	D49.0
lower	C03.1	C79.89	D00.03	D10.39	D37.09	D49.0
mandibular	C03.1	C79.89	D00.03	D10.39	D37.09	D49.0
maxillary	C03.0	C79.89	D00.03	D10.39	D37.09	D49.0
upper	C03.0	C79.89	D00.03	D10.39	D37.09	D49.0
gland, glandular (lymphatic) (system) (*see also* Neoplasm, lymph gland)						
endocrine NEC	C75.9	C79.89	D09.3	D35.9	D44.9	D49.7
salivary — *see* Neoplasm, salivary gland						
glans penis	C60.1	C79.82	D07.4	D29.0	D40.8	D49.59
globus pallidus	C71.0	C79.31	-	D33.0	D43.0	D49.6
glomus						
coccygeal	C49.5	C79.89	-	D21.5	D48.1	D49.2
jugularis	C75.5	C79.89	-	D35.6	D44.7	D49.7
glosso-epiglottic fold (s)	C10.1	C79.89	D00.08	D10.5	D37.05	D49.0
glossopalatine fold	C09.1	C79.89	D00.08	D10.5	D37.05	D49.0
glossopharyngeal sulcus	C09.0	C79.89	D00.08	D10.5	D37.05	D49.0
glottis	C32.0	C78.39	D02.0	D14.1	D38.0	D49.1
gluteal region	C76.3	C79.89	D04.5	D36.7	D48.7	D49.89
great vessels NEC	C49.3	C79.89	-	D21.3	D48.1	D49.2
groin NEC	C76.3	C79.89	D04.5	D36.7	D48.7	D49.89
gum	C03.9	C79.89	D00.03	D10.39	D37.09	D49.0
lower	C03.1	C79.89	D00.03	D10.39	D37.09	D49.0
upper	C03.0	C79.89	D00.03	D10.39	D37.09	D49.0
hand NEC	C76.4-	C79.89	D04.6-	D36.7	D48.7	D49.89
head NEC	C76.0	C79.89	D04.4	D36.7	D48.7	D49.89
heart	C38.0	C79.89	-	D15.1	D48.7	D49.89
heel NEC	C76.5-	C79.89	D04.7-	D36.7	D48.7	D49.89
helix (*see also* Neoplasm, skin, ear)	C44.20-	C79.2	D04.2-	D23.2-	D48.5	D49.2
hematopoietic, hemopoietic tissue NEC	C96.9	-	-	-	-	-
specified NEC	C96.Z	-	-	-	-	-
hemisphere, cerebral	C71.0	C79.31	-	D33.0	D43.0	D49.6
hemorrhoidal zone	C21.1	C78.5	D01.3	D12.9	D37.8	D49.0
hepatic (*see also* Index to disease, by histology)	C22.9	C78.7	D01.5	D13.4	D37.6	D49.0
duct (bile)	C24.0	C78.89	D01.5	D13.5	D37.6	D49.0
flexure (colon)	C18.3	C78.5	D01.0	D12.3	D37.4	D49.0
primary	C22.8	C78.7	D01.5	D13.4	D37.6	D49.0
hepatobiliary	C24.9	C78.89	D01.5	D13.5	D37.6	D49.0
hepatoblastoma	C22.2	C78.7	D01.5	D13.4	D37.6	D49.0
hepatoma	C22.0	C78.7	D01.5	D13.4	D37.6	D49.0
hilus of lung	C34.0-	C78.0-	D02.2-	D14.3-	D38.1	D49.1
hip NEC	C76.5-	C79.89	D04.7-	D36.7	D48.7	D49.89
hippocampus, brain	C71.2	C79.31	-	D33.0	D43.0	D49.6
humerus (any part)	C40.0-	C79.51	-	D16.0-	-	-
hymen	C52	C79.82	D07.2	D28.1	D39.8	D49.59
hypopharynx, hypopharyngeal NEC	C13.9	C79.89	D00.08	D10.7	D37.05	D49.0
overlapping lesion	C13.8	-	-	-	-	-
postcricoid region	C13.0	C79.89	D00.08	D10.7	D37.05	D49.0
posterior wall	C13.2	C79.89	D00.08	D10.7	D37.05	D49.0
pyriform fossa (sinus)	C12	C79.89	D00.08	D10.7	D37.05	D49.0
hypophysis	C75.1	C79.89	D09.3	D35.2	D44.3	D49.7
hypothalamus	C71.0	C79.31	-	D33.0	D43.0	D49.6
ileocecum, ileocecal (coil) (junction) (valve)	C18.0	C78.5	D01.0	D12.0	D37.4	D49.0
ileum	C17.2	C78.4	D01.49	D13.39	D37.2	D49.0
ilium	C41.4	C79.51	-	D16.8	D48.0	D49.2
immunoproliferative NEC	C88.9	-	-	-	-	-
infraclavicular (region)	C76.1	C79.89	D04.5	D36.7	D48.7	D49.89
inguinal (region)	C76.3	C79.89	D04.5	D36.7	D48.7	D49.89
insula	C71.0	C79.31	-	D33.0	D43.0	D49.6
insular tissue (pancreas)	C25.4	C78.89	D01.7	D13.7	D37.8	D49.0
brain	C71.0	C79.31	-	D33.0	D43.0	D49.6
interarytenoid fold	C13.1	C79.89	D00.08	D10.7	D37.05	D49.0
hypopharyngeal aspect	C13.1	C79.89	D00.08	D10.7	D37.05	D49.0
laryngeal aspect	C32.1	C78.39	D02.0	D14.1	D38.0	D49.1
marginal zone	C13.1	C79.89	D00.08	D10.7	D37.05	D49.0
interdental papillae	C03.9	C79.89	D00.03	D10.39	D37.09	D49.0
lower	C03.1	C79.89	D00.03	D10.39	D37.09	D49.0
upper	C03.0	C79.89	D00.03	D10.39	D37.09	D49.0
internal						
capsule	C71.0	C79.31	-	D33.0	D43.0	D49.6
os (cervix)	C53.0	C79.82	D06.0	D26.0	D39.0	D49.59
intervertebral cartilage or disc	C41.2	C79.51	-	D16.6	D48.0	D49.2
intestine, intestinal	C26.0	C78.80	D01.40	D13.9	D37.8	D49.0
large	C18.9	C78.5	D01.0	D12.6	D37.4	D49.0
appendix	C18.1	C78.5	D01.0	D12.1	D37.3	D49.0
caput coli	C18.0	C78.5	D01.0	D12.0	D37.4	D49.0
cecum	C18.0	C78.5	D01.0	D12.0	D37.4	D49.0
colon	C18.9	C78.5	D01.0	D12.6	D37.4	D49.0
and rectum	C19	C78.5	D01.1	D12.7	D37.5	D49.0
ascending	C18.2	C78.5	D01.0	D12.2	D37.4	D49.0
caput	C18.0	C78.5	D01.0	D12.0	D37.4	D49.0
descending	C18.6	C78.5	D01.0	D12.4	D37.4	D49.0
distal	C18.6	C78.5	D01.0	D12.4	D37.4	D49.0
left	C18.6	C78.5	D01.0	D12.4	D37.4	D49.0
overlapping lesion	C18.8	-	-	-	-	-
pelvic	C18.7	C78.5	D01.0	D12.5	D37.4	D49.0
right	C18.2	C78.5	D01.0	D12.2	D37.4	D49.0
sigmoid (flexure)	C18.7	C78.5	D01.0	D12.5	D37.4	D49.0
transverse	C18.4	C78.5	D01.0	D12.3	D37.4	D49.0
hepatic flexure	C18.3	C78.5	D01.0	D12.3	D37.4	D49.0
ileocecum, ileocecal (coil) (valve)	C18.0	C78.5	D01.0	D12.0	D37.4	D49.0
overlapping lesion	C18.8	-	-	-	-	-
sigmoid flexure (lower) (upper)	C18.7	C78.5	D01.0	D12.5	D37.4	D49.0
splenic flexure	C18.5	C78.5	D01.0	D12.3	D37.4	D49.0
small	C17.9	C78.4	D01.40	D13.30	D37.2	D49.0
duodenum	C17.0	C78.4	D01.49	D13.2	D37.2	D49.0
ileum	C17.2	C78.4	D01.49	D13.39	D37.2	D49.0
jejunum	C17.1	C78.4	D01.49	D13.39	D37.2	D49.0
overlapping lesion	C17.8	-	-	-	-	-
tract NEC	C26.0	C78.89	D01.40	D13.9	D37.8	D49.0
intra-abdominal	C76.2	C79.89	D09.8	D36.7	D48.7	D49.89
intracranial NEC	C71.9	C79.31	-	D33.2	D43.2	D49.6
intrahepatic (bile) duct	C22.1	C78.7	D01.5	D13.4	D37.6	D49.0
intraocular	C69.9-	C79.49	D09.2-	D31.9-	D48.7	D49.89
intraorbital	C69.6-	C79.49	D09.2-	D31.6-	D48.7	D49.89
intrasellar	C75.1	C79.89	D09.3	D35.2	D44.3	D49.7
intrathoracic (cavity) (organs)	C76.1	C79.89	D09.8	D15.9	D48.7	D49.89
specified NEC	C76.1	C79.89	D09.8	D15.7	-	-
iris	C69.4-	C79.49	D09.2-	D31.4-	D48.7	D49.89
ischiorectal (fossa)	C76.3	C79.89	D09.8	D36.7	D48.7	D49.89
ischium	C41.4	C79.51	-	D16.8	D48.0	D49.2
island of Reil	C71.0	C79.31	-	D33.0	D43.0	D49.6
islands or islets of Langerhans	C25.4	C78.89	D01.7	D13.7	D37.8	D49.0
isthmus uteri	C54.0	C79.82	D07.0	D26.1	D39.0	D49.59

filum - isthmus

ICD-10-CM TABLE OF NEOPLASMS

Neoplasm	Malignant Primary	Malignant Secondary	Ca in situ	Benign	Uncertain Behavior	Unspecified Behavior
jaw	C76.0	C79.89	D09.8	D36.7	D48.7	D49.89
bone	C41.1	C79.51	-	D16.5-	D48.0	D49.2
lower	C41.1	C79.51	-	D16.5-	-	-
upper	C41.0	C79.51	-	D16.4-	-	-
carcinoma (any type) (lower) (upper)	C76.0	C79.89	-	-	-	-
skin (*see also* Neoplasm, skin, face)	C44.309	C79.2	D04.39	D23.39	D48.5	D49.2
soft tissues	C03.9	C79.89	D00.03	D10.39	D37.09	D49.0
lower	C03.1	C79.89	D00.03	D10.39	D37.09	D49.0
upper	C03.0	C79.89	D00.03	D10.39	D37.09	D49.0
jejunum	C17.1	C78.4	D01.49	D13.39	D37.2	D49.0
joint NEC (*see also* Neoplasm, bone)	C41.9	C79.51	-	D16.9-	D48.0	D49.2
acromioclavicular	C40.0-	C79.51	-	D16.0-	-	-
bursa or synovial membrane — *see* Neoplasm, connective tissue						
costovertebral	C41.3	C79.51	-	D16.7	D48.0	D49.2
sternocostal	C41.3	C79.51	-	D16.7	D48.0	D49.2
temporomandibular	C41.1	C79.51	-	D16.5-	D48.0	D49.2
junction						
anorectal	C21.8	C78.5	D01.3	D12.9	D37.8	D49.0
cardioesophageal	C16.0	C78.89	D00.2	D13.1	D37.1	D49.0
esophagogastric	C16.0	C78.89	D00.2	D13.1	D37.1	D49.0
gastroesophageal	C16.0	C78.89	D00.2	D13.1	D37.1	D49.0
hard and soft palate	C05.9	C79.89	D00.00	D10.39	D37.09	D49.0
ileocecal	C18.0	C78.5	D01.0	D12.0	D37.4	D49.0
pelvirectal	C19	C78.5	D01.1	D12.7	D37.5	D49.0
pelviureteric	C65.-	C79.0-	D09.19	D30.1-	D41.1-	D49.59
rectosigmoid	C19	C78.5	D01.1	D12.7	D37.5	D49.0
squamocolumnar, of cervix	C53.8	C79.82	D06.7	D26.0	D39.0	D49.59
Kaposi's sarcoma — *see* Kaposi's, sarcoma						
kidney (parenchymal)	C64.-	C79.0-	D09.19	D30.0-	D41.0-	D49.51-
calyx	C65.-	C79.0-	D09.19	D30.1-	D41.1-	D49.51-
hilus	C65.-	C79.0-	D09.19	D30.1-	D41.1-	D49.51-
pelvis	C65.-	C79.0-	D09.19	D30.1-	D41.1-	D49.51-
knee NEC	C76.5-	C79.89	D04.7-	D36.7	D48.7	D49.89
labia (skin)	C51.9	C79.82	D07.1	D28.0	D39.8	D49.59
majora	C51.0	C79.82	D07.1	D28.0	D39.8	D49.59
minora	C51.1	C79.82	D07.1	D28.0	D39.8	D49.59
labial (*see also* Neoplasm, lip)	C00.9	C79.89	D00.01	D10.0	D37.01	D49.0
sulcus (lower) (upper)	C06.1	C79.89	D00.02	D10.39	D37.09	D49.0
labium (skin)	C51.9	C79.82	D07.1	D28.0	D39.8	D49.59
majus	C51.0	C79.82	D07.1	D28.0	D39.8	D49.59
minus	C51.1	C79.82	D07.1	D28.0	D39.8	D49.59
lacrimal						
canaliculi	C69.5-	C79.49	D09.2-	D31.5-	D48.7	D49.89
duct (nasal)	C69.5-	C79.49	D09.2-	D31.5-	D48.7	D49.89
gland	C69.5-	C79.49	D09.2-	D31.5-	D48.7	D49.89
punctum	C69.5-	C79.49	D09.2-	D31.5-	D48.7	D49.89
sac	C69.5-	C79.49	D09.2-	D31.5-	D48.7	D49.89
Langerhans, islands or islets	C25.4	C78.89	D01.7	D13.7	D37.8	D49.0
laryngopharynx	C13.9	C79.89	D00.08	D10.7	D37.05	D49.0
larynx, laryngeal NEC	C32.9	C78.39	D02.0	D14.1	D38.0	D49.1
aryepiglottic fold	C32.1	C78.39	D02.0	D14.1	D38.0	D49.1
cartilage (arytenoid) (cricoid) (cuneiform) (thyroid)	C32.3	C78.39	D02.0	D14.1	D38.0	D49.1
commissure (anterior) (posterior)	C32.0	C78.39	D02.0	D14.1	D38.0	D49.1
extrinsic NEC	C32.1	C78.39	D02.0	D14.1	D38.0	D49.1
meaning hypopharynx	C13.9	C79.89	D00.08	D10.7	D37.05	D49.0
interarytenoid fold	C32.1	C78.39	D02.0	D14.1	D38.0	D49.1
intrinsic	C32.0	C78.39	D02.0	D14.1	D38.0	D49.1
overlapping lesion	C32.8	-	-	-	-	-
ventricular band	C32.1	C78.39	D02.0	D14.1	D38.0	D49.1
leg NEC	C76.5-	C79.89	D04.7-	D36.7	D48.7	D49.89
lens, crystalline	C69.4-	C79.49	D09.2-	D31.4-	D48.7	D49.89
lid (lower) (upper)	C44.10-	C79.2	D04.1-	D23.1-	D48.5	D49.2
basal cell carcinoma	C44.11-	-	-	-	-	-
specified type NEC	C44.19-	-	-	-	-	-
squamous cell carcinoma	C44.12-	-	-	-	-	-
ligament (*see also* Neoplasm, connective tissue)						
broad	C57.1	C79.82	D07.39	D28.2	D39.8	D49.59
Mackenrodt's	C57.7	C79.82	D07.39	D28.7	D39.8	D49.59
non-uterine — *see* Neoplasm, connective tissue						
round	C57.2	C79.82	-	D28.2	D39.8	D49.59
sacro-uterine	C57.3	C79.82	-	D28.2	D39.8	D49.59
uterine	C57.3	C79.82	-	D28.2	D39.8	D49.59
utero-ovarian	C57.7	C79.82	D07.39	D28.2	D39.8	D49.59
uterosacral	C57.3	C79.82	-	D28.2	D39.8	D49.59
limb	C76.8	C79.89	D04.8	D36.7	D48.7	D49.89
lower	C76.5-	C79.89	D04.7-	D36.7	D48.7	D49.89
upper	C76.4-	C79.89	D04.6-	D36.7	D48.7	D49.89
limbus of cornea	C69.1-	C79.49	D09.2-	D31.1-	D48.7	D49.89
lingual NEC (*see also* Neoplasm, tongue)	C02.9	C79.89	D00.07	D10.1	D37.02	D49.0
lingula, lung	C34.1-	C78.0-	D02.2-	D14.3-	D38.1	D49.1
lip	C00.9	C79.89	D00.01	D10.0	D37.01	D49.0
buccal aspect — *see* Neoplasm, lip, internal						

Neoplasm	Malignant Primary	Malignant Secondary	Ca in situ	Benign	Uncertain Behavior	Unspecified Behavior
lip — *continued*						
commissure	C00.6	C79.89	D00.01	D10.0	D37.01	D49.0
external	C00.2	C79.89	D00.01	D10.0	D37.01	D49.0
lower	C00.1	C79.89	D00.01	D10.0	D37.01	D49.0
upper	C00.0	C79.89	D00.01	D10.0	D37.01	D49.0
frenulum — *see* Neoplasm, lip, internal						
inner aspect — *see* Neoplasm, lip, internal						
internal	C00.5	C79.89	D00.01	D10.0	D37.01	D49.0
lower	C00.4	C79.89	D00.01	D10.0	D37.01	D49.0
upper	C00.3	C79.89	D00.01	D10.0	D37.01	D49.0
lipstick area	C00.2	C79.89	D00.01	D10.0	D37.01	D49.0
lower	C00.1	C79.89	D00.01	D10.0	D37.01	D49.0
upper	C00.0	C79.89	D00.01	D10.0	D37.01	D49.0
lower	C00.1	C79.89	D00.01	D10.0	D37.01	D49.0
internal	C00.4	C79.89	D00.01	D10.0	D37.01	D49.0
mucosa — *see* Neoplasm, lip, internal						
oral aspect — *see* Neoplasm, lip, internal						
overlapping lesion	C00.8	-	-	-	-	-
with oral cavity or pharynx	C14.8	-	-	-	-	-
skin (commissure) (lower) (upper)	C44.00	C79.2	D04.0	D23.0	D48.5	D49.2
basal cell carcinoma	C44.01	-	-	-	-	-
specified type NEC	C44.09	-	-	-	-	-
squamous cell carcinoma	C44.02	-	-	-	-	-
upper	C00.0	C79.89	D00.01	D10.0	D37.01	D49.0
internal	C00.3	C79.89	D00.01	D10.0	D37.01	D49.0
vermilion border	C00.2	C79.89	D00.01	D10.0	D37.01	D49.0
lower	C00.1	C79.89	D00.01	D10.0	D37.01	D49.0
upper	C00.0	C79.89	D00.01	D10.0	D37.01	D49.0
lipomatous — *see* Lipoma, by site						
liver (*see also* Index to disease, by histology)	C22.9	C78.7	D01.5	D13.4	D37.6	D49.0
primary	C22.8	C78.7	D01.5	D13.4	D37.6	D49.0
lumbosacral plexus	C47.5	C79.89	-	D36.16	D48.2	D49.2
lung	C34.9-	C78.0-	D02.2-	D14.3-	D38.1	D49.1
azygos lobe	C34.1-	C78.0-	D02.2-	D14.3-	D38.1	D49.1
carina	C34.0-	C78.0-	D02.2-	D14.3-	D38.1	D49.1
hilus	C34.0-	C78.0-	D02.2-	D14.3-	D38.1	D49.1
lingula	C34.1-	C78.0-	D02.2-	D14.3-	D38.1	D49.1
lobe NEC	C34.9-	C78.0-	D02.2-	D14.3-	D38.1	D49.1
lower lobe	C34.3-	C78.0-	D02.2-	D14.3-	D38.1	D49.1
main bronchus	C34.0-	C78.0-	D02.2-	D14.3-	D38.1	D49.1
mesothelioma — *see* Mesothelioma						
middle lobe	C34.2	C78.0-	D02.21	D14.31	D38.1	D49.1
overlapping lesion	C34.8-	-	-	-	-	-
upper lobe	C34.1-	C78.0-	D02.2-	D14.3-	D38.1	D49.1
lymph, lymphatic channel NEC	C49.9	C79.89	-	D21.9	D48.1	D49.2
gland (secondary)	-	C77.9	-	D36.0	D48.7	D49.89
abdominal	-	C77.2	-	D36.0	D48.7	D49.89
aortic	-	C77.2	-	D36.0	D48.7	D49.89
arm	-	C77.3	-	D36.0	D48.7	D49.89
auricular (anterior) (posterior)	-	C77.0	-	D36.0	D48.7	D49.89
axilla, axillary	-	C77.3	-	D36.0	D48.7	D49.89
brachial	-	C77.3	-	D36.0	D48.7	D49.89
bronchial	-	C77.1	-	D36.0	D48.7	D49.89
bronchopulmonary	-	C77.1	-	D36.0	D48.7	D49.89
celiac	-	C77.2	-	D36.0	D48.7	D49.89
cervical	-	C77.0	-	D36.0	D48.7	D49.89
cervicofacial	-	C77.0	-	D36.0	D48.7	D49.89
Cloquet	-	C77.4	-	D36.0	D48.7	D49.89
colic	-	C77.2	-	D36.0	D48.7	D49.89
common duct	-	C77.2	-	D36.0	D48.7	D49.89
cubital	-	C77.3	-	D36.0	D48.7	D49.89
diaphragmatic	-	C77.1	-	D36.0	D48.7	D49.89
epigastric, inferior	-	C77.1	-	D36.0	D48.7	D49.89
epitrochlear	-	C77.3	-	D36.0	D48.7	D49.89
esophageal	-	C77.1	-	D36.0	D48.7	D49.89
face	-	C77.0	-	D36.0	D48.7	D49.89
femoral	-	C77.4	-	D36.0	D48.7	D49.89
gastric	-	C77.2	-	D36.0	D48.7	D49.89
groin	-	C77.4	-	D36.0	D48.7	D49.89
head	-	C77.0	-	D36.0	D48.7	D49.89
hepatic	-	C77.2	-	D36.0	D48.7	D49.89
hilar (pulmonary)	-	C77.1	-	D36.0	D48.7	D49.89
splenic	-	C77.2	-	D36.0	D48.7	D49.89
hypogastric	-	C77.5	-	D36.0	D48.7	D49.89
ileocolic	-	C77.2	-	D36.0	D48.7	D49.89
iliac	-	C77.5	-	D36.0	D48.7	D49.89
infraclavicular	-	C77.3	-	D36.0	D48.7	D49.89
inguina, inguinal	-	C77.4	-	D36.0	D48.7	D49.89
innominate	-	C77.1	-	D36.0	D48.7	D49.89
intercostal	-	C77.1	-	D36.0	D48.7	D49.89
intestinal	-	C77.2	-	D36.0	D48.7	D49.89
intrabdominal	-	C77.2	-	D36.0	D48.7	D49.89
intrapelvic	-	C77.5	-	D36.0	D48.7	D49.89
intrathoracic	-	C77.1	-	D36.0	D48.7	D49.89
jugular	-	C77.0	-	D36.0	D48.7	D49.89

Neoplasm	Malignant Primary	Malignant Secondary	Ca in situ	Benign	Uncertain Behavior	Unspecified Behavior
lymph — *continued*						
leg	-	C77.4	-	D36.0	D48.7	D49.89
limb						
lower	-	C77.4	-	D36.0	D48.7	D49.89
upper	-	C77.3	-	D36.0	D48.7	D49.89
lower limb	-	C77.4	-	D36.0	D48.7	D49.89
lumbar	-	C77.2	-	D36.0	D48.7	D49.89
mandibular	-	C77.0	-	D36.0	D48.7	D49.89
mediastinal	-	C77.1	-	D36.0	D48.7	D49.89
mesenteric (inferior) (superior)	-	C77.2	-	D36.0	D48.7	D49.89
midcolic	-	C77.2	-	D36.0	D48.7	D49.89
multiple sites in categories C77.0 - C77.5	-	C77.8	-	D36.0	D48.7	D49.89
neck	-	C77.0	-	D36.0	D48.7	D49.89
obturator	-	C77.5	-	D36.0	D48.7	D49.89
occipital	-	C77.0	-	D36.0	D48.7	D49.89
pancreatic	-	C77.2	-	D36.0	D48.7	D49.89
para-aortic	-	C77.2	-	D36.0	D48.7	D49.89
paracervical	-	C77.5	-	D36.0	D48.7	D49.89
parametrial	-	C77.5	-	D36.0	D48.7	D49.89
parasternal	-	C77.1	-	D36.0	D48.7	D49.89
parotid	-	C77.0	-	D36.0	D48.7	D49.89
pectoral	-	C77.3	-	D36.0	D48.7	D49.89
pelvic	-	C77.5	-	D36.0	D48.7	D49.89
peri-aortic	-	C77.2	-	D36.0	D48.7	D49.89
peripancreatic	-	C77.2	-	D36.0	D48.7	D49.89
popliteal	-	C77.4	-	D36.0	D48.7	D49.89
porta hepatis	-	C77.2	-	D36.0	D48.7	D49.89
portal	-	C77.2	-	D36.0	D48.7	D49.89
preauricular	-	C77.0	-	D36.0	D48.7	D49.89
prelaryngeal	-	C77.0	-	D36.0	D48.7	D49.89
presymphyseal	-	C77.5	-	D36.0	D48.7	D49.89
pretracheal	-	C77.0	-	D36.0	D48.7	D49.89
primary (any site) NEC	C96.9	-	-	-	-	-
pulmonary (hilar)	-	C77.1	-	D36.0	D48.7	D49.89
pyloric	-	C77.2	-	D36.0	D48.7	D49.89
retroperitoneal	-	C77.2	-	D36.0	D48.7	D49.89
retropharyngeal	-	C77.0	-	D36.0	D48.7	D49.89
Rosenmuller's	-	C77.4	-	D36.0	D48.7	D49.89
sacral	-	C77.5	-	D36.0	D48.7	D49.89
scalene	-	C77.0	-	D36.0	D48.7	D49.89
site NEC	-	C77.9	-	D36.0	D48.7	D49.89
splenic (hilar)	-	C77.2	-	D36.0	D48.7	D49.89
subclavicular	-	C77.3	-	D36.0	D48.7	D49.89
subinguinal	-	C77.4	-	D36.0	D48.7	D49.89
sublingual	-	C77.0	-	D36.0	D48.7	D49.89
submandibular	-	C77.0	-	D36.0	D48.7	D49.89
submaxillary	-	C77.0	-	D36.0	D48.7	D49.89
submental	-	C77.0	-	D36.0	D48.7	D49.89
subscapular	-	C77.3	-	D36.0	D48.7	D49.89
supraclavicular	-	C77.0	-	D36.0	D48.7	D49.89
thoracic	-	C77.1	-	D36.0	D48.7	D49.89
tibial	-	C77.4	-	D36.0	D48.7	D49.89
tracheal	-	C77.1	-	D36.0	D48.7	D49.89
tracheobronchial	-	C77.1	-	D36.0	D48.7	D49.89
upper limb	-	C77.3	-	D36.0	D48.7	D49.89
Virchow's	-	C77.0	-	D36.0	D48.7	D49.89
node (*see also* Neoplasm, lymph gland)						
primary NEC	C96.9	-	-	-	-	-
vessel (*see also* Neoplasm, connective tissue)	C49.9	C79.89	-	D21.9	D48.1	D49.2
Mackenrodt's ligament	C57.7	C79.82	D07.39	D28.7	D39.8	D49.59
malar	C41.0	C79.51	-	D16.4-	D48.0	D49.2
region — *see* Neoplasm, cheek						
mammary gland — *see* Neoplasm, breast						
mandible	C41.1	C79.51	-	D16.5-	D48.0	D49.2
alveolar						
mucosa (carcinoma)	C03.1	C79.89	D00.03	D10.39	D37.09	D49.0
ridge or process	C41.1	C79.51	-	D16.5-	D48.0	D49.2
marrow (bone) NEC	C96.9	C79.52	-	-	D47.9	D49.89
mastectomy site (skin) (*see also* Neoplasm, breast, skin)	C44.501	C79.2	-	-	-	-
specified as breast tissue	C50.8-	C79.81	-	-	-	-
mastoid (air cells) (antrum) (cavity)	C30.1	C78.39	D02.3	D14.0	D38.5	D49.1
bone or process	C41.0	C79.51	-	D16.4-	D48.0	D49.2
maxilla, maxillary (superior)	C41.0	C79.51	-	D16.4-	D48.0	D49.2
alveolar						
mucosa	C03.0	C79.89	D00.03	D10.39	D37.09	D49.0
ridge or process (carcinoma)	C41.0	C79.51	-	D16.4-	D48.0	D49.2
antrum	C31.0	C78.39	D02.3	D14.0	D38.5	D49.1
carcinoma	C03.0	C79.51	-	-	-	-
inferior — *see* Neoplasm, mandible						
sinus	C31.0	C78.39	D02.3	D14.0	D38.5	D49.1
meatus external (ear) (*see also* Neoplasm, skin, ear)	C44.20-	C79.2	D04.2-	D23.2-	D48.5	D49.2

Neoplasm	Malignant Primary	Malignant Secondary	Ca in situ	Benign	Uncertain Behavior	Unspecified Behavior
Meckel diverticulum, malignant	C17.3	C78.4	D01.49	D13.39	D37.2	D49.0
mediastinum, mediastinal	C38.3	C78.1	-	D15.2	D38.3	D49.89
anterior	C38.1	C78.1	-	D15.2	D38.3	D49.89
posterior	C38.2	C78.1	-	D15.2	D38.3	D49.89
medulla						
adrenal	C74.1-	C79.7-	D09.3	D35.0-	D44.1-	D49.7
oblongata	C71.7	C79.31	-	D33.1	D43.1	D49.6
meibomian gland	C44.10-	C79.2	D04.1-	D23.1-	D48.5	D49.2
basal cell carcinoma	C44.11-	-	-	-	-	-
specified type NEC	C44.19-	-	-	-	-	-
squamous cell carcinoma	C44.12-	-	-	-	-	-
melanoma — *see* Melanoma						
meninges	C70.9	C79.49	-	D32.9	D42.9	D49.7
brain	C70.0	C79.32	-	D32.0	D42.0	D49.7
cerebral	C70.0	C79.32	-	D32.0	D42.0	D49.7
crainial	C70.0	C79.32	-	D32.0	D42.0	D49.7
intracranial	C70.0	C79.32	-	D32.0	D42.0	D49.7
spinal (cord)	C70.1	C79.49	-	D32.1	D42.1	D49.7
meniscus, knee joint (lateral) (medial)	C40.2-	C79.51	-	D16.2-	D48.0	D49.2
Merkel cell — *see* Carcinoma, Merkel cell						
mesentery, mesenteric	C48.1	C78.6	-	D20.1	D48.4	D49.0
mesoappendix	C48.1	C78.6	-	D20.1	D48.4	D49.0
mesocolon	C48.1	C78.6	-	D20.1	D48.4	D49.0
mesopharynx — *see* Neoplasm, oropharynx						
mesosalpinx	C57.1	C79.82	D07.39	D28.2	D39.8	D49.59
mesothelial tissue — *see* Mesothelioma						
mesothelioma — *see* Mesothelioma						
mesovarium	C57.1	C79.82	D07.39	D28.2	D39.8	D49.59
metacarpus (any bone)	C40.1-	C79.51	-	D16.1-	-	-
metastatic NEC (*see also* Neoplasm, by site, secondary)	-	C79.9	-	-	-	-
metatarsus (any bone)	C40.3-	C79.51	-	D16.3-	-	-
midbrain	C71.7	C79.31	-	D33.1	D43.1	D49.6
milk duct — *see* Neoplasm, breast						
mons						
pubis	C51.9	C79.82	D07.1	D28.0	D39.8	D49.59
veneris	C51.9	C79.82	D07.1	D28.0	D39.8	D49.59
motor tract	C72.9	C79.49	-	D33.9	D43.9	D49.7
brain	C71.9	C79.31	-	D33.2	D43.2	D49.6
cauda equina	C72.1	C79.49	-	D33.4	D43.4	D49.7
spinal	C72.0	C79.49	-	D33.4	D43.4	D49.7
mouth	C06.9	C79.89	D00.00	D10.30	D37.09	D49.0
book-leaf	C06.89	C79.89	-	-	-	-
floor	C04.9	C79.89	D00.06	D10.2	D37.09	D49.0
anterior portion	C04.0	C79.89	D00.06	D10.2	D37.09	D49.0
lateral portion	C04.1	C79.89	D00.06	D10.2	D37.09	D49.0
overlapping lesion	C04.8	-	-	-	-	-
overlapping NEC	C06.80	-	-	-	-	-
roof	C05.9	C79.89	D00.00	D10.39	D37.09	D49.0
specified part NEC	C06.89	C79.89	D00.00	D10.39	D37.09	D49.0
vestibule	C06.1	C79.89	D00.00	D10.39	D37.09	D49.0
mucosa						
alveolar (ridge or process)	C03.9	C79.89	D00.03	D10.39	D37.09	D49.0
lower	C03.1	C79.89	D00.03	D10.39	D37.09	D49.0
upper	C03.0	C79.89	D00.03	D10.39	D37.09	D49.0
buccal	C06.0	C79.89	D00.02	D10.39	D37.09	D49.0
cheek	C06.0	C79.89	D00.02	D10.39	D37.09	D49.0
lip — *see* Neoplasm, lip, internal						
nasal	C30.0	C78.39	D02.3	D14.0	D38.5	D49.1
oral	C06.0	C79.89	D00.02	D10.39	D37.09	D49.0
Mullerian duct						
female	C57.7	C79.82	D07.39	D28.7	D39.8	D49.59
male	C63.7	C79.82	D07.69	D29.8	D40.8	D49.59
muscle (*see also* Neoplasm, connective tissue)						
extraocular	C69.6-	C79.49	D09.2-	D31.6-	D48.7	D49.89
myocardium	C38.0	C79.89	-	D15.1	D48.7	D49.89
myometrium	C54.2	C79.82	D07.0	D26.1	D39.0	D49.59
myopericardium	C38.0	C79.89	-	D15.1	D48.7	D49.89
nabothian gland (follicle)	C53.0	C79.82	D06.0	D26.0	D39.0	D49.59
nail (*see also* Neoplasm, skin, limb)	C44.90	C79.2	D04.9	D23.9	D48.5	D49.2
finger (*see also* Neoplasm, skin, limb, upper)	C44.60-	C79.2	D04.6-	D23.6-	D48.5	D49.2
toe (*see also* Neoplasm, skin, limb, lower)	C44.70-	C79.2	D04.7-	D23.7-	D48.5	D49.2
nares, naris (anterior) (posterior)	C30.0	C78.39	D02.3	D14.0	D38.5	D49.1
nasal — *see* Neoplasm, nose						
nasolabial groove (*see also* Neoplasm, skin, face)	C44.309	C79.2	D04.39	D23.39	D48.5	D49.2
nasolacrimal duct	C69.5-	C79.49	D09.2-	D31.5-	D48.7	D49.89
nasopharynx, nasopharyngeal	C11.9	C79.89	D00.08	D10.6	D37.05	D49.0
floor	C11.3	C79.89	D00.08	D10.6	D37.05	D49.0
overlapping lesion	C11.8	-	-	-	-	-
roof	C11.0	C79.89	D00.08	D10.6	D37.05	D49.0
wall	C11.9	C79.89	D00.08	D10.6	D37.05	D49.0
anterior	C11.3	C79.89	D00.08	D10.6	D37.05	D49.0

Neoplasm	Malignant Primary	Malignant Secondary	Ca in situ	Benign	Uncertain Behavior	Unspecified Behavior
nasopharynx, nasopharyngeal — *continued*						
wall — *continued*						
lateral	C11.2	C79.89	D00.08	D10.6	D37.05	D49.0
posterior	C11.1	C79.89	D00.08	D10.6	D37.05	D49.0
superior	C11.0	C79.89	D00.08	D10.6	D37.05	D49.0
nates (*see also* Neoplasm, skin, trunk)	C44.509	C79.2	D04.5	D23.5	D48.5	D49.2
neck NEC	C76.0	C79.89	D09.8	D36.7	D48.7	D49.89
skin	C44.40	-	-	-	-	-
basal cell carcinoma	C44.41	-	-	-	-	-
specified type NEC	C44.49	-	-	-	-	-
squamous cell carcinoma	C44.42	-	-	-	-	-
nerve (ganglion)	C47.9	C79.89	-	D36.10	D48.2	D49.2
abducens	C72.59	C79.49	-	D33.3	D43.3	D49.7
accessory (spinal)	C72.59	C79.49	-	D33.3	D43.3	D49.7
acoustic	C72.4-	C79.49	-	D33.3	D43.3	D49.7
auditory	C72.4-	C79.49	-	D33.3	D43.3	D49.7
autonomic NEC (*see also* Neoplasm, nerve, peripheral)	C47.9	C79.89	-	D36.10	D48.2	D49.2
brachial	C47.1-	C79.89	-	D36.12	D48.2	D49.2
cranial	C72.50	C79.49	-	D33.3	D43.3	D49.7
specified NEC	C72.59	C79.49	-	D33.3	D43.3	D49.7
facial	C72.59	C79.49	-	D33.3	D43.3	D49.7
femoral	C47.2-	C79.89	-	D36.13	D48.2	D49.2
ganglion NEC (*see also* Neoplasm, nerve, peripheral)	C47.9	C79.89	-	D36.10	D48.2	D49.2
glossopharyngeal	C72.59	C79.49	-	D33.3	D43.3	D49.7
hypoglossal	C72.59	C79.49	-	D33.3	D43.3	D49.7
intercostal	C47.3	C79.89	-	D36.14	D48.2	D49.2
lumbar	C47.6	C79.89	-	D36.17	D48.2	D49.2
median	C47.1-	C79.89	-	D36.12	D48.2	D49.2
obturator	C47.2-	C79.89	-	D36.13	D48.2	D49.2
oculomotor	C72.59	C79.49	-	D33.3	D43.3	D49.7
olfactory	C47.2-	C79.49	-	D33.3	D43.3	D49.7
optic	C72.3-	C79.49	-	D33.3	D43.3	D49.7
parasympathetic NEC	C47.9	C79.89	-	D36.10	D48.2	D49.2
peripheral NEC	C47.9	C79.89	-	D36.10	D48.2	D49.2
abdomen	C47.4	C79.89	-	D36.15	D48.2	D49.2
abdominal wall	C47.4	C79.89	-	D36.15	D48.2	D49.2
ankle	C47.2-	C79.89	-	D36.13	D48.2	D49.2
antecubital fossa or space	C47.1-	C79.89	-	D36.12	D48.2	D49.2
arm	C47.1-	C79.89	-	D36.12	D48.2	D49.2
auricle (ear)	C47.0	C79.89	-	D36.11	D48.2	D49.2
axilla	C47.3	C79.89	-	D36.12	D48.2	D49.2
back	C47.6	C79.89	-	D36.17	D48.2	D49.2
buttock	C47.5	C79.89	-	D36.16	D48.2	D49.2
calf	C47.2-	C79.89	-	D36.13	D48.2	D49.2
cervical region	C47.0	C79.89	-	D36.11	D48.2	D49.2
cheek	C47.0	C79.89	-	D36.11	D48.2	D49.2
chest (wall)	C47.3	C79.89	-	D36.14	D48.2	D49.2
chin	C47.0	C79.89	-	D36.11	D48.2	D49.2
ear (external)	C47.0	C79.89	-	D36.11	D48.2	D49.2
elbow	C47.1-	C79.89	-	D36.12	D48.2	D49.2
extrarectal	C47.5	C79.89	-	D36.16	D48.2	D49.2
extremity	C47.9	C79.89	-	D36.10	D48.2	D49.2
lower	C47.2-	C79.89	-	D36.13	D48.2	D49.2
upper	C47.1-	C79.89	-	D36.12	D48.2	D49.2
eyelid	C47.0	C79.89	-	D36.11	D48.2	D49.2
face	C47.0	C79.89	-	D36.11	D48.2	D49.2
finger	C47.1-	C79.89	-	D36.12	D48.2	D49.2
flank	C47.6	C79.89	-	D36.17	D48.2	D49.2
foot	C47.2-	C79.89	-	D36.13	D48.2	D49.2
forearm	C47.1-	C79.89	-	D36.12	D48.2	D49.2
forehead	C47.0	C79.89	-	D36.11	D48.2	D49.2
gluteal region	C47.5	C79.89	-	D36.16	D48.2	D49.2
groin	C47.5	C79.89	-	D36.16	D48.2	D49.2
hand	C47.1-	C79.89	-	D36.12	D48.2	D49.2
head	C47.0	C79.89	-	D36.11	D48.2	D49.2
heel	C47.2-	C79.89	-	D36.13	D48.2	D49.2
hip	C47.2-	C79.89	-	D36.13	D48.2	D49.2
infraclavicular region	C47.3	C79.89	-	D36.14	D48.2	D49.2
inguinal (canal) (region)	C47.5	C79.89	-	D36.16	D48.2	D49.2
intrathoracic	C47.3	C79.89	-	D36.14	D48.2	D49.2
ischiorectal fossa	C47.5	C79.89	-	D36.16	D48.2	D49.2
knee	C47.2-	C79.89	-	D36.13	D48.2	D49.2
leg	C47.2-	C79.89	-	D36.13	D48.2	D49.2
limb NEC	C47.9	C79.89	-	D36.10	D48.2	D49.2
lower	C47.2-	C79.89	-	D36.13	D48.2	D49.2
upper	C47.1-	C79.89	-	D36.12	D48.2	D49.2
nates	C47.5	C79.89	-	D36.16	D48.2	D49.2
neck	C47.0	C79.89	-	D36.11	D48.2	D49.2
orbit	C69.6-	C79.49	-	D31.6-	D48.7	D49.2
pararectal	C47.5	C79.89	-	D36.16	D48.2	D49.2
paraurethral	C47.5	C79.89	-	D36.16	D48.2	D49.2
paravaginal	C47.5	C79.89	-	D36.16	D48.2	D49.2
pelvis (floor)	C47.5	C79.89	-	D36.16	D48.2	D49.2
pelviabdominal	C47.8	C79.89	-	D36.17	D48.2	D49.2
perineum	C47.5	C79.89	-	D36.16	D48.2	D49.2
perirectal (tissue)	C47.5	C79.89	-	D36.16	D48.2	D49.2

Neoplasm	Malignant Primary	Malignant Secondary	Ca in situ	Benign	Uncertain Behavior	Unspecified Behavior
nerve — *continued*						
peripheral NEC — *continued*						
periurethral (tissue)	C47.5	C79.89	-	D36.16	D48.2	D49.2
popliteal fossa or space	C47.2-	C79.89	-	D36.13	D48.2	D49.2
presacral	C47.5	C79.89	-	D36.16	D48.2	D49.2
pterygoid fossa	C47.0	C79.89	-	D36.11	D48.2	D49.2
rectovaginal septum or wall	C47.5	C79.89	-	D36.16	D48.2	D49.2
rectovesical	C47.5	C79.89	-	D36.16	D48.2	D49.2
sacrococcygeal region	C47.5	C79.89	-	D36.16	D48.2	D49.2
scalp	C47.0	C79.89	-	D36.11	D48.2	D49.2
scapular region	C47.3	C79.89	-	D36.14	D48.2	D49.2
shoulder	C47.1-	C79.89	-	D36.12	D48.2	D49.2
submental	C47.0	C79.89	-	D36.11	D48.2	D49.2
supraclavicular region	C47.0	C79.89	-	D36.11	D48.2	D49.2
temple	C47.0	C79.89	-	D36.11	D48.2	D49.2
temporal region	C47.0	C79.89	-	D36.11	D48.2	D49.2
thigh	C47.2-	C79.89	-	D36.13	D48.2	D49.2
thoracic (duct) (wall)	C47.3	C79.89	-	D36.14	D48.2	D49.2
thorax	C47.3	C79.89	-	D36.14	D48.2	D49.2
thumb	C47.1-	C79.89	-	D36.12	D48.2	D49.2
toe	C47.2-	C79.89	-	D36.13	D48.2	D49.2
trunk	C47.6	C79.89	-	D36.17	D48.2	D49.2
umbilicus	C47.4	C79.89	-	D36.15	D48.2	D49.2
vesicorectal	C47.5	C79.89	-	D36.16	D48.2	D49.2
wrist	C47.1-	C79.89	-	D36.12	D48.2	D49.2
radial	C47.1-	C79.89	-	D36.12	D48.2	D49.2
sacral	C47.5	C79.89	-	D36.16	D48.2	D49.2
sciatic	C47.2-	C79.89	-	D36.13	D48.2	D49.2
spinal NEC	C47.9	C79.89	-	D36.10	D48.2	D49.2
accessory	C72.59	C79.49	-	D33.3	D43.3	D49.7
sympathetic NEC (*see also* Neoplasm, nerve, peripheral)	C47.9	C79.89	-	D36.10	D48.2	D49.2
trigeminal	C72.59	C79.49	-	D33.3	D43.3	D49.7
trochlear	C72.59	C79.49	-	D33.3	D43.3	D49.7
ulnar	C47.1-	C79.89	-	D36.12	D48.2	D49.2
vagus	C72.59	C79.49	-	D33.3	D43.3	D49.7
nervous system (central)	C72.9	C79.40	-	D33.9	D43.9	D49.7
autonomic — *see* Neoplasm, nerve, peripheral						
parasympathetic — *see* Neoplasm, nerve, peripheral						
specified site NEC	-	C79.49	-	D33.7	D43.8	-
sympathetic — *see* Neoplasm, nerve, peripheral						
nevus — *see* Nevus						
nipple	C50.0-	C79.81	D05.-	D24.-	-	-
nose, nasal	C76.0	C79.89	D09.8	D36.7	D48.7	D49.89
ala (external) (nasi) (*see also* Neoplasm, nose, skin)	C44.301	C79.2	D04.39	D23.39	D48.5	D49.2
bone	C41.0	C79.51	-	D16.4-	D48.0	D49.2
cartilage	C30.0	C78.39	D02.3	D14.0	D38.5	D49.1
cavity	C30.0	C78.39	D02.3	D14.0	D38.5	D49.1
choana	C11.3	C79.89	D00.08	D10.6	D37.05	D49.0
external (skin) (*see also* Neoplasm, nose, skin)	C44.301	C79.2	D04.39	D23.39	D48.5	D49.2
fossa	C30.0	C78.39	D02.3	D14.0	D38.5	D49.1
internal	C30.0	C78.39	D02.3	D14.0	D38.5	D49.1
mucosa	C30.0	C78.39	D02.3	D14.0	D38.5	D49.1
septum	C30.0	C78.39	D02.3	D14.0	D38.5	D49.1
posterior margin	C11.3	C79.89	D00.08	D10.6	D37.05	D49.0
sinus — *see* Neoplasm, sinus						
skin	C44.301	C79.2	D04.39	D23.39	D48.5	D49.2
basal cell carcinoma	C44.311	-	-	-	-	-
specified type NEC	C44.391	-	-	-	-	-
squamous cell carcinoma	C44.321	-	-	-	-	-
turbinate (mucosa)	C30.0	C78.39	D02.3	D14.0	D38.5	D49.1
bone	C41.0	C79.51	-	D16.4-	D48.0	D49.2
vestibule	C30.0	C78.39	D02.3	D14.0	D38.5	D49.1
nostril	C30.0	C78.39	D02.3	D14.0	D38.5	D49.1
nucleus pulposus	C41.2	C79.51	-	D16.6	D48.0	D49.2
occipital						
bone	C41.0	C79.51	-	D16.4-	D48.0	D49.2
lobe or pole, brain	C71.4	C79.31	-	D33.0	D43.0	D49.6
odontogenic — *see* Neoplasm, jaw bone						
olfactory nerve or bulb	C72.2-	C79.49	-	D33.3	D43.3	D49.7
olive (brain)	C71.7	C79.31	-	D33.1	D43.1	D49.6
omentum	C48.1	C78.6	-	D20.1	D48.4	D49.0
operculum (brain)	C71.0	C79.31	-	D33.0	D43.0	D49.6
optic nerve, chiasm, or tract	C72.3-	C79.49	-	D33.3	D43.3	D49.7
oral (cavity)	C06.9	C79.89	D00.00	D10.30	D37.09	D49.0
ill-defined	C14.8	C79.89	D00.00	D10.30	D37.09	D49.0
mucosa	C06.0	C79.89	D00.02	D10.39	D37.09	D49.0
orbit	C69.6-	C79.49	D09.2-	D31.6-	D48.7	D49.89
autonomic nerve	C69.6-	C79.49	-	D31.6-	D48.7	D49.2
bone	C41.0	C79.51	-	D16.4-	D48.0	D49.2
eye	C69.6-	C79.49	D09.2-	D31.6-	D48.7	D49.89
peripheral nerves	C69.6-	C79.49	-	D31.6-	D48.7	D49.2
soft parts	C69.6-	C79.49	D09.2-	D31.6-	D48.7	D49.89
organ of Zuckerkandl	C75.5	C79.89	-	D35.6	D44.7	D49.7

Neoplasm	Malignant Primary	Malignant Secondary	Ca in situ	Benign	Uncertain Behavior	Unspecified Behavior
oropharynx	C10.9	C79.89	D00.08	D10.5	D37.05	D49.0
branchial cleft (vestige)	C10.4	C79.89	D00.08	D10.5	D37.05	D49.0
junctional region	C10.8	C79.89	D00.08	D10.5	D37.05	D49.0
lateral wall	C10.2	C79.89	D00.08	D10.5	D37.05	D49.0
overlapping lesion	C10.8	-	-	-	-	-
pillars or fauces	C09.1	C79.89	D00.08	D10.5	D37.05	D49.0
posterior wall	C10.3	C79.89	D00.08	D10.5	D37.05	D49.0
vallecula	C10.0	C79.89	D00.08	D10.5	D37.05	D49.0
os						
external	C53.1	C79.82	D06.1	D26.0	D39.0	D49.59
internal	C53.0	C79.82	D06.0	D26.0	D39.0	D49.59
ovary	C56.-	C79.6-	D07.39	D27.-	D39.1-	D49.59
oviduct	C57.0-	C79.82	D07.39	D28.2	D39.8	D49.59
palate	C05.9	C79.89	D00.00	D10.39	D37.09	D49.0
hard	C05.0	C79.89	D00.05	D10.39	D37.09	D49.0
junction of hard and soft palate	C05.9	C79.89	D00.00	D10.39	D37.09	D49.0
overlapping lesions	C05.8	-	-	-	-	-
soft	C05.1	C79.89	D00.04	D10.39	D37.09	D49.0
nasopharyngeal surface	C11.3	C79.89	D00.08	D10.6	D37.05	D49.0
posterior surface	C11.3	C79.89	D00.08	D10.6	D37.05	D49.0
superior surface	C11.3	C79.89	D00.08	D10.6	D37.05	D49.0
palatoglossal arch	C09.1	C79.89	D00.00	D10.5	D37.09	D49.0
palatopharyngeal arch	C09.1	C79.89	D00.00	D10.5	D37.09	D49.0
pallium	C71.0	C79.31	-	D33.0	D43.0	D49.6
palpebra	C44.10-	C79.2	D04.1-	D23.1-	D48.5	D49.2
basal cell carcinoma	C44.11-	-	-	-	-	-
specified type NEC	C44.19-	-	-	-	-	-
squamous cell carcinoma	C44.12-	-	-	-	-	-
pancreas	C25.9	C78.89	D01.7	D13.6	D37.8	D49.0
body	C25.1	C78.89	D01.7	D13.6	D37.8	D49.0
duct (of Santorini) (of Wirsung)	C25.3	C78.89	D01.7	D13.6	D37.8	D49.0
ectopic tissue	C25.7	C78.89	-	D13.6	D37.8	D49.0
head	C25.0	C78.89	D01.7	D13.6	D37.8	D49.0
islet cells	C25.4	C78.89	D01.7	D13.7	D37.8	D49.0
neck	C25.7	C78.89	D01.7	D13.6	D37.8	D49.0
overlapping lesion	C25.8	-	-	-	-	-
tail	C25.2	C78.89	D01.7	D13.6	D37.8	D49.0
para-aortic body	C75.5	C79.89	-	D35.6	D44.7	D49.7
paraganglion NEC	C75.5	C79.89	-	D35.6	D44.7	D49.7
parametrium	C57.3	C79.82	-	D28.2	D39.8	D49.59
paranephric	C48.0	C78.6	-	D20.0	D48.3	D49.0
pararectal	C76.3	C79.89	-	D36.7	D48.7	D49.89
parasagittal (region)	C76.0	C79.89	D09.8	D36.7	D48.7	D49.89
parasellar	C72.9	C79.49	-	D33.9	D43.8	D49.7
parathyroid (gland)	C75.0	C79.89	D09.3	D35.1	D44.2	D49.7
paraurethral	C76.3	C79.89	-	D36.7	D48.7	D49.89
gland	C68.1	C79.19	D09.19	D30.8	D41.8	D49.59
paravaginal	C76.3	C79.89	-	D36.7	D48.7	D49.89
parenchyma, kidney	C64.-	C79.0-	D09.19	D30.0-	D41.0-	D49.51-
parietal						
bone	C41.0	C79.51	-	D16.4-	D48.0	D49.2
lobe, brain	C71.3	C79.31	-	D33.0	D43.0	D49.6
paroophoron	C57.1	C79.82	D07.39	D28.2	D39.8	D49.59
parotid (duct) (gland)	C07	C79.89	D00.00	D11.0	D37.030	D49.0
parovarium	C57.1	C79.82	D07.39	D28.2	D39.8	D49.59
patella	C40.20	C79.51	-	-	-	-
peduncle, cerebral	C71.7	C79.31	-	D33.1	D43.1	D49.6
pelvirectal junction	C19	C78.5	D01.1	D12.7	D37.5	D49.0
pelvis, pelvic	C76.3	C79.89	D09.8	D36.7	D48.7	D49.89
bone	C41.4	C79.51	-	D16.8	D48.0	D49.2
floor	C76.3	C79.89	D09.8	D36.7	D48.7	D49.89
renal	C65.-	C79.0-	D09.19	D30.1-	D41.1-	D49.51-
viscera	C76.3	C79.89	D09.8	D36.7	D48.7	D49.89
wall	C76.3	C79.89	D09.8	D36.7	D48.7	D49.89
pelvo-abdominal	C76.8	C79.89	D09.8	D36.7	D48.7	D49.89
penis	C60.9	C79.82	D07.4	D29.0	D40.8	D49.59
body	C60.2	C79.82	D07.4	D29.0	D40.8	D49.59
corpus (cavernosum)	C60.2	C79.82	D07.4	D29.0	D40.8	D49.59
glans	C60.1	C79.82	D07.4	D29.0	D40.8	D49.59
overlapping sites	C60.8	-	-	-	-	-
skin NEC	C60.9	C79.82	D07.4	D29.0	D40.8	D49.59
periadrenal (tissue)	C48.0	C78.6	-	D20.0	D48.3	D49.0
perianal (skin) (*see also* Neoplasm, anus, skin)	C44.500	C79.2	D04.5	D23.5	D48.5	D49.2
pericardium	C38.0	C79.89	-	D15.1	D48.7	D49.89
perinephric	C48.0	C78.6	-	D20.0	D48.3	D49.0
perineum	C76.3	C79.89	D09.8	D36.7	D48.7	D49.89
periodontal tissue NEC	C03.9	C79.89	D00.03	D10.39	D37.09	D49.0
periosteum — *see* Neoplasm, bone						
peripancreatic	C48.0	C78.6	-	D20.0	D48.3	D49.0
peripheral nerve NEC	C47.9	C79.89	-	D36.10	D48.2	D49.2
perirectal (tissue)	C76.3	C79.89	-	D36.7	D48.7	D49.89
perirenal (tissue)	C48.0	C78.6	-	D20.0	D48.3	D49.0
peritoneum, peritoneal (cavity)	C48.2	C78.6	-	D20.1	D48.4	D49.0
benign mesothelial tissue — *see* Mesothelioma, benign						
overlapping lesion	C48.8	-	-	-	-	-
with digestive organs	C26.9	-	-	-	-	-
parietal	C48.1	C78.6	-	D20.1	D48.4	D49.0
peritoneum — *continued*						
pelvic	C48.1	C78.6	-	D20.1	D48.4	D49.0
specified part NEC	C48.1	C78.6	-	D20.1	D48.4	D49.0
peritonsillar (tissue)	C76.0	C79.89	D09.8	D36.7	D48.7	D49.89
periurethral tissue	C76.3	C79.89	-	D36.7	D48.7	D49.89
phalanges						
foot	C40.3-	C79.51	-	D16.3-	-	-
hand	C40.1-	C79.51	-	D16.1-	-	-
pharynx, pharyngeal	C14.0	C79.89	D00.08	D10.9	D37.05	D49.0
bursa	C11.1	C79.89	D00.08	D10.6	D37.05	D49.0
fornix	C11.3	C79.89	D00.08	D10.6	D37.05	D49.0
recess	C11.2	C79.89	D00.08	D10.6	D37.05	D49.0
region	C14.0	C79.89	D00.08	D10.9	D37.05	D49.0
tonsil	C11.1	C79.89	D00.08	D10.6	D37.05	D49.0
wall (lateral) (posterior)	C14.0	C79.89	D00.08	D10.9	D37.05	D49.0
pia mater	C70.9	C79.40	-	D32.9	D42.9	D49.7
cerebral	C70.0	C79.32	-	D32.0	D42.0	D49.7
cranial	C70.0	C79.32	-	D32.0	D42.0	D49.7
spinal	C70.1	C79.49	-	D32.1	D42.1	D49.7
pillars of fauces	C09.1	C79.89	D00.08	D10.5	D37.05	D49.0
pineal (body) (gland)	C75.3	C79.89	D09.3	D35.4	D44.5	D49.7
pinna (ear) NEC (*see also* Neoplasm, skin, ear)	C44.20-	C79.2	D04.2-	D23.2-	D48.5	D49.2
piriform fossa or sinus	C12	C79.89	D00.08	D10.7	D37.05	D49.0
pituitary (body) (fossa) (gland) (lobe)	C75.1	C79.89	D09.3	D35.2	D44.3	D49.7
placenta	C58	C79.82	D07.0	D26.7	D39.2	D49.59
pleura, pleural (cavity)	C38.4	C78.2	-	D19.0	D38.2	D49.1
overlapping lesion with heart or mediastinum	C38.8	-	-	-	-	-
parietal	C38.4	C78.2	-	D19.0	D38.2	D49.1
visceral	C38.4	C78.2	-	D19.0	D38.2	D49.1
plexus						
brachial	C47.1-	C79.89	-	D36.12	D48.2	D49.2
cervical	C47.0	C79.89	-	D36.11	D48.2	D49.2
choroid	C71.5	C79.31	-	D33.0	D43.0	D49.6
lumbosacral	C47.5	C79.89	-	D36.16	D48.2	D49.2
sacral	C47.5	C79.89	-	D36.16	D48.2	D49.2
pluriendocrine	C75.8	C79.89	D09.3	D35.7	D44.9	D49.7
pole						
frontal	C71.1	C79.31	-	D33.0	D43.0	D49.6
occipital	C71.4	C79.31	-	D33.0	D43.0	D49.6
pons (varolii)	C71.7	C79.31	-	D33.1	D43.1	D49.6
popliteal fossa or space	C76.5-	C79.89	D04.7-	D36.7	D48.7	D49.89
postcricoid (region)	C13.0	C79.89	D00.08	D10.7	D37.05	D49.0
posterior fossa (cranial)	C71.9	C79.31	-	D33.2	D43.2	D49.6
postnasal space	C11.9	C79.89	D00.08	D10.6	D37.05	D49.0
prepuce	C60.0	C79.82	D07.4	D29.0	D40.8	D49.59
prepylorus	C16.4	C78.89	D00.2	D13.1	D37.1	D49.0
presacral (region)	C76.3	C79.89	-	D36.7	D48.7	D49.89
prostate (gland)	C61	C79.82	D07.5	D29.1	D40.0	D49.59
utricle	C68.0	C79.19	D09.19	D30.4	D41.3	D49.59
pterygoid fossa	C49.0	C79.89	-	D21.0	D48.1	D49.2
pubic bone	C41.4	C79.51	-	D16.8	D48.0	D49.2
pudenda, pudendum (female)	C51.9	C79.82	D07.1	D28.0	D39.8	D49.59
pulmonary (*see also* Neoplasm, lung)	C34.9-	C78.0-	D02.2-	D14.3-	D38.1	D49.1
putamen	C71.0	C79.31	-	D33.0	D43.0	D49.6
pyloric						
antrum	C16.3	C78.89	D00.2	D13.1	D37.1	D49.0
canal	C16.4	C78.89	D00.2	D13.1	D37.1	D49.0
pylorus	C16.4	C78.89	D00.2	D13.1	D37.1	D49.0
pyramid (brain)	C71.7	C79.31	-	D33.1	D43.1	D49.6
pyriform fossa or sinus	C12	C79.89	D00.08	D10.7	D37.05	D49.0
radius (any part)	C40.0-	C79.51	-	D16.0-	-	-
Rathke's pouch	C75.1	C79.89	D09.3	D35.2	D44.3	D49.7
rectosigmoid (junction)	C19	C78.5	D01.1	D12.7	D37.5	D49.0
overlapping lesion with anus or rectum	C21.8	-	-	-	-	-
rectouterine pouch	C48.1	C78.6	-	D20.1	D48.4	D49.0
rectovaginal septum or wall	C76.3	C79.89	D09.8	D36.7	D48.7	D49.89
rectovesical septum	C76.3	C79.89	D09.8	D36.7	D48.7	D49.89
rectum (ampulla)	C20	C78.5	D01.2	D12.8	D37.5	D49.0
and colon	C19	C78.5	D01.1	D12.7	D37.5	D49.0
overlapping lesion with anus or rectosigmoid junction	C21.8	-	-	-	-	-
renal	C64.-	C79.0-	D09.19	D30.0-	D41.0-	D49.51-
calyx	C65.-	C79.0-	D09.19	D30.1-	D41.1-	D49.51-
hilus	C65.-	C79.0-	D09.19	D30.1-	D41.1-	D49.51-
parenchyma	C64.-	C79.0-	D09.19	D30.0-	D41.0-	D49.51-
pelvis	C65.-	C79.0-	D09.19	D30.1-	D41.1-	D49.51-
respiratory						
organs or system NEC	C39.9	C78.30	D02.4	D14.4	D38.6	D49.1
tract NEC	C39.9	C78.30	D02.4	D14.4	D38.5	D49.1
upper	C39.0	C78.30	D02.4	D14.4	D38.5	D49.1
retina	C69.2-	C79.49	D09.2-	D31.2-	D48.7	D49.81
retrobulbar	C69.6-	C79.49	-	D31.6-	D48.7	D49.89
retrocecal	C48.0	C78.6	-	D20.0	D48.3	D49.0
retromolar (area) (triangle) (trigone)	C06.2	C79.89	D00.00	D10.39	D37.09	D49.0
retro-orbital	C76.0	C79.89	D09.8	D36.7	D48.7	D49.89
retroperitoneal (space) (tissue)	C48.0	C78.6	-	D20.0	D48.3	D49.0

retroperitoneum - skin

Neoplasm	Malignant Primary	Malignant Secondary	Ca in situ	Benign	Uncertain Behavior	Unspecified Behavior
retroperitoneum	C48.0	C78.6	-	D20.0	D48.3	D49.0
retropharyngeal	C14.0	C79.89	D00.08	D10.9	D37.05	D49.0
retrovesical (septum)	C76.3	C79.89	D09.8	D36.7	D48.7	D49.89
rhinencephalon	C71.0	C79.31	-	D33.0	D43.0	D49.6
rib	C41.3	C79.51	-	D16.7	D48.0	D49.2
Rosenmuller's fossa	C11.2	C79.89	D00.08	D10.6	D37.05	D49.0
round ligament	C57.2	C79.82	-	D28.2	D39.8	D49.59
sacrococcyx, sacrococcygeal	C41.4	C79.51	D16.8	D48.0	D49.2	
region	C76.3	C79.89	D09.8	D36.7	D48.7	D49.89
sacrouterine ligament	C57.3	C79.82	-	D28.2	D39.8	D49.59
sacrum, sacral (vertebra)	C41.4	C79.51	-	D16.8	D48.0	D49.2
salivary gland or duct (major)	C08.9	C79.89	D00.00	D11.9	D37.039	D49.0
minor NEC	C06.9	C79.89	D00.00	D10.39	D37.04	D49.0
overlapping lesion	C08.9	-	-	-	-	-
parotid	C07	C79.89	D00.00	D11.0	D37.030	D49.0
pluriglandular	C08.9	C79.89	D00.00	D11.9	D37.039	D49.0
sublingual	C08.1	C79.89	D00.00	D11.7	D37.031	D49.0
submandibular	C08.0	C79.89	D00.00	D11.7	D37.032	D49.0
submaxillary	C08.0	C79.89	D00.00	D11.7	D37.032	D49.0
salpinx (uterine)	C57.0-	C79.82	D07.39	D28.2	D39.8	D49.59
Santorini's duct	C25.3	C78.89	D01.7	D13.6	D37.8	D49.0
scalp	C44.40	C79.2	D04.4	D23.4	D48.5	D49.2
basal cell carcinoma	C44.41	-	-	-	-	-
specified type NEC	C44.49	-	-	-	-	-
squamous cell carcinoma	C44.42	-	-	-	-	-
scapula (any part)	C40.0-	C79.51	-	D16.0-	-	-
scapular region	C76.1	C79.89	D09.8	D36.7	D48.7	D49.89
scar NEC (*see also* Neoplasm, skin, by site)	C44.90	C79.2	D04.9	D23.9	D48.5	D49.2
sciatic nerve	C47.2-	C79.89	-	D36.13	D48.2	D49.2
sclera	C69.4-	C79.49	D09.2-	D31.4-	D48.7	D49.89
scrotum (skin)	C63.2	C79.82	D07.61	D29.4	D40.8	D49.59
sebaceous gland — *see* Neoplasm, skin						
sella turcica	C75.1	C79.89	D09.3	D35.2	D44.3	D49.7
bone	C41.0	C79.51	-	D16.4-	D48.0	D49.2
semilunar cartilage (knee)	C40.2-	C79.51	-	D16.2-	D48.0	D49.2
seminal vesicle	C63.7	C79.82	D07.69	D29.8	D40.8	D49.59
septum						
nasal	C30.0	C78.39	D02.3	D14.0	D38.5	D49.1
posterior margin	C11.3	C79.89	D00.08	D10.6	D37.05	D49.0
rectovaginal	C76.3	C79.89	D09.8	D36.7	D48.7	D49.89
rectovesical	C76.3	C79.89	D09.8	D36.7	D48.7	D49.89
urethrovaginal	C57.9	C79.82	D07.30	D28.9	D39.9	D49.59
vesicovaginal	C57.9	C79.82	D07.30	D28.9	D39.9	D49.59
shoulder NEC	C76.4-	C79.89	D04.6-	D36.7	D48.7	D49.89
sigmoid flexure (lower) (upper)	C18.7	C78.5	D01.0	D12.5	D37.4	D49.0
sinus (accessory)	C31.9	C78.39	D02.3	D14.0	D38.5	D49.1
bone (any)	C41.0	C79.51	-	D16.4-	D48.0	D49.2
ethmoidal	C31.1	C78.39	D02.3	D14.0	D38.5	D49.1
frontal	C31.2	C78.39	D02.3	D14.0	D38.5	D49.1
maxillary	C31.0	C78.39	D02.3	D14.0	D38.5	D49.1
nasal, paranasal NEC	C31.9	C78.39	D02.3	D14.0	D38.5	D49.1
overlapping lesion	C31.8	-	-	-	-	-
pyriform	C12	C79.89	D00.08	D10.7	D37.05	D49.0
sphenoid	C31.3	C78.39	D02.3	D14.0	D38.5	D49.1
skeleton, skeletal NEC	C41.9	C79.51	-	D16.9-	D48.0	D49.2
Skene's gland	C68.1	C79.19	D09.19	D30.8	D41.8	D49.59
skin NOS	C44.90	C79.2	D04.9	D23.9	D48.5	D49.2
abdominal wall	C44.509	C79.2	D04.5	D23.5	D48.5	D49.2
basal cell carcinoma	C44.519	-	-	-	-	-
specified type NEC	C44.599	-	-	-	-	-
squamous cell carcinoma	C44.529	-	-	-	-	-
ala nasi (*see also* Neoplasm, nose, skin)	C44.301	C79.2	D04.39	D23.39	D48.5	D49.2
ankle (*see also* Neoplasm, skin, limb, lower)	C44.70-	C79.2	D04.7-	D23.7-	D48.5	D49.2
antecubital space (*see also* Neoplasm, skin, limb, upper)	C44.60-	C79.2	D04.6-	D23.6-	D48.5	D49.2
anus	C44.500	C79.2	D04.5	D23.5	D48.5	D49.2
basal cell carcinoma	C44.510	-	-	-	-	-
specified type NEC	C44.590	-	-	-	-	-
squamous cell carcinoma	C44.520	-	-	-	-	-
arm (*see also* Neoplasm, skin, limb, upper)	C44.60-	C79.2	D04.6-	D23.6-	D48.5	D49.2
auditory canal (external) (*see also* Neoplasm, skin, ear)	C44.20-	C79.2	D04.2-	D23.2-	D48.5	D49.2
auricle (ear) (*see also* Neoplasm, skin, ear)	C44.20-	C79.2	D04.2-	D23.2-	D48.5	D49.2
auricular canal (external) (*see also* Neoplasm, skin, ear)	C44.20-	C79.2	D04.2-	D23.2-	D48.5	D49.2
axilla, axillary fold (*see also* Neoplasm, skin, trunk)	C44.509	C79.2	D04.5	D23.5	D48.5	D49.2
back (*see also* Neoplasm, skin, trunk)	C44.509	C79.2	D04.5	D23.5	D48.5	D49.2
basal cell carcinoma	C44.91					
breast	C44.501	C79.2	D04.5	D23.5	D48.5	D49.2
basal cell carcinoma	C44.511	-	-	-	-	-
specified type NEC	C44.591	-	-	-	-	-
squamous cell carcinoma	C44.521	-	-	-	-	-
brow (*see also* Neoplasm, skin, face)	C44.309	C79.2	D04.39	D23.39	D48.5	D49.2
skin NOS — *continued*						
buttock (*see also* Neoplasm, skin, trunk)	C44.509	C79.2	D04.5	D23.5	D48.5	D49.2
calf (*see also* Neoplasm, skin, limb, lower)	C44.70-	C79.2	D04.7-	D23.7-	D48.5	D49.2
canthus (eye) (inner) (outer)	C44.10-	C79.2	D04.1-	D23.1-	D48.5	D49.2
basal cell carcinoma	C44.11-	-	-	-	-	-
specified type NEC	C44.19-	-	-	-	-	-
squamous cell carcinoma	C44.12-	-	-	-	-	-
cervical region (*see also* Neoplasm, skin, neck)	C44.40	C79.2	D04.4	D23.4	D48.5	D49.2
cheek (external) (*see also* Neoplasm, skin, face)	C44.309	C79.2	D04.39	D23.39	D48.5	D49.2
chest (wall) (*see also* Neoplasm, skin, trunk)	C44.509	C79.2	D04.5	D23.5	D48.5	D49.2
chin (*see also* Neoplasm, skin, face)	C44.309	C79.2	D04.39	D23.39	D48.5	D49.2
clavicular area (*see also* Neoplasm, skin, trunk)	C44.509	C79.2	D04.5	D23.5	D48.5	D49.2
clitoris	C51.2	C79.82	D07.1	D28.0	D39.8	D49.59
columnella (*see also* Neoplasm, skin, face)	C44.309	C79.2	D04.39	D23.39	D48.5	D49.2
concha (*see also* Neoplasm, skin, ear)	C44.20-	C79.2	D04.2-	D23.2-	D48.5	D49.2
ear (external)	C44.20-	C79.2	D04.2-	D23.2-	D48.5	D49.2
basal cell carcinoma	C44.21-	-	-	-	-	-
specified type NEC	C44.29-	-	-	-	-	-
squamous cell carcinoma	C44.22-	-	-	-	-	-
elbow (*see also* Neoplasm, skin, limb, upper)	C44.60-	C79.2	D04.6-	D23.6-	D48.5	D49.2
eyebrow (*see also* Neoplasm, skin, face)	C44.309	C79.2	D04.39	D23.39	D48.5	D49.2
eyelid	C44.10-	C79.2	D04.1-	D23.1-	D48.5	D49.2
basal cell carcinoma	C44.11-	-	-	-	-	-
specified type NEC	C44.19-	-	-	-	-	-
squamous cell carcinoma	C44.12-	-	-	-	-	-
face NOS	C44.300	C79.2	D04.30	D23.30	D48.5	D49.2
basal cell carcinoma	C44.310	-	-	-	-	-
specified type NEC	C44.390	-	-	-	-	-
squamous cell carcinoma	C44.320	-	-	-	-	-
female genital organs (external)	C51.9	C79.82	D07.1	D28.0	D39.8	D49.59
clitoris	C51.2	C79.82	D07.1	D28.0	D39.8	D49.59
labium NEC	C51.9	C79.82	D07.1	D28.0	D39.8	D49.59
majus	C51.0	C79.82	D07.1	D28.0	D39.8	D49.59
minus	C51.1	C79.82	D07.1	D28.0	D39.8	D49.59
pudendum	C51.9	C79.82	D07.1	D28.0	D39.8	D49.59
vulva	C51.9	C79.82	D07.1	D28.0	D39.8	D49.59
finger (*see also* Neoplasm, skin, limb, upper)	C44.60-	C79.2	D04.6-	D23.6-	D48.5	D49.2
flank (*see also* Neoplasm, skin, trunk)	C44.509	C79.2	D04.5	D23.5	D48.5	D49.2
foot (*see also* Neoplasm, skin, limb, lower)	C44.70-	C79.2	D04.7-	D23.7-	D48.5	D49.2
forearm (*see also* Neoplasm, skin, limb, upper)	C44.60-	C79.2	D04.6-	D23.6-	D48.5	D49.2
forehead (*see also* Neoplasm, skin, face)	C44.309	C79.2	D04.39	D23.39	D48.5	D49.2
glabella (*see also* Neoplasm, skin, face)	C44.309	C79.2	D04.39	D23.39	D48.5	D49.2
gluteal region (*see also* Neoplasm, skin, trunk)	C44.509	C79.2	D04.5	D23.5	D48.5	D49.2
groin (*see also* Neoplasm, skin, trunk)	C44.509	C79.2	D04.5	D23.5	D48.5	D49.2
hand (*see also* Neoplasm, skin, limb, upper)	C44.60-	C79.2	D04.6-	D23.6-	D48.5	D49.2
head NEC (*see also* Neoplasm, skin, scalp)	C44.40	C79.2	D04.4	D23.4	D48.5	D49.2
heel (*see also* Neoplasm, skin, limb, lower)	C44.70-	C79.2	D04.7-	D23.7-	D48.5	D49.2
helix (*see also* Neoplasm, skin, ear)	C44.20-	C79.2	D04.2-	D23.2-	D48.5	D49.2
hip (*see also* Neoplasm, skin, limb, lower)	C44.70-	C79.2	D04.7-	D23.7-	D48.5	D49.2
infraclavicular region (*see also* Neoplasm, skin, trunk)	C44.509	C79.2	D04.5	D23.5	D48.5	D49.2
inguinal region (*see also* Neoplasm, skin, trunk)	C44.509	C79.2	D04.5	D23.5	D48.5	D49.2
jaw (*see also* Neoplasm, skin, face)	C44.309	C79.2	D04.39	D23.39	D48.5	D49.2
Kaposi's sarcoma — *see* Kaposi's, sarcoma, skin						
knee (*see also* Neoplasm, skin, limb, lower)	C44.70-	C79.2	D04.7-	D23.7-	D48.5	D49.2
labia						
majora	C51.0	C79.82	D07.1	D28.0	D39.8	D49.59
minora	C51.1	C79.82	D07.1	D28.0	D39.8	D49.59
leg (*see also* Neoplasm, skin, limb, lower)	C44.70-	C79.2	D04.7-	D23.7-	D48.5	D49.2
lid (lower) (upper)	C44.10-	C79.2	D04.1-	D23.1-	D48.5	D49.2
basal cell carcinoma	C44.11-	-	-	-	-	-
specified type NEC	C44.19-	-	-	-	-	-
squamous cell carcinoma	C44.12-	-	-	-	-	-
limb NEC	C44.90	C79.2	D04.9	D23.9	D48.5	D49.2

Neoplasm	Malignant Primary	Malignant Secondary	Ca in situ	Benign	Uncertain Behavior	Unspecified Behavior
skin NOS — *continued*						
limb NEC — *continued*						
basal cell carcinoma	C44.91					
lower	C44.70-	C79.2	D04.7-	D23.7-	D48.5	D49.2
basal cell carcinoma	C44.71-	-	-	-	-	-
specified type NEC	C44.79-	-	-	-	-	-
squamous cell carcinoma	C44.72-	-	-	-	-	-
upper	C44.60-	C79.2	D04.6-	D23.6-	D48.5	D49.2
basal cell carcinoma	C44.61-	-	-	-	-	-
specified type NEC	C44.69-	-	-	-	-	-
squamous cell carcinoma	C44.62-	-	-	-	-	-
lip (lower) (upper)	C44.00	C79.2	D04.0	D23.0	D48.5	D49.2
basal cell carcinoma	C44.01	-	-	-	-	-
specified type NEC	C44.09	-	-	-	-	-
squamous cell carcinoma	C44.02	-	-	-	-	-
male genital organs	C63.9	C79.82	D07.60	D29.9	D40.8	D49.59
penis	C60.9	C79.82	D07.4	D29.0	D40.8	D49.59
prepuce	C60.0	C79.82	D07.4	D29.0	D40.8	D49.59
scrotum	C63.2	C79.82	D07.61	D29.4	D40.8	D49.59
mastectomy site (skin) (*see also* Neoplasm, skin, breast)	C44.501	C79.2	-	-	-	-
specified as breast tissue	C50.8-	C79.81	-	-	-	-
meatus, acoustic (external) (*see also* Neoplasm, skin, ear)	C44.20-	C79.2	D04.2-	D23.2-	D48.5	D49.2
melanotic — *see* Melanoma						
Merkel cell — *see* Carcinoma, Merkel cell						
nates (*see also* Neoplasm, skin, trunk)	C44.509	C79.2	D04.5	D23.5	D48.5	D49.2
neck	C44.40	C79.2	D04.4	D23.4	D48.5	D49.2
basal cell carcinoma	C44.41	-	-	-	-	-
specified type NEC	C44.49	-	-	-	-	-
squamous cell carcinoma	C44.42	-	-	-	-	-
nevus — *see* Nevus, skin						
nose (external) (*see also* Neoplasm, nose, skin)	C44.301	C79.2	D04.39	D23.39	D48.5	D49.2
overlapping lesion	C44.80	-	-	-	-	-
basal cell carcinoma	C44.81	-	-	-	-	-
specified type NEC	C44.89	-	-	-	-	-
squamous cell carcinoma	C44.82	-	-	-	-	-
palm (*see also* Neoplasm, skin, limb, upper)	C44.60-	C79.2	D04.6-	D23.6-	D48.5	D49.2
palpebra	C44.10-	C79.2	D04.1-	D23.1-	D48.5	D49.2
basal cell carcinoma	C44.11-	-	-	-	-	-
specified type NEC	C44.19-	-	-	-	-	-
squamous cell carcinoma	C44.12-	-	-	-	-	-
penis NEC	C60.9	C79.82	D07.4	D29.0	D40.8	D49.59
perianal (*see also* Neoplasm, skin, anus)	C44.500	C79.2	D04.5	D23.5	D48.5	D49.2
perineum (*see also* Neoplasm, skin, anus)	C44.500	C79.2	D04.5	D23.5	D48.5	D49.2
pinna (*see also* Neoplasm, skin, ear)	C44.20-	C79.2	D04.2-	D23.2-	D48.5	D49.2
plantar (*see also* Neoplasm, skin, limb, lower)	C44.70-	C79.2	D04.7-	D23.7-	D48.5	D49.2
popliteal fossa or space (*see also* Neoplasm, skin, limb, lower)	C44.70-	C79.2	D04.7-	D23.7-	D48.5	D49.2
prepuce	C60.0	C79.82	D07.4	D29.0	D40.8	D49.59
pubes (*see also* Neoplasm, skin, trunk)	C44.509	C79.2	D04.5	D23.5	D48.5	D49.2
sacrococcygeal region (*see also* Neoplasm, skin, trunk)	C44.509	C79.2	D04.5	D23.5	D48.5	D49.2
scalp	C44.40	C79.2	D04.4	D23.4	D48.5	D49.2
basal cell carcinoma	C44.41	-	-	-	-	-
specified type NEC	C44.49	-	-	-	-	-
squamous cell carcinoma	C44.42	-	-	-	-	-
scapular region (*see also* Neoplasm, skin, trunk)	C44.509	C79.2	D04.5	D23.5	D48.5	D49.2
scrotum	C63.2	C79.82	D07.61	D29.4	D40.8	D49.59
shoulder (*see also* Neoplasm, skin, limb, upper)	C44.60-	C79.2	D04.6-	D23.6-	D48.5	D49.2
sole (foot) (*see also* Neoplasm, skin, limb, lower)	C44.70-	C79.2	D04.7-	D23.7-	D48.5	D49.2
specified sites NEC	C44.80	C79.2	D04.8	D23.9	D48.5	D49.2
basal cell carcinoma	C44.81	-	-	-	-	-
specified type NEC	C44.89	-	-	-	-	-
squamous cell carcinoma	C44.82	-	-	-	-	-
specified type NEC	C44.99	-	-	-	-	-
squamous cell carcinoma	C44.92	-	-	-	-	-
submammary fold (*see also* Neoplasm, skin, trunk)	C44.509	C79.2	D04.5	D23.5	D48.5	D49.2
supraclavicular region (*see also* Neoplasm, skin, neck)	C44.40	C79.2	D04.4	D23.4	D48.5	D49.2
temple (*see also* Neoplasm, skin, face)	C44.309	C79.2	D04.39	D23.39	D48.5	D49.2
thigh (*see also* Neoplasm, skin, limb, lower)	C44.70-	C79.2	D04.7-	D23.7-	D48.5	D49.2
thoracic wall (*see also* Neoplasm, skin, trunk)	C44.509	C79.2	D04.5	D23.5	D48.5	D49.2
thumb (*see also* Neoplasm, skin, limb, upper)	C44.60-	C79.2	D04.6-	D23.6-	D48.5	D49.2
skin NOS — *continued*						
toe (*see also* Neoplasm, skin, limb, lower)	C44.70-	C79.2	D04.7-	D23.7-	D48.5	D49.2
tragus (*see also* Neoplasm, skin, ear)	C44.20-	C79.2	D04.2-	D23.2-	D48.5	D49.2
trunk	C44.509	C79.2	D04.5	D23.5	D48.5	D49.2
basal cell carcinoma	C44.519	-	-	-	-	-
specified type NEC	C44.599	-	-	-	-	-
squamous cell carcinoma	C44.529	-	-	-	-	-
umbilicus (*see also* Neoplasm, skin, trunk)	C44.509	C79.2	D04.5	D23.5	D48.5	D49.2
vulva	C51.9	C79.82	D07.1	D28.0	D39.8	D49.59
overlapping lesion	C51.8	-	-	-	-	-
wrist (*see also* Neoplasm, skin, limb, upper)	C44.60-	C79.2	D04.6-	D23.6-	D48.5	D49.2
skull	C41.0	C79.51	-	D16.4-	D48.0	D49.2
soft parts or tissues — *see* Neoplasm, connective tissue						
specified site NEC	C76.8	C79.89	D09.8	D36.7	D48.7	D49.89
spermatic cord	C63.1-	C79.82	D07.69	D29.8	D40.8	D49.59
sphenoid	C31.3	C78.39	D02.3	D14.0	D38.5	D49.1
bone	C41.0	C79.51	-	D16.4-	D48.0	D49.2
sinus	C31.3	C78.39	D02.3	D14.0	D38.5	D49.1
sphincter						
anal	C21.1	C78.5	D01.3	D12.9	D37.8	D49.0
of Oddi	C24.0	C78.89	D01.5	D13.5	D37.6	D49.0
spine, spinal (column)	C41.2	C79.51	-	D16.6	D48.0	D49.2
bulb	C71.7	C79.31	-	D33.1	D43.1	D49.6
coccyx	C41.4	C79.51	-	D16.8	D48.0	D49.2
cord (cervical) (lumbar) (sacral) (thoracic)	C72.0	C79.49	-	D33.4	D43.4	D49.7
dura mater	C70.1	C79.49	-	D32.1	D42.1	D49.7
lumbosacral	C41.2	C79.51	-	D16.6	D48.0	D49.2
marrow NEC	C96.9	C79.52	-	-	D47.9	D49.89
membrane	C70.1	C79.49	-	D32.1	D42.1	D49.7
meninges	C70.1	C79.49	-	D32.1	D42.1	D49.7
nerve (root)	C47.9	C79.89	-	D36.10	D48.2	D49.2
pia mater	C70.1	C79.49	-	D32.1	D42.1	D49.7
root	C47.9	C79.89	-	D36.10	D48.2	D49.2
sacrum	C41.4	C79.51	-	D16.8	D48.0	D49.2
spleen, splenic NEC	C26.1	C78.89	D01.7	D13.9	D37.8	D49.0
flexure (colon)	C18.5	C78.5	D01.0	D12.3	D37.4	D49.0
stem, brain	C71.7	C79.31	-	D33.1	D43.1	D49.6
Stensen's duct	C07	C79.89	D00.00	D11.0	D37.030	D49.0
sternum	C41.3	C79.51	-	D16.7	D48.0	D49.2
stomach	C16.9	C78.89	D00.2	D13.1	D37.1	D49.0
antrum (pyloric)	C16.3	C78.89	D00.2	D13.1	D37.1	D49.0
body	C16.2	C78.89	D00.2	D13.1	D37.1	D49.0
cardia	C16.0	C78.89	D00.2	D13.1	D37.1	D49.0
cardiac orifice	C16.0	C78.89	D00.2	D13.1	D37.1	D49.0
corpus	C16.2	C78.89	D00.2	D13.1	D37.1	D49.0
fundus	C16.1	C78.89	D00.2	D13.1	D37.1	D49.0
greater curvature NEC	C16.6	C78.89	D00.2	D13.1	D37.1	D49.0
lesser curvature NEC	C16.5	C78.89	D00.2	D13.1	D37.1	D49.0
overlapping lesion	C16.8	-	-	-	-	-
prepylorus	C16.4	C78.89	D00.2	D13.1	D37.1	D49.0
pylorus	C16.4	C78.89	D00.2	D13.1	D37.1	D49.0
wall NEC	C16.9	C78.89	D00.2	D13.1	D37.1	D49.0
anterior NEC	C16.8	C78.89	D00.2	D13.1	D37.1	D49.0
posterior NEC	C16.8	C78.89	D00.2	D13.1	D37.1	D49.0
stroma, endometrial	C54.1	C79.82	D07.0	D26.1	D39.0	D49.59
stump, cervical	C53.8	C79.82	D06.7	D26.0	D39.0	D49.59
subcutaneous (nodule) (tissue) NEC — *see* Neoplasm, connective tissue						
subdural	C70.9	C79.32	-	D32.9	D42.9	D49.7
subglottis, subglottic	C32.2	C78.39	D02.0	D14.1	D38.0	D49.1
sublingual	C04.9	C79.89	D00.06	D10.2	D37.09	D49.0
gland or duct	C08.1	C79.89	D00.00	D11.7	D37.031	D49.0
submandibular gland	C08.0	C79.89	D00.00	D11.7	D37.032	D49.0
submaxillary gland or duct	C08.0	C79.89	D00.00	D11.7	D37.032	D49.0
submental	C76.0	C79.89	D09.8	D36.7	D48.7	D49.89
subpleural	C34.9-	C78.0-	D02.2-	D14.3-	D38.1	D49.1
substernal	C38.1	C78.1	-	D15.2	D38.3	D49.89
sudoriferous, sudoriparous gland, site unspecified	C44.90	C79.2	D04.9	D23.9	D48.5	D49.2
specified site — *see* Neoplasm, skin						
supraclavicular region	C76.0	C79.89	D09.8	D36.7	D48.7	D49.89
supraglottis	C32.1	C78.39	D02.0	D14.1	D38.0	D49.1
suprarenal	C74.9-	C79.7-	D09.3	D35.0-	D44.1-	D49.7
capsule	C74.9-	C79.7-	D09.3	D35.0-	D44.1-	D49.7
cortex	C74.0-	C79.7-	D09.3	D35.0-	D44.1-	D49.7
gland	C74.9-	C79.7-	D09.3	D35.0-	D44.1-	D49.7
medulla	C74.1-	C79.7-	D09.3	D35.0-	D44.1-	D49.7
suprasellar (region)	C71.9	C79.31	-	D33.2	D43.2	D49.6
supratentorial (brain) NEC	C71.0	C79.31	-	D33.0	D43.0	D49.6
sweat gland (apocrine) (eccrine), site unspecified	C44.90	C79.2	D04.9	D23.9	D48.5	D49.2
specified site — *see* Neoplasm, skin						
sympathetic nerve or nervous system NEC	C47.9	C79.89	-	D36.10	D48.2	D49.2

Neoplasm	Malignant Primary	Malignant Secondary	Ca in situ	Benign	Uncertain Behavior	Unspecified Behavior
symphysis pubis	C41.4	C79.51	-	D16.8	D48.0	D49.2
synovial membrane — *see* Neoplasm, connective tissue						
tapetum, brain	C71.8	C79.31	-	D33.2	D43.2	D49.6
tarsus (any bone)	C40.3-	C79.51	-	D16.3-	-	-
temple (skin) (*see also* Neoplasm, skin, face)	C44.309	C79.2	D04.39	D23.39	D48.5	D49.2
temporal						
bone	C41.0	C79.51	-	D16.4-	D48.0	D49.2
lobe or pole	C71.2	C79.31	-	D33.0	D43.0	D49.6
region	C76.0	C79.89	D09.8	D36.7	D48.7	D49.89
skin (*see also* Neoplasm, skin, face)	C44.309	C79.2	D04.39	D23.39	D48.5	D49.2
tendon (sheath) — *see* Neoplasm, connective tissue						
tentorium (cerebelli)	C70.0	C79.32	-	D32.0	D42.0	D49.7
testis, testes	C62.9-	C79.82	D07.69	D29.2-	D40.1-	D49.59
descended	C62.1-	C79.82	D07.69	D29.2-	D40.1-	D49.59
ectopic	C62.0-	C79.82	D07.69	D29.2-	D40.1-	D49.59
retained	C62.0-	C79.82	D07.69	D29.2-	D40.1-	D49.59
scrotal	C62.1-	C79.82	D07.69	D29.2-	D40.1-	D49.59
undescended	C62.0-	C79.82	D07.69	D29.2-	D40.1-	D49.59
unspecified whether descended or undescended	C62.9-	C79.82	D07.69	D29.2-	D40.1-	D49.59
thalamus	C71.0	C79.31	-	D33.0	D43.0	D49.6
thigh NEC	C76.5-	C79.89	D04.7-	D36.7	D48.7	D49.89
thorax, thoracic (cavity) (organs NEC)	C76.1	C79.89	D09.8	D36.7	D48.7	D49.89
duct	C49.3	C79.89	-	D21.3	D48.1	D49.2
wall NEC	C76.1	C79.89	D09.8	D36.7	D48.7	D49.89
throat	C14.0	C79.89	D00.08	D10.9	D37.05	D49.0
thumb NEC	C76.4-	C79.89	D04.6-	D36.7	D48.7	D49.89
thymus (gland)	C37	C79.89	D09.3	D15.0	D38.4	D49.89
thyroglossal duct	C73	C79.89	D09.3	D34	D44.0	D49.7
thyroid (gland)	C73	C79.89	D09.3	D34	D44.0	D49.7
cartilage	C32.3	C78.39	D02.0	D14.1	D38.0	D49.1
tibia (any part)	C40.2-	C79.51	-	D16.2-	-	-
toe NEC	C76.5-	C79.89	D04.7-	D36.7	D48.7	D49.89
tongue	C02.9	C79.89	D00.07	D10.1	D37.02	D49.0
anterior (two-thirds) NEC	C02.3	C79.89	D00.07	D10.1	D37.02	D49.0
dorsal surface	C02.0	C79.89	D00.07	D10.1	D37.02	D49.0
ventral surface	C02.2	C79.89	D00.07	D10.1	D37.02	D49.0
base (dorsal surface)	C01	C79.89	D00.07	D10.1	D37.02	D49.0
border (lateral)	C02.1	C79.89	D00.07	D10.1	D37.02	D49.0
dorsal surface NEC	C02.0	C79.89	D00.07	D10.1	D37.02	D49.0
fixed part NEC	C01	C79.89	D00.07	D10.1	D37.02	D49.0
foramen cecum	C02.0	C79.89	D00.07	D10.1	D37.02	D49.0
frenulum linguae	C02.2	C79.89	D00.07	D10.1	D37.02	D49.0
junctional zone	C02.8	C79.89	D00.07	D10.1	D37.02	D49.0
margin (lateral)	C02.1	C79.89	D00.07	D10.1	D37.02	D49.0
midline NEC	C02.0	C79.89	D00.07	D10.1	D37.02	D49.0
mobile part NEC	C02.3	C79.89	D00.07	D10.1	D37.02	D49.0
overlapping lesion	C02.8	-	-	-	-	-
posterior (third)	C01	C79.89	D00.07	D10.1	D37.02	D49.0
root	C01	C79.89	D00.07	D10.1	D37.02	D49.0
surface (dorsal)	C02.0	C79.89	D00.07	D10.1	D37.02	D49.0
base	C01	C79.89	D00.07	D10.1	D37.02	D49.0
ventral	C02.2	C79.89	D00.07	D10.1	D37.02	D49.0
tip	C02.1	C79.89	D00.07	D10.1	D37.02	D49.0
tonsil	C02.4	C79.89	D00.07	D10.1	D37.02	D49.0
tonsil	C09.9	C79.89	D00.08	D10.4	D37.05	D49.0
fauces, faucial	C09.9	C79.89	D00.08	D10.4	D37.05	D49.0
lingual	C02.4	C79.89	D00.07	D10.1	D37.02	D49.0
overlapping sites	C09.8	-	-	-	-	-
palatine	C09.9	C79.89	D00.08	D10.4	D37.05	D49.0
pharyngeal	C11.1	C79.89	D00.08	D10.6	D37.05	D49.0
pillar (anterior) (posterior)	C09.1	C79.89	D00.08	D10.5	D37.05	D49.0
tonsillar fossa	C09.0	C79.89	D00.08	D10.5	D37.05	D49.0
tooth socket NEC	C03.9	C79.89	D00.03	D10.39	D37.09	D49.0
trachea (cartilage) (mucosa)	C33	C78.39	D02.1	D14.2	D38.1	D49.1
overlapping lesion with bronchus or lung	C34.8-	-	-	-	-	-
tracheobronchial	C34.8-	C78.39	D02.1	D14.2	D38.1	D49.1
overlapping lesion with lung	C34.8-	-	-	-	-	-
tragus (*see also* Neoplasm, skin, ear)	C44.20-	C79.2	D04.2-	D23.2-	D48.5	D49.2
trunk NEC	C76.8	C79.89	D04.5	D36.7	D48.7	D49.89
tubo-ovarian	C57.8	C79.82	D07.39	D28.7	D39.8	D49.59
tunica vaginalis	C63.7	C79.82	D07.69	D29.8	D40.8	D49.59
turbinate (bone)	C41.0	C79.51	-	D16.4-	D48.0	D49.2
nasal	C30.0	C78.39	D02.3	D14.0	D38.5	D49.1
tympanic cavity	C30.1	C78.39	D02.3	D14.0	D38.5	D49.1
ulna (any part)	C40.0-	C79.51	-	D16.0-	-	-
umbilicus, umbilical (*see also* Neoplasm, skin, trunk)	C44.509	C79.2	D04.5	D23.5	D48.5	D49.2
uncus, brain	C71.2	C79.31	-	D33.0	D43.0	D49.6
unknown site or unspecified	C80.1	C79.9	D09.9	D36.9	D48.9	D49.9
urachus	C67.7	C79.11	D09.0	D30.3	D41.4	D49.4
ureter, ureteral	C66.-	C79.19	D09.19	D30.2-	D41.2-	D49.59
orifice (bladder)	C67.6	C79.11	D09.0	D30.3	D41.4	D49.4
ureter-bladder (junction)	C67.6	C79.11	D09.0	D30.3	D41.4	D49.4
urethra, urethral (gland)	C68.0	C79.19	D09.19	D30.4	D41.3	D49.59
orifice, internal	C67.5	C79.11	D09.0	D30.3	D41.4	D49.4
urethrovaginal (septum)	C57.9	C79.82	D07.30	D28.9	D39.8	D49.59
urinary organ or system	C68.9	C79.10	D09.10	D30.9	D41.9	D49.59
bladder — *see* Neoplasm, bladder						
overlapping lesion	C68.8	-	-	-	-	-
specified sites NEC	C68.8	C79.19	D09.19	D30.8	D41.8	D49.59
utero-ovarian	C57.8	C79.82	D07.39	D28.7	D39.8	D49.59
ligament	C57.1	C79.82	D07.39	D28.2	D39.8	D49.59
uterosacral ligament	C57.3	C79.82	-	D28.2	D39.8	D49.59
uterus, uteri, uterine	C55	C79.82	D07.0	D26.9	D39.0	D49.59
adnexa NEC	C57.4	C79.82	D07.39	D28.7	D39.8	D49.59
body	C54.9	C79.82	D07.0	D26.1	D39.0	D49.59
cervix	C53.9	C79.82	D06.9	D26.0	D39.0	D49.59
cornu	C54.9	C79.82	D07.0	D26.1	D39.0	D49.59
corpus	C54.9	C79.82	D07.0	D26.1	D39.0	D49.59
endocervix (canal) (gland)	C53.0	C79.82	D06.0	D26.0	D39.0	D49.59
endometrium	C54.1	C79.82	D07.0	D26.1	D39.0	D49.59
exocervix	C53.1	C79.82	D06.1	D26.0	D39.0	D49.59
external os	C53.1	C79.82	D06.1	D26.0	D39.0	D49.59
fundus	C54.3	C79.82	D07.0	D26.1	D39.0	D49.59
internal os	C53.0	C79.82	D06.0	D26.0	D39.0	D49.59
isthmus	C54.0	C79.82	D07.0	D26.1	D39.0	D49.59
ligament	C57.3	C79.82	-	D28.2	D39.8	D49.59
broad	C57.1	C79.82	D07.39	D28.2	D39.8	D49.59
round	C57.2	C79.82	-	D28.2	D39.8	D49.59
lower segment	C54.0	C79.82	D07.0	D26.1	D39.0	D49.59
myometrium	C54.2	C79.82	D07.0	D26.1	D39.0	D49.59
overlapping sites	C54.8	-	-	-	-	-
squamocolumnar junction	C53.8	C79.82	D06.7	D26.0	D39.0	D49.59
tube	C57.0-	C79.82	D07.39	D28.2	D39.8	D49.59
utricle, prostatic	C68.0	C79.19	D09.19	D30.4	D41.3	D49.59
uveal tract	C69.4-	C79.49	D09.2-	D31.4-	D48.7	D49.89
uvula	C05.2	C79.89	D00.04	D10.39	D37.09	D49.0
vagina, vaginal (fornix) (vault) (wall)	C52	C79.82	D07.2	D28.1	D39.8	D49.59
vaginovesical	C57.9	C79.82	D07.30	D28.9	D39.9	D49.59
septum	C57.9	C79.82	D07.30	D28.9	D39.9	D49.59
vallecula (epiglottis)	C10.0	C79.89	D00.08	D10.5	D37.05	D49.0
vas deferens	C63.1-	C79.82	D07.69	D29.8	D40.8	D49.59
vascular — *see* Neoplasm, connective tissue						
Vater's ampulla	C24.1	C78.89	D01.5	D13.5	D37.6	D49.0
vein, venous — *see* Neoplasm, connective tissue						
vena cava (abdominal) (inferior)	C49.4	C79.89	-	D21.4	D48.1	D49.2
superior	C49.3	C79.89	-	D21.3	D48.1	D49.2
ventricle (cerebral) (floor) (lateral) (third)	C71.5	C79.31	-	D33.0	D43.0	D49.6
cardiac (left) (right)	C38.0	C79.89	-	D15.1	D48.7	D49.89
fourth	C71.7	C79.31	-	D33.1	D43.1	D49.6
ventricular band of larynx	C32.1	C78.39	D02.0	D14.1	D38.0	D49.1
ventriculus — *see* Neoplasm, stomach						
vermillion border — *see* Neoplasm, lip						
vermis, cerebellum	C71.6	C79.31	-	D33.1	D43.1	D49.6
vertebra (column)	C41.2	C79.51	-	D16.6	D48.0	D49.2
coccyx	C41.4	C79.51	-	D16.8-	D48.0	D49.2
marrow NEC	C96.9	C79.52	-	-	D47.9	D49.89
sacrum	C41.4	C79.51	-	D16.8-	D48.0	D49.2
vesical — *see* Neoplasm, bladder						
vesicle, seminal	C63.7	C79.82	D07.69	D29.8	D40.8	D49.59
vesicocervical tissue	C57.9	C79.82	D07.30	D28.9	D39.9	D49.59
vesicorectal	C76.3	C79.82	D09.8	D36.7	D48.7	D49.89
vesicovaginal	C57.9	C79.82	D07.30	D28.9	D39.9	D49.59
septum	C57.9	C79.82	D07.30	D28.9	D39.8	D49.59
vessel (blood) — *see* Neoplasm, connective tissue						
vestibular gland, greater	C51.0	C79.82	D07.1	D28.0	D39.8	D49.59
vestibule						
mouth	C06.1	C79.89	D00.00	D10.39	D37.09	D49.0
nose	C30.0	C78.39	D02.3	D14.0	D38.5	D49.1
Virchow's gland	C77.0	C77.0	-	D36.0	D48.7	D49.89
viscera NEC	C76.8	C79.89	D09.8	D36.7	D48.7	D49.89
vocal cords (true)	C32.0	C78.39	D02.0	D14.1	D38.0	D49.1
false	C32.1	C78.39	D02.0	D14.1	D38.0	D49.1
vomer	C41.0	C79.51	-	D16.4-	D48.0	D49.2
vulva	C51.9	C79.82	D07.1	D28.0	D39.8	D49.59
vulvovaginal gland	C51.0	C79.82	D07.1	D28.0	D39.8	D49.59
Waldeyer's ring	C14.2	C79.89	D00.08	D10.9	D37.05	D49.0
Wharton's duct	C08.0	C79.89	D00.00	D11.7	D37.032	D49.0
white matter (central) (cerebral)	C71.0	C79.31	-	D33.0	D43.0	D49.6
windpipe	C33	C78.39	D02.1	D14.2	D38.1	D49.1
Wirsung's duct	C25.3	C78.89	D01.7	D13.6	D37.8	D49.0
wolffian (body) (duct)						
female	C57.7	C79.82	D07.39	D28.7	D39.8	D49.59
male	C63.7	C79.82	D07.69	D29.8	D40.8	D49.59
womb — *see* Neoplasm, uterus						
wrist NEC	C76.4-	C79.89	D04.6-	D36.7	D48.7	D49.89
xiphoid process	C41.3	C79.51	-	D16.7	D48.0	D49.2
Zuckerkandl organ	C75.5	C79.89	-	D35.6	D44.7	D49.7

ICD-10-CM Table of Drugs and Chemicals

Substance	Poisoning, Accidental unintentional	Poisoning, Intentional self-harm	Poisoning, Assault	Poisoning, Undetermined	Adverse effect	Underdosing
1-propanol	T51.3X1	T51.3X2	T51.3X3	T51.3X4	—	—
2-propanol	T51.2X1	T51.2X2	T51.2X3	T51.2X4	—	—
2,4-D (dichlorophen-oxyacetic acid)	T60.3X1	T60.3X2	T60.3X3	T60.3X4	—	—
2,4-toluene diisocyanate	T65.0X1	T65.0X2	T65.0X3	T65.0X4	—	—
2,4,5-T (trichloro-phenoxyacetic acid)	T60.1X1	T60.1X2	T60.1X3	T60.1X4	—	—
14-hydroxydihydro-morphinone	T40.2X1	T40.2X2	T40.2X3	T40.2X4	T40.2X5	T40.2X6
A						
ABOB	T37.5X1	T37.5X2	T37.5X3	T37.5X4	T37.5X5	T37.5X6
Abrine	T62.2X1	T62.2X2	T62.2X3	T62.2X4	—	—
Abrus (seed)	T62.2X1	T62.2X2	T62.2X3	T62.2X4	—	—
Absinthe	T51.0X1	T51.0X2	T51.0X3	T51.0X4	—	—
beverage	T51.0X1	T51.0X2	T51.0X3	T51.0X4	—	—
Acaricide	T60.8X1	T60.8X2	T60.8X3	T60.8X4	—	—
Acebutolol	T44.7X1	T44.7X2	T44.7X3	T44.7X4	T44.7X5	T44.7X6
Acecarbromal	T42.6X1	T42.6X2	T42.6X3	T42.6X4	T42.6X5	T42.6X6
Aceclidine	T44.1X1	T44.1X2	T44.1X3	T44.1X4	T44.1X5	T44.1X6
Acedapsone	T37.0X1	T37.0X2	T37.0X3	T37.0X4	T37.0X5	T37.0X6
Acefylline piperazine	T48.6X1	T48.6X2	T48.6X3	T48.6X4	T48.6X5	T48.6X6
Acemorphan	T40.2X1	T40.2X2	T40.2X3	T40.2X4	T40.2X5	T40.2X6
Acenocoumarin	T45.511	T45.512	T45.513	T45.514	T45.515	T45.516
Acenocoumarol	T45.511	T45.512	T45.513	T45.514	T45.515	T45.516
Acepifylline	T48.6X1	T48.6X2	T48.6X3	T48.6X4	T48.6X5	T48.6X6
Acepromazine	T43.3X1	T43.3X2	T43.3X3	T43.3X4	T43.3X5	T43.3X6
Acesulfamethoxypyridazine	T37.0X1	T37.0X2	T37.0X3	T37.0X4	T37.0X5	T37.0X6
Acetal	T52.8X1	T52.8X2	T52.8X3	T52.8X4	—	—
Acetaldehyde (vapor)	T52.8X1	T52.8X2	T52.8X3	T52.8X4	—	—
liquid	T65.891	T65.892	T65.893	T65.894	—	—
P-Acetamidophenol	T39.1X1	T39.1X2	T39.1X3	T39.1X4	T39.1X5	T39.1X6
Acetaminophen	T39.1X1	T39.1X2	T39.1X3	T39.1X4	T39.1X5	T39.1X6
Acetaminosalol	T39.1X1	T39.1X2	T39.1X3	T39.1X4	T39.1X5	T39.1X6
Acetanilide	T39.1X1	T39.1X2	T39.1X3	T39.1X4	T39.1X5	T39.1X6
Acetarsol	T37.3X1	T37.3X2	T37.3X3	T37.3X4	T37.3X5	T37.3X6
Acetazolamide	T50.2X1	T50.2X2	T50.2X3	T50.2X4	T50.2X5	T50.2X6
Acetiamine	T45.2X1	T45.2X2	T45.2X3	T45.2X4	T45.2X5	T45.2X6
Acetic						
acid	T54.2X1	T54.2X2	T54.2X3	T54.2X4	—	—
with sodium acetate (ointment)	T49.3X1	T49.3X2	T49.3X3	T49.3X4	T49.3X5	T49.3X6
ester (solvent) (vapor)	T52.8X1	T52.8X2	T52.8X3	T52.8X4	—	—
irrigating solution	T50.3X1	T50.3X2	T50.3X3	T50.3X4	T50.3X5	T50.3X6
medicinal (lotion)	T49.2X1	T49.2X2	T49.2X3	T49.2X4	T49.2X5	T49.2X6
anhydride	T65.891	T65.892	T65.893	T65.894	—	—
ether (vapor)	T52.8X1	T52.8X2	T52.8X3	T52.8X4	—	—
Acetohexamide	T38.3X1	T38.3X2	T38.3X3	T38.3X4	T38.3X5	T38.3X6
Acetohydroxamic acid	T50.991	T50.992	T50.993	T50.994	T50.995	T50.996
Acetomenaphthone	T45.7X1	T45.7X2	T45.7X3	T45.7X4	T45.7X5	T45.7X6
Acetomorphine	T40.1X1	T40.1X2	T40.1X3	T40.1X4	—	—
Acetone (oils)	T52.4X1	T52.4X2	T52.4X3	T52.4X4	—	—
chlorinated	T52.4X1	T52.4X2	T52.4X3	T52.4X4	—	—
vapor	T52.4X1	T52.4X2	T52.4X3	T52.4X4	—	—
Acetonitrile	T52.8X1	T52.8X2	T52.8X3	T52.8X4	—	—
Acetophenazine	T43.3X1	T43.3X2	T43.3X3	T43.3X4	T43.3X5	T43.3X6
Acetophenetedin	T39.1X1	T39.1X2	T39.1X3	T39.1X4	T39.1X5	T39.1X6
Acetophenone	T52.4X1	T52.4X2	T52.4X3	T52.4X4	—	—
Acetorphine	T40.2X1	T40.2X2	T40.2X3	T40.2X4	—	—
Acetosulfone (sodium)	T37.1X1	T37.1X2	T37.1X3	T37.1X4	T37.1X5	T37.1X6
Acetrizoate (sodium)	T50.8X1	T50.8X2	T50.8X3	T50.8X4	T50.8X5	T50.8X6
Acetrizoic acid	T50.8X1	T50.8X2	T50.8X3	T50.8X4	T50.8X5	T50.8X6
Acetyl						
bromide	T53.6X1	T53.6X2	T53.6X3	T53.6X4	—	—
chloride	T53.6X1	T53.6X2	T53.6X3	T53.6X4	—	—
Acetylcarbromal	T42.6X1	T42.6X2	T42.6X3	T42.6X4	T42.6X5	T42.6X6
Acetylcholine						
chloride	T44.1X1	T44.1X2	T44.1X3	T44.1X4	T44.1X5	T44.1X6
derivative	T44.1X1	T44.1X2	T44.1X3	T44.1X4	T44.1X5	T44.1X6
Acetylcysteine	T48.4X1	T48.4X2	T48.4X3	T48.4X4	T48.4X5	T48.4X6
Acetyldigitoxin	T46.0X1	T46.0X2	T46.0X3	T46.0X4	T46.0X5	T46.0X6
Acetyldigoxin	T46.0X1	T46.0X2	T46.0X3	T46.0X4	T46.0X5	T46.0X6
Acetyldihydrocodeine	T40.2X1	T40.2X2	T40.2X3	T40.2X4	—	—
Acetyldihydrocodeinone	T40.2X1	T40.2X2	T40.2X3	T40.2X4	—	—
Acetylene (gas)	T59.891	T59.892	T59.893	T59.894	—	—
dichloride	T53.6X1	T53.6X2	T53.6X3	T53.6X4	—	—
incomplete combustion of	T58.11	T58.12	T58.13	T58.14	—	—
industrial	T59.891	T59.892	T59.893	T59.894	—	—
tetrachloride	T53.6X1	T53.6X2	T53.6X3	T53.6X4	—	—
vapor	T53.6X1	T53.6X2	T53.6X3	T53.6X4	—	—

Substance	Poisoning, Accidental unintentional	Poisoning, Intentional self-harm	Poisoning, Assault	Poisoning, Undetermined	Adverse effect	Underdosing
Acetylpheneturide	T42.6X1	T42.6X2	T42.6X3	T42.6X4	T42.6X5	T42.6X6
Acetylphenylhydrazine	T39.8X1	T39.8X2	T39.8X3	T39.8X4	T39.8X5	T39.8X6
Acetylsalicylic acid (salts)	T39.011	T39.012	T39.013	T39.014	T39.015	T39.016
enteric coated	T39.011	T39.012	T39.013	T39.014	T39.015	T39.016
Acetylsulfamethoxypyri-dazine	T37.0X1	T37.0X2	T37.0X3	T37.0X4	T37.0X5	T37.0X6
Achromycin®	T36.4X1	T36.4X2	T36.4X3	T36.4X4	T36.4X5	T36.4X6
ophthalmic preparation	T49.5X1	T49.5X2	T49.5X3	T49.5X4	T49.5X5	T49.5X6
topical NEC	T49.0X1	T49.0X2	T49.0X3	T49.0X4	T49.0X5	T49.0X6
Aciclovir	T37.5X1	T37.5X2	T37.5X3	T37.5X4	T37.5X5	T37.5X6
Acid (corrosive) **NEC**	T54.2X1	T54.2X2	T54.2X3	T54.2X4	—	—
Acidifying agent NEC	T50.901	T50.902	T50.903	T50.904	T50.905	T50.906
Acipimox	T46.6X1	T46.6X2	T46.6X3	T46.6X4	T46.6X5	T46.6X6
Acitretin	T50.991	T50.992	T50.993	T50.994	T50.995	T50.996
Aclarubicin	T45.1X1	T45.1X2	T45.1X3	T45.1X4	T45.1X5	T45.1X6
Aclatonium napadisilate	T48.1X1	T48.1X2	T48.1X3	T48.1X4	T48.1X5	T48.1X6
Aconite (wild)	T46.991	T46.992	T46.993	T46.994	T46.995	T46.996
Aconitine	T46.991	T46.992	T46.993	T46.994	T46.995	T46.996
Aconitum ferox	T46.991	T46.992	T46.993	T46.994	T46.995	T46.996
Acridine	T65.6X1	T65.6X2	T65.6X3	T65.6X4	—	—
vapor	T59.891	T59.892	T59.893	T59.894	—	—
Acriflavine	T37.91	T37.92	T37.93	T37.94	T37.95	T37.96
Acriflavinium chloride	T49.0X1	T49.0X2	T49.0X3	T49.0X4	T49.0X5	T49.0X6
Acrinol	T49.0X1	T49.0X2	T49.0X3	T49.0X4	T49.0X5	T49.0X6
Acrisorcin	T49.0X1	T49.0X2	T49.0X3	T49.0X4	T49.0X5	T49.0X6
Acrivastine	T45.0X1	T45.0X2	T45.0X3	T45.0X4	T45.0X5	T45.0X6
Acrolein (gas)	T59.891	T59.892	T59.893	T59.894	—	—
liquid	T54.1X1	T54.1X2	T54.1X3	T54.1X4	—	—
Acrylamide	T65.891	T65.892	T65.893	T65.894	—	—
Acrylic resin	T49.3X1	T49.3X2	T49.3X3	T49.3X4	T49.3X5	T49.3X6
Acrylonitrile	T65.891	T65.892	T65.893	T65.894	—	—
Actaea spicata	T62.2X1	T62.2X2	T62.2X3	T62.2X4	—	—
berry	T62.1X1	T62.1X2	T62.1X3	T62.1X4	—	—
Acterol	T37.3X1	T37.3X2	T37.3X3	T37.3X4	T37.3X5	T37.3X6
ACTH	T38.811	T38.812	T38.813	T38.814	T38.815	T38.816
Actinomycin C	T45.1X1	T45.1X2	T45.1X3	T45.1X4	T45.1X5	T45.1X6
Actinomycin D	T45.1X1	T45.1X2	T45.1X3	T45.1X4	T45.1X5	T45.1X6
Activated charcoal — *see also Charcoal, medicinal*	T47.6X1	T47.6X2	T47.6X3	T47.6X4	T47.6X5	T47.6X6
Acyclovir	T37.5X1	T37.5X2	T37.5X3	T37.5X4	T37.5X5	T37.5X6
Adenine	T45.2X1	T45.2X2	T45.2X3	T45.2X4	T45.2X5	T45.2X6
arabinoside	T37.5X1	T37.5X2	T37.5X3	T37.5X4	T37.5X5	T37.5X6
Adenosine (phosphate)	T46.2X1	T46.2X2	T46.2X3	T46.2X4	T46.2X5	T46.2X6
ADH	T38.891	T38.892	T38.893	T38.894	T38.895	T38.896
Adhesive NEC	T65.891	T65.892	T65.893	T65.894	—	—
Adicillin	T36.0X1	T36.0X2	T36.0X3	T36.0X4	T36.0X5	T36.0X6
Adiphenine	T44.3X1	T44.3X2	T44.3X3	T44.3X4	T44.3X5	T44.3X6
Adipiodone	T50.8X1	T50.8X2	T50.8X3	T50.8X4	T50.8X5	T50.8X6
Adjunct, pharmaceutical	T50.901	T50.902	T50.903	T50.904	T50.905	T50.906
Adrenal (extract, cortex or medulla) (glucocorticoids) (hormones) (mineralocorticoids)	T38.0X1	T38.0X2	T38.0X3	T38.0X4	T38.0X5	T38.0X6
ENT agent	T49.6X1	T49.6X2	T49.6X3	T49.6X4	T49.6X5	T49.6X6
ophthalmic preparation	T49.5X1	T49.5X2	T49.5X3	T49.5X4	T49.5X5	T49.5X6
topical NEC	T49.0X1	T49.0X2	T49.0X3	T49.0X4	T49.0X5	T49.0X6
Adrenaline	T44.5X1	T44.5X2	T44.5X3	T44.5X4	T44.5X5	T44.5X6
Adrenalin — *see Adrenaline*						
Adrenergic NEC	T44.901	T44.902	T44.903	T44.904	T44.905	T44.906
blocking agent NEC	T44.8X1	T44.8X2	T44.8X3	T44.8X4	T44.8X5	T44.8X6
beta, heart	T44.7X1	T44.7X2	T44.7X3	T44.7X4	T44.7X5	T44.7X6
specified NEC	T44.991	T44.992	T44.993	T44.994	T44.995	T44.996
Adrenochrome						
(mono) semicarbazone	T46.991	T46.992	T46.993	T46.994	T46.995	T46.996
derivative	T46.991	T46.992	T46.993	T46.994	T46.995	T46.996
Adrenocorticotrophic hormone	T38.811	T38.812	T38.813	T38.814	T38.815	T38.816
Adrenocorticotrophin	T38.811	T38.812	T38.813	T38.814	T38.815	T38.816
Adriamycin®	T45.1X1	T45.1X2	T45.1X3	T45.1X4	T45.1X5	T45.1X6
Aerosol spray NEC	T65.91	T65.92	T65.93	T65.94	—	—
Aerosporin®	T36.8X1	T36.8X2	T36.8X3	T36.8X4	T36.8X5	T36.8X6
ENT agent	T49.6X1	T49.6X2	T49.6X3	T49.6X4	T49.6X5	T49.6X6
ophthalmic preparation	T49.5X1	T49.5X2	T49.5X3	T49.5X4	T49.5X5	T49.5X6
topical NEC	T49.0X1	T49.0X2	T49.0X3	T49.0X4	T49.0X5	T49.0X6
Aethusa cynapium	T62.2X1	T62.2X2	T62.2X3	T62.2X4	—	—
Afghanistan black	T40.7X1	T40.7X2	T40.7X3	T40.7X4	T40.7X5	T40.7X6
Aflatoxin	T64.01	T64.02	T64.03	T64.04	—	—
Afloqualone	T42.8X1	T42.8X2	T42.8X3	T42.8X4	T42.8X5	T42.8X6
African boxwood	T62.2X1	T62.2X2	T62.2X3	T62.2X4	—	—

Agar - Ambuphylline

Substance	Poisoning, Accidental unintentional	Poisoning, Intentional self-harm	Poisoning, Assault	Poisoning, Undetermined	Adverse effect	Underdosing
Agar	T47.4X1	T47.4X2	T47.4X3	T47.4X4	T47.4X5	T47.4X6
Agonist						
predominantly						
alpha-adrenoreceptor	T44.4X1	T44.4X2	T44.4X3	T44.4X4	T44.4X5	T44.4X6
beta-adrenoreceptor	T44.5X1	T44.5X2	T44.5X3	T44.5X4	T44.5X5	T44.5X6
Agricultural agent NEC	T65.91	T65.92	T65.93	T65.94	--	--
Agrypnal	T42.3X1	T42.3X2	T42.3X3	T42.3X4	T42.3X5	T42.3X6
AHLG	T50.Z11	T50.Z12	T50.Z13	T50.Z14	T50.Z15	T50.Z16
Air contaminant (s), **source/ type NOS**	T65.91	T65.92	T65.93	T65.94	--	--
Ajmaline	T46.2X1	T46.2X2	T46.2X3	T46.2X4	T46.2X5	T46.2X6
Akee	T62.1X1	T62.1X2	T62.1X3	T62.1X4	--	--
Akrinol®	T49.0X1	T49.0X2	T49.0X3	T49.0X4	T49.0X5	T49.0X6
Akritoin	T37.8X1	T37.8X2	T37.8X3	T37.8X4	T37.8X5	T37.8X6
Alacepril	T46.4X1	T46.4X2	T46.4X3	T46.4X4	T46.4X5	T46.4X6
Alantolactone	T37.4X1	T37.4X2	T37.4X3	T37.4X4	T37.4X5	T37.4X6
Albamycin®	T36.8X1	T36.8X2	T36.8X3	T36.8X4	T36.8X5	T36.8X6
Albendazole	T37.4X1	T37.4X2	T37.4X3	T37.4X4	T37.4X5	T37.4X6
Albumin						
bovine	T45.8X1	T45.8X2	T45.8X3	T45.8X4	T45.8X5	T45.8X6
human serum	T45.8X1	T45.8X2	T45.8X3	T45.8X4	T45.8X5	T45.8X6
salt-poor	T45.8X1	T45.8X2	T45.8X3	T45.8X4	T45.8X5	T45.8X6
normal human serum	T45.8X1	T45.8X2	T45.8X3	T45.8X4	T45.8X5	T45.8X6
Albuterol	T48.6X1	T48.6X2	T48.6X3	T48.6X4	T48.6X5	T48.6X6
Albutoin	T42.0X1	T42.0X2	T42.0X3	T42.0X4	T42.0X5	T42.0X6
Alclometasone	T49.0X1	T49.0X2	T49.0X3	T49.0X4	T49.0X5	T49.0X6
Alcohol	T51.91	T51.92	T51.93	T51.94	--	--
absolute	T51.0X1	T51.0X2	T51.0X3	T51.0X4	--	--
beverage	T51.0X1	T51.0X2	T51.0X3	T51.0X4	--	--
allyl	T51.8X1	T51.8X2	T51.8X3	T51.8X4	--	--
amyl	T51.3X1	T51.3X2	T51.3X3	T51.3X4	--	--
antifreeze	T51.1X1	T51.1X2	T51.1X3	T51.1X4	--	--
beverage	T51.0X1	T51.0X2	T51.0X3	T51.0X4	--	--
butyl	T51.3X1	T51.3X2	T51.3X3	T51.3X4	--	--
dehydrated	T51.0X1	T51.0X2	T51.0X3	T51.0X4	--	--
beverage	T51.0X1	T51.0X2	T51.0X3	T51.0X4	--	--
denatured	T51.0X1	T51.0X2	T51.0X3	T51.0X4	--	--
deterrent NEC	T50.6X1	T50.6X2	T50.6X3	T50.6X4	T50.6X5	T50.6X6
diagnostic (gastric function)	T50.8X1	T50.8X2	T50.8X3	T50.8X4	T50.8X5	T50.8X6
ethyl	T51.0X1	T51.0X2	T51.0X3	T51.0X4	--	--
beverage	T51.0X1	T51.0X2	T51.0X3	T51.0X4	--	--
grain	T51.0X1	T51.0X2	T51.0X3	T51.0X4	--	--
beverage	T51.0X1	T51.0X2	T51.0X3	T51.0X4	--	--
industrial	T51.0X1	T51.0X2	T51.0X3	T51.0X4	--	--
isopropyl	T51.2X1	T51.2X2	T51.2X3	T51.2X4	--	--
methyl	T51.1X1	T51.1X2	T51.1X3	T51.1X4	--	--
preparation for consumption	T51.0X1	T51.0X2	T51.0X3	T51.0X4	--	--
propyl	T51.3X1	T51.3X2	T51.3X3	T51.3X4	--	--
secondary	T51.2X1	T51.2X2	T51.2X3	T51.2X4	--	--
radiator	T51.1X1	T51.1X2	T51.1X3	T51.1X4	--	--
rubbing	T51.2X1	T51.2X2	T51.2X3	T51.2X4	--	--
specified type NEC	T51.8X1	T51.8X2	T51.8X3	T51.8X4	--	--
surgical	T51.0X1	T51.0X2	T51.0X3	T51.0X4	--	--
vapor (from any type of Alcohol)	T59.891	T59.892	T59.893	T59.894	--	--
wood	T51.1X1	T51.1X2	T51.1X3	T51.1X4	--	--
Alcuronium (chloride)	T48.1X1	T48.1X2	T48.1X3	T48.1X4	T48.1X5	T48.1X6
Aldactone	T50.0X1	T50.0X2	T50.0X3	T50.0X4	T50.0X5	T50.0X6
Aldesulfone sodium	T37.1X1	T37.1X2	T37.1X3	T37.1X4	T37.1X5	T37.1X6
Aldicarb	T60.0X1	T60.0X2	T60.0X3	T60.0X4	--	--
Aldomet®	T46.5X1	T46.5X2	T46.5X3	T46.5X4	T46.5X5	T46.5X6
Aldosterone	T50.0X1	T50.0X2	T50.0X3	T50.0X4	T50.0X5	T50.0X6
Aldrin (dust)	T60.1X1	T60.1X2	T60.1X3	T60.1X4	--	--
Aleve® — *see Naproxen*						
Alexitol sodium	T47.1X1	T47.1X2	T47.1X3	T47.1X4	T47.1X5	T47.1X6
Alfacalcidol	T45.2X1	T45.2X2	T45.2X3	T45.2X4	T45.2X5	T45.2X6
Alfadolone	T41.1X1	T41.1X2	T41.1X3	T41.1X4	T41.1X5	T41.1X6
Alfaxalone	T41.1X1	T41.1X2	T41.1X3	T41.1X4	T41.1X5	T41.1X6
Alfentanil	T40.4X1	T40.4X2	T40.4X3	T40.4X4	T40.4X5	T40.4X6
Alfuzosin (hydrochloride)	T44.8X1	T44.8X2	T44.8X3	T44.8X4	T44.8X5	T44.8X6
Algae (harmful) (toxin)	T65.821	T65.822	T65.823	T65.824	--	--
Algeldrate	T47.1X1	T47.1X2	T47.1X3	T47.1X4	T47.1X5	T47.1X6
Algin	T47.8X1	T47.8X2	T47.8X3	T47.8X4	T47.8X5	T47.8X6
Alglucerase	T45.3X1	T45.3X2	T45.3X3	T45.3X4	T45.3X5	T45.3X6
Alidase	T45.3X1	T45.3X2	T45.3X3	T45.3X4	T45.3X5	T45.3X6
Alimemazine	T43.3X1	T43.3X2	T43.3X3	T43.3X4	T43.3X5	T43.3X6
Aliphatic thiocyanates	T65.0X1	T65.0X2	T65.0X3	T65.0X4	--	--
Alizapride	T45.0X1	T45.0X2	T45.0X3	T45.0X4	T45.0X5	T45.0X6
Alkali (caustic)	T54.3X1	T54.3X2	T54.3X3	T54.3X4	--	--
Alkaline antiseptic solution (aromatic)	T49.6X1	T49.6X2	T49.6X3	T49.6X4	T49.6X5	T49.6X6
Alkalinizing agents (medicinal)	T50.901	T50.902	T50.903	T50.904	T50.905	T50.906
Alkalizing agent NEC	T50.901	T50.902	T50.903	T50.904	T50.905	T50.906
Alka-Seltzer®	T39.011	T39.012	T39.013	T39.014	T39.015	T39.016
Alkavervir	T46.5X1	T46.5X2	T46.5X3	T46.5X4	T46.5X5	T46.5X6
Alkonium (bromide)	T49.0X1	T49.0X2	T49.0X3	T49.0X4	T49.0X5	T49.0X6
Alkylating drug NEC	T45.1X1	T45.1X2	T45.1X3	T45.1X4	T45.1X5	T45.1X6
antimyeloproliferative	T45.1X1	T45.1X2	T45.1X3	T45.1X4	T45.1X5	T45.1X6
lymphatic	T45.1X1	T45.1X2	T45.1X3	T45.1X4	T45.1X5	T45.1X6
Alkylisocyanate	T65.0X1	T65.0X2	T65.0X3	T65.0X4	--	--
Allantoin	T49.4X1	T49.4X2	T49.4X3	T49.4X4	T49.4X5	T49.4X6
Allegron	T43.011	T43.012	T43.013	T43.014	T43.015	T43.016
Allethrin	T49.0X1	T49.0X2	T49.0X3	T49.0X4	T49.0X5	T49.0X6
Allobarbital	T42.3X1	T42.3X2	T42.3X3	T42.3X4	T42.3X5	T42.3X6
Allopurinol	T50.4X1	T50.4X2	T50.4X3	T50.4X4	T50.4X5	T50.4X6
Allyl						
Alcohol	T51.8X1	T51.8X2	T51.8X3	T51.8X4	--	--
disulfide	T46.6X1	T46.6X2	T46.6X3	T46.6X4	T46.6X5	T46.6X6
Allylestrenol	T38.5X1	T38.5X2	T38.5X3	T38.5X4	T38.5X5	T38.5X6
Allylisopropylacetylurea	T42.6X1	T42.6X2	T42.6X3	T42.6X4	T42.6X5	T42.6X6
Allylisopropylmalonylurea	T42.3X1	T42.3X2	T42.3X3	T42.3X4	T42.3X5	T42.3X6
Allylthiourea	T49.3X1	T49.3X2	T49.3X3	T49.3X4	T49.3X5	T49.3X6
Allyltribromide	T42.6X1	T42.6X2	T42.6X3	T42.6X4	T42.6X5	T42.6X6
Allypropymal	T42.3X1	T42.3X2	T42.3X3	T42.3X4	T42.3X5	T42.3X6
Almagate	T47.1X1	T47.1X2	T47.1X3	T47.1X4	T47.1X5	T47.1X6
Almasilate	T47.1X1	T47.1X2	T47.1X3	T47.1X4	T47.1X5	T47.1X6
Almitrine	T50.7X1	T50.7X2	T50.7X3	T50.7X4	T50.7X5	T50.7X6
Aloes	T47.2X1	T47.2X2	T47.2X3	T47.2X4	T47.2X5	T47.2X6
Aloglutamol	T47.1X1	T47.1X2	T47.1X3	T47.1X4	T47.1X5	T47.1X6
Aloin	T47.2X1	T47.2X2	T47.2X3	T47.2X4	T47.2X5	T47.2X6
Aloxidone	T42.2X1	T42.2X2	T42.2X3	T42.2X4	T42.2X5	T42.2X6
Alpha						
acetyldigoxin	T46.0X1	T46.0X2	T46.0X3	T46.0X4	T46.0X5	T46.0X6
adrenergic blocking drug	T44.6X1	T44.6X2	T44.6X3	T44.6X4	T44.6X5	T44.6X6
amylase	T45.3X1	T45.3X2	T45.3X3	T45.3X4	T45.3X5	T45.3X6
tocoferol (acetate)	T45.2X1	T45.2X2	T45.2X3	T45.2X4	T45.2X5	T45.2X6
tocopherol	T45.2X1	T45.2X2	T45.2X3	T45.2X4	T45.2X5	T45.2X6
Alphadolone	T41.1X1	T41.1X2	T41.1X3	T41.1X4	T41.1X5	T41.1X6
Alphaprodine	T40.4X1	T40.4X2	T40.4X3	T40.4X4	T40.4X5	T40.4X6
Alphaxalone	T41.1X1	T41.1X2	T41.1X3	T41.1X4	T41.1X5	T41.1X6
Alprazolam	T42.4X1	T42.4X2	T42.4X3	T42.4X4	T42.4X5	T42.4X6
Alprenolol	T44.7X1	T44.7X2	T44.7X3	T44.7X4	T44.7X5	T44.7X6
Alprostadil	T46.7X1	T46.7X2	T46.7X3	T46.7X4	T46.7X5	T46.7X6
Alsactide	T38.811	T38.812	T38.813	T38.814	T38.815	T38.816
Alseroxylon	T46.5X1	T46.5X2	T46.5X3	T46.5X4	T46.5X5	T46.5X6
Alteplase	T45.611	T45.612	T45.613	T45.614	T45.615	T45.616
Altizide	T50.2X1	T50.2X2	T50.2X3	T50.2X4	T50.2X5	T50.2X6
Altretamine	T45.1X1	T45.1X2	T45.1X3	T45.1X4	T45.1X5	T45.1X6
Alum (medicinal)	T49.4X1	T49.4X2	T49.4X3	T49.4X4	T49.4X5	T49.4X6
nonmedicinal (ammonium) (potassium)	T56.891	T56.892	T56.893	T56.894	--	--
Aluminium, aluminum						
acetate	T49.2X1	T49.2X2	T49.2X3	T49.2X4	T49.2X5	T49.2X6
solution	T49.0X1	T49.0X2	T49.0X3	T49.0X4	T49.0X5	T49.0X6
aspirin	T39.011	T39.012	T39.013	T39.014	T39.015	T39.016
bis (acetylsalicylate)	T39.011	T39.012	T39.013	T39.014	T39.015	T39.016
carbonate (gel, basic)	T47.1X1	T47.1X2	T47.1X3	T47.1X4	T47.1X5	T47.1X6
chlorhydroxide-complex	T47.1X1	T47.1X2	T47.1X3	T47.1X4	T47.1X5	T47.1X6
chloride	T49.2X1	T49.2X2	T49.2X3	T49.2X4	T49.2X5	T49.2X6
clofibrate	T46.6X1	T46.6X2	T46.6X3	T46.6X4	T46.6X5	T46.6X6
diacetate	T49.2X1	T49.2X2	T49.2X3	T49.2X4	T49.2X5	T49.2X6
glycinate	T47.1X1	T47.1X2	T47.1X3	T47.1X4	T47.1X5	T47.1X6
hydroxide (gel)	T47.1X1	T47.1X2	T47.1X3	T47.1X4	T47.1X5	T47.1X6
hydroxide-magnesium carb. gel	T47.1X1	T47.1X2	T47.1X3	T47.1X4	T47.1X5	T47.1X6
magnesium silicate	T47.1X1	T47.1X2	T47.1X3	T47.1X4	T47.1X5	T47.1X6
nicotinate	T46.7X1	T46.7X2	T46.7X3	T46.7X4	T46.7X5	T46.7X6
ointment (surgical) (topical)	T49.3X1	T49.3X2	T49.3X3	T49.3X4	T49.3X5	T49.3X6
phosphate	T47.1X1	T47.1X2	T47.1X3	T47.1X4	T47.1X5	T47.1X6
salicylate	T39.091	T39.092	T39.093	T39.094	T39.095	T39.096
silicate	T47.1X1	T47.1X2	T47.1X3	T47.1X4	T47.1X5	T47.1X6
sodium silicate	T47.1X1	T47.1X2	T47.1X3	T47.1X4	T47.1X5	T47.1X6
subacetate	T49.2X1	T49.2X2	T49.2X3	T49.2X4	T49.2X5	T49.2X6
sulfate	T49.0X1	T49.0X2	T49.0X3	T49.0X4	T49.0X5	T49.0X6
tannate	T47.6X1	T47.6X2	T47.6X3	T47.6X4	T47.6X5	T47.6X6
topical NEC	T49.3X1	T49.3X2	T49.3X3	T49.3X4	T49.3X5	T49.3X6
Alurate®	T42.3X1	T42.3X2	T42.3X3	T42.3X4	T42.3X5	T42.3X6
Alverine	T44.3X1	T44.3X2	T44.3X3	T44.3X4	T44.3X5	T44.3X6
Alvodine	T40.2X1	T40.2X2	T40.2X3	T40.2X4	T40.2X5	T40.2X6
Amanita phalloides	T62.0X1	T62.0X2	T62.0X3	T62.0X4	--	--
Amanitine	T62.0X1	T62.0X2	T62.0X3	T62.0X4	--	--
Amantadine	T42.8X1	T42.8X2	T42.8X3	T42.8X4	T42.8X5	T42.8X6
Ambazone	T49.6X1	T49.6X2	T49.6X3	T49.6X4	T49.6X5	T49.6X6
Ambenonium (chloride)	T44.0X1	T44.0X2	T44.0X3	T44.0X4	T44.0X5	T44.0X6
Ambroxol®	T48.4X1	T48.4X2	T48.4X3	T48.4X4	T48.4X5	T48.4X6
Ambuphylline	T48.6X1	T48.6X2	T48.6X3	T48.6X4	T48.6X5	T48.6X6

Substance	Poisoning, Accidental unintentional	Poisoning, Intentional self-harm	Poisoning, Assault	Poisoning, Undetermined	Adverse effect	Underdosing
Ambutonium bromide	T44.3X1	T44.3X2	T44.3X3	T44.3X4	T44.3X5	T44.3X6
Amcinonide	T49.0X1	T49.0X2	T49.0X3	T49.0X4	T49.0X5	T49.0X6
Amdinocilline	T36.0X1	T36.0X2	T36.0X3	T36.0X4	T36.0X5	T36.0X6
Ametazole	T50.8X1	T50.8X2	T50.8X3	T50.8X4	T50.8X5	T50.8X6
Amethocaine	T41.3X1	T41.3X2	T41.3X3	T41.3X4	T41.3X5	T41.3X6
regional	T41.3X1	T41.3X2	T41.3X3	T41.3X4	T41.3X5	T41.3X6
spinal	T41.3X1	T41.3X2	T41.3X3	T41.3X4	T41.3X5	T41.3X6
Amethopterin	T45.1X1	T45.1X2	T45.1X3	T45.1X4	T45.1X5	T45.1X6
Amezinium metilsulfate	T44.991	T44.992	T44.993	T44.994	T44.995	T44.996
Amfebutamone	T43.291	T43.292	T43.293	T43.294	T43.295	T43.296
Amfepramone	T50.5X1	T50.5X2	T50.5X3	T50.5X4	T50.5X5	T50.5X6
Amfetamine	T43.621	T43.622	T43.623	T43.624	T43.625	T43.626
Amfetaminil	T43.621	T43.622	T43.623	T43.624	T43.625	T43.626
Amfomycin	T36.8X1	T36.8X2	T36.8X3	T36.8X4	T36.8X5	T36.8X6
Amidefrine mesilate	T48.5X1	T48.5X2	T48.5X3	T48.5X4	T48.5X5	T48.5X6
Amidone	T40.3X1	T40.3X2	T40.3X3	T40.3X4	T40.3X5	T40.3X6
Amidopyrine	T39.2X1	T39.2X2	T39.2X3	T39.2X4	T39.2X5	T39.2X6
Amidotrizoate	T50.8X1	T50.8X2	T50.8X3	T50.8X4	T50.8X5	T50.8X6
Amiflamine	T43.1X1	T43.1X2	T43.1X3	T43.1X4	T43.1X5	T43.1X6
Amikacin	T36.5X1	T36.5X2	T36.5X3	T36.5X4	T36.5X5	T36.5X6
Amikhelline	T46.3X1	T46.3X2	T46.3X3	T46.3X4	T46.3X5	T46.3X6
Amiloride	T50.2X1	T50.2X2	T50.2X3	T50.2X4	T50.2X5	T50.2X6
Aminacrine	T49.0X1	T49.0X2	T49.0X3	T49.0X4	T49.0X5	T49.0X6
Amineptine	T43.011	T43.012	T43.013	T43.014	T43.015	T43.016
Aminitrozole	T37.3X1	T37.3X2	T37.3X3	T37.3X4	T37.3X5	T37.3X6
Amino acids	T50.3X1	T50.3X2	T50.3X3	T50.3X4	T50.3X5	T50.3X6
Aminoacetic acid (derivatives)	T50.3X1	T50.3X2	T50.3X3	T50.3X4	T50.3X5	T50.3X6
Aminoacridine	T49.0X1	T49.0X2	T49.0X3	T49.0X4	T49.0X5	T49.0X6
Aminobenzoic acid (-p)	T49.3X1	T49.3X2	T49.3X3	T49.3X4	T49.3X5	T49.3X6
4-Aminobutyric acid	T43.8X1	T43.8X2	T43.8X3	T43.8X4	T43.8X5	T43.8X6
Aminocaproic acid	T45.621	T45.622	T45.623	T45.624	T45.625	T45.626
Aminoethylisothiourium	T45.8X1	T45.8X2	T45.8X3	T45.8X4	T45.8X5	T45.8X6
Aminofenazone	T39.2X1	T39.2X2	T39.2X3	T39.2X4	T39.2X5	T39.2X6
Aminoglutethimide	T45.1X1	T45.1X2	T45.1X3	T45.1X4	T45.1X5	T45.1X6
Aminohippuric acid	T50.8X1	T50.8X2	T50.8X3	T50.8X4	T50.8X5	T50.8X6
Aminomethylbenzoic acid	T45.691	T45.692	T45.693	T45.694	T45.695	T45.696
Aminometradine	T50.2X1	T50.2X2	T50.2X3	T50.2X4	T50.2X5	T50.2X6
Aminopentamide	T44.3X1	T44.3X2	T44.3X3	T44.3X4	T44.3X5	T44.3X6
Aminophenazone	T39.2X1	T39.2X2	T39.2X3	T39.2X4	T39.2X5	T39.2X6
Aminophenol	T54.0X1	T54.0X2	T54.0X3	T54.0X4	--	--
4-Aminophenol derivatives	T39.1X1	T39.1X2	T39.1X3	T39.1X4	T39.1X5	T39.1X6
Aminophenylpyridone	T43.591	T43.592	T43.593	T43.594	T43.595	T43.596
Aminophylline	T48.6X1	T48.6X2	T48.6X3	T48.6X4	T48.6X5	T48.6X6
Aminopterin sodium	T45.1X1	T45.1X2	T45.1X3	T45.1X4	T45.1X5	T45.1X6
Aminopyrine	T39.2X1	T39.2X2	T39.2X3	T39.2X4	T39.2X5	T39.2X6
8-Aminoquinoline drugs	T37.2X1	T37.2X2	T37.2X3	T37.2X4	T37.2X5	T37.2X6
Aminorex	T50.5X1	T50.5X2	T50.5X3	T50.5X4	T50.5X5	T50.5X6
Aminosalicylic acid	T37.1X1	T37.1X2	T37.1X3	T37.1X4	T37.1X5	T37.1X6
Aminosalylum	T37.1X1	T37.1X2	T37.1X3	T37.1X4	T37.1X5	T37.1X6
Amiodarone	T46.2X1	T46.2X2	T46.2X3	T46.2X4	T46.2X5	T46.2X6
Amiphenazole	T50.7X1	T50.7X2	T50.7X3	T50.7X4	T50.7X5	T50.7X6
Amiquinsin	T46.5X1	T46.5X2	T46.5X3	T46.5X4	T46.5X5	T46.5X6
Amisometradine	T50.2X1	T50.2X2	T50.2X3	T50.2X4	T50.2X5	T50.2X6
Amisulpride	T43.591	T43.592	T43.593	T43.594	T43.595	T43.596
Amitriptyline	T43.011	T43.012	T43.013	T43.014	T43.015	T43.016
Amitriptylinoxide	T43.011	T43.012	T43.013	T43.014	T43.015	T43.016
Amlexanox	T48.6X1	T48.6X2	T48.6X3	T48.6X4	T48.6X5	T48.6X6
Ammonia (fumes) (gas) (vapor)	T59.891	T59.892	T59.893	T59.894	--	--
aromatic spirit	T48.991	T48.992	T48.993	T48.994	T48.995	T48.996
liquid (household)	T54.3X1	T54.3X2	T54.3X3	T54.3X4	--	--
Ammoniated mercury	T49.0X1	T49.0X2	T49.0X3	T49.0X4	T49.0X5	T49.0X6
Ammonium						
acid tartrate	T49.5X1	T49.5X2	T49.5X3	T49.5X4	T49.5X5	T49.5X6
bromide	T42.6X1	T42.6X2	T42.6X3	T42.6X4	T42.6X5	T42.6X6
carbonate	T54.3X1	T54.3X2	T54.3X3	T54.3X4	--	--
chloride	T50.991	T50.992	T50.993	T50.994	T50.995	T50.996
expectorant	T48.4X1	T48.4X2	T48.4X3	T48.4X4	T48.4X5	T48.4X6
compounds (household) NEC	T54.3X1	T54.3X2	T54.3X3	T54.3X4	--	--
fumes (any usage)	T59.891	T59.892	T59.893	T59.894	--	--
industrial	T54.3X1	T54.3X2	T54.3X3	T54.3X4	--	--
ichthyosulronate	T49.4X1	T49.4X2	T49.4X3	T49.4X4	T49.4X5	T49.4X6
mandelate	T37.91	T37.92	T37.93	T37.94	T37.95	T37.96
sulfamate	T60.3X1	T60.3X2	T60.3X3	T60.3X4	--	--
sulfonate resin	T47.8X1	T47.8X2	T47.8X3	T47.8X4	T47.8X5	T47.8X6
Amobarbital (sodium)	T42.3X1	T42.3X2	T42.3X3	T42.3X4	T42.3X5	T42.3X6
Amodiaquine	T37.2X1	T37.2X2	T37.2X3	T37.2X4	T37.2X5	T37.2X6
Amopyroquin (e)	T37.2X1	T37.2X2	T37.2X3	T37.2X4	T37.2X5	T37.2X6
Amoxapine	T43.011	T43.012	T43.013	T43.014	T43.015	T43.016
Amoxicillin	T36.0X1	T36.0X2	T36.0X3	T36.0X4	T36.0X5	T36.0X6
Amperozide	T43.591	T43.592	T43.593	T43.594	T43.595	T43.596
Amphenidone	T43.591	T43.592	T43.593	T43.594	T43.595	T43.596
Amphetamine NEC	T43.621	T43.622	T43.623	T43.624	T43.625	T43.626

Substance	Poisoning, Accidental unintentional	Poisoning, Intentional self-harm	Poisoning, Assault	Poisoning, Undetermined	Adverse effect	Underdosing
Amphomycin	T36.8X1	T36.8X2	T36.8X3	T36.8X4	T36.8X5	T36.8X6
Amphotalide	T37.4X1	T37.4X2	T37.4X3	T37.4X4	T37.4X5	T37.4X6
Amphotericin B	T36.7X1	T36.7X2	T36.7X3	T36.7X4	T36.7X5	T36.7X6
topical	T49.0X1	T49.0X2	T49.0X3	T49.0X4	T49.0X5	T49.0X6
Ampicillin	T36.0X1	T36.0X2	T36.0X3	T36.0X4	T36.0X5	T36.0X6
Amprotropine	T44.3X1	T44.3X2	T44.3X3	T44.3X4	T44.3X5	T44.3X6
Amsacrine	T45.1X1	T45.1X2	T45.1X3	T45.1X4	T45.1X5	T45.1X6
Amygdaline	T62.2X1	T62.2X2	T62.2X3	T62.2X4	--	--
Amyl						
acetate	T52.8X1	T52.8X2	T52.8X3	T52.8X4	--	--
vapor	T59.891	T59.892	T59.893	T59.894	--	--
alcohol	T51.3X1	T51.3X2	T51.3X3	T51.3X4	--	--
chloride	T53.6X1	T53.6X2	T53.6X3	T53.6X4	--	--
formate	T52.8X1	T52.8X2	T52.8X3	T52.8X4	--	--
nitrite	T46.3X1	T46.3X2	T46.3X3	T46.3X4	T46.3X5	T46.3X6
propionate	T65.891	T65.892	T65.893	T65.894	--	--
Amylase	T47.5X1	T47.5X2	T47.5X3	T47.5X4	T47.5X5	T47.5X6
Amyleine, regional	T41.3X1	T41.3X2	T41.3X3	T41.3X4	T41.3X5	T41.3X6
Amylene						
dichloride	T53.6X1	T53.6X2	T53.6X3	T53.6X4	--	--
hydrate	T51.3X1	T51.3X2	T51.3X3	T51.3X4	--	--
Amylmetacresol	T49.6X1	T49.6X2	T49.6X3	T49.6X4	T49.6X5	T49.6X6
Amylobarbitone	T42.3X1	T42.3X2	T42.3X3	T42.3X4	T42.3X5	T42.3X6
Amylocaine, regional	T41.3X1	T41.3X2	T41.3X3	T41.3X4	T41.3X5	T41.3X6
infiltration (subcutaneous)	T41.3X1	T41.3X2	T41.3X3	T41.3X4	T41.3X5	T41.3X6
nerve block (peripheral) (plexus)	T41.3X1	T41.3X2	T41.3X3	T41.3X4	T41.3X5	T41.3X6
spinal	T41.3X1	T41.3X2	T41.3X3	T41.3X4	T41.3X5	T41.3X6
topical (surface)	T41.3X1	T41.3X2	T41.3X3	T41.3X4	T41.3X5	T41.3X6
Amylopectin	T47.6X1	T47.6X2	T47.6X3	T47.6X4	T47.6X5	T47.6X6
Amytal (sodium)	T42.3X1	T42.3X2	T42.3X3	T42.3X4	T42.3X5	T42.3X6
Anabolic steroid	T38.7X1	T38.7X2	T38.7X3	T38.7X4	T38.7X5	T38.7X6
Analeptic NEC	T50.7X1	T50.7X2	T50.7X3	T50.7X4	T50.7X5	T50.7X6
Analgesic	T39.91	T39.92	T39.93	T39.94	T39.95	T39.96
anti-inflammatory NEC	T39.91	T39.92	T39.93	T39.94	T39.95	T39.96
propionic acid derivative	T39.311	T39.312	T39.313	T39.314	T39.315	T39.316
antirheumatic NEC	T39.4X1	T39.4X2	T39.4X3	T39.4X4	T39.4X5	T39.4X6
aromatic NEC	T39.1X1	T39.1X2	T39.1X3	T39.1X4	T39.1X5	T39.1X6
narcotic NEC	T40.601	T40.602	T40.603	T40.604	T40.605	T40.606
combination	T40.601	T40.602	T40.603	T40.604	T40.605	T40.606
obstetric	T40.601	T40.602	T40.603	T40.604	T40.605	T40.606
non-narcotic NEC	T39.91	T39.92	T39.93	T39.94	T39.95	T39.96
combination	T39.91	T39.92	T39.93	T39.94	T39.95	T39.96
pyrazole	T39.2X1	T39.2X2	T39.2X3	T39.2X4	T39.2X5	T39.2X6
specified NEC	T39.8X1	T39.8X2	T39.8X3	T39.8X4	T39.8X5	T39.8X6
Analgin	T39.2X1	T39.2X2	T39.2X3	T39.2X4	T39.2X5	T39.2X6
Anamirta cocculus	T62.1X1	T62.1X2	T62.1X3	T62.1X4	--	--
Ancillin	T36.0X1	T36.0X2	T36.0X3	T36.0X4	T36.0X5	T36.0X6
Ancrod	T45.691	T45.692	T45.693	T45.694	T45.695	T45.696
Androgen	T38.7X1	T38.7X2	T38.7X3	T38.7X4	T38.7X5	T38.7X6
Androgen-estrogen mixture	T38.7X1	T38.7X2	T38.7X3	T38.7X4	T38.7X5	T38.7X6
Androstalone	T38.7X1	T38.7X2	T38.7X3	T38.7X4	T38.7X5	T38.7X6
Androstanolone	T38.7X1	T38.7X2	T38.7X3	T38.7X4	T38.7X5	T38.7X6
Androsterone	T38.7X1	T38.7X2	T38.7X3	T38.7X4	T38.7X5	T38.7X6
Anemone pulsatilla	T62.2X1	T62.2X2	T62.2X3	T62.2X4	--	--
Anesthesia						
caudal	T41.3X1	T41.3X2	T41.3X3	T41.3X4	T41.3X5	T41.3X6
endotracheal	T41.0X1	T41.0X2	T41.0X3	T41.0X4	T41.0X5	T41.0X6
epidural	T41.3X1	T41.3X2	T41.3X3	T41.3X4	T41.3X5	T41.3X6
inhalation	T41.0X1	T41.0X2	T41.0X3	T41.0X4	T41.0X5	T41.0X6
local	T41.3X1	T41.3X2	T41.3X3	T41.3X4	T41.3X5	T41.3X6
mucosal	T41.3X1	T41.3X2	T41.3X3	T41.3X4	T41.3X5	T41.3X6
muscle relaxation	T48.1X1	T48.1X2	T48.1X3	T48.1X4	T48.1X5	T48.1X6
nerve blocking	T41.3X1	T41.3X2	T41.3X3	T41.3X4	T41.3X5	T41.3X6
plexus blocking	T41.3X1	T41.3X2	T41.3X3	T41.3X4	T41.3X5	T41.3X6
potentiated	T41.201	T41.202	T41.203	T41.204	T41.205	T41.206
rectal	T41.201	T41.202	T41.203	T41.204	T41.205	T41.206
general	T41.201	T41.202	T41.203	T41.204	T41.205	T41.206
local	T41.3X1	T41.3X2	T41.3X3	T41.3X4	T41.3X5	T41.3X6
regional	T41.3X1	T41.3X2	T41.3X3	T41.3X4	T41.3X5	T41.3X6
surface	T41.3X1	T41.3X2	T41.3X3	T41.3X4	T41.3X5	T41.3X6
Anesthetic NEC— *see also Anesthesia*	T41.41	T41.42	T41.43	T41.44	T41.45	T41.46
with muscle relaxant	T41.201	T41.202	T41.203	T41.204	T41.205	T41.206
general	T41.201	T41.202	T41.203	T41.204	T41.205	T41.206
local	T41.3X1	T41.3X2	T41.3X3	T41.3X4	T41.3X5	T41.3X6
gaseous NEC	T41.0X1	T41.0X2	T41.0X3	T41.0X4	T41.0X5	T41.0X6
general NEC	T41.201	T41.202	T41.203	T41.204	T41.205	T41.206
halogenated hydrocarbon derivatives NEC	T41.0X1	T41.0X2	T41.0X3	T41.0X4	T41.0X5	T41.0X6
infiltration NEC	T41.3X1	T41.3X2	T41.3X3	T41.3X4	T41.3X5	T41.3X6
intravenous NEC	T41.1X1	T41.1X2	T41.1X3	T41.1X4	T41.1X5	T41.1X6

Anesthetic NEC - Antihookworm drug

Substance	Poisoning, Accidental unintentional	Poisoning, Intentional self-harm	Poisoning, Assault	Poisoning, Undetermined	Adverse effect	Underdosing
Anesthetic NEC — *continued*						
local NEC	T41.3X1	T41.3X2	T41.3X3	T41.3X4	T41.3X5	T41.3X6
rectal	T41.201	T41.202	T41.203	T41.204	T41.205	T41.206
general	T41.201	T41.202	T41.203	T41.204	T41.205	T41.206
local	T41.3X1	T41.3X2	T41.3X3	T41.3X4	T41.3X5	T41.3X6
regional NEC	T41.3X1	T41.3X2	T41.3X3	T41.3X4	T41.3X5	T41.3X6
spinal NEC	T41.3X1	T41.3X2	T41.3X3	T41.3X4	T41.3X5	T41.3X6
thiobarbiturate	T41.1X1	T41.1X2	T41.1X3	T41.1X4	T41.1X5	T41.1X6
topical	T41.3X1	T41.3X2	T41.3X3	T41.3X4	T41.3X5	T41.3X6
Aneurine	T45.2X1	T45.2X2	T45.2X3	T45.2X4	T45.2X5	T45.2X6
Angio-Conray®	T50.8X1	T50.8X2	T50.8X3	T50.8X4	T50.8X5	T50.8X6
Angiotensin	T44.5X1	T44.5X2	T44.5X3	T44.5X4	T44.5X5	T44.5X6
Angiotensinamide	T44.991	T44.992	T44.993	T44.994	T44.995	T44.996
Anhydrohydroxy-progesterone	T38.5X1	T38.5X2	T38.5X3	T38.5X4	T38.5X5	T38.5X6
Anhydron	T50.2X1	T50.2X2	T50.2X3	T50.2X4	T50.2X5	T50.2X6
Anileridine	T40.4X1	T40.4X2	T40.4X3	T40.4X4	T40.4X5	T40.4X6
Aniline (dye) (liquid)	T65.3X1	T65.3X2	T65.3X3	T65.3X4	—	—
analgesic	T39.1X1	T39.1X2	T39.1X3	T39.1X4	T39.1X5	T39.1X6
derivatives, therapeutic NEC	T39.1X1	T39.1X2	T39.1X3	T39.1X4	T39.1X5	T39.1X6
vapor	T65.3X1	T65.3X2	T65.3X3	T65.3X4	—	—
Aniscoropine	T44.3X1	T44.3X2	T44.3X3	T44.3X4	T44.3X5	T44.3X6
Anise oil	T47.5X1	T47.5X2	T47.5X3	T47.5X4	T47.5X5	T47.5X6
Anisidine	T65.3X1	T65.3X2	T65.3X3	T65.3X4	—	—
Anisindione	T45.511	T45.512	T45.513	T45.514	T45.515	T45.516
Anisotropine methyl-bromide	T44.3X1	T44.3X2	T44.3X3	T44.3X4	T44.3X5	T44.3X6
Anistreplase	T45.611	T45.612	T45.613	T45.614	T45.615	T45.616
Anorexiant (central)	T50.5X1	T50.5X2	T50.5X3	T50.5X4	T50.5X5	T50.5X6
Anorexic agents	T50.5X1	T50.5X2	T50.5X3	T50.5X4	T50.5X5	T50.5X6
Ansamycin	T36.6X1	T36.6X2	T36.6X3	T36.6X4	T36.6X5	T36.6X6
Ant (bite) (sting)	T63.421	T63.422	T63.423	T63.424	—	—
Ant poison — *see Insecticide*						
Antabuse®	T50.6X1	T50.6X2	T50.6X3	T50.6X4	T50.6X5	T50.6X6
Antacid NEC	T47.1X1	T47.1X2	T47.1X3	T47.1X4	T47.1X5	T47.1X6
Antagonist						
Aldosterone	T50.0X1	T50.0X2	T50.0X3	T50.0X4	T50.0X5	T50.0X6
alpha-adrenoreceptor	T44.6X1	T44.6X2	T44.6X3	T44.6X4	T44.6X5	T44.6X6
anticoagulant	T45.7X1	T45.7X2	T45.7X3	T45.7X4	T45.7X5	T45.7X6
beta-adrenoreceptor	T44.7X1	T44.7X2	T44.7X3	T44.7X4	T44.7X5	T44.7X6
extrapyramidal NEC	T44.3X1	T44.3X2	T44.3X3	T44.3X4	T44.3X5	T44.3X6
folic acid	T45.1X1	T45.1X2	T45.1X3	T45.1X4	T45.1X5	T45.1X6
H2 receptor	T47.0X1	T47.0X2	T47.0X3	T47.0X4	T47.0X5	T47.0X6
heavy metal	T45.8X1	T45.8X2	T45.8X3	T45.8X4	T45.8X5	T45.8X6
narcotic analgesic	T50.7X1	T50.7X2	T50.7X3	T50.7X4	T50.7X5	T50.7X6
opiate	T50.7X1	T50.7X2	T50.7X3	T50.7X4	T50.7X5	T50.7X6
pyrimidine	T45.1X1	T45.1X2	T45.1X3	T45.1X4	T45.1X5	T45.1X6
serotonin	T46.5X1	T46.5X2	T46.5X3	T46.5X4	T46.5X5	T46.5X6
Antazolin (e)	T45.0X1	T45.0X2	T45.0X3	T45.0X4	T45.0X5	T45.0X6
Anterior pituitary hormone NEC	T38.811	T38.812	T38.813	T38.814	T38.815	T38.816
Anthelmintic NEC	T37.4X1	T37.4X2	T37.4X3	T37.4X4	T37.4X5	T37.4X6
Anthiolimine	T37.4X1	T37.4X2	T37.4X3	T37.4X4	T37.4X5	T37.4X6
Anthralin	T49.4X1	T49.4X2	T49.4X3	T49.4X4	T49.4X5	T49.4X6
Anthramycin	T45.1X1	T45.1X2	T45.1X3	T45.1X4	T45.1X5	T45.1X6
Antiadrenergic NEC	T44.8X1	T44.8X2	T44.8X3	T44.8X4	T44.8X5	T44.8X6
Antiallergic NEC	T45.0X1	T45.0X2	T45.0X3	T45.0X4	T45.0X5	T45.0X6
Anti-anemic (drug) (preparation)	T45.8X1	T45.8X2	T45.8X3	T45.8X4	T45.8X5	T45.8X6
Antiandrogen NEC	T38.6X1	T38.6X2	T38.6X3	T38.6X4	T38.6X5	T38.6X6
Antianxiety drug NEC	T43.501	T43.502	T43.503	T43.504	T43.505	T43.506
Antiaris toxicaria	T65.891	T65.892	T65.893	T65.894	—	—
Antiarteriosclerotic drug	T46.6X1	T46.6X2	T46.6X3	T46.6X4	T46.6X5	T46.6X6
Antiasthmatic drug NEC	T48.6X1	T48.6X2	T48.6X3	T48.6X4	T48.6X5	T48.6X6
Antibiotic NEC	T36.91	T36.92	T36.93	T36.94	T36.95	T36.96
aminoglycoside	T36.5X1	T36.5X2	T36.5X3	T36.5X4	T36.5X5	T36.5X6
anticancer	T45.1X1	T45.1X2	T45.1X3	T45.1X4	T45.1X5	T45.1X6
antifungal	T36.7X1	T36.7X2	T36.7X3	T36.7X4	T36.7X5	T36.7X6
antimycobacterial	T36.5X1	T36.5X2	T36.5X3	T36.5X4	T36.5X5	T36.5X6
antineoplastic	T45.1X1	T45.1X2	T45.1X3	T45.1X4	T45.1X5	T45.1X6
cephalosporin (group)	T36.1X1	T36.1X2	T36.1X3	T36.1X4	T36.1X5	T36.1X6
chloramphenicol (group)	T36.2X1	T36.2X2	T36.2X3	T36.2X4	T36.2X5	T36.2X6
ENT	T49.6X1	T49.6X2	T49.6X3	T49.6X4	T49.6X5	T49.6X6
eye	T49.5X1	T49.5X2	T49.5X3	T49.5X4	T49.5X5	T49.5X6
fungicidal (local)	T49.0X1	T49.0X2	T49.0X3	T49.0X4	T49.0X5	T49.0X6
intestinal	T36.8X1	T36.8X2	T36.8X3	T36.8X4	T36.8X5	T36.8X6
b-lactam NEC	T36.1X1	T36.1X2	T36.1X3	T36.1X4	T36.1X5	T36.1X6
local	T49.0X1	T49.0X2	T49.0X3	T49.0X4	T49.0X5	T49.0X6
macrolides	T36.3X1	T36.3X2	T36.3X3	T36.3X4	T36.3X5	T36.3X6
polypeptide	T36.8X1	T36.8X2	T36.8X3	T36.8X4	T36.8X5	T36.8X6
specified NEC	T36.8X1	T36.8X2	T36.8X3	T36.8X4	T36.8X5	T36.8X6
tetracycline (group)	T36.4X1	T36.4X2	T36.4X3	T36.4X4	T36.4X5	T36.4X6
throat	T49.6X1	T49.6X2	T49.6X3	T49.6X4	T49.6X5	T49.6X6
Anticancer agents NEC	T45.1X1	T45.1X2	T45.1X3	T45.1X4	T45.1X5	T45.1X6
Anticholesterolemic drug NEC	T46.6X1	T46.6X2	T46.6X3	T46.6X4	T46.6X5	T46.6X6
Anticholinergic NEC	T44.3X1	T44.3X2	T44.3X3	T44.3X4	T44.3X5	T44.3X6
Anticholinesterase	T44.0X1	T44.0X2	T44.0X3	T44.0X4	T44.0X5	T44.0X6
organophosphorus	T44.0X1	T44.0X2	T44.0X3	T44.0X4	T44.0X5	T44.0X6
insecticide	T60.0X1	T60.0X2	T60.0X3	T60.0X4	—	—
nerve gas	T59.891	T59.892	T59.893	T59.894	—	—
reversible	T44.0X1	T44.0X2	T44.0X3	T44.0X4	T44.0X5	T44.0X6
ophthalmological	T49.5X1	T49.5X2	T49.5X3	T49.5X4	T49.5X5	T49.5X6
Anticoagulant NEC	T45.511	T45.512	T45.513	T45.514	T45.515	T45.516
Antagonist	T45.7X1	T45.7X2	T45.7X3	T45.7X4	T45.7X5	T45.7X6
Anti-common-cold drug NEC	T48.5X1	T48.5X2	T48.5X3	T48.5X4	T48.5X5	T48.5X6
Anticonvulsant	T42.71	T42.72	T42.73	T42.74	T42.75	T42.76
barbiturate	T42.3X1	T42.3X2	T42.3X3	T42.3X4	T42.3X5	T42.3X6
combination (with barbiturate)	T42.3X1	T42.3X2	T42.3X3	T42.3X4	T42.3X5	T42.3X6
hydantoin	T42.0X1	T42.0X2	T42.0X3	T42.0X4	T42.0X5	T42.0X6
hypnotic NEC	T42.6X1	T42.6X2	T42.6X3	T42.6X4	T42.6X5	T42.6X6
oxazolidinedione	T42.2X1	T42.2X2	T42.2X3	T42.2X4	T42.2X5	T42.2X6
pyrimidinedione	T42.6X1	T42.6X2	T42.6X3	T42.6X4	T42.6X5	T42.6X6
specified NEC	T42.6X1	T42.6X2	T42.6X3	T42.6X4	T42.6X5	T42.6X6
succinimide	T42.2X1	T42.2X2	T42.2X3	T42.2X4	T42.2X5	T42.2X6
Anti-D immunoglobulin (human)	T50.Z11	T50.Z12	T50.Z13	T50.Z14	T50.Z15	T50.Z16
Antidepressant	T43.201	T43.202	T43.203	T43.204	T43.205	T43.206
monoamine oxidase inhibitor	T43.1X1	T43.1X2	T43.1X3	T43.1X4	T43.1X5	T43.1X6
selective serotonin norepinephrine reuptake inhibitor	T43.211	T43.212	T43.213	T43.214	T43.215	T43.216
selective serotonin reuptake inhibitor	T43.221	T43.222	T43.223	T43.224	T43.225	T43.226
specified NEC	T43.291	T43.292	T43.293	T43.294	T43.295	T43.296
tetracyclic	T43.021	T43.022	T43.023	T43.024	T43.025	T43.026
triazolopyridine	T43.211	T43.212	T43.213	T43.214	T43.215	T43.216
tricyclic	T43.011	T43.012	T43.013	T43.014	T43.015	T43.016
Antidiabetic NEC	T38.3X1	T38.3X2	T38.3X3	T38.3X4	T38.3X5	T38.3X6
biguanide	T38.3X1	T38.3X2	T38.3X3	T38.3X4	T38.3X5	T38.3X6
and sulfonyl combined	T38.3X1	T38.3X2	T38.3X3	T38.3X4	T38.3X5	T38.3X6
combined	T38.3X1	T38.3X2	T38.3X3	T38.3X4	T38.3X5	T38.3X6
sulfonylurea	T38.3X1	T38.3X2	T38.3X3	T38.3X4	T38.3X5	T38.3X6
Antidiarrheal drug NEC	T47.6X1	T47.6X2	T47.6X3	T47.6X4	T47.6X5	T47.6X6
absorbent	T47.6X1	T47.6X2	T47.6X3	T47.6X4	T47.6X5	T47.6X6
Antidiphtheria serum	T50.Z11	T50.Z12	T50.Z13	T50.Z14	T50.Z15	T50.Z16
Antidiuretic hormone	T38.891	T38.892	T38.893	T38.894	T38.895	T38.896
Antidote NEC	T50.6X1	T50.6X2	T50.6X3	T50.6X4	T50.6X5	T50.6X6
heavy metal	T45.8X1	T45.8X2	T45.8X3	T45.8X4	T45.8X5	T45.8X6
Antidysrhythmic NEC	T46.2X1	T46.2X2	T46.2X3	T46.2X4	T46.2X5	T46.2X6
Antiemetic drug	T45.0X1	T45.0X2	T45.0X3	T45.0X4	T45.0X5	T45.0X6
Antiepilepsy agent	T42.71	T42.72	T42.73	T42.74	T42.75	T42.76
combination	T42.5X1	T42.5X2	T42.5X3	T42.5X4	T42.5X5	T42.5X6
mixed	T42.5X1	T42.5X2	T42.5X3	T42.5X4	T42.5X5	T42.5X6
specified, NEC	T42.6X1	T42.6X2	T42.6X3	T42.6X4	T42.6X5	T42.6X6
Antiestrogen NEC	T38.6X1	T38.6X2	T38.6X3	T38.6X4	T38.6X5	T38.6X6
Antifertility pill	T38.4X1	T38.4X2	T38.4X3	T38.4X4	T38.4X5	T38.4X6
Antifibrinolytic drug	T45.621	T45.622	T45.623	T45.624	T45.625	T45.626
Antifilarial drug	T37.4X1	T37.4X2	T37.4X3	T37.4X4	T37.4X5	T37.4X6
Antiflatulent	T47.5X1	T47.5X2	T47.5X3	T47.5X4	T47.5X5	T47.5X6
Antifreeze	T65.91	T65.92	T65.93	T65.94	—	—
alcohol	T51.1X1	T51.1X2	T51.1X3	T51.1X4	—	—
ethylene glycol	T51.8X1	T51.8X2	T51.8X3	T51.8X4	—	—
Antifungal						
antibiotic (systemic)	T36.7X1	T36.7X2	T36.7X3	T36.7X4	T36.7X5	T36.7X6
anti-infective NEC	T37.91	T37.92	T37.93	T37.94	T37.95	T37.96
disinfectant, local	T49.0X1	T49.0X2	T49.0X3	T49.0X4	T49.0X5	T49.0X6
nonmedicinal (spray)	T60.3X1	T60.3X2	T60.3X3	T60.3X4	—	—
topical	T49.0X1	T49.0X2	T49.0X3	T49.0X4	T49.0X5	T49.0X6
Anti-gastric-secretion drug NEC	T47.1X1	T47.1X2	T47.1X3	T47.1X4	T47.1X5	T47.1X6
Antigonadotrophin NEC	T38.6X1	T38.6X2	T38.6X3	T38.6X4	T38.6X5	T38.6X6
Antihallucinogen	T43.501	T43.502	T43.503	T43.504	T43.505	T43.506
Antihelmintics	T37.4X1	T37.4X2	T37.4X3	T37.4X4	T37.4X5	T37.4X6
Antihemophilic						
factor	T45.8X1	T45.8X2	T45.8X3	T45.8X4	T45.8X5	T45.8X6
fraction	T45.8X1	T45.8X2	T45.8X3	T45.8X4	T45.8X5	T45.8X6
globulin concentrate	T45.7X1	T45.7X2	T45.7X3	T45.7X4	T45.7X5	T45.7X6
human plasma	T45.8X1	T45.8X2	T45.8X3	T45.8X4	T45.8X5	T45.8X6
plasma, dried	T45.7X1	T45.7X2	T45.7X3	T45.7X4	T45.7X5	T45.7X6
Antihemorrhoidal preparation	T49.2X1	T49.2X2	T49.2X3	T49.2X4	T49.2X5	T49.2X6
Antiheparin drug	T45.7X1	T45.7X2	T45.7X3	T45.7X4	T45.7X5	T45.7X6
Antihistamine	T45.0X1	T45.0X2	T45.0X3	T45.0X4	T45.0X5	T45.0X6
Antihookworm drug	T37.4X1	T37.4X2	T37.4X3	T37.4X4	T37.4X5	T37.4X6

Substance	Poisoning, Accidental unintentional	Poisoning, Intentional self-harm	Poisoning, Assault	Poisoning, Undetermined	Adverse effect	Underdosing
Anti-human lymphocytic globulin	T50.Z11	T50.Z12	T50.Z13	T50.Z14	T50.Z15	T50.Z16
Antihyperlipidemic drug	T46.6X1	T46.6X2	T46.6X3	T46.6X4	T46.6X5	T46.6X6
Antihypertensive drug NEC	T46.5X1	T46.5X2	T46.5X3	T46.5X4	T46.5X5	T46.5X6
Anti-infective NEC	T37.91	T37.92	T37.93	T37.94	T37.95	T37.96
anthelmintic	T37.4X1	T37.4X2	T37.4X3	T37.4X4	T37.4X5	T37.4X6
antibiotics	T36.91	T36.92	T36.93	T36.94	T36.95	T36.96
specified NEC	T36.8X1	T36.8X2	T36.8X3	T36.8X4	T36.8X5	T36.8X6
antimalarial	T37.2X1	T37.2X2	T37.2X3	T37.2X4	T37.2X5	T37.2X6
antimycobacterial NEC	T37.1X1	T37.1X2	T37.1X3	T37.1X4	T37.1X5	T37.1X6
antibiotics	T36.5X1	T36.5X2	T36.5X3	T36.5X4	T36.5X5	T36.5X6
antiprotozoal NEC	T37.3X1	T37.3X2	T37.3X3	T37.3X4	T37.3X5	T37.3X6
blood	T37.2X1	T37.2X2	T37.2X3	T37.2X4	T37.2X5	T37.2X6
antiviral	T37.5X1	T37.5X2	T37.5X3	T37.5X4	T37.5X5	T37.5X6
arsenical	T37.8X1	T37.8X2	T37.8X3	T37.8X4	T37.8X5	T37.8X6
bismuth, local	T49.0X1	T49.0X2	T49.0X3	T49.0X4	T49.0X5	T49.0X6
ENT	T49.6X1	T49.6X2	T49.6X3	T49.6X4	T49.6X5	T49.6X6
eye NEC	T49.5X1	T49.5X2	T49.5X3	T49.5X4	T49.5X5	T49.5X6
heavy metals NEC	T37.8X1	T37.8X2	T37.8X3	T37.8X4	T37.8X5	T37.8X6
local NEC	T49.0X1	T49.0X2	T49.0X3	T49.0X4	T49.0X5	T49.0X6
specified NEC	T49.0X1	T49.0X2	T49.0X3	T49.0X4	T49.0X5	T49.0X6
mixed	T37.91	T37.92	T37.93	T37.94	T37.95	T37.96
ophthalmic preparation	T49.5X1	T49.5X2	T49.5X3	T49.5X4	T49.5X5	T49.5X6
topical NEC	T49.0X1	T49.0X2	T49.0X3	T49.0X4	T49.0X5	T49.0X6
Anti-inflammatory drug NEC	T39.391	T39.392	T39.393	T39.394	T39.395	T39.396
local	T49.0X1	T49.0X2	T49.0X3	T49.0X4	T49.0X5	T49.0X6
nonsteroidal NEC	T39.391	T39.392	T39.393	T39.394	T39.395	T39.396
propionic acid derivative	T39.311	T39.312	T39.313	T39.314	T39.315	T39.316
specified NEC	T39.391	T39.392	T39.393	T39.394	T39.395	T39.396
Antikaluretic	T50.3X1	T50.3X2	T50.3X3	T50.3X4	T50.3X5	T50.3X6
Antiknock (tetraethyl lead)	T56.0X1	T56.0X2	T56.0X3	T56.0X4	—	—
Antilipemic drug NEC	T46.6X1	T46.6X2	T46.6X3	T46.6X4	T46.6X5	T46.6X6
Antimalarial	T37.2X1	T37.2X2	T37.2X3	T37.2X4	T37.2X5	T37.2X6
prophylactic NEC	T37.2X1	T37.2X2	T37.2X3	T37.2X4	T37.2X5	T37.2X6
pyrimidine derivative	T37.2X1	T37.2X2	T37.2X3	T37.2X4	T37.2X5	T37.2X6
Antimetabolite	T45.1X1	T45.1X2	T45.1X3	T45.1X4	T45.1X5	T45.1X6
Antimitotic agent	T45.1X1	T45.1X2	T45.1X3	T45.1X4	T45.1X5	T45.1X6
Antimony (compounds) (vapor) **NEC**	T56.891	T56.892	T56.893	T56.894	—	—
anti-infectives	T37.8X1	T37.8X2	T37.8X3	T37.8X4	T37.8X5	T37.8X6
dimercaptosuccinate	T37.3X1	T37.3X2	T37.3X3	T37.3X4	T37.3X5	T37.3X6
hydride	T56.891	T56.892	T56.893	T56.894	—	—
pesticide (vapor)	T60.8X1	T60.8X2	T60.8X3	T60.8X4	—	—
potassium (sodium) tartrate	T37.8X1	T37.8X2	T37.8X3	T37.8X4	T37.8X5	T37.8X6
sodium dimercaptosuccinate	T37.3X1	T37.3X2	T37.3X3	T37.3X4	T37.3X5	T37.3X6
tartrated	T37.8X1	T37.8X2	T37.8X3	T37.8X4	T37.8X5	T37.8X6
Antimuscarinic NEC	T44.3X1	T44.3X2	T44.3X3	T44.3X4	T44.3X5	T44.3X6
Antimycobacterial drug NEC	T37.1X1	T37.1X2	T37.1X3	T37.1X4	T37.1X5	T37.1X6
antibiotics	T36.5X1	T36.5X2	T36.5X3	T36.5X4	T36.5X5	T36.5X6
combination	T37.1X1	T37.1X2	T37.1X3	T37.1X4	T37.1X5	T37.1X6
Antinausea drug	T45.0X1	T45.0X2	T45.0X3	T45.0X4	T45.0X5	T45.0X6
Antinematode drug	T37.4X1	T37.4X2	T37.4X3	T37.4X4	T37.4X5	T37.4X6
Antineoplastic NEC	T45.1X1	T45.1X2	T45.1X3	T45.1X4	T45.1X5	T45.1X6
alkaloidal	T45.1X1	T45.1X2	T45.1X3	T45.1X4	T45.1X5	T45.1X6
antibiotics	T45.1X1	T45.1X2	T45.1X3	T45.1X4	T45.1X5	T45.1X6
combination	T45.1X1	T45.1X2	T45.1X3	T45.1X4	T45.1X5	T45.1X6
estrogen	T38.5X1	T38.5X2	T38.5X3	T38.5X4	T38.5X5	T38.5X6
steroid	T38.7X1	T38.7X2	T38.7X3	T38.7X4	T38.7X5	T38.7X6
Antiparasitic drug (systemic)	T37.91	T37.92	T37.93	T37.94	T37.95	T37.96
local	T49.0X1	T49.0X2	T49.0X3	T49.0X4	T49.0X5	T49.0X6
specified NEC	T37.8X1	T37.8X2	T37.8X3	T37.8X4	T37.8X5	T37.8X6
Antiparkinsonism drug NEC	T42.8X1	T42.8X2	T42.8X3	T42.8X4	T42.8X5	T42.8X6
Antiperspirant NEC	T49.2X1	T49.2X2	T49.2X3	T49.2X4	T49.2X5	T49.2X6
Antiphlogistic NEC	T39.4X1	T39.4X2	T39.4X3	T39.4X4	T39.4X5	T39.4X6
Antiplatyhelmintic drug	T37.4X1	T37.4X2	T37.4X3	T37.4X4	T37.4X5	T37.4X6
Antiprotozoal drug NEC	T37.3X1	T37.3X2	T37.3X3	T37.3X4	T37.3X5	T37.3X6
blood	T37.2X1	T37.2X2	T37.2X3	T37.2X4	T37.2X5	T37.2X6
local	T49.0X1	T49.0X2	T49.0X3	T49.0X4	T49.0X5	T49.0X6
Antipruritic drug NEC	T49.1X1	T49.1X2	T49.1X3	T49.1X4	T49.1X5	T49.1X6
Antipsychotic drug	T43.501	T43.502	T43.503	T43.504	T43.505	T43.506
specified NEC	T43.591	T43.592	T43.593	T43.594	T43.595	T43.596
Antipyretic	T39.91	T39.92	T39.93	T39.94	T39.95	T39.96
specified NEC	T39.8X1	T39.8X2	T39.8X3	T39.8X4	T39.8X5	T39.8X6
Antipyrine	T39.2X1	T39.2X2	T39.2X3	T39.2X4	T39.2X5	T39.2X6
Antirabies hyperimmune serum	T50.Z11	T50.Z12	T50.Z13	T50.Z14	T50.Z15	T50.Z16
Antirheumatic NEC	T39.4X1	T39.4X2	T39.4X3	T39.4X4	T39.4X5	T39.4X6
Antirigidity drug NEC	T42.8X1	T42.8X2	T42.8X3	T42.8X4	T42.8X5	T42.8X6
Antischistosomal drug	T37.4X1	T37.4X2	T37.4X3	T37.4X4	T37.4X5	T37.4X6
Antiscorpion sera	T50.Z11	T50.Z12	T50.Z13	T50.Z14	T50.Z15	T50.Z16
Antiseborrheics	T49.4X1	T49.4X2	T49.4X3	T49.4X4	T49.4X5	T49.4X6
Antiseptics (external) (medicinal)	T49.0X1	T49.0X2	T49.0X3	T49.0X4	T49.0X5	T49.0X6

Substance	Poisoning, Accidental unintentional	Poisoning, Intentional self-harm	Poisoning, Assault	Poisoning, Undetermined	Adverse effect	Underdosing
Antistine	T45.0X1	T45.0X2	T45.0X3	T45.0X4	T45.0X5	T45.0X6
Antitapeworm drug	T37.4X1	T37.4X2	T37.4X3	T37.4X4	T37.4X5	T37.4X6
Antitetanus immunoglobulin	T50.Z11	T50.Z12	T50.Z13	T50.Z14	T50.Z15	T50.Z16
Antithyroid drug NEC	T38.2X1	T38.2X2	T38.2X3	T38.2X4	T38.2X5	T38.2X6
Antitoxin	T50.Z11	T50.Z12	T50.Z13	T50.Z14	T50.Z15	T50.Z16
diphtheria	T50.Z11	T50.Z12	T50.Z13	T50.Z14	T50.Z15	T50.Z16
gas gangrene	T50.Z11	T50.Z12	T50.Z13	T50.Z14	T50.Z15	T50.Z16
tetanus	T50.Z11	T50.Z12	T50.Z13	T50.Z14	T50.Z15	T50.Z16
Antitrichomonal drug	T37.3X1	T37.3X2	T37.3X3	T37.3X4	T37.3X5	T37.3X6
Antituberculars	T37.1X1	T37.1X2	T37.1X3	T37.1X4	T37.1X5	T37.1X6
antibiotics	T36.5X1	T36.5X2	T36.5X3	T36.5X4	T36.5X5	T36.5X6
Antitussive NEC	T48.3X1	T48.3X2	T48.3X3	T48.3X4	T48.3X5	T48.3X6
codeine mixture	T40.2X1	T40.2X2	T40.2X3	T40.2X4	T40.2X5	T40.2X6
opiate	T40.2X1	T40.2X2	T40.2X3	T40.2X4	T40.2X5	T40.2X6
Antivaricose drug	T46.8X1	T46.8X2	T46.8X3	T46.8X4	T46.8X5	T46.8X6
Antivenin, antivenom (sera)	T50.Z11	T50.Z12	T50.Z13	T50.Z14	T50.Z15	T50.Z16
crotaline	T50.Z11	T50.Z12	T50.Z13	T50.Z14	T50.Z15	T50.Z16
spider bite	T50.Z11	T50.Z12	T50.Z13	T50.Z14	T50.Z15	T50.Z16
Antivertigo drug	T45.0X1	T45.0X2	T45.0X3	T45.0X4	T45.0X5	T45.0X6
Antiviral drug NEC	T37.5X1	T37.5X2	T37.5X3	T37.5X4	T37.5X5	T37.5X6
eye	T49.5X1	T49.5X2	T49.5X3	T49.5X4	T49.5X5	T49.5X6
Antiwhipworm drug	T37.4X1	T37.4X2	T37.4X3	T37.4X4	T37.4X5	T37.4X6
Antrol — *see also by specific chemical substance*	T60.91	T60.92	T60.93	T60.94	—	—
fungicide	T60.91	T60.92	T60.93	T60.94	—	—
ANTU (alpha naphthylthiourea)	T60.4X1	T60.4X2	T60.4X3	T60.4X4	—	—
Apalcillin	T36.0X1	T36.0X2	T36.0X3	T36.0X4	T36.0X5	T36.0X6
APC	T48.5X1	T48.5X2	T48.5X3	T48.5X4	T48.5X5	T48.5X6
Aplonidine	T44.4X1	T44.4X2	T44.4X3	T44.4X4	T44.4X5	T44.4X6
Apomorphine	T47.7X1	T47.7X2	T47.7X3	T47.7X4	T47.7X5	T47.7X6
Appetite depressants, central	T50.5X1	T50.5X2	T50.5X3	T50.5X4	T50.5X5	T50.5X6
Apraclonidine (hydrochloride)	T44.4X1	T44.4X2	T44.4X3	T44.4X4	T44.4X5	T44.4X6
Apresoline	T46.5X1	T46.5X2	T46.5X3	T46.5X4	T46.5X5	T46.5X6
Aprindine	T46.2X1	T46.2X2	T46.2X3	T46.2X4	T46.2X5	T46.2X6
Aprobarbital	T42.3X1	T42.3X2	T42.3X3	T42.3X4	T42.3X5	T42.3X6
Apronalide	T42.6X1	T42.6X2	T42.6X3	T42.6X4	T42.6X5	T42.6X6
Aprotinin	T45.621	T45.622	T45.623	T45.624	T45.625	T45.626
Aptocaine	T41.3X1	T41.3X2	T41.3X3	T41.3X4	T41.3X5	T41.3X6
Aqua fortis	T54.2X1	T54.2X2	T54.2X3	T54.2X4	—	—
Ara-A	T37.5X1	T37.5X2	T37.5X3	T37.5X4	T37.5X5	T37.5X6
Ara-C	T45.1X1	T45.1X2	T45.1X3	T45.1X4	T45.1X5	T45.1X6
Arachis oil	T49.3X1	T49.3X2	T49.3X3	T49.3X4	T49.3X5	T49.3X6
cathartic	T47.4X1	T47.4X2	T47.4X3	T47.4X4	T47.4X5	T47.4X6
Aralen	T37.2X1	T37.2X2	T37.2X3	T37.2X4	T37.2X5	T37.2X6
Arecoline	T44.1X1	T44.1X2	T44.1X3	T44.1X4	T44.1X5	T44.1X6
Arginine	T50.991	T50.992	T50.993	T50.994	T50.995	T50.996
glutamate	T50.991	T50.992	T50.993	T50.994	T50.995	T50.996
Argyrol®	T49.0X1	T49.0X2	T49.0X3	T49.0X4	T49.0X5	T49.0X6
ENT agent	T49.6X1	T49.6X2	T49.6X3	T49.6X4	T49.6X5	T49.6X6
ophthalmic preparation	T49.5X1	T49.5X2	T49.5X3	T49.5X4	T49.5X5	T49.5X6
Aristocort®	T38.0X1	T38.0X2	T38.0X3	T38.0X4	T38.0X5	T38.0X6
ENT agent	T49.6X1	T49.6X2	T49.6X3	T49.6X4	T49.6X5	T49.6X6
ophthalmic preparation	T49.5X1	T49.5X2	T49.5X3	T49.5X4	T49.5X5	T49.5X6
topical NEC	T49.0X1	T49.0X2	T49.0X3	T49.0X4	T49.0X5	T49.0X6
Aromatics, corrosive	T54.1X1	T54.1X2	T54.1X3	T54.1X4	—	—
disinfectants	T54.1X1	T54.1X2	T54.1X3	T54.1X4	—	—
Arsenate of lead	T57.0X1	T57.0X2	T57.0X3	T57.0X4	—	—
herbicide	T57.0X1	T57.0X2	T57.0X3	T57.0X4	—	—
Arsenic, arsenicals (compounds) (dust) (vapor) **NEC**	T57.0X1	T57.0X2	T57.0X3	T57.0X4	—	—
anti-infectives	T37.8X1	T37.8X2	T37.8X3	T37.8X4	T37.8X5	T37.8X6
pesticide (dust) (fumes)	T57.0X1	T57.0X2	T57.0X3	T57.0X4	—	—
Arsine (gas)	T57.0X1	T57.0X2	T57.0X3	T57.0X4	—	—
Arsphenamine (silver)	T37.8X1	T37.8X2	T37.8X3	T37.8X4	T37.8X5	T37.8X6
Arsthinol	T37.3X1	T37.3X2	T37.3X3	T37.3X4	T37.3X5	T37.3X6
Artane®	T44.3X1	T44.3X2	T44.3X3	T44.3X4	T44.3X5	T44.3X6
Arthropod (venomous) **NEC**	T63.481	T63.482	T63.483	T63.484	—	—
Articaine	T41.3X1	T41.3X2	T41.3X3	T41.3X4	T41.3X5	T41.3X6
Asbestos	T57.8X1	T57.8X2	T57.8X3	T57.8X4	—	—
Ascaridole	T37.4X1	T37.4X2	T37.4X3	T37.4X4	T37.4X5	T37.4X6
Ascorbic acid	T45.2X1	T45.2X2	T45.2X3	T45.2X4	T45.2X5	T45.2X6
Asiaticoside	T49.0X1	T49.0X2	T49.0X3	T49.0X4	T49.0X5	T49.0X6
Asparaginase	T45.1X1	T45.1X2	T45.1X3	T45.1X4	T45.1X5	T45.1X6
Aspidium (oleoresin)	T37.4X1	T37.4X2	T37.4X3	T37.4X4	T37.4X5	T37.4X6
Aspirin (aluminum) (soluble)	T39.011	T39.012	T39.013	T39.014	T39.015	T39.016
Aspoxicillin	T36.0X1	T36.0X2	T36.0X3	T36.0X4	T36.0X5	T36.0X6
Astemizole	T45.0X1	T45.0X2	T45.0X3	T45.0X4	T45.0X5	T45.0X6
Astringent (local)	T49.2X1	T49.2X2	T49.2X3	T49.2X4	T49.2X5	T49.2X6
specified NEC	T49.2X1	T49.2X2	T49.2X3	T49.2X4	T49.2X5	T49.2X6
Astromicin	T36.5X1	T36.5X2	T36.5X3	T36.5X4	T36.5X5	T36.5X6
Ataractic drug NEC	T43.501	T43.502	T43.503	T43.504	T43.505	T43.506
Atenolol	T44.7X1	T44.7X2	T44.7X3	T44.7X4	T44.7X5	T44.7X6
Atonia drug, intestinal	T47.4X1	T47.4X2	T47.4X3	T47.4X4	T47.4X5	T47.4X6
Atophan	T50.4X1	T50.4X2	T50.4X3	T50.4X4	T50.4X5	T50.4X6

Anti-human lymphocytic globulin - Atophan

ICD-10-CM TABLE OF DRUGS AND CHEMICALS

Atracurium besilate - Benzothiadiazides

Substance	Poisoning, Accidental unintentional	Poisoning, Intentional self-harm	Poisoning, Assault	Poisoning, Undetermined	Adverse effect	Underdosing
Atracurium besilate	T48.1X1	T48.1X2	T48.1X3	T48.1X4	T48.1X5	T48.1X6
Atropine	T44.3X1	T44.3X2	T44.3X3	T44.3X4	T44.3X5	T44.3X6
derivative	T44.3X1	T44.3X2	T44.3X3	T44.3X4	T44.3X5	T44.3X6
methonitrate	T44.3X1	T44.3X2	T44.3X3	T44.3X4	T44.3X5	T44.3X6
Attapulgite	T47.6X1	T47.6X2	T47.6X3	T47.6X4	T47.6X5	T47.6X6
Auramine	T65.891	T65.892	T65.893	T65.894	—	—
dye	T65.6X1	T65.6X2	T65.6X3	T65.6X4	—	—
fungicide	T60.3X1	T60.3X2	T60.3X3	T60.3X4	—	—
Auranofin	T39.4X1	T39.4X2	T39.4X3	T39.4X4	T39.4X5	T39.4X6
Aurantiin	T46.991	T46.992	T46.993	T46.994	T46.995	T46.996
Aureomycin®	T36.4X1	T36.4X2	T36.4X3	T36.4X4	T36.4X5	T36.4X6
ophthalmic preparation	T49.5X1	T49.5X2	T49.5X3	T49.5X4	T49.5X5	T49.5X6
topical NEC	T49.0X1	T49.0X2	T49.0X3	T49.0X4	T49.0X5	T49.0X6
Aurothioglucose	T39.4X1	T39.4X2	T39.4X3	T39.4X4	T39.4X5	T39.4X6
Aurothioglycanide	T39.4X1	T39.4X2	T39.4X3	T39.4X4	T39.4X5	T39.4X6
Aurothiomalate sodium	T39.4X1	T39.4X2	T39.4X3	T39.4X4	T39.4X5	T39.4X6
Aurotioprol	T39.4X1	T39.4X2	T39.4X3	T39.4X4	T39.4X5	T39.4X6
Automobile fuel	T52.0X1	T52.0X2	T52.0X3	T52.0X4	—	—
Autonomic nervous system agent NEC	T44.901	T44.902	T44.903	T44.904	T44.905	T44.906
Avlosulfon	T37.1X1	T37.1X2	T37.1X3	T37.1X4	T37.1X5	T37.1X6
Avomine	T42.6X1	T42.6X2	T42.6X3	T42.6X4	T42.6X5	T42.6X6
Axerophthol	T45.2X1	T45.2X2	T45.2X3	T45.2X4	T45.2X5	T45.2X6
Azacitidine	T45.1X1	T45.1X2	T45.1X3	T45.1X4	T45.1X5	T45.1X6
Azacyclonol	T43.591	T43.592	T43.593	T43.594	T43.595	T43.596
Azadirachta	T60.2X1	T60.2X2	T60.2X3	T60.2X4	—	—
Azanidazole	T37.3X1	T37.3X2	T37.3X3	T37.3X4	T37.3X5	T37.3X6
Azapetine	T46.7X1	T46.7X2	T46.7X3	T46.7X4	T46.7X5	T46.7X6
Azapropazone	T39.2X1	T39.2X2	T39.2X3	T39.2X4	T39.2X5	T39.2X6
Azaribine	T45.1X1	T45.1X2	T45.1X3	T45.1X4	T45.1X5	T45.1X6
Azaserine	T45.1X1	T45.1X2	T45.1X3	T45.1X4	T45.1X5	T45.1X6
Azatadine	T45.0X1	T45.0X2	T45.0X3	T45.0X4	T45.0X5	T45.0X6
Azatepa	T45.1X1	T45.1X2	T45.1X3	T45.1X4	T45.1X5	T45.1X6
Azathioprine	T45.1X1	T45.1X2	T45.1X3	T45.1X4	T45.1X5	T45.1X6
Azelaic acid	T49.0X1	T49.0X2	T49.0X3	T49.0X4	T49.0X5	T49.0X6
Azelastine	T45.0X1	T45.0X2	T45.0X3	T45.0X4	T45.0X5	T45.0X6
Azidocillin	T36.0X1	T36.0X2	T36.0X3	T36.0X4	T36.0X5	T36.0X6
Azidothymidine	T37.5X1	T37.5X2	T37.5X3	T37.5X4	T37.5X5	T37.5X6
Azinphos (ethyl) (methyl)	T60.0X1	T60.0X2	T60.0X3	T60.0X4	—	—
Aziridine (chelating)	T54.1X1	T54.1X2	T54.1X3	T54.1X4	—	—
Azithromycin	T36.3X1	T36.3X2	T36.3X3	T36.3X4	T36.3X5	T36.3X6
Azlocillin	T36.0X1	T36.0X2	T36.0X3	T36.0X4	T36.0X5	T36.0X6
Azobenzene smoke	T65.3X1	T65.3X2	T65.3X3	T65.3X4	—	—
acaricide	T60.8X1	T60.8X2	T60.8X3	T60.8X4	—	—
Azosulfamide	T37.0X1	T37.0X2	T37.0X3	T37.0X4	T37.0X5	T37.0X6
AZT	T37.5X1	T37.5X2	T37.5X3	T37.5X4	T37.5X5	T37.5X6
Aztreonam	T36.1X1	T36.1X2	T36.1X3	T36.1X4	T36.1X5	T36.1X6
Azulfidine	T37.0X1	T37.0X2	T37.0X3	T37.0X4	T37.0X5	T37.0X6
Azuresin	T50.8X1	T50.8X2	T50.8X3	T50.8X4	T50.8X5	T50.8X6
			B			
Bacampicillin	T36.0X1	T36.0X2	T36.0X3	T36.0X4	T36.0X5	T36.0X6
Bacillus						
lactobacillus	T47.8X1	T47.8X2	T47.8X3	T47.8X4	T47.8X5	T47.8X6
subtilis	T47.6X1	T47.6X2	T47.6X3	T47.6X4	T47.6X5	T47.6X6
Bacimycin®	T49.0X1	T49.0X2	T49.0X3	T49.0X4	T49.0X5	T49.0X6
ophthalmic preparation	T49.5X1	T49.5X2	T49.5X3	T49.5X4	T49.5X5	T49.5X6
Bacitracin zinc	T49.0X1	T49.0X2	T49.0X3	T49.0X4	T49.0X5	T49.0X6
with neomycin	T49.0X1	T49.0X2	T49.0X3	T49.0X4	T49.0X5	T49.0X6
ENT agent	T49.6X1	T49.6X2	T49.6X3	T49.6X4	T49.6X5	T49.6X6
ophthalmic preparation	T49.5X1	T49.5X2	T49.5X3	T49.5X4	T49.5X5	T49.5X6
topical NEC	T49.0X1	T49.0X2	T49.0X3	T49.0X4	T49.0X5	T49.0X6
Baclofen	T42.8X1	T42.8X2	T42.8X3	T42.8X4	T42.8X5	T42.8X6
Baking soda	T50.991	T50.992	T50.993	T50.994	T50.995	T50.996
BAL	T45.8X1	T45.8X2	T45.8X3	T45.8X4	T45.8X5	T45.8X6
Bambuterol	T48.6X1	T48.6X2	T48.6X3	T48.6X4	T48.6X5	T48.6X6
Bamethan (sulfate)	T46.7X1	T46.7X2	T46.7X3	T46.7X4	T46.7X5	T46.7X6
Bamifylline	T48.6X1	T48.6X2	T48.6X3	T48.6X4	T48.6X5	T48.6X6
Bamipine	T45.0X1	T45.0X2	T45.0X3	T45.0X4	T45.0X5	T45.0X6
Baneberry — *see Actaea spicata*						
Banewort — *see Belladonna*						
Barbenyl	T42.3X1	T42.3X2	T42.3X3	T42.3X4	T42.3X5	T42.3X6
Barbexaclone	T42.6X1	T42.6X2	T42.6X3	T42.6X4	T42.6X5	T42.6X6
Barbital	T42.3X1	T42.3X2	T42.3X3	T42.3X4	T42.3X5	T42.3X6
sodium	T42.3X1	T42.3X2	T42.3X3	T42.3X4	T42.3X5	T42.3X6
Barbitone	T42.3X1	T42.3X2	T42.3X3	T42.3X4	T42.3X5	T42.3X6
Barbiturate NEC	T42.3X1	T42.3X2	T42.3X3	T42.3X4	T42.3X5	T42.3X6
with tranquilizer	T42.3X1	T42.3X2	T42.3X3	T42.3X4	T42.3X5	T42.3X6
anesthetic (intravenous)	T41.1X1	T41.1X2	T41.1X3	T41.1X4	T41.1X5	T41.1X6
Barium (carbonate) (chloride) (sulfite)	T57.8X1	T57.8X2	T57.8X3	T57.8X4	—	—
diagnostic agent	T50.8X1	T50.8X2	T50.8X3	T50.8X4	T50.8X5	T50.8X6
pesticide	T60.4X1	T60.4X2	T60.4X3	T60.4X4	—	—
rodenticide	T60.4X1	T60.4X2	T60.4X3	T60.4X4	—	—
sulfate (medicinal)	T50.8X1	T50.8X2	T50.8X3	T50.8X4	T50.8X5	T50.8X6

Substance	Poisoning, Accidental unintentional	Poisoning, Intentional self-harm	Poisoning, Assault	Poisoning, Undetermined	Adverse effect	Underdosing
Barrier cream	T49.3X1	T49.3X2	T49.3X3	T49.3X4	T49.3X5	T49.3X6
Basic fuchsin	T49.0X1	T49.0X2	T49.0X3	T49.0X4	T49.0X5	T49.0X6
Battery acid or fluid	T54.2X1	T54.2X2	T54.2X3	T54.2X4	—	—
Bay rum	T51.8X1	T51.8X2	T51.8X3	T51.8X4	—	—
BCG (vaccine)	T50.A91	T50.A92	T50.A93	T50.A94	T50.A95	T50.A96
BCNU	T45.1X1	T45.1X2	T45.1X3	T45.1X4	T45.1X5	T45.1X6
Bearsfoot	T62.2X1	T62.2X2	T62.2X3	T62.2X4	—	—
Beclamide	T42.6X1	T42.6X2	T42.6X3	T42.6X4	T42.6X5	T42.6X6
Beclomethasone	T44.5X1	T44.5X2	T44.5X3	T44.5X4	T44.5X5	T44.5X6
Bee (sting) (venom)	T63.441	T63.442	T63.443	T63.444	—	—
Befunolol	T49.5X1	T49.5X2	T49.5X3	T49.5X4	T49.5X5	T49.5X6
Bekanamycin	T36.5X1	T36.5X2	T36.5X3	T36.5X4	T36.5X5	T36.5X6
Belladonna— *see also Nightshade*						
alkaloids	T44.3X1	T44.3X2	T44.3X3	T44.3X4	T44.3X5	T44.3X6
extract	T44.3X1	T44.3X2	T44.3X3	T44.3X4	T44.3X5	T44.3X6
herb	T44.3X1	T44.3X2	T44.3X3	T44.3X4	T44.3X5	T44.3X6
Bemegride	T50.7X1	T50.7X2	T50.7X3	T50.7X4	T50.7X5	T50.7X6
Benactyzine	T44.3X1	T44.3X2	T44.3X3	T44.3X4	T44.3X5	T44.3X6
Benadryl®	T45.0X1	T45.0X2	T45.0X3	T45.0X4	T45.0X5	T45.0X6
Benaprizine	T44.3X1	T44.3X2	T44.3X3	T44.3X4	T44.3X5	T44.3X6
Benazepril	T46.4X1	T46.4X2	T46.4X3	T46.4X4	T46.4X5	T46.4X6
Bencyclane	T46.7X1	T46.7X2	T46.7X3	T46.7X4	T46.7X5	T46.7X6
Bendazol	T46.3X1	T46.3X2	T46.3X3	T46.3X4	T46.3X5	T46.3X6
Bendrofluazide	T50.2X1	T50.2X2	T50.2X3	T50.2X4	T50.2X5	T50.2X6
Bendroflumethiazide	T50.2X1	T50.2X2	T50.2X3	T50.2X4	T50.2X5	T50.2X6
Benemid®	T50.4X1	T50.4X2	T50.4X3	T50.4X4	T50.4X5	T50.4X6
Benethamine penicillin	T36.0X1	T36.0X2	T36.0X3	T36.0X4	T36.0X5	T36.0X6
Benexate	T47.1X1	T47.1X2	T47.1X3	T47.1X4	T47.1X5	T47.1X6
Benfluorex	T46.6X1	T46.6X2	T46.6X3	T46.6X4	T46.6X5	T46.6X6
Benfotiamine	T45.2X1	T45.2X2	T45.2X3	T45.2X4	T45.2X5	T45.2X6
Benisone	T49.0X1	T49.0X2	T49.0X3	T49.0X4	T49.0X5	T49.0X6
Benomyl	T60.0X1	T60.0X2	T60.0X3	T60.0X4	—	—
Benoquin	T49.8X1	T49.8X2	T49.8X3	T49.8X4	T49.8X5	T49.8X6
Benoxinate	T41.3X1	T41.3X2	T41.3X3	T41.3X4	T41.3X5	T41.3X6
Benperidol	T43.4X1	T43.4X2	T43.4X3	T43.4X4	T43.4X5	T43.4X6
Benproperine	T48.3X1	T48.3X2	T48.3X3	T48.3X4	T48.3X5	T48.3X6
Benserazide	T42.8X1	T42.8X2	T42.8X3	T42.8X4	T42.8X5	T42.8X6
Bentazepam	T42.4X1	T42.4X2	T42.4X3	T42.4X4	T42.4X5	T42.4X6
Bentiromide	T50.8X1	T50.8X2	T50.8X3	T50.8X4	T50.8X5	T50.8X6
Bentonite	T49.3X1	T49.3X2	T49.3X3	T49.3X4	T49.3X5	T49.3X6
Benzalbutyramide	T46.6X1	T46.6X2	T46.6X3	T46.6X4	T46.6X5	T46.6X6
Benzalkonium (chloride)	T49.0X1	T49.0X2	T49.0X3	T49.0X4	T49.0X5	T49.0X6
ophthalmic preparation	T49.5X1	T49.5X2	T49.5X3	T49.5X4	T49.5X5	T49.5X6
Benzamidosalicylate (calcium)	T37.1X1	T37.1X2	T37.1X3	T37.1X4	T37.1X5	T37.1X6
Benzamine	T41.3X1	T41.3X2	T41.3X3	T41.3X4	T41.3X5	T41.3X6
lactate	T49.1X1	T49.1X2	T49.1X3	T49.1X4	T49.1X5	T49.1X6
Benzamphetamine	T50.5X1	T50.5X2	T50.5X3	T50.5X4	T50.5X5	T50.5X6
Benzapril hydrochloride	T46.5X1	T46.5X2	T46.5X3	T46.5X4	T46.5X5	T46.5X6
Benzathine benzylpenicillin	T36.0X1	T36.0X2	T36.0X3	T36.0X4	T36.0X5	T36.0X6
Benzathine penicillin	T36.0X1	T36.0X2	T36.0X3	T36.0X4	T36.0X5	T36.0X6
Benzatropine	T42.8X1	T42.8X2	T42.8X3	T42.8X4	T42.8X5	T42.8X6
Benzbromarone	T50.4X1	T50.4X2	T50.4X3	T50.4X4	T50.4X5	T50.4X6
Benzcarbimine	T45.1X1	T45.1X2	T45.1X3	T45.1X4	T45.1X5	T45.1X6
Benzedrex	T44.991	T44.992	T44.993	T44.994	T44.995	T44.996
Benzedrine (amphetamine)	T43.621	T43.622	T43.623	T43.624	T43.625	T43.626
Benzenamine	T65.3X1	T65.3X2	T65.3X3	T65.3X4	—	—
Benzene	T52.1X1	T52.1X2	T52.1X3	T52.1X4	—	—
homologues (acetyl) (dimethyl) (methyl) (solvent)	T52.2X1	T52.2X2	T52.2X3	T52.2X4	—	—
Benzethonium (chloride)	T49.0X1	T49.0X2	T49.0X3	T49.0X4	T49.0X5	T49.0X6
Benzfetamine	T50.5X1	T50.5X2	T50.5X3	T50.5X4	T50.5X5	T50.5X6
Benzhexol	T44.3X1	T44.3X2	T44.3X3	T44.3X4	T44.3X5	T44.3X6
Benzhydramine (chloride)	T45.0X1	T45.0X2	T45.0X3	T45.0X4	T45.0X5	T45.0X6
Benzidine	T65.891	T65.892	T65.893	T65.894	—	—
Benzilonium bromide	T44.3X1	T44.3X2	T44.3X3	T44.3X4	T44.3X5	T44.3X6
Benzimidazole	T60.3X1	T60.3X2	T60.3X3	T60.3X4	—	—
Benzin (e) — *see Ligroin*						
Benziodarone	T46.3X1	T46.3X2	T46.3X3	T46.3X4	T46.3X5	T46.3X6
Benznidazole	T37.3X1	T37.3X2	T37.3X3	T37.3X4	T37.3X5	T37.3X6
Benzocaine	T41.3X1	T41.3X2	T41.3X3	T41.3X4	T41.3X5	T41.3X6
Benzodiapin	T42.4X1	T42.4X2	T42.4X3	T42.4X4	T42.4X5	T42.4X6
Benzodiazepine NEC	T42.4X1	T42.4X2	T42.4X3	T42.4X4	T42.4X5	T42.4X6
Benzoic acid	T49.0X1	T49.0X2	T49.0X3	T49.0X4	T49.0X5	T49.0X6
with salicylic acid	T49.0X1	T49.0X2	T49.0X3	T49.0X4	T49.0X5	T49.0X6
Benzoin (tincture)	T48.5X1	T48.5X2	T48.5X3	T48.5X4	T48.5X5	T48.5X6
Benzol (benzene)	T52.1X1	T52.1X2	T52.1X3	T52.1X4	—	—
vapor	T52.0X1	T52.0X2	T52.0X3	T52.0X4	—	—
Benzomorphan	T40.2X1	T40.2X2	T40.2X3	T40.2X4	T40.2X5	T40.2X6
Benzonatate	T48.3X1	T48.3X2	T48.3X3	T48.3X4	T48.3X5	T48.3X6
Benzophenones	T49.3X1	T49.3X2	T49.3X3	T49.3X4	T49.3X5	T49.3X6
Benzopyrone	T46.991	T46.992	T46.993	T46.994	T46.995	T46.996
Benzothiadiazides	T50.2X1	T50.2X2	T50.2X3	T50.2X4	T50.2X5	T50.2X6

Substance	Poisoning, Accidental unintentional	Poisoning, Intentional self-harm	Poisoning, Assault	Poisoning, Undetermined	Adverse effect	Underdosing
Benzoxonium chloride	T49.0X1	T49.0X2	T49.0X3	T49.0X4	T49.0X5	T49.0X6
Benzoyl peroxide	T49.0X1	T49.0X2	T49.0X3	T49.0X4	T49.0X5	T49.0X6
Benzoylpas calcium	T37.1X1	T37.1X2	T37.1X3	T37.1X4	T37.1X5	T37.1X6
Benzperidin	T43.591	T43.592	T43.593	T43.594	T43.595	T43.596
Benzperidol	T43.591	T43.592	T43.593	T43.594	T43.595	T43.596
Benzphetamine	T50.5X1	T50.5X2	T50.5X3	T50.5X4	T50.5X5	T50.5X6
Benzpyrinium bromide	T44.1X1	T44.1X2	T44.1X3	T44.1X4	T44.1X5	T44.1X6
Benzquinamide	T45.0X1	T45.0X2	T45.0X3	T45.0X4	T45.0X5	T45.0X6
Benzthiazide	T50.2X1	T50.2X2	T50.2X3	T50.2X4	T50.2X5	T50.2X6
Benztropine						
anticholinergic	T44.3X1	T44.3X2	T44.3X3	T44.3X4	T44.3X5	T44.3X6
antiparkinson	T42.8X1	T42.8X2	T42.8X3	T42.8X4	T42.8X5	T42.8X6
Benzydamine	T49.0X1	T49.0X2	T49.0X3	T49.0X4	T49.0X5	T49.0X6
Benzyl						
acetate	T52.8X1	T52.8X2	T52.8X3	T52.8X4	--	--
alcohol	T49.0X1	T49.0X2	T49.0X3	T49.0X4	T49.0X5	T49.0X6
benzoate	T49.0X1	T49.0X2	T49.0X3	T49.0X4	T49.0X5	T49.0X6
Benzoic acid	T49.0X1	T49.0X2	T49.0X3	T49.0X4	T49.0X5	T49.0X6
morphine	T40.2X1	T40.2X2	T40.2X3	T40.2X4	--	--
nicotinate	T46.6X1	T46.6X2	T46.6X3	T46.6X4	T46.6X5	T46.6X6
penicillin	T36.0X1	T36.0X2	T36.0X3	T36.0X4	T36.0X5	T36.0X6
Benzylhydrochlorthia-zide	T50.2X1	T50.2X2	T50.2X3	T50.2X4	T50.2X5	T50.2X6
Benzylpenicillin	T36.0X1	T36.0X2	T36.0X3	T36.0X4	T36.0X5	T36.0X6
Benzylthiouracil	T38.2X1	T38.2X2	T38.2X3	T38.2X4	T38.2X5	T38.2X6
Bephenium hydroxy- naphthoate	T37.4X1	T37.4X2	T37.4X3	T37.4X4	T37.4X5	T37.4X6
Bepridil	T46.1X1	T46.1X2	T46.1X3	T46.1X4	T46.1X5	T46.1X6
Bergamot oil	T65.891	T65.892	T65.893	T65.894	--	--
Bergapten	T50.991	T50.992	T50.993	T50.994	T50.995	T50.996
Berries, poisonous	T62.1X1	T62.1X2	T62.1X3	T62.1X4	--	--
Beryllium (compounds)	T56.7X1	T56.7X2	T56.7X3	T56.7X4	--	--
b-acetyldigoxin	T46.0X1	T46.0X2	T46.0X3	T46.0X4	T46.0X5	T46.0X6
beta adrenergic blocking agent, heart	T44.7X1	T44.7X2	T44.7X3	T44.7X4	T44.7X5	T44.7X6
b-benzalbutyramide	T46.6X1	T46.6X2	T46.6X3	T46.6X4	T46.6X5	T46.6X6
Betacarotene	T45.2X1	T45.2X2	T45.2X3	T45.2X4	T45.2X5	T45.2X6
b-eucaine	T49.1X1	T49.1X2	T49.1X3	T49.1X4	T49.1X5	T49.1X6
Beta-Chlor®	T42.6X1	T42.6X2	T42.6X3	T42.6X4	T42.6X5	T42.6X6
b-galactosidase	T47.5X1	T47.5X2	T47.5X3	T47.5X4	T47.5X5	T47.5X6
Betahistine	T46.7X1	T46.7X2	T46.7X3	T46.7X4	T46.7X5	T46.7X6
Betaine	T47.5X1	T47.5X2	T47.5X3	T47.5X4	T47.5X5	T47.5X6
Betamethasone	T49.0X1	T49.0X2	T49.0X3	T49.0X4	T49.0X5	T49.0X6
topical	T49.0X1	T49.0X2	T49.0X3	T49.0X4	T49.0X5	T49.0X6
Betamicin	T36.8X1	T36.8X2	T36.8X3	T36.8X4	T36.8X5	T36.8X6
Betanidine	T46.5X1	T46.5X2	T46.5X3	T46.5X4	T46.5X5	T46.5X6
b-sitosterol (s)	T46.6X1	T46.6X2	T46.6X3	T46.6X4	T46.6X5	T46.6X6
Betaxolol	T44.7X1	T44.7X2	T44.7X3	T44.7X4	T44.7X5	T44.7X6
Betazole	T50.8X1	T50.8X2	T50.8X3	T50.8X4	T50.8X5	T50.8X6
Bethanechol	T44.1X1	T44.1X2	T44.1X3	T44.1X4	T44.1X5	T44.1X6
chloride	T44.1X1	T44.1X2	T44.1X3	T44.1X4	T44.1X5	T44.1X6
Bethanidine	T46.5X1	T46.5X2	T46.5X3	T46.5X4	T46.5X5	T46.5X6
Betoxycaine	T41.3X1	T41.3X2	T41.3X3	T41.3X4	T41.3X5	T41.3X6
Betula oil	T49.3X1	T49.3X2	T49.3X3	T49.3X4	T49.3X5	T49.3X6
Bevantolol	T44.7X1	T44.7X2	T44.7X3	T44.7X4	T44.7X5	T44.7X6
Bevonium metilsulfate	T44.3X1	T44.3X2	T44.3X3	T44.3X4	T44.3X5	T44.3X6
Bezafibrate	T46.6X1	T46.6X2	T46.6X3	T46.6X4	T46.6X5	T46.6X6
Bezitramide	T40.4X1	T40.4X2	T40.4X3	T40.4X4	T40.4X5	T40.4X6
BHA	T50.991	T50.992	T50.993	T50.994	T50.995	T50.996
Bhang	T40.7X1	T40.7X2	T40.7X3	T40.7X4	T40.7X5	T40.7X6
BHC (medicinal)	T49.0X1	T49.0X2	T49.0X3	T49.0X4	T49.0X5	T49.0X6
nonmedicinal (vapor)	T53.6X1	T53.6X2	T53.6X3	T53.6X4	--	--
Bialamicol	T37.3X1	T37.3X2	T37.3X3	T37.3X4	T37.3X5	T37.3X6
Bibenzonium bromide	T48.3X1	T48.3X2	T48.3X3	T48.3X4	T48.3X5	T48.3X6
Bibrocathol	T49.5X1	T49.5X2	T49.5X3	T49.5X4	T49.5X5	T49.5X6
Bichloride of mercury — *see Mercury, chloride*						
Bichromates (calcium) (potassium) (sodium) (crystals)	T57.8X1	T57.8X2	T57.8X3	T57.8X4	--	--
fumes	T56.2X1	T56.2X2	T56.2X3	T56.2X4	--	--
Biclotymol	T49.6X1	T49.6X2	T49.6X3	T49.6X4	T49.6X5	T49.6X6
Bicucculine	T50.7X1	T50.7X2	T50.7X3	T50.7X4	T50.7X5	T50.7X6
Bifemelane	T43.291	T43.292	T43.293	T43.294	T43.295	T43.296
Biguanide derivatives, oral	T38.3X1	T38.3X2	T38.3X3	T38.3X4	T38.3X5	T38.3X6
Bile salts	T47.5X1	T47.5X2	T47.5X3	T47.5X4	T47.5X5	T47.5X6
Biligrafin	T50.8X1	T50.8X2	T50.8X3	T50.8X4	T50.8X5	T50.8X6
Bilopaque	T50.8X1	T50.8X2	T50.8X3	T50.8X4	T50.8X5	T50.8X6
Binifibrate	T46.6X1	T46.6X2	T46.6X3	T46.6X4	T46.6X5	T46.6X6
Binitrobenzol	T65.3X1	T65.3X2	T65.3X3	T65.3X4	--	--
Bioflavonoid (s)	T46.991	T46.992	T46.993	T46.994	T46.995	T46.996
Biological substance NEC	T50.901	T50.902	T50.903	T50.904	T50.905	T50.906
Biotin	T45.2X1	T45.2X2	T45.2X3	T45.2X4	T45.2X5	T45.2X6
Biperiden	T44.3X1	T44.3X2	T44.3X3	T44.3X4	T44.3X5	T44.3X6
Bisacodyl	T47.2X1	T47.2X2	T47.2X3	T47.2X4	T47.2X5	T47.2X6

Substance	Poisoning, Accidental unintentional	Poisoning, Intentional self-harm	Poisoning, Assault	Poisoning, Undetermined	Adverse effect	Underdosing
Bisbentiamine	T45.2X1	T45.2X2	T45.2X3	T45.2X4	T45.2X5	T45.2X6
Bisbutiamine	T45.2X1	T45.2X2	T45.2X3	T45.2X4	T45.2X5	T45.2X6
Bisdequalinium (salts) (diacetate)	T49.6X1	T49.6X2	T49.6X3	T49.6X4	T49.6X5	T49.6X6
Bishydroxycoumarin	T45.511	T45.512	T45.513	T45.514	T45.515	T45.516
Bismarsen	T37.8X1	T37.8X2	T37.8X3	T37.8X4	T37.8X5	T37.8X6
Bismuth salts	T47.6X1	T47.6X2	T47.6X3	T47.6X4	T47.6X5	T47.6X6
aluminate	T47.1X1	T47.1X2	T47.1X3	T47.1X4	T47.1X5	T47.1X6
anti-infectives	T37.8X1	T37.8X2	T37.8X3	T37.8X4	T37.8X5	T37.8X6
formic iodide	T49.0X1	T49.0X2	T49.0X3	T49.0X4	T49.0X5	T49.0X6
glycolylarsenate	T49.0X1	T49.0X2	T49.0X3	T49.0X4	T49.0X5	T49.0X6
nonmedicinal (compounds) NEC	T65.91	T65.92	T65.93	T65.94	--	--
subcarbonate	T47.6X1	T47.6X2	T47.6X3	T47.6X4	T47.6X5	T47.6X6
subsalicylate	T37.8X1	T37.8X2	T37.8X3	T37.8X4	T37.8X5	T37.8X6
sulfarsphenamine	T37.8X1	T37.8X2	T37.8X3	T37.8X4	T37.8X5	T37.8X6
Bisoprolol	T44.7X1	T44.7X2	T44.7X3	T44.7X4	T44.7X5	T44.7X6
Bisoxatin	T47.2X1	T47.2X2	T47.2X3	T47.2X4	T47.2X5	T47.2X6
Bisulepin (hydrochloride)	T45.0X1	T45.0X2	T45.0X3	T45.0X4	T45.0X5	T45.0X6
Bithionol	T37.8X1	T37.8X2	T37.8X3	T37.8X4	T37.8X5	T37.8X6
anthelminthic	T37.4X1	T37.4X2	T37.4X3	T37.4X4	T37.4X5	T37.4X6
Bitolterol	T48.6X1	T48.6X2	T48.6X3	T48.6X4	T48.6X5	T48.6X6
Bitoscanate	T37.4X1	T37.4X2	T37.4X3	T37.4X4	T37.4X5	T37.4X6
Bitter almond oil	T62.8X1	T62.8X2	T62.8X3	T62.8X4	--	--
Bittersweet	T62.2X1	T62.2X2	T62.2X3	T62.2X4	--	--
Black						
flag	T60.91	T60.92	T60.93	T60.94	--	--
henbane	T62.2X1	T62.2X2	T62.2X3	T62.2X4	--	--
leaf (40)	T60.91	T60.92	T60.93	T60.94	--	--
widow spider (bite)	T63.311	T63.312	T63.313	T63.314	--	--
antivenin	T50.Z11	T50.Z12	T50.Z13	T50.Z14	T50.Z15	T50.Z16
Blast furnace gas (carbon monoxide from)	T58.8X1	T58.8X2	T58.8X3	T58.8X4	--	--
Bleach	T54.91	T54.92	T54.93	T54.94	--	--
Bleaching agent (medicinal)	T49.4X1	T49.4X2	T49.4X3	T49.4X4	T49.4X5	T49.4X6
Bleomycin	T45.1X1	T45.1X2	T45.1X3	T45.1X4	T45.1X5	T45.1X6
Blockain®	T41.3X1	T41.3X2	T41.3X3	T41.3X4	T41.3X5	T41.3X6
infiltration (subcutaneous)	T41.3X1	T41.3X2	T41.3X3	T41.3X4	T41.3X5	T41.3X6
nerve block (peripheral) (plexus)	T41.3X1	T41.3X2	T41.3X3	T41.3X4	T41.3X5	T41.3X6
topical (surface)	T41.3X1	T41.3X2	T41.3X3	T41.3X4	T41.3X5	T41.3X6
Blockers, calcium channel	T46.1X1	T46.1X2	T46.1X3	T46.1X4	T46.1X5	T46.1X6
Blood (derivatives) (natural) (plasma) (whole)	T45.8X1	T45.8X2	T45.8X3	T45.8X4	T45.8X5	T45.8X6
dried	T45.8X1	T45.8X2	T45.8X3	T45.8X4	T45.8X5	T45.8X6
drug affecting NEC	T45.91	T45.92	T45.93	T45.94	T45.95	T45.96
expander NEC	T45.8X1	T45.8X2	T45.8X3	T45.8X4	T45.8X5	T45.8X6
fraction NEC	T45.8X1	T45.8X2	T45.8X3	T45.8X4	T45.8X5	T45.8X6
substitute (macromolecular)	T45.8X1	T45.8X2	T45.8X3	T45.8X4	T45.8X5	T45.8X6
Blue velvet	T40.2X1	T40.2X2	T40.2X3	T40.2X4	--	--
Bone meal	T62.8X1	T62.8X2	T62.8X3	T62.8X4	--	--
Bonine	T45.0X1	T45.0X2	T45.0X3	T45.0X4	T45.0X5	T45.0X6
Bopindolol	T44.7X1	T44.7X2	T44.7X3	T44.7X4	T44.7X5	T44.7X6
Boracic acid	T49.0X1	T49.0X2	T49.0X3	T49.0X4	T49.0X5	T49.0X6
ENT agent	T49.6X1	T49.6X2	T49.6X3	T49.6X4	T49.6X5	T49.6X6
ophthalmic preparation	T49.5X1	T49.5X2	T49.5X3	T49.5X4	T49.5X5	T49.5X6
Borane complex	T57.8X1	T57.8X2	T57.8X3	T57.8X4	--	--
Borate (s)	T57.8X1	T57.8X2	T57.8X3	T57.8X4	--	--
buffer	T50.991	T50.992	T50.993	T50.994	T50.995	T50.996
cleanser	T54.91	T54.92	T54.93	T54.94	--	--
sodium	T57.8X1	T57.8X2	T57.8X3	T57.8X4	--	--
Borax (cleanser)	T54.91	T54.92	T54.93	T54.94	--	--
Bordeaux mixture	T60.3X1	T60.3X2	T60.3X3	T60.3X4	--	--
Boric acid	T49.0X1	T49.0X2	T49.0X3	T49.0X4	T49.0X5	T49.0X6
ENT agent	T49.6X1	T49.6X2	T49.6X3	T49.6X4	T49.6X5	T49.6X6
ophthalmic preparation	T49.5X1	T49.5X2	T49.5X3	T49.5X4	T49.5X5	T49.5X6
Bornaprine	T44.3X1	T44.3X2	T44.3X3	T44.3X4	T44.3X5	T44.3X6
Boron	T57.8X1	T57.8X2	T57.8X3	T57.8X4	--	--
hydride NEC	T57.8X1	T57.8X2	T57.8X3	T57.8X4	--	--
fumes or gas	T57.8X1	T57.8X2	T57.8X3	T57.8X4	--	--
trifluoride	T59.891	T59.892	T59.893	T59.894	--	--
Botox	T48.291	T48.292	T48.293	T48.294	T48.295	T48.296
Botulinus anti-toxin (type A, B)	T50.Z11	T50.Z12	T50.Z13	T50.Z14	T50.Z15	T50.Z16
Brake fluid vapor	T59.891	T59.892	T59.893	T59.894	--	--
Brallobarbital	T42.3X1	T42.3X2	T42.3X3	T42.3X4	T42.3X5	T42.3X6
Bran (wheat)	T47.4X1	T47.4X2	T47.4X3	T47.4X4	T47.4X5	T47.4X6
Brass (fumes)	T56.891	T56.892	T56.893	T56.894	--	--
Brasso	T52.0X1	T52.0X2	T52.0X3	T52.0X4	--	--
Bretylium tosilate	T46.2X1	T46.2X2	T46.2X3	T46.2X4	T46.2X5	T46.2X6
Brevital (sodium)	T41.1X1	T41.1X2	T41.1X3	T41.1X4	T41.1X5	T41.1X6
Brinase	T45.3X1	T45.3X2	T45.3X3	T45.3X4	T45.3X5	T45.3X6
British antilewisite	T45.8X1	T45.8X2	T45.8X3	T45.8X4	T45.8X5	T45.8X6

Substance	Poisoning, Accidental unintentional	Poisoning, Intentional self-harm	Poisoning, Assault	Poisoning, Undetermined	Adverse effect	Underdosing
Brodifacoum	T60.4X1	T60.4X2	T60.4X3	T60.4X4	--	--
Bromal (hydrate)	T42.6X1	T42.6X2	T42.6X3	T42.6X4	T42.6X5	T42.6X6
Bromazepam	T42.4X1	T42.4X2	T42.4X3	T42.4X4	T42.4X5	T42.4X6
Bromazine	T45.0X1	T45.0X2	T45.0X3	T45.0X4	T45.0X5	T45.0X6
Brombenzylcyanide	T59.3X1	T59.3X2	T59.3X3	T59.3X4	--	--
Bromelains	T45.3X1	T45.3X2	T45.3X3	T45.3X4	T45.3X5	T45.3X6
Bromethalin	T60.4X1	T60.4X2	T60.4X3	T60.4X4	--	--
Bromhexine	T48.4X1	T48.4X2	T48.4X3	T48.4X4	T48.4X5	T48.4X6
Bromide salts	T42.6X1	T42.6X2	T42.6X3	T42.6X4	T42.6X5	T42.6X6
Bromindione	T45.511	T45.512	T45.513	T45.514	T45.515	T45.516
Bromine						
compounds (medicinal)	T42.6X1	T42.6X2	T42.6X3	T42.6X4	T42.6X5	T42.6X6
sedative	T42.6X1	T42.6X2	T42.6X3	T42.6X4	T42.6X5	T42.6X6
vapor	T59.891	T59.892	T59.893	T59.894	--	--
Bromisoval	T42.6X1	T42.6X2	T42.6X3	T42.6X4	T42.6X5	T42.6X6
Bromisovalum	T42.6X1	T42.6X2	T42.6X3	T42.6X4	T42.6X5	T42.6X6
Bromobenzylcyanide	T59.3X1	T59.3X2	T59.3X3	T59.3X4	--	--
Bromochlorosalicylani-lide	T49.0X1	T49.0X2	T49.0X3	T49.0X4	T49.0X5	T49.0X6
Bromocriptine	T42.8X1	T42.8X2	T42.8X3	T42.8X4	T42.8X5	T42.8X6
Bromodiphenhydramine	T45.0X1	T45.0X2	T45.0X3	T45.0X4	T45.0X5	T45.0X6
Bromoform	T42.6X1	T42.6X2	T42.6X3	T42.6X4	T42.6X5	T42.6X6
Bromophenol blue reagent	T50.991	T50.992	T50.993	T50.994	T50.995	T50.996
Bromopride	T47.8X1	T47.8X2	T47.8X3	T47.8X4	T47.8X5	T47.8X6
Bromosalicylchloranitide	T49.0X1	T49.0X2	T49.0X3	T49.0X4	T49.0X5	T49.0X6
Bromosalicylhydroxamic acid	T37.1X1	T37.1X2	T37.1X3	T37.1X4	T37.1X5	T37.1X6
Bromo-seltzer	T39.1X1	T39.1X2	T39.1X3	T39.1X4	T39.1X5	T39.1X6
Bromoxynil	T60.3X1	T60.3X2	T60.3X3	T60.3X4	--	--
Bromperidol	T43.4X1	T43.4X2	T43.4X3	T43.4X4	T43.4X5	T43.4X6
Brompheniramine	T45.0X1	T45.0X2	T45.0X3	T45.0X4	T45.0X5	T45.0X6
Bromsulfophthalein	T50.8X1	T50.8X2	T50.8X3	T50.8X4	T50.8X5	T50.8X6
Bromural	T42.6X1	T42.6X2	T42.6X3	T42.6X4	T42.6X5	T42.6X6
Bromvaletone	T42.6X1	T42.6X2	T42.6X3	T42.6X4	T42.6X5	T42.6X6
Bronchodilator NEC	T48.6X1	T48.6X2	T48.6X3	T48.6X4	T48.6X5	T48.6X6
Brotizolam	T42.4X1	T42.4X2	T42.4X3	T42.4X4	T42.4X5	T42.4X6
Brovincamine	T46.7X1	T46.7X2	T46.7X3	T46.7X4	T46.7X5	T46.7X6
Brown recluse spider (bite) (venom)	T63.331	T63.332	T63.333	T63.334	--	--
Brown spider (bite) (venom)	T63.391	T63.392	T63.393	T63.394	--	--
Broxaterol	T48.6X1	T48.6X2	T48.6X3	T48.6X4	T48.6X5	T48.6X6
Broxuridine	T45.1X1	T45.1X2	T45.1X3	T45.1X4	T45.1X5	T45.1X6
Broxyquinoline	T37.8X1	T37.8X2	T37.8X3	T37.8X4	T37.8X5	T37.8X6
Bruceine	T48.291	T48.292	T48.293	T48.294	T48.295	T48.296
Brucia	T62.2X1	T62.2X2	T62.2X3	T62.2X4	--	--
Brucine	T65.1X1	T65.1X2	T65.1X3	T65.1X4	--	--
Brunswick green — *see Copper*						
Bruten — *see Ibuprofen*						
Bryonia	T47.2X1	T47.2X2	T47.2X3	T47.2X4	T47.2X5	T47.2X6
Buclizine	T45.0X1	T45.0X2	T45.0X3	T45.0X4	T45.0X5	T45.0X6
Buclosamide	T49.0X1	T49.0X2	T49.0X3	T49.0X4	T49.0X5	T49.0X6
Budesonide	T44.5X1	T44.5X2	T44.5X3	T44.5X4	T44.5X5	T44.5X6
Budralazine	T46.5X1	T46.5X2	T46.5X3	T46.5X4	T46.5X5	T46.5X6
Bufferin	T39.011	T39.012	T39.013	T39.014	T39.015	T39.016
Buflomedil	T46.7X1	T46.7X2	T46.7X3	T46.7X4	T46.7X5	T46.7X6
Buformin	T38.3X1	T38.3X2	T38.3X3	T38.3X4	T38.3X5	T38.3X6
Bufotenine	T40.991	T40.992	T40.993	T40.994	--	--
Bufrolin	T48.6X1	T48.6X2	T48.6X3	T48.6X4	T48.6X5	T48.6X6
Bufylline	T48.6X1	T48.6X2	T48.6X3	T48.6X4	T48.6X5	T48.6X6
Bulk filler	T50.5X1	T50.5X2	T50.5X3	T50.5X4	T50.5X5	T50.5X6
cathartic	T47.4X1	T47.4X2	T47.4X3	T47.4X4	T47.4X5	T47.4X6
Bumetanide	T50.1X1	T50.1X2	T50.1X3	T50.1X4	T50.1X5	T50.1X6
Bunaftine	T46.2X1	T46.2X2	T46.2X3	T46.2X4	T46.2X5	T46.2X6
Bunamiodyl	T50.8X1	T50.8X2	T50.8X3	T50.8X4	T50.8X5	T50.8X6
Bunazosin	T44.6X1	T44.6X2	T44.6X3	T44.6X4	T44.6X5	T44.6X6
Bunitrolol	T44.7X1	T44.7X2	T44.7X3	T44.7X4	T44.7X5	T44.7X6
Buphenine	T46.7X1	T46.7X2	T46.7X3	T46.7X4	T46.7X5	T46.7X6
Bupivacaine	T41.3X1	T41.3X2	T41.3X3	T41.3X4	T41.3X5	T41.3X6
infiltration (subcutaneous)	T41.3X1	T41.3X2	T41.3X3	T41.3X4	T41.3X5	T41.3X6
nerve block (peripheral) (plexus)	T41.3X1	T41.3X2	T41.3X3	T41.3X4	T41.3X5	T41.3X6
spinal	T41.3X1	T41.3X2	T41.3X3	T41.3X4	T41.3X5	T41.3X6
Bupranolol	T44.7X1	T44.7X2	T44.7X3	T44.7X4	T44.7X5	T44.7X6
Buprenorphine	T40.4X1	T40.4X2	T40.4X3	T40.4X4	T40.4X5	T40.4X6
Bupropion	T43.291	T43.292	T43.293	T43.294	T43.295	T43.296
Burimamide	T47.1X1	T47.1X2	T47.1X3	T47.1X4	T47.1X5	T47.1X6
Buserelin	T38.891	T38.892	T38.893	T38.894	T38.895	T38.896
Buspirone	T43.591	T43.592	T43.593	T43.594	T43.595	T43.596
Busulfan, busulphan	T45.1X1	T45.1X2	T45.1X3	T45.1X4	T45.1X5	T45.1X6
Butabarbital (sodium)	T42.3X1	T42.3X2	T42.3X3	T42.3X4	T42.3X5	T42.3X6
Butabarbitone	T42.3X1	T42.3X2	T42.3X3	T42.3X4	T42.3X5	T42.3X6
Butabarpal	T42.3X1	T42.3X2	T42.3X3	T42.3X4	T42.3X5	T42.3X6
Butacaine	T41.3X1	T41.3X2	T41.3X3	T41.3X4	T41.3X5	T41.3X6
Butalamine	T46.7X1	T46.7X2	T46.7X3	T46.7X4	T46.7X5	T46.7X6
Butalbital	T42.3X1	T42.3X2	T42.3X3	T42.3X4	T42.3X5	T42.3X6
Butallylonal	T42.3X1	T42.3X2	T42.3X3	T42.3X4	T42.3X5	T42.3X6
Butamben	T41.3X1	T41.3X2	T41.3X3	T41.3X4	T41.3X5	T41.3X6
Butamirate	T48.3X1	T48.3X2	T48.3X3	T48.3X4	T48.3X5	T48.3X6
Butane (distributed in mobile container)	T59.891	T59.892	T59.893	T59.894	--	--
distributed through pipes	T59.891	T59.892	T59.893	T59.894	--	--
incomplete combustion	T58.11	T58.12	T58.13	T58.14	--	--
Butanilicaine	T41.3X1	T41.3X2	T41.3X3	T41.3X4	T41.3X5	T41.3X6
Butanol	T51.3X1	T51.3X2	T51.3X3	T51.3X4	--	--
Butanone, 2-butanone	T52.4X1	T52.4X2	T52.4X3	T52.4X4	--	--
Butantrone	T49.4X1	T49.4X2	T49.4X3	T49.4X4	T49.4X5	T49.4X6
Butaperazine	T43.3X1	T43.3X2	T43.3X3	T43.3X4	T43.3X5	T43.3X6
Butazolidin	T39.2X1	T39.2X2	T39.2X3	T39.2X4	T39.2X5	T39.2X6
Butetamate	T48.6X1	T48.6X2	T48.6X3	T48.6X4	T48.6X5	T48.6X6
Butethal	T42.3X1	T42.3X2	T42.3X3	T42.3X4	T42.3X5	T42.3X6
Butethamate	T44.3X1	T44.3X2	T44.3X3	T44.3X4	T44.3X5	T44.3X6
Buthalitone (sodium)	T41.1X1	T41.1X2	T41.1X3	T41.1X4	T41.1X5	T41.1X6
Butisol (sodium)	T42.3X1	T42.3X2	T42.3X3	T42.3X4	T42.3X5	T42.3X6
Butizide	T50.2X1	T50.2X2	T50.2X3	T50.2X4	T50.2X5	T50.2X6
Butobarbital	T42.3X1	T42.3X2	T42.3X3	T42.3X4	T42.3X5	T42.3X6
sodium	T42.3X1	T42.3X2	T42.3X3	T42.3X4	T42.3X5	T42.3X6
Butobarbitone	T42.3X1	T42.3X2	T42.3X3	T42.3X4	T42.3X5	T42.3X6
Butoconazole (nitrate)	T49.0X1	T49.0X2	T49.0X3	T49.0X4	T49.0X5	T49.0X6
Butorphanol	T40.4X1	T40.4X2	T40.4X3	T40.4X4	T40.4X5	T40.4X6
Butriptyline	T43.011	T43.012	T43.013	T43.014	T43.015	T43.016
Butropium bromide	T44.3X1	T44.3X2	T44.3X3	T44.3X4	T44.3X5	T44.3X6
Butter of antimony — *see Antimony*						
Buttercups	T62.2X1	T62.2X2	T62.2X3	T62.2X4	--	--
Butyl						
acetate (secondary)	T52.8X1	T52.8X2	T52.8X3	T52.8X4	--	--
alcohol	T51.3X1	T51.3X2	T51.3X3	T51.3X4	--	--
aminobenzoate	T41.3X1	T41.3X2	T41.3X3	T41.3X4	T41.3X5	T41.3X6
butyrate	T52.8X1	T52.8X2	T52.8X3	T52.8X4	--	--
carbinol	T51.3X1	T51.3X2	T51.3X3	T51.3X4	--	--
carbitol	T52.3X1	T52.3X2	T52.3X3	T52.3X4	--	--
cellosolve	T52.3X1	T52.3X2	T52.3X3	T52.3X4	--	--
chloral (hydrate)	T42.6X1	T42.6X2	T42.6X3	T42.6X4	T42.6X5	T42.6X6
formate	T52.8X1	T52.8X2	T52.8X3	T52.8X4	--	--
lactate	T52.8X1	T52.8X2	T52.8X3	T52.8X4	--	--
propionate	T52.8X1	T52.8X2	T52.8X3	T52.8X4	--	--
scopolamine bromide	T44.3X1	T44.3X2	T44.3X3	T44.3X4	T44.3X5	T44.3X6
thiobarbital sodium	T41.1X1	T41.1X2	T41.1X3	T41.1X4	T41.1X5	T41.1X6
Butylated hydroxy-anisole	T50.991	T50.992	T50.993	T50.994	T50.995	T50.996
Butylchloral hydrate	T42.6X1	T42.6X2	T42.6X3	T42.6X4	T42.6X5	T42.6X6
Butyltoluene	T52.2X1	T52.2X2	T52.2X3	T52.2X4	--	--
Butyn	T41.3X1	T41.3X2	T41.3X3	T41.3X4	T41.3X5	T41.3X6
Butyrophenone (-based tranquilizers)	T43.4X1	T43.4X2	T43.4X3	T43.4X4	T43.4X5	T43.4X6
C						
Cabergoline	T42.8X1	T42.8X2	T42.8X3	T42.8X4	T42.8X5	T42.8X6
Cacodyl, cacodylic acid	T57.0X1	T57.0X2	T57.0X3	T57.0X4	--	--
Cactinomycin	T45.1X1	T45.1X2	T45.1X3	T45.1X4	T45.1X5	T45.1X6
Cade oil	T49.4X1	T49.4X2	T49.4X3	T49.4X4	T49.4X5	T49.4X6
Cadexomer iodine	T49.0X1	T49.0X2	T49.0X3	T49.0X4	T49.0X5	T49.0X6
Cadmium (chloride) (fumes) (oxide)	T56.3X1	T56.3X2	T56.3X3	T56.3X4	--	--
sulfide (medicinal) NEC	T49.4X1	T49.4X2	T49.4X3	T49.4X4	T49.4X5	T49.4X6
Cadralazine	T46.5X1	T46.5X2	T46.5X3	T46.5X4	T46.5X5	T46.5X6
Caffeine	T43.611	T43.612	T43.613	T43.614	T43.615	T43.616
Calabar bean	T62.2X1	T62.2X2	T62.2X3	T62.2X4	--	--
Caladium seguinum	T62.2X1	T62.2X2	T62.2X3	T62.2X4	--	--
Calamine (lotion)	T49.3X1	T49.3X2	T49.3X3	T49.3X4	T49.3X5	T49.3X6
Calcifediol	T45.2X1	T45.2X2	T45.2X3	T45.2X4	T45.2X5	T45.2X6
Calciferol	T45.2X1	T45.2X2	T45.2X3	T45.2X4	T45.2X5	T45.2X6
Calcitonin	T50.991	T50.992	T50.993	T50.994	T50.995	T50.996
Calcitriol	T45.2X1	T45.2X2	T45.2X3	T45.2X4	T45.2X5	T45.2X6
Calcium	T50.3X1	T50.3X2	T50.3X3	T50.3X4	T50.3X5	T50.3X6
actylsalicylate	T39.011	T39.012	T39.013	T39.014	T39.015	T39.016
benzamidosalicylate	T37.1X1	T37.1X2	T37.1X3	T37.1X4	T37.1X5	T37.1X6
bromide	T42.6X1	T42.6X2	T42.6X3	T42.6X4	T42.6X5	T42.6X6
bromolactobionate	T42.6X1	T42.6X2	T42.6X3	T42.6X4	T42.6X5	T42.6X6
carbaspirin	T39.011	T39.012	T39.013	T39.014	T39.015	T39.016
carbimide	T50.6X1	T50.6X2	T50.6X3	T50.6X4	T50.6X5	T50.6X6
carbonate	T47.1X1	T47.1X2	T47.1X3	T47.1X4	T47.1X5	T47.1X6
chloride	T50.991	T50.992	T50.993	T50.994	T50.995	T50.996
anhydrous	T50.991	T50.992	T50.993	T50.994	T50.995	T50.996
cyanide	T57.8X1	T57.8X2	T57.8X3	T57.8X4	--	--
dioctyl sulfosuccinate	T47.4X1	T47.4X2	T47.4X3	T47.4X4	T47.4X5	T47.4X6
disodium edathamil	T45.8X1	T45.8X2	T45.8X3	T45.8X4	T45.8X5	T45.8X6
disodium edetate	T45.8X1	T45.8X2	T45.8X3	T45.8X4	T45.8X5	T45.8X6
dobesilate	T46.991	T46.992	T46.993	T46.994	T46.995	T46.996
EDTA	T45.8X1	T45.8X2	T45.8X3	T45.8X4	T45.8X5	T45.8X6
ferrous citrate	T45.4X1	T45.4X2	T45.4X3	T45.4X4	T45.4X5	T45.4X6
folinate	T45.8X1	T45.8X2	T45.8X3	T45.8X4	T45.8X5	T45.8X6

Substance	Poisoning, Accidental unintentional	Poisoning, Intentional self-harm	Poisoning, Assault	Poisoning, Undetermined	Adverse effect	Underdosing
Calcium — *continued*						
glubionate	T50.3X1	T50.3X2	T50.3X3	T50.3X4	T50.3X5	T50.3X6
gluconate	T50.3X1	T50.3X2	T50.3X3	T50.3X4	T50.3X5	T50.3X6
gluconogalactogluc-onate	T50.3X1	T50.3X2	T50.3X3	T50.3X4	T50.3X5	T50.3X6
hydrate, hydroxide	T54.3X1	T54.3X2	T54.3X3	T54.3X4	—	—
hypochlorite	T54.3X1	T54.3X2	T54.3X3	T54.3X4	—	—
iodide	T48.4X1	T48.4X2	T48.4X3	T48.4X4	T48.4X5	T48.4X6
ipodate	T50.8X1	T50.8X2	T50.8X3	T50.8X4	T50.8X5	T50.8X6
lactate	T50.3X1	T50.3X2	T50.3X3	T50.3X4	T50.3X5	T50.3X6
leucovorin	T45.8X1	T45.8X2	T45.8X3	T45.8X4	T45.8X5	T45.8X6
mandelate	T37.91	T37.92	T37.93	T37.94	T37.95	T37.96
oxide	T54.3X1	T54.3X2	T54.3X3	T54.3X4	—	—
pantothenate	T45.2X1	T45.2X2	T45.2X3	T45.2X4	T45.2X5	T45.2X6
phosphate	T50.3X1	T50.3X2	T50.3X3	T50.3X4	T50.3X5	T50.3X6
salicylate	T39.091	T39.092	T39.093	T39.094	T39.095	T39.096
salts	T50.3X1	T50.3X2	T50.3X3	T50.3X4	T50.3X5	T50.3X6
Calculus-dissolving drug	T50.991	T50.992	T50.993	T50.994	T50.995	T50.996
Calomel	T49.0X1	T49.0X2	T49.0X3	T49.0X4	T49.0X5	T49.0X6
Caloric agent	T50.3X1	T50.3X2	T50.3X3	T50.3X4	T50.3X5	T50.3X6
Calusterone	T38.7X1	T38.7X2	T38.7X3	T38.7X4	T38.7X5	T38.7X6
Camazepam	T42.4X1	T42.4X2	T42.4X3	T42.4X4	T42.4X5	T42.4X6
Camomile	T49.0X1	T49.0X2	T49.0X3	T49.0X4	T49.0X5	T49.0X6
Camoquin	T37.2X1	T37.2X2	T37.2X3	T37.2X4	T37.2X5	T37.2X6
Camphor						
insecticide	T60.2X1	T60.2X2	T60.2X3	T60.2X4	—	—
medicinal	T49.8X1	T49.8X2	T49.8X3	T49.8X4	T49.8X5	T49.8X6
Camylofin	T44.3X1	T44.3X2	T44.3X3	T44.3X4	T44.3X5	T44.3X6
Cancer chemotherapy drug regimen	T45.1X1	T45.1X2	T45.1X3	T45.1X4	T45.1X5	T45.1X6
Candeptin	T49.0X1	T49.0X2	T49.0X3	T49.0X4	T49.0X5	T49.0X6
Candicidin	T49.0X1	T49.0X2	T49.0X3	T49.0X4	T49.0X5	T49.0X6
Cannabinol	T40.7X1	T40.7X2	T40.7X3	T40.7X4	T40.7X5	T40.7X6
Cannabis (derivatives)	T40.7X1	T40.7X2	T40.7X3	T40.7X4	T40.7X5	T40.7X6
Canned heat	T51.1X1	T51.1X2	T51.1X3	T51.1X4	—	—
Canrenoic acid	T50.0X1	T50.0X2	T50.0X3	T50.0X4	T50.0X5	T50.0X6
Canrenone	T50.0X1	T50.0X2	T50.0X3	T50.0X4	T50.0X5	T50.0X6
Cantharides, cantharidin, cantharis	T49.8X1	T49.8X2	T49.8X3	T49.8X4	T49.8X5	T49.8X6
Canthaxanthin	T50.991	T50.992	T50.993	T50.994	T50.995	T50.996
Capillary-active drug NEC	T46.901	T46.902	T46.903	T46.904	T46.905	T46.906
Capreomycin	T36.8X1	T36.8X2	T36.8X3	T36.8X4	T36.8X5	T36.8X6
Capsicum	T49.4X1	T49.4X2	T49.4X3	T49.4X4	T49.4X5	T49.4X6
Captafol	T60.3X1	T60.3X2	T60.3X3	T60.3X4	—	—
Captan	T60.3X1	T60.3X2	T60.3X3	T60.3X4	—	—
Captodiame, captodiamine	T43.591	T43.592	T43.593	T43.594	T43.595	T43.596
Captopril	T46.4X1	T46.4X2	T46.4X3	T46.4X4	T46.4X5	T46.4X6
Caramiphen	T44.3X1	T44.3X2	T44.3X3	T44.3X4	T44.3X5	T44.3X6
Carazolol	T44.7X1	T44.7X2	T44.7X3	T44.7X4	T44.7X5	T44.7X6
Carbachol	T44.1X1	T44.1X2	T44.1X3	T44.1X4	T44.1X5	T44.1X6
Carbacrylamine (resin)	T50.3X1	T50.3X2	T50.3X3	T50.3X4	T50.3X5	T50.3X6
Carbamate (insecticide)	T60.0X1	T60.0X2	T60.0X3	T60.0X4	—	—
Carbamate (sedative)	T42.6X1	T42.6X2	T42.6X3	T42.6X4	T42.6X5	T42.6X6
herbicide	T60.0X1	T60.0X2	T60.0X3	T60.0X4	—	—
insecticide	T60.0X1	T60.0X2	T60.0X3	T60.0X4	—	—
Carbamazepine	T42.1X1	T42.1X2	T42.1X3	T42.1X4	T42.1X5	T42.1X6
Carbamide	T47.3X1	T47.3X2	T47.3X3	T47.3X4	T47.3X5	T47.3X6
peroxide	T49.0X1	T49.0X2	T49.0X3	T49.0X4	T49.0X5	T49.0X6
topical	T49.8X1	T49.8X2	T49.8X3	T49.8X4	T49.8X5	T49.8X6
Carbamylcholine chloride	T44.1X1	T44.1X2	T44.1X3	T44.1X4	T44.1X5	T44.1X6
Carbaril	T60.0X1	T60.0X2	T60.0X3	T60.0X4	—	—
Carbarsone	T37.3X1	T37.3X2	T37.3X3	T37.3X4	T37.3X5	T37.3X6
Carbaryl	T60.0X1	T60.0X2	T60.0X3	T60.0X4	—	—
Carbaspirin	T39.011	T39.012	T39.013	T39.014	T39.015	T39.016
Carbazochrome (salicylate) (sodium sulfonate)	T49.4X1	T49.4X2	T49.4X3	T49.4X4	T49.4X5	T49.4X6
Carbenicillin	T36.0X1	T36.0X2	T36.0X3	T36.0X4	T36.0X5	T36.0X6
Carbenoxolone	T47.1X1	T47.1X2	T47.1X3	T47.1X4	T47.1X5	T47.1X6
Carbetapentane	T48.3X1	T48.3X2	T48.3X3	T48.3X4	T48.3X5	T48.3X6
Carbethyl salicylate	T39.091	T39.092	T39.093	T39.094	T39.095	T39.096
Carbidopa (with levodopa)	T42.8X1	T42.8X2	T42.8X3	T42.8X4	T42.8X5	T42.8X6
Carbimazole	T38.2X1	T38.2X2	T38.2X3	T38.2X4	T38.2X5	T38.2X6
Carbinol	T51.1X1	T51.1X2	T51.1X3	T51.1X4	—	—
Carbinoxamine	T45.0X1	T45.0X2	T45.0X3	T45.0X4	T45.0X5	T45.0X6
Carbiphene	T39.8X1	T39.8X2	T39.8X3	T39.8X4	T39.8X5	T39.8X6
Carbitol	T52.3X1	T52.3X2	T52.3X3	T52.3X4	—	—
Carbo medicinalis	T47.6X1	T47.6X2	T47.6X3	T47.6X4	T47.6X5	T47.6X6
Carbocaine	T41.3X1	T41.3X2	T41.3X3	T41.3X4	T41.3X5	T41.3X6
infiltration (subcutaneous)	T41.3X1	T41.3X2	T41.3X3	T41.3X4	T41.3X5	T41.3X6
nerve block (peripheral) (plexus)	T41.3X1	T41.3X2	T41.3X3	T41.3X4	T41.3X5	T41.3X6
topical (surface)	T41.3X1	T41.3X2	T41.3X3	T41.3X4	T41.3X5	T41.3X6
Carbocisteine	T48.4X1	T48.4X2	T48.4X3	T48.4X4	T48.4X5	T48.4X6
Carbocromen	T46.3X1	T46.3X2	T46.3X3	T46.3X4	T46.3X5	T46.3X6
Carbol fuchsin	T49.0X1	T49.0X2	T49.0X3	T49.0X4	T49.0X5	T49.0X6

Substance	Poisoning, Accidental unintentional	Poisoning, Intentional self-harm	Poisoning, Assault	Poisoning, Undetermined	Adverse effect	Underdosing
Carbolic acid — *see also Phenol*	T54.0X1	T54.0X2	T54.0X3	T54.0X4	—	—
Carbolonium (bromide)	T48.1X1	T48.1X2	T48.1X3	T48.1X4	T48.1X5	T48.1X6
Carbomycin	T36.8X1	T36.8X2	T36.8X3	T36.8X4	T36.8X5	T36.8X6
Carbon						
bisulfide (liquid)	T65.4X1	T65.4X2	T65.4X3	T65.4X4	—	—
vapor	T65.4X1	T65.4X2	T65.4X3	T65.4X4	—	—
dioxide (gas)	T59.7X1	T59.7X2	T59.7X3	T59.7X4	—	—
medicinal	T41.5X1	T41.5X2	T41.5X3	T41.5X4	T41.5X5	T41.5X6
nonmedicinal	T59.7X1	T59.7X2	T59.7X3	T59.7X4	—	—
snow	T49.4X1	T49.4X2	T49.4X3	T49.4X4	T49.4X5	T49.4X6
disulfide (liquid)	T65.4X1	T65.4X2	T65.4X3	T65.4X4	—	—
vapor	T65.4X1	T65.4X2	T65.4X3	T65.4X4	—	—
monoxide (from incomplete combustion)	T58.91	T58.92	T58.93	T58.94	—	—
blast furnace gas	T58.8X1	T58.8X2	T58.8X3	T58.8X4	—	—
butane (distributed in mobile container)	T58.11	T58.12	T58.13	T58.14	—	—
distributed through pipes	T58.11	T58.12	T58.13	T58.14	—	—
charcoal fumes	T58.2X1	T58.2X2	T58.2X3	T58.2X4	—	—
coal	T58.2X1	T58.2X2	T58.2X3	T58.2X4	—	—
coke (in domestic stoves, fireplaces)	T58.2X1	T58.2X2	T58.2X3	T58.2X4	—	—
gas (piped)	T58.11	T58.12	T58.13	T58.14	—	—
solid (in domestic stoves, fireplaces)	T58.2X1	T58.2X2	T58.2X3	T58.2X4	—	—
exhaust gas (motor) not in transit	T58.01	T58.02	T58.03	T58.04	—	—
combustion engine, any not in watercraft	T58.01	T58.02	T58.03	T58.04	—	—
farm tractor, not in transit	T58.01	T58.02	T58.03	T58.04	—	—
gas engine	T58.01	T58.02	T58.03	T58.04	—	—
motor pump	T58.01	T58.02	T58.03	T58.04	—	—
motor vehicle, not in transit	T58.01	T58.02	T58.03	T58.04	—	—
fuel (in domestic use)	T58.2X1	T58.2X2	T58.2X3	T58.2X4	—	—
gas (piped)	T58.11	T58.12	T58.13	T58.14	—	—
in mobile container	T58.11	T58.12	T58.13	T58.14	—	—
piped (natural)	T58.11	T58.12	T58.13	T58.14	—	—
utility	T58.11	T58.12	T58.13	T58.14	—	—
in mobile container	T58.11	T58.12	T58.13	T58.14	—	—
illuminating gas	T58.11	T58.12	T58.13	T58.14	—	—
industrial fuels or gases, any	T58.8X1	T58.8X2	T58.8X3	T58.8X4	—	—
kerosene (in domestic stoves, fireplaces)	T58.2X1	T58.2X2	T58.2X3	T58.2X4	—	—
kiln gas or vapor	T58.8X1	T58.8X2	T58.8X3	T58.8X4	—	—
motor exhaust gas, not in transit	T58.01	T58.02	T58.03	T58.04	—	—
piped gas (manufactured) (natural)	T58.11	T58.12	T58.13	T58.14	—	—
producer gas	T58.8X1	T58.8X2	T58.8X3	T58.8X4	—	—
propane (distributed in mobile container)	T58.11	T58.12	T58.13	T58.14	—	—
distributed through pipes	T58.11	T58.12	T58.13	T58.14	—	—
specified source NEC	T58.8X1	T58.8X2	T58.8X3	T58.8X4	—	—
stove gas	T58.11	T58.12	T58.13	T58.14	—	—
piped	T58.11	T58.12	T58.13	T58.14	—	—
utility gas	T58.11	T58.12	T58.13	T58.14	—	—
piped	T58.11	T58.12	T58.13	T58.14	—	—
water gas	T58.11	T58.12	T58.13	T58.14	—	—
wood (in domestic stoves, fireplaces)	T58.2X1	T58.2X2	T58.2X3	T58.2X4	—	—
tetrachloride (vapor) NEC	T53.0X1	T53.0X2	T53.0X3	T53.0X4	—	—
liquid (cleansing agent) NEC	T53.0X1	T53.0X2	T53.0X3	T53.0X4	—	—
solvent	T53.0X1	T53.0X2	T53.0X3	T53.0X4	—	—
Carbonic acid gas	T59.7X1	T59.7X2	T59.7X3	T59.7X4	—	—
anhydrase inhibitor NEC	T50.2X1	T50.2X2	T50.2X3	T50.2X4	T50.2X5	T50.2X6
Carbophenothion	T60.0X1	T60.0X2	T60.0X3	T60.0X4	—	—
Carboplatin	T45.1X1	T45.1X2	T45.1X3	T45.1X4	T45.1X5	T45.1X6
Carboprost	T48.0X1	T48.0X2	T48.0X3	T48.0X4	T48.0X5	T48.0X6
Carboquone	T45.1X1	T45.1X2	T45.1X3	T45.1X4	T45.1X5	T45.1X6
Carbowax	T49.3X1	T49.3X2	T49.3X3	T49.3X4	T49.3X5	T49.3X6
Carboxymethyl-cellulose	T47.4X1	T47.4X2	T47.4X3	T47.4X4	T47.4X5	T47.4X6
S-Carboxymethyl-cysteine	T48.4X1	T48.4X2	T48.4X3	T48.4X4	T48.4X5	T48.4X6
Carbrital	T42.3X1	T42.3X2	T42.3X3	T42.3X4	T42.3X5	T42.3X6
Carbromal	T42.6X1	T42.6X2	T42.6X3	T42.6X4	T42.6X5	T42.6X6

Carbutamide - Chalk, precipitated

Substance	Poisoning, Accidental unintentional	Poisoning, Intentional self-harm	Poisoning, Assault	Poisoning, Undetermined	Adverse effect	Underdosing
Carbutamide	T38.3X1	T38.3X2	T38.3X3	T38.3X4	T38.3X5	T38.3X6
Carbuterol	T48.6X1	T48.6X2	T48.6X3	T48.6X4	T48.6X5	T48.6X6
Cardiac						
depressants	T46.2X1	T46.2X2	T46.2X3	T46.2X4	T46.2X5	T46.2X6
rhythm regulator	T46.2X1	T46.2X2	T46.2X3	T46.2X4	T46.2X5	T46.2X6
specified NEC	T46.2X1	T46.2X2	T46.2X3	T46.2X4	T46.2X5	T46.2X6
Cardiografin	T50.8X1	T50.8X2	T50.8X3	T50.8X4	T50.8X5	T50.8X6
Cardio-green	T50.8X1	T50.8X2	T50.8X3	T50.8X4	T50.8X5	T50.8X6
Cardiotonic (glycoside) **NEC**	T46.0X1	T46.0X2	T46.0X3	T46.0X4	T46.0X5	T46.0X6
Cardiovascular drug NEC	T46.901	T46.902	T46.903	T46.904	T46.905	T46.906
Cardrase	T50.2X1	T50.2X2	T50.2X3	T50.2X4	T50.2X5	T50.2X6
Carfecillin	T36.0X1	T36.0X2	T36.0X3	T36.0X4	T36.0X5	T36.0X6
Carfenazine	T43.3X1	T43.3X2	T43.3X3	T43.3X4	T43.3X5	T43.3X6
Carfusin	T49.0X1	T49.0X2	T49.0X3	T49.0X4	T49.0X5	T49.0X6
Carindacillin	T36.0X1	T36.0X2	T36.0X3	T36.0X4	T36.0X5	T36.0X6
Carisoprodol	T42.8X1	T42.8X2	T42.8X3	T42.8X4	T42.8X5	T42.8X6
Carmellose	T47.4X1	T47.4X2	T47.4X3	T47.4X4	T47.4X5	T47.4X6
Carminative	T47.5X1	T47.5X2	T47.5X3	T47.5X4	T47.5X5	T47.5X6
Carmofur	T45.1X1	T45.1X2	T45.1X3	T45.1X4	T45.1X5	T45.1X6
Carmustine	T45.1X1	T45.1X2	T45.1X3	T45.1X4	T45.1X5	T45.1X6
Carotene	T45.2X1	T45.2X2	T45.2X3	T45.2X4	T45.2X5	T45.2X6
Carphenazine	T43.3X1	T43.3X2	T43.3X3	T43.3X4	T43.3X5	T43.3X6
Carpipramine	T42.4X1	T42.4X2	T42.4X3	T42.4X4	T42.4X5	T42.4X6
Carprofen	T39.311	T39.312	T39.313	T39.314	T39.315	T39.316
Carpronium chloride	T44.3X1	T44.3X2	T44.3X3	T44.3X4	T44.3X5	T44.3X6
Carrageenan	T47.8X1	T47.8X2	T47.8X3	T47.8X4	T47.8X5	T47.8X6
Carteolol	T44.7X1	T44.7X2	T44.7X3	T44.7X4	T44.7X5	T44.7X6
Carter's Little Pills	T47.2X1	T47.2X2	T47.2X3	T47.2X4	T47.2X5	T47.2X6
Cascara (sagrada)	T47.2X1	T47.2X2	T47.2X3	T47.2X4	T47.2X5	T47.2X6
Cassava	T62.2X1	T62.2X2	T62.2X3	T62.2X4	--	--
Castellani's paint	T49.0X1	T49.0X2	T49.0X3	T49.0X4	T49.0X5	T49.0X6
Castor						
bean	T62.2X1	T62.2X2	T62.2X3	T62.2X4	--	--
oil	T47.2X1	T47.2X2	T47.2X3	T47.2X4	T47.2X5	T47.2X6
Catalase	T45.3X1	T45.3X2	T45.3X3	T45.3X4	T45.3X5	T45.3X6
Caterpillar (sting)	T63.431	T63.432	T63.433	T63.434	--	--
Catha (edulis) (tea)	T43.691	T43.692	T43.693	T43.694	--	--
Cathartic NEC	T47.4X1	T47.4X2	T47.4X3	T47.4X4	T47.4X5	T47.4X6
anthacene derivative	T47.2X1	T47.2X2	T47.2X3	T47.2X4	T47.2X5	T47.2X6
bulk	T47.4X1	T47.4X2	T47.4X3	T47.4X4	T47.4X5	T47.4X6
contact	T47.2X1	T47.2X2	T47.2X3	T47.2X4	T47.2X5	T47.2X6
emollient NEC	T47.4X1	T47.4X2	T47.4X3	T47.4X4	T47.4X5	T47.4X6
irritant NEC	T47.2X1	T47.2X2	T47.2X3	T47.2X4	T47.2X5	T47.2X6
mucilage	T47.4X1	T47.4X2	T47.4X3	T47.4X4	T47.4X5	T47.4X6
saline	T47.3X1	T47.3X2	T47.3X3	T47.3X4	T47.3X5	T47.3X6
vegetable	T47.2X1	T47.2X2	T47.2X3	T47.2X4	T47.2X5	T47.2X6
Cathine	T50.5X1	T50.5X2	T50.5X3	T50.5X4	T50.5X5	T50.5X6
Cathomycin	T36.8X1	T36.8X2	T36.8X3	T36.8X4	T36.8X5	T36.8X6
Cation exchange resin	T50.3X1	T50.3X2	T50.3X3	T50.3X4	T50.3X5	T50.3X6
Caustic (s) **NEC**	T54.91	T54.92	T54.93	T54.94	--	--
alkali	T54.3X1	T54.3X2	T54.3X3	T54.3X4	--	--
hydroxide	T54.3X1	T54.3X2	T54.3X3	T54.3X4	--	--
potash	T54.3X1	T54.3X2	T54.3X3	T54.3X4	--	--
soda	T54.3X1	T54.3X2	T54.3X3	T54.3X4	--	--
specified NEC	T54.91	T54.92	T54.93	T54.94	--	--
Ceepryn	T49.0X1	T49.0X2	T49.0X3	T49.0X4	T49.0X5	T49.0X6
ENT agent	T49.6X1	T49.6X2	T49.6X3	T49.6X4	T49.6X5	T49.6X6
lozenges	T49.6X1	T49.6X2	T49.6X3	T49.6X4	T49.6X5	T49.6X6
Cefacetrile	T36.1X1	T36.1X2	T36.1X3	T36.1X4	T36.1X5	T36.1X6
Cefaclor	T36.1X1	T36.1X2	T36.1X3	T36.1X4	T36.1X5	T36.1X6
Cefadroxil	T36.1X1	T36.1X2	T36.1X3	T36.1X4	T36.1X5	T36.1X6
Cefalexin	T36.1X1	T36.1X2	T36.1X3	T36.1X4	T36.1X5	T36.1X6
Cefaloglycin	T36.1X1	T36.1X2	T36.1X3	T36.1X4	T36.1X5	T36.1X6
Cefaloridine	T36.1X1	T36.1X2	T36.1X3	T36.1X4	T36.1X5	T36.1X6
Cefalosporins	T36.1X1	T36.1X2	T36.1X3	T36.1X4	T36.1X5	T36.1X6
Cefalotin	T36.1X1	T36.1X2	T36.1X3	T36.1X4	T36.1X5	T36.1X6
Cefamandole	T36.1X1	T36.1X2	T36.1X3	T36.1X4	T36.1X5	T36.1X6
Cefamycin antibiotic	T36.1X1	T36.1X2	T36.1X3	T36.1X4	T36.1X5	T36.1X6
Cefapirin	T36.1X1	T36.1X2	T36.1X3	T36.1X4	T36.1X5	T36.1X6
Cefatrizine	T36.1X1	T36.1X2	T36.1X3	T36.1X4	T36.1X5	T36.1X6
Cefazedone	T36.1X1	T36.1X2	T36.1X3	T36.1X4	T36.1X5	T36.1X6
Cefazolin	T36.1X1	T36.1X2	T36.1X3	T36.1X4	T36.1X5	T36.1X6
Cefbuperazone	T36.1X1	T36.1X2	T36.1X3	T36.1X4	T36.1X5	T36.1X6
Cefetamet	T36.1X1	T36.1X2	T36.1X3	T36.1X4	T36.1X5	T36.1X6
Cefixime	T36.1X1	T36.1X2	T36.1X3	T36.1X4	T36.1X5	T36.1X6
Cefmenoxime	T36.1X1	T36.1X2	T36.1X3	T36.1X4	T36.1X5	T36.1X6
Cefmetazole	T36.1X1	T36.1X2	T36.1X3	T36.1X4	T36.1X5	T36.1X6
Cefminox	T36.1X1	T36.1X2	T36.1X3	T36.1X4	T36.1X5	T36.1X6
Cefonicid	T36.1X1	T36.1X2	T36.1X3	T36.1X4	T36.1X5	T36.1X6
Cefoperazone	T36.1X1	T36.1X2	T36.1X3	T36.1X4	T36.1X5	T36.1X6
Ceforanide	T36.1X1	T36.1X2	T36.1X3	T36.1X4	T36.1X5	T36.1X6
Cefotaxime	T36.1X1	T36.1X2	T36.1X3	T36.1X4	T36.1X5	T36.1X6
Cefotetan	T36.1X1	T36.1X2	T36.1X3	T36.1X4	T36.1X5	T36.1X6
Cefotiam	T36.1X1	T36.1X2	T36.1X3	T36.1X4	T36.1X5	T36.1X6
Cefoxitin	T36.1X1	T36.1X2	T36.1X3	T36.1X4	T36.1X5	T36.1X6
Cefpimizole	T36.1X1	T36.1X2	T36.1X3	T36.1X4	T36.1X5	T36.1X6
Cefpiramide	T36.1X1	T36.1X2	T36.1X3	T36.1X4	T36.1X5	T36.1X6
Cefradine	T36.1X1	T36.1X2	T36.1X3	T36.1X4	T36.1X5	T36.1X6
Cefroxadine	T36.1X1	T36.1X2	T36.1X3	T36.1X4	T36.1X5	T36.1X6
Cefsulodin	T36.1X1	T36.1X2	T36.1X3	T36.1X4	T36.1X5	T36.1X6
Ceftazidime	T36.1X1	T36.1X2	T36.1X3	T36.1X4	T36.1X5	T36.1X6
Cefteram	T36.1X1	T36.1X2	T36.1X3	T36.1X4	T36.1X5	T36.1X6
Ceftezole	T36.1X1	T36.1X2	T36.1X3	T36.1X4	T36.1X5	T36.1X6
Ceftizoxime	T36.1X1	T36.1X2	T36.1X3	T36.1X4	T36.1X5	T36.1X6
Ceftriaxone	T36.1X1	T36.1X2	T36.1X3	T36.1X4	T36.1X5	T36.1X6
Cefuroxime	T36.1X1	T36.1X2	T36.1X3	T36.1X4	T36.1X5	T36.1X6
Cefuzonam	T36.1X1	T36.1X2	T36.1X3	T36.1X4	T36.1X5	T36.1X6
Celestone	T38.0X1	T38.0X2	T38.0X3	T38.0X4	T38.0X5	T38.0X6
topical	T49.0X1	T49.0X2	T49.0X3	T49.0X4	T49.0X5	T49.0X6
Celiprolol	T44.7X1	T44.7X2	T44.7X3	T44.7X4	T44.7X5	T44.7X6
Cell stimulants and proliferants	T49.8X1	T49.8X2	T49.8X3	T49.8X4	T49.8X5	T49.8X6
Cellosolve	T52.91	T52.92	T52.93	T52.94	--	--
Cellulose						
cathartic	T47.4X1	T47.4X2	T47.4X3	T47.4X4	T47.4X5	T47.4X6
hydroxyethyl	T47.4X1	T47.4X2	T47.4X3	T47.4X4	T47.4X5	T47.4X6
nitrates (topical)	T49.3X1	T49.3X2	T49.3X3	T49.3X4	T49.3X5	T49.3X6
oxidized	T49.4X1	T49.4X2	T49.4X3	T49.4X4	T49.4X5	T49.4X6
Centipede (bite)	T63.411	T63.412	T63.413	T63.414	--	--
Central nervous system						
depressants	T42.71	T42.72	T42.73	T42.74	T42.75	T42.76
anesthetic (general) NEC	T41.201	T41.202	T41.203	T41.204	T41.205	T41.206
gases NEC	T41.0X1	T41.0X2	T41.0X3	T41.0X4	T41.0X5	T41.0X6
intravenous	T41.1X1	T41.1X2	T41.1X3	T41.1X4	T41.1X5	T41.1X6
barbiturates	T42.3X1	T42.3X2	T42.3X3	T42.3X4	T42.3X5	T42.3X6
benzodiazepines	T42.4X1	T42.4X2	T42.4X3	T42.4X4	T42.4X5	T42.4X6
bromides	T42.6X1	T42.6X2	T42.6X3	T42.6X4	T42.6X5	T42.6X6
cannabis sativa	T40.7X1	T40.7X2	T40.7X3	T40.7X4	T40.7X5	T40.7X6
chloral hydrate	T42.6X1	T42.6X2	T42.6X3	T42.6X4	T42.6X5	T42.6X6
ethanol	T51.0X1	T51.0X2	T51.0X3	T51.0X4	--	--
hallucinogenics	T40.901	T40.902	T40.903	T40.904	T40.905	T40.906
hypnotics	T42.71	T42.72	T42.73	T42.74	T42.75	T42.76
specified NEC	T42.6X1	T42.6X2	T42.6X3	T42.6X4	T42.6X5	T42.6X6
muscle relaxants	T42.8X1	T42.8X2	T42.8X3	T42.8X4	T42.8X5	T42.8X6
paraldehyde	T42.6X1	T42.6X2	T42.6X3	T42.6X4	T42.6X5	T42.6X6
sedatives; sedative-hypnotics	T42.71	T42.72	T42.73	T42.74	T42.75	T42.76
mixed NEC	T42.6X1	T42.6X2	T42.6X3	T42.6X4	T42.6X5	T42.6X6
specified NEC	T42.6X1	T42.6X2	T42.6X3	T42.6X4	T42.6X5	T42.6X6
muscle-tone depressants	T42.8X1	T42.8X2	T42.8X3	T42.8X4	T42.8X5	T42.8X6
stimulants	T43.601	T43.602	T43.603	T43.604	T43.605	T43.606
amphetamines	T43.621	T43.622	T43.623	T43.624	T43.625	T43.626
analeptics	T50.7X1	T50.7X2	T50.7X3	T50.7X4	T50.7X5	T50.7X6
antidepressants	T43.201	T43.202	T43.203	T43.204	T43.205	T43.206
opiate antagonists	T50.7X1	T50.7X2	T50.7X3	T50.7X4	T50.7X5	T50.7X6
specified NEC	T43.691	T43.692	T43.693	T43.694	T43.695	T43.696
Cephalexin	T36.1X1	T36.1X2	T36.1X3	T36.1X4	T36.1X5	T36.1X6
Cephaloglycin	T36.1X1	T36.1X2	T36.1X3	T36.1X4	T36.1X5	T36.1X6
Cephaloridine	T36.1X1	T36.1X2	T36.1X3	T36.1X4	T36.1X5	T36.1X6
Cephalosporins	T36.1X1	T36.1X2	T36.1X3	T36.1X4	T36.1X5	T36.1X6
N (adicillin)	T36.0X1	T36.0X2	T36.0X3	T36.0X4	T36.0X5	T36.0X6
Cephalothin	T36.1X1	T36.1X2	T36.1X3	T36.1X4	T36.1X5	T36.1X6
Cephalotin	T36.1X1	T36.1X2	T36.1X3	T36.1X4	T36.1X5	T36.1X6
Cephradine	T36.1X1	T36.1X2	T36.1X3	T36.1X4	T36.1X5	T36.1X6
Cerbera (odallam)	T62.2X1	T62.2X2	T62.2X3	T62.2X4	--	--
Cerberin	T46.0X1	T46.0X2	T46.0X3	T46.0X4	T46.0X5	T46.0X6
Cerebral stimulants	T43.601	T43.602	T43.603	T43.604	T43.605	T43.606
psychotherapeutic	T43.601	T43.602	T43.603	T43.604	T43.605	T43.606
specified NEC	T43.691	T43.692	T43.693	T43.694	T43.695	T43.696
Cerium oxalate	T45.0X1	T45.0X2	T45.0X3	T45.0X4	T45.0X5	T45.0X6
Cerous oxalate	T45.0X1	T45.0X2	T45.0X3	T45.0X4	T45.0X5	T45.0X6
Ceruletide	T50.8X1	T50.8X2	T50.8X3	T50.8X4	T50.8X5	T50.8X6
Cetalkonium (chloride)	T49.0X1	T49.0X2	T49.0X3	T49.0X4	T49.0X5	T49.0X6
Cethexonium chloride	T49.0X1	T49.0X2	T49.0X3	T49.0X4	T49.0X5	T49.0X6
Cetiedil	T46.7X1	T46.7X2	T46.7X3	T46.7X4	T46.7X5	T46.7X6
Cetirizine	T45.0X1	T45.0X2	T45.0X3	T45.0X4	T45.0X5	T45.0X6
Cetomacrogol	T50.991	T50.992	T50.993	T50.994	T50.995	T50.996
Cetotiamine	T45.2X1	T45.2X2	T45.2X3	T45.2X4	T45.2X5	T45.2X6
Cetoxime	T45.0X1	T45.0X2	T45.0X3	T45.0X4	T45.0X5	T45.0X6
Cetraxate	T47.1X1	T47.1X2	T47.1X3	T47.1X4	T47.1X5	T47.1X6
Cetrimide	T49.0X1	T49.0X2	T49.0X3	T49.0X4	T49.0X5	T49.0X6
Cetrimonium (bromide)	T49.0X1	T49.0X2	T49.0X3	T49.0X4	T49.0X5	T49.0X6
Cetylpyridinium chloride	T49.0X1	T49.0X2	T49.0X3	T49.0X4	T49.0X5	T49.0X6
ENT agent	T49.6X1	T49.6X2	T49.6X3	T49.6X4	T49.6X5	T49.6X6
lozenges	T49.6X1	T49.6X2	T49.6X3	T49.6X4	T49.6X5	T49.6X6
Cevadilla — *see Sabadilla*						
Cevitamic acid	T45.2X1	T45.2X2	T45.2X3	T45.2X4	T45.2X5	T45.2X6
Chalk, precipitated	T47.1X1	T47.1X2	T47.1X3	T47.1X4	T47.1X5	T47.1X6

Substance	Poisoning, Accidental unintentional	Poisoning, Intentional self-harm	Poisoning, Assault	Poisoning, Undetermined	Adverse effect	Underdosing
Chamomile	T49.0X1	T49.0X2	T49.0X3	T49.0X4	T49.0X5	T49.0X6
Ch'an su	T46.0X1	T46.0X2	T46.0X3	T46.0X4	T46.0X5	T46.0X6
Charcoal	T47.6X1	T47.6X2	T47.6X3	T47.6X4	T47.6X5	T47.6X6
activated— *see also Charcoal, medicinal*	T47.6X1	T47.6X2	T47.6X3	T47.6X4	T47.6X5	T47.6X6
fumes (Carbon monoxide)	T58.2X1	T58.2X2	T58.2X3	T58.2X4	--	--
industrial	T58.8X1	T58.8X2	T58.8X3	T58.8X4	--	--
medicinal (activated)	T47.6X1	T47.6X2	T47.6X3	T47.6X4	T47.6X5	T47.6X6
antidiarrheal	T47.6X1	T47.6X2	T47.6X3	T47.6X4	T47.6X5	T47.6X6
poison control	T47.8X1	T47.8X2	T47.8X3	T47.8X4	T47.8X5	T47.8X6
specified use other than for diarrhea	T47.8X1	T47.8X2	T47.8X3	T47.8X4	T47.8X5	T47.8X6
topical	T49.8X1	T49.8X2	T49.8X3	T49.8X4	T49.8X5	T49.8X6
Chaulmosulfone	T37.1X1	T37.1X2	T37.1X3	T37.1X4	T37.1X5	T37.1X6
Chelating agent NEC	T50.6X1	T50.6X2	T50.6X3	T50.6X4	T50.6X5	T50.6X6
Chelidonium majus	T62.2X1	T62.2X2	T62.2X3	T62.2X4	--	--
Chemical substance NEC	T65.91	T65.92	T65.93	T65.94	--	--
Chenodeoxycholic acid	T47.5X1	T47.5X2	T47.5X3	T47.5X4	T47.5X5	T47.5X6
Chenodiol	T47.5X1	T47.5X2	T47.5X3	T47.5X4	T47.5X5	T47.5X6
Chenopodium	T37.4X1	T37.4X2	T37.4X3	T37.4X4	T37.4X5	T37.4X6
Cherry laurel	T62.2X1	T62.2X2	T62.2X3	T62.2X4	--	--
Chinidin (e)	T46.2X1	T46.2X2	T46.2X3	T46.2X4	T46.2X5	T46.2X6
Chiniofon	T37.8X1	T37.8X2	T37.8X3	T37.8X4	T37.8X5	T37.8X6
Chlophedianol	T48.3X1	T48.3X2	T48.3X3	T48.3X4	T48.3X5	T48.3X6
Chloral	T42.6X1	T42.6X2	T42.6X3	T42.6X4	T42.6X5	T42.6X6
derivative	T42.6X1	T42.6X2	T42.6X3	T42.6X4	T42.6X5	T42.6X6
hydrate	T42.6X1	T42.6X2	T42.6X3	T42.6X4	T42.6X5	T42.6X6
Chloralamide	T42.6X1	T42.6X2	T42.6X3	T42.6X4	T42.6X5	T42.6X6
Chloralodol	T42.6X1	T42.6X2	T42.6X3	T42.6X4	T42.6X5	T42.6X6
Chloralose	T60.4X1	T60.4X2	T60.4X3	T60.4X4	--	--
Chlorambucil	T45.1X1	T45.1X2	T45.1X3	T45.1X4	T45.1X5	T45.1X6
Chloramine	T57.8X1	T57.8X2	T57.8X3	T57.8X4	--	--
T	T49.0X1	T49.0X2	T49.0X3	T49.0X4	T49.0X5	T49.0X6
topical	T49.0X1	T49.0X2	T49.0X3	T49.0X4	T49.0X5	T49.0X6
Chloramphenicol	T36.2X1	T36.2X2	T36.2X3	T36.2X4	T36.2X5	T36.2X6
ENT agent	T49.6X1	T49.6X2	T49.6X3	T49.6X4	T49.6X5	T49.6X6
ophthalmic preparation	T49.5X1	T49.5X2	T49.5X3	T49.5X4	T49.5X5	T49.5X6
topical NEC	T49.0X1	T49.0X2	T49.0X3	T49.0X4	T49.0X5	T49.0X6
Chlorate (potassium) (sodium) **NEC**	T60.3X1	T60.3X2	T60.3X3	T60.3X4	--	--
herbicide	T60.3X1	T60.3X2	T60.3X3	T60.3X4	--	--
Chlorazanil	T50.2X1	T50.2X2	T50.2X3	T50.2X4	T50.2X5	T50.2X6
Chlorbenzene, chlorbenzol	T53.7X1	T53.7X2	T53.7X3	T53.7X4	--	--
Chlorbenzoxamine	T44.3X1	T44.3X2	T44.3X3	T44.3X4	T44.3X5	T44.3X6
Chlorbutol	T42.6X1	T42.6X2	T42.6X3	T42.6X4	T42.6X5	T42.6X6
Chlorcyclizine	T45.0X1	T45.0X2	T45.0X3	T45.0X4	T45.0X5	T45.0X6
Chlordan (e) (dust)	T60.1X1	T60.1X2	T60.1X3	T60.1X4	--	--
Chlordantoin	T49.0X1	T49.0X2	T49.0X3	T49.0X4	T49.0X5	T49.0X6
Chlordiazepoxide	T42.4X1	T42.4X2	T42.4X3	T42.4X4	T42.4X5	T42.4X6
Chlordiethyl benzamide	T49.3X1	T49.3X2	T49.3X3	T49.3X4	T49.3X5	T49.3X6
Chloresium	T49.8X1	T49.8X2	T49.8X3	T49.8X4	T49.8X5	T49.8X6
Chlorethiazol	T42.6X1	T42.6X2	T42.6X3	T42.6X4	T42.6X5	T42.6X6
Chlorethyl — *see Ethyl chloride*						
Chloretone	T42.6X1	T42.6X2	T42.6X3	T42.6X4	T42.6X5	T42.6X6
Chlorex	T53.6X1	T53.6X2	T53.6X3	T53.6X4	--	--
insecticide	T60.1X1	T60.1X2	T60.1X3	T60.1X4	--	--
Chlorfenvinphos	T60.0X1	T60.0X2	T60.0X3	T60.0X4	--	--
Chlorhexadol	T42.6X1	T42.6X2	T42.6X3	T42.6X4	T42.6X5	T42.6X6
Chlorhexamide	T45.1X1	T45.1X2	T45.1X3	T45.1X4	T45.1X5	T45.1X6
Chlorhexidine	T49.0X1	T49.0X2	T49.0X3	T49.0X4	T49.0X5	T49.0X6
Chlorhydroxyquinolin	T49.0X1	T49.0X2	T49.0X3	T49.0X4	T49.0X5	T49.0X6
Chloride of lime (bleach)	T54.3X1	T54.3X2	T54.3X3	T54.3X4	--	--
Chlorimipramine	T43.011	T43.012	T43.013	T43.014	T43.015	T43.016
Chlorinated						
camphene	T53.6X1	T53.6X2	T53.6X3	T53.6X4	--	--
diphenyl	T53.7X1	T53.7X2	T53.7X3	T53.7X4	--	--
hydrocarbons NEC	T53.91	T53.92	T53.93	T53.94	--	--
solvents	T53.91	T53.92	T53.93	T53.94	--	--
lime (bleach)	T54.3X1	T54.3X2	T54.3X3	T54.3X4	--	--
and boric acid solution	T49.0X1	T49.0X2	T49.0X3	T49.0X4	T49.0X5	T49.0X6
naphthalene (insecticide)	T60.1X1	T60.1X2	T60.1X3	T60.1X4	--	--
industrial (non-pesticide)	T53.7X1	T53.7X2	T53.7X3	T53.7X4	--	--
pesticide NEC	T60.8X1	T60.8X2	T60.8X3	T60.8X4	--	--
soda — *see also sodium hypochlorite*						
solution	T49.0X1	T49.0X2	T49.0X3	T49.0X4	T49.0X5	T49.0X6
Chlorine (fumes) (gas)	T59.4X1	T59.4X2	T59.4X3	T59.4X4	--	--
bleach	T54.3X1	T54.3X2	T54.3X3	T54.3X4	--	--
compound gas NEC	T59.4X1	T59.4X2	T59.4X3	T59.4X4	--	--
disinfectant	T59.4X1	T59.4X2	T59.4X3	T59.4X4	--	--
releasing agents NEC	T59.4X1	T59.4X2	T59.4X3	T59.4X4	--	--
Chlorisondamine chloride	T46.991	T46.992	T46.993	T46.994	T46.995	T46.996
Chlormadinone	T38.5X1	T38.5X2	T38.5X3	T38.5X4	T38.5X5	T38.5X6
Chlormephos	T60.0X1	T60.0X2	T60.0X3	T60.0X4	--	--

Substance	Poisoning, Accidental unintentional	Poisoning, Intentional self-harm	Poisoning, Assault	Poisoning, Undetermined	Adverse effect	Underdosing
Chlormerodrin	T50.2X1	T50.2X2	T50.2X3	T50.2X4	T50.2X5	T50.2X6
Chlormethiazole	T42.6X1	T42.6X2	T42.6X3	T42.6X4	T42.6X5	T42.6X6
Chlormethine	T45.1X1	T45.1X2	T45.1X3	T45.1X4	T45.1X5	T45.1X6
Chlormethylenecycline	T36.4X1	T36.4X2	T36.4X3	T36.4X4	T36.4X5	T36.4X6
Chlormezanone	T42.6X1	T42.6X2	T42.6X3	T42.6X4	T42.6X5	T42.6X6
Chloroacetic acid	T60.3X1	T60.3X2	T60.3X3	T60.3X4	--	--
Chloroacetone	T59.3X1	T59.3X2	T59.3X3	T59.3X4	--	--
Chloroacetophenone	T59.3X1	T59.3X2	T59.3X3	T59.3X4	--	--
Chloroaniline	T53.7X1	T53.7X2	T53.7X3	T53.7X4	--	--
Chlorobenzene, chlorobenzol	T53.7X1	T53.7X2	T53.7X3	T53.7X4	--	--
Chlorobromomethane (fire extinguisher)	T53.6X1	T53.6X2	T53.6X3	T53.6X4	--	--
Chlorobutanol	T49.0X1	T49.0X2	T49.0X3	T49.0X4	T49.0X5	T49.0X6
Chlorocresol	T49.0X1	T49.0X2	T49.0X3	T49.0X4	T49.0X5	T49.0X6
Chlorodehydro-methyltestosterone	T38.7X1	T38.7X2	T38.7X3	T38.7X4	T38.7X5	T38.7X6
Chlorodinitrobenzene	T53.7X1	T53.7X2	T53.7X3	T53.7X4	--	--
dust or vapor	T53.7X1	T53.7X2	T53.7X3	T53.7X4	--	--
Chlorodiphenyl	T53.7X1	T53.7X2	T53.7X3	T53.7X4	--	--
Chloroethane — *see Ethyl chloride*						
Chloroethylene	T53.6X1	T53.6X2	T53.6X3	T53.6X4	--	--
Chlorofluorocarbons	T53.5X1	T53.5X2	T53.5X3	T53.5X4	--	--
Chloroform (fumes) (vapor)	T53.1X1	T53.1X2	T53.1X3	T53.1X4	--	--
anesthetic	T41.0X1	T41.0X2	T41.0X3	T41.0X4	T41.0X5	T41.0X6
solvent	T53.1X1	T53.1X2	T53.1X3	T53.1X4	--	--
water, concentrated	T41.0X1	T41.0X2	T41.0X3	T41.0X4	T41.0X5	T41.0X6
Chloroguanide	T37.2X1	T37.2X2	T37.2X3	T37.2X4	T37.2X5	T37.2X6
Chloromycetin	T36.2X1	T36.2X2	T36.2X3	T36.2X4	T36.2X5	T36.2X6
ENT agent	T49.6X1	T49.6X2	T49.6X3	T49.6X4	T49.6X5	T49.6X6
ophthalmic preparation	T49.5X1	T49.5X2	T49.5X3	T49.5X4	T49.5X5	T49.5X6
otic solution	T49.6X1	T49.6X2	T49.6X3	T49.6X4	T49.6X5	T49.6X6
topical NEC	T49.0X1	T49.0X2	T49.0X3	T49.0X4	T49.0X5	T49.0X6
Chloronitrobenzene	T53.7X1	T53.7X2	T53.7X3	T53.7X4	--	--
dust or vapor	T53.7X1	T53.7X2	T53.7X3	T53.7X4	--	--
Chlorophacinone	T60.4X1	T60.4X2	T60.4X3	T60.4X4	--	--
Chlorophenol	T53.7X1	T53.7X2	T53.7X3	T53.7X4	--	--
Chlorophenothane	T60.1X1	T60.1X2	T60.1X3	T60.1X4	--	--
Chlorophyll	T50.991	T50.992	T50.993	T50.994	T50.995	T50.996
Chloropicrin (fumes)	T53.6X1	T53.6X2	T53.6X3	T53.6X4	--	--
fumigant	T60.8X1	T60.8X2	T60.8X3	T60.8X4	--	--
fungicide	T60.3X1	T60.3X2	T60.3X3	T60.3X4	--	--
pesticide	T60.8X1	T60.8X2	T60.8X3	T60.8X4	--	--
Chloroprocaine	T41.3X1	T41.3X2	T41.3X3	T41.3X4	T41.3X5	T41.3X6
infiltration (subcutaneous)	T41.3X1	T41.3X2	T41.3X3	T41.3X4	T41.3X5	T41.3X6
nerve block (peripheral) (plexus)	T41.3X1	T41.3X2	T41.3X3	T41.3X4	T41.3X5	T41.3X6
spinal	T41.3X1	T41.3X2	T41.3X3	T41.3X4	T41.3X5	T41.3X6
Chloroptic	T49.5X1	T49.5X2	T49.5X3	T49.5X4	T49.5X5	T49.5X6
Chloropurine	T45.1X1	T45.1X2	T45.1X3	T45.1X4	T45.1X5	T45.1X6
Chloropyramine	T45.0X1	T45.0X2	T45.0X3	T45.0X4	T45.0X5	T45.0X6
Chloropyrifos	T60.0X1	T60.0X2	T60.0X3	T60.0X4	--	--
Chloropyrilene	T45.0X1	T45.0X2	T45.0X3	T45.0X4	T45.0X5	T45.0X6
Chloroquine	T37.2X1	T37.2X2	T37.2X3	T37.2X4	T37.2X5	T37.2X6
Chlorothalonil	T60.3X1	T60.3X2	T60.3X3	T60.3X4	--	--
Chlorothen	T45.0X1	T45.0X2	T45.0X3	T45.0X4	T45.0X5	T45.0X6
Chlorothiazide	T50.2X1	T50.2X2	T50.2X3	T50.2X4	T50.2X5	T50.2X6
Chlorothymol	T49.4X1	T49.4X2	T49.4X3	T49.4X4	T49.4X5	T49.4X6
Chlorotrianisene	T38.5X1	T38.5X2	T38.5X3	T38.5X4	T38.5X5	T38.5X6
Chlorovinyldichloro-arsine, not in war	T57.0X1	T57.0X2	T57.0X3	T57.0X4	--	--
Chloroxine	T49.4X1	T49.4X2	T49.4X3	T49.4X4	T49.4X5	T49.4X6
Chloroxylenol	T49.0X1	T49.0X2	T49.0X3	T49.0X4	T49.0X5	T49.0X6
Chlorphenamine	T45.0X1	T45.0X2	T45.0X3	T45.0X4	T45.0X5	T45.0X6
Chlorphenesin	T42.8X1	T42.8X2	T42.8X3	T42.8X4	T42.8X5	T42.8X6
topical (antifungal)	T49.0X1	T49.0X2	T49.0X3	T49.0X4	T49.0X5	T49.0X6
Chlorpheniramine	T45.0X1	T45.0X2	T45.0X3	T45.0X4	T45.0X5	T45.0X6
Chlorphenoxamine	T45.0X1	T45.0X2	T45.0X3	T45.0X4	T45.0X5	T45.0X6
Chlorphentermine	T50.5X1	T50.5X2	T50.5X3	T50.5X4	T50.5X5	T50.5X6
Chlorprocaine — *see Chloroprocaine*						
Chlorproguanil	T37.2X1	T37.2X2	T37.2X3	T37.2X4	T37.2X5	T37.2X6
Chlorpromazine	T43.3X1	T43.3X2	T43.3X3	T43.3X4	T43.3X5	T43.3X6
Chlorpropamide	T38.3X1	T38.3X2	T38.3X3	T38.3X4	T38.3X5	T38.3X6
Chlorprothixene	T43.4X1	T43.4X2	T43.4X3	T43.4X4	T43.4X5	T43.4X6
Chlorquinaldol	T49.0X1	T49.0X2	T49.0X3	T49.0X4	T49.0X5	T49.0X6
Chlorquinol	T49.0X1	T49.0X2	T49.0X3	T49.0X4	T49.0X5	T49.0X6
Chlortalidone	T50.2X1	T50.2X2	T50.2X3	T50.2X4	T50.2X5	T50.2X6
Chlortetracycline	T36.4X1	T36.4X2	T36.4X3	T36.4X4	T36.4X5	T36.4X6
Chlorthalidone	T50.2X1	T50.2X2	T50.2X3	T50.2X4	T50.2X5	T50.2X6
Chlorthiophos	T60.0X1	T60.0X2	T60.0X3	T60.0X4	--	--
Chlortrianisene	T38.5X1	T38.5X2	T38.5X3	T38.5X4	T38.5X5	T38.5X6
Chlor-Trimeton	T45.0X1	T45.0X2	T45.0X3	T45.0X4	T45.0X5	T45.0X6
Chlorthion	T60.0X1	T60.0X2	T60.0X3	T60.0X4	--	--

Chlorzoxazone - Cocaine

Substance	Poisoning, Accidental unintentional	Poisoning, Intentional self-harm	Poisoning, Assault	Poisoning, Undetermined	Adverse effect	Underdosing
Chlorzoxazone	T42.8X1	T42.8X2	T42.8X3	T42.8X4	T42.8X5	T42.8X6
Choke damp	T59.7X1	T59.7X2	T59.7X3	T59.7X4	—	—
Cholagogues	T47.5X1	T47.5X2	T47.5X3	T47.5X4	T47.5X5	T47.5X6
Cholebrine	T50.8X1	T50.8X2	T50.8X3	T50.8X4	T50.8X5	T50.8X6
Cholecalciferol	T45.2X1	T45.2X2	T45.2X3	T45.2X4	T45.2X5	T45.2X6
Cholecystokinin	T50.8X1	T50.8X2	T50.8X3	T50.8X4	T50.8X5	T50.8X6
Cholera vaccine	T50.A91	T50.A92	T50.A93	T50.A94	T50.A95	T50.A96
Choleretic	T47.5X1	T47.5X2	T47.5X3	T47.5X4	T47.5X5	T47.5X6
Cholesterol-lowering agents	T46.6X1	T46.6X2	T46.6X3	T46.6X4	T46.6X5	T46.6X6
Cholestyramine (resin)	T46.6X1	T46.6X2	T46.6X3	T46.6X4	T46.6X5	T46.6X6
Cholic acid	T47.5X1	T47.5X2	T47.5X3	T47.5X4	T47.5X5	T47.5X6
Choline	T48.6X1	T48.6X2	T48.6X3	T48.6X4	T48.6X5	T48.6X6
chloride	T50.991	T50.992	T50.993	T50.994	T50.995	T50.996
dihydrogen citrate	T50.991	T50.992	T50.993	T50.994	T50.995	T50.996
salicylate	T39.091	T39.092	T39.093	T39.094	T39.095	T39.096
theophyllinate	T48.6X1	T48.6X2	T48.6X3	T48.6X4	T48.6X5	T48.6X6
Cholinergic (drug) NEC	T44.1X1	T44.1X2	T44.1X3	T44.1X4	T44.1X5	T44.1X6
muscle tone enhancer	T44.1X1	T44.1X2	T44.1X3	T44.1X4	T44.1X5	T44.1X6
organophosphorus	T44.0X1	T44.0X2	T44.0X3	T44.0X4	T44.0X5	T44.0X6
insecticide	T60.0X1	T60.0X2	T60.0X3	T60.0X4	—	—
nerve gas	T59.891	T59.892	T59.893	T59.894	—	—
trimethyl ammonium propanediol	T44.1X1	T44.1X2	T44.1X3	T44.1X4	T44.1X5	T44.1X6
Cholinesterase reactivator	T50.6X1	T50.6X2	T50.6X3	T50.6X4	T50.6X5	T50.6X6
Cholografin	T50.8X1	T50.8X2	T50.8X3	T50.8X4	T50.8X5	T50.8X6
Chorionic gonadotropin	T38.891	T38.892	T38.893	T38.894	T38.895	T38.896
Chromate	T56.2X1	T56.2X2	T56.2X3	T56.2X4	—	—
dust or mist	T56.2X1	T56.2X2	T56.2X3	T56.2X4	—	—
lead— *see also lead*	T56.0X1	T56.0X2	T56.0X3	T56.0X4	—	—
paint	T56.0X1	T56.0X2	T56.0X3	T56.0X4	—	—
Chromic						
acid	T56.2X1	T56.2X2	T56.2X3	T56.2X4	—	—
dust or mist	T56.2X1	T56.2X2	T56.2X3	T56.2X4	—	—
phosphate 32P	T45.1X1	T45.1X2	T45.1X3	T45.1X4	T45.1X5	T45.1X6
Chromium	T56.2X1	T56.2X2	T56.2X3	T56.2X4	—	—
compounds — *see Chromate*						
sesquioxide	T50.8X1	T50.8X2	T50.8X3	T50.8X4	T50.8X5	T50.8X6
Chromomycin A3	T45.1X1	T45.1X2	T45.1X3	T45.1X4	T45.1X5	T45.1X6
Chromonar	T46.3X1	T46.3X2	T46.3X3	T46.3X4	T46.3X5	T46.3X6
Chromyl chloride	T56.2X1	T56.2X2	T56.2X3	T56.2X4	—	—
Chrysarobin	T49.4X1	T49.4X2	T49.4X3	T49.4X4	T49.4X5	T49.4X6
Chrysazin	T47.2X1	T47.2X2	T47.2X3	T47.2X4	T47.2X5	T47.2X6
Chymar	T45.3X1	T45.3X2	T45.3X3	T45.3X4	T45.3X5	T45.3X6
ophthalmic preparation	T49.5X1	T49.5X2	T49.5X3	T49.5X4	T49.5X5	T49.5X6
Chymopapain	T45.3X1	T45.3X2	T45.3X3	T45.3X4	T45.3X5	T45.3X6
Chymotrypsin	T45.3X1	T45.3X2	T45.3X3	T45.3X4	T45.3X5	T45.3X6
ophthalmic preparation	T49.5X1	T49.5X2	T49.5X3	T49.5X4	T49.5X5	T49.5X6
Cianidanol	T50.991	T50.992	T50.993	T50.994	T50.995	T50.996
Cianopramine	T43.011	T43.012	T43.013	T43.014	T43.015	T43.016
Cibenzoline	T46.2X1	T46.2X2	T46.2X3	T46.2X4	T46.2X5	T46.2X6
Ciclacillin	T36.0X1	T36.0X2	T36.0X3	T36.0X4	T36.0X5	T36.0X6
Ciclobarbital — *see Hexobarbital*						
Ciclonicate	T46.7X1	T46.7X2	T46.7X3	T46.7X4	T46.7X5	T46.7X6
Ciclopirox (olamine)	T49.0X1	T49.0X2	T49.0X3	T49.0X4	T49.0X5	T49.0X6
Ciclosporin	T45.1X1	T45.1X2	T45.1X3	T45.1X4	T45.1X5	T45.1X6
Cicuta maculata or virosa	T62.2X1	T62.2X2	T62.2X3	T62.2X4	—	—
Cicutoxin	T62.2X1	T62.2X2	T62.2X3	T62.2X4	—	—
Cigarette lighter fluid	T52.0X1	T52.0X2	T52.0X3	T52.0X4	—	—
Cigarettes (tobacco)	T65.221	T65.222	T65.223	T65.224	—	—
Ciguatoxin	T61.01	T61.02	T61.03	T61.04	—	—
Cilazapril	T46.4X1	T46.4X2	T46.4X3	T46.4X4	T46.4X5	T46.4X6
Cimetidine	T47.0X1	T47.0X2	T47.0X3	T47.0X4	T47.0X5	T47.0X6
Cimetropium bromide	T44.3X1	T44.3X2	T44.3X3	T44.3X4	T44.3X5	T44.3X6
Cinchocaine	T41.3X1	T41.3X2	T41.3X3	T41.3X4	T41.3X5	T41.3X6
topical (surface)	T41.3X1	T41.3X2	T41.3X3	T41.3X4	T41.3X5	T41.3X6
Cinchona	T37.2X1	T37.2X2	T37.2X3	T37.2X4	T37.2X5	T37.2X6
Cinchonine alkaloids	T37.2X1	T37.2X2	T37.2X3	T37.2X4	T37.2X5	T37.2X6
Cinchophen	T50.4X1	T50.4X2	T50.4X3	T50.4X4	T50.4X5	T50.4X6
Cinepazide	T46.7X1	T46.7X2	T46.7X3	T46.7X4	T46.7X5	T46.7X6
Cinnamedrine	T48.5X1	T48.5X2	T48.5X3	T48.5X4	T48.5X5	T48.5X6
Cinnarizine	T45.0X1	T45.0X2	T45.0X3	T45.0X4	T45.0X5	T45.0X6
Cinoxacin	T37.8X1	T37.8X2	T37.8X3	T37.8X4	T37.8X5	T37.8X6
Ciprofibrate	T46.6X1	T46.6X2	T46.6X3	T46.6X4	T46.6X5	T46.6X6
Ciprofloxacin	T36.8X1	T36.8X2	T36.8X3	T36.8X4	T36.8X5	T36.8X6
Cisapride	T47.8X1	T47.8X2	T47.8X3	T47.8X4	T47.8X5	T47.8X6
Cisplatin	T45.1X1	T45.1X2	T45.1X3	T45.1X4	T45.1X5	T45.1X6
Citalopram	T43.221	T43.222	T43.223	T43.224	T43.225	T43.226
Citanest	T41.3X1	T41.3X2	T41.3X3	T41.3X4	T41.3X5	T41.3X6
infiltration (subcutaneous)	T41.3X1	T41.3X2	T41.3X3	T41.3X4	T41.3X5	T41.3X6
nerve block (peripheral) (plexus)	T41.3X1	T41.3X2	T41.3X3	T41.3X4	T41.3X5	T41.3X6
Citric acid	T47.5X1	T47.5X2	T47.5X3	T47.5X4	T47.5X5	T47.5X6
Citrovorum (factor)	T45.8X1	T45.8X2	T45.8X3	T45.8X4	T45.8X5	T45.8X6
Claviceps purpurea	T62.2X1	T62.2X2	T62.2X3	T62.2X4	—	—

Substance	Poisoning, Accidental unintentional	Poisoning, Intentional self-harm	Poisoning, Assault	Poisoning, Undetermined	Adverse effect	Underdosing
Clavulanic acid	T36.1X1	T36.1X2	T36.1X3	T36.1X4	T36.1X5	T36.1X6
Cleaner, cleansing agent, type not specified	T65.891	T65.892	T65.893	T65.894	—	—
of paint or varnish	T52.91	T52.92	T52.93	T52.94	—	—
specified type NEC	T65.891	T65.892	T65.893	T65.894	—	—
Clebopride	T47.8X1	T47.8X2	T47.8X3	T47.8X4	T47.8X5	T47.8X6
Clefamide	T37.3X1	T37.3X2	T37.3X3	T37.3X4	T37.3X5	T37.3X6
Clemastine	T45.0X1	T45.0X2	T45.0X3	T45.0X4	T45.0X5	T45.0X6
Clematis vitalba	T62.2X1	T62.2X2	T62.2X3	T62.2X4	—	—
Clemizole	T45.0X1	T45.0X2	T45.0X3	T45.0X4	T45.0X5	T45.0X6
penicillin	T36.0X1	T36.0X2	T36.0X3	T36.0X4	T36.0X5	T36.0X6
Clenbuterol	T48.6X1	T48.6X2	T48.6X3	T48.6X4	T48.6X5	T48.6X6
Clidinium bromide	T44.3X1	T44.3X2	T44.3X3	T44.3X4	T44.3X5	T44.3X6
Clindamycin	T36.8X1	T36.8X2	T36.8X3	T36.8X4	T36.8X5	T36.8X6
Clinofibrate	T46.6X1	T46.6X2	T46.6X3	T46.6X4	T46.6X5	T46.6X6
Clioquinol	T37.8X1	T37.8X2	T37.8X3	T37.8X4	T37.8X5	T37.8X6
Cliradon	T40.2X1	T40.2X2	T40.2X3	T40.2X4	—	—
Clobazam	T42.4X1	T42.4X2	T42.4X3	T42.4X4	T42.4X5	T42.4X6
Clobenzorex	T50.5X1	T50.5X2	T50.5X3	T50.5X4	T50.5X5	T50.5X6
Clobetasol	T49.0X1	T49.0X2	T49.0X3	T49.0X4	T49.0X5	T49.0X6
Clobetasone	T49.0X1	T49.0X2	T49.0X3	T49.0X4	T49.0X5	T49.0X6
Clobutinol	T48.3X1	T48.3X2	T48.3X3	T48.3X4	T48.3X5	T48.3X6
Clocortolone	T38.0X1	T38.0X2	T38.0X3	T38.0X4	T38.0X5	T38.0X6
Clodantoin	T49.0X1	T49.0X2	T49.0X3	T49.0X4	T49.0X5	T49.0X6
Clodronic acid	T50.991	T50.992	T50.993	T50.994	T50.995	T50.996
Clofazimine	T37.1X1	T37.1X2	T37.1X3	T37.1X4	T37.1X5	T37.1X6
Clofedanol	T48.3X1	T48.3X2	T48.3X3	T48.3X4	T48.3X5	T48.3X6
Clofenamide	T50.2X1	T50.2X2	T50.2X3	T50.2X4	T50.2X5	T50.2X6
Clofenotane	T49.0X1	T49.0X2	T49.0X3	T49.0X4	T49.0X5	T49.0X6
Clofezone	T39.2X1	T39.2X2	T39.2X3	T39.2X4	T39.2X5	T39.2X6
Clofibrate	T46.6X1	T46.6X2	T46.6X3	T46.6X4	T46.6X5	T46.6X6
Clofibride	T46.6X1	T46.6X2	T46.6X3	T46.6X4	T46.6X5	T46.6X6
Cloforex	T50.5X1	T50.5X2	T50.5X3	T50.5X4	T50.5X5	T50.5X6
Clomethiazole	T42.6X1	T42.6X2	T42.6X3	T42.6X4	T42.6X5	T42.6X6
Clometocillin	T36.0X1	T36.0X2	T36.0X3	T36.0X4	T36.0X5	T36.0X6
Clomifene	T38.5X1	T38.5X2	T38.5X3	T38.5X4	T38.5X5	T38.5X6
Clomiphene	T38.5X1	T38.5X2	T38.5X3	T38.5X4	T38.5X5	T38.5X6
Clomipramine	T43.011	T43.012	T43.013	T43.014	T43.015	T43.016
Clomocycline	T36.4X1	T36.4X2	T36.4X3	T36.4X4	T36.4X5	T36.4X6
Clonazepam	T42.4X1	T42.4X2	T42.4X3	T42.4X4	T42.4X5	T42.4X6
Clonidine	T46.5X1	T46.5X2	T46.5X3	T46.5X4	T46.5X5	T46.5X6
Clonixin	T39.8X1	T39.8X2	T39.8X3	T39.8X4	T39.8X5	T39.8X6
Clopamide	T50.2X1	T50.2X2	T50.2X3	T50.2X4	T50.2X5	T50.2X6
Clopenthixol	T43.4X1	T43.4X2	T43.4X3	T43.4X4	T43.4X5	T43.4X6
Cloperastine	T48.3X1	T48.3X2	T48.3X3	T48.3X4	T48.3X5	T48.3X6
Clophedianol	T48.3X1	T48.3X2	T48.3X3	T48.3X4	T48.3X5	T48.3X6
Cloponone	T36.2X1	T36.2X2	T36.2X3	T36.2X4	T36.2X5	T36.2X6
Cloprednol	T38.0X1	T38.0X2	T38.0X3	T38.0X4	T38.0X5	T38.0X6
Cloral betaine	T42.6X1	T42.6X2	T42.6X3	T42.6X4	T42.6X5	T42.6X6
Cloramfenicol	T36.2X1	T36.2X2	T36.2X3	T36.2X4	T36.2X5	T36.2X6
Clorazepate (dipotassium)	T42.4X1	T42.4X2	T42.4X3	T42.4X4	T42.4X5	T42.4X6
Clorexolone	T50.2X1	T50.2X2	T50.2X3	T50.2X4	T50.2X5	T50.2X6
Clorfenamine	T45.0X1	T45.0X2	T45.0X3	T45.0X4	T45.0X5	T45.0X6
Clorgiline	T43.1X1	T43.1X2	T43.1X3	T43.1X4	T43.1X5	T43.1X6
Clorotepine	T44.3X1	T44.3X2	T44.3X3	T44.3X4	T44.3X5	T44.3X6
Clorox (bleach)	T54.91	T54.92	T54.93	T54.94	—	—
Clorprenaline	T48.6X1	T48.6X2	T48.6X3	T48.6X4	T48.6X5	T48.6X6
Clortermine	T50.5X1	T50.5X2	T50.5X3	T50.5X4	T50.5X5	T50.5X6
Clotiapine	T43.591	T43.592	T43.593	T43.594	T43.595	T43.596
Clotiazepam	T42.4X1	T42.4X2	T42.4X3	T42.4X4	T42.4X5	T42.4X6
Clotibric acid	T46.6X1	T46.6X2	T46.6X3	T46.6X4	T46.6X5	T46.6X6
Clotrimazole	T49.0X1	T49.0X2	T49.0X3	T49.0X4	T49.0X5	T49.0X6
Cloxacillin	T36.0X1	T36.0X2	T36.0X3	T36.0X4	T36.0X5	T36.0X6
Cloxazolam	T42.4X1	T42.4X2	T42.4X3	T42.4X4	T42.4X5	T42.4X6
Cloxiquine	T49.0X1	T49.0X2	T49.0X3	T49.0X4	T49.0X5	T49.0X6
Clozapine	T42.4X1	T42.4X2	T42.4X3	T42.4X4	T42.4X5	T42.4X6
Coagulant NEC	T45.7X1	T45.7X2	T45.7X3	T45.7X4	T45.7X5	T45.7X6
Coal (carbon monoxide from) — *see also Carbon, monoxide, coal*	T58.2X1	T58.2X2	T58.2X3	T58.2X4	—	—
oil — *see Kerosene*						
tar	T49.1X1	T49.1X2	T49.1X3	T49.1X4	T49.1X5	T49.1X6
fumes	T59.891	T59.892	T59.893	T59.894	—	—
medicinal (ointment)	T49.4X1	T49.4X2	T49.4X3	T49.4X4	T49.4X5	T49.4X6
analgesics NEC	T39.2X1	T39.2X2	T39.2X3	T39.2X4	T39.2X5	T39.2X6
naphtha (solvent)	T52.0X1	T52.0X2	T52.0X3	T52.0X4	—	—
Cobalamine	T45.2X1	T45.2X2	T45.2X3	T45.2X4	T45.2X5	T45.2X6
Cobalt (nonmedicinal) (fumes) (industrial)	T56.891	T56.892	T56.893	T56.894	—	—
medicinal (trace) (chloride)	T45.8X1	T45.8X2	T45.8X3	T45.8X4	T45.8X5	T45.8X6
Cobra (venom)	T63.041	T63.042	T63.043	T63.044	—	—
Coca (leaf)	T40.5X1	T40.5X2	T40.5X3	T40.5X4	T40.5X5	T40.5X6
Cocaine	T40.5X1	T40.5X2	T40.5X3	T40.5X4	T40.5X5	T40.5X6
topical anesthetic	T41.3X1	T41.3X2	T41.3X3	T41.3X4	T41.3X5	T41.3X6

Substance	Poisoning, Accidental unintentional	Poisoning, Intentional self-harm	Poisoning, Assault	Poisoning, Undetermined	Adverse effect	Underdosing
Cocarboxylase	T45.3X1	T45.3X2	T45.3X3	T45.3X4	T45.3X5	T45.3X6
Coccidioidin	T50.8X1	T50.8X2	T50.8X3	T50.8X4	T50.8X5	T50.8X6
Cocculus indicus	T62.1X1	T62.1X2	T62.1X3	T62.1X4	--	--
Cochineal	T65.6X1	T65.6X2	T65.6X3	T65.6X4	--	--
medicinal products	T50.991	T50.992	T50.993	T50.994	T50.995	T50.996
Codeine	T40.2X1	T40.2X2	T40.2X3	T40.2X4	T40.2X5	T40.2X6
Cod-liver oil	T45.2X1	T45.2X2	T45.2X3	T45.2X4	T45.2X5	T45.2X6
Coenzyme A	T50.991	T50.992	T50.993	T50.994	T50.995	T50.996
Coffee	T62.8X1	T62.8X2	T62.8X3	T62.8X4	--	--
Cogalactoiso-merase	T50.991	T50.992	T50.993	T50.994	T50.995	T50.996
Cogentin	T44.3X1	T44.3X2	T44.3X3	T44.3X4	T44.3X5	T44.3X6
Coke fumes or gas (carbon monoxide)	T58.2X1	T58.2X2	T58.2X3	T58.2X4	--	--
industrial use	T58.8X1	T58.8X2	T58.8X3	T58.8X4	--	--
Colace	T47.4X1	T47.4X2	T47.4X3	T47.4X4	T47.4X5	T47.4X6
Colaspase	T45.1X1	T45.1X2	T45.1X3	T45.1X4	T45.1X5	T45.1X6
Colchicine	T50.4X1	T50.4X2	T50.4X3	T50.4X4	T50.4X5	T50.4X6
Colchicum	T62.2X1	T62.2X2	T62.2X3	T62.2X4	--	--
Cold cream	T49.3X1	T49.3X2	T49.3X3	T49.3X4	T49.3X5	T49.3X6
Colecalciferol	T45.2X1	T45.2X2	T45.2X3	T45.2X4	T45.2X5	T45.2X6
Colestipol	T46.6X1	T46.6X2	T46.6X3	T46.6X4	T46.6X5	T46.6X6
Colestyramine	T46.6X1	T46.6X2	T46.6X3	T46.6X4	T46.6X5	T46.6X6
Colimycin	T36.8X1	T36.8X2	T36.8X3	T36.8X4	T36.8X5	T36.8X6
Colistimethate	T36.8X1	T36.8X2	T36.8X3	T36.8X4	T36.8X5	T36.8X6
Colistin	T36.8X1	T36.8X2	T36.8X3	T36.8X4	T36.8X5	T36.8X6
sulfate (eye preparation)	T49.5X1	T49.5X2	T49.5X3	T49.5X4	T49.5X5	T49.5X6
Collagen	T50.991	T50.992	T50.993	T50.994	T50.995	T50.996
Collagenase	T49.4X1	T49.4X2	T49.4X3	T49.4X4	T49.4X5	T49.4X6
Collodion	T49.3X1	T49.3X2	T49.3X3	T49.3X4	T49.3X5	T49.3X6
Colocynth	T47.2X1	T47.2X2	T47.2X3	T47.2X4	T47.2X5	T47.2X6
Colophony adhesive	T49.3X1	T49.3X2	T49.3X3	T49.3X4	T49.3X5	T49.3X6
Colorant — *see also Dye*	T50.991	T50.992	T50.993	T50.994	T50.995	T50.996
Coloring matter — *see Dye (s)*						
Combustion gas (after combustion) — *see Carbon, monoxide*						
prior to combustion	T59.891	T59.892	T59.893	T59.894	--	--
Compazine	T43.3X1	T43.3X2	T43.3X3	T43.3X4	T43.3X5	T43.3X6
Compound						
42 (warfarin)	T60.4X1	T60.4X2	T60.4X3	T60.4X4	--	--
269 (endrin)	T60.1X1	T60.1X2	T60.1X3	T60.1X4	--	--
497 (dieldrin)	T60.1X1	T60.1X2	T60.1X3	T60.1X4	--	--
1080 (sodium fluoroacetate)	T60.4X1	T60.4X2	T60.4X3	T60.4X4	--	--
3422 (parathion)	T60.0X1	T60.0X2	T60.0X3	T60.0X4	--	--
3911 (phorate)	T60.0X1	T60.0X2	T60.0X3	T60.0X4	--	--
3956 (toxaphene)	T60.1X1	T60.1X2	T60.1X3	T60.1X4	--	--
4049 (malathion)	T60.0X1	T60.0X2	T60.0X3	T60.0X4	--	--
4069 (malathion)	T60.0X1	T60.0X2	T60.0X3	T60.0X4	--	--
4124 (dicapthon)	T60.0X1	T60.0X2	T60.0X3	T60.0X4	--	--
E (cortisone)	T38.0X1	T38.0X2	T38.0X3	T38.0X4	T38.0X5	T38.0X6
F (hydrocortisone)	T38.0X1	T38.0X2	T38.0X3	T38.0X4	T38.0X5	T38.0X6
Congener, anabolic	T38.7X1	T38.7X2	T38.7X3	T38.7X4	T38.7X5	T38.7X6
Congo red	T50.8X1	T50.8X2	T50.8X3	T50.8X4	T50.8X5	T50.8X6
Coniine, conine	T62.2X1	T62.2X2	T62.2X3	T62.2X4	--	--
Conium (maculatum)	T62.2X1	T62.2X2	T62.2X3	T62.2X4	--	--
Conjugated estrogenic substances	T38.5X1	T38.5X2	T38.5X3	T38.5X4	T38.5X5	T38.5X6
Contac	T48.5X1	T48.5X2	T48.5X3	T48.5X4	T48.5X5	T48.5X6
Contact lens solution	T49.5X1	T49.5X2	T49.5X3	T49.5X4	T49.5X5	T49.5X6
Contraceptive (oral)	T38.4X1	T38.4X2	T38.4X3	T38.4X4	T38.4X5	T38.4X6
vaginal	T49.8X1	T49.8X2	T49.8X3	T49.8X4	T49.8X5	T49.8X6
Contrast medium, radiography	T50.8X1	T50.8X2	T50.8X3	T50.8X4	T50.8X5	T50.8X6
Convallaria glycosides	T46.0X1	T46.0X2	T46.0X3	T46.0X4	T46.0X5	T46.0X6
Convallaria majalis	T62.2X1	T62.2X2	T62.2X3	T62.2X4	--	--
berry	T62.1X1	T62.1X2	T62.1X3	T62.1X4	--	--
Copper (dust) (fumes) (nonmedicinal) **NEC**	T56.4X1	T56.4X2	T56.4X3	T56.4X4	--	--
arsenate, arsenite	T57.0X1	T57.0X2	T57.0X3	T57.0X4	--	--
insecticide	T60.2X1	T60.2X2	T60.2X3	T60.2X4	--	--
emetic	T47.7X1	T47.7X2	T47.7X3	T47.7X4	T47.7X5	T47.7X6
fungicide	T60.3X1	T60.3X2	T60.3X3	T60.3X4	--	--
gluconate	T49.0X1	T49.0X2	T49.0X3	T49.0X4	T49.0X5	T49.0X6
insecticide	T60.2X1	T60.2X2	T60.2X3	T60.2X4	--	--
medicinal (trace)	T45.8X1	T45.8X2	T45.8X3	T45.8X4	T45.8X5	T45.8X6
oleate	T49.0X1	T49.0X2	T49.0X3	T49.0X4	T49.0X5	T49.0X6
sulfate	T56.4X1	T56.4X2	T56.4X3	T56.4X4	--	--
cupric	T56.4X1	T56.4X2	T56.4X3	T56.4X4	--	--
fungicide	T60.3X1	T60.3X2	T60.3X3	T60.3X4	--	--
medicinal						
ear	T49.6X1	T49.6X2	T49.6X3	T49.6X4	T49.6X5	T49.6X6
Copper — *continued*						
sulfate — *continued*						
emetic	T47.7X1	T47.7X2	T47.7X3	T47.7X4	T47.7X5	T47.7X6
eye	T49.5X1	T49.5X2	T49.5X3	T49.5X4	T49.5X5	T49.5X6
cuprous	T56.4X1	T56.4X2	T56.4X3	T56.4X4	--	--
fungicide	T60.3X1	T60.3X2	T60.3X3	T60.3X4	--	--
medicinal						
ear	T49.6X1	T49.6X2	T49.6X3	T49.6X4	T49.6X5	T49.6X6
emetic	T47.7X1	T47.7X2	T47.7X3	T47.7X4	T47.7X5	T47.7X6
eye	T49.5X1	T49.5X2	T49.5X3	T49.5X4	T49.5X5	T49.5X6
Copperhead snake (bite) (venom)	T63.061	T63.062	T63.063	T63.064	--	--
Coral (sting)	T63.691	T63.692	T63.693	T63.694	--	--
snake (bite) (venom)	T63.021	T63.022	T63.023	T63.024	--	--
Corbadrine	T49.6X1	T49.6X2	T49.6X3	T49.6X4	T49.6X5	T49.6X6
Cordite	T65.891	T65.892	T65.893	T65.894	--	--
vapor	T59.891	T59.892	T59.893	T59.894	--	--
Cordran	T49.0X1	T49.0X2	T49.0X3	T49.0X4	T49.0X5	T49.0X6
Corn cures	T49.4X1	T49.4X2	T49.4X3	T49.4X4	T49.4X5	T49.4X6
Corn starch	T49.3X1	T49.3X2	T49.3X3	T49.3X4	T49.3X5	T49.3X6
Cornhusker's lotion	T49.3X1	T49.3X2	T49.3X3	T49.3X4	T49.3X5	T49.3X6
Coronary vasodilator NEC	T46.3X1	T46.3X2	T46.3X3	T46.3X4	T46.3X5	T46.3X6
Corrosive NEC	T54.91	T54.92	T54.93	T54.94	--	--
acid NEC	T54.2X1	T54.2X2	T54.2X3	T54.2X4	--	--
aromatics	T54.1X1	T54.1X2	T54.1X3	T54.1X4	--	--
disinfectant	T54.1X1	T54.1X2	T54.1X3	T54.1X4	--	--
fumes NEC	T54.91	T54.92	T54.93	T54.94	--	--
specified NEC	T54.91	T54.92	T54.93	T54.94	--	--
sublimate	T56.1X1	T56.1X2	T56.1X3	T56.1X4	--	--
Cortate	T38.0X1	T38.0X2	T38.0X3	T38.0X4	T38.0X5	T38.0X6
Cort-Dome	T38.0X1	T38.0X2	T38.0X3	T38.0X4	T38.0X5	T38.0X6
ENT agent	T49.6X1	T49.6X2	T49.6X3	T49.6X4	T49.6X5	T49.6X6
ophthalmic preparation	T49.5X1	T49.5X2	T49.5X3	T49.5X4	T49.5X5	T49.5X6
topical NEC	T49.0X1	T49.0X2	T49.0X3	T49.0X4	T49.0X5	T49.0X6
Cortef	T38.0X1	T38.0X2	T38.0X3	T38.0X4	T38.0X5	T38.0X6
ENT agent	T49.6X1	T49.6X2	T49.6X3	T49.6X4	T49.6X5	T49.6X6
ophthalmic preparation	T49.5X1	T49.5X2	T49.5X3	T49.5X4	T49.5X5	T49.5X6
topical NEC	T49.0X1	T49.0X2	T49.0X3	T49.0X4	T49.0X5	T49.0X6
Corticosteroid	T38.0X1	T38.0X2	T38.0X3	T38.0X4	T38.0X5	T38.0X6
ENT agent	T49.6X1	T49.6X2	T49.6X3	T49.6X4	T49.6X5	T49.6X6
mineral	T50.0X1	T50.0X2	T50.0X3	T50.0X4	T50.0X5	T50.0X6
ophthalmic	T49.5X1	T49.5X2	T49.5X3	T49.5X4	T49.5X5	T49.5X6
topical NEC	T49.0X1	T49.0X2	T49.0X3	T49.0X4	T49.0X5	T49.0X6
Corticotropin	T38.811	T38.812	T38.813	T38.814	T38.815	T38.816
Cortisol	T49.0X1	T49.0X2	T49.0X3	T49.0X4	T49.0X5	T49.0X6
ENT agent	T49.6X1	T49.6X2	T49.6X3	T49.6X4	T49.6X5	T49.6X6
ophthalmic preparation	T49.5X1	T49.5X2	T49.5X3	T49.5X4	T49.5X5	T49.5X6
topical NEC	T49.0X1	T49.0X2	T49.0X3	T49.0X4	T49.0X5	T49.0X6
Cortisone (acetate)	T38.0X1	T38.0X2	T38.0X3	T38.0X4	T38.0X5	T38.0X6
ENT agent	T49.6X1	T49.6X2	T49.6X3	T49.6X4	T49.6X5	T49.6X6
ophthalmic preparation	T49.5X1	T49.5X2	T49.5X3	T49.5X4	T49.5X5	T49.5X6
topical NEC	T49.0X1	T49.0X2	T49.0X3	T49.0X4	T49.0X5	T49.0X6
Cortivazol	T38.0X1	T38.0X2	T38.0X3	T38.0X4	T38.0X5	T38.0X6
Cortogen	T38.0X1	T38.0X2	T38.0X3	T38.0X4	T38.0X5	T38.0X6
ENT agent	T49.6X1	T49.6X2	T49.6X3	T49.6X4	T49.6X5	T49.6X6
ophthalmic preparation	T49.5X1	T49.5X2	T49.5X3	T49.5X4	T49.5X5	T49.5X6
Cortone	T38.0X1	T38.0X2	T38.0X3	T38.0X4	T38.0X5	T38.0X6
ENT agent	T49.6X1	T49.6X2	T49.6X3	T49.6X4	T49.6X5	T49.6X6
ophthalmic preparation	T49.5X1	T49.5X2	T49.5X3	T49.5X4	T49.5X5	T49.5X6
Cortril	T38.0X1	T38.0X2	T38.0X3	T38.0X4	T38.0X5	T38.0X6
ENT agent	T49.6X1	T49.6X2	T49.6X3	T49.6X4	T49.6X5	T49.6X6
ophthalmic preparation	T49.5X1	T49.5X2	T49.5X3	T49.5X4	T49.5X5	T49.5X6
topical NEC	T49.0X1	T49.0X2	T49.0X3	T49.0X4	T49.0X5	T49.0X6
Corynebacterium parvum	T45.1X1	T45.1X2	T45.1X3	T45.1X4	T45.1X5	T45.1X6
Cosmetic preparation	T49.8X1	T49.8X2	T49.8X3	T49.8X4	T49.8X5	T49.8X6
Cosmetics	T49.8X1	T49.8X2	T49.8X3	T49.8X4	T49.8X5	T49.8X6
Cosyntropin	T38.811	T38.812	T38.813	T38.814	T38.815	T38.816
Cotarnine	T45.7X1	T45.7X2	T45.7X3	T45.7X4	T45.7X5	T45.7X6
Co-trimoxazole	T36.8X1	T36.8X2	T36.8X3	T36.8X4	T36.8X5	T36.8X6
Cottonseed oil	T49.3X1	T49.3X2	T49.3X3	T49.3X4	T49.3X5	T49.3X6
Cough mixture (syrup)	T48.4X1	T48.4X2	T48.4X3	T48.4X4	T48.4X5	T48.4X6
containing opiates	T40.2X1	T40.2X2	T40.2X3	T40.2X4	T40.2X5	T40.2X6
expectorants	T48.4X1	T48.4X2	T48.4X3	T48.4X4	T48.4X5	T48.4X6
Coumadin	T45.511	T45.512	T45.513	T45.514	T45.515	T45.516
rodenticide	T60.4X1	T60.4X2	T60.4X3	T60.4X4	--	--
Coumaphos	T60.0X1	T60.0X2	T60.0X3	T60.0X4	--	--
Coumarin	T45.511	T45.512	T45.513	T45.514	T45.515	T45.516
Coumetarol	T45.511	T45.512	T45.513	T45.514	T45.515	T45.516
Cowbane	T62.2X1	T62.2X2	T62.2X3	T62.2X4	--	--
Cozyme	T45.2X1	T45.2X2	T45.2X3	T45.2X4	T45.2X5	T45.2X6
Crack	T40.5X1	T40.5X2	T40.5X3	T40.5X4	--	--
Crataegus extract	T46.0X1	T46.0X2	T46.0X3	T46.0X4	T46.0X5	T46.0X6
Creolin	T54.1X1	T54.1X2	T54.1X3	T54.1X4	--	--
disinfectant	T54.1X1	T54.1X2	T54.1X3	T54.1X4	--	--

Creosol - Demecolcine

Substance	Poisoning, Accidental unintentional	Poisoning, Intentional self-harm	Poisoning, Assault	Poisoning, Undetermined	Adverse effect	Underdosing
Creosol (compound)	T49.0X1	T49.0X2	T49.0X3	T49.0X4	T49.0X5	T49.0X6
Creosote (coal tar) (beechwood)	T49.0X1	T49.0X2	T49.0X3	T49.0X4	T49.0X5	T49.0X6
medicinal (expectorant)	T48.4X1	T48.4X2	T48.4X3	T48.4X4	T48.4X5	T48.4X6
syrup	T48.4X1	T48.4X2	T48.4X3	T48.4X4	T48.4X5	T48.4X6
Cresol (s)	T49.0X1	T49.0X2	T49.0X3	T49.0X4	T49.0X5	T49.0X6
and soap solution	T49.0X1	T49.0X2	T49.0X3	T49.0X4	T49.0X5	T49.0X6
Cresyl acetate	T49.0X1	T49.0X2	T49.0X3	T49.0X4	T49.0X5	T49.0X6
Cresylic acid	T49.0X1	T49.0X2	T49.0X3	T49.0X4	T49.0X5	T49.0X6
Crimidine	T60.4X1	T60.4X2	T60.4X3	T60.4X4	–	–
Croconazole	T37.8X1	T37.8X2	T37.8X3	T37.8X4	T37.8X5	T37.8X6
Cromoglicic acid	T48.6X1	T48.6X2	T48.6X3	T48.6X4	T48.6X5	T48.6X6
Cromolyn	T48.6X1	T48.6X2	T48.6X3	T48.6X4	T48.6X5	T48.6X6
Cromonar	T46.3X1	T46.3X2	T46.3X3	T46.3X4	T46.3X5	T46.3X6
Cropropamide	T39.8X1	T39.8X2	T39.8X3	T39.8X4	T39.8X5	T39.8X6
with crotethamide	T50.7X1	T50.7X2	T50.7X3	T50.7X4	T50.7X5	T50.7X6
Crotamiton	T49.0X1	T49.0X2	T49.0X3	T49.0X4	T49.0X5	T49.0X6
Crotethamide	T39.8X1	T39.8X2	T39.8X3	T39.8X4	T39.8X5	T39.8X6
with cropropamide	T50.7X1	T50.7X2	T50.7X3	T50.7X4	T50.7X5	T50.7X6
Croton (oil)	T47.2X1	T47.2X2	T47.2X3	T47.2X4	T47.2X5	T47.2X6
chloral	T42.6X1	T42.6X2	T42.6X3	T42.6X4	T42.6X5	T42.6X6
Crude oil	T52.0X1	T52.0X2	T52.0X3	T52.0X4	–	–
Cryogenine	T39.8X1	T39.8X2	T39.8X3	T39.8X4	T39.8X5	T39.8X6
Cryolite (vapor)	T60.1X1	T60.1X2	T60.1X3	T60.1X4	–	–
insecticide	T60.1X1	T60.1X2	T60.1X3	T60.1X4	–	–
Cryptenamine (tannates)	T46.5X1	T46.5X2	T46.5X3	T46.5X4	T46.5X5	T46.5X6
Crystal violet	T49.0X1	T49.0X2	T49.0X3	T49.0X4	T49.0X5	T49.0X6
Cuckoopint	T62.2X1	T62.2X2	T62.2X3	T62.2X4	–	–
Cumetharol	T45.511	T45.512	T45.513	T45.514	T45.515	T45.516
Cupric						
acetate	T60.3X1	T60.3X2	T60.3X3	T60.3X4	–	–
acetoarsenite	T57.0X1	T57.0X2	T57.0X3	T57.0X4	–	–
arsenate	T57.0X1	T57.0X2	T57.0X3	T57.0X4	–	–
gluconate	T49.0X1	T49.0X2	T49.0X3	T49.0X4	T49.0X5	T49.0X6
oleate	T49.0X1	T49.0X2	T49.0X3	T49.0X4	T49.0X5	T49.0X6
sulfate	T56.4X1	T56.4X2	T56.4X3	T56.4X4	–	–
Cuprous sulfate — *see also Copper sulfate*	T56.4X1	T56.4X2	T56.4X3	T56.4X4	–	–
Curare, curarine	T48.1X1	T48.1X2	T48.1X3	T48.1X4	T48.1X5	T48.1X6
Cyamemazine	T43.3X1	T43.3X2	T43.3X3	T43.3X4	T43.3X5	T43.3X6
Cyamopsis tetragono-loba	T46.6X1	T46.6X2	T46.6X3	T46.6X4	T46.6X5	T46.6X6
Cyanacetyl hydrazide	T37.1X1	T37.1X2	T37.1X3	T37.1X4	T37.1X5	T37.1X6
Cyanic acid (gas)	T59.891	T59.892	T59.893	T59.894	–	–
Cyanide (s) (compounds) (potassium) (sodium) **NEC**	T65.0X1	T65.0X2	T65.0X3	T65.0X4	–	–
dust or gas (inhalation) NEC	T57.3X1	T57.3X2	T57.3X3	T57.3X4	–	–
fumigant	T65.0X1	T65.0X2	T65.0X3	T65.0X4	–	–
hydrogen	T57.3X1	T57.3X2	T57.3X3	T57.3X4	–	–
mercuric — *see Mercury*						
pesticide (dust) (fumes)	T65.0X1	T65.0X2	T65.0X3	T65.0X4	–	–
Cyanoacrylate adhesive	T49.3X1	T49.3X2	T49.3X3	T49.3X4	T49.3X5	T49.3X6
Cyanocobalamin	T45.8X1	T45.8X2	T45.8X3	T45.8X4	T45.8X5	T45.8X6
Cyanogen (chloride) (gas) **NEC**	T59.891	T59.892	T59.893	T59.894	–	–
Cyclacillin	T36.0X1	T36.0X2	T36.0X3	T36.0X4	T36.0X5	T36.0X6
Cyclaine	T41.3X1	T41.3X2	T41.3X3	T41.3X4	T41.3X5	T41.3X6
Cyclamate	T50.991	T50.992	T50.993	T50.994	T50.995	T50.996
Cyclamen europaeum	T62.2X1	T62.2X2	T62.2X3	T62.2X4	–	–
Cyclandelate	T46.7X1	T46.7X2	T46.7X3	T46.7X4	T46.7X5	T46.7X6
Cyclazocine	T50.7X1	T50.7X2	T50.7X3	T50.7X4	T50.7X5	T50.7X6
Cyclizine	T45.0X1	T45.0X2	T45.0X3	T45.0X4	T45.0X5	T45.0X6
Cyclobarbital	T42.3X1	T42.3X2	T42.3X3	T42.3X4	T42.3X5	T42.3X6
Cyclobarbitone	T42.3X1	T42.3X2	T42.3X3	T42.3X4	T42.3X5	T42.3X6
Cyclobenzaprine	T48.1X1	T48.1X2	T48.1X3	T48.1X4	T48.1X5	T48.1X6
Cyclodrine	T44.3X1	T44.3X2	T44.3X3	T44.3X4	T44.3X5	T44.3X6
Cycloguanil embonate	T37.2X1	T37.2X2	T37.2X3	T37.2X4	T37.2X5	T37.2X6
Cyclohexane	T52.8X1	T52.8X2	T52.8X3	T52.8X4	–	–
Cyclohexanol	T51.8X1	T51.8X2	T51.8X3	T51.8X4	–	–
Cyclohexanone	T52.4X1	T52.4X2	T52.4X3	T52.4X4	–	–
Cycloheximide	T60.3X1	T60.3X2	T60.3X3	T60.3X4	–	–
Cyclohexyl acetate	T52.8X1	T52.8X2	T52.8X3	T52.8X4	–	–
Cycloleucin	T45.1X1	T45.1X2	T45.1X3	T45.1X4	T45.1X5	T45.1X6
Cyclomethycaine	T41.3X1	T41.3X2	T41.3X3	T41.3X4	T41.3X5	T41.3X6
Cyclopentamine	T44.4X1	T44.4X2	T44.4X3	T44.4X4	T44.4X5	T44.4X6
Cyclopenthiazide	T50.2X1	T50.2X2	T50.2X3	T50.2X4	T50.2X5	T50.2X6
Cyclopentolate	T44.3X1	T44.3X2	T44.3X3	T44.3X4	T44.3X5	T44.3X6
Cyclophosphamide	T45.1X1	T45.1X2	T45.1X3	T45.1X4	T45.1X5	T45.1X6
Cycloplegic drug	T49.5X1	T49.5X2	T49.5X3	T49.5X4	T49.5X5	T49.5X6
Cyclopropane	T41.291	T41.292	T41.293	T41.294	T41.295	T41.296
Cyclopyrabital	T39.8X1	T39.8X2	T39.8X3	T39.8X4	T39.8X5	T39.8X6
Cycloserine	T37.1X1	T37.1X2	T37.1X3	T37.1X4	T37.1X5	T37.1X6
Cyclosporin	T45.1X1	T45.1X2	T45.1X3	T45.1X4	T45.1X5	T45.1X6
Cyclothiazide	T50.2X1	T50.2X2	T50.2X3	T50.2X4	T50.2X5	T50.2X6
Cycrimine	T44.3X1	T44.3X2	T44.3X3	T44.3X4	T44.3X5	T44.3X6
Cyhalothrin	T60.1X1	T60.1X2	T60.1X3	T60.1X4	–	–

Substance	Poisoning, Accidental unintentional	Poisoning, Intentional self-harm	Poisoning, Assault	Poisoning, Undetermined	Adverse effect	Underdosing
Cymarin	T46.0X1	T46.0X2	T46.0X3	T46.0X4	T46.0X5	T46.0X6
Cypermethrin	T60.1X1	T60.1X2	T60.1X3	T60.1X4	–	–
Cyphenothrin	T60.2X1	T60.2X2	T60.2X3	T60.2X4	–	–
Cyproheptadine	T45.0X1	T45.0X2	T45.0X3	T45.0X4	T45.0X5	T45.0X6
Cyproterone	T38.6X1	T38.6X2	T38.6X3	T38.6X4	T38.6X5	T38.6X6
Cysteamine	T50.6X1	T50.6X2	T50.6X3	T50.6X4	T50.6X5	T50.6X6
Cytarabine	T45.1X1	T45.1X2	T45.1X3	T45.1X4	T45.1X5	T45.1X6
Cytisus						
laburnum	T62.2X1	T62.2X2	T62.2X3	T62.2X4	–	–
scoparius	T62.2X1	T62.2X2	T62.2X3	T62.2X4	–	–
Cytochrome C	T47.5X1	T47.5X2	T47.5X3	T47.5X4	T47.5X5	T47.5X6
Cytomel	T38.1X1	T38.1X2	T38.1X3	T38.1X4	T38.1X5	T38.1X6
Cytosine arabinoside	T45.1X1	T45.1X2	T45.1X3	T45.1X4	T45.1X5	T45.1X6
Cytoxan	T45.1X1	T45.1X2	T45.1X3	T45.1X4	T45.1X5	T45.1X6
Cytozyme	T45.7X1	T45.7X2	T45.7X3	T45.7X4	T45.7X5	T45.7X6
2,4-D	T60.3X1	T60.3X2	T60.3X3	T60.3X4	–	–
D						
Dacarbazine	T45.1X1	T45.1X2	T45.1X3	T45.1X4	T45.1X5	T45.1X6
Dactinomycin	T45.1X1	T45.1X2	T45.1X3	T45.1X4	T45.1X5	T45.1X6
DADPS	T37.1X1	T37.1X2	T37.1X3	T37.1X4	T37.1X5	T37.1X6
Dakin's solution	T49.0X1	T49.0X2	T49.0X3	T49.0X4	T49.0X5	T49.0X6
Dalapon (sodium)	T60.3X1	T60.3X2	T60.3X3	T60.3X4	–	–
Dalmane	T42.4X1	T42.4X2	T42.4X3	T42.4X4	T42.4X5	T42.4X6
Danazol	T38.6X1	T38.6X2	T38.6X3	T38.6X4	T38.6X5	T38.6X6
Danilone	T45.511	T45.512	T45.513	T45.514	T45.515	T45.516
Danthron	T47.2X1	T47.2X2	T47.2X3	T47.2X4	T47.2X5	T47.2X6
Dantrolene	T42.8X1	T42.8X2	T42.8X3	T42.8X4	T42.8X5	T42.8X6
Dantron	T47.2X1	T47.2X2	T47.2X3	T47.2X4	T47.2X5	T47.2X6
Daphne (gnidium) (mezereum)	T62.2X1	T62.2X2	T62.2X3	T62.2X4	–	–
berry	T62.1X1	T62.1X2	T62.1X3	T62.1X4	–	–
Dapsone	T37.1X1	T37.1X2	T37.1X3	T37.1X4	T37.1X5	T37.1X6
Daraprim	T37.2X1	T37.2X2	T37.2X3	T37.2X4	T37.2X5	T37.2X6
Darnel	T62.2X1	T62.2X2	T62.2X3	T62.2X4	–	–
Darvon	T39.8X1	T39.8X2	T39.8X3	T39.8X4	T39.8X5	T39.8X6
Daunomycin	T45.1X1	T45.1X2	T45.1X3	T45.1X4	T45.1X5	T45.1X6
Daunorubicin	T45.1X1	T45.1X2	T45.1X3	T45.1X4	T45.1X5	T45.1X6
DBI	T38.3X1	T38.3X2	T38.3X3	T38.3X4	T38.3X5	T38.3X6
D-Con	T60.91	T60.92	T60.93	T60.94	–	–
insecticide	T60.2X1	T60.2X2	T60.2X3	T60.2X4	–	–
rodenticide	T60.4X1	T60.4X2	T60.4X3	T60.4X4	–	–
DDAVP	T38.891	T38.892	T38.893	T38.894	T38.895	T38.896
DDE (bis (chlorophenyl)-dichloroethylene)	T60.2X1	T60.2X2	T60.2X3	T60.2X4	–	–
DDS	T37.1X1	T37.1X2	T37.1X3	T37.1X4	T37.1X5	T37.1X6
DDT (dust)	T60.1X1	T60.1X2	T60.1X3	T60.1X4	–	–
Deadly nightshade — *see also Belladonna*	T62.2X1	T62.2X2	T62.2X3	T62.2X4	–	–
berry	T62.1X1	T62.1X2	T62.1X3	T62.1X4	–	–
Deamino-D-arginine vasopressin	T38.891	T38.892	T38.893	T38.894	T38.895	T38.896
Deanol (aceglumate)	T50.991	T50.992	T50.993	T50.994	T50.995	T50.996
Debrisoquine	T46.5X1	T46.5X2	T46.5X3	T46.5X4	T46.5X5	T46.5X6
Decaborane	T57.8X1	T57.8X2	T57.8X3	T57.8X4	–	–
fumes	T59.891	T59.892	T59.893	T59.894	–	–
Decadron	T38.0X1	T38.0X2	T38.0X3	T38.0X4	T38.0X5	T38.0X6
ENT agent	T49.6X1	T49.6X2	T49.6X3	T49.6X4	T49.6X5	T49.6X6
ophthalmic preparation	T49.5X1	T49.5X2	T49.5X3	T49.5X4	T49.5X5	T49.5X6
topical NEC	T49.0X1	T49.0X2	T49.0X3	T49.0X4	T49.0X5	T49.0X6
Decahydronaphthalene	T52.8X1	T52.8X2	T52.8X3	T52.8X4	–	–
Decalin	T52.8X1	T52.8X2	T52.8X3	T52.8X4	–	–
Decamethonium (bromide)	T48.1X1	T48.1X2	T48.1X3	T48.1X4	T48.1X5	T48.1X6
Decholin	T47.5X1	T47.5X2	T47.5X3	T47.5X4	T47.5X5	T47.5X6
Declomycin	T36.4X1	T36.4X2	T36.4X3	T36.4X4	T36.4X5	T36.4X6
Decongestant, nasal (mucosa)	T48.5X1	T48.5X2	T48.5X3	T48.5X4	T48.5X5	T48.5X6
combination	T48.5X1	T48.5X2	T48.5X3	T48.5X4	T48.5X5	T48.5X6
Deet	T60.8X1	T60.8X2	T60.8X3	T60.8X4	–	–
Deferoxamine	T45.8X1	T45.8X2	T45.8X3	T45.8X4	T45.8X5	T45.8X6
Deflazacort	T38.0X1	T38.0X2	T38.0X3	T38.0X4	T38.0X5	T38.0X6
Deglycyrrhizinized extract of licorice	T48.4X1	T48.4X2	T48.4X3	T48.4X4	T48.4X5	T48.4X6
Dehydrocholic acid	T47.5X1	T47.5X2	T47.5X3	T47.5X4	T47.5X5	T47.5X6
Dehydroemetine	T37.3X1	T37.3X2	T37.3X3	T37.3X4	T37.3X5	T37.3X6
Dekalin	T52.8X1	T52.8X2	T52.8X3	T52.8X4	–	–
Delalutin	T38.5X1	T38.5X2	T38.5X3	T38.5X4	T38.5X5	T38.5X6
Delorazepam	T42.4X1	T42.4X2	T42.4X3	T42.4X4	T42.4X5	T42.4X6
Delphinium	T62.2X1	T62.2X2	T62.2X3	T62.2X4	–	–
Deltamethrin	T60.1X1	T60.1X2	T60.1X3	T60.1X4	–	–
Deltasone	T38.0X1	T38.0X2	T38.0X3	T38.0X4	T38.0X5	T38.0X6
Deltra	T38.0X1	T38.0X2	T38.0X3	T38.0X4	T38.0X5	T38.0X6
Delvinal	T42.3X1	T42.3X2	T42.3X3	T42.3X4	T42.3X5	T42.3X6
Demecarium (bromide)	T49.5X1	T49.5X2	T49.5X3	T49.5X4	T49.5X5	T49.5X6
Demeclocycline	T36.4X1	T36.4X2	T36.4X3	T36.4X4	T36.4X5	T36.4X6
Demecolcine	T45.1X1	T45.1X2	T45.1X3	T45.1X4	T45.1X5	T45.1X6

Substance	Poisoning, Accidental unintentional	Poisoning, Intentional self-harm	Poisoning, Assault	Poisoning, Undetermined	Adverse effect	Underdosing
Demegestone	T38.5X1	T38.5X2	T38.5X3	T38.5X4	T38.5X5	T38.5X6
Demelanizing agents	T49.8X1	T49.8X2	T49.8X3	T49.8X4	T49.8X5	T49.8X6
Demephion -O and -S	T60.0X1	T60.0X2	T60.0X3	T60.0X4	--	--
Demerol	T40.2X1	T40.2X2	T40.2X3	T40.2X4	T40.2X5	T40.2X6
Demethylchlortetracycline	T36.4X1	T36.4X2	T36.4X3	T36.4X4	T36.4X5	T36.4X6
Demethyltetracycline	T36.4X1	T36.4X2	T36.4X3	T36.4X4	T36.4X5	T36.4X6
Demeton -O and -S	T60.0X1	T60.0X2	T60.0X3	T60.0X4	--	--
Demulcent (external)	T49.3X1	T49.3X2	T49.3X3	T49.3X4	T49.3X5	T49.3X6
specified NEC	T49.3X1	T49.3X2	T49.3X3	T49.3X4	T49.3X5	T49.3X6
Demulen	T38.4X1	T38.4X2	T38.4X3	T38.4X4	T38.4X5	T38.4X6
Denatured alcohol	T51.0X1	T51.0X2	T51.0X3	T51.0X4	--	--
Dendrid	T49.5X1	T49.5X2	T49.5X3	T49.5X4	T49.5X5	T49.5X6
Dental drug, topical application NEC	T49.7X1	T49.7X2	T49.7X3	T49.7X4	T49.7X5	T49.7X6
Dentifrice	T49.7X1	T49.7X2	T49.7X3	T49.7X4	T49.7X5	T49.7X6
Deodorant spray (feminine hygiene)	T49.8X1	T49.8X2	T49.8X3	T49.8X4	T49.8X5	T49.8X6
Deoxycortone	T50.0X1	T50.0X2	T50.0X3	T50.0X4	T50.0X5	T50.0X6
2-Deoxy-5-fluorouridine	T45.1X1	T45.1X2	T45.1X3	T45.1X4	T45.1X5	T45.1X6
5-Deoxy-5-fluorouridine	T45.1X1	T45.1X2	T45.1X3	T45.1X4	T45.1X5	T45.1X6
Deoxyribonuclease (pancreatic)	T45.3X1	T45.3X2	T45.3X3	T45.3X4	T45.3X5	T45.3X6
Depilatory	T49.4X1	T49.4X2	T49.4X3	T49.4X4	T49.4X5	T49.4X6
Deprenalin	T42.8X1	T42.8X2	T42.8X3	T42.8X4	T42.8X5	T42.8X6
Deprenyl	T42.8X1	T42.8X2	T42.8X3	T42.8X4	T42.8X5	T42.8X6
Depressant, appetite	T50.5X1	T50.5X2	T50.5X3	T50.5X4	T50.5X5	T50.5X6
Depressant						
appetite (central)	T50.5X1	T50.5X2	T50.5X3	T50.5X4	T50.5X5	T50.5X6
cardiac	T46.2X1	T46.2X2	T46.2X3	T46.2X4	T46.2X5	T46.2X6
central nervous system (anesthetic) — *see also Central nervous system, depressants*	T42.71	T42.72	T42.73	T42.74	T42.75	T42.76
general anesthetic	T41.201	T41.202	T41.203	T41.204	T41.205	T41.206
muscle tone	T42.8X1	T42.8X2	T42.8X3	T42.8X4	T42.8X5	T42.8X6
muscle tone, central	T42.8X1	T42.8X2	T42.8X3	T42.8X4	T42.8X5	T42.8X6
psychotherapeutic	T43.501	T43.502	T43.503	T43.504	T43.505	T43.506
Deptropine	T45.0X1	T45.0X2	T45.0X3	T45.0X4	T45.0X5	T45.0X6
Dequalinium (chloride)	T49.0X1	T49.0X2	T49.0X3	T49.0X4	T49.0X5	T49.0X6
Derris root	T60.2X1	T60.2X2	T60.2X3	T60.2X4	--	--
Deserpidine	T46.5X1	T46.5X2	T46.5X3	T46.5X4	T46.5X5	T46.5X6
Desferrioxamine	T45.8X1	T45.8X2	T45.8X3	T45.8X4	T45.8X5	T45.8X6
Desipramine	T43.011	T43.012	T43.013	T43.014	T43.015	T43.016
Deslanoside	T46.0X1	T46.0X2	T46.0X3	T46.0X4	T46.0X5	T46.0X6
Desloughing agent	T49.4X1	T49.4X2	T49.4X3	T49.4X4	T49.4X5	T49.4X6
Desmethylimipramine	T43.011	T43.012	T43.013	T43.014	T43.015	T43.016
Desmopressin	T38.891	T38.892	T38.893	T38.894	T38.895	T38.896
Desocodeine	T40.2X1	T40.2X2	T40.2X3	T40.2X4	T40.2X5	T40.2X6
Desogestrel	T38.5X1	T38.5X2	T38.5X3	T38.5X4	T38.5X5	T38.5X6
Desomorphine	T40.2X1	T40.2X2	T40.2X3	T40.2X4	--	--
Desonide	T49.0X1	T49.0X2	T49.0X3	T49.0X4	T49.0X5	T49.0X6
Desoximetasone	T49.0X1	T49.0X2	T49.0X3	T49.0X4	T49.0X5	T49.0X6
Desoxycorticosteroid	T50.0X1	T50.0X2	T50.0X3	T50.0X4	T50.0X5	T50.0X6
Desoxycortone	T50.0X1	T50.0X2	T50.0X3	T50.0X4	T50.0X5	T50.0X6
Desoxyephedrine	T43.621	T43.622	T43.623	T43.624	T43.625	T43.626
Detaxtran	T46.6X1	T46.6X2	T46.6X3	T46.6X4	T46.6X5	T46.6X6
Detergent	T49.2X1	T49.2X2	T49.2X3	T49.2X4	T49.2X5	T49.2X6
external medication	T49.2X1	T49.2X2	T49.2X3	T49.2X4	T49.2X5	T49.2X6
local	T49.2X1	T49.2X2	T49.2X3	T49.2X4	T49.2X5	T49.2X6
medicinal	T49.2X1	T49.2X2	T49.2X3	T49.2X4	T49.2X5	T49.2X6
nonmedicinal	T55.1X1	T55.1X2	T55.1X3	T55.1X4	--	--
specified NEC	T55.1X1	T55.1X2	T55.1X3	T55.1X4	--	--
Deterrent, alcohol	T50.6X1	T50.6X2	T50.6X3	T50.6X4	T50.6X5	T50.6X6
Detoxifying agent	T50.6X1	T50.6X2	T50.6X3	T50.6X4	T50.6X5	T50.6X6
Detrothyronine	T38.1X1	T38.1X2	T38.1X3	T38.1X4	T38.1X5	T38.1X6
Dettol (external medication)	T49.0X1	T49.0X2	T49.0X3	T49.0X4	T49.0X5	T49.0X6
Dexamethasone	T38.0X1	T38.0X2	T38.0X3	T38.0X4	T38.0X5	T38.0X6
ENT agent	T49.6X1	T49.6X2	T49.6X3	T49.6X4	T49.6X5	T49.6X6
ophthalmic preparation	T49.5X1	T49.5X2	T49.5X3	T49.5X4	T49.5X5	T49.5X6
topical NEC	T49.0X1	T49.0X2	T49.0X3	T49.0X4	T49.0X5	T49.0X6
Dexamfetamine	T43.621	T43.622	T43.623	T43.624	T43.625	T43.626
Dexamphetamine	T43.621	T43.622	T43.623	T43.624	T43.625	T43.626
Dexbrompheniramine	T45.0X1	T45.0X2	T45.0X3	T45.0X4	T45.0X5	T45.0X6
Dexchlorpheniramine	T45.0X1	T45.0X2	T45.0X3	T45.0X4	T45.0X5	T45.0X6
Dexedrine	T43.621	T43.622	T43.623	T43.624	T43.625	T43.626
Dexetimide	T44.3X1	T44.3X2	T44.3X3	T44.3X4	T44.3X5	T44.3X6
Dexfenfluramine	T50.5X1	T50.5X2	T50.5X3	T50.5X4	T50.5X5	T50.5X6
Dexpanthenol	T45.2X1	T45.2X2	T45.2X3	T45.2X4	T45.2X5	T45.2X6
Dextran (40) (70) (150)	T45.8X1	T45.8X2	T45.8X3	T45.8X4	T45.8X5	T45.8X6
Dextriferron	T45.4X1	T45.4X2	T45.4X3	T45.4X4	T45.4X5	T45.4X6
Dextro calcium pantothenate	T45.2X1	T45.2X2	T45.2X3	T45.2X4	T45.2X5	T45.2X6
Dextro pantothenyl alcohol	T45.2X1	T45.2X2	T45.2X3	T45.2X4	T45.2X5	T45.2X6
Dextroamphetamine	T43.621	T43.622	T43.623	T43.624	T43.625	T43.626
Dextromethorphan	T48.3X1	T48.3X2	T48.3X3	T48.3X4	T48.3X5	T48.3X6
Dextromoramide	T40.4X1	T40.4X2	T40.4X3	T40.4X4	--	--
topical	T49.8X1	T49.8X2	T49.8X3	T49.8X4	T49.8X5	T49.8X6
Dextropropoxyphene	T40.4X1	T40.4X2	T40.4X3	T40.4X4	T40.4X5	T40.4X6
Dextrorphan	T40.2X1	T40.2X2	T40.2X3	T40.2X4	T40.2X5	T40.2X6
Dextrose	T50.3X1	T50.3X2	T50.3X3	T50.3X4	T50.3X5	T50.3X6
concentrated solution, intravenous	T46.8X1	T46.8X2	T46.8X3	T46.8X4	T46.8X5	T46.8X6
Dextrothyroxin	T38.1X1	T38.1X2	T38.1X3	T38.1X4	T38.1X5	T38.1X6
Dextrothyroxine sodium	T38.1X1	T38.1X2	T38.1X3	T38.1X4	T38.1X5	T38.1X6
DFP	T44.0X1	T44.0X2	T44.0X3	T44.0X4	T44.0X5	T44.0X6
DHE	T37.3X1	T37.3X2	T37.3X3	T37.3X4	T37.3X5	T37.3X6
45	T46.5X1	T46.5X2	T46.5X3	T46.5X4	T46.5X5	T46.5X6
Diabinese	T38.3X1	T38.3X2	T38.3X3	T38.3X4	T38.3X5	T38.3X6
Diacetone alcohol	T52.4X1	T52.4X2	T52.4X3	T52.4X4	--	--
Diacetyl monoxime	T50.991	T50.992	T50.993	T50.994	--	--
Diacetylmorphine	T40.1X1	T40.1X2	T40.1X3	T40.1X4	--	--
Diachylon plaster	T49.4X1	T49.4X2	T49.4X3	T49.4X4	T49.4X5	T49.4X6
Diaethylstilboestrolum	T38.5X1	T38.5X2	T38.5X3	T38.5X4	T38.5X5	T38.5X6
Diagnostic agent NEC	T50.8X1	T50.8X2	T50.8X3	T50.8X4	T50.8X5	T50.8X6
Dial (soap)	T49.2X1	T49.2X2	T49.2X3	T49.2X4	T49.2X5	T49.2X6
sedative	T42.3X1	T42.3X2	T42.3X3	T42.3X4	T42.3X5	T42.3X6
Dialkyl carbonate	T52.91	T52.92	T52.93	T52.94	--	--
Diallylbarbituric acid	T42.3X1	T42.3X2	T42.3X3	T42.3X4	T42.3X5	T42.3X6
Diallymal	T42.3X1	T42.3X2	T42.3X3	T42.3X4	T42.3X5	T42.3X6
Dialysis solution (intraperitoneal)	T50.3X1	T50.3X2	T50.3X3	T50.3X4	T50.3X5	T50.3X6
Diaminodiphenylsulfone	T37.1X1	T37.1X2	T37.1X3	T37.1X4	T37.1X5	T37.1X6
Diamorphine	T40.1X1	T40.1X2	T40.1X3	T40.1X4	--	--
Diamox	T50.2X1	T50.2X2	T50.2X3	T50.2X4	T50.2X5	T50.2X6
Diamthazole	T49.0X1	T49.0X2	T49.0X3	T49.0X4	T49.0X5	T49.0X6
Dianthone	T47.2X1	T47.2X2	T47.2X3	T47.2X4	T47.2X5	T47.2X6
Diaphenylsulfone	T37.0X1	T37.0X2	T37.0X3	T37.0X4	T37.0X5	T37.0X6
Diasone (sodium)	T37.1X1	T37.1X2	T37.1X3	T37.1X4	T37.1X5	T37.1X6
Diastase	T47.5X1	T47.5X2	T47.5X3	T47.5X4	T47.5X5	T47.5X6
Diatrizoate	T50.8X1	T50.8X2	T50.8X3	T50.8X4	T50.8X5	T50.8X6
Diazepam	T42.4X1	T42.4X2	T42.4X3	T42.4X4	T42.4X5	T42.4X6
Diazinon	T60.0X1	T60.0X2	T60.0X3	T60.0X4	--	--
Diazomethane (gas)	T59.891	T59.892	T59.893	T59.894	--	--
Diazoxide	T46.5X1	T46.5X2	T46.5X3	T46.5X4	T46.5X5	T46.5X6
Dibekacin	T36.5X1	T36.5X2	T36.5X3	T36.5X4	T36.5X5	T36.5X6
Dibenamine	T44.6X1	T44.6X2	T44.6X3	T44.6X4	T44.6X5	T44.6X6
Dibenzepin	T43.011	T43.012	T43.013	T43.014	T43.015	T43.016
Dibenzheptropine	T45.0X1	T45.0X2	T45.0X3	T45.0X4	T45.0X5	T45.0X6
Dibenzyline	T44.6X1	T44.6X2	T44.6X3	T44.6X4	T44.6X5	T44.6X6
Diborane (gas)	T59.891	T59.892	T59.893	T59.894	--	--
Dibromochloropropane	T60.8X1	T60.8X2	T60.8X3	T60.8X4	--	--
Dibromodulcitol	T45.1X1	T45.1X2	T45.1X3	T45.1X4	T45.1X5	T45.1X6
Dibromoethane	T53.6X1	T53.6X2	T53.6X3	T53.6X4	--	--
Dibromomannitol	T45.1X1	T45.1X2	T45.1X3	T45.1X4	T45.1X5	T45.1X6
Dibromopropamidine isethionate	T49.0X1	T49.0X2	T49.0X3	T49.0X4	T49.0X5	T49.0X6
Dibrompropamidine	T49.0X1	T49.0X2	T49.0X3	T49.0X4	T49.0X5	T49.0X6
Dibucaine	T41.3X1	T41.3X2	T41.3X3	T41.3X4	T41.3X5	T41.3X6
topical (surface)	T41.3X1	T41.3X2	T41.3X3	T41.3X4	T41.3X5	T41.3X6
Dibunate sodium	T48.3X1	T48.3X2	T48.3X3	T48.3X4	T48.3X5	T48.3X6
Dibutoline sulfate	T44.3X1	T44.3X2	T44.3X3	T44.3X4	T44.3X5	T44.3X6
Dicamba	T60.3X1	T60.3X2	T60.3X3	T60.3X4	--	--
Dicapthon	T60.0X1	T60.0X2	T60.0X3	T60.0X4	--	--
Dichlobenil	T60.3X1	T60.3X2	T60.3X3	T60.3X4	--	--
Dichlone	T60.3X1	T60.3X2	T60.3X3	T60.3X4	--	--
Dichloralphenozone	T42.6X1	T42.6X2	T42.6X3	T42.6X4	T42.6X5	T42.6X6
Dichlorbenzidine	T65.3X1	T65.3X2	T65.3X3	T65.3X4	--	--
Dichlorhydrin	T52.8X1	T52.8X2	T52.8X3	T52.8X4	--	--
Dichlorhydroxyquinoline	T37.8X1	T37.8X2	T37.8X3	T37.8X4	T37.8X5	T37.8X6
Dichlorobenzene	T53.7X1	T53.7X2	T53.7X3	T53.7X4	--	--
Dichlorobenzyl alcohol	T49.6X1	T49.6X2	T49.6X3	T49.6X4	T49.6X5	T49.6X6
Dichlorodifluoromethane	T53.5X1	T53.5X2	T53.5X3	T53.5X4	--	--
Dichloroethane	T52.8X1	T52.8X2	T52.8X3	T52.8X4	--	--
Sym-Dichloroethyl ether	T53.6X1	T53.6X2	T53.6X3	T53.6X4	--	--
Dichloroethyl sulfide, not in war	T59.891	T59.892	T59.893	T59.894	--	--
Dichloroethylene	T53.6X1	T53.6X2	T53.6X3	T53.6X4	--	--
Dichloroformoxine, not in war	T59.891	T59.892	T59.893	T59.894	--	--
Dichlorohydrin, alpha-dichlorohydrin	T52.8X1	T52.8X2	T52.8X3	T52.8X4	--	--
Dichloromethane (solvent)	T53.4X1	T53.4X2	T53.4X3	T53.4X4	--	--
vapor	T53.4X1	T53.4X2	T53.4X3	T53.4X4	--	--
Dichloronaphthoquinone	T60.3X1	T60.3X2	T60.3X3	T60.3X4	--	--
Dichlorophen	T37.4X1	T37.4X2	T37.4X3	T37.4X4	T37.4X5	T37.4X6
2,4-Dichlorophenoxyacetic acid	T60.3X1	T60.3X2	T60.3X3	T60.3X4	--	--
Dichloropropene	T60.3X1	T60.3X2	T60.3X3	T60.3X4	--	--
Dichloropropionic acid	T60.3X1	T60.3X2	T60.3X3	T60.3X4	--	--

Demegestone - Dichloropropionic acid

ICD-10-CM TABLE OF DRUGS AND CHEMICALS

Substance	Poisoning, Accidental unintentional	Poisoning, Intentional self-harm	Poisoning, Assault	Poisoning, Undetermined	Adverse effect	Underdosing
Dichlorphenamide	T50.2X1	T50.2X2	T50.2X3	T50.2X4	T50.2X5	T50.2X6
Dichlorvos	T60.0X1	T60.0X2	T60.0X3	T60.0X4	--	--
Diclofenac	T39.391	T39.392	T39.393	T39.394	T39.395	T39.396
Diclofenamide	T50.2X1	T50.2X2	T50.2X3	T50.2X4	T50.2X5	T50.2X6
Diclofensine	T43.291	T43.292	T43.293	T43.294	T43.295	T43.296
Diclonixine	T39.8X1	T39.8X2	T39.8X3	T39.8X4	T39.8X5	T39.8X6
Dicloxacillin	T36.0X1	T36.0X2	T36.0X3	T36.0X4	T36.0X5	T36.0X6
Dicophane	T49.0X1	T49.0X2	T49.0X3	T49.0X4	T49.0X5	T49.0X6
Dicoumarol, dicoumarin, dicumarol	T45.511	T45.512	T45.513	T45.514	T45.515	T45.516
Dicrotophos	T60.0X1	T60.0X2	T60.0X3	T60.0X4	--	--
Dicyanogen (gas)	T65.0X1	T65.0X2	T65.0X3	T65.0X4	--	--
Dicyclomine	T44.3X1	T44.3X2	T44.3X3	T44.3X4	T44.3X5	T44.3X6
Dicycloverine	T44.3X1	T44.3X2	T44.3X3	T44.3X4	T44.3X5	T44.3X6
Dideoxycytidine	T37.5X1	T37.5X2	T37.5X3	T37.5X4	T37.5X5	T37.5X6
Dideoxyinosine	T37.5X1	T37.5X2	T37.5X3	T37.5X4	T37.5X5	T37.5X6
Dieldrin (vapor)	T60.1X1	T60.1X2	T60.1X3	T60.1X4	--	--
Diemal	T42.3X1	T42.3X2	T42.3X3	T42.3X4	T42.3X5	T42.3X6
Dienestrol	T38.5X1	T38.5X2	T38.5X3	T38.5X4	T38.5X5	T38.5X6
Dienoestrol	T38.5X1	T38.5X2	T38.5X3	T38.5X4	T38.5X5	T38.5X6
Dietetic drug NEC	T50.901	T50.902	T50.903	T50.904	T50.905	T50.906
Diethazine	T42.8X1	T42.8X2	T42.8X3	T42.8X4	T42.8X5	T42.8X6
Diethyl						
barbituric acid	T42.3X1	T42.3X2	T42.3X3	T42.3X4	T42.3X5	T42.3X6
carbamazine	T37.4X1	T37.4X2	T37.4X3	T37.4X4	T37.4X5	T37.4X6
carbinol	T51.3X1	T51.3X2	T51.3X3	T51.3X4	--	--
carbonate	T52.8X1	T52.8X2	T52.8X3	T52.8X4	--	--
ether (vapor) — *see also ether*	T41.0X1	T41.0X2	T41.0X3	T41.0X4	T41.0X5	T41.0X6
oxide	T52.8X1	T52.8X2	T52.8X3	T52.8X4	--	--
propion	T50.5X1	T50.5X2	T50.5X3	T50.5X4	T50.5X5	T50.5X6
stilbestrol	T38.5X1	T38.5X2	T38.5X3	T38.5X4	T38.5X5	T38.5X6
toluamide (nonmedicinal)	T60.8X1	T60.8X2	T60.8X3	T60.8X4	--	--
medicinal	T49.3X1	T49.3X2	T49.3X3	T49.3X4	T49.3X5	T49.3X6
Diethylcarbamazine	T37.4X1	T37.4X2	T37.4X3	T37.4X4	T37.4X5	T37.4X6
Diethylene						
dioxide	T52.8X1	T52.8X2	T52.8X3	T52.8X4	--	--
glycol (monoacetate) (monobutyl ether) (monoethyl ether)	T52.3X1	T52.3X2	T52.3X3	T52.3X4	--	--
Diethylhexylphthalate	T65.891	T65.892	T65.893	T65.894	--	--
Diethylpropion	T50.5X1	T50.5X2	T50.5X3	T50.5X4	T50.5X5	T50.5X6
Diethylstilbestrol	T38.5X1	T38.5X2	T38.5X3	T38.5X4	T38.5X5	T38.5X6
Diethylstilboestrol	T38.5X1	T38.5X2	T38.5X3	T38.5X4	T38.5X5	T38.5X6
Diethylsulfone-diethylmethane	T42.6X1	T42.6X2	T42.6X3	T42.6X4	T42.6X5	T42.6X6
Diethyltoluamide	T49.0X1	T49.0X2	T49.0X3	T49.0X4	T49.0X5	T49.0X6
Diethyltryptamine (DET)	T40.991	T40.992	T40.993	T40.994	--	--
Difebarbamate	T42.3X1	T42.3X2	T42.3X3	T42.3X4	T42.3X5	T42.3X6
Difencloxazine	T40.2X1	T40.2X2	T40.2X3	T40.2X4	T40.2X5	T40.2X6
Difenidol	T45.0X1	T45.0X2	T45.0X3	T45.0X4	T45.0X5	T45.0X6
Difenoxin	T47.6X1	T47.6X2	T47.6X3	T47.6X4	T47.6X5	T47.6X6
Difetarsone	T37.3X1	T37.3X2	T37.3X3	T37.3X4	T37.3X5	T37.3X6
Diffusin	T45.3X1	T45.3X2	T45.3X3	T45.3X4	T45.3X5	T45.3X6
Diflorasone	T49.0X1	T49.0X2	T49.0X3	T49.0X4	T49.0X5	T49.0X6
Diflos	T44.0X1	T44.0X2	T44.0X3	T44.0X4	T44.0X5	T44.0X6
Diflubenzuron	T60.1X1	T60.1X2	T60.1X3	T60.1X4	--	--
Diflucortolone	T49.0X1	T49.0X2	T49.0X3	T49.0X4	T49.0X5	T49.0X6
Diflunisal	T39.091	T39.092	T39.093	T39.094	T39.095	T39.096
Difluoromethyldopa	T42.8X1	T42.8X2	T42.8X3	T42.8X4	T42.8X5	T42.8X6
Difluorophate	T44.0X1	T44.0X2	T44.0X3	T44.0X4	T44.0X5	T44.0X6
Digestant NEC	T47.5X1	T47.5X2	T47.5X3	T47.5X4	T47.5X5	T47.5X6
Digitalin (e)	T46.0X1	T46.0X2	T46.0X3	T46.0X4	T46.0X5	T46.0X6
Digitalis (leaf) (glycoside)	T46.0X1	T46.0X2	T46.0X3	T46.0X4	T46.0X5	T46.0X6
lanata	T46.0X1	T46.0X2	T46.0X3	T46.0X4	T46.0X5	T46.0X6
purpurea	T46.0X1	T46.0X2	T46.0X3	T46.0X4	T46.0X5	T46.0X6
Digitoxin	T46.0X1	T46.0X2	T46.0X3	T46.0X4	T46.0X5	T46.0X6
Digitoxose	T46.0X1	T46.0X2	T46.0X3	T46.0X4	T46.0X5	T46.0X6
Digoxin	T46.0X1	T46.0X2	T46.0X3	T46.0X4	T46.0X5	T46.0X6
Digoxine	T46.0X1	T46.0X2	T46.0X3	T46.0X4	T46.0X5	T46.0X6
Dihydralazine	T46.5X1	T46.5X2	T46.5X3	T46.5X4	T46.5X5	T46.5X6
Dihydrazine	T46.5X1	T46.5X2	T46.5X3	T46.5X4	T46.5X5	T46.5X6
Dihydrocodeine	T40.2X1	T40.2X2	T40.2X3	T40.2X4	T40.2X5	T40.2X6
Dihydrocodeinone	T40.2X1	T40.2X2	T40.2X3	T40.2X4	T40.2X5	T40.2X6
Dihydroergocornine	T46.7X1	T46.7X2	T46.7X3	T46.7X4	T46.7X5	T46.7X6
Dihydroergocristine (mesilate)	T46.7X1	T46.7X2	T46.7X3	T46.7X4	T46.7X5	T46.7X6
Dihydroergokryptine	T46.7X1	T46.7X2	T46.7X3	T46.7X4	T46.7X5	T46.7X6
Dihydroergotamine	T46.5X1	T46.5X2	T46.5X3	T46.5X4	T46.5X5	T46.5X6
Dihydroergotoxine	T46.7X1	T46.7X2	T46.7X3	T46.7X4	T46.7X5	T46.7X6
mesilate	T46.7X1	T46.7X2	T46.7X3	T46.7X4	T46.7X5	T46.7X6
Dihydrohydroxycodeinone	T40.2X1	T40.2X2	T40.2X3	T40.2X4	T40.2X5	T40.2X6
Dihydrohydroxymorphinone	T40.2X1	T40.2X2	T40.2X3	T40.2X4	T40.2X5	T40.2X6
Dihydroisocodeine	T40.2X1	T40.2X2	T40.2X3	T40.2X4	T40.2X5	T40.2X6
Dihydromorphine	T40.2X1	T40.2X2	T40.2X3	T40.2X4	--	--
Dihydromorphinone	T40.2X1	T40.2X2	T40.2X3	T40.2X4	T40.2X5	T40.2X6
Dihydrostreptomycin	T36.5X1	T36.5X2	T36.5X3	T36.5X4	T36.5X5	T36.5X6
Dihydrotachysterol	T45.2X1	T45.2X2	T45.2X3	T45.2X4	T45.2X5	T45.2X6
Dihydroxyaluminum aminoacetate	T47.1X1	T47.1X2	T47.1X3	T47.1X4	T47.1X5	T47.1X6
Dihydroxyaluminum sodium carbonate	T47.1X1	T47.1X2	T47.1X3	T47.1X4	T47.1X5	T47.1X6
Dihydroxyanthraquinone	T47.2X1	T47.2X2	T47.2X3	T47.2X4	T47.2X5	T47.2X6
Dihydroxycodeinone	T40.2X1	T40.2X2	T40.2X3	T40.2X4	T40.2X5	T40.2X6
Dihydroxypropyl theophylline	T50.2X1	T50.2X2	T50.2X3	T50.2X4	T50.2X5	T50.2X6
Diiodohydroxyquin	T37.8X1	T37.8X2	T37.8X3	T37.8X4	T37.8X5	T37.8X6
topical	T49.0X1	T49.0X2	T49.0X3	T49.0X4	T49.0X5	T49.0X6
Diiodohydroxyquinoline	T37.8X1	T37.8X2	T37.8X3	T37.8X4	T37.8X5	T37.8X6
Diiodotyrosine	T38.2X1	T38.2X2	T38.2X3	T38.2X4	T38.2X5	T38.2X6
Diisopromine	T44.3X1	T44.3X2	T44.3X3	T44.3X4	T44.3X5	T44.3X6
Diisopropylamine	T46.3X1	T46.3X2	T46.3X3	T46.3X4	T46.3X5	T46.3X6
Diisopropylfluorophos-phonate	T44.0X1	T44.0X2	T44.0X3	T44.0X4	T44.0X5	T44.0X6
Dilantin	T42.0X1	T42.0X2	T42.0X3	T42.0X4	T42.0X5	T42.0X6
Dilaudid	T40.2X1	T40.2X2	T40.2X3	T40.2X4	T40.2X5	T40.2X6
Dilazep	T46.3X1	T46.3X2	T46.3X3	T46.3X4	T46.3X5	T46.3X6
Dill	T47.5X1	T47.5X2	T47.5X3	T47.5X4	T47.5X5	T47.5X6
Diloxanide	T37.3X1	T37.3X2	T37.3X3	T37.3X4	T37.3X5	T37.3X6
Diltiazem	T46.1X1	T46.1X2	T46.1X3	T46.1X4	T46.1X5	T46.1X6
Dimazole	T49.0X1	T49.0X2	T49.0X3	T49.0X4	T49.0X5	T49.0X6
Dimefline	T50.7X1	T50.7X2	T50.7X3	T50.7X4	T50.7X5	T50.7X6
Dimefox	T60.0X1	T60.0X2	T60.0X3	T60.0X4	--	--
Dimemorfan	T48.3X1	T48.3X2	T48.3X3	T48.3X4	T48.3X5	T48.3X6
Dimenhydrinate	T45.0X1	T45.0X2	T45.0X3	T45.0X4	T45.0X5	T45.0X6
Dimercaprol (British anti-lewisite)	T45.8X1	T45.8X2	T45.8X3	T45.8X4	T45.8X5	T45.8X6
Dimercaptopropanol	T45.8X1	T45.8X2	T45.8X3	T45.8X4	T45.8X5	T45.8X6
Dimestrol	T38.5X1	T38.5X2	T38.5X3	T38.5X4	T38.5X5	T38.5X6
Dimetane	T45.0X1	T45.0X2	T45.0X3	T45.0X4	T45.0X5	T45.0X6
Dimethicone	T47.1X1	T47.1X2	T47.1X3	T47.1X4	T47.1X5	T47.1X6
Dimethindene	T45.0X1	T45.0X2	T45.0X3	T45.0X4	T45.0X5	T45.0X6
Dimethisoquin	T49.1X1	T49.1X2	T49.1X3	T49.1X4	T49.1X5	T49.1X6
Dimethisterone	T38.5X1	T38.5X2	T38.5X3	T38.5X4	T38.5X5	T38.5X6
Dimethoate	T60.0X1	T60.0X2	T60.0X3	T60.0X4	--	--
Dimethocaine	T41.3X1	T41.3X2	T41.3X3	T41.3X4	T41.3X5	T41.3X6
Dimethoxanate	T48.3X1	T48.3X2	T48.3X3	T48.3X4	T48.3X5	T48.3X6
Dimethyl						
arsine, arsinic acid	T57.0X1	T57.0X2	T57.0X3	T57.0X4	--	--
carbinol	T51.2X1	T51.2X2	T51.2X3	T51.2X4	--	--
carbonate	T52.8X1	T52.8X2	T52.8X3	T52.8X4	--	--
diguanide	T38.3X1	T38.3X2	T38.3X3	T38.3X4	T38.3X5	T38.3X6
ketone	T52.4X1	T52.4X2	T52.4X3	T52.4X4	--	--
vapor	T52.4X1	T52.4X2	T52.4X3	T52.4X4	--	--
meperidine	T40.2X1	T40.2X2	T40.2X3	T40.2X4	T40.2X5	T40.2X6
parathion	T60.0X1	T60.0X2	T60.0X3	T60.0X4	--	--
phthlate	T49.3X1	T49.3X2	T49.3X3	T49.3X4	T49.3X5	T49.3X6
polysiloxane	T47.8X1	T47.8X2	T47.8X3	T47.8X4	T47.8X5	T47.8X6
sulfate (fumes)	T59.891	T59.892	T59.893	T59.894	--	--
liquid	T65.891	T65.892	T65.893	T65.894	--	--
sulfoxide (nonmedicinal)	T52.8X1	T52.8X2	T52.8X3	T52.8X4	--	--
medicinal	T49.4X1	T49.4X2	T49.4X3	T49.4X4	T49.4X5	T49.4X6
tryptamine	T40.991	T40.992	T40.993	T40.994	--	--
tubocurarine	T48.1X1	T48.1X2	T48.1X3	T48.1X4	T48.1X5	T48.1X6
Dimethylamine sulfate	T49.4X1	T49.4X2	T49.4X3	T49.4X4	T49.4X5	T49.4X6
Dimethylformamide	T52.8X1	T52.8X2	T52.8X3	T52.8X4	--	--
Dimethyltubocurarinium chloride	T48.1X1	T48.1X2	T48.1X3	T48.1X4	T48.1X5	T48.1X6
Dimeticone	T47.1X1	T47.1X2	T47.1X3	T47.1X4	T47.1X5	T47.1X6
Dimetilan	T60.0X1	T60.0X2	T60.0X3	T60.0X4	--	--
Dimetindene	T45.0X1	T45.0X2	T45.0X3	T45.0X4	T45.0X5	T45.0X6
Dimetotiazine	T43.3X1	T43.3X2	T43.3X3	T43.3X4	T43.3X5	T43.3X6
Dimorpholamine	T50.7X1	T50.7X2	T50.7X3	T50.7X4	T50.7X5	T50.7X6
Dimoxyline	T46.3X1	T46.3X2	T46.3X3	T46.3X4	T46.3X5	T46.3X6
Dinitrobenzene	T65.3X1	T65.3X2	T65.3X3	T65.3X4	--	--
vapor	T59.891	T59.892	T59.893	T59.894	--	--
Dinitrobenzol	T65.3X1	T65.3X2	T65.3X3	T65.3X4	--	--
vapor	T59.891	T59.892	T59.893	T59.894	--	--
Dinitrobutylphenol	T65.3X1	T65.3X2	T65.3X3	T65.3X4	--	--
Dinitro (-ortho-)cresol (pesticide) (spray)	T65.3X1	T65.3X2	T65.3X3	T65.3X4	--	--
Dinitrocyclohexylphenol	T65.3X1	T65.3X2	T65.3X3	T65.3X4	--	--
Dinitrophenol	T65.3X1	T65.3X2	T65.3X3	T65.3X4	--	--
Dinoprost	T48.0X1	T48.0X2	T48.0X3	T48.0X4	T48.0X5	T48.0X6
Dinoprostone	T48.0X1	T48.0X2	T48.0X3	T48.0X4	T48.0X5	T48.0X6
Dinoseb	T60.3X1	T60.3X2	T60.3X3	T60.3X4	--	--

Substance	Poisoning, Accidental unintentional	Poisoning, Intentional self-harm	Poisoning, Assault	Poisoning, Undetermined	Adverse effect	Underdosing
Dioctyl sulfosuccinate (calcium) (sodium)	T47.4X1	T47.4X2	T47.4X3	T47.4X4	T47.4X5	T47.4X6
Diodone	T50.8X1	T50.8X2	T50.8X3	T50.8X4	T50.8X5	T50.8X6
Diodoquin	T37.8X1	T37.8X2	T37.8X3	T37.8X4	T37.8X5	T37.8X6
Dionin	T40.2X1	T40.2X2	T40.2X3	T40.2X4	T40.2X5	T40.2X6
Diosmin	T46.991	T46.992	T46.993	T46.994	T46.995	T46.996
Dioxane	T52.8X1	T52.8X2	T52.8X3	T52.8X4	--	--
Dioxathion	T60.0X1	T60.0X2	T60.0X3	T60.0X4	--	--
Dioxin	T53.7X1	T53.7X2	T53.7X3	T53.7X4	--	--
Dioxopromethazine	T43.3X1	T43.3X2	T43.3X3	T43.3X4	T43.3X5	T43.3X6
Dioxyline	T46.3X1	T46.3X2	T46.3X3	T46.3X4	T46.3X5	T46.3X6
Dipentene	T52.8X1	T52.8X2	T52.8X3	T52.8X4	--	--
Diperodon	T41.3X1	T41.3X2	T41.3X3	T41.3X4	T41.3X5	T41.3X6
Diphacinone	T60.4X1	T60.4X2	T60.4X3	T60.4X4	--	--
Diphemanil	T44.3X1	T44.3X2	T44.3X3	T44.3X4	T44.3X5	T44.3X6
metilsulfate	T44.3X1	T44.3X2	T44.3X3	T44.3X4	T44.3X5	T44.3X6
Diphenadione	T45.511	T45.512	T45.513	T45.514	T45.515	T45.516
rodenticide	T60.4X1	T60.4X2	T60.4X3	T60.4X4	--	--
Diphenhydramine	T45.0X1	T45.0X2	T45.0X3	T45.0X4	T45.0X5	T45.0X6
Diphenidol	T45.0X1	T45.0X2	T45.0X3	T45.0X4	T45.0X5	T45.0X6
Diphenoxylate	T47.6X1	T47.6X2	T47.6X3	T47.6X4	T47.6X5	T47.6X6
Diphenylamine	T65.3X1	T65.3X2	T65.3X3	T65.3X4	--	--
Diphenylbutazone	T39.2X1	T39.2X2	T39.2X3	T39.2X4	T39.2X5	T39.2X6
Diphenylchloroarsine, not in war	T57.0X1	T57.0X2	T57.0X3	T57.0X4	--	--
Diphenylhydantoin	T42.0X1	T42.0X2	T42.0X3	T42.0X4	T42.0X5	T42.0X6
Diphenylmethane dye	T52.1X1	T52.1X2	T52.1X3	T52.1X4	--	--
Diphenylpyraline	T45.0X1	T45.0X2	T45.0X3	T45.0X4	T45.0X5	T45.0X6
Diphtheria						
antitoxin	T50.Z11	T50.Z12	T50.Z13	T50.Z14	T50.Z15	T50.Z16
toxoid	T50.A91	T50.A92	T50.A93	T50.A94	T50.A95	T50.A96
with tetanus toxoid	T50.A21	T50.A22	T50.A23	T50.A24	T50.A25	T50.A26
with pertussis component	T50.A11	T50.A12	T50.A13	T50.A14	T50.A15	T50.A16
vaccine	T50.A91	T50.A92	T50.A93	T50.A94	T50.A95	T50.A96
combination						
including pertussis	T50.A11	T50.A12	T50.A13	T50.A14	T50.A15	T50.A16
without pertussis	T50.A21	T50.A22	T50.A23	T50.A24	T50.A25	T50.A26
Diphylline	T50.2X1	T50.2X2	T50.2X3	T50.2X4	T50.2X5	T50.2X6
Dipipanone	T40.4X1	T40.4X2	T40.4X3	T40.4X4	--	--
Dipivefrine	T49.5X1	T49.5X2	T49.5X3	T49.5X4	T49.5X5	T49.5X6
Diplovax	T50.B91	T50.B92	T50.B93	T50.B94	T50.B95	T50.B96
Diprophylline	T50.2X1	T50.2X2	T50.2X3	T50.2X4	T50.2X5	T50.2X6
Dipropyline	T48.291	T48.292	T48.293	T48.294	T48.295	T48.296
Dipyridamole	T46.3X1	T46.3X2	T46.3X3	T46.3X4	T46.3X5	T46.3X6
Dipyrone	T39.2X1	T39.2X2	T39.2X3	T39.2X4	T39.2X5	T39.2X6
Diquat (dibromide)	T60.3X1	T60.3X2	T60.3X3	T60.3X4	--	--
Disinfectant	T65.891	T65.892	T65.893	T65.894	--	--
alkaline	T54.3X1	T54.3X2	T54.3X3	T54.3X4	--	--
aromatic	T54.1X1	T54.1X2	T54.1X3	T54.1X4	--	--
intestinal	T37.8X1	T37.8X2	T37.8X3	T37.8X4	T37.8X5	T37.8X6
Disipal	T42.8X1	T42.8X2	T42.8X3	T42.8X4	T42.8X5	T42.8X6
Disodium edetate	T50.6X1	T50.6X2	T50.6X3	T50.6X4	T50.6X5	T50.6X6
Disoprofol	T41.291	T41.292	T41.293	T41.294	T41.295	T41.296
Disopyramide	T46.2X1	T46.2X2	T46.2X3	T46.2X4	T46.2X5	T46.2X6
Distigmine (bromide)	T44.0X1	T44.0X2	T44.0X3	T44.0X4	T44.0X5	T44.0X6
Disulfamide	T50.2X1	T50.2X2	T50.2X3	T50.2X4	T50.2X5	T50.2X6
Disulfanilamide	T37.0X1	T37.0X2	T37.0X3	T37.0X4	T37.0X5	T37.0X6
Disulfiram	T50.6X1	T50.6X2	T50.6X3	T50.6X4	T50.6X5	T50.6X6
Disulfoton	T60.0X1	T60.0X2	T60.0X3	T60.0X4	--	--
Dithiazanine iodide	T37.4X1	T37.4X2	T37.4X3	T37.4X4	T37.4X5	T37.4X6
Dithiocarbamate	T60.0X1	T60.0X2	T60.0X3	T60.0X4	--	--
Dithranol	T49.4X1	T49.4X2	T49.4X3	T49.4X4	T49.4X5	T49.4X6
Diucardin	T50.2X1	T50.2X2	T50.2X3	T50.2X4	T50.2X5	T50.2X6
Diupres	T50.2X1	T50.2X2	T50.2X3	T50.2X4	T50.2X5	T50.2X6
Diuretic NEC	T50.2X1	T50.2X2	T50.2X3	T50.2X4	T50.2X5	T50.2X6
benzothiadiazine	T50.2X1	T50.2X2	T50.2X3	T50.2X4	T50.2X5	T50.2X6
carbonic acid anhydrase inhibitors	T50.2X1	T50.2X2	T50.2X3	T50.2X4	T50.2X5	T50.2X6
furfuryl NEC	T50.2X1	T50.2X2	T50.2X3	T50.2X4	T50.2X5	T50.2X6
loop (high-ceiling)	T50.1X1	T50.1X2	T50.1X3	T50.1X4	T50.1X5	T50.1X6
mercurial NEC	T50.2X1	T50.2X2	T50.2X3	T50.2X4	T50.2X5	T50.2X6
osmotic	T50.2X1	T50.2X2	T50.2X3	T50.2X4	T50.2X5	T50.2X6
purine NEC	T50.2X1	T50.2X2	T50.2X3	T50.2X4	T50.2X5	T50.2X6
saluretic NEC	T50.2X1	T50.2X2	T50.2X3	T50.2X4	T50.2X5	T50.2X6
sulfonamide	T50.2X1	T50.2X2	T50.2X3	T50.2X4	T50.2X5	T50.2X6
thiazide NEC	T50.2X1	T50.2X2	T50.2X3	T50.2X4	T50.2X5	T50.2X6
xanthine	T50.2X1	T50.2X2	T50.2X3	T50.2X4	T50.2X5	T50.2X6
Diurgin	T50.2X1	T50.2X2	T50.2X3	T50.2X4	T50.2X5	T50.2X6
Diuril	T50.2X1	T50.2X2	T50.2X3	T50.2X4	T50.2X5	T50.2X6
Diuron	T60.3X1	T60.3X2	T60.3X3	T60.3X4	--	--
Divalproex	T42.6X1	T42.6X2	T42.6X3	T42.6X4	T42.6X5	T42.6X6
Divinyl ether	T41.0X1	T41.0X2	T41.0X3	T41.0X4	T41.0X5	T41.0X6
Dixanthogen	T49.0X1	T49.0X2	T49.0X3	T49.0X4	T49.0X5	T49.0X6
Dixyrazine	T43.3X1	T43.3X2	T43.3X3	T43.3X4	T43.3X5	T43.3X6
D-lysergic acid diethylamide	T40.8X1	T40.8X2	T40.8X3	T40.8X4	--	--
DMCT	T36.4X1	T36.4X2	T36.4X3	T36.4X4	T36.4X5	T36.4X6
DMSO — *see Dimethyl sulfoxide*						
DNBP	T60.3X1	T60.3X2	T60.3X3	T60.3X4	--	--
DNOC	T65.3X1	T65.3X2	T65.3X3	T65.3X4	--	--
Dobutamine	T44.5X1	T44.5X2	T44.5X3	T44.5X4	T44.5X5	T44.5X6
DOCA	T38.0X1	T38.0X2	T38.0X3	T38.0X4	T38.0X5	T38.0X6
Docusate sodium	T47.4X1	T47.4X2	T47.4X3	T47.4X4	T47.4X5	T47.4X6
Dodicin	T49.0X1	T49.0X2	T49.0X3	T49.0X4	T49.0X5	T49.0X6
Dofamium chloride	T49.0X1	T49.0X2	T49.0X3	T49.0X4	T49.0X5	T49.0X6
Dolophine	T40.3X1	T40.3X2	T40.3X3	T40.3X4	T40.3X5	T40.3X6
Doloxene	T39.8X1	T39.8X2	T39.8X3	T39.8X4	T39.8X5	T39.8X6
Domestic gas (after combustion) — *see Gas, utility*						
prior to combustion	T59.891	T59.892	T59.893	T59.894	--	--
Domiodol	T48.4X1	T48.4X2	T48.4X3	T48.4X4	T48.4X5	T48.4X6
Domiphen (bromide)	T49.0X1	T49.0X2	T49.0X3	T49.0X4	T49.0X5	T49.0X6
Domperidone	T45.0X1	T45.0X2	T45.0X3	T45.0X4	T45.0X5	T45.0X6
Dopa	T42.8X1	T42.8X2	T42.8X3	T42.8X4	T42.8X5	T42.8X6
Dopamine	T44.991	T44.992	T44.993	T44.994	T44.995	T44.996
Doriden	T42.6X1	T42.6X2	T42.6X3	T42.6X4	T42.6X5	T42.6X6
Dormiral	T42.3X1	T42.3X2	T42.3X3	T42.3X4	T42.3X5	T42.3X6
Dormison	T42.6X1	T42.6X2	T42.6X3	T42.6X4	T42.6X5	T42.6X6
Dornase	T48.4X1	T48.4X2	T48.4X3	T48.4X4	T48.4X5	T48.4X6
Dorsacaine	T41.3X1	T41.3X2	T41.3X3	T41.3X4	T41.3X5	T41.3X6
Dosulepin	T43.011	T43.012	T43.013	T43.014	T43.015	T43.016
Dothiepin	T43.011	T43.012	T43.013	T43.014	T43.015	T43.016
Doxantrazole	T48.6X1	T48.6X2	T48.6X3	T48.6X4	T48.6X5	T48.6X6
Doxapram	T50.7X1	T50.7X2	T50.7X3	T50.7X4	T50.7X5	T50.7X6
Doxazosin	T44.6X1	T44.6X2	T44.6X3	T44.6X4	T44.6X5	T44.6X6
Doxepin	T43.011	T43.012	T43.013	T43.014	T43.015	T43.016
Doxifluridine	T45.1X1	T45.1X2	T45.1X3	T45.1X4	T45.1X5	T45.1X6
Doxorubicin	T45.1X1	T45.1X2	T45.1X3	T45.1X4	T45.1X5	T45.1X6
Doxycycline	T36.4X1	T36.4X2	T36.4X3	T36.4X4	T36.4X5	T36.4X6
Doxylamine	T45.0X1	T45.0X2	T45.0X3	T45.0X4	T45.0X5	T45.0X6
Dramamine	T45.0X1	T45.0X2	T45.0X3	T45.0X4	T45.0X5	T45.0X6
Drano (drain cleaner)	T54.3X1	T54.3X2	T54.3X3	T54.3X4	--	--
Dressing, live pulp	T49.7X1	T49.7X2	T49.7X3	T49.7X4	T49.7X5	T49.7X6
Drocode	T40.2X1	T40.2X2	T40.2X3	T40.2X4	T40.2X5	T40.2X6
Dromoran	T40.2X1	T40.2X2	T40.2X3	T40.2X4	T40.2X5	T40.2X6
Dromostanolone	T38.7X1	T38.7X2	T38.7X3	T38.7X4	T38.7X5	T38.7X6
Dronabinol	T40.7X1	T40.7X2	T40.7X3	T40.7X4	T40.7X5	T40.7X6
Droperidol	T43.591	T43.592	T43.593	T43.594	T43.595	T43.596
Dropropizine	T48.3X1	T48.3X2	T48.3X3	T48.3X4	T48.3X5	T48.3X6
Drostanolone	T38.7X1	T38.7X2	T38.7X3	T38.7X4	T38.7X5	T38.7X6
Drotaverine	T44.3X1	T44.3X2	T44.3X3	T44.3X4	T44.3X5	T44.3X6
Drotrecogin alfa	T45.511	T45.512	T45.513	T45.514	T45.515	T45.516
Drug NEC	T50.901	T50.902	T50.903	T50.904	T50.905	T50.906
specified NEC	T50.991	T50.992	T50.993	T50.994	T50.995	T50.996
DTIC	T45.1X1	T45.1X2	T45.1X3	T45.1X4	T45.1X5	T45.1X6
Duboisine	T44.3X1	T44.3X2	T44.3X3	T44.3X4	T44.3X5	T44.3X6
Dulcolax	T47.2X1	T47.2X2	T47.2X3	T47.2X4	T47.2X5	T47.2X6
Duponol (C) (EP)	T49.2X1	T49.2X2	T49.2X3	T49.2X4	T49.2X5	T49.2X6
Durabolin	T38.7X1	T38.7X2	T38.7X3	T38.7X4	T38.7X5	T38.7X6
Dyclone	T41.3X1	T41.3X2	T41.3X3	T41.3X4	T41.3X5	T41.3X6
Dyclonine	T41.3X1	T41.3X2	T41.3X3	T41.3X4	T41.3X5	T41.3X6
Dydrogesterone	T38.5X1	T38.5X2	T38.5X3	T38.5X4	T38.5X5	T38.5X6
Dye NEC	T65.6X1	T65.6X2	T65.6X3	T65.6X4	--	--
antiseptic	T49.0X1	T49.0X2	T49.0X3	T49.0X4	T49.0X5	T49.0X6
diagnostic agents	T50.8X1	T50.8X2	T50.8X3	T50.8X4	T50.8X5	T50.8X6
pharmaceutical NEC	T50.901	T50.902	T50.903	T50.904	T50.905	T50.906
Dyflos	T44.0X1	T44.0X2	T44.0X3	T44.0X4	T44.0X5	T44.0X6
Dymelor	T38.3X1	T38.3X2	T38.3X3	T38.3X4	T38.3X5	T38.3X6
Dynamite	T65.3X1	T65.3X2	T65.3X3	T65.3X4	--	--
fumes	T59.891	T59.892	T59.893	T59.894	--	--
Dyphylline	T44.3X1	T44.3X2	T44.3X3	T44.3X4	T44.3X5	T44.3X6
E						
Ear drug NEC	T49.6X1	T49.6X2	T49.6X3	T49.6X4	T49.6X5	T49.6X6
Ear preparations	T49.6X1	T49.6X2	T49.6X3	T49.6X4	T49.6X5	T49.6X6
Echothiophate, echothiopate, ecothiopate	T49.5X1	T49.5X2	T49.5X3	T49.5X4	T49.5X5	T49.5X6
Econazole	T49.0X1	T49.0X2	T49.0X3	T49.0X4	T49.0X5	T49.0X6
Ecothiopate iodide	T49.5X1	T49.5X2	T49.5X3	T49.5X4	T49.5X5	T49.5X6
Ecstasy	T43.621	T43.622	T43.623	T43.624	T43.625	T43.626
Ectylurea	T42.6X1	T42.6X2	T42.6X3	T42.6X4	T42.6X5	T42.6X6
Edathamil disodium	T45.8X1	T45.8X2	T45.8X3	T45.8X4	T45.8X5	T45.8X6
Edecrin	T50.1X1	T50.1X2	T50.1X3	T50.1X4	T50.1X5	T50.1X6
Edetate, disodium (calcium)	T45.8X1	T45.8X2	T45.8X3	T45.8X4	T45.8X5	T45.8X6
Edoxudine	T49.5X1	T49.5X2	T49.5X3	T49.5X4	T49.5X5	T49.5X6
Edrophonium	T44.0X1	T44.0X2	T44.0X3	T44.0X4	T44.0X5	T44.0X6
chloride	T44.0X1	T44.0X2	T44.0X3	T44.0X4	T44.0X5	T44.0X6

EDTA - Ethocaine

Substance	Poisoning, Accidental unintentional	Poisoning, Intentional self-harm	Poisoning, Assault	Poisoning, Undetermined	Adverse effect	Underdosing
EDTA	T50.6X1	T50.6X2	T50.6X3	T50.6X4	T50.6X5	T50.6X6
Eflornithine	T37.2X1	T37.2X2	T37.2X3	T37.2X4	T37.2X5	T37.2X6
Efloxate	T46.3X1	T46.3X2	T46.3X3	T46.3X4	T46.3X5	T46.3X6
Elase	T49.8X1	T49.8X2	T49.8X3	T49.8X4	T49.8X5	T49.8X6
Elastase	T47.5X1	T47.5X2	T47.5X3	T47.5X4	T47.5X5	T47.5X6
Elaterium	T47.2X1	T47.2X2	T47.2X3	T47.2X4	T47.2X5	T47.2X6
Elcatonin	T50.991	T50.992	T50.993	T50.994	T50.995	T50.996
Elder	T62.2X1	T62.2X2	T62.2X3	T62.2X4	—	—
berry, (unripe)	T62.1X1	T62.1X2	T62.1X3	T62.1X4	—	—
Electrolyte balance drug	T50.3X1	T50.3X2	T50.3X3	T50.3X4	T50.3X5	T50.3X6
Electrolytes NEC	T50.3X1	T50.3X2	T50.3X3	T50.3X4	T50.3X5	T50.3X6
Electrolytic agent NEC	T50.3X1	T50.3X2	T50.3X3	T50.3X4	T50.3X5	T50.3X6
Elemental diet	T50.901	T50.902	T50.903	T50.904	T50.905	T50.906
Elliptinium acetate	T45.1X1	T45.1X2	T45.1X3	T45.1X4	T45.1X5	T45.1X6
Embramine	T45.0X1	T45.0X2	T45.0X3	T45.0X4	T45.0X5	T45.0X6
Emepronium (salts)	T44.3X1	T44.3X2	T44.3X3	T44.3X4	T44.3X5	T44.3X6
bromide	T44.3X1	T44.3X2	T44.3X3	T44.3X4	T44.3X5	T44.3X6
Emetic NEC	T47.7X1	T47.7X2	T47.7X3	T47.7X4	T47.7X5	T47.7X6
Emetine	T37.3X1	T37.3X2	T37.3X3	T37.3X4	T37.3X5	T37.3X6
Emollient NEC	T49.3X1	T49.3X2	T49.3X3	T49.3X4	T49.3X5	T49.3X6
Emorfazone	T39.8X1	T39.8X2	T39.8X3	T39.8X4	T39.8X5	T39.8X6
Emylcamate	T43.591	T43.592	T43.593	T43.594	T43.595	T43.596
Enalapril	T46.4X1	T46.4X2	T46.4X3	T46.4X4	T46.4X5	T46.4X6
Enalaprilat	T46.4X1	T46.4X2	T46.4X3	T46.4X4	T46.4X5	T46.4X6
Encainide	T46.2X1	T46.2X2	T46.2X3	T46.2X4	T46.2X5	T46.2X6
Endocaine	T41.3X1	T41.3X2	T41.3X3	T41.3X4	T41.3X5	T41.3X6
Endosulfan	T60.2X1	T60.2X2	T60.2X3	T60.2X4	—	—
Endothall	T60.3X1	T60.3X2	T60.3X3	T60.3X4	—	—
Endralazine	T46.5X1	T46.5X2	T46.5X3	T46.5X4	T46.5X5	T46.5X6
Endrin	T60.1X1	T60.1X2	T60.1X3	T60.1X4	—	—
Enflurane	T41.0X1	T41.0X2	T41.0X3	T41.0X4	T41.0X5	T41.0X6
Enhexymal	T42.3X1	T42.3X2	T42.3X3	T42.3X4	T42.3X5	T42.3X6
Enocitabine	T45.1X1	T45.1X2	T45.1X3	T45.1X4	T45.1X5	T45.1X6
Enovid	T38.4X1	T38.4X2	T38.4X3	T38.4X4	T38.4X5	T38.4X6
Enoxacin	T36.8X1	T36.8X2	T36.8X3	T36.8X4	T36.8X5	T36.8X6
Enoxaparin (sodium)	T45.511	T45.512	T45.513	T45.514	T45.515	T45.516
Enpiprazole	T43.591	T43.592	T43.593	T43.594	T43.595	T43.596
Enprofylline	T48.6X1	T48.6X2	T48.6X3	T48.6X4	T48.6X5	T48.6X6
Enprostil	T47.1X1	T47.1X2	T47.1X3	T47.1X4	T47.1X5	T47.1X6
ENT preparations (anti-infectives)	T49.6X1	T49.6X2	T49.6X3	T49.6X4	T49.6X5	T49.6X6
Enterogastrone	T38.891	T38.892	T38.893	T38.894	T38.895	T38.896
Enviomycin	T36.8X1	T36.8X2	T36.8X3	T36.8X4	T36.8X5	T36.8X6
Enzodase	T45.3X1	T45.3X2	T45.3X3	T45.3X4	T45.3X5	T45.3X6
Enzyme NEC	T45.3X1	T45.3X2	T45.3X3	T45.3X4	T45.3X5	T45.3X6
depolymerizing	T49.8X1	T49.8X2	T49.8X3	T49.8X4	T49.8X5	T49.8X6
fibrolytic	T45.3X1	T45.3X2	T45.3X3	T45.3X4	T45.3X5	T45.3X6
gastric	T47.5X1	T47.5X2	T47.5X3	T47.5X4	T47.5X5	T47.5X6
intestinal	T47.5X1	T47.5X2	T47.5X3	T47.5X4	T47.5X5	T47.5X6
local action	T49.4X1	T49.4X2	T49.4X3	T49.4X4	T49.4X5	T49.4X6
proteolytic	T49.4X1	T49.4X2	T49.4X3	T49.4X4	T49.4X5	T49.4X6
thrombolytic	T45.3X1	T45.3X2	T45.3X3	T45.3X4	T45.3X5	T45.3X6
EPAB	T41.3X1	T41.3X2	T41.3X3	T41.3X4	T41.3X5	T41.3X6
Epanutin	T42.0X1	T42.0X2	T42.0X3	T42.0X4	T42.0X5	T42.0X6
Ephedra	T44.991	T44.992	T44.993	T44.994	T44.995	T44.996
Ephedrine	T44.991	T44.992	T44.993	T44.994	T44.995	T44.996
Epichlorhydrin, epichlorohydrin	T52.8X1	T52.8X2	T52.8X3	T52.8X4	—	—
Epicillin	T36.0X1	T36.0X2	T36.0X3	T36.0X4	T36.0X5	T36.0X6
Epiestriol	T38.5X1	T38.5X2	T38.5X3	T38.5X4	T38.5X5	T38.5X6
Epilim — *see Sodium valproate*						
Epimestrol	T38.5X1	T38.5X2	T38.5X3	T38.5X4	T38.5X5	T38.5X6
Epinephrine	T44.5X1	T44.5X2	T44.5X3	T44.5X4	T44.5X5	T44.5X6
Epirubicin	T45.1X1	T45.1X2	T45.1X3	T45.1X4	T45.1X5	T45.1X6
Epitiostanol	T38.7X1	T38.7X2	T38.7X3	T38.7X4	T38.7X5	T38.7X6
Epitizide	T50.2X1	T50.2X2	T50.2X3	T50.2X4	T50.2X5	T50.2X6
EPN	T60.0X1	T60.0X2	T60.0X3	T60.0X4	—	—
EPO	T45.8X1	T45.8X2	T45.8X3	T45.8X4	T45.8X5	T45.8X6
Epoetin alpha	T45.8X1	T45.8X2	T45.8X3	T45.8X4	T45.8X5	T45.8X6
Epomediol	T50.991	T50.992	T50.993	T50.994	T50.995	T50.996
Epoprostenol	T45.521	T45.522	T45.523	T45.524	T45.525	T45.526
Epoxy resin	T65.891	T65.892	T65.893	T65.894	—	—
Eprazinone	T48.4X1	T48.4X2	T48.4X3	T48.4X4	T48.4X5	T48.4X6
Epsilon amino-caproic acid	T45.621	T45.622	T45.623	T45.624	T45.625	T45.626
Epsom salt	T47.3X1	T47.3X2	T47.3X3	T47.3X4	T47.3X5	T47.3X6
Eptazocine	T40.4X1	T40.4X2	T40.4X3	T40.4X4	T40.4X5	T40.4X6
Equanil	T43.591	T43.592	T43.593	T43.594	T43.595	T43.596
Equisetum	T62.2X1	T62.2X2	T62.2X3	T62.2X4	—	—
diuretic	T50.2X1	T50.2X2	T50.2X3	T50.2X4	T50.2X5	T50.2X6
Ergobasine	T48.0X1	T48.0X2	T48.0X3	T48.0X4	T48.0X5	T48.0X6
Ergocalciferol	T45.2X1	T45.2X2	T45.2X3	T45.2X4	T45.2X5	T45.2X6
Ergoloid mesylates	T46.7X1	T46.7X2	T46.7X3	T46.7X4	T46.7X5	T46.7X6
Ergometrine	T48.0X1	T48.0X2	T48.0X3	T48.0X4	T48.0X5	T48.0X6
Ergonovine	T48.0X1	T48.0X2	T48.0X3	T48.0X4	T48.0X5	T48.0X6
Ergot NEC	T64.81	T64.82	T64.83	T64.84	—	—
Ergot NEC — *continued*						
derivative	T48.0X1	T48.0X2	T48.0X3	T48.0X4	T48.0X5	T48.0X6
medicinal (alkaloids)	T48.0X1	T48.0X2	T48.0X3	T48.0X4	T48.0X5	T48.0X6
prepared	T48.0X1	T48.0X2	T48.0X3	T48.0X4	T48.0X5	T48.0X6
Ergotamine	T46.5X1	T46.5X2	T46.5X3	T46.5X4	T46.5X5	T46.5X6
Ergotocine	T48.0X1	T48.0X2	T48.0X3	T48.0X4	T48.0X5	T48.0X6
Ergotrate	T48.0X1	T48.0X2	T48.0X3	T48.0X4	T48.0X5	T48.0X6
Eritrityl tetranitrate	T46.3X1	T46.3X2	T46.3X3	T46.3X4	T46.3X5	T46.3X6
Erythrityl tetranitrate	T46.3X1	T46.3X2	T46.3X3	T46.3X4	T46.3X5	T46.3X6
Erythrol tetranitrate	T46.3X1	T46.3X2	T46.3X3	T46.3X4	T46.3X5	T46.3X6
Erythromycin (salts)	T36.3X1	T36.3X2	T36.3X3	T36.3X4	T36.3X5	T36.3X6
ophthalmic preparation	T49.5X1	T49.5X2	T49.5X3	T49.5X4	T49.5X5	T49.5X6
topical NEC	T49.0X1	T49.0X2	T49.0X3	T49.0X4	T49.0X5	T49.0X6
Erythropoietin	T45.8X1	T45.8X2	T45.8X3	T45.8X4	T45.8X5	T45.8X6
human	T45.8X1	T45.8X2	T45.8X3	T45.8X4	T45.8X5	T45.8X6
Escin	T46.991	T46.992	T46.993	T46.994	T46.995	T46.996
Esculin	T45.2X1	T45.2X2	T45.2X3	T45.2X4	T45.2X5	T45.2X6
Esculoside	T45.2X1	T45.2X2	T45.2X3	T45.2X4	T45.2X5	T45.2X6
ESDT (ether-soluble tar distillate)	T49.1X1	T49.1X2	T49.1X3	T49.1X4	T49.1X5	T49.1X6
Eserine	T49.5X1	T49.5X2	T49.5X3	T49.5X4	T49.5X5	T49.5X6
Esflurbiprofen	T39.311	T39.312	T39.313	T39.314	T39.315	T39.316
Eskabarb	T42.3X1	T42.3X2	T42.3X3	T42.3X4	T42.3X5	T42.3X6
Eskalith	T43.8X1	T43.8X2	T43.8X3	T43.8X4	T43.8X5	T43.8X6
Esmolol	T44.7X1	T44.7X2	T44.7X3	T44.7X4	T44.7X5	T44.7X6
Estanozolol	T38.7X1	T38.7X2	T38.7X3	T38.7X4	T38.7X5	T38.7X6
Estazolam	T42.4X1	T42.4X2	T42.4X3	T42.4X4	T42.4X5	T42.4X6
Estradiol	T38.5X1	T38.5X2	T38.5X3	T38.5X4	T38.5X5	T38.5X6
with testosterone	T38.7X1	T38.7X2	T38.7X3	T38.7X4	T38.7X5	T38.7X6
benzoate	T38.5X1	T38.5X2	T38.5X3	T38.5X4	T38.5X5	T38.5X6
Estramustine	T45.1X1	T45.1X2	T45.1X3	T45.1X4	T45.1X5	T45.1X6
Estriol	T38.5X1	T38.5X2	T38.5X3	T38.5X4	T38.5X5	T38.5X6
Estrogen	T38.5X1	T38.5X2	T38.5X3	T38.5X4	T38.5X5	T38.5X6
with progesterone	T38.5X1	T38.5X2	T38.5X3	T38.5X4	T38.5X5	T38.5X6
conjugated	T38.5X1	T38.5X2	T38.5X3	T38.5X4	T38.5X5	T38.5X6
Estrone	T38.5X1	T38.5X2	T38.5X3	T38.5X4	T38.5X5	T38.5X6
Estropipate	T38.5X1	T38.5X2	T38.5X3	T38.5X4	T38.5X5	T38.5X6
Etacrynate sodium	T50.1X1	T50.1X2	T50.1X3	T50.1X4	T50.1X5	T50.1X6
Etacrynic acid	T50.1X1	T50.1X2	T50.1X3	T50.1X4	T50.1X5	T50.1X6
Etafedrine	T48.6X1	T48.6X2	T48.6X3	T48.6X4	T48.6X5	T48.6X6
Etafenone	T46.3X1	T46.3X2	T46.3X3	T46.3X4	T46.3X5	T46.3X6
Etambutol	T37.1X1	T37.1X2	T37.1X3	T37.1X4	T37.1X5	T37.1X6
Etamiphyllin	T48.6X1	T48.6X2	T48.6X3	T48.6X4	T48.6X5	T48.6X6
Etamivan	T50.7X1	T50.7X2	T50.7X3	T50.7X4	T50.7X5	T50.7X6
Etamsylate	T45.7X1	T45.7X2	T45.7X3	T45.7X4	T45.7X5	T45.7X6
Etebenecid	T50.4X1	T50.4X2	T50.4X3	T50.4X4	T50.4X5	T50.4X6
Ethacridine	T49.0X1	T49.0X2	T49.0X3	T49.0X4	T49.0X5	T49.0X6
Ethacrynic acid	T50.1X1	T50.1X2	T50.1X3	T50.1X4	T50.1X5	T50.1X6
Ethadione	T42.2X1	T42.2X2	T42.2X3	T42.2X4	T42.2X5	T42.2X6
Ethambutol	T37.1X1	T37.1X2	T37.1X3	T37.1X4	T37.1X5	T37.1X6
Ethamide	T50.2X1	T50.2X2	T50.2X3	T50.2X4	T50.2X5	T50.2X6
Ethamivan	T50.7X1	T50.7X2	T50.7X3	T50.7X4	T50.7X5	T50.7X6
Ethamsylate	T45.7X1	T45.7X2	T45.7X3	T45.7X4	T45.7X5	T45.7X6
Ethanol	T51.0X1	T51.0X2	T51.0X3	T51.0X4	—	—
beverage	T51.0X1	T51.0X2	T51.0X3	T51.0X4	—	—
Ethanolamine oleate	T46.8X1	T46.8X2	T46.8X3	T46.8X4	T46.8X5	T46.8X6
Ethaverine	T44.3X1	T44.3X2	T44.3X3	T44.3X4	T44.3X5	T44.3X6
Ethchlorvynol	T42.6X1	T42.6X2	T42.6X3	T42.6X4	T42.6X5	T42.6X6
Ethebenecid	T50.4X1	T50.4X2	T50.4X3	T50.4X4	T50.4X5	T50.4X6
Ether (vapor)	T41.0X1	T41.0X2	T41.0X3	T41.0X4	T41.0X5	T41.0X6
anesthetic	T41.0X1	T41.0X2	T41.0X3	T41.0X4	T41.0X5	T41.0X6
divinyl	T41.0X1	T41.0X2	T41.0X3	T41.0X4	T41.0X5	T41.0X6
ethyl (medicinal)	T41.0X1	T41.0X2	T41.0X3	T41.0X4	T41.0X5	T41.0X6
nonmedicinal	T52.8X1	T52.8X2	T52.8X3	T52.8X4	—	—
petroleum — *see Ligroin*						
solvent	T52.8X1	T52.8X2	T52.8X3	T52.8X4	—	—
Ethiazide	T50.2X1	T50.2X2	T50.2X3	T50.2X4	T50.2X5	T50.2X6
Ethidium chloride (vapor)	T59.891	T59.892	T59.893	T59.894	—	—
Ethinamate	T42.6X1	T42.6X2	T42.6X3	T42.6X4	T42.6X5	T42.6X6
Ethinylestradiol, ethinyloestradiol	T38.5X1	T38.5X2	T38.5X3	T38.5X4	T38.5X5	T38.5X6
with						
levonorgestrel	T38.4X1	T38.4X2	T38.4X3	T38.4X4	T38.4X5	T38.4X6
norethisterone	T38.4X1	T38.4X2	T38.4X3	T38.4X4	T38.4X5	T38.4X6
Ethiodized oil (131 I)	T50.8X1	T50.8X2	T50.8X3	T50.8X4	T50.8X5	T50.8X6
Ethion	T60.0X1	T60.0X2	T60.0X3	T60.0X4	—	—
Ethionamide	T37.1X1	T37.1X2	T37.1X3	T37.1X4	T37.1X5	T37.1X6
Ethioniamide	T37.1X1	T37.1X2	T37.1X3	T37.1X4	T37.1X5	T37.1X6
Ethisterone	T38.5X1	T38.5X2	T38.5X3	T38.5X4	T38.5X5	T38.5X6
Ethobral	T42.3X1	T42.3X2	T42.3X3	T42.3X4	T42.3X5	T42.3X6
Ethocaine (infiltration) (topical)	T41.3X1	T41.3X2	T41.3X3	T41.3X4	T41.3X5	T41.3X6
nerve block (peripheral) (plexus)	T41.3X1	T41.3X2	T41.3X3	T41.3X4	T41.3X5	T41.3X6
spinal	T41.3X1	T41.3X2	T41.3X3	T41.3X4	T41.3X5	T41.3X6

Substance	Poisoning, Accidental unintentional	Poisoning, Intentional self-harm	Poisoning, Assault	Poisoning, Undetermined	Adverse effect	Underdosing
Ethoheptazine	T40.4X1	T40.4X2	T40.4X3	T40.4X4	T40.4X5	T40.4X6
Ethopropazine	T44.3X1	T44.3X2	T44.3X3	T44.3X4	T44.3X5	T44.3X6
Ethosuximide	T42.2X1	T42.2X2	T42.2X3	T42.2X4	T42.2X5	T42.2X6
Ethotoin	T42.0X1	T42.0X2	T42.0X3	T42.0X4	T42.0X5	T42.0X6
Ethoxazene	T37.91	T37.92	T37.93	T37.94	T37.95	T37.96
Ethoxazorutoside	T46.991	T46.992	T46.993	T46.994	T46.995	T46.996
2-Ethoxyethanol	T52.3X1	T52.3X2	T52.3X3	T52.3X4	--	--
Ethoxzolamide	T50.2X1	T50.2X2	T50.2X3	T50.2X4	T50.2X5	T50.2X6
Ethyl						
acetate	T52.8X1	T52.8X2	T52.8X3	T52.8X4	--	--
alcohol	T51.0X1	T51.0X2	T51.0X3	T51.0X4	--	--
beverage	T51.0X1	T51.0X2	T51.0X3	T51.0X4	--	--
aldehyde (vapor)	T59.891	T59.892	T59.893	T59.894	--	--
liquid	T52.8X1	T52.8X2	T52.8X3	T52.8X4	--	--
aminobenzoate	T41.3X1	T41.3X2	T41.3X3	T41.3X4	T41.3X5	T41.3X6
aminophenothiazine	T43.3X1	T43.3X2	T43.3X3	T43.3X4	T43.3X5	T43.3X6
benzoate	T52.8X1	T52.8X2	T52.8X3	T52.8X4	--	--
biscoumacetate	T45.511	T45.512	T45.513	T45.514	T45.515	T45.516
bromide (anesthetic)	T41.0X1	T41.0X2	T41.0X3	T41.0X4	T41.0X5	T41.0X6
carbamate	T45.1X1	T45.1X2	T45.1X3	T45.1X4	T45.1X5	T45.1X6
carbinol	T51.3X1	T51.3X2	T51.3X3	T51.3X4	--	--
carbonate	T52.8X1	T52.8X2	T52.8X3	T52.8X4	--	--
chaulmoograte	T37.1X1	T37.1X2	T37.1X3	T37.1X4	T37.1X5	T37.1X6
chloride (anesthetic)	T41.0X1	T41.0X2	T41.0X3	T41.0X4	T41.0X5	T41.0X6
anesthetic (local)	T41.3X1	T41.3X2	T41.3X3	T41.3X4	T41.3X5	T41.3X6
inhaled	T41.0X1	T41.0X2	T41.0X3	T41.0X4	T41.0X5	T41.0X6
local	T49.4X1	T49.4X2	T49.4X3	T49.4X4	T49.4X5	T49.4X6
solvent	T53.6X1	T53.6X2	T53.6X3	T53.6X4	--	--
dibunate	T48.3X1	T48.3X2	T48.3X3	T48.3X4	T48.3X5	T48.3X6
dichloroarsine (vapor)	T57.0X1	T57.0X2	T57.0X3	T57.0X4	--	--
estranol	T38.7X1	T38.7X2	T38.7X3	T38.7X4	T38.7X5	T38.7X6
ether — *see also ether*	T52.8X1	T52.8X2	T52.8X3	T52.8X4	--	--
formate NEC (solvent)	T52.0X1	T52.0X2	T52.0X3	T52.0X4	--	--
fumarate	T49.4X1	T49.4X2	T49.4X3	T49.4X4	T49.4X5	T49.4X6
hydroxyisobutyrate NEC (solvent)	T52.8X1	T52.8X2	T52.8X3	T52.8X4	--	--
iodoacetate	T59.3X1	T59.3X2	T59.3X3	T59.3X4	--	--
lactate NEC (solvent)	T52.8X1	T52.8X2	T52.8X3	T52.8X4	--	--
loflazepate	T42.4X1	T42.4X2	T42.4X3	T42.4X4	T42.4X5	T42.4X6
mercuric chloride	T56.1X1	T56.1X2	T56.1X3	T56.1X4	--	--
methylcarbinol	T51.8X1	T51.8X2	T51.8X3	T51.8X4	--	--
morphine	T40.2X1	T40.2X2	T40.2X3	T40.2X4	T40.2X5	T40.2X6
noradrenaline	T48.6X1	T48.6X2	T48.6X3	T48.6X4	T48.6X5	T48.6X6
oxybutyrate NEC (solvent)	T52.8X1	T52.8X2	T52.8X3	T52.8X4	--	--
Ethylene (gas)	T59.891	T59.892	T59.893	T59.894	--	--
anesthetic (general)	T41.0X1	T41.0X2	T41.0X3	T41.0X4	T41.0X5	T41.0X6
chlorohydrin	T52.8X1	T52.8X2	T52.8X3	T52.8X4	--	--
vapor	T53.6X1	T53.6X2	T53.6X3	T53.6X4	--	--
dichloride	T52.8X1	T52.8X2	T52.8X3	T52.8X4	--	--
vapor	T53.6X1	T53.6X2	T53.6X3	T53.6X4	--	--
dinitrate	T52.3X1	T52.3X2	T52.3X3	T52.3X4	--	--
glycol (s)	T52.8X1	T52.8X2	T52.8X3	T52.8X4	--	--
dinitrate	T52.3X1	T52.3X2	T52.3X3	T52.3X4	--	--
monobutyl ether	T52.3X1	T52.3X2	T52.3X3	T52.3X4	--	--
imine	T54.1X1	T54.1X2	T54.1X3	T54.1X4	--	--
oxide (fumigant) (nonmedicinal)	T59.891	T59.892	T59.893	T59.894	--	--
medicinal	T49.0X1	T49.0X2	T49.0X3	T49.0X4	T49.0X5	T49.0X6
Ethylenediamine theophylline	T48.6X1	T48.6X2	T48.6X3	T48.6X4	T48.6X5	T48.6X6
Ethylenediaminetetra-acetic acid	T50.6X1	T50.6X2	T50.6X3	T50.6X4	T50.6X5	T50.6X6
Ethylenedinitrilotetra-acetate	T50.6X1	T50.6X2	T50.6X3	T50.6X4	T50.6X5	T50.6X6
Ethylestrenol	T38.7X1	T38.7X2	T38.7X3	T38.7X4	T38.7X5	T38.7X6
Ethylhydroxycellulose	T47.4X1	T47.4X2	T47.4X3	T47.4X4	T47.4X5	T47.4X6
Ethylidene						
chloride NEC	T53.6X1	T53.6X2	T53.6X3	T53.6X4	--	--
diacetate	T60.3X1	T60.3X2	T60.3X3	T60.3X4	--	--
dicoumarin	T45.511	T45.512	T45.513	T45.514	T45.515	T45.516
dicoumarol	T45.511	T45.512	T45.513	T45.514	T45.515	T45.516
diethyl ether	T52.0X1	T52.0X2	T52.0X3	T52.0X4	--	--
Ethylmorphine	T40.2X1	T40.2X2	T40.2X3	T40.2X4	T40.2X5	T40.2X6
Ethylnorepinephrine	T48.6X1	T48.6X2	T48.6X3	T48.6X4	T48.6X5	T48.6X6
Ethylparachlorophen-oxyisobutyrate	T46.6X1	T46.6X2	T46.6X3	T46.6X4	T46.6X5	T46.6X6
Ethynodiol	T38.4X1	T38.4X2	T38.4X3	T38.4X4	T38.4X5	T38.4X6
with mestranol diacetate	T38.4X1	T38.4X2	T38.4X3	T38.4X4	T38.4X5	T38.4X6
Etidocaine	T41.3X1	T41.3X2	T41.3X3	T41.3X4	T41.3X5	T41.3X6
infiltration (subcutaneous)	T41.3X1	T41.3X2	T41.3X3	T41.3X4	T41.3X5	T41.3X6
nerve (peripheral) (plexus)	T41.3X1	T41.3X2	T41.3X3	T41.3X4	T41.3X5	T41.3X6
Etidronate	T50.991	T50.992	T50.993	T50.994	T50.995	T50.996
Etidronic acid (disodium salt)	T50.991	T50.992	T50.993	T50.994	T50.995	T50.996
Etifoxine	T42.6X1	T42.6X2	T42.6X3	T42.6X4	T42.6X5	T42.6X6
Etilefrine	T44.4X1	T44.4X2	T44.4X3	T44.4X4	T44.4X5	T44.4X6

Substance	Poisoning, Accidental unintentional	Poisoning, Intentional self-harm	Poisoning, Assault	Poisoning, Undetermined	Adverse effect	Underdosing
Etilfen	T42.3X1	T42.3X2	T42.3X3	T42.3X4	T42.3X5	T42.3X6
Etinodiol	T38.4X1	T38.4X2	T38.4X3	T38.4X4	T38.4X5	T38.4X6
Etiroxate	T46.6X1	T46.6X2	T46.6X3	T46.6X4	T46.6X5	T46.6X6
Etizolam	T42.4X1	T42.4X2	T42.4X3	T42.4X4	T42.4X5	T42.4X6
Etodolac	T39.391	T39.392	T39.393	T39.394	T39.395	T39.396
Etofamide	T37.3X1	T37.3X2	T37.3X3	T37.3X4	T37.3X5	T37.3X6
Etofibrate	T46.6X1	T46.6X2	T46.6X3	T46.6X4	T46.6X5	T46.6X6
Etofylline	T46.7X1	T46.7X2	T46.7X3	T46.7X4	T46.7X5	T46.7X6
clofibrate	T46.6X1	T46.6X2	T46.6X3	T46.6X4	T46.6X5	T46.6X6
Etoglucid	T45.1X1	T45.1X2	T45.1X3	T45.1X4	T45.1X5	T45.1X6
Etomidate	T41.1X1	T41.1X2	T41.1X3	T41.1X4	T41.1X5	T41.1X6
Etomide	T39.8X1	T39.8X2	T39.8X3	T39.8X4	T39.8X5	T39.8X6
Etomidoline	T44.3X1	T44.3X2	T44.3X3	T44.3X4	T44.3X5	T44.3X6
Etoposide	T45.1X1	T45.1X2	T45.1X3	T45.1X4	T45.1X5	T45.1X6
Etorphine	T40.2X1	T40.2X2	T40.2X3	T40.2X4	T40.2X5	T40.2X6
Etoval	T42.3X1	T42.3X2	T42.3X3	T42.3X4	T42.3X5	T42.3X6
Etozolin	T50.1X1	T50.1X2	T50.1X3	T50.1X4	T50.1X5	T50.1X6
Etretinate	T50.991	T50.992	T50.993	T50.994	T50.995	T50.996
Etryptamine	T43.691	T43.692	T43.693	T43.694	T43.695	T43.696
Etybenzatropine	T44.3X1	T44.3X2	T44.3X3	T44.3X4	T44.3X5	T44.3X6
Etynodiol	T38.4X1	T38.4X2	T38.4X3	T38.4X4	T38.4X5	T38.4X6
Eucaine	T41.3X1	T41.3X2	T41.3X3	T41.3X4	T41.3X5	T41.3X6
Eucalyptus oil	T49.7X1	T49.7X2	T49.7X3	T49.7X4	T49.7X5	T49.7X6
Eucatropine	T49.5X1	T49.5X2	T49.5X3	T49.5X4	T49.5X5	T49.5X6
Eucodal	T40.2X1	T40.2X2	T40.2X3	T40.2X4	T40.2X5	T40.2X6
Euneryl	T42.3X1	T42.3X2	T42.3X3	T42.3X4	T42.3X5	T42.3X6
Euphthalmine	T44.3X1	T44.3X2	T44.3X3	T44.3X4	T44.3X5	T44.3X6
Eurax	T49.0X1	T49.0X2	T49.0X3	T49.0X4	T49.0X5	T49.0X6
Euresol	T49.4X1	T49.4X2	T49.4X3	T49.4X4	T49.4X5	T49.4X6
Euthroid	T38.1X1	T38.1X2	T38.1X3	T38.1X4	T38.1X5	T38.1X6
Evans blue	T50.8X1	T50.8X2	T50.8X3	T50.8X4	T50.8X5	T50.8X6
Evipal	T42.3X1	T42.3X2	T42.3X3	T42.3X4	T42.3X5	T42.3X6
sodium	T41.1X1	T41.1X2	T41.1X3	T41.1X4	T41.1X5	T41.1X6
Evipan	T42.3X1	T42.3X2	T42.3X3	T42.3X4	T42.3X5	T42.3X6
sodium	T41.1X1	T41.1X2	T41.1X3	T41.1X4	T41.1X5	T41.1X6
Exalamide	T49.0X1	T49.0X2	T49.0X3	T49.0X4	T49.0X5	T49.0X6
Exalgin	T39.1X1	T39.1X2	T39.1X3	T39.1X4	T39.1X5	T39.1X6
Excipients, pharmaceutical	T50.901	T50.902	T50.903	T50.904	T50.905	T50.906
Exhaust gas (engine) (motor vehicle)	T58.01	T58.02	T58.03	T58.04	--	--
Ex-Lax (phenolphthalein)	T47.2X1	T47.2X2	T47.2X3	T47.2X4	T47.2X5	T47.2X6
Expectorant NEC	T48.4X1	T48.4X2	T48.4X3	T48.4X4	T48.4X5	T48.4X6
Extended insulin zinc suspension	T38.3X1	T38.3X2	T38.3X3	T38.3X4	T38.3X5	T38.3X6
External medications (skin) (mucous membrane)	T49.91	T49.92	T49.93	T49.94	T49.95	T49.96
dental agent	T49.7X1	T49.7X2	T49.7X3	T49.7X4	T49.7X5	T49.7X6
ENT agent	T49.6X1	T49.6X2	T49.6X3	T49.6X4	T49.6X5	T49.6X6
ophthalmic preparation	T49.5X1	T49.5X2	T49.5X3	T49.5X4	T49.5X5	T49.5X6
specified NEC	T49.8X1	T49.8X2	T49.8X3	T49.8X4	T49.8X5	T49.8X6
Extrapyramidal antagonist NEC	T44.3X1	T44.3X2	T44.3X3	T44.3X4	T44.3X5	T44.3X6
Eye agents (anti-infective)	T49.5X1	T49.5X2	T49.5X3	T49.5X4	T49.5X5	T49.5X6
Eye drug NEC	T49.5X1	T49.5X2	T49.5X3	T49.5X4	T49.5X5	T49.5X6
F						
FAC (fluorouracil + doxorubicin + cyclophosphamide)	T45.1X1	T45.1X2	T45.1X3	T45.1X4	T45.1X5	T45.1X6
Factor						
I (fibrinogen)	T45.8X1	T45.8X2	T45.8X3	T45.8X4	T45.8X5	T45.8X6
III (thromboplastin)	T45.8X1	T45.8X2	T45.8X3	T45.8X4	T45.8X5	T45.8X6
VIII (antihemophilic Factor) (concentrate)	T45.8X1	T45.8X2	T45.8X3	T45.8X4	T45.8X5	T45.8X6
IX complex	T45.7X1	T45.7X2	T45.7X3	T45.7X4	T45.7X5	T45.7X6
human	T45.8X1	T45.8X2	T45.8X3	T45.8X4	T45.8X5	T45.8X6
Famotidine	T47.0X1	T47.0X2	T47.0X3	T47.0X4	T47.0X5	T47.0X6
Fat suspension, intravenous	T50.991	T50.992	T50.993	T50.994	T50.995	T50.996
Fazadinium bromide	T48.1X1	T48.1X2	T48.1X3	T48.1X4	T48.1X5	T48.1X6
Febarbamate	T42.3X1	T42.3X2	T42.3X3	T42.3X4	T42.3X5	T42.3X6
Fecal softener	T47.4X1	T47.4X2	T47.4X3	T47.4X4	T47.4X5	T47.4X6
Fedrilate	T48.3X1	T48.3X2	T48.3X3	T48.3X4	T48.3X5	T48.3X6
Felodipine	T46.1X1	T46.1X2	T46.1X3	T46.1X4	T46.1X5	T46.1X6
Felypressin	T38.891	T38.892	T38.893	T38.894	T38.895	T38.896
Femoxetine	T43.221	T43.222	T43.223	T43.224	T43.225	T43.226
Fenalcomine	T46.3X1	T46.3X2	T46.3X3	T46.3X4	T46.3X5	T46.3X6
Fenamisal	T37.1X1	T37.1X2	T37.1X3	T37.1X4	T37.1X5	T37.1X6
Fenazone	T39.2X1	T39.2X2	T39.2X3	T39.2X4	T39.2X5	T39.2X6
Fenbendazole	T37.4X1	T37.4X2	T37.4X3	T37.4X4	T37.4X5	T37.4X6
Fenbutrazate	T50.5X1	T50.5X2	T50.5X3	T50.5X4	T50.5X5	T50.5X6
Fencamfamine	T43.691	T43.692	T43.693	T43.694	T43.695	T43.696
Fendiline	T46.1X1	T46.1X2	T46.1X3	T46.1X4	T46.1X5	T46.1X6
Fenetylline	T43.691	T43.692	T43.693	T43.694	T43.695	T43.696
Fenflumizole	T39.391	T39.392	T39.393	T39.394	T39.395	T39.396
Fenfluramine	T50.5X1	T50.5X2	T50.5X3	T50.5X4	T50.5X5	T50.5X6
Fenobarbital	T42.3X1	T42.3X2	T42.3X3	T42.3X4	T42.3X5	T42.3X6

Fenofibrate - Fominoben

Substance	Poisoning, Accidental unintentional	Poisoning, Intentional self-harm	Poisoning, Assault	Poisoning, Undetermined	Adverse effect	Underdosing
Fenofibrate	T46.6X1	T46.6X2	T46.6X3	T46.6X4	T46.6X5	T46.6X6
Fenoprofen	T39.311	T39.312	T39.313	T39.314	T39.315	T39.316
Fenoterol	T48.6X1	T48.6X2	T48.6X3	T48.6X4	T48.6X5	T48.6X6
Fenoverine	T44.3X1	T44.3X2	T44.3X3	T44.3X4	T44.3X5	T44.3X6
Fenoxazoline	T48.5X1	T48.5X2	T48.5X3	T48.5X4	T48.5X5	T48.5X6
Fenproporex	T50.5X1	T50.5X2	T50.5X3	T50.5X4	T50.5X5	T50.5X6
Fenquizone	T50.2X1	T50.2X2	T50.2X3	T50.2X4	T50.2X5	T50.2X6
Fentanyl	T40.4X1	T40.4X2	T40.4X3	T40.4X4	T40.4X5	T40.4X6
Fentazin	T43.3X1	T43.3X2	T43.3X3	T43.3X4	T43.3X5	T43.3X6
Fenthion	T60.0X1	T60.0X2	T60.0X3	T60.0X4	--	--
Fenticlor	T49.0X1	T49.0X2	T49.0X3	T49.0X4	T49.0X5	T49.0X6
Fenylbutazone	T39.2X1	T39.2X2	T39.2X3	T39.2X4	T39.2X5	T39.2X6
Feprazone	T39.2X1	T39.2X2	T39.2X3	T39.2X4	T39.2X5	T39.2X6
Fer de lance (bite) (venom)	T63.061	T63.062	T63.063	T63.064	--	--
Ferric — *see also Iron*						
chloride	T45.4X1	T45.4X2	T45.4X3	T45.4X4	T45.4X5	T45.4X6
citrate	T45.4X1	T45.4X2	T45.4X3	T45.4X4	T45.4X5	T45.4X6
hydroxide						
colloidal	T45.4X1	T45.4X2	T45.4X3	T45.4X4	T45.4X5	T45.4X6
polymaltose	T45.4X1	T45.4X2	T45.4X3	T45.4X4	T45.4X5	T45.4X6
pyrophosphate	T45.4X1	T45.4X2	T45.4X3	T45.4X4	T45.4X5	T45.4X6
Ferritin	T45.4X1	T45.4X2	T45.4X3	T45.4X4	T45.4X5	T45.4X6
Ferrocholinate	T45.4X1	T45.4X2	T45.4X3	T45.4X4	T45.4X5	T45.4X6
Ferrodextrane	T45.4X1	T45.4X2	T45.4X3	T45.4X4	T45.4X5	T45.4X6
Ferropolimaler	T45.4X1	T45.4X2	T45.4X3	T45.4X4	T45.4X5	T45.4X6
Ferrous — *see also Iron*						
phosphate	T45.4X1	T45.4X2	T45.4X3	T45.4X4	T45.4X5	T45.4X6
salt	T45.4X1	T45.4X2	T45.4X3	T45.4X4	T45.4X5	T45.4X6
with folic acid	T45.4X1	T45.4X2	T45.4X3	T45.4X4	T45.4X5	T45.4X6
Ferrous fumerate, gluconate, lactate, salt NEC, sulfate (medicinal)	T45.4X1	T45.4X2	T45.4X3	T45.4X4	T45.4X5	T45.4X6
Ferrovanadium (fumes)	T59.891	T59.892	T59.893	T59.894	--	--
Ferrum — *see Iron*						
Fertilizers NEC	T65.891	T65.892	T65.893	T65.894	--	--
with herbicide mixture	T60.3X1	T60.3X2	T60.3X3	T60.3X4	--	--
Fetoxilate	T47.6X1	T47.6X2	T47.6X3	T47.6X4	T47.6X5	T47.6X6
Fiber, dietary	T47.4X1	T47.4X2	T47.4X3	T47.4X4	T47.4X5	T47.4X6
Fiberglass	T65.831	T65.832	T65.833	T65.834	--	--
Fibrinogen (human)	T45.8X1	T45.8X2	T45.8X3	T45.8X4	T45.8X5	T45.8X6
Fibrinolysin (human)	T45.691	T45.692	T45.693	T45.694	T45.695	T45.696
Fibrinolysis						
affecting drug	T45.601	T45.602	T45.603	T45.604	T45.605	T45.606
inhibitor NEC	T45.621	T45.622	T45.623	T45.624	T45.625	T45.626
Fibrinolytic drug	T45.611	T45.612	T45.613	T45.614	T45.615	T45.616
Filix mas	T37.4X1	T37.4X2	T37.4X3	T37.4X4	T37.4X5	T37.4X6
Filtering cream	T49.3X1	T49.3X2	T49.3X3	T49.3X4	T49.3X5	T49.3X6
Fiorinal	T39.011	T39.012	T39.013	T39.014	T39.015	T39.016
Firedamp	T59.891	T59.892	T59.893	T59.894	--	--
Fish, noxious, nonbacterial	T61.91	T61.92	T61.93	T61.94	--	--
ciguatera	T61.01	T61.02	T61.03	T61.04	--	--
scombroid	T61.11	T61.12	T61.13	T61.14	--	--
shell	T61.781	T61.782	T61.783	T61.784	--	--
specified NEC	T61.771	T61.772	T61.773	T61.774	--	--
Flagyl	T37.3X1	T37.3X2	T37.3X3	T37.3X4	T37.3X5	T37.3X6
Flavine adenine dinucleotide	T45.2X1	T45.2X2	T45.2X3	T45.2X4	T45.2X5	T45.2X6
Flavodic acid	T46.991	T46.992	T46.993	T46.994	T46.995	T46.996
Flavoxate	T44.3X1	T44.3X2	T44.3X3	T44.3X4	T44.3X5	T44.3X6
Flaxedil	T48.1X1	T48.1X2	T48.1X3	T48.1X4	T48.1X5	T48.1X6
Flaxseed (medicinal)	T49.3X1	T49.3X2	T49.3X3	T49.3X4	T49.3X5	T49.3X6
Flecainide	T46.2X1	T46.2X2	T46.2X3	T46.2X4	T46.2X5	T46.2X6
Fleroxacin	T36.8X1	T36.8X2	T36.8X3	T36.8X4	T36.8X5	T36.8X6
Floctafenine	T39.8X1	T39.8X2	T39.8X3	T39.8X4	T39.8X5	T39.8X6
Flomax	T44.6X1	T44.6X2	T44.6X3	T44.6X4	T44.6X5	T44.6X6
Flomoxef	T36.1X1	T36.1X2	T36.1X3	T36.1X4	T36.1X5	T36.1X6
Flopropione	T44.3X1	T44.3X2	T44.3X3	T44.3X4	T44.3X5	T44.3X6
Florantyrone	T47.5X1	T47.5X2	T47.5X3	T47.5X4	T47.5X5	T47.5X6
Floraquin	T37.8X1	T37.8X2	T37.8X3	T37.8X4	T37.8X5	T37.8X6
Florinef	T38.0X1	T38.0X2	T38.0X3	T38.0X4	T38.0X5	T38.0X6
ENT agent	T49.6X1	T49.6X2	T49.6X3	T49.6X4	T49.6X5	T49.6X6
ophthalmic preparation	T49.5X1	T49.5X2	T49.5X3	T49.5X4	T49.5X5	T49.5X6
topical NEC	T49.0X1	T49.0X2	T49.0X3	T49.0X4	T49.0X5	T49.0X6
Flowers of sulfur	T49.4X1	T49.4X2	T49.4X3	T49.4X4	T49.4X5	T49.4X6
Floxuridine	T45.1X1	T45.1X2	T45.1X3	T45.1X4	T45.1X5	T45.1X6
Fluanisone	T43.4X1	T43.4X2	T43.4X3	T43.4X4	T43.4X5	T43.4X6
Flubendazole	T37.4X1	T37.4X2	T37.4X3	T37.4X4	T37.4X5	T37.4X6
Fluclorolone acetonide	T49.0X1	T49.0X2	T49.0X3	T49.0X4	T49.0X5	T49.0X6
Flucloxacillin	T36.0X1	T36.0X2	T36.0X3	T36.0X4	T36.0X5	T36.0X6
Fluconazole	T37.8X1	T37.8X2	T37.8X3	T37.8X4	T37.8X5	T37.8X6
Flucytosine	T37.8X1	T37.8X2	T37.8X3	T37.8X4	T37.8X5	T37.8X6
Fludeoxyglucose (18F)	T50.8X1	T50.8X2	T50.8X3	T50.8X4	T50.8X5	T50.8X6
Fludiazepam	T42.4X1	T42.4X2	T42.4X3	T42.4X4	T42.4X5	T42.4X6
Fludrocortisone	T50.0X1	T50.0X2	T50.0X3	T50.0X4	T50.0X5	T50.0X6
ENT agent	T49.6X1	T49.6X2	T49.6X3	T49.6X4	T49.6X5	T49.6X6
ophthalmic preparation	T49.5X1	T49.5X2	T49.5X3	T49.5X4	T49.5X5	T49.5X6
topical NEC	T49.0X1	T49.0X2	T49.0X3	T49.0X4	T49.0X5	T49.0X6
Fludroxycortide	T49.0X1	T49.0X2	T49.0X3	T49.0X4	T49.0X5	T49.0X6
Flufenamic acid	T39.391	T39.392	T39.393	T39.394	T39.395	T39.396
Fluindione	T45.511	T45.512	T45.513	T45.514	T45.515	T45.516
Flumequine	T37.8X1	T37.8X2	T37.8X3	T37.8X4	T37.8X5	T37.8X6
Flumethasone	T49.0X1	T49.0X2	T49.0X3	T49.0X4	T49.0X5	T49.0X6
Flumethiazide	T50.2X1	T50.2X2	T50.2X3	T50.2X4	T50.2X5	T50.2X6
Flumidin	T37.5X1	T37.5X2	T37.5X3	T37.5X4	T37.5X5	T37.5X6
Flunarizine	T46.7X1	T46.7X2	T46.7X3	T46.7X4	T46.7X5	T46.7X6
Flunidazole	T37.8X1	T37.8X2	T37.8X3	T37.8X4	T37.8X5	T37.8X6
Flunisolide	T48.6X1	T48.6X2	T48.6X3	T48.6X4	T48.6X5	T48.6X6
Flunitrazepam	T42.4X1	T42.4X2	T42.4X3	T42.4X4	T42.4X5	T42.4X6
Fluocinolone (acetonide)	T49.0X1	T49.0X2	T49.0X3	T49.0X4	T49.0X5	T49.0X6
Fluocinonide	T49.0X1	T49.0X2	T49.0X3	T49.0X4	T49.0X5	T49.0X6
Fluocortin (butyl)	T49.0X1	T49.0X2	T49.0X3	T49.0X4	T49.0X5	T49.0X6
Fluocortolone	T49.0X1	T49.0X2	T49.0X3	T49.0X4	T49.0X5	T49.0X6
Fluohydrocortisone	T38.0X1	T38.0X2	T38.0X3	T38.0X4	T38.0X5	T38.0X6
ENT agent	T49.6X1	T49.6X2	T49.6X3	T49.6X4	T49.6X5	T49.6X6
ophthalmic preparation	T49.5X1	T49.5X2	T49.5X3	T49.5X4	T49.5X5	T49.5X6
topical NEC	T49.0X1	T49.0X2	T49.0X3	T49.0X4	T49.0X5	T49.0X6
Fluonid	T49.0X1	T49.0X2	T49.0X3	T49.0X4	T49.0X5	T49.0X6
Fluopromazine	T43.3X1	T43.3X2	T43.3X3	T43.3X4	T43.3X5	T43.3X6
Fluoracetate	T60.8X1	T60.8X2	T60.8X3	T60.8X4	--	--
Fluorescein	T50.8X1	T50.8X2	T50.8X3	T50.8X4	T50.8X5	T50.8X6
Fluorhydrocortisone	T50.0X1	T50.0X2	T50.0X3	T50.0X4	T50.0X5	T50.0X6
Fluoride (nonmedicinal) (pesticide) (sodium) **NEC**	T60.8X1	T60.8X2	T60.8X3	T60.8X4	--	--
hydrogen — *see Hydrofluoric acid*						
medicinal NEC	T50.991	T50.992	T50.993	T50.994	T50.995	T50.996
dental use	T49.7X1	T49.7X2	T49.7X3	T49.7X4	T49.7X5	T49.7X6
not pesticide NEC	T54.91	T54.92	T54.93	T54.94	--	--
stannous	T49.7X1	T49.7X2	T49.7X3	T49.7X4	T49.7X5	T49.7X6
Fluorinated corticosteroids	T38.0X1	T38.0X2	T38.0X3	T38.0X4	T38.0X5	T38.0X6
Fluorine (gas)	T59.5X1	T59.5X2	T59.5X3	T59.5X4	--	--
salt — *see Fluoride (s)*						
Fluoristan	T49.7X1	T49.7X2	T49.7X3	T49.7X4	T49.7X5	T49.7X6
Fluormetholone	T49.0X1	T49.0X2	T49.0X3	T49.0X4	T49.0X5	T49.0X6
Fluoroacetate	T60.8X1	T60.8X2	T60.8X3	T60.8X4	--	--
Fluorocarbon monomer	T53.6X1	T53.6X2	T53.6X3	T53.6X4	--	--
Fluorocytosine	T37.8X1	T37.8X2	T37.8X3	T37.8X4	T37.8X5	T37.8X6
Fluorodeoxyuridine	T45.1X1	T45.1X2	T45.1X3	T45.1X4	T45.1X5	T45.1X6
Fluorometholone	T49.0X1	T49.0X2	T49.0X3	T49.0X4	T49.0X5	T49.0X6
ophthalmic preparation	T49.5X1	T49.5X2	T49.5X3	T49.5X4	T49.5X5	T49.5X6
Fluorophosphate insecticide	T60.0X1	T60.0X2	T60.0X3	T60.0X4	--	--
Fluorosol	T46.3X1	T46.3X2	T46.3X3	T46.3X4	T46.3X5	T46.3X6
Fluorouracil	T45.1X1	T45.1X2	T45.1X3	T45.1X4	T45.1X5	T45.1X6
Fluorphenylalanine	T49.5X1	T49.5X2	T49.5X3	T49.5X4	T49.5X5	T49.5X6
Fluothane	T41.0X1	T41.0X2	T41.0X3	T41.0X4	T41.0X5	T41.0X6
Fluoxetine	T43.221	T43.222	T43.223	T43.224	T43.225	T43.226
Fluoxymesterone	T38.7X1	T38.7X2	T38.7X3	T38.7X4	T38.7X5	T38.7X6
Flupenthixol	T43.4X1	T43.4X2	T43.4X3	T43.4X4	T43.4X5	T43.4X6
Flupentixol	T43.4X1	T43.4X2	T43.4X3	T43.4X4	T43.4X5	T43.4X6
Fluphenazine	T43.3X1	T43.3X2	T43.3X3	T43.3X4	T43.3X5	T43.3X6
Fluprednidene	T49.0X1	T49.0X2	T49.0X3	T49.0X4	T49.0X5	T49.0X6
Fluprednisolone	T38.0X1	T38.0X2	T38.0X3	T38.0X4	T38.0X5	T38.0X6
Fluradoline	T39.8X1	T39.8X2	T39.8X3	T39.8X4	T39.8X5	T39.8X6
Flurandrenolide	T49.0X1	T49.0X2	T49.0X3	T49.0X4	T49.0X5	T49.0X6
Flurandrenolone	T49.0X1	T49.0X2	T49.0X3	T49.0X4	T49.0X5	T49.0X6
Flurazepam	T42.4X1	T42.4X2	T42.4X3	T42.4X4	T42.4X5	T42.4X6
Flurbiprofen	T39.311	T39.312	T39.313	T39.314	T39.315	T39.316
Flurobate	T49.0X1	T49.0X2	T49.0X3	T49.0X4	T49.0X5	T49.0X6
Fluroxene	T41.0X1	T41.0X2	T41.0X3	T41.0X4	T41.0X5	T41.0X6
Fluspirilene	T43.591	T43.592	T43.593	T43.594	T43.595	T43.596
Flutamide	T38.6X1	T38.6X2	T38.6X3	T38.6X4	T38.6X5	T38.6X6
Flutazolam	T42.4X1	T42.4X2	T42.4X3	T42.4X4	T42.4X5	T42.4X6
Fluticasone propionate	T49.1X1	T49.1X2	T49.1X3	T49.1X4	T49.1X5	T49.1X6
Flutoprazepam	T42.4X1	T42.4X2	T42.4X3	T42.4X4	T42.4X5	T42.4X6
Flutropium bromide	T48.6X1	T48.6X2	T48.6X3	T48.6X4	T48.6X5	T48.6X6
Fluvoxamine	T43.221	T43.222	T43.223	T43.224	T43.225	T43.226
Folacin	T45.8X1	T45.8X2	T45.8X3	T45.8X4	T45.8X5	T45.8X6
Folic acid	T45.8X1	T45.8X2	T45.8X3	T45.8X4	T45.8X5	T45.8X6
with ferrous salt	T45.2X1	T45.2X2	T45.2X3	T45.2X4	T45.2X5	T45.2X6
antagonist	T45.1X1	T45.1X2	T45.1X3	T45.1X4	T45.1X5	T45.1X6
Folinic acid	T45.8X1	T45.8X2	T45.8X3	T45.8X4	T45.8X5	T45.8X6
Folium stramoniae	T48.6X1	T48.6X2	T48.6X3	T48.6X4	T48.6X5	T48.6X6
Follicle-stimulating hormone, human	T38.811	T38.812	T38.813	T38.814	T38.815	T38.816
Folpet	T60.3X1	T60.3X2	T60.3X3	T60.3X4	--	--
Fominoben	T48.3X1	T48.3X2	T48.3X3	T48.3X4	T48.3X5	T48.3X6

Substance	Poisoning, Accidental unintentional	Poisoning, Intentional self-harm	Poisoning, Assault	Poisoning, Undetermined	Adverse effect	Underdosing
Food, foodstuffs, noxious, nonbacterial, NEC	T62.91	T62.92	T62.93	T62.94	--	--
berries	T62.1X1	T62.1X2	T62.1X3	T62.1X4	--	--
fish — *see also Fish*	T61.91	T61.92	T61.93	T61.94	--	--
mushrooms	T62.0X1	T62.0X2	T62.0X3	T62.0X4	--	--
plants	T62.2X1	T62.2X2	T62.2X3	T62.2X4	--	--
seafood	T61.91	T61.92	T61.93	T61.94	--	--
specified NEC	T61.8X1	T61.8X2	T61.8X3	T61.8X4	--	--
seeds	T62.2X1	T62.2X2	T62.2X3	T62.2X4	--	--
shellfish	T61.781	T61.782	T61.783	T61.784	--	--
specified NEC	T62.8X1	T62.8X2	T62.8X3	T62.8X4	--	--
Fool's parsley	T62.2X1	T62.2X2	T62.2X3	T62.2X4	--	--
Formaldehyde (solution), **gas or vapor**	T59.2X1	T59.2X2	T59.2X3	T59.2X4	--	--
fungicide	T60.3X1	T60.3X2	T60.3X3	T60.3X4	--	--
Formalin	T59.2X1	T59.2X2	T59.2X3	T59.2X4	--	--
fungicide	T60.3X1	T60.3X2	T60.3X3	T60.3X4	--	--
vapor	T59.2X1	T59.2X2	T59.2X3	T59.2X4	--	--
Formic acid	T54.2X1	T54.2X2	T54.2X3	T54.2X4	--	--
vapor	T59.891	T59.892	T59.893	T59.894	--	--
Foscarnet sodium	T37.5X1	T37.5X2	T37.5X3	T37.5X4	T37.5X5	T37.5X6
Fosfestrol	T38.5X1	T38.5X2	T38.5X3	T38.5X4	T38.5X5	T38.5X6
Fosfomycin	T36.8X1	T36.8X2	T36.8X3	T36.8X4	T36.8X5	T36.8X6
Fosfonet sodium	T37.5X1	T37.5X2	T37.5X3	T37.5X4	T37.5X5	T37.5X6
Fosinopril	T46.4X1	T46.4X2	T46.4X3	T46.4X4	T46.4X5	T46.4X6
sodium	T46.4X1	T46.4X2	T46.4X3	T46.4X4	T46.4X5	T46.4X6
Fowler's solution	T57.0X1	T57.0X2	T57.0X3	T57.0X4	--	--
Foxglove	T62.2X1	T62.2X2	T62.2X3	T62.2X4	--	--
Framycetin	T36.5X1	T36.5X2	T36.5X3	T36.5X4	T36.5X5	T36.5X6
Frangula	T47.2X1	T47.2X2	T47.2X3	T47.2X4	T47.2X5	T47.2X6
extract	T47.2X1	T47.2X2	T47.2X3	T47.2X4	T47.2X5	T47.2X6
Frei antigen	T50.8X1	T50.8X2	T50.8X3	T50.8X4	T50.8X5	T50.8X6
Freon	T53.5X1	T53.5X2	T53.5X3	T53.5X4	--	--
Fructose	T50.3X1	T50.3X2	T50.3X3	T50.3X4	T50.3X5	T50.3X6
Frusemide	T50.1X1	T50.1X2	T50.1X3	T50.1X4	T50.1X5	T50.1X6
FSH	T38.811	T38.812	T38.813	T38.814	T38.815	T38.816
Ftorafur	T45.1X1	T45.1X2	T45.1X3	T45.1X4	T45.1X5	T45.1X6
Fuel						
automobile	T52.0X1	T52.0X2	T52.0X3	T52.0X4	--	--
exhaust gas, not in transit	T58.01	T58.02	T58.03	T58.04	--	--
vapor NEC	T52.0X1	T52.0X2	T52.0X3	T52.0X4	--	--
gas (domestic use) — *see also Carbon, monoxide, fuel, utility*	T59.891	T59.892	T59.893	T59.894	--	--
utility	T59.891	T59.892	T59.893	T59.894	--	--
in mobile container	T59.891	T59.892	T59.893	T59.894	--	--
incomplete combustion of — *see Carbon, monoxide, fuel, utility*						
piped (natural)	T59.891	T59.892	T59.893	T59.894	--	--
industrial, incomplete combustion	T58.8X1	T58.8X2	T58.8X3	T58.8X4	--	--
Fugillin	T36.8X1	T36.8X2	T36.8X3	T36.8X4	T36.8X5	T36.8X6
Fulminate of mercury	T56.1X1	T56.1X2	T56.1X3	T56.1X4	--	--
Fulvicin	T36.7X1	T36.7X2	T36.7X3	T36.7X4	T36.7X5	T36.7X6
Fumadil	T36.8X1	T36.8X2	T36.8X3	T36.8X4	T36.8X5	T36.8X6
Fumagillin	T36.8X1	T36.8X2	T36.8X3	T36.8X4	T36.8X5	T36.8X6
Fumaric acid	T49.4X1	T49.4X2	T49.4X3	T49.4X4	T49.4X5	T49.4X6
Fumes (from)	T59.91	T59.92	T59.93	T59.94	--	--
carbon monoxide — *see Carbon, monoxide*						
charcoal (domestic use) — *see Charcoal, fumes*						
chloroform — *see Chloroform*						
coke (in domestic stoves, fireplaces) — *see Coke fumes*						
corrosive NEC	T54.91	T54.92	T54.93	T54.94	--	--
ether — *see ether*						
freons	T53.5X1	T53.5X2	T53.5X3	T53.5X4	--	--
hydrocarbons	T59.891	T59.892	T59.893	T59.894	--	--
petroleum (liquefied)	T59.891	T59.892	T59.893	T59.894	--	--
distributed through pipes (pure or mixed with air)	T59.891	T59.892	T59.893	T59.894	--	--
lead — *see lead*						
metal — *see Metals, or the specified metal*						
nitrogen dioxide	T59.0X1	T59.0X2	T59.0X3	T59.0X4	--	--
pesticides — *see Pesticides*						

Substance	Poisoning, Accidental unintentional	Poisoning, Intentional self-harm	Poisoning, Assault	Poisoning, Undetermined	Adverse effect	Underdosing
Fumes — *continued*						
petroleum (liquefied)	T59.891	T59.892	T59.893	T59.894	--	--
distributed through pipes (pure or mixed with air)	T59.891	T59.892	T59.893	T59.894	--	--
polyester	T59.891	T59.892	T59.893	T59.894	--	--
specified source NEC — *see also substance specified*	T59.891	T59.892	T59.893	T59.894	--	--
sulfur dioxide	T59.1X1	T59.1X2	T59.1X3	T59.1X4	--	--
Fumigant NEC	T60.91	T60.92	T60.93	T60.94	--	--
Fungi, noxious, used as food	T62.0X1	T62.0X2	T62.0X3	T62.0X4	--	--
Fungicide NEC (nonmedicinal)	T60.3X1	T60.3X2	T60.3X3	T60.3X4	--	--
Fungizone	T36.7X1	T36.7X2	T36.7X3	T36.7X4	T36.7X5	T36.7X6
topical	T49.0X1	T49.0X2	T49.0X3	T49.0X4	T49.0X5	T49.0X6
Furacin	T49.0X1	T49.0X2	T49.0X3	T49.0X4	T49.0X5	T49.0X6
Furadantin	T37.91	T37.92	T37.93	T37.94	T37.95	T37.96
Furazolidone	T37.8X1	T37.8X2	T37.8X3	T37.8X4	T37.8X5	T37.8X6
Furazolium chloride	T49.0X1	T49.0X2	T49.0X3	T49.0X4	T49.0X5	T49.0X6
Furfural	T52.8X1	T52.8X2	T52.8X3	T52.8X4	--	--
Furnace (coal burning) (domestic), **gas from**	T58.2X1	T58.2X2	T58.2X3	T58.2X4	--	--
industrial	T58.8X1	T58.8X2	T58.8X3	T58.8X4	--	--
Furniture polish	T65.891	T65.892	T65.893	T65.894	--	--
Furosemide	T50.1X1	T50.1X2	T50.1X3	T50.1X4	T50.1X5	T50.1X6
Furoxone	T37.91	T37.92	T37.93	T37.94	T37.95	T37.96
Fursultiamine	T45.2X1	T45.2X2	T45.2X3	T45.2X4	T45.2X5	T45.2X6
Fusafungine	T36.8X1	T36.8X2	T36.8X3	T36.8X4	T36.8X5	T36.8X6
Fusel oil (any) (amyl) (butyl) (propyl), **vapor**	T51.3X1	T51.3X2	T51.3X3	T51.3X4	--	--
Fusidate (ethanolamine) (sodium)	T36.8X1	T36.8X2	T36.8X3	T36.8X4	T36.8X5	T36.8X6
Fusidic acid	T36.8X1	T36.8X2	T36.8X3	T36.8X4	T36.8X5	T36.8X6
Fytic acid, nonasodium	T50.6X1	T50.6X2	T50.6X3	T50.6X4	T50.6X5	T50.6X6
G						
GABA	T43.8X1	T43.8X2	T43.8X3	T43.8X4	T43.8X5	T43.8X6
Gadopentetic acid	T50.8X1	T50.8X2	T50.8X3	T50.8X4	T50.8X5	T50.8X6
Galactose	T50.3X1	T50.3X2	T50.3X3	T50.3X4	T50.3X5	T50.3X6
b-Galactosidase	T47.5X1	T47.5X2	T47.5X3	T47.5X4	T47.5X5	T47.5X6
Galantamine	T44.0X1	T44.0X2	T44.0X3	T44.0X4	T44.0X5	T44.0X6
Gallamine (triethiodide)	T48.1X1	T48.1X2	T48.1X3	T48.1X4	T48.1X5	T48.1X6
Gallium citrate	T50.991	T50.992	T50.993	T50.994	T50.995	T50.996
Gallopamil	T46.1X1	T46.1X2	T46.1X3	T46.1X4	T46.1X5	T46.1X6
Gamboge	T47.2X1	T47.2X2	T47.2X3	T47.2X4	T47.2X5	T47.2X6
Gamimune	T50.Z11	T50.Z12	T50.Z13	T50.Z14	T50.Z15	T50.Z16
Gamma globulin	T50.Z11	T50.Z12	T50.Z13	T50.Z14	T50.Z15	T50.Z16
Gamma-aminobutyric acid	T43.8X1	T43.8X2	T43.8X3	T43.8X4	T43.8X5	T43.8X6
Gamma-benzene hexachloride (medicinal)	T49.0X1	T49.0X2	T49.0X3	T49.0X4	T49.0X5	T49.0X6
nonmedicinal, vapor	T53.6X1	T53.6X2	T53.6X3	T53.6X4	--	--
Gamma-BHC (medicinal) — *see also Gamma-benzene hexachloride*	T49.0X1	T49.0X2	T49.0X3	T49.0X4	T49.0X5	T49.0X6
Gamulin	T50.Z11	T50.Z12	T50.Z13	T50.Z14	T50.Z15	T50.Z16
Ganciclovir (sodium)	T37.5X1	T37.5X2	T37.5X3	T37.5X4	T37.5X5	T37.5X6
Ganglionic blocking drug NEC	T44.2X1	T44.2X2	T44.2X3	T44.2X4	T44.2X5	T44.2X6
specified NEC	T44.2X1	T44.2X2	T44.2X3	T44.2X4	T44.2X5	T44.2X6
Ganja	T40.7X1	T40.7X2	T40.7X3	T40.7X4	T40.7X5	T40.7X6
Garamycin	T36.5X1	T36.5X2	T36.5X3	T36.5X4	T36.5X5	T36.5X6
ophthalmic preparation	T49.5X1	T49.5X2	T49.5X3	T49.5X4	T49.5X5	T49.5X6
topical NEC	T49.0X1	T49.0X2	T49.0X3	T49.0X4	T49.0X5	T49.0X6
Gardenal	T42.3X1	T42.3X2	T42.3X3	T42.3X4	T42.3X5	T42.3X6
Gardepanyl	T42.3X1	T42.3X2	T42.3X3	T42.3X4	T42.3X5	T42.3X6
Gas	T59.91	T59.92	T59.93	T59.94	--	--
acetylene	T59.891	T59.892	T59.893	T59.894	--	--
incomplete combustion of	T58.11	T58.12	T58.13	T58.14	--	--
air contaminants, source or type not specified	T59.91	T59.92	T59.93	T59.94	--	--
anesthetic	T41.0X1	T41.0X2	T41.0X3	T41.0X4	T41.0X5	T41.0X6
blast furnace	T58.8X1	T58.8X2	T58.8X3	T58.8X4	--	--
butane — *see butane*						
carbon monoxide — *see Carbon, monoxide*						
chlorine	T59.4X1	T59.4X2	T59.4X3	T59.4X4	--	--
coal	T58.2X1	T58.2X2	T58.2X3	T58.2X4	--	--
cyanide	T57.3X1	T57.3X2	T57.3X3	T57.3X4	--	--
dicyanogen	T65.0X1	T65.0X2	T65.0X3	T65.0X4	--	--
domestic — *see Domestic gas*						
exhaust	T58.01	T58.02	T58.03	T58.04	--	--

Substance	Poisoning, Accidental unintentional	Poisoning, Intentional self-harm	Poisoning, Assault	Poisoning, Undetermined	Adverse effect	Underdosing
Gas — *continued*						
from utility (for cooking, heating, or lighting) (after combustion) — *see Carbon, monoxide, fuel, utility*						
prior to combustion	T59.891	T59.892	T59.893	T59.894	--	--
from wood- or coal-burning stove or fireplace	T58.2X1	T58.2X2	T58.2X3	T58.2X4	--	--
fuel (domestic use) (after combustion) — *see also Carbon, monoxide, fuel*						
industrial use	T58.8X1	T58.8X2	T58.8X3	T58.8X4	--	--
prior to combustion	T59.891	T59.892	T59.893	T59.894	--	--
utility	T59.891	T59.892	T59.893	T59.894	--	--
in mobile container	T59.891	T59.892	T59.893	T59.894	--	--
incomplete combustion of — *see Carbon, monoxide, fuel, utility*						
piped (natural)	T59.891	T59.892	T59.893	T59.894	--	--
garage	T58.01	T58.02	T58.03	T58.04	--	--
hydrocarbon NEC	T59.891	T59.892	T59.893	T59.894	--	--
incomplete combustion of — *see Carbon, monoxide, fuel, utility*						
liquefied — *see butane*						
piped	T59.891	T59.892	T59.893	T59.894	--	--
hydrocyanic acid	T65.0X1	T65.0X2	T65.0X3	T65.0X4	--	--
illuminating (after combustion)	T58.11	T58.12	T58.13	T58.14	--	--
prior to combustion	T59.891	T59.892	T59.893	T59.894	--	--
incomplete combustion, any — *see Carbon, monoxide*						
kiln	T58.8X1	T58.8X2	T58.8X3	T58.8X4	--	--
lacrimogenic	T59.3X1	T59.3X2	T59.3X3	T59.3X4	--	--
liquefied petroleum — *see butane*						
marsh	T59.891	T59.892	T59.893	T59.894	--	--
motor exhaust, not in transit	T58.01	T58.02	T58.03	T58.04	--	--
mustard, not in war	T59.891	T59.892	T59.893	T59.894	--	--
natural	T59.891	T59.892	T59.893	T59.894	--	--
nerve, not in war	T59.91	T59.92	T59.93	T59.94	--	--
oil	T52.0X1	T52.0X2	T52.0X3	T52.0X4	--	--
petroleum (liquefied) (distributed in mobile containers)	T59.891	T59.892	T59.893	T59.894	--	--
piped (pure or mixed with air)	T59.891	T59.892	T59.893	T59.894	--	--
piped (manufactured) (natural) NEC	T59.891	T59.892	T59.893	T59.894	--	--
producer	T58.8X1	T58.8X2	T58.8X3	T58.8X4	--	--
propane — *see propane*						
refrigerant (chlorofluoro-carbon)	T53.5X1	T53.5X2	T53.5X3	T53.5X4	--	--
not chlorofluoro-carbon	T59.891	T59.892	T59.893	T59.894	--	--
sewer	T59.91	T59.92	T59.93	T59.94	--	--
specified source NEC	T59.91	T59.92	T59.93	T59.94	--	--
stove (after combustion)	T58.11	T58.12	T58.13	T58.14	--	--
prior to combustion	T59.891	T59.892	T59.893	T59.894	--	--
tear	T59.3X1	T59.3X2	T59.3X3	T59.3X4	--	--
therapeutic	T41.5X1	T41.5X2	T41.5X3	T41.5X4	T41.5X5	T41.5X6
utility (for cooking, heating, or lighting) (piped) NEC	T59.891	T59.892	T59.893	T59.894	--	--
in mobile container	T59.891	T59.892	T59.893	T59.894	--	--
incomplete combustion of — *see Carbon, monoxide, fuel, utilty*						
piped (natural)	T59.891	T59.892	T59.893	T59.894	--	--
water	T58.11	T58.12	T58.13	T58.14	--	--
incomplete combustion of — *see Carbon, monoxide, fuel, utility*						
Gaseous substance — *see Gas*						
Gasoline	T52.0X1	T52.0X2	T52.0X3	T52.0X4	--	--
vapor	T52.0X1	T52.0X2	T52.0X3	T52.0X4	--	--
Gastric enzymes	T47.5X1	T47.5X2	T47.5X3	T47.5X4	T47.5X5	T47.5X6
Gastrografin	T50.8X1	T50.8X2	T50.8X3	T50.8X4	T50.8X5	T50.8X6
Gastrointestinal drug	T47.91	T47.92	T47.93	T47.94	T47.95	T47.96
biological	T47.8X1	T47.8X2	T47.8X3	T47.8X4	T47.8X5	T47.8X6
specified NEC	T47.8X1	T47.8X2	T47.8X3	T47.8X4	T47.8X5	T47.8X6
Gaultheria procumbens	T62.2X1	T62.2X2	T62.2X3	T62.2X4	--	--
Gefarnate	T44.3X1	T44.3X2	T44.3X3	T44.3X4	T44.3X5	T44.3X6
Gelatin (intravenous)	T45.8X1	T45.8X2	T45.8X3	T45.8X4	T45.8X5	T45.8X6
absorbable (sponge)	T45.7X1	T45.7X2	T45.7X3	T45.7X4	T45.7X5	T45.7X6
Gelfilm	T49.8X1	T49.8X2	T49.8X3	T49.8X4	T49.8X5	T49.8X6
Gelfoam	T45.7X1	T45.7X2	T45.7X3	T45.7X4	T45.7X5	T45.7X6
Gelsemine	T50.991	T50.992	T50.993	T50.994	T50.995	T50.996
Gelsemium (sempervirens)	T62.2X1	T62.2X2	T62.2X3	T62.2X4	--	--
Gemeprost	T48.0X1	T48.0X2	T48.0X3	T48.0X4	T48.0X5	T48.0X6
Gemfibrozil	T46.6X1	T46.6X2	T46.6X3	T46.6X4	T46.6X5	T46.6X6
Gemonil	T42.3X1	T42.3X2	T42.3X3	T42.3X4	T42.3X5	T42.3X6
Gentamicin	T36.5X1	T36.5X2	T36.5X3	T36.5X4	T36.5X5	T36.5X6
ophthalmic preparation	T49.5X1	T49.5X2	T49.5X3	T49.5X4	T49.5X5	T49.5X6
topical NEC	T49.0X1	T49.0X2	T49.0X3	T49.0X4	T49.0X5	T49.0X6
Gentian	T47.5X1	T47.5X2	T47.5X3	T47.5X4	T47.5X5	T47.5X6
violet	T49.0X1	T49.0X2	T49.0X3	T49.0X4	T49.0X5	T49.0X6
Gepefrine	T44.4X1	T44.4X2	T44.4X3	T44.4X4	T44.4X5	T44.4X6
Gestonorone caproate	T38.5X1	T38.5X2	T38.5X3	T38.5X4	T38.5X5	T38.5X6
Gexane	T49.0X1	T49.0X2	T49.0X3	T49.0X4	T49.0X5	T49.0X6
Gila monster (venom)	T63.111	T63.112	T63.113	T63.114	--	--
Ginger	T47.5X1	T47.5X2	T47.5X3	T47.5X4	T47.5X5	T47.5X6
Jamaica — *see Jamaica, ginger*						
Gitalin	T46.0X1	T46.0X2	T46.0X3	T46.0X4	T46.0X5	T46.0X6
amorphous	T46.0X1	T46.0X2	T46.0X3	T46.0X4	T46.0X5	T46.0X6
Gitaloxin	T46.0X1	T46.0X2	T46.0X3	T46.0X4	T46.0X5	T46.0X6
Gitoxin	T46.0X1	T46.0X2	T46.0X3	T46.0X4	T46.0X5	T46.0X6
Glafenine	T39.8X1	T39.8X2	T39.8X3	T39.8X4	T39.8X5	T39.8X6
Glandular extract (medicinal) NEC	T50.Z91	T50.Z92	T50.Z93	T50.Z94	T50.Z95	T50.Z96
Glaucarubin	T37.3X1	T37.3X2	T37.3X3	T37.3X4	T37.3X5	T37.3X6
Glibenclamide	T38.3X1	T38.3X2	T38.3X3	T38.3X4	T38.3X5	T38.3X6
Glibornuride	T38.3X1	T38.3X2	T38.3X3	T38.3X4	T38.3X5	T38.3X6
Gliclazide	T38.3X1	T38.3X2	T38.3X3	T38.3X4	T38.3X5	T38.3X6
Glimidine	T38.3X1	T38.3X2	T38.3X3	T38.3X4	T38.3X5	T38.3X6
Glipizide	T38.3X1	T38.3X2	T38.3X3	T38.3X4	T38.3X5	T38.3X6
Gliquidone	T38.3X1	T38.3X2	T38.3X3	T38.3X4	T38.3X5	T38.3X6
Glisolamide	T38.3X1	T38.3X2	T38.3X3	T38.3X4	T38.3X5	T38.3X6
Glisoxepide	T38.3X1	T38.3X2	T38.3X3	T38.3X4	T38.3X5	T38.3X6
Globin zinc insulin	T38.3X1	T38.3X2	T38.3X3	T38.3X4	T38.3X5	T38.3X6
Globulin						
antilymphocytic	T50.Z11	T50.Z12	T50.Z13	T50.Z14	T50.Z15	T50.Z16
antirhesus	T50.Z11	T50.Z12	T50.Z13	T50.Z14	T50.Z15	T50.Z16
antivenin	T50.Z11	T50.Z12	T50.Z13	T50.Z14	T50.Z15	T50.Z16
antiviral	T50.Z11	T50.Z12	T50.Z13	T50.Z14	T50.Z15	T50.Z16
Glucagon	T38.3X1	T38.3X2	T38.3X3	T38.3X4	T38.3X5	T38.3X6
Glucocorticoids	T38.0X1	T38.0X2	T38.0X3	T38.0X4	T38.0X5	T38.0X6
Glucocorticosteroid	T38.0X1	T38.0X2	T38.0X3	T38.0X4	T38.0X5	T38.0X6
Gluconic acid	T50.991	T50.992	T50.993	T50.994	T50.995	T50.996
Glucosamine sulfate	T39.4X1	T39.4X2	T39.4X3	T39.4X4	T39.4X5	T39.4X6
Glucose	T50.3X1	T50.3X2	T50.3X3	T50.3X4	T50.3X5	T50.3X6
with sodium chloride	T50.3X1	T50.3X2	T50.3X3	T50.3X4	T50.3X5	T50.3X6
Glucosulfone sodium	T37.1X1	T37.1X2	T37.1X3	T37.1X4	T37.1X5	T37.1X6
Glucurolactone	T47.8X1	T47.8X2	T47.8X3	T47.8X4	T47.8X5	T47.8X6
Glue NEC	T52.8X1	T52.8X2	T52.8X3	T52.8X4	--	--
Glutamic acid	T47.5X1	T47.5X2	T47.5X3	T47.5X4	T47.5X5	T47.5X6
Glutaral (medicinal)	T49.0X1	T49.0X2	T49.0X3	T49.0X4	T49.0X5	T49.0X6
nonmedicinal	T65.891	T65.892	T65.893	T65.894	--	--
Glutaraldehyde (nonmedicinal)	T65.891	T65.892	T65.893	T65.894	--	--
medicinal	T49.0X1	T49.0X2	T49.0X3	T49.0X4	T49.0X5	T49.0X6
Glutathione	T50.6X1	T50.6X2	T50.6X3	T50.6X4	T50.6X5	T50.6X6
Glutethimide	T42.6X1	T42.6X2	T42.6X3	T42.6X4	T42.6X5	T42.6X6
Glyburide	T38.3X1	T38.3X2	T38.3X3	T38.3X4	T38.3X5	T38.3X6
Glycerin	T47.4X1	T47.4X2	T47.4X3	T47.4X4	T47.4X5	T47.4X6
Glycerol	T47.4X1	T47.4X2	T47.4X3	T47.4X4	T47.4X5	T47.4X6
borax	T49.6X1	T49.6X2	T49.6X3	T49.6X4	T49.6X5	T49.6X6
intravenous	T50.3X1	T50.3X2	T50.3X3	T50.3X4	T50.3X5	T50.3X6
iodinated	T48.4X1	T48.4X2	T48.4X3	T48.4X4	T48.4X5	T48.4X6
Glycerophosphate	T50.991	T50.992	T50.993	T50.994	T50.995	T50.996
Glyceryl						
gualacolate	T48.4X1	T48.4X2	T48.4X3	T48.4X4	T48.4X5	T48.4X6
nitrate	T46.3X1	T46.3X2	T46.3X3	T46.3X4	T46.3X5	T46.3X6
triacetate (topical)	T49.0X1	T49.0X2	T49.0X3	T49.0X4	T49.0X5	T49.0X6
trinitrate	T46.3X1	T46.3X2	T46.3X3	T46.3X4	T46.3X5	T46.3X6
Glycine	T50.3X1	T50.3X2	T50.3X3	T50.3X4	T50.3X5	T50.3X6
Glyclopyramide	T38.3X1	T38.3X2	T38.3X3	T38.3X4	T38.3X5	T38.3X6
Glycobiarsol	T37.3X1	T37.3X2	T37.3X3	T37.3X4	T37.3X5	T37.3X6
Glycols (ether)	T52.3X1	T52.3X2	T52.3X3	T52.3X4	--	--
Glyconiazide	T37.1X1	T37.1X2	T37.1X3	T37.1X4	T37.1X5	T37.1X6
Glycopyrrolate	T44.3X1	T44.3X2	T44.3X3	T44.3X4	T44.3X5	T44.3X6

Substance	Poisoning, Accidental unintentional	Poisoning, Intentional self-harm	Poisoning, Assault	Poisoning, Undetermined	Adverse effect	Underdosing
Glycopyrronium	T44.3X1	T44.3X2	T44.3X3	T44.3X4	T44.3X5	T44.3X6
bromide	T44.3X1	T44.3X2	T44.3X3	T44.3X4	T44.3X5	T44.3X6
Glycoside, cardiac (stimulant)	T46.0X1	T46.0X2	T46.0X3	T46.0X4	T46.0X5	T46.0X6
Glycyclamide	T38.3X1	T38.3X2	T38.3X3	T38.3X4	T38.3X5	T38.3X6
Glycyrrhiza extract	T48.4X1	T48.4X2	T48.4X3	T48.4X4	T48.4X5	T48.4X6
Glycyrrhizic acid	T48.4X1	T48.4X2	T48.4X3	T48.4X4	T48.4X5	T48.4X6
Glycyrrhizinate potassium	T48.4X1	T48.4X2	T48.4X3	T48.4X4	T48.4X5	T48.4X6
Glymidine sodium	T38.3X1	T38.3X2	T38.3X3	T38.3X4	T38.3X5	T38.3X6
Glyphosate	T60.3X1	T60.3X2	T60.3X3	T60.3X4	--	--
Glyphylline	T48.6X1	T48.6X2	T48.6X3	T48.6X4	T48.6X5	T48.6X6
Gold						
colloidal (I98Au)	T45.1X1	T45.1X2	T45.1X3	T45.1X4	T45.1X5	T45.1X6
salts	T39.4X1	T39.4X2	T39.4X3	T39.4X4	T39.4X5	T39.4X6
Golden sulfide of antimony	T56.891	T56.892	T56.893	T56.894	--	--
Goldylocks	T62.2X1	T62.2X2	T62.2X3	T62.2X4	--	--
Gonadal tissue extract	T38.901	T38.902	T38.903	T38.904	T38.905	T38.906
female	T38.5X1	T38.5X2	T38.5X3	T38.5X4	T38.5X5	T38.5X6
male	T38.7X1	T38.7X2	T38.7X3	T38.7X4	T38.7X5	T38.7X6
Gonadorelin	T38.891	T38.892	T38.893	T38.894	T38.895	T38.896
Gonadotropin	T38.891	T38.892	T38.893	T38.894	T38.895	T38.896
chorionic	T38.891	T38.892	T38.893	T38.894	T38.895	T38.896
pituitary	T38.811	T38.812	T38.813	T38.814	T38.815	T38.816
Goserelin	T45.1X1	T45.1X2	T45.1X3	T45.1X4	T45.1X5	T45.1X6
Grain alcohol	T51.0X1	T51.0X2	T51.0X3	T51.0X4	--	--
Gramicidin	T49.0X1	T49.0X2	T49.0X3	T49.0X4	T49.0X5	T49.0X6
Granisetron	T45.0X1	T45.0X2	T45.0X3	T45.0X4	T45.0X5	T45.0X6
Gratiola officinalis	T62.2X1	T62.2X2	T62.2X3	T62.2X4	--	--
Grease	T65.891	T65.892	T65.893	T65.894	--	--
Green hellebore	T62.2X1	T62.2X2	T62.2X3	T62.2X4	--	--
Green soap	T49.2X1	T49.2X2	T49.2X3	T49.2X4	T49.2X5	T49.2X6
Grifulvin	T36.7X1	T36.7X2	T36.7X3	T36.7X4	T36.7X5	T36.7X6
Griseofulvin	T36.7X1	T36.7X2	T36.7X3	T36.7X4	T36.7X5	T36.7X6
Growth hormone	T38.811	T38.812	T38.813	T38.814	T38.815	T38.816
Guaiac reagent	T50.991	T50.992	T50.993	T50.994	T50.995	T50.996
Guaiacol derivatives	T48.4X1	T48.4X2	T48.4X3	T48.4X4	T48.4X5	T48.4X6
Guaifenesin	T48.4X1	T48.4X2	T48.4X3	T48.4X4	T48.4X5	T48.4X6
Guaimesal	T48.4X1	T48.4X2	T48.4X3	T48.4X4	T48.4X5	T48.4X6
Guaiphenesin	T48.4X1	T48.4X2	T48.4X3	T48.4X4	T48.4X5	T48.4X6
Guamecycline	T36.4X1	T36.4X2	T36.4X3	T36.4X4	T36.4X5	T36.4X6
Guanabenz	T46.5X1	T46.5X2	T46.5X3	T46.5X4	T46.5X5	T46.5X6
Guanacline	T46.5X1	T46.5X2	T46.5X3	T46.5X4	T46.5X5	T46.5X6
Guanadrel	T46.5X1	T46.5X2	T46.5X3	T46.5X4	T46.5X5	T46.5X6
Guanatol	T37.2X1	T37.2X2	T37.2X3	T37.2X4	T37.2X5	T37.2X6
Guanethidine	T46.5X1	T46.5X2	T46.5X3	T46.5X4	T46.5X5	T46.5X6
Guanfacine	T46.5X1	T46.5X2	T46.5X3	T46.5X4	T46.5X5	T46.5X6
Guano	T65.891	T65.892	T65.893	T65.894	--	--
Guanochlor	T46.5X1	T46.5X2	T46.5X3	T46.5X4	T46.5X5	T46.5X6
Guanoclor	T46.5X1	T46.5X2	T46.5X3	T46.5X4	T46.5X5	T46.5X6
Guanoctine	T46.5X1	T46.5X2	T46.5X3	T46.5X4	T46.5X5	T46.5X6
Guanoxabenz	T46.5X1	T46.5X2	T46.5X3	T46.5X4	T46.5X5	T46.5X6
Guanoxan	T46.5X1	T46.5X2	T46.5X3	T46.5X4	T46.5X5	T46.5X6
Guar gum (medicinal)	T46.6X1	T46.6X2	T46.6X3	T46.6X4	T46.6X5	T46.6X6
H						
Hachimycin	T36.7X1	T36.7X2	T36.7X3	T36.7X4	T36.7X5	T36.7X6
Hair						
dye	T49.4X1	T49.4X2	T49.4X3	T49.4X4	T49.4X5	T49.4X6
preparation NEC	T49.4X1	T49.4X2	T49.4X3	T49.4X4	T49.4X5	T49.4X6
Halazepam	T42.4X1	T42.4X2	T42.4X3	T42.4X4	T42.4X5	T42.4X6
Halcinolone	T49.0X1	T49.0X2	T49.0X3	T49.0X4	T49.0X5	T49.0X6
Halcinonide	T49.0X1	T49.0X2	T49.0X3	T49.0X4	T49.0X5	T49.0X6
Halethazole	T49.0X1	T49.0X2	T49.0X3	T49.0X4	T49.0X5	T49.0X6
Hallucinogen NEC	T40.901	T40.902	T40.903	T40.904	T40.905	T40.906
Halofantrine	T37.2X1	T37.2X2	T37.2X3	T37.2X4	T37.2X5	T37.2X6
Halofenate	T46.6X1	T46.6X2	T46.6X3	T46.6X4	T46.6X5	T46.6X6
Halometasone	T49.0X1	T49.0X2	T49.0X3	T49.0X4	T49.0X5	T49.0X6
Haloperidol	T43.4X1	T43.4X2	T43.4X3	T43.4X4	T43.4X5	T43.4X6
Haloprogin	T49.0X1	T49.0X2	T49.0X3	T49.0X4	T49.0X5	T49.0X6
Halotex	T49.0X1	T49.0X2	T49.0X3	T49.0X4	T49.0X5	T49.0X6
Halothane	T41.0X1	T41.0X2	T41.0X3	T41.0X4	T41.0X5	T41.0X6
Haloxazolam	T42.4X1	T42.4X2	T42.4X3	T42.4X4	T42.4X5	T42.4X6
Halquinols	T49.0X1	T49.0X2	T49.0X3	T49.0X4	T49.0X5	T49.0X6
Hamamelis	T49.2X1	T49.2X2	T49.2X3	T49.2X4	T49.2X5	T49.2X6
Haptendextran	T45.8X1	T45.8X2	T45.8X3	T45.8X4	T45.8X5	T45.8X6
Harmonyl	T46.5X1	T46.5X2	T46.5X3	T46.5X4	T46.5X5	T46.5X6
Hartmann's solution	T50.3X1	T50.3X2	T50.3X3	T50.3X4	T50.3X5	T50.3X6
Hashish	T40.7X1	T40.7X2	T40.7X3	T40.7X4	T40.7X5	T40.7X6
Hawaiian Woodrose seeds	T40.991	T40.992	T40.993	T40.994	--	--
HCB	T60.3X1	T60.3X2	T60.3X3	T60.3X4	--	--
HCH	T53.6X1	T53.6X2	T53.6X3	T53.6X4	--	--
medicinal	T49.0X1	T49.0X2	T49.0X3	T49.0X4	T49.0X5	T49.0X6
HCN	T57.3X1	T57.3X2	T57.3X3	T57.3X4	--	--
Headache cures, drugs, powders NEC	T50.901	T50.902	T50.903	T50.904	T50.905	T50.906
Heavenly Blue (morning glory)	T40.991	T40.992	T40.993	T40.994	--	--

Substance	Poisoning, Accidental unintentional	Poisoning, Intentional self-harm	Poisoning, Assault	Poisoning, Undetermined	Adverse effect	Underdosing
Heavy metal antidote	T45.8X1	T45.8X2	T45.8X3	T45.8X4	T45.8X5	T45.8X6
Hedaquinium	T49.0X1	T49.0X2	T49.0X3	T49.0X4	T49.0X5	T49.0X6
Hedge hyssop	T62.2X1	T62.2X2	T62.2X3	T62.2X4	--	--
Heet	T49.8X1	T49.8X2	T49.8X3	T49.8X4	T49.8X5	T49.8X6
Helenin	T37.4X1	T37.4X2	T37.4X3	T37.4X4	T37.4X5	T37.4X6
Helium (nonmedicinal) **NEC**	T59.891	T59.892	T59.893	T59.894	--	--
medicinal	T48.991	T48.992	T48.993	T48.994	T48.995	T48.996
Hellebore (black) (green) (white)	T62.2X1	T62.2X2	T62.2X3	T62.2X4	--	--
Hematin	T45.8X1	T45.8X2	T45.8X3	T45.8X4	T45.8X5	T45.8X6
Hematinic preparation	T45.8X1	T45.8X2	T45.8X3	T45.8X4	T45.8X5	T45.8X6
Hematological agent	T45.91	T45.92	T45.93	T45.94	T45.95	T45.96
specified NEC	T45.8X1	T45.8X2	T45.8X3	T45.8X4	T45.8X5	T45.8X6
Hemlock	T62.2X1	T62.2X2	T62.2X3	T62.2X4	--	--
Hemostatic	T45.621	T45.622	T45.623	T45.624	T45.625	T45.626
drug, systemic	T45.621	T45.622	T45.623	T45.624	T45.625	T45.626
Hemostyptic	T49.4X1	T49.4X2	T49.4X3	T49.4X4	T49.4X5	T49.4X6
Henbane	T62.2X1	T62.2X2	T62.2X3	T62.2X4	--	--
Heparin (sodium)	T45.511	T45.512	T45.513	T45.514	T45.515	T45.516
action reverser	T45.7X1	T45.7X2	T45.7X3	T45.7X4	T45.7X5	T45.7X6
Heparin-fraction	T45.511	T45.512	T45.513	T45.514	T45.515	T45.516
Heparinoid (systemic)	T45.511	T45.512	T45.513	T45.514	T45.515	T45.516
Hepatic secretion stimulant	T47.8X1	T47.8X2	T47.8X3	T47.8X4	T47.8X5	T47.8X6
Hepatitis B						
immune globulin	T50.Z11	T50.Z12	T50.Z13	T50.Z14	T50.Z15	T50.Z16
vaccine	T50.B91	T50.B92	T50.B93	T50.B94	T50.B95	T50.B96
Hepronicate	T46.7X1	T46.7X2	T46.7X3	T46.7X4	T46.7X5	T46.7X6
Heptabarb	T42.3X1	T42.3X2	T42.3X3	T42.3X4	T42.3X5	T42.3X6
Heptabarbital	T42.3X1	T42.3X2	T42.3X3	T42.3X4	T42.3X5	T42.3X6
Heptabarbitone	T42.3X1	T42.3X2	T42.3X3	T42.3X4	T42.3X5	T42.3X6
Heptachlor	T60.1X1	T60.1X2	T60.1X3	T60.1X4	--	--
Heptalgin	T40.2X1	T40.2X2	T40.2X3	T40.2X4	T40.2X5	T40.2X6
Heptaminol	T46.3X1	T46.3X2	T46.3X3	T46.3X4	T46.3X5	T46.3X6
Herbicide NEC	T60.3X1	T60.3X2	T60.3X3	T60.3X4	--	--
Heroin	T40.1X1	T40.1X2	T40.1X3	T40.1X4	--	--
Herplex	T49.5X1	T49.5X2	T49.5X3	T49.5X4	T49.5X5	T49.5X6
HES	T45.8X1	T45.8X2	T45.8X3	T45.8X4	T45.8X5	T45.8X6
Hesperidin	T46.991	T46.992	T46.993	T46.994	T46.995	T46.996
Hetacillin	T36.0X1	T36.0X2	T36.0X3	T36.0X4	T36.0X5	T36.0X6
Hetastarch	T45.8X1	T45.8X2	T45.8X3	T45.8X4	T45.8X5	T45.8X6
HETP	T60.0X1	T60.0X2	T60.0X3	T60.0X4	--	--
Hexachlorobenzene (vapor)	T60.3X1	T60.3X2	T60.3X3	T60.3X4	--	--
Hexachlorocyclohexane	T53.6X1	T53.6X2	T53.6X3	T53.6X4	--	--
Hexachlorophene	T49.0X1	T49.0X2	T49.0X3	T49.0X4	T49.0X5	T49.0X6
Hexadiline	T46.3X1	T46.3X2	T46.3X3	T46.3X4	T46.3X5	T46.3X6
Hexadimethrine (bromide)	T45.7X1	T45.7X2	T45.7X3	T45.7X4	T45.7X5	T45.7X6
Hexadylamine	T46.3X1	T46.3X2	T46.3X3	T46.3X4	T46.3X5	T46.3X6
Hexaethyl tetraphos-phate	T60.0X1	T60.0X2	T60.0X3	T60.0X4	--	--
Hexafluorenium bromide	T48.1X1	T48.1X2	T48.1X3	T48.1X4	T48.1X5	T48.1X6
Hexafluronium (bromide)	T48.1X1	T48.1X2	T48.1X3	T48.1X4	T48.1X5	T48.1X6
Hexa-germ	T49.2X1	T49.2X2	T49.2X3	T49.2X4	T49.2X5	T49.2X6
Hexahydrobenzol	T52.8X1	T52.8X2	T52.8X3	T52.8X4	--	--
Hexahydrocresol (s)	T51.8X1	T51.8X2	T51.8X3	T51.8X4	--	--
arsenide	T57.0X1	T57.0X2	T57.0X3	T57.0X4	--	--
arseniurated	T57.0X1	T57.0X2	T57.0X3	T57.0X4	--	--
cyanide	T57.3X1	T57.3X2	T57.3X3	T57.3X4	--	--
gas	T59.891	T59.892	T59.893	T59.894	--	--
Fluoride (liquid)	T57.8X1	T57.8X2	T57.8X3	T57.8X4	--	--
vapor	T59.891	T59.892	T59.893	T59.894	--	--
phophorated	T60.0X1	T60.0X2	T60.0X3	T60.0X4	--	--
sulfate	T57.8X1	T57.8X2	T57.8X3	T57.8X4	--	--
sulfide (gas)	T59.6X1	T59.6X2	T59.6X3	T59.6X4	--	--
arseniurated	T57.0X1	T57.0X2	T57.0X3	T57.0X4	--	--
sulfurated	T57.8X1	T57.8X2	T57.8X3	T57.8X4	--	--
Hexahydrophenol	T51.8X1	T51.8X2	T51.8X3	T51.8X4	--	--
Hexalen	T51.8X1	T51.8X2	T51.8X3	T51.8X4	--	--
Hexamethonium bromide	T44.2X1	T44.2X2	T44.2X3	T44.2X4	T44.2X5	T44.2X6
Hexamethylene	T52.8X1	T52.8X2	T52.8X3	T52.8X4	--	--
Hexamethylmelamine	T45.1X1	T45.1X2	T45.1X3	T45.1X4	T45.1X5	T45.1X6
Hexamidine	T49.0X1	T49.0X2	T49.0X3	T49.0X4	T49.0X5	T49.0X6
Hexamine (mandelate)	T37.8X1	T37.8X2	T37.8X3	T37.8X4	T37.8X5	T37.8X6
Hexanone, 2-hexanone	T52.4X1	T52.4X2	T52.4X3	T52.4X4	--	--
Hexanuorenium	T48.1X1	T48.1X2	T48.1X3	T48.1X4	T48.1X5	T48.1X6
Hexapropymate	T42.6X1	T42.6X2	T42.6X3	T42.6X4	T42.6X5	T42.6X6
Hexasonium iodide	T44.3X1	T44.3X2	T44.3X3	T44.3X4	T44.3X5	T44.3X6
Hexcarbacholine bromide	T48.1X1	T48.1X2	T48.1X3	T48.1X4	T48.1X5	T48.1X6
Hexemal	T42.3X1	T42.3X2	T42.3X3	T42.3X4	T42.3X5	T42.3X6
Hexestrol	T38.5X1	T38.5X2	T38.5X3	T38.5X4	T38.5X5	T38.5X6
Hexethal (sodium)	T42.3X1	T42.3X2	T42.3X3	T42.3X4	T42.3X5	T42.3X6
Hexetidine	T37.8X1	T37.8X2	T37.8X3	T37.8X4	T37.8X5	T37.8X6
Hexobarbital	T42.3X1	T42.3X2	T42.3X3	T42.3X4	T42.3X5	T42.3X6
rectal	T41.291	T41.292	T41.293	T41.294	T41.295	T41.296
sodium	T41.1X1	T41.1X2	T41.1X3	T41.1X4	T41.1X5	T41.1X6
Hexobendine	T46.3X1	T46.3X2	T46.3X3	T46.3X4	T46.3X5	T46.3X6

Hexocyclium - Iloprost

Substance	Poisoning, Accidental unintentional	Poisoning, Intentional self-harm	Poisoning, Assault	Poisoning, Undetermined	Adverse effect	Underdosing
Hexocyclium	T44.3X1	T44.3X2	T44.3X3	T44.3X4	T44.3X5	T44.3X6
metilsulfate	T44.3X1	T44.3X2	T44.3X3	T44.3X4	T44.3X5	T44.3X6
Hexoestrol	T38.5X1	T38.5X2	T38.5X3	T38.5X4	T38.5X5	T38.5X6
Hexone	T52.4X1	T52.4X2	T52.4X3	T52.4X4	—	—
Hexoprenaline	T48.6X1	T48.6X2	T48.6X3	T48.6X4	T48.6X5	T48.6X6
Hexylcaine	T41.3X1	T41.3X2	T41.3X3	T41.3X4	T41.3X5	T41.3X6
Hexylresorcinol	T52.2X1	T52.2X2	T52.2X3	T52.2X4	—	—
HGH (human growth hormone)	T38.811	T38.812	T38.813	T38.814	T38.815	T38.816
Hinkle's pills	T47.2X1	T47.2X2	T47.2X3	T47.2X4	T47.2X5	T47.2X6
Histalog	T50.8X1	T50.8X2	T50.8X3	T50.8X4	T50.8X5	T50.8X6
Histamine (phosphate)	T50.8X1	T50.8X2	T50.8X3	T50.8X4	T50.8X5	T50.8X6
Histoplasmin	T50.8X1	T50.8X2	T50.8X3	T50.8X4	T50.8X5	T50.8X6
Holly berries	T62.2X1	T62.2X2	T62.2X3	T62.2X4	—	—
Homatropine	T44.3X1	T44.3X2	T44.3X3	T44.3X4	T44.3X5	T44.3X6
methylbromide	T44.3X1	T44.3X2	T44.3X3	T44.3X4	T44.3X5	T44.3X6
Homochlorcyclizine	T45.0X1	T45.0X2	T45.0X3	T45.0X4	T45.0X5	T45.0X6
Homosalate	T49.3X1	T49.3X2	T49.3X3	T49.3X4	T49.3X5	T49.3X6
Homo-tet	T50.Z11	T50.Z12	T50.Z13	T50.Z14	T50.Z15	T50.Z16
Hormone	T38.801	T38.802	T38.803	T38.804	T38.805	T38.806
adrenal cortical steroids	T38.0X1	T38.0X2	T38.0X3	T38.0X4	T38.0X5	T38.0X6
androgenic	T38.7X1	T38.7X2	T38.7X3	T38.7X4	T38.7X5	T38.7X6
anterior pituitary NEC	T38.811	T38.812	T38.813	T38.814	T38.815	T38.816
antidiabetic agents	T38.3X1	T38.3X2	T38.3X3	T38.3X4	T38.3X5	T38.3X6
antidiuretic	T38.891	T38.892	T38.893	T38.894	T38.895	T38.896
cancer therapy	T45.1X1	T45.1X2	T45.1X3	T45.1X4	T45.1X5	T45.1X6
follicle stimulating	T38.811	T38.812	T38.813	T38.814	T38.815	T38.816
gonadotropic	T38.891	T38.892	T38.893	T38.894	T38.895	T38.896
pituitary	T38.811	T38.812	T38.813	T38.814	T38.815	T38.816
growth	T38.811	T38.812	T38.813	T38.814	T38.815	T38.816
luteinizing	T38.811	T38.812	T38.813	T38.814	T38.815	T38.816
ovarian	T38.5X1	T38.5X2	T38.5X3	T38.5X4	T38.5X5	T38.5X6
oxytocic	T48.0X1	T48.0X2	T48.0X3	T48.0X4	T48.0X5	T48.0X6
parathyroid (derivatives)	T50.991	T50.992	T50.993	T50.994	T50.995	T50.996
pituitary (posterior) NEC	T38.891	T38.892	T38.893	T38.894	T38.895	T38.896
anterior	T38.811	T38.812	T38.813	T38.814	T38.815	T38.816
specified, NEC	T38.891	T38.892	T38.893	T38.894	T38.895	T38.896
thyroid	T38.1X1	T38.1X2	T38.1X3	T38.1X4	T38.1X5	T38.1X6
Hornet (sting)	T63.451	T63.452	T63.453	T63.454	—	—
Horse anti-human lymphocytic serum	T50.Z11	T50.Z12	T50.Z13	T50.Z14	T50.Z15	T50.Z16
Horticulture agent NEC	T65.91	T65.92	T65.93	T65.94	—	—
with pesticide	T60.91	T60.92	T60.93	T60.94	—	—
Human						
albumin	T45.8X1	T45.8X2	T45.8X3	T45.8X4	T45.8X5	T45.8X6
growth hormone (HGH)	T38.811	T38.812	T38.813	T38.814	T38.815	T38.816
immune serum	T50.Z11	T50.Z12	T50.Z13	T50.Z14	T50.Z15	T50.Z16
Hyaluronidase	T45.3X1	T45.3X2	T45.3X3	T45.3X4	T45.3X5	T45.3X6
Hyazyme	T45.3X1	T45.3X2	T45.3X3	T45.3X4	T45.3X5	T45.3X6
Hycodan	T40.2X1	T40.2X2	T40.2X3	T40.2X4	T40.2X5	T40.2X6
Hydantoin derivative NEC	T42.0X1	T42.0X2	T42.0X3	T42.0X4	T42.0X5	T42.0X6
Hydeltra	T38.0X1	T38.0X2	T38.0X3	T38.0X4	T38.0X5	T38.0X6
Hydergine	T44.6X1	T44.6X2	T44.6X3	T44.6X4	T44.6X5	T44.6X6
Hydrabamine penicillin	T36.0X1	T36.0X2	T36.0X3	T36.0X4	T36.0X5	T36.0X6
Hydralazine	T46.5X1	T46.5X2	T46.5X3	T46.5X4	T46.5X5	T46.5X6
Hydrargaphen	T49.0X1	T49.0X2	T49.0X3	T49.0X4	T49.0X5	T49.0X6
Hydrargyri amino-chloridum	T49.0X1	T49.0X2	T49.0X3	T49.0X4	T49.0X5	T49.0X6
Hydrastine	T48.291	T48.292	T48.293	T48.294	T48.295	T48.296
Hydrazine	T54.1X1	T54.1X2	T54.1X3	T54.1X4	—	—
monoamine oxidase inhibitors	T43.1X1	T43.1X2	T43.1X3	T43.1X4	T43.1X5	T43.1X6
Hydrazoic acid, azides	T54.2X1	T54.2X2	T54.2X3	T54.2X4	—	—
Hydriodic acid	T48.4X1	T48.4X2	T48.4X3	T48.4X4	T48.4X5	T48.4X6
Hydrocarbon gas	T59.891	T59.892	T59.893	T59.894	—	—
incomplete combustion of — *see Carbon, monoxide, fuel, utility*						
liquefied (mobile container)	T59.891	T59.892	T59.893	T59.894	—	—
piped (natural)	T59.891	T59.892	T59.893	T59.894	—	—
Hydrochloric acid (liquid)	T54.2X1	T54.2X2	T54.2X3	T54.2X4	—	—
medicinal (digestant)	T47.5X1	T47.5X2	T47.5X3	T47.5X4	T47.5X5	T47.5X6
vapor	T59.891	T59.892	T59.893	T59.894	—	—
Hydrochlorothiazide	T50.2X1	T50.2X2	T50.2X3	T50.2X4	T50.2X5	T50.2X6
Hydrocodone	T40.2X1	T40.2X2	T40.2X3	T40.2X4	T40.2X5	T40.2X6
Hydrocortisone (derivatives)	T38.0X1	T38.0X2	T38.0X3	T38.0X4	T38.0X5	T38.0X6
aceponate	T49.0X1	T49.0X2	T49.0X3	T49.0X4	T49.0X5	T49.0X6
ENT agent	T49.6X1	T49.6X2	T49.6X3	T49.6X4	T49.6X5	T49.6X6
ophthalmic preparation	T49.5X1	T49.5X2	T49.5X3	T49.5X4	T49.5X5	T49.5X6
topical NEC	T49.0X1	T49.0X2	T49.0X3	T49.0X4	T49.0X5	T49.0X6
Hydrocortone	T38.0X1	T38.0X2	T38.0X3	T38.0X4	T38.0X5	T38.0X6
ENT agent	T49.6X1	T49.6X2	T49.6X3	T49.6X4	T49.6X5	T49.6X6
ophthalmic preparation	T49.5X1	T49.5X2	T49.5X3	T49.5X4	T49.5X5	T49.5X6
topical NEC	T49.0X1	T49.0X2	T49.0X3	T49.0X4	T49.0X5	T49.0X6

Substance	Poisoning, Accidental unintentional	Poisoning, Intentional self-harm	Poisoning, Assault	Poisoning, Undetermined	Adverse effect	Underdosing
Hydrocyanic acid (liquid)	T57.3X1	T57.3X2	T57.3X3	T57.3X4	—	—
gas	T65.0X1	T65.0X2	T65.0X3	T65.0X4	—	—
Hydroflumethiazide	T50.2X1	T50.2X2	T50.2X3	T50.2X4	T50.2X5	T50.2X6
Hydrofluoric acid (liquid)	T54.2X1	T54.2X2	T54.2X3	T54.2X4	—	—
vapor	T59.891	T59.892	T59.893	T59.894	—	—
Hydrogen	T59.891	T59.892	T59.893	T59.894	—	—
arsenide	T57.0X1	T57.0X2	T57.0X3	T57.0X4	—	—
arseniureted	T57.0X1	T57.0X2	T57.0X3	T57.0X4	—	—
chloride	T57.8X1	T57.8X2	T57.8X3	T57.8X4	—	—
cyanide (salts)	T57.3X1	T57.3X2	T57.3X3	T57.3X4	—	—
gas	T57.3X1	T57.3X2	T57.3X3	T57.3X4	—	—
Fluoride	T59.5X1	T59.5X2	T59.5X3	T59.5X4	—	—
vapor	T59.5X1	T59.5X2	T59.5X3	T59.5X4	—	—
peroxide	T49.0X1	T49.0X2	T49.0X3	T49.0X4	T49.0X5	T49.0X6
phosphureted	T57.1X1	T57.1X2	T57.1X3	T57.1X4	—	—
sulfide	T59.6X1	T59.6X2	T59.6X3	T59.6X4	—	—
arseniureted	T57.0X1	T57.0X2	T57.0X3	T57.0X4	—	—
sulfureted	T59.6X1	T59.6X2	T59.6X3	T59.6X4	—	—
Hydromethylpyridine	T46.7X1	T46.7X2	T46.7X3	T46.7X4	T46.7X5	T46.7X6
Hydromorphinol	T40.2X1	T40.2X2	T40.2X3	T40.2X4	—	—
Hydromorphinone	T40.2X1	T40.2X2	T40.2X3	T40.2X4	T40.2X5	T40.2X6
Hydromorphone	T40.2X1	T40.2X2	T40.2X3	T40.2X4	T40.2X5	T40.2X6
Hydromox	T50.2X1	T50.2X2	T50.2X3	T50.2X4	T50.2X5	T50.2X6
Hydrophilic lotion	T49.3X1	T49.3X2	T49.3X3	T49.3X4	T49.3X5	T49.3X6
Hydroquinidine	T46.2X1	T46.2X2	T46.2X3	T46.2X4	T46.2X5	T46.2X6
Hydroquinone	T52.2X1	T52.2X2	T52.2X3	T52.2X4	—	—
vapor	T59.891	T59.892	T59.893	T59.894	—	—
Hydrosulfuric acid (gas)	T59.6X1	T59.6X2	T59.6X3	T59.6X4	—	—
Hydrotalcite	T47.1X1	T47.1X2	T47.1X3	T47.1X4	T47.1X5	T47.1X6
Hydrous wool fat	T49.3X1	T49.3X2	T49.3X3	T49.3X4	T49.3X5	T49.3X6
Hydroxide, caustic	T54.3X1	T54.3X2	T54.3X3	T54.3X4	—	—
Hydroxocobalamin	T45.8X1	T45.8X2	T45.8X3	T45.8X4	T45.8X5	T45.8X6
Hydroxyamphetamine	T49.5X1	T49.5X2	T49.5X3	T49.5X4	T49.5X5	T49.5X6
Hydroxycarbamide	T45.1X1	T45.1X2	T45.1X3	T45.1X4	T45.1X5	T45.1X6
Hydroxychloroquine	T37.8X1	T37.8X2	T37.8X3	T37.8X4	T37.8X5	T37.8X6
Hydroxydihydrocodeinone	T40.2X1	T40.2X2	T40.2X3	T40.2X4	T40.2X5	T40.2X6
Hydroxyestrone	T38.5X1	T38.5X2	T38.5X3	T38.5X4	T38.5X5	T38.5X6
Hydroxyethyl starch	T45.8X1	T45.8X2	T45.8X3	T45.8X4	T45.8X5	T45.8X6
Hydroxymethylpenta-none	T52.4X1	T52.4X2	T52.4X3	T52.4X4	—	—
Hydroxyphenamate	T43.591	T43.592	T43.593	T43.594	T43.595	T43.596
Hydroxyphenylbutazone	T39.2X1	T39.2X2	T39.2X3	T39.2X4	T39.2X5	T39.2X6
Hydroxyprogesterone	T38.5X1	T38.5X2	T38.5X3	T38.5X4	T38.5X5	T38.5X6
caproate	T38.5X1	T38.5X2	T38.5X3	T38.5X4	T38.5X5	T38.5X6
Hydroxyquinoline (derivatives) **NEC**	T37.8X1	T37.8X2	T37.8X3	T37.8X4	T37.8X5	T37.8X6
Hydroxystilbamidine	T37.3X1	T37.3X2	T37.3X3	T37.3X4	T37.3X5	T37.3X6
Hydroxytoluene (nonmedicinal)	T54.0X1	T54.0X2	T54.0X3	T54.0X4	—	—
medicinal	T49.0X1	T49.0X2	T49.0X3	T49.0X4	T49.0X5	T49.0X6
Hydroxyurea	T45.1X1	T45.1X2	T45.1X3	T45.1X4	T45.1X5	T45.1X6
Hydroxyzine	T43.591	T43.592	T43.593	T43.594	T43.595	T43.596
Hyoscine	T44.3X1	T44.3X2	T44.3X3	T44.3X4	T44.3X5	T44.3X6
Hyoscyamine	T44.3X1	T44.3X2	T44.3X3	T44.3X4	T44.3X5	T44.3X6
Hyoscyamus	T44.3X1	T44.3X2	T44.3X3	T44.3X4	T44.3X5	T44.3X6
dry extract	T44.3X1	T44.3X2	T44.3X3	T44.3X4	T44.3X5	T44.3X6
Hypaque	T50.8X1	T50.8X2	T50.8X3	T50.8X4	T50.8X5	T50.8X6
Hypertussis	T50.Z11	T50.Z12	T50.Z13	T50.Z14	T50.Z15	T50.Z16
Hypnotic	T42.71	T42.72	T42.73	T42.74	T42.75	T42.76
anticonvulsant	T42.71	T42.72	T42.73	T42.74	T42.75	T42.76
specified NEC	T42.6X1	T42.6X2	T42.6X3	T42.6X4	T42.6X5	T42.6X6
Hypochlorite	T49.0X1	T49.0X2	T49.0X3	T49.0X4	T49.0X5	T49.0X6
Hypophysis, posterior	T38.891	T38.892	T38.893	T38.894	T38.895	T38.896
Hypotensive NEC	T46.5X1	T46.5X2	T46.5X3	T46.5X4	T46.5X5	T46.5X6
Hypromellose	T49.5X1	T49.5X2	T49.5X3	T49.5X4	T49.5X5	T49.5X6
I						
Ibacitabine	T37.5X1	T37.5X2	T37.5X3	T37.5X4	T37.5X5	T37.5X6
Ibopamine	T44.991	T44.992	T44.993	T44.994	T44.995	T44.996
Ibufenac	T39.311	T39.312	T39.313	T39.314	T39.315	T39.316
Ibuprofen	T39.311	T39.312	T39.313	T39.314	T39.315	T39.316
Ibuproxam	T39.311	T39.312	T39.313	T39.314	T39.315	T39.316
Ibuterol	T48.6X1	T48.6X2	T48.6X3	T48.6X4	T48.6X5	T48.6X6
Ichthammol	T49.0X1	T49.0X2	T49.0X3	T49.0X4	T49.0X5	T49.0X6
Ichthyol	T49.4X1	T49.4X2	T49.4X3	T49.4X4	T49.4X5	T49.4X6
Idarubicin	T45.1X1	T45.1X2	T45.1X3	T45.1X4	T45.1X5	T45.1X6
Idrocilamide	T42.8X1	T42.8X2	T42.8X3	T42.8X4	T42.8X5	T42.8X6
Ifenprodil	T46.7X1	T46.7X2	T46.7X3	T46.7X4	T46.7X5	T46.7X6
Ifosfamide	T45.1X1	T45.1X2	T45.1X3	T45.1X4	T45.1X5	T45.1X6
Iletin	T38.3X1	T38.3X2	T38.3X3	T38.3X4	T38.3X5	T38.3X6
Ilex	T62.2X1	T62.2X2	T62.2X3	T62.2X4	—	—
Illuminating gas (after combustion)	T58.11	T58.12	T58.13	T58.14	—	—
prior to combustion	T59.891	T59.892	T59.893	T59.894	—	—
Ilopan	T45.2X1	T45.2X2	T45.2X3	T45.2X4	T45.2X5	T45.2X6
Iloprost	T46.7X1	T46.7X2	T46.7X3	T46.7X4	T46.7X5	T46.7X6

Substance	Poisoning, Accidental unintentional	Poisoning, Intentional self-harm	Poisoning, Assault	Poisoning, Undetermined	Adverse effect	Underdosing
Ilotycin	T36.3X1	T36.3X2	T36.3X3	T36.3X4	T36.3X5	T36.3X6
ophthalmic preparation	T49.5X1	T49.5X2	T49.5X3	T49.5X4	T49.5X5	T49.5X6
topical NEC	T49.0X1	T49.0X2	T49.0X3	T49.0X4	T49.0X5	T49.0X6
Imidazole-4-carboxamide	T45.1X1	T45.1X2	T45.1X3	T45.1X4	T45.1X5	T45.1X6
Imipenem	T36.0X1	T36.0X2	T36.0X3	T36.0X4	T36.0X5	T36.0X6
Imipramine	T43.011	T43.012	T43.013	T43.014	T43.015	T43.016
Iminostilbene	T42.1X1	T42.1X2	T42.1X3	T42.1X4	T42.1X5	T42.1X6
Immu-G	T50.Z11	T50.Z12	T50.Z13	T50.Z14	T50.Z15	T50.Z16
Immuglobin	T50.Z11	T50.Z12	T50.Z13	T50.Z14	T50.Z15	T50.Z16
Immune						
globulin	T50.Z11	T50.Z12	T50.Z13	T50.Z14	T50.Z15	T50.Z16
serum globulin	T50.Z11	T50.Z12	T50.Z13	T50.Z14	T50.Z15	T50.Z16
Immunoglobin human (intravenous) (normal)	T50.Z11	T50.Z12	T50.Z13	T50.Z14	T50.Z15	T50.Z16
unmodified	T50.Z11	T50.Z12	T50.Z13	T50.Z14	T50.Z15	T50.Z16
Immunosuppressive drug	T45.1X1	T45.1X2	T45.1X3	T45.1X4	T45.1X5	T45.1X6
Immu-tetanus	T50.Z11	T50.Z12	T50.Z13	T50.Z14	T50.Z15	T50.Z16
Indalpine	T43.221	T43.222	T43.223	T43.224	T43.225	T43.226
Indanazoline	T48.5X1	T48.5X2	T48.5X3	T48.5X4	T48.5X5	T48.5X6
Indandione (derivatives)	T45.511	T45.512	T45.513	T45.514	T45.515	T45.516
Indapamide	T46.5X1	T46.5X2	T46.5X3	T46.5X4	T46.5X5	T46.5X6
Indendione (derivatives)	T45.511	T45.512	T45.513	T45.514	T45.515	T45.516
Indenolol	T44.7X1	T44.7X2	T44.7X3	T44.7X4	T44.7X5	T44.7X6
Inderal	T44.7X1	T44.7X2	T44.7X3	T44.7X4	T44.7X5	T44.7X6
Indian						
hemp	T40.7X1	T40.7X2	T40.7X3	T40.7X4	T40.7X5	T40.7X6
tobacco	T62.2X1	T62.2X2	T62.2X3	T62.2X4	--	--
Indigo carmine	T50.8X1	T50.8X2	T50.8X3	T50.8X4	T50.8X5	T50.8X6
Indobufen	T45.521	T45.522	T45.523	T45.524	T45.525	T45.526
Indocin	T39.2X1	T39.2X2	T39.2X3	T39.2X4	T39.2X5	T39.2X6
Indocyanine green	T50.8X1	T50.8X2	T50.8X3	T50.8X4	T50.8X5	T50.8X6
Indometacin	T39.391	T39.392	T39.393	T39.394	T39.395	T39.396
Indomethacin	T39.391	T39.392	T39.393	T39.394	T39.395	T39.396
farnesil	T39.4X1	T39.4X2	T39.4X3	T39.4X4	T39.4X5	T39.4X6
Indoramin	T44.6X1	T44.6X2	T44.6X3	T44.6X4	T44.6X5	T44.6X6
Industrial						
alcohol	T51.0X1	T51.0X2	T51.0X3	T51.0X4	--	--
fumes	T59.891	T59.892	T59.893	T59.894	--	--
solvents (fumes) (vapors)	T52.91	T52.92	T52.93	T52.94	--	--
Influenza vaccine	T50.B91	T50.B92	T50.B93	T50.B94	T50.B95	T50.B96
Ingested substance NEC	T65.91	T65.92	T65.93	T65.94	--	--
INH	T37.1X1	T37.1X2	T37.1X3	T37.1X4	T37.1X5	T37.1X6
Inhalation, gas (noxious) — *see Gas*						
Inhibitor						
angiotensin-converting enzyme	T46.4X1	T46.4X2	T46.4X3	T46.4X4	T46.4X5	T46.4X6
carbonic anhydrase	T50.2X1	T50.2X2	T50.2X3	T50.2X4	T50.2X5	T50.2X6
fibrinolysis	T45.621	T45.622	T45.623	T45.624	T45.625	T45.626
monoamine oxidase NEC	T43.1X1	T43.1X2	T43.1X3	T43.1X4	T43.1X5	T43.1X6
hydrazine	T43.1X1	T43.1X2	T43.1X3	T43.1X4	T43.1X5	T43.1X6
postsynaptic	T43.8X1	T43.8X2	T43.8X3	T43.8X4	T43.8X5	T43.8X6
prothrombin synthesis	T45.511	T45.512	T45.513	T45.514	T45.515	T45.516
Ink	T65.891	T65.892	T65.893	T65.894	--	--
Inorganic substance NEC	T57.91	T57.92	T57.93	T57.94	--	--
Inosine pranobex	T37.5X1	T37.5X2	T37.5X3	T37.5X4	T37.5X5	T37.5X6
Inositol	T50.991	T50.992	T50.993	T50.994	T50.995	T50.996
nicotinate	T46.7X1	T46.7X2	T46.7X3	T46.7X4	T46.7X5	T46.7X6
Inproquone	T45.1X1	T45.1X2	T45.1X3	T45.1X4	T45.1X5	T45.1X6
Insect (sting), **venomous**	T63.481	T63.482	T63.483	T63.484	--	--
ant	T63.421	T63.422	T63.423	T63.424	--	--
bee	T63.441	T63.442	T63.443	T63.444	--	--
caterpillar	T63.431	T63.432	T63.433	T63.434	--	--
hornet	T63.451	T63.452	T63.453	T63.454	--	--
wasp	T63.461	T63.462	T63.463	T63.464	--	--
Insecticide NEC	T60.91	T60.92	T60.93	T60.94	--	--
carbamate	T60.0X1	T60.0X2	T60.0X3	T60.0X4	--	--
chlorinated	T60.1X1	T60.1X2	T60.1X3	T60.1X4	--	--
mixed	T60.91	T60.92	T60.93	T60.94	--	--
organochlorine	T60.1X1	T60.1X2	T60.1X3	T60.1X4	--	--
organophosphorus	T60.0X1	T60.0X2	T60.0X3	T60.0X4	--	--
Insular tissue extract	T38.3X1	T38.3X2	T38.3X3	T38.3X4	T38.3X5	T38.3X6
Insulin (amorphous) (globin) (isophane) (Lente) (NPH) (Semilente) (Ultralente)	T38.3X1	T38.3X2	T38.3X3	T38.3X4	T38.3X5	T38.3X6
defalan	T38.3X1	T38.3X2	T38.3X3	T38.3X4	T38.3X5	T38.3X6
human	T38.3X1	T38.3X2	T38.3X3	T38.3X4	T38.3X5	T38.3X6
injection, soluble	T38.3X1	T38.3X2	T38.3X3	T38.3X4	T38.3X5	T38.3X6
biphasic	T38.3X1	T38.3X2	T38.3X3	T38.3X4	T38.3X5	T38.3X6
intermediate acting	T38.3X1	T38.3X2	T38.3X3	T38.3X4	T38.3X5	T38.3X6
protamine zinc	T38.3X1	T38.3X2	T38.3X3	T38.3X4	T38.3X5	T38.3X6
slow acting	T38.3X1	T38.3X2	T38.3X3	T38.3X4	T38.3X5	T38.3X6
zinc						
protamine injection	T38.3X1	T38.3X2	T38.3X3	T38.3X4	T38.3X5	T38.3X6
suspension (amorphous) (crystalline)	T38.3X1	T38.3X2	T38.3X3	T38.3X4	T38.3X5	T38.3X6

Substance	Poisoning, Accidental unintentional	Poisoning, Intentional self-harm	Poisoning, Assault	Poisoning, Undetermined	Adverse effect	Underdosing
Interferon (alpha) (beta) (gamma)	T37.5X1	T37.5X2	T37.5X3	T37.5X4	T37.5X5	T37.5X6
Intestinal motility control drug	T47.6X1	T47.6X2	T47.6X3	T47.6X4	T47.6X5	T47.6X6
biological	T47.8X1	T47.8X2	T47.8X3	T47.8X4	T47.8X5	T47.8X6
Intranarcon	T41.1X1	T41.1X2	T41.1X3	T41.1X4	T41.1X5	T41.1X6
Intravenous						
amino acids	T50.991	T50.992	T50.993	T50.994	T50.995	T50.996
fat suspension	T50.991	T50.992	T50.993	T50.994	T50.995	T50.996
Inulin	T50.8X1	T50.8X2	T50.8X3	T50.8X4	T50.8X5	T50.8X6
Invert sugar	T50.3X1	T50.3X2	T50.3X3	T50.3X4	T50.3X5	T50.3X6
Inza — *see Naproxen*						
Iobenzamic acid	T50.8X1	T50.8X2	T50.8X3	T50.8X4	T50.8X5	T50.8X6
Iocarmic acid	T50.8X1	T50.8X2	T50.8X3	T50.8X4	T50.8X5	T50.8X6
Iocetamic acid	T50.8X1	T50.8X2	T50.8X3	T50.8X4	T50.8X5	T50.8X6
Iodamide	T50.8X1	T50.8X2	T50.8X3	T50.8X4	T50.8X5	T50.8X6
Iodide NEC — *see also Iodine*	T49.0X1	T49.0X2	T49.0X3	T49.0X4	T49.0X5	T49.0X6
mercury (ointment)	T49.0X1	T49.0X2	T49.0X3	T49.0X4	T49.0X5	T49.0X6
methylate	T49.0X1	T49.0X2	T49.0X3	T49.0X4	T49.0X5	T49.0X6
potassium (expectorant) NEC	T48.4X1	T48.4X2	T48.4X3	T48.4X4	T48.4X5	T48.4X6
Iodinated						
contrast medium	T50.8X1	T50.8X2	T50.8X3	T50.8X4	T50.8X5	T50.8X6
glycerol	T48.4X1	T48.4X2	T48.4X3	T48.4X4	T48.4X5	T48.4X6
human serum albumin (131I)	T50.8X1	T50.8X2	T50.8X3	T50.8X4	T50.8X5	T50.8X6
Iodine (antiseptic, external) (tincture) **NEC**	T49.0X1	T49.0X2	T49.0X3	T49.0X4	T49.0X5	T49.0X6
125 — *see also Radiation sickness, and Exposure to radioactivce isotopes*	T50.8X1	T50.8X2	T50.8X3	T50.8X4	T50.8X5	T50.8X6
therapeutic	T50.991	T50.992	T50.993	T50.994	T50.995	T50.996
131 — *see also Radiation sickness, and Exposure to radioactivce isotopes*	T50.8X1	T50.8X2	T50.8X3	T50.8X4	T50.8X5	T50.8X6
therapeutic	T38.2X1	T38.2X2	T38.2X3	T38.2X4	T38.2X5	T38.2X6
diagnostic	T50.8X1	T50.8X2	T50.8X3	T50.8X4	T50.8X5	T50.8X6
for thyroid conditions (antithyroid)	T38.2X1	T38.2X2	T38.2X3	T38.2X4	T38.2X5	T38.2X6
solution	T49.0X1	T49.0X2	T49.0X3	T49.0X4	T49.0X5	T49.0X6
vapor	T59.891	T59.892	T59.893	T59.894	--	--
Iodipamide	T50.8X1	T50.8X2	T50.8X3	T50.8X4	T50.8X5	T50.8X6
Iodized (poppy seed) **oil**	T50.8X1	T50.8X2	T50.8X3	T50.8X4	T50.8X5	T50.8X6
Iodobismitol	T37.8X1	T37.8X2	T37.8X3	T37.8X4	T37.8X5	T37.8X6
Iodochlorhydroxyquin	T37.8X1	T37.8X2	T37.8X3	T37.8X4	T37.8X5	T37.8X6
topical	T49.0X1	T49.0X2	T49.0X3	T49.0X4	T49.0X5	T49.0X6
Iodochlorhydroxyquinoline	T37.8X1	T37.8X2	T37.8X3	T37.8X4	T37.8X5	T37.8X6
Iodocholesterol (131I)	T50.8X1	T50.8X2	T50.8X3	T50.8X4	T50.8X5	T50.8X6
Iodoform	T49.0X1	T49.0X2	T49.0X3	T49.0X4	T49.0X5	T49.0X6
Iodohippuric acid	T50.8X1	T50.8X2	T50.8X3	T50.8X4	T50.8X5	T50.8X6
Iodopanoic acid	T50.8X1	T50.8X2	T50.8X3	T50.8X4	T50.8X5	T50.8X6
Iodophthalein (sodium)	T50.8X1	T50.8X2	T50.8X3	T50.8X4	T50.8X5	T50.8X6
Iodopyracet	T50.8X1	T50.8X2	T50.8X3	T50.8X4	T50.8X5	T50.8X6
Iodoquinol	T37.8X1	T37.8X2	T37.8X3	T37.8X4	T37.8X5	T37.8X6
Iodoxamic acid	T50.8X1	T50.8X2	T50.8X3	T50.8X4	T50.8X5	T50.8X6
Iofendylate	T50.8X1	T50.8X2	T50.8X3	T50.8X4	T50.8X5	T50.8X6
Ioglycamic acid	T50.8X1	T50.8X2	T50.8X3	T50.8X4	T50.8X5	T50.8X6
Iohexol	T50.8X1	T50.8X2	T50.8X3	T50.8X4	T50.8X5	T50.8X6
Ion exchange resin						
anion	T47.8X1	T47.8X2	T47.8X3	T47.8X4	T47.8X5	T47.8X6
cation	T50.3X1	T50.3X2	T50.3X3	T50.3X4	T50.3X5	T50.3X6
cholestyramine	T46.6X1	T46.6X2	T46.6X3	T46.6X4	T46.6X5	T46.6X6
intestinal	T47.8X1	T47.8X2	T47.8X3	T47.8X4	T47.8X5	T47.8X6
Iopamidol	T50.8X1	T50.8X2	T50.8X3	T50.8X4	T50.8X5	T50.8X6
Iopanoic acid	T50.8X1	T50.8X2	T50.8X3	T50.8X4	T50.8X5	T50.8X6
Iophenoic acid	T50.8X1	T50.8X2	T50.8X3	T50.8X4	T50.8X5	T50.8X6
Iopodate, sodium	T50.8X1	T50.8X2	T50.8X3	T50.8X4	T50.8X5	T50.8X6
Iopodic acid	T50.8X1	T50.8X2	T50.8X3	T50.8X4	T50.8X5	T50.8X6
Iopromide	T50.8X1	T50.8X2	T50.8X3	T50.8X4	T50.8X5	T50.8X6
Iopydol	T50.8X1	T50.8X2	T50.8X3	T50.8X4	T50.8X5	T50.8X6
Iotalamic acid	T50.8X1	T50.8X2	T50.8X3	T50.8X4	T50.8X5	T50.8X6
Iothalamate	T50.8X1	T50.8X2	T50.8X3	T50.8X4	T50.8X5	T50.8X6
Iothiouracil	T38.2X1	T38.2X2	T38.2X3	T38.2X4	T38.2X5	T38.2X6
Iotrol	T50.8X1	T50.8X2	T50.8X3	T50.8X4	T50.8X5	T50.8X6
Iotrolan	T50.8X1	T50.8X2	T50.8X3	T50.8X4	T50.8X5	T50.8X6
Iotroxate	T50.8X1	T50.8X2	T50.8X3	T50.8X4	T50.8X5	T50.8X6
Iotroxic acid	T50.8X1	T50.8X2	T50.8X3	T50.8X4	T50.8X5	T50.8X6
Ioversol	T50.8X1	T50.8X2	T50.8X3	T50.8X4	T50.8X5	T50.8X6
Ioxaglate	T50.8X1	T50.8X2	T50.8X3	T50.8X4	T50.8X5	T50.8X6
Ioxaglic acid	T50.8X1	T50.8X2	T50.8X3	T50.8X4	T50.8X5	T50.8X6
Ioxitalamic acid	T50.8X1	T50.8X2	T50.8X3	T50.8X4	T50.8X5	T50.8X6
Ipecac	T47.7X1	T47.7X2	T47.7X3	T47.7X4	T47.7X5	T47.7X6
Ipecacuanha	T48.4X1	T48.4X2	T48.4X3	T48.4X4	T48.4X5	T48.4X6

Ipodate, calcium - Lauryl sulfoacetate

Substance	Poisoning, Accidental unintentional	Poisoning, Intentional self-harm	Poisoning, Assault	Poisoning, Undetermined	Adverse effect	Underdosing
Ipodate, calcium	T50.8X1	T50.8X2	T50.8X3	T50.8X4	T50.8X5	T50.8X6
Ipral	T42.3X1	T42.3X2	T42.3X3	T42.3X4	T42.3X5	T42.3X6
Ipratropium (bromide)	T48.6X1	T48.6X2	T48.6X3	T48.6X4	T48.6X5	T48.6X6
Ipriflavone	T46.3X1	T46.3X2	T46.3X3	T46.3X4	T46.3X5	T46.3X6
Iprindole	T43.011	T43.012	T43.013	T43.014	T43.015	T43.016
Iproclozide	T43.1X1	T43.1X2	T43.1X3	T43.1X4	T43.1X5	T43.1X6
Iprofenin	T50.8X1	T50.8X2	T50.8X3	T50.8X4	T50.8X5	T50.8X6
Iproheptine	T49.2X1	T49.2X2	T49.2X3	T49.2X4	T49.2X5	T49.2X6
Iproniazid	T43.1X1	T43.1X2	T43.1X3	T43.1X4	T43.1X5	T43.1X6
Iproplatin	T45.1X1	T45.1X2	T45.1X3	T45.1X4	T45.1X5	T45.1X6
Iproveratril	T46.1X1	T46.1X2	T46.1X3	T46.1X4	T46.1X5	T46.1X6
Iron (compounds) (medicinal) NEC	T45.4X1	T45.4X2	T45.4X3	T45.4X4	T45.4X5	T45.4X6
ammonium	T45.4X1	T45.4X2	T45.4X3	T45.4X4	T45.4X5	T45.4X6
dextran injection	T45.4X1	T45.4X2	T45.4X3	T45.4X4	T45.4X5	T45.4X6
nonmedicinal	T56.891	T56.892	T56.893	T56.894	--	--
salts	T45.4X1	T45.4X2	T45.4X3	T45.4X4	T45.4X5	T45.4X6
sorbitex	T45.4X1	T45.4X2	T45.4X3	T45.4X4	T45.4X5	T45.4X6
sorbitol citric acid complex	T45.4X1	T45.4X2	T45.4X3	T45.4X4	T45.4X5	T45.4X6
Irrigating fluid (vaginal)	T49.8X1	T49.8X2	T49.8X3	T49.8X4	T49.8X5	T49.8X6
eye	T49.5X1	T49.5X2	T49.5X3	T49.5X4	T49.5X5	T49.5X6
Isepamicin	T36.5X1	T36.5X2	T36.5X3	T36.5X4	T36.5X5	T36.5X6
Isoaminile (citrate)	T48.3X1	T48.3X2	T48.3X3	T48.3X4	T48.3X5	T48.3X6
Isoamyl nitrite	T46.3X1	T46.3X2	T46.3X3	T46.3X4	T46.3X5	T46.3X6
Isobenzan	T60.1X1	T60.1X2	T60.1X3	T60.1X4	--	--
Isobutyl acetate	T52.8X1	T52.8X2	T52.8X3	T52.8X4	--	--
Isocarboxazid	T43.1X1	T43.1X2	T43.1X3	T43.1X4	T43.1X5	T43.1X6
Isoconazole	T49.0X1	T49.0X2	T49.0X3	T49.0X4	T49.0X5	T49.0X6
Isocyanate	T65.0X1	T65.0X2	T65.0X3	T65.0X4	--	--
Isoephedrine	T44.991	T44.992	T44.993	T44.994	T44.995	T44.996
Isoetarine	T48.6X1	T48.6X2	T48.6X3	T48.6X4	T48.6X5	T48.6X6
Isoethadione	T42.2X1	T42.2X2	T42.2X3	T42.2X4	T42.2X5	T42.2X6
Isoetharine	T44.5X1	T44.5X2	T44.5X3	T44.5X4	T44.5X5	T44.5X6
Isoflurane	T41.0X1	T41.0X2	T41.0X3	T41.0X4	T41.0X5	T41.0X6
Isoflurophate	T44.0X1	T44.0X2	T44.0X3	T44.0X4	T44.0X5	T44.0X6
Isomaltose, ferric complex	T45.4X1	T45.4X2	T45.4X3	T45.4X4	T45.4X5	T45.4X6
Isometheptene	T44.3X1	T44.3X2	T44.3X3	T44.3X4	T44.3X5	T44.3X6
Isoniazid	T37.1X1	T37.1X2	T37.1X3	T37.1X4	T37.1X5	T37.1X6
with						
rifampicin	T36.6X1	T36.6X2	T36.6X3	T36.6X4	T36.6X5	T36.6X6
thioacetazone	T37.1X1	T37.1X2	T37.1X3	T37.1X4	T37.1X5	T37.1X6
Isonicotinic acid hydrazide	T37.1X1	T37.1X2	T37.1X3	T37.1X4	T37.1X5	T37.1X6
Isonipecaine	T40.4X1	T40.4X2	T40.4X3	T40.4X4	T40.4X5	T40.4X6
Isopentaquine	T37.2X1	T37.2X2	T37.2X3	T37.2X4	T37.2X5	T37.2X6
Isophane insulin	T38.3X1	T38.3X2	T38.3X3	T38.3X4	T38.3X5	T38.3X6
Isophorone	T65.891	T65.892	T65.893	T65.894	--	--
Isophosphamide	T45.1X1	T45.1X2	T45.1X3	T45.1X4	T45.1X5	T45.1X6
Isopregnenone	T38.5X1	T38.5X2	T38.5X3	T38.5X4	T38.5X5	T38.5X6
Isoprenaline	T48.6X1	T48.6X2	T48.6X3	T48.6X4	T48.6X5	T48.6X6
Isopromethazine	T43.3X1	T43.3X2	T43.3X3	T43.3X4	T43.3X5	T43.3X6
Isopropamide	T44.3X1	T44.3X2	T44.3X3	T44.3X4	T44.3X5	T44.3X6
iodide	T44.3X1	T44.3X2	T44.3X3	T44.3X4	T44.3X5	T44.3X6
Isopropanol	T51.2X1	T51.2X2	T51.2X3	T51.2X4	--	--
Isopropyl						
acetate	T52.8X1	T52.8X2	T52.8X3	T52.8X4	--	--
alcohol	T51.2X1	T51.2X2	T51.2X3	T51.2X4	--	--
medicinal	T49.4X1	T49.4X2	T49.4X3	T49.4X4	T49.4X5	T49.4X6
ether	T52.8X1	T52.8X2	T52.8X3	T52.8X4	--	--
Isopropylaminophenazone	T39.2X1	T39.2X2	T39.2X3	T39.2X4	T39.2X5	T39.2X6
Isoproterenol	T48.6X1	T48.6X2	T48.6X3	T48.6X4	T48.6X5	T48.6X6
Isosorbide dinitrate	T46.3X1	T46.3X2	T46.3X3	T46.3X4	T46.3X5	T46.3X6
Isothipendyl	T45.0X1	T45.0X2	T45.0X3	T45.0X4	T45.0X5	T45.0X6
Isotretinoin	T50.991	T50.992	T50.993	T50.994	T50.995	T50.996
Isoxazolyl penicillin	T36.0X1	T36.0X2	T36.0X3	T36.0X4	T36.0X5	T36.0X6
Isoxicam	T39.391	T39.392	T39.393	T39.394	T39.395	T39.396
Isoxsuprine	T46.7X1	T46.7X2	T46.7X3	T46.7X4	T46.7X5	T46.7X6
Ispagula	T47.4X1	T47.4X2	T47.4X3	T47.4X4	T47.4X5	T47.4X6
husk	T47.4X1	T47.4X2	T47.4X3	T47.4X4	T47.4X5	T47.4X6
Isradipine	T46.1X1	T46.1X2	T46.1X3	T46.1X4	T46.1X5	T46.1X6
I-thyroxine sodium	T38.1X1	T38.1X2	T38.1X3	T38.1X4	T38.1X5	T38.1X6
Itraconazole	T37.8X1	T37.8X2	T37.8X3	T37.8X4	T37.8X5	T37.8X6
Itramin tosilate	T46.3X1	T46.3X2	T46.3X3	T46.3X4	T46.3X5	T46.3X6
Ivermectin	T37.4X1	T37.4X2	T37.4X3	T37.4X4	T37.4X5	T37.4X6
Izoniazid	T37.1X1	T37.1X2	T37.1X3	T37.1X4	T37.1X5	T37.1X6
with thioacetazone	T37.1X1	T37.1X2	T37.1X3	T37.1X4	T37.1X5	T37.1X6
J						
Jalap	T47.2X1	T47.2X2	T47.2X3	T47.2X4	T47.2X5	T47.2X6
Jamaica						
dogwood (bark)	T39.8X1	T39.8X2	T39.8X3	T39.8X4	T39.8X5	T39.8X6
ginger	T65.891	T65.892	T65.893	T65.894	--	--
root	T62.2X1	T62.2X2	T62.2X3	T62.2X4	--	--
Jatropha	T62.2X1	T62.2X2	T62.2X3	T62.2X4	--	--
curcas	T62.2X1	T62.2X2	T62.2X3	T62.2X4	--	--
Jectofer	T45.4X1	T45.4X2	T45.4X3	T45.4X4	T45.4X5	T45.4X6
Jellyfish (sting)	T63.621	T63.622	T63.623	T63.624	--	--
Jequirity (bean)	T62.2X1	T62.2X2	T62.2X3	T62.2X4	--	--
Jimson weed (stramonium)	T62.2X1	T62.2X2	T62.2X3	T62.2X4	--	--
seeds	T62.2X1	T62.2X2	T62.2X3	T62.2X4	--	--
Josamycin	T36.3X1	T36.3X2	T36.3X3	T36.3X4	T36.3X5	T36.3X6
Juniper tar	T49.1X1	T49.1X2	T49.1X3	T49.1X4	T49.1X5	T49.1X6
K						
Kallidinogenase	T46.7X1	T46.7X2	T46.7X3	T46.7X4	T46.7X5	T46.7X6
Kallikrein	T46.7X1	T46.7X2	T46.7X3	T46.7X4	T46.7X5	T46.7X6
Kanamycin	T36.5X1	T36.5X2	T36.5X3	T36.5X4	T36.5X5	T36.5X6
Kantrex	T36.5X1	T36.5X2	T36.5X3	T36.5X4	T36.5X5	T36.5X6
Kaolin	T47.6X1	T47.6X2	T47.6X3	T47.6X4	T47.6X5	T47.6X6
light	T47.6X1	T47.6X2	T47.6X3	T47.6X4	T47.6X5	T47.6X6
Karaya (gum)	T47.4X1	T47.4X2	T47.4X3	T47.4X4	T47.4X5	T47.4X6
Kebuzone	T39.2X1	T39.2X2	T39.2X3	T39.2X4	T39.2X5	T39.2X6
Kelevan	T60.1X1	T60.1X2	T60.1X3	T60.1X4	--	--
Kemithal	T41.1X1	T41.1X2	T41.1X3	T41.1X4	T41.1X5	T41.1X6
Kenacort	T38.0X1	T38.0X2	T38.0X3	T38.0X4	T38.0X5	T38.0X6
Keratolytic drug NEC	T49.4X1	T49.4X2	T49.4X3	T49.4X4	T49.4X5	T49.4X6
anthracene	T49.4X1	T49.4X2	T49.4X3	T49.4X4	T49.4X5	T49.4X6
Keratoplastic NEC	T49.4X1	T49.4X2	T49.4X3	T49.4X4	T49.4X5	T49.4X6
Kerosene, kerosine (fuel) (solvent) NEC	T52.0X1	T52.0X2	T52.0X3	T52.0X4	--	--
insecticide	T52.0X1	T52.0X2	T52.0X3	T52.0X4	--	--
vapor	T52.0X1	T52.0X2	T52.0X3	T52.0X4	--	--
Ketamine	T41.291	T41.292	T41.293	T41.294	T41.295	T41.296
Ketazolam	T42.4X1	T42.4X2	T42.4X3	T42.4X4	T42.4X5	T42.4X6
Ketazon	T39.2X1	T39.2X2	T39.2X3	T39.2X4	T39.2X5	T39.2X6
Ketobemidone	T40.4X1	T40.4X2	T40.4X3	T40.4X4	--	--
Ketoconazole	T49.0X1	T49.0X2	T49.0X3	T49.0X4	T49.0X5	T49.0X6
Ketols	T52.4X1	T52.4X2	T52.4X3	T52.4X4	--	--
Ketone oils	T52.4X1	T52.4X2	T52.4X3	T52.4X4	--	--
Ketoprofen	T39.311	T39.312	T39.313	T39.314	T39.315	T39.316
Ketorolac	T39.8X1	T39.8X2	T39.8X3	T39.8X4	T39.8X5	T39.8X6
Ketotifen	T45.0X1	T45.0X2	T45.0X3	T45.0X4	T45.0X5	T45.0X6
Khat	T43.691	T43.692	T43.693	T43.694	--	--
Khellin	T46.3X1	T46.3X2	T46.3X3	T46.3X4	T46.3X5	T46.3X6
Khelloside	T46.3X1	T46.3X2	T46.3X3	T46.3X4	T46.3X5	T46.3X6
Kiln gas or vapor (carbon monoxide)	T58.8X1	T58.8X2	T58.8X3	T58.8X4	--	--
Kitasamycin	T36.3X1	T36.3X2	T36.3X3	T36.3X4	T36.3X5	T36.3X6
Konsyl	T47.4X1	T47.4X2	T47.4X3	T47.4X4	T47.4X5	T47.4X6
Kosam seed	T62.2X1	T62.2X2	T62.2X3	T62.2X4	--	--
Krait (venom)	T63.091	T63.092	T63.093	T63.094	--	--
Kwell (insecticide)	T60.1X1	T60.1X2	T60.1X3	T60.1X4	--	--
anti-infective (topical)	T49.0X1	T49.0X2	T49.0X3	T49.0X4	T49.0X5	T49.0X6
L						
Labetalol	T44.8X1	T44.8X2	T44.8X3	T44.8X4	T44.8X5	T44.8X6
Laburnum (seeds)	T62.2X1	T62.2X2	T62.2X3	T62.2X4	--	--
leaves	T62.2X1	T62.2X2	T62.2X3	T62.2X4	--	--
Lachesine	T49.5X1	T49.5X2	T49.5X3	T49.5X4	T49.5X5	T49.5X6
Lacidipine	T46.5X1	T46.5X2	T46.5X3	T46.5X4	T46.5X5	T46.5X6
Lacquer	T65.6X1	T65.6X2	T65.6X3	T65.6X4	--	--
Lacrimogenic gas	T59.3X1	T59.3X2	T59.3X3	T59.3X4	--	--
Lactated potassic saline	T50.3X1	T50.3X2	T50.3X3	T50.3X4	T50.3X5	T50.3X6
Lactic acid	T49.8X1	T49.8X2	T49.8X3	T49.8X4	T49.8X5	T49.8X6
Lactobacillus						
acidophilus	T47.6X1	T47.6X2	T47.6X3	T47.6X4	T47.6X5	T47.6X6
compound	T47.6X1	T47.6X2	T47.6X3	T47.6X4	T47.6X5	T47.6X6
bifidus, lyophilized	T47.6X1	T47.6X2	T47.6X3	T47.6X4	T47.6X5	T47.6X6
bulgaricus	T47.6X1	T47.6X2	T47.6X3	T47.6X4	T47.6X5	T47.6X6
sporogenes	T47.6X1	T47.6X2	T47.6X3	T47.6X4	T47.6X5	T47.6X6
Lactoflavin	T45.2X1	T45.2X2	T45.2X3	T45.2X4	T45.2X5	T45.2X6
Lactose (as excipient)	T50.901	T50.902	T50.903	T50.904	T50.905	T50.906
Lactuca (virosa) (extract)	T42.6X1	T42.6X2	T42.6X3	T42.6X4	T42.6X5	T42.6X6
Lactucarium	T42.6X1	T42.6X2	T42.6X3	T42.6X4	T42.6X5	T42.6X6
Lactulose	T47.3X1	T47.3X2	T47.3X3	T47.3X4	T47.3X5	T47.3X6
Laevo — *see Levo-*						
Lanatosides	T46.0X1	T46.0X2	T46.0X3	T46.0X4	T46.0X5	T46.0X6
Lanolin	T49.3X1	T49.3X2	T49.3X3	T49.3X4	T49.3X5	T49.3X6
Largactil	T43.3X1	T43.3X2	T43.3X3	T43.3X4	T43.3X5	T43.3X6
Larkspur	T62.2X1	T62.2X2	T62.2X3	T62.2X4	--	--
Laroxyl	T43.011	T43.012	T43.013	T43.014	T43.015	T43.016
Lasix	T50.1X1	T50.1X2	T50.1X3	T50.1X4	T50.1X5	T50.1X6
Lassar's paste	T49.4X1	T49.4X2	T49.4X3	T49.4X4	T49.4X5	T49.4X6
Latamoxef	T36.1X1	T36.1X2	T36.1X3	T36.1X4	T36.1X5	T36.1X6
Latex	T65.811	T65.812	T65.813	T65.814	--	--
Lathyrus (seed)	T62.2X1	T62.2X2	T62.2X3	T62.2X4	--	--
Laudanum	T40.0X1	T40.0X2	T40.0X3	T40.0X4	T40.0X5	T40.0X6
Laudexium	T48.1X1	T48.1X2	T48.1X3	T48.1X4	T48.1X5	T48.1X6
Laughing gas	T41.0X1	T41.0X2	T41.0X3	T41.0X4	T41.0X5	T41.0X6
Laurel, black or cherry	T62.2X1	T62.2X2	T62.2X3	T62.2X4	--	--
Laurolinium	T49.0X1	T49.0X2	T49.0X3	T49.0X4	T49.0X5	T49.0X6
Lauryl sulfoacetate	T49.2X1	T49.2X2	T49.2X3	T49.2X4	T49.2X5	T49.2X6

Substance	Poisoning, Accidental unintentional	Poisoning, Intentional self-harm	Poisoning, Assault	Poisoning, Undetermined	Adverse effect	Underdosing
Laxative NEC	T47.4X1	T47.4X2	T47.4X3	T47.4X4	T47.4X5	T47.4X6
osmotic	T47.3X1	T47.3X2	T47.3X3	T47.3X4	T47.3X5	T47.3X6
saline	T47.3X1	T47.3X2	T47.3X3	T47.3X4	T47.3X5	T47.3X6
stimulant	T47.2X1	T47.2X2	T47.2X3	T47.2X4	T47.2X5	T47.2X6
L-dopa	T42.8X1	T42.8X2	T42.8X3	T42.8X4	T42.8X5	T42.8X6
Lead (dust) (fumes) (vapor) NEC	T56.0X1	T56.0X2	T56.0X3	T56.0X4	--	--
acetate	T49.2X1	T49.2X2	T49.2X3	T49.2X4	T49.2X5	T49.2X6
alkyl (fuel additive)	T56.0X1	T56.0X2	T56.0X3	T56.0X4	--	--
anti-infectives	T37.8X1	T37.8X2	T37.8X3	T37.8X4	T37.8X5	T37.8X6
antiknock compound (tetraethyl)	T56.0X1	T56.0X2	T56.0X3	T56.0X4	--	--
arsenate, arsenite (dust) (herbicide) (insecticide) (vapor)	T57.0X1	T57.0X2	T57.0X3	T57.0X4	--	--
carbonate	T56.0X1	T56.0X2	T56.0X3	T56.0X4	--	--
paint	T56.0X1	T56.0X2	T56.0X3	T56.0X4	--	--
chromate	T56.0X1	T56.0X2	T56.0X3	T56.0X4	--	--
paint	T56.0X1	T56.0X2	T56.0X3	T56.0X4	--	--
dioxide	T56.0X1	T56.0X2	T56.0X3	T56.0X4	--	--
inorganic	T56.0X1	T56.0X2	T56.0X3	T56.0X4	--	--
iodide	T56.0X1	T56.0X2	T56.0X3	T56.0X4	--	--
pigment (paint)	T56.0X1	T56.0X2	T56.0X3	T56.0X4	--	--
monoxide (dust)	T56.0X1	T56.0X2	T56.0X3	T56.0X4	--	--
paint	T56.0X1	T56.0X2	T56.0X3	T56.0X4	--	--
organic	T56.0X1	T56.0X2	T56.0X3	T56.0X4	--	--
oxide	T56.0X1	T56.0X2	T56.0X3	T56.0X4	--	--
paint	T56.0X1	T56.0X2	T56.0X3	T56.0X4	--	--
paint	T56.0X1	T56.0X2	T56.0X3	T56.0X4	--	--
salts	T56.0X1	T56.0X2	T56.0X3	T56.0X4	--	--
specified compound NEC	T56.0X1	T56.0X2	T56.0X3	T56.0X4	--	--
tetra-ethyl	T56.0X1	T56.0X2	T56.0X3	T56.0X4	--	--
Lebanese red	T40.7X1	T40.7X2	T40.7X3	T40.7X4	T40.7X5	T40.7X6
Lefetamine	T39.8X1	T39.8X2	T39.8X3	T39.8X4	T39.8X5	T39.8X6
Lenperone	T43.4X1	T43.4X2	T43.4X3	T43.4X4	T43.4X5	T43.4X6
Lente lietin (insulin)	T38.3X1	T38.3X2	T38.3X3	T38.3X4	T38.3X5	T38.3X6
Leptazol	T50.7X1	T50.7X2	T50.7X3	T50.7X4	T50.7X5	T50.7X6
Leptophos	T60.0X1	T60.0X2	T60.0X3	T60.0X4	--	--
Leritine	T40.2X1	T40.2X2	T40.2X3	T40.2X4	T40.2X5	T40.2X6
Letosteine	T48.4X1	T48.4X2	T48.4X3	T48.4X4	T48.4X5	T48.4X6
Letter	T38.1X1	T38.1X2	T38.1X3	T38.1X4	T38.1X5	T38.1X6
Lettuce opium	T42.6X1	T42.6X2	T42.6X3	T42.6X4	T42.6X5	T42.6X6
Leucinocaine	T41.3X1	T41.3X2	T41.3X3	T41.3X4	T41.3X5	T41.3X6
Leucocianidol	T46.991	T46.992	T46.993	T46.994	T46.995	T46.996
Leucovorin (factor)	T45.8X1	T45.8X2	T45.8X3	T45.8X4	T45.8X5	T45.8X6
Leukeran	T45.1X1	T45.1X2	T45.1X3	T45.1X4	T45.1X5	T45.1X6
Leuprolide	T38.891	T38.892	T38.893	T38.894	T38.895	T38.896
Levalbuterol	T48.6X1	T48.6X2	T48.6X3	T48.6X4	T48.6X5	T48.6X6
Levallorphan	T50.7X1	T50.7X2	T50.7X3	T50.7X4	T50.7X5	T50.7X6
Levamisole	T37.4X1	T37.4X2	T37.4X3	T37.4X4	T37.4X5	T37.4X6
Levanil	T42.6X1	T42.6X2	T42.6X3	T42.6X4	T42.6X5	T42.6X6
Levarterenol	T44.4X1	T44.4X2	T44.4X3	T44.4X4	T44.4X5	T44.4X6
Levdropropizine	T48.3X1	T48.3X2	T48.3X3	T48.3X4	T48.3X5	T48.3X6
Levobunolol	T49.5X1	T49.5X2	T49.5X3	T49.5X4	T49.5X5	T49.5X6
Levocabastine (hydrochloride)	T45.0X1	T45.0X2	T45.0X3	T45.0X4	T45.0X5	T45.0X6
Levocarnitine	T50.991	T50.992	T50.993	T50.994	T50.995	T50.996
Levodopa	T42.8X1	T42.8X2	T42.8X3	T42.8X4	T42.8X5	T42.8X6
with carbidopa	T42.8X1	T42.8X2	T42.8X3	T42.8X4	T42.8X5	T42.8X6
Levo-dromoran	T40.2X1	T40.2X2	T40.2X3	T40.2X4	T40.2X5	T40.2X6
Levoglutamide	T50.991	T50.992	T50.993	T50.994	T50.995	T50.996
Levoid	T38.1X1	T38.1X2	T38.1X3	T38.1X4	T38.1X5	T38.1X6
Levo-iso-methadone	T40.3X1	T40.3X2	T40.3X3	T40.3X4	T40.3X5	T40.3X6
Levomepromazine	T43.3X1	T43.3X2	T43.3X3	T43.3X4	T43.3X5	T43.3X6
Levonordefrin	T49.6X1	T49.6X2	T49.6X3	T49.6X4	T49.6X5	T49.6X6
Levonorgestrel	T38.4X1	T38.4X2	T38.4X3	T38.4X4	T38.4X5	T38.4X6
with ethinylestradiol	T38.5X1	T38.5X2	T38.5X3	T38.5X4	T38.5X5	T38.5X6
Levopromazine	T43.3X1	T43.3X2	T43.3X3	T43.3X4	T43.3X5	T43.3X6
Levoprome	T42.6X1	T42.6X2	T42.6X3	T42.6X4	T42.6X5	T42.6X6
Levopropoxyphene	T40.4X1	T40.4X2	T40.4X3	T40.4X4	T40.4X5	T40.4X6
Levopropylhexedrine	T50.5X1	T50.5X2	T50.5X3	T50.5X4	T50.5X5	T50.5X6
Levoproxyphylline	T48.6X1	T48.6X2	T48.6X3	T48.6X4	T48.6X5	T48.6X6
Levorphanol	T40.4X1	T40.4X2	T40.4X3	T40.4X4	T40.4X5	T40.4X6
Levothyroxine	T38.1X1	T38.1X2	T38.1X3	T38.1X4	T38.1X5	T38.1X6
sodium	T38.1X1	T38.1X2	T38.1X3	T38.1X4	T38.1X5	T38.1X6
Levsin	T44.3X1	T44.3X2	T44.3X3	T44.3X4	T44.3X5	T44.3X6
Levulose	T50.3X1	T50.3X2	T50.3X3	T50.3X4	T50.3X5	T50.3X6
Lewisite (gas), not in war	T57.0X1	T57.0X2	T57.0X3	T57.0X4	--	--
Librium	T42.4X1	T42.4X2	T42.4X3	T42.4X4	T42.4X5	T42.4X6
Lidex	T49.0X1	T49.0X2	T49.0X3	T49.0X4	T49.0X5	T49.0X6
Lidocaine	T41.3X1	T41.3X2	T41.3X3	T41.3X4	T41.3X5	T41.3X6
regional	T41.3X1	T41.3X2	T41.3X3	T41.3X4	T41.3X5	T41.3X6
spinal	T41.3X1	T41.3X2	T41.3X3	T41.3X4	T41.3X5	T41.3X6
Lidofenin	T50.8X1	T50.8X2	T50.8X3	T50.8X4	T50.8X5	T50.8X6
Lidoflazine	T46.1X1	T46.1X2	T46.1X3	T46.1X4	T46.1X5	T46.1X6
Lighter fluid	T52.0X1	T52.0X2	T52.0X3	T52.0X4	--	--
Lignin hemicellulose	T47.6X1	T47.6X2	T47.6X3	T47.6X4	T47.6X5	T47.6X6
Lignocaine	T41.3X1	T41.3X2	T41.3X3	T41.3X4	T41.3X5	T41.3X6
regional	T41.3X1	T41.3X2	T41.3X3	T41.3X4	T41.3X5	T41.3X6
spinal	T41.3X1	T41.3X2	T41.3X3	T41.3X4	T41.3X5	T41.3X6
Ligroin (e) (solvent)	T52.0X1	T52.0X2	T52.0X3	T52.0X4	--	--
vapor	T59.891	T59.892	T59.893	T59.894	--	--
Ligustrum vulgare	T62.2X1	T62.2X2	T62.2X3	T62.2X4	--	--
Lily of the valley	T62.2X1	T62.2X2	T62.2X3	T62.2X4	--	--
Lime (chloride)	T54.3X1	T54.3X2	T54.3X3	T54.3X4	--	--
Limonene	T52.8X1	T52.8X2	T52.8X3	T52.8X4	--	--
Lincomycin	T36.8X1	T36.8X2	T36.8X3	T36.8X4	T36.8X5	T36.8X6
Lindane (insecticide) (nonmedicinal) (vapor)	T53.6X1	T53.6X2	T53.6X3	T53.6X4	--	--
medicinal	T49.0X1	T49.0X2	T49.0X3	T49.0X4	T49.0X5	T49.0X6
Liniments NEC	T49.91	T49.92	T49.93	T49.94	T49.95	T49.96
Linoleic acid	T46.6X1	T46.6X2	T46.6X3	T46.6X4	T46.6X5	T46.6X6
Linolenic acid	T46.6X1	T46.6X2	T46.6X3	T46.6X4	T46.6X5	T46.6X6
Linseed	T47.4X1	T47.4X2	T47.4X3	T47.4X4	T47.4X5	T47.4X6
Liothyronine	T38.1X1	T38.1X2	T38.1X3	T38.1X4	T38.1X5	T38.1X6
Liotrix	T38.1X1	T38.1X2	T38.1X3	T38.1X4	T38.1X5	T38.1X6
Lipancreatin	T47.5X1	T47.5X2	T47.5X3	T47.5X4	T47.5X5	T47.5X6
Lipo-alprostadil	T46.7X1	T46.7X2	T46.7X3	T46.7X4	T46.7X5	T46.7X6
Lipo-Lutin	T38.5X1	T38.5X2	T38.5X3	T38.5X4	T38.5X5	T38.5X6
Lipotropic drug NEC	T50.901	T50.902	T50.903	T50.904	T50.905	T50.906
Liquefied petroleum gases	T59.891	T59.892	T59.893	T59.894	--	--
piped (pure or mixed with air)	T59.891	T59.892	T59.893	T59.894	--	--
Liquid						
paraffin	T47.4X1	T47.4X2	T47.4X3	T47.4X4	T47.4X5	T47.4X6
petrolatum	T47.4X1	T47.4X2	T47.4X3	T47.4X4	T47.4X5	T47.4X6
topical	T49.3X1	T49.3X2	T49.3X3	T49.3X4	T49.3X5	T49.3X6
specified NEC	T65.891	T65.892	T65.893	T65.894	--	--
substance	T65.91	T65.92	T65.93	T65.94	--	--
Liquor creosolis compositus	T65.891	T65.892	T65.893	T65.894	--	--
Liquorice	T48.4X1	T48.4X2	T48.4X3	T48.4X4	T48.4X5	T48.4X6
extract	T47.8X1	T47.8X2	T47.8X3	T47.8X4	T47.8X5	T47.8X6
Lisinopril	T46.4X1	T46.4X2	T46.4X3	T46.4X4	T46.4X5	T46.4X6
Lisuride	T42.8X1	T42.8X2	T42.8X3	T42.8X4	T42.8X5	T42.8X6
Lithane	T43.8X1	T43.8X2	T43.8X3	T43.8X4	T43.8X5	T43.8X6
Lithium	T56.891	T56.892	T56.893	T56.894	--	--
gluconate	T43.591	T43.592	T43.593	T43.594	T43.595	T43.596
salts (carbonate)	T43.591	T43.592	T43.593	T43.594	T43.595	T43.596
Lithonate	T43.8X1	T43.8X2	T43.8X3	T43.8X4	T43.8X5	T43.8X6
Liver						
extract	T45.8X1	T45.8X2	T45.8X3	T45.8X4	T45.8X5	T45.8X6
for parenteral use	T45.8X1	T45.8X2	T45.8X3	T45.8X4	T45.8X5	T45.8X6
fraction 1	T45.8X1	T45.8X2	T45.8X3	T45.8X4	T45.8X5	T45.8X6
hydrolysate	T45.8X1	T45.8X2	T45.8X3	T45.8X4	T45.8X5	T45.8X6
Lizard (bite) (venom)	T63.121	T63.122	T63.123	T63.124	--	--
LMD	T45.8X1	T45.8X2	T45.8X3	T45.8X4	T45.8X5	T45.8X6
Lobelia	T62.2X1	T62.2X2	T62.2X3	T62.2X4	--	--
Lobeline	T50.7X1	T50.7X2	T50.7X3	T50.7X4	T50.7X5	T50.7X6
Local action drug NEC	T49.8X1	T49.8X2	T49.8X3	T49.8X4	T49.8X5	T49.8X6
Locorten	T49.0X1	T49.0X2	T49.0X3	T49.0X4	T49.0X5	T49.0X6
Lofepramine	T43.011	T43.012	T43.013	T43.014	T43.015	T43.016
Lolium temulentum	T62.2X1	T62.2X2	T62.2X3	T62.2X4	--	--
Lomotil	T47.6X1	T47.6X2	T47.6X3	T47.6X4	T47.6X5	T47.6X6
Lomustine	T45.1X1	T45.1X2	T45.1X3	T45.1X4	T45.1X5	T45.1X6
Lonidamine	T45.1X1	T45.1X2	T45.1X3	T45.1X4	T45.1X5	T45.1X6
Loperamide	T47.6X1	T47.6X2	T47.6X3	T47.6X4	T47.6X5	T47.6X6
Loprazolam	T42.4X1	T42.4X2	T42.4X3	T42.4X4	T42.4X5	T42.4X6
Lorajmine	T46.2X1	T46.2X2	T46.2X3	T46.2X4	T46.2X5	T46.2X6
Loratidine	T45.0X1	T45.0X2	T45.0X3	T45.0X4	T45.0X5	T45.0X6
Lorazepam	T42.4X1	T42.4X2	T42.4X3	T42.4X4	T42.4X5	T42.4X6
Lorcainide	T46.2X1	T46.2X2	T46.2X3	T46.2X4	T46.2X5	T46.2X6
Lormetazepam	T42.4X1	T42.4X2	T42.4X3	T42.4X4	T42.4X5	T42.4X6
Lotions NEC	T49.91	T49.92	T49.93	T49.94	T49.95	T49.96
Lotusate	T42.3X1	T42.3X2	T42.3X3	T42.3X4	T42.3X5	T42.3X6
Lovastatin	T46.6X1	T46.6X2	T46.6X3	T46.6X4	T46.6X5	T46.6X6
Lowila	T49.2X1	T49.2X2	T49.2X3	T49.2X4	T49.2X5	T49.2X6
Loxapine	T43.591	T43.592	T43.593	T43.594	T43.595	T43.596
Lozenges (throat)	T49.6X1	T49.6X2	T49.6X3	T49.6X4	T49.6X5	T49.6X6
LSD	T40.8X1	T40.8X2	T40.8X3	T40.8X4	--	--
L-Tryptophan — *see amino acid*						
Lubricant, eye	T49.5X1	T49.5X2	T49.5X3	T49.5X4	T49.5X5	T49.5X6
Lubricating oil NEC	T52.0X1	T52.0X2	T52.0X3	T52.0X4	--	--
Lucanthone	T37.4X1	T37.4X2	T37.4X3	T37.4X4	T37.4X5	T37.4X6
Luminal	T42.3X1	T42.3X2	T42.3X3	T42.3X4	T42.3X5	T42.3X6
Lung irritant (gas) NEC	T59.91	T59.92	T59.93	T59.94	--	--
Luteinizing hormone	T38.811	T38.812	T38.813	T38.814	T38.815	T38.816
Lutocylol	T38.5X1	T38.5X2	T38.5X3	T38.5X4	T38.5X5	T38.5X6

Substance	Poisoning, Accidental unintentional	Poisoning, Intentional self-harm	Poisoning, Assault	Poisoning, Undetermined	Adverse effect	Underdosing
Lutromone	T38.5X1	T38.5X2	T38.5X3	T38.5X4	T38.5X5	T38.5X6
Lututrin	T48.291	T48.292	T48.293	T48.294	T48.295	T48.296
Lye (concentrated)	T54.3X1	T54.3X2	T54.3X3	T54.3X4	--	--
Lygranum (skin test)	T50.8X1	T50.8X2	T50.8X3	T50.8X4	T50.8X5	T50.8X6
Lymecycline	T36.4X1	T36.4X2	T36.4X3	T36.4X4	T36.4X5	T36.4X6
Lymphogranuloma venereum antigen	T50.8X1	T50.8X2	T50.8X3	T50.8X4	T50.8X5	T50.8X6
Lynestrenol	T38.4X1	T38.4X2	T38.4X3	T38.4X4	T38.4X5	T38.4X6
Lyovac Sodium Edecrin	T50.1X1	T50.1X2	T50.1X3	T50.1X4	T50.1X5	T50.1X6
Lypressin	T38.891	T38.892	T38.893	T38.894	T38.895	T38.896
Lysergic acid diethylamide	T40.8X1	T40.8X2	T40.8X3	T40.8X4	--	--
Lysergide	T40.8X1	T40.8X2	T40.8X3	T40.8X4	--	--
Lysine vasopressin	T38.891	T38.892	T38.893	T38.894	T38.895	T38.896
Lysol	T54.1X1	T54.1X2	T54.1X3	T54.1X4	--	--
Lysozyme	T49.0X1	T49.0X2	T49.0X3	T49.0X4	T49.0X5	T49.0X6
Lytta (vitatta)	T49.8X1	T49.8X2	T49.8X3	T49.8X4	T49.8X5	T49.8X6
M						
Mace	T59.3X1	T59.3X2	T59.3X3	T59.3X4	--	--
Macrogol	T50.991	T50.992	T50.993	T50.994	T50.995	T50.996
Macrolide						
anabolic drug	T38.7X1	T38.7X2	T38.7X3	T38.7X4	T38.7X5	T38.7X6
antibiotic	T36.3X1	T36.3X2	T36.3X3	T36.3X4	T36.3X5	T36.3X6
Mafenide	T49.0X1	T49.0X2	T49.0X3	T49.0X4	T49.0X5	T49.0X6
Magaldrate	T47.1X1	T47.1X2	T47.1X3	T47.1X4	T47.1X5	T47.1X6
Magic mushroom	T40.991	T40.992	T40.993	T40.994	--	--
Magnamycin	T36.8X1	T36.8X2	T36.8X3	T36.8X4	T36.8X5	T36.8X6
Magnesia magma	T47.1X1	T47.1X2	T47.1X3	T47.1X4	T47.1X5	T47.1X6
Magnesium NEC	T56.891	T56.892	T56.893	T56.894	--	--
carbonate	T47.1X1	T47.1X2	T47.1X3	T47.1X4	T47.1X5	T47.1X6
citrate	T47.4X1	T47.4X2	T47.4X3	T47.4X4	T47.4X5	T47.4X6
hydroxide	T47.1X1	T47.1X2	T47.1X3	T47.1X4	T47.1X5	T47.1X6
oxide	T47.1X1	T47.1X2	T47.1X3	T47.1X4	T47.1X5	T47.1X6
peroxide	T49.0X1	T49.0X2	T49.0X3	T49.0X4	T49.0X5	T49.0X6
salicylate	T39.091	T39.092	T39.093	T39.094	T39.095	T39.096
silicofluoride	T50.3X1	T50.3X2	T50.3X3	T50.3X4	T50.3X5	T50.3X6
sulfate	T47.4X1	T47.4X2	T47.4X3	T47.4X4	T47.4X5	T47.4X6
thiosulfate	T45.0X1	T45.0X2	T45.0X3	T45.0X4	T45.0X5	T45.0X6
trisilicate	T47.1X1	T47.1X2	T47.1X3	T47.1X4	T47.1X5	T47.1X6
Malathion (medicinal)	T49.0X1	T49.0X2	T49.0X3	T49.0X4	T49.0X5	T49.0X6
insecticide	T60.0X1	T60.0X2	T60.0X3	T60.0X4	--	--
Male fern extract	T37.4X1	T37.4X2	T37.4X3	T37.4X4	T37.4X5	T37.4X6
M-AMSA	T45.1X1	T45.1X2	T45.1X3	T45.1X4	T45.1X5	T45.1X6
Mandelic acid	T37.8X1	T37.8X2	T37.8X3	T37.8X4	T37.8X5	T37.8X6
Manganese (dioxide) (salts)	T57.2X1	T57.2X2	T57.2X3	T57.2X4	--	--
medicinal	T50.991	T50.992	T50.993	T50.994	T50.995	T50.996
Mannitol	T47.3X1	T47.3X2	T47.3X3	T47.3X4	T47.3X5	T47.3X6
hexanitrate	T46.3X1	T46.3X2	T46.3X3	T46.3X4	T46.3X5	T46.3X6
Mannomustine	T45.1X1	T45.1X2	T45.1X3	T45.1X4	T45.1X5	T45.1X6
MAO inhibitors	T43.1X1	T43.1X2	T43.1X3	T43.1X4	T43.1X5	T43.1X6
Mapharsen	T37.8X1	T37.8X2	T37.8X3	T37.8X4	T37.8X5	T37.8X6
Maphenide	T49.0X1	T49.0X2	T49.0X3	T49.0X4	T49.0X5	T49.0X6
Maprotiline	T43.021	T43.022	T43.023	T43.024	T43.025	T43.026
Marcaine	T41.3X1	T41.3X2	T41.3X3	T41.3X4	T41.3X5	T41.3X6
infiltration (subcutaneous)	T41.3X1	T41.3X2	T41.3X3	T41.3X4	T41.3X5	T41.3X6
nerve block (peripheral) (plexus)	T41.3X1	T41.3X2	T41.3X3	T41.3X4	T41.3X5	T41.3X6
Marezine	T45.0X1	T45.0X2	T45.0X3	T45.0X4	T45.0X5	T45.0X6
Marihuana	T40.7X1	T40.7X2	T40.7X3	T40.7X4	T40.7X5	T40.7X6
Marijuana	T40.7X1	T40.7X2	T40.7X3	T40.7X4	T40.7X5	T40.7X6
Marine (sting)	T63.691	T63.692	T63.693	T63.694	--	--
animals (sting)	T63.691	T63.692	T63.693	T63.694	--	--
plants (sting)	T63.711	T63.712	T63.713	T63.714	--	--
Marplan	T43.1X1	T43.1X2	T43.1X3	T43.1X4	T43.1X5	T43.1X6
Marsh gas	T59.891	T59.892	T59.893	T59.894	--	--
Marsilid	T43.1X1	T43.1X2	T43.1X3	T43.1X4	T43.1X5	T43.1X6
Matulane	T45.1X1	T45.1X2	T45.1X3	T45.1X4	T45.1X5	T45.1X6
Mazindol	T50.5X1	T50.5X2	T50.5X3	T50.5X4	T50.5X5	T50.5X6
MCPA	T60.3X1	T60.3X2	T60.3X3	T60.3X4	--	--
MDMA	T43.621	T43.622	T43.623	T43.624	T43.625	T43.626
Meadow saffron	T62.2X1	T62.2X2	T62.2X3	T62.2X4	--	--
Measles virus vaccine (attenuated)	T50.B91	T50.B92	T50.B93	T50.B94	T50.B95	T50.B96
Meat, noxious	T62.8X1	T62.8X2	T62.8X3	T62.8X4	--	--
Meballymal	T42.3X1	T42.3X2	T42.3X3	T42.3X4	T42.3X5	T42.3X6
Mebanazine	T43.1X1	T43.1X2	T43.1X3	T43.1X4	T43.1X5	T43.1X6
Mebaral	T42.3X1	T42.3X2	T42.3X3	T42.3X4	T42.3X5	T42.3X6
Mebendazole	T37.4X1	T37.4X2	T37.4X3	T37.4X4	T37.4X5	T37.4X6
Mebeverine	T44.3X1	T44.3X2	T44.3X3	T44.3X4	T44.3X5	T44.3X6
Mebhydrolin	T45.0X1	T45.0X2	T45.0X3	T45.0X4	T45.0X5	T45.0X6
Mebumal	T42.3X1	T42.3X2	T42.3X3	T42.3X4	T42.3X5	T42.3X6
Mebutamate	T43.591	T43.592	T43.593	T43.594	T43.595	T43.596
Mecamylamine	T44.2X1	T44.2X2	T44.2X3	T44.2X4	T44.2X5	T44.2X6
Mechlorethamine	T45.1X1	T45.1X2	T45.1X3	T45.1X4	T45.1X5	T45.1X6
Mecillinam	T36.0X1	T36.0X2	T36.0X3	T36.0X4	T36.0X5	T36.0X6
Meclizine (hydrochloride)	T45.0X1	T45.0X2	T45.0X3	T45.0X4	T45.0X5	T45.0X6
Meclocycline	T36.4X1	T36.4X2	T36.4X3	T36.4X4	T36.4X5	T36.4X6
Meclofenamate	T39.391	T39.392	T39.393	T39.394	T39.395	T39.396
Meclofenamic acid	T39.391	T39.392	T39.393	T39.394	T39.395	T39.396
Meclofenoxate	T43.691	T43.692	T43.693	T43.694	T43.695	T43.696
Meclozine	T45.0X1	T45.0X2	T45.0X3	T45.0X4	T45.0X5	T45.0X6
Mecobalamin	T45.8X1	T45.8X2	T45.8X3	T45.8X4	T45.8X5	T45.8X6
Mecoprop	T60.3X1	T60.3X2	T60.3X3	T60.3X4	--	--
Mecrilate	T49.3X1	T49.3X2	T49.3X3	T49.3X4	T49.3X5	T49.3X6
Mecysteine	T48.4X1	T48.4X2	T48.4X3	T48.4X4	T48.4X5	T48.4X6
Medazepam	T42.4X1	T42.4X2	T42.4X3	T42.4X4	T42.4X5	T42.4X6
Medicament NEC	T50.901	T50.902	T50.903	T50.904	T50.905	T50.906
Medinal	T42.3X1	T42.3X2	T42.3X3	T42.3X4	T42.3X5	T42.3X6
Medomin	T42.3X1	T42.3X2	T42.3X3	T42.3X4	T42.3X5	T42.3X6
Medrogestone	T38.5X1	T38.5X2	T38.5X3	T38.5X4	T38.5X5	T38.5X6
Medroxalol	T44.8X1	T44.8X2	T44.8X3	T44.8X4	T44.8X5	T44.8X6
Medroxyprogesterone acetate (depot)	T38.5X1	T38.5X2	T38.5X3	T38.5X4	T38.5X5	T38.5X6
Medrysone	T49.0X1	T49.0X2	T49.0X3	T49.0X4	T49.0X5	T49.0X6
Mefenamic acid	T39.391	T39.392	T39.393	T39.394	T39.395	T39.396
Mefenorex	T50.5X1	T50.5X2	T50.5X3	T50.5X4	T50.5X5	T50.5X6
Mefloquine	T37.2X1	T37.2X2	T37.2X3	T37.2X4	T37.2X5	T37.2X6
Mefruside	T50.2X1	T50.2X2	T50.2X3	T50.2X4	T50.2X5	T50.2X6
Megahallucinogen	T40.901	T40.902	T40.903	T40.904	T40.905	T40.906
Megestrol	T38.5X1	T38.5X2	T38.5X3	T38.5X4	T38.5X5	T38.5X6
Meglumine						
antimoniate	T37.8X1	T37.8X2	T37.8X3	T37.8X4	T37.8X5	T37.8X6
diatrizoate	T50.8X1	T50.8X2	T50.8X3	T50.8X4	T50.8X5	T50.8X6
iodipamide	T50.8X1	T50.8X2	T50.8X3	T50.8X4	T50.8X5	T50.8X6
iotroxate	T50.8X1	T50.8X2	T50.8X3	T50.8X4	T50.8X5	T50.8X6
MEK (methyl ethyl ketone)	T52.4X1	T52.4X2	T52.4X3	T52.4X4	--	--
Meladinin	T49.3X1	T49.3X2	T49.3X3	T49.3X4	T49.3X5	T49.3X6
Meladrazine	T44.3X1	T44.3X2	T44.3X3	T44.3X4	T44.3X5	T44.3X6
Melaleuca alternifolia oil	T49.0X1	T49.0X2	T49.0X3	T49.0X4	T49.0X5	T49.0X6
Melanizing agents	T49.3X1	T49.3X2	T49.3X3	T49.3X4	T49.3X5	T49.3X6
Melanocyte-stimulating hormone	T38.891	T38.892	T38.893	T38.894	T38.895	T38.896
Melarsonyl potassium	T37.3X1	T37.3X2	T37.3X3	T37.3X4	T37.3X5	T37.3X6
Melarsoprol	T37.3X1	T37.3X2	T37.3X3	T37.3X4	T37.3X5	T37.3X6
Melia azedarach	T62.2X1	T62.2X2	T62.2X3	T62.2X4	--	--
Melitracen	T43.011	T43.012	T43.013	T43.014	T43.015	T43.016
Mellaril	T43.3X1	T43.3X2	T43.3X3	T43.3X4	T43.3X5	T43.3X6
Meloxine	T49.3X1	T49.3X2	T49.3X3	T49.3X4	T49.3X5	T49.3X6
Melperone	T43.4X1	T43.4X2	T43.4X3	T43.4X4	T43.4X5	T43.4X6
Melphalan	T45.1X1	T45.1X2	T45.1X3	T45.1X4	T45.1X5	T45.1X6
Memantine	T43.8X1	T43.8X2	T43.8X3	T43.8X4	T43.8X5	T43.8X6
Menadiol	T45.7X1	T45.7X2	T45.7X3	T45.7X4	T45.7X5	T45.7X6
sodium sulfate	T45.7X1	T45.7X2	T45.7X3	T45.7X4	T45.7X5	T45.7X6
Menadione	T45.7X1	T45.7X2	T45.7X3	T45.7X4	T45.7X5	T45.7X6
sodium bisulfite	T45.7X1	T45.7X2	T45.7X3	T45.7X4	T45.7X5	T45.7X6
Menaphthone	T45.7X1	T45.7X2	T45.7X3	T45.7X4	T45.7X5	T45.7X6
Menaquinone	T45.7X1	T45.7X2	T45.7X3	T45.7X4	T45.7X5	T45.7X6
Menatetrenone	T45.7X1	T45.7X2	T45.7X3	T45.7X4	T45.7X5	T45.7X6
Meningococcal vaccine	T50.A91	T50.A92	T50.A93	T50.A94	T50.A95	T50.A96
Menningovax (-AC) (-C)	T50.A91	T50.A92	T50.A93	T50.A94	T50.A95	T50.A96
Menotropins	T38.811	T38.812	T38.813	T38.814	T38.815	T38.816
Menthol	T48.5X1	T48.5X2	T48.5X3	T48.5X4	T48.5X5	T48.5X6
Mepacrine	T37.2X1	T37.2X2	T37.2X3	T37.2X4	T37.2X5	T37.2X6
Meparfynol	T42.6X1	T42.6X2	T42.6X3	T42.6X4	T42.6X5	T42.6X6
Mepartricin	T36.7X1	T36.7X2	T36.7X3	T36.7X4	T36.7X5	T36.7X6
Mepazine	T43.3X1	T43.3X2	T43.3X3	T43.3X4	T43.3X5	T43.3X6
Mepenzolate	T44.3X1	T44.3X2	T44.3X3	T44.3X4	T44.3X5	T44.3X6
bromide	T44.3X1	T44.3X2	T44.3X3	T44.3X4	T44.3X5	T44.3X6
Meperidine	T40.4X1	T40.4X2	T40.4X3	T40.4X4	T40.4X5	T40.4X6
Mephebarbital	T42.3X1	T42.3X2	T42.3X3	T42.3X4	T42.3X5	T42.3X6
Mephenamin (e)	T42.8X1	T42.8X2	T42.8X3	T42.8X4	T42.8X5	T42.8X6
Mephenesin	T42.8X1	T42.8X2	T42.8X3	T42.8X4	T42.8X5	T42.8X6
Mephenhydramine	T45.0X1	T45.0X2	T45.0X3	T45.0X4	T45.0X5	T45.0X6
Mephenoxalone	T42.8X1	T42.8X2	T42.8X3	T42.8X4	T42.8X5	T42.8X6
Mephentermine	T44.991	T44.992	T44.993	T44.994	T44.995	T44.996
Mephenytoin	T42.0X1	T42.0X2	T42.0X3	T42.0X4	T42.0X5	T42.0X6
with phenobarbital	T42.3X1	T42.3X2	T42.3X3	T42.3X4	T42.3X5	T42.3X6
Mephobarbital	T42.3X1	T42.3X2	T42.3X3	T42.3X4	T42.3X5	T42.3X6
Mephosfolan	T60.0X1	T60.0X2	T60.0X3	T60.0X4	--	--
Mepindolol	T44.7X1	T44.7X2	T44.7X3	T44.7X4	T44.7X5	T44.7X6
Mepiperphenidol	T44.3X1	T44.3X2	T44.3X3	T44.3X4	T44.3X5	T44.3X6
Mepitiostane	T38.7X1	T38.7X2	T38.7X3	T38.7X4	T38.7X5	T38.7X6
Mepivacaine	T41.3X1	T41.3X2	T41.3X3	T41.3X4	T41.3X5	T41.3X6
epidural	T41.3X1	T41.3X2	T41.3X3	T41.3X4	T41.3X5	T41.3X6
Meprednisone	T38.0X1	T38.0X2	T38.0X3	T38.0X4	T38.0X5	T38.0X6
Meprobam	T43.591	T43.592	T43.593	T43.594	T43.595	T43.596
Meprobamate	T43.591	T43.592	T43.593	T43.594	T43.595	T43.596
Meproscillarin	T46.0X1	T46.0X2	T46.0X3	T46.0X4	T46.0X5	T46.0X6
Meprylcaine	T41.3X1	T41.3X2	T41.3X3	T41.3X4	T41.3X5	T41.3X6

Substance	Poisoning, Accidental unintentional	Poisoning, Intentional self-harm	Poisoning, Assault	Poisoning, Undetermined	Adverse effect	Underdosing
Meptazinol	T39.8X1	T39.8X2	T39.8X3	T39.8X4	T39.8X5	T39.8X6
Mepyramine	T45.0X1	T45.0X2	T45.0X3	T45.0X4	T45.0X5	T45.0X6
Mequitazine	T43.3X1	T43.3X2	T43.3X3	T43.3X4	T43.3X5	T43.3X6
Meralluride	T50.2X1	T50.2X2	T50.2X3	T50.2X4	T50.2X5	T50.2X6
Merbaphen	T50.2X1	T50.2X2	T50.2X3	T50.2X4	T50.2X5	T50.2X6
Merbromin	T49.0X1	T49.0X2	T49.0X3	T49.0X4	T49.0X5	T49.0X6
Mercaptobenzothiazole salts	T49.0X1	T49.0X2	T49.0X3	T49.0X4	T49.0X5	T49.0X6
Mercaptomerin	T50.2X1	T50.2X2	T50.2X3	T50.2X4	T50.2X5	T50.2X6
Mercaptopurine	T45.1X1	T45.1X2	T45.1X3	T45.1X4	T45.1X5	T45.1X6
Mercumatilin	T50.2X1	T50.2X2	T50.2X3	T50.2X4	T50.2X5	T50.2X6
Mercuramide	T50.2X1	T50.2X2	T50.2X3	T50.2X4	T50.2X5	T50.2X6
Mercurochrome	T49.0X1	T49.0X2	T49.0X3	T49.0X4	T49.0X5	T49.0X6
Mercurophylline	T50.2X1	T50.2X2	T50.2X3	T50.2X4	T50.2X5	T50.2X6
Mercury, mercurial, mercuric, mercurous (compounds) (cyanide) (fumes) (nonmedicinal) (vapor) **NEC**	T56.1X1	T56.1X2	T56.1X3	T56.1X4	--	--
ammoniated	T49.0X1	T49.0X2	T49.0X3	T49.0X4	T49.0X5	T49.0X6
anti-infective						
local	T49.0X1	T49.0X2	T49.0X3	T49.0X4	T49.0X5	T49.0X6
systemic	T37.8X1	T37.8X2	T37.8X3	T37.8X4	T37.8X5	T37.8X6
topical	T49.0X1	T49.0X2	T49.0X3	T49.0X4	T49.0X5	T49.0X6
chloride (ammoniated)	T49.0X1	T49.0X2	T49.0X3	T49.0X4	T49.0X5	T49.0X6
fungicide	T56.1X1	T56.1X2	T56.1X3	T56.1X4	--	--
diuretic NEC	T50.2X1	T50.2X2	T50.2X3	T50.2X4	T50.2X5	T50.2X6
fungicide	T56.1X1	T56.1X2	T56.1X3	T56.1X4	--	--
organic (fungicide)	T56.1X1	T56.1X2	T56.1X3	T56.1X4	--	--
oxide, yellow	T49.0X1	T49.0X2	T49.0X3	T49.0X4	T49.0X5	T49.0X6
Mersalyl	T50.2X1	T50.2X2	T50.2X3	T50.2X4	T50.2X5	T50.2X6
Merthiolate	T49.0X1	T49.0X2	T49.0X3	T49.0X4	T49.0X5	T49.0X6
ophthalmic preparation	T49.5X1	T49.5X2	T49.5X3	T49.5X4	T49.5X5	T49.5X6
Meruvax	T50.B91	T50.B92	T50.B93	T50.B94	T50.B95	T50.B96
Mesalazine	T47.8X1	T47.8X2	T47.8X3	T47.8X4	T47.8X5	T47.8X6
Mescal buttons	T40.991	T40.992	T40.993	T40.994	--	--
Mescaline	T40.991	T40.992	T40.993	T40.994	--	--
Mesna	T48.4X1	T48.4X2	T48.4X3	T48.4X4	T48.4X5	T48.4X6
Mesoglycan	T46.6X1	T46.6X2	T46.6X3	T46.6X4	T46.6X5	T46.6X6
Mesoridazine	T43.3X1	T43.3X2	T43.3X3	T43.3X4	T43.3X5	T43.3X6
Mestanolone	T38.7X1	T38.7X2	T38.7X3	T38.7X4	T38.7X5	T38.7X6
Mesterolone	T38.7X1	T38.7X2	T38.7X3	T38.7X4	T38.7X5	T38.7X6
Mestranol	T38.5X1	T38.5X2	T38.5X3	T38.5X4	T38.5X5	T38.5X6
Mesulergine	T42.8X1	T42.8X2	T42.8X3	T42.8X4	T42.8X5	T42.8X6
Mesulfen	T49.0X1	T49.0X2	T49.0X3	T49.0X4	T49.0X5	T49.0X6
Mesuximide	T42.2X1	T42.2X2	T42.2X3	T42.2X4	T42.2X5	T42.2X6
Metabutethamine	T41.3X1	T41.3X2	T41.3X3	T41.3X4	T41.3X5	T41.3X6
Metactesylacetate	T49.0X1	T49.0X2	T49.0X3	T49.0X4	T49.0X5	T49.0X6
Metacycline	T36.4X1	T36.4X2	T36.4X3	T36.4X4	T36.4X5	T36.4X6
Metaldehyde (snail killer) **NEC**	T60.8X1	T60.8X2	T60.8X3	T60.8X4	--	--
Metals (heavy) (nonmedicinal)	T56.91	T56.92	T56.93	T56.94	--	--
dust, fumes, or vapor NEC	T56.91	T56.92	T56.93	T56.94	--	--
light NEC	T56.91	T56.92	T56.93	T56.94	--	--
dust, fumes, or vapor NEC	T56.91	T56.92	T56.93	T56.94	--	--
specified NEC	T56.891	T56.892	T56.893	T56.894	--	--
thallium	T56.811	T56.812	T56.813	T56.814	--	--
Metamfetamine	T43.621	T43.622	T43.623	T43.624	T43.625	T43.626
Metamizole sodium	T39.2X1	T39.2X2	T39.2X3	T39.2X4	T39.2X5	T39.2X6
Metampicillin	T36.0X1	T36.0X2	T36.0X3	T36.0X4	T36.0X5	T36.0X6
Metamucil	T47.4X1	T47.4X2	T47.4X3	T47.4X4	T47.4X5	T47.4X6
Metandienone	T38.7X1	T38.7X2	T38.7X3	T38.7X4	T38.7X5	T38.7X6
Metandrostenolone	T38.7X1	T38.7X2	T38.7X3	T38.7X4	T38.7X5	T38.7X6
Metaphen	T49.0X1	T49.0X2	T49.0X3	T49.0X4	T49.0X5	T49.0X6
Metaphos	T60.0X1	T60.0X2	T60.0X3	T60.0X4	--	--
Metapramine	T43.011	T43.012	T43.013	T43.014	T43.015	T43.016
Metaproterenol	T48.291	T48.292	T48.293	T48.294	T48.295	T48.296
Metaraminol	T44.4X1	T44.4X2	T44.4X3	T44.4X4	T44.4X5	T44.4X6
Metaxalone	T42.8X1	T42.8X2	T42.8X3	T42.8X4	T42.8X5	T42.8X6
Metenolone	T38.7X1	T38.7X2	T38.7X3	T38.7X4	T38.7X5	T38.7X6
Metergoline	T42.8X1	T42.8X2	T42.8X3	T42.8X4	T42.8X5	T42.8X6
Metescufylline	T46.991	T46.992	T46.993	T46.994	T46.995	T46.996
Metetoin	T42.0X1	T42.0X2	T42.0X3	T42.0X4	T42.0X5	T42.0X6
Metformin	T38.3X1	T38.3X2	T38.3X3	T38.3X4	T38.3X5	T38.3X6
Methacholine	T44.1X1	T44.1X2	T44.1X3	T44.1X4	T44.1X5	T44.1X6
Methacycline	T36.4X1	T36.4X2	T36.4X3	T36.4X4	T36.4X5	T36.4X6
Methadone	T40.3X1	T40.3X2	T40.3X3	T40.3X4	T40.3X5	T40.3X6
Methallenestril	T38.5X1	T38.5X2	T38.5X3	T38.5X4	T38.5X5	T38.5X6
Methallenoestril	T38.5X1	T38.5X2	T38.5X3	T38.5X4	T38.5X5	T38.5X6
Methamphetamine	T43.621	T43.622	T43.623	T43.624	T43.625	T43.626
Methampyrone	T39.2X1	T39.2X2	T39.2X3	T39.2X4	T39.2X5	T39.2X6
Methandienone	T38.7X1	T38.7X2	T38.7X3	T38.7X4	T38.7X5	T38.7X6
Methandriol	T38.7X1	T38.7X2	T38.7X3	T38.7X4	T38.7X5	T38.7X6
Methandrostenolone	T38.7X1	T38.7X2	T38.7X3	T38.7X4	T38.7X5	T38.7X6
Methane	T59.891	T59.892	T59.893	T59.894	--	--
Methanethiol	T59.891	T59.892	T59.893	T59.894	--	--
Methaniazide	T37.1X1	T37.1X2	T37.1X3	T37.1X4	T37.1X5	T37.1X6
Methanol (vapor)	T51.1X1	T51.1X2	T51.1X3	T51.1X4	--	--
Methantheline	T44.3X1	T44.3X2	T44.3X3	T44.3X4	T44.3X5	T44.3X6
Methanthelinium bromide	T44.3X1	T44.3X2	T44.3X3	T44.3X4	T44.3X5	T44.3X6
Methaphenilene	T45.0X1	T45.0X2	T45.0X3	T45.0X4	T45.0X5	T45.0X6
Methapyrilene	T45.0X1	T45.0X2	T45.0X3	T45.0X4	T45.0X5	T45.0X6
Methaqualone (compound)	T42.6X1	T42.6X2	T42.6X3	T42.6X4	T42.6X5	T42.6X6
Metharbital	T42.3X1	T42.3X2	T42.3X3	T42.3X4	T42.3X5	T42.3X6
Methazolamide	T50.2X1	T50.2X2	T50.2X3	T50.2X4	T50.2X5	T50.2X6
Methdilazine	T43.3X1	T43.3X2	T43.3X3	T43.3X4	T43.3X5	T43.3X6
Methedrine	T43.621	T43.622	T43.623	T43.624	T43.625	T43.626
Methenamine (mandelate)	T37.8X1	T37.8X2	T37.8X3	T37.8X4	T37.8X5	T37.8X6
Methenolone	T38.7X1	T38.7X2	T38.7X3	T38.7X4	T38.7X5	T38.7X6
Methergine	T48.0X1	T48.0X2	T48.0X3	T48.0X4	T48.0X5	T48.0X6
Methetoin	T42.0X1	T42.0X2	T42.0X3	T42.0X4	T42.0X5	T42.0X6
Methiacil	T38.2X1	T38.2X2	T38.2X3	T38.2X4	T38.2X5	T38.2X6
Methicillin	T36.0X1	T36.0X2	T36.0X3	T36.0X4	T36.0X5	T36.0X6
Methimazole	T38.2X1	T38.2X2	T38.2X3	T38.2X4	T38.2X5	T38.2X6
Methiodal sodium	T50.8X1	T50.8X2	T50.8X3	T50.8X4	T50.8X5	T50.8X6
Methionine	T50.991	T50.992	T50.993	T50.994	T50.995	T50.996
Methisazone	T37.5X1	T37.5X2	T37.5X3	T37.5X4	T37.5X5	T37.5X6
Methisoprinol	T37.5X1	T37.5X2	T37.5X3	T37.5X4	T37.5X5	T37.5X6
Methitural	T42.3X1	T42.3X2	T42.3X3	T42.3X4	T42.3X5	T42.3X6
Methixene	T44.3X1	T44.3X2	T44.3X3	T44.3X4	T44.3X5	T44.3X6
Methobarbital, methobarbitone	T42.3X1	T42.3X2	T42.3X3	T42.3X4	T42.3X5	T42.3X6
Methocarbamol	T42.8X1	T42.8X2	T42.8X3	T42.8X4	T42.8X5	T42.8X6
skeletal muscle relaxant	T48.1X1	T48.1X2	T48.1X3	T48.1X4	T48.1X5	T48.1X6
Methohexital	T41.1X1	T41.1X2	T41.1X3	T41.1X4	T41.1X5	T41.1X6
Methohexitone	T41.1X1	T41.1X2	T41.1X3	T41.1X4	T41.1X5	T41.1X6
Methoin	T42.0X1	T42.0X2	T42.0X3	T42.0X4	T42.0X5	T42.0X6
Methopholine	T39.8X1	T39.8X2	T39.8X3	T39.8X4	T39.8X5	T39.8X6
Methopromazine	T43.3X1	T43.3X2	T43.3X3	T43.3X4	T43.3X5	T43.3X6
Methorate	T48.3X1	T48.3X2	T48.3X3	T48.3X4	T48.3X5	T48.3X6
Methoserpidine	T46.5X1	T46.5X2	T46.5X3	T46.5X4	T46.5X5	T46.5X6
Methotrexate	T45.1X1	T45.1X2	T45.1X3	T45.1X4	T45.1X5	T45.1X6
Methotrimeprazine	T43.3X1	T43.3X2	T43.3X3	T43.3X4	T43.3X5	T43.3X6
Methoxa-Dome	T49.3X1	T49.3X2	T49.3X3	T49.3X4	T49.3X5	T49.3X6
Methoxamine	T44.4X1	T44.4X2	T44.4X3	T44.4X4	T44.4X5	T44.4X6
Methoxsalen	T50.991	T50.992	T50.993	T50.994	T50.995	T50.996
Methoxyaniline	T65.3X1	T65.3X2	T65.3X3	T65.3X4	--	--
Methoxybenzyl penicillin	T36.0X1	T36.0X2	T36.0X3	T36.0X4	T36.0X5	T36.0X6
Methoxychlor	T53.7X1	T53.7X2	T53.7X3	T53.7X4	--	--
Methoxy-DDT	T53.7X1	T53.7X2	T53.7X3	T53.7X4	--	--
2-Methoxyethanol	T52.3X1	T52.3X2	T52.3X3	T52.3X4	--	--
Methoxyflurane	T41.0X1	T41.0X2	T41.0X3	T41.0X4	T41.0X5	T41.0X6
Methoxyphenamine	T48.6X1	T48.6X2	T48.6X3	T48.6X4	T48.6X5	T48.6X6
Methoxypromazine	T43.3X1	T43.3X2	T43.3X3	T43.3X4	T43.3X5	T43.3X6
5-Methoxypsoralen (5-MOP)	T50.991	T50.992	T50.993	T50.994	T50.995	T50.996
8-Methoxypsoralen (8-MOP)	T50.991	T50.992	T50.993	T50.994	T50.995	T50.996
Methscopolamine bromide	T44.3X1	T44.3X2	T44.3X3	T44.3X4	T44.3X5	T44.3X6
Methsuximide	T42.2X1	T42.2X2	T42.2X3	T42.2X4	T42.2X5	T42.2X6
Methyclothiazide	T50.2X1	T50.2X2	T50.2X3	T50.2X4	T50.2X5	T50.2X6
Methyl						
acetate	T52.4X1	T52.4X2	T52.4X3	T52.4X4	--	--
acetone	T52.4X1	T52.4X2	T52.4X3	T52.4X4	--	--
acrylate	T65.891	T65.892	T65.893	T65.894	--	--
alcohol	T51.1X1	T51.1X2	T51.1X3	T51.1X4	--	--
aminophenol	T65.3X1	T65.3X2	T65.3X3	T65.3X4	--	--
amphetamine	T43.621	T43.622	T43.623	T43.624	T43.625	T43.626
androstanolone	T38.7X1	T38.7X2	T38.7X3	T38.7X4	T38.7X5	T38.7X6
atropine	T44.3X1	T44.3X2	T44.3X3	T44.3X4	T44.3X5	T44.3X6
benzene	T52.2X1	T52.2X2	T52.2X3	T52.2X4	--	--
benzoate	T52.8X1	T52.8X2	T52.8X3	T52.8X4	--	--
benzol	T52.2X1	T52.2X2	T52.2X3	T52.2X4	--	--
bromide (gas)	T59.891	T59.892	T59.893	T59.894	--	--
fumigant	T60.8X1	T60.8X2	T60.8X3	T60.8X4	--	--
butanol	T51.3X1	T51.3X2	T51.3X3	T51.3X4	--	--
carbinol	T51.1X1	T51.1X2	T51.1X3	T51.1X4	--	--
carbonate	T52.8X1	T52.8X2	T52.8X3	T52.8X4	--	--
CCNU	T45.1X1	T45.1X2	T45.1X3	T45.1X4	T45.1X5	T45.1X6
cellosolve	T52.91	T52.92	T52.93	T52.94	--	--
cellulose	T47.4X1	T47.4X2	T47.4X3	T47.4X4	T47.4X5	T47.4X6
chloride (gas)	T59.891	T59.892	T59.893	T59.894	--	--
chloroformate	T59.3X1	T59.3X2	T59.3X3	T59.3X4	--	--
cyclohexane	T52.8X1	T52.8X2	T52.8X3	T52.8X4	--	--
cyclohexanol	T51.8X1	T51.8X2	T51.8X3	T51.8X4	--	--
cyclohexanone	T52.8X1	T52.8X2	T52.8X3	T52.8X4	--	--
cyclohexyl acetate	T52.8X1	T52.8X2	T52.8X3	T52.8X4	--	--
demeton	T60.0X1	T60.0X2	T60.0X3	T60.0X4	--	--
dihydromorphinone	T40.2X1	T40.2X2	T40.2X3	T40.2X4	T40.2X5	T40.2X6
ergometrine	T48.0X1	T48.0X2	T48.0X3	T48.0X4	T48.0X5	T48.0X6
ergonovine	T48.0X1	T48.0X2	T48.0X3	T48.0X4	T48.0X5	T48.0X6
ethyl ketone	T52.4X1	T52.4X2	T52.4X3	T52.4X4	--	--

Substance	Poisoning, Accidental unintentional	Poisoning, Intentional self-harm	Poisoning, Assault	Poisoning, Undetermined	Adverse effect	Underdosing
Methyl — *continued*						
glucamine antimonate	T37.8X1	T37.8X2	T37.8X3	T37.8X4	T37.8X5	T37.8X6
hydrazine	T65.891	T65.892	T65.893	T65.894	--	--
iodide	T65.891	T65.892	T65.893	T65.894	--	--
isobutyl ketone	T52.4X1	T52.4X2	T52.4X3	T52.4X4	--	--
isothiocyanate	T60.3X1	T60.3X2	T60.3X3	T60.3X4	--	--
mercaptan	T59.891	T59.892	T59.893	T59.894	--	--
morphine NEC	T40.2X1	T40.2X2	T40.2X3	T40.2X4	T40.2X5	T40.2X6
nicotinate	T49.4X1	T49.4X2	T49.4X3	T49.4X4	T49.4X5	T49.4X6
paraben	T49.0X1	T49.0X2	T49.0X3	T49.0X4	T49.0X5	T49.0X6
parafynol	T42.6X1	T42.6X2	T42.6X3	T42.6X4	T42.6X5	T42.6X6
parathion	T60.0X1	T60.0X2	T60.0X3	T60.0X4	--	--
peridol	T43.4X1	T43.4X2	T43.4X3	T43.4X4	T43.4X5	T43.4X6
phenidate	T43.631	T43.632	T43.633	T43.634	T43.635	T43.636
prednisolone	T38.0X1	T38.0X2	T38.0X3	T38.0X4	T38.0X5	T38.0X6
ENT agent	T49.6X1	T49.6X2	T49.6X3	T49.6X4	T49.6X5	T49.6X6
ophthalmic preparation	T49.5X1	T49.5X2	T49.5X3	T49.5X4	T49.5X5	T49.5X6
topical NEC	T49.0X1	T49.0X2	T49.0X3	T49.0X4	T49.0X5	T49.0X6
propylcarbinol	T51.3X1	T51.3X2	T51.3X3	T51.3X4	--	--
rosaniline NEC	T49.0X1	T49.0X2	T49.0X3	T49.0X4	T49.0X5	T49.0X6
salicylate	T49.2X1	T49.2X2	T49.2X3	T49.2X4	T49.2X5	T49.2X6
sulfate (fumes)	T59.891	T59.892	T59.893	T59.894	--	--
liquid	T52.8X1	T52.8X2	T52.8X3	T52.8X4	--	--
sulfonal	T42.6X1	T42.6X2	T42.6X3	T42.6X4	T42.6X5	T42.6X6
testosterone	T38.7X1	T38.7X2	T38.7X3	T38.7X4	T38.7X5	T38.7X6
thiouracil	T38.2X1	T38.2X2	T38.2X3	T38.2X4	T38.2X5	T38.2X6
Methylamphetamine	T43.621	T43.622	T43.623	T43.624	T43.625	T43.626
Methylated spirit	T51.1X1	T51.1X2	T51.1X3	T51.1X4	--	--
Methylatropine nitrate	T44.3X1	T44.3X2	T44.3X3	T44.3X4	T44.3X5	T44.3X6
Methylbenactyzium bromide	T44.3X1	T44.3X2	T44.3X3	T44.3X4	T44.3X5	T44.3X6
Methylbenzethonium chloride	T49.0X1	T49.0X2	T49.0X3	T49.0X4	T49.0X5	T49.0X6
Methylcellulose	T47.4X1	T47.4X2	T47.4X3	T47.4X4	T47.4X5	T47.4X6
laxative	T47.4X1	T47.4X2	T47.4X3	T47.4X4	T47.4X5	T47.4X6
Methylchlorophenoxy-acetic acid	T60.3X1	T60.3X2	T60.3X3	T60.3X4	--	--
Methyldopa	T46.5X1	T46.5X2	T46.5X3	T46.5X4	T46.5X5	T46.5X6
Methyldopate	T46.5X1	T46.5X2	T46.5X3	T46.5X4	T46.5X5	T46.5X6
Methylene						
blue	T50.6X1	T50.6X2	T50.6X3	T50.6X4	T50.6X5	T50.6X6
chloride or dichloride (solvent) NEC	T53.4X1	T53.4X2	T53.4X3	T53.4X4	--	--
Methylenedioxyamphet-amine	T43.621	T43.622	T43.623	T43.624	T43.625	T43.626
Methylenedioxymetham-phetamine	T43.621	T43.622	T43.623	T43.624	T43.625	T43.626
Methylergometrine	T48.0X1	T48.0X2	T48.0X3	T48.0X4	T48.0X5	T48.0X6
Methylergonovine	T48.0X1	T48.0X2	T48.0X3	T48.0X4	T48.0X5	T48.0X6
Methylestrenolone	T38.5X1	T38.5X2	T38.5X3	T38.5X4	T38.5X5	T38.5X6
Methylethyl cellulose	T50.991	T50.992	T50.993	T50.994	T50.995	T50.996
Methylhexabital	T42.3X1	T42.3X2	T42.3X3	T42.3X4	T42.3X5	T42.3X6
Methylmorphine	T40.2X1	T40.2X2	T40.2X3	T40.2X4	T40.2X5	T40.2X6
Methylparaben (ophthalmic)	T49.5X1	T49.5X2	T49.5X3	T49.5X4	T49.5X5	T49.5X6
Methylparafynol	T42.6X1	T42.6X2	T42.6X3	T42.6X4	T42.6X5	T42.6X6
Methylpentynol, methylpenthynol	T42.6X1	T42.6X2	T42.6X3	T42.6X4	T42.6X5	T42.6X6
Methylphenidate	T43.631	T43.632	T43.633	T43.634	T43.635	T43.636
Methylphenobarbital	T42.3X1	T42.3X2	T42.3X3	T42.3X4	T42.3X5	T42.3X6
Methylpolysiloxane	T47.1X1	T47.1X2	T47.1X3	T47.1X4	T47.1X5	T47.1X6
Methylprednisolone — *see Methyl, prednisolone*						
Methylrosaniline	T49.0X1	T49.0X2	T49.0X3	T49.0X4	T49.0X5	T49.0X6
Methylrosanilinium chloride	T49.0X1	T49.0X2	T49.0X3	T49.0X4	T49.0X5	T49.0X6
Methyltestosterone	T38.7X1	T38.7X2	T38.7X3	T38.7X4	T38.7X5	T38.7X6
Methylthionine chloride	T50.6X1	T50.6X2	T50.6X3	T50.6X4	T50.6X5	T50.6X6
Methylthioninium chloride	T50.6X1	T50.6X2	T50.6X3	T50.6X4	T50.6X5	T50.6X6
Methylthiouracil	T38.2X1	T38.2X2	T38.2X3	T38.2X4	T38.2X5	T38.2X6
Methyprylon	T42.6X1	T42.6X2	T42.6X3	T42.6X4	T42.6X5	T42.6X6
Methysergide	T46.5X1	T46.5X2	T46.5X3	T46.5X4	T46.5X5	T46.5X6
Metiamide	T47.1X1	T47.1X2	T47.1X3	T47.1X4	T47.1X5	T47.1X6
Meticillin	T36.0X1	T36.0X2	T36.0X3	T36.0X4	T36.0X5	T36.0X6
Meticrane	T50.2X1	T50.2X2	T50.2X3	T50.2X4	T50.2X5	T50.2X6
Metildigoxin	T46.0X1	T46.0X2	T46.0X3	T46.0X4	T46.0X5	T46.0X6
Metipranolol	T49.5X1	T49.5X2	T49.5X3	T49.5X4	T49.5X5	T49.5X6
Metirosine	T46.5X1	T46.5X2	T46.5X3	T46.5X4	T46.5X5	T46.5X6
Metisazone	T37.5X1	T37.5X2	T37.5X3	T37.5X4	T37.5X5	T37.5X6
Metixene	T44.3X1	T44.3X2	T44.3X3	T44.3X4	T44.3X5	T44.3X6
Metizoline	T48.5X1	T48.5X2	T48.5X3	T48.5X4	T48.5X5	T48.5X6
Metoclopramide	T45.0X1	T45.0X2	T45.0X3	T45.0X4	T45.0X5	T45.0X6
Metofenazate	T43.3X1	T43.3X2	T43.3X3	T43.3X4	T43.3X5	T43.3X6
Metofoline	T39.8X1	T39.8X2	T39.8X3	T39.8X4	T39.8X5	T39.8X6
Metolazone	T50.2X1	T50.2X2	T50.2X3	T50.2X4	T50.2X5	T50.2X6
Metopon	T40.2X1	T40.2X2	T40.2X3	T40.2X4	T40.2X5	T40.2X6
Metoprine	T45.1X1	T45.1X2	T45.1X3	T45.1X4	T45.1X5	T45.1X6

Substance	Poisoning, Accidental unintentional	Poisoning, Intentional self-harm	Poisoning, Assault	Poisoning, Undetermined	Adverse effect	Underdosing
Metoprolol	T44.7X1	T44.7X2	T44.7X3	T44.7X4	T44.7X5	T44.7X6
Metrifonate	T60.0X1	T60.0X2	T60.0X3	T60.0X4	--	--
Metrizamide	T50.8X1	T50.8X2	T50.8X3	T50.8X4	T50.8X5	T50.8X6
Metrizoic acid	T50.8X1	T50.8X2	T50.8X3	T50.8X4	T50.8X5	T50.8X6
Metronidazole	T37.8X1	T37.8X2	T37.8X3	T37.8X4	T37.8X5	T37.8X6
Metycaine	T41.3X1	T41.3X2	T41.3X3	T41.3X4	T41.3X5	T41.3X6
infiltration (subcutaneous)	T41.3X1	T41.3X2	T41.3X3	T41.3X4	T41.3X5	T41.3X6
nerve block (peripheral) (plexus)	T41.3X1	T41.3X2	T41.3X3	T41.3X4	T41.3X5	T41.3X6
topical (surface)	T41.3X1	T41.3X2	T41.3X3	T41.3X4	T41.3X5	T41.3X6
Metyrapone	T50.8X1	T50.8X2	T50.8X3	T50.8X4	T50.8X5	T50.8X6
Mevinphos	T60.0X1	T60.0X2	T60.0X3	T60.0X4	--	--
Mexazolam	T42.4X1	T42.4X2	T42.4X3	T42.4X4	T42.4X5	T42.4X6
Mexenone	T49.3X1	T49.3X2	T49.3X3	T49.3X4	T49.3X5	T49.3X6
Mexiletine	T46.2X1	T46.2X2	T46.2X3	T46.2X4	T46.2X5	T46.2X6
Mezereon	T62.2X1	T62.2X2	T62.2X3	T62.2X4	--	--
berries	T62.1X1	T62.1X2	T62.1X3	T62.1X4	--	--
Mezlocillin	T36.0X1	T36.0X2	T36.0X3	T36.0X4	T36.0X5	T36.0X6
Mianserin	T43.021	T43.022	T43.023	T43.024	T43.025	T43.026
Micatin	T49.0X1	T49.0X2	T49.0X3	T49.0X4	T49.0X5	T49.0X6
Miconazole	T49.0X1	T49.0X2	T49.0X3	T49.0X4	T49.0X5	T49.0X6
Micronomicin	T36.5X1	T36.5X2	T36.5X3	T36.5X4	T36.5X5	T36.5X6
Midazolam	T42.4X1	T42.4X2	T42.4X3	T42.4X4	T42.4X5	T42.4X6
Midecamycin	T36.3X1	T36.3X2	T36.3X3	T36.3X4	T36.3X5	T36.3X6
Mifepristone	T38.6X1	T38.6X2	T38.6X3	T38.6X4	T38.6X5	T38.6X6
Milk of magnesia	T47.1X1	T47.1X2	T47.1X3	T47.1X4	T47.1X5	T47.1X6
Millipede (tropical) (venomous)	T63.411	T63.412	T63.413	T63.414	--	--
Miltown	T43.591	T43.592	T43.593	T43.594	T43.595	T43.596
Milverine	T44.3X1	T44.3X2	T44.3X3	T44.3X4	T44.3X5	T44.3X6
Minaprine	T43.291	T43.292	T43.293	T43.294	T43.295	T43.296
Minaxolone	T41.291	T41.292	T41.293	T41.294	T41.295	T41.296
Mineral						
acids	T54.2X1	T54.2X2	T54.2X3	T54.2X4	--	--
oil (laxative) (medicinal)	T47.4X1	T47.4X2	T47.4X3	T47.4X4	T47.4X5	T47.4X6
emulsion	T47.2X1	T47.2X2	T47.2X3	T47.2X4	T47.2X5	T47.2X6
nonmedicinal	T52.0X1	T52.0X2	T52.0X3	T52.0X4	--	--
topical	T49.3X1	T49.3X2	T49.3X3	T49.3X4	T49.3X5	T49.3X6
salt NEC	T50.3X1	T50.3X2	T50.3X3	T50.3X4	T50.3X5	T50.3X6
spirits	T52.0X1	T52.0X2	T52.0X3	T52.0X4	--	--
Mineralocorticosteroid	T50.0X1	T50.0X2	T50.0X3	T50.0X4	T50.0X5	T50.0X6
Minocycline	T36.4X1	T36.4X2	T36.4X3	T36.4X4	T36.4X5	T36.4X6
Minoxidil	T46.7X1	T46.7X2	T46.7X3	T46.7X4	T46.7X5	T46.7X6
Miokamycin	T36.3X1	T36.3X2	T36.3X3	T36.3X4	T36.3X5	T36.3X6
Miotic drug	T49.5X1	T49.5X2	T49.5X3	T49.5X4	T49.5X5	T49.5X6
Mipafox	T60.0X1	T60.0X2	T60.0X3	T60.0X4	--	--
Mirex	T60.1X1	T60.1X2	T60.1X3	T60.1X4	--	--
Mirtazapine	T43.021	T43.022	T43.023	T43.024	T43.025	T43.026
Misonidazole	T37.3X1	T37.3X2	T37.3X3	T37.3X4	T37.3X5	T37.3X6
Misoprostol	T47.1X1	T47.1X2	T47.1X3	T47.1X4	T47.1X5	T47.1X6
Mithramycin	T45.1X1	T45.1X2	T45.1X3	T45.1X4	T45.1X5	T45.1X6
Mitobronitol	T45.1X1	T45.1X2	T45.1X3	T45.1X4	T45.1X5	T45.1X6
Mitoguazone	T45.1X1	T45.1X2	T45.1X3	T45.1X4	T45.1X5	T45.1X6
Mitolactol	T45.1X1	T45.1X2	T45.1X3	T45.1X4	T45.1X5	T45.1X6
Mitomycin	T45.1X1	T45.1X2	T45.1X3	T45.1X4	T45.1X5	T45.1X6
Mitopodozide	T45.1X1	T45.1X2	T45.1X3	T45.1X4	T45.1X5	T45.1X6
Mitotane	T45.1X1	T45.1X2	T45.1X3	T45.1X4	T45.1X5	T45.1X6
Mitoxantrone	T45.1X1	T45.1X2	T45.1X3	T45.1X4	T45.1X5	T45.1X6
Mivacurium chloride	T48.1X1	T48.1X2	T48.1X3	T48.1X4	T48.1X5	T48.1X6
Miyari bacteria	T47.6X1	T47.6X2	T47.6X3	T47.6X4	T47.6X5	T47.6X6
Moclobemide	T43.1X1	T43.1X2	T43.1X3	T43.1X4	T43.1X5	T43.1X6
Moderil	T46.5X1	T46.5X2	T46.5X3	T46.5X4	T46.5X5	T46.5X6
Mofebutazone	T39.2X1	T39.2X2	T39.2X3	T39.2X4	T39.2X5	T39.2X6
Mogadon — *see Nitrazepam*						
Molindone	T43.591	T43.592	T43.593	T43.594	T43.595	T43.596
Molsidomine	T46.3X1	T46.3X2	T46.3X3	T46.3X4	T46.3X5	T46.3X6
Mometasone	T49.0X1	T49.0X2	T49.0X3	T49.0X4	T49.0X5	T49.0X6
Monistat	T49.0X1	T49.0X2	T49.0X3	T49.0X4	T49.0X5	T49.0X6
Monkshood	T62.2X1	T62.2X2	T62.2X3	T62.2X4	--	--
Monoamine oxidase inhibitor NEC	T43.1X1	T43.1X2	T43.1X3	T43.1X4	T43.1X5	T43.1X6
hydrazine	T43.1X1	T43.1X2	T43.1X3	T43.1X4	T43.1X5	T43.1X6
Monobenzone	T49.4X1	T49.4X2	T49.4X3	T49.4X4	T49.4X5	T49.4X6
Monochloroacetic acid	T60.3X1	T60.3X2	T60.3X3	T60.3X4	--	--
Monochlorobenzene	T53.7X1	T53.7X2	T53.7X3	T53.7X4	--	--
Monoethanolamine	T46.8X1	T46.8X2	T46.8X3	T46.8X4	T46.8X5	T46.8X6
oleate	T46.8X1	T46.8X2	T46.8X3	T46.8X4	T46.8X5	T46.8X6
Monooctanoin	T50.991	T50.992	T50.993	T50.994	T50.995	T50.996
Monophenylbutazone	T39.2X1	T39.2X2	T39.2X3	T39.2X4	T39.2X5	T39.2X6
Monosodium glutamate	T65.891	T65.892	T65.893	T65.894	--	--
Monosulfiram	T49.0X1	T49.0X2	T49.0X3	T49.0X4	T49.0X5	T49.0X6
Monoxide, carbon — *see Carbon, monoxide*						
Monoxidine hydrochloride	T46.1X1	T46.1X2	T46.1X3	T46.1X4	T46.1X5	T46.1X6

Substance	Poisoning, Accidental unintentional	Poisoning, Intentional self-harm	Poisoning, Assault	Poisoning, Undetermined	Adverse effect	Underdosing
Monuron	T60.3X1	T60.3X2	T60.3X3	T60.3X4	--	--
Moperone	T43.4X1	T43.4X2	T43.4X3	T43.4X4	T43.4X5	T43.4X6
Mopidamol	T45.1X1	T45.1X2	T45.1X3	T45.1X4	T45.1X5	T45.1X6
MOPP (mechloreth-amine + vincristine + prednisone + procarba-zine)	T45.1X1	T45.1X2	T45.1X3	T45.1X4	T45.1X5	T45.1X6
Morfin	T40.2X1	T40.2X2	T40.2X3	T40.2X4	T40.2X5	T40.2X6
Morinamide	T37.1X1	T37.1X2	T37.1X3	T37.1X4	T37.1X5	T37.1X6
Morning glory seeds	T40.991	T40.992	T40.993	T40.994	--	--
Moroxydine	T37.5X1	T37.5X2	T37.5X3	T37.5X4	T37.5X5	T37.5X6
Morphazinamide	T37.1X1	T37.1X2	T37.1X3	T37.1X4	T37.1X5	T37.1X6
Morphine	T40.2X1	T40.2X2	T40.2X3	T40.2X4	T40.2X5	T40.2X6
antagonist	T50.7X1	T50.7X2	T50.7X3	T50.7X4	T50.7X5	T50.7X6
Morpholinylethylmorphine	T40.2X1	T40.2X2	T40.2X3	T40.2X4	--	--
Morsuximide	T42.2X1	T42.2X2	T42.2X3	T42.2X4	T42.2X5	T42.2X6
Mosapramine	T43.591	T43.592	T43.593	T43.594	T43.595	T43.596
Moth balls — *see also Pesticides*	T60.2X1	T60.2X2	T60.2X3	T60.2X4	--	--
naphthalene	T60.2X1	T60.2X2	T60.2X3	T60.2X4	--	--
paradichlorobenzene	T60.1X1	T60.1X2	T60.1X3	T60.1X4	--	--
Motor exhaust gas	T58.01	T58.02	T58.03	T58.04	--	--
Mouthwash (antiseptic) (zinc chloride)	T49.6X1	T49.6X2	T49.6X3	T49.6X4	T49.6X5	T49.6X6
Moxastine	T45.0X1	T45.0X2	T45.0X3	T45.0X4	T45.0X5	T45.0X6
Moxaverine	T44.3X1	T44.3X2	T44.3X3	T44.3X4	T44.3X5	T44.3X6
Moxisylyte	T46.7X1	T46.7X2	T46.7X3	T46.7X4	T46.7X5	T46.7X6
Mucilage, plant	T47.4X1	T47.4X2	T47.4X3	T47.4X4	T47.4X5	T47.4X6
Mucolytic drug	T48.4X1	T48.4X2	T48.4X3	T48.4X4	T48.4X5	T48.4X6
Mucomyst	T48.4X1	T48.4X2	T48.4X3	T48.4X4	T48.4X5	T48.4X6
Mucous membrane agents (external)	T49.91	T49.92	T49.93	T49.94	T49.95	T49.96
specified NEC	T49.8X1	T49.8X2	T49.8X3	T49.8X4	T49.8X5	T49.8X6
Mumps						
immune globulin (human)	T50.Z11	T50.Z12	T50.Z13	T50.Z14	T50.Z15	T50.Z16
skin test antigen	T50.8X1	T50.8X2	T50.8X3	T50.8X4	T50.8X5	T50.8X6
vaccine	T50.B91	T50.B92	T50.B93	T50.B94	T50.B95	T50.B96
Mumpsvax	T50.B91	T50.B92	T50.B93	T50.B94	T50.B95	T50.B96
Mupirocin	T49.0X1	T49.0X2	T49.0X3	T49.0X4	T49.0X5	T49.0X6
Muriatic acid — *see Hydrochloric acid*						
Muromonab-CD3	T45.1X1	T45.1X2	T45.1X3	T45.1X4	T45.1X5	T45.1X6
Muscle-action drug NEC	T48.201	T48.202	T48.203	T48.204	T48.205	T48.206
Muscle affecting agents NEC	T48.201	T48.202	T48.203	T48.204	T48.205	T48.206
oxytocic	T48.0X1	T48.0X2	T48.0X3	T48.0X4	T48.0X5	T48.0X6
relaxants	T48.201	T48.202	T48.203	T48.204	T48.205	T48.206
central nervous system	T42.8X1	T42.8X2	T42.8X3	T42.8X4	T42.8X5	T42.8X6
skeletal	T48.1X1	T48.1X2	T48.1X3	T48.1X4	T48.1X5	T48.1X6
smooth	T44.3X1	T44.3X2	T44.3X3	T44.3X4	T44.3X5	T44.3X6
Muscle relaxant — *see Relaxant, muscle*						
Muscle-tone depressant, central NEC	T42.8X1	T42.8X2	T42.8X3	T42.8X4	T42.8X5	T42.8X6
specified NEC	T42.8X1	T42.8X2	T42.8X3	T42.8X4	T42.8X5	T42.8X6
Mushroom, noxious	T62.0X1	T62.0X2	T62.0X3	T62.0X4	--	--
Mussel, noxious	T61.781	T61.782	T61.783	T61.784	--	--
Mustard (emetic)	T47.7X1	T47.7X2	T47.7X3	T47.7X4	T47.7X5	T47.7X6
black	T47.7X1	T47.7X2	T47.7X3	T47.7X4	T47.7X5	T47.7X6
gas, not in war	T59.91	T59.92	T59.93	T59.94	--	--
nitrogen	T45.1X1	T45.1X2	T45.1X3	T45.1X4	T45.1X5	T45.1X6
Mustine	T45.1X1	T45.1X2	T45.1X3	T45.1X4	T45.1X5	T45.1X6
M-vac	T45.1X1	T45.1X2	T45.1X3	T45.1X4	T45.1X5	T45.1X6
Mycifradin	T36.5X1	T36.5X2	T36.5X3	T36.5X4	T36.5X5	T36.5X6
topical	T49.0X1	T49.0X2	T49.0X3	T49.0X4	T49.0X5	T49.0X6
Mycitracin	T36.8X1	T36.8X2	T36.8X3	T36.8X4	T36.8X5	T36.8X6
ophthalmic preparation	T49.5X1	T49.5X2	T49.5X3	T49.5X4	T49.5X5	T49.5X6
Mycostatin	T36.7X1	T36.7X2	T36.7X3	T36.7X4	T36.7X5	T36.7X6
topical	T49.0X1	T49.0X2	T49.0X3	T49.0X4	T49.0X5	T49.0X6
Mycotoxins	T64.81	T64.82	T64.83	T64.84	--	--
aflatoxin	T64.01	T64.02	T64.03	T64.04	--	--
specified NEC	T64.81	T64.82	T64.83	T64.84	--	--
Mydriacyl	T44.3X1	T44.3X2	T44.3X3	T44.3X4	T44.3X5	T44.3X6
Mydriatic drug	T49.5X1	T49.5X2	T49.5X3	T49.5X4	T49.5X5	T49.5X6
Myelobromal	T45.1X1	T45.1X2	T45.1X3	T45.1X4	T45.1X5	T45.1X6
Myleran	T45.1X1	T45.1X2	T45.1X3	T45.1X4	T45.1X5	T45.1X6
Myochrysin (e)	T39.2X1	T39.2X2	T39.2X3	T39.2X4	T39.2X5	T39.2X6
Myoneural blocking agents	T48.1X1	T48.1X2	T48.1X3	T48.1X4	T48.1X5	T48.1X6
Myralact	T49.0X1	T49.0X2	T49.0X3	T49.0X4	T49.0X5	T49.0X6
Myristica fragrans	T62.2X1	T62.2X2	T62.2X3	T62.2X4	--	--
Myristicin	T65.891	T65.892	T65.893	T65.894	--	--
Mysoline	T42.3X1	T42.3X2	T42.3X3	T42.3X4	T42.3X5	T42.3X6
N						
Nabilone	T40.7X1	T40.7X2	T40.7X3	T40.7X4	T40.7X5	T40.7X6
Nabumetone	T39.391	T39.392	T39.393	T39.394	T39.395	T39.396
Nadolol	T44.7X1	T44.7X2	T44.7X3	T44.7X4	T44.7X5	T44.7X6
Nafcillin	T36.0X1	T36.0X2	T36.0X3	T36.0X4	T36.0X5	T36.0X6
Nafoxidine	T38.6X1	T38.6X2	T38.6X3	T38.6X4	T38.6X5	T38.6X6
Naftazone	T46.991	T46.992	T46.993	T46.994	T46.995	T46.996
Naftidrofuryl (oxalate)	T46.7X1	T46.7X2	T46.7X3	T46.7X4	T46.7X5	T46.7X6
Naftifine	T49.0X1	T49.0X2	T49.0X3	T49.0X4	T49.0X5	T49.0X6
Nail polish remover	T52.91	T52.92	T52.93	T52.94	--	--
Nalbuphine	T40.4X1	T40.4X2	T40.4X3	T40.4X4	T40.4X5	T40.4X6
Naled	T60.0X1	T60.0X2	T60.0X3	T60.0X4	--	--
Nalidixic acid	T37.8X1	T37.8X2	T37.8X3	T37.8X4	T37.8X5	T37.8X6
Nalorphine	T50.7X1	T50.7X2	T50.7X3	T50.7X4	T50.7X5	T50.7X6
Naloxone	T50.7X1	T50.7X2	T50.7X3	T50.7X4	T50.7X5	T50.7X6
Naltrexone	T50.7X1	T50.7X2	T50.7X3	T50.7X4	T50.7X5	T50.7X6
Namenda	T43.8X1	T43.8X2	T43.8X3	T43.8X4	T43.8X5	T43.8X6
Nandrolone	T38.7X1	T38.7X2	T38.7X3	T38.7X4	T38.7X5	T38.7X6
Naphazoline	T48.5X1	T48.5X2	T48.5X3	T48.5X4	T48.5X5	T48.5X6
Naphtha (painters') (petroleum)	T52.0X1	T52.0X2	T52.0X3	T52.0X4	--	--
solvent	T52.0X1	T52.0X2	T52.0X3	T52.0X4	--	--
vapor	T52.0X1	T52.0X2	T52.0X3	T52.0X4	--	--
Naphthalene (non-chlorinated)	T60.2X1	T60.2X2	T60.2X3	T60.2X4	--	--
chlorinated	T60.1X1	T60.1X2	T60.1X3	T60.1X4	--	--
vapor	T60.1X1	T60.1X2	T60.1X3	T60.1X4	--	--
insecticide or moth repellent	T60.2X1	T60.2X2	T60.2X3	T60.2X4	--	--
chlorinated	T60.1X1	T60.1X2	T60.1X3	T60.1X4	--	--
vapor	T60.2X1	T60.2X2	T60.2X3	T60.2X4	--	--
chlorinated	T60.1X1	T60.1X2	T60.1X3	T60.1X4	--	--
Naphthol	T65.891	T65.892	T65.893	T65.894	--	--
Naphthylamine	T65.891	T65.892	T65.893	T65.894	--	--
Naphthylthiourea (ANTU)	T60.4X1	T60.4X2	T60.4X3	T60.4X4	--	--
Naprosyn — *see Naproxen*						
Naproxen	T39.311	T39.312	T39.313	T39.314	T39.315	T39.316
Narcotic (drug)	T40.601	T40.602	T40.603	T40.604	T40.605	T40.606
analgesic NEC	T40.601	T40.602	T40.603	T40.604	T40.605	T40.606
antagonist	T50.7X1	T50.7X2	T50.7X3	T50.7X4	T50.7X5	T50.7X6
specified NEC	T40.691	T40.692	T40.693	T40.694	T40.695	T40.696
synthetic	T40.4X1	T40.4X2	T40.4X3	T40.4X4	T40.4X5	T40.4X6
Narcotine	T48.3X1	T48.3X2	T48.3X3	T48.3X4	T48.3X5	T48.3X6
Nardil	T43.1X1	T43.1X2	T43.1X3	T43.1X4	T43.1X5	T43.1X6
Nasal drug NEC	T49.6X1	T49.6X2	T49.6X3	T49.6X4	T49.6X5	T49.6X6
Natamycin	T49.0X1	T49.0X2	T49.0X3	T49.0X4	T49.0X5	T49.0X6
Natrium cyanide — *see Cyanide (s)*						
Natural						
blood (product)	T45.8X1	T45.8X2	T45.8X3	T45.8X4	T45.8X5	T45.8X6
gas (piped)	T59.891	T59.892	T59.893	T59.894	--	--
incomplete combustion	T58.11	T58.12	T58.13	T58.14	--	--
Nealbarbital	T42.3X1	T42.3X2	T42.3X3	T42.3X4	T42.3X5	T42.3X6
Nectadon	T48.3X1	T48.3X2	T48.3X3	T48.3X4	T48.3X5	T48.3X6
Nedocromil	T48.6X1	T48.6X2	T48.6X3	T48.6X4	T48.6X5	T48.6X6
Nefopam	T39.8X1	T39.8X2	T39.8X3	T39.8X4	T39.8X5	T39.8X6
Nematocyst (sting)	T63.691	T63.692	T63.693	T63.694	--	--
Nembutal	T42.3X1	T42.3X2	T42.3X3	T42.3X4	T42.3X5	T42.3X6
Nemonapride	T43.591	T43.592	T43.593	T43.594	T43.595	T43.596
Neoarsphenamine	T37.8X1	T37.8X2	T37.8X3	T37.8X4	T37.8X5	T37.8X6
Neocinchophen	T50.4X1	T50.4X2	T50.4X3	T50.4X4	T50.4X5	T50.4X6
Neomycin (derivatives)	T36.5X1	T36.5X2	T36.5X3	T36.5X4	T36.5X5	T36.5X6
with						
bacitracin	T49.0X1	T49.0X2	T49.0X3	T49.0X4	T49.0X5	T49.0X6
neostigmine	T44.0X1	T44.0X2	T44.0X3	T44.0X4	T44.0X5	T44.0X6
ENT agent	T49.6X1	T49.6X2	T49.6X3	T49.6X4	T49.6X5	T49.6X6
ophthalmic preparation	T49.5X1	T49.5X2	T49.5X3	T49.5X4	T49.5X5	T49.5X6
topical NEC	T49.0X1	T49.0X2	T49.0X3	T49.0X4	T49.0X5	T49.0X6
Neonal	T42.3X1	T42.3X2	T42.3X3	T42.3X4	T42.3X5	T42.3X6
Neoprontosil	T37.0X1	T37.0X2	T37.0X3	T37.0X4	T37.0X5	T37.0X6
Neosalvarsan	T37.8X1	T37.8X2	T37.8X3	T37.8X4	T37.8X5	T37.8X6
Neosilversalvarsan	T37.8X1	T37.8X2	T37.8X3	T37.8X4	T37.8X5	T37.8X6
Neosporin	T36.8X1	T36.8X2	T36.8X3	T36.8X4	T36.8X5	T36.8X6
ENT agent	T49.6X1	T49.6X2	T49.6X3	T49.6X4	T49.6X5	T49.6X6
opthalmic preparation	T49.5X1	T49.5X2	T49.5X3	T49.5X4	T49.5X5	T49.5X6
topical NEC	T49.0X1	T49.0X2	T49.0X3	T49.0X4	T49.0X5	T49.0X6
Neostigmine bromide	T44.0X1	T44.0X2	T44.0X3	T44.0X4	T44.0X5	T44.0X6
Neraval	T42.3X1	T42.3X2	T42.3X3	T42.3X4	T42.3X5	T42.3X6
Neravan	T42.3X1	T42.3X2	T42.3X3	T42.3X4	T42.3X5	T42.3X6
Nerium oleander	T62.2X1	T62.2X2	T62.2X3	T62.2X4	--	--
Nerve gas, not in war	T59.91	T59.92	T59.93	T59.94	--	--
Nesacaine	T41.3X1	T41.3X2	T41.3X3	T41.3X4	T41.3X5	T41.3X6
infiltration (subcutaneous)	T41.3X1	T41.3X2	T41.3X3	T41.3X4	T41.3X5	T41.3X6
nerve block (peripheral) (plexus)	T41.3X1	T41.3X2	T41.3X3	T41.3X4	T41.3X5	T41.3X6
Netilmicin	T36.5X1	T36.5X2	T36.5X3	T36.5X4	T36.5X5	T36.5X6
Neurobarb	T42.3X1	T42.3X2	T42.3X3	T42.3X4	T42.3X5	T42.3X6
Neuroleptic drug NEC	T43.501	T43.502	T43.503	T43.504	T43.505	T43.506

Neuromuscular blocking drug - Octotiamine

Substance	Poisoning, Accidental unintentional	Poisoning, Intentional self-harm	Poisoning, Assault	Poisoning, Undetermined	Adverse effect	Underdosing
Neuromuscular blocking drug	T48.1X1	T48.1X2	T48.1X3	T48.1X4	T48.1X5	T48.1X6
Neutral insulin injection	T38.3X1	T38.3X2	T38.3X3	T38.3X4	T38.3X5	T38.3X6
Neutral spirits	T51.0X1	T51.0X2	T51.0X3	T51.0X4	—	—
beverage	T51.0X1	T51.0X2	T51.0X3	T51.0X4	—	—
Niacin	T46.7X1	T46.7X2	T46.7X3	T46.7X4	T46.7X5	T46.7X6
Niacinamide	T45.2X1	T45.2X2	T45.2X3	T45.2X4	T45.2X5	T45.2X6
Nialamide	T43.1X1	T43.1X2	T43.1X3	T43.1X4	T43.1X5	T43.1X6
Niaprazine	T42.6X1	T42.6X2	T42.6X3	T42.6X4	T42.6X5	T42.6X6
Nicametate	T46.7X1	T46.7X2	T46.7X3	T46.7X4	T46.7X5	T46.7X6
Nicardipine	T46.1X1	T46.1X2	T46.1X3	T46.1X4	T46.1X5	T46.1X6
Nicergoline	T46.7X1	T46.7X2	T46.7X3	T46.7X4	T46.7X5	T46.7X6
Nickel (carbonyl) (tetra-carbonyl) (fumes) (vapor)	T56.891	T56.892	T56.893	T56.894	—	—
Nickelocene	T56.891	T56.892	T56.893	T56.894	—	—
Niclosamide	T37.4X1	T37.4X2	T37.4X3	T37.4X4	T37.4X5	T37.4X6
Nicofuranose	T46.7X1	T46.7X2	T46.7X3	T46.7X4	T46.7X5	T46.7X6
Nicomorphine	T40.2X1	T40.2X2	T40.2X3	T40.2X4	—	—
Nicorandil	T46.3X1	T46.3X2	T46.3X3	T46.3X4	T46.3X5	T46.3X6
Nicotiana (plant)	T62.2X1	T62.2X2	T62.2X3	T62.2X4	—	—
Nicotinamide	T45.2X1	T45.2X2	T45.2X3	T45.2X4	T45.2X5	T45.2X6
Nicotine (insecticide) (spray) (sulfate) **NEC**	T60.2X1	T60.2X2	T60.2X3	T60.2X4	—	—
from tobacco	T65.291	T65.292	T65.293	T65.294	—	—
cigarettes	T65.221	T65.222	T65.223	T65.224	—	—
not insecticide	T65.291	T65.292	T65.293	T65.294	—	—
Nicotinic acid	T46.7X1	T46.7X2	T46.7X3	T46.7X4	T46.7X5	T46.7X6
Nicotinyl alcohol	T46.7X1	T46.7X2	T46.7X3	T46.7X4	T46.7X5	T46.7X6
Nicoumalone	T45.511	T45.512	T45.513	T45.514	T45.515	T45.516
Nifedipine	T46.1X1	T46.1X2	T46.1X3	T46.1X4	T46.1X5	T46.1X6
Nifenazone	T39.2X1	T39.2X2	T39.2X3	T39.2X4	T39.2X5	T39.2X6
Nifuraldezone	T37.91	T37.92	T37.93	T37.94	T37.95	T37.96
Nifuratel	T37.8X1	T37.8X2	T37.8X3	T37.8X4	T37.8X5	T37.8X6
Nifurtimox	T37.3X1	T37.3X2	T37.3X3	T37.3X4	T37.3X5	T37.3X6
Nifurtoinol	T37.8X1	T37.8X2	T37.8X3	T37.8X4	T37.8X5	T37.8X6
Nightshade, deadly (solanum) — *see also Belladonna*	T62.2X1	T62.2X2	T62.2X3	T62.2X4	—	—
berry	T62.1X1	T62.1X2	T62.1X3	T62.1X4	—	—
Nikethamide	T50.7X1	T50.7X2	T50.7X3	T50.7X4	T50.7X5	T50.7X6
Nilstat	T36.7X1	T36.7X2	T36.7X3	T36.7X4	T36.7X5	T36.7X6
topical	T49.0X1	T49.0X2	T49.0X3	T49.0X4	T49.0X5	T49.0X6
Nilutamide	T38.6X1	T38.6X2	T38.6X3	T38.6X4	T38.6X5	T38.6X6
Nimesulide	T39.391	T39.392	T39.393	T39.394	T39.395	T39.396
Nimetazepam	T42.4X1	T42.4X2	T42.4X3	T42.4X4	T42.4X5	T42.4X6
Nimodipine	T46.1X1	T46.1X2	T46.1X3	T46.1X4	T46.1X5	T46.1X6
Nimorazole	T37.3X1	T37.3X2	T37.3X3	T37.3X4	T37.3X5	T37.3X6
Nimustine	T45.1X1	T45.1X2	T45.1X3	T45.1X4	T45.1X5	T45.1X6
Niridazole	T37.4X1	T37.4X2	T37.4X3	T37.4X4	T37.4X5	T37.4X6
Nisentil	T40.2X1	T40.2X2	T40.2X3	T40.2X4	T40.2X5	T40.2X6
Nisoldipine	T46.1X1	T46.1X2	T46.1X3	T46.1X4	T46.1X5	T46.1X6
Nitramine	T65.3X1	T65.3X2	T65.3X3	T65.3X4	—	—
Nitrate, organic	T46.3X1	T46.3X2	T46.3X3	T46.3X4	T46.3X5	T46.3X6
Nitrazepam	T42.4X1	T42.4X2	T42.4X3	T42.4X4	T42.4X5	T42.4X6
Nitrefazole	T50.6X1	T50.6X2	T50.6X3	T50.6X4	T50.6X5	T50.6X6
Nitrendipine	T46.1X1	T46.1X2	T46.1X3	T46.1X4	T46.1X5	T46.1X6
Nitric						
acid (liquid)	T54.2X1	T54.2X2	T54.2X3	T54.2X4	—	—
vapor	T59.891	T59.892	T59.893	T59.894	—	—
oxide (gas)	T59.0X1	T59.0X2	T59.0X3	T59.0X4	—	—
Nitrimidazine	T37.3X1	T37.3X2	T37.3X3	T37.3X4	T37.3X5	T37.3X6
Nitrite, amyl (medicinal) (vapor)	T46.3X1	T46.3X2	T46.3X3	T46.3X4	T46.3X5	T46.3X6
Nitroaniline	T65.3X1	T65.3X2	T65.3X3	T65.3X4	—	—
vapor	T59.891	T59.892	T59.893	T59.894	—	—
Nitrobenzene, nitrobenzol	T65.3X1	T65.3X2	T65.3X3	T65.3X4	—	—
vapor	T65.3X1	T65.3X2	T65.3X3	T65.3X4	—	—
Nitrocellulose	T65.891	T65.892	T65.893	T65.894	—	—
lacquer	T65.891	T65.892	T65.893	T65.894	—	—
Nitrodiphenyl	T65.3X1	T65.3X2	T65.3X3	T65.3X4	—	—
Nitrofural	T49.0X1	T49.0X2	T49.0X3	T49.0X4	T49.0X5	T49.0X6
Nitrofurantoin	T37.8X1	T37.8X2	T37.8X3	T37.8X4	T37.8X5	T37.8X6
Nitrofurazone	T49.0X1	T49.0X2	T49.0X3	T49.0X4	T49.0X5	T49.0X6
Nitrogen	T59.0X1	T59.0X2	T59.0X3	T59.0X4	—	—
mustard	T45.1X1	T45.1X2	T45.1X3	T45.1X4	T45.1X5	T45.1X6
Nitroglycerin, nitro-glycerol (medicinal)	T46.3X1	T46.3X2	T46.3X3	T46.3X4	T46.3X5	T46.3X6
nonmedicinal	T65.5X1	T65.5X2	T65.5X3	T65.5X4	—	—
fumes	T65.5X1	T65.5X2	T65.5X3	T65.5X4	—	—
Nitroglycol	T52.3X1	T52.3X2	T52.3X3	T52.3X4	—	—
Nitrohydrochloric acid	T54.2X1	T54.2X2	T54.2X3	T54.2X4	—	—
Nitromersol	T49.0X1	T49.0X2	T49.0X3	T49.0X4	T49.0X5	T49.0X6
Nitronaphthalene	T65.891	T65.892	T65.893	T65.894	—	—
Nitrophenol	T54.0X1	T54.0X2	T54.0X3	T54.0X4	—	—

Substance	Poisoning, Accidental unintentional	Poisoning, Intentional self-harm	Poisoning, Assault	Poisoning, Undetermined	Adverse effect	Underdosing
Nitropropane	T52.8X1	T52.8X2	T52.8X3	T52.8X4	—	—
Nitroprusside	T46.5X1	T46.5X2	T46.5X3	T46.5X4	T46.5X5	T46.5X6
Nitrosodimethylamine	T65.3X1	T65.3X2	T65.3X3	T65.3X4	—	—
Nitrothiazol	T37.4X1	T37.4X2	T37.4X3	T37.4X4	T37.4X5	T37.4X6
Nitrotoluene, nitrotoluol	T65.3X1	T65.3X2	T65.3X3	T65.3X4	—	—
vapor	T65.3X1	T65.3X2	T65.3X3	T65.3X4	—	—
Nitrous						
acid (liquid)	T54.2X1	T54.2X2	T54.2X3	T54.2X4	—	—
fumes	T59.891	T59.892	T59.893	T59.894	—	—
ether spirit	T46.3X1	T46.3X2	T46.3X3	T46.3X4	T46.3X5	T46.3X6
oxide	T41.0X1	T41.0X2	T41.0X3	T41.0X4	T41.0X5	T41.0X6
Nitroxoline	T37.8X1	T37.8X2	T37.8X3	T37.8X4	T37.8X5	T37.8X6
Nitrozone	T49.0X1	T49.0X2	T49.0X3	T49.0X4	T49.0X5	T49.0X6
Nizatidine	T47.0X1	T47.0X2	T47.0X3	T47.0X4	T47.0X5	T47.0X6
Nizofenone	T43.8X1	T43.8X2	T43.8X3	T43.8X4	T43.8X5	T43.8X6
Noctec	T42.6X1	T42.6X2	T42.6X3	T42.6X4	T42.6X5	T42.6X6
Noludar	T42.6X1	T42.6X2	T42.6X3	T42.6X4	T42.6X5	T42.6X6
Nomegestrol	T38.5X1	T38.5X2	T38.5X3	T38.5X4	T38.5X5	T38.5X6
Nomifensine	T43.291	T43.292	T43.293	T43.294	T43.295	T43.296
Nonoxinol	T49.8X1	T49.8X2	T49.8X3	T49.8X4	T49.8X5	T49.8X6
Nonylphenoxy (polyethoxy-ethanol)	T49.8X1	T49.8X2	T49.8X3	T49.8X4	T49.8X5	T49.8X6
Noptil	T42.3X1	T42.3X2	T42.3X3	T42.3X4	T42.3X5	T42.3X6
Noradrenaline	T44.4X1	T44.4X2	T44.4X3	T44.4X4	T44.4X5	T44.4X6
Noramidopyrine	T39.2X1	T39.2X2	T39.2X3	T39.2X4	T39.2X5	T39.2X6
methanesulfonate sodium	T39.2X1	T39.2X2	T39.2X3	T39.2X4	T39.2X5	T39.2X6
Norbormide	T60.4X1	T60.4X2	T60.4X3	T60.4X4	—	—
Nordazepam	T42.4X1	T42.4X2	T42.4X3	T42.4X4	T42.4X5	T42.4X6
Norepinephrine	T44.4X1	T44.4X2	T44.4X3	T44.4X4	T44.4X5	T44.4X6
Norethandrolone	T38.7X1	T38.7X2	T38.7X3	T38.7X4	T38.7X5	T38.7X6
Norethindrone	T38.4X1	T38.4X2	T38.4X3	T38.4X4	T38.4X5	T38.4X6
Norethisterone (acetate) (enantate)	T38.4X1	T38.4X2	T38.4X3	T38.4X4	T38.4X5	T38.4X6
with ethinylestradiol	T38.5X1	T38.5X2	T38.5X3	T38.5X4	T38.5X5	T38.5X6
Noretynodrel	T38.5X1	T38.5X2	T38.5X3	T38.5X4	T38.5X5	T38.5X6
Norfenefrine	T44.4X1	T44.4X2	T44.4X3	T44.4X4	T44.4X5	T44.4X6
Norfloxacin	T36.8X1	T36.8X2	T36.8X3	T36.8X4	T36.8X5	T36.8X6
Norgestrel	T38.4X1	T38.4X2	T38.4X3	T38.4X4	T38.4X5	T38.4X6
Norgestrienone	T38.4X1	T38.4X2	T38.4X3	T38.4X4	T38.4X5	T38.4X6
Norlestrin	T38.4X1	T38.4X2	T38.4X3	T38.4X4	T38.4X5	T38.4X6
Norlutin	T38.4X1	T38.4X2	T38.4X3	T38.4X4	T38.4X5	T38.4X6
Normal serum albumin (human), **salt-poor**	T45.8X1	T45.8X2	T45.8X3	T45.8X4	T45.8X5	T45.8X6
Normethandrone	T38.5X1	T38.5X2	T38.5X3	T38.5X4	T38.5X5	T38.5X6
Normison — *see Benzodiazepines*						
Normorphine	T40.2X1	T40.2X2	T40.2X3	T40.2X4	—	—
Norpseudoephedrine	T50.5X1	T50.5X2	T50.5X3	T50.5X4	T50.5X5	T50.5X6
Nortestosterone (furanpropionate)	T38.7X1	T38.7X2	T38.7X3	T38.7X4	T38.7X5	T38.7X6
Nortriptyline	T43.011	T43.012	T43.013	T43.014	T43.015	T43.016
Noscapine	T48.3X1	T48.3X2	T48.3X3	T48.3X4	T48.3X5	T48.3X6
Nose preparations	T49.6X1	T49.6X2	T49.6X3	T49.6X4	T49.6X5	T49.6X6
Novobiocin	T36.5X1	T36.5X2	T36.5X3	T36.5X4	T36.5X5	T36.5X6
Novocain (infiltration) (topical)	T41.3X1	T41.3X2	T41.3X3	T41.3X4	T41.3X5	T41.3X6
nerve block (peripheral) (plexus)	T41.3X1	T41.3X2	T41.3X3	T41.3X4	T41.3X5	T41.3X6
spinal	T41.3X1	T41.3X2	T41.3X3	T41.3X4	T41.3X5	T41.3X6
Noxious foodstuff	T62.91	T62.92	T62.93	T62.94	—	—
specified NEC	T62.8X1	T62.8X2	T62.8X3	T62.8X4	—	—
Noxiptiline	T43.011	T43.012	T43.013	T43.014	T43.015	T43.016
Noxytiolin	T49.0X1	T49.0X2	T49.0X3	T49.0X4	T49.0X5	T49.0X6
NPH Iletin (insulin)	T38.3X1	T38.3X2	T38.3X3	T38.3X4	T38.3X5	T38.3X6
Numorphan	T40.2X1	T40.2X2	T40.2X3	T40.2X4	T40.2X5	T40.2X6
Nunol	T42.3X1	T42.3X2	T42.3X3	T42.3X4	T42.3X5	T42.3X6
Nupercaine (spinal anesthetic)	T41.3X1	T41.3X2	T41.3X3	T41.3X4	T41.3X5	T41.3X6
topical (surface)	T41.3X1	T41.3X2	T41.3X3	T41.3X4	T41.3X5	T41.3X6
Nutmeg oil (liniment)	T49.3X1	T49.3X2	T49.3X3	T49.3X4	T49.3X5	T49.3X6
Nutritional supplement	T50.901	T50.902	T50.903	T50.904	T50.905	T50.906
Nux vomica	T65.1X1	T65.1X2	T65.1X3	T65.1X4	—	—
Nydrazid	T37.1X1	T37.1X2	T37.1X3	T37.1X4	T37.1X5	T37.1X6
Nylidrin	T46.7X1	T46.7X2	T46.7X3	T46.7X4	T46.7X5	T46.7X6
Nystatin	T36.7X1	T36.7X2	T36.7X3	T36.7X4	T36.7X5	T36.7X6
topical	T49.0X1	T49.0X2	T49.0X3	T49.0X4	T49.0X5	T49.0X6
Nytol	T45.0X1	T45.0X2	T45.0X3	T45.0X4	T45.0X5	T45.0X6
O						
Obidoxime chloride	T50.6X1	T50.6X2	T50.6X3	T50.6X4	T50.6X5	T50.6X6
Octafonium (chloride)	T49.3X1	T49.3X2	T49.3X3	T49.3X4	T49.3X5	T49.3X6
Octamethyl pyrophos-phoramide	T60.0X1	T60.0X2	T60.0X3	T60.0X4	—	—
Octanoin	T50.991	T50.992	T50.993	T50.994	T50.995	T50.996
Octatropine methyl-bromide	T44.3X1	T44.3X2	T44.3X3	T44.3X4	T44.3X5	T44.3X6
Octotiamine	T45.2X1	T45.2X2	T45.2X3	T45.2X4	T45.2X5	T45.2X6

Substance	Poisoning, Accidental unintentional	Poisoning, Intentional self-harm	Poisoning, Assault	Poisoning, Undetermined	Adverse effect	Underdosing
Octoxinol (9)	T49.8X1	T49.8X2	T49.8X3	T49.8X4	T49.8X5	T49.8X6
Octreotide	T38.991	T38.992	T38.993	T38.994	T38.995	T38.996
Octyl nitrite	T46.3X1	T46.3X2	T46.3X3	T46.3X4	T46.3X5	T46.3X6
Oestradiol	T38.5X1	T38.5X2	T38.5X3	T38.5X4	T38.5X5	T38.5X6
Oestriol	T38.5X1	T38.5X2	T38.5X3	T38.5X4	T38.5X5	T38.5X6
Oestrogen	T38.5X1	T38.5X2	T38.5X3	T38.5X4	T38.5X5	T38.5X6
Oestrone	T38.5X1	T38.5X2	T38.5X3	T38.5X4	T38.5X5	T38.5X6
Ofloxacin	T36.8X1	T36.8X2	T36.8X3	T36.8X4	T36.8X5	T36.8X6
Oil (of)	T65.891	T65.892	T65.893	T65.894	--	--
bitter almond	T62.8X1	T62.8X2	T62.8X3	T62.8X4	--	--
cloves	T49.7X1	T49.7X2	T49.7X3	T49.7X4	T49.7X5	T49.7X6
colors	T65.6X1	T65.6X2	T65.6X3	T65.6X4	--	--
fumes	T59.891	T59.892	T59.893	T59.894	--	--
lubricating	T52.0X1	T52.0X2	T52.0X3	T52.0X4	--	--
Niobe	T52.8X1	T52.8X2	T52.8X3	T52.8X4	--	--
vitriol (liquid)	T54.2X1	T54.2X2	T54.2X3	T54.2X4	--	--
fumes	T54.2X1	T54.2X2	T54.2X3	T54.2X4	--	--
wintergreen (bitter) NEC	T49.3X1	T49.3X2	T49.3X3	T49.3X4	T49.3X5	T49.3X6
Oily preparation (for skin)	T49.3X1	T49.3X2	T49.3X3	T49.3X4	T49.3X5	T49.3X6
Ointment NEC	T49.3X1	T49.3X2	T49.3X3	T49.3X4	T49.3X5	T49.3X6
Olanzapine	T43.591	T43.592	T43.593	T43.594	T43.595	T43.596
Oleander	T62.2X1	T62.2X2	T62.2X3	T62.2X4	--	--
Oleandomycin	T36.3X1	T36.3X2	T36.3X3	T36.3X4	T36.3X5	T36.3X6
Oleandrin	T46.0X1	T46.0X2	T46.0X3	T46.0X4	T46.0X5	T46.0X6
Oleic acid	T46.6X1	T46.6X2	T46.6X3	T46.6X4	T46.6X5	T46.6X6
Oleovitamin A	T45.2X1	T45.2X2	T45.2X3	T45.2X4	T45.2X5	T45.2X6
Oleum ricini	T47.2X1	T47.2X2	T47.2X3	T47.2X4	T47.2X5	T47.2X6
Olive oil (medicinal) **NEC**	T47.4X1	T47.4X2	T47.4X3	T47.4X4	T47.4X5	T47.4X6
Olivomycin	T45.1X1	T45.1X2	T45.1X3	T45.1X4	T45.1X5	T45.1X6
Olsalazine	T47.8X1	T47.8X2	T47.8X3	T47.8X4	T47.8X5	T47.8X6
Omeprazole	T47.1X1	T47.1X2	T47.1X3	T47.1X4	T47.1X5	T47.1X6
OMPA	T60.0X1	T60.0X2	T60.0X3	T60.0X4	--	--
Oncovin	T45.1X1	T45.1X2	T45.1X3	T45.1X4	T45.1X5	T45.1X6
Ondansetron	T45.0X1	T45.0X2	T45.0X3	T45.0X4	T45.0X5	T45.0X6
Ophthaine	T41.3X1	T41.3X2	T41.3X3	T41.3X4	T41.3X5	T41.3X6
Ophthetic	T41.3X1	T41.3X2	T41.3X3	T41.3X4	T41.3X5	T41.3X6
Opiate NEC	T40.601	T40.602	T40.603	T40.604	T40.605	T40.606
antagonists	T50.7X1	T50.7X2	T50.7X3	T50.7X4	T50.7X5	T50.7X6
Opioid NEC	T40.2X1	T40.2X2	T40.2X3	T40.2X4	T40.2X5	T40.2X6
Opipramol	T43.011	T43.012	T43.013	T43.014	T43.015	T43.016
Opium alkaloids (total)	T40.0X1	T40.0X2	T40.0X3	T40.0X4	T40.0X5	T40.0X6
standardized powdered	T40.0X1	T40.0X2	T40.0X3	T40.0X4	T40.0X5	T40.0X6
tincture (camphorated)	T40.0X1	T40.0X2	T40.0X3	T40.0X4	T40.0X5	T40.0X6
Oracon	T38.4X1	T38.4X2	T38.4X3	T38.4X4	T38.4X5	T38.4X6
Oragrafin	T50.8X1	T50.8X2	T50.8X3	T50.8X4	T50.8X5	T50.8X6
Oral contraceptives	T38.4X1	T38.4X2	T38.4X3	T38.4X4	T38.4X5	T38.4X6
Oral rehydration salts	T50.3X1	T50.3X2	T50.3X3	T50.3X4	T50.3X5	T50.3X6
Orazamide	T50.991	T50.992	T50.993	T50.994	T50.995	T50.996
Orciprenaline	T48.291	T48.292	T48.293	T48.294	T48.295	T48.296
Organidin	T48.4X1	T48.4X2	T48.4X3	T48.4X4	T48.4X5	T48.4X6
Organonitrate NEC	T46.3X1	T46.3X2	T46.3X3	T46.3X4	T46.3X5	T46.3X6
Organophosphates	T60.0X1	T60.0X2	T60.0X3	T60.0X4	--	--
Orimune	T50.B91	T50.B92	T50.B93	T50.B94	T50.B95	T50.B96
Orinase	T38.3X1	T38.3X2	T38.3X3	T38.3X4	T38.3X5	T38.3X6
Ormeloxifene	T38.6X1	T38.6X2	T38.6X3	T38.6X4	T38.6X5	T38.6X6
Ornidazole	T37.3X1	T37.3X2	T37.3X3	T37.3X4	T37.3X5	T37.3X6
Ornithine aspartate	T50.991	T50.992	T50.993	T50.994	T50.995	T50.996
Ornoprostil	T47.1X1	T47.1X2	T47.1X3	T47.1X4	T47.1X5	T47.1X6
Orphenadrine (hydrochloride)	T42.8X1	T42.8X2	T42.8X3	T42.8X4	T42.8X5	T42.8X6
Ortal (sodium)	T42.3X1	T42.3X2	T42.3X3	T42.3X4	T42.3X5	T42.3X6
Orthoboric acid	T49.0X1	T49.0X2	T49.0X3	T49.0X4	T49.0X5	T49.0X6
ENT agent	T49.6X1	T49.6X2	T49.6X3	T49.6X4	T49.6X5	T49.6X6
ophthalmic preparation	T49.5X1	T49.5X2	T49.5X3	T49.5X4	T49.5X5	T49.5X6
Orthocaine	T41.3X1	T41.3X2	T41.3X3	T41.3X4	T41.3X5	T41.3X6
Orthodichlorobenzene	T53.7X1	T53.7X2	T53.7X3	T53.7X4	--	--
Ortho-Novum	T38.4X1	T38.4X2	T38.4X3	T38.4X4	T38.4X5	T38.4X6
Orthotolidine (reagent)	T54.2X1	T54.2X2	T54.2X3	T54.2X4	--	--
Osmic acid (liquid)	T54.2X1	T54.2X2	T54.2X3	T54.2X4	--	--
fumes	T54.2X1	T54.2X2	T54.2X3	T54.2X4	--	--
Osmotic diuretics	T50.2X1	T50.2X2	T50.2X3	T50.2X4	T50.2X5	T50.2X6
Otilonium bromide	T44.3X1	T44.3X2	T44.3X3	T44.3X4	T44.3X5	T44.3X6
Otorhinolaryngological drug NEC	T49.6X1	T49.6X2	T49.6X3	T49.6X4	T49.6X5	T49.6X6
Ouabain (e)	T46.0X1	T46.0X2	T46.0X3	T46.0X4	T46.0X5	T46.0X6
Ovarian						
hormone	T38.5X1	T38.5X2	T38.5X3	T38.5X4	T38.5X5	T38.5X6
stimulant	T38.5X1	T38.5X2	T38.5X3	T38.5X4	T38.5X5	T38.5X6
Ovral	T38.4X1	T38.4X2	T38.4X3	T38.4X4	T38.4X5	T38.4X6
Ovulen	T38.4X1	T38.4X2	T38.4X3	T38.4X4	T38.4X5	T38.4X6
Oxacillin	T36.0X1	T36.0X2	T36.0X3	T36.0X4	T36.0X5	T36.0X6
Oxalic acid	T54.2X1	T54.2X2	T54.2X3	T54.2X4	--	--
ammonium salt	T50.991	T50.992	T50.993	T50.994	T50.995	T50.996
Oxamniquine	T37.4X1	T37.4X2	T37.4X3	T37.4X4	T37.4X5	T37.4X6
Oxanamide	T43.591	T43.592	T43.593	T43.594	T43.595	T43.596

Substance	Poisoning, Accidental unintentional	Poisoning, Intentional self-harm	Poisoning, Assault	Poisoning, Undetermined	Adverse effect	Underdosing
Oxandrolone	T38.7X1	T38.7X2	T38.7X3	T38.7X4	T38.7X5	T38.7X6
Oxantel	T37.4X1	T37.4X2	T37.4X3	T37.4X4	T37.4X5	T37.4X6
Oxapium iodide	T44.3X1	T44.3X2	T44.3X3	T44.3X4	T44.3X5	T44.3X6
Oxaprotiline	T43.021	T43.022	T43.023	T43.024	T43.025	T43.026
Oxaprozin	T39.311	T39.312	T39.313	T39.314	T39.315	T39.316
Oxatomide	T45.0X1	T45.0X2	T45.0X3	T45.0X4	T45.0X5	T45.0X6
Oxazepam	T42.4X1	T42.4X2	T42.4X3	T42.4X4	T42.4X5	T42.4X6
Oxazimedrine	T50.5X1	T50.5X2	T50.5X3	T50.5X4	T50.5X5	T50.5X6
Oxazolam	T42.4X1	T42.4X2	T42.4X3	T42.4X4	T42.4X5	T42.4X6
Oxazolidine derivatives	T42.2X1	T42.2X2	T42.2X3	T42.2X4	T42.2X5	T42.2X6
Oxazolidinedione (derivative)	T42.2X1	T42.2X2	T42.2X3	T42.2X4	T42.2X5	T42.2X6
Ox bile extract	T47.5X1	T47.5X2	T47.5X3	T47.5X4	T47.5X5	T47.5X6
Oxcarbazepine	T42.1X1	T42.1X2	T42.1X3	T42.1X4	T42.1X5	T42.1X6
Oxedrine	T44.4X1	T44.4X2	T44.4X3	T44.4X4	T44.4X5	T44.4X6
Oxeladin (citrate)	T48.3X1	T48.3X2	T48.3X3	T48.3X4	T48.3X5	T48.3X6
Oxendolone	T38.5X1	T38.5X2	T38.5X3	T38.5X4	T38.5X5	T38.5X6
Oxetacaine	T41.3X1	T41.3X2	T41.3X3	T41.3X4	T41.3X5	T41.3X6
Oxethazine	T41.3X1	T41.3X2	T41.3X3	T41.3X4	T41.3X5	T41.3X6
Oxetorone	T39.8X1	T39.8X2	T39.8X3	T39.8X4	T39.8X5	T39.8X6
Oxiconazole	T49.0X1	T49.0X2	T49.0X3	T49.0X4	T49.0X5	T49.0X6
Oxidizing agent NEC	T54.91	T54.92	T54.93	T54.94	--	--
Oxipurinol	T50.4X1	T50.4X2	T50.4X3	T50.4X4	T50.4X5	T50.4X6
Oxitriptan	T43.291	T43.292	T43.293	T43.294	T43.295	T43.296
Oxitropium bromide	T48.6X1	T48.6X2	T48.6X3	T48.6X4	T48.6X5	T48.6X6
Oxodipine	T46.1X1	T46.1X2	T46.1X3	T46.1X4	T46.1X5	T46.1X6
Oxolamine	T48.3X1	T48.3X2	T48.3X3	T48.3X4	T48.3X5	T48.3X6
Oxolinic acid	T37.8X1	T37.8X2	T37.8X3	T37.8X4	T37.8X5	T37.8X6
Oxomemazine	T43.3X1	T43.3X2	T43.3X3	T43.3X4	T43.3X5	T43.3X6
Oxophenarsine	T37.3X1	T37.3X2	T37.3X3	T37.3X4	T37.3X5	T37.3X6
Oxprenolol	T44.7X1	T44.7X2	T44.7X3	T44.7X4	T44.7X5	T44.7X6
Oxsoralen	T49.3X1	T49.3X2	T49.3X3	T49.3X4	T49.3X5	T49.3X6
Oxtriphylline	T48.6X1	T48.6X2	T48.6X3	T48.6X4	T48.6X5	T48.6X6
Oxybate sodium	T41.291	T41.292	T41.293	T41.294	T41.295	T41.296
Oxybuprocaine	T41.3X1	T41.3X2	T41.3X3	T41.3X4	T41.3X5	T41.3X6
Oxybutynin	T44.3X1	T44.3X2	T44.3X3	T44.3X4	T44.3X5	T44.3X6
Oxychlorosene	T49.0X1	T49.0X2	T49.0X3	T49.0X4	T49.0X5	T49.0X6
Oxycodone	T40.2X1	T40.2X2	T40.2X3	T40.2X4	T40.2X5	T40.2X6
Oxyfedrine	T46.3X1	T46.3X2	T46.3X3	T46.3X4	T46.3X5	T46.3X6
Oxygen	T41.5X1	T41.5X2	T41.5X3	T41.5X4	T41.5X5	T41.5X6
Oxylone	T49.0X1	T49.0X2	T49.0X3	T49.0X4	T49.0X5	T49.0X6
ophthalmic preparation	T49.5X1	T49.5X2	T49.5X3	T49.5X4	T49.5X5	T49.5X6
Oxymesterone	T38.7X1	T38.7X2	T38.7X3	T38.7X4	T38.7X5	T38.7X6
Oxymetazoline	T48.5X1	T48.5X2	T48.5X3	T48.5X4	T48.5X5	T48.5X6
Oxymetholone	T38.7X1	T38.7X2	T38.7X3	T38.7X4	T38.7X5	T38.7X6
Oxymorphone	T40.2X1	T40.2X2	T40.2X3	T40.2X4	T40.2X5	T40.2X6
Oxypertine	T43.591	T43.592	T43.593	T43.594	T43.595	T43.596
Oxyphenbutazone	T39.2X1	T39.2X2	T39.2X3	T39.2X4	T39.2X5	T39.2X6
Oxyphencyclimine	T44.3X1	T44.3X2	T44.3X3	T44.3X4	T44.3X5	T44.3X6
Oxyphenisatine	T47.2X1	T47.2X2	T47.2X3	T47.2X4	T47.2X5	T47.2X6
Oxyphenonium bromide	T44.3X1	T44.3X2	T44.3X3	T44.3X4	T44.3X5	T44.3X6
Oxypolygelatin	T45.8X1	T45.8X2	T45.8X3	T45.8X4	T45.8X5	T45.8X6
Oxyquinoline (derivatives)	T37.8X1	T37.8X2	T37.8X3	T37.8X4	T37.8X5	T37.8X6
Oxytetracycline	T36.4X1	T36.4X2	T36.4X3	T36.4X4	T36.4X5	T36.4X6
Oxytocic drug NEC	T48.0X1	T48.0X2	T48.0X3	T48.0X4	T48.0X5	T48.0X6
Oxytocin (synthetic)	T48.0X1	T48.0X2	T48.0X3	T48.0X4	T48.0X5	T48.0X6
Ozone	T59.891	T59.892	T59.893	T59.894	--	--
P						
PABA	T49.3X1	T49.3X2	T49.3X3	T49.3X4	T49.3X5	T49.3X6
Packed red cells	T45.8X1	T45.8X2	T45.8X3	T45.8X4	T45.8X5	T45.8X6
Padimate	T49.3X1	T49.3X2	T49.3X3	T49.3X4	T49.3X5	T49.3X6
Paint NEC	T65.6X1	T65.6X2	T65.6X3	T65.6X4	--	--
cleaner	T52.91	T52.92	T52.93	T52.94	--	--
fumes NEC	T59.891	T59.892	T59.893	T59.894	--	--
lead (fumes)	T56.0X1	T56.0X2	T56.0X3	T56.0X4	--	--
solvent NEC	T52.8X1	T52.8X2	T52.8X3	T52.8X4	--	--
stripper	T52.8X1	T52.8X2	T52.8X3	T52.8X4	--	--
Palfium	T40.2X1	T40.2X2	T40.2X3	T40.2X4	--	--
Palm kernel oil	T50.991	T50.992	T50.993	T50.994	T50.995	T50.996
Paludrine	T37.2X1	T37.2X2	T37.2X3	T37.2X4	T37.2X5	T37.2X6
PAM (pralidoxime)	T50.6X1	T50.6X2	T50.6X3	T50.6X4	T50.6X5	T50.6X6
Pamaquine (naphthoute)	T37.2X1	T37.2X2	T37.2X3	T37.2X4	T37.2X5	T37.2X6
Panadol	T39.1X1	T39.1X2	T39.1X3	T39.1X4	T39.1X5	T39.1X6
Pancreatic						
digestive secretion stimulant	T47.8X1	T47.8X2	T47.8X3	T47.8X4	T47.8X5	T47.8X6
dornase	T45.3X1	T45.3X2	T45.3X3	T45.3X4	T45.3X5	T45.3X6
Pancreatin	T47.5X1	T47.5X2	T47.5X3	T47.5X4	T47.5X5	T47.5X6
Pancrelipase	T47.5X1	T47.5X2	T47.5X3	T47.5X4	T47.5X5	T47.5X6
Pancuronium (bromide)	T48.1X1	T48.1X2	T48.1X3	T48.1X4	T48.1X5	T48.1X6
Pangamic acid	T45.2X1	T45.2X2	T45.2X3	T45.2X4	T45.2X5	T45.2X6
Panthenol	T45.2X1	T45.2X2	T45.2X3	T45.2X4	T45.2X5	T45.2X6
topical	T49.8X1	T49.8X2	T49.8X3	T49.8X4	T49.8X5	T49.8X6
Pantopon	T40.0X1	T40.0X2	T40.0X3	T40.0X4	T40.0X5	T40.0X6
Pantothenic acid	T45.2X1	T45.2X2	T45.2X3	T45.2X4	T45.2X5	T45.2X6

Substance	Poisoning, Accidental unintentional	Poisoning, Intentional self-harm	Poisoning, Assault	Poisoning, Undetermined	Adverse effect	Underdosing
Panwarfin	T45.511	T45.512	T45.513	T45.514	T45.515	T45.516
Papain	T47.5X1	T47.5X2	T47.5X3	T47.5X4	T47.5X5	T47.5X6
digestant	T47.5X1	T47.5X2	T47.5X3	T47.5X4	T47.5X5	T47.5X6
Papaveretum	T40.0X1	T40.0X2	T40.0X3	T40.0X4	T40.0X5	T40.0X6
Papaverine	T44.3X1	T44.3X2	T44.3X3	T44.3X4	T44.3X5	T44.3X6
Para-acetamidophenol	T39.1X1	T39.1X2	T39.1X3	T39.1X4	T39.1X5	T39.1X6
Para-aminobenzoic acid	T49.3X1	T49.3X2	T49.3X3	T49.3X4	T49.3X5	T49.3X6
Para-aminophenol derivatives	T39.1X1	T39.1X2	T39.1X3	T39.1X4	T39.1X5	T39.1X6
Para-aminosalicylic acid	T37.1X1	T37.1X2	T37.1X3	T37.1X4	T37.1X5	T37.1X6
Paracetaldehyde	T42.6X1	T42.6X2	T42.6X3	T42.6X4	T42.6X5	T42.6X6
Paracetamol	T39.1X1	T39.1X2	T39.1X3	T39.1X4	T39.1X5	T39.1X6
Parachlorophenol (camphorated)	T49.0X1	T49.0X2	T49.0X3	T49.0X4	T49.0X5	T49.0X6
Paracodin	T40.2X1	T40.2X2	T40.2X3	T40.2X4	T40.2X5	T40.2X6
Paradione	T42.2X1	T42.2X2	T42.2X3	T42.2X4	T42.2X5	T42.2X6
Paraffin (s) (wax)	T52.0X1	T52.0X2	T52.0X3	T52.0X4	--	--
liquid (medicinal)	T47.4X1	T47.4X2	T47.4X3	T47.4X4	T47.4X5	T47.4X6
nonmedicinal	T52.0X1	T52.0X2	T52.0X3	T52.0X4	--	--
Paraformaldehyde	T60.3X1	T60.3X2	T60.3X3	T60.3X4	--	--
Paraldehyde	T42.6X1	T42.6X2	T42.6X3	T42.6X4	T42.6X5	T42.6X6
Paramethadione	T42.2X1	T42.2X2	T42.2X3	T42.2X4	T42.2X5	T42.2X6
Paramethasone	T38.0X1	T38.0X2	T38.0X3	T38.0X4	T38.0X5	T38.0X6
acetate	T49.0X1	T49.0X2	T49.0X3	T49.0X4	T49.0X5	T49.0X6
Paraoxon	T60.0X1	T60.0X2	T60.0X3	T60.0X4	--	--
Paraquat	T60.3X1	T60.3X2	T60.3X3	T60.3X4	--	--
Parasympatholytic NEC	T44.3X1	T44.3X2	T44.3X3	T44.3X4	T44.3X5	T44.3X6
Parasympathomimetic drug NEC	T44.1X1	T44.1X2	T44.1X3	T44.1X4	T44.1X5	T44.1X6
Parathion	T60.0X1	T60.0X2	T60.0X3	T60.0X4	--	--
Parathormone	T50.991	T50.992	T50.993	T50.994	T50.995	T50.996
Parathyroid extract	T50.991	T50.992	T50.993	T50.994	T50.995	T50.996
Paratyphoid vaccine	T50.A91	T50.A92	T50.A93	T50.A94	T50.A95	T50.A96
Paredrine	T44.4X1	T44.4X2	T44.4X3	T44.4X4	T44.4X5	T44.4X6
Paregoric	T40.0X1	T40.0X2	T40.0X3	T40.0X4	T40.0X5	T40.0X6
Pargyline	T46.5X1	T46.5X2	T46.5X3	T46.5X4	T46.5X5	T46.5X6
Paris green	T57.0X1	T57.0X2	T57.0X3	T57.0X4	--	--
insecticide	T57.0X1	T57.0X2	T57.0X3	T57.0X4	--	--
Parnate	T43.1X1	T43.1X2	T43.1X3	T43.1X4	T43.1X5	T43.1X6
Paromomycin	T36.5X1	T36.5X2	T36.5X3	T36.5X4	T36.5X5	T36.5X6
Paroxypropione	T45.1X1	T45.1X2	T45.1X3	T45.1X4	T45.1X5	T45.1X6
Parzone	T40.2X1	T40.2X2	T40.2X3	T40.2X4	T40.2X5	T40.2X6
PAS	T37.1X1	T37.1X2	T37.1X3	T37.1X4	T37.1X5	T37.1X6
Pasiniazid	T37.1X1	T37.1X2	T37.1X3	T37.1X4	T37.1X5	T37.1X6
PBB (polybrominated biphenyls)	T65.891	T65.892	T65.893	T65.894	--	--
PCB	T65.891	T65.892	T65.893	T65.894	--	--
PCP						
meaning pentachlorophenol	T60.1X1	T60.1X2	T60.1X3	T60.1X4	--	--
fungicide	T60.3X1	T60.3X2	T60.3X3	T60.3X4	--	--
herbicide	T60.3X1	T60.3X2	T60.3X3	T60.3X4	--	--
insecticide	T60.1X1	T60.1X2	T60.1X3	T60.1X4	--	--
meaning phencyclidine	T40.991	T40.992	T40.993	T40.994	--	--
Peach kernel oil (emulsion)	T47.4X1	T47.4X2	T47.4X3	T47.4X4	T47.4X5	T47.4X6
Peanut oil (emulsion) **NEC**	T47.4X1	T47.4X2	T47.4X3	T47.4X4	T47.4X5	T47.4X6
topical	T49.3X1	T49.3X2	T49.3X3	T49.3X4	T49.3X5	T49.3X6
Pearly Gates (morning glory seeds)	T40.991	T40.992	T40.993	T40.994	--	--
Pecazine	T43.3X1	T43.3X2	T43.3X3	T43.3X4	T43.3X5	T43.3X6
Pectin	T47.6X1	T47.6X2	T47.6X3	T47.6X4	T47.6X5	T47.6X6
Pefloxacin	T37.8X1	T37.8X2	T37.8X3	T37.8X4	T37.8X5	T37.8X6
Pegademase, bovine	T50.Z91	T50.Z92	T50.Z93	T50.Z94	T50.Z95	T50.Z96
Pelletierine tannate	T37.4X1	T37.4X2	T37.4X3	T37.4X4	T37.4X5	T37.4X6
Pemirolast (potassium)	T48.6X1	T48.6X2	T48.6X3	T48.6X4	T48.6X5	T48.6X6
Pemoline	T50.7X1	T50.7X2	T50.7X3	T50.7X4	T50.7X5	T50.7X6
Pempidine	T44.2X1	T44.2X2	T44.2X3	T44.2X4	T44.2X5	T44.2X6
Penamecillin	T36.0X1	T36.0X2	T36.0X3	T36.0X4	T36.0X5	T36.0X6
Penbutolol	T44.7X1	T44.7X2	T44.7X3	T44.7X4	T44.7X5	T44.7X6
Penethamate	T36.0X1	T36.0X2	T36.0X3	T36.0X4	T36.0X5	T36.0X6
Penfluridol	T43.591	T43.592	T43.593	T43.594	T43.595	T43.596
Penflutizide	T50.2X1	T50.2X2	T50.2X3	T50.2X4	T50.2X5	T50.2X6
Pengitoxin	T46.0X1	T46.0X2	T46.0X3	T46.0X4	T46.0X5	T46.0X6
Penicillamine	T50.6X1	T50.6X2	T50.6X3	T50.6X4	T50.6X5	T50.6X6
Penicillin (any)	T36.0X1	T36.0X2	T36.0X3	T36.0X4	T36.0X5	T36.0X6
Penicillinase	T45.3X1	T45.3X2	T45.3X3	T45.3X4	T45.3X5	T45.3X6
Penicilloyl polylysine	T50.8X1	T50.8X2	T50.8X3	T50.8X4	T50.8X5	T50.8X6
Penimepicycline	T36.4X1	T36.4X2	T36.4X3	T36.4X4	T36.4X5	T36.4X6
Pentachloroethane	T53.6X1	T53.6X2	T53.6X3	T53.6X4	--	--
Pentachloronaphthalene	T53.7X1	T53.7X2	T53.7X3	T53.7X4	--	--
Pentachlorophenol (pesticide)	T60.1X1	T60.1X2	T60.1X3	T60.1X4	--	--
fungicide	T60.3X1	T60.3X2	T60.3X3	T60.3X4	--	--
herbicide	T60.3X1	T60.3X2	T60.3X3	T60.3X4	--	--
insecticide	T60.1X1	T60.1X2	T60.1X3	T60.1X4	--	--
Pentaerythritol	T46.3X1	T46.3X2	T46.3X3	T46.3X4	T46.3X5	T46.3X6
chloral	T42.6X1	T42.6X2	T42.6X3	T42.6X4	T42.6X5	T42.6X6
tetranitrate NEC	T46.3X1	T46.3X2	T46.3X3	T46.3X4	T46.3X5	T46.3X6
Pentaerythrityl tetranitrate	T46.3X1	T46.3X2	T46.3X3	T46.3X4	T46.3X5	T46.3X6
Pentagastrin	T50.8X1	T50.8X2	T50.8X3	T50.8X4	T50.8X5	T50.8X6
Pentalin	T53.6X1	T53.6X2	T53.6X3	T53.6X4	--	--
Pentamethonium bromide	T44.2X1	T44.2X2	T44.2X3	T44.2X4	T44.2X5	T44.2X6
Pentamidine	T37.3X1	T37.3X2	T37.3X3	T37.3X4	T37.3X5	T37.3X6
Pentanol	T51.3X1	T51.3X2	T51.3X3	T51.3X4	--	--
Pentapyrrolinium (bitartrate)	T44.2X1	T44.2X2	T44.2X3	T44.2X4	T44.2X5	T44.2X6
Pentaquine	T37.2X1	T37.2X2	T37.2X3	T37.2X4	T37.2X5	T37.2X6
Pentazocine	T40.4X1	T40.4X2	T40.4X3	T40.4X4	T40.4X5	T40.4X6
Pentetrazole	T50.7X1	T50.7X2	T50.7X3	T50.7X4	T50.7X5	T50.7X6
Penthienate bromide	T44.3X1	T44.3X2	T44.3X3	T44.3X4	T44.3X5	T44.3X6
Pentifylline	T46.7X1	T46.7X2	T46.7X3	T46.7X4	T46.7X5	T46.7X6
Pentobarbital	T42.3X1	T42.3X2	T42.3X3	T42.3X4	T42.3X5	T42.3X6
sodium	T42.3X1	T42.3X2	T42.3X3	T42.3X4	T42.3X5	T42.3X6
Pentobarbitone	T42.3X1	T42.3X2	T42.3X3	T42.3X4	T42.3X5	T42.3X6
Pentolonium tartrate	T44.2X1	T44.2X2	T44.2X3	T44.2X4	T44.2X5	T44.2X6
Pentosan polysulfate (sodium)	T39.8X1	T39.8X2	T39.8X3	T39.8X4	T39.8X5	T39.8X6
Pentostatin	T45.1X1	T45.1X2	T45.1X3	T45.1X4	T45.1X5	T45.1X6
Pentothal	T41.1X1	T41.1X2	T41.1X3	T41.1X4	T41.1X5	T41.1X6
Pentoxifylline	T46.7X1	T46.7X2	T46.7X3	T46.7X4	T46.7X5	T46.7X6
Pentoxyverine	T48.3X1	T48.3X2	T48.3X3	T48.3X4	T48.3X5	T48.3X6
Pentrinat	T46.3X1	T46.3X2	T46.3X3	T46.3X4	T46.3X5	T46.3X6
Pentylenetetrazole	T50.7X1	T50.7X2	T50.7X3	T50.7X4	T50.7X5	T50.7X6
Pentylsalicylamide	T37.1X1	T37.1X2	T37.1X3	T37.1X4	T37.1X5	T37.1X6
Pentymal	T42.3X1	T42.3X2	T42.3X3	T42.3X4	T42.3X5	T42.3X6
Peplomycin	T45.1X1	T45.1X2	T45.1X3	T45.1X4	T45.1X5	T45.1X6
Peppermint (oil)	T47.5X1	T47.5X2	T47.5X3	T47.5X4	T47.5X5	T47.5X6
Pepsin	T47.5X1	T47.5X2	T47.5X3	T47.5X4	T47.5X5	T47.5X6
digestant	T47.5X1	T47.5X2	T47.5X3	T47.5X4	T47.5X5	T47.5X6
Pepstatin	T47.1X1	T47.1X2	T47.1X3	T47.1X4	T47.1X5	T47.1X6
Peptavlon	T50.8X1	T50.8X2	T50.8X3	T50.8X4	T50.8X5	T50.8X6
Perazine	T43.3X1	T43.3X2	T43.3X3	T43.3X4	T43.3X5	T43.3X6
Percaine (spinal)	T41.3X1	T41.3X2	T41.3X3	T41.3X4	T41.3X5	T41.3X6
topical (surface)	T41.3X1	T41.3X2	T41.3X3	T41.3X4	T41.3X5	T41.3X6
Perchloroethylene	T53.3X1	T53.3X2	T53.3X3	T53.3X4	--	--
medicinal	T37.4X1	T37.4X2	T37.4X3	T37.4X4	T37.4X5	T37.4X6
vapor	T53.3X1	T53.3X2	T53.3X3	T53.3X4	--	--
Percodan	T40.2X1	T40.2X2	T40.2X3	T40.2X4	T40.2X5	T40.2X6
Percogesic — *see also acetaminophen*	T45.0X1	T45.0X2	T45.0X3	T45.0X4	T45.0X5	T45.0X6
Percorten	T38.0X1	T38.0X2	T38.0X3	T38.0X4	T38.0X5	T38.0X6
Pergolide	T42.8X1	T42.8X2	T42.8X3	T42.8X4	T42.8X5	T42.8X6
Pergonal	T38.811	T38.812	T38.813	T38.814	T38.815	T38.816
Perhexilene	T46.3X1	T46.3X2	T46.3X3	T46.3X4	T46.3X5	T46.3X6
Perhexiline (maleate)	T46.3X1	T46.3X2	T46.3X3	T46.3X4	T46.3X5	T46.3X6
Periactin	T45.0X1	T45.0X2	T45.0X3	T45.0X4	T45.0X5	T45.0X6
Periciazine	T43.3X1	T43.3X2	T43.3X3	T43.3X4	T43.3X5	T43.3X6
Periclor	T42.6X1	T42.6X2	T42.6X3	T42.6X4	T42.6X5	T42.6X6
Perindopril	T46.4X1	T46.4X2	T46.4X3	T46.4X4	T46.4X5	T46.4X6
Perisoxal	T39.8X1	T39.8X2	T39.8X3	T39.8X4	T39.8X5	T39.8X6
Peritoneal dialysis solution	T50.3X1	T50.3X2	T50.3X3	T50.3X4	T50.3X5	T50.3X6
Peritrate	T46.3X1	T46.3X2	T46.3X3	T46.3X4	T46.3X5	T46.3X6
Perlapine	T42.4X1	T42.4X2	T42.4X3	T42.4X4	T42.4X5	T42.4X6
Permanganate	T65.891	T65.892	T65.893	T65.894	--	--
Permethrin	T60.1X1	T60.1X2	T60.1X3	T60.1X4	--	--
Pernocton	T42.3X1	T42.3X2	T42.3X3	T42.3X4	T42.3X5	T42.3X6
Pernoston	T42.3X1	T42.3X2	T42.3X3	T42.3X4	T42.3X5	T42.3X6
Peronine	T40.2X1	T40.2X2	T40.2X3	T40.2X4	--	--
Perphenazine	T43.3X1	T43.3X2	T43.3X3	T43.3X4	T43.3X5	T43.3X6
Pertofrane	T43.011	T43.012	T43.013	T43.014	T43.015	T43.016
Pertussis						
immune serum (human)	T50.Z11	T50.Z12	T50.Z13	T50.Z14	T50.Z15	T50.Z16
vaccine (with diphtheria toxoid) (with tetanus toxoid)	T50.A11	T50.A12	T50.A13	T50.A14	T50.A15	T50.A16
Peruvian balsam	T49.0X1	T49.0X2	T49.0X3	T49.0X4	T49.0X5	T49.0X6
Peruvoside	T46.0X1	T46.0X2	T46.0X3	T46.0X4	T46.0X5	T46.0X6
Pesticide (dust) (fumes) (vapor) **NEC**	T60.91	T60.92	T60.93	T60.94	--	--
arsenic	T57.0X1	T57.0X2	T57.0X3	T57.0X4	--	--
chlorinated	T60.1X1	T60.1X2	T60.1X3	T60.1X4	--	--
cyanide	T65.0X1	T65.0X2	T65.0X3	T65.0X4	--	--
kerosene	T52.0X1	T52.0X2	T52.0X3	T52.0X4	--	--
mixture (of compounds)	T60.91	T60.92	T60.93	T60.94	--	--
naphthalene	T60.2X1	T60.2X2	T60.2X3	T60.2X4	--	--
organochlorine (compounds)	T60.1X1	T60.1X2	T60.1X3	T60.1X4	--	--
petroleum (distillate) (products) NEC	T60.8X1	T60.8X2	T60.8X3	T60.8X4	--	--
specified ingredient NEC	T60.8X1	T60.8X2	T60.8X3	T60.8X4	--	--
strychnine	T65.1X1	T65.1X2	T65.1X3	T65.1X4	--	--
thallium	T60.4X1	T60.4X2	T60.4X3	T60.4X4	--	--

Substance	Poisoning, Accidental unintentional	Poisoning, Intentional self-harm	Poisoning, Assault	Poisoning, Undetermined	Adverse effect	Underdosing
Pethidine	T40.4X1	T40.4X2	T40.4X3	T40.4X4	T40.4X5	T40.4X6
Petrichloral	T42.6X1	T42.6X2	T42.6X3	T42.6X4	T42.6X5	T42.6X6
Petrol	T52.0X1	T52.0X2	T52.0X3	T52.0X4	—	—
vapor	T52.0X1	T52.0X2	T52.0X3	T52.0X4	—	—
Petrolatum	T49.3X1	T49.3X2	T49.3X3	T49.3X4	T49.3X5	T49.3X6
hydrophilic	T49.3X1	T49.3X2	T49.3X3	T49.3X4	T49.3X5	T49.3X6
liquid	T47.4X1	T47.4X2	T47.4X3	T47.4X4	T47.4X5	T47.4X6
topical	T49.3X1	T49.3X2	T49.3X3	T49.3X4	T49.3X5	T49.3X6
nonmedicinal	T52.0X1	T52.0X2	T52.0X3	T52.0X4	—	—
red veterinary	T49.3X1	T49.3X2	T49.3X3	T49.3X4	T49.3X5	T49.3X6
white	T49.3X1	T49.3X2	T49.3X3	T49.3X4	T49.3X5	T49.3X6
Petroleum (products) **NEC**	T52.0X1	T52.0X2	T52.0X3	T52.0X4	—	—
benzine (s) — *see Ligroin*						
ether — *see Ligroin*						
jelly — *see Petrolatum*						
naphtha — *see Ligroin*						
pesticide	T60.8X1	T60.8X2	T60.8X3	T60.8X4	—	—
solids	T52.0X1	T52.0X2	T52.0X3	T52.0X4	—	—
solvents	T52.0X1	T52.0X2	T52.0X3	T52.0X4	—	—
vapor	T52.0X1	T52.0X2	T52.0X3	T52.0X4	—	—
Peyote	T40.991	T40.992	T40.993	T40.994	—	—
Phanodorm, phanodorn	T42.3X1	T42.3X2	T42.3X3	T42.3X4	T42.3X5	T42.3X6
Phanquinone	T37.3X1	T37.3X2	T37.3X3	T37.3X4	T37.3X5	T37.3X6
Phanquone	T37.3X1	T37.3X2	T37.3X3	T37.3X4	T37.3X5	T37.3X6
Pharmaceutical						
adjunct NEC	T50.901	T50.902	T50.903	T50.904	T50.905	T50.906
excipient NEC	T50.901	T50.902	T50.903	T50.904	T50.905	T50.906
sweetener	T50.901	T50.902	T50.903	T50.904	T50.905	T50.906
viscous agent	T50.901	T50.902	T50.903	T50.904	T50.905	T50.906
Phemitone	T42.3X1	T42.3X2	T42.3X3	T42.3X4	T42.3X5	T42.3X6
Phenacaine	T41.3X1	T41.3X2	T41.3X3	T41.3X4	T41.3X5	T41.3X6
Phenacemide	T42.6X1	T42.6X2	T42.6X3	T42.6X4	T42.6X5	T42.6X6
Phenacetin	T39.1X1	T39.1X2	T39.1X3	T39.1X4	T39.1X5	T39.1X6
Phenadoxone	T40.2X1	T40.2X2	T40.2X3	T40.2X4	—	—
Phenaglycodol	T43.591	T43.592	T43.593	T43.594	T43.595	T43.596
Phenantoin	T42.0X1	T42.0X2	T42.0X3	T42.0X4	T42.0X5	T42.0X6
Phenaphthazine reagent	T50.991	T50.992	T50.993	T50.994	T50.995	T50.996
Phenazocine	T40.4X1	T40.4X2	T40.4X3	T40.4X4	T40.4X5	T40.4X6
Phenazone	T39.2X1	T39.2X2	T39.2X3	T39.2X4	T39.2X5	T39.2X6
Phenazopyridine	T39.8X1	T39.8X2	T39.8X3	T39.8X4	T39.8X5	T39.8X6
Phenbenicillin	T36.0X1	T36.0X2	T36.0X3	T36.0X4	T36.0X5	T36.0X6
Phenbutrazate	T50.5X1	T50.5X2	T50.5X3	T50.5X4	T50.5X5	T50.5X6
Phencyclidine	T40.991	T40.992	T40.993	T40.994	T40.995	T40.996
Phendimetrazine	T50.5X1	T50.5X2	T50.5X3	T50.5X4	T50.5X5	T50.5X6
Phenelzine	T43.1X1	T43.1X2	T43.1X3	T43.1X4	T43.1X5	T43.1X6
Phenemal	T42.3X1	T42.3X2	T42.3X3	T42.3X4	T42.3X5	T42.3X6
Phenergan	T42.6X1	T42.6X2	T42.6X3	T42.6X4	T42.6X5	T42.6X6
Pheneticillin	T36.0X1	T36.0X2	T36.0X3	T36.0X4	T36.0X5	T36.0X6
Pheneturide	T42.6X1	T42.6X2	T42.6X3	T42.6X4	T42.6X5	T42.6X6
Phenformin	T38.3X1	T38.3X2	T38.3X3	T38.3X4	T38.3X5	T38.3X6
Phenglutarimide	T44.3X1	T44.3X2	T44.3X3	T44.3X4	T44.3X5	T44.3X6
Phenicarbazide	T39.8X1	T39.8X2	T39.8X3	T39.8X4	T39.8X5	T39.8X6
Phenindamine	T45.0X1	T45.0X2	T45.0X3	T45.0X4	T45.0X5	T45.0X6
Phenindione	T45.511	T45.512	T45.513	T45.514	T45.515	T45.516
Pheniprazine	T43.1X1	T43.1X2	T43.1X3	T43.1X4	T43.1X5	T43.1X6
Pheniramine	T45.0X1	T45.0X2	T45.0X3	T45.0X4	T45.0X5	T45.0X6
Phenisatin	T47.2X1	T47.2X2	T47.2X3	T47.2X4	T47.2X5	T47.2X6
Phenmetrazine	T50.5X1	T50.5X2	T50.5X3	T50.5X4	T50.5X5	T50.5X6
Phenobal	T42.3X1	T42.3X2	T42.3X3	T42.3X4	T42.3X5	T42.3X6
Phenobarbital	T42.3X1	T42.3X2	T42.3X3	T42.3X4	T42.3X5	T42.3X6
with						
mephenytoin	T42.3X1	T42.3X2	T42.3X3	T42.3X4	T42.3X5	T42.3X6
phenytoin	T42.3X1	T42.3X2	T42.3X3	T42.3X4	T42.3X5	T42.3X6
sodium	T42.3X1	T42.3X2	T42.3X3	T42.3X4	T42.3X5	T42.3X6
Phenobarbitone	T42.3X1	T42.3X2	T42.3X3	T42.3X4	T42.3X5	T42.3X6
Phenobutiodil	T50.8X1	T50.8X2	T50.8X3	T50.8X4	T50.8X5	T50.8X6
Phenoctide	T49.0X1	T49.0X2	T49.0X3	T49.0X4	T49.0X5	T49.0X6
Phenol	T49.0X1	T49.0X2	T49.0X3	T49.0X4	T49.0X5	T49.0X6
disinfectant	T54.0X1	T54.0X2	T54.0X3	T54.0X4	—	—
in oil injection	T46.8X1	T46.8X2	T46.8X3	T46.8X4	T46.8X5	T46.8X6
medicinal	T49.1X1	T49.1X2	T49.1X3	T49.1X4	T49.1X5	T49.1X6
nonmedicinal NEC	T54.0X1	T54.0X2	T54.0X3	T54.0X4	—	—
pesticide	T60.8X1	T60.8X2	T60.8X3	T60.8X4	—	—
red	T50.8X1	T50.8X2	T50.8X3	T50.8X4	T50.8X5	T50.8X6
Phenolic preparation	T49.1X1	T49.1X2	T49.1X3	T49.1X4	T49.1X5	T49.1X6
Phenolphthalein	T47.2X1	T47.2X2	T47.2X3	T47.2X4	T47.2X5	T47.2X6
Phenolsulfonphthalein	T50.8X1	T50.8X2	T50.8X3	T50.8X4	T50.8X5	T50.8X6
Phenomorphan	T40.2X1	T40.2X2	T40.2X3	T40.2X4	—	—
Phenonyl	T42.3X1	T42.3X2	T42.3X3	T42.3X4	T42.3X5	T42.3X6
Phenoperidine	T40.4X1	T40.4X2	T40.4X3	T40.4X4	—	—
Phenopyrazone	T46.991	T46.992	T46.993	T46.994	T46.995	T46.996
Phenoquin	T50.4X1	T50.4X2	T50.4X3	T50.4X4	T50.4X5	T50.4X6
Phenothiazine (psychotropic) **NEC**	T43.3X1	T43.3X2	T43.3X3	T43.3X4	T43.3X5	T43.3X6
insecticide	T60.2X1	T60.2X2	T60.2X3	T60.2X4	—	—
Phenothrin	T49.0X1	T49.0X2	T49.0X3	T49.0X4	T49.0X5	T49.0X6
Phenoxybenzamine	T46.7X1	T46.7X2	T46.7X3	T46.7X4	T46.7X5	T46.7X6
Phenoxyethanol	T49.0X1	T49.0X2	T49.0X3	T49.0X4	T49.0X5	T49.0X6
Phenoxymethyl penicillin	T36.0X1	T36.0X2	T36.0X3	T36.0X4	T36.0X5	T36.0X6
Phenprobamate	T42.8X1	T42.8X2	T42.8X3	T42.8X4	T42.8X5	T42.8X6
Phenprocoumon	T45.511	T45.512	T45.513	T45.514	T45.515	T45.516
Phensuximide	T42.2X1	T42.2X2	T42.2X3	T42.2X4	T42.2X5	T42.2X6
Phentermine	T50.5X1	T50.5X2	T50.5X3	T50.5X4	T50.5X5	T50.5X6
Phenthicillin	T36.0X1	T36.0X2	T36.0X3	T36.0X4	T36.0X5	T36.0X6
Phentolamine	T46.7X1	T46.7X2	T46.7X3	T46.7X4	T46.7X5	T46.7X6
Phenyl						
butazone	T39.2X1	T39.2X2	T39.2X3	T39.2X4	T39.2X5	T39.2X6
enediamine	T65.3X1	T65.3X2	T65.3X3	T65.3X4	—	—
hydrazine	T65.3X1	T65.3X2	T65.3X3	T65.3X4	—	—
antineoplastic	T45.1X1	T45.1X2	T45.1X3	T45.1X4	T45.1X5	T45.1X6
mercuric compounds — *see Mercury*						
salicylate	T49.3X1	T49.3X2	T49.3X3	T49.3X4	T49.3X5	T49.3X6
Phenylalanine mustard	T45.1X1	T45.1X2	T45.1X3	T45.1X4	T45.1X5	T45.1X6
Phenylbutazone	T39.2X1	T39.2X2	T39.2X3	T39.2X4	T39.2X5	T39.2X6
Phenylenediamine	T65.3X1	T65.3X2	T65.3X3	T65.3X4	—	—
Phenylephrine	T44.4X1	T44.4X2	T44.4X3	T44.4X4	T44.4X5	T44.4X6
Phenylethylbiguanide	T38.3X1	T38.3X2	T38.3X3	T38.3X4	T38.3X5	T38.3X6
Phenylmercuric						
acetate	T49.0X1	T49.0X2	T49.0X3	T49.0X4	T49.0X5	T49.0X6
borate	T49.0X1	T49.0X2	T49.0X3	T49.0X4	T49.0X5	T49.0X6
nitrate	T49.0X1	T49.0X2	T49.0X3	T49.0X4	T49.0X5	T49.0X6
Phenylmethylbarbitone	T42.3X1	T42.3X2	T42.3X3	T42.3X4	T42.3X5	T42.3X6
Phenylpropanol	T47.5X1	T47.5X2	T47.5X3	T47.5X4	T47.5X5	T47.5X6
Phenylpropanolamine	T44.991	T44.992	T44.993	T44.994	T44.995	T44.996
Phenylsulfthion	T60.0X1	T60.0X2	T60.0X3	T60.0X4	—	—
Phenyltoloxamine	T45.0X1	T45.0X2	T45.0X3	T45.0X4	T45.0X5	T45.0X6
Phenyramidol, phenyramidon	T39.8X1	T39.8X2	T39.8X3	T39.8X4	T39.8X5	T39.8X6
Phenytoin	T42.0X1	T42.0X2	T42.0X3	T42.0X4	T42.0X5	T42.0X6
with Phenobarbital	T42.3X1	T42.3X2	T42.3X3	T42.3X4	T42.3X5	T42.3X6
pHisoHex	T49.2X1	T49.2X2	T49.2X3	T49.2X4	T49.2X5	T49.2X6
Pholcodine	T48.3X1	T48.3X2	T48.3X3	T48.3X4	T48.3X5	T48.3X6
Pholedrine	T46.991	T46.992	T46.993	T46.994	T46.995	T46.996
Phorate	T60.0X1	T60.0X2	T60.0X3	T60.0X4	—	—
Phosdrin	T60.0X1	T60.0X2	T60.0X3	T60.0X4	—	—
Phosfolan	T60.0X1	T60.0X2	T60.0X3	T60.0X4	—	—
Phosgene (gas)	T59.891	T59.892	T59.893	T59.894	—	—
Phosphamidon	T60.0X1	T60.0X2	T60.0X3	T60.0X4	—	—
Phosphate	T65.891	T65.892	T65.893	T65.894	—	—
laxative	T47.4X1	T47.4X2	T47.4X3	T47.4X4	T47.4X5	T47.4X6
organic	T60.0X1	T60.0X2	T60.0X3	T60.0X4	—	—
solvent	T52.91	T52.92	T52.93	T52.94	—	—
tricresyl	T65.891	T65.892	T65.893	T65.894	—	—
Phosphine	T57.1X1	T57.1X2	T57.1X3	T57.1X4	—	—
fumigant	T57.1X1	T57.1X2	T57.1X3	T57.1X4	—	—
Phospholine	T49.5X1	T49.5X2	T49.5X3	T49.5X4	T49.5X5	T49.5X6
Phosphoric acid	T54.2X1	T54.2X2	T54.2X3	T54.2X4	—	—
Phosphorus (compound) **NEC**	T57.1X1	T57.1X2	T57.1X3	T57.1X4	—	—
pesticide	T60.0X1	T60.0X2	T60.0X3	T60.0X4	—	—
Phthalates	T65.891	T65.892	T65.893	T65.894	—	—
Phthalic anhydride	T65.891	T65.892	T65.893	T65.894	—	—
Phthalimidoglutarimide	T42.6X1	T42.6X2	T42.6X3	T42.6X4	T42.6X5	T42.6X6
Phthalylsulfathiazole	T37.0X1	T37.0X2	T37.0X3	T37.0X4	T37.0X5	T37.0X6
Phylloquinone	T45.7X1	T45.7X2	T45.7X3	T45.7X4	T45.7X5	T45.7X6
Physeptone	T40.3X1	T40.3X2	T40.3X3	T40.3X4	T40.3X5	T40.3X6
Physostigma venenosum	T62.2X1	T62.2X2	T62.2X3	T62.2X4	—	—
Physostigmine	T49.5X1	T49.5X2	T49.5X3	T49.5X4	T49.5X5	T49.5X6
Phytolacca decandra	T62.2X1	T62.2X2	T62.2X3	T62.2X4	—	—
berries	T62.1X1	T62.1X2	T62.1X3	T62.1X4	—	—
Phytomenadione	T45.7X1	T45.7X2	T45.7X3	T45.7X4	T45.7X5	T45.7X6
Phytonadione	T45.7X1	T45.7X2	T45.7X3	T45.7X4	T45.7X5	T45.7X6
Picoperine	T48.3X1	T48.3X2	T48.3X3	T48.3X4	T48.3X5	T48.3X6
Picosulfate (sodium)	T47.2X1	T47.2X2	T47.2X3	T47.2X4	T47.2X5	T47.2X6
Picric (acid)	T54.2X1	T54.2X2	T54.2X3	T54.2X4	—	—
Picrotoxin	T50.7X1	T50.7X2	T50.7X3	T50.7X4	T50.7X5	T50.7X6
Piketoprofen	T49.0X1	T49.0X2	T49.0X3	T49.0X4	T49.0X5	T49.0X6
Pilocarpine	T44.1X1	T44.1X2	T44.1X3	T44.1X4	T44.1X5	T44.1X6
Pilocarpus (jaborandi) **extract**	T44.1X1	T44.1X2	T44.1X3	T44.1X4	T44.1X5	T44.1X6
Pilsicainide (hydrochloride)	T46.2X1	T46.2X2	T46.2X3	T46.2X4	T46.2X5	T46.2X6
Pimaricin	T36.7X1	T36.7X2	T36.7X3	T36.7X4	T36.7X5	T36.7X6
Pimeclone	T50.7X1	T50.7X2	T50.7X3	T50.7X4	T50.7X5	T50.7X6
Pimelic ketone	T52.8X1	T52.8X2	T52.8X3	T52.8X4	—	—
Pimethixene	T45.0X1	T45.0X2	T45.0X3	T45.0X4	T45.0X5	T45.0X6
Piminodine	T40.2X1	T40.2X2	T40.2X3	T40.2X4	T40.2X5	T40.2X6
Pimozide	T43.591	T43.592	T43.593	T43.594	T43.595	T43.596
Pinacidil	T46.5X1	T46.5X2	T46.5X3	T46.5X4	T46.5X5	T46.5X6
Pinaverium bromide	T44.3X1	T44.3X2	T44.3X3	T44.3X4	T44.3X5	T44.3X6
Pinazepam	T42.4X1	T42.4X2	T42.4X3	T42.4X4	T42.4X5	T42.4X6
Pindolol	T44.7X1	T44.7X2	T44.7X3	T44.7X4	T44.7X5	T44.7X6

Substance	Poisoning, Accidental unintentional	Poisoning, Intentional self-harm	Poisoning, Assault	Poisoning, Undetermined	Adverse effect	Underdosing
Pindone	T60.4X1	T60.4X2	T60.4X3	T60.4X4	—	—
Pine oil (disinfectant)	T65.891	T65.892	T65.893	T65.894	—	—
Pinkroot	T37.4X1	T37.4X2	T37.4X3	T37.4X4	T37.4X5	T37.4X6
Pipadone	T40.2X1	T40.2X2	T40.2X3	T40.2X4	—	—
Pipamazine	T45.0X1	T45.0X2	T45.0X3	T45.0X4	T45.0X5	T45.0X6
Pipamperone	T43.4X1	T43.4X2	T43.4X3	T43.4X4	T43.4X5	T43.4X6
Pipazetate	T48.3X1	T48.3X2	T48.3X3	T48.3X4	T48.3X5	T48.3X6
Pipemidic acid	T37.8X1	T37.8X2	T37.8X3	T37.8X4	T37.8X5	T37.8X6
Pipenzolate bromide	T44.3X1	T44.3X2	T44.3X3	T44.3X4	T44.3X5	T44.3X6
Piperacetazine	T43.3X1	T43.3X2	T43.3X3	T43.3X4	T43.3X5	T43.3X6
Piperacillin	T36.0X1	T36.0X2	T36.0X3	T36.0X4	T36.0X5	T36.0X6
Piperazine	T37.4X1	T37.4X2	T37.4X3	T37.4X4	T37.4X5	T37.4X6
estrone sulfate	T38.5X1	T38.5X2	T38.5X3	T38.5X4	T38.5X5	T38.5X6
Piper cubeba	T62.2X1	T62.2X2	T62.2X3	T62.2X4	—	—
Piperidione	T48.3X1	T48.3X2	T48.3X3	T48.3X4	T48.3X5	T48.3X6
Piperidolate	T44.3X1	T44.3X2	T44.3X3	T44.3X4	T44.3X5	T44.3X6
Piperocaine	T41.3X1	T41.3X2	T41.3X3	T41.3X4	T41.3X5	T41.3X6
infiltration (subcutaneous)	T41.3X1	T41.3X2	T41.3X3	T41.3X4	T41.3X5	T41.3X6
nerve block (peripheral) (plexus)	T41.3X1	T41.3X2	T41.3X3	T41.3X4	T41.3X5	T41.3X6
topical (surface)	T41.3X1	T41.3X2	T41.3X3	T41.3X4	T41.3X5	T41.3X6
Piperonyl butoxide	T60.8X1	T60.8X2	T60.8X3	T60.8X4	—	—
Pipethanate	T44.3X1	T44.3X2	T44.3X3	T44.3X4	T44.3X5	T44.3X6
Pipobroman	T45.1X1	T45.1X2	T45.1X3	T45.1X4	T45.1X5	T45.1X6
Pipotiazine	T43.3X1	T43.3X2	T43.3X3	T43.3X4	T43.3X5	T43.3X6
Pipoxizine	T45.0X1	T45.0X2	T45.0X3	T45.0X4	T45.0X5	T45.0X6
Pipradrol	T43.691	T43.692	T43.693	T43.694	T43.695	T43.696
Piprinhydrinate	T45.0X1	T45.0X2	T45.0X3	T45.0X4	T45.0X5	T45.0X6
Pirarubicin	T45.1X1	T45.1X2	T45.1X3	T45.1X4	T45.1X5	T45.1X6
Pirazinamide	T37.1X1	T37.1X2	T37.1X3	T37.1X4	T37.1X5	T37.1X6
Pirbuterol	T48.6X1	T48.6X2	T48.6X3	T48.6X4	T48.6X5	T48.6X6
Pirenzepine	T47.1X1	T47.1X2	T47.1X3	T47.1X4	T47.1X5	T47.1X6
Piretanide	T50.1X1	T50.1X2	T50.1X3	T50.1X4	T50.1X5	T50.1X6
Piribedil	T42.8X1	T42.8X2	T42.8X3	T42.8X4	T42.8X5	T42.8X6
Piridoxilate	T46.3X1	T46.3X2	T46.3X3	T46.3X4	T46.3X5	T46.3X6
Piritramide	T40.4X1	T40.4X2	T40.4X3	T40.4X4	—	—
Piromidic acid	T37.8X1	T37.8X2	T37.8X3	T37.8X4	T37.8X5	T37.8X6
Piroxicam	T39.391	T39.392	T39.393	T39.394	T39.395	T39.396
beta-cyclodextrin complex	T39.8X1	T39.8X2	T39.8X3	T39.8X4	T39.8X5	T39.8X6
Pirozadil	T46.6X1	T46.6X2	T46.6X3	T46.6X4	T46.6X5	T46.6X6
Piscidia (bark) (erythrina)	T39.8X1	T39.8X2	T39.8X3	T39.8X4	T39.8X5	T39.8X6
Pitch	T65.891	T65.892	T65.893	T65.894	—	—
Pitkin's solution	T41.3X1	T41.3X2	T41.3X3	T41.3X4	T41.3X5	T41.3X6
Pitocin	T48.0X1	T48.0X2	T48.0X3	T48.0X4	T48.0X5	T48.0X6
Pitressin (tannate)	T38.891	T38.892	T38.893	T38.894	T38.895	T38.896
Pituitary extracts (posterior)	T38.891	T38.892	T38.893	T38.894	T38.895	T38.896
anterior	T38.811	T38.812	T38.813	T38.814	T38.815	T38.816
Pituitrin	T38.891	T38.892	T38.893	T38.894	T38.895	T38.896
Pivampicillin	T36.0X1	T36.0X2	T36.0X3	T36.0X4	T36.0X5	T36.0X6
Pivmecillinam	T36.0X1	T36.0X2	T36.0X3	T36.0X4	T36.0X5	T36.0X6
Placental hormone	T38.891	T38.892	T38.893	T38.894	T38.895	T38.896
Placidyl	T42.6X1	T42.6X2	T42.6X3	T42.6X4	T42.6X5	T42.6X6
Plague vaccine	T50.A91	T50.A92	T50.A93	T50.A94	T50.A95	T50.A96
Plant						
food or fertilizer NEC	T65.891	T65.892	T65.893	T65.894	—	—
containing herbicide	T60.3X1	T60.3X2	T60.3X3	T60.3X4	—	—
noxious, used as food	T62.2X1	T62.2X2	T62.2X3	T62.2X4	—	—
berries	T62.1X1	T62.1X2	T62.1X3	T62.1X4	—	—
seeds	T62.2X1	T62.2X2	T62.2X3	T62.2X4	—	—
specified type NEC	T62.2X1	T62.2X2	T62.2X3	T62.2X4	—	—
Plasma	T45.8X1	T45.8X2	T45.8X3	T45.8X4	T45.8X5	T45.8X6
expander NEC	T45.8X1	T45.8X2	T45.8X3	T45.8X4	T45.8X5	T45.8X6
protein fraction (human)	T45.8X1	T45.8X2	T45.8X3	T45.8X4	T45.8X5	T45.8X6
Plasmanate	T45.8X1	T45.8X2	T45.8X3	T45.8X4	T45.8X5	T45.8X6
Plasminogen (tissue) **activator**	T45.611	T45.612	T45.613	T45.614	T45.615	T45.616
Plaster dressing	T49.3X1	T49.3X2	T49.3X3	T49.3X4	T49.3X5	T49.3X6
Plastic dressing	T49.3X1	T49.3X2	T49.3X3	T49.3X4	T49.3X5	T49.3X6
Plegicil	T43.3X1	T43.3X2	T43.3X3	T43.3X4	T43.3X5	T43.3X6
Plicamycin	T45.1X1	T45.1X2	T45.1X3	T45.1X4	T45.1X5	T45.1X6
Podophyllotoxin	T49.8X1	T49.8X2	T49.8X3	T49.8X4	T49.8X5	T49.8X6
Podophyllum (resin)	T49.4X1	T49.4X2	T49.4X3	T49.4X4	T49.4X5	T49.4X6
Poison NEC	T65.91	T65.92	T65.93	T65.94	—	—
Poisonous berries	T62.1X1	T62.1X2	T62.1X3	T62.1X4	—	—
Pokeweed (any part)	T62.2X1	T62.2X2	T62.2X3	T62.2X4	—	—
Poldine metilsulfate	T44.3X1	T44.3X2	T44.3X3	T44.3X4	T44.3X5	T44.3X6
Polidexide (sulfate)	T46.6X1	T46.6X2	T46.6X3	T46.6X4	T46.6X5	T46.6X6
Polidocanol	T46.8X1	T46.8X2	T46.8X3	T46.8X4	T46.8X5	T46.8X6
Poliomyelitis vaccine	T50.B91	T50.B92	T50.B93	T50.B94	T50.B95	T50.B96
Polish (car) (floor) (furni-ture) (metal) (porcelain) (silver)	T65.891	T65.892	T65.893	T65.894	—	—
abrasive	T65.891	T65.892	T65.893	T65.894	—	—
porcelain	T65.891	T65.892	T65.893	T65.894	—	—
Poloxalkol	T47.4X1	T47.4X2	T47.4X3	T47.4X4	T47.4X5	T47.4X6
Poloxamer	T47.4X1	T47.4X2	T47.4X3	T47.4X4	T47.4X5	T47.4X6
Polyaminostyrene resins	T50.3X1	T50.3X2	T50.3X3	T50.3X4	T50.3X5	T50.3X6
Polycarbophil	T47.4X1	T47.4X2	T47.4X3	T47.4X4	T47.4X5	T47.4X6
Polychlorinated biphenyl	T65.891	T65.892	T65.893	T65.894	—	—
Polycycline	T36.4X1	T36.4X2	T36.4X3	T36.4X4	T36.4X5	T36.4X6
Polyester fumes	T59.891	T59.892	T59.893	T59.894	—	—
Polyester resin hardener	T52.91	T52.92	T52.93	T52.94	—	—
fumes	T59.891	T59.892	T59.893	T59.894	—	—
Polyestradiol phosphate	T38.5X1	T38.5X2	T38.5X3	T38.5X4	T38.5X5	T38.5X6
Polyethanolamine alkyl sulfate	T49.2X1	T49.2X2	T49.2X3	T49.2X4	T49.2X5	T49.2X6
Polyethylene adhesive	T49.3X1	T49.3X2	T49.3X3	T49.3X4	T49.3X5	T49.3X6
Polyferose	T45.4X1	T45.4X2	T45.4X3	T45.4X4	T45.4X5	T45.4X6
Polygeline	T45.8X1	T45.8X2	T45.8X3	T45.8X4	T45.8X5	T45.8X6
Polymyxin	T36.8X1	T36.8X2	T36.8X3	T36.8X4	T36.8X5	T36.8X6
B	T36.8X1	T36.8X2	T36.8X3	T36.8X4	T36.8X5	T36.8X6
ENT agent	T49.6X1	T49.6X2	T49.6X3	T49.6X4	T49.6X5	T49.6X6
ophthalmic preparation	T49.5X1	T49.5X2	T49.5X3	T49.5X4	T49.5X5	T49.5X6
topical NEC	T49.0X1	T49.0X2	T49.0X3	T49.0X4	T49.0X5	T49.0X6
E sulfate (eye preparation)	T49.5X1	T49.5X2	T49.5X3	T49.5X4	T49.5X5	T49.5X6
Polynoxylin	T49.0X1	T49.0X2	T49.0X3	T49.0X4	T49.0X5	T49.0X6
Polyoestradiol phosphate	T38.5X1	T38.5X2	T38.5X3	T38.5X4	T38.5X5	T38.5X6
Polyoxymethyleneurea	T49.0X1	T49.0X2	T49.0X3	T49.0X4	T49.0X5	T49.0X6
Polysilane	T47.8X1	T47.8X2	T47.8X3	T47.8X4	T47.8X5	T47.8X6
Polytetrafluoroethylene (inhaled)	T59.891	T59.892	T59.893	T59.894	—	—
Polythiazide	T50.2X1	T50.2X2	T50.2X3	T50.2X4	T50.2X5	T50.2X6
Polyvidone	T45.8X1	T45.8X2	T45.8X3	T45.8X4	T45.8X5	T45.8X6
Polyvinylpyrrolidone	T45.8X1	T45.8X2	T45.8X3	T45.8X4	T45.8X5	T45.8X6
Pontocaine (hydrochloride) (infiltration) (topical)	T41.3X1	T41.3X2	T41.3X3	T41.3X4	T41.3X5	T41.3X6
nerve block (peripheral) (plexus)	T41.3X1	T41.3X2	T41.3X3	T41.3X4	T41.3X5	T41.3X6
spinal	T41.3X1	T41.3X2	T41.3X3	T41.3X4	T41.3X5	T41.3X6
Porfiromycin	T45.1X1	T45.1X2	T45.1X3	T45.1X4	T45.1X5	T45.1X6
Posterior pituitary hormone NEC	T38.891	T38.892	T38.893	T38.894	T38.895	T38.896
Pot	T40.7X1	T40.7X2	T40.7X3	T40.7X4	T40.7X5	T40.7X6
Potash (caustic)	T54.3X1	T54.3X2	T54.3X3	T54.3X4	—	—
Potassic saline injection (lactated)	T50.3X1	T50.3X2	T50.3X3	T50.3X4	T50.3X5	T50.3X6
Potassium (salts) **NEC**	T50.3X1	T50.3X2	T50.3X3	T50.3X4	T50.3X5	T50.3X6
aminobenzoate	T45.8X1	T45.8X2	T45.8X3	T45.8X4	T45.8X5	T45.8X6
aminosalicylate	T37.1X1	T37.1X2	T37.1X3	T37.1X4	T37.1X5	T37.1X6
antimony 'tartrate'	T37.8X1	T37.8X2	T37.8X3	T37.8X4	T37.8X5	T37.8X6
arsenite (solution)	T57.0X1	T57.0X2	T57.0X3	T57.0X4	—	—
bichromate	T56.2X1	T56.2X2	T56.2X3	T56.2X4	—	—
bisulfate	T47.3X1	T47.3X2	T47.3X3	T47.3X4	T47.3X5	T47.3X6
bromide	T42.6X1	T42.6X2	T42.6X3	T42.6X4	T42.6X5	T42.6X6
canrenoate	T50.0X1	T50.0X2	T50.0X3	T50.0X4	T50.0X5	T50.0X6
carbonate	T54.3X1	T54.3X2	T54.3X3	T54.3X4	—	—
chlorate NEC	T65.891	T65.892	T65.893	T65.894	—	—
chloride	T50.3X1	T50.3X2	T50.3X3	T50.3X4	T50.3X5	T50.3X6
citrate	T50.991	T50.992	T50.993	T50.994	T50.995	T50.996
cyanide	T65.0X1	T65.0X2	T65.0X3	T65.0X4	—	—
ferric hexacyanoferrate (medicinal)	T50.6X1	T50.6X2	T50.6X3	T50.6X4	T50.6X5	T50.6X6
nonmedicinal	T65.891	T65.892	T65.893	T65.894	—	—
Fluoride	T57.8X1	T57.8X2	T57.8X3	T57.8X4	—	—
glucaldrate	T47.1X1	T47.1X2	T47.1X3	T47.1X4	T47.1X5	T47.1X6
hydroxide	T54.3X1	T54.3X2	T54.3X3	T54.3X4	—	—
iodate	T49.0X1	T49.0X2	T49.0X3	T49.0X4	T49.0X5	T49.0X6
iodide	T48.4X1	T48.4X2	T48.4X3	T48.4X4	T48.4X5	T48.4X6
nitrate	T57.8X1	T57.8X2	T57.8X3	T57.8X4	—	—
oxalate	T65.891	T65.892	T65.893	T65.894	—	—
perchlorate (nonmedicinal) NEC	T65.891	T65.892	T65.893	T65.894	—	—
antithyroid	T38.2X1	T38.2X2	T38.2X3	T38.2X4	T38.2X5	T38.2X6
medicinal	T38.2X1	T38.2X2	T38.2X3	T38.2X4	T38.2X5	T38.2X6
Permanganate (nonmedicinal)	T65.891	T65.892	T65.893	T65.894	—	—
medicinal	T49.0X1	T49.0X2	T49.0X3	T49.0X4	T49.0X5	T49.0X6
sulfate	T47.2X1	T47.2X2	T47.2X3	T47.2X4	T47.2X5	T47.2X6
Potassium-removing resin	T50.3X1	T50.3X2	T50.3X3	T50.3X4	T50.3X5	T50.3X6
Potassium-retaining drug	T50.3X1	T50.3X2	T50.3X3	T50.3X4	T50.3X5	T50.3X6
Povidone	T45.8X1	T45.8X2	T45.8X3	T45.8X4	T45.8X5	T45.8X6
iodine	T49.0X1	T49.0X2	T49.0X3	T49.0X4	T49.0X5	T49.0X6
Practolol	T44.7X1	T44.7X2	T44.7X3	T44.7X4	T44.7X5	T44.7X6
Prajmalium bitartrate	T46.2X1	T46.2X2	T46.2X3	T46.2X4	T46.2X5	T46.2X6
Pralidoxime (iodide)	T50.6X1	T50.6X2	T50.6X3	T50.6X4	T50.6X5	T50.6X6
chloride	T50.6X1	T50.6X2	T50.6X3	T50.6X4	T50.6X5	T50.6X6
Pramiverine	T44.3X1	T44.3X2	T44.3X3	T44.3X4	T44.3X5	T44.3X6
Pramocaine	T49.1X1	T49.1X2	T49.1X3	T49.1X4	T49.1X5	T49.1X6
Pramoxine	T49.1X1	T49.1X2	T49.1X3	T49.1X4	T49.1X5	T49.1X6

Substance	Poisoning, Accidental unintentional	Poisoning, Intentional self-harm	Poisoning, Assault	Poisoning, Undetermined	Adverse effect	Underdosing
Prasterone	T38.7X1	T38.7X2	T38.7X3	T38.7X4	T38.7X5	T38.7X6
Pravastatin	T46.6X1	T46.6X2	T46.6X3	T46.6X4	T46.6X5	T46.6X6
Prazepam	T42.4X1	T42.4X2	T42.4X3	T42.4X4	T42.4X5	T42.4X6
Praziquantel	T37.4X1	T37.4X2	T37.4X3	T37.4X4	T37.4X5	T37.4X6
Prazitone	T43.291	T43.292	T43.293	T43.294	T43.295	T43.296
Prazosin	T44.6X1	T44.6X2	T44.6X3	T44.6X4	T44.6X5	T44.6X6
Prednicarbate	T49.0X1	T49.0X2	T49.0X3	T49.0X4	T49.0X5	T49.0X6
Prednimustine	T45.1X1	T45.1X2	T45.1X3	T45.1X4	T45.1X5	T45.1X6
Prednisolone	T38.0X1	T38.0X2	T38.0X3	T38.0X4	T38.0X5	T38.0X6
ENT agent	T49.6X1	T49.6X2	T49.6X3	T49.6X4	T49.6X5	T49.6X6
ophthalmic preparation	T49.5X1	T49.5X2	T49.5X3	T49.5X4	T49.5X5	T49.5X6
steaglate	T49.0X1	T49.0X2	T49.0X3	T49.0X4	T49.0X5	T49.0X6
topical NEC	T49.0X1	T49.0X2	T49.0X3	T49.0X4	T49.0X5	T49.0X6
Prednisone	T38.0X1	T38.0X2	T38.0X3	T38.0X4	T38.0X5	T38.0X6
Prednylidene	T38.0X1	T38.0X2	T38.0X3	T38.0X4	T38.0X5	T38.0X6
Pregnandiol	T38.5X1	T38.5X2	T38.5X3	T38.5X4	T38.5X5	T38.5X6
Pregneninolone	T38.5X1	T38.5X2	T38.5X3	T38.5X4	T38.5X5	T38.5X6
Preludin	T43.691	T43.692	T43.693	T43.694	T43.695	T43.696
Premarin	T38.5X1	T38.5X2	T38.5X3	T38.5X4	T38.5X5	T38.5X6
Premedication anesthetic	T41.201	T41.202	T41.203	T41.204	T41.205	T41.206
Prenalterol	T44.5X1	T44.5X2	T44.5X3	T44.5X4	T44.5X5	T44.5X6
Prenoxdiazine	T48.3X1	T48.3X2	T48.3X3	T48.3X4	T48.3X5	T48.3X6
Prenylamine	T46.3X1	T46.3X2	T46.3X3	T46.3X4	T46.3X5	T46.3X6
Preparation H	T49.8X1	T49.8X2	T49.8X3	T49.8X4	T49.8X5	T49.8X6
Preparation, local	T49.4X1	T49.4X2	T49.4X3	T49.4X4	T49.4X5	T49.4X6
Preservative (nonmedicinal)	T65.891	T65.892	T65.893	T65.894	--	--
medicinal	T50.901	T50.902	T50.903	T50.904	T50.905	T50.906
wood	T60.91	T60.92	T60.93	T60.94	--	--
Prethcamide	T50.7X1	T50.7X2	T50.7X3	T50.7X4	T50.7X5	T50.7X6
Pride of China	T62.2X1	T62.2X2	T62.2X3	T62.2X4	--	--
Pridinol	T44.3X1	T44.3X2	T44.3X3	T44.3X4	T44.3X5	T44.3X6
Prifinium bromide	T44.3X1	T44.3X2	T44.3X3	T44.3X4	T44.3X5	T44.3X6
Prilocaine	T41.3X1	T41.3X2	T41.3X3	T41.3X4	T41.3X5	T41.3X6
infiltration (subcutaneous)	T41.3X1	T41.3X2	T41.3X3	T41.3X4	T41.3X5	T41.3X6
nerve block (peripheral) (plexus)	T41.3X1	T41.3X2	T41.3X3	T41.3X4	T41.3X5	T41.3X6
regional	T41.3X1	T41.3X2	T41.3X3	T41.3X4	T41.3X5	T41.3X6
Primaquine	T37.2X1	T37.2X2	T37.2X3	T37.2X4	T37.2X5	T37.2X6
Primidone	T42.6X1	T42.6X2	T42.6X3	T42.6X4	T42.6X5	T42.6X6
Primula (veris)	T62.2X1	T62.2X2	T62.2X3	T62.2X4	--	--
Prinadol	T40.2X1	T40.2X2	T40.2X3	T40.2X4	T40.2X5	T40.2X6
Priscol, Priscoline	T44.6X1	T44.6X2	T44.6X3	T44.6X4	T44.6X5	T44.6X6
Pristinamycin	T36.3X1	T36.3X2	T36.3X3	T36.3X4	T36.3X5	T36.3X6
Privet	T62.2X1	T62.2X2	T62.2X3	T62.2X4	--	--
berries	T62.1X1	T62.1X2	T62.1X3	T62.1X4	--	--
Privine	T44.4X1	T44.4X2	T44.4X3	T44.4X4	T44.4X5	T44.4X6
Pro-Banthine	T44.3X1	T44.3X2	T44.3X3	T44.3X4	T44.3X5	T44.3X6
Probarbital	T42.3X1	T42.3X2	T42.3X3	T42.3X4	T42.3X5	T42.3X6
Probenecid	T50.4X1	T50.4X2	T50.4X3	T50.4X4	T50.4X5	T50.4X6
Probucol	T46.6X1	T46.6X2	T46.6X3	T46.6X4	T46.6X5	T46.6X6
Procainamide	T46.2X1	T46.2X2	T46.2X3	T46.2X4	T46.2X5	T46.2X6
Procaine	T41.3X1	T41.3X2	T41.3X3	T41.3X4	T41.3X5	T41.3X6
benzylpenicillin	T36.0X1	T36.0X2	T36.0X3	T36.0X4	T36.0X5	T36.0X6
nerve block (periphreal) (plexus)	T41.3X1	T41.3X2	T41.3X3	T41.3X4	T41.3X5	T41.3X6
penicillin G	T36.0X1	T36.0X2	T36.0X3	T36.0X4	T36.0X5	T36.0X6
regional	T41.3X1	T41.3X2	T41.3X3	T41.3X4	T41.3X5	T41.3X6
spinal	T41.3X1	T41.3X2	T41.3X3	T41.3X4	T41.3X5	T41.3X6
Procalmidol	T43.591	T43.592	T43.593	T43.594	T43.595	T43.596
Procarbazine	T45.1X1	T45.1X2	T45.1X3	T45.1X4	T45.1X5	T45.1X6
Procaterol	T44.5X1	T44.5X2	T44.5X3	T44.5X4	T44.5X5	T44.5X6
Prochlorperazine	T43.3X1	T43.3X2	T43.3X3	T43.3X4	T43.3X5	T43.3X6
Procyclidine	T44.3X1	T44.3X2	T44.3X3	T44.3X4	T44.3X5	T44.3X6
Producer gas	T58.8X1	T58.8X2	T58.8X3	T58.8X4	--	--
Profadol	T40.4X1	T40.4X2	T40.4X3	T40.4X4	T40.4X5	T40.4X6
Profenamine	T44.3X1	T44.3X2	T44.3X3	T44.3X4	T44.3X5	T44.3X6
Profenil	T44.3X1	T44.3X2	T44.3X3	T44.3X4	T44.3X5	T44.3X6
Proflavine	T49.0X1	T49.0X2	T49.0X3	T49.0X4	T49.0X5	T49.0X6
Progabide	T42.6X1	T42.6X2	T42.6X3	T42.6X4	T42.6X5	T42.6X6
Progesterone	T38.5X1	T38.5X2	T38.5X3	T38.5X4	T38.5X5	T38.5X6
Progestin	T38.5X1	T38.5X2	T38.5X3	T38.5X4	T38.5X5	T38.5X6
oral contraceptive	T38.4X1	T38.4X2	T38.4X3	T38.4X4	T38.4X5	T38.4X6
Progestogen NEC	T38.5X1	T38.5X2	T38.5X3	T38.5X4	T38.5X5	T38.5X6
Progestone	T38.5X1	T38.5X2	T38.5X3	T38.5X4	T38.5X5	T38.5X6
Proglumide	T47.1X1	T47.1X2	T47.1X3	T47.1X4	T47.1X5	T47.1X6
Proguanil	T37.2X1	T37.2X2	T37.2X3	T37.2X4	T37.2X5	T37.2X6
Prolactin	T38.811	T38.812	T38.813	T38.814	T38.815	T38.816
Prolintane	T43.691	T43.692	T43.693	T43.694	T43.695	T43.696
Proloid	T38.1X1	T38.1X2	T38.1X3	T38.1X4	T38.1X5	T38.1X6
Proluton	T38.5X1	T38.5X2	T38.5X3	T38.5X4	T38.5X5	T38.5X6
Promacetin	T37.1X1	T37.1X2	T37.1X3	T37.1X4	T37.1X5	T37.1X6
Promazine	T43.3X1	T43.3X2	T43.3X3	T43.3X4	T43.3X5	T43.3X6
Promedol	T40.2X1	T40.2X2	T40.2X3	T40.2X4	--	--
Promegestone	T38.5X1	T38.5X2	T38.5X3	T38.5X4	T38.5X5	T38.5X6

Substance	Poisoning, Accidental unintentional	Poisoning, Intentional self-harm	Poisoning, Assault	Poisoning, Undetermined	Adverse effect	Underdosing
Promethazine (teoclate)	T43.3X1	T43.3X2	T43.3X3	T43.3X4	T43.3X5	T43.3X6
Promin	T37.1X1	T37.1X2	T37.1X3	T37.1X4	T37.1X5	T37.1X6
Pronase	T45.3X1	T45.3X2	T45.3X3	T45.3X4	T45.3X5	T45.3X6
Pronestyl (hydrochloride)	T46.2X1	T46.2X2	T46.2X3	T46.2X4	T46.2X5	T46.2X6
Pronetalol	T44.7X1	T44.7X2	T44.7X3	T44.7X4	T44.7X5	T44.7X6
Prontosil	T37.0X1	T37.0X2	T37.0X3	T37.0X4	T37.0X5	T37.0X6
Propachlor	T60.3X1	T60.3X2	T60.3X3	T60.3X4	--	--
Propafenone	T46.2X1	T46.2X2	T46.2X3	T46.2X4	T46.2X5	T46.2X6
Propallylonal	T42.3X1	T42.3X2	T42.3X3	T42.3X4	T42.3X5	T42.3X6
Propamidine	T49.0X1	T49.0X2	T49.0X3	T49.0X4	T49.0X5	T49.0X6
Propane (distributed in mobile container)	T59.891	T59.892	T59.893	T59.894	--	--
distributed through pipes	T59.891	T59.892	T59.893	T59.894	--	--
incomplete combustion	T58.11	T58.12	T58.13	T58.14	--	--
Propanidid	T41.291	T41.292	T41.293	T41.294	T41.295	T41.296
Propanil	T60.3X1	T60.3X2	T60.3X3	T60.3X4	--	--
1-Propanol	T51.3X1	T51.3X2	T51.3X3	T51.3X4	--	--
2-Propanol	T51.2X1	T51.2X2	T51.2X3	T51.2X4	--	--
Propantheline	T44.3X1	T44.3X2	T44.3X3	T44.3X4	T44.3X5	T44.3X6
bromide	T44.3X1	T44.3X2	T44.3X3	T44.3X4	T44.3X5	T44.3X6
Proparacaine	T41.3X1	T41.3X2	T41.3X3	T41.3X4	T41.3X5	T41.3X6
Propatylnitrate	T46.3X1	T46.3X2	T46.3X3	T46.3X4	T46.3X5	T46.3X6
Propicillin	T36.0X1	T36.0X2	T36.0X3	T36.0X4	T36.0X5	T36.0X6
Propiolactone	T49.0X1	T49.0X2	T49.0X3	T49.0X4	T49.0X5	T49.0X6
Propiomazine	T45.0X1	T45.0X2	T45.0X3	T45.0X4	T45.0X5	T45.0X6
Propionaldehyde (medicinal)	T42.6X1	T42.6X2	T42.6X3	T42.6X4	T42.6X5	T42.6X6
Propionate (calcium) (sodium)	T49.0X1	T49.0X2	T49.0X3	T49.0X4	T49.0X5	T49.0X6
Propion gel	T49.0X1	T49.0X2	T49.0X3	T49.0X4	T49.0X5	T49.0X6
Propitocaine	T41.3X1	T41.3X2	T41.3X3	T41.3X4	T41.3X5	T41.3X6
infiltration (subcutaneous)	T41.3X1	T41.3X2	T41.3X3	T41.3X4	T41.3X5	T41.3X6
nerve block (peripheral) (plexus)	T41.3X1	T41.3X2	T41.3X3	T41.3X4	T41.3X5	T41.3X6
Propofol	T41.291	T41.292	T41.293	T41.294	T41.295	T41.296
Propoxur	T60.0X1	T60.0X2	T60.0X3	T60.0X4	--	--
Propoxycaine	T41.3X1	T41.3X2	T41.3X3	T41.3X4	T41.3X5	T41.3X6
infiltration (subcutaneous)	T41.3X1	T41.3X2	T41.3X3	T41.3X4	T41.3X5	T41.3X6
nerve block (peripheral) (plexus)	T41.3X1	T41.3X2	T41.3X3	T41.3X4	T41.3X5	T41.3X6
topical (surface)	T41.3X1	T41.3X2	T41.3X3	T41.3X4	T41.3X5	T41.3X6
Propoxyphene	T40.4X1	T40.4X2	T40.4X3	T40.4X4	T40.4X5	T40.4X6
Propranolol	T44.7X1	T44.7X2	T44.7X3	T44.7X4	T44.7X5	T44.7X6
Propyl						
alcohol	T51.3X1	T51.3X2	T51.3X3	T51.3X4	--	--
carbinol	T51.3X1	T51.3X2	T51.3X3	T51.3X4	--	--
hexadrine	T44.4X1	T44.4X2	T44.4X3	T44.4X4	T44.4X5	T44.4X6
iodone	T50.8X1	T50.8X2	T50.8X3	T50.8X4	T50.8X5	T50.8X6
thiouracil	T38.2X1	T38.2X2	T38.2X3	T38.2X4	T38.2X5	T38.2X6
Propylaminopheno-thiazine	T43.3X1	T43.3X2	T43.3X3	T43.3X4	T43.3X5	T43.3X6
Propylene	T59.891	T59.892	T59.893	T59.894	--	--
Propylhexedrine	T48.5X1	T48.5X2	T48.5X3	T48.5X4	T48.5X5	T48.5X6
Propyliodone	T50.8X1	T50.8X2	T50.8X3	T50.8X4	T50.8X5	T50.8X6
Propylparaben (ophthalmic)	T49.5X1	T49.5X2	T49.5X3	T49.5X4	T49.5X5	T49.5X6
Propylthiouracil	T38.2X1	T38.2X2	T38.2X3	T38.2X4	T38.2X5	T38.2X6
Propyphenazone	T39.2X1	T39.2X2	T39.2X3	T39.2X4	T39.2X5	T39.2X6
Proquazone	T39.391	T39.392	T39.393	T39.394	T39.395	T39.396
Proscillaridin	T46.0X1	T46.0X2	T46.0X3	T46.0X4	T46.0X5	T46.0X6
Prostacyclin	T45.521	T45.522	T45.523	T45.524	T45.525	T45.526
Prostaglandin (I2)	T45.521	T45.522	T45.523	T45.524	T45.525	T45.526
E1	T46.7X1	T46.7X2	T46.7X3	T46.7X4	T46.7X5	T46.7X6
E2	T48.0X1	T48.0X2	T48.0X3	T48.0X4	T48.0X5	T48.0X6
F2 alpha	T48.0X1	T48.0X2	T48.0X3	T48.0X4	T48.0X5	T48.0X6
Prostigmin	T44.0X1	T44.0X2	T44.0X3	T44.0X4	T44.0X5	T44.0X6
Prosultiamine	T45.2X1	T45.2X2	T45.2X3	T45.2X4	T45.2X5	T45.2X6
Protamine sulfate	T45.7X1	T45.7X2	T45.7X3	T45.7X4	T45.7X5	T45.7X6
zinc insulin	T38.3X1	T38.3X2	T38.3X3	T38.3X4	T38.3X5	T38.3X6
Protease	T47.5X1	T47.5X2	T47.5X3	T47.5X4	T47.5X5	T47.5X6
Protectant, skin NEC	T49.3X1	T49.3X2	T49.3X3	T49.3X4	T49.3X5	T49.3X6
Protein hydrolysate	T50.991	T50.992	T50.993	T50.994	T50.995	T50.996
Prothiaden — *see Dothiepin hydrochloride*						
Prothionamide	T37.1X1	T37.1X2	T37.1X3	T37.1X4	T37.1X5	T37.1X6
Prothipendyl	T43.591	T43.592	T43.593	T43.594	T43.595	T43.596
Prothoate	T60.0X1	T60.0X2	T60.0X3	T60.0X4	--	--
Prothrombin						
activator	T45.7X1	T45.7X2	T45.7X3	T45.7X4	T45.7X5	T45.7X6
synthesis inhibitor	T45.511	T45.512	T45.513	T45.514	T45.515	T45.516
Protionamide	T37.1X1	T37.1X2	T37.1X3	T37.1X4	T37.1X5	T37.1X6
Protirelin	T38.891	T38.892	T38.893	T38.894	T38.895	T38.896
Protokylol	T48.6X1	T48.6X2	T48.6X3	T48.6X4	T48.6X5	T48.6X6
Protopam	T50.6X1	T50.6X2	T50.6X3	T50.6X4	T50.6X5	T50.6X6
Protoveratrine (s) (A) (B)	T46.5X1	T46.5X2	T46.5X3	T46.5X4	T46.5X5	T46.5X6
Protriptyline	T43.011	T43.012	T43.013	T43.014	T43.015	T43.016
Provera	T38.5X1	T38.5X2	T38.5X3	T38.5X4	T38.5X5	T38.5X6
Provitamin A	T45.2X1	T45.2X2	T45.2X3	T45.2X4	T45.2X5	T45.2X6

Substance	Poisoning, Accidental unintentional	Poisoning, Intentional self-harm	Poisoning, Assault	Poisoning, Undetermined	Adverse effect	Underdosing
Proxibarbal	T42.3X1	T42.3X2	T42.3X3	T42.3X4	T42.3X5	T42.3X6
Proxymetacaine	T41.3X1	T41.3X2	T41.3X3	T41.3X4	T41.3X5	T41.3X6
Proxyphylline	T48.6X1	T48.6X2	T48.6X3	T48.6X4	T48.6X5	T48.6X6
Prozac — *see Fluoxetine hydrochloride*						
Prunus						
laurocerasus	T62.2X1	T62.2X2	T62.2X3	T62.2X4	--	--
virginiana	T62.2X1	T62.2X2	T62.2X3	T62.2X4	--	--
Prussian blue						
commercial	T65.891	T65.892	T65.893	T65.894	--	--
therapeutic	T50.6X1	T50.6X2	T50.6X3	T50.6X4	T50.6X5	T50.6X6
Prussic acid	T65.0X1	T65.0X2	T65.0X3	T65.0X4	--	--
vapor	T57.3X1	T57.3X2	T57.3X3	T57.3X4	--	--
Pseudoephedrine	T44.991	T44.992	T44.993	T44.994	T44.995	T44.996
Psilocin	T40.991	T40.992	T40.993	T40.994	--	--
Psilocybin	T40.991	T40.992	T40.993	T40.994	--	--
Psilocybine	T40.991	T40.992	T40.993	T40.994	--	--
Psoralene (nonmedicinal)	T65.891	T65.892	T65.893	T65.894	--	--
Psoralens (medicinal)	T50.991	T50.992	T50.993	T50.994	T50.995	T50.996
PSP (phenolsulfonphthalein)	T50.8X1	T50.8X2	T50.8X3	T50.8X4	T50.8X5	T50.8X6
Psychodysleptic drug NEC	T40.901	T40.902	T40.903	T40.904	T40.905	T40.906
Psychostimulant	T43.601	T43.602	T43.603	T43.604	T43.605	T43.606
amphetamine	T43.621	T43.622	T43.623	T43.624	T43.625	T43.626
caffeine	T43.611	T43.612	T43.613	T43.614	T43.615	T43.616
methylphenidate	T43.631	T43.632	T43.633	T43.634	T43.635	T43.636
specified NEC	T43.691	T43.692	T43.693	T43.694	T43.695	T43.696
Psychotherapeutic drug NEC	T43.91	T43.92	T43.93	T43.94	T43.95	T43.96
antidepressants — *see also Antidepressant*	T43.201	T43.202	T43.203	T43.204	T43.205	T43.206
specified NEC	T43.8X1	T43.8X2	T43.8X3	T43.8X4	T43.8X5	T43.8X6
tranquilizers NEC	T43.501	T43.502	T43.503	T43.504	T43.505	T43.506
Psychotomimetic agents	T40.901	T40.902	T40.903	T40.904	T40.905	T40.906
Psychotropic drug NEC	T43.91	T43.92	T43.93	T43.94	T43.95	T43.96
specified NEC	T43.8X1	T43.8X2	T43.8X3	T43.8X4	T43.8X5	T43.8X6
Psyllium hydrophilic mucilloid	T47.4X1	T47.4X2	T47.4X3	T47.4X4	T47.4X5	T47.4X6
Pteroylglutamic acid	T45.8X1	T45.8X2	T45.8X3	T45.8X4	T45.8X5	T45.8X6
Pteroyltriglutamate	T45.1X1	T45.1X2	T45.1X3	T45.1X4	T45.1X5	T45.1X6
PTFE — *see Polytetrafluoroethylene*						
Pulp						
devitalizing paste	T49.7X1	T49.7X2	T49.7X3	T49.7X4	T49.7X5	T49.7X6
dressing	T49.7X1	T49.7X2	T49.7X3	T49.7X4	T49.7X5	T49.7X6
Pulsatilla	T62.2X1	T62.2X2	T62.2X3	T62.2X4	--	--
Pumpkin seed extract	T37.4X1	T37.4X2	T37.4X3	T37.4X4	T37.4X5	T37.4X6
Purex (bleach)	T54.91	T54.92	T54.93	T54.94	--	--
Purgative NEC — *see also Cathartic*	T47.4X1	T47.4X2	T47.4X3	T47.4X4	T47.4X5	T47.4X6
Purine analogue (antineoplastic)	T45.1X1	T45.1X2	T45.1X3	T45.1X4	T45.1X5	T45.1X6
Purine diuretics	T50.2X1	T50.2X2	T50.2X3	T50.2X4	T50.2X5	T50.2X6
Purinethol	T45.1X1	T45.1X2	T45.1X3	T45.1X4	T45.1X5	T45.1X6
PVP	T45.8X1	T45.8X2	T45.8X3	T45.8X4	T45.8X5	T45.8X6
Pyrabital	T39.8X1	T39.8X2	T39.8X3	T39.8X4	T39.8X5	T39.8X6
Pyramidon	T39.2X1	T39.2X2	T39.2X3	T39.2X4	T39.2X5	T39.2X6
Pyrantel	T37.4X1	T37.4X2	T37.4X3	T37.4X4	T37.4X5	T37.4X6
Pyrathiazine	T45.0X1	T45.0X2	T45.0X3	T45.0X4	T45.0X5	T45.0X6
Pyrazinamide	T37.1X1	T37.1X2	T37.1X3	T37.1X4	T37.1X5	T37.1X6
Pyrazinoic acid (amide)	T37.1X1	T37.1X2	T37.1X3	T37.1X4	T37.1X5	T37.1X6
Pyrazole (derivatives)	T39.2X1	T39.2X2	T39.2X3	T39.2X4	T39.2X5	T39.2X6
Pyrazolone analgesic NEC	T39.2X1	T39.2X2	T39.2X3	T39.2X4	T39.2X5	T39.2X6
Pyrethrin, pyrethrum (nonmedicinal)	T60.2X1	T60.2X2	T60.2X3	T60.2X4	--	--
Pyrethrum extract	T49.0X1	T49.0X2	T49.0X3	T49.0X4	T49.0X5	T49.0X6
Pyribenzamine	T45.0X1	T45.0X2	T45.0X3	T45.0X4	T45.0X5	T45.0X6
Pyridine	T52.8X1	T52.8X2	T52.8X3	T52.8X4	--	--
aldoxime methiodide	T50.6X1	T50.6X2	T50.6X3	T50.6X4	T50.6X5	T50.6X6
aldoxime methyl chloride	T50.6X1	T50.6X2	T50.6X3	T50.6X4	T50.6X5	T50.6X6
vapor	T59.891	T59.892	T59.893	T59.894	--	--
Pyridium	T39.8X1	T39.8X2	T39.8X3	T39.8X4	T39.8X5	T39.8X6
Pyridostigmine bromide	T44.0X1	T44.0X2	T44.0X3	T44.0X4	T44.0X5	T44.0X6
Pyridoxal phosphate	T45.2X1	T45.2X2	T45.2X3	T45.2X4	T45.2X5	T45.2X6
Pyridoxine	T45.2X1	T45.2X2	T45.2X3	T45.2X4	T45.2X5	T45.2X6
Pyrilamine	T45.0X1	T45.0X2	T45.0X3	T45.0X4	T45.0X5	T45.0X6
Pyrimethamine	T37.2X1	T37.2X2	T37.2X3	T37.2X4	T37.2X5	T37.2X6
with sulfadoxine	T37.2X1	T37.2X2	T37.2X3	T37.2X4	T37.2X5	T37.2X6
Pyrimidine antagonist	T45.1X1	T45.1X2	T45.1X3	T45.1X4	T45.1X5	T45.1X6
Pyriminil	T60.4X1	T60.4X2	T60.4X3	T60.4X4	--	--
Pyrithione zinc	T49.4X1	T49.4X2	T49.4X3	T49.4X4	T49.4X5	T49.4X6
Pyrithyldione	T42.6X1	T42.6X2	T42.6X3	T42.6X4	T42.6X5	T42.6X6
Pyrogallic acid	T49.0X1	T49.0X2	T49.0X3	T49.0X4	T49.0X5	T49.0X6
Pyrogallol	T49.0X1	T49.0X2	T49.0X3	T49.0X4	T49.0X5	T49.0X6
Pyroxylin	T49.3X1	T49.3X2	T49.3X3	T49.3X4	T49.3X5	T49.3X6
Pyrrobutamine	T45.0X1	T45.0X2	T45.0X3	T45.0X4	T45.0X5	T45.0X6
Pyrrolizidine alkaloids	T62.8X1	T62.8X2	T62.8X3	T62.8X4	--	--
Pyrvinium chloride	T37.4X1	T37.4X2	T37.4X3	T37.4X4	T37.4X5	T37.4X6
PZI	T38.3X1	T38.3X2	T38.3X3	T38.3X4	T38.3X5	T38.3X6
Q						
Quaalude	T42.6X1	T42.6X2	T42.6X3	T42.6X4	T42.6X5	T42.6X6
Quarternary ammonium						
anti-infective	T49.0X1	T49.0X2	T49.0X3	T49.0X4	T49.0X5	T49.0X6
ganglion blocking	T44.2X1	T44.2X2	T44.2X3	T44.2X4	T44.2X5	T44.2X6
parasympatholytic	T44.3X1	T44.3X2	T44.3X3	T44.3X4	T44.3X5	T44.3X6
Quazepam	T42.4X1	T42.4X2	T42.4X3	T42.4X4	T42.4X5	T42.4X6
Quicklime	T54.3X1	T54.3X2	T54.3X3	T54.3X4	--	--
Quillaja extract	T48.4X1	T48.4X2	T48.4X3	T48.4X4	T48.4X5	T48.4X6
Quinacrine	T37.2X1	T37.2X2	T37.2X3	T37.2X4	T37.2X5	T37.2X6
Quinaglute	T46.2X1	T46.2X2	T46.2X3	T46.2X4	T46.2X5	T46.2X6
Quinalbarbital	T42.3X1	T42.3X2	T42.3X3	T42.3X4	T42.3X5	T42.3X6
Quinalbarbitone sodium	T42.3X1	T42.3X2	T42.3X3	T42.3X4	T42.3X5	T42.3X6
Quinalphos	T60.0X1	T60.0X2	T60.0X3	T60.0X4	--	--
Quinapril	T46.4X1	T46.4X2	T46.4X3	T46.4X4	T46.4X5	T46.4X6
Quinestradiol	T38.5X1	T38.5X2	T38.5X3	T38.5X4	T38.5X5	T38.5X6
Quinestradol	T38.5X1	T38.5X2	T38.5X3	T38.5X4	T38.5X5	T38.5X6
Quinestrol	T38.5X1	T38.5X2	T38.5X3	T38.5X4	T38.5X5	T38.5X6
Quinethazone	T50.2X1	T50.2X2	T50.2X3	T50.2X4	T50.2X5	T50.2X6
Quingestanol	T38.4X1	T38.4X2	T38.4X3	T38.4X4	T38.4X5	T38.4X6
Quinidine	T46.2X1	T46.2X2	T46.2X3	T46.2X4	T46.2X5	T46.2X6
Quinine	T37.2X1	T37.2X2	T37.2X3	T37.2X4	T37.2X5	T37.2X6
Quiniobine	T37.8X1	T37.8X2	T37.8X3	T37.8X4	T37.8X5	T37.8X6
Quinisocaine	T49.1X1	T49.1X2	T49.1X3	T49.1X4	T49.1X5	T49.1X6
Quinocide	T37.2X1	T37.2X2	T37.2X3	T37.2X4	T37.2X5	T37.2X6
Quinoline (derivatives) **NEC**	T37.8X1	T37.8X2	T37.8X3	T37.8X4	T37.8X5	T37.8X6
Quinupramine	T43.011	T43.012	T43.013	T43.014	T43.015	T43.016
Quotane	T41.3X1	T41.3X2	T41.3X3	T41.3X4	T41.3X5	T41.3X6
R						
Rabies						
immune globulin (human)	T50.Z11	T50.Z12	T50.Z13	T50.Z14	T50.Z15	T50.Z16
vaccine	T50.B91	T50.B92	T50.B93	T50.B94	T50.B95	T50.B96
Racemoramide	T40.2X1	T40.2X2	T40.2X3	T40.2X4	--	--
Racemorphan	T40.2X1	T40.2X2	T40.2X3	T40.2X4	T40.2X5	T40.2X6
Racepinefrin	T44.5X1	T44.5X2	T44.5X3	T44.5X4	T44.5X5	T44.5X6
Raclopride	T43.591	T43.592	T43.593	T43.594	T43.595	T43.596
Radiator alcohol	T51.1X1	T51.1X2	T51.1X3	T51.1X4	--	--
Radioactive drug NEC	T50.8X1	T50.8X2	T50.8X3	T50.8X4	T50.8X5	T50.8X6
Radio-opaque (drugs) (materials)	T50.8X1	T50.8X2	T50.8X3	T50.8X4	T50.8X5	T50.8X6
Ramifenazone	T39.2X1	T39.2X2	T39.2X3	T39.2X4	T39.2X5	T39.2X6
Ramipril	T46.4X1	T46.4X2	T46.4X3	T46.4X4	T46.4X5	T46.4X6
Ranitidine	T47.0X1	T47.0X2	T47.0X3	T47.0X4	T47.0X5	T47.0X6
Ranunculus	T62.2X1	T62.2X2	T62.2X3	T62.2X4	--	--
Rat poison NEC	T60.4X1	T60.4X2	T60.4X3	T60.4X4	--	--
Rattlesnake (venom)	T63.011	T63.012	T63.013	T63.014	--	--
Raubasine	T46.7X1	T46.7X2	T46.7X3	T46.7X4	T46.7X5	T46.7X6
Raudixin	T46.5X1	T46.5X2	T46.5X3	T46.5X4	T46.5X5	T46.5X6
Rautensin	T46.5X1	T46.5X2	T46.5X3	T46.5X4	T46.5X5	T46.5X6
Rautina	T46.5X1	T46.5X2	T46.5X3	T46.5X4	T46.5X5	T46.5X6
Rautotal	T46.5X1	T46.5X2	T46.5X3	T46.5X4	T46.5X5	T46.5X6
Rauwiloid	T46.5X1	T46.5X2	T46.5X3	T46.5X4	T46.5X5	T46.5X6
Rauwoldin	T46.5X1	T46.5X2	T46.5X3	T46.5X4	T46.5X5	T46.5X6
Rauwolfia (alkaloids)	T46.5X1	T46.5X2	T46.5X3	T46.5X4	T46.5X5	T46.5X6
Razoxane	T45.1X1	T45.1X2	T45.1X3	T45.1X4	T45.1X5	T45.1X6
Realgar	T57.0X1	T57.0X2	T57.0X3	T57.0X4	--	--
Recombinant (R) — *see specific protein*						
Red blood cells, packed	T45.8X1	T45.8X2	T45.8X3	T45.8X4	T45.8X5	T45.8X6
Red squill (scilliroside)	T60.4X1	T60.4X2	T60.4X3	T60.4X4	--	--
Reducing agent, industrial NEC	T65.891	T65.892	T65.893	T65.894	--	--
Refrigerant gas (chlorofluoro-carbon)	T53.5X1	T53.5X2	T53.5X3	T53.5X4	--	--
not chlorofluoro-carbon	T59.891	T59.892	T59.893	T59.894	--	--
Regroton	T50.2X1	T50.2X2	T50.2X3	T50.2X4	T50.2X5	T50.2X6
Rehydration salts (oral)	T50.3X1	T50.3X2	T50.3X3	T50.3X4	T50.3X5	T50.3X6
Rela	T42.8X1	T42.8X2	T42.8X3	T42.8X4	T42.8X5	T42.8X6
Relaxant, muscle						
anesthetic	T48.1X1	T48.1X2	T48.1X3	T48.1X4	T48.1X5	T48.1X6
central nervous system	T42.8X1	T42.8X2	T42.8X3	T42.8X4	T42.8X5	T42.8X6
skeletal NEC	T48.1X1	T48.1X2	T48.1X3	T48.1X4	T48.1X5	T48.1X6
smooth NEC	T44.3X1	T44.3X2	T44.3X3	T44.3X4	T44.3X5	T44.3X6
Remoxipride	T43.591	T43.592	T43.593	T43.594	T43.595	T43.596
Renese	T50.2X1	T50.2X2	T50.2X3	T50.2X4	T50.2X5	T50.2X6
Renografin	T50.8X1	T50.8X2	T50.8X3	T50.8X4	T50.8X5	T50.8X6
Replacement solution	T50.3X1	T50.3X2	T50.3X3	T50.3X4	T50.3X5	T50.3X6
Reproterol	T48.6X1	T48.6X2	T48.6X3	T48.6X4	T48.6X5	T48.6X6
Rescinnamine	T46.5X1	T46.5X2	T46.5X3	T46.5X4	T46.5X5	T46.5X6
Reserpin (e)	T46.5X1	T46.5X2	T46.5X3	T46.5X4	T46.5X5	T46.5X6

Substance	Poisoning, Accidental unintentional	Poisoning, Intentional self-harm	Poisoning, Assault	Poisoning, Undetermined	Adverse effect	Underdosing
Resorcin, resorcinol (nonmedicinal)	T65.891	T65.892	T65.893	T65.894	--	--
medicinal	T49.4X1	T49.4X2	T49.4X3	T49.4X4	T49.4X5	T49.4X6
Respaire	T48.4X1	T48.4X2	T48.4X3	T48.4X4	T48.4X5	T48.4X6
Respiratory drug NEC	T48.901	T48.902	T48.903	T48.904	T48.905	T48.906
antiasthmatic NEC	T48.6X1	T48.6X2	T48.6X3	T48.6X4	T48.6X5	T48.6X6
anti-common-cold NEC	T48.5X1	T48.5X2	T48.5X3	T48.5X4	T48.5X5	T48.5X6
expectorant NEC	T48.4X1	T48.4X2	T48.4X3	T48.4X4	T48.4X5	T48.4X6
stimulant	T48.901	T48.902	T48.903	T48.904	T48.905	T48.906
Retinoic acid	T49.0X1	T49.0X2	T49.0X3	T49.0X4	T49.0X5	T49.0X6
Retinol	T45.2X1	T45.2X2	T45.2X3	T45.2X4	T45.2X5	T45.2X6
Rh (D) immune globulin (human)	T50.Z11	T50.Z12	T50.Z13	T50.Z14	T50.Z15	T50.Z16
Rhodine	T39.011	T39.012	T39.013	T39.014	T39.015	T39.016
RhoGAM	T50.Z11	T50.Z12	T50.Z13	T50.Z14	T50.Z15	T50.Z16
Rhubarb						
dry extract	T47.2X1	T47.2X2	T47.2X3	T47.2X4	T47.2X5	T47.2X6
tincture, compound	T47.2X1	T47.2X2	T47.2X3	T47.2X4	T47.2X5	T47.2X6
Ribavirin	T37.5X1	T37.5X2	T37.5X3	T37.5X4	T37.5X5	T37.5X6
Riboflavin	T45.2X1	T45.2X2	T45.2X3	T45.2X4	T45.2X5	T45.2X6
Ribostamycin	T36.5X1	T36.5X2	T36.5X3	T36.5X4	T36.5X5	T36.5X6
Ricin	T62.2X1	T62.2X2	T62.2X3	T62.2X4	--	--
Ricinus communis	T62.2X1	T62.2X2	T62.2X3	T62.2X4	--	--
Rickettsial vaccine NEC	T50.A91	T50.A92	T50.A93	T50.A94	T50.A95	T50.A96
Rifabutin	T36.6X1	T36.6X2	T36.6X3	T36.6X4	T36.6X5	T36.6X6
Rifamide	T36.6X1	T36.6X2	T36.6X3	T36.6X4	T36.6X5	T36.6X6
Rifampicin	T36.6X1	T36.6X2	T36.6X3	T36.6X4	T36.6X5	T36.6X6
with isoniazid	T37.1X1	T37.1X2	T37.1X3	T37.1X4	T37.1X5	T37.1X6
Rifampin	T36.6X1	T36.6X2	T36.6X3	T36.6X4	T36.6X5	T36.6X6
Rifamycin	T36.6X1	T36.6X2	T36.6X3	T36.6X4	T36.6X5	T36.6X6
Rifaximin	T36.6X1	T36.6X2	T36.6X3	T36.6X4	T36.6X5	T36.6X6
Rimantadine	T37.5X1	T37.5X2	T37.5X3	T37.5X4	T37.5X5	T37.5X6
Rimazolium metilsulfate	T39.8X1	T39.8X2	T39.8X3	T39.8X4	T39.8X5	T39.8X6
Rimifon	T37.1X1	T37.1X2	T37.1X3	T37.1X4	T37.1X5	T37.1X6
Rimiterol	T48.6X1	T48.6X2	T48.6X3	T48.6X4	T48.6X5	T48.6X6
Ringer (lactate) **solution**	T50.3X1	T50.3X2	T50.3X3	T50.3X4	T50.3X5	T50.3X6
Ristocetin	T36.8X1	T36.8X2	T36.8X3	T36.8X4	T36.8X5	T36.8X6
Ritalin	T43.631	T43.632	T43.633	T43.634	T43.635	T43.636
Ritodrine	T44.5X1	T44.5X2	T44.5X3	T44.5X4	T44.5X5	T44.5X6
Roach killer — *see Insecticide*						
Rociverine	T44.3X1	T44.3X2	T44.3X3	T44.3X4	T44.3X5	T44.3X6
Rocky Mountain spotted fever vaccine	T50.A91	T50.A92	T50.A93	T50.A94	T50.A95	T50.A96
Rodenticide NEC	T60.4X1	T60.4X2	T60.4X3	T60.4X4	--	--
Rohypnol	T42.4X1	T42.4X2	T42.4X3	T42.4X4	T42.4X5	T42.4X6
Rokitamycin	T36.3X1	T36.3X2	T36.3X3	T36.3X4	T36.3X5	T36.3X6
Rolaids	T47.1X1	T47.1X2	T47.1X3	T47.1X4	T47.1X5	T47.1X6
Rolitetracycline	T36.4X1	T36.4X2	T36.4X3	T36.4X4	T36.4X5	T36.4X6
Romilar	T48.3X1	T48.3X2	T48.3X3	T48.3X4	T48.3X5	T48.3X6
Ronifibrate	T46.6X1	T46.6X2	T46.6X3	T46.6X4	T46.6X5	T46.6X6
Rosaprostol	T47.1X1	T47.1X2	T47.1X3	T47.1X4	T47.1X5	T47.1X6
Rose bengal sodium (131I)	T50.8X1	T50.8X2	T50.8X3	T50.8X4	T50.8X5	T50.8X6
Rose water ointment	T49.3X1	T49.3X2	T49.3X3	T49.3X4	T49.3X5	T49.3X6
Rosoxacin	T37.8X1	T37.8X2	T37.8X3	T37.8X4	T37.8X5	T37.8X6
Rotenone	T60.2X1	T60.2X2	T60.2X3	T60.2X4	--	--
Rotoxamine	T45.0X1	T45.0X2	T45.0X3	T45.0X4	T45.0X5	T45.0X6
Rough-on-rats	T60.4X1	T60.4X2	T60.4X3	T60.4X4	--	--
Roxatidine	T47.0X1	T47.0X2	T47.0X3	T47.0X4	T47.0X5	T47.0X6
Roxithromycin	T36.3X1	T36.3X2	T36.3X3	T36.3X4	T36.3X5	T36.3X6
Rt-PA	T45.611	T45.612	T45.613	T45.614	T45.615	T45.616
Rubbing alcohol	T51.2X1	T51.2X2	T51.2X3	T51.2X4	--	--
Rubefacient	T49.4X1	T49.4X2	T49.4X3	T49.4X4	T49.4X5	T49.4X6
Rubella vaccine	T50.B91	T50.B92	T50.B93	T50.B94	T50.B95	T50.B96
Rubeola vaccine	T50.B91	T50.B92	T50.B93	T50.B94	T50.B95	T50.B96
Rubidium chloride Rb82	T50.8X1	T50.8X2	T50.8X3	T50.8X4	T50.8X5	T50.8X6
Rubidomycin	T45.1X1	T45.1X2	T45.1X3	T45.1X4	T45.1X5	T45.1X6
Rue	T62.2X1	T62.2X2	T62.2X3	T62.2X4	--	--
Rufocromomycin	T45.1X1	T45.1X2	T45.1X3	T45.1X4	T45.1X5	T45.1X6
Russel's viper venin	T45.7X1	T45.7X2	T45.7X3	T45.7X4	T45.7X5	T45.7X6
Ruta (graveolens)	T62.2X1	T62.2X2	T62.2X3	T62.2X4	--	--
Rutinum	T46.991	T46.992	T46.993	T46.994	T46.995	T46.996
Rutoside	T46.991	T46.992	T46.993	T46.994	T46.995	T46.996
S						
Sabadilla (plant)	T62.2X1	T62.2X2	T62.2X3	T62.2X4	--	--
pesticide	T60.2X1	T60.2X2	T60.2X3	T60.2X4	--	--
Saccharated iron oxide	T45.8X1	T45.8X2	T45.8X3	T45.8X4	T45.8X5	T45.8X6
Saccharin	T50.901	T50.902	T50.903	T50.904	T50.905	T50.906
Saccharomyces boulardii	T47.6X1	T47.6X2	T47.6X3	T47.6X4	T47.6X5	T47.6X6
Safflower oil	T46.6X1	T46.6X2	T46.6X3	T46.6X4	T46.6X5	T46.6X6
Safrazine	T43.1X1	T43.1X2	T43.1X3	T43.1X4	T43.1X5	T43.1X6
Salazosulfapyridine	T37.0X1	T37.0X2	T37.0X3	T37.0X4	T37.0X5	T37.0X6
Salbutamol	T48.6X1	T48.6X2	T48.6X3	T48.6X4	T48.6X5	T48.6X6
Salicylamide	T39.091	T39.092	T39.093	T39.094	T39.095	T39.096
Salicylate NEC	T39.091	T39.092	T39.093	T39.094	T39.095	T39.096
methyl	T49.3X1	T49.3X2	T49.3X3	T49.3X4	T49.3X5	T49.3X6
theobromine calcium	T50.2X1	T50.2X2	T50.2X3	T50.2X4	T50.2X5	T50.2X6

Substance	Poisoning, Accidental unintentional	Poisoning, Intentional self-harm	Poisoning, Assault	Poisoning, Undetermined	Adverse effect	Underdosing
Salicylazosulfapyridine	T37.0X1	T37.0X2	T37.0X3	T37.0X4	T37.0X5	T37.0X6
Salicylhydroxamic acid	T49.0X1	T49.0X2	T49.0X3	T49.0X4	T49.0X5	T49.0X6
Salicylic acid	T49.4X1	T49.4X2	T49.4X3	T49.4X4	T49.4X5	T49.4X6
with benzoic acid	T49.4X1	T49.4X2	T49.4X3	T49.4X4	T49.4X5	T49.4X6
congeners	T39.091	T39.092	T39.093	T39.094	T39.095	T39.096
derivative	T39.091	T39.092	T39.093	T39.094	T39.095	T39.096
salts	T39.091	T39.092	T39.093	T39.094	T39.095	T39.096
Salinazid	T37.1X1	T37.1X2	T37.1X3	T37.1X4	T37.1X5	T37.1X6
Salmeterol	T48.6X1	T48.6X2	T48.6X3	T48.6X4	T48.6X5	T48.6X6
Salol	T49.3X1	T49.3X2	T49.3X3	T49.3X4	T49.3X5	T49.3X6
Salsalate	T39.091	T39.092	T39.093	T39.094	T39.095	T39.096
Salt substitute	T50.901	T50.902	T50.903	T50.904	T50.905	T50.906
Salt-replacing drug	T50.901	T50.902	T50.903	T50.904	T50.905	T50.906
Salt-retaining mineralocorticoid	T50.0X1	T50.0X2	T50.0X3	T50.0X4	T50.0X5	T50.0X6
Saluretic NEC	T50.2X1	T50.2X2	T50.2X3	T50.2X4	T50.2X5	T50.2X6
Saluron	T50.2X1	T50.2X2	T50.2X3	T50.2X4	T50.2X5	T50.2X6
Salvarsan 606 (neosilver) (silver)	T37.8X1	T37.8X2	T37.8X3	T37.8X4	T37.8X5	T37.8X6
Sambucus canadensis	T62.2X1	T62.2X2	T62.2X3	T62.2X4	--	--
berry	T62.1X1	T62.1X2	T62.1X3	T62.1X4	--	--
Sandril	T46.5X1	T46.5X2	T46.5X3	T46.5X4	T46.5X5	T46.5X6
Sanguinaria canadensis	T62.2X1	T62.2X2	T62.2X3	T62.2X4	--	--
Saniflush (cleaner)	T54.2X1	T54.2X2	T54.2X3	T54.2X4	--	--
Santonin	T37.4X1	T37.4X2	T37.4X3	T37.4X4	T37.4X5	T37.4X6
Santyl	T49.8X1	T49.8X2	T49.8X3	T49.8X4	T49.8X5	T49.8X6
Saralasin	T46.5X1	T46.5X2	T46.5X3	T46.5X4	T46.5X5	T46.5X6
Sarcolysin	T45.1X1	T45.1X2	T45.1X3	T45.1X4	T45.1X5	T45.1X6
Sarkomycin	T45.1X1	T45.1X2	T45.1X3	T45.1X4	T45.1X5	T45.1X6
Saroten	T43.011	T43.012	T43.013	T43.014	T43.015	T43.016
Saturnine — *see Lead*						
Savin (oil)	T49.4X1	T49.4X2	T49.4X3	T49.4X4	T49.4X5	T49.4X6
Scammony	T47.2X1	T47.2X2	T47.2X3	T47.2X4	T47.2X5	T47.2X6
Scarlet red	T49.8X1	T49.8X2	T49.8X3	T49.8X4	T49.8X5	T49.8X6
Scheele's green	T57.0X1	T57.0X2	T57.0X3	T57.0X4	--	--
insecticide	T57.0X1	T57.0X2	T57.0X3	T57.0X4	--	--
Schizontozide (blood) (tissue)	T37.2X1	T37.2X2	T37.2X3	T37.2X4	T37.2X5	T37.2X6
Schradan	T60.0X1	T60.0X2	T60.0X3	T60.0X4	--	--
Schweinfurth green	T57.0X1	T57.0X2	T57.0X3	T57.0X4	--	--
insecticide	T57.0X1	T57.0X2	T57.0X3	T57.0X4	--	--
Scilla, rat poison	T60.4X1	T60.4X2	T60.4X3	T60.4X4	--	--
Scillaren	T60.4X1	T60.4X2	T60.4X3	T60.4X4	--	--
Sclerosing agent	T46.8X1	T46.8X2	T46.8X3	T46.8X4	T46.8X5	T46.8X6
Scombrotoxin	T61.11	T61.12	T61.13	T61.14	--	--
Scopolamine	T44.3X1	T44.3X2	T44.3X3	T44.3X4	T44.3X5	T44.3X6
Scopolia extract	T44.3X1	T44.3X2	T44.3X3	T44.3X4	T44.3X5	T44.3X6
Scouring powder	T65.891	T65.892	T65.893	T65.894	--	--
Sea						
anemone (sting)	T63.631	T63.632	T63.633	T63.634	--	--
cucumber (sting)	T63.691	T63.692	T63.693	T63.694	--	--
snake (bite) (venom)	T63.091	T63.092	T63.093	T63.094	--	--
urchin spine (puncture)	T63.691	T63.692	T63.693	T63.694	--	--
Seafood	T61.91	T61.92	T61.93	T61.94	--	--
specified NEC	T61.8X1	T61.8X2	T61.8X3	T61.8X4	--	--
Secbutabarbital	T42.3X1	T42.3X2	T42.3X3	T42.3X4	T42.3X5	T42.3X6
Secbutabarbitone	T42.3X1	T42.3X2	T42.3X3	T42.3X4	T42.3X5	T42.3X6
Secnidazole	T37.3X1	T37.3X2	T37.3X3	T37.3X4	T37.3X5	T37.3X6
Secobarbital	T42.3X1	T42.3X2	T42.3X3	T42.3X4	T42.3X5	T42.3X6
Seconal	T42.3X1	T42.3X2	T42.3X3	T42.3X4	T42.3X5	T42.3X6
Secretin	T50.8X1	T50.8X2	T50.8X3	T50.8X4	T50.8X5	T50.8X6
Sedative NEC	T42.71	T42.72	T42.73	T42.74	T42.75	T42.76
mixed NEC	T42.6X1	T42.6X2	T42.6X3	T42.6X4	T42.6X5	T42.6X6
Sedormid	T42.6X1	T42.6X2	T42.6X3	T42.6X4	T42.6X5	T42.6X6
Seed disinfectant or dressing	T60.8X1	T60.8X2	T60.8X3	T60.8X4	--	--
Seeds (poisonous)	T62.2X1	T62.2X2	T62.2X3	T62.2X4	--	--
Selegiline	T42.8X1	T42.8X2	T42.8X3	T42.8X4	T42.8X5	T42.8X6
Selenium NEC	T56.891	T56.892	T56.893	T56.894	--	--
disulfide or sulfide	T49.4X1	T49.4X2	T49.4X3	T49.4X4	T49.4X5	T49.4X6
fumes	T59.891	T59.892	T59.893	T59.894	--	--
sulfide	T49.4X1	T49.4X2	T49.4X3	T49.4X4	T49.4X5	T49.4X6
Selenomethionine (75Se)	T50.8X1	T50.8X2	T50.8X3	T50.8X4	T50.8X5	T50.8X6
Selsun	T49.4X1	T49.4X2	T49.4X3	T49.4X4	T49.4X5	T49.4X6
Semustine	T45.1X1	T45.1X2	T45.1X3	T45.1X4	T45.1X5	T45.1X6
Senega syrup	T48.4X1	T48.4X2	T48.4X3	T48.4X4	T48.4X5	T48.4X6
Senna	T47.2X1	T47.2X2	T47.2X3	T47.2X4	T47.2X5	T47.2X6
Sennoside A+B	T47.2X1	T47.2X2	T47.2X3	T47.2X4	T47.2X5	T47.2X6
Septisol	T49.2X1	T49.2X2	T49.2X3	T49.2X4	T49.2X5	T49.2X6
Seractide	T38.811	T38.812	T38.813	T38.814	T38.815	T38.816
Serax	T42.4X1	T42.4X2	T42.4X3	T42.4X4	T42.4X5	T42.4X6
Serenesil	T42.6X1	T42.6X2	T42.6X3	T42.6X4	T42.6X5	T42.6X6
Serenium (hydrochloride)	T37.91	T37.92	T37.93	T37.94	T37.95	T37.96
Serepax — *see Oxazepam*						
Sermorelin	T38.891	T38.892	T38.893	T38.894	T38.895	T38.896
Sernyl	T41.1X1	T41.1X2	T41.1X3	T41.1X4	T41.1X5	T41.1X6

Substance	Poisoning, Accidental unintentional	Poisoning, Intentional self-harm	Poisoning, Assault	Poisoning, Undetermined	Adverse effect	Underdosing
Serotonin	T50.991	T50.992	T50.993	T50.994	T50.995	T50.996
Serpasil	T46.5X1	T46.5X2	T46.5X3	T46.5X4	T46.5X5	T46.5X6
Serrapeptase	T45.3X1	T45.3X2	T45.3X3	T45.3X4	T45.3X5	T45.3X6
Serum						
antibotulinus	T50.Z11	T50.Z12	T50.Z13	T50.Z14	T50.Z15	T50.Z16
anticytotoxic	T50.Z11	T50.Z12	T50.Z13	T50.Z14	T50.Z15	T50.Z16
antidiphtheria	T50.Z11	T50.Z12	T50.Z13	T50.Z14	T50.Z15	T50.Z16
antimeningococcus	T50.Z11	T50.Z12	T50.Z13	T50.Z14	T50.Z15	T50.Z16
anti-Rh	T50.Z11	T50.Z12	T50.Z13	T50.Z14	T50.Z15	T50.Z16
anti-snake-bite	T50.Z11	T50.Z12	T50.Z13	T50.Z14	T50.Z15	T50.Z16
antitetanic	T50.Z11	T50.Z12	T50.Z13	T50.Z14	T50.Z15	T50.Z16
antitoxic	T50.Z11	T50.Z12	T50.Z13	T50.Z14	T50.Z15	T50.Z16
complement (inhibitor)	T45.8X1	T45.8X2	T45.8X3	T45.8X4	T45.8X5	T45.8X6
convalescent	T50.Z11	T50.Z12	T50.Z13	T50.Z14	T50.Z15	T50.Z16
hemolytic complement	T45.8X1	T45.8X2	T45.8X3	T45.8X4	T45.8X5	T45.8X6
immune (human)	T50.Z11	T50.Z12	T50.Z13	T50.Z14	T50.Z15	T50.Z16
protective NEC	T50.Z11	T50.Z12	T50.Z13	T50.Z14	T50.Z15	T50.Z16
Setastine	T45.0X1	T45.0X2	T45.0X3	T45.0X4	T45.0X5	T45.0X6
Setoperone	T43.591	T43.592	T43.593	T43.594	T43.595	T43.596
Sewer gas	T59.91	T59.92	T59.93	T59.94	--	--
Shampoo	T55.0X1	T55.0X2	T55.0X3	T55.0X4	--	--
Shellfish, noxious, nonbacterial	T61.781	T61.782	T61.783	T61.784	--	--
Sildenafil	T46.7X1	T46.7X2	T46.7X3	T46.7X4	T46.7X5	T46.7X6
Silibinin	T50.991	T50.992	T50.993	T50.994	T50.995	T50.996
Silicone NEC	T65.891	T65.892	T65.893	T65.894	--	--
medicinal	T49.3X1	T49.3X2	T49.3X3	T49.3X4	T49.3X5	T49.3X6
Silvadene	T49.0X1	T49.0X2	T49.0X3	T49.0X4	T49.0X5	T49.0X6
Silver	T49.0X1	T49.0X2	T49.0X3	T49.0X4	T49.0X5	T49.0X6
anti-infectives	T49.0X1	T49.0X2	T49.0X3	T49.0X4	T49.0X5	T49.0X6
arsphenamine	T37.8X1	T37.8X2	T37.8X3	T37.8X4	T37.8X5	T37.8X6
colloidal	T49.0X1	T49.0X2	T49.0X3	T49.0X4	T49.0X5	T49.0X6
nitrate	T49.0X1	T49.0X2	T49.0X3	T49.0X4	T49.0X5	T49.0X6
ophthalmic preparation	T49.5X1	T49.5X2	T49.5X3	T49.5X4	T49.5X5	T49.5X6
toughened (keratolytic)	T49.4X1	T49.4X2	T49.4X3	T49.4X4	T49.4X5	T49.4X6
nonmedicinal (dust)	T56.891	T56.892	T56.893	T56.894	--	--
protein	T49.5X1	T49.5X2	T49.5X3	T49.5X4	T49.5X5	T49.5X6
salvarsan	T37.8X1	T37.8X2	T37.8X3	T37.8X4	T37.8X5	T37.8X6
sulfadiazine	T49.4X1	T49.4X2	T49.4X3	T49.4X4	T49.4X5	T49.4X6
Silymarin	T50.991	T50.992	T50.993	T50.994	T50.995	T50.996
Simaldrate	T47.1X1	T47.1X2	T47.1X3	T47.1X4	T47.1X5	T47.1X6
Simazine	T60.3X1	T60.3X2	T60.3X3	T60.3X4	--	--
Simethicone	T47.1X1	T47.1X2	T47.1X3	T47.1X4	T47.1X5	T47.1X6
Simfibrate	T46.6X1	T46.6X2	T46.6X3	T46.6X4	T46.6X5	T46.6X6
Simvastatin	T46.6X1	T46.6X2	T46.6X3	T46.6X4	T46.6X5	T46.6X6
Sincalide	T50.8X1	T50.8X2	T50.8X3	T50.8X4	T50.8X5	T50.8X6
Sinequan	T43.011	T43.012	T43.013	T43.014	T43.015	T43.016
Singoserp	T46.5X1	T46.5X2	T46.5X3	T46.5X4	T46.5X5	T46.5X6
Sintrom	T45.511	T45.512	T45.513	T45.514	T45.515	T45.516
Sisomicin	T36.5X1	T36.5X2	T36.5X3	T36.5X4	T36.5X5	T36.5X6
Sitosterols	T46.6X1	T46.6X2	T46.6X3	T46.6X4	T46.6X5	T46.6X6
Skeletal muscle relaxants	T48.1X1	T48.1X2	T48.1X3	T48.1X4	T48.1X5	T48.1X6
Skin						
agents (external)	T49.91	T49.92	T49.93	T49.94	T49.95	T49.96
specified NEC	T49.8X1	T49.8X2	T49.8X3	T49.8X4	T49.8X5	T49.8X6
test antigen	T50.8X1	T50.8X2	T50.8X3	T50.8X4	T50.8X5	T50.8X6
Sleep-eze	T45.0X1	T45.0X2	T45.0X3	T45.0X4	T45.0X5	T45.0X6
Sleeping draught, pill	T42.71	T42.72	T42.73	T42.74	T42.75	T42.76
Smallpox vaccine	T50.B11	T50.B12	T50.B13	T50.B14	T50.B15	T50.B16
Smelter fumes NEC	T56.91	T56.92	T56.93	T56.94	--	--
Smog	T59.1X1	T59.1X2	T59.1X3	T59.1X4	--	--
Smoke NEC	T59.811	T59.812	T59.813	T59.814	--	--
Smooth muscle relaxant	T44.3X1	T44.3X2	T44.3X3	T44.3X4	T44.3X5	T44.3X6
Snail killer NEC	T60.8X1	T60.8X2	T60.8X3	T60.8X4	--	--
Snake venom or bite	T63.001	T63.002	T63.003	T63.004	--	--
hemocoagulase	T45.7X1	T45.7X2	T45.7X3	T45.7X4	T45.7X5	T45.7X6
Snuff	T65.211	T65.212	T65.213	T65.214	--	--
Soap (powder) (product)	T55.0X1	T55.0X2	T55.0X3	T55.0X4	--	--
enema	T47.4X1	T47.4X2	T47.4X3	T47.4X4	T47.4X5	T47.4X6
medicinal, soft	T49.2X1	T49.2X2	T49.2X3	T49.2X4	T49.2X5	T49.2X6
superfatted	T49.2X1	T49.2X2	T49.2X3	T49.2X4	T49.2X5	T49.2X6
Sobrerol	T48.4X1	T48.4X2	T48.4X3	T48.4X4	T48.4X5	T48.4X6
Soda (caustic)	T54.3X1	T54.3X2	T54.3X3	T54.3X4	--	--
bicarb	T47.1X1	T47.1X2	T47.1X3	T47.1X4	T47.1X5	T47.1X6
chlorinated — *see Sodium, hypochlorite*						
Sodium						
acetosulfone	T37.1X1	T37.1X2	T37.1X3	T37.1X4	T37.1X5	T37.1X6
acetrizoate	T50.8X1	T50.8X2	T50.8X3	T50.8X4	T50.8X5	T50.8X6
acid phosphate	T50.3X1	T50.3X2	T50.3X3	T50.3X4	T50.3X5	T50.3X6
alginate	T47.8X1	T47.8X2	T47.8X3	T47.8X4	T47.8X5	T47.8X6
amidotrizoate	T50.8X1	T50.8X2	T50.8X3	T50.8X4	T50.8X5	T50.8X6
aminopterin	T45.1X1	T45.1X2	T45.1X3	T45.1X4	T45.1X5	T45.1X6
amylosulfate	T47.8X1	T47.8X2	T47.8X3	T47.8X4	T47.8X5	T47.8X6
Sodium — *continued*						
amytal	T42.3X1	T42.3X2	T42.3X3	T42.3X4	T42.3X5	T42.3X6
antimony gluconate	T37.3X1	T37.3X2	T37.3X3	T37.3X4	T37.3X5	T37.3X6
arsenate	T57.0X1	T57.0X2	T57.0X3	T57.0X4	--	--
aurothiomalate	T39.4X1	T39.4X2	T39.4X3	T39.4X4	T39.4X5	T39.4X6
aurothiosulfate	T39.4X1	T39.4X2	T39.4X3	T39.4X4	T39.4X5	T39.4X6
barbiturate	T42.3X1	T42.3X2	T42.3X3	T42.3X4	T42.3X5	T42.3X6
basic phosphate	T47.4X1	T47.4X2	T47.4X3	T47.4X4	T47.4X5	T47.4X6
bicarbonate	T47.1X1	T47.1X2	T47.1X3	T47.1X4	T47.1X5	T47.1X6
bichromate	T57.8X1	T57.8X2	T57.8X3	T57.8X4	--	--
biphosphate	T50.3X1	T50.3X2	T50.3X3	T50.3X4	T50.3X5	T50.3X6
bisulfate	T65.891	T65.892	T65.893	T65.894	--	--
borate						
cleanser	T57.8X1	T57.8X2	T57.8X3	T57.8X4	--	--
eye	T49.5X1	T49.5X2	T49.5X3	T49.5X4	T49.5X5	T49.5X6
therapeutic	T49.8X1	T49.8X2	T49.8X3	T49.8X4	T49.8X5	T49.8X6
bromide	T42.6X1	T42.6X2	T42.6X3	T42.6X4	T42.6X5	T42.6X6
cacodylate (nonmedicinal) NEC	T50.8X1	T50.8X2	T50.8X3	T50.8X4	T50.8X5	T50.8X6
anti-infective	T37.8X1	T37.8X2	T37.8X3	T37.8X4	T37.8X5	T37.8X6
herbicide	T60.3X1	T60.3X2	T60.3X3	T60.3X4	--	--
calcium edetate	T45.8X1	T45.8X2	T45.8X3	T45.8X4	T45.8X5	T45.8X6
carbonate NEC	T54.3X1	T54.3X2	T54.3X3	T54.3X4	--	--
chlorate NEC	T65.891	T65.892	T65.893	T65.894	--	--
herbicide	T54.91	T54.92	T54.93	T54.94	--	--
chloride	T50.3X1	T50.3X2	T50.3X3	T50.3X4	T50.3X5	T50.3X6
with glucose	T50.3X1	T50.3X2	T50.3X3	T50.3X4	T50.3X5	T50.3X6
chromate	T65.891	T65.892	T65.893	T65.894	--	--
citrate	T50.991	T50.992	T50.993	T50.994	T50.995	T50.996
cromoglicate	T48.6X1	T48.6X2	T48.6X3	T48.6X4	T48.6X5	T48.6X6
cyanide	T65.0X1	T65.0X2	T65.0X3	T65.0X4	--	--
cyclamate	T50.3X1	T50.3X2	T50.3X3	T50.3X4	T50.3X5	T50.3X6
dehydrocholate	T45.8X1	T45.8X2	T45.8X3	T45.8X4	T45.8X5	T45.8X6
diatrizoate	T50.8X1	T50.8X2	T50.8X3	T50.8X4	T50.8X5	T50.8X6
dibunate	T48.4X1	T48.4X2	T48.4X3	T48.4X4	T48.4X5	T48.4X6
dioctyl sulfosuccinate	T47.4X1	T47.4X2	T47.4X3	T47.4X4	T47.4X5	T47.4X6
dipantoyl ferrate	T45.8X1	T45.8X2	T45.8X3	T45.8X4	T45.8X5	T45.8X6
edetate	T45.8X1	T45.8X2	T45.8X3	T45.8X4	T45.8X5	T45.8X6
ethacrynate	T50.1X1	T50.1X2	T50.1X3	T50.1X4	T50.1X5	T50.1X6
feredetate	T45.8X1	T45.8X2	T45.8X3	T45.8X4	T45.8X5	T45.8X6
Fluoride — *see Fluoride*						
fluoroacetate (dust) (pesticide)	T60.4X1	T60.4X2	T60.4X3	T60.4X4	--	--
free salt	T50.3X1	T50.3X2	T50.3X3	T50.3X4	T50.3X5	T50.3X6
fusidate	T36.8X1	T36.8X2	T36.8X3	T36.8X4	T36.8X5	T36.8X6
glucaldrate	T47.1X1	T47.1X2	T47.1X3	T47.1X4	T47.1X5	T47.1X6
glucosulfone	T37.1X1	T37.1X2	T37.1X3	T37.1X4	T37.1X5	T37.1X6
glutamate	T45.8X1	T45.8X2	T45.8X3	T45.8X4	T45.8X5	T45.8X6
hydrogen carbonate	T50.3X1	T50.3X2	T50.3X3	T50.3X4	T50.3X5	T50.3X6
hydroxide	T54.3X1	T54.3X2	T54.3X3	T54.3X4	--	--
hypochlorite (bleach) NEC	T54.3X1	T54.3X2	T54.3X3	T54.3X4	--	--
disinfectant	T54.3X1	T54.3X2	T54.3X3	T54.3X4	--	--
medicinal (anti-infective) (external)	T49.0X1	T49.0X2	T49.0X3	T49.0X4	T49.0X5	T49.0X6
vapor	T54.3X1	T54.3X2	T54.3X3	T54.3X4	--	--
hyposulfite	T49.0X1	T49.0X2	T49.0X3	T49.0X4	T49.0X5	T49.0X6
indigotin disulfonate	T50.8X1	T50.8X2	T50.8X3	T50.8X4	T50.8X5	T50.8X6
iodide	T50.991	T50.992	T50.993	T50.994	T50.995	T50.996
I-131	T50.8X1	T50.8X2	T50.8X3	T50.8X4	T50.8X5	T50.8X6
therapeutic	T38.2X1	T38.2X2	T38.2X3	T38.2X4	T38.2X5	T38.2X6
iodohippurate (131I)	T50.8X1	T50.8X2	T50.8X3	T50.8X4	T50.8X5	T50.8X6
iopodate	T50.8X1	T50.8X2	T50.8X3	T50.8X4	T50.8X5	T50.8X6
iothalamate	T50.8X1	T50.8X2	T50.8X3	T50.8X4	T50.8X5	T50.8X6
iron edetate	T45.4X1	T45.4X2	T45.4X3	T45.4X4	T45.4X5	T45.4X6
lactate (compound solution)	T45.8X1	T45.8X2	T45.8X3	T45.8X4	T45.8X5	T45.8X6
lauryl (sulfate)	T49.2X1	T49.2X2	T49.2X3	T49.2X4	T49.2X5	T49.2X6
L-triiodothyronine	T38.1X1	T38.1X2	T38.1X3	T38.1X4	T38.1X5	T38.1X6
magnesium citrate	T50.991	T50.992	T50.993	T50.994	T50.995	T50.996
mersalate	T50.2X1	T50.2X2	T50.2X3	T50.2X4	T50.2X5	T50.2X6
metasilicate	T65.891	T65.892	T65.893	T65.894	--	--
metrizoate	T50.8X1	T50.8X2	T50.8X3	T50.8X4	T50.8X5	T50.8X6
monofluoroacetate (pesticide)	T60.1X1	T60.1X2	T60.1X3	T60.1X4	--	--
morrhuate	T46.8X1	T46.8X2	T46.8X3	T46.8X4	T46.8X5	T46.8X6
nafcillin	T36.0X1	T36.0X2	T36.0X3	T36.0X4	T36.0X5	T36.0X6
nitrate (oxidizing agent)	T65.891	T65.892	T65.893	T65.894	--	--
nitrite	T50.6X1	T50.6X2	T50.6X3	T50.6X4	T50.6X5	T50.6X6
nitroferricyanide	T46.5X1	T46.5X2	T46.5X3	T46.5X4	T46.5X5	T46.5X6
nitroprusside	T46.5X1	T46.5X2	T46.5X3	T46.5X4	T46.5X5	T46.5X6
oxalate	T65.891	T65.892	T65.893	T65.894	--	--
oxide/peroxide	T65.891	T65.892	T65.893	T65.894	--	--
oxybate	T41.291	T41.292	T41.293	T41.294	T41.295	T41.296
para-aminohippurate	T50.8X1	T50.8X2	T50.8X3	T50.8X4	T50.8X5	T50.8X6

Substance	Poisoning, Accidental unintentional	Poisoning, Intentional self-harm	Poisoning, Assault	Poisoning, Undetermined	Adverse effect	Underdosing
Sodium — *continued*						
perborate (nonmedicinal) NEC	T65.891	T65.892	T65.893	T65.894	--	--
medicinal	T49.0X1	T49.0X2	T49.0X3	T49.0X4	T49.0X5	T49.0X6
soap	T55.0X1	T55.0X2	T55.0X3	T55.0X4	--	--
percarbonate — *see Sodium, perborate*						
pertechnetate Tc99m	T50.8X1	T50.8X2	T50.8X3	T50.8X4	T50.8X5	T50.8X6
phosphate						
cellulose	T45.8X1	T45.8X2	T45.8X3	T45.8X4	T45.8X5	T45.8X6
dibasic	T47.2X1	T47.2X2	T47.2X3	T47.2X4	T47.2X5	T47.2X6
monobasic	T47.2X1	T47.2X2	T47.2X3	T47.2X4	T47.2X5	T47.2X6
phytate	T50.6X1	T50.6X2	T50.6X3	T50.6X4	T50.6X5	T50.6X6
picosulfate	T47.2X1	T47.2X2	T47.2X3	T47.2X4	T47.2X5	T47.2X6
polyhydroxyaluminium monocarbonate	T47.1X1	T47.1X2	T47.1X3	T47.1X4	T47.1X5	T47.1X6
polystyrene sulfonate	T50.3X1	T50.3X2	T50.3X3	T50.3X4	T50.3X5	T50.3X6
propionate	T49.0X1	T49.0X2	T49.0X3	T49.0X4	T49.0X5	T49.0X6
propyl hydroxybenzoate	T50.991	T50.992	T50.993	T50.994	T50.995	T50.996
psylliate	T46.8X1	T46.8X2	T46.8X3	T46.8X4	T46.8X5	T46.8X6
removing resins	T50.3X1	T50.3X2	T50.3X3	T50.3X4	T50.3X5	T50.3X6
salicylate	T39.091	T39.092	T39.093	T39.094	T39.095	T39.096
salt NEC	T50.3X1	T50.3X2	T50.3X3	T50.3X4	T50.3X5	T50.3X6
selenate	T60.2X1	T60.2X2	T60.2X3	T60.2X4	--	--
stibogluconate	T37.3X1	T37.3X2	T37.3X3	T37.3X4	T37.3X5	T37.3X6
sulfate	T47.4X1	T47.4X2	T47.4X3	T47.4X4	T47.4X5	T47.4X6
sulfoxone	T37.1X1	T37.1X2	T37.1X3	T37.1X4	T37.1X5	T37.1X6
tetradecyl sulfate	T46.8X1	T46.8X2	T46.8X3	T46.8X4	T46.8X5	T46.8X6
thiopental	T41.1X1	T41.1X2	T41.1X3	T41.1X4	T41.1X5	T41.1X6
thiosalicylate	T39.091	T39.092	T39.093	T39.094	T39.095	T39.096
thiosulfate	T50.6X1	T50.6X2	T50.6X3	T50.6X4	T50.6X5	T50.6X6
tolbutamide	T38.3X1	T38.3X2	T38.3X3	T38.3X4	T38.3X5	T38.3X6
(L)-triiodothyronine	T38.1X1	T38.1X2	T38.1X3	T38.1X4	T38.1X5	T38.1X6
tyropanoate	T50.8X1	T50.8X2	T50.8X3	T50.8X4	T50.8X5	T50.8X6
valproate	T42.6X1	T42.6X2	T42.6X3	T42.6X4	T42.6X5	T42.6X6
versenate	T50.6X1	T50.6X2	T50.6X3	T50.6X4	T50.6X5	T50.6X6
Sodium-free salt	T50.901	T50.902	T50.903	T50.904	T50.905	T50.906
Sodium-removing resin	T50.3X1	T50.3X2	T50.3X3	T50.3X4	T50.3X5	T50.3X6
Soft soap	T55.0X1	T55.0X2	T55.0X3	T55.0X4	--	--
Solanine	T62.2X1	T62.2X2	T62.2X3	T62.2X4	--	--
berries	T62.1X1	T62.1X2	T62.1X3	T62.1X4	--	--
Solanum dulcamara	T62.2X1	T62.2X2	T62.2X3	T62.2X4	--	--
berries	T62.1X1	T62.1X2	T62.1X3	T62.1X4	--	--
Solapsone	T37.1X1	T37.1X2	T37.1X3	T37.1X4	T37.1X5	T37.1X6
Solar lotion	T49.3X1	T49.3X2	T49.3X3	T49.3X4	T49.3X5	T49.3X6
Solasulfone	T37.1X1	T37.1X2	T37.1X3	T37.1X4	T37.1X5	T37.1X6
Soldering fluid	T65.891	T65.892	T65.893	T65.894	--	--
Solid substance	T65.91	T65.92	T65.93	T65.94	--	--
specified NEC	T65.891	T65.892	T65.893	T65.894	--	--
Solvent, industrial NEC	T52.91	T52.92	T52.93	T52.94	--	--
naphtha	T52.0X1	T52.0X2	T52.0X3	T52.0X4	--	--
petroleum	T52.0X1	T52.0X2	T52.0X3	T52.0X4	--	--
specified NEC	T52.8X1	T52.8X2	T52.8X3	T52.8X4	--	--
Soma	T42.8X1	T42.8X2	T42.8X3	T42.8X4	T42.8X5	T42.8X6
Somatorelin	T38.891	T38.892	T38.893	T38.894	T38.895	T38.896
Somatostatin	T38.991	T38.992	T38.993	T38.994	T38.995	T38.996
Somatotropin	T38.811	T38.812	T38.813	T38.814	T38.815	T38.816
Somatrem	T38.811	T38.812	T38.813	T38.814	T38.815	T38.816
Somatropin	T38.811	T38.812	T38.813	T38.814	T38.815	T38.816
Sominex	T45.0X1	T45.0X2	T45.0X3	T45.0X4	T45.0X5	T45.0X6
Somnos	T42.6X1	T42.6X2	T42.6X3	T42.6X4	T42.6X5	T42.6X6
Somonal	T42.3X1	T42.3X2	T42.3X3	T42.3X4	T42.3X5	T42.3X6
Soneryl	T42.3X1	T42.3X2	T42.3X3	T42.3X4	T42.3X5	T42.3X6
Soothing syrup	T50.901	T50.902	T50.903	T50.904	T50.905	T50.906
Sopor	T42.6X1	T42.6X2	T42.6X3	T42.6X4	T42.6X5	T42.6X6
Soporific	T42.71	T42.72	T42.73	T42.74	T42.75	T42.76
Soporific drug	T42.71	T42.72	T42.73	T42.74	T42.75	T42.76
specified type NEC	T42.6X1	T42.6X2	T42.6X3	T42.6X4	T42.6X5	T42.6X6
Sorbide nitrate	T46.3X1	T46.3X2	T46.3X3	T46.3X4	T46.3X5	T46.3X6
Sorbitol	T47.4X1	T47.4X2	T47.4X3	T47.4X4	T47.4X5	T47.4X6
Sotalol	T44.7X1	T44.7X2	T44.7X3	T44.7X4	T44.7X5	T44.7X6
Sotradecol	T46.8X1	T46.8X2	T46.8X3	T46.8X4	T46.8X5	T46.8X6
Soysterol	T46.6X1	T46.6X2	T46.6X3	T46.6X4	T46.6X5	T46.6X6
Spacoline	T44.3X1	T44.3X2	T44.3X3	T44.3X4	T44.3X5	T44.3X6
Spanish fly	T49.8X1	T49.8X2	T49.8X3	T49.8X4	T49.8X5	T49.8X6
Sparine	T43.3X1	T43.3X2	T43.3X3	T43.3X4	T43.3X5	T43.3X6
Sparteine	T48.0X1	T48.0X2	T48.0X3	T48.0X4	T48.0X5	T48.0X6
Spasmolytic						
anticholinergics	T44.3X1	T44.3X2	T44.3X3	T44.3X4	T44.3X5	T44.3X6
autonomic	T44.3X1	T44.3X2	T44.3X3	T44.3X4	T44.3X5	T44.3X6
bronchial NEC	T48.6X1	T48.6X2	T48.6X3	T48.6X4	T48.6X5	T48.6X6
quaternary ammonium	T44.3X1	T44.3X2	T44.3X3	T44.3X4	T44.3X5	T44.3X6
skeletal muscle NEC	T48.1X1	T48.1X2	T48.1X3	T48.1X4	T48.1X5	T48.1X6
Spectinomycin	T36.5X1	T36.5X2	T36.5X3	T36.5X4	T36.5X5	T36.5X6

Substance	Poisoning, Accidental unintentional	Poisoning, Intentional self-harm	Poisoning, Assault	Poisoning, Undetermined	Adverse effect	Underdosing
Speed	T43.621	T43.622	T43.623	T43.624	T43.625	T43.626
Spermicide	T49.8X1	T49.8X2	T49.8X3	T49.8X4	T49.8X5	T49.8X6
Spider (bite) (venom)	T63.391	T63.392	T63.393	T63.394	--	--
antivenin	T50.Z11	T50.Z12	T50.Z13	T50.Z14	T50.Z15	T50.Z16
Spigelia (root)	T37.4X1	T37.4X2	T37.4X3	T37.4X4	T37.4X5	T37.4X6
Spindle inactivator	T50.4X1	T50.4X2	T50.4X3	T50.4X4	T50.4X5	T50.4X6
Spiperone	T43.4X1	T43.4X2	T43.4X3	T43.4X4	T43.4X5	T43.4X6
Spiramycin	T36.3X1	T36.3X2	T36.3X3	T36.3X4	T36.3X5	T36.3X6
Spirapril	T46.4X1	T46.4X2	T46.4X3	T46.4X4	T46.4X5	T46.4X6
Spirilene	T43.591	T43.592	T43.593	T43.594	T43.595	T43.596
Spirit (s) (neutral) **NEC**	T51.0X1	T51.0X2	T51.0X3	T51.0X4	--	--
beverage	T51.0X1	T51.0X2	T51.0X3	T51.0X4	--	--
industrial	T51.0X1	T51.0X2	T51.0X3	T51.0X4	--	--
mineral	T52.0X1	T52.0X2	T52.0X3	T52.0X4	--	--
of salt — *see Hydrochloric acid*						
surgical	T51.0X1	T51.0X2	T51.0X3	T51.0X4	--	--
Spironolactone	T50.0X1	T50.0X2	T50.0X3	T50.0X4	T50.0X5	T50.0X6
Spiroperidol	T43.4X1	T43.4X2	T43.4X3	T43.4X4	T43.4X5	T43.4X6
Sponge, absorbable (gelatin)	T45.7X1	T45.7X2	T45.7X3	T45.7X4	T45.7X5	T45.7X6
Sporostacin	T49.0X1	T49.0X2	T49.0X3	T49.0X4	T49.0X5	T49.0X6
Spray (aerosol)	T65.91	T65.92	T65.93	T65.94	--	--
cosmetic	T65.891	T65.892	T65.893	T65.894	--	--
medicinal NEC	T50.901	T50.902	T50.903	T50.904	T50.905	T50.906
pesticides — *see Pesticides*						
specified content — *see specific substance*						
Spurge flax	T62.2X1	T62.2X2	T62.2X3	T62.2X4	--	--
Spurges	T62.2X1	T62.2X2	T62.2X3	T62.2X4	--	--
Sputum viscosity-lowering drug	T48.4X1	T48.4X2	T48.4X3	T48.4X4	T48.4X5	T48.4X6
Squill	T46.0X1	T46.0X2	T46.0X3	T46.0X4	T46.0X5	T46.0X6
rat poison	T60.4X1	T60.4X2	T60.4X3	T60.4X4	--	--
Squirting cucumber (cathartic)	T47.2X1	T47.2X2	T47.2X3	T47.2X4	T47.2X5	T47.2X6
Stains	T65.6X1	T65.6X2	T65.6X3	T65.6X4	--	--
Stannous fluoride	T49.7X1	T49.7X2	T49.7X3	T49.7X4	T49.7X5	T49.7X6
Stanolone	T38.7X1	T38.7X2	T38.7X3	T38.7X4	T38.7X5	T38.7X6
Stanozolol	T38.7X1	T38.7X2	T38.7X3	T38.7X4	T38.7X5	T38.7X6
Staphisagria or stavesacre (pediculicide)	T49.0X1	T49.0X2	T49.0X3	T49.0X4	T49.0X5	T49.0X6
Starch	T50.901	T50.902	T50.903	T50.904	T50.905	T50.906
Stelazine	T43.3X1	T43.3X2	T43.3X3	T43.3X4	T43.3X5	T43.3X6
Stemetil	T43.3X1	T43.3X2	T43.3X3	T43.3X4	T43.3X5	T43.3X6
Stepronin	T48.4X1	T48.4X2	T48.4X3	T48.4X4	T48.4X5	T48.4X6
Sterculia	T47.4X1	T47.4X2	T47.4X3	T47.4X4	T47.4X5	T47.4X6
Sternutator gas	T59.891	T59.892	T59.893	T59.894	--	--
Steroid	T38.0X1	T38.0X2	T38.0X3	T38.0X4	T38.0X5	T38.0X6
anabolic	T38.7X1	T38.7X2	T38.7X3	T38.7X4	T38.7X5	T38.7X6
androgenic	T38.7X1	T38.7X2	T38.7X3	T38.7X4	T38.7X5	T38.7X6
antineoplastic, hormone	T38.7X1	T38.7X2	T38.7X3	T38.7X4	T38.7X5	T38.7X6
estrogen	T38.5X1	T38.5X2	T38.5X3	T38.5X4	T38.5X5	T38.5X6
ENT agent	T49.6X1	T49.6X2	T49.6X3	T49.6X4	T49.6X5	T49.6X6
ophthalmic preparation	T49.5X1	T49.5X2	T49.5X3	T49.5X4	T49.5X5	T49.5X6
topical NEC	T49.0X1	T49.0X2	T49.0X3	T49.0X4	T49.0X5	T49.0X6
Stibine	T56.891	T56.892	T56.893	T56.894	--	--
Stibogluconate	T37.3X1	T37.3X2	T37.3X3	T37.3X4	T37.3X5	T37.3X6
Stibophen	T37.4X1	T37.4X2	T37.4X3	T37.4X4	T37.4X5	T37.4X6
Stilbamidine (isetionate)	T37.3X1	T37.3X2	T37.3X3	T37.3X4	T37.3X5	T37.3X6
Stilbestrol	T38.5X1	T38.5X2	T38.5X3	T38.5X4	T38.5X5	T38.5X6
Stilboestrol	T38.5X1	T38.5X2	T38.5X3	T38.5X4	T38.5X5	T38.5X6
Stimulant						
central nervous system — *see also Psychostimulant*	T43.601	T43.602	T43.603	T43.604	T43.605	T43.606
analeptics	T50.7X1	T50.7X2	T50.7X3	T50.7X4	T50.7X5	T50.7X6
opiate antagonist	T50.7X1	T50.7X2	T50.7X3	T50.7X4	T50.7X5	T50.7X6
psychotherapeutic NEC — *see also Psychotherapeutic drug*	T43.601	T43.602	T43.603	T43.604	T43.605	T43.606
specified NEC	T43.691	T43.692	T43.693	T43.694	T43.695	T43.696
respiratory	T48.901	T48.902	T48.903	T48.904	T48.905	T48.906
Stone-dissolving drug	T50.901	T50.902	T50.903	T50.904	T50.905	T50.906
Storage battery (cells) (acid)	T54.2X1	T54.2X2	T54.2X3	T54.2X4	--	--
Stovaine	T41.3X1	T41.3X2	T41.3X3	T41.3X4	T41.3X5	T41.3X6
infiltration (subcutaneous)	T41.3X1	T41.3X2	T41.3X3	T41.3X4	T41.3X5	T41.3X6
nerve block (peripheral) (plexus)	T41.3X1	T41.3X2	T41.3X3	T41.3X4	T41.3X5	T41.3X6
spinal	T41.3X1	T41.3X2	T41.3X3	T41.3X4	T41.3X5	T41.3X6
topical (surface)	T41.3X1	T41.3X2	T41.3X3	T41.3X4	T41.3X5	T41.3X6
Stovarsal	T37.8X1	T37.8X2	T37.8X3	T37.8X4	T37.8X5	T37.8X6
Stove gas — *see Gas, stove*						
Stoxil	T49.5X1	T49.5X2	T49.5X3	T49.5X4	T49.5X5	T49.5X6

Substance	Poisoning, Accidental unintentional	Poisoning, Intentional self-harm	Poisoning, Assault	Poisoning, Undetermined	Adverse effect	Underdosing
Stramonium	T48.6X1	T48.6X2	T48.6X3	T48.6X4	T48.6X5	T48.6X6
natural state	T62.2X1	T62.2X2	T62.2X3	T62.2X4	—	—
Streptodornase	T45.3X1	T45.3X2	T45.3X3	T45.3X4	T45.3X5	T45.3X6
Streptoduocin	T36.5X1	T36.5X2	T36.5X3	T36.5X4	T36.5X5	T36.5X6
Streptokinase	T45.611	T45.612	T45.613	T45.614	T45.615	T45.616
Streptomycin (derivative)	T36.5X1	T36.5X2	T36.5X3	T36.5X4	T36.5X5	T36.5X6
Streptonivicin	T36.5X1	T36.5X2	T36.5X3	T36.5X4	T36.5X5	T36.5X6
Streptovarycin	T36.5X1	T36.5X2	T36.5X3	T36.5X4	T36.5X5	T36.5X6
Streptozocin	T45.1X1	T45.1X2	T45.1X3	T45.1X4	T45.1X5	T45.1X6
Streptozotocin	T45.1X1	T45.1X2	T45.1X3	T45.1X4	T45.1X5	T45.1X6
Stripper (paint) (solvent)	T52.8X1	T52.8X2	T52.8X3	T52.8X4	—	—
Strobane	T60.1X1	T60.1X2	T60.1X3	T60.1X4	—	—
Strofantina	T46.0X1	T46.0X2	T46.0X3	T46.0X4	T46.0X5	T46.0X6
Strophanthin (g) (k)	T46.0X1	T46.0X2	T46.0X3	T46.0X4	T46.0X5	T46.0X6
Strophanthus	T46.0X1	T46.0X2	T46.0X3	T46.0X4	T46.0X5	T46.0X6
Strophantin	T46.0X1	T46.0X2	T46.0X3	T46.0X4	T46.0X5	T46.0X6
Strophantin-g	T46.0X1	T46.0X2	T46.0X3	T46.0X4	T46.0X5	T46.0X6
Strychnine (nonmedicinal) (pesticide) (salts)	T65.1X1	T65.1X2	T65.1X3	T65.1X4	—	—
medicinal	T48.291	T48.292	T48.293	T48.294	T48.295	T48.296
Strychnos (ignatii) — *see Strychnine*						
Styramate	T42.8X1	T42.8X2	T42.8X3	T42.8X4	T42.8X5	T42.8X6
Styrene	T65.891	T65.892	T65.893	T65.894	—	—
Succinimide, antiepileptic or anticonvulsant	T42.2X1	T42.2X2	T42.2X3	T42.2X4	T42.2X5	T42.2X6
mercuric — *see Mercury*						
Succinylcholine	T48.1X1	T48.1X2	T48.1X3	T48.1X4	T48.1X5	T48.1X6
Succinylsulfathiazole	T37.0X1	T37.0X2	T37.0X3	T37.0X4	T37.0X5	T37.0X6
Sucralfate	T47.1X1	T47.1X2	T47.1X3	T47.1X4	T47.1X5	T47.1X6
Sucrose	T50.3X1	T50.3X2	T50.3X3	T50.3X4	T50.3X5	T50.3X6
Sufentanil	T40.4X1	T40.4X2	T40.4X3	T40.4X4	T40.4X5	T40.4X6
Sulbactam	T36.0X1	T36.0X2	T36.0X3	T36.0X4	T36.0X5	T36.0X6
Sulbenicillin	T36.0X1	T36.0X2	T36.0X3	T36.0X4	T36.0X5	T36.0X6
Sulbentine	T49.0X1	T49.0X2	T49.0X3	T49.0X4	T49.0X5	T49.0X6
Sulfacetamide	T49.0X1	T49.0X2	T49.0X3	T49.0X4	T49.0X5	T49.0X6
ophthalmic preparation	T49.5X1	T49.5X2	T49.5X3	T49.5X4	T49.5X5	T49.5X6
Sulfachlorpyridazine	T37.0X1	T37.0X2	T37.0X3	T37.0X4	T37.0X5	T37.0X6
Sulfacitine	T37.0X1	T37.0X2	T37.0X3	T37.0X4	T37.0X5	T37.0X6
Sulfadiasulfone sodium	T37.0X1	T37.0X2	T37.0X3	T37.0X4	T37.0X5	T37.0X6
Sulfadiazine	T37.0X1	T37.0X2	T37.0X3	T37.0X4	T37.0X5	T37.0X6
silver (topical)	T49.0X1	T49.0X2	T49.0X3	T49.0X4	T49.0X5	T49.0X6
Sulfadimethoxine	T37.0X1	T37.0X2	T37.0X3	T37.0X4	T37.0X5	T37.0X6
Sulfadimidine	T37.0X1	T37.0X2	T37.0X3	T37.0X4	T37.0X5	T37.0X6
Sulfadoxine	T37.0X1	T37.0X2	T37.0X3	T37.0X4	T37.0X5	T37.0X6
with pyrimethamine	T37.2X1	T37.2X2	T37.2X3	T37.2X4	T37.2X5	T37.2X6
Sulfaethidole	T37.0X1	T37.0X2	T37.0X3	T37.0X4	T37.0X5	T37.0X6
Sulfafurazole	T37.0X1	T37.0X2	T37.0X3	T37.0X4	T37.0X5	T37.0X6
Sulfaguanidine	T37.0X1	T37.0X2	T37.0X3	T37.0X4	T37.0X5	T37.0X6
Sulfalene	T37.0X1	T37.0X2	T37.0X3	T37.0X4	T37.0X5	T37.0X6
Sulfaloxate	T37.0X1	T37.0X2	T37.0X3	T37.0X4	T37.0X5	T37.0X6
Sulfaloxic acid	T37.0X1	T37.0X2	T37.0X3	T37.0X4	T37.0X5	T37.0X6
Sulfamazone	T39.2X1	T39.2X2	T39.2X3	T39.2X4	T39.2X5	T39.2X6
Sulfamerazine	T37.0X1	T37.0X2	T37.0X3	T37.0X4	T37.0X5	T37.0X6
Sulfameter	T37.0X1	T37.0X2	T37.0X3	T37.0X4	T37.0X5	T37.0X6
Sulfamethazine	T37.0X1	T37.0X2	T37.0X3	T37.0X4	T37.0X5	T37.0X6
Sulfamethizole	T37.0X1	T37.0X2	T37.0X3	T37.0X4	T37.0X5	T37.0X6
Sulfamethoxazole	T37.0X1	T37.0X2	T37.0X3	T37.0X4	T37.0X5	T37.0X6
with trimethoprim	T36.8X1	T36.8X2	T36.8X3	T36.8X4	T36.8X5	T36.8X6
Sulfamethoxydiazine	T37.0X1	T37.0X2	T37.0X3	T37.0X4	T37.0X5	T37.0X6
Sulfamethoxypyridazine	T37.0X1	T37.0X2	T37.0X3	T37.0X4	T37.0X5	T37.0X6
Sulfamethylthiazole	T37.0X1	T37.0X2	T37.0X3	T37.0X4	T37.0X5	T37.0X6
Sulfametoxydiazine	T37.0X1	T37.0X2	T37.0X3	T37.0X4	T37.0X5	T37.0X6
Sulfamidopyrine	T39.2X1	T39.2X2	T39.2X3	T39.2X4	T39.2X5	T39.2X6
Sulfamonomethoxine	T37.0X1	T37.0X2	T37.0X3	T37.0X4	T37.0X5	T37.0X6
Sulfamoxole	T37.0X1	T37.0X2	T37.0X3	T37.0X4	T37.0X5	T37.0X6
Sulfamylon	T49.0X1	T49.0X2	T49.0X3	T49.0X4	T49.0X5	T49.0X6
Sulfan blue (diagnostic dye)	T50.8X1	T50.8X2	T50.8X3	T50.8X4	T50.8X5	T50.8X6
Sulfanilamide	T37.0X1	T37.0X2	T37.0X3	T37.0X4	T37.0X5	T37.0X6
Sulfanilylguanidine	T37.0X1	T37.0X2	T37.0X3	T37.0X4	T37.0X5	T37.0X6
Sulfaperin	T37.0X1	T37.0X2	T37.0X3	T37.0X4	T37.0X5	T37.0X6
Sulfaphenazole	T37.0X1	T37.0X2	T37.0X3	T37.0X4	T37.0X5	T37.0X6
Sulfaphenylthiazole	T37.0X1	T37.0X2	T37.0X3	T37.0X4	T37.0X5	T37.0X6
Sulfaproxyline	T37.0X1	T37.0X2	T37.0X3	T37.0X4	T37.0X5	T37.0X6
Sulfapyridine	T37.0X1	T37.0X2	T37.0X3	T37.0X4	T37.0X5	T37.0X6
Sulfapyrimidine	T37.0X1	T37.0X2	T37.0X3	T37.0X4	T37.0X5	T37.0X6
Sulfarsphenamine	T37.8X1	T37.8X2	T37.8X3	T37.8X4	T37.8X5	T37.8X6
Sulfasalazine	T37.0X1	T37.0X2	T37.0X3	T37.0X4	T37.0X5	T37.0X6
Sulfasuxidine	T37.0X1	T37.0X2	T37.0X3	T37.0X4	T37.0X5	T37.0X6
Sulfasymazine	T37.0X1	T37.0X2	T37.0X3	T37.0X4	T37.0X5	T37.0X6
Sulfated amylopectin	T47.8X1	T47.8X2	T47.8X3	T47.8X4	T47.8X5	T47.8X6
Sulfathiazole	T37.0X1	T37.0X2	T37.0X3	T37.0X4	T37.0X5	T37.0X6
Sulfatostearate	T49.2X1	T49.2X2	T49.2X3	T49.2X4	T49.2X5	T49.2X6
Sulfinpyrazone	T50.4X1	T50.4X2	T50.4X3	T50.4X4	T50.4X5	T50.4X6
Sulfiram	T49.0X1	T49.0X2	T49.0X3	T49.0X4	T49.0X5	T49.0X6
Sulfisomidine	T37.0X1	T37.0X2	T37.0X3	T37.0X4	T37.0X5	T37.0X6
Sulfisoxazole	T37.0X1	T37.0X2	T37.0X3	T37.0X4	T37.0X5	T37.0X6
ophthalmic preparation	T49.5X1	T49.5X2	T49.5X3	T49.5X4	T49.5X5	T49.5X6
Sulfobromophthalein (sodium)	T50.8X1	T50.8X2	T50.8X3	T50.8X4	T50.8X5	T50.8X6
Sulfobromphthalein	T50.8X1	T50.8X2	T50.8X3	T50.8X4	T50.8X5	T50.8X6
Sulfogaiacol	T48.4X1	T48.4X2	T48.4X3	T48.4X4	T48.4X5	T48.4X6
Sulfomyxin	T36.8X1	T36.8X2	T36.8X3	T36.8X4	T36.8X5	T36.8X6
Sulfonal	T42.6X1	T42.6X2	T42.6X3	T42.6X4	T42.6X5	T42.6X6
Sulfonamide NEC	T37.0X1	T37.0X2	T37.0X3	T37.0X4	T37.0X5	T37.0X6
eye	T49.5X1	T49.5X2	T49.5X3	T49.5X4	T49.5X5	T49.5X6
Sulfonazide	T37.1X1	T37.1X2	T37.1X3	T37.1X4	T37.1X5	T37.1X6
Sulfones	T37.1X1	T37.1X2	T37.1X3	T37.1X4	T37.1X5	T37.1X6
Sulfonethylmethane	T42.6X1	T42.6X2	T42.6X3	T42.6X4	T42.6X5	T42.6X6
Sulfonmethane	T42.6X1	T42.6X2	T42.6X3	T42.6X4	T42.6X5	T42.6X6
Sulfonphthal, sulfonphthol	T50.8X1	T50.8X2	T50.8X3	T50.8X4	T50.8X5	T50.8X6
Sulfonylurea derivatives, oral	T38.3X1	T38.3X2	T38.3X3	T38.3X4	T38.3X5	T38.3X6
Sulforidazine	T43.3X1	T43.3X2	T43.3X3	T43.3X4	T43.3X5	T43.3X6
Sulfoxone	T37.1X1	T37.1X2	T37.1X3	T37.1X4	T37.1X5	T37.1X6
Sulfur, sulfurated, sulfuric, sulfurous, sulfuryl (compounds NEC) (medicinal)	T49.4X1	T49.4X2	T49.4X3	T49.4X4	T49.4X5	T49.4X6
acid	T54.2X1	T54.2X2	T54.2X3	T54.2X4	—	—
dioxide (gas)	T59.1X1	T59.1X2	T59.1X3	T59.1X4	—	—
ether — *see Ether (s)*						
hydrogen	T59.6X1	T59.6X2	T59.6X3	T59.6X4	—	—
medicinal (keratolytic) (ointment) NEC	T49.4X1	T49.4X2	T49.4X3	T49.4X4	T49.4X5	T49.4X6
ointment	T49.0X1	T49.0X2	T49.0X3	T49.0X4	T49.0X5	T49.0X6
pesticide (vapor)	T60.91	T60.92	T60.93	T60.94	—	—
vapor NEC	T59.891	T59.892	T59.893	T59.894	—	—
Sulfuric acid	T54.2X1	T54.2X2	T54.2X3	T54.2X4	—	—
Sulglicotide	T47.1X1	T47.1X2	T47.1X3	T47.1X4	T47.1X5	T47.1X6
Sulindac	T39.391	T39.392	T39.393	T39.394	T39.395	T39.396
Sulisatin	T47.2X1	T47.2X2	T47.2X3	T47.2X4	T47.2X5	T47.2X6
Sulisobenzone	T49.3X1	T49.3X2	T49.3X3	T49.3X4	T49.3X5	T49.3X6
Sulkowitch's reagent	T50.8X1	T50.8X2	T50.8X3	T50.8X4	T50.8X5	T50.8X6
Sulmetozine	T44.3X1	T44.3X2	T44.3X3	T44.3X4	T44.3X5	T44.3X6
Suloctidil	T46.7X1	T46.7X2	T46.7X3	T46.7X4	T46.7X5	T46.7X6
Sulph- — *see also Sulf-*						
Sulphadiazine	T37.0X1	T37.0X2	T37.0X3	T37.0X4	T37.0X5	T37.0X6
Sulphadimethoxine	T37.0X1	T37.0X2	T37.0X3	T37.0X4	T37.0X5	T37.0X6
Sulphadimidine	T37.0X1	T37.0X2	T37.0X3	T37.0X4	T37.0X5	T37.0X6
Sulphadione	T37.1X1	T37.1X2	T37.1X3	T37.1X4	T37.1X5	T37.1X6
Sulphafurazole	T37.0X1	T37.0X2	T37.0X3	T37.0X4	T37.0X5	T37.0X6
Sulphamethizole	T37.0X1	T37.0X2	T37.0X3	T37.0X4	T37.0X5	T37.0X6
Sulphamethoxazole	T37.0X1	T37.0X2	T37.0X3	T37.0X4	T37.0X5	T37.0X6
Sulphan blue	T50.8X1	T50.8X2	T50.8X3	T50.8X4	T50.8X5	T50.8X6
Sulphaphenazole	T37.0X1	T37.0X2	T37.0X3	T37.0X4	T37.0X5	T37.0X6
Sulphapyridine	T37.0X1	T37.0X2	T37.0X3	T37.0X4	T37.0X5	T37.0X6
Sulphasalazine	T37.0X1	T37.0X2	T37.0X3	T37.0X4	T37.0X5	T37.0X6
Sulphinpyrazone	T50.4X1	T50.4X2	T50.4X3	T50.4X4	T50.4X5	T50.4X6
Sulpiride	T43.591	T43.592	T43.593	T43.594	T43.595	T43.596
Sulprostone	T48.0X1	T48.0X2	T48.0X3	T48.0X4	T48.0X5	T48.0X6
Sulpyrine	T39.2X1	T39.2X2	T39.2X3	T39.2X4	T39.2X5	T39.2X6
Sultamicillin	T36.0X1	T36.0X2	T36.0X3	T36.0X4	T36.0X5	T36.0X6
Sulthiame	T42.6X1	T42.6X2	T42.6X3	T42.6X4	T42.6X5	T42.6X6
Sultiame	T42.6X1	T42.6X2	T42.6X3	T42.6X4	T42.6X5	T42.6X6
Sultopride	T43.591	T43.592	T43.593	T43.594	T43.595	T43.596
Sumatriptan	T39.8X1	T39.8X2	T39.8X3	T39.8X4	T39.8X5	T39.8X6
Sunflower seed oil	T46.6X1	T46.6X2	T46.6X3	T46.6X4	T46.6X5	T46.6X6
Superinone	T48.4X1	T48.4X2	T48.4X3	T48.4X4	T48.4X5	T48.4X6
Suprofen	T39.311	T39.312	T39.313	T39.314	T39.315	T39.316
Suramin (sodium)	T37.4X1	T37.4X2	T37.4X3	T37.4X4	T37.4X5	T37.4X6
Surfacaine	T41.3X1	T41.3X2	T41.3X3	T41.3X4	T41.3X5	T41.3X6
Surital	T41.1X1	T41.1X2	T41.1X3	T41.1X4	T41.1X5	T41.1X6
Sutilains	T45.3X1	T45.3X2	T45.3X3	T45.3X4	T45.3X5	T45.3X6
Suxamethonium (chloride)	T48.1X1	T48.1X2	T48.1X3	T48.1X4	T48.1X5	T48.1X6
Suxethonium (chloride)	T48.1X1	T48.1X2	T48.1X3	T48.1X4	T48.1X5	T48.1X6
Suxibuzone	T39.2X1	T39.2X2	T39.2X3	T39.2X4	T39.2X5	T39.2X6
Sweet niter spirit	T46.3X1	T46.3X2	T46.3X3	T46.3X4	T46.3X5	T46.3X6
Sweet oil (birch)	T49.3X1	T49.3X2	T49.3X3	T49.3X4	T49.3X5	T49.3X6
Sweetener	T50.901	T50.902	T50.903	T50.904	T50.905	T50.906
Sym-dichloroethyl ether	T53.6X1	T53.6X2	T53.6X3	T53.6X4	—	—
Sympatholytic NEC	T44.8X1	T44.8X2	T44.8X3	T44.8X4	T44.8X5	T44.8X6
haloalkylamine	T44.8X1	T44.8X2	T44.8X3	T44.8X4	T44.8X5	T44.8X6
Sympathomimetic NEC	T44.901	T44.902	T44.903	T44.904	T44.905	T44.906
anti-common-cold	T48.5X1	T48.5X2	T48.5X3	T48.5X4	T48.5X5	T48.5X6
bronchodilator	T48.6X1	T48.6X2	T48.6X3	T48.6X4	T48.6X5	T48.6X6
specified NEC	T44.991	T44.992	T44.993	T44.994	T44.995	T44.996
Synagis	T50.B91	T50.B92	T50.B93	T50.B94	T50.B95	T50.B96
Synalar	T49.0X1	T49.0X2	T49.0X3	T49.0X4	T49.0X5	T49.0X6
Synthroid	T38.1X1	T38.1X2	T38.1X3	T38.1X4	T38.1X5	T38.1X6
Syntocinon	T48.0X1	T48.0X2	T48.0X3	T48.0X4	T48.0X5	T48.0X6
Syrosingopine	T46.5X1	T46.5X2	T46.5X3	T46.5X4	T46.5X5	T46.5X6

Substance	Poisoning, Accidental unintentional	Poisoning, Intentional self-harm	Poisoning, Assault	Poisoning, Undetermined	Adverse effect	Underdosing
Systemic drug	T45.91	T45.92	T45.93	T45.94	T45.95	T45.96
specified NEC	T45.8X1	T45.8X2	T45.8X3	T45.8X4	T45.8X5	T45.8X6
2,4,5-T	T60.3X1	T60.3X2	T60.3X3	T60.3X4	—	—
T						
Tablets — *see also specified substance*	T50.901	T50.902	T50.903	T50.904	T50.905	T50.906
Tace	T38.5X1	T38.5X2	T38.5X3	T38.5X4	T38.5X5	T38.5X6
Tacrine	T44.0X1	T44.0X2	T44.0X3	T44.0X4	T44.0X5	T44.0X6
Tadalafil	T46.7X1	T46.7X2	T46.7X3	T46.7X4	T46.7X5	T46.7X6
Talampicillin	T36.0X1	T36.0X2	T36.0X3	T36.0X4	T36.0X5	T36.0X6
Talbutal	T42.3X1	T42.3X2	T42.3X3	T42.3X4	T42.3X5	T42.3X6
Talc powder	T49.3X1	T49.3X2	T49.3X3	T49.3X4	T49.3X5	T49.3X6
Talcum	T49.3X1	T49.3X2	T49.3X3	T49.3X4	T49.3X5	T49.3X6
Taleranol	T38.6X1	T38.6X2	T38.6X3	T38.6X4	T38.6X5	T38.6X6
Tamoxifen	T38.6X1	T38.6X2	T38.6X3	T38.6X4	T38.6X5	T38.6X6
Tamsulosin	T44.6X1	T44.6X2	T44.6X3	T44.6X4	T44.6X5	T44.6X6
Tandearil, tanderil	T39.2X1	T39.2X2	T39.2X3	T39.2X4	T39.2X5	T39.2X6
Tannic acid	T49.2X1	T49.2X2	T49.2X3	T49.2X4	T49.2X5	T49.2X6
medicinal (astringent)	T49.2X1	T49.2X2	T49.2X3	T49.2X4	T49.2X5	T49.2X6
Tannin — *see Tannic acid*						
Tansy	T62.2X1	T62.2X2	T62.2X3	T62.2X4	—	—
TAO	T36.3X1	T36.3X2	T36.3X3	T36.3X4	T36.3X5	T36.3X6
Tapazole	T38.2X1	T38.2X2	T38.2X3	T38.2X4	T38.2X5	T38.2X6
Tar NEC	T52.0X1	T52.0X2	T52.0X3	T52.0X4	—	—
camphor	T60.1X1	T60.1X2	T60.1X3	T60.1X4	—	—
distillate	T49.1X1	T49.1X2	T49.1X3	T49.1X4	T49.1X5	T49.1X6
fumes	T59.891	T59.892	T59.893	T59.894	—	—
medicinal	T49.1X1	T49.1X2	T49.1X3	T49.1X4	T49.1X5	T49.1X6
ointment	T49.1X1	T49.1X2	T49.1X3	T49.1X4	T49.1X5	T49.1X6
Taractan	T43.591	T43.592	T43.593	T43.594	T43.595	T43.596
Tarantula (venomous)	T63.321	T63.322	T63.323	T63.324	—	—
Tartar emetic	T37.8X1	T37.8X2	T37.8X3	T37.8X4	T37.8X5	T37.8X6
Tartaric acid	T65.891	T65.892	T65.893	T65.894	—	—
Tartrate, laxative	T47.4X1	T47.4X2	T47.4X3	T47.4X4	T47.4X5	T47.4X6
Tartrated antimony (anti-infective)	T37.8X1	T37.8X2	T37.8X3	T37.8X4	T37.8X5	T37.8X6
Tauromustine	T45.1X1	T45.1X2	T45.1X3	T45.1X4	T45.1X5	T45.1X6
TCA — *see Trichloroacetic acid*						
TCDD	T53.7X1	T53.7X2	T53.7X3	T53.7X4	—	—
TDI (vapor)	T65.0X1	T65.0X2	T65.0X3	T65.0X4	—	—
Tear						
gas	T59.3X1	T59.3X2	T59.3X3	T59.3X4	—	—
solution	T49.5X1	T49.5X2	T49.5X3	T49.5X4	T49.5X5	T49.5X6
Teclothiazide	T50.2X1	T50.2X2	T50.2X3	T50.2X4	T50.2X5	T50.2X6
Teclozan	T37.3X1	T37.3X2	T37.3X3	T37.3X4	T37.3X5	T37.3X6
Tegafur	T45.1X1	T45.1X2	T45.1X3	T45.1X4	T45.1X5	T45.1X6
Tegretol	T42.1X1	T42.1X2	T42.1X3	T42.1X4	T42.1X5	T42.1X6
Teicoplanin	T36.8X1	T36.8X2	T36.8X3	T36.8X4	T36.8X5	T36.8X6
Telepaque	T50.8X1	T50.8X2	T50.8X3	T50.8X4	T50.8X5	T50.8X6
Tellurium	T56.891	T56.892	T56.893	T56.894	—	—
fumes	T56.891	T56.892	T56.893	T56.894	—	—
TEM	T45.1X1	T45.1X2	T45.1X3	T45.1X4	T45.1X5	T45.1X6
Temazepam	T42.4X1	T42.4X2	T42.4X3	T42.4X4	T42.4X5	T42.4X6
Temocillin	T36.0X1	T36.0X2	T36.0X3	T36.0X4	T36.0X5	T36.0X6
Tenamfetamine	T43.621	T43.622	T43.623	T43.624	T43.625	T43.626
Teniposide	T45.1X1	T45.1X2	T45.1X3	T45.1X4	T45.1X5	T45.1X6
Tenitramine	T46.3X1	T46.3X2	T46.3X3	T46.3X4	T46.3X5	T46.3X6
Tenoglicin	T48.4X1	T48.4X2	T48.4X3	T48.4X4	T48.4X5	T48.4X6
Tenonitrozole	T37.3X1	T37.3X2	T37.3X3	T37.3X4	T37.3X5	T37.3X6
Tenoxicam	T39.391	T39.392	T39.393	T39.394	T39.395	T39.396
TEPA	T45.1X1	T45.1X2	T45.1X3	T45.1X4	T45.1X5	T45.1X6
TEPP	T60.0X1	T60.0X2	T60.0X3	T60.0X4	—	—
Teprotide	T46.5X1	T46.5X2	T46.5X3	T46.5X4	T46.5X5	T46.5X6
Terazosin	T44.6X1	T44.6X2	T44.6X3	T44.6X4	T44.6X5	T44.6X6
Terbufos	T60.0X1	T60.0X2	T60.0X3	T60.0X4	—	—
Terbutaline	T48.6X1	T48.6X2	T48.6X3	T48.6X4	T48.6X5	T48.6X6
Terconazole	T49.0X1	T49.0X2	T49.0X3	T49.0X4	T49.0X5	T49.0X6
Terfenadine	T45.0X1	T45.0X2	T45.0X3	T45.0X4	T45.0X5	T45.0X6
Teriparatide (acetate)	T50.991	T50.992	T50.993	T50.994	T50.995	T50.996
Terizidone	T37.1X1	T37.1X2	T37.1X3	T37.1X4	T37.1X5	T37.1X6
Terlipressin	T38.891	T38.892	T38.893	T38.894	T38.895	T38.896
Terodiline	T46.3X1	T46.3X2	T46.3X3	T46.3X4	T46.3X5	T46.3X6
Teroxalene	T37.4X1	T37.4X2	T37.4X3	T37.4X4	T37.4X5	T37.4X6
Terpin (cis) hydrate	T48.4X1	T48.4X2	T48.4X3	T48.4X4	T48.4X5	T48.4X6
Terramycin	T36.4X1	T36.4X2	T36.4X3	T36.4X4	T36.4X5	T36.4X6
Tertatolol	T44.7X1	T44.7X2	T44.7X3	T44.7X4	T44.7X5	T44.7X6
Tessalon	T48.3X1	T48.3X2	T48.3X3	T48.3X4	T48.3X5	T48.3X6
Testolactone	T38.7X1	T38.7X2	T38.7X3	T38.7X4	T38.7X5	T38.7X6
Testosterone	T38.7X1	T38.7X2	T38.7X3	T38.7X4	T38.7X5	T38.7X6
Tetanus toxoid or vaccine	T50.A91	T50.A92	T50.A93	T50.A94	T50.A95	T50.A96
antitoxin	T50.Z11	T50.Z12	T50.Z13	T50.Z14	T50.Z15	T50.Z16
immune globulin (human)	T50.Z11	T50.Z12	T50.Z13	T50.Z14	T50.Z15	T50.Z16
toxoid	T50.A91	T50.A92	T50.A93	T50.A94	T50.A95	T50.A96
with diphtheria toxoid	T50.A21	T50.A22	T50.A23	T50.A24	T50.A25	T50.A26
with pertussis	T50.A11	T50.A12	T50.A13	T50.A14	T50.A15	T50.A16
Tetrabenazine	T43.591	T43.592	T43.593	T43.594	T43.595	T43.596
Tetracaine	T41.3X1	T41.3X2	T41.3X3	T41.3X4	T41.3X5	T41.3X6
nerve block (peripheral) (plexus)	T41.3X1	T41.3X2	T41.3X3	T41.3X4	T41.3X5	T41.3X6
regional	T41.3X1	T41.3X2	T41.3X3	T41.3X4	T41.3X5	T41.3X6
spinal	T41.3X1	T41.3X2	T41.3X3	T41.3X4	T41.3X5	T41.3X6
Tetrachlorethylene — *see Tetrachloroethylene*						
Tetrachlormethiazide	T50.2X1	T50.2X2	T50.2X3	T50.2X4	T50.2X5	T50.2X6
2,3,7,8-Tetrachlorodibenzo-p-dioxin	T53.7X1	T53.7X2	T53.7X3	T53.7X4	—	—
Tetrachloroethane	T53.6X1	T53.6X2	T53.6X3	T53.6X4	—	—
vapor	T53.6X1	T53.6X2	T53.6X3	T53.6X4	—	—
paint or varnish	T53.6X1	T53.6X2	T53.6X3	T53.6X4	—	—
Tetrachloroethylene (liquid)	T53.3X1	T53.3X2	T53.3X3	T53.3X4	—	—
medicinal	T37.4X1	T37.4X2	T37.4X3	T37.4X4	T37.4X5	T37.4X6
vapor	T53.3X1	T53.3X2	T53.3X3	T53.3X4	—	—
Tetrachloromethane — *see Carbon tetrachloride*						
Tetracosactide	T38.811	T38.812	T38.813	T38.814	T38.815	T38.816
Tetracosactrin	T38.811	T38.812	T38.813	T38.814	T38.815	T38.816
Tetracycline	T36.4X1	T36.4X2	T36.4X3	T36.4X4	T36.4X5	T36.4X6
ophthalmic preparation	T49.5X1	T49.5X2	T49.5X3	T49.5X4	T49.5X5	T49.5X6
topical NEC	T49.0X1	T49.0X2	T49.0X3	T49.0X4	T49.0X5	T49.0X6
Tetradifon	T60.8X1	T60.8X2	T60.8X3	T60.8X4	—	—
Tetradotoxin	T61.771	T61.772	T61.773	T61.774	—	—
Tetraethyl						
lead	T56.0X1	T56.0X2	T56.0X3	T56.0X4	—	—
pyrophosphate	T60.0X1	T60.0X2	T60.0X3	T60.0X4	—	—
Tetraethylammonium chloride	T44.2X1	T44.2X2	T44.2X3	T44.2X4	T44.2X5	T44.2X6
Tetraethylthiuram disulfide	T50.6X1	T50.6X2	T50.6X3	T50.6X4	T50.6X5	T50.6X6
Tetrahydroaminoacridine	T44.0X1	T44.0X2	T44.0X3	T44.0X4	T44.0X5	T44.0X6
Tetrahydrocannabinol	T40.7X1	T40.7X2	T40.7X3	T40.7X4	T40.7X5	T40.7X6
Tetrahydrofuran	T52.8X1	T52.8X2	T52.8X3	T52.8X4	—	—
Tetrahydronaphthalene	T52.8X1	T52.8X2	T52.8X3	T52.8X4	—	—
Tetrahydrozoline	T49.5X1	T49.5X2	T49.5X3	T49.5X4	T49.5X5	T49.5X6
Tetralin	T52.8X1	T52.8X2	T52.8X3	T52.8X4	—	—
Tetramethrin	T60.2X1	T60.2X2	T60.2X3	T60.2X4	—	—
Tetramethylthiuram (disulfide) **NEC**	T60.3X1	T60.3X2	T60.3X3	T60.3X4	—	—
medicinal	T49.0X1	T49.0X2	T49.0X3	T49.0X4	T49.0X5	T49.0X6
Tetramisole	T37.4X1	T37.4X2	T37.4X3	T37.4X4	T37.4X5	T37.4X6
Tetranicotinoyl fructose	T46.7X1	T46.7X2	T46.7X3	T46.7X4	T46.7X5	T46.7X6
Tetrazepam	T42.4X1	T42.4X2	T42.4X3	T42.4X4	T42.4X5	T42.4X6
Tetronal	T42.6X1	T42.6X2	T42.6X3	T42.6X4	T42.6X5	T42.6X6
Tetryl	T65.3X1	T65.3X2	T65.3X3	T65.3X4	—	—
Tetrylammonium chloride	T44.2X1	T44.2X2	T44.2X3	T44.2X4	T44.2X5	T44.2X6
Tetryzoline	T49.5X1	T49.5X2	T49.5X3	T49.5X4	T49.5X5	T49.5X6
Thalidomide	T45.1X1	T45.1X2	T45.1X3	T45.1X4	T45.1X5	T45.1X6
Thallium (compounds) (dust) **NEC**	T56.811	T56.812	T56.813	T56.814	—	—
pesticide	T60.4X1	T60.4X2	T60.4X3	T60.4X4	—	—
THC	T40.7X1	T40.7X2	T40.7X3	T40.7X4	T40.7X5	T40.7X6
Thebacon	T48.3X1	T48.3X2	T48.3X3	T48.3X4	T48.3X5	T48.3X6
Thebaine	T40.2X1	T40.2X2	T40.2X3	T40.2X4	T40.2X5	T40.2X6
Thenoic acid	T49.6X1	T49.6X2	T49.6X3	T49.6X4	T49.6X5	T49.6X6
Thenyldiamine	T45.0X1	T45.0X2	T45.0X3	T45.0X4	T45.0X5	T45.0X6
Theobromine (calcium salicylate)	T48.6X1	T48.6X2	T48.6X3	T48.6X4	T48.6X5	T48.6X6
sodium salicylate	T48.6X1	T48.6X2	T48.6X3	T48.6X4	T48.6X5	T48.6X6
Theophyllamine	T48.6X1	T48.6X2	T48.6X3	T48.6X4	T48.6X5	T48.6X6
Theophylline	T48.6X1	T48.6X2	T48.6X3	T48.6X4	T48.6X5	T48.6X6
aminobenzoic acid	T48.6X1	T48.6X2	T48.6X3	T48.6X4	T48.6X5	T48.6X6
ethylenediamine	T48.6X1	T48.6X2	T48.6X3	T48.6X4	T48.6X5	T48.6X6
piperazine p-aminobenzoate	T48.6X1	T48.6X2	T48.6X3	T48.6X4	T48.6X5	T48.6X6
Thiabendazole	T37.4X1	T37.4X2	T37.4X3	T37.4X4	T37.4X5	T37.4X6
Thialbarbital	T41.1X1	T41.1X2	T41.1X3	T41.1X4	T41.1X5	T41.1X6
Thiamazole	T38.2X1	T38.2X2	T38.2X3	T38.2X4	T38.2X5	T38.2X6
Thiambutosine	T37.1X1	T37.1X2	T37.1X3	T37.1X4	T37.1X5	T37.1X6
Thiamine	T45.2X1	T45.2X2	T45.2X3	T45.2X4	T45.2X5	T45.2X6
Thiamphenicol	T36.2X1	T36.2X2	T36.2X3	T36.2X4	T36.2X5	T36.2X6
Thiamylal	T41.1X1	T41.1X2	T41.1X3	T41.1X4	T41.1X5	T41.1X6
sodium	T41.1X1	T41.1X2	T41.1X3	T41.1X4	T41.1X5	T41.1X6
Thiazesim	T43.291	T43.292	T43.293	T43.294	T43.295	T43.296
Thiazides (diuretics)	T50.2X1	T50.2X2	T50.2X3	T50.2X4	T50.2X5	T50.2X6
Thiazinamium metilsulfate	T43.3X1	T43.3X2	T43.3X3	T43.3X4	T43.3X5	T43.3X6
Thiethylperazine	T43.3X1	T43.3X2	T43.3X3	T43.3X4	T43.3X5	T43.3X6
Thimerosal	T49.0X1	T49.0X2	T49.0X3	T49.0X4	T49.0X5	T49.0X6
ophthalmic preparation	T49.5X1	T49.5X2	T49.5X3	T49.5X4	T49.5X5	T49.5X6
Thioacetazone	T37.1X1	T37.1X2	T37.1X3	T37.1X4	T37.1X5	T37.1X6
with isoniazid	T37.1X1	T37.1X2	T37.1X3	T37.1X4	T37.1X5	T37.1X6

Thiobarbital sodium - Tranquilizer NEC

Substance	Poisoning, Accidental unintentional	Poisoning, Intentional self-harm	Poisoning, Assault	Poisoning, Undetermined	Adverse effect	Underdosing
Thiobarbital sodium	T41.1X1	T41.1X2	T41.1X3	T41.1X4	T41.1X5	T41.1X6
Thiobarbiturate anesthetic	T41.1X1	T41.1X2	T41.1X3	T41.1X4	T41.1X5	T41.1X6
Thiobismol	T37.8X1	T37.8X2	T37.8X3	T37.8X4	T37.8X5	T37.8X6
Thiobutabarbital sodium	T41.1X1	T41.1X2	T41.1X3	T41.1X4	T41.1X5	T41.1X6
Thiocarbamate (insecticide)	T60.0X1	T60.0X2	T60.0X3	T60.0X4	--	--
Thiocarbamide	T38.2X1	T38.2X2	T38.2X3	T38.2X4	T38.2X5	T38.2X6
Thiocarbarsone	T37.8X1	T37.8X2	T37.8X3	T37.8X4	T37.8X5	T37.8X6
Thiocarlide	T37.1X1	T37.1X2	T37.1X3	T37.1X4	T37.1X5	T37.1X6
Thioctamide	T50.991	T50.992	T50.993	T50.994	T50.995	T50.996
Thioctic acid	T50.991	T50.992	T50.993	T50.994	T50.995	T50.996
Thiofos	T60.0X1	T60.0X2	T60.0X3	T60.0X4	--	--
Thioglycolate	T49.4X1	T49.4X2	T49.4X3	T49.4X4	T49.4X5	T49.4X6
Thioglycolic acid	T65.891	T65.892	T65.893	T65.894	--	--
Thioguanine	T45.1X1	T45.1X2	T45.1X3	T45.1X4	T45.1X5	T45.1X6
Thiomercaptomerin	T50.2X1	T50.2X2	T50.2X3	T50.2X4	T50.2X5	T50.2X6
Thiomerin	T50.2X1	T50.2X2	T50.2X3	T50.2X4	T50.2X5	T50.2X6
Thiomersal	T49.0X1	T49.0X2	T49.0X3	T49.0X4	T49.0X5	T49.0X6
Thionazin	T60.0X1	T60.0X2	T60.0X3	T60.0X4	--	--
Thiopental (sodium)	T41.1X1	T41.1X2	T41.1X3	T41.1X4	T41.1X5	T41.1X6
Thiopentone (sodium)	T41.1X1	T41.1X2	T41.1X3	T41.1X4	T41.1X5	T41.1X6
Thiopropazate	T43.3X1	T43.3X2	T43.3X3	T43.3X4	T43.3X5	T43.3X6
Thioproperazine	T43.3X1	T43.3X2	T43.3X3	T43.3X4	T43.3X5	T43.3X6
Thioridazine	T43.3X1	T43.3X2	T43.3X3	T43.3X4	T43.3X5	T43.3X6
Thiosinamine	T49.3X1	T49.3X2	T49.3X3	T49.3X4	T49.3X5	T49.3X6
Thiotepa	T45.1X1	T45.1X2	T45.1X3	T45.1X4	T45.1X5	T45.1X6
Thiothixene	T43.4X1	T43.4X2	T43.4X3	T43.4X4	T43.4X5	T43.4X6
Thiouracil (benzyl) (methyl) (propyl)	T38.2X1	T38.2X2	T38.2X3	T38.2X4	T38.2X5	T38.2X6
Thiourea	T38.2X1	T38.2X2	T38.2X3	T38.2X4	T38.2X5	T38.2X6
Thiphenamil	T44.3X1	T44.3X2	T44.3X3	T44.3X4	T44.3X5	T44.3X6
Thiram	T60.3X1	T60.3X2	T60.3X3	T60.3X4	--	--
medicinal	T49.2X1	T49.2X2	T49.2X3	T49.2X4	T49.2X5	T49.2X6
Thonzylamine (systemic)	T45.0X1	T45.0X2	T45.0X3	T45.0X4	T45.0X5	T45.0X6
mucosal decongestant	T48.5X1	T48.5X2	T48.5X3	T48.5X4	T48.5X5	T48.5X6
Thorazine	T43.3X1	T43.3X2	T43.3X3	T43.3X4	T43.3X5	T43.3X6
Thorium dioxide suspension	T50.8X1	T50.8X2	T50.8X3	T50.8X4	T50.8X5	T50.8X6
Thornapple	T62.2X1	T62.2X2	T62.2X3	T62.2X4	--	--
Throat drug NEC	T49.6X1	T49.6X2	T49.6X3	T49.6X4	T49.6X5	T49.6X6
Thrombin	T45.7X1	T45.7X2	T45.7X3	T45.7X4	T45.7X5	T45.7X6
Thrombolysin	T45.611	T45.612	T45.613	T45.614	T45.615	T45.616
Thromboplastin	T45.7X1	T45.7X2	T45.7X3	T45.7X4	T45.7X5	T45.7X6
Thurfyl nicotinate	T46.7X1	T46.7X2	T46.7X3	T46.7X4	T46.7X5	T46.7X6
Thymol	T49.0X1	T49.0X2	T49.0X3	T49.0X4	T49.0X5	T49.0X6
Thymopentin	T37.5X1	T37.5X2	T37.5X3	T37.5X4	T37.5X5	T37.5X6
Thymoxamine	T46.7X1	T46.7X2	T46.7X3	T46.7X4	T46.7X5	T46.7X6
Thymus extract	T38.891	T38.892	T38.893	T38.894	T38.895	T38.896
Thyreotrophic hormone	T38.811	T38.812	T38.813	T38.814	T38.815	T38.816
Thyroglobulin	T38.1X1	T38.1X2	T38.1X3	T38.1X4	T38.1X5	T38.1X6
Thyroid (hormone)	T38.1X1	T38.1X2	T38.1X3	T38.1X4	T38.1X5	T38.1X6
Thyrolar	T38.1X1	T38.1X2	T38.1X3	T38.1X4	T38.1X5	T38.1X6
Thyrotrophin	T38.811	T38.812	T38.813	T38.814	T38.815	T38.816
Thyrotropic hormone	T38.811	T38.812	T38.813	T38.814	T38.815	T38.816
Thyroxine	T38.1X1	T38.1X2	T38.1X3	T38.1X4	T38.1X5	T38.1X6
Tiabendazole	T37.4X1	T37.4X2	T37.4X3	T37.4X4	T37.4X5	T37.4X6
Tiamizide	T50.2X1	T50.2X2	T50.2X3	T50.2X4	T50.2X5	T50.2X6
Tianeptine	T43.291	T43.292	T43.293	T43.294	T43.295	T43.296
Tiapamil	T46.1X1	T46.1X2	T46.1X3	T46.1X4	T46.1X5	T46.1X6
Tiapride	T43.591	T43.592	T43.593	T43.594	T43.595	T43.596
Tiaprofenic acid	T39.311	T39.312	T39.313	T39.314	T39.315	T39.316
Tiaramide	T39.8X1	T39.8X2	T39.8X3	T39.8X4	T39.8X5	T39.8X6
Ticarcillin	T36.0X1	T36.0X2	T36.0X3	T36.0X4	T36.0X5	T36.0X6
Ticlatone	T49.0X1	T49.0X2	T49.0X3	T49.0X4	T49.0X5	T49.0X6
Ticlopidine	T45.521	T45.522	T45.523	T45.524	T45.525	T45.526
Ticrynafen	T50.1X1	T50.1X2	T50.1X3	T50.1X4	T50.1X5	T50.1X6
Tidiacic	T50.991	T50.992	T50.993	T50.994	T50.995	T50.996
Tiemonium	T44.3X1	T44.3X2	T44.3X3	T44.3X4	T44.3X5	T44.3X6
iodide	T44.3X1	T44.3X2	T44.3X3	T44.3X4	T44.3X5	T44.3X6
Tienilic acid	T50.1X1	T50.1X2	T50.1X3	T50.1X4	T50.1X5	T50.1X6
Tifenamil	T44.3X1	T44.3X2	T44.3X3	T44.3X4	T44.3X5	T44.3X6
Tigan	T45.0X1	T45.0X2	T45.0X3	T45.0X4	T45.0X5	T45.0X6
Tigloidine	T44.3X1	T44.3X2	T44.3X3	T44.3X4	T44.3X5	T44.3X6
Tilactase	T47.5X1	T47.5X2	T47.5X3	T47.5X4	T47.5X5	T47.5X6
Tiletamine	T41.291	T41.292	T41.293	T41.294	T41.295	T41.296
Tilidine	T40.4X1	T40.4X2	T40.4X3	T40.4X4	--	--
Timepidium bromide	T44.3X1	T44.3X2	T44.3X3	T44.3X4	T44.3X5	T44.3X6
Timiperone	T43.4X1	T43.4X2	T43.4X3	T43.4X4	T43.4X5	T43.4X6
Timolol	T44.7X1	T44.7X2	T44.7X3	T44.7X4	T44.7X5	T44.7X6
Tin (chloride) (dust) (oxide) NEC	T56.6X1	T56.6X2	T56.6X3	T56.6X4	--	--
anti-infectives	T37.8X1	T37.8X2	T37.8X3	T37.8X4	T37.8X5	T37.8X6
Tincture, iodine — *see Iodine*						
Tindal	T43.3X1	T43.3X2	T43.3X3	T43.3X4	T43.3X5	T43.3X6
Tinidazole	T37.3X1	T37.3X2	T37.3X3	T37.3X4	T37.3X5	T37.3X6
Tinoridine	T39.8X1	T39.8X2	T39.8X3	T39.8X4	T39.8X5	T39.8X6
Tiocarlide	T37.1X1	T37.1X2	T37.1X3	T37.1X4	T37.1X5	T37.1X6
Tioclomarol	T45.511	T45.512	T45.513	T45.514	T45.515	T45.516
Tioconazole	T49.0X1	T49.0X2	T49.0X3	T49.0X4	T49.0X5	T49.0X6
Tioguanine	T45.1X1	T45.1X2	T45.1X3	T45.1X4	T45.1X5	T45.1X6
Tiopronin	T50.991	T50.992	T50.993	T50.994	T50.995	T50.996
Tiotixene	T43.4X1	T43.4X2	T43.4X3	T43.4X4	T43.4X5	T43.4X6
Tioxolone	T49.4X1	T49.4X2	T49.4X3	T49.4X4	T49.4X5	T49.4X6
Tipepidine	T48.3X1	T48.3X2	T48.3X3	T48.3X4	T48.3X5	T48.3X6
Tiquizium bromide	T44.3X1	T44.3X2	T44.3X3	T44.3X4	T44.3X5	T44.3X6
Tiratricol	T38.1X1	T38.1X2	T38.1X3	T38.1X4	T38.1X5	T38.1X6
Tisopurine	T50.4X1	T50.4X2	T50.4X3	T50.4X4	T50.4X5	T50.4X6
Titanium (compounds) (vapor)	T56.891	T56.892	T56.893	T56.894	--	--
dioxide	T49.3X1	T49.3X2	T49.3X3	T49.3X4	T49.3X5	T49.3X6
ointment	T49.3X1	T49.3X2	T49.3X3	T49.3X4	T49.3X5	T49.3X6
oxide	T49.3X1	T49.3X2	T49.3X3	T49.3X4	T49.3X5	T49.3X6
tetrachloride	T56.891	T56.892	T56.893	T56.894	--	--
Titanocene	T56.891	T56.892	T56.893	T56.894	--	--
Titroid	T38.1X1	T38.1X2	T38.1X3	T38.1X4	T38.1X5	T38.1X6
Tizanidine	T42.8X1	T42.8X2	T42.8X3	T42.8X4	T42.8X5	T42.8X6
TMTD	T60.3X1	T60.3X2	T60.3X3	T60.3X4	--	--
TNT (fumes)	T65.3X1	T65.3X2	T65.3X3	T65.3X4	--	--
Toadstool	T62.0X1	T62.0X2	T62.0X3	T62.0X4	--	--
Tobacco NEC	T65.291	T65.292	T65.293	T65.294	--	--
cigarettes	T65.221	T65.222	T65.223	T65.224	--	--
Indian	T62.2X1	T62.2X2	T62.2X3	T62.2X4	--	--
smoke, second-hand	T65.221	T65.222	T65.223	T65.224	--	--
Tobramycin	T36.5X1	T36.5X2	T36.5X3	T36.5X4	T36.5X5	T36.5X6
Tocainide	T46.2X1	T46.2X2	T46.2X3	T46.2X4	T46.2X5	T46.2X6
Tocoferol	T45.2X1	T45.2X2	T45.2X3	T45.2X4	T45.2X5	T45.2X6
Tocopherol	T45.2X1	T45.2X2	T45.2X3	T45.2X4	T45.2X5	T45.2X6
acetate	T45.2X1	T45.2X2	T45.2X3	T45.2X4	T45.2X5	T45.2X6
Tocosamine	T48.0X1	T48.0X2	T48.0X3	T48.0X4	T48.0X5	T48.0X6
Todralazine	T46.5X1	T46.5X2	T46.5X3	T46.5X4	T46.5X5	T46.5X6
Tofisopam	T42.4X1	T42.4X2	T42.4X3	T42.4X4	T42.4X5	T42.4X6
Tofranil	T43.011	T43.012	T43.013	T43.014	T43.015	T43.016
Toilet deodorizer	T65.891	T65.892	T65.893	T65.894	--	--
Tolamolol	T44.7X1	T44.7X2	T44.7X3	T44.7X4	T44.7X5	T44.7X6
Tolazamide	T38.3X1	T38.3X2	T38.3X3	T38.3X4	T38.3X5	T38.3X6
Tolazoline	T46.7X1	T46.7X2	T46.7X3	T46.7X4	T46.7X5	T46.7X6
Tolbutamide (sodium)	T38.3X1	T38.3X2	T38.3X3	T38.3X4	T38.3X5	T38.3X6
Tolciclate	T49.0X1	T49.0X2	T49.0X3	T49.0X4	T49.0X5	T49.0X6
Tolmetin	T39.391	T39.392	T39.393	T39.394	T39.395	T39.396
Tolnaftate	T49.0X1	T49.0X2	T49.0X3	T49.0X4	T49.0X5	T49.0X6
Tolonidine	T46.5X1	T46.5X2	T46.5X3	T46.5X4	T46.5X5	T46.5X6
Toloxatone	T42.6X1	T42.6X2	T42.6X3	T42.6X4	T42.6X5	T42.6X6
Tolperisone	T44.3X1	T44.3X2	T44.3X3	T44.3X4	T44.3X5	T44.3X6
Tolserol	T42.8X1	T42.8X2	T42.8X3	T42.8X4	T42.8X5	T42.8X6
Toluene (liquid)	T52.2X1	T52.2X2	T52.2X3	T52.2X4	--	--
diisocyanate	T65.0X1	T65.0X2	T65.0X3	T65.0X4	--	--
Toluidine	T65.891	T65.892	T65.893	T65.894	--	--
vapor	T59.891	T59.892	T59.893	T59.894	--	--
Toluol (liquid)	T52.2X1	T52.2X2	T52.2X3	T52.2X4	--	--
vapor	T52.2X1	T52.2X2	T52.2X3	T52.2X4	--	--
Toluylenediamine	T65.3X1	T65.3X2	T65.3X3	T65.3X4	--	--
Tolylene-2,4-diisocyanate	T65.0X1	T65.0X2	T65.0X3	T65.0X4	--	--
Tonic NEC	T50.901	T50.902	T50.903	T50.904	T50.905	T50.906
Topical action drug NEC	T49.91	T49.92	T49.93	T49.94	T49.95	T49.96
ear, nose or throat	T49.6X1	T49.6X2	T49.6X3	T49.6X4	T49.6X5	T49.6X6
eye	T49.5X1	T49.5X2	T49.5X3	T49.5X4	T49.5X5	T49.5X6
skin	T49.91	T49.92	T49.93	T49.94	T49.95	T49.96
specified NEC	T49.8X1	T49.8X2	T49.8X3	T49.8X4	T49.8X5	T49.8X6
Toquizine	T44.3X1	T44.3X2	T44.3X3	T44.3X4	T44.3X5	T44.3X6
Toremifene	T38.6X1	T38.6X2	T38.6X3	T38.6X4	T38.6X5	T38.6X6
Tosylchloramide sodium	T49.8X1	T49.8X2	T49.8X3	T49.8X4	T49.8X5	T49.8X6
Toxaphene (dust) (spray)	T60.1X1	T60.1X2	T60.1X3	T60.1X4	--	--
Toxin, diphtheria (Schick Test)	T50.8X1	T50.8X2	T50.8X3	T50.8X4	T50.8X5	T50.8X6
Toxoid						
combined	T50.A21	T50.A22	T50.A23	T50.A24	T50.A25	T50.A26
diphtheria	T50.A91	T50.A92	T50.A93	T50.A94	T50.A95	T50.A96
tetanus	T50.A91	T50.A92	T50.A93	T50.A94	T50.A95	T50.A96
Trace element NEC	T45.8X1	T45.8X2	T45.8X3	T45.8X4	T45.8X5	T45.8X6
Tractor fuel NEC	T52.0X1	T52.0X2	T52.0X3	T52.0X4	--	--
Tragacanth	T50.991	T50.992	T50.993	T50.994	T50.995	T50.996
Tramadol	T40.4X1	T40.4X2	T40.4X3	T40.4X4	T40.4X5	T40.4X6
Tramazoline	T48.5X1	T48.5X2	T48.5X3	T48.5X4	T48.5X5	T48.5X6
Tranexamic acid	T45.621	T45.622	T45.623	T45.624	T45.625	T45.626
Tranilast	T45.0X1	T45.0X2	T45.0X3	T45.0X4	T45.0X5	T45.0X6
Tranquilizer NEC	T43.501	T43.502	T43.503	T43.504	T43.505	T43.506
with hypnotic or sedative	T42.6X1	T42.6X2	T42.6X3	T42.6X4	T42.6X5	T42.6X6
benzodiazepine NEC	T42.4X1	T42.4X2	T42.4X3	T42.4X4	T42.4X5	T42.4X6
butyrophenone NEC	T43.4X1	T43.4X2	T43.4X3	T43.4X4	T43.4X5	T43.4X6
carbamate	T43.591	T43.592	T43.593	T43.594	T43.595	T43.596
dimethylamine	T43.3X1	T43.3X2	T43.3X3	T43.3X4	T43.3X5	T43.3X6
ethylamine	T43.3X1	T43.3X2	T43.3X3	T43.3X4	T43.3X5	T43.3X6

Substance	Poisoning, Accidental unintentional	Poisoning, Intentional self-harm	Poisoning, Assault	Poisoning, Undetermined	Adverse effect	Underdosing
Tranquilizer NEC — *continued*						
hydroxyzine	T43.591	T43.592	T43.593	T43.594	T43.595	T43.596
major NEC	T43.501	T43.502	T43.503	T43.504	T43.505	T43.506
penothiazine NEC	T43.3X1	T43.3X2	T43.3X3	T43.3X4	T43.3X5	T43.3X6
phenothiazine-based	T43.3X1	T43.3X2	T43.3X3	T43.3X4	T43.3X5	T43.3X6
piperazine NEC	T43.3X1	T43.3X2	T43.3X3	T43.3X4	T43.3X5	T43.3X6
piperidine	T43.3X1	T43.3X2	T43.3X3	T43.3X4	T43.3X5	T43.3X6
propylamine	T43.3X1	T43.3X2	T43.3X3	T43.3X4	T43.3X5	T43.3X6
specified NEC	T43.591	T43.592	T43.593	T43.594	T43.595	T43.596
thioxanthene NEC	T43.591	T43.592	T43.593	T43.594	T43.595	T43.596
Tranxene	T42.4X1	T42.4X2	T42.4X3	T42.4X4	T42.4X5	T42.4X6
Tranylcypromine	T43.1X1	T43.1X2	T43.1X3	T43.1X4	T43.1X5	T43.1X6
Trapidil	T46.3X1	T46.3X2	T46.3X3	T46.3X4	T46.3X5	T46.3X6
Trasentine	T44.3X1	T44.3X2	T44.3X3	T44.3X4	T44.3X5	T44.3X6
Travert	T50.3X1	T50.3X2	T50.3X3	T50.3X4	T50.3X5	T50.3X6
Trazodone	T43.211	T43.212	T43.213	T43.214	T43.215	T43.216
Trecator	T37.1X1	T37.1X2	T37.1X3	T37.1X4	T37.1X5	T37.1X6
Treosulfan	T45.1X1	T45.1X2	T45.1X3	T45.1X4	T45.1X5	T45.1X6
Tretamine	T45.1X1	T45.1X2	T45.1X3	T45.1X4	T45.1X5	T45.1X6
Tretinoin	T49.0X1	T49.0X2	T49.0X3	T49.0X4	T49.0X5	T49.0X6
Tretoquinol	T48.6X1	T48.6X2	T48.6X3	T48.6X4	T48.6X5	T48.6X6
Triacetin	T49.0X1	T49.0X2	T49.0X3	T49.0X4	T49.0X5	T49.0X6
Triacetoxyanthracene	T49.4X1	T49.4X2	T49.4X3	T49.4X4	T49.4X5	T49.4X6
Triacetyloleandomycin	T36.3X1	T36.3X2	T36.3X3	T36.3X4	T36.3X5	T36.3X6
Triamcinolone	T49.0X1	T49.0X2	T49.0X3	T49.0X4	T49.0X5	T49.0X6
ENT agent	T49.6X1	T49.6X2	T49.6X3	T49.6X4	T49.6X5	T49.6X6
hexacetonide	T49.0X1	T49.0X2	T49.0X3	T49.0X4	T49.0X5	T49.0X6
ophthalmic preparation	T49.5X1	T49.5X2	T49.5X3	T49.5X4	T49.5X5	T49.5X6
topical NEC	T49.0X1	T49.0X2	T49.0X3	T49.0X4	T49.0X5	T49.0X6
Triampyzine	T44.3X1	T44.3X2	T44.3X3	T44.3X4	T44.3X5	T44.3X6
Triamterene	T50.2X1	T50.2X2	T50.2X3	T50.2X4	T50.2X5	T50.2X6
Triazine (herbicide)	T60.3X1	T60.3X2	T60.3X3	T60.3X4	--	--
Triaziquone	T45.1X1	T45.1X2	T45.1X3	T45.1X4	T45.1X5	T45.1X6
Triazolam	T42.4X1	T42.4X2	T42.4X3	T42.4X4	T42.4X5	T42.4X6
Triazole (herbicide)	T60.3X1	T60.3X2	T60.3X3	T60.3X4	--	--
Tribenoside	T46.991	T46.992	T46.993	T46.994	T46.995	T46.996
Tribromacetaldehyde	T42.6X1	T42.6X2	T42.6X3	T42.6X4	T42.6X5	T42.6X6
Tribromoethanol, rectal	T41.291	T41.292	T41.293	T41.294	T41.295	T41.296
Tribromomethane	T42.6X1	T42.6X2	T42.6X3	T42.6X4	T42.6X5	T42.6X6
Trichlorethane	T53.2X1	T53.2X2	T53.2X3	T53.2X4	--	--
Trichlorethylene	T53.2X1	T53.2X2	T53.2X3	T53.2X4	--	--
Trichlorfon	T60.0X1	T60.0X2	T60.0X3	T60.0X4	--	--
Trichlormethiazide	T50.2X1	T50.2X2	T50.2X3	T50.2X4	T50.2X5	T50.2X6
Trichlormethine	T45.1X1	T45.1X2	T45.1X3	T45.1X4	T45.1X5	T45.1X6
Trichloroacetic acid, Trichloracetic acid	T54.2X1	T54.2X2	T54.2X3	T54.2X4	--	--
medicinal	T49.4X1	T49.4X2	T49.4X3	T49.4X4	T49.4X5	T49.4X6
Trichloroethane	T53.2X1	T53.2X2	T53.2X3	T53.2X4	--	--
Trichloroethanol	T42.6X1	T42.6X2	T42.6X3	T42.6X4	T42.6X5	T42.6X6
Trichloroethyl phosphate	T42.6X1	T42.6X2	T42.6X3	T42.6X4	T42.6X5	T42.6X6
Trichloroethylene (liquid) (vapor)	T53.2X1	T53.2X2	T53.2X3	T53.2X4	--	--
anesthetic (gas)	T41.0X1	T41.0X2	T41.0X3	T41.0X4	T41.0X5	T41.0X6
vapor NEC	T53.2X1	T53.2X2	T53.2X3	T53.2X4	--	--
Trichlorofluoromethane NEC	T53.5X1	T53.5X2	T53.5X3	T53.5X4	--	--
Trichloronate	T60.0X1	T60.0X2	T60.0X3	T60.0X4	--	--
2,4,5-Trichlorophen-oxyacetic acid	T60.3X1	T60.3X2	T60.3X3	T60.3X4	--	--
Trichloropropane	T53.6X1	T53.6X2	T53.6X3	T53.6X4	--	--
Trichlorotriethylamine	T45.1X1	T45.1X2	T45.1X3	T45.1X4	T45.1X5	T45.1X6
Trichomonacides NEC	T37.3X1	T37.3X2	T37.3X3	T37.3X4	T37.3X5	T37.3X6
Trichomycin	T36.7X1	T36.7X2	T36.7X3	T36.7X4	T36.7X5	T36.7X6
Triclobisonium chloride	T49.0X1	T49.0X2	T49.0X3	T49.0X4	T49.0X5	T49.0X6
Triclocarban	T49.0X1	T49.0X2	T49.0X3	T49.0X4	T49.0X5	T49.0X6
Triclofos	T42.6X1	T42.6X2	T42.6X3	T42.6X4	T42.6X5	T42.6X6
Triclosan	T49.0X1	T49.0X2	T49.0X3	T49.0X4	T49.0X5	T49.0X6
Tricresyl phosphate	T65.891	T65.892	T65.893	T65.894	--	--
solvent	T52.91	T52.92	T52.93	T52.94	--	--
Tricyclamol chloride	T44.3X1	T44.3X2	T44.3X3	T44.3X4	T44.3X5	T44.3X6
Tridesilon	T49.0X1	T49.0X2	T49.0X3	T49.0X4	T49.0X5	T49.0X6
Tridihexethyl iodide	T44.3X1	T44.3X2	T44.3X3	T44.3X4	T44.3X5	T44.3X6
Tridione	T42.2X1	T42.2X2	T42.2X3	T42.2X4	T42.2X5	T42.2X6
Trientine	T45.8X1	T45.8X2	T45.8X3	T45.8X4	T45.8X5	T45.8X6
Triethanolamine NEC	T54.3X1	T54.3X2	T54.3X3	T54.3X4	--	--
detergent	T54.3X1	T54.3X2	T54.3X3	T54.3X4	--	--
trinitrate (biphosphate)	T46.3X1	T46.3X2	T46.3X3	T46.3X4	T46.3X5	T46.3X6
Triethanomelamine	T45.1X1	T45.1X2	T45.1X3	T45.1X4	T45.1X5	T45.1X6
Triethylenemelamine	T45.1X1	T45.1X2	T45.1X3	T45.1X4	T45.1X5	T45.1X6
Triethylenephosphoramide	T45.1X1	T45.1X2	T45.1X3	T45.1X4	T45.1X5	T45.1X6
Triethylenethiophosphoramide	T45.1X1	T45.1X2	T45.1X3	T45.1X4	T45.1X5	T45.1X6
Trifluoperazine	T43.3X1	T43.3X2	T43.3X3	T43.3X4	T43.3X5	T43.3X6
Trifluoroethyl vinyl ether	T41.0X1	T41.0X2	T41.0X3	T41.0X4	T41.0X5	T41.0X6
Trifluperidol	T43.4X1	T43.4X2	T43.4X3	T43.4X4	T43.4X5	T43.4X6
Triflupromazine	T43.3X1	T43.3X2	T43.3X3	T43.3X4	T43.3X5	T43.3X6
Trifluridine	T37.5X1	T37.5X2	T37.5X3	T37.5X4	T37.5X5	T37.5X6

Substance	Poisoning, Accidental unintentional	Poisoning, Intentional self-harm	Poisoning, Assault	Poisoning, Undetermined	Adverse effect	Underdosing
Triflusal	T45.521	T45.522	T45.523	T45.524	T45.525	T45.526
Trihexyphenidyl	T44.3X1	T44.3X2	T44.3X3	T44.3X4	T44.3X5	T44.3X6
Triiodothyronine	T38.1X1	T38.1X2	T38.1X3	T38.1X4	T38.1X5	T38.1X6
Trilene	T41.0X1	T41.0X2	T41.0X3	T41.0X4	T41.0X5	T41.0X6
Trilostane	T38.991	T38.992	T38.993	T38.994	T38.995	T38.996
Trimebutine	T44.3X1	T44.3X2	T44.3X3	T44.3X4	T44.3X5	T44.3X6
Trimecaine	T41.3X1	T41.3X2	T41.3X3	T41.3X4	T41.3X5	T41.3X6
Trimeprazine (tartrate)	T44.3X1	T44.3X2	T44.3X3	T44.3X4	T44.3X5	T44.3X6
Trimetaphan camsilate	T44.2X1	T44.2X2	T44.2X3	T44.2X4	T44.2X5	T44.2X6
Trimetazidine	T46.7X1	T46.7X2	T46.7X3	T46.7X4	T46.7X5	T46.7X6
Trimethadione	T42.2X1	T42.2X2	T42.2X3	T42.2X4	T42.2X5	T42.2X6
Trimethaphan	T44.2X1	T44.2X2	T44.2X3	T44.2X4	T44.2X5	T44.2X6
Trimethidinium	T44.2X1	T44.2X2	T44.2X3	T44.2X4	T44.2X5	T44.2X6
Trimethobenzamide	T45.0X1	T45.0X2	T45.0X3	T45.0X4	T45.0X5	T45.0X6
Trimethoprim	T37.8X1	T37.8X2	T37.8X3	T37.8X4	T37.8X5	T37.8X6
with sulfamethoxazole	T36.8X1	T36.8X2	T36.8X3	T36.8X4	T36.8X5	T36.8X6
Trimethylcarbinol	T51.3X1	T51.3X2	T51.3X3	T51.3X4	--	--
Trimethylpsoralen	T49.3X1	T49.3X2	T49.3X3	T49.3X4	T49.3X5	T49.3X6
Trimeton	T45.0X1	T45.0X2	T45.0X3	T45.0X4	T45.0X5	T45.0X6
Trimetrexate	T45.1X1	T45.1X2	T45.1X3	T45.1X4	T45.1X5	T45.1X6
Trimipramine	T43.011	T43.012	T43.013	T43.014	T43.015	T43.016
Trimustine	T45.1X1	T45.1X2	T45.1X3	T45.1X4	T45.1X5	T45.1X6
Trinitrine	T46.3X1	T46.3X2	T46.3X3	T46.3X4	T46.3X5	T46.3X6
Trinitrobenzol	T65.3X1	T65.3X2	T65.3X3	T65.3X4	--	--
Trinitrophenol	T65.3X1	T65.3X2	T65.3X3	T65.3X4	--	--
Trinitrotoluene (fumes)	T65.3X1	T65.3X2	T65.3X3	T65.3X4	--	--
Trional	T42.6X1	T42.6X2	T42.6X3	T42.6X4	T42.6X5	T42.6X6
Triorthocresyl phosphate	T65.891	T65.892	T65.893	T65.894	--	--
Trioxide of arsenic	T57.0X1	T57.0X2	T57.0X3	T57.0X4	--	--
Trioxysalen	T49.4X1	T49.4X2	T49.4X3	T49.4X4	T49.4X5	T49.4X6
Tripamide	T50.2X1	T50.2X2	T50.2X3	T50.2X4	T50.2X5	T50.2X6
Triparanol	T46.6X1	T46.6X2	T46.6X3	T46.6X4	T46.6X5	T46.6X6
Tripelennamine	T45.0X1	T45.0X2	T45.0X3	T45.0X4	T45.0X5	T45.0X6
Triperiden	T44.3X1	T44.3X2	T44.3X3	T44.3X4	T44.3X5	T44.3X6
Triperidol	T43.4X1	T43.4X2	T43.4X3	T43.4X4	T43.4X5	T43.4X6
Triphenylphosphate	T65.891	T65.892	T65.893	T65.894	--	--
Triple						
bromides	T42.6X1	T42.6X2	T42.6X3	T42.6X4	T42.6X5	T42.6X6
carbonate	T47.1X1	T47.1X2	T47.1X3	T47.1X4	T47.1X5	T47.1X6
vaccine						
DPT	T50.A11	T50.A12	T50.A13	T50.A14	T50.A15	T50.A16
including pertussis	T50.A11	T50.A12	T50.A13	T50.A14	T50.A15	T50.A16
MMR	T50.B91	T50.B92	T50.B93	T50.B94	T50.B95	T50.B96
Triprolidine	T45.0X1	T45.0X2	T45.0X3	T45.0X4	T45.0X5	T45.0X6
Trisodium hydrogen edetate	T50.6X1	T50.6X2	T50.6X3	T50.6X4	T50.6X5	T50.6X6
Trisoralen	T49.3X1	T49.3X2	T49.3X3	T49.3X4	T49.3X5	T49.3X6
Trisulfapyrimidines	T37.0X1	T37.0X2	T37.0X3	T37.0X4	T37.0X5	T37.0X6
Trithiozine	T44.3X1	T44.3X2	T44.3X3	T44.3X4	T44.3X5	T44.3X6
Tritiozine	T44.3X1	T44.3X2	T44.3X3	T44.3X4	T44.3X5	T44.3X6
Tritoqualine	T45.0X1	T45.0X2	T45.0X3	T45.0X4	T45.0X5	T45.0X6
Trofosfamide	T45.1X1	T45.1X2	T45.1X3	T45.1X4	T45.1X5	T45.1X6
Troleandomycin	T36.3X1	T36.3X2	T36.3X3	T36.3X4	T36.3X5	T36.3X6
Trolnitrate (phosphate)	T46.3X1	T46.3X2	T46.3X3	T46.3X4	T46.3X5	T46.3X6
Tromantadine	T37.5X1	T37.5X2	T37.5X3	T37.5X4	T37.5X5	T37.5X6
Trometamol	T50.2X1	T50.2X2	T50.2X3	T50.2X4	T50.2X5	T50.2X6
Tromethamine	T50.2X1	T50.2X2	T50.2X3	T50.2X4	T50.2X5	T50.2X6
Tronothane	T41.3X1	T41.3X2	T41.3X3	T41.3X4	T41.3X5	T41.3X6
Tropacine	T44.3X1	T44.3X2	T44.3X3	T44.3X4	T44.3X5	T44.3X6
Tropatepine	T44.3X1	T44.3X2	T44.3X3	T44.3X4	T44.3X5	T44.3X6
Tropicamide	T44.3X1	T44.3X2	T44.3X3	T44.3X4	T44.3X5	T44.3X6
Trospium chloride	T44.3X1	T44.3X2	T44.3X3	T44.3X4	T44.3X5	T44.3X6
Troxerutin	T46.991	T46.992	T46.993	T46.994	T46.995	T46.996
Troxidone	T42.2X1	T42.2X2	T42.2X3	T42.2X4	T42.2X5	T42.2X6
Tryparsamide	T37.3X1	T37.3X2	T37.3X3	T37.3X4	T37.3X5	T37.3X6
Trypsin	T45.3X1	T45.3X2	T45.3X3	T45.3X4	T45.3X5	T45.3X6
Tryptizol	T43.011	T43.012	T43.013	T43.014	T43.015	T43.016
TSH	T38.811	T38.812	T38.813	T38.814	T38.815	T38.816
Tuaminoheptane	T48.5X1	T48.5X2	T48.5X3	T48.5X4	T48.5X5	T48.5X6
Tuberculin, purified protein derivative (PPD)	T50.8X1	T50.8X2	T50.8X3	T50.8X4	T50.8X5	T50.8X6
Tubocurare	T48.1X1	T48.1X2	T48.1X3	T48.1X4	T48.1X5	T48.1X6
Tubocurarine (chloride)	T48.1X1	T48.1X2	T48.1X3	T48.1X4	T48.1X5	T48.1X6
Tulobuterol	T48.6X1	T48.6X2	T48.6X3	T48.6X4	T48.6X5	T48.6X6
Turpentine (spirits of)	T52.8X1	T52.8X2	T52.8X3	T52.8X4	--	--
vapor	T52.8X1	T52.8X2	T52.8X3	T52.8X4	--	--
Tybamate	T43.591	T43.592	T43.593	T43.594	T43.595	T43.596
Tyloxapol	T48.4X1	T48.4X2	T48.4X3	T48.4X4	T48.4X5	T48.4X6
Tymazoline	T48.5X1	T48.5X2	T48.5X3	T48.5X4	T48.5X5	T48.5X6
Typhoid-paratyphoid vaccine	T50.A91	T50.A92	T50.A93	T50.A94	T50.A95	T50.A96
Typhus vaccine	T50.A91	T50.A92	T50.A93	T50.A94	T50.A95	T50.A96
Tyropanoate	T50.8X1	T50.8X2	T50.8X3	T50.8X4	T50.8X5	T50.8X6
Tyrothricin	T49.6X1	T49.6X2	T49.6X3	T49.6X4	T49.6X5	T49.6X6
ENT agent	T49.6X1	T49.6X2	T49.6X3	T49.6X4	T49.6X5	T49.6X6
ophthalmic preparation	T49.5X1	T49.5X2	T49.5X3	T49.5X4	T49.5X5	T49.5X6

Substance	Poisoning, Accidental unintentional	Poisoning, Intentional self-harm	Poisoning, Assault	Poisoning, Undetermined	Adverse effect	Underdosing
U						
Ufenamate	T39.391	T39.392	T39.393	T39.394	T39.395	T39.396
Ultraviolet light protectant	T49.3X1	T49.3X2	T49.3X3	T49.3X4	T49.3X5	T49.3X6
Undecenoic acid	T49.0X1	T49.0X2	T49.0X3	T49.0X4	T49.0X5	T49.0X6
Undecoylium	T49.0X1	T49.0X2	T49.0X3	T49.0X4	T49.0X5	T49.0X6
Undecylenic acid (derivatives)	T49.0X1	T49.0X2	T49.0X3	T49.0X4	T49.0X5	T49.0X6
Unna's boot	T49.3X1	T49.3X2	T49.3X3	T49.3X4	T49.3X5	T49.3X6
Unsaturated fatty acid	T46.6X1	T46.6X2	T46.6X3	T46.6X4	T46.6X5	T46.6X6
Uracil mustard	T45.1X1	T45.1X2	T45.1X3	T45.1X4	T45.1X5	T45.1X6
Uramustine	T45.1X1	T45.1X2	T45.1X3	T45.1X4	T45.1X5	T45.1X6
Urapidil	T46.5X1	T46.5X2	T46.5X3	T46.5X4	T46.5X5	T46.5X6
Urari	T48.1X1	T48.1X2	T48.1X3	T48.1X4	T48.1X5	T48.1X6
Urate oxidase	T50.4X1	T50.4X2	T50.4X3	T50.4X4	T50.4X5	T50.4X6
Urea	T47.3X1	T47.3X2	T47.3X3	T47.3X4	T47.3X5	T47.3X6
peroxide	T49.0X1	T49.0X2	T49.0X3	T49.0X4	T49.0X5	T49.0X6
stibamine	T37.4X1	T37.4X2	T37.4X3	T37.4X4	T37.4X5	T37.4X6
topical	T49.8X1	T49.8X2	T49.8X3	T49.8X4	T49.8X5	T49.8X6
Urethane	T45.1X1	T45.1X2	T45.1X3	T45.1X4	T45.1X5	T45.1X6
Urginea (maritima) (scilla) — *see Squill*						
Uric acid metabolism drug NEC	T50.4X1	T50.4X2	T50.4X3	T50.4X4	T50.4X5	T50.4X6
Uricosuric agent	T50.4X1	T50.4X2	T50.4X3	T50.4X4	T50.4X5	T50.4X6
Urinary anti-infective	T37.8X1	T37.8X2	T37.8X3	T37.8X4	T37.8X5	T37.8X6
Urofollitropin	T38.811	T38.812	T38.813	T38.814	T38.815	T38.816
Urokinase	T45.611	T45.612	T45.613	T45.614	T45.615	T45.616
Urokon	T50.8X1	T50.8X2	T50.8X3	T50.8X4	T50.8X5	T50.8X6
Ursodeoxycholic acid	T50.991	T50.992	T50.993	T50.994	T50.995	T50.996
Ursodiol	T50.991	T50.992	T50.993	T50.994	T50.995	T50.996
Urtica	T62.2X1	T62.2X2	T62.2X3	T62.2X4	--	--
Utility gas — *see Gas, utility*						
V						
Vaccine NEC	T50.Z91	T50.Z92	T50.Z93	T50.Z94	T50.Z95	T50.Z96
antineoplastic	T50.Z91	T50.Z92	T50.Z93	T50.Z94	T50.Z95	T50.Z96
bacterial NEC	T50.A91	T50.A92	T50.A93	T50.A94	T50.A95	T50.A96
with						
other bacterial component	T50.A21	T50.A22	T50.A23	T50.A24	T50.A25	T50.A26
pertussis component	T50.A11	T50.A12	T50.A13	T50.A14	T50.A15	T50.A16
viral-rickettsial component	T50.A21	T50.A22	T50.A23	T50.A24	T50.A25	T50.A26
mixed NEC	T50.A21	T50.A22	T50.A23	T50.A24	T50.A25	T50.A26
BCG	T50.A91	T50.A92	T50.A93	T50.A94	T50.A95	T50.A96
cholera	T50.A91	T50.A92	T50.A93	T50.A94	T50.A95	T50.A96
diphtheria	T50.A91	T50.A92	T50.A93	T50.A94	T50.A95	T50.A96
with tetanus	T50.A21	T50.A22	T50.A23	T50.A24	T50.A25	T50.A26
and pertussis	T50.A11	T50.A12	T50.A13	T50.A14	T50.A15	T50.A16
influenza	T50.B91	T50.B92	T50.B93	T50.B94	T50.B95	T50.B96
measles	T50.B91	T50.B92	T50.B93	T50.B94	T50.B95	T50.B96
with mumps and rubella	T50.B91	T50.B92	T50.B93	T50.B94	T50.B95	T50.B96
meningococcal	T50.A91	T50.A92	T50.A93	T50.A94	T50.A95	T50.A96
mumps	T50.B91	T50.B92	T50.B93	T50.B94	T50.B95	T50.B96
paratyphoid	T50.A91	T50.A92	T50.A93	T50.A94	T50.A95	T50.A96
pertussis	T50.A11	T50.A12	T50.A13	T50.A14	T50.A15	T50.A16
with diphtheria	T50.A11	T50.A12	T50.A13	T50.A14	T50.A15	T50.A16
and tetanus	T50.A11	T50.A12	T50.A13	T50.A14	T50.A15	T50.A16
with other component	T50.A11	T50.A12	T50.A13	T50.A14	T50.A15	T50.A16
plague	T50.A91	T50.A92	T50.A93	T50.A94	T50.A95	T50.A96
poliomyelitis	T50.B91	T50.B92	T50.B93	T50.B94	T50.B95	T50.B96
poliovirus	T50.B91	T50.B92	T50.B93	T50.B94	T50.B95	T50.B96
rabies	T50.B91	T50.B92	T50.B93	T50.B94	T50.B95	T50.B96
respiratory syncytial virus	T50.B91	T50.B92	T50.B93	T50.B94	T50.B95	T50.B96
rickettsial NEC	T50.A91	T50.A92	T50.A93	T50.A94	T50.A95	T50.A96
with						
bacterial component	T50.A21	T50.A22	T50.A23	T50.A24	T50.A25	T50.A26
Rocky Mountain spotted fever	T50.A91	T50.A92	T50.A93	T50.A94	T50.A95	T50.A96
rubella	T50.B91	T50.B92	T50.B93	T50.B94	T50.B95	T50.B96
sabin oral	T50.B91	T50.B92	T50.B93	T50.B94	T50.B95	T50.B96
smallpox	T50.B11	T50.B12	T50.B13	T50.B14	T50.B15	T50.B16
TAB	T50.A91	T50.A92	T50.A93	T50.A94	T50.A95	T50.A96
tetanus	T50.A91	T50.A92	T50.A93	T50.A94	T50.A95	T50.A96
typhoid	T50.A91	T50.A92	T50.A93	T50.A94	T50.A95	T50.A96
typhus	T50.A91	T50.A92	T50.A93	T50.A94	T50.A95	T50.A96
viral NEC	T50.B91	T50.B92	T50.B93	T50.B94	T50.B95	T50.B96
yellow fever	T50.B91	T50.B92	T50.B93	T50.B94	T50.B95	T50.B96
Vaccinia immune globulin	T50.Z11	T50.Z12	T50.Z13	T50.Z14	T50.Z15	T50.Z16
Vaginal contraceptives	T49.8X1	T49.8X2	T49.8X3	T49.8X4	T49.8X5	T49.8X6
Valerian						
root	T42.6X1	T42.6X2	T42.6X3	T42.6X4	T42.6X5	T42.6X6
tincture	T42.6X1	T42.6X2	T42.6X3	T42.6X4	T42.6X5	T42.6X6
Valethamate bromide	T44.3X1	T44.3X2	T44.3X3	T44.3X4	T44.3X5	T44.3X6
Valisone	T49.0X1	T49.0X2	T49.0X3	T49.0X4	T49.0X5	T49.0X6
Valium	T42.4X1	T42.4X2	T42.4X3	T42.4X4	T42.4X5	T42.4X6
Valmid	T42.6X1	T42.6X2	T42.6X3	T42.6X4	T42.6X5	T42.6X6
Valnoctamide	T42.6X1	T42.6X2	T42.6X3	T42.6X4	T42.6X5	T42.6X6
Valproate (sodium)	T42.6X1	T42.6X2	T42.6X3	T42.6X4	T42.6X5	T42.6X6
Valproic acid	T42.6X1	T42.6X2	T42.6X3	T42.6X4	T42.6X5	T42.6X6
Valpromide	T42.6X1	T42.6X2	T42.6X3	T42.6X4	T42.6X5	T42.6X6
Vanadium	T56.891	T56.892	T56.893	T56.894	--	--
Vancomycin	T36.8X1	T36.8X2	T36.8X3	T36.8X4	T36.8X5	T36.8X6
Vapor — *see also Gas*	T59.91	T59.92	T59.93	T59.94	--	--
kiln (carbon monoxide)	T58.8X1	T58.8X2	T58.8X3	T58.8X4	--	--
lead — *see lead*						
specified source NEC	T59.891	T59.892	T59.893	T59.894	--	--
Vardenafil	T46.7X1	T46.7X2	T46.7X3	T46.7X4	T46.7X5	T46.7X6
Varicose reduction drug	T46.8X1	T46.8X2	T46.8X3	T46.8X4	T46.8X5	T46.8X6
Varnish	T65.4X1	T65.4X2	T65.4X3	T65.4X4	--	--
cleaner	T52.91	T52.92	T52.93	T52.94	--	--
Vaseline	T49.3X1	T49.3X2	T49.3X3	T49.3X4	T49.3X5	T49.3X6
Vasodilan	T46.7X1	T46.7X2	T46.7X3	T46.7X4	T46.7X5	T46.7X6
Vasodilator						
coronary NEC	T46.3X1	T46.3X2	T46.3X3	T46.3X4	T46.3X5	T46.3X6
peripheral NEC	T46.7X1	T46.7X2	T46.7X3	T46.7X4	T46.7X5	T46.7X6
Vasopressin	T38.891	T38.892	T38.893	T38.894	T38.895	T38.896
Vasopressor drugs	T38.891	T38.892	T38.893	T38.894	T38.895	T38.896
Vecuronium bromide	T48.1X1	T48.1X2	T48.1X3	T48.1X4	T48.1X5	T48.1X6
Vegetable extract, astringent	T49.2X1	T49.2X2	T49.2X3	T49.2X4	T49.2X5	T49.2X6
Venlafaxine	T43.211	T43.212	T43.213	T43.214	T43.215	T43.216
Venom, venomous (bite) (sting)	T63.91	T63.92	T63.93	T63.94	--	--
amphibian NEC	T63.831	T63.832	T63.833	T63.834	--	--
animal NEC	T63.891	T63.892	T63.893	T63.894	--	--
ant	T63.421	T63.422	T63.423	T63.424	--	--
arthropod NEC	T63.481	T63.482	T63.483	T63.484	--	--
bee	T63.441	T63.442	T63.443	T63.444	--	--
centipede	T63.411	T63.412	T63.413	T63.414	--	--
fish	T63.591	T63.592	T63.593	T63.594	--	--
frog	T63.811	T63.812	T63.813	T63.814	--	--
hornet	T63.451	T63.452	T63.453	T63.454	--	--
insect NEC	T63.481	T63.482	T63.483	T63.484	--	--
lizard	T63.121	T63.122	T63.123	T63.124	--	--
marine						
animals	T63.691	T63.692	T63.693	T63.694	--	--
bluebottle	T63.611	T63.612	T63.613	T63.614	--	--
jellyfish NEC	T63.621	T63.622	T63.623	T63.624	--	--
Portugese Man-o-war	T63.611	T63.612	T63.613	T63.614	--	--
sea anemone	T63.631	T63.632	T63.633	T63.634	--	--
specified NEC	T63.691	T63.692	T63.693	T63.694	--	--
fish	T63.591	T63.592	T63.593	T63.594	--	--
plants	T63.711	T63.712	T63.713	T63.714	--	--
sting ray	T63.511	T63.512	T63.513	T63.514	--	--
millipede (tropical)	T63.411	T63.412	T63.413	T63.414	--	--
plant NEC	T63.791	T63.792	T63.793	T63.794	--	--
marine	T63.711	T63.712	T63.713	T63.714	--	--
reptile	T63.191	T63.192	T63.193	T63.194	--	--
gila monster	T63.111	T63.112	T63.113	T63.114	--	--
lizard NEC	T63.121	T63.122	T63.123	T63.124	--	--
scorpion	T63.2X1	T63.2X2	T63.2X3	T63.2X4	--	--
snake	T63.001	T63.002	T63.003	T63.004	--	--
African NEC	T63.081	T63.082	T63.083	T63.084	--	--
American (North) (South) NEC	T63.061	T63.062	T63.063	T63.064	--	--
Asian	T63.081	T63.082	T63.083	T63.084	--	--
Australian	T63.071	T63.072	T63.073	T63.074	--	--
cobra	T63.041	T63.042	T63.043	T63.044	--	--
coral snake	T63.021	T63.022	T63.023	T63.024	--	--
rattlesnake	T63.011	T63.012	T63.013	T63.014	--	--
specified NEC	T63.091	T63.092	T63.093	T63.094	--	--
taipan	T63.031	T63.032	T63.033	T63.034	--	--
specified NEC	T63.891	T63.892	T63.893	T63.894	--	--
spider	T63.301	T63.302	T63.303	T63.304	--	--
black widow	T63.311	T63.312	T63.313	T63.314	--	--
brown recluse	T63.331	T63.332	T63.333	T63.334	--	--
specified NEC	T63.391	T63.392	T63.393	T63.394	--	--
tarantula	T63.321	T63.322	T63.323	T63.324	--	--
sting ray	T63.511	T63.512	T63.513	T63.514	--	--
toad	T63.821	T63.822	T63.823	T63.824	--	--
wasp	T63.461	T63.462	T63.463	T63.464	--	--
Venous sclerosing drug NEC	T46.8X1	T46.8X2	T46.8X3	T46.8X4	T46.8X5	T46.8X6
Ventolin — *see Albuterol*						
Veramon	T42.3X1	T42.3X2	T42.3X3	T42.3X4	T42.3X5	T42.3X6
Verapamil	T46.1X1	T46.1X2	T46.1X3	T46.1X4	T46.1X5	T46.1X6
Veratrine	T46.5X1	T46.5X2	T46.5X3	T46.5X4	T46.5X5	T46.5X6
Veratrum						
album	T62.2X1	T62.2X2	T62.2X3	T62.2X4	--	--
alkaloids	T46.5X1	T46.5X2	T46.5X3	T46.5X4	T46.5X5	T46.5X6
viride	T62.2X1	T62.2X2	T62.2X3	T62.2X4	--	--

Substance	Poisoning, Accidental unintentional	Poisoning, Intentional self-harm	Poisoning, Assault	Poisoning, Undetermined	Adverse effect	Underdosing
Verdigris	T60.3X1	T60.3X2	T60.3X3	T60.3X4	--	--
Veronal	T42.3X1	T42.3X2	T42.3X3	T42.3X4	T42.3X5	T42.3X6
Veroxil	T37.4X1	T37.4X2	T37.4X3	T37.4X4	T37.4X5	T37.4X6
Versenate	T50.6X1	T50.6X2	T50.6X3	T50.6X4	T50.6X5	T50.6X6
Versidyne	T39.8X1	T39.8X2	T39.8X3	T39.8X4	T39.8X5	T39.8X6
Vetrabutine	T48.0X1	T48.0X2	T48.0X3	T48.0X4	T48.0X5	T48.0X6
Vidarabine	T37.5X1	T37.5X2	T37.5X3	T37.5X4	T37.5X5	T37.5X6
Vienna						
green	T57.0X1	T57.0X2	T57.0X3	T57.0X4	--	--
insecticide	T60.2X1	T60.2X2	T60.2X3	T60.2X4	--	--
red	T57.0X1	T57.0X2	T57.0X3	T57.0X4	--	--
pharmaceutical dye	T50.991	T50.992	T50.993	T50.994	T50.995	T50.996
Vigabatrin	T42.6X1	T42.6X2	T42.6X3	T42.6X4	T42.6X5	T42.6X6
Viloxazine	T43.291	T43.292	T43.293	T43.294	T43.295	T43.296
Viminol	T39.8X1	T39.8X2	T39.8X3	T39.8X4	T39.8X5	T39.8X6
Vinbarbital, vinbarbitone	T42.3X1	T42.3X2	T42.3X3	T42.3X4	T42.3X5	T42.3X6
Vinblastine	T45.1X1	T45.1X2	T45.1X3	T45.1X4	T45.1X5	T45.1X6
Vinburnine	T46.7X1	T46.7X2	T46.7X3	T46.7X4	T46.7X5	T46.7X6
Vincamine	T45.1X1	T45.1X2	T45.1X3	T45.1X4	T45.1X5	T45.1X6
Vincristine	T45.1X1	T45.1X2	T45.1X3	T45.1X4	T45.1X5	T45.1X6
Vindesine	T45.1X1	T45.1X2	T45.1X3	T45.1X4	T45.1X5	T45.1X6
Vinesthene, vinethene	T41.0X1	T41.0X2	T41.0X3	T41.0X4	T41.0X5	T41.0X6
Vinorelbine tartrate	T45.1X1	T45.1X2	T45.1X3	T45.1X4	T45.1X5	T45.1X6
Vinpocetine	T46.7X1	T46.7X2	T46.7X3	T46.7X4	T46.7X5	T46.7X6
Vinyl						
acetate	T65.891	T65.892	T65.893	T65.894	--	--
bital	T42.3X1	T42.3X2	T42.3X3	T42.3X4	T42.3X5	T42.3X6
bromide	T65.891	T65.892	T65.893	T65.894	--	--
chloride	T59.891	T59.892	T59.893	T59.894	--	--
ether	T41.0X1	T41.0X2	T41.0X3	T41.0X4	T41.0X5	T41.0X6
Vinylbital	T42.3X1	T42.3X2	T42.3X3	T42.3X4	T42.3X5	T42.3X6
Vinylidene chloride	T65.891	T65.892	T65.893	T65.894	--	--
Vioform	T37.8X1	T37.8X2	T37.8X3	T37.8X4	T37.8X5	T37.8X6
topical	T49.0X1	T49.0X2	T49.0X3	T49.0X4	T49.0X5	T49.0X6
Viomycin	T36.8X1	T36.8X2	T36.8X3	T36.8X4	T36.8X5	T36.8X6
Viosterol	T45.2X1	T45.2X2	T45.2X3	T45.2X4	T45.2X5	T45.2X6
Viper (venom)	T63.091	T63.092	T63.093	T63.094	--	--
Viprynium	T37.4X1	T37.4X2	T37.4X3	T37.4X4	T37.4X5	T37.4X6
Viquidil	T46.7X1	T46.7X2	T46.7X3	T46.7X4	T46.7X5	T46.7X6
Viral vaccine NEC	T50.B91	T50.B92	T50.B93	T50.B94	T50.B95	T50.B96
Virginiamycin	T36.8X1	T36.8X2	T36.8X3	T36.8X4	T36.8X5	T36.8X6
Virugon	T37.5X1	T37.5X2	T37.5X3	T37.5X4	T37.5X5	T37.5X6
Viscous agent	T50.901	T50.902	T50.903	T50.904	T50.905	T50.906
Visine	T49.5X1	T49.5X2	T49.5X3	T49.5X4	T49.5X5	T49.5X6
Visnadine	T46.3X1	T46.3X2	T46.3X3	T46.3X4	T46.3X5	T46.3X6
Vitamin NEC	T45.2X1	T45.2X2	T45.2X3	T45.2X4	T45.2X5	T45.2X6
A	T45.2X1	T45.2X2	T45.2X3	T45.2X4	T45.2X5	T45.2X6
B NEC	T45.2X1	T45.2X2	T45.2X3	T45.2X4	T45.2X5	T45.2X6
nicotinic acid	T46.7X1	T46.7X2	T46.7X3	T46.7X4	T46.7X5	T46.7X6
B1	T45.2X1	T45.2X2	T45.2X3	T45.2X4	T45.2X5	T45.2X6
B2	T45.2X1	T45.2X2	T45.2X3	T45.2X4	T45.2X5	T45.2X6
B6	T45.2X1	T45.2X2	T45.2X3	T45.2X4	T45.2X5	T45.2X6
B12	T45.2X1	T45.2X2	T45.2X3	T45.2X4	T45.2X5	T45.2X6
B15	T45.2X1	T45.2X2	T45.2X3	T45.2X4	T45.2X5	T45.2X6
C	T45.2X1	T45.2X2	T45.2X3	T45.2X4	T45.2X5	T45.2X6
D	T45.2X1	T45.2X2	T45.2X3	T45.2X4	T45.2X5	T45.2X6
D2	T45.2X1	T45.2X2	T45.2X3	T45.2X4	T45.2X5	T45.2X6
D3	T45.2X1	T45.2X2	T45.2X3	T45.2X4	T45.2X5	T45.2X6
E	T45.2X1	T45.2X2	T45.2X3	T45.2X4	T45.2X5	T45.2X6
E acetate	T45.2X1	T45.2X2	T45.2X3	T45.2X4	T45.2X5	T45.2X6
hematopoietic	T45.8X1	T45.8X2	T45.8X3	T45.8X4	T45.8X5	T45.8X6
K NEC	T45.7X1	T45.7X2	T45.7X3	T45.7X4	T45.7X5	T45.7X6
K1	T45.7X1	T45.7X2	T45.7X3	T45.7X4	T45.7X5	T45.7X6
K2	T45.7X1	T45.7X2	T45.7X3	T45.7X4	T45.7X5	T45.7X6
PP	T45.2X1	T45.2X2	T45.2X3	T45.2X4	T45.2X5	T45.2X6
ulceroprotectant	T47.1X1	T47.1X2	T47.1X3	T47.1X4	T47.1X5	T47.1X6
Vleminckx's solution	T49.4X1	T49.4X2	T49.4X3	T49.4X4	T49.4X5	T49.4X6
Voltaren — *see Diclofenac sodium*						
W						
Warfarin	T45.511	T45.512	T45.513	T45.514	T45.515	T45.516
rodenticide	T60.4X1	T60.4X2	T60.4X3	T60.4X4	--	--
sodium	T60.4X1	T60.4X2	T60.4X3	T60.4X4	--	--
Wasp (sting)	T63.461	T63.462	T63.463	T63.464	--	--
Water						
balance drug	T50.3X1	T50.3X2	T50.3X3	T50.3X4	T50.3X5	T50.3X6
distilled	T50.3X1	T50.3X2	T50.3X3	T50.3X4	T50.3X5	T50.3X6
gas — *see Gas, water*						
incomplete combustion of — *see Carbon, monoxide, fuel, utility*						
hemlock	T62.2X1	T62.2X2	T62.2X3	T62.2X4	--	--
moccasin (venom)	T63.061	T63.062	T63.063	T63.064	--	--
purified	T50.3X1	T50.3X2	T50.3X3	T50.3X4	T50.3X5	T50.3X6
Wax (paraffin) (petroleum)	T52.0X1	T52.0X2	T52.0X3	T52.0X4	--	--
automobile	T65.891	T65.892	T65.893	T65.894	--	--
floor	T52.0X1	T52.0X2	T52.0X3	T52.0X4	--	--
Weed killers NEC	T60.3X1	T60.3X2	T60.3X3	T60.3X4	--	--
Welldorm	T42.6X1	T42.6X2	T42.6X3	T42.6X4	T42.6X5	T42.6X6
White						
arsenic	T57.0X1	T57.0X2	T57.0X3	T57.0X4	--	--
hellebore	T62.2X1	T62.2X2	T62.2X3	T62.2X4	--	--
lotion (keratolytic)	T49.4X1	T49.4X2	T49.4X3	T49.4X4	T49.4X5	T49.4X6
spirit	T52.0X1	T52.0X2	T52.0X3	T52.0X4	--	--
Whitewash	T65.891	T65.892	T65.893	T65.894	--	--
Whole blood (human)	T45.8X1	T45.8X2	T45.8X3	T45.8X4	T45.8X5	T45.8X6
Wild						
black cherry	T62.2X1	T62.2X2	T62.2X3	T62.2X4	--	--
poisonous plants NEC	T62.2X1	T62.2X2	T62.2X3	T62.2X4	--	--
Window cleaning fluid	T65.891	T65.892	T65.893	T65.894	--	--
Wintergreen (oil)	T49.3X1	T49.3X2	T49.3X3	T49.3X4	T49.3X5	T49.3X6
Wisterine	T62.2X1	T62.2X2	T62.2X3	T62.2X4	--	--
Witch hazel	T49.2X1	T49.2X2	T49.2X3	T49.2X4	T49.2X5	T49.2X6
Wood alcohol or spirit	T51.1X1	T51.1X2	T51.1X3	T51.1X4	--	--
Wool fat (hydrous)	T49.3X1	T49.3X2	T49.3X3	T49.3X4	T49.3X5	T49.3X6
Woorali	T48.1X1	T48.1X2	T48.1X3	T48.1X4	T48.1X5	T48.1X6
Wormseed, American	T37.4X1	T37.4X2	T37.4X3	T37.4X4	T37.4X5	T37.4X6
X						
Xamoterol	T44.5X1	T44.5X2	T44.5X3	T44.5X4	T44.5X5	T44.5X6
Xanthine diuretics	T50.2X1	T50.2X2	T50.2X3	T50.2X4	T50.2X5	T50.2X6
Xanthinol nicotinate	T46.7X1	T46.7X2	T46.7X3	T46.7X4	T46.7X5	T46.7X6
Xanthotoxin	T49.3X1	T49.3X2	T49.3X3	T49.3X4	T49.3X5	T49.3X6
Xantinol nicotinate	T46.7X1	T46.7X2	T46.7X3	T46.7X4	T46.7X5	T46.7X6
Xantocillin	T36.0X1	T36.0X2	T36.0X3	T36.0X4	T36.0X5	T36.0X6
Xenon (127Xe) (133Xe)	T50.8X1	T50.8X2	T50.8X3	T50.8X4	T50.8X5	T50.8X6
Xenysalate	T49.4X1	T49.4X2	T49.4X3	T49.4X4	T49.4X5	T49.4X6
Xibornol	T37.8X1	T37.8X2	T37.8X3	T37.8X4	T37.8X5	T37.8X6
Xigris	T45.511	T45.512	T45.513	T45.514	T45.515	T45.516
Xipamide	T50.2X1	T50.2X2	T50.2X3	T50.2X4	T50.2X5	T50.2X6
Xylene (vapor)	T52.2X1	T52.2X2	T52.2X3	T52.2X4	--	--
Xylocaine (infiltration) (topical)	T41.3X1	T41.3X2	T41.3X3	T41.3X4	T41.3X5	T41.3X6
nerve block (peripheral) (plexus)	T41.3X1	T41.3X2	T41.3X3	T41.3X4	T41.3X5	T41.3X6
spinal	T41.3X1	T41.3X2	T41.3X3	T41.3X4	T41.3X5	T41.3X6
Xylol (vapor)	T52.2X1	T52.2X2	T52.2X3	T52.2X4	--	--
Xylometazoline	T48.5X1	T48.5X2	T48.5X3	T48.5X4	T48.5X5	T48.5X6
Y						
Yeast	T45.2X1	T45.2X2	T45.2X3	T45.2X4	T45.2X5	T45.2X6
dried	T45.2X1	T45.2X2	T45.2X3	T45.2X4	T45.2X5	T45.2X6
Yellow						
fever vaccine	T50.B91	T50.B92	T50.B93	T50.B94	T50.B95	T50.B96
jasmine	T62.2X1	T62.2X2	T62.2X3	T62.2X4	--	--
phenolphthalein	T47.2X1	T47.2X2	T47.2X3	T47.2X4	T47.2X5	T47.2X6
Yew	T62.2X1	T62.2X2	T62.2X3	T62.2X4	--	--
Yohimbic acid	T40.991	T40.992	T40.993	T40.994	T40.995	T40.996
Z						
Zactane	T39.8X1	T39.8X2	T39.8X3	T39.8X4	T39.8X5	T39.8X6
Zalcitabine	T37.5X1	T37.5X2	T37.5X3	T37.5X4	T37.5X5	T37.5X6
Zaroxolyn	T50.2X1	T50.2X2	T50.2X3	T50.2X4	T50.2X5	T50.2X6
Zephiran (topical)	T49.0X1	T49.0X2	T49.0X3	T49.0X4	T49.0X5	T49.0X6
ophthalmic preparation	T49.5X1	T49.5X2	T49.5X3	T49.5X4	T49.5X5	T49.5X6
Zeranol	T38.7X1	T38.7X2	T38.7X3	T38.7X4	T38.7X5	T38.7X6
Zerone	T51.1X1	T51.1X2	T51.1X3	T51.1X4	--	--
Zidovudine	T37.5X1	T37.5X2	T37.5X3	T37.5X4	T37.5X5	T37.5X6
Zimeldine	T43.221	T43.222	T43.223	T43.224	T43.225	T43.226
Zinc (compounds) (fumes) (vapor) **NEC**	T56.5X1	T56.5X2	T56.5X3	T56.5X4	--	--
anti-infectives	T49.0X1	T49.0X2	T49.0X3	T49.0X4	T49.0X5	T49.0X6
antivaricose	T46.8X1	T46.8X2	T46.8X3	T46.8X4	T46.8X5	T46.8X6
bacitracin	T49.0X1	T49.0X2	T49.0X3	T49.0X4	T49.0X5	T49.0X6
chloride (mouthwash)	T49.6X1	T49.6X2	T49.6X3	T49.6X4	T49.6X5	T49.6X6
chromate	T56.5X1	T56.5X2	T56.5X3	T56.5X4	--	--
gelatin	T49.3X1	T49.3X2	T49.3X3	T49.3X4	T49.3X5	T49.3X6
oxide	T49.3X1	T49.3X2	T49.3X3	T49.3X4	T49.3X5	T49.3X6
plaster	T49.3X1	T49.3X2	T49.3X3	T49.3X4	T49.3X5	T49.3X6
peroxide	T49.0X1	T49.0X2	T49.0X3	T49.0X4	T49.0X5	T49.0X6
pesticides	T56.5X1	T56.5X2	T56.5X3	T56.5X4	--	--
phosphide	T60.4X1	T60.4X2	T60.4X3	T60.4X4	--	--
pyrithionate	T49.4X1	T49.4X2	T49.4X3	T49.4X4	T49.4X5	T49.4X6
stearate	T49.3X1	T49.3X2	T49.3X3	T49.3X4	T49.3X5	T49.3X6
sulfate	T49.5X1	T49.5X2	T49.5X3	T49.5X4	T49.5X5	T49.5X6
ENT agent	T49.6X1	T49.6X2	T49.6X3	T49.6X4	T49.6X5	T49.6X6
ophthalmic solution	T49.5X1	T49.5X2	T49.5X3	T49.5X4	T49.5X5	T49.5X6
topical NEC	T49.0X1	T49.0X2	T49.0X3	T49.0X4	T49.0X5	T49.0X6
undecylenate	T49.0X1	T49.0X2	T49.0X3	T49.0X4	T49.0X5	T49.0X6
Zineb	T60.0X1	T60.0X2	T60.0X3	T60.0X4	--	--
Zinostatin	T45.1X1	T45.1X2	T45.1X3	T45.1X4	T45.1X5	T45.1X6

Verdigris - Zinostatin

ICD-10-CM TABLE OF DRUGS AND CHEMICALS

Zipeprol - Zyprexa

Substance	Poisoning, Accidental unintentional	Poisoning, Intentional self-harm	Poisoning, Assault	Poisoning, Undetermined	Adverse effect	Underdosing
Zipeprol	T48.3X1	T48.3X2	T48.3X3	T48.3X4	T48.3X5	T48.3X6
Zofenopril	T46.4X1	T46.4X2	T46.4X3	T46.4X4	T46.4X5	T46.4X6
Zolpidem	T42.6X1	T42.6X2	T42.6X3	T42.6X4	T42.6X5	T42.6X6
Zomepirac	T39.391	T39.392	T39.393	T39.394	T39.395	T39.396
Zopiclone	T42.6X1	T42.6X2	T42.6X3	T42.6X4	T42.6X5	T42.6X6
Zorubicin	T45.1X1	T45.1X2	T45.1X3	T45.1X4	T45.1X5	T45.1X6
Zotepine	T43.591	T43.592	T43.593	T43.594	T43.595	T43.596
Zovant	T45.511	T45.512	T45.513	T45.514	T45.515	T45.516
Zoxazolamine	T42.8X1	T42.8X2	T42.8X3	T42.8X4	T42.8X5	T42.8X6
Zuclopenthixol	T43.4X1	T43.4X2	T43.4X3	T43.4X4	T43.4X5	T43.4X6
Zygadenus (venenosus)	T62.2X1	T62.2X2	T62.2X3	T62.2X4	--	--
Zyprexa	T43.591	T43.592	T43.593	T43.594	T43.595	T43.596

ICD-10-CM Index to External Causes of Injuries

A

Abandonment (causing exposure to weather conditions) (with intent to injure or kill) NEC X58 ☑

Abuse (adult) (child) (mental) (physical) (sexual) X58 ☑

Accident (to) X58 ☑
- aircraft (in transit) (powered) (*see also* Accident, transport, aircraft)
  - due to, caused by cataclysm — *see* Forces of nature, by type
- animal-rider — *see* Accident, transport, animal-rider
- animal-drawn vehicle — *see* Accident, transport, animal-drawn vehicle occupant
- automobile — *see* Accident, transport, car occupant
- bare foot water skier V94.4 ☑
- boat, boating (*see also* Accident, watercraft)
  - striking swimmer
    - powered V94.11 ☑
    - unpowered V94.12 ☑
- bus — *see* Accident, transport, bus occupant
- cable car, not on rails V98.0 ☑
  - on rails — *see* Accident, transport, streetcar occupant
- car — *see* Accident, transport, car occupant
- caused by, due to
  - animal NEC W64 ☑
  - chain hoist W24.0 ☑
  - cold (excessive) — *see* Exposure, cold
  - corrosive liquid, substance — *see* Table of Drugs and Chemicals
  - cutting or piercing instrument — *see* Contact, with, by type of instrument
  - drive belt W24.0 ☑
  - electric
    - current — *see* Exposure, electric current
    - motor (*see also* Contact, with, by type of machine) W31.3 ☑
      - current (of) W86.8 ☑
  - environmental factor NEC X58 ☑
  - explosive material — *see* Explosion
  - fire, flames — *see* Exposure, fire
  - firearm missile — *see* Discharge, firearm by type
  - heat (excessive) — *see* Heat
  - hot — *see* Contact, with, hot
  - ignition — *see* Ignition
  - lifting device W24.0 ☑
  - lightning — *see* subcategory T75.0
    - causing fire — *see* Exposure, fire
  - machine, machinery — *see* Contact, with, by type of machine
  - natural factor NEC X58 ☑
  - pulley (block) W24.0 ☑
  - radiation — *see* Radiation
  - steam X13.1 ☑
    - inhalation X13.0 ☑
    - pipe X16 ☑
  - thunderbolt — *see* subcategory T75.0
    - causing fire — *see* Exposure, fire
  - transmission device W24.1 ☑
- coach — *see* Accident, transport, bus occupant
- coal car — *see* Accident, transport, industrial vehicle occupant
- diving (*see also* Fall, into, water)
  - with
    - drowning or submersion — *see* Drowning
- forklift — *see* Accident, transport, industrial vehicle occupant
- heavy transport vehicle NOS — *see* Accident, transport, truck occupant
- ice yacht V98.2 ☑
- in
  - medical, surgical procedure
    - as, or due to misadventure — *see* Misadventure
    - causing an abnormal reaction or later complication without mention of misadventure (*see also* Complication of or following, by type of procedure) Y84.9
- land yacht V98.1 ☑
- late effect of — *see* W00-X58 with 7th character S

Accident — *continued*
- logging car — *see* Accident, transport, industrial vehicle occupant
- machine, machinery (*see also* Contact, with, by type of machine)
  - on board watercraft V93.69 ☑
    - explosion — *see* Explosion, in, watercraft
    - fire — *see* Burn, on board watercraft
    - powered craft V93.63 ☑
      - ferry boat V93.61 ☑
      - fishing boat V93.62 ☑
      - jet skis V93.63 ☑
      - liner V93.61 ☑
      - merchant ship V93.60 ☑
      - passenger ship V93.61 ☑
      - sailboat V93.64 ☑
- mine tram — *see* Accident, transport, industrial vehicle occupant
- mobility scooter (motorized) — *see* Accident, transport, pedestrian, conveyance, specified type NEC
- motor scooter — *see* Accident, transport, motorcyclist
- motor vehicle NOS (traffic) (*see also* Accident, transport) V89.2 ☑
  - nontraffic V89.0 ☑
  - three-wheeled NOS — *see* Accident, transport, three-wheeled motor vehicle occupant
- motorcycle NOS — *see* Accident, transport, motorcyclist
- nonmotor vehicle NOS (nontraffic) (*see also* Accident, transport) V89.1 ☑
  - traffic NOS V89.3 ☑
- nontraffic (victim's mode of transport NOS) V88.9 ☑
  - collision (between) V88.7 ☑
    - bus and truck V88.5 ☑
    - car and:
      - bus V88.3 ☑
      - pickup V88.2 ☑
      - three-wheeled motor vehicle V88.0 ☑
      - train V88.6 ☑
      - truck V88.4 ☑
      - two-wheeled motor vehicle V88.0 ☑
      - van V88.2 ☑
    - specified vehicle NEC and:
      - three-wheeled motor vehicle V88.1 ☑
      - two-wheeled motor vehicle V88.1 ☑
  - known mode of transport — *see* Accident, transport, by type of vehicle
  - noncollision V88.8 ☑
- on board watercraft V93.89 ☑
  - powered craft V93.83 ☑
    - ferry boat V93.81 ☑
    - fishing boat V93.82 ☑
    - jet skis V93.83 ☑
    - liner V93.81 ☑
    - merchant ship V93.80 ☑
    - passenger ship V93.81 ☑
  - unpowered craft V93.88 ☑
    - canoe V93.85 ☑
    - inflatable V93.86 ☑
      - in tow
        - recreational V94.31 ☑
        - specified NEC V94.32 ☑
    - kayak V93.85 ☑
    - sailboat V93.84 ☑
    - surf-board V93.88 ☑
    - water skis V93.87 ☑
    - windsurfer V93.88 ☑
- parachutist V97.29 ☑
  - entangled in object V97.21 ☑
  - injured on landing V97.22 ☑
- pedal cycle — *see* Accident, transport, pedal cyclist
- pedestrian (on foot)
  - with
    - another pedestrian W51 ☑
      - with fall W03 ☑
        - due to ice or snow W00.0 ☑
      - on pedestrian conveyance NEC V00.09 ☑
    - roller skater (in-line) V00.01 ☑
    - skate boarder V00.02 ☑
    - transport vehicle — *see* Accident, transport
  - on pedestrian conveyance — *see* Accident, transport, pedestrian, conveyance
- pick-up truck or van — *see* Accident, transport, pickup truck occupant

Accident — *continued*
- quarry truck — *see* Accident, transport, industrial vehicle occupant
- railway vehicle (any) (in motion) — *see* Accident, transport, railway vehicle occupant
  - due to cataclysm — *see* Forces of nature, by type
- scooter (non-motorized) — *see* Accident, transport, pedestrian, conveyance, scooter
- sequelae of — *see* W00-X58 with 7th character S
- skateboard — *see* Accident, transport, pedestrian, conveyance, skateboard
- ski (ing) — *see* Accident, transport, pedestrian, conveyance
  - lift V98.3 ☑
- specified cause NEC X58 ☑
- streetcar — *see* Accident, transport, streetcar occupant
- traffic (victim's mode of transport NOS) V87.9 ☑
  - collision (between) V87.7 ☑
    - bus and truck V87.5 ☑
    - car and:
      - bus V87.3 ☑
      - pickup V87.2 ☑
      - three-wheeled motor vehicle V87.0 ☑
      - train V87.6 ☑
      - truck V87.4 ☑
      - two-wheeled motor vehicle V87.0 ☑
      - van V87.2 ☑
    - specified vehicle NEC and:
      - three-wheeled motor vehicle V87.1 ☑
      - two-wheeled motor vehicle V87.1 ☑
  - known mode of transport — *see* Accident, transport, by type of vehicle
  - noncollision V87.8 ☑
- transport (involving injury to) V99 ☑
  - 18 wheeler — *see* Accident, transport, truck occupant
  - agricultural vehicle occupant (nontraffic) V84.9 ☑
    - driver V84.5 ☑
    - hanger-on V84.7 ☑
    - passenger V84.6 ☑
    - traffic V84.3 ☑
      - driver V84.0 ☑
      - hanger-on V84.2 ☑
      - passenger V84.1 ☑
    - while boarding or alighting V84.4 ☑
  - aircraft NEC V97.89 ☑
    - military NEC V97.818 ☑
      - with civilian aircraft V97.810 ☑
      - civilian injured by V97.811 ☑
    - occupant injured (in)
      - nonpowered craft accident V96.9 ☑
        - balloon V96.00 ☑
          - collision V96.03 ☑
          - crash V96.01 ☑
          - explosion V96.05 ☑
          - fire V96.04 ☑
          - forced landing V96.02 ☑
          - specified type NEC V96.09 ☑
        - glider V96.20 ☑
          - collision V96.23 ☑
          - crash V96.21 ☑
          - explosion V96.25 ☑
          - fire V96.24 ☑
          - forced landing V96.22 ☑
          - specified type NEC V96.29 ☑
        - hang glider V96.10 ☑
          - collision V96.13 ☑
          - crash V96.11 ☑
          - explosion V96.15 ☑
          - fire V96.14 ☑
          - forced landing V96.12 ☑
          - specified type NEC V96.19 ☑
        - specified craft NEC V96.8 ☑
      - powered craft accident V95.9 ☑
        - fixed wing NEC
          - commercial V95.30 ☑
            - collision V95.33 ☑
            - crash V95.31 ☑
            - explosion V95.35 ☑
            - fire V95.34 ☑
            - forced landing V95.32 ☑
            - specified type NEC V95.39 ☑
          - private V95.20 ☑
            - collision V95.23 ☑
            - crash V95.21 ☑

- **Accident** — *continued*
  - transport — *continued*
              - explosion V95.25 ☑
              - fire V95.24 ☑
              - forced landing V95.22 ☑
              - specified type NEC V95.29 ☑
          - glider V95.10 ☑
            - collision V95.13 ☑
            - crash V95.11 ☑
            - explosion V95.15 ☑
            - fire V95.14 ☑
            - forced landing V95.12 ☑
            - specified type NEC V95.19 ☑
          - helicopter V95.00 ☑
            - collision V95.03 ☑
            - crash V95.01 ☑
            - explosion V95.05 ☑
            - fire V95.04 ☑
            - forced landing V95.02 ☑
            - specified type NEC V95.09 ☑
          - spacecraft V95.40 ☑
            - collision V95.43 ☑
            - crash V95.41 ☑
            - explosion V95.45 ☑
            - fire V95.44 ☑
            - forced landing V95.42 ☑
            - specified type NEC V95.49 ☑
          - specified craft NEC V95.8 ☑
          - ultralight V95.10 ☑
            - collision V95.13 ☑
            - crash V95.11 ☑
            - explosion V95.15 ☑
            - fire V95.14 ☑
            - forced landing V95.12 ☑
            - specified type NEC V95.19 ☑
        - specified accident NEC V97.0 ☑
        - while boarding or alighting V97.1 ☑
      - person (injured by)
        - falling from, in or on aircraft V97.0 ☑
        - machinery on aircraft V97.89 ☑
        - on ground with aircraft involvement V97.39 ☑
        - rotating propeller V97.32 ☑
        - struck by object falling from aircraft V97.31 ☑
        - sucked into aircraft jet V97.33 ☑
        - while boarding or alighting aircraft V97.1 ☑
    - airport (battery-powered) passenger vehicle — *see* Accident, transport, industrial vehicle occupant
    - all-terrain vehicle occupant (nontraffic) V86.99 ☑
      - driver V86.59 ☑
      - dune buggy — *see* Accident, transport, dune buggy occupant
      - hanger-on V86.79 ☑
      - passenger V86.69 ☑
      - snowmobile — *see* Accident, transport, snowmobile occupant
      - traffic V86.39 ☑
        - driver V86.09 ☑
        - hanger-on V86.29 ☑
        - passenger V86.19 ☑
      - while boarding or alighting V86.49 ☑
    - ambulance occupant (traffic) V86.31 ☑
      - driver V86.01 ☑
      - hanger-on V86.21 ☑
      - nontraffic V86.91 ☑
        - driver V86.51 ☑
        - hanger-on V86.71 ☑
        - passenger V86.61 ☑
      - passenger V86.11 ☑
      - while boarding or alighting V86.41 ☑
    - animal-drawn vehicle occupant (in) V80.929 ☑
      - collision (with)
        - animal V80.12 ☑
          - being ridden V80.711 ☑
        - animal-drawn vehicle V80.721 ☑
        - bus V80.42 ☑
        - car V80.42 ☑
        - fixed or stationary object V80.82 ☑
        - military vehicle V80.920 ☑
        - nonmotor vehicle V80.791 ☑
        - pedal cycle V80.22 ☑
        - pedestrian V80.12 ☑
        - pickup V80.42 ☑
        - railway train or vehicle V80.62 ☑
        - specified motor vehicle NEC V80.52 ☑
        - streetcar V80.731 ☑
        - truck V80.42 ☑

- **Accident** — *continued*
  - transport — *continued*
        - two- or three-wheeled motor vehicle V80.32 ☑
        - van V80.42 ☑
      - noncollision V80.02 ☑
      - specified circumstance NEC V80.928 ☑
    - animal-rider V80.919 ☑
      - collision (with)
        - animal V80.11 ☑
          - being ridden V80.710 ☑
        - animal-drawn vehicle V80.720 ☑
        - bus V80.41 ☑
        - car V80.41 ☑
        - fixed or stationary object V80.81 ☑
        - military vehicle V80.910 ☑
        - nonmotor vehicle V80.790 ☑
        - pedal cycle V80.21 ☑
        - pedestrian V80.11 ☑
        - pickup V80.41 ☑
        - railway train or vehicle V80.61 ☑
        - specified motor vehicle NEC V80.51 ☑
        - streetcar V80.730 ☑
        - truck V80.41 ☑
        - two- or three-wheeled motor vehicle V80.31 ☑
        - van V80.41 ☑
      - noncollision V80.018 ☑
        - specified as horse rider V80.010 ☑
      - specified circumstance NEC V80.918 ☑
    - armored car — *see* Accident, transport, truck occupant
    - battery-powered truck (baggage) (mail) — *see* Accident, transport, industrial vehicle occupant
    - bus occupant V79.9 ☑
      - collision (with)
        - animal (traffic) V70.9 ☑
          - being ridden (traffic) V76.9 ☑
            - nontraffic V76.3 ☑
            - while boarding or alighting V76.4 ☑
          - nontraffic V70.3 ☑
          - while boarding or alighting V70.4 ☑
        - animal-drawn vehicle (traffic) V76.9 ☑
          - nontraffic V76.3 ☑
          - while boarding or alighting V76.4 ☑
        - bus (traffic) V74.9 ☑
          - nontraffic V74.3 ☑
          - while boarding or alighting V74.4 ☑
        - car (traffic) V73.9 ☑
          - nontraffic V73.3 ☑
          - while boarding or alighting V73.4 ☑
        - motor vehicle NOS (traffic) V79.60 ☑
          - nontraffic V79.20 ☑
          - specified type NEC (traffic) V79.69 ☑
            - nontraffic V79.29 ☑
        - pedal cycle (traffic) V71.9 ☑
          - nontraffic V71.3 ☑
          - while boarding or alighting V71.4 ☑
        - pickup truck (traffic) V73.9 ☑
          - nontraffic V73.3 ☑
          - while boarding or alighting V73.4 ☑
        - railway vehicle (traffic) V75.9 ☑
          - nontraffic V75.3 ☑
          - while boarding or alighting V75.4 ☑
        - specified vehicle NEC (traffic) V76.9 ☑
          - nontraffic V76.3 ☑
          - while boarding or alighting V76.4 ☑
        - stationary object (traffic) V77.9 ☑
          - nontraffic V77.3 ☑
          - while boarding or alighting V77.4 ☑
        - streetcar (traffic) V76.9 ☑
          - nontraffic V76.3 ☑
          - while boarding or alighting V76.4 ☑
        - three wheeled motor vehicle (traffic) V72.9 ☑
          - nontraffic V72.3 ☑
          - while boarding or alighting V72.4 ☑
        - truck (traffic) V74.9 ☑
          - nontraffic V74.3 ☑
          - while boarding or alighting V74.4 ☑
        - two wheeled motor vehicle (traffic) V72.9 ☑
          - nontraffic V72.3 ☑
          - while boarding or alighting V72.4 ☑
        - van (traffic) V73.9 ☑
          - nontraffic V73.3 ☑
          - while boarding or alighting V73.4 ☑
      - driver
        - collision (with)
          - animal (traffic) V70.5 ☑
            - being ridden (traffic) V76.5 ☑

- **Accident** — *continued*
  - transport — *continued*
              - nontraffic V76.0 ☑
            - nontraffic V70.0 ☑
          - animal-drawn vehicle (traffic) V76.5 ☑
            - nontraffic V76.0 ☑
          - bus (traffic) V74.5 ☑
            - nontraffic V74.0 ☑
          - car (traffic) V73.5 ☑
            - nontraffic V73.0 ☑
          - motor vehicle NOS (traffic) V79.40 ☑
            - nontraffic V79.00 ☑
            - specified type NEC (traffic) V79.49 ☑
              - nontraffic V79.09 ☑
          - pedal cycle (traffic) V71.5 ☑
            - nontraffic V71.0 ☑
          - pickup truck (traffic) V73.5 ☑
            - nontraffic V73.0 ☑
          - railway vehicle (traffic) V75.5 ☑
            - nontraffic V75.0 ☑
          - specified vehicle NEC (traffic) V76.5 ☑
            - nontraffic V76.0 ☑
          - stationary object (traffic) V77.5 ☑
            - nontraffic V77.0 ☑
          - streetcar (traffic) V76.5 ☑
            - nontraffic V76.0 ☑
          - three wheeled motor vehicle (traffic) V72.5 ☑
            - nontraffic V72.0 ☑
          - truck (traffic) V74.5 ☑
            - nontraffic V74.0 ☑
          - two wheeled motor vehicle (traffic) V72.5 ☑
            - nontraffic V72.0 ☑
          - van (traffic) V73.5 ☑
            - nontraffic V73.0 ☑
        - noncollision accident (traffic) V78.5 ☑
          - nontraffic V78.0 ☑
      - noncollision accident (traffic) V78.9 ☑
        - nontraffic V78.3 ☑
        - while boarding or alighting V78.4 ☑
      - nontraffic V79.3 ☑
      - hanger-on
        - collision (with)
          - animal (traffic) V70.7 ☑
            - being ridden (traffic) V76.7 ☑
              - nontraffic V76.2 ☑
            - nontraffic V70.2 ☑
          - animal-drawn vehicle (traffic) V76.7 ☑
            - nontraffic V76.2 ☑
          - bus (traffic) V74.7 ☑
            - nontraffic V74.2 ☑
          - car (traffic) V73.7 ☑
            - nontraffic V73.2 ☑
          - pedal cycle (traffic) V71.7 ☑
            - nontraffic V71.2 ☑
          - pickup truck (traffic) V73.7 ☑
            - nontraffic V73.2 ☑
          - railway vehicle (traffic) V75.7 ☑
            - nontraffic V75.2 ☑
          - specified vehicle NEC (traffic) V76.7 ☑
            - nontraffic V76.2 ☑
          - stationary object (traffic) V77.7 ☑
            - nontraffic V77.2 ☑
          - streetcar (traffic) V76.7 ☑
            - nontraffic V76.2 ☑
          - three wheeled motor vehicle (traffic) V72.7 ☑
            - nontraffic V72.2 ☑
          - truck (traffic) V74.7 ☑
            - nontraffic V74.2 ☑
          - two wheeled motor vehicle (traffic) V72.7 ☑
            - nontraffic V72.2 ☑
          - van (traffic) V73.7 ☑
            - nontraffic V73.2 ☑
        - noncollision accident (traffic) V78.7 ☑
          - nontraffic V78.2 ☑
      - passenger
        - collision (with)
          - animal (traffic) V70.6 ☑
            - being ridden (traffic) V76.6 ☑
              - nontraffic V76.1 ☑
            - nontraffic V70.1 ☑
          - animal-drawn vehicle (traffic) V76.6 ☑
            - nontraffic V76.1 ☑
          - bus (traffic) V74.6 ☑
            - nontraffic V74.1 ☑
          - car (traffic) V73.6 ☑
            - nontraffic V73.1 ☑
          - motor vehicle NOS (traffic) V79.50 ☑
            - nontraffic V79.10 ☑

- **Accident** — *continued*
  - transport — *continued*
        - bus or heavy transport V04.99 ☑
          - nontraffic V04.09 ☑
          - traffic V04.19 ☑
        - car V03.99 ☑
          - nontraffic V03.09 ☑
          - traffic V03.19 ☑
        - pedal cycle V01.99 ☑
          - nontraffic V01.09 ☑
          - traffic V01.19 ☑
        - pick-up truck or van V03.99 ☑
          - nontraffic V03.09 ☑
          - traffic V03.19 ☑
        - railway (train) (vehicle) V05.99 ☑
          - nontraffic V05.09 ☑
          - traffic V05.19 ☑
        - stationary object V00.282 ☑
        - streetcar V06.99 ☑
          - nontraffic V06.09 ☑
          - traffic V06.19 ☑
        - two- or three-wheeled motor vehicle V02.99 ☑
          - nontraffic V02.09 ☑
          - traffic V02.19 ☑
        - vehicle V09.9 ☑
          - animal-drawn V06.99 ☑
            - nontraffic V06.09 ☑
            - traffic V06.19 ☑
          - motor
            - nontraffic V09.00 ☑
            - traffic V09.20 ☑
      - fall V00.281 ☑
      - heelies — *see* Accident, transport, pedestrian, conveyance, heelies
      - ice skate — *see* Accident, transport, pedestrian, conveyance, ice skate
      - nontraffic V09.1 ☑
        - involving motor vehicle NEC V09.00 ☑
      - sled — *see* Accident, transport, pedestrian, conveyance, sled
      - traffic V09.3 ☑
        - involving motor vehicle NEC V09.20 ☑
        - wheelies — *see* Accident, transport, pedestrian, conveyance, heelies
    - heelies V00.158 ☑
      - colliding with stationary object V00.152 ☑
      - fall V00.151 ☑
    - ice skates V00.218 ☑
      - collision (with) V09.9 ☑
        - animal being ridden or animal drawn vehicle V06.99 ☑
          - nontraffic V06.09 ☑
          - traffic V06.19 ☑
        - bus or heavy transport V04.99 ☑
          - nontraffic V04.09 ☑
          - traffic V04.19 ☑
        - car V03.99 ☑
          - nontraffic V03.09 ☑
          - traffic V03.19 ☑
        - pedal cycle V01.99 ☑
          - nontraffic V01.09 ☑
          - traffic V01.19 ☑
        - pick-up truck or van V03.99 ☑
          - nontraffic V03.09 ☑
          - traffic V03.19 ☑
        - railway (train) (vehicle) V05.99 ☑
          - nontraffic V05.09 ☑
          - traffic V05.19 ☑
        - streetcar V06.99 ☑
          - nontraffic V06.09 ☑
          - traffic V06.19 ☑
        - stationary object V00.212 ☑
        - two- or three-wheeled motor vehicle V02.99 ☑
          - nontraffic V02.09 ☑
          - traffic V02.19 ☑
        - vehicle V09.9 ☑
          - animal-drawn V06.99 ☑
            - nontraffic V06.09 ☑
            - traffic V06.19 ☑
          - motor
            - nontraffic V09.00 ☑
            - traffic V09.20 ☑
      - fall V00.211 ☑
      - nontraffic V09.1 ☑
        - involving motor vehicle NEC V09.00 ☑
      - traffic V09.3 ☑
        - involving motor vehicle NEC V09.20 ☑
    - motorized mobility scooter V00.838 ☑

- **Accident** — *continued*
  - transport — *continued*
      - collision with stationary object V00.832 ☑
      - fall from V00.831 ☑
    - nontraffic V09.1 ☑
      - involving motor vehicle V09.00 ☑
        - military V09.01 ☑
        - specified type NEC V09.09 ☑
    - roller skates (non in-line) V00.128 ☑
      - collision (with) V09.9 ☑
        - animal being ridden or animal drawn vehicle V06.91 ☑
          - nontraffic V06.01 ☑
          - traffic V06.11 ☑
        - bus or heavy transport V04.91 ☑
          - nontraffic V04.01 ☑
          - traffic V04.11 ☑
        - car V03.91 ☑
          - nontraffic V03.01 ☑
          - traffic V03.11 ☑
        - pedal cycle V01.91 ☑
          - nontraffic V01.01 ☑
          - traffic V01.11 ☑
        - pick-up truck or van V03.91 ☑
          - nontraffic V03.01 ☑
          - traffic V03.11 ☑
        - railway (train) (vehicle) V05.91 ☑
          - nontraffic V05.01 ☑
          - traffic V05.11 ☑
        - streetcar V06.91 ☑
          - nontraffic V06.01 ☑
          - traffic V06.11 ☑
        - stationary object V00.122 ☑
        - two- or three-wheeled motor vehicle V02.91 ☑
          - nontraffic V02.01 ☑
          - traffic V02.11 ☑
        - vehicle V09.9 ☑
          - animal-drawn V06.91 ☑
            - nontraffic V06.01 ☑
            - traffic V06.11 ☑
          - motor
            - nontraffic V09.00 ☑
            - traffic V09.20 ☑
      - fall V00.121 ☑
      - in-line V00.118 ☑
        - collision- — *see* also Accident, transport, pedestrian, conveyance occupant, roller skates, collision
          - with stationary object V00.112 ☑
        - fall V00.111 ☑
      - nontraffic V09.1 ☑
        - involving motor vehicle NEC V09.00 ☑
      - traffic V09.3 ☑
        - involving motor vehicle NEC V09.20 ☑
    - rolling shoes V00.158 ☑
      - colliding with stationary object V00.152 ☑
      - fall V00.151 ☑
    - rolling type NEC V00.188 ☑
      - collision (with) V09.9 ☑
        - animal being ridden or animal drawn vehicle V06.99 ☑
          - nontraffic V06.09 ☑
          - traffic V06.19 ☑
        - bus or heavy transport V04.99 ☑
          - nontraffic V04.09 ☑
          - traffic V04.19 ☑
        - car V03.99 ☑
          - nontraffic V03.09 ☑
          - traffic V03.19 ☑
        - pedal cycle V01.99 ☑
          - nontraffic V01.09 ☑
          - traffic V01.19 ☑
        - pick-up truck or van V03.99 ☑
          - nontraffic V03.09 ☑
          - traffic V03.19 ☑
        - railway (train) (vehicle) V05.99 ☑
          - nontraffic V05.09 ☑
          - traffic V05.19 ☑
        - stationary object V00.182 ☑
        - streetcar V06.99 ☑
          - nontraffic V06.09 ☑
          - traffic V06.19 ☑
        - two- or three-wheeled motor vehicle V02.99 ☑
          - nontraffic V02.09 ☑
          - traffic V02.19 ☑
        - vehicle V09.9 ☑
          - animal-drawn V06.99 ☑
            - nontraffic V06.09 ☑

- **Accident** — *continued*
  - transport — *continued*
            - traffic V06.19 ☑
          - motor
            - nontraffic V09.00 ☑
            - traffic V09.20 ☑
      - fall V00.181 ☑
      - in-line roller skate — *see* Accident, transport, pedestrian, conveyance, roller skate, in-line
      - nontraffic V09.1 ☑
        - involving motor vehicle NEC V09.00 ☑
      - roller skate — *see* Accident, transport, pedestrian, conveyance, roller skate
      - scooter (non-motorized) — *see* Accident, transport, pedestrian, conveyance, scooter
      - skateboard — *see* Accident, transport, pedestrian, conveyance, skateboard
      - traffic V09.3 ☑
        - involving motor vehicle NEC V09.20 ☑
    - scooter (non-motorized) V00.148 ☑
      - collision (with) V09.9 ☑
        - animal being ridden or animal drawn vehicle V06.99 ☑
          - nontraffic V06.09 ☑
          - traffic V06.19 ☑
        - bus or heavy transport V04.99 ☑
          - nontraffic V04.09 ☑
          - traffic V04.19 ☑
        - car V03.99 ☑
          - nontraffic V03.09 ☑
          - traffic V03.19 ☑
        - pedal cycle V01.99 ☑
          - nontraffic V01.09 ☑
          - traffic V01.19 ☑
        - pick-up truck or van V03.99 ☑
          - nontraffic V03.09 ☑
          - traffic V03.19 ☑
        - railway (train) (vehicle) V05.99 ☑
          - nontraffic V05.09 ☑
          - traffic V05.19 ☑
        - streetcar V06.99 ☑
          - nontraffic V06.09 ☑
          - traffic V06.19 ☑
        - stationary object V00.142 ☑
        - two- or three-wheeled motor vehicle V02.99 ☑
          - nontraffic V02.09 ☑
          - traffic V02.19 ☑
        - vehicle V09.9 ☑
          - animal-drawn V06.99 ☑
            - nontraffic V06.09 ☑
            - traffic V06.19 ☑
          - motor
            - nontraffic V09.00 ☑
            - traffic V09.20 ☑
      - fall V00.141 ☑
      - nontraffic V09.1 ☑
        - involving motor vehicle NEC V09.00 ☑
      - traffic V09.3 ☑
        - involving motor vehicle NEC V09.20 ☑
    - skate board V00.138 ☑
      - collision (with) V09.9 ☑
        - animal being ridden or animal drawn vehicle V06.92 ☑
          - nontraffic V06.02 ☑
          - traffic V06.12 ☑
        - bus or heavy transport V04.92 ☑
          - nontraffic V04.02 ☑
          - traffic V04.12 ☑
        - car V03.92 ☑
          - nontraffic V03.02 ☑
          - traffic V03.12 ☑
        - pedal cycle V01.92 ☑
          - nontraffic V01.02 ☑
          - traffic V01.12 ☑
        - pick-up truck or van V03.92 ☑
          - nontraffic V03.02 ☑
          - traffic V03.12 ☑
        - railway (train) (vehicle) V05.92 ☑
          - nontraffic V05.02 ☑
          - traffic V05.12 ☑
        - streetcar V06.92 ☑
          - nontraffic V06.02 ☑
          - traffic V06.12 ☑
        - stationary object V00.132 ☑
        - two- or three-wheeled motor vehicle V02.92 ☑
          - nontraffic V02.02 ☑
          - traffic V02.12 ☑
        - vehicle V09.9 ☑

- **Accident** — *continued*
  - transport — *continued*
            - animal-drawn V06.92 ☑
              - nontraffic V06.02 ☑
              - traffic V06.12 ☑
            - motor
              - nontraffic V09.00 ☑
              - traffic V09.20 ☑
        - fall V00.131 ☑
        - nontraffic V09.1 ☑
          - involving motor vehicle NEC V09.00 ☑
        - traffic V09.3 ☑
          - involving motor vehicle NEC V09.20 ☑
      - sled V00.228 ☑
        - collision (with) V09.9 ☑
          - animal being ridden or animal drawn vehicle V06.99 ☑
            - nontraffic V06.09 ☑
            - traffic V06.19 ☑
          - bus or heavy transport V04.99 ☑
            - nontraffic V04.09 ☑
            - traffic V04.19 ☑
          - car V03.99 ☑
            - nontraffic V03.09 ☑
            - traffic V03.19 ☑
          - pedal cycle V01.99 ☑
            - nontraffic V01.09 ☑
            - traffic V01.19 ☑
          - pick-up truck or van V03.99 ☑
            - nontraffic V03.09 ☑
            - traffic V03.19 ☑
          - railway (train) (vehicle) V05.99 ☑
            - nontraffic V05.09 ☑
            - traffic V05.19 ☑
          - streetcar V06.99 ☑
            - nontraffic V06.09 ☑
            - traffic V06.19 ☑
          - stationary object V00.222 ☑
          - two- or three-wheeled motor vehicle V02.99 ☑
            - nontraffic V02.09 ☑
            - traffic V02.19 ☑
          - vehicle V09.9 ☑
            - animal-drawn V06.99 ☑
              - nontraffic V06.09 ☑
              - traffic V06.19 ☑
            - motor
              - nontraffic V09.00 ☑
              - traffic V09.20 ☑
        - fall V00.221 ☑
        - nontraffic V09.1 ☑
          - involving motor vehicle NEC V09.00 ☑
        - traffic V09.3 ☑
          - involving motor vehicle NEC V09.20 ☑
      - skis (snow) V00.328 ☑
        - collision (with) V09.9 ☑
          - animal being ridden or animal drawn vehicle V06.99 ☑
            - nontraffic V06.09 ☑
            - traffic V06.19 ☑
          - bus or heavy transport V04.99 ☑
            - nontraffic V04.09 ☑
            - traffic V04.19 ☑
          - car V03.99 ☑
            - nontraffic V03.09 ☑
            - traffic V03.19 ☑
          - pedal cycle V01.99 ☑
            - nontraffic V01.09 ☑
            - traffic V01.19 ☑
          - pick-up truck or van V03.99 ☑
            - nontraffic V03.09 ☑
            - traffic V03.19 ☑
          - railway (train) (vehicle) V05.99 ☑
            - nontraffic V05.09 ☑
            - traffic V05.19 ☑
          - streetcar V06.99 ☑
            - nontraffic V06.09 ☑
            - traffic V06.19 ☑
          - stationary object V00.322 ☑
          - two- or three-wheeled motor vehicle V02.99 ☑
            - nontraffic V02.09 ☑
            - traffic V02.19 ☑
          - vehicle V09.9 ☑
            - animal-drawn V06.99 ☑
              - nontraffic V06.09 ☑
              - traffic V06.19 ☑
            - motor
              - nontraffic V09.00 ☑
              - traffic V09.20 ☑
        - fall V00.321 ☑
        - nontraffic V09.1 ☑

- **Accident** — *continued*
  - transport — *continued*
          - involving motor vehicle NEC V09.00 ☑
        - traffic V09.3 ☑
          - involving motor vehicle NEC V09.20 ☑
      - snow board V00.318 ☑
        - collision (with) V09.9 ☑
          - animal being ridden or animal drawn vehicle V06.99 ☑
            - nontraffic V06.09 ☑
            - traffic V06.19 ☑
          - bus or heavy transport V04.99 ☑
            - nontraffic V04.09 ☑
            - traffic V04.19 ☑
          - car V03.99 ☑
            - nontraffic V03.09 ☑
            - traffic V03.19 ☑
          - pedal cycle V01.99 ☑
            - nontraffic V01.09 ☑
            - traffic V01.19 ☑
          - pick-up truck or van V03.99 ☑
            - nontraffic V03.09 ☑
            - traffic V03.19 ☑
          - railway (train) (vehicle) V05.99 ☑
            - nontraffic V05.09 ☑
            - traffic V05.19 ☑
          - streetcar V06.99 ☑
            - nontraffic V06.09 ☑
            - traffic V06.19 ☑
          - stationary object V00.312 ☑
          - two- or three-wheeled motor vehicle V02.99 ☑
            - nontraffic V02.09 ☑
            - traffic V02.19 ☑
          - vehicle V09.9 ☑
            - animal-drawn V06.99 ☑
              - nontraffic V06.09 ☑
              - traffic V06.19 ☑
            - motor
              - nontraffic V09.00 ☑
              - traffic V09.20 ☑
        - fall V00.311 ☑
        - nontraffic V09.1 ☑
          - involving motor vehicle NEC V09.00 ☑
        - traffic V09.3 ☑
          - involving motor vehicle NEC V09.20 ☑
      - specified type NEC V00.898 ☑
        - collision (with) V09.9 ☑
          - animal being ridden or animal drawn vehicle V06.99 ☑
            - nontraffic V06.09 ☑
            - traffic V06.19 ☑
          - bus or heavy transport V04.99 ☑
            - nontraffic V04.09 ☑
            - traffic V04.19 ☑
          - car V03.99 ☑
            - nontraffic V03.09 ☑
            - traffic V03.19 ☑
          - pedal cycle V01.99 ☑
            - nontraffic V01.09 ☑
            - traffic V01.19 ☑
          - pick-up truck or van V03.99 ☑
            - nontraffic V03.09 ☑
            - traffic V03.19 ☑
          - railway (train) (vehicle) V05.99 ☑
            - nontraffic V05.09 ☑
            - traffic V05.19 ☑
          - streetcar V06.99 ☑
            - nontraffic V06.09 ☑
            - traffic V06.19 ☑
          - stationary object V00.892 ☑
          - two- or three-wheeled motor vehicle V02.99 ☑
            - nontraffic V02.09 ☑
            - traffic V02.19 ☑
          - vehicle V09.9 ☑
            - animal-drawn V06.99 ☑
              - nontraffic V06.09 ☑
              - traffic V06.19 ☑
            - motor
              - nontraffic V09.00 ☑
              - traffic V09.20 ☑
        - fall V00.891 ☑
        - nontraffic V09.1 ☑
          - involving motor vehicle NEC V09.00 ☑
        - traffic V09.3 ☑
          - involving motor vehicle NEC V09.20 ☑
      - traffic V09.3 ☑
        - involving motor vehicle V09.20 ☑
          - military V09.21 ☑
          - specified type NEC V09.29 ☑
      - wheelchair (powered) V00.818 ☑

- **Accident** — *continued*
  - transport — *continued*
        - collision (with) V09.9 ☑
          - animal being ridden or animal drawn vehicle V06.99 ☑
            - nontraffic V06.09 ☑
            - traffic V06.19 ☑
          - bus or heavy transport V04.99 ☑
            - nontraffic V04.09 ☑
            - traffic V04.19 ☑
          - car V03.99 ☑
            - nontraffic V03.09 ☑
            - traffic V03.19 ☑
          - pedal cycle V01.99 ☑
            - nontraffic V01.09 ☑
            - traffic V01.19 ☑
          - pick-up truck or van V03.99 ☑
            - nontraffic V03.09 ☑
            - traffic V03.19 ☑
          - railway (train) (vehicle) V05.99 ☑
            - nontraffic V05.09 ☑
            - traffic V05.19 ☑
          - streetcar V06.99 ☑
            - nontraffic V06.09 ☑
            - traffic V06.19 ☑
          - stationary object V00.812 ☑
          - two- or three-wheeled motor vehicle V02.99 ☑
            - nontraffic V02.09 ☑
            - traffic V02.19 ☑
          - vehicle V09.9 ☑
            - animal-drawn V06.99 ☑
              - nontraffic V06.09 ☑
              - traffic V06.19 ☑
            - motor
              - nontraffic V09.00 ☑
              - traffic V09.20 ☑
        - fall V00.811 ☑
        - nontraffic V09.1 ☑
          - involving motor vehicle NEC V09.00 ☑
        - traffic V09.3 ☑
          - involving motor vehicle NEC V09.20 ☑
      - wheeled shoe V00.158 ☑
        - colliding with stationary object V00.152 ☑
        - fall V00.151 ☑
    - on foot (*see also* Accident, pedestrian)
      - collision (with)
        - animal being ridden or animal drawn vehicle V06.90 ☑
          - nontraffic V06.00 ☑
          - traffic V06.10 ☑
        - bus or heavy transport V04.90 ☑
          - nontraffic V04.00 ☑
          - traffic V04.10 ☑
        - car V03.90 ☑
          - nontraffic V03.00 ☑
          - traffic V03.10 ☑
        - pedal cycle V01.90 ☑
          - nontraffic V01.00 ☑
          - traffic V01.10 ☑
        - pick-up truck or van V03.90 ☑
          - nontraffic V03.00 ☑
          - traffic V03.10 ☑
        - railway (train) (vehicle) V05.90 ☑
          - nontraffic V05.00 ☑
          - traffic V05.10 ☑
        - streetcar V06.90 ☑
          - nontraffic V06.00 ☑
          - traffic V06.10 ☑
        - two- or three-wheeled motor vehicle V02.90 ☑
          - nontraffic V02.00 ☑
          - traffic V02.10 ☑
        - vehicle V09.9 ☑
          - animal-drawn V06.90 ☑
            - nontraffic V06.00 ☑
            - traffic V06.10 ☑
          - motor
            - nontraffic V09.00 ☑
            - traffic V09.20 ☑
      - nontraffic V09.1 ☑
        - involving motor vehicle V09.00 ☑
          - military V09.01 ☑
          - specified type NEC V09.09 ☑
      - traffic V09.3 ☑
        - involving motor vehicle V09.20 ☑
          - military V09.21 ☑
          - specified type NEC V09.29 ☑
    - person NEC (unknown way or transportation) V99 ☑
      - collision (between)

- **Accident** — *continued*
  - transport — *continued*
        - bus (with)
          - heavy transport vehicle (traffic) V87.5 ☑
            - nontraffic V88.5 ☑
        - car (with)
          - nontraffic V88.5 ☑
          - bus (traffic) V87.3 ☑
            - nontraffic V88.3 ☑
          - heavy transport vehicle (traffic) V87.4 ☑
            - nontraffic V88.4 ☑
          - pick-up truck or van (traffic) V87.2 ☑
            - nontraffic V88.2 ☑
          - train or railway vehicle (traffic) V87.6 ☑
            - nontraffic V88.6 ☑
          - two-or three-wheeled motor vehicle (traffic) V87.0 ☑
            - nontraffic V88.0 ☑
        - motor vehicle (traffic) NEC V87.7 ☑
          - nontraffic V88.7 ☑
        - two-or three-wheeled vehicle (with) (traffic)
          - motor vehicle NEC V87.1 ☑
            - nontraffic V88.1 ☑
      - nonmotor vehicle (collision) (noncollision) (traffic) V87.9 ☑
        - nontraffic V88.9 ☑
    - pickup truck occupant V59.9 ☑
      - collision (with)
        - animal (traffic) V50.9 ☑
          - being ridden (traffic) V56.9 ☑
            - nontraffic V56.3 ☑
            - while boarding or alighting V56.4 ☑
          - nontraffic V50.3 ☑
          - while boarding or alighting V50.4 ☑
        - animal-drawn vehicle (traffic) V56.9 ☑
          - nontraffic V56.3 ☑
          - while boarding or alighting V56.4 ☑
        - bus (traffic) V54.9 ☑
          - nontraffic V54.3 ☑
          - while boarding or alighting V54.4 ☑
        - car (traffic) V53.9 ☑
          - nontraffic V53.3 ☑
          - while boarding or alighting V53.4 ☑
        - motor vehicle NOS (traffic) V59.60 ☑
          - nontraffic V59.20 ☑
          - specified type NEC (traffic) V59.69 ☑
            - nontraffic V59.29 ☑
        - pedal cycle (traffic) V51.9 ☑
          - nontraffic V51.3 ☑
          - while boarding or alighting V51.4 ☑
        - pickup truck (traffic) V53.9 ☑
          - nontraffic V53.3 ☑
          - while boarding or alighting V53.4 ☑
        - railway vehicle (traffic) V55.9 ☑
          - nontraffic V55.3 ☑
          - while boarding or alighting V55.4 ☑
        - specified vehicle NEC (traffic) V56.9 ☑
          - nontraffic V56.3 ☑
          - while boarding or alighting V56.4 ☑
        - stationary object (traffic) V57.9 ☑
          - nontraffic V57.3 ☑
          - while boarding or alighting V57.4 ☑
        - streetcar (traffic) V56.9 ☑
          - nontraffic V56.3 ☑
          - while boarding or alighting V56.4 ☑
        - three wheeled motor vehicle (traffic) V52.9 ☑
          - nontraffic V52.3 ☑
          - while boarding or alighting V52.4 ☑
        - truck (traffic) V54.9 ☑
          - nontraffic V54.3 ☑
          - while boarding or alighting V54.4 ☑
        - two wheeled motor vehicle (traffic) V52.9 ☑
          - nontraffic V52.3 ☑
          - while boarding or alighting V52.4 ☑
        - van (traffic) V53.9 ☑
          - nontraffic V53.3 ☑
          - while boarding or alighting V53.4 ☑
      - driver
        - collision (with)
          - animal (traffic) V50.5 ☑
            - being ridden (traffic) V56.5 ☑
              - nontraffic V56.0 ☑
            - nontraffic V50.0 ☑
          - animal-drawn vehicle (traffic) V56.5 ☑
            - nontraffic V56.0 ☑
          - bus (traffic) V54.5 ☑
            - nontraffic V54.0 ☑
          - car (traffic) V53.5 ☑
            - nontraffic V53.0 ☑
          - motor vehicle NOS (traffic) V59.40 ☑
            - nontraffic V59.00 ☑
            - specified type NEC (traffic) V59.49 ☑
              - nontraffic V59.09 ☑
          - pedal cycle (traffic) V51.5 ☑
            - nontraffic V51.0 ☑
          - pickup truck (traffic) V53.5 ☑
            - nontraffic V53.0 ☑
          - railway vehicle (traffic) V55.5 ☑
            - nontraffic V55.0 ☑
          - specified vehicle NEC (traffic) V56.5 ☑
            - nontraffic V56.0 ☑
          - stationary object (traffic) V57.5 ☑
            - nontraffic V57.0 ☑
          - streetcar (traffic) V56.5 ☑
            - nontraffic V56.0 ☑
          - three wheeled motor vehicle (traffic) V52.5 ☑
            - nontraffic V52.0 ☑
          - truck (traffic) V54.5 ☑
            - nontraffic V54.0 ☑
          - two wheeled motor vehicle (traffic) V52.5 ☑
            - nontraffic V52.0 ☑
          - van (traffic) V53.5 ☑
            - nontraffic V53.0 ☑
        - noncollision accident (traffic) V58.5 ☑
          - nontraffic V58.0 ☑
      - noncollision accident (traffic) V58.9 ☑
        - nontraffic V58.3 ☑
        - while boarding or alighting V58.4 ☑
      - nontraffic V59.3 ☑
      - hanger-on
        - collision (with)
          - animal (traffic) V50.7 ☑
            - being ridden (traffic) V56.7 ☑
              - nontraffic V56.2 ☑
            - nontraffic V50.2 ☑
          - animal-drawn vehicle (traffic) V56.7 ☑
            - nontraffic V56.2 ☑
          - bus (traffic) V54.7 ☑
            - nontraffic V54.2 ☑
          - car (traffic) V53.7 ☑
            - nontraffic V53.2 ☑
          - pedal cycle (traffic) V51.7 ☑
            - nontraffic V51.2 ☑
          - pickup truck (traffic) V53.7 ☑
            - nontraffic V53.2 ☑
          - railway vehicle (traffic) V55.7 ☑
            - nontraffic V55.2 ☑
          - specified vehicle NEC (traffic) V56.7 ☑
            - nontraffic V56.2 ☑
          - stationary object (traffic) V57.7 ☑
            - nontraffic V57.2 ☑
          - streetcar (traffic) V56.7 ☑
            - nontraffic V56.2 ☑
          - three wheeled motor vehicle (traffic) V52.7 ☑
            - nontraffic V52.2 ☑
          - truck (traffic) V54.7 ☑
            - nontraffic V54.2 ☑
          - two wheeled motor vehicle (traffic) V52.7 ☑
            - nontraffic V52.2 ☑
          - van (traffic) V53.7 ☑
            - nontraffic V53.2 ☑
        - noncollision accident (traffic) V58.7 ☑
          - nontraffic V58.2 ☑
      - passenger
        - collision (with)
          - animal (traffic) V50.6 ☑
            - being ridden (traffic) V56.6 ☑
              - nontraffic V56.1 ☑
            - nontraffic V50.1 ☑
          - animal-drawn vehicle (traffic) V56.6 ☑
            - nontraffic V56.1 ☑
          - bus (traffic) V54.6 ☑
            - nontraffic V54.1 ☑
          - car (traffic) V53.6 ☑
            - nontraffic V53.1 ☑
          - motor vehicle NOS (traffic) V59.50 ☑
            - nontraffic V59.10 ☑
            - specified type NEC (traffic) V59.59 ☑
              - nontraffic V59.19 ☑
          - pedal cycle (traffic) V51.6 ☑
            - nontraffic V51.1 ☑
          - pickup truck (traffic) V53.6 ☑
            - nontraffic V53.1 ☑
          - railway vehicle (traffic) V55.6 ☑
            - nontraffic V55.1 ☑
          - specified vehicle NEC (traffic) V56.6 ☑
            - nontraffic V56.1 ☑
          - stationary object (traffic) V57.6 ☑
            - nontraffic V57.1 ☑
          - streetcar (traffic) V56.6 ☑
            - nontraffic V56.1 ☑
          - three wheeled motor vehicle (traffic) V52.6 ☑
            - nontraffic V52.1 ☑
          - truck (traffic) V54.6 ☑
            - nontraffic V54.1 ☑
          - two wheeled motor vehicle (traffic) V52.6 ☑
            - nontraffic V52.1 ☑
          - van (traffic) V53.6 ☑
            - nontraffic V53.1 ☑
        - noncollision accident (traffic) V58.6 ☑
          - nontraffic V58.1 ☑
      - specified type NEC V59.88 ☑
        - military vehicle V59.81 ☑
    - quarry truck — *see* Accident, transport, industrial vehicle occupant
    - race car — *see* Accident, transport, motor vehicle NEC occupant
    - railway vehicle occupant V81.9 ☑
      - collision (with) V81.3 ☑
        - motor vehicle (non-military) (traffic) V81.1 ☑
          - military V81.83 ☑
          - nontraffic V81.0 ☑
        - rolling stock V81.2 ☑
        - specified object NEC V81.3 ☑
      - during derailment V81.7 ☑
        - with antecedent collision — *see* Accident, transport, railway vehicle occupant, collision
      - explosion V81.81 ☑
      - fall (in railway vehicle) V81.5 ☑
        - during derailment V81.7 ☑
          - with antecedent collision — *see* Accident, transport, railway vehicle occupant, collision
        - from railway vehicle V81.6 ☑
          - during derailment V81.7 ☑
            - with antecedent collision — *see* Accident, transport, railway vehicle occupant, collision
        - while boarding or alighting V81.4 ☑
      - fire V81.81 ☑
      - object falling onto train V81.82 ☑
      - specified type NEC V81.89 ☑
      - while boarding or alighting V81.4 ☑
    - ski lift V98.3 ☑
    - snowmobile occupant (nontraffic) V86.92 ☑
      - driver V86.52 ☑
      - hanger-on V86.72 ☑
      - passenger V86.62 ☑
      - traffic V86.32 ☑
        - driver V86.02 ☑
        - hanger-on V86.22 ☑
        - passenger V86.12 ☑
      - while boarding or alighting V86.42 ☑
    - specified NEC V98.8 ☑
    - sport utility vehicle occupant (*see also* Accident, transport, pickup truck occupant)
    - streetcar occupant V82.9 ☑
      - collision (with) V82.3 ☑
        - motor vehicle (traffic) V82.1 ☑
          - nontraffic V82.0 ☑
        - rolling stock V82.2 ☑
      - during derailment V82.7 ☑
        - with antecedent collision — *see* Accident, transport, streetcar occupant, collision
      - fall (in streetcar) V82.5 ☑
        - during derailment V82.7 ☑
          - with antecedent collision — *see* Accident, transport, streetcar occupant, collision
        - from streetcar V82.6 ☑
          - during derailment V82.7 ☑
            - with antecedent collision — *see* Accident, transport, streetcar occupant, collision
          - while boarding or alighting V82.4 ☑
        - while boarding or alighting V82.4 ☑
      - specified type NEC V82.8 ☑
      - while boarding or alighting V82.4 ☑
    - three-wheeled motor vehicle occupant V39.9 ☑
      - collision (with)

- **Accident** — *continued*
  - transport — *continued*
        - animal (traffic) V30.9 ☑
          - being ridden (traffic) V36.9 ☑
            - nontraffic V36.3 ☑
            - while boarding or alighting V36.4 ☑
          - nontraffic V30.3 ☑
          - while boarding or alighting V30.4 ☑
        - animal-drawn vehicle (traffic) V36.9 ☑
          - nontraffic V36.3 ☑
          - while boarding or alighting V36.4 ☑
        - bus (traffic) V34.9 ☑
          - nontraffic V34.3 ☑
          - while boarding or alighting V34.4 ☑
        - car (traffic) V33.9 ☑
          - nontraffic V33.3 ☑
          - while boarding or alighting V33.4 ☑
        - motor vehicle NOS (traffic) V39.60 ☑
          - nontraffic V39.20 ☑
          - specified type NEC (traffic) V39.69 ☑
            - nontraffic V39.29 ☑
        - pedal cycle (traffic) V31.9 ☑
          - nontraffic V31.3 ☑
          - while boarding or alighting V31.4 ☑
        - pickup truck (traffic) V33.9 ☑
          - nontraffic V33.3 ☑
          - while boarding or alighting V33.4 ☑
        - railway vehicle (traffic) V35.9 ☑
          - nontraffic V35.3 ☑
          - while boarding or alighting V35.4 ☑
        - specified vehicle NEC (traffic) V36.9 ☑
          - nontraffic V36.3 ☑
          - while boarding or alighting V36.4 ☑
        - stationary object (traffic) V37.9 ☑
          - nontraffic V37.3 ☑
          - while boarding or alighting V37.4 ☑
        - streetcar (traffic) V36.9 ☑
          - nontraffic V36.3 ☑
          - while boarding or alighting V36.4 ☑
        - three wheeled motor vehicle (traffic) V32.9 ☑
          - nontraffic V32.3 ☑
          - while boarding or alighting V32.4 ☑
        - truck (traffic) V34.9 ☑
          - nontraffic V34.3 ☑
          - while boarding or alighting V34.4 ☑
        - two wheeled motor vehicle (traffic) V32.9 ☑
          - nontraffic V32.3 ☑
          - while boarding or alighting V32.4 ☑
        - van (traffic) V33.9 ☑
          - nontraffic V33.3 ☑
          - while boarding or alighting V33.4 ☑
      - driver
        - collision (with)
          - animal (traffic) V30.5 ☑
            - being ridden (traffic) V36.5 ☑
              - nontraffic V36.0 ☑
            - nontraffic V30.0 ☑
          - animal-drawn vehicle (traffic) V36.5 ☑
            - nontraffic V36.0 ☑
          - bus (traffic) V34.5 ☑
            - nontraffic V34.0 ☑
          - car (traffic) V33.5 ☑
            - nontraffic V33.0 ☑
          - motor vehicle NOS (traffic) V39.40 ☑
            - nontraffic V39.00 ☑
            - specified type NEC (traffic) V39.49 ☑
              - nontraffic V39.09 ☑
          - pedal cycle (traffic) V31.5 ☑
            - nontraffic V31.0 ☑
          - pickup truck (traffic) V33.5 ☑
            - nontraffic V33.0 ☑
          - railway vehicle (traffic) V35.5 ☑
            - nontraffic V35.0 ☑
          - specified vehicle NEC (traffic) V36.5 ☑
            - nontraffic V36.0 ☑
          - stationary object (traffic) V37.5 ☑
            - nontraffic V37.0 ☑
          - streetcar (traffic) V36.5 ☑
            - nontraffic V36.0 ☑
          - three wheeled motor vehicle (traffic) V32.5 ☑
            - nontraffic V32.0 ☑
          - truck (traffic) V34.5 ☑
            - nontraffic V34.0 ☑
          - two wheeled motor vehicle (traffic) V32.5 ☑
            - nontraffic V32.0 ☑
          - van (traffic) V33.5 ☑
            - nontraffic V33.0 ☑
        - noncollision accident (traffic) V38.5 ☑

- **Accident** — *continued*
  - transport — *continued*
          - nontraffic V38.0 ☑
      - noncollision accident (traffic) V38.9 ☑
        - nontraffic V38.3 ☑
        - while boarding or alighting V38.4 ☑
      - nontraffic V39.3 ☑
      - hanger-on
        - collision (with)
          - animal (traffic) V30.7 ☑
            - being ridden (traffic) V36.7 ☑
              - nontraffic V36.2 ☑
            - nontraffic V30.2 ☑
          - animal-drawn vehicle (traffic) V36.7 ☑
            - nontraffic V36.2 ☑
          - bus (traffic) V34.7 ☑
            - nontraffic V34.2 ☑
          - car (traffic) V33.7 ☑
            - nontraffic V33.2 ☑
          - pedal cycle (traffic) V31.7 ☑
            - nontraffic V31.2 ☑
          - pickup truck (traffic) V33.7 ☑
            - nontraffic V33.2 ☑
          - railway vehicle (traffic) V35.7 ☑
            - nontraffic V35.2 ☑
          - specified vehicle NEC (traffic) V36.7 ☑
            - nontraffic V36.2 ☑
          - stationary object (traffic) V37.7 ☑
            - nontraffic V37.2 ☑
          - streetcar (traffic) V36.7 ☑
            - nontraffic V36.2 ☑
          - three wheeled motor vehicle (traffic) V32.7 ☑
            - nontraffic V32.2 ☑
          - truck (traffic) V34.7 ☑
            - nontraffic V34.2 ☑
          - two wheeled motor vehicle (traffic) V32.7 ☑
            - nontraffic V32.2 ☑
          - van (traffic) V33.7 ☑
            - nontraffic V33.2 ☑
        - noncollision accident (traffic) V38.7 ☑
          - nontraffic V38.2 ☑
      - passenger
        - collision (with)
          - animal (traffic) V30.6 ☑
            - being ridden (traffic) V36.6 ☑
              - nontraffic V36.1 ☑
            - nontraffic V30.1 ☑
          - animal-drawn vehicle (traffic) V36.6 ☑
            - nontraffic V36.1 ☑
          - bus (traffic) V34.6 ☑
            - nontraffic V34.1 ☑
          - car (traffic) V33.6 ☑
            - nontraffic V33.1 ☑
          - motor vehicle NOS (traffic) V39.50 ☑
            - nontraffic V39.10 ☑
            - specified type NEC (traffic) V39.59 ☑
              - nontraffic V39.19 ☑
          - pedal cycle (traffic) V31.6 ☑
            - nontraffic V31.1 ☑
          - pickup truck (traffic) V33.6 ☑
            - nontraffic V33.1 ☑
          - railway vehicle (traffic) V35.6 ☑
            - nontraffic V35.1 ☑
          - specified vehicle NEC (traffic) V36.6 ☑
            - nontraffic V36.1 ☑
          - stationary object (traffic) V37.6 ☑
            - nontraffic V37.1 ☑
          - streetcar (traffic) V36.6 ☑
            - nontraffic V36.1 ☑
          - three wheeled motor vehicle (traffic) V32.6 ☑
            - nontraffic V32.1 ☑
          - truck (traffic) V34.6 ☑
            - nontraffic V34.1 ☑
          - two wheeled motor vehicle (traffic) V32.6 ☑
            - nontraffic V32.1 ☑
          - van (traffic) V33.6 ☑
            - nontraffic V33.1 ☑
        - noncollision accident (traffic) V38.6 ☑
          - nontraffic V38.1 ☑
      - specified type NEC V39.89 ☑
        - military vehicle V39.81 ☑
    - tractor (farm) (and trailer) — *see* Accident, transport, agricultural vehicle occupant
    - tram — *see* Accident, transport, streetcar
      - in mine or quarry — *see* Accident, transport, industrial vehicle occupant
    - trolley — *see* Accident, transport, streetcar

- **Accident** — *continued*
  - transport — *continued*
      - in mine or quarry — *see* Accident, transport, industrial vehicle occupant
    - truck (heavy) occupant V69.9 ☑
      - collision (with)
        - animal (traffic) V60.9 ☑
          - being ridden (traffic) V66.9 ☑
            - nontraffic V66.3 ☑
            - while boarding or alighting V66.4 ☑
          - nontraffic V60.3 ☑
          - while boarding or alighting V60.4 ☑
        - animal-drawn vehicle (traffic) V66.9 ☑
          - nontraffic V66.3 ☑
          - while boarding or alighting V66.4 ☑
        - bus (traffic) V64.9 ☑
          - nontraffic V64.3 ☑
          - while boarding or alighting V64.4 ☑
        - car (traffic) V63.9 ☑
          - nontraffic V63.3 ☑
          - while boarding or alighting V63.4 ☑
        - motor vehicle NOS (traffic) V69.60 ☑
          - nontraffic V69.20 ☑
          - specified type NEC (traffic) V69.69 ☑
            - nontraffic V69.29 ☑
        - pedal cycle (traffic) V61.9 ☑
          - nontraffic V61.3 ☑
          - while boarding or alighting V61.4 ☑
        - pickup truck (traffic) V63.9 ☑
          - nontraffic V63.3 ☑
          - while boarding or alighting V63.4 ☑
        - railway vehicle (traffic) V65.9 ☑
          - nontraffic V65.3 ☑
          - while boarding or alighting V65.4 ☑
        - specified vehicle NEC (traffic) V66.9 ☑
          - nontraffic V66.3 ☑
          - while boarding or alighting V66.4 ☑
        - stationary object (traffic) V67.9 ☑
          - nontraffic V67.3 ☑
          - while boarding or alighting V67.4 ☑
        - streetcar (traffic) V66.9 ☑
          - nontraffic V66.3 ☑
          - while boarding or alighting V66.4 ☑
        - three wheeled motor vehicle (traffic) V62.9 ☑
          - nontraffic V62.3 ☑
          - while boarding or alighting V62.4 ☑
        - truck (traffic) V64.9 ☑
          - nontraffic V64.3 ☑
          - while boarding or alighting V64.4 ☑
        - two wheeled motor vehicle (traffic) V62.9 ☑
          - nontraffic V62.3 ☑
          - while boarding or alighting V62.4 ☑
        - van (traffic) V63.9 ☑
          - nontraffic V63.3 ☑
          - while boarding or alighting V63.4 ☑
      - driver
        - collision (with)
          - animal (traffic) V60.5 ☑
            - being ridden (traffic) V66.5 ☑
              - nontraffic V66.0 ☑
            - nontraffic V60.0 ☑
          - animal-drawn vehicle (traffic) V66.5 ☑
            - nontraffic V66.0 ☑
          - bus (traffic) V64.5 ☑
            - nontraffic V64.0 ☑
          - car (traffic) V63.5 ☑
            - nontraffic V63.0 ☑
          - motor vehicle NOS (traffic) V69.40 ☑
            - nontraffic V69.00 ☑
            - specified type NEC (traffic) V69.49 ☑
              - nontraffic V69.09 ☑
          - pedal cycle (traffic) V61.5 ☑
            - nontraffic V61.0 ☑
          - pickup truck (traffic) V63.5 ☑
            - nontraffic V63.0 ☑
          - railway vehicle (traffic) V65.5 ☑
            - nontraffic V65.0 ☑
          - specified vehicle NEC (traffic) V66.5 ☑
            - nontraffic V66.0 ☑
          - stationary object (traffic) V67.5 ☑
            - nontraffic V67.0 ☑
          - streetcar (traffic) V66.5 ☑
            - nontraffic V66.0 ☑
          - three wheeled motor vehicle (traffic) V62.5 ☑
            - nontraffic V62.0 ☑
          - truck (traffic) V64.5 ☑
            - nontraffic V64.0 ☑
          - two wheeled motor vehicle (traffic) V62.5 ☑

Accident

- **Accident** — *continued*
  - transport — *continued*
          - nontraffic V62.0 ☑
        - van (traffic) V63.5 ☑
          - nontraffic V63.0 ☑
      - noncollision accident (traffic) V68.5 ☑
        - nontraffic V68.0 ☑
    - dump — *see* Accident, transport, construction vehicle occupant
    - hanger-on
      - collision (with)
        - animal (traffic) V60.7 ☑
          - being ridden (traffic) V66.7 ☑
            - nontraffic V66.2 ☑
          - nontraffic V60.2 ☑
        - animal-drawn vehicle (traffic) V66.7 ☑
          - nontraffic V66.2 ☑
        - bus (traffic) V64.7 ☑
          - nontraffic V64.2 ☑
        - car (traffic) V63.7 ☑
          - nontraffic V63.2 ☑
        - pedal cycle (traffic) V61.7 ☑
          - nontraffic V61.2 ☑
        - pickup truck (traffic) V63.7 ☑
          - nontraffic V63.2 ☑
        - railway vehicle (traffic) V65.7 ☑
          - nontraffic V65.2 ☑
        - specified vehicle NEC (traffic) V66.7 ☑
          - nontraffic V66.2 ☑
        - stationary object (traffic) V67.7 ☑
          - nontraffic V67.2 ☑
        - streetcar (traffic) V66.7 ☑
          - nontraffic V66.2 ☑
        - three wheeled motor vehicle (traffic) V62.7 ☑
          - nontraffic V62.2 ☑
        - truck (traffic) V64.7 ☑
          - nontraffic V64.2 ☑
        - two wheeled motor vehicle (traffic) V62.7 ☑
          - nontraffic V62.2 ☑
        - van (traffic) V63.7 ☑
          - nontraffic V63.2 ☑
      - noncollision accident (traffic) V68.7 ☑
        - nontraffic V68.2 ☑
    - noncollision accident (traffic) V68.9 ☑
      - nontraffic V68.3 ☑
      - while boarding or alighting V68.4 ☑
    - nontraffic V69.3 ☑
    - passenger
      - collision (with)
        - animal (traffic) V60.6 ☑
          - being ridden (traffic) V66.6 ☑
            - nontraffic V66.1 ☑
          - nontraffic V60.1 ☑
        - animal-drawn vehicle (traffic) V66.6 ☑
          - nontraffic V66.1 ☑
        - bus (traffic) V64.6 ☑
          - nontraffic V64.1 ☑
        - car (traffic) V63.6 ☑
          - nontraffic V63.1 ☑
        - motor vehicle NOS (traffic) V69.50 ☑
          - nontraffic V69.10 ☑
          - specified type NEC (traffic) V69.59 ☑
            - nontraffic V69.19 ☑
        - pedal cycle (traffic) V61.6 ☑
          - nontraffic V61.1 ☑
        - pickup truck (traffic) V63.6 ☑
          - nontraffic V63.1 ☑
        - railway vehicle (traffic) V65.6 ☑
          - nontraffic V65.1 ☑
        - specified vehicle NEC (traffic) V66.6 ☑
          - nontraffic V66.1 ☑
        - stationary object (traffic) V67.6 ☑
          - nontraffic V67.1 ☑
        - streetcar (traffic) V66.6 ☑
          - nontraffic V66.1 ☑
        - three wheeled motor vehicle (traffic) V62.6 ☑
          - nontraffic V62.1 ☑
        - truck (traffic) V64.6 ☑
          - nontraffic V64.1 ☑
        - two wheeled motor vehicle (traffic) V62.6 ☑
          - nontraffic V62.1 ☑
        - van (traffic) V63.6 ☑
          - nontraffic V63.1 ☑
      - noncollision accident (traffic) V68.6 ☑
        - nontraffic V68.1 ☑
    - pickup — *see* Accident, transport, pickup truck occupant
    - specified type NEC V69.88 ☑

- **Accident** — *continued*
  - transport — *continued*
        - military vehicle V69.81 ☑
    - van occupant V59.9 ☑
      - collision (with)
        - animal (traffic) V50.9 ☑
          - being ridden (traffic) V56.9 ☑
            - nontraffic V56.3 ☑
            - while boarding or alighting V56.4 ☑
          - nontraffic V50.3 ☑
          - while boarding or alighting V50.4 ☑
        - animal-drawn vehicle (traffic) V56.9 ☑
          - nontraffic V56.3 ☑
          - while boarding or alighting V56.4 ☑
        - bus (traffic) V54.9 ☑
          - nontraffic V54.3 ☑
          - while boarding or alighting V54.4 ☑
        - car (traffic) V53.9 ☑
          - nontraffic V53.3 ☑
          - while boarding or alighting V53.4 ☑
        - motor vehicle NOS (traffic) V59.60 ☑
          - nontraffic V59.20 ☑
          - specified type NEC (traffic) V59.69 ☑
            - nontraffic V59.29 ☑
        - pedal cycle (traffic) V51.9 ☑
          - nontraffic V51.3 ☑
          - while boarding or alighting V51.4 ☑
        - pickup truck (traffic) V53.9 ☑
          - nontraffic V53.3 ☑
          - while boarding or alighting V53.4 ☑
        - railway vehicle (traffic) V55.9 ☑
          - nontraffic V55.3 ☑
          - while boarding or alighting V55.4 ☑
        - specified vehicle NEC (traffic) V56.9 ☑
          - nontraffic V56.3 ☑
          - while boarding or alighting V56.4 ☑
        - stationary object (traffic) V57.9 ☑
          - nontraffic V57.3 ☑
          - while boarding or alighting V57.4 ☑
        - streetcar (traffic) V56.9 ☑
          - nontraffic V56.3 ☑
          - while boarding or alighting V56.4 ☑
        - three wheeled motor vehicle (traffic) V52.9 ☑
          - nontraffic V52.3 ☑
          - while boarding or alighting V52.4 ☑
        - truck (traffic) V54.9 ☑
          - nontraffic V54.3 ☑
          - while boarding or alighting V54.4 ☑
        - two wheeled motor vehicle (traffic) V52.9 ☑
          - nontraffic V52.3 ☑
          - while boarding or alighting V52.4 ☑
        - van (traffic) V53.9 ☑
          - nontraffic V53.3 ☑
          - while boarding or alighting V53.4 ☑
      - driver
        - collision (with)
          - animal (traffic) V50.5 ☑
            - being ridden (traffic) V56.5 ☑
              - nontraffic V56.0 ☑
            - nontraffic V50.0 ☑
          - animal-drawn vehicle (traffic) V56.5 ☑
            - nontraffic V56.0 ☑
          - bus (traffic) V54.5 ☑
            - nontraffic V54.0 ☑
          - car (traffic) V53.5 ☑
            - nontraffic V53.0 ☑
          - motor vehicle NOS (traffic) V59.40 ☑
            - nontraffic V59.00 ☑
            - specified type NEC (traffic) V59.49 ☑
              - nontraffic V59.09 ☑
          - pedal cycle (traffic) V51.5 ☑
            - nontraffic V51.0 ☑
          - pickup truck (traffic) V53.5 ☑
            - nontraffic V53.0 ☑
          - railway vehicle (traffic) V55.5 ☑
            - nontraffic V55.0 ☑
          - specified vehicle NEC (traffic) V56.5 ☑
            - nontraffic V56.0 ☑
          - stationary object (traffic) V57.5 ☑
            - nontraffic V57.0 ☑
          - streetcar (traffic) V56.5 ☑
            - nontraffic V56.0 ☑
          - three wheeled motor vehicle (traffic) V52.5 ☑
            - nontraffic V52.0 ☑
          - truck (traffic) V54.5 ☑
            - nontraffic V54.0 ☑
          - two wheeled motor vehicle (traffic) V52.5 ☑
            - nontraffic V52.0 ☑

- **Accident** — *continued*
  - transport — *continued*
          - van (traffic) V53.5 ☑
            - nontraffic V53.0 ☑
        - noncollision accident (traffic) V58.5 ☑
          - nontraffic V58.0 ☑
      - noncollision accident (traffic) V58.9 ☑
        - nontraffic V58.3 ☑
        - while boarding or alighting V58.4 ☑
      - nontraffic V59.3 ☑
      - hanger-on
        - collision (with)
          - animal (traffic) V50.7 ☑
            - being ridden (traffic) V56.7 ☑
              - nontraffic V56.2 ☑
            - nontraffic V50.2 ☑
          - animal-drawn vehicle (traffic) V56.7 ☑
            - nontraffic V56.2 ☑
          - bus (traffic) V54.7 ☑
            - nontraffic V54.2 ☑
          - car (traffic) V53.7 ☑
            - nontraffic V53.2 ☑
          - pedal cycle (traffic) V51.7 ☑
            - nontraffic V51.2 ☑
          - pickup truck (traffic) V53.7 ☑
            - nontraffic V53.2 ☑
          - railway vehicle (traffic) V55.7 ☑
            - nontraffic V55.2 ☑
          - specified vehicle NEC (traffic) V56.7 ☑
            - nontraffic V56.2 ☑
          - stationary object (traffic) V57.7 ☑
            - nontraffic V57.2 ☑
          - streetcar (traffic) V56.7 ☑
            - nontraffic V56.2 ☑
          - three wheeled motor vehicle (traffic) V52.7 ☑
            - nontraffic V52.2 ☑
          - truck (traffic) V54.7 ☑
            - nontraffic V54.2 ☑
          - two wheeled motor vehicle (traffic) V52.7 ☑
            - nontraffic V52.2 ☑
          - van (traffic) V53.7 ☑
            - nontraffic V53.2 ☑
        - noncollision accident (traffic) V58.7 ☑
          - nontraffic V58.2 ☑
      - passenger
        - collision (with)
          - animal (traffic) V50.6 ☑
            - being ridden (traffic) V56.6 ☑
              - nontraffic V56.1 ☑
            - nontraffic V50.1 ☑
          - animal-drawn vehicle (traffic) V56.6 ☑
            - nontraffic V56.1 ☑
          - bus (traffic) V54.6 ☑
            - nontraffic V54.1 ☑
          - car (traffic) V53.6 ☑
            - nontraffic V53.1 ☑
          - motor vehicle NOS (traffic) V59.50 ☑
            - nontraffic V59.10 ☑
            - specified type NEC (traffic) V59.59 ☑
              - nontraffic V59.19 ☑
          - pedal cycle (traffic) V51.6 ☑
            - nontraffic V51.1 ☑
          - pickup truck (traffic) V53.6 ☑
            - nontraffic V53.1 ☑
          - railway vehicle (traffic) V55.6 ☑
            - nontraffic V55.1 ☑
          - specified vehicle NEC (traffic) V56.6 ☑
            - nontraffic V56.1 ☑
          - stationary object (traffic) V57.6 ☑
            - nontraffic V57.1 ☑
          - streetcar (traffic) V56.6 ☑
            - nontraffic V56.1 ☑
          - three wheeled motor vehicle (traffic) V52.6 ☑
            - nontraffic V52.1 ☑
          - truck (traffic) V54.6 ☑
            - nontraffic V54.1 ☑
          - two wheeled motor vehicle (traffic) V52.6 ☑
            - nontraffic V52.1 ☑
          - van (traffic) V53.6 ☑
            - nontraffic V53.1 ☑
        - noncollision accident (traffic) V58.6 ☑
          - nontraffic V58.1 ☑
      - specified type NEC V59.88 ☑
        - military vehicle V59.81 ☑
    - watercraft occupant — *see* Accident, watercraft
  - vehicle NEC V89.9 ☑
    - animal-drawn NEC — *see* Accident, transport, animal-drawn vehicle occupant

- **Accident** — *continued*
  - vehicle NEC — *continued*
    - special
      - agricultural — *see* Accident, transport, agricultural vehicle occupant
      - construction — *see* Accident, transport, construction vehicle occupant
      - industrial — *see* Accident, transport, industrial vehicle occupant
    - three-wheeled NEC (motorized) — *see* Accident, transport, three-wheeled motor vehicle occupant
  - watercraft V94.9 ☑
    - causing
      - drowning — *see* Drowning, due to, accident to, watercraft
      - injury NEC V91.89 ☑
        - crushed between craft and object V91.19 ☑
          - powered craft V91.13 ☑
            - ferry boat V91.11 ☑
            - fishing boat V91.12 ☑
            - jet skis V91.13 ☑
            - liner V91.11 ☑
            - merchant ship V91.10 ☑
            - passenger ship V91.11 ☑
          - unpowered craft V91.18 ☑
            - canoe V91.15 ☑
            - inflatable V91.16 ☑
            - kayak V91.15 ☑
            - sailboat V91.14 ☑
            - surf-board V91.18 ☑
            - windsurfer V91.18 ☑
        - fall on board V91.29 ☑
          - powered craft V91.23 ☑
            - ferry boat V91.21 ☑
            - fishing boat V91.22 ☑
            - jet skis V91.23 ☑
            - liner V91.21 ☑
            - merchant ship V91.20 ☑
            - passenger ship V91.21 ☑
          - unpowered craft
            - canoe V91.25 ☑
            - inflatable V91.26 ☑
            - kayak V91.25 ☑
            - sailboat V91.24 ☑
        - fire on board causing burn V91.09 ☑
          - powered craft V91.03 ☑
            - ferry boat V91.01 ☑
            - fishing boat V91.02 ☑
            - jet skis V91.03 ☑
            - liner V91.01 ☑
            - merchant ship V91.00 ☑
            - passenger ship V91.01 ☑
          - unpowered craft V91.08 ☑
            - canoe V91.05 ☑
            - inflatable V91.06 ☑
            - kayak V91.05 ☑
            - sailboat V91.04 ☑
            - surf-board V91.08 ☑
            - water skis V91.07 ☑
            - windsurfer V91.08 ☑
        - hit by falling object V91.39 ☑
          - powered craft V91.33 ☑
            - ferry boat V91.31 ☑
            - fishing boat V91.32 ☑
            - jet skis V91.33 ☑
            - liner V91.31 ☑
            - merchant ship V91.30 ☑
            - passenger ship V91.31 ☑
          - unpowered craft V91.38 ☑
            - canoe V91.35 ☑
            - inflatable V91.36 ☑
            - kayak V91.35 ☑
            - sailboat V91.34 ☑
            - surf-board V91.38 ☑
            - water skis V91.37 ☑
            - windsurfer V91.38 ☑
        - specified type NEC V91.89 ☑
          - powered craft V91.83 ☑
            - ferry boat V91.81 ☑
            - fishing boat V91.82 ☑
            - jet skis V91.83 ☑
            - liner V91.81 ☑
            - merchant ship V91.80 ☑
            - passenger ship V91.81 ☑
          - unpowered craft V91.88 ☑
            - canoe V91.85 ☑
            - inflatable V91.86 ☑
            - kayak V91.85 ☑
            - sailboat V91.84 ☑
            - surf-board V91.88 ☑

- **Accident** — *continued*
  - watercraft — *continued*
    - water skis V91.87 ☑
    - windsurfer V91.88 ☑
    - due to, caused by cataclysm — *see* Forces of nature, by type
    - military NEC V94.818 ☑
      - with civilian watercraft V94.810 ☑
      - civilian in water injured by V94.811 ☑
    - nonpowered, struck by
      - nonpowered vessel V94.22 ☑
      - powered vessel V94.21 ☑
    - specified type NEC V94.89 ☑
    - striking swimmer
      - powered V94.11 ☑
      - unpowered V94.12 ☑
- **Acid** throwing (assault) Y08.89 ☑
- **Activity** (involving) (of victim at time of event) Y93.9
  - aerobic and step exercise (class) Y93.A3
  - alpine skiing Y93.23
  - animal care NEC Y93.K9
  - arts and handcrafts NEC Y93.D9
  - athletics NEC Y93.79
  - athletics played as a team or group NEC Y93.69
  - athletics played individually NEC Y93.59
  - baking Y93.G3
  - ballet Y93.41
  - barbells Y93.B3
  - BASE (Building, Antenna, Span, Earth) jumping Y93.33
  - baseball Y93.64
  - basketball Y93.67
  - bathing (personal) Y93.E1
  - beach volleyball Y93.68
  - bike riding Y93.55
  - blackout game Y93.85
  - boogie boarding Y93.18
  - bowling Y93.54
  - boxing Y93.71
  - brass instrument playing Y93.J4
  - building construction Y93.H3
  - bungee jumping Y93.34
  - calisthenics Y93.A2
  - canoeing (in calm and turbulent water) Y93.16
  - capture the flag Y93.6A
  - cardiorespiratory exercise NEC Y93.A9
  - caregiving (providing) NEC Y93.F9
    - bathing Y93.F1
    - lifting Y93.F2
  - cellular
    - communication device Y93.C2
    - telephone Y93.C2
  - challenge course Y93.A5
  - cheerleading Y93.45
  - choking game Y93.85
  - circuit training Y93.A4
  - cleaning
    - floor Y93.E5
  - climbing NEC Y93.39
    - mountain Y93.31
    - rock Y93.31
    - wall Y93.31
  - clothing care and maintenance NEC Y93.E9
  - combatives Y93.75
  - computer
    - keyboarding Y93.C1
    - technology NEC Y93.C9
  - confidence course Y93.A5
  - construction (building) Y93.H3
  - cooking and baking Y93.G3
  - cool down exercises Y93.A2
  - cricket Y93.69
  - crocheting Y93.D1
  - cross country skiing Y93.24
  - dancing (all types) Y93.41
  - digging
    - dirt Y93.H1
  - dirt digging Y93.H1
  - dishwashing Y93.G1
  - diving (platform) (springboard) Y93.12
    - underwater Y93.15
  - dodge ball Y93.6A
  - downhill skiing Y93.23
  - drum playing Y93.J2
  - dumbbells Y93.B3
  - electronic
    - devices NEC Y93.C9
      - hand held interactive Y93.C2
    - game playing (using) (with)
      - interactive device Y93.C2
      - keyboard or other stationary device Y93.C1

- **Activity** — *continued*
  - elliptical machine Y93.A1
  - exercise (s)
    - machines ((primarily) for)
      - cardiorespiratory conditioning Y93.A1
      - muscle strengthening Y93.B1
    - muscle strengthening (non-machine) NEC Y93.B9
  - external motion NEC Y93.I9
    - rollercoaster Y93.I1
  - fainting game Y93.85
  - field hockey Y93.65
  - figure skating (pairs) (singles) Y93.21
  - flag football Y93.62
  - floor mopping and cleaning Y93.E5
  - food preparation and clean up Y93.G1
  - football (American) NOS Y93.61
    - flag Y93.62
    - tackle Y93.61
    - touch Y93.62
  - four square Y93.6A
  - free weights Y93.B3
  - frisbee (ultimate) Y93.74
  - furniture
    - building Y93.D3
    - finishing Y93.D3
    - repair Y93.D3
  - game playing (electronic)
    - using keyboard or other stationary device Y93.C1
    - using interactive device Y93.C2
  - gardening Y93.H2
  - golf Y93.53
  - grass drills Y93.A6
  - grilling and smoking food Y93.G2
  - grooming and shearing an animal Y93.K3
  - guerilla drills Y93.A6
  - gymnastics (rhythmic) Y93.43
  - handball Y93.73
  - handcrafts NEC Y93.D9
  - hand held interactive electronic device Y93.C2
  - hang gliding Y93.35
  - hiking (on level or elevated terrain) Y93.01
  - hockey (ice) Y93.22
    - field Y93.65
  - horseback riding Y93.52
  - household (interior) maintenance NEC Y93.E9
  - ice NEC Y93.29
    - dancing Y93.21
    - hockey Y93.22
    - skating Y93.21
  - inline roller skating Y93.51
  - ironing Y93.E4
  - judo Y93.75
  - jumping (off) NEC Y93.39
    - BASE (Building, Antenna, Span, Earth) Y93.33
    - bungee Y93.34
    - jacks Y93.A2
    - rope Y93.56
  - jumping jacks Y93.A2
  - jumping rope Y93.56
  - karate Y93.75
  - kayaking (in calm and turbulent water) Y93.16
  - keyboarding (computer) Y93.C1
  - kickball Y93.6A
  - knitting Y93.D1
  - lacrosse Y93.65
  - land maintenance NEC Y93.H9
  - landscaping Y93.H2
  - laundry Y93.E2
  - machines (exercise)
    - primarily for cardiorespiratory conditioning Y93.A1
    - primarily for muscle strengthening Y93.B1
  - maintenance
    - exterior building NEC Y93.H9
    - household (interior) NEC Y93.E9
    - land Y93.H9
    - property Y93.H9
  - marching (on level or elevated terrain) Y93.01
  - martial arts Y93.75
  - microwave oven Y93.G3
  - milking an animal Y93.K2
  - mopping (floor) Y93.E5
  - mountain climbing Y93.31
  - muscle strengthening
    - exercises (non-machine) NEC Y93.B9
    - machines Y93.B1
  - musical keyboard (electronic) playing Y93.J1
  - Nordic skiing Y93.24
  - obstacle course Y93.A5
  - oven (microwave) Y93.G3

Activity - Assault

Activity — *continued*
- packing up and unpacking in moving to a new residence Y93.E6
- parasailing Y93.19
- pass out game Y93.85
- percussion instrument playing NEC Y93.J2
- personal
  - bathing and showering Y93.E1
  - hygiene NEC Y93.E8
  - showering Y93.E1
- physical games generally associated with school recess, summer camp and children Y93.6A
- physical training NEC Y93.A9
- piano playing Y93.J1
- Pilates Y93.B4
- platform diving Y93.12
- playing musical instrument
  - brass instrument Y93.J4
  - drum Y93.J2
  - musical keyboard (electronic) Y93.J1
  - percussion instrument NEC Y93.J2
  - piano Y93.J1
  - string instrument Y93.J3
  - winds instrument Y93.J4
- property maintenance
  - exterior NEC Y93.H9
  - interior NEC Y93.E9
- pruning (garden and lawn) Y93.H2
- pull-ups Y93.B2
- push-ups Y93.B2
- racquetball Y93.73
- rafting (in calm and turbulent water) Y93.16
- raking (leaves) Y93.H1
- rappelling Y93.32
- refereeing a sports activity Y93.81
- residential relocation Y93.E6
- rhythmic gymnastics Y93.43
- rhythmic movement NEC Y93.49
- riding
  - horseback Y93.52
  - rollercoaster Y93.I1
- rock climbing Y93.31
- rollercoaster riding Y93.I1
- roller skating (inline) Y93.51
- rough housing and horseplay Y93.83
- rowing (in calm and turbulent water) Y93.16
- rugby Y93.63
- running Y93.02
- SCUBA diving Y93.15
- sewing Y93.D2
- shoveling Y93.H1
  - dirt Y93.H1
  - snow Y93.H1
- showering (personal) Y93.E1
- sit-ups Y93.B2
- skateboarding Y93.51
- skating (ice) Y93.21
  - roller Y93.51
- skiing (alpine) (downhill) Y93.23
  - cross country Y93.24
  - nordic Y93.24
  - water Y93.17
- sledding (snow) Y93.23
- sleeping (sleep) Y93.84
- smoking and grilling food Y93.G2
- snorkeling Y93.15
- snow NEC Y93.29
  - boarding Y93.23
  - shoveling Y93.H1
  - sledding Y93.23
  - tubing Y93.23
- soccer Y93.66
- softball Y93.64
- specified NEC Y93.89
- spectator at an event Y93.82
- sports NEC Y93.79
  - sports played as a team or group NEC Y93.69
  - sports played individually NEC Y93.59
- springboard diving Y93.12
- squash Y93.73
- stationary bike Y93.A1
- step (stepping) exercise (class) Y93.A3
- stepper machine Y93.A1
- stove Y93.G3
- string instrument playing Y93.J3
- surfing Y93.18
  - wind Y93.18
- swimming Y93.11
- tackle football Y93.61
- tap dancing Y93.41
- tennis Y93.73
- tobogganing Y93.23

Activity — *continued*
- touch football Y93.62
- track and field events (non-running) Y93.57
  - running Y93.02
- trampoline Y93.44
- treadmill Y93.A1
- trimming shrubs Y93.H2
- tubing (in calm and turbulent water) Y93.16
  - snow Y93.23
- ultimate frisbee Y93.74
- underwater diving Y93.15
- unpacking in moving to a new residence Y93.E6
- use of stove, oven and microwave oven Y93.G3
- vacuuming Y93.E3
- volleyball (beach) (court) Y93.68
- wake boarding Y93.17
- walking an animal Y93.K1
- walking (on level or elevated terrain) Y93.01
  - an animal Y93.K1
- wall climbing Y93.31
- warm up and cool down exercises Y93.A2
- water NEC Y93.19
  - aerobics Y93.14
  - craft NEC Y93.19
  - exercise Y93.14
  - polo Y93.13
  - skiing Y93.17
  - sliding Y93.18
  - survival training and testing Y93.19
- weeding (garden and lawn) Y93.H2
- wind instrument playing Y93.J4
- windsurfing Y93.18
- wrestling Y93.72
- yoga Y93.42

Adverse effect of drugs — *see* Table of Drugs and Chemicals

Aerosinusitis - — *see* Air, pressure

After-effect, late — *see* Sequelae

Air
- blast in war operations — *see* War operations, air blast
- pressure
  - change, rapid
    - during
      - ascent W94.29 ☑
        - while (in) (surfacing from)
          - aircraft W94.23 ☑
          - deep water diving W94.21 ☑
          - underground W94.22 ☑
      - descent W94.39 ☑
        - in
          - aircraft W94.31 ☑
          - water W94.32 ☑
  - high, prolonged W94.0 ☑
  - low, prolonged W94.12 ☑
    - due to residence or long visit at high altitude W94.11 ☑

Alpine sickness W94.11 ☑

Altitude sickness W94.11 ☑

Anaphylactic shock, anaphylaxis — *see* Table of Drugs and Chemicals

Andes disease W94.11 ☑

Arachnidism, arachnoidism X58 ☑

Arson (with intent to injure or kill) X97 ☑

Asphyxia, asphyxiation
- by
  - food (bone) (seed) — *see* categories T17 and T18 ☑
  - gas (*see also* Table of Drugs and Chemicals)
    - legal
      - execution — *see* Legal, intervention, gas
      - intervention — *see* Legal, intervention, gas
- from
  - fire (*see also* Exposure, fire)
    - in war operations — *see* War operations, fire
  - ignition — *see* Ignition
  - vomitus T17.81 ☑
- in war operations — *see* War operations, restriction of airway

Aspiration
- food (any type) (into respiratory tract) (with asphyxia, obstruction respiratory tract, suffocation) — *see* categories T17 and T18 ☑
- foreign body — *see* Foreign body, aspiration
- vomitus (with asphyxia, obstruction respiratory tract, suffocation) T17.81 ☑

Assassination (attempt) — *see* Assault

Assault (homicidal) (by) (in) Y09
- arson X97 ☑
- bite (of human being) Y04.1 ☑
- bodily force Y04.8 ☑
  - bite Y04.1 ☑

Assault — *continued*
- bodily force — *continued*
  - bumping into Y04.2 ☑
  - sexual — *see* subcategories T74.0, T76.0 ☑
  - unarmed fight Y04.0 ☑
- bomb X96.9 ☑
  - antipersonnel X96.0 ☑
  - fertilizer X96.3 ☑
  - gasoline X96.1 ☑
  - letter X96.2 ☑
  - petrol X96.1 ☑
  - pipe X96.3 ☑
  - specified NEC X96.8 ☑
- brawl (hand) (fists) (foot) (unarmed) Y04.0 ☑
- burning, burns (by fire) NEC X97 ☑
  - acid Y08.89 ☑
  - caustic, corrosive substance Y08.89 ☑
  - chemical from swallowing caustic, corrosive substance — *see* Table of Drugs and Chemicals
  - cigarette (s) X97 ☑
  - hot object X98.9 ☑
    - fluid NEC X98.2 ☑
    - household appliance X98.3 ☑
    - specified NEC X98.8 ☑
    - steam X98.0 ☑
    - tap water X98.1 ☑
    - vapors X98.0 ☑
  - scalding — *see* Assault, burning
  - steam X98.0 ☑
  - vitriol Y08.89 ☑
- caustic, corrosive substance (gas) Y08.89 ☑
- crashing of
  - aircraft Y08.81 ☑
  - motor vehicle Y03.8 ☑
    - pushed in front of Y02.0 ☑
    - run over Y03.0 ☑
    - specified NEC Y03.8 ☑
- cutting or piercing instrument X99.9 ☑
  - dagger X99.2 ☑
  - glass X99.0 ☑
  - knife X99.1 ☑
  - specified NEC X99.8 ☑
  - sword X99.2 ☑
- dagger X99.2 ☑
- drowning (in) X92.9 ☑
  - bathtub X92.0 ☑
  - natural water X92.3 ☑
  - specified NEC X92.8 ☑
  - swimming pool X92.1 ☑
    - following fall X92.2 ☑
- dynamite X96.8 ☑
- explosive (s) (material) X96.9 ☑
- fight (hand) (fists) (foot) (unarmed) Y04.0 ☑
  - with weapon — *see* Assault, by type of weapon
- fire X97 ☑
- firearm X95.9 ☑
  - airgun X95.01 ☑
  - handgun X93 ☑
  - hunting rifle X94.1 ☑
  - larger X94.9 ☑
    - specified NEC X94.8 ☑
  - machine gun X94.2 ☑
  - shotgun X94.0 ☑
  - specified NEC X95.8 ☑
- gunshot (wound) NEC — *see* Assault, firearm, by type
- incendiary device X97 ☑
- injury Y09
  - to child due to criminal abortion attempt NEC Y08.89 ☑
- knife X99.1 ☑
- late effect of — *see* X92-Y08 with 7th character S
- placing before moving object NEC Y02.8 ☑
  - motor vehicle Y02.0 ☑
- poisoning — *see* categories T36-T65 with 7th character S
- puncture, any part of body — *see* Assault, cutting or piercing instrument
- pushing
  - before moving object NEC Y02.8 ☑
    - motor vehicle Y02.0 ☑
    - subway train Y02.1 ☑
    - train Y02.1 ☑
  - from high place Y01 ☑
- rape T74.2 ☑
- scalding — *see* Assault, burning
- sequelae of — *see* X92-Y08 with 7th character S
- sexual (by bodily force) T74.2 ☑
- shooting — *see* Assault, firearm
- specified means NEC Y08.89 ☑

- **Assault** — *continued*
  - stab, any part of body — *see* Assault, cutting or piercing instrument
  - steam X98.0 ☑
  - striking against
    - other person Y04.2 ☑
    - sports equipment Y08.09 ☑
      - baseball bat Y08.02 ☑
      - hockey stick Y08.01 ☑
  - struck by
    - sports equipment Y08.09 ☑
      - baseball bat Y08.02 ☑
      - hockey stick Y08.01 ☑
  - submersion — *see* Assault, drowning
  - violence Y09
  - weapon Y09
    - blunt Y00 ☑
    - cutting or piercing — *see* Assault, cutting or piercing instrument
    - firearm — *see* Assault, firearm
  - wound Y09
    - cutting — *see* Assault, cutting or piercing instrument
    - gunshot — *see* Assault, firearm
    - knife X99.1 ☑
    - piercing — *see* Assault, cutting or piercing instrument
    - puncture — *see* Assault, cutting or piercing instrument
    - stab — *see* Assault, cutting or piercing instrument
- **Attack** by mammals NEC W55.89 ☑
- **Avalanche** — *see* Landslide
- **Aviator**'s disease - — *see* Air, pressure

B

- **Barotitis**, barodontalgia, barosinusitis, barotrauma (otitic) (sinus) - — *see* Air, pressure
- **Battered** (baby) (child) (person) (syndrome) X58 ☑
- **Bayonet** wound W26.1 ☑
  - in
    - legal intervention — *see* Legal, intervention, sharp object, bayonet
    - war operations — *see* War operations, combat
  - stated as undetermined whether accidental or intentional Y28.8 ☑
  - suicide (attempt) X78.2 ☑
- **Bean** in nose — *see* categories T17 and T18 ☑
- **Bed** set on fire NEC — *see* Exposure, fire, uncontrolled, building, bed
- **Beheading** (by guillotine)
  - homicide X99.9 ☑
  - legal execution — *see* Legal, intervention
- **Bending**, injury in (prolonged) (static) X50.1 ☑
- **Bends** - — *see* Air, pressure, change
- **Bite**, bitten by
  - alligator W58.01 ☑
  - arthropod (nonvenomous) NEC W57 ☑
  - bull W55.21 ☑
  - cat W55.01 ☑
  - cow W55.21 ☑
  - crocodile W58.11 ☑
  - dog W54.0 ☑
  - goat W55.31 ☑
  - hoof stock NEC W55.31 ☑
  - horse W55.11 ☑
  - human being (accidentally) W50.3 ☑
    - with intent to injure or kill Y04.1 ☑
    - as, or caused by, a crowd or human stampede (with fall) W52 ☑
    - assault Y04.1 ☑
    - homicide (attempt) Y04.1 ☑
    - in
      - fight Y04.1 ☑
  - insect (nonvenomous) W57 ☑
  - lizard (nonvenomous) W59.01 ☑
  - mammal NEC W55.81 ☑
    - marine W56.31 ☑
  - marine animal (nonvenomous) W56.81 ☑
  - millipede W57 ☑
  - moray eel W56.51 ☑
  - mouse W53.01 ☑
  - person (s) (accidentally) W50.3 ☑
    - with intent to injure or kill Y04.1 ☑
    - as, or caused by, a crowd or human stampede (with fall) W52 ☑
    - assault Y04.1 ☑
    - homicide (attempt) Y04.1 ☑
    - in
      - fight Y04.1 ☑
- **Bite**, bitten by — *continued*
  - pig W55.41 ☑
  - raccoon W55.51 ☑
  - rat W53.11 ☑
  - reptile W59.81 ☑
    - lizard W59.01 ☑
    - snake W59.11 ☑
    - turtle W59.21 ☑
      - terrestrial W59.81 ☑
  - rodent W53.81 ☑
    - mouse W53.01 ☑
    - rat W53.11 ☑
    - specified NEC W53.81 ☑
    - squirrel W53.21 ☑
  - shark W56.41 ☑
  - sheep W55.31 ☑
  - snake (nonvenomous) W59.11 ☑
  - spider (nonvenomous) W57 ☑
  - squirrel W53.21 ☑
- **Blast** (air) in war operations — *see* War operations, blast
- **Blizzard** X37.2 ☑
- **Blood** alcohol level Y90.9
  - less than 20mg/100ml Y90.0
  - presence in blood, level not specified Y90.9
  - 20-39mg/100ml Y90.1
  - 40-59mg/100ml Y90.2
  - 60-79mg/100ml Y90.3
  - 80-99mg/100ml Y90.4
  - 100-119mg/100ml Y90.5
  - 120-199mg/100ml Y90.6
  - 200-239mg/100ml Y90.7
- **Blow** X58 ☑
  - by law-enforcing agent, police (on duty) — *see* Legal, intervention, manhandling
    - blunt object — *see* Legal, intervention, blunt object
- **Blowing** up — *see* Explosion
- **Brawl** (hand) (fists) (foot) Y04.0 ☑
- **Breakage** (accidental) (part of)
  - ladder (causing fall) W11 ☑
  - scaffolding (causing fall) W12 ☑
- **Broken**
  - glass, contact with — *see* Contact, with, glass
  - power line (causing electric shock) W85 ☑
- **Bumping** against, into (accidentally)
  - object NEC W22.8 ☑
    - with fall — *see* Fall, due to, bumping against, object
    - caused by crowd or human stampede (with fall) W52 ☑
    - sports equipment W21.9 ☑
  - person (s) W51 ☑
    - with fall W03 ☑
      - due to ice or snow W00.0 ☑
    - assault Y04.2 ☑
    - caused by, a crowd or human stampede (with fall) W52 ☑
    - homicide (attempt) Y04.2 ☑
  - sports equipment W21.9 ☑
- **Burn**, burned, burning (accidental) (by) (from) (on)
  - acid NEC — *see* Table of Drugs and Chemicals
  - bed linen — *see* Exposure, fire, uncontrolled, in building, bed
  - blowtorch X08.8 ☑
    - with ignition of clothing NEC X06.2 ☑
      - nightwear X05 ☑
  - bonfire, campfire (controlled) (*see also* Exposure, fire, controlled, not in building)
    - uncontrolled — *see* Exposure, fire, uncontrolled, not in building
  - candle X08.8 ☑
    - with ignition of clothing NEC X06.2 ☑
      - nightwear X05 ☑
  - caustic liquid, substance (external) (internal) NEC — *see* Table of Drugs and Chemicals
  - chemical (external) (internal) (*see also* Table of Drugs and Chemicals)
    - in war operations — *see* War operations. fire
  - cigar (s) or cigarette (s) X08.8 ☑
    - with ignition of clothing NEC X06.2 ☑
      - nightwear X05 ☑
  - clothes, clothing NEC (from controlled fire) X06.2 ☑
    - with conflagration — *see* Exposure, fire, uncontrolled, building
      - not in building or structure — *see* Exposure, fire, uncontrolled, not in building
  - cooker (hot) X15.8 ☑
    - stated as undetermined whether accidental or intentional Y27.3 ☑
    - suicide (attempt) X77.3 ☑
- **Burn** — *continued*
  - electric blanket X16 ☑
  - engine (hot) X17 ☑
  - fire, flames — *see* Exposure, fire
  - flare, Very pistol — *see* Discharge, firearm NEC
  - heat
    - from appliance (electrical) (household) X15.8 ☑
      - cooker X15.8 ☑
      - hotplate X15.2 ☑
      - kettle X15.8 ☑
      - light bulb X15.8 ☑
      - saucepan X15.3 ☑
      - skillet X15.3 ☑
      - stove X15.0 ☑
      - stated as undetermined whether accidental or intentional Y27.3 ☑
      - suicide (attempt) X77.3 ☑
      - toaster X15.1 ☑
    - in local application or packing during medical or surgical procedure Y63.5
  - heating
    - appliance, radiator or pipe X16 ☑
  - homicide (attempt) — *see* Assault, burning
  - hot
    - air X14.1 ☑
    - cooker X15.8 ☑
    - drink X10.0 ☑
    - engine X17 ☑
    - fat X10.2 ☑
    - fluid NEC X12 ☑
    - food X10.1 ☑
    - gases X14.1 ☑
    - heating appliance X16 ☑
    - household appliance NEC X15.8 ☑
    - kettle X15.8 ☑
    - liquid NEC X12 ☑
    - machinery X17 ☑
    - metal (molten) (liquid) NEC X18 ☑
    - object (not producing fire or flames) NEC X19 ☑
    - oil (cooking) X10.2 ☑
    - pipe (s) X16 ☑
    - radiator X16 ☑
    - saucepan (glass) (metal) X15.3 ☑
    - stove (kitchen) X15.0 ☑
    - substance NEC X19 ☑
      - caustic or corrosive NEC — *see* Table of Drugs and Chemicals
    - toaster X15.1 ☑
    - tool X17 ☑
    - vapor X13.1 ☑
    - water (tap) — *see* Contact, with, hot, tap water
  - hotplate X15.2 ☑
    - suicide (attempt) X77.3 ☑
  - ignition — *see* Ignition
  - in war operations — *see* War operations, fire
  - inflicted by other person X97 ☑
    - by hot objects, hot vapor, and steam — *see* Assault, burning, hot object
  - internal, from swallowed caustic, corrosive liquid, substance — *see* Table of Drugs and Chemicals
  - iron (hot) X15.8 ☑
    - stated as undetermined whether accidental or intentional Y27.3 ☑
    - suicide (attempt) X77.3 ☑
  - kettle (hot) X15.8 ☑
    - stated as undetermined whether accidental or intentional Y27.3 ☑
    - suicide (attempt) X77.3 ☑
  - lamp (flame) X08.8 ☑
    - with ignition of clothing NEC X06.2 ☑
      - nightwear X05 ☑
  - lighter (cigar) (cigarette) X08.8 ☑
    - with ignition of clothing NEC X06.2 ☑
      - nightwear X05 ☑
  - lightning — *see* subcategory T75.0
    - causing fire — *see* Exposure, fire
  - liquid (boiling) (hot) NEC X12 ☑
    - stated as undetermined whether accidental or intentional Y27.2 ☑
    - suicide (attempt) X77.2 ☑
  - local application of externally applied substance in medical or surgical care Y63.5
  - on board watercraft
    - due to
      - accident to watercraft V91.09 ☑
        - powered craft V91.03 ☑
          - ferry boat V91.01 ☑
          - fishing boat V91.02 ☑
          - jet skis V91.03 ☑

Burn - Compression

- **Burn** — *continued*
  - on board watercraft — *continued*
          - liner V91.01 ☑
          - merchant ship V91.00 ☑
          - passenger ship V91.01 ☑
        - unpowered craft V91.08 ☑
          - canoe V91.05 ☑
          - inflatable V91.06 ☑
          - kayak V91.05 ☑
          - sailboat V91.04 ☑
          - surf-board V91.08 ☑
          - water skis V91.07 ☑
          - windsurfer V91.08 ☑
      - fire on board V93.09 ☑
        - ferry boat V93.01 ☑
        - fishing boat V93.02 ☑
        - jet skis V93.03 ☑
        - liner V93.01 ☑
        - merchant ship V93.00 ☑
        - passenger ship V93.01 ☑
        - powered craft NEC V93.03 ☑
        - sailboat V93.04 ☑
      - specified heat source NEC on board V93.19 ☑
        - ferry boat V93.11 ☑
        - fishing boat V93.12 ☑
        - jet skis V93.13 ☑
        - liner V93.11 ☑
        - merchant ship V93.10 ☑
        - passenger ship V93.11 ☑
        - powered craft NEC V93.13 ☑
        - sailboat V93.14 ☑
  - machinery (hot) X17 ☑
  - matches X08.8 ☑
    - with ignition of clothing NEC X06.2 ☑
      - nightwear X05 ☑
  - mattress — *see* Exposure, fire, uncontrolled, building, bed
  - medicament, externally applied Y63.5
  - metal (hot) (liquid) (molten) NEC X18 ☑
  - nightwear (nightclothes, nightdress, gown, pajamas, robe) X05 ☑
  - object (hot) NEC X19 ☑
  - pipe (hot) X16 ☑
    - smoking X08.8 ☑
      - with ignition of clothing NEC X06.2 ☑
        - nightwear X05 ☑
  - powder — *see* Powder burn
  - radiator (hot) X16 ☑
  - saucepan (hot) (glass) (metal) X15.3 ☑
    - stated as undetermined whether accidental or intentional Y27.3 ☑
    - suicide (attempt) X77.3 ☑
  - self-inflicted X76 ☑
    - stated as undetermined whether accidental or intentional Y26 ☑
  - steam X13.1 ☑
    - pipe X16 ☑
      - stated as undetermined whether accidental or intentional Y27.8 ☑
    - stated as undetermined whether accidental or intentional Y27.0 ☑
    - suicide (attempt) X77.0 ☑
  - stove (hot) (kitchen) X15.0 ☑
    - stated as undetermined whether accidental or intentional Y27.3 ☑
    - suicide (attempt) X77.3 ☑
  - substance (hot) NEC X19 ☑
    - boiling X12 ☑
      - stated as undetermined whether accidental or intentional Y27.2 ☑
      - suicide (attempt) X77.2 ☑
    - molten (metal) X18 ☑
  - suicide (attempt) NEC X76 ☑
    - hot
      - household appliance X77.3 ☑
      - object X77.9 ☑
  - stated as undetermined whether accidental or intentional Y27.0 ☑
  - therapeutic misadventure
    - heat in local application or packing during medical or surgical procedure Y63.5
    - overdose of radiation Y63.2
  - toaster (hot) X15.1 ☑
    - stated as undetermined whether accidental or intentional Y27.3 ☑
    - suicide (attempt) X77.3 ☑
  - tool (hot) X17 ☑
  - torch, welding X08.8 ☑
    - with ignition of clothing NEC X06.2 ☑
      - nightwear X05 ☑

- **Burn** — *continued*
  - trash fire (controlled) — *see* Exposure, fire, controlled, not in building
    - uncontrolled — *see* Exposure, fire, uncontrolled, not in building
  - vapor (hot) X13.1 ☑
    - stated as undetermined whether accidental or intentional Y27.0 ☑
    - suicide (attempt) X77.0 ☑
  - Very pistol — *see* Discharge, firearm NEC
- **Butted** by animal W55.82 ☑
  - bull W55.22 ☑
  - cow W55.22 ☑
  - goat W55.32 ☑
  - horse W55.12 ☑
  - pig W55.42 ☑
  - sheep W55.32 ☑

C

- **Caisson** disease - — *see* Air, pressure, change
- **Campfire** (exposure to) (controlled) (*see also* Exposure, fire, controlled, not in building)
  - uncontrolled — *see* Exposure, fire, uncontrolled, not in building
- **Capital** punishment (any means) — *see* Legal, intervention
- **Car** sickness T75.3 ☑
- **Casualty** (not due to war) NEC X58 ☑
  - war — *see* War operations
- **Cat**
  - bite W55.01 ☑
  - scratch W55.03 ☑
- **Cataclysm,** cataclysmic (any injury) NEC — *see* Forces of nature
- **Catching** fire — *see* Exposure, fire
- **Caught**
  - between
    - folding object W23.0 ☑
    - objects (moving) (stationary and moving) W23.0 ☑
      - and machinery — *see* Contact, with, by type of machine
      - stationary W23.1 ☑
    - sliding door and door frame W23.0 ☑
  - by, in
    - machinery (moving parts of) — *see* Contact, with, by type of machine
    - washing-machine wringer W23.0 ☑
  - under packing crate (due to losing grip) W23.1 ☑
- **Cave-in** caused by cataclysmic earth surface movement or eruption — *see* Landslide
- **Change** (s) in air pressure - — *see* Air, pressure, change
- **Choked,** choking (on) (any object except food or vomitus)
  - food (bone) (seed) — *see* categories T17 and T18 ☑
  - vomitus T17.81 ☑
- **Civil** insurrection — *see* War operations
- **Cloudburst** (any injury) X37.8 ☑
- **Cold,** exposure to (accidental) (excessive) (extreme) (natural) (place) NEC — *see* Exposure, cold
- **Collapse**
  - building W20.1 ☑
    - burning (uncontrolled fire) X00.2 ☑
  - dam or man-made structure (causing earth movement) X36.0 ☑
  - machinery — *see* Contact, with, by type of machine
  - structure W20.1 ☑
    - burning (uncontrolled fire) X00.2 ☑
- **Collision** (accidental) NEC (*see also* Accident, transport) V89.9 ☑
  - pedestrian W51 ☑
    - with fall W03 ☑
      - due to ice or snow W00.0 ☑
      - involving pedestrian conveyance — *see* Accident, transport, pedestrian, conveyance
    - and
      - crowd or human stampede (with fall) W52 ☑
      - object W22.8 ☑
        - with fall — *see* Fall, due to, bumping against, object
  - person (s) — *see* Collision, pedestrian
  - transport vehicle NEC V89.9 ☑
    - and
      - avalanche, fallen or not moving — *see* Accident, transport

- **Collision** — *continued*
  - transport vehicle NEC — *continued*
        - falling or moving — *see* Landslide
      - landslide, fallen or not moving — *see* Accident, transport
        - falling or moving — *see* Landslide
    - due to cataclysm — *see* Forces of nature, by type
    - intentional, purposeful suicide (attempt) — *see* Suicide, collision
- **Combustion,** spontaneous — *see* Ignition
- **Complication** (delayed) of or following (medical or surgical procedure) Y84.9
  - with misadventure — *see* Misadventure
  - amputation of limb (s) Y83.5
  - anastomosis (arteriovenous) (blood vessel) (gastrojejunal) (tendon) (natural or artificial material) Y83.2
  - aspiration (of fluid) Y84.4
    - tissue Y84.8
  - biopsy Y84.8
  - blood
    - sampling Y84.7
    - transfusion
      - procedure Y84.8
  - bypass Y83.2
  - catheterization (urinary) Y84.6
    - cardiac Y84.0
  - colostomy Y83.3
  - cystostomy Y83.3
  - dialysis (kidney) Y84.1
  - drug — *see* Table of Drugs and Chemicals
  - due to misadventure — *see* Misadventure
  - duodenostomy Y83.3
  - electroshock therapy Y84.3
  - external stoma, creation of Y83.3
  - formation of external stoma Y83.3
  - gastrostomy Y83.3
  - graft Y83.2
  - hypothermia (medically-induced) Y84.8
  - implant, implantation (of)
    - artificial
      - internal device (cardiac pacemaker) (electrodes in brain) (heart valve prosthesis) (orthopedic) Y83.1
      - material or tissue (for anastomosis or bypass) Y83.2
        - with creation of external stoma Y83.3
    - natural tissues (for anastomosis or bypass) Y83.2
      - with creation of external stoma Y83.3
  - infusion
    - procedure Y84.8
  - injection — *see* Table of Drugs and Chemicals
    - procedure Y84.8
  - insertion of gastric or duodenal sound Y84.5
  - insulin-shock therapy Y84.3
  - paracentesis (abdominal) (thoracic) (aspirative) Y84.4
  - procedures other than surgical operation — *see* Complication of or following, by type of procedure
  - radiological procedure or therapy Y84.2
  - removal of organ (partial) (total) NEC Y83.6
  - sampling
    - blood Y84.7
    - fluid NEC Y84.4
    - tissue Y84.8
  - shock therapy Y84.3
  - surgical operation NEC (*see also* Complication of or following, by type of operation) Y83.9
    - reconstructive NEC Y83.4
      - with
        - anastomosis, bypass or graft Y83.2
        - formation of external stoma Y83.3
    - specified NEC Y83.8
  - transfusion (*see also* Table of Drugs and Chemicals)
    - procedure Y84.8
  - transplant, transplantation (heart) (kidney) (liver) (whole organ, any) Y83.0
    - partial organ Y83.4
  - ureterostomy Y83.3
  - vaccination (*see also* Table of Drugs and Chemicals)
    - procedure Y84.8
- **Compression**
  - divers' squeeze - — *see* Air, pressure, change
  - trachea by
    - food (lodged in esophagus) — *see* categories T17 and T18 ☑
    - vomitus (lodged in esophagus) T17.81 ☑

- **Contact** — *continued*
  - with — *continued*
    - splinter W45.8 ☑
    - sports equipment W21.9 ☑
    - staple gun (powered) W29.8 ☑
    - steam X13.1 ☑
      - engine W31.3 ☑
      - inhalation X13.0 ☑
      - pipe X16 ☑
      - shovel W31.89 ☑
    - stove (hot) (kitchen) X15.0 ☑
    - substance, hot NEC X19 ☑
      - molten (metal) X18 ☑
    - sword W26.1 ☑
      - assault X99.2 ☑
      - stated as undetermined whether accidental or intentional Y28.2 ☑
      - suicide (attempt) X78.2 ☑
    - tarantula X58 ☑
    - thresher W30.0 ☑
    - tin can lid W26.8 ☑
    - toad W62.1 ☑
    - toaster (hot) X15.1 ☑
    - tool W27.8 ☑
      - hand (not powered) W27.8 ☑
        - auger W27.0 ☑
        - axe W27.0 ☑
        - can opener W27.4 ☑
        - chisel W27.0 ☑
        - fork W27.4 ☑
        - garden W27.1 ☑
        - handsaw W27.0 ☑
        - hoe W27.1 ☑
        - ice-pick W27.4 ☑
        - kitchen utensil W27.4 ☑
        - manual
          - lawn mower W27.1 ☑
          - sewing machine W27.8 ☑
        - meat grinder W27.4 ☑
        - needle (sewing) W27.3 ☑
          - hypodermic W46.0 ☑
            - contaminated W46.1 ☑
        - paper cutter W27.5 ☑
        - pitchfork W27.1 ☑
        - rake W27.1 ☑
        - scissors W27.2 ☑
        - screwdriver W27.0 ☑
        - specified NEC W27.8 ☑
        - workbench W27.0 ☑
      - hot X17 ☑
      - powered W29.8 ☑
        - blender W29.0 ☑
          - commercial W31.82 ☑
        - can opener W29.0 ☑
          - commercial W31.82 ☑
        - chainsaw W29.3 ☑
        - clothes dryer W29.2 ☑
          - commercial W31.82 ☑
        - dishwasher W29.2 ☑
          - commercial W31.82 ☑
        - edger W29.3 ☑
        - electric fan W29.2 ☑
          - commercial W31.82 ☑
        - electric knife W29.1 ☑
        - food processor W29.0 ☑
          - commercial W31.82 ☑
        - garbage disposal W29.0 ☑
          - commercial W31.82 ☑
        - garden tool W29.3 ☑
        - hedge trimmer W29.3 ☑
        - ice maker W29.0 ☑
          - commercial W31.82 ☑
        - kitchen appliance W29.0 ☑
          - commercial W31.82 ☑
        - lawn mower W28 ☑
        - meat grinder W29.0 ☑
          - commercial W31.82 ☑
        - mixer W29.0 ☑
          - commercial W31.82 ☑
        - Rototiller® W29.3 ☑
        - sewing machine W29.2 ☑
          - commercial W31.82 ☑
        - washing machine W29.2 ☑
          - commercial W31.82 ☑
    - transmission device (belt, cable, chain, gear, pinion, shaft) W24.1 ☑
      - agricultural operations W30.89 ☑
    - turbine (gas) (water-driven) W31.3 ☑
    - turkey W61.49 ☑
      - peck W61.43 ☑
      - strike W61.42 ☑
    - turtle (nonvenomous) W59.29 ☑
      - bite W59.21 ☑
      - strike W59.22 ☑
      - terrestrial W59.89 ☑
        - bite W59.81 ☑
        - crushing W59.83 ☑
        - strike W59.82 ☑
    - under-cutter W31.0 ☑
    - urine — *see* Contact, with, by type of animal
    - vehicle
      - agricultural use (transport) — *see* Accident, transport, agricultural vehicle
        - not on public highway W30.81 ☑
      - industrial use (transport) — *see* Accident, transport, industrial vehicle
        - not on public highway W31.83 ☑
      - off-road use (transport) — *see* Accident, transport, all-terrain or off-road vehicle
        - not on public highway W31.83 ☑
      - special construction use (transport) — *see* Accident, transport, construction vehicle
        - not on public highway W31.83 ☑
    - venomous
      - animal X58 ☑
      - arthropods X58 ☑
      - lizard X58 ☑
      - marine animal NEC X58 ☑
      - marine plant NEC X58 ☑
      - millipedes (tropical) X58 ☑
      - plant (s) X58 ☑
      - snake X58 ☑
      - spider X58 ☑
    - viper X58 ☑
    - washing-machine (powered) W29.2 ☑
    - wasp X58 ☑
    - weaving-machine W31.89 ☑
    - winch W24.0 ☑
      - agricultural operations W30.89 ☑
    - wire NEC W24.0 ☑
      - agricultural operations W30.89 ☑
    - wood slivers W45.8 ☑
    - yellow jacket X58 ☑
    - zebra — *see* Contact, with, hoof stock NEC
  - pressure X50.9 ☑
  - stress X50.9 ☑
- **Coup de soleil** X32 ☑
- **Crash**
  - aircraft (in transit) (powered) V95.9 ☑
    - balloon V96.01 ☑
    - fixed wing NEC (private) V95.21 ☑
      - commercial V95.31 ☑
    - glider V96.21 ☑
      - hang V96.11 ☑
      - powered V95.11 ☑
    - helicopter V95.01 ☑
    - in war operations — *see* War operations, destruction of aircraft
    - microlight V95.11 ☑
    - nonpowered V96.9 ☑
      - specified NEC V96.8 ☑
    - powered NEC V95.8 ☑
    - stated as
      - homicide (attempt) Y08.81 ☑
      - suicide (attempt) X83.0 ☑
    - ultralight V95.11 ☑
  - spacecraft V95.41 ☑
  - transport vehicle NEC (*see also* Accident, transport) V89.9 ☑
    - homicide (attempt) Y03.8 ☑
    - motor NEC (traffic) V89.2 ☑
      - homicide (attempt) Y03.8 ☑
      - suicide (attempt) — *see* Suicide, collision
- **Cruelty** (mental) (physical) (sexual) X58 ☑
- **Crushed** (accidentally) X58 ☑
  - between objects (moving) (stationary and moving) W23.0 ☑
    - stationary W23.1 ☑
  - by
    - alligator W58.03 ☑
    - avalanche NEC — *see* Landslide
    - cave-in W20.0 ☑
      - caused by cataclysmic earth surface movement — *see* Landslide
    - crocodile W58.13 ☑
    - crowd or human stampede W52 ☑
    - falling
      - aircraft V97.39 ☑
        - in war operations — *see* War operations, destruction of aircraft
      - earth, material W20.0 ☑
        - caused by cataclysmic earth surface movement — *see* Landslide
      - object NEC W20.8 ☑
    - landslide NEC — *see* Landslide
    - lizard (nonvenomous) W59.09 ☑
    - machinery — *see* Contact, with, by type of machine
    - reptile NEC W59.89 ☑
    - snake (nonvenomous) W59.13 ☑
  - in
    - machinery — *see* Contact, with, by type of machine
- **Cut, cutting** (any part of body) (accidental) (*see also* Contact, with, by object or machine)
  - during medical or surgical treatment as misadventure — *see* Index to Diseases and Injuries, Complications
  - homicide (attempt) — *see* Assault, cutting or piercing instrument
  - inflicted by other person — *see* Assault, cutting or piercing instrument
  - legal
    - execution — *see* Legal, intervention
    - intervention — *see* Legal, intervention, sharp object
  - machine NEC (*see also* Contact, with, by type of machine) W31.9 ☑
  - self-inflicted — *see* Suicide, cutting or piercing instrument
  - suicide (attempt) — *see* Suicide, cutting or piercing instrument
- **Cyclone** (any injury) X37.1 ☑

D

- **Decapitation** (accidental circumstances) NEC X58 ☑
  - homicide X99.9 ☑
  - legal execution — *see* Legal, intervention
- **Dehydration** from lack of water X58 ☑
- **Deprivation** X58 ☑
- **Derailment** (accidental)
  - railway (rolling stock) (train) (vehicle) (without antecedent collision) V81.7 ☑
    - with antecedent collision — *see* Accident, transport, railway vehicle occupant
  - streetcar (without antecedent collision) V82.7 ☑
    - with antecedent collision — *see* Accident, transport, streetcar occupant
- **Descent**
  - parachute (voluntary) (without accident to aircraft) V97.29 ☑
    - due to accident to aircraft — *see* Accident, transport, aircraft
- **Desertion** X58 ☑
- **Destitution** X58 ☑
- **Disability,** late effect or sequela of injury — *see* Sequelae
- **Discharge** (accidental)
  - airgun W34.010 ☑
    - assault X95.01 ☑
    - homicide (attempt) X95.01 ☑
    - stated as undetermined whether accidental or intentional Y24.0 ☑
    - suicide (attempt) X74.01 ☑
  - BB gun — *see* Discharge, airgun
  - firearm (accidental) W34.00 ☑
    - assault X95.9 ☑
    - handgun (pistol) (revolver) W32.0 ☑
      - assault X93 ☑
      - homicide (attempt) X93 ☑
      - legal intervention — *see* Legal, intervention, firearm, handgun
      - stated as undetermined whether accidental or intentional Y22 ☑
      - suicide (attempt) X72 ☑
    - homicide (attempt) X95.9 ☑
    - hunting rifle W33.02 ☑
      - assault X94.1 ☑
      - homicide (attempt) X94.1 ☑
      - legal intervention
        - injuring
          - bystander Y35.032 ☑
          - law enforcement personnel Y35.031 ☑
          - suspect Y35.033 ☑
      - stated as undetermined whether accidental or intentional Y23.1 ☑
      - suicide (attempt) X73.1 ☑
    - larger W33.00 ☑

- **Discharge** — *continued*
  - firearm — *continued*
      - assault X94.9 ☑
      - homicide (attempt) X94.9 ☑
      - hunting rifle — *see* Discharge, firearm, hunting rifle
      - legal intervention — *see* Legal, intervention, firearm by type of firearm
      - machine gun — *see* Discharge, firearm, machine gun
      - shotgun — *see* Discharge, firearm, shotgun
      - specified NEC W33.09 ☑
        - assault X94.8 ☑
        - homicide (attempt) X94.8 ☑
        - legal intervention
          - injuring
            - bystander Y35.092 ☑
            - law enforcement personnel Y35.091 ☑
            - suspect Y35.093 ☑
        - stated as undetermined whether accidental or intentional Y23.8 ☑
        - suicide (attempt) X73.8 ☑
      - stated as undetermined whether accidental or intentional Y23.9 ☑
      - suicide (attempt) X73.9 ☑
    - legal intervention
      - injuring
        - bystander Y35.002 ☑
        - law enforcement personnel Y35.001 ☑
        - suspect Y35.03 ☑
      - using rubber bullet
        - injuring
          - bystander Y35.042 ☑
          - law enforcement personnel Y35.041 ☑
          - suspect Y35.043 ☑
    - machine gun W33.03 ☑
      - assault X94.2 ☑
      - homicide (attempt) X94.2 ☑
      - legal intervention — *see* Legal, intervention, firearm, machine gun
      - stated as undetermined whether accidental or intentional Y23.3 ☑
      - suicide (attempt) X73.2 ☑
    - pellet gun — *see* Discharge, airgun
    - shotgun W33.01 ☑
      - assault X94.0 ☑
      - homicide (attempt) X94.0 ☑
      - legal intervention — *see* Legal, intervention, firearm, specified NEC
      - stated as undetermined whether accidental or intentional Y23.0 ☑
      - suicide (attempt) X73.0 ☑
    - specified NEC W34.09 ☑
      - assault X95.8 ☑
      - homicide (attempt) X95.8 ☑
      - legal intervention — *see* Legal, intervention, firearm, specified NEC
      - stated as undetermined whether accidental or intentional Y24.8 ☑
      - suicide (attempt) X74.8 ☑
    - stated as undetermined whether accidental or intentional Y24.9 ☑
    - suicide (attempt) X74.9 ☑
    - Very pistol W34.09 ☑
      - assault X95.8 ☑
      - homicide (attempt) X95.8 ☑
      - stated as undetermined whether accidental or intentional Y24.8 ☑
      - suicide (attempt) X74.8 ☑
  - firework (s) W39 ☑
    - stated as undetermined whether accidental or intentional Y25 ☑
  - gas-operated gun NEC W34.018 ☑
    - airgun — *see* Discharge, airgun
    - assault X95.09 ☑
    - homicide (attempt) X95.09 ☑
    - paintball gun — *see* Discharge, paintball gun
    - stated as undetermined whether accidental or intentional Y24.8 ☑
    - suicide (attempt) X74.09 ☑
  - gun NEC (*see also* Discharge, firearm NEC)
    - air — *see* Discharge, airgun
    - BB — *see* Discharge, airgun
    - for single hand use — *see* Discharge, firearm, handgun
    - hand — *see* Discharge, firearm, handgun
    - machine — *see* Discharge, firearm, machine gun
    - other specified — *see* Discharge, firearm NEC
    - paintball — *see* Discharge, paintball gun
    - pellet — *see* Discharge, airgun

- **Discharge** — *continued*
  - handgun — *see* Discharge, firearm, handgun
  - machine gun — *see* Discharge, firearm, machine gun
  - paintball gun W34.011 ☑
    - assault X95.02 ☑
    - homicide (attempt) X95.02 ☑
    - stated as undetermined whether accidental or intentional Y24.8 ☑
    - suicide (attempt) X74.02 ☑
  - pistol — *see* Discharge, firearm, handgun
    - flare — *see* Discharge, firearm, Very pistol
    - pellet — *see* Discharge, airgun
    - Very — *see* Discharge, firearm, Very pistol
  - revolver — *see* Discharge, firearm, handgun
  - rifle (hunting) — *see* Discharge, firearm, hunting rifle
  - shotgun — *see* Discharge, firearm, shotgun
  - spring-operated gun NEC W34.018 ☑
    - assault X95.09 ☑
    - homicide (attempt) X95.09 ☑
    - stated as undetermined whether accidental or intentional Y24.8 ☑
    - suicide (attempt) X74.09 ☑
- **Disease**
  - Andes W94.11 ☑
  - aviator's - — *see* Air, pressure
  - range W94.11 ☑
- **Diver's** disease, palsy, paralysis, squeeze - — *see* Air, pressure
- **Diving** (into water) — *see* Accident, diving
- **Dog** bite W54.0 ☑
- **Dragged** by transport vehicle NEC (*see also* Accident, transport) V09.9 ☑
- **Drinking** poison (accidental) — *see* Table of Drugs and Chemicals
- **Dropped** (accidentally) while being carried or supported by other person W04 ☑
- **Drowning** (accidental) W74 ☑
  - assault X92.9 ☑
  - due to
    - accident (to)
      - machinery — *see* Contact, with, by type of machine
      - watercraft V90.89 ☑
        - burning V90.29 ☑
          - powered V90.23 ☑
            - merchant ship V90.20 ☑
            - passenger ship V90.21 ☑
            - fishing boat V90.22 ☑
            - jet skis V90.23 ☑
          - unpowered V90.28 ☑
            - canoe V90.25 ☑
            - inflatable V90.26 ☑
            - kayak V90.25 ☑
            - sailboat V90.24 ☑
            - water skis V90.27 ☑
        - crushed V90.39 ☑
          - powered V90.33 ☑
            - merchant ship V90.30 ☑
            - passenger ship V90.31 ☑
            - fishing boat V90.32 ☑
            - jet skis V90.33 ☑
          - unpowered V90.38 ☑
            - canoe V90.35 ☑
            - inflatable V90.36 ☑
            - kayak V90.35 ☑
            - sailboat V90.34 ☑
            - water skis V90.37 ☑
        - overturning V90.09 ☑
          - powered V90.03 ☑
            - merchant ship V90.00 ☑
            - passenger ship V90.01 ☑
            - fishing boat V90.02 ☑
            - jet skis V90.03 ☑
          - unpowered V90.08 ☑
            - canoe V90.05 ☑
            - inflatable V90.06 ☑
            - kayak V90.05 ☑
            - sailboat V90.04 ☑
        - sinking V90.19 ☑
          - powered V90.13 ☑
            - merchant ship V90.10 ☑
            - passenger ship V90.11 ☑
            - fishing boat V90.12 ☑
            - jet skis V90.13 ☑
          - unpowered V90.18 ☑
            - canoe V90.15 ☑
            - inflatable V90.16 ☑
            - kayak V90.15 ☑
            - sailboat V90.14 ☑
        - specified type NEC V90.89 ☑

- **Drowning** — *continued*
  - due to — *continued*
          - powered V90.83 ☑
            - merchant ship V90.80 ☑
            - passenger ship V90.81 ☑
            - fishing boat V90.82 ☑
            - jet skis V90.83 ☑
          - unpowered V90.88 ☑
            - canoe V90.85 ☑
            - inflatable V90.86 ☑
            - kayak V90.85 ☑
            - sailboat V90.84 ☑
            - water skis V90.87 ☑
    - avalanche — *see* Landslide
    - cataclysmic
      - earth surface movement NEC — *see* Forces of nature, earth movement
      - storm — *see* Forces of nature, cataclysmic storm
    - cloudburst X37.8 ☑
    - cyclone X37.1 ☑
    - fall overboard (from) V92.09 ☑
      - powered craft V92.03 ☑
        - ferry boat V92.01 ☑
        - liner V92.01 ☑
        - merchant ship V92.00 ☑
        - passenger ship V92.01 ☑
        - fishing boat V92.02 ☑
        - jet skis V92.03 ☑
      - unpowered craft V92.08 ☑
        - canoe V92.05 ☑
        - inflatable V92.06 ☑
        - kayak V92.05 ☑
        - sailboat V92.04 ☑
        - surf-board V92.08 ☑
        - water skis V92.07 ☑
        - windsurfer V92.08 ☑
      - resulting from
        - accident to watercraft — *see* Drowning, due to, accident to, watercraft
        - being washed overboard (from) V92.29 ☑
          - powered craft V92.23 ☑
            - ferry boat V92.21 ☑
            - liner V92.21 ☑
            - merchant ship V92.20 ☑
            - passenger ship V92.21 ☑
            - fishing boat V92.22 ☑
            - jet skis V92.23 ☑
          - unpowered craft V92.28 ☑
            - canoe V92.25 ☑
            - inflatable V92.26 ☑
            - kayak V92.25 ☑
            - sailboat V92.24 ☑
            - surf-board V92.28 ☑
            - water skis V92.27 ☑
            - windsurfer V92.28 ☑
        - motion of watercraft V92.19 ☑
          - powered craft V92.13 ☑
            - ferry boat V92.11 ☑
            - liner V92.11 ☑
            - merchant ship V92.10 ☑
            - passenger ship V92.11 ☑
            - fishing boat V92.12 ☑
            - jet skis V92.13 ☑
          - unpowered craft
            - canoe V92.15 ☑
            - inflatable V92.16 ☑
            - kayak V92.15 ☑
            - sailboat V92.14 ☑
    - hurricane X37.0 ☑
    - jumping into water from watercraft (involved in accident) (*see also* Drowning, due to, accident to, watercraft)
      - without accident to or on watercraft W16.711 ☑
    - tidal wave NEC — *see* Forces of nature, tidal wave
    - torrential rain X37.8 ☑
  - following
    - fall
      - into
        - bathtub W16.211 ☑
        - bucket W16.221 ☑
        - fountain — *see* Drowning, following, fall, into, water, specified NEC
        - quarry — *see* Drowning, following, fall, into, water, specified NEC
        - reservoir — *see* Drowning, following, fall, into, water, specified NEC
        - swimming-pool W16.011 ☑
          - striking
            - bottom W16.021 ☑

- **Drowning** — *continued*
  - following — *continued*
            - wall W16.031 ☑
          - stated as undetermined whether accidental or intentional Y21.3 ☑
          - suicide (attempt) X71.2 ☑
        - water NOS W16.41 ☑
          - natural (lake) (open sea) (river) (stream) (pond) W16.111 ☑
            - striking
              - bottom W16.121 ☑
              - side W16.131 ☑
          - specified NEC W16.311 ☑
            - striking
              - bottom W16.321 ☑
              - wall W16.331 ☑
      - overboard NEC — *see* Drowning, due to, fall overboard
    - jump or dive
      - from boat W16.711 ☑
        - striking bottom W16.721 ☑
      - into
        - fountain — *see* Drowning, following, jump or dive, into, water, specified NEC
        - quarry — *see* Drowning, following, jump or dive, into, water, specified NEC
        - reservoir — *see* Drowning, following, jump or dive, into, water, specified NEC
        - swimming-pool W16.511 ☑
          - striking
            - bottom W16.521 ☑
            - wall W16.531 ☑
          - suicide (attempt) X71.2 ☑
        - water NOS W16.91 ☑
          - natural (lake) (open sea) (river) (stream) (pond) W16.611 ☑
          - specified NEC W16.811 ☑
            - striking
              - bottom W16.821 ☑
              - wall W16.831 ☑
          - striking bottom W16.621 ☑
  - homicide (attempt) X92.9 ☑
  - in
    - bathtub (accidental) W65 ☑
      - assault X92.0 ☑
      - following fall W16.211 ☑
        - stated as undetermined whether accidental or intentional Y21.1 ☑
      - stated as undetermined whether accidental or intentional Y21.0 ☑
      - suicide (attempt) X71.0 ☑
    - lake — *see* Drowning, in, natural water
    - natural water (lake) (open sea) (river) (stream) (pond) W69 ☑
      - assault X92.3 ☑
      - following
        - dive or jump W16.611 ☑
          - striking bottom W16.621 ☑
        - fall W16.111 ☑
          - striking
            - bottom W16.121 ☑
            - side W16.131 ☑
      - stated as undetermined whether accidental or intentional Y21.4 ☑
      - suicide (attempt) X71.3 ☑
    - quarry — *see* Drowning, in, specified place NEC
    - quenching tank — *see* Drowning, in, specified place NEC
    - reservoir — *see* Drowning, in, specified place NEC
    - river — *see* Drowning, in, natural water
    - sea — *see* Drowning, in, natural water
    - specified place NEC W73 ☑
      - assault X92.8 ☑
      - following
        - dive or jump W16.811 ☑
          - striking
            - bottom W16.821 ☑
            - wall W16.831 ☑
        - fall W16.311 ☑
          - striking
            - bottom W16.321 ☑
            - wall W16.331 ☑
      - stated as undetermined whether accidental or intentional Y21.8 ☑
      - suicide (attempt) X71.8 ☑
    - stream — *see* Drowning, in, natural water
    - swimming-pool W67 ☑
      - assault X92.1 ☑
        - following fall X92.2 ☑
      - following
        - dive or jump W16.511 ☑

- **Drowning** — *continued*
  - in — *continued*
          - striking
            - bottom W16.521 ☑
            - wall W16.531 ☑
        - fall W16.011 ☑
          - striking
            - bottom W16.021 ☑
            - wall W16.031 ☑
      - stated as undetermined whether accidental or intentional Y21.2 ☑
        - following fall Y21.3 ☑
      - suicide (attempt) X71.1 ☑
        - following fall X71.2 ☑
    - war operations — *see* War operations, restriction of airway
  - resulting from accident to watercraft — *see* Drowning, due to, accident, watercraft
  - self-inflicted X71.9 ☑
  - stated as undetermined whether accidental or intentional Y21.9 ☑
  - suicide (attempt) X71.9 ☑

E

- **Earth** (surface) movement NEC — *see* Forces of nature, earth movement
- **Earth** falling (on) W20.0 ☑
  - caused by cataclysmic earth surface movement or eruption — *see* Landslide
- **Earthquake** (any injury) X34 ☑
- **Effect** (s) (adverse) of
  - air pressure (any) - — *see* Air, pressure
  - cold, excessive (exposure to) — *see* Exposure, cold
  - heat (excessive) — *see* Heat
  - hot place (weather) — *see* Heat
  - insolation X30 ☑
  - late — *see* Sequelae
  - motion — *see* Motion
  - nuclear explosion or weapon in war operations — *see* War operations, nuclear weapon
  - radiation — *see* Radiation
  - travel — *see* Travel
- **Electric** shock (accidental) (by) (in) — *see* Exposure, electric current
- **Electrocution** (accidental) — *see* Exposure, electric current
- **Endotracheal** tube wrongly placed during anesthetic procedure
- **Entanglement**
  - in
    - bed linen, causing suffocation T71
    - wheel of pedal cycle V19.88 ☑
- **Entry** of foreign body or material — *see* Foreign body
- **Environmental** pollution related condition- see Z57 ☑
- **Execution**, legal (any method) — *see* Legal, intervention
- **Exhaustion**
  - cold — *see* Exposure, cold
  - due to excessive exertion (*see also* Overexertion) X50.9 ☑
  - heat — *see* Heat
- **Explosion** (accidental) (of) (with secondary fire) W40.9 ☑
  - acetylene W40.1 ☑
  - aerosol can W36.1 ☑
  - air tank (compressed) (in machinery) W36.2 ☑
  - aircraft (in transit) (powered) NEC V95.9 ☑
    - balloon V96.05 ☑
    - fixed wing NEC (private) V95.25 ☑
      - commercial V95.35 ☑
    - glider V96.25 ☑
      - hang V96.15 ☑
      - powered V95.15 ☑
    - helicopter V95.05 ☑
    - in war operations — *see* War operations, destruction of aircraft
    - microlight V95.15 ☑
    - nonpowered V96.9 ☑
      - specified NEC V96.8 ☑
    - powered NEC V95.8 ☑
    - stated as
      - homicide (attempt) Y03.8 ☑
      - suicide (attempt) X83.0 ☑
    - ultralight V95.15 ☑
  - anesthetic gas in operating room W40.1 ☑
  - antipersonnel bomb W40.8 ☑

- **Explosion** — *continued*
  - antipersonnel bomb — *continued*
    - assault X96.0 ☑
    - homicide (attempt) X96.0 ☑
    - suicide (attempt) X75 ☑
  - assault X96.9 ☑
  - bicycle tire W37.0 ☑
  - blasting (cap) (materials) W40.0 ☑
  - boiler (machinery), not on transport vehicle W35 ☑
    - on watercraft — *see* Explosion, in, watercraft
  - butane W40.1 ☑
  - caused by other person X96.9 ☑
  - coal gas W40.1 ☑
  - detonator W40.0 ☑
  - dump (munitions) W40.8 ☑
  - dynamite W40.0 ☑
    - in
      - assault X96.8 ☑
      - homicide (attempt) X96.8 ☑
      - legal intervention
        - injuring
          - bystander Y35.112 ☑
          - law enforcement personnel Y35.111 ☑
          - suspect Y35.113 ☑
      - suicide (attempt) X75 ☑
  - explosive (material) W40.9 ☑
    - gas W40.1 ☑
    - in blasting operation W40.0 ☑
    - specified NEC W40.8 ☑
      - in
        - assault X96.8 ☑
        - homicide (attempt) X96.8 ☑
        - legal intervention
          - injuring
            - bystander Y35.192 ☑
            - law enforcement personnel Y35.191 ☑
            - suspect Y35.193 ☑
        - suicide (attempt) X75 ☑
  - factory (munitions) W40.8 ☑
  - fertilizer bomb W40.8 ☑
    - assault X96.3 ☑
    - homicide (attempt) X96.3 ☑
    - suicide (attempt) X75 ☑
  - firearm (parts) NEC W34.19 ☑
    - airgun W34.110 ☑
    - BB gun W34.110 ☑
    - gas, air or spring-operated gun NEC W34.118 ☑
    - handgun W32.1 ☑
    - hunting rifle W33.12 ☑
    - larger firearm W33.10 ☑
      - specified NEC W33.19 ☑
    - machine gun W33.13 ☑
    - paintball gun W34.111 ☑
    - pellet gun W34.110 ☑
    - shotgun W33.11 ☑
    - Very pistol [flare] W34.19 ☑
  - fire-damp W40.1 ☑
  - fireworks W39 ☑
  - gas (coal) (explosive) W40.1 ☑
    - cylinder W36.9 ☑
      - aerosol can W36.1 ☑
      - air tank W36.2 ☑
      - pressurized W36.3 ☑
      - specified NEC W36.8 ☑
  - gasoline (fumes) (tank) not in moving motor vehicle W40.1 ☑
    - bomb W40.8 ☑
      - assault X96.1 ☑
      - homicide (attempt) X96.1 ☑
      - suicide (attempt) X75 ☑
    - in motor vehicle — *see* Accident, transport, by type of vehicle
  - grain store W40.8 ☑
  - grenade W40.8 ☑
    - in
      - assault X96.8 ☑
      - homicide (attempt) X96.8 ☑
      - legal intervention
        - injuring
          - bystander Y35.192 ☑
          - law enforcement personnel Y35.191 ☑
          - suspect Y35.193 ☑
      - suicide (attempt) X75 ☑
  - handgun (parts) — *see* Explosion, firearm, handgun (parts)
  - homicide (attempt) X96.9 ☑
    - antipersonnel bomb — *see* Explosion, antipersonnel bomb
    - fertilizer bomb — *see* Explosion, fertilizer bomb

Explosion - Exposure

- **Explosion** — *continued*
  - homicide — *continued*
    - gasoline bomb — *see* Explosion, gasoline bomb
    - letter bomb — *see* Explosion, letter bomb
    - pipe bomb — *see* Explosion, pipe bomb
    - specified NEC X96.8 ☑
  - hose, pressurized W37.8 ☑
  - hot water heater, tank (in machinery) W35 ☑
    - on watercraft — *see* Explosion, in, watercraft
  - in, on
    - dump W40.8 ☑
    - factory W40.8 ☑
    - mine (of explosive gases) NEC W40.1 ☑
    - watercraft V93.59 ☑
      - powered craft V93.53 ☑
        - ferry boat V93.51 ☑
        - fishing boat V93.52 ☑
        - jet skis V93.53 ☑
        - liner V93.51 ☑
        - merchant ship V93.50 ☑
        - passenger ship V93.51 ☑
        - sailboat V93.54 ☑
  - letter bomb W40.8 ☑
    - assault X96.2 ☑
    - homicide (attempt) X96.2 ☑
    - suicide (attempt) X75 ☑
  - machinery (*see also* Contact, with, by type of machine)
    - on board watercraft — *see* Explosion, in, watercraft
    - pressure vessel — *see* Explosion, by type of vessel
  - methane W40.1 ☑
  - mine W40.1 ☑
  - missile NEC W40.8 ☑
  - mortar bomb W40.8 ☑
    - in
      - assault X96.8 ☑
      - homicide (attempt) X96.8 ☑
      - legal intervention
        - injuring
          - bystander Y35.192 ☑
          - law enforcement personnel Y35.191 ☑
          - suspect Y35.193 ☑
      - suicide (attempt) X75 ☑
  - munitions (dump) (factory) W40.8 ☑
  - pipe, pressurized W37.8 ☑
    - bomb W40.8 ☑
      - assault X96.4 ☑
      - homicide (attempt) X96.4 ☑
      - suicide (attempt) X75 ☑
  - pressure, pressurized
    - cooker W38 ☑
    - gas tank (in machinery) W36.3 ☑
    - hose W37.8 ☑
    - pipe W37.8 ☑
    - specified device NEC W38 ☑
    - tire W37.8 ☑
      - bicycle W37.0 ☑
    - vessel (in machinery) W38 ☑
  - propane W40.1 ☑
  - self-inflicted X75 ☑
  - shell (artillery) NEC W40.8 ☑
    - during war operations — *see* War operations, explosion
    - in
      - legal intervention
        - injuring
          - bystander Y35.122 ☑
          - law enforcement personnel Y35.121 ☑
          - suspect Y35.123 ☑
      - war — *see* War operations, explosion
  - spacecraft V95.45 ☑
  - steam or water lines (in machinery) W37.8 ☑
  - stove W40.9 ☑
  - stated as undetermined whether accidental or intentional Y25 ☑
  - suicide (attempt) X75 ☑
  - tire, pressurized W37.8 ☑
    - bicycle W37.0 ☑
  - undetermined whether accidental or intentional Y25 ☑
  - vehicle tire NEC W37.8 ☑
    - bicycle W37.0 ☑
  - war operations — *see* War operations, explosion
- **Exposure** (to) X58 ☑
  - air pressure change — *see* Air, pressure
  - cold (accidental) (excessive) (extreme) (natural) (place) X31 ☑
    - assault Y08.89 ☑
    - due to
- **Exposure** — *continued*
  - cold — *continued*
      - man-made conditions W93.8 ☑
        - dry ice (contact) W93.01 ☑
          - inhalation W93.02 ☑
        - liquid air (contact) (hydrogen) (nitrogen) W93.11 ☑
          - inhalation W93.12 ☑
        - refrigeration unit (deep freeze) W93.2 ☑
        - suicide (attempt) X83.2 ☑
      - weather (conditions) X31 ☑
    - homicide (attempt) Y08.89 ☑
    - self-inflicted X83.2 ☑
  - due to abandonment or neglect X58 ☑
  - electric current W86.8 ☑
    - appliance (faulty) W86.8 ☑
      - domestic W86.0 ☑
    - caused by other person Y08.89 ☑
    - conductor (faulty) W86.1 ☑
    - control apparatus (faulty) W86.1 ☑
    - electric power generating plant, distribution station W86.1 ☑
    - electroshock gun — *see* Exposure, electric current, taser
    - high-voltage cable W85 ☑
    - homicide (attempt) Y08.89 ☑
    - legal execution — *see* Legal, intervention, specified means NEC
    - lightning — *see* subcategory T75.0
    - live rail W86.8 ☑
    - misadventure in medical or surgical procedure in electroshock therapy Y63.4
    - motor (electric) (faulty) W86.8 ☑
      - domestic W86.0 ☑
    - self-inflicted X83.1 ☑
    - specified NEC W86.8 ☑
      - domestic W86.0 ☑
    - stun gun — *see* Exposure, electric current, taser
    - suicide (attempt) X83.1 ☑
    - taser W86.8 ☑
      - assault Y08.89 ☑
      - legal intervention Y35
      - self-harm (intentional) X83.8 ☑
      - undetermined intent Y33 ☑
    - third rail W86.8 ☑
    - transformer (faulty) W86.1 ☑
    - transmission lines W85 ☑
  - environmental tobacco smoke X58 ☑
  - excessive
    - cold — *see* Exposure, cold
    - heat (natural) NEC X30 ☑
      - man-made W92 ☑
  - factor (s) NOS X58 ☑
    - environmental NEC X58 ☑
      - man-made NEC W99 ☑
      - natural NEC — *see* Forces of nature
    - specified NEC X58 ☑
  - fire, flames (accidental) X08.8 ☑
    - assault X97 ☑
    - campfire — *see* Exposure, fire, controlled, not in building
    - controlled (in)
      - with ignition (of) clothing (*see also* Ignition, clothes) X06.2 ☑
        - nightwear X05 ☑
      - bonfire — *see* Exposure, fire, controlled, not in building
      - brazier (in building or structure) (*see also* Exposure, fire, controlled, building)
        - not in building or structure — *see* Exposure, fire, controlled, not in building
      - building or structure X02.0 ☑
        - with
          - fall from building X02.3 ☑
          - injury due to building collapse X02.2 ☑
          - from building X02.5 ☑
          - smoke inhalation X02.1 ☑
        - hit by object from building X02.4 ☑
        - specified mode of injury NEC X02.8 ☑
      - fireplace, furnace or stove — *see* Exposure, fire, controlled, building
      - not in building or structure X03.0 ☑
        - with
          - fall X03.3 ☑
          - smoke inhalation X03.1 ☑
        - hit by object X03.4 ☑
        - specified mode of injury NEC X03.8 ☑
      - trash — *see* Exposure, fire, controlled, not in building
    - fireplace — *see* Exposure, fire, controlled, building
- **Exposure** — *continued*
  - fire, flames — *continued*
    - fittings or furniture (in building or structure) (uncontrolled) — *see* Exposure, fire, uncontrolled, building
    - forest (uncontrolled) — *see* Exposure, fire, uncontrolled, not in building
    - grass (uncontrolled) — *see* Exposure, fire, uncontrolled, not in building
    - hay (uncontrolled) — *see* Exposure, fire, uncontrolled, not in building
    - homicide (attempt) X97 ☑
    - ignition of highly flammable material X04 ☑
    - in, of, on, starting in
      - machinery — *see* Contact, with, by type of machine
      - motor vehicle (in motion) (*see also* Accident, transport, occupant by type of vehicle) V87.8 ☑
        - with collision — *see* Collision
      - railway rolling stock, train, vehicle V81.81 ☑
        - with collision — *see* Accident, transport, railway vehicle occupant
      - street car (in motion) V82.8 ☑
        - with collision — *see* Accident, transport, streetcar occupant
      - transport vehicle NEC (*see also* Accident, transport)
        - with collision — *see* Collision
      - war operations (*see also* War operations, fire)
        - from nuclear explosion — *see* War operations, nuclear weapons
      - watercraft (in transit) (not in transit) V91.09 ☑
        - localized — *see* Burn, on board watercraft, due to, fire on board
        - powered craft V91.03 ☑
          - ferry boat V91.01 ☑
          - fishing boat V91.02 ☑
          - jet skis V91.03 ☑
          - liner V91.01 ☑
          - merchant ship V91.00 ☑
          - passenger ship V91.01 ☑
        - unpowered craft V91.08 ☑
          - canoe V91.05 ☑
          - inflatable V91.06 ☑
          - kayak V91.05 ☑
          - sailboat V91.04 ☑
          - surf-board V91.08 ☑
          - water skis V91.07 ☑
          - windsurfer V91.08 ☑
    - lumber (uncontrolled) — *see* Exposure, fire, uncontrolled, not in building
    - mine (uncontrolled) — *see* Exposure, fire, uncontrolled, not in building
    - prairie (uncontrolled) — *see* Exposure, fire, uncontrolled, not in building
    - resulting from
      - explosion — *see* Explosion
      - lightning X08.8 ☑
    - self-inflicted X76 ☑
    - specified NEC X08.8 ☑
    - started by other person X97 ☑
    - stove — *see* Exposure, fire, controlled, building
    - stated as undetermined whether accidental or intentional Y26 ☑
    - suicide (attempt) X76 ☑
    - tunnel (uncontrolled) — *see* Exposure, fire, uncontrolled, not in building
    - uncontrolled
      - in building or structure X00.0 ☑
        - with
          - fall from building X00.3 ☑
          - injury due to building collapse X00.2 ☑
          - jump from building X00.5 ☑
          - smoke inhalation X00.1 ☑
        - bed X08.00 ☑
          - due to
            - cigarette X08.01 ☑
            - specified material NEC X08.09 ☑
        - furniture NEC X08.20 ☑
          - due to
            - cigarette X08.21 ☑
            - specified material NEC X08.29 ☑
        - hit by object from building X00.4 ☑
        - sofa X08.10 ☑
          - due to
            - cigarette X08.11 ☑
            - specified material NEC X08.19 ☑
        - specified mode of injury NEC X00.8 ☑
      - not in building or structure (any) X01.0 ☑
        - with

F

- **Fall**, falling — *continued*
  - in, on — *continued*
    - jungle gym W09.2 ☑
    - slide W09.0 ☑
    - swing W09.1 ☑
  - ramp W10.2 ☑
  - scaffolding W12 ☑
  - shower W18.2 ☑
    - causing drowning W16.211 ☑
  - staircase, stairs, steps W10.9 ☑
    - curb W10.1 ☑
    - due to ice or snow W00.1 ☑
    - escalator W10.0 ☑
    - incline W10.2 ☑
    - specified NEC W10.8 ☑
  - streetcar (without antecedent collision) V82.5 ☑
    - with antecedent collision — *see* Accident, transport, streetcar occupant
    - while boarding or alighting V82.4 ☑
  - train (without antecedent collision) V81.5 ☑
    - with antecedent collision — *see* Accident, transport, railway vehicle occupant
    - during derailment (without antecedent collision) V81.7 ☑
      - with antecedent collision — *see* Accident, transport, railway vehicle occupant
    - while boarding or alighting V81.4 ☑
  - transport vehicle after collision — *see* Accident, transport, by type of vehicle, collision
  - watercraft V93.39 ☑
    - due to
      - accident to craft V91.29 ☑
        - powered craft V91.23 ☑
          - ferry boat V91.21 ☑
          - fishing boat V91.22 ☑
          - jet skis V91.23 ☑
          - liner V91.21 ☑
          - merchant ship V91.20 ☑
          - passenger ship V91.21 ☑
        - unpowered craft
          - canoe V91.25 ☑
          - inflatable V91.26 ☑
          - kayak V91.25 ☑
          - sailboat V91.24 ☑
    - powered craft V93.33 ☑
      - ferry boat V93.31 ☑
      - fishing boat V93.32 ☑
      - jet skis V93.33 ☑
      - liner V93.31 ☑
      - merchant ship V93.30 ☑
      - passenger ship V93.31 ☑
    - unpowered craft V93.38 ☑
      - canoe V93.35 ☑
      - inflatable V93.36 ☑
      - kayak V93.35 ☑
      - sailboat V93.34 ☑
      - surf-board V93.38 ☑
      - windsurfer V93.38 ☑
  - into
    - cavity W17.2 ☑
    - dock W17.4 ☑
    - fire — *see* Exposure, fire, by type
    - haystack W17.89 ☑
    - hole W17.2 ☑
    - lake — *see* Fall, into, water
    - manhole W17.1 ☑
    - moving part of machinery — *see* Contact, with, by type of machine
    - ocean — *see* Fall, into, water
    - opening in surface NEC W17.89 ☑
    - pit W17.2 ☑
    - pond — *see* Fall, into, water
    - quarry W17.89 ☑
    - river — *see* Fall, into, water
    - shaft W17.89 ☑
    - storm drain W17.1 ☑
    - stream — *see* Fall, into, water
    - swimming pool (*see also* Fall, into, water, in, swimming pool)
      - empty W17.3 ☑
    - tank W17.89 ☑
    - water W16.42 ☑
      - causing drowning W16.41 ☑
      - from watercraft — *see* Drowning, due to, fall overboard
      - hitting diving board W21.4 ☑
      - in
        - bathtub W16.212 ☑
          - causing drowning W16.211 ☑
        - bucket W16.222 ☑
          - causing drowning W16.221 ☑

- **Fall**, falling — *continued*
  - into — *continued*
        - natural body of water W16.112 ☑
          - causing drowning W16.111 ☑
          - striking
            - bottom W16.122 ☑
              - causing drowning W16.121 ☑
            - side W16.132 ☑
              - causing drowning W16.131 ☑
        - specified water NEC W16.312 ☑
          - causing drowning W16.311 ☑
          - striking
            - bottom W16.322 ☑
              - causing drowning W16.321 ☑
            - wall W16.332 ☑
              - causing drowning W16.331 ☑
        - swimming pool W16.012 ☑
          - causing drowning W16.011 ☑
          - striking
            - bottom W16.022 ☑
              - causing drowning W16.021 ☑
            - wall W16.032 ☑
              - causing drowning W16.031 ☑
        - utility bucket W16.222 ☑
          - causing drowning W16.221 ☑
    - well W17.0 ☑
  - involving
    - bed W06 ☑
    - chair W07 ☑
    - furniture NEC W08 ☑
    - glass — *see* Fall, by type
    - playground equipment W09.8 ☑
      - jungle gym W09.2 ☑
      - slide W09.0 ☑
      - swing W09.1 ☑
    - roller blades — *see* Accident, transport, pedestrian, conveyance
    - skateboard (s) — *see* Accident, transport, pedestrian, conveyance
    - skates (ice) (in line) (roller) — *see* Accident, transport, pedestrian, conveyance
    - skis — *see* Accident, transport, pedestrian, conveyance
    - table W08 ☑
    - wheelchair, non-moving W05.0 ☑
      - powered — *see* Accident, transport, pedestrian, conveyance, specified type NEC
  - object — *see* Struck by, object, falling
  - off
    - toilet W18.11 ☑
      - with subsequent striking against object W18.12 ☑
  - on same level W18.30 ☑
    - due to
      - specified NEC W18.39 ☑
      - stepping on an object W18.31 ☑
  - out of
    - bed W06 ☑
    - building NEC W13.8 ☑
    - chair W07 ☑
    - furniture NEC W08 ☑
    - wheelchair, non-moving W05.0 ☑
      - powered — *see* Accident, transport, pedestrian, conveyance, specified type NEC
    - window W13.4 ☑
  - over
    - animal W01.0 ☑
    - cliff W15 ☑
    - embankment W17.81 ☑
    - small object W01.0 ☑
  - rock W20.8 ☑
  - same level W18.30 ☑
    - from
      - being crushed, pushed, or stepped on by a crowd or human stampede W52 ☑
      - collision, pushing, shoving, by or with other person W03 ☑
      - slipping, stumbling, tripping W01.0 ☑
    - involving ice or snow W00.0 ☑
      - involving skates (ice) (roller), skateboard, skis — *see* Accident, transport, pedestrian, conveyance
  - snowslide (avalanche) — *see* Landslide
  - stone W20.8 ☑
  - structure W20.1 ☑
    - burning (uncontrolled fire) X00.3 ☑
  - through
    - bridge W13.1 ☑
    - floor W13.3 ☑
    - roof W13.2 ☑

- **Fall**, falling — *continued*
  - through — *continued*
    - wall W13.8 ☑
    - window W13.4 ☑
  - timber W20.8 ☑
  - tree (caused by lightning) W20.8 ☑
  - while being carried or supported by other person (s) W04 ☑
- **Fallen** on by
  - animal (not being ridden) NEC W55.89 ☑
- **Felo-de-se** — *see* Suicide
- **Fight** (hand) (fists) (foot) — *see* Assault, fight
- **Fire** (accidental) — *see* Exposure, fire
- **Firearm** discharge — *see* Discharge, firearm
- **Fireball** effects from nuclear explosion in war operations — *see* War operations, nuclear weapons
- **Fireworks** (explosion) W39 ☑
- **Flash** burns from explosion — *see* Explosion
- **Flood** (any injury) (caused by) X38 ☑
  - collapse of man-made structure causing earth movement X36.0 ☑
  - tidal wave — *see* Forces of nature, tidal wave
- **Food** (any type) in
  - air passages (with asphyxia, obstruction, or suffocation) — *see* categories T17 and T18 ☑
  - alimentary tract causing asphyxia (due to compression of trachea) — *see* categories T17 and T18 ☑
- **Forces** of nature X39.8 ☑
  - avalanche X36.1 ☑
    - causing transport accident — *see* Accident, transport, by type of vehicle
  - blizzard X37.2 ☑
  - cataclysmic storm X37.9 ☑
    - with flood X38 ☑
    - blizzard X37.2 ☑
    - cloudburst X37.8 ☑
    - cyclone X37.1 ☑
    - dust storm X37.3 ☑
    - hurricane X37.0 ☑
    - specified storm NEC X37.8 ☑
    - storm surge X37.0 ☑
    - tornado X37.1 ☑
    - twister X37.1 ☑
    - typhoon X37.0 ☑
  - cloudburst X37.8 ☑
  - cold (natural) X31 ☑
  - cyclone X37.1 ☑
  - dam collapse causing earth movement X36.0 ☑
  - dust storm X37.3 ☑
  - earth movement X36.1 ☑
    - earthquake X34 ☑
    - caused by dam or structure collapse X36.0 ☑
  - earthquake X34 ☑
  - flood (caused by) X38 ☑
    - dam collapse X36.0 ☑
    - tidal wave — *see* Forces of nature, tidal wave
  - heat (natural) X30 ☑
  - hurricane X37.0 ☑
  - landslide X36.1 ☑
    - causing transport accident — *see* Accident, transport, by type of vehicle
  - lightning — *see* subcategory T75.0
    - causing fire — *see* Exposure, fire
  - mudslide X36.1 ☑
    - causing transport accident — *see* Accident, transport, by type of vehicle
  - radiation (natural) X39.08 ☑
    - radon X39.01 ☑
  - radon X39.01 ☑
  - specified force NEC X39.8 ☑
  - storm surge X37.0 ☑
  - structure collapse causing earth movement X36.0 ☑
  - sunlight X32 ☑
  - tidal wave X37.41 ☑
    - due to
      - earthquake X37.41 ☑
      - landslide X37.43 ☑
      - storm X37.42 ☑
      - volcanic eruption X37.41 ☑
  - tornado X37.1 ☑
  - tsunami X37.41 ☑
  - twister X37.1 ☑
  - typhoon X37.0 ☑
  - volcanic eruption X35 ☑
- **Foreign** body
  - aspiration — *see* Index to Diseases and Injuries, Foreign body, respiratory tract
  - embedded in skin W45 ☑

Foreign body — *continued*
- entering through skin W45.8 ☑
  - can lid W26.8 ☑
  - nail W45.0 ☑
  - paper W26.2 ☑
  - specified NEC W45.8 ☑
  - splinter W45.8 ☑

Forest fire (exposure to) — *see* Exposure, fire, uncontrolled, not in building

Found injured X58 ☑
- from exposure (to) — *see* Exposure
- on
  - highway, road (way), street V89.9 ☑
  - railway right of way V81.9 ☑

Fracture (circumstances unknown or unspecified) X58 ☑
- due to specified cause NEC X58 ☑

Freezing — *see* Exposure, cold

Frostbite X31 ☑
- due to man-made conditions — *see* Exposure, cold, man-made

Frozen — *see* Exposure, cold

G

Gored by bull W55.22 ☑

Gunshot wound W34.00 ☑

H

Hailstones, injured by X39.8 ☑

Hanged herself or himself — *see* Hanging, self-inflicted

Hanging (accidental) (*see also* category) T71 ☑
- legal execution — *see* Legal, intervention, specified means NEC

Heat (effects of) (excessive) X30 ☑
- due to
  - man-made conditions W92 ☑
    - on board watercraft V93.29 ☑
      - fishing boat V93.22 ☑
      - merchant ship V93.20 ☑
      - passenger ship V93.21 ☑
      - sailboat V93.24 ☑
      - specified powered craft NEC V93.23 ☑
  - weather (conditions) X30 ☑
- from
  - electric heating apparatus causing burning X16 ☑
  - nuclear explosion in war operations — *see* War operations, nuclear weapons
- inappropriate in local application or packing in medical or surgical procedure Y63.5

Hemorrhage
- delayed following medical or surgical treatment without mention of misadventure — *see* Index to Diseases and Injuries, Complication (s)
- during medical or surgical treatment as misadventure — *see* Index to Diseases and Injuries, Complication (s)

High
- altitude (effects) - — *see* Air, pressure, low
- level of radioactivity, effects — *see* Radiation
- pressure (effects) - — *see* Air, pressure, high
- temperature, effects — *see* Heat

Hit, hitting (accidental) by — *see* Struck by

Hitting against — *see* Striking against

Homicide (attempt) (justifiable) — *see* Assault

Hot
- place, effects (*see also* Heat)
- weather, effects X30 ☑

House fire (uncontrolled) — *see* Exposure, fire, uncontrolled, building

Humidity, causing problem X39.8 ☑

Hunger X58 ☑

Hurricane (any injury) X37.0 ☑

Hypobarism, hypobaropathy - — *see* Air, pressure, low

I

Ictus
- caloris (*see also* Heat)
- solaris X30 ☑

Ignition (accidental) (*see also* Exposure, fire) X08.8 ☑
- anesthetic gas in operating room W40.1 ☑
- apparel X06.2 ☑
  - from highly flammable material X04 ☑
  - nightwear X05 ☑
- bed linen (sheets) (spreads) (pillows) (mattress) — *see* Exposure, fire, uncontrolled, building, bed
- benzine X04 ☑
- clothes, clothing NEC (from controlled fire) X06.2 ☑
  - from
    - highly flammable material X04 ☑
- ether X04 ☑
  - in operating room W40.1 ☑
- explosive material — *see* Explosion
- gasoline X04 ☑
- jewelry (plastic) (any) X06.0 ☑
- kerosene X04 ☑
- material
  - explosive — *see* Explosion
  - highly flammable with secondary explosion X04 ☑
- nightwear X05 ☑
- paraffin X04 ☑
- petrol X04 ☑

Immersion (accidental) (*see also* Drowning)
- hand or foot due to cold (excessive) X31 ☑

Implantation of quills of porcupine W55.89 ☑

Inanition (from) (hunger) X58 ☑
- thirst X58 ☑

Inappropriate operation performed
- correct operation on wrong side or body part (wrong side) (wrong site) Y65.53
- operation intended for another patient done on wrong patient Y65.52
- wrong operation performed on correct patient Y65.51

Inattention after, at birth (homicidal intent) (infanticidal intent) X58 ☑

Incident, adverse
- device
  - anesthesiology Y70.8
    - accessory Y70.2
    - diagnostic Y70.0
    - miscellaneous Y70.8
    - monitoring Y70.0
    - prosthetic Y70.2
    - rehabilitative Y70.1
    - surgical Y70.3
    - therapeutic Y70.1
  - cardiovascular Y71.8
    - accessory Y71.2
    - diagnostic Y71.0
    - miscellaneous Y71.8
    - monitoring Y71.0
    - prosthetic Y71.2
    - rehabilitative Y71.1
    - surgical Y71.3
    - therapeutic Y71.1
  - gastroenterology Y73.8
    - accessory Y73.2
    - diagnostic Y73.0
    - miscellaneous Y73.8
    - monitoring Y73.0
    - prosthetic Y73.2
    - rehabilitative Y73.1
    - surgical Y73.3
    - therapeutic Y73.1
  - general
    - hospital Y74.8
      - accessory Y74.2
      - diagnostic Y74.0
      - miscellaneous Y74.8
      - monitoring Y74.0
      - prosthetic Y74.2
      - rehabilitative Y74.1
      - surgical Y74.3
      - therapeutic Y74.1
    - surgical Y81.8
      - accessory Y81.2
      - diagnostic Y81.0
      - miscellaneous Y81.8
      - monitoring Y81.0
      - prosthetic Y81.2
      - rehabilitative Y81.1
      - surgical Y81.3
      - therapeutic Y81.1
  - gynecological Y76.8
    - accessory Y76.2
    - diagnostic Y76.0
    - miscellaneous Y76.8

Incident, adverse — *continued*
- device — *continued*
    - monitoring Y76.0
    - prosthetic Y76.2
    - rehabilitative Y76.1
    - surgical Y76.3
    - therapeutic Y76.1
  - medical Y82.9
    - specified type NEC Y82.8
  - neurological Y75.8
    - accessory Y75.2
    - diagnostic Y75.0
    - miscellaneous Y75.8
    - monitoring Y75.0
    - prosthetic Y75.2
    - rehabilitative Y75.1
    - surgical Y75.3
    - therapeutic Y75.1
  - obstetrical Y76.8
    - accessory Y76.2
    - diagnostic Y76.0
    - miscellaneous Y76.8
    - monitoring Y76.0
    - prosthetic Y76.2
    - rehabilitative Y76.1
    - surgical Y76.3
    - therapeutic Y76.1
  - ophthalmic Y77.8
    - accessory Y77.2
    - diagnostic Y77.0
    - miscellaneous Y77.8
    - monitoring Y77.0
    - prosthetic Y77.2
    - rehabilitative Y77.1
    - surgical Y77.3
    - therapeutic Y77.1
  - orthopedic Y79.8
    - accessory Y79.2
    - diagnostic Y79.0
    - miscellaneous Y79.8
    - monitoring Y79.0
    - prosthetic Y79.2
    - rehabilitative Y79.1
    - surgical Y79.3
    - therapeutic Y79.1
  - otorhinolaryngological Y72.8
    - accessory Y72.2
    - diagnostic Y72.0
    - miscellaneous Y72.8
    - monitoring Y72.0
    - prosthetic Y72.2
    - rehabilitative Y72.1
    - surgical Y72.3
    - therapeutic Y72.1
  - personal use Y74.8
    - accessory Y74.2
    - diagnostic Y74.0
    - miscellaneous Y74.8
    - monitoring Y74.0
    - prosthetic Y74.2
    - rehabilitative Y74.1
    - surgical Y74.3
    - therapeutic Y74.1
  - physical medicine Y80.8
    - accessory Y80.2
    - diagnostic Y80.0
    - miscellaneous Y80.8
    - monitoring Y80.0
    - prosthetic Y80.2
    - rehabilitative Y80.1
    - surgical Y80.3
    - therapeutic Y80.1
  - plastic surgical Y81.8
    - accessory Y81.2
    - diagnostic Y81.0
    - miscellaneous Y81.8
    - monitoring Y81.0
    - prosthetic Y81.2
    - rehabilitative Y81.1
    - surgical Y81.3
    - therapeutic Y81.1
  - radiological Y78.8
    - accessory Y78.2
    - diagnostic Y78.0
    - miscellaneous Y78.8
    - monitoring Y78.0
    - prosthetic Y78.2
    - rehabilitative Y78.1
    - surgical Y78.3
    - therapeutic Y78.1
  - urology Y73.8
    - accessory Y73.2

- **Incident,** adverse — *continued*
  - device — *continued*
    - diagnostic Y73.0
    - miscellaneous Y73.8
    - monitoring Y73.0
    - prosthetic Y73.2
    - rehabilitative Y73.1
    - surgical Y73.3
    - therapeutic Y73.1
- **Incineration** (accidental) — *see* Exposure, fire
- **Infanticide** — *see* Assault
- **Infrasound** waves (causing injury) W49.9 ☑
- **Ingestion**
  - foreign body (causing injury) (with obstruction) — *see* Foreign body, alimentary canal
  - poisonous
    - plant (s) X58 ☑
    - substance NEC — *see* Table of Drugs and Chemicals
- **Inhalation**
  - excessively cold substance, man-made — *see* Exposure, cold, man-made
  - food (any type) (into respiratory tract) (with asphyxia, obstruction respiratory tract, suffocation) — *see* categories T17 and T18 ☑
  - foreign body — *see* Foreign body, aspiration
  - gastric contents (with asphyxia, obstruction respiratory passage, suffocation) T17.81 ☑
  - hot air or gases X14.0 ☑
  - liquid air, hydrogen, nitrogen W93.12 ☑
    - suicide (attempt) X83.2 ☑
  - steam X13.0 ☑
    - assault X98.0 ☑
    - stated as undetermined whether accidental or intentional Y27.0 ☑
    - suicide (attempt) X77.0 ☑
  - toxic gas — *see* Table of Drugs and Chemicals
  - vomitus (with asphyxia, obstruction respiratory passage, suffocation) T17.81 ☑
- **Injury,** injured (accidental (ly)) NOS X58 ☑
  - by, caused by, from
    - assault — *see* Assault
    - law-enforcing agent, police, in course of legal intervention — *see* Legal intervention
    - suicide (attempt) X83.8 ☑
  - due to, in
    - civil insurrection — *see* War operations
    - fight (*see also* Assault, fight) Y04.0 ☑
    - war operations — *see* War operations
  - homicide (*see also* Assault) Y09
  - inflicted (by)
    - in course of arrest (attempted), suppression of disturbance, maintenance of order, by law-enforcing agents — *see* Legal intervention
    - other person
      - stated as
        - accidental X58 ☑
        - intentional, homicide (attempt) — *see* Assault
        - undetermined whether accidental or intentional Y33 ☑
  - purposely (inflicted) by other person (s) — *see* Assault
  - self-inflicted X83.8 ☑
    - stated as accidental X58 ☑
  - specified cause NEC X58 ☑
  - undetermined whether accidental or intentional Y33 ☑
- **Insolation,** effects X30 ☑
- **Insufficient** nourishment X58 ☑
- **Interruption** of respiration (by)
  - food (lodged in esophagus) — *see* categories T17 and T18 ☑
  - vomitus (lodged in esophagus) T17.81 ☑
- **Intervention,** legal — *see* Legal intervention
- **Intoxication**
  - drug — *see* Table of Drugs and Chemicals
  - poison — *see* Table of Drugs and Chemicals

J

- **Jammed** (accidentally)
  - between objects (moving) (stationary and moving) W23.0 ☑
    - stationary W23.1 ☑
- **Jumped,** jumping
  - before moving object NEC X81.8 ☑
    - motor vehicle X81.0 ☑
    - subway train X81.1 ☑
    - train X81.1 ☑
- **Jumped,** jumping — *continued*
  - before moving object NEC — *continued*
    - undetermined whether accidental or intentional Y31 ☑
  - from
    - boat (into water) voluntarily, without accident (to or on boat) W16.712 ☑
      - with
        - accident to or on boat — *see* Accident, watercraft
        - drowning or submersion W16.711 ☑
          - suicide (attempt) X71.3 ☑
      - striking bottom W16.722 ☑
        - causing drowning W16.721 ☑
    - building (*see also* Jumped, from, high place) W13.9 ☑
      - burning (uncontrolled fire) X00.5 ☑
    - high place NEC W17.89 ☑
      - suicide (attempt) X80 ☑
      - undetermined whether accidental or intentional Y30 ☑
    - structure (*see also* Jumped, from, high place) W13.9 ☑
      - burning (uncontrolled fire) X00.5 ☑
  - into water W16.92 ☑
    - causing drowning W16.91 ☑
    - from, off watercraft — *see* Jumped, from, boat
    - in
      - natural body W16.612 ☑
        - causing drowning W16.611 ☑
        - striking bottom W16.622 ☑
          - causing drowning W16.621 ☑
      - specified place NEC W16.812 ☑
        - causing drowning W16.811 ☑
        - striking
          - bottom W16.822 ☑
            - causing drowning W16.821 ☑
          - wall W16.832 ☑
            - causing drowning W16.831 ☑
      - swimming pool W16.512 ☑
        - causing drowning W16.511 ☑
        - striking
          - bottom W16.522 ☑
            - causing drowning W16.521 ☑
          - wall W16.532 ☑
            - causing drowning W16.531 ☑
    - suicide (attempt) X71.3 ☑

K

- **Kicked** by
  - animal NEC W55.82 ☑
  - person (s) (accidentally) W50.1 ☑
    - with intent to injure or kill Y04.0 ☑
    - as, or caused by, a crowd or human stampede (with fall) W52 ☑
    - assault Y04.0 ☑
    - homicide (attempt) Y04.0 ☑
    - in
      - fight Y04.0 ☑
      - legal intervention
        - injuring
          - bystander Y35.812 ☑
          - law enforcement personnel Y35.811 ☑
          - suspect Y35.813 ☑
- **Kicking**
  - against
    - object W22.8 ☑
      - sports equipment W21.9 ☑
      - stationary W22.09 ☑
        - sports equipment W21.89 ☑
    - person — *see* Striking against, person
    - sports equipment W21.9 ☑
  - carpet stretcher with knee X50.3 ☑
- **Killed,** killing (accidentally) NOS (*see also* Injury) X58 ☑
  - in
    - action — *see* War operations
    - brawl, fight (hand) (fists) (foot) Y04.0 ☑
      - by weapon (*see also* Assault)
        - cutting, piercing — *see* Assault, cutting or piercing instrument
        - firearm — *see* Discharge, firearm, by type, homicide
  - self
    - stated as
      - accident NOS X58 ☑
      - suicide — *see* Suicide
      - undetermined whether accidental or intentional Y33 ☑
- **Kneeling** (prolonged) (static) X50.1 ☑
- **Knocked** down (accidentally) (by) NOS X58 ☑
  - animal (not being ridden) NEC (*see also* Struck by, by type of animal)
  - crowd or human stampede W52 ☑
  - person W51 ☑
    - in brawl, fight Y04.0 ☑
  - transport vehicle NEC (*see also* Accident, transport) V09.9 ☑

L

- **Laceration** NEC — *see* Injury
- **Lack** of
  - care (helpless person) (infant) (newborn) X58 ☑
  - food except as result of abandonment or neglect X58 ☑
    - due to abandonment or neglect X58 ☑
  - water except as result of transport accident X58 ☑
    - due to transport accident — *see* Accident, transport, by type
  - helpless person, infant, newborn X58 ☑
- **Landslide** (falling on transport vehicle) X36.1 ☑
  - caused by collapse of man-made structure X36.0 ☑
- **Late** effect — *see* Sequelae
- **Legal**
  - execution (any method) — *see* Legal, intervention
  - intervention (by)
    - baton — *see* Legal, intervention, blunt object, baton
    - bayonet — *see* Legal, intervention, sharp object, bayonet
    - blow — *see* Legal, intervention, manhandling
    - blunt object
      - baton
        - injuring
          - bystander Y35.312 ☑
          - law enforcement personnel Y35.311 ☑
          - suspect Y35.313 ☑
      - injuring
        - bystander Y35.302 ☑
        - law enforcement personnel Y35.301 ☑
        - suspect Y35.303 ☑
      - specified NEC
        - injuring
          - bystander Y35.392 ☑
          - law enforcement personnel Y35.391 ☑
          - suspect Y35.393 ☑
      - stave
        - injuring
          - bystander Y35.392 ☑
          - law enforcement personnel Y35.391 ☑
          - suspect Y35.393 ☑
    - bomb — *see* Legal, intervention, explosive
    - cutting or piercing instrument — *see* Legal, intervention, sharp object
    - dynamite — *see* Legal, intervention, explosive, dynamite
    - explosive (s)
      - dynamite
        - injuring
          - bystander Y35.112 ☑
          - law enforcement personnel Y35.111 ☑
          - suspect Y35.113 ☑
      - grenade
        - injuring
          - bystander Y35.192 ☑
          - law enforcement personnel Y35.191 ☑
          - suspect Y35.193 ☑
      - injuring
        - bystander Y35.102 ☑
        - law enforcement personnel Y35.101 ☑
        - suspect Y35.103 ☑
      - mortar bomb
        - injuring
          - bystander Y35.192 ☑
          - law enforcement personnel Y35.191 ☑
          - suspect Y35.193 ☑
      - shell
        - injuring
          - bystander Y35.122 ☑
          - law enforcement personnel Y35.121 ☑
          - suspect Y35.123 ☑
      - specified NEC
        - injuring
          - bystander Y35.192 ☑
          - law enforcement personnel Y35.191 ☑

- **Legal** — *continued*
  - intervention — *continued*
        - suspect Y35.193 ☑
    - firearm (s) (discharge)
      - handgun
        - injuring
          - bystander Y35.022 ☑
          - law enforcement personnel Y35.021 ☑
          - suspect Y35.023 ☑
      - injuring
        - bystander Y35.002 ☑
        - law enforcement personnel Y35.001 ☑
        - suspect Y35.003 ☑
      - machine gun
        - injuring
          - bystander Y35.012 ☑
          - law enforcement personnel Y35.011 ☑
          - suspect Y35.013 ☑
      - rifle pellet
        - injuring
          - bystander Y35.032 ☑
          - law enforcement personnel Y35.031 ☑
          - suspect Y35.033 ☑
      - rubber bullet
        - injuring
          - bystander Y35.042 ☑
          - law enforcement personnel Y35.041 ☑
          - suspect Y35.043 ☑
      - shotgun — *see* Legal, intervention, firearm, specified NEC
      - specified NEC
        - injuring
          - bystander Y35.092 ☑
          - law enforcement personnel Y35.091 ☑
          - suspect Y35.093 ☑
    - gas (asphyxiation) (poisoning)
      - injuring
        - bystander Y35.202 ☑
        - law enforcement personnel Y35.201 ☑
        - suspect Y35.203 ☑
      - specified NEC
        - injuring
          - bystander Y35.292 ☑
          - law enforcement personnel Y35.291 ☑
          - suspect Y35.293 ☑
      - tear gas
        - injuring
          - bystander Y35.212 ☑
          - law enforcement personnel Y35.211 ☑
          - suspect Y35.213 ☑
    - grenade — *see* Legal, intervention, explosive, grenade
    - injuring
      - bystander Y35.92 ☑
      - law enforcement personnel Y35.91 ☑
      - suspect Y35.93 ☑
    - late effect (of) — *see* with 7th character S Y35 ☑
    - manhandling
      - injuring
        - bystander Y35.812 ☑
        - law enforcement personnel Y35.811 ☑
        - suspect Y35.813 ☑
    - sequelae (of) — *see* with 7th character S Y35 ☑
    - sharp objects
      - bayonet
        - injuring
          - bystander Y35.412 ☑
          - law enforcement personnel Y35.411 ☑
          - suspect Y35.413 ☑
      - injuring
        - bystander Y35.402 ☑
        - law enforcement personnel Y35.401 ☑
        - suspect Y35.403 ☑
      - specified NEC
        - injuring
          - bystander Y35.492 ☑
          - law enforcement personnel Y35.491 ☑
          - suspect Y35.493 ☑
    - specified means NEC
      - injuring
        - bystander Y35.892 ☑
        - law enforcement personnel Y35.891 ☑
        - suspect Y35.893 ☑
    - stabbing — *see* Legal, intervention, sharp object
    - stave — *see* Legal, intervention, blunt object, stave
    - tear gas — *see* Legal, intervention, gas, tear gas
    - truncheon — *see* Legal, intervention, blunt object, stave
- **Lifting** (*see also* Overexertion)
  - heavy objects X50.0 ☑
  - weights X50.0 ☑
- **Lightning** (shock) (stroke) (struck by) — *see* subcategory T75.0
  - causing fire — *see* Exposure, fire
- **Loss** of control (transport vehicle) NEC — *see* Accident, transport
- **Lost** at sea NOS — *see* Drowning, due to, fall overboard
- **Low**
  - pressure (effects) - — *see* Air, pressure, low
  - temperature (effects) — *see* Exposure, cold
- **Lying** before train, vehicle or other moving object X81.8 ☑
  - subway train X81.1 ☑
  - train X81.1 ☑
  - undetermined whether accidental or intentional Y31 ☑
- **Lynching** — *see* Assault

M

- **Malfunction** (mechanism or component) (of)
  - firearm W34.10 ☑
    - airgun W34.110 ☑
    - BB gun W34.110 ☑
    - gas, air or spring-operated gun NEC W34.118 ☑
    - handgun W32.1 ☑
    - hunting rifle W33.12 ☑
    - larger firearm W33.10 ☑
      - specified NEC W33.19 ☑
    - machine gun W33.13 ☑
    - paintball gun W34.111 ☑
    - pellet gun W34.110 ☑
    - shotgun W33.11 ☑
    - specified NEC W34.19 ☑
    - Very pistol [flare] W34.19 ☑
  - handgun — *see* Malfunction, firearm, handgun
- **Maltreatment** — *see* Perpetrator
- **Mangled** (accidentally) NOS X58 ☑
- **Manhandling** (in brawl, fight) Y04.0 ☑
  - legal intervention — *see* Legal, intervention, manhandling
- **Manslaughter** (nonaccidental) — *see* Assault
- **Mauled** by animal NEC W55.89 ☑
- **Medical** procedure, complication of (delayed or as an abnormal reaction without mention of misadventure) — *see* Complication of or following, by specified type of procedure
  - due to or as a result of misadventure — *see* Misadventure
- **Melting** (due to fire) (*see also* Exposure, fire)
  - apparel NEC X06.3 ☑
  - clothes, clothing NEC X06.3 ☑
    - nightwear X05 ☑
  - fittings or furniture (burning building) (uncontrolled fire) X00.8 ☑
  - nightwear X05 ☑
  - plastic jewelry X06.1 ☑
- **Mental** cruelty X58 ☑
- **Military** operations (injuries to military and civilians occurring during peacetime on military property and during routine military exercises and operations) (by) (from) (involving) Y37.90 ☑
  - air blast Y37.20 ☑
  - aircraft
    - destruction — *see* Military operations, destruction of aircraft
  - airway restriction — *see* Military operations, restriction of airways
  - asphyxiation — *see* Military operations, restriction of airways
  - biological weapons Y37.6X ☑
  - blast Y37.20 ☑
  - blast fragments Y37.20 ☑
  - blast wave Y37.20 ☑
  - blast wind Y37.20 ☑
  - bomb Y37.20 ☑
    - dirty Y37.50 ☑
    - gasoline Y37.31 ☑
    - incendiary Y37.31 ☑
    - petrol Y37.31 ☑
  - bullet Y37.43 ☑
    - incendiary Y37.32 ☑
    - rubber Y37.41 ☑
  - chemical weapons Y37.7X ☑
  - combat
    - hand to hand (unarmed) combat Y37.44 ☑
    - using blunt or piercing object Y37.45 ☑
- **Military,** operations— *continued*
  - conflagration — *see* Military operations, fire
  - conventional warfare NEC Y37.49 ☑
  - depth-charge Y37.01 ☑
  - destruction of aircraft Y37.10 ☑
    - due to
      - air to air missile Y37.11 ☑
      - collision with other aircraft Y37.12 ☑
      - detonation (accidental) of onboard munitions and explosives Y37.14 ☑
      - enemy fire or explosives Y37.11 ☑
      - explosive placed on aircraft Y37.11 ☑
      - onboard fire Y37.13 ☑
      - rocket propelled grenade [RPG] Y37.11 ☑
      - small arms fire Y37.11 ☑
      - surface to air missile Y37.11 ☑
    - specified NEC Y37.19 ☑
  - detonation (accidental) of
    - onboard marine weapons Y37.05 ☑
    - own munitions or munitions launch device Y37.24 ☑
  - dirty bomb Y37.50 ☑
  - explosion (of) Y37.20 ☑
    - aerial bomb Y37.21 ☑
    - bomb NOS (*see also* Military operations, bomb (s)) Y37.20 ☑
    - own munitions or munitions launch device (accidental) Y37.24 ☑
    - fragments Y37.20 ☑
    - grenade Y37.29 ☑
    - guided missile Y37.22 ☑
    - improvised explosive device [IED] (person-borne) (roadside) (vehicle-borne) Y37.23 ☑
    - land mine Y37.29 ☑
    - marine mine (at sea) (in harbor) Y37.02 ☑
    - marine weapon Y37.00 ☑
      - specified NEC Y37.09 ☑
    - sea-based artillery shell Y37.03 ☑
    - specified NEC Y37.29 ☑
    - torpedo Y37.04 ☑
  - fire Y37.30 ☑
    - specified NEC Y37.39 ☑
  - firearms
    - discharge Y37.43 ☑
    - pellets Y37.42 ☑
  - flamethrower Y37.33 ☑
  - fragments (from) (of)
    - improvised explosive device [IED] (person-borne) (roadside) (vehicle-borne) Y37.26 ☑
    - munitions Y37.25 ☑
    - specified NEC Y37.29 ☑
    - weapons Y37.27 ☑
  - friendly fire Y37.92 ☑
  - hand to hand (unarmed) combat Y37.44 ☑
  - hot substances — *see* Military operations, fire
  - incendiary bullet Y37.32 ☑
  - nuclear weapon (effects of) Y37.50 ☑
    - acute radiation exposure Y37.54 ☑
    - blast pressure Y37.51 ☑
    - direct blast Y37.51 ☑
    - direct heat Y37.53 ☑
    - fallout exposure Y37.54 ☑
    - fireball Y37.53 ☑
    - indirect blast (struck or crushed by blast debris) (being thrown by blast) Y37.52 ☑
    - ionizing radiation (immediate exposure) Y37.54 ☑
    - nuclear radiation Y37.54 ☑
    - radiation
      - ionizing (immediate exposure) Y37.54 ☑
      - nuclear Y37.54 ☑
      - thermal Y37.53 ☑
    - specified NEC Y37.59 ☑
    - secondary effects Y37.54 ☑
    - thermal radiation Y37.53 ☑
  - restriction of air (airway)
    - intentional Y37.46 ☑
    - unintentional Y37.47 ☑
  - rubber bullets Y37.41 ☑
  - shrapnel NOS Y37.29 ☑
  - suffocation — *see* Military operations, restriction of airways
  - unconventional warfare NEC Y37.7X ☑
  - underwater blast NOS Y37.00 ☑
  - warfare
    - conventional NEC Y37.49 ☑
    - unconventional NEC Y37.7X ☑
  - weapons
    - biological weapons Y37.6X ☑
    - chemical Y37.7X ☑
    - nuclear (effects of) Y37.50 ☑
      - acute radiation exposure Y37.54 ☑

N

O

P

Puncture, puncturing — *continued*
- during medical or surgical treatment as misadventure — *see* Index to Diseases and Injuries, Complication (s)

Pushed, pushing (accidental) (injury in)
- by other person (s) (accidental) W51 ☑
  - with fall W03 ☑
    - due to ice or snow W00.0 ☑
  - as, or caused by, a crowd or human stampede (with fall) W52 ☑
  - before moving object NEC Y02.8 ☑
    - motor vehicle Y02.0 ☑
    - subway train Y02.1 ☑
    - train Y02.1 ☑
  - from
    - high place NEC
      - in accidental circumstances W17.89 ☑
      - stated as
        - intentional, homicide (attempt) Y01 ☑
        - undetermined whether accidental or intentional Y30 ☑
    - transport vehicle NEC (*see also* Accident, transport) V89.9 ☑
      - stated as
        - intentional, homicide (attempt) Y08.89 ☑
- overexertion X50.9 ☑

R

Radiation (exposure to)
- arc lamps W89.0 ☑
- atomic power plant (malfunction) NEC W88.1 ☑
- complication of or abnormal reaction to medical radiotherapy Y84.2
- electromagnetic, ionizing W88.0 ☑
- gamma rays W88.1 ☑
- in
  - war operations (from or following nuclear explosion) — *see* War operations
- inadvertent exposure of patient (receiving test or therapy) Y63.3
- infrared (heaters and lamps) W90.1 ☑
  - excessive heat from W92 ☑
- ionized, ionizing (particles, artificially accelerated)
  - radioisotopes W88.1 ☑
  - specified NEC W88.8 ☑
  - x-rays W88.0 ☑
- isotopes, radioactive — *see* Radiation, radioactive isotopes
- laser (s) W90.2 ☑
  - in war operations — *see* War operations
  - misadventure in medical care Y63.2
- light sources (man-made visible and ultraviolet) W89.9 ☑
  - natural X32 ☑
  - specified NEC W89.8 ☑
  - tanning bed W89.1 ☑
  - welding light W89.0 ☑
- man-made visible light W89.9 ☑
  - specified NEC W89.8 ☑
  - tanning bed W89.1 ☑
  - welding light W89.0 ☑
- microwave W90.8 ☑
- misadventure in medical or surgical procedure Y63.2
- natural NEC X39.08 ☑
  - radon X39.01 ☑
- overdose (in medical or surgical procedure) Y63.2
- radar W90.0 ☑
- radioactive isotopes (any) W88.1 ☑
  - atomic power plant malfunction W88.1 ☑
  - misadventure in medical or surgical treatment Y63.2
- radiofrequency W90.0 ☑
- radium NEC W88.1 ☑
- sun X32 ☑
- ultraviolet (light) (man-made) W89.9 ☑
  - natural X32 ☑
  - specified NEC W89.8 ☑
  - tanning bed W89.1 ☑
  - welding light W89.0 ☑
- welding arc, torch, or light W89.0 ☑
  - excessive heat from W92 ☑
- x-rays (hard) (soft) W88.0 ☑

Range disease W94.11 ☑

Rape (attempted) T74.2 ☑

Rat bite W53.11 ☑

Reaching (prolonged) (static) X50.1 ☑

Reaction, abnormal to medical procedure (*see also* Complication of or following, by type of procedure) Y84.9
- with misadventure — *see* Misadventure
- biologicals — *see* Table of Drugs and Chemicals
- drugs — *see* Table of Drugs and Chemicals
- vaccine — *see* Table of Drugs and Chemicals

Recoil
- airgun W34.110 ☑
- BB gun W34.110 ☑
- firearm NEC W34.19 ☑
- gas, air or spring-operated gun NEC W34.118 ☑
- handgun W32.1 ☑
- hunting rifle W33.12 ☑
- larger firearm W33.10 ☑
  - specified NEC W33.19 ☑
- machine gun W33.13 ☑
- paintball gun W34.111 ☑
- pellet W34.110 ☑
- shotgun W33.11 ☑
- Very pistol [flare] W34.19 ☑

Reduction in
- atmospheric pressure - — *see* Air, pressure, change

Rock falling on or hitting (accidentally) (person) W20.8 ☑
- in cave-in W20.0 ☑

Run over (accidentally) (by)
- animal (not being ridden) NEC W55.89 ☑
- machinery — *see* Contact, with, by specified type of machine
- transport vehicle NEC (*see also* Accident, transport) V09.9 ☑
  - intentional homicide (attempt) Y03.0 ☑
  - motor NEC V09.20 ☑
    - intentional homicide (attempt) Y03.0 ☑

Running
- before moving object X81.8 ☑
  - motor vehicle X81.0 ☑

Running off, away
- animal (being ridden) (*see also* Accident, transport) V80.918 ☑
  - not being ridden W55.89 ☑
- animal-drawn vehicle NEC (*see also* Accident, transport) V80.928 ☑
- highway, road (way), street
  - transport vehicle NEC (*see also* Accident, transport) V89.9 ☑

Rupture pressurized devices — *see* Explosion, by type of device

S

Saturnism — *see* Table of Drugs and Chemicals, lead

Scald, scalding (accidental) (by) (from) (in) X19 ☑
- air (hot) X14.1 ☑
- gases (hot) X14.1 ☑
- homicide (attempt) — *see* Assault, burning, hot object
- inflicted by other person
  - stated as intentional, homicide (attempt) — *see* Assault, burning, hot object
- liquid (boiling) (hot) NEC X12 ☑
  - stated as undetermined whether accidental or intentional Y27.2 ☑
  - suicide (attempt) X77.2 ☑
- local application of externally applied substance in medical or surgical care Y63.5
- metal (molten) (liquid) (hot) NEC X18 ☑
- self-inflicted X77.9 ☑
- stated as undetermined whether accidental or intentional Y27.8 ☑
- steam X13.1 ☑
  - assault X98.0 ☑
  - stated as undetermined whether accidental or intentional Y27.0 ☑
  - suicide (attempt) X77.0 ☑
- suicide (attempt) X77.9 ☑
- vapor (hot) X13.1 ☑
  - assault X98.0 ☑
  - stated as undetermined whether accidental or intentional Y27.0 ☑
  - suicide (attempt) X77.0 ☑

Scratched by
- cat W55.03 ☑
- person (s) (accidentally) W50.4 ☑
  - with intent to injure or kill Y04.0 ☑
  - as, or caused by, a crowd or human stampede (with fall) W52 ☑
  - assault Y04.0 ☑

Scratched by — *continued*
- person — *continued*
  - homicide (attempt) Y04.0 ☑
  - in
    - fight Y04.0 ☑
    - legal intervention
      - injuring
        - bystander Y35.892 ☑
        - law enforcement personnel Y35.891 ☑
        - suspect Y35.893 ☑

Seasickness T75.3 ☑

Self-harm NEC (*see also* External cause by type, undetermined whether accidental or intentional)
- intentional — *see* Suicide
- poisoning NEC — *see* Table of drugs and biologicals, accident

Self-inflicted (injury) NEC (*see also* External cause by type, undetermined whether accidental or intentional)
- intentional — *see* Suicide
- poisoning NEC — *see* Table of drugs and biologicals, accident

Sequelae (of)
- accident NEC — *see* W00-X58 with 7th character S
- assault (homicidal) (any means) — *see* X92-Y08 with 7th character S
- homicide, attempt (any means) — *see* X92-Y08 with 7th character S
- injury undetermined whether accidentally or purposely inflicted — *see* Y21-Y33 with 7th character S
- intentional self-harm (classifiable to X71-X83) — *see* X71-X83 with 7th character S
- legal intervention — *see* with 7th character S Y35 ☑
- motor vehicle accident — *see* V00-V99 with 7th character S
- suicide, attempt (any means) — *see* X71-X83 with 7th character S
- transport accident — *see* V00-V99 with 7th character S
- war operations — *see* War operations

Shock
- electric — *see* Exposure, electric current
- from electric appliance (any) (faulty) W86.8 ☑
  - domestic W86.0 ☑
  - suicide (attempt) X83.1 ☑

Shooting, shot (accidental (ly)) (*see also* Discharge, firearm, by type)
- herself or himself — *see* Discharge, firearm by type, self-inflicted
- homicide (attempt) — *see* Discharge, firearm by type, homicide
- in war operations — *see* War operations
- inflicted by other person — *see* Discharge, firearm by type, homicide
  - accidental — *see* Discharge, firearm, by type of firearm
- legal
  - execution — *see* Legal, intervention, firearm
  - intervention — *see* Legal, intervention, firearm
- self-inflicted — *see* Discharge, firearm by type, suicide
  - accidental — *see* Discharge, firearm, by type of firearm
- suicide (attempt) — *see* Discharge, firearm by type, suicide

Shoving (accidentally) by other person — *see* Pushed, by other person

Sickness
- alpine W94.11 ☑
- motion — *see* Motion
- mountain W94.11 ☑

Sinking (accidental)
- watercraft (causing drowning, submersion) (*see also* Drowning, due to, accident to, watercraft, sinking)
  - causing injury except drowning or submersion — *see* Accident, watercraft, causing, injury NEC

Siriasis X32 ☑

Sitting (prolonged) (static) X50.1 ☑

Slashed wrists — *see* Cut, self-inflicted

Slipping (accidental) (on same level) (with fall) W01.0 ☑
- on
  - ice W00.0 ☑
    - with skates — *see* Accident, transport, pedestrian, conveyance
  - mud W01.0 ☑
  - oil W01.0 ☑

- **Slipping** — *continued*
  - on — *continued*
    - snow W00.0 ☑
      - with skis — *see* Accident, transport, pedestrian, conveyance
    - surface (slippery) (wet) NEC W01.0 ☑
  - without fall W18.40 ☑
    - due to
      - specified NEC W18.49 ☑
      - stepping from one level to another W18.43 ☑
      - stepping into hole or opening W18.42 ☑
      - stepping on object W18.41 ☑
- **Sliver,** wood, contact with W45.8 ☑
- **Smoldering** (due to fire) — *see* Exposure, fire
- **Sodomy** (attempted) by force T74.2 ☑
- **Sound** waves (causing injury) W42.9 ☑
  - supersonic W42.0 ☑
- **Splinter**, contact with W45.8 ☑
- **Stab**, stabbing — *see* Cut
- **Standing** (prolonged) (static) X50.1 ☑
- **Starvation** X58 ☑
- **Status** of external cause Y99.9
  - child assisting in compensated work for family Y99.8
  - civilian activity done for financial or other compensation Y99.0
  - civilian activity done for income or pay Y99.0
  - family member assisting in compensated work for other family member Y99.8
  - hobby not done for income Y99.8
  - leisure activity Y99.8
  - military activity Y99.1
  - off-duty activity of military personnel Y99.8
  - recreation or sport not for income or while a student Y99.8
  - specified NEC Y99.8
  - student activity Y99.8
  - volunteer activity Y99.2
- **Stepped** on
  - by
    - animal (not being ridden) NEC W55.89 ☑
    - crowd or human stampede W52 ☑
    - person W50.0 ☑
- **Stepping** on
  - object W22.8 ☑
    - with fall W18.31 ☑
    - sports equipment W21.9 ☑
    - stationary W22.09 ☑
      - sports equipment W21.89 ☑
  - person W51 ☑
    - by crowd or human stampede W52 ☑
  - sports equipment W21.9 ☑
- **Sting**
  - arthropod, nonvenomous W57 ☑
  - insect, nonvenomous W57 ☑
- **Storm** (cataclysmic) — *see* Forces of nature, cataclysmic storm
- **Straining,** excessive (*see also* Overexertion) X50.9 ☑
- **Strangling** — *see* Strangulation
- **Strangulation** (accidental) T71
- **Strenuous** movements (*see also* Overexertion) X50.9 ☑
- **Striking** against
  - airbag (automobile) W22.10 ☑
    - driver side W22.11 ☑
    - front passenger side W22.12 ☑
    - specified NEC W22.19 ☑
  - bottom when
    - diving or jumping into water (in) W16.822 ☑
      - causing drowning W16.821 ☑
      - from boat W16.722 ☑
        - causing drowning W16.721 ☑
      - natural body W16.622 ☑
        - causing drowning W16.821 ☑
      - swimming pool W16.522 ☑
        - causing drowning W16.521 ☑
    - falling into water (in) W16.322 ☑
      - causing drowning W16.321 ☑
      - fountain — *see* Striking against, bottom when, falling into water, specified NEC
      - natural body W16.122 ☑
        - causing drowning W16.121 ☑
      - reservoir — *see* Striking against, bottom when, falling into water, specified NEC
      - specified NEC W16.322 ☑
        - causing drowning W16.321 ☑
      - swimming pool W16.022 ☑
        - causing drowning W16.021 ☑
  - diving board (swimming-pool) W21.4 ☑
  - object W22.8 ☑
    - with

- **Striking** against — *continued*
  - object — *continued*
    - with — *continued*
      - drowning or submersion — *see* Drowning
      - fall — *see* Fall, due to, bumping against, object
    - caused by crowd or human stampede (with fall) W52 ☑
    - furniture W22.03 ☑
    - lamppost W22.02 ☑
    - sports equipment W21.9 ☑
    - stationary W22.09 ☑
      - sports equipment W21.89 ☑
    - wall W22.01 ☑
  - person (s) W51 ☑
    - with fall W03 ☑
      - due to ice or snow W00.0 ☑
    - as, or caused by, a crowd or human stampede (with fall) W52 ☑
    - assault Y04.2 ☑
    - homicide (attempt) Y04.2 ☑
  - sports equipment W21.9 ☑
  - wall (when) W22.01 ☑
    - diving or jumping into water (in) W16.832 ☑
      - causing drowning W16.831 ☑
      - swimming pool W16.532 ☑
        - causing drowning W16.531 ☑
    - falling into water (in) W16.332 ☑
      - causing drowning W16.331 ☑
      - fountain — *see* Striking against, wall when, falling into water, specified NEC
      - natural body W16.132 ☑
        - causing drowning W16.131 ☑
      - reservoir — *see* Striking against, wall when, falling into water, specified NEC
      - specified NEC W16.332 ☑
        - causing drowning W16.331 ☑
      - swimming pool W16.032 ☑
        - causing drowning W16.031 ☑
    - swimming pool (when) W22.042 ☑
      - causing drowning W22.041 ☑
      - diving or jumping into water W16.532 ☑
        - causing drowning W16.531 ☑
      - falling into water W16.032 ☑
        - causing drowning W16.031 ☑
- **Struck** (accidentally) by
  - airbag (automobile) W22.10 ☑
    - driver side W22.11 ☑
    - front passenger side W22.12 ☑
    - specified NEC W22.19 ☑
  - alligator W58.02 ☑
  - animal (not being ridden) NEC W55.89 ☑
  - avalanche — *see* Landslide
  - ball (hit) (thrown) W21.00 ☑
    - assault Y08.09 ☑
    - baseball W21.03 ☑
    - basketball W21.05 ☑
    - golf ball W21.04 ☑
    - football W21.01 ☑
    - soccer W21.02 ☑
    - softball W21.07 ☑
    - specified NEC W21.09 ☑
    - volleyball W21.06 ☑
  - bat or racquet
    - baseball bat W21.11 ☑
      - assault Y08.02 ☑
    - golf club W21.13 ☑
      - assault Y08.09 ☑
    - specified NEC W21.19 ☑
      - assault Y08.09 ☑
    - tennis racquet W21.12 ☑
      - assault Y08.09 ☑
  - bullet (*see also* Discharge, firearm by type)
    - in war operations — *see* War operations
  - crocodile W58.12 ☑
  - dog W54.1 ☑
  - flare, Very pistol — *see* Discharge, firearm NEC
  - hailstones X39.8 ☑
  - hockey (ice)
    - field
      - puck W21.221 ☑
      - stick W21.211 ☑
    - puck W21.220 ☑
    - stick W21.210 ☑
      - assault Y08.01 ☑
  - landslide — *see* Landslide
  - law-enforcement agent (on duty) — *see* Legal, intervention, manhandling
    - with blunt object — *see* Legal, intervention, blunt object
  - lightning — *see* subcategory T75.0
    - causing fire — *see* Exposure, fire
  - machine — *see* Contact, with, by type of machine
  - mammal NEC W55.89 ☑
    - marine W56.32 ☑

- **Struck** by — *continued*
  - marine animal W56.82 ☑
  - missile
    - firearm — *see* Discharge, firearm by type
    - in war operations — *see* War operations, missile
  - object W22.8 ☑
    - blunt W22.8 ☑
      - assault Y00 ☑
      - suicide (attempt) X79 ☑
      - undetermined whether accidental or intentional Y29 ☑
    - falling W20.8 ☑
      - from, in, on
        - building W20.1 ☑
          - burning (uncontrolled fire) X00.4 ☑
        - cataclysmic
          - earth surface movement NEC — *see* Landslide
          - storm — *see* Forces of nature, cataclysmic storm
        - cave-in W20.0 ☑
        - earthquake X34 ☑
        - machine (in operation) — *see* Contact, with, by type of machine
        - structure W20.1 ☑
          - burning X00.4 ☑
        - transport vehicle (in motion) — *see* Accident, transport, by type of vehicle
        - watercraft V93.49 ☑
          - due to
            - accident to craft V91.39 ☑
              - powered craft V91.33 ☑
                - ferry boat V91.31 ☑
                - fishing boat V91.32 ☑
                - jet skis V91.33 ☑
                - liner V91.31 ☑
                - merchant ship V91.30 ☑
                - passenger ship V91.31 ☑
              - unpowered craft V91.38 ☑
                - canoe V91.35 ☑
                - inflatable V91.36 ☑
                - kayak V91.35 ☑
                - sailboat V91.34 ☑
                - surf-board V91.38 ☑
                - windsurfer V91.38 ☑
          - powered craft V93.43 ☑
            - ferry boat V93.41 ☑
            - fishing boat V93.42 ☑
            - jet skis V93.43 ☑
            - liner V93.41 ☑
            - merchant ship V93.40 ☑
            - passenger ship V93.41 ☑
          - unpowered craft V93.48 ☑
            - sailboat V93.44 ☑
            - surf-board V93.48 ☑
            - windsurfer V93.48 ☑
    - moving NEC W20.8 ☑
    - projected W20.8 ☑
      - assault Y00 ☑
      - in sports W21.9 ☑
        - assault Y08.09 ☑
        - ball W21.00 ☑
          - baseball W21.03 ☑
          - basketball W21.05 ☑
          - football W21.01 ☑
          - golf ball W21.04 ☑
          - soccer W21.02 ☑
          - softball W21.07 ☑
          - specified NEC W21.09 ☑
          - volleyball W21.06 ☑
        - bat or racquet
          - baseball bat W21.11 ☑
            - assault Y08.02 ☑
          - golf club W21.13 ☑
            - assault Y08.09 ☑
          - specified NEC W21.19 ☑
            - assault Y08.09 ☑
          - tennis racquet W21.12 ☑
            - assault Y08.09 ☑
        - hockey (ice)
          - field
            - puck W21.221 ☑
            - stick W21.211 ☑
          - puck W21.220 ☑
          - stick W21.210 ☑
            - assault Y08.01 ☑
        - specified NEC W21.89 ☑
    - set in motion by explosion — *see* Explosion
    - thrown W20.8 ☑
      - assault Y00 ☑
      - in sports W21.9 ☑

- **Struck** by — *continued*
  - object — *continued*
    - assault Y08.09 ☑
    - ball W21.00 ☑
      - baseball W21.03 ☑
      - basketball W21.05 ☑
      - football W21.01 ☑
      - golf ball W21.04 ☑
      - soccer W21.02 ☑
      - soft ball W21.07 ☑
      - specified NEC W21.09 ☑
      - volleyball W21.06 ☑
    - bat or racquet
      - baseball bat W21.11 ☑
        - assault Y08.02 ☑
      - golf club W21.13 ☑
        - assault Y08.09 ☑
      - specified NEC W21.19 ☑
        - assault Y08.09 ☑
      - tennis racquet W21.12 ☑
        - assault Y08.09 ☑
    - hockey (ice)
      - field
        - puck W21.221 ☑
        - stick W21.211 ☑
      - puck W21.220 ☑
      - stick W21.210 ☑
        - assault Y08.01 ☑
    - specified NEC W21.89 ☑
  - other person (s) W50.0 ☑
    - with
      - blunt object W22.8 ☑
        - intentional, homicide (attempt) Y00 ☑
        - sports equipment W21.9 ☑
        - undetermined whether accidental or intentional Y29 ☑
      - fall W03 ☑
        - due to ice or snow W00.0 ☑
    - as, or caused by, a crowd or human stampede (with fall) W52 ☑
    - assault Y04.2 ☑
    - homicide (attempt) Y04.2 ☑
    - in legal intervention
      - injuring
        - bystander Y35.812 ☑
        - law enforcement personnel Y35.811 ☑
        - suspect Y35.813 ☑
    - sports equipment W21.9 ☑
  - police (on duty) — *see* Legal, intervention, manhandling
    - with blunt object — *see* Legal, intervention, blunt object
  - sports equipment W21.9 ☑
    - assault Y08.09 ☑
    - ball W21.00 ☑
      - baseball W21.03 ☑
      - basketball W21.05 ☑
      - football W21.01 ☑
      - golf ball W21.04 ☑
      - soccer W21.02 ☑
      - soft ball W21.07 ☑
      - specified NEC W21.09 ☑
      - volleyball W21.06 ☑
    - bat or racquet
      - baseball bat W21.11 ☑
        - assault Y08.02 ☑
      - golf club W21.13 ☑
        - assault Y08.09 ☑
      - specified NEC W21.19 ☑
      - tennis racquet W21.12 ☑
        - assault Y08.09 ☑
    - cleats (shoe) W21.31 ☑
    - foot wear NEC W21.39 ☑
    - football helmet W21.81 ☑
    - hockey (ice)
      - field
        - puck W21.221 ☑
        - stick W21.211 ☑
      - puck W21.220 ☑
      - stick W21.210 ☑
        - assault Y08.01 ☑
    - skate blades W21.32 ☑
    - specified NEC W21.89 ☑
      - assault Y08.09 ☑
  - thunderbolt — *see* subcategory T75.0
    - causing fire — *see* Exposure, fire
  - transport vehicle NEC (*see also* Accident, transport) V09.9 ☑
    - intentional, homicide (attempt) Y03.0 ☑
    - motor NEC (*see also* Accident, transport) V09.20 ☑
      - homicide Y03.0 ☑

- **Struck** by — *continued*
  - vehicle (transport) NEC — *see* Accident, transport, by type of vehicle
    - stationary (falling from jack, hydraulic lift, ramp) W20.8 ☑
- **Stumbling**
  - over
    - animal NEC W01.0 ☑
      - with fall W18.09 ☑
    - carpet, rug or (small) object W22.8 ☑
      - with fall W18.09 ☑
    - person W51 ☑
      - with fall W03 ☑
        - due to ice or snow W00.0 ☑
  - without fall W18.40 ☑
    - due to
      - specified NEC W18.49 ☑
      - stepping from one level to another W18.43 ☑
      - stepping into hole or opening W18.42 ☑
      - stepping on object W18.41 ☑
- **Submersion** (accidental) — *see* Drowning
- **Suffocation** (accidental) (by external means) (by pressure) (mechanical) (*see also* category) T71 ☑
  - due to, by
    - avalanche — *see* Landslide
    - explosion — *see* Explosion
    - fire — *see* Exposure, fire
    - food, any type (aspiration) (ingestion) (inhalation) — *see* categories T17 and T18 ☑
    - ignition — *see* Ignition
    - landslide — *see* Landslide
    - machine (ry) — *see* Contact, with, by type of machine
    - vomitus (aspiration) (inhalation) T17.81 ☑
  - in
    - burning building X00.8 ☑
- **Suicide**, suicidal (attempted) (by) X83.8 ☑
  - blunt object X79 ☑
  - burning, burns X76 ☑
    - hot object X77.9 ☑
      - fluid NEC X77.2 ☑
      - household appliance X77.3 ☑
      - specified NEC X77.8 ☑
      - steam X77.0 ☑
      - tap water X77.1 ☑
      - vapors X77.0 ☑
  - caustic substance — *see* Table of Drugs and Chemicals
  - cold, extreme X83.2 ☑
  - collision of motor vehicle with
    - motor vehicle X82.0 ☑
    - specified NEC X82.8 ☑
    - train X82.1 ☑
    - tree X82.2 ☑
  - crashing of aircraft X83.0 ☑
  - cut (any part of body) X78.9 ☑
  - cutting or piercing instrument X78.9 ☑
    - dagger X78.2 ☑
    - glass X78.0 ☑
    - knife X78.1 ☑
    - specified NEC X78.8 ☑
    - sword X78.2 ☑
  - drowning (in) X71.9 ☑
    - bathtub X71.0 ☑
    - natural water X71.3 ☑
    - specified NEC X71.8 ☑
    - swimming pool X71.1 ☑
      - following fall X71.2 ☑
  - electrocution X83.1 ☑
  - explosive (s) (material) X75 ☑
  - fire, flames X76 ☑
  - firearm X74.9 ☑
    - airgun X74.01 ☑
    - handgun X72 ☑
    - hunting rifle X73.1 ☑
    - larger X73.9 ☑
      - specified NEC X73.8 ☑
    - machine gun X73.2 ☑
    - shotgun X73.0 ☑
    - specified NEC X74.8 ☑
  - hanging X83.8 ☑
  - hot object — *see* Suicide, burning, hot object
  - jumping
    - before moving object X81.8 ☑
      - motor vehicle X81.0 ☑
      - subway train X81.1 ☑
      - train X81.1 ☑
    - from high place X80 ☑
  - late effect of attempt — *see* X71-X83 with 7th character S

- **Suicide**, suicidal — *continued*
  - lying before moving object, train, vehicle X81.8 ☑
  - poisoning — *see* Table of Drugs and Chemicals
  - puncture (any part of body) — *see* Suicide, cutting or piercing instrument
  - scald — *see* Suicide, burning, hot object
  - sequelae of attempt — *see* X71-X83 with 7th character S
  - sharp object (any) — *see* Suicide, cutting or piercing instrument
  - shooting — *see* Suicide, firearm
  - specified means NEC X83.8 ☑
  - stab (any part of body) — *see* Suicide, cutting or piercing instrument
  - steam, hot vapors X77.0 ☑
  - strangulation X83.8 ☑
  - submersion — *see* Suicide, drowning
  - suffocation X83.8 ☑
  - wound NEC X83.8 ☑
- **Sunstroke** X32 ☑
- **Supersonic** waves (causing injury) W42.0 ☑
- **Surgical** procedure, complication of (delayed or as an abnormal reaction without mention of misadventure) (*see also* Complication of or following, by type of procedure)
  - due to or as a result of misadventure — *see* Misadventure
- **Swallowed**, swallowing
  - foreign body — *see* Foreign body, alimentary canal
  - poison — *see* Table of Drugs and Chemicals
  - substance
    - caustic or corrosive — *see* Table of Drugs and Chemicals
    - poisonous — *see* Table of Drugs and Chemicals

T

- **Tackle** in sport W03 ☑
- **Terrorism** (involving) Y38.80 ☑
  - biological weapons Y38.6X ☑
  - chemical weapons Y38.7X ☑
  - conflagration Y38.3X ☑
  - drowning and submersion Y38.89 ☑
  - explosion Y38.2X ☑
    - destruction of aircraft Y38.1X ☑
    - marine weapons Y38.0X ☑
  - fire Y38.3X ☑
  - firearms Y38.4X ☑
  - hot substances Y38.3X ☑
  - lasers Y38.89 ☑
  - nuclear weapons Y38.5X ☑
  - piercing or stabbing instruments Y38.89 ☑
  - secondary effects Y38.9X ☑
  - specified method NEC Y38.89 ☑
  - suicide bomber Y38.81 ☑
- **Thirst** X58 ☑
- **Threat** to breathing
  - aspiration — *see* Aspiration
  - due to cave-in, falling earth or substance NEC T71
- **Thrown** (accidentally)
  - against part (any) of or object in transport vehicle (in motion) NEC (*see also* Accident, transport)
  - from
    - high place, homicide (attempt) Y01 ☑
    - machinery — *see* Contact, with, by type of machine
    - transport vehicle NEC (*see also* Accident, transport) V89.9 ☑
  - off — *see* Thrown, from
- **Thunderbolt** — *see* subcategory T75.0
  - causing fire — *see* Exposure, fire
- **Tidal** wave (any injury) NEC — *see* Forces of nature, tidal wave
- **Took**
  - overdose (drug) — *see* Table of Drugs and Chemicals
  - poison — *see* Table of Drugs and Chemicals
- **Tornado** (any injury) X37.1 ☑
- **Torrential** rain (any injury) X37.8 ☑
- **Torture** X58 ☑
- **Trampled** by animal NEC W55.89 ☑
- **Trapped** (accidentally)
  - between objects (moving) (stationary and moving) — *see* Caught
  - by part (any) of
    - motorcycle V29.88 ☑
    - pedal cycle V19.88 ☑
    - transport vehicle NEC (*see also* Accident, transport) V89.9 ☑

Travel (effects) (sickness) T75.3 ☑

Tree falling on or hitting (accidentally) (person) W20.8 ☑

Tripping
- over
  - animal W01.0 ☑
    - with fall W01.0 ☑
  - carpet, rug or (small) object W22.8 ☑
    - with fall W18.09 ☑
  - person W51 ☑
    - with fall W03 ☑
      - due to ice or snow W00.0 ☑
- without fall W18.40 ☑
  - due to
    - specified NEC W18.49 ☑
    - stepping from one level to another W18.43 ☑
    - stepping into hole or opening W18.42 ☑
    - stepping on object W18.41 ☑

Twisted by person (s) (accidentally) W50.2 ☑
- with intent to injure or kill Y04.0 ☑
- as, or caused by, a crowd or human stampede (with fall) W52 ☑
- assault Y04.0 ☑
- homicide (attempt) Y04.0 ☑
- in
  - fight Y04.0 ☑
  - legal intervention — *see* Legal, intervention, manhandling

Twisting (prolonged) (static) X50.1 ☑

U

Underdosing of necessary drugs, medicaments or biological substances Y63.6

Undetermined intent (contact) (exposure)
- automobile collision Y32 ☑
- blunt object Y29 ☑
- drowning (submersion) (in) Y21.9 ☑
  - bathtub Y21.0 ☑
    - after fall Y21.1 ☑
  - natural water (lake) (ocean) (pond) (river) (stream) Y21.4 ☑
  - specified place NEC Y21.8 ☑
  - swimming pool Y21.2 ☑
    - after fall Y21.3 ☑
- explosive material Y25 ☑
- fall, jump or push from high place Y30 ☑
- falling, lying or running before moving object Y31 ☑
- fire Y26 ☑
- firearm discharge Y24.9 ☑
  - airgun (BB) (pellet) Y24.0 ☑
  - handgun (pistol) (revolver) Y22 ☑
  - hunting rifle Y23.1 ☑
  - larger Y23.9 ☑
    - hunting rifle Y23.1 ☑
    - machine gun Y23.3 ☑
    - military Y23.2 ☑
    - shotgun Y23.0 ☑
    - specified type NEC Y23.8 ☑
  - machine gun Y23.3 ☑
  - military Y23.2 ☑
  - shotgun Y23.0 ☑
  - specified type NEC Y24.8 ☑
  - Very pistol Y24.8 ☑
- hot object Y27.9 ☑
  - fluid NEC Y27.2 ☑
  - household appliance Y27.3 ☑
  - specified object NEC Y27.8 ☑
  - steam Y27.0 ☑
  - tap water Y27.1 ☑
  - vapor Y27.0 ☑
- jump, fall or push from high place Y30 ☑
- lying, falling or running before moving object Y31 ☑
- motor vehicle crash Y32 ☑
- push, fall or jump from high place Y30 ☑
- running, falling or lying before moving object Y31 ☑
- sharp object Y28.9 ☑
  - dagger Y28.2 ☑
  - glass Y28.0 ☑
  - knife Y28.1 ☑
  - specified object NEC Y28.8 ☑
  - sword Y28.2 ☑
- smoke Y26 ☑
- specified event NEC Y33 ☑

Use of hand as hammer X50.3 ☑

V

Vibration (causing injury) W49.9 ☑

Victim (of)
- avalanche — *see* Landslide
- earth movements NEC — *see* Forces of nature, earth movement
- earthquake X34 ☑
- flood — *see* Flood
- landslide — *see* Landslide
- lightning — *see* subcategory T75.0
  - causing fire — *see* Exposure, fire
- storm (cataclysmic) NEC — *see* Forces of nature, cataclysmic storm
- volcanic eruption X35 ☑

Volcanic eruption (any injury) X35 ☑

Vomitus, gastric contents in air passages (with asphyxia, obstruction or suffocation) T17.81 ☑

W

Walked into stationary object (any) W22.09 ☑
- furniture W22.03 ☑
- lamppost W22.02 ☑
- wall W22.01 ☑

War operations (injuries to military personnel and civilians during war, civil insurrection and peacekeeping missions) (by) (from) (involving) Y36.90 ☑
- after cessation of hostilities Y36.89 ☑
  - explosion (of)
    - bomb placed during war operations Y36.82 ☑
    - mine placed during war operations Y36.81 ☑
  - specified NEC Y36.88 ☑
- air blast Y36.20 ☑
- aircraft
  - destruction — *see* War operations, destruction of aircraft
- airway restriction — *see* War operations, restriction of airways
- asphyxiation — *see* War operations, restriction of airways
- biological weapons Y36.6X ☑
- blast Y36.20 ☑
- blast fragments Y36.20 ☑
- blast wave Y36.20 ☑
- blast wind Y36.20 ☑
- bomb Y36.20 ☑
  - dirty Y36.50 ☑
  - gasoline Y36.31 ☑
  - incendiary Y36.31 ☑
  - petrol Y36.31 ☑
- bullet Y36.43 ☑
  - incendiary Y36.32 ☑
  - rubber Y36.41 ☑
- chemical weapons Y36.7X ☑
- combat
  - hand to hand (unarmed) combat Y36.44 ☑
  - using blunt or piercing object Y36.45 ☑
- conflagration — *see* War operations, fire
- conventional warfare NEC Y36.49 ☑
- depth-charge Y36.01 ☑
- destruction of aircraft Y36.10 ☑
  - due to
    - air to air missile Y36.11 ☑
    - collision with other aircraft Y36.12 ☑
    - detonation (accidental) of onboard munitions and explosives Y36.14 ☑
    - enemy fire or explosives Y36.11 ☑
    - explosive placed on aircraft Y36.11 ☑
    - onboard fire Y36.13 ☑
    - rocket propelled grenade [RPG] Y36.11 ☑
    - small arms fire Y36.11 ☑
    - surface to air missile Y36.11 ☑
  - specified NEC Y36.19 ☑
- detonation (accidental) of
  - onboard marine weapons Y36.05 ☑
  - own munitions or munitions launch device Y36.24 ☑
- dirty bomb Y36.50 ☑
- explosion (of) Y36.20 ☑
  - after cessation of hostilities
    - bomb placed during war operations Y36.82 ☑
    - mine placed during war operations Y36.81 ☑
  - aerial bomb Y36.21 ☑
  - bomb NOS (*see also* War operations, bomb (s)) Y36.20 ☑
  - own munitions or munitions launch device (accidental) Y36.24 ☑
  - fragments Y36.20 ☑
  - grenade Y36.29 ☑
  - guided missile Y36.22 ☑
  - improvised explosive device [IED] (person-borne) (roadside) (vehicle-borne) Y36.23 ☑

War operations — *continued*
- explosion — *continued*
  - land mine Y36.29 ☑
  - marine mine (at sea) (in harbor) Y36.02 ☑
  - marine weapon Y36.00 ☑
    - specified NEC Y36.09 ☑
  - sea-based artillery shell Y36.03 ☑
  - specified NEC Y36.29 ☑
  - torpedo Y36.04 ☑
- fire Y36.30 ☑
  - specified NEC Y36.39 ☑
- firearms
  - discharge Y36.43 ☑
  - pellets Y36.42 ☑
- flamethrower Y36.33 ☑
- fragments (from) (of)
  - improvised explosive device [IED] (person-borne) (roadside) (vehicle-borne) Y36.26 ☑
  - munitions Y36.25 ☑
  - specified NEC Y36.29 ☑
  - weapons Y36.27 ☑
- friendly fire Y36.92 ☑
- hand to hand (unarmed) combat Y36.44 ☑
- hot substances — *see* War operations, fire
- incendiary bullet Y36.32 ☑
- nuclear weapon (effects of) Y36.50 ☑
  - acute radiation exposure Y36.54 ☑
  - blast pressure Y36.51 ☑
  - direct blast Y36.51 ☑
  - direct heat Y36.53 ☑
  - fallout exposure Y36.54 ☑
  - fireball Y36.53 ☑
  - indirect blast (struck or crushed by blast debris) (being thrown by blast) Y36.52 ☑
  - ionizing radiation (immediate exposure) Y36.54 ☑
  - nuclear radiation Y36.54 ☑
  - radiation
    - ionizing (immediate exposure) Y36.54 ☑
    - nuclear Y36.54 ☑
    - thermal Y36.53 ☑
  - specified NEC Y36.59 ☑
  - secondary effects Y36.54 ☑
  - thermal radiation Y36.53 ☑
- restriction of air (airway)
  - intentional Y36.46 ☑
  - unintentional Y36.47 ☑
- rubber bullets Y36.41 ☑
- shrapnel NOS Y36.29 ☑
- suffocation — *see* War operations, restriction of airways
- unconventional warfare NEC Y36.7X ☑
- underwater blast NOS Y36.00 ☑
- warfare
  - conventional NEC Y36.49 ☑
  - unconventional NEC Y36.7X ☑
- weapons
  - biological weapons Y36.6X ☑
  - chemical Y36.7X ☑
  - nuclear (effects of) Y36.50 ☑
    - acute radiation exposure Y36.54 ☑
    - blast pressure Y36.51 ☑
    - direct blast Y36.51 ☑
    - direct heat Y36.53 ☑
    - fallout exposure Y36.54 ☑
    - fireball Y36.53 ☑
    - indirect blast (struck or crushed by blast debris) (being thrown by blast) Y36.52 ☑
    - radiation
      - ionizing (immediate exposure) Y36.54 ☑
      - nuclear Y36.54 ☑
      - thermal Y36.53 ☑
    - secondary effects Y36.54 ☑
    - specified NEC Y36.59 ☑
  - of mass destruction [WMD] Y36.91 ☑
- weapon of mass destruction [WMD] Y36.91 ☑

Washed
- away by flood — *see* Flood
- off road by storm (transport vehicle) — *see* Forces of nature, cataclysmic storm

Weather exposure NEC — *see* Forces of nature

Weightlessness (causing injury) (effects of) (in spacecraft, real or simulated) X52 ☑

Work related condition Y99.0

Wound (accidental) NEC (*see also* Injury) X58 ☑
- battle (*see also* War operations) Y36.90 ☑
- gunshot — *see* Discharge, firearm by type

Wreck transport vehicle NEC (*see also* Accident, transport) V89.9 ☑

Wrong
- device implanted into correct surgical site Y65.51
- fluid in infusion Y65.1
- procedure (operation) on correct patient Y65.51
- patient, procedure performed on Y65.52

Chapter 1: Certain Infectious and Parasitic Diseases (A00-B99)

Guidelines for Assigning Codes From This Chapter

Chapter 1 of ICD-10-CM includes a long list of infectious and parasitic diseases. Everything from cholera and bubonic plague to toxoplasmosis has a home here. But as you code, keep in mind that ICD-10-CM may list infections in the chapters for their specific anatomic area instead of in Chapter 1. Each time you code, search the index and then confirm your code choice in the tabular list.

List of Sections

- A00-A09: Intestinal infectious diseases
- A15-A19: Tuberculosis
- A20-A28: Certain zoonotic bacterial diseases
- A30-A49: Other bacterial diseases
- A50-A64: Infections with a predominantly sexual mode of transmission
- A65-A69: Other spirochetal diseases
- A70-A74: Other diseases caused by chlamydiae
- A75-A79: Rickettsioses
- A80-A89: Viral and prion infections of the central nervous system
- A90-A99: Arthropod-borne viral fevers and viral hemorrhagic fevers
- B00-B09: Viral infections characterized by skin and mucous membrane lesions
- B10: Other human herpesviruses
- B15-B19: Viral hepatitis
- B20: Human immunodeficiency virus [HIV] disease
- B25-B34: Other viral diseases
- B35-B49: Mycoses
- B50-B64: Protozoal diseases
- B65-B83: Helminthiases
- B85-B89: Pediculosis, acariasis and other infestations
- B90-B94: Sequelae of infectious and parasitic diseases
- B95-B97: Bacterial and viral infectious agents
- B99: Other infectious diseases

Highlights From the ICD-10-CM Official Guidelines for Coding and Reporting

The ICD-10-CM Official Guidelines for Coding and Reporting for Chapter 1 keep the focus on proper coding for HIV, infection agents as the cause of diseases classified to other chapters, infectious resistant to antibiotics, sepsis and shock, and methicillin-resistant *Staphylococcus aureus* (MRSA) conditions. The information below covers the major points of Section I.C.1 of the 2017 Official Guidelines.

Guidelines Provide Crucial Answers for Coders Reporting HIV

The Official Guidelines give you practical coding guidance for a variety of HIV-related scenarios.

First, you must use B20 (*Human immunodeficiency virus [HIV] disease*) to report only confirmed cases of HIV. A diagnostic statement from the provider that the patient is positive for HIV or has an HIV-related illness counts as confirmation.

Sequencing: Whether you use B20 as the first-listed (or principal) diagnosis depends on the nature of the patient's visit.

Use B20 as the principal diagnosis for a patient admitted for an HIV-related condition (unless the patient is pregnant or recently gave birth, as explained below). You also should report additional diagnoses for the HIV-related conditions documented for the patient.

On the other hand, if the provider admits the patient for a condition unrelated to HIV, you should choose your principal diagnosis based on the reason for admission. Then report B20 and codes for the patient's other HIV-related conditions.

The guidelines indicate the above sequencing rules apply regardless of whether the patient is newly diagnosed or has had previous encounters for HIV-related conditions.

B20 Isn't the Only Possibility for HIV Encounters

Asymptomatic: When documentation doesn't record any symptoms, but it does show the patient is HIV positive, you should use Z21 (*Asymptomatic human immunodeficiency virus [HIV] infection status*) rather than B20. However, if the provider documents AIDS, treatment for an HIV-related illness, or one or more conditions caused by being HIV-positive, then you should use B20.

Inconclusive serology: When a patient with no definitive diagnosis or manifestations of HIV has an inconclusive HIV serology, you should not use B20. You should use R75 (*Inconclusive laboratory evidence of human immunodeficiency virus [HIV]*).

Note that you should never use Z21 or R75 if the patient has ever been diagnosed with an HIV illness that falls under B20. You always should use B20 for patients who have had an HIV-related illness.

Pregnancy, puerperium: When a patient presents with an HIV-related illness during pregnancy, childbirth, or the puerperium, your first-listed (or principal) code must be from O98.7- (*Human immunodeficiency [HIV] disease complicating pregnancy, childbirth, and the puerperium*). Then report B20 and the code or codes for the patient's HIV-related illnesses. Sequence the conditions that ICD-10 indexes to Chapter 16, Certain Conditions Originating in the Perinatal Period (O00-P96), first.

If the patient's status is asymptomatic HIV, report O98.7- and Z21.

HIV Test Codes Vary Based on Circumstances

The codes you report when a patient presents for determination of HIV status depends on the patient's specific case.

- You should use the screening code Z11.4 (*Encounter for screening for human immunodeficiency virus [HIV]*) as the primary code.
- For patients without symptoms who are in a high-risk group for HIV, you should use additional codes for any associated high-risk behaviors.
- When a patient has an HIV test because of signs or symptoms, you should report the code(s) for the signs and symptoms. If the patient has counseling at the same session, report Z71.7 (*Human immunodeficiency virus [HIV] counseling*), too.
  - ➢ Code Z71.7 is also the appropriate code to use when a patient returns for the test results and learns she is HIV negative. If the test shows the patient is HIV positive, report either Z21 for an asymptomatic patient or B20 for a symptomatic patient. For symptomatic patients, you also should add codes for the symptoms or confirmed HIV-related diagnoses.

An Additional Code for an Organism May be Necessary

For patients with infections classified in chapters other than Chapter 1 but with no organism identified in the infection code, you should assign an additional code from Chapter 1, B95-B97 (*Bacterial and viral infectious agents*), to identify the organism.

Look for the instructional note with the infection code advising you to assign an additional code for the organism.

Identify Infections Resistant to Antibiotics

You must always report a bacterial infection's resistance to antibiotics. If the infection code does not specify drug resistance, report both the infection code and a code from category Z16 (*Resistance to antimicrobial drugs*).

Sort Through Sepsis, Severe Sepsis, and Shock

Sepsis is the body's overwhelming and life-threatening response to an infection which can lead to tissue damage, organ failure, and death. Septic shock refers to circulatory failure associated with severe sepsis and represents a type of acute organ dysfunction.

To report sepsis correctly, assign the code for the underlying systemic infection. Assign A41.9 (*Sepsis, unspecified organism*) when the causal organism isn't known.

Report a code from subcategory R65.2 (*Severe sepsis*) only when the provider documents severe sepsis or associated organ dysfunction. If the patient has multiple organ dysfunction (MOD), follow the instructions for reporting severe sepsis. If acute organ dysfunction is due to a condition other than sepsis, do not assign a code from R65.2.

Caution: Query the provider when a patient with clinical signs of sepsis has negative or inconclusive blood cultures or if the term *urosepsis* is used. Urosepsis is not synonymous with sepsis.

Remember Sequencing Rules for Severe Sepsis and Septic Shock

To report sepsis correctly, you should report a minimum of two codes, in this order:

- The systemic infection code
- A code from subcategory R65.2; note that you may not assign R65.2 as a principal diagnosis
- A41.9 (*Sepsis, unspecified organism*), if the causal organism is not documented
- Additional codes for acute organ dysfunction, if appropriate

If severe sepsis was not present on admission, the systemic infection code and a code from R65.2 should be associated as secondary diagnoses. Query the provider if the documentation if it isn't clear when severe sepsis developed.

When the documentation indicates septic shock, report codes in this order:

- The systemic infection code
- A septic shock code, either R65.21 (*Severe sepsis with septic shock*) or code T81.12 (*Postprocedural septic shock*)
- Additional codes for acute organ dysfunction

Note that septic shock cannot be assigned as a principal diagnosis.

Lock Down Proper Coding When Patient Has Localized Infection, Too

If the provider documents both sepsis or severe sepsis and a localized infection, such as pneumonia or cellulitis, as reasons for admission, assign codes in this order:

- The systemic infection code
- The appropriate code from R65.2, if severe sepsis is present on admission
- The localized infection code

Caution: If severe sepsis develops after admission, assign the localized infection code first and then the appropriate sepsis or severe sepsis code.

Postprocedural Sepsis Coding Has Variations to Watch

When documentation reveals postprocedural sepsis, you should report your codes in the following order:

- The complication code, such as T81.4 (*Infection following a procedure*) or O86.0 (*Infection of obstetrical surgical wound*)
- The sepsis code, R65.20
- The code for the systemic infection

Your coding will change a bit if postprocedural infection leads to severe sepsis and postprocedural septic shock:

- Complication code
- T81.12- (*Postprocedural septic shock*)
- The code for the systemic infection

Don't Assume Infection Caused the Sepsis

When sepsis or severe sepsis result from something other than infection, use the following order for your codes:

- The code for the noninfectious condition, such as the appropriate burn or injury code, assuming this condition meets the definition of a principal diagnosis
- The code for the systemic infection
- A severe sepsis code from R65.2, if present
- Codes for any acute organ dysfunction for severe sepsis

You won't assign a code from R65.1 (*Systemic inflammatory response syndrome [SIRS] of noninfectious origin*).

Note that if the sepsis meets the principal diagnosis requirements, you should report the systemic infection and sepsis/severe sepsis codes followed by the code for the noninfectious condition. You may report either the noninfectious condition or the sepsis as principal if both meet the definition of principal diagnosis.

Caution: When a patient has a noninfectious condition that results in an infection that then leads to severe sepsis, you should report a code from R65.2. You should not also report a code from R65.1 (*Systemic inflammatory response syndrome [SIRS] of noninfectious origin*).

Note: See Chapter 15 to report sepsis and septic shock related to abortion, pregnancy, childbirth, and the puerperium. See Chapter 16 to report bacterial sepsis involving a newborn.

MRSA Conditions Often Feature Combination Codes

ICD-10-CM offers combination codes for certain methicillin resistant *Staphylococcus aureus* (MRSA) diagnoses. In those cases, you should report the combination code that describes the complete condition rather than reporting the individual elements.

Example 1: The patient has sepsis caused by MRSA. You should report A41.02 (*Sepsis due to methicillin-resistant Staphylococcus aureus*).

Example 2: The patient has pneumonia due to MRSA. You should report J15.212 (*Pneumonia due to methicillin-resistant Staphylococcus aureus*).

Do not report: When combination codes apply, you should not report B95.62 (*Methicillin-resistant Staphylococcus aureus infection as the cause of diseases classified elsewhere*). You also should not report Z16.11 (*Resistance to penicillins*).

Double Up on the Codes When Necessary

You won't always have the option of using a combination code for a current MRSA infection. In those cases, you should report the condition as well as MRSA code B95.62. You shouldn't report Z16.11 as an additional code.

Distinguish Between Colonization and Infection

A person may have MRSA or methicillin-susceptible *Staphylococcus aureus* (MSSA) on or in the body without being sick. In these cases, you may see the documentation refer to colonization, carriage, carrier, MRSA screen positive, or MRSA nasal swab positive.

How to code: When documentation shows MSSA colonization, you should report Z22.321 (*Carrier or suspected carrier of methicillin-susceptible Staphylococcus aureus*).

For MRSA colonization, use Z22.322 (*Carrier or suspected carrier of methicillin-resistant staphylococcus aureus*). When the patient has both MRSA colonization and MRSA infection documented, you may report codes for both.

Certain infectious and parasitic diseases (A00-B99)

INCLUDES *diseases generally recognized as communicable or transmissible*

Use additional code to identify resistance to antimicrobial drugs (Z16.-)

EXCLUDES1 *certain localized infections - see body system-related chapters*

EXCLUDES2 *carrier or suspected carrier of infectious disease (Z22.-)*
infectious and parasitic diseases complicating pregnancy, childbirth and the puerperium (O98.-)
infectious and parasitic diseases specific to the perinatal period (P35-P39)
influenza and other acute respiratory infections (J00-J22)

This chapter contains the following blocks:

A00-A09 Intestinal infectious diseases
A15-A19 Tuberculosis
A20-A28 Certain zoonotic bacterial diseases
A30-A49 Other bacterial diseases
A50-A64 Infections with a predominantly sexual mode of transmission
A65-A69 Other spirochetal diseases
A70-A74 Other diseases caused by chlamydiae
A75-A79 Rickettsioses
A80-A89 Viral and prion infections of the central nervous system
A90-A99 Arthropod-borne viral fevers and viral hemorrhagic fevers
B00-B09 Viral infections characterized by skin and mucous membrane lesions
B10 Other human herpesviruses
B15-B19 Viral hepatitis
B20 Human immunodeficiency virus [HIV] disease
B25-B34 Other viral diseases
B35-B49 Mycoses
B50-B64 Protozoal diseases
B65-B83 Helminthiases
B85-B89 Pediculosis, acariasis and other infestations
B90-B94 Sequelae of infectious and parasitic diseases
B95-B97 Bacterial and viral infectious agents
B99 Other infectious diseases

Intestinal infectious diseases (A00-A09)

A00 Cholera
- **A00.0 Cholera due to Vibrio cholerae 01, biovar cholerae** CC
  Classical cholera
- **A00.1 Cholera due to Vibrio cholerae 01, biovar El Tor** CC
  Cholera El Tor
- **A00.9 Cholera, unspecified** CC

A01 Typhoid and paratyphoid fevers
- **A01.0 Typhoid fever**
  Infection due to Salmonella typhi
  - **A01.00 Typhoid fever, unspecified** CC
  - **A01.01 Typhoid meningitis** CC
  - **A01.02 Typhoid fever with heart involvement** CC
    Typhoid endocarditis
    Typhoid myocarditis
  - **A01.03 Typhoid pneumonia** CC
  - **A01.04 Typhoid arthritis** CC
  - **A01.05 Typhoid osteomyelitis** CC
  - **A01.09 Typhoid fever with other complications** CC
- **A01.1 Paratyphoid fever A** CC
- **A01.2 Paratyphoid fever B** CC
- **A01.3 Paratyphoid fever C** CC
- **A01.4 Paratyphoid fever, unspecified** CC
  Infection due to Salmonella paratyphi NOS

A02 Other salmonella infections

INCLUDES *infection or food-borne intoxication due to any Salmonella species other than S. typhi and S. paratyphi*
- **A02.0 Salmonella enteritis** CC
  Salmonellosis
- **A02.1 Salmonella sepsis** MCC
- **A02.2 Localized salmonella infections**
  - **A02.20 Localized salmonella infection, unspecified**
  - **A02.21 Salmonella meningitis** MCC
  - **A02.22 Salmonella pneumonia** MCC
  - **A02.23 Salmonella arthritis** CC
  - **A02.24 Salmonella osteomyelitis** CC
  - **A02.25 Salmonella pyelonephritis** CC
    Salmonella tubulo-interstitial nephropathy
  - **A02.29 Salmonella with other localized infection** CC
- **A02.8 Other specified salmonella infections** CC
- **A02.9 Salmonella infection, unspecified** CC

A03 Shigellosis
- **A03.0 Shigellosis due to Shigella dysenteriae** CC
  Group A shigellosis [Shiga-Kruse dysentery]
- **A03.1 Shigellosis due to Shigella flexneri**
  Group B shigellosis
- **A03.2 Shigellosis due to Shigella boydii**
  Group C shigellosis
- **A03.3 Shigellosis due to Shigella sonnei**
  Group D shigellosis
- **A03.8 Other shigellosis**
- **A03.9 Shigellosis, unspecified**
  Bacillary dysentery NOS

A04 Other bacterial intestinal infections

EXCLUDES1 *bacterial food-borne intoxications, NEC (A05.-)*
tuberculous enteritis (A18.32)
- **A04.0 Enteropathogenic Escherichia coli infection** CC
- **A04.1 Enterotoxigenic Escherichia coli infection** CC
- **A04.2 Enteroinvasive Escherichia coli infection** CC
- **A04.3 Enterohemorrhagic Escherichia coli infection** CC
- **A04.4 Other intestinal Escherichia coli infections** CC
  Escherichia coli enteritis NOS
- **A04.5 Campylobacter enteritis** CC
- **A04.6 Enteritis due to Yersinia enterocolitica** CC
  EXCLUDES1 *extraintestinal yersiniosis (A28.2)*
- **A04.7 Enterocolitis due to Clostridium difficile** CC
  Food-borne intoxication by Clostridium difficile
  Pseudomembranous colitis
- **A04.8 Other specified bacterial intestinal infections** CC
- **A04.9 Bacterial intestinal infection, unspecified** CC
  Bacterial enteritis NOS

A05 Other bacterial food-borne intoxications, not elsewhere classified

EXCLUDES1 *Clostridium difficile food-borne intoxication and infection (A04.7)*
Escherichia coli infection (A04.0-A04.4)
listeriosis (A32.-)
salmonella food-borne intoxication and infection (A02.-)
toxic effect of noxious foodstuffs (T61-T62)
- **A05.0 Food-borne staphylococcal intoxication** CC
- **A05.1 Botulism food poisoning** CC
  Botulism NOS
  Classical food-borne intoxication due to Clostridium botulinum
  EXCLUDES1 *infant botulism (A48.51)*
  wound botulism (A48.52)
- **A05.2 Food-borne Clostridium perfringens [Clostridium welchii] intoxication** CC
  Enteritis necroticans
  Pig-bel
- **A05.3 Food-borne Vibrio parahaemolyticus intoxication** CC
- **A05.4 Food-borne Bacillus cereus intoxication** CC
- **A05.5 Food-borne Vibrio vulnificus intoxication** CC
- **A05.8 Other specified bacterial food-borne intoxications** CC
- **A05.9 Bacterial food-borne intoxication, unspecified**

A06 Amebiasis

INCLUDES *infection due to Entamoeba histolytica*

EXCLUDES1 *other protozoal intestinal diseases (A07.-)*

EXCLUDES2 *acanthamebiasis (B60.1-)*
Naegleriasis (B60.2)
- **A06.0 Acute amebic dysentery** CC
  Acute amebiasis
  Intestinal amebiasis NOS
- **A06.1 Chronic intestinal amebiasis** CC
- **A06.2 Amebic nondysenteric colitis** CC
- **A06.3 Ameboma of intestine** CC
  Ameboma NOS
- **A06.4 Amebic liver abscess** MCC
  Hepatic amebiasis
- **A06.5 Amebic lung abscess** MCC
  Amebic abscess of lung (and liver)

Unspecified Code | Other Specified Code | Manifestation Code | N Newborn | P Pediatric | M Maternity | A Adult | ♂ Male | ♀ Female
● New Code | ▲ Revised Code Title | ►◄ Revised Text | NOTES | INCLUDES | EXCLUDES1 Not coded here | EXCLUDES2 Not included here
4th character required | 5th character required | 6th character required | 7th character required
Extension 'X' Alert | HAC Hospital-acquired condition (HAC) alert | AHA AHA Coding Clinic©

A06.6 **Amebic brain abscess** MCC
Amebic abscess of brain (and liver) (and lung)
A06.7 **Cutaneous amebiasis**
5th A06.8 **Amebic infection of other sites**
A06.81 **Amebic cystitis** CC
A06.82 **Other amebic genitourinary infections** CC
Amebic balanitis
Amebic vesiculitis
Amebic vulvovaginitis
A06.89 **Other amebic infections** CC
Amebic appendicitis
Amebic splenic abscess
A06.9 **Amebiasis, unspecified**

4th A07 **Other protozoal intestinal diseases**
A07.0 **Balantidiasis**
Balantidial dysentery
A07.1 **Giardiasis [lambliasis]** CC
A07.2 **Cryptosporidiosis** CC
A07.3 **Isosporiasis** CC
Infection due to Isospora belli and Isospora hominis
Intestinal coccidiosis
Isosporosis
A07.4 **Cyclosporiasis** CC
A07.8 **Other specified protozoal intestinal diseases** CC
Intestinal microsporidiosis
Intestinal trichomoniasis
Sarcocystosis
Sarcosporidiosis
A07.9 **Protozoal intestinal disease, unspecified** CC
Flagellate diarrhea
Protozoal colitis
Protozoal diarrhea
Protozoal dysentery

4th A08 **Viral and other specified intestinal infections**
EXCLUDES1 *influenza with involvement of gastrointestinal tract (J09.X3, J10.2, J11.2)*
A08.0 **Rotaviral enteritis** CC
5th A08.1 **Acute gastroenteropathy due to Norwalk agent and other small round viruses**
A08.11 **Acute gastroenteropathy due to Norwalk agent** CC
Acute gastroenteropathy due to Norovirus
Acute gastroenteropathy due to Norwalk-like agent
A08.19 **Acute gastroenteropathy due to other small round viruses** CC
Acute gastroenteropathy due to small round virus [SRV] NOS
A08.2 **Adenoviral enteritis** CC
5th A08.3 **Other viral enteritis**
A08.31 **Calicivirus enteritis** CC
A08.32 **Astrovirus enteritis** CC
A08.39 **Other viral enteritis** CC
Coxsackie virus enteritis
Echovirus enteritis
Enterovirus enteritis NEC
Torovirus enteritis
A08.4 **Viral intestinal infection, unspecified**
Viral enteritis NOS
Viral gastroenteritis NOS
Viral gastroenteropathy NOS
A08.8 **Other specified intestinal infections**

A09 **Infectious gastroenteritis and colitis, unspecified** CC
Infectious colitis NOS
Infectious enteritis NOS
Infectious gastroenteritis NOS
EXCLUDES1 *colitis NOS (K52.9)*
diarrhea NOS (R19.7)
enteritis NOS (K52.9)
gastroenteritis NOS (K52.9)
noninfective gastroenteritis and colitis, unspecified (K52.9)

Tuberculosis (A15-A19)

INCLUDES *infections due to Mycobacterium tuberculosis and Mycobacterium bovis*
EXCLUDES1 *congenital tuberculosis (P37.0)*
nonspecific reaction to test for tuberculosis without active tuberculosis (R76.1-)
pneumoconiosis associated with tuberculosis, any type in A15 (J65)
positive PPD (R76.11)
positive tuberculin skin test without active tuberculosis (R76.11)
sequelae of tuberculosis (B90.-)
silicotuberculosis (J65)

Capillary
Macrophage
Inside an alveolus
Ingested bacteria
1. Tubercle bacilli ingested by macrophages but survive inside
2. Inflammation response brings more defensive cells to the area. Alveolar walls damaged by cytokines
Living lymphocytes
Dead macrophages releasing bacteria
3. Tubercle formed with caseous center
4. Tubercle ruptures, bacteria spread to other parts of lungs and other organs

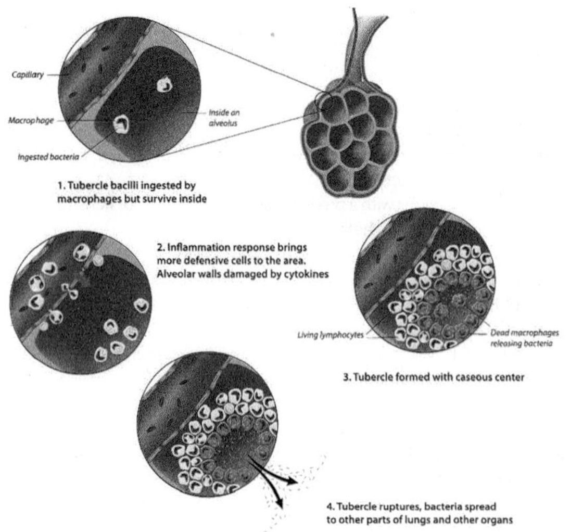

Figure 1.1 Progression of tuberculosis

4th A15 **Respiratory tuberculosis**
A15.0 **Tuberculosis of lung** CC
Tuberculous bronchiectasis
Tuberculous fibrosis of lung
Tuberculous pneumonia
Tuberculous pneumothorax
A15.4 **Tuberculosis of intrathoracic lymph nodes** CC
Tuberculosis of hilar lymph nodes
Tuberculosis of mediastinal lymph nodes
Tuberculosis of tracheobronchial lymph nodes
EXCLUDES1 *tuberculosis specified as primary (A15.7)*
A15.5 **Tuberculosis of larynx, trachea and bronchus** CC
Tuberculosis of bronchus
Tuberculosis of glottis
Tuberculosis of larynx
Tuberculosis of trachea
A15.6 **Tuberculous pleurisy** CC
Tuberculosis of pleura Tuberculous empyema
EXCLUDES1 *primary respiratory tuberculosis (A15.7)*
A15.7 **Primary respiratory tuberculosis** CC
A15.8 **Other respiratory tuberculosis** CC
Mediastinal tuberculosis
Nasopharyngeal tuberculosis
Tuberculosis of nose
Tuberculosis of sinus [any nasal]
A15.9 **Respiratory tuberculosis unspecified** CC

4th A17 **Tuberculosis of nervous system**
A17.0 **Tuberculous meningitis** MCC
Tuberculosis of meninges (cerebral)(spinal)
Tuberculous leptomeningitis
EXCLUDES1 *tuberculous meningoencephalitis (A17.82)*
A17.1 **Meningeal tuberculoma** MCC
Tuberculoma of meninges (cerebral) (spinal)
EXCLUDES2 *tuberculoma of brain and spinal cord (A17.81)*
5th A17.8 **Other tuberculosis of nervous system**
A17.81 **Tuberculoma of brain and spinal cord** MCC
Tuberculous abscess of brain and spinal cord
A17.82 **Tuberculous meningoencephalitis** MCC
Tuberculous myelitis
A17.83 **Tuberculous neuritis** MCC
Tuberculous mononeuropathy

PDx Unacceptable principal diagnosis symbol per Medicare code edits POA Code exempt from diagnosis present on admission requirement
Q Questionable admission CC Complication or comorbidity CC/MCC Exc CC/MCC exclusion MCC Major complication or comorbidity
PDx CC Principal diagnosis as its own CC PDx MCC Principal diagnosis as its own MCC Z1 Z code as first-listed diagnosis

A17.89 **Other tuberculosis of nervous system** MCC
Tuberculous polyneuropathy
A17.9 **Tuberculosis of nervous system, unspecified** CC

A18 **Tuberculosis of other organs**
A18.0 **Tuberculosis of bones and joints**
A18.01 **Tuberculosis of spine** CC
Pott's disease or curvature of spine
Tuberculous arthritis
Tuberculous osteomyelitis of spine
Tuberculous spondylitis
A18.02 **Tuberculous arthritis of other joints** CC
Tuberculosis of hip (joint)
Tuberculosis of knee (joint)
A18.03 **Tuberculosis of other bones** CC
Tuberculous mastoiditis
Tuberculous osteomyelitis
A18.09 **Other musculoskeletal tuberculosis** CC
Tuberculous myositis
Tuberculous synovitis
Tuberculous tenosynovitis
A18.1 **Tuberculosis of genitourinary system**
A18.10 **Tuberculosis of genitourinary system, unspecified** CC
A18.11 **Tuberculosis of kidney and ureter** CC
A18.12 **Tuberculosis of bladder** CC
A18.13 **Tuberculosis of other urinary organs** CC
Tuberculous urethritis
A18.14 **Tuberculosis of prostate** A CC ♂
A18.15 **Tuberculosis of other male genital organs** CC ♂
A18.16 **Tuberculosis of cervix** CC ♀
A18.17 **Tuberculous female pelvic inflammatory disease** CC ♀
Tuberculous endometritis
Tuberculous oophoritis and salpingitis
A18.18 **Tuberculosis of other female genital organs** CC ♀
Tuberculous ulceration of vulva
A18.2 **Tuberculous peripheral lymphadenopathy** CC
Tuberculous adenitis
EXCLUDES2 *tuberculosis of bronchial and mediastinal lymph nodes (A15.4)*
tuberculosis of mesenteric and retroperitoneal lymph nodes (A18.39)
tuberculous tracheobronchial adenopathy (A15.4)
A18.3 **Tuberculosis of intestines, peritoneum and mesenteric glands**
A18.31 **Tuberculous peritonitis** MCC
Tuberculous ascites
A18.32 **Tuberculous enteritis** CC
Tuberculosis of anus and rectum
Tuberculosis of intestine (large) (small)
A18.39 **Retroperitoneal tuberculosis** CC
Tuberculosis of mesenteric glands
Tuberculosis of retroperitoneal (lymph glands)
A18.4 **Tuberculosis of skin and subcutaneous tissue** CC
Erythema induratum, tuberculous
Lupus exedens
Lupus vulgaris NOS
Lupus vulgaris of eyelid
Scrofuloderma
Tuberculosis of external ear
EXCLUDES2 *lupus erythematosus (L93.-)*
lupus NOS (M32.9)
systemic (M32.-)
A18.5 **Tuberculosis of eye**
EXCLUDES2 *lupus vulgaris of eyelid (A18.4)*
A18.50 **Tuberculosis of eye, unspecified** CC
A18.51 **Tuberculous episcleritis** CC
A18.52 **Tuberculous keratitis** CC
Tuberculous interstitial keratitis
Tuberculous keratoconjunctivitis (interstitial) (phlyctenular)
A18.53 **Tuberculous chorioretinitis** CC
A18.54 **Tuberculous iridocyclitis** CC
A18.59 **Other tuberculosis of eye** CC
Tuberculous conjunctivitis
A18.6 **Tuberculosis of (inner) (middle) ear** CC
Tuberculous otitis media
EXCLUDES2 *tuberculosis of external ear (A18.4)*
tuberculous mastoiditis (A18.03)
A18.7 **Tuberculosis of adrenal glands** CC
Tuberculous Addison's disease
A18.8 **Tuberculosis of other specified organs**
A18.81 **Tuberculosis of thyroid gland** CC
A18.82 **Tuberculosis of other endocrine glands** CC
Tuberculosis of pituitary gland
Tuberculosis of thymus gland
A18.83 **Tuberculosis of digestive tract organs, not elsewhere classified** CC
EXCLUDES1 *tuberculosis of intestine (A18.32)*
A18.84 **Tuberculosis of heart** CC
Tuberculous cardiomyopathy
Tuberculous endocarditis
Tuberculous myocarditis
Tuberculous pericarditis
A18.85 **Tuberculosis of spleen** CC
A18.89 **Tuberculosis of other sites** CC
Tuberculosis of muscle
Tuberculous cerebral arteritis

A19 **Miliary tuberculosis**
INCLUDES *disseminated tuberculosis*
generalized tuberculosis
tuberculous polyserositis
A19.0 **Acute miliary tuberculosis of a single specified site** MCC
A19.1 **Acute miliary tuberculosis of multiple sites** MCC
A19.2 **Acute miliary tuberculosis, unspecified** MCC
A19.8 **Other miliary tuberculosis** MCC
A19.9 **Miliary tuberculosis, unspecified** MCC

Certain zoonotic bacterial diseases (A20-A28)

A20 **Plague**
INCLUDES *infection due to Yersinia pestis*
A20.0 **Bubonic plague** MCC
A20.1 **Cellulocutaneous plague** MCC
A20.2 **Pneumonic plague** MCC
A20.3 **Plague meningitis** MCC
A20.7 **Septicemic plague** MCC
A20.8 **Other forms of plague** MCC
Abortive plague
Asymptomatic plague
Pestis minor
A20.9 **Plague, unspecified** MCC

A21 **Tularemia**
INCLUDES *deer-fly fever*
infection due to Francisella tularensis
rabbit fever
A21.0 **Ulceroglandular tularemia** CC
A21.1 **Oculoglandular tularemia** CC
Ophthalmic tularemia
A21.2 **Pulmonary tularemia** CC
A21.3 **Gastrointestinal tularemia** CC
Abdominal tularemia
A21.7 **Generalized tularemia** CC
A21.8 **Other forms of tularemia** CC
A21.9 **Tularemia, unspecified** CC

A22 **Anthrax**
INCLUDES *infection due to Bacillus anthracis*
A22.0 **Cutaneous anthrax** CC
Malignant carbuncle
Malignant pustule
A22.1 **Pulmonary anthrax** MCC
Inhalation anthrax
Ragpicker's disease
Woolsorter's disease
A22.2 **Gastrointestinal anthrax** CC
A22.7 **Anthrax sepsis** MCC PDx MCC
A22.8 **Other forms of anthrax** CC
Anthrax meningitis
A22.9 **Anthrax, unspecified** CC

Unspecified Code | Other Specified Code | Manifestation Code | N Newborn | P Pediatric | M Maternity | A Adult | ♂ Male | ♀ Female
● New Code | ▲ Revised Code Title | ►◄ Revised Text | NOTES | INCLUDES | EXCLUDES1 Not coded here | EXCLUDES2 Not included here
4th character required | 5th character required | 6th character required | 7th character required
Extension 'X' Alert | HAC Hospital-acquired condition (HAC) alert | AHA AHA Coding Clinic®

When symbols appear on a code that requires a 7th character extension, refer to Appendix D to identify applicable 7th character codes.

A23 Brucellosis
INCLUDES *Malta fever*
Mediterranean fever
undulant fever
A23.0 **Brucellosis due to Brucella melitensis**
A23.1 **Brucellosis due to Brucella abortus**
A23.2 **Brucellosis due to Brucella suis**
A23.3 **Brucellosis due to Brucella canis**
A23.8 **Other brucellosis** CC
A23.9 **Brucellosis, unspecified** CC
A24 Glanders and melioidosis
A24.0 **Glanders** CC
Infection due to Pseudomonas mallei
Malleus
A24.1 **Acute and fulminating melioidosis** CC
Melioidosis pneumonia
Melioidosis sepsis
A24.2 **Subacute and chronic melioidosis** CC
A24.3 **Other melioidosis** CC
A24.9 **Melioidosis, unspecified** CC
Infection due to Pseudomonas pseudomallei NOS
Whitmore's disease
A25 Rat-bite fevers
A25.0 **Spirillosis** CC
Sodoku
A25.1 **Streptobacillosis** CC
Epidemic arthritic erythema
Haverhill fever
Streptobacillary rat-bite fever
A25.9 **Rat-bite fever, unspecified** CC
A26 Erysipeloid
A26.0 **Cutaneous erysipeloid**
Erythema migrans
A26.7 **Erysipelothrix sepsis** MCC PDx MCC
A26.8 **Other forms of erysipeloid**
A26.9 **Erysipeloid, unspecified**
A27 Leptospirosis
A27.0 **Leptospirosis icterohemorrhagica** CC
Leptospiral or spirochetal jaundice (hemorrhagic)
Weil's disease
A27.8 **Other forms of leptospirosis**
A27.81 **Aseptic meningitis in leptospirosis** MCC
A27.89 **Other forms of leptospirosis** CC
A27.9 **Leptospirosis, unspecified** CC
A28 Other zoonotic bacterial diseases, not elsewhere classified
A28.0 **Pasteurellosis** CC
A28.1 **Cat-scratch disease** CC
Cat-scratch fever
A28.2 **Extraintestinal yersiniosis** CC
EXCLUDES1 *enteritis due to Yersinia enterocolitica (A04.6)*
plague (A20.-)
A28.8 **Other specified zoonotic bacterial diseases, not elsewhere classified** CC
A28.9 **Zoonotic bacterial disease, unspecified** CC

Other bacterial diseases (A30-A49)

A30 Leprosy [Hansen's disease]
INCLUDES *infection due to Mycobacterium leprae*
EXCLUDES1 *sequelae of leprosy (B92)*
A30.0 **Indeterminate leprosy** CC
I leprosy
A30.1 **Tuberculoid leprosy** CC
TT leprosy
A30.2 **Borderline tuberculoid leprosy** CC
BT leprosy
A30.3 **Borderline leprosy** CC
BB leprosy
A30.4 **Borderline lepromatous leprosy** CC
BL leprosy
A30.5 **Lepromatous leprosy** CC
LL leprosy
A30.8 **Other forms of leprosy** CC
A30.9 **Leprosy, unspecified** CC
A31 Infection due to other mycobacteria
EXCLUDES2 *leprosy (A30.-)*
tuberculosis (A15-A19)
A31.0 **Pulmonary mycobacterial infection** CC
Infection due to Mycobacterium avium
Infection due to Mycobacterium intracellulare [Battey bacillus]
Infection due to Mycobacterium kansasii
A31.1 **Cutaneous mycobacterial infection** CC
Buruli ulcer
Infection due to Mycobacterium marinum
Infection due to Mycobacterium ulcerans
A31.2 **Disseminated mycobacterium avium-intracellulare complex (DMAC)** CC
MAC sepsis
A31.8 **Other mycobacterial infections** CC
A31.9 **Mycobacterial infection, unspecified** CC
Atypical mycobacterial infection NOS
Mycobacteriosis NOS
A32 Listeriosis
INCLUDES *listerial food-borne infection*
EXCLUDES1 *neonatal (disseminated) listeriosis (P37.2)*
A32.0 **Cutaneous listeriosis** CC
A32.1 **Listerial meningitis and meningoencephalitis**
A32.11 **Listerial meningitis** CC
A32.12 **Listerial meningoencephalitis** CC
A32.7 **Listerial sepsis** MCC PDx MCC
A32.8 **Other forms of listeriosis**
A32.81 **Oculoglandular listeriosis** CC
A32.82 **Listerial endocarditis** CC
A32.89 **Other forms of listeriosis** CC
Listerial cerebral arteritis
A32.9 **Listeriosis, unspecified** CC
A33 **Tetanus neonatorum** N MCC
A34 **Obstetrical tetanus** M CC ♀
A35 **Other tetanus** MCC
Tetanus NOS
EXCLUDES1 *obstetrical tetanus (A34)*
tetanus neonatorum (A33)
A36 Diphtheria
A36.0 **Pharyngeal diphtheria** CC
Diphtheritic membranous angina
Tonsillar diphtheria
A36.1 **Nasopharyngeal diphtheria** CC
A36.2 **Laryngeal diphtheria** CC
Diphtheritic laryngotracheitis
A36.3 **Cutaneous diphtheria** CC
EXCLUDES2 *erythrasma (L08.1)*
A36.8 **Other diphtheria**
A36.81 **Diphtheritic cardiomyopathy** CC
Diphtheritic myocarditis
A36.82 **Diphtheritic radiculomyelitis** CC
A36.83 **Diphtheritic polyneuritis** CC
A36.84 **Diphtheritic tubulo-interstitial nephropathy** CC
A36.85 **Diphtheritic cystitis** CC
A36.86 **Diphtheritic conjunctivitis** CC
A36.89 **Other diphtheritic complications** CC
Diphtheritic peritonitis
A36.9 **Diphtheria, unspecified** CC
A37 Whooping cough
A37.0 **Whooping cough due to Bordetella pertussis**
A37.00 **Whooping cough due to Bordetella pertussis without pneumonia** CC
A37.01 **Whooping cough due to Bordetella pertussis with pneumonia** MCC PDx MCC
A37.1 **Whooping cough due to Bordetella parapertussis**
A37.10 **Whooping cough due to Bordetella parapertussis without pneumonia** CC
A37.11 **Whooping cough due to Bordetella parapertussis with pneumonia** MCC PDx MCC
A37.8 **Whooping cough due to other Bordetella species**
A37.80 **Whooping cough due to other Bordetella species without pneumonia** CC

PDx Unacceptable principal diagnosis symbol per Medicare code edits | POA Code exempt from diagnosis present on admission requirement
? Questionable admission | CC Complication or comorbidity | CC/MCC Exc CC/MCC exclusion | MCC Major complication or comorbidity
PDx CC Principal diagnosis as its own CC | PDx MCC Principal diagnosis as its own MCC | Z Z code as first-listed diagnosis

 When symbols appear on a code that requires a 7th character extension, refer to Appendix D to identify applicable 7th character codes.

A37.81 **Whooping cough due to other Bordetella species with pneumonia** MCC PDx MCC

A37.9 **Whooping cough, unspecified species**

A37.90 **Whooping cough, unspecified species without pneumonia** CC

A37.91 **Whooping cough, unspecified species with pneumonia** MCC PDx MCC

A38 **Scarlet fever**

INCLUDES *scarlatina*

EXCLUDES2 *streptococcal sore throat (J02.0)*

A38.0 **Scarlet fever** with otitis media CC

A38.1 **Scarlet fever** with myocarditis CC

A38.8 **Scarlet fever** with other complications CC

A38.9 **Scarlet fever,** uncomplicated CC

Scarlet fever, NOS

A39 Meningococcal **infection**

A39.0 **Meningococcal** meningitis MCC

A39.1 **Waterhouse-Friderichsen syndrome** MCC

Meningococcal hemorrhagic adrenalitis

Meningococcic adrenal syndrome

A39.2 Acute **meningococcemia** MCC

A39.3 Chronic **meningococcemia** MCC

A39.4 **Meningococcemia, unspecified** MCC

A39.5 **Meningococcal** heart disease

A39.50 **Meningococcal carditis, unspecified** MCC

A39.51 **Meningococcal** endocarditis MCC

A39.52 **Meningococcal** myocarditis MCC

A39.53 **Meningococcal** pericarditis MCC

A39.8 **Other meningococcal infections**

A39.81 **Meningococcal** encephalitis MCC

A39.82 **Meningococcal** retrobulbar neuritis CC

A39.83 **Meningococcal** arthritis CC

A39.84 Postmeningococcal **arthritis** CC

A39.89 **Other meningococcal infections** CC

Meningococcal conjunctivitis

A39.9 **Meningococcal infection, unspecified** CC

Meningococcal disease NOS

A40 **Streptococcal** sepsis

Code first postprocedural streptococcal sepsis (▶T81.4-◀)

streptococcal sepsis during labor (O75.3)

streptococcal sepsis following abortion or ectopic or molar pregnancy (O03-O07, O08.0)

streptococcal sepsis following immunization (T88.0)

streptococcal sepsis following infusion, transfusion or therapeutic injection (T80.2-)

EXCLUDES1 *neonatal (P36.0-P36.1)*

puerperal sepsis (O85)

sepsis due to Streptococcus, group D (A41.81)

A40.0 **Sepsis due to streptococcus,** group A MCC

A40.1 **Sepsis due to streptococcus,** group B MCC

A40.3 **Sepsis due to Streptococcus** pneumoniae MCC

Pneumococcal sepsis

A40.8 **Other streptococcal sepsis** MCC

A40.9 **Streptococcal sepsis, unspecified** MCC

A41 Other **sepsis**

Code first postprocedural sepsis (▶T81.4-◀)

sepsis during labor (O75.3)

sepsis following abortion, ectopic or molar pregnancy (O03-O07, O08.0)

sepsis following immunization (T88.0)

sepsis following infusion, transfusion or therapeutic injection (T80.2-)

EXCLUDES1 *bacteremia NOS (R78.81)*

neonatal (P36.-)

puerperal sepsis (O85)

streptococcal sepsis (A40.-)

EXCLUDES2 *sepsis (due to) (in) actinomycotic (A42.7)*

sepsis (due to) (in) anthrax (A22.7)

sepsis (due to) (in) candidal (B37.7)

sepsis (due to) (in) Erysipelothrix (A26.7)

sepsis (due to) (in) extraintestinal yersiniosis (A28.2)

sepsis (due to) (in) gonococcal (A54.86)

sepsis (due to) (in) herpesviral (B00.7)

sepsis (due to) (in) listerial (A32.7)

sepsis (due to) (in) melioidosis (A24.1)

sepsis (due to) (in) meningococcal (A39.2-A39.4)

sepsis (due to) (in) plague (A20.7)

sepsis (due to) (in) tularemia (A21.7)

toxic shock syndrome (A48.3)

AHA: Q1, 2016

A41.0 **Sepsis** due to Staphylococcus aureus

A41.01 **Sepsis due to** Methicillin susceptible **Staphylococcus aureus** MCC

MSSA sepsis

Staphylococcus aureus sepsis NOS

A41.02 **Sepsis due to** Methicillin resistant **Staphylococcus aureus** MCC

A41.1 **Sepsis due to other specified staphylococcus** MCC

Coagulase negative staphylococcus sepsis

A41.2 **Sepsis due to unspecified staphylococcus** MCC

A41.3 **Sepsis** due to Haemophilus influenzae MCC

A41.4 **Sepsis** due to anaerobes MCC

EXCLUDES1 *gas gangrene (A48.0)*

A41.5 **Sepsis due to** other Gram-negative organisms

A41.50 **Gram-negative sepsis, unspecified** MCC

Gram-negative sepsis NOS

A41.51 **Sepsis due to** Escherichia **coli [E. coli]** MCC

A41.52 **Sepsis due to** Pseudomonas MCC

Pseudomonas aeruginosa

A41.53 **Sepsis due to** Serratia MCC

A41.59 **Other Gram-negative sepsis** MCC

A41.8 **Other specified sepsis**

A41.81 **Sepsis due to** Enterococcus MCC

A41.89 **Other specified sepsis** MCC

A41.9 **Sepsis, unspecified organism** MCC

Septicemia NOS

A42 **Actinomycosis**

EXCLUDES1 *actinomycetoma (B47.1)*

A42.0 Pulmonary **actinomycosis** CC

A42.1 Abdominal **actinomycosis** CC

A42.2 Cervicofacial **actinomycosis** CC

A42.7 **Actinomycotic** sepsis MCC

A42.8 **Other forms of actinomycosis**

A42.81 **Actinomycotic** meningitis CC

A42.82 **Actinomycotic** encephalitis CC

A42.89 **Other forms of actinomycosis** CC

A42.9 **Actinomycosis, unspecified** CC

A43 **Nocardiosis**

A43.0 Pulmonary **nocardiosis** CC

A43.1 Cutaneous **nocardiosis** CC

A43.8 Other forms **of nocardiosis** CC

A43.9 **Nocardiosis, unspecified** CC

A44 **Bartonellosis**

A44.0 Systemic **bartonellosis** CC

Oroya fever

A44.1 Cutaneous and mucocutaneous **bartonellosis** CC

Verruga peruana

A44.8 Other forms **of bartonellosis** CC

A44.9 **Bartonellosis, unspecified** CC

A46 **Erysipelas**

EXCLUDES1 *postpartum or puerperal erysipelas (O86.89)*

A48 **Other bacterial diseases, not elsewhere classified**

EXCLUDES1 *actinomycetoma (B47.1)*

A48.0 **Gas gangrene** MCC

Clostridial cellulitis

Clostridial myonecrosis

A48.1 **Legionnaires' disease** MCC

A48.2 **Nonpneumonic Legionnaires' disease [Pontiac fever]**

A48.3 **Toxic shock syndrome** MCC

Use additional code to identify the organism (B95, B96)

EXCLUDES1 *endotoxic shock NOS (R57.8)*

sepsis NOS (A41.9)

A48.4 **Brazilian purpuric fever**

Systemic Haemophilus aegyptius infection

Unspecified Code | Other Specified Code | Manifestation Code | N Newborn | P Pediatric | M Maternity | A Adult | ♂ Male | ♀ Female
● New Code ▲ Revised Code Title ▶◀ Revised Text NOTES INCLUDES EXCLUDES1 Not coded here EXCLUDES2 Not included here
4th character required 5th character required 6th character required 7th character required
Extension 'X' Alert HAC Hospital-acquired condition (HAC) alert AHA AHA Coding Clinic®

A48.5 Other specified botulism
Non-food-borne intoxication due to toxins of Clostridium botulinum [C. botulinum]
EXCLUDES1 *food poisoning due to toxins of Clostridium botulinum (A05.1)*
A48.51 Infant botulism
A48.52 Wound botulism
Non-food-borne botulism NOS
Use additional code for associated wound
A48.8 Other specified bacterial diseases

A49 Bacterial infection of unspecified site
EXCLUDES1 *bacterial agents as the cause of diseases classified elsewhere (B95-B96)*
chlamydial infection NOS (A74.9)
meningococcal infection NOS (A39.9)
rickettsial infection NOS (A79.9)
spirochetal infection NOS (A69.9)

A49.0 Staphylococcal infection, unspecified site
A49.01 Methicillin susceptible Staphylococcus aureus infection, unspecified site
Methicillin susceptible Staphylococcus aureus (MSSA) infection
Staphylococcus aureus infection NOS
A49.02 Methicillin resistant Staphylococcus aureus infection, unspecified site
Methicillin resistant Staphylococcus aureus (MRSA) infection
A49.1 Streptococcal infection, unspecified site
A49.2 Haemophilus influenzae infection, unspecified site
A49.3 Mycoplasma infection, unspecified site
A49.8 Other bacterial infections of unspecified site
A49.9 Bacterial infection, unspecified
EXCLUDES1 *bacteremia NOS (R78.81)*

Infections with a predominantly sexual mode of transmission (A50-A64)

EXCLUDES1 *human immunodeficiency virus [HIV] disease (B20)*
nonspecific and nongonococcal urethritis (N34.1)
Reiter's disease (M02.3-)

A50 Congenital syphilis

A50.0 Early congenital syphilis, symptomatic
Any congenital syphilitic condition specified as early or manifest less than two years after birth.
A50.01 Early congenital syphilitic oculopathy
A50.02 Early congenital syphilitic osteochondropathy
A50.03 Early congenital syphilitic pharyngitis
Early congenital syphilitic laryngitis
A50.04 Early congenital syphilitic pneumonia
A50.05 Early congenital syphilitic rhinitis
A50.06 Early cutaneous congenital syphilis
A50.07 Early mucocutaneous congenital syphilis
A50.08 Early visceral congenital syphilis
A50.09 Other early congenital syphilis, symptomatic
A50.1 Early congenital syphilis, latent
Congenital syphilis without clinical manifestations, with positive serological reaction and negative spinal fluid test, less than two years after birth.
A50.2 Early congenital syphilis, unspecified
Congenital syphilis NOS less than two years after birth.

A50.3 Late congenital syphilitic oculopathy
EXCLUDES1 *Hutchinson's triad (A50.53)*
A50.30 Late congenital syphilitic oculopathy, unspecified
A50.31 Late congenital syphilitic interstitial keratitis
A50.32 Late congenital syphilitic chorioretinitis
A50.39 Other late congenital syphilitic oculopathy

A50.4 Late congenital neurosyphilis [juvenile neurosyphilis]
Use additional code to identify any associated mental disorder
EXCLUDES1 *Hutchinson's triad (A50.53)*
A50.40 Late congenital neurosyphilis, unspecified
Juvenile neurosyphilis NOS
A50.41 Late congenital syphilitic meningitis
A50.42 Late congenital syphilitic encephalitis
A50.43 Late congenital syphilitic polyneuropathy
A50.44 Late congenital syphilitic optic nerve atrophy
A50.45 Juvenile general paresis
Dementia paralytica juvenilis
Juvenile tabetoparetic neurosyphilis
A50.49 Other late congenital neurosyphilis
Juvenile tabes dorsalis

A50.5 Other late congenital syphilis, symptomatic
Any congenital syphilitic condition specified as late or manifest two years or more after birth.
A50.51 Clutton's joints
A50.52 Hutchinson's teeth
A50.53 Hutchinson's triad
A50.54 Late congenital cardiovascular syphilis
A50.55 Late congenital syphilitic arthropathy
A50.56 Late congenital syphilitic osteochondropathy
A50.57 Syphilitic saddle nose
A50.59 Other late congenital syphilis, symptomatic
A50.6 Late congenital syphilis, latent
Congenital syphilis without clinical manifestations, with positive serological reaction and negative spinal fluid test, two years or more after birth.
A50.7 Late congenital syphilis, unspecified
Congenital syphilis NOS two years or more after birth.
A50.9 Congenital syphilis, unspecified

A51 Early syphilis
A51.0 Primary genital syphilis
Syphilitic chancre NOS
A51.1 Primary anal syphilis
A51.2 Primary syphilis of other sites

A51.3 Secondary syphilis of skin and mucous membranes
A51.31 Condyloma latum
A51.32 Syphilitic alopecia
A51.39 Other secondary syphilis of skin
Syphilitic leukoderma
Syphilitic mucous patch
EXCLUDES1 *late syphilitic leukoderma (A52.79)*

A51.4 Other secondary syphilis
A51.41 Secondary syphilitic meningitis
A51.42 Secondary syphilitic female pelvic disease
A51.43 Secondary syphilitic oculopathy
Secondary syphilitic chorioretinitis
Secondary syphilitic iridocyclitis, iritis
Secondary syphilitic uveitis
A51.44 Secondary syphilitic nephritis
A51.45 Secondary syphilitic hepatitis
A51.46 Secondary syphilitic osteopathy
A51.49 Other secondary syphilitic conditions
Secondary syphilitic lymphadenopathy
Secondary syphilitic myositis
A51.5 Early syphilis, latent
Syphilis (acquired) without clinical manifestations, with positive serological reaction and negative spinal fluid test, less than two years after infection.
A51.9 Early syphilis, unspecified

A52 Late syphilis

A52.0 Cardiovascular and cerebrovascular syphilis
A52.00 Cardiovascular syphilis, unspecified
A52.01 Syphilitic aneurysm of aorta
A52.02 Syphilitic aortitis
A52.03 Syphilitic endocarditis
Syphilitic aortic valve incompetence or stenosis
Syphilitic mitral valve stenosis
Syphilitic pulmonary valve regurgitation
A52.04 Syphilitic cerebral arteritis

Unacceptable principal diagnosis symbol per Medicare code edits; Code exempt from diagnosis present on admission requirement; Questionable admission; Complication or comorbidity; CC/MCC exclusion; Major complication or comorbidity; Principal diagnosis as its own CC; Principal diagnosis as its own MCC; Z code as first-listed diagnosis

 When symbols appear on a code that requires a 7th character extension, refer to Appendix D to identify applicable 7th character codes.

A52.05 Other cerebrovascular syphilis CC
Syphilitic cerebral aneurysm (ruptured) (non-ruptured)
Syphilitic cerebral thrombosis
A52.06 Other syphilitic heart involvement CC
Syphilitic coronary artery disease
Syphilitic myocarditis
Syphilitic pericarditis
A52.09 Other cardiovascular syphilis CC
A52.1 Symptomatic neurosyphilis
A52.10 Symptomatic neurosyphilis, unspecified CC
A52.11 Tabes dorsalis CC
Locomotor ataxia (progressive)
Tabetic neurosyphilis
A52.12 Other cerebrospinal syphilis CC
A52.13 Late syphilitic meningitis MCC
A52.14 Late syphilitic encephalitis MCC
A52.15 Late syphilitic neuropathy CC
Late syphilitic acoustic neuritis
Late syphilitic optic (nerve) atrophy
Late syphilitic polyneuropathy
Late syphilitic retrobulbar neuritis
A52.16 Charcôt's arthropathy (tabetic) CC
A52.17 General paresis CC
Dementia paralytica
A52.19 Other symptomatic neurosyphilis CC
Syphilitic parkinsonism
A52.2 Asymptomatic neurosyphilis CC
A52.3 Neurosyphilis, unspecified CC
Gumma (syphilitic)
Syphilis (late)
Syphiloma
A52.7 Other symptomatic late syphilis
A52.71 Late syphilitic oculopathy CC
Late syphilitic chorioretinitis
Late syphilitic episcleritis
A52.72 Syphilis of lung and bronchus CC
A52.73 Symptomatic late syphilis of other respiratory organs CC
A52.74 Syphilis of liver and other viscera CC
Late syphilitic peritonitis
A52.75 Syphilis of kidney and ureter CC
Syphilitic glomerular disease
A52.76 Other genitourinary symptomatic late syphilis CC
Late syphilitic female pelvic inflammatory disease
A52.77 Syphilis of bone and joint CC
A52.78 Syphilis of other musculoskeletal tissue CC
Late syphilitic bursitis
Syphilis [stage unspecified] of bursa
Syphilis [stage unspecified] of muscle
Syphilis [stage unspecified] of synovium
Syphilis [stage unspecified] of tendon
A52.79 Other symptomatic late syphilis CC
Late syphilitic leukoderma
Syphilis of adrenal gland
Syphilis of pituitary gland
Syphilis of thyroid gland
Syphilitic splenomegaly
EXCLUDES1 *syphilitic leukoderma (secondary) (A51.39)*
A52.8 Late syphilis, latent
Syphilis (acquired) without clinical manifestations, with positive serological reaction and negative spinal fluid test, two years or more after infection
A52.9 Late syphilis, unspecified
A53 Other and unspecified syphilis
A53.0 Latent syphilis, unspecified as early or late
Latent syphilis NOS
Positive serological reaction for syphilis
A53.9 Syphilis, unspecified
Infection due to Treponema pallidum NOS
Syphilis (acquired) NOS
EXCLUDES1 *syphilis NOS under two years of age (A50.2)*
A54 Gonococcal infection
A54.0 Gonococcal infection of lower genitourinary tract without periurethral or accessory gland abscess
EXCLUDES1 *gonococcal infection with genitourinary gland abscess (A54.1)*
gonococcal infection with periurethral abscess (A54.1)
A54.00 Gonococcal infection of lower genitourinary tract, unspecified CC
A54.01 Gonococcal cystitis and urethritis, unspecified CC
A54.02 Gonococcal vulvovaginitis, unspecified CC ♀
A54.03 Gonococcal cervicitis, unspecified CC ♀
A54.09 Other gonococcal infection of lower genitourinary tract CC
A54.1 Gonococcal infection of lower genitourinary tract with periurethral and accessory gland abscess CC
Gonococcal Bartholin's gland abscess
A54.2 Gonococcal pelviperitonitis and other gonococcal genitourinary infection
A54.21 Gonococcal infection of kidney and ureter CC
A54.22 Gonococcal prostatitis CC ♂
A54.23 Gonococcal infection of other male genital organs CC ♂
Gonococcal epididymitis
Gonococcal orchitis
A54.24 Gonococcal female pelvic inflammatory disease CC ♀
Gonococcal pelviperitonitis
EXCLUDES1 *gonococcal peritonitis (A54.85)*
A54.29 Other gonococcal genitourinary infections CC
A54.3 Gonococcal infection of eye
A54.30 Gonococcal infection of eye, unspecified CC
A54.31 Gonococcal conjunctivitis CC
Ophthalmia neonatorum due to gonococcus
A54.32 Gonococcal iridocyclitis CC
A54.33 Gonococcal keratitis CC
A54.39 Other gonococcal eye infection CC
Gonococcal endophthalmia
A54.4 Gonococcal infection of musculoskeletal system
A54.40 Gonococcal infection of musculoskeletal system, unspecified CC
A54.41 Gonococcal spondylopathy CC
A54.42 Gonococcal arthritis CC
EXCLUDES2 *gonococcal infection of spine (A54.41)*
A54.43 Gonococcal osteomyelitis CC
EXCLUDES2 *gonococcal infection of spine (A54.41)*
A54.49 Gonococcal infection of other musculoskeletal tissue CC
Gonococcal bursitis
Gonococcal myositis
Gonococcal synovitis
Gonococcal tenosynovitis
A54.5 Gonococcal pharyngitis
A54.6 Gonococcal infection of anus and rectum
A54.8 Other gonococcal infections
A54.81 Gonococcal meningitis MCC
A54.82 Gonococcal brain abscess CC
A54.83 Gonococcal heart infection CC
Gonococcal endocarditis
Gonococcal myocarditis
Gonococcal pericarditis
A54.84 Gonococcal pneumonia CC
A54.85 Gonococcal peritonitis CC
EXCLUDES1 *gonococcal pelviperitonitis (A54.24)*
A54.86 Gonococcal sepsis MCC PDx MCC
A54.89 Other gonococcal infections CC
Gonococcal keratoderma
Gonococcal lymphadenitis
A54.9 Gonococcal infection, unspecified CC
A55 Chlamydial lymphogranuloma (venereum)
Climatic or tropical bubo
Durand-Nicolas-Favre disease
Esthiomene
Lymphogranuloma inguinale
A56 Other sexually transmitted chlamydial diseases
INCLUDES *sexually transmitted diseases due to Chlamydia trachomatis*

Unspecified Code | Other Specified Code | Manifestation Code | N Newborn | P Pediatric | M Maternity | A Adult | ♂ Male | ♀ Female
● New Code | ▲ Revised Code Title | ►◄ Revised Text | NOTES | INCLUDES | EXCLUDES1 Not coded here | EXCLUDES2 Not included here
4th character required | 5th character required | 6th character required | 7th character required
Extension 'X' Alert | HAC Hospital-acquired condition (HAC) alert | AHA AHA Coding Clinic©

EXCLUDES1 *neonatal chlamydial conjunctivitis (P39.1)*
neonatal chlamydial pneumonia (P23.1)
EXCLUDES2 *chlamydial lymphogranuloma (A55)*
conditions classified to A74.-

A56.0 Chlamydial infection of lower genitourinary tract
- **A56.00 Chlamydial infection of lower genitourinary tract, unspecified**
- **A56.01 Chlamydial cystitis and urethritis**
- **A56.02 Chlamydial vulvovaginitis** ♀
- **A56.09 Other chlamydial infection of lower genitourinary tract**
  Chlamydial cervicitis

A56.1 Chlamydial infection of pelviperitoneum and other genitourinary organs
- **A56.11 Chlamydial female pelvic inflammatory disease** ♀
- **A56.19 Other chlamydial genitourinary infection**
  Chlamydial epididymitis
  Chlamydial orchitis

A56.2 Chlamydial infection of genitourinary tract, unspecified
A56.3 Chlamydial infection of anus and rectum
A56.4 Chlamydial infection of pharynx
A56.8 Sexually transmitted chlamydial infection of other sites

A57 Chancroid
Ulcus molle

A58 Granuloma inguinale
Donovanosis

A59 Trichomoniasis
EXCLUDES2 *intestinal trichomoniasis (A07.8)*

A59.0 Urogenital trichomoniasis
- **A59.00 Urogenital trichomoniasis, unspecified**
  Fluor (vaginalis) due to Trichomonas
  Leukorrhea (vaginalis) due to Trichomonas
- **A59.01 Trichomonal vulvovaginitis** ♀
- **A59.02 Trichomonal prostatitis** ♂
- **A59.03 Trichomonal cystitis and urethritis**
- **A59.09 Other urogenital trichomoniasis**
  Trichomonas cervicitis

A59.8 Trichomoniasis of other sites
A59.9 Trichomoniasis, unspecified

A60 Anogenital herpesviral [herpes simplex] infections

A60.0 Herpesviral infection of genitalia and urogenital tract
- **A60.00 Herpesviral infection of urogenital system, unspecified**
- **A60.01 Herpesviral infection of penis** ♂
- **A60.02 Herpesviral infection of other male genital organs** ♂
- **A60.03 Herpesviral cervicitis** ♀
- **A60.04 Herpesviral vulvovaginitis** ♀
  Herpesviral [herpes simplex] ulceration
  Herpesviral [herpes simplex] vaginitis
  Herpesviral [herpes simplex] vulvitis
- **A60.09 Herpesviral infection of other urogenital tract**

A60.1 Herpesviral infection of perianal skin and rectum
A60.9 Anogenital herpesviral infection, unspecified

A63 Other predominantly sexually transmitted diseases, not elsewhere classified
EXCLUDES2 *molluscum contagiosum (B08.1)*
papilloma of cervix (D26.0)

A63.0 Anogenital (venereal) warts
Anogenital warts due to (human) papillomavirus [HPV]
Condyloma acuminatum
A63.8 Other specified predominantly sexually transmitted diseases

A64 Unspecified sexually transmitted disease

Other spirochetal diseases (A65-A69)

EXCLUDES2 *leptospirosis (A27.-)*
syphilis (A50-A53)

A65 Nonvenereal syphilis
Bejel
Endemic syphilis
Njovera

A66 Yaws
INCLUDES *bouba*
frambesia (tropica)
pian

A66.0 Initial lesions of yaws
Chancre of yaws
Frambesia, initial or primary
Initial frambesial ulcer
Mother yaw

A66.1 Multiple papillomata and wet crab yaws
Frambesioma
Pianoma
Plantar or palmar papilloma of yaws

A66.2 Other early skin lesions of yaws
Cutaneous yaws, less than five years after infection
Early yaws (cutaneous)(macular)(maculopapular)(micropapular)(papular)
Frambeside of early yaws

A66.3 Hyperkeratosis of yaws
Ghoul hand
Hyperkeratosis, palmar or plantar (early) (late) due to yaws
Worm-eaten soles

A66.4 Gummata and ulcers of yaws
Gummatous frambeside
Nodular late yaws (ulcerated)

A66.5 Gangosa
Rhinopharyngitis mutilans

A66.6 Bone and joint lesions of yaws
Yaws ganglion
Yaws goundou
Yaws gumma, bone
Yaws gummatous osteitis or periostitis
Yaws hydrarthrosis
Yaws osteitis
Yaws periostitis (hypertrophic)

A66.7 Other manifestations of yaws
Juxta-articular nodules of yaws
Mucosal yaws

A66.8 Latent yaws
Yaws without clinical manifestations, with positive serology

A66.9 Yaws, unspecified

A67 Pinta [carate]

A67.0 Primary lesions of pinta
Chancre (primary) of pinta
Papule (primary) of pinta

A67.1 Intermediate lesions of pinta
Erythematous plaques of pinta
Hyperchromic lesions of pinta
Hyperkeratosis of pinta
Pintids

A67.2 Late lesions of pinta
Achromic skin lesions of pinta
Cicatricial skin lesions of pinta
Dyschromic skin lesions of pinta

A67.3 Mixed lesions of pinta
Achromic with hyperchromic skin lesions of pinta [carate]

A67.9 Pinta, unspecified

A68 Relapsing fevers
INCLUDES *recurrent fever*
EXCLUDES2 *Lyme disease (A69.2-)*

A68.0 Louse-borne relapsing fever CC
Relapsing fever due to Borrelia recurrentis

A68.1 Tick-borne relapsing fever CC
Relapsing fever due to any Borrelia species other than Borrelia recurrentis

A68.9 Relapsing fever, unspecified CC

A69 Other spirochetal infections

A69.0 Necrotizing ulcerative stomatitis
Cancrum oris
Fusospirochetal gangrene
Noma
Stomatitis gangrenosa

A69.1 Other Vincent's infections CC
Fusospirochetal pharyngitis
Necrotizing ulcerative (acute) gingivitis
Necrotizing ulcerative (acute) gingivostomatitis
Spirochetal stomatitis
Trench mouth
Vincent's angina
Vincent's gingivitis

Unacceptable principal diagnosis symbol per Medicare code edits | Code exempt from diagnosis present on admission requirement
Questionable admission | Complication or comorbidity | CC/MCC exclusion | Major complication or comorbidity
Principal diagnosis as its own CC | Principal diagnosis as its own MCC | Z code as first-listed diagnosis

When symbols appear on a code that requires a 7th character extension, refer to Appendix D to identify applicable 7th character codes.

A69.2 Lyme disease
Erythema chronicum migrans due to Borrelia burgdorferi
A69.20 Lyme disease, unspecified CC
A69.21 Meningitis due to Lyme disease CC
A69.22 Other neurologic disorders in Lyme disease CC
Cranial neuritis
Meningoencephalitis
Polyneuropathy
A69.23 Arthritis due to Lyme disease CC
A69.29 Other conditions associated with Lyme disease CC
Myopericarditis due to Lyme disease
A69.8 Other specified spirochetal infections
A69.9 Spirochetal infection, unspecified

Other diseases caused by chlamydiae (A70-A74)

EXCLUDES1 *sexually transmitted chlamydial diseases (A55-A56)*

A70 Chlamydia psittaci infections CC
Ornithosis
Parrot fever
Psittacosis
A71 Trachoma
EXCLUDES1 *sequelae of trachoma (B94.0)*
A71.0 Initial stage of trachoma
Trachoma dubium
A71.1 Active stage of trachoma
Granular conjunctivitis (trachomatous)
Trachomatous follicular conjunctivitis
Trachomatous pannus
A71.9 Trachoma, unspecified
A74 Other diseases caused by chlamydiae
EXCLUDES1 *neonatal chlamydial conjunctivitis (P39.1)*
neonatal chlamydial pneumonia (P23.1)
Reiter's disease (M02.3-)
sexually transmitted chlamydial diseases (A55-A56)
EXCLUDES2 *chlamydial pneumonia (J16.0)*
A74.0 Chlamydial conjunctivitis
Paratrachoma
A74.8 Other chlamydial diseases
A74.81 Chlamydial peritonitis
A74.89 Other chlamydial diseases
A74.9 Chlamydial infection, unspecified
Chlamydiosis NOS

Rickettsioses (A75-A79)

A75 Typhus fever
EXCLUDES1 *rickettsiosis due to Ehrlichia sennetsu (A79.81)*
A75.0 Epidemic louse-borne typhus fever due to Rickettsia prowazekii CC
Classical typhus (fever)
Epidemic (louse-borne) typhus
A75.1 Recrudescent typhus [Brill's disease] CC
Brill-Zinsser disease
A75.2 Typhus fever due to Rickettsia typhi CC
Murine (flea-borne) typhus
A75.3 Typhus fever due to Rickettsia tsutsugamushi CC
Scrub (mite-borne) typhus
Tsutsugamushi fever
A75.9 Typhus fever, unspecified CC
Typhus (fever) NOS
A77 Spotted fever [tick-borne rickettsioses]
A77.0 Spotted fever due to Rickettsia rickettsii CC
Rocky Mountain spotted fever
Sao Paulo fever
A77.1 Spotted fever due to Rickettsia conorii CC
African tick typhus
Boutonneuse fever
India tick typhus
Kenya tick typhus
Marseilles fever
Mediterranean tick fever
A77.2 Spotted fever due to Rickettsia siberica CC
North Asian tick fever
Siberian tick typhus
A77.3 Spotted fever due to Rickettsia australis CC
Queensland tick typhus
A77.4 Ehrlichiosis
EXCLUDES1 *Rickettsiosis due to Ehrlichia sennetsu (A79.81)*
A77.40 Ehrlichiosis, unspecified CC
A77.41 Ehrlichiosis chafeensis [E. chafeensis] CC
A77.49 Other ehrlichiosis CC
A77.8 Other spotted fevers CC
A77.9 Spotted fever, unspecified CC
Tick-borne typhus NOS
A78 Q fever CC
Infection due to Coxiella burnetii
Nine Mile fever
Quadrilateral fever
A79 Other rickettsioses
A79.0 Trench fever CC
Quintan fever
Wolhynian fever
A79.1 Rickettsialpox due to Rickettsia akari CC
Kew Garden fever
Vesicular rickettsiosis
A79.8 Other specified rickettsioses
A79.81 Rickettsiosis due to Ehrlichia sennetsu CC
A79.89 Other specified rickettsioses CC
A79.9 Rickettsiosis, unspecified CC
Rickettsial infection NOS

Viral and prion infections of the central nervous system (A80-A89)

EXCLUDES1 *postpolio syndrome (G14)*
sequelae of poliomyelitis (B91)
sequelae of viral encephalitis (B94.1)

A80 Acute poliomyelitis
A80.0 Acute paralytic poliomyelitis, vaccine-associated MCC
A80.1 Acute paralytic poliomyelitis, wild virus, imported MCC
A80.2 Acute paralytic poliomyelitis, wild virus, indigenous MCC
A80.3 Acute paralytic poliomyelitis, other and unspecified
A80.30 Acute paralytic poliomyelitis, unspecified MCC
A80.39 Other acute paralytic poliomyelitis MCC
A80.4 Acute nonparalytic poliomyelitis
A80.9 Acute poliomyelitis, unspecified
A81 Atypical virus infections of central nervous system
INCLUDES *diseases of the central nervous system caused by prions*
Use additional code to identify:
dementia with behavioral disturbance (F02.81)
dementia without behavioral disturbance (F02.80)
A81.0 Creutzfeldt-Jakob disease
A81.00 Creutzfeldt-Jakob disease, unspecified CC
Jakob-Creutzfeldt disease, unspecified
A81.01 Variant Creutzfeldt-Jakob disease CC
vCJD
A81.09 Other Creutzfeldt-Jakob disease CC
CJD
Familial Creutzfeldt-Jakob disease
Iatrogenic Creutzfeldt-Jakob disease
Sporadic Creutzfeldt-Jakob disease
Subacute spongiform encephalopathy (with dementia)
A81.1 Subacute sclerosing panencephalitis CC
Dawson's inclusion body encephalitis
Van Bogaert's sclerosing leukoencephalopathy
A81.2 Progressive multifocal leukoencephalopathy CC
Multifocal leukoencephalopathy NOS
A81.8 Other atypical virus infections of central nervous system
A81.81 Kuru CC
A81.82 Gerstmann-Sträussler-Scheinker syndrome CC
GSS syndrome
A81.83 Fatal familial insomnia CC
FFI
A81.89 Other atypical virus infections of central nervous system CC

Unspecified Code Other Specified Code Manifestation Code N Newborn P Pediatric M Maternity A Adult ♂ Male ♀ Female
● New Code ▲ Revised Code Title ►◄ Revised Text NOTES INCLUDES EXCLUDES1 Not coded here EXCLUDES2 Not included here
4th character required 5th character required 6th character required 7th character required
Extension 'X' Alert HAC Hospital-acquired condition (HAC) alert AHA AHA Coding Clinic®

When symbols appear on a code that requires a 7th character extension, refer to Appendix D to identify applicable 7th character codes.

A81.9 Atypical virus infection of central nervous system, unspecified CC
Prion diseases of the central nervous system NOS

A82 Rabies
A82.0 Sylvatic rabies CC
A82.1 Urban rabies CC
A82.9 Rabies, unspecified CC

A83 Mosquito-borne viral encephalitis
INCLUDES *mosquito-borne viral meningoencephalitis*
EXCLUDES2 *Venezuelan equine encephalitis (A92.2)*
West Nile fever (A92.3-)
West Nile virus (A92.3-)
A83.0 Japanese encephalitis MCC
A83.1 Western equine encephalitis MCC
A83.2 Eastern equine encephalitis MCC
A83.3 St Louis encephalitis MCC
A83.4 Australian encephalitis MCC
Kunjin virus disease
A83.5 California encephalitis MCC
California meningoencephalitis
La Crosse encephalitis
A83.6 Rocio virus disease MCC
A83.8 Other mosquito-borne viral encephalitis MCC
A83.9 Mosquito-borne viral encephalitis, unspecified MCC

A84 Tick-borne viral encephalitis
INCLUDES *tick-borne viral meningoencephalitis*
A84.0 Far Eastern tick-borne encephalitis [Russian spring-summer encephalitis] MCC
A84.1 Central European tick-borne encephalitis MCC
A84.8 Other tick-borne viral encephalitis MCC
Louping ill
Powassan virus disease
A84.9 Tick-borne viral encephalitis, unspecified MCC

A85 Other viral encephalitis, not elsewhere classified
INCLUDES *specified viral encephalomyelitis NEC*
specified viral meningoencephalitis NEC
EXCLUDES1 *benign myalgic encephalomyelitis (G93.3)*
encephalitis due to cytomegalovirus (B25.8)
encephalitis due to herpesvirus NEC (B10.0-)
encephalitis due to herpesvirus [herpes simplex] (B00.4)
encephalitis due to measles virus (B05.0)
encephalitis due to mumps virus (B26.2)
encephalitis due to poliomyelitis virus (A80.-)
encephalitis due to zoster (B02.0)
lymphocytic choriomeningitis (A87.2)
A85.0 Enteroviral encephalitis CC
Enteroviral encephalomyelitis
A85.1 Adenoviral encephalitis CC
Adenoviral meningoencephalitis
A85.2 Arthropod-borne viral encephalitis, unspecified MCC
EXCLUDES1 *West Nile virus with encephalitis (A92.31)*
A85.8 Other specified viral encephalitis CC
Encephalitis lethargica
Von Economo-Cruchet disease

A86 Unspecified viral encephalitis CC
Viral encephalomyelitis NOS
Viral meningoencephalitis NOS

A87 Viral meningitis
EXCLUDES1 *meningitis due to herpesvirus [herpes simplex] (B00.3)*
meningitis due to herpesvirus [herpes simplex] (B00.3)
meningitis due to measles virus (B05.1)
meningitis due to mumps virus (B26.1)
meningitis due to poliomyelitis virus (A80.-)
meningitis due to zoster (B02.1)
A87.0 Enteroviral meningitis CC
Coxsackievirus meningitis
Echovirus meningitis
A87.1 Adenoviral meningitis CC
A87.2 Lymphocytic choriomeningitis CC
Lymphocytic meningoencephalitis
A87.8 Other viral meningitis CC
A87.9 Viral meningitis, unspecified CC

A88 Other viral infections of central nervous system, not elsewhere classified
EXCLUDES1 *viral encephalitis NOS (A86)*
viral meningitis NOS (A87.9)
A88.0 Enteroviral exanthematous fever [Boston exanthem] CC
A88.1 Epidemic vertigo
A88.8 Other specified viral infections of central nervous system CC

A89 Unspecified viral infection of central nervous system CC

Arthropod-borne viral fevers and viral hemorrhagic fevers (A90-A99)

A90 Dengue fever [classical dengue] CC
EXCLUDES1 *dengue hemorrhagic fever (A91)*

A91 Dengue hemorrhagic fever CC

A92 Other mosquito-borne viral fevers
EXCLUDES1 *Ross River disease (B33.1)*
A92.0 Chikungunya virus disease CC
Chikungunya (hemorrhagic) fever
A92.1 O'nyong-nyong fever CC
A92.2 Venezuelan equine fever CC
Venezuelan equine encephalitis
Venezuelan equine encephalomyelitis virus disease
A92.3 West Nile virus infection
West Nile fever
A92.30 West Nile virus infection, unspecified MCC
West Nile fever NOS
West Nile fever without complications
West Nile virus NOS
A92.31 West Nile virus infection with encephalitis MCC
West Nile encephalitis
West Nile encephalomyelitis
A92.32 West Nile virus infection with other neurologic manifestation MCC
Use additional code to specify the neurologic manifestation
A92.39 West Nile virus infection with other complications MCC
Use additional code to specify the other conditions
A92.4 Rift Valley fever CC
● A92.5 Zika virus disease
Zika virus fever
Zika virus infection
Zika NOS
A92.8 Other specified mosquito-borne viral fevers CC
A92.9 Mosquito-borne viral fever, unspecified CC

A93 Other arthropod-borne viral fevers, not elsewhere classified
A93.0 Oropouche virus disease CC
Oropouche fever
A93.1 Sandfly fever CC
Pappataci fever
Phlebotomus fever
A93.2 Colorado tick fever CC
A93.8 Other specified arthropod-borne viral fevers CC
Piry virus disease
Vesicular stomatitis virus disease [Indiana fever]

A94 Unspecified arthropod-borne viral fever CC
Arboviral fever NOS
Arbovirus infection NOS

A95 Yellow fever
A95.0 Sylvatic yellow fever CC
Jungle yellow fever
A95.1 Urban yellow fever CC
A95.9 Yellow fever, unspecified CC

A96 Arenaviral hemorrhagic fever
A96.0 Junin hemorrhagic fever CC
Argentinian hemorrhagic fever
A96.1 Machupo hemorrhagic fever CC
Bolivian hemorrhagic fever
A96.2 Lassa fever CC
A96.8 Other arenaviral hemorrhagic fevers CC
A96.9 Arenaviral hemorrhagic fever, unspecified CC

PDx Unacceptable principal diagnosis symbol per Medicare code edits | POA Code exempt from diagnosis present on admission requirement
Q Questionable admission | CC Complication or comorbidity | CC/MCC Excl CC/MCC exclusion | MCC Major complication or comorbidity
PDx CC Principal diagnosis as its own CC | PDx MCC Principal diagnosis as its own MCC | Z1 Z code as first-listed diagnosis

A98 Other viral hemorrhagic fevers, not elsewhere classified
EXCLUDES1 *chikungunya hemorrhagic fever (A92.0)*
dengue hemorrhagic fever (A91)
A98.0 Crimean-Congo hemorrhagic fever CC
Central Asian hemorrhagic fever
A98.1 Omsk hemorrhagic fever CC
A98.2 Kyasanur Forest disease CC
A98.3 Marburg virus disease
A98.4 Ebola virus disease
A98.5 Hemorrhagic fever with renal syndrome CC
Epidemic hemorrhagic fever
Korean hemorrhagic fever
Russian hemorrhagic fever
Hantaan virus disease
Hantavirus disease with renal manifestations
Nephropathia epidemica
Songo fever
EXCLUDES1 *hantavirus (cardio)-pulmonary syndrome (B33.4)*
A98.8 Other specified viral hemorrhagic fevers CC
A99 Unspecified viral hemorrhagic fever CC

Viral infections characterized by skin and mucous membrane lesions (B00-B09)

B00 Herpesviral [herpes simplex] infections
EXCLUDES1 *congenital herpesviral infections (P35.2)*
EXCLUDES2 *anogenital herpesviral infection (A60.-)*
gammaherpesviral mononucleosis (B27.0-)
herpangina (B08.5)
B00.0 Eczema herpeticum
Kaposi's varicelliform eruption
B00.1 Herpesviral vesicular dermatitis
Herpes simplex facialis
Herpes simplex labialis
Herpes simplex otitis externa
Vesicular dermatitis of ear
Vesicular dermatitis of lip
B00.2 Herpesviral gingivostomatitis and pharyngotonsillitis CC
Herpesviral pharyngitis
B00.3 Herpesviral meningitis MCC
B00.4 Herpesviral encephalitis MCC
Herpesviral meningoencephalitis
Simian B disease
EXCLUDES1 *herpesviral encephalitis due to herpesvirus 6 and 7 (B10.01, B10.09)*
non-simplex herpesviral encephalitis (B10.0-)
B00.5 Herpesviral ocular disease
B00.50 Herpesviral ocular disease, unspecified CC
B00.51 Herpesviral iridocyclitis CC
Herpesviral iritis
Herpesviral uveitis, anterior
B00.52 Herpesviral keratitis CC
Herpesviral keratoconjunctivitis
B00.53 Herpesviral conjunctivitis CC
B00.59 Other herpesviral disease of eye CC
Herpesviral dermatitis of eyelid
B00.7 Disseminated herpesviral disease MCC
Herpesviral sepsis
B00.8 Other forms of herpesviral infections
B00.81 Herpesviral hepatitis CC
B00.82 Herpes simplex myelitis MCC
B00.89 Other herpesviral infection CC
Herpesviral whitlow
B00.9 Herpesviral infection, unspecified
Herpes simplex infection NOS
B01 Varicella [chickenpox]
B01.0 Varicella meningitis CC
B01.1 Varicella encephalitis, myelitis and encephalomyelitis
Postchickenpox encephalitis, myelitis and encephalomyelitis
B01.11 Varicella encephalitis and encephalomyelitis MCC
Postchickenpox encephalitis and encephalomyelitis
B01.12 Varicella myelitis MCC
Postchickenpox myelitis
B01.2 Varicella pneumonia MCC
B01.8 Varicella with other complications
B01.81 Varicella keratitis CC
B01.89 Other varicella complications CC
B01.9 Varicella without complication CC
Varicella NOS

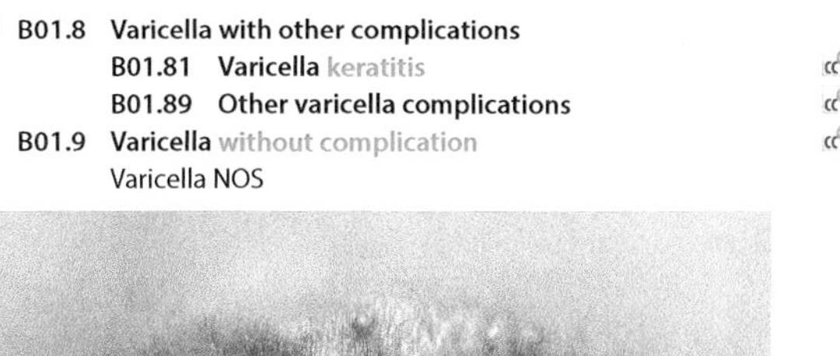
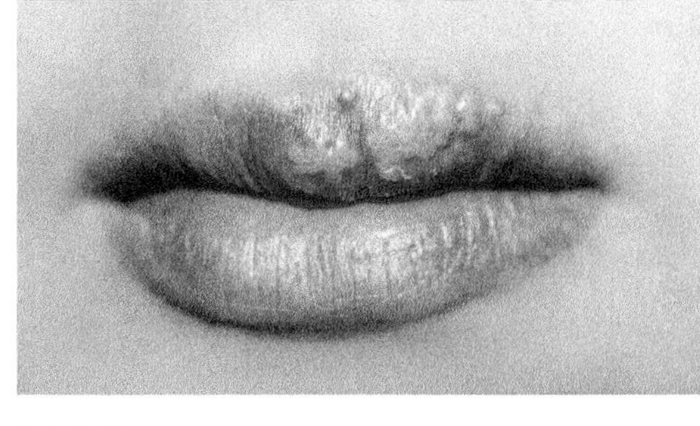

Figure 1.2 Oral herpes

B02 Zoster [herpes zoster]
INCLUDES *shingles*
zona
B02.0 Zoster encephalitis CC
Zoster meningoencephalitis
B02.1 Zoster meningitis MCC
B02.2 Zoster with other nervous system involvement
B02.21 Postherpetic geniculate ganglionitis CC
B02.22 Postherpetic trigeminal neuralgia CC
B02.23 Postherpetic polyneuropathy CC
B02.24 Postherpetic myelitis MCC
Herpes zoster myelitis
B02.29 Other postherpetic nervous system involvement CC
Postherpetic radiculopathy
B02.3 Zoster ocular disease
B02.30 Zoster ocular disease, unspecified CC
B02.31 Zoster conjunctivitis CC
B02.32 Zoster iridocyclitis CC
B02.33 Zoster keratitis CC
Herpes zoster keratoconjunctivitis
B02.34 Zoster scleritis CC
B02.39 Other herpes zoster eye disease CC
Zoster blepharitis
B02.7 Disseminated zoster CC
B02.8 Zoster with other complications CC
Herpes zoster otitis externa
B02.9 Zoster without complications
Zoster NOS
B03 Smallpox CC
NOTES In 1980 the 33rd World Health Assembly declared that smallpox had been eradicated.
The classification is maintained for surveillance purposes.
B04 Monkeypox CC
B05 Measles
INCLUDES *morbilli*
EXCLUDES1 *subacute sclerosing panencephalitis (A81.1)*
B05.0 Measles complicated by encephalitis MCC
Postmeasles encephalitis
B05.1 Measles complicated by meningitis CC
Postmeasles meningitis
B05.2 Measles complicated by pneumonia MCC
Postmeasles pneumonia
B05.3 Measles complicated by otitis media
Postmeasles otitis media
B05.4 Measles with intestinal complications CC
B05.8 Measles with other complications
B05.81 Measles keratitis and keratoconjunctivitis CC
B05.89 Other measles complications CC
B05.9 Measles without complication
Measles NOS
B06 Rubella [German measles]
EXCLUDES1 *congenital rubella (P35.0)*
B06.0 Rubella with neurological complications

Unspecified Code Other Specified Code Manifestation Code N Newborn P Pediatric M Maternity A Adult ♂ Male ♀ Female
● New Code ▲ Revised Code Title ►◄ Revised Text NOTES INCLUDES EXCLUDES1 Not coded here EXCLUDES2 Not included here
4th character required 5th character required 6th character required 7th character required
Extension 'X' Alert HAC Hospital-acquired condition (HAC) alert AHA AHA Coding Clinic©

 When symbols appear on a code that requires a 7th character extension, refer to Appendix D to identify applicable 7th character codes.

B06.00 Rubella with neurological complication, unspecified CC
B06.01 Rubella encephalitis MCC
Rubella meningoencephalitis
B06.02 Rubella meningitis CC
B06.09 Other neurological complications of rubella CC
B06.8 Rubella with other complications
B06.81 Rubella pneumonia CC
B06.82 Rubella arthritis CC
B06.89 Other rubella complications CC
B06.9 Rubella without complication
Rubella NOS

B07 Viral warts
INCLUDES *verruca simplex*
verruca vulgaris
viral warts due to human papillomavirus
EXCLUDES2 *anogenital (venereal) warts (A63.0)*
papilloma of bladder (D41.4)
papilloma of cervix (D26.0)
papilloma larynx (D14.1)
B07.0 Plantar wart
Verruca plantaris
B07.8 Other viral warts
Common wart
Flat wart
Verruca plana
B07.9 Viral wart, unspecified

B08 Other viral infections characterized by skin and mucous membrane lesions, not elsewhere classified
EXCLUDES1 *vesicular stomatitis virus disease (A93.8)*
B08.0 Other orthopoxvirus infections
EXCLUDES2 *monkeypox (B04)*
B08.01 Cowpox and vaccinia not from vaccine
B08.010 Cowpox
B08.011 Vaccinia not from vaccine
EXCLUDES1 *vaccinia (from vaccination) (generalized) (T88.1)*
B08.02 Orf virus disease
Contagious pustular dermatitis
Ecthyma contagiosum
B08.03 Pseudocowpox [milker's node]
B08.04 Paravaccinia, unspecified
B08.09 Other orthopoxvirus infections
Orthopoxvirus infection NOS
B08.1 Molluscum contagiosum
B08.2 Exanthema subitum [sixth disease]
Roseola infantum
B08.20 Exanthema subitum [sixth disease], unspecified Q
Roseola infantum, unspecified
B08.21 Exanthema subitum [sixth disease] due to human herpesvirus 6 Q
Roseola infantum due to human herpesvirus 6
B08.22 Exanthema subitum [sixth disease] due to human herpesvirus 7 Q
Roseola infantum due to human herpesvirus 7
B08.3 Erythema infectiosum [fifth disease] CC
B08.4 Enteroviral vesicular stomatitis with exanthem
Hand, foot and mouth disease
B08.5 Enteroviral vesicular pharyngitis
Herpangina
B08.6 Parapoxvirus infections
B08.60 Parapoxvirus infection, unspecified
B08.61 Bovine stomatitis
B08.62 Sealpox
B08.69 Other parapoxvirus infections
B08.7 Yatapoxvirus infections
B08.70 Yatapoxvirus infection, unspecified
B08.71 Tanapox virus disease CC
B08.72 Yaba pox virus disease
Yaba monkey tumor disease
B08.79 Other yatapoxvirus infections
B08.8 Other specified viral infections characterized by skin and mucous membrane lesions
Enteroviral lymphonodular pharyngitis
Foot-and-mouth disease
Poxvirus NEC

B09 Unspecified viral infection characterized by skin and mucous membrane lesions
Viral enanthema NOS
Viral exanthema NOS

Other human herpesviruses (B10)

B10 Other human herpesviruses
EXCLUDES2 *cytomegalovirus (B25.9)*
Epstein-Barr virus (B27.0-)
herpes NOS (B00.9)
herpes simplex (B00.-)
herpes zoster (B02.-)
human herpesvirus NOS (B00.-)
human herpesvirus 1 and 2 (B00.-)
human herpesvirus 3 (B01.-, B02.-)
human herpesvirus 4 (B27.0-)
human herpesvirus 5 (B25.-)
varicella (B01.-)
zoster (B02.-)
B10.0 Other human herpesvirus encephalitis
EXCLUDES2 *herpes encephalitis NOS (B00.4)*
herpes simplex encephalitis (B00.4)
human herpesvirus encephalitis (B00.4)
simian B herpes virus encephalitis (B00.4)
B10.01 Human herpesvirus 6 encephalitis MCC
B10.09 Other human herpesvirus encephalitis MCC
Human herpesvirus 7 encephalitis
B10.8 Other human herpesvirus infection
B10.81 Human herpesvirus 6 infection
B10.82 Human herpesvirus 7 infection
B10.89 Other human herpesvirus infection
Human herpesvirus 8 infection
Kaposi's sarcoma-associated herpesvirus infection

Viral hepatitis (B15-B19)

EXCLUDES1 *sequelae of viral hepatitis (B94.2)*
EXCLUDES2 *cytomegaloviral hepatitis (B25.1)*
herpesviral [herpes simplex] hepatitis (B00.81)

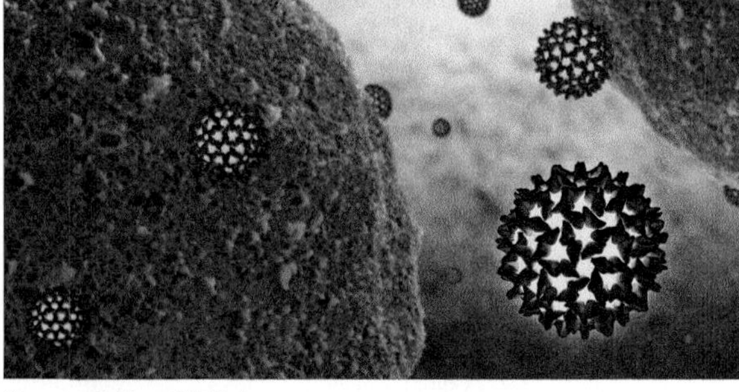

Figure 1.3 Hepatitis B virus

B15 Acute hepatitis A
B15.0 Hepatitis A with hepatic coma MCC
B15.9 Hepatitis A without hepatic coma CC
Hepatitis A (acute)(viral) NOS

B16 Acute hepatitis B
B16.0 Acute hepatitis B with delta-agent with hepatic coma MCC
B16.1 Acute hepatitis B with delta-agent without hepatic coma CC
B16.2 Acute hepatitis B without delta-agent with hepatic coma MCC
B16.9 Acute hepatitis B without delta-agent and without hepatic coma CC
Hepatitis B (acute) (viral) NOS

PDx Unacceptable principal diagnosis symbol per Medicare code edits — POA Code exempt from diagnosis present on admission requirement
Q Questionable admission — CC Complication or comorbidity — CC/MCC Exc CC/MCC exclusion — MCC Major complication or comorbidity
PDx CC Principal diagnosis as its own CC — PDx MCC Principal diagnosis as its own MCC — Z1 Z code as first-listed diagnosis

B17 Other acute viral hepatitis
B17.0 Acute delta-(super) infection of hepatitis B carrier CC
B17.1 Acute hepatitis C
B17.10 Acute hepatitis C without hepatic coma CC
Acute hepatitis C NOS
B17.11 Acute hepatitis C with hepatic coma MCC
B17.2 Acute hepatitis E CC
B17.8 Other specified acute viral hepatitis CC
Hepatitis non-A non-B (acute) (viral) NEC
B17.9 Acute viral hepatitis, unspecified CC
Acute hepatitis NOS
Acute infectious hepatitis NOS

B18 Chronic viral hepatitis
INCLUDES *Carrier of viral hepatitis*
B18.0 Chronic viral hepatitis B with delta-agent CC
B18.1 Chronic viral hepatitis B without delta-agent CC
Carrier of viral hepatitis B
Chronic (viral) hepatitis B
B18.2 Chronic viral hepatitis C
Carrier of viral hepatitis C
B18.8 Other chronic viral hepatitis CC
Carrier of other viral hepatitis
B18.9 Chronic viral hepatitis, unspecified CC
Carrier of unspecified viral hepatitis

B19 Unspecified viral hepatitis
B19.0 Unspecified viral hepatitis with hepatic coma MCC
B19.1 Unspecified viral hepatitis B
B19.10 Unspecified viral hepatitis B without hepatic coma CC
Unspecified viral hepatitis B NOS
B19.11 Unspecified viral hepatitis B with hepatic coma MCC
B19.2 Unspecified viral hepatitis C
B19.20 Unspecified viral hepatitis C without hepatic coma
Viral hepatitis C NOS
B19.21 Unspecified viral hepatitis C with hepatic coma MCC
B19.9 Unspecified viral hepatitis without hepatic coma CC
Viral hepatitis NOS

Human immunodeficiency virus [HIV] disease (B20)

B20 Human immunodeficiency virus [HIV] disease MCC
INCLUDES *acquired immune deficiency syndrome [AIDS]*
AIDS-related complex [ARC]
HIV infection, symptomatic
Code first Human immunodeficiency virus [HIV] disease complicating pregnancy, childbirth and the puerperium, if applicable (O98.7-)
Use additional code(s) to identify all manifestations of HIV infection
EXCLUDES1 *asymptomatic human immunodeficiency virus [HIV] infection status (Z21)*
exposure to HIV virus (Z20.6)
inconclusive serologic evidence of HIV (R75)

Other viral diseases (B25-B34)

B25 Cytomegaloviral disease
EXCLUDES1 *congenital cytomegalovirus infection (P35.1)*
cytomegaloviral mononucleosis (B27.1-)
B25.0 Cytomegaloviral pneumonitis MCC PDx
B25.1 Cytomegaloviral hepatitis CC PDx
B25.2 Cytomegaloviral pancreatitis MCC PDx
B25.8 Other cytomegaloviral diseases CC
Cytomegaloviral encephalitis
B25.9 Cytomegaloviral disease, unspecified CC

B26 Mumps
INCLUDES *epidemic parotitis*
infectious parotitis
B26.0 Mumps orchitis CC ♂
B26.1 Mumps meningitis MCC
B26.2 Mumps encephalitis MCC
B26.3 Mumps pancreatitis CC
B26.8 Mumps with other complications
B26.81 Mumps hepatitis CC
B26.82 Mumps myocarditis CC
B26.83 Mumps nephritis CC
B26.84 Mumps polyneuropathy CC
B26.85 Mumps arthritis CC
B26.89 Other mumps complications CC
B26.9 Mumps without complication
Mumps NOS
Mumps parotitis NOS

B27 Infectious mononucleosis
INCLUDES *glandular fever*
monocytic angina
Pfeiffer's disease
B27.0 Gammaherpesviral mononucleosis
Mononucleosis due to Epstein-Barr virus
B27.00 Gammaherpesviral mononucleosis without complication
B27.01 Gammaherpesviral mononucleosis with polyneuropathy
B27.02 Gammaherpesviral mononucleosis with meningitis
B27.09 Gammaherpesviral mononucleosis with other complications
Hepatomegaly in gammaherpesviral mononucleosis
B27.1 Cytomegaloviral mononucleosis
B27.10 Cytomegaloviral mononucleosis without complications
B27.11 Cytomegaloviral mononucleosis with polyneuropathy
B27.12 Cytomegaloviral mononucleosis with meningitis
B27.19 Cytomegaloviral mononucleosis with other complication
Hepatomegaly in cytomegaloviral mononucleosis
B27.8 Other infectious mononucleosis
B27.80 Other infectious mononucleosis without complication
B27.81 Other infectious mononucleosis with polyneuropathy
B27.82 Other infectious mononucleosis with meningitis
B27.89 Other infectious mononucleosis with other complication
Hepatomegaly in other infectious mononucleosis

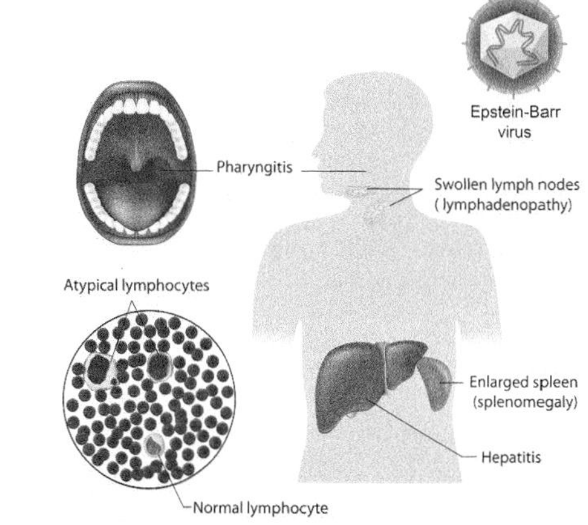

Figure 1.4 Infectious mononucleosis

B27.9 Infectious mononucleosis, unspecified
B27.90 Infectious mononucleosis, unspecified without complication
B27.91 Infectious mononucleosis, unspecified with polyneuropathy
B27.92 Infectious mononucleosis, unspecified with meningitis
B27.99 Infectious mononucleosis, unspecified with other complication
Hepatomegaly in unspecified infectious mononucleosis

B30 Viral conjunctivitis
EXCLUDES1 *herpesviral [herpes simplex] ocular disease (B00.5)*
ocular zoster (B02.3)

Unspecified Code | Other Specified Code | Manifestation Code | N Newborn | P Pediatric | M Maternity | A Adult | ♂ Male | ♀ Female
● New Code ▲ Revised Code Title ►◄ Revised Text NOTES INCLUDES EXCLUDES1 Not coded here EXCLUDES2 Not included here
4th character required 5th character required 6th character required 7th character required
Extension 'X' Alert HAC Hospital-acquired condition (HAC) alert AHA AHA Coding Clinic©

B30.0 Keratoconjunctivitis due to adenovirus
Epidemic keratoconjunctivitis
Shipyard eye
B30.1 Conjunctivitis due to adenovirus
Acute adenoviral follicular conjunctivitis
Swimming-pool conjunctivitis
B30.2 Viral pharyngoconjunctivitis
B30.3 Acute epidemic hemorrhagic conjunctivitis (enteroviral)
Conjunctivitis due to coxsackievirus 24
Conjunctivitis due to enterovirus 70
Hemorrhagic conjunctivitis (acute)(epidemic)
B30.8 Other viral conjunctivitis
Newcastle conjunctivitis
B30.9 Viral conjunctivitis, unspecified

B33 Other viral diseases, not elsewhere classified
B33.0 Epidemic myalgia
Bornholm disease
B33.1 Ross River disease CC
Epidemic polyarthritis and exanthema
Ross River fever
B33.2 Viral carditis
Coxsackie (virus) carditis
B33.20 Viral carditis, unspecified CC
B33.21 Viral endocarditis CC
B33.22 Viral myocarditis CC
B33.23 Viral pericarditis CC
B33.24 Viral cardiomyopathy
B33.3 Retrovirus infections, not elsewhere classified
Retrovirus infection NOS
B33.4 Hantavirus (cardio)-pulmonary syndrome [HPS] [HCPS] CC
Hantavirus disease with pulmonary manifestations
Sin nombre virus disease
Use additional code to identify any associated acute kidney failure (N17.9)
EXCLUDES1 *hantavirus disease with renal manifestations (A98.5)*
hemorrhagic fever with renal manifestations (A98.5)
B33.8 Other specified viral diseases
EXCLUDES1 *anogenital human papillomavirus infection (A63.0)*
viral warts due to human papillomavirus infection (B07)

B34 Viral infection of unspecified site
EXCLUDES1 *anogenital human papillomavirus infection (A63.0)*
cytomegaloviral disease NOS (B25.9)
herpesvirus [herpes simplex] infection NOS (B00.9)
retrovirus infection NOS (B33.3)
viral agents as the cause of diseases classified elsewhere (B97.-)
viral warts due to human papillomavirus infection (B07)
B34.0 Adenovirus infection, unspecified
B34.1 Enterovirus infection, unspecified
Coxsackievirus infection NOS
Echovirus infection NOS
B34.2 Coronavirus infection, unspecified
EXCLUDES1 *pneumonia due to SARS-associated coronavirus (J12.81)*
B34.3 Parvovirus infection, unspecified CC
B34.4 Papovavirus infection, unspecified
B34.8 Other viral infections of unspecified site
B34.9 Viral infection, unspecified
Viremia NOS

Mycoses (B35-B49)

EXCLUDES2 *hypersensitivity pneumonitis due to organic dust (J67.-)*
mycosis fungoides (C84.0-)

B35 Dermatophytosis
INCLUDES *favus*
infections due to species of Epidermophyton, Microsporum and Trichophyton
tinea, any type except those in B36.-
B35.0 Tinea barbae and tinea capitis
Beard ringworm
Kerion
Scalp ringworm
Sycosis, mycotic
B35.1 Tinea unguium
Dermatophytic onychia
Dermatophytosis of nail
Onychomycosis
Ringworm of nails
B35.2 Tinea manuum
Dermatophytosis of hand
Hand ringworm
B35.3 Tinea pedis
Athlete's foot
Dermatophytosis of foot
Foot ringworm
B35.4 Tinea corporis
Ringworm of the body
B35.5 Tinea imbricata
Tokelau
B35.6 Tinea cruris
Dhobi itch
Groin ringworm
Jock itch
B35.8 Other dermatophytoses
Disseminated dermatophytosis
Granulomatous dermatophytosis
B35.9 Dermatophytosis, unspecified
Ringworm NOS

B36 Other superficial mycoses
B36.0 Pityriasis versicolor
Tinea flava
Tinea versicolor
B36.1 Tinea nigra
Keratomycosis nigricans palmaris
Microsporosis nigra
Pityriasis nigra
B36.2 White piedra
Tinea blanca
B36.3 Black piedra
B36.8 Other specified superficial mycoses
B36.9 Superficial mycosis, unspecified

B37 Candidiasis
INCLUDES *candidosis*
moniliasis
EXCLUDES1 *neonatal candidiasis (P37.5)*
B37.0 Candidal stomatitis CC
Oral thrush
B37.1 Pulmonary candidiasis MCC
Candidal bronchitis
Candidal pneumonia
B37.2 Candidiasis of skin and nail
Candidal onychia
Candidal paronychia
EXCLUDES2 *diaper dermatitis (L22)*
B37.3 Candidiasis of vulva and vagina ♀
Candidal vulvovaginitis
Monilial vulvovaginitis
Vaginal thrush
B37.4 Candidiasis of other urogenital sites
B37.41 Candidal cystitis and urethritis CC
B37.42 Candidal balanitis
B37.49 Other urogenital candidiasis CC
Candidal pyelonephritis
B37.5 Candidal meningitis MCC
B37.6 Candidal endocarditis MCC
B37.7 Candidal sepsis MCC PDx MCC
Disseminated candidiasis
Systemic candidiasis
B37.8 Candidiasis of other sites
B37.81 Candidal esophagitis CC
B37.82 Candidal enteritis CC
Candidal proctitis
B37.83 Candidal cheilitis CC
B37.84 Candidal otitis externa CC
B37.89 Other sites of candidiasis CC
Candidal osteomyelitis
B37.9 Candidiasis, unspecified
Thrush NOS

PDx Unacceptable principal diagnosis symbol per Medicare code edits POA Code exempt from diagnosis present on admission requirement
? Questionable admission CC Complication or comorbidity CC/MCC Exc CC/MCC exclusion MCC Major complication or comorbidity
PDx CC Principal diagnosis as its own CC PDx MCC Principal diagnosis as its own MCC Z1 Z code as first-listed diagnosis

B38 Coccidioidomycosis
B38.0 Acute pulmonary coccidioidomycosis
B38.1 Chronic pulmonary coccidioidomycosis
B38.2 Pulmonary coccidioidomycosis, unspecified
B38.3 Cutaneous coccidioidomycosis
B38.4 Coccidioidomycosis meningitis
B38.7 Disseminated coccidioidomycosis
Generalized coccidioidomycosis
B38.8 Other forms of coccidioidomycosis
B38.81 Prostatic coccidioidomycosis ♂
B38.89 Other forms of coccidioidomycosis
B38.9 Coccidioidomycosis, unspecified
B39 Histoplasmosis
Code first associated AIDS (B20)
Use additional code for any associated manifestations, such as:
endocarditis (I39)
meningitis (G02)
pericarditis (I32)
retinitits (H32)
B39.0 Acute pulmonary histoplasmosis capsulati
B39.1 Chronic pulmonary histoplasmosis capsulati
B39.2 Pulmonary histoplasmosis capsulati, unspecified
B39.3 Disseminated histoplasmosis capsulati
Generalized histoplasmosis capsulati
B39.4 Histoplasmosis capsulati, unspecified
American histoplasmosis
B39.5 Histoplasmosis duboisii
African histoplasmosis
B39.9 Histoplasmosis, unspecified
B40 Blastomycosis
EXCLUDES1 *Brazilian blastomycosis (B41.-)*
keloidal blastomycosis (B48.0)
B40.0 Acute pulmonary blastomycosis
B40.1 Chronic pulmonary blastomycosis
B40.2 Pulmonary blastomycosis, unspecified
B40.3 Cutaneous blastomycosis
B40.7 Disseminated blastomycosis
Generalized blastomycosis
B40.8 Other forms of blastomycosis
B40.81 Blastomycotic meningoencephalitis
Meningomyelitis due to blastomycosis
B40.89 Other forms of blastomycosis
B40.9 Blastomycosis, unspecified
B41 Paracoccidioidomycosis
INCLUDES *Brazilian blastomycosis*
Lutz' disease
B41.0 Pulmonary paracoccidioidomycosis
B41.7 Disseminated paracoccidioidomycosis
Generalized paracoccidioidomycosis
B41.8 Other forms of paracoccidioidomycosis
B41.9 Paracoccidioidomycosis, unspecified
B42 Sporotrichosis
B42.0 Pulmonary sporotrichosis
B42.1 Lymphocutaneous sporotrichosis
B42.7 Disseminated sporotrichosis
Generalized sporotrichosis
B42.8 Other forms of sporotrichosis
B42.81 Cerebral sporotrichosis
Meningitis due to sporotrichosis
B42.82 Sporotrichosis arthritis
B42.89 Other forms of sporotrichosis
B42.9 Sporotrichosis, unspecified
B43 Chromomycosis and pheomycotic abscess
B43.0 Cutaneous chromomycosis
Dermatitis verrucosa
B43.1 Pheomycotic brain abscess
Cerebral chromomycosis
B43.2 Subcutaneous pheomycotic abscess and cyst
B43.8 Other forms of chromomycosis
B43.9 Chromomycosis, unspecified
B44 Aspergillosis
INCLUDES *aspergilloma*
B44.0 Invasive pulmonary aspergillosis
B44.1 Other pulmonary aspergillosis
B44.2 Tonsillar aspergillosis
B44.7 Disseminated aspergillosis
Generalized aspergillosis
B44.8 Other forms of aspergillosis
B44.81 Allergic bronchopulmonary aspergillosis
B44.89 Other forms of aspergillosis
B44.9 Aspergillosis, unspecified
B45 Cryptococcosis
B45.0 Pulmonary cryptococcosis
B45.1 Cerebral cryptococcosis
Cryptococcal meningitis
Cryptococcosis meningocerebralis
B45.2 Cutaneous cryptococcosis
B45.3 Osseous cryptococcosis
B45.7 Disseminated cryptococcosis
Generalized cryptococcosis
B45.8 Other forms of cryptococcosis
B45.9 Cryptococcosis, unspecified
B46 Zygomycosis
B46.0 Pulmonary mucormycosis
B46.1 Rhinocerebral mucormycosis
B46.2 Gastrointestinal mucormycosis
B46.3 Cutaneous mucormycosis
Subcutaneous mucormycosis
B46.4 Disseminated mucormycosis
Generalized mucormycosis
B46.5 Mucormycosis, unspecified
B46.8 Other zygomycoses
Entomophthoromycosis
B46.9 Zygomycosis, unspecified
Phycomycosis NOS
B47 Mycetoma
B47.0 Eumycetoma
Madura foot, mycotic
Maduromycosis
B47.1 Actinomycetoma
B47.9 Mycetoma, unspecified
Madura foot NOS
B48 Other mycoses, not elsewhere classified
B48.0 Lobomycosis
Keloidal blastomycosis
Lobo's disease
B48.1 Rhinosporidiosis
B48.2 Allescheriasis
Infection due to Pseudallescheria boydii
EXCLUDES1 *eumycetoma (B47.0)*
B48.3 Geotrichosis
Geotrichum stomatitis
B48.4 Penicillosis
B48.8 Other specified mycoses
Adiaspiromycosis
Infection of tissue and organs by Alternaria
Infection of tissue and organs by Drechslera
Infection of tissue and organs by Fusarium
Infection of tissue and organs by saprophytic fungi NEC
B49 Unspecified mycosis
Fungemia NOS

Protozoal diseases (B50-B64)

EXCLUDES1 *amebiasis (A06.-)*
other protozoal intestinal diseases (A07.-)

B50 Plasmodium falciparum malaria
INCLUDES *mixed infections of Plasmodium falciparum with any other Plasmodium species*
B50.0 Plasmodium falciparum malaria with cerebral complications
Cerebral malaria NOS
B50.8 Other severe and complicated Plasmodium falciparum malaria
Severe or complicated Plasmodium falciparum malaria NOS
B50.9 Plasmodium falciparum malaria, unspecified

Unspecified Code Other Specified Code Manifestation Code N Newborn P Pediatric M Maternity A Adult ♂ Male ♀ Female
● New Code ▲ Revised Code Title ►◄ Revised Text NOTES INCLUDES EXCLUDES1 Not coded here EXCLUDES2 Not included here
4th character required 5th character required 6th character required 7th character required
Extension 'X' Alert HAC Hospital-acquired condition (HAC) alert AHA AHA Coding Clinic©

B51 Plasmodium vivax malaria
INCLUDES *mixed infections of Plasmodium vivax with other Plasmodium species, except Plasmodium falciparum*
EXCLUDES1 *plasmodium vivax with Plasmodium falciparum (B50.-)*
B51.0 **Plasmodium vivax malaria** with rupture of spleen
B51.8 **Plasmodium vivax malaria** with other complications
B51.9 **Plasmodium vivax malaria** without complication
Plasmodium vivax malaria NOS

B52 Plasmodium malariae malaria
INCLUDES *mixed infections of Plasmodium malariae with other Plasmodium species, except Plasmodium falciparum and Plasmodium vivax*
EXCLUDES1 *Plasmodium falciparum (B50.-)*
Plasmodium vivax (B51.-)
B52.0 **Plasmodium malariae malaria** with nephropathy
B52.8 **Plasmodium malariae malaria** with other complications
B52.9 **Plasmodium malariae malaria** without complication
Plasmodium malariae malaria NOS

B53 Other specified malaria
B53.0 **Plasmodium** ovale **malaria**
EXCLUDES1 *Plasmodium ovale with Plasmodium falciparum (B50.-)*
Plasmodium ovale with Plasmodium malariae (B52.-)
Plasmodium ovale with Plasmodium vivax (B51.-)
B53.1 **Malaria due to** simian plasmodia
EXCLUDES1 *Malaria due to simian plasmodia with Plasmodium falciparum (B50.-)*
Malaria due to simian plasmodia with Plasmodium malariae (B52.-)
Malaria due to simian plasmodia with Plasmodium ovale (B53.0)
Malaria due to simian plasmodia with Plasmodium vivax (B51.-)
B53.8 **Other malaria, not elsewhere classified**

B54 Unspecified **malaria**

B55 Leishmaniasis
B55.0 Visceral **leishmaniasis**
Kala-azar
Post-kala-azar dermal leishmaniasis
B55.1 Cutaneous **leishmaniasis**
B55.2 Mucocutaneous **leishmaniasis**
B55.9 **Leishmaniasis, unspecified**

B56 African trypanosomiasis
B56.0 Gambiense **trypanosomiasis**
Infection due to Trypanosoma brucei gambiense
West African sleeping sickness
B56.1 Rhodesiense **trypanosomiasis**
East African sleeping sickness
Infection due to Trypanosoma brucei rhodesiense
B56.9 **African trypanosomiasis, unspecified**
Sleeping sickness NOS

B57 Chagas' disease
INCLUDES *American trypanosomiasis*
infection due to Trypanosoma cruzi
B57.0 Acute **Chagas' disease** with heart involvement
Acute Chagas' disease with myocarditis
B57.1 Acute **Chagas' disease** without heart involvement
Acute Chagas' disease NOS
B57.2 **Chagas' disease** (chronic) with heart involvement
American trypanosomiasis NOS
Chagas' disease (chronic) NOS
Chagas' disease (chronic) with myocarditis
Trypanosomiasis NOS
B57.3 **Chagas' disease** (chronic) with digestive system involvement
B57.30 **Chagas' disease with digestive system involvement, unspecified**
B57.31 Megaesophagus **in Chagas' disease**
B57.32 Megacolon **in Chagas' disease**
B57.39 **Other digestive system involvement in Chagas' disease**
B57.4 **Chagas' disease (chronic)** with nervous system involvement
B57.40 **Chagas' disease with nervous system involvement, unspecified**
B57.41 Meningitis **in Chagas' disease**
B57.42 Meningoencephalitis **in Chagas' disease**
B57.49 **Other nervous system involvement in Chagas' disease**
B57.5 **Chagas' disease (chronic) with other organ involvement**

B58 Toxoplasmosis
INCLUDES *infection due to Toxoplasma gondii*
EXCLUDES1 *congenital toxoplasmosis (P37.1)*
B58.0 **Toxoplasma** oculopathy
B58.00 **Toxoplasma oculopathy,** unspecified
B58.01 **Toxoplasma** chorioretinitis
B58.09 Other **toxoplasma oculopathy**
Toxoplasma uveitis
B58.1 **Toxoplasma** hepatitis
B58.2 **Toxoplasma** meningoencephalitis
B58.3 Pulmonary **toxoplasmosis**
B58.8 **Toxoplasmosis** with other organ involvement
B58.81 **Toxoplasma** myocarditis
B58.82 **Toxoplasma** myositis
B58.83 **Toxoplasma** tubulo-interstitial nephropathy
Toxoplasma pyelonephritis
B58.89 **Toxoplasmosis with other organ involvement**
B58.9 **Toxoplasmosis, unspecified**

B59 Pneumocystosis
Pneumonia due to Pneumocystis carinii
Pneumonia due to Pneumocystis jiroveci

B60 Other protozoal diseases, not elsewhere classified
EXCLUDES1 *cryptosporidiosis (A07.2)*
intestinal microsporidiosis (A07.8)
isosporiasis (A07.3)
B60.0 **Babesiosis**
Piroplasmosis
B60.1 **Acanthamebiasis**
B60.10 **Acanthamebiasis, unspecified**
B60.11 Meningoencephalitis **due to Acanthamoeba (culbertsoni)**
B60.12 Conjunctivitis **due to Acanthamoeba**
B60.13 Keratoconjunctivitis **due to Acanthamoeba**
B60.19 **Other acanthamebic disease**
B60.2 **Naegleriasis**
Primary amebic meningoencephalitis
B60.8 **Other specified protozoal diseases**
Microsporidiosis

B64 Unspecified protozoal disease

Helminthiases (B65-B83)

B65 Schistosomiasis [bilharziasis]
INCLUDES *snail fever*
B65.0 **Schistosomiasis due to Schistosoma** haematobium **[urinary schistosomiasis]**
B65.1 **Schistosomiasis due to Schistosoma** mansoni **[intestinal schistosomiasis]**
B65.2 **Schistosomiasis due to Schistosoma** japonicum
Asiatic schistosomiasis
B65.3 **Cercarial dermatitis**
Swimmer's itch
B65.8 **Other schistosomiasis**
Infection due to Schistosoma intercalatum
Infection due to Schistosoma mattheei
Infection due to Schistosoma mekongi
B65.9 **Schistosomiasis, unspecified**

B66 Other fluke infections
B66.0 **Opisthorchiasis**
Infection due to cat liver fluke
Infection due to Opisthorchis (felineus)(viverrini)
B66.1 **Clonorchiasis**
Chinese liver fluke disease
Infection due to Clonorchis sinensis
Oriental liver fluke disease
B66.2 **Dicroceliasis**
Infection due to Dicrocoelium dendriticum
Lancet fluke infection

Unacceptable principal diagnosis symbol per Medicare code edits | Code exempt from diagnosis present on admission requirement | Questionable admission | Complication or comorbidity | CC/MCC exclusion | Major complication or comorbidity | Principal diagnosis as its own CC | Principal diagnosis as its own MCC | Z code as first-listed diagnosis

B66.3 **Fascioliasis**
Infection due to Fasciola gigantica
Infection due to Fasciola hepatica
Infection due to Fasciola indica
Sheep liver fluke disease
B66.4 **Paragonimiasis**
Infection due to Paragonimus species
Lung fluke disease
Pulmonary distomiasis
B66.5 **Fasciolopsiasis**
Infection due to Fasciolopsis buski
Intestinal distomiasis
B66.8 **Other specified fluke infections**
Echinostomiasis
Heterophyiasis
Metagonimiasis
Nanophyetiasis
Watsoniasis
B66.9 **Fluke infection, unspecified**

B67 **Echinococcosis**
INCLUDES *hydatidosis*
B67.0 **Echinococcus granulosus infection of liver**
B67.1 **Echinococcus granulosus infection of lung**
B67.2 **Echinococcus granulosus infection of bone**
B67.3 **Echinococcus granulosus infection, other and multiple sites**
B67.31 **Echinococcus granulosus infection, thyroid gland**
B67.32 **Echinococcus granulosus infection, multiple sites**
B67.39 **Echinococcus granulosus infection, other sites**
B67.4 **Echinococcus granulosus infection, unspecified**
Dog tapeworm (infection)
B67.5 **Echinococcus multilocularis infection of liver**
B67.6 **Echinococcus multilocularis infection, other and multiple sites**
B67.61 **Echinococcus multilocularis infection, multiple sites**
B67.69 **Echinococcus multilocularis infection, other sites**
B67.7 **Echinococcus multilocularis infection, unspecified**
B67.8 **Echinococcosis, unspecified, of liver**
B67.9 **Echinococcosis, other and unspecified**
B67.90 **Echinococcosis, unspecified**
Echinococcosis NOS
B67.99 **Other echinococcosis**

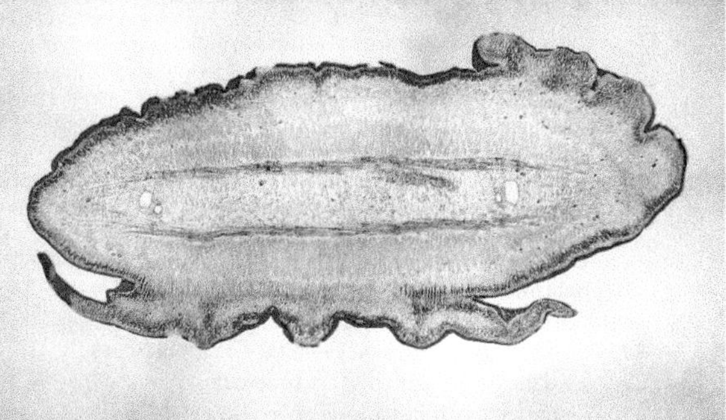

Figure 1.5 Taeniasis

B68 **Taeniasis**
EXCLUDES1 *cysticercosis (B69.-)*
B68.0 **Taenia solium taeniasis**
Pork tapeworm (infection)
B68.1 **Taenia saginata taeniasis**
Beef tapeworm (infection)
Infection due to adult tapeworm Taenia saginata
B68.9 **Taeniasis, unspecified**

B69 **Cysticercosis**
INCLUDES *cysticerciasis infection due to larval form of Taenia solium*
B69.0 **Cysticercosis of central nervous system**
B69.1 **Cysticercosis of eye**
B69.8 **Cysticercosis of other sites**
B69.81 **Myositis in cysticercosis**
B69.89 **Cysticercosis of other sites**
B69.9 **Cysticercosis, unspecified**

B70 **Diphyllobothriasis and sparganosis**
B70.0 **Diphyllobothriasis**
Diphyllobothrium (adult) (latum) (pacificum) infection
Fish tapeworm (infection)
EXCLUDES2 *larval diphyllobothriasis (B70.1)*
B70.1 **Sparganosis**
Infection due to Sparganum (mansoni) (proliferum)
Infection due to Spirometra larva
Larval diphyllobothriasis
Spirometrosis

B71 **Other cestode infections**
B71.0 **Hymenolepiasis**
Dwarf tapeworm infection
Rat tapeworm (infection)
B71.1 **Dipylidiasis**
B71.8 **Other specified cestode infections**
Coenurosis
B71.9 **Cestode infection, unspecified**
Tapeworm (infection) NOS

B72 **Dracunculiasis**
INCLUDES *guinea worm infection*
infection due to Dracunculus medinensis

B73 **Onchocerciasis**
INCLUDES *Onchocerca volvulus infection*
onchocercosis
river blindness
B73.0 **Onchocerciasis with eye disease**
B73.00 **Onchocerciasis with eye involvement, unspecified**
B73.01 **Onchocerciasis with endophthalmitis**
B73.02 **Onchocerciasis with glaucoma**
B73.09 **Onchocerciasis with other eye involvement**
Infestation of eyelid due to onchocerciasis
B73.1 **Onchocerciasis without eye disease**

B74 **Filariasis**
EXCLUDES2 *onchocerciasis (B73)*
tropical (pulmonary) eosinophilia NOS (J82)
B74.0 **Filariasis due to Wuchereria bancrofti**
Bancroftian elephantiasis
Bancroftian filariasis
B74.1 **Filariasis due to Brugia malayi**
B74.2 **Filariasis due to Brugia timori**
B74.3 **Loiasis**
Calabar swelling
Eyeworm disease of Africa
Loa loa infection
B74.4 **Mansonelliasis**
Infection due to Mansonella ozzardi
Infection due to Mansonella perstans
Infection due to Mansonella streptocerca
B74.8 **Other filariases**
Dirofilariasis
B74.9 **Filariasis, unspecified**

B75 **Trichinellosis**
INCLUDES *infection due to Trichinella species*
trichiniasis

B76 **Hookworm diseases**
INCLUDES *uncinariasis*
B76.0 **Ancylostomiasis**
Infection due to Ancylostoma species
B76.1 **Necatoriasis**
Infection due to Necator americanus
B76.8 **Other hookworm diseases**
B76.9 **Hookworm disease, unspecified**
Cutaneous larva migrans NOS

B77 **Ascariasis**
INCLUDES *ascaridiasis*
roundworm infection
B77.0 **Ascariasis with intestinal complications**
B77.8 **Ascariasis with other complications**
B77.81 **Ascariasis pneumonia** MCC PDx
B77.89 **Ascariasis with other complications**
B77.9 **Ascariasis, unspecified**

Unspecified Code | Other Specified Code | Manifestation Code | N Newborn | P Pediatric | M Maternity | A Adult | ♂ Male | ♀ Female
● New Code ▲ Revised Code Title ►◄ Revised Text NOTES INCLUDES EXCLUDES1 Not coded here EXCLUDES2 Not included here
4th character required 5th character required 6th character required 7th character required
Extension 'X' Alert HAC Hospital-acquired condition (HAC) alert AHA AHA Coding Clinic©

B78 Strongyloidiasis
EXCLUDES1 *trichostrongyliasis (B81.2)*
B78.0 Intestinal strongyloidiasis
B78.1 Cutaneous strongyloidiasis
B78.7 Disseminated strongyloidiasis
B78.9 Strongyloidiasis, unspecified

B79 Trichuriasis
INCLUDES *trichocephaliasis*
whipworm (disease)(infection)

B80 Enterobiasis
INCLUDES *oxyuriasis*
pinworm infection
threadworm infection

B81 Other intestinal helminthiases, not elsewhere classified
EXCLUDES1 *angiostrongyliasis due to Parastrongylus cantonensis (B83.2)*
B81.0 Anisakiasis
Infection due to Anisakis larva
B81.1 Intestinal capillariasis
Capillariasis NOS
Infection due to Capillaria philippinensis
EXCLUDES2 *hepatic capillariasis (B83.8)*
B81.2 Trichostrongyliasis
B81.3 Intestinal angiostrongyliasis
Angiostrongyliasis due to Parastrongylus costaricensis
B81.4 Mixed intestinal helminthiases
Infection due to intestinal helminths classified to more than one of the categories B65.0-B81.3 and B81.8
Mixed helminthiasis NOS
B81.8 Other specified intestinal helminthiases
Infection due to Oesophagostomum species [esophagostomiasis]
Infection due to Ternidens diminutus [ternidensiasis]

B82 Unspecified intestinal parasitism
B82.0 Intestinal helminthiasis, unspecified
B82.9 Intestinal parasitism, unspecified

B83 Other helminthiases
EXCLUDES1 *capillariasis NOS (B81.1)*
EXCLUDES2 *intestinal capillariasis (B81.1)*
B83.0 Visceral larva migrans
Toxocariasis
B83.1 Gnathostomiasis
Wandering swelling
B83.2 Angiostrongyliasis due to Parastrongylus cantonensis
Eosinophilic meningoencephalitis due to Parastrongylus cantonensis
EXCLUDES2 *intestinal angiostrongyliasis (B81.3)*
B83.3 Syngamiasis
Syngamosis
B83.4 Internal hirudiniasis
EXCLUDES2 *external hirudiniasis (B88.3)*
B83.8 Other specified helminthiases
Acanthocephaliasis
Gongylonemiasis
Hepatic capillariasis
Metastrongyliasis
Thelaziasis
B83.9 Helminthiasis, unspecified
Worms NOS
EXCLUDES1 *intestinal helminthiasis NOS (B82.0)*

Pediculosis, acariasis and other infestations (B85-B89)

B85 Pediculosis and phthiriasis
B85.0 Pediculosis due to Pediculus humanus capitis
Head-louse infestation
B85.1 Pediculosis due to Pediculus humanus corporis
Body-louse infestation
B85.2 Pediculosis, unspecified
B85.3 Phthiriasis
Infestation by crab-louse
Infestation by Phthirus pubis
B85.4 Mixed pediculosis and phthiriasis
Infestation classifiable to more than one of the categories B85.0-B85.3

B86 Scabies
Sarcoptic itch

B87 Myiasis
INCLUDES *infestation by larva of flies*
B87.0 Cutaneous myiasis
Creeping myiasis
B87.1 Wound myiasis
Traumatic myiasis
B87.2 Ocular myiasis
B87.3 Nasopharyngeal myiasis
Laryngeal myiasis
B87.4 Aural myiasis
B87.8 Myiasis of other sites
B87.81 Genitourinary myiasis
B87.82 Intestinal myiasis
B87.89 Myiasis of other sites
B87.9 Myiasis, unspecified

B88 Other infestations
B88.0 Other acariasis
Acarine dermatitis
Dermatitis due to Demodex species
Dermatitis due to Dermanyssus gallinae
Dermatitis due to Liponyssoides sanguineus
Trombiculosis
EXCLUDES2 *scabies (B86)*
B88.1 Tungiasis [sandflea infestation]
B88.2 Other arthropod infestations
Scarabiasis
B88.3 External hirudiniasis
Leech infestation NOS
EXCLUDES2 *internal hirudiniasis (B83.4)*
B88.8 Other specified infestations
Ichthyoparasitism due to Vandellia cirrhosa
Linguatulosis
Porocephaliasis
B88.9 Infestation, unspecified
Infestation (skin) NOS
Infestation by mites NOS
Skin parasites NOS

B89 Unspecified parasitic disease

Sequelae of infectious and parasitic diseases (B90-B94)

NOTES Categories B90-B94 are to be used to indicate conditions in categories A00-B89 as the cause of sequelae, which are themselves classified elsewhere. The 'sequelae' include conditions specified as such; they also include residuals of diseases classifiable to the above categories if there is evidence that the disease itself is no longer present. Codes from these categories are not to be used for chronic infections. Code chronic current infections to active infectious disease as appropriate.
Code first condition resulting from (sequela) the infectious or parasitic disease

B90 Sequelae of tuberculosis
B90.0 Sequelae of central nervous system tuberculosis
B90.1 Sequelae of genitourinary tuberculosis
B90.2 Sequelae of tuberculosis of bones and joints
B90.8 Sequelae of tuberculosis of other organs
EXCLUDES2 *sequelae of respiratory tuberculosis (B90.9)*
B90.9 Sequelae of respiratory and unspecified tuberculosis
Sequelae of tuberculosis NOS

B91 Sequelae of poliomyelitis
EXCLUDES1 *postpolio syndrome (G14)*

B92 Sequelae of leprosy

B94 Sequelae of other and unspecified infectious and parasitic diseases
B94.0 Sequelae of trachoma
B94.1 Sequelae of viral encephalitis
B94.2 Sequelae of viral hepatitis
B94.8 Sequelae of other specified infectious and parasitic diseases
B94.9 Sequelae of unspecified infectious and parasitic disease

Unacceptable principal diagnosis symbol per Medicare code edits; Code exempt from diagnosis present on admission requirement; Questionable admission; Complication or comorbidity; CC/MCC exclusion; Major complication or comorbidity; Principal diagnosis as its own CC; Principal diagnosis as its own MCC; Z code as first-listed diagnosis

 When symbols appear on a code that requires a 7th character extension, refer to Appendix D to identify applicable 7th character codes.

Bacterial and viral infectious agents (B95-B97)

NOTES These categories are provided for use as supplementary or additional codes to identify the infectious agent(s) in diseases classified elsewhere.

B95 Streptococcus, Staphylococcus, and Enterococcus as the cause of diseases classified elsewhere
- **B95.0 Streptococcus, group A, as the cause of diseases classified elsewhere**
- **B95.1 Streptococcus, group B, as the cause of diseases classified elsewhere**
- **B95.2 Enterococcus as the cause of diseases classified elsewhere**
- **B95.3 Streptococcus pneumoniae as the cause of diseases classified elsewhere**
- **B95.4 Other streptococcus as the cause of diseases classified elsewhere**
- **B95.5 Unspecified streptococcus as the cause of diseases classified elsewhere**
- **B95.6 Staphylococcus aureus as the cause of diseases classified elsewhere**
  - **B95.61 Methicillin susceptible Staphylococcus aureus infection as the cause of diseases classified elsewhere**
    Methicillin susceptible Staphylococcus aureus (MSSA) infection as the cause of diseases classified elsewhere
    Staphylococcus aureus infection NOS as the cause of diseases classified elsewhere
  - **B95.62 Methicillin resistant Staphylococcus aureus infection as the cause of diseases classified elsewhere**
    Methicillin resistant staphylococcus aureus (MRSA) infection as the cause of diseases classified elsewhere
    AHA: Q1, 2016
- **B95.7 Other staphylococcus as the cause of diseases classified elsewhere**
- **B95.8 Unspecified staphylococcus as the cause of diseases classified elsewhere**

B96 Other bacterial agents as the cause of diseases classified elsewhere
- **B96.0 Mycoplasma pneumoniae [M. pneumoniae] as the cause of diseases classified elsewhere**
  Pleuro-pneumonia-like-organism [PPLO]
- **B96.1 Klebsiella pneumoniae [K. pneumoniae] as the cause of diseases classified elsewhere**
- **B96.2 Escherichia coli [E. coli] as the cause of diseases classified elsewhere**
  - **B96.20 Unspecified Escherichia coli [E. coli] as the cause of diseases classified elsewhere**
    Escherichia coli [E. coli] NOS
  - **B96.21 Shiga toxin-producing Escherichia coli [E. coli] (STEC) O157 as the cause of diseases classified elsewhere**
    E. coli O157:H- (nonmotile) with confirmation of Shiga toxin
    E. coli O157 with confirmation of Shiga toxin when H antigen is unknown, or is not H7
    O157:H7 Escherichia coli [E. coli] with or without confirmation of Shiga toxin-production
    Shiga toxin-producing Escherichia coli [E. coli] O157:H7 with or without confirmation of Shiga toxin-production
    STEC O157:H7 with or without confirmation of Shiga toxin-production
  - **B96.22 Other specified Shiga toxin-producing Escherichia coli [E. coli] (STEC) as the cause of diseases classified elsewhere**
    Non-O157 Shiga toxin-producing Escherichia coli [E. coli]
    Non-O157 Shiga toxin-producing Escherichia coli [E. coli] with known O group
  - **B96.23 Unspecified Shiga toxin-producing Escherichia coli [E. coli] (STEC) as the cause of diseases classified elsewhere**
    Shiga toxin-producing Escherichia coli [E. coli] with unspecified O group
    STEC NOS
  - **B96.29 Other Escherichia coli [E. coli] as the cause of diseases classified elsewhere**
    Non-Shiga toxin-producing E. coli
- **B96.3 Haemophilus influenzae [H. influenzae] as the cause of diseases classified elsewhere**
- **B96.4 Proteus (mirabilis) (morganii) as the cause of diseases classified elsewhere**
- **B96.5 Pseudomonas (aeruginosa) (mallei) (pseudomallei) as the cause of diseases classified elsewhere**
  AHA: Q1, 2015
- **B96.6 Bacteroides fragilis [B. fragilis] as the cause of diseases classified elsewhere**
- **B96.7 Clostridium perfringens [C. perfringens] as the cause of diseases classified elsewhere**
- **B96.8 Other specified bacterial agents as the cause of diseases classified elsewhere**
  - **B96.81 Helicobacter pylori [H. pylori] as the cause of diseases classified elsewhere**
  - **B96.82 Vibrio vulnificus as the cause of diseases classified elsewhere**
  - **B96.89 Other specified bacterial agents as the cause of diseases classified elsewhere**

B97 Viral agents as the cause of diseases classified elsewhere
- **B97.0 Adenovirus as the cause of diseases classified elsewhere**
- **B97.1 Enterovirus as the cause of diseases classified elsewhere**
  - **B97.10 Unspecified enterovirus as the cause of diseases classified elsewhere**
  - **B97.11 Coxsackievirus as the cause of diseases classified elsewhere**
  - **B97.12 Echovirus as the cause of diseases classified elsewhere**
  - **B97.19 Other enterovirus as the cause of diseases classified elsewhere**
- **B97.2 Coronavirus as the cause of diseases classified elsewhere**
  - **B97.21 SARS-associated coronavirus as the cause of diseases classified elsewhere**
    EXCLUDES1 *pneumonia due to SARS-associated coronavirus (J12.81)*
  - **B97.29 Other coronavirus as the cause of diseases classified elsewhere**
- **B97.3 Retrovirus as the cause of diseases classified elsewhere**
  EXCLUDES1 *Human immunodeficiency virus [HIV] disease (B20)*
  - **B97.30 Unspecified retrovirus as the cause of diseases classified elsewhere**
  - **B97.31 Lentivirus as the cause of diseases classified elsewhere**
  - **B97.32 Oncovirus as the cause of diseases classified elsewhere**
  - **B97.33 Human T-cell lymphotrophic virus, type I [HTLV-I] as the cause of diseases classified elsewhere**
  - **B97.34 Human T-cell lymphotrophic virus, type II [HTLV-II] as the cause of diseases classified elsewhere**
  - **B97.35 Human immunodeficiency virus, type 2 [HIV 2] as the cause of diseases classified elsewhere**
  - **B97.39 Other retrovirus as the cause of diseases classified elsewhere**
- **B97.4 Respiratory syncytial virus as the cause of diseases classified elsewhere**
- **B97.5 Reovirus as the cause of diseases classified elsewhere**
- **B97.6 Parvovirus as the cause of diseases classified elsewhere**
- **B97.7 Papillomavirus as the cause of diseases classified elsewhere**
- **B97.8 Other viral agents as the cause of diseases classified elsewhere**
  - **B97.81 Human metapneumovirus as the cause of diseases classified elsewhere**
  - **B97.89 Other viral agents as the cause of diseases classified elsewhere**

Other infectious diseases (B99)

B99 Other and unspecified infectious diseases
- **B99.8 Other infectious disease**
- **B99.9 Unspecified infectious disease**

Unspecified Code | Other Specified Code | Manifestation Code | N Newborn | P Pediatric | M Maternity | A Adult | ♂ Male | ♀ Female
● New Code | ▲ Revised Code Title | ►◄ Revised Text | NOTES | INCLUDES | EXCLUDES1 Not coded here | EXCLUDES2 Not included here
4th character required | 5th character required | 6th character required | 7th character required
Extension 'X' Alert | HAC Hospital-acquired condition (HAC) alert | AHA AHA Coding Clinic©

This page intentionally left blank

Chapter 2: Neoplasms (C00-D49)

Guidelines for Assigning Codes From This Chapter

A neoplasm is a new, abnormal growth of tissue. Although you may often hear the term neoplasm in relation to cancerous tumors, which are malignant, not all neoplasms are malignant. ICD-10-CM includes codes in this chapter for all the following:

- Malignant neoplasms, which may be primary (at the point of origin) or secondary (the result of metastasis, or the location where the malignancy has spread)
- Benign neoplasms, which are cancer free
- Neuroendocrine tumors, which may be either malignant or benign, and form from hormone-releasing cells
- Carcinomas in situ, which are abnormal cells that stay in their original location but may later develop into invasive cancer
- Neoplasms of uncertain behavior, a specific histology type that the pathologist identifies when a neoplasm is transitioning from benign to malignant
- behavior neoplasms for which the documentation doesn't specify the nature of the neoplasm

List of Sections

- C00-C96: Malignant neoplasms
- D00-D09: In situ neoplasms
- D3A: Benign neuroendocrine tumors
- D10-D36: Benign neoplasms, except benign neuroendocrine tumors
- D37-D48: Neoplasms of uncertain behavior, polycythemia vera and myelodysplastic syndromes
- D49: Neoplasms of unspecified behavior

Highlights From the ICD-10-CM Official Guidelines for Coding and Reporting

The ICD-10-CM Official Guidelines for Coding and Reporting for Chapter 2 offer insights into proper coding for patients with neoplasms, particularly as it relates to sequencing the codes. The information below is from Section I.C.2 of the 2017 Official Guidelines.

General Information

The Official Guidelines explain that Chapter 2 includes the codes available for all malignant neoplasms and most benign neoplasms. In some cases, ICD-10-CM lists the codes for benign neoplasms in the chapters for their specific body systems instead of in Chapter 2.

To code a neoplasm, you must determine from the documentation if the neoplasm is benign, in situ, malignant or of uncertain histologic behavior. For malignant neoplasms, take note of any secondary, or metastatic, sites.

Use .8 for overlapping sites: If a primary malignant neoplasm overlaps two or more adjacent (contiguous) sites, select the overlapping lesion code, .8, unless there a specific combination code exists. If there are multiple neoplasms as the same site that are noncontiguous, such as tumors in different quadrants of the same breast, report individual codes for each site.

- ➢ A patient with more than one malignant tumor in the same organ may have either different primaries or metastatic disease. Query the provider as to the status of each tumor so you can assign the correct codes.

Code the site of origin: Malignant neoplasms of ectopic tissue, which is tissue outside of its normal location, code the site of origin. For example, report C25. 9 *(Malignant neoplasm of pancreas, unspecified)* for malignant pancreatic neoplasms involving the stomach.

The guidelines offer advice on how to start the search for the proper neoplasm code in the Index. Typically, you'll start by looking at the table located at the Index's Neoplasm entry. But when the documentation includes the histology of the neoplasm (such as adenoma), you should look up that term in the Index and start your search there.

Begin With the Sequencing Basics

The Official Guidelines explain the proper code order when the patient presents for treatment of a malignancy.

- **Primary malignancy treated:** The guidelines start by saying that for treatment of the primary malignancy, you should report the malignancy as the principal diagnosis.
  - ➢ But the guidelines quickly add an exception that "if a patient admission/encounter is solely for the administration of chemotherapy, immunotherapy or radiation therapy, assign the appropriate Z51.-- code as the first-listed or principal diagnosis, and the diagnosis or problem for which the service is being performed as a secondary diagnosis."
    - ➢ You should remember this rule about using the encounter code before the neoplasm code as you read through the other rules and as you code for neoplasm treatment.
  - ➢ Don't report symptoms, signs, and abnormal findings listed in Chapter 18 to replace the malignancy as the principal diagnosis, regardless of the number of admissions or encounters.
- **Secondary site treated:** When the purpose of an encounter is to treat only a secondary neoplasm, you should sequence the secondary neoplasm before the primary neoplasm.

Understand How Variations Alter Code Order

Patients with neoplasms may present for multiple treatments or have multiple diagnoses that apply to the same encounter. The following guidelines help with coding those situations:

- **Chemotherapy/radiation in addition to main reason:** When a single episode of care involves surgical neoplasm removal AND chemotherapy or radiation treatment, you should assign the neoplasm code first. Similarly, if the reason the patient presents is a procedure like paracentesis or to determine the malignancy's extent, you should report the malignancy first even when the patient has chemotherapy or radiation, too.
  - ➢ **Note:** that if the sole reason for the encounter is chemotherapy or radiation treatment, you should assign the appropriate Z code representing the chemotherapy or radiation as the first-listed code.
- **Complications develop:** When complications occur during a session for chemotherapy, immunotherapy, or radiation therapy, you should report the appropriate Z51.- encounter code first with the complications as additional codes.
- **Pregnancy:** If the patient is pregnant, assign first a code from subcategory O9A.1- (Malignant neoplasm complicating pregnancy, childbirth, and the puerperium) followed by the malignancy code from Chapter 2.

Use C80 Unspecified Codes Sparingly

Code C80.0 (*Disseminated malignant neoplasm, unspecified*) only for cases of advanced metastatic disease with no known primary or secondary sites specified. You should never assign this code if either the primary site or any secondary sites are known.

Code C80.1 (*Malignant [primary] neoplasm, unspecified*) means a determination cannot be made as to the site of the primary malignancy and should rarely be used in an inpatient setting.

Base Anemia Code Choice on Cause

The general rule for coding complications is that if the encounter is aimed at treating the complication, you should report the complication before the neoplasm. Here's how the Official Guidelines apply that rule to anemia:

- **Anemia from malignancy:** When the patient presents for treatment of anemia due to malignancy, and only for the anemia, list the code for the malignancy as the primary diagnosis code followed by the appropriate code for the anemia. The typical anemia code in this situation is D63.0 (*Anemia in neoplastic disease*). *Note that this is an exception to the general practice of listing the code for the condition being treated as the primary diagnosis.*
- **Anemia from therapy:** When the patient presents for treatment of only anemia due to chemotherapy, immunotherapy, or radiotherapy, you should report the appropriate anemia code first followed by the malignancy code and the adverse effect, such as T45.1X5 (*Adverse effect of antineoplastic and immunosuppressive drugs*) *or Y84.2* (*Radiological procedure and radiotherapy as the cause of abnormal reaction of the*

patient, or of later complication, without mention of misadventure at the time of the procedure).

Follow the Rules for Dehydration, Surgical Complications, and Pathologic Fractures

Dehydration: In some cases a patient with a malignancy may report for treatment only of dehydration. A typical example involves a patient who is suffering from nausea and vomiting as a result of chemotherapy at an earlier encounter. In those cases, you should report the dehydration first and then the malignancy.

Surgical complication: By now you know the sequencing rule: If the encounter is for treatment of a surgical complication, you should report the complication first.

Pathologic fractures: A neoplasm can result in a fracture. If the fracture is the primary reason for the treatment, assign a code from M84.5 (*Pathological fracture in neoplastic disease*) first, followed by the code for the neoplasm. If the neoplasm is the primary reason for the treatment, sequence the neoplasm code first, followed by the M84.5 code.

Master When to Switch to Personal History Z Code

A key element of coding for neoplasms is knowing when to swap from a neoplasm code to a code from Z85 (*Personal history of malignant neoplasm*).

The rule: You should use a personal history Z code only when documentation shows there is no evidence of the primary malignancy AND the patient is no longer receiving treatment aimed at that site.

In some cases, the patient will still have secondary neoplasms even after treatment eradicates the primary malignancy. You may report the secondary neoplasm first followed by the appropriate Z85 code for the personal history of the primary neoplasm.

Remission vs. personal history: Leukemia codes and category C90 (Multiple myeloma and malignant plasma cell neoplasms) indicate whether or not the patient is in remission. There are also codes Z85.6 (*Personal history of leukemia*) and Z85.79 (*Personal history of other malignant neoplasms of lymphoid, hematopoietic and related tissues*). Query the provider if the documentation doesn't specify remission for these conditions.

Tackle Transplanted Organ Neoplasm Using T86.-

The Official Guidelines also offer instructions on how to code when a patient develops a malignant neoplasm of a transplanted organ. In that situation, report a complication code first, T86.- (*Complications of transplanted organs and tissue*) and then C80.2 (*Malignant neoplasm associated with transplanted organ*). Use an additional code for the specific malignancy.

Note: See Chapter 6 to report neoplasm pain control and management. For aftercare, follow-up care, and prophylactic organ removal for prevention of malignancy, see Chapter 21.

Neoplasms (C00-D49)

This chapter contains the following blocks:

C00-C14	Malignant neoplasms of lip, oral cavity and pharynx
C15-C26	Malignant neoplasms of digestive organs
C30-C39	Malignant neoplasms of respiratory and intrathoracic organs
C40-C41	Malignant neoplasms of bone and articular cartilage
C43-C44	Melanoma and other malignant neoplasms of skin
C45-C49	Malignant neoplasms of mesothelial and soft tissue
C50	Malignant neoplasms of breast
C51-C58	Malignant neoplasms of female genital organs
C60-C63	Malignant neoplasms of male genital organs
C64-C68	Malignant neoplasms of urinary tract
C69-C72	Malignant neoplasms of eye, brain and other parts of central nervous system
C73-C75	Malignant neoplasms of thyroid and other endocrine glands
C7A	Malignant neuroendocrine tumors
C7B	Secondary neuroendocrine tumors
C76-C80	Malignant neoplasms of ill-defined, other secondary and unspecified sites
C81-C96	Malignant neoplasms of lymphoid, hematopoietic and related tissue
D00-D09	In situ neoplasms
D10-D36	Benign neoplasms, except benign neuroendocrine tumors
D3A	Benign neuroendocrine tumors
D37-D48	Neoplasms of uncertain behavior, polycythemia vera and myelodysplastic syndromes
D49	Neoplasms of unspecified behavior

NOTES **Functional activity**
All neoplasms are classified in this chapter, whether they are functionally active or not. An additional code from Chapter 4 may be used, to identify functional activity associated with any neoplasm.
Morphology [Histology]
Chapter 2 classifies neoplasms primarily by site (topography), with broad groupings for behavior, malignant, in situ, benign, etc. The Table of Neoplasms should be used to identify the correct topography code. In a few cases, such as for malignant melanoma and certain neuroendocrine tumors, the morphology (histologic type) is included in the category and codes.
Primary malignant neoplasms overlapping site boundaries
A primary malignant neoplasm that overlaps two or more contiguous (next to each other) sites should be classified to the subcategory/code .8 ('overlapping lesion'), unless the combination is specifically indexed elsewhere. For multiple neoplasms of the same site that are not contiguous, such as tumors in different quadrants of the same breast, codes for each site should be assigned.
Malignant neoplasm of ectopic tissue
Malignant neoplasms of ectopic tissue are to be coded to the site mentioned, e.g., ectopic pancreatic malignant neoplasms are coded to pancreas, unspecified (C25.9).

Malignant neoplasms (C00-C96)

Malignant neoplasms, stated or presumed to be primary (of specified sites), and certain specified histologies, except neuroendocrine, and of lymphoid, hematopoietic and related tissue (C00-C75)

Malignant neoplasms of lip, oral cavity and pharynx (C00-C14)

④ C00 Malignant neoplasm of lip
Use additional code to identify:
alcohol abuse and dependence (F10.-)
history of tobacco ▶dependence◀ (Z87.891)
tobacco dependence (F17.-)
tobacco use (Z72.0)
EXCLUDES1 *malignant melanoma of lip (C43.0)*
Merkel cell carcinoma of lip (C4A.0)
other and unspecified malignant neoplasm of skin of lip (C44.0-)

C00.0 **Malignant neoplasm of external upper lip**
Malignant neoplasm of lipstick area of upper lip
Malignant neoplasm of upper lip NOS
Malignant neoplasm of vermilion border of upper lip

C00.1 **Malignant neoplasm of external lower lip**
Malignant neoplasm of lower lip NOS
Malignant neoplasm of lipstick area of lower lip
Malignant neoplasm of vermilion border of lower lip

C00.2 **Malignant neoplasm of external lip, unspecified**
Malignant neoplasm of vermilion border of lip NOS

C00.3 **Malignant neoplasm of upper lip, inner aspect**
Malignant neoplasm of buccal aspect of upper lip
Malignant neoplasm of frenulum of upper lip
Malignant neoplasm of mucosa of upper lip
Malignant neoplasm of oral aspect of upper lip

C00.4 **Malignant neoplasm of lower lip, inner aspect**
Malignant neoplasm of buccal aspect of lower lip
Malignant neoplasm of frenulum of lower lip
Malignant neoplasm of mucosa of lower lip
Malignant neoplasm of oral aspect of lower lip

C00.5 **Malignant neoplasm of lip, unspecified, inner aspect**
Malignant neoplasm of buccal aspect of lip, unspecified
Malignant neoplasm of frenulum of lip, unspecified
Malignant neoplasm of mucosa of lip, unspecified
Malignant neoplasm of oral aspect of lip, unspecified

C00.6 **Malignant neoplasm of commissure of lip, unspecified**

C00.8 **Malignant neoplasm of overlapping sites of lip**

C00.9 **Malignant neoplasm of lip, unspecified**

C01 **Malignant neoplasm of base of tongue**
Malignant neoplasm of dorsal surface of base of tongue
Malignant neoplasm of fixed part of tongue NOS
Malignant neoplasm of posterior third of tongue
Use additional code to identify:
alcohol abuse and dependence (F10.-)
history of tobacco ▶dependence◀ (Z87.891)
tobacco dependence (F17.-)
tobacco use (Z72.0)

④ C02 **Malignant neoplasm of other and unspecified parts of tongue**
Use additional code to identify:
alcohol abuse and dependence (F10.-)
history of tobacco ▶dependence◀ (Z87.891)
tobacco dependence (F17.-)
tobacco use (Z72.0)

C02.0 **Malignant neoplasm of dorsal surface of tongue**
Malignant neoplasm of anterior two-thirds of tongue, dorsal surface
EXCLUDES2 *malignant neoplasm of dorsal surface of base of tongue (C01)*

C02.1 **Malignant neoplasm of border of tongue**
Malignant neoplasm of tip of tongue

C02.2 **Malignant neoplasm of ventral surface of tongue**
Malignant neoplasm of anterior two-thirds of tongue, ventral surface
Malignant neoplasm of frenulum linguae

C02.3 **Malignant neoplasm of anterior two-thirds of tongue, part unspecified**
Malignant neoplasm of middle third of tongue NOS
Malignant neoplasm of mobile part of tongue NOS

C02.4 **Malignant neoplasm of lingual tonsil**
EXCLUDES2 *malignant neoplasm of tonsil NOS (C09.9)*

C02.8 **Malignant neoplasm of overlapping sites of tongue**
Malignant neoplasm of two or more contiguous sites of tongue

C02.9 **Malignant neoplasm of tongue, unspecified**

④ C03 **Malignant neoplasm of gum**
INCLUDES *malignant neoplasm of alveolar (ridge) mucosa*
malignant neoplasm of gingiva
Use additional code to identify:
alcohol abuse and dependence (F10.-)
history of tobacco ▶dependence◀ (Z87.891)
tobacco dependence (F17.-)
tobacco use (Z72.0)
EXCLUDES2 *malignant odontogenic neoplasms (C41.0-C41.1)*

C03.0 **Malignant neoplasm of upper gum**

C03.1 **Malignant neoplasm of lower gum**

C03.9 **Malignant neoplasm of gum, unspecified**

Unspecified Code | Other Specified Code | Manifestation Code | N Newborn | P Pediatric | M Maternity | A Adult | ♂ Male | ♀ Female
● New Code | ▲ Revised Code Title | ▶◀ Revised Text | NOTES | INCLUDES | EXCLUDES1 Not coded here | EXCLUDES2 Not included here
④ 4th character required | ⑤ 5th character required | ⑥ 6th character required | ⑦ 7th character required
Ⓧ Extension 'X' Alert | HAC Hospital-acquired condition (HAC) alert | AHA AHA Coding Clinic©

C04 Malignant neoplasm of floor of mouth
Use additional code to identify:
alcohol abuse and dependence (F10.-)
history of tobacco ▶dependence◀ (Z87.891)
tobacco dependence (F17.-)
tobacco use (Z72.0)

C04.0 Malignant neoplasm of anterior floor of mouth
Malignant neoplasm of anterior to the premolar-canine junction

C04.1 Malignant neoplasm of lateral floor of mouth

C04.8 Malignant neoplasm of overlapping sites of floor of mouth

C04.9 Malignant neoplasm of floor of mouth, unspecified

C05 Malignant neoplasm of palate
Use additional code to identify:
alcohol abuse and dependence (F10.-)
history of tobacco ▶dependence◀ (Z87.891)
tobacco dependence (F17.-)
tobacco use (Z72.0)

EXCLUDES1 *Kaposi's sarcoma of palate (C46.2)*

C05.0 Malignant neoplasm of hard palate

C05.1 Malignant neoplasm of soft palate
EXCLUDES2 *malignant neoplasm of nasopharyngeal surface of soft palate (C11.3)*

C05.2 Malignant neoplasm of uvula

C05.8 Malignant neoplasm of overlapping sites of palate

C05.9 Malignant neoplasm of palate, unspecified
Malignant neoplasm of roof of mouth

C06 Malignant neoplasm of other and unspecified parts of mouth
Use additional code to identify:
alcohol abuse and dependence (F10.-)
history of tobacco ▶dependence◀ (Z87.891)
tobacco dependence (F17.-)
tobacco use (Z72.0)

C06.0 Malignant neoplasm of cheek mucosa
Malignant neoplasm of buccal mucosa NOS
Malignant neoplasm of internal cheek

C06.1 Malignant neoplasm of vestibule of mouth
Malignant neoplasm of buccal sulcus (upper) (lower)
Malignant neoplasm of labial sulcus (upper) (lower)

C06.2 Malignant neoplasm of retromolar area

C06.8 Malignant neoplasm of overlapping sites of other and unspecified parts of mouth

C06.80 Malignant neoplasm of overlapping sites of unspecified parts of mouth

C06.89 Malignant neoplasm of overlapping sites of other parts of mouth
'book leaf' neoplasm [ventral surface of tongue and floor of mouth]

C06.9 Malignant neoplasm of mouth, unspecified
Malignant neoplasm of minor salivary gland, unspecified site
Malignant neoplasm of oral cavity NOS

C07 Malignant neoplasm of parotid gland
Use additional code to identify:
alcohol abuse and dependence (F10.-)
exposure to environmental tobacco smoke (Z77.22)
exposure to tobacco smoke in the perinatal period (P96.81)
history of tobacco ▶dependence◀ (Z87.891)
occupational exposure to environmental tobacco smoke (Z57.31)
tobacco dependence (F17.-)
tobacco use (Z72.0)

C08 Malignant neoplasm of other and unspecified major salivary glands
INCLUDES *malignant neoplasm of salivary ducts*
Use additional code to identify:
alcohol abuse and dependence (F10.-)
exposure to environmental tobacco smoke (Z77.22)
exposure to tobacco smoke in the perinatal period (P96.81)
history of tobacco ▶dependence◀ (Z87.891)
occupational exposure to environmental tobacco smoke (Z57.31)
tobacco dependence (F17.-)
tobacco use (Z72.0)

EXCLUDES1 *malignant neoplasms of specified minor salivary glands which are classified according to their anatomical location*
EXCLUDES2 *malignant neoplasms of minor salivary glands NOS (C06.9)*
malignant neoplasm of parotid gland (C07)

C08.0 Malignant neoplasm of submandibular gland
Malignant neoplasm of submaxillary gland

C08.1 Malignant neoplasm of sublingual gland

C08.9 Malignant neoplasm of major salivary gland, unspecified
Malignant neoplasm of salivary gland (major) NOS

C09 Malignant neoplasm of tonsil
Use additional code to identify:
alcohol abuse and dependence (F10.-)
exposure to environmental tobacco smoke (Z77.22)
exposure to tobacco smoke in the perinatal period (P96.81)
history of tobacco ▶dependence◀ (Z87.891)
occupational exposure to environmental tobacco smoke (Z57.31)
tobacco dependence (F17.-)
tobacco use (Z72.0)

EXCLUDES2 *malignant neoplasm of lingual tonsil (C02.4)*
malignant neoplasm of pharyngeal tonsil (C11.1)

C09.0 Malignant neoplasm of tonsillar fossa

C09.1 Malignant neoplasm of tonsillar pillar (anterior) (posterior)

C09.8 Malignant neoplasm of overlapping sites of tonsil

C09.9 Malignant neoplasm of tonsil, unspecified
Malignant neoplasm of tonsil NOS
Malignant neoplasm of faucial tonsils
Malignant neoplasm of palatine tonsils

C10 Malignant neoplasm of oropharynx
Use additional code to identify:
alcohol abuse and dependence (F10.-)
exposure to environmental tobacco smoke (Z77.22)
exposure to tobacco smoke in the perinatal period (P96.81)
history of tobacco ▶dependence◀ (Z87.891)
occupational exposure to environmental tobacco smoke (Z57.31)
tobacco dependence (F17.-)
tobacco use (Z72.0)

EXCLUDES2 *malignant neoplasm of tonsil (C09.-)*

C10.0 Malignant neoplasm of vallecula

C10.1 Malignant neoplasm of anterior surface of epiglottis
Malignant neoplasm of epiglottis, free border [margin]
Malignant neoplasm of glossoepiglottic fold(s)
EXCLUDES2 *malignant neoplasm of epiglottis (suprahyoid portion) NOS (C32.1)*

C10.2 Malignant neoplasm of lateral wall of oropharynx

C10.3 Malignant neoplasm of posterior wall of oropharynx

C10.4 Malignant neoplasm of branchial cleft
Malignant neoplasm of branchial cyst [site of neoplasm]

C10.8 Malignant neoplasm of overlapping sites of oropharynx
Malignant neoplasm of junctional region of oropharynx

C10.9 Malignant neoplasm of oropharynx, unspecified

C11 Malignant neoplasm of nasopharynx
Use additional code to identify:
exposure to environmental tobacco smoke (Z77.22)
exposure to tobacco smoke in the perinatal period (P96.81)
history of tobacco ▶dependence◀ (Z87.891)
occupational exposure to environmental tobacco smoke (Z57.31)
tobacco dependence (F17.-)
tobacco use (Z72.0)

C11.0 Malignant neoplasm of superior wall of nasopharynx
Malignant neoplasm of roof of nasopharynx

C11.1 Malignant neoplasm of posterior wall of nasopharynx
Malignant neoplasm of adenoid
Malignant neoplasm of pharyngeal tonsil

C11.2 Malignant neoplasm of lateral wall of nasopharynx
Malignant neoplasm of fossa of Rosenmüller
Malignant neoplasm of opening of auditory tube
Malignant neoplasm of pharyngeal recess

C11.3 Malignant neoplasm of anterior wall of nasopharynx
Malignant neoplasm of floor of nasopharynx
Malignant neoplasm of nasopharyngeal (anterior) (posterior) surface of soft palate
Malignant neoplasm of posterior margin of nasal choana
Malignant neoplasm of posterior margin of nasal septum

C11.8 Malignant neoplasm of overlapping sites of nasopharynx

C11.9 Malignant neoplasm of nasopharynx, unspecified
Malignant neoplasm of nasopharyngeal wall NOS

Unacceptable principal diagnosis symbol per Medicare code edits · Code exempt from diagnosis present on admission requirement
Questionable admission · Complication or comorbidity · CC/MCC exclusion · Major complication or comorbidity
Principal diagnosis as its own CC · Principal diagnosis as its own MCC · Z code as first-listed diagnosis

C12 Malignant neoplasm of pyriform sinus
Malignant neoplasm of pyriform fossa
Use additional code to identify:
exposure to environmental tobacco smoke (Z77.22)
exposure to tobacco smoke in the perinatal period (P96.81)
history of tobacco ▶dependence◀ (Z87.891)
occupational exposure to environmental tobacco smoke (Z57.31)
tobacco dependence (F17.-)
tobacco use (Z72.0)

C13 Malignant neoplasm of hypopharynx
Use additional code to identify:
exposure to environmental tobacco smoke (Z77.22)
exposure to tobacco smoke in the perinatal period (P96.81)
history of tobacco ▶dependence◀ (Z87.891)
occupational exposure to environmental tobacco smoke (Z57.31)
tobacco dependence (F17.-)
tobacco use (Z72.0)
EXCLUDES2 *malignant neoplasm of pyriform sinus (C12)*
C13.0 Malignant neoplasm of postcricoid region
C13.1 Malignant neoplasm of aryepiglottic fold, hypopharyngeal aspect
Malignant neoplasm of aryepiglottic fold, marginal zone
Malignant neoplasm of aryepiglottic fold NOS
Malignant neoplasm of interarytenoid fold, marginal zone
Malignant neoplasm of interarytenoid fold NOS
EXCLUDES2 *malignant neoplasm of aryepiglottic fold or interarytenoid fold, laryngeal aspect (C32.1)*
C13.2 Malignant neoplasm of posterior wall of hypopharynx
C13.8 Malignant neoplasm of overlapping sites of hypopharynx
C13.9 Malignant neoplasm of hypopharynx, unspecified
Malignant neoplasm of hypopharyngeal wall NOS

C14 Malignant neoplasm of other and ill-defined sites in the lip, oral cavity and pharynx
Use additional code to identify:
alcohol abuse and dependence (F10.-)
exposure to environmental tobacco smoke (Z77.22)
exposure to tobacco smoke in the perinatal period (P96.81)
history of tobacco ▶dependence◀ (Z87.891)
occupational exposure to environmental tobacco smoke (Z57.31)
tobacco dependence (F17.-)
tobacco use (Z72.0)
EXCLUDES1 *malignant neoplasm of oral cavity NOS (C06.9)*
C14.0 Malignant neoplasm of pharynx, unspecified
C14.2 Malignant neoplasm of Waldeyer's ring
C14.8 Malignant neoplasm of overlapping sites of lip, oral cavity and pharynx
Primary malignant neoplasm of two or more contiguous sites of lip, oral cavity and pharynx
EXCLUDES1 *'book leaf' neoplasm [ventral surface of tongue and floor of mouth] (C06.89)*

Malignant neoplasms of digestive organs (C15-C26)

EXCLUDES1 *Kaposi's sarcoma of gastrointestinal sites (C46.4)*
EXCLUDES2 *gastrointestinal stromal tumors (C49.A-)*

C15 Malignant neoplasm of esophagus
Use additional code to identify:
alcohol abuse and dependence (F10.-)
C15.3 Malignant neoplasm of upper third of esophagus
C15.4 Malignant neoplasm of middle third of esophagus
C15.5 Malignant neoplasm of lower third of esophagus
EXCLUDES1 *malignant neoplasm of cardio-esophageal junction (C16.0)*
C15.8 Malignant neoplasm of overlapping sites of esophagus
C15.9 Malignant neoplasm of esophagus, unspecified

C16 Malignant neoplasm of stomach
Use additional code to identify:
alcohol abuse and dependence (F10.-)
EXCLUDES2 *malignant carcinoid tumor of the stomach (C7A.092)*
C16.0 Malignant neoplasm of cardia
Malignant neoplasm of cardiac orifice
Malignant neoplasm of cardio-esophageal junction
Malignant neoplasm of esophagus and stomach
Malignant neoplasm of gastro-esophageal junction
C16.1 Malignant neoplasm of fundus of stomach
C16.2 Malignant neoplasm of body of stomach
C16.3 Malignant neoplasm of pyloric antrum
Malignant neoplasm of gastric antrum
C16.4 Malignant neoplasm of pylorus
Malignant neoplasm of prepylorus
Malignant neoplasm of pyloric canal
C16.5 Malignant neoplasm of lesser curvature of stomach, unspecified
Malignant neoplasm of lesser curvature of stomach, not classifiable to C16.1-C16.4
C16.6 Malignant neoplasm of greater curvature of stomach, unspecified
Malignant neoplasm of greater curvature of stomach, not classifiable to C16.0-C16.4
C16.8 Malignant neoplasm of overlapping sites of stomach
C16.9 Malignant neoplasm of stomach, unspecified
Gastric cancer NOS

C17 Malignant neoplasm of small intestine
EXCLUDES1 *malignant carcinoid tumors of the small intestine (C7A.01)*
C17.0 Malignant neoplasm of duodenum
C17.1 Malignant neoplasm of jejunum
C17.2 Malignant neoplasm of ileum
EXCLUDES1 *malignant neoplasm of ileocecal valve (C18.0)*
C17.3 Meckel's diverticulum, malignant
EXCLUDES1 *Meckel's diverticulum, congenital (Q43.0)*
C17.8 Malignant neoplasm of overlapping sites of small intestine
C17.9 Malignant neoplasm of small intestine, unspecified

C18 Malignant neoplasm of colon
EXCLUDES1 *malignant carcinoid tumors of the colon (C7A.02-)*
C18.0 Malignant neoplasm of cecum
Malignant neoplasm of ileocecal valve
C18.1 Malignant neoplasm of appendix
C18.2 Malignant neoplasm of ascending colon
C18.3 Malignant neoplasm of hepatic flexure
C18.4 Malignant neoplasm of transverse colon
C18.5 Malignant neoplasm of splenic flexure
C18.6 Malignant neoplasm of descending colon
C18.7 Malignant neoplasm of sigmoid colon
Malignant neoplasm of sigmoid (flexure)
EXCLUDES1 *malignant neoplasm of rectosigmoid junction (C19)*
C18.8 Malignant neoplasm of overlapping sites of colon
C18.9 Malignant neoplasm of colon, unspecified
Malignant neoplasm of large intestine NOS

C19 Malignant neoplasm of rectosigmoid junction
Malignant neoplasm of colon with rectum
Malignant neoplasm of rectosigmoid (colon)
EXCLUDES1 *malignant carcinoid tumors of the colon (C7A.02-)*

C20 Malignant neoplasm of rectum
Malignant neoplasm of rectal ampulla
EXCLUDES1 *malignant carcinoid tumor of the rectum (C7A.026)*

C21 Malignant neoplasm of anus and anal canal
EXCLUDES2 *malignant carcinoid tumors of the colon (C7A.02-)*
malignant melanoma of anal margin (C43.51)
malignant melanoma of anal skin (C43.51)
malignant melanoma of perianal skin (C43.51)
other and unspecified malignant neoplasm of anal margin (C44.500, C44.510, C44.520, C44.590)
other and unspecified malignant neoplasm of anal skin (C44.500, C44.510, C44.520, C44.590)
other and unspecified malignant neoplasm of perianal skin (C44.500, C44.510, C44.520, C44.590)
C21.0 Malignant neoplasm of anus, unspecified
C21.1 Malignant neoplasm of anal canal
Malignant neoplasm of anal sphincter
C21.2 Malignant neoplasm of cloacogenic zone
C21.8 Malignant neoplasm of overlapping sites of rectum, anus and anal canal
Malignant neoplasm of anorectal junction
Malignant neoplasm of anorectum
Primary malignant neoplasm of two or more contiguous sites of rectum, anus and anal canal

Unspecified Code | Other Specified Code | Manifestation Code | N Newborn | P Pediatric | M Maternity | A Adult | ♂ Male | ♀ Female
● New Code | ▲ Revised Code Title | ▶◀ Revised Text | NOTES | INCLUDES | EXCLUDES1 Not coded here | EXCLUDES2 Not included here
4th character required | 5th character required | 6th character required | 7th character required
Extension 'X' Alert | HAC Hospital-acquired condition (HAC) alert | AHA AHA Coding Clinic©

C22 Malignant neoplasm of liver and intrahepatic bile ducts
EXCLUDES1 *malignant neoplasm of biliary tract NOS (C24.9)*
secondary malignant neoplasm of liver and intrahepatic bile duct (C78.7)
Use additional code to identify:
alcohol abuse and dependence (F10.-)
hepatitis B (B16.-, B18.0-B18.1)
hepatitis C (B17.1-, B18.2)
C22.0 **Liver cell carcinoma** CC
Hepatocellular carcinoma
Hepatoma
AHA: Q1, 2016
C22.1 **Intrahepatic bile duct carcinoma** CC
Cholangiocarcinoma
EXCLUDES1 *malignant neoplasm of hepatic duct (C24.0)*
C22.2 **Hepatoblastoma** CC
C22.3 **Angiosarcoma of liver** CC
Kupffer cell sarcoma
C22.4 **Other sarcomas of liver** CC
C22.7 **Other specified carcinomas of liver** CC
C22.8 **Malignant neoplasm of liver, primary, unspecified as to type** CC
C22.9 **Malignant neoplasm of liver, not specified as primary or secondary** CC
C23 **Malignant neoplasm of gallbladder** CC
C24 **Malignant neoplasm of other and unspecified parts of biliary tract**
EXCLUDES1 *malignant neoplasm of intrahepatic bile duct (C22.1)*
C24.0 **Malignant neoplasm of extrahepatic bile duct** CC
Malignant neoplasm of biliary duct or passage NOS
Malignant neoplasm of common bile duct
Malignant neoplasm of cystic duct
Malignant neoplasm of hepatic duct
C24.1 **Malignant neoplasm of ampulla of Vater** CC
C24.8 **Malignant neoplasm of overlapping sites of biliary tract** CC
Malignant neoplasm involving both intrahepatic and extrahepatic bile ducts
Primary malignant neoplasm of two or more contiguous sites of biliary tract
C24.9 **Malignant neoplasm of biliary tract, unspecified** CC
C25 **Malignant neoplasm of pancreas**
Code also exocrine pancreatic insufficiency (K86.81)
Use additional code to identify:
alcohol abuse and dependence (F10.-)
C25.0 **Malignant neoplasm of head of pancreas** CC
C25.1 **Malignant neoplasm of body of pancreas** CC
C25.2 **Malignant neoplasm of tail of pancreas** CC
C25.3 **Malignant neoplasm of pancreatic duct** CC
C25.4 **Malignant neoplasm of endocrine pancreas** CC
Malignant neoplasm of islets of Langerhans
Use additional code to identify any functional activity.
C25.7 **Malignant neoplasm of other parts of pancreas** CC
Malignant neoplasm of neck of pancreas
C25.8 **Malignant neoplasm of overlapping sites of pancreas** CC
C25.9 **Malignant neoplasm of pancreas, unspecified** CC
C26 **Malignant neoplasm of other and ill-defined digestive organs**
EXCLUDES1 *malignant neoplasm of peritoneum and retroperitoneum (C48.-)*
C26.0 **Malignant neoplasm of intestinal tract, part unspecified**
Malignant neoplasm of intestine NOS
C26.1 **Malignant neoplasm of spleen**
EXCLUDES1 *Hodgkin lymphoma (C81.-)*
non-Hodgkin lymphoma (C82-C85)
C26.9 **Malignant neoplasm of ill-defined sites within the digestive system**
Malignant neoplasm of alimentary canal or tract NOS
Malignant neoplasm of gastrointestinal tract NOS
EXCLUDES1 *malignant neoplasm of abdominal NOS (C76.2)*
malignant neoplasm of intra-abdominal NOS (C76.2)

Malignant neoplasms of respiratory and intrathoracic organs (C30-C39)

INCLUDES *malignant neoplasm of middle ear*
EXCLUDES1 *mesothelioma (C45.-)*
C30 **Malignant neoplasm of nasal cavity and middle ear**
C30.0 **Malignant neoplasm of nasal cavity**
Malignant neoplasm of cartilage of nose
Malignant neoplasm of nasal concha
Malignant neoplasm of internal nose
Malignant neoplasm of septum of nose
Malignant neoplasm of vestibule of nose
EXCLUDES1 *malignant neoplasm of nasal bone (C41.0)*
malignant neoplasm of nose NOS (C76.0)
malignant neoplasm of olfactory bulb (C72.2-)
malignant neoplasm of posterior margin of nasal septum and choana (C11.3)
malignant melanoma of skin of nose (C43.31)
malignant neoplasm of turbinates (C41.0)
other and unspecified malignant neoplasm of skin of nose C44.301, C44.311, C44.321, C44.391)
C30.1 **Malignant neoplasm of middle ear**
Malignant neoplasm of antrum tympanicum
Malignant neoplasm of auditory tube
Malignant neoplasm of eustachian tube
Malignant neoplasm of inner ear
Malignant neoplasm of mastoid air cells
Malignant neoplasm of tympanic cavity
EXCLUDES1 *malignant neoplasm of auricular canal (external) (C43.2-,C44.2-)*
malignant neoplasm of bone of ear (meatus) (C41.0)
malignant neoplasm of cartilage of ear (C49.0)
malignant melanoma of skin of (external) ear (C43.2-)
other and unspecified malignant neoplasm of skin of (external) ear (C44.2-)
C31 **Malignant neoplasm of accessory sinuses**
C31.0 **Malignant neoplasm of maxillary sinus**
Malignant neoplasm of antrum (Highmore) (maxillary)
C31.1 **Malignant neoplasm of ethmoidal sinus**
C31.2 **Malignant neoplasm of frontal sinus**
C31.3 **Malignant neoplasm of sphenoid sinus**
C31.8 **Malignant neoplasm of overlapping sites of accessory sinuses**
C31.9 **Malignant neoplasm of accessory sinus, unspecified**
C32 **Malignant neoplasm of larynx**
Use additional code to identify:
alcohol abuse and dependence (F10.-)
exposure to environmental tobacco smoke (Z77.22)
exposure to tobacco smoke in the perinatal period (P96.81)
history of tobacco ▶dependence◀ (Z87.891)
occupational exposure to environmental tobacco smoke (Z57.31)
tobacco dependence (F17.-)
tobacco use (Z72.0)
C32.0 **Malignant neoplasm of glottis**
Malignant neoplasm of intrinsic larynx
Malignant neoplasm of laryngeal commissure (anterior) (posterior)
Malignant neoplasm of vocal cord (true) NOS
C32.1 **Malignant neoplasm of supraglottis**
Malignant neoplasm of aryepiglottic fold or interarytenoid fold, laryngeal aspect
Malignant neoplasm of epiglottis (suprahyoid portion) NOS
Malignant neoplasm of extrinsic larynx
Malignant neoplasm of false vocal cord
Malignant neoplasm of posterior (laryngeal) surface of epiglottis
Malignant neoplasm of ventricular bands
EXCLUDES2 *malignant neoplasm of anterior surface of epiglottis (C10.1)*
malignant neoplasm of aryepiglottic fold or interarytenoid fold, hypopharyngeal aspect (C13.1)
malignant neoplasm of aryepiglottic fold or interarytenoid fold, marginal zone (C13.1)
malignant neoplasm of aryepiglottic fold or interarytenoid fold NOS (C13.1)

Unacceptable principal diagnosis symbol per Medicare code edits · Code exempt from diagnosis present on admission requirement
Questionable admission · CC Complication or comorbidity · CC/MCC exclusion · MCC Major complication or comorbidity
Principal diagnosis as its own CC · Principal diagnosis as its own MCC · Z code as first-listed diagnosis

When symbols appear on a code that requires a 7th character extension, refer to Appendix D to identify applicable 7th character codes.

C32.2 Malignant neoplasm of subglottis

C32.3 Malignant neoplasm of laryngeal cartilage

C32.8 Malignant neoplasm of overlapping sites of larynx

C32.9 Malignant neoplasm of larynx, unspecified

C33 Malignant neoplasm of trachea

Use additional code to identify:
exposure to environmental tobacco smoke (Z77.22)
exposure to tobacco smoke in the perinatal period (P96.81)
history of tobacco ▶dependence◀ (Z87.891)
occupational exposure to environmental tobacco smoke (Z57.31)
tobacco dependence (F17.-)
tobacco use (Z72.0)

C34 Malignant neoplasm of bronchus and lung

Use additional code to identify:
exposure to environmental tobacco smoke (Z77.22)
exposure to tobacco smoke in the perinatal period (P96.81)
history of tobacco ▶dependence◀ (Z87.891)
occupational exposure to environmental tobacco smoke (Z57.31)
tobacco dependence (F17.-)
tobacco use (Z72.0)

EXCLUDES1 *Kaposi's sarcoma of lung (C46.5-)*
malignant carcinoid tumor of the bronchus and lung (C7A.090)

C34.0 Malignant neoplasm of main bronchus
Malignant neoplasm of carina
Malignant neoplasm of hilus (of lung)

C34.00 Malignant neoplasm of unspecified main bronchus

C34.01 Malignant neoplasm of right main bronchus

C34.02 Malignant neoplasm of left main bronchus

C34.1 Malignant neoplasm of upper lobe, bronchus or lung

C34.10 Malignant neoplasm of upper lobe, unspecified bronchus or lung

C34.11 Malignant neoplasm of upper lobe, right bronchus or lung

C34.12 Malignant neoplasm of upper lobe, left bronchus or lung

C34.2 Malignant neoplasm of middle lobe, bronchus or lung

C34.3 Malignant neoplasm of lower lobe, bronchus or lung

C34.30 Malignant neoplasm of lower lobe, unspecified bronchus or lung

C34.31 Malignant neoplasm of lower lobe, right bronchus or lung

C34.32 Malignant neoplasm of lower lobe, left bronchus or lung

C34.8 Malignant neoplasm of overlapping sites of bronchus and lung

C34.80 Malignant neoplasm of overlapping sites of unspecified bronchus and lung

C34.81 Malignant neoplasm of overlapping sites of right bronchus and lung

C34.82 Malignant neoplasm of overlapping sites of left bronchus and lung

C34.9 Malignant neoplasm of unspecified part of bronchus or lung

C34.90 Malignant neoplasm of unspecified part of unspecified bronchus or lung
Lung cancer NOS

C34.91 Malignant neoplasm of unspecified part of right bronchus or lung

C34.92 Malignant neoplasm of unspecified part of left bronchus or lung

C37 Malignant neoplasm of thymus

EXCLUDES1 *malignant carcinoid tumor of the thymus (C7A.091)*

C38 Malignant neoplasm of heart, mediastinum and pleura

EXCLUDES1 *mesothelioma (C45.-)*

C38.0 Malignant neoplasm of heart
Malignant neoplasm of pericardium
EXCLUDES1 *malignant neoplasm of great vessels (C49.3)*

C38.1 Malignant neoplasm of anterior mediastinum

C38.2 Malignant neoplasm of posterior mediastinum

C38.3 Malignant neoplasm of mediastinum, part unspecified

C38.4 Malignant neoplasm of pleura

C38.8 Malignant neoplasm of overlapping sites of heart, mediastinum and pleura

C39 Malignant neoplasm of other and ill-defined sites in the respiratory system and intrathoracic organs

Use additional code to identify:
exposure to environmental tobacco smoke (Z77.22)
exposure to tobacco smoke in the perinatal period (P96.81)
history of tobacco ▶dependence◀ (Z87.891)
occupational exposure to environmental tobacco smoke (Z57.31)
tobacco dependence (F17.-)
tobacco use (Z72.0)

EXCLUDES1 *intrathoracic malignant neoplasm NOS (C76.1)*
thoracic malignant neoplasm NOS (C76.1)

C39.0 Malignant neoplasm of upper respiratory tract, part unspecified

C39.9 Malignant neoplasm of lower respiratory tract, part unspecified
Malignant neoplasm of respiratory tract NOS

Malignant neoplasms of bone and articular cartilage (C40-C41)

INCLUDES *malignant neoplasm of cartilage (articular) (joint)*
malignant neoplasm of periosteum

EXCLUDES1 *malignant neoplasm of bone marrow NOS (C96.9)*
malignant neoplasm of synovia (C49.-)

C40 Malignant neoplasm of bone and articular cartilage of limbs

Use additional code to identify major osseous defect, if applicable (M89.7-)

C40.0 Malignant neoplasm of scapula and long bones of upper limb

C40.00 Malignant neoplasm of scapula and long bones of unspecified upper limb

C40.01 Malignant neoplasm of scapula and long bones of right upper limb

C40.02 Malignant neoplasm of scapula and long bones of left upper limb

C40.1 Malignant neoplasm of short bones of upper limb

C40.10 Malignant neoplasm of short bones of unspecified upper limb

C40.11 Malignant neoplasm of short bones of right upper limb

C40.12 Malignant neoplasm of short bones of left upper limb

C40.2 Malignant neoplasm of long bones of lower limb

C40.20 Malignant neoplasm of long bones of unspecified lower limb

C40.21 Malignant neoplasm of long bones of right lower limb

C40.22 Malignant neoplasm of long bones of left lower limb

C40.3 Malignant neoplasm of short bones of lower limb

C40.30 Malignant neoplasm of short bones of unspecified lower limb

C40.31 Malignant neoplasm of short bones of right lower limb

C40.32 Malignant neoplasm of short bones of left lower limb

C40.8 Malignant neoplasm of overlapping sites of bone and articular cartilage of limb

C40.80 Malignant neoplasm of overlapping sites of bone and articular cartilage of unspecified limb

C40.81 Malignant neoplasm of overlapping sites of bone and articular cartilage of right limb

C40.82 Malignant neoplasm of overlapping sites of bone and articular cartilage of left limb

C40.9 Malignant neoplasm of unspecified bones and articular cartilage of limb

C40.90 Malignant neoplasm of unspecified bones and articular cartilage of unspecified limb

C40.91 Malignant neoplasm of unspecified bones and articular cartilage of right limb

C40.92 Malignant neoplasm of unspecified bones and articular cartilage of left limb

C41 Malignant neoplasm of bone and articular cartilage of other and unspecified sites

EXCLUDES1 *malignant neoplasm of bones of limbs (C40.-)*
malignant neoplasm of cartilage of ear (C49.0)

Unspecified Code Other Specified Code Manifestation Code N Newborn P Pediatric M Maternity A Adult ♂ Male ♀ Female
● New Code ▲ Revised Code Title ▶◀ Revised Text NOTES INCLUDES EXCLUDES1 Not coded here EXCLUDES2 Not included here
4th character required 5th character required 6th character required 7th character required
Extension 'X' Alert HAC Hospital-acquired condition (HAC) alert AHA AHA Coding Clinic©

When symbols appear on a code that requires a 7th character extension, refer to Appendix D to identify applicable 7th character codes.

malignant neoplasm of cartilage of eyelid (C49.0)
malignant neoplasm of cartilage of larynx (C32.3)
malignant neoplasm of cartilage of limbs (C40.-)
malignant neoplasm of cartilage of nose (C30.0)

C41.0 Malignant neoplasm of bones of skull and face CC
Malignant neoplasm of maxilla (superior)
Malignant neoplasm of orbital bone
EXCLUDES2 *carcinoma, any type except intraosseous or odontogenic of:*
maxillary sinus (C31.0)
upper jaw (C03.0)
malignant neoplasm of jaw bone (lower) (C41.1)

C41.1 Malignant neoplasm of mandible CC
Malignant neoplasm of inferior maxilla
Malignant neoplasm of lower jaw bone
EXCLUDES2 *carcinoma, any type except intraosseous or odontogenic of:*
jaw NOS (C03.9)
lower (C03.1)
malignant neoplasm of upper jaw bone (C41.0)

C41.2 Malignant neoplasm of vertebral column CC
EXCLUDES1 *malignant neoplasm of sacrum and coccyx (C41.4)*

C41.3 Malignant neoplasm of ribs, sternum and clavicle CC

C41.4 Malignant neoplasm of pelvic bones, sacrum and coccyx CC

C41.9 Malignant neoplasm of bone and articular cartilage, unspecified CC

Melanoma and other malignant neoplasms of skin (C43-C44)

4th C43 Malignant melanoma of skin
EXCLUDES1 *melanoma in situ (D03.-)*
EXCLUDES2 *malignant melanoma of skin of genital organs (C51-C52, C60.-, C63.-)*
Merkel cell carcinoma (C4A.-)
sites other than skin-code to malignant neoplasm of the site

C43.0 Malignant melanoma of lip
EXCLUDES1 *malignant neoplasm of vermilion border of lip (C00.0-C00.2)*

5th C43.1 Malignant melanoma of eyelid, including canthus
- **C43.10 Malignant melanoma of unspecified eyelid, including canthus**
- **C43.11 Malignant melanoma of right eyelid, including canthus**
- **C43.12 Malignant melanoma of left eyelid, including canthus**

5th C43.2 Malignant melanoma of ear and external auricular canal
- **C43.20 Malignant melanoma of unspecified ear and external auricular canal**
- **C43.21 Malignant melanoma of right ear and external auricular canal**
- **C43.22 Malignant melanoma of left ear and external auricular canal**

5th C43.3 Malignant melanoma of other and unspecified parts of face
- **C43.30 Malignant melanoma of unspecified part of face**
- **C43.31 Malignant melanoma of nose**
- **C43.39 Malignant melanoma of other parts of face**

C43.4 Malignant melanoma of scalp and neck

5th C43.5 Malignant melanoma of trunk
EXCLUDES2 *malignant neoplasm of anus NOS (C21.0)*
malignant neoplasm of scrotum (C63.2)
- **C43.51 Malignant melanoma of anal skin**
  Malignant melanoma of anal margin
  Malignant melanoma of perianal skin
- **C43.52 Malignant melanoma of skin of breast**
- **C43.59 Malignant melanoma of other part of trunk**

5th C43.6 Malignant melanoma of upper limb, including shoulder
- **C43.60 Malignant melanoma of unspecified upper limb, including shoulder**
- **C43.61 Malignant melanoma of right upper limb, including shoulder**
- **C43.62 Malignant melanoma of left upper limb, including shoulder**

5th C43.7 Malignant melanoma of lower limb, including hip
- **C43.70 Malignant melanoma of unspecified lower limb, including hip**
- **C43.71 Malignant melanoma of right lower limb, including hip**
- **C43.72 Malignant melanoma of left lower limb, including hip**

C43.8 Malignant melanoma of overlapping sites of skin

C43.9 Malignant melanoma of skin, unspecified
Malignant melanoma of unspecified site of skin
Melanoma (malignant) NOS

4th C4A Merkel cell carcinoma

C4A.0 Merkel cell carcinoma of lip
EXCLUDES1 *malignant neoplasm of vermilion border of lip (C00.0-C00.2)*

5th C4A.1 Merkel cell carcinoma of eyelid, including canthus
- **C4A.10 Merkel cell carcinoma of unspecified eyelid, including canthus**
- **C4A.11 Merkel cell carcinoma of right eyelid, including canthus**
- **C4A.12 Merkel cell carcinoma of left eyelid, including canthus**

5th C4A.2 Merkel cell carcinoma of ear and external auricular canal
- **C4A.20 Merkel cell carcinoma of unspecified ear and external auricular canal**
- **C4A.21 Merkel cell carcinoma of right ear and external auricular canal**
- **C4A.22 Merkel cell carcinoma of left ear and external auricular canal**

5th C4A.3 Merkel cell carcinoma of other and unspecified parts of face
- **C4A.30 Merkel cell carcinoma of unspecified part of face**
- **C4A.31 Merkel cell carcinoma of nose**
- **C4A.39 Merkel cell carcinoma of other parts of face**

C4A.4 Merkel cell carcinoma of scalp and neck

5th C4A.5 Merkel cell carcinoma of trunk
EXCLUDES2 *malignant neoplasm of anus NOS (C21.0)*
malignant neoplasm of scrotum (C63.2)
- **C4A.51 Merkel cell carcinoma of anal skin**
  Merkel cell carcinoma of anal margin
  Merkel cell carcinoma of perianal skin
- **C4A.52 Merkel cell carcinoma of skin of breast**
- **C4A.59 Merkel cell carcinoma of other part of trunk**

5th C4A.6 Merkel cell carcinoma of upper limb, including shoulder
- **C4A.60 Merkel cell carcinoma of unspecified upper limb, including shoulder**
- **C4A.61 Merkel cell carcinoma of right upper limb, including shoulder**
- **C4A.62 Merkel cell carcinoma of left upper limb, including shoulder**

5th C4A.7 Merkel cell carcinoma of lower limb, including hip
- **C4A.70 Merkel cell carcinoma of unspecified lower limb, including hip**
- **C4A.71 Merkel cell carcinoma of right lower limb, including hip**
- **C4A.72 Merkel cell carcinoma of left lower limb, including hip**

C4A.8 Merkel cell carcinoma of overlapping sites

C4A.9 Merkel cell carcinoma, unspecified
Merkel cell carcinoma of unspecified site
Merkel cell carcinoma NOS

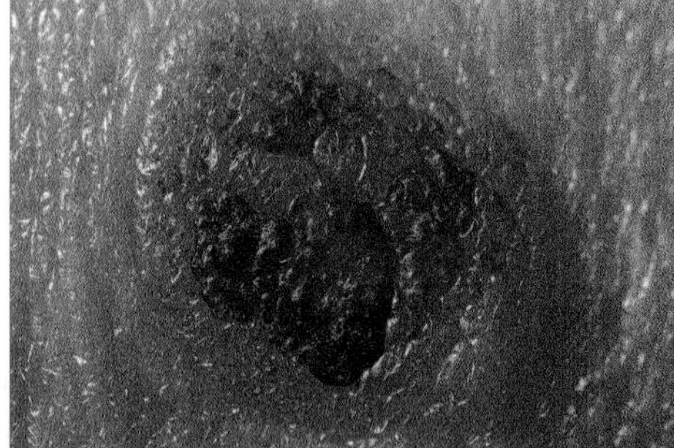

Figure 2.1 Malignant neoplasm of skin

PDx Unacceptable principal diagnosis symbol per Medicare code edits | POA Code exempt from diagnosis present on admission requirement
? Questionable admission | CC Complication or comorbidity | CC/MCC Exc CC/MCC exclusion | MCC Major complication or comorbidity
PDx CC Principal diagnosis as its own CC | PDx MCC Principal diagnosis as its own MCC | Z1 Z code as first-listed diagnosis

When symbols appear on a code that requires a 7th character extension, refer to Appendix D to identify applicable 7th character codes.

C44 Other and unspecified malignant neoplasm of skin
INCLUDES *malignant neoplasm of sebaceous glands*
malignant neoplasm of sweat glands
EXCLUDES1 *Kaposi's sarcoma of skin (C46.0)*
malignant melanoma of skin (C43.-)
malignant neoplasm of skin of genital organs (C51-C52, C60.-, C63.2)
Merkel cell carcinoma (C4A.-)

C44.0 Other and unspecified malignant neoplasm of skin of lip
EXCLUDES1 *malignant neoplasm of lip (C00.-)*
C44.00 Unspecified malignant neoplasm of skin of lip
C44.01 Basal cell carcinoma of skin of lip
C44.02 Squamous cell carcinoma of skin of lip
C44.09 Other specified malignant neoplasm of skin of lip

C44.1 Other and unspecified malignant neoplasm of skin of eyelid, including canthus
EXCLUDES1 *connective tissue of eyelid (C49.0)*
C44.10 Unspecified malignant neoplasm of skin of eyelid, including canthus
C44.101 Unspecified malignant neoplasm of skin of unspecified eyelid, including canthus
C44.102 Unspecified malignant neoplasm of skin of right eyelid, including canthus
C44.109 Unspecified malignant neoplasm of skin of left eyelid, including canthus
C44.11 Basal cell carcinoma of skin of eyelid, including canthus
C44.111 Basal cell carcinoma of skin of unspecified eyelid, including canthus
C44.112 Basal cell carcinoma of skin of right eyelid, including canthus
C44.119 Basal cell carcinoma of skin of left eyelid, including canthus
C44.12 Squamous cell carcinoma of skin of eyelid, including canthus
C44.121 Squamous cell carcinoma of skin of unspecified eyelid, including canthus
C44.122 Squamous cell carcinoma of skin of right eyelid, including canthus
C44.129 Squamous cell carcinoma of skin of left eyelid, including canthus
C44.19 Other specified malignant neoplasm of skin of eyelid, including canthus
C44.191 Other specified malignant neoplasm of skin of unspecified eyelid, including canthus
C44.192 Other specified malignant neoplasm of skin of right eyelid, including canthus
C44.199 Other specified malignant neoplasm of skin of left eyelid, including canthus

C44.2 Other and unspecified malignant neoplasm of skin of ear and external auricular canal
EXCLUDES1 *connective tissue of ear (C49.0)*
C44.20 Unspecified malignant neoplasm of skin of ear and external auricular canal
C44.201 Unspecified malignant neoplasm of skin of unspecified ear and external auricular canal
C44.202 Unspecified malignant neoplasm of skin of right ear and external auricular canal
C44.209 Unspecified malignant neoplasm of skin of left ear and external auricular canal
C44.21 Basal cell carcinoma of skin of ear and external auricular canal
C44.211 Basal cell carcinoma of skin of unspecified ear and external auricular canal
C44.212 Basal cell carcinoma of skin of right ear and external auricular canal
C44.219 Basal cell carcinoma of skin of left ear and external auricular canal
C44.22 Squamous cell carcinoma of skin of ear and external auricular canal
C44.221 Squamous cell carcinoma of skin of unspecified ear and external auricular canal
C44.222 Squamous cell carcinoma of skin of right ear and external auricular canal
C44.229 Squamous cell carcinoma of skin of left ear and external auricular canal
C44.29 Other specified malignant neoplasm of skin of ear and external auricular canal
C44.291 Other specified malignant neoplasm of skin of unspecified ear and external auricular canal
C44.292 Other specified malignant neoplasm of skin of right ear and external auricular canal
C44.299 Other specified malignant neoplasm of skin of left ear and external auricular canal

C44.3 Other and unspecified malignant neoplasm of skin of other and unspecified parts of face
C44.30 Unspecified malignant neoplasm of skin of other and unspecified parts of face
C44.300 Unspecified malignant neoplasm of skin of unspecified part of face
C44.301 Unspecified malignant neoplasm of skin of nose
C44.309 Unspecified malignant neoplasm of skin of other parts of face
C44.31 Basal cell carcinoma of skin of other and unspecified parts of face
C44.310 Basal cell carcinoma of skin of unspecified parts of face
C44.311 Basal cell carcinoma of skin of nose
C44.319 Basal cell carcinoma of skin of other parts of face
C44.32 Squamous cell carcinoma of skin of other and unspecified parts of face
C44.320 Squamous cell carcinoma of skin of unspecified parts of face
C44.321 Squamous cell carcinoma of skin of nose
C44.329 Squamous cell carcinoma of skin of other parts of face
C44.39 Other specified malignant neoplasm of skin of other and unspecified parts of face
C44.390 Other specified malignant neoplasm of skin of unspecified parts of face
C44.391 Other specified malignant neoplasm of skin of nose
C44.399 Other specified malignant neoplasm of skin of other parts of face

C44.4 Other and unspecified malignant neoplasm of skin of scalp and neck
C44.40 Unspecified malignant neoplasm of skin of scalp and neck
C44.41 Basal cell carcinoma of skin of scalp and neck
C44.42 Squamous cell carcinoma of skin of scalp and neck
C44.49 Other specified malignant neoplasm of skin of scalp and neck

C44.5 Other and unspecified malignant neoplasm of skin of trunk
EXCLUDES1 *anus NOS (C21.0)*
scrotum (C63.2)
C44.50 Unspecified malignant neoplasm of skin of trunk
C44.500 Unspecified malignant neoplasm of anal skin
Unspecified malignant neoplasm of anal margin
Unspecified malignant neoplasm of perianal skin
C44.501 Unspecified malignant neoplasm of skin of breast
C44.509 Unspecified malignant neoplasm of skin of other part of trunk
C44.51 Basal cell carcinoma of skin of trunk
C44.510 Basal cell carcinoma of anal skin
Basal cell carcinoma of anal margin
Basal cell carcinoma of perianal skin
C44.511 Basal cell carcinoma of skin of breast

C44.519 Basal cell carcinoma of skin of other part of trunk

C44.52 Squamous cell carcinoma of skin of trunk

C44.520 Squamous cell carcinoma of anal skin
Squamous cell carcinoma of anal margin
Squamous cell carcinoma of perianal skin

C44.521 Squamous cell carcinoma of skin of breast

C44.529 Squamous cell carcinoma of skin of other part of trunk

C44.59 Other specified malignant neoplasm of skin of trunk

C44.590 Other specified malignant neoplasm of anal skin
Other specified malignant neoplasm of anal margin
Other specified malignant neoplasm of perianal skin

C44.591 Other specified malignant neoplasm of skin of breast

C44.599 Other specified malignant neoplasm of skin of other part of trunk

C44.6 Other and unspecified malignant neoplasm of skin of upper limb, including shoulder

C44.60 Unspecified malignant neoplasm of skin of upper limb, including shoulder

C44.601 Unspecified malignant neoplasm of skin of unspecified upper limb, including shoulder

C44.602 Unspecified malignant neoplasm of skin of right upper limb, including shoulder

C44.609 Unspecified malignant neoplasm of skin of left upper limb, including shoulder

C44.61 Basal cell carcinoma of skin of upper limb, including shoulder

C44.611 Basal cell carcinoma of skin of unspecified upper limb, including shoulder

C44.612 Basal cell carcinoma of skin of right upper limb, including shoulder

C44.619 Basal cell carcinoma of skin of left upper limb, including shoulder

C44.62 Squamous cell carcinoma of skin of upper limb, including shoulder

C44.621 Squamous cell carcinoma of skin of unspecified upper limb, including shoulder

C44.622 Squamous cell carcinoma of skin of right upper limb, including shoulder

C44.629 Squamous cell carcinoma of skin of left upper limb, including shoulder

C44.69 Other specified malignant neoplasm of skin of upper limb, including shoulder

C44.691 Other specified malignant neoplasm of skin of unspecified upper limb, including shoulder

C44.692 Other specified malignant neoplasm of skin of right upper limb, including shoulder

C44.699 Other specified malignant neoplasm of skin of left upper limb, including shoulder

C44.7 Other and unspecified malignant neoplasm of skin of lower limb, including hip

C44.70 Unspecified malignant neoplasm of skin of lower limb, including hip

C44.701 Unspecified malignant neoplasm of skin of unspecified lower limb, including hip

C44.702 Unspecified malignant neoplasm of skin of right lower limb, including hip

C44.709 Unspecified malignant neoplasm of skin of left lower limb, including hip

C44.71 Basal cell carcinoma of skin of lower limb, including hip

C44.711 Basal cell carcinoma of skin of unspecified lower limb, including hip

C44.712 Basal cell carcinoma of skin of right lower limb, including hip

C44.719 Basal cell carcinoma of skin of left lower limb, including hip

C44.72 Squamous cell carcinoma of skin of lower limb, including hip

C44.721 Squamous cell carcinoma of skin of unspecified lower limb, including hip

C44.722 Squamous cell carcinoma of skin of right lower limb, including hip

C44.729 Squamous cell carcinoma of skin of left lower limb, including hip

C44.79 Other specified malignant neoplasm of skin of lower limb, including hip

C44.791 Other specified malignant neoplasm of skin of unspecified lower limb, including hip

C44.792 Other specified malignant neoplasm of skin of right lower limb, including hip

C44.799 Other specified malignant neoplasm of skin of left lower limb, including hip

C44.8 Other and unspecified malignant neoplasm of overlapping sites of skin

C44.80 Unspecified malignant neoplasm of overlapping sites of skin

C44.81 Basal cell carcinoma of overlapping sites of skin

C44.82 Squamous cell carcinoma of overlapping sites of skin

C44.89 Other specified malignant neoplasm of overlapping sites of skin

C44.9 Other and unspecified malignant neoplasm of skin, unspecified

C44.90 Unspecified malignant neoplasm of skin, unspecified
Malignant neoplasm of unspecified site of skin

C44.91 Basal cell carcinoma of skin, unspecified

C44.92 Squamous cell carcinoma of skin, unspecified

C44.99 Other specified malignant neoplasm of skin, unspecified

Malignant neoplasms of mesothelial and soft tissue (C45-C49)

C45 Mesothelioma

C45.0 Mesothelioma of pleura CC
EXCLUDES1 *other malignant neoplasm of pleura (C38.4)*

C45.1 Mesothelioma of peritoneum CC
Mesothelioma of cul-de-sac
Mesothelioma of mesentery
Mesothelioma of mesocolon
Mesothelioma of omentum
Mesothelioma of peritoneum (parietal) (pelvic)
EXCLUDES1 *other malignant neoplasm of soft tissue of peritoneum (C48.-)*

C45.2 Mesothelioma of pericardium CC
EXCLUDES1 *other malignant neoplasm of pericardium (C38.0)*

C45.7 Mesothelioma of other sites

C45.9 Mesothelioma, unspecified

C46 Kaposi's sarcoma
Code first any human immunodeficiency virus [HIV] disease (B20)

C46.0 Kaposi's sarcoma of skin CC

C46.1 Kaposi's sarcoma of soft tissue CC
Kaposi's sarcoma of blood vessel
Kaposi's sarcoma of connective tissue
Kaposi's sarcoma of fascia
Kaposi's sarcoma of ligament
Kaposi's sarcoma of lymphatic(s) NEC
Kaposi's sarcoma of muscle
EXCLUDES2 *Kaposi's sarcoma of lymph glands and nodes (C46.3)*

C46.2 Kaposi's sarcoma of palate CC

C46.3 Kaposi's sarcoma of lymph nodes CC

C46.4 Kaposi's sarcoma of gastrointestinal sites CC

C46.5 Kaposi's sarcoma of lung

C46.50 Kaposi's sarcoma of unspecified lung CC

C46.51 Kaposi's sarcoma of right lung CC

C46.52 Kaposi's sarcoma of left lung CC

C46.7 Kaposi's sarcoma of other sites CC

C46.9 Kaposi's sarcoma, unspecified CC
Kaposi's sarcoma of unspecified site

Unacceptable principal diagnosis symbol per Medicare code edits — Code exempt from diagnosis present on admission requirement — Questionable admission — Complication or comorbidity — CC/MCC exclusion — Major complication or comorbidity — Principal diagnosis as its own CC — Principal diagnosis as its own MCC — Z code as first-listed diagnosis

C47 Malignant neoplasm of peripheral nerves and autonomic nervous system
INCLUDES *malignant neoplasm of sympathetic and parasympathetic nerves and ganglia*
EXCLUDES1 *Kaposi's sarcoma of soft tissue (C46.1)*
C47.0 **Malignant neoplasm of peripheral nerves of head, face and neck**
EXCLUDES1 *malignant neoplasm of peripheral nerves of orbit (C69.6-)*
C47.1 **Malignant neoplasm of peripheral nerves of upper limb, including shoulder**
C47.10 **Malignant neoplasm of peripheral nerves of unspecified upper limb, including shoulder**
C47.11 **Malignant neoplasm of peripheral nerves of right upper limb, including shoulder**
C47.12 **Malignant neoplasm of peripheral nerves of left upper limb, including shoulder**
C47.2 **Malignant neoplasm of peripheral nerves of lower limb, including hip**
C47.20 **Malignant neoplasm of peripheral nerves of unspecified lower limb, including hip**
C47.21 **Malignant neoplasm of peripheral nerves of right lower limb, including hip**
C47.22 **Malignant neoplasm of peripheral nerves of left lower limb, including hip**
C47.3 **Malignant neoplasm of peripheral nerves of thorax**
C47.4 **Malignant neoplasm of peripheral nerves of abdomen**
C47.5 **Malignant neoplasm of peripheral nerves of pelvis**
C47.6 **Malignant neoplasm of peripheral nerves of trunk, unspecified**
Malignant neoplasm of peripheral nerves of unspecified part of trunk
C47.8 **Malignant neoplasm of overlapping sites of peripheral nerves and autonomic nervous system**
C47.9 **Malignant neoplasm of peripheral nerves and autonomic nervous system, unspecified**
Malignant neoplasm of unspecified site of peripheral nerves and autonomic nervous system

C48 **Malignant neoplasm of retroperitoneum and peritoneum**
EXCLUDES1 *Kaposi's sarcoma of connective tissue (C46.1)*
mesothelioma (C45.-)
C48.0 **Malignant neoplasm of retroperitoneum**
C48.1 **Malignant neoplasm of specified parts of peritoneum**
Malignant neoplasm of cul-de-sac
Malignant neoplasm of mesentery
Malignant neoplasm of mesocolon
Malignant neoplasm of omentum
Malignant neoplasm of parietal peritoneum
Malignant neoplasm of pelvic peritoneum
C48.2 **Malignant neoplasm of peritoneum, unspecified**
C48.8 **Malignant neoplasm of overlapping sites of retroperitoneum and peritoneum**

C49 **Malignant neoplasm of other connective and soft tissue**
INCLUDES *malignant neoplasm of blood vessel*
malignant neoplasm of bursa
malignant neoplasm of cartilage
malignant neoplasm of fascia
malignant neoplasm of fat
malignant neoplasm of ligament, except uterine
malignant neoplasm of lymphatic vessel
malignant neoplasm of muscle
malignant neoplasm of synovia
malignant neoplasm of tendon (sheath)
EXCLUDES1 *malignant neoplasm of cartilage (of):*
articular (C40-C41)
larynx (C32.3)
nose (C30.0)
malignant neoplasm of connective tissue of breast (C50.-)
EXCLUDES2 *Kaposi's sarcoma of soft tissue (C46.1)*
malignant neoplasm of heart (C38.0)
malignant neoplasm of peripheral nerves and autonomic nervous system (C47.-)
malignant neoplasm of peritoneum (C48.2)
malignant neoplasm of retroperitoneum (C48.0)
malignant neoplasm of uterine ligament (C57.3)
mesothelioma (C45.-)
C49.0 **Malignant neoplasm of connective and soft tissue of head, face and neck**
Malignant neoplasm of connective tissue of ear
Malignant neoplasm of connective tissue of eyelid
EXCLUDES1 *connective tissue of orbit (C69.6-)*
C49.1 **Malignant neoplasm of connective and soft tissue of upper limb, including shoulder**
C49.10 **Malignant neoplasm of connective and soft tissue of unspecified upper limb, including shoulder**
C49.11 **Malignant neoplasm of connective and soft tissue of right upper limb, including shoulder**
C49.12 **Malignant neoplasm of connective and soft tissue of left upper limb, including shoulder**
C49.2 **Malignant neoplasm of connective and soft tissue of lower limb, including hip**
C49.20 **Malignant neoplasm of connective and soft tissue of unspecified lower limb, including hip**
C49.21 **Malignant neoplasm of connective and soft tissue of right lower limb, including hip**
C49.22 **Malignant neoplasm of connective and soft tissue of left lower limb, including hip**
C49.3 **Malignant neoplasm of connective and soft tissue of thorax**
Malignant neoplasm of axilla
Malignant neoplasm of diaphragm
Malignant neoplasm of great vessels
EXCLUDES1 *malignant neoplasm of breast (C50.-)*
malignant neoplasm of heart (C38.0)
malignant neoplasm of mediastinum (C38.1-C38.3)
malignant neoplasm of thymus (C37)
AHA: Q3, 2015
C49.4 **Malignant neoplasm of connective and soft tissue of abdomen**
Malignant neoplasm of abdominal wall
Malignant neoplasm of hypochondrium
C49.5 **Malignant neoplasm of connective and soft tissue of pelvis**
Malignant neoplasm of buttock
Malignant neoplasm of groin
Malignant neoplasm of perineum
C49.6 **Malignant neoplasm of connective and soft tissue of trunk, unspecified**
Malignant neoplasm of back NOS
C49.8 **Malignant neoplasm of overlapping sites of connective and soft tissue**
Primary malignant neoplasm of two or more contiguous sites of connective and soft tissue
C49.9 **Malignant neoplasm of connective and soft tissue, unspecified**
● C49.A Gastrointestinal stromal tumor
● C49.A0 **Gastrointestinal stromal tumor, unspecified site**
● C49.A1 **Gastrointestinal stromal tumor of esophagus**
● C49.A2 **Gastrointestinal stromal tumor of stomach**
● C49.A3 **Gastrointestinal stromal tumor of small intestine**
● C49.A4 **Gastrointestinal stromal tumor of large intestine**
● C49.A5 **Gastrointestinal stromal tumor of rectum**
● C49.A9 **Gastrointestinal stromal tumor of other sites**

Unspecified Code Other Specified Code Manifestation Code N Newborn P Pediatric M Maternity A Adult ♂ Male ♀ Female
● New Code ▲ Revised Code Title ►◄ Revised Text NOTES INCLUDES EXCLUDES1 Not coded here EXCLUDES2 Not included here
4th character required 5th character required 6th character required 7th character required
Extension 'X' Alert HAC Hospital-acquired condition (HAC) alert AHA AHA Coding Clinic©

When symbols appear on a code that requires a 7th character extension, refer to Appendix D to identify applicable 7th character codes.

Malignant neoplasms of breast (C50)

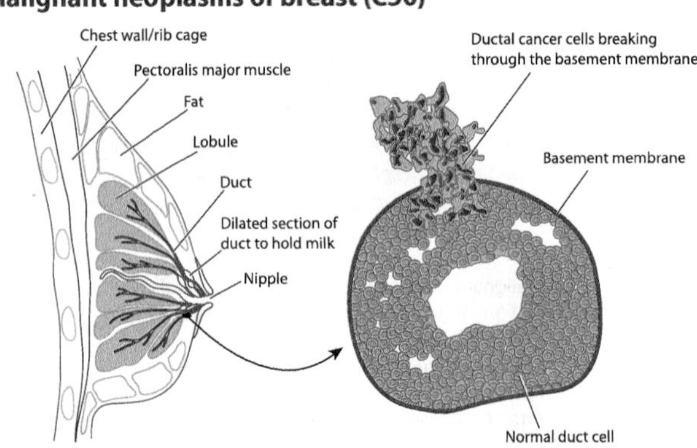

Figure 2.2 Breast cancer cells

C50 Malignant neoplasm of breast
INCLUDES *connective tissue of breast*
Paget's disease of breast
Paget's disease of nipple
Use additional code to identify estrogen receptor status (Z17.0, Z17.1)
EXCLUDES1 *skin of breast (C44.501, C44.511, C44.521, C44.591)*

C50.0 Malignant neoplasm of nipple and areola
C50.01 Malignant neoplasm of nipple and areola, female
C50.011 Malignant neoplasm of nipple and areola, right female breast ♀
C50.012 Malignant neoplasm of nipple and areola, left female breast ♀
C50.019 Malignant neoplasm of nipple and areola, unspecified female breast ♀
C50.02 Malignant neoplasm of nipple and areola, male
C50.021 Malignant neoplasm of nipple and areola, right male breast ♂
C50.022 Malignant neoplasm of nipple and areola, left male breast ♂
C50.029 Malignant neoplasm of nipple and areola, unspecified male breast ♂

C50.1 Malignant neoplasm of central portion of breast
C50.11 Malignant neoplasm of central portion of breast, female
C50.111 Malignant neoplasm of central portion of right female breast ♀
C50.112 Malignant neoplasm of central portion of left female breast ♀
C50.119 Malignant neoplasm of central portion of unspecified female breast ♀
C50.12 Malignant neoplasm of central portion of breast, male
C50.121 Malignant neoplasm of central portion of right male breast ♂
C50.122 Malignant neoplasm of central portion of left male breast ♂
C50.129 Malignant neoplasm of central portion of unspecified male breast ♂

C50.2 Malignant neoplasm of upper-inner quadrant of breast
C50.21 Malignant neoplasm of upper-inner quadrant of breast, female
C50.211 Malignant neoplasm of upper-inner quadrant of right female breast ♀
C50.212 Malignant neoplasm of upper-inner quadrant of left female breast ♀
C50.219 Malignant neoplasm of upper-inner quadrant of unspecified female breast ♀
C50.22 Malignant neoplasm of upper-inner quadrant of breast, male
C50.221 Malignant neoplasm of upper-inner quadrant of right male breast ♂
C50.222 Malignant neoplasm of upper-inner quadrant of left male breast ♂
C50.229 Malignant neoplasm of upper-inner quadrant of unspecified male breast ♂

C50.3 Malignant neoplasm of lower-inner quadrant of breast
C50.31 Malignant neoplasm of lower-inner quadrant of breast, female
C50.311 Malignant neoplasm of lower-inner quadrant of right female breast ♀
C50.312 Malignant neoplasm of lower-inner quadrant of left female breast ♀
C50.319 Malignant neoplasm of lower-inner quadrant of unspecified female breast ♀
C50.32 Malignant neoplasm of lower-inner quadrant of breast, male
C50.321 Malignant neoplasm of lower-inner quadrant of right male breast ♂
C50.322 Malignant neoplasm of lower-inner quadrant of left male breast ♂
C50.329 Malignant neoplasm of lower-inner quadrant of unspecified male breast ♂

C50.4 Malignant neoplasm of upper-outer quadrant of breast
C50.41 Malignant neoplasm of upper-outer quadrant of breast, female
C50.411 Malignant neoplasm of upper-outer quadrant of right female breast ♀
C50.412 Malignant neoplasm of upper-outer quadrant of left female breast ♀
C50.419 Malignant neoplasm of upper-outer quadrant of unspecified female breast ♀
C50.42 Malignant neoplasm of upper-outer quadrant of breast, male
C50.421 Malignant neoplasm of upper-outer quadrant of right male breast ♂
C50.422 Malignant neoplasm of upper-outer quadrant of left male breast ♂
C50.429 Malignant neoplasm of upper-outer quadrant of unspecified male breast ♂

C50.5 Malignant neoplasm of lower-outer quadrant of breast
C50.51 Malignant neoplasm of lower-outer quadrant of breast, female
C50.511 Malignant neoplasm of lower-outer quadrant of right female breast ♀
C50.512 Malignant neoplasm of lower-outer quadrant of left female breast ♀
C50.519 Malignant neoplasm of lower-outer quadrant of unspecified female breast ♀
C50.52 Malignant neoplasm of lower-outer quadrant of breast, male
C50.521 Malignant neoplasm of lower-outer quadrant of right male breast ♂
C50.522 Malignant neoplasm of lower-outer quadrant of left male breast ♂
C50.529 Malignant neoplasm of lower-outer quadrant of unspecified male breast ♂

C50.6 Malignant neoplasm of axillary tail of breast
C50.61 Malignant neoplasm of axillary tail of breast, female
C50.611 Malignant neoplasm of axillary tail of right female breast ♀
C50.612 Malignant neoplasm of axillary tail of left female breast ♀
C50.619 Malignant neoplasm of axillary tail of unspecified female breast ♀
C50.62 Malignant neoplasm of axillary tail of breast, male
C50.621 Malignant neoplasm of axillary tail of right male breast ♂
C50.622 Malignant neoplasm of axillary tail of left male breast ♂
C50.629 Malignant neoplasm of axillary tail of unspecified male breast ♂

C50.8 Malignant neoplasm of overlapping sites of breast
C50.81 Malignant neoplasm of overlapping sites of breast, female
C50.811 Malignant neoplasm of overlapping sites of right female breast ♀

Unacceptable principal diagnosis symbol per Medicare code edits · Code exempt from diagnosis present on admission requirement
Questionable admission · Complication or comorbidity · CC/MCC exclusion · Major complication or comorbidity
Principal diagnosis as its own CC · Principal diagnosis as its own MCC · Z code as first-listed diagnosis

C50.812 **Malignant neoplasm of overlapping sites of left female breast** ♀
C50.819 **Malignant neoplasm of overlapping sites of unspecified female breast** ♀
C50.82 **Malignant neoplasm of overlapping sites of breast, male**
C50.821 **Malignant neoplasm of overlapping sites of right male breast** ♂
C50.822 **Malignant neoplasm of overlapping sites of left male breast** ♂
C50.829 **Malignant neoplasm of overlapping sites of unspecified male breast** ♂
C50.9 **Malignant neoplasm of breast of unspecified site**
C50.91 **Malignant neoplasm of breast of unspecified site, female**
C50.911 **Malignant neoplasm of unspecified site of right female breast** ♀
C50.912 **Malignant neoplasm of unspecified site of left female breast** ♀
C50.919 **Malignant neoplasm of unspecified site of unspecified female breast** ♀
C50.92 **Malignant neoplasm of breast of unspecified site, male**
C50.921 **Malignant neoplasm of unspecified site of right male breast** ♂
C50.922 **Malignant neoplasm of unspecified site of left male breast** ♂
C50.929 **Malignant neoplasm of unspecified site of unspecified male breast** ♂

Malignant neoplasms of female genital organs (C51-C58)

INCLUDES *malignant neoplasm of skin of female genital organs*

C51 **Malignant neoplasm of vulva**
EXCLUDES1 *carcinoma in situ of vulva (D07.1)*
C51.0 **Malignant neoplasm of labium majus** ♀
Malignant neoplasm of Bartholin's [greater vestibular] gland
C51.1 **Malignant neoplasm of labium minus** ♀
C51.2 **Malignant neoplasm of clitoris** ♀
C51.8 **Malignant neoplasm of overlapping sites of vulva** ♀
C51.9 **Malignant neoplasm of vulva, unspecified** ♀
Malignant neoplasm of external female genitalia NOS
Malignant neoplasm of pudendum
C52 **Malignant neoplasm of vagina** ♀
EXCLUDES1 *carcinoma in situ of vagina (D07.2)*
C53 **Malignant neoplasm of cervix uteri**
EXCLUDES1 *carcinoma in situ of cervix uteri (D06.-)*
C53.0 **Malignant neoplasm of endocervix** ♀
C53.1 **Malignant neoplasm of exocervix** ♀
C53.8 **Malignant neoplasm of overlapping sites of cervix uteri** ♀
C53.9 **Malignant neoplasm of cervix uteri, unspecified** ♀
C54 **Malignant neoplasm of corpus uteri**
C54.0 **Malignant neoplasm of isthmus uteri** ♀
Malignant neoplasm of lower uterine segment
C54.1 **Malignant neoplasm of endometrium** ♀
C54.2 **Malignant neoplasm of myometrium** ♀
C54.3 **Malignant neoplasm of fundus uteri** ♀
C54.8 **Malignant neoplasm of overlapping sites of corpus uteri** ♀
C54.9 **Malignant neoplasm of corpus uteri, unspecified** ♀
C55 **Malignant neoplasm of uterus, part unspecified** ♀
C56 **Malignant neoplasm of ovary**
Use additional code to identify any functional activity
C56.1 **Malignant neoplasm of right ovary** ♀
C56.2 **Malignant neoplasm of left ovary** ♀
C56.9 **Malignant neoplasm of unspecified ovary** ♀
C57 **Malignant neoplasm of other and unspecified female genital organs**
C57.0 **Malignant neoplasm of fallopian tube**
Malignant neoplasm of oviduct
Malignant neoplasm of uterine tube
C57.00 **Malignant neoplasm of unspecified fallopian tube** ♀
C57.01 **Malignant neoplasm of right fallopian tube** ♀
C57.02 **Malignant neoplasm of left fallopian tube** ♀
C57.1 **Malignant neoplasm of broad ligament**
C57.10 **Malignant neoplasm of unspecified broad ligament** ♀
C57.11 **Malignant neoplasm of right broad ligament** ♀
C57.12 **Malignant neoplasm of left broad ligament** ♀
C57.2 **Malignant neoplasm of round ligament**
C57.20 **Malignant neoplasm of unspecified round ligament** ♀
C57.21 **Malignant neoplasm of right round ligament** ♀
C57.22 **Malignant neoplasm of left round ligament** ♀
C57.3 **Malignant neoplasm of parametrium** ♀
Malignant neoplasm of uterine ligament NOS
C57.4 **Malignant neoplasm of uterine adnexa, unspecified** ♀
C57.7 **Malignant neoplasm of other specified female genital organs** ♀
Malignant neoplasm of wolffian body or duct
C57.8 **Malignant neoplasm of overlapping sites of female genital organs** ♀
Primary malignant neoplasm of two or more contiguous sites of the female genital organs whose point of origin cannot be determined
Primary tubo-ovarian malignant neoplasm whose point of origin cannot be determined
Primary utero-ovarian malignant neoplasm whose point of origin cannot be determined
C57.9 **Malignant neoplasm of female genital organ, unspecified** ♀
Malignant neoplasm of female genitourinary tract NOS
C58 **Malignant neoplasm of placenta** ♀
INCLUDES *choriocarcinoma NOS*
chorionepithelioma NOS
EXCLUDES1 *chorioadenoma (destruens) (D39.2)*
hydatidiform mole NOS (O01.9)
invasive hydatidiform mole (D39.2)
male choriocarcinoma NOS (C62.9-)
malignant hydatidiform mole (D39.2)

Malignant neoplasms of male genital organs (C60-C63)

INCLUDES *malignant neoplasm of skin of male genital organs*

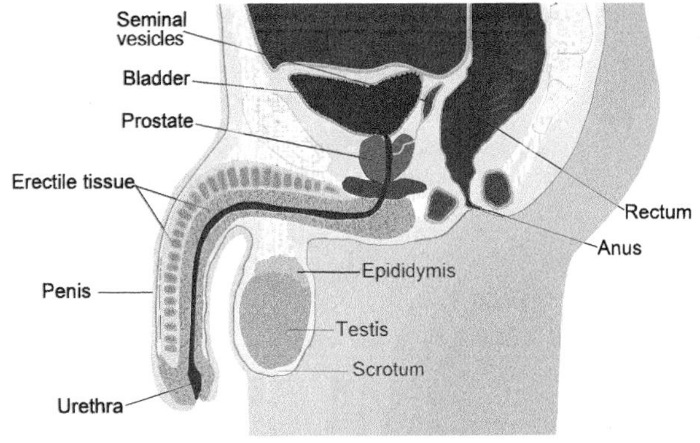

Figure 2.3 Male reproductive tract

C60 **Malignant neoplasm of penis**
C60.0 **Malignant neoplasm of prepuce** ♂
Malignant neoplasm of foreskin
C60.1 **Malignant neoplasm of glans penis** ♂
C60.2 **Malignant neoplasm of body of penis** ♂
Malignant neoplasm of corpus cavernosum
C60.8 **Malignant neoplasm of overlapping sites of penis** ♂
C60.9 **Malignant neoplasm of penis, unspecified** ♂
Malignant neoplasm of skin of penis NOS
C61 **Malignant neoplasm of prostate** ♂
Use additional code to identify:
hormone sensitivity status (Z19.1-Z19.2)
rising PSA following treatment for malignant neoplasm of prostate (R97.21)
EXCLUDES1 *malignant neoplasm of seminal vesicle (C63.7)*

Unspecified Code | Other Specified Code | Manifestation Code | N Newborn | P Pediatric | M Maternity | A Adult | ♂ Male | ♀ Female
● New Code ▲ Revised Code Title ►◄ Revised Text NOTES INCLUDES EXCLUDES1 Not coded here EXCLUDES2 Not included here
4th character required 5th character required 6th character required 7th character required
Extension 'X' Alert HAC Hospital-acquired condition (HAC) alert AHA AHA Coding Clinic©

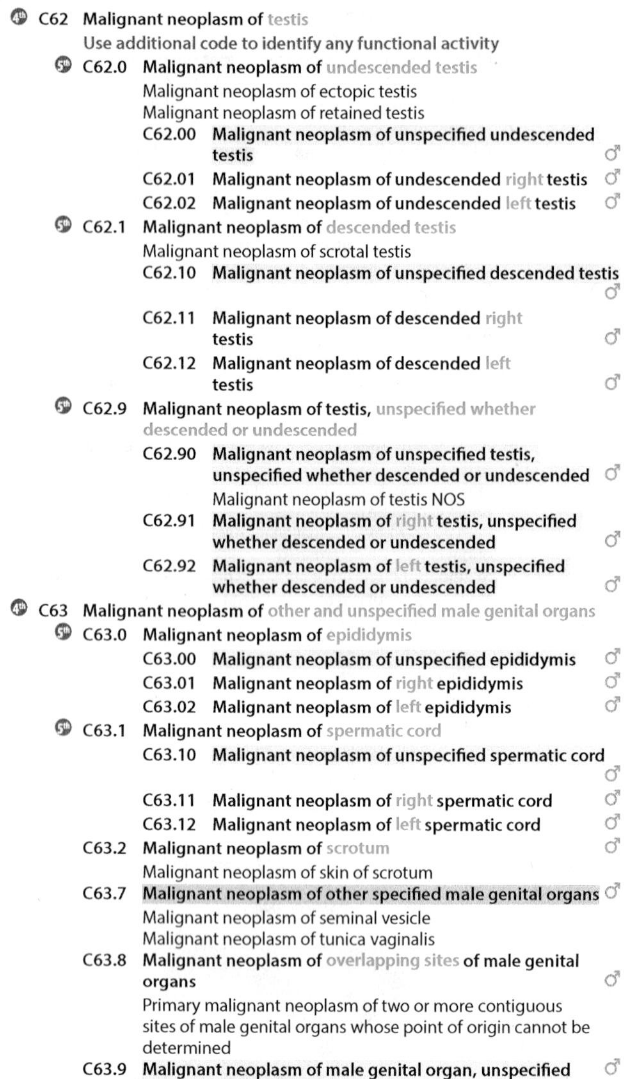

C62 Malignant neoplasm of testis
Use additional code to identify any functional activity

- **C62.0 Malignant neoplasm of undescended testis**
  Malignant neoplasm of ectopic testis
  Malignant neoplasm of retained testis
  - **C62.00 Malignant neoplasm of unspecified undescended testis** ♂
  - **C62.01 Malignant neoplasm of undescended right testis** ♂
  - **C62.02 Malignant neoplasm of undescended left testis** ♂
- **C62.1 Malignant neoplasm of descended testis**
  Malignant neoplasm of scrotal testis
  - **C62.10 Malignant neoplasm of unspecified descended testis** ♂
  - **C62.11 Malignant neoplasm of descended right testis** ♂
  - **C62.12 Malignant neoplasm of descended left testis** ♂
- **C62.9 Malignant neoplasm of testis, unspecified whether descended or undescended**
  - **C62.90 Malignant neoplasm of unspecified testis, unspecified whether descended or undescended** ♂
    Malignant neoplasm of testis NOS
  - **C62.91 Malignant neoplasm of right testis, unspecified whether descended or undescended** ♂
  - **C62.92 Malignant neoplasm of left testis, unspecified whether descended or undescended** ♂

C63 Malignant neoplasm of other and unspecified male genital organs

- **C63.0 Malignant neoplasm of epididymis**
  - **C63.00 Malignant neoplasm of unspecified epididymis** ♂
  - **C63.01 Malignant neoplasm of right epididymis** ♂
  - **C63.02 Malignant neoplasm of left epididymis** ♂
- **C63.1 Malignant neoplasm of spermatic cord**
  - **C63.10 Malignant neoplasm of unspecified spermatic cord** ♂
  - **C63.11 Malignant neoplasm of right spermatic cord** ♂
  - **C63.12 Malignant neoplasm of left spermatic cord** ♂
- **C63.2 Malignant neoplasm of scrotum** ♂
  Malignant neoplasm of skin of scrotum
- **C63.7 Malignant neoplasm of other specified male genital organs** ♂
  Malignant neoplasm of seminal vesicle
  Malignant neoplasm of tunica vaginalis
- **C63.8 Malignant neoplasm of overlapping sites of male genital organs** ♂
  Primary malignant neoplasm of two or more contiguous sites of male genital organs whose point of origin cannot be determined
- **C63.9 Malignant neoplasm of male genital organ, unspecified** ♂
  Malignant neoplasm of male genitourinary tract NOS

Malignant neoplasms of urinary tract (C64-C68)

C64 Malignant neoplasm of kidney, except renal pelvis

EXCLUDES1 *malignant carcinoid tumor of the kidney (C7A.093)*
malignant neoplasm of renal calyces (C65.-)
malignant neoplasm of renal pelvis (C65.-)

- **C64.1 Malignant neoplasm of right kidney, except renal pelvis** CC
- **C64.2 Malignant neoplasm of left kidney, except renal pelvis** CC
- **C64.9 Malignant neoplasm of unspecified kidney, except renal pelvis** CC

C65 Malignant neoplasm of renal pelvis

INCLUDES *malignant neoplasm of pelviureteric junction*
malignant neoplasm of renal calyces

- **C65.1 Malignant neoplasm of right renal pelvis** CC
- **C65.2 Malignant neoplasm of left renal pelvis** CC
- **C65.9 Malignant neoplasm of unspecified renal pelvis** CC

C66 Malignant neoplasm of ureter

EXCLUDES1 *malignant neoplasm of ureteric orifice of bladder (C67.6)*

- **C66.1 Malignant neoplasm of right ureter** CC
- **C66.2 Malignant neoplasm of left ureter** CC
- **C66.9 Malignant neoplasm of unspecified ureter** CC

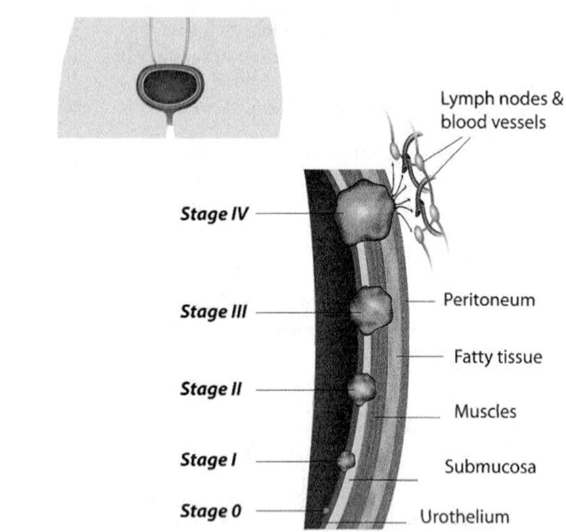

Figure 2.4 Urinary bladder cancer

C67 Malignant neoplasm of bladder

- **C67.0 Malignant neoplasm of trigone of bladder**
- **C67.1 Malignant neoplasm of dome of bladder**
- **C67.2 Malignant neoplasm of lateral wall of bladder**
- **C67.3 Malignant neoplasm of anterior wall of bladder**
- **C67.4 Malignant neoplasm of posterior wall of bladder**
- **C67.5 Malignant neoplasm of bladder neck**
  Malignant neoplasm of internal urethral orifice
- **C67.6 Malignant neoplasm of ureteric orifice**
- **C67.7 Malignant neoplasm of urachus**
- **C67.8 Malignant neoplasm of overlapping sites of bladder**
- **C67.9 Malignant neoplasm of bladder, unspecified**
  AHA: Q1, 2016

C68 Malignant neoplasm of other and unspecified urinary organs

EXCLUDES1 *malignant neoplasm of female genitourinary tract NOS (C57.9)*
malignant neoplasm of male genitourinary tract NOS (C63.9)

- **C68.0 Malignant neoplasm of urethra** CC
  EXCLUDES1 *malignant neoplasm of urethral orifice of bladder (C67.5)*
- **C68.1 Malignant neoplasm of paraurethral glands** CC
- **C68.8 Malignant neoplasm of overlapping sites of urinary organs** CC
  Primary malignant neoplasm of two or more contiguous sites of urinary organs whose point of origin cannot be determined
- **C68.9 Malignant neoplasm of urinary organ, unspecified** CC
  Malignant neoplasm of urinary system NOS

Malignant neoplasms of eye, brain and other parts of central nervous system (C69-C72)

C69 Malignant neoplasm of eye and adnexa

EXCLUDES1 *malignant neoplasm of connective tissue of eyelid (C49.0)*
malignant neoplasm of eyelid (skin) (C43.1-, C44.1-)
malignant neoplasm of optic nerve (C72.3-)

- **C69.0 Malignant neoplasm of conjunctiva**
  - **C69.00 Malignant neoplasm of unspecified conjunctiva**
  - **C69.01 Malignant neoplasm of right conjunctiva**
  - **C69.02 Malignant neoplasm of left conjunctiva**
- **C69.1 Malignant neoplasm of cornea**
  - **C69.10 Malignant neoplasm of unspecified cornea**
  - **C69.11 Malignant neoplasm of right cornea**
  - **C69.12 Malignant neoplasm of left cornea**
- **C69.2 Malignant neoplasm of retina**
  EXCLUDES1 *dark area on retina (D49.81)*
  neoplasm of unspecified behavior of retina and choroid (D49.81)
  retinal freckle (D49.81)
  - **C69.20 Malignant neoplasm of unspecified retina**
  - **C69.21 Malignant neoplasm of right retina**

PDx Unacceptable principal diagnosis symbol per Medicare code edits · POA Code exempt from diagnosis present on admission requirement
Q Questionable admission · CC Complication or comorbidity · CC/MCC Exc CC/MCC exclusion · MCC Major complication or comorbidity
PDx CC Principal diagnosis as its own CC · PDx MCC Principal diagnosis as its own MCC · Z Z code as first-listed diagnosis

C69.22 Malignant neoplasm of left retina
C69.3 Malignant neoplasm of choroid
C69.30 Malignant neoplasm of unspecified choroid
C69.31 Malignant neoplasm of right choroid
C69.32 Malignant neoplasm of left choroid
C69.4 Malignant neoplasm of ciliary body
C69.40 Malignant neoplasm of unspecified ciliary body
C69.41 Malignant neoplasm of right ciliary body
C69.42 Malignant neoplasm of left ciliary body
C69.5 Malignant neoplasm of lacrimal gland and duct
Malignant neoplasm of lacrimal sac
Malignant neoplasm of nasolacrimal duct
C69.50 Malignant neoplasm of unspecified lacrimal gland and duct
C69.51 Malignant neoplasm of right lacrimal gland and duct
C69.52 Malignant neoplasm of left lacrimal gland and duct
C69.6 Malignant neoplasm of orbit
Malignant neoplasm of connective tissue of orbit
Malignant neoplasm of extraocular muscle
Malignant neoplasm of peripheral nerves of orbit
Malignant neoplasm of retrobulbar tissue
Malignant neoplasm of retro-ocular tissue
EXCLUDES1 *malignant neoplasm of orbital bone (C41.0)*
C69.60 Malignant neoplasm of unspecified orbit
C69.61 Malignant neoplasm of right orbit
C69.62 Malignant neoplasm of left orbit
C69.8 Malignant neoplasm of overlapping sites of eye and adnexa
C69.80 Malignant neoplasm of overlapping sites of unspecified eye and adnexa
C69.81 Malignant neoplasm of overlapping sites of right eye and adnexa
C69.82 Malignant neoplasm of overlapping sites of left eye and adnexa
C69.9 Malignant neoplasm of unspecified site of eye
Malignant neoplasm of eyeball
C69.90 Malignant neoplasm of unspecified site of unspecified eye
C69.91 Malignant neoplasm of unspecified site of right eye
C69.92 Malignant neoplasm of unspecified site of left eye
C70 Malignant neoplasm of meninges
C70.0 Malignant neoplasm of cerebral meninges
C70.1 Malignant neoplasm of spinal meninges
C70.9 Malignant neoplasm of meninges, unspecified
C71 Malignant neoplasm of brain
EXCLUDES1 *malignant neoplasm of cranial nerves (C72.2-C72.5)*
retrobulbar malignant neoplasm (C69.6-)
C71.0 Malignant neoplasm of cerebrum, except lobes and ventricles
Malignant neoplasm of supratentorial NOS
C71.1 Malignant neoplasm of frontal lobe
C71.2 Malignant neoplasm of temporal lobe
C71.3 Malignant neoplasm of parietal lobe
C71.4 Malignant neoplasm of occipital lobe
C71.5 Malignant neoplasm of cerebral ventricle
EXCLUDES1 *malignant neoplasm of fourth cerebral ventricle (C71.7)*
C71.6 Malignant neoplasm of cerebellum
C71.7 Malignant neoplasm of brain stem
Malignant neoplasm of fourth cerebral ventricle
Infratentorial malignant neoplasm NOS
C71.8 Malignant neoplasm of overlapping sites of brain
C71.9 Malignant neoplasm of brain, unspecified
C72 Malignant neoplasm of spinal cord, cranial nerves and other parts of central nervous system
EXCLUDES1 *malignant neoplasm of meninges (C70.-)*
malignant neoplasm of peripheral nerves and autonomic nervous system (C47.-)
C72.0 Malignant neoplasm of spinal cord
C72.1 Malignant neoplasm of cauda equina
C72.2 Malignant neoplasm of olfactory nerve
Malignant neoplasm of olfactory bulb
C72.20 Malignant neoplasm of unspecified olfactory nerve
C72.21 Malignant neoplasm of right olfactory nerve
C72.22 Malignant neoplasm of left olfactory nerve
C72.3 Malignant neoplasm of optic nerve
C72.30 Malignant neoplasm of unspecified optic nerve
C72.31 Malignant neoplasm of right optic nerve
C72.32 Malignant neoplasm of left optic nerve
C72.4 Malignant neoplasm of acoustic nerve
C72.40 Malignant neoplasm of unspecified acoustic nerve
C72.41 Malignant neoplasm of right acoustic nerve
C72.42 Malignant neoplasm of left acoustic nerve
C72.5 Malignant neoplasm of other and unspecified cranial nerves
C72.50 Malignant neoplasm of unspecified cranial nerve
Malignant neoplasm of cranial nerve NOS
C72.59 Malignant neoplasm of other cranial nerves
C72.9 Malignant neoplasm of central nervous system, unspecified
Malignant neoplasm of unspecified site of central nervous system
Malignant neoplasm of nervous system NOS

Malignant neoplasms of thyroid and other endocrine glands (C73-C75)

C73 Malignant neoplasm of thyroid gland
Use additional code to identify any functional activity
C74 Malignant neoplasm of adrenal gland
C74.0 Malignant neoplasm of cortex of adrenal gland
C74.00 Malignant neoplasm of cortex of unspecified adrenal gland
C74.01 Malignant neoplasm of cortex of right adrenal gland
C74.02 Malignant neoplasm of cortex of left adrenal gland
C74.1 Malignant neoplasm of medulla of adrenal gland
C74.10 Malignant neoplasm of medulla of unspecified adrenal gland
C74.11 Malignant neoplasm of medulla of right adrenal gland
C74.12 Malignant neoplasm of medulla of left adrenal gland
C74.9 Malignant neoplasm of unspecified part of adrenal gland
C74.90 Malignant neoplasm of unspecified part of unspecified adrenal gland
C74.91 Malignant neoplasm of unspecified part of right adrenal gland
C74.92 Malignant neoplasm of unspecified part of left adrenal gland
C75 Malignant neoplasm of other endocrine glands and related structures
EXCLUDES1 *malignant carcinoid tumors (C7A.0-)*
malignant neoplasm of adrenal gland (C74.-)
malignant neoplasm of endocrine pancreas (C25.4)
malignant neoplasm of islets of Langerhans (C25.4)
malignant neoplasm of ovary (C56.-)
malignant neoplasm of testis (C62.-)
malignant neoplasm of thymus (C37)
malignant neoplasm of thyroid gland (C73)
malignant neuroendocrine tumors (C7A.-)
C75.0 Malignant neoplasm of parathyroid gland
C75.1 Malignant neoplasm of pituitary gland
C75.2 Malignant neoplasm of craniopharyngeal duct
C75.3 Malignant neoplasm of pineal gland
C75.4 Malignant neoplasm of carotid body
C75.5 Malignant neoplasm of aortic body and other paraganglia
C75.8 Malignant neoplasm with pluriglandular involvement, unspecified
C75.9 Malignant neoplasm of endocrine gland, unspecified

Malignant neuroendocrine tumors (C7A)

C7A Malignant neuroendocrine tumors
Code also any associated multiple endocrine neoplasia [MEN] syndromes (E31.2-)

Unspecified Code Other Specified Code Manifestation Code N Newborn P Pediatric M Maternity A Adult ♂ Male ♀ Female
● New Code ▲ Revised Code Title ►◄ Revised Text NOTES INCLUDES EXCLUDES1 Not coded here EXCLUDES2 Not included here
4th character required 5th character required 6th character required 7th character required
Extension 'X' Alert HAC Hospital-acquired condition (HAC) alert AHA AHA Coding Clinic©

Use additional code to identify any associated endocrine syndrome, such as:
carcinoid syndrome (E34.0)

EXCLUDES2 *malignant pancreatic islet cell tumors (C25.4)*
Merkel cell carcinoma (C4A.-)

C7A.0 **Malignant carcinoid tumors**
C7A.00 **Malignant carcinoid tumor of unspecified site**
C7A.01 **Malignant carcinoid tumors of the small intestine**
C7A.010 **Malignant carcinoid tumor of the duodenum**
C7A.011 **Malignant carcinoid tumor of the jejunum**
C7A.012 **Malignant carcinoid tumor of the ileum**
C7A.019 **Malignant carcinoid tumor of the small intestine, unspecified portion**
C7A.02 **Malignant carcinoid tumors of the appendix, large intestine, and rectum**
C7A.020 **Malignant carcinoid tumor of the appendix**
C7A.021 **Malignant carcinoid tumor of the cecum**
C7A.022 **Malignant carcinoid tumor of the ascending colon**
C7A.023 **Malignant carcinoid tumor of the transverse colon**
C7A.024 **Malignant carcinoid tumor of the descending colon**
C7A.025 **Malignant carcinoid tumor of the sigmoid colon**
C7A.026 **Malignant carcinoid tumor of the rectum**
C7A.029 **Malignant carcinoid tumor of the large intestine, unspecified portion**
Malignant carcinoid tumor of the colon NOS
C7A.09 **Malignant carcinoid tumors of other sites**
C7A.090 **Malignant carcinoid tumor of the bronchus and lung**
C7A.091 **Malignant carcinoid tumor of the thymus**
C7A.092 **Malignant carcinoid tumor of the stomach**
C7A.093 **Malignant carcinoid tumor of the kidney**
▲ C7A.094 **Malignant carcinoid tumor of the foregut, ▶unspecified◀**
▲ C7A.095 **Malignant carcinoid tumor of the midgut, ▶unspecified◀**
▲ C7A.096 **Malignant carcinoid tumor of the hindgut, ▶unspecified◀**
C7A.098 **Malignant carcinoid tumors of other sites**

C7A.1 **Malignant poorly differentiated neuroendocrine tumors**
Malignant poorly differentiated neuroendocrine tumor NOS
Malignant poorly differentiated neuroendocrine carcinoma, any site
High grade neuroendocrine carcinoma, any site
C7A.8 **Other malignant neuroendocrine tumors**

Secondary neuroendocrine tumors (C7B)

C7B **Secondary neuroendocrine tumors**
Use additional code to identify any functional activity
C7B.0 **Secondary carcinoid tumors**
C7B.00 **Secondary carcinoid tumors, unspecified site**
C7B.01 **Secondary carcinoid tumors of distant lymph nodes**
C7B.02 **Secondary carcinoid tumors of liver**
C7B.03 **Secondary carcinoid tumors of bone**
C7B.04 **Secondary carcinoid tumors of peritoneum**
Mesentery metastasis of carcinoid tumor
C7B.09 **Secondary carcinoid tumors of other sites**
C7B.1 **Secondary Merkel cell carcinoma**
Merkel cell carcinoma nodal presentation
Merkel cell carcinoma visceral metastatic presentation
C7B.8 **Other secondary neuroendocrine tumors**

Malignant neoplasms of ill-defined, other secondary and unspecified sites (C76-C80)

C76 **Malignant neoplasm of other and ill-defined sites**

EXCLUDES1 *malignant neoplasm of female genitourinary tract NOS (C57.9)*
malignant neoplasm of male genitourinary tract NOS (C63.9)
malignant neoplasm of lymphoid, hematopoietic and related tissue (C81-C96)
malignant neoplasm of skin (C44.-)
malignant neoplasm of unspecified site NOS (C80.1)

C76.0 **Malignant neoplasm of head, face and neck**
Malignant neoplasm of cheek NOS
Malignant neoplasm of nose NOS
C76.1 **Malignant neoplasm of thorax**
Intrathoracic malignant neoplasm NOS
Malignant neoplasm of axilla NOS
Thoracic malignant neoplasm NOS
C76.2 **Malignant neoplasm of abdomen**
C76.3 **Malignant neoplasm of pelvis**
Malignant neoplasm of groin NOS
Malignant neoplasm of sites overlapping systems within the pelvis
Rectovaginal (septum) malignant neoplasm
Rectovesical (septum) malignant neoplasm
C76.4 **Malignant neoplasm of upper limb**
C76.40 **Malignant neoplasm of unspecified upper limb**
C76.41 **Malignant neoplasm of right upper limb**
C76.42 **Malignant neoplasm of left upper limb**
C76.5 **Malignant neoplasm of lower limb**
C76.50 **Malignant neoplasm of unspecified lower limb**
C76.51 **Malignant neoplasm of right lower limb**
C76.52 **Malignant neoplasm of left lower limb**
C76.8 **Malignant neoplasm of other specified ill-defined sites**
Malignant neoplasm of overlapping ill-defined sites

C77 **Secondary and unspecified malignant neoplasm of lymph nodes**

EXCLUDES1 *malignant neoplasm of lymph nodes, specified as primary (C81-C86, C88, C96.-)*
Mesentery metastasis of carcinoid tumor (C7B.04)
secondary carcinoid tumors of distant lymph nodes (C7B.01)

C77.0 **Secondary and unspecified malignant neoplasm of lymph nodes of head, face and neck**
Secondary and unspecified malignant neoplasm of supraclavicular lymph nodes
C77.1 **Secondary and unspecified malignant neoplasm of intrathoracic lymph nodes**
C77.2 **Secondary and unspecified malignant neoplasm of intra-abdominal lymph nodes**
C77.3 **Secondary and unspecified malignant neoplasm of axilla and upper limb lymph nodes**
Secondary and unspecified malignant neoplasm of pectoral lymph nodes
C77.4 **Secondary and unspecified malignant neoplasm of inguinal and lower limb lymph nodes**
C77.5 **Secondary and unspecified malignant neoplasm of intrapelvic lymph nodes**
C77.8 **Secondary and unspecified malignant neoplasm of lymph nodes of multiple regions**
C77.9 **Secondary and unspecified malignant neoplasm of lymph node, unspecified**

C78 **Secondary malignant neoplasm of respiratory and digestive organs**

EXCLUDES1 *secondary carcinoid tumors of liver (C7B.02)*
secondary carcinoid tumors of peritoneum (C7B.04)

EXCLUDES2 *lymph node metastases (C77.0)*

C78.0 **Secondary malignant neoplasm of lung**
C78.00 **Secondary malignant neoplasm of unspecified lung**
C78.01 **Secondary malignant neoplasm of right lung**
C78.02 **Secondary malignant neoplasm of left lung**
C78.1 **Secondary malignant neoplasm of mediastinum**

Unacceptable principal diagnosis symbol per Medicare code edits · Code exempt from diagnosis present on admission requirement
Questionable admission · Complication or comorbidity · CC/MCC exclusion · Major complication or comorbidity
Principal diagnosis as its own CC · Principal diagnosis as its own MCC · Z code as first-listed diagnosis

 When symbols appear on a code that requires a 7th character extension, refer to Appendix D to identify applicable 7th character codes.

C78.2 Secondary malignant neoplasm of pleura
C78.3 Secondary malignant neoplasm of other and unspecified respiratory organs
C78.30 Secondary malignant neoplasm of unspecified respiratory organ
C78.39 Secondary malignant neoplasm of other respiratory organs
C78.4 Secondary malignant neoplasm of small intestine
C78.5 Secondary malignant neoplasm of large intestine and rectum
C78.6 Secondary malignant neoplasm of retroperitoneum and peritoneum
C78.7 Secondary malignant neoplasm of liver and intrahepatic bile duct
C78.8 Secondary malignant neoplasm of other and unspecified digestive organs
C78.80 Secondary malignant neoplasm of unspecified digestive organ
C78.89 Secondary malignant neoplasm of other digestive organs
Code also exocrine pancreatic insufficiency (K86.81)

C79 Secondary malignant neoplasm of other and unspecified sites
EXCLUDES1 *secondary carcinoid tumors (C7B.-)*
secondary neuroendocrine tumors (C7B.-)
EXCLUDES2 *lymph node metastases (C77.0)*
C79.0 Secondary malignant neoplasm of kidney and renal pelvis
C79.00 Secondary malignant neoplasm of unspecified kidney and renal pelvis
C79.01 Secondary malignant neoplasm of right kidney and renal pelvis
C79.02 Secondary malignant neoplasm of left kidney and renal pelvis
C79.1 Secondary malignant neoplasm of bladder and other and unspecified urinary organs
C79.10 Secondary malignant neoplasm of unspecified urinary organs
C79.11 Secondary malignant neoplasm of bladder
C79.19 Secondary malignant neoplasm of other urinary organs
C79.2 Secondary malignant neoplasm of skin
EXCLUDES1 *secondary Merkel cell carcinoma (C7B.1)*
C79.3 Secondary malignant neoplasm of brain and cerebral meninges
C79.31 Secondary malignant neoplasm of brain
C79.32 Secondary malignant neoplasm of cerebral meninges
C79.4 Secondary malignant neoplasm of other and unspecified parts of nervous system
C79.40 Secondary malignant neoplasm of unspecified part of nervous system
C79.49 Secondary malignant neoplasm of other parts of nervous system
C79.5 Secondary malignant neoplasm of bone and bone marrow
EXCLUDES1 *secondary carcinoid tumors of bone (C7B.03)*
C79.51 Secondary malignant neoplasm of bone
C79.52 Secondary malignant neoplasm of bone marrow
C79.6 Secondary malignant neoplasm of ovary
C79.60 Secondary malignant neoplasm of unspecified ovary ♀
C79.61 Secondary malignant neoplasm of right ovary ♀
C79.62 Secondary malignant neoplasm of left ovary ♀
C79.7 Secondary malignant neoplasm of adrenal gland
C79.70 Secondary malignant neoplasm of unspecified adrenal gland
C79.71 Secondary malignant neoplasm of right adrenal gland
C79.72 Secondary malignant neoplasm of left adrenal gland
C79.8 Secondary malignant neoplasm of other specified sites
C79.81 Secondary malignant neoplasm of breast
C79.82 Secondary malignant neoplasm of genital organs
C79.89 Secondary malignant neoplasm of other specified sites
C79.9 Secondary malignant neoplasm of unspecified site
Metastatic cancer NOS
Metastatic disease NOS
EXCLUDES1 *carcinomatosis NOS (C80.0)*
generalized cancer NOS (C80.0)
malignant (primary) neoplasm of unspecified site (C80.1)

C80 Malignant neoplasm without specification of site
EXCLUDES1 *malignant carcinoid tumor of unspecified site (C7A.00)*
malignant neoplasm of specified multiple sites- code to each site
C80.0 Disseminated malignant neoplasm, unspecified
Carcinomatosis NOS
Generalized cancer, unspecified site (primary) (secondary)
Generalized malignancy, unspecified site (primary) (secondary)
C80.1 Malignant (primary) neoplasm, unspecified
Cancer NOS
Cancer unspecified site (primary)
Carcinoma unspecified site (primary)
Malignancy unspecified site (primary)
EXCLUDES1 *secondary malignant neoplasm of unspecified site (C79.9)*
C80.2 Malignant neoplasm associated with transplanted organ PDx
Code first complication of transplanted organ (T86.-)
Use additional code to identify the specific malignancy

Malignant neoplasms of lymphoid, hematopoietic and related tissue (C81-C96)

EXCLUDES2 *Kaposi's sarcoma of lymph nodes (C46.3)*
secondary and unspecified neoplasm of lymph nodes (C77.-)
secondary neoplasm of bone marrow (C79.52)
secondary neoplasm of spleen (C78.89)

C81 Hodgkin lymphoma
EXCLUDES1 *personal history of Hodgkin lymphoma (Z85.71)*
C81.0 Nodular lymphocyte predominant Hodgkin lymphoma
C81.00 Nodular lymphocyte predominant Hodgkin lymphoma, unspecified site
C81.01 Nodular lymphocyte predominant Hodgkin lymphoma, lymph nodes of head, face, and neck
C81.02 Nodular lymphocyte predominant Hodgkin lymphoma, intrathoracic lymph nodes
C81.03 Nodular lymphocyte predominant Hodgkin lymphoma, intra-abdominal lymph nodes
C81.04 Nodular lymphocyte predominant Hodgkin lymphoma, lymph nodes of axilla and upper limb
C81.05 Nodular lymphocyte predominant Hodgkin lymphoma, lymph nodes of inguinal region and lower limb
C81.06 Nodular lymphocyte predominant Hodgkin lymphoma, intrapelvic lymph nodes
C81.07 Nodular lymphocyte predominant Hodgkin lymphoma, spleen
C81.08 Nodular lymphocyte predominant Hodgkin lymphoma, lymph nodes of multiple sites
C81.09 Nodular lymphocyte predominant Hodgkin lymphoma, extranodal and solid organ sites
▲ C81.1 Nodular ▶sclerosis Hodgkin◀ lymphoma
Nodular sclerosis classical Hodgkin lymphoma
▲ C81.10 Nodular ▶sclerosis Hodgkin◀ lymphoma, unspecified site
▲ C81.11 Nodular ▶sclerosis Hodgkin◀ lymphoma, lymph nodes of head, face, and neck
▲ C81.12 Nodular ▶sclerosis Hodgkin◀ lymphoma, intrathoracic lymph nodes
▲ C81.13 Nodular ▶sclerosis Hodgkin◀ lymphoma, intra-abdominal lymph nodes
▲ C81.14 Nodular ▶sclerosis Hodgkin◀ lymphoma, lymph nodes of axilla and upper limb
▲ C81.15 Nodular ▶sclerosis Hodgkin◀ lymphoma, lymph nodes of inguinal region and lower limb
▲ C81.16 Nodular ▶sclerosis Hodgkin◀ lymphoma, intrapelvic lymph nodes
▲ C81.17 Nodular ▶sclerosis Hodgkin◀ lymphoma, spleen

Unspecified Code Other Specified Code Manifestation Code N Newborn P Pediatric M Maternity A Adult ♂ Male ♀ Female
● New Code ▲ Revised Code Title ▶◀ Revised Text NOTES INCLUDES EXCLUDES1 Not coded here EXCLUDES2 Not included here
4th character required 5th character required 6th character required 7th character required
Extension 'X' Alert HAC Hospital-acquired condition (HAC) alert AHA AHA Coding Clinic©

▲ C81.18 Nodular ▶sclerosis Hodgkin◀ lymphoma, lymph nodes of multiple sites CC
▲ C81.19 Nodular ▶sclerosis Hodgkin◀ lymphoma, extranodal and solid organ sites CC

▲ C81.2 Mixed ▶cellularity Hodgkin◀ lymphoma
Mixed cellularity classical Hodgkin lymphoma
▲ C81.20 Mixed ▶cellularity Hodgkin◀ lymphoma, unspecified site CC
▲ C81.21 Mixed ▶cellularity Hodgkin◀ lymphoma, lymph nodes of head, face, and neck CC
▲ C81.22 Mixed ▶cellularity Hodgkin◀ lymphoma, intrathoracic lymph nodes CC
▲ C81.23 Mixed ▶cellularity Hodgkin◀ lymphoma, intra-abdominal lymph nodes CC
▲ C81.24 Mixed ▶cellularity Hodgkin◀ lymphoma, lymph nodes of axilla and upper limb CC
▲ C81.25 Mixed ▶cellularity Hodgkin◀ lymphoma, lymph nodes of inguinal region and lower limb CC
▲ C81.26 Mixed ▶cellularity Hodgkin◀ lymphoma, intrapelvic lymph nodes CC
▲ C81.27 Mixed ▶cellularity Hodgkin◀ lymphoma, spleen CC
▲ C81.28 Mixed ▶cellularity Hodgkin◀ lymphoma, lymph nodes of multiple sites CC
▲ C81.29 Mixed ▶cellularity Hodgkin◀ lymphoma, extranodal and solid organ sites CC

▲ C81.3 Lymphocyte ▶depleted Hodgkin◀ lymphoma
Lymphocyte depleted classical Hodgkin lymphoma
▲ C81.30 Lymphocyte ▶depleted Hodgkin◀ lymphoma, unspecified site CC
▲ C81.31 Lymphocyte ▶depleted Hodgkin◀ lymphoma, lymph nodes of head, face, and neck CC
▲ C81.32 Lymphocyte ▶depleted Hodgkin◀ lymphoma, intrathoracic lymph nodes CC
▲ C81.33 Lymphocyte ▶depleted Hodgkin◀ lymphoma, intra-abdominal lymph nodes CC
▲ C81.34 Lymphocyte ▶depleted Hodgkin◀ lymphoma, lymph nodes of axilla and upper limb CC
▲ C81.35 Lymphocyte ▶depleted Hodgkin◀ lymphoma, lymph nodes of inguinal region and lower limb CC
▲ C81.36 Lymphocyte ▶depleted Hodgkin◀ lymphoma, intrapelvic lymph nodes CC
▲ C81.37 Lymphocyte ▶depleted Hodgkin◀ lymphoma, spleen CC
▲ C81.38 Lymphocyte ▶depleted Hodgkin◀ lymphoma, lymph nodes of multiple sites CC
▲ C81.39 Lymphocyte depleted Hodgkin lymphoma, extranodal and solid organ sites CC

▲ C81.4 Lymphocyte-▶rich Hodgkin◀ lymphoma
Lymphocyte-rich classical Hodgkin lymphoma
EXCLUDES1 *nodular lymphocyte predominant Hodgkin lymphoma (C81.0-)*
▲ C81.40 Lymphocyte-▶rich Hodgkin◀ lymphoma, unspecified site CC
▲ C81.41 Lymphocyte-▶rich Hodgkin◀ lymphoma, lymph nodes of head, face, and neck CC
▲ C81.42 Lymphocyte-▶rich Hodgkin◀ lymphoma, intrathoracic lymph nodes CC
▲ C81.43 Lymphocyte-▶rich Hodgkin◀ lymphoma, intra-abdominal lymph nodes CC
▲ C81.44 Lymphocyte-▶rich Hodgkin◀ lymphoma, lymph nodes of axilla and upper limb CC
▲ C81.45 Lymphocyte-▶rich Hodgkin◀ lymphoma, lymph nodes of inguinal region and lower limb CC
▲ C81.46 Lymphocyte-▶rich Hodgkin◀ lymphoma, intrapelvic lymph nodes CC
▲ C81.47 Lymphocyte-▶rich Hodgkin◀ lymphoma, spleen CC
▲ C81.48 Lymphocyte-▶rich Hodgkin◀ lymphoma, lymph nodes of multiple sites CC
▲ C81.49 Lymphocyte-▶rich Hodgkin◀ lymphoma, extranodal and solid organ sites CC

▲ C81.7 ▶Other Hodgkin◀ lymphoma
Classical Hodgkin lymphoma NOS
Other classical Hodgkin lymphoma
▲ C81.70 ▶Other Hodgkin◀ lymphoma, unspecified site CC
▲ C81.71 ▶Other Hodgkin◀ lymphoma, lymph nodes of head, face, and neck CC
▲ C81.72 ▶Other Hodgkin◀ lymphoma, intrathoracic lymph nodes CC
▲ C81.73 ▶Other Hodgkin◀ lymphoma, intra-abdominal lymph nodes CC
▲ C81.74 ▶Other Hodgkin◀ lymphoma, lymph nodes of axilla and upper limb CC
▲ C81.75 ▶Other Hodgkin◀ lymphoma, lymph nodes of inguinal region and lower limb CC
▲ C81.76 ▶Other Hodgkin◀ lymphoma, intrapelvic lymph nodes CC
▲ C81.77 ▶Other Hodgkin◀ lymphoma, spleen CC
▲ C81.78 ▶Other Hodgkin◀ lymphoma, lymph nodes of multiple sites CC
▲ C81.79 ▶Other Hodgkin◀ lymphoma, extranodal and solid organ sites CC

C81.9 Hodgkin lymphoma, unspecified
C81.90 Hodgkin lymphoma, unspecified, unspecified site CC
C81.91 Hodgkin lymphoma, unspecified, lymph nodes of head, face, and neck CC
C81.92 Hodgkin lymphoma, unspecified, intrathoracic lymph nodes CC
C81.93 Hodgkin lymphoma, unspecified, intra-abdominal lymph nodes CC
C81.94 Hodgkin lymphoma, unspecified, lymph nodes of axilla and upper limb CC
C81.95 Hodgkin lymphoma, unspecified, lymph nodes of inguinal region and lower limb CC
C81.96 Hodgkin lymphoma, unspecified, intrapelvic lymph nodes CC
C81.97 Hodgkin lymphoma, unspecified, spleen CC
C81.98 Hodgkin lymphoma, unspecified, lymph nodes of multiple sites CC
C81.99 Hodgkin lymphoma, unspecified, extranodal and solid organ sites CC

C82 Follicular lymphoma
INCLUDES *follicular lymphoma with or without diffuse areas*
EXCLUDES1 *mature T/NK-cell lymphomas (C84.-)*
personal history of non-Hodgkin lymphoma (Z85.72)

C82.0 Follicular lymphoma grade I
C82.00 Follicular lymphoma grade I, unspecified site CC
C82.01 Follicular lymphoma grade I, lymph nodes of head, face, and neck CC
C82.02 Follicular lymphoma grade I, intrathoracic lymph nodes CC
C82.03 Follicular lymphoma grade I, intra-abdominal lymph nodes CC
C82.04 Follicular lymphoma grade I, lymph nodes of axilla and upper limb CC
C82.05 Follicular lymphoma grade I, lymph nodes of inguinal region and lower limb CC
C82.06 Follicular lymphoma grade I, intrapelvic lymph nodes CC
C82.07 Follicular lymphoma grade I, spleen CC
C82.08 Follicular lymphoma grade I, lymph nodes of multiple sites CC
C82.09 Follicular lymphoma grade I, extranodal and solid organ sites CC

C82.1 Follicular lymphoma grade II
C82.10 Follicular lymphoma grade II, unspecified site CC
C82.11 Follicular lymphoma grade II, lymph nodes of head, face, and neck CC
C82.12 Follicular lymphoma grade II, intrathoracic lymph nodes CC
C82.13 Follicular lymphoma grade II, intra-abdominal lymph nodes CC
C82.14 Follicular lymphoma grade II, lymph nodes of axilla and upper limb CC
C82.15 Follicular lymphoma grade II, lymph nodes of inguinal region and lower limb CC
C82.16 Follicular lymphoma grade II, intrapelvic lymph nodes CC
C82.17 Follicular lymphoma grade II, spleen CC
C82.18 Follicular lymphoma grade II, lymph nodes of multiple sites CC

Unacceptable principal diagnosis symbol per Medicare code edits · Code exempt from diagnosis present on admission requirement
Questionable admission · Complication or comorbidity · CC/MCC exclusion · Major complication or comorbidity
Principal diagnosis as its own CC · Principal diagnosis as its own MCC · Z code as first-listed diagnosis

C82.19 Follicular lymphoma grade II, extranodal and solid organ sites

C82.2 Follicular lymphoma grade III, unspecified
- C82.20 Follicular lymphoma grade III, unspecified, unspecified site
- C82.21 Follicular lymphoma grade III, unspecified, lymph nodes of head, face, and neck
- C82.22 Follicular lymphoma grade III, unspecified, intrathoracic lymph nodes
- C82.23 Follicular lymphoma grade III, unspecified, intra-abdominal lymph nodes
- C82.24 Follicular lymphoma grade III, unspecified, lymph nodes of axilla and upper limb
- C82.25 Follicular lymphoma grade III, unspecified, lymph nodes of inguinal region and lower limb
- C82.26 Follicular lymphoma grade III, unspecified, intrapelvic lymph nodes
- C82.27 Follicular lymphoma grade III, unspecified, spleen
- C82.28 Follicular lymphoma grade III, unspecified, lymph nodes of multiple sites
- C82.29 Follicular lymphoma grade III, unspecified, extranodal and solid organ sites

C82.3 Follicular lymphoma grade IIIa
- C82.30 Follicular lymphoma grade IIIa, unspecified site
- C82.31 Follicular lymphoma grade IIIa, lymph nodes of head, face, and neck
- C82.32 Follicular lymphoma grade IIIa, intrathoracic lymph nodes
- C82.33 Follicular lymphoma grade IIIa, intra-abdominal lymph nodes
- C82.34 Follicular lymphoma grade IIIa, lymph nodes of axilla and upper limb
- C82.35 Follicular lymphoma grade IIIa, lymph nodes of inguinal region and lower limb
- C82.36 Follicular lymphoma grade IIIa, intrapelvic lymph nodes
- C82.37 Follicular lymphoma grade IIIa, spleen
- C82.38 Follicular lymphoma grade IIIa, lymph nodes of multiple sites
- C82.39 Follicular lymphoma grade IIIa, extranodal and solid organ sites

C82.4 Follicular lymphoma grade IIIb
- C82.40 Follicular lymphoma grade IIIb, unspecified site
- C82.41 Follicular lymphoma grade IIIb, lymph nodes of head, face, and neck
- C82.42 Follicular lymphoma grade IIIb, intrathoracic lymph nodes
- C82.43 Follicular lymphoma grade IIIb, intra-abdominal lymph nodes
- C82.44 Follicular lymphoma grade IIIb, lymph nodes of axilla and upper limb
- C82.45 Follicular lymphoma grade IIIb, lymph nodes of inguinal region and lower limb
- C82.46 Follicular lymphoma grade IIIb, intrapelvic lymph nodes
- C82.47 Follicular lymphoma grade IIIb, spleen
- C82.48 Follicular lymphoma grade IIIb, lymph nodes of multiple sites
- C82.49 Follicular lymphoma grade IIIb, extranodal and solid organ sites

C82.5 Diffuse follicle center lymphoma
- C82.50 Diffuse follicle center lymphoma, unspecified site
- C82.51 Diffuse follicle center lymphoma, lymph nodes of head, face, and neck
- C82.52 Diffuse follicle center lymphoma, intrathoracic lymph nodes
- C82.53 Diffuse follicle center lymphoma, intra-abdominal lymph nodes
- C82.54 Diffuse follicle center lymphoma, lymph nodes of axilla and upper limb
- C82.55 Diffuse follicle center lymphoma, lymph nodes of inguinal region and lower limb
- C82.56 Diffuse follicle center lymphoma, intrapelvic lymph nodes
- C82.57 Diffuse follicle center lymphoma, spleen
- C82.58 Diffuse follicle center lymphoma, lymph nodes of multiple sites
- C82.59 Diffuse follicle center lymphoma, extranodal and solid organ sites

C82.6 Cutaneous follicle center lymphoma
- C82.60 Cutaneous follicle center lymphoma, unspecified site
- C82.61 Cutaneous follicle center lymphoma, lymph nodes of head, face, and neck
- C82.62 Cutaneous follicle center lymphoma, intrathoracic lymph nodes
- C82.63 Cutaneous follicle center lymphoma, intra-abdominal lymph nodes
- C82.64 Cutaneous follicle center lymphoma, lymph nodes of axilla and upper limb
- C82.65 Cutaneous follicle center lymphoma, lymph nodes of inguinal region and lower limb
- C82.66 Cutaneous follicle center lymphoma, intrapelvic lymph nodes
- C82.67 Cutaneous follicle center lymphoma, spleen
- C82.68 Cutaneous follicle center lymphoma, lymph nodes of multiple sites
- C82.69 Cutaneous follicle center lymphoma, extranodal and solid organ sites

C82.8 Other types of follicular lymphoma
- C82.80 Other types of follicular lymphoma, unspecified site
- C82.81 Other types of follicular lymphoma, lymph nodes of head, face, and neck
- C82.82 Other types of follicular lymphoma, intrathoracic lymph nodes
- C82.83 Other types of follicular lymphoma, intra-abdominal lymph nodes
- C82.84 Other types of follicular lymphoma, lymph nodes of axilla and upper limb
- C82.85 Other types of follicular lymphoma, lymph nodes of inguinal region and lower limb
- C82.86 Other types of follicular lymphoma, intrapelvic lymph nodes
- C82.87 Other types of follicular lymphoma, spleen
- C82.88 Other types of follicular lymphoma, lymph nodes of multiple sites
- C82.89 Other types of follicular lymphoma, extranodal and solid organ sites

C82.9 Follicular lymphoma, unspecified
- C82.90 Follicular lymphoma, unspecified, unspecified site
- C82.91 Follicular lymphoma, unspecified, lymph nodes of head, face, and neck
- C82.92 Follicular lymphoma, unspecified, intrathoracic lymph nodes
- C82.93 Follicular lymphoma, unspecified, intra-abdominal lymph nodes
- C82.94 Follicular lymphoma, unspecified, lymph nodes of axilla and upper limb
- C82.95 Follicular lymphoma, unspecified, lymph nodes of inguinal region and lower limb
- C82.96 Follicular lymphoma, unspecified, intrapelvic lymph nodes
- C82.97 Follicular lymphoma, unspecified, spleen
- C82.98 Follicular lymphoma, unspecified, lymph nodes of multiple sites
- C82.99 Follicular lymphoma, unspecified, extranodal and solid organ sites

C83 Non-follicular lymphoma

EXCLUDES1 *personal history of non-Hodgkin lymphoma (Z85.72)*

C83.0 Small cell B-cell lymphoma

Lymphoplasmacytic lymphoma
Nodal marginal zone lymphoma
Non-leukemic variant of B-CLL
Splenic marginal zone lymphoma

EXCLUDES1 *chronic lymphocytic leukemia (C91.1)*
mature T/NK-cell lymphomas (C84.-)
Waldenström macroglobulinemia (C88.0)

- C83.00 Small cell B-cell lymphoma, unspecified site

Unspecified Code | Other Specified Code | Manifestation Code | N Newborn | P Pediatric | M Maternity | A Adult | ♂ Male | ♀ Female
● New Code ▲ Revised Code Title ►◄ Revised Text NOTES INCLUDES EXCLUDES1 Not coded here EXCLUDES2 Not included here
4th character required | 5th character required | 6th character required | 7th character required
Extension 'X' Alert | HAC Hospital-acquired condition (HAC) alert | AHA AHA Coding Clinic©

C83.01 **Small cell B-cell lymphoma, lymph nodes of head, face, and neck**
C83.02 **Small cell B-cell lymphoma, intrathoracic lymph nodes**
C83.03 **Small cell B-cell lymphoma, intra-abdominal lymph nodes**
C83.04 **Small cell B-cell lymphoma, lymph nodes of axilla and upper limb**
C83.05 **Small cell B-cell lymphoma, lymph nodes of inguinal region and lower limb**
C83.06 **Small cell B-cell lymphoma, intrapelvic lymph nodes**
C83.07 **Small cell B-cell lymphoma, spleen**
C83.08 **Small cell B-cell lymphoma, lymph nodes of multiple sites**
C83.09 **Small cell B-cell lymphoma, extranodal and solid organ sites**

C83.1 **Mantle cell lymphoma**
Centrocytic lymphoma
Malignant lymphomatous polyposis
C83.10 **Mantle cell lymphoma, unspecified site**
C83.11 **Mantle cell lymphoma, lymph nodes of head, face, and neck**
C83.12 **Mantle cell lymphoma, intrathoracic lymph nodes**
C83.13 **Mantle cell lymphoma, intra-abdominal lymph nodes**
C83.14 **Mantle cell lymphoma, lymph nodes of axilla and upper limb**
C83.15 **Mantle cell lymphoma, lymph nodes of inguinal region and lower limb**
C83.16 **Mantle cell lymphoma, intrapelvic lymph nodes**
C83.17 **Mantle cell lymphoma, spleen**
C83.18 **Mantle cell lymphoma, lymph nodes of multiple sites**
C83.19 **Mantle cell lymphoma, extranodal and solid organ sites**

C83.3 **Diffuse large B-cell lymphoma**
Anaplastic diffuse large B-cell lymphoma
CD30-positive diffuse large B-cell lymphoma
Centroblastic diffuse large B-cell lymphoma
Diffuse large B-cell lymphoma, subtype not specified
Immunoblastic diffuse large B-cell lymphoma
Plasmablastic diffuse large B-cell lymphoma
Diffuse large B-cell lymphoma, subtype not specified
T-cell rich diffuse large B-cell lymphoma
EXCLUDES1 *mediastinal (thymic) large B-cell lymphoma (C85.2-)*
mature T/NK-cell lymphomas (C84.-)
C83.30 **Diffuse large B-cell lymphoma, unspecified site**
C83.31 **Diffuse large B-cell lymphoma, lymph nodes of head, face, and neck**
C83.32 **Diffuse large B-cell lymphoma, intrathoracic lymph nodes**
C83.33 **Diffuse large B-cell lymphoma, intra-abdominal lymph nodes**
C83.34 **Diffuse large B-cell lymphoma, lymph nodes of axilla and upper limb**
C83.35 **Diffuse large B-cell lymphoma, lymph nodes of inguinal region and lower limb**
C83.36 **Diffuse large B-cell lymphoma, intrapelvic lymph nodes**
C83.37 **Diffuse large B-cell lymphoma, spleen**
C83.38 **Diffuse large B-cell lymphoma, lymph nodes of multiple sites**
C83.39 **Diffuse large B-cell lymphoma, extranodal and solid organ sites**

C83.5 **Lymphoblastic (diffuse) lymphoma**
B-precursor lymphoma
Lymphoblastic B-cell lymphoma
Lymphoblastic lymphoma NOS
Lymphoblastic T-cell lymphoma
T-precursor lymphoma
C83.50 **Lymphoblastic (diffuse) lymphoma, unspecified site**
C83.51 **Lymphoblastic (diffuse) lymphoma, lymph nodes of head, face, and neck**
C83.52 **Lymphoblastic (diffuse) lymphoma, intrathoracic lymph nodes**
C83.53 **Lymphoblastic (diffuse) lymphoma, intra-abdominal lymph nodes**
C83.54 **Lymphoblastic (diffuse) lymphoma, lymph nodes of axilla and upper limb**
C83.55 **Lymphoblastic (diffuse) lymphoma, lymph nodes of inguinal region and lower limb**
C83.56 **Lymphoblastic (diffuse) lymphoma, intrapelvic lymph nodes**
C83.57 **Lymphoblastic (diffuse) lymphoma, spleen**
C83.58 **Lymphoblastic (diffuse) lymphoma, lymph nodes of multiple sites**
C83.59 **Lymphoblastic (diffuse) lymphoma, extranodal and solid organ sites**

C83.7 **Burkitt lymphoma**
Atypical Burkitt lymphoma
Burkitt-like lymphoma
EXCLUDES1 *mature B-cell leukemia Burkitt type (C91.A-)*
C83.70 **Burkitt lymphoma, unspecified site**
C83.71 **Burkitt lymphoma, lymph nodes of head, face, and neck**
C83.72 **Burkitt lymphoma, intrathoracic lymph nodes**
C83.73 **Burkitt lymphoma, intra-abdominal lymph nodes**
C83.74 **Burkitt lymphoma, lymph nodes of axilla and upper limb**
C83.75 **Burkitt lymphoma, lymph nodes of inguinal region and lower limb**
C83.76 **Burkitt lymphoma, intrapelvic lymph nodes**
C83.77 **Burkitt lymphoma, spleen**
C83.78 **Burkitt lymphoma, lymph nodes of multiple sites**
C83.79 **Burkitt lymphoma, extranodal and solid organ sites**

C83.8 **Other non-follicular lymphoma**
Intravascular large B-cell lymphoma
Lymphoid granulomatosis
Primary effusion B-cell lymphoma
EXCLUDES1 *mediastinal (thymic) large B-cell lymphoma (C85.2-)*
T-cell rich B-cell lymphoma (C83.3-)
C83.80 **Other non-follicular lymphoma, unspecified site**
C83.81 **Other non-follicular lymphoma, lymph nodes of head, face, and neck**
C83.82 **Other non-follicular lymphoma, intrathoracic lymph nodes**
C83.83 **Other non-follicular lymphoma, intra-abdominal lymph nodes**
C83.84 **Other non-follicular lymphoma, lymph nodes of axilla and upper limb**
C83.85 **Other non-follicular lymphoma, lymph nodes of inguinal region and lower limb**
C83.86 **Other non-follicular lymphoma, intrapelvic lymph nodes**
C83.87 **Other non-follicular lymphoma, spleen**
C83.88 **Other non-follicular lymphoma, lymph nodes of multiple sites**
C83.89 **Other non-follicular lymphoma, extranodal and solid organ sites**

C83.9 **Non-follicular (diffuse) lymphoma, unspecified**
C83.90 **Non-follicular (diffuse) lymphoma, unspecified, unspecified site**
C83.91 **Non-follicular (diffuse) lymphoma, unspecified, lymph nodes of head, face, and neck**
C83.92 **Non-follicular (diffuse) lymphoma, unspecified, intrathoracic lymph nodes**
C83.93 **Non-follicular (diffuse) lymphoma, unspecified, intra-abdominal lymph nodes**
C83.94 **Non-follicular (diffuse) lymphoma, unspecified, lymph nodes of axilla and upper limb**
C83.95 **Non-follicular (diffuse) lymphoma, unspecified, lymph nodes of inguinal region and lower limb**
C83.96 **Non-follicular (diffuse) lymphoma, unspecified, intrapelvic lymph nodes**
C83.97 **Non-follicular (diffuse) lymphoma, unspecified, spleen**

Unacceptable principal diagnosis symbol per Medicare code edits — Code exempt from diagnosis present on admission requirement
Questionable admission — Complication or comorbidity — CC/MCC exclusion — Major complication or comorbidity
Principal diagnosis as its own CC — Principal diagnosis as its own MCC — Z code as first-listed diagnosis

 When symbols appear on a code that requires a 7th character extension, refer to Appendix D to identify applicable 7th character codes.

C83.98 Non-follicular (diffuse) lymphoma, unspecified, lymph nodes of multiple sites
C83.99 Non-follicular (diffuse) lymphoma, unspecified, extranodal and solid organ sites

C84 Mature T/NK-cell lymphomas
EXCLUDES1 *personal history of non-Hodgkin lymphoma (Z85.72)*

C84.0 Mycosis fungoides
EXCLUDES1 *peripheral T-cell lymphoma, not classified (C84.4-)*
C84.00 Mycosis fungoides, unspecified site
C84.01 Mycosis fungoides, lymph nodes of head, face, and neck
C84.02 Mycosis fungoides, intrathoracic lymph nodes
C84.03 Mycosis fungoides, intra-abdominal lymph nodes
C84.04 Mycosis fungoides, lymph nodes of axilla and upper limb
C84.05 Mycosis fungoides, lymph nodes of inguinal region and lower limb
C84.06 Mycosis fungoides, intrapelvic lymph nodes
C84.07 Mycosis fungoides, spleen
C84.08 Mycosis fungoides, lymph nodes of multiple sites
C84.09 Mycosis fungoides, extranodal and solid organ sites

C84.1 Sézary disease
C84.10 Sézary disease, unspecified site
C84.11 Sézary disease, lymph nodes of head, face, and neck
C84.12 Sézary disease, intrathoracic lymph nodes
C84.13 Sézary disease, intra-abdominal lymph nodes
C84.14 Sézary disease, lymph nodes of axilla and upper limb
C84.15 Sézary disease, lymph nodes of inguinal region and lower limb
C84.16 Sézary disease, intrapelvic lymph nodes
C84.17 Sézary disease, spleen
C84.18 Sézary disease, lymph nodes of multiple sites
C84.19 Sézary disease, extranodal and solid organ sites

C84.4 Peripheral T-cell lymphoma, not classified
Lennert's lymphoma
Lymphoepithelioid lymphoma
Mature T-cell lymphoma, not elsewhere classified
C84.40 Peripheral T-cell lymphoma, not classified, unspecified site
C84.41 Peripheral T-cell lymphoma, not classified, lymph nodes of head, face, and neck
C84.42 Peripheral T-cell lymphoma, not classified, intrathoracic lymph nodes
C84.43 Peripheral T-cell lymphoma, not classified, intra-abdominal lymph nodes
C84.44 Peripheral T-cell lymphoma, not classified, lymph nodes of axilla and upper limb
C84.45 Peripheral T-cell lymphoma, not classified, lymph nodes of inguinal region and lower limb
C84.46 Peripheral T-cell lymphoma, not classified, intrapelvic lymph nodes
C84.47 Peripheral T-cell lymphoma, not classified, spleen
C84.48 Peripheral T-cell lymphoma, not classified, lymph nodes of multiple sites
C84.49 Peripheral T-cell lymphoma, not classified, extranodal and solid organ sites

C84.6 Anaplastic large cell lymphoma, ALK-positive
Anaplastic large cell lymphoma, CD30-positive
C84.60 Anaplastic large cell lymphoma, ALK-positive, unspecified site
C84.61 Anaplastic large cell lymphoma, ALK-positive, lymph nodes of head, face, and neck
C84.62 Anaplastic large cell lymphoma, ALK-positive, intrathoracic lymph nodes
C84.63 Anaplastic large cell lymphoma, ALK-positive, intra-abdominal lymph nodes
C84.64 Anaplastic large cell lymphoma, ALK-positive, lymph nodes of axilla and upper limb
C84.65 Anaplastic large cell lymphoma, ALK-positive, lymph nodes of inguinal region and lower limb
C84.66 Anaplastic large cell lymphoma, ALK-positive, intrapelvic lymph nodes
C84.67 Anaplastic large cell lymphoma, ALK-positive, spleen
C84.68 Anaplastic large cell lymphoma, ALK-positive, lymph nodes of multiple sites
C84.69 Anaplastic large cell lymphoma, ALK-positive, extranodal and solid organ sites

C84.7 Anaplastic large cell lymphoma, ALK-negative
EXCLUDES1 *primary cutaneous CD30-positive T-cell proliferations (C86.6-)*
C84.70 Anaplastic large cell lymphoma, ALK-negative, unspecified site
C84.71 Anaplastic large cell lymphoma, ALK-negative, lymph nodes of head, face, and neck
C84.72 Anaplastic large cell lymphoma, ALK-negative, intrathoracic lymph nodes
C84.73 Anaplastic large cell lymphoma, ALK-negative, intra-abdominal lymph nodes
C84.74 Anaplastic large cell lymphoma, ALK-negative, lymph nodes of axilla and upper limb
C84.75 Anaplastic large cell lymphoma, ALK-negative, lymph nodes of inguinal region and lower limb
C84.76 Anaplastic large cell lymphoma, ALK-negative, intrapelvic lymph nodes
C84.77 Anaplastic large cell lymphoma, ALK-negative, spleen
C84.78 Anaplastic large cell lymphoma, ALK-negative, lymph nodes of multiple sites
C84.79 Anaplastic large cell lymphoma, ALK-negative, extranodal and solid organ sites

C84.A Cutaneous T-cell lymphoma, unspecified
C84.A0 Cutaneous T-cell lymphoma, unspecified, unspecified site
C84.A1 Cutaneous T-cell lymphoma, unspecified lymph nodes of head, face, and neck
C84.A2 Cutaneous T-cell lymphoma, unspecified, intrathoracic lymph nodes
C84.A3 Cutaneous T-cell lymphoma, unspecified, intra-abdominal lymph nodes
C84.A4 Cutaneous T-cell lymphoma, unspecified, lymph nodes of axilla and upper limb
C84.A5 Cutaneous T-cell lymphoma, unspecified, lymph nodes of inguinal region and lower limb
C84.A6 Cutaneous T-cell lymphoma, unspecified, intrapelvic lymph nodes
C84.A7 Cutaneous T-cell lymphoma, unspecified, spleen
C84.A8 Cutaneous T-cell lymphoma, unspecified, lymph nodes of multiple sites
C84.A9 Cutaneous T-cell lymphoma, unspecified, extranodal and solid organ sites

C84.Z Other mature T/NK-cell lymphomas
NOTES If T-cell lineage or involvement is mentioned in conjunction with a specific lymphoma, code to the more specific description.
EXCLUDES1 *angioimmunoblastic T-cell lymphoma (C86.5)*
blastic NK-cell lymphoma (C86.4)
enteropathy-type T-cell lymphoma (C86.2)
extranodal NK-cell lymphoma, nasal type (C86.0)
hepatosplenic T-cell lymphoma (C86.1)
primary cutaneous CD30-positive T-cell proliferations (C86.6)
subcutaneous panniculitis-like T-cell lymphoma (C86.3)
T-cell leukemia (C91.1-)
C84.Z0 Other mature T/NK-cell lymphomas, unspecified site
C84.Z1 Other mature T/NK-cell lymphomas, lymph nodes of head, face, and neck
C84.Z2 Other mature T/NK-cell lymphomas, intrathoracic lymph nodes
C84.Z3 Other mature T/NK-cell lymphomas, intra-abdominal lymph nodes

Unspecified Code | Other Specified Code | Manifestation Code | N Newborn | P Pediatric | M Maternity | A Adult | ♂ Male | ♀ Female
● New Code | ▲ Revised Code Title | ►◄ Revised Text | NOTES | INCLUDES | EXCLUDES1 Not coded here | EXCLUDES2 Not included here
4th character required | 5th character required | 6th character required | 7th character required
Extension 'X' Alert | HAC Hospital-acquired condition (HAC) alert | AHA AHA Coding Clinic©

C84.Z4 Other mature T/NK-cell lymphomas, lymph nodes of axilla and upper limb
C84.Z5 Other mature T/NK-cell lymphomas, lymph nodes of inguinal region and lower limb
C84.Z6 Other mature T/NK-cell lymphomas, intrapelvic lymph nodes
C84.Z7 Other mature T/NK-cell lymphomas, spleen
C84.Z8 Other mature T/NK-cell lymphomas, lymph nodes of multiple sites
C84.Z9 Other mature T/NK-cell lymphomas, extranodal and solid organ sites

C84.9 Mature T/NK-cell lymphomas, unspecified
NK/T cell lymphoma NOS
EXCLUDES1 *mature T-cell lymphoma, not elsewhere classified (C84.4-)*
C84.90 Mature T/NK-cell lymphomas, unspecified, unspecified site
C84.91 Mature T/NK-cell lymphomas, unspecified, lymph nodes of head, face, and neck
C84.92 Mature T/NK-cell lymphomas, unspecified, intrathoracic lymph nodes
C84.93 Mature T/NK-cell lymphomas, unspecified, intra-abdominal lymph nodes
C84.94 Mature T/NK-cell lymphomas, unspecified, lymph nodes of axilla and upper limb
C84.95 Mature T/NK-cell lymphomas, unspecified, lymph nodes of inguinal region and lower limb
C84.96 Mature T/NK-cell lymphomas, unspecified, intrapelvic lymph nodes
C84.97 Mature T/NK-cell lymphomas, unspecified, spleen
C84.98 Mature T/NK-cell lymphomas, unspecified, lymph nodes of multiple sites
C84.99 Mature T/NK-cell lymphomas, unspecified, extranodal and solid organ sites

C85 Other specified and unspecified types of non-Hodgkin lymphoma
EXCLUDES1 *other specified types of T/NK-cell lymphoma (C86.-)*
personal history of non-Hodgkin lymphoma (Z85.72)

C85.1 Unspecified B-cell lymphoma
NOTES If B-cell lineage or involvement is mentioned in conjunction with a specific lymphoma, code to the more specific description.
C85.10 Unspecified B-cell lymphoma, unspecified site
C85.11 Unspecified B-cell lymphoma, lymph nodes of head, face, and neck
C85.12 Unspecified B-cell lymphoma, intrathoracic lymph nodes
C85.13 Unspecified B-cell lymphoma, intra-abdominal lymph nodes
C85.14 Unspecified B-cell lymphoma, lymph nodes of axilla and upper limb
C85.15 Unspecified B-cell lymphoma, lymph nodes of inguinal region and lower limb
C85.16 Unspecified B-cell lymphoma, intrapelvic lymph nodes
C85.17 Unspecified B-cell lymphoma, spleen
C85.18 Unspecified B-cell lymphoma, lymph nodes of multiple sites
C85.19 Unspecified B-cell lymphoma, extranodal and solid organ sites

C85.2 Mediastinal (thymic) large B-cell lymphoma
C85.20 Mediastinal (thymic) large B-cell lymphoma, unspecified site
C85.21 Mediastinal (thymic) large B-cell lymphoma, lymph nodes of head, face, and neck
C85.22 Mediastinal (thymic) large B-cell lymphoma, intrathoracic lymph nodes
C85.23 Mediastinal (thymic) large B-cell lymphoma, intra-abdominal lymph nodes
C85.24 Mediastinal (thymic) large B-cell lymphoma, lymph nodes of axilla and upper limb
C85.25 Mediastinal (thymic) large B-cell lymphoma, lymph nodes of inguinal region and lower limb
C85.26 Mediastinal (thymic) large B-cell lymphoma, intrapelvic lymph nodes
C85.27 Mediastinal (thymic) large B-cell lymphoma, spleen
C85.28 Mediastinal (thymic) large B-cell lymphoma, lymph nodes of multiple sites
C85.29 Mediastinal (thymic) large B-cell lymphoma, extranodal and solid organ sites

C85.8 Other specified types of non-Hodgkin lymphoma
C85.80 Other specified types of non-Hodgkin lymphoma, unspecified site
C85.81 Other specified types of non-Hodgkin lymphoma, lymph nodes of head, face, and neck
C85.82 Other specified types of non-Hodgkin lymphoma, intrathoracic lymph nodes
C85.83 Other specified types of non-Hodgkin lymphoma, intra-abdominal lymph nodes
C85.84 Other specified types of non-Hodgkin lymphoma, lymph nodes of axilla and upper limb
C85.85 Other specified types of non-Hodgkin lymphoma, lymph nodes of inguinal region and lower limb
C85.86 Other specified types of non-Hodgkin lymphoma, intrapelvic lymph nodes
C85.87 Other specified types of non-Hodgkin lymphoma, spleen
C85.88 Other specified types of non-Hodgkin lymphoma, lymph nodes of multiple sites
C85.89 Other specified types of non-Hodgkin lymphoma, extranodal and solid organ sites

C85.9 Non-Hodgkin lymphoma, unspecified
Lymphoma NOS
Malignant lymphoma NOS
Non-Hodgkin lymphoma NOS
C85.90 Non-Hodgkin lymphoma, unspecified, unspecified site
C85.91 Non-Hodgkin lymphoma, unspecified, lymph nodes of head, face, and neck
C85.92 Non-Hodgkin lymphoma, unspecified, intrathoracic lymph nodes
C85.93 Non-Hodgkin lymphoma, unspecified, intra-abdominal lymph nodes
C85.94 Non-Hodgkin lymphoma, unspecified, lymph nodes of axilla and upper limb
C85.95 Non-Hodgkin lymphoma, unspecified, lymph nodes of inguinal region and lower limb
C85.96 Non-Hodgkin lymphoma, unspecified, intrapelvic lymph nodes
C85.97 Non-Hodgkin lymphoma, unspecified, spleen
C85.98 Non-Hodgkin lymphoma, unspecified, lymph nodes of multiple sites
C85.99 Non-Hodgkin lymphoma, unspecified, extranodal and solid organ sites

C86 Other specified types of T/NK-cell lymphoma
EXCLUDES1 *anaplastic large cell lymphoma, ALK negative (C84.7-)*
anaplastic large cell lymphoma, ALK positive (C84.6-)
mature T/NK-cell lymphomas (C84.-)
other specified types of non-Hodgkin lymphoma (C85.8-)
C86.0 Extranodal NK/T-cell lymphoma, nasal type
C86.1 Hepatosplenic T-cell lymphoma
Alpha-beta and gamma delta types
C86.2 Enteropathy-type (intestinal) T-cell lymphoma
Enteropathy associated T-cell lymphoma
C86.3 Subcutaneous panniculitis-like T-cell lymphoma
C86.4 Blastic NK-cell lymphoma
C86.5 Angioimmunoblastic T-cell lymphoma
Angioimmunoblastic lymphadenopathy with dysproteinemia (AILD)
C86.6 Primary cutaneous CD30-positive T-cell proliferations
Lymphomatoid papulosis
Primary cutaneous anaplastic large cell lymphoma
Primary cutaneous CD30-positive large T-cell lymphoma

C88 Malignant immunoproliferative diseases and certain other B-cell lymphomas
EXCLUDES1 *B-cell lymphoma, unspecified (C85.1-)*
personal history of other malignant neoplasms of lymphoid, hematopoietic and related tissues (Z85.79)

Unacceptable principal diagnosis symbol per Medicare code edits · Code exempt from diagnosis present on admission requirement · Questionable admission · Complication or comorbidity · CC/MCC exclusion · Major complication or comorbidity · Principal diagnosis as its own CC · Principal diagnosis as its own MCC · Z code as first-listed diagnosis

C88.0 **Waldenström macroglobulinemia**
Lymphoplasmacytic lymphoma with IgM-production
Macroglobulinemia (idiopathic) (primary)
EXCLUDES1 *small cell B-cell lymphoma (C83.0)*

C88.2 **Heavy chain disease**
Franklin disease
Gamma heavy chain disease
Mu heavy chain disease

C88.3 **Immunoproliferative small intestinal disease**
Alpha heavy chain disease
Mediterranean lymphoma

C88.4 **Extranodal marginal zone B-cell lymphoma of mucosa-associated lymphoid tissue [MALT-lymphoma]**
Lymphoma of skin-associated lymphoid tissue [SALT-lymphoma]
Lymphoma of bronchial-associated lymphoid tissue [BALT-lymphoma]
EXCLUDES1 *high malignant (diffuse large B-cell) lymphoma (C83.3-)*

C88.8 **Other malignant immunoproliferative diseases**

C88.9 **Malignant immunoproliferative disease, unspecified**
Immunoproliferative disease NOS

C90 **Multiple myeloma and malignant plasma cell neoplasms**
EXCLUDES1 *personal history of other malignant neoplasms of lymphoid, hematopoietic and related tissues (Z85.79)*

C90.0 **Multiple myeloma**
Kahler's disease
Medullary plasmacytoma
Myelomatosis
Plasma cell myeloma
EXCLUDES1 *solitary myeloma (C90.3-)*
solitary plasmactyoma (C90.3-)

C90.00 **Multiple myeloma** not having achieved remission
Multiple myeloma with failed remission
Multiple myeloma NOS

C90.01 **Multiple myeloma** in remission

C90.02 **Multiple myeloma** in relapse

C90.1 **Plasma cell leukemia**
Plasmacytic leukemia

C90.10 **Plasma cell leukemia** not having achieved remission
Plasma cell leukemia with failed remission
Plasma cell leukemia NOS

C90.11 **Plasma cell leukemia** in remission

C90.12 **Plasma cell leukemia** in relapse

C90.2 **Extramedullary plasmacytoma**

C90.20 **Extramedullary plasmacytoma** not having achieved remission
Extramedullary plasmacytoma with failed remission
Extramedullary plasmacytoma NOS

C90.21 **Extramedullary plasmacytoma** in remission

C90.22 **Extramedullary plasmacytoma** in relapse

C90.3 **Solitary plasmacytoma**
Localized malignant plasma cell tumor NOS
Plasmacytoma NOS
Solitary myeloma

C90.30 **Solitary plasmacytoma** not having achieved remission
Solitary plasmacytoma with failed remission
Solitary plasmacytoma NOS

C90.31 **Solitary plasmacytoma** in remission

C90.32 **Solitary plasmacytoma** in relapse

C91 **Lymphoid leukemia**
EXCLUDES1 *personal history of leukemia (Z85.6)*

C91.0 Acute lymphoblastic **leukemia [ALL]**
NOTES Code C91.0 should only be used for T-cell and B-cell precursor leukemia

C91.00 **Acute lymphoblastic leukemia** not having achieved remission
Acute lymphoblastic leukemia with failed remission
Acute lymphoblastic leukemia NOS

C91.01 **Acute lymphoblastic leukemia,** in remission

C91.02 **Acute lymphoblastic leukemia,** in relapse

C91.1 Chronic lymphocytic **leukemia of** B-cell type
Lymphoplasmacytic leukemia
Richter syndrome
EXCLUDES1 *lymphoplasmacytic lymphoma (C83.0-)*

C91.10 **Chronic lymphocytic leukemia of B-cell type** not having achieved remission
Chronic lymphocytic leukemia of B-cell type with failed remission
Chronic lymphocytic leukemia of B-cell type NOS

C91.11 **Chronic lymphocytic leukemia of B-cell type** in remission

C91.12 **Chronic lymphocytic leukemia of B-cell type** in relapse

C91.3 Prolymphocytic **leukemia of** B-cell type

C91.30 **Prolymphocytic leukemia of B-cell type** not having achieved remission
Prolymphocytic leukemia of B-cell type with failed remission
Prolymphocytic leukemia of B-cell type NOS

C91.31 **Prolymphocytic leukemia of B-cell type,** in remission

C91.32 **Prolymphocytic leukemia of B-cell type,** in relapse

C91.4 Hairy cell **leukemia**
Leukemic reticuloendotheliosis

C91.40 **Hairy cell leukemia** not having achieved remission
Hairy cell leukemia with failed remission
Hairy cell leukemia NOS

C91.41 **Hairy cell leukemia,** in remission

C91.42 **Hairy cell leukemia,** in relapse

C91.5 Adult T-cell **lymphoma/leukemia (HTLV-1-associated)**
Acute variant of adult T-cell lymphoma/leukemia (HTLV-1-associated)
Chronic variant of adult T-cell lymphoma/leukemia (HTLV-1-associated)
Lymphomatoid variant of adult T-cell lymphoma/leukemia (HTLV-1-associated)
Smouldering variant of adult T-cell lymphoma/leukemia (HTLV-1-associated)

C91.50 **Adult T-cell lymphoma/leukemia (HTLV-1-associated)** not having achieved remission A
Adult T-cell lymphoma/leukemia (HTLV-1-associated) with failed remission
Adult T-cell lymphoma/leukemia (HTLV-1-associated) NOS

C91.51 **Adult T-cell lymphoma/leukemia (HTLV-1-associated),** in remission A

C91.52 **Adult T-cell lymphoma/leukemia (HTLV-1-associated),** in relapse A

C91.6 Prolymphocytic **leukemia of** T-cell type

C91.60 **Prolymphocytic leukemia of T-cell type** not having achieved remission
Prolymphocytic leukemia of T-cell type with failed remission
Prolymphocytic leukemia of T-cell type NOS

C91.61 **Prolymphocytic leukemia of T-cell type,** in remission

C91.62 **Prolymphocytic leukemia of T-cell type,** in relapse

C91.A Mature B-cell **leukemia** Burkitt-type
EXCLUDES1 *Burkitt lymphoma (C83.7-)*

C91.A0 **Mature B-cell leukemia Burkitt-type** not having achieved remission
Mature B-cell leukemia Burkitt-type with failed remission
Mature B-cell leukemia Burkitt-type NOS

C91.A1 **Mature B-cell leukemia Burkitt-type,** in remission

C91.A2 **Mature B-cell leukemia Burkitt-type,** in relapse

C91.Z Other **lymphoid leukemia**
T-cell large granular lymphocytic leukemia (associated with rheumatoid arthritis)

C91.Z0 **Other lymphoid leukemia** not having achieved remission
Other lymphoid leukemia with failed remission
Other lymphoid leukemia NOS

C91.Z1 **Other lymphoid leukemia,** in remission

C91.Z2 **Other lymphoid leukemia,** in relapse

C91.9 **Lymphoid leukemia,** unspecified

C91.90 **Lymphoid leukemia, unspecified** not having achieved remission
Lymphoid leukemia with failed remission
Lymphoid leukemia NOS

Unspecified Code | Other Specified Code | Manifestation Code | N Newborn | P Pediatric | M Maternity | A Adult | ♂ Male | ♀ Female
● New Code | ▲ Revised Code Title | ►◄ Revised Text | NOTES | INCLUDES | EXCLUDES1 Not coded here | EXCLUDES2 Not included here
4th character required | 5th character required | 6th character required | 7th character required
Extension 'X' Alert | HAC Hospital-acquired condition (HAC) alert | AHA AHA Coding Clinic©

When symbols appear on a code that requires a 7th character extension, refer to Appendix D to identify applicable 7th character codes.

C91.91 **Lymphoid leukemia, unspecified,** in remission CC
C91.92 **Lymphoid leukemia, unspecified,** in relapse CC

C92 Myeloid leukemia

INCLUDES *granulocytic leukemia*
myelogenous leukemia

EXCLUDES1 *personal history of leukemia (Z85.6)*

C92.0 Acute myeloblastic **leukemia**

Acute myeloblastic leukemia, minimal differentiation
Acute myeloblastic leukemia (with maturation)
Acute myeloblastic leukemia 1/ETO
Acute myeloblastic leukemia M0
Acute myeloblastic leukemia M1
Acute myeloblastic leukemia M2
Acute myeloblastic leukemia with t(8;21)
Acute myeloblastic leukemia (without a FAB classification) NOS
Refractory anemia with excess blasts in transformation [RAEB T]

EXCLUDES1 *acute exacerbation of chronic myeloid leukemia (C92.10)*
refractory anemia with excess of blasts not in transformation (D46.2-)

C92.00 **Acute myeloblastic leukemia,** not having achieved remission CC
Acute myeloblastic leukemia with failed remission
Acute myeloblastic leukemia NOS
C92.01 **Acute myeloblastic leukemia,** in remission CC
C92.02 **Acute myeloblastic leukemia,** in relapse CC

C92.1 Chronic myeloid **leukemia,** BCR/ABL-positive

Chronic myelogenous leukemia, Philadelphia chromosome (Ph1) positive
Chronic myelogenous leukemia, t(9;22) (q34;q11)
Chronic myelogenous leukemia with crisis of blast cells

EXCLUDES1 *atypical chronic myeloid leukemia BCR/ABL-negative (C92.2-)*
chronic myelomonocytic leukemia (C93.1-)
chronic myeloproliferative disease (D47.1)

C92.10 **Chronic myeloid leukemia, BCR/ABL-positive,** not having achieved remission CC
Chronic myeloid leukemia, BCR/ABL-positive with failed remission
Chronic myeloid leukemia, BCR/ABL-positive NOS
C92.11 **Chronic myeloid leukemia, BCR/ABL-positive,** in remission CC
C92.12 **Chronic myeloid leukemia, BCR/ABL-positive,** in relapse CC

C92.2 Atypical chronic **myeloid leukemia,** BCR/ABL-negative

C92.20 **Atypical chronic myeloid leukemia, BCR/ABL-negative,** not having achieved remission CC
Atypical chronic myeloid leukemia, BCR/ABL-negative with failed remission
Atypical chronic myeloid leukemia, BCR/ABL-negative NOS
C92.21 **Atypical chronic myeloid leukemia, BCR/ABL-negative,** in remission CC
C92.22 **Atypical chronic myeloid leukemia, BCR/ABL-negative,** in relapse CC

C92.3 Myeloid sarcoma

A malignant tumor of immature myeloid cells
Chloroma
Granulocytic sarcoma

C92.30 **Myeloid sarcoma,** not having achieved remission CC
Myeloid sarcoma with failed remission
Myeloid sarcoma NOS
C92.31 **Myeloid sarcoma,** in remission CC
C92.32 **Myeloid sarcoma,** in relapse CC

C92.4 Acute promyelocytic **leukemia**

AML M3
AML Me with t(15;17) and variants

C92.40 **Acute promyelocytic leukemia,** not having achieved remission CC
Acute promyelocytic leukemia with failed remission
Acute promyelocytic leukemia NOS
C92.41 **Acute promyelocytic leukemia,** in remission CC
C92.42 **Acute promyelocytic leukemia,** in relapse CC

C92.5 Acute myelomonocytic **leukemia**

AML M4
AML M4 Eo with inv(16) or t(16;16)

C92.50 **Acute myelomonocytic leukemia,** not having achieved remission CC
Acute myelomonocytic leukemia with failed remission
Acute myelomonocytic leukemia NOS
C92.51 **Acute myelomonocytic leukemia,** in remission CC
C92.52 **Acute myelomonocytic leukemia,** in relapse CC

C92.6 Acute myeloid **leukemia with** 11q23-abnormality

Acute myeloid leukemia with variation of MLL-gene

C92.60 **Acute myeloid leukemia with 11q23-abnormality** not having achieved remission CC
Acute myeloid leukemia with 11q23-abnormality with failed remission
Acute myeloid leukemia with 11q23-abnormality NOS
C92.61 **Acute myeloid leukemia with 11q23-abnormality** in remission CC
C92.62 **Acute myeloid leukemia with 11q23-abnormality** in relapse CC

C92.A Acute myeloid **leukemia with** multilineage dysplasia

Acute myeloid leukemia with dysplasia of remaining hematopoiesis and/or myelodysplastic disease in its history

C92.A0 **Acute myeloid leukemia with multilineage dysplasia,** not having achieved remission CC
Acute myeloid leukemia with multilineage dysplasia with failed remission
Acute myeloid leukemia with multilineage dysplasia NOS
C92.A1 **Acute myeloid leukemia with multilineage dysplasia,** in remission CC
C92.A2 **Acute myeloid leukemia with multilineage dysplasia,** in relapse CC

C92.Z Other **myeloid leukemia**

C92.Z0 **Other myeloid leukemia** not having achieved remission CC
Myeloid leukemia NEC with failed remission
Myeloid leukemia NEC
C92.Z1 **Other myeloid leukemia,** in remission CC
C92.Z2 **Other myeloid leukemia,** in relapse CC

C92.9 **Myeloid leukemia,** unspecified

C92.90 **Myeloid leukemia, unspecified,** not having achieved remission CC
Myeloid leukemia, unspecified with failed remission
Myeloid leukemia, unspecified NOS
C92.91 **Myeloid leukemia, unspecified** in remission CC
C92.92 **Myeloid leukemia, unspecified** in relapse CC

C93 Monocytic leukemia

INCLUDES *monocytoid leukemia*

EXCLUDES1 *personal history of leukemia (Z85.6)*

C93.0 Acute **monoblastic/monocytic leukemia**

AML M5
AML M5a
AML M5b

C93.00 **Acute monoblastic/monocytic leukemia,** not having achieved remission CC
Acute monoblastic/monocytic leukemia with failed remission
Acute monoblastic/monocytic leukemia NOS
C93.01 **Acute monoblastic/monocytic leukemia,** in remission CC
C93.02 **Acute monoblastic/monocytic leukemia,** in relapse CC

C93.1 Chronic **myelomonocytic leukemia**

Chronic monocytic leukemia
CMML-1
CMML-2
CMML with eosinophilia

C93.10 **Chronic myelomonocytic leukemia** not having achieved remission CC
Chronic myelomonocytic leukemia with failed remission
Chronic myelomonocytic leukemia NOS
C93.11 **Chronic myelomonocytic leukemia,** in remission CC
C93.12 **Chronic myelomonocytic leukemia,** in relapse CC

C93.3 Juvenile **myelomonocytic leukemia**

PDx Unacceptable principal diagnosis symbol per Medicare code edits POA Code exempt from diagnosis present on admission requirement
Q Questionable admission CC Complication or comorbidity CC/MCC Exc CC/MCC exclusion MCC Major complication or comorbidity
PDx CC Principal diagnosis as its own CC PDx MCC Principal diagnosis as its own MCC Z1 Z code as first-listed diagnosis

C93.30 **Juvenile myelomonocytic leukemia,** not having achieved remission
Juvenile myelomonocytic leukemia with failed remission
Juvenile myelomonocytic leukemia NOS
C93.31 **Juvenile myelomonocytic leukemia,** in remission
C93.32 **Juvenile myelomonocytic leukemia,** in relapse
C93.Z Other **monocytic leukemia**
C93.Z0 **Other monocytic leukemia,** not having achieved remission
Other monocytic leukemia NOS
C93.Z1 **Other monocytic leukemia,** in remission
C93.Z2 **Other monocytic leukemia,** in relapse
C93.9 **Monocytic leukemia,** unspecified
C93.90 **Monocytic leukemia, unspecified,** not having achieved remission
Monocytic leukemia, unspecified with failed remission
Monocytic leukemia, unspecified NOS
C93.91 **Monocytic leukemia, unspecified** in remission
C93.92 **Monocytic leukemia, unspecified** in relapse

C94 Other **leukemias of** specified cell type
EXCLUDES1 *leukemic reticuloendotheliosis (C91.4-)*
myelodysplastic syndromes (D46.-)
personal history of leukemia (Z85.6)
plasma cell leukemia (C90.1-)
C94.0 Acute erythroid **leukemia**
Acute myeloid leukemia M6(a)(b)
Erythroleukemia
C94.00 **Acute erythroid leukemia,** not having achieved remission
Acute erythroid leukemia with failed remission
Acute erythroid leukemia NOS
C94.01 **Acute erythroid leukemia,** in remission
C94.02 **Acute erythroid leukemia,** in relapse
C94.2 Acute megakaryoblastic **leukemia**
Acute myeloid leukemia M7
Acute megakaryocytic leukemia
C94.20 **Acute megakaryoblastic leukemia** not having achieved remission
Acute megakaryoblastic leukemia with ▶failed◀ remission
Acute megakaryoblastic leukemia NOS
C94.21 **Acute megakaryoblastic leukemia,** in remission
C94.22 **Acute megakaryoblastic leukemia,** in relapse
C94.3 Mast cell **leukemia**
C94.30 **Mast cell leukemia** not having achieved remission
Mast cell leukemia with failed remission
Mast cell leukemia NOS
C94.31 **Mast cell leukemia,** in remission
C94.32 **Mast cell leukemia,** in relapse
C94.4 Acute panmyelosis **with** myelofibrosis
Acute myelofibrosis
EXCLUDES1 *myelofibrosis NOS (D75.81)*
secondary myelofibrosis NOS (D75.81)
C94.40 **Acute panmyelosis with myelofibrosis** not having achieved remission
Acute myelofibrosis NOS
Acute panmyelosis with myelofibrosis with failed remission
Acute panmyelosis NOS
C94.41 **Acute panmyelosis with myelofibrosis,** in remission
C94.42 **Acute panmyelosis with myelofibrosis,** in relapse
C94.6 **Myelodysplastic disease, not classified**
Myeloproliferative disease, not classified
C94.8 **Other specified leukemias**
Aggressive NK-cell leukemia
Acute basophilic leukemia
C94.80 **Other specified leukemias** not having achieved remission
Other specified leukemia with failed remission
Other specified leukemias NOS
C94.81 **Other specified leukemias,** in remission
C94.82 **Other specified leukemias,** in relapse

C95 **Leukemia of** unspecified cell type
EXCLUDES1 *personal history of leukemia (Z85.6)*
C95.0 Acute leukemia **of unspecified cell type**
Acute bilineal leukemia
Acute mixed lineage leukemia
Biphenotypic acute leukemia
Stem cell leukemia of unclear lineage
EXCLUDES1 *acute exacerbation of unspecified chronic leukemia (C95.10)*
C95.00 **Acute leukemia of unspecified cell type** not having achieved remission
Acute leukemia of unspecified cell type with failed remission
Acute leukemia NOS
C95.01 **Acute leukemia of unspecified cell type,** in remission
C95.02 **Acute leukemia of unspecified cell type,** in relapse
C95.1 Chronic leukemia **of unspecified cell type**
C95.10 **Chronic leukemia of unspecified cell type** not having achieved remission
Chronic leukemia of unspecified cell type with failed remission
Chronic leukemia NOS
C95.11 **Chronic leukemia of unspecified cell type,** in remission
C95.12 **Chronic leukemia of unspecified cell type,** in relapse
C95.9 **Leukemia,** unspecified
C95.90 **Leukemia, unspecified** not having achieved remission
Leukemia, unspecified with failed remission
Leukemia NOS
C95.91 **Leukemia, unspecified,** in remission
C95.92 **Leukemia, unspecified,** in relapse

C96 **Other and unspecified malignant neoplasms of lymphoid, hematopoietic and related tissue**
EXCLUDES1 *personal history of other malignant neoplasms of lymphoid, hematopoietic and related tissues (Z85.79)*
C96.0 **Multifocal and multisystemic (disseminated) Langerhans-cell histiocytosis**
Histiocytosis X, multisystemic
Letterer-Siwe disease
EXCLUDES1 *adult pulmonary Langerhans cell histiocytosis (J84.82)*
multifocal and unisystemic Langerhans-cell histiocytosis (C96.5)
unifocal Langerhans-cell histiocytosis (C96.6)
C96.2 **Malignant mast cell tumor**
Aggressive systemic mastocytosis
Mast cell sarcoma
EXCLUDES1 *indolent mastocytosis (D47.0)*
mast cell leukemia (C94.30)
mastocytosis (congenital) (cutaneous) (Q82.2)
C96.4 **Sarcoma of dendritic cells (accessory cells)**
Follicular dendritic cell sarcoma
Interdigitating dendritic cell sarcoma
Langerhans cell sarcoma
C96.5 **Multifocal and unisystemic Langerhans-cell histiocytosis**
Hand-Schüller-Christian disease
Histiocytosis X, multifocal
EXCLUDES1 *multifocal and multisystemic (disseminated) Langerhans-cell histiocytosis (C96.0)*
unifocal Langerhans-cell histiocytosis (C96.6)
C96.6 **Unifocal Langerhans-cell histiocytosis**
Eosinophilic granuloma
Histiocytosis X, unifocal
Histiocytosis X NOS
Langerhans-cell histiocytosis NOS
EXCLUDES1 *multifocal and multisystemic (disseminated) Langerhans-cell histiocytosis (C96.0)*
multifocal and unisystemic Langerhans-cell histiocytosis (C96.5)
C96.A **Histiocytic sarcoma**
Malignant histiocytosis

Unspecified Code Other Specified Code Manifestation Code N Newborn P Pediatric M Maternity A Adult ♂ Male ♀ Female
● New Code ▲ Revised Code Title ▶◀ Revised Text NOTES INCLUDES EXCLUDES1 Not coded here EXCLUDES2 Not included here
4th character required 5th character required 6th character required 7th character required
Extension 'X' Alert HAC Hospital-acquired condition (HAC) alert AHA AHA Coding Clinic©

C96.Z Other specified malignant neoplasms of lymphoid, hematopoietic and related tissue
C96.9 Malignant neoplasm of lymphoid, hematopoietic and related tissue, unspecified

In situ neoplasms (D00-D09)

INCLUDES *Bowen's disease*
erythroplasia
grade III intraepithelial neoplasia
Queyrat's erythroplasia

D00 Carcinoma in situ of oral cavity, esophagus and stomach
EXCLUDES1 *melanoma in situ (D03.-)*

D00.0 Carcinoma in situ of lip, oral cavity and pharynx
Use additional code to identify:
exposure to environmental tobacco smoke (Z77.22)
exposure to tobacco smoke in the perinatal period (P96.81)
history of tobacco ▶dependence◀ (Z87.891)
occupational exposure to environmental tobacco smoke (Z57.31)
tobacco dependence (F17.-)
tobacco use (Z72.0)
EXCLUDES1 *carcinoma in situ of aryepiglottic fold or interarytenoid fold, laryngeal aspect (D02.0)*
carcinoma in situ of epiglottis NOS (D02.0)
carcinoma in situ of epiglottis suprahyoid portion (D02.0)
carcinoma in situ of skin of lip (D03.0, D04.0)

D00.00 Carcinoma in situ of oral cavity, unspecified site
D00.01 Carcinoma in situ of labial mucosa and vermilion border
D00.02 Carcinoma in situ of buccal mucosa
D00.03 Carcinoma in situ of gingiva and edentulous alveolar ridge
D00.04 Carcinoma in situ of soft palate
D00.05 Carcinoma in situ of hard palate
D00.06 Carcinoma in situ of floor of mouth
D00.07 Carcinoma in situ of tongue
D00.08 Carcinoma in situ of pharynx
Carcinoma in situ of aryepiglottic fold NOS
Carcinoma in situ of hypopharyngeal aspect of aryepiglottic fold
Carcinoma in situ of marginal zone of aryepiglottic fold

D00.1 Carcinoma in situ of esophagus
D00.2 Carcinoma in situ of stomach

D01 Carcinoma in situ of other and unspecified digestive organs
EXCLUDES1 *melanoma in situ (D03.-)*

D01.0 Carcinoma in situ of colon
EXCLUDES1 *carcinoma in situ of rectosigmoid junction (D01.1)*
D01.1 Carcinoma in situ of rectosigmoid junction
D01.2 Carcinoma in situ of rectum
D01.3 Carcinoma in situ of anus and anal canal
Anal intraepithelial neoplasia III [AIN III]
Severe dysplasia of anus
EXCLUDES1 *anal intraepithelial neoplasia I and II [AIN I and AIN II] (K62.82)*
carcinoma in situ of anal margin (D04.5)
carcinoma in situ of anal skin (D04.5)
carcinoma in situ of perianal skin (D04.5)
D01.4 Carcinoma in situ of other and unspecified parts of intestine
EXCLUDES1 *carcinoma in situ of ampulla of Vater (D01.5)*
D01.40 Carcinoma in situ of unspecified part of intestine
D01.49 Carcinoma in situ of other parts of intestine
D01.5 Carcinoma in situ of liver, gallbladder and bile ducts
Carcinoma in situ of ampulla of Vater
D01.7 Carcinoma in situ of other specified digestive organs
Carcinoma in situ of pancreas
D01.9 Carcinoma in situ of digestive organ, unspecified

D02 Carcinoma in situ of middle ear and respiratory system
Use additional code to identify:
exposure to environmental tobacco smoke (Z77.22)
exposure to tobacco smoke in the perinatal period (P96.81)
history of tobacco ▶dependence◀ (Z87.891)
occupational exposure to environmental tobacco smoke (Z57.31)
tobacco dependence (F17.-)
tobacco use (Z72.0)
EXCLUDES1 *melanoma in situ (D03.-)*

D02.0 Carcinoma in situ of larynx
Carcinoma in situ of aryepiglottic fold or interarytenoid fold, laryngeal aspect
Carcinoma in situ of epiglottis (suprahyoid portion)
EXCLUDES1 *carcinoma in situ of aryepiglottic fold or interarytenoid fold NOS (D00.08)*
carcinoma in situ of hypopharyngeal aspect (D00.08)
carcinoma in situ of marginal zone (D00.08)
D02.1 Carcinoma in situ of trachea
D02.2 Carcinoma in situ of bronchus and lung
D02.20 Carcinoma in situ of unspecified bronchus and lung
D02.21 Carcinoma in situ of right bronchus and lung
D02.22 Carcinoma in situ of left bronchus and lung
D02.3 Carcinoma in situ of other parts of respiratory system
Carcinoma in situ of accessory sinuses
Carcinoma in situ of middle ear
Carcinoma in situ of nasal cavities
EXCLUDES1 *carcinoma in situ of ear (external) (skin) (D04.2-)*
carcinoma in situ of nose NOS D09.8
carcinoma in situ of skin of nose (D04.3)
D02.4 Carcinoma in situ of respiratory system, unspecified

D03 Melanoma in situ
D03.0 Melanoma in situ of lip
D03.1 Melanoma in situ of eyelid, including canthus
D03.10 Melanoma in situ of unspecified eyelid, including canthus
D03.11 Melanoma in situ of right eyelid, including canthus
D03.12 Melanoma in situ of left eyelid, including canthus
D03.2 Melanoma in situ of ear and external auricular canal
D03.20 Melanoma in situ of unspecified ear and external auricular canal
D03.21 Melanoma in situ of right ear and external auricular canal
D03.22 Melanoma in situ of left ear and external auricular canal
D03.3 Melanoma in situ of other and unspecified parts of face
D03.30 Melanoma in situ of unspecified part of face
D03.39 Melanoma in situ of other parts of face
D03.4 Melanoma in situ of scalp and neck
D03.5 Melanoma in situ of trunk
D03.51 Melanoma in situ of anal skin
Melanoma in situ of anal margin
Melanoma in situ of perianal skin
D03.52 Melanoma in situ of breast (skin) (soft tissue)
D03.59 Melanoma in situ of other part of trunk
D03.6 Melanoma in situ of upper limb, including shoulder
D03.60 Melanoma in situ of unspecified upper limb, including shoulder
D03.61 Melanoma in situ of right upper limb, including shoulder
D03.62 Melanoma in situ of left upper limb, including shoulder
D03.7 Melanoma in situ of lower limb, including hip
D03.70 Melanoma in situ of unspecified lower limb, including hip
D03.71 Melanoma in situ of right lower limb, including hip
D03.72 Melanoma in situ of left lower limb, including hip
D03.8 Melanoma in situ of other sites
Melanoma in situ of scrotum
EXCLUDES1 *carcinoma in situ of scrotum (D07.61)*
D03.9 Melanoma in situ, unspecified

D04 Carcinoma in situ of skin
EXCLUDES1 *erythroplasia of Queyrat (penis) NOS (D07.4)*
melanoma in situ (D03.-)
D04.0 Carcinoma in situ of skin of lip
EXCLUDES1 *carcinoma in situ of vermilion border of lip (D00.01)*
D04.1 Carcinoma in situ of skin of eyelid, including canthus

Unacceptable principal diagnosis symbol per Medicare code edits | Code exempt from diagnosis present on admission requirement | Questionable admission | Complication or comorbidity | CC/MCC exclusion | Major complication or comorbidity | Principal diagnosis as its own CC | Principal diagnosis as its own MCC | Z code as first-listed diagnosis

D04.10 Carcinoma in situ of skin of unspecified eyelid, including canthus
D04.11 Carcinoma in situ of skin of right eyelid, including canthus
D04.12 Carcinoma in situ of skin of left eyelid, including canthus
D04.2 Carcinoma in situ of skin of ear and external auricular canal
D04.20 Carcinoma in situ of skin of unspecified ear and external auricular canal
D04.21 Carcinoma in situ of skin of right ear and external auricular canal
D04.22 Carcinoma in situ of skin of left ear and external auricular canal
D04.3 Carcinoma in situ of skin of other and unspecified parts of face
D04.30 Carcinoma in situ of skin of unspecified part of face
D04.39 Carcinoma in situ of skin of other parts of face
D04.4 Carcinoma in situ of skin of scalp and neck
D04.5 Carcinoma in situ of skin of trunk
Carcinoma in situ of anal margin
Carcinoma in situ of anal skin
Carcinoma in situ of perianal skin
Carcinoma in situ of skin of breast
EXCLUDES1 *carcinoma in situ of anus NOS (D01.3)*
carcinoma in situ of scrotum (D07.61)
carcinoma in situ of skin of genital organs (D07.-)
D04.6 Carcinoma in situ of skin of upper limb, including shoulder
D04.60 Carcinoma in situ of skin of unspecified upper limb, including shoulder
D04.61 Carcinoma in situ of skin of right upper limb, including shoulder
D04.62 Carcinoma in situ of skin of left upper limb, including shoulder
D04.7 Carcinoma in situ of skin of lower limb, including hip
D04.70 Carcinoma in situ of skin of unspecified lower limb, including hip
D04.71 Carcinoma in situ of skin of right lower limb, including hip
D04.72 Carcinoma in situ of skin of left lower limb, including hip
D04.8 Carcinoma in situ of skin of other sites
D04.9 Carcinoma in situ of skin, unspecified
D05 Carcinoma in situ of breast
EXCLUDES1 *carcinoma in situ of skin of breast (D04.5)*
melanoma in situ of breast (skin) (D03.5)
Paget's disease of breast or nipple (C50.-)
D05.0 Lobular carcinoma in situ of breast
D05.00 Lobular carcinoma in situ of unspecified breast
D05.01 Lobular carcinoma in situ of right breast
D05.02 Lobular carcinoma in situ of left breast
D05.1 Intraductal carcinoma in situ of breast
D05.10 Intraductal carcinoma in situ of unspecified breast
D05.11 Intraductal carcinoma in situ of right breast
D05.12 Intraductal carcinoma in situ of left breast
D05.8 Other specified type of carcinoma in situ of breast
D05.80 Other specified type of carcinoma in situ of unspecified breast
D05.81 Other specified type of carcinoma in situ of right breast
D05.82 Other specified type of carcinoma in situ of left breast
D05.9 Unspecified type of carcinoma in situ of breast
D05.90 Unspecified type of carcinoma in situ of unspecified breast
D05.91 Unspecified type of carcinoma in situ of right breast
D05.92 Unspecified type of carcinoma in situ of left breast
D06 Carcinoma in situ of cervix uteri
INCLUDES *cervical adenocarcinoma in situ*
cervical intraepithelial glandular neoplasia
cervical intraepithelial neoplasia III [CIN III]
severe dysplasia of cervix uteri
EXCLUDES1 *cervical intraepithelial neoplasia II [CIN II] (N87.1)*
cytologic evidence of malignancy of cervix without histologic confirmation (R87.614)
high grade squamous intraepithelial lesion (HGSIL) of cervix (R87.613)
melanoma in situ of cervix (D03.5)
moderate cervical dysplasia (N87.1)
D06.0 Carcinoma in situ of endocervix ♀
D06.1 Carcinoma in situ of exocervix ♀
D06.7 Carcinoma in situ of other parts of cervix ♀
D06.9 Carcinoma in situ of cervix, unspecified ♀
D07 Carcinoma in situ of other and unspecified genital organs
EXCLUDES1 *melanoma in situ of trunk (D03.5)*
D07.0 Carcinoma in situ of endometrium ♀
D07.1 Carcinoma in situ of vulva ♀
Severe dysplasia of vulva
Vulvar intraepithelial neoplasia III [VIN III]
EXCLUDES1 *moderate dysplasia of vulva (N90.1)*
vulvar intraepithelial neoplasia II [VIN II] (N90.1)
D07.2 Carcinoma in situ of vagina ♀
Severe dysplasia of vagina
Vaginal intraepithelial neoplasia III [VAIN III]
EXCLUDES1 *moderate dysplasia of vagina (N89.1)*
vaginal intraepithelial neoplasia II [VIN II] (N89.1)
D07.3 Carcinoma in situ of other and unspecified female genital organs
D07.30 Carcinoma in situ of unspecified female genital organs ♀
D07.39 Carcinoma in situ of other female genital organs ♀
D07.4 Carcinoma in situ of penis ♂
Erythroplasia of Queyrat NOS
D07.5 Carcinoma in situ of prostate ♂
Prostatic intraepithelial neoplasia III (PIN III)
Severe dysplasia of prostate
EXCLUDES1 *dysplasia (mild) (moderate) of prostate ▶(N42.3-)◀*
prostatic intraepithelial neoplasia II [PIN II] (N42.3-)
D07.6 Carcinoma in situ of other and unspecified male genital organs
D07.60 Carcinoma in situ of unspecified male genital organs ♂
D07.61 Carcinoma in situ of scrotum ♂
D07.69 Carcinoma in situ of other male genital organs ♂
D09 Carcinoma in situ of other and unspecified sites
EXCLUDES1 *melanoma in situ (D03.-)*
D09.0 Carcinoma in situ of bladder
D09.1 Carcinoma in situ of other and unspecified urinary organs
D09.10 Carcinoma in situ of unspecified urinary organ
D09.19 Carcinoma in situ of other urinary organs
D09.2 Carcinoma in situ of eye
EXCLUDES1 *carcinoma in situ of skin of eyelid (D04.1-)*
D09.20 Carcinoma in situ of unspecified eye
D09.21 Carcinoma in situ of right eye
D09.22 Carcinoma in situ of left eye
D09.3 Carcinoma in situ of thyroid and other endocrine glands
EXCLUDES1 *carcinoma in situ of endocrine pancreas (D01.7)*
carcinoma in situ of ovary (D07.39)
carcinoma in situ of testis (D07.69)
D09.8 Carcinoma in situ of other specified sites
D09.9 Carcinoma in situ, unspecified

Benign neoplasms, except benign neuroendocrine tumors (D10-D36)

D10 Benign neoplasm of mouth and pharynx
D10.0 Benign neoplasm of lip
Benign neoplasm of lip (frenulum) (inner aspect) (mucosa) (vermilion border)
EXCLUDES1 *benign neoplasm of skin of lip (D22.0, D23.0)*
D10.1 Benign neoplasm of tongue
Benign neoplasm of lingual tonsil
D10.2 Benign neoplasm of floor of mouth
▲ D10.3 ▶Benign neoplasm of◀ other and unspecified parts of mouth

Unspecified Code | Other Specified Code | Manifestation Code | N Newborn | P Pediatric | M Maternity | A Adult | ♂ Male | ♀ Female
● New Code | ▲ Revised Code Title | ▶◀ Revised Text | NOTES | INCLUDES | EXCLUDES1 Not coded here | EXCLUDES2 Not included here
4th character required | 5th character required | 6th character required | 7th character required
Extension 'X' Alert | HAC Hospital-acquired condition (HAC) alert | AHA AHA Coding Clinic©

D10.30 **Benign neoplasm of unspecified part of mouth**
D10.39 **Benign neoplasm of other parts of mouth**
Benign neoplasm of minor salivary gland NOS
EXCLUDES1 *benign odontogenic neoplasms (D16.4-D16.5)*
benign neoplasm of mucosa of lip (D10.0)
benign neoplasm of nasopharyngeal surface of soft palate (D10.6)

D10.4 **Benign neoplasm of tonsil**
Benign neoplasm of tonsil (faucial) (palatine)
EXCLUDES1 *benign neoplasm of lingual tonsil (D10.1)*
benign neoplasm of pharyngeal tonsil (D10.6)
benign neoplasm of tonsillar fossa (D10.5)
benign neoplasm of tonsillar pillars (D10.5)

D10.5 **Benign neoplasm of other parts of oropharynx**
Benign neoplasm of epiglottis, anterior aspect
Benign neoplasm of tonsillar fossa
Benign neoplasm of tonsillar pillars
Benign neoplasm of vallecula
EXCLUDES1 *benign neoplasm of epiglottis NOS (D14.1)*
benign neoplasm of epiglottis, suprahyoid portion (D14.1)

D10.6 **Benign neoplasm of nasopharynx**
Benign neoplasm of pharyngeal tonsil
Benign neoplasm of posterior margin of septum and choanae

D10.7 **Benign neoplasm of hypopharynx**
D10.9 **Benign neoplasm of pharynx, unspecified**

4th D11 **Benign neoplasm of major salivary glands**
EXCLUDES1 *benign neoplasms of specified minor salivary glands which are classified according to their anatomical location*
benign neoplasms of minor salivary glands NOS (D10.39)

D11.0 **Benign neoplasm of parotid gland**
D11.7 **Benign neoplasm of other major salivary glands**
Benign neoplasm of sublingual salivary gland
Benign neoplasm of submandibular salivary gland
D11.9 **Benign neoplasm of major salivary gland, unspecified**

4th D12 **Benign neoplasm of colon, rectum, anus and anal canal**
EXCLUDES1 *benign carcinoid tumors of the large intestine, and rectum (D3A.02-)*

D12.0 **Benign neoplasm of cecum**
Benign neoplasm of ileocecal valve
D12.1 **Benign neoplasm of appendix**
EXCLUDES1 *benign carcinoid tumor of the appendix (D3A.020)*
D12.2 **Benign neoplasm of ascending colon**
D12.3 **Benign neoplasm of transverse colon**
Benign neoplasm of hepatic flexure
Benign neoplasm of splenic flexure
D12.4 **Benign neoplasm of descending colon**
D12.5 **Benign neoplasm of sigmoid colon**
D12.6 **Benign neoplasm of colon, unspecified**
Adenomatosis of colon
Benign neoplasm of large intestine NOS
Polyposis (hereditary) of colon
EXCLUDES1 *inflammatory polyp of colon (K51.4-)*
polyp of colon NOS (K63.5)
D12.7 **Benign neoplasm of rectosigmoid junction**
D12.8 **Benign neoplasm of rectum**
EXCLUDES1 *benign carcinoid tumor of the rectum (D3A.026)*
D12.9 **Benign neoplasm of anus and anal canal**
Benign neoplasm of anus NOS
EXCLUDES1 *benign neoplasm of anal margin (D22.5, D23.5)*
benign neoplasm of anal skin (D22.5, D23.5)
benign neoplasm of perianal skin (D22.5, D23.5)

4th D13 **Benign neoplasm of other and ill-defined parts of digestive system**
EXCLUDES1 *benign stromal tumors of digestive system (D21.4)*

D13.0 **Benign neoplasm of esophagus**
D13.1 **Benign neoplasm of stomach**
EXCLUDES1 *benign carcinoid tumor of the stomach (D3A.092)*
D13.2 **Benign neoplasm of duodenum**
EXCLUDES1 *benign carcinoid tumor of the duodenum (D3A.010)*
5th D13.3 **Benign neoplasm of other and unspecified parts of small intestine**
EXCLUDES1 *benign carcinoid tumors of the small intestine(D3A.01-)*
benign neoplasm of ileocecal valve (D12.0)
D13.30 **Benign neoplasm of unspecified part of small intestine**
D13.39 **Benign neoplasm of other parts of small intestine**
D13.4 **Benign neoplasm of liver**
Benign neoplasm of intrahepatic bile ducts
D13.5 **Benign neoplasm of extrahepatic bile ducts**
D13.6 **Benign neoplasm of pancreas**
EXCLUDES1 *benign neoplasm of endocrine pancreas (D13.7)*
D13.7 **Benign neoplasm of endocrine pancreas**
Islet cell tumor
Benign neoplasm of islets of Langerhans
Use additional code to identify any functional activity.
D13.9 **Benign neoplasm of ill-defined sites within the digestive system**
Benign neoplasm of digestive system NOS
Benign neoplasm of intestine NOS
Benign neoplasm of spleen

4th D14 **Benign neoplasm of middle ear and respiratory system**
D14.0 **Benign neoplasm of middle ear, nasal cavity and accessory sinuses**
Benign neoplasm of cartilage of nose
EXCLUDES1 *benign neoplasm of auricular canal (external) (D22.2-, D23.2-)*
benign neoplasm of bone of ear (D16.4)
benign neoplasm of bone of nose (D16.4)
benign neoplasm of cartilage of ear (D21.0)
benign neoplasm of ear (external)(skin) (D22.2-, D23.2-)
benign neoplasm of nose NOS (D36.7)
benign neoplasm of skin of nose (D22.39, D23.39)
benign neoplasm of olfactory bulb (D33.3)
benign neoplasm of posterior margin of septum and choanae (D10.6)
polyp of accessory sinus (J33.8)
polyp of ear (middle) (H74.4)
polyp of nasal (cavity) (J33.-)
D14.1 **Benign neoplasm of larynx**
Adenomatous polyp of larynx
Benign neoplasm of epiglottis (suprahyoid portion)
EXCLUDES1 *benign neoplasm of epiglottis, anterior aspect (D10.5)*
polyp (nonadenomatous) of vocal cord or larynx (J38.1)
D14.2 **Benign neoplasm of trachea**
5th D14.3 **Benign neoplasm of bronchus and lung**
EXCLUDES1 *benign carcinoid tumor of the bronchus and lung (D3A.090)*
D14.30 **Benign neoplasm of unspecified bronchus and lung**
D14.31 **Benign neoplasm of right bronchus and lung**
D14.32 **Benign neoplasm of left bronchus and lung**
D14.4 **Benign neoplasm of respiratory system, unspecified**

4th D15 **Benign neoplasm of other and unspecified intrathoracic organs**
EXCLUDES1 *benign neoplasm of mesothelial tissue (D19.-)*
D15.0 **Benign neoplasm of thymus**
EXCLUDES1 *benign carcinoid tumor of the thymus (D3A.091)*
D15.1 **Benign neoplasm of heart**
EXCLUDES1 *benign neoplasm of great vessels (D21.3)*
D15.2 **Benign neoplasm of mediastinum**
D15.7 **Benign neoplasm of other specified intrathoracic organs**
D15.9 **Benign neoplasm of intrathoracic organ, unspecified**

4th D16 **Benign neoplasm of bone and articular cartilage**
EXCLUDES1 *benign neoplasm of connective tissue of ear (D21.0)*
benign neoplasm of connective tissue of eyelid (D21.0)
benign neoplasm of connective tissue of larynx (D14.1)
benign neoplasm of connective tissue of nose (D14.0)
benign neoplasm of synovia (D21.-)
5th D16.0 **Benign neoplasm of scapula and long bones of upper limb**
D16.00 **Benign neoplasm of scapula and long bones of unspecified upper limb**
D16.01 **Benign neoplasm of scapula and long bones of right upper limb**

Unacceptable principal diagnosis symbol per Medicare code edits · Code exempt from diagnosis present on admission requirement
Questionable admission · Complication or comorbidity · CC/MCC exclusion · Major complication or comorbidity
Principal diagnosis as its own CC · Principal diagnosis as its own MCC · Z code as first-listed diagnosis

D16.02 Benign neoplasm of scapula and long bones of left upper limb
D16.1 Benign neoplasm of short bones of upper limb
D16.10 Benign neoplasm of short bones of unspecified upper limb
D16.11 Benign neoplasm of short bones of right upper limb
D16.12 Benign neoplasm of short bones of left upper limb
D16.2 Benign neoplasm of long bones of lower limb
D16.20 Benign neoplasm of long bones of unspecified lower limb
D16.21 Benign neoplasm of long bones of right lower limb
D16.22 Benign neoplasm of long bones of left lower limb
D16.3 Benign neoplasm of short bones of lower limb
D16.30 Benign neoplasm of short bones of unspecified lower limb
D16.31 Benign neoplasm of short bones of right lower limb
D16.32 Benign neoplasm of short bones of left lower limb
D16.4 Benign neoplasm of bones of skull and face
Benign neoplasm of maxilla (superior)
Benign neoplasm of orbital bone
Keratocyst of maxilla
Keratocystic odontogenic tumor of maxilla
EXCLUDES2 *benign neoplasm of lower jaw bone (D16.5)*
D16.5 Benign neoplasm of lower jaw bone
Keratocyst of mandible
Keratocystic odontogenic tumor of mandible
D16.6 Benign neoplasm of vertebral column
EXCLUDES1 *benign neoplasm of sacrum and coccyx (D16.8)*
D16.7 Benign neoplasm of ribs, sternum and clavicle
D16.8 Benign neoplasm of pelvic bones, sacrum and coccyx
D16.9 Benign neoplasm of bone and articular cartilage, unspecified
D17 Benign lipomatous neoplasm
D17.0 Benign lipomatous neoplasm of skin and subcutaneous tissue of head, face and neck
D17.1 Benign lipomatous neoplasm of skin and subcutaneous tissue of trunk
D17.2 Benign lipomatous neoplasm of skin and subcutaneous tissue of limb
D17.20 Benign lipomatous neoplasm of skin and subcutaneous tissue of unspecified limb
D17.21 Benign lipomatous neoplasm of skin and subcutaneous tissue of right arm
D17.22 Benign lipomatous neoplasm of skin and subcutaneous tissue of left arm
D17.23 Benign lipomatous neoplasm of skin and subcutaneous tissue of right leg
D17.24 Benign lipomatous neoplasm of skin and subcutaneous tissue of left leg
D17.3 Benign lipomatous neoplasm of skin and subcutaneous tissue of other and unspecified sites
D17.30 Benign lipomatous neoplasm of skin and subcutaneous tissue of unspecified sites
D17.39 Benign lipomatous neoplasm of skin and subcutaneous tissue of other sites
D17.4 Benign lipomatous neoplasm of intrathoracic organs
D17.5 Benign lipomatous neoplasm of intra-abdominal organs
EXCLUDES1 *benign lipomatous neoplasm of peritoneum and retroperitoneum (D17.79)*
D17.6 Benign lipomatous neoplasm of spermatic cord ♂
D17.7 Benign lipomatous neoplasm of other sites
D17.71 Benign lipomatous neoplasm of kidney
D17.72 Benign lipomatous neoplasm of other genitourinary organ
D17.79 Benign lipomatous neoplasm of other sites
Benign lipomatous neoplasm of peritoneum
Benign lipomatous neoplasm of retroperitoneum
D17.9 Benign lipomatous neoplasm, unspecified
Lipoma NOS
D18 Hemangioma and lymphangioma, any site
EXCLUDES1 *benign neoplasm of glomus jugulare (D35.6)*
blue or pigmented nevus (D22.-)
nevus NOS (D22.-)
vascular nevus (Q82.5)
D18.0 Hemangioma
Angioma NOS
Cavernous nevus
D18.00 Hemangioma unspecified site
D18.01 Hemangioma of skin and subcutaneous tissue
D18.02 Hemangioma of intracranial structures
D18.03 Hemangioma of intra-abdominal structures
D18.09 Hemangioma of other sites
D18.1 Lymphangioma, any site
D19 Benign neoplasm of mesothelial tissue
D19.0 Benign neoplasm of mesothelial tissue of pleura
D19.1 Benign neoplasm of mesothelial tissue of peritoneum
D19.7 Benign neoplasm of mesothelial tissue of other sites
D19.9 Benign neoplasm of mesothelial tissue, unspecified
Benign mesothelioma NOS
D20 Benign neoplasm of soft tissue of retroperitoneum and peritoneum
EXCLUDES1 *benign lipomatous neoplasm of peritoneum and retroperitoneum (D17.79)*
benign neoplasm of mesothelial tissue (D19.-)
D20.0 Benign neoplasm of soft tissue of retroperitoneum
D20.1 Benign neoplasm of soft tissue of peritoneum
D21 Other benign neoplasms of connective and other soft tissue
INCLUDES *benign neoplasm of blood vessel*
benign neoplasm of bursa
benign neoplasm of cartilage
benign neoplasm of fascia
benign neoplasm of fat
benign neoplasm of ligament, except uterine
benign neoplasm of lymphatic channel
benign neoplasm of muscle
benign neoplasm of synovia
benign neoplasm of tendon (sheath)
benign stromal tumors
EXCLUDES1 *benign neoplasm of articular cartilage (D16.-)*
benign neoplasm of cartilage of larynx (D14.1)
benign neoplasm of cartilage of nose (D14.0)
benign neoplasm of connective tissue of breast (D24.-)
benign neoplasm of peripheral nerves and autonomic nervous system (D36.1-)
benign neoplasm of peritoneum (D20.1)
benign neoplasm of retroperitoneum (D20.0)
benign neoplasm of uterine ligament, any (D28.2)
benign neoplasm of vascular tissue (D18.-)
hemangioma (D18.0-)
lipomatous neoplasm (D17.-)
lymphangioma (D18.1)
uterine leiomyoma (D25.-)
D21.0 Benign neoplasm of connective and other soft tissue of head, face and neck
Benign neoplasm of connective tissue of ear
Benign neoplasm of connective tissue of eyelid
EXCLUDES1 *benign neoplasm of connective tissue of orbit (D31.6-)*
D21.1 Benign neoplasm of connective and other soft tissue of upper limb, including shoulder
D21.10 Benign neoplasm of connective and other soft tissue of unspecified upper limb, including shoulder
D21.11 Benign neoplasm of connective and other soft tissue of right upper limb, including shoulder
D21.12 Benign neoplasm of connective and other soft tissue of left upper limb, including shoulder
D21.2 Benign neoplasm of connective and other soft tissue of lower limb, including hip
D21.20 Benign neoplasm of connective and other soft tissue of unspecified lower limb, including hip
D21.21 Benign neoplasm of connective and other soft tissue of right lower limb, including hip
D21.22 Benign neoplasm of connective and other soft tissue of left lower limb, including hip

Unspecified Code Other Specified Code Manifestation Code N Newborn P Pediatric M Maternity A Adult ♂ Male ♀ Female
● New Code ▲ Revised Code Title ►◄ Revised Text NOTES INCLUDES EXCLUDES1 Not coded here EXCLUDES2 Not included here
4th character required 5th character required 6th character required 7th character required
Extension 'X' Alert HAC Hospital-acquired condition (HAC) alert AHA AHA Coding Clinic©

D21.3 Benign neoplasm of connective and other soft tissue of thorax
Benign neoplasm of axilla
Benign neoplasm of diaphragm
Benign neoplasm of great vessels
EXCLUDES1 *benign neoplasm of heart (D15.1)*
benign neoplasm of mediastinum (D15.2)
benign neoplasm of thymus (D15.0)

D21.4 Benign neoplasm of connective and other soft tissue of abdomen
Benign stromal tumors of abdomen

D21.5 Benign neoplasm of connective and other soft tissue of pelvis
EXCLUDES1 *benign neoplasm of any uterine ligament (D28.2)*
uterine leiomyoma (D25.-)

D21.6 Benign neoplasm of connective and other soft tissue of trunk, unspecified
Benign neoplasm of back NOS

D21.9 Benign neoplasm of connective and other soft tissue, unspecified

4th D22 Melanocytic nevi
INCLUDES *atypical nevus*
blue hairy pigmented nevus
nevus NOS

D22.0 Melanocytic nevi of lip
5th D22.1 Melanocytic nevi of eyelid, including canthus
D22.10 Melanocytic nevi of unspecified eyelid, including canthus
D22.11 Melanocytic nevi of right eyelid, including canthus
D22.12 Melanocytic nevi of left eyelid, including canthus
5th D22.2 Melanocytic nevi of ear and external auricular canal
D22.20 Melanocytic nevi of unspecified ear and external auricular canal
D22.21 Melanocytic nevi of right ear and external auricular canal
D22.22 Melanocytic nevi of left ear and external auricular canal
5th D22.3 Melanocytic nevi of other and unspecified parts of face
D22.30 Melanocytic nevi of unspecified part of face
D22.39 Melanocytic nevi of other parts of face
D22.4 Melanocytic nevi of scalp and neck
D22.5 Melanocytic nevi of trunk
Melanocytic nevi of anal margin
Melanocytic nevi of anal skin
Melanocytic nevi of perianal skin
Melanocytic nevi of skin of breast
5th D22.6 Melanocytic nevi of upper limb, including shoulder
D22.60 Melanocytic nevi of unspecified upper limb, including shoulder
D22.61 Melanocytic nevi of right upper limb, including shoulder
D22.62 Melanocytic nevi of left upper limb, including shoulder
5th D22.7 Melanocytic nevi of lower limb, including hip
D22.70 Melanocytic nevi of unspecified lower limb, including hip
D22.71 Melanocytic nevi of right lower limb, including hip
D22.72 Melanocytic nevi of left lower limb, including hip
D22.9 Melanocytic nevi, unspecified

4th D23 Other benign neoplasms of skin
INCLUDES *benign neoplasm of hair follicles*
benign neoplasm of sebaceous glands
benign neoplasm of sweat glands
EXCLUDES1 *benign lipomatous neoplasms of skin (D17.0-D17.3)*
melanocytic nevi (D22.-)

D23.0 Other benign neoplasm of skin of lip
EXCLUDES1 *benign neoplasm of vermilion border of lip (D10.0)*
5th D23.1 Other benign neoplasm of skin of eyelid, including canthus
D23.10 Other benign neoplasm of skin of unspecified eyelid, including canthus
D23.11 Other benign neoplasm of skin of right eyelid, including canthus
D23.12 Other benign neoplasm of skin of left eyelid, including canthus
5th D23.2 Other benign neoplasm of skin of ear and external auricular canal
D23.20 Other benign neoplasm of skin of unspecified ear and external auricular canal
D23.21 Other benign neoplasm of skin of right ear and external auricular canal
D23.22 Other benign neoplasm of skin of left ear and external auricular canal
5th D23.3 Other benign neoplasm of skin of other and unspecified parts of face
D23.30 Other benign neoplasm of skin of unspecified part of face
D23.39 Other benign neoplasm of skin of other parts of face
D23.4 Other benign neoplasm of skin of scalp and neck
D23.5 Other benign neoplasm of skin of trunk
Other benign neoplasm of anal margin
Other benign neoplasm of anal skin
Other benign neoplasm of perianal skin
Other benign neoplasm of skin of breast
EXCLUDES1 *benign neoplasm of anus NOS (D12.9)*
5th D23.6 Other benign neoplasm of skin of upper limb, including shoulder
D23.60 Other benign neoplasm of skin of unspecified upper limb, including shoulder
D23.61 Other benign neoplasm of skin of right upper limb, including shoulder
D23.62 Other benign neoplasm of skin of left upper limb, including shoulder
5th D23.7 Other benign neoplasm of skin of lower limb, including hip
D23.70 Other benign neoplasm of skin of unspecified lower limb, including hip
D23.71 Other benign neoplasm of skin of right lower limb, including hip
D23.72 Other benign neoplasm of skin of left lower limb, including hip
D23.9 Other benign neoplasm of skin, unspecified

4th D24 Benign neoplasm of breast
INCLUDES *benign neoplasm of connective tissue of breast*
benign neoplasm of soft parts of breast
fibroadenoma of breast
EXCLUDES2 *adenofibrosis of breast (N60.2)*
benign cyst of breast (N60.-)
benign mammary dysplasia (N60.-)
benign neoplasm of skin of breast (D22.5, D23.5)
fibrocystic disease of breast (N60.-)

D24.1 Benign neoplasm of right breast
D24.2 Benign neoplasm of left breast
D24.9 Benign neoplasm of unspecified breast

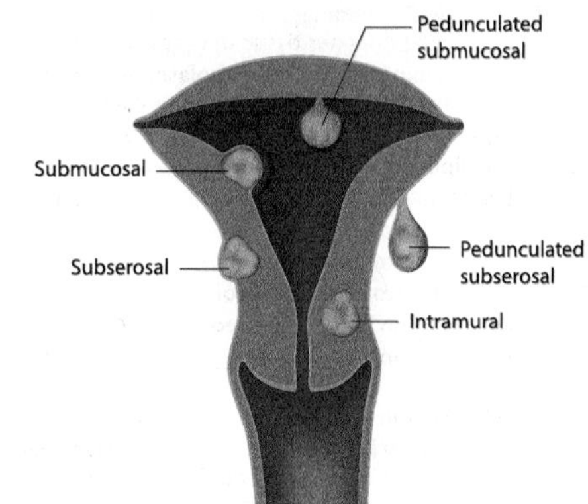

Figure 2.5 Uterine fibroids

4th D25 Leiomyoma of uterus
INCLUDES *uterine fibroid*
uterine fibromyoma
uterine myoma

D25.0 Submucous leiomyoma of uterus ♀

Unacceptable principal diagnosis symbol per Medicare code edits · Code exempt from diagnosis present on admission requirement · Questionable admission · Complication or comorbidity · CC/MCC exclusion · Major complication or comorbidity · Principal diagnosis as its own CC · Principal diagnosis as its own MCC · Z code as first-listed diagnosis

D25.1 Intramural leiomyoma of uterus ♀
Interstitial leiomyoma of uterus
D25.2 Subserosal leiomyoma of uterus ♀
Subperitoneal leiomyoma of uterus
D25.9 **Leiomyoma of uterus, unspecified** ♀

D26 Other benign neoplasms of uterus
D26.0 Other benign neoplasm of cervix uteri ♀
D26.1 Other benign neoplasm of corpus uteri ♀
D26.7 Other benign neoplasm of other parts of uterus ♀
D26.9 **Other benign neoplasm of uterus, unspecified** ♀

D27 Benign neoplasm of ovary
Use additional code to identify any functional activity.
EXCLUDES2 *corpus albicans cyst ▶(N83.2-)◀*
corpus luteum cyst ▶(N83.1-)◀
endometrial cyst ▶(N80.1)◀
follicular (atretic) cyst ▶(N83.0-)◀
graafian follicle cyst ▶(N83.0-)◀
ovarian cyst NEC ▶(N83.2-)◀
ovarian retention cyst ▶(N83.2-)◀
D27.0 Benign neoplasm of right ovary ♀
D27.1 Benign neoplasm of left ovary ♀
D27.9 **Benign neoplasm of unspecified ovary** ♀

D28 Benign neoplasm of other and unspecified female genital organs
INCLUDES *adenomatous polyp*
benign neoplasm of skin of female genital organs
benign teratoma
EXCLUDES1 *epoophoron cyst (Q50.5)*
fimbrial cyst (Q50.4)
Gartner's duct cyst (Q52.4)
parovarian cyst (Q50.5)
D28.0 Benign neoplasm of vulva ♀
D28.1 Benign neoplasm of vagina ♀
D28.2 Benign neoplasm of uterine tubes and ligaments ♀
Benign neoplasm of fallopian tube
Benign neoplasm of uterine ligament (broad) (round)
D28.7 Benign neoplasm of other specified female genital organs ♀
D28.9 **Benign neoplasm of female genital organ, unspecified** ♀

D29 Benign neoplasm of male genital organs
INCLUDES *benign neoplasm of skin of male genital organs*
D29.0 Benign neoplasm of penis ♂
D29.1 Benign neoplasm of prostate ♂
EXCLUDES1 *enlarged prostate (N40.-)*
D29.2 Benign neoplasm of testis
Use additional code to identify any functional activity.
D29.20 **Benign neoplasm of unspecified testis** ♂
D29.21 Benign neoplasm of right testis ♂
D29.22 Benign neoplasm of left testis ♂
D29.3 Benign neoplasm of epididymis
D29.30 **Benign neoplasm of unspecified epididymis** ♂
D29.31 Benign neoplasm of right epididymis ♂
D29.32 Benign neoplasm of left epididymis ♂
D29.4 Benign neoplasm of scrotum ♂
Benign neoplasm of skin of scrotum
D29.8 Benign neoplasm of other specified male genital organs ♂
Benign neoplasm of seminal vesicle
Benign neoplasm of spermatic cord
Benign neoplasm of tunica vaginalis
D29.9 **Benign neoplasm of male genital organ, unspecified** ♂

D30 Benign neoplasm of urinary organs
D30.0 Benign neoplasm of kidney
EXCLUDES1 *benign carcinoid tumor of the kidney (D3A.093)*
benign neoplasm of renal calyces (D30.1-)
benign neoplasm of renal pelvis (D30.1-)
D30.00 **Benign neoplasm of unspecified kidney**
D30.01 Benign neoplasm of right kidney
D30.02 Benign neoplasm of left kidney
D30.1 Benign neoplasm of renal pelvis
D30.10 **Benign neoplasm of unspecified renal pelvis**
D30.11 Benign neoplasm of right renal pelvis
D30.12 Benign neoplasm of left renal pelvis
D30.2 Benign neoplasm of ureter
EXCLUDES1 *benign neoplasm of ureteric orifice of bladder (D30.3)*
D30.20 **Benign neoplasm of unspecified ureter**
D30.21 Benign neoplasm of right ureter
D30.22 Benign neoplasm of left ureter
D30.3 Benign neoplasm of bladder
Benign neoplasm of ureteric orifice of bladder
Benign neoplasm of urethral orifice of bladder
D30.4 Benign neoplasm of urethra
EXCLUDES1 *benign neoplasm of urethral orifice of bladder (D30.3)*
D30.8 Benign neoplasm of other specified urinary organs
Benign neoplasm of paraurethral glands
D30.9 **Benign neoplasm of urinary organ, unspecified**
Benign neoplasm of urinary system NOS

D31 Benign neoplasm of eye and adnexa
EXCLUDES1 *benign neoplasm of connective tissue of eyelid (D21.0)*
benign neoplasm of optic nerve (D33.3)
benign neoplasm of skin of eyelid (D22.1-, D23.1-)
D31.0 Benign neoplasm of conjunctiva
D31.00 **Benign neoplasm of unspecified conjunctiva**
D31.01 Benign neoplasm of right conjunctiva
D31.02 Benign neoplasm of left conjunctiva
D31.1 Benign neoplasm of cornea
D31.10 **Benign neoplasm of unspecified cornea**
D31.11 Benign neoplasm of right cornea
D31.12 Benign neoplasm of left cornea
D31.2 Benign neoplasm of retina
EXCLUDES1 *dark area on retina (D49.81)*
hemangioma of retina (D49.81)
neoplasm of unspecified behavior of retina and choroid (D49.81)
retinal freckle (D49.81)
D31.20 **Benign neoplasm of unspecified retina**
D31.21 Benign neoplasm of right retina
D31.22 Benign neoplasm of left retina
D31.3 Benign neoplasm of choroid
D31.30 **Benign neoplasm of unspecified choroid**
D31.31 Benign neoplasm of right choroid
D31.32 Benign neoplasm of left choroid
D31.4 Benign neoplasm of ciliary body
D31.40 **Benign neoplasm of unspecified ciliary body**
D31.41 Benign neoplasm of right ciliary body
D31.42 Benign neoplasm of left ciliary body
D31.5 Benign neoplasm of lacrimal gland and duct
Benign neoplasm of lacrimal sac
Benign neoplasm of nasolacrimal duct
D31.50 **Benign neoplasm of unspecified lacrimal gland and duct**
D31.51 Benign neoplasm of right lacrimal gland and duct
D31.52 Benign neoplasm of left lacrimal gland and duct
D31.6 Benign neoplasm of unspecified site of orbit
Benign neoplasm of connective tissue of orbit
Benign neoplasm of extraocular muscle
Benign neoplasm of peripheral nerves of orbit
Benign neoplasm of retrobulbar tissue
Benign neoplasm of retro-ocular tissue
EXCLUDES1 *benign neoplasm of orbital bone (D16.4)*
D31.60 **Benign neoplasm of unspecified site of unspecified orbit**
D31.61 Benign neoplasm of unspecified site of right orbit
D31.62 Benign neoplasm of unspecified site of left orbit
D31.9 Benign neoplasm of unspecified part of eye
Benign neoplasm of eyeball
D31.90 **Benign neoplasm of unspecified part of unspecified eye**
D31.91 Benign neoplasm of unspecified part of right eye
D31.92 Benign neoplasm of unspecified part of left eye

D32 Benign neoplasm of meninges
D32.0 Benign neoplasm of cerebral meninges
D32.1 Benign neoplasm of spinal meninges
D32.9 **Benign neoplasm of meninges, unspecified**
Meningioma NOS

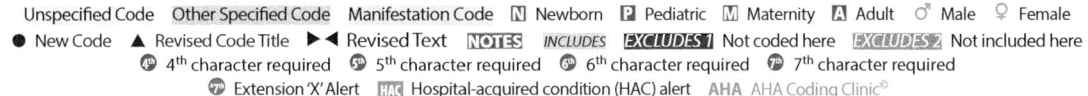

Unspecified Code | Other Specified Code | Manifestation Code | N Newborn | P Pediatric | M Maternity | A Adult | ♂ Male | ♀ Female
● New Code ▲ Revised Code Title ▶◀ Revised Text NOTES INCLUDES EXCLUDES1 Not coded here EXCLUDES2 Not included here
4th character required | 5th character required | 6th character required | 7th character required
Extension 'X' Alert | HAC Hospital-acquired condition (HAC) alert | AHA AHA Coding Clinic©

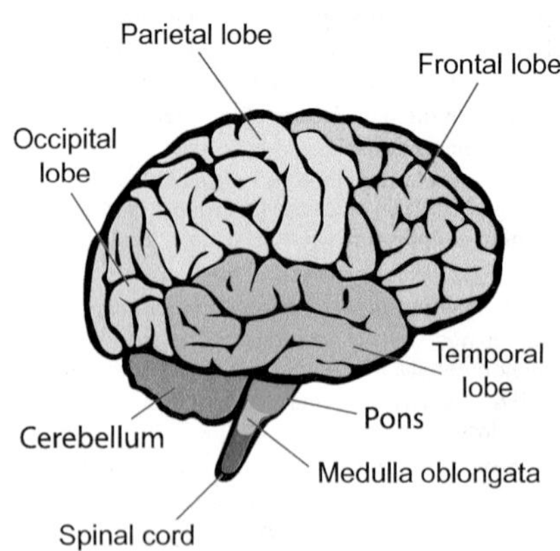

Figure 2.6 Brain lobes

D33 **Benign neoplasm of brain and other parts of central nervous system**
EXCLUDES1 *angioma (D18.0-)*
benign neoplasm of meninges (D32.-)
benign neoplasm of peripheral nerves and autonomic nervous system (D36.1-)
hemangioma (D18.0-)
neurofibromatosis (Q85.0-)
retro-ocular benign neoplasm (D31.6-)

D33.0 **Benign neoplasm of brain, supratentorial**
Benign neoplasm of cerebral ventricle
Benign neoplasm of cerebrum
Benign neoplasm of frontal lobe
Benign neoplasm of occipital lobe
Benign neoplasm of parietal lobe
Benign neoplasm of temporal lobe
EXCLUDES1 *benign neoplasm of fourth ventricle (D33.1)*

D33.1 **Benign neoplasm of brain, infratentorial**
Benign neoplasm of brain stem
Benign neoplasm of cerebellum
Benign neoplasm of fourth ventricle

D33.2 **Benign neoplasm of brain, unspecified**

D33.3 **Benign neoplasm of cranial nerves**
Benign neoplasm of olfactory bulb

D33.4 **Benign neoplasm of spinal cord**

D33.7 **Benign neoplasm of other specified parts of central nervous system**

D33.9 **Benign neoplasm of central nervous system, unspecified**
Benign neoplasm of nervous system (central) NOS

D34 **Benign neoplasm of thyroid gland**
Use additional code to identify any functional activity

D35 **Benign neoplasm of other and unspecified endocrine glands**
Use additional code to identify any functional activity
EXCLUDES1 *benign neoplasm of endocrine pancreas (D13.7)*
benign neoplasm of ovary (D27.-)
benign neoplasm of testis (D29.2.-)
benign neoplasm of thymus (D15.0)

D35.0 **Benign neoplasm of adrenal gland**
D35.00 **Benign neoplasm of unspecified adrenal gland**
D35.01 **Benign neoplasm of right adrenal gland**
D35.02 **Benign neoplasm of left adrenal gland**

D35.1 **Benign neoplasm of parathyroid gland**
D35.2 **Benign neoplasm of pituitary gland**
D35.3 **Benign neoplasm of craniopharyngeal duct**
D35.4 **Benign neoplasm of pineal gland**
D35.5 **Benign neoplasm of carotid body**
D35.6 **Benign neoplasm of aortic body and other paraganglia**
Benign tumor of glomus jugulare
D35.7 **Benign neoplasm of other specified endocrine glands**
D35.9 **Benign neoplasm of endocrine gland, unspecified**
Benign neoplasm of unspecified endocrine gland

D36 **Benign neoplasm of other and unspecified sites**
D36.0 **Benign neoplasm of lymph nodes**
EXCLUDES1 *lymphangioma (D18.1)*

D36.1 **Benign neoplasm of peripheral nerves and autonomic nervous system**
EXCLUDES1 *benign neoplasm of peripheral nerves of orbit (D31.6-)*
neurofibromatosis (Q85.0-)
D36.10 **Benign neoplasm of peripheral nerves and autonomic nervous system, unspecified**
D36.11 **Benign neoplasm of peripheral nerves and autonomic nervous system of face, head, and neck**
D36.12 **Benign neoplasm of peripheral nerves and autonomic nervous system, upper limb, including shoulder**
D36.13 **Benign neoplasm of peripheral nerves and autonomic nervous system of lower limb, including hip**
D36.14 **Benign neoplasm of peripheral nerves and autonomic nervous system of thorax**
D36.15 **Benign neoplasm of peripheral nerves and autonomic nervous system of abdomen**
D36.16 **Benign neoplasm of peripheral nerves and autonomic nervous system of pelvis**
D36.17 **Benign neoplasm of peripheral nerves and autonomic nervous system of trunk, unspecified**

D36.7 **Benign neoplasm of other specified sites**
Benign neoplasm of nose NOS
D36.9 **Benign neoplasm, unspecified site**

Benign neuroendocrine tumors (D3A)

D3A **Benign neuroendocrine tumors**
Code also any associated multiple endocrine neoplasia [MEN] syndromes (E31.2-)
Use additional code to identify any associated endocrine syndrome, such as:
carcinoid syndrome (E34.0)
EXCLUDES2 *benign pancreatic islet cell tumors (D13.7)*

D3A.0 **Benign carcinoid tumors**
D3A.00 **Benign carcinoid tumor of unspecified site**
Carcinoid tumor NOS
D3A.01 **Benign carcinoid tumors of the small intestine**
D3A.010 **Benign carcinoid tumor of the duodenum**
D3A.011 **Benign carcinoid tumor of the jejunum**
D3A.012 **Benign carcinoid tumor of the ileum**
D3A.019 **Benign carcinoid tumor of the small intestine, unspecified portion**
D3A.02 **Benign carcinoid tumors of the appendix, large intestine, and rectum**
D3A.020 **Benign carcinoid tumor of the appendix**
D3A.021 **Benign carcinoid tumor of the cecum**
D3A.022 **Benign carcinoid tumor of the ascending colon**
D3A.023 **Benign carcinoid tumor of the transverse colon**
D3A.024 **Benign carcinoid tumor of the descending colon**
D3A.025 **Benign carcinoid tumor of the sigmoid colon**
D3A.026 **Benign carcinoid tumor of the rectum**
D3A.029 **Benign carcinoid tumor of the large intestine, unspecified portion**
Benign carcinoid tumor of the colon NOS
D3A.09 **Benign carcinoid tumors of other sites**
D3A.090 **Benign carcinoid tumor of the bronchus and lung**
D3A.091 **Benign carcinoid tumor of the thymus**
D3A.092 **Benign carcinoid tumor of the stomach**
D3A.093 **Benign carcinoid tumor of the kidney**
▲ D3A.094 **Benign carcinoid tumor of the foregut, ▶unspecified◀**
▲ D3A.095 **Benign carcinoid tumor of the midgut, ▶unspecified◀**
▲ D3A.096 **Benign carcinoid tumor of the hindgut, ▶unspecified◀**
D3A.098 **Benign carcinoid tumors of other sites**

D3A.8 **Other benign neuroendocrine tumors**
Neuroendocrine tumor NOS

Unacceptable principal diagnosis symbol per Medicare code edits | Code exempt from diagnosis present on admission requirement
Questionable admission | Complication or comorbidity | CC/MCC exclusion | Major complication or comorbidity
Principal diagnosis as its own CC | Principal diagnosis as its own MCC | Z code as first-listed diagnosis

 When symbols appear on a code that requires a 7th character extension, refer to Appendix D to identify applicable 7th character codes.

Neoplasms of uncertain behavior, polycythemia vera and myelodysplastic syndromes (D37-D48)

NOTES Categories D37-D44, and D48 classify by site neoplasms of uncertain behavior, i.e., histologic confirmation whether the neoplasm is malignant or benign cannot be made.

EXCLUDES1 *neoplasms of unspecified behavior (D49.-)*

④ **D37 Neoplasm of uncertain behavior of oral cavity and digestive organs**

EXCLUDES1 *stromal tumors of uncertain behavior of digestive system (D48.1)*

⑤ **D37.0 Neoplasm of uncertain behavior of lip, oral cavity and pharynx**

EXCLUDES1 *neoplasm of uncertain behavior of aryepiglottic fold or interarytenoid fold, laryngeal aspect (D38.0)*
neoplasm of uncertain behavior of epiglottis NOS (D38.0)
neoplasm of uncertain behavior of skin of lip (D48.5)
neoplasm of uncertain behavior of suprahyoid portion of epiglottis (D38.0)

D37.01 Neoplasm of uncertain behavior of lip
Neoplasm of uncertain behavior of vermilion border of lip

D37.02 Neoplasm of uncertain behavior of tongue

⑥ **D37.03 Neoplasm of uncertain behavior of the major salivary glands**

D37.030 Neoplasm of uncertain behavior of the parotid salivary glands

D37.031 Neoplasm of uncertain behavior of the sublingual salivary glands

D37.032 Neoplasm of uncertain behavior of the submandibular salivary glands

D37.039 Neoplasm of uncertain behavior of the major salivary glands, unspecified

D37.04 Neoplasm of uncertain behavior of the minor salivary glands
Neoplasm of uncertain behavior of submucosal salivary glands of lip
Neoplasm of uncertain behavior of submucosal salivary glands of cheek
Neoplasm of uncertain behavior of submucosal salivary glands of hard palate
Neoplasm of uncertain behavior of submucosal salivary glands of soft palate

D37.05 Neoplasm of uncertain behavior of pharynx
Neoplasm of uncertain behavior of aryepiglottic fold of pharynx NOS
Neoplasm of uncertain behavior of hypopharyngeal aspect of aryepiglottic fold of pharynx
Neoplasm of uncertain behavior of marginal zone of aryepiglottic fold of pharynx

D37.09 Neoplasm of uncertain behavior of other specified sites of the oral cavity

D37.1 Neoplasm of uncertain behavior of stomach

D37.2 Neoplasm of uncertain behavior of small intestine

D37.3 Neoplasm of uncertain behavior of appendix

D37.4 Neoplasm of uncertain behavior of colon

D37.5 Neoplasm of uncertain behavior of rectum
Neoplasm of uncertain behavior of rectosigmoid junction

D37.6 Neoplasm of uncertain behavior of liver, gallbladder and bile ducts
Neoplasm of uncertain behavior of ampulla of Vater

D37.8 Neoplasm of uncertain behavior of other specified digestive organs
Neoplasm of uncertain behavior of anal canal
Neoplasm of uncertain behavior of anal sphincter
Neoplasm of uncertain behavior of anus NOS
Neoplasm of uncertain behavior of esophagus
Neoplasm of uncertain behavior of intestine NOS
Neoplasm of uncertain behavior of pancreas

EXCLUDES1 *neoplasm of uncertain behavior of anal margin (D48.5)*
neoplasm of uncertain behavior of anal skin (D48.5)
neoplasm of uncertain behavior of perianal skin (D48.5)

D37.9 Neoplasm of uncertain behavior of digestive organ, unspecified

④ **D38 Neoplasm of uncertain behavior of middle ear and respiratory and intrathoracic organs**

EXCLUDES1 *neoplasm of uncertain behavior of heart (D48.7)*

D38.0 Neoplasm of uncertain behavior of larynx
Neoplasm of uncertain behavior of aryepiglottic fold or interarytenoid fold, laryngeal aspect
Neoplasm of uncertain behavior of epiglottis (suprahyoid portion)

EXCLUDES1 *neoplasm of uncertain behavior of aryepiglottic fold or interarytenoid fold NOS (D37.05)*
neoplasm of uncertain behavior of hypopharyngeal aspect of aryepiglottic fold (D37.05)
neoplasm of uncertain behavior of marginal zone of aryepiglottic fold (D37.05)

D38.1 Neoplasm of uncertain behavior of trachea, bronchus and lung

D38.2 Neoplasm of uncertain behavior of pleura

D38.3 Neoplasm of uncertain behavior of mediastinum

D38.4 Neoplasm of uncertain behavior of thymus

D38.5 Neoplasm of uncertain behavior of other respiratory organs
Neoplasm of uncertain behavior of accessory sinuses
Neoplasm of uncertain behavior of cartilage of nose
Neoplasm of uncertain behavior of middle ear
Neoplasm of uncertain behavior of nasal cavities

EXCLUDES1 *neoplasm of uncertain behavior of ear (external) (skin) (D48.5)*
neoplasm of uncertain behavior of nose NOS (D48.7)
neoplasm of uncertain behavior of skin of nose (D48.5)

D38.6 Neoplasm of uncertain behavior of respiratory organ, unspecified

④ **D39 Neoplasm of uncertain behavior of female genital organs**

D39.0 Neoplasm of uncertain behavior of uterus ♀

⑤ **D39.1 Neoplasm of uncertain behavior of ovary**
Use additional code to identify any functional activity.

D39.10 Neoplasm of uncertain behavior of unspecified ovary ♀

D39.11 Neoplasm of uncertain behavior of right ovary ♀

D39.12 Neoplasm of uncertain behavior of left ovary ♀

D39.2 Neoplasm of uncertain behavior of placenta ♀
Chorioadenoma destruens
Invasive hydatidiform mole
Malignant hydatidiform mole

EXCLUDES1 *hydatidiform mole NOS (O01.9)*

D39.8 Neoplasm of uncertain behavior of other specified female genital organs ♀
Neoplasm of uncertain behavior of skin of female genital organs

D39.9 Neoplasm of uncertain behavior of female genital organ, unspecified ♀

④ **D40 Neoplasm of uncertain behavior of male genital organs**

D40.0 Neoplasm of uncertain behavior of prostate ♂

⑤ **D40.1 Neoplasm of uncertain behavior of testis**

D40.10 Neoplasm of uncertain behavior of unspecified testis ♂

D40.11 Neoplasm of uncertain behavior of right testis ♂

D40.12 Neoplasm of uncertain behavior of left testis ♂

D40.8 Neoplasm of uncertain behavior of other specified male genital organs ♂
Neoplasm of uncertain behavior of skin of male genital organs

D40.9 Neoplasm of uncertain behavior of male genital organ, unspecified ♂

④ **D41 Neoplasm of uncertain behavior of urinary organs**

⑤ **D41.0 Neoplasm of uncertain behavior of kidney**

EXCLUDES1 *neoplasm of uncertain behavior of renal pelvis (D41.1-)*

D41.00 Neoplasm of uncertain behavior of unspecified kidney

D41.01 Neoplasm of uncertain behavior of right kidney

D41.02 Neoplasm of uncertain behavior of left kidney

⑤ **D41.1 Neoplasm of uncertain behavior of renal pelvis**

D41.10 Neoplasm of uncertain behavior of unspecified renal pelvis

D41.11 Neoplasm of uncertain behavior of right renal pelvis

D41.12 Neoplasm of uncertain behavior of left renal pelvis

⑤ **D41.2 Neoplasm of uncertain behavior of ureter**

Unspecified Code Other Specified Code Manifestation Code N Newborn P Pediatric M Maternity A Adult ♂ Male ♀ Female
● New Code ▲ Revised Code Title ►◄ Revised Text NOTES INCLUDES EXCLUDES1 Not coded here EXCLUDES2 Not included here
④ 4th character required ⑤ 5th character required ⑥ 6th character required ⑦ 7th character required
Ⓧ Extension 'X' Alert HAC Hospital-acquired condition (HAC) alert AHA AHA Coding Clinic©

D41.20 Neoplasm of uncertain behavior of unspecified ureter
D41.21 Neoplasm of uncertain behavior of right ureter
D41.22 Neoplasm of uncertain behavior of left ureter
D41.3 Neoplasm of uncertain behavior of urethra
D41.4 Neoplasm of uncertain behavior of bladder
D41.8 Neoplasm of uncertain behavior of other specified urinary organs
D41.9 Neoplasm of uncertain behavior of unspecified urinary organ

D42 Neoplasm of uncertain behavior of meninges
D42.0 Neoplasm of uncertain behavior of cerebral meninges
D42.1 Neoplasm of uncertain behavior of spinal meninges
D42.9 Neoplasm of uncertain behavior of meninges, unspecified

D43 Neoplasm of uncertain behavior of brain and central nervous system
EXCLUDES1 *neoplasm of uncertain behavior of peripheral nerves and autonomic nervous system (D48.2)*
D43.0 Neoplasm of uncertain behavior of brain, supratentorial
Neoplasm of uncertain behavior of cerebral ventricle
Neoplasm of uncertain behavior of cerebrum
Neoplasm of uncertain behavior of frontal lobe
Neoplasm of uncertain behavior of occipital lobe
Neoplasm of uncertain behavior of parietal lobe
Neoplasm of uncertain behavior of temporal lobe
EXCLUDES1 *neoplasm of uncertain behavior of fourth ventricle (D43.1)*
D43.1 Neoplasm of uncertain behavior of brain, infratentorial
Neoplasm of uncertain behavior of brain stem
Neoplasm of uncertain behavior of cerebellum
Neoplasm of uncertain behavior of fourth ventricle
D43.2 Neoplasm of uncertain behavior of brain, unspecified
D43.3 Neoplasm of uncertain behavior of cranial nerves
D43.4 Neoplasm of uncertain behavior of spinal cord
D43.8 Neoplasm of uncertain behavior of other specified parts of central nervous system
D43.9 Neoplasm of uncertain behavior of central nervous system, unspecified
Neoplasm of uncertain behavior of nervous system (central) NOS

D44 Neoplasm of uncertain behavior of endocrine glands
EXCLUDES1 *multiple endocrine adenomatosis (E31.2-)*
multiple endocrine neoplasia (E31.2-)
neoplasm of uncertain behavior of endocrine pancreas (D37.8)
neoplasm of uncertain behavior of ovary (D39.1-)
neoplasm of uncertain behavior of testis (D40.1-)
neoplasm of uncertain behavior of thymus (D38.4)
D44.0 Neoplasm of uncertain behavior of thyroid gland
D44.1 Neoplasm of uncertain behavior of adrenal gland
Use additional code to identify any functional activity.
D44.10 Neoplasm of uncertain behavior of unspecified adrenal gland
D44.11 Neoplasm of uncertain behavior of right adrenal gland
D44.12 Neoplasm of uncertain behavior of left adrenal gland
D44.2 Neoplasm of uncertain behavior of parathyroid gland
D44.3 Neoplasm of uncertain behavior of pituitary gland
Use additional code to identify any functional activity.
D44.4 Neoplasm of uncertain behavior of craniopharyngeal duct
D44.5 Neoplasm of uncertain behavior of pineal gland
D44.6 Neoplasm of uncertain behavior of carotid body
D44.7 Neoplasm of uncertain behavior of aortic body and other paraganglia
D44.9 Neoplasm of uncertain behavior of unspecified endocrine gland

D45 Polycythemia vera
EXCLUDES1 *familial polycythemia (D75.0)*
secondary polycythemia (D75.1)

D46 Myelodysplastic syndromes
Use additional code for adverse effect, if applicable, to identify drug (T36-T50 with fifth or sixth character 5)
EXCLUDES2 *drug-induced aplastic anemia (D61.1)*
D46.0 Refractory anemia without ring sideroblasts, so stated
Refractory anemia without sideroblasts, without excess of blasts
D46.1 Refractory anemia with ring sideroblasts
RARS
▲ D46.2 Refractory anemia with excess of blasts [▶RAEB◀]
D46.20 Refractory anemia with excess of blasts, unspecified
RAEB NOS
D46.21 Refractory anemia with excess of blasts 1
RAEB 1
D46.22 Refractory anemia with excess of blasts 2 CC
RAEB 2
D46.A Refractory cytopenia with multilineage dysplasia
D46.B Refractory cytopenia with multilineage dysplasia and ring sideroblasts
RCMD RS
D46.C Myelodysplastic syndrome with isolated del(5q) chromosomal abnormality CC
Myelodysplastic syndrome with 5q deletion
5q minus syndrome NOS
D46.4 Refractory anemia, unspecified
D46.Z Other myelodysplastic syndromes
EXCLUDES1 *chronic myelomonocytic leukemia (C93.1-)*
D46.9 Myelodysplastic syndrome, unspecified
Myelodysplasia NOS

D47 Other neoplasms of uncertain behavior of lymphoid, hematopoietic and related tissue
D47.0 Histiocytic and mast cell tumors of uncertain behavior CC
Indolent systemic mastocytosis
Mast cell tumor NOS
Mastocytoma NOS
EXCLUDES1 *malignant mast cell tumor (C96.2)*
mastocytosis (congenital) (cutaneous) (Q82.2)
D47.1 Chronic myeloproliferative disease CC
Chronic neutrophilic leukemia
Myeloproliferative disease, unspecified
EXCLUDES1 *atypical chronic myeloid leukemia BCR/ABL-negative (C92.2-)*
chronic myeloid leukemia BCR/ABL-positive (C92.1-)
myelofibrosis NOS (D75.81)
myelophthisic anemia (D61.82)
myelophthisis (D61.82)
secondary myelofibrosis NOS (D75.81)
D47.2 Monoclonal gammopathy
Monoclonal gammopathy of undetermined significance [MGUS]
D47.3 Essential (hemorrhagic) thrombocythemia
Essential thrombocytosis
Idiopathic hemorrhagic thrombocythemia
D47.4 Osteomyelofibrosis
Chronic idiopathic myelofibrosis
Myelofibrosis (idiopathic) (with myeloid metaplasia)
Myelosclerosis (megakaryocytic) with myeloid metaplasia
Secondary myelofibrosis in myeloproliferative disease
EXCLUDES1 *acute myelofibrosis (C94.4-)*
D47.Z Other specified neoplasms of uncertain behavior of lymphoid, hematopoietic and related tissue
D47.Z1 Post-transplant lymphoproliferative disorder (PTLD) CC PDx
Code first complications of transplanted organs and tissue (T86.-)
● D47.Z2 Castleman disease
Code also if applicable human herpesvirus 8 infection (B10.89)
EXCLUDES2 *Kaposi's sarcoma (C46-)*
D47.Z9 Other specified neoplasms of uncertain behavior of lymphoid, hematopoietic and related tissue CC
Histiocytic tumors of uncertain behavior
D47.9 Neoplasm of uncertain behavior of lymphoid, hematopoietic and related tissue, unspecified CC
Lymphoproliferative disease NOS

D48 Neoplasm of uncertain behavior of other and unspecified sites
EXCLUDES1 *neurofibromatosis (nonmalignant) (Q85.0-)*
D48.0 Neoplasm of uncertain behavior of bone and articular cartilage
EXCLUDES1 *neoplasm of uncertain behavior of cartilage of ear (D48.1)*
neoplasm of uncertain behavior of cartilage of larynx (D38.0)

PDx Unacceptable principal diagnosis symbol per Medicare code edits · POA Code exempt from diagnosis present on admission requirement
? Questionable admission · CC Complication or comorbidity · CC/MCC Excl CC/MCC exclusion · MCC Major complication or comorbidity
PDx CC Principal diagnosis as its own CC · PDx MCC Principal diagnosis as its own MCC · Z1 Z code as first-listed diagnosis

neoplasm of uncertain behavior of cartilage of nose (D38.5)
neoplasm of uncertain behavior of connective tissue of eyelid (D48.1)
neoplasm of uncertain behavior of synovia (D48.1)

D48.1 Neoplasm of uncertain behavior of connective and other soft tissue
Neoplasm of uncertain behavior of connective tissue of ear
Neoplasm of uncertain behavior of connective tissue of eyelid
Stromal tumors of uncertain behavior of digestive system
EXCLUDES1 *neoplasm of uncertain behavior of articular cartilage (D48.0)*
neoplasm of uncertain behavior of cartilage of larynx (D38.0)
neoplasm of uncertain behavior of cartilage of nose (D38.5)
neoplasm of uncertain behavior of connective tissue of breast (D48.6-)

D48.2 Neoplasm of uncertain behavior of peripheral nerves and autonomic nervous system
EXCLUDES1 *neoplasm of uncertain behavior of peripheral nerves of orbit (D48.7)*

D48.3 Neoplasm of uncertain behavior of retroperitoneum
D48.4 Neoplasm of uncertain behavior of peritoneum
D48.5 Neoplasm of uncertain behavior of skin
Neoplasm of uncertain behavior of anal margin
Neoplasm of uncertain behavior of anal skin
Neoplasm of uncertain behavior of perianal skin
Neoplasm of uncertain behavior of skin of breast
EXCLUDES1 *neoplasm of uncertain behavior of anus NOS (D37.8)*
neoplasm of uncertain behavior of skin of genital organs (D39.8, D40.8)
neoplasm of uncertain behavior of vermilion border of lip (D37.0)

(5th) **D48.6 Neoplasm of uncertain behavior of breast**
Neoplasm of uncertain behavior of connective tissue of breast
Cystosarcoma phyllodes
EXCLUDES1 *neoplasm of uncertain behavior of skin of breast (D48.5)*
D48.60 Neoplasm of uncertain behavior of unspecified breast
D48.61 Neoplasm of uncertain behavior of right breast
D48.62 Neoplasm of uncertain behavior of left breast

D48.7 Neoplasm of uncertain behavior of other specified sites
Neoplasm of uncertain behavior of eye
Neoplasm of uncertain behavior of heart
Neoplasm of uncertain behavior of peripheral nerves of orbit
EXCLUDES1 *neoplasm of uncertain behavior of connective tissue (D48.1)*
neoplasm of uncertain behavior of skin of eyelid (D48.5)

D48.9 Neoplasm of uncertain behavior, unspecified

Neoplasms of unspecified behavior (D49)

(4th) **D49 Neoplasms of unspecified behavior**
NOTES Category D49 classifies by site neoplasms of unspecified morphology and behavior. The term 'mass', unless otherwise stated, is not to be regarded as a neoplastic growth.
INCLUDES *'growth' NOS*
neoplasm NOS
new growth NOS
tumor NOS
EXCLUDES1 *neoplasms of uncertain behavior (D37-D44, D48)*

D49.0 Neoplasm of unspecified behavior of digestive system
EXCLUDES1 *neoplasm of unspecified behavior of margin of anus (D49.2)*
neoplasm of unspecified behavior of perianal skin (D49.2)
neoplasm of unspecified behavior of skin of anus (D49.2)

D49.1 Neoplasm of unspecified behavior of respiratory system

D49.2 Neoplasm of unspecified behavior of bone, soft tissue, and skin
EXCLUDES1 *neoplasm of unspecified behavior of anal canal (D49.0)*
neoplasm of unspecified behavior of anus NOS (D49.0)
neoplasm of unspecified behavior of bone marrow (D49.89)
neoplasm of unspecified behavior of cartilage of larynx (D49.1)
neoplasm of unspecified behavior of cartilage of nose (D49.1)
neoplasm of unspecified behavior of connective tissue of breast (D49.3)
neoplasm of unspecified behavior of skin of genital organs ►(D49.59)◄
neoplasm of unspecified behavior of vermilion border of lip (D49.0)

D49.3 Neoplasm of unspecified behavior of breast
EXCLUDES1 *neoplasm of unspecified behavior of skin of breast (D49.2)*

D49.4 Neoplasm of unspecified behavior of bladder

● (5th) **D49.5 Neoplasm of unspecified behavior of other genitourinary organs**
● (6th) **D49.51 Neoplasm of unspecified behavior of kidney**
● **D49.511 Neoplasm of unspecified behavior of right kidney** CC/MCC Exc
● **D49.512 Neoplasm of unspecified behavior of left kidney** CC/MCC Exc
● **D49.519 Neoplasm of unspecified behavior of unspecified kidney** CC/MCC Exc
● **D49.59 Neoplasm of unspecified behavior of other genitourinary organ** CC/MCC Exc

D49.6 Neoplasm of unspecified behavior of brain
EXCLUDES1 *neoplasm of unspecified behavior of cerebral meninges (D49.7)*
neoplasm of unspecified behavior of cranial nerves (D49.7)

D49.7 Neoplasm of unspecified behavior of endocrine glands and other parts of nervous system
EXCLUDES1 *neoplasm of unspecified behavior of peripheral, sympathetic, and parasympathetic nerves and ganglia (D49.2)*

(5th) **D49.8 Neoplasm of unspecified behavior of other specified sites**
EXCLUDES1 *neoplasm of unspecified behavior of eyelid (skin) (D49.2)*
neoplasm of unspecified behavior of eyelid cartilage (D49.2)
neoplasm of unspecified behavior of great vessels (D49.2)
neoplasm of unspecified behavior of optic nerve (D49.7)
D49.81 Neoplasm of unspecified behavior of retina and choroid
Dark area on retina
Retinal freckle
D49.89 Neoplasm of unspecified behavior of other specified sites

D49.9 Neoplasm of unspecified behavior of unspecified site

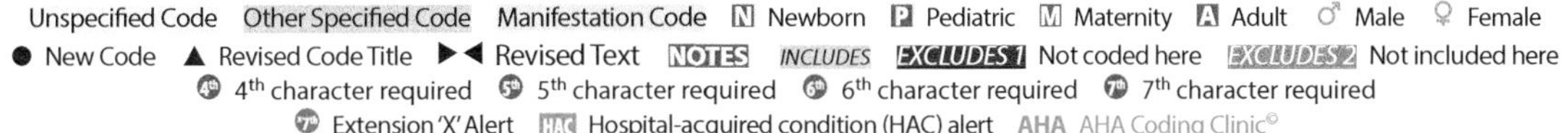

Unspecified Code Other Specified Code Manifestation Code N Newborn P Pediatric M Maternity A Adult ♂ Male ♀ Female
● New Code ▲ Revised Code Title ►◄ Revised Text NOTES INCLUDES EXCLUDES1 Not coded here EXCLUDES2 Not included here
4th character required 5th character required 6th character required 7th character required
Extension 'X' Alert HAC Hospital-acquired condition (HAC) alert AHA AHA Coding Clinic©

This page intentionally left blank

Chapter 3: Disease of the Blood and Blood-forming Organs and Certain Disorders Involving the Immune Mechanism (D50-D89)

Guidelines for Assigning Codes From This Chapter

Chapter 3 includes conditions affecting the blood and related anatomic structures, such as the spleen and bone marrow. Some of the diagnoses you'll find in this chapter include anemias, coagulation defects, hemorrhagic conditions, white blood cell disorders, and spleen disorders. You'll also find immune disorders, including various immunodeficiency syndromes and graft-versus-host disease.

List of Sections

- D50-D53: Nutritional anemias
- D55-D59: Hemolytic anemias
- D60-D64: Aplastic and other anemias and other bone marrow failure syndromes
- D65-D69: Coagulation defects, purpura and other hemorrhagic conditions
- D70-D77: Other disorders of blood and blood-forming organs
- D78: Intraoperative and postprocedural complications of the spleen
- D80-D89: Certain disorders involving the immune mechanism

Highlights From the ICD-10-CM Official Guidelines for Coding and Reporting

The 2017 version of ICD-10-CM Official Guidelines for Coding and Reporting does not include specific guidelines for Chapter 3, stating that the section is reserved for future expansion.

Still, as with every ICD-10-CM chapter, you should be sure to review and apply the guidelines and instructions included in the manual with the codes and code ranges. Below are some key areas to watch for anemia codes:

CKD: When the patient has anemia due to chronic kidney disease (CKD), you must report a code from N18.- (*Chronic kidney disease*) in addition to D63.1 (*Anemia in chronic kidney disease*). Codes from N18.- indicate the stage of the illness.

> ➢ **Example:** Documentation shows the patient presented for treatment of stage 3 CKD. The provider also addresses the CKD-caused anemia during the encounter. You should report N18.3 (*Chronic kidney disease, stage 3 [moderate]*) followed by D63.1 for the anemia.

Neoplastic disease: In cases where the patient has anemia due to a neoplasm, you should report the proper neoplasm code followed by D63.0 (*Anemia in neoplastic disease*). However, if a patient has anemia caused by his chemotherapy, immunotherapy, or radiotherapy, and he presents for treatment of the anemia only, your first-listed code should be the anemia code followed by the neoplasm and adverse effect codes.

> ➢ **Example:** The patient presents for treatment of anemia caused by treatment of colon cancer with overlapping neoplasms, C18.8 (*Malignant neoplasm of contiguous or overlapping sites of colon whose point of origin cannot be determined*). You should report D63.0 followed by C18.8 and T45.1X5 (*Adverse effect of antineoplastic and immunosuppressive drugs*) or Y84.2 (*Radiological procedure and radiotherapy as the cause of abnormal reaction of the patient, or of later complication, without mention of misadventure at the time of the procedure*).

Assign Additional Codes for Drug-induced Anemias

Autoimmune hemolytic anemia (AIHA) is caused by autoantibody-induced hemolysis (the premature destruction of circulating red blood cells). It is usually idiopathic but can be associated with infection, lymphoproliferative disorders, autoimmune diseases, and some drugs. Category D59 contains codes used to report the different types of hemolytic anemias. D59.0 (Drug-induced autoimmune hemolytic anemia) and D59.1 (Other autoimmune hemolytic anemias) codes require an additional code to identify the drug. Select a code from T36-T50 with fifth or sixth character 5.

Diseases of the blood and blood-forming organs and certain disorders involving the immune mechanism (D50-D89)

EXCLUDES2 *autoimmune disease (systemic) NOS (M35.9)*
certain conditions originating in the perinatal period (P00-P96)
complications of pregnancy, childbirth and the puerperium (O00-O9A)
congenital malformations, deformations and chromosomal abnormalities (Q00-Q99)
endocrine, nutritional and metabolic diseases (E00-E88)
human immunodeficiency virus [HIV] disease (B20)
injury, poisoning and certain other consequences of external causes (S00-T88)
neoplasms (C00-D49)
symptoms, signs and abnormal clinical and laboratory findings, not elsewhere classified (R00-R94)

This chapter contains the following blocks:

D50-D53	Nutritional anemias
D55-D59	Hemolytic anemias
D60-D64	Aplastic and other anemias and other bone marrow failure syndromes
D65-D69	Coagulation defects, purpura and other hemorrhagic conditions
D70-D77	Other disorders of blood and blood-forming organs
D78	Intraoperative and postprocedural complications of the spleen
D80-D89	Certain disorders involving the immune mechanism

Nutritional anemias (D50-D53)

D50 Iron deficiency anemia
INCLUDES *asiderotic anemia*
hypochromic anemia

D50.0 Iron deficiency anemia secondary to blood loss (chronic)
Posthemorrhagic anemia (chronic)
EXCLUDES1 *acute posthemorrhagic anemia (D62)*
congenital anemia from fetal blood loss (P61.3)

D50.1 Sideropenic dysphagia
Kelly-Paterson syndrome
Plummer-Vinson syndrome

D50.8 Other iron deficiency anemias
Iron deficiency anemia due to inadequate dietary iron intake

D50.9 Iron deficiency anemia, unspecified

D51 Vitamin B12 deficiency anemia
EXCLUDES1 *vitamin B12 deficiency (E53.8)*

D51.0 Vitamin B12 deficiency anemia due to intrinsic factor deficiency
Addison anemia
Biermer anemia
Pernicious (congenital) anemia
Congenital intrinsic factor deficiency

D51.1 Vitamin B12 deficiency anemia due to selective vitamin B12 malabsorption with proteinuria
Imerslund (Grasbeck) syndrome
Megaloblastic hereditary anemia

D51.2 Transcobalamin II deficiency

D51.3 Other dietary vitamin B12 deficiency anemia
Vegan anemia

D51.8 Other vitamin B12 deficiency anemias

D51.9 Vitamin B12 deficiency anemia, unspecified

D52 Folate deficiency anemia
EXCLUDES1 *folate deficiency without anemia (E53.8)*

D52.0 Dietary folate deficiency anemia
Nutritional megaloblastic anemia

D52.1 Drug-induced folate deficiency anemia
Use additional code for adverse effect, if applicable, to identify drug (T36-T50 with fifth or sixth character 5)

D52.8 Other folate deficiency anemias

D52.9 Folate deficiency anemia, unspecified
Folic acid deficiency anemia NOS

D53 Other nutritional anemias
INCLUDES *megaloblastic anemia unresponsive to vitamin B12 or folate therapy*

D53.0 Protein deficiency anemia
Amino-acid deficiency anemia
Orotaciduric anemia
EXCLUDES1 *Lesch-Nyhan syndrome (E79.1)*

D53.1 Other megaloblastic anemias, not elsewhere classified
Megaloblastic anemia NOS
EXCLUDES1 *Di Guglielmo's disease (C94.0)*

D53.2 Scorbutic anemia
EXCLUDES1 *scurvy (E54)*

D53.8 Other specified nutritional anemias
Anemia associated with deficiency of copper
Anemia associated with deficiency of molybdenum
Anemia associated with deficiency of zinc
EXCLUDES1 *nutritional deficiencies without anemia, such as:*
copper deficiency NOS (E61.0)
molybdenum deficiency NOS (E61.5)
zinc deficiency NOS (E60)

D53.9 Nutritional anemia, unspecified
Simple chronic anemia
EXCLUDES1 *anemia NOS (D64.9)*

Hemolytic anemias (D55-D59)

D55 Anemia due to enzyme disorders
EXCLUDES1 *drug-induced enzyme deficiency anemia (D59.2)*

D55.0 Anemia due to glucose-6-phosphate dehydrogenase [G6PD] deficiency
Favism
G6PD deficiency anemia

D55.1 Anemia due to other disorders of glutathione metabolism
Anemia (due to) enzyme deficiencies, except G6PD, related to the hexose monophosphate [HMP] shunt pathway
Anemia (due to) hemolytic nonspherocytic (hereditary), type I

D55.2 Anemia due to disorders of glycolytic enzymes
Hemolytic nonspherocytic (hereditary) anemia, type II
Hexokinase deficiency anemia
Pyruvate kinase [PK] deficiency anemia
Triose-phosphate isomerase deficiency anemia
EXCLUDES1 *disorders of glycolysis not associated with anemia (E74.8)*

D55.3 Anemia due to disorders of nucleotide metabolism

D55.8 Other anemias due to enzyme disorders

D55.9 Anemia due to enzyme disorder, unspecified

D56 Thalassemia
EXCLUDES1 *sickle-cell thalassemia (D57.4-)*

D56.0 Alpha thalassemia
Alpha thalassemia major
Hemoglobin H Constant Spring
Hemoglobin H disease
Hydrops fetalis due to alpha thalassemia
Severe alpha thalassemia
Triple gene defect alpha thalassemia
Use additional code, if applicable, for hydrops fetalis due to alpha thalassemia (P56.99)
EXCLUDES1 *alpha thalassemia trait or minor (D56.3)*
asymptomatic alpha thalassemia (D56.3)
hydrops fetalis due to isoimmunization (P56.0)
hydrops fetalis not due to immune hemolysis (P83.2)

D56.1 Beta thalassemia
Beta thalassemia major
Cooley's anemia
Homozygous beta thalassemia
Severe beta thalassemia
Thalassemia intermedia
Thalassemia major
EXCLUDES1 *beta thalassemia minor (D56.3)*
beta thalassemia trait (D56.3)
delta-beta thalassemia (D56.2)
hemoglobin E-beta thalassemia (D56.5)
sickle-cell beta thalassemia (D57.4-)

D56.2 Delta-beta thalassemia
Homozygous delta-beta thalassemia
EXCLUDES1 *delta-beta thalassemia minor (D56.3)*
delta-beta thalassemia trait (D56.3)

Unacceptable principal diagnosis symbol per Medicare code edits — Code exempt from diagnosis present on admission requirement — Questionable admission — Complication or comorbidity — CC/MCC exclusion — Major complication or comorbidity — Principal diagnosis as its own CC — Principal diagnosis as its own MCC — Z code as first-listed diagnosis

When symbols appear on a code that requires a 7th character extension, refer to Appendix D to identify applicable 7th character codes.

D56.3 Thalassemia minor
Alpha thalassemia minor
Alpha thalassemia silent carrier
Alpha thalassemia trait
Beta thalassemia minor
Beta thalassemia trait
Delta-beta thalassemia minor
Delta-beta thalassemia trait
Thalassemia trait NOS
EXCLUDES1 *alpha thalassemia (D56.0)*
beta thalassemia (D56.1)
delta-beta thalassemia (D56.2)
hemoglobin E-beta thalassemia (D56.5)
sickle-cell trait (D57.3)

D56.4 Hereditary persistence of fetal hemoglobin [HPFH]

D56.5 Hemoglobin E-beta thalassemia
EXCLUDES1 *beta thalassemia (D56.1)*
beta thalassemia minor (D56.3)
beta thalassemia trait (D56.3)
delta-beta thalassemia (D56.2)
delta-beta thalassemia trait (D56.3)
hemoglobin E disease (D58.2)
other hemoglobinopathies (D58.2)
sickle-cell beta thalassemia (D57.4-)

D56.8 Other thalassemias
Dominant thalassemia
Hemoglobin C thalassemia
Mixed thalassemia
Thalassemia with other hemoglobinopathy
EXCLUDES1 *hemoglobin C disease (D58.2)*
hemoglobin E disease (D58.2)
other hemoglobinopathies (D58.2)
sickle-cell anemia (D57.-)
sickle-cell thalassemia (D57.4)

D56.9 Thalassemia, unspecified
Mediterranean anemia (with other hemoglobinopathy)

D57 Sickle-cell disorders (4th)
Use additional code for any associated fever (R50.81)
EXCLUDES1 *other hemoglobinopathies (D58.-)*

D57.0 Hb-SS disease with crisis (5th)
Sickle-cell disease NOS with crisis
Hb-SS disease with vasoocclusive pain
D57.00 Hb-SS disease with crisis, unspecified MCC
D57.01 Hb-SS disease with acute chest syndrome MCC
D57.02 Hb-SS disease with splenic sequestration MCC

D57.1 Sickle-cell disease without crisis
Hb-SS disease without crisis
Sickle-cell anemia NOS
Sickle-cell disease NOS
Sickle-cell disorder NOS

D57.2 Sickle-cell/Hb-C disease (5th)
Hb-SC disease
Hb-S/Hb-C disease
D57.20 Sickle-cell/Hb-C disease without crisis
D57.21 Sickle-cell/Hb-C disease with crisis (6th)
D57.211 Sickle-cell/Hb-C disease with acute chest syndrome MCC PDx
D57.212 Sickle-cell/Hb-C disease with splenic sequestration MCC
D57.219 Sickle-cell/Hb-C disease with crisis, unspecified MCC
Sickle-cell/Hb-C disease with crisis NOS

D57.3 Sickle-cell trait
Hb-S trait
Heterozygous hemoglobin S

D57.4 Sickle-cell thalassemia (5th)
Sickle-cell beta thalassemia
Thalassemia Hb-S disease
D57.40 Sickle-cell thalassemia without crisis
Microdrepanocytosis
Sickle-cell thalassemia NOS
D57.41 Sickle-cell thalassemia with crisis (6th)
Sickle-cell thalassemia with vasoocclusive pain
D57.411 Sickle-cell thalassemia with acute chest syndrome MCC PDx
D57.412 Sickle-cell thalassemia with splenic sequestration MCC
D57.419 Sickle-cell thalassemia with crisis, unspecified MCC
Sickle-cell thalassemia with crisis NOS

D57.8 Other sickle-cell disorders (5th)
Hb-SD disease
Hb-SE disease
D57.80 Other sickle-cell disorders without crisis
D57.81 Other sickle-cell disorders with crisis (6th)
D57.811 Other sickle-cell disorders with acute chest syndrome MCC
D57.812 Other sickle-cell disorders with splenic sequestration MCC
D57.819 Other sickle-cell disorders with crisis, unspecified MCC
Other sickle-cell disorders with crisis NOS

D58 Other hereditary hemolytic anemias (4th)
EXCLUDES1 *hemolytic anemia of the newborn (P55.-)*

D58.0 Hereditary spherocytosis
Acholuric (familial) jaundice
Congenital (spherocytic) hemolytic icterus
Minkowski-Chauffard syndrome

D58.1 Hereditary elliptocytosis
Elliptocytosis (congenital)
Ovalocytosis (congenital) (hereditary)

D58.2 Other hemoglobinopathies
Abnormal hemoglobin NOS
Congenital Heinz body anemia
Hb-C disease
Hb-D disease
Hb-E disease
Hemoglobinopathy NOS
Unstable hemoglobin hemolytic disease
EXCLUDES1 *familial polycythemia (D75.0)*
Hb-M disease (D74.0)
hemoglobin E-beta thalassemia (D56.5)
hereditary persistence of fetal hemoglobin [HPFH] (D56.4)
high-altitude polycythemia (D75.1)
methemoglobinemia (D74.-)
other hemoglobinopathies with thalassemia (D56.8)

D58.8 Other specified hereditary hemolytic anemias CC
Stomatocytosis

D58.9 Hereditary hemolytic anemia, unspecified CC

D59 Acquired hemolytic anemia (4th)

D59.0 Drug-induced autoimmune hemolytic anemia CC
Use additional code for adverse effect, if applicable, to identify drug (T36-T50 with fifth or sixth character 5)

D59.1 Other autoimmune hemolytic anemias CC
Autoimmune hemolytic disease (cold type) (warm type)
Chronic cold hemagglutinin disease
Cold agglutinin disease
Cold agglutinin hemoglobinuria
Cold type (secondary) (symptomatic) hemolytic anemia
Warm type (secondary) (symptomatic) hemolytic anemia
EXCLUDES1 *Evans syndrome (D69.41)*
hemolytic disease of newborn (P55.-)
paroxysmal cold hemoglobinuria (D59.6)

D59.2 Drug-induced nonautoimmune hemolytic anemia CC
Drug-induced enzyme deficiency anemia
Use additional code for adverse effect, if applicable, to identify drug (T36-T50 with fifth or sixth character 5)

D59.3 Hemolytic-uremic syndrome MCC
Use additional code to identify associated:
E. coli infection (B96.2-)
Pneumococcal pneumonia (J13)
Shigella dysenteriae (A03.9)

D59.4 Other nonautoimmune hemolytic anemias CC
Mechanical hemolytic anemia
Microangiopathic hemolytic anemia
Toxic hemolytic anemia

Unspecified Code | Other Specified Code | Manifestation Code | N Newborn | P Pediatric | M Maternity | A Adult | ♂ Male | ♀ Female
● New Code | ▲ Revised Code Title | ►◄ Revised Text | NOTES | INCLUDES | EXCLUDES1 Not coded here | EXCLUDES2 Not included here
4th character required | 5th character required | 6th character required | 7th character required
Extension 'X' Alert | HAC Hospital-acquired condition (HAC) alert | AHA AHA Coding Clinic©

D59.5 Paroxysmal nocturnal hemoglobinuria [Marchiafava-Micheli]
EXCLUDES1 *hemoglobinuria NOS (R82.3)*

D59.6 Hemoglobinuria due to hemolysis from other external causes
Hemoglobinuria from exertion
March hemoglobinuria
Paroxysmal cold hemoglobinuria
Use additional code (Chapter 20) to identify external cause
EXCLUDES1 *hemoglobinuria NOS (R82.3)*

D59.8 Other acquired hemolytic anemias

D59.9 Acquired hemolytic anemia, unspecified CC
Idiopathic hemolytic anemia, chronic

Aplastic and other anemias and other bone marrow failure syndromes (D60-D64)

4th D60 **Acquired pure red cell aplasia [erythroblastopenia]**
INCLUDES *red cell aplasia (acquired) (adult) (with thymoma)*
EXCLUDES1 *congenital red cell aplasia (D61.01)*

D60.0 Chronic **acquired pure red cell aplasia** MCC
D60.1 Transient **acquired pure red cell aplasia** MCC
D60.8 **Other acquired pure red cell aplasias** MCC
D60.9 **Acquired pure red cell aplasia, unspecified** MCC

4th D61 **Other aplastic anemias and other bone marrow failure syndromes**
EXCLUDES1 *neutropenia (D70.-)*

5th D61.0 Constitutional **aplastic anemia**

D61.01 **Constitutional (pure) red blood cell aplasia** CC
Blackfan-Diamond syndrome
Congenital (pure) red cell aplasia
Familial hypoplastic anemia
Primary (pure) red cell aplasia
Red cell (pure) aplasia of infants
EXCLUDES1 *acquired red cell aplasia (D60.9)*

D61.09 **Other constitutional aplastic anemia** CC
Fanconi's anemia
Pancytopenia with malformations

D61.1 Drug-induced **aplastic anemia** MCC
Use additional code for adverse effect, if applicable, to identify drug (T36-T50 with fifth or sixth character 5)

D61.2 **Aplastic anemia due to other** external agents MCC
Code first , if applicable, toxic effects of substances chiefly nonmedicinal as to source (T51-T65)

D61.3 Idiopathic **aplastic anemia** MCC

5th D61.8 **Other specified aplastic anemias and other bone marrow failure syndromes**

6th D61.81 **Pancytopenia**
EXCLUDES1 *pancytopenia (due to) (with) aplastic anemia (D61.9)*
pancytopenia (due to) (with) bone marrow infiltration (D61.82)
pancytopenia (due to) (with) congenital (pure) red cell aplasia (D61.01)
pancytopenia (due to) (with) hairy cell leukemia (C91.4-)
pancytopenia (due to) (with) human immunodeficiency virus disease (B20.-)
pancytopenia (due to) (with) leukoerythroblastic anemia (D61.82)
pancytopenia (due to) (with) myeloproliferative disease (D47.1)
EXCLUDES2 *pancytopenia (due to) (with) myelodysplastic syndromes (D46.-)*

D61.810 Antineoplastic chemotherapy **induced pancytopenia** MCC
EXCLUDES2 *aplastic anemia due to antineoplastic chemotherapy (D61.1)*

D61.811 **Other** drug-induced **pancytopenia** MCC
EXCLUDES2 *aplastic anemia due to drugs (D61.1)*

D61.818 **Other pancytopenia** CC

D61.82 **Myelophthisis** CC
Leukoerythroblastic anemia
Myelophthisic anemia
Panmyelophthisis
Code also the underlying disorder, such as:
malignant neoplasm of breast (C50.-)
tuberculosis (A15.-)
EXCLUDES1 *idiopathic myelofibrosis (D47.1)*
myelofibrosis NOS (D75.81)
myelofibrosis with myeloid metaplasia (D47.4)
primary myelofibrosis (D47.1)
secondary myelofibrosis (D75.81)

D61.89 **Other specified aplastic anemias and other bone marrow failure syndromes** MCC

D61.9 **Aplastic anemia, unspecified** CC
Hypoplastic anemia NOS
Medullary hypoplasia

D62 **Acute posthemorrhagic anemia** CC
EXCLUDES1 *anemia due to chronic blood loss (D50.0)*
blood loss anemia NOS (D50.0)
congenital anemia from fetal blood loss (P61.3)

4th D63 **Anemia in chronic diseases classified elsewhere**

D63.0 **Anemia in** neoplastic disease
Code first neoplasm (C00-D49)
EXCLUDES1 *anemia due to antineoplastic chemotherapy (D64.81)*
aplastic anemia due to antineoplastic chemotherapy (D61.1)

D63.1 **Anemia in** chronic kidney disease
Erythropoietin resistant anemia (EPO resistant anemia)
Code first underlying chronic kidney disease (CKD) (N18.-)

D63.8 **Anemia in other** chronic diseases classified elsewhere
Code first underlying disease, such as:
diphyllobothriasis (B70.0)
hookworm disease (B76.0-B76.9)
hypothyroidism (E00.0-E03.9)
malaria (B50.0-B54)
symptomatic late syphilis (A52.79)
tuberculosis (A18.89)

4th D64 **Other anemias**
EXCLUDES1 *refractory anemia (D46.-)*
refractory anemia with excess blasts in transformation [RAEB T] (C92.0-)

D64.0 Hereditary sideroblastic **anemia**
Sex-linked hypochromic sideroblastic anemia

D64.1 Secondary sideroblastic **anemia** due to disease
Code first underlying disease

D64.2 Secondary sideroblastic **anemia** due to drugs and toxins
Code first poisoning due to drug or toxin, if applicable (T36-T65 with fifth or sixth character 1-4 or 6)
Use additional code for adverse effect, if applicable, to identify drug (T36-T50 with fifth or sixth character 5)

D64.3 **Other** sideroblastic **anemias**
Sideroblastic anemia NOS
Pyridoxine-responsive sideroblastic anemia NEC

D64.4 Congenital dyserythropoietic **anemia**
Dyshematopoietic anemia (congenital)
EXCLUDES1 *Blackfan-Diamond syndrome (D61.01)*
Di Guglielmo's disease (C94.0)

5th D64.8 **Other specified anemias**

D64.81 **Anemia due to** antineoplastic chemotherapy
Antineoplastic chemotherapy induced anemia
EXCLUDES1 *aplastic anemia due to antineoplastic chemotherapy (D61.1)*
EXCLUDES2 *anemia in neoplastic disease (D63.0)*

D64.89 **Other specified anemias**
Infantile pseudoleukemia

D64.9 **Anemia, unspecified**

PDx Unacceptable principal diagnosis symbol per Medicare code edits; POA Code exempt from diagnosis present on admission requirement
? Questionable admission; CC Complication or comorbidity; CC/MCC Exc CC/MCC exclusion; MCC Major complication or comorbidity
PDx CC Principal diagnosis as its own CC; PDx MCC Principal diagnosis as its own MCC; Z1 Z code as first-listed diagnosis

When symbols appear on a code that requires a 7th character extension, refer to Appendix D to identify applicable 7th character codes.

Coagulation defects, purpura and other hemorrhagic conditions (D65-D69)

D65 Disseminated intravascular coagulation [defibrination syndrome] MCC
Afibrinogenemia, acquired
Consumption coagulopathy
Diffuse or disseminated intravascular coagulation [DIC]
Fibrinolytic hemorrhage, acquired
Fibrinolytic purpura
Purpura fulminans
EXCLUDES1 *disseminated intravascular coagulation (complicating):*
abortion or ectopic or molar pregnancy (O00-O07, O08.1)
in newborn (P60)
pregnancy, childbirth and the puerperium (O45.0, O46.0, O67.0, O72.3)

D66 Hereditary factor VIII deficiency MCC
Classical hemophilia
Deficiency factor VIII (with functional defect)
Hemophilia NOS
Hemophilia A
EXCLUDES1 *factor VIII deficiency with vascular defect (D68.0)*

D67 Hereditary factor IX deficiency MCC
Christmas disease
Factor IX deficiency (with functional defect)
Hemophilia B
Plasma thromboplastin component [PTC] deficiency

D68 Other coagulation defects
EXCLUDES1 *abnormal coagulation profile (R79.1)*
coagulation defects complicating abortion or ectopic or molar pregnancy (O00-O07, O08.1)
coagulation defects complicating pregnancy, childbirth and the puerperium (O45.0, O46.0, O67.0, O72.3)
AHA: Q1, 2016

D68.0 Von Willebrand's disease CC
Angiohemophilia
Factor VIII deficiency with vascular defect
Vascular hemophilia
EXCLUDES1 *capillary fragility (hereditary) (D69.8)*
factor VIII deficiency NOS (D66)
factor VIII deficiency with functional defect (D66)

D68.1 Hereditary factor XI deficiency CC
Hemophilia C
Plasma thromboplastin antecedent [PTA] deficiency
Rosenthal's disease

D68.2 Hereditary deficiency of other clotting factors CC
AC globulin deficiency
Congenital afibrinogenemia
Deficiency of factor I [fibrinogen]
Deficiency of factor II [prothrombin]
Deficiency of factor V [labile]
Deficiency of factor VII [stable]
Deficiency of factor X [Stuart-Prower]
Deficiency of factor XII [Hageman]
Deficiency of factor XIII [fibrin stabilizing]
Dysfibrinogenemia (congenital)
Hypoproconvertinemia
Owren's disease
Proaccelerin deficiency

D68.3 Hemorrhagic disorder due to circulating anticoagulants

D68.31 Hemorrhagic disorder due to intrinsic circulating anticoagulants, antibodies, or inhibitors

D68.311 Acquired hemophilia CC
Autoimmune hemophilia
Autoimmune inhibitors to clotting factors
Secondary hemophilia

D68.312 Antiphospholipid antibody with hemorrhagic disorder CC
Lupus anticoagulant (LAC) with hemorrhagic disorder
Systemic lupus erythematosus [SLE] inhibitor with hemorrhagic disorder
EXCLUDES1 *antiphospholipid antibody, finding without diagnosis (R76.0)*
antiphospholipid antibody syndrome (D68.61)
antiphospholipid antibody with hypercoagulable state (D68.61)
lupus anticoagulant (LAC) finding without diagnosis (R76.0)
lupus anticoagulant (LAC) with hypercoagulable state (D68.62)
systemic lupus erythematosus [SLE] inhibitor finding without diagnosis (R76.0)
systemic lupus erythematosus [SLE] inhibitor with hypercoagulable state (D68.62)

D68.318 Other hemorrhagic disorder due to intrinsic circulating anticoagulants, antibodies, or inhibitors CC
Antithromboplastinemia
Antithromboplastinogenemia
Hemorrhagic disorder due to intrinsic increase in antithrombin
Hemorrhagic disorder due to intrinsic increase in anti-VIIIa
Hemorrhagic disorder due to intrinsic increase in anti-IXa
Hemorrhagic disorder due to intrinsic increase in anti-XIa

D68.32 Hemorrhagic disorder due to extrinsic circulating anticoagulants CC
Drug-induced hemorrhagic disorder
Hemorrhagic disorder due to increase in anti-IIa
Hemorrhagic disorder due to increase in anti-Xa
Hyperheparinemia
Use additional code for adverse effect, if applicable, to identify drug (T45.515, T45.525)
AHA: Q1, 2016

D68.4 Acquired coagulation factor deficiency CC
Deficiency of coagulation factor due to liver disease
Deficiency of coagulation factor due to vitamin K deficiency
EXCLUDES1 *vitamin K deficiency of newborn (P53)*

D68.5 Primary thrombophilia
Primary hypercoagulable states
EXCLUDES1 *antiphospholipid syndrome (D68.61)*
lupus anticoagulant (D68.62)
secondary activated protein C resistance (D68.69)
secondary antiphospholipid antibody syndrome (D68.69)
secondary lupus anticoagulant with hypercoagulable state (D68.69)
secondary systemic lupus erythematosus [SLE] inhibitor with hypercoagulable state (D68.69)
systemic lupus erythematosus [SLE] inhibitor finding without diagnosis (R76.0)
systemic lupus erythematosus [SLE] inhibitor with hemorrhagic disorder (D68.312)
thrombotic thrombocytopenic purpura (M31.1)

D68.51 Activated protein C resistance CC
Factor V Leiden mutation

D68.52 Prothrombin gene mutation CC

D68.59 Other primary thrombophilia CC
Antithrombin III deficiency
Hypercoagulable state NOS
Primary hypercoagulable state NEC
Primary thrombophilia NEC
Protein C deficiency
Protein S deficiency
Thrombophilia NOS

D68.6 Other thrombophilia
Other hypercoagulable states
EXCLUDES1 *diffuse or disseminated intravascular coagulation [DIC] (D65)*
heparin induced thrombocytopenia (HIT) (D75.82)
hyperhomocysteinemia (E72.11)

D68.61 Antiphospholipid syndrome CC
Anticardiolipin syndrome
Antiphospholipid antibody syndrome

Unspecified Code | Other Specified Code | Manifestation Code | N Newborn | P Pediatric | M Maternity | A Adult | ♂ Male | ♀ Female
● New Code ▲ Revised Code Title ►◄ Revised Text NOTES INCLUDES EXCLUDES1 Not coded here EXCLUDES2 Not included here
4th character required 5th character required 6th character required 7th character required
Extension 'X' Alert HAC Hospital-acquired condition (HAC) alert AHA AHA Coding Clinic®

EXCLUDES1 *anti-phospholipid antibody, finding without diagnosis (R76.0)*
anti-phospholipid antibody with hemorrhagic disorder (D68.312)
lupus anticoagulant syndrome (D68.62)

D68.62 Lupus anticoagulant syndrome
Lupus anticoagulant
Presence of systemic lupus erythematosus [SLE] inhibitor
EXCLUDES1 *anticardiolipin syndrome (D68.61)*
antiphospholipid syndrome (D68.61)
lupus anticoagulant (LAC) finding without diagnosis ▶(R76.0)◀
lupus anticoagulant (LAC) with hemorrhagic disorder (D68.312)

D68.69 Other thrombophilia
Hypercoagulable states NEC
Secondary hypercoagulable state NOS

D68.8 Other specified coagulation defects
EXCLUDES1 *hemorrhagic disease of newborn (P53)*

D68.9 Coagulation defect, unspecified

D69 Purpura and other hemorrhagic conditions
EXCLUDES1 *benign hypergammaglobulinemic purpura (D89.0)*
cryoglobulinemic purpura (D89.1)
essential (hemorrhagic) thrombocythemia (D47.3)
hemorrhagic thrombocythemia (D47.3)
purpura fulminans (D65)
thrombotic thrombocytopenic purpura (M31.1)
Waldenström hypergammaglobulinemic purpura (D89.0)

D69.0 Allergic purpura
Allergic vasculitis
Nonthrombocytopenic hemorrhagic purpura
Nonthrombocytopenic idiopathic purpura
Purpura anaphylactoid
Purpura Henoch(-Schönlein)
Purpura rheumatica
Vascular purpura
EXCLUDES1 *thrombocytopenic hemorrhagic purpura (D69.3)*

D69.1 Qualitative platelet defects
Bernard-Soulier [giant platelet] syndrome
Glanzmann's disease
Grey platelet syndrome
Thromboasthenia (hemorrhagic) (hereditary)
Thrombocytopathy
EXCLUDES1 *von Willebrand's disease (D68.0)*

D69.2 Other nonthrombocytopenic purpura
Purpura NOS
Purpura simplex
Senile purpura

D69.3 Immune thrombocytopenic purpura
Hemorrhagic (thrombocytopenic) purpura
Idiopathic thrombocytopenic purpura
Tidal platelet dysgenesis

D69.4 Other primary thrombocytopenia
EXCLUDES1 *transient neonatal thrombocytopenia (P61.0)*
Wiskott-Aldrich syndrome (D82.0)

D69.41 Evans syndrome

D69.42 Congenital and hereditary thrombocytopenia purpura
Congenital thrombocytopenia
Hereditary thrombocytopenia
Code first congenital or hereditary disorder, such as: thrombocytopenia with absent radius (TAR syndrome) (Q87.2)

D69.49 Other primary thrombocytopenia
Megakaryocytic hypoplasia
Primary thrombocytopenia NOS

D69.5 Secondary thrombocytopenia
EXCLUDES1 *heparin induced thrombocytopenia (HIT) (D75.82)*
transient thrombocytopenia of newborn (P61.0)

D69.51 Posttransfusion purpura
Posttransfusion purpura from whole blood (fresh) or blood products
PTP

D69.59 Other secondary thrombocytopenia

D69.6 Thrombocytopenia, unspecified

D69.8 Other specified hemorrhagic conditions
Capillary fragility (hereditary)
Vascular pseudohemophilia

D69.9 Hemorrhagic condition, unspecified

Other disorders of blood and blood-forming organs (D70-D77)

D70 Neutropenia
INCLUDES *agranulocytosis*
decreased absolute neutrophil count (ANC)
Use additional code for any associated:
fever (R50.81)
mucositis (J34.81, K12.3-, K92.81, N76.81)
EXCLUDES1 *neutropenic splenomegaly (D73.81)*
transient neonatal neutropenia (P61.5)

D70.0 Congenital agranulocytosis
Congenital neutropenia
Infantile genetic agranulocytosis
Kostmann's disease

D70.1 Agranulocytosis secondary to cancer chemotherapy
Code also underlying neoplasm
Use additional code for adverse effect, if applicable, to identify drug (T45.1X5)

D70.2 Other drug-induced agranulocytosis
Use additional code for adverse effect, if applicable, to identify drug (T36-T50 with fifth or sixth character 5)

D70.3 Neutropenia due to infection

D70.4 Cyclic neutropenia
Cyclic hematopoiesis
Periodic neutropenia

D70.8 Other neutropenia

D70.9 Neutropenia, unspecified

D71 Functional disorders of polymorphonuclear neutrophils
Cell membrane receptor complex [CR3] defect
Chronic (childhood) granulomatous disease
Congenital dysphagocytosis
Progressive septic granulomatosis

D72 Other disorders of white blood cells
EXCLUDES1 *basophilia (D72.824)*
immunity disorders (D80-D89)
neutropenia (D70)
preleukemia (syndrome) (D46.9)

D72.0 Genetic anomalies of leukocytes
Alder (granulation) (granulocyte) anomaly
Alder syndrome
Hereditary leukocytic hypersegmentation
Hereditary leukocytic hyposegmentation
Hereditary leukomelanopathy
May-Hegglin (granulation) (granulocyte) anomaly
May-Hegglin syndrome
Pelger-Huët (granulation) (granulocyte) anomaly
Pelger-Huët syndrome
EXCLUDES1 *Chédiak (-Steinbrinck)-Higashi syndrome (E70.330)*

D72.1 Eosinophilia
Allergic eosinophilia
Hereditary eosinophilia
EXCLUDES1 *Löffler's syndrome (J82)*
pulmonary eosinophilia (J82)

D72.8 Other specified disorders of white blood cells
EXCLUDES1 *leukemia (C91-C95)*

D72.81 Decreased white blood cell count
EXCLUDES1 *neutropenia (D70.-)*

D72.810 Lymphocytopenia
Decreased lymphocytes

D72.818 Other decreased white blood cell count
Basophilic leukopenia
Eosinophilic leukopenia
Monocytopenia
Other decreased leukocytes
Plasmacytopenia

Unacceptable principal diagnosis symbol per Medicare code edits · Code exempt from diagnosis present on admission requirement
Questionable admission · CC Complication or comorbidity · CC/MCC exclusion · MCC Major complication or comorbidity
Principal diagnosis as its own CC · Principal diagnosis as its own MCC · Z code as first-listed diagnosis

D72.819 Decreased white blood cell count, unspecified
Decreased leukocytes, unspecified
Leukocytopenia, unspecified
Leukopenia
EXCLUDES1 *malignant leukopenia (D70.9)*

D72.82 Elevated white blood cell count
EXCLUDES1 *eosinophilia (D72.1)*

D72.820 Lymphocytosis (symptomatic)
Elevated lymphocytes

D72.821 Monocytosis (symptomatic)
EXCLUDES1 *infectious mononucleosis (B27.-)*

D72.822 Plasmacytosis

D72.823 Leukemoid reaction
Basophilic leukemoid reaction
Leukemoid reaction NOS
Lymphocytic leukemoid reaction
Monocytic leukemoid reaction
Myelocytic leukemoid reaction
Neutrophilic leukemoid reaction

D72.824 Basophilia

D72.825 Bandemia
Bandemia without diagnosis of specific infection
EXCLUDES1 *confirmed infection - code to infection*
leukemia (C91.-, C92.-, C93.-, C94.-, C95.-)

D72.828 Other elevated white blood cell count

D72.829 Elevated white blood cell count, unspecified
Elevated leukocytes, unspecified
Leukocytosis, unspecified

D72.89 Other specified disorders of white blood cells
Abnormality of white blood cells NEC

D72.9 Disorder of white blood cells, unspecified
Abnormal leukocyte differential NOS

D73 Diseases of spleen

D73.0 Hyposplenism
Atrophy of spleen
EXCLUDES1 *asplenia (congenital) (Q89.01)*
postsurgical absence of spleen (Z90.81)

D73.1 Hypersplenism
EXCLUDES1 *neutropenic splenomegaly (D73.81)*
primary splenic neutropenia (D73.81)
splenitis, splenomegaly in late syphilis (A52.79)
splenitis, splenomegaly in tuberculosis (A18.85)
splenomegaly NOS (R16.1)
splenomegaly congenital (Q89.0)

D73.2 Chronic congestive splenomegaly

D73.3 Abscess of spleen

D73.4 Cyst of spleen

D73.5 Infarction of spleen
Splenic rupture, nontraumatic
Torsion of spleen
EXCLUDES1 *rupture of spleen due to Plasmodium vivax malaria (B51.0)*
traumatic rupture of spleen (S36.03-)

D73.8 Other diseases of spleen

D73.81 Neutropenic splenomegaly
Werner-Schultz disease

D73.89 Other diseases of spleen
Fibrosis of spleen NOS
Perisplenitis
Splenitis NOS

D73.9 Disease of spleen, unspecified

D74 Methemoglobinemia

D74.0 Congenital methemoglobinemia
Congenital NADH-methemoglobin reductase deficiency
Hemoglobin-M [Hb-M] disease
Methemoglobinemia, hereditary

D74.8 Other methemoglobinemias
Acquired methemoglobinemia (with sulfhemoglobinemia)
Toxic methemoglobinemia

D74.9 Methemoglobinemia, unspecified

D75 Other and unspecified diseases of blood and blood-forming organs
EXCLUDES2 *acute lymphadenitis (L04.-)*
chronic lymphadenitis (I88.1)
enlarged lymph nodes (R59.-)
hypergammaglobulinemia NOS (D89.2)
lymphadenitis NOS (I88.9)
mesenteric lymphadenitis (acute) (chronic) (I88.0)

D75.0 Familial erythrocytosis
Benign polycythemia
Familial polycythemia
EXCLUDES1 *hereditary ovalocytosis (D58.1)*

D75.1 Secondary polycythemia
Acquired polycythemia
Emotional polycythemia
Erythrocytosis NOS
Hypoxemic polycythemia
Nephrogenous polycythemia
Polycythemia due to erythropoietin
Polycythemia due to fall in plasma volume
Polycythemia due to high altitude
Polycythemia due to stress
Polycythemia NOS
Relative polycythemia
EXCLUDES1 *polycythemia neonatorum (P61.1)*
polycythemia vera (D45)

D75.8 Other specified diseases of blood and blood-forming organs

D75.81 Myelofibrosis
Myelofibrosis NOS
Secondary myelofibrosis NOS
Code first the underlying disorder, such as:
malignant neoplasm of breast (C50.-)
Use additional code, if applicable, for associated therapy-related myelodysplastic syndrome (D46.-)
Use additional code for adverse effect, if applicable, to identify drug (T45.1X5)
EXCLUDES1 *acute myelofibrosis (C94.4-)*
idiopathic myelofibrosis (D47.1)
leukoerythroblastic anemia (D61.82)
myelofibrosis with myeloid metaplasia (D47.4)
myelophthisic anemia (D61.82)
myelophthisis (D61.82)
primary myelofibrosis (D47.1)

D75.82 Heparin induced thrombocytopenia (HIT)

D75.89 Other specified diseases of blood and blood-forming organs

D75.9 Disease of blood and blood-forming organs, unspecified

D76 Other specified diseases with participation of lymphoreticular and reticulohistiocytic tissue
EXCLUDES1 *(Abt-) Letterer-Siwe disease (C96.0)*
eosinophilic granuloma (C96.6)
Hand-Schüller-Christian disease (C96.5)
histiocytic medullary reticulosis (C96.9)
histiocytic sarcoma (C96.A)
histiocytosis X, multifocal (C96.5)
histiocytosis X, unifocal (C96.6)
Langerhans-cell histiocytosis, multifocal (C96.5)
Langerhans-cell histiocytosis NOS (C96.6)
Langerhans-cell histiocytosis, unifocal (C96.6)
leukemic reticuloendotheliosis (C91.4-)
lipomelanotic reticulosis (I89.8)
malignant histiocytosis (C96.A)
malignant reticulosis (C86.0)
nonlipid reticuloendotheliosis (C96.0)

D76.1 Hemophagocytic lymphohistiocytosis
Familial hemophagocytic reticulosis
Histiocytoses of mononuclear phagocytes

D76.2 Hemophagocytic syndrome, infection-associated
Use additional code to identify infectious agent or disease.

Unspecified Code | Other Specified Code | Manifestation Code | N Newborn | P Pediatric | M Maternity | A Adult | ♂ Male | ♀ Female
● New Code | ▲ Revised Code Title | ►◄ Revised Text | NOTES | INCLUDES | EXCLUDES1 Not coded here | EXCLUDES2 Not included here
4th character required | 5th character required | 6th character required | 7th character required
Extension 'X' Alert | HAC Hospital-acquired condition (HAC) alert | AHA AHA Coding Clinic©

D76.3 **Other histiocytosis syndromes**
Reticulohistiocytoma (giant-cell)
Sinus histiocytosis with massive lymphadenopathy
Xanthogranuloma

D77 **Other disorders of blood and blood-forming organs in diseases classified elsewhere**
Code first underlying disease, such as:
amyloidosis (E85.-)
congenital early syphilis (A50.0)
echinococcosis (B67.0-B67.9)
malaria (B50.0-B54)
schistosomiasis [bilharziasis] (B65.0-B65.9)
vitamin C deficiency (E54)
EXCLUDES1 *rupture of spleen due to Plasmodium vivax malaria (B51.0)*
splenitis, splenomegaly in late syphilis (A52.79)
splenitis, splenomegaly in tuberculosis (A18.85)

Intraoperative and postprocedural complications of the spleen (D78)

D78 **Intraoperative and postprocedural complications of the spleen**
D78.0 **Intraoperative hemorrhage and hematoma of the spleen complicating a procedure**
EXCLUDES1 *intraoperative hemorrhage and hematoma of the spleen due to accidental puncture or laceration during a procedure (D78.1-)*
D78.01 **Intraoperative hemorrhage and hematoma of the spleen complicating a procedure on the spleen**
D78.02 **Intraoperative hemorrhage and hematoma of the spleen complicating other procedure**
D78.1 **Accidental puncture and laceration of the spleen during a procedure**
D78.11 **Accidental puncture and laceration of the spleen during a procedure on the spleen**
D78.12 **Accidental puncture and laceration of the spleen during other procedure**
▲ D78.2 **Postprocedural ▶hemorrhage of◀ the spleen following a procedure**
▲ D78.21 **Postprocedural ▶hemorrhage of◀ the spleen following a procedure on the spleen**
▲ D78.22 **Postprocedural ▶hemorrhage of◀ the spleen following other procedure**
● D78.3 **Postprocedural hematoma and seroma of the spleen following a procedure**
● D78.31 **Postprocedural hematoma of the spleen following a procedure on the spleen**
● D78.32 **Postprocedural hematoma of the spleen following other procedure**
● D78.33 **Postprocedural seroma of the spleen following a procedure on the spleen**
● D78.34 **Postprocedural seroma of the spleen following other procedure**
D78.8 **Other intraoperative and postprocedural complications of the spleen**
Use additional code, if applicable, to further specify disorder
D78.81 **Other intraoperative complications of the spleen**
D78.89 **Other postprocedural complications of the spleen**

Certain disorders involving the immune mechanism (D80-D89)

INCLUDES *defects in the complement system*
immunodeficiency disorders, except human immunodeficiency virus [HIV] disease
sarcoidosis
EXCLUDES1 *autoimmune disease (systemic) NOS (M35.9)*
functional disorders of polymorphonuclear neutrophils (D71)
human immunodeficiency virus [HIV] disease (B20)

D80 **Immunodeficiency with predominantly antibody defects**
D80.0 **Hereditary hypogammaglobulinemia**
Autosomal recessive agammaglobulinemia (Swiss type)
X-linked agammaglobulinemia [Bruton] (with growth hormone deficiency)
D80.1 **Nonfamilial hypogammaglobulinemia**
Agammaglobulinemia with immunoglobulin-bearing B-lymphocytes
Common variable agammaglobulinemia [CVAgamma]
Hypogammaglobulinemia NOS
D80.2 **Selective deficiency of immunoglobulin A [IgA]**
D80.3 **Selective deficiency of immunoglobulin G [IgG] subclasses**
D80.4 **Selective deficiency of immunoglobulin M [IgM]**
D80.5 **Immunodeficiency with increased immunoglobulin M [IgM]**
D80.6 **Antibody deficiency with near-normal immunoglobulins or with hyperimmunoglobulinemia**
D80.7 **Transient hypogammaglobulinemia of infancy**
D80.8 **Other immunodeficiencies with predominantly antibody defects**
Kappa light chain deficiency
D80.9 **Immunodeficiency with predominantly antibody defects, unspecified**

D81 **Combined immunodeficiencies**
EXCLUDES1 *autosomal recessive agammaglobulinemia (Swiss type) (D80.0)*
D81.0 **Severe combined immunodeficiency [SCID] with reticular dysgenesis**
D81.1 **Severe combined immunodeficiency [SCID] with low T- and B-cell numbers**
D81.2 **Severe combined immunodeficiency [SCID] with low or normal B-cell numbers**
D81.3 **Adenosine deaminase [ADA] deficiency**
D81.4 **Nezelof's syndrome**
D81.5 **Purine nucleoside phosphorylase [PNP] deficiency**
D81.6 **Major histocompatibility complex class I deficiency**
Bare lymphocyte syndrome
D81.7 **Major histocompatibility complex class II deficiency**
D81.8 **Other combined immunodeficiencies**
D81.81 **Biotin-dependent carboxylase deficiency**
Multiple carboxylase deficiency
EXCLUDES1 *biotin-dependent carboxylase deficiency due to dietary deficiency of biotin (E53.8)*
D81.810 **Biotinidase deficiency**
D81.818 **Other biotin-dependent carboxylase deficiency**
Holocarboxylase synthetase deficiency
Other multiple carboxylase deficiency
D81.819 **Biotin-dependent carboxylase deficiency, unspecified**
Multiple carboxylase deficiency, unspecified
D81.89 **Other combined immunodeficiencies**
D81.9 **Combined immunodeficiency, unspecified**
Severe combined immunodeficiency disorder [SCID] NOS

D82 **Immunodeficiency associated with other major defects**
EXCLUDES1 *ataxia telangiectasia [Louis-Bar] (G11.3)*
D82.0 **Wiskott-Aldrich syndrome**
Immunodeficiency with thrombocytopenia and eczema
D82.1 **Di George's syndrome**
Pharyngeal pouch syndrome
Thymic alymphoplasia
Thymic aplasia or hypoplasia with immunodeficiency
D82.2 **Immunodeficiency with short-limbed stature**
D82.3 **Immunodeficiency following hereditary defective response to Epstein-Barr virus**
X-linked lymphoproliferative disease
D82.4 **Hyperimmunoglobulin E [IgE] syndrome**
D82.8 **Immunodeficiency associated with other specified major defects**
D82.9 **Immunodeficiency associated with major defect, unspecified**

D83 **Common variable immunodeficiency**
D83.0 **Common variable immunodeficiency with predominant abnormalities of B-cell numbers and function**
D83.1 **Common variable immunodeficiency with predominant immunoregulatory T-cell disorders**
D83.2 **Common variable immunodeficiency with autoantibodies to B- or T-cells**
D83.8 **Other common variable immunodeficiencies**
D83.9 **Common variable immunodeficiency, unspecified**

D84 **Other immunodeficiencies**

Unacceptable principal diagnosis symbol per Medicare code edits · Code exempt from diagnosis present on admission requirement
Questionable admission · Complication or comorbidity · CC/MCC exclusion · Major complication or comorbidity
Principal diagnosis as its own CC · Principal diagnosis as its own MCC · Z code as first-listed diagnosis

When symbols appear on a code that requires a 7th character extension, refer to Appendix D to identify applicable 7th character codes.

D84.0 Lymphocyte function antigen-1 [LFA-1] defect
D84.1 Defects in the complement system
C1 esterase inhibitor [C1-INH] deficiency
D84.8 Other specified immunodeficiencies CC
D84.9 Immunodeficiency, unspecified CC

D86 Sarcoidosis
D86.0 Sarcoidosis of lung
D86.1 Sarcoidosis of lymph nodes
D86.2 Sarcoidosis of lung with sarcoidosis of lymph nodes
D86.3 Sarcoidosis of skin
D86.8 Sarcoidosis of other sites
D86.81 Sarcoid meningitis
D86.82 Multiple cranial nerve palsies in sarcoidosis
D86.83 Sarcoid iridocyclitis
D86.84 Sarcoid pyelonephritis
Tubulo-interstitial nephropathy in sarcoidosis
D86.85 Sarcoid myocarditis
D86.86 Sarcoid arthropathy
Polyarthritis in sarcoidosis
D86.87 Sarcoid myositis
D86.89 Sarcoidosis of other sites
Hepatic granuloma
Uveoparotid fever [Heerfordt]
D86.9 Sarcoidosis, unspecified

D89 Other disorders involving the immune mechanism, not elsewhere classified
EXCLUDES1 *hyperglobulinemia NOS (R77.1)*
monoclonal gammopathy (of undetermined significance) (D47.2)
EXCLUDES2 *transplant failure and rejection (T86.-)*
D89.0 Polyclonal hypergammaglobulinemia
Benign hypergammaglobulinemic purpura
Polyclonal gammopathy NOS
D89.1 Cryoglobulinemia
Cryoglobulinemic purpura
Cryoglobulinemic vasculitis
Essential cryoglobulinemia
Idiopathic cryoglobulinemia
Mixed cryoglobulinemia
Primary cryoglobulinemia
Secondary cryoglobulinemia
D89.2 Hypergammaglobulinemia, unspecified
D89.3 Immune reconstitution syndrome
Immune reconstitution inflammatory syndrome [IRIS]
Use additional code for adverse effect, if applicable, to identify drug (T36-T50 with fifth or sixth character 5)
● D89.4 Mast cell activation syndrome and related disorders
EXCLUDES1 *aggressive systemic mastocytosis (C96.2)*
cutaneous mastocytosis (Q82.2)
indolent systemic mastocytosis (D47.0)
malignant mastocytoma (C96.2)
mast cell leukemia (C94.3-)
mastocytoma (D47.0)
systemic mastocytosis associated with a clonal hematologic non-mast cell lineage disease (SM-AHNMD) (D47.0)
● D89.40 Mast cell activation, unspecified
Mast cell activation disorder, unspecified
Mast cell activation syndrome, NOS
● D89.41 Monoclonal mast cell activation syndrome
● D89.42 Idiopathic mast cell activation syndrome
● D89.43 Secondary mast cell activation
Secondary mast cell activation syndrome
Code also underlying etiology, if known
● D89.49 Other mast cell activation disorder
Other mast cell activation syndrome

D89.8 Other specified disorders involving the immune mechanism, not elsewhere classified
D89.81 Graft-versus-host disease
Code first underlying cause, such as:
complications of transplanted organs and tissue (T86.-)
complications of blood transfusion (T80.89)
Use additional code to identify associated manifestations, such as:
desquamative dermatitis (L30.8)
diarrhea (R19.7)
elevated bilirubin (R17)
hair loss (L65.9)
D89.810 Acute graft-versus-host disease CC PDx
D89.811 Chronic graft-versus-host disease CC PDx
D89.812 Acute on chronic graft-versus-host disease CC PDx
D89.813 Graft-versus-host disease, unspecified CC PDx
D89.82 Autoimmune lymphoproliferative syndrome [ALPS]
D89.89 Other specified disorders involving the immune mechanism, not elsewhere classified
EXCLUDES1 *human immunodeficiency virus disease (B20)*
D89.9 Disorder involving the immune mechanism, unspecified
Immune disease NOS
AHA: Q3, 2015

Unspecified Code | Other Specified Code | Manifestation Code | N Newborn | P Pediatric | M Maternity | A Adult | ♂ Male | ♀ Female
● New Code | ▲ Revised Code Title | ►◄ Revised Text | NOTES | INCLUDES | EXCLUDES1 Not coded here | EXCLUDES2 Not included here
4th character required | 5th character required | 6th character required | 7th character required
Extension 'X' Alert | HAC Hospital-acquired condition (HAC) alert | AHA AHA Coding Clinic©

This page intentionally left blank

Chapter 4: Endocrine, Nutritional and Metabolic Diseases (E00-E89)

Guidelines for Assigning Codes From This Chapter

List of Sections

- E00-E07: Disorders of thyroid gland
- E08-E13: Diabetes mellitus
- E15-E16: Other disorders of glucose regulation and pancreatic internal secretion
- E20-E35: Disorders of other endocrine glands
- E36: Intraoperative complications of endocrine system
- E40-E46: Malnutrition
- E50-E64: Other nutritional deficiencies
- E65-E68: Overweight, obesity and other hyperalimentation
- E70-E88: Metabolic disorders
- E89: Postprocedural endocrine and metabolic complications and disorders, not elsewhere classified

Highlights From the ICD-10-CM Official Guidelines for Coding and Reporting

The Chapter 4 section of the ICD-10-CM Official Guidelines for Coding and Reporting is all about diabetes. The information below summarizes the key points from Section I.C.4 of the 2017 Official Guidelines.

Get to Know Combination Codes

Diabetes mellitus codes are combination codes that specify the type of diabetes mellitus, the body system affected, and the complications affecting that body system. You should report as many codes within a particular category as necessary to describe all complications of the disease. Sequence the codes based on the reason for the encounter. Assign as many codes from categories E08-E13 as needed to identify all associated conditions.

Begin by Establishing the Type of Diabetes

Diabetes mellitus has two main types. Type 1 involves the body not producing insulin and usually develops in children and young adults. Type 1 is often called juvenile diabetes and is the least common form. In type 2, the most common form of diabetes, the body does not produce adequate insulin or resists the effects of insulin it has produced, which results in high levels of glucose in the blood.

Age can be misleading. Don't let the patient's age determine your code selection as either type of diabetes can occur at almost any age. Look to the documentation. If the type of diabetes mellitus is not documented, the default is E11.- (*Type 2 diabetes mellitus*).

Insulin usage provides a clue. If the documentation in a medical record does not indicate the type of diabetes but indicates the patient uses insulin, assign both E11 (*Type 2 diabetes mellitus*) and Z79.4 (*Long-term [current] use of insulin*). Note that Z79.4 should not be assigned if insulin is given temporarily to bring a type 2 patient's blood sugar under control during an encounter.

T85.6 is Your First Stop for Insulin Pump Malfunctions

Insulin pump malfunctions may result in underdosing or overdosing.

- **Underdosing:** Specify the type of malfunction with a code from subcategory T85.6 (*Mechanical complication of other specified internal and external prosthetic devices, implants and grafts*) as the principal or first-listed code, followed by code T38.3X6- (*Underdosing of insulin and oral hypoglycemic [antidiabetic] drugs*). You should then assign additional codes for the type of diabetes mellitus and any associated complications due to the underdosing.
- **Overdosing:** Look again to T85.6 when overdosing results from an insulin pump malfunction. Then assign T38.3X1- (*Poisoning by insulin and oral hypoglycemic [antidiabetic] drugs, accidental [unintentional]*).

Code the Cause for Secondary Diabetes

When reporting secondary diabetes with codes under categories E08 (*Diabetes mellitus due to underlying condition*), E09 (*Drug or chemical induced diabetes mellitus*), and E13 (*Other specified diabetes mellitus*), you'll follow rules similar to those for diabetes mellitus. But secondary diabetes results from another condition, so you have to add coding that condition to the mix. You should choose the condition that triggered the encounter as the principal diagnosis.

Don't miss: For secondary diabetes due to removal of the pancreas or due to adverse effects from ingesting a substance, you should apply slightly different guidelines.

- For postpancreatectomy diabetes mellitus, you should report E89.1 (Postprocedural hypoinsulinemia). You should also assign a code from category E13 and a code from subcategory Z90.41-(Acquired absence of pancreas) as additional codes.
- To determine proper coding for diabetes due to adverse effect of medication or poisoning, look to Chapter 19 and Chapter 20.

Note: See chapter 15 for coding diabetes mellitus in pregnancy and gestational (pregnancy-induced) diabetes.

Anatomy of the Endocrine System

1. **An Outline of the Endocrine System**
   a) The endocrine system is primarily responsible for maintaining the body's homeostasis through various hormones.
   b) The endocrine system is based on the ductless endocrine glands that secrete their hormones directly into the blood stream. These hormones are further carried to the target organs through the blood stream.
   c) The pituitary gland (or hypophysis) is regarded as the master gland of the endocrine system. This gland is monitored and controlled by the hypothalamus of the brain.

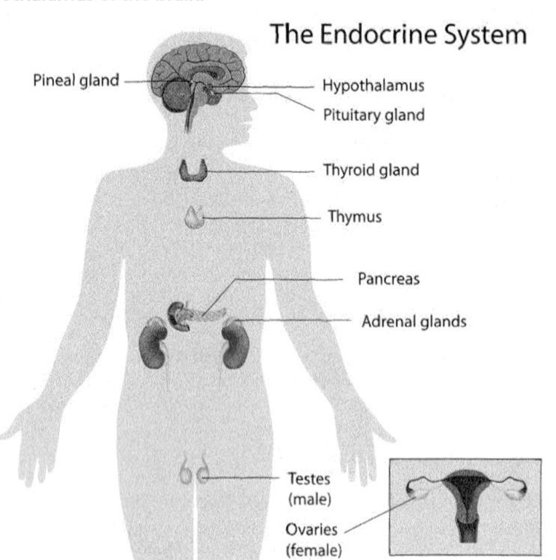

2. **The Endocrine Hormones**
   a) The names of various endocrine hormones of the body are as follows:
      i) epinephrine
      ii) norepinephrine
      iii) oxytocin
      iv) vasopressin
      v) insulin
      vi) growth hormone
      vii) cortisol
      viii) estrogen
      ix) testosterone
   b) The hormones monitor and control the processes of cellular respiration, growth, reproduction and electrolyte balances of the body. They also regulate the reproductive cycles, growth and the secretion of other hormones.
3. **The Hypothalamus (of the Brain)**
   a) The hypothalamus controls the secretions of the pituitary gland.
   b) The hypothalamus controls and monitors the secretions of the endocrine system.
   c) The endocrine system can influence the functions of the hypothalamus via negative feedback mechanisms.
4. **The Major Endocrine Glands**
   a) The names of the major endocrine glands are as follows:
      i) anterior pituitary gland
      ii) posterior pituitary gland
      iii) pineal gland
      iv) thyroid gland
      v) parathyroid gland
      vi) thymus
      vii) adrenal gland
      viii) pancreatic islets
      ix) ovaries
      x) testes
5. **The Anatomy of the Anterior Pituitary Gland**
   The anterior pituitary gland is constituted by the glandular epithelium and generates the following hormones, which are listed below:
   a) Growth Hormone

      The growth hormone stimulates cell metabolism and growth of bones and muscles.
   b) Thyroid Stimulating Hormone (TSH)

      The TSH stimulates the thyroid gland for the production of T3, T4 and calcitonin hormones.
   c) Adrenocorticotropic Hormone (ACTH)

      The ACTH stimulates the adrenal cortex for the secretion of the hormone cortisol.
   d) Melanocyte Stimulating Hormone (MSH)

      The MSH stimulates melanocytes for the production of melanin, which causes darkening of the skin.
   e) Luteinizing Hormone (LH)

      The LH stimulates the production of testosterone in males and progesterone in females.
   f) Prolactin

      The Prolactin provides stimulation for milk production in the mammary glands of female after child birth.
6. **The Anatomy of the Posterior Pituitary Gland**
   The posterior pituitary gland is also known as neurohypophysis. It is made up of the posterior lobe of the pituitary gland. The hormones of the posterior pituitary gland are listed below:
   a) Antidiuretic Hormone (ADH)/Vasopressin

      Function of vasopressin is to enhance water re-absorption in the kidney tubules. Deficiency of vasopressin can cause Diabetes insipidus.
   b) Oxytocin

      Oxytocin facilitates childbirth by causing the contraction of uterine smooth muscles. It also facilitates lactation by causing constriction of the mammary glands during breastfeeding.
7. **The Anatomy of the Thyroid Gland**
   a) The thyroid gland is located below the thyroid cartilage in the neck region. It is one of the largest endocrine glands in the body.
   b) The overactive thyroid gland causes excessive secretion of thyroid hormone or hyperthyroidism.
   c) The underactive thyroid gland causes a condition of lack of thyroid hormone, which is known as the hypothyroidism.
   d) The hormone calcitonin is secreted by the extrafollicular cells of the thyroid gland. It causes an increased excretion of the calcium and phosphate ions via the kidneys.
8. **The Anatomy of the Parathyroid Glands**
   a) The parathyroid glands are four in number and remain embedded in the posterior surface of the thyroid gland in the neck region. These glands secrete parathyroid hormone or parathormone (PTH).
   b) PTH stimulates the bone cells to release calcium and phosphate into the blood stream.
   c) A deficiency of PTH causes hypoparathyroidism.
   d) The high levels of PTH can result in the condition of hyperparathyroidism.
9. **The Anatomy of Adrenal Glands**
   a) The adrenal (or suprarenal) glands are located on top of each kidney.
   b) The adrenal gland is divided into the following components:
      i) adrenal medulla (or the inner portion)
      ii) adrenal cortex (or the outer portion)
   c) The hormones epinephrine (or adrenalin) and norepinephrine (or noradrenalin) are produced by the adrenal medulla.
   d) The adrenal cortex is divided into the following three layers:
      i) outer layer of adrenal cortex secretes aldosterone, which is a mineralocorticoid hormone and regulates sodium reabsorption and potassium excretion by the kidney.
      ii) hormone cortisol (or hydrocortisone) is secreted by the middle layer of adrenal cortex. It stimulates the liver to manufacture glucose from the circulating amino acids. The cortisol also possesses anti-inflammatory properties.

iii) adrenal male sex hormones (or androgens) are produced by the inner layer of the adrenal cortex. These hormones enhance the male sex characteristics. The androgens are also the precursors of all estrogens (or the female sex hormones) and stimulate the female sex drive. Testosterone is the primary and most well-known androgen.

e) A deficit of adrenal cortex hormones causes Addison's disease.

f) An increased secretion of adrenal cortex causes Cushing's syndrome.

10. The Anatomy of the Pancreas

a) The pancreas is a glandular organ of both digestive and endocrine systems.

b) The islets of Langerhans of pancreas constitute its endocrine portion, and produce insulin and glucagon hormones for the regulation of blood glucose levels.

c) The blood glucose concentration is regulated by the negative feedback mechanism.

d) The clinical abnormality of diabetes mellitus is caused by the insufficient production of insulin.

11. The Anatomy of the Testes and Ovaries

a) Each of the two testes is the component of the reproductive and endocrine systems and produces the male sex hormone, testosterone.

b) Testosterone is responsible for the development of secondary male sex characteristics, which include facial and chest hairs, narrow hips, broad shoulders and deep voice.

c) Each of the two ovaries is an ovum-producing reproductive organ and secretes estrogen and progesterone, which are the female sex hormones.

d) Estrogen and progesterone are responsible for the development of the female reproductive organs and the development of secondary female sex characteristics, which include the fat deposition on thighs, hips and legs, high-pitched voice, broad hips and breast enlargement.

12. The Anatomy of the Thymus Gland

a) The thymus gland is regarded as a specialized organ of the immune system that produces the hormone thymosin.

b) Thymosin stimulates the production of the T-lymphocyte white blood cells (or T cells) that are critical cells of the adaptive immune system and protect the body against the invasion of foreign microbes.

13. The Anatomy of the Pineal Gland

a) The pineal gland is also known as the pineal body, epiphysis cerebri or epiphysis. It is a small endocrine gland located near the thalamus inside the human brain.

b) The pineal gland secretes the following hormones:

i) melatonin, which regulates the body rhythms (wake and sleep patterns) and inhibits the functions of the reproductive system.

ii) serotonin, which acts as a neurotransmitter and vasoconstrictor.

Common Pathologies

Adrenal Insufficiency

This is a condition in which the production of steroid hormones such as cortisol and aldosterone becomes low. Symptoms include fatigue, stomach upset, dehydration, and skin changes. Addison's disease is a type of adrenal insufficiency.

Cushing's Syndrome

This is a condition in which overproduction of a pituitary gland hormone (ACTH) leads to an overactive adrenal gland. A similar condition called Cushing's disease may occur in people, particularly children, who take high doses of corticosteroid medications.

Gigantism (acromegaly) and other growth hormone problems

This is a condition in which, if the pituitary gland produces too much growth hormone, a child's bones and body parts may grow abnormally fast. If growth hormone levels are too low, a child can stop growing in height.

Hyperthyroidism

This is a condition in which the thyroid gland produces too much thyroid hormone, leading to weight loss, fast heart rate, sweating, and nervousness. The most common cause for an overactive thyroid is an autoimmune disorder called Grave's disease.

Hypothyroidism

This is a condition in which, the thyroid gland does not produce enough thyroid hormone, leading to fatigue, constipation, dry skin, and depression. The underactive gland can cause slowed development in children. Some types of hypothyroidism are present at birth.

Hypopituitarism

This is a condition in which the pituitary gland releases little or no hormones. It may be caused by a number of different diseases. Women with this condition may stop getting their periods.

Polycystic Ovary Syndrome (PCOS)

This is a condition in which overproduction of androgens interfere with the development of eggs and their release from the female ovaries. PCOS is a leading cause of infertility.

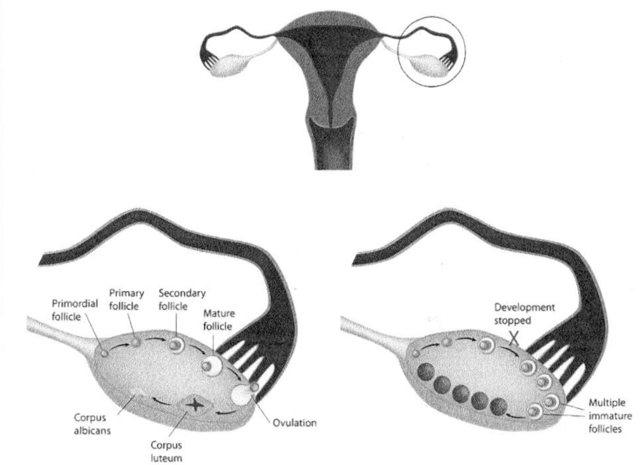

Normal Ovary *Polycystic Ovary*

Precocious Puberty

This is a condition in which abnormally early puberty occurs when glands tell the body to release sex hormones too soon in life.

Endocrine, nutritional and metabolic diseases (E00-E89)

NOTES All neoplasms, whether functionally active or not, are classified in Chapter 2. Appropriate codes in this chapter (i.e. E05.8, E07.0, E16-E31, E34.-) may be used as additional codes to indicate either functional activity by neoplasms and ectopic endocrine tissue or hyperfunction and hypofunction of endocrine glands associated with neoplasms and other conditions classified elsewhere.

EXCLUDES1 *transitory endocrine and metabolic disorders specific to newborn (P70-P74)*

This chapter contains the following blocks:

- E00-E07 Disorders of thyroid gland
- E08-E13 Diabetes mellitus
- E15-E16 Other disorders of glucose regulation and pancreatic internal secretion
- E20-E35 Disorders of other endocrine glands
- E36 Intraoperative complications of endocrine system
- E40-E46 Malnutrition
- E50-E64 Other nutritional deficiencies
- E65-E68 Overweight, obesity and other hyperalimentation
- E70-E88 Metabolic disorders
- E89 Postprocedural endocrine and metabolic complications and disorders, not elsewhere classified

Disorders of thyroid gland (E00-E07)

E00 Congenital iodine-deficiency syndrome
Use additional code (F70-F79) to identify associated intellectual disabilities.
EXCLUDES1 *subclinical iodine-deficiency hypothyroidism (E02)*

E00.0 Congenital iodine-deficiency syndrome, neurological type
Endemic cretinism, neurological type

E00.1 Congenital iodine-deficiency syndrome, myxedematous type
Endemic hypothyroid cretinism
Endemic cretinism, myxedematous type

E00.2 Congenital iodine-deficiency syndrome, mixed type
Endemic cretinism, mixed type

E00.9 Congenital iodine-deficiency syndrome, unspecified
Congenital iodine-deficiency hypothyroidism NOS
Endemic cretinism NOS

E01 Iodine-deficiency related thyroid disorders and allied conditions
EXCLUDES1 *congenital iodine-deficiency syndrome (E00.-)*
subclinical iodine-deficiency hypothyroidism (E02)

E01.0 Iodine-deficiency related diffuse (endemic) **goiter**

E01.1 Iodine-deficiency related multinodular (endemic) **goiter**
Iodine-deficiency related nodular goiter

E01.2 Iodine-deficiency related (endemic) goiter, unspecified
Endemic goiter NOS

E01.8 Other iodine-deficiency related thyroid disorders and allied conditions
Acquired iodine-deficiency hypothyroidism NOS

E02 Subclinical iodine-deficiency hypothyroidism

E03 Other hypothyroidism
EXCLUDES1 *iodine-deficiency related hypothyroidism (E00-E02)*
postprocedural hypothyroidism (E89.0)

E03.0 Congenital hypothyroidism with diffuse goiter
Congenital parenchymatous goiter (nontoxic)
Congenital goiter (nontoxic) NOS
EXCLUDES1 *transitory congenital goiter with normal function (P72.0)*

E03.1 Congenital hypothyroidism without goiter
Aplasia of thyroid (with myxedema)
Congenital atrophy of thyroid
Congenital hypothyroidism NOS

E03.2 Hypothyroidism due to medicaments and other exogenous substances
Code first poisoning due to drug or toxin, if applicable (T36-T65 with fifth or sixth character 1-4 or 6)
Use additional code for adverse effect, if applicable, to identify drug (T36-T50 with fifth or sixth character 5)

E03.3 Postinfectious **hypothyroidism**

E03.4 Atrophy **of thyroid (acquired)**
EXCLUDES1 *congenital atrophy of thyroid (E03.1)*

E03.5 Myxedema coma MCC

E03.8 Other specified hypothyroidism

E03.9 Hypothyroidism, unspecified
Myxedema NOS

E04 Other nontoxic goiter
EXCLUDES1 *congenital goiter (NOS) (diffuse) (parenchymatous) (E03.0)*
iodine-deficiency related goiter (E00-E02)

E04.0 Nontoxic diffuse **goiter**
Diffuse (colloid) nontoxic goiter
Simple nontoxic goiter

E04.1 Nontoxic single **thyroid nodule**
Colloid nodule (cystic) (thyroid)
Nontoxic uninodular goiter
Thyroid (cystic) nodule NOS

E04.2 Nontoxic multinodular **goiter**
Cystic goiter NOS
Multinodular (cystic) goiter NOS

E04.8 Other specified nontoxic goiter

E04.9 Nontoxic goiter, unspecified
Goiter NOS
Nodular goiter (nontoxic) NOS

E05 Thyrotoxicosis [hyperthyroidism]
EXCLUDES1 *chronic thyroiditis with transient thyrotoxicosis (E06.2)*
neonatal thyrotoxicosis (P72.1)

E05.0 Thyrotoxicosis with diffuse goiter
Exophthalmic or toxic goiter NOS
Graves' disease
Toxic diffuse goiter

E05.00 Thyrotoxicosis with diffuse goiter without thyrotoxic crisis or storm

E05.01 Thyrotoxicosis with diffuse goiter with thyrotoxic crisis or storm MCC

E05.1 Thyrotoxicosis with toxic single thyroid nodule
Thyrotoxicosis with toxic uninodular goiter

E05.10 Thyrotoxicosis with toxic single thyroid nodule without thyrotoxic crisis or storm

E05.11 Thyrotoxicosis with toxic single thyroid nodule with thyrotoxic crisis or storm MCC

E05.2 Thyrotoxicosis with toxic multinodular goiter
Toxic nodular goiter NOS

E05.20 Thyrotoxicosis with toxic multinodular goiter without thyrotoxic crisis or storm

E05.21 Thyrotoxicosis with toxic multinodular goiter with thyrotoxic crisis or storm MCC

E05.3 Thyrotoxicosis from ectopic thyroid tissue

E05.30 Thyrotoxicosis from ectopic thyroid tissue without thyrotoxic crisis or storm

E05.31 Thyrotoxicosis from ectopic thyroid tissue with thyrotoxic crisis or storm MCC

E05.4 Thyrotoxicosis factitia

E05.40 Thyrotoxicosis factitia without thyrotoxic crisis or storm

E05.41 Thyrotoxicosis factitia with thyrotoxic crisis or storm MCC

E05.8 Other thyrotoxicosis
Overproduction of thyroid-stimulating hormone

E05.80 Other thyrotoxicosis without thyrotoxic crisis or storm

E05.81 Other thyrotoxicosis with thyrotoxic crisis or storm MCC

E05.9 Thyrotoxicosis, unspecified
Hyperthyroidism NOS

E05.90 Thyrotoxicosis, unspecified without thyrotoxic crisis or storm

E05.91 Thyrotoxicosis, unspecified with thyrotoxic crisis or storm MCC

E06 Thyroiditis
EXCLUDES1 *postpartum thyroiditis (O90.5)*

E06.0 Acute **thyroiditis** CC
Abscess of thyroid
Pyogenic thyroiditis
Suppurative thyroiditis
Use additional code (B95-B97) to identify infectious agent.

E06.1 Subacute **thyroiditis**
de Quervain thyroiditis
Giant-cell thyroiditis
Granulomatous thyroiditis
Nonsuppurative thyroiditis
Viral thyroiditis
EXCLUDES1 *autoimmune thyroiditis (E06.3)*

Unacceptable principal diagnosis symbol per Medicare code edits | Code exempt from diagnosis present on admission requirement
Questionable admission | Complication or comorbidity | CC/MCC exclusion | Major complication or comorbidity
Principal diagnosis as its own CC | Principal diagnosis as its own MCC | Z code as first-listed diagnosis

 When symbols appear on a code that requires a 7th character extension, refer to Appendix D to identify applicable 7th character codes.

E06.2 Chronic **thyroiditis** with transient thyrotoxicosis
EXCLUDES1 *autoimmune thyroiditis (E06.3)*

E06.3 Autoimmune **thyroiditis**
Hashimoto's thyroiditis
Hashitoxicosis (transient)
Lymphadenoid goiter
Lymphocytic thyroiditis
Struma lymphomatosa

E06.4 Drug-induced **thyroiditis**
Use additional code for adverse effect, if applicable, to identify drug (T36-T50 with fifth or sixth character 5)

E06.5 **Other chronic thyroiditis**
Chronic fibrous thyroiditis
Chronic thyroiditis NOS
Ligneous thyroiditis
Riedel thyroiditis

E06.9 **Thyroiditis, unspecified**

E07 **Other disorders of thyroid**

E07.0 **Hypersecretion of calcitonin**
C-cell hyperplasia of thyroid
Hypersecretion of thyrocalcitonin

E07.1 **Dyshormogenetic goiter**
Familial dyshormogenetic goiter
Pendred's syndrome
EXCLUDES1 *transitory congenital goiter with normal function (P72.0)*

E07.8 **Other specified disorders of thyroid**

E07.81 **Sick-euthyroid syndrome**
Euthyroid sick-syndrome

E07.89 **Other specified disorders of thyroid**
Abnormality of thyroid-binding globulin
Hemorrhage of thyroid
Infarction of thyroid

E07.9 **Disorder of thyroid, unspecified**

Diabetes mellitus (E08-E13)

E08 **Diabetes mellitus** due to underlying condition
Code first the underlying condition, such as:
congenital rubella (P35.0)
Cushing's syndrome (E24.-)
cystic fibrosis (E84.-)
malignant neoplasm (C00-C96)
malnutrition (E40-E46)
pancreatitis and other diseases of the pancreas (K85-K86.-)
Use additional code to identify ▶control using:◀
insulin (Z79.4)
oral antidiabetic drugs (Z79.84)
oral hypoglycemic drugs (Z79.84)
EXCLUDES1 *drug or chemical induced diabetes mellitus (E09.-)*
gestational diabetes (O24.4-)
neonatal diabetes mellitus (P70.2)
postpancreatectomy diabetes mellitus (E13.-)
postprocedural diabetes mellitus (E13.-)
secondary diabetes mellitus NEC (E13.-)
type 1 diabetes mellitus (E10.-)
type 2 diabetes mellitus (E11.-)

E08.0 **Diabetes mellitus due to underlying condition with** hyperosmolarity

E08.00 **Diabetes mellitus due to underlying condition with hyperosmolarity** without nonketotic hyperglycemic-hyperosmolar coma (NKHHC) HAC MCC

E08.01 **Diabetes mellitus due to underlying condition with hyperosmolarity** with coma HAC MCC

E08.1 **Diabetes mellitus due to underlying condition with** ketoacidosis

E08.10 **Diabetes mellitus due to underlying condition with ketoacidosis** without coma HAC MCC

E08.11 **Diabetes mellitus due to underlying condition with ketoacidosis** with coma MCC

E08.2 **Diabetes mellitus due to underlying condition with** kidney complications

E08.21 **Diabetes mellitus due to underlying condition with diabetic** nephropathy
Diabetes mellitus due to underlying condition with intercapillary glomerulosclerosis
Diabetes mellitus due to underlying condition with intracapillary glomerulonephrosis
Diabetes mellitus due to underlying condition with Kimmelstiel-Wilson disease

E08.22 **Diabetes mellitus due to underlying condition with diabetic** chronic kidney disease
Use additional code to identify stage of chronic kidney disease (N18.1-N18.6)

E08.29 **Diabetes mellitus due to underlying condition with other diabetic kidney complication**
Renal tubular degeneration in diabetes mellitus due to underlying condition

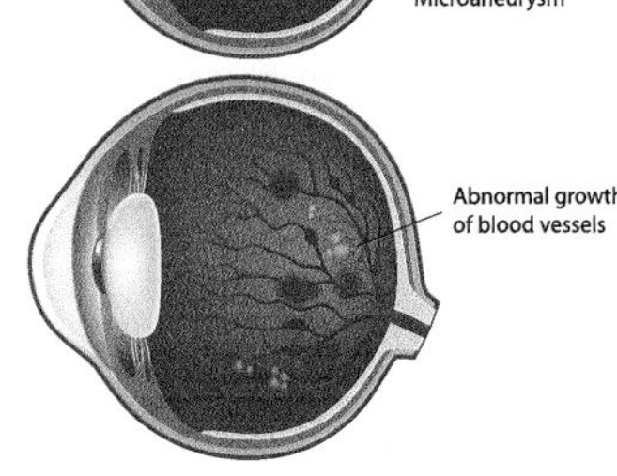

Figure 4.1 Diabetic retinopathy

E08.3 **Diabetes mellitus due to underlying condition with** ophthalmic complications

E08.31 **Diabetes mellitus due to underlying condition with unspecified** diabetic retinopathy

E08.311 **Diabetes mellitus due to underlying condition with unspecified diabetic retinopathy** with macular edema

E08.319 **Diabetes mellitus due to underlying condition with unspecified diabetic retinopathy** without macular edema

E08.32 **Diabetes mellitus due to underlying condition** with mild nonproliferative diabetic retinopathy
Diabetes mellitus due to underlying condition with nonproliferative diabetic retinopathy NOS
One of the following 7th characters is to be assigned to codes in subcategory E08.32 to designate laterality of the disease:
1 = right eye
2 = left eye
3 = bilateral
9 = unspecified eye

E08.321 **Diabetes mellitus due to underlying condition with mild nonproliferative diabetic retinopathy** with macular edema CC/MCC Exc

E08.329 **Diabetes mellitus due to underlying condition with mild nonproliferative diabetic retinopathy** without macular edema CC/MCC Exc

Unspecified Code | Other Specified Code | Manifestation Code | N Newborn | P Pediatric | M Maternity | A Adult | ♂ Male | ♀ Female
● New Code ▲ Revised Code Title ▶◀ Revised Text NOTES INCLUDES EXCLUDES1 Not coded here EXCLUDES2 Not included here
4th character required 5th character required 6th character required 7th character required
Extension 'X' Alert HAC Hospital-acquired condition (HAC) alert AHA AHA Coding Clinic©

E08.33 Diabetes mellitus due to underlying condition with moderate nonproliferative diabetic retinopathy
One of the following 7th characters is to be assigned to codes in subcategory E08.33 to designate laterality of the disease:
1 = right eye
2 = left eye
3 = bilateral
9 = unspecified eye
E08.331 Diabetes mellitus due to underlying condition with moderate nonproliferative diabetic retinopathy with macular edema
E08.339 Diabetes mellitus due to underlying condition with moderate nonproliferative diabetic retinopathy without macular edema
E08.34 Diabetes mellitus due to underlying condition with severe nonproliferative diabetic retinopathy
One of the following 7th characters is to be assigned to codes in subcategory E08.34 to designate laterality of the disease:
1 = right eye
2 = left eye
3 = bilateral
9 = unspecified eye
E08.341 Diabetes mellitus due to underlying condition with severe nonproliferative diabetic retinopathy with macular edema
E08.349 Diabetes mellitus due to underlying condition with severe nonproliferative diabetic retinopathy without macular edema
E08.35 Diabetes mellitus due to underlying condition with proliferative diabetic retinopathy
One of the following 7th characters is to be assigned to codes in subcategory E08.35 to designate laterality of the disease:
1 = right eye
2 = left eye
3 = bilateral
9 = unspecified eye
E08.351 Diabetes mellitus due to underlying condition with proliferative diabetic retinopathy with macular edema
E08.352 Diabetes mellitus due to underlying condition with proliferative diabetic retinopathy with traction retinal detachment involving the macula
E08.353 Diabetes mellitus due to underlying condition with proliferative diabetic retinopathy with traction retinal detachment not involving the macula
E08.354 Diabetes mellitus due to underlying condition with proliferative diabetic retinopathy with combined traction retinal detachment and rhegmatogenous retinal detachment
E08.355 Diabetes mellitus due to underlying condition with stable proliferative diabetic retinopathy
E08.359 Diabetes mellitus due to underlying condition with proliferative diabetic retinopathy without macular edema
E08.36 Diabetes mellitus due to underlying condition with diabetic cataract
E08.37 Diabetes mellitus due to underlying condition with diabetic macular edema, resolved following treatment
One of the following 7th characters is to be assigned to code E08.37 to designate laterality of the disease:
1 = right eye
2 = left eye
3 = bilateral
9 = unspecified eye

E08.39 Diabetes mellitus due to underlying condition with other diabetic ophthalmic complication
Use additional code to identify manifestation, such as: diabetic glaucoma (H40-H42)
E08.4 Diabetes mellitus due to underlying condition with neurological complications
E08.40 Diabetes mellitus due to underlying condition with diabetic neuropathy, unspecified
E08.41 Diabetes mellitus due to underlying condition with diabetic mononeuropathy
E08.42 Diabetes mellitus due to underlying condition with diabetic polyneuropathy
Diabetes mellitus due to underlying condition with diabetic neuralgia
E08.43 Diabetes mellitus due to underlying condition with diabetic autonomic (poly)neuropathy
Diabetes mellitus due to underlying condition with diabetic gastroparesis
AHA: Q4, 2013
E08.44 Diabetes mellitus due to underlying condition with diabetic amyotrophy
E08.49 Diabetes mellitus due to underlying condition with other diabetic neurological complication
E08.5 Diabetes mellitus due to underlying condition with circulatory complications
E08.51 Diabetes mellitus due to underlying condition with diabetic peripheral angiopathy without gangrene
E08.52 Diabetes mellitus due to underlying condition with diabetic peripheral angiopathy with gangrene
Diabetes mellitus due to underlying condition with diabetic gangrene
E08.59 Diabetes mellitus due to underlying condition with other circulatory complications
E08.6 Diabetes mellitus due to underlying condition with other specified complications
E08.61 Diabetes mellitus due to underlying condition with diabetic arthropathy
E08.610 Diabetes mellitus due to underlying condition with diabetic neuropathic arthropathy
Diabetes mellitus due to underlying condition with Charcôt's joints
E08.618 Diabetes mellitus due to underlying condition with other diabetic arthropathy
E08.62 Diabetes mellitus due to underlying condition with skin complications
E08.620 Diabetes mellitus due to underlying condition with diabetic dermatitis
Diabetes mellitus due to underlying condition with diabetic necrobiosis lipoidica
E08.621 Diabetes mellitus due to underlying condition with foot ulcer
Use additional code to identify site of ulcer (L97.4-, L97.5-)
E08.622 Diabetes mellitus due to underlying condition with other skin ulcer
Use additional code to identify site of ulcer (L97.1-L97.9, L98.41-L98.49)
E08.628 Diabetes mellitus due to underlying condition with other skin complications
E08.63 Diabetes mellitus due to underlying condition with oral complications
E08.630 Diabetes mellitus due to underlying condition with periodontal disease
E08.638 Diabetes mellitus due to underlying condition with other oral complications
E08.64 Diabetes mellitus due to underlying condition with hypoglycemia
E08.641 Diabetes mellitus due to underlying condition with hypoglycemia with coma
E08.649 Diabetes mellitus due to underlying condition with hypoglycemia without coma
E08.65 Diabetes mellitus due to underlying condition with hyperglycemia

Unacceptable principal diagnosis symbol per Medicare code edits; Code exempt from diagnosis present on admission requirement; Questionable admission; Complication or comorbidity; CC/MCC exclusion; Major complication or comorbidity; Principal diagnosis as its own CC; Principal diagnosis as its own MCC; Z code as first-listed diagnosis

E08.69 Diabetes mellitus due to underlying condition with other specified complication
Use additional code to identify complication

E08.8 Diabetes mellitus due to underlying condition with unspecified complications

E08.9 Diabetes mellitus due to underlying condition without complications

E09 Drug or chemical induced diabetes mellitus
Code first poisoning due to drug or toxin, if applicable (T36-T65 with fifth or sixth character 1-4 or 6)
Use additional code for adverse effect, if applicable, to identify drug (T36-T50 with fifth or sixth character 5)
Use additional code to identify ▶control using:◀
insulin (Z79.4)
oral antidiabetic drugs (Z79.84)
oral hypoglycemic drugs (Z79.84)

EXCLUDES1 *diabetes mellitus due to underlying condition (E08.-)*
gestational diabetes (O24.4-)
neonatal diabetes mellitus (P70.2)
postpancreatectomy diabetes mellitus (E13.-)
postprocedural diabetes mellitus (E13.-)
secondary diabetes mellitus NEC (E13.-)
type 1 diabetes mellitus (E10.-)
type 2 diabetes mellitus (E11.-)

E09.0 Drug or chemical induced diabetes mellitus with hyperosmolarity

E09.00 Drug or chemical induced diabetes mellitus with hyperosmolarity without nonketotic hyperglycemic-hyperosmolar coma (NKHHC) HAC MCC

E09.01 Drug or chemical induced diabetes mellitus with hyperosmolarity with coma HAC MCC

E09.1 Drug or chemical induced diabetes mellitus with ketoacidosis

E09.10 Drug or chemical induced diabetes mellitus with ketoacidosis without coma HAC MCC

E09.11 Drug or chemical induced diabetes mellitus with ketoacidosis with coma MCC

E09.2 Drug or chemical induced diabetes mellitus with kidney complications

E09.21 Drug or chemical induced diabetes mellitus with diabetic nephropathy
Drug or chemical induced diabetes mellitus with intercapillary glomerulosclerosis
Drug or chemical induced diabetes mellitus with intracapillary glomerulonephrosis
Drug or chemical induced diabetes mellitus with Kimmelstiel-Wilson disease

E09.22 Drug or chemical induced diabetes mellitus with diabetic chronic kidney disease
Use additional code to identify stage of chronic kidney disease (N18.1-N18.6)

E09.29 Drug or chemical induced diabetes mellitus with other diabetic kidney complication
Drug or chemical induced diabetes mellitus with renal tubular degeneration

E09.3 Drug or chemical induced diabetes mellitus with ophthalmic complications

E09.31 Drug or chemical induced diabetes mellitus with unspecified diabetic retinopathy

E09.311 Drug or chemical induced diabetes mellitus with unspecified diabetic retinopathy with macular edema

E09.319 Drug or chemical induced diabetes mellitus with unspecified diabetic retinopathy without macular edema

E09.32 Drug or chemical induced diabetes mellitus with mild nonproliferative diabetic retinopathy
Drug or chemical induced diabetes mellitus with nonproliferative diabetic retinopathy NOS
One of the following 7th characters is to be assigned to codes in subcategory E09.32 to designate laterality of the disease:
1 = right eye
2 = left eye
3 = bilateral
9 = unspecified eye

E09.321 Drug or chemical induced diabetes mellitus with mild nonproliferative diabetic retinopathy with macular edema CC/MCC Exc

E09.329 Drug or chemical induced diabetes mellitus with mild nonproliferative diabetic retinopathy without macular edema CC/MCC Exc

E09.33 Drug or chemical induced diabetes mellitus with moderate nonproliferative diabetic retinopathy
One of the following 7th characters is to be assigned to codes in subcategory E09.33 to designate laterality of the disease:
1 = right eye
2 = left eye
3 = bilateral
9 = unspecified eye

E09.331 Drug or chemical induced diabetes mellitus with moderate nonproliferative diabetic retinopathy with macular edema CC/MCC Exc

E09.339 Drug or chemical induced diabetes mellitus with moderate nonproliferative diabetic retinopathy without macular edema CC/MCC Exc

E09.34 Drug or chemical induced diabetes mellitus with severe nonproliferative diabetic retinopathy
One of the following 7th characters is to be assigned to codes in subcategory E09.34 to designate laterality of the disease:
1 = right eye
2 = left eye
3 = bilateral
9 = unspecified eye

E09.341 Drug or chemical induced diabetes mellitus with severe nonproliferative diabetic retinopathy with macular edema CC/MCC Exc

E09.349 Drug or chemical induced diabetes mellitus with severe nonproliferative diabetic retinopathy without macular edema CC/MCC Exc

E09.35 Drug or chemical induced diabetes mellitus with proliferative diabetic retinopathy
One of the following 7th characters is to be assigned to codes in subcategory E09.35 to designate laterality of the disease:
1 = right eye
2 = left eye
3 = bilateral
9 = unspecified eye

E09.351 Drug or chemical induced diabetes mellitus with proliferative diabetic retinopathy with macular edema CC/MCC Exc

● E09.352 Drug or chemical induced diabetes mellitus with proliferative diabetic retinopathy with traction retinal detachment involving the macula CC/MCC Exc

● E09.353 Drug or chemical induced diabetes mellitus with proliferative diabetic retinopathy with traction retinal detachment not involving the macula CC/MCC Exc

● E09.354 Drug or chemical induced diabetes mellitus with proliferative diabetic retinopathy with combined traction retinal detachment and rhegmatogenous retinal detachment CC/MCC Exc

● E09.355 Drug or chemical induced diabetes mellitus with stable proliferative diabetic retinopathy CC/MCC Exc

E09.359 Drug or chemical induced diabetes mellitus with proliferative diabetic retinopathy without macular edema CC/MCC Exc

E09.36 Drug or chemical induced diabetes mellitus with diabetic cataract

Unspecified Code | Other Specified Code | Manifestation Code | N Newborn | P Pediatric | M Maternity | A Adult | ♂ Male | ♀ Female
● New Code | ▲ Revised Code Title | ▶◀ Revised Text | NOTES | INCLUDES | EXCLUDES1 Not coded here | EXCLUDES2 Not included here
4th character required | 5th character required | 6th character required | 7th character required
Extension 'X' Alert | HAC Hospital-acquired condition (HAC) alert | AHA AHA Coding Clinic©

● E09.37 Drug or chemical induced diabetes mellitus with diabetic macular edema, resolved following treatment CC/MCC Exc

One of the following 7th characters is to be assigned to code E09.37 to designate laterality of the disease:
- 1 = right eye
- 2 = left eye
- 3 = bilateral
- 9 = unspecified eye

E09.39 Drug or chemical induced diabetes mellitus with other diabetic ophthalmic complication
Use additional code to identify manifestation, such as:
diabetic glaucoma (H40-H42)

E09.4 Drug or chemical induced diabetes mellitus with neurological complications

E09.40 Drug or chemical induced diabetes mellitus with neurological complications with diabetic neuropathy, unspecified

E09.41 Drug or chemical induced diabetes mellitus with neurological complications with diabetic mononeuropathy

E09.42 Drug or chemical induced diabetes mellitus with neurological complications with diabetic polyneuropathy
Drug or chemical induced diabetes mellitus with diabetic neuralgia

E09.43 Drug or chemical induced diabetes mellitus with neurological complications with diabetic autonomic (poly)neuropathy
Drug or chemical induced diabetes mellitus with diabetic gastroparesis
AHA: Q4, 2013

E09.44 Drug or chemical induced diabetes mellitus with neurological complications with diabetic amyotrophy

E09.49 Drug or chemical induced diabetes mellitus with neurological complications with other diabetic neurological complication

E09.5 Drug or chemical induced diabetes mellitus with circulatory complications

E09.51 Drug or chemical induced diabetes mellitus with diabetic peripheral angiopathy without gangrene

E09.52 Drug or chemical induced diabetes mellitus with diabetic peripheral angiopathy with gangrene CC PDx CC
Drug or chemical induced diabetes mellitus with diabetic gangrene

E09.59 Drug or chemical induced diabetes mellitus with other circulatory complications

E09.6 Drug or chemical induced diabetes mellitus with other specified complications

E09.61 Drug or chemical induced diabetes mellitus with diabetic arthropathy

E09.610 Drug or chemical induced diabetes mellitus with diabetic neuropathic arthropathy
Drug or chemical induced diabetes mellitus with Charcôt's joints

E09.618 Drug or chemical induced diabetes mellitus with other diabetic arthropathy

E09.62 Drug or chemical induced diabetes mellitus with skin complications

E09.620 Drug or chemical induced diabetes mellitus with diabetic dermatitis
Drug or chemical induced diabetes mellitus with diabetic necrobiosis lipoidica

E09.621 Drug or chemical induced diabetes mellitus with foot ulcer
Use additional code to identify site of ulcer (L97.4-, L97.5-)

E09.622 Drug or chemical induced diabetes mellitus with other skin ulcer
Use additional code to identify site of ulcer (L97.1-L97.9, L98.41-L98.49)

E09.628 Drug or chemical induced diabetes mellitus with other skin complications

E09.63 Drug or chemical induced diabetes mellitus with oral complications

E09.630 Drug or chemical induced diabetes mellitus with periodontal disease

E09.638 Drug or chemical induced diabetes mellitus with other oral complications

E09.64 Drug or chemical induced diabetes mellitus with hypoglycemia

E09.641 Drug or chemical induced diabetes mellitus with hypoglycemia with coma MCC

E09.649 Drug or chemical induced diabetes mellitus with hypoglycemia without coma

E09.65 Drug or chemical induced diabetes mellitus with hyperglycemia

E09.69 Drug or chemical induced diabetes mellitus with other specified complication
Use additional code to identify complication

E09.8 Drug or chemical induced diabetes mellitus with unspecified complications

E09.9 Drug or chemical induced diabetes mellitus without complications

E10 Type 1 diabetes mellitus

INCLUDES
brittle diabetes (mellitus)
diabetes (mellitus) due to autoimmune process
diabetes (mellitus) due to immune mediated pancreatic islet beta-cell destruction
idiopathic diabetes (mellitus)
juvenile onset diabetes (mellitus)
ketosis-prone diabetes (mellitus)

EXCLUDES1
diabetes mellitus due to underlying condition (E08.-)
drug or chemical induced diabetes mellitus (E09.-)
gestational diabetes (O24.4-)
hyperglycemia NOS (R73.9)
neonatal diabetes mellitus (P70.2)
postpancreatectomy diabetes mellitus (E13.-)
postprocedural diabetes mellitus (E13.-)
secondary diabetes mellitus NEC (E13.-)
type 2 diabetes mellitus (E11.-)

E10.1 Type 1 diabetes mellitus with ketoacidosis

E10.10 Type 1 diabetes mellitus with ketoacidosis without coma HAC MCC
AHA: Q3, 2013

E10.11 Type 1 diabetes mellitus with ketoacidosis with coma MCC

E10.2 Type 1 diabetes mellitus with kidney complications

E10.21 Type 1 diabetes mellitus with diabetic nephropathy
Type 1 diabetes mellitus with intercapillary glomerulosclerosis
Type 1 diabetes mellitus with intracapillary glomerulonephrosis
Type 1 diabetes mellitus with Kimmelstiel-Wilson disease

E10.22 Type 1 diabetes mellitus with diabetic chronic kidney disease
Use additional code to identify stage of chronic kidney disease (N18.1-N18.6)

E10.29 Type 1 diabetes mellitus with other diabetic kidney complication
Type 1 diabetes mellitus with renal tubular degeneration
AHA: Q1, 2016

E10.3 Type 1 diabetes mellitus with ophthalmic complications

E10.31 Type 1 diabetes mellitus with unspecified diabetic retinopathy

E10.311 Type 1 diabetes mellitus with unspecified diabetic retinopathy with macular edema

E10.319 Type 1 diabetes mellitus with unspecified diabetic retinopathy without macular edema

PDx Unacceptable principal diagnosis symbol per Medicare code edits; POA Code exempt from diagnosis present on admission requirement; ? Questionable admission; CC Complication or comorbidity; CC/MCC Exc CC/MCC exclusion; MCC Major complication or comorbidity; PDx CC Principal diagnosis as its own CC; PDx MCC Principal diagnosis as its own MCC; Z Z code as first-listed diagnosis

E10.32 Type 1 diabetes mellitus with mild nonproliferative diabetic retinopathy
Type 1 diabetes mellitus with nonproliferative diabetic retinopathy NOS
One of the following 7th characters is to be assigned to codes in subcategory E10.32 to designate laterality of the disease:
1 = right eye
2 = left eye
3 = bilateral
9 = unspecified eye
E10.321 Type 1 diabetes mellitus with mild nonproliferative diabetic retinopathy with macular edema CC/MCC Exc
E10.329 Type 1 diabetes mellitus with mild nonproliferative diabetic retinopathy without macular edema CC/MCC Exc
E10.33 Type 1 diabetes mellitus with moderate nonproliferative diabetic retinopathy
One of the following 7th characters is to be assigned to codes in subcategory E10.33 to designate laterality of the disease:
1 = right eye
2 = left eye
3 = bilateral
9 = unspecified eye
E10.331 Type 1 diabetes mellitus with moderate nonproliferative diabetic retinopathy with macular edema CC/MCC Exc
E10.339 Type 1 diabetes mellitus with moderate nonproliferative diabetic retinopathy without macular edema CC/MCC Exc
E10.34 Type 1 diabetes mellitus with severe nonproliferative diabetic retinopathy
One of the following 7th characters is to be assigned to codes in subcategory E10.34 to designate laterality of the disease:
1 = right eye
2 = left eye
3 = bilateral
9 = unspecified eye
E10.341 Type 1 diabetes mellitus with severe nonproliferative diabetic retinopathy with macular edema CC/MCC Exc
E10.349 Type 1 diabetes mellitus with severe nonproliferative diabetic retinopathy without macular edema CC/MCC Exc
E10.35 Type 1 diabetes mellitus with proliferative diabetic retinopathy
One of the following 7th characters is to be assigned to codes in subcategory E10.35 to designate laterality of the disease:
1 = right eye
2 = left eye
3 = bilateral
9 = unspecified eye
E10.351 Type 1 diabetes mellitus with proliferative diabetic retinopathy with macular edema CC/MCC Exc
● E10.352 Type 1 diabetes mellitus with proliferative diabetic retinopathy with traction retinal detachment involving the macula CC/MCC Exc
● E10.353 Type 1 diabetes mellitus with proliferative diabetic retinopathy with traction retinal detachment not involving the macula CC/MCC Exc
● E10.354 Type 1 diabetes mellitus with proliferative diabetic retinopathy with combined traction retinal detachment and rhegmatogenous retinal detachment CC/MCC Exc
● E10.355 Type 1 diabetes mellitus with stable proliferative diabetic retinopathy CC/MCC Exc
E10.359 Type 1 diabetes mellitus with proliferative diabetic retinopathy without macular edema CC/MCC Exc

E10.36 Type 1 diabetes mellitus with diabetic cataract
● E10.37 Type 1 diabetes mellitus with diabetic macular edema, resolved following treatment CC/MCC Exc
One of the following 7th characters is to be assigned to code E10.37 to designate laterality of the disease:
1 = right eye
2 = left eye
3 = bilateral
9 = unspecified eye
E10.39 Type 1 diabetes mellitus with other diabetic ophthalmic complication
Use additional code to identify manifestation, such as:
diabetic glaucoma (H40-H42)
E10.4 Type 1 diabetes mellitus with neurological complications
E10.40 Type 1 diabetes mellitus with diabetic neuropathy, unspecified
E10.41 Type 1 diabetes mellitus with diabetic mononeuropathy
E10.42 Type 1 diabetes mellitus with diabetic polyneuropathy
Type 1 diabetes mellitus with diabetic neuralgia
E10.43 Type 1 diabetes mellitus with diabetic autonomic (poly)neuropathy
Type 1 diabetes mellitus with diabetic gastroparesis
AHA: Q4, 2013
E10.44 Type 1 diabetes mellitus with diabetic amyotrophy
E10.49 Type 1 diabetes mellitus with other diabetic neurological complication
E10.5 Type 1 diabetes mellitus with circulatory complications
E10.51 Type 1 diabetes mellitus with diabetic peripheral angiopathy without gangrene
E10.52 Type 1 diabetes mellitus with diabetic peripheral angiopathy with gangrene CC PDx
Type 1 diabetes mellitus with diabetic gangrene
E10.59 Type 1 diabetes mellitus with other circulatory complications
E10.6 Type 1 diabetes mellitus with other specified complications
E10.61 Type 1 diabetes mellitus with diabetic arthropathy
E10.610 Type 1 diabetes mellitus with diabetic neuropathic arthropathy
Type 1 diabetes mellitus with Charcôt's joints
E10.618 Type 1 diabetes mellitus with other diabetic arthropathy
E10.62 Type 1 diabetes mellitus with skin complications
E10.620 Type 1 diabetes mellitus with diabetic dermatitis
Type 1 diabetes mellitus with diabetic necrobiosis lipoidica
E10.621 Type 1 diabetes mellitus with foot ulcer
Use additional code to identify site of ulcer (L97.4-, L97.5-)
E10.622 Type 1 diabetes mellitus with other skin ulcer
Use additional code to identify site of ulcer (L97.1-L97.9, L98.41-L98.49)
E10.628 Type 1 diabetes mellitus with other skin complications
E10.63 Type 1 diabetes mellitus with oral complications
E10.630 Type 1 diabetes mellitus with periodontal disease
E10.638 Type 1 diabetes mellitus with other oral complications
E10.64 Type 1 diabetes mellitus with hypoglycemia
E10.641 Type 1 diabetes mellitus with hypoglycemia with coma MCC
E10.649 Type 1 diabetes mellitus with hypoglycemia without coma
AHA: Q1, 2016
E10.65 Type 1 diabetes mellitus with hyperglycemia
AHA: Q3, 2013
E10.69 Type 1 diabetes mellitus with other specified complication
Use additional code to identify complication
E10.8 Type 1 diabetes mellitus with unspecified complications
E10.9 Type 1 diabetes mellitus without complications

Unspecified Code Other Specified Code Manifestation Code N Newborn P Pediatric M Maternity A Adult ♂ Male ♀ Female
● New Code ▲ Revised Code Title ►◄ Revised Text NOTES INCLUDES EXCLUDES1 Not coded here EXCLUDES2 Not included here
4th character required 5th character required 6th character required 7th character required
Extension 'X' Alert HAC Hospital-acquired condition (HAC) alert AHA AHA Coding Clinic©

E11 Type 2 diabetes mellitus

INCLUDES *diabetes (mellitus) due to insulin secretory defect*
diabetes NOS
insulin resistant diabetes (mellitus)

Use additional code to identify ▶control using: ◀
insulin (Z79.4)
oral antidiabetic drugs (Z79.84)
oral hypoglycemic drugs (Z79.84)

EXCLUDES1 *diabetes mellitus due to underlying condition (E08.-)*
drug or chemical induced diabetes mellitus (E09.-)
gestational diabetes (O24.4-)
neonatal diabetes mellitus (P70.2)
postpancreatectomy diabetes mellitus (E13.-)
postprocedural diabetes mellitus (E13.-)
secondary diabetes mellitus NEC (E13.-)
type 1 diabetes mellitus (E10.-)

E11.0 Type 2 diabetes mellitus with hyperosmolarity

E11.00 Type 2 diabetes mellitus with hyperosmolarity without nonketotic hyperglycemic-hyperosmolar coma (NKHHC) HAC MCC

E11.01 Type 2 diabetes mellitus with hyperosmolarity with coma HAC MCC

E11.2 Type 2 diabetes mellitus with kidney complications

E11.21 Type 2 diabetes mellitus with diabetic nephropathy
Type 2 diabetes mellitus with intercapillary glomerulosclerosis
Type 2 diabetes mellitus with intracapillary glomerulonephrosis
Type 2 diabetes mellitus with Kimmelstiel-Wilson disease

E11.22 Type 2 diabetes mellitus with diabetic chronic kidney disease
Use additional code to identify stage of chronic kidney disease (N18.1-N18.6)
AHA: Q1, 2016

E11.29 Type 2 diabetes mellitus with other diabetic kidney complication
Type 2 diabetes mellitus with renal tubular degeneration

E11.3 Type 2 diabetes mellitus with ophthalmic complications

E11.31 Type 2 diabetes mellitus with unspecified diabetic retinopathy

E11.311 Type 2 diabetes mellitus with unspecified diabetic retinopathy with macular edema

E11.319 Type 2 diabetes mellitus with unspecified diabetic retinopathy without macular edema
AHA: Q3, 2013

E11.32 Type 2 diabetes mellitus with mild nonproliferative diabetic retinopathy
Type 2 diabetes mellitus with nonproliferative diabetic retinopathy NOS
One of the following 7th characters is to be assigned to codes in subcategory E11.32 to designate laterality of the disease:
1 = right eye
2 = left eye
3 = bilateral
9 = unspecified eye

E11.321 Type 2 diabetes mellitus with mild nonproliferative diabetic retinopathy with macular edema CC/MCC Exc

E11.329 Type 2 diabetes mellitus with mild nonproliferative diabetic retinopathy without macular edema CC/MCC Exc

E11.33 Type 2 diabetes mellitus with moderate nonproliferative diabetic retinopathy
One of the following 7th characters is to be assigned to codes in subcategory E11.33 to designate laterality of the disease:
1 = right eye
2 = left eye
3 = bilateral
9 = unspecified eye

E11.331 Type 2 diabetes mellitus with moderate nonproliferative diabetic retinopathy with macular edema CC/MCC Exc

E11.339 Type 2 diabetes mellitus with moderate nonproliferative diabetic retinopathy without macular edema CC/MCC Exc

E11.34 Type 2 diabetes mellitus with severe nonproliferative diabetic retinopathy
One of the following 7th characters is to be assigned to codes in subcategory E11.34 to designate laterality of the disease:
1 = right eye
2 = left eye
3 = bilateral
9 = unspecified eye

E11.341 Type 2 diabetes mellitus with severe nonproliferative diabetic retinopathy with macular edema CC/MCC Exc

E11.349 Type 2 diabetes mellitus with severe nonproliferative diabetic retinopathy without macular edema CC/MCC Exc

E11.35 Type 2 diabetes mellitus with proliferative diabetic retinopathy
One of the following 7th characters is to be assigned to codes in subcategory E11.35 to designate laterality of the disease:
1 = right eye
2 = left eye
3 = bilateral
9 = unspecified eye

E11.351 Type 2 diabetes mellitus with proliferative diabetic retinopathy with macular edema CC/MCC Exc

● **E11.352 Type 2 diabetes mellitus with proliferative diabetic retinopathy with traction retinal detachment involving the macula** CC/MCC Exc

● **E11.353 Type 2 diabetes mellitus with proliferative diabetic retinopathy with traction retinal detachment not involving the macula** CC/MCC Exc

● **E11.354 Type 2 diabetes mellitus with proliferative diabetic retinopathy with combined traction retinal detachment and rhegmatogenous retinal detachment** CC/MCC Exc

● **E11.355 Type 2 diabetes mellitus with stable proliferative diabetic retinopathy** CC/MCC Exc

E11.359 Type 2 diabetes mellitus with proliferative diabetic retinopathy without macular edema CC/MCC Exc

E11.36 Type 2 diabetes mellitus with diabetic cataract
AHA: Q2, 2016

● **E11.37 Type 2 diabetes mellitus with diabetic macular edema, resolved following treatment** CC/MCC Exc
One of the following 7th characters is to be assigned to code E11.37 to designate laterality of the disease:
1 = right eye
2 = left eye
3 = bilateral
9 = unspecified eye

E11.39 Type 2 diabetes mellitus with other diabetic ophthalmic complication
Use additional code to identify manifestation, such as:
diabetic glaucoma (H40-H42)

E11.4 Type 2 diabetes mellitus with neurological complications

E11.40 Type 2 diabetes mellitus with diabetic neuropathy, unspecified
AHA: Q4, 2013

E11.41 Type 2 diabetes mellitus with diabetic mononeuropathy

E11.42 Type 2 diabetes mellitus with diabetic polyneuropathy
Type 2 diabetes mellitus with diabetic neuralgia
AHA: Q1, 2016

Unacceptable principal diagnosis symbol per Medicare code edits | Code exempt from diagnosis present on admission requirement | Questionable admission | Complication or comorbidity | CC/MCC exclusion | Major complication or comorbidity | Principal diagnosis as its own CC | Principal diagnosis as its own MCC | Z code as first-listed diagnosis

E11.43 Type 2 diabetes mellitus with diabetic autonomic (poly)neuropathy
Type 2 diabetes mellitus with diabetic gastroparesis
AHA: Q4, 2013

E11.44 Type 2 diabetes mellitus with diabetic amyotrophy
AHA: Q2, 2016

E11.49 Type 2 diabetes mellitus with other diabetic neurological complication

E11.5 Type 2 diabetes mellitus with circulatory complications

E11.51 Type 2 diabetes mellitus with diabetic peripheral angiopathy without gangrene

E11.52 Type 2 diabetes mellitus with diabetic peripheral angiopathy with gangrene CC PDx
Type 2 diabetes mellitus with diabetic gangrene

E11.59 Type 2 diabetes mellitus with other circulatory complications

E11.6 Type 2 diabetes mellitus with other specified complications

E11.61 Type 2 diabetes mellitus with diabetic arthropathy

E11.610 Type 2 diabetes mellitus with diabetic neuropathic arthropathy
Type 2 diabetes mellitus with Charcôt's joints
AHA: Q2, 2016

E11.618 Type 2 diabetes mellitus with other diabetic arthropathy
AHA: Q2, 2016

E11.62 Type 2 diabetes mellitus with skin complications

E11.620 Type 2 diabetes mellitus with diabetic dermatitis
Type 2 diabetes mellitus with diabetic necrobiosis lipoidica

E11.621 Type 2 diabetes mellitus with foot ulcer
Use additional code to identify site of ulcer (L97.4-, L97.5-)
AHA: Q1, 2016

E11.622 Type 2 diabetes mellitus with other skin ulcer
Use additional code to identify site of ulcer (L97.1-L97.9, L98.41-L98.49)

E11.628 Type 2 diabetes mellitus with other skin complications

E11.63 Type 2 diabetes mellitus with oral complications

E11.630 Type 2 diabetes mellitus with periodontal disease

E11.638 Type 2 diabetes mellitus with other oral complications

E11.64 Type 2 diabetes mellitus with hypoglycemia

E11.641 Type 2 diabetes mellitus with hypoglycemia with coma MCC

E11.649 Type 2 diabetes mellitus with hypoglycemia without coma
AHA: Q3, 2015

E11.65 Type 2 diabetes mellitus with hyperglycemia
AHA: Q3, 2013

E11.69 Type 2 diabetes mellitus with other specified complication
Use additional code to identify complication

E11.8 Type 2 diabetes mellitus with unspecified complications

E11.9 Type 2 diabetes mellitus without complications
AHA: Q4, 2013

E13 Other specified diabetes mellitus

INCLUDES *diabetes mellitus due to genetic defects of beta-cell function*
diabetes mellitus due to genetic defects in insulin action
postpancreatectomy diabetes mellitus
postprocedural diabetes mellitus
secondary diabetes mellitus NEC

Use additional code to identify ▶control using:◀
insulin (Z79.4)
oral antidiabetic drugs (Z79.84)
oral hypoglycemic drugs (Z79.84)

EXCLUDES1 *diabetes (mellitus) due to autoimmune process (E10.-)*
diabetes (mellitus) due to immune mediated pancreatic islet beta-cell destruction (E10.-)
diabetes mellitus due to underlying condition (E08.-)
drug or chemical induced diabetes mellitus (E09.-)
gestational diabetes (O24.4-)
neonatal diabetes mellitus (P70.2)
type 1 diabetes mellitus (E10.-)
type 2 diabetes mellitus (E11.-)

E13.0 Other specified diabetes mellitus with hyperosmolarity

E13.00 Other specified diabetes mellitus with hyperosmolarity without nonketotic hyperglycemic-hyperosmolar coma (NKHHC) HAC MCC

E13.01 Other specified diabetes mellitus with hyperosmolarity with coma HAC MCC

E13.1 Other specified diabetes mellitus with ketoacidosis

E13.10 Other specified diabetes mellitus with ketoacidosis without coma HAC MCC
AHA: Q1, 2013

E13.11 Other specified diabetes mellitus with ketoacidosis with coma MCC

E13.2 Other specified diabetes mellitus with kidney complications

E13.21 Other specified diabetes mellitus with diabetic nephropathy
Other specified diabetes mellitus with intercapillary glomerulosclerosis
Other specified diabetes mellitus with intracapillary glomerulonephrosis
Other specified diabetes mellitus with Kimmelstiel-Wilson disease

E13.22 Other specified diabetes mellitus with diabetic chronic kidney disease
Use additional code to identify stage of chronic kidney disease (N18.1-N18.6)

E13.29 Other specified diabetes mellitus with other diabetic kidney complication
Other specified diabetes mellitus with renal tubular degeneration

E13.3 Other specified diabetes mellitus with ophthalmic complications

E13.31 Other specified diabetes mellitus with unspecified diabetic retinopathy

E13.311 Other specified diabetes mellitus with unspecified diabetic retinopathy with macular edema

E13.319 Other specified diabetes mellitus with unspecified diabetic retinopathy without macular edema

E13.32 Other specified diabetes mellitus with mild nonproliferative diabetic retinopathy
Other specified diabetes mellitus with nonproliferative diabetic retinopathy NOS
One of the following 7th characters is to be assigned to codes in subcategory E13.32 to designate laterality of the disease:
1 = right eye
2 = left eye
3 = bilateral
9 = unspecified eye

E13.321 Other specified diabetes mellitus with mild nonproliferative diabetic retinopathy with macular edema CC/MCC Exc

E13.329 Other specified diabetes mellitus with mild nonproliferative diabetic retinopathy without macular edema CC/MCC Exc

E13.33 Other specified diabetes mellitus with moderate nonproliferative diabetic retinopathy
One of the following 7th characters is to be assigned to codes in subcategory E13.33 to designate laterality of the disease:
1 = right eye
2 = left eye
3 = bilateral
9 = unspecified eye

E13.331 Other specified diabetes mellitus with moderate nonproliferative diabetic retinopathy with macular edema CC/MCC Exc

Unspecified Code | Other Specified Code | Manifestation Code | N Newborn | P Pediatric | M Maternity | A Adult | ♂ Male | ♀ Female
● New Code | ▲ Revised Code Title | ▶◀ Revised Text | NOTES | INCLUDES | EXCLUDES1 Not coded here | EXCLUDES2 Not included here
4th character required | 5th character required | 6th character required | 7th character required
Extension 'X' Alert | HAC Hospital-acquired condition (HAC) alert | AHA AHA Coding Clinic©

E11.43 - E13.331
CHAPTER 4: ENDOCRINE, NUTRITIONAL AND METABOLIC DISEASES (E00-E89)

E13.339 Other specified diabetes mellitus with moderate nonproliferative diabetic retinopathy without macular edema

E13.34 Other specified diabetes mellitus with severe nonproliferative diabetic retinopathy

One of the following 7th characters is to be assigned to codes in subcategory E13.34 to designate laterality of the disease:

1 = right eye
2 = left eye
3 = bilateral
9 = unspecified eye

E13.341 Other specified diabetes mellitus with severe nonproliferative diabetic retinopathy with macular edema

E13.349 Other specified diabetes mellitus with severe nonproliferative diabetic retinopathy without macular edema

E13.35 Other specified diabetes mellitus with proliferative diabetic retinopathy

One of the following 7th characters is to be assigned to codes in subcategory E13.35 to designate laterality of the disease:

1 = right eye
2 = left eye
3 = bilateral
9 = unspecified eye

E13.351 Other specified diabetes mellitus with proliferative diabetic retinopathy with macular edema

● E13.352 Other specified diabetes mellitus with proliferative diabetic retinopathy with traction retinal detachment involving the macula

● E13.353 Other specified diabetes mellitus with proliferative diabetic retinopathy with traction retinal detachment not involving the macula

● E13.354 Other specified diabetes mellitus with proliferative diabetic retinopathy with combined traction retinal detachment and rhegmatogenous retinal detachment

● E13.355 Other specified diabetes mellitus with stable proliferative diabetic retinopathy

E13.359 Other specified diabetes mellitus with proliferative diabetic retinopathy without macular edema

E13.36 Other specified diabetes mellitus with diabetic cataract

● E13.37 Other specified diabetes mellitus with diabetic macular edema, resolved following treatment

One of the following 7th characters is to be assigned to code E13.37 to designate laterality of the disease:

1 = right eye
2 = left eye
3 = bilateral
9 = unspecified eye

E13.39 Other specified diabetes mellitus with other diabetic ophthalmic complication

Use additional code to identify manifestation, such as:

diabetic glaucoma (H40-H42)

E13.4 Other specified diabetes mellitus with neurological complications

E13.40 Other specified diabetes mellitus with diabetic neuropathy, unspecified

E13.41 Other specified diabetes mellitus with diabetic mononeuropathy

E13.42 Other specified diabetes mellitus with diabetic polyneuropathy

Other specified diabetes mellitus with diabetic neuralgia

E13.43 Other specified diabetes mellitus with diabetic autonomic (poly)neuropathy

Other specified diabetes mellitus with diabetic gastroparesis

AHA: Q4, 2013

E13.44 Other specified diabetes mellitus with diabetic amyotrophy

E13.49 Other specified diabetes mellitus with other diabetic neurological complication

E13.5 Other specified diabetes mellitus with circulatory complications

E13.51 Other specified diabetes mellitus with diabetic peripheral angiopathy without gangrene

E13.52 Other specified diabetes mellitus with diabetic peripheral angiopathy with gangrene

Other specified diabetes mellitus with diabetic gangrene

E13.59 Other specified diabetes mellitus with other circulatory complications

E13.6 Other specified diabetes mellitus with other specified complications

E13.61 Other specified diabetes mellitus with diabetic arthropathy

E13.610 Other specified diabetes mellitus with diabetic neuropathic arthropathy

Other specified diabetes mellitus with Charcôt's joints

E13.618 Other specified diabetes mellitus with other diabetic arthropathy

E13.62 Other specified diabetes mellitus with skin complications

E13.620 Other specified diabetes mellitus with diabetic dermatitis

Other specified diabetes mellitus with diabetic necrobiosis lipoidica

E13.621 Other specified diabetes mellitus with foot ulcer

Use additional code to identify site of ulcer (L97.4-, L97.5-)

E13.622 Other specified diabetes mellitus with other skin ulcer

Use additional code to identify site of ulcer (L97.1-L97.9, L98.41-L98.49)

E13.628 Other specified diabetes mellitus with other skin complications

E13.63 Other specified diabetes mellitus with oral complications

E13.630 Other specified diabetes mellitus with periodontal disease

E13.638 Other specified diabetes mellitus with other oral complications

E13.64 Other specified diabetes mellitus with hypoglycemia

E13.641 Other specified diabetes mellitus with hypoglycemia with coma

E13.649 Other specified diabetes mellitus with hypoglycemia without coma

E13.65 Other specified diabetes mellitus with hyperglycemia

E13.69 Other specified diabetes mellitus with other specified complication

Use additional code to identify complication

E13.8 Other specified diabetes mellitus with unspecified complications

E13.9 Other specified diabetes mellitus without complications

Other disorders of glucose regulation and pancreatic internal secretion (E15-E16)

E15 Nondiabetic hypoglycemic coma

INCLUDES *drug-induced insulin coma in nondiabetic*
hyperinsulinism with hypoglycemic coma
hypoglycemic coma NOS

E16 Other disorders of pancreatic internal secretion

E16.0 Drug-induced hypoglycemia without coma

EXCLUDES1 *diabetes with hypoglycemia without coma (E09.692)*

Use additional code for adverse effect, if applicable, to identify drug (T36-T50 with fifth or sixth character 5)

Unacceptable principal diagnosis symbol per Medicare code edits | Code exempt from diagnosis present on admission requirement | Questionable admission | Complication or comorbidity | CC/MCC exclusion | Major complication or comorbidity | Principal diagnosis as its own CC | Principal diagnosis as its own MCC | Z code as first-listed diagnosis

E16.1 **Other hypoglycemia**
Functional hyperinsulinism
Functional nonhyperinsulinemic hypoglycemia
Hyperinsulinism NOS
Hyperplasia of pancreatic islet beta cells NOS
EXCLUDES1 *diabetes with hypoglycemia (E08.649, E10.649, E11.649, E13.649)*
hypoglycemia in infant of diabetic mother (P70.1)
neonatal hypoglycemia (P70.4)

E16.2 **Hypoglycemia, unspecified**
EXCLUDES1 *diabetes with hypoglycemia (E08.649, E10.649, E11.649, E13.649)*

E16.3 **Increased secretion of glucagon**
Hyperplasia of pancreatic endocrine cells with glucagon excess

E16.4 **Increased secretion of gastrin**
Hypergastrinemia
Hyperplasia of pancreatic endocrine cells with gastrin excess
Zollinger-Ellison syndrome

E16.8 **Other specified disorders of pancreatic internal secretion**
Increased secretion from endocrine pancreas of growth hormone-releasing hormone
Increased secretion from endocrine pancreas of pancreatic polypeptide
Increased secretion from endocrine pancreas of somatostatin
Increased secretion from endocrine pancreas of vasoactive-intestinal polypeptide

E16.9 **Disorder of pancreatic internal secretion, unspecified**
Islet-cell hyperplasia NOS
Pancreatic endocrine cell hyperplasia NOS

Disorders of other endocrine glands (E20-E35)

EXCLUDES1 *galactorrhea (N64.3)*
gynecomastia (N62)

E20 **Hypoparathyroidism**
EXCLUDES1 *Di George's syndrome (D82.1)*
postprocedural hypoparathyroidism (E89.2)
tetany NOS (R29.0)
transitory neonatal hypoparathyroidism (P71.4)

E20.0 Idiopathic **hypoparathyroidism**
E20.1 Pseudohypoparathyroidism
E20.8 **Other hypoparathyroidism**
E20.9 **Hypoparathyroidism, unspecified**
Parathyroid tetany

E21 **Hyperparathyroidism and other disorders of parathyroid gland**
EXCLUDES1 *adult osteomalacia (M83.-)*
ectopic hyperparathyroidism (E34.2)
familial hypocalciuric hypercalcemia (E83.52)
hungry bone syndrome (E83.81)
infantile and juvenile osteomalacia (E55.0)

E21.0 Primary **hyperparathyroidism**
Hyperplasia of parathyroid
Osteitis fibrosa cystica generalisata [von Recklinghausen's disease of bone]

E21.1 Secondary **hyperparathyroidism, not elsewhere classified**
EXCLUDES1 *secondary hyperparathyroidism of renal origin (N25.81)*

E21.2 **Other hyperparathyroidism**
Tertiary hyperparathyroidism
EXCLUDES1 *familial hypocalciuric hypercalcemia (E83.52)*

E21.3 **Hyperparathyroidism, unspecified**
E21.4 **Other specified disorders of parathyroid gland**
E21.5 **Disorder of parathyroid gland, unspecified**

E22 **Hyperfunction of pituitary gland**
EXCLUDES1 *Cushing's syndrome (E24.-)*
Nelson's syndrome (E24.1)
overproduction of ACTH not associated with Cushing's disease (E27.0)
overproduction of pituitary ACTH (E24.0)
overproduction of thyroid-stimulating hormone (E05.8-)

E22.0 **Acromegaly and pituitary gigantism**
Overproduction of growth hormone
EXCLUDES1 *constitutional gigantism (E34.4)*
constitutional tall stature (E34.4)
increased secretion from endocrine pancreas of growth hormone-releasing hormone (E16.8)

E22.1 **Hyperprolactinemia**
Use additional code for adverse effect, if applicable, to identify drug (T36-T50 with fifth or sixth character 5)

E22.2 **Syndrome of inappropriate secretion of antidiuretic hormone**
E22.8 **Other hyperfunction of pituitary gland**
Central precocious puberty
E22.9 **Hyperfunction of pituitary gland, unspecified**

E23 **Hypofunction and other disorders of the pituitary gland**
INCLUDES *the listed conditions whether the disorder is in the pituitary or the hypothalamus*
EXCLUDES1 *postprocedural hypopituitarism (E89.3)*

E23.0 **Hypopituitarism**
Fertile eunuch syndrome
Hypogonadotropic hypogonadism
Idiopathic growth hormone deficiency
Isolated deficiency of gonadotropin
Isolated deficiency of growth hormone
Isolated deficiency of pituitary hormone
Kallmann's syndrome
Lorain-Levi short stature
Necrosis of pituitary gland (postpartum)
Panhypopituitarism
Pituitary cachexia
Pituitary insufficiency NOS
Pituitary short stature
Sheehan's syndrome
Simmonds' disease

E23.1 **Drug-induced hypopituitarism**
Use additional code for adverse effect, if applicable, to identify drug (T36-T50 with fifth or sixth character 5)

E23.2 **Diabetes insipidus**
EXCLUDES1 *nephrogenic diabetes insipidus (N25.1)*

E23.3 **Hypothalamic dysfunction, not elsewhere classified**
EXCLUDES1 *Prader-Willi syndrome (Q87.1)*
Russell-Silver syndrome (Q87.1)

E23.6 **Other disorders of pituitary gland**
Abscess of pituitary
Adiposogenital dystrophy
E23.7 **Disorder of pituitary gland, unspecified**

E24 **Cushing's syndrome**
EXCLUDES1 *congenital adrenal hyperplasia (E25.0)*

E24.0 Pituitary-dependent **Cushing's disease**
Overproduction of pituitary ACTH
Pituitary-dependent hypercorticalism
E24.1 Nelson's syndrome
E24.2 Drug-induced **Cushing's syndrome**
Use additional code for adverse effect, if applicable, to identify drug (T36-T50 with fifth or sixth character 5)
E24.3 Ectopic ACTH syndrome
E24.4 Alcohol-induced pseudo-**Cushing's syndrome**
E24.8 **Other Cushing's syndrome**
E24.9 **Cushing's syndrome, unspecified**

E25 **Adrenogenital disorders**
INCLUDES *adrenogenital syndromes, virilizing or feminizing, whether acquired or due to adrenal hyperplasia consequent on inborn enzyme defects in hormone synthesis*
Female adrenal pseudohermaphroditism
Female heterosexual precocious pseudopuberty
Male isosexual precocious pseudopuberty
Male macrogenitosomia praecox
Male sexual precocity with adrenal hyperplasia
Male virilization (female)
EXCLUDES1 *indeterminate sex and pseudohermaphroditism (Q56)*
chromosomal abnormalities (Q90-Q99)

E25.0 Congenital **adrenogenital disorders** associated with enzyme deficiency
Congenital adrenal hyperplasia
21-Hydroxylase deficiency
Salt-losing congenital adrenal hyperplasia

Unspecified Code | Other Specified Code | Manifestation Code | N Newborn | P Pediatric | M Maternity | A Adult | ♂ Male | ♀ Female
● New Code | ▲ Revised Code Title | ►◄ Revised Text | NOTES | INCLUDES | EXCLUDES1 Not coded here | EXCLUDES2 Not included here
4th character required | 5th character required | 6th character required | 7th character required
Extension 'X' Alert | HAC Hospital-acquired condition (HAC) alert | AHA AHA Coding Clinic©

E25.8 **Other adrenogenital disorders**
Idiopathic adrenogenital disorder
Use additional code for adverse effect, if applicable, to identify drug (T36-T50 with fifth or sixth character 5)

E25.9 **Adrenogenital disorder, unspecified**
Adrenogenital syndrome NOS

E26 **Hyperaldosteronism**

E26.0 Primary **hyperaldosteronism**

E26.01 **Conn's syndrome**
Code also adrenal adenoma (D35.0-)

E26.02 **Glucocorticoid-remediable aldosteronism**
Familial aldosteronism type I

E26.09 **Other primary hyperaldosteronism**
Primary aldosteronism due to adrenal hyperplasia (bilateral)

E26.1 Secondary **hyperaldosteronism**

E26.8 **Other hyperaldosteronism**

E26.81 **Bartter's syndrome**

E26.89 **Other hyperaldosteronism**

E26.9 **Hyperaldosteronism, unspecified**
Aldosteronism NOS
Hyperaldosteronism NOS

E27 **Other disorders of adrenal gland**

E27.0 **Other adrenocortical overactivity** CC
Overproduction of ACTH, not associated with Cushing's disease
Premature adrenarche
EXCLUDES1 *Cushing's syndrome (E24.-)*

E27.1 **Primary adrenocortical insufficiency** CC
Addison's disease
Autoimmune adrenalitis
EXCLUDES1 *Addison only phenotype adrenoleukodystrophy (E71.528)*
amyloidosis (E85.-)
tuberculous Addison's disease (A18.7)
Waterhouse-Friderichsen syndrome (A39.1)

E27.2 **Addisonian crisis** CC
Adrenal crisis
Adrenocortical crisis

E27.3 **Drug-induced adrenocortical insufficiency** CC
Use additional code for adverse effect, if applicable, to identify drug (T36-T50 with fifth or sixth character 5)

E27.4 **Other and unspecified adrenocortical insufficiency**
EXCLUDES1 *adrenoleukodystrophy [Addison-Schilder] (E71.528)*
Waterhouse-Friderichsen syndrome (A39.1)

E27.40 **Unspecified adrenocortical insufficiency** CC
Adrenocortical insufficiency NOS
Hypoaldosteronism

E27.49 **Other adrenocortical insufficiency** CC
Adrenal hemorrhage
Adrenal infarction

E27.5 **Adrenomedullary hyperfunction** CC
Adrenomedullary hyperplasia
Catecholamine hypersecretion

E27.8 **Other specified disorders of adrenal gland**
Abnormality of cortisol-binding globulin

E27.9 **Disorder of adrenal gland, unspecified**

E28 **Ovarian dysfunction**
EXCLUDES1 *isolated gonadotropin deficiency (E23.0)*
postprocedural ovarian failure (E89.4-)

E28.0 **Estrogen excess** ♀
Use additional code for adverse effect, if applicable, to identify drug (T36-T50 with fifth or sixth character 5)

E28.1 **Androgen excess** ♀
Hypersecretion of ovarian androgens
Use additional code for adverse effect, if applicable, to identify drug (T36-T50 with fifth or sixth character 5)

E28.2 **Polycystic ovarian syndrome** ♀
Sclerocystic ovary syndrome
Stein-Leventhal syndrome

E28.3 **Primary ovarian failure**
EXCLUDES1 *pure gonadal dysgenesis (Q99.1)*
Turner's syndrome (Q96.-)

E28.31 Premature **menopause**

E28.310 Symptomatic **premature menopause** A ♀
Symptoms such as flushing, sleeplessness, headache, lack of concentration, associated with premature menopause

E28.319 Asymptomatic **premature menopause** A ♀
Premature menopause NOS

E28.39 **Other primary ovarian failure** ♀
Decreased estrogen
Resistant ovary syndrome

E28.8 **Other ovarian dysfunction** ♀
Ovarian hyperfunction NOS
EXCLUDES1 *postprocedural ovarian failure (E89.4-)*

E28.9 **Ovarian dysfunction, unspecified** ♀

E29 **Testicular dysfunction**
EXCLUDES1 *androgen insensitivity syndrome (E34.5-)*
azoospermia or oligospermia NOS (N46.0-N46.1)
isolated gonadotropin deficiency (E23.0)
Klinefelter's syndrome (▶Q98.0-Q98.1◀, Q98.4)

E29.0 **Testicular** hyperfunction ♂
Hypersecretion of testicular hormones

E29.1 **Testicular** hypofunction ♂
Defective biosynthesis of testicular androgen NOS
5-delta-Reductase deficiency (with male pseudohermaphroditism)
Testicular hypogonadism NOS
Use additional code for adverse effect, if applicable, to identify drug (T36-T50 with fifth or sixth character 5)
EXCLUDES1 *postprocedural testicular hypofunction (E89.5)*

E29.8 **Other testicular dysfunction** ♂

E29.9 **Testicular dysfunction, unspecified** ♂

E30 **Disorders of puberty, not elsewhere classified**

E30.0 Delayed **puberty**
Constitutional delay of puberty
Delayed sexual development

E30.1 Precocious **puberty** Q
Precocious menstruation
EXCLUDES1 *Albright (-McCune) (-Sternberg) syndrome (Q78.1)*
central precocious puberty (E22.8)
congenital adrenal hyperplasia (E25.0)
female heterosexual precocious pseudopuberty (E25.-)
male isosexual precocious pseudopuberty (E25.-)

E30.8 **Other disorders of puberty** Q
Premature thelarche

E30.9 **Disorder of puberty, unspecified**

E31 **Polyglandular dysfunction**
EXCLUDES1 *ataxia telangiectasia [Louis-Bar] (G11.3)*
dystrophia myotonica [Steinert] (G71.11)
pseudohypoparathyroidism (E20.1)

E31.0 Autoimmune **polyglandular failure**
Schmidt's syndrome

E31.1 **Polyglandular** hyperfunction
EXCLUDES1 *multiple endocrine adenomatosis (E31.2-)*
multiple endocrine neoplasia (E31.2-)

E31.2 Multiple endocrine neoplasia [MEN] syndromes
Multiple endocrine adenomatosis
Code also any associated malignancies and other conditions associated with the syndromes

E31.20 **Multiple endocrine neoplasia [MEN] syndrome, unspecified**
Multiple endocrine adenomatosis NOS
Multiple endocrine neoplasia [MEN] syndrome NOS

E31.21 **Multiple endocrine neoplasia [MEN]** type I
Wermer's syndrome

E31.22 **Multiple endocrine neoplasia [MEN]** type IIA
Sipple's syndrome

E31.23 **Multiple endocrine neoplasia [MEN]** type IIB

E31.8 **Other polyglandular dysfunction**

E31.9 **Polyglandular dysfunction, unspecified**

E32 **Diseases of thymus**
EXCLUDES1 *aplasia or hypoplasia of thymus with immunodeficiency (D82.1)*
myasthenia gravis (G70.0)

PDx Unacceptable principal diagnosis symbol per Medicare code edits | POA Code exempt from diagnosis present on admission requirement
Q Questionable admission | CC Complication or comorbidity | CC/MCC Exc CC/MCC exclusion | MCC Major complication or comorbidity
PDx CC Principal diagnosis as its own CC | PDx MCC Principal diagnosis as its own MCC | Z1 Z code as first-listed diagnosis

When symbols appear on a code that requires a 7th character extension, refer to Appendix D to identify applicable 7th character codes.

E32.0 Persistent hyperplasia **of thymus**
Hypertrophy of thymus
E32.1 Abscess **of thymus** CC
E32.8 **Other diseases of thymus**
EXCLUDES1 *aplasia or hypoplasia with immunodeficiency (D82.1)*
thymoma (D15.0)
E32.9 **Disease of thymus, unspecified**
E34 **Other endocrine disorders**
EXCLUDES1 *pseudohypoparathyroidism (E20.1)*
E34.0 **Carcinoid syndrome** CC
NOTES May be used as an additional code to identify functional activity associated with a carcinoid tumor.
E34.1 **Other hypersecretion of intestinal hormones**
E34.2 **Ectopic hormone secretion, not elsewhere classified**
EXCLUDES1 *ectopic ACTH syndrome (E24.3)*
E34.3 **Short stature due to endocrine disorder**
Constitutional short stature
Laron-type short stature
EXCLUDES1 *achondroplastic short stature (Q77.4)*
hypochondroplastic short stature (Q77.4)
nutritional short stature (E45)
pituitary short stature (E23.0)
progeria (E34.8)
renal short stature (N25.0)
Russell-Silver syndrome (Q87.1)
short-limbed stature with immunodeficiency (D82.2)
short stature in specific dysmorphic syndromes - code to syndrome - see Alphabetical Index
short stature NOS (R62.52)
E34.4 **Constitutional tall stature**
Constitutional gigantism
E34.5 **Androgen insensitivity syndrome**
E34.50 **Androgen insensitivity syndrome, unspecified**
Androgen insensitivity NOS
E34.51 Complete **androgen insensitivity syndrome**
Complete androgen insensitivity
de Quervain syndrome
Goldberg-Maxwell syndrome
E34.52 Partial **androgen insensitivity syndrome**
Partial androgen insensitivity
Reifenstein syndrome
E34.8 **Other specified endocrine disorders**
Pineal gland dysfunction
Progeria
EXCLUDES2 *pseudohypoparathyroidism (E20.1)*
E34.9 **Endocrine disorder, unspecified**
Endocrine disturbance NOS
Hormone disturbance NOS
E35 **Disorders of endocrine glands in diseases classified elsewhere**
Code first underlying disease, such as:
late congenital syphilis of thymus gland [Dubois disease] (A50.5)
Use additional code , if applicable, to identify:
sequelae of tuberculosis of other organs (B90.8)
EXCLUDES1 *Echinococcus granulosus infection of thyroid gland (B67.3)*
meningococcal hemorrhagic adrenalitis (A39.1)
syphilis of endocrine gland (A52.79)
tuberculosis of adrenal gland, except calcification (A18.7)
tuberculosis of endocrine gland NEC (A18.82)
tuberculosis of thyroid gland (A18.81)
Waterhouse-Friderichsen syndrome (A39.1)

Intraoperative complications of endocrine system (E36)

E36 **Intraoperative complications of endocrine system**
EXCLUDES2 *postprocedural endocrine and metabolic complications and disorders, not elsewhere classified (E89.-)*
E36.0 Intraoperative hemorrhage and hematoma **of an endocrine system organ or structure complicating a procedure**
EXCLUDES1 *intraoperative hemorrhage and hematoma of an endocrine system organ or structure due to accidental puncture or laceration during a procedure (E36.1-)*
E36.01 **Intraoperative hemorrhage and hematoma of an endocrine system organ or structure complicating an** endocrine system procedure CC
E36.02 **Intraoperative hemorrhage and hematoma of an endocrine system organ or structure complicating** other procedure CC
E36.1 Accidental puncture and laceration **of an endocrine system organ or structure during a procedure**
E36.11 **Accidental puncture and laceration of an endocrine system organ or structure during an** endocrine system procedure CC
E36.12 **Accidental puncture and laceration of an endocrine system organ or structure during** other procedure CC
E36.8 **Other intraoperative complications of endocrine system**
Use additional code, if applicable, to further specify disorder

Malnutrition (E40-E46)

EXCLUDES1 *intestinal malabsorption (K90.-)*
sequelae of protein-calorie malnutrition (E64.0)
EXCLUDES2 *nutritional anemias (D50-D53)*
starvation (T73.0)
E40 **Kwashiorkor** MCC
Severe malnutrition with nutritional edema with dyspigmentation of skin and hair
EXCLUDES1 *marasmic kwashiorkor (E42)*
E41 **Nutritional marasmus** MCC
Severe malnutrition with marasmus
EXCLUDES1 *marasmic kwashiorkor (E42)*
E42 **Marasmic kwashiorkor** MCC
Intermediate form severe protein-calorie malnutrition
Severe protein-calorie malnutrition with signs of both kwashiorkor and marasmus
E43 **Unspecified severe protein-calorie malnutrition** MCC
Starvation edema
E44 **Protein-calorie malnutrition of moderate and mild degree**
E44.0 Moderate **protein-calorie malnutrition** CC
E44.1 Mild **protein-calorie malnutrition** CC
E45 **Retarded development following protein-calorie malnutrition** CC
Nutritional short stature
Nutritional stunting
Physical retardation due to malnutrition
E46 **Unspecified protein-calorie malnutrition** CC
Malnutrition NOS
Protein-calorie imbalance NOS
EXCLUDES1 *nutritional deficiency NOS (E63.9)*

Other nutritional deficiencies (E50-E64)

EXCLUDES2 *nutritional anemias (D50-D53)*
E50 Vitamin A **deficiency**
EXCLUDES1 *sequelae of vitamin A deficiency (E64.1)*
E50.0 **Vitamin A deficiency with** conjunctival xerosis
E50.1 **Vitamin A deficiency with** Bitot's spot and conjunctival xerosis
Bitot's spot in the young child
E50.2 **Vitamin A deficiency with** corneal xerosis
E50.3 **Vitamin A deficiency with** corneal ulceration and xerosis
E50.4 **Vitamin A deficiency with** keratomalacia
E50.5 **Vitamin A deficiency with** night blindness
E50.6 **Vitamin A deficiency with** xerophthalmic scars of cornea
E50.7 Other ocular manifestations **of vitamin A deficiency**
Xerophthalmia NOS
E50.8 **Other manifestations of vitamin A deficiency**
Follicular keratosis
Xeroderma
E50.9 **Vitamin A deficiency, unspecified**
Hypovitaminosis A NOS
E51 Thiamine **deficiency**
EXCLUDES1 *sequelae of thiamine deficiency (E64.8)*
E51.1 Beriberi
E51.11 Dry **beriberi** CC
Beriberi NOS
Beriberi with polyneuropathy

Unspecified Code Other Specified Code Manifestation Code N Newborn P Pediatric M Maternity A Adult ♂ Male ♀ Female
● New Code ▲ Revised Code Title ►◄ Revised Text NOTES INCLUDES EXCLUDES1 Not coded here EXCLUDES2 Not included here
4th character required 5th character required 6th character required 7th character required
Extension 'X' Alert HAC Hospital-acquired condition (HAC) alert AHA AHA Coding Clinic©

E51.12 Wet beriberi
Beriberi with cardiovascular manifestations
Cardiovascular beriberi
Shoshin disease
E51.2 Wernicke's encephalopathy
E51.8 Other manifestations of thiamine deficiency
E51.9 Thiamine deficiency, unspecified

E52 Niacin deficiency [pellagra]
Niacin (-tryptophan) deficiency
Nicotinamide deficiency
Pellagra (alcoholic)
EXCLUDES1 *sequelae of niacin deficiency (E64.8)*

E53 Deficiency of other B group vitamins
EXCLUDES1 *sequelae of vitamin B deficiency (E64.8)*
E53.0 Riboflavin deficiency
Ariboflavinosis
Vitamin B2 deficiency
E53.1 Pyridoxine deficiency
Vitamin B6 deficiency
EXCLUDES1 *pyridoxine-responsive sideroblastic anemia (D64.3)*
E53.8 Deficiency of other specified B group vitamins
Biotin deficiency
Cyanocobalamin deficiency
Folate deficiency
Folic acid deficiency
Pantothenic acid deficiency
Vitamin B12 deficiency
EXCLUDES1 *folate deficiency anemia (D52.-)*
vitamin B12 deficiency anemia (D51.-)
E53.9 Vitamin B deficiency, unspecified

E54 Ascorbic acid deficiency
Deficiency of vitamin C
Scurvy
EXCLUDES1 *scorbutic anemia (D53.2)*
sequelae of vitamin C deficiency (E64.2)

E55 Vitamin D deficiency
EXCLUDES1 *adult osteomalacia (M83.-)*
osteoporosis (M80.-)
sequelae of rickets (E64.3)
E55.0 Rickets, active
Infantile osteomalacia
Juvenile osteomalacia
EXCLUDES1 *celiac rickets (K90.0)*
Crohn's rickets (K50.-)
hereditary vitamin D-dependent rickets (E83.32)
inactive rickets (E64.3)
renal rickets (N25.0)
sequelae of rickets (E64.3)
vitamin D-resistant rickets (E83.31)
E55.9 Vitamin D deficiency, unspecified
Avitaminosis D

E56 Other vitamin deficiencies
EXCLUDES1 *sequelae of other vitamin deficiencies (E64.8)*
E56.0 Deficiency of vitamin E
E56.1 Deficiency of vitamin K
EXCLUDES1 *deficiency of coagulation factor due to vitamin K deficiency (D68.4)*
vitamin K deficiency of newborn (P53)
E56.8 Deficiency of other vitamins
E56.9 Vitamin deficiency, unspecified

E58 Dietary calcium deficiency
EXCLUDES1 *disorders of calcium metabolism (E83.5-)*
sequelae of calcium deficiency (E64.8)

E59 Dietary selenium deficiency
Keshan disease
EXCLUDES1 *sequelae of selenium deficiency (E64.8)*

E60 Dietary zinc deficiency

E61 Deficiency of other nutrient elements
Use additional code for adverse effect, if applicable, to identify drug (T36-T50 with fifth or sixth character 5)
EXCLUDES1 *disorders of mineral metabolism (E83.-)*
iodine deficiency related thyroid disorders (E00-E02)
sequelae of malnutrition and other nutritional deficiencies (E64.-)
E61.0 Copper deficiency
E61.1 Iron deficiency
EXCLUDES1 *iron deficiency anemia (D50.-)*
E61.2 Magnesium deficiency
E61.3 Manganese deficiency
E61.4 Chromium deficiency
E61.5 Molybdenum deficiency
E61.6 Vanadium deficiency
E61.7 Deficiency of multiple nutrient elements
E61.8 Deficiency of other specified nutrient elements
E61.9 Deficiency of nutrient element, unspecified

E63 Other nutritional deficiencies
EXCLUDES1 *dehydration (E86.0)*
failure to thrive, adult (R62.7)
failure to thrive, child (R62.51)
feeding problems in newborn (P92.-)
sequelae of malnutrition and other nutritional deficiencies (E64.-)
E63.0 Essential fatty acid [EFA] deficiency
E63.1 Imbalance of constituents of food intake
E63.8 Other specified nutritional deficiencies
E63.9 Nutritional deficiency, unspecified

E64 Sequelae of malnutrition and other nutritional deficiencies
NOTES This category is to be used to indicate conditions in categories E43, E44, E46, E50-E63 as the cause of sequelae, which are themselves classified elsewhere. The 'sequelae' include conditions specified as such; they also include the late effects of diseases classifiable to the above categories if the disease itself is no longer present
Code first condition resulting from (sequela) of malnutrition and other nutritional deficiencies
E64.0 Sequelae of protein-calorie malnutrition
EXCLUDES2 *retarded development following protein-calorie malnutrition (E45)*
E64.1 Sequelae of vitamin A deficiency
E64.2 Sequelae of vitamin C deficiency
E64.3 Sequelae of rickets
E64.8 Sequelae of other nutritional deficiencies
E64.9 Sequelae of unspecified nutritional deficiency

Overweight, obesity and other hyperalimentation (E65-E68)

E65 Localized adiposity
Fat pad

E66 Overweight and obesity
Code first obesity complicating pregnancy, childbirth and the puerperium, if applicable (O99.21-)
Use additional code to identify body mass index (BMI), if known (Z68.-)
EXCLUDES1 *adiposogenital dystrophy (E23.6)*
lipomatosis NOS (E88.2)
lipomatosis dolorosa [Dercum] (E88.2)
Prader-Willi syndrome (Q87.1)
E66.0 Obesity due to excess calories
E66.01 Morbid (severe) obesity due to excess calories
EXCLUDES1 *morbid (severe) obesity with alveolar hypoventilation (E66.2)*
E66.09 Other obesity due to excess calories
E66.1 Drug-induced obesity
Use additional code for adverse effect, if applicable, to identify drug (T36-T50 with fifth or sixth character 5)
E66.2 Morbid (severe) obesity with alveolar hypoventilation
Obesity hypoventilation syndrome (OHS)
Pickwickian syndrome
E66.3 Overweight
E66.8 Other obesity
E66.9 Obesity, unspecified
Obesity NOS
AHA: Q4, 2013

Unacceptable principal diagnosis symbol per Medicare code edits · Code exempt from diagnosis present on admission requirement · Questionable admission · Complication or comorbidity · CC/MCC exclusion · Major complication or comorbidity · Principal diagnosis as its own CC · Principal diagnosis as its own MCC · Z code as first-listed diagnosis

E67 Other hyperalimentation
EXCLUDES1 *hyperalimentation NOS (R63.2)*
sequelae of hyperalimentation (E68)
E67.0 Hypervitaminosis A
E67.1 Hypercarotinemia
E67.2 Megavitamin-B6 syndrome
E67.3 Hypervitaminosis D
E67.8 Other specified hyperalimentation
E68 Sequelae of hyperalimentation
Code first condition resulting from (sequela) of hyperalimentation

Metabolic disorders (E70-E88)

EXCLUDES1 *androgen insensitivity syndrome (E34.5-)*
congenital adrenal hyperplasia (E25.0)
Ehlers-Danlos syndrome (Q79.6)
hemolytic anemias attributable to enzyme disorders (D55.-)
Marfan's syndrome (Q87.4)
5-alpha-reductase deficiency (E29.1)

E70 Disorders of aromatic amino-acid metabolism
E70.0 Classical phenylketonuria
E70.1 Other hyperphenylalaninemias
E70.2 Disorders of tyrosine metabolism
EXCLUDES1 *transitory tyrosinemia of newborn (P74.5)*
E70.20 Disorder of tyrosine metabolism, unspecified
E70.21 Tyrosinemia
Hypertyrosinemia
E70.29 Other disorders of tyrosine metabolism
Alkaptonuria
Ochronosis
E70.3 Albinism
E70.30 Albinism, unspecified
E70.31 Ocular albinism
E70.310 X-linked ocular albinism
E70.311 Autosomal recessive ocular albinism
E70.318 Other ocular albinism
E70.319 Ocular albinism, unspecified
E70.32 Oculocutaneous albinism
EXCLUDES1 *Chediak-Higashi syndrome (E70.330)*
Hermansky-Pudlak syndrome (E70.331)
E70.320 Tyrosinase negative oculocutaneous albinism
Albinism I
Oculocutaneous albinism ty-neg
E70.321 Tyrosinase positive oculocutaneous albinism
Albinism II
Oculocutaneous albinism ty-pos
E70.328 Other oculocutaneous albinism
Cross syndrome
E70.329 Oculocutaneous albinism, unspecified
E70.33 Albinism with hematologic abnormality
E70.330 Chediak-Higashi syndrome
E70.331 Hermansky-Pudlak syndrome
E70.338 Other albinism with hematologic abnormality
E70.339 Albinism with hematologic abnormality, unspecified
E70.39 Other specified albinism
Piebaldism
E70.4 Disorders of histidine metabolism
E70.40 Disorders of histidine metabolism, unspecified
E70.41 Histidinemia
E70.49 Other disorders of histidine metabolism
E70.5 Disorders of tryptophan metabolism
E70.8 Other disorders of aromatic amino-acid metabolism
E70.9 Disorder of aromatic amino-acid metabolism, unspecified
E71 Disorders of branched-chain amino-acid metabolism and fatty-acid metabolism
E71.0 Maple-syrup-urine disease
E71.1 Other disorders of branched-chain amino-acid metabolism
E71.11 Branched-chain organic acidurias
E71.110 Isovaleric acidemia
E71.111 3 -methylglutaconic aciduria
E71.118 Other branched-chain organic acidurias
E71.12 Disorders of propionate metabolism
E71.120 Methylmalonic acidemia
E71.121 Propionic acidemia
E71.128 Other disorders of propionate metabolism
E71.19 Other disorders of branched-chain amino-acid metabolism
Hyperleucine-isoleucinemia
Hypervalinemia
E71.2 Disorder of branched-chain amino-acid metabolism, unspecified
E71.3 Disorders of fatty-acid metabolism
EXCLUDES1 *peroxisomal disorders (E71.5)*
Refsum's disease (G60.1)
Schilder's disease (G37.0)
EXCLUDES2 *carnitine deficiency due to inborn error of metabolism (E71.42)*
E71.30 Disorder of fatty-acid metabolism, unspecified
E71.31 Disorders of fatty-acid oxidation
E71.310 Long chain/very long chain acyl CoA dehydrogenase deficiency
LCAD
VLCAD
E71.311 Medium chain acyl CoA dehydrogenase deficiency
MCAD
E71.312 Short chain acyl CoA dehydrogenase deficiency
SCAD
E71.313 Glutaric aciduria type II
Glutaric aciduria type II A
Glutaric aciduria type II B
Glutaric aciduria type II C
EXCLUDES1 *glutaric aciduria (type 1) NOS (E72.3)*
E71.314 Muscle carnitine palmitoyltransferase deficiency
E71.318 Other disorders of fatty-acid oxidation
E71.32 Disorders of ketone metabolism
E71.39 Other disorders of fatty-acid metabolism
E71.4 Disorders of carnitine metabolism
EXCLUDES1 *Muscle carnitine palmitoyltransferase deficiency (E71.314)*
E71.40 Disorder of carnitine metabolism, unspecified
E71.41 Primary carnitine deficiency
E71.42 Carnitine deficiency due to inborn errors of metabolism
Code also associated inborn error or metabolism
E71.43 Iatrogenic carnitine deficiency
Carnitine deficiency due to hemodialysis
Carnitine deficiency due to Valproic acid therapy
E71.44 Other secondary carnitine deficiency
E71.440 Ruvalcaba-Myhre-Smith syndrome
E71.448 Other secondary carnitine deficiency
E71.5 Peroxisomal disorders
EXCLUDES1 *Schilder's disease (G37.0)*
E71.50 Peroxisomal disorder, unspecified
E71.51 Disorders of peroxisome biogenesis
Group 1 peroxisomal disorders
EXCLUDES1 *Refsum's disease (G60.1)*
E71.510 Zellweger syndrome
E71.511 Neonatal adrenoleukodystrophy N
EXCLUDES1 *X-linked adrenoleukodystrophy (E71.42-)*
E71.518 Other disorders of peroxisome biogenesis
E71.52 X-linked adrenoleukodystrophy
E71.520 Childhood cerebral X-linked adrenoleukodystrophy

Unspecified Code | Other Specified Code | Manifestation Code | N Newborn | P Pediatric | M Maternity | A Adult | ♂ Male | ♀ Female
● New Code | ▲ Revised Code Title | ►◄ Revised Text | NOTES | INCLUDES | EXCLUDES1 Not coded here | EXCLUDES2 Not included here
4th character required | 5th character required | 6th character required | 7th character required
Extension 'X' Alert | HAC Hospital-acquired condition (HAC) alert | AHA AHA Coding Clinic©

E71.521 Adolescent X-linked adrenoleukodystrophy
E71.522 Adrenomyeloneuropathy
E71.528 Other X-linked adrenoleukodystrophy
Addison only phenotype adrenoleukodystrophy
Addison-Schilder adrenoleukodystrophy
E71.529 X-linked adrenoleukodystrophy, unspecified type
E71.53 Other group 2 peroxisomal disorders
E71.54 Other peroxisomal disorders
E71.540 Rhizomelic chondrodysplasia punctata
EXCLUDES1 *chondrodysplasia punctata NOS (Q77.3)*
E71.541 Zellweger-like syndrome
E71.542 Other group 3 peroxisomal disorders
E71.548 Other peroxisomal disorders

E72 Other disorders of amino-acid metabolism
EXCLUDES1 *disorders of:*
aromatic amino-acid metabolism (E70.-)
branched-chain amino-acid metabolism (E71.0-E71.2)
fatty-acid metabolism (E71.3)
purine and pyrimidine metabolism (E79.-)
gout (M1A.-, M10.-)

E72.0 Disorders of amino-acid transport
EXCLUDES1 *disorders of tryptophan metabolism (E70.5)*
E72.00 Disorders of amino-acid transport, unspecified
E72.01 Cystinuria
E72.02 Hartnup's disease
E72.03 Lowe's syndrome
Use additional code for associated glaucoma (H42)
E72.04 Cystinosis
Fanconi (-de Toni) (-Debré) syndrome with cystinosis
EXCLUDES1 *Fanconi (-de Toni) (-Debré) syndrome without cystinosis (E72.09)*
E72.09 Other disorders of amino-acid transport
Fanconi (-de Toni) (-Debré) syndrome, unspecified

E72.1 Disorders of sulfur-bearing amino-acid metabolism
EXCLUDES1 *cystinosis (E72.04)*
cystinuria (E72.01)
transcobalamin II deficiency (D51.2)
E72.10 Disorders of sulfur-bearing amino-acid metabolism, unspecified
E72.11 Homocystinuria
Cystathionine synthase deficiency
E72.12 Methylenetetrahydrofolate reductase deficiency
E72.19 Other disorders of sulfur-bearing amino-acid metabolism
Cystathioninuria
Methioninemia
Sulfite oxidase deficiency

E72.2 Disorders of urea cycle metabolism
EXCLUDES1 *disorders of ornithine metabolism (E72.4)*
E72.20 Disorder of urea cycle metabolism, unspecified
Hyperammonemia
EXCLUDES1 *hyperammonemia-hyperornithinemia-homocitrullinemia syndrome E72.4*
transient hyperammonemia of newborn (P74.6)
E72.21 Argininemia
E72.22 Arginosuccinic aciduria
E72.23 Citrullinemia
E72.29 Other disorders of urea cycle metabolism

E72.3 Disorders of lysine and hydroxylysine metabolism
Glutaric aciduria NOS
Glutaric aciduria (type I)
Hydroxylysinemia
Hyperlysinemia
EXCLUDES1 *glutaric aciduria type II (E71.313)*
Refsum's disease (G60.1)
Zellweger syndrome (E71.510)

E72.4 Disorders of ornithine metabolism
Hyperammonemia-Hyperornithinemia-Homocitrullinemia syndrome
Ornithinemia (types I, II)
Ornithine transcarbamylase deficiency
EXCLUDES1 *hereditary choroidal dystrophy (H31.2-)*

E72.5 Disorders of glycine metabolism
E72.50 Disorder of glycine metabolism, unspecified
E72.51 Non-ketotic hyperglycinemia
E72.52 Trimethylaminuria
E72.53 Hyperoxaluria
Oxalosis
Oxaluria
E72.59 Other disorders of glycine metabolism
D-glycericacidemia
Hyperhydroxyprolinemia
Hyperprolinemia (types I, II)
Sarcosinemia

E72.8 Other specified disorders of amino-acid metabolism
Disorders of beta-amino-acid metabolism
Disorders of gamma-glutamyl cycle

E72.9 Disorder of amino-acid metabolism, unspecified

E73 Lactose intolerance
E73.0 Congenital lactase deficiency
E73.1 Secondary lactase deficiency
E73.8 Other lactose intolerance
E73.9 Lactose intolerance, unspecified

E74 Other disorders of carbohydrate metabolism
EXCLUDES1 *diabetes mellitus (E08-E13)*
hypoglycemia NOS (E16.2)
increased secretion of glucagon (E16.3)
mucopolysaccharidosis (E76.0-E76.3)

E74.0 Glycogen storage disease
E74.00 Glycogen storage disease, unspecified
E74.01 von Gierke disease
Type I glycogen storage disease
E74.02 Pompe disease
Cardiac glycogenosis
Type II glycogen storage disease
E74.03 Cori disease
Forbes disease
Type III glycogen storage disease
E74.04 McArdle disease
Type V glycogen storage disease
E74.09 Other glycogen storage disease
Andersen disease
Hers disease
Tauri disease
Glycogen storage disease, types 0, IV, VI-XI
Liver phosphorylase deficiency
Muscle phosphofructokinase deficiency

E74.1 Disorders of fructose metabolism
EXCLUDES1 *muscle phosphofructokinase deficiency (E74.09)*
E74.10 Disorder of fructose metabolism, unspecified
E74.11 Essential fructosuria
Fructokinase deficiency
E74.12 Hereditary fructose intolerance
Fructosemia
E74.19 Other disorders of fructose metabolism
Fructose-1, 6-diphosphatase deficiency

E74.2 Disorders of galactose metabolism
E74.20 Disorders of galactose metabolism, unspecified
E74.21 Galactosemia
E74.29 Other disorders of galactose metabolism
Galactokinase deficiency

E74.3 Other disorders of intestinal carbohydrate absorption
EXCLUDES2 *lactose intolerance (E73.-)*
E74.31 Sucrase-isomaltase deficiency
E74.39 Other disorders of intestinal carbohydrate absorption
Disorder of intestinal carbohydrate absorption NOS
Glucose-galactose malabsorption
Sucrase deficiency

Unacceptable principal diagnosis symbol per Medicare code edits · Code exempt from diagnosis present on admission requirement
Questionable admission · Complication or comorbidity · CC/MCC exclusion · Major complication or comorbidity
Principal diagnosis as its own CC · Principal diagnosis as its own MCC · Z code as first-listed diagnosis

E74.4 **Disorders of pyruvate metabolism and gluconeogenesis** CC
Deficiency of phosphoenolpyruvate carboxykinase
Deficiency of pyruvate carboxylase
Deficiency of pyruvate dehydrogenase
EXCLUDES1 *disorders of pyruvate metabolism and gluconeogenesis with anemia (D55.-)*
Leigh's syndrome (G31.82)

E74.8 **Other specified disorders of carbohydrate metabolism** CC
Essential pentosuria
Renal glycosuria

E74.9 **Disorder of carbohydrate metabolism, unspecified**

E75 Disorders of sphingolipid metabolism and other lipid storage disorders
EXCLUDES1 *mucolipidosis, types I-III (E77.0-E77.1)*
Refsum's disease (G60.1)

E75.0 **GM2 gangliosidosis**
- E75.00 **GM2 gangliosidosis, unspecified** CC
- E75.01 **Sandhoff disease** CC
- E75.02 **Tay-Sachs disease** CC
- E75.09 **Other GM2 gangliosidosis** CC
  Adult GM2 gangliosidosis
  Juvenile GM2 gangliosidosis

E75.1 **Other and unspecified gangliosidosis**
- E75.10 **Unspecified gangliosidosis** CC
  Gangliosidosis NOS
- E75.11 **Mucolipidosis IV** CC
- E75.19 **Other gangliosidosis** CC
  GM1 gangliosidosis
  GM3 gangliosidosis

E75.2 **Other sphingolipidosis**
EXCLUDES1 *adrenoleukodystrophy [Addison-Schilder] (E71.528)*
- E75.21 **Fabry (-Anderson) disease**
- E75.22 **Gaucher disease**
- E75.23 **Krabbe disease** CC
- E75.24 **Niemann-Pick disease**
  - E75.240 **Niemann-Pick disease type A**
  - E75.241 **Niemann-Pick disease type B**
  - E75.242 **Niemann-Pick disease type C**
  - E75.243 **Niemann-Pick disease type D**
  - E75.248 **Other Niemann-Pick disease**
  - E75.249 **Niemann-Pick disease, unspecified**
- E75.25 **Metachromatic leukodystrophy** CC
- E75.29 **Other sphingolipidosis** CC
  Farber's syndrome
  Sulfatase deficiency
  Sulfatide lipidosis

E75.3 **Sphingolipidosis, unspecified**

E75.4 **Neuronal ceroid lipofuscinosis** CC
Batten disease
Bielschowsky-Jansky disease
Kufs disease
Spielmeyer-Vogt disease

E75.5 **Other lipid storage disorders**
Cerebrotendinous cholesterosis [van Bogaert-Scherer-Epstein]
Wolman's disease

E75.6 **Lipid storage disorder, unspecified**

E76 Disorders of glycosaminoglycan metabolism

E76.0 **Mucopolysaccharidosis, type I**
- E76.01 **Hurler's syndrome** CC
- E76.02 **Hurler-Scheie syndrome** CC
- E76.03 **Scheie's syndrome** CC

E76.1 **Mucopolysaccharidosis, type II** CC
Hunter's syndrome

E76.2 **Other mucopolysaccharidoses**
- E76.21 **Morquio mucopolysaccharidoses**
  - E76.210 **Morquio A mucopolysaccharidoses** CC
    Classic Morquio syndrome
    Morquio syndrome A
    Mucopolysaccharidosis, type IVA
  - E76.211 **Morquio B mucopolysaccharidoses** CC
    Morquio-like mucopolysaccharidoses
    Morquio-like syndrome
    Morquio syndrome B
    Mucopolysaccharidosis, type IVB
  - E76.219 **Morquio mucopolysaccharidoses, unspecified** CC
    Morquio syndrome
    Mucopolysaccharidosis, type IV
- E76.22 **Sanfilippo mucopolysaccharidoses** CC
  Mucopolysaccharidosis, type III (A) (B) (C) (D)
  Sanfilippo A syndrome
  Sanfilippo B syndrome
  Sanfilippo C syndrome
  Sanfilippo D syndrome
- E76.29 **Other mucopolysaccharidoses** CC
  beta-Glucuronidase deficiency
  Maroteaux-Lamy (mild) (severe) syndrome
  Mucopolysaccharidosis, types VI, VII

E76.3 **Mucopolysaccharidosis, unspecified** CC

E76.8 **Other disorders of glucosaminoglycan metabolism** CC

E76.9 **Glucosaminoglycan metabolism disorder, unspecified** CC

E77 Disorders of glycoprotein metabolism

E77.0 **Defects in post-translational modification of lysosomal enzymes**
Mucolipidosis II [I-cell disease]
Mucolipidosis III [pseudo-Hurler polydystrophy]

E77.1 **Defects in glycoprotein degradation**
Aspartylglucosaminuria
Fucosidosis
Mannosidosis
Sialidosis [mucolipidosis I]

E77.8 **Other disorders of glycoprotein metabolism**

E77.9 **Disorder of glycoprotein metabolism, unspecified**

E78 Disorders of lipoprotein metabolism and other lipidemias
EXCLUDES1 *sphingolipidosis (E75.0-E75.3)*

E78.0 **Pure hypercholesterolemia**
- ● E78.00 **Pure hypercholesterolemia, unspecified** CC/MCC Exc
  Fredrickson's hyperlipoproteinemia, type IIa
  Hyperbetalipoproteinemia
  Low-density-lipoprotein-type [LDL] hyperlipoproteinemia
- ● E78.01 **Familial hypercholesterolemia** CC/MCC Exc

E78.1 **Pure hyperglyceridemia**
Elevated fasting triglycerides
Endogenous hyperglyceridemia
Fredrickson's hyperlipoproteinemia, type IV
Hyperlipidemia, group B
Hyperprebetalipoproteinemia
Very-low-density-lipoprotein-type [VLDL] hyperlipoproteinemia

E78.2 **Mixed hyperlipidemia**
Broad- or floating-betalipoproteinemia
Combined hyperlipidemia NOS
Elevated cholesterol with elevated triglycerides NEC
Fredrickson's hyperlipoproteinemia, type IIb or III
Hyperbetalipoproteinemia with prebetalipoproteinemia
Hypercholesteremia with endogenous hyperglyceridemia
Hyperlipidemia, group C
Tubo-eruptive xanthoma
Xanthoma tuberosum
EXCLUDES1 *cerebrotendinous cholesterosis [van Bogaert-Scherer-Epstein] (E75.5)*
familial combined hyperlipidemia (E78.4)

E78.3 **Hyperchylomicronemia**
Chylomicron retention disease
Fredrickson's hyperlipoproteinemia, type I or V
Hyperlipidemia, group D
Mixed hyperglyceridemia

E78.4 **Other hyperlipidemia**
Familial combined hyperlipidemia

E78.5 **Hyperlipidemia, unspecified**

E78.6 **Lipoprotein deficiency**
Abetalipoproteinemia
Depressed HDL cholesterol
High-density lipoprotein deficiency
Hypoalphalipoproteinemia
Hypobetalipoproteinemia (familial)
Lecithin cholesterol acyltransferase deficiency
Tangier disease

Unspecified Code Other Specified Code Manifestation Code N Newborn P Pediatric M Maternity A Adult ♂ Male ♀ Female
● New Code ▲ Revised Code Title ►◄ Revised Text NOTES INCLUDES EXCLUDES1 Not coded here EXCLUDES2 Not included here
4th character required 5th character required 6th character required 7th character required
Extension 'X' Alert HAC Hospital-acquired condition (HAC) alert AHA AHA Coding Clinic©

 When symbols appear on a code that requires a 7th character extension, refer to Appendix D to identify applicable 7th character codes.

E78.7 Disorders of bile acid and cholesterol metabolism
EXCLUDES1 *Niemann-Pick disease type C (E75.242)*
E78.70 Disorder of bile acid and cholesterol metabolism, unspecified
E78.71 Barth syndrome
E78.72 Smith-Lemli-Opitz syndrome
E78.79 Other disorders of bile acid and cholesterol metabolism
E78.8 Other disorders of lipoprotein metabolism
E78.81 Lipoid dermatoarthritis
E78.89 Other lipoprotein metabolism disorders
E78.9 Disorder of lipoprotein metabolism, unspecified
E79 Disorders of purine and pyrimidine metabolism
EXCLUDES1 *Ataxia-telangiectasia (Q87.1)*
Bloom's syndrome (Q82.8)
Cockayne's syndrome (Q87.1)
calculus of kidney (N20.0)
combined immunodeficiency disorders (D81.-)
Fanconi's anemia (D61.09)
gout (M1A.-, M10.-)
orotaciduric anemia (D53.0)
progeria (E34.8)
Werner's syndrome (E34.8)
xeroderma pigmentosum (Q82.1)
E79.0 Hyperuricemia without signs of inflammatory arthritis and tophaceous disease
Asymptomatic hyperuricemia
E79.1 Lesch-Nyhan syndrome
HGPRT deficiency
E79.2 Myoadenylate deaminase deficiency
E79.8 Other disorders of purine and pyrimidine metabolism
Hereditary xanthinuria
E79.9 Disorder of purine and pyrimidine metabolism, unspecified
E80 Disorders of porphyrin and bilirubin metabolism
INCLUDES *defects of catalase and peroxidase*
E80.0 Hereditary erythropoietic porphyria
Congenital erythropoietic porphyria
Erythropoietic protoporphyria
E80.1 Porphyria cutanea tarda
E80.2 Other and unspecified porphyria
E80.20 Unspecified porphyria
Porphyria NOS
E80.21 Acute intermittent (hepatic) porphyria
E80.29 Other porphyria
Hereditary coproporphyria
E80.3 Defects of catalase and peroxidase
Acatalasia [Takahara]
E80.4 Gilbert syndrome
E80.5 Crigler-Najjar syndrome
E80.6 Other disorders of bilirubin metabolism
Dubin-Johnson syndrome
Rotor's syndrome
E80.7 Disorder of bilirubin metabolism, unspecified
E83 Disorders of mineral metabolism
EXCLUDES1 *dietary mineral deficiency (E58-E61)*
parathyroid disorders (E20-E21)
vitamin D deficiency (E55.-)
E83.0 Disorders of copper metabolism
E83.00 Disorder of copper metabolism, unspecified
E83.01 Wilson's disease
Code also associated Kayser Fleischer ring (H18.04-)
E83.09 Other disorders of copper metabolism
Menkes' (kinky hair) (steely hair) disease
E83.1 Disorders of iron metabolism
EXCLUDES1 *iron deficiency anemia (D50.-)*
sideroblastic anemia (D64.0-D64.3)
E83.10 Disorder of iron metabolism, unspecified
E83.11 Hemochromatosis
E83.110 Hereditary hemochromatosis
Bronzed diabetes
Pigmentary cirrhosis (of liver)
Primary (hereditary) hemochromatosis
E83.111 Hemochromatosis due to repeated red blood cell transfusions
Iron overload due to repeated red blood cell transfusions
Transfusion (red blood cell) associated hemochromatosis
E83.118 Other hemochromatosis
E83.119 Hemochromatosis, unspecified
E83.19 Other disorders of iron metabolism
Use additional code, if applicable, for idiopathic pulmonary hemosiderosis (J84.03)
E83.2 Disorders of zinc metabolism
Acrodermatitis enteropathica
E83.3 Disorders of phosphorus metabolism and phosphatases
EXCLUDES1 *adult osteomalacia (M83.-)*
osteoporosis (M80.-)
E83.30 Disorder of phosphorus metabolism, unspecified
E83.31 Familial hypophosphatemia
Vitamin D-resistant osteomalacia
Vitamin D-resistant rickets
EXCLUDES1 *vitamin D-deficiency rickets (E55.0)*
E83.32 Hereditary vitamin D-dependent rickets (type 1) (type 2)
25-hydroxyvitamin D 1-alpha-hydroxylase deficiency
Pseudovitamin D deficiency
Vitamin D receptor defect
E83.39 Other disorders of phosphorus metabolism
Acid phosphatase deficiency
Hypophosphatasia
E83.4 Disorders of magnesium metabolism
E83.40 Disorders of magnesium metabolism, unspecified
E83.41 Hypermagnesemia
E83.42 Hypomagnesemia
E83.49 Other disorders of magnesium metabolism
E83.5 Disorders of calcium metabolism
EXCLUDES1 *chondrocalcinosis (M11.1-M11.2)*
hungry bone syndrome (E83.81)
hyperparathyroidism (E21.0-E21.3)
E83.50 Unspecified disorder of calcium metabolism
E83.51 Hypocalcemia
E83.52 Hypercalcemia
Familial hypocalciuric hypercalcemia
E83.59 Other disorders of calcium metabolism
Idiopathic hypercalciuria
E83.8 Other disorders of mineral metabolism
E83.81 Hungry bone syndrome
E83.89 Other disorders of mineral metabolism
E83.9 Disorder of mineral metabolism, unspecified
E84 Cystic fibrosis
INCLUDES *mucoviscidosis*
Code also exocrine pancreatic insufficiency (K86.81)
E84.0 Cystic fibrosis with pulmonary manifestations
Use additional code to identify any infectious organism present, such as:
Pseudomonas (B96.5)
E84.1 Cystic fibrosis with intestinal manifestations
E84.11 Meconium ileus in cystic fibrosis
EXCLUDES1 *meconium ileus not due to cystic fibrosis (P76.0)*
E84.19 Cystic fibrosis with other intestinal manifestations
Distal intestinal obstruction syndrome
E84.8 Cystic fibrosis with other manifestations
E84.9 Cystic fibrosis, unspecified
E85 Amyloidosis
EXCLUDES1 *Alzheimer's disease (G30.0-)*
E85.0 Non-neuropathic heredofamilial amyloidosis
Hereditary amyloid nephropathy
E85.1 Neuropathic heredofamilial amyloidosis
Amyloid polyneuropathy (Portuguese)
E85.2 Heredofamilial amyloidosis, unspecified
E85.3 Secondary systemic amyloidosis
Hemodialysis-associated amyloidosis

Unacceptable principal diagnosis symbol per Medicare code edits · Code exempt from diagnosis present on admission requirement
Questionable admission · Complication or comorbidity · CC/MCC exclusion · Major complication or comorbidity
Principal diagnosis as its own CC · Principal diagnosis as its own MCC · Z code as first-listed diagnosis

When symbols appear on a code that requires a 7th character extension, refer to Appendix D to identify applicable 7th character codes.

E85.4 Organ-limited **amyloidosis**
Localized amyloidosis
E85.8 Other amyloidosis
E85.9 Amyloidosis, unspecified

E86 Volume depletion
Use additional code(s) for any associated disorders of electrolyte and acid-base balance (E87.-)
EXCLUDES1 *dehydration of newborn (P74.1)*
hypovolemic shock NOS (R57.1)
postprocedural hypovolemic shock (T81.19)
traumatic hypovolemic shock (T79.4)
E86.0 Dehydration
E86.1 Hypovolemia
Depletion of volume of plasma
E86.9 Volume depletion, unspecified

E87 Other disorders of fluid, electrolyte and acid-base balance
EXCLUDES1 *diabetes insipidus (E23.2)*
electrolyte imbalance associated with hyperemesis gravidarum (O21.1)
electrolyte imbalance following ectopic or molar pregnancy (O08.5)
familial periodic paralysis (G72.3)
E87.0 Hyperosmolality and hypernatremia
Sodium [Na] excess
Sodium [Na] overload
E87.1 Hypo-osmolality and hyponatremia
Sodium [Na] deficiency
EXCLUDES1 *syndrome of inappropriate secretion of antidiuretic hormone (E22.2)*
E87.2 Acidosis
Acidosis NOS
Lactic acidosis
Metabolic acidosis
Respiratory acidosis
EXCLUDES1 *diabetic acidosis - see categories E08-E10, E13 with ketoacidosis*
E87.3 Alkalosis
Alkalosis NOS
Metabolic alkalosis
Respiratory alkalosis
E87.4 Mixed disorder of acid-base balance
E87.5 Hyperkalemia
Potassium [K] excess
Potassium [K] overload
E87.6 Hypokalemia
Potassium [K] deficiency
E87.7 Fluid overload
EXCLUDES1 *edema NOS (R60.9)*
fluid retention (R60.9)
E87.70 Fluid overload, unspecified
E87.71 Transfusion associated **circulatory overload**
Fluid overload due to transfusion (blood) (blood components)
TACO
E87.79 Other fluid overload
E87.8 Other disorders of electrolyte and fluid balance, not elsewhere classified
Electrolyte imbalance NOS
Hyperchloremia
Hypochloremia

E88 Other and unspecified metabolic disorders
Use additional codes for associated conditions
EXCLUDES1 *histiocytosis X (chronic) (C96.6)*
E88.0 Disorders of plasma-protein metabolism, not elsewhere classified
EXCLUDES1 *disorder of lipoprotein metabolism (E78.-)*
monoclonal gammopathy (of undetermined significance) (D47.2)
polyclonal hypergammaglobulinemia (D89.0)
Waldenström macroglobulinemia (C88.0)
E88.01 Alpha-1-antitrypsin deficiency
AAT deficiency
E88.09 Other disorders of plasma-protein metabolism, not elsewhere classified
Bisalbuminemia
E88.1 Lipodystrophy, not elsewhere classified
Lipodystrophy NOS
EXCLUDES1 *Whipple's disease (K90.81)*
E88.2 Lipomatosis, not elsewhere classified
Lipomatosis NOS
Lipomatosis (Check) dolorosa [Dercum]
E88.3 Tumor lysis syndrome MCC
Tumor lysis syndrome (spontaneous)
Tumor lysis syndrome following antineoplastic drug chemotherapy
Use additional code for adverse effect, if applicable, to identify drug (T45.1X5)
E88.4 Mitochondrial metabolism disorders
EXCLUDES1 *disorders of pyruvate metabolism (E74.4)*
Kearns-Sayre syndrome (H49.81)
Leber's disease (H47.22)
Leigh's encephalopathy (G31.82)
Mitochondrial myopathy, NEC (G71.3)
Reye's syndrome (G93.7)
E88.40 Mitochondrial metabolism disorder, unspecified
E88.41 MELAS syndrome
Mitochondrial myopathy, encephalopathy, lactic acidosis and stroke-like episodes
E88.42 MERRF syndrome
Myoclonic epilepsy associated with ragged-red fibers
Code also ▶progressive◀ myoclonic epilepsy (G40.3-)
E88.49 Other mitochondrial metabolism disorders
E88.8 Other specified metabolic disorders
E88.81 Metabolic syndrome
Dysmetabolic syndrome X
Use additional codes for associated manifestations, such as:
obesity (E66.-)
E88.89 Other specified metabolic disorders
Launois-Bensaude adenolipomatosis
EXCLUDES1 *adult pulmonary Langerhans cell histiocytosis (J84.82)*
E88.9 Metabolic disorder, unspecified

Postprocedural endocrine and metabolic complications and disorders, not elsewhere classified (E89)

E89 Postprocedural endocrine and metabolic complications and disorders, not elsewhere classified
EXCLUDES2 *intraoperative complications of endocrine system organ or structure (E36.0-, E36.1-, E36.8)*
E89.0 Postprocedural hypothyroidism
Postirradiation hypothyroidism
Postsurgical hypothyroidism
E89.1 Postprocedural hypoinsulinemia
Postpancreatectomy hyperglycemia
Postsurgical hypoinsulinemia
Use additional code, if applicable, to identify:
acquired absence of pancreas (Z90.41-)
diabetes mellitus (postpancreatectomy) (postprocedural) (E13.-)
insulin use (Z79.4)
EXCLUDES1 *transient postprocedural hyperglycemia (R73.9)*
transient postprocedural hypoglycemia (E16.2)
E89.2 Postprocedural hypoparathyroidism
Parathyroprival tetany
E89.3 Postprocedural hypopituitarism
Postirradiation hypopituitarism
E89.4 Postprocedural ovarian failure
E89.40 Asymptomatic **postprocedural ovarian failure** ♀
Postprocedural ovarian failure NOS
E89.41 Symptomatic **postprocedural ovarian failure** ♀
Symptoms such as flushing, sleeplessness, headache, lack of concentration, associated with postprocedural menopause

Unspecified Code | Other Specified Code | Manifestation Code | N Newborn | P Pediatric | M Maternity | A Adult | ♂ Male | ♀ Female
● New Code | ▲ Revised Code Title | ▶◀ Revised Text | NOTES | INCLUDES | EXCLUDES1 Not coded here | EXCLUDES2 Not included here
4th character required | 5th character required | 6th character required | 7th character required
Extension 'X' Alert | HAC Hospital-acquired condition (HAC) alert | AHA AHA Coding Clinic©

E89.5 Postprocedural testicular hypofunction ♂

E89.6 Postprocedural adrenocortical (-medullary) hypofunction CC

E89.8 Other postprocedural endocrine and metabolic complications and disorders

▲ E89.81 Postprocedural ▶hemorrhage of◀ an endocrine system organ or structure following a procedure

▲ E89.810 Postprocedural ▶hemorrhage of◀ an endocrine system organ or structure following an endocrine system procedure CC

▲ E89.811 Postprocedural ▶hemorrhage of◀ an endocrine system organ or structure following other procedure CC

● E89.82 Postprocedural hematoma and seroma of an endocrine system organ or structure

● E89.820 Postprocedural hematoma of an endocrine system organ or structure following an endocrine system procedure CC CC/MCC Exc

● E89.821 Postprocedural hematoma of an endocrine system organ or structure following other procedure CC CC/MCC Exc

● E89.822 Postprocedural seroma of an endocrine system organ or structure following an endocrine system procedure

● E89.823 Postprocedural seroma of an endocrine system organ or structure following other procedure

E89.89 Other postprocedural endocrine and metabolic complications and disorders CC

Use additional code, if applicable, to further specify disorder

PDx Unacceptable principal diagnosis symbol per Medicare code edits POA Code exempt from diagnosis present on admission requirement
? Questionable admission CC Complication or comorbidity CC/MCC Exc CC/MCC exclusion MCC Major complication or comorbidity
PDx CC Principal diagnosis as its own CC PDx MCC Principal diagnosis as its own MCC Z1 Z code as first-listed diagnosis

Chapter 5: Mental, Behavioral and Neurodevelopmental Disorders (F01-F99)

Guidelines for Assigning Codes From This Chapter

Chapter 5 includes codes for both organic psychotic conditions, such as senile dementia, and other psychotic conditions, such as schizophrenia. You'll also find codes for a variety of nonpsychotic disorders, such as anxiety disorders, psychosexual disorders, and drug abuse. Intellectual disabilities also land in this chapter.

List of Sections

- F01-F09: Mental disorders due to known physiological conditions
- F10-F19: Mental and behavioral disorders due to psychoactive substance use
- F20-F29: Schizophrenia, schizotypal, delusional, and other non-mood psychotic disorders
- F30-F39: Mood [affective] disorders
- F40-F48: Anxiety, dissociative, stress-related, somatoform and other nonpsychotic mental disorders
- F50-F59: Behavioral syndromes associated with physiological disturbances and physical factors
- F60-F69: Disorders of adult personality and behavior
- F70-F79: Intellectual Disabilities
- F80-F89: Pervasive and specific developmental disorders
- F90-F98: Behavioral and emotional disorders with onset usually occurring in childhood and adolescence
- F99: Unspecified mental disorder

Highlights From the ICD-10-CM Official Guidelines for Coding and Reporting

The ICD-10-CM Official Guidelines for Coding and Reporting for Chapter 5 focus on pain disorders of psychological origin and mental and behavioral disorders due to psychoactive substance use. The information below is from the 2017 Official Guidelines.

Keep Pain Disorders Related to Psychological Factors Under Control

- When pain is exclusively related to psychological disorders, assign code F45.41 (*Pain disorder exclusively related to psychological factors*). This type of pain disorder is also known as a persistent somatoform disorder.
- An Excludes1 note with category G89 (Pain, not elsewhere classified), in Chapter 6, reminds you not to assign a G89 code with code F45.41.
- Do assign a code from category G89 with F45.42 (*Pain disorders with related psychological factors*) if the documentation demonstrates a psychological component with acute or chronic pain.

Watch for Psychoactive Substance Use in Remission

If a patient's mental or behavioral disorder due to psychoactive substance abuse is in remission, you will choose a code from categories F10-F19 (*Mental and behavioral disorders due to psychoactive substance use*) that ends in .21. Rely on the provider's documentation to determine if a remission code is appropriate.

Use a Single Code to Classify the Pattern of Use

When the documentation refers to use, abuse, and dependence of the same substance, such as alcohol or cannabis or opioid, assign only a single code to identify the pattern of use. Use these criteria to make your selection:

- If both use and abuse are documented, assign only the code for abuse
- If both abuse and dependence are documented, assign only the code for dependence
- If use, abuse and dependence are all documented, assign only the code for dependence
- If both use and dependence are documented, assign only the code for dependence.

Note: Report codes for psychoactive substance abuse only when the psychoactive substance use is associated with a mental or behavioral disorder and this relationship is documented by the provider.

Mental, behavioral and neurodevelopmental disorders (F01-F99)

INCLUDES *disorders of psychological development*

EXCLUDES2 *symptoms, signs and abnormal clinical laboratory findings, not elsewhere classified (R00-R99)*

This chapter contains the following blocks:

- F01-F09 Mental disorders due to known physiological conditions
- F10-F19 Mental and behavioral disorders due to psychoactive substance use
- F20-F29 Schizophrenia, schizotypal, delusional, and other non-mood psychotic disorders
- F30-F39 Mood [affective] disorders
- F40-F48 Anxiety, dissociative, stress-related, somatoform and other nonpsychotic mental disorders
- F50-F59 Behavioral syndromes associated with physiological disturbances and physical factors
- F60-F69 Disorders of adult personality and behavior
- F70-F79 Intellectual disabilities
- F80-F89 Pervasive and specific developmental disorders
- F90-F98 Behavioral and emotional disorders with onset usually occurring in childhood and adolescence
- F99 Unspecified mental disorder

Mental disorders due to known physiological conditions (F01-F09)

NOTES This block comprises a range of mental disorders grouped together on the basis of their having in common a demonstrable etiology in cerebral disease, brain injury, or other insult leading to cerebral dysfunction. The dysfunction may be primary, as in diseases, injuries, and insults that affect the brain directly and selectively; or secondary, as in systemic diseases and disorders that attack the brain only as one of the multiple organs or systems of the body that are involved.

F01 Vascular dementia

Vascular dementia as a result of infarction of the brain due to vascular disease, including hypertensive cerebrovascular disease.

INCLUDES *arteriosclerotic dementia*

Code first the underlying physiological condition or sequelae of cerebrovascular disease.

F01.5 Vascular dementia

F01.50 Vascular dementia without behavioral disturbance A

Major neurocognitive disorder without behavioral disturbance

F01.51 Vascular dementia with behavioral disturbance A CC

Major neurocognitive disorder due to vascular disease, with behavioral disturbance
Major neurocognitive disorder with aggressive behavior
Major neurocognitive disorder with combative behavior
Major neurocognitive disorder with violent behavior
Vascular dementia with aggressive behavior
Vascular dementia with combative behavior
Vascular dementia with violent behavior
Use additional code, if applicable, to identify wandering in vascular dementia (Z91.83)

F02 Dementia in other diseases classified elsewhere

INCLUDES *Major neurocognitive disorder in other diseases classified elsewhere*

Code first the underlying physiological condition, such as:
Alzheimer's (G30.-)
cerebral lipidosis (E75.4)
Creutzfeldt-Jakob disease (A81.0-)
dementia with Lewy bodies (G31.83)
dementia with Parkinsonism (G31.83)
epilepsy and recurrent seizures (G40.-)
frontotemporal dementia (G31.09)
hepatolenticular degeneration (E83.0)
human immunodeficiency virus [HIV] disease (B20)
Huntington's disease (G10)
hypercalcemia (E83.52)
hypothyroidism, acquired (E00-E03.-)
intoxications (T36-T65)
Jakob-Creutzfeldt disease (A81.0-)
multiple sclerosis (G35)
neurosyphilis (A52.17)
niacin deficiency [pellagra] (E52)
Parkinson's disease (G20)
Pick's disease (G31.01)
polyarteritis nodosa (M30.0)
prion disease (A81.9)
systemic lupus erythematosus (M32.-)
traumatic brain injury (S06.-)
trypanosomiasis (B56.-, B57.-)
vitamin B deficiency (E53.8)

EXCLUDES2 *dementia in alcohol and psychoactive substance disorders (F10-F19, with .17, .27, .97)*
vascular dementia (F01.5-)

F02.8 Dementia in other diseases classified elsewhere

F02.80 Dementia in other diseases classified elsewhere without behavioral disturbance

Dementia in other diseases classified elsewhere NOS
Major neurocognitive disorder in other diseases classified elsewhere
AHA: Q2, 2016

F02.81 Dementia in other diseases classified elsewhere with behavioral disturbance CC

Dementia in other diseases classified elsewhere with aggressive behavior
Dementia in other diseases classified elsewhere with combative behavior
Dementia in other diseases classified elsewhere with violent behavior
Major neurocognitive disorder in other diseases classified elsewhere with aggressive behavior
Major neurocognitive disorder in other diseases classified elsewhere with combative behavior
Major neurocognitive disorder in other diseases classified elsewhere with violent behavior
Use additional code, if applicable, to identify wandering in dementia in conditions classified elsewhere (Z91.83)

F03 Unspecified dementia

Presenile dementia NOS
Presenile psychosis NOS
Primary degenerative dementia NOS
Senile dementia NOS
Senile dementia depressed or paranoid type
Senile psychosis NOS

EXCLUDES1 *senility NOS (R41.81)*

EXCLUDES2 *mild memory disturbance due to known physiological condition (F06.8)*
senile dementia with delirium or acute confusional state (F05)

F03.9 Unspecified dementia

F03.90 Unspecified dementia without behavioral disturbance A

Dementia NOS

F03.91 Unspecified dementia with behavioral disturbance A CC

Unspecified dementia with aggressive behavior
Unspecified dementia with combative behavior
Unspecified dementia with violent behavior
Use additional code, if applicable, to identify wandering in unspecified dementia (Z91.83)

F04 Amnestic disorder due to known physiological condition

Korsakov's psychosis or syndrome, nonalcoholic
Code first the underlying physiological condition

EXCLUDES1 *amnesia NOS (R41.3)*
anterograde amnesia (R41.1)
dissociative amnesia (F44.0)
retrograde amnesia (R41.2)

EXCLUDES2 *alcohol-induced or unspecified Korsakov's syndrome (F10.26, F10.96)*
Korsakov's syndrome induced by other psychoactive substances (F13.26, F13.96, F19.16, F19.26, F19.96)

Unacceptable principal diagnosis symbol per Medicare code edits · Code exempt from diagnosis present on admission requirement
Questionable admission · Complication or comorbidity · CC/MCC exclusion · Major complication or comorbidity
Principal diagnosis as its own CC · Principal diagnosis as its own MCC · Z code as first-listed diagnosis

When symbols appear on a code that requires a 7th character extension, refer to Appendix D to identify applicable 7th character codes.

F05 Delirium due to known physiological condition
Acute or subacute brain syndrome
Acute or subacute confusional state (nonalcoholic)
Acute or subacute infective psychosis
Acute or subacute organic reaction
Acute or subacute psycho-organic syndrome
Delirium of mixed etiology
Delirium superimposed on dementia
Sundowning
Code first the underlying physiological condition
EXCLUDES1 *delirium NOS (R41.0)*
EXCLUDES2 *delirium tremens alcohol-induced or unspecified (F10.231, F10.921)*

F06 Other mental disorders due to known physiological condition
INCLUDES *mental disorders due to endocrine disorder*
mental disorders due to exogenous hormone
mental disorders due to exogenous toxic substance
mental disorders due to primary cerebral disease
mental disorders due to somatic illness
mental disorders due to systemic disease affecting the brain
Code first the underlying physiological condition
EXCLUDES1 *unspecified dementia (F03)*
EXCLUDES2 *delirium due to known physiological condition (F05)*
dementia as classified in F01-F02
other mental disorders associated with alcohol and other psychoactive substances (F10-F19)

F06.0 Psychotic disorder with hallucinations due to known physiological condition
Organic hallucinatory state (nonalcoholic)
EXCLUDES2 *hallucinations and perceptual disturbance induced by alcohol and other psychoactive substances (F10-F19 with .151, .251, .951)*
schizophrenia (F20.-)

F06.1 Catatonic disorder due to known physiological condition
Catatonia associated with another mental disorder
Catatonia NOS
EXCLUDES1 *catatonic stupor (R40.1)*
stupor NOS (R40.1)
EXCLUDES2 *catatonic schizophrenia (F20.2)*
dissociative stupor (F44.2)

F06.2 Psychotic disorder with delusions due to known physiological condition
Paranoid and paranoid-hallucinatory organic states
Schizophrenia-like psychosis in epilepsy
EXCLUDES2 *alcohol and drug-induced psychotic disorder (F10-F19 with .150, .250, .950)*
brief psychotic disorder (F23)
delusional disorder (F22)
schizophrenia (F20.-)

F06.3 Mood disorder due to known physiological condition
EXCLUDES2 *mood disorders due to alcohol and other psychoactive substances (F10-F19 with .14, .24, .94)*
mood disorders, not due to known physiological condition or unspecified (F30-F39)

F06.30 Mood disorder due to known physiological condition, unspecified
F06.31 Mood disorder due to known physiological condition with depressive features
F06.32 Mood disorder due to known physiological condition with major depressive-like episode
F06.33 Mood disorder due to known physiological condition with manic features
F06.34 Mood disorder due to known physiological condition with mixed features

F06.4 Anxiety disorder due to known physiological condition
EXCLUDES2 *anxiety disorders due to alcohol and other psychoactive substances (F10-F19 with .180, .280, .980)*
anxiety disorders, not due to known physiological condition or unspecified (F40.-, F41.-)

F06.8 Other specified mental disorders due to known physiological condition
Epileptic psychosis NOS
Organic dissociative disorder
Organic emotionally labile [asthenic] disorder

F07 Personality and behavioral disorders due to known physiological condition
Code first the underlying physiological condition

F07.0 Personality change due to known physiological condition
Frontal lobe syndrome
Limbic epilepsy personality syndrome
Lobotomy syndrome
Organic personality disorder
Organic pseudopsychopathic personality
Organic pseudoretarded personality
Postleucotomy syndrome
Code first underlying physiological condition
EXCLUDES1 *mild cognitive impairment (G31.84)*
postconcussional syndrome (F07.81)
postencephalitic syndrome (F07.89)
signs and symptoms involving emotional state (R45.-)
EXCLUDES2 *specific personality disorder (F60.-)*

F07.8 Other personality and behavioral disorders due to known physiological condition

F07.81 Postconcussional syndrome
Postcontusional syndrome (encephalopathy)
Post-traumatic brain syndrome, nonpsychotic
Use additional code to identify associated post-traumatic headache, if applicable (G44.3-)
EXCLUDES1 *current concussion (brain) (S06.0-)*
postencephalitic syndrome (F07.89)

F07.89 Other personality and behavioral disorders due to known physiological condition
Postencephalitic syndrome
Right hemispheric organic affective disorder

F07.9 Unspecified personality and behavioral disorder due to known physiological condition
Organic psychosyndrome

F09 Unspecified mental disorder due to known physiological condition
Mental disorder NOS due to known physiological condition
Organic brain syndrome NOS
Organic mental disorder NOS
Organic psychosis NOS
Symptomatic psychosis NOS
Code first the underlying physiological condition
EXCLUDES1 *psychosis NOS (F29)*

Mental and behavioral disorders due to psychoactive substance use (F10-F19)

F10 Alcohol related disorders
Use additional code for blood alcohol level, if applicable (Y90.-)

F10.1 Alcohol abuse
EXCLUDES1 *alcohol dependence (F10.2-)*
alcohol use, unspecified (F10.9-)

F10.10 Alcohol abuse, uncomplicated
Alcohol use disorder, mild

F10.12 Alcohol abuse with intoxication
F10.120 Alcohol abuse with intoxication, uncomplicated
F10.121 Alcohol abuse with intoxication delirium
F10.129 Alcohol abuse with intoxication, unspecified

F10.14 Alcohol abuse with alcohol-induced mood disorder
Alcohol use disorder, mild, with alcohol-induced bipolar or related disorder
Alcohol use disorder, mild, with alcohol-induced depressive disorder

F10.15 Alcohol abuse with alcohol-induced psychotic disorder
F10.150 Alcohol abuse with alcohol-induced psychotic disorder with delusions
F10.151 Alcohol abuse with alcohol-induced psychotic disorder with hallucinations
F10.159 Alcohol abuse with alcohol-induced psychotic disorder, unspecified

Unspecified Code Other Specified Code Manifestation Code N Newborn P Pediatric M Maternity A Adult ♂ Male ♀ Female
● New Code ▲ Revised Code Title ►◄ Revised Text NOTES INCLUDES EXCLUDES1 Not coded here EXCLUDES2 Not included here
4th character required 5th character required 6th character required 7th character required
Extension 'X' Alert HAC Hospital-acquired condition (HAC) alert AHA AHA Coding Clinic©

F10.18 Alcohol abuse with other alcohol-induced disorders
- F10.180 Alcohol abuse with alcohol-induced anxiety disorder CC
- F10.181 Alcohol abuse with alcohol-induced sexual dysfunction CC
- F10.182 Alcohol abuse with alcohol-induced sleep disorder
- F10.188 Alcohol abuse with other alcohol-induced disorder CC

F10.19 Alcohol abuse with unspecified alcohol-induced disorder CC

F10.2 Alcohol dependence

EXCLUDES1 *alcohol abuse (F10.1-)*
alcohol use, unspecified (F10.9-)

EXCLUDES2 *toxic effect of alcohol (T51.0-)*

F10.20 Alcohol dependence, uncomplicated
Alcohol use disorder, moderate
Alcohol use disorder, severe

F10.21 Alcohol dependence, in remission

F10.22 Alcohol dependence with intoxication
Acute drunkenness (in alcoholism)
EXCLUDES2 *alcohol dependence with withdrawal (F10.23-)*
- F10.220 Alcohol dependence with intoxication, uncomplicated
- F10.221 Alcohol dependence with intoxication delirium CC
- F10.229 Alcohol dependence with intoxication, unspecified

F10.23 Alcohol dependence with withdrawal
EXCLUDES2 *Alcohol dependence with intoxication (F10.22-)*
- F10.230 Alcohol dependence with withdrawal, uncomplicated CC
- F10.231 Alcohol dependence with withdrawal delirium CC
- F10.232 Alcohol dependence with withdrawal with perceptual disturbance CC
- F10.239 Alcohol dependence with withdrawal, unspecified CC

F10.24 Alcohol dependence with alcohol-induced mood disorder CC
Alcohol use disorder, moderate, with alcohol-induced bipolar or related disorder
Alcohol use disorder, moderate, with alcohol-induced depressive disorder
Alcohol use disorder, severe, with alcohol-induced bipolar or related disorder
Alcohol use disorder, severe, with alcohol-induced depressive disorder

F10.25 Alcohol dependence with alcohol-induced psychotic disorder
- F10.250 Alcohol dependence with alcohol-induced psychotic disorder with delusions
- F10.251 Alcohol dependence with alcohol-induced psychotic disorder with hallucinations CC
- F10.259 Alcohol dependence with alcohol-induced psychotic disorder, unspecified CC

F10.26 Alcohol dependence with alcohol-induced persisting amnestic disorder
Alcohol use disorder, moderate, with alcohol-induced major neurocognitive disorder, amnestic-confabulatory type
Alcohol use disorder, severe, with alcohol-induced major neurocognitive disorder, amnestic-confabulatory type

F10.27 Alcohol dependence with alcohol-induced persisting dementia CC
Alcohol use disorder, moderate, with alcohol-induced major neurocognitive disorder, nonamnestic-confabulatory type
Alcohol use disorder, severe, with alcohol-induced major neurocognitive disorder, nonamnestic-confabulatory type

F10.28 Alcohol dependence with other alcohol-induced disorders
- F10.280 Alcohol dependence with alcohol-induced anxiety disorder CC
- F10.281 Alcohol dependence with alcohol-induced sexual dysfunction CC
- F10.282 Alcohol dependence with alcohol-induced sleep disorder
- F10.288 Alcohol dependence with other alcohol-induced disorder CC
  Alcohol use disorder, moderate, with alcohol-induced mild neurocognitive disorder
  Alcohol use disorder, severe, with alcohol-induced mild neurocognitive disorder

F10.29 Alcohol dependence with unspecified alcohol-induced disorder CC

F10.9 Alcohol use , unspecified

EXCLUDES1 *alcohol abuse (F10.1-)*
alcohol dependence (F10.2-)

F10.92 Alcohol use, unspecified with intoxication
- F10.920 Alcohol use, unspecified with intoxication, uncomplicated
- F10.921 Alcohol use, unspecified with intoxication delirium CC
- F10.929 Alcohol use, unspecified with intoxication, unspecified

F10.94 Alcohol use, unspecified with alcohol-induced mood disorder CC
Alcohol induced bipolar or related disorder, without use disorder
Alcohol induced depressive disorder, without use disorder

F10.95 Alcohol use, unspecified with alcohol-induced psychotic disorder
- F10.950 Alcohol use, unspecified with alcohol-induced psychotic disorder with delusions
- F10.951 Alcohol use, unspecified with alcohol-induced psychotic disorder with hallucinations CC
- F10.959 Alcohol use, unspecified with alcohol-induced psychotic disorder, unspecified CC
  Alcohol-induced psychotic disorder without use disorder

F10.96 Alcohol use, unspecified with alcohol-induced persisting amnestic disorder
Alcohol-induced major neurocognitive disorder, amnestic-confabulatory type, without use disorder

F10.97 Alcohol use, unspecified with alcohol-induced persisting dementia
Alcohol-induced major neurocognitive disorder, nonamnestic-confabulatory type, without use disorder

F10.98 Alcohol use, unspecified with other alcohol-induced disorders
- F10.980 Alcohol use, unspecified with alcohol-induced anxiety disorder CC
  Alcohol induced anxiety disorder, without use disorder
- F10.981 Alcohol use, unspecified with alcohol-induced sexual dysfunction CC
  Alcohol induced sexual dysfunction, without use disorder
- F10.982 Alcohol use, unspecified with alcohol-induced sleep disorder
  Alcohol induced sleep disorder, without use disorder
- F10.988 Alcohol use, unspecified with other alcohol-induced disorder CC
  Alcohol induced mild neurocognitive disorder, without use disorder

F10.99 Alcohol use, unspecified with unspecified alcohol-induced disorder CC

F11 Opioid related disorders

F11.1 Opioid abuse

EXCLUDES1 *opioid dependence (F11.2-)*
opioid use, unspecified (F11.9-)

F11.10 Opioid abuse, uncomplicated
Opioid use disorder, mild

F11.12 Opioid abuse with intoxication

Unacceptable principal diagnosis symbol per Medicare code edits · Code exempt from diagnosis present on admission requirement · Questionable admission · Complication or comorbidity · CC/MCC exclusion · Major complication or comorbidity · Principal diagnosis as its own CC · Principal diagnosis as its own MCC · Z code as first-listed diagnosis

F11.120 Opioid abuse with intoxication, uncomplicated
F11.121 Opioid abuse with intoxication delirium
F11.122 Opioid abuse with intoxication with perceptual disturbance
F11.129 Opioid abuse with intoxication, unspecified
F11.14 Opioid abuse with opioid-induced mood disorder
Opioid use disorder, mild, with opioid-induced depressive disorder
F11.15 Opioid abuse with opioid-induced psychotic disorder
F11.150 Opioid abuse with opioid-induced psychotic disorder with delusions
F11.151 Opioid abuse with opioid-induced psychotic disorder with hallucinations
F11.159 Opioid abuse with opioid-induced psychotic disorder, unspecified
F11.18 Opioid abuse with other opioid-induced disorder
F11.181 Opioid abuse with opioid-induced sexual dysfunction
F11.182 Opioid abuse with opioid-induced sleep disorder
F11.188 Opioid abuse with other opioid-induced disorder
F11.19 Opioid abuse with unspecified opioid-induced disorder
F11.2 Opioid dependence
EXCLUDES1 *opioid abuse (F11.1-)*
opioid use, unspecified (F11.9-)
EXCLUDES2 *opioid poisoning (T40.0-T40.2-)*
F11.20 Opioid dependence, uncomplicated
Opioid use disorder, moderate
Opioid use disorder, severe
F11.21 Opioid dependence, in remission
F11.22 Opioid dependence with intoxication
EXCLUDES1 *opioid dependence with withdrawal (F11.23)*
F11.220 Opioid dependence with intoxication, uncomplicated
F11.221 Opioid dependence with intoxication delirium
F11.222 Opioid dependence with intoxication with perceptual disturbance
F11.229 Opioid dependence with intoxication, unspecified
F11.23 Opioid dependence with withdrawal
EXCLUDES1 *opioid dependence with intoxication (F11.22-)*
F11.24 Opioid dependence with opioid-induced mood disorder
Opioid use disorder, moderate, with opioid induced depressive disorder
F11.25 Opioid dependence with opioid-induced psychotic disorder
F11.250 Opioid dependence with opioid-induced psychotic disorder with delusions
F11.251 Opioid dependence with opioid-induced psychotic disorder with hallucinations
F11.259 Opioid dependence with opioid-induced psychotic disorder, unspecified
F11.28 Opioid dependence with other opioid-induced disorder
F11.281 Opioid dependence with opioid-induced sexual dysfunction
F11.282 Opioid dependence with opioid-induced sleep disorder
F11.288 Opioid dependence with other opioid-induced disorder
F11.29 Opioid dependence with unspecified opioid-induced disorder
F11.9 Opioid use, unspecified
EXCLUDES1 *opioid abuse (F11.1-)*
opioid dependence (F11.2-)
F11.90 Opioid use, unspecified, uncomplicated
F11.92 Opioid use, unspecified with intoxication
EXCLUDES1 *opioid use, unspecified with withdrawal (F11.93)*
F11.920 Opioid use, unspecified with intoxication, uncomplicated
F11.921 Opioid use, unspecified with intoxication delirium
Opioid-induced delirium
F11.922 Opioid use, unspecified with intoxication with perceptual disturbance
F11.929 Opioid use, unspecified with intoxication, unspecified
F11.93 Opioid use, unspecified with withdrawal
EXCLUDES1 *opioid use, unspecified with intoxication (F11.92-)*
F11.94 Opioid use, unspecified with opioid-induced mood disorder
Opioid induced depressive disorder, without use disorder
F11.95 Opioid use, unspecified with opioid-induced psychotic disorder
F11.950 Opioid use, unspecified with opioid-induced psychotic disorder with delusions
F11.951 Opioid use, unspecified with opioid-induced psychotic disorder with hallucinations
F11.959 Opioid use, unspecified with opioid-induced psychotic disorder, unspecified
F11.98 Opioid use, unspecified with other specified opioid-induced disorder
F11.981 Opioid use, unspecified with opioid-induced sexual dysfunction
Opioid induced sexual dysfunction, without use disorder
F11.982 Opioid use, unspecified with opioid-induced sleep disorder
Opioid induced sleep disorder, without use disorder
F11.988 Opioid use, unspecified with other opioid-induced disorder
Opioid induced anxiety disorder, without use disorder
F11.99 Opioid use, unspecified with unspecified opioid-induced disorder
F12 Cannabis related disorders
INCLUDES *marijuana*
F12.1 Cannabis abuse
EXCLUDES1 *cannabis dependence (F12.2-)*
cannabis use, unspecified (F12.9-)
F12.10 Cannabis abuse, uncomplicated
Cannabis use disorder, mild
F12.12 Cannabis abuse with intoxication
F12.120 Cannabis abuse with intoxication, uncomplicated
F12.121 Cannabis abuse with intoxication delirium
F12.122 Cannabis abuse with intoxication with perceptual disturbance
F12.129 Cannabis abuse with intoxication, unspecified
F12.15 Cannabis abuse with psychotic disorder
F12.150 Cannabis abuse with psychotic disorder with delusions
F12.151 Cannabis abuse with psychotic disorder with hallucinations
F12.159 Cannabis abuse with psychotic disorder, unspecified
F12.18 Cannabis abuse with other cannabis-induced disorder
F12.180 Cannabis abuse with cannabis-induced anxiety disorder
F12.188 Cannabis abuse with other cannabis-induced disorder
Cannabis use disorder, mild, with cannabis-induced sleep disorder

Unspecified Code | Other Specified Code | Manifestation Code | N Newborn | P Pediatric | M Maternity | A Adult | ♂ Male | ♀ Female
● New Code ▲ Revised Code Title ►◄ Revised Text NOTES INCLUDES EXCLUDES1 Not coded here EXCLUDES2 Not included here
4th character required | 5th character required | 6th character required | 7th character required
Extension 'X' Alert | HAC Hospital-acquired condition (HAC) alert | AHA AHA Coding Clinic©

F12.19 **Cannabis abuse with unspecified cannabis-induced disorder**

F12.2 Cannabis dependence

EXCLUDES1 *cannabis abuse (F12.1-)*
cannabis use, unspecified (F12.9-)

EXCLUDES2 *cannabis poisoning (T40.7-)*

F12.20 **Cannabis dependence, uncomplicated**
Cannabis use disorder, moderate
Cannabis use disorder, severe

F12.21 **Cannabis dependence, in remission**

F12.22 Cannabis dependence with intoxication

F12.220 **Cannabis dependence with intoxication, uncomplicated**

F12.221 **Cannabis dependence with intoxication delirium** CC

F12.222 **Cannabis dependence with intoxication with perceptual disturbance**

F12.229 **Cannabis dependence with intoxication, unspecified**

F12.25 Cannabis dependence with psychotic disorder

F12.250 **Cannabis dependence with psychotic disorder with delusions** CC

F12.251 **Cannabis dependence with psychotic disorder with hallucinations** CC

F12.259 **Cannabis dependence with psychotic disorder, unspecified**

F12.28 Cannabis dependence with other cannabis-induced disorder

F12.280 **Cannabis dependence with cannabis-induced anxiety disorder**

F12.288 **Cannabis dependence with other cannabis-induced disorder**
Cannabis use disorder, moderate, with cannabis-induced sleep disorder
Cannabis use disorder, severe, with cannabis-induced sleep disorder
Cannabis withdrawal

F12.29 **Cannabis dependence with unspecified cannabis-induced disorder**

F12.9 Cannabis use, unspecified

EXCLUDES1 *cannabis abuse (F12.1-)*
cannabis dependence (F12.2-)

F12.90 **Cannabis use, unspecified, uncomplicated**

F12.92 Cannabis use, unspecified with intoxication

F12.920 **Cannabis use, unspecified with intoxication, uncomplicated**

F12.921 **Cannabis use, unspecified with intoxication delirium** CC

F12.922 **Cannabis use, unspecified with intoxication with perceptual disturbance**

F12.929 **Cannabis use, unspecified with intoxication, unspecified**

F12.95 Cannabis use, unspecified with psychotic disorder

F12.950 **Cannabis use, unspecified with psychotic disorder with delusions** CC

F12.951 **Cannabis use, unspecified with psychotic disorder with hallucinations** CC

F12.959 **Cannabis use, unspecified with psychotic disorder, unspecified**
Cannabis induced psychotic disorder, without use disorder

F12.98 Cannabis use, unspecified with other cannabis-induced disorder

F12.980 **Cannabis use, unspecified with anxiety disorder**
Cannabis induced anxiety disorder, without use disorder

F12.988 **Cannabis use, unspecified with other cannabis-induced disorder**
Cannabis induced sleep disorder, without use disorder

F12.99 **Cannabis use, unspecified with unspecified cannabis-induced disorder**

F13 Sedative, hypnotic, or anxiolytic related disorders

F13.1 Sedative, hypnotic or anxiolytic-related abuse

EXCLUDES1 *sedative, hypnotic or anxiolytic-related dependence (F13.2-)*
sedative, hypnotic, or anxiolytic use, unspecified (F13.9-)

F13.10 **Sedative, hypnotic or anxiolytic abuse, uncomplicated**
Sedative, hypnotic, or anxiolytic use disorder, mild

F13.12 Sedative, hypnotic or anxiolytic abuse with intoxication

F13.120 **Sedative, hypnotic or anxiolytic abuse with intoxication, uncomplicated**

F13.121 **Sedative, hypnotic or anxiolytic abuse with intoxication delirium** CC

F13.129 **Sedative, hypnotic or anxiolytic abuse with intoxication, unspecified**

F13.14 **Sedative, hypnotic or anxiolytic abuse with sedative, hypnotic or anxiolytic-induced mood disorder**
Sedative, hypnotic, or anxiolytic use disorder, mild, with sedative, hypnotic, or anxiolytic induced bipolar or related disorder
Sedative, hypnotic, or anxiolytic use disorder, mild, with sedative, hypnotic, or anxiolytic induced depressive disorder

F13.15 Sedative, hypnotic or anxiolytic abuse with sedative, hypnotic or anxiolytic-induced psychotic disorder

F13.150 **Sedative, hypnotic or anxiolytic abuse with sedative, hypnotic or anxiolytic-induced psychotic disorder with delusions** CC

F13.151 **Sedative, hypnotic or anxiolytic abuse with sedative, hypnotic or anxiolytic-induced psychotic disorder with hallucinations** CC

F13.159 **Sedative, hypnotic or anxiolytic abuse with sedative, hypnotic or anxiolytic-induced psychotic disorder, unspecified**

F13.18 Sedative, hypnotic or anxiolytic abuse with other sedative, hypnotic or anxiolytic-induced disorders

F13.180 **Sedative, hypnotic or anxiolytic abuse with sedative, hypnotic or anxiolytic-induced anxiety disorder**

F13.181 **Sedative, hypnotic or anxiolytic abuse with sedative, hypnotic or anxiolytic-induced sexual dysfunction**

F13.182 **Sedative, hypnotic or anxiolytic abuse with sedative, hypnotic or anxiolytic-induced sleep disorder**

F13.188 **Sedative, hypnotic or anxiolytic abuse with other sedative, hypnotic or anxiolytic-induced disorder**

F13.19 **Sedative, hypnotic or anxiolytic abuse with unspecified sedative, hypnotic or anxiolytic-induced disorder**

F13.2 Sedative, hypnotic or anxiolytic-related dependence

EXCLUDES1 *sedative, hypnotic or anxiolytic-related abuse (F13.1-)*
sedative, hypnotic, or anxiolytic use, unspecified (F13.9-)

EXCLUDES2 *sedative, hypnotic, or anxiolytic poisoning (T42.-)*

F13.20 **Sedative, hypnotic or anxiolytic dependence, uncomplicated** CC

F13.21 **Sedative, hypnotic or anxiolytic dependence, in remission**

F13.22 Sedative, hypnotic or anxiolytic dependence with intoxication

EXCLUDES1 *sedative, hypnotic or anxiolytic dependence with withdrawal (F13.23-)*

F13.220 **Sedative, hypnotic or anxiolytic dependence with intoxication, uncomplicated**

F13.221 **Sedative, hypnotic or anxiolytic dependence with intoxication delirium** CC

F13.229 **Sedative, hypnotic or anxiolytic dependence with intoxication, unspecified**

Unacceptable principal diagnosis symbol per Medicare code edits · Code exempt from diagnosis present on admission requirement
Questionable admission · CC Complication or comorbidity · CC/MCC exclusion · MCC Major complication or comorbidity
Principal diagnosis as its own CC · Principal diagnosis as its own MCC · Z code as first-listed diagnosis

F13.23 **Sedative, hypnotic or anxiolytic dependence with withdrawal**
Sedative, hypnotic, or anxiolytic use disorder, moderate
Sedative, hypnotic, or anxiolytic use disorder, severe
EXCLUDES1 *sedative, hypnotic or anxiolytic dependence with intoxication (F13.22-)*
F13.230 **Sedative, hypnotic or anxiolytic dependence with withdrawal, uncomplicated**
F13.231 **Sedative, hypnotic or anxiolytic dependence with withdrawal delirium**
F13.232 **Sedative, hypnotic or anxiolytic dependence with withdrawal with perceptual disturbance**
Sedative, hypnotic, or anxiolytic withdrawal with perceptual disturbances
F13.239 **Sedative, hypnotic or anxiolytic dependence with withdrawal, unspecified**
Sedative, hypnotic, or anxiolytic withdrawal without perceptual disturbances

F13.24 **Sedative, hypnotic or anxiolytic dependence with sedative, hypnotic or anxiolytic-induced mood disorder**
Sedative, hypnotic, or anxiolytic use disorder, moderate, with sedative, hypnotic, or anxiolytic induced bipolar or related disorder
Sedative, hypnotic, or anxiolytic use disorder, moderate, with sedative, hypnotic, or anxiolytic induced depressive disorder
Sedative, hypnotic, or anxiolytic use disorder, severe, with sedative, hypnotic, or anxiolytic-induced bipolar or related disorder
Sedative, hypnotic, or anxiolytic use disorder, severe, with sedative, hypnotic, or anxiolytic induced depressive disorder

F13.25 **Sedative, hypnotic or anxiolytic dependence with sedative, hypnotic or anxiolytic-induced psychotic disorder**
F13.250 **Sedative, hypnotic or anxiolytic dependence with sedative, hypnotic or anxiolytic-induced psychotic disorder with delusions**
F13.251 **Sedative, hypnotic or anxiolytic dependence with sedative, hypnotic or anxiolytic-induced psychotic disorder with hallucinations**
F13.259 **Sedative, hypnotic or anxiolytic dependence with sedative, hypnotic or anxiolytic-induced psychotic disorder, unspecified**

F13.26 **Sedative, hypnotic or anxiolytic dependence with sedative, hypnotic or anxiolytic-induced persisting amnestic disorder**

F13.27 **Sedative, hypnotic or anxiolytic dependence with sedative, hypnotic or anxiolytic-induced persisting dementia**
Sedative, hypnotic, or anxiolytic use disorder, moderate, with sedative, hypnotic, or anxiolytic induced major neurocognitive disorder
Sedative, hypnotic, or anxiolytic use disorder, severe, with sedative, hypnotic, or anxiolytic-induced major neurocognitive disorder

F13.28 **Sedative, hypnotic or anxiolytic dependence with other sedative, hypnotic or anxiolytic-induced disorders**
F13.280 **Sedative, hypnotic or anxiolytic dependence with sedative, hypnotic or anxiolytic-induced anxiety disorder**
F13.281 **Sedative, hypnotic or anxiolytic dependence with sedative, hypnotic or anxiolytic-induced sexual dysfunction**
F13.282 **Sedative, hypnotic or anxiolytic dependence with sedative, hypnotic or anxiolytic-induced sleep disorder**
F13.288 **Sedative, hypnotic or anxiolytic dependence with other sedative, hypnotic or anxiolytic-induced disorder**
Sedative, hypnotic, or anxiolytic use disorder, moderate, with sedative, hypnotic, or anxiolytic induced mild neurocognitive disorder
Sedative, hypnotic, or anxiolytic use disorder, severe, with sedative, hypnotic, or anxiolytic induced mild neurocognitive disorder

F13.29 **Sedative, hypnotic or anxiolytic dependence with unspecified sedative, hypnotic or anxiolytic-induced disorder**

F13.9 **Sedative, hypnotic or anxiolytic-related use, unspecified**
EXCLUDES1 *sedative, hypnotic or anxiolytic-related abuse (F13.1-)*
sedative, hypnotic or anxiolytic-related dependence (F13.2-)

F13.90 **Sedative, hypnotic, or anxiolytic use, unspecified, uncomplicated**

F13.92 **Sedative, hypnotic or anxiolytic use, unspecified with intoxication**
EXCLUDES1 *sedative, hypnotic or anxiolytic use, unspecified with withdrawal (F13.93-)*
F13.920 **Sedative, hypnotic or anxiolytic use, unspecified with intoxication, uncomplicated**
F13.921 **Sedative, hypnotic or anxiolytic use, unspecified with intoxication delirium**
Sedative, hypnotic, or anxiolytic-induced delirium
F13.929 **Sedative, hypnotic or anxiolytic use, unspecified with intoxication, unspecified**

F13.93 **Sedative, hypnotic or anxiolytic use, unspecified with withdrawal**
EXCLUDES1 *sedative, hypnotic or anxiolytic use, unspecified with intoxication (F13.92-)*
F13.930 **Sedative, hypnotic or anxiolytic use, unspecified with withdrawal, uncomplicated**
F13.931 **Sedative, hypnotic or anxiolytic use, unspecified with withdrawal delirium**
F13.932 **Sedative, hypnotic or anxiolytic use, unspecified with withdrawal with perceptual disturbances**
F13.939 **Sedative, hypnotic or anxiolytic use, unspecified with withdrawal, unspecified**

F13.94 **Sedative, hypnotic or anxiolytic use, unspecified with sedative, hypnotic or anxiolytic-induced mood disorder**
Sedative, hypnotic, or anxiolytic-induced bipolar or related disorder, without use disorder
Sedative, hypnotic, or anxiolytic-induced depressive disorder, without use disorder

F13.95 **Sedative, hypnotic or anxiolytic use, unspecified with sedative, hypnotic or anxiolytic-induced psychotic disorder**
F13.950 **Sedative, hypnotic or anxiolytic use, unspecified with sedative, hypnotic or anxiolytic-induced psychotic disorder with delusions**
F13.951 **Sedative, hypnotic or anxiolytic use, unspecified with sedative, hypnotic or anxiolytic-induced psychotic disorder with hallucinations**
F13.959 **Sedative, hypnotic or anxiolytic use, unspecified with sedative, hypnotic or anxiolytic-induced psychotic disorder, unspecified**
Sedative, hypnotic, or anxiolytic induced psychotic disorder, without use disorder

F13.96 **Sedative, hypnotic or anxiolytic use, unspecified with sedative, hypnotic or anxiolytic-induced persisting amnestic disorder**

F13.97 **Sedative, hypnotic or anxiolytic use, unspecified with sedative, hypnotic or anxiolytic-induced persisting dementia**
Sedative, hypnotic, or anxiolytic induced major neurocognitive disorder, without use disorder

Unspecified Code Other Specified Code Manifestation Code N Newborn P Pediatric M Maternity A Adult ♂ Male ♀ Female
● New Code ▲ Revised Code Title ►◄ Revised Text NOTES INCLUDES EXCLUDES1 Not coded here EXCLUDES2 Not included here
4th character required 5th character required 6th character required 7th character required
Extension 'X' Alert HAC Hospital-acquired condition (HAC) alert AHA AHA Coding Clinic©

F13.98 Sedative, hypnotic or anxiolytic use, unspecified with other sedative, hypnotic or anxiolytic-induced disorders
- F13.980 **Sedative, hypnotic or anxiolytic use, unspecified with sedative, hypnotic or anxiolytic-induced anxiety disorder**
  Sedative, hypnotic, or anxiolytic induced anxiety disorder, without use disorder
- F13.981 **Sedative, hypnotic or anxiolytic use, unspecified with sedative, hypnotic or anxiolytic-induced sexual dysfunction**
  Sedative, hypnotic, or anxiolytic induced sexual dysfunction disorder, without use disorder
- F13.982 **Sedative, hypnotic or anxiolytic use, unspecified with sedative, hypnotic or anxiolytic-induced sleep disorder**
  Sedative, hypnotic, or anxiolytic induced sleep disorder, without use disorder
- F13.988 **Sedative, hypnotic or anxiolytic use, unspecified with other sedative, hypnotic or anxiolytic-induced disorder**
  Sedative, hypnotic, or anxiolytic induced mild neurocognitive disorder

F13.99 **Sedative, hypnotic or anxiolytic use, unspecified with unspecified sedative, hypnotic or anxiolytic-induced disorder**

F14 Cocaine related disorders

EXCLUDES2 *other stimulant-related disorders (F15.-)*

F14.1 Cocaine abuse

EXCLUDES1 *cocaine dependence (F14.2-)*
cocaine use, unspecified (F14.9-)

F14.10 **Cocaine abuse, uncomplicated**
Cocaine use disorder, mild

F14.12 **Cocaine abuse with intoxication**
- F14.120 **Cocaine abuse with intoxication, uncomplicated**
- F14.121 **Cocaine abuse with intoxication with delirium** CC
- F14.122 **Cocaine abuse with intoxication with perceptual disturbance**
- F14.129 **Cocaine abuse with intoxication, unspecified**

F14.14 **Cocaine abuse with cocaine-induced mood disorder**
Cocaine use disorder, mild, with cocaine-induced bipolar or related disorder
Cocaine use disorder, mild, with cocaine-induced depressive disorder

F14.15 **Cocaine abuse with cocaine-induced psychotic disorder**
- F14.150 **Cocaine abuse with cocaine-induced psychotic disorder with delusions** CC
- F14.151 **Cocaine abuse with cocaine-induced psychotic disorder with hallucinations** CC
- F14.159 **Cocaine abuse with cocaine-induced psychotic disorder, unspecified**

F14.18 **Cocaine abuse with other cocaine-induced disorder**
- F14.180 **Cocaine abuse with cocaine-induced anxiety disorder**
- F14.181 **Cocaine abuse with cocaine-induced sexual dysfunction**
- F14.182 **Cocaine abuse with cocaine-induced sleep disorder**
- F14.188 **Cocaine abuse with other cocaine-induced disorder**
  Cocaine use disorder, mild, with cocaine-induced obsessive compulsive or related disorder

F14.19 **Cocaine abuse with unspecified cocaine-induced disorder**

F14.2 Cocaine dependence

EXCLUDES1 *cocaine abuse (F14.1-)*
cocaine use, unspecified (F14.9-)

EXCLUDES2 *cocaine poisoning (T40.5-)*

F14.20 **Cocaine dependence, uncomplicated** CC
Cocaine use disorder, moderate
Cocaine use disorder, severe

F14.21 **Cocaine dependence, in remission**

F14.22 **Cocaine dependence with intoxication**

EXCLUDES1 *cocaine dependence with withdrawal (F14.23)*

- F14.220 **Cocaine dependence with intoxication, uncomplicated**
- F14.221 **Cocaine dependence with intoxication delirium** CC
- F14.222 **Cocaine dependence with intoxication with perceptual disturbance** CC
- F14.229 **Cocaine dependence with intoxication, unspecified** CC

F14.23 **Cocaine dependence with withdrawal** CC

EXCLUDES1 *cocaine dependence with intoxication (F14.22-)*

F14.24 **Cocaine dependence with cocaine-induced mood disorder**
Cocaine use disorder, moderate, with cocaine-induced bipolar or related disorder
Cocaine use disorder, moderate, with cocaine-induced depressive disorder
Cocaine use disorder, severe, with cocaine-induced bipolar or related disorder
Cocaine use disorder, severe, with cocaine-induced depressive disorder

F14.25 **Cocaine dependence with cocaine-induced psychotic disorder**
- F14.250 **Cocaine dependence with cocaine-induced psychotic disorder with delusions** CC
- F14.251 **Cocaine dependence with cocaine-induced psychotic disorder with hallucinations** CC
- F14.259 **Cocaine dependence with cocaine-induced psychotic disorder, unspecified** CC

F14.28 **Cocaine dependence with other cocaine-induced disorder**
- F14.280 **Cocaine dependence with cocaine-induced anxiety disorder** CC
- F14.281 **Cocaine dependence with cocaine-induced sexual dysfunction** CC
- F14.282 **Cocaine dependence with cocaine-induced sleep disorder** CC
- F14.288 **Cocaine dependence with other cocaine-induced disorder** CC
  Cocaine use disorder, moderate, with cocaine-induced obsessive compulsive or related disorder
  Cocaine use disorder, severe, with cocaine-induced obsessive compulsive or related disorder

F14.29 **Cocaine dependence with unspecified cocaine-induced disorder**

F14.9 Cocaine use, unspecified

EXCLUDES1 *cocaine abuse (F14.1-)*
cocaine dependence (F14.2-)

F14.90 **Cocaine use, unspecified, uncomplicated**

F14.92 **Cocaine use, unspecified with intoxication**
- F14.920 **Cocaine use, unspecified with intoxication, uncomplicated**
- F14.921 **Cocaine use, unspecified with intoxication delirium** CC
- F14.922 **Cocaine use, unspecified with intoxication with perceptual disturbance**
- F14.929 **Cocaine use, unspecified with intoxication, unspecified**

F14.94 **Cocaine use, unspecified with cocaine-induced mood disorder**
Cocaine induced bipolar or related disorder, without use disorder
Cocaine induced depressive disorder, without use disorder

F14.95 **Cocaine use, unspecified with cocaine-induced psychotic disorder**
- F14.950 **Cocaine use, unspecified with cocaine-induced psychotic disorder with delusions** CC

Unacceptable principal diagnosis symbol per Medicare code edits · Code exempt from diagnosis present on admission requirement · Questionable admission · CC Complication or comorbidity · CC/MCC exclusion · MCC Major complication or comorbidity · Principal diagnosis as its own CC · Principal diagnosis as its own MCC · Z code as first-listed diagnosis

F14.951 **Cocaine use, unspecified with cocaine-induced psychotic disorder with hallucinations**

F14.959 **Cocaine use, unspecified with cocaine-induced psychotic disorder, unspecified**
Cocaine induced psychotic disorder, without use disorder

F14.98 **Cocaine use, unspecified with other specified cocaine-induced disorder**

F14.980 **Cocaine use, unspecified with cocaine-induced anxiety disorder**
Cocaine induced anxiety disorder, without use disorder

F14.981 **Cocaine use, unspecified with cocaine-induced sexual dysfunction**
Cocaine induced sexual dysfunction, without use disorder

F14.982 **Cocaine use, unspecified with cocaine-induced sleep disorder**
Cocaine induced sleep disorder, without use disorder

F14.988 **Cocaine use, unspecified with other cocaine-induced disorder**
Cocaine induced obsessive compulsive or related disorder

F14.99 **Cocaine use, unspecified with unspecified cocaine-induced disorder**

F15 **Other stimulant related disorders**
INCLUDES *amphetamine-related disorders*
caffeine
EXCLUDES2 *cocaine-related disorders (F14.-)*

F15.1 **Other stimulant abuse**
EXCLUDES1 *other stimulant dependence (F15.2-)*
other stimulant use, unspecified (F15.9-)

F15.10 **Other stimulant abuse, uncomplicated**
Amphetamine type substance use disorder, mild
Other or unspecified stimulant use disorder, mild

F15.12 **Other stimulant abuse with intoxication**

F15.120 **Other stimulant abuse with intoxication, uncomplicated**

F15.121 **Other stimulant abuse with intoxication delirium**

F15.122 **Other stimulant abuse with intoxication with perceptual disturbance**
Amphetamine or other stimulant use disorder, mild, with amphetamine or other stimulant intoxication, with perceptual disturbances

F15.129 **Other stimulant abuse with intoxication, unspecified**
Amphetamine or other stimulant use disorder, mild, with amphetamine or other stimulant intoxication, without perceptual disturbances

F15.14 **Other stimulant abuse with stimulant-induced mood disorder**
Amphetamine or other stimulant use disorder, mild, with amphetamine or other stimulant induced bipolar or related disorder
Amphetamine or other stimulant use disorder, mild, with amphetamine or other stimulant induced depressive disorder

F15.15 **Other stimulant abuse with stimulant-induced psychotic disorder**

F15.150 **Other stimulant abuse with stimulant-induced psychotic disorder with delusions**

F15.151 **Other stimulant abuse with stimulant-induced psychotic disorder with hallucinations**

F15.159 **Other stimulant abuse with stimulant-induced psychotic disorder, unspecified**

F15.18 **Other stimulant abuse with other stimulant-induced disorder**

F15.180 **Other stimulant abuse with stimulant-induced anxiety disorder**

F15.181 **Other stimulant abuse with stimulant-induced sexual dysfunction**

F15.182 **Other stimulant abuse with stimulant-induced sleep disorder**

F15.188 **Other stimulant abuse with other stimulant-induced disorder**
Amphetamine or other stimulant use disorder, mild, with amphetamine or other stimulant induced obsessive-compulsive or related disorder

F15.19 **Other stimulant abuse with unspecified stimulant-induced disorder**

F15.2 **Other stimulant dependence**
EXCLUDES1 *other stimulant abuse (F15.1-)*
other stimulant use, unspecified (F15.9-)

F15.20 **Other stimulant dependence, uncomplicated**
Amphetamine type substance use disorder, moderate
Amphetamine type substance use disorder, severe
Other or unspecified stimulant use disorder, moderate
Other or unspecified stimulant use disorder, severe

F15.21 **Other stimulant dependence, in remission**

F15.22 **Other stimulant dependence with intoxication**
EXCLUDES1 *other stimulant dependence with withdrawal (F15.23)*

F15.220 **Other stimulant dependence with intoxication, uncomplicated**

F15.221 **Other stimulant dependence with intoxication delirium**

F15.222 **Other stimulant dependence with intoxication with perceptual disturbance**
Amphetamine or other stimulant use disorder, moderate, with amphetamine or other stimulant intoxication, with perceptual disturbances
Amphetamine or other stimulant use disorder, severe, with amphetamine or other stimulant intoxication, with perceptual disturbances

F15.229 **Other stimulant dependence with intoxication, unspecified**
Amphetamine or other stimulant use disorder, moderate, with amphetamine or other stimulant intoxication, without perceptual disturbances
Amphetamine or other stimulant use disorder, severe, with amphetamine or other stimulant intoxication, without perceptual disturbances

F15.23 **Other stimulant dependence with withdrawal**
Amphetamine or other stimulant withdrawal
EXCLUDES1 *other stimulant dependence with intoxication (F15.22-)*

F15.24 **Other stimulant dependence with stimulant-induced mood disorder**
Amphetamine or other stimulant use disorder, moderate, with amphetamine or other stimulant-induced bipolar or related disorder
Amphetamine or other stimulant use disorder, moderate, with amphetamine or other stimulant induced depressive disorder
Amphetamine or other stimulant use disorder, severe, with amphetamine or other stimulant-induced bipolar or related disorder
Amphetamine or other stimulant use disorder, severe, with amphetamine or other stimulant-induced depressive disorder

F15.25 **Other stimulant dependence with stimulant-induced psychotic disorder**

F15.250 **Other stimulant dependence with stimulant-induced psychotic disorder with delusions**

F15.251 **Other stimulant dependence with stimulant-induced psychotic disorder with hallucinations**

F15.259 **Other stimulant dependence with stimulant-induced psychotic disorder, unspecified**

Unspecified Code Other Specified Code Manifestation Code N Newborn P Pediatric M Maternity A Adult ♂ Male ♀ Female
● New Code ▲ Revised Code Title ►◄ Revised Text NOTES INCLUDES EXCLUDES1 Not coded here EXCLUDES2 Not included here
4th character required 5th character required 6th character required 7th character required
Extension 'X' Alert HAC Hospital-acquired condition (HAC) alert AHA AHA Coding Clinic©

F15.28 Other stimulant dependence with other stimulant-induced disorder

F15.280 Other stimulant dependence with stimulant-induced anxiety disorder

F15.281 Other stimulant dependence with stimulant-induced sexual dysfunction

F15.282 Other stimulant dependence with stimulant-induced sleep disorder

F15.288 Other stimulant dependence with other stimulant-induced disorder

Amphetamine or other stimulant use disorder, moderate, with amphetamine or other stimulant induced obsessive compulsive or related disorder
Amphetamine or other stimulant use disorder, severe, with amphetamine or other stimulant induced obsessive compulsive or related disorder

F15.29 Other stimulant dependence with unspecified stimulant-induced disorder

F15.9 Other stimulant use, unspecified

EXCLUDES1 *other stimulant abuse (F15.1-)*
other stimulant dependence (F15.2-)

F15.90 Other stimulant use, unspecified, uncomplicated

F15.92 Other stimulant use, unspecified with intoxication

EXCLUDES1 *other stimulant use, unspecified with withdrawal (F15.93)*

F15.920 Other stimulant use, unspecified with intoxication, uncomplicated

F15.921 Other stimulant use, unspecified with intoxication delirium

Amphetamine or other stimulant-induced delirium

F15.922 Other stimulant use, unspecified with intoxication with perceptual disturbance

F15.929 Other stimulant use, unspecified with intoxication, unspecified

Caffeine intoxication

F15.93 Other stimulant use, unspecified with withdrawal

Caffeine withdrawal

EXCLUDES1 *other stimulant use, unspecified with intoxication (F15.92-)*

F15.94 Other stimulant use, unspecified with stimulant-induced mood disorder

Amphetamine or other stimulant-induced bipolar or related disorder, without use disorder
Amphetamine or other stimulant-induced depressive disorder, without use disorder

F15.95 Other stimulant use, unspecified with stimulant-induced psychotic disorder

F15.950 Other stimulant use, unspecified with stimulant-induced psychotic disorder with delusions

F15.951 Other stimulant use, unspecified with stimulant-induced psychotic disorder with hallucinations

F15.959 Other stimulant use, unspecified with stimulant-induced psychotic disorder, unspecified

Amphetamine or other stimulant-induced induced psychotic disorder, without use disorder

F15.98 Other stimulant use, unspecified with other stimulant-induced disorder

F15.980 Other stimulant use, unspecified with stimulant-induced anxiety disorder

Amphetamine or other stimulant-induced anxiety disorder, without use disorder
Caffeine induced anxiety disorder, without use disorder

F15.981 Other stimulant use, unspecified with stimulant-induced sexual dysfunction

Amphetamine or other stimulant-induced sexual dysfunction, without use disorder

F15.982 Other stimulant use, unspecified with stimulant-induced sleep disorder

Amphetamine or other stimulant-induced sleep disorder, without use disorder
Caffeine induced sleep disorder, without use disorder

F15.988 Other stimulant use, unspecified with other stimulant-induced disorder

Amphetamine or other stimulant-induced obsessive compulsive or related disorder, without use disorder

F15.99 Other stimulant use, unspecified with unspecified stimulant-induced disorder

F16 Hallucinogen related disorders

INCLUDES *ecstasy*
PCP
phencyclidine

F16.1 Hallucinogen abuse

EXCLUDES1 *hallucinogen dependence (F16.2-)*
hallucinogen use, unspecified (F16.9-)

F16.10 Hallucinogen abuse, uncomplicated

Other hallucinogen use disorder, mild
Phencyclidine use disorder, mild

F16.12 Hallucinogen abuse with intoxication

F16.120 Hallucinogen abuse with intoxication, uncomplicated

F16.121 Hallucinogen abuse with intoxication with delirium

F16.122 Hallucinogen abuse with intoxication with perceptual disturbance

F16.129 Hallucinogen abuse with intoxication, unspecified

F16.14 Hallucinogen abuse with hallucinogen-induced mood disorder

Other hallucinogen use disorder, mild, with other hallucinogen induced bipolar or related disorder
Other hallucinogen use disorder, mild, with other hallucinogen induced depressive disorder
Phencyclidine use disorder, mild, with phencyclidine induced bipolar or related disorder
Phencyclidine use disorder, mild, with phencyclidine induced depressive disorder

F16.15 Hallucinogen abuse with hallucinogen-induced psychotic disorder

F16.150 Hallucinogen abuse with hallucinogen-induced psychotic disorder with delusions

F16.151 Hallucinogen abuse with hallucinogen-induced psychotic disorder with hallucinations

F16.159 Hallucinogen abuse with hallucinogen-induced psychotic disorder, unspecified

F16.18 Hallucinogen abuse with other hallucinogen-induced disorder

F16.180 Hallucinogen abuse with hallucinogen-induced anxiety disorder

F16.183 Hallucinogen abuse with hallucinogen persisting perception disorder (flashbacks)

F16.188 Hallucinogen abuse with other hallucinogen-induced disorder

F16.19 Hallucinogen abuse with unspecified hallucinogen-induced disorder

F16.2 Hallucinogen dependence

EXCLUDES1 *hallucinogen abuse (F16.1-)*
hallucinogen use, unspecified (F16.9-)

F16.20 Hallucinogen dependence, uncomplicated

Other hallucinogen use disorder, moderate
Other hallucinogen use disorder, severe
Phencyclidine use disorder, moderate
Phencyclidine use disorder, severe

F16.21 Hallucinogen dependence, in remission

F16.22 Hallucinogen dependence with intoxication

F16.220 Hallucinogen dependence with intoxication, uncomplicated

F16.221 Hallucinogen dependence with intoxication with delirium

Unacceptable principal diagnosis symbol per Medicare code edits · Code exempt from diagnosis present on admission requirement · Questionable admission · Complication or comorbidity · CC/MCC exclusion · Major complication or comorbidity · Principal diagnosis as its own CC · Principal diagnosis as its own MCC · Z code as first-listed diagnosis

F16.229 **Hallucinogen dependence with intoxication, unspecified**

F16.24 **Hallucinogen dependence with hallucinogen-induced mood disorder**
Other hallucinogen use disorder, moderate, with other hallucinogen induced bipolar or related disorder
Other hallucinogen use disorder, moderate, with other hallucinogen induced depressive disorder
Other hallucinogen use disorder, severe, with other hallucinogen-induced bipolar or related disorder
Other hallucinogen use disorder, severe, with other hallucinogen-induced depressive disorder
Phencyclidine use disorder, moderate, with phencyclidine induced bipolar or related disorder
Phencyclidine use disorder, moderate, with phencyclidine induced depressive disorder
Phencyclidine use disorder, severe, with phencyclidine induced bipolar or related disorder
Phencyclidine use disorder, severe, with phencyclidine-induced depressive disorder

F16.25 **Hallucinogen dependence with hallucinogen-induced psychotic disorder**
F16.250 **Hallucinogen dependence with hallucinogen-induced psychotic disorder with delusions** CC
F16.251 **Hallucinogen dependence with hallucinogen-induced psychotic disorder with hallucinations** CC
F16.259 **Hallucinogen dependence with hallucinogen-induced psychotic disorder, unspecified** CC

F16.28 **Hallucinogen dependence with other hallucinogen-induced disorder**
F16.280 **Hallucinogen dependence with hallucinogen-induced anxiety disorder** CC
F16.283 **Hallucinogen dependence with hallucinogen persisting perception disorder (flashbacks)** CC
F16.288 **Hallucinogen dependence with other hallucinogen-induced disorder** CC

F16.29 **Hallucinogen dependence with unspecified hallucinogen-induced disorder**

F16.9 **Hallucinogen use, unspecified**
EXCLUDES1 *hallucinogen abuse (F16.1-)*
hallucinogen dependence (F16.2-)

F16.90 **Hallucinogen use, unspecified, uncomplicated**

F16.92 **Hallucinogen use, unspecified with intoxication**
F16.920 **Hallucinogen use, unspecified with intoxication, uncomplicated**
F16.921 **Hallucinogen use, unspecified with intoxication with delirium** CC
Other hallucinogen intoxication delirium
F16.929 **Hallucinogen use, unspecified with intoxication, unspecified**

F16.94 **Hallucinogen use, unspecified with hallucinogen-induced mood disorder**
Other hallucinogen induced bipolar or related disorder, without use disorder
Other hallucinogen induced depressive disorder, without use disorder
Phencyclidine induced bipolar or related disorder, without use disorder
Phencyclidine induced depressive disorder, without use disorder

F16.95 **Hallucinogen use, unspecified with hallucinogen-induced psychotic disorder**
F16.950 **Hallucinogen use, unspecified with hallucinogen-induced psychotic disorder with delusions** CC
F16.951 **Hallucinogen use, unspecified with hallucinogen-induced psychotic disorder with hallucinations** CC
F16.959 **Hallucinogen use, unspecified with hallucinogen-induced psychotic disorder, unspecified**
Other hallucinogen induced psychotic disorder, without use disorder
Phencyclidine induced psychotic disorder, without use disorder

F16.98 **Hallucinogen use, unspecified with other specified hallucinogen-induced disorder**
F16.980 **Hallucinogen use, unspecified with hallucinogen-induced anxiety disorder**
Other hallucinogen-induced anxiety disorder, without use disorder
Phencyclidine induced anxiety disorder, without use disorder
F16.983 **Hallucinogen use, unspecified with hallucinogen persisting perception disorder (flashbacks)**
F16.988 **Hallucinogen use, unspecified with other hallucinogen-induced disorder**

F16.99 **Hallucinogen use, unspecified with unspecified hallucinogen-induced disorder**

F17 **Nicotine dependence**
EXCLUDES1 *history of tobacco dependence (Z87.891)*
tobacco use NOS (Z72.0)
EXCLUDES2 *tobacco use (smoking) during pregnancy, childbirth and the puerperium (O99.33-)*
toxic effect of nicotine (T65.2-)

F17.2 **Nicotine dependence**

F17.20 **Nicotine dependence, unspecified**
F17.200 **Nicotine dependence, unspecified, uncomplicated** PDx
Tobacco use disorder, mild
Tobacco use disorder, moderate
Tobacco use disorder, severe
AHA: Q4, 2013
F17.201 **Nicotine dependence, unspecified, in remission** PDx
F17.203 **Nicotine dependence unspecified, with withdrawal** CC
Tobacco withdrawal
F17.208 **Nicotine dependence, unspecified, with other nicotine-induced disorders**
F17.209 **Nicotine dependence, unspecified, with unspecified nicotine-induced disorders**

F17.21 **Nicotine dependence, cigarettes**
F17.210 **Nicotine dependence, cigarettes, uncomplicated** PDx
AHA: Q4, 2013
F17.211 **Nicotine dependence, cigarettes, in remission** PDx
F17.213 **Nicotine dependence, cigarettes, with withdrawal** CC
F17.218 **Nicotine dependence, cigarettes, with other nicotine-induced disorders**
AHA: Q4, 2013
F17.219 **Nicotine dependence, cigarettes, with unspecified nicotine-induced disorders**

F17.22 **Nicotine dependence, chewing tobacco**
F17.220 **Nicotine dependence, chewing tobacco, uncomplicated** PDx
F17.221 **Nicotine dependence, chewing tobacco, in remission** PDx
F17.223 **Nicotine dependence, chewing tobacco, with withdrawal** CC
F17.228 **Nicotine dependence, chewing tobacco, with other nicotine-induced disorders**
F17.229 **Nicotine dependence, chewing tobacco, with unspecified nicotine-induced disorders**

F17.29 **Nicotine dependence, other tobacco product**
F17.290 **Nicotine dependence, other tobacco product, uncomplicated** PDx
F17.291 **Nicotine dependence, other tobacco product, in remission** PDx
F17.293 **Nicotine dependence, other tobacco product, with withdrawal** CC
F17.298 **Nicotine dependence, other tobacco product, with other nicotine-induced disorders**

Unspecified Code | Other Specified Code | Manifestation Code | N Newborn | P Pediatric | M Maternity | A Adult | ♂ Male | ♀ Female
● New Code | ▲ Revised Code Title | ►◄ Revised Text | NOTES | INCLUDES | EXCLUDES1 Not coded here | EXCLUDES2 Not included here
4th character required | 5th character required | 6th character required | 7th character required
Extension 'X' Alert | HAC Hospital-acquired condition (HAC) alert | AHA AHA Coding Clinic®

F17.299 **Nicotine dependence, other tobacco product, with unspecified nicotine-induced disorders**

F18 Inhalant related disorders

INCLUDES *volatile solvents*

F18.1 Inhalant abuse

EXCLUDES1 *inhalant dependence (F18.2-)*
inhalant use, unspecified (F18.9-)

F18.10 **Inhalant abuse, uncomplicated**
Inhalant use disorder, mild

F18.12 **Inhalant abuse with intoxication**

F18.120 **Inhalant abuse with intoxication, uncomplicated**

F18.121 **Inhalant abuse with intoxication delirium** CC

F18.129 **Inhalant abuse with intoxication, unspecified**

F18.14 **Inhalant abuse with inhalant-induced mood disorder**
Inhalant use disorder, mild, with inhalant induced depressive disorder

F18.15 **Inhalant abuse with inhalant-induced psychotic disorder**

F18.150 **Inhalant abuse with inhalant-induced psychotic disorder with delusions** CC

F18.151 **Inhalant abuse with inhalant-induced psychotic disorder with hallucinations** CC

F18.159 **Inhalant abuse with inhalant-induced psychotic disorder, unspecified**

F18.17 **Inhalant abuse with inhalant-induced dementia** CC
Inhalant use disorder, mild, with inhalant induced major neurocognitive disorder

F18.18 **Inhalant abuse with other inhalant-induced disorders**

F18.180 **Inhalant abuse with inhalant-induced anxiety disorder**

F18.188 **Inhalant abuse with other inhalant-induced disorder**
Inhalant use disorder, mild, with inhalant induced mild neurocognitive disorder

F18.19 **Inhalant abuse with unspecified inhalant-induced disorder**

F18.2 Inhalant dependence

EXCLUDES1 *inhalant abuse (F18.1-)*
inhalant use, unspecified (F18.9-)

F18.20 **Inhalant dependence, uncomplicated** CC
Inhalant use disorder, moderate
Inhalant use disorder, severe

F18.21 **Inhalant dependence, in remission**

F18.22 **Inhalant dependence with intoxication**

F18.220 **Inhalant dependence with intoxication, uncomplicated**

F18.221 **Inhalant dependence with intoxication delirium** CC

F18.229 **Inhalant dependence with intoxication, unspecified**

F18.24 **Inhalant dependence with inhalant-induced mood disorder**
Inhalant use disorder, moderate, with inhalant induced depressive disorder
Inhalant use disorder, severe, with inhalant induced depressive disorder

F18.25 **Inhalant dependence with inhalant-induced psychotic disorder**

F18.250 **Inhalant dependence with inhalant-induced psychotic disorder with delusions** CC

F18.251 **Inhalant dependence with inhalant-induced psychotic disorder with hallucinations** CC

F18.259 **Inhalant dependence with inhalant-induced psychotic disorder, unspecified** CC

F18.27 **Inhalant dependence with inhalant-induced dementia** CC
Inhalant use disorder, moderate, with inhalant induced major neurocognitive disorder
Inhalant use disorder, severe, with inhalant induced major neurocognitive disorder

F18.28 **Inhalant dependence with other inhalant-induced disorders**

F18.280 **Inhalant dependence with inhalant-induced anxiety disorder** CC

F18.288 **Inhalant dependence with other inhalant-induced disorder** CC
Inhalant use disorder, moderate, with inhalant-induced mild neurocognitive disorder
Inhalant use disorder, severe, with inhalant-induced mild neurocognitive disorder

F18.29 **Inhalant dependence with unspecified inhalant-induced disorder**

F18.9 Inhalant use, unspecified

EXCLUDES1 *inhalant abuse (F18.1-)*
inhalant dependence (F18.2-)

F18.90 **Inhalant use, unspecified, uncomplicated**

F18.92 **Inhalant use, unspecified with intoxication**

F18.920 **Inhalant use, unspecified with intoxication, uncomplicated**

F18.921 **Inhalant use, unspecified with intoxication with delirium** CC

F18.929 **Inhalant use, unspecified with intoxication, unspecified**

F18.94 **Inhalant use, unspecified with inhalant-induced mood disorder**
Inhalant induced depressive disorder

F18.95 **Inhalant use, unspecified with inhalant-induced psychotic disorder**

F18.950 **Inhalant use, unspecified with inhalant-induced psychotic disorder with delusions** CC

F18.951 **Inhalant use, unspecified with inhalant-induced psychotic disorder with hallucinations** CC

F18.959 **Inhalant use, unspecified with inhalant-induced psychotic disorder, unspecified**

F18.97 **Inhalant use, unspecified with inhalant-induced persisting dementia** CC
Inhalant-induced major neurocognitive disorder

F18.98 **Inhalant use, unspecified with other inhalant-induced disorders**

F18.980 **Inhalant use, unspecified with inhalant-induced anxiety disorder**

F18.988 **Inhalant use, unspecified with other inhalant-induced disorder**
Inhalant-induced mild neurocognitive disorder

F18.99 **Inhalant use, unspecified with unspecified inhalant-induced disorder**

F19 Other psychoactive substance related disorders

INCLUDES *polysubstance drug use (indiscriminate drug use)*

F19.1 Other psychoactive substance abuse

EXCLUDES1 *other psychoactive substance dependence (F19.2-)*
other psychoactive substance use, unspecified (F19.9-)

F19.10 **Other psychoactive substance abuse, uncomplicated**
Other (or unknown) substance use disorder, mild

F19.12 **Other psychoactive substance abuse with intoxication**

F19.120 **Other psychoactive substance abuse with intoxication, uncomplicated**

F19.121 **Other psychoactive substance abuse with intoxication delirium** CC

F19.122 **Other psychoactive substance abuse with intoxication with perceptual disturbances**

F19.129 **Other psychoactive substance abuse with intoxication, unspecified**

F19.14 **Other psychoactive substance abuse with psychoactive substance-induced mood disorder**
Other (or unknown) substance use disorder, mild, with other (or unknown) substance-induced bipolar or related disorder
Other (or unknown) substance use disorder, mild, with other (or unknown) substance-induced depressive disorder

Unacceptable principal diagnosis symbol per Medicare code edits; Code exempt from diagnosis present on admission requirement; Questionable admission; CC Complication or comorbidity; CC/MCC exclusion; MCC Major complication or comorbidity; Principal diagnosis as its own CC; Principal diagnosis as its own MCC; Z code as first-listed diagnosis

When symbols appear on a code that requires a 7th character extension, refer to Appendix D to identify applicable 7th character codes.

F19.15 Other psychoactive substance abuse with psychoactive substance-induced psychotic disorder
- F19.150 Other psychoactive substance abuse with psychoactive substance-induced psychotic disorder with delusions
- F19.151 Other psychoactive substance abuse with psychoactive substance-induced psychotic disorder with hallucinations
- F19.159 Other psychoactive substance abuse with psychoactive substance-induced psychotic disorder, unspecified

F19.16 Other psychoactive substance abuse with psychoactive substance-induced persisting amnestic disorder

F19.17 Other psychoactive substance abuse with psychoactive substance-induced persisting dementia
Other (or unknown) substance use disorder, mild, with other (or unknown) substance-induced major neurocognitive disorder

F19.18 Other psychoactive substance abuse with other psychoactive substance-induced disorders
- F19.180 Other psychoactive substance abuse with psychoactive substance-induced anxiety disorder
- F19.181 Other psychoactive substance abuse with psychoactive substance-induced sexual dysfunction
- F19.182 Other psychoactive substance abuse with psychoactive substance-induced sleep disorder
- F19.188 Other psychoactive substance abuse with other psychoactive substance-induced disorder
  Other (or unknown) substance use disorder, mild, with other (or unknown) substance induced mild neurocognitive disorder
  Other (or unknown) substance use disorder, mild, with other (or unknown) substance induced obsessive-compulsive or related disorder

F19.19 Other psychoactive substance abuse with unspecified psychoactive substance-induced disorder

F19.2 Other psychoactive substance dependence
EXCLUDES1 *other psychoactive substance abuse (F19.1-)*
other psychoactive substance use, unspecified (F19.9-)

F19.20 Other psychoactive substance dependence, uncomplicated
Other (or unknown) substance use disorder, moderate
Other (or unknown) substance use disorder, severe

F19.21 Other psychoactive substance dependence, in remission

F19.22 Other psychoactive substance dependence with intoxication
EXCLUDES1 *other psychoactive substance dependence with withdrawal (F19.23-)*
- F19.220 Other psychoactive substance dependence with intoxication, uncomplicated
- F19.221 Other psychoactive substance dependence with intoxication delirium
- F19.222 Other psychoactive substance dependence with intoxication with perceptual disturbance
- F19.229 Other psychoactive substance dependence with intoxication, unspecified

F19.23 Other psychoactive substance dependence with withdrawal
EXCLUDES1 *other psychoactive substance dependence with intoxication (F19.22-)*
- F19.230 Other psychoactive substance dependence with withdrawal, uncomplicated
- F19.231 Other psychoactive substance dependence with withdrawal delirium
- F19.232 Other psychoactive substance dependence with withdrawal with perceptual disturbance
- F19.239 Other psychoactive substance dependence with withdrawal, unspecified

F19.24 Other psychoactive substance dependence with psychoactive substance-induced mood disorder
Other (or unknown) substance use disorder, moderate, with other (or unknown) substance induced bipolar or related disorder
Other (or unknown) substance use disorder, moderate, with other (or unknown) substance induced depressive disorder
Other (or unknown) substance use disorder, severe, with other (or unknown) substance induced bipolar or related disorder
Other (or unknown) substance use disorder, severe, with other (or unknown) substance induced depressive disorder

F19.25 Other psychoactive substance dependence with psychoactive substance-induced psychotic disorder
- F19.250 Other psychoactive substance dependence with psychoactive substance-induced psychotic disorder with delusions
- F19.251 Other psychoactive substance dependence with psychoactive substance-induced psychotic disorder with hallucinations
- F19.259 Other psychoactive substance dependence with psychoactive substance-induced psychotic disorder, unspecified

F19.26 Other psychoactive substance dependence with psychoactive substance-induced persisting amnestic disorder

F19.27 Other psychoactive substance dependence with psychoactive substance-induced persisting dementia
Other (or unknown) substance use disorder, moderate, with other (or unknown) substance induced major neurocognitive disorder
Other (or unknown) substance use disorder, severe, with other (or unknown) substance induced major neurocognitive disorder

F19.28 Other psychoactive substance dependence with other psychoactive substance-induced disorders
- F19.280 Other psychoactive substance dependence with psychoactive substance-induced anxiety disorder
- F19.281 Other psychoactive substance dependence with psychoactive substance-induced sexual dysfunction
- F19.282 Other psychoactive substance dependence with psychoactive substance-induced sleep disorder
- F19.288 Other psychoactive substance dependence with other psychoactive substance-induced disorder
  Other (or unknown) substance use disorder, moderate, with other (or unknown) substance induced mild neurocognitive disorder
  Other (or unknown) substance use disorder, severe, with other (or unknown) substance induced mild neurocognitive disorder
  Other (or unknown) substance use disorder, moderate, with other (or unknown) substance induced obsessive compulsive or related disorder
  Other (or unknown) substance use disorder, severe, with other (or unknown) substance induced obsessive-compulsive or related disorder

F19.29 Other psychoactive substance dependence with unspecified psychoactive substance-induced disorder

Unspecified Code Other Specified Code Manifestation Code N Newborn P Pediatric M Maternity A Adult ♂ Male ♀ Female
● New Code ▲ Revised Code Title ►◄ Revised Text NOTES INCLUDES EXCLUDES1 Not coded here EXCLUDES2 Not included here
4th character required 5th character required 6th character required 7th character required
Extension 'X' Alert HAC Hospital-acquired condition (HAC) alert AHA AHA Coding Clinic©

F19.9 Other psychoactive substance use, unspecified
EXCLUDES1 *other psychoactive substance abuse (F19.1-)*
other psychoactive substance dependence (F19.2-)
F19.90 Other psychoactive substance use, unspecified, uncomplicated
F19.92 Other psychoactive substance use, unspecified with intoxication
EXCLUDES1 *other psychoactive substance use, unspecified with withdrawal (F19.93)*
F19.920 Other psychoactive substance use, unspecified with intoxication, uncomplicated
F19.921 Other psychoactive substance use, unspecified with intoxication with delirium CC
Other (or unknown) substance-induced delirium
F19.922 Other psychoactive substance use, unspecified with intoxication with perceptual disturbance
F19.929 Other psychoactive substance use, unspecified with intoxication, unspecified
F19.93 Other psychoactive substance use, unspecified with withdrawal
EXCLUDES1 *other psychoactive substance use, unspecified with intoxication (F19.92-)*
F19.930 Other psychoactive substance use, unspecified with withdrawal, uncomplicated CC
F19.931 Other psychoactive substance use, unspecified with withdrawal delirium CC
F19.932 Other psychoactive substance use, unspecified with withdrawal with perceptual disturbance CC
F19.939 Other psychoactive substance use, unspecified with withdrawal, unspecified CC
F19.94 Other psychoactive substance use, unspecified with psychoactive substance-induced mood disorder
Other (or unknown) substance-induced bipolar or related disorder, without use disorder
Other (or unknown) substance-induced depressive disorder, without use disorder
F19.95 Other psychoactive substance use, unspecified with psychoactive substance-induced psychotic disorder
F19.950 Other psychoactive substance use, unspecified with psychoactive substance-induced psychotic disorder with delusions CC
F19.951 Other psychoactive substance use, unspecified with psychoactive substance-induced psychotic disorder with hallucinations CC
F19.959 Other psychoactive substance use, unspecified with psychoactive substance-induced psychotic disorder, unspecified
Other or unknown substance-induced psychotic disorder, without use disorder
F19.96 Other psychoactive substance use, unspecified with psychoactive substance-induced persisting amnestic disorder
F19.97 Other psychoactive substance use, unspecified with psychoactive substance-induced persisting dementia CC
Other (or unknown) substance-induced major neurocognitive disorder, without use disorder
F19.98 Other psychoactive substance use, unspecified with other psychoactive substance-induced disorders
F19.980 Other psychoactive substance use, unspecified with psychoactive substance-induced anxiety disorder
Other (or unknown) substance-induced anxiety disorder, without use disorder
F19.981 Other psychoactive substance use, unspecified with psychoactive substance-induced sexual dysfunction
Other (or unknown) substance-induced sexual dysfunction, without use disorder
F19.982 Other psychoactive substance use, unspecified with psychoactive substance-induced sleep disorder
Other (or unknown) substance-induced sleep disorder, without use disorder
F19.988 Other psychoactive substance use, unspecified with other psychoactive substance-induced disorder
Other (or unknown) substance-induced mild neurocognitive disorder, without use disorder
Other (or unknown) substance-induced obsessive-compulsive or related disorder, without use disorder
F19.99 Other psychoactive substance use, unspecified with unspecified psychoactive substance-induced disorder

Schizophrenia, schizotypal, delusional, and other non-mood psychotic disorders (F20-F29)

F20 Schizophrenia
EXCLUDES1 *brief psychotic disorder (F23)*
cyclic schizophrenia (F25.0)
mood [affective] disorders with psychotic symptoms (F30.2, F31.2, F31.5, F31.64, F32.3, F33.3)
schizoaffective disorder (F25.-)
schizophrenic reaction NOS (F23)
EXCLUDES2 *schizophrenic reaction in:*
alcoholism (F10.15-, F10.25-, F10.95-)
brain disease (F06.2)
epilepsy (F06.2)
psychoactive drug use (F11-F19 with .15. .25, .95)
schizotypal disorder (F21)
F20.0 Paranoid schizophrenia CC
Paraphrenic schizophrenia
EXCLUDES1 *involutional paranoid state (F22)*
paranoia (F22)
F20.1 Disorganized schizophrenia CC
Hebephrenic schizophrenia
Hebephrenia
F20.2 Catatonic schizophrenia CC
Schizophrenic catalepsy
Schizophrenic catatonia
Schizophrenic flexibilitas cerea
EXCLUDES1 *catatonic stupor (R40.1)*
F20.3 Undifferentiated schizophrenia
Atypical schizophrenia
EXCLUDES1 *acute schizophrenia-like psychotic disorder (F23)*
EXCLUDES2 *post-schizophrenic depression ►(F32.89)◄*
F20.5 Residual schizophrenia CC
Restzustand (schizophrenic)
Schizophrenic residual state
F20.8 Other schizophrenia
F20.81 Schizophreniform disorder CC
Schizophreniform psychosis NOS
F20.89 Other schizophrenia CC
Cenesthopathic schizophrenia
Simple schizophrenia
F20.9 Schizophrenia, unspecified
F21 Schizotypal disorder
Borderline schizophrenia
Latent schizophrenia
Latent schizophrenic reaction
Prepsychotic schizophrenia
Prodromal schizophrenia
Pseudoneurotic schizophrenia
Pseudopsychopathic schizophrenia
Schizotypal personality disorder
EXCLUDES2 *Asperger's syndrome (F84.5)*
schizoid personality disorder (F60.1)

Unacceptable principal diagnosis symbol per Medicare code edits | Code exempt from diagnosis present on admission requirement | Questionable admission | Complication or comorbidity | CC/MCC exclusion | Major complication or comorbidity | Principal diagnosis as its own CC | Principal diagnosis as its own MCC | Z code as first-listed diagnosis

F22 **Delusional disorders**
Delusional dysmorphophobia
Involutional paranoid state
Paranoia
Paranoia querulans
Paranoid psychosis
Paranoid state
Paraphrenia (late)
Sensitiver Beziehungswahn
EXCLUDES1 *mood [affective] disorders with psychotic symptoms (F30.2, F31.2, F31.5, F31.64, F32.3, F33.3)*
paranoid schizophrenia (F20.0)
EXCLUDES2 *paranoid personality disorder (F60.0)*
paranoid psychosis, psychogenic (F23)
paranoid reaction (F23)

F23 **Brief psychotic disorder**
Paranoid reaction
Psychogenic paranoid psychosis
EXCLUDES2 *mood [affective] disorders with psychotic symptoms (F30.2, F31.2, F31.5, F31.64, F32.3, F33.3)*

F24 **Shared psychotic disorder**
Folie à deux
Induced paranoid disorder
Induced psychotic disorder

F25 **Schizoaffective disorders**
EXCLUDES1 *mood [affective] disorders with psychotic symptoms (F30.2, F31.2, F31.5, F31.64, F32.3, F33.3)*
schizophrenia (F20.-)

F25.0 **Schizoaffective disorder, bipolar type**
Cyclic schizophrenia
Schizoaffective disorder, manic type
Schizoaffective disorder, mixed type
Schizoaffective psychosis, bipolar type
Schizophreniform psychosis, manic type

F25.1 **Schizoaffective disorder, depressive type**
Schizoaffective psychosis, depressive type
Schizophreniform psychosis, depressive type

F25.8 **Other schizoaffective disorders**

F25.9 **Schizoaffective disorder, unspecified**
Schizoaffective psychosis NOS

F28 **Other psychotic disorder not due to a substance or known physiological condition**
Chronic hallucinatory psychosis

F29 **Unspecified psychosis not due to a substance or known physiological condition**
Psychosis NOS
EXCLUDES1 *mental disorder NOS (F99)*
unspecified mental disorder due to known physiological condition (F09)

Mood [affective] disorders (F30-F39)

F30 **Manic episode**
INCLUDES *bipolar disorder, single manic episode*
mixed affective episode
EXCLUDES1 *bipolar disorder (F31.-)*
major depressive disorder, single episode (F32.-)
major depressive disorder, recurrent (F33.-)

F30.1 **Manic episode without psychotic symptoms**

F30.10 **Manic episode without psychotic symptoms, unspecified**

F30.11 **Manic episode without psychotic symptoms, mild**

F30.12 **Manic episode without psychotic symptoms, moderate**

F30.13 **Manic episode, severe, without psychotic symptoms**

F30.2 **Manic episode, severe with psychotic symptoms**
Manic stupor
Mania with mood-congruent psychotic symptoms
Mania with mood-incongruent psychotic symptoms

F30.3 **Manic episode in partial remission**

F30.4 **Manic episode in full remission**

F30.8 **Other manic episodes**
Hypomania

F30.9 **Manic episode, unspecified**
Mania NOS

F31 **Bipolar disorder**
INCLUDES *manic-depressive illness*
manic-depressive psychosis
manic-depressive reaction
EXCLUDES1 *bipolar disorder, single manic episode (F30.-)*
major depressive disorder, single episode (F32.-)
major depressive disorder, recurrent (F33.-)
EXCLUDES2 *cyclothymia (F34.0)*

F31.0 **Bipolar disorder, current episode hypomanic**

F31.1 **Bipolar disorder, current episode manic without psychotic features**

F31.10 **Bipolar disorder, current episode manic without psychotic features, unspecified**

F31.11 **Bipolar disorder, current episode manic without psychotic features, mild**

F31.12 **Bipolar disorder, current episode manic without psychotic features, moderate**

F31.13 **Bipolar disorder, current episode manic without psychotic features, severe**

F31.2 **Bipolar disorder, current episode manic severe with psychotic features**
Bipolar disorder, current episode manic with mood-congruent psychotic symptoms
Bipolar disorder, current episode manic with mood-incongruent psychotic symptoms

F31.3 **Bipolar disorder, current episode depressed, mild or moderate severity**

F31.30 **Bipolar disorder, current episode depressed, mild or moderate severity, unspecified**

F31.31 **Bipolar disorder, current episode depressed, mild**

F31.32 **Bipolar disorder, current episode depressed, moderate**

F31.4 **Bipolar disorder, current episode depressed, severe, without psychotic features**

F31.5 **Bipolar disorder, current episode depressed, severe, with psychotic features**
Bipolar disorder, current episode depressed with mood-incongruent psychotic symptoms
Bipolar disorder, current episode depressed with mood-congruent psychotic symptoms

F31.6 **Bipolar disorder, current episode mixed**

F31.60 **Bipolar disorder, current episode mixed, unspecified**

F31.61 **Bipolar disorder, current episode mixed, mild**

F31.62 **Bipolar disorder, current episode mixed, moderate**

F31.63 **Bipolar disorder, current episode mixed, severe, without psychotic features**

F31.64 **Bipolar disorder, current episode mixed, severe, with psychotic features**
Bipolar disorder, current episode mixed with mood-congruent psychotic symptoms
Bipolar disorder, current episode mixed with mood-incongruent psychotic symptoms

F31.7 **Bipolar disorder, currently in remission**

F31.70 **Bipolar disorder, currently in remission, most recent episode unspecified**

F31.71 **Bipolar disorder, in partial remission, most recent episode hypomanic**

F31.72 **Bipolar disorder, in full remission, most recent episode hypomanic**

F31.73 **Bipolar disorder, in partial remission, most recent episode manic**

F31.74 **Bipolar disorder, in full remission, most recent episode manic**

F31.75 **Bipolar disorder, in partial remission, most recent episode depressed**

F31.76 **Bipolar disorder, in full remission, most recent episode depressed**

F31.77 **Bipolar disorder, in partial remission, most recent episode mixed**

F31.78 **Bipolar disorder, in full remission, most recent episode mixed**

Unspecified Code Other Specified Code Manifestation Code N Newborn P Pediatric M Maternity A Adult ♂ Male ♀ Female
● New Code ▲ Revised Code Title ►◄ Revised Text NOTES INCLUDES EXCLUDES1 Not coded here EXCLUDES2 Not included here
4th character required 5th character required 6th character required 7th character required
Extension 'X' Alert HAC Hospital-acquired condition (HAC) alert AHA AHA Coding Clinic©

F31.8 Other bipolar disorders
F31.81 Bipolar II disorder
F31.89 Other bipolar disorder
Recurrent manic episodes NOS
F31.9 Bipolar disorder, unspecified

F32 Major depressive disorder, single episode

INCLUDES *single episode of agitated depression*
single episode of depressive reaction
single episode of major depression
single episode of psychogenic depression
single episode of reactive depression
single episode of vital depression

EXCLUDES1 *bipolar disorder (F31.-)*
manic episode (F30.-)
recurrent depressive disorder (F33.-)

EXCLUDES2 *adjustment disorder (F43.2)*

F32.0 Major depressive disorder, single episode, mild
F32.1 Major depressive disorder, single episode, moderate
F32.2 Major depressive disorder, single episode, severe without psychotic features
F32.3 Major depressive disorder, single episode, severe with psychotic features
Single episode of major depression with mood-congruent psychotic symptoms
Single episode of major depression with mood-incongruent psychotic symptoms
Single episode of major depression with psychotic symptoms
Single episode of psychogenic depressive psychosis
Single episode of psychotic depression
Single episode of reactive depressive psychosis
F32.4 Major depressive disorder, single episode, in partial remission
F32.5 Major depressive disorder, single episode, in full remission
F32.8 Other depressive episodes
● F32.81 Premenstrual dysphoric disorder
EXCLUDES1 *premenstrual tension syndrome (N94.3)*
● F32.89 Other specified depressive episodes
Atypical depression
Post-schizophrenic depression
Single episode of 'masked' depression NOS
F32.9 Major depressive disorder, single episode, unspecified
Depression NOS
Depressive disorder NOS
Major depression NOS
AHA: Q4, 2013

F33 Major depressive disorder, recurrent

INCLUDES *recurrent episodes of depressive reaction*
recurrent episodes of endogenous depression
recurrent episodes of major depression
recurrent episodes of psychogenic depression
recurrent episodes of reactive depression
recurrent episodes of seasonal depressive disorder
recurrent episodes of vital depression

EXCLUDES1 *bipolar disorder (F31.-)*
manic episode (F30.-)

F33.0 Major depressive disorder, recurrent, mild
F33.1 Major depressive disorder, recurrent, moderate
F33.2 Major depressive disorder, recurrent severe without psychotic features
F33.3 Major depressive disorder, recurrent, severe with psychotic symptoms
Endogenous depression with psychotic symptoms
Recurrent severe episodes of major depression with mood-congruent psychotic symptoms
Recurrent severe episodes of major depression with mood-incongruent psychotic symptoms
Recurrent severe episodes of major depression with psychotic symptoms
Recurrent severe episodes of psychogenic depressive psychosis
Recurrent severe episodes of psychotic depression
Recurrent severe episodes of reactive depressive psychosis
F33.4 Major depressive disorder, recurrent, in remission
F33.40 Major depressive disorder, recurrent, in remission, unspecified
F33.41 Major depressive disorder, recurrent, in partial remission
F33.42 Major depressive disorder, recurrent, in full remission
F33.8 Other recurrent depressive disorders
Recurrent brief depressive episodes
F33.9 Major depressive disorder, recurrent, unspecified
Monopolar depression NOS

F34 Persistent mood [affective] disorders

F34.0 Cyclothymic disorder
Affective personality disorder
Cycloid personality
Cyclothymia
Cyclothymic personality
F34.1 Dysthymic disorder
Depressive neurosis
Depressive personality disorder
Dysthymia
Neurotic depression
Persistent anxiety depression
Persistent depressive disorder
EXCLUDES2 *anxiety depression (mild or not persistent) (F41.8)*
F34.8 Other persistent mood [affective] disorders
● F34.81 Disruptive mood dysregulation disorder
● F34.89 Other specified persistent mood disorders
F34.9 Persistent mood [affective] disorder, unspecified

F39 Unspecified mood [affective] disorder

Affective psychosis NOS

Anxiety, dissociative, stress-related, somatoform and other nonpsychotic mental disorders (F40-F48)

F40 Phobic anxiety disorders

F40.0 Agoraphobia
F40.00 Agoraphobia, unspecified
F40.01 Agoraphobia with panic disorder
Panic disorder with agoraphobia
EXCLUDES1 *panic disorder without agoraphobia (F41.0)*
F40.02 Agoraphobia without panic disorder
F40.1 Social phobias
Anthropophobia
Social anxiety disorder of childhood
Social neurosis
F40.10 Social phobia, unspecified
F40.11 Social phobia, generalized
F40.2 Specific (isolated) phobias
EXCLUDES2 *dysmorphophobia (nondelusional) (F45.22)*
nosophobia (F45.22)
F40.21 Animal type phobia
F40.210 Arachnophobia
Fear of spiders
F40.218 Other animal type phobia
F40.22 Natural environment type phobia
F40.220 Fear of thunderstorms
F40.228 Other natural environment type phobia
F40.23 Blood, injection, injury type phobia
F40.230 Fear of blood
F40.231 Fear of injections and transfusions
F40.232 Fear of other medical care
F40.233 Fear of injury
F40.24 Situational type phobia
F40.240 Claustrophobia
F40.241 Acrophobia
F40.242 Fear of bridges
F40.243 Fear of flying
F40.248 Other situational type phobia
F40.29 Other specified phobia
F40.290 Androphobia
Fear of men
F40.291 Gynephobia
Fear of women
F40.298 Other specified phobia
F40.8 Other phobic anxiety disorders
Phobic anxiety disorder of childhood

Unacceptable principal diagnosis symbol per Medicare code edits | Code exempt from diagnosis present on admission requirement
Questionable admission | Complication or comorbidity | CC/MCC exclusion | Major complication or comorbidity
Principal diagnosis as its own CC | Principal diagnosis as its own MCC | Z code as first-listed diagnosis

When symbols appear on a code that requires a 7th character extension, refer to Appendix D to identify applicable 7th character codes.

F40.9 **Phobic anxiety disorder, unspecified**
Phobia NOS
Phobic state NOS

F41 **Other anxiety disorders**
EXCLUDES2 *anxiety in:*
acute stress reaction (F43.0)
transient adjustment reaction (F43.2)
neurasthenia (F48.8)
psychophysiologic disorders (F45.-)
separation anxiety (F93.0)

F41.0 **Panic disorder [episodic paroxysmal anxiety] without agoraphobia**
Panic attack
Panic state
EXCLUDES1 *panic disorder with agoraphobia (F40.01)*

F41.1 **Generalized anxiety disorder**
Anxiety neurosis
Anxiety reaction
Anxiety state
Overanxious disorder
EXCLUDES2 *neurasthenia (F48.8)*

F41.3 **Other mixed anxiety disorders**

F41.8 **Other specified anxiety disorders**
Anxiety depression (mild or not persistent)
Anxiety hysteria
Mixed anxiety and depressive disorder

F41.9 **Anxiety disorder, unspecified**
Anxiety NOS

F42 **Obsessive-compulsive disorder**
EXCLUDES2 *obsessive-compulsive personality (disorder) (F60.5)*
obsessive-compulsive symptoms occurring in depression (F32-F33)
obsessive-compulsive symptoms occurring in schizophrenia (F20.-)

● F42.2 **Mixed obsessional thoughts and acts** CC/MCC Exc
● F42.3 **Hoarding disorder** CC/MCC Exc
● F42.4 **Excoriation (skin-picking) disorder** CC/MCC Exc
EXCLUDES1 *factitial dermatitis (L98.1)*
other specified behavioral and emotional disorders with onset usually occurring in early childhood and adolescence (F98.8)

● F42.8 **Other obsessive-compulsive disorder** CC/MCC Exc
Anancastic neurosis
Obsessive-compulsive neurosis

● F42.9 **Obsessive-compulsive disorder, unspecified** CC/MCC Exc

F43 **Reaction to severe stress, and adjustment disorders**

F43.0 **Acute stress reaction**
Acute crisis reaction
Acute reaction to stress
Combat and operational stress reaction
Combat fatigue
Crisis state
Psychic shock

F43.1 **Post-traumatic stress disorder (PTSD)**
Traumatic neurosis
F43.10 **Post-traumatic stress disorder, unspecified**
F43.11 **Post-traumatic stress disorder, acute**
F43.12 **Post-traumatic stress disorder, chronic**

F43.2 **Adjustment disorders**
Culture shock
Grief reaction
Hospitalism in children
EXCLUDES2 *separation anxiety disorder of childhood (F93.0)*
F43.20 **Adjustment disorder, unspecified**
F43.21 **Adjustment disorder with depressed mood**
F43.22 **Adjustment disorder with anxiety**
F43.23 **Adjustment disorder with mixed anxiety and depressed mood**
F43.24 **Adjustment disorder with disturbance of conduct**
F43.25 **Adjustment disorder with mixed disturbance of emotions and conduct**
F43.29 **Adjustment disorder with other symptoms**

F43.8 **Other reactions to severe stress**
Other specified trauma and stressor-related disorder

F43.9 **Reaction to severe stress, unspecified**
Trauma and stressor-related disorder, NOS

F44 **Dissociative and conversion disorders**
INCLUDES *conversion hysteria*
conversion reaction
hysteria
hysterical psychosis
EXCLUDES2 *malingering [conscious simulation] (Z76.5)*

F44.0 **Dissociative amnesia**
EXCLUDES1 *amnesia NOS (R41.3)*
anterograde amnesia (R41.1)
dissociative amnesia with dissociative fugue (F44.1)
retrograde amnesia (R41.2)
EXCLUDES2 *alcohol-or other psychoactive substance-induced amnestic disorder (F10, F13, F19 with .26, .96)*
amnestic disorder due to known physiological condition (F04)
postictal amnesia in epilepsy (G40.-)

F44.1 **Dissociative fugue**
Dissociative amnesia with dissociative fugue
EXCLUDES2 *postictal fugue in epilepsy (G40.-)*

F44.2 **Dissociative stupor**
EXCLUDES1 *catatonic stupor (R40.1)*
stupor NOS (R40.1)
EXCLUDES2 *catatonic disorder due to known physiological condition (F06.1)*
depressive stupor (F32, F33)
manic stupor (F30, F31)

F44.4 **Conversion disorder with motor symptom or deficit**
Dissociative motor disorders
Psychogenic aphonia
Psychogenic dysphonia

F44.5 **Conversion disorder with seizures or convulsions**
Dissociative convulsions

F44.6 **Conversion disorder with sensory symptom or deficit**
Dissociative anesthesia and sensory loss
Psychogenic deafness

F44.7 **Conversion disorder with mixed symptom presentation**

F44.8 **Other dissociative and conversion disorders**
F44.81 **Dissociative identity disorder**
Multiple personality disorder
F44.89 **Other dissociative and conversion disorders**
Ganser's syndrome
Psychogenic confusion
Psychogenic twilight state
Trance and possession disorders

F44.9 **Dissociative and conversion disorder, unspecified**
Dissociative disorder NOS

F45 **Somatoform disorders**
EXCLUDES2 *dissociative and conversion disorders (F44.-)*
factitious disorders (F68.1-)
hair-plucking (F63.3)
lalling (F80.0)
lisping (F80.0)
malingering [conscious simulation] (Z76.5)
nail-biting (F98.8)
psychological or behavioral factors associated with disorders or diseases classified elsewhere (F54)
sexual dysfunction, not due to a substance or known physiological condition (F52.-)
thumb-sucking (F98.8)
tic disorders (in childhood and adolescence) (F95.-)
Tourette's syndrome (F95.2)
trichotillomania (F63.3)

F45.0 **Somatization disorder**
Briquet's disorder
Multiple psychosomatic disorder

F45.1 **Undifferentiated somatoform disorder**
Somatic symptom disorder
Undifferentiated psychosomatic disorder

Unspecified Code | Other Specified Code | Manifestation Code | N Newborn | P Pediatric | M Maternity | A Adult | ♂ Male | ♀ Female
● New Code | ▲ Revised Code Title | ►◄ Revised Text | NOTES | INCLUDES | EXCLUDES1 Not coded here | EXCLUDES2 Not included here
4th character required | 5th character required | 6th character required | 7th character required
Extension 'X' Alert | HAC Hospital-acquired condition (HAC) alert | AHA AHA Coding Clinic©

F45.2 Hypochondriacal disorders
EXCLUDES2 *delusional dysmorphophobia (F22)*
fixed delusions about bodily functions or shape (F22)
F45.20 **Hypochondriacal disorder, unspecified**
F45.21 **Hypochondriasis**
Hypochondriacal neurosis
Illness anxiety disorder
F45.22 **Body dysmorphic disorder**
Dysmorphophobia (nondelusional)
Nosophobia
F45.29 **Other hypochondriacal disorders**

F45.4 **Pain disorders related to psychological factors**
EXCLUDES1 *pain NOS (R52)*
F45.41 **Pain disorder exclusively related to psychological factors**
Somatoform pain disorder (persistent)
F45.42 **Pain disorder with related psychological factors**
Code also associated acute or chronic pain (G89.-)

F45.8 **Other somatoform disorders**
Psychogenic dysmenorrhea
Psychogenic dysphagia, including 'globus hystericus'
Psychogenic pruritus
Psychogenic torticollis
Somatoform autonomic dysfunction
Teeth grinding
EXCLUDES1 *sleep related teeth grinding (G47.63)*
F45.9 **Somatoform disorder, unspecified**
Psychosomatic disorder NOS

F48 **Other nonpsychotic mental disorders**
F48.1 **Depersonalization-derealization syndrome**
F48.2 **Pseudobulbar affect**
Involuntary emotional expression disorder
Code first underlying cause, if known, such as:
amyotrophic lateral sclerosis (G12.21)
multiple sclerosis (G35)
sequelae of cerebrovascular disease (I69.-)
sequelae of traumatic intracranial injury (S06.-)
F48.8 **Other specified nonpsychotic mental disorders**
Dhat syndrome
Neurasthenia
Occupational neurosis, including writer's cramp
Psychasthenia
Psychasthenic neurosis
Psychogenic syncope
F48.9 **Nonpsychotic mental disorder, unspecified**
Neurosis NOS

Behavioral syndromes associated with physiological disturbances and physical factors (F50-F59)

F50 **Eating disorders**
EXCLUDES1 *anorexia NOS (R63.0)*
feeding difficulties (R63.3)
polyphagia (R63.2)
EXCLUDES2 *feeding disorder in infancy or childhood (F98.2-)*

F50.0 Anorexia nervosa
EXCLUDES1 *loss of appetite (R63.0)*
psychogenic loss of appetite ▶(F50.89)◀
F50.00 **Anorexia nervosa, unspecified** CC
F50.01 **Anorexia nervosa,** restricting type CC
F50.02 **Anorexia nervosa,** binge eating/purging type CC
EXCLUDES1 *bulimia nervosa (F50.2)*
F50.2 Bulimia **nervosa** CC
Bulimia NOS
Hyperorexia nervosa
EXCLUDES1 *anorexia nervosa, binge eating/purging type (F50.02)*
F50.8 **Other eating disorders**
EXCLUDES2 *pica of infancy and childhood (F98.3)*
● F50.81 Binge **eating disorder** CC/MCC Exc
● F50.89 **Other specified eating disorder** CC/MCC Exc
Pica in adults
Psychogenic loss of appetite
F50.9 **Eating disorder, unspecified**

Atypical anorexia nervosa
Atypical bulimia nervosa

F51 **Sleep disorders not due to a substance or known physiological condition**
EXCLUDES2 *organic sleep disorders (G47.-)*

F51.0 Insomnia **not due to a substance or known physiological condition**
EXCLUDES2 *alcohol related insomnia (F10.182, F10.282, F10.982)*
drug-related insomnia (F11.182, F11.282, F11.982, F13.182, F13.282, F13.982, F14.182, F14.282, F14.982, F15.182, F15.282, F15.982, F19.182, F19.282, F19.982)
insomnia NOS (G47.0-)
insomnia due to known physiological condition (G47.0-)
organic insomnia (G47.0-)
sleep deprivation (Z72.820)
F51.01 Primary **insomnia**
Idiopathic insomnia
F51.02 Adjustment **insomnia**
F51.03 Paradoxical **insomnia**
F51.04 Psychophysiologic **insomnia**
F51.05 **Insomnia** due to other mental disorder
Code also associated mental disorder
F51.09 **Other insomnia not due to a substance or known physiological condition**

F51.1 Hypersomnia **not due to a substance or known physiological condition**
EXCLUDES2 *alcohol related hypersomnia (F10.182, F10.282, F10.982)*
drug-related hypersomnia (F11.182, F11.282, F11.982, F13.182, F13.282, F13.982, F14.182, F14.282, F14.982, F15.182, F15.282, F15.982, F19.182, F19.282, F19.982)
hypersomnia NOS (G47.10)
hypersomnia due to known physiological condition (G47.10)
idiopathic hypersomnia (G47.11, G47.12)
narcolepsy (G47.4-)
F51.11 Primary **hypersomnia**
F51.12 Insufficient sleep syndrome
EXCLUDES1 *sleep deprivation (Z72.820)*
F51.13 **Hypersomnia due to other mental disorder**
Code also associated mental disorder
F51.19 **Other hypersomnia not due to a substance or known physiological condition**
F51.3 **Sleepwalking [somnambulism]**
F51.4 **Sleep terrors [night terrors]**
F51.5 **Nightmare disorder**
Dream anxiety disorder
F51.8 **Other sleep disorders not due to a substance or known physiological condition**
F51.9 **Sleep disorder not due to a substance or known physiological condition, unspecified**
Emotional sleep disorder NOS

F52 Sexual dysfunction **not due to a substance or known physiological condition**
EXCLUDES2 *Dhat syndrome (F48.8)*
F52.0 **Hypoactive sexual** desire **disorder**
Lack or loss of sexual desire
Sexual anhedonia
EXCLUDES1 *decreased libido (R68.82)*
F52.1 **Sexual** aversion **disorder**
Sexual aversion and lack of sexual enjoyment
F52.2 **Sexual arousal disorders**
Failure of genital response
F52.21 Male **erectile disorder** ♂
Psychogenic impotence
EXCLUDES1 *impotence of organic origin (N52.-)*
impotence NOS (N52.-)
F52.22 Female **sexual arousal disorder** ♀
F52.3 Orgasmic **disorder**
Inhibited orgasm
Psychogenic anorgasmy
F52.31 Female **orgasmic disorder** ♀

Unacceptable principal diagnosis symbol per Medicare code edits — Code exempt from diagnosis present on admission requirement
Questionable admission — CC Complication or comorbidity — CC/MCC exclusion — MCC Major complication or comorbidity
Principal diagnosis as its own CC — Principal diagnosis as its own MCC — Z code as first-listed diagnosis

F52.32 Male orgasmic disorder ♂
Delayed ejaculation
F52.4 Premature ejaculation ♂
F52.5 Vaginismus not due to a substance or known physiological condition ♀
Psychogenic vaginismus
EXCLUDES2 *vaginismus (due to a known physiological condition) (N94.2)*
F52.6 Dyspareunia not due to a substance or known physiological condition ♀
Genito-pelvic pain penetration disorder
Psychogenic dyspareunia
EXCLUDES2 *dyspareunia (due to a known physiological condition) ▶(N94.1-)◀*
F52.8 Other sexual dysfunction not due to a substance or known physiological condition
Excessive sexual drive
Nymphomania
Satyriasis
F52.9 Unspecified sexual dysfunction not due to a substance or known physiological condition PDx♀
Sexual dysfunction NOS
F53 Puerperal psychosis ♀
Postpartum depression
EXCLUDES1 *mood disorders with psychotic features (F30.2, F31.2, F31.5, F31.64, F32.3, F33.3)*
postpartum dysphoria (O90.6)
psychosis in schizophrenia, schizotypal, delusional, and other psychotic disorders (F20-F29)
F54 Psychological and behavioral factors associated with disorders or diseases classified elsewhere
Psychological factors affecting physical conditions
Code first the associated physical disorder, such as:
asthma (J45.-)
dermatitis (L23-L25)
gastric ulcer (K25.-)
mucous colitis (K58.-)
ulcerative colitis (K51.-)
urticaria (L50.-)
EXCLUDES2 *tension-type headache (G44.2)*
④ F55 Abuse of non-psychoactive substances
EXCLUDES2 *abuse of psychoactive substances (F10-F19)*
F55.0 Abuse of antacids
F55.1 Abuse of herbal or folk remedies
F55.2 Abuse of laxatives
F55.3 Abuse of steroids or hormones
F55.4 Abuse of vitamins
F55.8 Abuse of other non-psychoactive substances
F59 Unspecified behavioral syndromes associated with physiological disturbances and physical factors
Psychogenic physiological dysfunction NOS

Disorders of adult personality and behavior (F60-F69)

④ F60 Specific personality disorders
F60.0 Paranoid personality disorder
Expansive paranoid personality (disorder)
Fanatic personality (disorder)
Querulant personality (disorder)
Paranoid personality (disorder)
Sensitive paranoid personality (disorder)
EXCLUDES2 *paranoia (F22)*
paranoia querulans (F22)
paranoid psychosis (F22)
paranoid schizophrenia (F20.0)
paranoid state (F22)
F60.1 Schizoid personality disorder
EXCLUDES2 *Asperger's syndrome (F84.5)*
delusional disorder (F22)
schizoid disorder of childhood (F84.5)
schizophrenia (F20.-)
schizotypal disorder (F21)
F60.2 Antisocial personality disorder
Amoral personality (disorder)
Asocial personality (disorder)
Dissocial personality disorder
Psychopathic personality (disorder)
Sociopathic personality (disorder)
EXCLUDES1 *conduct disorders (F91.-)*
EXCLUDES2 *borderline personality disorder (F60.3)*
F60.3 Borderline personality disorder
Aggressive personality (disorder)
Emotionally unstable personality disorder
Explosive personality (disorder)
EXCLUDES2 *antisocial personality disorder (F60.2)*
F60.4 Histrionic personality disorder
Hysterical personality (disorder)
Psychoinfantile personality (disorder)
F60.5 Obsessive-compulsive personality disorder
Anankastic personality (disorder)
Compulsive personality (disorder)
Obsessional personality (disorder)
EXCLUDES2 *obsessive-compulsive disorder ▶(F42-)◀*
F60.6 Avoidant personality disorder
Anxious personality disorder
F60.7 Dependent personality disorder
Asthenic personality (disorder)
Inadequate personality (disorder)
Passive personality (disorder)
⑤ F60.8 Other specific personality disorders
F60.81 Narcissistic personality disorder
F60.89 Other specific personality disorders
Eccentric personality disorder
'Haltlose' type personality disorder
Immature personality disorder
Passive-aggressive personality disorder
Psychoneurotic personality disorder
Self-defeating personality disorder
F60.9 Personality disorder, unspecified
Character disorder NOS
Character neurosis NOS
Pathological personality NOS
④ F63 Impulse disorders
EXCLUDES2 *habitual excessive use of alcohol or psychoactive substances (F10-F19)*
impulse disorders involving sexual behavior (F65.-)
F63.0 Pathological gambling
Compulsive gambling
EXCLUDES1 *gambling and betting NOS (Z72.6)*
EXCLUDES2 *excessive gambling by manic patients (F30, F31)*
gambling in antisocial personality disorder (F60.2)
F63.1 Pyromania
Pathological fire-setting
EXCLUDES2 *fire-setting (by) (in):*
adult with antisocial personality disorder (F60.2)
alcohol or psychoactive substance intoxication (F10-F19)
conduct disorders (F91.-)
mental disorders due to known physiological condition (F01-F09)
schizophrenia (F20.-)
F63.2 Kleptomania
Pathological stealing
EXCLUDES1 *shoplifting as the reason for observation for suspected mental disorder (Z03.8)*
EXCLUDES2 *depressive disorder with stealing (F31-F33)*
stealing due to underlying mental condition-code to mental condition
stealing in mental disorders due to known physiological condition (F01-F09)
F63.3 Trichotillomania
Hair plucking
EXCLUDES2 *other stereotyped movement disorder (F98.4)*
⑤ F63.8 Other impulse disorders
F63.81 Intermittent explosive disorder
F63.89 Other impulse disorders

Unspecified Code Other Specified Code Manifestation Code N Newborn P Pediatric M Maternity A Adult ♂ Male ♀ Female
● New Code ▲ Revised Code Title ▶◀ Revised Text NOTES INCLUDES EXCLUDES1 Not coded here EXCLUDES2 Not included here
④ 4th character required ⑤ 5th character required ⑥ 6th character required ⑦ 7th character required
⊗ Extension 'X' Alert HAC Hospital-acquired condition (HAC) alert AHA AHA Coding Clinic©

F63.9 **Impulse disorder, unspecified**
Impulse control disorder NOS

F64 **Gender identity disorders**

F64.0 Transsexualism
Gender identity disorder in adolescence and adulthood
Gender dysphoria in adolescents and adults

F64.1 ▶Dual role transvestism◀
Use additional code to identify sex reassignment status (Z87.890)
EXCLUDES1 *gender identity disorder in childhood (F64.2)*
EXCLUDES2 *fetishistic transvestism (F65.1)*

F64.2 **Gender identity disorder of childhood**
Gender dysphoria in children
EXCLUDES1 *gender identity disorder in adolescence and adulthood ▶(F64.0)◀*
EXCLUDES2 *sexual maturation disorder (F66)*

F64.8 **Other gender identity disorders**

F64.9 **Gender identity disorder, unspecified**
Gender-role disorder NOS

F65 **Paraphilias**

F65.0 **Fetishism**

F65.1 **Transvestic fetishism**
Fetishistic transvestism

F65.2 **Exhibitionism**

F65.3 **Voyeurism**

F65.4 **Pedophilia**

F65.5 **Sadomasochism**

F65.50 **Sadomasochism, unspecified**

F65.51 **Sexual masochism**

F65.52 **Sexual sadism**

F65.8 **Other paraphilias**

F65.81 **Frotteurism**

F65.89 **Other paraphilias**
Necrophilia

F65.9 **Paraphilia, unspecified**
Sexual deviation NOS

F66 **Other sexual disorders**
Sexual maturation disorder
Sexual relationship disorder

F68 **Other disorders of adult personality and behavior**

F68.1 **Factitious disorder**
Compensation neurosis
Elaboration of physical symptoms for psychological reasons
Hospital hopper syndrome
Münchausen's syndrome
Peregrinating patient
EXCLUDES2 *factitial dermatitis (L98.1)*
person feigning illness (with obvious motivation) (Z76.5)

F68.10 **Factitious disorder, unspecified** CC

F68.11 **Factitious disorder with predominantly psychological signs and symptoms**

F68.12 **Factitious disorder with predominantly physical signs and symptoms** CC

F68.13 **Factitious disorder with combined psychological and physical signs and symptoms**

F68.8 **Other specified disorders of adult personality and behavior**

F69 **Unspecified disorder of adult personality and behavior**

Intellectual Disabilities (F70-F79)

Code first any associated physical or developmental disorders
EXCLUDES1 *borderline intellectual functioning, IQ above 70 to 84 (R41.83)*

F70 **Mild intellectual disabilities**
IQ level 50-55 to approximately 70
Mild mental subnormality

F71 **Moderate intellectual disabilities**
IQ level 35-40 to 50-55
Moderate mental subnormality

F72 **Severe intellectual disabilities** CC
IQ 20-25 to 35-40
Severe mental subnormality

F73 **Profound intellectual disabilities** CC
IQ level below 20-25
Profound mental subnormality

F78 **Other intellectual disabilities**

F79 **Unspecified intellectual disabilities**
Mental deficiency NOS
Mental subnormality NOS

Pervasive and specific developmental disorders (F80-F89)

F80 **Specific developmental disorders of speech and language**

F80.0 **Phonological disorder**
Dyslalia
Functional speech articulation disorder
Lalling
Lisping
Phonological developmental disorder
Speech articulation developmental disorder
Speech-sound disorder
EXCLUDES1 *speech articulation impairment due to aphasia NOS (R47.01)*
speech articulation impairment due to apraxia (R48.2)
EXCLUDES2 *speech articulation impairment due to hearing loss (F80.4)*
speech articulation impairment due to intellectual disabilities (F70-F79)
speech articulation impairment with expressive language developmental disorder (F80.1)
speech articulation impairment with mixed receptive expressive language developmental disorder (F80.2)

F80.1 **Expressive language disorder**
Developmental dysphasia or aphasia, expressive type
EXCLUDES1 *mixed receptive-expressive language disorder (F80.2)*
dysphasia and aphasia NOS (R47.-)
EXCLUDES2 *acquired aphasia with epilepsy [Landau-Kleffner] (G40.80-)*
selective mutism (F94.0)
intellectual disabilities (F70-F79)
pervasive developmental disorders (F84.-)

F80.2 **Mixed receptive-expressive language disorder**
Developmental dysphasia or aphasia, receptive type
Developmental Wernicke's aphasia
EXCLUDES1 *central auditory processing disorder (H93.25)*
dysphasia or aphasia NOS (R47.-)
expressive language disorder (F80.1)
expressive type dysphasia or aphasia (F80.1)
word deafness (H93.25)
EXCLUDES2 *acquired aphasia with epilepsy [Landau-Kleffner] (G40.80-)*
pervasive developmental disorders (F84.-)
selective mutism (F94.0)
intellectual disabilities (F70-F79)

F80.4 **Speech and language development delay due to hearing loss**
Code also type of hearing loss (H90.-, H91.-)

F80.8 **Other developmental disorders of speech and language**

F80.81 **Childhood onset fluency disorder**
Cluttering NOS
Stuttering NOS
EXCLUDES1 *adult onset fluency disorder (F98.5)*
fluency disorder in conditions classified elsewhere (R47.82)
fluency disorder (stuttering) following cerebrovascular disease (I69. with final characters -23)

F80.82 **Social pragmatic communication disorder** CC/MCC Exc
EXCLUDES1 *Asperger's syndrome (F84.5)*
autistic disorder (F84.0)

F80.89 **Other developmental disorders of speech and language**

F80.9 **Developmental disorder of speech and language, unspecified**
Communication disorder NOS
Language disorder NOS

Unacceptable principal diagnosis symbol per Medicare code edits — Code exempt from diagnosis present on admission requirement
Questionable admission — Complication or comorbidity — CC/MCC exclusion — Major complication or comorbidity
Principal diagnosis as its own CC — Principal diagnosis as its own MCC — Z code as first-listed diagnosis

F81 Specific developmental disorders of scholastic skills

F81.0 Specific reading disorder
'Backward reading'
Developmental dyslexia
Specific reading retardation
EXCLUDES1 *alexia NOS (R48.0)*
dyslexia NOS (R48.0)

F81.2 Mathematics disorder
Developmental acalculia
Developmental arithmetical disorder
Developmental Gerstmann's syndrome
EXCLUDES1 *acalculia NOS (R48.8)*
EXCLUDES2 *arithmetical difficulties associated with a reading disorder (F81.0)*
arithmetical difficulties associated with a spelling disorder (F81.81)
arithmetical difficulties due to inadequate teaching (Z55.8)

F81.8 Other developmental disorders of scholastic skills

F81.81 Disorder of written expression
Specific spelling disorder

F81.89 Other developmental disorders of scholastic skills

F81.9 Developmental disorder of scholastic skills, unspecified
Knowledge acquisition disability NOS
Learning disability NOS
Learning disorder NOS

F82 Specific developmental disorder of motor function
Clumsy child syndrome
Developmental coordination disorder
Developmental dyspraxia
EXCLUDES1 *abnormalities of gait and mobility (R26.-)*
lack of coordination (R27.-)
EXCLUDES2 *lack of coordination secondary to intellectual disabilities (F70-F79)*

F84 Pervasive developmental disorders
Use additional code to identify any associated medical condition and intellectual disabilities.

F84.0 Autistic disorder
Autism spectrum disorder
Infantile autism
Infantile psychosis
Kanner's syndrome
EXCLUDES1 *Asperger's syndrome (F84.5)*

F84.2 Rett's syndrome
EXCLUDES1 *Asperger's syndrome (F84.5)*
Autistic disorder (F84.0)
Other childhood disintegrative disorder (F84.3)

F84.3 Other childhood disintegrative disorder P
Dementia infantilis
Disintegrative psychosis
Heller's syndrome
Symbiotic psychosis
Use additional code to identify any associated neurological condition.
EXCLUDES1 *Asperger's syndrome (F84.5)*
Autistic disorder (F84.0)
Rett's syndrome (F84.2)

F84.5 Asperger's syndrome
Asperger's disorder
Autistic psychopathy
Schizoid disorder of childhood

F84.8 Other pervasive developmental disorders
Overactive disorder associated with intellectual disabilities and stereotyped movements

F84.9 Pervasive developmental disorder, unspecified
Atypical autism

F88 Other disorders of psychological development
Developmental agnosia
Global developmental delay
Other specified neurodevelopmental disorder

F89 Unspecified disorder of psychological development
Developmental disorder NOS
Neurodevelopmental disorder NOS

Behavioral and emotional disorders with onset usually occurring in childhood and adolescence (F90-F98)

NOTES Codes within categories F90-F98 may be used regardless of the age of a patient. These disorders generally have onset within the childhood or adolescent years, but may continue throughout life or not be diagnosed until adulthood

F90 Attention-deficit hyperactivity disorders
INCLUDES *attention deficit disorder with hyperactivity*
attention deficit syndrome with hyperactivity
EXCLUDES2 *anxiety disorders (F40.-, F41.-)*
mood [affective] disorders (F30-F39)
pervasive developmental disorders (F84.-)
schizophrenia (F20.-)

F90.0 Attention-deficit hyperactivity disorder, predominantly inattentive type

F90.1 Attention-deficit hyperactivity disorder, predominantly hyperactive type

F90.2 Attention-deficit hyperactivity disorder, combined type

F90.8 Attention-deficit hyperactivity disorder, other type

F90.9 Attention-deficit hyperactivity disorder, unspecified type
Attention-deficit hyperactivity disorder of childhood or adolescence NOS
Attention-deficit hyperactivity disorder NOS

F91 Conduct disorders
EXCLUDES1 *antisocial behavior (Z72.81-)*
antisocial personality disorder (F60.2)
EXCLUDES2 *conduct problems associated with attention-deficit hyperactivity disorder (F90.-)*
mood [affective] disorders (F30-F39)
pervasive developmental disorders (F84.-)
schizophrenia (F20.-)

F91.0 Conduct disorder confined to family context

F91.1 Conduct disorder, childhood-onset type
Unsocialized conduct disorder
Conduct disorder, solitary aggressive type
Unsocialized aggressive disorder

F91.2 Conduct disorder, adolescent-onset type
Socialized conduct disorder
Conduct disorder, group type

F91.3 Oppositional defiant disorder

F91.8 Other conduct disorders
Other specified conduct disorder
Other specified disruptive disorder

F91.9 Conduct disorder, unspecified
Behavioral disorder NOS
Conduct disorder NOS
Disruptive behavior disorder NOS
Disruptive disorder NOS

F93 Emotional disorders with onset specific to childhood

F93.0 Separation anxiety disorder of childhood P
EXCLUDES2 *mood [affective] disorders (F30-F39)*
nonpsychotic mental disorders (F40-F48)
phobic anxiety disorder of childhood (F40.8)
social phobia (F40.1)

F93.8 Other childhood emotional disorders P
Identity disorder
EXCLUDES2 *gender identity disorder of childhood (F64.2)*

F93.9 Childhood emotional disorder, unspecified P

F94 Disorders of social functioning with onset specific to childhood and adolescence

F94.0 Selective mutism
Elective mutism
EXCLUDES2 *pervasive developmental disorders (F84.-)*
schizophrenia (F20.-)
specific developmental disorders of speech and language (F80.-)
transient mutism as part of separation anxiety in young children (F93.0)

Unspecified Code Other Specified Code Manifestation Code N Newborn P Pediatric M Maternity A Adult ♂ Male ♀ Female
● New Code ▲ Revised Code Title ►◄ Revised Text NOTES INCLUDES EXCLUDES1 Not coded here EXCLUDES2 Not included here
4th character required 5th character required 6th character required 7th character required
Extension 'X' Alert HAC Hospital-acquired condition (HAC) alert AHA AHA Coding Clinic©

F94.1 Reactive attachment disorder of childhood P
Use additional code to identify any associated failure to thrive or growth retardation
EXCLUDES1 *disinhibited attachment disorder of childhood (F94.2)*
normal variation in pattern of selective attachment
EXCLUDES2 *Asperger's syndrome (F84.5)*
maltreatment syndromes (T74.-)
sexual or physical abuse in childhood, resulting in psychosocial problems (Z62.81-)

F94.2 Disinhibited attachment disorder of childhood P
Affectionless psychopathy
Institutional syndrome
EXCLUDES1 *reactive attachment disorder of childhood (F94.1)*
EXCLUDES2 *Asperger's syndrome (F84.5)*
attention-deficit hyperactivity disorders (F90.-)
hospitalism in children (F43.2-)

F94.8 Other childhood disorders of social functioning P

F94.9 Childhood disorder of social functioning, unspecified P

F95 Tic disorder

F95.0 Transient tic disorder
Provisional tic disorder

F95.1 Chronic motor or vocal tic disorder

F95.2 Tourette's disorder
Combined vocal and multiple motor tic disorder [de la Tourette]
Tourette's syndrome

F95.8 Other tic disorders

F95.9 Tic disorder, unspecified
Tic NOS

F98 Other behavioral and emotional disorders with onset usually occurring in childhood and adolescence
EXCLUDES2 *breath-holding spells (R06.89)*
gender identity disorder of childhood (F64.2)
Kleine-Levin syndrome (G47.13)
obsessive-compulsive disorder ▶(F42-)◀
sleep disorders not due to a substance or known physiological condition (F51.-)

F98.0 Enuresis not due to a substance or known physiological condition
Enuresis (primary) (secondary) of nonorganic origin
Functional enuresis
Psychogenic enuresis
Urinary incontinence of nonorganic origin
EXCLUDES1 *enuresis NOS (R32)*

F98.1 Encopresis not due to a substance or known physiological condition
Functional encopresis
Incontinence of feces of nonorganic origin
Psychogenic encopresis
Use additional code to identify the cause of any coexisting constipation.
EXCLUDES1 *encopresis NOS (R15.-)*

F98.2 Other feeding disorders of infancy and childhood
EXCLUDES1 *feeding difficulties (R63.3)*
EXCLUDES2 *anorexia nervosa and other eating disorders (F50.-)*
feeding problems of newborn (P92.-)
pica of infancy or childhood (F98.3)

F98.21 Rumination disorder of infancy P

F98.29 Other feeding disorders of infancy and early childhood P

F98.3 Pica of infancy and childhood P

F98.4 Stereotyped movement disorders
Stereotype/habit disorder
EXCLUDES1 *abnormal involuntary movements (R25.-)*
EXCLUDES2 *compulsions in obsessive-compulsive disorder ▶(F42-)◀*
hair plucking (F63.3)
movement disorders of organic origin (G20-G25)
nail-biting (F98.8)
nose-picking (F98.8)
stereotypies that are part of a broader psychiatric condition (F01-F95)
thumb-sucking (F98.8)
tic disorders (F95.-)
trichotillomania (F63.3)

F98.5 Adult onset fluency disorder
EXCLUDES1 *childhood onset fluency disorder (F80.81)*
dysphasia (R47.02)
fluency disorder in conditions classified elsewhere (R47.82)
fluency disorder (stuttering) following cerebrovascular disease (I69. with final characters -23)
tic disorders (F95.-)

F98.8 Other specified behavioral and emotional disorders with onset usually occurring in childhood and adolescence P
Excessive masturbation
Nail-biting
Nose-picking
Thumb-sucking

F98.9 Unspecified behavioral and emotional disorders with onset usually occurring in childhood and adolescence P

Unspecified mental disorder (F99)

F99 Mental disorder, not otherwise specified
Mental illness NOS
EXCLUDES1 *unspecified mental disorder due to known physiological condition (F09)*

Unacceptable principal diagnosis symbol per Medicare code edits — Code exempt from diagnosis present on admission requirement
Questionable admission — Complication or comorbidity — CC/MCC exclusion — Major complication or comorbidity
Principal diagnosis as its own CC — Principal diagnosis as its own MCC — Z code as first-listed diagnosis

Chapter 6: Diseases of the Nervous System (G00-G99)

Guidelines for Assigning Codes From This Chapter

Chapter 6 features diseases of the nervous system, which includes a central nervous system and a peripheral nervous system. The central nervous system includes the brain and spinal cord, while the peripheral nervous system includes other nerve tissue responsible for tasks such as sending signals to muscles and sending sensory information to the central nervous system.

List of Sections

- G00-G09: Inflammatory diseases of the central nervous system
- G10-G14: Systemic atrophies primarily affecting the central nervous system
- G20-G26: Extrapyramidal and movement disorders
- G30-G32: Other degenerative diseases of the nervous system
- G35-G37: Demyelinating diseases of the central nervous system
- G40-G47: Episodic and paroxysmal disorders
- G50-G59: Nerve, nerve root and plexus disorders
- G60-G65: Polyneuropathies and other disorders of the peripheral nervous system
- G70-G73: Diseases of myoneural junction and muscle
- G80-G83: Cerebral palsy and other paralytic syndromes
- G89-G99: Other disorders of the nervous system

Highlights From the ICD-10-CM Official Guidelines for Coding and Reporting

The Official Guidelines for Chapter 6 offer a lot of information on pain. It also provides guidance on distinguishing between the dominant and nondominant side, a concept used in coding weakness and paralysis. The advice that follows is from the 2017 Official Guidelines.

Clear Up Confusion Over Dominant vs. Nondominant Side

Before you can assign codes from category G81 (*Hemiplegia and hemiparesis*) and subcategories G83.1 (*Monoplegia of lower limb*), G83.2 (*Monoplegia of upper limb*), and G83.3 (*Monoplegia, unspecified*), you need to know if the affected side of the body is dominant or nondominant. The provider may document the affected side but not specify if the side is dominant or nondominant. Tabular notes may direct you to choose a particular dominance as the default choice for some codes, when the documentation does not specify one or the other. If a default choice isn't provided, use the following guidelines to make your selection:

- For ambidextrous patients, the default is dominant.
- If the left side is affected, the default is nondominant.
- If the right side is affected, the default is dominant.

Practice Proper Pain Coding Using These Guidelines

Among the various pain guidelines, you'll find help with sequencing. The general rule is that the code you report first should be the one that explains the reason for the encounter.

Pain control/management: You may sequence a code from G89 (Pain, not elsewhere classified) first when the patient presents for pain control or management. Also report the underlying cause of the pain if the documentation includes the cause.

Underlying condition treatment: When a patient presents for treatment of the condition causing the pain, you should report the condition in the primary spot. You should not assign a pain code from G89.

Neurostimulator insertion: You should put the pain code first when the patient is admitted for insertion of a neurostimulator to control pain. But if the patient is admitted to treat the underlying condition and happens to also have a neurostimulator inserted, report the underlying condition first followed by the pain code.

With site-specific pain codes: If adding a code from G89 would add information (such as acute, chronic, etc.) to a site-specific pain code, you may report both codes. Again your sequencing depends on the reason for the encounter. For pain control or management, report the G89 code followed by the site-specific code. For an encounter for any other reason, report the definitive diagnosis related to the visit. If there is no definitive diagnosis documented, report the site-specific pain code followed by the G89 code.

Postoperative pain: You'll find options for postsurgical pain in G89.1- (*Acute pain, not elsewhere classified*) and G89.2- (*Chronic pain, not elsewhere classified*). The guidelines make it clear that you should not use those codes for the typical levels of pain that occur right after an operation.

Note that when a specific complication causes the pain, you should report the appropriate complication code and can include G89.18 (*Other acute postoperative pain*) or G89.28 (*Other chronic postprocedural pain*), if applicable. If the patient with the complication presents for control of the related pain, report the G89.- code first.

Chronic pain and chronic pain syndrome: The Official Guidelines do not define a time frame for when to classify pain as chronic, G89.2 (*Chronic pain, not elsewhere classified*). Instead use the provider's documentation to make your choice. Similarly, only report G89.0 (*Central pain syndrome*) and G89.4 (*Chronic pain syndrome*) when the provider specifically documents the syndrome.

Neoplasm-related pain: When coding for neoplasm-related pain, you should apply the same basic rules that are listed above. You should report G89.3 (*Neoplasm related pain [acute] [chronic]*) first when the patient presents for pain control or management. Then add the neoplasm code after that. But when the patient presents for neoplasm treatment, limit the pain code to being an additional diagnosis when documented.

Anatomy of the Nervous System

The nervous system constitutes the body's control center and the communication network and directs the functions of multiple body organs and systems. It helps the individual to interpret external environmental events and respond to various environmental stimuli. The nervous system includes the following types and components:

1. **The Central Nervous System (CNS)**
   The central nervous system is regarded as the control center of the entire nervous system. It is composed of the brain and the spinal cord. The CNS receives the body's sensations and information about the external environmental changes via receptors and sense organs, and directs the body to act accordingly in response to these external environmental stimuli.

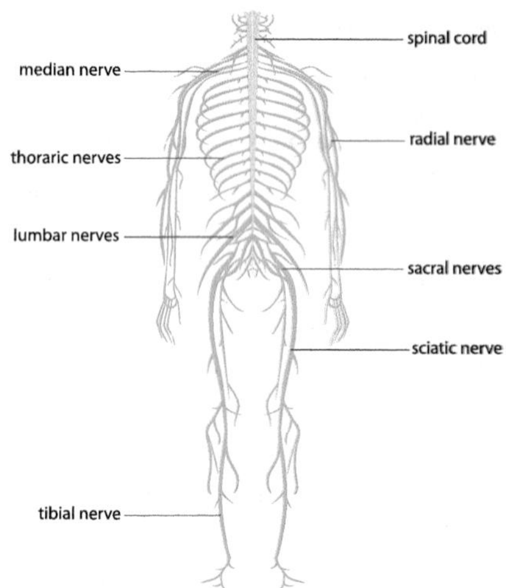

2. **The Peripheral Nervous System (PNS)**
   The peripheral nervous system is composed of the nerves that connect the brain and spinal cord with the glands, muscles and sensory receptors. The PNS can be further divided into the following subcategories:
   a) The Afferent Peripheral System

      The afferent peripheral system is composed of sensory (or afferent) neurons that transfer information to the brain and spinal cord via peripheral receptors.
   b) The Efferent Peripheral System

      The efferent peripheral system consists of the motor (or efferent) neurons that form a communication channel (for information transfer) between the brain, spinal cord, muscles and glands. This system of neurons is further divided into the following subcategories:
      i) Somatic Nervous System

         The somatic nervous system helps the individual to respond to the changes in the external environment by conducting the impulses from the brain and spinal cord to the skeletal muscle.
      ii) Autonomic Nervous System

         The autonomic nervous system (ANS) is an involuntary system of nerves that conduct impulses from the brain and spinal cord to the smooth muscles of the intestine, the cardiac muscles of the heart, and the endocrine glands. The organs of this particular system receive nerve fibers from the following divisions of the ANS:
         (a) Sympathetic Division

             The sympathetic division acts to mobilize the body's resources and induce the fight-or-flight response. This system uses norepinephrine as a neurotransmitter to speed up its activity through energy expenditure.
         (b) Parasympathetic Division

             The parasympathetic division facilitates the vegetative activities of human body (like digestion, urination and defecation).
3. **The Spinal Cord (or Medulla Spinalis)**
   The spinal cord initiates as a continuation of the medulla oblongata of the brainstem. Its length varies between 16 to 18 inches and is made up of a series of 31 segments, each of which gives rise to a pair of spinal nerves.

   The human spinal cord is further protected by a series of connective tissue membranes that are known as the spinal meninges.
4. **The Brain or Encephalon**
   The brain is regarded as one of the largest organs of the body and weighs about 3 pounds in an average adult. The major parts of the human brain are described as follows:
   a) The Brainstem

      The brainstem is regarded as the posterior portion of the brain, which is structurally continuous with the spinal cord. It is composed of the medulla oblongata, the pons Varolii, and the midbrain.
   b) The Diencephalon

      The diencephalon is located between the two cerebral hemispheres, and superiorly to the midbrain. It surrounds the third ventricle of the brain and consists of the thalamus and hypothalamus regions.
   c) The Cerebrum (or Telencephalon)

      The cerebrum constitutes the bulk of the brain and is composed of the gray matter (or cerebral cortex), longitudinal fissure, and the right and left cerebral hemispheres. It is further subdivided into the frontal, parietal, occipital and temporal lobes.
   d) The Cerebellum

      The cerebellum is regarded as the second largest portion of the brain. It is located under the occipital lobes of the cerebrum, and behind the pons and medulla oblongata of brainstem. The two partially separated hemispheres of the cerebellum are connected together by a centrally constricted structure, which is known as the vermis. The cerebellum is constituted primarily by the white matter and a thin layer of gray matter on its surface, which is known as the cerebellar cortex. The cerebrospinal fluid (CSF) is a colorless fluid that fills up the subarachnoid space (or interval between the arachnoid membrane and pia mater) and the ventricular system inside and around the spinal cord and brain.

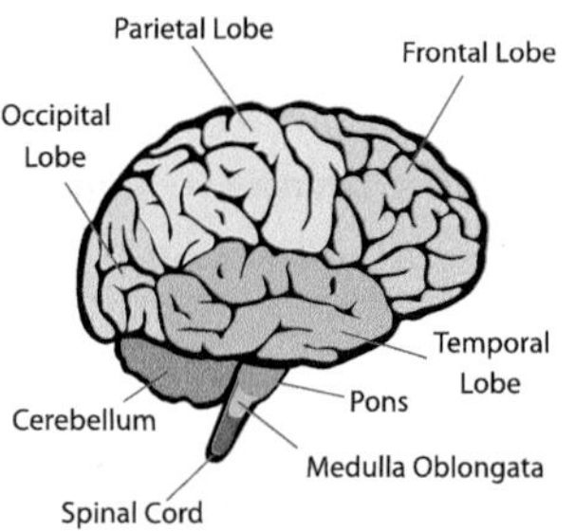

5. **The Cranial Nerves**
   The cranial nerves are based on 12 pairs that remain attached to the brain and leave the skull through various foramina in the cranial base. The names of the various cranial nerves are listed below:
   a) Olfactory (1st cranial nerve)
   b) Optic (2nd cranial nerve)
   c) Oculomotor (3rd cranial nerve)
   d) Trochlear (4th cranial nerve)
   e) Trigeminal (5th cranial nerve)
   f) Abducens (6th cranial nerve)
   g) The Facial (7th cranial nerve)
   h) Acoustic (8th cranial nerve)
   i) Glossopharyngeal (9th cranial nerve)
   j) Vagus/Pneumogastric (10th cranial nerve)
   k) Accessory (11th cranial nerve)
   l) Hypoglossal (12th cranial nerve)

The Cranial Nerves

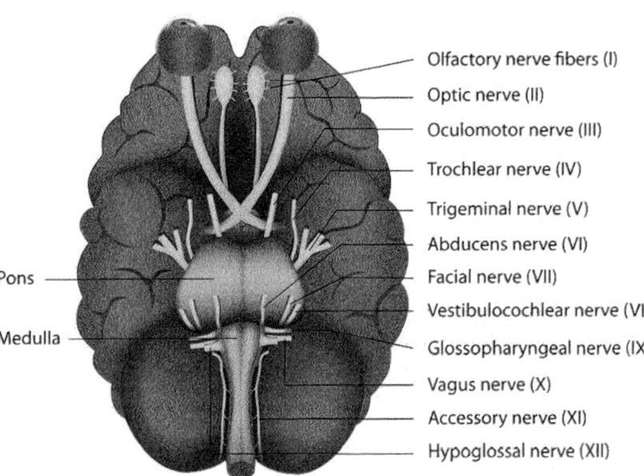

6. **The Spinal Nerves**
   The 31 pairs of spinal nerves originate from the integration of the dorsal and ventral roots of the spinal nerves. These nerves carry the motor, sensory and the autonomic signals between the spinal cord and the body. They are also called mixed nerves as they consist of both motor and sensory fibers. The spinal nerves exit the vertebral column between the adjacent vertebrae. The naming convention of the spinal nerves is based on the region and level of the spinal cord from which these nerves arise. The division of the spinal nerves is documented below:
   a) 8 pairs of cervical nerves (C1-C8)
   b) 12 pairs of thoracic nerves (T1-T12)
   c) 5 pairs of lumbar nerves (L1-L5)
   d) 5 pairs of sacral nerves (S1-S5)
   e) 1 pair of coccygeal nerves (Cx)
7. **The Sympathetic Nerves**
   The sympathetic nerves are a part of the sympathetic nervous system, which innervates the striated muscles of the heart, the smooth muscles, and multiple glands of the body. The sympathetic nervous system is that division of the autonomic nervous system which prepares the body for stressful conditions requiring energy expenditure. The nerve fibers of this system originate from the thoracic and lumbar regions of the spinal cord. The axons of these nerves leave the spinal cord via the anterior root. They further pass near the spinal ganglion and integrate with the anterior rami of the spinal nerves.

Common Pathologies

Muscular dystrophy (MD)

This is characterized by progressive muscle weakness, abnormal muscle protein, and death of muscle tissues and cells.

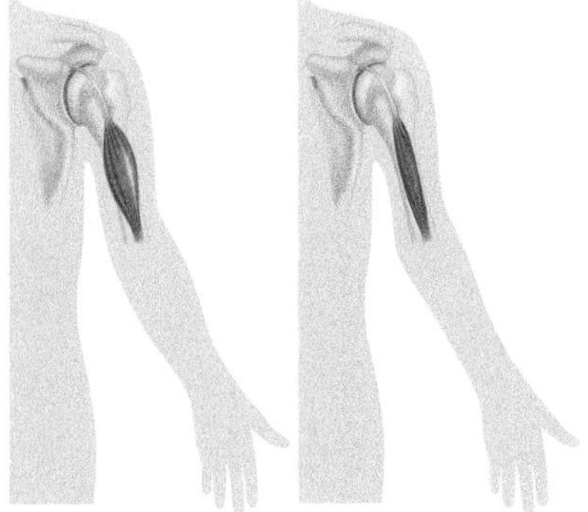

Spina Bifida
This is a type of birth defect of the brain, spine, or spinal cord, also known as the neural tube defect. It happens if the spinal column of the fetus doesn't close completely during the first month of pregnancy.

Parkinson's Disease (PD)
This is a progressive disorder of the nervous system that affects the movement and is known as a movement disorder.

Alzheimer's Disease (AD)
This is a brain disorder that seriously affects a person's ability to carry out daily activities. Alzheimer's disease is the most common form of dementia.

Strokes
This is a condition in which, due to lack of oxygen, the sudden death of brain cells occurs and can be caused by an obstruction in the blood flow to the brain. The more common kind, called ischemic stroke, is caused by a blood clot that blocks or plugs a blood vessel in the brain. The other kind, called hemorrhagic stroke, is caused by a blood vessel that breaks and bleeds into the brain. "Mini-strokes" or transient ischemic attacks (TIAs), occur when the blood supply to the brain is briefly interrupted.

Hemorrhagic Stroke

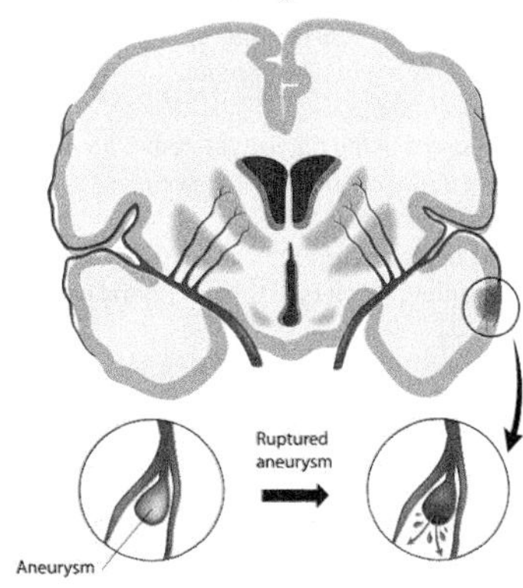

Malignant Brain Tumor
Cancer of the brain is usually called a malignant brain tumor.

Meningitis
The inflammation of the thin tissue that surrounds the brain and spinal cord, called the meninges, is known as Meningitis.

Epilepsy
This is a neurological condition that affects the nervous system. Epilepsy is also known as a seizure disorder that causes people to have recurring seizures.

Bell's Palsy
This condition occurs due to compression of a facial nerve.

Diseases of the nervous system (G00-G99)

EXCLUDES2 *certain conditions originating in the perinatal period (P04-P96)*
certain infectious and parasitic diseases (A00-B99)
complications of pregnancy, childbirth and the puerperium (O00-O9A)
congenital malformations, deformations, and chromosomal abnormalities (Q00-Q99)
endocrine, nutritional and metabolic diseases (E00-E88)
injury, poisoning and certain other consequences of external causes (S00-T88)
neoplasms (C00-D49)
symptoms, signs and abnormal clinical and laboratory findings, not elsewhere classified (R00-R94)

This chapter contains the following blocks:

G00-G09	Inflammatory diseases of the central nervous system
G10-G14	Systemic atrophies primarily affecting the central nervous system
G20-G26	Extrapyramidal and movement disorders
G30-G32	Other degenerative diseases of the nervous system
G35-G37	Demyelinating diseases of the central nervous system
G40-G47	Episodic and paroxysmal disorders
G50-G59	Nerve, nerve root and plexus disorders
G60-G65	Polyneuropathies and other disorders of the peripheral nervous system
G70-G73	Diseases of myoneural junction and muscle
G80-G83	Cerebral palsy and other paralytic syndromes
G89-G99	Other disorders of the nervous system

Inflammatory diseases of the central nervous system (G00-G09)

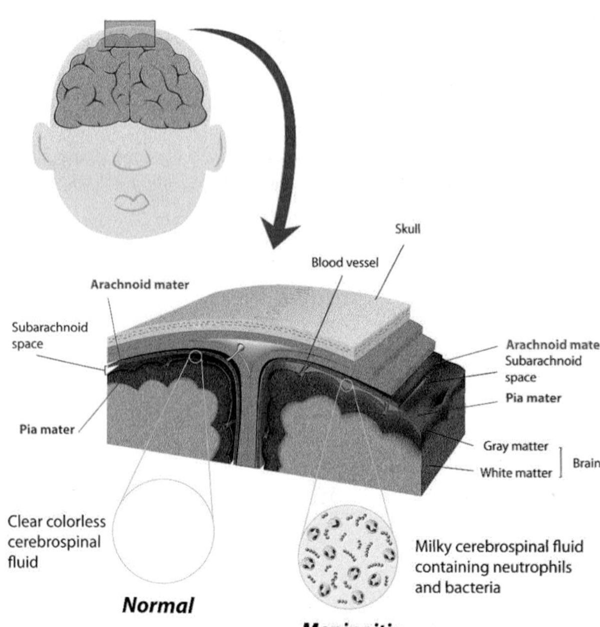

Figure 6.1 Meningitis

4th **G00 Bacterial meningitis, not elsewhere classified**
INCLUDES *bacterial arachnoiditis*
bacterial leptomeningitis
bacterial meningitis
bacterial pachymeningitis
EXCLUDES1 *bacterial:*
meningoencephalitis (G04.2)
meningomyelitis (G04.2)

G00.0 Hemophilus meningitis MCC
Meningitis due to Hemophilus influenzae

G00.1 Pneumococcal meningitis MCC
Meningitis due to Streptococcal pneumoniae

G00.2 Streptococcal meningitis MCC
Use additional code to further identify organism (B95.0-B95.5)

G00.3 Staphylococcal meningitis MCC
Use additional code to further identify organism (B95.61-B95.8)

G00.8 Other bacterial meningitis MCC
Meningitis due to Escherichia coli
Meningitis due to Friedländer's bacillus
Meningitis due to Klebsiella
Use additional code to further identify organism (B96.-)

G00.9 Bacterial meningitis, unspecified MCC
Meningitis due to gram-negative bacteria, unspecified
Purulent meningitis NOS
Pyogenic meningitis NOS
Suppurative meningitis NOS

G01 Meningitis in bacterial diseases classified elsewhere MCC
Code first underlying disease
EXCLUDES1 *meningitis (in):*
gonococcal (A54.81)
leptospirosis (A27.81)
listeriosis (A32.11)
Lyme disease (A69.21)
meningococcal (A39.0)
neurosyphilis (A52.13)
tuberculosis (A17.0)
meningoencephalitis and meningomyelitis in bacterial diseases classified elsewhere (G05)

G02 Meningitis in other infectious and parasitic diseases classified elsewhere MCC
Code first underlying disease, such as:
African trypanosomiasis (B56.-)
poliovirus infection (A80.-)
EXCLUDES1 *candidal meningitis (B37.5)*
coccidioidomycosis meningitis (B38.4)
cryptococcal meningitis (B45.1)
herpesviral [herpes simplex] meningitis (B00.3)
infectious mononucleosis complicated by meningitis (B27.- with fourth character 2)
measles complicated by meningitis (B05.1)
meningoencephalitis and meningomyelitis in other infectious and parasitic diseases classified elsewhere (G05)
mumps meningitis (B26.1)
rubella meningitis (B06.02)
varicella [chickenpox] meningitis (B01.0)
zoster meningitis (B02.1)

4th **G03 Meningitis due to other and unspecified causes**
INCLUDES *arachnoiditis NOS*
leptomeningitis NOS
meningitis NOS
pachymeningitis NOS
EXCLUDES1 *meningoencephalitis (G04.-)*
meningomyelitis (G04.-)

G03.0 Nonpyogenic meningitis MCC
Aseptic meningitis
Nonbacterial meningitis

G03.1 Chronic meningitis CC

G03.2 Benign recurrent meningitis [Mollaret] CC

G03.8 Meningitis due to other specified causes MCC

G03.9 Meningitis, unspecified MCC
Arachnoiditis (spinal) NOS

4th **G04 Encephalitis, myelitis and encephalomyelitis**
INCLUDES *acute ascending myelitis*
meningoencephalitis
meningomyelitis
EXCLUDES1 *encephalopathy NOS (G93.40)*
EXCLUDES2 *acute transverse myelitis (G37.3-)*
alcoholic encephalopathy (G31.2)
benign myalgic encephalomyelitis (G93.3)
multiple sclerosis (G35)

PDx Unacceptable principal diagnosis symbol per Medicare code edits · POA Code exempt from diagnosis present on admission requirement
? Questionable admission · CC Complication or comorbidity · CC/MCC Exc CC/MCC exclusion · MCC Major complication or comorbidity
PDx CC Principal diagnosis as its own CC · PDx MCC Principal diagnosis as its own MCC · Z1 Z code as first-listed diagnosis

 When symbols appear on a code that requires a 7th character extension, refer to Appendix D to identify applicable 7th character codes.

subacute necrotizing myelitis (G37.4)
toxic encephalitis (G92)
toxic encephalopathy (G92)

G04.0 Acute disseminated encephalitis and encephalomyelitis (ADEM)
EXCLUDES1 *acute necrotizing hemorrhagic encephalopathy (G04.3-)*
other noninfectious acute disseminated encephalomyelitis (noninfectious ADEM) (G04.81)

G04.00 Acute disseminated encephalitis and encephalomyelitis, unspecified MCC

G04.01 Postinfectious acute disseminated encephalitis and encephalomyelitis (postinfectious ADEM) MCC
EXCLUDES1 *post chickenpox encephalitis (B01.1)*
post measles encephalitis (B05.0)
post measles myelitis (B05.1)

G04.02 Postimmunization acute disseminated encephalitis, myelitis and encephalomyelitis MCC
Encephalitis, post immunization
Encephalomyelitis, post immunization
Use additional code to identify the vaccine (T50.A-, T50.B-, T50.Z-)

G04.1 Tropical spastic paraplegia CC

G04.2 Bacterial meningoencephalitis and meningomyelitis, not elsewhere classified MCC

G04.3 Acute necrotizing hemorrhagic encephalopathy
EXCLUDES1 *acute disseminated encephalitis and encephalomyelitis (G04.0-)*

G04.30 Acute necrotizing hemorrhagic encephalopathy, unspecified MCC

G04.31 Postinfectious acute necrotizing hemorrhagic encephalopathy MCC

G04.32 Postimmunization acute necrotizing hemorrhagic encephalopathy MCC
Use additional code to identify the vaccine (T50.A-, T50.B-, T50.Z-)

G04.39 Other acute necrotizing hemorrhagic encephalopathy MCC
Code also underlying etiology, if applicable

G04.8 Other encephalitis, myelitis and encephalomyelitis
Code also any associated seizure (G40.-, R56.9)

G04.81 Other encephalitis and encephalomyelitis MCC
Noninfectious acute disseminated encephalomyelitis (noninfectious ADEM)

G04.89 Other myelitis MCC

G04.9 Encephalitis, myelitis and encephalomyelitis, unspecified

G04.90 Encephalitis and encephalomyelitis, unspecified MCC
Ventriculitis (cerebral) NOS

G04.91 Myelitis, unspecified MCC

G05 Encephalitis, myelitis and encephalomyelitis in diseases classified elsewhere
Code first underlying disease, such as:
human immunodeficiency virus [HIV] disease (B20)
poliovirus (A80.-)
suppurative otitis media (H66.01-H66.4)
trichinellosis (B75)
EXCLUDES1 *adenoviral encephalitis, myelitis and encephalomyelitis (A85.1)*
congenital toxoplasmosis encephalitis, myelitis and encephalomyelitis (P37.1)
cytomegaloviral encephalitis, myelitis and encephalomyelitis (B25.8)
encephalitis, myelitis and encephalomyelitis (in) measles (B05.0)
encephalitis, myelitis and encephalomyelitis (in) systemic lupus erythematosus (M32.19)
enteroviral encephalitis, myelitis and encephalomyelitis (A85.0)
eosinophilic meningoencephalitis (B83.2)
herpesviral [herpes simplex] encephalitis, myelitis and encephalomyelitis (B00.4)
listerial encephalitis, myelitis and encephalomyelitis (A32.12)
meningococcal encephalitis, myelitis and encephalomyelitis (A39.81)
mumps encephalitis, myelitis and encephalomyelitis (B26.2)
postchickenpox encephalitis, myelitis and encephalomyelitis (B01.1-)
rubella encephalitis, myelitis and encephalomyelitis (B06.01)
toxoplasmosis encephalitis, myelitis and encephalomyelitis (B58.2)
zoster encephalitis, myelitis and encephalomyelitis (B02.0)

G05.3 Encephalitis and encephalomyelitis in diseases classified elsewhere MCC
Meningoencephalitis in diseases classified elsewhere

G05.4 Myelitis in diseases classified elsewhere MCC
Meningomyelitis in diseases classified elsewhere

G06 Intracranial and intraspinal abscess and granuloma
Use additional code (B95-B97) to identify infectious agent.

G06.0 Intracranial abscess and granuloma MCC
Brain [any part] abscess (embolic)
Cerebellar abscess (embolic)
Cerebral abscess (embolic)
Intracranial epidural abscess or granuloma
Intracranial extradural abscess or granuloma
Intracranial subdural abscess or granuloma
Otogenic abscess (embolic)
EXCLUDES1 *tuberculous intracranial abscess and granuloma (A17.81)*

G06.1 Intraspinal abscess and granuloma MCC
Abscess (embolic) of spinal cord [any part]
Intraspinal epidural abscess or granuloma
Intraspinal extradural abscess or granuloma
Intraspinal subdural abscess or granuloma
EXCLUDES1 *tuberculous intraspinal abscess and granuloma (A17.81)*

G06.2 Extradural and subdural abscess, unspecified MCC

G07 Intracranial and intraspinal abscess and granuloma in diseases classified elsewhere MCC
Code first underlying disease, such as:
schistosomiasis granuloma of brain (B65.-)
EXCLUDES1 *abscess of brain:*
amebic (A06.6)
chromomycotic (B43.1)
gonococcal (A54.82)
tuberculous (A17.81)
tuberculoma of meninges (A17.1)

G08 Intracranial and intraspinal phlebitis and thrombophlebitis MCC
Septic embolism of intracranial or intraspinal venous sinuses and veins
Septic endophlebitis of intracranial or intraspinal venous sinuses and veins
Septic phlebitis of intracranial or intraspinal venous sinuses and veins
Septic thrombophlebitis of intracranial or intraspinal venous sinuses and veins
Septic thrombosis of intracranial or intraspinal venous sinuses and veins
EXCLUDES1 *intracranial phlebitis and thrombophlebitis complicating:*
abortion, ectopic or molar pregnancy (O00-O07, O08.7)
pregnancy, childbirth and the puerperium (O22.5, O87.3)
nonpyogenic intracranial phlebitis and thrombophlebitis (I67.6)
EXCLUDES2 *intracranial phlebitis and thrombophlebitis complicating nonpyogenic intraspinal phlebitis and thrombophlebitis (G95.1)*

G09 Sequelae of inflammatory diseases of central nervous system
NOTES Category G09 is to be used to indicate conditions whose primary classification is to G00-G08 as the cause of sequelae, themselves classifiable elsewhere. The 'sequelae' include conditions specified as residuals.
Code first condition resulting from (sequela) of inflammatory diseases of central nervous system

Systemic atrophies primarily affecting the central nervous system (G10-G14)

G10 Huntington's disease CC
Huntington's chorea
Huntington's dementia

G11 Hereditary ataxia
EXCLUDES2 *cerebral palsy (G80.-)*
hereditary and idiopathic neuropathy (G60.-)
metabolic disorders (E70-E88)

Unspecified Code Other Specified Code Manifestation Code N Newborn P Pediatric M Maternity A Adult ♂ Male ♀ Female
● New Code ▲ Revised Code Title ►◄ Revised Text NOTES INCLUDES EXCLUDES1 Not coded here EXCLUDES2 Not included here
4th character required 5th character required 6th character required 7th character required
Extension 'X' Alert HAC Hospital-acquired condition (HAC) alert AHA AHA Coding Clinic©

G11.0 Congenital nonprogressive ataxia

G11.1 Early-onset cerebellar ataxia
Early-onset cerebellar ataxia with essential tremor
Early-onset cerebellar ataxia with myoclonus [Hunt's ataxia]
Early-onset cerebellar ataxia with retained tendon reflexes
Friedreich's ataxia (autosomal recessive)
X-linked recessive spinocerebellar ataxia

G11.2 Late-onset cerebellar ataxia

G11.3 Cerebellar ataxia with defective DNA repair
Ataxia telangiectasia [Louis-Bar]
EXCLUDES2 *Cockayne's syndrome (Q87.1)*
other disorders of purine and pyrimidine metabolism (E79.-)
xeroderma pigmentosum (Q82.1)

G11.4 Hereditary spastic paraplegia

G11.8 Other hereditary ataxias

G11.9 Hereditary ataxia, unspecified
Hereditary cerebellar ataxia NOS
Hereditary cerebellar degeneration
Hereditary cerebellar disease
Hereditary cerebellar syndrome

G12 Spinal muscular atrophy and related syndromes

G12.0 Infantile spinal muscular atrophy, type I [Werdnig-Hoffman]

G12.1 Other inherited spinal muscular atrophy
Adult form spinal muscular atrophy
Childhood form, type II spinal muscular atrophy
Distal spinal muscular atrophy
Juvenile form, type III spinal muscular atrophy [Kugelberg-Welander]
Progressive bulbar palsy of childhood [Fazio-Londe]
Scapuloperoneal form spinal muscular atrophy

G12.2 Motor neuron disease

G12.20 Motor neuron disease, unspecified

G12.21 Amyotrophic lateral sclerosis
Progressive spinal muscle atrophy

G12.22 Progressive bulbar palsy

G12.29 Other motor neuron disease
Familial motor neuron disease
Primary lateral sclerosis

G12.8 Other spinal muscular atrophies and related syndromes

G12.9 Spinal muscular atrophy, unspecified

G13 Systemic atrophies primarily affecting central nervous system in diseases classified elsewhere

G13.0 Paraneoplastic neuromyopathy and neuropathy
Carcinomatous neuromyopathy
Sensorial paraneoplastic neuropathy [Denny Brown]
Code first underlying neoplasm (C00-D49)

G13.1 Other systemic atrophy primarily affecting central nervous system in neoplastic disease
Paraneoplastic limbic encephalopathy
Code first underlying neoplasm (C00-D49)

G13.2 Systemic atrophy primarily affecting the central nervous system in myxedema
Code first underlying disease, such as:
hypothyroidism (E03.-)
myxedematous congenital iodine deficiency (E00.1)

G13.8 Systemic atrophy primarily affecting central nervous system in other diseases classified elsewhere
Code first underlying disease

G14 Postpolio syndrome
INCLUDES *postpolio myelitic syndrome*
EXCLUDES1 *sequelae of poliomyelitis (B91)*

Extrapyramidal and movement disorders (G20-G26)

G20 Parkinson's disease
Hemiparkinsonism
Idiopathic Parkinsonism or Parkinson's disease
Paralysis agitans
Parkinsonism or Parkinson's disease NOS
Primary Parkinsonism or Parkinson's disease
EXCLUDES1 *dementia with Parkinsonism (G31.83)*
AHA: Q2, 2016

G21 Secondary parkinsonism
EXCLUDES1 *dementia with Parkinsonism (G31.83)*
Huntington's disease (G10)
Shy-Drager syndrome (G90.3)
syphilitic Parkinsonism (A52.19)

G21.0 Malignant neuroleptic syndrome
Use additional code for adverse effect, if applicable, to identify drug (T43.3X5, T43.4X5, T43.505, T43.595)
EXCLUDES1 *neuroleptic induced parkinsonism (G21.11)*

G21.1 Other drug-induced secondary parkinsonism

G21.11 Neuroleptic induced parkinsonism
Use additional code for adverse effect, if applicable, to identify drug (T43.3X5, T43.4X5, T43.505, T43.595)
EXCLUDES1 *malignant neuroleptic syndrome (G21.0)*

G21.19 Other drug induced secondary parkinsonism
Use additional code for adverse effect, if applicable, to identify drug (T36-T50 with fifth or sixth character 5)

G21.2 Secondary parkinsonism due to other external agents
Code first (T51-T65) to identify external agent

G21.3 Postencephalitic parkinsonism

G21.4 Vascular parkinsonism

G21.8 Other secondary parkinsonism

G21.9 Secondary parkinsonism, unspecified

G23 Other degenerative diseases of basal ganglia
EXCLUDES2 *multi-system degeneration of the autonomic nervous system (G90.3)*

G23.0 Hallervorden-Spatz disease
Pigmentary pallidal degeneration

G23.1 Progressive supranuclear ophthalmoplegia [Steele-Richardson-Olszewski]
Progressive supranuclear palsy

G23.2 Striatonigral degeneration

G23.8 Other specified degenerative diseases of basal ganglia
Calcification of basal ganglia

G23.9 Degenerative disease of basal ganglia, unspecified

G24 Dystonia
INCLUDES *dyskinesia*
EXCLUDES2 *athetoid cerebral palsy (G80.3)*

G24.0 Drug induced dystonia
Use additional code for adverse effect, if applicable, to identify drug (T36-T50 with fifth or sixth character 5)

G24.01 Drug induced subacute dyskinesia
Drug induced blepharospasm
Drug induced orofacial dyskinesia
Neuroleptic induced tardive dyskinesia
Tardive dyskinesia

G24.02 Drug induced acute dystonia
Acute dystonic reaction to drugs
Neuroleptic induced acute dystonia

G24.09 Other drug induced dystonia

G24.1 Genetic torsion dystonia
Dystonia deformans progressiva
Dystonia musculorum deformans
Familial torsion dystonia
Idiopathic familial dystonia
Idiopathic (torsion) dystonia NOS
(Schwalbe-) Ziehen-Oppenheim disease

G24.2 Idiopathic nonfamilial dystonia

G24.3 Spasmodic torticollis
EXCLUDES1 *congenital torticollis (Q68.0)*
hysterical torticollis (F44.4)
ocular torticollis (R29.891)
psychogenic torticollis (F45.8)
torticollis NOS (M43.6)
traumatic recurrent torticollis (S13.4)

G24.4 Idiopathic orofacial dystonia
Orofacial dyskinesia
EXCLUDES1 *drug induced orofacial dyskinesia (G24.01)*

G24.5 Blepharospasm
EXCLUDES1 *drug induced blepharospasm (G24.01)*

Unacceptable principal diagnosis symbol per Medicare code edits · Code exempt from diagnosis present on admission requirement
Questionable admission · Complication or comorbidity · CC/MCC exclusion · Major complication or comorbidity
Principal diagnosis as its own CC · Principal diagnosis as its own MCC · Z code as first-listed diagnosis

G24.8 Other dystonia
Acquired torsion dystonia NOS
G24.9 Dystonia, unspecified
Dyskinesia NOS

G25 Other extrapyramidal and movement disorders
EXCLUDES2 *sleep related movement disorders (G47.6-)*
G25.0 Essential tremor
Familial tremor
EXCLUDES1 *tremor NOS (R25.1)*
G25.1 Drug-induced tremor
Use additional code for adverse effect, if applicable, to identify drug (T36-T50 with fifth or sixth character 5)
G25.2 Other specified forms of tremor
Intention tremor
G25.3 Myoclonus
Drug-induced myoclonus
Palatal myoclonus
Use additional code for adverse effect, if applicable, to identify drug (T36-T50 with fifth or sixth character 5)
EXCLUDES1 *facial myokymia (G51.4)*
myoclonic epilepsy (G40.-)
G25.4 Drug-induced chorea
Use additional code for adverse effect, if applicable, to identify drug (T36-T50 with fifth or sixth character 5)
G25.5 Other chorea
Chorea NOS
EXCLUDES1 *chorea NOS with heart involvement (I02.0)*
Huntington's chorea (G10)
rheumatic chorea (I02.-)
Sydenham's chorea (I02.-)
G25.6 Drug induced tics and other tics of organic origin
G25.61 Drug induced tics
Use additional code for adverse effect, if applicable, to identify drug (T36-T50 with fifth or sixth character 5)
G25.69 Other tics of organic origin
EXCLUDES1 *habit spasm (F95.9)*
tic NOS (F95.9)
Tourette's syndrome (F95.2)
G25.7 Other and unspecified drug induced movement disorders
Use additional code for adverse effect, if applicable, to identify drug (T36-T50 with fifth or sixth character 5)
G25.70 Drug induced movement disorder, unspecified.
G25.71 Drug induced akathisia
Drug induced acathisia
Neuroleptic induced acute akathisia
G25.79 Other drug induced movement disorders
G25.8 Other specified extrapyramidal and movement disorders
G25.81 Restless legs syndrome
G25.82 Stiff-man syndrome
G25.83 Benign shuddering attacks
G25.89 Other specified extrapyramidal and movement disorders
G25.9 Extrapyramidal and movement disorder, unspecified

G26 Extrapyramidal and movement disorders in diseases classified elsewhere
Code first underlying disease

Other degenerative diseases of the nervous system (G30-G32)

G30 Alzheimer's disease
INCLUDES *Alzheimer's dementia senile and presenile forms*
Use additional code to identify:
delirium, if applicable (F05)
dementia with behavioral disturbance (F02.81)
dementia without behavioral disturbance (F02.80)
EXCLUDES1 *senile degeneration of brain NEC (G31.1)*
senile dementia NOS (F03)
senility NOS (R41.81)
G30.0 Alzheimer's disease with early onset
G30.1 Alzheimer's disease with late onset A
G30.8 Other Alzheimer's disease
G30.9 Alzheimer's disease, unspecified
AHA: Q4, 2012

G31 Other degenerative diseases of nervous system, not elsewhere classified
Use additional code to identify:
dementia with behavioral disturbance (F02.81)
dementia without behavioral disturbance (F02.80)
EXCLUDES2 *Reye's syndrome (G93.7)*
G31.0 Frontotemporal dementia
G31.01 Pick's disease
Primary progressive aphasia
Progressive isolated aphasia
G31.09 Other frontotemporal dementia
Frontal dementia
G31.1 Senile degeneration of brain, not elsewhere classified
EXCLUDES1 *Alzheimer's disease (G30.-)*
senility NOS (R41.81)
G31.2 Degeneration of nervous system due to alcohol
Alcoholic cerebellar ataxia
Alcoholic cerebellar degeneration
Alcoholic cerebral degeneration
Alcoholic encephalopathy
Dysfunction of the autonomic nervous system due to alcohol
Code also associated alcoholism (F10.-)
G31.8 Other specified degenerative diseases of nervous system
G31.81 Alpers disease
Grey-matter degeneration
G31.82 Leigh's disease
Subacute necrotizing encephalopathy
G31.83 Dementia with Lewy bodies
Dementia with Parkinsonism
Lewy body dementia
Lewy body disease
G31.84 Mild cognitive impairment, so stated
EXCLUDES1 *age related cognitive decline (R41.81)*
altered mental status (R41.82)
cerebral degeneration (G31.9)
change in mental status (R41.82)
cognitive deficits following (sequelae of) cerebral hemorrhage or infarction ▶(I69.01-, I69.11-, I69.21-, I69.31-, I69.81-, I69.91-)◀
cognitive impairment due to intracranial or head injury (S06.-)
dementia (F01.-, F02.-, F03)
mild memory disturbance (F06.8)
neurologic neglect syndrome (R41.4)
personality change, nonpsychotic (F68.8)
G31.85 Corticobasal degeneration
G31.89 Other specified degenerative diseases of nervous system
G31.9 Degenerative disease of nervous system, unspecified

G32 Other degenerative disorders of nervous system in diseases classified elsewhere
G32.0 Subacute combined degeneration of spinal cord in diseases classified elsewhere
Dana-Putnam syndrome
Sclerosis of spinal cord (combined) (dorsolateral) (posterolateral)
Code first underlying disease, such as:
anemia (D51.9)
dietary (D51.3)
pernicious (D51.0)
vitamin B12 deficiency (E53.8)
EXCLUDES1 *syphilitic combined degeneration of spinal cord (A52.11)*
G32.8 Other specified degenerative disorders of nervous system in diseases classified elsewhere
Code first underlying disease, such as:
amyloidosis cerebral degeneration (E85.-)
cerebral degeneration (due to) hypothyroidism (E00.0-E03.9)
cerebral degeneration (due to) neoplasm (C00-D49)
cerebral degeneration (due to) vitamin B deficiency, except thiamine (E52-E53.-)

Unspecified Code | Other Specified Code | Manifestation Code | N Newborn | P Pediatric | M Maternity | A Adult | ♂ Male | ♀ Female
● New Code | ▲ Revised Code Title | ▶◀ Revised Text | NOTES | INCLUDES | EXCLUDES1 Not coded here | EXCLUDES2 Not included here
4th character required | 5th character required | 6th character required | 7th character required
Extension 'X' Alert | HAC Hospital-acquired condition (HAC) alert | AHA AHA Coding Clinic©

EXCLUDES1 *superior hemorrhagic polioencephalitis [Wernicke's encephalopathy] (E51.2)*

G32.81 **Cerebellar ataxia in diseases classified elsewhere** CC

Code first underlying disease, such as:
celiac disease (with gluten ataxia) (K90.0)
cerebellar ataxia (in) neoplastic disease (paraneoplastic cerebellar degeneration) (C00-D49)
non-celiac gluten ataxia (M35.9)

EXCLUDES1 *systemic atrophy primarily affecting the central nervous system in alcoholic cerebellar ataxia (G31.2)*
systemic atrophy primarily affecting the central nervous system in myxedema (G13.2)

G32.89 **Other specified degenerative disorders of nervous system in diseases classified elsewhere**

Degenerative encephalopathy in diseases classified elsewhere

Demyelinating diseases of the central nervous system (G35-G37)

G35 **Multiple sclerosis**

Disseminated multiple sclerosis
Generalized multiple sclerosis
Multiple sclerosis NOS
Multiple sclerosis of brain stem
Multiple sclerosis of cord

G36 **Other acute disseminated demyelination**

EXCLUDES1 *postinfectious encephalitis and encephalomyelitis NOS (G04.01)*

G36.0 **Neuromyelitis optica [Devic]** CC

Demyelination in optic neuritis

EXCLUDES1 *optic neuritis NOS (H46)*

G36.1 **Acute and subacute hemorrhagic leukoencephalitis [Hurst]** CC

G36.8 **Other specified acute disseminated demyelination** CC

G36.9 **Acute disseminated demyelination, unspecified** CC

G37 **Other demyelinating diseases of central nervous system**

G37.0 **Diffuse sclerosis of central nervous system** CC

Periaxial encephalitis
Schilder's disease

EXCLUDES1 *X linked adrenoleukodystrophy (E71.52-)*

G37.1 **Central demyelination of corpus callosum** CC

G37.2 **Central pontine myelinolysis** CC

G37.3 **Acute transverse myelitis in demyelinating disease of central nervous system** CC

Acute transverse myelitis NOS
Acute transverse myelopathy

EXCLUDES1 *multiple sclerosis (G35)*
neuromyelitis optica [Devic] (G36.0)

G37.4 **Subacute necrotizing myelitis of central nervous system** MCC

G37.5 **Concentric sclerosis [Balo] of central nervous system** CC

G37.8 **Other specified demyelinating diseases of central nervous system** CC

G37.9 **Demyelinating disease of central nervous system, unspecified** CC

Episodic and paroxysmal disorders (G40-G47)

G40 **Epilepsy and recurrent seizures**

NOTES The following terms are to be considered equivalent to intractable: pharmacoresistant (pharmacologically resistant), treatment resistant, refractory (medically) and poorly controlled

EXCLUDES1 *conversion disorder with seizures (F44.5)*
convulsions NOS (R56.9)
post traumatic seizures (R56.1)
seizure (convulsive) NOS (R56.9)
seizure of newborn (P90)

EXCLUDES2 *hippocampal sclerosis (G93.81)*
mesial temporal sclerosis (G93.81)
temporal sclerosis (G93.81)
Todd's paralysis (G83.84)

G40.0 **Localization-related (focal) (partial) idiopathic epilepsy and epileptic syndromes** with seizures of localized onset

Benign childhood epilepsy with centrotemporal EEG spikes
Childhood epilepsy with occipital EEG paroxysms

EXCLUDES1 *adult onset localization-related epilepsy (G40.1-, G40.2-)*

G40.00 **Localization-related (focal) (partial) idiopathic epilepsy and epileptic syndromes with seizures of localized onset,** not intractable

Localization-related (focal) (partial) idiopathic epilepsy and epileptic syndromes with seizures of localized onset without intractability

G40.001 **Localization-related (focal) (partial) idiopathic epilepsy and epileptic syndromes with seizures of localized onset, not intractable,** with status epilepticus CC

G40.009 **Localization-related (focal) (partial) idiopathic epilepsy and epileptic syndromes with seizures of localized onset, not intractable,** without status epilepticus CC

Localization-related (focal) (partial) idiopathic epilepsy and epileptic syndromes with seizures of localized onset NOS

G40.01 **Localization-related (focal) (partial) idiopathic epilepsy and epileptic syndromes with seizures of localized onset,** intractable

G40.011 **Localization-related (focal) (partial) idiopathic epilepsy and epileptic syndromes with seizures of localized onset, intractable,** with status epilepticus CC

G40.019 **Localization-related (focal) (partial) idiopathic epilepsy and epileptic syndromes with seizures of localized onset, intractable,** without status epilepticus CC

G40.1 **Localization-related (focal) (partial) symptomatic epilepsy and epileptic syndromes** with simple partial seizures

Attacks without alteration of consciousness
Epilepsia partialis continua [Kozhevnikov]
Simple partial seizures developing into secondarily generalized seizures

G40.10 **Localization-related (focal) (partial) symptomatic epilepsy and epileptic syndromes with simple partial seizures,** not intractable

Localization-related (focal) (partial) symptomatic epilepsy and epileptic syndromes with simple partial seizures without intractability

G40.101 **Localization-related (focal) (partial) symptomatic epilepsy and epileptic syndromes with simple partial seizures, not intractable,** with status epilepticus CC

G40.109 **Localization-related (focal) (partial) symptomatic epilepsy and epileptic syndromes with simple partial seizures, not intractable,** without status epilepticus CC

Localization-related (focal) (partial) symptomatic epilepsy and epileptic syndromes with simple partial seizures NOS

G40.11 **Localization-related (focal) (partial) symptomatic epilepsy and epileptic syndromes with simple partial seizures,** intractable

G40.111 **Localization-related (focal) (partial) symptomatic epilepsy and epileptic syndromes with simple partial seizures, intractable,** with status epilepticus CC

G40.119 **Localization-related (focal) (partial) symptomatic epilepsy and epileptic syndromes with simple partial seizures, intractable,** without status epilepticus CC

G40.2 **Localization-related (focal) (partial) symptomatic epilepsy and epileptic syndromes** with complex partial seizures

Attacks with alteration of consciousness, often with automatisms
Complex partial seizures developing into secondarily generalized seizures

Unacceptable principal diagnosis symbol per Medicare code edits — Code exempt from diagnosis present on admission requirement
Questionable admission — CC Complication or comorbidity — CC/MCC exclusion — MCC Major complication or comorbidity
Principal diagnosis as its own CC — Principal diagnosis as its own MCC — Z code as first-listed diagnosis

G40.20 Localization-related (focal) (partial) symptomatic epilepsy and epileptic syndromes with complex partial seizures, not intractable
Localization-related (focal) (partial) symptomatic epilepsy and epileptic syndromes with complex partial seizures without intractability
G40.201 Localization-related (focal) (partial) symptomatic epilepsy and epileptic syndromes with complex partial seizures, not intractable, with status epilepticus CC
G40.209 Localization-related (focal) (partial) symptomatic epilepsy and epileptic syndromes with complex partial seizures, not intractable, without status epilepticus CC
Localization-related (focal) (partial) symptomatic epilepsy and epileptic syndromes with complex partial seizures NOS
G40.21 Localization-related (focal) (partial) symptomatic epilepsy and epileptic syndromes with complex partial seizures, intractable
G40.211 Localization-related (focal) (partial) symptomatic epilepsy and epileptic syndromes with complex partial seizures, intractable, with status epilepticus CC
G40.219 Localization-related (focal) (partial) symptomatic epilepsy and epileptic syndromes with complex partial seizures, intractable, without status epilepticus CC
G40.3 Generalized idiopathic epilepsy and epileptic syndromes
Code also MERRF syndrome, if applicable (E88.42)
G40.30 Generalized idiopathic epilepsy and epileptic syndromes, not intractable
Generalized idiopathic epilepsy and epileptic syndromes without intractability
G40.301 Generalized idiopathic epilepsy and epileptic syndromes, not intractable, with status epilepticus MCC
G40.309 Generalized idiopathic epilepsy and epileptic syndromes, not intractable, without status epilepticus
Generalized idiopathic epilepsy and epileptic syndromes NOS
G40.31 Generalized idiopathic epilepsy and epileptic syndromes, intractable
G40.311 Generalized idiopathic epilepsy and epileptic syndromes, intractable, with status epilepticus MCC
G40.319 Generalized idiopathic epilepsy and epileptic syndromes, intractable, without status epilepticus MCC
G40.A Absence epileptic syndrome
Childhood absence epilepsy [pyknolepsy]
Juvenile absence epilepsy
Absence epileptic syndrome, NOS
G40.A0 Absence epileptic syndrome, not intractable
G40.A01 Absence epileptic syndrome, not intractable, with status epilepticus
G40.A09 Absence epileptic syndrome, not intractable, without status epilepticus
G40.A1 Absence epileptic syndrome, intractable
G40.A11 Absence epileptic syndrome, intractable, with status epilepticus CC
G40.A19 Absence epileptic syndrome, intractable, without status epilepticus CC
G40.B Juvenile myoclonic epilepsy [impulsive petit mal]
G40.B0 Juvenile myoclonic epilepsy, not intractable
G40.B01 Juvenile myoclonic epilepsy, not intractable, with status epilepticus CC
G40.B09 Juvenile myoclonic epilepsy, not intractable, without status epilepticus CC
G40.B1 Juvenile myoclonic epilepsy, intractable
G40.B11 Juvenile myoclonic epilepsy, intractable, with status epilepticus CC
G40.B19 Juvenile myoclonic epilepsy, intractable, without status epilepticus CC

G40.4 Other generalized epilepsy and epileptic syndromes
Epilepsy with grand mal seizures on awakening
Epilepsy with myoclonic absences
Epilepsy with myoclonic-astatic seizures
Grand mal seizure NOS
Nonspecific atonic epileptic seizures
Nonspecific clonic epileptic seizures
Nonspecific myoclonic epileptic seizures
Nonspecific tonic epileptic seizures
Nonspecific tonic-clonic epileptic seizures
Symptomatic early myoclonic encephalopathy
G40.40 Other generalized epilepsy and epileptic syndromes, not intractable
Other generalized epilepsy and epileptic syndromes without intractability
Other generalized epilepsy and epileptic syndromes NOS
G40.401 Other generalized epilepsy and epileptic syndromes, not intractable, with status epilepticus
G40.409 Other generalized epilepsy and epileptic syndromes, not intractable, without status epilepticus
G40.41 Other generalized epilepsy and epileptic syndromes, intractable
G40.411 Other generalized epilepsy and epileptic syndromes, intractable, with status epilepticus CC
G40.419 Other generalized epilepsy and epileptic syndromes, intractable, without status epilepticus CC
G40.5 Epileptic seizures related to external causes
Epileptic seizures related to alcohol
Epileptic seizures related to drugs
Epileptic seizures related to hormonal changes
Epileptic seizures related to sleep deprivation
Epileptic seizures related to stress
Code also , if applicable, associated epilepsy and recurrent seizures (G40.-)
Use additional code for adverse effect, if applicable, to identify drug (T36-T50 with fifth or sixth character 5)
G40.50 Epileptic seizures related to external causes, not intractable
G40.501 Epileptic seizures related to external causes, not intractable, with status epilepticus CC
G40.509 Epileptic seizures related to external causes, not intractable, without status epilepticus CC
Epileptic seizures related to external causes, NOS
G40.8 Other epilepsy and recurrent seizures
Epilepsies and epileptic syndromes undetermined as to whether they are focal or generalized
Landau-Kleffner syndrome
G40.80 Other epilepsy
G40.801 Other epilepsy, not intractable, with status epilepticus CC
Other epilepsy without intractability with status epilepticus
G40.802 Other epilepsy, not intractable, without status epilepticus CC
Other epilepsy NOS
Other epilepsy without intractability without status epilepticus
G40.803 Other epilepsy, intractable, with status epilepticus CC
G40.804 Other epilepsy, intractable, without status epilepticus CC
G40.81 Lennox-Gastaut syndrome
G40.811 Lennox-Gastaut syndrome, not intractable, with status epilepticus CC
G40.812 Lennox-Gastaut syndrome, not intractable, without status epilepticus CC
G40.813 Lennox-Gastaut syndrome, intractable, with status epilepticus CC
G40.814 Lennox-Gastaut syndrome, intractable, without status epilepticus CC

G40.82 Epileptic spasms
Infantile spasms
Salaam attacks
West's syndrome
G40.821 **Epileptic spasms, not intractable,** with status epilepticus CC
G40.822 **Epileptic spasms, not intractable,** without status epilepticus CC
G40.823 **Epileptic spasms, intractable,** with status epilepticus CC
G40.824 **Epileptic spasms, intractable,** without status epilepticus CC
G40.89 **Other seizures** CC
EXCLUDES1 *post traumatic seizures (R56.1)*
recurrent seizures NOS (G40.909)
seizure NOS (R56.9)

G40.9 **Epilepsy, unspecified**
G40.90 **Epilepsy, unspecified,** not intractable
Epilepsy, unspecified, without intractability
G40.901 **Epilepsy, unspecified, not intractable,** with status epilepticus
G40.909 **Epilepsy, unspecified, not intractable,** without status epilepticus
Epilepsy NOS
Epileptic convulsions NOS
Epileptic fits NOS
Epileptic seizures NOS
Recurrent seizures NOS
Seizure disorder NOS
G40.91 **Epilepsy, unspecified,** intractable
Intractable seizure disorder NOS
G40.911 **Epilepsy, unspecified, intractable,** with status epilepticus CC
G40.919 **Epilepsy, unspecified, intractable,** without status epilepticus CC

G43 **Migraine**
NOTES The following terms are to be considered equivalent to intractable: pharmacoresistant (pharmacologically resistant), treatment resistant, refractory (medically) and poorly controlled
Use additional code for adverse effect, if applicable, to identify drug (T36-T50 with fifth or sixth character 5)
EXCLUDES1 *headache NOS (R51)*
lower half migraine (G44.00)
EXCLUDES2 *headache syndromes (G44.-)*

G43.0 **Migraine** without aura
Common migraine
EXCLUDES1 *chronic migraine without aura (G43.7-)*
G43.00 **Migraine without aura,** not intractable
Migraine without aura without mention of refractory migraine
G43.001 **Migraine without aura, not intractable,** with status migrainosus
G43.009 **Migraine without aura, not intractable,** without status migrainosus
Migraine without aura NOS
G43.01 **Migraine without aura,** intractable
Migraine without aura with refractory migraine
G43.011 **Migraine without aura, intractable,** with status migrainosus
G43.019 **Migraine without aura, intractable,** without status migrainosus

G43.1 **Migraine** with aura
Basilar migraine
Classical migraine
Migraine equivalents
Migraine preceded or accompanied by transient focal neurological phenomena
Migraine triggered seizures
Migraine with acute-onset aura
Migraine with aura without headache (migraine equivalents)
Migraine with prolonged aura
Migraine with typical aura
Retinal migraine
Code also any associated seizure (G40.-, R56.9)
EXCLUDES1 *persistent migraine aura (G43.5-, G43.6-)*
G43.10 **Migraine with aura,** not intractable
Migraine with aura without mention of refractory migraine
G43.101 **Migraine with aura, not intractable,** with status migrainosus
G43.109 **Migraine with aura, not intractable,** without status migrainosus
Migraine with aura NOS
G43.11 **Migraine with aura,** intractable
Migraine with aura with refractory migraine
G43.111 **Migraine with aura, intractable,** with status migrainosus
G43.119 **Migraine with aura, intractable,** without status migrainosus

G43.4 Hemiplegic **migraine**
Familial migraine
Sporadic migraine
G43.40 **Hemiplegic migraine,** not intractable
Hemiplegic migraine without refractory migraine
G43.401 **Hemiplegic migraine, not intractable,** with status migrainosus
G43.409 **Hemiplegic migraine, not intractable,** without status migrainosus
Hemiplegic migraine NOS
G43.41 **Hemiplegic migraine,** intractable
Hemiplegic migraine with refractory migraine
G43.411 **Hemiplegic migraine, intractable,** with status migrainosus
G43.419 **Hemiplegic migraine, intractable,** without status migrainosus

G43.5 Persistent **migraine aura** without cerebral infarction
G43.50 **Persistent migraine aura without cerebral infarction,** not intractable
Persistent migraine aura without cerebral infarction, without refractory migraine
G43.501 **Persistent migraine aura without cerebral infarction, not intractable,** with status migrainosus
G43.509 **Persistent migraine aura without cerebral infarction, not intractable,** without status migrainosus
Persistent migraine aura NOS
G43.51 **Persistent migraine aura without cerebral infarction,** intractable
Persistent migraine aura without cerebral infarction, with refractory migraine
G43.511 **Persistent migraine aura without cerebral infarction, intractable,** with status migrainosus
G43.519 **Persistent migraine aura without cerebral infarction, intractable,** without status migrainosus

G43.6 **Persistent migraine aura** with cerebral infarction
Code also the type of cerebral infarction (I63.-)
G43.60 **Persistent migraine aura with cerebral infarction,** not intractable
Persistent migraine aura with cerebral infarction, without refractory migraine
G43.601 **Persistent migraine aura with cerebral infarction, not intractable,** with status migrainosus CC
G43.609 **Persistent migraine aura with cerebral infarction, not intractable,** without status migrainosus CC
G43.61 **Persistent migraine aura with cerebral infarction,** intractable
Persistent migraine aura with cerebral infarction, with refractory migraine
G43.611 **Persistent migraine aura with cerebral infarction, intractable,** with status migrainosus CC
G43.619 **Persistent migraine aura with cerebral infarction, intractable,** without status migrainosus CC

G43.7 Chronic **migraine** without aura
Transformed migraine
EXCLUDES1 *migraine without aura (G43.0-)*

Unacceptable principal diagnosis symbol per Medicare code edits | Code exempt from diagnosis present on admission requirement
Questionable admission | CC Complication or comorbidity | CC/MCC exclusion | MCC Major complication or comorbidity
Principal diagnosis as its own CC | Principal diagnosis as its own MCC | Z code as first-listed diagnosis

G43.70 **Chronic migraine without aura,** not intractable
Chronic migraine without aura, without refractory migraine
G43.701 **Chronic migraine without aura, not intractable,** with status migrainosus
G43.709 **Chronic migraine without aura, not intractable,** without status migrainosus
Chronic migraine without aura NOS
G43.71 **Chronic migraine without aura,** intractable
Chronic migraine without aura, with refractory migraine
G43.711 **Chronic migraine without aura, intractable,** with status migrainosus
G43.719 **Chronic migraine without aura, intractable,** without status migrainosus
G43.A Cyclical vomiting
G43.A0 **Cyclical vomiting,** not intractable
Cyclical vomiting, without refractory migraine
G43.A1 **Cyclical vomiting,** intractable
Cyclical vomiting, with refractory migraine
G43.B Ophthalmoplegic **migraine**
G43.B0 **Ophthalmoplegic migraine,** not intractable
Ophthalmoplegic migraine, without refractory migraine
G43.B1 **Ophthalmoplegic migraine,** intractable
Ophthalmoplegic migraine, with refractory migraine
G43.C Periodic headache **syndromes in** child or adult
G43.C0 **Periodic headache syndromes in child or adult,** not intractable
Periodic headache syndromes in child or adult, without refractory migraine
G43.C1 **Periodic headache syndromes in child or adult,** intractable
Periodic headache syndromes in child or adult, with refractory migraine
G43.D Abdominal **migraine**
G43.D0 **Abdominal migraine,** not intractable
Abdominal migraine, without refractory migraine
G43.D1 **Abdominal migraine,** intractable
Abdominal migraine, with refractory migraine
G43.8 Other **migraine**
G43.80 **Other migraine,** not intractable
Other migraine, without refractory migraine
G43.801 **Other migraine, not intractable,** with status migrainosus
G43.809 **Other migraine, not intractable,** without status migrainosus
G43.81 **Other migraine,** intractable
Other migraine, with refractory migraine
G43.811 **Other migraine, intractable,** with status migrainosus
G43.819 **Other migraine, intractable,** without status migrainosus
G43.82 **Menstrual migraine,** not intractable
Menstrual headache, not intractable
Menstrual migraine, without refractory migraine
Menstrually related migraine, not intractable
Pre-menstrual headache, not intractable
Pre-menstrual migraine, not intractable
Pure menstrual migraine, not intractable
Code also associated premenstrual tension syndrome (N94.3)
G43.821 **Menstrual migraine, not intractable,** with status migrainosus ♀
G43.829 **Menstrual migraine, not intractable,** without status migrainosus ♀
Menstrual migraine NOS
G43.83 **Menstrual migraine,** intractable
Menstrual headache, intractable
Menstrual migraine, with refractory migraine
Menstrually related migraine, intractable
Pre-menstrual headache, intractable
Pre-menstrual migraine, intractable
Pure menstrual migraine, intractable
Code also associated premenstrual tension syndrome (N94.3)
G43.831 **Menstrual migraine, intractable,** with status migrainosus ♀
G43.839 **Menstrual migraine, intractable,** without status migrainosus ♀
G43.9 **Migraine,** unspecified
G43.90 **Migraine, unspecified,** not intractable
Migraine, unspecified, without refractory migraine
G43.901 **Migraine, unspecified, not intractable,** with status migrainosus
Status migrainosus NOS
G43.909 **Migraine, unspecified, not intractable,** without status migrainosus
Migraine NOS
G43.91 **Migraine, unspecified,** intractable
Migraine, unspecified, with refractory migraine
G43.911 **Migraine, unspecified, intractable,** with status migrainosus
G43.919 **Migraine, unspecified, intractable,** without status migrainosus

G44 Other **headache syndromes**
EXCLUDES1 *headache NOS (R51)*
EXCLUDES2 *atypical facial pain (G50.1)*
headache due to lumbar puncture (G97.1)
migraines (G43.-)
trigeminal neuralgia (G50.0)

G44.0 **Cluster headaches and other trigeminal autonomic cephalgias (TAC)**
G44.00 **Cluster headache syndrome,** unspecified
Ciliary neuralgia
Cluster headache NOS
Histamine cephalgia
Lower half migraine
Migrainous neuralgia
G44.001 **Cluster headache syndrome, unspecified,** intractable
G44.009 **Cluster headache syndrome, unspecified,** not intractable
Cluster headache syndrome NOS
G44.01 Episodic **cluster headache**
G44.011 **Episodic cluster headache,** intractable
G44.019 **Episodic cluster headache,** not intractable
Episodic cluster headache NOS
G44.02 Chronic **cluster headache**
G44.021 **Chronic cluster headache,** intractable
G44.029 **Chronic cluster headache,** not intractable
Chronic cluster headache NOS
G44.03 Episodic paroxysmal hemicrania
Paroxysmal hemicrania NOS
G44.031 **Episodic paroxysmal hemicrania,** intractable
G44.039 **Episodic paroxysmal hemicrania,** not intractable
Episodic paroxysmal hemicrania NOS
G44.04 Chronic **paroxysmal hemicrania**
G44.041 **Chronic paroxysmal hemicrania,** intractable
G44.049 **Chronic paroxysmal hemicrania,** not intractable
Chronic paroxysmal hemicrania NOS
G44.05 **Short lasting unilateral neuralgiform headache** with conjunctival injection and tearing (SUNCT)
G44.051 **Short lasting unilateral neuralgiform headache with conjunctival injection and tearing (SUNCT),** intractable
G44.059 **Short lasting unilateral neuralgiform headache with conjunctival injection and tearing (SUNCT),** not intractable
Short lasting unilateral neuralgiform headache with conjunctival injection and tearing (SUNCT) NOS
G44.09 Other **trigeminal autonomic cephalgias (TAC)**
G44.091 **Other trigeminal autonomic cephalgias (TAC),** intractable
G44.099 **Other trigeminal autonomic cephalgias (TAC),** not intractable

Unspecified Code Other Specified Code Manifestation Code N Newborn P Pediatric M Maternity A Adult ♂ Male ♀ Female
● New Code ▲ Revised Code Title ►◄ Revised Text NOTES INCLUDES EXCLUDES1 Not coded here EXCLUDES2 Not included here
4th character required 5th character required 6th character required 7th character required
Extension 'X' Alert HAC Hospital-acquired condition (HAC) alert AHA AHA Coding Clinic©

G44.1 Vascular headache, not elsewhere classified
EXCLUDES2 *cluster headache (G44.0)*
complicated headache syndromes (G44.5-)
drug-induced headache (G44.4-)
migraine (G43.-)
other specified headache syndromes (G44.8-)
post-traumatic headache (G44.3-)
tension-type headache (G44.2-)

G44.2 Tension-type headache
G44.20 Tension-type headache, unspecified
G44.201 Tension-type headache, unspecified, intractable
G44.209 Tension-type headache, unspecified, not intractable
Tension headache NOS
G44.21 Episodic tension-type headache
G44.211 Episodic tension-type headache, intractable
G44.219 Episodic tension-type headache, not intractable
Episodic tension-type headache NOS
G44.22 Chronic tension-type headache
G44.221 Chronic tension-type headache, intractable
G44.229 Chronic tension-type headache, not intractable
Chronic tension-type headache NOS

G44.3 Post-traumatic headache
G44.30 Post-traumatic headache, unspecified
G44.301 Post-traumatic headache, unspecified, intractable
G44.309 Post-traumatic headache, unspecified, not intractable
Post-traumatic headache NOS
G44.31 Acute post-traumatic headache
G44.311 Acute post-traumatic headache, intractable
G44.319 Acute post-traumatic headache, not intractable
Acute post-traumatic headache NOS
G44.32 Chronic post-traumatic headache
G44.321 Chronic post-traumatic headache, intractable
G44.329 Chronic post-traumatic headache, not intractable
Chronic post-traumatic headache NOS

G44.4 Drug-induced headache, not elsewhere classified
Medication overuse headache
Use additional code for adverse effect, if applicable, to identify drug (T36-T50 with fifth or sixth character 5)
G44.40 Drug-induced headache, not elsewhere classified, not intractable
G44.41 Drug-induced headache, not elsewhere classified, intractable

G44.5 Complicated headache syndromes
G44.51 Hemicrania continua
G44.52 New daily persistent headache (NDPH)
G44.53 Primary thunderclap headache
G44.59 Other complicated headache syndrome

G44.8 Other specified headache syndromes
G44.81 Hypnic headache
G44.82 Headache associated with sexual activity
Orgasmic headache
Preorgasmic headache
G44.83 Primary cough headache
G44.84 Primary exertional headache
G44.85 Primary stabbing headache
G44.89 Other headache syndrome

G45 Transient cerebral ischemic attacks and related syndromes
EXCLUDES1 *neonatal cerebral ischemia (P91.0)*
transient retinal artery occlusion (H34.0-)
G45.0 Vertebro-basilar artery syndrome CC
G45.1 Carotid artery syndrome (hemispheric) CC
G45.2 Multiple and bilateral precerebral artery syndromes CC
G45.3 Amaurosis fugax CC
G45.4 Transient global amnesia
EXCLUDES1 *amnesia NOS (R41.3)*
G45.8 Other transient cerebral ischemic attacks and related syndromes CC
G45.9 Transient cerebral ischemic attack, unspecified CC
Spasm of cerebral artery
TIA
Transient cerebral ischemia NOS

G46 Vascular syndromes of brain in cerebrovascular diseases
Code first underlying cerebrovascular disease (I60-I69)
G46.0 Middle cerebral artery syndrome CC
G46.1 Anterior cerebral artery syndrome CC
G46.2 Posterior cerebral artery syndrome CC
G46.3 Brain stem stroke syndrome
Benedikt syndrome
Claude syndrome
Foville syndrome
Millard-Gubler syndrome
Wallenberg syndrome
Weber syndrome
G46.4 Cerebellar stroke syndrome
G46.5 Pure motor lacunar syndrome
G46.6 Pure sensory lacunar syndrome
G46.7 Other lacunar syndromes
G46.8 Other vascular syndromes of brain in cerebrovascular diseases

G47 Sleep disorders
EXCLUDES2 *nightmares (F51.5)*
nonorganic sleep disorders (F51.-)
sleep terrors (F51.4)
sleepwalking (F51.3)

G47.0 Insomnia
EXCLUDES2 *alcohol related insomnia (F10.182, F10.282, F10.982)*
drug-related insomnia (F11.182, F11.282, F11.982, F13.182, F13.282, F13.982, F14.182, F14.282, F14.982, F15.182, F15.282, F15.982, F19.182, F19.282, F19.982)
idiopathic insomnia (F51.01)
insomnia due to a mental disorder (F51.05)
insomnia not due to a substance or known physiological condition (F51.0-)
nonorganic insomnia (F51.0-)
primary insomnia (F51.01)
sleep apnea (G47.3-)
G47.00 Insomnia, unspecified
Insomnia NOS
G47.01 Insomnia due to medical condition
Code also associated medical condition
G47.09 Other insomnia

G47.1 Hypersomnia
EXCLUDES2 *alcohol-related hypersomnia (F10.182, F10.282, F10.982)*
drug-related hypersomnia (F11.182, F11.282, F11.982, F13.182, F13.282, F13.982, F14.182, F14.282, F14.982, F15.182, F15.282, F15.982, F19.182, F19.282, F19.982)
hypersomnia due to a mental disorder (F51.13)
hypersomnia not due to a substance or known physiological condition (F51.1-)
primary hypersomnia (F51.11)
sleep apnea (G47.3-)
G47.10 Hypersomnia, unspecified
Hypersomnia NOS
G47.11 Idiopathic hypersomnia with long sleep time
Idiopathic hypersomnia NOS
G47.12 Idiopathic hypersomnia without long sleep time
G47.13 Recurrent hypersomnia
Kleine-Levin syndrome
Menstrual related hypersomnia
G47.14 Hypersomnia due to medical condition
Code also associated medical condition
G47.19 Other hypersomnia

PDx Unacceptable principal diagnosis symbol per Medicare code edits · POA Code exempt from diagnosis present on admission requirement
Q Questionable admission · CC Complication or comorbidity · CC/MCC Excl CC/MCC exclusion · MCC Major complication or comorbidity
PDx CC Principal diagnosis as its own CC · PDx MCC Principal diagnosis as its own MCC · Z Z code as first-listed diagnosis

 When symbols appear on a code that requires a 7th character extension, refer to Appendix D to identify applicable 7th character codes.

G47.2 Circadian rhythm sleep disorders
Disorders of the sleep wake schedule
Inversion of nyctohemeral rhythm
Inversion of sleep rhythm
G47.20 **Circadian rhythm sleep disorder, unspecified type**
Sleep wake schedule disorder NOS
G47.21 **Circadian rhythm sleep disorder, delayed sleep phase type**
Delayed sleep phase syndrome
G47.22 **Circadian rhythm sleep disorder, advanced sleep phase type**
G47.23 **Circadian rhythm sleep disorder, irregular sleep wake type**
Irregular sleep-wake pattern
G47.24 **Circadian rhythm sleep disorder, free running type**
G47.25 **Circadian rhythm sleep disorder, jet lag type**
G47.26 **Circadian rhythm sleep disorder, shift work type**
G47.27 **Circadian rhythm sleep disorder in conditions classified elsewhere**
Code first underlying condition
G47.29 **Other circadian rhythm sleep disorder**

G47.3 Sleep apnea
Code also any associated underlying condition
EXCLUDES1 *apnea NOS (R06.81)*
Cheyne-Stokes breathing (R06.3)
pickwickian syndrome (E66.2)
sleep apnea of newborn (P28.3)
G47.30 **Sleep apnea, unspecified**
Sleep apnea NOS
G47.31 **Primary central sleep apnea**
G47.32 **High altitude periodic breathing**
G47.33 **Obstructive sleep apnea (adult) (pediatric)**
EXCLUDES1 *obstructive sleep apnea of newborn (P28.3)*
G47.34 **Idiopathic sleep related nonobstructive alveolar hypoventilation**
Sleep related hypoxia
G47.35 **Congenital central alveolar hypoventilation syndrome**
G47.36 **Sleep related hypoventilation in conditions classified elsewhere**
Sleep related hypoxemia in conditions classified elsewhere
Code first underlying condition
G47.37 **Central sleep apnea in conditions classified elsewhere**
Code first underlying condition
G47.39 **Other sleep apnea**

G47.4 Narcolepsy and cataplexy
G47.41 Narcolepsy
G47.411 **Narcolepsy with cataplexy**
G47.419 **Narcolepsy without cataplexy**
Narcolepsy NOS
G47.42 Narcolepsy in conditions classified elsewhere
Code first underlying condition
G47.421 **Narcolepsy in conditions classified elsewhere with cataplexy**
G47.429 **Narcolepsy in conditions classified elsewhere without cataplexy**

G47.5 Parasomnia
EXCLUDES1 *alcohol induced parasomnia (F10.182, F10.282, F10.982)*
drug induced parasomnia (F11.182, F11.282, F11.982, F13.182, F13.282, F13.982, F14.182, F14.282, F14.982, F15.182, F15.282, F15.982, F19.182, F19.282, F19.982)
parasomnia not due to a substance or known physiological condition (F51.8)
G47.50 **Parasomnia, unspecified**
Parasomnia NOS
G47.51 **Confusional arousals**
G47.52 **REM sleep behavior disorder**
G47.53 **Recurrent isolated sleep paralysis**
G47.54 **Parasomnia in conditions classified elsewhere**
Code first underlying condition
G47.59 **Other parasomnia**

G47.6 Sleep related movement disorders
EXCLUDES2 *restless legs syndrome (G25.81)*
G47.61 **Periodic limb movement disorder**
Periodic limb movement disorder
G47.62 **Sleep related leg cramps**
G47.63 **Sleep related bruxism**
EXCLUDES1 *psychogenic bruxism (F45.8)*
G47.69 **Other sleep related movement disorders**
G47.8 **Other sleep disorders**
G47.9 **Sleep disorder, unspecified**
Sleep disorder NOS

Nerve, nerve root and plexus disorders (G50-G59)

EXCLUDES1 *current traumatic nerve, nerve root and plexus disorders - see Injury, nerve by body region*
neuralgia NOS (M79.2)
neuritis NOS (M79.2)
peripheral neuritis in pregnancy (O26.82-)
radiculitis NOS (M54.1-)

G50 Disorders of trigeminal nerve
INCLUDES *disorders of 5th cranial nerve*
G50.0 **Trigeminal neuralgia**
Syndrome of paroxysmal facial pain
Tic douloureux
G50.1 **Atypical facial pain**
G50.8 **Other disorders of trigeminal nerve**
G50.9 **Disorder of trigeminal nerve, unspecified**

G51 Facial nerve disorders
INCLUDES *disorders of 7th cranial nerve*
G51.0 **Bell's palsy**
Facial palsy
G51.1 **Geniculate ganglionitis**
EXCLUDES1 *postherpetic geniculate ganglionitis (B02.21)*
G51.2 **Melkersson's syndrome**
Melkersson-Rosenthal syndrome
G51.3 **Clonic hemifacial spasm**
G51.4 **Facial myokymia**
G51.8 **Other disorders of facial nerve**
G51.9 **Disorder of facial nerve, unspecified**

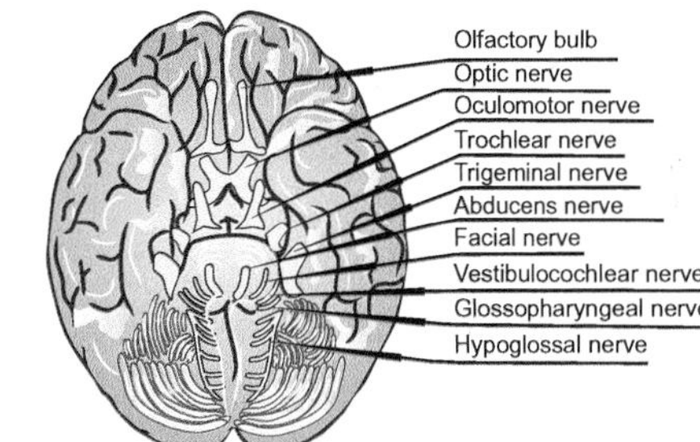

Figure 6.2 The Cranial nerves

G52 Disorders of other cranial nerves
EXCLUDES2 *disorders of acoustic [8th] nerve (H93.3)*
disorders of optic [2nd] nerve (H46, H47.0)
paralytic strabismus due to nerve palsy (H49.0-H49.2)
G52.0 **Disorders of olfactory nerve**
Disorders of 1st cranial nerve
G52.1 **Disorders of glossopharyngeal nerve**
Disorder of 9th cranial nerve
Glossopharyngeal neuralgia
G52.2 **Disorders of vagus nerve**
Disorders of pneumogastric [10th] nerve
G52.3 **Disorders of hypoglossal nerve**
Disorders of 12th cranial nerve
G52.7 **Disorders of multiple cranial nerves**
Polyneuritis cranialis
G52.8 **Disorders of other specified cranial nerves**
G52.9 **Cranial nerve disorder, unspecified**

Unspecified Code Other Specified Code Manifestation Code N Newborn P Pediatric M Maternity A Adult ♂ Male ♀ Female
● New Code ▲ Revised Code Title ►◄ Revised Text NOTES INCLUDES EXCLUDES1 Not coded here EXCLUDES2 Not included here
4th character required 5th character required 6th character required 7th character required
Extension 'X' Alert HAC Hospital-acquired condition (HAC) alert AHA AHA Coding Clinic©

G53 **Cranial nerve disorders in diseases classified elsewhere**
Code first underlying disease, such as:
neoplasm (C00-D49)
EXCLUDES1 *multiple cranial nerve palsy in sarcoidosis (D86.82)*
multiple cranial nerve palsy in syphilis (A52.15)
postherpetic geniculate ganglionitis (B02.21)
postherpetic trigeminal neuralgia (B02.22)

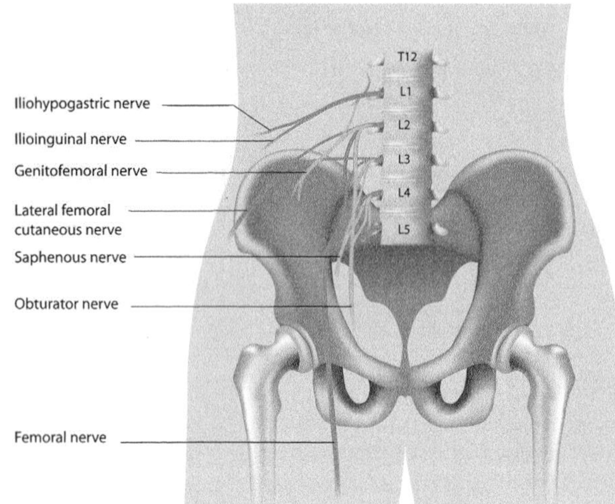

Figure 6.3 The Lumbar plexus

G54 **Nerve root and plexus disorders**
EXCLUDES1 *current traumatic nerve root and plexus disorders - see nerve injury by body region*
intervertebral disc disorders (M50-M51)
neuralgia or neuritis NOS (M79.2)
neuritis or radiculitis brachial NOS (M54.13)
neuritis or radiculitis lumbar NOS (M54.16)
neuritis or radiculitis lumbosacral NOS (M54.17)
neuritis or radiculitis thoracic NOS (M54.14)
radiculitis NOS (M54.10)
radiculopathy NOS (M54.10)
spondylosis (M47.-)

G54.0 **Brachial plexus disorders**
Thoracic outlet syndrome
G54.1 **Lumbosacral plexus disorders**
G54.2 **Cervical root disorders, not elsewhere classified**
G54.3 **Thoracic root disorders, not elsewhere classified** PDx
G54.4 **Lumbosacral root disorders, not elsewhere classified**
G54.5 **Neuralgic amyotrophy**
Parsonage-Aldren-Turner syndrome
Shoulder-girdle neuritis
EXCLUDES1 *neuralgic amyotrophy in diabetes mellitus (E08-E13 with .44)*
G54.6 **Phantom limb syndrome with pain**
G54.7 **Phantom limb syndrome without pain**
Phantom limb syndrome NOS
G54.8 **Other nerve root and plexus disorders**
G54.9 **Nerve root and plexus disorder, unspecified**

G55 **Nerve root and plexus compressions in diseases classified elsewhere**
Code first underlying disease, such as:
neoplasm (C00-D49)
EXCLUDES1 *nerve root compression (due to) (in) ankylosing spondylitis (M45.-)*
nerve root compression (due to) (in) dorsopathies (M53.-, M54.-)
nerve root compression (due to) (in) intervertebral disc disorders (M50.1.-, M51.1.-)
nerve root compression (due to) (in) spondylopathies (M46.-, M48.-)
nerve root compression (due to) (in) spondylosis (M47.0-M47.2.-)

G56 **Mononeuropathies of upper limb**
EXCLUDES1 *current traumatic nerve disorder - see nerve injury by body region*

G56.0 **Carpal tunnel syndrome**
G56.00 **Carpal tunnel syndrome, unspecified upper limb**
G56.01 **Carpal tunnel syndrome, right upper limb**
G56.02 **Carpal tunnel syndrome, left upper limb**
● G56.03 **Carpal tunnel syndrome, bilateral upper limbs** CC/MCC Exc

G56.1 **Other lesions of median nerve**
G56.10 **Other lesions of median nerve, unspecified upper limb**
G56.11 **Other lesions of median nerve, right upper limb**
G56.12 **Other lesions of median nerve, left upper limb**
● G56.13 **Other lesions of median nerve, bilateral upper limbs** CC/MCC Exc

G56.2 **Lesion of ulnar nerve**
Tardy ulnar nerve palsy
G56.20 **Lesion of ulnar nerve, unspecified upper limb**
G56.21 **Lesion of ulnar nerve, right upper limb**
G56.22 **Lesion of ulnar nerve, left upper limb**
● G56.23 **Lesion of ulnar nerve, bilateral upper limbs** CC/MCC Exc

G56.3 **Lesion of radial nerve**
G56.30 **Lesion of radial nerve, unspecified upper limb**
G56.31 **Lesion of radial nerve, right upper limb**
G56.32 **Lesion of radial nerve, left upper limb**
● G56.33 **Lesion of radial nerve, bilateral upper limbs** CC/MCC Exc

G56.4 **Causalgia of upper limb**
Complex regional pain syndrome II of upper limb
EXCLUDES1 *complex regional pain syndrome I of lower limb (G90.52-)*
complex regional pain syndrome I of upper limb (G90.51-)
complex regional pain syndrome II of lower limb (G57.7-)
reflex sympathetic dystrophy of lower limb (G90.52-)
reflex sympathetic dystrophy of upper limb (G90.51-)
G56.40 **Causalgia of unspecified upper limb**
G56.41 **Causalgia of right upper limb**
G56.42 **Causalgia of left upper limb**
● G56.43 **Causalgia of bilateral upper limbs** CC/MCC Exc

G56.8 **Other specified mononeuropathies of upper limb**
Interdigital neuroma of upper limb
G56.80 **Other specified mononeuropathies of unspecified upper limb**
G56.81 **Other specified mononeuropathies of right upper limb**
G56.82 **Other specified mononeuropathies of left upper limb**
● G56.83 **Other specified mononeuropathies of bilateral upper limbs** CC/MCC Exc

G56.9 **Unspecified mononeuropathy of upper limb**
G56.90 **Unspecified mononeuropathy of unspecified upper limb**
G56.91 **Unspecified mononeuropathy of right upper limb**
G56.92 **Unspecified mononeuropathy of left upper limb**
● G56.93 **Unspecified mononeuropathy of bilateral upper limbs** CC/MCC Exc

G57 **Mononeuropathies of lower limb**
EXCLUDES1 *current traumatic nerve disorder - see nerve injury by body region*

G57.0 **Lesion of sciatic nerve**
EXCLUDES1 *sciatica NOS (M54.3-)*
EXCLUDES2 *sciatica attributed to intervertebral disc disorder (M51.1.-)*
G57.00 **Lesion of sciatic nerve, unspecified lower limb**
G57.01 **Lesion of sciatic nerve, right lower limb**
G57.02 **Lesion of sciatic nerve, left lower limb**
● G57.03 **Lesion of sciatic nerve, bilateral lower limbs** CC/MCC Exc

PDx Unacceptable principal diagnosis symbol per Medicare code edits · POA Code exempt from diagnosis present on admission requirement
Q Questionable admission · CC Complication or comorbidity · CC/MCC Exc CC/MCC exclusion · MCC Major complication or comorbidity
PDx CC Principal diagnosis as its own CC · PDx MCC Principal diagnosis as its own MCC · Z Z code as first-listed diagnosis

 When symbols appear on a code that requires a 7th character extension, refer to Appendix D to identify applicable 7th character codes.

G57.1 Meralgia paresthetica
Lateral cutaneous nerve of thigh syndrome
- G57.10 **Meralgia paresthetica, unspecified lower limb**
- G57.11 **Meralgia paresthetica, right lower limb**
- G57.12 **Meralgia paresthetica, left lower limb**
- ● G57.13 **Meralgia paresthetica, bilateral lower limbs** CC/MCC Exc

G57.2 Lesion of femoral nerve
- G57.20 **Lesion of femoral nerve, unspecified lower limb**
- G57.21 **Lesion of femoral nerve, right lower limb**
- G57.22 **Lesion of femoral nerve, left lower limb**
- ● G57.23 **Lesion of femoral nerve, bilateral lower limbs** CC/MCC Exc

G57.3 Lesion of lateral popliteal nerve
Peroneal nerve palsy
- G57.30 **Lesion of lateral popliteal nerve, unspecified lower limb**
- G57.31 **Lesion of lateral popliteal nerve, right lower limb**
- G57.32 **Lesion of lateral popliteal nerve, left lower limb**
- ● G57.33 **Lesion of lateral popliteal nerve, bilateral lower limbs** CC/MCC Exc

G57.4 Lesion of medial popliteal nerve
- G57.40 **Lesion of medial popliteal nerve, unspecified lower limb**
- G57.41 **Lesion of medial popliteal nerve, right lower limb**
- G57.42 **Lesion of medial popliteal nerve, left lower limb**
- ● G57.43 **Lesion of medial popliteal nerve, bilateral lower limbs** CC/MCC Exc

G57.5 Tarsal tunnel syndrome
- G57.50 **Tarsal tunnel syndrome, unspecified lower limb**
- G57.51 **Tarsal tunnel syndrome, right lower limb**
- G57.52 **Tarsal tunnel syndrome, left lower limb**
- ● G57.53 **Tarsal tunnel syndrome, bilateral lower limbs** CC/MCC Exc

G57.6 Lesion of plantar nerve
Morton's metatarsalgia
- G57.60 **Lesion of plantar nerve, unspecified lower limb**
- G57.61 **Lesion of plantar nerve, right lower limb**
- G57.62 **Lesion of plantar nerve, left lower limb**
- ● G57.63 **Lesion of plantar nerve, bilateral lower limbs** CC/MCC Exc

G57.7 Causalgia of lower limb
Complex regional pain syndrome II of lower limb
EXCLUDES1 *complex regional pain syndrome I of lower limb (G90.52-)*
complex regional pain syndrome I of upper limb (G90.51-)
complex regional pain syndrome II of upper limb (G56.4-)
reflex sympathetic dystrophy of lower limb (G90.52-)
reflex sympathetic dystrophy of upper limb (G90.51-)
- G57.70 **Causalgia of unspecified lower limb**
- G57.71 **Causalgia of right lower limb**
- G57.72 **Causalgia of left lower limb**
- ● G57.73 **Causalgia of bilateral lower limbs** CC/MCC Exc

G57.8 Other specified mononeuropathies of lower limb
Interdigital neuroma of lower limb
- G57.80 **Other specified mononeuropathies of unspecified lower limb**
- G57.81 **Other specified mononeuropathies of right lower limb**
- G57.82 **Other specified mononeuropathies of left lower limb**
- ● G57.83 **Other specified mononeuropathies of bilateral lower limbs** CC/MCC Exc

G57.9 Unspecified mononeuropathy of lower limb
- G57.90 **Unspecified mononeuropathy of unspecified lower limb**
- G57.91 **Unspecified mononeuropathy of right lower limb**
- G57.92 **Unspecified mononeuropathy of left lower limb**
- ● G57.93 **Unspecified mononeuropathy of bilateral lower limbs** CC/MCC Exc

G58 Other mononeuropathies
- G58.0 **Intercostal neuropathy**
- G58.7 **Mononeuritis multiplex**
- G58.8 **Other specified mononeuropathies**
- G58.9 **Mononeuropathy, unspecified**

G59 **Mononeuropathy in diseases classified elsewhere**
Code first underlying disease
EXCLUDES1 *diabetic mononeuropathy (E08-E13 with .41)*
syphilitic nerve paralysis (A52.19)
syphilitic neuritis (A52.15)
tuberculous mononeuropathy (A17.83)

Polyneuropathies and other disorders of the peripheral nervous system (G60-G65)

EXCLUDES1 *neuralgia NOS (M79.2)*
neuritis NOS (M79.2)
peripheral neuritis in pregnancy (O26.82-)
radiculitis NOS (M54.10)

G60 Hereditary and idiopathic neuropathy
- G60.0 **Hereditary motor and sensory neuropathy**
  Charcot-Marie-Tooth disease
  Déjérine-Sottas disease
  Hereditary motor and sensory neuropathy, types I-IV
  Hypertrophic neuropathy of infancy
  Peroneal muscular atrophy (axonal type) (hypertrophic type)
  Roussy-Levy syndrome
- G60.1 **Refsum's disease** CC
  Infantile Refsum disease
- G60.2 **Neuropathy in association with hereditary ataxia**
- G60.3 **Idiopathic progressive neuropathy**
- G60.8 **Other hereditary and idiopathic neuropathies**
  Dominantly inherited sensory neuropathy
  Morvan's disease
  Nelaton's syndrome
  Recessively inherited sensory neuropathy
- G60.9 **Hereditary and idiopathic neuropathy, unspecified**

G61 Inflammatory polyneuropathy
- G61.0 **Guillain-Barre syndrome** CC
  Acute (post-)infective polyneuritis
  Miller Fisher Syndrome
- G61.1 **Serum neuropathy**
  Use additional code for adverse effect, if applicable, to identify serum (T50.-)
- G61.8 **Other inflammatory polyneuropathies**
  - G61.81 **Chronic inflammatory demyelinating polyneuritis** CC
  - ● G61.82 **Multifocal motor neuropathy** CC/MCC Exc
    MMN
  - G61.89 **Other inflammatory polyneuropathies**
- G61.9 **Inflammatory polyneuropathy, unspecified**

G62 Other and unspecified polyneuropathies
- G62.0 **Drug-induced polyneuropathy**
  Use additional code for adverse effect, if applicable, to identify drug (T36-T50 with fifth or sixth character 5)
- G62.1 **Alcoholic polyneuropathy**
- G62.2 **Polyneuropathy due to other toxic agents**
  Code first (T51-T65) to identify toxic agent
- G62.8 **Other specified polyneuropathies**
  - G62.81 **Critical illness polyneuropathy** CC
    Acute motor neuropathy
  - G62.82 **Radiation-induced polyneuropathy**
    Use additional external cause code (W88-W90, X39.0-) to identify cause
  - G62.89 **Other specified polyneuropathies**
    AHA: Q2, 2016
- G62.9 **Polyneuropathy, unspecified**
  Neuropathy NOS

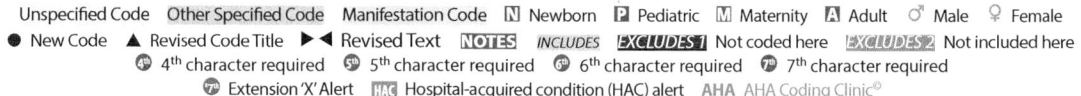

Unspecified Code | Other Specified Code | Manifestation Code | N Newborn | P Pediatric | M Maternity | A Adult | ♂ Male | ♀ Female
● New Code | ▲ Revised Code Title | ►◄ Revised Text | NOTES | INCLUDES | EXCLUDES1 Not coded here | EXCLUDES2 Not included here
4th character required | 5th character required | 6th character required | 7th character required
Extension 'X' Alert | HAC Hospital-acquired condition (HAC) alert | AHA AHA Coding Clinic®

G63 **Polyneuropathy in diseases classified elsewhere**
Code first underlying disease, such as:
amyloidosis (E85.-)
endocrine disease, except diabetes (E00-E07, E15-E16, E20-E34)
metabolic diseases (E70-E88)
neoplasm (C00-D49)
nutritional deficiency (E40-E64)
EXCLUDES1 *polyneuropathy (in):*
diabetes mellitus (E08-E13 with .42)
diphtheria (A36.83)
infectious mononucleosis (B27.0-B27.9 with 1)
Lyme disease (A69.22)
mumps (B26.84)
postherpetic (B02.23)
rheumatoid arthritis (M05.33)
scleroderma (M34.83)
systemic lupus erythematosus (M32.19)
AHA: Q4, 2012

G64 **Other disorders of peripheral nervous system**
Disorder of peripheral nervous system NOS

G65 **Sequelae of inflammatory and toxic polyneuropathies**
Code first condition resulting from (sequela) of inflammatory and toxic polyneuropathies
G65.0 **Sequelae of Guillain-Barré syndrome**
G65.1 **Sequelae of other inflammatory polyneuropathy**
G65.2 **Sequelae of toxic polyneuropathy**

Diseases of myoneural junction and muscle (G70-G73)

G70 **Myasthenia gravis and other myoneural disorders**
EXCLUDES1 *botulism (A05.1, A48.51-A48.52)*
transient neonatal myasthenia gravis (P94.0)
G70.0 **Myasthenia gravis**
G70.00 **Myasthenia gravis without (acute) exacerbation**
Myasthenia gravis NOS
G70.01 **Myasthenia gravis with (acute) exacerbation** MCC
Myasthenia gravis in crisis
G70.1 **Toxic myoneural disorders**
Code first (T51-T65) to identify toxic agent
G70.2 **Congenital and developmental myasthenia**
G70.8 **Other specified myoneural disorders**
G70.80 **Lambert-Eaton syndrome, unspecified** CC
Lambert-Eaton syndrome NOS
G70.81 **Lambert-Eaton syndrome in disease classified elsewhere** CC
Code first underlying disease
EXCLUDES1 *Lambert-Eaton syndrome in neoplastic disease (G73.1)*
G70.89 **Other specified myoneural disorders**
G70.9 **Myoneural disorder, unspecified**

G71 **Primary disorders of muscles**
EXCLUDES2 *arthrogryposis multiplex congenita (Q74.3)*
metabolic disorders (E70-E88)
myositis (M60.-)
G71.0 **Muscular dystrophy** CC
Autosomal recessive, childhood type, muscular dystrophy resembling Duchenne or Becker muscular dystrophy
Benign [Becker] muscular dystrophy
Benign scapuloperoneal muscular dystrophy with early contractures [Emery-Dreifuss]
Congenital muscular dystrophy NOS
Congenital muscular dystrophy with specific morphological abnormalities of the muscle fiber
Distal muscular dystrophy
Facioscapulohumeral muscular dystrophy
Limb-girdle muscular dystrophy
Ocular muscular dystrophy
Oculopharyngeal muscular dystrophy
Scapuloperoneal muscular dystrophy
Severe [Duchenne] muscular dystrophy
G71.1 **Myotonic disorders**
G71.11 **Myotonic muscular dystrophy**
Dystrophia myotonica [Steinert]
Myotonia atrophica
Myotonic dystrophy
Proximal myotonic myopathy (PROMM)
Steinert disease
G71.12 **Myotonia congenita**
Acetazolamide responsive myotonia congenita
Dominant myotonia congenita [Thomsen disease]
Myotonia levior
Recessive myotonia congenita [Becker disease]
G71.13 **Myotonic chondrodystrophy**
Chondrodystrophic myotonia
Congenital myotonic chondrodystrophy
Schwartz-Jampel disease
G71.14 **Drug induced myotonia**
Use additional code for adverse effect, if applicable, to identify drug (T36-T50 with fifth or sixth character 5)
G71.19 **Other specified myotonic disorders**
Myotonia fluctuans
Myotonia permanens
Neuromyotonia [Isaacs]
Paramyotonia congenita (of von Eulenburg)
Pseudomyotonia
Symptomatic myotonia
G71.2 **Congenital myopathies** CC
Central core disease
Fiber-type disproportion
Minicore disease
Multicore disease
Myotubular (centronuclear) myopathy
Nemaline myopathy
EXCLUDES1 *arthrogryposis multiplex congenita (Q74.3)*
G71.3 **Mitochondrial myopathy, not elsewhere classified**
EXCLUDES1 *Kearns-Sayre syndrome (H49.81)*
Leber's disease (H47.21)
Leigh's encephalopathy (G31.82)
mitochondrial metabolism disorders (E88.4.-)
Reye's syndrome (G93.7)
G71.8 **Other primary disorders of muscles**
G71.9 **Primary disorder of muscle, unspecified**
Hereditary myopathy NOS

G72 **Other and unspecified myopathies**
EXCLUDES1 *arthrogryposis multiplex congenita (Q74.3)*
dermatopolymyositis (M33.-)
ischemic infarction of muscle (M62.2-)
myositis (M60.-)
polymyositis (M33.2.-)
G72.0 **Drug-induced myopathy** CC
Use additional code for adverse effect, if applicable, to identify drug (T36-T50 with fifth or sixth character 5)
G72.1 **Alcoholic myopathy** CC
Use additional code to identify alcoholism (F10.-)
G72.2 **Myopathy due to other toxic agents** CC
Code first (T51-T65) to identify toxic agent
G72.3 **Periodic paralysis**
Familial periodic paralysis
Hyperkalemic periodic paralysis (familial)
Hypokalemic periodic paralysis (familial)
Myotonic periodic paralysis (familial)
Normokalemic paralysis (familial)
Potassium sensitive periodic paralysis
EXCLUDES1 *paramyotonia congenita (of von Eulenburg) (G71.19)*
G72.4 **Inflammatory and immune myopathies, not elsewhere classified**
G72.41 **Inclusion body myositis [IBM]**
G72.49 **Other inflammatory and immune myopathies, not elsewhere classified**
Inflammatory myopathy NOS
G72.8 **Other specified myopathies**
G72.81 **Critical illness myopathy** CC
Acute necrotizing myopathy
Acute quadriplegic myopathy
Intensive care (ICU) myopathy
Myopathy of critical illness

PDx Unacceptable principal diagnosis symbol per Medicare code edits; POA Code exempt from diagnosis present on admission requirement; Q Questionable admission; CC Complication or comorbidity; CC/MCC Exc CC/MCC exclusion; MCC Major complication or comorbidity; Principal diagnosis as its own CC; Principal diagnosis as its own MCC; Z code as first-listed diagnosis

 When symbols appear on a code that requires a 7th character extension, refer to Appendix D to identify applicable 7th character codes.

G72.89 Other specified myopathies

G72.9 Myopathy, unspecified

G73 Disorders of myoneural junction and muscle in diseases classified elsewhere

G73.1 Lambert-Eaton syndrome in neoplastic disease
Code first underlying neoplasm (C00-D49)
EXCLUDES1 *Lambert-Eaton syndrome not associated with neoplasm (G70.80-G70.81)*

G73.3 Myasthenic syndromes in other diseases classified elsewhere
Code first underlying disease, such as:
neoplasm (C00-D49)
thyrotoxicosis (E05.-)

G73.7 Myopathy in diseases classified elsewhere
Code first underlying disease, such as:
hyperparathyroidism (E21.0, E21.3)
hypoparathyroidism (E20.-)
glycogen storage disease (E74.0)
lipid storage disorders (E75.-)
EXCLUDES1 *myopathy in:*
rheumatoid arthritis (M05.32)
sarcoidosis (D86.87)
scleroderma (M34.82)
sicca syndrome Sjögren (M35.03)
systemic lupus erythematosus (M32.19)

Cerebral palsy and other paralytic syndromes (G80-G83)

G80 Cerebral palsy
EXCLUDES1 *hereditary spastic paraplegia (G11.4)*

G80.0 Spastic quadriplegic cerebral palsy
Congenital spastic paralysis (cerebral)

G80.1 Spastic diplegic cerebral palsy
Spastic cerebral palsy NOS

G80.2 Spastic hemiplegic cerebral palsy

G80.3 Athetoid cerebral palsy
Double athetosis (syndrome)
Dyskinetic cerebral palsy
Dystonic cerebral palsy
Vogt disease

G80.4 Ataxic cerebral palsy

G80.8 Other cerebral palsy
Mixed cerebral palsy syndromes

G80.9 Cerebral palsy, unspecified
Cerebral palsy NOS

G81 Hemiplegia and hemiparesis
NOTES This category is to be used only when hemiplegia (complete) (incomplete) is reported without further specification, or is stated to be old or longstanding but of unspecified cause. The category is also for use in multiple coding to identify these types of hemiplegia resulting from any cause.
EXCLUDES1 *congenital cerebral palsy (G80.-)*
hemiplegia and hemiparesis due to sequela of cerebrovascular disease (I69.05-, I69.15-, I69.25-, I69.35-, I69.85-, I69.95-)

G81.0 Flaccid hemiplegia

G81.00 Flaccid hemiplegia affecting unspecified side

G81.01 Flaccid hemiplegia affecting right dominant side

G81.02 Flaccid hemiplegia affecting left dominant side

G81.03 Flaccid hemiplegia affecting right nondominant side

G81.04 Flaccid hemiplegia affecting left nondominant side

G81.1 Spastic hemiplegia

G81.10 Spastic hemiplegia affecting unspecified side

G81.11 Spastic hemiplegia affecting right dominant side

G81.12 Spastic hemiplegia affecting left dominant side

G81.13 Spastic hemiplegia affecting right nondominant side

G81.14 Spastic hemiplegia affecting left nondominant side

G81.9 Hemiplegia, unspecified

G81.90 Hemiplegia, unspecified affecting unspecified side

G81.91 Hemiplegia, unspecified affecting right dominant side

G81.92 Hemiplegia, unspecified affecting left dominant side

G81.93 Hemiplegia, unspecified affecting right nondominant side

G81.94 Hemiplegia, unspecified affecting left nondominant side
AHA: Q1, 2015

G82 Paraplegia (paraparesis) and quadriplegia (quadriparesis)
NOTES This category is to be used only when the listed conditions are reported without further specification, or are stated to be old or longstanding but of unspecified cause. The category is also for use in multiple coding to identify these conditions resulting from any cause
EXCLUDES1 *congenital cerebral palsy (G80.-)*
functional quadriplegia (R53.2)
hysterical paralysis (F44.4)

G82.2 Paraplegia
Paralysis of both lower limbs NOS
Paraparesis (lower) NOS
Paraplegia (lower) NOS

G82.20 Paraplegia, unspecified

G82.21 Paraplegia, complete

G82.22 Paraplegia, incomplete

G82.5 Quadriplegia

G82.50 Quadriplegia, unspecified

G82.51 Quadriplegia, C1-C4 complete

G82.52 Quadriplegia, C1-C4 incomplete

G82.53 Quadriplegia, C5-C7 complete

G82.54 Quadriplegia, C5-C7 incomplete

G83 Other paralytic syndromes
NOTES This category is to be used only when the listed conditions are reported without further specification, or are stated to be old or longstanding but of unspecified cause. The category is also for use in multiple coding to identify these conditions resulting from any cause.
INCLUDES *paralysis (complete) (incomplete), except as in G80-G82*

G83.0 Diplegia of upper limbs
Diplegia (upper)
Paralysis of both upper limbs

G83.1 Monoplegia of lower limb
Paralysis of lower limb
EXCLUDES1 *monoplegia of lower limbs due to sequela of cerebrovascular disease (I69.04-, I69.14-, I69.24-, I69.34-, I69.84-, I69.94-)*

G83.10 Monoplegia of lower limb affecting unspecified side

G83.11 Monoplegia of lower limb affecting right dominant side

G83.12 Monoplegia of lower limb affecting left dominant side

G83.13 Monoplegia of lower limb affecting right nondominant side

G83.14 Monoplegia of lower limb affecting left nondominant side

G83.2 Monoplegia of upper limb
Paralysis of upper limb
EXCLUDES1 *monoplegia of upper limbs due to sequela of cerebrovascular disease (I69.03-, I69.13-, I69.23-, I69.33-, I69.83-, I69.93-)*

G83.20 Monoplegia of upper limb affecting unspecified side

G83.21 Monoplegia of upper limb affecting right dominant side

G83.22 Monoplegia of upper limb affecting left dominant side

G83.23 Monoplegia of upper limb affecting right nondominant side

G83.24 Monoplegia of upper limb affecting left nondominant side

G83.3 Monoplegia, unspecified

G83.30 Monoplegia, unspecified affecting unspecified side

G83.31 Monoplegia, unspecified affecting right dominant side

Unspecified Code | Other Specified Code | Manifestation Code | N Newborn | P Pediatric | M Maternity | A Adult | ♂ Male | ♀ Female
● New Code | ▲ Revised Code Title | ▶◀ Revised Text | NOTES | INCLUDES | EXCLUDES1 Not coded here | EXCLUDES2 Not included here
4th character required | 5th character required | 6th character required | 7th character required
Extension 'X' Alert | HAC Hospital-acquired condition (HAC) alert | AHA AHA Coding Clinic©

G83.32 **Monoplegia, unspecified affecting left dominant side**
G83.33 **Monoplegia, unspecified affecting right nondominant side**
G83.34 **Monoplegia, unspecified affecting left nondominant side**
G83.4 **Cauda equina syndrome**
Neurogenic bladder due to cauda equina syndrome
EXCLUDES1 *cord bladder NOS (G95.89)*
neurogenic bladder NOS (N31.9)
G83.5 **Locked-in state**
G83.8 **Other specified paralytic syndromes**
EXCLUDES1 *paralytic syndromes due to current spinal cord injury-code to spinal cord injury (S14, S24, S34)*
G83.81 **Brown-Séquard syndrome**
G83.82 **Anterior cord syndrome**
G83.83 **Posterior cord syndrome**
G83.84 **Todd's paralysis (postepileptic)**
G83.89 **Other specified paralytic syndromes**
G83.9 **Paralytic syndrome, unspecified**

Other disorders of the nervous system (G89-G99)

G89 **Pain, not elsewhere classified**
Code also related psychological factors associated with pain (F45.42)
EXCLUDES1 *generalized pain NOS (R52)*
pain disorders exclusively related to psychological factors (F45.41)
pain NOS (R52)
EXCLUDES2 *atypical face pain (G50.1)*
headache syndromes (G44.-)
localized pain, unspecified type - code to pain by site, such as:
abdomen pain (R10.-)
back pain (M54.9)
breast pain (N64.4)
chest pain (R07.1-R07.9)
ear pain (H92.0-)
eye pain (H57.1)
headache (R51)
joint pain (M25.5-)
limb pain (M79.6-)
lumbar region pain (M54.5)
painful urination (R30.9)
pelvic and perineal pain (R10.2)
shoulder pain (M25.51-)
spine pain (M54.-)
throat pain (R07.0)
tongue pain (K14.6)
tooth pain (K08.8)
renal colic (N23)
migraines (G43.-)
myalgia (M79.1)
pain from prosthetic devices, implants, and grafts(T82.84, T83.84, T84.84, ▶T85.84-◀)
phantom limb syndrome with pain (G54.6)
vulvar vestibulitis (N94.810)
vulvodynia (N94.81-)
G89.0 **Central pain syndrome**
Déjérine-Roussy syndrome
Myelopathic pain syndrome
Thalamic pain syndrome (hyperesthetic)
G89.1 **Acute pain, not elsewhere classified**
G89.11 **Acute pain due to trauma**
G89.12 **Acute post-thoracotomy pain**
Post-thoracotomy pain NOS
G89.18 **Other acute postprocedural pain**
Postoperative pain NOS
Postprocedural pain NOS
G89.2 **Chronic pain, not elsewhere classified**
EXCLUDES1 *causalgia, lower limb (G57.7-)*
causalgia, upper limb (G56.4-)
central pain syndrome (G89.0)
chronic pain syndrome (G89.4)
complex regional pain syndrome II, lower limb (G57.7-)
complex regional pain syndrome II, upper limb (G56.4-)
neoplasm related chronic pain (G89.3)
reflex sympathetic dystrophy (G90.5-)
G89.21 **Chronic pain due to trauma**
G89.22 **Chronic post-thoracotomy pain**
G89.28 **Other chronic postprocedural pain**
Other chronic postoperative pain
G89.29 **Other chronic pain**
G89.3 **Neoplasm related pain (acute) (chronic)**
Cancer associated pain
Pain due to malignancy (primary) (secondary)
Tumor associated pain
G89.4 **Chronic pain syndrome**
Chronic pain associated with significant psychosocial dysfunction
G90 **Disorders of autonomic nervous system**
EXCLUDES1 *dysfunction of the autonomic nervous system due to alcohol (G31.2)*
G90.0 **Idiopathic peripheral autonomic neuropathy**
G90.01 **Carotid sinus syncope**
Carotid sinus syndrome
G90.09 **Other idiopathic peripheral autonomic neuropathy**
Idiopathic peripheral autonomic neuropathy NOS
G90.1 **Familial dysautonomia [Riley-Day]**
G90.2 **Horner's syndrome**
Bernard(-Horner) syndrome
Cervical sympathetic dystrophy or paralysis
G90.3 **Multi-system degeneration of the autonomic nervous system**
Neurogenic orthostatic hypotension [Shy-Drager]
EXCLUDES1 *orthostatic hypotension NOS (I95.1)*
G90.4 **Autonomic dysreflexia**
Use additional code to identify the cause, such as:
fecal impaction (K56.41)
pressure ulcer (pressure area) (L89.-)
urinary tract infection (N39.0)
G90.5 **Complex regional pain syndrome I (CRPS I)**
Reflex sympathetic dystrophy
EXCLUDES1 *causalgia of lower limb (G57.7-)*
causalgia of upper limb (G56.4-)
complex regional pain syndrome II of lower limb (G57.7-)
complex regional pain syndrome II of upper limb (G56.4-)
G90.50 **Complex regional pain syndrome I, unspecified**
G90.51 **Complex regional pain syndrome I of upper limb**
G90.511 **Complex regional pain syndrome I of right upper limb**
G90.512 **Complex regional pain syndrome I of left upper limb**
G90.513 **Complex regional pain syndrome I of upper limb, bilateral**
G90.519 **Complex regional pain syndrome I of unspecified upper limb**
G90.52 **Complex regional pain syndrome I of lower limb**
G90.521 **Complex regional pain syndrome I of right lower limb**
G90.522 **Complex regional pain syndrome I of left lower limb**
G90.523 **Complex regional pain syndrome I of lower limb, bilateral**
G90.529 **Complex regional pain syndrome I of unspecified lower limb**
G90.59 **Complex regional pain syndrome I of other specified site**
G90.8 **Other disorders of autonomic nervous system**
G90.9 **Disorder of the autonomic nervous system, unspecified**
G91 **Hydrocephalus**
INCLUDES *acquired hydrocephalus*
EXCLUDES1 *Arnold-Chiari syndrome with hydrocephalus (Q07.-)*
congenital hydrocephalus (Q03.-)
spina bifida with hydrocephalus (Q05.-)

Unacceptable principal diagnosis symbol per Medicare code edits; Code exempt from diagnosis present on admission requirement
Questionable admission; Complication or comorbidity; CC/MCC exclusion; Major complication or comorbidity
Principal diagnosis as its own CC; Principal diagnosis as its own MCC; Z code as first-listed diagnosis

When symbols appear on a code that requires a 7th character extension, refer to Appendix D to identify applicable 7th character codes.

G91.0 Communicating hydrocephalus CC
Secondary normal pressure hydrocephalus
G91.1 Obstructive hydrocephalus CC
G91.2 (Idiopathic) normal pressure hydrocephalus CC
Normal pressure hydrocephalus NOS
G91.3 Post-traumatic hydrocephalus, unspecified CC
G91.4 Hydrocephalus in diseases classified elsewhere
Code first underlying condition, such as:
congenital syphilis (A50.4-)
neoplasm (C00-D49)
EXCLUDES1 *hydrocephalus due to congenital toxoplasmosis (P37.1)*
G91.8 Other hydrocephalus CC
G91.9 Hydrocephalus, unspecified CC

G92 Toxic encephalopathy MCC
Toxic encephalitis
Toxic metabolic encephalopathy
Code first (T51-T65) to identify toxic agent

G93 Other disorders of brain
G93.0 Cerebral cysts
Arachnoid cyst
Porencephalic cyst, acquired
EXCLUDES1 *acquired periventricular cysts of newborn (P91.1)*
congenital cerebral cysts (Q04.6)
G93.1 Anoxic brain damage, not elsewhere classified CC
EXCLUDES1 *cerebral anoxia due to anesthesia during labor and delivery (O74.3)*
cerebral anoxia due to anesthesia during the puerperium (O89.2)
neonatal anoxia (P84)
G93.2 Benign intracranial hypertension
EXCLUDES1 *hypertensive encephalopathy (I67.4)*
G93.3 Postviral fatigue syndrome
Benign myalgic encephalomyelitis
EXCLUDES1 *chronic fatigue syndrome NOS (R53.82)*
G93.4 Other and unspecified encephalopathy
EXCLUDES1 *alcoholic encephalopathy (G31.2)*
encephalopathy in diseases classified elsewhere (G94)
hypertensive encephalopathy (I67.4)
toxic (metabolic) encephalopathy (G92)
G93.40 Encephalopathy, unspecified MCC
G93.41 Metabolic encephalopathy MCC
AHA: Q3, 2015
Septic encephalopathy
G93.49 Other encephalopathy MCC
Encephalopathy NEC
G93.5 Compression of brain MCC
Arnold-Chiari type 1 compression of brain
Compression of brain (stem)
Herniation of brain (stem)
EXCLUDES1 *diffuse traumatic compression of brain (S06.2-)*
focal traumatic compression of brain (S06.3-)
G93.6 Cerebral edema MCC
EXCLUDES1 *cerebral edema due to birth injury (P11.0)*
traumatic cerebral edema (S06.1-)
G93.7 Reye's syndrome P MCC
Code first (T39.0-), if salicylates-induced
G93.8 Other specified disorders of brain
G93.81 Temporal sclerosis
Hippocampal sclerosis
Mesial temporal sclerosis
G93.82 Brain death MCC
G93.89 Other specified disorders of brain
Postradiation encephalopathy
G93.9 Disorder of brain, unspecified

G94 Other disorders of brain in diseases classified elsewhere
Code first underlying disease
EXCLUDES1 *encephalopathy in congenital syphilis (A50.49)*
encephalopathy in influenza (J09.X9, J10.81, J11.81)
encephalopathy in syphilis (A52.19)
hydrocephalus in diseases classified elsewhere (G91.4)

G95 Other and unspecified diseases of spinal cord
EXCLUDES2 *myelitis (G04.-)*
G95.0 Syringomyelia and syringobulbia CC
G95.1 Vascular myelopathies
EXCLUDES2 *intraspinal phlebitis and thrombophlebitis, except non-pyogenic (G08)*
G95.11 Acute infarction of spinal cord (embolic) (nonembolic) MCC
Anoxia of spinal cord
Arterial thrombosis of spinal cord
G95.19 Other vascular myelopathies MCC
Edema of spinal cord
Hematomyelia
Nonpyogenic intraspinal phlebitis and thrombophlebitis
Subacute necrotic myelopathy
G95.2 Other and unspecified cord compression
G95.20 Unspecified cord compression CC
G95.29 Other cord compression CC
G95.8 Other specified diseases of spinal cord
EXCLUDES1 *neurogenic bladder NOS (N31.9)*
neurogenic bladder due to cauda equina syndrome (G83.4)
neuromuscular dysfunction of bladder without spinal cord lesion (N31.-)
G95.81 Conus medullaris syndrome CC
G95.89 Other specified diseases of spinal cord CC
Cord bladder NOS
Drug-induced myelopathy
Radiation-induced myelopathy
EXCLUDES1 *myelopathy NOS (G95.9)*
G95.9 Disease of spinal cord, unspecified CC
Myelopathy NOS

G96 Other disorders of central nervous system
G96.0 Cerebrospinal fluid leak CC
EXCLUDES1 *cerebrospinal fluid leak from spinal puncture (G97.0)*
G96.1 Disorders of meninges, not elsewhere classified
G96.11 Dural tear CC
EXCLUDES1 *accidental puncture or laceration of dura during a procedure (G97.41)*
G96.12 Meningeal adhesions (cerebral) (spinal)
G96.19 Other disorders of meninges, not elsewhere classified
G96.8 Other specified disorders of central nervous system
G96.9 Disorder of central nervous system, unspecified

G97 Intraoperative and postprocedural complications and disorders of nervous system, not elsewhere classified
EXCLUDES2 *intraoperative and postprocedural cerebrovascular infarction (I97.81-, I97.82-)*
G97.0 Cerebrospinal fluid leak from spinal puncture CC
G97.1 Other reaction to spinal and lumbar puncture
Headache due to lumbar puncture
G97.2 Intracranial hypotension following ventricular shunting CC
G97.3 Intraoperative hemorrhage and hematoma of a nervous system organ or structure complicating a procedure
EXCLUDES1 *intraoperative hemorrhage and hematoma of a nervous system organ or structure due to accidental puncture and laceration during a procedure (G97.4-)*
G97.31 Intraoperative hemorrhage and hematoma of a nervous system organ or structure complicating a nervous system procedure CC
G97.32 Intraoperative hemorrhage and hematoma of a nervous system organ or structure complicating other procedure CC
G97.4 Accidental puncture and laceration of a nervous system organ or structure during a procedure
G97.41 Accidental puncture or laceration of dura during a procedure CC
Incidental (inadvertent) durotomy
G97.48 Accidental puncture and laceration of other nervous system organ or structure during a nervous system procedure CC
G97.49 Accidental puncture and laceration of other nervous system organ or structure during other procedure CC

Unspecified Code | Other Specified Code | Manifestation Code | N Newborn | P Pediatric | M Maternity | A Adult | ♂ Male | ♀ Female
● New Code | ▲ Revised Code Title | ►◄ Revised Text | NOTES | INCLUDES | EXCLUDES1 Not coded here | EXCLUDES2 Not included here
4th character required | 5th character required | 6th character required | 7th character required
Extension 'X' Alert | HAC Hospital-acquired condition (HAC) alert | AHA AHA Coding Clinic©

▲ G97.5 Postprocedural ▶hemorrhage of◀ a nervous system organ or structure following a procedure

▲ G97.51 Postprocedural ▶hemorrhage of◀ a nervous system organ or structure following a nervous system procedure

▲ G97.52 Postprocedural ▶hemorrhage of◀ a nervous system organ or structure following other procedure

● G97.6 Postprocedural hematoma and seroma of a nervous system organ or structure following a procedure

● G97.61 Postprocedural hematoma of a nervous system organ or structure following a nervous system procedure

● G97.62 Postprocedural hematoma of a nervous system organ or structure following other procedure

● G97.63 Postprocedural seroma of a nervous system organ or structure following a nervous system procedure

● G97.64 Postprocedural seroma of a nervous system organ or structure following other procedure

G97.8 Other intraoperative and postprocedural complications and disorders of nervous system

Use additional code to further specify disorder

G97.81 Other intraoperative complications of nervous system

G97.82 Other postprocedural complications and disorders of nervous system

G98 Other disorders of nervous system not elsewhere classified

INCLUDES *nervous system disorder NOS*

G98.0 Neurogenic arthritis, not elsewhere classified

Nonsyphilitic neurogenic arthropathy NEC
Nonsyphilitic neurogenic spondylopathy NEC

EXCLUDES1 *spondylopathy (in):*
syringomyelia and syringobulbia (G95.0)
tabes dorsalis (A52.11)

G98.8 Other disorders of nervous system

Nervous system disorder NOS

G99 Other disorders of nervous system in diseases classified elsewhere

G99.0 Autonomic neuropathy in diseases classified elsewhere

Code first underlying disease, such as:
amyloidosis (E85.-)
gout (M1A.-, M10.-)
hyperthyroidism (E05.-)

EXCLUDES1 *diabetic autonomic neuropathy (E08-E13 with .43)*

G99.2 Myelopathy in diseases classified elsewhere

Code first underlying disease, such as:
neoplasm (C00-D49)

EXCLUDES1 *myelopathy in:*
intervertebral disease (M50.0-, M51.0-)
spondylosis (M47.0-, M47.1-)

G99.8 Other specified disorders of nervous system in diseases classified elsewhere

Code first underlying disorder, such as:
amyloidosis (E85.-)
avitaminosis (E56.9)

EXCLUDES1 *nervous system involvement in:*
cysticercosis (B69.0)
rubella (B06.0-)
syphilis (A52.1-)

Unacceptable principal diagnosis symbol per Medicare code edits · Code exempt from diagnosis present on admission requirement
Questionable admission · Complication or comorbidity · CC/MCC exclusion · Major complication or comorbidity
Principal diagnosis as its own CC · Principal diagnosis as its own MCC · Z code as first-listed diagnosis

Chapter 7: Diseases of the Eye and Adnexa (H00-H59)

Guidelines for Assigning Codes From This Chapter

Chapter 7 features diseases of the eye and adnexal structures. The adnexa refers to the adjoining, or accessory, portions of the eye, such as the ocular muscles and eyelids. The eye itself consists of the cornea, anterior chamber, iris, lens, vitreous body, retina, and the optic nerve. Also included in this section are the conjunctiva, which is the membrane that covers the eye and lines the eyelids, and the lacrimal system, or tear ducts.

List of Sections

- H00-H05: Disorders of eyelid, lacrimal system and orbit
- H10-H11: Disorders of conjunctiva
- H15-H22: Disorders of sclera, cornea, iris and ciliary body
- H25-H28: Disorders of lens
- H30-H36: Disorders of choroid and retina
- H40-H42: Glaucoma
- H43-H44: Disorders of vitreous body and globe
- H46-H47: Disorders of optic nerve and visual pathways
- H49-H52: Disorders of ocular muscles, binocular movement, accommodation and refraction
- H53-H54: Visual disturbances and blindness
- H55-H57: Other disorders of eye and adnexa
- H59: Intraoperative and postprocedural complications and disorders of eye and adnexa, not elsewhere classified

Highlights From the ICD-10-CM Official Guidelines for Coding and Reporting

The Official Guidelines for Chapter 7 help you with questions you may face when a patient has glaucoma in both eyes. You'll also find important tips for coding when the stage of the glaucoma changes during a patient's admission and how to tell the difference between the codes for indeterminate and unspecified stages. The information that follows is from the 2017 Official Guidelines.

Master Coding for Glaucoma Type and Stage

Glaucoma refers to a group of diseases that damage the optic nerve, leading to vision loss and blindness. You can assign as many codes from category H40 (Glaucoma) as you need to identify the type of glaucoma, the affected eye, and the stage of the disease.

Bilateral, same type/stage: When the patient has glaucoma in both eyes documented as the same type and stage, and there is a code for bilateral glaucoma, report only the one code for the type of glaucoma, bilateral, and select the seventh character for the stage. If the classification does not provide a code for bilateral glaucoma, such as H40.10 (*Unspecified open-angle glaucoma*), H40.11 (*Primary open-angle glaucoma*), and H40.20 (*Unspecified primary angle-closure glaucoma*), report only one code for the type of glaucoma and choose the seventh character to represent the stage.

Bilateral, same type/different stages: When documentation shows the same type of glaucoma in each eye but with different stages, and the classification does not specify laterality, i.e., H40.10, H40.11, and H40.20, you should report one code for the type of glaucoma for each eye with the seventh character for the specific glaucoma stage documented for each eye.

Bilateral, different types/stages: For a patient who has bilateral glaucoma with a different type and a different stage for each eye and the classification specifies laterality, you should report a code for each eye instead of the code for bilateral glaucoma. If the classification does not specify laterality, report one code for each type of glaucoma with the seventh character indicating the stage.

Evolving: If the patient's glaucoma gets worse during the patient's stay, report the code for the highest documented stage.

Indeterminate vs. unspecified: ICD-10-CM offers a seventh character of "4" for "indeterminate stage" and "0" for unspecified," which can be confusing. Use "0" only when the provider doesn't document the stage. Use "4" when the provider documents she can't determine the stage clinically.

Anatomy of the Eye

1. **The Organ of Sight**
Eyes are regarded as the organs of sight. They are located in the orbits of the skull. The eyelids and eyelashes serve to protect the eyes from foreign objects. Blinking of the eyelids lubricates the surface of the eye by spreading tears that are produced by the lacrimal gland. A typical human eye is in the form of a sphere and filled with the following two fluids:
   a) Aqueous Humor

      The frontal portion of the lens of the eye is known as the anterior compartment that remains filled with fluid, which is called the aqueous humor.

   b) Vitreous Humor

      The portion behind the lens of the eye is known as the posterior compartment that is filled with a fluid called the vitreous humor.

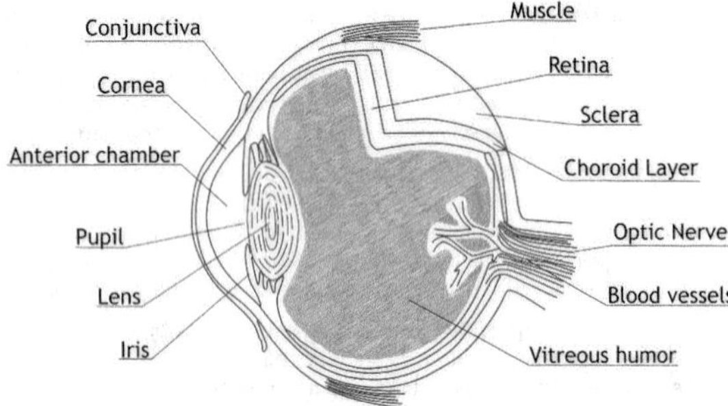

2. **The Other Parts of the Eye:**
   a) **Ciliary Body and Muscle:** This is a ring of striated smooth muscle in the middle layer eye (vascular layer). It is triangular in the horizontal section and is coated by a double layer, the ciliary epithelium. The inner layer is transparent and covers the vitreous body and is a continuation of neural tissue of the retina. The outer layer is continuous with the retinal pigment epithelium and constitutes the cells of the dilator muscle.
   b) **Suspensory Ligament:** A series of fibers that connect the ciliary body of the eye with the lens, holding it in place. Suspensory ligaments are thin fibers that connect the ciliary body of the lens with the receptors. It is a thickening of Tenon's capsule, the dense connective tissue capsule surrounding the globe and separating it from orbital fat. Suspensory ligaments in the eye lens allow easy focusing.
   c) **Iris:** A thin, circular structure in the eye which covers the sclera. It is responsible for controlling the diameter and size of the pupils and thus the amount of light reaching the retina. In response to the amount of light entering the eye, muscles attached to the iris expand or contract the aperture at the center of the iris, known as the pupil.
   d) **Pupil:** The dark center opening in the middle of the iris is called the pupil. The pupil is a hole located in the center of the iris of the eye that allows light to enter the retina. The pupil changes size to adjust for the amount of light available.
   e) **Cornea:** The cornea is transparent and comprises the front part of the eye that covers the iris, pupil and anterior chamber. Together with the lens, the cornea refracts light accounting for approximately two-thirds of the eye's total optical power.
   f) **Lens:** The crystalline lens is a biconvex structure and is suspended behind the colored iris. The lens is behind the covering known as the cornea. The lens is more flat on its anterior side than on its posterior side.
   g) **Retina:** The vertebrate retina is 0.5 mm thick and lines the back of the eye. It is a light-sensitive layer of tissue, lining the inner surface of the eye. The optic nerve contains the ganglion cell axons running to the brain.
   h) **Retinal Arteries and Veins:** The retinal arteries and veins emerge from the nasal side of the optic disc. Vessels directed temporally have an arching course; those directed nasally have a radial course. Arteries are brighter red and narrower than veins.
   i) **Fovea Centralis:** The fovea is the depression in the inner retinal surface, about 1.5 mm wide and is specialized for maximum visual acuity. This is the thickest part of the retina. This part has the highest density of cones in the eye.
   j) **Optic Nerve:** The optic nerve is the second of twelve paired cranial nerves, but is considered to be part of the central nervous system as it is derived from an out-pouching of the diencephalon during embryonic development. It consists mainly of fibers derived from the ganglionic cells of the retina. Its fibers are covered with myelin produced by oligodendrocytes rather than Schwann cells.
   k) **Choroid Coat:** The choroid, also known as the choroidea or choroid coat, is the vascular layer of the eye containing connective tissue and lies between the retina and the sclera. It contains the retinal pigmented epithelial cells and provides oxygen and nourishment to the retina.
   l) **Sclera:** The posterior five-sixths of the connective tissue coat of the ocular globe is formed by sclera. It maintains the shape of the globe and provides an attachment for the extraocular muscle insertions. The sclera is perforated by many nerves and vessels passing through the posterior scleral foramen, the hole that is formed by the optic nerve. The inner layer of the sclera (lamina fusca) blends with the suprachoroidal and supraciliary lamellae of the uveal tract.
   m) **Blind Spot:** This is a small portion of the visual field of each eye where the optic nerve and blood vessels pass through to connect to the back of the eye and is also called an optic disk. There are no photoreceptors in the optic disk, therefore there is no image detection in this area. The blind spot of the right eye is located to the right of the center of vision and vice versa in the left eye.
   n) **Hyaloid Canal (or Cloquet's/Stilling's Canal):** This is a small transparent canal running through the vitreous body from the optical nerve disc to the lens. It is formed by pouch of the hyaloid membrane, which encloses the vitreous body. It is filled with lymph.

Common Pathologies

Cataract

Cataracts are an eye disorder in which clouding of the lens occurs, which leads to blurry vision. It is an aging disorder. This disorder leads to dimness in eye vision, and if not treated can lead to blindness.

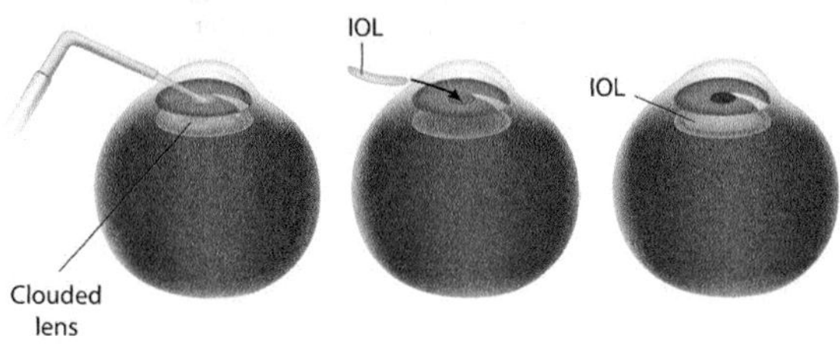

Glaucoma

In this disease, damage occurs to optic nerves due to increased intraocular pressure and leads to blindness.

Development of Glaucoma

Healthy eye

Vitreous body

Flow of aqueous humour

Drainage canal

Glaucoma

1. Drainage canal blocked; build-up of fluid

2. Increased pressure damages blood vessels and optic nerve

Strabismus

A condition of eye in which there is nonalignment between both eyes. This condition is commonly called squint.

Strabismus

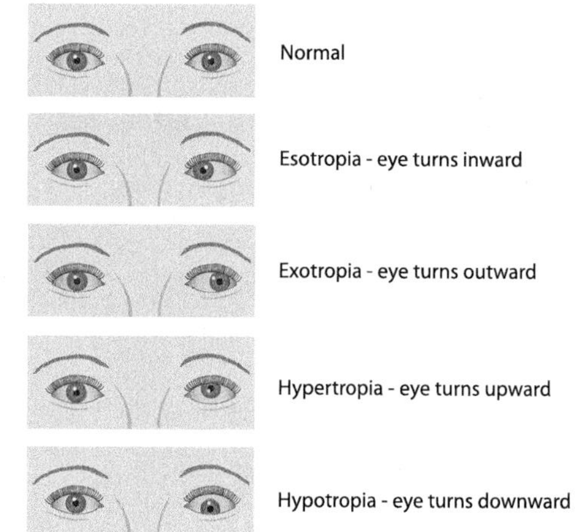

Macular Degeneration

This condition occurs because of degeneration in the macula of the eye due to aging and leads to blurry vision. It is a disease that destroys sharp, central vision. Central vision is required to see objects clearly and to do tasks such as reading and driving.

Conjunctivitis

An infection in the eye. The conjunctiva in the eye gets exposed to bacteria and other allergic irritants, which can lead to inflammation and infection. It is also known as pinkeye.

Optic Neuritis

This disorder occurs due to inflammation of the optic nerve. Pain and temporary vision loss are common.

Diseases of the eye and adnexa (H00-H59)

NOTES Use an external cause code following the code for the eye condition, if applicable, to identify the cause of the eye condition

EXCLUDES2 *certain conditions originating in the perinatal period (P04-P96)*
certain infectious and parasitic diseases (A00-B99)
complications of pregnancy, childbirth and the puerperium (O00-O9A)
congenital malformations, deformations, and chromosomal abnormalities (Q00-Q99)
diabetes mellitus related eye conditions (E09.3-, E10.3-, E11.3-, E13.3-)
endocrine, nutritional and metabolic diseases (E00-E88)
injury (trauma) of eye and orbit (S05.-)
injury, poisoning and certain other consequences of external causes (S00-T88)
neoplasms (C00-D49)
symptoms, signs and abnormal clinical and laboratory findings, not elsewhere classified (R00-R94)
syphilis related eye disorders (A50.01, A50.3-, A51.43, A52.71)

This chapter contains the following blocks:

H00-H05	Disorders of eyelid, lacrimal system and orbit
H10-H11	Disorders of conjunctiva
H15-H22	Disorders of sclera, cornea, iris and ciliary body
H25-H28	Disorders of lens
H30-H36	Disorders of choroid and retina
H40-H42	Glaucoma
H43-H44	Disorders of vitreous body and globe
H46-H47	Disorders of optic nerve and visual pathways
H49-H52	Disorders of ocular muscles, binocular movement, accommodation and refraction
H53-H54	Visual disturbances and blindness
H55-H57	Other disorders of eye and adnexa
H59	Intraoperative and postprocedural complications and disorders of eye and adnexa, not elsewhere classified

Disorders of eyelid, lacrimal system and orbit (H00-H05)

EXCLUDES2 *open wound of eyelid (S01.1-)*
superficial injury of eyelid (S00.1-, S00.2-)

H00 Hordeolum and chalazion
- **H00.0 Hordeolum (externum) (internum) of eyelid**
  - **H00.01 Hordeolum externum**
    Hordeolum NOS
    Stye
    - H00.011 **Hordeolum externum right upper eyelid**
    - H00.012 **Hordeolum externum right lower eyelid**
    - H00.013 **Hordeolum externum right eye, unspecified eyelid**
    - H00.014 **Hordeolum externum left upper eyelid**
    - H00.015 **Hordeolum externum left lower eyelid**
    - H00.016 **Hordeolum externum left eye, unspecified eyelid**
    - H00.019 **Hordeolum externum unspecified eye, unspecified eyelid**
  - **H00.02 Hordeolum internum**
    Infection of meibomian gland
    - H00.021 **Hordeolum internum right upper eyelid**
    - H00.022 **Hordeolum internum right lower eyelid**
    - H00.023 **Hordeolum internum right eye, unspecified eyelid**
    - H00.024 **Hordeolum internum left upper eyelid**
    - H00.025 **Hordeolum internum left lower eyelid**
    - H00.026 **Hordeolum internum left eye, unspecified eyelid**
    - H00.029 **Hordeolum internum unspecified eye, unspecified eyelid**
  - **H00.03 Abscess of eyelid**
    Furuncle of eyelid
    - H00.031 **Abscess of right upper eyelid**
    - H00.032 **Abscess of right lower eyelid**
    - H00.033 **Abscess of eyelid right eye, unspecified eyelid**
    - H00.034 **Abscess of left upper eyelid**
    - H00.035 **Abscess of left lower eyelid**
    - H00.036 **Abscess of eyelid left eye, unspecified eyelid**
    - H00.039 **Abscess of eyelid unspecified eye, unspecified eyelid**
- **H00.1 Chalazion**
  Meibomian (gland) cyst
  EXCLUDES2 *infected meibomian gland (H00.02-)*
  - H00.11 **Chalazion right upper eyelid**
  - H00.12 **Chalazion right lower eyelid**
  - H00.13 **Chalazion right eye, unspecified eyelid**
  - H00.14 **Chalazion left upper eyelid**
  - H00.15 **Chalazion left lower eyelid**
  - H00.16 **Chalazion left eye, unspecified eyelid**
  - H00.19 **Chalazion unspecified eye, unspecified eyelid**

H01 Other inflammation of eyelid

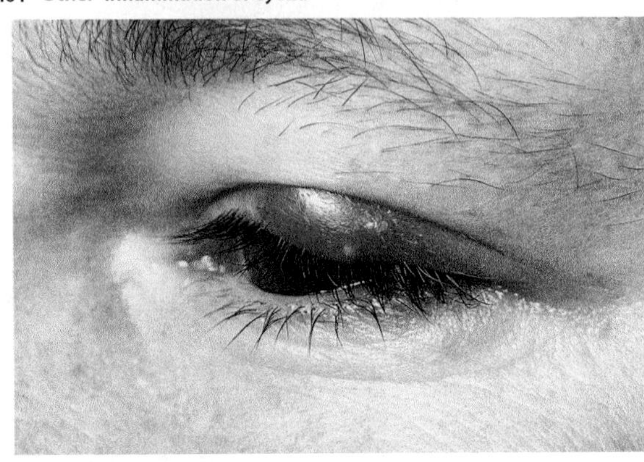

Figure 7.1 Blepharitis

- **H01.0 Blepharitis**
  EXCLUDES1 *blepharoconjunctivitis (H10.5-)*
  - **H01.00 Unspecified blepharitis**
    - H01.001 **Unspecified blepharitis right upper eyelid**
    - H01.002 **Unspecified blepharitis right lower eyelid**
    - H01.003 **Unspecified blepharitis right eye, unspecified eyelid**
    - H01.004 **Unspecified blepharitis left upper eyelid**
    - H01.005 **Unspecified blepharitis left lower eyelid**
    - H01.006 **Unspecified blepharitis left eye, unspecified eyelid**
    - H01.009 **Unspecified blepharitis unspecified eye, unspecified eyelid**
  - **H01.01 Ulcerative blepharitis**
    - H01.011 **Ulcerative blepharitis right upper eyelid**
    - H01.012 **Ulcerative blepharitis right lower eyelid**
    - H01.013 **Ulcerative blepharitis right eye, unspecified eyelid**
    - H01.014 **Ulcerative blepharitis left upper eyelid**
    - H01.015 **Ulcerative blepharitis left lower eyelid**
    - H01.016 **Ulcerative blepharitis left eye, unspecified eyelid**
    - H01.019 **Ulcerative blepharitis unspecified eye, unspecified eyelid**
  - **H01.02 Squamous blepharitis**
    - H01.021 **Squamous blepharitis right upper eyelid**
    - H01.022 **Squamous blepharitis right lower eyelid**
    - H01.023 **Squamous blepharitis right eye, unspecified eyelid**
    - H01.024 **Squamous blepharitis left upper eyelid**
    - H01.025 **Squamous blepharitis left lower eyelid**
    - H01.026 **Squamous blepharitis left eye, unspecified eyelid**
    - H01.029 **Squamous blepharitis unspecified eye, unspecified eyelid**
- **H01.1 Noninfectious dermatoses of eyelid**
  - **H01.11 Allergic dermatitis of eyelid**
    Contact dermatitis of eyelid

Unacceptable principal diagnosis symbol per Medicare code edits · Code exempt from diagnosis present on admission requirement · Questionable admission · Complication or comorbidity · CC/MCC exclusion · Major complication or comorbidity · Principal diagnosis as its own CC · Principal diagnosis as its own MCC · Z code as first-listed diagnosis

H01.111 Allergic dermatitis of right upper eyelid
H01.112 Allergic dermatitis of right lower eyelid
H01.113 Allergic dermatitis of right eye, unspecified eyelid
H01.114 Allergic dermatitis of left upper eyelid
H01.115 Allergic dermatitis of left lower eyelid
H01.116 Allergic dermatitis of left eye, unspecified eyelid
H01.119 Allergic dermatitis of unspecified eye, unspecified eyelid

H01.12 Discoid lupus erythematosus of eyelid
H01.121 Discoid lupus erythematosus of right upper eyelid
H01.122 Discoid lupus erythematosus of right lower eyelid
H01.123 Discoid lupus erythematosus of right eye, unspecified eyelid
H01.124 Discoid lupus erythematosus of left upper eyelid
H01.125 Discoid lupus erythematosus of left lower eyelid
H01.126 Discoid lupus erythematosus of left eye, unspecified eyelid
H01.129 Discoid lupus erythematosus of unspecified eye, unspecified eyelid

H01.13 Eczematous dermatitis of eyelid
H01.131 Eczematous dermatitis of right upper eyelid
H01.132 Eczematous dermatitis of right lower eyelid
H01.133 Eczematous dermatitis of right eye, unspecified eyelid
H01.134 Eczematous dermatitis of left upper eyelid
H01.135 Eczematous dermatitis of left lower eyelid
H01.136 Eczematous dermatitis of left eye, unspecified eyelid
H01.139 Eczematous dermatitis of unspecified eye, unspecified eyelid

H01.14 Xeroderma of eyelid
H01.141 Xeroderma of right upper eyelid
H01.142 Xeroderma of right lower eyelid
H01.143 Xeroderma of right eye, unspecified eyelid
H01.144 Xeroderma of left upper eyelid
H01.145 Xeroderma of left lower eyelid
H01.146 Xeroderma of left eye, unspecified eyelid
H01.149 Xeroderma of unspecified eye, unspecified eyelid

H01.8 Other specified inflammations of eyelid
H01.9 Unspecified inflammation of eyelid
Inflammation of eyelid NOS

H02 Other disorders of eyelid
EXCLUDES1 *congenital malformations of eyelid (Q10.0-Q10.3)*

H02.0 Entropion and trichiasis of eyelid
H02.00 Unspecified entropion of eyelid
H02.001 Unspecified entropion of right upper eyelid
H02.002 Unspecified entropion of right lower eyelid
H02.003 Unspecified entropion of right eye, unspecified eyelid
H02.004 Unspecified entropion of left upper eyelid
H02.005 Unspecified entropion of left lower eyelid
H02.006 Unspecified entropion of left eye, unspecified eyelid
H02.009 Unspecified entropion of unspecified eye, unspecified eyelid

H02.01 Cicatricial entropion of eyelid
H02.011 Cicatricial entropion of right upper eyelid
H02.012 Cicatricial entropion of right lower eyelid
H02.013 Cicatricial entropion of right eye, unspecified eyelid
H02.014 Cicatricial entropion of left upper eyelid
H02.015 Cicatricial entropion of left lower eyelid
H02.016 Cicatricial entropion of left eye, unspecified eyelid
H02.019 Cicatricial entropion of unspecified eye, unspecified eyelid

H02.02 Mechanical entropion of eyelid
H02.021 Mechanical entropion of right upper eyelid
H02.022 Mechanical entropion of right lower eyelid
H02.023 Mechanical entropion of right eye, unspecified eyelid
H02.024 Mechanical entropion of left upper eyelid
H02.025 Mechanical entropion of left lower eyelid
H02.026 Mechanical entropion of left eye, unspecified eyelid
H02.029 Mechanical entropion of unspecified eye, unspecified eyelid

H02.03 Senile entropion of eyelid
H02.031 Senile entropion of right upper eyelid A
H02.032 Senile entropion of right lower eyelid A
H02.033 Senile entropion of right eye, unspecified eyelid A
H02.034 Senile entropion of left upper eyelid A
H02.035 Senile entropion of left lower eyelid A
H02.036 Senile entropion of left eye, unspecified eyelid A
H02.039 Senile entropion of unspecified eye, unspecified eyelid A

H02.04 Spastic entropion of eyelid
H02.041 Spastic entropion of right upper eyelid
H02.042 Spastic entropion of right lower eyelid
H02.043 Spastic entropion of right eye, unspecified eyelid
H02.044 Spastic entropion of left upper eyelid
H02.045 Spastic entropion of left lower eyelid
H02.046 Spastic entropion of left eye, unspecified eyelid
H02.049 Spastic entropion of unspecified eye, unspecified eyelid

H02.05 Trichiasis without entropion
H02.051 Trichiasis without entropion right upper eyelid
H02.052 Trichiasis without entropion right lower eyelid
H02.053 Trichiasis without entropion right eye, unspecified eyelid
H02.054 Trichiasis without entropion left upper eyelid
H02.055 Trichiasis without entropion left lower eyelid
H02.056 Trichiasis without entropion left eye, unspecified eyelid
H02.059 Trichiasis without entropion unspecified eye, unspecified eyelid

H02.1 Ectropion of eyelid
H02.10 Unspecified ectropion of eyelid
H02.101 Unspecified ectropion of right upper eyelid
H02.102 Unspecified ectropion of right lower eyelid
H02.103 Unspecified ectropion of right eye, unspecified eyelid
H02.104 Unspecified ectropion of left upper eyelid
H02.105 Unspecified ectropion of left lower eyelid
H02.106 Unspecified ectropion of left eye, unspecified eyelid
H02.109 Unspecified ectropion of unspecified eye, unspecified eyelid

H02.11 Cicatricial ectropion of eyelid
H02.111 Cicatricial ectropion of right upper eyelid
H02.112 Cicatricial ectropion of right lower eyelid
H02.113 Cicatricial ectropion of right eye, unspecified eyelid
H02.114 Cicatricial ectropion of left upper eyelid

Unspecified Code | Other Specified Code | Manifestation Code | N Newborn | P Pediatric | M Maternity | A Adult | ♂ Male | ♀ Female
● New Code ▲ Revised Code Title ►◄ Revised Text NOTES INCLUDES EXCLUDES1 Not coded here EXCLUDES2 Not included here
4th character required 5th character required 6th character required 7th character required
Extension 'X' Alert HAC Hospital-acquired condition (HAC) alert AHA AHA Coding Clinic©

H02.115 Cicatricial ectropion of left lower eyelid
H02.116 Cicatricial ectropion of left eye, unspecified eyelid
H02.119 Cicatricial ectropion of unspecified eye, unspecified eyelid

H02.12 Mechanical ectropion of eyelid
H02.121 Mechanical ectropion of right upper eyelid
H02.122 Mechanical ectropion of right lower eyelid
H02.123 Mechanical ectropion of right eye, unspecified eyelid
H02.124 Mechanical ectropion of left upper eyelid
H02.125 Mechanical ectropion of left lower eyelid
H02.126 Mechanical ectropion of left eye, unspecified eyelid
H02.129 Mechanical ectropion of unspecified eye, unspecified eyelid

H02.13 Senile ectropion of eyelid
H02.131 Senile ectropion of right upper eyelid A
H02.132 Senile ectropion of right lower eyelid A
H02.133 Senile ectropion of right eye, unspecified eyelid A
H02.134 Senile ectropion of left upper eyelid A
H02.135 Senile ectropion of left lower eyelid A
H02.136 Senile ectropion of left eye, unspecified eyelid A
H02.139 Senile ectropion of unspecified eye, unspecified eyelid A

H02.14 Spastic ectropion of eyelid
H02.141 Spastic ectropion of right upper eyelid
H02.142 Spastic ectropion of right lower eyelid
H02.143 Spastic ectropion of right eye, unspecified eyelid
H02.144 Spastic ectropion of left upper eyelid
H02.145 Spastic ectropion of left lower eyelid
H02.146 Spastic ectropion of left eye, unspecified eyelid
H02.149 Spastic ectropion of unspecified eye, unspecified eyelid

H02.2 Lagophthalmos

H02.20 Unspecified lagophthalmos
H02.201 Unspecified lagophthalmos right upper eyelid
H02.202 Unspecified lagophthalmos right lower eyelid
H02.203 Unspecified lagophthalmos right eye, unspecified eyelid
H02.204 Unspecified lagophthalmos left upper eyelid
H02.205 Unspecified lagophthalmos left lower eyelid
H02.206 Unspecified lagophthalmos left eye, unspecified eyelid
H02.209 Unspecified lagophthalmos unspecified eye, unspecified eyelid

H02.21 Cicatricial lagophthalmos
H02.211 Cicatricial lagophthalmos right upper eyelid
H02.212 Cicatricial lagophthalmos right lower eyelid
H02.213 Cicatricial lagophthalmos right eye, unspecified eyelid
H02.214 Cicatricial lagophthalmos left upper eyelid
H02.215 Cicatricial lagophthalmos left lower eyelid
H02.216 Cicatricial lagophthalmos left eye, unspecified eyelid
H02.219 Cicatricial lagophthalmos unspecified eye, unspecified eyelid

H02.22 Mechanical lagophthalmos
H02.221 Mechanical lagophthalmos right upper eyelid
H02.222 Mechanical lagophthalmos right lower eyelid
H02.223 Mechanical lagophthalmos right eye, unspecified eyelid
H02.224 Mechanical lagophthalmos left upper eyelid
H02.225 Mechanical lagophthalmos left lower eyelid
H02.226 Mechanical lagophthalmos left eye, unspecified eyelid
H02.229 Mechanical lagophthalmos unspecified eye, unspecified eyelid

H02.23 Paralytic lagophthalmos
H02.231 Paralytic lagophthalmos right upper eyelid
H02.232 Paralytic lagophthalmos right lower eyelid
H02.233 Paralytic lagophthalmos right eye, unspecified eyelid
H02.234 Paralytic lagophthalmos left upper eyelid
H02.235 Paralytic lagophthalmos left lower eyelid
H02.236 Paralytic lagophthalmos left eye, unspecified eyelid
H02.239 Paralytic lagophthalmos unspecified eye, unspecified eyelid

H02.3 Blepharochalasis
Pseudoptosis
H02.30 Blepharochalasis unspecified eye, unspecified eyelid
H02.31 Blepharochalasis right upper eyelid
H02.32 Blepharochalasis right lower eyelid
H02.33 Blepharochalasis right eye, unspecified eyelid
H02.34 Blepharochalasis left upper eyelid
H02.35 Blepharochalasis left lower eyelid
H02.36 Blepharochalasis left eye, unspecified eyelid

H02.4 Ptosis of eyelid

H02.40 Unspecified ptosis of eyelid
H02.401 Unspecified ptosis of right eyelid
H02.402 Unspecified ptosis of left eyelid
H02.403 Unspecified ptosis of bilateral eyelids
H02.409 Unspecified ptosis of unspecified eyelid

H02.41 Mechanical ptosis of eyelid
H02.411 Mechanical ptosis of right eyelid
H02.412 Mechanical ptosis of left eyelid
H02.413 Mechanical ptosis of bilateral eyelids
H02.419 Mechanical ptosis of unspecified eyelid

H02.42 Myogenic ptosis of eyelid
H02.421 Myogenic ptosis of right eyelid
H02.422 Myogenic ptosis of left eyelid
H02.423 Myogenic ptosis of bilateral eyelids
H02.429 Myogenic ptosis of unspecified eyelid

H02.43 Paralytic ptosis of eyelid
Neurogenic ptosis of eyelid
H02.431 Paralytic ptosis of right eyelid
H02.432 Paralytic ptosis of left eyelid
H02.433 Paralytic ptosis of bilateral eyelids
H02.439 Paralytic ptosis unspecified eyelid

H02.5 Other disorders affecting eyelid function
EXCLUDES2 *blepharospasm (G24.5)*
organic tic (G25.69)
psychogenic tic (F95.-)

H02.51 Abnormal innervation syndrome
H02.511 Abnormal innervation syndrome right upper eyelid
H02.512 Abnormal innervation syndrome right lower eyelid
H02.513 Abnormal innervation syndrome right eye, unspecified eyelid
H02.514 Abnormal innervation syndrome left upper eyelid
H02.515 Abnormal innervation syndrome left lower eyelid
H02.516 Abnormal innervation syndrome left eye, unspecified eyelid

Unacceptable principal diagnosis symbol per Medicare code edits; Code exempt from diagnosis present on admission requirement; Questionable admission; Complication or comorbidity; CC/MCC exclusion; Major complication or comorbidity; Principal diagnosis as its own CC; Principal diagnosis as its own MCC; Z code as first-listed diagnosis

H02.519 Abnormal innervation syndrome unspecified eye, unspecified eyelid
H02.52 Blepharophimosis
Ankyloblepharon
H02.521 Blepharophimosis right upper eyelid
H02.522 Blepharophimosis right lower eyelid
H02.523 Blepharophimosis right eye, unspecified eyelid
H02.524 Blepharophimosis left upper eyelid
H02.525 Blepharophimosis left lower eyelid
H02.526 Blepharophimosis left eye, unspecified eyelid
H02.529 Blepharophimosis unspecified eye, unspecified lid
H02.53 Eyelid retraction
Eyelid lag
H02.531 Eyelid retraction right upper eyelid
H02.532 Eyelid retraction right lower eyelid
H02.533 Eyelid retraction right eye, unspecified eyelid
H02.534 Eyelid retraction left upper eyelid
H02.535 Eyelid retraction left lower eyelid
H02.536 Eyelid retraction left eye, unspecified eyelid
H02.539 Eyelid retraction unspecified eye, unspecified lid
H02.59 Other disorders affecting eyelid function
Deficient blink reflex
Sensory disorders
H02.6 Xanthelasma of eyelid
H02.60 Xanthelasma of unspecified eye, unspecified eyelid
H02.61 Xanthelasma of right upper eyelid
H02.62 Xanthelasma of right lower eyelid
H02.63 Xanthelasma of right eye, unspecified eyelid
H02.64 Xanthelasma of left upper eyelid
H02.65 Xanthelasma of left lower eyelid
H02.66 Xanthelasma of left eye, unspecified eyelid
H02.7 Other and unspecified degenerative disorders of eyelid and periocular area
H02.70 Unspecified degenerative disorders of eyelid and periocular area
H02.71 Chloasma of eyelid and periocular area
Dyspigmentation of eyelid
Hyperpigmentation of eyelid
H02.711 Chloasma of right upper eyelid and periocular area
H02.712 Chloasma of right lower eyelid and periocular area
H02.713 Chloasma of right eye, unspecified eyelid and periocular area
H02.714 Chloasma of left upper eyelid and periocular area
H02.715 Chloasma of left lower eyelid and periocular area
H02.716 Chloasma of left eye, unspecified eyelid and periocular area
H02.719 Chloasma of unspecified eye, unspecified eyelid and periocular area
H02.72 Madarosis of eyelid and periocular area
Hypotrichosis of eyelid
H02.721 Madarosis of right upper eyelid and periocular area
H02.722 Madarosis of right lower eyelid and periocular area
H02.723 Madarosis of right eye, unspecified eyelid and periocular area
H02.724 Madarosis of left upper eyelid and periocular area
H02.725 Madarosis of left lower eyelid and periocular area
H02.726 Madarosis of left eye, unspecified eyelid and periocular area
H02.729 Madarosis of unspecified eye, unspecified eyelid and periocular area
H02.73 Vitiligo of eyelid and periocular area
Hypopigmentation of eyelid
H02.731 Vitiligo of right upper eyelid and periocular area
H02.732 Vitiligo of right lower eyelid and periocular area
H02.733 Vitiligo of right eye, unspecified eyelid and periocular area
H02.734 Vitiligo of left upper eyelid and periocular area
H02.735 Vitiligo of left lower eyelid and periocular area
H02.736 Vitiligo of left eye, unspecified eyelid and periocular area
H02.739 Vitiligo of unspecified eye, unspecified eyelid and periocular area
H02.79 Other degenerative disorders of eyelid and periocular area
H02.8 Other specified disorders of eyelid
H02.81 Retained foreign body in eyelid
Use additional code to identify the type of retained foreign body (Z18.-)
EXCLUDES1 *laceration of eyelid with foreign body (S01.12-)*
retained intraocular foreign body (H44.6-, H44.7-)
superficial foreign body of eyelid and periocular area (S00.25-)
H02.811 Retained foreign body in right upper eyelid
H02.812 Retained foreign body in right lower eyelid
H02.813 Retained foreign body in right eye, unspecified eyelid
H02.814 Retained foreign body in left upper eyelid
H02.815 Retained foreign body in left lower eyelid
H02.816 Retained foreign body in left eye, unspecified eyelid
H02.819 Retained foreign body in unspecified eye, unspecified eyelid
H02.82 Cysts of eyelid
Sebaceous cyst of eyelid
H02.821 Cysts of right upper eyelid
H02.822 Cysts of right lower eyelid
H02.823 Cysts of right eye, unspecified eyelid
H02.824 Cysts of left upper eyelid
H02.825 Cysts of left lower eyelid
H02.826 Cysts of left eye, unspecified eyelid
H02.829 Cysts of unspecified eye, unspecified eyelid
H02.83 Dermatochalasis of eyelid
H02.831 Dermatochalasis of right upper eyelid
H02.832 Dermatochalasis of right lower eyelid
H02.833 Dermatochalasis of right eye, unspecified eyelid
H02.834 Dermatochalasis of left upper eyelid
H02.835 Dermatochalasis of left lower eyelid
H02.836 Dermatochalasis of left eye, unspecified eyelid
H02.839 Dermatochalasis of unspecified eye, unspecified eyelid
H02.84 Edema of eyelid
Hyperemia of eyelid
H02.841 Edema of right upper eyelid
H02.842 Edema of right lower eyelid
H02.843 Edema of right eye, unspecified eyelid
H02.844 Edema of left upper eyelid
H02.845 Edema of left lower eyelid
H02.846 Edema of left eye, unspecified eyelid
H02.849 Edema of unspecified eye, unspecified eyelid
H02.85 Elephantiasis of eyelid
H02.851 Elephantiasis of right upper eyelid
H02.852 Elephantiasis of right lower eyelid

Unspecified Code Other Specified Code Manifestation Code N Newborn P Pediatric M Maternity A Adult ♂ Male ♀ Female
● New Code ▲ Revised Code Title ►◄ Revised Text NOTES INCLUDES EXCLUDES1 Not coded here EXCLUDES2 Not included here
4th character required 5th character required 6th character required 7th character required
Extension 'X' Alert HAC Hospital-acquired condition (HAC) alert AHA AHA Coding Clinic©

H02.853 Elephantiasis of right eye, unspecified eyelid
H02.854 Elephantiasis of left upper eyelid
H02.855 Elephantiasis of left lower eyelid
H02.856 Elephantiasis of left eye, unspecified eyelid
H02.859 Elephantiasis of unspecified eye, unspecified eyelid

H02.86 Hypertrichosis of eyelid
H02.861 Hypertrichosis of right upper eyelid
H02.862 Hypertrichosis of right lower eyelid
H02.863 Hypertrichosis of right eye, unspecified eyelid
H02.864 Hypertrichosis of left upper eyelid
H02.865 Hypertrichosis of left lower eyelid
H02.866 Hypertrichosis of left eye, unspecified eyelid
H02.869 Hypertrichosis of unspecified eye, unspecified eyelid

H02.87 Vascular anomalies of eyelid
H02.871 Vascular anomalies of right upper eyelid
H02.872 Vascular anomalies of right lower eyelid
H02.873 Vascular anomalies of right eye, unspecified eyelid
H02.874 Vascular anomalies of left upper eyelid
H02.875 Vascular anomalies of left lower eyelid
H02.876 Vascular anomalies of left eye, unspecified eyelid
H02.879 Vascular anomalies of unspecified eye, unspecified eyelid

H02.89 Other specified disorders of eyelid
Hemorrhage of eyelid

H02.9 Unspecified disorder of eyelid
Disorder of eyelid NOS

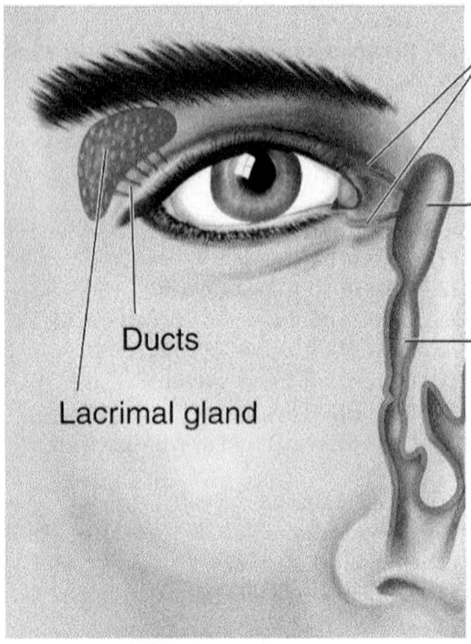

Figure 7.2 Lacrimal system

H04 Disorders of lacrimal system
EXCLUDES1 *congenital malformations of lacrimal system (Q10.4-Q10.6)*

H04.0 Dacryoadenitis

H04.00 Unspecified dacryoadenitis
H04.001 Unspecified dacryoadenitis, right lacrimal gland
H04.002 Unspecified dacryoadenitis, left lacrimal gland
H04.003 Unspecified dacryoadenitis, bilateral lacrimal glands
H04.009 Unspecified dacryoadenitis, unspecified lacrimal gland

H04.01 Acute dacryoadenitis
H04.011 Acute dacryoadenitis, right lacrimal gland
H04.012 Acute dacryoadenitis, left lacrimal gland
H04.013 Acute dacryoadenitis, bilateral lacrimal glands
H04.019 Acute dacryoadenitis, unspecified lacrimal gland

H04.02 Chronic dacryoadenitis
H04.021 Chronic dacryoadenitis, right lacrimal gland
H04.022 Chronic dacryoadenitis, left lacrimal gland
H04.023 Chronic dacryoadenitis, bilateral lacrimal gland
H04.029 Chronic dacryoadenitis, unspecified lacrimal gland

H04.03 Chronic enlargement of lacrimal gland
H04.031 Chronic enlargement of right lacrimal gland
H04.032 Chronic enlargement of left lacrimal gland
H04.033 Chronic enlargement of bilateral lacrimal glands
H04.039 Chronic enlargement of unspecified lacrimal gland

H04.1 Other disorders of lacrimal gland

H04.11 Dacryops
H04.111 Dacryops of right lacrimal gland
H04.112 Dacryops of left lacrimal gland
H04.113 Dacryops of bilateral lacrimal glands
H04.119 Dacryops of unspecified lacrimal gland

H04.12 Dry eye syndrome
Tear film insufficiency, NOS
H04.121 Dry eye syndrome of right lacrimal gland
H04.122 Dry eye syndrome of left lacrimal gland
H04.123 Dry eye syndrome of bilateral lacrimal glands
H04.129 Dry eye syndrome of unspecified lacrimal gland

H04.13 Lacrimal cyst
Lacrimal cystic degeneration
H04.131 Lacrimal cyst, right lacrimal gland
H04.132 Lacrimal cyst, left lacrimal gland
H04.133 Lacrimal cyst, bilateral lacrimal glands
H04.139 Lacrimal cyst, unspecified lacrimal gland

H04.14 Primary lacrimal gland atrophy
H04.141 Primary lacrimal gland atrophy, right lacrimal gland
H04.142 Primary lacrimal gland atrophy, left lacrimal gland
H04.143 Primary lacrimal gland atrophy, bilateral lacrimal glands
H04.149 Primary lacrimal gland atrophy, unspecified lacrimal gland

H04.15 Secondary lacrimal gland atrophy
H04.151 Secondary lacrimal gland atrophy, right lacrimal gland
H04.152 Secondary lacrimal gland atrophy, left lacrimal gland
H04.153 Secondary lacrimal gland atrophy, bilateral lacrimal glands
H04.159 Secondary lacrimal gland atrophy, unspecified lacrimal gland

H04.16 Lacrimal gland dislocation
H04.161 Lacrimal gland dislocation, right lacrimal gland
H04.162 Lacrimal gland dislocation, left lacrimal gland
H04.163 Lacrimal gland dislocation, bilateral lacrimal glands
H04.169 Lacrimal gland dislocation, unspecified lacrimal gland

H04.19 Other specified disorders of lacrimal gland

H04.2 Epiphora

H04.20 Unspecified epiphora
H04.201 Unspecified epiphora, right lacrimal gland
H04.202 Unspecified epiphora, left lacrimal gland
H04.203 Unspecified epiphora, bilateral lacrimal glands

Unacceptable principal diagnosis symbol per Medicare code edits — Code exempt from diagnosis present on admission requirement
Questionable admission — Complication or comorbidity — CC/MCC exclusion — Major complication or comorbidity
Principal diagnosis as its own CC — Principal diagnosis as its own MCC — Z code as first-listed diagnosis

H04.209 Unspecified epiphora, unspecified lacrimal gland

H04.21 Epiphora due to excess lacrimation
- H04.211 Epiphora due to excess lacrimation, right lacrimal gland
- H04.212 Epiphora due to excess lacrimation, left lacrimal gland
- H04.213 Epiphora due to excess lacrimation, bilateral lacrimal glands
- H04.219 Epiphora due to excess lacrimation, unspecified lacrimal gland

H04.22 Epiphora due to insufficient drainage
- H04.221 Epiphora due to insufficient drainage, right lacrimal gland
- H04.222 Epiphora due to insufficient drainage, left lacrimal gland
- H04.223 Epiphora due to insufficient drainage, bilateral lacrimal glands
- H04.229 Epiphora due to insufficient drainage, unspecified lacrimal gland

H04.3 Acute and unspecified inflammation of lacrimal passages

EXCLUDES1 *neonatal dacryocystitis (P39.1)*

H04.30 Unspecified dacryocystitis
- H04.301 Unspecified dacryocystitis of right lacrimal passage
- H04.302 Unspecified dacryocystitis of left lacrimal passage
- H04.303 Unspecified dacryocystitis of bilateral lacrimal passages
- H04.309 Unspecified dacryocystitis of unspecified lacrimal passage

H04.31 Phlegmonous dacryocystitis
- H04.311 Phlegmonous dacryocystitis of right lacrimal passage
- H04.312 Phlegmonous dacryocystitis of left lacrimal passage
- H04.313 Phlegmonous dacryocystitis of bilateral lacrimal passages
- H04.319 Phlegmonous dacryocystitis of unspecified lacrimal passage

H04.32 Acute dacryocystitis

Acute dacryopericystitis
- H04.321 Acute dacryocystitis of right lacrimal passage
- H04.322 Acute dacryocystitis of left lacrimal passage
- H04.323 Acute dacryocystitis of bilateral lacrimal passages
- H04.329 Acute dacryocystitis of unspecified lacrimal passage

H04.33 Acute lacrimal canaliculitis
- H04.331 Acute lacrimal canaliculitis of right lacrimal passage
- H04.332 Acute lacrimal canaliculitis of left lacrimal passage
- H04.333 Acute lacrimal canaliculitis of bilateral lacrimal passages
- H04.339 Acute lacrimal canaliculitis of unspecified lacrimal passage

H04.4 Chronic inflammation of lacrimal passages

H04.41 Chronic dacryocystitis
- H04.411 Chronic dacryocystitis of right lacrimal passage
- H04.412 Chronic dacryocystitis of left lacrimal passage
- H04.413 Chronic dacryocystitis of bilateral lacrimal passages
- H04.419 Chronic dacryocystitis of unspecified lacrimal passage

H04.42 Chronic lacrimal canaliculitis
- H04.421 Chronic lacrimal canaliculitis of right lacrimal passage
- H04.422 Chronic lacrimal canaliculitis of left lacrimal passage
- H04.423 Chronic lacrimal canaliculitis of bilateral lacrimal passages
- H04.429 Chronic lacrimal canaliculitis of unspecified lacrimal passage

H04.43 Chronic lacrimal mucocele
- H04.431 Chronic lacrimal mucocele of right lacrimal passage
- H04.432 Chronic lacrimal mucocele of left lacrimal passage
- H04.433 Chronic lacrimal mucocele of bilateral lacrimal passages
- H04.439 Chronic lacrimal mucocele of unspecified lacrimal passage

H04.5 Stenosis and insufficiency of lacrimal passages

H04.51 Dacryolith
- H04.511 Dacryolith of right lacrimal passage
- H04.512 Dacryolith of left lacrimal passage
- H04.513 Dacryolith of bilateral lacrimal passages
- H04.519 Dacryolith of unspecified lacrimal passage

H04.52 Eversion of lacrimal punctum
- H04.521 Eversion of right lacrimal punctum
- H04.522 Eversion of left lacrimal punctum
- H04.523 Eversion of bilateral lacrimal punctum
- H04.529 Eversion of unspecified lacrimal punctum

H04.53 Neonatal obstruction of nasolacrimal duct

EXCLUDES1 *congenital stenosis and stricture of lacrimal duct (Q10.5)*
- H04.531 Neonatal obstruction of right nasolacrimal duct N
- H04.532 Neonatal obstruction of left nasolacrimal duct N
- H04.533 Neonatal obstruction of bilateral nasolacrimal duct N
- H04.539 Neonatal obstruction of unspecified nasolacrimal duct N

H04.54 Stenosis of lacrimal canaliculi
- H04.541 Stenosis of right lacrimal canaliculi
- H04.542 Stenosis of left lacrimal canaliculi
- H04.543 Stenosis of bilateral lacrimal canaliculi
- H04.549 Stenosis of unspecified lacrimal canaliculi

H04.55 Acquired stenosis of nasolacrimal duct
- H04.551 Acquired stenosis of right nasolacrimal duct
- H04.552 Acquired stenosis of left nasolacrimal duct
- H04.553 Acquired stenosis of bilateral nasolacrimal duct
- H04.559 Acquired stenosis of unspecified nasolacrimal duct

H04.56 Stenosis of lacrimal punctum
- H04.561 Stenosis of right lacrimal punctum
- H04.562 Stenosis of left lacrimal punctum
- H04.563 Stenosis of bilateral lacrimal punctum
- H04.569 Stenosis of unspecified lacrimal punctum

H04.57 Stenosis of lacrimal sac
- H04.571 Stenosis of right lacrimal sac
- H04.572 Stenosis of left lacrimal sac
- H04.573 Stenosis of bilateral lacrimal sac
- H04.579 Stenosis of unspecified lacrimal sac

H04.6 Other changes of lacrimal passages

H04.61 Lacrimal fistula
- H04.611 Lacrimal fistula right lacrimal passage
- H04.612 Lacrimal fistula left lacrimal passage
- H04.613 Lacrimal fistula bilateral lacrimal passages
- H04.619 Lacrimal fistula unspecified lacrimal passage

H04.69 Other changes of lacrimal passages

H04.8 Other disorders of lacrimal system

H04.81 Granuloma of lacrimal passages
- H04.811 Granuloma of right lacrimal passage
- H04.812 Granuloma of left lacrimal passage
- H04.813 Granuloma of bilateral lacrimal passages
- H04.819 Granuloma of unspecified lacrimal passage

H04.89 Other disorders of lacrimal system

Unspecified Code Other Specified Code Manifestation Code N Newborn P Pediatric M Maternity A Adult ♂ Male ♀ Female
● New Code ▲ Revised Code Title ►◄ Revised Text NOTES INCLUDES EXCLUDES1 Not coded here EXCLUDES2 Not included here
4th character required 5th character required 6th character required 7th character required
Extension 'X' Alert HAC Hospital-acquired condition (HAC) alert AHA AHA Coding Clinic©

When symbols appear on a code that requires a 7th character extension, refer to Appendix D to identify applicable 7th character codes.

H04.9 Disorder of lacrimal system, unspecified

H05 Disorders of orbit

EXCLUDES1 *congenital malformation of orbit (Q10.7)*

H05.0 Acute inflammation of orbit

H05.00 Unspecified acute inflammation of orbit

H05.01 Cellulitis of orbit

Abscess of orbit

H05.011 Cellulitis of right orbit CC

H05.012 Cellulitis of left orbit CC

H05.013 Cellulitis of bilateral orbits CC

H05.019 Cellulitis of unspecified orbit CC

H05.02 Osteomyelitis of orbit

H05.021 Osteomyelitis of right orbit CC

H05.022 Osteomyelitis of left orbit CC

H05.023 Osteomyelitis of bilateral orbits CC

H05.029 Osteomyelitis of unspecified orbit CC

H05.03 Periostitis of orbit

H05.031 Periostitis of right orbit CC

H05.032 Periostitis of left orbit CC

H05.033 Periostitis of bilateral orbits CC

H05.039 Periostitis of unspecified orbit CC

H05.04 Tenonitis of orbit

H05.041 Tenonitis of right orbit

H05.042 Tenonitis of left orbit

H05.043 Tenonitis of bilateral orbits

H05.049 Tenonitis of unspecified orbit

H05.1 Chronic inflammatory disorders of orbit

H05.10 Unspecified chronic inflammatory disorders of orbit

H05.11 Granuloma of orbit

Pseudotumor (inflammatory) of orbit

H05.111 Granuloma of right orbit

H05.112 Granuloma of left orbit

H05.113 Granuloma of bilateral orbits

H05.119 Granuloma of unspecified orbit

H05.12 Orbital myositis

H05.121 Orbital myositis, right orbit

H05.122 Orbital myositis, left orbit

H05.123 Orbital myositis, bilateral

H05.129 Orbital myositis, unspecified orbit

H05.2 Exophthalmic conditions

H05.20 Unspecified exophthalmos

H05.21 Displacement (lateral) of globe

H05.211 Displacement (lateral) of globe, right eye

H05.212 Displacement (lateral) of globe, left eye

H05.213 Displacement (lateral) of globe, bilateral

H05.219 Displacement (lateral) of globe, unspecified eye

H05.22 Edema of orbit

Orbital congestion

H05.221 Edema of right orbit

H05.222 Edema of left orbit

H05.223 Edema of bilateral orbit

H05.229 Edema of unspecified orbit

H05.23 Hemorrhage of orbit

H05.231 Hemorrhage of right orbit

H05.232 Hemorrhage of left orbit

H05.233 Hemorrhage of bilateral orbit

H05.239 Hemorrhage of unspecified orbit

H05.24 Constant exophthalmos

H05.241 Constant exophthalmos, right eye

H05.242 Constant exophthalmos, left eye

H05.243 Constant exophthalmos, bilateral

H05.249 Constant exophthalmos, unspecified eye

H05.25 Intermittent exophthalmos

H05.251 Intermittent exophthalmos, right eye

H05.252 Intermittent exophthalmos, left eye

H05.253 Intermittent exophthalmos, bilateral

H05.259 Intermittent exophthalmos, unspecified eye

H05.26 Pulsating exophthalmos

H05.261 Pulsating exophthalmos, right eye

H05.262 Pulsating exophthalmos, left eye

H05.263 Pulsating exophthalmos, bilateral

H05.269 Pulsating exophthalmos, unspecified eye

H05.3 Deformity of orbit

EXCLUDES1 *congenital deformity of orbit (Q10.7)*
hypertelorism (Q75.2)

H05.30 Unspecified deformity of orbit

H05.31 Atrophy of orbit

H05.311 Atrophy of right orbit

H05.312 Atrophy of left orbit

H05.313 Atrophy of bilateral orbit

H05.319 Atrophy of unspecified orbit

H05.32 Deformity of orbit due to bone disease

Code also associated bone disease

H05.321 Deformity of right orbit due to bone disease

H05.322 Deformity of left orbit due to bone disease

H05.323 Deformity of bilateral orbits due to bone disease

H05.329 Deformity of unspecified orbit due to bone disease

H05.33 Deformity of orbit due to trauma or surgery

H05.331 Deformity of right orbit due to trauma or surgery

H05.332 Deformity of left orbit due to trauma or surgery

H05.333 Deformity of bilateral orbits due to trauma or surgery

H05.339 Deformity of unspecified orbit due to trauma or surgery

H05.34 Enlargement of orbit

H05.341 Enlargement of right orbit

H05.342 Enlargement of left orbit

H05.343 Enlargement of bilateral orbits

H05.349 Enlargement of unspecified orbit

H05.35 Exostosis of orbit

H05.351 Exostosis of right orbit

H05.352 Exostosis of left orbit

H05.353 Exostosis of bilateral orbits

H05.359 Exostosis of unspecified orbit

H05.4 Enophthalmos

H05.40 Unspecified enophthalmos

H05.401 Unspecified enophthalmos, right eye

H05.402 Unspecified enophthalmos, left eye

H05.403 Unspecified enophthalmos, bilateral

H05.409 Unspecified enophthalmos, unspecified eye

H05.41 Enophthalmos due to atrophy of orbital tissue

H05.411 Enophthalmos due to atrophy of orbital tissue, right eye

H05.412 Enophthalmos due to atrophy of orbital tissue, left eye

H05.413 Enophthalmos due to atrophy of orbital tissue, bilateral

H05.419 Enophthalmos due to atrophy of orbital tissue, unspecified eye

H05.42 Enophthalmos due to trauma or surgery

H05.421 Enophthalmos due to trauma or surgery, right eye

H05.422 Enophthalmos due to trauma or surgery, left eye

H05.423 Enophthalmos due to trauma or surgery, bilateral

H05.429 Enophthalmos due to trauma or surgery, unspecified eye

H05.5 Retained (old) foreign body following penetrating wound of orbit

Retrobulbar foreign body

Use additional code to identify the type of retained foreign body (Z18.-)

EXCLUDES1 *current penetrating wound of orbit (S05.4-)*

EXCLUDES2 *retained foreign body of eyelid (H02.81-)*
retained intraocular foreign body (H44.6-, H44.7-)

Unacceptable principal diagnosis symbol per Medicare code edits · Code exempt from diagnosis present on admission requirement · Questionable admission · CC Complication or comorbidity · CC/MCC exclusion · Major complication or comorbidity · Principal diagnosis as its own CC · Principal diagnosis as its own MCC · Z code as first-listed diagnosis

When symbols appear on a code that requires a 7th character extension, refer to Appendix D to identify applicable 7th character codes.

H05.50 Retained (old) foreign body following penetrating wound of unspecified orbit
H05.51 Retained (old) foreign body following penetrating wound of right orbit
H05.52 Retained (old) foreign body following penetrating wound of left orbit
H05.53 Retained (old) foreign body following penetrating wound of bilateral orbits
H05.8 Other disorders of orbit
H05.81 Cyst of orbit
Encephalocele of orbit
H05.811 Cyst of right orbit
H05.812 Cyst of left orbit
H05.813 Cyst of bilateral orbits
H05.819 Cyst of unspecified orbit
H05.82 Myopathy of extraocular muscles
H05.821 Myopathy of extraocular muscles, right orbit
H05.822 Myopathy of extraocular muscles, left orbit
H05.823 Myopathy of extraocular muscles, bilateral
H05.829 Myopathy of extraocular muscles, unspecified orbit
H05.89 Other disorders of orbit
H05.9 Unspecified disorder of orbit

Disorders of conjunctiva (H10-H11)

H10 Conjunctivitis
EXCLUDES1 *keratoconjunctivitis (H16.2-)*
H10.0 Mucopurulent conjunctivitis
H10.01 Acute follicular conjunctivitis
H10.011 Acute follicular conjunctivitis, right eye
H10.012 Acute follicular conjunctivitis, left eye
H10.013 Acute follicular conjunctivitis, bilateral
H10.019 Acute follicular conjunctivitis, unspecified eye
H10.02 Other mucopurulent conjunctivitis
H10.021 Other mucopurulent conjunctivitis, right eye
H10.022 Other mucopurulent conjunctivitis, left eye
H10.023 Other mucopurulent conjunctivitis, bilateral
H10.029 Other mucopurulent conjunctivitis, unspecified eye
H10.1 Acute atopic conjunctivitis
Acute papillary conjunctivitis
H10.10 Acute atopic conjunctivitis, unspecified eye
H10.11 Acute atopic conjunctivitis, right eye
H10.12 Acute atopic conjunctivitis, left eye
H10.13 Acute atopic conjunctivitis, bilateral
H10.2 Other acute conjunctivitis
H10.21 Acute toxic conjunctivitis
Acute chemical conjunctivitis
Code first (T51-T65) to identify chemical and intent
EXCLUDES1 *burn and corrosion of eye and adnexa (T26.-)*
H10.211 Acute toxic conjunctivitis, right eye
H10.212 Acute toxic conjunctivitis, left eye
H10.213 Acute toxic conjunctivitis, bilateral
H10.219 Acute toxic conjunctivitis, unspecified eye
H10.22 Pseudomembranous conjunctivitis
H10.221 Pseudomembranous conjunctivitis, right eye
H10.222 Pseudomembranous conjunctivitis, left eye
H10.223 Pseudomembranous conjunctivitis, bilateral
H10.229 Pseudomembranous conjunctivitis, unspecified eye
H10.23 Serous conjunctivitis, except viral
EXCLUDES1 *viral conjunctivitis (B30.-)*
H10.231 Serous conjunctivitis, except viral, right eye
H10.232 Serous conjunctivitis, except viral, left eye
H10.233 Serous conjunctivitis, except viral, bilateral
H10.239 Serous conjunctivitis, except viral, unspecified eye
H10.3 Unspecified acute conjunctivitis
EXCLUDES1 *ophthalmia neonatorum NOS (P39.1)*
H10.30 Unspecified acute conjunctivitis, unspecified eye
H10.31 Unspecified acute conjunctivitis, right eye
H10.32 Unspecified acute conjunctivitis, left eye
H10.33 Unspecified acute conjunctivitis, bilateral
H10.4 Chronic conjunctivitis
H10.40 Unspecified chronic conjunctivitis
H10.401 Unspecified chronic conjunctivitis, right eye
H10.402 Unspecified chronic conjunctivitis, left eye
H10.403 Unspecified chronic conjunctivitis, bilateral
H10.409 Unspecified chronic conjunctivitis, unspecified eye
H10.41 Chronic giant papillary conjunctivitis
H10.411 Chronic giant papillary conjunctivitis, right eye
H10.412 Chronic giant papillary conjunctivitis, left eye
H10.413 Chronic giant papillary conjunctivitis, bilateral
H10.419 Chronic giant papillary conjunctivitis, unspecified eye
H10.42 Simple chronic conjunctivitis
H10.421 Simple chronic conjunctivitis, right eye
H10.422 Simple chronic conjunctivitis, left eye
H10.423 Simple chronic conjunctivitis, bilateral
H10.429 Simple chronic conjunctivitis, unspecified eye
H10.43 Chronic follicular conjunctivitis
H10.431 Chronic follicular conjunctivitis, right eye
H10.432 Chronic follicular conjunctivitis, left eye
H10.433 Chronic follicular conjunctivitis, bilateral
H10.439 Chronic follicular conjunctivitis, unspecified eye
H10.44 Vernal conjunctivitis
EXCLUDES1 *vernal keratoconjunctivitis with limbal and corneal involvement (H16.26-)*
H10.45 Other chronic allergic conjunctivitis
H10.5 Blepharoconjunctivitis
H10.50 Unspecified blepharoconjunctivitis
H10.501 Unspecified blepharoconjunctivitis, right eye
H10.502 Unspecified blepharoconjunctivitis, left eye
H10.503 Unspecified blepharoconjunctivitis, bilateral
H10.509 Unspecified blepharoconjunctivitis, unspecified eye
H10.51 Ligneous conjunctivitis
H10.511 Ligneous conjunctivitis, right eye
H10.512 Ligneous conjunctivitis, left eye
H10.513 Ligneous conjunctivitis, bilateral
H10.519 Ligneous conjunctivitis, unspecified eye
H10.52 Angular blepharoconjunctivitis
H10.521 Angular blepharoconjunctivitis, right eye
H10.522 Angular blepharoconjunctivitis, left eye
H10.523 Angular blepharoconjunctivitis, bilateral
H10.529 Angular blepharoconjunctivitis, unspecified eye
H10.53 Contact blepharoconjunctivitis
H10.531 Contact blepharoconjunctivitis, right eye
H10.532 Contact blepharoconjunctivitis, left eye
H10.533 Contact blepharoconjunctivitis, bilateral
H10.539 Contact blepharoconjunctivitis, unspecified eye

Unspecified Code Other Specified Code Manifestation Code N Newborn P Pediatric M Maternity A Adult ♂ Male ♀ Female
● New Code ▲ Revised Code Title ►◄ Revised Text NOTES INCLUDES EXCLUDES1 Not coded here EXCLUDES2 Not included here
4th character required 5th character required 6th character required 7th character required
Extension 'X' Alert HAC Hospital-acquired condition (HAC) alert AHA AHA Coding Clinic©

H10.8 Other conjunctivitis
H10.81 Pingueculitis
EXCLUDES1 *pinguecula (H11.15-)*
H10.811 Pingueculitis, right eye
H10.812 Pingueculitis, left eye
H10.813 Pingueculitis, bilateral
H10.819 **Pingueculitis, unspecified eye**
H10.89 Other conjunctivitis
H10.9 Unspecified conjunctivitis
H11 Other disorders of conjunctiva
EXCLUDES1 *keratoconjunctivitis (H16.2-)*

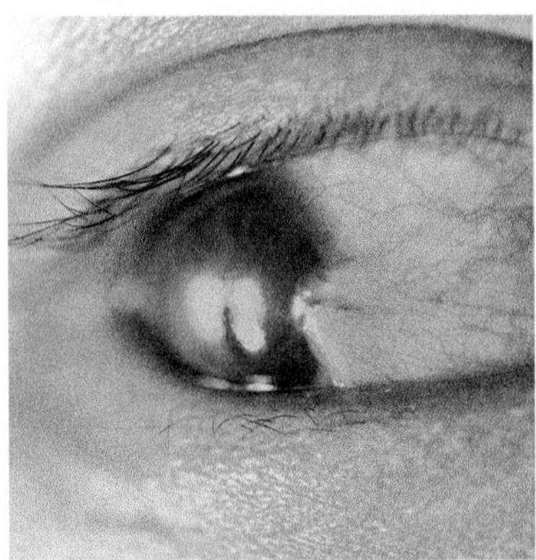

Figure 7.3 Pterygium

H11.0 Pterygium of eye
EXCLUDES1 *pseudopterygium (H11.81-)*
H11.00 Unspecified pterygium of eye
H11.001 Unspecified pterygium of right eye
H11.002 Unspecified pterygium of left eye
H11.003 Unspecified pterygium of eye, bilateral
H11.009 **Unspecified pterygium of unspecified eye**
H11.01 Amyloid pterygium
H11.011 Amyloid pterygium of right eye
H11.012 Amyloid pterygium of left eye
H11.013 Amyloid pterygium of eye, bilateral
H11.019 **Amyloid pterygium of unspecified eye**
H11.02 Central pterygium of eye
H11.021 Central pterygium of right eye
H11.022 Central pterygium of left eye
H11.023 Central pterygium of eye, bilateral
H11.029 **Central pterygium of unspecified eye**
H11.03 Double pterygium of eye
H11.031 Double pterygium of right eye
H11.032 Double pterygium of left eye
H11.033 Double pterygium of eye, bilateral
H11.039 **Double pterygium of unspecified eye**
H11.04 Peripheral pterygium of eye, stationary
H11.041 Peripheral pterygium, stationary, right eye
H11.042 Peripheral pterygium, stationary, left eye
H11.043 Peripheral pterygium, stationary, bilateral
H11.049 **Peripheral pterygium, stationary, unspecified eye**
H11.05 Peripheral pterygium of eye, progressive
H11.051 Peripheral pterygium, progressive, right eye
H11.052 Peripheral pterygium, progressive, left eye
H11.053 Peripheral pterygium, progressive, bilateral
H11.059 **Peripheral pterygium, progressive, unspecified eye**
H11.06 Recurrent pterygium of eye
H11.061 Recurrent pterygium of right eye
H11.062 Recurrent pterygium of left eye
H11.063 Recurrent pterygium of eye, bilateral
H11.069 **Recurrent pterygium of unspecified eye**

H11.1 Conjunctival degenerations and deposits
EXCLUDES2 *pseudopterygium (H11.81)*
H11.10 **Unspecified conjunctival degenerations**
H11.11 Conjunctival deposits
H11.111 Conjunctival deposits, right eye
H11.112 Conjunctival deposits, left eye
H11.113 Conjunctival deposits, bilateral
H11.119 **Conjunctival deposits, unspecified eye**
H11.12 Conjunctival concretions
H11.121 Conjunctival concretions, right eye
H11.122 Conjunctival concretions, left eye
H11.123 Conjunctival concretions, bilateral
H11.129 **Conjunctival concretions, unspecified eye**
H11.13 Conjunctival pigmentations
Conjunctival argyrosis [argyria]
H11.131 Conjunctival pigmentations, right eye
H11.132 Conjunctival pigmentations, left eye
H11.133 Conjunctival pigmentations, bilateral
H11.139 **Conjunctival pigmentations, unspecified eye**
H11.14 Conjunctival xerosis, unspecified
EXCLUDES1 *xerosis of conjunctiva due to vitamin A deficiency (E50.0, E50.1)*
H11.141 Conjunctival xerosis, unspecified, right eye
H11.142 Conjunctival xerosis, unspecified, left eye
H11.143 Conjunctival xerosis, unspecified, bilateral
H11.149 **Conjunctival xerosis, unspecified, unspecified eye**
H11.15 Pinguecula
EXCLUDES1 *pingueculitis (H10.81-)*
H11.151 Pinguecula, right eye
H11.152 Pinguecula, left eye
H11.153 Pinguecula, bilateral
H11.159 **Pinguecula, unspecified eye**
H11.2 Conjunctival scars
H11.21 Conjunctival adhesions and strands (localized)
H11.211 Conjunctival adhesions and strands (localized), right eye
H11.212 Conjunctival adhesions and strands (localized), left eye
H11.213 Conjunctival adhesions and strands (localized), bilateral
H11.219 **Conjunctival adhesions and strands (localized), unspecified eye**
H11.22 Conjunctival granuloma
H11.221 Conjunctival granuloma, right eye
H11.222 Conjunctival granuloma, left eye
H11.223 Conjunctival granuloma, bilateral
H11.229 **Conjunctival granuloma, unspecified**
H11.23 Symblepharon
H11.231 Symblepharon, right eye
H11.232 Symblepharon, left eye
H11.233 Symblepharon, bilateral
H11.239 **Symblepharon, unspecified eye**
H11.24 Scarring of conjunctiva
H11.241 Scarring of conjunctiva, right eye
H11.242 Scarring of conjunctiva, left eye
H11.243 Scarring of conjunctiva, bilateral
H11.249 **Scarring of conjunctiva, unspecified eye**
H11.3 Conjunctival hemorrhage
Subconjunctival hemorrhage
H11.30 **Conjunctival hemorrhage, unspecified eye**
H11.31 Conjunctival hemorrhage, right eye
H11.32 Conjunctival hemorrhage, left eye
H11.33 Conjunctival hemorrhage, bilateral
H11.4 Other conjunctival vascular disorders and cysts
H11.41 Vascular abnormalities of conjunctiva
Conjunctival aneurysm
H11.411 Vascular abnormalities of conjunctiva, right eye
H11.412 Vascular abnormalities of conjunctiva, left eye

Unacceptable principal diagnosis symbol per Medicare code edits — Code exempt from diagnosis present on admission requirement
Questionable admission — Complication or comorbidity — CC/MCC exclusion — Major complication or comorbidity
Principal diagnosis as its own CC — Principal diagnosis as its own MCC — Z code as first-listed diagnosis

When symbols appear on a code that requires a 7th character extension, refer to Appendix D to identify applicable 7th character codes.

H11.413 Vascular abnormalities of conjunctiva, bilateral
H11.419 Vascular abnormalities of conjunctiva, unspecified eye
H11.42 Conjunctival edema
H11.421 Conjunctival edema, right eye
H11.422 Conjunctival edema, left eye
H11.423 Conjunctival edema, bilateral
H11.429 Conjunctival edema, unspecified eye
H11.43 Conjunctival hyperemia
H11.431 Conjunctival hyperemia, right eye
H11.432 Conjunctival hyperemia, left eye
H11.433 Conjunctival hyperemia, bilateral
H11.439 Conjunctival hyperemia, unspecified eye
H11.44 Conjunctival cysts
H11.441 Conjunctival cysts, right eye
H11.442 Conjunctival cysts, left eye
H11.443 Conjunctival cysts, bilateral
H11.449 Conjunctival cysts, unspecified eye
H11.8 Other specified disorders of conjunctiva
H11.81 Pseudopterygium of conjunctiva
H11.811 Pseudopterygium of conjunctiva, right eye
H11.812 Pseudopterygium of conjunctiva, left eye
H11.813 Pseudopterygium of conjunctiva, bilateral
H11.819 Pseudopterygium of conjunctiva, unspecified eye
H11.82 Conjunctivochalasis
H11.821 Conjunctivochalasis, right eye
H11.822 Conjunctivochalasis, left eye
H11.823 Conjunctivochalasis, bilateral
H11.829 Conjunctivochalasis, unspecified eye
H11.89 Other specified disorders of conjunctiva
H11.9 Unspecified disorder of conjunctiva

Disorders of sclera, cornea, iris and ciliary body (H15-H22)

H15 Disorders of sclera
H15.0 Scleritis
H15.00 Unspecified scleritis
H15.001 Unspecified scleritis, right eye
H15.002 Unspecified scleritis, left eye
H15.003 Unspecified scleritis, bilateral
H15.009 Unspecified scleritis, unspecified eye
H15.01 Anterior scleritis
H15.011 Anterior scleritis, right eye
H15.012 Anterior scleritis, left eye
H15.013 Anterior scleritis, bilateral
H15.019 Anterior scleritis, unspecified eye
H15.02 Brawny scleritis
H15.021 Brawny scleritis, right eye
H15.022 Brawny scleritis, left eye
H15.023 Brawny scleritis, bilateral
H15.029 Brawny scleritis, unspecified eye
H15.03 Posterior scleritis
Sclerotenonitis
H15.031 Posterior scleritis, right eye
H15.032 Posterior scleritis, left eye
H15.033 Posterior scleritis, bilateral
H15.039 Posterior scleritis, unspecified eye
H15.04 Scleritis with corneal involvement
H15.041 Scleritis with corneal involvement, right eye
H15.042 Scleritis with corneal involvement, left eye
H15.043 Scleritis with corneal involvement, bilateral
H15.049 Scleritis with corneal involvement, unspecified eye
H15.05 Scleromalacia perforans
H15.051 Scleromalacia perforans, right eye
H15.052 Scleromalacia perforans, left eye
H15.053 Scleromalacia perforans, bilateral
H15.059 Scleromalacia perforans, unspecified eye
H15.09 Other scleritis
Scleral abscess
H15.091 Other scleritis, right eye
H15.092 Other scleritis, left eye
H15.093 Other scleritis, bilateral
H15.099 Other scleritis, unspecified eye
H15.1 Episcleritis
H15.10 Unspecified episcleritis
H15.101 Unspecified episcleritis, right eye
H15.102 Unspecified episcleritis, left eye
H15.103 Unspecified episcleritis, bilateral
H15.109 Unspecified episcleritis, unspecified eye
H15.11 Episcleritis periodica fugax
H15.111 Episcleritis periodica fugax, right eye
H15.112 Episcleritis periodica fugax, left eye
H15.113 Episcleritis periodica fugax, bilateral
H15.119 Episcleritis periodica fugax, unspecified eye
H15.12 Nodular episcleritis
H15.121 Nodular episcleritis, right eye
H15.122 Nodular episcleritis, left eye
H15.123 Nodular episcleritis, bilateral
H15.129 Nodular episcleritis, unspecified eye
H15.8 Other disorders of sclera
EXCLUDES2 *blue sclera (Q13.5)*
degenerative myopia (H44.2-)
H15.81 Equatorial staphyloma
H15.811 Equatorial staphyloma, right eye
H15.812 Equatorial staphyloma, left eye
H15.813 Equatorial staphyloma, bilateral
H15.819 Equatorial staphyloma, unspecified eye
H15.82 Localized anterior staphyloma
H15.821 Localized anterior staphyloma, right eye
H15.822 Localized anterior staphyloma, left eye
H15.823 Localized anterior staphyloma, bilateral
H15.829 Localized anterior staphyloma, unspecified eye
H15.83 Staphyloma posticum
H15.831 Staphyloma posticum, right eye
H15.832 Staphyloma posticum, left eye
H15.833 Staphyloma posticum, bilateral
H15.839 Staphyloma posticum, unspecified eye
H15.84 Scleral ectasia
H15.841 Scleral ectasia, right eye
H15.842 Scleral ectasia, left eye
H15.843 Scleral ectasia, bilateral
H15.849 Scleral ectasia, unspecified eye
H15.85 Ring staphyloma
H15.851 Ring staphyloma, right eye
H15.852 Ring staphyloma, left eye
H15.853 Ring staphyloma, bilateral
H15.859 Ring staphyloma, unspecified eye
H15.89 Other disorders of sclera
H15.9 Unspecified disorder of sclera
H16 Keratitis
H16.0 Corneal ulcer
H16.00 Unspecified corneal ulcer
H16.001 Unspecified corneal ulcer, right eye
H16.002 Unspecified corneal ulcer, left eye
H16.003 Unspecified corneal ulcer, bilateral
H16.009 Unspecified corneal ulcer, unspecified eye
H16.01 Central corneal ulcer
H16.011 Central corneal ulcer, right eye
H16.012 Central corneal ulcer, left eye
H16.013 Central corneal ulcer, bilateral
H16.019 Central corneal ulcer, unspecified eye
H16.02 Ring corneal ulcer
H16.021 Ring corneal ulcer, right eye
H16.022 Ring corneal ulcer, left eye
H16.023 Ring corneal ulcer, bilateral
H16.029 Ring corneal ulcer, unspecified eye
H16.03 Corneal ulcer with hypopyon

Unspecified Code · Other Specified Code · Manifestation Code · N Newborn · P Pediatric · M Maternity · A Adult · ♂ Male · ♀ Female
● New Code · ▲ Revised Code Title · ►◄ Revised Text · NOTES · INCLUDES · EXCLUDES1 Not coded here · EXCLUDES2 Not included here
4th character required · 5th character required · 6th character required · 7th character required
Extension 'X' Alert · HAC Hospital-acquired condition (HAC) alert · AHA AHA Coding Clinic©

H16.031 Corneal ulcer with hypopyon, right eye
H16.032 Corneal ulcer with hypopyon, left eye
H16.033 Corneal ulcer with hypopyon, bilateral
H16.039 Corneal ulcer with hypopyon, unspecified eye

H16.04 Marginal corneal ulcer
H16.041 Marginal corneal ulcer, right eye
H16.042 Marginal corneal ulcer, left eye
H16.043 Marginal corneal ulcer, bilateral
H16.049 Marginal corneal ulcer, unspecified eye

H16.05 Mooren's corneal ulcer
H16.051 Mooren's corneal ulcer, right eye
H16.052 Mooren's corneal ulcer, left eye
H16.053 Mooren's corneal ulcer, bilateral
H16.059 Mooren's corneal ulcer, unspecified eye

H16.06 Mycotic corneal ulcer
H16.061 Mycotic corneal ulcer, right eye
H16.062 Mycotic corneal ulcer, left eye
H16.063 Mycotic corneal ulcer, bilateral
H16.069 Mycotic corneal ulcer, unspecified eye

H16.07 Perforated corneal ulcer
H16.071 Perforated corneal ulcer, right eye
H16.072 Perforated corneal ulcer, left eye
H16.073 Perforated corneal ulcer, bilateral
H16.079 Perforated corneal ulcer, unspecified eye

H16.1 Other and unspecified superficial keratitis without conjunctivitis

H16.10 Unspecified superficial keratitis
H16.101 Unspecified superficial keratitis, right eye
H16.102 Unspecified superficial keratitis, left eye
H16.103 Unspecified superficial keratitis, bilateral
H16.109 Unspecified superficial keratitis, unspecified eye

H16.11 Macular keratitis
Areolar keratitis
Nummular keratitis
Stellate keratitis
Striate keratitis
H16.111 Macular keratitis, right eye
H16.112 Macular keratitis, left eye
H16.113 Macular keratitis, bilateral
H16.119 Macular keratitis, unspecified eye

H16.12 Filamentary keratitis
H16.121 Filamentary keratitis, right eye
H16.122 Filamentary keratitis, left eye
H16.123 Filamentary keratitis, bilateral
H16.129 Filamentary keratitis, unspecified eye

H16.13 Photokeratitis
Snow blindness
Welders keratitis
H16.131 Photokeratitis, right eye
H16.132 Photokeratitis, left eye
H16.133 Photokeratitis, bilateral
H16.139 Photokeratitis, unspecified eye

H16.14 Punctate keratitis
H16.141 Punctate keratitis, right eye
H16.142 Punctate keratitis, left eye
H16.143 Punctate keratitis, bilateral
H16.149 Punctate keratitis, unspecified eye

H16.2 Keratoconjunctivitis

H16.20 Unspecified keratoconjunctivitis
Superficial keratitis with conjunctivitis NOS
H16.201 Unspecified keratoconjunctivitis, right eye
H16.202 Unspecified keratoconjunctivitis, left eye
H16.203 Unspecified keratoconjunctivitis, bilateral
H16.209 Unspecified keratoconjunctivitis, unspecified eye

H16.21 Exposure keratoconjunctivitis
H16.211 Exposure keratoconjunctivitis, right eye
H16.212 Exposure keratoconjunctivitis, left eye
H16.213 Exposure keratoconjunctivitis, bilateral
H16.219 Exposure keratoconjunctivitis, unspecified eye

H16.22 Keratoconjunctivitis sicca, not specified as Sjögren's
EXCLUDES1 *Sjögren's syndrome (M35.01)*
H16.221 Keratoconjunctivitis sicca, not specified as Sjögren's, right eye
H16.222 Keratoconjunctivitis sicca, not specified as Sjögren's, left eye
H16.223 Keratoconjunctivitis sicca, not specified as Sjögren's, bilateral
H16.229 Keratoconjunctivitis sicca, not specified as Sjögren's, unspecified eye

H16.23 Neurotrophic keratoconjunctivitis
H16.231 Neurotrophic keratoconjunctivitis, right eye
H16.232 Neurotrophic keratoconjunctivitis, left eye
H16.233 Neurotrophic keratoconjunctivitis, bilateral
H16.239 Neurotrophic keratoconjunctivitis, unspecified eye

H16.24 Ophthalmia nodosa
H16.241 Ophthalmia nodosa, right eye
H16.242 Ophthalmia nodosa, left eye
H16.243 Ophthalmia nodosa, bilateral
H16.249 Ophthalmia nodosa, unspecified eye

H16.25 Phlyctenular keratoconjunctivitis
H16.251 Phlyctenular keratoconjunctivitis, right eye
H16.252 Phlyctenular keratoconjunctivitis, left eye
H16.253 Phlyctenular keratoconjunctivitis, bilateral
H16.259 Phlyctenular keratoconjunctivitis, unspecified eye

H16.26 Vernal keratoconjunctivitis, with limbal and corneal involvement
EXCLUDES1 *vernal conjunctivitis without limbal and corneal involvement (H10.44)*
H16.261 Vernal keratoconjunctivitis, with limbal and corneal involvement, right eye
H16.262 Vernal keratoconjunctivitis, with limbal and corneal involvement, left eye
H16.263 Vernal keratoconjunctivitis, with limbal and corneal involvement, bilateral
H16.269 Vernal keratoconjunctivitis, with limbal and corneal involvement, unspecified eye

H16.29 Other keratoconjunctivitis
H16.291 Other keratoconjunctivitis, right eye
H16.292 Other keratoconjunctivitis, left eye
H16.293 Other keratoconjunctivitis, bilateral
H16.299 Other keratoconjunctivitis, unspecified eye

H16.3 Interstitial and deep keratitis

H16.30 Unspecified interstitial keratitis
H16.301 Unspecified interstitial keratitis, right eye
H16.302 Unspecified interstitial keratitis, left eye
H16.303 Unspecified interstitial keratitis, bilateral
H16.309 Unspecified interstitial keratitis, unspecified eye

H16.31 Corneal abscess
H16.311 Corneal abscess, right eye
H16.312 Corneal abscess, left eye
H16.313 Corneal abscess, bilateral
H16.319 Corneal abscess, unspecified eye

H16.32 Diffuse interstitial keratitis
Cogan's syndrome
H16.321 Diffuse interstitial keratitis, right eye
H16.322 Diffuse interstitial keratitis, left eye
H16.323 Diffuse interstitial keratitis, bilateral
H16.329 Diffuse interstitial keratitis, unspecified eye

H16.33 Sclerosing keratitis
H16.331 Sclerosing keratitis, right eye
H16.332 Sclerosing keratitis, left eye
H16.333 Sclerosing keratitis, bilateral
H16.339 Sclerosing keratitis, unspecified eye

Unacceptable principal diagnosis symbol per Medicare code edits; Code exempt from diagnosis present on admission requirement
Questionable admission; Complication or comorbidity; CC/MCC exclusion; Major complication or comorbidity
Principal diagnosis as its own CC; Principal diagnosis as its own MCC; Z code as first-listed diagnosis

H16.39 Other interstitial and deep keratitis
H16.391 Other interstitial and deep keratitis, right eye
H16.392 Other interstitial and deep keratitis, left eye
H16.393 Other interstitial and deep keratitis, bilateral
H16.399 Other interstitial and deep keratitis, unspecified eye
H16.4 Corneal neovascularization
H16.40 Unspecified corneal neovascularization
H16.401 Unspecified corneal neovascularization, right eye
H16.402 Unspecified corneal neovascularization, left eye
H16.403 Unspecified corneal neovascularization, bilateral
H16.409 Unspecified corneal neovascularization, unspecified eye
H16.41 Ghost vessels (corneal)
H16.411 Ghost vessels (corneal), right eye
H16.412 Ghost vessels (corneal), left eye
H16.413 Ghost vessels (corneal), bilateral
H16.419 Ghost vessels (corneal), unspecified eye
H16.42 Pannus (corneal)
H16.421 Pannus (corneal), right eye
H16.422 Pannus (corneal), left eye
H16.423 Pannus (corneal), bilateral
H16.429 Pannus (corneal), unspecified eye
H16.43 Localized vascularization of cornea
H16.431 Localized vascularization of cornea, right eye
H16.432 Localized vascularization of cornea, left eye
H16.433 Localized vascularization of cornea, bilateral
H16.439 Localized vascularization of cornea, unspecified eye
H16.44 Deep vascularization of cornea
H16.441 Deep vascularization of cornea, right eye
H16.442 Deep vascularization of cornea, left eye
H16.443 Deep vascularization of cornea, bilateral
H16.449 Deep vascularization of cornea, unspecified eye
H16.8 Other keratitis PDx
H16.9 Unspecified keratitis
H17 Corneal scars and opacities
H17.0 Adherent leukoma
H17.00 Adherent leukoma, unspecified eye
H17.01 Adherent leukoma, right eye
H17.02 Adherent leukoma, left eye
H17.03 Adherent leukoma, bilateral
H17.1 Central corneal opacity
H17.10 Central corneal opacity, unspecified eye
H17.11 Central corneal opacity, right eye
H17.12 Central corneal opacity, left eye
H17.13 Central corneal opacity, bilateral
H17.8 Other corneal scars and opacities
H17.81 Minor opacity of cornea
Corneal nebula
H17.811 Minor opacity of cornea, right eye
H17.812 Minor opacity of cornea, left eye
H17.813 Minor opacity of cornea, bilateral
H17.819 Minor opacity of cornea, unspecified eye
H17.82 Peripheral opacity of cornea
H17.821 Peripheral opacity of cornea, right eye
H17.822 Peripheral opacity of cornea, left eye
H17.823 Peripheral opacity of cornea, bilateral
H17.829 Peripheral opacity of cornea, unspecified eye
H17.89 Other corneal scars and opacities
H17.9 Unspecified corneal scar and opacity
H18 Other disorders of cornea
H18.0 Corneal pigmentations and deposits
H18.00 Unspecified corneal deposit
H18.001 Unspecified corneal deposit, right eye
H18.002 Unspecified corneal deposit, left eye
H18.003 Unspecified corneal deposit, bilateral
H18.009 Unspecified corneal deposit, unspecified eye
H18.01 Anterior corneal pigmentations
Staehli's line
H18.011 Anterior corneal pigmentations, right eye
H18.012 Anterior corneal pigmentations, left eye
H18.013 Anterior corneal pigmentations, bilateral
H18.019 Anterior corneal pigmentations, unspecified eye
H18.02 Argentous corneal deposits
H18.021 Argentous corneal deposits, right eye
H18.022 Argentous corneal deposits, left eye
H18.023 Argentous corneal deposits, bilateral
H18.029 Argentous corneal deposits, unspecified eye
H18.03 Corneal deposits in metabolic disorders
Code also associated metabolic disorder
H18.031 Corneal deposits in metabolic disorders, right eye
H18.032 Corneal deposits in metabolic disorders, left eye
H18.033 Corneal deposits in metabolic disorders, bilateral
H18.039 Corneal deposits in metabolic disorders, unspecified eye
H18.04 Kayser-Fleischer ring
Code also associated Wilson's disease (E83.01)
H18.041 Kayser-Fleischer ring, right eye
H18.042 Kayser-Fleischer ring, left eye
H18.043 Kayser-Fleischer ring, bilateral
H18.049 Kayser-Fleischer ring, unspecified eye
H18.05 Posterior corneal pigmentations
Krukenberg's spindle
H18.051 Posterior corneal pigmentations, right eye
H18.052 Posterior corneal pigmentations, left eye
H18.053 Posterior corneal pigmentations, bilateral
H18.059 Posterior corneal pigmentations, unspecified eye
H18.06 Stromal corneal pigmentations
Hematocornea
H18.061 Stromal corneal pigmentations, right eye
H18.062 Stromal corneal pigmentations, left eye
H18.063 Stromal corneal pigmentations, bilateral
H18.069 Stromal corneal pigmentations, unspecified eye
H18.1 Bullous keratopathy
H18.10 Bullous keratopathy, unspecified eye
H18.11 Bullous keratopathy, right eye
H18.12 Bullous keratopathy, left eye
H18.13 Bullous keratopathy, bilateral
H18.2 Other and unspecified corneal edema
H18.20 Unspecified corneal edema
H18.21 Corneal edema secondary to contact lens
EXCLUDES2 *other corneal disorders due to contact lens (H18.82-)*
H18.211 Corneal edema secondary to contact lens, right eye
H18.212 Corneal edema secondary to contact lens, left eye
H18.213 Corneal edema secondary to contact lens, bilateral
H18.219 Corneal edema secondary to contact lens, unspecified eye
H18.22 Idiopathic corneal edema
H18.221 Idiopathic corneal edema, right eye
H18.222 Idiopathic corneal edema, left eye
H18.223 Idiopathic corneal edema, bilateral
H18.229 Idiopathic corneal edema, unspecified eye
H18.23 Secondary corneal edema

Unspecified Code Other Specified Code Manifestation Code N Newborn P Pediatric M Maternity A Adult ♂ Male ♀ Female
● New Code ▲ Revised Code Title ►◄ Revised Text NOTES INCLUDES EXCLUDES1 Not coded here EXCLUDES2 Not included here
4th character required 5th character required 6th character required 7th character required
Extension 'X' Alert HAC Hospital-acquired condition (HAC) alert AHA AHA Coding Clinic©

H18.231 Secondary corneal edema, right eye
H18.232 Secondary corneal edema, left eye
H18.233 Secondary corneal edema, bilateral
H18.239 Secondary corneal edema, unspecified eye

H18.3 Changes of corneal membranes
H18.30 Unspecified corneal membrane change
H18.31 Folds and rupture in Bowman's membrane
H18.311 Folds and rupture in Bowman's membrane, right eye
H18.312 Folds and rupture in Bowman's membrane, left eye
H18.313 Folds and rupture in Bowman's membrane, bilateral
H18.319 Folds and rupture in Bowman's membrane, unspecified eye
H18.32 Folds in Descemet's membrane
H18.321 Folds in Descemet's membrane, right eye
H18.322 Folds in Descemet's membrane, left eye
H18.323 Folds in Descemet's membrane, bilateral
H18.329 Folds in Descemet's membrane, unspecified eye
H18.33 Rupture in Descemet's membrane
H18.331 Rupture in Descemet's membrane, right eye
H18.332 Rupture in Descemet's membrane, left eye
H18.333 Rupture in Descemet's membrane, bilateral
H18.339 Rupture in Descemet's membrane, unspecified eye

H18.4 Corneal degeneration
EXCLUDES1 *Mooren's ulcer (H16.0-)*
recurrent erosion of cornea (H18.83-)
H18.40 Unspecified corneal degeneration
H18.41 Arcus senilis
Senile corneal changes
H18.411 Arcus senilis, right eye
H18.412 Arcus senilis, left eye
H18.413 Arcus senilis, bilateral
H18.419 Arcus senilis, unspecified eye
H18.42 Band keratopathy
H18.421 Band keratopathy, right eye
H18.422 Band keratopathy, left eye
H18.423 Band keratopathy, bilateral
H18.429 Band keratopathy, unspecified eye
H18.43 Other calcerous corneal degeneration
H18.44 Keratomalacia
EXCLUDES1 *keratomalacia due to vitamin A deficiency (E50.4)*
H18.441 Keratomalacia, right eye
H18.442 Keratomalacia, left eye
H18.443 Keratomalacia, bilateral
H18.449 Keratomalacia, unspecified eye
H18.45 Nodular corneal degeneration
H18.451 Nodular corneal degeneration, right eye
H18.452 Nodular corneal degeneration, left eye
H18.453 Nodular corneal degeneration, bilateral
H18.459 Nodular corneal degeneration, unspecified eye
H18.46 Peripheral corneal degeneration
H18.461 Peripheral corneal degeneration, right eye
H18.462 Peripheral corneal degeneration, left eye
H18.463 Peripheral corneal degeneration, bilateral
H18.469 Peripheral corneal degeneration, unspecified eye
H18.49 Other corneal degeneration

H18.5 Hereditary corneal dystrophies
H18.50 Unspecified hereditary corneal dystrophies
H18.51 Endothelial corneal dystrophy
Fuchs' dystrophy
H18.52 Epithelial (juvenile) corneal dystrophy
H18.53 Granular corneal dystrophy
H18.54 Lattice corneal dystrophy
H18.55 Macular corneal dystrophy
H18.59 Other hereditary corneal dystrophies

H18.6 Keratoconus
H18.60 Keratoconus, unspecified
H18.601 Keratoconus, unspecified, right eye
H18.602 Keratoconus, unspecified, left eye
H18.603 Keratoconus, unspecified, bilateral
H18.609 Keratoconus, unspecified, unspecified eye
H18.61 Keratoconus, stable
H18.611 Keratoconus, stable, right eye
H18.612 Keratoconus, stable, left eye
H18.613 Keratoconus, stable, bilateral
H18.619 Keratoconus, stable, unspecified eye
H18.62 Keratoconus, unstable
Acute hydrops
H18.621 Keratoconus, unstable, right eye
H18.622 Keratoconus, unstable, left eye
H18.623 Keratoconus, unstable, bilateral
H18.629 Keratoconus, unstable, unspecified eye

H18.7 Other and unspecified corneal deformities
EXCLUDES1 *congenital malformations of cornea (Q13.3-Q13.4)*
H18.70 Unspecified corneal deformity
H18.71 Corneal ectasia
H18.711 Corneal ectasia, right eye
H18.712 Corneal ectasia, left eye
H18.713 Corneal ectasia, bilateral
H18.719 Corneal ectasia, unspecified eye
H18.72 Corneal staphyloma
H18.721 Corneal staphyloma, right eye
H18.722 Corneal staphyloma, left eye
H18.723 Corneal staphyloma, bilateral
H18.729 Corneal staphyloma, unspecified eye
H18.73 Descemetocele
H18.731 Descemetocele, right eye
H18.732 Descemetocele, left eye
H18.733 Descemetocele, bilateral
H18.739 Descemetocele, unspecified eye
H18.79 Other corneal deformities
H18.791 Other corneal deformities, right eye
H18.792 Other corneal deformities, left eye
H18.793 Other corneal deformities, bilateral
H18.799 Other corneal deformities, unspecified eye

H18.8 Other specified disorders of cornea
H18.81 Anesthesia and hypoesthesia of cornea
H18.811 Anesthesia and hypoesthesia of cornea, right eye
H18.812 Anesthesia and hypoesthesia of cornea, left eye
H18.813 Anesthesia and hypoesthesia of cornea, bilateral
H18.819 Anesthesia and hypoesthesia of cornea, unspecified eye
H18.82 Corneal disorder due to contact lens
EXCLUDES2 *corneal edema due to contact lens (H18.21-)*
H18.821 Corneal disorder due to contact lens, right eye
H18.822 Corneal disorder due to contact lens, left eye
H18.823 Corneal disorder due to contact lens, bilateral
H18.829 Corneal disorder due to contact lens, unspecified eye
H18.83 Recurrent erosion of cornea
H18.831 Recurrent erosion of cornea, right eye
H18.832 Recurrent erosion of cornea, left eye
H18.833 Recurrent erosion of cornea, bilateral
H18.839 Recurrent erosion of cornea, unspecified eye
H18.89 Other specified disorders of cornea

Unacceptable principal diagnosis symbol per Medicare code edits · Code exempt from diagnosis present on admission requirement
Questionable admission · Complication or comorbidity · CC/MCC exclusion · Major complication or comorbidity
Principal diagnosis as its own CC · Principal diagnosis as its own MCC · Z code as first-listed diagnosis

H18.891 Other specified disorders of cornea, right eye
H18.892 Other specified disorders of cornea, left eye
H18.893 Other specified disorders of cornea, bilateral
H18.899 Other specified disorders of cornea, unspecified eye
H18.9 Unspecified disorder of cornea

H20 Iridocyclitis

H20.0 Acute and subacute iridocyclitis
Acute anterior uveitis
Acute cyclitis
Acute iritis
Subacute anterior uveitis
Subacute cyclitis
Subacute iritis

EXCLUDES1 *iridocyclitis, iritis, uveitis (due to) (in) diabetes mellitus (E08-E13 with .39)*
iridocyclitis, iritis, uveitis (due to) (in) diphtheria (A36.89)
iridocyclitis, iritis, uveitis (due to) (in) gonococcal (A54.32)
iridocyclitis, iritis, uveitis (due to) (in) herpes (simplex) (B00.51)
iridocyclitis, iritis, uveitis (due to) (in) herpes zoster (B02.32)
iridocyclitis, iritis, uveitis (due to) (in) late congenital syphilis (A50.39)
iridocyclitis, iritis, uveitis (due to) (in) late syphilis (A52.71)
iridocyclitis, iritis, uveitis (due to) (in) sarcoidosis (D86.83)
iridocyclitis, iritis, uveitis (due to) (in) syphilis (A51.43)
iridocyclitis, iritis, uveitis (due to) (in) toxoplasmosis (B58.09)
iridocyclitis, iritis, uveitis (due to) (in) tuberculosis (A18.54)

H20.00 Unspecified acute and subacute iridocyclitis CC

H20.01 Primary iridocyclitis
H20.011 Primary iridocyclitis, right eye CC
H20.012 Primary iridocyclitis, left eye CC
H20.013 Primary iridocyclitis, bilateral CC
H20.019 Primary iridocyclitis, unspecified eye CC

H20.02 Recurrent acute iridocyclitis
H20.021 Recurrent acute iridocyclitis, right eye CC
H20.022 Recurrent acute iridocyclitis, left eye CC
H20.023 Recurrent acute iridocyclitis, bilateral CC
H20.029 Recurrent acute iridocyclitis, unspecified eye CC

H20.03 Secondary infectious iridocyclitis
H20.031 Secondary infectious iridocyclitis, right eye CC
H20.032 Secondary infectious iridocyclitis, left eye CC
H20.033 Secondary infectious iridocyclitis, bilateral CC
H20.039 Secondary infectious iridocyclitis, unspecified eye CC

H20.04 Secondary noninfectious iridocyclitis
H20.041 Secondary noninfectious iridocyclitis, right eye
H20.042 Secondary noninfectious iridocyclitis, left eye
H20.043 Secondary noninfectious iridocyclitis, bilateral
H20.049 Secondary noninfectious iridocyclitis, unspecified eye

H20.05 Hypopyon
H20.051 Hypopyon, right eye
H20.052 Hypopyon, left eye
H20.053 Hypopyon, bilateral
H20.059 Hypopyon, unspecified eye

H20.1 Chronic iridocyclitis
Use additional code for any associated cataract (H26.21-)
EXCLUDES2 *posterior cyclitis (H30.2-)*
H20.10 Chronic iridocyclitis, unspecified eye
H20.11 Chronic iridocyclitis, right eye
H20.12 Chronic iridocyclitis, left eye
H20.13 Chronic iridocyclitis, bilateral

H20.2 Lens-induced iridocyclitis
H20.20 Lens-induced iridocyclitis, unspecified eye
H20.21 Lens-induced iridocyclitis, right eye
H20.22 Lens-induced iridocyclitis, left eye
H20.23 Lens-induced iridocyclitis, bilateral

H20.8 Other iridocyclitis
EXCLUDES2 *glaucomatocyclitis crises (H40.4-)*
posterior cyclitis (H30.2-)
sympathetic uveitis (H44.13-)

H20.81 Fuchs' heterochromic cyclitis
H20.811 Fuchs' heterochromic cyclitis, right eye
H20.812 Fuchs' heterochromic cyclitis, left eye
H20.813 Fuchs' heterochromic cyclitis, bilateral
H20.819 Fuchs' heterochromic cyclitis, unspecified eye

H20.82 Vogt-Koyanagi syndrome
H20.821 Vogt-Koyanagi syndrome, right eye
H20.822 Vogt-Koyanagi syndrome, left eye
H20.823 Vogt-Koyanagi syndrome, bilateral
H20.829 Vogt-Koyanagi syndrome, unspecified eye

H20.9 Unspecified iridocyclitis CC
Uveitis NOS

H21 Other disorders of iris and ciliary body
EXCLUDES2 *sympathetic uveitis (H44.1-)*

H21.0 Hyphema
EXCLUDES1 *traumatic hyphema (S05.1-)*
H21.00 Hyphema, unspecified eye
H21.01 Hyphema, right eye
H21.02 Hyphema, left eye
H21.03 Hyphema, bilateral

H21.1 Other vascular disorders of iris and ciliary body
Neovascularization of iris or ciliary body
Rubeosis iridis
Rubeosis of iris

H21.1X Other vascular disorders of iris and ciliary body
H21.1X1 Other vascular disorders of iris and ciliary body, right eye
H21.1X2 Other vascular disorders of iris and ciliary body, left eye
H21.1X3 Other vascular disorders of iris and ciliary body, bilateral
H21.1X9 Other vascular disorders of iris and ciliary body, unspecified eye

H21.2 Degeneration of iris and ciliary body

H21.21 Degeneration of chamber angle
H21.211 Degeneration of chamber angle, right eye
H21.212 Degeneration of chamber angle, left eye
H21.213 Degeneration of chamber angle, bilateral
H21.219 Degeneration of chamber angle, unspecified eye

H21.22 Degeneration of ciliary body
H21.221 Degeneration of ciliary body, right eye
H21.222 Degeneration of ciliary body, left eye
H21.223 Degeneration of ciliary body, bilateral
H21.229 Degeneration of ciliary body, unspecified eye

H21.23 Degeneration of iris (pigmentary)
Translucency of iris
H21.231 Degeneration of iris (pigmentary), right eye
H21.232 Degeneration of iris (pigmentary), left eye
H21.233 Degeneration of iris (pigmentary), bilateral
H21.239 Degeneration of iris (pigmentary), unspecified eye

H21.24 Degeneration of pupillary margin
H21.241 Degeneration of pupillary margin, right eye

Unspecified Code Other Specified Code Manifestation Code N Newborn P Pediatric M Maternity A Adult ♂ Male ♀ Female
● New Code ▲ Revised Code Title ►◄ Revised Text NOTES INCLUDES EXCLUDES1 Not coded here EXCLUDES2 Not included here
4th character required 5th character required 6th character required 7th character required
Extension 'X' Alert HAC Hospital-acquired condition (HAC) alert AHA AHA Coding Clinic©

H21.242 Degeneration of pupillary margin, left eye
H21.243 Degeneration of pupillary margin, bilateral
H21.249 Degeneration of pupillary margin, unspecified eye

H21.25 Iridoschisis
H21.251 Iridoschisis, right eye
H21.252 Iridoschisis, left eye
H21.253 Iridoschisis, bilateral
H21.259 Iridoschisis, unspecified eye

H21.26 Iris atrophy (essential) (progressive)
H21.261 Iris atrophy (essential) (progressive), right eye
H21.262 Iris atrophy (essential) (progressive), left eye
H21.263 Iris atrophy (essential) (progressive), bilateral
H21.269 Iris atrophy (essential) (progressive), unspecified eye

H21.27 Miotic pupillary cyst
H21.271 Miotic pupillary cyst, right eye
H21.272 Miotic pupillary cyst, left eye
H21.273 Miotic pupillary cyst, bilateral
H21.279 Miotic pupillary cyst, unspecified eye

H21.29 Other iris atrophy

H21.3 Cyst of iris, ciliary body and anterior chamber
EXCLUDES2 *miotic pupillary cyst (H21.27-)*

H21.30 Idiopathic cysts of iris, ciliary body or anterior chamber
Cyst of iris, ciliary body or anterior chamber NOS
H21.301 Idiopathic cysts of iris, ciliary body or anterior chamber, right eye
H21.302 Idiopathic cysts of iris, ciliary body or anterior chamber, left eye
H21.303 Idiopathic cysts of iris, ciliary body or anterior chamber, bilateral
H21.309 Idiopathic cysts of iris, ciliary body or anterior chamber, unspecified eye

H21.31 Exudative cysts of iris or anterior chamber
H21.311 Exudative cysts of iris or anterior chamber, right eye
H21.312 Exudative cysts of iris or anterior chamber, left eye
H21.313 Exudative cysts of iris or anterior chamber, bilateral
H21.319 Exudative cysts of iris or anterior chamber, unspecified eye

H21.32 Implantation cysts of iris, ciliary body or anterior chamber
H21.321 Implantation cysts of iris, ciliary body or anterior chamber, right eye
H21.322 Implantation cysts of iris, ciliary body or anterior chamber, left eye
H21.323 Implantation cysts of iris, ciliary body or anterior chamber, bilateral
H21.329 Implantation cysts of iris, ciliary body or anterior chamber, unspecified eye

H21.33 Parasitic cyst of iris, ciliary body or anterior chamber
H21.331 Parasitic cyst of iris, ciliary body or anterior chamber, right eye CC
H21.332 Parasitic cyst of iris, ciliary body or anterior chamber, left eye CC
H21.333 Parasitic cyst of iris, ciliary body or anterior chamber, bilateral CC
H21.339 Parasitic cyst of iris, ciliary body or anterior chamber, unspecified eye CC

H21.34 Primary cyst of pars plana
H21.341 Primary cyst of pars plana, right eye
H21.342 Primary cyst of pars plana, left eye
H21.343 Primary cyst of pars plana, bilateral
H21.349 Primary cyst of pars plana, unspecified eye

H21.35 Exudative cyst of pars plana
H21.351 Exudative cyst of pars plana, right eye
H21.352 Exudative cyst of pars plana, left eye
H21.353 Exudative cyst of pars plana, bilateral
H21.359 Exudative cyst of pars plana, unspecified eye

H21.4 Pupillary membranes
Iris bombé
Pupillary occlusion
Pupillary seclusion
EXCLUDES1 *congenital pupillary membranes (Q13.8)*
H21.40 Pupillary membranes, unspecified eye
H21.41 Pupillary membranes, right eye
H21.42 Pupillary membranes, left eye
H21.43 Pupillary membranes, bilateral

H21.5 Other and unspecified adhesions and disruptions of iris and ciliary body
EXCLUDES1 *corectopia (Q13.2)*

H21.50 Unspecified adhesions of iris
Synechia (iris) NOS
H21.501 Unspecified adhesions of iris, right eye
H21.502 Unspecified adhesions of iris, left eye
H21.503 Unspecified adhesions of iris, bilateral
H21.509 Unspecified adhesions of iris and ciliary body, unspecified eye

H21.51 Anterior synechiae (iris)
H21.511 Anterior synechiae (iris), right eye
H21.512 Anterior synechiae (iris), left eye
H21.513 Anterior synechiae (iris), bilateral
H21.519 Anterior synechiae (iris), unspecified eye

H21.52 Goniosynechiae
H21.521 Goniosynechiae, right eye
H21.522 Goniosynechiae, left eye
H21.523 Goniosynechiae, bilateral
H21.529 Goniosynechiae, unspecified eye

H21.53 Iridodialysis
H21.531 Iridodialysis, right eye
H21.532 Iridodialysis, left eye
H21.533 Iridodialysis, bilateral
H21.539 Iridodialysis, unspecified eye

H21.54 Posterior synechiae (iris)
H21.541 Posterior synechiae (iris), right eye
H21.542 Posterior synechiae (iris), left eye
H21.543 Posterior synechiae (iris), bilateral
H21.549 Posterior synechiae (iris), unspecified eye

H21.55 Recession of chamber angle
H21.551 Recession of chamber angle, right eye
H21.552 Recession of chamber angle, left eye
H21.553 Recession of chamber angle, bilateral
H21.559 Recession of chamber angle, unspecified eye

H21.56 Pupillary abnormalities
Deformed pupil
Ectopic pupil
Rupture of sphincter, pupil
EXCLUDES1 *congenital deformity of pupil (Q13.2-)*
H21.561 Pupillary abnormality, right eye
H21.562 Pupillary abnormality, left eye
H21.563 Pupillary abnormality, bilateral
H21.569 Pupillary abnormality, unspecified eye

H21.8 Other specified disorders of iris and ciliary body
H21.81 Floppy iris syndrome
Intraoperative floppy iris syndrome (IFIS)
Use additional code for adverse effect, if applicable, to identify drug (T36-T50 with fifth or sixth character 5)
H21.82 Plateau iris syndrome (post-iridectomy) (postprocedural)
H21.89 Other specified disorders of iris and ciliary body

H21.9 Unspecified disorder of iris and ciliary body

H22 Disorders of iris and ciliary body in diseases classified elsewhere
Code first underlying disease, such as:
gout (M1A.-, M10.-)
leprosy (A30.-)
parasitic disease (B89)

Unacceptable principal diagnosis symbol per Medicare code edits; Code exempt from diagnosis present on admission requirement; Questionable admission; Complication or comorbidity; CC/MCC exclusion; Major complication or comorbidity; Principal diagnosis as its own CC; Principal diagnosis as its own MCC; Z code as first-listed diagnosis

When symbols appear on a code that requires a 7th character extension, refer to Appendix D to identify applicable 7th character codes.

Disorders of lens (H25-H28)

H25 Age-related cataract
Senile cataract
EXCLUDES2 *capsular glaucoma with pseudoexfoliation of lens (H40.1-)*
- H25.0 Age-related incipient cataract
  - H25.01 Cortical age-related cataract
    - H25.011 Cortical age-related cataract, right eye A
    - H25.012 Cortical age-related cataract, left eye A
    - H25.013 Cortical age-related cataract, bilateral A
    - H25.019 Cortical age-related cataract, unspecified eye A
  - H25.03 Anterior subcapsular polar age-related cataract
    - H25.031 Anterior subcapsular polar age-related cataract, right eye A
    - H25.032 Anterior subcapsular polar age-related cataract, left eye A
    - H25.033 Anterior subcapsular polar age-related cataract, bilateral A
    - H25.039 Anterior subcapsular polar age-related cataract, unspecified eye A
  - H25.04 Posterior subcapsular polar age-related cataract
    - H25.041 Posterior subcapsular polar age-related cataract, right eye A
    - H25.042 Posterior subcapsular polar age-related cataract, left eye A
    - H25.043 Posterior subcapsular polar age-related cataract, bilateral A
    - H25.049 Posterior subcapsular polar age-related cataract, unspecified eye A
  - H25.09 Other age-related incipient cataract
    Coronary age-related cataract
    Punctate age-related cataract
    Water clefts
    - H25.091 Other age-related incipient cataract, right eye A
    - H25.092 Other age-related incipient cataract, left eye A
    - H25.093 Other age-related incipient cataract, bilateral A
    - H25.099 Other age-related incipient cataract, unspecified eye A
- H25.1 Age-related nuclear cataract
  Cataracta brunescens
  Nuclear sclerosis cataract
  - H25.10 Age-related nuclear cataract, unspecified eye A
  - H25.11 Age-related nuclear cataract, right eye A
  - H25.12 Age-related nuclear cataract, left eye A
    AHA: Q1, 2016
  - H25.13 Age-related nuclear cataract, bilateral A
    AHA: Q1, 2016
- H25.2 Age-related cataract, morgagnian type
  Age-related hypermature cataract
  - H25.20 Age-related cataract, morgagnian type, unspecified eye A
  - H25.21 Age-related cataract, morgagnian type, right eye A
  - H25.22 Age-related cataract, morgagnian type, left eye A
  - H25.23 Age-related cataract, morgagnian type, bilateral A
- H25.8 Other age-related cataract
  - H25.81 Combined forms of age-related cataract
    - H25.811 Combined forms of age-related cataract, right eye A
    - H25.812 Combined forms of age-related cataract, left eye A
    - H25.813 Combined forms of age-related cataract, bilateral A
    - H25.819 Combined forms of age-related cataract, unspecified eye A
  - H25.89 Other age-related cataract A
- H25.9 Unspecified age-related cataract A

H26 Other cataract
EXCLUDES1 *congenital cataract (Q12.0)*
- H26.0 Infantile and juvenile cataract
  - H26.00 Unspecified infantile and juvenile cataract
    - H26.001 Unspecified infantile and juvenile cataract, right eye P
    - H26.002 Unspecified infantile and juvenile cataract, left eye P
    - H26.003 Unspecified infantile and juvenile cataract, bilateral P
    - H26.009 Unspecified infantile and juvenile cataract, unspecified eye P
  - H26.01 Infantile and juvenile cortical, lamellar, or zonular cataract
    - H26.011 Infantile and juvenile cortical, lamellar, or zonular cataract, right eye P
    - H26.012 Infantile and juvenile cortical, lamellar, or zonular cataract, left eye P
    - H26.013 Infantile and juvenile cortical, lamellar, or zonular cataract, bilateral P
    - H26.019 Infantile and juvenile cortical, lamellar, or zonular cataract, unspecified eye P
  - H26.03 Infantile and juvenile nuclear cataract
    - H26.031 Infantile and juvenile nuclear cataract, right eye P
    - H26.032 Infantile and juvenile nuclear cataract, left eye P
    - H26.033 Infantile and juvenile nuclear cataract, bilateral P
    - H26.039 Infantile and juvenile nuclear cataract, unspecified eye P
  - H26.04 Anterior subcapsular polar infantile and juvenile cataract
    - H26.041 Anterior subcapsular polar infantile and juvenile cataract, right eye P
    - H26.042 Anterior subcapsular polar infantile and juvenile cataract, left eye P
    - H26.043 Anterior subcapsular polar infantile and juvenile cataract, bilateral P
    - H26.049 Anterior subcapsular polar infantile and juvenile cataract, unspecified eye P
  - H26.05 Posterior subcapsular polar infantile and juvenile cataract
    - H26.051 Posterior subcapsular polar infantile and juvenile cataract, right eye P
    - H26.052 Posterior subcapsular polar infantile and juvenile cataract, left eye P
    - H26.053 Posterior subcapsular polar infantile and juvenile cataract, bilateral P
    - H26.059 Posterior subcapsular polar infantile and juvenile cataract, unspecified eye P
  - H26.06 Combined forms of infantile and juvenile cataract
    - H26.061 Combined forms of infantile and juvenile cataract, right eye P
    - H26.062 Combined forms of infantile and juvenile cataract, left eye P
    - H26.063 Combined forms of infantile and juvenile cataract, bilateral P
    - H26.069 Combined forms of infantile and juvenile cataract, unspecified eye P
  - H26.09 Other infantile and juvenile cataract P
- H26.1 Traumatic cataract
  Use additional code (Chapter 20) to identify external cause
  - H26.10 Unspecified traumatic cataract
    - H26.101 Unspecified traumatic cataract, right eye
    - H26.102 Unspecified traumatic cataract, left eye
    - H26.103 Unspecified traumatic cataract, bilateral
    - H26.109 Unspecified traumatic cataract, unspecified eye
  - H26.11 Localized traumatic opacities
    - H26.111 Localized traumatic opacities, right eye
    - H26.112 Localized traumatic opacities, left eye
    - H26.113 Localized traumatic opacities, bilateral
    - H26.119 Localized traumatic opacities, unspecified eye
  - H26.12 Partially resolved traumatic cataract
    - H26.121 Partially resolved traumatic cataract, right eye

Unspecified Code | Other Specified Code | Manifestation Code | N Newborn | P Pediatric | M Maternity | A Adult | ♂ Male | ♀ Female
● New Code | ▲ Revised Code Title | ►◄ Revised Text | NOTES | INCLUDES | EXCLUDES1 Not coded here | EXCLUDES2 Not included here
4th character required | 5th character required | 6th character required | 7th character required
Extension 'X' Alert | HAC Hospital-acquired condition (HAC) alert | AHA AHA Coding Clinic©

H26.122 **Partially resolved traumatic cataract, left eye**
H26.123 **Partially resolved traumatic cataract, bilateral**
H26.129 **Partially resolved traumatic cataract, unspecified eye**
H26.13 **Total traumatic cataract**
H26.131 **Total traumatic cataract, right eye**
H26.132 **Total traumatic cataract, left eye**
H26.133 **Total traumatic cataract, bilateral**
H26.139 **Total traumatic cataract, unspecified eye**
H26.2 **Complicated cataract**
H26.20 **Unspecified complicated cataract**
Cataracta complicata NOS
H26.21 **Cataract with neovascularization**
Code also associated condition, such as:
chronic iridocyclitis (H20.1-)
H26.211 **Cataract with neovascularization, right eye**
H26.212 **Cataract with neovascularization, left eye**
H26.213 **Cataract with neovascularization, bilateral**
H26.219 **Cataract with neovascularization, unspecified eye**
H26.22 **Cataract secondary to ocular disorders (degenerative) (inflammatory)**
Code also associated ocular disorder
H26.221 **Cataract secondary to ocular disorders (degenerative) (inflammatory), right eye**
H26.222 **Cataract secondary to ocular disorders (degenerative) (inflammatory), left eye**
H26.223 **Cataract secondary to ocular disorders (degenerative) (inflammatory), bilateral**
H26.229 **Cataract secondary to ocular disorders (degenerative) (inflammatory), unspecified eye**
H26.23 **Glaucomatous flecks (subcapsular)**
Code first underlying glaucoma (H40-H42)
H26.231 **Glaucomatous flecks (subcapsular), right eye**
H26.232 **Glaucomatous flecks (subcapsular), left eye**
H26.233 **Glaucomatous flecks (subcapsular), bilateral**
H26.239 **Glaucomatous flecks (subcapsular), unspecified eye**
H26.3 **Drug-induced cataract**
Toxic cataract
Use additional code for adverse effect, if applicable, to identify drug (T36-T50 with fifth or sixth character 5)
H26.30 **Drug-induced cataract, unspecified eye**
H26.31 **Drug-induced cataract, right eye**
H26.32 **Drug-induced cataract, left eye**
H26.33 **Drug-induced cataract, bilateral**
H26.4 **Secondary cataract**
H26.40 **Unspecified secondary cataract**
H26.41 **Soemmering's ring**
H26.411 **Soemmering's ring, right eye**
H26.412 **Soemmering's ring, left eye**
H26.413 **Soemmering's ring, bilateral**
H26.419 **Soemmering's ring, unspecified eye**
H26.49 **Other secondary cataract**
H26.491 **Other secondary cataract, right eye**
H26.492 **Other secondary cataract, left eye**
H26.493 **Other secondary cataract, bilateral**
H26.499 **Other secondary cataract, unspecified eye**
H26.8 **Other specified cataract**
H26.9 **Unspecified cataract**
H27 **Other disorders of lens**
EXCLUDES1 *congenital lens malformations (Q12.-)*
mechanical complications of intraocular lens implant (T85.2)
pseudophakia (Z96.1)
H27.0 **Aphakia**
Acquired absence of lens
Acquired aphakia
Aphakia due to trauma
EXCLUDES1 *cataract extraction status (Z98.4-)*
congenital absence of lens (Q12.3)
congenital aphakia (Q12.3)
H27.00 **Aphakia, unspecified eye**
H27.01 **Aphakia, right eye**
H27.02 **Aphakia, left eye**
H27.03 **Aphakia, bilateral**
H27.1 **Dislocation of lens**
H27.10 **Unspecified dislocation of lens**
H27.11 **Subluxation of lens**
H27.111 **Subluxation of lens, right eye**
H27.112 **Subluxation of lens, left eye**
H27.113 **Subluxation of lens, bilateral**
H27.119 **Subluxation of lens, unspecified eye**
H27.12 **Anterior dislocation of lens**
H27.121 **Anterior dislocation of lens, right eye**
H27.122 **Anterior dislocation of lens, left eye**
H27.123 **Anterior dislocation of lens, bilateral**
H27.129 **Anterior dislocation of lens, unspecified eye**
H27.13 **Posterior dislocation of lens**
H27.131 **Posterior dislocation of lens, right eye**
H27.132 **Posterior dislocation of lens, left eye**
H27.133 **Posterior dislocation of lens, bilateral**
H27.139 **Posterior dislocation of lens, unspecified eye**
H27.8 **Other specified disorders of lens**
H27.9 **Unspecified disorder of lens**
H28 **Cataract in diseases classified elsewhere**
Code first underlying disease, such as:
hypoparathyroidism (E20.-)
myotonia (G71.1-)
myxedema (E03.-)
protein-calorie malnutrition (E40-E46)
EXCLUDES1 *cataract in diabetes mellitus (E08.36, E09.36, E10.36, E11.36, E13.36)*

Disorders of choroid and retina (H30-H36)

H30 **Chorioretinal inflammation**
H30.0 **Focal chorioretinal inflammation**
Focal chorioretinitis
Focal choroiditis
Focal retinitis
Focal retinochoroiditis
H30.00 **Unspecified focal chorioretinal inflammation**
Focal chorioretinitis NOS
Focal choroiditis NOS
Focal retinitis NOS
Focal retinochoroiditis NOS
H30.001 **Unspecified focal chorioretinal inflammation, right eye**
H30.002 **Unspecified focal chorioretinal inflammation, left eye**
H30.003 **Unspecified focal chorioretinal inflammation, bilateral**
H30.009 **Unspecified focal chorioretinal inflammation, unspecified eye**
H30.01 **Focal chorioretinal inflammation, juxtapapillary**
H30.011 **Focal chorioretinal inflammation, juxtapapillary, right eye**
H30.012 **Focal chorioretinal inflammation, juxtapapillary, left eye**
H30.013 **Focal chorioretinal inflammation, juxtapapillary, bilateral**
H30.019 **Focal chorioretinal inflammation, juxtapapillary, unspecified eye**
H30.02 **Focal chorioretinal inflammation of posterior pole**
H30.021 **Focal chorioretinal inflammation of posterior pole, right eye**
H30.022 **Focal chorioretinal inflammation of posterior pole, left eye**

Unacceptable principal diagnosis symbol per Medicare code edits | Code exempt from diagnosis present on admission requirement
Questionable admission | Complication or comorbidity | CC/MCC exclusion | Major complication or comorbidity
Principal diagnosis as its own CC | Principal diagnosis as its own MCC | Z code as first-listed diagnosis

H30.023 Focal chorioretinal inflammation of posterior pole, bilateral
H30.029 Focal chorioretinal inflammation of posterior pole, unspecified eye
H30.03 Focal chorioretinal inflammation, peripheral
H30.031 Focal chorioretinal inflammation, peripheral, right eye
H30.032 Focal chorioretinal inflammation, peripheral, left eye
H30.033 Focal chorioretinal inflammation, peripheral, bilateral
H30.039 Focal chorioretinal inflammation, peripheral, unspecified eye
H30.04 Focal chorioretinal inflammation, macular or paramacular
H30.041 Focal chorioretinal inflammation, macular or paramacular, right eye
H30.042 Focal chorioretinal inflammation, macular or paramacular, left eye
H30.043 Focal chorioretinal inflammation, macular or paramacular, bilateral
H30.049 Focal chorioretinal inflammation, macular or paramacular, unspecified eye
H30.1 Disseminated chorioretinal inflammation
Disseminated chorioretinitis
Disseminated choroiditis
Disseminated retinitis
Disseminated retinochoroiditis
EXCLUDES2 *exudative retinopathy (H35.02-)*
H30.10 Unspecified disseminated chorioretinal inflammation
Disseminated chorioretinitis NOS
Disseminated choroiditis NOS
Disseminated retinitis NOS
Disseminated retinochoroiditis NOS
H30.101 Unspecified disseminated chorioretinal inflammation, right eye
H30.102 Unspecified disseminated chorioretinal inflammation, left eye
H30.103 Unspecified disseminated chorioretinal inflammation, bilateral
H30.109 Unspecified disseminated chorioretinal inflammation, unspecified eye
H30.11 Disseminated chorioretinal inflammation of posterior pole
H30.111 Disseminated chorioretinal inflammation of posterior pole, right eye
H30.112 Disseminated chorioretinal inflammation of posterior pole, left eye
H30.113 Disseminated chorioretinal inflammation of posterior pole, bilateral
H30.119 Disseminated chorioretinal inflammation of posterior pole, unspecified eye
H30.12 Disseminated chorioretinal inflammation, peripheral
H30.121 Disseminated chorioretinal inflammation, peripheral right eye
H30.122 Disseminated chorioretinal inflammation, peripheral, left eye
H30.123 Disseminated chorioretinal inflammation, peripheral, bilateral
H30.129 Disseminated chorioretinal inflammation, peripheral, unspecified eye
H30.13 Disseminated chorioretinal inflammation, generalized
H30.131 Disseminated chorioretinal inflammation, generalized, right eye
H30.132 Disseminated chorioretinal inflammation, generalized, left eye
H30.133 Disseminated chorioretinal inflammation, generalized, bilateral
H30.139 Disseminated chorioretinal inflammation, generalized, unspecified eye
H30.14 Acute posterior multifocal placoid pigment epitheliopathy
H30.141 Acute posterior multifocal placoid pigment epitheliopathy, right eye
H30.142 Acute posterior multifocal placoid pigment epitheliopathy, left eye
H30.143 Acute posterior multifocal placoid pigment epitheliopathy, bilateral
H30.149 Acute posterior multifocal placoid pigment epitheliopathy, unspecified eye
H30.2 Posterior cyclitis
Pars planitis
H30.20 Posterior cyclitis, unspecified eye
H30.21 Posterior cyclitis, right eye
H30.22 Posterior cyclitis, left eye
H30.23 Posterior cyclitis, bilateral
H30.8 Other chorioretinal inflammations
H30.81 Harada's disease
H30.811 Harada's disease, right eye
H30.812 Harada's disease, left eye
H30.813 Harada's disease, bilateral
H30.819 Harada's disease, unspecified eye
H30.89 Other chorioretinal inflammations
H30.891 Other chorioretinal inflammations, right eye
H30.892 Other chorioretinal inflammations, left eye
H30.893 Other chorioretinal inflammations, bilateral
H30.899 Other chorioretinal inflammations, unspecified eye
H30.9 Unspecified chorioretinal inflammation
Chorioretinitis NOS
Choroiditis NOS
Neuroretinitis NOS
Retinitis NOS
Retinochoroiditis NOS
H30.90 Unspecified chorioretinal inflammation, unspecified eye
H30.91 Unspecified chorioretinal inflammation, right eye
H30.92 Unspecified chorioretinal inflammation, left eye
H30.93 Unspecified chorioretinal inflammation, bilateral
H31 Other disorders of choroid
H31.0 Chorioretinal scars
EXCLUDES2 *postsurgical chorioretinal scars (H59.81-)*
H31.00 Unspecified chorioretinal scars
H31.001 Unspecified chorioretinal scars, right eye
H31.002 Unspecified chorioretinal scars, left eye
H31.003 Unspecified chorioretinal scars, bilateral
H31.009 Unspecified chorioretinal scars, unspecified eye
H31.01 Macula scars of posterior pole (postinflammatory) (post-traumatic)
EXCLUDES1 *postprocedural chorioretinal scar (H59.81-)*
H31.011 Macula scars of posterior pole (postinflammatory) (post-traumatic), right eye
H31.012 Macula scars of posterior pole (postinflammatory) (post-traumatic), left eye
H31.013 Macula scars of posterior pole (postinflammatory) (post-traumatic), bilateral
H31.019 Macula scars of posterior pole (postinflammatory) (post-traumatic), unspecified eye
H31.02 Solar retinopathy
H31.021 Solar retinopathy, right eye
H31.022 Solar retinopathy, left eye
H31.023 Solar retinopathy, bilateral
H31.029 Solar retinopathy, unspecified eye
H31.09 Other chorioretinal scars
H31.091 Other chorioretinal scars, right eye
H31.092 Other chorioretinal scars, left eye
H31.093 Other chorioretinal scars, bilateral
H31.099 Other chorioretinal scars, unspecified eye
H31.1 Choroidal degeneration
EXCLUDES2 *angioid streaks of macula (H35.33)*

Unspecified Code | Other Specified Code | Manifestation Code | N Newborn | P Pediatric | M Maternity | A Adult | ♂ Male | ♀ Female
● New Code | ▲ Revised Code Title | ►◄ Revised Text | NOTES | INCLUDES | EXCLUDES1 Not coded here | EXCLUDES2 Not included here
4th character required | 5th character required | 6th character required | 7th character required
Extension 'X' Alert | HAC Hospital-acquired condition (HAC) alert | AHA AHA Coding Clinic©

H31.10 Unspecified choroidal degeneration
Choroidal sclerosis NOS
H31.101 Choroidal degeneration, unspecified, right eye
H31.102 Choroidal degeneration, unspecified, left eye
H31.103 Choroidal degeneration, unspecified, bilateral
H31.109 Choroidal degeneration, unspecified, unspecified eye
H31.11 Age-related choroidal atrophy
H31.111 Age-related choroidal atrophy, right eye A
H31.112 Age-related choroidal atrophy, left eye A
H31.113 Age-related choroidal atrophy, bilateral A
H31.119 Age-related choroidal atrophy, unspecified eye A
H31.12 Diffuse secondary atrophy of choroid
H31.121 Diffuse secondary atrophy of choroid, right eye
H31.122 Diffuse secondary atrophy of choroid, left eye
H31.123 Diffuse secondary atrophy of choroid, bilateral
H31.129 Diffuse secondary atrophy of choroid, unspecified eye
H31.2 Hereditary choroidal dystrophy
EXCLUDES2 *hyperornithinemia (E72.4)*
ornithinemia (E72.4)
H31.20 Hereditary choroidal dystrophy, unspecified
H31.21 Choroideremia
H31.22 Choroidal dystrophy (central areolar) (generalized) (peripapillary)
H31.23 Gyrate atrophy, choroid
H31.29 Other hereditary choroidal dystrophy
H31.3 Choroidal hemorrhage and rupture
H31.30 Unspecified choroidal hemorrhage
H31.301 Unspecified choroidal hemorrhage, right eye
H31.302 Unspecified choroidal hemorrhage, left eye
H31.303 Unspecified choroidal hemorrhage, bilateral
H31.309 Unspecified choroidal hemorrhage, unspecified eye
H31.31 Expulsive choroidal hemorrhage
H31.311 Expulsive choroidal hemorrhage, right eye
H31.312 Expulsive choroidal hemorrhage, left eye
H31.313 Expulsive choroidal hemorrhage, bilateral
H31.319 Expulsive choroidal hemorrhage, unspecified eye
H31.32 Choroidal rupture
H31.321 Choroidal rupture, right eye CC
H31.322 Choroidal rupture, left eye CC
H31.323 Choroidal rupture, bilateral CC
H31.329 Choroidal rupture, unspecified eye CC
H31.4 Choroidal detachment
H31.40 Unspecified choroidal detachment
H31.401 Unspecified choroidal detachment, right eye CC
H31.402 Unspecified choroidal detachment, left eye CC
H31.403 Unspecified choroidal detachment, bilateral CC
H31.409 Unspecified choroidal detachment, unspecified eye CC
H31.41 Hemorrhagic choroidal detachment
H31.411 Hemorrhagic choroidal detachment, right eye CC
H31.412 Hemorrhagic choroidal detachment, left eye CC
H31.413 Hemorrhagic choroidal detachment, bilateral CC
H31.419 Hemorrhagic choroidal detachment, unspecified eye CC
H31.42 Serous choroidal detachment
H31.421 Serous choroidal detachment, right eye CC
H31.422 Serous choroidal detachment, left eye CC
H31.423 Serous choroidal detachment, bilateral CC
H31.429 Serous choroidal detachment, unspecified eye CC
H31.8 Other specified disorders of choroid
H31.9 Unspecified disorder of choroid
H32 Chorioretinal disorders in diseases classified elsewhere
Code first underlying disease, such as:
congenital toxoplasmosis (P37.1)
histoplasmosis (B39.-)
leprosy (A30.-)
EXCLUDES1 *chorioretinitis (in):*
toxoplasmosis (acquired) (B58.01)
tuberculosis (A18.53)
H33 Retinal detachments and breaks
EXCLUDES1 *detachment of retinal pigment epithelium (H35.72-, H35.73-)*
H33.0 Retinal detachment with retinal break
Rhegmatogenous retinal detachment
EXCLUDES1 *serous retinal detachment (without retinal break) (H33.2-)*
H33.00 Unspecified retinal detachment with retinal break
H33.001 Unspecified retinal detachment with retinal break, right eye
H33.002 Unspecified retinal detachment with retinal break, left eye
H33.003 Unspecified retinal detachment with retinal break, bilateral
H33.009 Unspecified retinal detachment with retinal break, unspecified eye
H33.01 Retinal detachment with single break
H33.011 Retinal detachment with single break, right eye
H33.012 Retinal detachment with single break, left eye
H33.013 Retinal detachment with single break, bilateral
H33.019 Retinal detachment with single break, unspecified eye
H33.02 Retinal detachment with multiple breaks
H33.021 Retinal detachment with multiple breaks, right eye
H33.022 Retinal detachment with multiple breaks, left eye
H33.023 Retinal detachment with multiple breaks, bilateral
H33.029 Retinal detachment with multiple breaks, unspecified eye
H33.03 Retinal detachment with giant retinal tear
H33.031 Retinal detachment with giant retinal tear, right eye
H33.032 Retinal detachment with giant retinal tear, left eye
H33.033 Retinal detachment with giant retinal tear, bilateral
H33.039 Retinal detachment with giant retinal tear, unspecified eye
H33.04 Retinal detachment with retinal dialysis
H33.041 Retinal detachment with retinal dialysis, right eye
H33.042 Retinal detachment with retinal dialysis, left eye
H33.043 Retinal detachment with retinal dialysis, bilateral
H33.049 Retinal detachment with retinal dialysis, unspecified eye
H33.05 Total retinal detachment
H33.051 Total retinal detachment, right eye
H33.052 Total retinal detachment, left eye
H33.053 Total retinal detachment, bilateral
H33.059 Total retinal detachment, unspecified eye

Unacceptable principal diagnosis symbol per Medicare code edits; Code exempt from diagnosis present on admission requirement
Questionable admission; CC Complication or comorbidity; CC/MCC exclusion; MCC Major complication or comorbidity
Principal diagnosis as its own CC; Principal diagnosis as its own MCC; Z code as first-listed diagnosis

H33.1 Retinoschisis and retinal cysts
EXCLUDES1 *congenital retinoschisis (Q14.1)*
microcystoid degeneration of retina (H35.42-)
H33.10 Unspecified retinoschisis
H33.101 Unspecified retinoschisis, right eye
H33.102 Unspecified retinoschisis, left eye
H33.103 Unspecified retinoschisis, bilateral
H33.109 Unspecified retinoschisis, unspecified eye
H33.11 Cyst of ora serrata
H33.111 Cyst of ora serrata, right eye
H33.112 Cyst of ora serrata, left eye
H33.113 Cyst of ora serrata, bilateral
H33.119 Cyst of ora serrata, unspecified eye
H33.12 Parasitic cyst of retina
H33.121 Parasitic cyst of retina, right eye
H33.122 Parasitic cyst of retina, left eye
H33.123 Parasitic cyst of retina, bilateral
H33.129 Parasitic cyst of retina, unspecified eye
H33.19 Other retinoschisis and retinal cysts
Pseudocyst of retina
H33.191 Other retinoschisis and retinal cysts, right eye
H33.192 Other retinoschisis and retinal cysts, left eye
H33.193 Other retinoschisis and retinal cysts, bilateral
H33.199 Other retinoschisis and retinal cysts, unspecified eye
H33.2 Serous retinal detachment
Retinal detachment NOS
Retinal detachment without retinal break
EXCLUDES1 *central serous chorioretinopathy (H35.71-)*
H33.20 Serous retinal detachment, unspecified eye
H33.21 Serous retinal detachment, right eye
H33.22 Serous retinal detachment, left eye
H33.23 Serous retinal detachment, bilateral
H33.3 Retinal breaks without detachment
EXCLUDES1 *chorioretinal scars after surgery for detachment (H59.81-)*
peripheral retinal degeneration without break (H35.4-)
H33.30 Unspecified retinal break
H33.301 Unspecified retinal break, right eye
H33.302 Unspecified retinal break, left eye
H33.303 Unspecified retinal break, bilateral
H33.309 Unspecified retinal break, unspecified eye
H33.31 Horseshoe tear of retina without detachment
Operculum of retina without detachment
H33.311 Horseshoe tear of retina without detachment, right eye
H33.312 Horseshoe tear of retina without detachment, left eye
H33.313 Horseshoe tear of retina without detachment, bilateral
H33.319 Horseshoe tear of retina without detachment, unspecified eye
H33.32 Round hole of retina without detachment
H33.321 Round hole, right eye
H33.322 Round hole, left eye
H33.323 Round hole, bilateral
H33.329 Round hole, unspecified eye
H33.33 Multiple defects of retina without detachment
H33.331 Multiple defects of retina without detachment, right eye
H33.332 Multiple defects of retina without detachment, left eye
H33.333 Multiple defects of retina without detachment, bilateral
H33.339 Multiple defects of retina without detachment, unspecified eye
H33.4 Traction detachment of retina
Proliferative vitreo-retinopathy with retinal detachment
H33.40 Traction detachment of retina, unspecified eye
H33.41 Traction detachment of retina, right eye
H33.42 Traction detachment of retina, left eye
H33.43 Traction detachment of retina, bilateral
H33.8 Other retinal detachments
H34 Retinal vascular occlusions
EXCLUDES1 *amaurosis fugax (G45.3)*
H34.0 Transient retinal artery occlusion
H34.00 Transient retinal artery occlusion, unspecified eye
H34.01 Transient retinal artery occlusion, right eye
H34.02 Transient retinal artery occlusion, left eye
H34.03 Transient retinal artery occlusion, bilateral
H34.1 Central retinal artery occlusion
H34.10 Central retinal artery occlusion, unspecified eye
H34.11 Central retinal artery occlusion, right eye
H34.12 Central retinal artery occlusion, left eye
H34.13 Central retinal artery occlusion, bilateral
H34.2 Other retinal artery occlusions
H34.21 Partial retinal artery occlusion
Hollenhorst's plaque
Retinal microembolism
H34.211 Partial retinal artery occlusion, right eye
H34.212 Partial retinal artery occlusion, left eye
H34.213 Partial retinal artery occlusion, bilateral
H34.219 Partial retinal artery occlusion, unspecified eye
H34.23 Retinal artery branch occlusion
H34.231 Retinal artery branch occlusion, right eye
H34.232 Retinal artery branch occlusion, left eye
H34.233 Retinal artery branch occlusion, bilateral
H34.239 Retinal artery branch occlusion, unspecified eye
H34.8 Other retinal vascular occlusions
H34.81 Central retinal vein occlusion
One of the following 7th characters is to be assigned to codes in subcategory H34.81 to designate the severity of the occlusion:
0 = with macular edema
1 = with retinal neovascularization
2 = stableOld central retinal vein occlusion
H34.811 Central retinal vein occlusion, right eye
H34.812 Central retinal vein occlusion, left eye
H34.813 Central retinal vein occlusion, bilateral
H34.819 Central retinal vein occlusion, unspecified eye
H34.82 Venous engorgement
Incipient retinal vein occlusion
Partial retinal vein occlusion
H34.821 Venous engorgement, right eye
H34.822 Venous engorgement, left eye
H34.823 Venous engorgement, bilateral
H34.829 Venous engorgement, unspecified eye
H34.83 Tributary (branch) retinal vein occlusion
One of the following 7th characters is to be assigned to codes in subcategory H34.83 to designate the severity of the occlusion:
0 = with macular edema
1 = with retinal neovascularization
2 = stableOld tributary (branch) retinal vein occlusion
H34.831 Tributary (branch) retinal vein occlusion, right eye
H34.832 Tributary (branch) retinal vein occlusion, left eye
H34.833 Tributary (branch) retinal vein occlusion, bilateral
H34.839 Tributary (branch) retinal vein occlusion, unspecified eye

Unspecified Code | Other Specified Code | Manifestation Code | N Newborn | P Pediatric | M Maternity | A Adult | ♂ Male | ♀ Female
● New Code | ▲ Revised Code Title | ►◄ Revised Text | NOTES | INCLUDES | EXCLUDES1 Not coded here | EXCLUDES2 Not included here
4th character required | 5th character required | 6th character required | 7th character required
Extension 'X' Alert | HAC Hospital-acquired condition (HAC) alert | AHA AHA Coding Clinic©

When symbols appear on a code that requires a 7th character extension, refer to Appendix D to identify applicable 7th character codes.

H34.9 Unspecified retinal vascular occlusion

H35 Other retinal disorders

EXCLUDES2 *diabetic retinal disorders (E08.311-E08.359, E09.311-E09.359, E10.311-E10.359, E11.311-E11.359, E13.311-E13.359)*

H35.0 Background retinopathy and retinal vascular changes
Code also any associated hypertension (I10.-)

H35.00 Unspecified background retinopathy

H35.01 Changes in retinal vascular appearance
Retinal vascular sheathing

H35.011 Changes in retinal vascular appearance, right eye
H35.012 Changes in retinal vascular appearance, left eye
H35.013 Changes in retinal vascular appearance, bilateral
H35.019 Changes in retinal vascular appearance, unspecified eye

H35.02 Exudative retinopathy
Coats retinopathy

H35.021 Exudative retinopathy, right eye
H35.022 Exudative retinopathy, left eye
H35.023 Exudative retinopathy, bilateral
H35.029 Exudative retinopathy, unspecified eye

H35.03 Hypertensive retinopathy

H35.031 Hypertensive retinopathy, right eye
H35.032 Hypertensive retinopathy, left eye
H35.033 Hypertensive retinopathy, bilateral
H35.039 Hypertensive retinopathy, unspecified eye

H35.04 Retinal micro-aneurysms, unspecified

H35.041 Retinal micro-aneurysms, unspecified, right eye
H35.042 Retinal micro-aneurysms, unspecified, left eye
H35.043 Retinal micro-aneurysms, unspecified, bilateral
H35.049 Retinal micro-aneurysms, unspecified, unspecified eye

H35.05 Retinal neovascularization, unspecified

H35.051 Retinal neovascularization, unspecified, right eye
H35.052 Retinal neovascularization, unspecified, left eye
H35.053 Retinal neovascularization, unspecified, bilateral
H35.059 Retinal neovascularization, unspecified, unspecified eye

H35.06 Retinal vasculitis
Eales disease
Retinal perivasculitis

H35.061 Retinal vasculitis, right eye
H35.062 Retinal vasculitis, left eye
H35.063 Retinal vasculitis, bilateral
H35.069 Retinal vasculitis, unspecified eye

H35.07 Retinal telangiectasis

H35.071 Retinal telangiectasis, right eye
H35.072 Retinal telangiectasis, left eye
H35.073 Retinal telangiectasis, bilateral
H35.079 Retinal telangiectasis, unspecified eye

H35.09 Other intraretinal microvascular abnormalities
Retinal varices

H35.1 Retinopathy of prematurity

H35.10 Retinopathy of prematurity, unspecified
Retinopathy of prematurity NOS

H35.101 Retinopathy of prematurity, unspecified, right eye
H35.102 Retinopathy of prematurity, unspecified, left eye
H35.103 Retinopathy of prematurity, unspecified, bilateral
H35.109 Retinopathy of prematurity, unspecified, unspecified eye

H35.11 Retinopathy of prematurity, stage 0

H35.111 Retinopathy of prematurity, stage 0, right eye
H35.112 Retinopathy of prematurity, stage 0, left eye
H35.113 Retinopathy of prematurity, stage 0, bilateral
H35.119 Retinopathy of prematurity, stage 0, unspecified eye

H35.12 Retinopathy of prematurity, stage 1

H35.121 Retinopathy of prematurity, stage 1, right eye
H35.122 Retinopathy of prematurity, stage 1, left eye
H35.123 Retinopathy of prematurity, stage 1, bilateral
H35.129 Retinopathy of prematurity, stage 1, unspecified eye

H35.13 Retinopathy of prematurity, stage 2

H35.131 Retinopathy of prematurity, stage 2, right eye
H35.132 Retinopathy of prematurity, stage 2, left eye
H35.133 Retinopathy of prematurity, stage 2, bilateral
H35.139 Retinopathy of prematurity, stage 2, unspecified eye

H35.14 Retinopathy of prematurity, stage 3

H35.141 Retinopathy of prematurity, stage 3, right eye
H35.142 Retinopathy of prematurity, stage 3, left eye
H35.143 Retinopathy of prematurity, stage 3, bilateral
H35.149 Retinopathy of prematurity, stage 3, unspecified eye

H35.15 Retinopathy of prematurity, stage 4

H35.151 Retinopathy of prematurity, stage 4, right eye
H35.152 Retinopathy of prematurity, stage 4, left eye
H35.153 Retinopathy of prematurity, stage 4, bilateral
H35.159 Retinopathy of prematurity, stage 4, unspecified eye

H35.16 Retinopathy of prematurity, stage 5

H35.161 Retinopathy of prematurity, stage 5, right eye
H35.162 Retinopathy of prematurity, stage 5, left eye
H35.163 Retinopathy of prematurity, stage 5, bilateral
H35.169 Retinopathy of prematurity, stage 5, unspecified eye

H35.17 Retrolental fibroplasia

H35.171 Retrolental fibroplasia, right eye
H35.172 Retrolental fibroplasia, left eye
H35.173 Retrolental fibroplasia, bilateral
H35.179 Retrolental fibroplasia, unspecified eye

H35.2 Other non-diabetic proliferative retinopathy
Proliferative vitreo-retinopathy

EXCLUDES1 *proliferative vitreo-retinopathy with retinal detachment (H33.4-)*

H35.20 Other non-diabetic proliferative retinopathy, unspecified eye
H35.21 Other non-diabetic proliferative retinopathy, right eye
H35.22 Other non-diabetic proliferative retinopathy, left eye
H35.23 Other non-diabetic proliferative retinopathy, bilateral

H35.3 Degeneration of macula and posterior pole

H35.30 Unspecified macular degeneration
Age-related macular degeneration

Unacceptable principal diagnosis symbol per Medicare code edits — Code exempt from diagnosis present on admission requirement — Questionable admission — Complication or comorbidity — CC/MCC exclusion — Major complication or comorbidity — Principal diagnosis as its own CC — Principal diagnosis as its own MCC — Z code as first-listed diagnosis

When symbols appear on a code that requires a 7th character extension, refer to Appendix D to identify applicable 7th character codes.

H35.31 Nonexudative age-related macular degeneration
Atrophic age-related macular degeneration
Dry age-related macular degeneration
One of the following 7th characters is to be assigned to codes in subcategory H35.31 to designate the stage of the disease:
0 = stage unspecified
1 = early dry stage
2 = intermediate dry stage
3 = advanced atrophic without subfoveal involvementadvanced dry stage
4 = advanced atrophic with subfoveal involvement
● H35.311 Nonexudative age-related macular degeneration, right eye
● H35.312 Nonexudative age-related macular degeneration, left eye
● H35.313 Nonexudative age-related macular degeneration, bilateral
● H35.319 Nonexudative age-related macular degeneration, unspecified eye
H35.32 Exudative age-related macular degeneration
Wet age-related macular degeneration
One of the following 7th characters is to be assigned to codes in subcategory H35.32 to designate the stage of the disease:
0 = stage unspecified
1 = with active choroidal neovascularization
2 = with inactive choroidal neovascularization with involuted or regressed neovascularization
3 = with inactive scar
● H35.321 Exudative age-related macular degeneration, right eye
● H35.322 Exudative age-related macular degeneration, left eye
● H35.323 Exudative age-related macular degeneration, bilateral
● H35.329 Exudative age-related macular degeneration, unspecified eye
H35.33 Angioid streaks of macula
H35.34 Macular cyst, hole, or pseudohole
H35.341 Macular cyst, hole, or pseudohole, right eye
H35.342 Macular cyst, hole, or pseudohole, left eye
H35.343 Macular cyst, hole, or pseudohole, bilateral
H35.349 Macular cyst, hole, or pseudohole, unspecified eye
H35.35 Cystoid macular degeneration
EXCLUDES1 *cystoid macular edema following cataract surgery (H59.03-)*
H35.351 Cystoid macular degeneration, right eye
H35.352 Cystoid macular degeneration, left eye
H35.353 Cystoid macular degeneration, bilateral
H35.359 Cystoid macular degeneration, unspecified eye
H35.36 Drusen (degenerative) of macula
H35.361 Drusen (degenerative) of macula, right eye
H35.362 Drusen (degenerative) of macula, left eye
H35.363 Drusen (degenerative) of macula, bilateral
H35.369 Drusen (degenerative) of macula, unspecified eye
H35.37 Puckering of macula
H35.371 Puckering of macula, right eye
H35.372 Puckering of macula, left eye
H35.373 Puckering of macula, bilateral
H35.379 Puckering of macula, unspecified eye
H35.38 Toxic maculopathy
Code first poisoning due to drug or toxin, if applicable (T36-T65 with fifth or sixth character 1-4 or 6)
Use additional code for adverse effect, if applicable, to identify drug (T36-T50 with fifth or sixth character 5)
H35.381 Toxic maculopathy, right eye
H35.382 Toxic maculopathy, left eye
H35.383 Toxic maculopathy, bilateral
H35.389 Toxic maculopathy, unspecified eye
H35.4 Peripheral retinal degeneration
EXCLUDES1 *hereditary retinal degeneration (dystrophy) (H35.5-)*
peripheral retinal degeneration with retinal break (H33.3-)
H35.40 Unspecified peripheral retinal degeneration
H35.41 Lattice degeneration of retina
Palisade degeneration of retina
H35.411 Lattice degeneration of retina, right eye
H35.412 Lattice degeneration of retina, left eye
H35.413 Lattice degeneration of retina, bilateral
H35.419 Lattice degeneration of retina, unspecified eye
H35.42 Microcystoid degeneration of retina
H35.421 Microcystoid degeneration of retina, right eye
H35.422 Microcystoid degeneration of retina, left eye
H35.423 Microcystoid degeneration of retina, bilateral
H35.429 Microcystoid degeneration of retina, unspecified eye
H35.43 Paving stone degeneration of retina
H35.431 Paving stone degeneration of retina, right eye
H35.432 Paving stone degeneration of retina, left eye
H35.433 Paving stone degeneration of retina, bilateral
H35.439 Paving stone degeneration of retina, unspecified eye
H35.44 Age-related reticular degeneration of retina
H35.441 Age-related reticular degeneration of retina, right eye A
H35.442 Age-related reticular degeneration of retina, left eye A
H35.443 Age-related reticular degeneration of retina, bilateral A
H35.449 Age-related reticular degeneration of retina, unspecified eye A
H35.45 Secondary pigmentary degeneration
H35.451 Secondary pigmentary degeneration, right eye
H35.452 Secondary pigmentary degeneration, left eye
H35.453 Secondary pigmentary degeneration, bilateral
H35.459 Secondary pigmentary degeneration, unspecified eye
H35.46 Secondary vitreoretinal degeneration
H35.461 Secondary vitreoretinal degeneration, right eye
H35.462 Secondary vitreoretinal degeneration, left eye
H35.463 Secondary vitreoretinal degeneration, bilateral
H35.469 Secondary vitreoretinal degeneration, unspecified eye
H35.5 Hereditary retinal dystrophy
EXCLUDES1 *dystrophies primarily involving Bruch's membrane (H31.1-)*
H35.50 Unspecified hereditary retinal dystrophy
H35.51 Vitreoretinal dystrophy
H35.52 Pigmentary retinal dystrophy
Albipunctate retinal dystrophy
Retinitis pigmentosa
Tapetoretinal dystrophy
H35.53 Other dystrophies primarily involving the sensory retina
Stargardt's disease

Unspecified Code | Other Specified Code | Manifestation Code | N Newborn | P Pediatric | M Maternity | A Adult | ♂ Male | ♀ Female
● New Code | ▲ Revised Code Title | ►◄ Revised Text | NOTES | INCLUDES | EXCLUDES1 Not coded here | EXCLUDES2 Not included here
4th character required | 5th character required | 6th character required | 7th character required
Extension 'X' Alert | HAC Hospital-acquired condition (HAC) alert | AHA AHA Coding Clinic©

H35.54 Dystrophies primarily involving the retinal pigment epithelium
Vitelliform retinal dystrophy

H35.6 Retinal hemorrhage
H35.60 Retinal hemorrhage, unspecified eye
H35.61 Retinal hemorrhage, right eye
H35.62 Retinal hemorrhage, left eye
H35.63 Retinal hemorrhage, bilateral

H35.7 Separation of retinal layers
EXCLUDES1 *retinal detachment (serous) (H33.2-)*
rhegmatogenous retinal detachment (H33.0-)
H35.70 Unspecified separation of retinal layers CC
H35.71 Central serous chorioretinopathy
H35.711 Central serous chorioretinopathy, right eye
H35.712 Central serous chorioretinopathy, left eye
H35.713 Central serous chorioretinopathy, bilateral
H35.719 Central serous chorioretinopathy, unspecified eye
H35.72 Serous detachment of retinal pigment epithelium
H35.721 Serous detachment of retinal pigment epithelium, right eye CC
H35.722 Serous detachment of retinal pigment epithelium, left eye CC
H35.723 Serous detachment of retinal pigment epithelium, bilateral CC
H35.729 Serous detachment of retinal pigment epithelium, unspecified eye CC
H35.73 Hemorrhagic detachment of retinal pigment epithelium
H35.731 Hemorrhagic detachment of retinal pigment epithelium, right eye CC
H35.732 Hemorrhagic detachment of retinal pigment epithelium, left eye CC
H35.733 Hemorrhagic detachment of retinal pigment epithelium, bilateral CC
H35.739 Hemorrhagic detachment of retinal pigment epithelium, unspecified eye CC

H35.8 Other specified retinal disorders
EXCLUDES2 *retinal hemorrhage (H35.6-)*
H35.81 Retinal edema
Retinal cotton wool spots
H35.82 Retinal ischemia CC
H35.89 Other specified retinal disorders

H35.9 Unspecified retinal disorder

H36 Retinal disorders in diseases classified elsewhere
Code first underlying disease, such as:
lipid storage disorders (E75.-)
sickle-cell disorders (D57.-)
EXCLUDES1 *arteriosclerotic retinopathy (H35.0-)*
diabetic retinopathy (E08.3-, E09.3-, E10.3-, E11.3-, E13.3-)

Glaucoma (H40-H42)

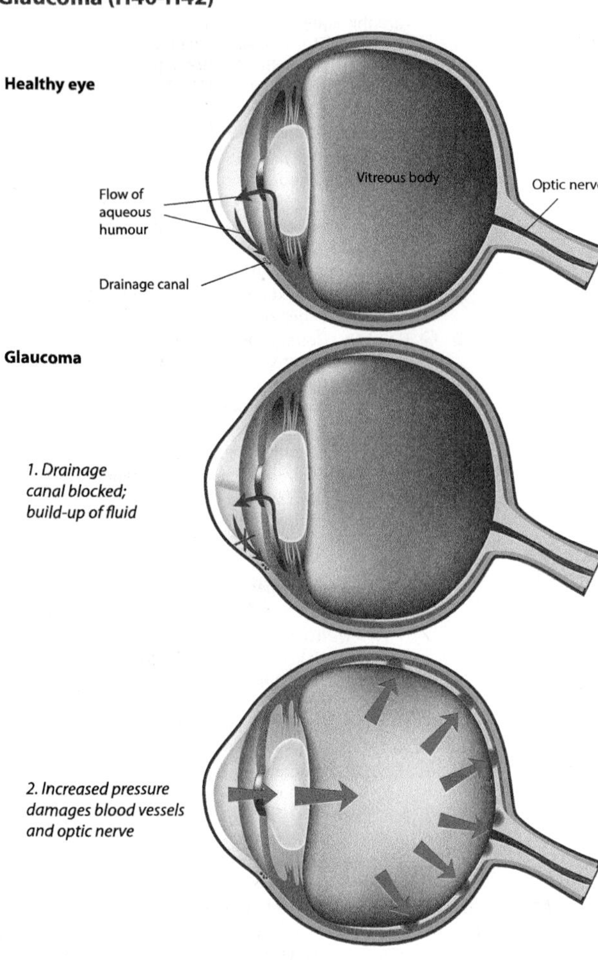

Figure 7.4 Development of glaucoma

H40 Glaucoma
EXCLUDES1 *absolute glaucoma (H44.51-)*
congenital glaucoma (Q15.0)
traumatic glaucoma due to birth injury (P15.3)

H40.0 Glaucoma suspect
H40.00 Preglaucoma, unspecified
H40.001 Preglaucoma, unspecified, right eye
H40.002 Preglaucoma, unspecified, left eye
H40.003 Preglaucoma, unspecified, bilateral
H40.009 Preglaucoma, unspecified, unspecified eye
H40.01 Open angle with borderline findings, low risk
Open angle, low risk
H40.011 Open angle with borderline findings, low risk, right eye
H40.012 Open angle with borderline findings, low risk, left eye
H40.013 Open angle with borderline findings, low risk, bilateral
H40.019 Open angle with borderline findings, low risk, unspecified eye
H40.02 Open angle with borderline findings, high risk
Open angle, high risk
H40.021 Open angle with borderline findings, high risk, right eye
H40.022 Open angle with borderline findings, high risk, left eye
H40.023 Open angle with borderline findings, high risk, bilateral

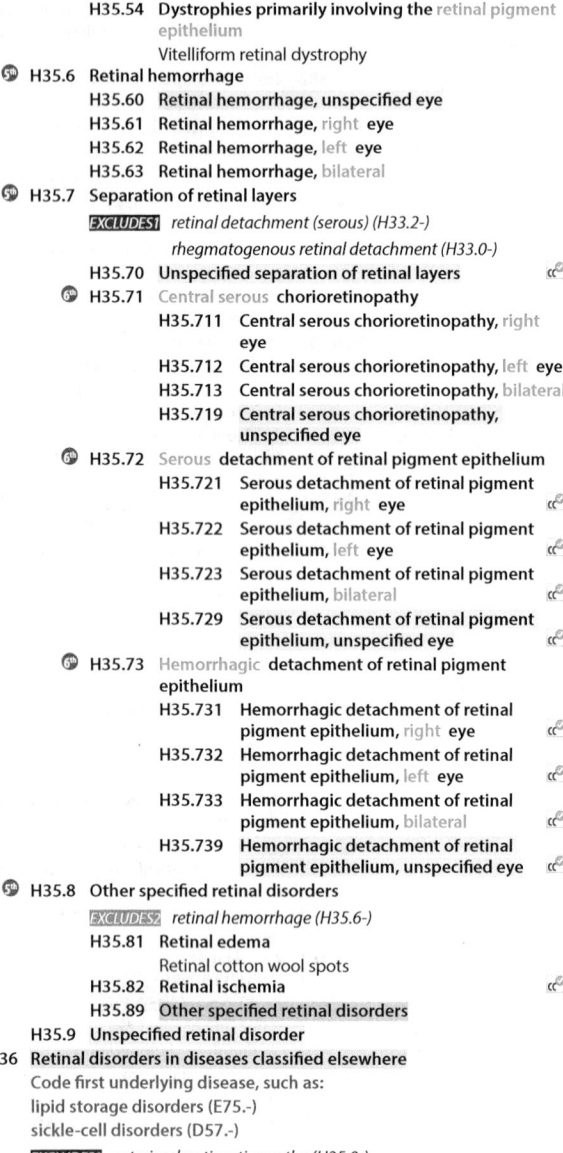

Unacceptable principal diagnosis symbol per Medicare code edits · Code exempt from diagnosis present on admission requirement
Questionable admission · Complication or comorbidity · CC/MCC exclusion · Major complication or comorbidity
Principal diagnosis as its own CC · Principal diagnosis as its own MCC · Z code as first-listed diagnosis

When symbols appear on a code that requires a 7th character extension, refer to Appendix D to identify applicable 7th character codes.

H40.029 Open angle with borderline findings, high risk, unspecified eye

H40.03 Anatomical narrow angle
Primary angle closure suspect
H40.031 Anatomical narrow angle, right eye
H40.032 Anatomical narrow angle, left eye
H40.033 Anatomical narrow angle, bilateral
H40.039 Anatomical narrow angle, unspecified eye

H40.04 Steroid responder
H40.041 Steroid responder, right eye
H40.042 Steroid responder, left eye
H40.043 Steroid responder, bilateral
H40.049 Steroid responder, unspecified eye

H40.05 Ocular hypertension
H40.051 Ocular hypertension, right eye
H40.052 Ocular hypertension, left eye
H40.053 Ocular hypertension, bilateral
H40.059 Ocular hypertension, unspecified eye

H40.06 Primary angle closure without glaucoma damage
H40.061 Primary angle closure without glaucoma damage, right eye
H40.062 Primary angle closure without glaucoma damage, left eye
H40.063 Primary angle closure without glaucoma damage, bilateral
H40.069 Primary angle closure without glaucoma damage, unspecified eye

H40.1 Open-angle glaucoma

H40.10 Unspecified open-angle glaucoma
One of the following 7th characters is to be assigned to code H40.10 to designate the stage of glaucoma
0 = stage unspecified
1 = mild stage
2 = moderate stage
3 = severe stage
4 = indeterminate stage

H40.11 Primary open-angle glaucoma
Chronic simple glaucoma
One of the following 7th characters is to be assigned to ▶each code in subcategory◀ H40.11 to designate the stage of glaucoma
0 = stage unspecified
1 = mild stage
2 = moderate stage
3 = severe stage
4 = indeterminate stage
● H40.111 Primary open-angle glaucoma, right eye
● H40.112 Primary open-angle glaucoma, left eye
● H40.113 Primary open-angle glaucoma, bilateral
● H40.119 Primary open-angle glaucoma, unspecified eye

H40.12 Low-tension glaucoma
One of the following 7th characters is to be assigned to each code in subcategory H40.12 to designate the stage of glaucoma
0 = stage unspecified
1 = mild stage
2 = moderate stage
3 = severe stage
4 = indeterminate stage
H40.121 Low-tension glaucoma, right eye PDx
H40.122 Low-tension glaucoma, left eye PDx
H40.123 Low-tension glaucoma, bilateral PDx
H40.129 Low-tension glaucoma, unspecified eye PDx

H40.13 Pigmentary glaucoma
One of the following 7th characters is to be assigned to each code in subcategory H40.13 to designate the stage of glaucoma
0 = stage unspecified
1 = mild stage
2 = moderate stage
3 = severe stage
4 = indeterminate stage
H40.131 Pigmentary glaucoma, right eye PDx
H40.132 Pigmentary glaucoma, left eye PDx
H40.133 Pigmentary glaucoma, bilateral PDx
H40.139 Pigmentary glaucoma, unspecified eye PDx

H40.14 Capsular glaucoma with pseudoexfoliation of lens
One of the following 7th characters is to be assigned to each code in subcategory H40.14 to designate the stage of glaucoma
0 = stage unspecified
1 = mild stage
2 = moderate stage
3 = severe stage
4 = indeterminate stage
H40.141 Capsular glaucoma with pseudoexfoliation of lens, right eye
H40.142 Capsular glaucoma with pseudoexfoliation of lens, left eye
H40.143 Capsular glaucoma with pseudoexfoliation of lens, bilateral
H40.149 Capsular glaucoma with pseudoexfoliation of lens, unspecified eye

H40.15 Residual stage of open-angle glaucoma
H40.151 Residual stage of open-angle glaucoma, right eye PDx
H40.152 Residual stage of open-angle glaucoma, left eye PDx
H40.153 Residual stage of open-angle glaucoma, bilateral PDx
H40.159 Residual stage of open-angle glaucoma, unspecified eye PDx

H40.2 Primary angle-closure glaucoma
EXCLUDES1 *aqueous misdirection (H40.83-)*
malignant glaucoma (H40.83-)

H40.20 Unspecified primary angle-closure glaucoma
One of the following 7th characters is to be assigned to code H40.20 to designate the stage of glaucoma
0 = stage unspecified
1 = mild stage
2 = moderate stage
3 = severe stage
4 = indeterminate stage

H40.21 Acute angle-closure glaucoma
Acute angle-closure glaucoma attack
Acute angle-closure glaucoma crisis
H40.211 Acute angle-closure glaucoma, right eye CC
H40.212 Acute angle-closure glaucoma, left eye CC
H40.213 Acute angle-closure glaucoma, bilateral CC
H40.219 Acute angle-closure glaucoma, unspecified eye CC

H40.22 Chronic angle-closure glaucoma
Chronic primary angle closure glaucoma
One of the following 7th characters is to be assigned to each code in subcategory H40.22 to designate the stage of glaucoma
0 = stage unspecified
1 = mild stage
2 = moderate stage
3 = severe stage
4 = indeterminate stage
H40.221 Chronic angle-closure glaucoma, right eye
H40.222 Chronic angle-closure glaucoma, left eye
H40.223 Chronic angle-closure glaucoma, bilateral
H40.229 Chronic angle-closure glaucoma, unspecified eye

H40.23 Intermittent angle-closure glaucoma
H40.231 Intermittent angle-closure glaucoma, right eye
H40.232 Intermittent angle-closure glaucoma, left eye
H40.233 Intermittent angle-closure glaucoma, bilateral

Unspecified Code Other Specified Code Manifestation Code N Newborn P Pediatric M Maternity A Adult ♂ Male ♀ Female
● New Code ▲ Revised Code Title ▶◀ Revised Text NOTES INCLUDES EXCLUDES1 Not coded here EXCLUDES2 Not included here
4th character required 5th character required 6th character required 7th character required
Extension 'X' Alert HAC Hospital-acquired condition (HAC) alert AHA AHA Coding Clinic©

H40.239 Intermittent angle-closure glaucoma, unspecified eye

H40.24 Residual stage of angle-closure glaucoma

H40.241 Residual stage of angle-closure glaucoma, right eye

H40.242 Residual stage of angle-closure glaucoma, left eye

H40.243 Residual stage of angle-closure glaucoma, bilateral

H40.249 Residual stage of angle-closure glaucoma, unspecified eye

H40.3 Glaucoma secondary to eye trauma

Code also underlying condition

One of the following 7th characters is to be assigned to each code in subcategory H40.3 to designate the stage of glaucoma

0 = stage unspecified
1 = mild stage
2 = moderate stage
3 = severe stage
4 = indeterminate stage

H40.30 Glaucoma secondary to eye trauma, unspecified eye

H40.31 Glaucoma secondary to eye trauma, right eye

H40.32 Glaucoma secondary to eye trauma, left eye

H40.33 Glaucoma secondary to eye trauma, bilateral

H40.4 Glaucoma secondary to eye inflammation

Code also underlying condition

One of the following 7th characters is to be assigned to each code in subcategory H40.4 to designate the stage of glaucoma

0 = stage unspecified
1 = mild stage
2 = moderate stage
3 = severe stage
4 = indeterminate stage

H40.40 Glaucoma secondary to eye inflammation, unspecified eye

H40.41 Glaucoma secondary to eye inflammation, right eye

H40.42 Glaucoma secondary to eye inflammation, left eye

H40.43 Glaucoma secondary to eye inflammation, bilateral

H40.5 Glaucoma secondary to other eye disorders

Code also underlying eye disorder

One of the following 7th characters is to be assigned to each code in subcategory H40.5 to designate the stage of glaucoma

0 = stage unspecified
1 = mild stage
2 = moderate stage
3 = severe stage
4 = indeterminate stage

H40.50 Glaucoma secondary to other eye disorders, unspecified eye

H40.51 Glaucoma secondary to other eye disorders, right eye

H40.52 Glaucoma secondary to other eye disorders, left eye

H40.53 Glaucoma secondary to other eye disorders, bilateral

H40.6 Glaucoma secondary to drugs

Use additional code for adverse effect, if applicable, to identify drug (T36-T50 with fifth or sixth character 5)

One of the following 7th characters is to be assigned to each code in subcategory H40.6 to designate the stage of glaucoma

0 = stage unspecified
1 = mild stage
2 = moderate stage
3 = severe stage
4 = indeterminate stage

H40.60 Glaucoma secondary to drugs, unspecified eye

H40.61 Glaucoma secondary to drugs, right eye

H40.62 Glaucoma secondary to drugs, left eye

H40.63 Glaucoma secondary to drugs, bilateral

H40.8 Other glaucoma

H40.81 Glaucoma with increased episcleral venous pressure

H40.811 Glaucoma with increased episcleral venous pressure, right eye

H40.812 Glaucoma with increased episcleral venous pressure, left eye

H40.813 Glaucoma with increased episcleral venous pressure, bilateral

H40.819 Glaucoma with increased episcleral venous pressure, unspecified eye

H40.82 Hypersecretion glaucoma

H40.821 Hypersecretion glaucoma, right eye

H40.822 Hypersecretion glaucoma, left eye

H40.823 Hypersecretion glaucoma, bilateral

H40.829 Hypersecretion glaucoma, unspecified eye

H40.83 Aqueous misdirection

Malignant glaucoma

H40.831 Aqueous misdirection, right eye

H40.832 Aqueous misdirection, left eye

H40.833 Aqueous misdirection, bilateral

H40.839 Aqueous misdirection, unspecified eye

H40.89 Other specified glaucoma

H40.9 Unspecified glaucoma

H42 Glaucoma in diseases classified elsewhere

Code first underlying condition, such as:
amyloidosis (E85.-)
aniridia (Q13.1)
Lowe's syndrome (E72.03)
Reiger's anomaly (Q13.81)
specified metabolic disorder (E70-E88)

EXCLUDES1 *glaucoma (in) ►onchocerciasis (B73.02)◄*
►glaucoma (in)◄ syphilis (A52.71)
►glaucoma (in)◄ tuberculous (A18.59)

EXCLUDES2 *glaucoma (in) diabetes mellitus (E08.39, E09.39, E10.39, E11.39, E13.39)*

Disorders of vitreous body and globe (H43-H44)

H43 Disorders of vitreous body

H43.0 Vitreous prolapse

EXCLUDES1 *vitreous syndrome following cataract surgery (H59.0-)*
traumatic vitreous prolapse (S05.2-)

H43.00 Vitreous prolapse, unspecified eye

H43.01 Vitreous prolapse, right eye

H43.02 Vitreous prolapse, left eye

H43.03 Vitreous prolapse, bilateral

H43.1 Vitreous hemorrhage

H43.10 Vitreous hemorrhage, unspecified eye

H43.11 Vitreous hemorrhage, right eye

H43.12 Vitreous hemorrhage, left eye

H43.13 Vitreous hemorrhage, bilateral

H43.2 Crystalline deposits in vitreous body

H43.20 Crystalline deposits in vitreous body, unspecified eye

H43.21 Crystalline deposits in vitreous body, right eye

H43.22 Crystalline deposits in vitreous body, left eye

H43.23 Crystalline deposits in vitreous body, bilateral

H43.3 Other vitreous opacities

H43.31 Vitreous membranes and strands

H43.311 Vitreous membranes and strands, right eye

H43.312 Vitreous membranes and strands, left eye

H43.313 Vitreous membranes and strands, bilateral

H43.319 Vitreous membranes and strands, unspecified eye

H43.39 Other vitreous opacities

Vitreous floaters

H43.391 Other vitreous opacities, right eye

H43.392 Other vitreous opacities, left eye

H43.393 Other vitreous opacities, bilateral

H43.399 Other vitreous opacities, unspecified eye

H43.8 Other disorders of vitreous body

EXCLUDES1 *proliferative vitreo-retinopathy with retinal detachment (H33.4-)*

EXCLUDES2 *vitreous abscess (H44.02-)*

Unacceptable principal diagnosis symbol per Medicare code edits; Code exempt from diagnosis present on admission requirement; Questionable admission; Complication or comorbidity; CC/MCC exclusion; Major complication or comorbidity; Principal diagnosis as its own CC; Principal diagnosis as its own MCC; Z code as first-listed diagnosis

When symbols appear on a code that requires a 7th character extension, refer to Appendix D to identify applicable 7th character codes.

H43.81 Vitreous degeneration
Vitreous detachment
H43.811 Vitreous degeneration, right eye
H43.812 Vitreous degeneration, left eye
H43.813 Vitreous degeneration, bilateral
H43.819 Vitreous degeneration, unspecified eye
H43.82 Vitreomacular adhesion
Vitreomacular traction
H43.821 Vitreomacular adhesion, right eye A
H43.822 Vitreomacular adhesion, left eye A
H43.823 Vitreomacular adhesion, bilateral A
H43.829 Vitreomacular adhesion, unspecified eye A
H43.89 Other disorders of vitreous body
H43.9 Unspecified disorder of vitreous body
H44 Disorders of globe
INCLUDES *disorders affecting multiple structures of eye*
H44.0 Purulent endophthalmitis
Use additional code to identify organism
EXCLUDES1 *bleb associated endophthalmitis (H59.4-)*
H44.00 Unspecified purulent endophthalmitis
H44.001 Unspecified purulent endophthalmitis, right eye
H44.002 Unspecified purulent endophthalmitis, left eye
H44.003 Unspecified purulent endophthalmitis, bilateral
H44.009 Unspecified purulent endophthalmitis, unspecified eye
H44.01 Panophthalmitis (acute)
H44.011 Panophthalmitis (acute), right eye
H44.012 Panophthalmitis (acute), left eye
H44.013 Panophthalmitis (acute), bilateral
H44.019 Panophthalmitis (acute), unspecified eye
H44.02 Vitreous abscess (chronic)
H44.021 Vitreous abscess (chronic), right eye
H44.022 Vitreous abscess (chronic), left eye
H44.023 Vitreous abscess (chronic), bilateral
H44.029 Vitreous abscess (chronic), unspecified eye
H44.1 Other endophthalmitis
EXCLUDES1 *bleb associated endophthalmitis (H59.4-)*
EXCLUDES2 *ophthalmia nodosa (H16.2-)*
H44.11 Panuveitis
H44.111 Panuveitis, right eye
H44.112 Panuveitis, left eye
H44.113 Panuveitis, bilateral
H44.119 Panuveitis, unspecified eye
H44.12 Parasitic endophthalmitis, unspecified
H44.121 Parasitic endophthalmitis, unspecified, right eye
H44.122 Parasitic endophthalmitis, unspecified, left eye
H44.123 Parasitic endophthalmitis, unspecified, bilateral
H44.129 Parasitic endophthalmitis, unspecified, unspecified eye
H44.13 Sympathetic uveitis
H44.131 Sympathetic uveitis, right eye
H44.132 Sympathetic uveitis, left eye
H44.133 Sympathetic uveitis, bilateral
H44.139 Sympathetic uveitis, unspecified eye
H44.19 Other endophthalmitis
H44.2 Degenerative myopia
Malignant myopia
H44.20 Degenerative myopia, unspecified eye
H44.21 Degenerative myopia, right eye
H44.22 Degenerative myopia, left eye
H44.23 Degenerative myopia, bilateral
H44.3 Other and unspecified degenerative disorders of globe
H44.30 Unspecified degenerative disorder of globe
H44.31 Chalcosis
H44.311 Chalcosis, right eye
H44.312 Chalcosis, left eye
H44.313 Chalcosis, bilateral
H44.319 Chalcosis, unspecified eye
H44.32 Siderosis of eye
H44.321 Siderosis of eye, right eye
H44.322 Siderosis of eye, left eye
H44.323 Siderosis of eye, bilateral
H44.329 Siderosis of eye, unspecified eye
H44.39 Other degenerative disorders of globe
H44.391 Other degenerative disorders of globe, right eye
H44.392 Other degenerative disorders of globe, left eye
H44.393 Other degenerative disorders of globe, bilateral
H44.399 Other degenerative disorders of globe, unspecified eye
H44.4 Hypotony of eye
H44.40 Unspecified hypotony of eye
H44.41 Flat anterior chamber hypotony of eye
H44.411 Flat anterior chamber hypotony of right eye
H44.412 Flat anterior chamber hypotony of left eye
H44.413 Flat anterior chamber hypotony of eye, bilateral
H44.419 Flat anterior chamber hypotony of unspecified eye
H44.42 Hypotony of eye due to ocular fistula
H44.421 Hypotony of right eye due to ocular fistula
H44.422 Hypotony of left eye due to ocular fistula
H44.423 Hypotony of eye due to ocular fistula, bilateral
H44.429 Hypotony of unspecified eye due to ocular fistula
H44.43 Hypotony of eye due to other ocular disorders
H44.431 Hypotony of eye due to other ocular disorders, right eye
H44.432 Hypotony of eye due to other ocular disorders, left eye
H44.433 Hypotony of eye due to other ocular disorders, bilateral
H44.439 Hypotony of eye due to other ocular disorders, unspecified eye
H44.44 Primary hypotony of eye
H44.441 Primary hypotony of right eye
H44.442 Primary hypotony of left eye
H44.443 Primary hypotony of eye, bilateral
H44.449 Primary hypotony of unspecified eye
H44.5 Degenerated conditions of globe
H44.50 Unspecified degenerated conditions of globe
H44.51 Absolute glaucoma
H44.511 Absolute glaucoma, right eye
H44.512 Absolute glaucoma, left eye
H44.513 Absolute glaucoma, bilateral
H44.519 Absolute glaucoma, unspecified eye
H44.52 Atrophy of globe
Phthisis bulbi
H44.521 Atrophy of globe, right eye
H44.522 Atrophy of globe, left eye
H44.523 Atrophy of globe, bilateral
H44.529 Atrophy of globe, unspecified eye
H44.53 Leucocoria
H44.531 Leucocoria, right eye
H44.532 Leucocoria, left eye
H44.533 Leucocoria, bilateral
H44.539 Leucocoria, unspecified eye

Unspecified Code Other Specified Code Manifestation Code N Newborn P Pediatric M Maternity A Adult ♂ Male ♀ Female
● New Code ▲ Revised Code Title ►◄ Revised Text NOTES INCLUDES EXCLUDES1 Not coded here EXCLUDES2 Not included here
4th character required 5th character required 6th character required 7th character required
Extension 'X' Alert HAC Hospital-acquired condition (HAC) alert AHA AHA Coding Clinic©

H44.6 Retained (old) intraocular foreign body, magnetic
Use additional code to identify magnetic foreign body (Z18.11)
EXCLUDES1 *current intraocular foreign body (S05.-)*
EXCLUDES2 *retained foreign body in eyelid (H02.81-)*
retained (old) foreign body following penetrating wound of orbit (H05.5-)
retained (old) intraocular foreign body, nonmagnetic (H44.7-)

H44.60 Unspecified retained (old) intraocular foreign body, magnetic
- H44.601 Unspecified retained (old) intraocular foreign body, magnetic, right eye
- H44.602 Unspecified retained (old) intraocular foreign body, magnetic, left eye
- H44.603 Unspecified retained (old) intraocular foreign body, magnetic, bilateral
- H44.609 Unspecified retained (old) intraocular foreign body, magnetic, unspecified eye

H44.61 Retained (old) magnetic foreign body in anterior chamber
- H44.611 Retained (old) magnetic foreign body in anterior chamber, right eye
- H44.612 Retained (old) magnetic foreign body in anterior chamber, left eye
- H44.613 Retained (old) magnetic foreign body in anterior chamber, bilateral
- H44.619 Retained (old) magnetic foreign body in anterior chamber, unspecified eye

H44.62 Retained (old) magnetic foreign body in iris or ciliary body
- H44.621 Retained (old) magnetic foreign body in iris or ciliary body, right eye
- H44.622 Retained (old) magnetic foreign body in iris or ciliary body, left eye
- H44.623 Retained (old) magnetic foreign body in iris or ciliary body, bilateral
- H44.629 Retained (old) magnetic foreign body in iris or ciliary body, unspecified eye

H44.63 Retained (old) magnetic foreign body in lens
- H44.631 Retained (old) magnetic foreign body in lens, right eye
- H44.632 Retained (old) magnetic foreign body in lens, left eye
- H44.633 Retained (old) magnetic foreign body in lens, bilateral
- H44.639 Retained (old) magnetic foreign body in lens, unspecified eye

H44.64 Retained (old) magnetic foreign body in posterior wall of globe
- H44.641 Retained (old) magnetic foreign body in posterior wall of globe, right eye
- H44.642 Retained (old) magnetic foreign body in posterior wall of globe, left eye
- H44.643 Retained (old) magnetic foreign body in posterior wall of globe, bilateral
- H44.649 Retained (old) magnetic foreign body in posterior wall of globe, unspecified eye

H44.65 Retained (old) magnetic foreign body in vitreous body
- H44.651 Retained (old) magnetic foreign body in vitreous body, right eye
- H44.652 Retained (old) magnetic foreign body in vitreous body, left eye
- H44.653 Retained (old) magnetic foreign body in vitreous body, bilateral
- H44.659 Retained (old) magnetic foreign body in vitreous body, unspecified eye

H44.69 Retained (old) intraocular foreign body, magnetic, in other or multiple sites
- H44.691 Retained (old) intraocular foreign body, magnetic, in other or multiple sites, right eye
- H44.692 Retained (old) intraocular foreign body, magnetic, in other or multiple sites, left eye
- H44.693 Retained (old) intraocular foreign body, magnetic, in other or multiple sites, bilateral
- H44.699 Retained (old) intraocular foreign body, magnetic, in other or multiple sites, unspecified eye

H44.7 Retained (old) intraocular foreign body, nonmagnetic
Use additional code to identify nonmagnetic foreign body (Z18.01-Z18.10, Z18.12, Z18.2-Z18.9)
EXCLUDES1 *current intraocular foreign body (S05.-)*
EXCLUDES2 *retained foreign body in eyelid (H02.81-)*
retained (old) foreign body following penetrating wound of orbit (H05.5-)
retained (old) intraocular foreign body, magnetic (H44.6-)

H44.70 Unspecified retained (old) intraocular foreign body, nonmagnetic
- H44.701 Unspecified retained (old) intraocular foreign body, nonmagnetic, right eye
- H44.702 Unspecified retained (old) intraocular foreign body, nonmagnetic, left eye
- H44.703 Unspecified retained (old) intraocular foreign body, nonmagnetic, bilateral
- H44.709 Unspecified retained (old) intraocular foreign body, nonmagnetic, unspecified eye
  Retained (old) intraocular foreign body NOS

H44.71 Retained (nonmagnetic) (old) foreign body in anterior chamber
- H44.711 Retained (nonmagnetic) (old) foreign body in anterior chamber, right eye
- H44.712 Retained (nonmagnetic) (old) foreign body in anterior chamber, left eye
- H44.713 Retained (nonmagnetic) (old) foreign body in anterior chamber, bilateral
- H44.719 Retained (nonmagnetic) (old) foreign body in anterior chamber, unspecified eye

H44.72 Retained (nonmagnetic) (old) foreign body in iris or ciliary body
- H44.721 Retained (nonmagnetic) (old) foreign body in iris or ciliary body, right eye
- H44.722 Retained (nonmagnetic) (old) foreign body in iris or ciliary body, left eye
- H44.723 Retained (nonmagnetic) (old) foreign body in iris or ciliary body, bilateral
- H44.729 Retained (nonmagnetic) (old) foreign body in iris or ciliary body, unspecified eye

H44.73 Retained (nonmagnetic) (old) foreign body in lens
- H44.731 Retained (nonmagnetic) (old) foreign body in lens, right eye
- H44.732 Retained (nonmagnetic) (old) foreign body in lens, left eye
- H44.733 Retained (nonmagnetic) (old) foreign body in lens, bilateral
- H44.739 Retained (nonmagnetic) (old) foreign body in lens, unspecified eye

H44.74 Retained (nonmagnetic) (old) foreign body in posterior wall of globe
- H44.741 Retained (nonmagnetic) (old) foreign body in posterior wall of globe, right eye
- H44.742 Retained (nonmagnetic) (old) foreign body in posterior wall of globe, left eye
- H44.743 Retained (nonmagnetic) (old) foreign body in posterior wall of globe, bilateral
- H44.749 Retained (nonmagnetic) (old) foreign body in posterior wall of globe, unspecified eye

H44.75 Retained (nonmagnetic) (old) foreign body in vitreous body
- H44.751 Retained (nonmagnetic) (old) foreign body in vitreous body, right eye
- H44.752 Retained (nonmagnetic) (old) foreign body in vitreous body, left eye
- H44.753 Retained (nonmagnetic) (old) foreign body in vitreous body, bilateral

Unacceptable principal diagnosis symbol per Medicare code edits — Code exempt from diagnosis present on admission requirement
Questionable admission — Complication or comorbidity — CC/MCC exclusion — Major complication or comorbidity
Principal diagnosis as its own CC — Principal diagnosis as its own MCC — Z code as first-listed diagnosis

H44.759 Retained (nonmagnetic) (old) foreign body in vitreous body, unspecified eye
H44.79 Retained (old) intraocular foreign body, nonmagnetic, in other or multiple sites
H44.791 Retained (old) intraocular foreign body, nonmagnetic, in other or multiple sites, right eye
H44.792 Retained (old) intraocular foreign body, nonmagnetic, in other or multiple sites, left eye
H44.793 Retained (old) intraocular foreign body, nonmagnetic, in other or multiple sites, bilateral
H44.799 Retained (old) intraocular foreign body, nonmagnetic, in other or multiple sites, unspecified eye
H44.8 Other disorders of globe
H44.81 Hemophthalmos
H44.811 Hemophthalmos, right eye
H44.812 Hemophthalmos, left eye
H44.813 Hemophthalmos, bilateral
H44.819 Hemophthalmos, unspecified eye
H44.82 Luxation of globe
H44.821 Luxation of globe, right eye
H44.822 Luxation of globe, left eye
H44.823 Luxation of globe, bilateral
H44.829 Luxation of globe, unspecified eye
H44.89 Other disorders of globe
H44.9 Unspecified disorder of globe

Disorders of optic nerve and visual pathways (H46-H47)

H46 Optic neuritis
EXCLUDES2 *ischemic optic neuropathy (H47.01-)*
neuromyelitis optica [Devic] (G36.0)
H46.0 Optic papillitis
H46.00 Optic papillitis, unspecified eye
H46.01 Optic papillitis, right eye
H46.02 Optic papillitis, left eye
H46.03 Optic papillitis, bilateral
H46.1 Retrobulbar neuritis
Retrobulbar neuritis NOS
EXCLUDES1 *syphilitic retrobulbar neuritis (A52.15)*
H46.10 Retrobulbar neuritis, unspecified eye
H46.11 Retrobulbar neuritis, right eye
H46.12 Retrobulbar neuritis, left eye
H46.13 Retrobulbar neuritis, bilateral
H46.2 Nutritional optic neuropathy
H46.3 Toxic optic neuropathy
Code first (T51-T65) to identify cause
H46.8 Other optic neuritis
H46.9 Unspecified optic neuritis
H47 Other disorders of optic [2nd] nerve and visual pathways
H47.0 Disorders of optic nerve, not elsewhere classified
H47.01 Ischemic optic neuropathy
H47.011 Ischemic optic neuropathy, right eye
H47.012 Ischemic optic neuropathy, left eye
H47.013 Ischemic optic neuropathy, bilateral
H47.019 Ischemic optic neuropathy, unspecified eye
H47.02 Hemorrhage in optic nerve sheath
H47.021 Hemorrhage in optic nerve sheath, right eye
H47.022 Hemorrhage in optic nerve sheath, left eye
H47.023 Hemorrhage in optic nerve sheath, bilateral
H47.029 Hemorrhage in optic nerve sheath, unspecified eye
H47.03 Optic nerve hypoplasia
H47.031 Optic nerve hypoplasia, right eye
H47.032 Optic nerve hypoplasia, left eye
H47.033 Optic nerve hypoplasia, bilateral
H47.039 Optic nerve hypoplasia, unspecified eye
H47.09 Other disorders of optic nerve, not elsewhere classified
Compression of optic nerve
H47.091 Other disorders of optic nerve, not elsewhere classified, right eye
H47.092 Other disorders of optic nerve, not elsewhere classified, left eye
H47.093 Other disorders of optic nerve, not elsewhere classified, bilateral
H47.099 Other disorders of optic nerve, not elsewhere classified, unspecified eye
H47.1 Papilledema
H47.10 Unspecified papilledema
H47.11 Papilledema associated with increased intracranial pressure
H47.12 Papilledema associated with decreased ocular pressure
H47.13 Papilledema associated with retinal disorder
H47.14 Foster-Kennedy syndrome
H47.141 Foster-Kennedy syndrome, right eye
H47.142 Foster-Kennedy syndrome, left eye
H47.143 Foster-Kennedy syndrome, bilateral
H47.149 Foster-Kennedy syndrome, unspecified eye
H47.2 Optic atrophy
H47.20 Unspecified optic atrophy
H47.21 Primary optic atrophy
H47.211 Primary optic atrophy, right eye
H47.212 Primary optic atrophy, left eye
H47.213 Primary optic atrophy, bilateral
H47.219 Primary optic atrophy, unspecified eye
H47.22 Hereditary optic atrophy
Leber's optic atrophy
H47.23 Glaucomatous optic atrophy
H47.231 Glaucomatous optic atrophy, right eye
H47.232 Glaucomatous optic atrophy, left eye
H47.233 Glaucomatous optic atrophy, bilateral
H47.239 Glaucomatous optic atrophy, unspecified eye
H47.29 Other optic atrophy
Temporal pallor of optic disc
H47.291 Other optic atrophy, right eye
H47.292 Other optic atrophy, left eye
H47.293 Other optic atrophy, bilateral
H47.299 Other optic atrophy, unspecified eye
H47.3 Other disorders of optic disc
H47.31 Coloboma of optic disc
H47.311 Coloboma of optic disc, right eye
H47.312 Coloboma of optic disc, left eye
H47.313 Coloboma of optic disc, bilateral
H47.319 Coloboma of optic disc, unspecified eye
H47.32 Drusen of optic disc
H47.321 Drusen of optic disc, right eye
H47.322 Drusen of optic disc, left eye
H47.323 Drusen of optic disc, bilateral
H47.329 Drusen of optic disc, unspecified eye
H47.33 Pseudopapilledema of optic disc
H47.331 Pseudopapilledema of optic disc, right eye
H47.332 Pseudopapilledema of optic disc, left eye
H47.333 Pseudopapilledema of optic disc, bilateral
H47.339 Pseudopapilledema of optic disc, unspecified eye
H47.39 Other disorders of optic disc
H47.391 Other disorders of optic disc, right eye
H47.392 Other disorders of optic disc, left eye
H47.393 Other disorders of optic disc, bilateral
H47.399 Other disorders of optic disc, unspecified eye
H47.4 Disorders of optic chiasm
Code also underlying condition
H47.41 Disorders of optic chiasm in (due to) inflammatory disorders

Unspecified Code Other Specified Code Manifestation Code N Newborn P Pediatric M Maternity A Adult ♂ Male ♀ Female
● New Code ▲ Revised Code Title ►◄ Revised Text NOTES INCLUDES EXCLUDES1 Not coded here EXCLUDES2 Not included here
4th character required 5th character required 6th character required 7th character required
Extension 'X' Alert HAC Hospital-acquired condition (HAC) alert AHA AHA Coding Clinic©

H47.42 Disorders of optic chiasm in (due to) neoplasm
H47.43 Disorders of optic chiasm in (due to) vascular disorders
H47.49 Disorders of optic chiasm in (due to) other disorders

H47.5 Disorders of other visual pathways
Disorders of optic tracts, geniculate nuclei and optic radiations
Code also underlying condition

H47.51 Disorders of visual pathways in (due to) inflammatory disorders
H47.511 Disorders of visual pathways in (due to) inflammatory disorders, right side
H47.512 Disorders of visual pathways in (due to) inflammatory disorders, left side
H47.519 Disorders of visual pathways in (due to) inflammatory disorders, unspecified side

H47.52 Disorders of visual pathways in (due to) neoplasm
H47.521 Disorders of visual pathways in (due to) neoplasm, right side
H47.522 Disorders of visual pathways in (due to) neoplasm, left side
H47.529 Disorders of visual pathways in (due to) neoplasm, unspecified side

H47.53 Disorders of visual pathways in (due to) vascular disorders
H47.531 Disorders of visual pathways in (due to) vascular disorders, right side
H47.532 Disorders of visual pathways in (due to) vascular disorders, left side
H47.539 Disorders of visual pathways in (due to) vascular disorders, unspecified side

H47.6 Disorders of visual cortex
Code also underlying condition
EXCLUDES1 *injury to visual cortex S04.04*

H47.61 Cortical blindness
H47.611 Cortical blindness, right side of brain
H47.612 Cortical blindness, left side of brain
H47.619 Cortical blindness, unspecified side of brain

H47.62 Disorders of visual cortex in (due to) inflammatory disorders
H47.621 Disorders of visual cortex in (due to) inflammatory disorders, right side of brain
H47.622 Disorders of visual cortex in (due to) inflammatory disorders, left side of brain
H47.629 Disorders of visual cortex in (due to) inflammatory disorders, unspecified side of brain

H47.63 Disorders of visual cortex in (due to) neoplasm
H47.631 Disorders of visual cortex in (due to) neoplasm, right side of brain
H47.632 Disorders of visual cortex in (due to) neoplasm, left side of brain
H47.639 Disorders of visual cortex in (due to) neoplasm, unspecified side of brain

H47.64 Disorders of visual cortex in (due to) vascular disorders
H47.641 Disorders of visual cortex in (due to) vascular disorders, right side of brain
H47.642 Disorders of visual cortex in (due to) vascular disorders, left side of brain
H47.649 Disorders of visual cortex in (due to) vascular disorders, unspecified side of brain

H47.9 Unspecified disorder of visual pathways

Disorders of ocular muscles, binocular movement, accommodation and refraction (H49-H52)

EXCLUDES2 *nystagmus and other irregular eye movements (H55)*

H49 Paralytic strabismus
EXCLUDES2 *internal ophthalmoplegia (H52.51-)*
internuclear ophthalmoplegia (H51.2-)
progressive supranuclear ophthalmoplegia (G23.1)

H49.0 Third [oculomotor] nerve palsy
H49.00 Third [oculomotor] nerve palsy, unspecified eye
H49.01 Third [oculomotor] nerve palsy, right eye
H49.02 Third [oculomotor] nerve palsy, left eye
H49.03 Third [oculomotor] nerve palsy, bilateral

H49.1 Fourth [trochlear] nerve palsy
H49.10 Fourth [trochlear] nerve palsy, unspecified eye
H49.11 Fourth [trochlear] nerve palsy, right eye
H49.12 Fourth [trochlear] nerve palsy, left eye
H49.13 Fourth [trochlear] nerve palsy, bilateral

H49.2 Sixth [abducent] nerve palsy
H49.20 Sixth [abducent] nerve palsy, unspecified eye
H49.21 Sixth [abducent] nerve palsy, right eye
H49.22 Sixth [abducent] nerve palsy, left eye
H49.23 Sixth [abducent] nerve palsy, bilateral

H49.3 Total (external) ophthalmoplegia
H49.30 Total (external) ophthalmoplegia, unspecified eye
H49.31 Total (external) ophthalmoplegia, right eye
H49.32 Total (external) ophthalmoplegia, left eye
H49.33 Total (external) ophthalmoplegia, bilateral

H49.4 Progressive external ophthalmoplegia
EXCLUDES1 *Kearns-Sayre syndrome (H49.81-)*
H49.40 Progressive external ophthalmoplegia, unspecified eye
H49.41 Progressive external ophthalmoplegia, right eye
H49.42 Progressive external ophthalmoplegia, left eye
H49.43 Progressive external ophthalmoplegia, bilateral

H49.8 Other paralytic strabismus

H49.81 Kearns-Sayre syndrome
Progressive external ophthalmoplegia with pigmentary retinopathy
Use additional code for other manifestation, such as: heart block (I45.9)
H49.811 Kearns-Sayre syndrome, right eye
H49.812 Kearns-Sayre syndrome, left eye
H49.813 Kearns-Sayre syndrome, bilateral
H49.819 Kearns-Sayre syndrome, unspecified eye

H49.88 Other paralytic strabismus
External ophthalmoplegia NOS
H49.881 Other paralytic strabismus, right eye
H49.882 Other paralytic strabismus, left eye
H49.883 Other paralytic strabismus, bilateral
H49.889 Other paralytic strabismus, unspecified eye

H49.9 Unspecified paralytic strabismus

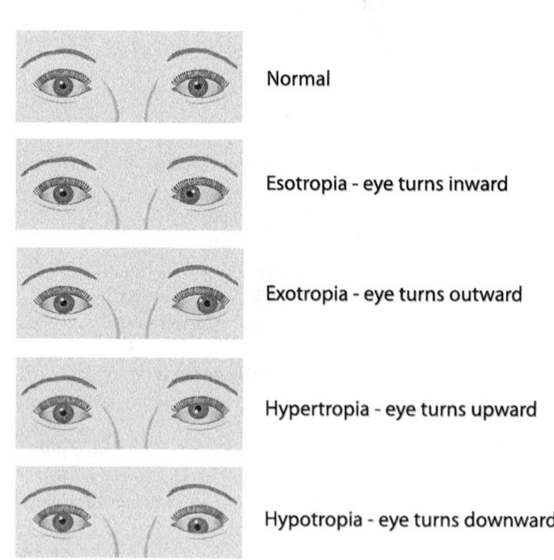

Figure 7.5 Types of Strabismus

H50 Other strabismus

H50.0 Esotropia
Convergent concomitant strabismus
EXCLUDES1 *intermittent esotropia (H50.31-, H50.32)*

Unacceptable principal diagnosis symbol per Medicare code edits | Code exempt from diagnosis present on admission requirement | Questionable admission | Complication or comorbidity | CC/MCC exclusion | Major complication or comorbidity | Principal diagnosis as its own CC | Principal diagnosis as its own MCC | Z code as first-listed diagnosis

H50.00 Unspecified esotropia
H50.01 Monocular esotropia
H50.011 Monocular esotropia, right eye
H50.012 Monocular esotropia, left eye
H50.02 Monocular esotropia with A pattern
H50.021 Monocular esotropia with A pattern, right eye
H50.022 Monocular esotropia with A pattern, left eye
H50.03 Monocular esotropia with V pattern
H50.031 Monocular esotropia with V pattern, right eye
H50.032 Monocular esotropia with V pattern, left eye
H50.04 Monocular esotropia with other noncomitancies
H50.041 Monocular esotropia with other noncomitancies, right eye
H50.042 Monocular esotropia with other noncomitancies, left eye
H50.05 Alternating esotropia
H50.06 Alternating esotropia with A pattern
H50.07 Alternating esotropia with V pattern
H50.08 Alternating esotropia with other noncomitancies
H50.1 Exotropia
Divergent concomitant strabismus
EXCLUDES1 *intermittent exotropia (H50.33-, H50.34)*
H50.10 Unspecified exotropia
H50.11 Monocular exotropia
H50.111 Monocular exotropia, right eye
H50.112 Monocular exotropia, left eye
H50.12 Monocular exotropia with A pattern
H50.121 Monocular exotropia with A pattern, right eye
H50.122 Monocular exotropia with A pattern, left eye
H50.13 Monocular exotropia with V pattern
H50.131 Monocular exotropia with V pattern, right eye
H50.132 Monocular exotropia with V pattern, left eye
H50.14 Monocular exotropia with other noncomitancies
H50.141 Monocular exotropia with other noncomitancies, right eye
H50.142 Monocular exotropia with other noncomitancies, left eye
H50.15 Alternating exotropia
H50.16 Alternating exotropia with A pattern
H50.17 Alternating exotropia with V pattern
H50.18 Alternating exotropia with other noncomitancies
H50.2 Vertical strabismus
Hypertropia
H50.21 Vertical strabismus, right eye
H50.22 Vertical strabismus, left eye
H50.3 Intermittent heterotropia
H50.30 Unspecified intermittent heterotropia
H50.31 Intermittent monocular esotropia
H50.311 Intermittent monocular esotropia, right eye
H50.312 Intermittent monocular esotropia, left eye
H50.32 Intermittent alternating esotropia
H50.33 Intermittent monocular exotropia
H50.331 Intermittent monocular exotropia, right eye
H50.332 Intermittent monocular exotropia, left eye
H50.34 Intermittent alternating exotropia
H50.4 Other and unspecified heterotropia
H50.40 Unspecified heterotropia
H50.41 Cyclotropia
H50.411 Cyclotropia, right eye
H50.412 Cyclotropia, left eye
H50.42 Monofixation syndrome
H50.43 Accommodative component in esotropia
H50.5 Heterophoria
H50.50 Unspecified heterophoria
H50.51 Esophoria
H50.52 Exophoria
H50.53 Vertical heterophoria
H50.54 Cyclophoria
H50.55 Alternating heterophoria
H50.6 Mechanical strabismus
H50.60 Mechanical strabismus, unspecified
H50.61 Brown's sheath syndrome
H50.611 Brown's sheath syndrome, right eye
H50.612 Brown's sheath syndrome, left eye
H50.69 Other mechanical strabismus
Strabismus due to adhesions
Traumatic limitation of duction of eye muscle
H50.8 Other specified strabismus
H50.81 Duane's syndrome
H50.811 Duane's syndrome, right eye
H50.812 Duane's syndrome, left eye
H50.89 Other specified strabismus
H50.9 Unspecified strabismus
H51 Other disorders of binocular movement
H51.0 Palsy (spasm) of conjugate gaze
H51.1 Convergence insufficiency and excess
H51.11 Convergence insufficiency
H51.12 Convergence excess
H51.2 Internuclear ophthalmoplegia
H51.20 Internuclear ophthalmoplegia, unspecified eye
H51.21 Internuclear ophthalmoplegia, right eye
H51.22 Internuclear ophthalmoplegia, left eye
H51.23 Internuclear ophthalmoplegia, bilateral
H51.8 Other specified disorders of binocular movement
H51.9 Unspecified disorder of binocular movement
H52 Disorders of refraction and accommodation
H52.0 Hypermetropia
H52.00 Hypermetropia, unspecified eye
H52.01 Hypermetropia, right eye
H52.02 Hypermetropia, left eye
H52.03 Hypermetropia, bilateral
H52.1 Myopia
EXCLUDES1 *degenerative myopia (H44.2-)*
H52.10 Myopia, unspecified eye
H52.11 Myopia, right eye
H52.12 Myopia, left eye
H52.13 Myopia, bilateral
H52.2 Astigmatism
H52.20 Unspecified astigmatism
H52.201 Unspecified astigmatism, right eye
H52.202 Unspecified astigmatism, left eye
H52.203 Unspecified astigmatism, bilateral
H52.209 Unspecified astigmatism, unspecified eye
H52.21 Irregular astigmatism
H52.211 Irregular astigmatism, right eye
H52.212 Irregular astigmatism, left eye
H52.213 Irregular astigmatism, bilateral
H52.219 Irregular astigmatism, unspecified eye
H52.22 Regular astigmatism
H52.221 Regular astigmatism, right eye
H52.222 Regular astigmatism, left eye
H52.223 Regular astigmatism, bilateral
H52.229 Regular astigmatism, unspecified eye
H52.3 Anisometropia and aniseikonia
H52.31 Anisometropia
H52.32 Aniseikonia
H52.4 Presbyopia
H52.5 Disorders of accommodation
H52.51 Internal ophthalmoplegia (complete) (total)
H52.511 Internal ophthalmoplegia (complete) (total), right eye
H52.512 Internal ophthalmoplegia (complete) (total), left eye

H50.00 - H52.512

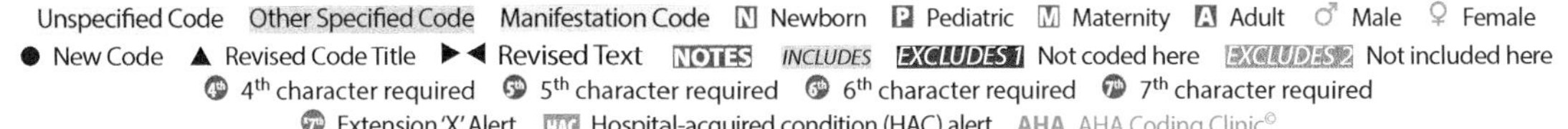

H52.513 Internal ophthalmoplegia (complete) (total), bilateral
H52.519 Internal ophthalmoplegia (complete) (total), unspecified eye
H52.52 Paresis of accommodation
H52.521 Paresis of accommodation, right eye
H52.522 Paresis of accommodation, left eye
H52.523 Paresis of accommodation, bilateral
H52.529 Paresis of accommodation, unspecified eye
H52.53 Spasm of accommodation
H52.531 Spasm of accommodation, right eye
H52.532 Spasm of accommodation, left eye
H52.533 Spasm of accommodation, bilateral
H52.539 Spasm of accommodation, unspecified eye
H52.6 Other disorders of refraction
H52.7 Unspecified disorder of refraction

Visual disturbances and blindness (H53-H54)

H53 Visual disturbances
H53.0 Amblyopia ex anopsia
EXCLUDES1 *amblyopia due to vitamin A deficiency (E50.5)*
H53.00 Unspecified amblyopia
H53.001 Unspecified amblyopia, right eye
H53.002 Unspecified amblyopia, left eye
H53.003 Unspecified amblyopia, bilateral
H53.009 Unspecified amblyopia, unspecified eye
H53.01 Deprivation amblyopia
H53.011 Deprivation amblyopia, right eye
H53.012 Deprivation amblyopia, left eye
H53.013 Deprivation amblyopia, bilateral
H53.019 Deprivation amblyopia, unspecified eye
H53.02 Refractive amblyopia
H53.021 Refractive amblyopia, right eye
H53.022 Refractive amblyopia, left eye
H53.023 Refractive amblyopia, bilateral
H53.029 Refractive amblyopia, unspecified eye
H53.03 Strabismic amblyopia
EXCLUDES1 *strabismus (H50.-)*
H53.031 Strabismic amblyopia, right eye
H53.032 Strabismic amblyopia, left eye
H53.033 Strabismic amblyopia, bilateral
H53.039 Strabismic amblyopia, unspecified eye
● H53.04 Amblyopia suspect
● H53.041 Amblyopia suspect, right eye
● H53.042 Amblyopia suspect, left eye
● H53.043 Amblyopia suspect, bilateral
● H53.049 Amblyopia suspect, unspecified eye
H53.1 Subjective visual disturbances
EXCLUDES1 *subjective visual disturbances due to vitamin A deficiency (E50.5)*
visual hallucinations (R44.1)
H53.10 Unspecified subjective visual disturbances
H53.11 Day blindness
Hemeralopia
H53.12 Transient visual loss
Scintillating scotoma
EXCLUDES1 *amaurosis fugax (G45.3-)*
transient retinal artery occlusion (H34.0-)
H53.121 Transient visual loss, right eye CC
H53.122 Transient visual loss, left eye CC
H53.123 Transient visual loss, bilateral CC
H53.129 Transient visual loss, unspecified eye CC
H53.13 Sudden visual loss
H53.131 Sudden visual loss, right eye CC
H53.132 Sudden visual loss, left eye CC
H53.133 Sudden visual loss, bilateral CC
H53.139 Sudden visual loss, unspecified eye CC
H53.14 Visual discomfort
Asthenopia
Photophobia
H53.141 Visual discomfort, right eye
H53.142 Visual discomfort, left eye
H53.143 Visual discomfort, bilateral
H53.149 Visual discomfort, unspecified
H53.15 Visual distortions of shape and size
Metamorphopsia
H53.16 Psychophysical visual disturbances
H53.19 Other subjective visual disturbances
Visual halos
H53.2 Diplopia
Double vision
H53.3 Other and unspecified disorders of binocular vision
H53.30 Unspecified disorder of binocular vision
H53.31 Abnormal retinal correspondence
H53.32 Fusion with defective stereopsis
H53.33 Simultaneous visual perception without fusion
H53.34 Suppression of binocular vision
H53.4 Visual field defects
H53.40 Unspecified visual field defects
H53.41 Scotoma involving central area
Central scotoma
H53.411 Scotoma involving central area, right eye
H53.412 Scotoma involving central area, left eye
H53.413 Scotoma involving central area, bilateral
H53.419 Scotoma involving central area, unspecified eye
H53.42 Scotoma of blind spot area
Enlarged blind spot
H53.421 Scotoma of blind spot area, right eye
H53.422 Scotoma of blind spot area, left eye
H53.423 Scotoma of blind spot area, bilateral
H53.429 Scotoma of blind spot area, unspecified eye
H53.43 Sector or arcuate defects
Arcuate scotoma
Bjerrum scotoma
H53.431 Sector or arcuate defects, right eye
H53.432 Sector or arcuate defects, left eye
H53.433 Sector or arcuate defects, bilateral
H53.439 Sector or arcuate defects, unspecified eye
H53.45 Other localized visual field defect
Peripheral visual field defect
Ring scotoma NOS
Scotoma NOS
H53.451 Other localized visual field defect, right eye
H53.452 Other localized visual field defect, left eye
H53.453 Other localized visual field defect, bilateral
H53.459 Other localized visual field defect, unspecified eye
H53.46 Homonymous bilateral field defects
Homonymous hemianopia
Homonymous hemianopsia
Quadrant anopia
Quadrant anopsia
H53.461 Homonymous bilateral field defects, right side
H53.462 Homonymous bilateral field defects, left side
H53.469 Homonymous bilateral field defects, unspecified side
Homonymous bilateral field defects NOS
H53.47 Heteronymous bilateral field defects
Heteronymous hemianop(s)ia
H53.48 Generalized contraction of visual field
H53.481 Generalized contraction of visual field, right eye
H53.482 Generalized contraction of visual field, left eye
H53.483 Generalized contraction of visual field, bilateral
H53.489 Generalized contraction of visual field, unspecified eye

Unacceptable principal diagnosis symbol per Medicare code edits | Code exempt from diagnosis present on admission requirement
Questionable admission | Complication or comorbidity | CC/MCC exclusion | Major complication or comorbidity
Principal diagnosis as its own CC | Principal diagnosis as its own MCC | Z code as first-listed diagnosis

H53.5 Color vision deficiencies
Color blindness
EXCLUDES2 *day blindness (H53.11)*
H53.50 **Unspecified color vision deficiencies**
Color blindness NOS
H53.51 **Achromatopsia**
H53.52 **Acquired color vision deficiency**
H53.53 **Deuteranomaly**
Deuteranopia
H53.54 **Protanomaly**
Protanopia
H53.55 **Tritanomaly**
Tritanopia
H53.59 **Other color vision deficiencies**

H53.6 **Night blindness**
EXCLUDES1 *night blindness due to vitamin A deficiency (E50.5)*
H53.60 **Unspecified night blindness**
H53.61 **Abnormal dark adaptation curve**
H53.62 **Acquired night blindness**
H53.63 **Congenital night blindness**
H53.69 **Other night blindness**

H53.7 **Vision sensitivity deficiencies**
H53.71 **Glare sensitivity**
H53.72 **Impaired contrast sensitivity**
H53.8 **Other visual disturbances**
H53.9 **Unspecified visual disturbance**

H54 **Blindness and low vision**
NOTES For definition of visual impairment categories see table below
Code first any associated underlying cause of the blindness
EXCLUDES1 *amaurosis fugax (G45.3)*
H54.0 **Blindness, both eyes**
Visual impairment categories 3, 4, 5 in both eyes.
H54.1 **Blindness, one eye, low vision other eye**
Visual impairment categories 3, 4, 5 in one eye, with categories 1 or 2 in the other eye.
H54.10 **Blindness, one eye, low vision other eye, unspecified eyes**
H54.11 **Blindness, right eye, low vision left eye**
H54.12 **Blindness, left eye, low vision right eye**
H54.2 **Low vision, both eyes**
Visual impairment categories 1 or 2 in both eyes.
H54.3 **Unqualified visual loss, both eyes**
Visual impairment category 9 in both eyes.
H54.4 **Blindness, one eye**
Visual impairment categories 3, 4, 5 in one eye [normal vision in other eye]
H54.40 **Blindness, one eye, unspecified eye**
H54.41 **Blindness, right eye, normal vision left eye**
H54.42 **Blindness, left eye, normal vision right eye**
H54.5 **Low vision, one eye**
Visual impairment categories 1 or 2 in one eye [normal vision in other eye].
H54.50 **Low vision, one eye, unspecified eye**
H54.51 **Low vision, right eye, normal vision left eye**
H54.52 **Low vision, left eye, normal vision right eye**
H54.6 **Unqualified visual loss, one eye**
Visual impairment category 9 in one eye [normal vision in other eye].
H54.60 **Unqualified visual loss, one eye, unspecified**
H54.61 **Unqualified visual loss, right eye, normal vision left eye**
H54.62 **Unqualified visual loss, left eye, normal vision right eye**
H54.7 **Unspecified visual loss** PDx
Visual impairment category 9 NOS
H54.8 **Legal blindness, as defined in USA**
Blindness NOS according to USA definition
EXCLUDES1 *legal blindness with specification of impairment level (H54.0-H54.7)*
NOTES The table below gives a classification of severity of visual impairment recommended by a WHO Study Group on the Prevention of Blindness, Geneva, 6-10 November 1972.
The term 'low vision' in category H54 comprises categories 1 and 2 of the table, the term 'blindness' categories 3, 4 and 5, and the term 'unqualified visual loss' category 9.
If the extent of the visual field is taken into account, patients with a field no greater than 10 but greater than 5 around central fixation should be placed in category 3 and patients with a field no greater than 5 around central fixation should be placed in category 4, even if the central acuity is not impaired.

Category of visual impairment	Visual acuity with best possible correction	
	Maximum less than:	Minimum equal to or better than:
	6/18	6/60
3/10(0.3)	1/10(0.1)	-
20/70	20/200	-
	6/60	3/60
1/10(0.1)	1/20(0.05)	-
20/200	20/400	-
	3/60	1/60 (finger counting at one meter)
1/20(0.05)	1/50(0.02)	-
20/400	5/300(20/1200)	-
	1/60 (finger counting at one meter)	Light perception
1/50(0.02)		-
5/300		-
	No light perception	-
	Undetermined or unspecified	-

Other disorders of eye and adnexa (H55-H57)

H55 **Nystagmus and other irregular eye movements**
H55.0 **Nystagmus**
H55.00 **Unspecified nystagmus**
H55.01 **Congenital nystagmus**
H55.02 **Latent nystagmus**
H55.03 **Visual deprivation nystagmus**
H55.04 **Dissociated nystagmus**
H55.09 **Other forms of nystagmus**
H55.8 **Other irregular eye movements**
H55.81 **Saccadic eye movements**
H55.89 **Other irregular eye movements**

H57 **Other disorders of eye and adnexa**
H57.0 **Anomalies of pupillary function**
H57.00 **Unspecified anomaly of pupillary function**
H57.01 **Argyll Robertson pupil, atypical**
EXCLUDES1 *syphilitic Argyll Robertson pupil (A52.19)*
H57.02 **Anisocoria**
H57.03 **Miosis**
H57.04 **Mydriasis**
H57.05 **Tonic pupil**
H57.051 **Tonic pupil, right eye**
H57.052 **Tonic pupil, left eye**
H57.053 **Tonic pupil, bilateral**
H57.059 **Tonic pupil, unspecified eye**
H57.09 **Other anomalies of pupillary function**
H57.1 **Ocular pain**
H57.10 **Ocular pain, unspecified eye**
H57.11 **Ocular pain, right eye**
H57.12 **Ocular pain, left eye**
H57.13 **Ocular pain, bilateral**
H57.8 **Other specified disorders of eye and adnexa**
H57.9 **Unspecified disorder of eye and adnexa** PDx

Intraoperative and postprocedural complications and disorders of eye and adnexa, not elsewhere classified (H59)

H59 **Intraoperative and postprocedural complications and disorders of eye and adnexa, not elsewhere classified**
EXCLUDES1 *mechanical complication of intraocular lens (T85.2)*
mechanical complication of other ocular prosthetic devices, implants and grafts (T85.3)
pseudophakia (Z96.1)
secondary cataracts (H26.4-)

H59.0 Disorders of the eye following cataract surgery

H59.01 Keratopathy (bullous aphakic) following cataract surgery
Vitreal corneal syndrome
Vitreous (touch) syndrome

H59.011 Keratopathy (bullous aphakic) following cataract surgery, right eye

H59.012 Keratopathy (bullous aphakic) following cataract surgery, left eye

H59.013 Keratopathy (bullous aphakic) following cataract surgery, bilateral

H59.019 Keratopathy (bullous aphakic) following cataract surgery, unspecified eye

H59.02 Cataract (lens) fragments in eye following cataract surgery

H59.021 Cataract (lens) fragments in eye following cataract surgery, right eye

H59.022 Cataract (lens) fragments in eye following cataract surgery, left eye

H59.023 Cataract (lens) fragments in eye following cataract surgery, bilateral

H59.029 Cataract (lens) fragments in eye following cataract surgery, unspecified eye

H59.03 Cystoid macular edema following cataract surgery

H59.031 Cystoid macular edema following cataract surgery, right eye

H59.032 Cystoid macular edema following cataract surgery, left eye

H59.033 Cystoid macular edema following cataract surgery, bilateral

H59.039 Cystoid macular edema following cataract surgery, unspecified eye

H59.09 Other disorders of the eye following cataract surgery

H59.091 Other disorders of the right eye following cataract surgery

H59.092 Other disorders of the left eye following cataract surgery

H59.093 Other disorders of the eye following cataract surgery, bilateral

H59.099 Other disorders of unspecified eye following cataract surgery

H59.1 Intraoperative hemorrhage and hematoma of eye and adnexa complicating a procedure

EXCLUDES1 *intraoperative hemorrhage and hematoma of eye and adnexa due to accidental puncture or laceration during a procedure (H59.2-)*

H59.11 Intraoperative hemorrhage and hematoma of eye and adnexa complicating an ophthalmic procedure

H59.111 Intraoperative hemorrhage and hematoma of right eye and adnexa complicating an ophthalmic procedure

H59.112 Intraoperative hemorrhage and hematoma of left eye and adnexa complicating an ophthalmic procedure

H59.113 Intraoperative hemorrhage and hematoma of eye and adnexa complicating an ophthalmic procedure, bilateral

H59.119 Intraoperative hemorrhage and hematoma of unspecified eye and adnexa complicating an ophthalmic procedure

H59.12 Intraoperative hemorrhage and hematoma of eye and adnexa complicating other procedure

H59.121 Intraoperative hemorrhage and hematoma of right eye and adnexa complicating other procedure

H59.122 Intraoperative hemorrhage and hematoma of left eye and adnexa complicating other procedure

H59.123 Intraoperative hemorrhage and hematoma of eye and adnexa complicating other procedure, bilateral

H59.129 Intraoperative hemorrhage and hematoma of unspecified eye and adnexa complicating other procedure

H59.2 Accidental puncture and laceration of eye and adnexa during a procedure

H59.21 Accidental puncture and laceration of eye and adnexa during an ophthalmic procedure

H59.211 Accidental puncture and laceration of right eye and adnexa during an ophthalmic procedure

H59.212 Accidental puncture and laceration of left eye and adnexa during an ophthalmic procedure

H59.213 Accidental puncture and laceration of eye and adnexa during an ophthalmic procedure, bilateral

H59.219 Accidental puncture and laceration of unspecified eye and adnexa during an ophthalmic procedure

H59.22 Accidental puncture and laceration of eye and adnexa during other procedure

H59.221 Accidental puncture and laceration of right eye and adnexa during other procedure

H59.222 Accidental puncture and laceration of left eye and adnexa during other procedure

H59.223 Accidental puncture and laceration of eye and adnexa during other procedure, bilateral

H59.229 Accidental puncture and laceration of unspecified eye and adnexa during other procedure

▲ H59.3 Postprocedural hemorrhage, ▶hematoma, and seroma◀ of eye and adnexa following a procedure

▲ H59.31 Postprocedural ▶hemorrhage of◀ eye and adnexa following an ophthalmic procedure

▲ H59.311 Postprocedural ▶hemorrhage of◀ right eye and adnexa following an ophthalmic procedure

▲ H59.312 Postprocedural ▶hemorrhage of◀ left eye and adnexa following an ophthalmic procedure

▲ H59.313 Postprocedural ▶hemorrhage of◀ eye and adnexa following an ophthalmic procedure, bilateral

▲ H59.319 Postprocedural ▶hemorrhage of◀ unspecified eye and adnexa following an ophthalmic procedure

▲ H59.32 Postprocedural ▶hemorrhage of◀ eye and adnexa following other procedure

▲ H59.321 Postprocedural ▶hemorrhage of◀ right eye and adnexa following other procedure

▲ H59.322 Postprocedural ▶hemorrhage of◀ left eye and adnexa following other procedure

▲ H59.323 Postprocedural ▶hemorrhage of◀ eye and adnexa following other procedure, bilateral

▲ H59.329 Postprocedural ▶hemorrhage of◀ unspecified eye and adnexa following other procedure

● H59.33 Postprocedural hematoma of eye and adnexa following an ophthalmic procedure

● H59.331 Postprocedural hematoma of right eye and adnexa following an ophthalmic procedure

● H59.332 Postprocedural hematoma of left eye and adnexa following an ophthalmic procedure

● H59.333 Postprocedural hematoma of eye and adnexa following an ophthalmic procedure, bilateral

● H59.339 Postprocedural hematoma of unspecified eye and adnexa following an ophthalmic procedure

● H59.34 Postprocedural hematoma of eye and adnexa following other procedure

Unacceptable principal diagnosis symbol per Medicare code edits | Code exempt from diagnosis present on admission requirement | Questionable admission | Complication or comorbidity | CC/MCC exclusion | Major complication or comorbidity | Principal diagnosis as its own CC | Principal diagnosis as its own MCC | Z code as first-listed diagnosis

● H59.341 Postprocedural hematoma of right eye and adnexa following other procedure CC CC/MCC Exc

● H59.342 Postprocedural hematoma of left eye and adnexa following other procedure CC CC/MCC Exc

● H59.343 Postprocedural hematoma of eye and adnexa following other procedure, bilateral CC CC/MCC Exc

● H59.349 Postprocedural hematoma of unspecified eye and adnexa following other procedure CC CC/MCC Exc

● 6th H59.35 Postprocedural seroma of eye and adnexa following an ophthalmic procedure

● H59.351 Postprocedural seroma of right eye and adnexa following an ophthalmic procedure

● H59.352 Postprocedural seroma of left eye and adnexa following an ophthalmic procedure

● H59.353 Postprocedural seroma of eye and adnexa following an ophthalmic procedure, bilateral

● H59.359 Postprocedural seroma of unspecified eye and adnexa following an ophthalmic procedure

● 6th H59.36 Postprocedural seroma of eye and adnexa following other procedure

● H59.361 Postprocedural seroma of right eye and adnexa following other procedure

● H59.362 Postprocedural seroma of left eye and adnexa following other procedure

● H59.363 Postprocedural seroma of eye and adnexa following other procedure, bilateral

● H59.369 Postprocedural seroma of unspecified eye and adnexa following other procedure

5th H59.4 Inflammation (infection) of postprocedural bleb

Postprocedural blebitis

EXCLUDES1 *filtering (vitreous) bleb after glaucoma surgery status (Z98.83)*

H59.40 Inflammation (infection) of postprocedural bleb, unspecified

H59.41 Inflammation (infection) of postprocedural bleb, stage 1

H59.42 Inflammation (infection) of postprocedural bleb, stage 2

H59.43 Inflammation (infection) of postprocedural bleb, stage 3

Bleb endophthalmitis

5th H59.8 Other intraoperative and postprocedural complications and disorders of eye and adnexa, not elsewhere classified

6th H59.81 Chorioretinal scars after surgery for detachment

H59.811 Chorioretinal scars after surgery for detachment, right eye CC

H59.812 Chorioretinal scars after surgery for detachment, left eye CC

H59.813 Chorioretinal scars after surgery for detachment, bilateral CC

H59.819 Chorioretinal scars after surgery for detachment, unspecified eye CC

H59.88 Other intraoperative complications of eye and adnexa, not elsewhere classified CC

H59.89 Other postprocedural complications and disorders of eye and adnexa, not elsewhere classified CC

Unspecified Code Other Specified Code Manifestation Code N Newborn P Pediatric M Maternity A Adult ♂ Male ♀ Female
● New Code ▲ Revised Code Title ►◄ Revised Text NOTES INCLUDES EXCLUDES1 Not coded here EXCLUDES2 Not included here
4th 4th character required 5th 5th character required 6th 6th character required 7th 7th character required
X Extension 'X' Alert HAC Hospital-acquired condition (HAC) alert AHA AHA Coding Clinic©

This page intentionally left blank

Chapter 8: Diseases of the Ear and Mastoid Process (H60-H95)

Guidelines for Assigning Codes From This Chapter

Chapter 8 covers the ear, the organ of hearing, and the mastoid process, the bony projection at the base of the temporal bone, behind each ear, which serves as the site of attachment for the neck muscles. The ear consists of the external ear, the middle ear, and the inner ear. The tympanic membrane, or ear drum, divides the outer and middle ear. The inner ear is responsible for both hearing and balance.

List of Sections

- H60-H62: Diseases of external ear
- H65-H75: Diseases of middle ear and mastoid
- H80-H83: Diseases of inner ear
- H90-H94: Other disorders of ear
- H95: Intraoperative and postprocedural complications and disorders of ear and mastoid process, not elsewhere classified

Highlights From the ICD-10-CM Official Guidelines for Coding and Reporting

The 2017 version of the ICD-10-CM Official Guidelines for Coding and Reporting does not include specific guidelines for Chapter 8, stating that the section is reserved for future expansion.

As with every ICD-10-CM chapter, you should be sure to review and apply the guidelines and instructions included in the manual with the codes and code ranges. Below are some key areas to watch:

Learn the Ins and Outs of Otitis Media

Start with the basics: With more than 80 codes for otitis media, zeroing in the right code can be a challenge. For you to code appropriately, look for documentation that indicates the otitis media is:

- Nonsuppurative or suppurative
- Acute, acute recurrent, or chronic
- Tubotympanic or atticoantral, if appropriate
- Left, right, or bilateral

You'll typically choose between categories H65 (Nonsuppurative otitis media) and H66 (Suppurative and unspecified otitis media). Watch for whether the case is serous, allergic, or another type and whether there is documentation of a spontaneous rupture of the ear drum to aid you in code selection.

Use additional codes: You'll use an additional code to identify tobacco use and exposure for codes in categories H65 and H66. If the patient has a perforated ear drum, use an additional code from category H72 (*Perforation of tympanic membrane*) for an associated perforated tympanic membrane.

In diseases classified elsewhere: You also should stay alert for times when you should use category H67 (*Otitis media in diseases classified elsewhere*). As usual, you'll code the underlying disease first, but don't miss the Excludes1 note for influenza, measles, scarlet fever, and tuberculosis.

Helpful Hints for Hearing Loss

Conductive: Conductive hearing loss occurs because of a mechanical problem in the outer or middle ear. Sound does not carry, or conduct, efficiently through the outer ear canal to the eardrum and the tiny bones (called ossicles) of the middle ear.

Sensorineural: Sensorineural hearing loss originates in the vestibulocochlear nerve, the inner ear, or central processing centers of the brain. Sensorineural hearing loss can be mild, moderate, or severe, including total deafness.

Follow the documentation: To correctly report a code from category H90 (*Conductive and sensorineural hearing loss*), the documentation must designate the hearing loss as conductive, sensorineural, or mixed and whether the hearing loss is in the right ear, left ear, or is bilateral.

Don't overlook: You can report unilateral hearing loss with unrestricted hearing in the opposite ear with a code from H90.4 (Sensorineural hearing loss, unilateral with unrestricted hearing on the contralateral side). Keep an eye on the Excludes1 nodes for all of category H90 and for H90.5 (*Unspecified sensorineural hearing loss*).

Anatomy of the Ear

The Organ of Hearing

The external, inner and middle ear contain the organs of hearing and balance. The external ear extends from outside of the head to the eardrum. The middle ear is the air-filled chamber and located medially to the eardrum. It contains the auditory ossicles (the malleus, incus, and stapes). The external and middle ears are primarily involved in the process of hearing. The inner ear comprises of fluid-filled chambers, which serve to maintain balance (or equilibrium) and hearing. The various organs of a typical human ear are listed below:

1. **The External Ear**
   a) Auricle (or Pinna)
   b) External Auditory (or Auricular) Canal (or Ear Canal/External Auditory Meatus/External Acoustic Meatus)
   c) Surface of Eardrum
2. **The Middle Ear**
   a) Malleus
   b) Incus
   c) Stapes
   d) Tympanic Membrane (or Eardrum)
   e) Auditory/Eustachian Tube (or Pharyngotympanic Tube)
3. **The Inner Ear**
   a) Cochlea
   b) Vestibule
   c) Semicircular Canals

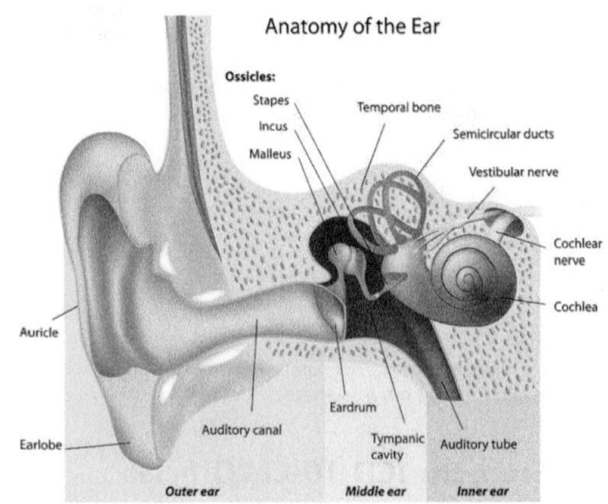

Common Pathologies

Swimmer's ear

Swimmer's ear is an inflammation, irritation, or infection of the outer ear and ear canal. The medical term for swimmer's ear is otitis externa. Acute external otitis is commonly a bacterial infection caused by streptococcus, staphylococcus, or pseudomonas types of bacteria.

Otitis media

Otitis media is the medical term for middle ear infection. One symptom of acute otitis media is ear pain; other possible symptoms include fever and irritability (in infants) often with drainage of purulent material. After an acute infection, fluid (an effusion) may remain behind the ear drum (tympanic membrane) leading to otitis media with effusion chronic suppurative otitis media.

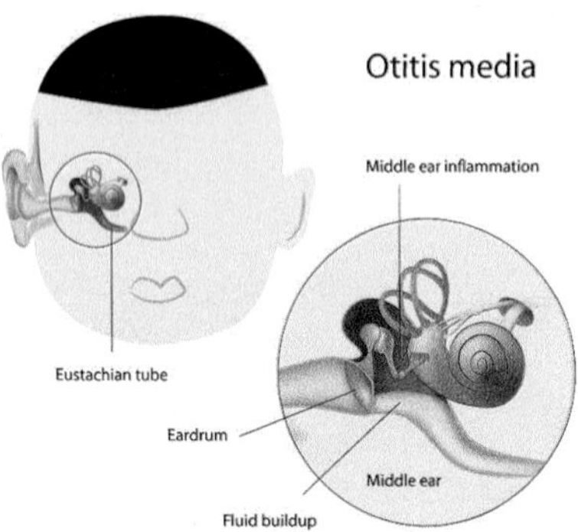

Ménière's disease

Ménière's disease is a disorder of the inner ear that can affect hearing. It causes severe dizziness and a feeling of ear pressure or pain. It is characterized by episodes of vertigo, low-pitched tinnitus, and hearing loss. It usually affects just one ear. It may occur when the pressure of the fluid in part of the inner ear gets too high. The inner ear contains fluid-filled tubes called semicircular canals. These canals help to maintain position and balance.

Vestibular neuritis

Vestibular neuritis is a disorder resulting from an acute infection of the nerves in the inner ear. This disrupts transmission of sensory information. Its main symptom is vertigo, which appears suddenly, often with nausea and vomiting. This can be made worse by head movement. Vertigo usually lasts for several days or weeks. In rare cases it can take months to go away entirely. Vestibular neuritis does not lead to loss of hearing.

Cholesteatoma

Cholesteatoma can be congenital, but it more commonly occurs as a complication of chronic ear infection. An abnormal skin growth in the middle ear behind the eardrum is called cholesteatoma. Poor function in the eustachian tube leads to negative pressure in the middle ear. Over time, the cholesteatoma can increase in size and destroy the surrounding delicate bones of the middle ear leading to hearing loss.

Otosclerosis

Otosclerosis is an abnormal bone growth in the middle ear that causes hearing loss. This bone prevents structures within the ear from working properly and causes hearing loss. It is a condition that mainly affects the stapes, one of the tiny bony ossicles in the middle ear. It significantly involves the bone that surrounds the inner ear, called the otic capsule, and a sensory-type hearing loss occurs.

Acoustic Neuroma

An acoustic neuroma is a benign tumor of the nerve that connects the ear to the brain. This nerve is called the vestibular cochlear nerve. It is also called vestibular schwannoma. The cause is generally unknown. If an acoustic tumor becomes large it will push on the surface of the brainstem but not really grow into brain tissue. Symptoms of acoustic neuroma are loss of hearing on one side, ringing in ears, dizziness and balance problems.

Acoustic Neuroma

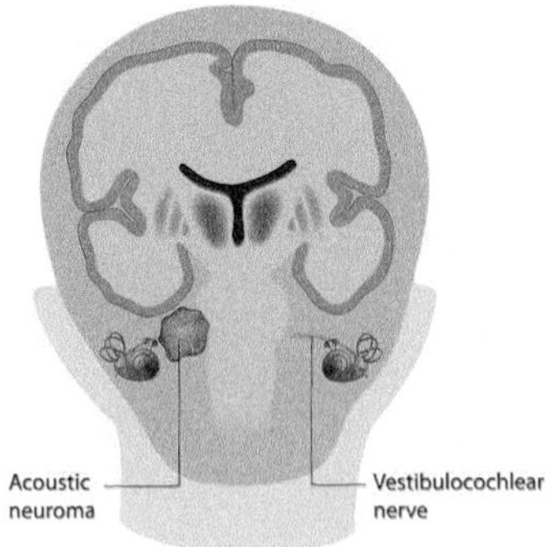

Diseases of the ear and mastoid process (H60-H95)

NOTES Use an external cause code following the code for the ear condition, if applicable, to identify the cause of the ear condition

EXCLUDES2 *certain conditions originating in the perinatal period (P04-P96)*
certain infectious and parasitic diseases (A00-B99)
complications of pregnancy, childbirth and the puerperium (O00-O9A)
congenital malformations, deformations and chromosomal abnormalities (Q00-Q99)
endocrine, nutritional and metabolic diseases (E00-E88)
injury, poisoning and certain other consequences of external causes (S00-T88)
neoplasms (C00-D49)
symptoms, signs and abnormal clinical and laboratory findings, not elsewhere classified (R00-R94)

This chapter contains the following blocks:

H60-H62	Diseases of external ear
H65-H75	Diseases of middle ear and mastoid
H80-H83	Diseases of inner ear
H90-H94	Other disorders of ear
H95	Intraoperative and postprocedural complications and disorders of ear and mastoid process, not elsewhere classified

Diseases of external ear (H60-H62)

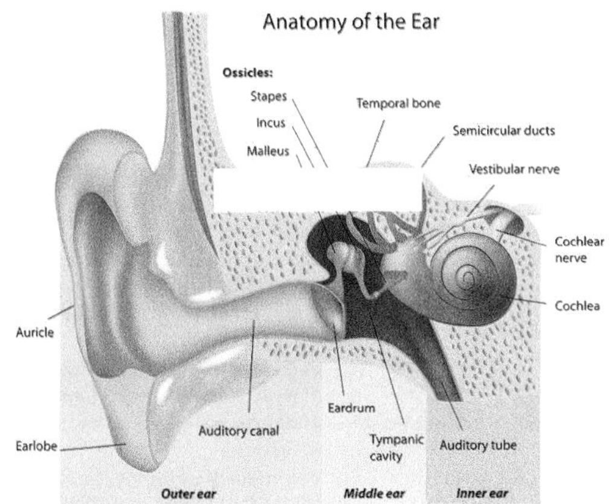

Figure 8.1 Anatomy of the ear

H60 Otitis externa
- **H60.0 Abscess of external ear**
  Boil of external ear
  Carbuncle of auricle or external auditory canal
  Furuncle of external ear
  - **H60.00 Abscess of external ear, unspecified ear**
  - **H60.01 Abscess of right external ear**
  - **H60.02 Abscess of left external ear**
  - **H60.03 Abscess of external ear, bilateral**
- **H60.1 Cellulitis of external ear**
  Cellulitis of auricle
  Cellulitis of external auditory canal
  - **H60.10 Cellulitis of external ear, unspecified ear**
  - **H60.11 Cellulitis of right external ear**
  - **H60.12 Cellulitis of left external ear**
  - **H60.13 Cellulitis of external ear, bilateral**
- **H60.2 Malignant otitis externa**
  - **H60.20 Malignant otitis externa, unspecified ear** CC
  - **H60.21 Malignant otitis externa, right ear** CC
  - **H60.22 Malignant otitis externa, left ear** CC
  - **H60.23 Malignant otitis externa, bilateral** CC
- **H60.3 Other infective otitis externa**
  - **H60.31 Diffuse otitis externa**
    - **H60.311 Diffuse otitis externa, right ear**
    - **H60.312 Diffuse otitis externa, left ear**
    - **H60.313 Diffuse otitis externa, bilateral**
    - **H60.319 Diffuse otitis externa, unspecified ear**
  - **H60.32 Hemorrhagic otitis externa**
    - **H60.321 Hemorrhagic otitis externa, right ear**
    - **H60.322 Hemorrhagic otitis externa, left ear**
    - **H60.323 Hemorrhagic otitis externa, bilateral**
    - **H60.329 Hemorrhagic otitis externa, unspecified ear**
  - **H60.33 Swimmer's ear**
    - **H60.331 Swimmer's ear, right ear**
    - **H60.332 Swimmer's ear, left ear**
    - **H60.333 Swimmer's ear, bilateral**
    - **H60.339 Swimmer's ear, unspecified ear**
  - **H60.39 Other infective otitis externa**
    - **H60.391 Other infective otitis externa, right ear**
    - **H60.392 Other infective otitis externa, left ear**
    - **H60.393 Other infective otitis externa, bilateral**
    - **H60.399 Other infective otitis externa, unspecified ear**
- **H60.4 Cholesteatoma of external ear**
  Keratosis obturans of external ear (canal)
  EXCLUDES2 *cholesteatoma of middle ear (H71.-)*
  recurrent cholesteatoma of postmastoidectomy cavity (H95.0-)
  - **H60.40 Cholesteatoma of external ear, unspecified ear**
  - **H60.41 Cholesteatoma of right external ear**
  - **H60.42 Cholesteatoma of left external ear**
  - **H60.43 Cholesteatoma of external ear, bilateral**
- **H60.5 Acute noninfective otitis externa**
  - **H60.50 Unspecified acute noninfective otitis externa**
    Acute otitis externa NOS
    - **H60.501 Unspecified acute noninfective otitis externa, right ear**
    - **H60.502 Unspecified acute noninfective otitis externa, left ear**
    - **H60.503 Unspecified acute noninfective otitis externa, bilateral**
    - **H60.509 Unspecified acute noninfective otitis externa, unspecified ear**
  - **H60.51 Acute actinic otitis externa**
    - **H60.511 Acute actinic otitis externa, right ear**
    - **H60.512 Acute actinic otitis externa, left ear**
    - **H60.513 Acute actinic otitis externa, bilateral**
    - **H60.519 Acute actinic otitis externa, unspecified ear**
  - **H60.52 Acute chemical otitis externa**
    - **H60.521 Acute chemical otitis externa, right ear**
    - **H60.522 Acute chemical otitis externa, left ear**
    - **H60.523 Acute chemical otitis externa, bilateral**
    - **H60.529 Acute chemical otitis externa, unspecified ear**
  - **H60.53 Acute contact otitis externa**
    - **H60.531 Acute contact otitis externa, right ear**
    - **H60.532 Acute contact otitis externa, left ear**
    - **H60.533 Acute contact otitis externa, bilateral**
    - **H60.539 Acute contact otitis externa, unspecified ear**
  - **H60.54 Acute eczematoid otitis externa**
    - **H60.541 Acute eczematoid otitis externa, right ear**
    - **H60.542 Acute eczematoid otitis externa, left ear**
    - **H60.543 Acute eczematoid otitis externa, bilateral**
    - **H60.549 Acute eczematoid otitis externa, unspecified ear**
  - **H60.55 Acute reactive otitis externa**
    - **H60.551 Acute reactive otitis externa, right ear**
    - **H60.552 Acute reactive otitis externa, left ear**
    - **H60.553 Acute reactive otitis externa, bilateral**
    - **H60.559 Acute reactive otitis externa, unspecified ear**
  - **H60.59 Other noninfective acute otitis externa**
    - **H60.591 Other noninfective acute otitis externa, right ear**
    - **H60.592 Other noninfective acute otitis externa, left ear**
    - **H60.593 Other noninfective acute otitis externa, bilateral**

Unspecified Code Other Specified Code Manifestation Code N Newborn P Pediatric M Maternity A Adult ♂ Male ♀ Female
● New Code ▲ Revised Code Title ►◄ Revised Text NOTES INCLUDES EXCLUDES1 Not coded here EXCLUDES2 Not included here
4th character required 5th character required 6th character required 7th character required
Extension 'X' Alert HAC Hospital-acquired condition (HAC) alert AHA AHA Coding Clinic©

H60.599 Other noninfective acute otitis externa, unspecified ear
H60.6 Unspecified chronic otitis externa
H60.60 Unspecified chronic otitis externa, unspecified ear
H60.61 Unspecified chronic otitis externa, right ear
H60.62 Unspecified chronic otitis externa, left ear
H60.63 Unspecified chronic otitis externa, bilateral
H60.8 Other otitis externa
H60.8X Other otitis externa
H60.8X1 Other otitis externa, right ear
H60.8X2 Other otitis externa, left ear
H60.8X3 Other otitis externa, bilateral
H60.8X9 Other otitis externa, unspecified ear
H60.9 Unspecified otitis externa
H60.90 Unspecified otitis externa, unspecified ear
H60.91 Unspecified otitis externa, right ear
H60.92 Unspecified otitis externa, left ear
H60.93 Unspecified otitis externa, bilateral
H61 Other disorders of external ear
H61.0 Chondritis and perichondritis of external ear
Chondrodermatitis nodularis chronica helicis
Perichondritis of auricle
Perichondritis of pinna
H61.00 Unspecified perichondritis of external ear
H61.001 Unspecified perichondritis of right external ear
H61.002 Unspecified perichondritis of left external ear
H61.003 Unspecified perichondritis of external ear, bilateral
H61.009 Unspecified perichondritis of external ear, unspecified ear
H61.01 Acute perichondritis of external ear
H61.011 Acute perichondritis of right external ear
H61.012 Acute perichondritis of left external ear
H61.013 Acute perichondritis of external ear, bilateral
H61.019 Acute perichondritis of external ear, unspecified ear
H61.02 Chronic perichondritis of external ear
H61.021 Chronic perichondritis of right external ear
H61.022 Chronic perichondritis of left external ear
H61.023 Chronic perichondritis of external ear, bilateral
H61.029 Chronic perichondritis of external ear, unspecified ear
H61.03 Chondritis of external ear
Chondritis of auricle
Chondritis of pinna
H61.031 Chondritis of right external ear
H61.032 Chondritis of left external ear
H61.033 Chondritis of external ear, bilateral
H61.039 Chondritis of external ear, unspecified ear
H61.1 Noninfective disorders of pinna
EXCLUDES2 *cauliflower ear (M95.1-)*
gouty tophi of ear (M1A.-)
H61.10 Unspecified noninfective disorders of pinna
Disorder of pinna NOS
H61.101 Unspecified noninfective disorders of pinna, right ear
H61.102 Unspecified noninfective disorders of pinna, left ear
H61.103 Unspecified noninfective disorders of pinna, bilateral
H61.109 Unspecified noninfective disorders of pinna, unspecified ear
H61.11 Acquired deformity of pinna
Acquired deformity of auricle
EXCLUDES2 *cauliflower ear (M95.1-)*
H61.111 Acquired deformity of pinna, right ear
H61.112 Acquired deformity of pinna, left ear
H61.113 Acquired deformity of pinna, bilateral
H61.119 Acquired deformity of pinna, unspecified ear
H61.12 Hematoma of pinna
Hematoma of auricle
H61.121 Hematoma of pinna, right ear
H61.122 Hematoma of pinna, left ear
H61.123 Hematoma of pinna, bilateral
H61.129 Hematoma of pinna, unspecified ear
H61.19 Other noninfective disorders of pinna
H61.191 Noninfective disorders of pinna, right ear
H61.192 Noninfective disorders of pinna, left ear
H61.193 Noninfective disorders of pinna, bilateral
H61.199 Noninfective disorders of pinna, unspecified ear
H61.2 Impacted cerumen
Wax in ear
H61.20 Impacted cerumen, unspecified ear
H61.21 Impacted cerumen, right ear
H61.22 Impacted cerumen, left ear
H61.23 Impacted cerumen, bilateral
H61.3 Acquired stenosis of external ear canal
Collapse of external ear canal
EXCLUDES1 *postprocedural stenosis of external ear canal (H95.81-)*
H61.30 Acquired stenosis of external ear canal, unspecified
H61.301 Acquired stenosis of right external ear canal, unspecified
H61.302 Acquired stenosis of left external ear canal, unspecified
H61.303 Acquired stenosis of external ear canal, unspecified, bilateral
H61.309 Acquired stenosis of external ear canal, unspecified, unspecified ear
H61.31 Acquired stenosis of external ear canal secondary to trauma
H61.311 Acquired stenosis of right external ear canal secondary to trauma
H61.312 Acquired stenosis of left external ear canal secondary to trauma
H61.313 Acquired stenosis of external ear canal secondary to trauma, bilateral
H61.319 Acquired stenosis of external ear canal secondary to trauma, unspecified ear
H61.32 Acquired stenosis of external ear canal secondary to inflammation and infection
H61.321 Acquired stenosis of right external ear canal secondary to inflammation and infection
H61.322 Acquired stenosis of left external ear canal secondary to inflammation and infection
H61.323 Acquired stenosis of external ear canal secondary to inflammation and infection, bilateral
H61.329 Acquired stenosis of external ear canal secondary to inflammation and infection, unspecified ear
H61.39 Other acquired stenosis of external ear canal
H61.391 Other acquired stenosis of right external ear canal
H61.392 Other acquired stenosis of left external ear canal
H61.393 Other acquired stenosis of external ear canal, bilateral
H61.399 Other acquired stenosis of external ear canal, unspecified ear
H61.8 Other specified disorders of external ear
H61.81 Exostosis of external canal
H61.811 Exostosis of right external canal
H61.812 Exostosis of left external canal
H61.813 Exostosis of external canal, bilateral
H61.819 Exostosis of external canal, unspecified ear
H61.89 Other specified disorders of external ear
H61.891 Other specified disorders of right external ear

Unacceptable principal diagnosis symbol per Medicare code edits; Code exempt from diagnosis present on admission requirement; Questionable admission; Complication or comorbidity; CC/MCC exclusion; Major complication or comorbidity; Principal diagnosis as its own CC; Principal diagnosis as its own MCC; Z code as first-listed diagnosis

 When symbols appear on a code that requires a 7th character extension, refer to Appendix D to identify applicable 7th character codes.

H61.892 Other specified disorders of left external ear
H61.893 Other specified disorders of external ear, bilateral
H61.899 Other specified disorders of external ear, unspecified ear
H61.9 Disorder of external ear, unspecified
H61.90 Disorder of external ear, unspecified, unspecified ear
H61.91 Disorder of right external ear, unspecified
H61.92 Disorder of left external ear, unspecified
H61.93 Disorder of external ear, unspecified, bilateral
H62 Disorders of external ear in diseases classified elsewhere
H62.4 Otitis externa in other diseases classified elsewhere
Code first underlying disease, such as:
erysipelas (A46)
impetigo (L01.0)
EXCLUDES1 *otitis externa (in):*
candidiasis (B37.84)
herpes viral [herpes simplex] (B00.1)
herpes zoster (B02.8)
H62.40 Otitis externa in other diseases classified elsewhere, unspecified ear
H62.41 Otitis externa in other diseases classified elsewhere, right ear
H62.42 Otitis externa in other diseases classified elsewhere, left ear
H62.43 Otitis externa in other diseases classified elsewhere, bilateral
H62.8 Other disorders of external ear in diseases classified elsewhere
Code first underlying disease, such as:
gout (M1A.-, M10.-)
H62.8X Other disorders of external ear in diseases classified elsewhere
H62.8X1 Other disorders of right external ear in diseases classified elsewhere
H62.8X2 Other disorders of left external ear in diseases classified elsewhere
H62.8X3 Other disorders of external ear in diseases classified elsewhere, bilateral
H62.8X9 Other disorders of external ear in diseases classified elsewhere, unspecified ear

Diseases of middle ear and mastoid (H65-H75)

H65 Nonsuppurative otitis media
INCLUDES *nonsuppurative otitis media with myringitis*
Use additional code for any associated perforated tympanic membrane (H72.-)
Use additional code to identify:
exposure to environmental tobacco smoke (Z77.22)
exposure to tobacco smoke in the perinatal period (P96.81)
history of tobacco ▶dependence◀ (Z87.891)
occupational exposure to environmental tobacco smoke (Z57.31)
tobacco dependence (F17.-)
tobacco use (Z72.0)
H65.0 Acute serous otitis media
Acute and subacute secretory otitis
H65.00 Acute serous otitis media, unspecified ear
H65.01 Acute serous otitis media, right ear
H65.02 Acute serous otitis media, left ear
H65.03 Acute serous otitis media, bilateral
H65.04 Acute serous otitis media, recurrent, right ear
H65.05 Acute serous otitis media, recurrent, left ear
H65.06 Acute serous otitis media, recurrent, bilateral
H65.07 Acute serous otitis media, recurrent, unspecified ear
H65.1 Other acute nonsuppurative otitis media
EXCLUDES1 *otitic barotrauma (T70.0)*
otitis media (acute) NOS (H66.9)
H65.11 Acute and subacute allergic otitis media (mucoid) (sanguinous) (serous)
H65.111 Acute and subacute allergic otitis media (mucoid) (sanguinous) (serous), right ear
H65.112 Acute and subacute allergic otitis media (mucoid) (sanguinous) (serous), left ear
H65.113 Acute and subacute allergic otitis media (mucoid) (sanguinous) (serous), bilateral
H65.114 Acute and subacute allergic otitis media (mucoid) (sanguinous) (serous), recurrent, right ear
H65.115 Acute and subacute allergic otitis media (mucoid) (sanguinous) (serous), recurrent, left ear
H65.116 Acute and subacute allergic otitis media (mucoid) (sanguinous) (serous), recurrent, bilateral
H65.117 Acute and subacute allergic otitis media (mucoid) (sanguinous) (serous), recurrent, unspecified ear
H65.119 Acute and subacute allergic otitis media (mucoid) (sanguinous) (serous), unspecified ear
H65.19 Other acute nonsuppurative otitis media
Acute and subacute mucoid otitis media
Acute and subacute nonsuppurative otitis media NOS
Acute and subacute sanguinous otitis media
Acute and subacute seromucinous otitis media
H65.191 Other acute nonsuppurative otitis media, right ear
H65.192 Other acute nonsuppurative otitis media, left ear
H65.193 Other acute nonsuppurative otitis media, bilateral
H65.194 Other acute nonsuppurative otitis media, recurrent, right ear
H65.195 Other acute nonsuppurative otitis media, recurrent, left ear
H65.196 Other acute nonsuppurative otitis media, recurrent, bilateral
H65.197 Other acute nonsuppurative otitis media recurrent, unspecified ear
H65.199 Other acute nonsuppurative otitis media, unspecified ear
H65.2 Chronic serous otitis media
Chronic tubotympanal catarrh
H65.20 Chronic serous otitis media, unspecified ear
H65.21 Chronic serous otitis media, right ear
H65.22 Chronic serous otitis media, left ear
H65.23 Chronic serous otitis media, bilateral
H65.3 Chronic mucoid otitis media
Chronic mucinous otitis media
Chronic secretory otitis media
Chronic transudative otitis media
Glue ear
EXCLUDES1 *adhesive middle ear disease (H74.1)*
H65.30 Chronic mucoid otitis media, unspecified ear
H65.31 Chronic mucoid otitis media, right ear
H65.32 Chronic mucoid otitis media, left ear
H65.33 Chronic mucoid otitis media, bilateral
H65.4 Other chronic nonsuppurative otitis media
H65.41 Chronic allergic otitis media
H65.411 Chronic allergic otitis media, right ear
H65.412 Chronic allergic otitis media, left ear
H65.413 Chronic allergic otitis media, bilateral
H65.419 Chronic allergic otitis media, unspecified ear
H65.49 Other chronic nonsuppurative otitis media
Chronic exudative otitis media
Chronic nonsuppurative otitis media NOS
Chronic otitis media with effusion (nonpurulent)
Chronic seromucinous otitis media
H65.491 Other chronic nonsuppurative otitis media, right ear
H65.492 Other chronic nonsuppurative otitis media, left ear
H65.493 Other chronic nonsuppurative otitis media, bilateral
H65.499 Other chronic nonsuppurative otitis media, unspecified ear

Unspecified Code Other Specified Code Manifestation Code N Newborn P Pediatric M Maternity A Adult ♂ Male ♀ Female
● New Code ▲ Revised Code Title ▶◀ Revised Text NOTES INCLUDES EXCLUDES1 Not coded here EXCLUDES2 Not included here
4th character required 5th character required 6th character required 7th character required
Extension 'X' Alert HAC Hospital-acquired condition (HAC) alert AHA AHA Coding Clinic©

H65.9 **Unspecified nonsuppurative otitis media**
Allergic otitis media NOS
Catarrhal otitis media NOS
Exudative otitis media NOS
Mucoid otitis media NOS
Otitis media with effusion (nonpurulent) NOS
Secretory otitis media NOS
Seromucinous otitis media NOS
Serous otitis media NOS
Transudative otitis media NOS
H65.90 **Unspecified nonsuppurative otitis media, unspecified ear**
H65.91 **Unspecified nonsuppurative otitis media, right ear**
H65.92 **Unspecified nonsuppurative otitis media, left ear**
H65.93 **Unspecified nonsuppurative otitis media, bilateral**

H66 **Suppurative and unspecified otitis media**
INCLUDES *suppurative and unspecified otitis media with myringitis*
Use additional code to identify:
exposure to environmental tobacco smoke (Z77.22)
exposure to tobacco smoke in the perinatal period (P96.81)
history of tobacco ▶dependence◀ (Z87.891)
occupational exposure to environmental tobacco smoke (Z57.31)
tobacco dependence (F17.-)
tobacco use (Z72.0)

H66.0 **Acute suppurative otitis media**
H66.00 **Acute suppurative otitis media without spontaneous rupture of ear drum**
H66.001 **Acute suppurative otitis media without spontaneous rupture of ear drum, right ear**
AHA: Q1, 2016
H66.002 **Acute suppurative otitis media without spontaneous rupture of ear drum, left ear**
H66.003 **Acute suppurative otitis media without spontaneous rupture of ear drum, bilateral**
H66.004 **Acute suppurative otitis media without spontaneous rupture of ear drum, recurrent, right ear**
H66.005 **Acute suppurative otitis media without spontaneous rupture of ear drum, recurrent, left ear**
H66.006 **Acute suppurative otitis media without spontaneous rupture of ear drum, recurrent, bilateral**
H66.007 **Acute suppurative otitis media without spontaneous rupture of ear drum, recurrent, unspecified ear**
H66.009 **Acute suppurative otitis media without spontaneous rupture of ear drum, unspecified ear**
H66.01 **Acute suppurative otitis media with spontaneous rupture of ear drum**
H66.011 **Acute suppurative otitis media with spontaneous rupture of ear drum, right ear**
H66.012 **Acute suppurative otitis media with spontaneous rupture of ear drum, left ear**
H66.013 **Acute suppurative otitis media with spontaneous rupture of ear drum, bilateral**
H66.014 **Acute suppurative otitis media with spontaneous rupture of ear drum, recurrent, right ear**
H66.015 **Acute suppurative otitis media with spontaneous rupture of ear drum, recurrent, left ear**
H66.016 **Acute suppurative otitis media with spontaneous rupture of ear drum, recurrent, bilateral**
H66.017 **Acute suppurative otitis media with spontaneous rupture of ear drum, recurrent, unspecified ear**
H66.019 **Acute suppurative otitis media with spontaneous rupture of ear drum, unspecified ear**

H66.1 **Chronic tubotympanic suppurative otitis media**
Benign chronic suppurative otitis media
Chronic tubotympanic disease
Use additional code for any associated perforated tympanic membrane (H72.-)
H66.10 **Chronic tubotympanic suppurative otitis media, unspecified**
H66.11 **Chronic tubotympanic suppurative otitis media, right ear**
H66.12 **Chronic tubotympanic suppurative otitis media, left ear**
H66.13 **Chronic tubotympanic suppurative otitis media, bilateral**

H66.2 **Chronic atticoantral suppurative otitis media**
Chronic atticoantral disease
Use additional code for any associated perforated tympanic membrane (H72.-)
H66.20 **Chronic atticoantral suppurative otitis media, unspecified ear**
H66.21 **Chronic atticoantral suppurative otitis media, right ear**
H66.22 **Chronic atticoantral suppurative otitis media, left ear**
H66.23 **Chronic atticoantral suppurative otitis media, bilateral**

H66.3 **Other chronic suppurative otitis media**
Chronic suppurative otitis media NOS
Use additional code for any associated perforated tympanic membrane (H72.-)
EXCLUDES1 *tuberculous otitis media (A18.6)*
H66.3X **Other chronic suppurative otitis media**
H66.3X1 **Other chronic suppurative otitis media, right ear**
H66.3X2 **Other chronic suppurative otitis media, left ear**
H66.3X3 **Other chronic suppurative otitis media, bilateral**
H66.3X9 **Other chronic suppurative otitis media, unspecified ear**

H66.4 **Suppurative otitis media, unspecified**
Purulent otitis media NOS
Use additional code for any associated perforated tympanic membrane (H72.-)
H66.40 **Suppurative otitis media, unspecified, unspecified ear**
H66.41 **Suppurative otitis media, unspecified, right ear**
H66.42 **Suppurative otitis media, unspecified, left ear**
H66.43 **Suppurative otitis media, unspecified, bilateral**

H66.9 **Otitis media, unspecified**
Otitis media NOS
Acute otitis media NOS
Chronic otitis media NOS
Use additional code for any associated perforated tympanic membrane (H72.-)
H66.90 **Otitis media, unspecified, unspecified ear**
H66.91 **Otitis media, unspecified, right ear**
H66.92 **Otitis media, unspecified, left ear**
H66.93 **Otitis media, unspecified, bilateral**

H67 **Otitis media in diseases classified elsewhere**
Code first underlying disease, such as:
viral disease NEC (B00-B34)
Use additional code for any associated perforated tympanic membrane (H72.-)
EXCLUDES1 *otitis media in:*
influenza (J09.X9, J10.83, J11.83)
measles (B05.3)
scarlet fever (A38.0)
tuberculosis (A18.6)
H67.1 **Otitis media in diseases classified elsewhere, right ear**
H67.2 **Otitis media in diseases classified elsewhere, left ear**
H67.3 **Otitis media in diseases classified elsewhere, bilateral**
H67.9 **Otitis media in diseases classified elsewhere, unspecified ear**

H68 **Eustachian salpingitis and obstruction**

Unacceptable principal diagnosis symbol per Medicare code edits — Code exempt from diagnosis present on admission requirement
Questionable admission — Complication or comorbidity — CC/MCC exclusion — Major complication or comorbidity
Principal diagnosis as its own CC — Principal diagnosis as its own MCC — Z code as first-listed diagnosis

H68.0 Eustachian salpingitis
H68.00 Unspecified Eustachian salpingitis
H68.001 Unspecified Eustachian salpingitis, right ear
H68.002 Unspecified Eustachian salpingitis, left ear
H68.003 Unspecified Eustachian salpingitis, bilateral
H68.009 Unspecified Eustachian salpingitis, unspecified ear
H68.01 Acute Eustachian salpingitis
H68.011 Acute Eustachian salpingitis, right ear
H68.012 Acute Eustachian salpingitis, left ear
H68.013 Acute Eustachian salpingitis, bilateral
H68.019 Acute Eustachian salpingitis, unspecified ear
H68.02 Chronic Eustachian salpingitis
H68.021 Chronic Eustachian salpingitis, right ear
H68.022 Chronic Eustachian salpingitis, left ear
H68.023 Chronic Eustachian salpingitis, bilateral
H68.029 Chronic Eustachian salpingitis, unspecified ear
H68.1 Obstruction of Eustachian tube
Stenosis of Eustachian tube
Stricture of Eustachian tube
H68.10 Unspecified obstruction of Eustachian tube
H68.101 Unspecified obstruction of Eustachian tube, right ear
H68.102 Unspecified obstruction of Eustachian tube, left ear
H68.103 Unspecified obstruction of Eustachian tube, bilateral
H68.109 Unspecified obstruction of Eustachian tube, unspecified ear
H68.11 Osseous obstruction of Eustachian tube
H68.111 Osseous obstruction of Eustachian tube, right ear
H68.112 Osseous obstruction of Eustachian tube, left ear
H68.113 Osseous obstruction of Eustachian tube, bilateral
H68.119 Osseous obstruction of Eustachian tube, unspecified ear
H68.12 Intrinsic cartilagenous obstruction of Eustachian tube
H68.121 Intrinsic cartilagenous obstruction of Eustachian tube, right ear
H68.122 Intrinsic cartilagenous obstruction of Eustachian tube, left ear
H68.123 Intrinsic cartilagenous obstruction of Eustachian tube, bilateral
H68.129 Intrinsic cartilagenous obstruction of Eustachian tube, unspecified ear
H68.13 Extrinsic cartilagenous obstruction of Eustachian tube
Compression of Eustachian tube
H68.131 Extrinsic cartilagenous obstruction of Eustachian tube, right ear
H68.132 Extrinsic cartilagenous obstruction of Eustachian tube, left ear
H68.133 Extrinsic cartilagenous obstruction of Eustachian tube, bilateral
H68.139 Extrinsic cartilagenous obstruction of Eustachian tube, unspecified ear
H69 Other and unspecified disorders of Eustachian tube
H69.0 Patulous Eustachian tube
H69.00 Patulous Eustachian tube, unspecified ear
H69.01 Patulous Eustachian tube, right ear
H69.02 Patulous Eustachian tube, left ear
H69.03 Patulous Eustachian tube, bilateral
H69.8 Other specified disorders of Eustachian tube
H69.80 Other specified disorders of Eustachian tube, unspecified ear
H69.81 Other specified disorders of Eustachian tube, right ear
H69.82 Other specified disorders of Eustachian tube, left ear
H69.83 Other specified disorders of Eustachian tube, bilateral
H69.9 Unspecified Eustachian tube disorder
H69.90 Unspecified Eustachian tube disorder, unspecified ear
H69.91 Unspecified Eustachian tube disorder, right ear
H69.92 Unspecified Eustachian tube disorder, left ear
H69.93 Unspecified Eustachian tube disorder, bilateral
H70 Mastoiditis and related conditions
H70.0 Acute mastoiditis
Abscess of mastoid
Empyema of mastoid
H70.00 Acute mastoiditis without complications
H70.001 Acute mastoiditis without complications, right ear
H70.002 Acute mastoiditis without complications, left ear
H70.003 Acute mastoiditis without complications, bilateral
H70.009 Acute mastoiditis without complications, unspecified ear
H70.01 Subperiosteal abscess of mastoid
H70.011 Subperiosteal abscess of mastoid, right ear
H70.012 Subperiosteal abscess of mastoid, left ear
H70.013 Subperiosteal abscess of mastoid, bilateral
H70.019 Subperiosteal abscess of mastoid, unspecified ear
H70.09 Acute mastoiditis with other complications
H70.091 Acute mastoiditis with other complications, right ear
H70.092 Acute mastoiditis with other complications, left ear
H70.093 Acute mastoiditis with other complications, bilateral
H70.099 Acute mastoiditis with other complications, unspecified ear
H70.1 Chronic mastoiditis
Caries of mastoid
Fistula of mastoid
EXCLUDES1 *tuberculous mastoiditis (A18.03)*
H70.10 Chronic mastoiditis, unspecified ear
H70.11 Chronic mastoiditis, right ear
H70.12 Chronic mastoiditis, left ear
H70.13 Chronic mastoiditis, bilateral
H70.2 Petrositis
Inflammation of petrous bone
H70.20 Unspecified petrositis
H70.201 Unspecified petrositis, right ear
H70.202 Unspecified petrositis, left ear
H70.203 Unspecified petrositis, bilateral
H70.209 Unspecified petrositis, unspecified ear
H70.21 Acute petrositis
H70.211 Acute petrositis, right ear
H70.212 Acute petrositis, left ear
H70.213 Acute petrositis, bilateral
H70.219 Acute petrositis, unspecified ear
H70.22 Chronic petrositis
H70.221 Chronic petrositis, right ear
H70.222 Chronic petrositis, left ear
H70.223 Chronic petrositis, bilateral
H70.229 Chronic petrositis, unspecified ear
H70.8 Other mastoiditis and related conditions
EXCLUDES1 *preauricular sinus and cyst (Q18.1)*
sinus, fistula, and cyst of branchial cleft (Q18.0)
H70.81 Postauricular fistula
H70.811 Postauricular fistula, right ear
H70.812 Postauricular fistula, left ear
H70.813 Postauricular fistula, bilateral
H70.819 Postauricular fistula, unspecified ear
H70.89 Other mastoiditis and related conditions

Unspecified Code | Other Specified Code | Manifestation Code | N Newborn | P Pediatric | M Maternity | A Adult | ♂ Male | ♀ Female
● New Code | ▲ Revised Code Title | ►◄ Revised Text | NOTES | INCLUDES | EXCLUDES1 Not coded here | EXCLUDES2 Not included here
4th character required | 5th character required | 6th character required | 7th character required
Extension 'X' Alert | HAC Hospital-acquired condition (HAC) alert | AHA AHA Coding Clinic©

H70.891 Other mastoiditis and related conditions, right ear
H70.892 Other mastoiditis and related conditions, left ear
H70.893 Other mastoiditis and related conditions, bilateral
H70.899 Other mastoiditis and related conditions, unspecified ear

H70.9 Unspecified mastoiditis
H70.90 Unspecified mastoiditis, unspecified ear
H70.91 Unspecified mastoiditis, right ear
H70.92 Unspecified mastoiditis, left ear
H70.93 Unspecified mastoiditis, bilateral

H71 Cholesteatoma of middle ear
EXCLUDES2 *cholesteatoma of external ear (H60.4-)*
recurrent cholesteatoma of postmastoidectomy cavity (H95.0-)

H71.0 Cholesteatoma of attic
H71.00 Cholesteatoma of attic, unspecified ear
H71.01 Cholesteatoma of attic, right ear
H71.02 Cholesteatoma of attic, left ear
H71.03 Cholesteatoma of attic, bilateral

H71.1 Cholesteatoma of tympanum
H71.10 Cholesteatoma of tympanum, unspecified ear
H71.11 Cholesteatoma of tympanum, right ear
H71.12 Cholesteatoma of tympanum, left ear
H71.13 Cholesteatoma of tympanum, bilateral

H71.2 Cholesteatoma of mastoid
H71.20 Cholesteatoma of mastoid, unspecified ear
H71.21 Cholesteatoma of mastoid, right ear
H71.22 Cholesteatoma of mastoid, left ear
H71.23 Cholesteatoma of mastoid, bilateral

H71.3 Diffuse cholesteatosis
H71.30 Diffuse cholesteatosis, unspecified ear
H71.31 Diffuse cholesteatosis, right ear
H71.32 Diffuse cholesteatosis, left ear
H71.33 Diffuse cholesteatosis, bilateral

H71.9 Unspecified cholesteatoma
H71.90 Unspecified cholesteatoma, unspecified ear
H71.91 Unspecified cholesteatoma, right ear
H71.92 Unspecified cholesteatoma, left ear
H71.93 Unspecified cholesteatoma, bilateral

H72 Perforation of tympanic membrane
INCLUDES *persistent post-traumatic perforation of ear drum*
postinflammatory perforation of ear drum
Code first any associated otitis media (H65.-, H66.1-, H66.2-, H66.3-, H66.4-, H66.9-, H67.-)
EXCLUDES1 *acute suppurative otitis media with rupture of the tympanic membrane (H66.01-)*
traumatic rupture of ear drum (S09.2-)

H72.0 Central perforation of tympanic membrane
H72.00 Central perforation of tympanic membrane, unspecified ear
H72.01 Central perforation of tympanic membrane, right ear
H72.02 Central perforation of tympanic membrane, left ear
H72.03 Central perforation of tympanic membrane, bilateral

H72.1 Attic perforation of tympanic membrane
Perforation of pars flaccida
H72.10 Attic perforation of tympanic membrane, unspecified ear
H72.11 Attic perforation of tympanic membrane, right ear
H72.12 Attic perforation of tympanic membrane, left ear
H72.13 Attic perforation of tympanic membrane, bilateral

H72.2 Other marginal perforations of tympanic membrane
H72.2X Other marginal perforations of tympanic membrane
H72.2X1 Other marginal perforations of tympanic membrane, right ear
H72.2X2 Other marginal perforations of tympanic membrane, left ear
H72.2X3 Other marginal perforations of tympanic membrane, bilateral
H72.2X9 Other marginal perforations of tympanic membrane, unspecified ear

H72.8 Other perforations of tympanic membrane
H72.81 Multiple perforations of tympanic membrane
H72.811 Multiple perforations of tympanic membrane, right ear
H72.812 Multiple perforations of tympanic membrane, left ear
H72.813 Multiple perforations of tympanic membrane, bilateral
H72.819 Multiple perforations of tympanic membrane, unspecified ear
H72.82 Total perforations of tympanic membrane
H72.821 Total perforations of tympanic membrane, right ear
H72.822 Total perforations of tympanic membrane, left ear
H72.823 Total perforations of tympanic membrane, bilateral
H72.829 Total perforations of tympanic membrane, unspecified ear

H72.9 Unspecified perforation of tympanic membrane
H72.90 Unspecified perforation of tympanic membrane, unspecified ear
H72.91 Unspecified perforation of tympanic membrane, right ear
H72.92 Unspecified perforation of tympanic membrane, left ear
H72.93 Unspecified perforation of tympanic membrane, bilateral

H73 Other disorders of tympanic membrane

H73.0 Acute myringitis
EXCLUDES1 *acute myringitis with otitis media (H65, H66)*
H73.00 Unspecified acute myringitis
Acute tympanitis NOS
H73.001 Acute myringitis, right ear
H73.002 Acute myringitis, left ear
H73.003 Acute myringitis, bilateral
H73.009 Acute myringitis, unspecified ear
H73.01 Bullous myringitis
H73.011 Bullous myringitis, right ear
H73.012 Bullous myringitis, left ear
H73.013 Bullous myringitis, bilateral
H73.019 Bullous myringitis, unspecified ear
H73.09 Other acute myringitis
H73.091 Other acute myringitis, right ear
H73.092 Other acute myringitis, left ear
H73.093 Other acute myringitis, bilateral
H73.099 Other acute myringitis, unspecified ear

H73.1 Chronic myringitis
Chronic tympanitis
EXCLUDES1 *chronic myringitis with otitis media (H65, H66)*
H73.10 Chronic myringitis, unspecified ear
H73.11 Chronic myringitis, right ear
H73.12 Chronic myringitis, left ear
H73.13 Chronic myringitis, bilateral

H73.2 Unspecified myringitis
H73.20 Unspecified myringitis, unspecified ear
H73.21 Unspecified myringitis, right ear
H73.22 Unspecified myringitis, left ear
H73.23 Unspecified myringitis, bilateral

H73.8 Other specified disorders of tympanic membrane
H73.81 Atrophic flaccid tympanic membrane
H73.811 Atrophic flaccid tympanic membrane, right ear
H73.812 Atrophic flaccid tympanic membrane, left ear
H73.813 Atrophic flaccid tympanic membrane, bilateral
H73.819 Atrophic flaccid tympanic membrane, unspecified ear
H73.82 Atrophic nonflaccid tympanic membrane
H73.821 Atrophic nonflaccid tympanic membrane, right ear
H73.822 Atrophic nonflaccid tympanic membrane, left ear

Unacceptable principal diagnosis symbol per Medicare code edits · Code exempt from diagnosis present on admission requirement
Questionable admission · Complication or comorbidity · CC/MCC exclusion · Major complication or comorbidity
Principal diagnosis as its own CC · Principal diagnosis as its own MCC · Z code as first-listed diagnosis

H73.823 Atrophic nonflaccid tympanic membrane, bilateral
H73.829 Atrophic nonflaccid tympanic membrane, unspecified ear
H73.89 Other specified disorders of tympanic membrane
H73.891 Other specified disorders of tympanic membrane, right ear
H73.892 Other specified disorders of tympanic membrane, left ear
H73.893 Other specified disorders of tympanic membrane, bilateral
H73.899 Other specified disorders of tympanic membrane, unspecified ear
H73.9 Unspecified disorder of tympanic membrane
H73.90 Unspecified disorder of tympanic membrane, unspecified ear
H73.91 Unspecified disorder of tympanic membrane, right ear
H73.92 Unspecified disorder of tympanic membrane, left ear
H73.93 Unspecified disorder of tympanic membrane, bilateral

H74 Other disorders of middle ear mastoid
EXCLUDES2 *mastoiditis (H70.-)*
H74.0 Tympanosclerosis
H74.01 Tympanosclerosis, right ear
H74.02 Tympanosclerosis, left ear
H74.03 Tympanosclerosis, bilateral
H74.09 Tympanosclerosis, unspecified ear
H74.1 Adhesive middle ear disease
Adhesive otitis
EXCLUDES1 *glue ear (H65.3-)*
H74.11 Adhesive right middle ear disease
H74.12 Adhesive left middle ear disease
H74.13 Adhesive middle ear disease, bilateral
H74.19 Adhesive middle ear disease, unspecified ear
H74.2 Discontinuity and dislocation of ear ossicles
H74.20 Discontinuity and dislocation of ear ossicles, unspecified ear
H74.21 Discontinuity and dislocation of right ear ossicles
H74.22 Discontinuity and dislocation of left ear ossicles
H74.23 Discontinuity and dislocation of ear ossicles, bilateral
H74.3 Other acquired abnormalities of ear ossicles
H74.31 Ankylosis of ear ossicles
H74.311 Ankylosis of ear ossicles, right ear
H74.312 Ankylosis of ear ossicles, left ear
H74.313 Ankylosis of ear ossicles, bilateral
H74.319 Ankylosis of ear ossicles, unspecified ear
H74.32 Partial loss of ear ossicles
H74.321 Partial loss of ear ossicles, right ear
H74.322 Partial loss of ear ossicles, left ear
H74.323 Partial loss of ear ossicles, bilateral
H74.329 Partial loss of ear ossicles, unspecified ear
H74.39 Other acquired abnormalities of ear ossicles
H74.391 Other acquired abnormalities of right ear ossicles
H74.392 Other acquired abnormalities of left ear ossicles
H74.393 Other acquired abnormalities of ear ossicles, bilateral
H74.399 Other acquired abnormalities of ear ossicles, unspecified ear
H74.4 Polyp of middle ear
H74.40 Polyp of middle ear, unspecified ear
H74.41 Polyp of right middle ear
H74.42 Polyp of left middle ear
H74.43 Polyp of middle ear, bilateral
H74.8 Other specified disorders of middle ear and mastoid
H74.8X Other specified disorders of middle ear and mastoid
H74.8X1 Other specified disorders of right middle ear and mastoid
H74.8X2 Other specified disorders of left middle ear and mastoid
H74.8X3 Other specified disorders of middle ear and mastoid, bilateral
H74.8X9 Other specified disorders of middle ear and mastoid, unspecified ear
H74.9 Unspecified disorder of middle ear and mastoid
H74.90 Unspecified disorder of middle ear and mastoid, unspecified ear
H74.91 Unspecified disorder of right middle ear and mastoid
H74.92 Unspecified disorder of left middle ear and mastoid
H74.93 Unspecified disorder of middle ear and mastoid, bilateral

H75 Other disorders of middle ear and mastoid in diseases classified elsewhere
Code first underlying disease
H75.0 Mastoiditis in infectious and parasitic diseases classified elsewhere
EXCLUDES1 *mastoiditis (in):*
syphilis (A52.77)
tuberculosis (A18.03)
H75.00 Mastoiditis in infectious and parasitic diseases classified elsewhere, unspecified ear
H75.01 Mastoiditis in infectious and parasitic diseases classified elsewhere, right ear
H75.02 Mastoiditis in infectious and parasitic diseases classified elsewhere, left ear
H75.03 Mastoiditis in infectious and parasitic diseases classified elsewhere, bilateral
H75.8 Other specified disorders of middle ear and mastoid in diseases classified elsewhere
H75.80 Other specified disorders of middle ear and mastoid in diseases classified elsewhere, unspecified ear
H75.81 Other specified disorders of right middle ear and mastoid in diseases classified elsewhere
H75.82 Other specified disorders of left middle ear and mastoid in diseases classified elsewhere
H75.83 Other specified disorders of middle ear and mastoid in diseases classified elsewhere, bilateral

Diseases of inner ear (H80-H83)

H80 Otosclerosis
INCLUDES *Otospongiosis*
H80.0 Otosclerosis involving oval window, nonobliterative
H80.00 Otosclerosis involving oval window, nonobliterative, unspecified ear
H80.01 Otosclerosis involving oval window, nonobliterative, right ear
H80.02 Otosclerosis involving oval window, nonobliterative, left ear
H80.03 Otosclerosis involving oval window, nonobliterative, bilateral
H80.1 Otosclerosis involving oval window, obliterative
H80.10 Otosclerosis involving oval window, obliterative, unspecified ear
H80.11 Otosclerosis involving oval window, obliterative, right ear
H80.12 Otosclerosis involving oval window, obliterative, left ear
H80.13 Otosclerosis involving oval window, obliterative, bilateral
H80.2 Cochlear otosclerosis
Otosclerosis involving otic capsule
Otosclerosis involving round window
H80.20 Cochlear otosclerosis, unspecified ear
H80.21 Cochlear otosclerosis, right ear
H80.22 Cochlear otosclerosis, left ear
H80.23 Cochlear otosclerosis, bilateral
H80.8 Other otosclerosis
H80.80 Other otosclerosis, unspecified ear
H80.81 Other otosclerosis, right ear
H80.82 Other otosclerosis, left ear
H80.83 Other otosclerosis, bilateral
H80.9 Unspecified otosclerosis
H80.90 Unspecified otosclerosis, unspecified ear

H80.91 Unspecified otosclerosis, right ear
H80.92 Unspecified otosclerosis, left ear
H80.93 Unspecified otosclerosis, bilateral

H81 Disorders of vestibular function
EXCLUDES1 *epidemic vertigo (A88.1)*
vertigo NOS (R42)

H81.0 Ménière's disease
Labyrinthine hydrops
Ménière's syndrome or vertigo
H81.01 Ménière's disease, right ear
H81.02 Ménière's disease, left ear
H81.03 Ménière's disease, bilateral
H81.09 Ménière's disease, unspecified ear

H81.1 Benign paroxysmal vertigo
H81.10 Benign paroxysmal vertigo, unspecified ear
H81.11 Benign paroxysmal vertigo, right ear
H81.12 Benign paroxysmal vertigo, left ear
H81.13 Benign paroxysmal vertigo, bilateral

H81.2 Vestibular neuronitis
H81.20 Vestibular neuronitis, unspecified ear
H81.21 Vestibular neuronitis, right ear
H81.22 Vestibular neuronitis, left ear
H81.23 Vestibular neuronitis, bilateral

H81.3 Other peripheral vertigo
H81.31 Aural vertigo
H81.311 Aural vertigo, right ear
H81.312 Aural vertigo, left ear
H81.313 Aural vertigo, bilateral
H81.319 Aural vertigo, unspecified ear
H81.39 Other peripheral vertigo
Lermoyez' syndrome
Otogenic vertigo
Peripheral vertigo NOS
H81.391 Other peripheral vertigo, right ear
H81.392 Other peripheral vertigo, left ear
H81.393 Other peripheral vertigo, bilateral
H81.399 Other peripheral vertigo, unspecified ear

H81.4 Vertigo of central origin
Central positional nystagmus
H81.41 Vertigo of central origin, right ear
H81.42 Vertigo of central origin, left ear
H81.43 Vertigo of central origin, bilateral
H81.49 Vertigo of central origin, unspecified ear

H81.8 Other disorders of vestibular function
H81.8X Other disorders of vestibular function
H81.8X1 Other disorders of vestibular function, right ear
H81.8X2 Other disorders of vestibular function, left ear
H81.8X3 Other disorders of vestibular function, bilateral
H81.8X9 Other disorders of vestibular function, unspecified ear

H81.9 Unspecified disorder of vestibular function
Vertiginous syndrome NOS
H81.90 Unspecified disorder of vestibular function, unspecified ear
H81.91 Unspecified disorder of vestibular function, right ear
H81.92 Unspecified disorder of vestibular function, left ear
H81.93 Unspecified disorder of vestibular function, bilateral

H82 Vertiginous syndromes in diseases classified elsewhere
Code first underlying disease
EXCLUDES1 *epidemic vertigo (A88.1)*
H82.1 Vertiginous syndromes in diseases classified elsewhere, right ear
H82.2 Vertiginous syndromes in diseases classified elsewhere, left ear
H82.3 Vertiginous syndromes in diseases classified elsewhere, bilateral
H82.9 Vertiginous syndromes in diseases classified elsewhere, unspecified ear

H83 Other diseases of inner ear
H83.0 Labyrinthitis
H83.01 Labyrinthitis, right ear
H83.02 Labyrinthitis, left ear
H83.03 Labyrinthitis, bilateral
H83.09 Labyrinthitis, unspecified ear

H83.1 Labyrinthine fistula
H83.11 Labyrinthine fistula, right ear
H83.12 Labyrinthine fistula, left ear
H83.13 Labyrinthine fistula, bilateral
H83.19 Labyrinthine fistula, unspecified ear

H83.2 Labyrinthine dysfunction
Labyrinthine hypersensitivity
Labyrinthine hypofunction
Labyrinthine loss of function
H83.2X Labyrinthine dysfunction
H83.2X1 Labyrinthine dysfunction, right ear
H83.2X2 Labyrinthine dysfunction, left ear
H83.2X3 Labyrinthine dysfunction, bilateral
H83.2X9 Labyrinthine dysfunction, unspecified ear

H83.3 Noise effects on inner ear
Acoustic trauma of inner ear
Noise-induced hearing loss of inner ear
H83.3X Noise effects on inner ear
H83.3X1 Noise effects on right inner ear
H83.3X2 Noise effects on left inner ear
H83.3X3 Noise effects on inner ear, bilateral
H83.3X9 Noise effects on inner ear, unspecified ear

H83.8 Other specified diseases of inner ear
H83.8X Other specified diseases of inner ear
H83.8X1 Other specified diseases of right inner ear
H83.8X2 Other specified diseases of left inner ear
H83.8X3 Other specified diseases of inner ear, bilateral
H83.8X9 Other specified diseases of inner ear, unspecified ear

H83.9 Unspecified disease of inner ear
H83.90 Unspecified disease of inner ear, unspecified ear
H83.91 Unspecified disease of right inner ear
H83.92 Unspecified disease of left inner ear
H83.93 Unspecified disease of inner ear, bilateral

Other disorders of ear (H90-H94)

H90 Conductive and sensorineural hearing loss
EXCLUDES1 *deaf nonspeaking NEC (H91.3)*
deafness NOS (H91.9-)
hearing loss NOS (H91.9-)
noise-induced hearing loss (H83.3-)
ototoxic hearing loss (H91.0-)
sudden (idiopathic) hearing loss (H91.2-)

H90.0 Conductive hearing loss, bilateral
H90.1 Conductive hearing loss, unilateral with unrestricted hearing on the contralateral side
H90.11 Conductive hearing loss, unilateral, right ear, with unrestricted hearing on the contralateral side
H90.12 Conductive hearing loss, unilateral, left ear, with unrestricted hearing on the contralateral side
H90.2 Conductive hearing loss, unspecified
Conductive deafness NOS
H90.3 Sensorineural hearing loss, bilateral
H90.4 Sensorineural hearing loss, unilateral with unrestricted hearing on the contralateral side
H90.41 Sensorineural hearing loss, unilateral, right ear, with unrestricted hearing on the contralateral side
H90.42 Sensorineural hearing loss, unilateral, left ear, with unrestricted hearing on the contralateral side
H90.5 Unspecified sensorineural hearing loss
Central hearing loss NOS
Congenital deafness NOS
Neural hearing loss NOS
Perceptive hearing loss NOS
Sensorineural deafness NOS
Sensory hearing loss NOS
EXCLUDES1 *abnormal auditory perception (H93.2-)*
psychogenic deafness (F44.6)
H90.6 Mixed conductive and sensorineural hearing loss, bilateral

Unacceptable principal diagnosis symbol per Medicare code edits — Code exempt from diagnosis present on admission requirement
Questionable admission — Complication or comorbidity — CC/MCC exclusion — Major complication or comorbidity
Principal diagnosis as its own CC — Principal diagnosis as its own MCC — Z code as first-listed diagnosis

H90.7 Mixed conductive and sensorineural hearing loss, unilateral with unrestricted hearing on the contralateral side
H90.71 Mixed conductive and sensorineural hearing loss, unilateral, right ear, with unrestricted hearing on the contralateral side
H90.72 Mixed conductive and sensorineural hearing loss, unilateral, left ear, with unrestricted hearing on the contralateral side
H90.8 Mixed conductive and sensorineural hearing loss, unspecified
● H90.A Conductive and sensorineural hearing loss with restricted hearing on the contralateral side
● H90.A1 Conductive hearing loss, unilateral, with restricted hearing on the contralateral side
● H90.A11 Conductive hearing loss, unilateral, right ear with restricted hearing on the contralateral side
● H90.A12 Conductive hearing loss, unilateral, left ear with restricted hearing on the contralateral side
● H90.A2 Sensorineural hearing loss, unilateral, with restricted hearing on the contralateral side
● H90.A21 Sensorineural hearing loss, unilateral, right ear, with restricted hearing on the contralateral side
● H90.A22 Sensorineural hearing loss, unilateral, left ear, with restricted hearing on the contralateral side
● H90.A3 Mixed conductive and sensorineural hearing loss, unilateral with restricted hearing on the contralateral side
● H90.A31 Mixed conductive and sensorineural hearing loss, unilateral, right ear with restricted hearing on the contralateral side
● H90.A32 Mixed conductive and sensorineural hearing loss, unilateral, left ear with restricted hearing on the contralateral side

H91 Other and unspecified hearing loss
EXCLUDES1 *abnormal auditory perception (H93.2-)*
hearing loss as classified in H90.-
impacted cerumen (H61.2-)
noise-induced hearing loss (H83.3-)
psychogenic deafness (F44.6)
transient ischemic deafness (H93.01-)
H91.0 Ototoxic hearing loss
Code first poisoning due to drug or toxin, if applicable (T36-T65 with fifth or sixth character 1-4 or 6)
Use additional code for adverse effect, if applicable, to identify drug (T36-T50 with fifth or sixth character 5)
H91.01 Ototoxic hearing loss, right ear
H91.02 Ototoxic hearing loss, left ear
H91.03 Ototoxic hearing loss, bilateral
H91.09 Ototoxic hearing loss, unspecified ear
H91.1 Presbycusis
Presbyacusia
H91.10 Presbycusis, unspecified ear
H91.11 Presbycusis, right ear
H91.12 Presbycusis, left ear
H91.13 Presbycusis, bilateral
H91.2 Sudden idiopathic hearing loss
Sudden hearing loss NOS
H91.20 Sudden idiopathic hearing loss, unspecified ear
H91.21 Sudden idiopathic hearing loss, right ear
H91.22 Sudden idiopathic hearing loss, left ear
H91.23 Sudden idiopathic hearing loss, bilateral
H91.3 Deaf nonspeaking, not elsewhere classified
H91.8 Other specified hearing loss
H91.8X Other specified hearing loss
H91.8X1 Other specified hearing loss, right ear
H91.8X2 Other specified hearing loss, left ear
H91.8X3 Other specified hearing loss, bilateral
H91.8X9 Other specified hearing loss, unspecified ear
H91.9 Unspecified hearing loss
Deafness NOS
High frequency deafness
Low frequency deafness
H91.90 Unspecified hearing loss, unspecified ear
H91.91 Unspecified hearing loss, right ear
H91.92 Unspecified hearing loss, left ear
H91.93 Unspecified hearing loss, bilateral

H92 Otalgia and effusion of ear
H92.0 Otalgia
H92.01 Otalgia, right ear
H92.02 Otalgia, left ear
H92.03 Otalgia, bilateral
H92.09 Otalgia, unspecified ear
H92.1 Otorrhea
EXCLUDES1 *leakage of cerebrospinal fluid through ear (G96.0)*
H92.10 Otorrhea, unspecified ear
H92.11 Otorrhea, right ear
H92.12 Otorrhea, left ear
H92.13 Otorrhea, bilateral
H92.2 Otorrhagia
EXCLUDES1 *traumatic otorrhagia - code to injury*
H92.20 Otorrhagia, unspecified ear
H92.21 Otorrhagia, right ear
H92.22 Otorrhagia, left ear
H92.23 Otorrhagia, bilateral

H93 Other disorders of ear, not elsewhere classified
H93.0 Degenerative and vascular disorders of ear
EXCLUDES1 *presbycusis (H91.1)*
H93.01 Transient ischemic deafness
H93.011 Transient ischemic deafness, right ear
H93.012 Transient ischemic deafness, left ear
H93.013 Transient ischemic deafness, bilateral
H93.019 Transient ischemic deafness, unspecified ear
H93.09 Unspecified degenerative and vascular disorders of ear
H93.091 Unspecified degenerative and vascular disorders of right ear
H93.092 Unspecified degenerative and vascular disorders of left ear
H93.093 Unspecified degenerative and vascular disorders of ear, bilateral
H93.099 Unspecified degenerative and vascular disorders of unspecified ear
H93.1 Tinnitus
H93.11 Tinnitus, right ear
H93.12 Tinnitus, left ear
H93.13 Tinnitus, bilateral
H93.19 Tinnitus, unspecified ear
● H93.A Pulsatile tinnitus
● H93.A1 Pulsatile tinnitus, right ear
● H93.A2 Pulsatile tinnitus, left ear
● H93.A3 Pulsatile tinnitus, bilateral
● H93.A9 Pulsatile tinnitus, unspecified ear
H93.2 Other abnormal auditory perceptions
EXCLUDES2 *auditory hallucinations (R44.0)*
H93.21 Auditory recruitment
H93.211 Auditory recruitment, right ear
H93.212 Auditory recruitment, left ear
H93.213 Auditory recruitment, bilateral
H93.219 Auditory recruitment, unspecified ear
H93.22 Diplacusis
H93.221 Diplacusis, right ear
H93.222 Diplacusis, left ear
H93.223 Diplacusis, bilateral
H93.229 Diplacusis, unspecified ear
H93.23 Hyperacusis
H93.231 Hyperacusis, right ear
H93.232 Hyperacusis, left ear
H93.233 Hyperacusis, bilateral
H93.239 Hyperacusis, unspecified ear

Unspecified Code Other Specified Code Manifestation Code N Newborn P Pediatric M Maternity A Adult ♂ Male ♀ Female
● New Code ▲ Revised Code Title ►◄ Revised Text NOTES INCLUDES EXCLUDES1 Not coded here EXCLUDES2 Not included here
4th character required 5th character required 6th character required 7th character required
Extension 'X' Alert HAC Hospital-acquired condition (HAC) alert AHA AHA Coding Clinic©

When symbols appear on a code that requires a 7th character extension, refer to Appendix D to identify applicable 7th character codes.

H93.24 Temporary auditory threshold shift
H93.241 Temporary auditory threshold shift, right ear
H93.242 Temporary auditory threshold shift, left ear
H93.243 Temporary auditory threshold shift, bilateral
H93.249 Temporary auditory threshold shift, unspecified ear
H93.25 Central auditory processing disorder
Congenital auditory imperception
Word deafness
EXCLUDES1 *mixed receptive-expressive language disorder (F80.2)*
H93.29 Other abnormal auditory perceptions
H93.291 Other abnormal auditory perceptions, right ear
H93.292 Other abnormal auditory perceptions, left ear
H93.293 Other abnormal auditory perceptions, bilateral
H93.299 Other abnormal auditory perceptions, unspecified ear
H93.3 Disorders of acoustic nerve
Disorder of 8th cranial nerve
EXCLUDES1 *acoustic neuroma (D33.3)*
syphilitic acoustic neuritis (A52.15)
H93.3X Disorders of acoustic nerve
H93.3X1 Disorders of right acoustic nerve
H93.3X2 Disorders of left acoustic nerve
H93.3X3 Disorders of bilateral acoustic nerves
H93.3X9 Disorders of unspecified acoustic nerve
H93.8 Other specified disorders of ear
H93.8X Other specified disorders of ear
H93.8X1 Other specified disorders of right ear
H93.8X2 Other specified disorders of left ear
H93.8X3 Other specified disorders of ear, bilateral
H93.8X9 Other specified disorders of ear, unspecified ear
H93.9 Unspecified disorder of ear
H93.90 Unspecified disorder of ear, unspecified ear PDx
H93.91 Unspecified disorder of right ear PDx
H93.92 Unspecified disorder of left ear PDx
H93.93 Unspecified disorder of ear, bilateral PDx
H94 Other disorders of ear in diseases classified elsewhere
H94.0 Acoustic neuritis in infectious and parasitic diseases classified elsewhere
Code first underlying disease, such as:
parasitic disease (B65-B89)
EXCLUDES1 *acoustic neuritis (in):*
herpes zoster (B02.29)
syphilis (A52.15)
H94.00 Acoustic neuritis in infectious and parasitic diseases classified elsewhere, unspecified ear
H94.01 Acoustic neuritis in infectious and parasitic diseases classified elsewhere, right ear
H94.02 Acoustic neuritis in infectious and parasitic diseases classified elsewhere, left ear
H94.03 Acoustic neuritis in infectious and parasitic diseases classified elsewhere, bilateral
H94.8 Other specified disorders of ear in diseases classified elsewhere
Code first underlying disease, such as:
congenital syphilis (A50.0)
EXCLUDES1 *aural myiasis (B87.4)*
syphilitic labyrinthitis (A52.79)
H94.80 Other specified disorders of ear in diseases classified elsewhere, unspecified ear
H94.81 Other specified disorders of right ear in diseases classified elsewhere
H94.82 Other specified disorders of left ear in diseases classified elsewhere
H94.83 Other specified disorders of ear in diseases classified elsewhere, bilateral

Intraoperative and postprocedural complications and disorders of ear and mastoid process, not elsewhere classified (H95)

H95 Intraoperative and postprocedural complications and disorders of ear and mastoid process, not elsewhere classified
H95.0 Recurrent cholesteatoma of postmastoidectomy cavity
H95.00 Recurrent cholesteatoma of postmastoidectomy cavity, unspecified ear
H95.01 Recurrent cholesteatoma of postmastoidectomy cavity, right ear
H95.02 Recurrent cholesteatoma of postmastoidectomy cavity, left ear
H95.03 Recurrent cholesteatoma of postmastoidectomy cavity, bilateral ears
H95.1 Other disorders of ear and mastoid process following mastoidectomy
H95.11 Chronic inflammation of postmastoidectomy cavity
H95.111 Chronic inflammation of postmastoidectomy cavity, right ear
H95.112 Chronic inflammation of postmastoidectomy cavity, left ear
H95.113 Chronic inflammation of postmastoidectomy cavity, bilateral ears
H95.119 Chronic inflammation of postmastoidectomy cavity, unspecified ear
H95.12 Granulation of postmastoidectomy cavity
H95.121 Granulation of postmastoidectomy cavity, right ear
H95.122 Granulation of postmastoidectomy cavity, left ear
H95.123 Granulation of postmastoidectomy cavity, bilateral ears
H95.129 Granulation of postmastoidectomy cavity, unspecified ear
H95.13 Mucosal cyst of postmastoidectomy cavity
H95.131 Mucosal cyst of postmastoidectomy cavity, right ear
H95.132 Mucosal cyst of postmastoidectomy cavity, left ear
H95.133 Mucosal cyst of postmastoidectomy cavity, bilateral ears
H95.139 Mucosal cyst of postmastoidectomy cavity, unspecified ear
H95.19 Other disorders following mastoidectomy
H95.191 Other disorders following mastoidectomy, right ear
H95.192 Other disorders following mastoidectomy, left ear
H95.193 Other disorders following mastoidectomy, bilateral ears
H95.199 Other disorders following mastoidectomy, unspecified ear
H95.2 Intraoperative hemorrhage and hematoma of ear and mastoid process complicating a procedure
EXCLUDES1 *intraoperative hemorrhage and hematoma of ear and mastoid process due to accidental puncture or laceration during a procedure (H95.3-)*
H95.21 Intraoperative hemorrhage and hematoma of ear and mastoid process complicating a procedure on the ear and mastoid process CC
H95.22 Intraoperative hemorrhage and hematoma of ear and mastoid process complicating other procedure CC
H95.3 Accidental puncture and laceration of ear and mastoid process during a procedure
H95.31 Accidental puncture and laceration of the ear and mastoid process during a procedure on the ear and mastoid process CC
H95.32 Accidental puncture and laceration of the ear and mastoid process during other procedure CC
▲ H95.4 Postprocedural ▶hemorrhage of◀ ear and mastoid process following a procedure

PDx Unacceptable principal diagnosis symbol per Medicare code edits POA Code exempt from diagnosis present on admission requirement
? Questionable admission CC Complication or comorbidity CC/MCC Exc CC/MCC exclusion MCC Major complication or comorbidity
Principal diagnosis as its own CC Principal diagnosis as its own MCC Z code as first-listed diagnosis

▲ H95.41 Postprocedural ▶hemorrhage of◀ ear and mastoid process following a procedure on the ear and mastoid process CC

▲ H95.42 Postprocedural ▶hemorrhage of◀ ear and mastoid process following other procedure CC

● 5th H95.5 Postprocedural hematoma and seroma of ear and mastoid process following a procedure

● H95.51 Postprocedural hematoma of ear and mastoid process following a procedure on the ear and mastoid process CC CC/MCC Exc

● H95.52 Postprocedural hematoma of ear and mastoid process following other procedure CC CC/MCC Exc

● H95.53 Postprocedural seroma of ear and mastoid process following a procedure on the ear and mastoid process

● H95.54 Postprocedural seroma of ear and mastoid process following other procedure

5th H95.8 Other intraoperative and postprocedural complications and disorders of the ear and mastoid process, not elsewhere classified

EXCLUDES2 *postprocedural complications and disorders following mastoidectomy (H95.0-, H95.1-)*

6th H95.81 Postprocedural stenosis of external ear canal

H95.811 Postprocedural stenosis of right external ear canal CC

H95.812 Postprocedural stenosis of left external ear canal CC

H95.813 Postprocedural stenosis of external ear canal, bilateral CC

H95.819 Postprocedural stenosis of unspecified external ear canal CC

H95.88 Other intraoperative complications and disorders of the ear and mastoid process, not elsewhere classified CC

Use additional code , if applicable, to further specify disorder

H95.89 Other postprocedural complications and disorders of the ear and mastoid process, not elsewhere classified CC

Use additional code, if applicable, to further specify disorder

This page intentionally left blank

Chapter 9: Diseases of the Circulatory System (I00-I99)

Guidelines for Assigning Codes From This Chapter

Chapter 9 is where you'll find codes related to diseases of the heart, blood vessels, and certain lymph conditions, too. ICD-10-CM includes codes from all over the body in this chapter, from cerebral artery occlusions to hemorrhoids to hypertension.

List of Sections

- I00-I02: Acute rheumatic fever
- I05-I09: Chronic rheumatic heart diseases
- I10-I15: Hypertensive diseases
- I20-I25: Ischemic heart diseases
- I26-I28: Pulmonary heart disease and diseases of pulmonary circulation
- I30-I52: Other forms of heart disease
- I60-I69: Cerebrovascular diseases
- I70-I79: Diseases of arteries, arterioles and capillaries
- I80-I89: Diseases of veins, lymphatic vessels and lymph nodes, not elsewhere classified
- I95-I99: Other and unspecified disorders of the circulatory system

Highlights From the ICD-10-CM Official Guidelines for Coding and Reporting

The part of the ICD-10-CM Official Guidelines for Coding and Reporting dedicated to Chapter 9 give you coding rules for hypertension (HTN), atherosclerotic coronary artery disease and angina, cerebrovascular accident (CVA), cerebrovascular disease, and acute myocardial infarction (AMI). The following material summarizes the major pointers for this chapter from the 2017 Official Guidelines.

Hang on to These Hypertension Coding Tips for Accurate Claims

To keep your coding compliant, apply these rules for coding hypertension diagnoses.

Hypertension + heart disease: Unless the documentation clearly indicates that a patient's hypertension and heart disease are *not* related, *assume a causal relationship exists and assign codes accordingly*. The terms hypertension and heart involvement are linked by the word "with" in the Alphabetic Index. Documentation must link conditions not specifically associated with hypertension by words such as "with" or "due to" in the classification in order to code them as related.

Assign a code from category I11 (*Hypertensive heart disease*) for hypertension with heart conditions classified to I50.- or I51.4-I51.9. For patients with heart failure, identify the type with an additional code from I50 (*Heart failure*). If the provider specifically documents a *different* cause, code hypertension separately from I50.- and I51.4-I51.9).

The reason for the admission/encounter determines the sequence of the codes.

Assume HTN and CKD are connected: ICD-10-CM also presumes a causal relationship between HTN and chronic kidney disease (CKD).

So if documentation shows a patient has HTN and a condition that falls under N18 (*Chronic kidney disease*), then you should report a code from I12 (*Hypertensive chronic kidney disease*), even if there's no indication one caused the other. You also should report the relevant N18 code to indicate the CKD stage.

Be on the watch for acute renal failure in the documentation, too, because that merits an additional code when present.

Simplify coding for hypertensive heart and CKD: A single code from I13 (*Hypertensive heart and chronic kidney disease*) indicates the patient has both hypertensive heart disease and hypertensive CKD. You again should assume a relationship between the HTN and CKD.

When the patient has hypertensive heart disease and CKD, you should choose a code from I13. You should not report I11 (*Hypertensive heart disease*) and I12 (*Hypertensive chronic kidney disease*) together.

To fully describe the patient's medical status, pay attention to the ICD-10-CM instructions to report more than the I13.- code. If the patient has heart failure, you should assign an additional code from I50 (*Heart failure*) to indicate the type.

You'll also need to add a code from N18 (*Chronic kidney disease*) to show the CKD stage.

Think 2 codes for head diagnoses: Not all hypertensive diseases have combination codes that instruct you to keep a separate HTN code off your claim.

When the patient is diagnosed with hypertensive cerebrovascular disease, you should report the appropriate code from I60-I69 (*Cerebrovascular diseases*) first, and then report the correct hypertension code, I10-I15 (*Hypertensive diseases*).

Similarly, for hypertensive retinopathy, guidelines instruct you first to report a code from subcategory H35.0 (*Background retinopathy and retinal vascular changes*) and then the appropriate HTN code from I10-I15. Sequence the codes based on the reason for the encounter.

I15 applies when there's another cause: In some cases, an underlying condition can be the cause of the patient's HTN. When documentation reveals that situation, the HTN is known as secondary HTN.

To report this patient's diagnoses, you'll need one code to report the underlying condition (etiology) and a code from I15 (*Secondary hypertension*) to report the HTN. Your sequencing will depend on the reason for the admission or encounter.

Understand the meaning of uncontrolled: Providers may document HTN using the terms controlled and uncontrolled. Controlled usually means the therapy being used is keeping the patient's HTN under control. Uncontrolled may mean either the HTN is untreated or that the current regimen isn't keeping the HTN under control.

In either case, you should choose the appropriate code from I10-I15 (*Hypertensive diseases*) to provide the appropriate hypertension codes.

Elevated or transient doesn't equal HTN: If documentation shows only elevated blood pressure, you should not use a code from I10.-

Code R03.0 (*Elevated blood pressure reading without diagnosis of hypertension*) is appropriate when documentation doesn't establish HTN definitively.

If the patient is pregnant, look instead to O13.- (*Gestational [pregnancy-induced] hypertension without significant proteinuria*) or O14.- (*Pre-eclampsia*) for transient HTN of pregnancy.

Get to Know Combination Codes for Atherosclerotic Coronary Artery Disease and Angina

ICD-10-CM offers combination codes for atherosclerotic heart disease with angina pectoris. You will find these combination code in subcategories I25.11 (*Atherosclerotic heart disease of native coronary artery with angina pectoris*) and I25.7 (*Atherosclerosis of coronary artery bypass graft[s] and coronary artery of transplanted heart with angina pectoris*). Don't assign an additional code for angina pectoris when using one of these combination codes.

Assume a causal relationship: When a patient has atherosclerosis and angina pectoris, you can assume the angina is due to the atherosclerosis unless the documentation indicates otherwise.

Sequencing tip: If a patient with coronary artery disease is admitted due to an acute myocardial infarction (AMI), report the AMI first, before the coronary artery disease.

Know the Facts About Intervention-related CVA Options

The Official Guidelines emphasize that documentation must clearly specify the cause-and-effect relationship between a medical procedure and a cerebrovascular accident (CVA) before you can assign a code for intraoperative or postprocedural CVA. To make a proper code assignment, you need to know if the CVA is due to infarction (obstruction of blood supply that leads to tissue death) or hemorrhage (profuse bleeding) and whether it occurred intraoperatively (during the procedure) or postoperatively (after the procedure).

For a patient who suffers a cerebral hemorrhage, code assignment depends on the type of procedure performed.

Master Coding for Sequelae of Cerebrovascular Disease

Codes from I69 (*Sequelae of cerebrovascular disease*) allow you to code for neurologic deficits that cerebrovascular diseases cause either at onset of the disease or at any time after. Keep in mind that you should use I69.- codes only for sequelae, or late effects, and not for deficits that are part of a current acute CVA.

However, if the patient has an acute CVA and also has late effects from a previous event, you may report the late effect and acute diagnoses (I60-I69) together.

In some cases, a patient may have an event and not suffer from late effects. Codes from I69 would not be appropriate for those patients. Instead use Z86.73 (*Personal history of transient ischemic attack [TIA], and cerebral infarction*).

Dominant or nondominant side: Codes from I69 that specify hemiplegia, hemiparesis, and monoplegia identify whether the dominant or nondominant side is affected. Tabular notes may direct you to choose a particular dominance as the default choice for some codes, when the documentation does not specify one or the other. If a default choice isn't provided, use the following guidelines to make your selection:

- For ambidextrous patients, the default is dominant.
- If the left side is affected, the default is nondominant.
- If the right side is affected, the default is dominant.

Keep the Focus on STEMI vs. NSTEMI for Acute Myocardial Infarction (AMI) Coding

The Official Guidelines for AMI coding stress that there are separate options for ST elevation myocardial infarction (STEMI) and non-STEMI (NSTEMI).

- It might help to explain that "ST" refers to a specific portion of an electrocardiogram (ECG). ST elevated away from the baseline suggests a heart attack is occurring (STEMI). But this elevation won't appear on ECGs for many patients experiencing an MI, so the provider will classify those as NSTEMI.

Use subcategories I21.0-I21.2 and I21.3 for STEMI. Turn to I21.4 for NSTEMI and nontransmural MIs.

- Nontransmural means not (non) through (trans) the wall (mural), indicating the heart muscle death due to restricted blood flow does not extend through the full thickness of the myocardial wall segment.

STEMI overrides NSTEMI: One thing you need to watch out for is that if NSTEMI evolves to STEMI, you should assign the STEMI code. What's more, you also should use a STEMI code when STEMI converts to NSTEMI due to thrombolytic therapy. So in both cases, whether NSTEMI becomes STEMI, or STEMI becomes NSTEMI, you should use the appropriate STEMI code.

NSTEMI and site documented: Another area to watch is that you may see documentation of a nontransmural or subendocardial infarction along with a documented site. If an AMI is documented as nontransmural or subendocardial, but the site is provided, it is still coded as a subendocardial AMI.

Unspecified MI: Report I21.3 (*ST elevation [STEMI] myocardial infarction of unspecified site*) as the default code for an unspecified MI. If the provider doesn't specify the site but does document a STEMI or transmural MI, you should assign I21.3.

Hold off on aftercare coding for up to 4 weeks: You can continue to report codes for I21 (*ST elevation [STEMI] and non-ST elevation [NSTEMI] myocardial infarction*) for all MI-related encounters up to four weeks old. If the patient is still receiving care related to the MI after four weeks, look to aftercare codes and not I21.-. For old or healed MIs not requiring further care, you may assign I25.2 (*Old myocardial infarction*).

Anatomy of the Cardiovascular System

Introduction

The human vascular system comprises a series of tubes (which are known as vessels) that travel in almost all parts of the human body. It is categorized into the following two classes:

1. **Blood Vascular System**
   The blood vascular system includes the heart and blood vessels required to facilitate the circulation of the colored fluid (blood) inside the body.

   a) The Structure of Arteries

   The arteries possess stronger and thicker walls than the corresponding veins and are based on the following components:

   i) Tunica Intima

   ii) Tunica Media

   iii) Tunica Externa

   b. The Structure of Veins

   The veins have a similar structure as that of the arteries. The components of a typical vein are described below:

   i) Tunica Intima

   ii) Tunica Media

   iii) Tunica Externa

   c. The Blood

   The blood is considered a uniquely specialized connective tissue that is composed of the formed elements (or the blood cells) and the fluid portion (or plasma). The formed elements of blood are based on the red blood cells (RBCs or erythrocytes), the white blood cells (WBCs or leukocytes) and the platelets (or thrombocytes). The blood contributes to about 8% of total body weight. The quantity of blood in an average human varies between 5 to 6 liters. The elements of blood are categorized below:

   d. Erythrocytes or Red Blood Cells: The red blood cells are the most common type of blood cells that contribute to about 95% of the blood cell volume.

   e. Leukocytes or White Blood Cells: The white blood cells can be divided into the following subcategories:

   f. Granular Leukocytes- The granular leukocytes contain granules in their cytoplasm and can be further classified into the following three types:

   i) neutrophils constitute about 60% to 70% of the white blood cells.

   ii) eosinophils constitute about 2% to 4% of the white blood cells.

   iii) basophils constitute about 0.5% to 1% of the white blood cells.

   g. Agranular Leukocytes: The agranular leukocytes do not contain granules in their cytoplasm and can be further classified into the following two types:

   i) monocytes constitute about 3% to 8% of the white blood cells.

   ii) lymphocytes constitute about 20% to 25% of the white blood cells.

   h. Thrombocytes or Platelets: The platelets are small cell fragments that do not contain nucleus in their cytoplasm.

   i. Blood Plasma

   The plasma is the fluid component of blood in which the blood cells usually remain suspended. The blood plasma is composed of 91% water, 7% proteins, and 2% solutes.

2. **Lymph Vascular System**
   The lymph vascular system includes the lymph glands and lymphatic vessels for circulating the colorless fluid (lymph) throughout the human body. Both of the blood vascular and the lymph vascular systems work in close association with each other for sustaining the human life cycle.

3. **The Thoracic Cavity**
   The thoracic cavity is enclosed by the thoracic wall and primarily contains the structures of the cardiovascular and respiratory systems.

   a) The Pericardium

   The heart and the roots of the great vessels are contained within the conical and fibro-serous sac, which is known as the pericardium. It is composed of two closely connected sacs, which are known as the fibrous pericardium (or the outer sac) and the serous pericardium (the inner sac).

   b) The Heart

   The heart is a hollow muscular organ that remains enclosed in the fibro-serous sac (or the pericardium) and is regarded as the central organ of the cardiovascular system. It lies between the lungs in the middle mediastinum and receives blood from the veins.

CIRCULATION OF BLOOD THROUGH THE HEART

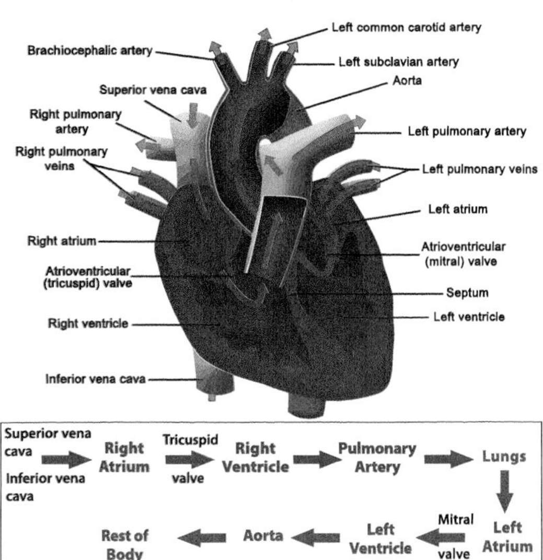

4. **The Chambers of the Heart**
   The human heart is based on the following four chambers:

   a) The Right Atrium: The right border of the human heart is formed by the right atrium. The superior vena cava, inferior vena cava and coronary sinus provide venous blood supply to the right atrium of the heart.

   The right atrium contains the following elements inside it:

   i) Sinus Venarum

   ii) Pectinate Muscles

   iii) Opening of Superior Vena Cava

   iv) Opening of Inferior Vena Cava

   v) Opening of Coronary Sinus

   vi) The Right Atrioventricular Orifice

   vii) Interatrial Septum

   b) The Right Ventricle: The inferior border of the human heart is constituted by the right ventricle.

   c) The Left Atrium: The left atrium chiefly constitutes the base of the heart and utilizes the mitral valve to pump the oxygenated blood received from the pulmonary veins into the left ventricle of the heart. The interior of the left atrium is based on the following components:

   i) Two superior and two inferior pulmonary veins that enter the posterior wall of the left atrium.

   ii) A posteriorly directed interatrial septum that separates the right atrium from the left atrium of the heart.

   iii) A smooth walled portion and a muscular auricle containing pectinate muscles.

   iv) A comparatively thicker wall than the corresponding right atrium.

   v) A left atrioventricular orifice that facilitates the discharge of oxygenated blood into the left ventricle.

   d) The Left Ventricle: The left ventricle pumps the oxygenated blood (through the aortic valve) to the whole body through the aorta. The interior of the left ventricle is based on the following elements:

   i) a double-leaflet/dual-flap mitral (bicuspid or left atrioventricular) valve, which is located between the left atrium and ventricle for guarding the left atrioventricular orifice.

   ii) walls of the left ventricle, which are comparatively thicker than the corresponding right ventricle.

   iii) conical cavity of the left ventricle that is comparatively longer than the corresponding right ventricle.

   iv) anterior and posterior left ventricular papillary muscles that get attached to the cusps of the mitral valve through the tendinous cords (or the chordae tendineae).

   v) aortic vestibule, which is a smooth-walled, nonmuscular, superoanterior outflow portion of the left ventricle that lies inferior to the aortic orifice and possesses fibrous walls.

vi) aortic orifice (or opening) is an opening of the left ventricle into the aorta. This valve is usually tricuspid (with three leaflets) and located posterior to the left side of the sternum at the level of the third intercostal space.

vii) inner surface of the left ventricle gives rise to the irregular, rounded and thick muscular ridges that are termed as the trabeculae carneae.

5. **The Cardiac Cycle:**
The cardiac cycle is based on the synchronous pumping of the right and left chambers of the heart.

a) The Arterial Supply of the Heart

The heart is supplied by the following arteries:

i) right coronary artery (RCA)
ii) sino-atrial nodal artery
iii) right marginal artery
iv) posterior interventricular artery
v) atrio-ventricular nodal artery
vi) left coronary artery
vii) anterior interventricular artery (or Left Anterior Descending Artery)
viii) circumflex artery
ix) left marginal artery
x) posterior interventricular artery

b) The Arteries

The major types of arteries are described below:

i) pulmonary arteries- pulmonary arteries carry the oxygen deficient blood from the heart to the lungs for attaining oxygen.
ii) systemic arteries- systemic arteries transport the oxygenated blood to the rest of the body.

c) The Aorta

The aorta is divided into the following components:

i) ascending aorta
ii) arch of aorta
iii) descending aorta

d) Thoracic Aorta

i) aortic intercostal arteries (nine pairs)
ii) left bronchial arteries (two in number)
iii) posterior mediastinal arteries
iv) pericardial arteries
v) superior phrenic arteries

e) The Abdominal Aorta

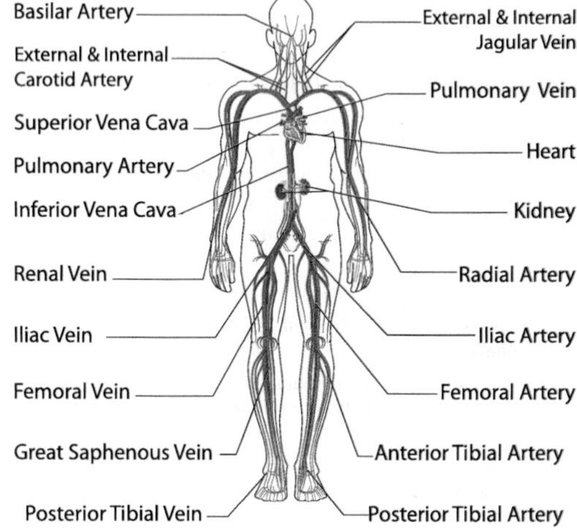

6. **The Arteries of the Head and Neck**
The major arteries that supply blood to the head and neck regions are the two common carotid arteries. These arteries travel through the neck and each one of them gets divided into the following branches:

a) External Carotid Arteries

b) Ascending Pharyngeal Artery

c) Occipital Artery

i) muscular branches
ii) sternocleidomastoid branch/sternocleidomastoid artery
iii) auricular branch
iv) meningeal or dural branch
v) descending branch

d) Posterior Auricular Artery

i) stylomastoid branch/stylomastoid artery
ii) auricular branch
iii) occipital branch

e) Superior Thyroid Artery

i) hyoid branch
ii) sternocleidomastoid branch/sternocleidomastoid artery
iii) superior laryngeal branch/superior laryngeal artery
iv) cricothyroid branch

f) Lingual Artery

i) hyoid branch
ii) dorsal lingual branches
iii) sublingual branch/sublingual artery
iv) deep lingual branch/deep lingual artery

g) Facial (or External Maxillary) Artery

Cervical Branches	Facial Branches
i) ascending palatine artery	i) inferior labial artery
ii) tonsillar branch	ii) superior labial artery
iii) glandular branches	iii) lateral nasal branch
iv) submental artery	iv) angular artery
v) muscular branches	v) muscular branches

7. **The Internal Carotid Arteries:** The internal carotid arteries are the direct continuation of the common carotid arteries. However, the other portions of these arteries extend into the following arterial branches:

a) The petrous portion of the internal carotid arteries gives rise to the following branches:

i) caroticotympanic artery
ii) artery of the pterygoid canal (or vidian artery)

b) The cavernous portion of the internal carotid arteries gives rise to the following branches:

i) cavernous artery
ii) hypophyseal artery
iii) semilunar arterial branches
iv) anterior meningeal artery
v) ophthalmic artery

c) Anterior Cerebral Artery

i) anteromedial ganglionic branches
ii) inferior branches
iii) anterior branches
iv) middle branches
v) posterior branches

d) The Middle Cerebral Artery

i) anterolateral ganglionic branches
ii) inferior lateral frontal branch
iii) ascending frontal branch
iv) ascending parietal branch
v) parietotemporal branch
vi) temporal branches

e) Posterior Communicating Artery

f) Anterior Choroidal Artery (or Choroid Artery)

8. **The Arteries of the Upper Extremity:** The Subclavian Artery divides into the following branches:

a) Vertebral Artery: The vertebral artery is divided into the following branches:

Cervical Branches	Cranial Branches
i) spinal branches	i) posterior meningeal branch
ii) muscular branches	ii) posterior/dorsal spinal artery
	iii) anterior/ventral spinal artery
	iv) posterior inferior cerebellar artery
	v) medullary arteries

b) Internal Thoracic (or Internal Mammary) Artery
   i) pericardiacophrenic artery
   ii) anterior mediastinal arteries
   iii) pericardial branches
   iv) sternal branches
   v) anterior intercostal arteries
   vi) perforating branches
   vii) musculophrenic artery
   viii) superior epigastric artery

c) Thyrocervical trunk (or Thyroid axis)
   i) inferior thyroid artery
   ii) inferior laryngeal artery
   iii) esophageal branches
   iv) tracheal artery
   v) ascending cervical artery
   vi) muscular branches

d) Suprascapular (or Transverse Scapular) Artery
   i) suprasternal branch
   ii) acromial branch

e) Transverse Cervical Artery (or Transverse Artery of Neck)
   i) ascending branch
   ii) descending branch

f) The costocervical trunk is the highest intercostal artery (superior intercostal), and it includes:
   i) first posterior intercostal artery
   ii) second posterior intercostal artery
   iii) deep cervical artery
   iv) third arterial part

g) Axillary Artery
   i) first part
   ii) second part
   iii) third part

h) Brachial Artery
   i) muscular branches
   ii) human nutrient artery
   iii) profunda brachii artery (deep artery of the arm/superior profunda artery)
   iv) superior ulnar collateral artery (or inferior profunda artery)
   v) inferior ulnar collateral artery (or anastomotica magna artery)

i) Radial Artery

Branches of the Radial Artery in Forearm	**Branches of the Radial Artery in Wrist**	**Branches of the Radial Artery in Hand**
The Radial Recurrent Artery	The Posterior Radial Carpal Artery (The Dorsal Carpal Branch)	The Princeps Pollicis Artery
The Muscular (Arterial) Branches	The First Dorsal Metacarpal Artery	The Radialis Indicis Artery
The Anterior Radial Carpal Artery (The Volar Carpal Branch)		The Deep Palmar/ Volar Arch
The Superficial Volar Artery (The Superficial Palmar Branch of Radial Artery)		The Palmar Interosseous (or Volar Metacarpal) Arteries
		The Perforating (Arterial) Branches
		The Recurrent (Arterial) Branches

j) Ulnar Artery- The ulnar artery originates from the brachial artery and runs along the medial aspect (or ulnar side) of the forearm. A tabular representation of the arterial branches of ulnar artery is provided below:

Branches of the Ulnar Artery in Forearm	**Branches of the Ulnar Artery in Wrist**	**Branches of the Ulnar Artery in Hand**
The Anterior Ulnar Recurrent Artery	The Volar Carpal Branch (or Anterior Ulnar Carpal Artery)	The Deep Volar Branch (or Profunda Branch)
The Posterior Ulnar Recurrent Artery	The Dorsal Carpal Branch (or Posterior Ulnar Carpal Artery)	The Superficial Volar Arch (or Superficial Palmar Arch)
The Common Interosseous Artery (divides into the following two branches) ➲ The Volar Interosseous Artery (or Anterior Interosseous Artery) ➲ The Dorsal Interosseous Artery (or Posterior Interosseous Artery)		
The Muscular (Arterial) Branches		

9. Arteries of the Trunk

Arteries of the trunk are based on the following arteries:

a) The Descending Aorta
   i) thoracic aorta
   ii) abdominal aorta

b) The Common Iliac Arteries

c) Internal Iliac (or Hypogastric) Artery

The Anterior Trunk	**The Posterior Trunk**
The Superior Vesical Artery The Middle Vesical Artery The Inferior Vesical Artery	The Iliolumbar Artery-with the following branches: - The Lumbar (Arterial) Branch - The Iliac (Arterial) Branch
The Middle Hemorrhoidal Artery The Uterine Artery (In Female)	The Superior and Inferior Lateral Sacral Arteries
The Vaginal Artery (In Female) The Obturator Artery	The Superior Gluteal Artery (or Gluteal Artery)-with the following branches: - The Superficial (Arterial) Branch - The Deep (Arterial) Branch

The Internal Pudendal Artery (Internal Pubic Artery)-with the following branches: The Muscular (Arterial) Branches The Inferior Hemorrhoidal Artery The Perineal (or Superficial Perineal) Artery The Artery of the Urethral Bulb The Urethral Artery The Deep Artery of the Penis (or Artery to the Corpus Cavernosum) The Dorsal Artery of the Penis	
The Inferior Gluteal Artery (Sciatic Artery)-with the following branches: The Muscular (Arterial) Branches The Coccygeal (Arterial) Branches The Arteria Comitans Nervi Ischiadici The Anastomotic (Arterial) Branch The Articular (Arterial) Branch The Cutaneous (Arterial) Branches	

d) The External Iliac Artery divides into the inferior epigastric artery, which includes:
   i) muscular branches
   ii) cutaneous branches
   iii) external spermatic branch (in males) and artery of round ligament of uterus (in females)
   iv) pubic branch

e) Deep Iliac Circumflex Artery
   i) muscular branch
   ii) cutaneous branch

10. The Arteries of the Lower Extremity

a) Femoral Artery- The branches of the femoral artery are presented below in a tabular format:

The Branches of the Femoral Artery		
The Superficial Epigastric Artery		
The Superficial Iliac Circumflex Artery		
The Superficial External Pudendal Artery (or Superficial External Pubic Artery)		
The Deep External Pudendal Artery (or Deep External Pubic Artery)		
The Muscular (Arterial) Branches		
The Profunda Femoris Artery (or Deep Femoral Artery)		
Branches and Subordinate Branches of the Profunda Femoris Artery	The Lateral Femoral Circumflex Artery	
	Sub-Branches	The Ascending (Arterial) Branch
		The Descending (Arterial) Branch
		The Transverse (Arterial) Branch
	The Medial Femoral Circumflex Artery (or Internal Circumflex Artery)	
	Sub-Branches	The Superficial (Arterial) Branch
		The Deep (Arterial) Branch
		The Acetabular (Arterial) Branch
	The Perforating Arteries	
	Sub-Branches	The First Perforating Artery
		The Second Perforating Artery
		The Third Perforating Artery
	The Muscular (Arterial) Branches	

The Highest Genicular Artery (or Anastomotica Magna Artery)	
Branches of the Highest Genicular Artery	The Saphenous (Arterial) Branch
	The Musculoarticular (Arterial) Branch

b) Popliteal Artery- A tabular presentation of the branches of the popliteal artery is given below:

Branches of the Popliteal Artery	
The Superior Muscular Branches	
The Sural Arteries (or Inferior Muscular Arteries)	
The Cutaneous Branches	
The Superior Genicular Arteries (or Superior Articular Arteries)	
Branches of the Superior Genicular Arteries	The Medial Superior Genicular Artery
	The Lateral Superior Genicular Artery
The Middle Genicular Artery (or Azygos Articular Artery)	
The Inferior Genicular Arteries (or Inferior Articular Arteries)	
Branches of the Inferior Genicular Arteries	The Medial Inferior Genicular Artery
	The Lateral Inferior Genicular Artery

c) Anterior Tibial Artery
   i) Posterior Tibial Recurrent Artery
   ii) Fibular Artery
   iii) Anterior Tibial Recurrent Artery
   iv) Muscular (Arterial) Branches
   v) Anterior Medial Malleolar Artery (or Internal Malleolar Artery)
   vi) Anterior Lateral Malleolar Artery (or External Malleolar Artery)

d) Dorsalis Pedis Artery (or Dorsal Artery of Foot)- A tabular presentation of the branches of the dorsalis pedis artery is given below:

Branches of the Dorsalis Pedis Artery	
The lateral Tarsal Artery (or Tarsal Artery)	
The Medial Tarsal Arteries	
The Arcuate Artery (or Metatarsal Artery)	
Branches of Arcuate Artery	The Second Dorsal Metatarsal Artery
	The Third Dorsal Metatarsal Artery
	The Fourth Dorsal Metatarsal Artery
The First Dorsal Metatarsal Artery	
The Deep Plantar Artery (or Communicating Artery)	

e) Posterior Tibial Artery- The branching tree of the posterior tibial artery is presented below:

Branches of the Posterior Tibial Artery	
The Peroneal Artery	
Branches of Peroneal Artery	The Muscular (Arterial) Branches
	The Nutrient Artery of Fibula
	The Perforating Branch (or Anterior Peroneal Artery)
	The Communicating Branch of Peroneal Artery
	The Lateral Calcaneal Arteries (or External Calcaneal Arteries)
The Nutrient Artery of Tibia	
The Muscular Branches of the Posterior Tibial Artery	
The Posterior Medial Malleolar Artery (or Internal Malleolar Artery)	
The Communicating Branch of Posterior Tibial Artery	
The Medial Calcaneal Arteries (or Internal Calcaneal Arteries)	
The Medial Plantar Artery (or Internal Plantar Artery)	
The Lateral Plantar Artery (or External Plantar Artery)	

11. The Veins

The veins are the blood vessels that carry deoxygenated blood from the body tissues towards the heart via capillaries. The veins can be categorized into the following classes:

a) Pulmonary Veins: The pulmonary veins carry oxygenated blood from the lungs to the left atrium of the heart. The pulmonary veins are of the following types:
   i) right inferior pulmonary vein
   ii) right superior pulmonary vein
   iii) left inferior pulmonary vein
   iv) left superior pulmonary vein

b) Systemic Veins: The systemic veins deliver deoxygenated blood from the body tissues to the right atrium of the human heart.

c) Superficial (or Cutaneous) Veins: The superficial veins are found immediately beneath the skin between the layers of the superficial fascia.

d) Deep Veins: The deep veins are located under the deep fascia with their corresponding arteries.

e) Systemic Veins

   The systemic veins are divided into the following groups:
   i) veins of the heart
   ii) veins of the head and neck
   iii) veins of the upper extremity and thorax
   iv) veins of the lower extremity, abdomen, and pelvis

f) Veins of the Heart
   i) great cardiac vein
   ii) small cardiac vein
   iii) middle cardiac vein
   iv) posterior vein of the left ventricle
   v) oblique vein of the left atrium

g) Veins of the Head and Neck
   i) frontal vein (or supratrochlear vein)
   ii) supraorbital vein
   iii) angular vein
   iv) anterior facial vein (or facial vein)
   v) superficial temporal vein
   vi) parotid veins
   vii) articular veins (from temporomandibular joint)
   viii) anterior auricular veins
   ix) transverse facial veins
   x) internal maxillary vein
   xi) posterior facial vein (or temporomaxillary vein)
   xii) posterior auricular vein
   xiii) occipital vein

h) Veins of the Neck
   i) external jugular vein
   ii) posterior external jugular vein
   iii) anterior jugular vein
   iv) internal jugular vein
   v) vertebral vein
   vi) diploic veins
      (a) frontal diploic vein
      (b) anterior temporal diploic vein
      (c) posterior temporal diploic vein
      (d) occipital diploic vein

12. Veins of the Brain

a) External Cerebral Veins
   i) superior cerebral veins
   ii) middle cerebral vein (or superficial sylvian vein)
   iii) inferior cerebral veins

b) Internal Cerebral Veins (or deep cerebral veins)

c) Terminal Vein

d) Great Cerebral Veins (or Great Vein of Galen)

e) Cerebellar Veins
   i) superior cerebellar veins
   ii) inferior cerebellar veins

f) Ophthalmic and Emissary Veins
   i) Ophthalmic veins are the veins that serve to perform the venous drainage of the orbit and pass through the superior orbital fissure to enter into the cavernous sinus.
   ii) superior ophthalmic veins
   iii) inferior ophthalmic veins
   iv) Emissary veins are those valveless veins that connect the dural venous sinuses with veins outside the cranium.

g) Sinuses of the Dura Mater
   i) posterosuperior sinuses
   ii) superior sagittal sinus (or superior longitudinal sinus)
   iii) inferior sagittal sinus (or inferior sagittal sinus)
   iv) straight sinus (or tentorial sinus)
   v) transverse sinuses (or lateral sinuses)

h) Occipital Sinuses
   i) anteroinferior sinuses
   ii) cavernous sinuses
   iii) intercavernous sinuses
   iv) superior petrosal sinuses
   v) inferior petrosal sinuses
   vi) basilar plexus (or transverse/basilar sinus)

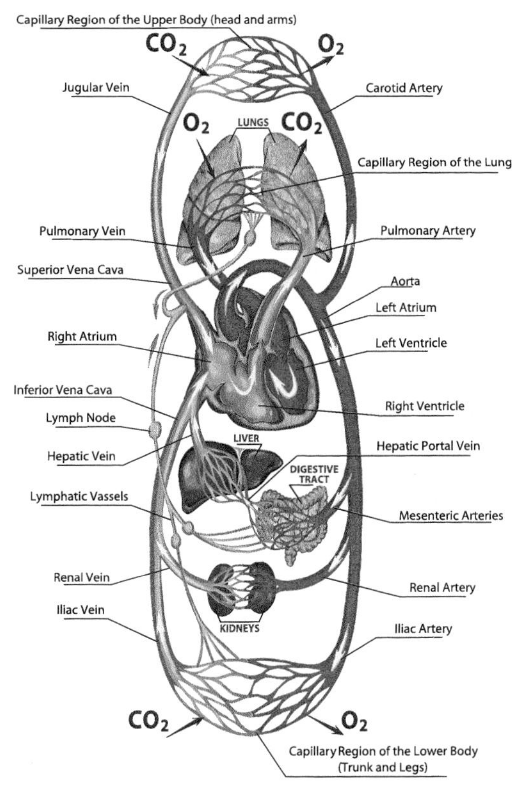

13. Veins of the Upper Extremity, Thorax and Vertebral Column

The veins of the upper extremity are divided into the following two major groups:

a) Superficial Veins of the Upper Extremity
   i) cephalic vein (or antecubital vein)
   ii) accessory cephalic vein
   iii) median cubital vein (or median basilic vein/antecubital vein)
   iv) basilic vein
   v) median antebrachial vein
   vi) dorsal venous network of the hand

vii) intercapitular veins
viii) dorsal metacarpal veins
ix) dorsal digital veins

b) Deep Veins of the Upper Extremity
i) radial veins
ii) ulnar veins
iii) brachial veins
iv) axillary veins
v) subclavian veins
vi) deep palmar venous arch

c) Veins of the thorax
i) innominate veins (or brachiocephalic veins)
ii) internal mammary veins (or internal thoracic veins)
iii) inferior thyroid veins
iv) highest intercostal vein (or superior intercostal vein)
v) right superior intercostal vein
vi) left superior intercostal vein
vii) superior vena cava
viii) azygos vein
ix) hemiazygos vein
x) accessory hemiazygos vein (or vena azygos minor superior)
xi) bronchial veins

d) Veins of the vertebral column
i) external vertebral venous plexuses (or extraspinal veins)
ii) anterior external vertebral plexuses
iii) posterior external vertebral plexuses
iv) internal vertebral venous plexus (or intraspinal veins)
v) basivertebral veins
vi) intervertebral veins
vii) veins of the medulla spinalis (or veins of spinal cord)

14. Veins of the Lower Extremity, Abdomen, and Pelvis
The veins of the lower extremity are arranged into the following groups:

a. Superficial Veins of the Lower Extremity
i) great saphenous vein
ii) small saphenous vein (or lesser saphenous vein)

b. Deep Veins of the Lower Extremity
i) posterior tibial veins
ii) peroneal veins
iii) tibioperoneal trunk
iv) anterior tibial veins
v) popliteal vein
vi) femoral vein
vii) deep femoral vein (or profunda femoris vein)
viii) common femoral vein
ix) external iliac vein

b) Major Veins of Abdomen and Pelvis
i) ascending lumbar vein
ii) left gastric vein
iii) right gastric vein
iv) left gastro-omental vein
v) right gastro-omental vein
vi) left hepatic vein
vii) middle hepatic vein
viii) right hepatic vein
ix) superior mesenteric vein
x) inferior phrenic veins
xi) inferior vena cava
xii) left renal vein
xiii) right renal vein
xiv) splenic vein
xv) suprarenal veins
xvi) deep dorsal vein of clitoris
xvii) deep dorsal vein of penis
xviii) external pudendal veins
xix) internal pudendal vein
xx) ovarian vein
xxi) pampiniform venous plexus
xxii) prostatic venous plexus
xxiii) rectal venous plexus
xxiv) uterine venous plexus
xxv) vaginal venous plexus
xxvi) common iliac veins
xxvii) middle sacral veins
xxviii) vesical venous plexus

15. The Portal System of Veins
The hepatic portal system of the veins is responsible for the portal circulation, which denotes the passage of blood from the gastrointestinal tract and spleen through the portal vein to the liver.

The tributaries and sub-tributaries of the portal vein are presented below:

<table>
<tr><th colspan="3">The Tributaries and Subtributaries of the Portal Vein</th></tr>
<tr><td colspan="3">The Lienal Vein</td></tr>
<tr><td rowspan="6">The Tributaries of Lienal Vein</td><td colspan="2">The Short Gastric Veins</td></tr>
<tr><td colspan="2">The Left Gastroepiploic Vein</td></tr>
<tr><td colspan="2">The Pancreatic Veins</td></tr>
<tr><td colspan="2">The Inferior Mesenteric Vein</td></tr>
<tr><td rowspan="2">The Tributaries of Inferior Mesenteric Vein</td><td>The Sigmoid Veins</td></tr>
<tr><td>The Left Colic Vein</td></tr>
<tr><td colspan="3">The Superior Mesenteric Vein</td></tr>
<tr><td rowspan="2">The Tributaries of Superior Mesenteric Vein</td><td colspan="2">The Right Gastroepiploic Vein</td></tr>
<tr><td colspan="2">The Pancreaticoduodenal Veins</td></tr>
<tr><td colspan="3">The Coronary Vein</td></tr>
<tr><td colspan="3">The Pyloric Vein</td></tr>
<tr><td colspan="3">The Cystic Vein</td></tr>
<tr><td colspan="3">The Paraumbilical Veins</td></tr>
</table>

Common Pathologies

Angina pectoris
Commonly known as angina, angina pectoris chest pain is due to ischemia of the heart muscle, generally due to obstruction or spasm of the coronary arteries. The main cause of angina pectoris is coronary artery disease, due to atherosclerosis of the arteries feeding the heart.

Cardiomyopathy
Cardiomyopathy is a chronic disease of the heart muscle, in which the muscle is abnormally enlarged, thickened, and/or stiffened. The weakened heart muscle loses the ability to pump blood effectively, resulting in irregular heartbeats (arrhythmias) and possibly even heart failure.

Rheumatic Heart Disease
Rheumatic heart disease is a condition in which permanent damage to heart valves is caused by rheumatic fever. The heart valve is damaged by a disease process that generally begins with a strep throat caused by bacteria called Streptococcus, and may eventually cause rheumatic fever.

Arrhythmia
An arrhythmia is an abnormal rate or rhythm of the heart beat. It can beat too fast, too slow, or with an irregular rhythm. If the heart beat is fast it is called tachycardia and if is too slow, it is referred to as bradycardia.

Congenital Heart Defects

Congenital heart defects are abnormalities in the morphological or physiological functioning of the heart that are present at the time of birth. The primary cause is the incomplete or abnormal development of the fetal heart during the early weeks of pregnancy.

Hypertension

Hypertension, also referred to as high blood pressure, is a condition in which the arteries have persistently elevated blood pressure. Every time the human heart beats, it pumps blood to the whole body through the arteries. The pumping through the narrowed vessel consistently increases the systolic and diastolic pressure above normal reference range.

Main complications of hypertension

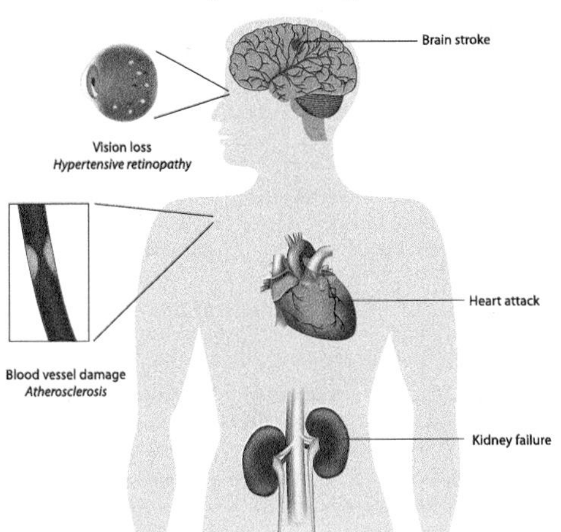

Aortic Aneurysm

An aneurysm is an abnormal bulging or swelling of a portion of a blood vessel. The aorta, which can develop these abnormal bulges, is the large blood vessel that carries oxygen-rich blood away from the heart to the rest of the body.

Atherosclerosis

Atherosclerosis is a disease of the arterial blood vessels (arteries), in which the walls of the blood vessels become thickened and hardened by "plaques." The plaques are composed of cholesterol and other lipids, inflammatory cells, and calcium deposits.

STAGES OF ATHEROSCLEROSIS

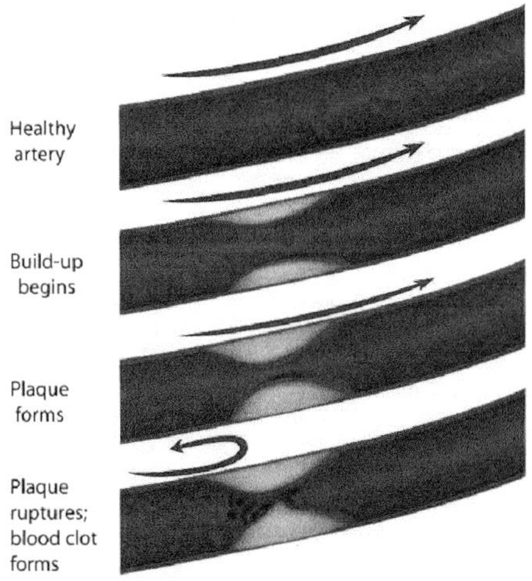

Deep Vein Thrombosis

Deep vein thrombosis (DVT) is a blood clot in a major vein that usually develops in the legs and/or pelvis.

Coronary Artery Disease

Coronary artery disease (CAD) is one of the common vascular diseases marked by accumulation of atherosclerotic plaque in the coronary blood vessels. As the plaque thickens, secondary changes may take place like enlargement of size and calcification that may lead to complete occlusion of the lumen of the coronary artery, resulting in inadequate supply of oxygen to the heart muscle.

Peripheral Vascular Disease

Peripheral vascular disease is a narrowing of blood vessels that restricts blood flow. It mostly occurs in the legs, but is sometimes seen in the arms.

Hypercholesterolemia

Hypercholesterolemia is the presence of high levels of cholesterol in the blood. It is a form of "hyperlipidemia" (elevated levels of lipids in the blood) and "hyperlipoproteinemia" (elevated levels of lipoproteins in the blood).

Lymphedema

A condition in which excess fluid collects in tissue and causes swelling. Lymphedema may occur in the arm or leg after lymph vessels or lymph nodes in the underarm or groin are removed.

Hodgkin's Lymphoma

This is a type of cancer of the lymphatic system. It can start almost anywhere in the body. It's believed to be caused by HIV, Epstein-Barr Syndrome, age, and family history.

Non-Hodgkin's Lymphoma

Non-Hodgkin's lymphoma is a cancer of the lymphoid system. It is divided into three types: high-grade, intermediate-grade and low-grade.

Lymphangitis

Lymphangitis is an inflammation of the lymphatics (lymph channels) due to an infection by a microbe or some chemical irritant. It occurs when an infection or inflammation occurs somewhere else and the microbe or the irritant is transported along with lymph fluid through the lymphatics.

Splenomegaly

Splenomegaly is a condition in which the spleen becomes enlarged, tender and painful. It can occur due to a number of reasons, ranging from certain infections to cancers.

Anatomy of the Lymphatic System

1. **Introduction**
The human lymphatic system is closely linked with the blood and the vascular system. Both of these systems work in an intimate association with each other and transport vital fluids throughout the body via a system of vessels. The lymph capillaries and lymphatics are the special vessels that serve to transport a fluid (called lymph). The human lymphatic system consists of the below mentioned components:
   a) The Lymph
   b) The Lymph Vessels
   c) The Lymph Nodes
   d) The Tonsils, Spleen, Thymus Gland and Peyer's Patches

   The most important function of the lymphatic system is to drain the protein containing fluid from the tissue spaces. The entire lymphatics of the body converge into one of the following major channels:
      i) thoracic duct (or the main collecting channel)
      ii) right lymphatic duct
   e) The lymph nodes (or lymph glands) are oval structures that are found along the length of lymphatics at various intervals. The lymph trunk is a specific lymph vessel containing lymph. The various types of lymph trunks are documented below:
      i) jugular lymph trunk
      ii) subclavian lymph trunk
      iii) bronchomediastinal lymph trunk
      iv) lumbar lymph trunk
      v) intestinal lymph trunk

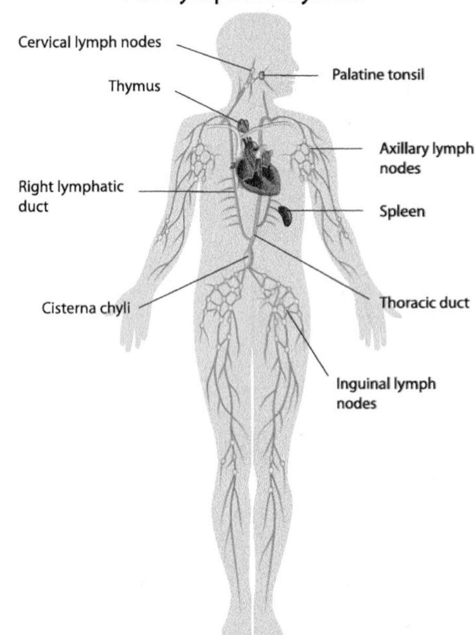

2. **Thoracic Duct**
The thoracic duct is the largest lymphatic vessel in the body and constitutes an essential part of the lymphatic system. It is also called the alimentary duct, chyliferous duct, left lymphatic duct or Van Hoorne's canal.
3. **Lymphatics of the Head, Face and Neck**
The entire lymph glands of the head are mostly extra-cranial, and arranged in the following groups:
   a) Occipital Lymph Glands: The occipital lymph glands are two or three in number and located on the back of the head.
   b) Posterior Auricular Lymph Glands (or Mastoid Glands): The posterior auricular lymph glands are two in number and exist on the upper part of the sternomastoid muscle and mastoid portion of the temporal bone.
   c) Anterior Auricular Lymph Glands (or Superficial Parotid/Preauricular Glands): The superficial parotid glands are present on the lateral surface of the parotid gland.
   d) Parotid Lymph Glands (or Deep Parotid Glands): The parotid lymph glands remain embedded in the deeper portions of the parotid gland.
   e) Superficial Facial Lymph Glands: The superficial facial lymph glands are based on several lymph glands in the region of face. However, the major ones are described below:
      i) Infraorbital Lymph Glands (or Maxillary Glands): The infraorbital lymph glands remain scattered along the angle between the nose and cheek, and below the margin of the orbit.
      ii) Buccinator Lymph Glands: The buccinator lymph glands are found on the superficial surface of the anterior part of buccinator muscle, opposite to the angle of the mouth.
      iii) Supramandibular Lymph Glands: The supramandibular lymph glands lie on the outer surface of the mandible at the anterior border of the masseter muscle, between the external maxillary artery and the anterior facial vein.
   f) The Deep Facial Lymph Glands (or Internal Maxillary Glands): The deep facial lymph glands are found in association with the internal maxillary artery, on the outer surface of the external pterygoid muscle.
   g) The Lingual Lymph Glands: The lingual lymph glands are based on two or three small nodules that exist on the lateral surfaces of the hypoglossal and genioglossus muscles.
   h) The Retropharyngeal Glands: The retropharyngeal glands are located in the buccopharyngeal fascia behind the upper part of the pharynx.
4. **The Lymph Glands of the Neck:** The lymph glands of the neck are divided into the following major groups:
   a) The Submaxillary Glands: The submaxillary glands are a pair of salivary glands located on each side under the body of the mandible.
   b) The Submental (or Suprahyoid Glands): The submental glands are located beneath the chin, and between the anterior bellies of the two digastric muscles.
   c) The Superficial Cervical Glands: The superficial cervical glands remain embedded in the deep fascia along the course of the external jugular vein, and superficial to the sternomastoid muscle.
5. **The Anterior Cervical Glands:** The lymph glands of the anterior neck region are divisible into the following two groups:
   a) Superficial Anterior Cervical Lymph Glands- The superficial anterior cervical lymph glands exist in association with the anterior jugular veins.
   b) Deep Anterior Cervical Lymph Glands: The deep anterior cervical lymph glands are divisible into the following groups/types:
      i) infrahyoid glands obtain lymph fluid from the region of epiglottis and transport it to the deep cervical glands.
      ii) prelaryngeal gland obtains lymph from the anterior portion of the larynx, the isthmus, and the portions of the right and left lobes of the thyroid gland.
      iii) pretracheal lymph glands are the numerous small nodules that follow the course of the inferior thyroid veins.
      iv) paratracheal lymph glands lie in association with the branches of the superior and inferior thyroid arteries and the recurrent nerves.
   c) Deep Cervical Glands: The deep cervical glands are the intercommunicating lymph vessels that remain positioned in the anterior and posterior triangles of the neck, and under the cover of the sternomastoid muscle. These glands are divisible into the following groups:
      i) superior deep cervical glands are located under the cover of the sternomastoid muscle, and lie in close association with the accessory nerve and internal jugular vein.
      ii) inferior deep cervical glands are located below the level of the omohyoid muscle.
   d) Lymphatic vessels of the scalp are distributed in the soft tissue envelope of the frontal, temporoparietal and the occipital regions of the cranium.
   e) Lymphatic Vessels of the Ear divide into upper and lateral portions of the auricle and terminate into the anterior auricular glands.
   f) Lymphatic vessels of the face are more widely distributed than the scalp vessels, and can be divided into the following groups:
6. **Lymphatic Vessels of the Eyelids and Conjunctiva:** The lymphatic vessels of the eyelids and conjunctiva form the following two groups:

a) Medial Lymph Vessels: The medial lymph vessels travel from the medial portions of the superior and inferior eyelids, and terminate to the submaxillary lymph glands.

b) Lateral Lymph Vessels: The lateral lymph vessels arise from the lateral parts of the eyelids, and terminate into the anterior auricular and the parotid lymph glands.

c) Lymphatic Vessels of the Cheeks: The superficial and deep lymphatic vessels of the cheeks usually communicate with the submaxillary glands.

d) Lymphatic Vessels of the Lips: The lymphatic vessels of the lips drain lymph fluid to the submental and submaxillary glands.

e) Lymphatic Vessels of the Nose: The lymphatic vessels from the external part of the nose drain lymph fluid to the anterior auricular and submaxillary glands.

f) Lymphatic Vessels of the Nasal Cavities: The lymphatic vessels from the anterior and posterior portions of the nasal cavities drain lymph fluid to the submaxillary, the retropharyngeal, and the superior deep cervical glands.

g) Lymphatic Vessels of the Mouth: The lymphatic vessels of the mouth can be divided into the following groups:

h) Lymphatic Vessels of the Palatine Tonsil: The lymphatic vessels of the palatine tonsil arise from the buccopharyngeal fascia and constrictor pharyngis superior and meet with the superior deep cervical glands.

i) Lymphatic Vessels of the Tongue: The lymphatic vessels of the tongue are divided into the following three groups:

   i) anterior lymph vessels of the tongue drain lymph fluid from the tip and lower surface of the tongue to the submental glands.

   ii) middle lymph vessels of the tongue drain lymph fluid from the anterior two third portion of the tongue to the submaxillary and medial superior deep cervical glands.

   iii) posterior lymph vessels of the tongue drain lymph fluid from the portion of the tongue, which lies in the anterior wall of pharynx.

j) Lymphatic Vessels of the Gums: The lymph vessels of the anterior portion of mandibular gum drain lymph fluid to the submandibular gland. The lymph vessels from the inner portion of the mandibular gum also drain lymph fluid to the submaxillary glands.

k) Lymphatic Vessels of the Teeth: The lymph vessels of the teeth and mandible transport lymph fluid to the sub maxillary or the superior deep cervical glands.

7. **The Lymphatics of the Upper Extremity:** The lymph glands of the upper extremity are divisible into the following two groups:

   a) The Superficial Lymph Glands- The superficial lymph glands of the upper extremity are of the following types:

      i) supratrochlear lymph glands are situated above the medial epicondyle of humerus, and drain lymph fluid from the middle, ring and little fingers, and the portions of the hand and forearm.

      ii) deltoideopectoral lymph glands are located in the groove between the pectoralis major and deltoid muscles.

   b) The Deep Lymph Glands: The deep lymph glands are chiefly found in the axillary region, where they constitute several constant as well as variable groups.

      i) lateral group of axillary lymph glands lies along the line of the great axillary vessels. These glands drain lymph fluid from the greater part of the upper extremity to the central and inferior deep cervical glands.

      ii) anterior group of axillary lymph glands travels from third to sixth intercostal space, along the line of the lateral thoracic artery.

      iii) posterior group of axillary lymph glands lies along the posterior wall of axilla, and follow the course of the subscapular vessels.

      iv) central group of axillary lymph glands are located in the central part of the axilla, and along the line of the intercosto-brachial nerve.

      v) infra-clavicular group of axillary lymph glands is found between the upper border of the pectoralis minor muscle and the clavicle, along the medial side of the axillary artery.

   c) The Lymphatic Vessels of the Upper Extremity: The lymphatic vessels of the upper extremity are divisible into the following two groups:

      i) superficial lymph vessels of the upper extremity are located in the skin and subcutaneous tissues, and commence in the cutaneous plexuses on the volar aspects of the fingers and hand.

      ii) deep lymph vessels of the upper extremity follow the course of the deeper blood vessels in the regions of the forearm and hand.

8. **Lymphatics of the Lower Extremity:** The lymph glands of the lower extremity are divisible into the following groups:

   a) The Superficial Lymph Glands- superficial lymph glands are found in the superficial fascia in subinguinal and inguinal regions. These glands are separable into the following groups:

      i) inguinal lymph glands are located above the level of the inguinal ligament.

      ii) superficial sublingual lymph glands are divisible into the proximal and distal groups.

   b) Deep Lymph Glands: The deep lymph glands of the inferior extremity are divided into the following two groups:

      i) popliteal lymph glands are located in the popliteal fossa.

      ii) deep sublingual lymph glands are located in the femoral trigone.

   c) Lymphatic Vessels of the Lower Extremity: The lymphatic vessels of the lower extremity are based on the following two groups:

      i) superficial lymphatic vessels are located in the superficial fascia and divided into vessels of the medial group arises on the tibial side and dorsum of the foot, and terminates in the distal group of superficial subinguinal glands and vessels of the lateral group commences from the fibular side of the foot.

      ii) deep lymphatic vessels of the lower extremity follow the course of the deep blood vessels, and terminate into the deep subinguinal and hypogastric glands.

9. **The Lymphatics of the Abdomen and Pelvis:** The lymph glands of the abdomen and pelvis are divisible into parietal lymph glands and visceral lymph glands.

   a) External Iliac Glands: The external iliac group of glands pertains to the pelvic region, located along the course of the external iliac vessels, and constitutes the lateral, intermediate and medial chains.

   b) Common Iliac Glands: The common iliac glands of the pelvis are located on the sides of the common iliac artery and below the bifurcation of aorta.

   c) Epigastric Glands: The epigastric glands of the anterior abdominal wall are divisible into the following types:

      i) superior epigastric gland is located in the superficial fascia of the median part of the epigastric region.

      ii) inferior epigastric glands are located along the course of the inferior epigastric artery.

   d) Circumflex Iliac Glands: The circumflex iliac glands of the anterior abdominal wall follow the course of the deep circumflex iliac artery in the lateral aspect of groin.

   e) Hypogastric Glands: The hypogastric glands of the pelvis are located along the course of the hypogastric vessels.

      i) gluteal lymph glands

      ii) pubo-gluteal lymph glands

      iii) middle hemorrhoidal gland

      iv) inter-iliac glands

      v) obturator gland

   f) Sacral Glands: The sacral lymph glands of the pelvis are located along the anterior aspect of sacrum, between the anterior sacral foramina.

   g) Lumbar Glands: The lumbar lymph glands are located behind the peritoneum of the posterior wall of the abdomen. The lumbar lymph glands are further separable into the following groups:

      i) right lateral aortic glands

      ii) left lateral aortic glands

      iii) preaortic glands

      iv) retroaortic glands

   h) Superior Gastric Glands: The superior gastric glands exist in association with the left gastric artery and constitute the following subdivisions:

      i) anterior left gastric glands (or lower coronary glands)

      ii) right paracardial glands

      iii) left paracardial glands

      iv) posterior paracardial glands

      v) posterior left gastric glands (or upper coronary glands)

      vi) right gastric gland (or pyloric gland)

      vii) left suprapancreatic glands

      viii) right suprapancreatic glands

      ix) subpyloric glands

      x) biliary lymph glands

i) Inferior Gastric Glands (or Right Gastroepiploic Glands): The inferior gastric glands are associated with the greater curvature of the stomach and follow the course of the right gastroepiploic artery.

j) Hepatic Glands: The hepatic lymph glands exist in the region of porta hepatis (or transverse fissure of the liver), between the layers of the lesser omentum.

k) Pancreaticolienal Glands (or Splenic Glands): The pancreaticolienal glands are positioned in relation to the posterior surface and upper border of pancreas, and follow the course of the lienal (or splenic) artery.

l) Mesenteric Glands: The mesenteric lymph glands are located between the layers of the mesentery.

m) Ileocolic glands: The ileocolic glands are located around the ileocolic artery and form the following major groups:

 i) ileal glands
 ii) anterior ileocolic glands
 iii) posterior ileocolic glands
 iv) right colic glands

n) Mesocolic Glands: The mesocolic glands exist in close association with the transverse colon.

o) Inferior Mesenteric Glands- The inferior mesenteric glands are located on the branches of the left colic and sigmoid arteries, the superior hemorrhoidal artery, and the muscular coat of the rectum.

10. The Lymphatic Vessels of the Abdominal Viscera and the Superior and Posterior Walls of the Abdomen

a) Lymphatic Vessels of the Abdominal Part of the Alimentary Canal
b) Lymphatic Vessels of the Stomach
c) Lymphatic Vessels of the Duodenum
d) Lymphatic Vessels of the Jejunum and Ileum (or the Lacteals)
e) Lymphatic Vessels of the Cecum, Vermiform Process, and the Ascending Colon
f) Lymphatic Vessels of the Right Colic Flexure and the Transverse Colon
g) Lymphatic Vessels of the Left Colic Flexure, Descending Colon, Iliac Colon, and Pelvic Colon
h) Lymphatic Vessels of the Liver
i) Lymphatic Vessels of the Gall Bladder
j) Lymphatic Vessels of the Pancreas
k) Lymphatic Vessels of the Spleen
l) Lymphatic Vessels of the Kidneys
m) Lymphatic Vessels of the Ureters
n) Lymphatic Vessels of the Suprarenal Glands
o) Lymphatic Vessels of the Diaphragm

11. The Lymphatic Vessels of the Pelvic Viscera

a) lymphatic Vessels of the Male Urethra
b) Lymphatic Vessels of the Prostate
c) Lymphatic Vessels of the Female Urethra
d) Lymphatic Vessels of the Seminal Vesicle
e) Lymphatic Vessels of the Ductus Deferens
f) Lymphatic Vessels of the Urinary Bladder
g) Lymphatic Vessels of the Ureter
h) Lymphatic Vessels of the Vagina
i) Lymphatic Vessels of the Uterus
j) Lymphatic Vessels of the Uterine Tube
k) Lymphatic Vessels of the Ovaries
l) Lymphatic Vessels of the Testis and Epididymis
m) Lymphatic Vessels of the Anus, Anal Canal and Rectum

12. The Lymphatics of the Thorax

The Lymph Glands of the thorax are separable into the following groups:

a) Sternal Lymph Glands- The sternal lymph glands are located at the margins of the sternum along the side of the internal mammary artery.

b) Intercostal Lymph Glands- The intercostal lymph glands are situated in the posterior portions of the intercostal spaces (in relation to the intercostal vessels), and in front of the heads of the ribs.

c) Anterior Mediastinal Lymph Glands- The anterior mediastinal lymph glands are located in the lower portion of the anterior mediastinum, and the anterior part of the superior mediastinal cavity.

d) Posterior Mediastinal Lymph Glands- The posterior mediastinal lymph glands exist along the thoracic part of the esophagus and the descending thoracic aorta.

e) Bronchial Lymph Glands- The bronchial lymph glands lie along the walls of the intrathoracic of the trachea, the bronchi and their intrapulmonary branches. These glands are further categorized into the following groups:

 i) tracheobronchial lymph glands
 ii) lymph glands of the bifurcation (or intertracheobronchial lymph glands)
 iii) bronchopulmonary lymph glands
 iv) pulmonary lymph glands

13. The Lymphatic Vessels of the Thorax

These vessels are divisible into the following groups:

a) Intercostal Lymph Vessels
b) Lymph Vessels of the Diaphragm
c) Lymphatic Vessels of the Contents of the Thorax: The lymphatic vessels of the contents of the thorax are divisible into the following groups:

 i) lymph vessels of the heart
 ii) lymph vessels of the pericardium
 iii) lymph vessels of the thymus
 iv) lymph vessels of the thoracic part of esophagus
 v) lymph vessels of the pleura
 vi) lymph vessels of the lungs

Diseases of the circulatory system (I00-I99)

EXCLUDES2 *certain conditions originating in the perinatal period (P04-P96)*
certain infectious and parasitic diseases (A00-B99)
complications of pregnancy, childbirth and the puerperium (O00-O9A)
congenital malformations, deformations, and chromosomal abnormalities (Q00-Q99)
endocrine, nutritional and metabolic diseases (E00-E88)
injury, poisoning and certain other consequences of external causes (S00-T88)
neoplasms (C00-D49)
symptoms, signs and abnormal clinical and laboratory findings, not elsewhere classified (R00-R94)
systemic connective tissue disorders (M30-M36)
transient cerebral ischemic attacks and related syndromes (G45.-)

This chapter contains the following blocks:

I00-I02	Acute rheumatic fever
I05-I09	Chronic rheumatic heart diseases
▶I10-I16◀	Hypertensive diseases
I20-I25	Ischemic heart diseases
I26-I28	Pulmonary heart disease and diseases of pulmonary circulation
I30-I52	Other forms of heart disease
I60-I69	Cerebrovascular diseases
I70-I79	Diseases of arteries, arterioles and capillaries
I80-I89	Diseases of veins, lymphatic vessels and lymph nodes, not elsewhere classified
I95-I99	Other and unspecified disorders of the circulatory system

Acute rheumatic fever (I00-I02)

I00 **Rheumatic fever** without heart involvement
INCLUDES *arthritis, rheumatic, acute or subacute*
EXCLUDES1 *rheumatic fever with heart involvement (I01.0 -I01.9)*

④ I01 **Rheumatic fever** with heart involvement
EXCLUDES1 *chronic diseases of rheumatic origin (I05-I09) unless rheumatic fever is also present or there is evidence of reactivation or activity of the rheumatic process.*

I01.0 **Acute rheumatic** pericarditis CC
Any condition in I00 with pericarditis
Rheumatic pericarditis (acute)
EXCLUDES1 *acute pericarditis not specified as rheumatic (I30.-)*

I01.1 **Acute rheumatic** endocarditis CC
Any condition in I00 with endocarditis or valvulitis
Acute rheumatic valvulitis

I01.2 **Acute rheumatic** myocarditis CC
Any condition in I00 with myocarditis

I01.8 **Other acute rheumatic heart disease** CC
Any condition in I00 with other or multiple types of heart involvement
Acute rheumatic pancarditis

I01.9 **Acute rheumatic heart disease, unspecified** CC
Any condition in I00 with unspecified type of heart involvement
Rheumatic carditis, acute
Rheumatic heart disease, active or acute

④ I02 **Rheumatic** chorea
INCLUDES *Sydenham's chorea*
EXCLUDES1 *chorea NOS (G25.5)*
Huntington's chorea (G10)

I02.0 **Rheumatic chorea** with heart involvement CC
Chorea NOS with heart involvement
Rheumatic chorea with heart involvement of any type classifiable under I01.-

I02.9 **Rheumatic chorea** without heart involvement CC
Rheumatic chorea NOS

Chronic rheumatic heart diseases (I05-I09)

④ I05 **Rheumatic** mitral valve **diseases**
INCLUDES *conditions classifiable to both I05.0 and I05.2-I05.9, whether specified as rheumatic or not*
EXCLUDES1 *mitral valve disease specified as nonrheumatic (I34.-)*
mitral valve disease with aortic and/or tricuspid valve involvement (I08.-)

I05.0 **Rheumatic mitral** stenosis
Mitral (valve) obstruction (rheumatic)

I05.1 **Rheumatic mitral** insufficiency
Rheumatic mitral incompetence
Rheumatic mitral regurgitation
EXCLUDES1 *mitral insufficiency not specified as rheumatic (I34.0)*

I05.2 **Rheumatic mitral** stenosis with insufficiency
Rheumatic mitral stenosis with incompetence or regurgitation

I05.8 **Other rheumatic mitral valve diseases**
Rheumatic mitral (valve) failure

I05.9 **Rheumatic mitral valve disease, unspecified**
Rheumatic mitral (valve) disorder (chronic) NOS

④ I06 **Rheumatic** aortic valve **diseases**
EXCLUDES1 *aortic valve disease not specified as rheumatic (I35.-)*
aortic valve disease with mitral and/or tricuspid valve involvement (I08.-)

I06.0 **Rheumatic aortic** stenosis
Rheumatic aortic (valve) obstruction

I06.1 **Rheumatic aortic** insufficiency
Rheumatic aortic incompetence
Rheumatic aortic regurgitation

I06.2 **Rheumatic aortic** stenosis with insufficiency
Rheumatic aortic stenosis with incompetence or regurgitation

I06.8 **Other rheumatic aortic valve diseases**

I06.9 **Rheumatic aortic valve disease, unspecified**
Rheumatic aortic (valve) disease NOS

④ I07 **Rheumatic** tricuspid valve **diseases**
INCLUDES *rheumatic tricuspid valve diseases specified as rheumatic or unspecified*
EXCLUDES1 *tricuspid valve disease specified as nonrheumatic (I36.-)*
tricuspid valve disease with aortic and/or mitral valve involvement (I08.-)

I07.0 **Rheumatic tricuspid** stenosis
Tricuspid (valve) stenosis (rheumatic)

I07.1 **Rheumatic tricuspid** insufficiency
Tricuspid (valve) insufficiency (rheumatic)

I07.2 **Rheumatic tricuspid** stenosis and insufficiency

I07.8 **Other rheumatic tricuspid valve diseases**

I07.9 **Rheumatic tricuspid valve disease, unspecified**
Rheumatic tricuspid valve disorder NOS

④ I08 Multiple valve **diseases**
INCLUDES *multiple valve diseases specified as rheumatic or unspecified*
EXCLUDES1 *endocarditis, valve unspecified (I38)*
multiple valve disease specified a nonrheumatic (I34.-, I35.-, I36.-, I37.-, I38.-, Q22.-, Q23.-, Q24.8-)
rheumatic valve disease NOS (I09.1)

I08.0 **Rheumatic disorders of both** mitral **and** aortic **valves**
Involvement of both mitral and aortic valves specified as rheumatic or unspecified

I08.1 **Rheumatic disorders of both** mitral **and** tricuspid **valves**

I08.2 **Rheumatic disorders of both** aortic **and** tricuspid **valves**

I08.3 **Combined rheumatic disorders of** mitral , aortic **and** tricuspid **valves**

I08.8 **Other rheumatic multiple valve diseases**

I08.9 **Rheumatic multiple valve disease, unspecified**

④ I09 **Other rheumatic heart diseases**

I09.0 **Rheumatic** myocarditis CC
EXCLUDES1 *myocarditis not specified as rheumatic (I51.4)*

I09.1 **Rheumatic diseases of endocardium, valve unspecified**
Rheumatic endocarditis (chronic)
Rheumatic valvulitis (chronic)
EXCLUDES1 *endocarditis, valve unspecified (I38)*

I09.2 Chronic **rheumatic** pericarditis CC
Adherent pericardium, rheumatic
Chronic rheumatic mediastinopericarditis
Chronic rheumatic myopericarditis
EXCLUDES1 *chronic pericarditis not specified as rheumatic (I31.-)*

⑤ I09.8 **Other specified rheumatic heart diseases**

I09.81 **Rheumatic heart failure** CC
Use additional code to identify type of heart failure (I50.-)

I09.89 **Other specified rheumatic heart diseases**
Rheumatic disease of pulmonary valve

Unspecified Code | Other Specified Code | Manifestation Code | N Newborn | P Pediatric | M Maternity | A Adult | ♂ Male | ♀ Female
● New Code | ▲ Revised Code Title | ▶◀ Revised Text | NOTES | INCLUDES | EXCLUDES1 Not coded here | EXCLUDES2 Not included here
④ 4th character required | ⑤ 5th character required | ⑥ 6th character required | ⑦ 7th character required
Extension 'X' Alert | HAC Hospital-acquired condition (HAC) alert | AHA AHA Coding Clinic©

I09.9 Rheumatic heart disease, unspecified
Rheumatic carditis
EXCLUDES1 *rheumatoid carditis (M05.31)*

Hypertensive diseases (I10-I16)

Use additional code to identify:
exposure to environmental tobacco smoke (Z77.22)
history of tobacco dependence (Z87.891)
occupational exposure to environmental tobacco smoke (Z57.31)
tobacco dependence (F17.-)
tobacco use (Z72.0)

EXCLUDES1 *neonatal hypertension (P29.2)*
primary pulmonary hypertension (I27.0)

EXCLUDES2 *hypertensive disease complicating pregnancy, childbirth and the puerperium (O10-O11, O13-O16)*

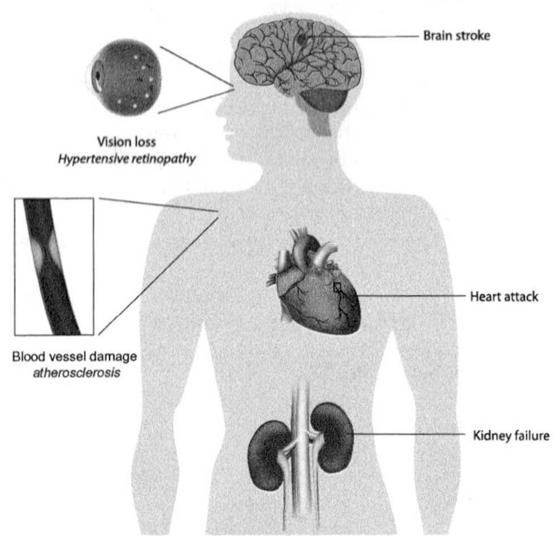

Figure 9.1 Main complications of hypertension

I10 Essential (primary) hypertension ?
INCLUDES *high blood pressure*
hypertension (arterial) (benign) (essential) (malignant) (primary) (systemic)
EXCLUDES1 *hypertensive disease complicating pregnancy, childbirth and the puerperium (O10-O11, O13-O16)*
EXCLUDES2 *essential (primary) hypertension involving vessels of brain (I60-I69)*
essential (primary) hypertension involving vessels of eye (H35.0-)
AHA: Q4, 2013

4th **I11 Hypertensive heart disease**
INCLUDES *any condition in I51.4-I51.9 due to hypertension*
I11.0 Hypertensive heart disease with heart failure
Hypertensive heart failure
Use additional code to identify type of heart failure (I50.-)
I11.9 Hypertensive heart disease without heart failure
Hypertensive heart disease NOS

4th **I12 Hypertensive chronic kidney disease**
INCLUDES *any condition in N18 and N26 - due to hypertension*
arteriosclerosis of kidney
arteriosclerotic nephritis (chronic) (interstitial)
hypertensive nephropathy
nephrosclerosis
EXCLUDES1 *hypertension due to kidney disease (I15.0, I15.1)*
renovascular hypertension (I15.0)
secondary hypertension (I15.-)
EXCLUDES2 *acute kidney failure (N17.-)*
I12.0 Hypertensive chronic kidney disease with stage 5 chronic kidney disease or end stage renal disease CC
Use additional code to identify the stage of chronic kidney disease (N18.5, N18.6)
I12.9 Hypertensive chronic kidney disease with stage 1 through stage 4 chronic kidney disease, or unspecified chronic kidney disease
Hypertensive chronic kidney disease NOS
Hypertensive renal disease NOS
Use additional code to identify the stage of chronic kidney disease (N18.1-N18.4, N18.9)

4th **I13 Hypertensive heart and chronic kidney disease**
INCLUDES *any condition in I11.- with any condition in I12.-*
cardiorenal disease
cardiovascular renal disease
I13.0 Hypertensive heart and chronic kidney disease with heart failure and stage 1 through stage 4 chronic kidney disease, or unspecified chronic kidney disease CC
Use additional code to identify type of heart failure (I50.-)
Use additional code to identify stage of chronic kidney disease (N18.1-N18.4, N18.9)
5th **I13.1 Hypertensive heart and chronic kidney disease without heart failure**
I13.10 Hypertensive heart and chronic kidney disease without heart failure, with stage 1 through stage 4 chronic kidney disease, or unspecified chronic kidney disease
Hypertensive heart disease and hypertensive chronic kidney disease NOS
Use additional code to identify the stage of chronic kidney disease (N18.1-N18.4, N18.9)
I13.11 Hypertensive heart and chronic kidney disease without heart failure, with stage 5 chronic kidney disease, or end stage renal disease CC
Use additional code to identify the stage of chronic kidney disease (N18.5, N18.6)
I13.2 Hypertensive heart and chronic kidney disease with heart failure and with stage 5 chronic kidney disease, or end stage renal disease CC
Use additional code to identify type of heart failure (I50.-)
Use additional code to identify the stage of chronic kidney disease (N18.5, N18.6)

4th **I15 Secondary hypertension**
Code also underlying condition
EXCLUDES1 *postprocedural hypertension (I97.3)*
EXCLUDES2 *secondary hypertension involving vessels of brain (I60-I69)*
secondary hypertension involving vessels of eye (H35.0-)
I15.0 Renovascular hypertension
I15.1 Hypertension secondary to other renal disorders
I15.2 Hypertension secondary to endocrine disorders
I15.8 Other secondary hypertension
I15.9 Secondary hypertension, unspecified

● 4th **I16 Hypertensive crisis**
Code also any identified hypertensive disease (I10-I15)
● **I16.0 Hypertensive urgency**
● **I16.1 Hypertensive emergency**
● **I16.9 Hypertensive crisis, unspecified**

Ischemic heart diseases (I20-I25)

Use additional code to identify presence of hypertension ▶(I10-I16)◀

4th **I20 Angina pectoris**
Use additional code to identify:
exposure to environmental tobacco smoke (Z77.22)
history of tobacco ▶dependence◀ (Z87.891)
occupational exposure to environmental tobacco smoke (Z57.31)
tobacco dependence (F17.-)
tobacco use (Z72.0)
EXCLUDES1 *angina pectoris with atherosclerotic heart disease of native coronary arteries (I25.1-)*
atherosclerosis of coronary artery bypass graft(s) and coronary artery of transplanted heart with angina pectoris (I25.7-)
postinfarction angina (I23.7)

Unacceptable principal diagnosis symbol per Medicare code edits | Code exempt from diagnosis present on admission requirement
Questionable admission | Complication or comorbidity | CC/MCC exclusion | Major complication or comorbidity
Principal diagnosis as its own CC | Principal diagnosis as its own MCC | Z code as first-listed diagnosis

 When symbols appear on a code that requires a 7th character extension, refer to Appendix D to identify applicable 7th character codes.

I20.0 Unstable angina
Accelerated angina
Crescendo angina
De novo effort angina
Intermediate coronary syndrome
Preinfarction syndrome
Worsening effort angina

I20.1 Angina pectoris with documented spasm
Angiospastic angina
Prinzmetal angina
Spasm-induced angina
Variant angina

I20.8 Other forms of angina pectoris
Angina equivalent
Angina of effort
Coronary slow flow syndrome
Stenocardia
Stable angina
Use additional code(s) for symptoms associated with angina equivalent

I20.9 Angina pectoris, unspecified
Angina NOS
Anginal syndrome
Cardiac angina
Ischemic chest pain

I21 ST elevation (STEMI) and non-ST elevation (NSTEMI) myocardial infarction

INCLUDES *cardiac infarction*
coronary (artery) embolism
coronary (artery) occlusion
coronary (artery) rupture
coronary (artery) thrombosis
infarction of heart, myocardium, or ventricle
myocardial infarction specified as acute or with a stated duration of 4 weeks (28 days) or less from onset

Use additional code, if applicable, to identify:
exposure to environmental tobacco smoke (Z77.22)
history of tobacco ▶dependence◀ (Z87.891)
occupational exposure to environmental tobacco smoke (Z57.31)
status post administration of tPA (rtPA) in a different facility within the last 24 hours prior to admission to current facility (Z92.82)
tobacco dependence (F17.-)
tobacco use (Z72.0)

EXCLUDES2 *old myocardial infarction (I25.2)*
postmyocardial infarction syndrome (I24.1)
subsequent myocardial infarction (I22.-)

AHA: Q1, 2013

I21.0 ST elevation (STEMI) myocardial infarction of anterior wall

I21.01 ST elevation (STEMI) myocardial infarction involving left main coronary artery MCC

I21.02 ST elevation (STEMI) myocardial infarction involving left anterior descending coronary artery MCC
ST elevation (STEMI) myocardial infarction involving diagonal coronary artery
AHA: Q1, 2013

I21.09 ST elevation (STEMI) myocardial infarction involving other coronary artery of anterior wall MCC
Acute transmural myocardial infarction of anterior wall
Anteroapical transmural (Q wave) infarction (acute)
Anterolateral transmural (Q wave) infarction (acute)
Anteroseptal transmural (Q wave) infarction (acute)
Transmural (Q wave) infarction (acute) (of) anterior (wall) NOS
AHA: Q4, 2012

I21.1 ST elevation (STEMI) myocardial infarction of inferior wall

I21.11 ST elevation (STEMI) myocardial infarction involving right coronary artery MCC
Inferoposterior transmural (Q wave) infarction (acute)

I21.19 ST elevation (STEMI) myocardial infarction involving other coronary artery of inferior wall MCC
Acute transmural myocardial infarction of inferior wall
Inferolateral transmural (Q wave) infarction (acute)
Transmural (Q wave) infarction (acute) (of) diaphragmatic wall
Transmural (Q wave) infarction (acute) (of) inferior (wall) NOS

EXCLUDES2 *ST elevation (STEMI) myocardial infarction involving left circumflex coronary artery (I21.21)*

AHA: Q4, 2012

I21.2 ST elevation (STEMI) myocardial infarction of other sites

I21.21 ST elevation (STEMI) myocardial infarction involving left circumflex coronary artery MCC
ST elevation (STEMI) myocardial infarction involving oblique marginal coronary artery

I21.29 ST elevation (STEMI) myocardial infarction involving other sites MCC
Acute transmural myocardial infarction of other sites
Apical-lateral transmural (Q wave) infarction (acute)
Basal-lateral transmural (Q wave) infarction (acute)
High lateral transmural (Q wave) infarction (acute)
Lateral (wall) NOS transmural (Q wave) infarction (acute)
Posterior (true) transmural (Q wave) infarction (acute)
Posterobasal transmural (Q wave) infarction (acute)
Posterolateral transmural (Q wave) infarction (acute)
Posteroseptal transmural (Q wave) infarction (acute)
Septal transmural (Q wave) infarction (acute) NOS

I21.3 ST elevation (STEMI) myocardial infarction of unspecified site MCC
Acute transmural myocardial infarction of unspecified site
Myocardial infarction (acute) NOS
Transmural (Q wave) myocardial infarction NOS
AHA: Q1, 2013

I21.4 Non-ST elevation (NSTEMI) myocardial infarction MCC
Acute subendocardial myocardial infarction
Non-Q wave myocardial infarction NOS
Nontransmural myocardial infarction NOS

I22 Subsequent ST elevation (STEMI) and non-ST elevation (NSTEMI) myocardial infarction

INCLUDES *acute myocardial infarction occurring within four weeks (28 days) of a previous acute myocardial infarction, regardless of site*
cardiac infarction
coronary (artery) embolism
coronary (artery) occlusion
coronary (artery) rupture
coronary (artery) thrombosis
infarction of heart, myocardium, or ventricle
recurrent myocardial infarction
reinfarction of myocardium
rupture of heart, myocardium, or ventricle

Use additional code, if applicable, to identify:
exposure to environmental tobacco smoke (Z77.22)
history of tobacco ▶dependence◀ (Z87.891)
occupational exposure to environmental tobacco smoke (Z57.31)
status post administration of tPA (rtPA) in a different facility within the last 24 hours prior to admission to current facility (Z92.82)
tobacco dependence (F17.-)
tobacco use (Z72.0)
AHA: Q1, 2013

I22.0 Subsequent ST elevation (STEMI) myocardial infarction of anterior wall MCC
Subsequent acute transmural myocardial infarction of anterior wall
Subsequent transmural (Q wave) infarction (acute)(of) anterior (wall) NOS
Subsequent anteroapical transmural (Q wave) infarction (acute)
Subsequent anterolateral transmural (Q wave) infarction (acute)
Subsequent anteroseptal transmural (Q wave) infarction (acute)

I22.1 Subsequent ST elevation (STEMI) myocardial infarction of inferior wall MCC
Subsequent acute transmural myocardial infarction of inferior wall
Subsequent transmural (Q wave) infarction (acute)(of) diaphragmatic wall
Subsequent transmural (Q wave) infarction (acute)(of) inferior (wall) NOS
Subsequent inferolateral transmural (Q wave) infarction (acute)
Subsequent inferoposterior transmural (Q wave) infarction (acute)
AHA: Q4, 2012

Unspecified Code | Other Specified Code | Manifestation Code | N Newborn | P Pediatric | M Maternity | A Adult | ♂ Male | ♀ Female
● New Code | ▲ Revised Code Title | ▶◀ Revised Text | NOTES | INCLUDES | EXCLUDES1 Not coded here | EXCLUDES2 Not included here
4th character required | 5th character required | 6th character required | 7th character required
Extension 'X' Alert | HAC Hospital-acquired condition (HAC) alert | AHA AHA Coding Clinic©

I22.2 **Subsequent non-ST elevation (NSTEMI) myocardial infarction** MCC
Subsequent acute subendocardial myocardial infarction
Subsequent non-Q wave myocardial infarction NOS
Subsequent nontransmural myocardial infarction NOS

I22.8 **Subsequent ST elevation (STEMI) myocardial infarction of other sites** MCC
Subsequent acute transmural myocardial infarction of other sites
Subsequent apical-lateral transmural (Q wave) myocardial infarction (acute)
Subsequent basal-lateral transmural (Q wave) myocardial infarction (acute)
Subsequent high lateral transmural (Q wave) myocardial infarction (acute)
Subsequent transmural (Q wave) myocardial infarction (acute) (of) lateral (wall) NOS
Subsequent posterior (true)transmural (Q wave) myocardial infarction (acute)
Subsequent posterobasal transmural (Q wave) myocardial infarction (acute)
Subsequent posterolateral transmural (Q wave) myocardial infarction (acute)
Subsequent posteroseptal transmural (Q wave) myocardial infarction (acute)
Subsequent septal NOS transmural (Q wave) myocardial infarction (acute)

I22.9 **Subsequent ST elevation (STEMI) myocardial infarction of unspecified site** MCC
Subsequent acute myocardial infarction of unspecified site
Subsequent myocardial infarction (acute) NOS

I23 **Certain current complications following ST elevation (STEMI) and non-ST elevation (NSTEMI) myocardial infarction (within the 28 day period)**

I23.0 **Hemopericardium as current complication following acute myocardial infarction** A CC
EXCLUDES1 *hemopericardium not specified as current complication following acute myocardial infarction (I31.2)*

I23.1 **Atrial septal defect as current complication following acute myocardial infarction** A CC
EXCLUDES1 *acquired atrial septal defect not specified as current complication following acute myocardial infarction (I51.0)*

I23.2 **Ventricular septal defect as current complication following acute myocardial infarction** A CC
EXCLUDES1 *acquired ventricular septal defect not specified as current complication following acute myocardial infarction (I51.0)*

I23.3 **Rupture of cardiac wall without hemopericardium as current complication following acute myocardial infarction** A CC

I23.4 **Rupture of chordae tendineae as current complication following acute myocardial infarction** MCC
EXCLUDES1 *rupture of chordae tendineae not specified as current complication following acute myocardial infarction (I51.1)*

I23.5 **Rupture of papillary muscle as current complication following acute myocardial infarction** MCC
EXCLUDES1 *rupture of papillary muscle not specified as current complication following acute myocardial infarction (I51.2)*

I23.6 **Thrombosis of atrium, auricular appendage, and ventricle as current complications following acute myocardial infarction** A CC
EXCLUDES1 *thrombosis of atrium, auricular appendage, and ventricle not specified as current complication following acute myocardial infarction (I51.3)*

I23.7 **Postinfarction angina** A CC

I23.8 **Other current complications following acute myocardial infarction** A CC

I24 **Other acute ischemic heart diseases**
EXCLUDES1 *angina pectoris (I20.-)*
transient myocardial ischemia in newborn (P29.4)

I24.0 **Acute coronary thrombosis not resulting in myocardial infarction** CC
Acute coronary (artery) (vein) embolism not resulting in myocardial infarction
Acute coronary (artery) (vein) occlusion not resulting in myocardial infarction
Acute coronary (artery) (vein) thromboembolism not resulting in myocardial infarction
EXCLUDES1 *atherosclerotic heart disease (I25.1-)*
AHA: Q1, 2013

I24.1 **Dressler's syndrome** CC
Postmyocardial infarction syndrome
EXCLUDES1 *postinfarction angina (I23.7)*

I24.8 **Other forms of acute ischemic heart disease** CC

I24.9 **Acute ischemic heart disease, unspecified** CC
EXCLUDES1 *ischemic heart disease (chronic) NOS (I25.9)*

I25 **Chronic ischemic heart disease**
Use additional code to identify:
chronic total occlusion of coronary artery (I25.82)
exposure to environmental tobacco smoke (Z77.22)
history of tobacco ▶dependence◀ (Z87.891)
occupational exposure to environmental tobacco smoke (Z57.31)
tobacco dependence (F17.-)
tobacco use (Z72.0)

I25.1 **Atherosclerotic heart disease of native coronary artery**
Atherosclerotic cardiovascular disease
Coronary (artery) atheroma
Coronary (artery) atherosclerosis
Coronary (artery) disease
Coronary (artery) sclerosis
Use additional code, if applicable, to identify:
coronary atherosclerosis due to calcified coronary lesion (I25.84)
coronary atherosclerosis due to lipid rich plaque (I25.83)
EXCLUDES2 *atheroembolism (I75.-)*
atherosclerosis of coronary artery bypass graft(s) and transplanted heart (I25.7-)

I25.10 **Atherosclerotic heart disease of native coronary artery without angina pectoris** A
Atherosclerotic heart disease NOS
AHA: Q4, 2013

I25.11 **Atherosclerotic heart disease of native coronary artery with angina pectoris**

I25.110 **Atherosclerotic heart disease of native coronary artery with unstable angina pectoris** A CC PDx
EXCLUDES1 *unstable angina without atherosclerotic heart disease (I20.0)*

I25.111 **Atherosclerotic heart disease of native coronary artery with angina pectoris with documented spasm** A
EXCLUDES1 *angina pectoris with documented spasm without atherosclerotic heart disease (I20.1)*

I25.118 **Atherosclerotic heart disease of native coronary artery with other forms of angina pectoris** A
EXCLUDES1 *other forms of angina pectoris without atherosclerotic heart disease (I20.8)*

I25.119 **Atherosclerotic heart disease of native coronary artery with unspecified angina pectoris** A
Atherosclerotic heart disease with angina NOS
Atherosclerotic heart disease with ischemic chest pain
EXCLUDES1 *unspecified angina pectoris without atherosclerotic heart disease (I20.9)*

I25.2 **Old myocardial infarction** POA
Healed myocardial infarction
Past myocardial infarction diagnosed by ECG or other investigation, but currently presenting no symptoms

I25.3 **Aneurysm of heart** CC
Mural aneurysm
Ventricular aneurysm

I25.4 **Coronary artery aneurysm and dissection**

Unacceptable principal diagnosis symbol per Medicare code edits — Code exempt from diagnosis present on admission requirement
Questionable admission — CC Complication or comorbidity — CC/MCC exclusion — MCC Major complication or comorbidity
Principal diagnosis as its own CC — Principal diagnosis as its own MCC — Z code as first-listed diagnosis

I25.41 Coronary artery aneurysm
Coronary arteriovenous fistula, acquired
EXCLUDES1 *congenital coronary (artery) aneurysm (Q24.5)*

I25.42 Coronary artery dissection MCC

I25.5 Ischemic cardiomyopathy
EXCLUDES2 *coronary atherosclerosis (I25.1-, I25.7-)*

I25.6 Silent myocardial ischemia

I25.7 Atherosclerosis of coronary artery bypass graft (s) and coronary artery of transplanted heart with angina pectoris
Use additional code, if applicable, to identify:
coronary atherosclerosis due to calcified coronary lesion (I25.84)
coronary atherosclerosis due to lipid rich plaque (I25.83)
EXCLUDES1 *atherosclerosis of bypass graft(s) of transplanted heart without angina pectoris (I25.812)*
atherosclerosis of coronary artery bypass graft(s) without angina pectoris (I25.810)
atherosclerosis of native coronary artery of transplanted heart without angina pectoris (I25.811)
embolism or thrombus of coronary artery bypass graft(s) (T82.8-)

I25.70 Atherosclerosis of coronary artery bypass graft(s), unspecified , with angina pectoris

I25.700 Atherosclerosis of coronary artery bypass graft(s), unspecified, with unstable angina pectoris A CC PDx
EXCLUDES1 *unstable angina pectoris without atherosclerosis of coronary artery bypass graft (I20.0)*

I25.701 Atherosclerosis of coronary artery bypass graft(s), unspecified, with angina pectoris with documented spasm A
EXCLUDES1 *angina pectoris with documented spasm without atherosclerosis of coronary artery bypass graft (I20.1)*

I25.708 Atherosclerosis of coronary artery bypass graft(s), unspecified, with other forms of angina pectoris A
EXCLUDES1 *other forms of angina pectoris without atherosclerosis of coronary artery bypass graft (I20.8)*

I25.709 Atherosclerosis of coronary artery bypass graft(s), unspecified, with unspecified angina pectoris A
EXCLUDES1 *unspecified angina pectoris without atherosclerosis of coronary artery bypass graft (I20.9)*

I25.71 Atherosclerosis of autologous vein coronary artery bypass graft(s) with angina pectoris

I25.710 Atherosclerosis of autologous vein coronary artery bypass graft(s) with unstable angina pectoris A CC PDx
EXCLUDES1 *unstable angina without atherosclerosis of autologous vein coronary artery bypass graft(s) (I20.0)*

I25.711 Atherosclerosis of autologous vein coronary artery bypass graft(s) with angina pectoris with documented spasm A CC
EXCLUDES1 *angina pectoris with documented spasm without atherosclerosis of autologous vein coronary artery bypass graft(s) (I20.1)*

I25.718 Atherosclerosis of autologous vein coronary artery bypass graft(s) with other forms of angina pectoris A CC
EXCLUDES1 *other forms of angina pectoris without atherosclerosis of autologous vein coronary artery bypass graft(s) (I20.8)*

I25.719 Atherosclerosis of autologous vein coronary artery bypass graft(s) with unspecified angina pectoris A CC
EXCLUDES1 *unspecified angina pectoris without atherosclerosis of autologous vein coronary artery bypass graft(s) (I20.9)*

I25.72 Atherosclerosis of autologous artery coronary artery bypass graft(s) with angina pectoris
Atherosclerosis of internal mammary artery graft with angina pectoris

I25.720 Atherosclerosis of autologous artery coronary artery bypass graft(s) with unstable angina pectoris A CC PDx
EXCLUDES1 *unstable angina without atherosclerosis of autologous artery coronary artery bypass graft(s) (I20.0)*

I25.721 Atherosclerosis of autologous artery coronary artery bypass graft(s) with angina pectoris with documented spasm A CC
EXCLUDES1 *angina pectoris with documented spasm without atherosclerosis of autologous artery coronary artery bypass graft(s) (I20.1)*

I25.728 Atherosclerosis of autologous artery coronary artery bypass graft(s) with other forms of angina pectoris A CC
EXCLUDES1 *other forms of angina pectoris without atherosclerosis of autologous artery coronary artery bypass graft(s) (I20.8)*

I25.729 Atherosclerosis of autologous artery coronary artery bypass graft(s) with unspecified angina pectoris A CC
EXCLUDES1 *unspecified angina pectoris without atherosclerosis of autologous artery coronary artery bypass graft(s) (I20.9)*

I25.73 Atherosclerosis of nonautologous biological coronary artery bypass graft(s) with angina pectoris

I25.730 Atherosclerosis of nonautologous biological coronary artery bypass graft(s) with unstable angina pectoris A CC PDx
EXCLUDES1 *unstable angina without atherosclerosis of nonautologous biological coronary artery bypass graft(s) (I20.0)*

I25.731 Atherosclerosis of nonautologous biological coronary artery bypass graft(s) with angina pectoris with documented spasm A CC
EXCLUDES1 *angina pectoris with documented spasm without atherosclerosis of nonautologous biological coronary artery bypass graft(s) (I20.1)*

I25.738 Atherosclerosis of nonautologous biological coronary artery bypass graft(s) with other forms of angina pectoris A CC
EXCLUDES1 *other forms of angina pectoris without atherosclerosis of nonautologous biological coronary artery bypass graft(s) (I20.8)*

I25.739 Atherosclerosis of nonautologous biological coronary artery bypass graft(s) with unspecified angina pectoris A CC
EXCLUDES1 *unspecified angina pectoris without atherosclerosis of nonautologous biological coronary artery bypass graft(s) (I20.9)*

I25.75 Atherosclerosis of native coronary artery of transplanted heart with angina pectoris
EXCLUDES1 *atherosclerosis of native coronary artery of transplanted heart without angina pectoris (I25.811)*

Unspecified Code Other Specified Code Manifestation Code N Newborn P Pediatric M Maternity A Adult ♂ Male ♀ Female
● New Code ▲ Revised Code Title ►◄ Revised Text NOTES INCLUDES EXCLUDES1 Not coded here EXCLUDES2 Not included here
4th character required 5th character required 6th character required 7th character required
Extension 'X' Alert HAC Hospital-acquired condition (HAC) alert AHA AHA Coding Clinic©

I25.750 **Atherosclerosis of native coronary artery of transplanted heart with unstable angina**

I25.751 **Atherosclerosis of native coronary artery of transplanted heart with angina pectoris with documented spasm**

I25.758 **Atherosclerosis of native coronary artery of transplanted heart with other forms of angina pectoris**

I25.759 **Atherosclerosis of native coronary artery of transplanted heart with unspecified angina pectoris**

I25.76 **Atherosclerosis of bypass graft of coronary artery of transplanted heart with angina pectoris**

EXCLUDES1 *atherosclerosis of bypass graft of coronary artery of transplanted heart without angina pectoris (I25.812)*

I25.760 **Atherosclerosis of bypass graft of coronary artery of transplanted heart with unstable angina**

I25.761 **Atherosclerosis of bypass graft of coronary artery of transplanted heart with angina pectoris with documented spasm**

I25.768 **Atherosclerosis of bypass graft of coronary artery of transplanted heart with other forms of angina pectoris**

I25.769 **Atherosclerosis of bypass graft of coronary artery of transplanted heart with unspecified angina pectoris**

I25.79 **Atherosclerosis of other coronary artery bypass graft(s) with angina pectoris**

I25.790 **Atherosclerosis of other coronary artery bypass graft(s) with unstable angina pectoris**

EXCLUDES1 *unstable angina without atherosclerosis of other coronary artery bypass graft(s) (I20.0)*

I25.791 **Atherosclerosis of other coronary artery bypass graft(s) with angina pectoris with documented spasm**

EXCLUDES1 *angina pectoris with documented spasm without atherosclerosis of other coronary artery bypass graft(s) (I20.1)*

I25.798 **Atherosclerosis of other coronary artery bypass graft(s) with other forms of angina pectoris**

EXCLUDES1 *other forms of angina pectoris without atherosclerosis of other coronary artery bypass graft(s) (I20.8)*

I25.799 **Atherosclerosis of other coronary artery bypass graft(s) with unspecified angina pectoris**

EXCLUDES1 *unspecified angina pectoris without atherosclerosis of other coronary artery bypass graft(s) (I20.9)*

I25.8 **Other forms of chronic ischemic heart disease**

I25.81 **Atherosclerosis of other coronary vessels without angina pectoris**

Use additional code, if applicable, to identify:

coronary atherosclerosis due to calcified coronary lesion (I25.84)

coronary atherosclerosis due to lipid rich plaque (I25.83)

EXCLUDES1 *atherosclerotic heart disease of native coronary artery without angina pectoris (I25.10)*

I25.810 **Atherosclerosis of coronary artery bypass graft(s) without angina pectoris**

Atherosclerosis of coronary artery bypass graft NOS

EXCLUDES1 *atherosclerosis of coronary bypass graft(s) with angina pectoris (I25.70-I25.73-, I25.79-)*

I25.811 **Atherosclerosis of native coronary artery of transplanted heart without angina pectoris**

Atherosclerosis of native coronary artery of transplanted heart NOS

EXCLUDES1 *atherosclerosis of native coronary artery of transplanted heart with angina pectoris (I25.75-)*

I25.812 **Atherosclerosis of bypass graft of coronary artery of transplanted heart without angina pectoris**

Atherosclerosis of bypass graft of transplanted heart NOS

EXCLUDES1 *atherosclerosis of bypass graft of transplanted heart with angina pectoris (I25.76)*

I25.82 **Chronic total occlusion of coronary artery**

Complete occlusion of coronary artery

Total occlusion of coronary artery

Code first coronary atherosclerosis (I25.1-, I25.7-, I25.81-)

EXCLUDES1 *acute coronary occlusion with myocardial infarction (I21.-, I22.-)*

acute coronary occlusion without myocardial infarction (I24.0)

I25.83 **Coronary atherosclerosis due to lipid rich plaque**

Code first coronary atherosclerosis (I25.1-, I25.7-, I25.81-)

I25.84 **Coronary atherosclerosis due to calcified coronary lesion**

Coronary atherosclerosis due to severely calcified coronary lesion

Code first coronary atherosclerosis (I25.1-, I25.7-, I25.81-)

I25.89 **Other forms of chronic ischemic heart disease**

I25.9 **Chronic ischemic heart disease, unspecified**

Ischemic heart disease (chronic) NOS

Pulmonary heart disease and diseases of pulmonary circulation (I26-I28)

I26 **Pulmonary embolism**

INCLUDES *pulmonary (acute) (artery)(vein) infarction*

pulmonary (acute) (artery)(vein) thromboembolism

pulmonary (acute) (artery)(vein) thrombosis

EXCLUDES2 *chronic pulmonary embolism (I27.82)*

personal history of pulmonary embolism (Z86.711)

pulmonary embolism complicating abortion, ectopic or molar pregnancy (O00-O07, O08.2)

pulmonary embolism complicating pregnancy, childbirth and the puerperium (O88.-)

pulmonary embolism due to trauma (T79.0, T79.1)

pulmonary embolism due to complications of surgical and medical care (T80.0, T81.7-, T82.8-)

septic (non-pulmonary) arterial embolism (I76)

I26.0 **Pulmonary embolism with acute cor pulmonale**

I26.01 **Septic pulmonary embolism with acute cor pulmonale**

Code first underlying infection

I26.02 **Saddle embolus of pulmonary artery with acute cor pulmonale**

I26.09 **Other pulmonary embolism with acute cor pulmonale**

Acute cor pulmonale NOS

I26.9 **Pulmonary embolism without acute cor pulmonale**

I26.90 **Septic pulmonary embolism without acute cor pulmonale**

Code first underlying infection

I26.92 **Saddle embolus of pulmonary artery without acute cor pulmonale**

I26.99 **Other pulmonary embolism without acute cor pulmonale**

Acute pulmonary embolism NOS

Pulmonary embolism NOS

Unacceptable principal diagnosis symbol per Medicare code edits | Code exempt from diagnosis present on admission requirement | Questionable admission | Complication or comorbidity | CC/MCC exclusion | Major complication or comorbidity | Principal diagnosis as its own CC | Principal diagnosis as its own MCC | Z code as first-listed diagnosis

I27 Other pulmonary heart diseases

I27.0 Primary pulmonary hypertension
EXCLUDES1 *pulmonary hypertension NOS (I27.2)*
secondary pulmonary hypertension (I27.2)

I27.1 Kyphoscoliotic heart disease

I27.2 Other secondary pulmonary hypertension
Pulmonary hypertension NOS
Code also associated underlying condition
AHA: Q2, 2016

I27.8 Other specified pulmonary heart diseases

I27.81 Cor pulmonale (chronic)
Cor pulmonale NOS
EXCLUDES1 *acute cor pulmonale (I26.0-)*

I27.82 Chronic pulmonary embolism
Use additional code, if applicable, for associated long-term (current) use of anticoagulants (Z79.01)
EXCLUDES1 *personal history of pulmonary embolism (Z86.711)*

I27.89 Other specified pulmonary heart diseases
Eisenmenger's complex
Eisenmenger's syndrome
EXCLUDES1 *Eisenmenger's defect (Q21.8)*

I27.9 Pulmonary heart disease, unspecified
Chronic cardiopulmonary disease

I28 Other diseases of pulmonary vessels

I28.0 Arteriovenous fistula of pulmonary vessels
EXCLUDES1 *congenital arteriovenous fistula (Q25.72)*

I28.1 Aneurysm of pulmonary artery
EXCLUDES1 *congenital aneurysm (Q25.79)*
congenital arteriovenous aneurysm (Q25.72)

I28.8 Other diseases of pulmonary vessels
Pulmonary arteritis
Pulmonary endarteritis
Rupture of pulmonary vessels
Stenosis of pulmonary vessels
Stricture of pulmonary vessels

I28.9 Disease of pulmonary vessels, unspecified

Other forms of heart disease (I30-I52)

I30 Acute pericarditis
INCLUDES *acute mediastinopericarditis*
acute myopericarditis
acute pericardial effusion
acute pleuropericarditis
acute pneumopericarditis
EXCLUDES1 *Dressler's syndrome (I24.1)*
rheumatic pericarditis (acute) (I01.0)

I30.0 Acute nonspecific idiopathic pericarditis

I30.1 Infective pericarditis
Pneumococcal pericarditis
Pneumopyopericardium
Purulent pericarditis
Pyopericarditis
Pyopericardium
Pyopneumopericardium
Staphylococcal pericarditis
Streptococcal pericarditis
Suppurative pericarditis
Viral pericarditis
Use additional code (B95-B97) to identify infectious agent

I30.8 Other forms of acute pericarditis

I30.9 Acute pericarditis, unspecified

I31 Other diseases of pericardium
EXCLUDES1 *diseases of pericardium specified as rheumatic (I09.2)*
postcardiotomy syndrome (I97.0)
traumatic injury to pericardium (S26.-)

I31.0 Chronic adhesive pericarditis
Accretio cordis
Adherent pericardium
Adhesive mediastinopericarditis

I31.1 Chronic constrictive pericarditis
Concretio cordis
Pericardial calcification

I31.2 Hemopericardium, not elsewhere classified
EXCLUDES1 *hemopericardium as current complication following acute myocardial infarction (I23.0)*

I31.3 Pericardial effusion (noninflammatory)
Chylopericardium
EXCLUDES1 *acute pericardial effusion (I30.9)*

I31.4 Cardiac tamponade
Code first underlying cause

I31.8 Other specified diseases of pericardium
Epicardial plaques
Focal pericardial adhesions

I31.9 Disease of pericardium, unspecified
Pericarditis (chronic) NOS

I32 Pericarditis in diseases classified elsewhere
Code first underlying disease
EXCLUDES1 *pericarditis (in):*
coxsackie (virus) (B33.23)
gonococcal (A54.83)
meningococcal (A39.53)
rheumatoid (arthritis) (M05.31)
syphilitic (A52.06)
systemic lupus erythematosus (M32.12)
tuberculosis (A18.84)

I33 Acute and subacute endocarditis
EXCLUDES1 *acute rheumatic endocarditis (I01.1)*
endocarditis NOS (I38)

I33.0 Acute and subacute infective endocarditis
Bacterial endocarditis (acute) (subacute)
Infective endocarditis (acute) (subacute) NOS
Endocarditis lenta (acute) (subacute)
Malignant endocarditis (acute) (subacute)
Purulent endocarditis (acute) (subacute)
Septic endocarditis (acute) (subacute)
Ulcerative endocarditis (acute) (subacute)
Vegetative endocarditis (acute) (subacute)
Use additional code (B95-B97) to identify infectious agent

I33.9 Acute and subacute endocarditis, unspecified
Acute endocarditis NOS
Acute myoendocarditis NOS
Acute periendocarditis NOS
Subacute endocarditis NOS
Subacute myoendocarditis NOS
Subacute periendocarditis NOS

I34 Nonrheumatic mitral valve disorders
EXCLUDES1 *mitral valve disease (I05.9)*
mitral valve failure (I05.8)
mitral valve stenosis (I05.0)
mitral valve disorder of unspecified cause with diseases of aortic and/or tricuspid valve(s) (I08.-)
mitral valve disorder of unspecified cause with mitral stenosis or obstruction (I05.0)
mitral valve disorder specified as congenital (Q23.2, Q23.3)
mitral valve disorder specified as rheumatic (I05.-)

I34.0 Nonrheumatic mitral (valve) insufficiency
Nonrheumatic mitral (valve) incompetence NOS
Nonrheumatic mitral (valve) regurgitation NOS

I34.1 Nonrheumatic mitral (valve) prolapse
Floppy nonrheumatic mitral valve syndrome
EXCLUDES1 *Marfan's syndrome (Q87.4-)*

I34.2 Nonrheumatic mitral (valve) stenosis

I34.8 Other nonrheumatic mitral valve disorders

I34.9 Nonrheumatic mitral valve disorder, unspecified

I35 Nonrheumatic aortic valve disorders
EXCLUDES1 *aortic valve disorder of unspecified cause but with diseases of mitral and/or tricuspid valve(s) (I08.-)*
aortic valve disorder specified as congenital (Q23.0, Q23.1)
aortic valve disorder specified as rheumatic (I06.-)
hypertrophic subaortic stenosis (I42.1)

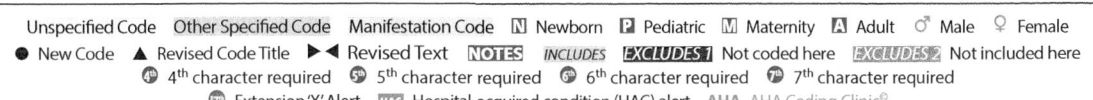

Unspecified Code | Other Specified Code | Manifestation Code | N Newborn | P Pediatric | M Maternity | A Adult | ♂ Male | ♀ Female
● New Code ▲ Revised Code Title ►◄ Revised Text NOTES INCLUDES EXCLUDES1 Not coded here EXCLUDES2 Not included here
4th character required | 5th character required | 6th character required | 7th character required
Extension 'X' Alert | HAC Hospital-acquired condition (HAC) alert | AHA AHA Coding Clinic©

I35.0 **Nonrheumatic aortic (valve) stenosis**
I35.1 **Nonrheumatic aortic (valve) insufficiency**
Nonrheumatic aortic (valve) incompetence NOS
Nonrheumatic aortic (valve) regurgitation NOS
I35.2 **Nonrheumatic aortic (valve) stenosis with insufficiency**
I35.8 **Other nonrheumatic aortic valve disorders**
I35.9 **Nonrheumatic aortic valve disorder, unspecified**

I36 **Nonrheumatic tricuspid valve disorders**
EXCLUDES1 *tricuspid valve disorders of unspecified cause (I07.-)*
tricuspid valve disorders specified as congenital (Q22.4, Q22.8, Q22.9)
tricuspid valve disorders specified as rheumatic (I07.-)
tricuspid valve disorders with aortic and/or mitral valve involvement (I08.-)
I36.0 **Nonrheumatic tricuspid (valve) stenosis**
I36.1 **Nonrheumatic tricuspid (valve) insufficiency**
Nonrheumatic tricuspid (valve) incompetence
Nonrheumatic tricuspid (valve) regurgitation
I36.2 **Nonrheumatic tricuspid (valve) stenosis with insufficiency**
I36.8 **Other nonrheumatic tricuspid valve disorders**
I36.9 **Nonrheumatic tricuspid valve disorder, unspecified**

I37 **Nonrheumatic pulmonary valve disorders**
EXCLUDES1 *pulmonary valve disorder specified as congenital (Q22.1, Q22.2, Q22.3)*
pulmonary valve disorder specified as rheumatic (I09.89)
I37.0 **Nonrheumatic pulmonary valve stenosis**
I37.1 **Nonrheumatic pulmonary valve insufficiency**
Nonrheumatic pulmonary valve incompetence
Nonrheumatic pulmonary valve regurgitation
I37.2 **Nonrheumatic pulmonary valve stenosis with insufficiency**
I37.8 **Other nonrheumatic pulmonary valve disorders**
I37.9 **Nonrheumatic pulmonary valve disorder, unspecified**

I38 **Endocarditis, valve unspecified** CC
INCLUDES *endocarditis (chronic) NOS*
valvular incompetence NOS
valvular insufficiency NOS
valvular regurgitation NOS
valvular stenosis NOS
valvulitis (chronic) NOS
EXCLUDES1 *congenital insufficiency of cardiac valve NOS (Q24.8)*
congenital stenosis of cardiac valve NOS (Q24.8)
endocardial fibroelastosis (I42.4)
endocarditis specified as rheumatic (I09.1)

I39 **Endocarditis and heart valve disorders in diseases classified elsewhere** CC
Code first underlying disease, such as:
Q fever (A78)
EXCLUDES1 *endocardial involvement in:*
candidiasis (B37.6)
gonococcal infection (A54.83)
Libman-Sacks disease (M32.11)
listerosis (A32.82)
meningococcal infection (A39.51)
rheumatoid arthritis (M05.31)
syphilis (A52.03)
tuberculosis (A18.84)
typhoid fever (A01.02)

I40 **Acute myocarditis**
INCLUDES *subacute myocarditis*
EXCLUDES1 *acute rheumatic myocarditis (I01.2)*
I40.0 **Infective myocarditis** MCC
Septic myocarditis
Use additional code (B95-B97) to identify infectious agent
I40.1 **Isolated myocarditis** MCC
Fiedler's myocarditis
Giant cell myocarditis
Idiopathic myocarditis
I40.8 **Other acute myocarditis** MCC
I40.9 **Acute myocarditis, unspecified** MCC

I41 **Myocarditis in diseases classified elsewhere** MCC
Code first underlying disease, such as:
typhus (A75.0-A75.9)
EXCLUDES1 *myocarditis (in):*
Chagas' disease (chronic) (B57.2)
acute (B57.0)
coxsackie (virus) infection (B33.22)
diphtheritic (A36.81)
gonococcal (A54.83)
influenzal (J09.X9, J10.82, J11.82)
meningococcal (A39.52)
mumps (B26.82)
rheumatoid arthritis (M05.31)
sarcoid (D86.85)
syphilis (A52.06)
toxoplasmosis (B58.81)
tuberculous (A18.84)

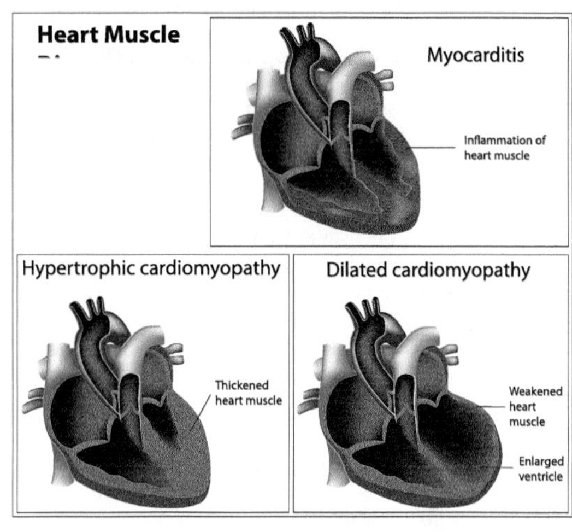

Figure 9.2 Heart muscle disease

I42 **Cardiomyopathy**
INCLUDES *myocardiopathy*
Code first pre-existing cardiomyopathy complicating pregnancy and puerperium (O99.4)
EXCLUDES2 *ischemic cardiomyopathy (I25.5)*
peripartum cardiomyopathy (O90.3)
ventricular hypertrophy (I51.7)
I42.0 **Dilated cardiomyopathy** CC
Congestive cardiomyopathy
I42.1 **Obstructive hypertrophic cardiomyopathy** CC
Hypertrophic subaortic stenosis (idiopathic)
I42.2 **Other hypertrophic cardiomyopathy** CC
Nonobstructive hypertrophic cardiomyopathy
I42.3 **Endomyocardial (eosinophilic) disease** CC
Endomyocardial (tropical) fibrosis
Löffler's endocarditis
I42.4 **Endocardial fibroelastosis** CC
Congenital cardiomyopathy
Elastomyofibrosis
I42.5 **Other restrictive cardiomyopathy** CC
Constrictive cardiomyopathy NOS
I42.6 **Alcoholic cardiomyopathy** CC
Code also presence of alcoholism (F10.-)
I42.7 **Cardiomyopathy due to drug and external agent** CC
Code first poisoning due to drug or toxin, if applicable (T36-T65 with fifth or sixth character 1-4 or 6)
Use additional code for adverse effect, if applicable, to identify drug (T36-T50 with fifth or sixth character 5)
I42.8 **Other cardiomyopathies** CC
I42.9 **Cardiomyopathy, unspecified** CC
Cardiomyopathy (primary) (secondary) NOS

I43 **Cardiomyopathy in diseases classified elsewhere** CC
Code first underlying disease, such as:
amyloidosis (E85.-)
glycogen storage disease (E74.0)

Unacceptable principal diagnosis symbol per Medicare code edits | Code exempt from diagnosis present on admission requirement
Questionable admission | CC Complication or comorbidity | CC/MCC exclusion | MCC Major complication or comorbidity
Principal diagnosis as its own CC | Principal diagnosis as its own MCC | Z code as first-listed diagnosis

When symbols appear on a code that requires a 7th character extension, refer to Appendix D to identify applicable 7th character codes.

gout (M10.0-)
thyrotoxicosis (E05.0-E05.9-)

EXCLUDES1 *cardiomyopathy (in):*
coxsackie (virus) (B33.24)
diphtheria (A36.81)
sarcoidosis (D86.85)
tuberculosis (A18.84)

I44 Atrioventricular and left bundle-branch block
- **I44.0 Atrioventricular block, first degree**
- **I44.1 Atrioventricular block, second degree**
  Atrioventricular block, type I and II
  Möbitz block, type I and II
  Second degree block, type I and II
  Wenckebach's block
- **I44.2 Atrioventricular block, complete** CC
  Complete heart block NOS
  Third degree block
- **I44.3 Other and unspecified atrioventricular block**
  Atrioventricular block NOS
  - **I44.30 Unspecified atrioventricular block**
  - **I44.39 Other atrioventricular block**
- **I44.4 Left anterior fascicular block** P
- **I44.5 Left posterior fascicular block** P
- **I44.6 Other and unspecified fascicular block**
  - **I44.60 Unspecified fascicular block** P
    Left bundle-branch hemiblock NOS
  - **I44.69 Other fascicular block** P
- **I44.7 Left bundle-branch block, unspecified** P

I45 Other conduction disorders
- **I45.0 Right fascicular block** P
- **I45.1 Other and unspecified right bundle-branch block**
  - **I45.10 Unspecified right bundle-branch block** P
    Right bundle-branch block NOS
  - **I45.19 Other right bundle-branch block** P
- **I45.2 Bifascicular block** CC
- **I45.3 Trifascicular block** CC
- **I45.4 Nonspecific intraventricular block**
  Bundle-branch block NOS
- **I45.5 Other specified heart block**
  Sinoatrial block
  Sinoauricular block
  EXCLUDES1 *heart block NOS (I45.9)*
- **I45.6 Pre-excitation syndrome**
  Accelerated atrioventricular conduction
  Accessory atrioventricular conduction
  Anomalous atrioventricular excitation
  Lown-Ganong-Levine syndrome
  Pre-excitation atrioventricular conduction
  Wolff-Parkinson-White syndrome
- **I45.8 Other specified conduction disorders**
  - **I45.81 Long QT syndrome**
  - **I45.89 Other specified conduction disorders** CC
    Atrioventricular [AV] dissociation
    Interference dissociation
    Isorhythmic dissociation
    Nonparoxysmal AV nodal tachycardia
- **I45.9 Conduction disorder, unspecified**
  Heart block NOS
  Stokes-Adams syndrome

I46 Cardiac arrest
EXCLUDES1 *cardiogenic shock (R57.0)*
- **I46.2 Cardiac arrest due to underlying cardiac condition** MCC
  Code first underlying cardiac condition
- **I46.8 Cardiac arrest due to other underlying condition** MCC
  Code first underlying condition
- **I46.9 Cardiac arrest, cause unspecified** MCC

I47 Paroxysmal tachycardia
Code first tachycardia complicating:
abortion or ectopic or molar pregnancy (O00-O07, O08.8)
obstetric surgery and procedures (O75.4)
EXCLUDES1 *tachycardia NOS (R00.0)*
sinoauricular tachycardia NOS (R00.0)
sinus [sinusal] tachycardia NOS (R00.0)
- **I47.0 Re-entry ventricular arrhythmia** CC
- **I47.1 Supraventricular tachycardia** CC
  Atrial (paroxysmal) tachycardia
  Atrioventricular [AV] (paroxysmal) tachycardia
  Atrioventricular re-entrant (nodal) tachycardia [AVNRT] [AVRT]
  Junctional (paroxysmal) tachycardia
  Nodal (paroxysmal) tachycardia
- **I47.2 Ventricular tachycardia** CC
  AHA: Q3, 2013
- **I47.9 Paroxysmal tachycardia, unspecified**
  Bouveret (-Hoffman) syndrome

I48 Atrial fibrillation and flutter
- **I48.0 Paroxysmal atrial fibrillation**
- **I48.1 Persistent atrial fibrillation** CC
- **I48.2 Chronic atrial fibrillation**
  Permanent atrial fibrillation
  AHA: Q4, 2013
- **I48.3 Typical atrial flutter** CC
  Type I atrial flutter
- **I48.4 Atypical atrial flutter** CC
  Type II atrial flutter
- **I48.9 Unspecified atrial fibrillation and atrial flutter**
  - **I48.91 Unspecified atrial fibrillation**
  - **I48.92 Unspecified atrial flutter** CC

I49 Other cardiac arrhythmias
Code first cardiac arrhythmia complicating:
abortion or ectopic or molar pregnancy (O00-O07, O08.8)
obstetric surgery and procedures (O75.4)
EXCLUDES1 *bradycardia NOS (R00.1)*
neonatal dysrhythmia (P29.1-)
sinoatrial bradycardia (R00.1)
sinus bradycardia (R00.1)
vagal bradycardia (R00.1)
- **I49.0 Ventricular fibrillation and flutter**
  - **I49.01 Ventricular fibrillation** MCC
  - **I49.02 Ventricular flutter** MCC
- **I49.1 Atrial premature depolarization**
  Atrial premature beats
- **I49.2 Junctional premature depolarization** CC
- **I49.3 Ventricular premature depolarization**
- **I49.4 Other and unspecified premature depolarization**
  - **I49.40 Unspecified premature depolarization**
    Premature beats NOS
  - **I49.49 Other premature depolarization**
    Ectopic beats
    Extrasystoles
    Extrasystolic arrhythmias
    Premature contractions
- **I49.5 Sick sinus syndrome**
  Tachycardia-bradycardia syndrome
- **I49.8 Other specified cardiac arrhythmias**
  Coronary sinus rhythm disorder
  Ectopic rhythm disorder
  Nodal rhythm disorder
- **I49.9 Cardiac arrhythmia, unspecified**
  Arrhythmia (cardiac) NOS

I50 Heart failure
Code first heart failure complicating abortion or ectopic or molar pregnancy (O00-O07, O08.8)
heart failure due to hypertension (I11.0)
heart failure due to hypertension with chronic kidney disease (I13.-)
heart failure following surgery (I97.13-)
obstetric surgery and procedures (O75.4)
rheumatic heart failure (I09.81)
EXCLUDES1 *neonatal cardiac failure (P29.0)*
EXCLUDES2 *cardiac arrest (I46.-)*
- **I50.1 Left ventricular failure** CC
  Cardiac asthma
  Edema of lung with heart disease NOS
  Edema of lung with heart failure
  Left heart failure
  Pulmonary edema with heart disease NOS
  Pulmonary edema with heart failure
  EXCLUDES1 *edema of lung without heart disease or heart failure (J81.-)*
  pulmonary edema without heart disease or failure (J81.-)

Unspecified Code | Other Specified Code | Manifestation Code | N Newborn | P Pediatric | M Maternity | A Adult | ♂ Male | ♀ Female
● New Code ▲ Revised Code Title ►◄ Revised Text NOTES INCLUDES EXCLUDES1 Not coded here EXCLUDES2 Not included here
4th character required 5th character required 6th character required 7th character required
Extension 'X' Alert HAC Hospital-acquired condition (HAC) alert AHA AHA Coding Clinic©

I50.2 Systolic (congestive) heart failure

EXCLUDES1 *combined systolic (congestive) and diastolic (congestive) heart failure (I50.4-)*

- I50.20 **Unspecified systolic (congestive) heart failure** CC
- I50.21 **Acute systolic (congestive) heart failure** MCC
- I50.22 **Chronic systolic (congestive) heart failure** CC
- I50.23 **Acute on chronic systolic (congestive) heart failure** MCC

I50.3 Diastolic (congestive) heart failure

EXCLUDES1 *combined systolic (congestive) and diastolic (congestive) heart failure (I50.4-)*

- I50.30 **Unspecified diastolic (congestive) heart failure** CC
- I50.31 **Acute diastolic (congestive) heart failure** MCC
- I50.32 **Chronic diastolic (congestive) heart failure** CC
- I50.33 **Acute on chronic diastolic (congestive) heart failure** MCC

I50.4 Combined systolic (congestive) and diastolic (congestive) heart failure

- I50.40 **Unspecified combined systolic (congestive) and diastolic (congestive) heart failure** CC
- I50.41 Acute **combined systolic (congestive) and diastolic (congestive) heart failure** MCC
- I50.42 Chronic **combined systolic (congestive) and diastolic (congestive) heart failure** CC
- I50.43 Acute on chronic **combined systolic (congestive) and diastolic (congestive) heart failure** MCC

I50.9 **Heart failure, unspecified**

Biventricular (heart) failure NOS
Cardiac, heart or myocardial failure NOS
Congestive heart disease
Congestive heart failure NOS
Right ventricular failure (secondary to left heart failure)

EXCLUDES2 *fluid overload (E87.70)*

I51 **Complications and ill-defined descriptions of heart disease**

EXCLUDES1 *any condition in I51.4-I51.9 due to hypertension (I11.-)*
any condition in I51.4-I51.9 due to hypertension and chronic kidney disease (I13.-)
heart disease specified as rheumatic (I00-I09)

I51.0 **Cardiac septal defect, acquired** A CC

Acquired septal atrial defect (old)
Acquired septal auricular defect (old)
Acquired septal ventricular defect (old)

EXCLUDES1 *cardiac septal defect as current complication following acute myocardial infarction (I23.1, I23.2)*

I51.1 **Rupture of chordae tendineae, not elsewhere classified** MCC

EXCLUDES1 *rupture of chordae tendineae as current complication following acute myocardial infarction (I23.4)*

I51.2 **Rupture of papillary muscle, not elsewhere classified** MCC

EXCLUDES1 *rupture of papillary muscle as current complication following acute myocardial infarction (I23.5)*

I51.3 **Intracardiac thrombosis, not elsewhere classified**

Apical thrombosis (old)
Atrial thrombosis (old)
Auricular thrombosis (old)
Mural thrombosis (old)
Ventricular thrombosis (old)

EXCLUDES1 *intracardiac thrombosis as current complication following acute myocardial infarction (I23.6)*

AHA: Q1, 2013

I51.4 **Myocarditis, unspecified**

Chronic (interstitial) myocarditis
Myocardial fibrosis
Myocarditis NOS

EXCLUDES1 *acute or subacute myocarditis (I40.-)*

I51.5 **Myocardial degeneration**

Fatty degeneration of heart or myocardium
Myocardial disease
Senile degeneration of heart or myocardium

I51.7 **Cardiomegaly**

Cardiac dilatation
Cardiac hypertrophy
Ventricular dilatation

I51.8 **Other ill-defined heart diseases**

- I51.81 **Takotsubo syndrome** CC

  Reversible left ventricular dysfunction following sudden emotional stress
  Stress induced cardiomyopathy
  Takotsubo cardiomyopathy
  Transient left ventricular apical ballooning syndrome

- I51.89 **Other ill-defined heart diseases**

  Carditis (acute)(chronic)
  Pancarditis (acute)(chronic)

I51.9 **Heart disease, unspecified**

I52 **Other heart disorders in diseases classified elsewhere**

Code first underlying disease, such as:
congenital syphilis (A50.5)
mucopolysaccharidosis (E76.3)
schistosomiasis (B65.0-B65.9)

EXCLUDES1 *heart disease (in):*
gonococcal infection (A54.83)
meningococcal infection (A39.50)
rheumatoid arthritis (M05.31)
syphilis (A52.06)

Cerebrovascular diseases (I60-I69)

Use additional code to identify presence of:
alcohol abuse and dependence (F10.-)
exposure to environmental tobacco smoke (Z77.22)
history of tobacco ▶dependence◀ (Z87.891)
hypertension (I10-I15)
occupational exposure to environmental tobacco smoke (Z57.31)
tobacco dependence (F17.-)
tobacco use (Z72.0)

EXCLUDES1 *transient cerebral ischemic attacks and related syndromes (G45.-)*
traumatic intracranial hemorrhage (S06.-)

I60 **Nontraumatic** subarachnoid **hemorrhage**

INCLUDES *ruptured cerebral aneurysm*

EXCLUDES1 *syphilitic ruptured cerebral aneurysm (A52.05)*

EXCLUDES2 *sequelae of subarachnoid hemorrhage (I69.0-)*

AHA: Q4, 2015

I60.0 **Nontraumatic subarachnoid hemorrhage from** carotid siphon and bifurcation

- I60.00 **Nontraumatic subarachnoid hemorrhage from** unspecified **carotid siphon and bifurcation** MCC
- I60.01 **Nontraumatic subarachnoid hemorrhage from** right **carotid siphon and bifurcation** MCC
- I60.02 **Nontraumatic subarachnoid hemorrhage from** left **carotid siphon and bifurcation** MCC

I60.1 **Nontraumatic subarachnoid hemorrhage from** middle cerebral artery

- I60.10 **Nontraumatic subarachnoid hemorrhage from** unspecified **middle cerebral artery** MCC
- I60.11 **Nontraumatic subarachnoid hemorrhage from** right **middle cerebral artery** MCC
- I60.12 **Nontraumatic subarachnoid hemorrhage from** left **middle cerebral artery** MCC

I60.2 **Nontraumatic subarachnoid hemorrhage** from anterior communicating artery MCC CC/MCC Exc

I60.3 **Nontraumatic subarachnoid hemorrhage from** posterior communicating artery

- I60.30 **Nontraumatic subarachnoid hemorrhage from** unspecified **posterior communicating artery** MCC
- I60.31 **Nontraumatic subarachnoid hemorrhage from** right **posterior communicating artery** MCC
- I60.32 **Nontraumatic subarachnoid hemorrhage from** left **posterior communicating artery** MCC

I60.4 **Nontraumatic subarachnoid hemorrhage from basilar artery** MCC

I60.5 **Nontraumatic subarachnoid hemorrhage from** vertebral artery

- I60.50 **Nontraumatic subarachnoid hemorrhage from** unspecified **vertebral artery** MCC
- I60.51 **Nontraumatic subarachnoid hemorrhage from** right **vertebral artery** MCC
- I60.52 **Nontraumatic subarachnoid hemorrhage from** left **vertebral artery** MCC

PDx Unacceptable principal diagnosis symbol per Medicare code edits — POA Code exempt from diagnosis present on admission requirement
Q Questionable admission — CC Complication or comorbidity — CC/MCC Exc CC/MCC exclusion — MCC Major complication or comorbidity
PDx CC Principal diagnosis as its own CC — PDx MCC Principal diagnosis as its own MCC — Z Z code as first-listed diagnosis

I60.6 **Nontraumatic subarachnoid hemorrhage from other intracranial arteries** MCC
I60.7 **Nontraumatic subarachnoid hemorrhage from unspecified intracranial artery** MCC
Ruptured (congenital) berry aneurysm
Ruptured (congenital) cerebral aneurysm
Subarachnoid hemorrhage (nontraumatic) from cerebral artery NOS
Subarachnoid hemorrhage (nontraumatic) from communicating artery NOS
EXCLUDES1 *berry aneurysm, nonruptured (I67.1)*
I60.8 **Other nontraumatic subarachnoid hemorrhage** MCC
Meningeal hemorrhage
Rupture of cerebral arteriovenous malformation
I60.9 **Nontraumatic subarachnoid hemorrhage, unspecified** MCC

I61 **Nontraumatic intracerebral hemorrhage**
EXCLUDES2 *sequelae of intracerebral hemorrhage (I69.1-)*
I61.0 **Nontraumatic intracerebral hemorrhage in hemisphere, subcortical** MCC
Deep intracerebral hemorrhage (nontraumatic)
I61.1 **Nontraumatic intracerebral hemorrhage in hemisphere, cortical** MCC
Cerebral lobe hemorrhage (nontraumatic)
Superficial intracerebral hemorrhage (nontraumatic)
I61.2 **Nontraumatic intracerebral hemorrhage in hemisphere, unspecified** MCC
I61.3 **Nontraumatic intracerebral hemorrhage in brain stem** MCC
I61.4 **Nontraumatic intracerebral hemorrhage in cerebellum** MCC
I61.5 **Nontraumatic intracerebral hemorrhage, intraventricular** MCC
I61.6 **Nontraumatic intracerebral hemorrhage, multiple localized** MCC
I61.8 **Other nontraumatic intracerebral hemorrhage** MCC
I61.9 **Nontraumatic intracerebral hemorrhage, unspecified** MCC

I62 **Other and unspecified nontraumatic intracranial hemorrhage**
EXCLUDES2 *sequelae of intracranial hemorrhage (I69.2)*
I62.0 **Nontraumatic subdural hemorrhage**
I62.00 **Nontraumatic subdural hemorrhage, unspecified** MCC
I62.01 **Nontraumatic acute subdural hemorrhage** MCC
I62.02 **Nontraumatic subacute subdural hemorrhage** MCC
I62.03 **Nontraumatic chronic subdural hemorrhage** MCC
I62.1 **Nontraumatic extradural hemorrhage** MCC
Nontraumatic epidural hemorrhage
I62.9 **Nontraumatic intracranial hemorrhage, unspecified** CC

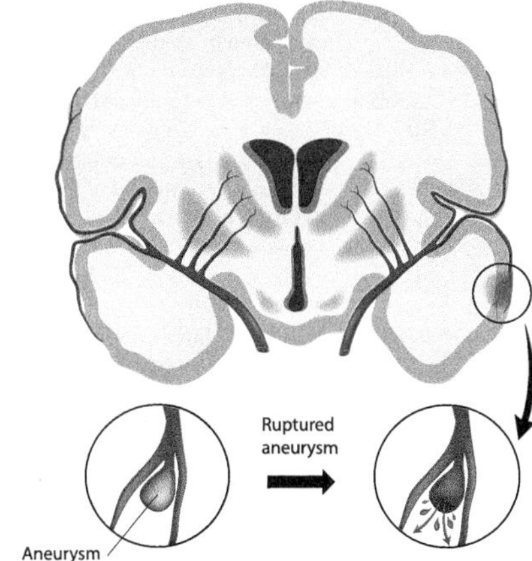

Figure 9.3 Hemorrhagic stroke

I63 **Cerebral infarction**
INCLUDES *occlusion and stenosis of cerebral and precerebral arteries, resulting in cerebral infarction*
Use additional code, if applicable, to identify status post administration of tPA (rtPA) in a different facility within the last 24 hours prior to admission to current facility (Z92.82)
Use additional code, if known, to indicate National Institutes of Health Stroke Scale (NIHSS) score (R29.7-)
EXCLUDES2 *sequelae of cerebral infarction (I69.3-)*
I63.0 **Cerebral infarction due to thrombosis of precerebral arteries**
I63.00 **Cerebral infarction due to thrombosis of unspecified precerebral artery** MCC
I63.01 **Cerebral infarction due to thrombosis of vertebral artery**
I63.011 **Cerebral infarction due to thrombosis of right vertebral artery** MCC
I63.012 **Cerebral infarction due to thrombosis of left vertebral artery** MCC
● I63.013 **Cerebral infarction due to thrombosis of bilateral vertebral arteries** CC/MCC Exc MCC
I63.019 **Cerebral infarction due to thrombosis of unspecified vertebral artery** MCC
I63.02 **Cerebral infarction due to thrombosis of basilar artery** MCC
I63.03 **Cerebral infarction due to thrombosis of carotid artery**
I63.031 **Cerebral infarction due to thrombosis of right carotid artery** MCC
I63.032 **Cerebral infarction due to thrombosis of left carotid artery** MCC
● I63.033 **Cerebral infarction due to thrombosis of bilateral carotid arteries** CC/MCC Exc MCC
I63.039 **Cerebral infarction due to thrombosis of unspecified carotid artery** MCC
I63.09 **Cerebral infarction due to thrombosis of other precerebral artery** MCC
I63.1 **Cerebral infarction due to embolism of precerebral arteries**
I63.10 **Cerebral infarction due to embolism of unspecified precerebral artery** MCC
I63.11 **Cerebral infarction due to embolism of vertebral artery**
I63.111 **Cerebral infarction due to embolism of right vertebral artery** MCC
I63.112 **Cerebral infarction due to embolism of left vertebral artery** MCC
● I63.113 **Cerebral infarction due to embolism of bilateral vertebral arteries** CC/MCC Exc MCC
I63.119 **Cerebral infarction due to embolism of unspecified vertebral artery** MCC
I63.12 **Cerebral infarction due to embolism of basilar artery** MCC
I63.13 **Cerebral infarction due to embolism of carotid artery**
I63.131 **Cerebral infarction due to embolism of right carotid artery** MCC
I63.132 **Cerebral infarction due to embolism of left carotid artery** MCC
● I63.133 **Cerebral infarction due to embolism of bilateral carotid arteries** CC/MCC Exc MCC
I63.139 **Cerebral infarction due to embolism of unspecified carotid artery** MCC
I63.19 **Cerebral infarction due to embolism of other precerebral artery** MCC
I63.2 **Cerebral infarction due to unspecified occlusion or stenosis of precerebral arteries**
I63.20 **Cerebral infarction due to unspecified occlusion or stenosis of unspecified precerebral arteries** MCC
I63.21 **Cerebral infarction due to unspecified occlusion or stenosis of vertebral arteries**
I63.211 **Cerebral infarction due to unspecified occlusion or stenosis of right vertebral arteries** MCC
I63.212 **Cerebral infarction due to unspecified occlusion or stenosis of left vertebral arteries** MCC
● I63.213 **Cerebral infarction due to unspecified occlusion or stenosis of bilateral vertebral arteries** CC/MCC Exc MCC
I63.219 **Cerebral infarction due to unspecified occlusion or stenosis of unspecified vertebral arteries** MCC
I63.22 **Cerebral infarction due to unspecified occlusion or stenosis of basilar arteries** MCC
I63.23 **Cerebral infarction due to unspecified occlusion or stenosis of carotid arteries**

Unspecified Code | Other Specified Code | Manifestation Code | N Newborn | P Pediatric | M Maternity | A Adult | ♂ Male | ♀ Female
● New Code | ▲ Revised Code Title | ►◄ Revised Text | NOTES | INCLUDES | EXCLUDES1 Not coded here | EXCLUDES2 Not included here
4th character required | 5th character required | 6th character required | 7th character required
Extension 'X' Alert | HAC Hospital-acquired condition (HAC) alert | AHA AHA Coding Clinic®

I63.231 Cerebral infarction due to unspecified occlusion or stenosis of right carotid arteries MCC

I63.232 Cerebral infarction due to unspecified occlusion or stenosis of left carotid arteries MCC

● I63.233 Cerebral infarction due to unspecified occlusion or stenosis of bilateral carotid arteries CC/MCC Exc MCC

I63.239 Cerebral infarction due to unspecified occlusion or stenosis of unspecified carotid arteries MCC

I63.29 Cerebral infarction due to unspecified occlusion or stenosis of other precerebral arteries MCC

5th I63.3 Cerebral infarction due to thrombosis of cerebral arteries

I63.30 Cerebral infarction due to thrombosis of unspecified cerebral artery MCC

6th I63.31 Cerebral infarction due to thrombosis of middle cerebral artery

I63.311 Cerebral infarction due to thrombosis of right middle cerebral artery MCC

I63.312 Cerebral infarction due to thrombosis of left middle cerebral artery MCC

● I63.313 Cerebral infarction due to thrombosis of bilateral middle cerebral arteries CC/MCC Exc MCC

I63.319 Cerebral infarction due to thrombosis of unspecified middle cerebral artery MCC

6th I63.32 Cerebral infarction due to thrombosis of anterior cerebral artery

I63.321 Cerebral infarction due to thrombosis of right anterior cerebral artery MCC

I63.322 Cerebral infarction due to thrombosis of left anterior cerebral artery MCC

● I63.323 Cerebral infarction due to thrombosis of bilateral anterior arteries CC/MCC Exc MCC

I63.329 Cerebral infarction due to thrombosis of unspecified anterior cerebral artery MCC

6th I63.33 Cerebral infarction due to thrombosis of posterior cerebral artery

I63.331 Cerebral infarction due to thrombosis of right posterior cerebral artery MCC

I63.332 Cerebral infarction due to thrombosis of left posterior cerebral artery MCC

● I63.333 Cerebral infarction to thrombosis of bilateral posterior arteries CC/MCC Exc MCC

I63.339 Cerebral infarction due to thrombosis of unspecified posterior cerebral artery MCC

6th I63.34 Cerebral infarction due to thrombosis of cerebellar artery

I63.341 Cerebral infarction due to thrombosis of right cerebellar artery MCC

I63.342 Cerebral infarction due to thrombosis of left cerebellar artery MCC

● I63.343 Cerebral infarction to thrombosis of bilateral cerebellar arteries CC/MCC Exc MCC

I63.349 Cerebral infarction due to thrombosis of unspecified cerebellar artery MCC

I63.39 Cerebral infarction due to thrombosis of other cerebral artery MCC

5th I63.4 Cerebral infarction due to embolism of cerebral arteries

I63.40 Cerebral infarction due to embolism of unspecified cerebral artery MCC

6th I63.41 Cerebral infarction due to embolism of middle cerebral artery

I63.411 Cerebral infarction due to embolism of right middle cerebral artery MCC

I63.412 Cerebral infarction due to embolism of left middle cerebral artery MCC

● I63.413 Cerebral infarction due to embolism of bilateral middle cerebral arteries CC/MCC Exc MCC

I63.419 Cerebral infarction due to embolism of unspecified middle cerebral artery MCC

6th I63.42 Cerebral infarction due to embolism of anterior cerebral artery

I63.421 Cerebral infarction due to embolism of right anterior cerebral artery MCC

I63.422 Cerebral infarction due to embolism of left anterior cerebral artery MCC

● I63.423 Cerebral infarction due to embolism of bilateral anterior cerebral arteries CC/MCC Exc MCC

I63.429 Cerebral infarction due to embolism of unspecified anterior cerebral artery MCC

6th I63.43 Cerebral infarction due to embolism of posterior cerebral artery

I63.431 Cerebral infarction due to embolism of right posterior cerebral artery MCC

I63.432 Cerebral infarction due to embolism of left posterior cerebral artery MCC

● I63.433 Cerebral infarction due to embolism of bilateral posterior cerebral arteries CC/MCC Exc MCC

I63.439 Cerebral infarction due to embolism of unspecified posterior cerebral artery MCC

6th I63.44 Cerebral infarction due to embolism of cerebellar artery

I63.441 Cerebral infarction due to embolism of right cerebellar artery MCC

I63.442 Cerebral infarction due to embolism of left cerebellar artery MCC

● I63.443 Cerebral infarction due to embolism of bilateral cerebellar arteries CC/MCC Exc MCC

I63.449 Cerebral infarction due to embolism of unspecified cerebellar artery MCC

I63.49 Cerebral infarction due to embolism of other cerebral artery MCC

5th I63.5 Cerebral infarction due to unspecified occlusion or stenosis of cerebral arteries

I63.50 Cerebral infarction due to unspecified occlusion or stenosis of unspecified cerebral artery MCC

6th I63.51 Cerebral infarction due to unspecified occlusion or stenosis of middle cerebral artery

I63.511 Cerebral infarction due to unspecified occlusion or stenosis of right middle cerebral artery MCC

I63.512 Cerebral infarction due to unspecified occlusion or stenosis of left middle cerebral artery MCC

● I63.513 Cerebral infarction due to unspecified occlusion or stenosis of bilateral middle arteries CC/MCC Exc MCC

I63.519 Cerebral infarction due to unspecified occlusion or stenosis of unspecified middle cerebral artery MCC

6th I63.52 Cerebral infarction due to unspecified occlusion or stenosis of anterior cerebral artery

I63.521 Cerebral infarction due to unspecified occlusion or stenosis of right anterior cerebral artery MCC

I63.522 Cerebral infarction due to unspecified occlusion or stenosis of left anterior cerebral artery MCC

● I63.523 Cerebral infarction due to unspecified occlusion or stenosis of bilateral anterior arteries CC/MCC Exc MCC

I63.529 Cerebral infarction due to unspecified occlusion or stenosis of unspecified anterior cerebral artery MCC

6th I63.53 Cerebral infarction due to unspecified occlusion or stenosis of posterior cerebral artery

I63.531 Cerebral infarction due to unspecified occlusion or stenosis of right posterior cerebral artery MCC

I63.532 Cerebral infarction due to unspecified occlusion or stenosis of left posterior cerebral artery MCC

● I63.533 Cerebral infarction due to unspecified occlusion or stenosis of bilateral posterior arteries CC/MCC Exc MCC

I63.539 Cerebral infarction due to unspecified occlusion or stenosis of unspecified posterior cerebral artery MCC

PDx Unacceptable principal diagnosis symbol per Medicare code edits; POA Code exempt from diagnosis present on admission requirement
Q Questionable admission; CC Complication or comorbidity; CC/MCC Exc CC/MCC exclusion; MCC Major complication or comorbidity
PDx CC Principal diagnosis as its own CC; PDx MCC Principal diagnosis as its own MCC; Z1 Z code as first-listed diagnosis

When symbols appear on a code that requires a 7th character extension, refer to Appendix D to identify applicable 7th character codes.

I63.54 Cerebral infarction due to unspecified occlusion or stenosis of cerebellar artery
- I63.541 Cerebral infarction due to unspecified occlusion or stenosis of right cerebellar artery MCC
- I63.542 Cerebral infarction due to unspecified occlusion or stenosis of left cerebellar artery MCC
- ● I63.543 Cerebral infarction due to unspecified occlusion or stenosis of bilateral cerebellar arteries CC/MCC Exc MCC
- I63.549 Cerebral infarction due to unspecified occlusion or stenosis of unspecified cerebellar artery MCC

I63.59 Cerebral infarction due to unspecified occlusion or stenosis of other cerebral artery MCC

I63.6 Cerebral infarction due to cerebral venous thrombosis, nonpyogenic MCC

I63.8 Other cerebral infarction MCC

I63.9 Cerebral infarction, unspecified MCC
Stroke NOS

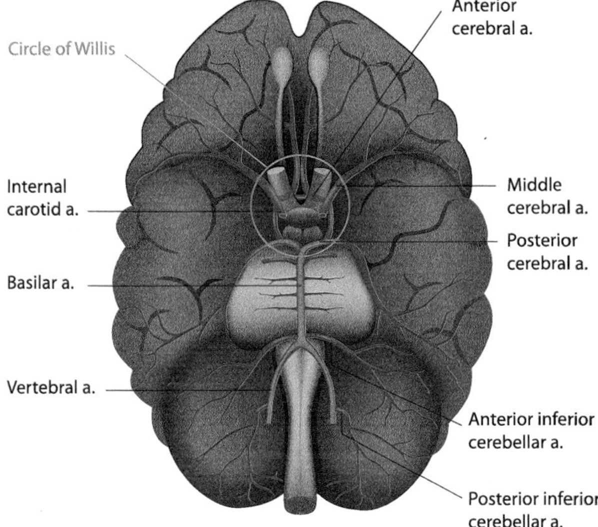

Figure 9.4 Blood supply of the brain

I65 Occlusion and stenosis of precerebral arteries, not resulting in cerebral infarction

INCLUDES *embolism of precerebral artery*
narrowing of precerebral artery
obstruction (complete) (partial) of precerebral artery
thrombosis of precerebral artery

EXCLUDES1 *insufficiency, NOS, of precerebral artery (G45.-)*
insufficiency of precerebral arteries causing cerebral infarction (I63.0-I63.2)

I65.0 Occlusion and stenosis of vertebral artery
- I65.01 Occlusion and stenosis of right vertebral artery
- I65.02 Occlusion and stenosis of left vertebral artery
- I65.03 Occlusion and stenosis of bilateral vertebral arteries
- I65.09 Occlusion and stenosis of unspecified vertebral artery

I65.1 Occlusion and stenosis of basilar artery

I65.2 Occlusion and stenosis of carotid artery
- I65.21 Occlusion and stenosis of right carotid artery
- I65.22 Occlusion and stenosis of left carotid artery
- I65.23 Occlusion and stenosis of bilateral carotid arteries
- I65.29 Occlusion and stenosis of unspecified carotid artery

I65.8 Occlusion and stenosis of other precerebral arteries

I65.9 Occlusion and stenosis of unspecified precerebral artery
Occlusion and stenosis of precerebral artery NOS

I66 Occlusion and stenosis of cerebral arteries, not resulting in cerebral infarction

INCLUDES *embolism of cerebral artery*
narrowing of cerebral artery
obstruction (complete) (partial) of cerebral artery
thrombosis of cerebral artery

EXCLUDES1 *Occlusion and stenosis of cerebral artery causing cerebral infarction (I63.3-I63.5)*

I66.0 Occlusion and stenosis of middle cerebral artery
- I66.01 Occlusion and stenosis of right middle cerebral artery
- I66.02 Occlusion and stenosis of left middle cerebral artery
- I66.03 Occlusion and stenosis of bilateral middle cerebral arteries
- I66.09 Occlusion and stenosis of unspecified middle cerebral artery

I66.1 Occlusion and stenosis of anterior cerebral artery
- I66.11 Occlusion and stenosis of right anterior cerebral artery
- I66.12 Occlusion and stenosis of left anterior cerebral artery
- I66.13 Occlusion and stenosis of bilateral anterior cerebral arteries
- I66.19 Occlusion and stenosis of unspecified anterior cerebral artery

I66.2 Occlusion and stenosis of posterior cerebral artery
- I66.21 Occlusion and stenosis of right posterior cerebral artery
- I66.22 Occlusion and stenosis of left posterior cerebral artery
- I66.23 Occlusion and stenosis of bilateral posterior cerebral arteries
- I66.29 Occlusion and stenosis of unspecified posterior cerebral artery

I66.3 Occlusion and stenosis of cerebellar arteries

I66.8 Occlusion and stenosis of other cerebral arteries
Occlusion and stenosis of perforating arteries

I66.9 Occlusion and stenosis of unspecified cerebral artery

I67 Other cerebrovascular diseases

EXCLUDES2 *sequelae of the listed conditions (I69.8)*

I67.0 Dissection of cerebral arteries, nonruptured MCC
EXCLUDES1 *ruptured cerebral arteries (I60.7)*

I67.1 Cerebral aneurysm, nonruptured
Cerebral aneurysm NOS
Cerebral arteriovenous fistula, acquired
Internal carotid artery aneurysm, intracranial portion
Internal carotid artery aneurysm, NOS
EXCLUDES1 *congenital cerebral aneurysm, nonruptured (Q28.-)*
ruptured cerebral aneurysm (I60.7)

I67.2 Cerebral atherosclerosis A
Atheroma of cerebral and precerebral arteries

I67.3 Progressive vascular leukoencephalopathy CC
Binswanger's disease

I67.4 Hypertensive encephalopathy CC

I67.5 Moyamoya disease CC

I67.6 Nonpyogenic thrombosis of intracranial venous system CC
Nonpyogenic thrombosis of cerebral vein
Nonpyogenic thrombosis of intracranial venous sinus
EXCLUDES1 *nonpyogenic thrombosis of intracranial venous system causing infarction (I63.6)*

I67.7 Cerebral arteritis, not elsewhere classified CC
Granulomatous angiitis of the nervous system
EXCLUDES1 *allergic granulomatous angiitis (M30.1)*

I67.8 Other specified cerebrovascular diseases
- I67.81 Acute cerebrovascular insufficiency CC
  Acute cerebrovascular insufficiency unspecified as to location or reversibility
- I67.82 Cerebral ischemia CC
  Chronic cerebral ischemia
- I67.83 Posterior reversible encephalopathy syndrome MCC
  PRES

Unspecified Code | Other Specified Code | Manifestation Code | N Newborn | P Pediatric | M Maternity | A Adult | ♂ Male | ♀ Female
● New Code | ▲ Revised Code Title | ►◄ Revised Text | NOTES | INCLUDES | EXCLUDES1 Not coded here | EXCLUDES2 Not included here
4th character required | 5th character required | 6th character required | 7th character required
Extension 'X' Alert | HAC Hospital-acquired condition (HAC) alert | AHA AHA Coding Clinic©

I67.84 Cerebral vasospasm and vasoconstriction

I67.841 Reversible cerebrovascular vasoconstriction syndrome

Call-Fleming syndrome

Code first underlying condition, if applicable, such as eclampsia (O15.00-O15.9)

I67.848 Other cerebrovascular vasospasm and vasoconstriction

I67.89 Other cerebrovascular disease

I67.9 Cerebrovascular disease, unspecified

I68 Cerebrovascular disorders in diseases classified elsewhere

I68.0 Cerebral amyloid angiopathy

Code first underlying amyloidosis (E85.-)

I68.2 Cerebral arteritis in other diseases classified elsewhere

Code first underlying disease

EXCLUDES1 *cerebral arteritis (in):*

listerosis (A32.89)

systemic lupus erythematosus (M32.19)

syphilis (A52.04)

tuberculosis (A18.89)

I68.8 Other cerebrovascular disorders in diseases classified elsewhere

Code first underlying disease

EXCLUDES1 *syphilitic cerebral aneurysm (A52.05)*

I69 Sequelae of cerebrovascular disease

NOTES Category I69 is to be used to indicate conditions in I60-I67 as the cause of sequelae. The 'sequelae' include conditions specified as such or as residuals which may occur at any time after the onset of the causal condition

EXCLUDES1 *personal history of cerebral infarction without residual deficit (Z86.73)*

personal history of prolonged reversible ischemic neurologic deficit (PRIND) (Z86.73)

personal history of reversible ischemic neurological deficit (RIND) (Z86.73)

sequelae of traumatic intracranial injury (S06.-)

transient ischemic attack (TIA) (G45.9)

AHA: Q4, 2013

I69.0 Sequelae of nontraumatic subarachnoid hemorrhage

I69.00 Unspecified sequelae of nontraumatic subarachnoid hemorrhage

I69.01 Cognitive deficits following nontraumatic subarachnoid hemorrhage

- I69.010 Attention and concentration deficit following nontraumatic subarachnoid hemorrhage
- I69.011 Memory deficit following nontraumatic subarachnoid hemorrhage
- I69.012 Visuospatial deficit and spatial neglect following nontraumatic subarachnoid hemorrhage
- I69.013 Psychomotor deficit following nontraumatic subarachnoid hemorrhage
- I69.014 Frontal lobe and executive function deficit following nontraumatic subarachnoid hemorrhage
- I69.015 Cognitive social or emotional deficit following nontraumatic subarachnoid hemorrhage
- I69.018 Other symptoms and signs involving cognitive functions following nontraumatic subarachnoid hemorrhage
- I69.019 Unspecified symptoms and signs involving cognitive functions following nontraumatic subarachnoid hemorrhage

I69.02 Speech and language deficits following nontraumatic subarachnoid hemorrhage

I69.020 Aphasia following nontraumatic subarachnoid hemorrhage

I69.021 Dysphasia following nontraumatic subarachnoid hemorrhage

I69.022 Dysarthria following nontraumatic subarachnoid hemorrhage

I69.023 Fluency disorder following nontraumatic subarachnoid hemorrhage

Stuttering following nontraumatic subarachnoid hemorrhage

I69.028 Other speech and language deficits following nontraumatic subarachnoid hemorrhage

I69.03 Monoplegia of upper limb following nontraumatic subarachnoid hemorrhage

AHA: Q4, 2012

I69.031 Monoplegia of upper limb following nontraumatic subarachnoid hemorrhage affecting right dominant side

I69.032 Monoplegia of upper limb following nontraumatic subarachnoid hemorrhage affecting left dominant side

I69.033 Monoplegia of upper limb following nontraumatic subarachnoid hemorrhage affecting right non-dominant side

I69.034 Monoplegia of upper limb following nontraumatic subarachnoid hemorrhage affecting left non-dominant side

I69.039 Monoplegia of upper limb following nontraumatic subarachnoid hemorrhage affecting unspecified side

I69.04 Monoplegia of lower limb following nontraumatic subarachnoid hemorrhage

AHA: Q4, 2012

I69.041 Monoplegia of lower limb following nontraumatic subarachnoid hemorrhage affecting right dominant side

I69.042 Monoplegia of lower limb following nontraumatic subarachnoid hemorrhage affecting left dominant side

I69.043 Monoplegia of lower limb following nontraumatic subarachnoid hemorrhage affecting right non-dominant side

I69.044 Monoplegia of lower limb following nontraumatic subarachnoid hemorrhage affecting left non-dominant side

I69.049 Monoplegia of lower limb following nontraumatic subarachnoid hemorrhage affecting unspecified side

I69.05 Hemiplegia and hemiparesis following nontraumatic subarachnoid hemorrhage

I69.051 Hemiplegia and hemiparesis following nontraumatic subarachnoid hemorrhage affecting right dominant side

I69.052 Hemiplegia and hemiparesis following nontraumatic subarachnoid hemorrhage affecting left dominant side

I69.053 Hemiplegia and hemiparesis following nontraumatic subarachnoid hemorrhage affecting right non-dominant side

I69.054 Hemiplegia and hemiparesis following nontraumatic subarachnoid hemorrhage affecting left non-dominant side

I69.059 Hemiplegia and hemiparesis following nontraumatic subarachnoid hemorrhage affecting unspecified side

I69.06 Other paralytic syndrome following nontraumatic subarachnoid hemorrhage

Use additional code to identify type of paralytic syndrome, such as:

locked-in state (G83.5)

quadriplegia (G82.5-)

EXCLUDES1 *hemiplegia/hemiparesis following nontraumatic subarachnoid hemorrhage (I69.05-)*

monoplegia of lower limb following nontraumatic subarachnoid hemorrhage (I69.04-)

monoplegia of upper limb following nontraumatic subarachnoid hemorrhage (I69.03-)

PDx Unacceptable principal diagnosis symbol per Medicare code edits · POA Code exempt from diagnosis present on admission requirement · Q Questionable admission · CC Complication or comorbidity · CC/MCC Excl CC/MCC exclusion · MCC Major complication or comorbidity · PDx CC Principal diagnosis as its own CC · PDx MCC Principal diagnosis as its own MCC · Z Z code as first-listed diagnosis

When symbols appear on a code that requires a 7th character extension, refer to Appendix D to identify applicable 7th character codes.

I69.061 Other paralytic syndrome following nontraumatic subarachnoid hemorrhage affecting right dominant side POA

I69.062 Other paralytic syndrome following nontraumatic subarachnoid hemorrhage affecting left dominant side POA

I69.063 Other paralytic syndrome following nontraumatic subarachnoid hemorrhage affecting right non-dominant side POA

I69.064 Other paralytic syndrome following nontraumatic subarachnoid hemorrhage affecting left non-dominant side POA

I69.065 Other paralytic syndrome following nontraumatic subarachnoid hemorrhage, bilateral POA

I69.069 Other paralytic syndrome following nontraumatic subarachnoid hemorrhage affecting unspecified side POA

(6th) I69.09 Other sequelae of nontraumatic subarachnoid hemorrhage

I69.090 Apraxia following nontraumatic subarachnoid hemorrhage POA

I69.091 Dysphagia following nontraumatic subarachnoid hemorrhage POA

Use additional code to identify the type of dysphagia, if known (R13.1-)

I69.092 Facial weakness following nontraumatic subarachnoid hemorrhage POA

Facial droop following nontraumatic subarachnoid hemorrhage

I69.093 Ataxia following nontraumatic subarachnoid hemorrhage POA

I69.098 Other sequelae following nontraumatic subarachnoid hemorrhage POA

Alterations of sensation following nontraumatic subarachnoid hemorrhage

Disturbance of vision following nontraumatic subarachnoid hemorrhage

Use additional code to identify the sequelae

(5th) I69.1 Sequelae of nontraumatic intracerebral hemorrhage

I69.10 Unspecified sequelae of nontraumatic intracerebral hemorrhage POA

(6th) I69.11 Cognitive deficits following nontraumatic intracerebral hemorrhage

● I69.110 Attention and concentration deficit following nontraumatic intracerebral hemorrhage

● I69.111 Memory deficit following nontraumatic intracerebral hemorrhage

● I69.112 Visuospatial deficit and spatial neglect following nontraumatic intracerebral hemorrhage

● I69.113 Psychomotor deficit following nontraumatic intracerebral hemorrhage

● I69.114 Frontal lobe and executive function deficit following nontraumatic intracerebral hemorrhage

● I69.115 Cognitive social or emotional deficit following nontraumatic intracerebral hemorrhage

● I69.118 Other symptoms and signs involving cognitive functions following nontraumatic intracerebral hemorrhage

● I69.119 Unspecified symptoms and signs involving cognitive functions following nontraumatic intracerebral hemorrhage

(6th) I69.12 Speech and language deficits following nontraumatic intracerebral hemorrhage

I69.120 Aphasia following nontraumatic intracerebral hemorrhage POA

I69.121 Dysphasia following nontraumatic intracerebral hemorrhage POA

I69.122 Dysarthria following nontraumatic intracerebral hemorrhage POA

I69.123 Fluency disorder following nontraumatic intracerebral hemorrhage POA

Stuttering following nontraumatic ▶intracerebral◀ hemorrhage

I69.128 Other speech and language deficits following nontraumatic intracerebral hemorrhage POA

(6th) I69.13 Monoplegia of upper limb following nontraumatic intracerebral hemorrhage

AHA: Q4, 2012

I69.131 Monoplegia of upper limb following nontraumatic intracerebral hemorrhage affecting right dominant side POA

I69.132 Monoplegia of upper limb following nontraumatic intracerebral hemorrhage affecting left dominant side POA

I69.133 Monoplegia of upper limb following nontraumatic intracerebral hemorrhage affecting right non-dominant side POA

I69.134 Monoplegia of upper limb following nontraumatic intracerebral hemorrhage affecting left non-dominant side POA

I69.139 Monoplegia of upper limb following nontraumatic intracerebral hemorrhage affecting unspecified side POA

(6th) I69.14 Monoplegia of lower limb following nontraumatic intracerebral hemorrhage

AHA: Q4, 2012

I69.141 Monoplegia of lower limb following nontraumatic intracerebral hemorrhage affecting right dominant side POA

I69.142 Monoplegia of lower limb following nontraumatic intracerebral hemorrhage affecting left dominant side POA

I69.143 Monoplegia of lower limb following nontraumatic intracerebral hemorrhage affecting right non-dominant side POA

I69.144 Monoplegia of lower limb following nontraumatic intracerebral hemorrhage affecting left non-dominant side POA

I69.149 Monoplegia of lower limb following nontraumatic intracerebral hemorrhage affecting unspecified side POA

(6th) I69.15 Hemiplegia and hemiparesis following nontraumatic intracerebral hemorrhage

I69.151 Hemiplegia and hemiparesis following nontraumatic intracerebral hemorrhage affecting right dominant side CC POA

I69.152 Hemiplegia and hemiparesis following nontraumatic intracerebral hemorrhage affecting left dominant side CC POA

I69.153 Hemiplegia and hemiparesis following nontraumatic intracerebral hemorrhage affecting right non-dominant side CC POA

I69.154 Hemiplegia and hemiparesis following nontraumatic intracerebral hemorrhage affecting left non-dominant side CC POA

I69.159 Hemiplegia and hemiparesis following nontraumatic intracerebral hemorrhage affecting unspecified side CC POA

(6th) I69.16 Other paralytic syndrome following nontraumatic intracerebral hemorrhage

Use additional code to identify type of paralytic syndrome, such as:

locked-in state (G83.5)

quadriplegia (G82.5-)

EXCLUDES1 *hemiplegia/hemiparesis following nontraumatic intracerebral hemorrhage (I69.15-)*

monoplegia of lower limb following nontraumatic intracerebral hemorrhage (I69.14-)

monoplegia of upper limb following nontraumatic intracerebral hemorrhage (I69.13-)

I69.161 Other paralytic syndrome following nontraumatic intracerebral hemorrhage affecting right dominant side POA

Unspecified Code | Other Specified Code | Manifestation Code | N Newborn | P Pediatric | M Maternity | A Adult | ♂ Male | ♀ Female
● New Code | ▲ Revised Code Title | ▶◀ Revised Text | NOTES | INCLUDES | EXCLUDES1 Not coded here | EXCLUDES2 Not included here
(4th) 4th character required | (5th) 5th character required | (6th) 6th character required | (7th) 7th character required
(X) Extension 'X' Alert | HAC Hospital-acquired condition (HAC) alert | AHA AHA Coding Clinic©

I69.162 Other paralytic syndrome following nontraumatic intracerebral hemorrhage affecting left dominant side

I69.163 Other paralytic syndrome following nontraumatic intracerebral hemorrhage affecting right non-dominant side

I69.164 Other paralytic syndrome following nontraumatic intracerebral hemorrhage affecting left non-dominant side

I69.165 Other paralytic syndrome following nontraumatic intracerebral hemorrhage, bilateral

I69.169 Other paralytic syndrome following nontraumatic intracerebral hemorrhage affecting unspecified side

I69.19 Other sequelae of nontraumatic intracerebral hemorrhage

I69.190 Apraxia following nontraumatic intracerebral hemorrhage

I69.191 Dysphagia following nontraumatic intracerebral hemorrhage
Use additional code to identify the type of dysphagia, if known (R13.1-)

I69.192 Facial weakness following nontraumatic intracerebral hemorrhage
Facial droop following nontraumatic intracerebral hemorrhage

I69.193 Ataxia following nontraumatic intracerebral hemorrhage

I69.198 Other sequelae of nontraumatic intracerebral hemorrhage
Alteration of sensations following nontraumatic intracerebral hemorrhage
Disturbance of vision following nontraumatic intracerebral hemorrhage
Use additional code to identify the sequelae

I69.2 Sequelae of other nontraumatic intracranial hemorrhage

I69.20 Unspecified sequelae of other nontraumatic intracranial hemorrhage

I69.21 Cognitive deficits following other nontraumatic intracranial hemorrhage

- I69.210 Attention and concentration deficit following other nontraumatic intracranial hemorrhage
- I69.211 Memory deficit following other nontraumatic intracranial hemorrhage
- I69.212 Visuospatial deficit and spatial neglect following other nontraumatic intracranial hemorrhage
- I69.213 Psychomotor deficit following other nontraumatic intracranial hemorrhage
- I69.214 Frontal lobe and executive function deficit following other nontraumatic intracranial hemorrhage
- I69.215 Cognitive social or emotional deficit following other nontraumatic intracranial hemorrhage
- I69.218 Other symptoms and signs involving cognitive functions following other nontraumatic intracranial hemorrhage
- I69.219 Unspecified symptoms and signs involving cognitive functions following other nontraumatic intracranial hemorrhage

I69.22 Speech and language deficits following other nontraumatic intracranial hemorrhage

I69.220 Aphasia following other nontraumatic intracranial hemorrhage

I69.221 Dysphasia following other nontraumatic intracranial hemorrhage

I69.222 Dysarthria following other nontraumatic intracranial hemorrhage

I69.223 Fluency disorder following other nontraumatic intracranial hemorrhage
Stuttering following ▶other nontraumatic intracranial◀ hemorrhage

I69.228 Other speech and language deficits following other nontraumatic intracranial hemorrhage

I69.23 Monoplegia of upper limb following other nontraumatic intracranial hemorrhage

I69.231 Monoplegia of upper limb following other nontraumatic intracranial hemorrhage affecting right dominant side

I69.232 Monoplegia of upper limb following other nontraumatic intracranial hemorrhage affecting left dominant side

I69.233 Monoplegia of upper limb following other nontraumatic intracranial hemorrhage affecting right non-dominant side

I69.234 Monoplegia of upper limb following other nontraumatic intracranial hemorrhage affecting left non-dominant side

I69.239 Monoplegia of upper limb following other nontraumatic intracranial hemorrhage affecting unspecified side

I69.24 Monoplegia of lower limb following other nontraumatic intracranial hemorrhage

I69.241 Monoplegia of lower limb following other nontraumatic intracranial hemorrhage affecting right dominant side

I69.242 Monoplegia of lower limb following other nontraumatic intracranial hemorrhage affecting left dominant side

I69.243 Monoplegia of lower limb following other nontraumatic intracranial hemorrhage affecting right non-dominant side

I69.244 Monoplegia of lower limb following other nontraumatic intracranial hemorrhage affecting left non-dominant side

I69.249 Monoplegia of lower limb following other nontraumatic intracranial hemorrhage affecting unspecified side

I69.25 Hemiplegia and hemiparesis following other nontraumatic intracranial hemorrhage

I69.251 Hemiplegia and hemiparesis following other nontraumatic intracranial hemorrhage affecting right dominant side CC

I69.252 Hemiplegia and hemiparesis following other nontraumatic intracranial hemorrhage affecting left dominant side CC

I69.253 Hemiplegia and hemiparesis following other nontraumatic intracranial hemorrhage affecting right non-dominant side CC

I69.254 Hemiplegia and hemiparesis following other nontraumatic intracranial hemorrhage affecting left non-dominant side CC

I69.259 Hemiplegia and hemiparesis following other nontraumatic intracranial hemorrhage affecting unspecified side CC

I69.26 Other paralytic syndrome following other nontraumatic intracranial hemorrhage
Use additional code to identify type of paralytic syndrome, such as:
locked-in state (G83.5)
quadriplegia (G82.5-)

EXCLUDES1 *hemiplegia/hemiparesis following other nontraumatic intracranial hemorrhage (I69.25-)*
monoplegia of lower limb following other nontraumatic intracranial hemorrhage (I69.24-)
monoplegia of upper limb following other nontraumatic intracranial hemorrhage (I69.23-)

I69.261 Other paralytic syndrome following other nontraumatic intracranial hemorrhage affecting right dominant side

Unacceptable principal diagnosis symbol per Medicare code edits · Code exempt from diagnosis present on admission requirement · Questionable admission · CC Complication or comorbidity · CC/MCC exclusion · MCC Major complication or comorbidity · Principal diagnosis as its own CC · Principal diagnosis as its own MCC · Z code as first-listed diagnosis

I69.262 Other paralytic syndrome following other nontraumatic intracranial hemorrhage affecting left dominant side POA
I69.263 Other paralytic syndrome following other nontraumatic intracranial hemorrhage affecting right non-dominant side POA
I69.264 Other paralytic syndrome following other nontraumatic intracranial hemorrhage affecting left non-dominant side POA
I69.265 Other paralytic syndrome following other nontraumatic intracranial hemorrhage, bilateral POA
I69.269 Other paralytic syndrome following other nontraumatic intracranial hemorrhage affecting unspecified side POA

I69.29 Other sequelae of other nontraumatic intracranial hemorrhage
I69.290 Apraxia following other nontraumatic intracranial hemorrhage POA
I69.291 Dysphagia following other nontraumatic intracranial hemorrhage POA
Use additional code to identify the type of dysphagia, if known (R13.1-)
I69.292 Facial weakness following other nontraumatic intracranial hemorrhage POA
Facial droop following other nontraumatic intracranial hemorrhage
I69.293 Ataxia following other nontraumatic intracranial hemorrhage POA
I69.298 Other sequelae of other nontraumatic intracranial hemorrhage POA
Alteration of sensation following other nontraumatic intracranial hemorrhage
Disturbance of vision following other nontraumatic intracranial hemorrhage
Use additional code to identify the sequelae

I69.3 Sequelae of cerebral infarction
Sequelae of stroke NOS
AHA: Q4, 2013

I69.30 Unspecified sequelae of cerebral infarction POA

I69.31 Cognitive deficits following cerebral infarction
● I69.310 Attention and concentration deficit following cerebral infarction
● I69.311 Memory deficit following cerebral infarction
● I69.312 Visuospatial deficit and spatial neglect following cerebral infarction
● I69.313 Psychomotor deficit following cerebral infarction
● I69.314 Frontal lobe and executive function deficit following cerebral infarction
● I69.315 Cognitive social or emotional deficit following cerebral infarction
● I69.318 Other symptoms and signs involving cognitive functions following cerebral infarction
● I69.319 Unspecified symptoms and signs involving cognitive functions following cerebral infarction

I69.32 Speech and language deficits following cerebral infarction
I69.320 Aphasia following cerebral infarction POA
AHA: Q4, 2013
I69.321 Dysphasia following cerebral infarction POA
I69.322 Dysarthria following cerebral infarction POA
I69.323 Fluency disorder following cerebral infarction POA
Stuttering following ►cerebral infarction◄
I69.328 Other speech and language deficits following cerebral infarction POA

I69.33 Monoplegia of upper limb following cerebral infarction
I69.331 Monoplegia of upper limb following cerebral infarction affecting right dominant side POA
I69.332 Monoplegia of upper limb following cerebral infarction affecting left dominant side POA
I69.333 Monoplegia of upper limb following cerebral infarction affecting right non-dominant side POA
I69.334 Monoplegia of upper limb following cerebral infarction affecting left non-dominant side POA
I69.339 Monoplegia of upper limb following cerebral infarction affecting unspecified side POA

I69.34 Monoplegia of lower limb following cerebral infarction
I69.341 Monoplegia of lower limb following cerebral infarction affecting right dominant side POA
I69.342 Monoplegia of lower limb following cerebral infarction affecting left dominant side POA
I69.343 Monoplegia of lower limb following cerebral infarction affecting right non-dominant side POA
I69.344 Monoplegia of lower limb following cerebral infarction affecting left non-dominant side POA
I69.349 Monoplegia of lower limb following cerebral infarction affecting unspecified side POA

I69.35 Hemiplegia and hemiparesis following cerebral infarction
I69.351 Hemiplegia and hemiparesis following cerebral infarction affecting right dominant side CC POA
AHA: Q4, 2013
I69.352 Hemiplegia and hemiparesis following cerebral infarction affecting left dominant side CC POA
I69.353 Hemiplegia and hemiparesis following cerebral infarction affecting right non-dominant side CC POA
I69.354 Hemiplegia and hemiparesis following cerebral infarction affecting left non-dominant side CC POA
I69.359 Hemiplegia and hemiparesis following cerebral infarction affecting unspecified side CC POA

I69.36 Other paralytic syndrome following cerebral infarction
Use additional code to identify type of paralytic syndrome, such as:
locked-in state (G83.5)
quadriplegia (G82.5-)
EXCLUDES1 *hemiplegia/hemiparesis following cerebral infarction (I69.35-)*
monoplegia of lower limb following cerebral infarction (I69.34-)
monoplegia of upper limb following cerebral infarction (I69.33-)
I69.361 Other paralytic syndrome following cerebral infarction affecting right dominant side POA
I69.362 Other paralytic syndrome following cerebral infarction affecting left dominant side POA
I69.363 Other paralytic syndrome following cerebral infarction affecting right non-dominant side POA
I69.364 Other paralytic syndrome following cerebral infarction affecting left non-dominant side POA
I69.365 Other paralytic syndrome following cerebral infarction, bilateral POA
I69.369 Other paralytic syndrome following cerebral infarction affecting unspecified side POA

I69.39 Other sequelae of cerebral infarction
I69.390 Apraxia following cerebral infarction POA

Unspecified Code | Other Specified Code | Manifestation Code | N Newborn | P Pediatric | M Maternity | A Adult | ♂ Male | ♀ Female
● New Code ▲ Revised Code Title ►◄ Revised Text NOTES INCLUDES EXCLUDES1 Not coded here EXCLUDES2 Not included here
4th character required | 5th character required | 6th character required | 7th character required
Extension 'X' Alert | HAC Hospital-acquired condition (HAC) alert | AHA AHA Coding Clinic©

I69.391 Dysphagia following cerebral infarction
Use additional code to identify the type of dysphagia, if known (R13.1-)

I69.392 Facial weakness following cerebral infarction
Facial droop following cerebral infarction

I69.393 Ataxia following cerebral infarction

I69.398 Other sequelae of cerebral infarction
Alteration of sensation following cerebral infarction
Disturbance of vision following cerebral infarction
Use additional code to identify the sequelae

I69.8 Sequelae of other cerebrovascular diseases
EXCLUDES1 *sequelae of traumatic intracranial injury (S06.-)*

I69.80 Unspecified sequelae of other cerebrovascular disease

I69.81 Cognitive deficits following other cerebrovascular disease

● I69.810 Attention and concentration deficit following other cerebrovascular disease

● I69.811 Memory deficit following other cerebrovascular disease

● I69.812 Visuospatial deficit and spatial neglect following other cerebrovascular disease

● I69.813 Psychomotor deficit following other cerebrovascular disease

● I69.814 Frontal lobe and executive function deficit following other cerebrovascular disease

● I69.815 Cognitive social or emotional deficit following other cerebrovascular disease

● I69.818 Other symptoms and signs involving cognitive functions following other cerebrovascular disease

● I69.819 Unspecified symptoms and signs involving cognitive functions following other cerebrovascular disease

I69.82 Speech and language deficits following other cerebrovascular disease

I69.820 Aphasia following other cerebrovascular disease

I69.821 Dysphasia following other cerebrovascular disease

I69.822 Dysarthria following other cerebrovascular disease

I69.823 Fluency disorder following other cerebrovascular disease
Stuttering following ▶other cerebrovascular disease◀

I69.828 Other speech and language deficits following other cerebrovascular disease

I69.83 Monoplegia of upper limb following other cerebrovascular disease

I69.831 Monoplegia of upper limb following other cerebrovascular disease affecting right dominant side

I69.832 Monoplegia of upper limb following other cerebrovascular disease affecting left dominant side

I69.833 Monoplegia of upper limb following other cerebrovascular disease affecting right non-dominant side

I69.834 Monoplegia of upper limb following other cerebrovascular disease affecting left non-dominant side

I69.839 Monoplegia of upper limb following other cerebrovascular disease affecting unspecified side

I69.84 Monoplegia of lower limb following other cerebrovascular disease

I69.841 Monoplegia of lower limb following other cerebrovascular disease affecting right dominant side

I69.842 Monoplegia of lower limb following other cerebrovascular disease affecting left dominant side

I69.843 Monoplegia of lower limb following other cerebrovascular disease affecting right non-dominant side

I69.844 Monoplegia of lower limb following other cerebrovascular disease affecting left non-dominant side

I69.849 Monoplegia of lower limb following other cerebrovascular disease affecting unspecified side

I69.85 Hemiplegia and hemiparesis following other cerebrovascular disease

I69.851 Hemiplegia and hemiparesis following other cerebrovascular disease affecting right dominant side

I69.852 Hemiplegia and hemiparesis following other cerebrovascular disease affecting left dominant side

I69.853 Hemiplegia and hemiparesis following other cerebrovascular disease affecting right non-dominant side

I69.854 Hemiplegia and hemiparesis following other cerebrovascular disease affecting left non-dominant side

I69.859 Hemiplegia and hemiparesis following other cerebrovascular disease affecting unspecified side

I69.86 Other paralytic syndrome following other cerebrovascular disease
Use additional code to identify type of paralytic syndrome, such as:
locked-in state (G83.5)
quadriplegia (G82.5-)
EXCLUDES1 *hemiplegia/hemiparesis following other cerebrovascular disease (I69.85-)*
monoplegia of lower limb following other cerebrovascular disease (I69.84-)
monoplegia of upper limb following other cerebrovascular disease (I69.83-)

I69.861 Other paralytic syndrome following other cerebrovascular disease affecting right dominant side

I69.862 Other paralytic syndrome following other cerebrovascular disease affecting left dominant side

I69.863 Other paralytic syndrome following other cerebrovascular disease affecting right non-dominant side

I69.864 Other paralytic syndrome following other cerebrovascular disease affecting left non-dominant side

I69.865 Other paralytic syndrome following other cerebrovascular disease, bilateral

I69.869 Other paralytic syndrome following other cerebrovascular disease affecting unspecified side

I69.89 Other sequelae of other cerebrovascular disease

I69.890 Apraxia following other cerebrovascular disease

I69.891 Dysphagia following other cerebrovascular disease
Use additional code to identify the type of dysphagia, if known (R13.1-)

I69.892 Facial weakness following other cerebrovascular disease
Facial droop following other cerebrovascular disease

I69.893 Ataxia following other cerebrovascular disease

I69.898 Other sequelae of other cerebrovascular disease
Alteration of sensation following other cerebrovascular disease
Disturbance of vision following other cerebrovascular disease
Use additional code to identify the sequelae

Unacceptable principal diagnosis symbol per Medicare code edits · Code exempt from diagnosis present on admission requirement · Questionable admission · Complication or comorbidity · CC/MCC exclusion · Major complication or comorbidity · Principal diagnosis as its own CC · Principal diagnosis as its own MCC · Z code as first-listed diagnosis

When symbols appear on a code that requires a 7th character extension, refer to Appendix D to identify applicable 7th character codes.

I69.9 Sequelae of unspecified cerebrovascular diseases
EXCLUDES1 *sequelae of stroke (I69.3)*
sequelae of traumatic intracranial injury (S06.-)

I69.90 Unspecified sequelae of unspecified cerebrovascular disease POA

I69.91 Cognitive deficits following unspecified cerebrovascular disease

● I69.910 Attention and concentration deficit following unspecified cerebrovascular disease

● I69.911 Memory deficit following unspecified cerebrovascular disease

● I69.912 Visuospatial deficit and spatial neglect following unspecified cerebrovascular disease

● I69.913 Psychomotor deficit following unspecified cerebrovascular disease

● I69.914 Frontal lobe and executive function deficit following unspecified cerebrovascular disease

● I69.915 Cognitive social or emotional deficit following unspecified cerebrovascular disease

● I69.918 Other symptoms and signs involving cognitive functions following unspecified cerebrovascular disease

● I69.919 Unspecified symptoms and signs involving cognitive functions following unspecified cerebrovascular disease

I69.92 Speech and language deficits following unspecified cerebrovascular disease

I69.920 Aphasia following unspecified cerebrovascular disease POA

I69.921 Dysphasia following unspecified cerebrovascular disease POA

I69.922 Dysarthria following unspecified cerebrovascular disease POA

I69.923 Fluency disorder following unspecified cerebrovascular disease POA
Stuttering following ▶unspecified cerebrovascular disease◀

I69.928 Other speech and language deficits following unspecified cerebrovascular disease POA

I69.93 Monoplegia of upper limb following unspecified cerebrovascular disease

I69.931 Monoplegia of upper limb following unspecified cerebrovascular disease affecting right dominant side POA

I69.932 Monoplegia of upper limb following unspecified cerebrovascular disease affecting left dominant side POA

I69.933 Monoplegia of upper limb following unspecified cerebrovascular disease affecting right non-dominant side POA

I69.934 Monoplegia of upper limb following unspecified cerebrovascular disease affecting left non-dominant side POA

I69.939 Monoplegia of upper limb following unspecified cerebrovascular disease affecting unspecified side POA

I69.94 Monoplegia of lower limb following unspecified cerebrovascular disease

I69.941 Monoplegia of lower limb following unspecified cerebrovascular disease affecting right dominant side POA

I69.942 Monoplegia of lower limb following unspecified cerebrovascular disease affecting left dominant side POA

I69.943 Monoplegia of lower limb following unspecified cerebrovascular disease affecting right non-dominant side POA

I69.944 Monoplegia of lower limb following unspecified cerebrovascular disease affecting left non-dominant side POA

I69.949 Monoplegia of lower limb following unspecified cerebrovascular disease affecting unspecified side POA

I69.95 Hemiplegia and hemiparesis following unspecified cerebrovascular disease

I69.951 Hemiplegia and hemiparesis following unspecified cerebrovascular disease affecting right dominant side CC POA

I69.952 Hemiplegia and hemiparesis following unspecified cerebrovascular disease affecting left dominant side CC POA

I69.953 Hemiplegia and hemiparesis following unspecified cerebrovascular disease affecting right non-dominant side CC POA

I69.954 Hemiplegia and hemiparesis following unspecified cerebrovascular disease affecting left non-dominant side CC POA

I69.959 Hemiplegia and hemiparesis following unspecified cerebrovascular disease affecting unspecified side CC POA

I69.96 Other paralytic syndrome following unspecified cerebrovascular disease
Use additional code to identify type of paralytic syndrome, such as:
locked-in state (G83.5)
quadriplegia (G82.5-)
EXCLUDES1 *hemiplegia/hemiparesis following unspecified cerebrovascular disease (I69.95-)*
monoplegia of lower limb following unspecified cerebrovascular disease (I69.94-)
monoplegia of upper limb following unspecified cerebrovascular disease (I69.93-)

I69.961 Other paralytic syndrome following unspecified cerebrovascular disease affecting right dominant side POA

I69.962 Other paralytic syndrome following unspecified cerebrovascular disease affecting left dominant side POA

I69.963 Other paralytic syndrome following unspecified cerebrovascular disease affecting right non-dominant side POA

I69.964 Other paralytic syndrome following unspecified cerebrovascular disease affecting left non-dominant side POA

I69.965 Other paralytic syndrome following unspecified cerebrovascular disease, bilateral POA

I69.969 Other paralytic syndrome following unspecified cerebrovascular disease affecting unspecified side POA

I69.99 Other sequelae of unspecified cerebrovascular disease

I69.990 Apraxia following unspecified cerebrovascular disease POA

I69.991 Dysphagia following unspecified cerebrovascular disease POA
Use additional code to identify the type of dysphagia, if known (R13.1-)

I69.992 Facial weakness following unspecified cerebrovascular disease POA
Facial droop following unspecified cerebrovascular disease

I69.993 Ataxia following unspecified cerebrovascular disease POA

I69.998 Other sequelae following unspecified cerebrovascular disease POA
Alteration in sensation following unspecified cerebrovascular disease
Disturbance of vision following unspecified cerebrovascular disease
Use additional code to identify the sequelae

Unspecified Code | Other Specified Code | Manifestation Code | N Newborn | P Pediatric | M Maternity | A Adult | ♂ Male | ♀ Female
● New Code | ▲ Revised Code Title | ▶◀ Revised Text | NOTES | INCLUDES | EXCLUDES1 Not coded here | EXCLUDES2 Not included here
4th character required | 5th character required | 6th character required | 7th character required
Extension 'X' Alert | HAC Hospital-acquired condition (HAC) alert | AHA AHA Coding Clinic©

Diseases of arteries, arterioles and capillaries (I70-I79)

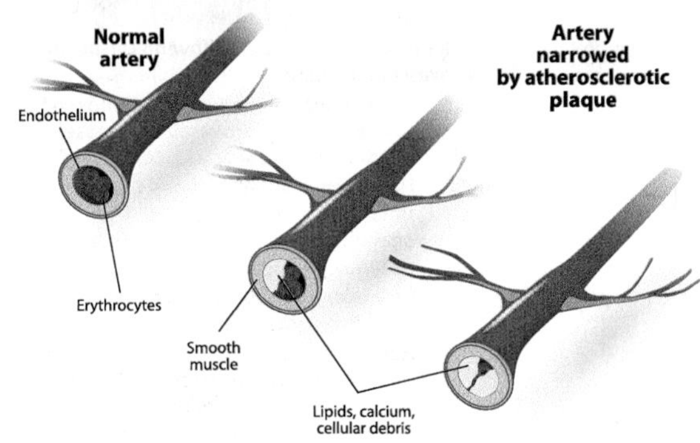

Figure 9.5 Atherosclerosis

I70 Atherosclerosis

INCLUDES *arteriolosclerosis*
arterial degeneration
arteriosclerosis
arteriosclerotic vascular disease
arteriovascular degeneration
atheroma
endarteritis deformans or obliterans
senile arteritis
senile endarteritis
vascular degeneration

Use additional code to identify:
exposure to environmental tobacco smoke (Z77.22)
history of tobacco ▶dependence◀ (Z87.891)
occupational exposure to environmental tobacco smoke (Z57.31)
tobacco dependence (F17.-)
tobacco use (Z72.0)

EXCLUDES2 *arteriosclerotic cardiovascular disease (I25.1-)*
arteriosclerotic heart disease (I25.1-)
atheroembolism (I75.-)
cerebral atherosclerosis (I67.2)
coronary atherosclerosis (I25.1-)
mesenteric atherosclerosis (K55.1)
precerebral atherosclerosis (I67.2)
primary pulmonary atherosclerosis (I27.0)

I70.0 Atherosclerosis of aorta A

I70.1 Atherosclerosis of renal artery A
Goldblatt's kidney
EXCLUDES2 *atherosclerosis of renal arterioles (I12.-)*

I70.2 Atherosclerosis of native arteries of the extremities
Mönckeberg's (medial) sclerosis
Use additional code, if applicable, to identify chronic total occlusion of artery of extremity (I70.92)
EXCLUDES2 *atherosclerosis of bypass graft of extremities (I70.30-I70.79)*

I70.20 Unspecified atherosclerosis of native arteries of extremities

I70.201 Unspecified atherosclerosis of native arteries of extremities, right leg A

I70.202 Unspecified atherosclerosis of native arteries of extremities, left leg A

I70.203 Unspecified atherosclerosis of native arteries of extremities, bilateral legs A

I70.208 Unspecified atherosclerosis of native arteries of extremities, other extremity A

I70.209 Unspecified atherosclerosis of native arteries of extremities, unspecified extremity A

I70.21 Atherosclerosis of native arteries of extremities with intermittent claudication

I70.211 Atherosclerosis of native arteries of extremities with intermittent claudication, right leg A

I70.212 Atherosclerosis of native arteries of extremities with intermittent claudication, left leg A

I70.213 Atherosclerosis of native arteries of extremities with intermittent claudication, bilateral legs A

I70.218 Atherosclerosis of native arteries of extremities with intermittent claudication, other extremity A

I70.219 Atherosclerosis of native arteries of extremities with intermittent claudication, unspecified extremity A

I70.22 Atherosclerosis of native arteries of extremities with rest pain
INCLUDES *any condition classifiable to I70.21-*

I70.221 Atherosclerosis of native arteries of extremities with rest pain, right leg A

I70.222 Atherosclerosis of native arteries of extremities with rest pain, left leg A

I70.223 Atherosclerosis of native arteries of extremities with rest pain, bilateral legs A

I70.228 Atherosclerosis of native arteries of extremities with rest pain, other extremity A

I70.229 Atherosclerosis of native arteries of extremities with rest pain, unspecified extremity A

I70.23 Atherosclerosis of native arteries of right leg with ulceration
INCLUDES *any condition classifiable to I70.211 and I70.221*
Use additional code to identify severity of ulcer (L97.-)

I70.231 Atherosclerosis of native arteries of right leg with ulceration of thigh A

I70.232 Atherosclerosis of native arteries of right leg with ulceration of calf A

I70.233 Atherosclerosis of native arteries of right leg with ulceration of ankle A

I70.234 Atherosclerosis of native arteries of right leg with ulceration of heel and midfoot A
Atherosclerosis of native arteries of right leg with ulceration of plantar surface of midfoot

I70.235 Atherosclerosis of native arteries of right leg with ulceration of other part of foot A
Atherosclerosis of native arteries of right leg extremities with ulceration of toe

I70.238 Atherosclerosis of native arteries of right leg with ulceration of other part of lower right leg A

I70.239 Atherosclerosis of native arteries of right leg with ulceration of unspecified site A

I70.24 Atherosclerosis of native arteries of left leg with ulceration
INCLUDES *any condition classifiable to I70.212 and I70.222*
Use additional code to identify severity of ulcer (L97.-)

I70.241 Atherosclerosis of native arteries of left leg with ulceration of thigh A

I70.242 Atherosclerosis of native arteries of left leg with ulceration of calf A

I70.243 Atherosclerosis of native arteries of left leg with ulceration of ankle A

I70.244 Atherosclerosis of native arteries of left leg with ulceration of heel and midfoot A
Atherosclerosis of native arteries of left leg with ulceration of plantar surface of midfoot

I70.245 Atherosclerosis of native arteries of left leg with ulceration of other part of foot A
Atherosclerosis of native arteries of left leg extremities with ulceration of toe

Unacceptable principal diagnosis symbol per Medicare code edits · Code exempt from diagnosis present on admission requirement
Questionable admission · Complication or comorbidity · CC/MCC exclusion · Major complication or comorbidity
Principal diagnosis as its own CC · Principal diagnosis as its own MCC · Z code as first-listed diagnosis

 When symbols appear on a code that requires a 7th character extension, refer to Appendix D to identify applicable 7th character codes.

I70.248 Atherosclerosis of native arteries of left leg with ulceration of other part of lower left leg A

I70.249 Atherosclerosis of native arteries of left leg with ulceration of unspecified site A

● I70.25 Atherosclerosis of native arteries of other extremities with ulceration A

INCLUDES *any condition classifiable to I70.218 and I70.228*

Use additional code to identify the severity of the ulcer (L98.49-)

I70.26 Atherosclerosis of native arteries of extremities with gangrene

INCLUDES *any condition classifiable to I70.21-, I70.22-, I70.23-, I70.24-, and I70.25-*

Use additional code to identify the severity of any ulcer (L97.-, L98.49-), if applicable

I70.261 Atherosclerosis of native arteries of extremities with gangrene, right leg A cc

I70.262 Atherosclerosis of native arteries of extremities with gangrene, left leg A cc

I70.263 Atherosclerosis of native arteries of extremities with gangrene, bilateral legs A cc

I70.268 Atherosclerosis of native arteries of extremities with gangrene, other extremity A cc

I70.269 Atherosclerosis of native arteries of extremities with gangrene, unspecified extremity A cc

I70.29 Other atherosclerosis of native arteries of extremities

I70.291 Other atherosclerosis of native arteries of extremities, right leg A

I70.292 Other atherosclerosis of native arteries of extremities, left leg A

I70.293 Other atherosclerosis of native arteries of extremities, bilateral legs A

I70.298 Other atherosclerosis of native arteries of extremities, other extremity A

I70.299 Other atherosclerosis of native arteries of extremities, unspecified extremity A

I70.3 Atherosclerosis of unspecified type of bypass graft(s) of the extremities

Use additional code, if applicable, to identify chronic total occlusion of artery of extremity (I70.92)

EXCLUDES1 *embolism or thrombus of bypass graft(s) of extremities (T82.8-)*

I70.30 Unspecified atherosclerosis of unspecified type of bypass graft(s) of the extremities

I70.301 Unspecified atherosclerosis of unspecified type of bypass graft(s) of the extremities, right leg A

I70.302 Unspecified atherosclerosis of unspecified type of bypass graft(s) of the extremities, left leg A

I70.303 Unspecified atherosclerosis of unspecified type of bypass graft(s) of the extremities, bilateral legs A

I70.308 Unspecified atherosclerosis of unspecified type of bypass graft(s) of the extremities, other extremity A

I70.309 Unspecified atherosclerosis of unspecified type of bypass graft(s) of the extremities, unspecified extremity A

I70.31 Atherosclerosis of unspecified type of bypass graft(s) of the extremities with intermittent claudication

I70.311 Atherosclerosis of unspecified type of bypass graft(s) of the extremities with intermittent claudication, right leg A

I70.312 Atherosclerosis of unspecified type of bypass graft(s) of the extremities with intermittent claudication, left leg A

I70.313 Atherosclerosis of unspecified type of bypass graft(s) of the extremities with intermittent claudication, bilateral legs A

I70.318 Atherosclerosis of unspecified type of bypass graft(s) of the extremities with intermittent claudication, other extremity A

I70.319 Atherosclerosis of unspecified type of bypass graft(s) of the extremities with intermittent claudication, unspecified extremity A

I70.32 Atherosclerosis of unspecified type of bypass graft(s) of the extremities with rest pain

INCLUDES *any condition classifiable to I70.31-*

I70.321 Atherosclerosis of unspecified type of bypass graft(s) of the extremities with rest pain, right leg A

I70.322 Atherosclerosis of unspecified type of bypass graft(s) of the extremities with rest pain, left leg A

I70.323 Atherosclerosis of unspecified type of bypass graft(s) of the extremities with rest pain, bilateral legs A

I70.328 Atherosclerosis of unspecified type of bypass graft(s) of the extremities with rest pain, other extremity A

I70.329 Atherosclerosis of unspecified type of bypass graft(s) of the extremities with rest pain, unspecified extremity A

I70.33 Atherosclerosis of unspecified type of bypass graft(s) of the right leg with ulceration

INCLUDES *any condition classifiable to I70.311 and I70.321*

Use additional code to identify severity of ulcer (L97.-)

I70.331 Atherosclerosis of unspecified type of bypass graft(s) of the right leg with ulceration of thigh A cc PDx

I70.332 Atherosclerosis of unspecified type of bypass graft(s) of the right leg with ulceration of calf A cc PDx

I70.333 Atherosclerosis of unspecified type of bypass graft(s) of the right leg with ulceration of ankle A cc PDx

I70.334 Atherosclerosis of unspecified type of bypass graft(s) of the right leg with ulceration of heel and midfoot A cc PDx

Atherosclerosis of unspecified type of bypass graft(s) of right leg with ulceration of plantar surface of midfoot

I70.335 Atherosclerosis of unspecified type of bypass graft(s) of the right leg with ulceration of other part of foot A

Atherosclerosis of unspecified type of bypass graft(s) of the right leg with ulceration of toe

I70.338 Atherosclerosis of unspecified type of bypass graft(s) of the right leg with ulceration of other part of lower leg A cc PDx

I70.339 Atherosclerosis of unspecified type of bypass graft(s) of the right leg with ulceration of unspecified site A cc PDx

I70.34 Atherosclerosis of unspecified type of bypass graft(s) of the left leg with ulceration

INCLUDES *any condition classifiable to I70.312 and I70.322*

Use additional code to identify severity of ulcer (L97.-)

I70.341 Atherosclerosis of unspecified type of bypass graft(s) of the left leg with ulceration of thigh A cc PDx

I70.342 Atherosclerosis of unspecified type of bypass graft(s) of the left leg with ulceration of calf A cc PDx

I70.343 Atherosclerosis of unspecified type of bypass graft(s) of the left leg with ulceration of ankle A cc PDx

Unspecified Code Other Specified Code Manifestation Code N Newborn P Pediatric M Maternity A Adult ♂ Male ♀ Female
● New Code ▲ Revised Code Title ►◄ Revised Text NOTES INCLUDES EXCLUDES1 Not coded here EXCLUDES2 Not included here
4th character required 5th character required 6th character required 7th character required
Extension 'X' Alert HAC Hospital-acquired condition (HAC) alert AHA AHA Coding Clinic©

I70.344 **Atherosclerosis of unspecified type of bypass graft(s) of the left leg with ulceration of heel and midfoot** A CC PDx
Atherosclerosis of unspecified type of bypass graft(s) of left leg with ulceration of plantar surface of midfoot

I70.345 **Atherosclerosis of unspecified type of bypass graft(s) of the left leg with ulceration of other part of foot** A
Atherosclerosis of unspecified type of bypass graft(s) of the left leg with ulceration of toe

I70.348 **Atherosclerosis of unspecified type of bypass graft(s) of the left leg with ulceration of other part of lower leg** A CC PDx

I70.349 **Atherosclerosis of unspecified type of bypass graft(s) of the left leg with ulceration of unspecified site** A CC PDx

I70.35 **Atherosclerosis of unspecified type of bypass graft(s) of other extremity with ulceration** A
INCLUDES *any condition classifiable to I70.318 and I70.328*
Use additional code to identify severity of ulcer (L98.49-)

I70.36 **Atherosclerosis of unspecified type of bypass graft(s) of the extremities with gangrene**
INCLUDES *any condition classifiable to I70.31-, I70.32-, I70.33-, I70.34-, I70.35*
Use additional code to identify the severity of any ulcer (L97.-, L98.49-), if applicable

I70.361 **Atherosclerosis of unspecified type of bypass graft(s) of the extremities with gangrene, right leg** A CC PDx

I70.362 **Atherosclerosis of unspecified type of bypass graft(s) of the extremities with gangrene, left leg** A CC PDx

I70.363 **Atherosclerosis of unspecified type of bypass graft(s) of the extremities with gangrene, bilateral legs** A CC PDx

I70.368 **Atherosclerosis of unspecified type of bypass graft(s) of the extremities with gangrene, other extremity** A CC PDx

I70.369 **Atherosclerosis of unspecified type of bypass graft(s) of the extremities with gangrene, unspecified extremity** A CC PDx

I70.39 **Other atherosclerosis of unspecified type of bypass graft(s) of the extremities**

I70.391 **Other atherosclerosis of unspecified type of bypass graft(s) of the extremities, right leg** A

I70.392 **Other atherosclerosis of unspecified type of bypass graft(s) of the extremities, left leg** A

I70.393 **Other atherosclerosis of unspecified type of bypass graft(s) of the extremities, bilateral legs** A

I70.398 **Other atherosclerosis of unspecified type of bypass graft(s) of the extremities, other extremity** A

I70.399 **Other atherosclerosis of unspecified type of bypass graft(s) of the extremities, unspecified extremity** A

I70.4 **Atherosclerosis of autologous vein bypass graft(s) of the extremities**
Use additional code, if applicable, to identify chronic total occlusion of artery of extremity (I70.92)

I70.40 **Unspecified atherosclerosis of autologous vein bypass graft(s) of the extremities**

I70.401 **Unspecified atherosclerosis of autologous vein bypass graft(s) of the extremities, right leg** A

I70.402 **Unspecified atherosclerosis of autologous vein bypass graft(s) of the extremities, left leg** A

I70.403 **Unspecified atherosclerosis of autologous vein bypass graft(s) of the extremities, bilateral legs** A

I70.408 **Unspecified atherosclerosis of autologous vein bypass graft(s) of the extremities, other extremity** A

I70.409 **Unspecified atherosclerosis of autologous vein bypass graft(s) of the extremities, unspecified extremity** A

I70.41 **Atherosclerosis of autologous vein bypass graft(s) of the extremities with intermittent claudication**

I70.411 **Atherosclerosis of autologous vein bypass graft(s) of the extremities with intermittent claudication, right leg** A

I70.412 **Atherosclerosis of autologous vein bypass graft(s) of the extremities with intermittent claudication, left leg** A

I70.413 **Atherosclerosis of autologous vein bypass graft(s) of the extremities with intermittent claudication, bilateral legs** A

I70.418 **Atherosclerosis of autologous vein bypass graft(s) of the extremities with intermittent claudication, other extremity** A

I70.419 **Atherosclerosis of autologous vein bypass graft(s) of the extremities with intermittent claudication, unspecified extremity** A

I70.42 **Atherosclerosis of autologous vein bypass graft(s) of the extremities with rest pain**
INCLUDES *any condition classifiable to I70.41-*

I70.421 **Atherosclerosis of autologous vein bypass graft(s) of the extremities with rest pain, right leg** A

I70.422 **Atherosclerosis of autologous vein bypass graft(s) of the extremities with rest pain, left leg** A

I70.423 **Atherosclerosis of autologous vein bypass graft(s) of the extremities with rest pain, bilateral legs** A

I70.428 **Atherosclerosis of autologous vein bypass graft(s) of the extremities with rest pain, other extremity** A

I70.429 **Atherosclerosis of autologous vein bypass graft(s) of the extremities with rest pain, unspecified extremity** A

I70.43 **Atherosclerosis of autologous vein bypass graft(s) of the right leg with ulceration**
INCLUDES *any condition classifiable to I70.411 and I70.421*
Use additional code to identify severity of ulcer (L97.-)

I70.431 **Atherosclerosis of autologous vein bypass graft(s) of the right leg with ulceration of thigh** A CC PDx

I70.432 **Atherosclerosis of autologous vein bypass graft(s) of the right leg with ulceration of calf** A CC PDx

I70.433 **Atherosclerosis of autologous vein bypass graft(s) of the right leg with ulceration of ankle** A CC PDx

I70.434 **Atherosclerosis of autologous vein bypass graft(s) of the right leg with ulceration of heel and midfoot** A CC PDx
Atherosclerosis of autologous vein bypass graft(s) of right leg with ulceration of plantar surface of midfoot

I70.435 **Atherosclerosis of autologous vein bypass graft(s) of the right leg with ulceration of other part of foot** A
Atherosclerosis of autologous vein bypass graft(s) of right leg with ulceration of toe

I70.438 **Atherosclerosis of autologous vein bypass graft(s) of the right leg with ulceration of other part of lower leg** A CC PDx

I70.439 **Atherosclerosis of autologous vein bypass graft(s) of the right leg with ulceration of unspecified site** A CC PDx

PDx Unacceptable principal diagnosis symbol per Medicare code edits · POA Code exempt from diagnosis present on admission requirement
? Questionable admission · CC Complication or comorbidity · CC/MCC Exc CC/MCC exclusion · MCC Major complication or comorbidity
PDx CC Principal diagnosis as its own CC · PDx MCC Principal diagnosis as its own MCC · Z1 Z code as first-listed diagnosis

I70.44 Atherosclerosis of autologous vein bypass graft(s) of the left leg with ulceration
INCLUDES any condition classifiable to I70.412 and I70.422
Use additional code to identify severity of ulcer (L97.-)
I70.441 Atherosclerosis of autologous vein bypass graft(s) of the left leg with ulceration of thigh
I70.442 Atherosclerosis of autologous vein bypass graft(s) of the left leg with ulceration of calf
I70.443 Atherosclerosis of autologous vein bypass graft(s) of the left leg with ulceration of ankle
I70.444 Atherosclerosis of autologous vein bypass graft(s) of the left leg with ulceration of heel and midfoot
Atherosclerosis of autologous vein bypass graft(s) of left leg with ulceration of plantar surface of midfoot
I70.445 Atherosclerosis of autologous vein bypass graft(s) of the left leg with ulceration of other part of foot
Atherosclerosis of autologous vein bypass graft(s) of left leg with ulceration of toe
I70.448 Atherosclerosis of autologous vein bypass graft(s) of the left leg with ulceration of other part of lower leg
I70.449 Atherosclerosis of autologous vein bypass graft(s) of the left leg with ulceration of unspecified site
I70.45 Atherosclerosis of autologous vein bypass graft(s) of other extremity with ulceration
INCLUDES any condition classifiable to I70.418, I70.428, and I70.438
Use additional code to identify severity of ulcer (L98.49)
I70.46 Atherosclerosis of autologous vein bypass graft(s) of the extremities with gangrene
INCLUDES any condition classifiable to I70.41-, I70.42-, and I70.43-, I70.44-, I70.45
Use additional code to identify the severity of any ulcer (L97.-, L98.49-), if applicable
I70.461 Atherosclerosis of autologous vein bypass graft(s) of the extremities with gangrene, right leg
I70.462 Atherosclerosis of autologous vein bypass graft(s) of the extremities with gangrene, left leg
I70.463 Atherosclerosis of autologous vein bypass graft(s) of the extremities with gangrene, bilateral legs
I70.468 Atherosclerosis of autologous vein bypass graft(s) of the extremities with gangrene, other extremity
I70.469 Atherosclerosis of autologous vein bypass graft(s) of the extremities with gangrene, unspecified extremity
I70.49 Other atherosclerosis of autologous vein bypass graft(s) of the extremities
I70.491 Other atherosclerosis of autologous vein bypass graft(s) of the extremities, right leg
I70.492 Other atherosclerosis of autologous vein bypass graft(s) of the extremities, left leg
I70.493 Other atherosclerosis of autologous vein bypass graft(s) of the extremities, bilateral legs
I70.498 Other atherosclerosis of autologous vein bypass graft(s) of the extremities, other extremity
I70.499 Other atherosclerosis of autologous vein bypass graft(s) of the extremities, unspecified extremity

I70.5 Atherosclerosis of nonautologous biological bypass graft(s) of the extremities
Use additional code, if applicable, to identify chronic total occlusion of artery of extremity (I70.92)
I70.50 Unspecified atherosclerosis of nonautologous biological bypass graft(s) of the extremities
I70.501 Unspecified atherosclerosis of nonautologous biological bypass graft(s) of the extremities, right leg
I70.502 Unspecified atherosclerosis of nonautologous biological bypass graft(s) of the extremities, left leg
I70.503 Unspecified atherosclerosis of nonautologous biological bypass graft(s) of the extremities, bilateral legs
I70.508 Unspecified atherosclerosis of nonautologous biological bypass graft(s) of the extremities, other extremity
I70.509 Unspecified atherosclerosis of nonautologous biological bypass graft(s) of the extremities, unspecified extremity
I70.51 Atherosclerosis of nonautologous biological bypass graft(s) of the extremities intermittent claudication
I70.511 Atherosclerosis of nonautologous biological bypass graft(s) of the extremities with intermittent claudication, right leg
I70.512 Atherosclerosis of nonautologous biological bypass graft(s) of the extremities with intermittent claudication, left leg
I70.513 Atherosclerosis of nonautologous biological bypass graft(s) of the extremities with intermittent claudication, bilateral legs
I70.518 Atherosclerosis of nonautologous biological bypass graft(s) of the extremities with intermittent claudication, other extremity
I70.519 Atherosclerosis of nonautologous biological bypass graft(s) of the extremities with intermittent claudication, unspecified extremity
I70.52 Atherosclerosis of nonautologous biological bypass graft(s) of the extremities with rest pain
INCLUDES any condition classifiable to I70.51-
I70.521 Atherosclerosis of nonautologous biological bypass graft(s) of the extremities with rest pain, right leg
I70.522 Atherosclerosis of nonautologous biological bypass graft(s) of the extremities with rest pain, left leg
I70.523 Atherosclerosis of nonautologous biological bypass graft(s) of the extremities with rest pain, bilateral legs
I70.528 Atherosclerosis of nonautologous biological bypass graft(s) of the extremities with rest pain, other extremity
I70.529 Atherosclerosis of nonautologous biological bypass graft(s) of the extremities with rest pain, unspecified extremity
I70.53 Atherosclerosis of nonautologous biological bypass graft(s) of the right leg with ulceration
INCLUDES any condition classifiable to I70.511 and I70.521
Use additional code to identify severity of ulcer (L97.-)
I70.531 Atherosclerosis of nonautologous biological bypass graft(s) of the right leg with ulceration of thigh
I70.532 Atherosclerosis of nonautologous biological bypass graft(s) of the right leg with ulceration of calf

Unspecified Code Other Specified Code Manifestation Code N Newborn P Pediatric M Maternity A Adult ♂ Male ♀ Female
● New Code ▲ Revised Code Title ►◄ Revised Text NOTES INCLUDES EXCLUDES 1 Not coded here EXCLUDES 2 Not included here
4th character required 5th character required 6th character required 7th character required
Extension 'X' Alert HAC Hospital-acquired condition (HAC) alert AHA AHA Coding Clinic©

When symbols appear on a code that requires a 7th character extension, refer to Appendix D to identify applicable 7th character codes.

I70.533 Atherosclerosis of nonautologous biological bypass graft(s) of the right leg with ulceration of ankle

I70.534 Atherosclerosis of nonautologous biological bypass graft(s) of the right leg with ulceration of heel and midfoot
Atherosclerosis of nonautologous biological bypass graft(s) of right leg with ulceration of plantar surface of midfoot

I70.535 Atherosclerosis of nonautologous biological bypass graft(s) of the right leg with ulceration of other part of foot
Atherosclerosis of nonautologous biological bypass graft(s) of the right leg with ulceration of toe

I70.538 Atherosclerosis of nonautologous biological bypass graft(s) of the right leg with ulceration of other part of lower leg

I70.539 Atherosclerosis of nonautologous biological bypass graft(s) of the right leg with ulceration of unspecified site

I70.54 Atherosclerosis of nonautologous biological bypass graft(s) of the left leg with ulceration
INCLUDES *any condition classifiable to I70.512 and I70.522*
Use additional code to identify severity of ulcer (L97.-)

I70.541 Atherosclerosis of nonautologous biological bypass graft(s) of the left leg with ulceration of thigh

I70.542 Atherosclerosis of nonautologous biological bypass graft(s) of the left leg with ulceration of calf

I70.543 Atherosclerosis of nonautologous biological bypass graft(s) of the left leg with ulceration of ankle

I70.544 Atherosclerosis of nonautologous biological bypass graft(s) of the left leg with ulceration of heel and midfoot
Atherosclerosis of nonautologous biological bypass graft(s) of left leg with ulceration of plantar surface of midfoot

I70.545 Atherosclerosis of nonautologous biological bypass graft(s) of the left leg with ulceration of other part of foot
Atherosclerosis of nonautologous biological bypass graft(s) of the left leg with ulceration of toe

I70.548 Atherosclerosis of nonautologous biological bypass graft(s) of the left leg with ulceration of other part of lower leg

I70.549 Atherosclerosis of nonautologous biological bypass graft(s) of the left leg with ulceration of unspecified site

I70.55 Atherosclerosis of nonautologous biological bypass graft(s) of other extremity with ulceration
INCLUDES *any condition classifiable to I70.518, I70.528, and I70.538*
Use additional code to identify severity of ulcer (L98.49)

I70.56 Atherosclerosis of nonautologous biological bypass graft(s) of the extremities with gangrene
INCLUDES *any condition classifiable to I70.51-, I70.52-, and I70.53-, I70.54-, I70.55*
Use additional code to identify the severity of any ulcer (L97.-, L98.49-), if applicable

I70.561 Atherosclerosis of nonautologous biological bypass graft(s) of the extremities with gangrene, right leg

I70.562 Atherosclerosis of nonautologous biological bypass graft(s) of the extremities with gangrene, left leg

I70.563 Atherosclerosis of nonautologous biological bypass graft(s) of the extremities with gangrene, bilateral legs

I70.568 Atherosclerosis of nonautologous biological bypass graft(s) of the extremities with gangrene, other extremity

I70.569 Atherosclerosis of nonautologous biological bypass graft(s) of the extremities with gangrene, unspecified extremity

I70.59 Other atherosclerosis of nonautologous biological bypass graft(s) of the extremities

I70.591 Other atherosclerosis of nonautologous biological bypass graft(s) of the extremities, right leg

I70.592 Other atherosclerosis of nonautologous biological bypass graft(s) of the extremities, left leg

I70.593 Other atherosclerosis of nonautologous biological bypass graft(s) of the extremities, bilateral legs

I70.598 Other atherosclerosis of nonautologous biological bypass graft(s) of the extremities, other extremity

I70.599 Other atherosclerosis of nonautologous biological bypass graft(s) of the extremities, unspecified extremity

I70.6 Atherosclerosis of nonbiological bypass graft(s) of the extremities
Use additional code, if applicable, to identify chronic total occlusion of artery of extremity (I70.92)

I70.60 Unspecified atherosclerosis of nonbiological bypass graft(s) of the extremities

I70.601 Unspecified atherosclerosis of nonbiological bypass graft(s) of the extremities, right leg

I70.602 Unspecified atherosclerosis of nonbiological bypass graft(s) of the extremities, left leg

I70.603 Unspecified atherosclerosis of nonbiological bypass graft(s) of the extremities, bilateral legs

I70.608 Unspecified atherosclerosis of nonbiological bypass graft(s) of the extremities, other extremity

I70.609 Unspecified atherosclerosis of nonbiological bypass graft(s) of the extremities, unspecified extremity

I70.61 Atherosclerosis of nonbiological bypass graft(s) of the extremities with intermittent claudication

I70.611 Atherosclerosis of nonbiological bypass graft(s) of the extremities with intermittent claudication, right leg

I70.612 Atherosclerosis of nonbiological bypass graft(s) of the extremities with intermittent claudication, left leg

I70.613 Atherosclerosis of nonbiological bypass graft(s) of the extremities with intermittent claudication, bilateral legs

I70.618 Atherosclerosis of nonbiological bypass graft(s) of the extremities with intermittent claudication, other extremity

I70.619 Atherosclerosis of nonbiological bypass graft(s) of the extremities with intermittent claudication, unspecified extremity

I70.62 Atherosclerosis of nonbiological bypass graft(s) of the extremities with rest pain
INCLUDES *any condition classifiable to I70.61-*

I70.621 Atherosclerosis of nonbiological bypass graft(s) of the extremities with rest pain, right leg

I70.622 Atherosclerosis of nonbiological bypass graft(s) of the extremities with rest pain, left leg

Unacceptable principal diagnosis symbol per Medicare code edits — Code exempt from diagnosis present on admission requirement
Questionable admission — Complication or comorbidity — CC/MCC exclusion — Major complication or comorbidity
Principal diagnosis as its own CC — Principal diagnosis as its own MCC — Z code as first-listed diagnosis

I70.623 Atherosclerosis of nonbiological bypass graft(s) of the extremities with rest pain, bilateral legs A

I70.628 Atherosclerosis of nonbiological bypass graft(s) of the extremities with rest pain, other extremity A

I70.629 Atherosclerosis of nonbiological bypass graft(s) of the extremities with rest pain, unspecified extremity A

I70.63 Atherosclerosis of nonbiological bypass graft(s) of the right leg with ulceration

INCLUDES *any condition classifiable to I70.611 and I70.621*

Use additional code to identify severity of ulcer (L97.-)

I70.631 Atherosclerosis of nonbiological bypass graft(s) of the right leg with ulceration of thigh A CC PDx

I70.632 Atherosclerosis of nonbiological bypass graft(s) of the right leg with ulceration of calf A CC PDx

I70.633 Atherosclerosis of nonbiological bypass graft(s) of the right leg with ulceration of ankle A CC PDx

I70.634 Atherosclerosis of nonbiological bypass graft(s) of the right leg with ulceration of heel and midfoot A CC PDx
Atherosclerosis of nonbiological bypass graft(s) of right leg with ulceration of plantar surface of midfoot

I70.635 Atherosclerosis of nonbiological bypass graft(s) of the right leg with ulceration of other part of foot A
Atherosclerosis of nonbiological bypass graft(s) of the right leg with ulceration of toe

I70.638 Atherosclerosis of nonbiological bypass graft(s) of the right leg with ulceration of other part of lower leg A CC PDx

I70.639 Atherosclerosis of nonbiological bypass graft(s) of the right leg with ulceration of unspecified site A CC PDx

I70.64 Atherosclerosis of nonbiological bypass graft(s) of the left leg with ulceration

INCLUDES *any condition classifiable to I70.612 and I70.622*

Use additional code to identify severity of ulcer (L97.-)

I70.641 Atherosclerosis of nonbiological bypass graft(s) of the left leg with ulceration of thigh A CC PDx

I70.642 Atherosclerosis of nonbiological bypass graft(s) of the left leg with ulceration of calf A CC PDx

I70.643 Atherosclerosis of nonbiological bypass graft(s) of the left leg with ulceration of ankle A CC PDx

I70.644 Atherosclerosis of nonbiological bypass graft(s) of the left leg with ulceration of heel and midfoot A CC PDx
Atherosclerosis of nonbiological bypass graft(s) of left leg with ulceration of plantar surface of midfoot

I70.645 Atherosclerosis of nonbiological bypass graft(s) of the left leg with ulceration of other part of foot A
Atherosclerosis of nonbiological bypass graft(s) of the left leg with ulceration of toe

I70.648 Atherosclerosis of nonbiological bypass graft(s) of the left leg with ulceration of other part of lower leg A CC PDx

I70.649 Atherosclerosis of nonbiological bypass graft(s) of the left leg with ulceration of unspecified site A CC PDx

I70.65 Atherosclerosis of nonbiological bypass graft(s) of other extremity with ulceration A

INCLUDES *any condition classifiable to I70.618 and I70.628*

Use additional code to identify severity of ulcer (L98.49)

I70.66 Atherosclerosis of nonbiological bypass graft(s) of the extremities with gangrene

INCLUDES *any condition classifiable to I70.61-, I70.62-, I70.63-, I70.64-, I70.65*

Use additional code to identify the severity of any ulcer (L97.-, L98.49-), if applicable

I70.661 Atherosclerosis of nonbiological bypass graft(s) of the extremities with gangrene, right leg A CC PDx

I70.662 Atherosclerosis of nonbiological bypass graft(s) of the extremities with gangrene, left leg A CC PDx

I70.663 Atherosclerosis of nonbiological bypass graft(s) of the extremities with gangrene, bilateral legs A CC PDx

I70.668 Atherosclerosis of nonbiological bypass graft(s) of the extremities with gangrene, other extremity A CC PDx

I70.669 Atherosclerosis of nonbiological bypass graft(s) of the extremities with gangrene, unspecified extremity A CC PDx

I70.69 Other atherosclerosis of nonbiological bypass graft(s) of the extremities

I70.691 Other atherosclerosis of nonbiological bypass graft(s) of the extremities, right leg A

I70.692 Other atherosclerosis of nonbiological bypass graft(s) of the extremities, left leg A

I70.693 Other atherosclerosis of nonbiological bypass graft(s) of the extremities, bilateral legs A

I70.698 Other atherosclerosis of nonbiological bypass graft(s) of the extremities, other extremity A

I70.699 Other atherosclerosis of nonbiological bypass graft(s) of the extremities, unspecified extremity A

I70.7 Atherosclerosis of other type of bypass graft(s) of the extremities

Use additional code, if applicable, to identify chronic total occlusion of artery of extremity (I70.92)

I70.70 Unspecified atherosclerosis of other type of bypass graft(s) of the extremities

I70.701 Unspecified atherosclerosis of other type of bypass graft(s) of the extremities, right leg A

I70.702 Unspecified atherosclerosis of other type of bypass graft(s) of the extremities, left leg A

I70.703 Unspecified atherosclerosis of other type of bypass graft(s) of the extremities, bilateral legs A

I70.708 Unspecified atherosclerosis of other type of bypass graft(s) of the extremities, other extremity A

I70.709 Unspecified atherosclerosis of other type of bypass graft(s) of the extremities, unspecified extremity A

I70.71 Atherosclerosis of other type of bypass graft(s) of the extremities with intermittent claudication

I70.711 Atherosclerosis of other type of bypass graft(s) of the extremities with intermittent claudication, right leg A

I70.712 Atherosclerosis of other type of bypass graft(s) of the extremities with intermittent claudication, left leg A

I70.713 Atherosclerosis of other type of bypass graft(s) of the extremities with intermittent claudication, bilateral legs A

I70.718 Atherosclerosis of other type of bypass graft(s) of the extremities with intermittent claudication, other extremity A

Unspecified Code Other Specified Code Manifestation Code N Newborn P Pediatric M Maternity A Adult ♂ Male ♀ Female
● New Code ▲ Revised Code Title ►◄ Revised Text NOTES INCLUDES EXCLUDES1 Not coded here EXCLUDES2 Not included here
4th character required 5th character required 6th character required 7th character required
Extension 'X' Alert HAC Hospital-acquired condition (HAC) alert AHA AHA Coding Clinic©

I70.719 **Atherosclerosis of other type of bypass graft(s) of the extremities with intermittent claudication, unspecified extremity** A

I70.72 **Atherosclerosis of other type of bypass graft(s) of the extremities with rest pain**

INCLUDES *any condition classifiable to I70.71-*

I70.721 **Atherosclerosis of other type of bypass graft(s) of the extremities with rest pain, right leg** A

I70.722 **Atherosclerosis of other type of bypass graft(s) of the extremities with rest pain, left leg** A

I70.723 **Atherosclerosis of other type of bypass graft(s) of the extremities with rest pain, bilateral legs** A

I70.728 **Atherosclerosis of other type of bypass graft(s) of the extremities with rest pain, other extremity** A

I70.729 **Atherosclerosis of other type of bypass graft(s) of the extremities with rest pain, unspecified extremity** A

I70.73 **Atherosclerosis of other type of bypass graft(s) of the right leg with ulceration**

INCLUDES *any condition classifiable to I70.711 and I70.721*

Use additional code to identify severity of ulcer (L97.-)

I70.731 **Atherosclerosis of other type of bypass graft(s) of the right leg with ulceration of thigh** A CC PDx

I70.732 **Atherosclerosis of other type of bypass graft(s) of the right leg with ulceration of calf** A CC PDx

I70.733 **Atherosclerosis of other type of bypass graft(s) of the right leg with ulceration of ankle** A CC PDx

I70.734 **Atherosclerosis of other type of bypass graft(s) of the right leg with ulceration of heel and midfoot** A CC PDx

Atherosclerosis of other type of bypass graft(s) of right leg with ulceration of plantar surface of midfoot

I70.735 **Atherosclerosis of other type of bypass graft(s) of the right leg with ulceration of other part of foot** A

Atherosclerosis of other type of bypass graft(s) of right leg with ulceration of toe

I70.738 **Atherosclerosis of other type of bypass graft(s) of the right leg with ulceration of other part of lower leg** A CC PDx

I70.739 **Atherosclerosis of other type of bypass graft(s) of the right leg with ulceration of unspecified site** A CC PDx

I70.74 **Atherosclerosis of other type of bypass graft(s) of the left leg with ulceration**

INCLUDES *any condition classifiable to I70.712 and I70.722*

Use additional code to identify severity of ulcer (L97.-)

I70.741 **Atherosclerosis of other type of bypass graft(s) of the left leg with ulceration of thigh** A CC PDx

I70.742 **Atherosclerosis of other type of bypass graft(s) of the left leg with ulceration of calf** A CC PDx

I70.743 **Atherosclerosis of other type of bypass graft(s) of the left leg with ulceration of ankle** A CC PDx

I70.744 **Atherosclerosis of other type of bypass graft(s) of the left leg with ulceration of heel and midfoot** A CC PDx

Atherosclerosis of other type of bypass graft(s) of left leg with ulceration of plantar surface of midfoot

I70.745 **Atherosclerosis of other type of bypass graft(s) of the left leg with ulceration of other part of foot** A

Atherosclerosis of other type of bypass graft(s) of left leg with ulceration of toe

I70.748 **Atherosclerosis of other type of bypass graft(s) of the left leg with ulceration of other part of lower leg** A CC PDx

I70.749 **Atherosclerosis of other type of bypass graft(s) of the left leg with ulceration of unspecified site** A CC PDx

I70.75 **Atherosclerosis of other type of bypass graft(s) of other extremity with ulceration** A

INCLUDES *any condition classifiable to I70.718 and I70.728*

Use additional code to identify severity of ulcer (L98.49)

I70.76 **Atherosclerosis of other type of bypass graft(s) of the extremities with gangrene**

INCLUDES *any condition classifiable to I70.71-, I70.72-, I70.73-, I70.74-, I70.75*

Use additional code to identify the severity of any ulcer (L97.-, L98.49-), if applicable

I70.761 **Atherosclerosis of other type of bypass graft(s) of the extremities with gangrene, right leg** A CC PDx

I70.762 **Atherosclerosis of other type of bypass graft(s) of the extremities with gangrene, left leg** A CC PDx

I70.763 **Atherosclerosis of other type of bypass graft(s) of the extremities with gangrene, bilateral legs** A CC PDx

I70.768 **Atherosclerosis of other type of bypass graft(s) of the extremities with gangrene, other extremity** A CC PDx

I70.769 **Atherosclerosis of other type of bypass graft(s) of the extremities with gangrene, unspecified extremity** A CC PDx

I70.79 **Other atherosclerosis of other type of bypass graft(s) of the extremities**

I70.791 **Other atherosclerosis of other type of bypass graft(s) of the extremities, right leg** A

I70.792 **Other atherosclerosis of other type of bypass graft(s) of the extremities, left leg** A

I70.793 **Other atherosclerosis of other type of bypass graft(s) of the extremities, bilateral legs** A

I70.798 **Other atherosclerosis of other type of bypass graft(s) of the extremities, other extremity** A

I70.799 **Other atherosclerosis of other type of bypass graft(s) of the extremities, unspecified extremity** A

I70.8 **Atherosclerosis of other arteries** A

I70.9 **Other and unspecified atherosclerosis**

I70.90 **Unspecified atherosclerosis** A

I70.91 **Generalized atherosclerosis** A

I70.92 **Chronic total occlusion of artery of the extremities** A CC PDxIn

Complete occlusion of artery of the extremities
Total occlusion of artery of the extremities
Code first atherosclerosis of arteries of the extremities (I70.2-, I70.3-, I70.4-, I70.5-, I70.6-, I70.7-)

PDxIn Unacceptable principal diagnosis symbol per Medicare code edits; POA Code exempt from diagnosis present on admission requirement; ? Questionable admission; CC Complication or comorbidity; CC/MCC Exc CC/MCC exclusion; MCC Major complication or comorbidity; PDx CC Principal diagnosis as its own CC; PDx MCC Principal diagnosis as its own MCC; Z1 Z code as first-listed diagnosis

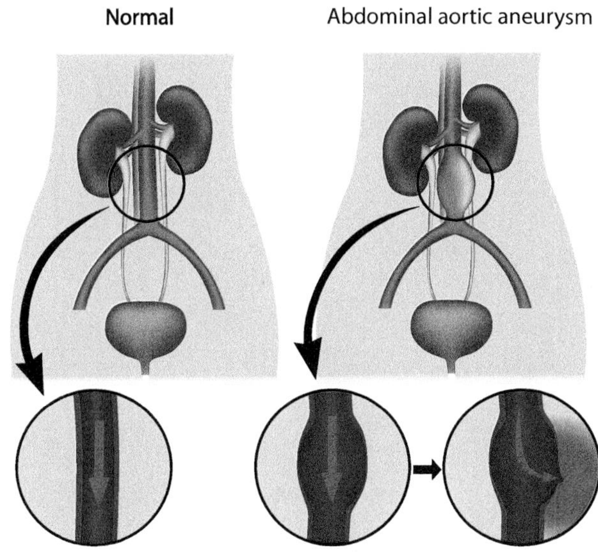

Figure 9.6 Abdominal aortic aneurysm

I71 Aortic aneurysm and dissection
EXCLUDES1 *aortic ectasia (I77.81-)*
syphilitic aortic aneurysm (A52.01)
traumatic aortic aneurysm (S25.09, S35.09)

I71.0 Dissection of aorta
- **I71.00 Dissection of unspecified site of aorta** MCC
- **I71.01 Dissection of thoracic aorta** MCC
- **I71.02 Dissection of abdominal aorta** MCC
- **I71.03 Dissection of thoracoabdominal aorta** MCC

I71.1 Thoracic aortic aneurysm, ruptured MCC
I71.2 Thoracic aortic aneurysm, without rupture
I71.3 Abdominal aortic aneurysm, ruptured MCC
I71.4 Abdominal aortic aneurysm, without rupture
I71.5 Thoracoabdominal aortic aneurysm, ruptured MCC
I71.6 Thoracoabdominal aortic aneurysm, without rupture
I71.8 Aortic aneurysm of unspecified site, ruptured MCC
Rupture of aorta NOS
I71.9 Aortic aneurysm of unspecified site, without rupture
Aneurysm of aorta
Dilatation of aorta
Hyaline necrosis of aorta

I72 Other aneurysm
INCLUDES *aneurysm (cirsoid) (false) (ruptured)*
EXCLUDES2 *acquired aneurysm (I77.0)*
aneurysm (of) aorta (I71.-)
aneurysm (of) arteriovenous NOS (Q27.3-)
carotid artery dissection (I77.71)
cerebral (nonruptured) aneurysm (I67.1)
coronary aneurysm (I25.4)
coronary artery dissection (I25.42)
dissection of artery NEC (I77.79)
dissection of precerebral artery, congenital (nonruptured) (Q28.1)
heart aneurysm (I25.3)
iliac artery dissection (I77.72)
pulmonary artery aneurysm (I28.1)
renal artery dissection (I77.73)
retinal aneurysm (H35.0)
ruptured cerebral aneurysm (I60.7)
varicose aneurysm (I77.0)
vertebral artery dissection (I77.74)

I72.0 Aneurysm of carotid artery
Aneurysm of common carotid artery
Aneurysm of external carotid artery
Aneurysm of internal carotid artery, extracranial portion
EXCLUDES1 *aneurysm of internal carotid artery, intracranial portion (I67.1)*
aneurysm of internal carotid artery NOS (I67.1)
I72.1 Aneurysm of artery of upper extremity
I72.2 Aneurysm of renal artery
I72.3 Aneurysm of iliac artery
I72.4 Aneurysm of artery of lower extremity
● **I72.5 Aneurysm of other precerebral arteries**
Aneurysm of basilar artery (trunk)
EXCLUDES2 *aneurysm of carotid artery (I72.0)*
aneurysm of vertebral artery (I72.6)
dissection of carotid artery (I77.71)
dissection of other precerebral arteries (I77.75)
dissection of vertebral artery (I77.74)
● **I72.6 Aneurysm of vertebral artery**
EXCLUDES2 *dissection of vertebral artery (I77.74)*
I72.8 Aneurysm of other specified arteries
I72.9 Aneurysm of unspecified site

I73 Other peripheral vascular diseases
EXCLUDES2 *chilblains (T69.1)*
frostbite (T33-T34)
immersion hand or foot (T69.0-)
spasm of cerebral artery (G45.9)

I73.0 Raynaud's syndrome
Raynaud's disease
Raynaud's phenomenon (secondary)
- **I73.00 Raynaud's syndrome without gangrene**
- **I73.01 Raynaud's syndrome with gangrene** CC PDx

I73.1 Thromboangiitis obliterans [Buerger's disease]
I73.8 Other specified peripheral vascular diseases
EXCLUDES1 *diabetic (peripheral) angiopathy (E08-E13 with .51-.52)*
- **I73.81 Erythromelalgia**
- **I73.89 Other specified peripheral vascular diseases**
  Acrocyanosis
  Erythrocyanosis
  Simple acroparesthesia [Schultze's type]
  Vasomotor acroparesthesia [Nothnagel's type]

I73.9 Peripheral vascular disease, unspecified
Intermittent claudication
Peripheral angiopathy NOS
Spasm of artery
EXCLUDES1 *atherosclerosis of the extremities (I70.2--I70.7-)*

I74 Arterial embolism and thrombosis
INCLUDES *embolic infarction*
embolic occlusion
thrombotic infarction
thrombotic occlusion
Code first embolism and thrombosis complicating abortion or ectopic or molar pregnancy (O00-O07, O08.2)
embolism and thrombosis complicating pregnancy, childbirth and the puerperium (O88.-)
EXCLUDES2 *atheroembolism (I75.-)*
basilar embolism and thrombosis (I63.0-I63.2, I65.1)
carotid embolism and thrombosis (I63.0-I63.2, I65.2)
cerebral embolism and thrombosis (I63.3-I63.5, I66.-)
coronary embolism and thrombosis (I21-I25)
mesenteric embolism and thrombosis ▶(K55.0-)◀
ophthalmic embolism and thrombosis (H34.-)
precerebral embolism and thrombosis NOS (I63.0-I63.2, I65.9)
pulmonary embolism and thrombosis (I26.-)
renal embolism and thrombosis (N28.0)
retinal embolism and thrombosis (H34.-)
septic embolism and thrombosis (I76)
vertebral embolism and thrombosis (I63.0-I63.2, I65.0)

I74.0 Embolism and thrombosis of abdominal aorta
- **I74.01 Saddle embolus of abdominal aorta** MCC
- **I74.09 Other arterial embolism and thrombosis of abdominal aorta** CC
  Aortic bifurcation syndrome
  Aortoiliac obstruction
  Leriche's syndrome

Unspecified Code Other Specified Code Manifestation Code N Newborn P Pediatric M Maternity A Adult ♂ Male ♀ Female
● New Code ▲ Revised Code Title ▶◀ Revised Text NOTES INCLUDES EXCLUDES1 Not coded here EXCLUDES2 Not included here
4th character required 5th character required 6th character required 7th character required
Extension 'X' Alert HAC Hospital-acquired condition (HAC) alert AHA AHA Coding Clinic®

I74.1 Embolism and thrombosis of other and unspecified parts of aorta
- I74.10 Embolism and thrombosis of unspecified parts of aorta CC
- I74.11 Embolism and thrombosis of thoracic aorta CC
- I74.19 Embolism and thrombosis of other parts of aorta CC

I74.2 Embolism and thrombosis of arteries of the upper extremities CC

I74.3 Embolism and thrombosis of arteries of the lower extremities CC

I74.4 Embolism and thrombosis of arteries of extremities, unspecified CC
Peripheral arterial embolism NOS

I74.5 Embolism and thrombosis of iliac artery CC

I74.8 Embolism and thrombosis of other arteries CC

I74.9 Embolism and thrombosis of unspecified artery CC

I75 Atheroembolism

INCLUDES *atherothrombotic microembolism*
cholesterol embolism

I75.0 Atheroembolism of extremities
- I75.01 Atheroembolism of upper extremity
  - I75.011 Atheroembolism of right upper extremity CC
  - I75.012 Atheroembolism of left upper extremity CC
  - I75.013 Atheroembolism of bilateral upper extremities CC
  - I75.019 Atheroembolism of unspecified upper extremity CC
- I75.02 Atheroembolism of lower extremity
  - I75.021 Atheroembolism of right lower extremity CC
  - I75.022 Atheroembolism of left lower extremity CC
  - I75.023 Atheroembolism of bilateral lower extremities CC
  - I75.029 Atheroembolism of unspecified lower extremity CC

I75.8 Atheroembolism of other sites
- I75.81 Atheroembolism of kidney CC
  Use additional code for any associated acute kidney failure and chronic kidney disease (N17.-, N18.-)
- I75.89 Atheroembolism of other site CC

I76 Septic arterial embolism CC PDx
Code first underlying infection, such as:
infective endocarditis (I33.0)
lung abscess (J85.-)
Use additional code to identify the site of the embolism (I74.-)

EXCLUDES2 *septic pulmonary embolism (I26.01, I26.90)*

I77 Other disorders of arteries and arterioles

EXCLUDES2 *collagen (vascular) diseases (M30-M36)*
hypersensitivity angiitis (M31.0)
pulmonary artery (I28.-)

I77.0 Arteriovenous fistula, acquired
Aneurysmal varix
Arteriovenous aneurysm, acquired
EXCLUDES1 *arteriovenous aneurysm NOS (Q27.3-)*
presence of arteriovenous shunt (fistula) for dialysis (Z99.2)
traumatic - see injury of blood vessel by body region
EXCLUDES2 *cerebral (I67.1)*
coronary (I25.4)

I77.1 Stricture of artery
Narrowing of artery

I77.2 Rupture of artery CC
Erosion of artery
Fistula of artery
Ulcer of artery
EXCLUDES1 *traumatic rupture of artery - see injury of blood vessel by body region*

I77.3 Arterial fibromuscular dysplasia
Fibromuscular hyperplasia (of) carotid artery
Fibromuscular hyperplasia (of) renal artery

I77.4 Celiac artery compression syndrome CC

I77.5 Necrosis of artery CC

I77.6 Arteritis, unspecified
Aortitis NOS
Endarteritis NOS
EXCLUDES1 *arteritis or endarteritis:*
aortic arch (M31.4)
cerebral NEC (I67.7)
coronary (I25.89)
deformans (I70.-)
giant cell (M31.5., M31.6)
obliterans (I70.-)
senile (I70.-)

I77.7 Other arterial dissection
EXCLUDES2 *dissection of aorta (I71.0-)*
dissection of coronary artery (I25.42)
- ● I77.70 Dissection of unspecified artery CC/MCC Exc MCC
- I77.71 Dissection of carotid artery MCC
- I77.72 Dissection of iliac artery MCC
- I77.73 Dissection of renal artery MCC
- I77.74 Dissection of vertebral artery MCC
  EXCLUDES2 *aneurysm of vertebral artery (I72.6)*
- ● I77.75 Dissection of other precerebral arteries CC/MCC Exc MCC
  Dissection of basilar artery (trunk)
  EXCLUDES2 *aneurysm of carotid artery (I72.0)*
  aneurysm of other precerebral arteries (I72.5)
  aneurysm of vertebral artery (I72.6)
  dissection of carotid artery (I77.71)
  dissection of vertebral artery (I77.74)
- ● I77.76 Dissection of artery of upper extremity CC/MCC Exc MCC
- ● I77.77 Dissection of artery of lower extremity CC/MCC Exc MCC
- ▲ I77.79 Dissection of other uspecifiedt artery MCC

I77.8 Other specified disorders of arteries and arterioles
- I77.81 Aortic ectasia
  Ectatic aorta
  EXCLUDES1 *aortic aneurysm and dissection (I71.0-)*
  - I77.810 Thoracic aortic ectasia
  - I77.811 Abdominal aortic ectasia
  - I77.812 Thoracoabdominal aortic ectasia
  - I77.819 Aortic ectasia, unspecified site
- I77.89 Other specified disorders of arteries and arterioles

I77.9 Disorder of arteries and arterioles, unspecified

I78 Diseases of capillaries

I78.0 Hereditary hemorrhagic telangiectasia
Rendu-Osler-Weber disease

I78.1 Nevus, non-neoplastic
Araneus nevus
Senile nevus
Spider nevus
Stellar nevus
EXCLUDES1 *nevus NOS (D22.-)*
vascular NOS (Q82.5)
EXCLUDES2 *blue nevus (D22.-)*
flammeus nevus (Q82.5)
hairy nevus (D22.-)
melanocytic nevus (D22.-)
pigmented nevus (D22.-)
portwine nevus (Q82.5)
sanguineous nevus (Q82.5)
strawberry nevus (Q82.5)
verrucous nevus (Q82.5)

I78.8 Other diseases of capillaries

I78.9 Disease of capillaries, unspecified

I79 Disorders of arteries, arterioles and capillaries in diseases classified elsewhere

I79.0 Aneurysm of aorta in diseases classified elsewhere
Code first underlying disease
EXCLUDES1 *syphilitic aneurysm (A52.01)*

I79.1 Aortitis in diseases classified elsewhere
Code first underlying disease
EXCLUDES1 *syphilitic aortitis (A52.02)*

PDx Unacceptable principal diagnosis symbol per Medicare code edits; POA Code exempt from diagnosis present on admission requirement
? Questionable admission; CC Complication or comorbidity; CC/MCC Exc CC/MCC exclusion; MCC Major complication or comorbidity
PDx CC Principal diagnosis as its own CC; PDx MCC Principal diagnosis as its own MCC; Z1 Z code as first-listed diagnosis

I79.8 **Other disorders of arteries, arterioles and capillaries in diseases classified elsewhere**
Code first underlying disease, such as:
amyloidosis (E85.-)
EXCLUDES1 *diabetic (peripheral) angiopathy (E08-E13 with .51-.52)*
syphilitic endarteritis (A52.09)
tuberculous endarteritis (A18.89)

Diseases of veins, lymphatic vessels and lymph nodes, not elsewhere classified (I80-I89)

I80 Phlebitis and thrombophlebitis
INCLUDES *endophlebitis*
inflammation, vein
periphlebitis
suppurative phlebitis
Code first phlebitis and thrombophlebitis complicating abortion, ectopic or molar pregnancy (O00-O07, O08.7)
phlebitis and thrombophlebitis complicating pregnancy, childbirth and the puerperium (O22.-, O87.-)
EXCLUDES1 *venous embolism and thrombosis of lower extremities (I82.4-, I82.5-, I82.81-)*

I80.0 Phlebitis and thrombophlebitis of superficial vessels of lower extremities
Phlebitis and thrombophlebitis of femoropopliteal vein
I80.00 **Phlebitis and thrombophlebitis of superficial vessels of unspecified lower extremity**
I80.01 **Phlebitis and thrombophlebitis of superficial vessels of right lower extremity**
I80.02 **Phlebitis and thrombophlebitis of superficial vessels of left lower extremity**
I80.03 **Phlebitis and thrombophlebitis of superficial vessels of lower extremities, bilateral**

I80.1 Phlebitis and thrombophlebitis of femoral vein
I80.10 **Phlebitis and thrombophlebitis of unspecified femoral vein** CC
I80.11 **Phlebitis and thrombophlebitis of right femoral vein** CC
I80.12 **Phlebitis and thrombophlebitis of left femoral vein** CC
I80.13 **Phlebitis and thrombophlebitis of femoral vein, bilateral** CC

I80.2 Phlebitis and thrombophlebitis of other and unspecified deep vessels of lower extremities
I80.20 **Phlebitis and thrombophlebitis of unspecified deep vessels of lower extremities**
I80.201 **Phlebitis and thrombophlebitis of unspecified deep vessels of right lower extremity** CC
I80.202 **Phlebitis and thrombophlebitis of unspecified deep vessels of left lower extremity** CC
I80.203 **Phlebitis and thrombophlebitis of unspecified deep vessels of lower extremities, bilateral** CC
I80.209 **Phlebitis and thrombophlebitis of unspecified deep vessels of unspecified lower extremity** CC
I80.21 **Phlebitis and thrombophlebitis of iliac vein**
I80.211 **Phlebitis and thrombophlebitis of right iliac vein** CC
I80.212 **Phlebitis and thrombophlebitis of left iliac vein** CC
I80.213 **Phlebitis and thrombophlebitis of iliac vein, bilateral** CC
I80.219 **Phlebitis and thrombophlebitis of unspecified iliac vein** CC
I80.22 **Phlebitis and thrombophlebitis of popliteal vein**
I80.221 **Phlebitis and thrombophlebitis of right popliteal vein** CC
I80.222 **Phlebitis and thrombophlebitis of left popliteal vein** CC
I80.223 **Phlebitis and thrombophlebitis of popliteal vein, bilateral** CC
I80.229 **Phlebitis and thrombophlebitis of unspecified popliteal vein** CC
I80.23 **Phlebitis and thrombophlebitis of tibial vein**
I80.231 **Phlebitis and thrombophlebitis of right tibial vein** CC
I80.232 **Phlebitis and thrombophlebitis of left tibial vein** CC
I80.233 **Phlebitis and thrombophlebitis of tibial vein, bilateral** CC
I80.239 **Phlebitis and thrombophlebitis of unspecified tibial vein** CC
I80.29 **Phlebitis and thrombophlebitis of other deep vessels of lower extremities**
I80.291 **Phlebitis and thrombophlebitis of other deep vessels of right lower extremity** CC
I80.292 **Phlebitis and thrombophlebitis of other deep vessels of left lower extremity** CC
I80.293 **Phlebitis and thrombophlebitis of other deep vessels of lower extremity, bilateral** CC
I80.299 **Phlebitis and thrombophlebitis of other deep vessels of unspecified lower extremity** CC
I80.3 **Phlebitis and thrombophlebitis of lower extremities, unspecified**
I80.8 **Phlebitis and thrombophlebitis of other sites**
I80.9 **Phlebitis and thrombophlebitis of unspecified site**

I81 **Portal vein thrombosis** MCC
Portal (vein) obstruction
EXCLUDES2 *hepatic vein thrombosis (I82.0)*
phlebitis of portal vein (K75.1)

I82 Other venous embolism and thrombosis
Code first venous embolism and thrombosis complicating:
abortion, ectopic or molar pregnancy (O00-O07, O08.7)
pregnancy, childbirth and the puerperium (O22.-, O87.-)
EXCLUDES2 *venous embolism and thrombosis (of):*
cerebral (I63.6, I67.6)
coronary (I21-I25)
intracranial and intraspinal, septic or NOS (G08)
intracranial, nonpyogenic (I67.6)
intraspinal, nonpyogenic (G95.1)
mesenteric ►(K55.0-)◄
portal (I81)
pulmonary (I26.-)
I82.0 **Budd-Chiari syndrome** MCC
Hepatic vein thrombosis
I82.1 **Thrombophlebitis migrans** CC
I82.2 **Embolism and thrombosis of vena cava and other thoracic veins**
I82.21 **Embolism and thrombosis of superior vena cava**
I82.210 **Acute embolism and thrombosis of superior vena cava** CC
Embolism and thrombosis of superior vena cava NOS
I82.211 **Chronic embolism and thrombosis of superior vena cava** CC
I82.22 **Embolism and thrombosis of inferior vena cava**
I82.220 **Acute embolism and thrombosis of inferior vena cava** MCC
Embolism and thrombosis of inferior vena cava NOS
I82.221 **Chronic embolism and thrombosis of inferior vena cava** MCC
I82.29 **Embolism and thrombosis of other thoracic veins**
Embolism and thrombosis of brachiocephalic (innominate) vein
I82.290 **Acute embolism and thrombosis of other thoracic veins** CC
I82.291 **Chronic embolism and thrombosis of other thoracic veins** CC
I82.3 **Embolism and thrombosis of renal vein** CC
I82.4 **Acute embolism and thrombosis of deep veins of lower extremity**

Unspecified Code Other Specified Code Manifestation Code N Newborn P Pediatric M Maternity A Adult ♂ Male ♀ Female
● New Code ▲ Revised Code Title ►◄ Revised Text NOTES INCLUDES EXCLUDES1 Not coded here EXCLUDES2 Not included here
4th character required 5th character required 6th character required 7th character required
Extension 'X' Alert HAC Hospital-acquired condition (HAC) alert AHA AHA Coding Clinic®

I82.40 Acute embolism and thrombosis of unspecified deep veins of lower extremity
Deep vein thrombosis NOS
DVT NOS
EXCLUDES1 *acute embolism and thrombosis of unspecified deep veins of distal lower extremity (I82.4Z-)*
acute embolism and thrombosis of unspecified deep veins of proximal lower extremity (I82.4Y-)
- I82.401 **Acute embolism and thrombosis of unspecified deep veins of right lower extremity** CC HAC
- I82.402 **Acute embolism and thrombosis of unspecified deep veins of left lower extremity** CC HAC
- I82.403 **Acute embolism and thrombosis of unspecified deep veins of lower extremity, bilateral** CC HAC
- I82.409 **Acute embolism and thrombosis of unspecified deep veins of unspecified lower extremity** CC HAC

I82.41 Acute embolism and thrombosis of femoral vein
- I82.411 **Acute embolism and thrombosis of right femoral vein** CC HAC
- I82.412 **Acute embolism and thrombosis of left femoral vein** CC HAC
- I82.413 **Acute embolism and thrombosis of femoral vein, bilateral** CC HAC
- I82.419 **Acute embolism and thrombosis of unspecified femoral vein** CC HAC

I82.42 Acute embolism and thrombosis of iliac vein
- I82.421 **Acute embolism and thrombosis of right iliac vein** CC HAC
- I82.422 **Acute embolism and thrombosis of left iliac vein** CC HAC
- I82.423 **Acute embolism and thrombosis of iliac vein, bilateral** CC HAC
- I82.429 **Acute embolism and thrombosis of unspecified iliac vein** CC HAC

I82.43 Acute embolism and thrombosis of popliteal vein
- I82.431 **Acute embolism and thrombosis of right popliteal vein** CC HAC
- I82.432 **Acute embolism and thrombosis of left popliteal vein** CC HAC
- I82.433 **Acute embolism and thrombosis of popliteal vein, bilateral** CC HAC
- I82.439 **Acute embolism and thrombosis of unspecified popliteal vein** CC HAC

I82.44 Acute embolism and thrombosis of tibial vein
- I82.441 **Acute embolism and thrombosis of right tibial vein** CC HAC
- I82.442 **Acute embolism and thrombosis of left tibial vein** CC HAC
- I82.443 **Acute embolism and thrombosis of tibial vein, bilateral** CC HAC
- I82.449 **Acute embolism and thrombosis of unspecified tibial vein** CC HAC

I82.49 Acute embolism and thrombosis of other specified deep vein of lower extremity
- I82.491 **Acute embolism and thrombosis of other specified deep vein of right lower extremity** CC HAC
- I82.492 **Acute embolism and thrombosis of other specified deep vein of left lower extremity** CC HAC
- I82.493 **Acute embolism and thrombosis of other specified deep vein of lower extremity, bilateral** CC HAC
- I82.499 **Acute embolism and thrombosis of other specified deep vein of unspecified lower extremity** CC HAC

I82.4Y Acute embolism and thrombosis of unspecified deep veins of proximal lower extremity
Acute embolism and thrombosis of deep vein of thigh NOS
Acute embolism and thrombosis of deep vein of upper leg NOS
- I82.4Y1 **Acute embolism and thrombosis of unspecified deep veins of right proximal lower extremity** CC HAC
- I82.4Y2 **Acute embolism and thrombosis of unspecified deep veins of left proximal lower extremity** CC HAC
- I82.4Y3 **Acute embolism and thrombosis of unspecified deep veins of proximal lower extremity, bilateral** CC HAC
- I82.4Y9 **Acute embolism and thrombosis of unspecified deep veins of unspecified proximal lower extremity** CC HAC

I82.4Z Acute embolism and thrombosis of unspecified deep veins of distal lower extremity
Acute embolism and thrombosis of deep vein of calf NOS
Acute embolism and thrombosis of deep vein of lower leg NOS
- I82.4Z1 **Acute embolism and thrombosis of unspecified deep veins of right distal lower extremity** CC HAC
- I82.4Z2 **Acute embolism and thrombosis of unspecified deep veins of left distal lower extremity** CC HAC
- I82.4Z3 **Acute embolism and thrombosis of unspecified deep veins of distal lower extremity, bilateral** CC HAC
- I82.4Z9 **Acute embolism and thrombosis of unspecified deep veins of unspecified distal lower extremity** CC HAC

I82.5 Chronic embolism and thrombosis of deep veins of lower extremity
Use additional code, if applicable, for associated long-term (current) use of anticoagulants (Z79.01)
EXCLUDES1 *personal history of venous embolism and thrombosis (Z86.718)*

I82.50 Chronic embolism and thrombosis of unspecified deep veins of lower extremity
EXCLUDES1 *chronic embolism and thrombosis of unspecified deep veins of distal lower extremity (I82.5Z-)*
chronic embolism and thrombosis of unspecified deep veins of proximal lower extremity (I82.5Y-)
- I82.501 **Chronic embolism and thrombosis of unspecified deep veins of right lower extremity** CC
- I82.502 **Chronic embolism and thrombosis of unspecified deep veins of left lower extremity** CC
- I82.503 **Chronic embolism and thrombosis of unspecified deep veins of lower extremity, bilateral** CC
- I82.509 **Chronic embolism and thrombosis of unspecified deep veins of unspecified lower extremity** CC

I82.51 Chronic embolism and thrombosis of femoral vein
- I82.511 **Chronic embolism and thrombosis of right femoral vein** CC
- I82.512 **Chronic embolism and thrombosis of left femoral vein** CC
- I82.513 **Chronic embolism and thrombosis of femoral vein, bilateral** CC
- I82.519 **Chronic embolism and thrombosis of unspecified femoral vein** CC

I82.52 Chronic embolism and thrombosis of iliac vein
- I82.521 **Chronic embolism and thrombosis of right iliac vein** CC
- I82.522 **Chronic embolism and thrombosis of left iliac vein** CC
- I82.523 **Chronic embolism and thrombosis of iliac vein, bilateral** CC
- I82.529 **Chronic embolism and thrombosis of unspecified iliac vein** CC

I82.53 Chronic embolism and thrombosis of popliteal vein

PDx Unacceptable principal diagnosis symbol per Medicare code edits; POA Code exempt from diagnosis present on admission requirement; ? Questionable admission; CC Complication or comorbidity; CC/MCC Excl CC/MCC exclusion; MCC Major complication or comorbidity; PDx CC Principal diagnosis as its own CC; PDx MCC Principal diagnosis as its own MCC; Z1 Z code as first-listed diagnosis

When symbols appear on a code that requires a 7th character extension, refer to Appendix D to identify applicable 7th character codes.

I82.531 Chronic embolism and thrombosis of right popliteal vein
I82.532 Chronic embolism and thrombosis of left popliteal vein
I82.533 Chronic embolism and thrombosis of popliteal vein, bilateral
I82.539 Chronic embolism and thrombosis of unspecified popliteal vein

I82.54 Chronic embolism and thrombosis of tibial vein
I82.541 Chronic embolism and thrombosis of right tibial vein
I82.542 Chronic embolism and thrombosis of left tibial vein
I82.543 Chronic embolism and thrombosis of tibial vein, bilateral
I82.549 Chronic embolism and thrombosis of unspecified tibial vein

I82.59 Chronic embolism and thrombosis of other specified deep vein of lower extremity
I82.591 Chronic embolism and thrombosis of other specified deep vein of right lower extremity
I82.592 Chronic embolism and thrombosis of other specified deep vein of left lower extremity
I82.593 Chronic embolism and thrombosis of other specified deep vein of lower extremity, bilateral
I82.599 Chronic embolism and thrombosis of other specified deep vein of unspecified lower extremity

I82.5Y Chronic embolism and thrombosis of unspecified deep veins of proximal lower extremity
Chronic embolism and thrombosis of deep veins of thigh NOS
Chronic embolism and thrombosis of deep veins of upper leg NOS
I82.5Y1 Chronic embolism and thrombosis of unspecified deep veins of right proximal lower extremity
I82.5Y2 Chronic embolism and thrombosis of unspecified deep veins of left proximal lower extremity
I82.5Y3 Chronic embolism and thrombosis of unspecified deep veins of proximal lower extremity, bilateral
I82.5Y9 Chronic embolism and thrombosis of unspecified deep veins of unspecified proximal lower extremity

I82.5Z Chronic embolism and thrombosis of unspecified deep veins of distal lower extremity
Chronic embolism and thrombosis of deep veins of calf NOS
Chronic embolism and thrombosis of deep veins of lower leg NOS
I82.5Z1 Chronic embolism and thrombosis of unspecified deep veins of right distal lower extremity
I82.5Z2 Chronic embolism and thrombosis of unspecified deep veins of left distal lower extremity
I82.5Z3 Chronic embolism and thrombosis of unspecified deep veins of distal lower extremity, bilateral
I82.5Z9 Chronic embolism and thrombosis of unspecified deep veins of unspecified distal lower extremity

I82.6 Acute embolism and thrombosis of veins of upper extremity

I82.60 Acute embolism and thrombosis of unspecified veins of upper extremity
I82.601 Acute embolism and thrombosis of unspecified veins of right upper extremity
I82.602 Acute embolism and thrombosis of unspecified veins of left upper extremity
I82.603 Acute embolism and thrombosis of unspecified veins of upper extremity, bilateral
I82.609 Acute embolism and thrombosis of unspecified veins of unspecified upper extremity

I82.61 Acute embolism and thrombosis of superficial veins of upper extremity
Acute embolism and thrombosis of antecubital vein
Acute embolism and thrombosis of basilic vein
Acute embolism and thrombosis of cephalic vein
I82.611 Acute embolism and thrombosis of superficial veins of right upper extremity
I82.612 Acute embolism and thrombosis of superficial veins of left upper extremity
I82.613 Acute embolism and thrombosis of superficial veins of upper extremity, bilateral
I82.619 Acute embolism and thrombosis of superficial veins of unspecified upper extremity

I82.62 Acute embolism and thrombosis of deep veins of upper extremity
Acute embolism and thrombosis of brachial vein
Acute embolism and thrombosis of radial vein
Acute embolism and thrombosis of ulnar vein
I82.621 Acute embolism and thrombosis of deep veins of right upper extremity
I82.622 Acute embolism and thrombosis of deep veins of left upper extremity
I82.623 Acute embolism and thrombosis of deep veins of upper extremity, bilateral
I82.629 Acute embolism and thrombosis of deep veins of unspecified upper extremity

I82.7 Chronic embolism and thrombosis of veins of upper extremity
Use additional code, if applicable, for associated long-term (current) use of anticoagulants (Z79.01)
EXCLUDES1 *personal history of venous embolism and thrombosis (Z86.718)*

I82.70 Chronic embolism and thrombosis of unspecified veins of upper extremity
I82.701 Chronic embolism and thrombosis of unspecified veins of right upper extremity
I82.702 Chronic embolism and thrombosis of unspecified veins of left upper extremity
I82.703 Chronic embolism and thrombosis of unspecified veins of upper extremity, bilateral
I82.709 Chronic embolism and thrombosis of unspecified veins of unspecified upper extremity

I82.71 Chronic embolism and thrombosis of superficial veins of upper extremity
Chronic embolism and thrombosis of antecubital vein
Chronic embolism and thrombosis of basilic vein
Chronic embolism and thrombosis of cephalic vein
I82.711 Chronic embolism and thrombosis of superficial veins of right upper extremity
I82.712 Chronic embolism and thrombosis of superficial veins of left upper extremity
I82.713 Chronic embolism and thrombosis of superficial veins of upper extremity, bilateral
I82.719 Chronic embolism and thrombosis of superficial veins of unspecified upper extremity

I82.72 Chronic embolism and thrombosis of deep veins of upper extremity
Chronic embolism and thrombosis of brachial vein
Chronic embolism and thrombosis of radial vein
Chronic embolism and thrombosis of ulnar vein
I82.721 Chronic embolism and thrombosis of deep veins of right upper extremity

Unspecified Code | Other Specified Code | Manifestation Code | N Newborn | P Pediatric | M Maternity | A Adult | ♂ Male | ♀ Female
● New Code | ▲ Revised Code Title | ►◄ Revised Text | NOTES | INCLUDES | EXCLUDES1 Not coded here | EXCLUDES2 Not included here
4th character required | 5th character required | 6th character required | 7th character required
Extension 'X' Alert | HAC Hospital-acquired condition (HAC) alert | AHA AHA Coding Clinic©

When symbols appear on a code that requires a 7th character extension, refer to Appendix D to identify applicable 7th character codes.

I82.722 Chronic embolism and thrombosis of deep veins of left upper extremity CC
I82.723 Chronic embolism and thrombosis of deep veins of upper extremity, bilateral CC
I82.729 Chronic embolism and thrombosis of deep veins of unspecified upper extremity CC

5th I82.A Embolism and thrombosis of axillary vein
6th I82.A1 Acute embolism and thrombosis of axillary vein
I82.A11 Acute embolism and thrombosis of right axillary vein CC
I82.A12 Acute embolism and thrombosis of left axillary vein CC
I82.A13 Acute embolism and thrombosis of axillary vein, bilateral CC
I82.A19 Acute embolism and thrombosis of unspecified axillary vein CC
6th I82.A2 Chronic embolism and thrombosis of axillary vein
I82.A21 Chronic embolism and thrombosis of right axillary vein CC
I82.A22 Chronic embolism and thrombosis of left axillary vein CC
I82.A23 Chronic embolism and thrombosis of axillary vein, bilateral CC
I82.A29 Chronic embolism and thrombosis of unspecified axillary vein CC

5th I82.B Embolism and thrombosis of subclavian vein
6th I82.B1 Acute embolism and thrombosis of subclavian vein
I82.B11 Acute embolism and thrombosis of right subclavian vein CC
I82.B12 Acute embolism and thrombosis of left subclavian vein CC
I82.B13 Acute embolism and thrombosis of subclavian vein, bilateral CC
I82.B19 Acute embolism and thrombosis of unspecified subclavian vein CC
6th I82.B2 Chronic embolism and thrombosis of subclavian vein
I82.B21 Chronic embolism and thrombosis of right subclavian vein CC
I82.B22 Chronic embolism and thrombosis of left subclavian vein CC
I82.B23 Chronic embolism and thrombosis of subclavian vein, bilateral CC
I82.B29 Chronic embolism and thrombosis of unspecified subclavian vein CC

5th I82.C Embolism and thrombosis of internal jugular vein
6th I82.C1 Acute embolism and thrombosis of internal jugular vein
I82.C11 Acute embolism and thrombosis of right internal jugular vein CC
I82.C12 Acute embolism and thrombosis of left internal jugular vein CC
I82.C13 Acute embolism and thrombosis of internal jugular vein, bilateral CC
I82.C19 Acute embolism and thrombosis of unspecified internal jugular vein CC
6th I82.C2 Chronic embolism and thrombosis of internal jugular vein
I82.C21 Chronic embolism and thrombosis of right internal jugular vein CC
I82.C22 Chronic embolism and thrombosis of left internal jugular vein CC
I82.C23 Chronic embolism and thrombosis of internal jugular vein, bilateral CC
I82.C29 Chronic embolism and thrombosis of unspecified internal jugular vein CC

5th I82.8 Embolism and thrombosis of other specified veins
Use additional code, if applicable, for associated long-term (current) use of anticoagulants (Z79.01)
6th I82.81 Embolism and thrombosis of superficial veins of lower extremities
Embolism and thrombosis of saphenous vein (greater) (lesser)
I82.811 Embolism and thrombosis of superficial veins of right lower extremities CC
I82.812 Embolism and thrombosis of superficial veins of left lower extremities CC
I82.813 Embolism and thrombosis of superficial veins of lower extremities, bilateral CC
I82.819 Embolism and thrombosis of superficial veins of unspecified lower extremities CC
6th I82.89 Embolism and thrombosis of other specified veins
I82.890 Acute embolism and thrombosis of other specified veins CC
I82.891 Chronic embolism and thrombosis of other specified veins CC

5th I82.9 Embolism and thrombosis of unspecified vein
I82.90 Acute embolism and thrombosis of unspecified vein CC
Embolism of vein NOS
Thrombosis (vein) NOS
I82.91 Chronic embolism and thrombosis of unspecified vein CC

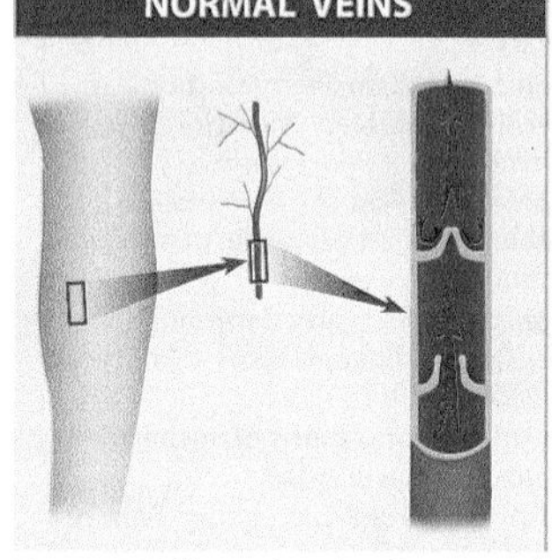

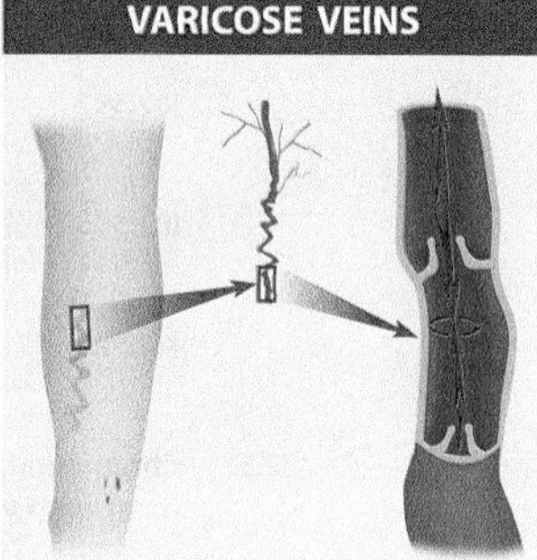

Figure 9.7 Illustration showing normal and varicose veins

4th I83 Varicose veins of lower extremities
EXCLUDES1 *varicose veins complicating pregnancy (O22.0-)*
varicose veins complicating the puerperium (O87.4)

5th I83.0 Varicose veins of lower extremities with ulcer
Use additional code to identify severity of ulcer (L97.-)
6th I83.00 Varicose veins of unspecified lower extremity with ulcer
I83.001 Varicose veins of unspecified lower extremity with ulcer of thigh A
I83.002 Varicose veins of unspecified lower extremity with ulcer of calf A
I83.003 Varicose veins of unspecified lower extremity with ulcer of ankle A
I83.004 Varicose veins of unspecified lower extremity with ulcer of heel and midfoot A
Varicose veins of unspecified lower extremity with ulcer of plantar surface of midfoot
I83.005 Varicose veins of unspecified lower extremity with ulcer other part of foot A
Varicose veins of unspecified lower extremity with ulcer of toe
I83.008 Varicose veins of unspecified lower extremity with ulcer other part of lower leg A
I83.009 Varicose veins of unspecified lower extremity with ulcer of unspecified site A
6th I83.01 Varicose veins of right lower extremity with ulcer
I83.011 Varicose veins of right lower extremity with ulcer of thigh A
I83.012 Varicose veins of right lower extremity with ulcer of calf A
I83.013 Varicose veins of right lower extremity with ulcer of ankle A
I83.014 Varicose veins of right lower extremity with ulcer of heel and midfoot A
Varicose veins of right lower extremity with ulcer of plantar surface of midfoot
I83.015 Varicose veins of right lower extremity with ulcer other part of foot A

PDx Unacceptable principal diagnosis symbol per Medicare code edits   POA Code exempt from diagnosis present on admission requirement
Q Questionable admission   CC Complication or comorbidity   CC/MCC Exc CC/MCC exclusion   MCC Major complication or comorbidity
PDx CC Principal diagnosis as its own CC   PDx MCC Principal diagnosis as its own MCC   Z Z code as first-listed diagnosis

Varicose veins of right lower extremity with ulcer of toe

I83.018 **Varicose veins of right lower extremity with ulcer other part of lower leg** A

I83.019 **Varicose veins of right lower extremity with ulcer of unspecified site** A

I83.02 **Varicose veins of left lower extremity with ulcer**

I83.021 **Varicose veins of left lower extremity with ulcer of thigh** A

I83.022 **Varicose veins of left lower extremity with ulcer of calf** A

I83.023 **Varicose veins of left lower extremity with ulcer of ankle** A

I83.024 **Varicose veins of left lower extremity with ulcer of heel and midfoot** A

Varicose veins of left lower extremity with ulcer of plantar surface of midfoot

I83.025 **Varicose veins of left lower extremity with ulcer other part of foot** A

Varicose veins of left lower extremity with ulcer of toe

I83.028 **Varicose veins of left lower extremity with ulcer other part of lower leg** A

I83.029 **Varicose veins of left lower extremity with ulcer of unspecified site** A

I83.1 **Varicose veins of lower extremities with inflammation**

I83.10 **Varicose veins of unspecified lower extremity with inflammation** A

I83.11 **Varicose veins of right lower extremity with inflammation** A

I83.12 **Varicose veins of left lower extremity with inflammation** A

I83.2 **Varicose veins of lower extremities with both ulcer and inflammation**

Use additional code to identify severity of ulcer (L97.-)

I83.20 **Varicose veins of unspecified lower extremity with both ulcer and inflammation**

I83.201 **Varicose veins of unspecified lower extremity with both ulcer of thigh and inflammation** A cc

I83.202 **Varicose veins of unspecified lower extremity with both ulcer of calf and inflammation** A cc

I83.203 **Varicose veins of unspecified lower extremity with both ulcer of ankle and inflammation** A cc

I83.204 **Varicose veins of unspecified lower extremity with both ulcer of heel and midfoot and inflammation** A cc

Varicose veins of unspecified lower extremity with both ulcer of plantar surface of midfoot and inflammation

I83.205 **Varicose veins of unspecified lower extremity with both ulcer other part of foot and inflammation** A cc

Varicose veins of unspecified lower extremity with both ulcer of toe and inflammation

I83.208 **Varicose veins of unspecified lower extremity with both ulcer of other part of lower extremity and inflammation** A cc

I83.209 **Varicose veins of unspecified lower extremity with both ulcer of unspecified site and inflammation** A cc

I83.21 **Varicose veins of right lower extremity with both ulcer and inflammation**

I83.211 **Varicose veins of right lower extremity with both ulcer of thigh and inflammation** A cc

I83.212 **Varicose veins of right lower extremity with both ulcer of calf and inflammation** A cc

I83.213 **Varicose veins of right lower extremity with both ulcer of ankle and inflammation** A cc

I83.214 **Varicose veins of right lower extremity with both ulcer of heel and midfoot and inflammation** A cc

Varicose veins of right lower extremity with both ulcer of plantar surface of midfoot and inflammation

I83.215 **Varicose veins of right lower extremity with both ulcer other part of foot and inflammation** A cc

Varicose veins of right lower extremity with both ulcer of toe and inflammation

I83.218 **Varicose veins of right lower extremity with both ulcer of other part of lower extremity and inflammation** A cc

I83.219 **Varicose veins of right lower extremity with both ulcer of unspecified site and inflammation** A cc

I83.22 **Varicose veins of left lower extremity with both ulcer and inflammation**

I83.221 **Varicose veins of left lower extremity with both ulcer of thigh and inflammation** A cc

I83.222 **Varicose veins of left lower extremity with both ulcer of calf and inflammation** A cc

I83.223 **Varicose veins of left lower extremity with both ulcer of ankle and inflammation** A cc

I83.224 **Varicose veins of left lower extremity with both ulcer of heel and midfoot and inflammation** A cc

Varicose veins of left lower extremity with both ulcer of plantar surface of midfoot and inflammation

I83.225 **Varicose veins of left lower extremity with both ulcer other part of foot and inflammation** A cc

Varicose veins of left lower extremity with both ulcer of toe and inflammation

I83.228 **Varicose veins of left lower extremity with both ulcer of other part of lower extremity and inflammation** A cc

I83.229 **Varicose veins of left lower extremity with both ulcer of unspecified site and inflammation** A cc

I83.8 **Varicose veins of lower extremities with other complications**

I83.81 **Varicose veins of lower extremities with pain**

I83.811 **Varicose veins of right lower extremities with pain** A

I83.812 **Varicose veins of left lower extremities with pain** A

I83.813 **Varicose veins of bilateral lower extremities with pain** A

I83.819 **Varicose veins of unspecified lower extremities with pain** A

I83.89 **Varicose veins of lower extremities with other complications**

Varicose veins of lower extremities with edema
Varicose veins of lower extremities with swelling

I83.891 **Varicose veins of right lower extremities with other complications** A

I83.892 **Varicose veins of left lower extremities with other complications** A

I83.893 **Varicose veins of bilateral lower extremities with other complications** A

I83.899 **Varicose veins of unspecified lower extremities with other complications** A

I83.9 **Asymptomatic varicose veins of lower extremities**

Phlebectasia of lower extremities
Varicose veins of lower extremities
Varix of lower extremities

I83.90 **Asymptomatic varicose veins of unspecified lower extremity** A

Varicose veins NOS

I83.91 **Asymptomatic varicose veins of right lower extremity** A

I83.92 **Asymptomatic varicose veins of left lower extremity** A

I83.93 **Asymptomatic varicose veins of bilateral lower extremities** A

Unspecified Code | Other Specified Code | Manifestation Code | N Newborn | P Pediatric | M Maternity | A Adult | ♂ Male | ♀ Female
● New Code ▲ Revised Code Title ▶◀ Revised Text NOTES INCLUDES EXCLUDES1 Not coded here EXCLUDES2 Not included here
4th character required 5th character required 6th character required 7th character required
Extension 'X' Alert HAC Hospital-acquired condition (HAC) alert AHA AHA Coding Clinic®

When symbols appear on a code that requires a 7th character extension, refer to Appendix D to identify applicable 7th character codes.

I85 Esophageal varices
Use additional code to identify:
alcohol abuse and dependence (F10.-)
I85.0 Esophageal varices
Idiopathic esophageal varices
Primary esophageal varices
I85.00 Esophageal varices without bleeding CC
Esophageal varices NOS
I85.01 Esophageal varices with bleeding MCC
I85.1 Secondary esophageal varices
Esophageal varices secondary to alcoholic liver disease
Esophageal varices secondary to cirrhosis of liver
Esophageal varices secondary to schistosomiasis
Esophageal varices secondary to toxic liver disease
Code first underlying disease
I85.10 Secondary esophageal varices without bleeding CC
I85.11 Secondary esophageal varices with bleeding MCC
I86 Varicose veins of other sites
EXCLUDES1 *varicose veins of unspecified site (I83.9-)*
EXCLUDES2 *retinal varices (H35.0-)*
I86.0 Sublingual varices
I86.1 Scrotal varices ♂
Varicocele
I86.2 Pelvic varices
I86.3 Vulval varices ♀
EXCLUDES1 *vulval varices complicating childbirth and the puerperium (O87.8)*
vulval varices complicating pregnancy (O22.1-)
I86.4 Gastric varices
I86.8 Varicose veins of other specified sites A
Varicose ulcer of nasal septum
I87 Other disorders of veins
I87.0 Postthrombotic syndrome
Chronic venous hypertension due to deep vein thrombosis
Postphlebitic syndrome
EXCLUDES1 *chronic venous hypertension without deep vein thrombosis (I87.3-)*
I87.00 Postthrombotic syndrome without complications
Asymptomatic Postthrombotic syndrome
I87.001 Postthrombotic syndrome without complications of right lower extremity
I87.002 Postthrombotic syndrome without complications of left lower extremity
I87.003 Postthrombotic syndrome without complications of bilateral lower extremity
I87.009 Postthrombotic syndrome without complications of unspecified extremity
Postthrombotic syndrome NOS
I87.01 Postthrombotic syndrome with ulcer
Use additional code to specify site and severity of ulcer (L97.-)
I87.011 Postthrombotic syndrome with ulcer of right lower extremity CC
I87.012 Postthrombotic syndrome with ulcer of left lower extremity CC
I87.013 Postthrombotic syndrome with ulcer of bilateral lower extremity CC
I87.019 Postthrombotic syndrome with ulcer of unspecified lower extremity CC
I87.02 Postthrombotic syndrome with inflammation
I87.021 Postthrombotic syndrome with inflammation of right lower extremity
I87.022 Postthrombotic syndrome with inflammation of left lower extremity
I87.023 Postthrombotic syndrome with inflammation of bilateral lower extremity
I87.029 Postthrombotic syndrome with inflammation of unspecified lower extremity
I87.03 Postthrombotic syndrome with ulcer and inflammation
Use additional code to specify site and severity of ulcer (L97.-)
I87.031 Postthrombotic syndrome with ulcer and inflammation of right lower extremity CC
I87.032 Postthrombotic syndrome with ulcer and inflammation of left lower extremity CC
I87.033 Postthrombotic syndrome with ulcer and inflammation of bilateral lower extremity CC
I87.039 Postthrombotic syndrome with ulcer and inflammation of unspecified lower extremity CC
I87.09 Postthrombotic syndrome with other complications
I87.091 Postthrombotic syndrome with other complications of right lower extremity
I87.092 Postthrombotic syndrome with other complications of left lower extremity
I87.093 Postthrombotic syndrome with other complications of bilateral lower extremity
I87.099 Postthrombotic syndrome with other complications of unspecified lower extremity
I87.1 Compression of vein CC
Stricture of vein
Vena cava syndrome (inferior) (superior)
EXCLUDES2 *compression of pulmonary vein (I28.8)*
I87.2 Venous insufficiency (chronic) (peripheral)
Stasis dermatitis
EXCLUDES1 *stasis dermatitis with varicose veins of lower extremities (I83.1-, I83.2-)*
I87.3 Chronic venous hypertension (idiopathic)
Stasis edema
EXCLUDES1 *chronic venous hypertension due to deep vein thrombosis (I87.0-)*
varicose veins of lower extremities (I83.-)
I87.30 Chronic venous hypertension (idiopathic) without complications
Asymptomatic chronic venous hypertension (idiopathic)
I87.301 Chronic venous hypertension (idiopathic) without complications of right lower extremity
I87.302 Chronic venous hypertension (idiopathic) without complications of left lower extremity
I87.303 Chronic venous hypertension (idiopathic) without complications of bilateral lower extremity
I87.309 Chronic venous hypertension (idiopathic) without complications of unspecified lower extremity
Chronic venous hypertension NOS
I87.31 Chronic venous hypertension (idiopathic) with ulcer
Use additional code to specify site and severity of ulcer (L97.-)
I87.311 Chronic venous hypertension (idiopathic) with ulcer of right lower extremity CC
I87.312 Chronic venous hypertension (idiopathic) with ulcer of left lower extremity CC
I87.313 Chronic venous hypertension (idiopathic) with ulcer of bilateral lower extremity CC
I87.319 Chronic venous hypertension (idiopathic) with ulcer of unspecified lower extremity CC
I87.32 Chronic venous hypertension (idiopathic) with inflammation
I87.321 Chronic venous hypertension (idiopathic) with inflammation of right lower extremity
I87.322 Chronic venous hypertension (idiopathic) with inflammation of left lower extremity
I87.323 Chronic venous hypertension (idiopathic) with inflammation of bilateral lower extremity
I87.329 Chronic venous hypertension (idiopathic) with inflammation of unspecified lower extremity
I87.33 Chronic venous hypertension (idiopathic) with ulcer and inflammation
Use additional code to specify site and severity of ulcer (L97.-)

Unacceptable principal diagnosis symbol per Medicare code edits · Code exempt from diagnosis present on admission requirement · Questionable admission · CC Complication or comorbidity · CC/MCC exclusion · MCC Major complication or comorbidity · Principal diagnosis as its own CC · Principal diagnosis as its own MCC · Z code as first-listed diagnosis

When symbols appear on a code that requires a 7th character extension, refer to Appendix D to identify applicable 7th character codes.

I87.331 Chronic venous hypertension (idiopathic) with ulcer and inflammation of right lower extremity
I87.332 Chronic venous hypertension (idiopathic) with ulcer and inflammation of left lower extremity
I87.333 Chronic venous hypertension (idiopathic) with ulcer and inflammation of bilateral lower extremity
I87.339 Chronic venous hypertension (idiopathic) with ulcer and inflammation of unspecified lower extremity

I87.39 Chronic venous hypertension (idiopathic) with other complications
I87.391 Chronic venous hypertension (idiopathic) with other complications of right lower extremity
I87.392 Chronic venous hypertension (idiopathic) with other complications of left lower extremity
I87.393 Chronic venous hypertension (idiopathic) with other complications of bilateral lower extremity
I87.399 Chronic venous hypertension (idiopathic) with other complications of unspecified lower extremity

I87.8 Other specified disorders of veins
Phlebosclerosis
Venofibrosis

I87.9 Disorder of vein, unspecified

I88 Nonspecific lymphadenitis
EXCLUDES1 *acute lymphadenitis, except mesenteric (L04.-)*
enlarged lymph nodes NOS (R59.-)
human immunodeficiency virus [HIV] disease resulting in generalized lymphadenopathy (B20)

I88.0 Nonspecific mesenteric lymphadenitis
Mesenteric lymphadenitis (acute)(chronic)

I88.1 Chronic lymphadenitis, except mesenteric
Adenitis
Lymphadenitis

I88.8 Other nonspecific lymphadenitis

I88.9 Nonspecific lymphadenitis, unspecified
Lymphadenitis NOS

I89 Other noninfective disorders of lymphatic vessels and lymph nodes
EXCLUDES1 *chylocele, tunica vaginalis (nonfilarial) NOS ▶(N50.89)◀*
enlarged lymph nodes NOS (R59.-)
filarial chylocele (B74.-)
hereditary lymphedema (Q82.0)

I89.0 Lymphedema, not elsewhere classified
Elephantiasis (nonfilarial) NOS
Lymphangiectasis
Obliteration, lymphatic vessel
Praecox lymphedema
Secondary lymphedema
EXCLUDES1 *postmastectomy lymphedema (I97.2)*

I89.1 Lymphangitis
Chronic lymphangitis
Lymphangitis NOS
Subacute lymphangitis
EXCLUDES1 *acute lymphangitis (L03.-)*

I89.8 Other specified noninfective disorders of lymphatic vessels and lymph nodes
Chylocele (nonfilarial)
Chylous ascites
Chylous cyst
Lipomelanotic reticulosis
Lymph node or vessel fistula
Lymph node or vessel infarction
Lymph node or vessel rupture

I89.9 Noninfective disorder of lymphatic vessels and lymph nodes, unspecified
Disease of lymphatic vessels NOS

Other and unspecified disorders of the circulatory system (I95-I99)

I95 Hypotension
EXCLUDES1 *cardiovascular collapse (R57.9)*
maternal hypotension syndrome (O26.5-)
nonspecific low blood pressure reading NOS (R03.1)

I95.0 Idiopathic hypotension

I95.1 Orthostatic hypotension
Hypotension, postural
EXCLUDES1 *neurogenic orthostatic hypotension [Shy-Drager] (G90.3)*
orthostatic hypotension due to drugs (I95.2)

I95.2 Hypotension due to drugs
Orthostatic hypotension due to drugs
Use additional code for adverse effect, if applicable, to identify drug (T36-T50 with fifth or sixth character 5)

I95.3 Hypotension of hemodialysis
Intra-dialytic hypotension

I95.8 Other hypotension
I95.81 Postprocedural hypotension
I95.89 Other hypotension
Chronic hypotension

I95.9 Hypotension, unspecified

I96 Gangrene, not elsewhere classified
Gangrenous cellulitis
EXCLUDES1 *gangrene in atherosclerosis of native arteries of the extremities (I70.26)*
gangrene in diabetes mellitus (E08-E13 ▶with .52◀)
gangrene in hernia (K40.1, K40.4, K41.1, K41.4, K42.1, K43.1-, K44.1, K45.1, K46.1)
gangrene in other peripheral vascular diseases (I73.-)
gangrene of certain specified sites - see Alphabetical Index
gas gangrene (A48.0)
pyoderma gangrenosum (L88)

I97 Intraoperative and postprocedural complications and disorders of circulatory system, not elsewhere classified
EXCLUDES2 *postprocedural shock (T81.1-)*

I97.0 Postcardiotomy syndrome

I97.1 Other postprocedural cardiac functional disturbances
EXCLUDES2 *acute pulmonary insufficiency following thoracic surgery (J95.1)*
intraoperative cardiac functional disturbances (I97.7-)

I97.11 Postprocedural cardiac insufficiency
I97.110 Postprocedural cardiac insufficiency following cardiac surgery
I97.111 Postprocedural cardiac insufficiency following other surgery

I97.12 Postprocedural cardiac arrest
I97.120 Postprocedural cardiac arrest following cardiac surgery
I97.121 Postprocedural cardiac arrest following other surgery

I97.13 Postprocedural heart failure
Use additional code to identify the heart failure (I50.-)
I97.130 Postprocedural heart failure following cardiac surgery
I97.131 Postprocedural heart failure following other surgery

I97.19 Other postprocedural cardiac functional disturbances
Use additional code, if applicable, to further specify disorder
I97.190 Other postprocedural cardiac functional disturbances following cardiac surgery
I97.191 Other postprocedural cardiac functional disturbances following other surgery

I97.2 Postmastectomy lymphedema syndrome A
Elephantiasis due to mastectomy
Obliteration of lymphatic vessels

I97.3 Postprocedural hypertension

I97.4 Intraoperative hemorrhage and hematoma of a circulatory system organ or structure complicating a procedure
- EXCLUDES1 *intraoperative hemorrhage and hematoma of a circulatory system organ or structure due to accidental puncture and laceration during a procedure (I97.5-)*
- EXCLUDES2 *intraoperative cerebrovascular hemorrhage complicating a procedure (G97.3-)*

I97.41 Intraoperative hemorrhage and hematoma of a circulatory system organ or structure complicating a circulatory system procedure
- I97.410 Intraoperative hemorrhage and hematoma of a circulatory system organ or structure complicating a cardiac catheterization CC
- I97.411 Intraoperative hemorrhage and hematoma of a circulatory system organ or structure complicating a cardiac bypass CC
- I97.418 Intraoperative hemorrhage and hematoma of a circulatory system organ or structure complicating other circulatory system procedure CC

I97.42 Intraoperative hemorrhage and hematoma of a circulatory system organ or structure complicating other procedure CC

I97.5 Accidental puncture and laceration of a circulatory system organ or structure during a procedure
- EXCLUDES2 *accidental puncture and laceration of brain during a procedure (G97.4-)*

I97.51 Accidental puncture and laceration of a circulatory system organ or structure during a circulatory system procedure CC

I97.52 Accidental puncture and laceration of a circulatory system organ or structure during other procedure CC

▲ I97.6 Postprocedural hemorrhage, ▶hematoma and seroma◀ of a circulatory system organ or structure following a procedure
- EXCLUDES2 *postprocedural cerebrovascular hemorrhage complicating a procedure (G97.5-)*

▲ I97.61 Postprocedural ▶hemorrhage of◀ a circulatory system organ or structure following a circulatory system procedure
- ▲ I97.610 Postprocedural ▶hemorrhage of◀ a circulatory system organ or structure following a cardiac catheterization CC
- ▲ I97.611 Postprocedural ▶hemorrhage of◀ a circulatory system organ or structure following cardiac bypass CC
- ▲ I97.618 Postprocedural ▶hemorrhage of◀ a circulatory system organ or structure following other circulatory system procedure CC

▲ I97.62 Postprocedural hemorrhage, ▶hematoma and seroma◀ of a circulatory system organ or structure following other procedure
- ● I97.620 Postprocedural hemorrhage of a circulatory system organ or structure following other procedure CC CC/MCC Exc
- ● I97.621 Postprocedural hematoma of a circulatory system organ or structure following other procedure CC CC/MCC Exc
- ● I97.622 Postprocedural seroma of a circulatory system organ or structure following other procedure

● I97.63 Postprocedural hematoma of a circulatory system organ or structure following a circulatory system procedure
- ● I97.630 Postprocedural hematoma of a circulatory system organ or structure following a cardiac catheterization CC CC/MCC Exc
- ● I97.631 Postprocedural hematoma of a circulatory system organ or structure following cardiac bypass CC CC/MCC Exc
- ● I97.638 Postprocedural hematoma of a circulatory system organ or structure following other circulatory system procedure CC CC/MCC Exc

● I97.64 Postprocedural seroma of a circulatory system organ or structure following a circulatory system procedure
- ● I97.640 Postprocedural seroma of a circulatory system organ or structure following a cardiac catheterization
- ● I97.641 Postprocedural seroma of a circulatory system organ or structure following cardiac bypass
- ● I97.648 Postprocedural seroma of a circulatory system organ or structure following other circulatory system procedure

I97.7 Intraoperative cardiac functional disturbances
- EXCLUDES2 *acute pulmonary insufficiency following thoracic surgery (J95.1)*
- *postprocedural cardiac functional disturbances (I97.1-)*

I97.71 Intraoperative cardiac arrest
- I97.710 Intraoperative cardiac arrest during cardiac surgery CC
- I97.711 Intraoperative cardiac arrest during other surgery CC

I97.79 Other intraoperative cardiac functional disturbances
Use additional code, if applicable, to further specify disorder
- I97.790 Other intraoperative cardiac functional disturbances during cardiac surgery CC
- I97.791 Other intraoperative cardiac functional disturbances during other surgery CC

I97.8 Other intraoperative and postprocedural complications and disorders of the circulatory system, not elsewhere classified
Use additional code, if applicable, to further specify disorder

I97.81 Intraoperative cerebrovascular infarction
- I97.810 Intraoperative cerebrovascular infarction during cardiac surgery CC
- I97.811 Intraoperative cerebrovascular infarction during other surgery CC

I97.82 Postprocedural cerebrovascular infarction
- ▲ I97.820 Postprocedural cerebrovascular infarction ▶following◀ cardiac surgery CC
- ▲ I97.821 Postprocedural cerebrovascular infarction ▶following◀ other surgery CC

I97.88 Other intraoperative complications of the circulatory system, not elsewhere classified CC

I97.89 Other postprocedural complications and disorders of the circulatory system, not elsewhere classified CC

I99 Other and unspecified disorders of circulatory system
- I99.8 Other disorder of circulatory system
- I99.9 Unspecified disorder of circulatory system

PDx Unacceptable principal diagnosis symbol per Medicare code edits · POA Code exempt from diagnosis present on admission requirement
Q Questionable admission · CC Complication or comorbidity · CC/MCC Exc CC/MCC exclusion · MCC Major complication or comorbidity
PDx CC Principal diagnosis as its own CC · PDx MCC Principal diagnosis as its own MCC · Z1 Z code as first-listed diagnosis

When symbols appear on a code that requires a 7th character extension, refer to Appendix D to identify applicable 7th character codes.

Chapter 10: Diseases of the Respiratory System (J00-J99)

Guidelines for Assigning Codes From This Chapter

The respiratory system includes those organs that help you breathe, and those are the areas you'll find covered in Chapter 10. Many of the diagnoses relate to infections, but you'll also find other breathing-related conditions in this chapter, such as asthma and disorders caused by environmental toxins.

List of Sections

- J00-J06: Acute upper respiratory infections
- J09-J18: Influenza and pneumonia
- J20-J22: Other acute lower respiratory infections
- J30-J39: Other diseases of upper respiratory tract
- J40-J47: Chronic lower respiratory diseases
- J60-J70: Lung diseases due to external agents
- J80-J84: Other respiratory diseases principally affecting the interstitium
- J85-J86: Suppurative and necrotic conditions of the lower respiratory tract
- J90-J94: Other diseases of the pleura
- J95: Intraoperative and postprocedural complications and disorders of respiratory system, not elsewhere classified
- J96-J99: Other diseases of the respiratory system

Highlights From the ICD-10-CM Official Guidelines for Coding and Reporting

The ICD-10-CM Official Guidelines for Coding and Reporting for Chapter 10 reveal proper coding solutions for four areas: chronic obstructive pulmonary disease (COPD) and asthma, acute respiratory failure, influenza due to certain viruses, and ventilator-associated pneumonia. The information that follows covers the major points from Section I.C.10 of the 2017 Official Guidelines.

Focus on the COPD and Asthma Coding Fundamentals

Proper code selection in categories J44 (Other chronic obstructive pulmonary diseases) and J45 (Asthma) requires you to distinguish between uncomplicated cases and those in acute exacerbation. An acute exacerbation is a worsening or a decompensation of a chronic condition. Although an exacerbation can be triggered by an infection, avoid assuming that a respiratory infection in a patient with chronic lung disease is equivalent to an acute exacerbation.

Determine Proper Place for Acute Respiratory Failure

Primary: The guidelines allow you to report codes from J96.0 (*Acute respiratory failure*) or J96.2 (*Acute and chronic respiratory failure*) as a principal diagnosis, but they do stress the need to confirm it was the chief reason for the admission. Also, if other guidelines have related sequencing instructions, you should follow those before choosing acute respiratory failure as the principal diagnosis.

Secondary: Acute respiratory failure also can be a secondary diagnosis. You'd choose this sequencing when the diagnosis either wasn't present on admission or the diagnosis otherwise doesn't qualify as the principal diagnosis.

More sequencing rules: A patient may have more than one acute condition present on admission. To choose the principal diagnosis, you need to know which diagnosis is chiefly responsible for the admission and whether any ICD-10-CM sequencing rules affect those diagnoses. If multiple conditions share the same level of responsibility for admission, then inpatient facilities should follow the rules in Section II.C of the Official Guidelines, which state you may sequence any of the diagnoses first.

Inpatient Coders Need to Check This Influenza Rule

The guidelines for influenza hold an important exception for facility coders. The guidelines state that you should report only confirmed cases of influenza due to certain identified influenza virus from category J09 (*Influenza due to certain identified influenza viruses*) and J10 (*Influenza due to other identified influenza virus*). This is an exception to hospital inpatient guideline Section II, H. (*Uncertain Diagnosis*). Facilities should be sure to mark this exception with a reminder that even inpatient coders should report only confirmed cases using the specific influenza diagnoses listed above.

Note that "confirmed" simply means the provider must document that the patient has one of the listed types of influenza. You don't have to have a positive lab test to report the code.

What if it's not confirmed? For cases of these influenza diagnoses that are not confirmed, you should choose a code from J11 (*Influenza due to unidentified virus*).Terms you may see related to unconfirmed diagnoses include suspected, possible, and probable.

Take the Guesswork out of Ventilator-associated Pneumonia

Ventilator-associated pneumonia, or VAP, is a life-threatening lung infection that affects patients who are already critically ill. As with all procedural or postprocedural complications, code assignment is based on the provider's documentation of the relationship between the condition and the procedure.

Let the provider connect the dots: Don't assume that a patient on a mechanical ventilator who develops pneumonia has ventilator-associated pneumonia. You should report J95.851 (*Ventilator-associated pneumonia*) only when the provider documents this specific condition. If the documentation is unclear as to whether the patient has a pneumonia that is a complication attributable to the mechanical ventilator, query the provider.

You won't need an additional code from categories J12-J18 to identify the type of pneumonia, but remember to report an additional code to identify the organism, e.g., B96.5 (*Pseudomonas aeruginosa*).

VAP after admission: A patient with another type of pneumonia, such as J13 (*Pneumonia due to Streptococcus pneumonia*), may develop VAP after admission. You should assign the appropriate code from categories J12-J18 for the pneumonia diagnosed at the time of admission as the principal diagnosis. When VAP is documented, assign it as an additional diagnosis.

Anatomy of the Respiratory System

1. **An Outline of the Respiratory System**
   a) The human respiratory system is based on the following organs:
      i) nose
      ii) pharynx
      iii) larynx
      iv) trachea
      v) bronchi
      vi) lungs
   b) The process of respiration involves the exchange of oxygen and carbon dioxide between the atmosphere, blood and cells.

The Respiratory System

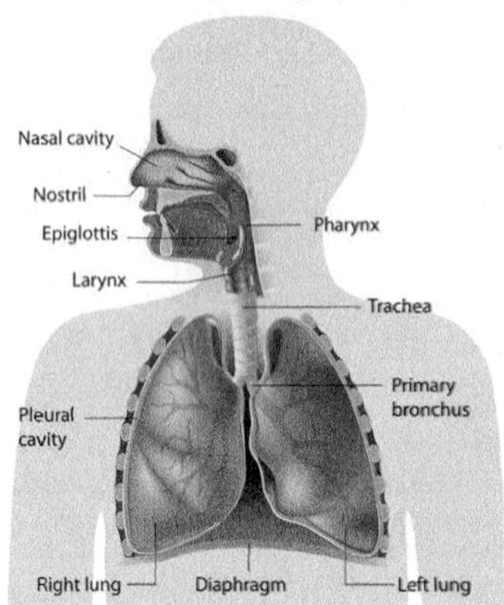

2. **The Anatomy of the Nose**
   a) The nostrils or external nares are openings into the external nose.
   b) The internal nares serve to connect the internal nose with the throat or pharynx.
   c) The nasal septum divides the nose into the right and left nasal cavities.
   d) The internal nose contains three turbinate bones (superior, middle and inferior meatus).
   e) The olfactory receptors are located in the superior meatus.
3. **The Anatomy of the Pharynx**
   a) The pharynx is a resonating chamber for speech sounds and also provides a passage to both air and food.
   b) The nasopharynx, oropharynx and laryngopharynx are the parts of the pharynx.
   c) The nasopharynx surrounds the pharyngeal tonsils. It contains two internal nares and the openings of the eustachian tubes.
   d) The oropharynx surrounds the palatine and lingual tonsils and its opening (or fauces) provides connection to the mouth.
   e) The laryngopharynx gets connected with the larynx on anterior aspect and the esophagus posteriorly.
4. **The Anatomy of the Larynx**
   a) The larynx is also known as the voice box.
   b) The skeleton of the larynx is made up of nine cartilages. Three of them are single (thyroid, cricoid, and epiglottis) and the remaining three (arytenoid, corniculate, and cuneiform) are paired cartilages.
   c) The thyroid cartilage is also known as the Adam's apple. It is the largest single cartilage of the laryngeal skeleton.
   d) The cricoid cartilage connects with the first tracheal ring and is made up of a single ring of cartilage.
   e) The epiglottis is a large and single leaf-shaped flap of elastic cartilage. It is lined with the mucous membrane and remains attached to the entrance of larynx. It pulls down over the glottis during the process of swallowing to obstruct the entrance of the fluids and food in the trachea.
   f) The arytenoid cartilages are formed by a pair of three ladle-shaped pyramids that remain attached to the laryngeal muscles and the vocal cords.
   g) The corniculate cartilages are based on two cone-shaped nodules of yellow elastic cartilage.
   h) The cuneiform cartilages are also known as the cartilages of Wrisberg. They are based on two rod-shaped pieces of yellow elastic cartilage.
   i) The mucous membrane of the larynx is divided into two pairs of folds. The vestibular folds (or false vocal cords) constitute the upper pair, while the vocal folds (or true vocal cords) form the lower pair of fold.
   j) The opening over the true vocal cords is known as the glottis.
5. **The Anatomy of the Trachea**
   a) The trachea is also known as the windpipe and located anteriorly to the esophagus.
   b) It begins at the larynx and gets divided into primary bronchi at the level of T4/T5 vertebrae.
   c) The trachea is lined by the respiratory epithelium and consists of a series of incomplete C-shaped cartilaginous rings.
6. **The Anatomy of the Bronchial Tree**
   a) The bronchial tree is based on right and left primary bronchi, secondary and tertiary bronchi, and the bronchioles.
   b) The right and left primary bronchi emanate from the trachea and merge with the right and left lungs.
   c) The primary bronchi further get branched into the secondary (or lobar) bronchi that penetrate into the lobes of the lungs.
   d) The secondary bronchi further get divided into the tertiary or segmental bronchi that penetrate into the segments of the lobes of the lungs.
   e) The bronchioles are the branches that emanate from the tertiary bronchi.
7. **The Anatomy of the Lungs**
   a) The lungs are the human organs of respiration.
   b) The right and left lungs are based on multiple lobes. The right lung contains three lobes, while the left lung is based on two lobes.
   c) The lungs are protected by the pleural membrane. The pleural membrane is further made up of two layers of serous membranes. The outer layer is known as the parietal pleura, while the inner layer is termed as the visceral pleura.
   d) The bronchopulmonary segment is a segment of lung tissue that is supplied by each of the tertiary bronchi. It is divided into multiple lobules that remain covered with the elastic connective tissue.
   e) A terminal bronchiole exists at the end of the conducting zone of the respiratory system.
   f) The microscopic respiratory bronchioles are the subdivisions of the terminal bronchioles. The atria or the alveolar ducts emanate from these respiratory bronchioles.
   g) The alveoli and alveolar sacs lie around the circumference of the alveolar ducts.
   h) The alveolar sac is made up of two or more alveoli with a common opening.
   i) The respiratory (or the alveolar capillary) membrane is a membrane that provides a medium for the movement of respiratory gases.
8. **The Process of Respiration**
   a) The respiration in humans is based on the following stages:
      i) Ventilation is also known as the breathing, which involves the movement of the ambient air into the alveoli of the lungs.
      ii) The process of pulmonary gas exchange is based on the exchange of respiratory gases between the alveoli and the pulmonary capillaries.
      iii) The gas process involves the transport of respiratory gases from the pulmonary capillaries to the peripheral capillaries in the organs via circulation.
      iv) Peripheral gas exchange is the process of exchange of respiratory gases between the tissue capillaries and the cells and mitochondria.
   b) Nasal breathing is the process of respiration that involves the inhalation and exhalation of the respiratory gases through the nose.

Common Pathologies

Sinusitis
Inflammation of mucous membrane lining that lines the paranasal sinuses. This inflammation dries out the sinuses and can also cause dizziness and difficulty breathing. Using a humidifier can alleviate symptoms

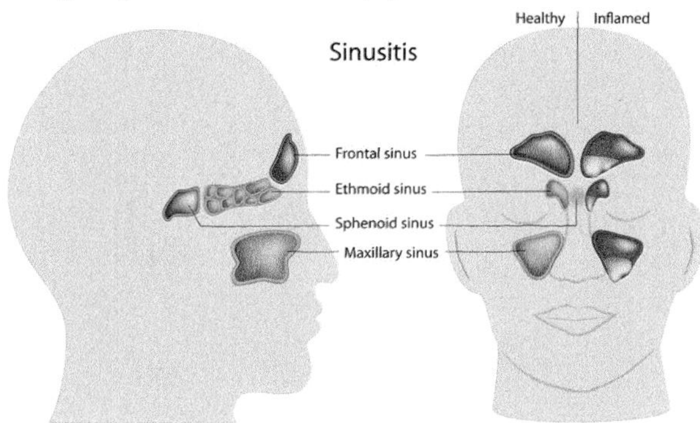

Epiglottitis

Inflammation of the epiglottis caused by H. Influenzae type B; characterized by fever and a severe sore throat and difficulty in swallowing.

Laryngitis
Inflammation of the larynx and vocal cords resulting in hoarseness of the voice (Dysphonia), and difficulty in swallowing (Dysphagia).

Pharyngitis
Inflammation of the pharynx, usually causing a sore throat. Acute Pharyngitis is a sudden, severe inflammation of the pharynx. Chronic Pharyngitis is a persistent throat inflammation that may be associated with the lymphoid granules in the pharyngeal mucosa.

Acute Bronchitis
Inflammation of the mucous membrane lining the bronchus, involves the trachea resulting in tracheobronchitis, chest tightness, fever, and a cough that progresses from nonproductive to productive.

Chronic Bronchitis
Inflammation of the bronchial mucous membrane characterized by cough, hyper-secretion of mucus, and expectoration of sputum over a long period of time and associated with increased vulnerability to bronchial infection.

Influenza
Influenza is a highly infectious respiratory disease. The disease is caused by certain strains of the influenza virus.

Pneumonia
Pneumonia is an infection of the lung that can be caused by nearly any class of organism known to cause human infections. These include bacteria, amoebae, viruses, fungi, and parasites.

Alveoli Changes in Lung Diseases

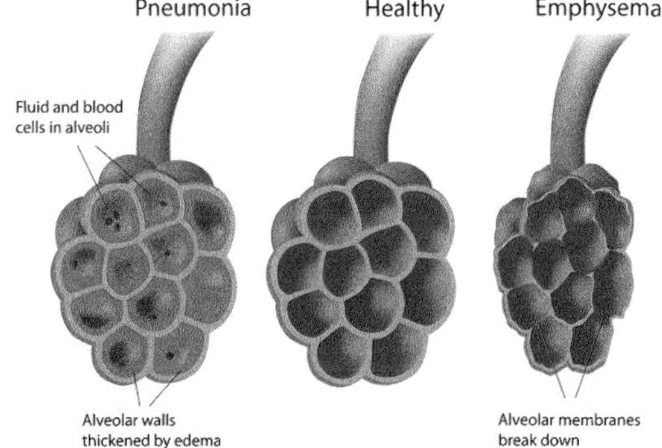

Pulmonary Abscess
Lung abscess that is a collection of infectious material contained within a capsule in the lung, which results in coughing of bloody or foul-smelling sputum (breath foul-smelling). The most important preventative measure to avoid pulmonary abscess is to prevent aspiration.

Pulmonary TB

Pulmonary tuberculosis is an infection (inflammation) caused by mycobacterium tuberculosis.Pathologic changes depend on the type of infection or "exposure" given below:Primary pulmonary TB (Primary Exposure), Secondary pulmonary TB(Reactivation) and Progressive pulmonary TB.

Progression of Tuberculosis

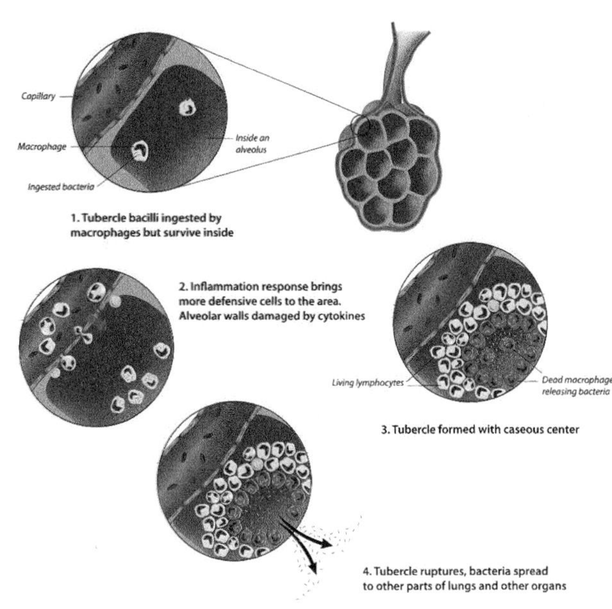

Asthma
Asthma is a common chronic inflammatory disease of the airways characterized by variable and recurring symptoms, reversible airflow obstruction, and bronchospasm. Common symptoms include wheezing, coughing, chest tightness, and shortness of breath.

Pathology of Asthma

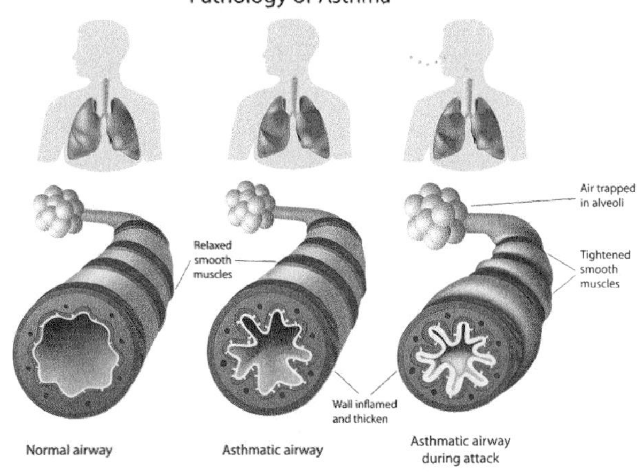

Cystic Fibrosis
Cystic Fibrosis is an autosomal recessive genetic disorder that affects most critically the lungs, and also the pancreas, liver, and intestine. It is characterized by abnormal transport of chloride and sodium across an epithelium, leading to thick, viscous secretions.

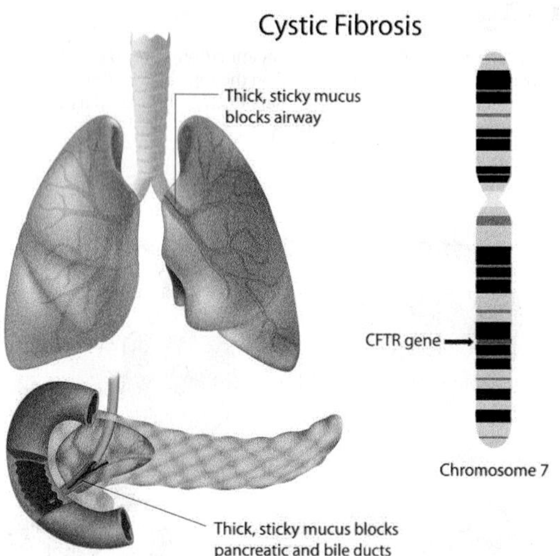

Chronic Obstructive Pulmonary Disease (COPD)

Chronic obstructive pulmonary disease (COPD) is a lung disease characterized by chronic obstruction of lung airflow that interferes with normal breathing and is not fully reversible. The more familiar terms 'chronic bronchitis' and 'emphysema' are no longer used, but are now included within the COPD diagnosis.

Emphysema

Emphysema is a chronic lung disease caused by damage to the alveoli, the tiny air sacs in the lung where exchange of oxygen and carbon dioxide takes place. With emphysema, damage to the alveoli results in air becoming trapped, causing them to expand and rupture.

Bronchiectasis

Bronchiectasis is a disease state defined by localized, irreversible dilation of part of the bronchial tree caused by destruction of the muscle and elastic tissue. It is classified as an obstructive lung disease, along with emphysema, bronchitis, asthma, and cystic fibrosis.

Diseases of the respiratory system (J00-J99)

NOTES When a respiratory condition is described as occurring in more than one site and is not specifically indexed, it should be classified to the lower anatomic site (e.g. tracheobronchitis to bronchitis in J40).

Use additional code, where applicable, to identify:
exposure to environmental tobacco smoke (Z77.22)
exposure to tobacco smoke in the perinatal period (P96.81)
history of tobacco ▶dependence◀ (Z87.891)
occupational exposure to environmental tobacco smoke (Z57.31)
tobacco dependence (F17.-)
tobacco use (Z72.0)

EXCLUDES2 *certain conditions originating in the perinatal period (P04-P96)*
certain infectious and parasitic diseases (A00-B99)
complications of pregnancy, childbirth and the puerperium (O00-O9A)
congenital malformations, deformations and chromosomal abnormalities (Q00-Q99)
endocrine, nutritional and metabolic diseases (E00-E88)
injury, poisoning and certain other consequences of external causes (S00-T88)
neoplasms (C00-D49)
smoke inhalation (T59.81-)
symptoms, signs and abnormal clinical and laboratory findings, not elsewhere classified (R00-R94)

This chapter contains the following blocks:

J00-J06	Acute upper respiratory infections
J09-J18	Influenza and pneumonia
J20-J22	Other acute lower respiratory infections
J30-J39	Other diseases of upper respiratory tract
J40-J47	Chronic lower respiratory diseases
J60-J70	Lung diseases due to external agents
J80-J84	Other respiratory diseases principally affecting the interstitium
J85-J86	Suppurative and necrotic conditions of the lower respiratory tract
J90-J94	Other diseases of the pleura
J95	Intraoperative and postprocedural complications and disorders of respiratory system, not elsewhere classified
J96-J99	Other diseases of the respiratory system

Acute upper respiratory infections (J00-J06)

EXCLUDES1 *chronic obstructive pulmonary disease with acute lower respiratory infection (J44.0)*
influenza virus with other respiratory manifestations (J09.X2, J10.1, J11.1)

J00 Acute nasopharyngitis [common cold]
Acute rhinitis
Coryza (acute)
Infective nasopharyngitis NOS
Infective rhinitis
Nasal catarrh, acute
Nasopharyngitis NOS
EXCLUDES1 *acute pharyngitis (J02.-)*
acute sore throat NOS (J02.9)
pharyngitis NOS (J02.9)
rhinitis NOS (J31.0)
sore throat NOS (J02.9)
EXCLUDES2 *allergic rhinitis (J30.1-J30.9)*
chronic pharyngitis (J31.2)
chronic rhinitis (J31.0)
chronic sore throat (J31.2)
nasopharyngitis, chronic (J31.1)
vasomotor rhinitis (J30.0)

④ **J01 Acute sinusitis**
INCLUDES *acute abscess of sinus*
acute empyema of sinus
acute infection of sinus
acute inflammation of sinus
acute suppuration of sinus
Use additional code (B95-B97) to identify infectious agent.
EXCLUDES1 *sinusitis NOS (J32.9)*
EXCLUDES2 *chronic sinusitis (J32.0-J32.8)*

⑤ **J01.0 Acute maxillary sinusitis**
Acute antritis
J01.00 Acute maxillary sinusitis, unspecified
J01.01 Acute recurrent maxillary sinusitis

⑤ **J01.1 Acute frontal sinusitis**
J01.10 Acute frontal sinusitis, unspecified
J01.11 Acute recurrent frontal sinusitis

⑤ **J01.2 Acute ethmoidal sinusitis**
J01.20 Acute ethmoidal sinusitis, unspecified
J01.21 Acute recurrent ethmoidal sinusitis

⑤ **J01.3 Acute sphenoidal sinusitis**
J01.30 Acute sphenoidal sinusitis, unspecified
J01.31 Acute recurrent sphenoidal sinusitis

⑤ **J01.4 Acute pansinusitis**
J01.40 Acute pansinusitis, unspecified
J01.41 Acute recurrent pansinusitis

⑤ **J01.8 Other acute sinusitis**
J01.80 Other acute sinusitis
Acute sinusitis involving more than one sinus but not pansinusitis
J01.81 Other acute recurrent sinusitis
Acute recurrent sinusitis involving more than one sinus but not pansinusitis

⑤ **J01.9 Acute sinusitis, unspecified**
J01.90 Acute sinusitis, unspecified
J01.91 Acute recurrent sinusitis, unspecified

④ **J02 Acute pharyngitis**
INCLUDES *acute sore throat*
EXCLUDES1 *acute laryngopharyngitis (J06.0)*
peritonsillar abscess (J36)
pharyngeal abscess (J39.1)
retropharyngeal abscess (J39.0)
EXCLUDES2 *chronic pharyngitis (J31.2)*

J02.0 Streptococcal pharyngitis
Septic pharyngitis
Streptococcal sore throat
EXCLUDES2 *scarlet fever (A38.-)*

J02.8 Acute pharyngitis due to other specified organisms
Use additional code (B95-B97) to identify infectious agent
EXCLUDES1 *acute pharyngitis due to coxsackie virus (B08.5)*
acute pharyngitis due to gonococcus (A54.5)
acute pharyngitis due to herpes [simplex] virus (B00.2)
acute pharyngitis due to infectious mononucleosis (B27.-)
enteroviral vesicular pharyngitis (B08.5)

J02.9 Acute pharyngitis, unspecified
Gangrenous pharyngitis (acute)
Infective pharyngitis (acute) NOS
Pharyngitis (acute) NOS
Sore throat (acute) NOS
Suppurative pharyngitis (acute)
Ulcerative pharyngitis (acute)

④ **J03 Acute tonsillitis**
EXCLUDES1 *acute sore throat (J02.-)*
hypertrophy of tonsils (J35.1)
peritonsillar abscess (J36)
sore throat NOS (J02.9)
streptococcal sore throat (J02.0)
EXCLUDES2 *chronic tonsillitis (J35.0)*

⑤ **J03.0 Streptococcal tonsillitis**
J03.00 Acute streptococcal tonsillitis, unspecified
J03.01 Acute recurrent streptococcal tonsillitis

⑤ **J03.8 Acute tonsillitis due to other specified organisms**
Use additional code (B95-B97) to identify infectious agent.
EXCLUDES1 *diphtheritic tonsillitis (A36.0)*
herpesviral pharyngotonsillitis (B00.2)
streptococcal tonsillitis (J03.0)
tuberculous tonsillitis (A15.8)
Vincent's tonsillitis (A69.1)

Unspecified Code · Other Specified Code · Manifestation Code · N Newborn · P Pediatric · M Maternity · A Adult · ♂ Male · ♀ Female
● New Code · ▲ Revised Code Title · ▶◀ Revised Text · NOTES · INCLUDES · EXCLUDES1 Not coded here · EXCLUDES2 Not included here
④ 4th character required · ⑤ 5th character required · ⑥ 6th character required · ⑦ 7th character required
⑦ Extension 'X' Alert · HAC Hospital-acquired condition (HAC) alert · AHA AHA Coding Clinic©

J03.80 **Acute tonsillitis due to other specified organisms**

J03.81 **Acute recurrent tonsillitis due to other specified organisms**

J03.9 **Acute tonsillitis, unspecified**
Follicular tonsillitis (acute)
Gangrenous tonsillitis (acute)
Infective tonsillitis (acute)
Tonsillitis (acute) NOS
Ulcerative tonsillitis (acute)

J03.90 **Acute tonsillitis, unspecified**

J03.91 **Acute recurrent tonsillitis, unspecified**

J04 **Acute laryngitis and tracheitis**
Use additional code (B95-B97) to identify infectious agent.
EXCLUDES1 *acute obstructive laryngitis [croup] and epiglottitis (J05.-)*
EXCLUDES2 *laryngismus (stridulus) (J38.5)*

J04.0 **Acute laryngitis**
Edematous laryngitis (acute)
Laryngitis (acute) NOS
Subglottic laryngitis (acute)
Suppurative laryngitis (acute)
Ulcerative laryngitis (acute)
EXCLUDES1 *acute obstructive laryngitis (J05.0)*
EXCLUDES2 *chronic laryngitis (J37.0)*

J04.1 **Acute tracheitis**
Acute viral tracheitis
Catarrhal tracheitis (acute)
Tracheitis (acute) NOS
EXCLUDES2 *chronic tracheitis (J42)*

J04.10 **Acute tracheitis without obstruction**

J04.11 **Acute tracheitis with obstruction** MCC

J04.2 **Acute laryngotracheitis**
Laryngotracheitis NOS
Tracheitis (acute) with laryngitis (acute)
EXCLUDES1 *acute obstructive laryngotracheitis (J05.0)*
EXCLUDES2 *chronic laryngotracheitis (J37.1)*

J04.3 **Supraglottitis, unspecified**

J04.30 **Supraglottitis, unspecified, without obstruction**

J04.31 **Supraglottitis, unspecified, with obstruction** MCC

J05 **Acute obstructive laryngitis [croup] and epiglottitis**
Use additional code (B95-B97) to identify infectious agent.

J05.0 **Acute obstructive laryngitis [croup]**
Obstructive laryngitis (acute) NOS
Obstructive laryngotracheitis NOS

J05.1 **Acute epiglottitis**
EXCLUDES2 *epiglottitis, chronic (J37.0)*

J05.10 **Acute epiglottitis without obstruction** CC
Epiglottitis NOS

J05.11 **Acute epiglottitis with obstruction** MCC

J06 **Acute upper respiratory infections of multiple and unspecified sites**
EXCLUDES1 *acute respiratory infection NOS (J22)*
streptococcal pharyngitis (J02.0)

J06.0 **Acute laryngopharyngitis**

J06.9 **Acute upper respiratory infection, unspecified**
Upper respiratory disease, acute
Upper respiratory infection NOS

Influenza and pneumonia (J09-J18)

EXCLUDES2 *allergic or eosinophilic pneumonia (J82)*
aspiration pneumonia NOS (J69.0)
meconium pneumonia (P24.01)
neonatal aspiration pneumonia (P24.-)
pneumonia due to solids and liquids (J69.-)
congenital pneumonia (P23.9)
lipid pneumonia (J69.1)
rheumatic pneumonia (I00)
ventilator associated pneumonia (J95.851)

J09 **Influenza due to certain identified influenza viruses**
EXCLUDES1 *influenza due to other identified influenza virus (J10.-)*
influenza due to unidentified influenza virus (J11.-)
seasonal influenza due to other identified influenza virus (J10.-)
seasonal influenza due to unidentified influenza virus (J11.-)

J09.X **Influenza due to identified novel influenza A virus**
Avian influenza
Bird influenza
Influenza A/H5N1
Influenza of other animal origin, not bird or swine
Swine influenza virus (viruses that normally cause infections in pigs)

J09.X1 **Influenza due to identified novel influenza A virus with pneumonia** MCC
Code also , if applicable, associated:
lung abscess (J85.1)
other specified type of pneumonia

J09.X2 **Influenza due to identified novel influenza A virus with other respiratory manifestations**
Influenza due to identified novel influenza A virus NOS
Influenza due to identified novel influenza A virus with laryngitis
Influenza due to identified novel influenza A virus with pharyngitis
Influenza due to identified novel influenza A virus with upper respiratory symptoms
Use additional code, if applicable, for associated:
pleural effusion (J91.8)
sinusitis (J01.-)

J09.X3 **Influenza due to identified novel influenza A virus with gastrointestinal manifestations**
Influenza due to identified novel influenza A virus gastroenteritis
EXCLUDES1 *'intestinal flu' [viral gastroenteritis] (A08.-)*

J09.X9 **Influenza due to identified novel influenza A virus with other manifestations**
Influenza due to identified novel influenza A virus with encephalopathy
Influenza due to identified novel influenza A virus with myocarditis
Influenza due to identified novel influenza A virus with otitis media
Use additional code to identify manifestation

J10 **Influenza due to other identified influenza virus**
EXCLUDES1 *influenza due to avian influenza virus (J09.X-)*
influenza due to swine flu (J09.X-)
influenza due to unidentified influenza virus (J11.-)

J10.0 **Influenza due to other identified influenza virus with pneumonia**
Code also associated lung abscess, if applicable (J85.1)

J10.00 **Influenza due to other identified influenza virus with unspecified type of pneumonia** MCC

J10.01 **Influenza due to other identified influenza virus with the same other identified influenza virus pneumonia** MCC

J10.08 **Influenza due to other identified influenza virus with other specified pneumonia** MCC
Code also other specified type of pneumonia

J10.1 **Influenza due to other identified influenza virus with other respiratory manifestations**
Influenza due to other identified influenza virus NOS
Influenza due to other identified influenza virus with laryngitis
Influenza due to other identified influenza virus with pharyngitis
Influenza due to other identified influenza virus with upper respiratory symptoms
Use additional code for associated pleural effusion, if applicable (J91.8)
Use additional code for associated sinusitis, if applicable (J01.-)

J10.2 **Influenza due to other identified influenza virus with gastrointestinal manifestations**
Influenza due to other identified influenza virus gastroenteritis
EXCLUDES1 *'intestinal flu' [viral gastroenteritis] (A08.-)*

J10.8 **Influenza due to other identified influenza virus with other manifestations**

J10.81 **Influenza due to other identified influenza virus with encephalopathy**

J10.82 **Influenza due to other identified influenza virus with myocarditis**

PDx Unacceptable principal diagnosis symbol per Medicare code edits · POA Code exempt from diagnosis present on admission requirement · ? Questionable admission · CC Complication or comorbidity · CC/MCC Exc CC/MCC exclusion · MCC Major complication or comorbidity · PDx CC Principal diagnosis as its own CC · PDx MCC Principal diagnosis as its own MCC · Z1 Z code as first-listed diagnosis

J10.83 **Influenza due to other identified influenza virus** with otitis media
Use additional code for any associated perforated tympanic membrane (H72.-)

J10.89 **Influenza due to other identified influenza virus** with other manifestations
Use additional codes to identify the manifestations

J11 **Influenza due to** unidentified influenza virus

J11.0 **Influenza due to unidentified influenza virus** with pneumonia
Code also associated lung abscess, if applicable (J85.1)

J11.00 **Influenza due to unidentified influenza virus** with unspecified type of pneumonia MCC
Influenza with pneumonia NOS

J11.08 **Influenza due to unidentified influenza virus** with specified pneumonia MCC
Code also other specified type of pneumonia

J11.1 **Influenza due to unidentified influenza virus** with other respiratory manifestations
Influenza NOS
Influenzal laryngitis NOS
Influenzal pharyngitis NOS
Influenza with upper respiratory symptoms NOS
Use additional code for associated pleural effusion, if applicable (J91.8)
Use additional code for associated sinusitis, if applicable (J01.-)

J11.2 **Influenza due to unidentified influenza virus** with gastrointestinal manifestations
Influenza gastroenteritis NOS
EXCLUDES1 *'intestinal flu' [viral gastroenteritis] (A08.-)*

J11.8 **Influenza due to unidentified influenza virus** with other manifestations

J11.81 **Influenza due to unidentified influenza virus** with encephalopathy
Influenzal encephalopathy NOS

J11.82 **Influenza due to unidentified influenza virus** with myocarditis
Influenzal myocarditis NOS

J11.83 **Influenza due to unidentified influenza virus** with otitis media
Influenzal otitis media NOS
Use additional code for any associated perforated tympanic membrane (H72.-)

J11.89 **Influenza due to unidentified influenza virus** with other manifestations
Use additional codes to identify the manifestations

J12 Viral pneumonia**, not elsewhere classified**
INCLUDES *bronchopneumonia due to viruses other than influenza viruses*
Code first associated influenza, if applicable (J09.X1, J10.0-, J11.0-)
Code also associated abscess, if applicable (J85.1)
EXCLUDES1 *aspiration pneumonia due to anesthesia during labor and delivery (O74.0)*
aspiration pneumonia due to anesthesia during pregnancy (O29)
aspiration pneumonia due to anesthesia during puerperium (O89.0)
aspiration pneumonia due to solids and liquids (J69.-)
aspiration pneumonia NOS (J69.0)
congenital pneumonia (P23.0)
congenital rubella pneumonitis (P35.0)
interstitial pneumonia NOS (J84.9)
lipid pneumonia (J69.1)
neonatal aspiration pneumonia (P24.-)

J12.0 Adenoviral **pneumonia** MCC
J12.1 Respiratory syncytial virus **pneumonia** MCC
J12.2 Parainfluenza virus **pneumonia** MCC
J12.3 Human metapneumovirus **pneumonia** MCC
J12.8 Other **viral pneumonia**

J12.81 **Pneumonia** due to SARS-associated coronavirus MCC
Severe acute respiratory syndrome NOS

J12.89 Other **viral pneumonia** MCC

J12.9 **Viral pneumonia, unspecified** MCC

J13 **Pneumonia due to** Streptococcus pneumoniae MCC
Bronchopneumonia due to S. pneumoniae
Code first associated influenza, if applicable (J09.X1, J10.0-, J11.0-)
Code also associated abscess, if applicable (J85.1)
EXCLUDES1 *congenital pneumonia due to S. pneumoniae (P23.6)*
lobar pneumonia, unspecified organism (J18.1)
pneumonia due to other streptococci (J15.3-J15.4)

J14 **Pneumonia due to** Hemophilus influenzae MCC
Bronchopneumonia due to H. influenzae
Code first associated influenza, if applicable (J09.X1, J10.0-, J11.0-)
Code also associated abscess, if applicable (J85.1)
EXCLUDES1 *congenital pneumonia due to H. influenzae (P23.6)*

J15 Bacterial **pneumonia, not elsewhere classified**
INCLUDES *bronchopneumonia due to bacteria other than S. pneumoniae and H. influenzae*
Code first associated influenza, if applicable (J09.X1, J10.0-, J11.0-)
Code also associated abscess, if applicable (J85.1)
EXCLUDES1 *chlamydial pneumonia (J16.0)*
congenital pneumonia (P23.-)
Legionnaires' disease (A48.1)
spirochetal pneumonia (A69.8)

J15.0 **Pneumonia due to** Klebsiella pneumoniae MCC
J15.1 **Pneumonia due to** Pseudomonas MCC
J15.2 **Pneumonia due to** staphylococcus

J15.20 **Pneumonia due to staphylococcus,** unspecified MCC
J15.21 **Pneumonia due to** staphylococcus aureus

J15.211 **Pneumonia due to** Methicillin susceptible Staphylococcus aureus MCC
MSSA pneumonia
Pneumonia due to Staphylococcus aureus NOS

J15.212 **Pneumonia due to** Methicillin resistant Staphylococcus aureus MCC

J15.29 **Pneumonia due to other** staphylococcus MCC

J15.3 **Pneumonia due to** streptococcus, group B MCC
J15.4 **Pneumonia due to** other streptococci MCC
EXCLUDES1 *pneumonia due to streptococcus, group B (J15.3)*
pneumonia due to Streptococcus pneumoniae (J13)

J15.5 **Pneumonia due to** Escherichia coli MCC
J15.6 **Pneumonia due to** other aerobic Gram-negative bacteria MCC
Pneumonia due to Serratia marcescens
J15.7 **Pneumonia due to** Mycoplasma pneumoniae MCC
J15.8 **Pneumonia due to** other specified bacteria MCC
J15.9 **Unspecified bacterial pneumonia** MCC
Pneumonia due to gram-positive bacteria

J16 **Pneumonia due to** other infectious organisms**, not elsewhere classified**
Code first associated influenza, if applicable (J09.X1, J10.0-, J11.0-)
Code also associated abscess, if applicable (J85.1)
EXCLUDES1 *congenital pneumonia (P23.-)*
ornithosis (A70)
pneumocystosis (B59)
pneumonia NOS (J18.9)

J16.0 Chlamydial **pneumonia** MCC
J16.8 **Pneumonia due to other specified infectious organisms** MCC

J17 **Pneumonia in diseases classified elsewhere** MCC
Code first underlying disease, such as:
Q fever (A78)
rheumatic fever (I00)
schistosomiasis (B65.0-B65.9)
EXCLUDES1 *candidal pneumonia (B37.1)*
chlamydial pneumonia (J16.0)
gonorrheal pneumonia (A54.84)
histoplasmosis pneumonia (B39.0-B39.2)
measles pneumonia (B05.2)
nocardiosis pneumonia (A43.0)
pneumocystosis (B59)
pneumonia due to Pneumocystis carinii (B59)
pneumonia due to Pneumocystis jiroveci (B59)
pneumonia in actinomycosis (A42.0)
pneumonia in anthrax (A22.1)
pneumonia in ascariasis (B77.81)

Unspecified Code Other Specified Code Manifestation Code N Newborn P Pediatric M Maternity A Adult ♂ Male ♀ Female
● New Code ▲ Revised Code Title ►◄ Revised Text NOTES INCLUDES EXCLUDES1 Not coded here EXCLUDES2 Not included here
4th character required 5th character required 6th character required 7th character required
Extension 'X' Alert HAC Hospital-acquired condition (HAC) alert AHA AHA Coding Clinic®

pneumonia in aspergillosis (B44.0-B44.1)
pneumonia in coccidioidomycosis (B38.0-B38.2)
pneumonia in cytomegalovirus disease (B25.0)
pneumonia in toxoplasmosis (B58.3)
rubella pneumonia (B06.81)
salmonella pneumonia (A02.22)
spirochetal infection NEC with pneumonia (A69.8)
tularemia pneumonia (A21.2)
typhoid fever with pneumonia (A01.03)
varicella pneumonia (B01.2)
whooping cough with pneumonia (A37 with fifth-character 1)

J18 Pneumonia, unspecified organism
Code first associated influenza, if applicable (J09.X1, J10.0-, J11.0-)
EXCLUDES1 *abscess of lung with pneumonia (J85.1)*
aspiration pneumonia due to anesthesia during labor and delivery (O74.0)
aspiration pneumonia due to anesthesia during pregnancy (O29)
aspiration pneumonia due to anesthesia during puerperium (O89.0)
aspiration pneumonia due to solids and liquids (J69.-)
aspiration pneumonia NOS (J69.0)
congenital pneumonia (P23.0)
drug-induced interstitial lung disorder (J70.2-J70.4)
interstitial pneumonia NOS (J84.9)
lipid pneumonia (J69.1)
neonatal aspiration pneumonia (P24.-)
pneumonitis due to external agents (J67-J70)
pneumonitis due to fumes and vapors (J68.0)
usual interstitial pneumonia (J84.17)

J18.0 Bronchopneumonia, unspecified organism MCC
EXCLUDES1 *hypostatic bronchopneumonia (J18.2)*
lipid pneumonia (J69.1)
EXCLUDES2 *acute bronchiolitis (J21.-)*
chronic bronchiolitis (J44.9)

J18.1 Lobar pneumonia, unspecified organism MCC
J18.2 Hypostatic pneumonia, unspecified organism CC
Hypostatic bronchopneumonia
Passive pneumonia
J18.8 Other pneumonia, unspecified organism MCC
J18.9 Pneumonia, unspecified organism MCC
AHA: Q4, 2013

Other acute lower respiratory infections (J20-J22)

EXCLUDES2 *chronic obstructive pulmonary disease with acute lower respiratory infection (J44.0)*

J20 Acute bronchitis
INCLUDES *acute and subacute bronchitis (with) bronchospasm*
acute and subacute bronchitis (with) tracheitis
acute and subacute bronchitis (with) tracheobronchitis, acute
acute and subacute fibrinous bronchitis
acute and subacute membranous bronchitis
acute and subacute purulent bronchitis
acute and subacute septic bronchitis
EXCLUDES1 *bronchitis NOS (J40)*
tracheobronchitis NOS (J40)
EXCLUDES2 *acute bronchitis with bronchiectasis (J47.0)*
acute bronchitis with chronic obstructive asthma (J44.0)
acute bronchitis with chronic obstructive pulmonary disease (J44.0)
allergic bronchitis NOS (J45.909-)
bronchitis due to chemicals, fumes and vapors (J68.0)
chronic bronchitis NOS (J42)
chronic mucopurulent bronchitis (J41.1)
chronic obstructive bronchitis (J44.-)
chronic obstructive tracheobronchitis (J44.-)
chronic simple bronchitis (J41.0)
chronic tracheobronchitis (J42)

J20.0 Acute bronchitis due to Mycoplasma pneumoniae
J20.1 Acute bronchitis due to Hemophilus influenzae
J20.2 Acute bronchitis due to streptococcus
J20.3 Acute bronchitis due to coxsackievirus
J20.4 Acute bronchitis due to parainfluenza virus
J20.5 Acute bronchitis due to respiratory syncytial virus
J20.6 Acute bronchitis due to rhinovirus
J20.7 Acute bronchitis due to echovirus
J20.8 Acute bronchitis due to other specified organisms
J20.9 Acute bronchitis, unspecified

J21 Acute bronchiolitis
INCLUDES *acute bronchiolitis with bronchospasm*
EXCLUDES2 *respiratory bronchiolitis interstitial lung disease (J84.115)*
J21.0 Acute bronchiolitis due to respiratory syncytial virus CC
J21.1 Acute bronchiolitis due to human metapneumovirus CC
J21.8 Acute bronchiolitis due to other specified organisms CC
J21.9 Acute bronchiolitis, unspecified CC
Bronchiolitis (acute)
EXCLUDES1 *chronic bronchiolitis (J44.-)*

J22 Unspecified acute lower respiratory infection
Acute (lower) respiratory (tract) infection NOS
EXCLUDES1 *upper respiratory infection (acute) (J06.9)*

Other diseases of upper respiratory tract (J30-J39)

J30 Vasomotor and allergic rhinitis
INCLUDES *spasmodic rhinorrhea*
EXCLUDES1 *allergic rhinitis with asthma (bronchial) (J45.909)*
rhinitis NOS (J31.0)
J30.0 Vasomotor rhinitis
J30.1 Allergic rhinitis due to pollen
Allergy NOS due to pollen
Hay fever
Pollinosis
J30.2 Other seasonal allergic rhinitis
J30.5 Allergic rhinitis due to food
J30.8 Other allergic rhinitis
J30.81 Allergic rhinitis due to animal (cat) (dog) hair and dander
J30.89 Other allergic rhinitis
Perennial allergic rhinitis
J30.9 Allergic rhinitis, unspecified

J31 Chronic rhinitis, nasopharyngitis and pharyngitis
Use additional code to identify:
exposure to environmental tobacco smoke (Z77.22)
exposure to tobacco smoke in the perinatal period (P96.81)
history of tobacco ▶dependence◀ (Z87.891)
occupational exposure to environmental tobacco smoke (Z57.31)
tobacco dependence (F17.-)
tobacco use (Z72.0)
J31.0 Chronic rhinitis
Atrophic rhinitis (chronic)
Granulomatous rhinitis (chronic)
Hypertrophic rhinitis (chronic)
Obstructive rhinitis (chronic)
Ozena
Purulent rhinitis (chronic)
Rhinitis (chronic) NOS
Ulcerative rhinitis (chronic)
EXCLUDES1 *allergic rhinitis (J30.1-J30.9)*
vasomotor rhinitis (J30.0)
J31.1 Chronic nasopharyngitis
EXCLUDES2 *acute nasopharyngitis (J00)*
J31.2 Chronic pharyngitis
Chronic sore throat
Atrophic pharyngitis (chronic)
Granular pharyngitis (chronic)
Hypertrophic pharyngitis (chronic)
EXCLUDES2 *acute pharyngitis (J02.9)*

PDx Unacceptable principal diagnosis symbol per Medicare code edits; POA Code exempt from diagnosis present on admission requirement
? Questionable admission; CC Complication or comorbidity; CC/MCC Excl CC/MCC exclusion; MCC Major complication or comorbidity
PDx CC Principal diagnosis as its own CC; PDx MCC Principal diagnosis as its own MCC; Z1 Z code as first-listed diagnosis

 When symbols appear on a code that requires a 7th character extension, refer to Appendix D to identify applicable 7th character codes.

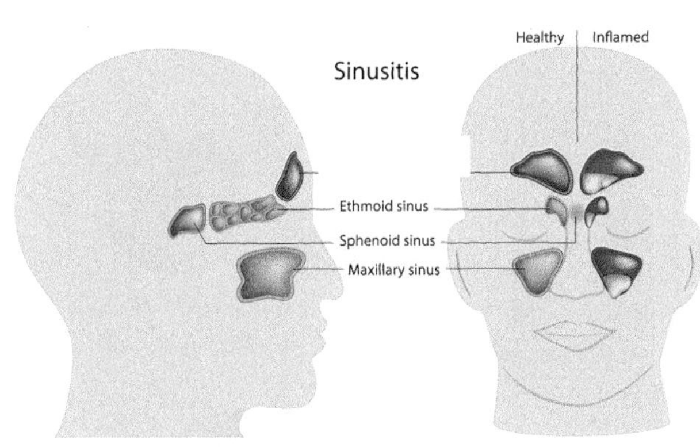

Figure 10.1 Sinusitis

J32 Chronic sinusitis
INCLUDES sinus abscess
sinus empyema
sinus infection
sinus suppuration
Use additional code to identify:
exposure to environmental tobacco smoke (Z77.22)
exposure to tobacco smoke in the perinatal period (P96.81)
history of tobacco ▶dependence◀ (Z87.891)
infectious agent (B95-B97)
occupational exposure to environmental tobacco smoke (Z57.31)
tobacco dependence (F17.-)
tobacco use (Z72.0)
EXCLUDES2 *acute sinusitis (J01.-)*

J32.0 Chronic maxillary sinusitis
Antritis (chronic)
Maxillary sinusitis NOS

J32.1 Chronic frontal sinusitis
Frontal sinusitis NOS

J32.2 Chronic ethmoidal sinusitis
Ethmoidal sinusitis NOS
EXCLUDES1 *Woakes' ethmoiditis (J33.1)*

J32.3 Chronic sphenoidal sinusitis
Sphenoidal sinusitis NOS

J32.4 Chronic pansinusitis
Pansinusitis NOS

J32.8 Other chronic sinusitis
Sinusitis (chronic) involving more than one sinus but not pansinusitis

J32.9 Chronic sinusitis, unspecified
Sinusitis (chronic) NOS

J33 Nasal polyp
Use additional code to identify:
exposure to environmental tobacco smoke (Z77.22)
exposure to tobacco smoke in the perinatal period (P96.81)
history of tobacco ▶dependence◀ (Z87.891)
occupational exposure to environmental tobacco smoke (Z57.31)
tobacco dependence (F17.-)
tobacco use (Z72.0)
EXCLUDES1 *adenomatous polyps (D14.0)*

J33.0 Polyp of nasal cavity
Choanal polyp
Nasopharyngeal polyp

J33.1 Polypoid sinus degeneration
Woakes' syndrome or ethmoiditis

J33.8 Other polyp of sinus
Accessory polyp of sinus
Ethmoidal polyp of sinus
Maxillary polyp of sinus
Sphenoidal polyp of sinus

J33.9 Nasal polyp, unspecified

J34 Other and unspecified disorders of nose and nasal sinuses
EXCLUDES2 *varicose ulcer of nasal septum (I86.8)*

J34.0 Abscess, furuncle and carbuncle of nose
Cellulitis of nose
Necrosis of nose
Ulceration of nose

J34.1 Cyst and mucocele of nose and nasal sinus

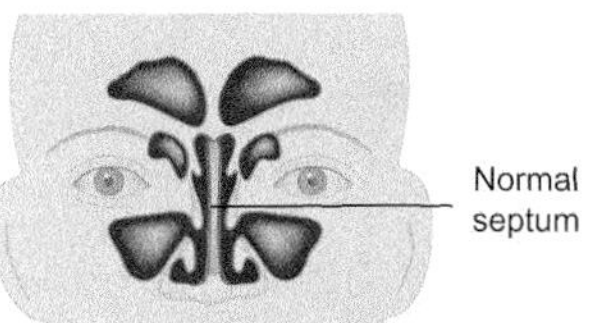

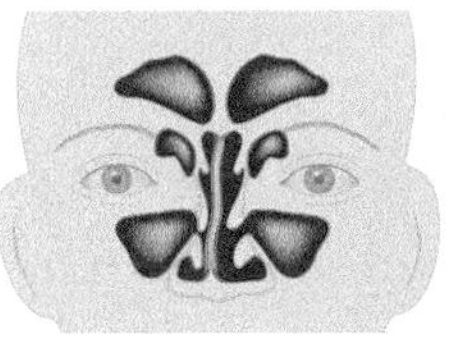

Figure 10.2 Deviated nasal septum

J34.2 Deviated nasal septum
Deflection or deviation of septum (nasal) (acquired)
EXCLUDES1 *congenital deviated nasal septum (Q67.4)*

J34.3 Hypertrophy of nasal turbinates

J34.8 Other specified disorders of nose and nasal sinuses

J34.81 Nasal mucositis (ulcerative)
Code also type of associated therapy, such as:
antineoplastic and immunosuppressive drugs (T45.1X-)
radiological procedure and radiotherapy (Y84.2)
EXCLUDES2 *gastrointestinal mucositis (ulcerative) (K92.81)*
mucositis (ulcerative) of vagina and vulva (N76.81)
oral mucositis (ulcerative) (K12.3-)

J34.89 Other specified disorders of nose and nasal sinuses
Perforation of nasal septum NOS
Rhinolith

J34.9 Unspecified disorder of nose and nasal sinuses

J35 Chronic diseases of tonsils and adenoids
Use additional code to identify:
exposure to environmental tobacco smoke (Z77.22)
exposure to tobacco smoke in the perinatal period (P96.81)
history of tobacco ▶dependence◀ (Z87.891)
occupational exposure to environmental tobacco smoke (Z57.31)
tobacco dependence (F17.-)
tobacco use (Z72.0)

J35.0 Chronic tonsillitis and adenoiditis
EXCLUDES2 *acute tonsillitis (J03.-)*

J35.01 Chronic tonsillitis

J35.02 Chronic adenoiditis

J35.03 Chronic tonsillitis and adenoiditis

J35.1 Hypertrophy of tonsils
Enlargement of tonsils
EXCLUDES1 *hypertrophy of tonsils with tonsillitis (J35.0-)*

Unspecified Code | Other Specified Code | Manifestation Code | N Newborn | P Pediatric | M Maternity | A Adult | ♂ Male | ♀ Female
● New Code | ▲ Revised Code Title | ▶◀ Revised Text | NOTES | INCLUDES | EXCLUDES1 Not coded here | EXCLUDES2 Not included here
4th character required | 5th character required | 6th character required | 7th character required
Extension 'X' Alert | HAC Hospital-acquired condition (HAC) alert | AHA AHA Coding Clinic©

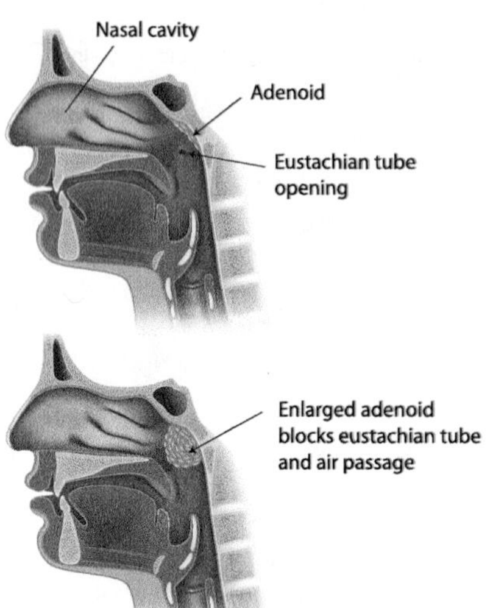

Figure 10.3 Adenoid hypertrophy

J35.2 **Hypertrophy of adenoids**
Enlargement of adenoids
EXCLUDES1 *hypertrophy of adenoids with adenoiditis (J35.0-)*

J35.3 **Hypertrophy of tonsils with hypertrophy of adenoids**
EXCLUDES1 *hypertrophy of tonsils and adenoids with tonsillitis and adenoiditis (J35.03)*

J35.8 **Other chronic diseases of tonsils and adenoids**
Adenoid vegetations
Amygdalolith
Calculus, tonsil
Cicatrix of tonsil (and adenoid)
Tonsillar tag
Ulcer of tonsil

J35.9 **Chronic disease of tonsils and adenoids, unspecified**
Disease (chronic) of tonsils and adenoids NOS

J36 **Peritonsillar abscess** CC
INCLUDES *abscess of tonsil*
peritonsillar cellulitis
quinsy
Use additional code (B95-B97) to identify infectious agent.
EXCLUDES1 *acute tonsillitis (J03.-)*
chronic tonsillitis (J35.0)
retropharyngeal abscess (J39.0)
tonsillitis NOS (J03.9-)

J37 **Chronic laryngitis and laryngotracheitis**
Use additional code to identify:
exposure to environmental tobacco smoke (Z77.22)
exposure to tobacco smoke in the perinatal period (P96.81)
history of tobacco ▶dependence◀ (Z87.891)
infectious agent (B95-B97)
occupational exposure to environmental tobacco smoke (Z57.31)
tobacco dependence (F17.-)
tobacco use (Z72.0)

J37.0 **Chronic laryngitis**
Catarrhal laryngitis
Hypertrophic laryngitis
Sicca laryngitis
EXCLUDES2 *acute laryngitis (J04.0)*
obstructive (acute) laryngitis (J05.0)

J37.1 **Chronic laryngotracheitis**
Laryngitis, chronic, with tracheitis (chronic)
Tracheitis, chronic, with laryngitis
EXCLUDES1 *chronic tracheitis (J42)*
EXCLUDES2 *acute laryngotracheitis (J04.2)*
acute tracheitis (J04.1)

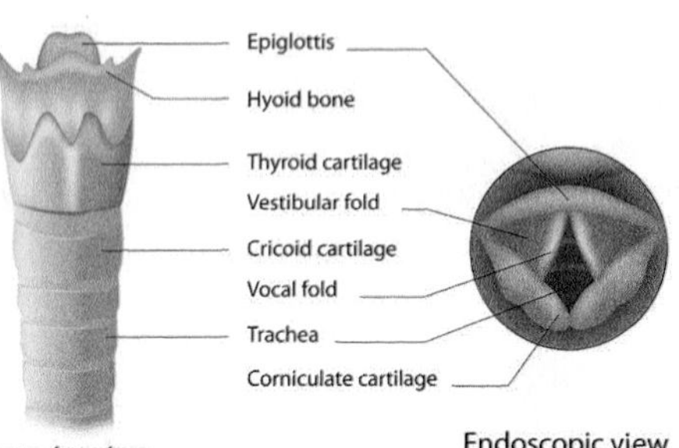

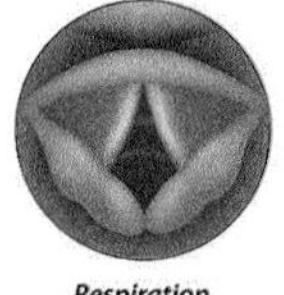

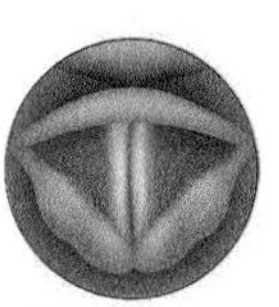

Figure 10.4 Larynx

J38 **Diseases of vocal cords and larynx, not elsewhere classified**
Use additional code to identify:
exposure to environmental tobacco smoke (Z77.22)
exposure to tobacco smoke in the perinatal period (P96.81)
history of tobacco ▶dependence◀ (Z87.891)
occupational exposure to environmental tobacco smoke (Z57.31)
tobacco dependence (F17.-)
tobacco use (Z72.0)
EXCLUDES1 *congenital laryngeal stridor (P28.89)*
obstructive laryngitis (acute) (J05.0)
postprocedural subglottic stenosis (J95.5)
stridor (R06.1)
ulcerative laryngitis (J04.0)

J38.0 **Paralysis of vocal cords and larynx**
Laryngoplegia
Paralysis of glottis
J38.00 **Paralysis of vocal cords and larynx, unspecified**
J38.01 **Paralysis of vocal cords and larynx, unilateral**
J38.02 **Paralysis of vocal cords and larynx, bilateral**

J38.1 **Polyp of vocal cord and larynx**
EXCLUDES1 *adenomatous polyps (D14.1)*

J38.2 **Nodules of vocal cords**
Chorditis (fibrinous)(nodosa)(tuberosa)
Singer's nodes
Teacher's nodes

J38.3 **Other diseases of vocal cords**
Abscess of vocal cords
Cellulitis of vocal cords
Granuloma of vocal cords
Leukokeratosis of vocal cords
Leukoplakia of vocal cords

J38.4 **Edema of larynx**
Edema (of) glottis
Subglottic edema
Supraglottic edema
EXCLUDES1 *acute obstructive laryngitis [croup] (J05.0)*
edematous laryngitis (J04.0)

J38.5 **Laryngeal spasm**
Laryngismus (stridulus)

J38.6 **Stenosis of larynx**

J38.7 **Other diseases of larynx**
Abscess of larynx
Cellulitis of larynx
Disease of larynx NOS
Necrosis of larynx
Pachyderma of larynx
Perichondritis of larynx
Ulcer of larynx

PDx Unacceptable principal diagnosis symbol per Medicare code edits   POA Code exempt from diagnosis present on admission requirement
? Questionable admission   CC Complication or comorbidity   CC/MCC Exc CC/MCC exclusion   MCC Major complication or comorbidity
PDx CC Principal diagnosis as its own CC   PDx MCC Principal diagnosis as its own MCC   Z1 Z code as first-listed diagnosis

J39 Other diseases of upper respiratory tract
EXCLUDES1 *acute respiratory infection NOS (J22)*
acute upper respiratory infection (J06.9)
upper respiratory inflammation due to chemicals, gases, fumes or vapors (J68.2)

J39.0 **Retropharyngeal and parapharyngeal abscess**
Peripharyngeal abscess
EXCLUDES1 *peritonsillar abscess (J36)*

J39.1 **Other abscess of pharynx**
Cellulitis of pharynx
Nasopharyngeal abscess

J39.2 **Other diseases of pharynx**
Cyst of pharynx
Edema of pharynx
EXCLUDES2 *chronic pharyngitis (J31.2)*
ulcerative pharyngitis (J02.9)

J39.3 **Upper respiratory tract hypersensitivity reaction, site unspecified**
EXCLUDES1 *hypersensitivity reaction of upper respiratory tract, such as:*
extrinsic allergic alveolitis (J67.9)
pneumoconiosis (J60-J67.9)

J39.8 **Other specified diseases of upper respiratory tract**

J39.9 **Disease of upper respiratory tract, unspecified**

Chronic lower respiratory diseases (J40-J47)

EXCLUDES1 *bronchitis due to chemicals, gases, fumes and vapors (J68.0)*
EXCLUDES2 *cystic fibrosis (E84.-)*

J40 **Bronchitis, not specified as acute or chronic**
Bronchitis NOS
Bronchitis with tracheitis NOS
Catarrhal bronchitis
Tracheobronchitis NOS
Use additional code to identify:
exposure to environmental tobacco smoke (Z77.22)
exposure to tobacco smoke in the perinatal period (P96.81)
history of tobacco ▶dependence◀ (Z87.891)
occupational exposure to environmental tobacco smoke (Z57.31)
tobacco dependence (F17.-)
tobacco use (Z72.0)
EXCLUDES1 *acute bronchitis (J20.-)*
allergic bronchitis NOS (J45.909-)
asthmatic bronchitis NOS (J45.9-)
bronchitis due to chemicals, gases, fumes and vapors (J68.0)

J41 **Simple and mucopurulent chronic bronchitis**
Use additional code to identify:
exposure to environmental tobacco smoke (Z77.22)
exposure to tobacco smoke in the perinatal period (P96.81)
history of tobacco ▶dependence◀ (Z87.891)
occupational exposure to environmental tobacco smoke (Z57.31)
tobacco dependence (F17.-)
tobacco use (Z72.0)
EXCLUDES1 *chronic bronchitis NOS (J42)*
chronic obstructive bronchitis (J44.-)

J41.0 **Simple chronic bronchitis**

J41.1 **Mucopurulent chronic bronchitis**

J41.8 **Mixed simple and mucopurulent chronic bronchitis**

J42 **Unspecified chronic bronchitis**
Chronic bronchitis NOS
Chronic tracheitis
Chronic tracheobronchitis
Use additional code to identify:
exposure to environmental tobacco smoke (Z77.22)
exposure to tobacco smoke in the perinatal period (P96.81)
history of tobacco ▶dependence◀ (Z87.891)
occupational exposure to environmental tobacco smoke (Z57.31)
tobacco dependence (F17.-)
tobacco use (Z72.0)
EXCLUDES1 *chronic asthmatic bronchitis (J44.-)*
chronic bronchitis with airways obstruction (J44.-)
chronic emphysematous bronchitis (J44.-)
chronic obstructive pulmonary disease NOS (J44.9)
simple and mucopurulent chronic bronchitis (J41.-)

J43 **Emphysema**
Use additional code to identify:
exposure to environmental tobacco smoke (Z77.22)
history of tobacco ▶dependence◀ (Z87.891)
occupational exposure to environmental tobacco smoke (Z57.31)
tobacco dependence (F17.-)
tobacco use (Z72.0)
EXCLUDES1 *compensatory emphysema (J98.3)*
emphysema due to inhalation of chemicals, gases, fumes or vapors (J68.4)
emphysema with chronic (obstructive) bronchitis (J44.-)
emphysematous (obstructive) bronchitis (J44.-)
interstitial emphysema (J98.2)
mediastinal emphysema (J98.2)
neonatal interstitial emphysema (P25.0)
surgical (subcutaneous) emphysema (T81.82)
traumatic subcutaneous emphysema (T79.7)

J43.0 **Unilateral pulmonary emphysema [MacLeod's syndrome]**
Swyer-James syndrome
Unilateral emphysema
Unilateral hyperlucent lung
Unilateral pulmonary artery functional hypoplasia
Unilateral transparency of lung

J43.1 **Panlobular emphysema**
Panacinar emphysema

J43.2 **Centrilobular emphysema**

J43.8 **Other emphysema**

J43.9 **Emphysema, unspecified**
Bullous emphysema (lung)(pulmonary)
Emphysema (lung)(pulmonary) NOS
Emphysematous bleb
Vesicular emphysema (lung)(pulmonary)

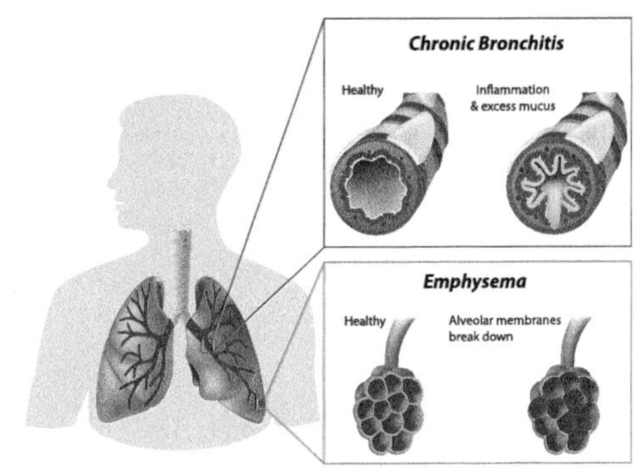

Figure 10.5 Chronic obstructive pulmonary disease (COPD): chronic bronchitis and emphysema

J44 **Other chronic obstructive pulmonary disease**
INCLUDES *asthma with chronic obstructive pulmonary disease*
chronic asthmatic (obstructive) bronchitis
chronic bronchitis with airways obstruction
chronic bronchitis with emphysema
chronic emphysematous bronchitis
chronic obstructive asthma
chronic obstructive bronchitis
chronic obstructive tracheobronchitis
Code also type of asthma, if applicable (J45.-)
Use additional code to identify:
exposure to environmental tobacco smoke (Z77.22)
history of tobacco ▶dependence◀ (Z87.891)
occupational exposure to environmental tobacco smoke (Z57.31)
tobacco dependence (F17.-)
tobacco use (Z72.0)
EXCLUDES1 *bronchiectasis (J47.-)*
chronic bronchitis NOS (J42)

Unspecified Code Other Specified Code Manifestation Code N Newborn P Pediatric M Maternity A Adult ♂ Male ♀ Female
● New Code ▲ Revised Code Title ▶◀ Revised Text NOTES INCLUDES EXCLUDES1 Not coded here EXCLUDES2 Not included here
4th character required 5th character required 6th character required 7th character required
Extension 'X' Alert HAC Hospital-acquired condition (HAC) alert AHA AHA Coding Clinic©

chronic simple and mucopurulent bronchitis (J41.-)
chronic tracheitis (J42)
chronic tracheobronchitis (J42)
emphysema without chronic bronchitis (J43.-)
EXCLUDES2 *lung diseases due to external agents (J60-J70)*

J44.0 **Chronic obstructive pulmonary disease** with acute lower respiratory infection CC
Use additional code to identify the infection

J44.1 **Chronic obstructive pulmonary disease** with (acute) exacerbation CC
Decompensated COPD
Decompensated COPD with (acute) exacerbation
EXCLUDES2 *chronic obstructive pulmonary disease [COPD] with acute bronchitis (J44.0)*

J44.9 **Chronic obstructive pulmonary disease, unspecified**
Chronic obstructive airway disease NOS
Chronic obstructive lung disease NOS
AHA: Q4, 2013

4th J45 **Asthma**
INCLUDES *allergic (predominantly) asthma*
allergic bronchitis NOS
allergic rhinitis with asthma
atopic asthma
extrinsic allergic asthma
hay fever with asthma
idiosyncratic asthma
intrinsic nonallergic asthma
nonallergic asthma
Use additional code to identify:
exposure to environmental tobacco smoke (Z77.22)
exposure to tobacco smoke in the perinatal period (P96.81)
history of tobacco ▶dependence◀ (Z87.891)
occupational exposure to environmental tobacco smoke (Z57.31)
tobacco dependence (F17.-)
tobacco use (Z72.0)
EXCLUDES1 *detergent asthma (J69.8)*
eosinophilic asthma (J82)
lung diseases due to external agents (J60-J70)
miner's asthma (J60)
wheezing NOS (R06.2)
wood asthma (J67.8)
EXCLUDES2 *asthma with chronic obstructive pulmonary disease (J44.9)*
chronic asthmatic (obstructive) bronchitis (J44.9)
chronic obstructive asthma (J44.9)

5th J45.2 Mild intermittent **asthma**
J45.20 **Mild intermittent asthma,** uncomplicated
Mild intermittent asthma NOS
J45.21 **Mild intermittent asthma** with (acute) exacerbation CC
J45.22 **Mild intermittent asthma** with status asthmaticus CC

5th J45.3 Mild persistent **asthma**
J45.30 **Mild persistent asthma,** uncomplicated
Mild persistent asthma NOS
J45.31 **Mild persistent asthma** with (acute) exacerbation CC
J45.32 **Mild persistent asthma** with status asthmaticus CC

5th J45.4 Moderate persistent **asthma**
J45.40 **Moderate persistent asthma,** uncomplicated
Moderate persistent asthma NOS
J45.41 **Moderate persistent asthma** with (acute) exacerbation CC
J45.42 **Moderate persistent asthma** with status asthmaticus CC

5th J45.5 Severe persistent **asthma**
J45.50 **Severe persistent asthma,** uncomplicated
Severe persistent asthma NOS
J45.51 **Severe persistent asthma** with (acute) exacerbation CC
J45.52 **Severe persistent asthma** with status asthmaticus CC

5th J45.9 Other and unspecified **asthma**
6th J45.90 Unspecified **asthma**
Asthmatic bronchitis NOS
Childhood asthma NOS
Late onset asthma
J45.901 **Unspecified asthma** with (acute) exacerbation CC
J45.902 **Unspecified asthma** with status asthmaticus CC
J45.909 **Unspecified asthma, uncomplicated**
Asthma NOS
6th J45.99 **Other asthma**
J45.990 Exercise induced **bronchospasm**
J45.991 Cough variant **asthma**
J45.998 Other **asthma**

4th J47 **Bronchiectasis**
INCLUDES *bronchiolectasis*
Use additional code to identify:
exposure to environmental tobacco smoke (Z77.22)
exposure to tobacco smoke in the perinatal period (P96.81)
history of tobacco ▶dependence◀ (Z87.891)
occupational exposure to environmental tobacco smoke (Z57.31)
tobacco dependence (F17.-)
tobacco use (Z72.0)
EXCLUDES1 *congenital bronchiectasis (Q33.4)*
tuberculous bronchiectasis (current disease) (A15.0)
J47.0 **Bronchiectasis** with acute lower respiratory infection CC
Bronchiectasis with acute bronchitis
Use additional code to identify the infection
J47.1 **Bronchiectasis** with (acute) exacerbation CC
J47.9 **Bronchiectasis,** uncomplicated
Bronchiectasis NOS

Lung diseases due to external agents (J60-J70)

EXCLUDES2 *asthma (J45.-)*
malignant neoplasm of bronchus and lung (C34.-)

J60 **Coalworker's pneumoconiosis** A
Anthracosilicosis
Anthracosis
Black lung disease
Coalworker's lung
EXCLUDES1 *coalworker pneumoconiosis with tuberculosis, any type in A15 (J65)*

J61 **Pneumoconiosis** due to asbestos and other mineral fibers A
Asbestosis
EXCLUDES1 *pleural plaque with asbestosis (J92.0)*
pneumoconiosis with tuberculosis, any type in A15 (J65)

4th J62 **Pneumoconiosis** due to dust containing silica
INCLUDES *silicotic fibrosis (massive) of lung*
EXCLUDES1 *pneumoconiosis with tuberculosis, any type in A15 (J65)*
J62.0 **Pneumoconiosis due to** talc dust
J62.8 **Pneumoconiosis due to** other dust containing silica
Silicosis NOS

4th J63 **Pneumoconiosis due to** other inorganic dusts
EXCLUDES1 *pneumoconiosis with tuberculosis, any type in A15 (J65)*
J63.0 Aluminosis **(of lung)**
J63.1 Bauxite fibrosis **(of lung)**
J63.2 Berylliosis
J63.3 Graphite fibrosis **(of lung)**
J63.4 Siderosis
J63.5 Stannosis
J63.6 **Pneumoconiosis due to** other specified inorganic dusts

J64 **Unspecified pneumoconiosis**
EXCLUDES1 *pneumonoconiosis with tuberculosis, any type in A15 (J65)*

J65 **Pneumoconiosis associated with tuberculosis**
Any condition in J60-J64 with tuberculosis, any type in A15
Silicotuberculosis

4th J66 **Airway disease due to specific organic dust**
EXCLUDES2 *allergic alveolitis (J67.-)*
asbestosis (J61)
bagassosis (J67.1)
farmer's lung (J67.0)
hypersensitivity pneumonitis due to organic dust (J67.-)
reactive airways dysfunction syndrome (J68.3)

PDx Unacceptable principal diagnosis symbol per Medicare code edits · POA Code exempt from diagnosis present on admission requirement · Q Questionable admission · CC Complication or comorbidity · CC/MCC Exc CC/MCC exclusion · MCC Major complication or comorbidity · PDx CC Principal diagnosis as its own CC · PDx MCC Principal diagnosis as its own MCC · Z1 Z code as first-listed diagnosis

J66.0 **Byssinosis**
Airway disease due to cotton dust
J66.1 **Flax-dressers' disease**
J66.2 **Cannabinosis**
J66.8 **Airway disease due to other specific organic dusts**

J67 Hypersensitivity pneumonitis due to organic dust
INCLUDES *allergic alveolitis and pneumonitis due to inhaled organic dust and particles of fungal, actinomycetic or other origin*
EXCLUDES1 *pneumonitis due to inhalation of chemicals, gases, fumes or vapors (J68.0)*

J67.0 **Farmer's lung**
Harvester's lung
Haymaker's lung
Moldy hay disease
J67.1 **Bagassosis**
Bagasse disease
Bagasse pneumonitis
J67.2 **Bird fancier's lung**
Budgerigar fancier's disease or lung
Pigeon fancier's disease or lung
J67.3 **Suberosis**
Corkhandler's disease or lung
Corkworker's disease or lung
J67.4 **Maltworker's lung**
Alveolitis due to Aspergillus clavatus
J67.5 **Mushroom-worker's lung**
J67.6 **Maple-bark-stripper's lung**
Alveolitis due to Cryptostroma corticale
Cryptostromosis
J67.7 **Air conditioner and humidifier lung** CC
Allergic alveolitis due to fungal, thermophilic actinomycetes and other organisms growing in ventilation [air conditioning] systems
J67.8 **Hypersensitivity pneumonitis due to other organic dusts** CC
Cheese-washer's lung
Coffee-worker's lung
Fish-meal worker's lung
Furrier's lung
Sequoiosis
J67.9 **Hypersensitivity pneumonitis due to unspecified organic dust** CC
Allergic alveolitis (extrinsic) NOS
Hypersensitivity pneumonitis NOS

J68 Respiratory conditions due to inhalation of chemicals, gases, fumes and vapors
Code first (T51-T65) to identify cause
Use additional code to identify associated respiratory conditions, such as:
acute respiratory failure (J96.0-)

J68.0 **Bronchitis and pneumonitis due to chemicals, gases, fumes and vapors** CC
Chemical bronchitis (acute)
J68.1 **Pulmonary edema due to chemicals, gases, fumes and vapors** MCC
Chemical pulmonary edema (acute) (chronic)
EXCLUDES1 *pulmonary edema (acute) (chronic) NOS (J81.-)*
J68.2 **Upper respiratory inflammation due to chemicals, gases, fumes and vapors, not elsewhere classified**
J68.3 **Other acute and subacute respiratory conditions due to chemicals, gases, fumes and vapors**
Reactive airways dysfunction syndrome
J68.4 **Chronic respiratory conditions due to chemicals, gases, fumes and vapors**
Emphysema (diffuse) (chronic) due to inhalation of chemicals, gases, fumes and vapors
Obliterative bronchiolitis (chronic) (subacute) due to inhalation of chemicals, gases, fumes and vapors
Pulmonary fibrosis (chronic) due to inhalation of chemicals, gases, fumes and vapors
EXCLUDES1 *chronic pulmonary edema due to chemicals, gases, fumes and vapors (J68.1)*
J68.8 **Other respiratory conditions due to chemicals, gases, fumes and vapors**
J68.9 **Unspecified respiratory condition due to chemicals, gases, fumes and vapors**

J69 Pneumonitis due to solids and liquids
EXCLUDES1 *neonatal aspiration syndromes (P24.-)*
postprocedural pneumonitis (J95.4)

J69.0 **Pneumonitis due to inhalation of food and vomit** MCC
Aspiration pneumonia NOS
Aspiration pneumonia (due to) food (regurgitated)
Aspiration pneumonia (due to) gastric secretions
Aspiration pneumonia (due to) milk
Aspiration pneumonia (due to) vomit
Code also any associated foreign body in respiratory tract (T17.-)
EXCLUDES1 *chemical pneumonitis due to anesthesia (J95.4)*
obstetric aspiration pneumonitis (O74.0)
J69.1 **Pneumonitis due to inhalation of oils and essences** MCC
Exogenous lipoid pneumonia
Lipid pneumonia NOS
Code first (T51-T65) to identify substance
EXCLUDES1 *endogenous lipoid pneumonia (J84.89)*
J69.8 **Pneumonitis due to inhalation of other solids and liquids** MCC
Pneumonitis due to aspiration of blood
Pneumonitis due to aspiration of detergent
Code first (T51-T65) to identify substance

J70 Respiratory conditions due to other external agents

J70.0 **Acute pulmonary manifestations due to radiation** CC
Radiation pneumonitis
Use additional code (W88-W90, X39.0-) to identify the external cause
J70.1 **Chronic and other pulmonary manifestations due to radiation** CC
Fibrosis of lung following radiation
Use additional code (W88-W90, X39.0-) to identify the external cause
J70.2 **Acute drug-induced interstitial lung disorders**
Use additional code for adverse effect, if applicable, to identify drug (T36-T50 with fifth or sixth character 5)
EXCLUDES1 *interstitial pneumonia NOS (J84.9)*
lymphoid interstitial pneumonia (J84.2)
J70.3 **Chronic drug-induced interstitial lung disorders**
Use additional code for adverse effect, if applicable, to identify drug (T36-T50 with fifth or sixth character 5)
EXCLUDES1 *interstitial pneumonia NOS (J84.9)*
lymphoid interstitial pneumonia (J84.2)
J70.4 **Drug-induced interstitial lung disorders, unspecified**
Use additional code for adverse effect, if applicable, to identify drug (T36-T50 with fifth or sixth character 5)
EXCLUDES1 *interstitial pneumonia NOS (J84.9)*
lymphoid interstitial pneumonia (J84.2)
J70.5 **Respiratory conditions due to smoke inhalation**
Smoke inhalation NOS
EXCLUDES1 *smoke inhalation due to chemicals, gases, fumes and vapors (J68.9)*
AHA: Q4, 2013
J70.8 **Respiratory conditions due to other specified external agents**
Code first (T51-T65) to identify the external agent
J70.9 **Respiratory conditions due to unspecified external agent**
Code first (T51-T65) to identify the external agent

Unspecified Code Other Specified Code Manifestation Code N Newborn P Pediatric M Maternity A Adult ♂ Male ♀ Female
● New Code ▲ Revised Code Title ►◄ Revised Text NOTES INCLUDES EXCLUDES1 Not coded here EXCLUDES2 Not included here
4th character required 5th character required 6th character required 7th character required
Extension 'X' Alert HAC Hospital-acquired condition (HAC) alert AHA AHA Coding Clinic©

Other respiratory diseases principally affecting the interstitium (J80-J84)

J80 Acute respiratory distress syndrome CC
Acute respiratory distress syndrome in adult or child
Adult hyaline membrane disease
EXCLUDES1 *respiratory distress syndrome in newborn (perinatal) (P22.0)*

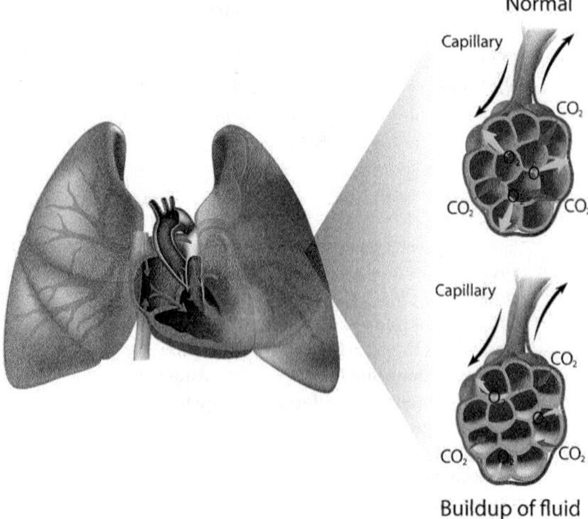

Figure 10.6 Pulmonary edema

4th **J81 Pulmonary edema**
Use additional code to identify:
exposure to environmental tobacco smoke (Z77.22)
history of tobacco ▶dependence◀ (Z87.891)
occupational exposure to environmental tobacco smoke (Z57.31)
tobacco dependence (F17.-)
tobacco use (Z72.0)
EXCLUDES1 *chemical (acute) pulmonary edema (J68.1)*
hypostatic pneumonia (J18.2)
passive pneumonia (J18.2)
pulmonary edema due to external agents (J60-J70)
pulmonary edema with heart disease NOS (I50.1)
pulmonary edema with heart failure (I50.1)

J81.0 **Acute pulmonary edema** MCC
Acute edema of lung

J81.1 **Chronic pulmonary edema** CC
Pulmonary congestion (chronic) (passive)
Pulmonary edema NOS

J82 Pulmonary eosinophilia, not elsewhere classified CC
Allergic pneumonia
Eosinophilic asthma
Eosinophilic pneumonia
Löffler's pneumonia
Tropical (pulmonary) eosinophilia NOS
EXCLUDES1 *pulmonary eosinophilia due to aspergillosis (B44.-)*
pulmonary eosinophilia due to drugs (J70.2-J70.4)
pulmonary eosinophilia due to specified parasitic infection (B50-B83)
pulmonary eosinophilia due to systemic connective tissue disorders (M30-M36)
pulmonary infiltrate NOS (R91.8)

4th **J84 Other interstitial pulmonary diseases**
EXCLUDES1 *drug-induced interstitial lung disorders (J70.2-J70.4)*
interstitial emphysema (J98.2)
lung diseases due to external agents (J60-J70)

5th J84.0 **Alveolar and parieto-alveolar conditions**

J84.01 **Alveolar proteinosis** CC

J84.02 **Pulmonary alveolar microlithiasis** CC

J84.03 **Idiopathic pulmonary hemosiderosis** CC
Essential brown induration of lung
Code first underlying disease, such as:
disorders of iron metabolism (E83.1-)
EXCLUDES1 *acute idiopathic pulmonary hemorrhage in infants [AIPHI] (R04.81)*

J84.09 **Other alveolar and parieto-alveolar conditions** CC

5th J84.1 **Other interstitial pulmonary diseases with fibrosis**
EXCLUDES1 *pulmonary fibrosis (chronic) due to inhalation of chemicals, gases, fumes or vapors (J68.4)*
pulmonary fibrosis (chronic) following radiation (J70.1)

J84.10 **Pulmonary fibrosis, unspecified**
Capillary fibrosis of lung
Cirrhosis of lung (chronic) NOS
Fibrosis of lung (atrophic) (chronic) (confluent) (massive) (perialveolar) (peribronchial) NOS
Induration of lung (chronic) NOS
Postinflammatory pulmonary fibrosis

6th J84.11 **Idiopathic interstitial pneumonia**
EXCLUDES1 *lymphoid interstitial pneumonia (J84.2)*
pneumocystis pneumonia (B59)

J84.111 **Idiopathic interstitial pneumonia, not otherwise specified**

J84.112 **Idiopathic pulmonary fibrosis**
Cryptogenic fibrosing alveolitis
Idiopathic fibrosing alveolitis

J84.113 **Idiopathic non-specific interstitial pneumonitis**
EXCLUDES1 *non-specific interstitial pneumonia NOS, or due to known underlying cause (J84.89)*

J84.114 **Acute interstitial pneumonitis** CC
Hamman-Rich syndrome
EXCLUDES1 *pneumocystis pneumonia (B59)*

J84.115 **Respiratory bronchiolitis interstitial lung disease**

J84.116 **Cryptogenic organizing pneumonia** CC
EXCLUDES1 *organizing pneumonia NOS, or due to known underlying cause (J84.89)*

J84.117 **Desquamative interstitial pneumonia** CC

J84.17 **Other interstitial pulmonary diseases with fibrosis in diseases classified elsewhere**
Interstitial pneumonia (nonspecific) (usual) due to collagen vascular disease
Interstitial pneumonia (nonspecific) (usual) in diseases classified elsewhere
Organizing pneumonia due to collagen vascular disease
Organizing pneumonia in diseases classified elsewhere
Code first underlying disease, such as:
progressive systemic sclerosis (M34.0)
rheumatoid arthritis (M05.00-M06.9)
systemic lupus erythematosis (M32.0-M32.9)

J84.2 **Lymphoid interstitial pneumonia** CC
Lymphoid interstitial pneumonitis

5th J84.8 **Other specified interstitial pulmonary diseases**
EXCLUDES1 *exogenous lipoid pneumonia (J69.1)*
unspecified lipoid pneumonia (J69.1)

J84.81 **Lymphangioleiomyomatosis** MCC ♀
Lymphangiomyomatosis

J84.82 **Adult pulmonary Langerhans cell histiocytosis** A CC
Adult PLCH

J84.83 **Surfactant mutations of the lung** MCC

6th J84.84 **Other interstitial lung diseases of childhood**

J84.841 **Neuroendocrine cell hyperplasia of infancy** MCC

J84.842 **Pulmonary interstitial glycogenosis** MCC

J84.843 **Alveolar capillary dysplasia with vein misalignment** MCC

J84.848 **Other interstitial lung diseases of childhood** MCC

J84.89 **Other specified interstitial pulmonary diseases**
Endogenous lipoid pneumonia
Interstitial pneumonitis
Non-specific interstitial pneumonitis NOS
Organizing pneumonia NOS
Code first , if applicable:

PDx Unacceptable principal diagnosis symbol per Medicare code edits   POA Code exempt from diagnosis present on admission requirement
Q Questionable admission   CC Complication or comorbidity   CC/MCC Exc CC/MCC exclusion   MCC Major complication or comorbidity
PDx CC Principal diagnosis as its own CC   PDx MCC Principal diagnosis as its own MCC   Z1 Z code as first-listed diagnosis

poisoning due to drug or toxin (T51-T65 with fifth or sixth character to indicate intent), for toxic pneumonopathy
underlying cause of pneumonopathy, if known
Use additional code, for adverse effect, to identify drug (T36-T50 with fifth or sixth character 5), if drug-induced
EXCLUDES1 *cryptogenic organizing pneumonia (J84.116)*
idiopathic non-specific interstitial pneumonitis (J84.113)
lipoid pneumonia, exogenous or unspecified (J69.1)
lymphoid interstitial pneumonia (J84.2)

J84.9 **Interstitial pulmonary disease, unspecified** CC
Interstitial pneumonia NOS

Suppurative and necrotic conditions of the lower respiratory tract (J85-J86)

J85 **Abscess of lung and mediastinum**
Use additional code (B95-B97) to identify infectious agent.
J85.0 Gangrene **and** necrosis **of lung** MCC
J85.1 Abscess **of lung** with pneumonia MCC
Code also the type of pneumonia
J85.2 **Abscess of lung** without pneumonia MCC
Abscess of lung NOS
J85.3 **Abscess of** mediastinum MCC

J86 Pyothorax
Use additional code (B95-B97) to identify infectious agent.
EXCLUDES1 *abscess of lung (J85.-)*
pyothorax due to tuberculosis (A15.6)
J86.0 **Pyothorax** with fistula MCC
Bronchocutaneous fistula
Bronchopleural fistula
Hepatopleural fistula
Mediastinal fistula
Pleural fistula
Thoracic fistula
Any condition classifiable to J86.9 with fistula
J86.9 **Pyothorax** without fistula MCC
Abscess of pleura
Abscess of thorax
Empyema (chest) (lung) (pleura)
Fibrinopurulent pleurisy
Purulent pleurisy
Pyopneumothorax
Septic pleurisy
Seropurulent pleurisy
Suppurative pleurisy

Other diseases of the pleura (J90-J94)

J90 Pleural effusion**, not elsewhere classified** CC
Encysted pleurisy
Pleural effusion NOS
Pleurisy with effusion (exudative) (serous)
EXCLUDES1 *chylous (pleural) effusion (J94.0)*
malignant pleural effusion (J91.0))
pleurisy NOS (R09.1)
tuberculous pleural effusion (A15.6)

J91 **Pleural effusion in conditions classified elsewhere**
EXCLUDES2 *pleural effusion in heart failure (I50.-)*
pleural effusion in systemic lupus erythematosus (M32.13)
J91.0 **Malignant pleural effusion** CC
Code first underlying neoplasm
J91.8 **Pleural effusion in other conditions classified elsewhere** CC
Code first underlying disease, such as:
filariasis (B74.0-B74.9)
influenza (J09.X2, J10.1, J11.1)

J92 **Pleural plaque**
INCLUDES *pleural thickening*
J92.0 **Pleural plaque with presence of asbestos**
J92.9 **Pleural plaque without asbestos**
Pleural plaque NOS

J93 **Pneumothorax and air leak**
EXCLUDES1 *congenital or perinatal pneumothorax (P25.1)*
postprocedural air leak (J95.812)
postprocedural pneumothorax (J95.811)
traumatic pneumothorax (S27.0)
tuberculous (current disease) pneumothorax (A15.-)
pyopneumothorax (J86.-)
J93.0 **Spontaneous tension pneumothorax** MCC
J93.1 **Other** spontaneous pneumothorax
J93.11 Primary **spontaneous pneumothorax** CC
J93.12 Secondary **spontaneous pneumothorax** CC PDx
Code first underlying condition, such as:
catamenial pneumothorax due to endometriosis (N80.8)
cystic fibrosis (E84.-)
eosinophilic pneumonia (J82)
lymphangioleiomyomatosis (J84.81)
malignant neoplasm of bronchus and lung (C34.-)
Marfan's syndrome (Q87.4)
pneumonia due to Pneumocystis carinii (B59)
secondary malignant neoplasm of lung (C78.0-)
spontaneous rupture of the esophagus (K22.3)
J93.8 **Other pneumothorax and air leak**
J93.81 Chronic **pneumothorax** CC
J93.82 Other air leak CC
Persistent air leak
J93.83 Other **pneumothorax** CC
Acute pneumothorax
Spontaneous pneumothorax NOS
J93.9 **Pneumothorax, unspecified** CC
Pneumothorax NOS

J94 Other **pleural conditions**
EXCLUDES1 *pleurisy NOS (R09.1)*
traumatic hemopneumothorax (S27.2)
traumatic hemothorax (S27.1)
tuberculous pleural conditions (current disease) (A15.-)
J94.0 **Chylous effusion** CC
Chyliform effusion
J94.1 **Fibrothorax**
J94.2 **Hemothorax** CC
Hemopneumothorax
J94.8 **Other specified pleural conditions** CC
Hydropneumothorax
Hydrothorax
J94.9 **Pleural condition, unspecified**

Intraoperative and postprocedural complications and disorders of respiratory system, not elsewhere classified (J95)

J95 Intraoperative and postprocedural **complications and disorders of respiratory system, not elsewhere classified**
EXCLUDES2 *aspiration pneumonia (J69.-)*
emphysema (subcutaneous) resulting from a procedure (T81.82)
hypostatic pneumonia (J18.2)
pulmonary manifestations due to radiation (J70.0-J70.1)
J95.0 Tracheostomy **complications**
J95.00 **Unspecified tracheostomy complication** CC
J95.01 Hemorrhage **from tracheostomy stoma** CC
J95.02 Infection **of tracheostomy stoma** CC
Use additional code to identify type of infection, such as:
cellulitis of neck (L03.8)
sepsis (A40, A41.-)
J95.03 Malfunction **of tracheostomy stoma** CC
Mechanical complication of tracheostomy stoma
Obstruction of tracheostomy airway
Tracheal stenosis due to tracheostomy
J95.04 Tracheo-esophageal fistula **following tracheostomy** CC
J95.09 Other **tracheostomy complication** CC

Unspecified Code Other Specified Code Manifestation Code N Newborn P Pediatric M Maternity A Adult ♂ Male ♀ Female
● New Code ▲ Revised Code Title ►◄ Revised Text NOTES INCLUDES EXCLUDES1 Not coded here EXCLUDES2 Not included here
4th character required 5th character required 6th character required 7th character required
Extension 'X' Alert HAC Hospital-acquired condition (HAC) alert AHA AHA Coding Clinic®

J95.1 Acute pulmonary insufficiency following thoracic surgery
EXCLUDES2 *Functional disturbances following cardiac surgery (I97.0, I97.1-)*

J95.2 Acute pulmonary insufficiency following nonthoracic surgery
EXCLUDES2 *Functional disturbances following cardiac surgery (I97.0, I97.1-)*

J95.3 Chronic pulmonary insufficiency following surgery
EXCLUDES2 *Functional disturbances following cardiac surgery (I97.0, I97.1-)*

J95.4 Chemical pneumonitis due to anesthesia
Mendelson's syndrome
Postprocedural aspiration pneumonia
Use additional code for adverse effect, if applicable, to identify drug (T41.- with fifth or sixth character 5)
EXCLUDES1 *aspiration pneumonitis due to anesthesia complicating labor and delivery (O74.0)*
aspiration pneumonitis due to anesthesia complicating pregnancy (O29)
aspiration pneumonitis due to anesthesia complicating the puerperium (O89.01)

J95.5 Postprocedural subglottic stenosis

J95.6 Intraoperative hemorrhage and hematoma of a respiratory system organ or structure complicating a procedure
EXCLUDES1 *intraoperative hemorrhage and hematoma of a respiratory system organ or structure due to accidental puncture and laceration during procedure (J95.7-)*
J95.61 Intraoperative hemorrhage and hematoma of a respiratory system organ or structure complicating a respiratory system procedure
J95.62 Intraoperative hemorrhage and hematoma of a respiratory system organ or structure complicating other procedure

J95.7 Accidental puncture and laceration of a respiratory system organ or structure during a procedure
EXCLUDES2 *postprocedural pneumothorax (J95.811)*
J95.71 Accidental puncture and laceration of a respiratory system organ or structure during a respiratory system procedure
J95.72 Accidental puncture and laceration of a respiratory system organ or structure during other procedure

J95.8 Other intraoperative and postprocedural complications and disorders of respiratory system, not elsewhere classified
J95.81 Postprocedural pneumothorax and air leak
J95.811 Postprocedural pneumothorax HAC
J95.812 Postprocedural air leak
J95.82 Postprocedural respiratory failure
EXCLUDES1 *Respiratory failure in other conditions (J96.-)*
J95.821 Acute postprocedural respiratory failure
Postprocedural respiratory failure NOS
J95.822 Acute and chronic postprocedural respiratory failure
▲ J95.83 Postprocedural ▶hemorrhage of◀ a respiratory system organ or structure following a procedure
▲ J95.830 Postprocedural ▶hemorrhage of◀ a respiratory system organ or structure following a respiratory system procedure
▲ J95.831 Postprocedural ▶hemorrhage of◀ a respiratory system organ or structure following other procedure
J95.84 Transfusion-related acute lung injury (TRALI)
J95.85 Complication of respirator [ventilator]
J95.850 Mechanical complication of respirator
EXCLUDES1 *encounter for respirator [ventilator] dependence during power failure (Z99.12)*
J95.851 Ventilator associated pneumonia
Ventilator associated pneumonitis
Use additional code to identify the organism, if known (B95.-, B96.-, B97.-)
EXCLUDES1 *ventilator lung in newborn (P27.8)*
J95.859 Other complication of respirator [ventilator]
● J95.86 Postprocedural hematoma and seroma of a respiratory system organ or structure following a procedure
● J95.860 Postprocedural hematoma of a respiratory system organ or structure following a respiratory system procedure
● J95.861 Postprocedural hematoma of a respiratory system organ or structure following other procedure
● J95.862 Postprocedural seroma of a respiratory system organ or structure following a respiratory system procedure
● J95.863 Postprocedural seroma of a respiratory system organ or structure following other procedure
J95.88 Other intraoperative complications of respiratory system, not elsewhere classified
J95.89 Other postprocedural complications and disorders of respiratory system, not elsewhere classified
Use additional code to identify disorder, such as:
aspiration pneumonia (J69.-)
bacterial or viral pneumonia (J12-J18)
EXCLUDES2 *acute pulmonary insufficiency following thoracic surgery (J95.1)*
postprocedural subglottic stenosis (J95.5)

Other diseases of the respiratory system (J96-J99)

J96 Respiratory failure, not elsewhere classified
EXCLUDES1 *acute respiratory distress syndrome (J80)*
cardiorespiratory failure (R09.2)
newborn respiratory distress syndrome (P22.0)
postprocedural respiratory failure (J95.82-)
respiratory arrest (R09.2)
respiratory arrest of newborn (P28.81)
respiratory failure of newborn (P28.5)

J96.0 Acute respiratory failure
J96.00 Acute respiratory failure, unspecified whether with hypoxia or hypercapnia
AHA: Q4, 2013
J96.01 Acute respiratory failure with hypoxia
J96.02 Acute respiratory failure with hypercapnia

J96.1 Chronic respiratory failure
J96.10 Chronic respiratory failure, unspecified whether with hypoxia or hypercapnia
AHA: Q1, 2015
J96.11 Chronic respiratory failure with hypoxia
AHA: Q4, 2013
J96.12 Chronic respiratory failure with hypercapnia

J96.2 Acute and chronic respiratory failure
Acute on chronic respiratory failure
J96.20 Acute and chronic respiratory failure, unspecified whether with hypoxia or hypercapnia
J96.21 Acute and chronic respiratory failure with hypoxia
J96.22 Acute and chronic respiratory failure with hypercapnia

J96.9 Respiratory failure, unspecified
J96.90 Respiratory failure, unspecified, unspecified whether with hypoxia or hypercapnia
J96.91 Respiratory failure, unspecified with hypoxia
J96.92 Respiratory failure, unspecified with hypercapnia

J98 Other respiratory disorders
Use additional code to identify:
exposure to environmental tobacco smoke (Z77.22)
exposure to tobacco smoke in the perinatal period (P96.81)
history of tobacco ▶dependence◀ (Z87.891)
occupational exposure to environmental tobacco smoke (Z57.31)
tobacco dependence (F17.-)
tobacco use (Z72.0)
EXCLUDES1 *newborn apnea (P28.4)*
newborn sleep apnea (P28.3)
EXCLUDES2 *apnea NOS (R06.81)*
sleep apnea (G47.3-)

Unacceptable principal diagnosis symbol per Medicare code edits | Code exempt from diagnosis present on admission requirement
Questionable admission | Complication or comorbidity | CC/MCC exclusion | Major complication or comorbidity
Principal diagnosis as its own CC | Principal diagnosis as its own MCC | Z code as first-listed diagnosis

J98.0 Diseases of bronchus, not elsewhere classified

J98.01 Acute bronchospasm

EXCLUDES1 *acute bronchiolitis with bronchospasm (J21.-)*
acute bronchitis with bronchospasm (J20.-)
asthma (J45.-)
exercise induced bronchospasm (J45.990)

J98.09 Other diseases of bronchus, not elsewhere classified

Broncholithiasis
Calcification of bronchus
Stenosis of bronchus
Tracheobronchial collapse
Tracheobronchial dyskinesia
Ulcer of bronchus

J98.1 Pulmonary collapse

EXCLUDES1 *therapeutic collapse of lung status (Z98.3)*

J98.11 Atelectasis CC

EXCLUDES1 *newborn atelectasis*
tuberculous atelectasis (current disease) (A15)

J98.19 Other pulmonary collapse CC

J98.2 Interstitial emphysema

Mediastinal emphysema

EXCLUDES1 *emphysema NOS (J43.9)*
emphysema in newborn (P25.0)
surgical emphysema (subcutaneous) (T81.82)
traumatic subcutaneous emphysema (T79.7)

J98.3 Compensatory emphysema

J98.4 Other disorders of lung

Calcification of lung
Cystic lung disease (acquired)
Lung disease NOS
Pulmolithiasis

EXCLUDES1 *acute interstitial pneumonitis (J84.114)*
pulmonary insufficiency following surgery (J95.1-J95.2)

J98.5 Diseases of mediastinum, not elsewhere classified

EXCLUDES2 *abscess of mediastinum (J85.3)*

● J98.51 Mediastinitis MCC

Code first underlying condition, if applicable, such as postoperative mediastinitis (T81.-)

● J98.59 Other diseases of mediastinum, not elsewhere classified MCC

Fibrosis of mediastinum
Hernia of mediastinum
Retraction of mediastinum

J98.6 Disorders of diaphragm

Diaphragmatitis
Paralysis of diaphragm
Relaxation of diaphragm

EXCLUDES1 *congenital malformation of diaphragm NEC (Q79.1)*
congenital diaphragmatic hernia (Q79.0)

EXCLUDES2 *diaphragmatic hernia (K44.-)*

J98.8 Other specified respiratory disorders

J98.9 Respiratory disorder, unspecified

Respiratory disease (chronic) NOS

J99 Respiratory disorders in diseases classified elsewhere

Code first underlying disease, such as:
amyloidosis (E85.-)
ankylosing spondylitis (M45)
congenital syphilis (A50.5)
cryoglobulinemia (D89.1)
early congenital syphilis (A50.0)
schistosomiasis (B65.0-B65.9)

EXCLUDES1 *respiratory disorders in:*
amebiasis (A06.5)
blastomycosis (B40.0-B40.2)
candidiasis (B37.1)
coccidioidomycosis (B38.0-B38.2)
cystic fibrosis with pulmonary manifestations (E84.0)
dermatomyositis (M33.01, M33.11)
histoplasmosis (B39.0-B39.2)
late syphilis (A52.72, A52.73)
polymyositis (M33.21)
sicca syndrome (M35.02)
systemic lupus erythematosus (M32.13)
systemic sclerosis (M34.81)
Wegener's granulomatosis (M31.30-M31.31)

This page intentionally left blank

Chapter 11: Diseases of the Digestive System (K00-K95)

Guidelines for Assigning Codes From This Chapter

The first six sections of Chapter 11 codes cover mostly the digestive system from beginning to end, starting with the mouth and jaws and going to the intestines. The next section for digestive system diseases covers abdominal structures (peritoneum and retroperitoneum), the next two sections relate to diseases involving the organs, including many liver, gallbladder, biliary tract, and pancreas disorders. The final section identifies other diseases that do not fit into the first nine sections.

List of Sections

- K00-K14 Diseases of oral cavity and salivary glands
- K20-K31 Diseases of esophagus, stomach and duodenum
- K35-K38 Diseases of appendix
- K40-K46 Hernia
- K50-K52 Noninfective enteritis and colitis
- K55-K64 Other diseases of intestines
- K65-K68 Diseases of peritoneum and retroperitoneum
- K70-K77 Diseases of liver
- K80-K87 Disorders of gallbladder, biliary tract and pancreas
- K90-K95 Other diseases of the digestive system

Highlights From the ICD-10-CM Official Guidelines for Coding and Reporting

The 2017 version of the ICD-10-CM Official Guidelines for Coding and Reporting do not include specific guidelines for Chapter 11, stating that the section is reserved for future expansion.

Still, as with every ICD-10-CM chapter, you should be sure to review and apply the guidelines and instructions included in the manual with the codes and code ranges. Below are some key areas to watch:

- **Ulcers:** When reporting esophageal (K22.1-), gastric (K25.-), duodenal (K26.-), and peptic (K27.-) ulcers, keep an eye out for an instruction specific to drug-induced ulcers. When the medical record shows a drug caused the ulcer, you should report a code from the T36-T50 range with fifth or sixth character of 5 to identify the drug. In addition, if the ulcer is caused by a corrosive substance, there is a code first note that instructs you to code for the chemical involved in a chemical-caused ulcer (T51-T65).
- **Bariatric complications:** Two of the codes in the range K95.- (*Complications of bariatric procedures*) include an instruction to report an additional code to identify the specific infection if the complication is a result of infection. In other words, you should report more than just the existence of a complication. When reporting K95.01 (*Infection due to gastric band procedure*) and K95.81 (*Infection due to other bariatric procedure*), you should check the documentation for the specific infective agent and report that code as well.
- **Diaphragmatic hernia:** The Excludes note with K44 (*Diaphragmatic hernia*) states that you should not use it for a congenital diaphragmatic hernia or a congenital hiatal hernia. Instead you should use Q79.0 (*Congenital diaphragmatic hernia*). Similarly, although K44 includes hiatal hernias, you should use Q40.1 (*Congenital hiatus hernia*) for congenital hiatal hernias.
  - ➢ This Excludes note serves as a reminder that ICD-10-CM often uses separate codes for acquired and congenital disorders. The definition of the acquired condition code may not specify "acquired," making it difficult to know whether the code only applies to an acquired condition. When coding a congenital condition, keep the likelihood of a distinct code in mind as you check the index and tabular list for the proper code.
- **Portal hypertension:** When documentation shows a complication related to portal hypertension, an instruction with K76.6 (*Portal hypertension*) states that you should report the complication as an additional diagnosis. The example ICD-10-CM gives is K31.89 (*Portal hypertensive gastropathy*), but this is not the only possibility. You should choose your codes based on the documentation for the specific case you're coding.

Anatomy of the Digestive System

1. **An Overview of the Digestive System**
   a) The process of digestion involves the breaking down of food into the simpler substances that can be utilized by multiple cells of the body for producing high energy (or ATP) molecules.
   b) The digestive system is based on the processes of ingestion, peristalsis, digestion, absorption and defecation.
   c) The mouth, pharynx, esophagus, stomach, small and large intestines, and anus are regarded as the organs of the digestive tract.
   d) The teeth, tongue, salivary glands, liver, gall bladder and pancreas are known as the accessory or subordinate organs of the digestive tract.
   e) The mucosa, submucosa, muscularis and adventitia (or serosa) are the coats (or tunics) of the digestive tract.
2. **The Anatomy of the Oral Cavity**
   a) The oral cavity is also known as the mouth and is the first portion of the alimentary canal that receives food and saliva.
   b) The functions of the oral cavity are listed below:
      i) taste (through the taste buds on tongue).
      ii) mechanical breakdown of the food by the teeth.
      iii) chemical digestion of carbohydrates by the salivary enzyme amylase.
   c) The oral cavity is composed of the following components:
      i) mucus membrane that lines the oral cavity.
      ii) tongue that forms the floor of the oral cavity.
      iii) hard and soft palate that forms the roof of the oral cavity.
      iv) cheeks that form the sides of the oral cavity.
   d) The salivary glands are the exocrine glands that produce saliva. The parotid, submandibular (or submaxillary) and the sublingual glands are the three pairs of salivary glands.
   e) A typical human tooth is made up of dentin and consists of the following components:
      i) crown, which remains covered with enamel.
      ii) neck (or cervix).
      iii) root.
      iv) periodontal ligament, which fixates the tooth into its alveolar socket.

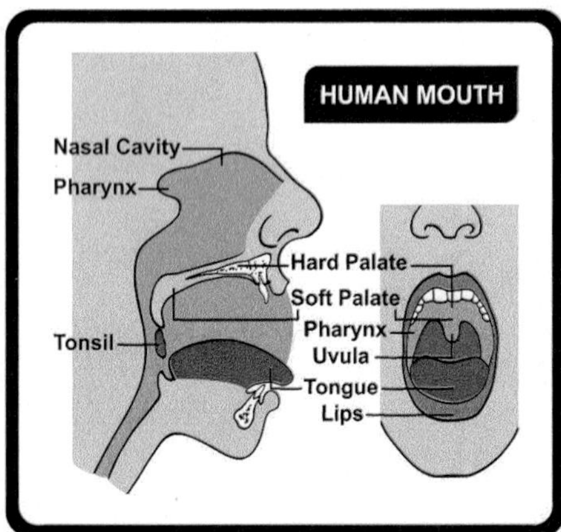

3. **The Anatomy of the Pharynx**
   a) The pharynx is the part of the throat that remains situated behind the nasal cavity and mouth and is a common passageway for food and air.
   b) The nasopharynx, oropharynx and laryngopharynx are the three parts of the pharynx.
   c) The pharynx is a part of both the digestive and respiratory systems and facilitates the process of speech production and swallowing (or deglutition).

The Salivary Glands

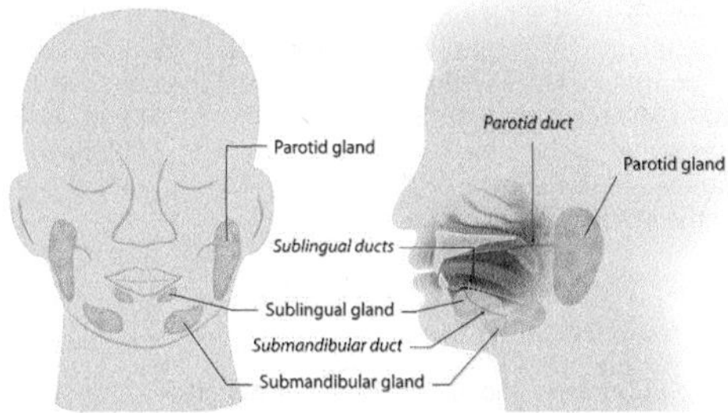

4. **The Anatomy of the Esophagus**
   a) The esophagus is a muscular tube for transporting the food from the pharynx to the stomach through the esophageal hiatus (or opening in the diaphragm).
   b) The food is propelled into the stomach via the lower esophageal sphincter. The movement of food is caused by the peristalsis (or symmetrical contraction and relaxation) of the smooth muscles.
5. **The Anatomy of the Stomach**
   a) The stomach is a muscular and hollow organ of the digestive tract and facilitates the second phase of digestion. It is positioned between the esophagus and the small intestine.
   b) The stomach aids in the digestion of food by performing the chemical breakdown of proteins through the protein-digesting enzyme pepsin.
   c) The stomach is based on the following four parts:
      i) cardia
      ii) fundus
      iii) body
      iv) pylorus
   d) The partially digested food (or chyme) is transported to the small intestine from the stomach.
   e) There are three kind of secretory cells in the gastric glands of the stomach mucosa.
      i) zymogenic cells, which secrete pepsinogen.
      ii) parietal cells, which secrete hydrochloric acid.
      iii) mucous cells, which secrete mucus.
   f) The stomach contains the below mentioned two sphincters (to retain the food contents inside it):
      i) esophageal sphincter, which is located in the cardiac region of the stomach.
      ii) pyloric sphincter, which demarcates the stomach from the small intestine.
6. **The Anatomy of the Pancreas**
   a) The pancreas is a glandular organ of both the digestive and endocrine systems.
   b) The pancreas is an endocrine as well as exocrine gland, and secretes hormones (like insulin, glucagon, and somatostatin) and the pancreatic juice (which contains several digestive enzymes). The digestive enzymes of the pancreatic juice facilitate the breakdown of the carbohydrates, proteins, and lipids in the chyme (or the partially digested food).
   c) The pancreas contains two types of the parenchymal tissues:
      i) pancreatic acini, which produce the digestive enzymes into the duodenum of the small intestine.
      ii) pancreatic islets of Langerhans, which secrete insulin and glucagon hormones into the blood for maintaining blood sugar levels.
7. **The Anatomy of the Liver**
   a) The liver is the largest glandular organ of the human body. It weighs about 1500g and is divided into the right and left lobes.
   b) The lobules are the functional units of the liver.
   c) The primary function of the liver is the storage of glycogen and secretion of bile. It also produces heparin, prothrombin, and thrombin.
   d) The Kupffer cells (or stellate macrophages) of the liver perform phagocytosis of the bacteria and the worn out blood cells.
   e) The liver stores various elements like copper, iron, and vitamins A, D, E, and K. It also helps to detoxify the poisonous substances in the human body, and produces bile salts for the emulsification (or break down) of the body fats.

f) The liver lobules facilitate the production of bile, which is then stored and concentrated in gall bladder.

g) The common bile duct carries the bile from the liver and gallbladder to the duodenum. It is formed by the union of the cystic and hepatic ducts.

h) The porta hepatis is a transverse fissure in the middle visceral surface of the liver that gives passage to the hepatic portal vein, hepatic artery, hepatic nerve plexus, hepatic ducts, and the lymphatic vessels.

Liver Anatomy

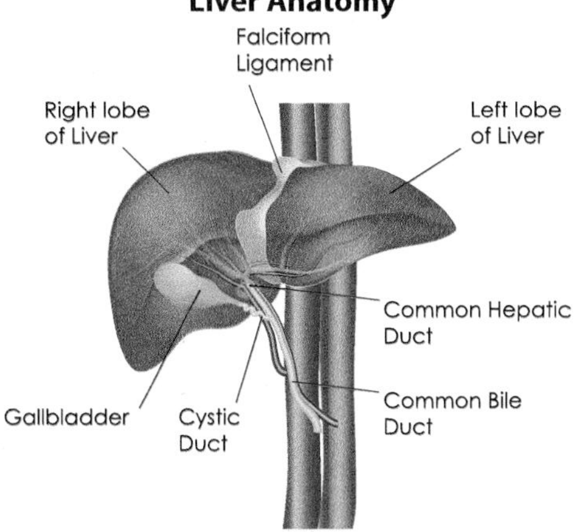

8. **The Anatomy of the Small Intestine**
   a) The small intestine extends from the pylorus of the stomach to the ileocecal junction. It is divided into the duodenum, jejunum and ileum.
   b) The ileocecal valve serves to connect the small intestine with the large intestine.
   c) The small intestine is involved in the completion of absorption of the digested food through the intestinal digestive enzymes, which are secreted by the intestinal glands (or the crypts of Lieberkuhn).
   d) The Brunner's glands (or pancreal glands/duodenal glands) are the compound tubular submucosal glands of the duodenum that secrete alkaline mucus.

9. **The Anatomy of the Large Intestine**
   a) The large intestine performs the following functions:
      i) reabsorption of water.
      ii) absorption and manufacture of vitamins.
      iii) formation and expulsion of feces.
   b) The large intestine is based on cecum, colon, rectum, and anus.
   c) The colon is divided into the following parts:
      i) ascending colon
      ii) right colic (or hepatic) flexure
      iii) transverse colon
      iv) left colic (or splenic) flexure
      v) descending colon
      vi) sigmoid colon
   d) The rectum terminates at the anus. The dilated portion of the rectum where feces are stored (before their elimination through the anal canal) is termed as the rectal ampulla.

Common Pathologies

Appendicitis
Inflammation of the appendix, which is usually acute and caused by the blocking of the appendix.

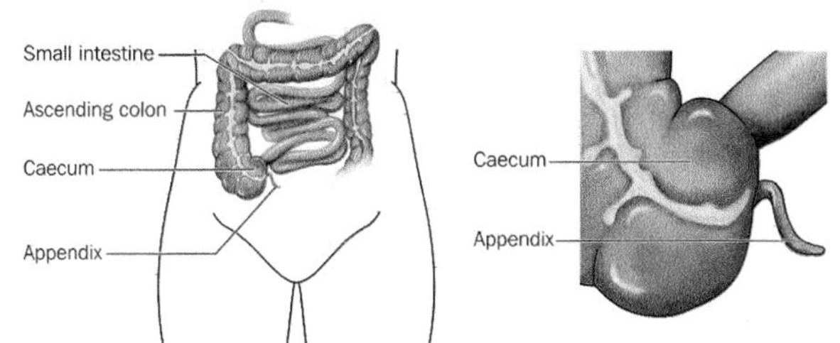

Ascites
Condition of abnormal accumulation of serous fluid in the peritoneal cavity.

Cirrhosis of Liver
This is a chronic liver disease, which is characterized by destruction of liver cells that ultimately leads to ineffective liver function and jaundice.

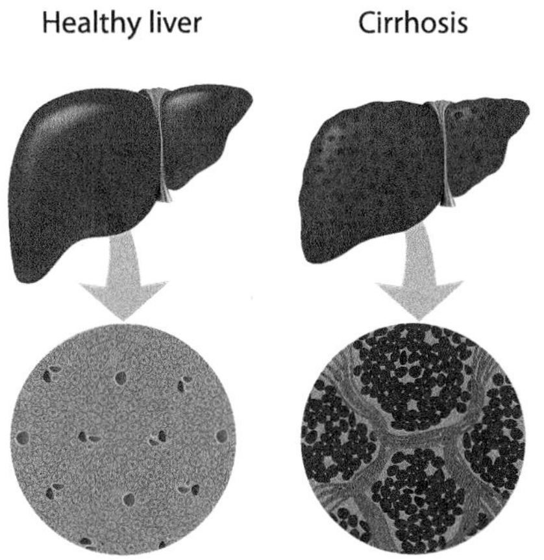

Diverticular Disease
This is a condition in which bulging pouches (known as diverticula) in the gastrointestinal (GI) tract push the mucosal lining through the surrounding muscle.

Dysentery
This is a condition that leads to inflammation of the intestine, especially of the colon, which may be caused by chemical irritants, bacteria, protozoa, or parasites.

Fistula
This is a condition in which there is an abnormal passage from one organ to another, or from a hollow organ to the surface.

Gastroesophageal Reflux Disease (GERD)
This is a condition that causes backflow (reflux) of gastric contents into the esophagus due to malfunction of the lower esophageal sphincter (LES).

Hematochezia
This is a condition marked by the passage of stools containing bright red blood.

Hemorrhoid
This is a condition that causes a mass of enlarged, twisted varicose veins in the mucous membrane inside (internal) or just outside (external) the rectum; also known as piles.

Hemorrhoid

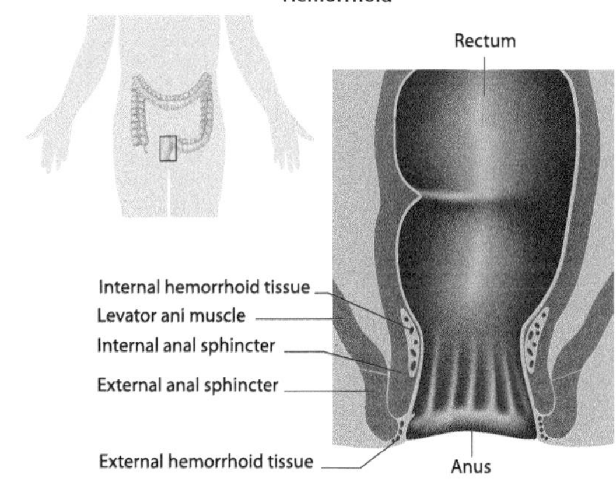

Hernia
This is a condition caused by the protrusion or projection of an organ or a part of an organ through the wall of the cavity that normally contains it.

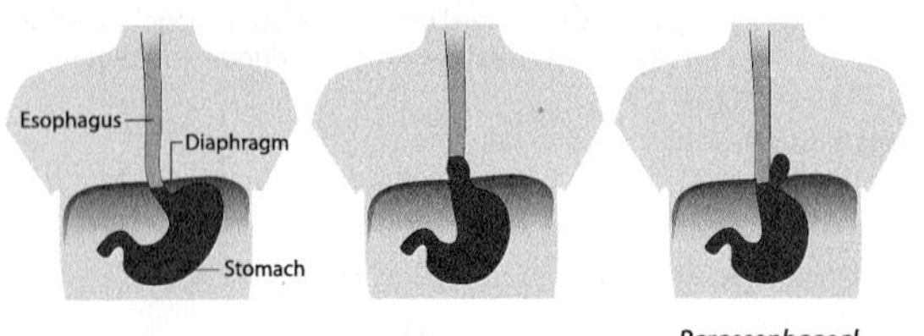

Inflammatory Bowel Disease (IBD)
This is a condition in which ulceration of the colon mucosa occurs.Ulcerative colitis and Crohn's disease are forms of IBD.

Crohn's Disease
This is the condition of chronic IBD that usually affects the ileum but may affect any portion of the intestinal tract.

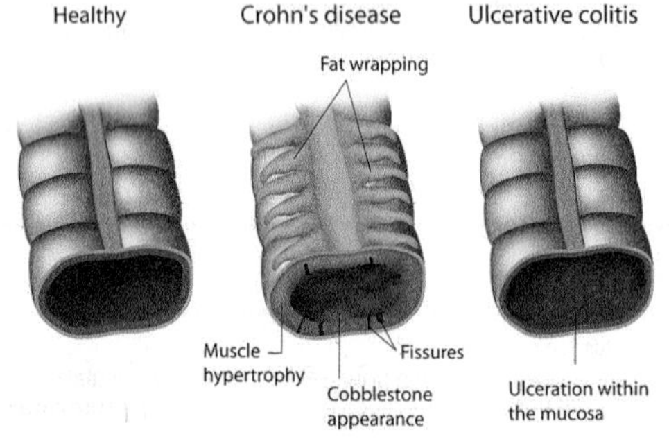

Ulcerative Colitis
This is the condition of chronic IBD of the colon characterized by episodes of diarrhea, rectal bleeding, and pain.

Irritable Bowel Syndrome (IBS)
This is the condition characterized by gastrointestinal signs and symptoms, including constipation, diarrhea, gas, and bloating, all in the absence of organic pathology; also called spastic colon.

Jaundice
This is the condition in which yellow discoloration of the skin, mucous membranes, and sclerae of the eyes is caused by excessive levels of bilirubin in the blood (hyperbilirubinemia).

Obesity
This is the condition in which a person accumulates an amount of fat that exceeds the body's skeletal and physical standards, usually an increase of 20 percent or more above ideal body weight.

Morbid Obesity
Condition of more severe obesity in which a person has a body mass index (BMI) of 40 or greater, which is generally 100 or more pounds over ideal body weight.

Polyp
A polyp is a small tumorlike, benign growth that projects from a mucous membrane surface.

Polyposis
This is a condition in which polyps develop in the intestinal tract.

Peptic Ulcer
This condition is also known as peptic ulcer disease; these are the painful ulcers that usually arise in duodenum.

Volvulus

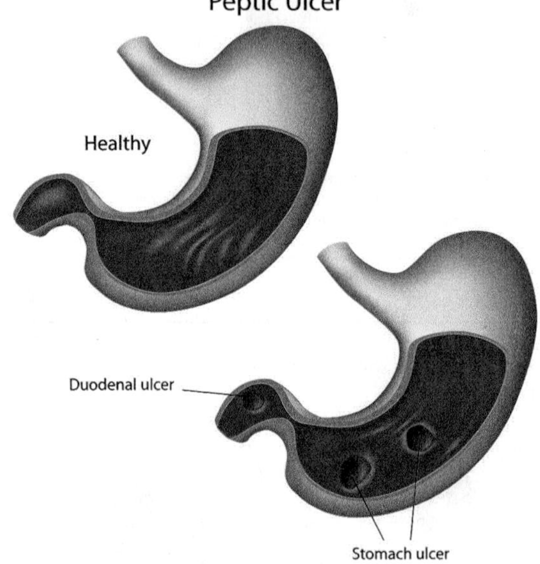

This is a condition in which the bowel twists on itself, causing obstruction.

Diseases of the digestive system (K00-K95)

EXCLUDES2 *certain conditions originating in the perinatal period (P04-P96)*
certain infectious and parasitic diseases (A00-B99)
complications of pregnancy, childbirth and the puerperium (O00-O9A)
congenital malformations, deformations and chromosomal abnormalities (Q00-Q99)
endocrine, nutritional and metabolic diseases (E00-E88)
injury, poisoning and certain other consequences of external causes (S00-T88)
neoplasms (C00-D49)
symptoms, signs and abnormal clinical and laboratory findings, not elsewhere classified (R00-R94)

This chapter contains the following blocks:

K00-K14 Diseases of oral cavity and salivary glands
K20-K31 Diseases of esophagus, stomach and duodenum
K35-K38 Diseases of appendix
K40-K46 Hernia
K50-K52 Noninfective enteritis and colitis
K55-K64 Other diseases of intestines
K65-K68 Diseases of peritoneum and retroperitoneum
K70-K77 Diseases of liver
K80-K87 Disorders of gallbladder, biliary tract and pancreas
K90-K95 Other diseases of the digestive system

Diseases of oral cavity and salivary glands (K00-K14)

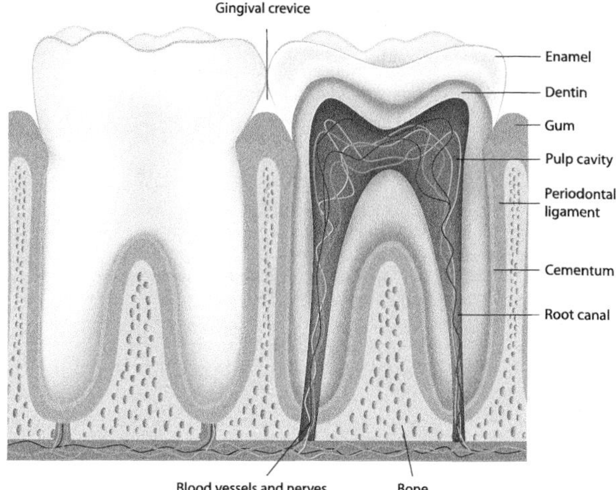

Figure 11.1 Tooth anatomy

K00 Disorders of tooth development and eruption
EXCLUDES2 *embedded and impacted teeth (K01.-)*

K00.0 Anodontia
Hypodontia
Oligodontia
EXCLUDES1 *acquired absence of teeth (K08.1-)*

K00.1 Supernumerary teeth
Distomolar
Fourth molar
Mesiodens
Paramolar
Supplementary teeth
EXCLUDES2 *supernumerary roots (K00.2)*

K00.2 Abnormalities of size and form of teeth
Concrescence of teeth
Fusion of teeth
Gemination of teeth
Dens evaginatus
Dens in dente
Dens invaginatus
Enamel pearls
Macrodontia
Microdontia
Peg-shaped [conical] teeth
Supernumerary roots
Taurodontism
Tuberculum paramolare
EXCLUDES1 *abnormalities of teeth due to congenital syphilis (A50.5)*
tuberculum Carabelli, which is regarded as a normal variation and should not be coded

K00.3 Mottled teeth
Dental fluorosis
Mottling of enamel
Nonfluoride enamel opacities
EXCLUDES2 *deposits [accretions] on teeth (K03.6)*

K00.4 Disturbances in tooth formation
Aplasia and hypoplasia of cementum
Dilaceration of tooth
Enamel hypoplasia (neonatal) (postnatal) (prenatal)
Regional odontodysplasia
Turner's tooth
EXCLUDES1 *Hutchinson's teeth and mulberry molars in congenital syphilis (A50.5)*
EXCLUDES2 *mottled teeth (K00.3)*

K00.5 Hereditary disturbances in tooth structure, not elsewhere classified
Amelogenesis imperfecta
Dentinogenesis imperfecta
Odontogenesis imperfecta
Dentinal dysplasia
Shell teeth

K00.6 Disturbances in tooth eruption
Dentia praecox
Natal tooth
Neonatal tooth
Premature eruption of tooth
Premature shedding of primary [deciduous] tooth
Prenatal teeth
Retained [persistent] primary tooth
EXCLUDES2 *embedded and impacted teeth (K01.-)*

K00.7 Teething syndrome

K00.8 Other disorders of tooth development
Color changes during tooth formation
Intrinsic staining of teeth NOS
EXCLUDES2 *posteruptive color changes (K03.7)*

K00.9 Disorder of tooth development, unspecified
Disorder of odontogenesis NOS

K01 Embedded and impacted teeth
EXCLUDES1 *abnormal position of fully erupted teeth (M26.3-)*

K01.0 Embedded teeth

K01.1 Impacted teeth

K02 Dental caries
INCLUDES *caries of dentine*
dental cavities
early childhood caries
pre-eruptive caries
recurrent caries (dentino enamel junction) (enamel) (to the pulp)
tooth decay

K02.3 Arrested dental caries
Arrested coronal and root caries

K02.5 Dental caries on pit and fissure surface
Dental caries on chewing surface of tooth

K02.51 Dental caries on pit and fissure surface limited to enamel
White spot lesions [initial caries] on pit and fissure surface of tooth

K02.52 Dental caries on pit and fissure surface penetrating into dentin
Primary dental caries, cervical origin

K02.53 Dental caries on pit and fissure surface penetrating into pulp

Unspecified Code Other Specified Code Manifestation Code N Newborn P Pediatric M Maternity A Adult ♂ Male ♀ Female
● New Code ▲ Revised Code Title ►◄ Revised Text NOTES INCLUDES EXCLUDES1 Not coded here EXCLUDES2 Not included here
4th character required 5th character required 6th character required 7th character required
Extension 'X' Alert HAC Hospital-acquired condition (HAC) alert AHA AHA Coding Clinic©

K02.6 Dental caries on smooth surface
- K02.61 **Dental caries on smooth surface limited to enamel**
  White spot lesions [initial caries] on smooth surface of tooth
- K02.62 **Dental caries on smooth surface penetrating into dentin**
- K02.63 **Dental caries on smooth surface penetrating into pulp**

K02.7 **Dental root caries**
K02.9 **Dental caries, unspecified**

K03 Other diseases of hard tissues of teeth
EXCLUDES2 *bruxism (F45.8)*
dental caries (K02.-)
teeth-grinding NOS (F45.8)

K03.0 **Excessive attrition of teeth**
Approximal wear of teeth
Occlusal wear of teeth

K03.1 **Abrasion of teeth**
Dentifrice abrasion of teeth
Habitual abrasion of teeth
Occupational abrasion of teeth
Ritual abrasion of teeth
Traditional abrasion of teeth
Wedge defect NOS

K03.2 **Erosion of teeth**
Erosion of teeth due to diet
Erosion of teeth due to drugs and medicaments
Erosion of teeth due to persistent vomiting
Erosion of teeth NOS
Idiopathic erosion of teeth
Occupational erosion of teeth

K03.3 **Pathological resorption of teeth**
Internal granuloma of pulp
Resorption of teeth (external)

K03.4 **Hypercementosis**
Cementation hyperplasia

K03.5 **Ankylosis of teeth**

K03.6 **Deposits [accretions] on teeth**
Betel deposits [accretions] on teeth
Black deposits [accretions] on teeth
Extrinsic staining of teeth NOS
Green deposits [accretions] on teeth
Materia alba deposits [accretions] on teeth
Orange deposits [accretions] on teeth
Staining of teeth NOS
Subgingival dental calculus
Supragingival dental calculus
Tobacco deposits [accretions] on teeth

K03.7 **Posteruptive color changes of dental hard tissues**
EXCLUDES2 *deposits [accretions] on teeth (K03.6)*

K03.8 **Other specified diseases of hard tissues of teeth**
- K03.81 **Cracked tooth**
  EXCLUDES1 *asymptomatic craze lines in enamel - omit code*
  broken or fractured tooth due to trauma (S02.5)
- K03.89 **Other specified diseases of hard tissues of teeth**

K03.9 **Disease of hard tissues of teeth, unspecified**

K04 Diseases of pulp and periapical tissues

K04.0 **Pulpitis**
Acute pulpitis
Chronic (hyperplastic) (ulcerative) pulpitis
- ● K04.01 **Reversible pulpitis** CC CC/MCC Exc
- ● K04.02 **Irreversible pulpitis** CC CC/MCC Exc

K04.1 **Necrosis of pulp**
Pulpal gangrene

K04.2 **Pulp degeneration**
Denticles
Pulpal calcifications
Pulpal stones

K04.3 **Abnormal hard tissue formation in pulp**
Secondary or irregular dentine

K04.4 **Acute apical periodontitis of pulpal origin** CC
Acute apical periodontitis NOS
EXCLUDES1 *acute periodontitis (K05.2-)*

K04.5 **Chronic apical periodontitis**
Apical or periapical granuloma
Apical periodontitis NOS
EXCLUDES1 *chronic periodontitis (K05.3-)*

K04.6 **Periapical abscess with sinus**
Dental abscess with sinus
Dentoalveolar abscess with sinus

K04.7 **Periapical abscess without sinus**
Dental abscess without sinus
Dentoalveolar abscess without sinus
Periapical abscess without sinus

K04.8 **Radicular cyst**
Apical (periodontal) cyst
Periapical cyst
Residual radicular cyst
EXCLUDES2 *lateral periodontal cyst (K09.0)*

K04.9 **Other and unspecified diseases of pulp and periapical tissues**
- K04.90 **Unspecified diseases of pulp and periapical tissues**
- K04.99 **Other diseases of pulp and periapical tissues**

K05 Gingivitis and periodontal diseases
Use additional code to identify:
alcohol abuse and dependence (F10.-)
exposure to environmental tobacco smoke (Z77.22)
exposure to tobacco smoke in the perinatal period (P96.81)
history of tobacco ▶dependence◀ (Z87.891)
occupational exposure to environmental tobacco smoke (Z57.31)
tobacco dependence (F17.-)
tobacco use (Z72.0)

K05.0 **Acute gingivitis**
EXCLUDES1 *acute necrotizing ulcerative gingivitis (A69.1)*
herpesviral [herpes simplex] gingivostomatitis (B00.2)
- K05.00 **Acute gingivitis, plaque induced**
  Acute gingivitis NOS
  Plaque induced gingival disease
- K05.01 **Acute gingivitis, non-plaque induced**

K05.1 **Chronic gingivitis**
Desquamative gingivitis (chronic)
Gingivitis (chronic) NOS
Hyperplastic gingivitis (chronic)
Pregnancy associated gingivitis
Simple marginal gingivitis (chronic)
Ulcerative gingivitis (chronic)
Code first, if applicable, diseases of the digestive system complicating pregnancy (O99.61-)
- K05.10 **Chronic gingivitis, plaque induced**
  Chronic gingivitis NOS
  Gingivitis NOS
- K05.11 **Chronic gingivitis, non-plaque induced**

K05.2 **Aggressive periodontitis**
Acute pericoronitis
EXCLUDES1 *acute apical periodontitis (K04.4)*
periapical abscess (K04.7)
periapical abscess with sinus (K04.6)
- K05.20 **Aggressive periodontitis, unspecified**
- K05.21 **Aggressive periodontitis, localized**
  Periodontal abscess
  - ● K05.211 **Aggressive periodontitis, localized, slight** CC/MCC Exc
  - ● K05.212 **Aggressive periodontitis, localized, moderate** CC/MCC Exc
  - ● K05.213 **Aggressive periodontitis, localized, severe** CC/MCC Exc
  - ● K05.219 **Aggressive periodontitis, localized, unspecified severity** CC/MCC Exc
- K05.22 **Aggressive periodontitis, generalized**
  - ● K05.221 **Aggressive periodontitis, generalized, slight** CC/MCC Exc
  - ● K05.222 **Aggressive periodontitis, generalized, moderate** CC/MCC Exc
  - ● K05.223 **Aggressive periodontitis, generalized, severe** CC/MCC Exc
  - ● K05.229 **Aggressive periodontitis, generalized, unspecified severity** CC/MCC Exc

PDx Unacceptable principal diagnosis symbol per Medicare code edits | POA Code exempt from diagnosis present on admission requirement
? Questionable admission | CC Complication or comorbidity | CC/MCC Exc CC/MCC exclusion | MCC Major complication or comorbidity
PDx CC Principal diagnosis as its own CC | PDx MCC Principal diagnosis as its own MCC | Z1 Z code as first-listed diagnosis

K05.3 Chronic periodontitis
Chronic pericoronitis
Complex periodontitis
Periodontitis NOS
Simplex periodontitis
EXCLUDES1 *chronic apical periodontitis (K04.5)*

K05.30 **Chronic periodontitis, unspecified**

K05.31 Chronic periodontitis, localized

- K05.311 **Chronic periodontitis, localized, slight** CC/MCC Exc
- K05.312 **Chronic periodontitis, localized, moderate** CC/MCC Exc
- K05.313 **Chronic periodontitis, localized, severe** CC/MCC Exc
- K05.319 **Chronic periodontitis, localized, unspecified severity** CC/MCC Exc

K05.32 Chronic periodontitis, generalized

- K05.321 **Chronic periodontitis, generalized, slight** CC/MCC Exc
- K05.322 **Chronic periodontitis, generalized, moderate** CC/MCC Exc
- K05.323 **Chronic periodontitis, generalized, severe** CC/MCC Exc
- K05.329 **Chronic periodontitis, generalized, unspecified severity** CC/MCC Exc

K05.4 **Periodontosis**
Juvenile periodontosis

K05.5 **Other periodontal diseases**
Combined periodontic-endodontic lesion
Narrow gingival width (of periodontal soft tissue)
EXCLUDES2 *leukoplakia of gingiva (K13.21)*

K05.6 **Periodontal disease, unspecified**

K06 **Other disorders of gingiva and edentulous alveolar ridge**
EXCLUDES2 *acute gingivitis (K05.0)*
atrophy of edentulous alveolar ridge (K08.2)
chronic gingivitis (K05.1)
gingivitis NOS (K05.1)

K06.0 **Gingival recession**
Gingival recession (generalized) (localized) (postinfective) (postprocedural)

K06.1 **Gingival enlargement**
Gingival fibromatosis

K06.2 **Gingival and edentulous alveolar ridge lesions associated with trauma**
Irritative hyperplasia of edentulous ridge [denture hyperplasia]
Use additional code (Chapter 20) to identify external cause or denture status (Z97.2)

- K06.3 **Horizontal alveolar bone loss** CC/MCC Exc

K06.8 **Other specified disorders of gingiva and edentulous alveolar ridge**
Fibrous epulis
Flabby alveolar ridge
Giant cell epulis
Peripheral giant cell granuloma of gingiva
Pyogenic granuloma of gingiva
Vertical ridge deficiency
EXCLUDES2 *gingival cyst (K09.0)*

K06.9 **Disorder of gingiva and edentulous alveolar ridge, unspecified**

K08 **Other disorders of teeth and supporting structures**
EXCLUDES2 *dentofacial anomalies [including malocclusion] (M26.-)*
disorders of jaw (M27.-)

K08.0 **Exfoliation of teeth due to systemic causes**
Code also underlying systemic condition

K08.1 **Complete loss of teeth**
Acquired loss of teeth, complete
EXCLUDES1 *congenital absence of teeth (K00.0)*
exfoliation of teeth due to systemic causes (K08.0)
partial loss of teeth (K08.4-)

K08.10 **Complete loss of teeth, unspecified cause**

K08.101 **Complete loss of teeth, unspecified cause, class I**
K08.102 **Complete loss of teeth, unspecified cause, class II**
K08.103 **Complete loss of teeth, unspecified cause, class III**
K08.104 **Complete loss of teeth, unspecified cause, class IV**
K08.109 **Complete loss of teeth, unspecified cause, unspecified class**
Edentulism NOS

K08.11 **Complete loss of teeth due to trauma**

K08.111 **Complete loss of teeth due to trauma, class I**
K08.112 **Complete loss of teeth due to trauma, class II**
K08.113 **Complete loss of teeth due to trauma, class III**
K08.114 **Complete loss of teeth due to trauma, class IV**
K08.119 **Complete loss of teeth due to trauma, unspecified class**

K08.12 **Complete loss of teeth due to periodontal diseases**

K08.121 **Complete loss of teeth due to periodontal diseases, class I**
K08.122 **Complete loss of teeth due to periodontal diseases, class II**
K08.123 **Complete loss of teeth due to periodontal diseases, class III**
K08.124 **Complete loss of teeth due to periodontal diseases, class IV**
K08.129 **Complete loss of teeth due to periodontal diseases, unspecified class**

K08.13 **Complete loss of teeth due to caries**

K08.131 **Complete loss of teeth due to caries, class I**
K08.132 **Complete loss of teeth due to caries, class II**
K08.133 **Complete loss of teeth due to caries, class III**
K08.134 **Complete loss of teeth due to caries, class IV**
K08.139 **Complete loss of teeth due to caries, unspecified class**

K08.19 **Complete loss of teeth due to other specified cause**

K08.191 **Complete loss of teeth due to other specified cause, class I**
K08.192 **Complete loss of teeth due to other specified cause, class II**
K08.193 **Complete loss of teeth due to other specified cause, class III**
K08.194 **Complete loss of teeth due to other specified cause, class IV**
K08.199 **Complete loss of teeth due to other specified cause, unspecified class**

K08.2 **Atrophy of edentulous alveolar ridge**

K08.20 **Unspecified atrophy of edentulous alveolar ridge**
Atrophy of the mandible NOS
Atrophy of the maxilla NOS

K08.21 **Minimal atrophy of the mandible**
Minimal atrophy of the edentulous mandible

K08.22 **Moderate atrophy of the mandible**
Moderate atrophy of the edentulous mandible

K08.23 **Severe atrophy of the mandible**
Severe atrophy of the edentulous mandible

K08.24 **Minimal atrophy of maxilla**
Minimal atrophy of the edentulous maxilla

K08.25 **Moderate atrophy of the maxilla**
Moderate atrophy of the edentulous maxilla

K08.26 **Severe atrophy of the maxilla**
Severe atrophy of the edentulous maxilla

K08.3 **Retained dental root**

K08.4 **Partial loss of teeth**
Acquired loss of teeth, partial
EXCLUDES1 *complete loss of teeth (K08.1-)*
congenital absence of teeth (K00.0)
EXCLUDES2 *exfoliation of teeth due to systemic causes (K08.0)*

Unspecified Code | Other Specified Code | Manifestation Code | N Newborn | P Pediatric | M Maternity | A Adult | ♂ Male | ♀ Female
● New Code | ▲ Revised Code Title | ►◄ Revised Text | NOTES | INCLUDES | EXCLUDES1 Not coded here | EXCLUDES2 Not included here
4th character required | 5th character required | 6th character required | 7th character required
Extension 'X' Alert | HAC Hospital-acquired condition (HAC) alert | AHA AHA Coding Clinic©

K08.40 Partial loss of teeth, unspecified cause
- K08.401 **Partial loss of teeth, unspecified cause, class I**
- K08.402 **Partial loss of teeth, unspecified cause, class II**
- K08.403 **Partial loss of teeth, unspecified cause, class III**
- K08.404 **Partial loss of teeth, unspecified cause, class IV**
- K08.409 **Partial loss of teeth, unspecified cause, unspecified class**
  Tooth extraction status NOS

K08.41 Partial loss of teeth due to trauma
- K08.411 **Partial loss of teeth due to trauma, class I**
- K08.412 **Partial loss of teeth due to trauma, class II**
- K08.413 **Partial loss of teeth due to trauma, class III**
- K08.414 **Partial loss of teeth due to trauma, class IV**
- K08.419 **Partial loss of teeth due to trauma, unspecified class**

K08.42 Partial loss of teeth due to periodontal diseases
- K08.421 **Partial loss of teeth due to periodontal diseases, class I**
- K08.422 **Partial loss of teeth due to periodontal diseases, class II**
- K08.423 **Partial loss of teeth due to periodontal diseases, class III**
- K08.424 **Partial loss of teeth due to periodontal diseases, class IV**
- K08.429 **Partial loss of teeth due to periodontal diseases, unspecified class**

K08.43 Partial loss of teeth due to caries
- K08.431 **Partial loss of teeth due to caries, class I**
- K08.432 **Partial loss of teeth due to caries, class II**
- K08.433 **Partial loss of teeth due to caries, class III**
- K08.434 **Partial loss of teeth due to caries, class IV**
- K08.439 **Partial loss of teeth due to caries, unspecified class**

K08.49 Partial loss of teeth due to other specified cause
- K08.491 **Partial loss of teeth due to other specified cause, class I**
- K08.492 **Partial loss of teeth due to other specified cause, class II**
- K08.493 **Partial loss of teeth due to other specified cause, class III**
- K08.494 **Partial loss of teeth due to other specified cause, class IV**
- K08.499 **Partial loss of teeth due to other specified cause, unspecified class**

K08.5 Unsatisfactory restoration of tooth

Defective bridge, crown, filling
Defective dental restoration

EXCLUDES1 *dental restoration status (Z98.811)*

EXCLUDES2 *endosseous dental implant failure (M27.6-)*
unsatisfactory endodontic treatment (M27.5-)

- K08.50 **Unsatisfactory restoration of tooth, unspecified**
  Defective dental restoration NOS
- K08.51 **Open restoration margins of tooth**
  Dental restoration failure of marginal integrity
  Open margin on tooth restoration
  Poor gingival margin to tooth restoration
- K08.52 **Unrepairable overhanging of dental restorative materials**
  Overhanging of tooth restoration
- K08.53 **Fractured dental restorative material**
  EXCLUDES1 *cracked tooth (K03.81)*
  traumatic fracture of tooth (S02.5)
  - K08.530 **Fractured dental restorative material without loss of material**
  - K08.531 **Fractured dental restorative material with loss of material**
  - K08.539 **Fractured dental restorative material, unspecified**
- K08.54 **Contour of existing restoration of tooth biologically incompatible with oral health**
  Dental restoration failure of periodontal anatomical integrity
  Unacceptable contours of existing restoration of tooth
  Unacceptable morphology of existing restoration of tooth
- K08.55 **Allergy to existing dental restorative material**
  Use additional code to identify the specific type of allergy
- K08.56 **Poor aesthetic of existing restoration of tooth**
  Dental restoration aesthetically inadequate or displeasing
- K08.59 **Other unsatisfactory restoration of tooth**
  Other defective dental restoration

K08.8 Other specified disorders of teeth and supporting structures
- ● K08.81 **Primary occlusal trauma** CC/MCC Exc
- ● K08.82 **Secondary occlusal trauma** CC/MCC Exc
- ● K08.89 **Other specified disorders of teeth and supporting structures** CC/MCC Exc
  Enlargement of alveolar ridge NOS
  Insufficient anatomic crown height
  Insufficient clinical crown length
  Irregular alveolar process
  Toothache NOS

K08.9 Disorder of teeth and supporting structures, unspecified

K09 Cysts of oral region, not elsewhere classified

INCLUDES *lesions showing histological features both of aneurysmal cyst and of another fibro-osseous lesion*

EXCLUDES2 *cysts of jaw (M27.0-, M27.4-)*
radicular cyst (K04.8)

K09.0 Developmental odontogenic cysts
Dentigerous cyst
Eruption cyst
Follicular cyst
Gingival cyst
Lateral periodontal cyst
Primordial cyst
EXCLUDES2 *keratocysts (D16.4, D16.5)*
odontogenic keratocystic tumors (D16.4, D16.5)

K09.1 Developmental (nonodontogenic) cysts of oral region
Cyst (of) incisive canal
Cyst (of) palatine of papilla
Globulomaxillary cyst
Median palatal cyst
Nasoalveolar cyst
Nasolabial cyst
Nasopalatine duct cyst

K09.8 Other cysts of oral region, not elsewhere classified
Dermoid cyst
Epidermoid cyst
Lymphoepithelial cyst
Epstein's pearl

K09.9 Cyst of oral region, unspecified

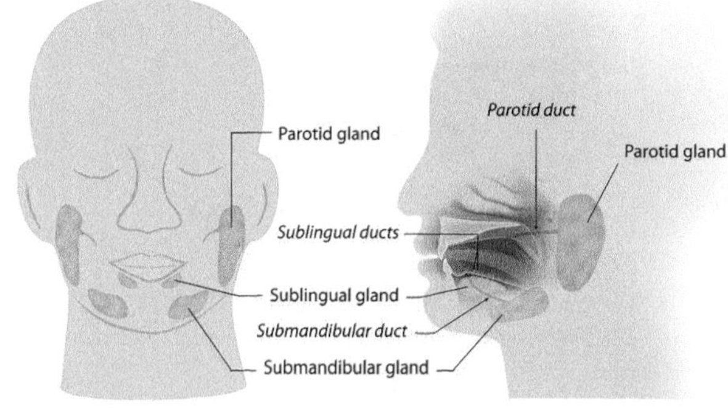

Figure 11.2 Salivary glands

Unacceptable principal diagnosis symbol per Medicare code edits | Code exempt from diagnosis present on admission requirement | Questionable admission | Complication or comorbidity | CC/MCC exclusion | Major complication or comorbidity | Principal diagnosis as its own CC | Principal diagnosis as its own MCC | Z code as first-listed diagnosis

When symbols appear on a code that requires a 7th character extension, refer to Appendix D to identify applicable 7th character codes.

K11 Diseases of salivary glands
Use additional code to identify:
alcohol abuse and dependence (F10.-)
exposure to environmental tobacco smoke (Z77.22)
exposure to tobacco smoke in the perinatal period (P96.81)
history of tobacco ▶dependence◀ (Z87.891)
occupational exposure to environmental tobacco smoke (Z57.31)
tobacco dependence (F17.-)
tobacco use (Z72.0)

K11.0 Atrophy of salivary gland
K11.1 Hypertrophy of salivary gland
K11.2 Sialoadenitis
Parotitis
EXCLUDES1 *epidemic parotitis (B26.-)*
mumps (B26.-)
uveoparotid fever [Heerfordt] (D86.89)
K11.20 Sialoadenitis, unspecified
K11.21 Acute sialoadenitis
EXCLUDES1 *acute recurrent sialoadenitis (K11.22)*
K11.22 Acute recurrent sialoadenitis
K11.23 Chronic sialoadenitis
K11.3 Abscess of salivary gland
K11.4 Fistula of salivary gland
EXCLUDES1 *congenital fistula of salivary gland (Q38.4)*
K11.5 Sialolithiasis
Calculus of salivary gland or duct
Stone of salivary gland or duct
K11.6 Mucocele of salivary gland
Mucous extravasation cyst of salivary gland
Mucous retention cyst of salivary gland
Ranula
K11.7 Disturbances of salivary secretion
Hypoptyalism
Ptyalism
Xerostomia
EXCLUDES2 *dry mouth NOS (R68.2)*
K11.8 Other diseases of salivary glands
Benign lymphoepithelial lesion of salivary gland
Mikulicz' disease
Necrotizing sialometaplasia
Sialectasia
Stenosis of salivary duct
Stricture of salivary duct
EXCLUDES1 *sicca syndrome [Sjögren] (M35.0-)*
K11.9 Disease of salivary gland, unspecified
Sialoadenopathy NOS

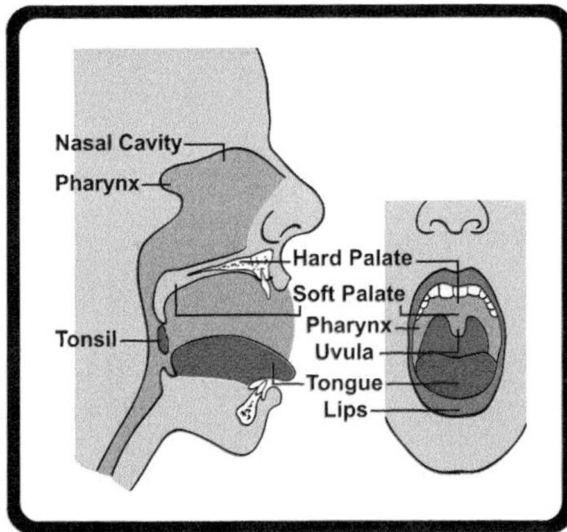

Figure 11.3 Mouth

K12 Stomatitis and related lesions
Use additional code to identify:
alcohol abuse and dependence (F10.-)
exposure to environmental tobacco smoke (Z77.22)
exposure to tobacco smoke in the perinatal period (P96.81)
history of tobacco ▶dependence◀ (Z87.891)
occupational exposure to environmental tobacco smoke (Z57.31)
tobacco dependence (F17.-)
tobacco use (Z72.0)
EXCLUDES1 *cancrum oris (A69.0)*
cheilitis (K13.0)
gangrenous stomatitis (A69.0)
herpesviral [herpes simplex] gingivostomatitis (B00.2)
noma (A69.0)

K12.0 Recurrent oral aphthae
Aphthous stomatitis (major) (minor)
Bednar's aphthae
Periadenitis mucosa necrotica recurrens
Recurrent aphthous ulcer
Stomatitis herpetiformis
K12.1 Other forms of stomatitis
Stomatitis NOS
Denture stomatitis
Ulcerative stomatitis
Vesicular stomatitis
EXCLUDES1 *acute necrotizing ulcerative stomatitis (A69.1)*
Vincent's stomatitis (A69.1)
K12.2 Cellulitis and abscess of mouth
Cellulitis of mouth (floor)
Submandibular abscess
EXCLUDES2 *abscess of salivary gland (K11.3)*
abscess of tongue (K14.0)
periapical abscess (K04.6-K04.7)
periodontal abscess (K05.21)
peritonsillar abscess (J36)
K12.3 Oral mucositis (ulcerative)
Mucositis (oral) (oropharyngeal)
EXCLUDES2 *gastrointestinal mucositis (ulcerative) (K92.81)*
mucositis (ulcerative) of vagina and vulva (N76.81)
nasal mucositis (ulcerative) (J34.81)
K12.30 Oral mucositis (ulcerative), unspecified
K12.31 Oral mucositis (ulcerative) due to antineoplastic therapy
Use additional code for adverse effect, if applicable, to identify antineoplastic and immunosuppressive drugs (T45.1X5)
Use additional code for other antineoplastic therapy, such as:
radiological procedure and radiotherapy (Y84.2)
K12.32 Oral mucositis (ulcerative) due to other drugs
Use additional code for adverse effect, if applicable, to identify drug (T36-T50 with fifth or sixth character 5)
K12.33 Oral mucositis (ulcerative) due to radiation
Use additional external cause code (W88-W90, X39.0-) to identify cause
K12.39 Other oral mucositis (ulcerative)
Viral oral mucositis (ulcerative)

K13 Other diseases of lip and oral mucosa
INCLUDES *epithelial disturbances of tongue*
Use additional code to identify:
alcohol abuse and dependence (F10.-)
exposure to environmental tobacco smoke (Z77.22)
exposure to tobacco smoke in the perinatal period (P96.81)
history of tobacco ▶dependence◀ (Z87.891)
occupational exposure to environmental tobacco smoke (Z57.31)
tobacco dependence (F17.-)
tobacco use (Z72.0)
EXCLUDES2 *certain disorders of gingiva and edentulous alveolar ridge (K05-K06)*
cysts of oral region (K09.-)
diseases of tongue (K14.-)
stomatitis and related lesions (K12.-)

Unspecified Code Other Specified Code Manifestation Code N Newborn P Pediatric M Maternity A Adult ♂ Male ♀ Female
● New Code ▲ Revised Code Title ▶◀ Revised Text NOTES INCLUDES EXCLUDES1 Not coded here EXCLUDES2 Not included here
4th character required 5th character required 6th character required 7th character required
Extension 'X' Alert HAC Hospital-acquired condition (HAC) alert AHA AHA Coding Clinic©

K13.0 **Diseases of lips**
Abscess of lips
Angular cheilitis
Cellulitis of lips
Cheilitis NOS
Cheilodynia
Cheilosis
Exfoliative cheilitis
Fistula of lips
Glandular cheilitis
Hypertrophy of lips
Perlèche NEC
EXCLUDES1 *ariboflavinosis (E53.0)*
cheilitis due to radiation-related disorders (L55-L59)
congenital fistula of lips (Q38.0)
congenital hypertrophy of lips (Q18.6)
Perlèche due to candidiasis (B37.83)
Perlèche due to riboflavin deficiency (E53.0)

K13.1 **Cheek and lip biting**

K13.2 **Leukoplakia and other disturbances of oral epithelium, including tongue**
EXCLUDES1 *carcinoma in situ of oral epithelium (D00.0-)*
hairy leukoplakia (K13.3)

K13.21 **Leukoplakia of oral mucosa, including tongue**
Leukokeratosis of oral mucosa
Leukoplakia of gingiva, lips, tongue
EXCLUDES1 *hairy leukoplakia (K13.3)*
leukokeratosis nicotina palati (K13.24)

K13.22 **Minimal keratinized residual ridge mucosa**
Minimal keratinization of alveolar ridge mucosa

K13.23 **Excessive keratinized residual ridge mucosa**
Excessive keratinization of alveolar ridge mucosa

K13.24 **Leukokeratosis nicotina palati**
Smoker's palate

K13.29 **Other disturbances of oral epithelium, including tongue**
Erythroplakia of mouth or tongue
Focal epithelial hyperplasia of mouth or tongue
Leukoedema of mouth or tongue
Other oral epithelium disturbances

K13.3 **Hairy leukoplakia**

K13.4 **Granuloma and granuloma-like lesions of oral mucosa**
Eosinophilic granuloma
Granuloma pyogenicum
Verrucous xanthoma

K13.5 **Oral submucous fibrosis**
Submucous fibrosis of tongue

K13.6 **Irritative hyperplasia of oral mucosa**
EXCLUDES2 *irritative hyperplasia of edentulous ridge [denture hyperplasia] (K06.2)*

K13.7 **Other and unspecified lesions of oral mucosa**

K13.70 **Unspecified lesions of oral mucosa**

K13.79 **Other lesions of oral mucosa**
Focal oral mucinosis

K14 **Diseases of tongue**
Use additional code to identify:
alcohol abuse and dependence (F10.-)
exposure to environmental tobacco smoke (Z77.22)
history of tobacco ▶dependence◀ (Z87.891)
occupational exposure to environmental tobacco smoke (Z57.31)
tobacco dependence (F17.-)
tobacco use (Z72.0)
EXCLUDES2 *erythroplakia (K13.29)*
focal epithelial hyperplasia (K13.29)
leukedema of tongue (K13.29)
leukoplakia of tongue (K13.21)
hairy leukoplakia (K13.3)
macroglossia (congenital) (Q38.2)
submucous fibrosis of tongue (K13.5)

K14.0 **Glossitis**
Abscess of tongue
Ulceration (traumatic) of tongue
EXCLUDES1 *atrophic glossitis (K14.4)*

K14.1 **Geographic tongue**
Benign migratory glossitis
Glossitis areata exfoliativa

K14.2 **Median rhomboid glossitis**

K14.3 **Hypertrophy of tongue papillae**
Black hairy tongue
Coated tongue
Hypertrophy of foliate papillae
Lingua villosa nigra

K14.4 **Atrophy of tongue papillae**
Atrophic glossitis

K14.5 **Plicated tongue**
Fissured tongue
Furrowed tongue
Scrotal tongue
EXCLUDES1 *fissured tongue, congenital (Q38.3)*

K14.6 **Glossodynia**
Glossopyrosis
Painful tongue

K14.8 **Other diseases of tongue**
Atrophy of tongue
Crenated tongue
Enlargement of tongue
Glossocele
Glossoptosis
Hypertrophy of tongue

K14.9 **Disease of tongue, unspecified**
Glossopathy NOS

Diseases of esophagus, stomach and duodenum (K20-K31)

EXCLUDES2 *hiatus hernia (K44.-)*

K20 **Esophagitis**
Use additional code to identify:
alcohol abuse and dependence (F10.-)
EXCLUDES1 *erosion of esophagus (K22.1-)*
esophagitis with gastro-esophageal reflux disease (K21.0)
reflux esophagitis (K21.0)
ulcerative esophagitis (K22.1-)
EXCLUDES2 *eosinophilic gastritis or gastroenteritis (K52.81)*

K20.0 **Eosinophilic esophagitis**

K20.8 **Other esophagitis**
Abscess of esophagus

K20.9 **Esophagitis, unspecified**
Esophagitis NOS

K21 **Gastro-esophageal reflux disease**
EXCLUDES1 *newborn esophageal reflux (P78.83)*

K21.0 **Gastro-esophageal reflux disease with esophagitis**
Reflux esophagitis

K21.9 **Gastro-esophageal reflux disease without esophagitis**
Esophageal reflux NOS
AHA: Q1, 2016

K22 **Other diseases of esophagus**
EXCLUDES2 *esophageal varices (I85.-)*

K22.0 **Achalasia of cardia**
Achalasia NOS
Cardiospasm
EXCLUDES1 *congenital cardiospasm (Q39.5)*

K22.1 **Ulcer of esophagus**
Barrett's ulcer
Erosion of esophagus
Fungal ulcer of esophagus
Peptic ulcer of esophagus
Ulcer of esophagus due to ingestion of chemicals
Ulcer of esophagus due to ingestion of drugs and medicaments
Ulcerative esophagitis
Code first poisoning due to drug or toxin, if applicable (T36-T65 with fifth or sixth character 1-4 or 6)
Use additional code for adverse effect, if applicable, to identify drug (T36-T50 with fifth or sixth character 5)
EXCLUDES1 *Barrett's esophagus (K22.7-)*

K22.10 **Ulcer of esophagus without bleeding** CC
Ulcer of esophagus NOS

K22.11 **Ulcer of esophagus with bleeding** MCC
EXCLUDES2 *bleeding esophageal varices (I85.01, I85.11)*

Unacceptable principal diagnosis symbol per Medicare code edits · Code exempt from diagnosis present on admission requirement
Questionable admission · Complication or comorbidity · CC/MCC exclusion · Major complication or comorbidity
Principal diagnosis as its own CC · Principal diagnosis as its own MCC · Z code as first-listed diagnosis

K22.2 **Esophageal obstruction**
Compression of esophagus
Constriction of esophagus
Stenosis of esophagus
Stricture of esophagus
EXCLUDES1 *congenital stenosis or stricture of esophagus (Q39.3)*

K22.3 **Perforation of esophagus** MCC
Rupture of esophagus
EXCLUDES1 *traumatic perforation of (thoracic) esophagus (S27.8-)*

K22.4 **Dyskinesia of esophagus**
Corkscrew esophagus
Diffuse esophageal spasm
Spasm of esophagus
EXCLUDES1 *cardiospasm (K22.0)*

K22.5 **Diverticulum of esophagus, acquired**
Esophageal pouch, acquired
EXCLUDES1 *diverticulum of esophagus (congenital) (Q39.6)*

K22.6 **Gastro-esophageal laceration-hemorrhage syndrome** MCC
Mallory-Weiss syndrome

K22.7 **Barrett's esophagus** (5th)
Barrett's disease
Barrett's syndrome
EXCLUDES1 *Barrett's ulcer (K22.1)*
malignant neoplasm of esophagus (C15.-)

K22.70 **Barrett's esophagus without dysplasia**
Barrett's esophagus NOS

K22.71 **Barrett's esophagus with dysplasia** (6th)

K22.710 **Barrett's esophagus with low grade dysplasia**

K22.711 **Barrett's esophagus with high grade dysplasia**

K22.719 **Barrett's esophagus with dysplasia, unspecified**

K22.8 **Other specified diseases of esophagus**
Hemorrhage of esophagus NOS
EXCLUDES2 *esophageal varices (I85.-)*
Paterson-Kelly syndrome (D50.1)

K22.9 **Disease of esophagus, unspecified**

K23 **Disorders of esophagus in diseases classified elsewhere**
Code first underlying disease, such as:
congenital syphilis (A50.5)
EXCLUDES1 *late syphilis (A52.79)*
megaesophagus due to Chagas' disease (B57.31)
tuberculosis (A18.83)

K25 **Gastric ulcer** (4th)
INCLUDES *erosion (acute) of stomach*
pylorus ulcer (peptic)
stomach ulcer (peptic)
Use additional code to identify:
alcohol abuse and dependence (F10.-)
EXCLUDES1 *acute gastritis (K29.0-)*
peptic ulcer NOS (K27.-)

K25.0 **Acute gastric ulcer with hemorrhage** MCC
K25.1 **Acute gastric ulcer with perforation** MCC
K25.2 **Acute gastric ulcer with both hemorrhage and perforation** MCC
K25.3 **Acute gastric ulcer without hemorrhage or perforation** CC
K25.4 **Chronic or unspecified gastric ulcer with hemorrhage** MCC
K25.5 **Chronic or unspecified gastric ulcer with perforation** MCC
K25.6 **Chronic or unspecified gastric ulcer with both hemorrhage and perforation** MCC
K25.7 **Chronic gastric ulcer without hemorrhage or perforation**
K25.9 **Gastric ulcer, unspecified as acute or chronic, without hemorrhage or perforation**

K26 **Duodenal ulcer** (4th)
INCLUDES *erosion (acute) of duodenum*
duodenum ulcer (peptic)
postpyloric ulcer (peptic)
Use additional code to identify:
alcohol abuse and dependence (F10.-)
EXCLUDES1 *peptic ulcer NOS (K27.-)*

K26.0 **Acute duodenal ulcer with hemorrhage** MCC
K26.1 **Acute duodenal ulcer with perforation** MCC
K26.2 **Acute duodenal ulcer with both hemorrhage and perforation** MCC
K26.3 **Acute duodenal ulcer without hemorrhage or perforation** CC
K26.4 **Chronic or unspecified duodenal ulcer with hemorrhage** MCC
K26.5 **Chronic or unspecified duodenal ulcer with perforation** MCC
K26.6 **Chronic or unspecified duodenal ulcer with both hemorrhage and perforation**
K26.7 **Chronic duodenal ulcer without hemorrhage or perforation**
K26.9 **Duodenal ulcer, unspecified as acute or chronic, without hemorrhage or perforation**

K27 **Peptic ulcer, site unspecified** (4th)
INCLUDES *gastroduodenal ulcer NOS*
peptic ulcer NOS
Use additional code to identify:
alcohol abuse and dependence (F10.-)
EXCLUDES1 *peptic ulcer of newborn (P78.82)*

K27.0 **Acute peptic ulcer, site unspecified, with hemorrhage** MCC
K27.1 **Acute peptic ulcer, site unspecified, with perforation** MCC
K27.2 **Acute peptic ulcer, site unspecified, with both hemorrhage and perforation** MCC
K27.3 **Acute peptic ulcer, site unspecified, without hemorrhage or perforation** CC
K27.4 **Chronic or unspecified peptic ulcer, site unspecified, with hemorrhage** MCC
K27.5 **Chronic or unspecified peptic ulcer, site unspecified, with perforation** MCC
K27.6 **Chronic or unspecified peptic ulcer, site unspecified, with both hemorrhage and perforation** MCC
K27.7 **Chronic peptic ulcer, site unspecified, without hemorrhage or perforation**
K27.9 **Peptic ulcer, site unspecified, unspecified as acute or chronic, without hemorrhage or perforation**

K28 **Gastrojejunal ulcer** (4th)
INCLUDES *anastomotic ulcer (peptic) or erosion*
gastrocolic ulcer (peptic) or erosion
gastrointestinal ulcer (peptic) or erosion
gastrojejunal ulcer (peptic) or erosion
jejunal ulcer (peptic) or erosion
marginal ulcer (peptic) or erosion
stomal ulcer (peptic) or erosion
Use additional code to identify:
alcohol abuse and dependence (F10.-)
EXCLUDES1 *primary ulcer of small intestine (K63.3)*

K28.0 **Acute gastrojejunal ulcer with hemorrhage** MCC
K28.1 **Acute gastrojejunal ulcer with perforation** MCC
K28.2 **Acute gastrojejunal ulcer with both hemorrhage and perforation** MCC
K28.3 **Acute gastrojejunal ulcer without hemorrhage or perforation** CC
K28.4 **Chronic or unspecified gastrojejunal ulcer with hemorrhage** MCC
K28.5 **Chronic or unspecified gastrojejunal ulcer with perforation** MCC
K28.6 **Chronic or unspecified gastrojejunal ulcer with both hemorrhage and perforation** MCC
K28.7 **Chronic gastrojejunal ulcer without hemorrhage or perforation**
K28.9 **Gastrojejunal ulcer, unspecified as acute or chronic, without hemorrhage or perforation**

K29 **Gastritis and duodenitis** (4th)
EXCLUDES1 *eosinophilic gastritis or gastroenteritis (K52.81)*
Zollinger-Ellison syndrome (E16.4)

K29.0 **Acute gastritis** (5th)
Use additional code to identify:
alcohol abuse and dependence (F10.-)
EXCLUDES1 *erosion (acute) of stomach (K25.-)*

K29.00 **Acute gastritis without bleeding**
K29.01 **Acute gastritis with bleeding** MCC

K29.2 **Alcoholic gastritis** (5th)
Use additional code to identify:
alcohol abuse and dependence (F10.-)

Unspecified Code | Other Specified Code | Manifestation Code | N Newborn | P Pediatric | M Maternity | A Adult | ♂ Male | ♀ Female
● New Code | ▲ Revised Code Title | ►◄ Revised Text | NOTES | INCLUDES | EXCLUDES1 Not coded here | EXCLUDES2 Not included here
4th character required | 5th character required | 6th character required | 7th character required
Extension 'X' Alert | HAC Hospital-acquired condition (HAC) alert | AHA AHA Coding Clinic©

K29.20 Alcoholic gastritis without bleeding
K29.21 Alcoholic gastritis with bleeding MCC

K29.3 Chronic superficial gastritis
K29.30 Chronic superficial gastritis without bleeding
K29.31 Chronic superficial gastritis with bleeding MCC

K29.4 Chronic atrophic gastritis
Gastric atrophy
K29.40 Chronic atrophic gastritis without bleeding
K29.41 Chronic atrophic gastritis with bleeding MCC

K29.5 Unspecified chronic gastritis
Chronic antral gastritis
Chronic fundal gastritis
K29.50 Unspecified chronic gastritis without bleeding
K29.51 Unspecified chronic gastritis with bleeding MCC

K29.6 Other gastritis
Giant hypertrophic gastritis
Granulomatous gastritis
Ménétrier's disease
K29.60 Other gastritis without bleeding
K29.61 Other gastritis with bleeding MCC

K29.7 Gastritis, unspecified
K29.70 Gastritis, unspecified, without bleeding
K29.71 Gastritis, unspecified, with bleeding MCC

K29.8 Duodenitis
K29.80 Duodenitis without bleeding
K29.81 Duodenitis with bleeding MCC

K29.9 Gastroduodenitis, unspecified
K29.90 Gastroduodenitis, unspecified, without bleeding
K29.91 Gastroduodenitis, unspecified, with bleeding MCC

K30 Functional dyspepsia
Indigestion
EXCLUDES1 *dyspepsia NOS (R10.13)*
heartburn (R12)
nervous dyspepsia (F45.8)
neurotic dyspepsia (F45.8)
psychogenic dyspepsia (F45.8)

K31 Other diseases of stomach and duodenum
INCLUDES *functional disorders of stomach*
EXCLUDES2 *diabetic gastroparesis (E08.43, E09.43, E10.43, E11.43, E13.43)*
diverticulum of duodenum (K57.00-K57.13)

K31.0 Acute dilatation of stomach CC
Acute distention of stomach

K31.1 Adult hypertrophic pyloric stenosis A CC
Pyloric stenosis NOS
EXCLUDES1 *congenital or infantile pyloric stenosis (Q40.0)*

K31.2 Hourglass stricture and stenosis of stomach
EXCLUDES1 *congenital hourglass stomach (Q40.2)*
hourglass contraction of stomach (K31.89)

K31.3 Pylorospasm, not elsewhere classified
EXCLUDES1 *congenital or infantile pylorospasm (Q40.0)*
neurotic pylorospasm (F45.8)
psychogenic pylorospasm (F45.8)

K31.4 Gastric diverticulum
EXCLUDES1 *congenital diverticulum of stomach (Q40.2)*

K31.5 Obstruction of duodenum CC
Constriction of duodenum
Duodenal ileus (chronic)
Stenosis of duodenum
Stricture of duodenum
Volvulus of duodenum
EXCLUDES1 *congenital stenosis of duodenum (Q41.0)*

K31.6 Fistula of stomach and duodenum CC
Gastrocolic fistula
Gastrojejunocolic fistula

K31.7 Polyp of stomach and duodenum
EXCLUDES1 *adenomatous polyp of stomach (D13.1)*

K31.8 Other specified diseases of stomach and duodenum
K31.81 Angiodysplasia of stomach and duodenum
K31.811 Angiodysplasia of stomach and duodenum with bleeding MCC
K31.819 Angiodysplasia of stomach and duodenum without bleeding
Angiodysplasia of stomach and duodenum NOS

K31.82 Dieulafoy lesion (hemorrhagic) of stomach and duodenum MCC
EXCLUDES2 *Dieulafoy lesion of intestine (K63.81)*
K31.83 Achlorhydria
K31.84 Gastroparesis
Gastroparalysis
Code first underlying disease, if known, such as:
anorexia nervosa (F50.0-)
diabetes mellitus (E08.43, E09.43, E10.43, E11.43, E13.43)
scleroderma (M34.-)
AHA: Q4, 2013
K31.89 Other diseases of stomach and duodenum

K31.9 Disease of stomach and duodenum, unspecified

Diseases of appendix (K35-K38)

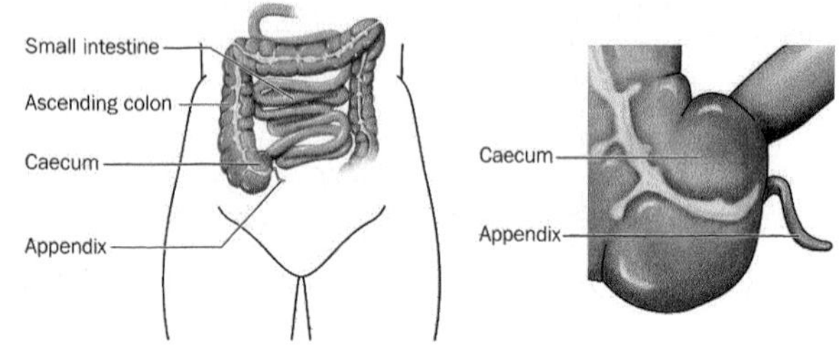

Figure 11.4 Vermiform appendix

K35 Acute appendicitis
K35.2 Acute appendicitis with generalized peritonitis MCC
Appendicitis (acute) with generalized (diffuse) peritonitis following rupture or perforation of appendix
Perforated appendix NOS
Ruptured appendix NOS
K35.3 Acute appendicitis with localized peritonitis MCC
Acute appendicitis with or without perforation or rupture ▶with peritonitis◀ NOS
Acute appendicitis with or without perforation or rupture with localized peritonitis
Acute appendicitis with peritoneal abscess
K35.8 Other and unspecified acute appendicitis
K35.80 Unspecified acute appendicitis CC
Acute appendicitis NOS
Acute appendicitis without (localized) (generalized) peritonitis
K35.89 Other acute appendicitis CC

K36 Other appendicitis
Chronic appendicitis
Recurrent appendicitis

K37 Unspecified appendicitis
EXCLUDES1 *-unspecified appendicitis with peritonitis (K35.2-K35.3)*

K38 Other diseases of appendix
K38.0 Hyperplasia of appendix
K38.1 Appendicular concretions
Fecalith of appendix
Stercolith of appendix
K38.2 Diverticulum of appendix
K38.3 Fistula of appendix
K38.8 Other specified diseases of appendix
Intussusception of appendix
K38.9 Disease of appendix, unspecified

Hernia (K40-K46)

NOTES Hernia with both gangrene and obstruction is classified to hernia with gangrene.
INCLUDES *acquired hernia*
congenital [except diaphragmatic or hiatus] hernia
recurrent hernia

PDx Unacceptable principal diagnosis symbol per Medicare code edits; POA Code exempt from diagnosis present on admission requirement
Q Questionable admission; CC Complication or comorbidity; CC/MCC Exc CC/MCC exclusion; MCC Major complication or comorbidity
PDx CC Principal diagnosis as its own CC; PDx MCC Principal diagnosis as its own MCC; Z1 Z code as first-listed diagnosis

K40 Inguinal hernia
INCLUDES *bubonocele*
direct inguinal hernia
double inguinal hernia
indirect inguinal hernia
inguinal hernia NOS
oblique inguinal hernia
scrotal hernia

K40.0 Bilateral inguinal hernia, with obstruction, without gangrene
Inguinal hernia (bilateral) causing obstruction without gangrene
Incarcerated inguinal hernia (bilateral) without gangrene
Irreducible inguinal hernia (bilateral) without gangrene
Strangulated inguinal hernia (bilateral) without gangrene

K40.00 Bilateral inguinal hernia, with obstruction, without gangrene, not specified as recurrent CC
Bilateral inguinal hernia, with obstruction, without gangrene NOS

K40.01 Bilateral inguinal hernia, with obstruction, without gangrene, recurrent CC

K40.1 Bilateral inguinal hernia, with gangrene

K40.10 Bilateral inguinal hernia, with gangrene, not specified as recurrent MCC
Bilateral inguinal hernia, with gangrene NOS

K40.11 Bilateral inguinal hernia, with gangrene, recurrent MCC

K40.2 Bilateral inguinal hernia, without obstruction or gangrene

K40.20 Bilateral inguinal hernia, without obstruction or gangrene, not specified as recurrent
Bilateral inguinal hernia NOS

K40.21 Bilateral inguinal hernia, without obstruction or gangrene, recurrent

K40.3 Unilateral inguinal hernia, with obstruction, without gangrene
Inguinal hernia (unilateral) causing obstruction without gangrene
Incarcerated inguinal hernia (unilateral) without gangrene
Irreducible inguinal hernia (unilateral) without gangrene
Strangulated inguinal hernia (unilateral) without gangrene

K40.30 Unilateral inguinal hernia, with obstruction, without gangrene, not specified as recurrent CC
Inguinal hernia, with obstruction NOS
Unilateral inguinal hernia, with obstruction, without gangrene NOS

K40.31 Unilateral inguinal hernia, with obstruction, without gangrene, recurrent CC

K40.4 Unilateral inguinal hernia, with gangrene

K40.40 Unilateral inguinal hernia, with gangrene, not specified as recurrent MCC
Inguinal hernia with gangrene NOS
Unilateral inguinal hernia with gangrene NOS

K40.41 Unilateral inguinal hernia, with gangrene, recurrent MCC

K40.9 Unilateral inguinal hernia, without obstruction or gangrene

K40.90 Unilateral inguinal hernia, without obstruction or gangrene, not specified as recurrent
Inguinal hernia NOS
Unilateral inguinal hernia NOS

K40.91 Unilateral inguinal hernia, without obstruction or gangrene, recurrent

K41 Femoral hernia

K41.0 Bilateral femoral hernia, with obstruction, without gangrene
Femoral hernia (bilateral) causing obstruction, without gangrene
Incarcerated femoral hernia (bilateral), without gangrene
Irreducible femoral hernia (bilateral), without gangrene
Strangulated femoral hernia (bilateral), without gangrene

K41.00 Bilateral femoral hernia, with obstruction, without gangrene, not specified as recurrent CC
Bilateral femoral hernia, with obstruction, without gangrene NOS

K41.01 Bilateral femoral hernia, with obstruction, without gangrene, recurrent CC

K41.1 Bilateral femoral hernia, with gangrene

K41.10 Bilateral femoral hernia, with gangrene, not specified as recurrent MCC
Bilateral femoral hernia, with gangrene NOS

K41.11 Bilateral femoral hernia, with gangrene, recurrent MCC

K41.2 Bilateral femoral hernia, without obstruction or gangrene

K41.20 Bilateral femoral hernia, without obstruction or gangrene, not specified as recurrent
Bilateral femoral hernia NOS

K41.21 Bilateral femoral hernia, without obstruction or gangrene, recurrent

K41.3 Unilateral femoral hernia, with obstruction, without gangrene
Femoral hernia (unilateral) causing obstruction, without gangrene
Incarcerated femoral hernia (unilateral), without gangrene
Irreducible femoral hernia (unilateral), without gangrene
Strangulated femoral hernia (unilateral), without gangrene

K41.30 Unilateral femoral hernia, with obstruction, without gangrene, not specified as recurrent CC
Femoral hernia, with obstruction NOS
Unilateral femoral hernia, with obstruction NOS

K41.31 Unilateral femoral hernia, with obstruction, without gangrene, recurrent CC

K41.4 Unilateral femoral hernia, with gangrene

K41.40 Unilateral femoral hernia, with gangrene, not specified as recurrent MCC
Femoral hernia, with gangrene NOS
Unilateral femoral hernia, with gangrene NOS

K41.41 Unilateral femoral hernia, with gangrene, recurrent MCC

K41.9 Unilateral femoral hernia, without obstruction or gangrene

K41.90 Unilateral femoral hernia, without obstruction or gangrene, not specified as recurrent
Femoral hernia NOS
Unilateral femoral hernia NOS

K41.91 Unilateral femoral hernia, without obstruction or gangrene, recurrent

K42 Umbilical hernia
INCLUDES *paraumbilical hernia*
EXCLUDES1 *omphalocele (Q79.2)*

K42.0 Umbilical hernia with obstruction, without gangrene CC
Umbilical hernia causing obstruction, without gangrene
Incarcerated umbilical hernia, without gangrene
Irreducible umbilical hernia, without gangrene
Strangulated umbilical hernia, without gangrene

K42.1 Umbilical hernia with gangrene MCC
Gangrenous umbilical hernia

K42.9 Umbilical hernia without obstruction or gangrene
Umbilical hernia NOS

K43 Ventral hernia

K43.0 Incisional hernia with obstruction, without gangrene CC
Incisional hernia causing obstruction, without gangrene
Incarcerated incisional hernia, without gangrene
Irreducible incisional hernia, without gangrene
Strangulated incisional hernia, without gangrene

K43.1 Incisional hernia with gangrene MCC
Gangrenous incisional hernia

K43.2 Incisional hernia without obstruction or gangrene
Incisional hernia NOS

K43.3 Parastomal hernia with obstruction, without gangrene CC
Incarcerated parastomal hernia, without gangrene
Irreducible parastomal hernia, without gangrene
Parastomal hernia causing obstruction, without gangrene
Strangulated parastomal hernia, without gangrene

K43.4 Parastomal hernia with gangrene MCC
Gangrenous parastomal hernia

K43.5 Parastomal hernia without obstruction or gangrene
Parastomal hernia NOS

K43.6 Other and unspecified ventral hernia with obstruction, without gangrene CC
Epigastric hernia causing obstruction, without gangrene
Hypogastric hernia causing obstruction, without gangrene
Incarcerated epigastric hernia without gangrene
Incarcerated hypogastric hernia without gangrene
Incarcerated midline hernia without gangrene
Incarcerated spigelian hernia without gangrene
Incarcerated subxiphoid hernia without gangrene
Irreducible epigastric hernia without gangrene
Irreducible hypogastric hernia without gangrene
Irreducible midline hernia without gangrene

Irreducible spigelian hernia without gangrene
Irreducible subxiphoid hernia without gangrene
Midline hernia causing obstruction, without gangrene
Spigelian hernia causing obstruction, without gangrene
Strangulated epigastric hernia without gangrene
Strangulated hypogastric hernia without gangrene
Strangulated midline hernia without gangrene
Strangulated spigelian hernia without gangrene
Strangulated subxiphoid hernia without gangrene
Subxiphoid hernia causing obstruction, without gangrene

K43.7 **Other and unspecified ventral hernia with gangrene** MCC
Any condition listed under K43.6 specified as gangrenous

K43.9 **Ventral hernia without obstruction or gangrene**
Epigastric hernia
Ventral hernia NOS

4th K44 **Diaphragmatic hernia**
INCLUDES *hiatus hernia (esophageal) (sliding)*
paraesophageal hernia
EXCLUDES1 *congenital diaphragmatic hernia (Q79.0)*
congenital hiatus hernia (Q40.1)

K44.0 **Diaphragmatic hernia with obstruction, without gangrene** CC
Diaphragmatic hernia causing obstruction
Incarcerated diaphragmatic hernia
Irreducible diaphragmatic hernia
Strangulated diaphragmatic hernia

K44.1 **Diaphragmatic hernia with gangrene** MCC
Gangrenous diaphragmatic hernia

K44.9 **Diaphragmatic hernia without obstruction or gangrene**
Diaphragmatic hernia NOS

4th K45 **Other abdominal hernia**
INCLUDES *abdominal hernia, specified site NEC*
lumbar hernia
obturator hernia
pudendal hernia
retroperitoneal hernia
sciatic hernia

K45.0 **Other specified abdominal hernia with obstruction, without gangrene** CC
Other specified abdominal hernia causing obstruction
Other specified incarcerated abdominal hernia
Other specified irreducible abdominal hernia
Other specified strangulated abdominal hernia

K45.1 **Other specified abdominal hernia with gangrene** MCC
Any condition listed under K45 specified as gangrenous

K45.8 **Other specified abdominal hernia without obstruction or gangrene**

4th K46 **Unspecified abdominal hernia**
INCLUDES *enterocele*
epiplocele
hernia NOS
interstitial hernia
intestinal hernia
intra-abdominal hernia
EXCLUDES1 *vaginal enterocele (N81.5)*

K46.0 **Unspecified abdominal hernia with obstruction, without gangrene** CC
Unspecified abdominal hernia causing obstruction
Unspecified incarcerated abdominal hernia
Unspecified irreducible abdominal hernia
Unspecified strangulated abdominal hernia

K46.1 **Unspecified abdominal hernia with gangrene** MCC
Any condition listed under K46 specified as gangrenous

K46.9 **Unspecified abdominal hernia without obstruction or gangrene**
Abdominal hernia NOS

Noninfective enteritis and colitis (K50-K52)

INCLUDES *noninfective inflammatory bowel disease*
EXCLUDES1 *irritable bowel syndrome (K58.-)*
megacolon ►(K59.3-)◄

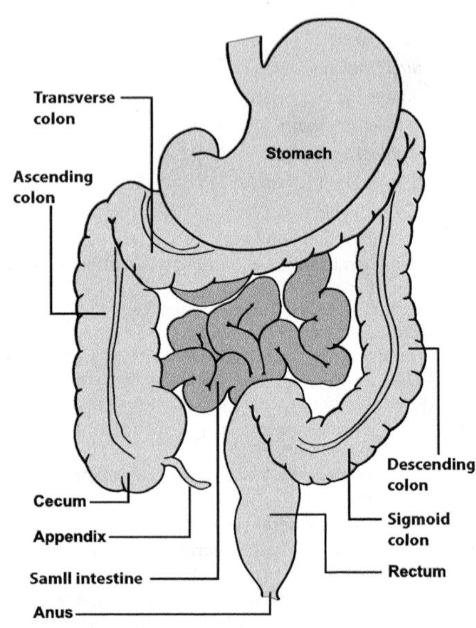

Figure 11.5 Large and small intestine

4th K50 **Crohn's disease [regional enteritis]**
INCLUDES *granulomatous enteritis*
Use additional code to identify manifestations, such as:
pyoderma gangrenosum (L88)
EXCLUDES1 *ulcerative colitis (K51.-)*

5th K50.0 **Crohn's disease of small intestine**
Crohn's disease [regional enteritis] of duodenum
Crohn's disease [regional enteritis] of ileum
Crohn's disease [regional enteritis] of jejunum
Regional ileitis
Terminal ileitis
EXCLUDES1 *Crohn's disease of both small and large intestine (K50.8-)*

K50.00 **Crohn's disease of small intestine without complications** CC

6th K50.01 **Crohn's disease of small intestine with complications**

K50.011 **Crohn's disease of small intestine with rectal bleeding** CC

K50.012 **Crohn's disease of small intestine with intestinal obstruction** CC PDx

K50.013 **Crohn's disease of small intestine with fistula** CC PDx

K50.014 **Crohn's disease of small intestine with abscess** CC PDx
AHA: Q4, 2012

K50.018 **Crohn's disease of small intestine with other complication** CC

K50.019 **Crohn's disease of small intestine with unspecified complications** CC

5th K50.1 **Crohn's disease of large intestine**
Crohn's disease [regional enteritis] of colon
Crohn's disease [regional enteritis] of large bowel
Crohn's disease [regional enteritis] of rectum
Granulomatous colitis
Regional colitis
EXCLUDES1 *Crohn's disease of both small and large intestine (K50.8)*

K50.10 **Crohn's disease of large intestine without complications** CC

6th K50.11 **Crohn's disease of large intestine with complications**

K50.111 **Crohn's disease of large intestine with rectal bleeding** CC

K50.112 **Crohn's disease of large intestine with intestinal obstruction** CC PDx

K50.113 **Crohn's disease of large intestine with fistula** CC PDx

K50.114 **Crohn's disease of large intestine with abscess** CC PDx
AHA: Q4, 2012

PDx Unacceptable principal diagnosis symbol per Medicare code edits · POA Code exempt from diagnosis present on admission requirement
Q Questionable admission · CC Complication or comorbidity · CC/MCC Excl CC/MCC exclusion · MCC Major complication or comorbidity
PDx CC Principal diagnosis as its own CC · PDx MCC Principal diagnosis as its own MCC · Z1 Z code as first-listed diagnosis

K50.118 Crohn's disease of large intestine with other complication
K50.119 Crohn's disease of large intestine with unspecified complications
K50.8 Crohn's disease of both small and large intestine
K50.80 Crohn's disease of both small and large intestine without complications
K50.81 Crohn's disease of both small and large intestine with complications
K50.811 Crohn's disease of both small and large intestine with rectal bleeding
K50.812 Crohn's disease of both small and large intestine with intestinal obstruction
K50.813 Crohn's disease of both small and large intestine with fistula
K50.814 Crohn's disease of both small and large intestine with abscess
AHA: Q4, 2012
K50.818 Crohn's disease of both small and large intestine with other complication
K50.819 Crohn's disease of both small and large intestine with unspecified complications
K50.9 Crohn's disease, unspecified
K50.90 Crohn's disease, unspecified, without complications
Crohn's disease NOS
Regional enteritis NOS
K50.91 Crohn's disease, unspecified, with complications
K50.911 Crohn's disease, unspecified, with rectal bleeding
K50.912 Crohn's disease, unspecified, with intestinal obstruction
K50.913 Crohn's disease, unspecified, with fistula
K50.914 Crohn's disease, unspecified, with abscess
AHA: Q4, 2012
K50.918 Crohn's disease, unspecified, with other complication
K50.919 Crohn's disease, unspecified, with unspecified complications
K51 Ulcerative colitis
Use additional code to identify manifestations, such as: pyoderma gangrenosum (L88)
EXCLUDES1 *Crohn's disease [regional enteritis] (K50.-)*
K51.0 Ulcerative (chronic) pancolitis
Backwash ileitis
K51.00 Ulcerative (chronic) pancolitis without complications
Ulcerative (chronic) pancolitis NOS
K51.01 Ulcerative (chronic) pancolitis with complications
K51.011 Ulcerative (chronic) pancolitis with rectal bleeding
K51.012 Ulcerative (chronic) pancolitis with intestinal obstruction
K51.013 Ulcerative (chronic) pancolitis with fistula
K51.014 Ulcerative (chronic) pancolitis with abscess
K51.018 Ulcerative (chronic) pancolitis with other complication
K51.019 Ulcerative (chronic) pancolitis with unspecified complications
K51.2 Ulcerative (chronic) proctitis
K51.20 Ulcerative (chronic) proctitis without complications
Ulcerative (chronic) proctitis NOS
K51.21 Ulcerative (chronic) proctitis with complications
K51.211 Ulcerative (chronic) proctitis with rectal bleeding
K51.212 Ulcerative (chronic) proctitis with intestinal obstruction
K51.213 Ulcerative (chronic) proctitis with fistula
K51.214 Ulcerative (chronic) proctitis with abscess
K51.218 Ulcerative (chronic) proctitis with other complication
K51.219 Ulcerative (chronic) proctitis with unspecified complications
K51.3 Ulcerative (chronic) rectosigmoiditis
K51.30 Ulcerative (chronic) rectosigmoiditis without complications
Ulcerative (chronic) rectosigmoiditis NOS
K51.31 Ulcerative (chronic) rectosigmoiditis with complications
K51.311 Ulcerative (chronic) rectosigmoiditis with rectal bleeding
K51.312 Ulcerative (chronic) rectosigmoiditis with intestinal obstruction
K51.313 Ulcerative (chronic) rectosigmoiditis with fistula
K51.314 Ulcerative (chronic) rectosigmoiditis with abscess
K51.318 Ulcerative (chronic) rectosigmoiditis with other complication
K51.319 Ulcerative (chronic) rectosigmoiditis with unspecified complications
K51.4 Inflammatory polyps of colon
EXCLUDES1 *adenomatous polyp of colon (D12.6)*
polyposis of colon (D12.6)
polyps of colon NOS (K63.5)
K51.40 Inflammatory polyps of colon without complications
Inflammatory polyps of colon NOS
K51.41 Inflammatory polyps of colon with complications
K51.411 Inflammatory polyps of colon with rectal bleeding
K51.412 Inflammatory polyps of colon with intestinal obstruction
K51.413 Inflammatory polyps of colon with fistula
K51.414 Inflammatory polyps of colon with abscess
K51.418 Inflammatory polyps of colon with other complication
K51.419 Inflammatory polyps of colon with unspecified complications
K51.5 Left sided colitis
Left hemicolitis
K51.50 Left sided colitis without complications
Left sided colitis NOS
K51.51 Left sided colitis with complications
K51.511 Left sided colitis with rectal bleeding
K51.512 Left sided colitis with intestinal obstruction
K51.513 Left sided colitis with fistula
K51.514 Left sided colitis with abscess
K51.518 Left sided colitis with other complication
K51.519 Left sided colitis with unspecified complications
K51.8 Other ulcerative colitis
K51.80 Other ulcerative colitis without complications
K51.81 Other ulcerative colitis with complications
K51.811 Other ulcerative colitis with rectal bleeding
K51.812 Other ulcerative colitis with intestinal obstruction
K51.813 Other ulcerative colitis with fistula
K51.814 Other ulcerative colitis with abscess
K51.818 Other ulcerative colitis with other complication
K51.819 Other ulcerative colitis with unspecified complications
K51.9 Ulcerative colitis, unspecified
K51.90 Ulcerative colitis, unspecified, without complications
K51.91 Ulcerative colitis, unspecified, with complications

Unspecified Code Other Specified Code Manifestation Code N Newborn P Pediatric M Maternity A Adult ♂ Male ♀ Female
● New Code ▲ Revised Code Title ►◄ Revised Text NOTES INCLUDES EXCLUDES1 Not coded here EXCLUDES2 Not included here
4th character required 5th character required 6th character required 7th character required
Extension 'X' Alert HAC Hospital-acquired condition (HAC) alert AHA AHA Coding Clinic©

K51.911 **Ulcerative colitis, unspecified with rectal bleeding** CC

K51.912 **Ulcerative colitis, unspecified with intestinal obstruction** CC PDx

K51.913 **Ulcerative colitis, unspecified with fistula** CC PDx

K51.914 **Ulcerative colitis, unspecified with abscess** CC PDx

K51.918 **Ulcerative colitis, unspecified with other complication** CC

K51.919 **Ulcerative colitis, unspecified with unspecified complications** CC

4th K52 **Other and unspecified noninfective gastroenteritis and colitis**

K52.0 **Gastroenteritis and colitis due to radiation** CC

K52.1 **Toxic gastroenteritis and colitis** CC
Drug-induced gastroenteritis and colitis
Code first (T51-T65) to identify toxic agent
Use additional code for adverse effect, if applicable, to identify drug (T36-T50 with fifth or sixth character 5)

5th K52.2 **Allergic and dietetic gastroenteritis and colitis**
Food hypersensitivity gastroenteritis or colitis
Use additional code to identify type of food allergy (Z91.01-, Z91.02-)
EXCLUDES2 *allergic eosinophilic colitis (K52.82)*
allergic eosinophilic esophagitis (K20.0)
allergic eosinophilic gastritis (K52.81)
allergic eosinophilic gastroenteritis (K52.81)
food protein-induced proctocolitis (K52.82)

● K52.21 **Food protein-induced enterocolitis syndrome** CC/MCC Exc
Use additional code for hypovolemic shock, if present (R57.1)

● K52.22 **Food protein-induced enteropathy** CC/MCC Exc

● K52.29 **Other allergic and dietetic gastroenteritis and colitis** CC/MCC Exc
Food hypersensitivity gastroenteritis or colitis
Immediate gastrointestinal hypersensitivity

● K52.3 **Indeterminate colitis** CC/MCC Exc
Colonic inflammatory bowel disease unclassified (IBDU)
EXCLUDES1 *unspecified colitis (K52.9)*

5th K52.8 **Other specified noninfective gastroenteritis and colitis**

K52.81 **Eosinophilic gastritis or gastroenteritis**
Eosinophilic enteritis
EXCLUDES2 *eosinophilic esophagitis (K20.0)*

K52.82 **Eosinophilic colitis**
Allergic proctocolitis
Food-induced eosinophilic proctocolitis
Food protein-induced proctocolitis
Milk protein-induced proctocolitis

● 6th K52.83 **Microscopic colitis**

● K52.831 **Collagenous colitis** CC/MCC Exc

● K52.832 **Lymphocytic colitis** CC/MCC Exc

● K52.838 **Other microscopic colitis** CC/MCC Exc

● K52.839 **Microscopic colitis, unspecified** CC/MCC Exc

K52.89 **Other specified noninfective gastroenteritis and colitis**

K52.9 **Noninfective gastroenteritis and colitis, unspecified**
Colitis NOS
Enteritis NOS
Gastroenteritis NOS
Ileitis NOS
Jejunitis NOS
Sigmoiditis NOS
EXCLUDES1 *diarrhea NOS (R19.7)*
functional diarrhea (K59.1)
infectious gastroenteritis and colitis NOS (A09)
neonatal diarrhea (noninfective) (P78.3)
psychogenic diarrhea (F45.8)

Other diseases of intestines (K55-K64)

4th K55 **Vascular disorders of intestine**
EXCLUDES1 *necrotizing enterocolitis of newborn (P77.-)*

5th K55.0 **Acute vascular disorders of intestine**
Infarction of appendices epiploicae
Mesenteric (artery) (vein) embolism
Mesenteric (artery) (vein) infarction
Mesenteric (artery) (vein) thrombosis

● 6th K55.01 **Acute (reversible) ischemia of small intestine**

● K55.011 **Focal (segmental) acute (reversible) ischemia of small intestine** CC/MCC Exc MCC

● K55.012 **Diffuse acute (reversible) ischemia of small intestine** CC/MCC Exc MCC

● K55.019 **Acute (reversible) ischemia of small intestine, extent unspecified** CC/MCC Exc MCC

● 6th K55.02 **Acute infarction of small intestine**
Gangrene of small intestine
Necrosis of small intestine

● K55.021 **Focal (segmental) acute infarction of small intestine** CC/MCC Exc MCC

● K55.022 **Diffuse acute infarction of small intestine** CC/MCC Exc MCC

● K55.029 **Acute infarction of small intestine, extent unspecified** CC/MCC Exc MCC

● 6th K55.03 **Acute (reversible) ischemia of large intestine**
Acute fulminant ischemic colitis
Subacute ischemic colitis

● K55.031 **Focal (segmental) acute (reversible) ischemia of large intestine** CC/MCC Exc MCC

● K55.032 **Diffuse acute (reversible) ischemia of large intestine** CC/MCC Exc MCC

● K55.039 **Acute (reversible) ischemia of large intestine, extent unspecified** CC/MCC Exc MCC

● 6th K55.04 **Acute infarction of large intestine**
Gangrene of large intestine
Necrosis of large intestine

● K55.041 **Focal (segmental) acute infarction of large intestine** CC/MCC Exc MCC

● K55.042 **Diffuse acute infarction of large intestine** CC/MCC Exc MCC

● K55.049 **Acute infarction of large intestine, extent unspecified** CC/MCC Exc MCC

● 6th K55.05 **Acute (reversible) ischemia of intestine, part unspecified**

● K55.051 **Focal (segmental) acute (reversible) ischemia of intestine, part unspecified** CC/MCC Exc MCC

● K55.052 **Diffuse acute (reversible) ischemia of intestine, part unspecified** CC/MCC Exc MCC

● K55.059 **Acute (reversible) ischemia of intestine, part and extent unspecified** CC/MCC Exc MCC

● 6th K55.06 **Acute infarction of intestine, part unspecified**
Acute intestinal infarction
Gangrene of intestine
Necrosis of intestine

● K55.061 **Focal (segmental) acute infarction of intestine, part unspecified** CC/MCC Exc MCC

● K55.062 **Diffuse acute infarction of intestine, part unspecified** CC/MCC Exc MCC

● K55.069 **Acute infarction of intestine, part and extent unspecified** CC/MCC Exc MCC

K55.1 **Chronic vascular disorders of intestine** CC
Chronic ischemic colitis
Chronic ischemic enteritis
Chronic ischemic enterocolitis
Ischemic stricture of intestine
Mesenteric atherosclerosis
Mesenteric vascular insufficiency

5th K55.2 **Angiodysplasia of colon**

K55.20 **Angiodysplasia of colon without hemorrhage**

K55.21 **Angiodysplasia of colon with hemorrhage** MCC

● 5th K55.3 **Necrotizing enterocolitis**
EXCLUDES1 *necrotizing enterocolitis of newborn (P77.-)*
EXCLUDES2 *necrotizing enterocolitis due to Clostridium difficile (A04.7)*

● K55.30 **Necrotizing enterocolitis, unspecified** CC/MCC Exc MCC
Necrotizing enterocolitis, NOS

● K55.31 **Stage 1 necrotizing enterocolitis** CC/MCC Exc MCC
Necrotizing enterocolitis without pneumatosis, without perforation

● K55.32 **Stage 2 necrotizing enterocolitis** CC/MCC Exc MCC
Necrotizing enterocolitis with pneumatosis, without perforation

PDxExc Unacceptable principal diagnosis symbol per Medicare code edits · POA Code exempt from diagnosis present on admission requirement
? Questionable admission · CC Complication or comorbidity · CC/MCC Exc CC/MCC exclusion · MCC Major complication or comorbidity
PDx CC Principal diagnosis as its own CC · PDx MCC Principal diagnosis as its own MCC · Z1 Z code as first-listed diagnosis

● K55.33 Stage 3 **necrotizing enterocolitis** CC/MCC Exc MCC
Necrotizing enterocolitis with perforation
Necrotizing enterocolitis with pneumatosis and perforation

K55.8 Other vascular disorders of intestine CC

K55.9 Vascular disorder of intestine, unspecified CC
Ischemic colitis
Ischemic enteritis
Ischemic enterocolitis

K56 Paralytic ileus and intestinal obstruction without hernia
EXCLUDES1 *congenital stricture or stenosis of intestine (Q41-Q42)*
cystic fibrosis with meconium ileus (E84.11)
ischemic stricture of intestine (K55.1)
meconium ileus NOS (P76.0)
neonatal intestinal obstructions classifiable to P76.-
obstruction of duodenum (K31.5)
postprocedural intestinal obstruction (K91.3)
stenosis of anus or rectum (K62.4)
intestinal obstruction with hernia (K40-K46)

K56.0 Paralytic ileus CC
Paralysis of bowel
Paralysis of colon
Paralysis of intestine
EXCLUDES1 *gallstone ileus (K56.3)*
ileus NOS (K56.7)
obstructive ileus NOS (K56.69)

K56.1 Intussusception CC
Intussusception or invagination of bowel
Intussusception or invagination of colon
Intussusception or invagination of intestine
Intussusception or invagination of rectum
EXCLUDES2 *intussusception of appendix (K38.8)*

K56.2 Volvulus MCC
Strangulation of colon or intestine
Torsion of colon or intestine
Twist of colon or intestine
EXCLUDES2 *volvulus of duodenum (K31.5)*

K56.3 Gallstone ileus CC
Obstruction of intestine by gallstone

K56.4 Other impaction of intestine

K56.41 Fecal impaction
EXCLUDES1 *constipation (K59.0-)*
incomplete defecation (R15.0)

K56.49 Other impaction of intestine CC

K56.5 Intestinal adhesions [bands] with obstruction (postprocedural) (postinfection) CC
Abdominal hernia due to adhesions with obstruction
Peritoneal adhesions [bands] with intestinal obstruction (postprocedural) (postinfection)

K56.6 Other and unspecified intestinal obstruction

K56.60 Unspecified intestinal obstruction CC
Intestinal obstruction NOS
EXCLUDES1 *intestinal obstruction due to specified condition-code to condition*

K56.69 Other intestinal obstruction CC
Enterostenosis NOS
Obstructive ileus NOS
Occlusion of colon or intestine NOS
Stenosis of colon or intestine NOS
Stricture of colon or intestine NOS
EXCLUDES1 *intestinal obstruction due to specified condition-code to condition*

K56.7 Ileus, unspecified CC
EXCLUDES1 *obstructive ileus (K56.69)*

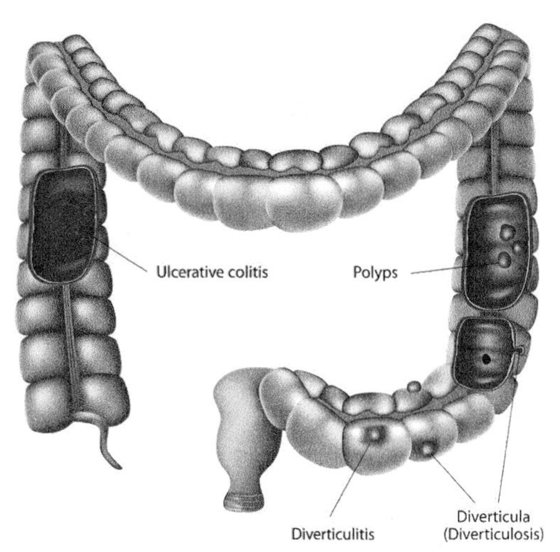

Figure 11.6 Noncancerous colon disorders

K57 Diverticular disease of intestine
EXCLUDES1 *congenital diverticulum of intestine (Q43.8)*
Meckel's diverticulum (Q43.0)
EXCLUDES2 *diverticulum of appendix (K38.2)*

K57.0 Diverticulitis of small intestine with perforation and abscess
Diverticulitis of small intestine with peritonitis
EXCLUDES1 *diverticulitis of both small and large intestine with perforation and abscess (K57.4-)*

K57.00 Diverticulitis of small intestine with perforation and abscess without bleeding CC PDx

K57.01 Diverticulitis of small intestine with perforation and abscess with bleeding MCC PDx

K57.1 Diverticular disease of small intestine without perforation or abscess
EXCLUDES1 *diverticular disease of both small and large intestine without perforation or abscess (K57.5-)*

K57.10 Diverticulosis **of small intestine without perforation or abscess** without bleeding
Diverticular disease of small intestine NOS

K57.11 Diverticulosis **of small intestine without perforation or abscess** with bleeding MCC

K57.12 Diverticulitis **of small intestine without perforation or abscess** without bleeding CC

K57.13 Diverticulitis **of small intestine without perforation or abscess** with bleeding MCC

K57.2 Diverticulitis of large intestine with perforation and abscess
Diverticulitis of colon with peritonitis
EXCLUDES1 *diverticulitis of both small and large intestine with perforation and abscess (K57.4-)*

K57.20 Diverticulitis of large intestine with perforation and abscess without bleeding CC PDx

K57.21 Diverticulitis of large intestine with perforation and abscess with bleeding MCC PDx

K57.3 Diverticular disease of large intestine without perforation or abscess
EXCLUDES1 *diverticular disease of both small and large intestine without perforation or abscess (K57.5-)*

K57.30 Diverticulosis **of large intestine without perforation or abscess** without bleeding
Diverticular disease of colon NOS

K57.31 Diverticulosis **of large intestine without perforation or abscess** with bleeding MCC

K57.32 Diverticulitis **of large intestine without perforation or abscess** without bleeding CC

K57.33 Diverticulitis **of large intestine without perforation or abscess** with bleeding MCC

K57.4 Diverticulitis of both small and large intestine with perforation and abscess
Diverticulitis of both small and large intestine with peritonitis

K57.40 Diverticulitis of both small and large intestine with perforation and abscess without bleeding CC PDx

Unspecified Code | Other Specified Code | Manifestation Code | N Newborn | P Pediatric | M Maternity | A Adult | ♂ Male | ♀ Female
● New Code ▲ Revised Code Title ►◄ Revised Text NOTES INCLUDES EXCLUDES1 Not coded here EXCLUDES2 Not included here
4th character required | 5th character required | 6th character required | 7th character required
Extension 'X' Alert | HAC Hospital-acquired condition (HAC) alert | AHA AHA Coding Clinic©

When symbols appear on a code that requires a 7th character extension, refer to Appendix D to identify applicable 7th character codes.

K57.41 **Diverticulitis of both small and large intestine with perforation and abscess with bleeding** MCC PDx

K57.5 **Diverticular disease of both small and large intestine without perforation or abscess**

K57.50 **Diverticulosis of both small and large intestine without perforation or abscess without bleeding**
Diverticular disease of both small and large intestine NOS

K57.51 **Diverticulosis of both small and large intestine without perforation or abscess with bleeding** MCC

K57.52 **Diverticulitis of both small and large intestine without perforation or abscess without bleeding** CC PDx

K57.53 **Diverticulitis of both small and large intestine without perforation or abscess with bleeding** MCC

K57.8 **Diverticulitis of intestine, part unspecified, with perforation and abscess**
Diverticulitis of intestine NOS with peritonitis

K57.80 **Diverticulitis of intestine, part unspecified, with perforation and abscess without bleeding** CC PDx

K57.81 **Diverticulitis of intestine, part unspecified, with perforation and abscess with bleeding** MCC PDx

K57.9 **Diverticular disease of intestine, part unspecified, without perforation or abscess**

K57.90 **Diverticulosis of intestine, part unspecified, without perforation or abscess without bleeding**
Diverticular disease of intestine NOS

K57.91 **Diverticulosis of intestine, part unspecified, without perforation or abscess with bleeding** MCC

K57.92 **Diverticulitis of intestine, part unspecified, without perforation or abscess without bleeding** CC

K57.93 **Diverticulitis of intestine, part unspecified, without perforation or abscess with bleeding** MCC

K58 **Irritable bowel syndrome**
INCLUDES *irritable colon*
spastic colon

K58.0 **Irritable bowel syndrome with diarrhea**
● K58.1 **Irritable bowel syndrome with constipation** CC/MCC Exc
● K58.2 **Mixed irritable bowel syndrome** CC/MCC Exc
● K58.8 **Other irritable bowel syndrome** CC/MCC Exc
K58.9 **Irritable bowel syndrome without diarrhea**
Irritable bowel syndrome NOS

K59 **Other functional intestinal disorders**
EXCLUDES1 *change in bowel habit NOS (R19.4)*
intestinal malabsorption (K90.-)
psychogenic intestinal disorders (F45.8)
EXCLUDES2 *functional disorders of stomach (K31.-)*

K59.0 **Constipation**
Use additional code for adverse effect, if applicable, to identify drug (T36-T50 with fifth or sixth character 5)
EXCLUDES1 *fecal impaction (K56.41)*
incomplete defecation (R15.0)

K59.00 **Constipation, unspecified**
K59.01 **Slow transit constipation**
K59.02 **Outlet dysfunction constipation**
● K59.03 **Drug induced constipation**
Use additional code for adverse effect, if applicable, to identify drug (T36-T50 with fifth or sixth character 5)
● K59.04 **Chronic idiopathic constipation**
Functional constipation
K59.09 **Other constipation**
Chronic constipation

K59.1 **Functional diarrhea**
EXCLUDES1 *diarrhea NOS (R19.7)*
irritable bowel syndrome with diarrhea (K58.0)

K59.2 **Neurogenic bowel, not elsewhere classified** CC

K59.3 **Megacolon, not elsewhere classified**
Dilatation of colon
Code first , ►if applicable◄ (T51-T65) to identify toxic agent
EXCLUDES1 *congenital megacolon (aganglionic) (Q43.1)*
megacolon (due to) (in) Chagas' disease (B57.32)
megacolon (due to) (in) Clostridium difficile (A04.7)
megacolon (due to) (in) Hirschsprung's disease (Q43.1)

● K59.31 **Toxic megacolon** CC CC/MCC Exc
● K59.39 **Other megacolon** CC CC/MCC Exc
Megacolon NOS

K59.4 **Anal spasm**
Proctalgia fugax

K59.8 **Other specified functional intestinal disorders**
Atony of colon
Pseudo-obstruction (acute) (chronic) of intestine

K59.9 **Functional intestinal disorder, unspecified**

Internal hemorrhoids
External hemorrhoids
Anal fistula
Anal fissures
Anal abscess

Figure 11.7 Anal disorders

K60 **Fissure and fistula of anal and rectal regions**
EXCLUDES1 *fissure and fistula of anal and rectal regions with abscess or cellulitis (K61.-)*
EXCLUDES2 *anal sphincter tear (healed) (nontraumatic) (old) (K62.81)*

K60.0 **Acute anal fissure**
K60.1 **Chronic anal fissure**
K60.2 **Anal fissure, unspecified**
K60.3 **Anal fistula**
K60.4 **Rectal fistula**
Fistula of rectum to skin
EXCLUDES1 *rectovaginal fistula (N82.3)*
vesicorectal fistula (N32.1)
K60.5 **Anorectal fistula**

K61 **Abscess of anal and rectal regions**
INCLUDES *abscess of anal and rectal regions*
cellulitis of anal and rectal regions

K61.0 **Anal abscess** CC
Perianal abscess
EXCLUDES1 *intrasphincteric abscess (K61.4)*

K61.1 **Rectal abscess** CC
Perirectal abscess
EXCLUDES1 *ischiorectal abscess (K61.3)*
AHA: Q4, 2012

K61.2 **Anorectal abscess** CC
K61.3 **Ischiorectal abscess** CC
Abscess of ischiorectal fossa
K61.4 **Intrasphincteric abscess** CC

K62 **Other diseases of anus and rectum**
INCLUDES *anal canal*
EXCLUDES2 *colostomy and enterostomy malfunction (K94.0-, K94.1-)*
fecal incontinence (R15.-)
hemorrhoids (K64.-)

K62.0 **Anal polyp**
K62.1 **Rectal polyp**
EXCLUDES1 *adenomatous polyp (D12.8)*
K62.2 **Anal prolapse**
Prolapse of anal canal
K62.3 **Rectal prolapse**
Prolapse of rectal mucosa
K62.4 **Stenosis of anus and rectum**
Stricture of anus (sphincter)
K62.5 **Hemorrhage of anus and rectum** CC
EXCLUDES1 *gastrointestinal bleeding NOS (K92.2)*
melena (K92.1)
neonatal rectal hemorrhage (P54.2)

PDx Unacceptable principal diagnosis symbol per Medicare code edits POA Code exempt from diagnosis present on admission requirement
Q Questionable admission CC Complication or comorbidity CC/MCC Exc CC/MCC exclusion MCC Major complication or comorbidity
PDx CC Principal diagnosis as its own CC PDx MCC Principal diagnosis as its own MCC Z Z code as first-listed diagnosis

K62.6 **Ulcer of anus and rectum**
Solitary ulcer of anus and rectum
Stercoral ulcer of anus and rectum
EXCLUDES1 *fissure and fistula of anus and rectum (K60.-)*
ulcerative colitis (K51.-)

K62.7 **Radiation proctitis**
Use additional code to identify the type of radiation (W90.-)

K62.8 **Other specified diseases of anus and rectum**
EXCLUDES2 *ulcerative proctitis (K51.2)*

K62.81 **Anal sphincter tear (healed) (nontraumatic) (old)**
Tear of anus, nontraumatic
Use additional code for any associated fecal incontinence (R15.-)
EXCLUDES2 *anal fissure (K60.-)*
anal sphincter tear (healed) (old) complicating delivery (O34.7-)
traumatic tear of anal sphincter (S31.831)

K62.82 **Dysplasia of anus**
Anal intraepithelial neoplasia I and II (AIN I and II) (histologically confirmed)
Dysplasia of anus NOS
Mild and moderate dysplasia of anus (histologically confirmed)
EXCLUDES1 *abnormal results from anal cytologic examination without histologic confirmation (R85.61-)*
anal intraepithelial neoplasia III (D01.3)
carcinoma in situ of anus (D01.3)
HGSIL of anus (R85.613)
severe dysplasia of anus (D01.3)

K62.89 **Other specified diseases of anus and rectum**
Proctitis NOS
Use additional code for any associated fecal incontinence (R15.-)

K62.9 **Disease of anus and rectum, unspecified**

K63 **Other diseases of intestine**

K63.0 **Abscess of intestine**
EXCLUDES1 *abscess of intestine with Crohn's disease (K50.014, K50.114, K50.814, K50.914,)*
abscess of intestine with diverticular disease (K57.0, K57.2, K57.4, K57.8)
abscess of intestine with ulcerative colitis (K51.014, K51.214, K51.314, K51.414, K51.514, K51.814, K51.914)
EXCLUDES2 *abscess of anal and rectal regions (K61.-)*
abscess of appendix (K35.3)

K63.1 **Perforation of intestine (nontraumatic)**
Perforation (nontraumatic) of rectum
EXCLUDES1 *perforation (nontraumatic) of duodenum (K26.-)*
perforation (nontraumatic) of intestine with diverticular disease (K57.0, K57.2, K57.4, K57.8)
EXCLUDES2 *perforation (nontraumatic) of appendix (K35.2, K35.3)*

K63.2 **Fistula of intestine**
EXCLUDES1 *fistula of duodenum (K31.6)*
fistula of intestine with Crohn's disease (K50.013, K50.113, K50.813, K50.913,)
fistula of intestine with ulcerative colitis (K51.013, K51.213, K51.313, K51.413, K51.513, K51.813, K51.913)
EXCLUDES2 *fistula of anal and rectal regions (K60.-)*
fistula of appendix (K38.3)
intestinal-genital fistula, female (N82.2-N82.4)
vesicointestinal fistula (N32.1)

K63.3 **Ulcer of intestine**
Primary ulcer of small intestine
EXCLUDES1 *duodenal ulcer (K26.-)*
gastrointestinal ulcer (K28.-)
gastrojejunal ulcer (K28.-)
jejunal ulcer (K28.-)
peptic ulcer, site unspecified (K27.-)
ulcer of intestine with perforation (K63.1)
ulcer of anus or rectum (K62.6)
ulcerative colitis (K51.-)

K63.4 **Enteroptosis**

K63.5 **Polyp of colon**
EXCLUDES1 *adenomatous polyp of colon (D12.6)*
inflammatory polyp of colon (K51.4-)
polyposis of colon (D12.6)

K63.8 **Other specified diseases of intestine**

K63.81 **Dieulafoy lesion of intestine**
EXCLUDES2 *Dieulafoy lesion of stomach and duodenum (K31.82)*

K63.89 **Other specified diseases of intestine**

K63.9 **Disease of intestine, unspecified**

K64 **Hemorrhoids and perianal venous thrombosis**
INCLUDES *piles*
EXCLUDES1 *hemorrhoids complicating childbirth and the puerperium (O87.2)*
hemorrhoids complicating pregnancy (O22.4)

K64.0 **First degree hemorrhoids**
Grade/stage I hemorrhoids
Hemorrhoids (bleeding) without prolapse outside of anal canal

K64.1 **Second degree hemorrhoids**
Grade/stage II hemorrhoids
Hemorrhoids (bleeding) that prolapse with straining, but retract spontaneously

K64.2 **Third degree hemorrhoids**
Grade/stage III hemorrhoids
Hemorrhoids (bleeding) that prolapse with straining and require manual replacement back inside anal canal

K64.3 **Fourth degree hemorrhoids**
Grade/stage IV hemorrhoids
Hemorrhoids (bleeding) with prolapsed tissue that cannot be manually replaced

K64.4 **Residual hemorrhoidal skin tags**
External hemorrhoids, NOS
Skin tags of anus

K64.5 **Perianal venous thrombosis**
External hemorrhoids with thrombosis
Perianal hematoma
Thrombosed hemorrhoids NOS

K64.8 **Other hemorrhoids**
Internal hemorrhoids, without mention of degree
Prolapsed hemorrhoids, degree not specified

K64.9 **Unspecified hemorrhoids**
Hemorrhoids (bleeding) NOS
Hemorrhoids (bleeding) without mention of degree

Diseases of peritoneum and retroperitoneum (K65-K68)

K65 **Peritonitis**
Use additional code (B95-B97), to identify infectious agent
EXCLUDES1 *acute appendicitis with generalized peritonitis (K35.2)*
aseptic peritonitis (T81.6)
benign paroxysmal peritonitis (E85.0)
chemical peritonitis (T81.6)
diverticulitis of both small and large intestine with peritonitis (K57.4-)
diverticulitis of colon with peritonitis (K57.2-)
diverticulitis of intestine, NOS, with peritonitis (K57.8-)
diverticulitis of small intestine with peritonitis (K57.0-)
gonococcal peritonitis (A54.85)
neonatal peritonitis (P78.0-P78.1)
pelvic peritonitis, female (N73.3-N73.5)
periodic familial peritonitis (E85.0)
peritonitis due to talc or other foreign substance (T81.6)
peritonitis in chlamydia (A74.81)
peritonitis in diphtheria (A36.89)
peritonitis in syphilis (late) (A52.74)
peritonitis in tuberculosis (A18.31)
peritonitis with or following abortion or ectopic or molar pregnancy (O00-O07, O08.0)
peritonitis with or following appendicitis (K35.-)
peritonitis with or following diverticular disease of intestine (K57.-)
puerperal peritonitis (O85)
retroperitoneal infections (K68.-)

Unspecified Code | Other Specified Code | Manifestation Code | N Newborn | P Pediatric | M Maternity | A Adult | ♂ Male | ♀ Female
● New Code | ▲ Revised Code Title | ►◄ Revised Text | NOTES | INCLUDES | EXCLUDES1 Not coded here | EXCLUDES2 Not included here
4th character required | 5th character required | 6th character required | 7th character required
Extension 'X' Alert | HAC Hospital-acquired condition (HAC) alert | AHA AHA Coding Clinic©

When symbols appear on a code that requires a 7th character extension, refer to Appendix D to identify applicable 7th character codes.

K65.0 Generalized (acute) peritonitis MCC
Pelvic peritonitis (acute), male
Subphrenic peritonitis (acute)
Suppurative peritonitis (acute)

K65.1 Peritoneal abscess MCC
Abdominopelvic abscess
Abscess (of) omentum
Abscess (of) peritoneum
Mesenteric abscess
Retrocecal abscess
Subdiaphragmatic abscess
Subhepatic abscess
Subphrenic abscess

K65.2 Spontaneous bacterial peritonitis MCC
EXCLUDES1 *bacterial peritonitis NOS (K65.9)*

K65.3 Choleperitonitis MCC
Peritonitis due to bile

K65.4 Sclerosing mesenteritis CC
Fat necrosis of peritoneum
(Idiopathic) sclerosing mesenteric fibrosis
Mesenteric lipodystrophy
Mesenteric panniculitis
Retractile mesenteritis

K65.8 Other peritonitis MCC
Chronic proliferative peritonitis
Peritonitis due to urine

K65.9 **Peritonitis, unspecified** MCC
Bacterial peritonitis NOS

K66 Other disorders of peritoneum
EXCLUDES2 *ascites (R18.-)*
peritoneal effusion (chronic) (R18.8)

K66.0 Peritoneal adhesions (postprocedural) (postinfection)
Adhesions (of) abdominal (wall)
Adhesions (of) diaphragm
Adhesions (of) intestine
Adhesions (of) male pelvis
Adhesions (of) omentum
Adhesions (of) stomach
Adhesive bands
Mesenteric adhesions
EXCLUDES1 *female pelvic adhesions [bands] (N73.6)*
peritoneal adhesions with intestinal obstruction (K56.5)

K66.1 Hemoperitoneum MCC
EXCLUDES1 *traumatic hemoperitoneum (S36.8-)*

K66.8 Other specified disorders of peritoneum

K66.9 Disorder of peritoneum, unspecified

K67 Disorders of peritoneum in infectious diseases classified elsewhere MCC
Code first underlying disease, such as :
congenital syphilis (A50.0)
helminthiasis (B65.0 -B83.9)
EXCLUDES1 *peritonitis in chlamydia (A74.81)*
peritonitis in diphtheria (A36.89)
peritonitis in gonococcal (A54.85)
peritonitis in syphilis (late) (A52.74)
peritonitis in tuberculosis (A18.31)

K68 Disorders of retroperitoneum

K68.1 Retroperitoneal abscess

K68.11 Postprocedural retroperitoneal abscess CC HAC

K68.12 Psoas muscle abscess MCC

K68.19 Other retroperitoneal abscess MCC

K68.9 Other disorders of retroperitoneum MCC

Diseases of liver (K70-K77)

EXCLUDES1 *jaundice NOS (R17)*
EXCLUDES2 *hemochromatosis (E83.11-)*
Reye's syndrome (G93.7)
viral hepatitis (B15-B19)
Wilson's disease (E83.0)

K70 Alcoholic liver disease
Use additional code to identify:
alcohol abuse and dependence (F10.-)

K70.0 Alcoholic fatty liver A

K70.1 Alcoholic hepatitis

K70.10 Alcoholic hepatitis without ascites A

K70.11 Alcoholic hepatitis with ascites A

K70.2 Alcoholic fibrosis and sclerosis of liver A

K70.3 Alcoholic cirrhosis of liver
Alcoholic cirrhosis NOS

K70.30 Alcoholic cirrhosis of liver without ascites A

K70.31 Alcoholic cirrhosis of liver with ascites A

K70.4 Alcoholic hepatic failure
Acute alcoholic hepatic failure
Alcoholic hepatic failure NOS
Chronic alcoholic hepatic failure
Subacute alcoholic hepatic failure

K70.40 Alcoholic hepatic failure without coma A

K70.41 Alcoholic hepatic failure with coma A MCC PDx MCC

K70.9 Alcoholic liver disease, unspecified A

K71 Toxic liver disease
INCLUDES *drug-induced idiosyncratic (unpredictable) liver disease*
drug-induced toxic (predictable) liver disease
Code first poisoning due to drug or toxin, if applicable (T36-T65 with fifth or sixth character 1-4 or 6)
Use additional code for adverse effect, if applicable, to identify drug (T36-T50 with fifth or sixth character 5)
EXCLUDES2 *alcoholic liver disease (K70.-)*
Budd-Chiari syndrome (I82.0)

K71.0 Toxic liver disease with cholestasis
Cholestasis with hepatocyte injury
'Pure' cholestasis

K71.1 Toxic liver disease with hepatic necrosis
Hepatic failure (acute) (chronic) due to drugs

K71.10 Toxic liver disease with hepatic necrosis, without coma

K71.11 Toxic liver disease with hepatic necrosis, with coma MCC PDx MCC

K71.2 Toxic liver disease with acute hepatitis

K71.3 Toxic liver disease with chronic persistent hepatitis

K71.4 Toxic liver disease with chronic lobular hepatitis

K71.5 Toxic liver disease with chronic active hepatitis
Toxic liver disease with lupoid hepatitis

K71.50 Toxic liver disease with chronic active hepatitis without ascites

K71.51 Toxic liver disease with chronic active hepatitis with ascites

K71.6 Toxic liver disease with hepatitis, not elsewhere classified

K71.7 Toxic liver disease with fibrosis and cirrhosis of liver

K71.8 Toxic liver disease with other disorders of liver
Toxic liver disease with focal nodular hyperplasia
Toxic liver disease with hepatic granulomas
Toxic liver disease with peliosis hepatis
Toxic liver disease with veno-occlusive disease of liver

K71.9 Toxic liver disease, unspecified

K72 Hepatic failure, not elsewhere classified
INCLUDES *fulminant hepatitis NEC, with hepatic failure*
hepatic encephalopathy NOS
liver (cell) necrosis with hepatic failure
malignant hepatitis NEC, with hepatic failure
yellow liver atrophy or dystrophy
EXCLUDES1 *alcoholic hepatic failure (K70.4)*
hepatic failure with toxic liver disease (K71.1-)
icterus of newborn (P55-P59)
postprocedural hepatic failure (K91.82)
EXCLUDES2 *hepatic failure complicating abortion or ectopic or molar pregnancy (O00-O07, O08.8)*
hepatic failure complicating pregnancy, childbirth and the puerperium (O26.6-)
viral hepatitis with hepatic coma (B15-B19)

K72.0 Acute and subacute hepatic failure
Acute non-viral hepatitis NOS

K72.00 Acute and subacute hepatic failure without coma MCC

K72.01 Acute and subacute hepatic failure with coma MCC PDx MCC

K72.1 Chronic hepatic failure

K72.10 Chronic hepatic failure without coma

K72.11 Chronic hepatic failure with coma MCC PDx MCC

PDx Unacceptable principal diagnosis symbol per Medicare code edits · POA Code exempt from diagnosis present on admission requirement
Q Questionable admission · CC Complication or comorbidity · CC/MCC Exc CC/MCC exclusion · MCC Major complication or comorbidity
PDx CC Principal diagnosis as its own CC · PDx MCC Principal diagnosis as its own MCC · Z1 Z code as first-listed diagnosis

K72.9 Hepatic failure, unspecified
K72.90 Hepatic failure, unspecified without coma
AHA: Q2, 2016
K72.91 Hepatic failure, unspecified with coma MCC
Hepatic coma NOS

K73 Chronic hepatitis, not elsewhere classified
EXCLUDES1 *alcoholic hepatitis (chronic) (K70.1-)*
drug-induced hepatitis (chronic) (K71.-)
granulomatous hepatitis (chronic) NEC (K75.3)
reactive, nonspecific hepatitis (chronic) (K75.2)
viral hepatitis (chronic) (B15-B19)
K73.0 Chronic persistent hepatitis, not elsewhere classified
K73.1 Chronic lobular hepatitis, not elsewhere classified
K73.2 Chronic active hepatitis, not elsewhere classified
K73.8 Other chronic hepatitis, not elsewhere classified
K73.9 Chronic hepatitis, unspecified

Healthy liver
Cirrhosis

Figure 11.8 Cirrhosis of the liver

K74 Fibrosis and cirrhosis of liver
Code also, if applicable, viral hepatitis (acute) (chronic) (B15-B19)
EXCLUDES1 *alcoholic cirrhosis (of liver) (K70.3)*
alcoholic fibrosis of liver (K70.2)
cardiac sclerosis of liver (K76.1)
cirrhosis (of liver) with toxic liver disease (K71.7)
congenital cirrhosis (of liver) (P78.81)
pigmentary cirrhosis (of liver) (E83.110)
K74.0 Hepatic fibrosis
K74.1 Hepatic sclerosis
K74.2 Hepatic fibrosis with hepatic sclerosis
K74.3 Primary biliary cirrhosis
Chronic nonsuppurative destructive cholangitis
K74.4 Secondary biliary cirrhosis
K74.5 Biliary cirrhosis, unspecified
K74.6 Other and unspecified cirrhosis of liver
K74.60 Unspecified cirrhosis of liver
Cirrhosis (of liver) NOS
K74.69 Other cirrhosis of liver
Cryptogenic cirrhosis (of liver)
Macronodular cirrhosis (of liver)
Micronodular cirrhosis (of liver)
Mixed type cirrhosis (of liver)
Portal cirrhosis (of liver)
Postnecrotic cirrhosis (of liver)

K75 Other inflammatory liver diseases
EXCLUDES2 *toxic liver disease (K71.-)*
K75.0 Abscess of liver MCC
Cholangitic hepatic abscess
Hematogenic hepatic abscess
Hepatic abscess NOS
Lymphogenic hepatic abscess
Pylephlebitic hepatic abscess
EXCLUDES1 *amebic liver abscess (A06.4)*
cholangitis without liver abscess (K83.0)
pylephlebitis without liver abscess (K75.1)
EXCLUDES2 *acute or subacute hepatitis NOS (B17.9)*
acute or subacute non-viral hepatitis (K72.0)
chronic hepatitis NEC (K73.8)
K75.1 Phlebitis of portal vein MCC
Pylephlebitis
EXCLUDES1 *pylephlebitic liver abscess (K75.0)*
K75.2 Nonspecific reactive hepatitis
EXCLUDES1 *acute or subacute hepatitis (K72.0-)*
chronic hepatitis NEC (K73.-)
viral hepatitis (B15-B19)
K75.3 Granulomatous hepatitis, not elsewhere classified
EXCLUDES1 *acute or subacute hepatitis (K72.0-)*
chronic hepatitis NEC (K73.-)
viral hepatitis (B15-B19)
K75.4 Autoimmune hepatitis
Lupoid hepatitis NEC
K75.8 Other specified inflammatory liver diseases
K75.81 Nonalcoholic steatohepatitis (NASH)
K75.89 Other specified inflammatory liver diseases
K75.9 Inflammatory liver disease, unspecified
Hepatitis NOS
EXCLUDES1 *acute or subacute hepatitis (K72.0-)*
chronic hepatitis NEC (K73.-)
viral hepatitis (B15-B19)

K76 Other diseases of liver
EXCLUDES2 *alcoholic liver disease (K70.-)*
amyloid degeneration of liver (E85.-)
cystic disease of liver (congenital) (Q44.6)
hepatic vein thrombosis (I82.0)
hepatomegaly NOS (R16.0)
pigmentary cirrhosis (of liver) (E83.110)
portal vein thrombosis (I81)
toxic liver disease (K71.-)
K76.0 Fatty (change of) liver, not elsewhere classified
Nonalcoholic fatty liver disease (NAFLD)
EXCLUDES1 *nonalcoholic steatohepatitis (NASH) (K75.81)*
K76.1 Chronic passive congestion of liver
Cardiac cirrhosis
Cardiac sclerosis
K76.2 Central hemorrhagic necrosis of liver MCC
EXCLUDES1 *liver necrosis with hepatic failure (K72.-)*
K76.3 Infarction of liver MCC
K76.4 Peliosis hepatis
Hepatic angiomatosis
K76.5 Hepatic veno-occlusive disease
EXCLUDES1 *Budd-Chiari syndrome (I82.0)*
K76.6 Portal hypertension CC
Use additional code for any associated complications, such as:
portal hypertensive gastropathy (K31.89)
K76.7 Hepatorenal syndrome MCC
EXCLUDES1 *hepatorenal syndrome following labor and delivery (O90.4)*
postprocedural hepatorenal syndrome ▶(K91.83)◀
K76.8 Other specified diseases of liver
K76.81 Hepatopulmonary syndrome PDx
Code first underlying liver disease, such as:
alcoholic cirrhosis of liver (K70.3-)
cirrhosis of liver without mention of alcohol (K74.6-)
K76.89 Other specified diseases of liver
Cyst (simple) of liver
Focal nodular hyperplasia of liver
Hepatoptosis
K76.9 Liver disease, unspecified

Unspecified Code Other Specified Code Manifestation Code N Newborn P Pediatric M Maternity A Adult ♂ Male ♀ Female
● New Code ▲ Revised Code Title ▶◀ Revised Text NOTES INCLUDES EXCLUDES1 Not coded here EXCLUDES2 Not included here
4th character required 5th character required 6th character required 7th character required
Extension 'X' Alert HAC Hospital-acquired condition (HAC) alert AHA AHA Coding Clinic©

K77 **Liver disorders in diseases classified elsewhere**
Code first underlying disease, such as:
amyloidosis (E85.-)
congenital syphilis (A50.0, A50.5)
congenital toxoplasmosis (P37.1)
schistosomiasis (B65.0-B65.9)
EXCLUDES1 *alcoholic hepatitis (K70.1-)*
alcoholic liver disease (K70.-)
cytomegaloviral hepatitis (B25.1)
herpesviral [herpes simplex] hepatitis (B00.81)
infectious mononucleosis with liver disease (B27.0-B27.9 with .9)
mumps hepatitis (B26.81)
sarcoidosis with liver disease (D86.89)
secondary syphilis with liver disease (A51.45)
syphilis (late) with liver disease (A52.74)
toxoplasmosis (acquired) hepatitis (B58.1)
tuberculosis with liver disease (A18.83)

Disorders of gallbladder, biliary tract and pancreas (K80-K87)

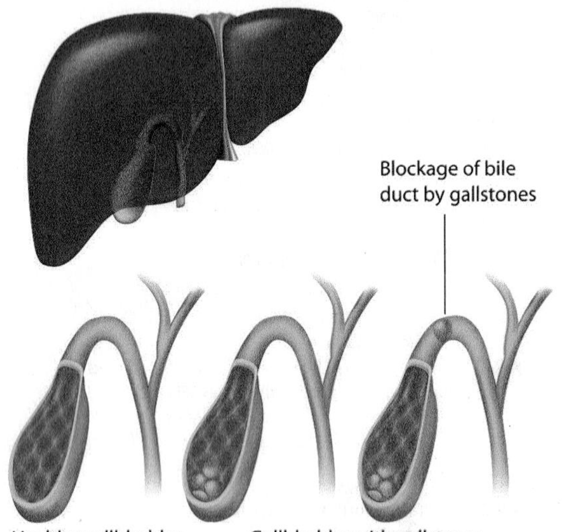

Figure 11.9 Illustration showing normal and obstructed gallbladder

K80 **Cholelithiasis**
EXCLUDES1 *retained cholelithiasis following cholecystectomy (K91.86)*

K80.0 Calculus of gallbladder with acute cholecystitis
Any condition listed in K80.2 with acute cholecystitis
K80.00 **Calculus of gallbladder with acute cholecystitis** without obstruction
K80.01 **Calculus of gallbladder with acute cholecystitis** with obstruction

K80.1 Calculus of gallbladder with other cholecystitis
K80.10 **Calculus of gallbladder with** chronic **cholecystitis** without obstruction
Cholelithiasis with cholecystitis NOS
K80.11 **Calculus of gallbladder with** chronic **cholecystitis** with obstruction
K80.12 **Calculus of gallbladder with** acute and chronic **cholecystitis** without obstruction
K80.13 **Calculus of gallbladder with** acute and chronic **cholecystitis** with obstruction
K80.18 **Calculus of gallbladder with other cholecystitis** without obstruction
K80.19 **Calculus of gallbladder with other cholecystitis** with obstruction

K80.2 Calculus of gallbladder without cholecystitis
Cholecystolithiasis without cholecystitis
Cholelithiasis (without cholecystitis)
Colic (recurrent) of gallbladder (without cholecystitis)
Gallstone (impacted) of cystic duct (without cholecystitis)
Gallstone (impacted) of gallbladder (without cholecystitis)
K80.20 **Calculus of gallbladder without cholecystitis** without obstruction
K80.21 **Calculus of gallbladder without cholecystitis** with obstruction

K80.3 Calculus of bile duct with cholangitis
Any condition listed in K80.5 with cholangitis
K80.30 **Calculus of bile duct with cholangitis, unspecified,** without obstruction
K80.31 **Calculus of bile duct with cholangitis, unspecified,** with obstruction
K80.32 **Calculus of bile duct with** acute **cholangitis** without obstruction
K80.33 **Calculus of bile duct with** acute **cholangitis** with obstruction
K80.34 **Calculus of bile duct with** chronic **cholangitis** without obstruction
K80.35 **Calculus of bile duct with** chronic **cholangitis** with obstruction
K80.36 **Calculus of bile duct with** acute and chronic **cholangitis** without obstruction
K80.37 **Calculus of bile duct with** acute and chronic **cholangitis** with obstruction

K80.4 Calculus of bile duct with cholecystitis
Any condition listed in K80.5 with cholecystitis (with cholangitis)
K80.40 **Calculus of bile duct with cholecystitis, unspecified,** without obstruction
K80.41 **Calculus of bile duct with cholecystitis, unspecified,** with obstruction
K80.42 **Calculus of bile duct with** acute **cholecystitis** without obstruction
K80.43 **Calculus of bile duct with** acute **cholecystitis** with obstruction
K80.44 **Calculus of bile duct with** chronic **cholecystitis** without obstruction
K80.45 **Calculus of bile duct with** chronic **cholecystitis** with obstruction
K80.46 **Calculus of bile duct with** acute and chronic **cholecystitis** without obstruction
K80.47 **Calculus of bile duct with** acute and chronic **cholecystitis** with obstruction

K80.5 Calculus of bile duct without cholangitis or cholecystitis
Choledocholithiasis (without cholangitis or cholecystitis)
Gallstone (impacted) of bile duct NOS (without cholangitis or cholecystitis)
Gallstone (impacted) of common duct (without cholangitis or cholecystitis)
Gallstone (impacted) of hepatic duct (without cholangitis or cholecystitis)
Hepatic cholelithiasis (without cholangitis or cholecystitis)
Hepatic colic (recurrent) (without cholangitis or cholecystitis)
K80.50 **Calculus of bile duct without cholangitis or cholecystitis** without obstruction
K80.51 **Calculus of bile duct without cholangitis or cholecystitis** with obstruction

K80.6 Calculus of gallbladder and bile duct with cholecystitis
K80.60 **Calculus of gallbladder and bile duct with cholecystitis, unspecified,** without obstruction
K80.61 **Calculus of gallbladder and bile duct with cholecystitis, unspecified,** with obstruction
K80.62 **Calculus of gallbladder and bile duct with** acute **cholecystitis** without obstruction
K80.63 **Calculus of gallbladder and bile duct with** acute **cholecystitis** with obstruction
K80.64 **Calculus of gallbladder and bile duct with** chronic **cholecystitis** without obstruction
K80.65 **Calculus of gallbladder and bile duct with** chronic **cholecystitis** with obstruction
K80.66 **Calculus of gallbladder and bile duct with** acute and chronic **cholecystitis** without obstruction
K80.67 **Calculus of gallbladder and bile duct with** acute and chronic **cholecystitis** with obstruction

Unacceptable principal diagnosis symbol per Medicare code edits | Code exempt from diagnosis present on admission requirement
Questionable admission | Complication or comorbidity | CC/MCC exclusion | Major complication or comorbidity
Principal diagnosis as its own CC | Principal diagnosis as its own MCC | Z code as first-listed diagnosis

K80.7 Calculus of gallbladder and bile duct without cholecystitis
K80.70 Calculus of gallbladder and bile duct without cholecystitis without obstruction
K80.71 Calculus of gallbladder and bile duct without cholecystitis with obstruction CC

K80.8 Other cholelithiasis
K80.80 Other cholelithiasis without obstruction
K80.81 Other cholelithiasis with obstruction CC

K81 Cholecystitis
EXCLUDES1 *cholecystitis with cholelithiasis (K80.-)*
K81.0 Acute cholecystitis CC
Abscess of gallbladder
Angiocholecystitis
Emphysematous (acute) cholecystitis
Empyema of gallbladder
Gangrene of gallbladder
Gangrenous cholecystitis
Suppurative cholecystitis
K81.1 Chronic cholecystitis
K81.2 Acute cholecystitis with chronic cholecystitis CC
K81.9 Cholecystitis, unspecified

K82 Other diseases of gallbladder
EXCLUDES1 *nonvisualization of gallbladder (R93.2)*
postcholecystectomy syndrome (K91.5)
K82.0 Obstruction of gallbladder CC
Occlusion of cystic duct or gallbladder without cholelithiasis
Stenosis of cystic duct or gallbladder without cholelithiasis
Stricture of cystic duct or gallbladder without cholelithiasis
EXCLUDES1 *obstruction of gallbladder with cholelithiasis (K80.-)*
K82.1 Hydrops of gallbladder CC
Mucocele of gallbladder
K82.2 Perforation of gallbladder MCC
Rupture of cystic duct or gallbladder
K82.3 Fistula of gallbladder CC
Cholecystocolic fistula
Cholecystoduodenal fistula
K82.4 Cholesterolosis of gallbladder
Strawberry gallbladder
EXCLUDES1 *cholesterolosis of gallbladder with cholecystitis (K81.-)*
cholesterolosis of gallbladder with cholelithiasis (K80.-)
K82.8 Other specified diseases of gallbladder
Adhesions of cystic duct or gallbladder
Atrophy of cystic duct or gallbladder
Cyst of cystic duct or gallbladder
Dyskinesia of cystic duct or gallbladder
Hypertrophy of cystic duct or gallbladder
Nonfunctioning of cystic duct or gallbladder
Ulcer of cystic duct or gallbladder
K82.9 Disease of gallbladder, unspecified

K83 Other diseases of biliary tract
EXCLUDES1 *postcholecystectomy syndrome (K91.5)*
EXCLUDES2 *conditions involving the gallbladder (K81-K82)*
conditions involving the cystic duct (K81-K82)
K83.0 Cholangitis CC
Ascending cholangitis
Cholangitis NOS
Primary cholangitis
Recurrent cholangitis
Sclerosing cholangitis
Secondary cholangitis
Stenosing cholangitis
Suppurative cholangitis
EXCLUDES1 *cholangitic liver abscess (K75.0)*
cholangitis with choledocholithiasis (K80.3-, K80.4-)
chronic nonsuppurative destructive cholangitis (K74.3)
K83.1 Obstruction of bile duct MCC
Occlusion of bile duct without cholelithiasis
Stenosis of bile duct without cholelithiasis
Stricture of bile duct without cholelithiasis
EXCLUDES1 *congenital obstruction of bile duct (Q44.3)*
obstruction of bile duct with cholelithiasis (K80.-)
AHA: Q1, 2016
K83.2 Perforation of bile duct MCC
Rupture of bile duct
K83.3 Fistula of bile duct CC
Choledochoduodenal fistula
K83.4 Spasm of sphincter of Oddi
K83.5 Biliary cyst
K83.8 Other specified diseases of biliary tract
Adhesions of biliary tract
Atrophy of biliary tract
Hypertrophy of biliary tract
Ulcer of biliary tract
K83.9 Disease of biliary tract, unspecified

Figure 11.10 Acute pancreatitis

K85 Acute pancreatitis
INCLUDES *acute (recurrent) pancreatitis*
subacute pancreatitis
K85.0 Idiopathic acute pancreatitis
● K85.00 Idiopathic acute pancreatitis without necrosis or infection CC/MCC Exc MCC
● K85.01 Idiopathic acute pancreatitis with uninfected necrosis CC/MCC Exc MCC
● K85.02 Idiopathic acute pancreatitis with infected necrosis CC/MCC Exc MCC
K85.1 Biliary acute pancreatitis
Gallstone pancreatitis
● K85.10 Biliary acute pancreatitis without necrosis or infection CC/MCC Exc MCC
● K85.11 Biliary acute pancreatitis with uninfected necrosis CC/MCC Exc MCC
● K85.12 Biliary acute pancreatitis with infected necrosis CC/MCC Exc MCC
K85.2 Alcohol induced acute pancreatitis
EXCLUDES2 *alcohol induced chronic pancreatitis (K86.0)*
● K85.20 Alcohol induced acute pancreatitis without necrosis or infection CC/MCC Exc MCC
● K85.21 Alcohol induced acute pancreatitis with uninfected necrosis CC/MCC Exc MCC
● K85.22 Alcohol induced acute pancreatitis with infected necrosis CC/MCC Exc MCC
K85.3 Drug induced acute pancreatitis
Use additional code for adverse effect, if applicable, to identify drug (T36-T50 with fifth or sixth character 5)
Use additional code to identify drug abuse and dependence (F11.-F17.-)
● K85.30 Drug induced acute pancreatitis without necrosis or infection CC/MCC Exc MCC
● K85.31 Drug induced acute pancreatitis with uninfected necrosis CC/MCC Exc MCC
● K85.32 Drug induced acute pancreatitis with infected necrosis CC/MCC Exc MCC
K85.8 Other acute pancreatitis

Unspecified Code Other Specified Code Manifestation Code N Newborn P Pediatric M Maternity A Adult ♂ Male ♀ Female
● New Code ▲ Revised Code Title ►◄ Revised Text NOTES INCLUDES EXCLUDES1 Not coded here EXCLUDES2 Not included here
4th character required 5th character required 6th character required 7th character required
Extension 'X' Alert HAC Hospital-acquired condition (HAC) alert AHA AHA Coding Clinic©

- ● K85.80 **Other acute pancreatitis** without necrosis or infection
- ● K85.81 **Other acute pancreatitis** with uninfected necrosis
- ● K85.82 **Other acute pancreatitis** with infected necrosis

K85.9 **Acute pancreatitis, unspecified**
Pancreatitis NOS

- ● K85.90 **Acute pancreatitis** without necrosis or infection, **unspecified**
- ● K85.91 **Acute pancreatitis** with uninfected necrosis, **unspecified**
- ● K85.92 **Acute pancreatitis** with infected necrosis, **unspecified**

K86 Other diseases of pancreas
EXCLUDES2 *fibrocystic disease of pancreas (E84.-)*
islet cell tumor (of pancreas) (D13.7)
pancreatic steatorrhea (K90.3)

K86.0 **Alcohol-induced chronic pancreatitis**
Use additional code to identify:
alcohol abuse and dependence (F10.-)
Code also exocrine pancreatic insufficiency (K86.81)
EXCLUDES2 *alcohol induced acute pancreatitis ▶(K85.2-)◀*

K86.1 **Other chronic pancreatitis**
Chronic pancreatitis NOS
Infectious chronic pancreatitis
Recurrent chronic pancreatitis
Relapsing chronic pancreatitis
Code also exocrine pancreatic insufficiency (K86.81)

K86.2 **Cyst of pancreas**
K86.3 **Pseudocyst of pancreas**
K86.8 **Other specified diseases of pancreas**

- ● K86.81 Exocrine pancreatic insufficiency
- ● K86.89 **Other specified diseases of pancreas**
  Aseptic pancreatic necrosis, unrelated to acute pancreatitis
  Atrophy of pancreas
  Calculus of pancreas
  Cirrhosis of pancreas
  Fibrosis of pancreas
  Pancreatic fat necrosis, unrelated to acute pancreatitis
  Pancreatic infantilism
  Pancreatic necrosis NOS, unrelated to acute pancreatitis

K86.9 **Disease of pancreas, unspecified**

K87 Disorders of gallbladder, biliary tract and pancreas in diseases classified elsewhere
Code first underlying disease
EXCLUDES1 *cytomegaloviral pancreatitis(B25.2)*
mumps pancreatitis (B26.3)
syphilitic gallbladder (A52.74)
syphilitic pancreas (A52.74)
tuberculosis of gallbladder (A18.83)
tuberculosis of pancreas (A18.83)

Other diseases of the digestive system (K90-K95)

K90 Intestinal malabsorption
EXCLUDES1 *intestinal malabsorption following gastrointestinal surgery (K91.2)*

K90.0 **Celiac disease**
Celiac disease with steatorrhea
Gluten-sensitive enteropathy
Nontropical sprue
Use additional code for associated disorders including:
dermatitis herpetiformis (L13.0)
gluten ataxia (G32.81)
Code also exocrine pancreatic insufficiency (K86.81)

K90.1 **Tropical sprue**
Sprue NOS
Tropical steatorrhea

K90.2 **Blind loop syndrome, not elsewhere classified**
Blind loop syndrome NOS
EXCLUDES1 *congenital blind loop syndrome (Q43.8)*
postsurgical blind loop syndrome (K91.2)

K90.3 **Pancreatic steatorrhea**
▲ K90.4 **▶Other malabsorption** due to intolerance◀
EXCLUDES2 *gluten-sensitive enteropathy (K90.0)*
lactose intolerance (E73.-)

- ● K90.41 Non-celiac gluten sensitivity
  Gluten sensitivity NOS
  Non-celiac gluten sensitive enteropathy
- ● K90.49 **Malabsorption due to intolerance,** not elsewhere classified
  Malabsorption due to intolerance to carbohydrate
  Malabsorption due to intolerance to fat
  Malabsorption due to intolerance to protein
  Malabsorption due to intolerance to starch

K90.8 **Other intestinal malabsorption**
K90.81 **Whipple's disease**
K90.89 **Other intestinal malabsorption**
K90.9 **Intestinal malabsorption, unspecified**

K91 Intraoperative and postprocedural complications and disorders of digestive system, not elsewhere classified
EXCLUDES2 *complications of artificial opening of digestive system (K94.-)*
complications of bariatric procedures (K95.-)
gastrojejunal ulcer (K28.-)
postprocedural (radiation) retroperitoneal abscess (K68.11)
radiation colitis (K52.0)
radiation gastroenteritis (K52.0)
radiation proctitis (K62.7)

K91.0 **Vomiting following gastrointestinal surgery**
K91.1 **Postgastric surgery syndromes**
Dumping syndrome
Postgastrectomy syndrome
Postvagotomy syndrome

K91.2 **Postsurgical malabsorption, not elsewhere classified**
Postsurgical blind loop syndrome
EXCLUDES1 *malabsorption osteomalacia in adults (M83.2)*
malabsorption osteoporosis, postsurgical (M80.8-, M81.8)

K91.3 **Postprocedural intestinal obstruction**
K91.5 **Postcholecystectomy syndrome**
K91.6 Intraoperative hemorrhage and hematoma **of a digestive system organ or structure complicating a procedure**
EXCLUDES1 *intraoperative hemorrhage and hematoma of a digestive system organ or structure due to accidental puncture and laceration during a procedure (K91.7-)*

- ▲ K91.61 **Intraoperative hemorrhage and hematoma of a digestive system organ or structure complicating a** digestive **▶**system**◀ procedure**
- K91.62 **Intraoperative hemorrhage and hematoma of a digestive system organ or structure complicating** other **procedure**

K91.7 Accidental puncture and laceration **of a digestive system organ or structure** during a procedure

- K91.71 **Accidental puncture and laceration of a digestive system organ or structure during a** digestive system procedure
- K91.72 **Accidental puncture and laceration of a digestive system organ or structure during** other procedure

K91.8 Other **intraoperative and postprocedural complications and disorders of digestive system**

- K91.81 **Other** intraoperative **complications of digestive system**
- K91.82 **Postprocedural** hepatic failure
- K91.83 **Postprocedural** hepatorenal syndrome
- ▲ K91.84 **Postprocedural ▶**hemorrhage of**◀ a digestive system organ or structure** following a procedure
  - ▲ K91.840 **Postprocedural ▶hemorrhage of◀ a digestive system organ or structure following a** digestive system procedure
    AHA: Q1, 2016
  - ▲ K91.841 **Postprocedural ▶hemorrhage of◀ a digestive system organ or structure following** other procedure

Unacceptable principal diagnosis symbol per Medicare code edits — Code exempt from diagnosis present on admission requirement — Questionable admission — Complication or comorbidity — CC/MCC exclusion — Major complication or comorbidity — Principal diagnosis as its own CC — Principal diagnosis as its own MCC — Z code as first-listed diagnosis

K91.85 Complications of intestinal pouch
K91.850 Pouchitis
Inflammation of internal ileoanal pouch
K91.858 Other complications of intestinal pouch
K91.86 Retained cholelithiasis following cholecystectomy
● K91.87 Postprocedural hematoma and seroma of a digestive system organ or structure following a procedure
● K91.870 Postprocedural hematoma of a digestive system organ or structure following a digestive system procedure
● K91.871 Postprocedural hematoma of a digestive system organ or structure following other procedure
● K91.872 Postprocedural seroma of a digestive system organ or structure following a digestive system procedure
● K91.873 Postprocedural seroma of a digestive system organ or structure following other procedure
K91.89 Other postprocedural complications and disorders of digestive system
Use additional code, if applicable, to further specify disorder
EXCLUDES2 *postprocedural retroperitoneal abscess (K68.11)*

K92 Other diseases of digestive system
EXCLUDES1 *neonatal gastrointestinal hemorrhage (P54.0-P54.3)*
K92.0 Hematemesis
K92.1 Melena
EXCLUDES1 *occult blood in feces (R19.5)*
K92.2 Gastrointestinal hemorrhage, unspecified
Gastric hemorrhage NOS
Intestinal hemorrhage NOS
EXCLUDES1 *acute hemorrhagic gastritis (K29.01)*
hemorrhage of anus and rectum (K62.5)
angiodysplasia of stomach with hemorrhage (K31.811)
diverticular disease with hemorrhage (K57.-)
gastritis and duodenitis with hemorrhage (K29.-)
peptic ulcer with hemorrhage (K25-K28)
K92.8 Other specified diseases of the digestive system
K92.81 Gastrointestinal mucositis (ulcerative)
Code also type of associated therapy, such as:
antineoplastic and immunosuppressive drugs (T45.1X-)
radiological procedure and radiotherapy (Y84.2)
EXCLUDES2 *mucositis (ulcerative) of vagina and vulva (N76.81)*
nasal mucositis (ulcerative) (J34.81)
oral mucositis (ulcerative) (K12.3-)
K92.89 Other specified diseases of the digestive system
K92.9 Disease of digestive system, unspecified

K94 Complications of artificial openings of the digestive system
K94.0 Colostomy complications
K94.00 Colostomy complication, unspecified
K94.01 Colostomy hemorrhage
K94.02 Colostomy infection
Use additional code to specify type of infection, such as:
cellulitis of abdominal wall (L03.311)
sepsis (A40.-, A41.-)
K94.03 Colostomy malfunction
Mechanical complication of colostomy
K94.09 Other complications of colostomy
K94.1 Enterostomy complications
K94.10 Enterostomy complication, unspecified
K94.11 Enterostomy hemorrhage
K94.12 Enterostomy infection
Use additional code to specify type of infection, such as:
cellulitis of abdominal wall (L03.311)
sepsis (A40.-, A41.-)
K94.13 Enterostomy malfunction
Mechanical complication of enterostomy
K94.19 Other complications of enterostomy
K94.2 Gastrostomy complications
K94.20 Gastrostomy complication, unspecified
K94.21 Gastrostomy hemorrhage
K94.22 Gastrostomy infection
Use additional code to specify type of infection, such as:
cellulitis of abdominal wall (L03.311)
sepsis (A40.-, A41.-)
K94.23 Gastrostomy malfunction
Mechanical complication of gastrostomy
K94.29 Other complications of gastrostomy
K94.3 Esophagostomy complications
K94.30 Esophagostomy complications, unspecified
K94.31 Esophagostomy hemorrhage
K94.32 Esophagostomy infection
Use additional code to identify the infection
K94.33 Esophagostomy malfunction
Mechanical complication of esophagostomy
K94.39 Other complications of esophagostomy

K95 Complications of bariatric procedures
K95.0 Complications of gastric band procedure
K95.01 Infection due to gastric band procedure HAC
Use additional code to specify type of infection or organism, such as:
bacterial and viral infectious agents (B95.-, B96.-)
cellulitis of abdominal wall (L03.311)
sepsis (A40.-, A41.-)
K95.09 Other complications of gastric band procedure
Use additional code, if applicable, to further specify complication
K95.8 Complications of other bariatric procedure
EXCLUDES1 *complications of gastric band surgery (K95.0-)*
K95.81 Infection due to other bariatric procedure HAC
Use additional code to specify type of infection or organism, such as:
bacterial and viral infectious agents (B95.-, B96.-)
cellulitis of abdominal wall (L03.311)
sepsis (A40.-, A41.-)
K95.89 Other complications of other bariatric procedure
Use additional code, if applicable, to further specify complication

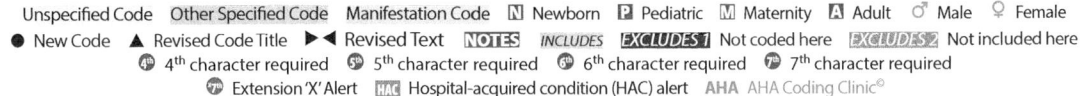

Unspecified Code Other Specified Code Manifestation Code N Newborn P Pediatric M Maternity A Adult ♂ Male ♀ Female
● New Code ▲ Revised Code Title ►◄ Revised Text NOTES INCLUDES EXCLUDES1 Not coded here EXCLUDES2 Not included here
4th character required 5th character required 6th character required 7th character required
Extension 'X' Alert HAC Hospital-acquired condition (HAC) alert AHA AHA Coding Clinic©

This page intentionally left blank

Chapter 12: Diseases of the Skin and Subcutaneous Tissue (L00-L99)

Guidelines for Assigning Codes From This Chapter

For a diagnosis involving the skin or the fatty subcutaneous tissue just under the skin, you'll likely find your code in Chapter 12. Cellulitis, dermatitis, psoriasis, corns, and hives are just some of the diagnoses you'll find here. You may be surprised to learn that this chapter also includes codes for diseases of the nails and hair.

But remember to always start your diagnosis code search in the Index. The codes for skin cancers such as melanoma and basal cell carcinoma are not in Chapter 12, and the Index will help you find the proper code.

List of Sections

- L00-L08: Infections of the skin and subcutaneous tissue
- L10-L14: Bullous disorders
- L20-L30: Dermatitis and eczema
- L40-L45: Papulosquamous disorders
- L49-L54: Urticaria and erythema
- L55-L59: Radiation-related disorders of the skin and subcutaneous tissue
- L60-L75: Disorders of skin appendages
- L76: Intraoperative and postprocedural complications of skin and subcutaneous tissue
- L80-L99: Other disorders of the skin and subcutaneous tissue

Highlights From the ICD-10-CM Official Guidelines for Coding and Reporting

The ICD-10-CM Official Guidelines for Coding and Reporting for Chapter 12 focus on coding for pressure ulcers (L89.-). The information below is from Section I.C.12 of the 2017 Official Guidelines.

Take note: I-10 codes for pressure ulcers are combination codes that specify both the site and the stage in a single code. If the patient has more than one pressure ulcer, you would assign as many codes as needed to identify all the involved sites.

Stages: There are four stages (1-4) used to identify the degree of severity of pressure ulcers. There are also codes for unstageable and unspecified. Choose the correct stage based on the clinical documentation. Go to "Ulcer, pressure" in the Alphabetic Index for key terms that you can look for in the documentation to determine the correct stage. If the ulcer stage has not been documented or the ulcer is not described well, query the provider. There is no code that can be assigned for a pressure ulcer documented as healed.

Separate Unstageable From Unspecified Stage

Do not confuse an unstageable pressure ulcer (L89.--0) with an unspecified stage pressure ulcer (L89.--9). Sometimes, a provider cannot determine the stage of a pressure ulcer because a skin or muscle graft has been applied over the ulcer, the ulcer is covered with eschar (scabbed over), or the ulcer is documented as a deep tissue injury but without documentation of trauma. You must analyze the documentation to see if any of these situations apply before assigning L89.--0. Use unspecified (L89.--9) only when the documentation fails to identify the stage.

Don't Confuse Healed With Healing

When the documentation for the patient's admission records a healed ulcer, you should not include a code for the ulcer. However, when the record mentions a healing ulcer, you should report the site and the ulcer stage documented. If the record fails to provide enough information to determine the stage of a healing pressure ulcer, report the code for an unspecified stage for that site. If the record does not make it clear whether the pressure ulcer is new or healing, you should ask the provider to clarify.

Report the Highest Stage for Progressing Ulcer

Finally, the guidelines offer instructions on what to do when a patient has a pressure ulcer that is one stage at admission, but it evolves to a higher stage during the stay. You should report the code for the highest stage when that situation occurs.

Anatomy of the Integumentary System

The Common Integument

The integumentary system is composed of the common integument (or skin) and its appendages. The skin covers the body and proves to be an effective barrier to most harmful chemicals that can cause damage to our internal body system. It contains the peripheral endings of various sensory nerves and plays an important role in the regulation of our body temperature. The various layers/components of the skin (from outside to inside) are listed below:

1. **The Epidermis**
   a) Stratum Corneum
   b) Stratum Lucidum
   c) Stratum Granulosum
   d) Stratum Spinosum
   e) Stratum Germinativum (or Basal Layer/Stratum Basale)
2. **The Dermis (or Corium)**
   a) Papillary Layer of Dermis
   b) Reticular Layer of Dermis
3. **The Subcutaneous Tissue/Superficial Fascia (or Hypodermis)**
4. **The Appendages of the Skin**
   a) Hair (for protection and sensation)
   b) Nails (for protection)
   c) Sebaceous Glands (or the glands that secrete sebum onto hair follicle)
   d) Sweat Glands (or the glands that secrete sweat) and ducts
      i) eccrine sweat glands (or the glands secreting sweat with faint odor)
      ii) apocrine sweat glands (or the glands secreting sweat with strong odor)
   e) Arrector Pili (or smooth muscles that pull hairs straight)

Common Pathologies

Cellulitis
It is a noncontiguous inflammation of the skin and deeper tissues. It causes diffuse inflammation of connective tissue with severe inflammation of dermal and subcutaneous layers of the skin. Skin in the infected area will become red, hot, irritated and painful. Group A strep (streptococcal) bacteria are the most common cause of cellulitis.

Impetigo
Impetigo is a highly contagious skin infection which causes sores and blisters. This contagious superficial skin infection is generally caused by one of two bacteria: Staphylococcus aureus or Streptococcus pyogenes. Symptoms start with red or pimple-like sores surrounded by red skin.

Folliculitis
It is the infection and inflammation of one or more hair follicles. It usually is caused by bacteria. It can occur anywhere on the skin. Numerous smooth little red bumps form around hair follicles and are most commonly seen on the chest, back, buttocks and legs.

Acne
Acne vulgaris is a common human skin disease. Human skin has pores which connect to oil glands located under the skin. A small hair grows through the follicle out of the skin. Pimples form when hair follicles under the skin clog up. Acne lesions heal slowly, and when one begins to resolve, others seem to crop up.

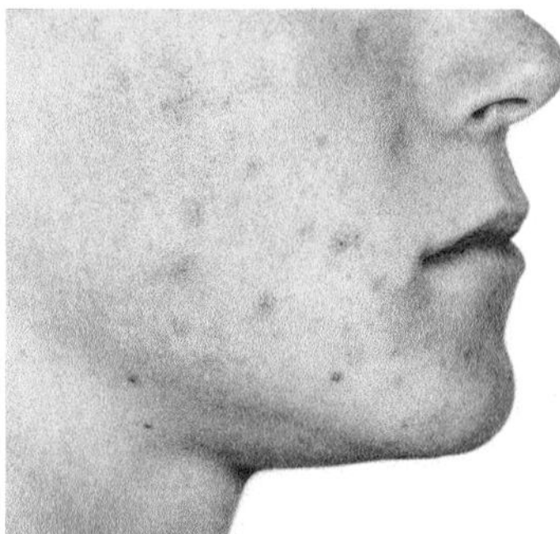

Herpes simplex
Herpes is an infection that is caused by a herpes simplex virus (HSV). Oral herpes is the most common form of infection followed by genital herpes. Main symptoms of herpes are tingling, itching and burning.

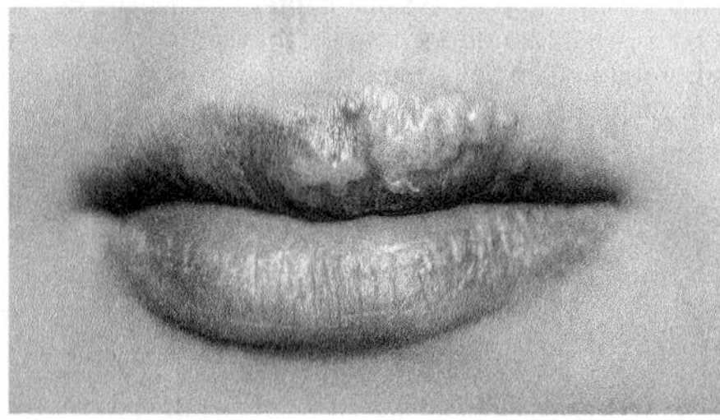

Chicken pox
Chicken pox is a viral infection in which extremely itchy blisters develop all over the body. It is a highly contagious disease caused by primary infection with varicella zoster virus. The classic symptoms of this disease are an uncomfortable itchy rash, fever, headache, tiredness and loss of appetite. The rash turns into fluid-filled blisters and eventually into scabs. It usually shows up on the face, chest, and back and then spreads to the rest of the body. If the virus becomes active again, it can cause a painful infection called shingles.

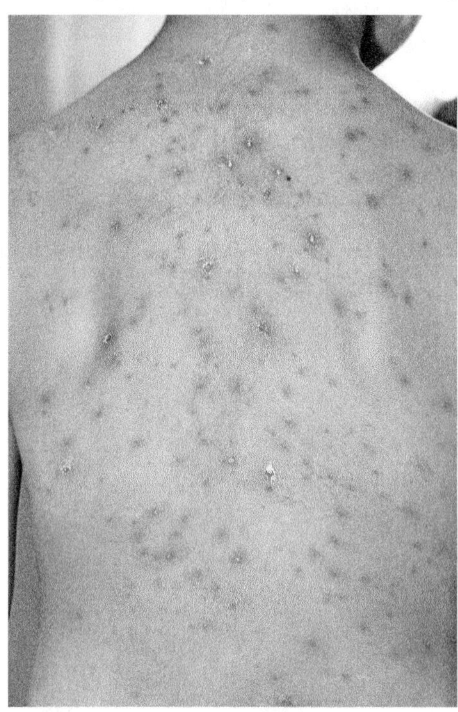

Verrucae
A verruca is a type of wart that is found on the soles of your feet, though they can also appear around the toes. Warts are rough lumps that often develop on the skin of the hands and feet. It is a small growth on the sole of the foot often with tiny black dots on the surface.

Scabies
Scabies is a contagious and itchy skin infection caused by the mite Sarcoptes scabiei. The mite is a tiny and usually not directly visible parasite which burrows under the patient's skin, causing intense allergic itching. Direct skin-to-skin contact is the mode of transmission. Scabies can also be spread by sharing towels, bed sheets, and other personal belongings. Scabies causes severe itching that is usually worse at night and a rash with tiny blisters. It spreads quickly in crowded conditions.

Psoriasis
Psoriasis is a chronic skin problem that causes skin cells to grow too quickly, resulting in thick, white, silvery patches of skin. This occurs when the immune system mistakenly attacks and destroys healthy body tissue. Bacteria or viral infections, stress, dry air, injury to the skin and some medicines may trigger the

condition. It is a noncontagious skin condition that produces red papules that merge together into plaques of thickened scaling skin. Psoriasis commonly affects the skin of the elbows, knees, and scalp. Psoriasis symptoms improve or can go into remission.

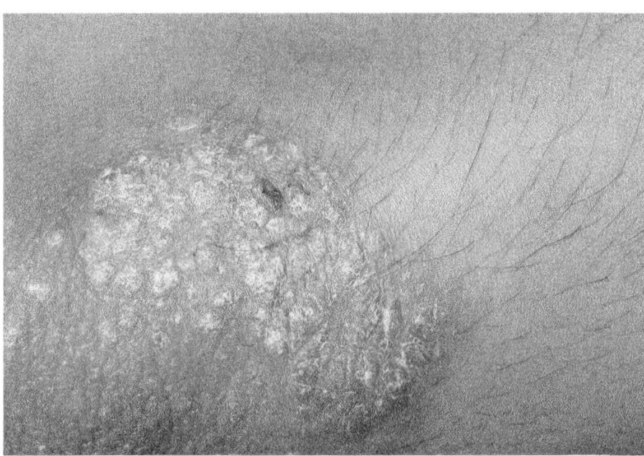

Ringworm

Ringworm is a type of fungal skin infection which is caused by fungi called tinea. It is a common highly contagious skin infection that causes a ring-like red rash on the skin. The rash can appear almost anywhere on the body, with the scalp, feet and groin being most common sites.

Diseases of the skin and subcutaneous tissue (L00-L99)

EXCLUDES2 *certain conditions originating in the perinatal period (P04-P96)*
certain infectious and parasitic diseases (A00-B99)
complications of pregnancy, childbirth and the puerperium (O00-O9A)
congenital malformations, deformations, and chromosomal abnormalities (Q00-Q99)
endocrine, nutritional and metabolic diseases (E00-E88)
lipomelanotic reticulosis (I89.8)
neoplasms (C00-D49)
symptoms, signs and abnormal clinical and laboratory findings, not elsewhere classified (R00-R94)
systemic connective tissue disorders (M30-M36)
viral warts (B07.-)

This chapter contains the following blocks:

- L00-L08 Infections of the skin and subcutaneous tissue
- L10-L14 Bullous disorders
- L20-L30 Dermatitis and eczema
- L40-L45 Papulosquamous disorders
- L49-L54 Urticaria and erythema
- L55-L59 Radiation-related disorders of the skin and subcutaneous tissue
- L60-L75 Disorders of skin appendages
- L76 Intraoperative and postprocedural complications of skin and subcutaneous tissue
- L80-L99 Other disorders of the skin and subcutaneous tissue

Infections of the skin and subcutaneous tissue (L00-L08)

Use additional code (B95-B97) to identify infectious agent.

EXCLUDES2 *hordeolum (H00.0)*
infective dermatitis (L30.3)
local infections of skin classified in Chapter 1
lupus panniculitis (L93.2)
panniculitis NOS (M79.3)
panniculitis of neck and back (M54.0-)
Perlèche NOS (K13.0)
Perlèche due to candidiasis (B37.0)
Perlèche due to riboflavin deficiency (E53.0)
pyogenic granuloma (L98.0)
relapsing panniculitis [Weber-Christian] (M35.6)
viral warts (B07.-)
zoster (B02.-)

L00 Staphylococcal scalded skin syndromee
Ritter's disease
Use additional code to identify percentage of skin exfoliation (L49.-)
EXCLUDES1 *bullous impetigo (L01.03)*
pemphigus neonatorum (L01.03)
toxic epidermal necrolysis [Lyell] (L51.2)

4th **L01 Impetigo**
EXCLUDES1 *impetigo herpetiformis (L40.1)*

5th **L01.0 Impetigo**
Impetigo contagiosa
Impetigo vulgaris
L01.00 Impetigo, unspecified
Impetigo NOS
L01.01 Non-bullous impetigo
L01.02 Bockhart's impetigo
Impetigo follicularis
Perifolliculitis NOS
Superficial pustular perifolliculitis
L01.03 Bullous impetigo
Impetigo neonatorum
Pemphigus neonatorum
L01.09 Other impetigo
Ulcerative impetigo

L01.1 Impetiginization of other dermatoses

4th **L02 Cutaneous abscess, furuncle and carbuncle**
Use additional code to identify organism (B95-B96)
EXCLUDES2 *abscess of anus and rectal regions (K61.-)*
abscess of female genital organs (external) (N76.4)
abscess of male genital organs (external) (N48.2, N49.-)

5th **L02.0 Cutaneous abscess, furuncle and carbuncle of face**
EXCLUDES2 *abscess of ear, external (H60.0)*
abscess of eyelid (H00.0)
abscess of head [any part, except face] (L02.8)
abscess of lacrimal gland (H04.0)
abscess of lacrimal passages (H04.3)
abscess of mouth (K12.2)
abscess of nose (J34.0)
abscess of orbit (H05.0)
submandibular abscess (K12.2)
L02.01 Cutaneous abscess of face CC
L02.02 Furuncle of face
Boil of face
Folliculitis of face
L02.03 Carbuncle of face

5th **L02.1 Cutaneous abscess, furuncle and carbuncle of neck**
L02.11 Cutaneous abscess of neck CC
L02.12 Furuncle of neck
Boil of neck
Folliculitis of neck
L02.13 Carbuncle of neck

5th **L02.2 Cutaneous abscess, furuncle and carbuncle of trunk**
EXCLUDES1 *non-newborn omphalitis (L08.82)*
omphalitis of newborn (P38.-)
EXCLUDES2 *abscess of breast ►(N61.1)◄*
abscess of buttocks (L02.3)
abscess of female external genital organs (N76.4)
abscess of male external genital organs (N48.2, N49.-)
abscess of hip (L02.4)

6th **L02.21 Cutaneous abscess of trunk**
L02.211 Cutaneous abscess of abdominal wall CC
L02.212 Cutaneous abscess of back [any part, except buttock] CC
L02.213 Cutaneous abscess of chest wall CC
L02.214 Cutaneous abscess of groin CC
L02.215 Cutaneous abscess of perineum CC
L02.216 Cutaneous abscess of umbilicus CC
L02.219 Cutaneous abscess of trunk, unspecified CC

6th **L02.22 Furuncle of trunk**
Boil of trunk
Folliculitis of trunk
L02.221 Furuncle of abdominal wall
L02.222 Furuncle of back [any part, except buttock]
L02.223 Furuncle of chest wall
L02.224 Furuncle of groin
L02.225 Furuncle of perineum
L02.226 Furuncle of umbilicus
L02.229 Furuncle of trunk, unspecified

6th **L02.23 Carbuncle of trunk**
L02.231 Carbuncle of abdominal wall
L02.232 Carbuncle of back [any part, except buttock]
L02.233 Carbuncle of chest wall
L02.234 Carbuncle of groin
L02.235 Carbuncle of perineum
L02.236 Carbuncle of umbilicus
L02.239 Carbuncle of trunk, unspecified

5th **L02.3 Cutaneous abscess, furuncle and carbuncle of buttock**
EXCLUDES1 *pilonidal cyst with abscess (L05.01)*
L02.31 Cutaneous abscess of buttock CC
Cutaneous abscess of gluteal region
L02.32 Furuncle of buttock
Boil of buttock
Folliculitis of buttock
Furuncle of gluteal region
L02.33 Carbuncle of buttock
Carbuncle of gluteal region

PDx Unacceptable principal diagnosis symbol per Medicare code edits · POA Code exempt from diagnosis present on admission requirement · Questionable admission · CC Complication or comorbidity · CC/MCC EXC CC/MCC exclusion · MCC Major complication or comorbidity · PDx CC Principal diagnosis as its own CC · PDx MCC Principal diagnosis as its own MCC · Z1 Z code as first-listed diagnosis

When symbols appear on a code that requires a 7th character extension, refer to Appendix D to identify applicable 7th character codes.

L02.4 Cutaneous abscess, furuncle and carbuncle of limb
EXCLUDES2 *Cutaneous abscess, furuncle and carbuncle of groin (L02.214, L02.224, L02.234)*
Cutaneous abscess, furuncle and carbuncle of hand (L02.5-)
Cutaneous abscess, furuncle and carbuncle of foot (L02.6-)

L02.41 Cutaneous abscess of limb
L02.411 Cutaneous abscess of right axilla
L02.412 Cutaneous abscess of left axilla
L02.413 Cutaneous abscess of right upper limb
L02.414 Cutaneous abscess of left upper limb
L02.415 Cutaneous abscess of right lower limb
L02.416 Cutaneous abscess of left lower limb
L02.419 Cutaneous abscess of limb, unspecified

L02.42 Furuncle of limb
Boil of limb
Folliculitis of limb
L02.421 Furuncle of right axilla
L02.422 Furuncle of left axilla
L02.423 Furuncle of right upper limb
L02.424 Furuncle of left upper limb
L02.425 Furuncle of right lower limb
L02.426 Furuncle of left lower limb
L02.429 Furuncle of limb, unspecified

L02.43 Carbuncle of limb
L02.431 Carbuncle of right axilla
L02.432 Carbuncle of left axilla
L02.433 Carbuncle of right upper limb
L02.434 Carbuncle of left upper limb
L02.435 Carbuncle of right lower limb
L02.436 Carbuncle of left lower limb
L02.439 Carbuncle of limb, unspecified

L02.5 Cutaneous abscess, furuncle and carbuncle of hand

L02.51 Cutaneous abscess of hand
L02.511 Cutaneous abscess of right hand
L02.512 Cutaneous abscess of left hand
L02.519 Cutaneous abscess of unspecified hand

L02.52 Furuncle hand
Boil of hand
Folliculitis of hand
L02.521 Furuncle right hand
L02.522 Furuncle left hand
L02.529 Furuncle unspecified hand

L02.53 Carbuncle of hand
L02.531 Carbuncle of right hand
L02.532 Carbuncle of left hand
L02.539 Carbuncle of unspecified hand

L02.6 Cutaneous abscess, furuncle and carbuncle of foot

L02.61 Cutaneous abscess of foot
L02.611 Cutaneous abscess of right foot
L02.612 Cutaneous abscess of left foot
L02.619 Cutaneous abscess of unspecified foot

L02.62 Furuncle of foot
Boil of foot
Folliculitis of foot
L02.621 Furuncle of right foot
L02.622 Furuncle of left foot
L02.629 Furuncle of unspecified foot

L02.63 Carbuncle of foot
L02.631 Carbuncle of right foot
L02.632 Carbuncle of left foot
L02.639 Carbuncle of unspecified foot

L02.8 Cutaneous abscess, furuncle and carbuncle of other sites

L02.81 Cutaneous abscess of other sites
L02.811 Cutaneous abscess of head [any part, except face]
L02.818 Cutaneous abscess of other sites

L02.82 Furuncle of other sites
Boil of other sites
Folliculitis of other sites
L02.821 Furuncle of head [any part, except face]
L02.828 Furuncle of other sites

L02.83 Carbuncle of other sites
L02.831 Carbuncle of head [any part, except face]
L02.838 Carbuncle of other sites

L02.9 Cutaneous abscess, furuncle and carbuncle, unspecified
L02.91 Cutaneous abscess, unspecified
L02.92 Furuncle, unspecified
Boil NOS
Furunculosis NOS
L02.93 Carbuncle, unspecified

L03 Cellulitis and acute lymphangitis
EXCLUDES2 *cellulitis of anal and rectal region (K61.-)*
cellulitis of external auditory canal (H60.1)
cellulitis of eyelid (H00.0)
cellulitis of female external genital organs (N76.4)
cellulitis of lacrimal apparatus (H04.3)
cellulitis of male external genital organs (N48.2, N49.-)
cellulitis of mouth (K12.2)
cellulitis of nose (J34.0)
eosinophilic cellulitis [Wells] (L98.3)
febrile neutrophilic dermatosis [Sweet] (L98.2)
lymphangitis (chronic) (subacute) (I89.1)

L03.0 Cellulitis and acute lymphangitis of finger and toe
Infection of nail
Onychia
Paronychia
Perionychia

L03.01 Cellulitis of finger
Felon
Whitlow
EXCLUDES1 *herpetic whitlow (B00.89)*
L03.011 Cellulitis of right finger
L03.012 Cellulitis of left finger
L03.019 Cellulitis of unspecified finger

L03.02 Acute lymphangitis of finger
Hangnail with lymphangitis of finger
L03.021 Acute lymphangitis of right finger
L03.022 Acute lymphangitis of left finger
L03.029 Acute lymphangitis of unspecified finger

L03.03 Cellulitis of toe
L03.031 Cellulitis of right toe
L03.032 Cellulitis of left toe
L03.039 Cellulitis of unspecified toe

L03.04 Acute lymphangitis of toe
Hangnail with lymphangitis of toe
L03.041 Acute lymphangitis of right toe
L03.042 Acute lymphangitis of left toe
L03.049 Acute lymphangitis of unspecified toe

L03.1 Cellulitis and acute lymphangitis of other parts of limb

L03.11 Cellulitis of other parts of limb
EXCLUDES2 *cellulitis of fingers (L03.01-)*
cellulitis of toes (L03.03-)
groin (L03.314)
L03.111 Cellulitis of right axilla
L03.112 Cellulitis of left axilla
L03.113 Cellulitis of right upper limb
L03.114 Cellulitis of left upper limb
L03.115 Cellulitis of right lower limb
L03.116 Cellulitis of left lower limb
L03.119 Cellulitis of unspecified part of limb

L03.12 Acute lymphangitis of other parts of limb
EXCLUDES2 *acute lymphangitis of fingers (L03.2-)*
acute lymphangitis of toes (L03.04-)
acute lymphangitis of groin (L03.324)
L03.121 Acute lymphangitis of right axilla
L03.122 Acute lymphangitis of left axilla
L03.123 Acute lymphangitis of right upper limb
L03.124 Acute lymphangitis of left upper limb
L03.125 Acute lymphangitis of right lower limb
L03.126 Acute lymphangitis of left lower limb
L03.129 Acute lymphangitis of unspecified part of limb

Unspecified Code | Other Specified Code | Manifestation Code | N Newborn | P Pediatric | M Maternity | A Adult | ♂ Male | ♀ Female
● New Code | ▲ Revised Code Title | ►◄ Revised Text | NOTES | INCLUDES | EXCLUDES1 Not coded here | EXCLUDES2 Not included here
4th character required | 5th character required | 6th character required | 7th character required
Extension 'X' Alert | HAC Hospital-acquired condition (HAC) alert | AHA AHA Coding Clinic©

L03.2 Cellulitis and acute lymphangitis of face and neck
- L03.21 Cellulitis and acute lymphangitis of face
  - L03.211 Cellulitis of face
    - EXCLUDES2 *abscess of orbit (H05.01-)*
      - *cellulitis of ear (H60.1-)*
      - *cellulitis of eyelid (H00.0-)*
      - *cellulitis of head (L03.81)*
      - *cellulitis of lacrimal apparatus (H04.3)*
      - *cellulitis of lip (K13.0)*
      - *cellulitis of mouth (K12.2)*
      - *cellulitis of nose (internal) (J34.0)*
      - *cellulitis of orbit ►(H05.01-)◄*
      - *cellulitis of scalp (L03.81)*
    - AHA: Q4, 2013
  - L03.212 Acute lymphangitis of face
  - ● L03.213 Periorbital cellulitis
    - Preseptal cellulitis
- L03.22 Cellulitis and acute lymphangitis of neck
  - L03.221 Cellulitis of neck
  - L03.222 Acute lymphangitis of neck

L03.3 Cellulitis and acute lymphangitis of trunk
- L03.31 Cellulitis of trunk
  - EXCLUDES2 *cellulitis of anal and rectal regions (K61.-)*
    - *cellulitis of breast NOS ►(N61.0)◄*
    - *cellulitis of female external genital organs (N76.4)*
    - *cellulitis of male external genital organs (N48.2, N49.-)*
    - *omphalitis of newborn (P38.-)*
    - *puerperal cellulitis of breast (O91.2)*
  - L03.311 Cellulitis of abdominal wall
    - EXCLUDES2 *cellulitis of umbilicus (L03.316)*
      - *cellulitis of groin (L03.314)*
  - L03.312 Cellulitis of back [any part except buttock]
  - L03.313 Cellulitis of chest wall
  - L03.314 Cellulitis of groin
  - L03.315 Cellulitis of perineum
  - L03.316 Cellulitis of umbilicus
  - L03.317 Cellulitis of buttock
  - L03.319 Cellulitis of trunk, unspecified
- L03.32 Acute lymphangitis of trunk
  - L03.321 Acute lymphangitis of abdominal wall
  - L03.322 Acute lymphangitis of back [any part except buttock]
  - L03.323 Acute lymphangitis of chest wall
  - L03.324 Acute lymphangitis of groin
  - L03.325 Acute lymphangitis of perineum
  - L03.326 Acute lymphangitis of umbilicus
  - L03.327 Acute lymphangitis of buttock
  - L03.329 Acute lymphangitis of trunk, unspecified

L03.8 Cellulitis and acute lymphangitis of other sites
- L03.81 Cellulitis of other sites
  - L03.811 Cellulitis of head [any part, except face]
    - Cellulitis of scalp
    - EXCLUDES2 *cellulitis of face (L03.211)*
  - L03.818 Cellulitis of other sites
- L03.89 Acute lymphangitis of other sites
  - L03.891 Acute lymphangitis of head [any part, except face]
  - L03.898 Acute lymphangitis of other sites

L03.9 Cellulitis and acute lymphangitis, unspecified
- L03.90 Cellulitis, unspecified
- L03.91 Acute lymphangitis, unspecified
  - EXCLUDES1 *lymphangitis NOS (I89.1)*

L04 Acute lymphadenitis
- INCLUDES *abscess (acute) of lymph nodes, except mesenteric*
  - *acute lymphadenitis, except mesenteric*
- EXCLUDES1 *chronic or subacute lymphadenitis, except mesenteric (I88.1)*
  - *enlarged lymph nodes (R59.-)*
  - *human immunodeficiency virus [HIV] disease resulting in generalized lymphadenopathy (B20)*
  - *lymphadenitis NOS (I88.9)*
  - *nonspecific mesenteric lymphadenitis (I88.0)*
- L04.0 Acute lymphadenitis of face, head and neck
- L04.1 Acute lymphadenitis of trunk
- L04.2 Acute lymphadenitis of upper limb
  - Acute lymphadenitis of axilla
  - Acute lymphadenitis of shoulder
- L04.3 Acute lymphadenitis of lower limb
  - Acute lymphadenitis of hip
  - EXCLUDES2 *acute lymphadenitis of groin (L04.1)*
- L04.8 Acute lymphadenitis of other sites
- L04.9 Acute lymphadenitis, unspecified

L05 Pilonidal cyst and sinus
- L05.0 Pilonidal cyst and sinus with abscess
  - L05.01 Pilonidal cyst with abscess
    - Pilonidal abscess
    - Pilonidal dimple with abscess
    - Postanal dimple with abscess
    - EXCLUDES2 *congenital sacral dimple (Q82.6)*
      - *parasacral dimple (Q82.6)*
  - L05.02 Pilonidal sinus with abscess
    - Coccygeal fistula with abscess
    - Coccygeal sinus with abscess
    - Pilonidal fistula with abscess
- L05.9 Pilonidal cyst and sinus without abscess
  - L05.91 Pilonidal cyst without abscess
    - Pilonidal dimple
    - Postanal dimple
    - Pilonidal cyst NOS
    - EXCLUDES2 *congenital sacral dimple (Q82.6)*
      - *parasacral dimple (Q82.6)*
  - L05.92 Pilonidal sinus without abscess
    - Coccygeal fistula
    - Coccygeal sinus without abscess
    - Pilonidal fistula

L08 Other local infections of skin and subcutaneous tissue
- L08.0 Pyoderma
  - Dermatitis gangrenosa
  - Purulent dermatitis
  - Septic dermatitis
  - Suppurative dermatitis
  - EXCLUDES1 *pyoderma gangrenosum (L88)*
    - *pyoderma vegetans (L08.81)*
- L08.1 Erythrasma
- L08.8 Other specified local infections of the skin and subcutaneous tissue
  - L08.81 Pyoderma vegetans
    - EXCLUDES1 *pyoderma gangrenosum (L88)*
      - *pyoderma NOS (L08.0)*
  - L08.82 Omphalitis not of newborn
    - EXCLUDES1 *omphalitis of newborn (P38.-)*
  - L08.89 Other specified local infections of the skin and subcutaneous tissue
- L08.9 Local infection of the skin and subcutaneous tissue, unspecified

Bullous disorders (L10-L14)

EXCLUDES1 *benign familial pemphigus [Hailey-Hailey] (Q82.8)*
- *staphylococcal scalded skin syndromee (L00)*
- *toxic epidermal necrolysis [Lyell] (L51.2)*

L10 Pemphigus
- EXCLUDES1 *pemphigus neonatorum (L01.03)*
- L10.0 Pemphigus vulgaris
- L10.1 Pemphigus vegetans

Unacceptable principal diagnosis symbol per Medicare code edits · Code exempt from diagnosis present on admission requirement · Questionable admission · Complication or comorbidity · CC/MCC exclusion · Major complication or comorbidity · Principal diagnosis as its own CC · Principal diagnosis as its own MCC · Z code as first-listed diagnosis

When symbols appear on a code that requires a 7th character extension, refer to Appendix D to identify applicable 7th character codes.

L10.2 **Pemphigus** foliaceous
L10.3 Brazilian **pemphigus [fogo selvagem]**
L10.4 **Pemphigus** erythematosus
Senear-Usher syndromee
L10.5 Drug-induced **pemphigus**
Use additional code for adverse effect, if applicable, to identify drug (T36-T50 with fifth or sixth character 5)
L10.8 Other **pemphigus**
L10.81 Paraneoplastic **pemphigus**
L10.89 **Other pemphigus**
L10.9 **Pemphigus, unspecified**

L11 Other **acantholytic disorders**
L11.0 **Acquired keratosis follicularis**
EXCLUDES1 *keratosis follicularis (congenital) [Darier-White] (Q82.8)*
L11.1 **Transient acantholytic dermatosis [Grover]**
L11.8 **Other specified acantholytic disorders**
L11.9 **Acantholytic disorder, unspecified**

L12 **Pemphigoid**
EXCLUDES1 *herpes gestationis (O26.4-)*
impetigo herpetiformis (L40.1)
L12.0 Bullous **pemphigoid**
L12.1 Cicatricial **pemphigoid**
Benign mucous membrane pemphigoid
L12.2 **Chronic bullous disease of childhood**
Juvenile dermatitis herpetiformis
L12.3 Acquired epidermolysis **bullosa**
EXCLUDES1 *epidermolysis bullosa (congenital) (Q81.-)*
L12.30 **Acquired epidermolysis bullosa, unspecified**
L12.31 **Epidermolysis bullosa due to drug**
Use additional code for adverse effect, if applicable, to identify drug (T36-T50 with fifth or sixth character 5)
L12.35 **Other acquired epidermolysis bullosa**
L12.8 **Other pemphigoid**
L12.9 **Pemphigoid, unspecified**

L13 Other **bullous disorders**
L13.0 **Dermatitis herpetiformis**
Duhring's disease
Hydroa herpetiformis
EXCLUDES1 *juvenile dermatitis herpetiformis (L12.2)*
senile dermatitis herpetiformis (L12.0)
L13.1 Subcorneal pustular **dermatitis**
Sneddon-Wilkinson disease
L13.8 **Other specified bullous disorders**
L13.9 **Bullous disorder, unspecified**

L14 **Bullous disorders in diseases classified elsewhere**
Code first underlying disease

Dermatitis and eczema (L20-L30)

NOTES In this block the terms dermatitis and eczema are used synonymously and interchangeably.
EXCLUDES2 *chronic (childhood) granulomatous disease (D71)*
dermatitis gangrenosa (L08.0)
dermatitis herpetiformis (L13.0)
dry skin dermatitis (L85.3)
factitial dermatitis (L98.1)
perioral dermatitis (L71.0)
radiation-related disorders of the skin and subcutaneous tissue (L55-L59)
stasis dermatitis ▶(I87.2)◀

L20 Atopic **dermatitis**
L20.0 **Besnier's prurigo**
L20.8 **Other atopic dermatitis**
EXCLUDES2 *circumscribed neurodermatitis (L28.0)*
L20.81 **Atopic** neurodermatitis
Diffuse neurodermatitis
L20.82 Flexural **eczema**
L20.83 Infantile (acute) (chronic) **eczema**
L20.84 Intrinsic (allergic) **eczema**
L20.89 **Other atopic dermatitis**
L20.9 **Atopic dermatitis, unspecified**

L21 Seborrheic **dermatitis**
EXCLUDES2 *infective dermatitis (L30.3)*
seborrheic keratosis (L82.-)
L21.0 **Seborrhea** capitis
Cradle cap
L21.1 **Seborrheic** infantile dermatitis
L21.8 **Other seborrheic dermatitis**
L21.9 **Seborrheic dermatitis, unspecified**
Seborrhea NOS

L22 Diaper **dermatitis**
Diaper erythema
Diaper rash
Psoriasiform diaper rash

L23 Allergic contact **dermatitis**
EXCLUDES1 *allergy NOS (T78.40)*
contact dermatitis NOS (L25.9)
dermatitis NOS (L30.9)
EXCLUDES2 *dermatitis due to substances taken internally (L27.-)*
dermatitis of eyelid (H01.1-)
diaper dermatitis (L22)
eczema of external ear (H60.5-)
irritant contact dermatitis (L24.-)
perioral dermatitis (L71.0)
radiation-related disorders of the skin and subcutaneous tissue (L55-L59)
L23.0 **Allergic contact dermatitis** due to metals
Allergic contact dermatitis due to chromium
Allergic contact dermatitis due to nickel
L23.1 **Allergic contact dermatitis** due to adhesives
L23.2 **Allergic contact dermatitis** due to cosmetics
L23.3 **Allergic contact dermatitis** due to drugs in contact with skin
Use additional code for adverse effect, if applicable, to identify drug (T36-T50 with fifth or sixth character 5)
EXCLUDES2 *dermatitis due to ingested drugs and medicaments (L27.0-L27.1)*
L23.4 **Allergic contact dermatitis** due to dyes
L23.5 **Allergic contact dermatitis** due to other chemical products
Allergic contact dermatitis due to cement
Allergic contact dermatitis due to insecticide
Allergic contact dermatitis due to plastic
Allergic contact dermatitis due to rubber
L23.6 **Allergic contact dermatitis** due to food in contact with the skin
EXCLUDES2 *dermatitis due to ingested food (L27.2)*
L23.7 **Allergic contact dermatitis** due to plants, except food
EXCLUDES2 *allergy NOS due to pollen (J30.1)*
L23.8 **Allergic contact dermatitis** due to other agents
L23.81 **Allergic contact dermatitis** due to animal (cat) (dog) dander
Allergic contact dermatitis due to animal (cat) (dog) hair
L23.89 **Allergic contact dermatitis** due to other agents
L23.9 **Allergic contact dermatitis, unspecified cause**
Allergic contact eczema NOS

L24 **Irritant contact dermatitis**
EXCLUDES1 *allergy NOS (T78.40)*
contact dermatitis NOS (L25.9)
dermatitis NOS (L30.9)
EXCLUDES2 *allergic contact dermatitis (L23.-)*
dermatitis due to substances taken internally (L27.-)
dermatitis of eyelid (H01.1-)
diaper dermatitis (L22)
eczema of external ear (H60.5-)
perioral dermatitis (L71.0)
radiation-related disorders of the skin and subcutaneous tissue (L55-L59)
L24.0 **Irritant contact dermatitis** due to detergents
L24.1 **Irritant contact dermatitis** due to oils and greases
L24.2 **Irritant contact dermatitis** due to solvents
Irritant contact dermatitis due to chlorocompound
Irritant contact dermatitis due to cyclohexane
Irritant contact dermatitis due to ester

Unspecified Code | Other Specified Code | Manifestation Code | N Newborn | P Pediatric | M Maternity | A Adult | ♂ Male | ♀ Female
● New Code ▲ Revised Code Title ▶◀ Revised Text NOTES INCLUDES EXCLUDES1 Not coded here EXCLUDES2 Not included here
4th character required | 5th character required | 6th character required | 7th character required
Extension 'X' Alert | HAC Hospital-acquired condition (HAC) alert | AHA AHA Coding Clinic©

Irritant contact dermatitis due to glycol
Irritant contact dermatitis due to hydrocarbon
Irritant contact dermatitis due to ketone

L24.3 **Irritant contact dermatitis** due to cosmetics

L24.4 **Irritant contact dermatitis** due to drugs in contact with skin
Use additional code for adverse effect, if applicable, to identify drug (T36-T50 with fifth or sixth character 5)

L24.5 **Irritant contact dermatitis** due to other chemical products
Irritant contact dermatitis due to cement
Irritant contact dermatitis due to insecticide
Irritant contact dermatitis due to plastic
Irritant contact dermatitis due to rubber

L24.6 **Irritant contact dermatitis** due to food in contact with skin
EXCLUDES2 *dermatitis due to ingested food (L27.2)*

L24.7 **Irritant contact dermatitis** due to plants, except food
EXCLUDES2 *allergy NOS to pollen (J30.1)*

5th L24.8 **Irritant contact dermatitis** due to other agents

L24.81 **Irritant contact dermatitis** due to metals
Irritant contact dermatitis due to chromium
Irritant contact dermatitis due to nickel

L24.89 **Irritant contact dermatitis due to other agents**
Irritant contact dermatitis due to dyes

L24.9 **Irritant contact dermatitis, unspecified cause**
Irritant contact eczema NOS

4th L25 **Unspecified contact dermatitis**
EXCLUDES1 *allergic contact dermatitis (L23.-)*
allergy NOS (T78.40)
dermatitis NOS (L30.9)
irritant contact dermatitis (L24.-)
EXCLUDES2 *dermatitis due to ingested substances (L27.-)*
dermatitis of eyelid (H01.1-)
eczema of external ear (H60.5-)
perioral dermatitis (L71.0)
radiation-related disorders of the skin and subcutaneous tissue (L55-L59)

L25.0 **Unspecified contact dermatitis** due to cosmetics

L25.1 **Unspecified contact dermatitis** due to drugs in contact with skin
Use additional code for adverse effect, if applicable, to identify drug (T36-T50 with fifth or sixth character 5)
EXCLUDES2 *dermatitis due to ingested drugs and medicaments (L27.0-L27.1)*

L25.2 **Unspecified contact dermatitis** due to dyes

L25.3 **Unspecified contact dermatitis** due to other chemical products
Unspecified contact dermatitis due to cement
Unspecified contact dermatitis due to insecticide

L25.4 **Unspecified contact dermatitis** due to food in contact with skin
EXCLUDES2 *dermatitis due to ingested food (L27.2)*

L25.5 **Unspecified contact dermatitis** due to plants, except food
EXCLUDES1 *nettle rash (L50.9)*
EXCLUDES2 *allergy NOS due to pollen (J30.1)*

L25.8 **Unspecified contact dermatitis** due to other agents

L25.9 **Unspecified contact dermatitis, unspecified cause**
Contact dermatitis (occupational) NOS
Contact eczema (occupational) NOS

L26 **Exfoliative dermatitis**
Hebra's pityriasis
EXCLUDES1 *Ritter's disease (L00)*

4th L27 **Dermatitis due to** substances taken internally
EXCLUDES1 *allergy NOS (T78.40)*
EXCLUDES2 *adverse food reaction, except dermatitis (T78.0-T78.1)*
contact dermatitis (L23-L25)
drug photoallergic response (L56.1)
drug phototoxic response (L56.0)
urticaria (L50.-)

L27.0 Generalized skin eruption **due to drugs and medicaments taken internally**
Use additional code for adverse effect, if applicable, to identify drug (T36-T50 with fifth or sixth character 5)

L27.1 Localized skin eruption **due to drugs and medicaments taken internally**
Use additional code for adverse effect, if applicable, to identify drug (T36-T50 with fifth or sixth character 5)

L27.2 Dermatitis **due to ingested food**
EXCLUDES2 *dermatitis due to food in contact with skin (L23.6, L24.6, L25.4)*

L27.8 **Dermatitis due to other substances taken internally**

L27.9 **Dermatitis due to unspecified substance taken internally**

4th L28 **Lichen simplex chronicus and prurigo**

L28.0 Lichen simplex chronicus
Circumscribed neurodermatitis
Lichen NOS

L28.1 Prurigo nodularis

L28.2 **Other prurigo**
Prurigo NOS
Prurigo Hebra
Prurigo mitis
Urticaria papulosa

4th L29 **Pruritus**
EXCLUDES1 *neurotic excoriation (L98.1)*
psychogenic pruritus (F45.8)

L29.0 **Pruritus** ani

L29.1 **Pruritus** scroti ♂

L29.2 **Pruritus** vulvae ♀

L29.3 Anogenital **pruritus, unspecified**

L29.8 **Other pruritus**

L29.9 **Pruritus, unspecified**
Itch NOS

4th L30 Other and unspecified **dermatitis**
EXCLUDES2 *contact dermatitis (L23-L25)*
dry skin dermatitis (L85.3)
small plaque parapsoriasis (L41.3)
stasis dermatitis ►(I87.2)◄

L30.0 Nummular **dermatitis**

L30.1 Dyshidrosis [pompholyx]

L30.2 Cutaneous autosensitization
Candidid [levurid]
Dermatophytid
Eczematoid

L30.3 Infective **dermatitis**
Infectious eczematoid dermatitis

L30.4 Erythema intertrigo

L30.5 Pityriasis alba

L30.8 **Other specified dermatitis**

L30.9 **Dermatitis, unspecified**
Eczema NOS

Papulosquamous disorders (L40-L45)

4th L40 **Psoriasis**

L40.0 **Psoriasis** vulgaris
Nummular psoriasis
Plaque psoriasis

L40.1 Generalized pustular **psoriasis**
Impetigo herpetiformis
Von Zumbusch's disease

L40.2 Acrodermatitis continua

L40.3 Pustulosis palmaris et plantaris

L40.4 Guttate **psoriasis**

5th L40.5 Arthropathic **psoriasis**

L40.50 **Arthropathic psoriasis, unspecified**

L40.51 Distal interphalangeal **psoriatic arthropathy**

L40.52 **Psoriatic arthritis** mutilans

L40.53 **Psoriatic** spondylitis

L40.54 **Psoriatic** juvenile **arthropathy**

L40.59 **Other psoriatic arthropathy**

L40.8 **Other psoriasis**
Flexural psoriasis

L40.9 **Psoriasis, unspecified**

4th L41 **Parapsoriasis**
EXCLUDES1 *poikiloderma vasculare atrophicans (L94.5)*

L41.0 Pityriasis lichenoides et varioliformis acuta
Mucha-Habermann disease

PDx Unacceptable principal diagnosis symbol per Medicare code edits POA Code exempt from diagnosis present on admission requirement
? Questionable admission CC Complication or comorbidity CC/MCC Exc CC/MCC exclusion MCC Major complication or comorbidity
PDx CC Principal diagnosis as its own CC PDx MCC Principal diagnosis as its own MCC Z Z code as first-listed diagnosis

When symbols appear on a code that requires a 7th character extension, refer to Appendix D to identify applicable 7th character codes.

L41.1 Pityriasis lichenoides chronica
L41.3 Small plaque parapsoriasis
L41.4 Large plaque parapsoriasis
L41.5 Retiform parapsoriasis
L41.8 Other parapsoriasis
L41.9 Parapsoriasis, unspecified

L42 Pityriasis rosea

L43 Lichen planus

EXCLUDES1 *lichen planopilaris (L66.1)*

L43.0 Hypertrophic lichen planus
L43.1 Bullous lichen planus
L43.2 Lichenoid drug reaction
Use additional code for adverse effect, if applicable, to identify drug (T36-T50 with fifth or sixth character 5)
L43.3 Subacute (active) lichen planus
Lichen planus tropicus
L43.8 Other lichen planus
L43.9 Lichen planus, unspecified

L44 Other papulosquamous disorders

L44.0 Pityriasis rubra pilaris
L44.1 Lichen nitidus
L44.2 Lichen striatus
L44.3 Lichen ruber moniliformis
L44.4 Infantile papular acrodermatitis [Gianotti-Crosti] P
L44.8 Other specified papulosquamous disorders
L44.9 Papulosquamous disorder, unspecified

L45 Papulosquamous disorders in diseases classified elsewhere
Code first underlying disease.

Urticaria and erythema (L49-L54)

EXCLUDES1 *Lyme disease (A69.2-)*
rosacea (L71.-)

L49 Exfoliation due to erythematous conditions according to extent of body surface involved
Code first erythematous condition causing exfoliation, such as:
Ritter's disease (L00)
(Staphylococcal) scalded skin syndrome (L00)
Stevens-Johnson syndromee (L51.1)
Stevens-Johnson syndromee-toxic epidermal necrolysis overlap syndromee (L51.3)
Toxic epidermal necrolysis (L51.2)

L49.0 Exfoliation due to erythematous condition involving less than 10 percent of body surface PDx
Exfoliation due to erythematous condition NOS
L49.1 Exfoliation due to erythematous condition involving 10-19 percent of body surface PDx
L49.2 Exfoliation due to erythematous condition involving 20-29 percent of body surface PDx
L49.3 Exfoliation due to erythematous condition involving 30-39 percent of body surface CC PDx
L49.4 Exfoliation due to erythematous condition involving 40-49 percent of body surface CC PDx
L49.5 Exfoliation due to erythematous condition involving 50-59 percent of body surface CC PDx
L49.6 Exfoliation due to erythematous condition involving 60-69 percent of body surface CC PDx
L49.7 Exfoliation due to erythematous condition involving 70-79 percent of body surface CC PDx
L49.8 Exfoliation due to erythematous condition involving 80-89 percent of body surface CC PDx
L49.9 Exfoliation due to erythematous condition involving 90 or more percent of body surface CC PDx

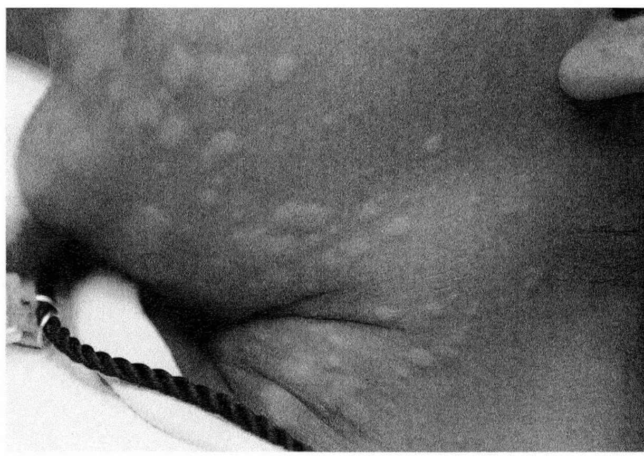

Figure 12.1 Urticaria

L50 Urticaria

EXCLUDES1 *allergic contact dermatitis (L23.-)*
angioneurotic edema (T78.3)
giant urticaria (T78.3)
hereditary angio-edema (D84.1)
Quincke's edema (T78.3)
serum urticaria (T80.6-)
solar urticaria (L56.3)
urticaria neonatorum (P83.8)
urticaria papulosa (L28.2)
urticaria pigmentosa (Q82.2)

L50.0 Allergic urticaria
L50.1 Idiopathic urticaria
L50.2 Urticaria due to cold and heat
EXCLUDES2 *familial cold urticaria (M04.2)*
L50.3 Dermatographic urticaria
L50.4 Vibratory urticaria
L50.5 Cholinergic urticaria
L50.6 Contact urticaria
L50.8 Other urticaria
Chronic urticaria
Recurrent periodic urticaria
L50.9 Urticaria, unspecified

L51 Erythema multiforme
Use additional code for adverse effect, if applicable, to identify drug (T36-T50 with fifth or sixth character 5)
Use additional code to identify associated manifestations, such as:
arthropathy associated with dermatological disorders (M14.8-)
conjunctival edema (H11.42)
conjunctivitis (H10.22-)
corneal scars and opacities (H17.-)
corneal ulcer (H16.0-)
edema of eyelid (H02.84)
inflammation of eyelid (H01.8)
keratoconjunctivitis sicca (H16.22-)
mechanical lagophthalmos (H02.22-)
stomatitis (K12.-)
symblepharon (H11.23-)
Use additional code to identify percentage of skin exfoliation (L49.-)

EXCLUDES1 *staphylococcal scalded skin syndromee (L00)*
Ritter's disease (L00)

L51.0 Nonbullous erythema multiforme
L51.1 Stevens-Johnson syndromee CC
L51.2 Toxic epidermal necrolysis [Lyell] CC
L51.3 Stevens-Johnson syndromee-toxic epidermal necrolysis overlap syndromee CC
SJS-TEN overlap syndromee
L51.8 Other erythema multiforme
L51.9 Erythema multiforme, unspecified
Erythema iris
Erythema multiforme major NOS
Erythema multiforme minor NOS
Herpes iris

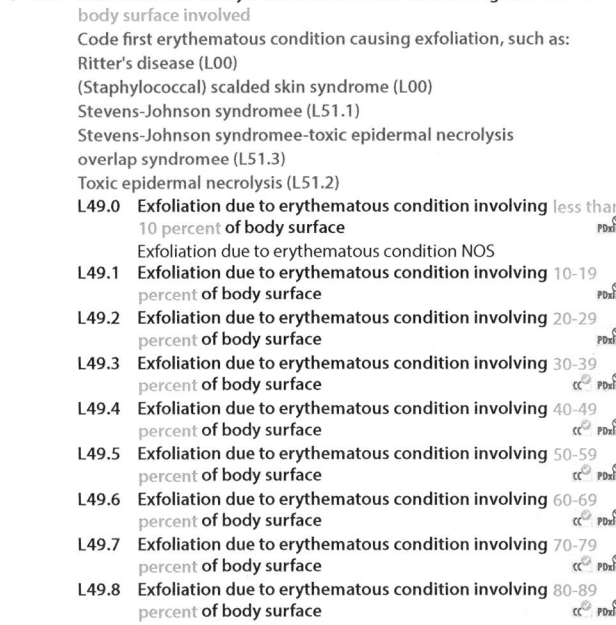

Unspecified Code | Other Specified Code | Manifestation Code | N Newborn | P Pediatric | M Maternity | A Adult | ♂ Male | ♀ Female
● New Code | ▲ Revised Code Title | ►◄ Revised Text | NOTES | INCLUDES | EXCLUDES1 Not coded here | EXCLUDES2 Not included here
4th character required | 5th character required | 6th character required | 7th character required
Extension 'X' Alert | HAC Hospital-acquired condition (HAC) alert | AHA AHA Coding Clinic©

L52 Erythema nodosum
EXCLUDES1 *tuberculous erythema nodosum (A18.4)*

L53 Other erythematous conditions
EXCLUDES1 *erythema ab igne (L59.0)*
erythema due to external agents in contact with skin (L23-L25)
erythema intertrigo (L30.4)

L53.0 Toxic erythema
Code first poisoning due to drug or toxin, if applicable (T36-T65 with fifth or sixth character 1-4 or 6)
Use additional code for adverse effect, if applicable, to identify drug (T36-T50 with fifth or sixth character 5)
EXCLUDES1 *neonatal erythema toxicum (P83.1)*

L53.1 Erythema annulare centrifugum
L53.2 Erythema marginatum
L53.3 Other chronic figurate erythema
L53.8 Other specified erythematous conditions
L53.9 Erythematous condition, unspecified
Erythema NOS
Erythroderma NOS

L54 Erythema in diseases classified elsewhere
Code first underlying disease.

Radiation-related disorders of the skin and subcutaneous tissue (L55-L59)

L55 Sunburn
L55.0 Sunburn of first degree
L55.1 Sunburn of second degree
L55.2 Sunburn of third degree
L55.9 Sunburn, unspecified

L56 Other acute skin changes due to ultraviolet radiation
Use additional code to identify the source of the ultraviolet radiation (W89, X32)
L56.0 Drug phototoxic response
Use additional code for adverse effect, if applicable, to identify drug (T36-T50 with fifth or sixth character 5)
L56.1 Drug photoallergic response
Use additional code for adverse effect, if applicable, to identify drug (T36-T50 with fifth or sixth character 5)
L56.2 Photocontact dermatitis [berloque dermatitis]
L56.3 Solar urticaria
L56.4 Polymorphous light eruption
L56.5 Disseminated superficial actinic porokeratosis (DSAP)
L56.8 Other specified acute skin changes due to ultraviolet radiation
L56.9 Acute skin change due to ultraviolet radiation, unspecified

L57 Skin changes due to chronic exposure to nonionizing radiation
Use additional code to identify the source of the ultraviolet radiation (W89, X32)
L57.0 Actinic keratosis
Keratosis NOS
Senile keratosis
Solar keratosis
L57.1 Actinic reticuloid
L57.2 Cutis rhomboidalis nuchae
L57.3 Poikiloderma of Civatte
L57.4 Cutis laxa senilis
Elastosis senilis
L57.5 Actinic granuloma
L57.8 Other skin changes due to chronic exposure to nonionizing radiation
Farmer's skin
Sailor's skin
Solar dermatitis
L57.9 Skin changes due to chronic exposure to nonionizing radiation, unspecified

L58 Radiodermatitis
Use additional code to identify the source of the radiation (W88, W90)
L58.0 Acute radiodermatitis
L58.1 Chronic radiodermatitis
L58.9 Radiodermatitis, unspecified

L59 Other disorders of skin and subcutaneous tissue related to radiation
L59.0 Erythema ab igne [dermatitis ab igne]
L59.8 Other specified disorders of the skin and subcutaneous tissue related to radiation
L59.9 Disorder of the skin and subcutaneous tissue related to radiation, unspecified

Disorders of skin appendages (L60-L75)

EXCLUDES1 *congenital malformations of integument (Q84.-)*

L60 Nail disorders
EXCLUDES2 *clubbing of nails (R68.3)*
onychia and paronychia (L03.0-)
L60.0 Ingrowing nail
L60.1 Onycholysis
L60.2 Onychogryphosis
L60.3 Nail dystrophy
L60.4 Beau's lines
L60.5 Yellow nail syndromee
L60.8 Other nail disorders
L60.9 Nail disorder, unspecified

L62 Nail disorders in diseases classified elsewhere
Code first underlying disease, such as:
pachydermoperiostosis (M89.4-)

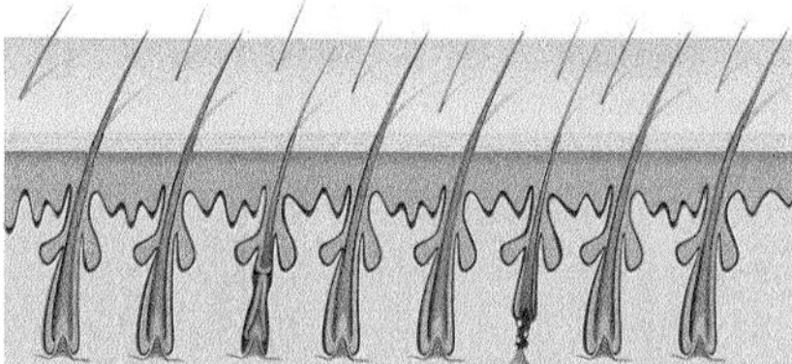
Healthy

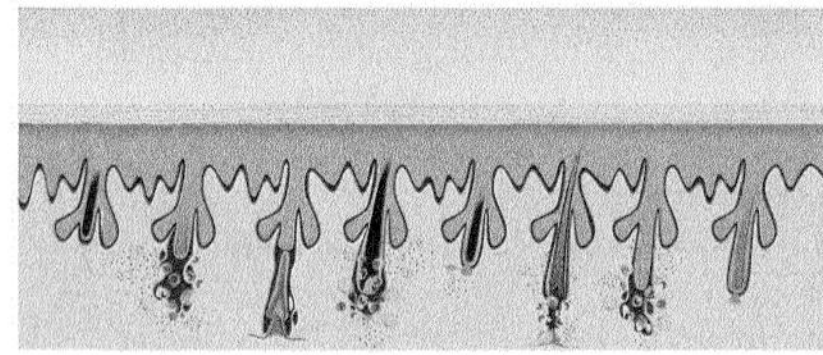
Unhealthy hair roots and follicles

Figure 12.2 Alopecia areata

L63 Alopecia areata
L63.0 Alopecia (capitis) totalis
L63.1 Alopecia universalis
L63.2 Ophiasis
L63.8 Other alopecia areata
L63.9 Alopecia areata, unspecified

L64 Androgenic alopecia
INCLUDES *male-pattern baldness*
L64.0 Drug-induced androgenic alopecia
Use additional code for adverse effect, if applicable, to identify drug (T36-T50 with fifth or sixth character 5)
L64.8 Other androgenic alopecia
L64.9 Androgenic alopecia, unspecified

L65 Other nonscarring hair loss
Use additional code for adverse effect, if applicable, to identify drug (T36-T50 with fifth or sixth character 5)
EXCLUDES1 *trichotillomania (F63.3)*
L65.0 Telogen effluvium
L65.1 Anagen effluvium
L65.2 Alopecia mucinosa
L65.8 Other specified nonscarring hair loss
L65.9 Nonscarring hair loss, unspecified
Alopecia NOS

L66 Cicatricial alopecia [scarring hair loss]
L66.0 Pseudopelade
L66.1 Lichen planopilaris
Follicular lichen planus
L66.2 Folliculitis decalvans

Unacceptable principal diagnosis symbol per Medicare code edits · Code exempt from diagnosis present on admission requirement · Questionable admission · Complication or comorbidity · CC/MCC exclusion · Major complication or comorbidity · Principal diagnosis as its own CC · Principal diagnosis as its own MCC · Z code as first-listed diagnosis

L66.3 Perifolliculitis capitis abscedens
L66.4 Folliculitis ulerythematosa reticulata
L66.8 Other cicatricial alopecia
L66.9 Cicatricial alopecia, unspecified

L67 Hair color and hair shaft abnormalities
EXCLUDES1 *monilethrix (Q84.1)*
pili annulati (Q84.1)
telogen effluvium (L65.0)
L67.0 Trichorrhexis nodosa
L67.1 Variations in hair color
Canities
Greyness, hair (premature)
Heterochromia of hair
Poliosis circumscripta, acquired
Poliosis NOS
L67.8 Other hair color and hair shaft abnormalities
Fragilitas crinium
L67.9 Hair color and hair shaft abnormality, unspecified

L68 Hypertrichosis
INCLUDES *excess hair*
EXCLUDES1 *congenital hypertrichosis (Q84.2)*
persistent lanugo (Q84.2)
L68.0 Hirsutism
L68.1 Acquired hypertrichosis lanuginosa
L68.2 Localized hypertrichosis
L68.3 Polytrichia
L68.8 Other hypertrichosis
L68.9 Hypertrichosis, unspecified

L70 Acne
EXCLUDES2 *acne keloid (L73.0)*
L70.0 Acne vulgaris
L70.1 Acne conglobata
L70.2 Acne varioliformis
Acne necrotica miliaris
L70.3 Acne tropica
L70.4 Infantile acne P
▲ L70.5 Acné ▶excoriée◀
Acné excoriée des jeunes filles
Picker's acne
L70.8 Other acne
L70.9 Acne, unspecified

L71 Rosacea
Use additional code for adverse effect, if applicable, to identify drug (T36-T50 with fifth or sixth character 5)
L71.0 Perioral dermatitis
L71.1 Rhinophyma
L71.8 Other rosacea
L71.9 Rosacea, unspecified

L72 Follicular cysts of skin and subcutaneous tissue
L72.0 Epidermal cyst
L72.1 Pilar and trichodermal cyst
L72.11 Pilar cyst
L72.12 Trichodermal cyst
Trichilemmal (proliferating) cyst
L72.2 Steatocystoma multiplex
L72.3 Sebaceous cyst
EXCLUDES2 *pilar cyst (L72.11)*
trichilemmal (proliferating) cyst (L72.12)
L72.8 Other follicular cysts of the skin and subcutaneous tissue
L72.9 Follicular cyst of the skin and subcutaneous tissue, unspecified

L73 Other follicular disorders
L73.0 Acne keloid
L73.1 Pseudofolliculitis barbae
L73.2 Hidradenitis suppurativa
L73.8 Other specified follicular disorders
Sycosis barbae
L73.9 Follicular disorder, unspecified

L74 Eccrine sweat disorders
EXCLUDES2 *generalized hyperhidrosis (R61)*
L74.0 Miliaria rubra
L74.1 Miliaria crystallina
L74.2 Miliaria profunda
Miliaria tropicalis
L74.3 Miliaria, unspecified
L74.4 Anhidrosis
Hypohidrosis
L74.5 Focal hyperhidrosis
L74.51 Primary focal hyperhidrosis
L74.510 Primary focal hyperhidrosis, axilla
L74.511 Primary focal hyperhidrosis, face
L74.512 Primary focal hyperhidrosis, palms
L74.513 Primary focal hyperhidrosis, soles
L74.519 Primary focal hyperhidrosis, unspecified
L74.52 Secondary focal hyperhidrosis
Frey's syndromee
L74.8 Other eccrine sweat disorders
L74.9 Eccrine sweat disorder, unspecified
Sweat gland disorder NOS

L75 Apocrine sweat disorders
EXCLUDES1 *dyshidrosis (L30.1)*
hidradenitis suppurativa (L73.2)
L75.0 Bromhidrosis
L75.1 Chromhidrosis
L75.2 Apocrine miliaria
Fox-Fordyce disease
L75.8 Other apocrine sweat disorders
L75.9 Apocrine sweat disorder, unspecified

Intraoperative and postprocedural complications of skin and subcutaneous tissue (L76)

L76 Intraoperative and postprocedural complications of skin and subcutaneous tissue
L76.0 Intraoperative hemorrhage and hematoma of skin and subcutaneous tissue complicating a procedure
EXCLUDES1 *intraoperative hemorrhage and hematoma of skin and subcutaneous tissue due to accidental puncture and laceration during a procedure (L76.1-)*
L76.01 Intraoperative hemorrhage and hematoma of skin and subcutaneous tissue complicating a dermatologic procedure CC
L76.02 Intraoperative hemorrhage and hematoma of skin and subcutaneous tissue complicating other procedure CC
L76.1 Accidental puncture and laceration of skin and subcutaneous tissue during a procedure
L76.11 Accidental puncture and laceration of skin and subcutaneous tissue during a dermatologic procedure CC
L76.12 Accidental puncture and laceration of skin and subcutaneous tissue during other procedure CC
▲ L76.2 Postprocedural ▶hemorrhage of◀ skin and subcutaneous tissue following a procedure
▲ L76.21 Postprocedural ▶hemorrhage of◀ skin and subcutaneous tissue following a dermatologic procedure CC
▲ L76.22 Postprocedural ▶hemorrhage of◀ skin and subcutaneous tissue following other procedure CC
● L76.3 Postprocedural hematoma and seroma of skin and subcutaneous tissue following a procedure
● L76.31 Postprocedural hematoma of skin and subcutaneous tissue following a dermatologic procedure CC CC/MCC Exc
● L76.32 Postprocedural hematoma of skin and subcutaneous tissue following other procedure CC CC/MCC Exc
● L76.33 Postprocedural seroma of skin and subcutaneous tissue following a dermatologic procedure
● L76.34 Postprocedural seroma of skin and subcutaneous tissue following other procedure
L76.8 Other intraoperative and postprocedural complications of skin and subcutaneous tissue
Use additional code, if applicable, to further specify disorder
L76.81 Other intraoperative complications of skin and subcutaneous tissue
L76.82 Other postprocedural complications of skin and subcutaneous tissue

Unspecified Code · Other Specified Code · Manifestation Code · N Newborn · P Pediatric · M Maternity · A Adult · ♂ Male · ♀ Female
● New Code · ▲ Revised Code Title · ▶◀ Revised Text · NOTES · INCLUDES · EXCLUDES1 Not coded here · EXCLUDES2 Not included here
4th character required · 5th character required · 6th character required · 7th character required
Extension 'X' Alert · HAC Hospital-acquired condition (HAC) alert · AHA AHA Coding Clinic©

Other disorders of the skin and subcutaneous tissue (L80-L99)

L80 Vitiligo
EXCLUDES2 *vitiligo of eyelids (H02.73-)*
vitiligo of vulva (N90.89)

L81 Other disorders of pigmentation
EXCLUDES1 *birthmark NOS (Q82.5)*
Peutz-Jeghers syndromee (Q85.8)
EXCLUDES2 *nevus - see Alphabetical Index*
L81.0 Postinflammatory hyperpigmentation
L81.1 Chloasma
L81.2 Freckles
L81.3 Café au lait spots
L81.4 Other melanin hyperpigmentation
Lentigo
L81.5 Leukoderma, not elsewhere classified
L81.6 Other disorders of diminished melanin formation
L81.7 Pigmented purpuric dermatosis
Angioma serpiginosum
L81.8 Other specified disorders of pigmentation
Iron pigmentation
Tattoo pigmentation
L81.9 Disorder of pigmentation, unspecified

L82 Seborrheic keratosis
INCLUDES *basal cell papilloma*
dermatosis papulosa nigra
Leser-Trélat disease
EXCLUDES2 *seborrheic dermatitis (L21.-)*
L82.0 Inflamed seborrheic keratosis
L82.1 Other seborrheic keratosis
Seborrheic keratosis NOS

L83 Acanthosis nigricans
Confluent and reticulated papillomatosis

L84 Corns and callosities
Callus
Clavus

L85 Other epidermal thickening
EXCLUDES2 *hypertrophic disorders of the skin (L91.-)*
L85.0 Acquired ichthyosis
EXCLUDES1 *congenital ichthyosis (Q80.-)*
L85.1 Acquired keratosis [keratoderma] palmaris et plantaris
EXCLUDES1 *inherited keratosis palmaris et plantaris (Q82.8)*
L85.2 Keratosis punctata (palmaris et plantaris)
L85.3 Xerosis cutis
Dry skin dermatitis
L85.8 Other specified epidermal thickening
Cutaneous horn
L85.9 Epidermal thickening, unspecified

L86 Keratoderma in diseases classified elsewhere
Code first underlying disease, such as:
Reiter's disease (M02.3-)
EXCLUDES1 *gonococcal keratoderma (A54.89)*
gonococcal keratosis (A54.89)
keratoderma due to vitamin A deficiency (E50.8)
keratosis due to vitamin A deficiency (E50.8)
xeroderma due to vitamin A deficiency (E50.8)

L87 Transepidermal elimination disorders
EXCLUDES1 *granuloma annulare (perforating) (L92.0)*
L87.0 Keratosis follicularis et parafollicularis in cutem penetrans
Kyrle disease
Hyperkeratosis follicularis penetrans
L87.1 Reactive perforating collagenosis
L87.2 Elastosis perforans serpiginosa
L87.8 Other transepidermal elimination disorders
L87.9 Transepidermal elimination disorder, unspecified

L88 Pyoderma gangrenosum CC
Phagedenic pyoderma
EXCLUDES1 *dermatitis gangrenosa (L08.0)*

L89 Pressure ulcer
INCLUDES *bed sore*
decubitus ulcer
plaster ulcer
pressure area
pressure sore
Code first any associated gangrene (I96)
EXCLUDES2 *decubitus (trophic) ulcer of cervix (uteri) (N86)*
diabetic ulcers (E08.621, E08.622, E09.621, E09.622, E10.621, E10.622, E11.621, E11.622, E13.621, E13.622)
non-pressure chronic ulcer of skin (L97.-)
skin infections (L00-L08)
varicose ulcer (I83.0, I83.2)

L89.0 Pressure ulcer of elbow
L89.00 Pressure ulcer of unspecified elbow
L89.000 Pressure ulcer of unspecified elbow, unstageable
L89.001 Pressure ulcer of unspecified elbow, stage 1
Healing pressure ulcer of unspecified elbow, stage 1
Pressure pre-ulcer skin changes limited to persistent focal edema, unspecified elbow
L89.002 Pressure ulcer of unspecified elbow, stage 2
Healing pressure ulcer of unspecified elbow, stage 2
Pressure ulcer with abrasion, blister, partial thickness skin loss involving epidermis and/or dermis, unspecified elbow
L89.003 Pressure ulcer of unspecified elbow, stage 3 HAC MCC PDx
Healing pressure ulcer of unspecified elbow, stage 3
Pressure ulcer with full thickness skin loss involving damage or necrosis of subcutaneous tissue, unspecified elbow
L89.004 Pressure ulcer of unspecified elbow, stage 4 HAC MCC PDx
Healing pressure ulcer of unspecified elbow, stage 4
Pressure ulcer with necrosis of soft tissues through to underlying muscle, tendon, or bone, unspecified elbow
L89.009 Pressure ulcer of unspecified elbow, unspecified stage
Healing pressure ulcer of elbow NOS
Healing pressure ulcer of unspecified elbow, unspecified stage
L89.01 Pressure ulcer of right elbow
L89.010 Pressure ulcer of right elbow, unstageable
L89.011 Pressure ulcer of right elbow, stage 1
Healing pressure ulcer of right elbow, stage 1
Pressure pre-ulcer skin changes limited to persistent focal edema, right elbow
L89.012 Pressure ulcer of right elbow, stage 2
Healing pressure ulcer of right elbow, stage 2
Pressure ulcer with abrasion, blister, partial thickness skin loss involving epidermis and/or dermis, right elbow
L89.013 Pressure ulcer of right elbow, stage 3 HAC MCC PDx
Healing pressure ulcer of right elbow, stage 3
Pressure ulcer with full thickness skin loss involving damage or necrosis of subcutaneous tissue, right elbow
L89.014 Pressure ulcer of right elbow, stage 4 HAC MCC PDx
Healing pressure ulcer of right elbow, stage 4
Pressure ulcer with necrosis of soft tissues through to underlying muscle, tendon, or bone, right elbow
L89.019 Pressure ulcer of right elbow, unspecified stage
Healing pressure right of elbow NOS
Healing pressure ulcer of unspecified elbow, unspecified stage
L89.02 Pressure ulcer of left elbow
L89.020 Pressure ulcer of left elbow, unstageable

PDx Unacceptable principal diagnosis symbol per Medicare code edits · POA Code exempt from diagnosis present on admission requirement · ? Questionable admission · CC Complication or comorbidity · CC/MCC Exc CC/MCC exclusion · MCC Major complication or comorbidity · PDx CC Principal diagnosis as its own CC · PDx MCC Principal diagnosis as its own MCC · Z Z code as first-listed diagnosis

L89.021 Pressure ulcer of left elbow, stage 1
Healing pressure ulcer of left elbow, stage 1
Pressure pre-ulcer skin changes limited to persistent focal edema, left elbow

L89.022 Pressure ulcer of left elbow, stage 2
Healing pressure ulcer of left elbow, stage 2
Pressure ulcer with abrasion, blister, partial thickness skin loss involving epidermis and/or dermis, left elbow

L89.023 Pressure ulcer of left elbow, stage 3 HAC MCC PDx MCC
Healing pressure ulcer of left elbow, stage 3
Pressure ulcer with full thickness skin loss involving damage or necrosis of subcutaneous tissue, left elbow

L89.024 Pressure ulcer of left elbow, stage 4 HAC MCC PDx MCC
Healing pressure ulcer of left elbow, stage 4
Pressure ulcer with necrosis of soft tissues through to underlying muscle, tendon, or bone, left elbow

L89.029 Pressure ulcer of left **elbow,** unspecified stage
Healing pressure ulcer of left of elbow NOS
Healing pressure ulcer of unspecified elbow, unspecified stage

5th **L89.1 Pressure ulcer of** back

6th **L89.10 Pressure ulcer of** unspecified part **of back**

L89.100 Pressure ulcer of unspecified part of back, unstageable

L89.101 Pressure ulcer of unspecified part of back, stage 1
Healing pressure ulcer of unspecified part of back, stage 1
Pressure pre-ulcer skin changes limited to persistent focal edema, unspecified part of back

L89.102 Pressure ulcer of unspecified part of back, stage 2
Healing pressure ulcer of unspecified part of back, stage 2
Pressure ulcer with abrasion, blister, partial thickness skin loss involving epidermis and/or dermis, unspecified part of back

L89.103 Pressure ulcer of unspecified part of back, stage 3 HAC MCC PDx MCC
Healing pressure ulcer of unspecified part of back, stage 3
Pressure ulcer with full thickness skin loss involving damage or necrosis of subcutaneous tissue, unspecified part of back

L89.104 Pressure ulcer of unspecified part of back, stage 4 HAC MCC PDx MCC
Healing pressure ulcer of unspecified part of back, stage 4
Pressure ulcer with necrosis of soft tissues through to underlying muscle, tendon, or bone, unspecified part of back

L89.109 Pressure ulcer of unspecified part of back, unspecified stage
Healing pressure ulcer of unspecified part of back NOS
Healing pressure ulcer of unspecified part of back, unspecified stage

6th **L89.11 Pressure ulcer of** right upper back
Pressure ulcer of right shoulder blade

L89.110 Pressure ulcer of right upper back, unstageable

L89.111 Pressure ulcer of right upper back, stage 1
Healing pressure ulcer of right upper back, stage 1
Pressure pre-ulcer skin changes limited to persistent focal edema, right upper back

L89.112 Pressure ulcer of right upper back, stage 2
Healing pressure ulcer of right upper back, stage 2
Pressure ulcer with abrasion, blister, partial thickness skin loss involving epidermis and/or dermis, right upper back

L89.113 Pressure ulcer of right upper back, stage 3 HAC MCC PDx MCC
Healing pressure ulcer of right upper back, stage 3
Pressure ulcer with full thickness skin loss involving damage or necrosis of subcutaneous tissue, right upper back

L89.114 Pressure ulcer of right upper back, stage 4 HAC MCC PDx MCC
Healing pressure ulcer of right upper back, stage 4
Pressure ulcer with necrosis of soft tissues through to underlying muscle, tendon, or bone, right upper back

L89.119 Pressure ulcer of right upper back, unspecified stage
Healing pressure ulcer of right upper back NOS
Healing pressure ulcer of right upper back, unspecified stage

6th **L89.12 Pressure ulcer of** left upper back
Pressure ulcer of left shoulder blade

L89.120 Pressure ulcer of left upper back, unstageable

L89.121 Pressure ulcer of left upper back, stage 1
Healing pressure ulcer of left upper back, stage 1
Pressure pre-ulcer skin changes limited to persistent focal edema, left upper back

L89.122 Pressure ulcer of left upper back, stage 2
Healing pressure ulcer of left upper back, stage 2
Pressure ulcer with abrasion, blister, partial thickness skin loss involving epidermis and/or dermis, left upper back

L89.123 Pressure ulcer of left upper back, stage 3 HAC MCC PDx MCC
Healing pressure ulcer of left upper back, stage 3
Pressure ulcer with full thickness skin loss involving damage or necrosis of subcutaneous tissue, left upper back

L89.124 Pressure ulcer of left upper back, stage 4 HAC MCC PDx MCC
Healing pressure ulcer of left upper back, stage 4
Pressure ulcer with necrosis of soft tissues through to underlying muscle, tendon, or bone, left upper back

L89.129 Pressure ulcer of left upper back, unspecified stage
Healing pressure ulcer of left upper back NOS
Healing pressure ulcer of left upper back, unspecified stage

6th **L89.13 Pressure ulcer of** right lower back

L89.130 Pressure ulcer of right lower back, unstageable

L89.131 Pressure ulcer of right lower back, stage 1
Healing pressure ulcer of right lower back, stage 1
Pressure pre-ulcer skin changes limited to persistent focal edema, right lower back

L89.132 Pressure ulcer of right lower back, stage 2
Healing pressure ulcer of right lower back, stage 2
Pressure ulcer with abrasion, blister, partial thickness skin loss involving epidermis and/or dermis, right lower back

L89.133 Pressure ulcer of right lower back, stage 3 HAC MCC PDx MCC
Healing pressure ulcer of right lower back, stage 3
Pressure ulcer with full thickness skin loss involving damage or necrosis of subcutaneous tissue, right lower back

Unspecified Code | Other Specified Code | Manifestation Code | N Newborn | P Pediatric | M Maternity | A Adult | ♂ Male | ♀ Female
● New Code | ▲ Revised Code Title | ►◄ Revised Text | NOTES | INCLUDES | EXCLUDES 1 Not coded here | EXCLUDES 2 Not included here
4th 4th character required | 5th 5th character required | 6th 6th character required | 7th 7th character required
Extension 'X' Alert | HAC Hospital-acquired condition (HAC) alert | AHA AHA Coding Clinic©

L89.134 **Pressure ulcer of right lower back,** stage 4 HAC MCC PDx MCC
Healing pressure ulcer of right lower back, stage 4
Pressure ulcer with necrosis of soft tissues through to underlying muscle, tendon, or bone, right lower back

L89.139 **Pressure ulcer of right lower back,** unspecified stage
Healing pressure ulcer of right lower back NOS
Healing pressure ulcer of right lower back, unspecified stage

6th L89.14 Pressure ulcer of left lower back

L89.140 **Pressure ulcer of left lower back,** unstageable

L89.141 **Pressure ulcer of left lower back,** stage 1
Healing pressure ulcer of left lower back, stage 1
Pressure pre-ulcer skin changes limited to persistent focal edema, left lower back

L89.142 **Pressure ulcer of left lower back,** stage 2
Healing pressure ulcer of left lower back, stage 2
Pressure ulcer with abrasion, blister, partial thickness skin loss involving epidermis and/or dermis, left lower back

L89.143 **Pressure ulcer of left lower back,** stage 3 HAC MCC PDx MCC
Healing pressure ulcer of left lower back, stage 3
Pressure ulcer with full thickness skin loss involving damage or necrosis of subcutaneous tissue, left lower back

L89.144 **Pressure ulcer of left lower back,** stage 4 HAC MCC PDx MCC
Healing pressure ulcer of left lower back, stage 4
Pressure ulcer with necrosis of soft tissues through to underlying muscle, tendon, or bone, left lower back

L89.149 **Pressure ulcer of left lower back,** unspecified stage
Healing pressure ulcer of left lower back NOS
Healing pressure ulcer of left lower back, unspecified stage

6th L89.15 Pressure ulcer of sacral region
Pressure ulcer of coccyx
Pressure ulcer of tailbone

L89.150 **Pressure ulcer of sacral region,** unstageable

L89.151 **Pressure ulcer of sacral region,** stage 1
Healing pressure ulcer of sacral region, stage 1
Pressure pre-ulcer skin changes limited to persistent focal edema, sacral region

L89.152 **Pressure ulcer of sacral region,** stage 2
Healing pressure ulcer of sacral region, stage 2
Pressure ulcer with abrasion, blister, partial thickness skin loss involving epidermis and/or dermis, sacral region

L89.153 **Pressure ulcer of sacral region,** stage 3 HAC MCC PDx MCC
Healing pressure ulcer of sacral region, stage 3
Pressure ulcer with full thickness skin loss involving damage or necrosis of subcutaneous tissue, sacral region

L89.154 **Pressure ulcer of sacral region,** stage 4 HAC MCC PDx MCC
Healing pressure ulcer of sacral region, stage 4
Pressure ulcer with necrosis of soft tissues through to underlying muscle, tendon, or bone, sacral region

L89.159 **Pressure ulcer of sacral region,** unspecified stage
Healing pressure ulcer of sacral region NOS
Healing pressure ulcer of sacral region, unspecified stage

5th L89.2 Pressure ulcer of hip

6th L89.20 Pressure ulcer of unspecified hip

L89.200 **Pressure ulcer of unspecified hip,** unstageable

L89.201 **Pressure ulcer of unspecified hip,** stage 1
Healing pressure ulcer of unspecified hip back, stage 1
Pressure pre-ulcer skin changes limited to persistent focal edema, unspecified hip

L89.202 **Pressure ulcer of unspecified hip,** stage 2
Healing pressure ulcer of unspecified hip, stage 2
Pressure ulcer with abrasion, blister, partial thickness skin loss involving epidermis and/or dermis, unspecified hip

L89.203 **Pressure ulcer of unspecified hip,** stage 3 HAC MCC PDx MCC
Healing pressure ulcer of unspecified hip, stage 3
Pressure ulcer with full thickness skin loss involving damage or necrosis of subcutaneous tissue, unspecified hip

L89.204 **Pressure ulcer of unspecified hip,** stage 4 HAC MCC PDx MCC
Healing pressure ulcer of unspecified hip, stage 4
Pressure ulcer with necrosis of soft tissues through to underlying muscle, tendon, or bone, unspecified hip

L89.209 **Pressure ulcer of unspecified hip,** unspecified stage
Healing pressure ulcer of unspecified hip NOS
Healing pressure ulcer of unspecified hip, unspecified stage

6th L89.21 Pressure ulcer of right hip

L89.210 **Pressure ulcer of right hip,** unstageable

L89.211 **Pressure ulcer of right hip,** stage 1
Healing pressure ulcer of right hip back, stage 1
Pressure pre-ulcer skin changes limited to persistent focal edema, right hip

L89.212 **Pressure ulcer of right hip,** stage 2
Healing pressure ulcer of right hip, stage 2
Pressure ulcer with abrasion, blister, partial thickness skin loss involving epidermis and/or dermis, right hip

L89.213 **Pressure ulcer of right hip,** stage 3 HAC MCC PDx MCC
Healing pressure ulcer of right hip, stage 3
Pressure ulcer with full thickness skin loss involving damage or necrosis of subcutaneous tissue, right hip

L89.214 **Pressure ulcer of right hip,** stage 4 HAC MCC PDx MCC
Healing pressure ulcer of right hip, stage 4
Pressure ulcer with necrosis of soft tissues through to underlying muscle, tendon, or bone, right hip

L89.219 **Pressure ulcer of right hip,** unspecified stage
Healing pressure ulcer of right hip NOS
Healing pressure ulcer of right hip, unspecified stage

6th L89.22 Pressure ulcer of left hip

L89.220 **Pressure ulcer of left hip,** unstageable

L89.221 **Pressure ulcer of left hip,** stage 1
Healing pressure ulcer of left hip back, stage 1
Pressure pre-ulcer skin changes limited to persistent focal edema, left hip

L89.222 **Pressure ulcer of left hip,** stage 2
Healing pressure ulcer of left hip, stage 2
Pressure ulcer with abrasion, blister, partial thickness skin loss involving epidermis and/or dermis, left hip

PDx Unacceptable principal diagnosis symbol per Medicare code edits · POA Code exempt from diagnosis present on admission requirement
? Questionable admission · CC Complication or comorbidity · CC/MCC Exc CC/MCC exclusion · MCC Major complication or comorbidity
PDx CC Principal diagnosis as its own CC · PDx MCC Principal diagnosis as its own MCC · Z-1 Z code as first-listed diagnosis

L89.223 **Pressure ulcer of left hip,** stage 3 HAC MCC PDx
Healing pressure ulcer of left hip, stage 3
Pressure ulcer with full thickness skin loss involving damage or necrosis of subcutaneous tissue, left hip

L89.224 **Pressure ulcer of left hip,** stage 4 HAC MCC PDx
Healing pressure ulcer of left hip, stage 4
Pressure ulcer with necrosis of soft tissues through to underlying muscle, tendon, or bone, left hip

L89.229 **Pressure ulcer of left hip,** unspecified stage
Healing pressure ulcer of left hip NOS
Healing pressure ulcer of left hip, unspecified stage

L89.3 Pressure ulcer of buttock

L89.30 Pressure ulcer of unspecified buttock

L89.300 **Pressure ulcer of unspecified buttock,** unstageable

L89.301 **Pressure ulcer of unspecified buttock,** stage 1
Healing pressure ulcer of unspecified buttock, stage 1
Pressure pre-ulcer skin changes limited to persistent focal edema, unspecified buttock

L89.302 **Pressure ulcer of unspecified buttock,** stage 2
Healing pressure ulcer of unspecified buttock, stage 2
Pressure ulcer with abrasion, blister, partial thickness skin loss involving epidermis and/or dermis, unspecified buttock

L89.303 **Pressure ulcer of unspecified buttock,** stage 3 HAC MCC PDx
Healing pressure ulcer of unspecified buttock, stage 3
Pressure ulcer with full thickness skin loss involving damage or necrosis of subcutaneous tissue, unspecified buttock

L89.304 **Pressure ulcer of unspecified buttock,** stage 4 HAC MCC PDx
Healing pressure ulcer of unspecified buttock, stage 4
Pressure ulcer with necrosis of soft tissues through to underlying muscle, tendon, or bone, unspecified buttock

L89.309 **Pressure ulcer of unspecified buttock,** unspecified stage
Healing pressure ulcer of unspecified buttock NOS
Healing pressure ulcer of unspecified buttock, unspecified stage

L89.31 Pressure ulcer of right buttock

L89.310 **Pressure ulcer of right buttock,** unstageable

L89.311 **Pressure ulcer of right buttock,** stage 1
Healing pressure ulcer of right buttock, stage 1
Pressure pre-ulcer skin changes limited to persistent focal edema, right buttock

L89.312 **Pressure ulcer of right buttock,** stage 2
Healing pressure ulcer of right buttock, stage 2
Pressure ulcer with abrasion, blister, partial thickness skin loss involving epidermis and/or dermis, right buttock

L89.313 **Pressure ulcer of right buttock,** stage 3 HAC MCC PDx
Healing pressure ulcer of right buttock, stage 3
Pressure ulcer with full thickness skin loss involving damage or necrosis of subcutaneous tissue, right buttock

L89.314 **Pressure ulcer of right buttock,** stage 4 HAC MCC PDx
Healing pressure ulcer of right buttock, stage 4
Pressure ulcer with necrosis of soft tissues through to underlying muscle, tendon, or bone, right buttock

L89.319 **Pressure ulcer of right buttock,** unspecified stage
Healing pressure ulcer of right buttock NOS
Healing pressure ulcer of right buttock, unspecified stage

L89.32 Pressure ulcer of left buttock

L89.320 **Pressure ulcer of left buttock,** unstageable

L89.321 **Pressure ulcer of left buttock,** stage 1
Healing pressure ulcer of left buttock, stage 1
Pressure pre-ulcer skin changes limited to persistent focal edema, left buttock

L89.322 **Pressure ulcer of left buttock,** stage 2
Healing pressure ulcer of left buttock, stage 2
Pressure ulcer with abrasion, blister, partial thickness skin loss involving epidermis and/or dermis, left buttock

L89.323 **Pressure ulcer of left buttock,** stage 3 HAC MCC PDx
Healing pressure ulcer of left buttock, stage 3
Pressure ulcer with full thickness skin loss involving damage or necrosis of subcutaneous tissue, left buttock

L89.324 **Pressure ulcer of left buttock,** stage 4 HAC MCC PDx
Healing pressure ulcer of left buttock, stage 4
Pressure ulcer with necrosis of soft tissues through to underlying muscle, tendon, or bone, left buttock

L89.329 **Pressure ulcer of left buttock,** unspecified stage
Healing pressure ulcer of left buttock NOS
Healing pressure ulcer of left buttock, unspecified stage

L89.4 Pressure ulcer of contiguous site of back, buttock and hip

L89.40 **Pressure ulcer of contiguous site of back, buttock and hip,** unspecified stage
Healing pressure ulcer of contiguous site of back, buttock and hip NOS
Healing pressure ulcer of contiguous site of back, buttock and hip, unspecified stage

L89.41 **Pressure ulcer of contiguous site of back, buttock and hip,** stage 1
Healing pressure ulcer of contiguous site of back, buttock and hip, stage 1
Pressure pre-ulcer skin changes limited to persistent focal edema, contiguous site of back, buttock and hip

L89.42 **Pressure ulcer of contiguous site of back, buttock and hip,** stage 2
Healing pressure ulcer of contiguous site of back, buttock and hip, stage 2
Pressure ulcer with abrasion, blister, partial thickness skin loss involving epidermis and/or dermis, contiguous site of back, buttock and hip

L89.43 **Pressure ulcer of contiguous site of back, buttock and hip,** stage 3 HAC MCC PDx
Healing pressure ulcer of contiguous site of back, buttock and hip, stage 3
Pressure ulcer with full thickness skin loss involving damage or necrosis of subcutaneous tissue, contiguous site of back, buttock and hip

L89.44 **Pressure ulcer of contiguous site of back, buttock and hip,** stage 4 HAC MCC PDx
Healing pressure ulcer of contiguous site of back, buttock and hip, stage 4
Pressure ulcer with necrosis of soft tissues through to underlying muscle, tendon, or bone, contiguous site of back, buttock and hip

L89.45 **Pressure ulcer of contiguous site of back, buttock and hip,** unstageable

L89.5 Pressure ulcer of ankle

L89.50 Pressure ulcer of unspecified ankle

Unspecified Code Other Specified Code Manifestation Code N Newborn P Pediatric M Maternity A Adult ♂ Male ♀ Female
● New Code ▲ Revised Code Title ►◄ Revised Text NOTES INCLUDES EXCLUDES 1 Not coded here EXCLUDES 2 Not included here
4th character required 5th character required 6th character required 7th character required
Extension 'X' Alert HAC Hospital-acquired condition (HAC) alert AHA AHA Coding Clinic©

L89.500 **Pressure ulcer of unspecified ankle,** unstageable

L89.501 **Pressure ulcer of unspecified ankle,** stage 1
Healing pressure ulcer of unspecified ankle, stage 1
Pressure pre-ulcer skin changes limited to persistent focal edema, unspecified ankle

L89.502 **Pressure ulcer of unspecified ankle,** stage 2
Healing pressure ulcer of unspecified ankle, stage 2
Pressure ulcer with abrasion, blister, partial thickness skin loss involving epidermis and/or dermis, unspecified ankle

L89.503 **Pressure ulcer of unspecified ankle,** stage 3 HAC MCC PDx
Healing pressure ulcer of unspecified ankle, stage 3
Pressure ulcer with full thickness skin loss involving damage or necrosis of subcutaneous tissue, unspecified ankle

L89.504 **Pressure ulcer of unspecified ankle,** stage 4 HAC MCC PDx
Healing pressure ulcer of unspecified ankle, stage 4
Pressure ulcer with necrosis of soft tissues through to underlying muscle, tendon, or bone, unspecified ankle

L89.509 **Pressure ulcer of unspecified ankle,** unspecified stage
Healing pressure ulcer of unspecified ankle NOS
Healing pressure ulcer of unspecified ankle, unspecified stage

6th L89.51 Pressure ulcer of right ankle

L89.510 **Pressure ulcer of right ankle,** unstageable

L89.511 **Pressure ulcer of right ankle,** stage 1
Healing pressure ulcer of right ankle, stage 1
Pressure pre-ulcer skin changes limited to persistent focal edema, right ankle

L89.512 **Pressure ulcer of right ankle,** stage 2
Healing pressure ulcer of right ankle, stage 2
Pressure ulcer with abrasion, blister, partial thickness skin loss involving epidermis and/or dermis, right ankle

L89.513 **Pressure ulcer of right ankle,** stage 3 HAC MCC PDx
Healing pressure ulcer of right ankle, stage 3
Pressure ulcer with full thickness skin loss involving damage or necrosis of subcutaneous tissue, right ankle

L89.514 **Pressure ulcer of right ankle,** stage 4 HAC MCC PDx
Healing pressure ulcer of right ankle, stage 4
Pressure ulcer with necrosis of soft tissues through to underlying muscle, tendon, or bone, right ankle

L89.519 **Pressure ulcer of right ankle,** unspecified stage
Healing pressure ulcer of right ankle NOS
Healing pressure ulcer of right ankle, unspecified stage

6th L89.52 Pressure ulcer of left ankle

L89.520 **Pressure ulcer of left ankle,** unstageable

L89.521 **Pressure ulcer of left ankle,** stage 1
Healing pressure ulcer of left ankle, stage 1
Pressure pre-ulcer skin changes limited to ►persistent◄ focal edema, left ankle

L89.522 **Pressure ulcer of left ankle,** stage 2
Healing pressure ulcer of left ankle, stage 2
Pressure ulcer with abrasion, blister, partial thickness skin loss involving epidermis and/or dermis, left ankle

L89.523 **Pressure ulcer of left ankle,** stage 3 HAC MCC PDx
Healing pressure ulcer of left ankle, stage 3
Pressure ulcer with full thickness skin loss involving damage or necrosis of subcutaneous tissue, left ankle

L89.524 **Pressure ulcer of left ankle,** stage 4 HAC MCC PDx
Healing pressure ulcer of left ankle, stage 4
Pressure ulcer with necrosis of soft tissues through to underlying muscle, tendon, or bone, left ankle

L89.529 **Pressure ulcer of left ankle,** unspecified stage
Healing pressure ulcer of left ankle NOS
Healing pressure ulcer of left ankle, unspecified stage

5th L89.6 Pressure ulcer of heel

6th L89.60 Pressure ulcer of unspecified heel

L89.600 **Pressure ulcer of unspecified heel,** unstageable

L89.601 **Pressure ulcer of unspecified heel,** stage 1
Healing pressure ulcer of unspecified heel, stage 1
Pressure pre-ulcer skin changes limited to persistent focal edema, unspecified heel

L89.602 **Pressure ulcer of unspecified heel,** stage 2
Healing pressure ulcer of unspecified heel, stage 2
Pressure ulcer with abrasion, blister, partial thickness skin loss involving epidermis and/or dermis, unspecified heel

L89.603 **Pressure ulcer of unspecified heel,** stage 3 HAC MCC PDx
Healing pressure ulcer of unspecified heel, stage 3
Pressure ulcer with full thickness skin loss involving damage or necrosis of subcutaneous tissue, unspecified heel

L89.604 **Pressure ulcer of unspecified heel,** stage 4 HAC MCC PDx
Healing pressure ulcer of unspecified heel, stage 4
Pressure ulcer with necrosis of soft tissues through to underlying muscle, tendon, or bone, unspecified heel

L89.609 **Pressure ulcer of unspecified heel,** unspecified stage
Healing pressure ulcer of unspecified heel NOS
Healing pressure ulcer of unspecified heel, unspecified stage

6th L89.61 Pressure ulcer of right heel

L89.610 **Pressure ulcer of right heel,** unstageable

L89.611 **Pressure ulcer of right heel,** stage 1
Healing pressure ulcer of right heel, stage 1
Pressure pre-ulcer skin changes limited to persistent focal edema, right heel

L89.612 **Pressure ulcer of right heel,** stage 2
Healing pressure ulcer of right heel, stage 2
Pressure ulcer with abrasion, blister, partial thickness skin loss involving epidermis and/or dermis, right heel

L89.613 **Pressure ulcer of right heel,** stage 3 HAC MCC PDx
Healing pressure ulcer of right heel, stage 3
Pressure ulcer with full thickness skin loss involving damage or necrosis of subcutaneous tissue, right heel

L89.614 **Pressure ulcer of right heel,** stage 4 HAC MCC PDx
Healing pressure ulcer of right heel, stage 4
Pressure ulcer with necrosis of soft tissues through to underlying muscle, tendon, or bone, right heel

L89.619 **Pressure ulcer of right heel,** unspecified stage
Healing pressure ulcer of right heel NOS
Healing pressure ulcer of unspecified heel, right stage

6th L89.62 Pressure ulcer of left heel

L89.620 **Pressure ulcer of left heel,** unstageable

L89.621 **Pressure ulcer of left heel,** stage 1
Healing pressure ulcer of left heel, stage 1
Pressure pre-ulcer skin changes limited to persistent focal edema, left heel

PDx Unacceptable principal diagnosis symbol per Medicare code edits; POA Code exempt from diagnosis present on admission requirement
? Questionable admission; CC Complication or comorbidity; CC/MCC Exc CC/MCC exclusion; MCC Major complication or comorbidity
PDx CC Principal diagnosis as its own CC; PDx MCC Principal diagnosis as its own MCC; Z1 Z code as first-listed diagnosis

When symbols appear on a code that requires a 7th character extension, refer to Appendix D to identify applicable 7th character codes.

L89.622 **Pressure ulcer of left heel,** stage 2
Healing pressure ulcer of left heel, stage 2
Pressure ulcer with abrasion, blister, partial thickness skin loss involving epidermis and/ or dermis, left heel

L89.623 **Pressure ulcer of left heel,** stage 3 HAC MCC PDx
Healing pressure ulcer of left heel, stage 3
Pressure ulcer with full thickness skin loss involving damage or necrosis of subcutaneous tissue, left heel

L89.624 **Pressure ulcer of left heel,** stage 4 HAC MCC PDx
Healing pressure ulcer of left heel, stage 4
Pressure ulcer with necrosis of soft tissues through to underlying muscle, tendon, or bone, left heel

L89.629 **Pressure ulcer of left heel,** unspecified stage
Healing pressure ulcer of left heel NOS
Healing pressure ulcer of left heel, unspecified stage

L89.8 **Pressure ulcer of** other site

L89.81 **Pressure ulcer of** head
Pressure ulcer of face

L89.810 **Pressure ulcer of head,** unstageable

L89.811 **Pressure ulcer of head,** stage 1
Healing pressure ulcer of head, stage 1
Pressure pre-ulcer skin changes limited to persistent focal edema, head

L89.812 **Pressure ulcer of head,** stage 2
Healing pressure ulcer of head, stage 2
Pressure ulcer with abrasion, blister, partial thickness skin loss involving epidermis and/ or dermis, head

L89.813 **Pressure ulcer of head,** stage 3 HAC MCC PDx
Healing pressure ulcer of head, stage 3
Pressure ulcer with full thickness skin loss involving damage or necrosis of subcutaneous tissue, head

L89.814 **Pressure ulcer of head,** stage 4 HAC MCC PDx
Healing pressure ulcer of head, stage 4
Pressure ulcer with necrosis of soft tissues through to underlying muscle, tendon, or bone, head

L89.819 **Pressure ulcer of head, unspecified stage**
Healing pressure ulcer of head NOS
Healing pressure ulcer of head, unspecified stage

L89.89 **Pressure ulcer of** other site

L89.890 **Pressure ulcer of other site,** unstageable

L89.891 **Pressure ulcer of other site,** stage 1
Healing pressure ulcer of other site, stage 1
Pressure pre-ulcer skin changes limited to persistent focal edema, other site

L89.892 **Pressure ulcer of other site,** stage 2
Healing pressure ulcer of other site, stage 2
Pressure ulcer with abrasion, blister, partial thickness skin loss involving epidermis and/ or dermis, other site

L89.893 **Pressure ulcer of other site,** stage 3 HAC MCC PDx
Healing pressure ulcer of other site, stage 3
Pressure ulcer with full thickness skin loss involving damage or necrosis of subcutaneous tissue, other site

L89.894 **Pressure ulcer of other site,** stage 4 HAC MCC PDx
Healing pressure ulcer of other site, stage 4
Pressure ulcer with necrosis of soft tissues through to underlying muscle, tendon, or bone, other site

L89.899 **Pressure ulcer of other site, unspecified stage**
Healing pressure ulcer of other site NOS
Healing pressure ulcer of other site, unspecified stage

L89.9 **Pressure ulcer of** unspecified site

L89.90 **Pressure ulcer of unspecified site,** unspecified stage
Healing pressure ulcer of unspecified site NOS
Healing pressure ulcer of unspecified site, unspecified stage

L89.91 **Pressure ulcer of unspecified site,** stage 1
Healing pressure ulcer of unspecified site, stage 1
Pressure pre-ulcer skin changes limited to persistent focal edema, unspecified site

L89.92 **Pressure ulcer of unspecified site,** stage 2
Healing pressure ulcer of unspecified site, stage 2
Pressure ulcer with abrasion, blister, partial thickness skin loss involving epidermis and/or dermis, unspecified site

L89.93 **Pressure ulcer of unspecified site,** stage 3 HAC MCC PDx
Healing pressure ulcer of unspecified site, stage 3
Pressure ulcer with full thickness skin loss involving damage or necrosis of subcutaneous tissue, unspecified site

L89.94 **Pressure ulcer of unspecified site,** stage 4 HAC MCC PDx
Healing pressure ulcer of unspecified site, stage 4
Pressure ulcer with necrosis of soft tissues through to underlying muscle, tendon, or bone, unspecified site

L89.95 **Pressure ulcer of unspecified site,** unstageable

L90 **Atrophic disorders of skin**

L90.0 **Lichen sclerosus et atrophicus**
EXCLUDES2 *lichen sclerosus of external female genital organs (N90.4)*
lichen sclerosus of external male genital organs (N48.0)

L90.1 **Anetoderma of Schweninger-Buzzi**

L90.2 **Anetoderma of Jadassohn-Pellizzari**

L90.3 **Atrophoderma of Pasini and Pierini**

L90.4 **Acrodermatitis chronica atrophicans**

L90.5 **Scar conditions and fibrosis of skin**
Adherent scar (skin)
Cicatrix
Disfigurement of skin due to scar
Fibrosis of skin NOS
Scar NOS
EXCLUDES2 *hypertrophic scar (L91.0)*
keloid scar (L91.0)
AHA: Q1, 2015

L90.6 **Striae atrophicae**

L90.8 **Other atrophic disorders of skin**

L90.9 **Atrophic disorder of skin, unspecified**

L91 **Hypertrophic disorders of skin**

L91.0 **Hypertrophic scar**
Keloid
Keloid scar
EXCLUDES2 *acne keloid (L73.0)*
scar NOS (L90.5)

L91.8 **Other hypertrophic disorders of the skin**

L91.9 **Hypertrophic disorder of the skin, unspecified**

L92 **Granulomatous disorders of skin and subcutaneous tissue**
EXCLUDES2 *actinic granuloma (L57.5)*

L92.0 **Granuloma annulare**
Perforating granuloma annulare

L92.1 **Necrobiosis lipoidica, not elsewhere classified**
EXCLUDES1 *necrobiosis lipoidica associated with diabetes mellitus (E08-E13 with .620)*

L92.2 **Granuloma faciale [eosinophilic granuloma of skin]**

L92.3 **Foreign body granuloma of the skin and subcutaneous tissue**
Use additional code to identify the type of retained foreign body (Z18.-)

L92.8 **Other granulomatous disorders of the skin and subcutaneous tissue**

L92.9 **Granulomatous disorder of the skin and subcutaneous tissue, unspecified**

L93 **Lupus erythematosus**
Use additional code for adverse effect, if applicable, to identify drug (T36-T50 with fifth or sixth character 5)
EXCLUDES1 *lupus exedens (A18.4)*
lupus vulgaris (A18.4)
scleroderma (M34.-)
systemic lupus erythematosus (M32.-)

Unspecified Code Other Specified Code Manifestation Code N Newborn P Pediatric M Maternity A Adult ♂ Male ♀ Female
● New Code ▲ Revised Code Title ►◄ Revised Text NOTES INCLUDES EXCLUDES1 Not coded here EXCLUDES2 Not included here
4th character required 5th character required 6th character required 7th character required
Extension 'X' Alert HAC Hospital-acquired condition (HAC) alert AHA AHA Coding Clinic©

L93.0 **Discoid lupus erythematosus**
Lupus erythematosus NOS
L93.1 **Subacute cutaneous lupus erythematosus**
L93.2 **Other local lupus erythematosus**
Lupus erythematosus profundus
Lupus panniculitis

L94 **Other localized connective tissue disorders**
EXCLUDES1 *systemic connective tissue disorders (M30-M36)*
L94.0 **Localized scleroderma [morphea]**
Circumscribed scleroderma
L94.1 **Linear scleroderma**
En coup de sabre lesion
L94.2 **Calcinosis cutis**
L94.3 **Sclerodactyly**
L94.4 **Gottron's papules**
L94.5 **Poikiloderma vasculare atrophicans**
L94.6 **Ainhum**
L94.8 **Other specified localized connective tissue disorders**
L94.9 **Localized connective tissue disorder, unspecified**

L95 **Vasculitis limited to skin, not elsewhere classified**
EXCLUDES1 *angioma serpiginosum (L81.7)*
Henoch(-Schönlein) purpura (D69.0)
hypersensitivity angiitis (M31.0)
lupus panniculitis (L93.2)
panniculitis NOS (M79.3)
panniculitis of neck and back (M54.0-)
polyarteritis nodosa (M30.0)
relapsing panniculitis (M35.6)
rheumatoid vasculitis (M05.2)
serum sickness (T80.6-)
urticaria (L50.-)
Wegener's granulomatosis (M31.3-)
L95.0 **Livedoid vasculitis**
Atrophie blanche (en plaque)
L95.1 **Erythema elevatum diutinum**
L95.8 **Other vasculitis limited to the skin**
L95.9 **Vasculitis limited to the skin, unspecified**

L97 **Non-pressure chronic ulcer of lower limb, not elsewhere classified**
INCLUDES *chronic ulcer of skin of lower limb NOS*
non-healing ulcer of skin
non-infected sinus of skin
trophic ulcer NOS
tropical ulcer NOS
ulcer of skin of lower limb NOS
Code first any associated underlying condition, such as:
any associated gangrene (I96)
atherosclerosis of the lower extremities (I70.23-, I70.24-, I70.33-, I70.34-, I70.43-, I70.44-, I70.53-, I70.54-, I70.63-, I70.64-, I70.73-, I70.74-)
chronic venous hypertension (I87.31-, I87.33-)
diabetic ulcers (E08.621, E08.622, E09.621, E09.622, E10.621, E10.622, E11.621, E11.622, E13.621, E13.622)
postphlebitic syndromee (I87.01-, I87.03-)
postthrombotic syndromee (I87.01-, I87.03-)
varicose ulcer (I83.0-, I83.2-)
EXCLUDES2 *pressure ulcer (pressure area) (L89.-)*
skin infections (L00-L08)
specific infections classified to A00-B99

L97.1 **Non-pressure chronic ulcer of thigh**
L97.10 **Non-pressure chronic ulcer of unspecified thigh**
L97.101 **Non-pressure chronic ulcer of unspecified thigh limited to breakdown of skin** CC
L97.102 **Non-pressure chronic ulcer of unspecified thigh with fat layer exposed** CC
L97.103 **Non-pressure chronic ulcer of unspecified thigh with necrosis of muscle** CC
L97.104 **Non-pressure chronic ulcer of unspecified thigh with necrosis of bone** CC
L97.109 **Non-pressure chronic ulcer of unspecified thigh with unspecified severity** CC
L97.11 **Non-pressure chronic ulcer of right thigh**
L97.111 **Non-pressure chronic ulcer of right thigh limited to breakdown of skin** CC
L97.112 **Non-pressure chronic ulcer of right thigh with fat layer exposed** CC
L97.113 **Non-pressure chronic ulcer of right thigh with necrosis of muscle** CC
L97.114 **Non-pressure chronic ulcer of right thigh with necrosis of bone** CC
L97.119 **Non-pressure chronic ulcer of right thigh with unspecified severity** CC
L97.12 **Non-pressure chronic ulcer of left thigh**
L97.121 **Non-pressure chronic ulcer of left thigh limited to breakdown of skin** CC
L97.122 **Non-pressure chronic ulcer of left thigh with fat layer exposed** CC
L97.123 **Non-pressure chronic ulcer of left thigh with necrosis of muscle** CC
L97.124 **Non-pressure chronic ulcer of left thigh with necrosis of bone** CC
L97.129 **Non-pressure chronic ulcer of left thigh with unspecified severity** CC

L97.2 **Non-pressure chronic ulcer of calf**
L97.20 **Non-pressure chronic ulcer of unspecified calf**
L97.201 **Non-pressure chronic ulcer of unspecified calf limited to breakdown of skin** CC
L97.202 **Non-pressure chronic ulcer of unspecified calf with fat layer exposed** CC
L97.203 **Non-pressure chronic ulcer of unspecified calf with necrosis of muscle** CC
L97.204 **Non-pressure chronic ulcer of unspecified calf with necrosis of bone** CC
L97.209 **Non-pressure chronic ulcer of unspecified calf with unspecified severity** CC
L97.21 **Non-pressure chronic ulcer of right calf**
L97.211 **Non-pressure chronic ulcer of right calf limited to breakdown of skin** CC
L97.212 **Non-pressure chronic ulcer of right calf with fat layer exposed** CC
L97.213 **Non-pressure chronic ulcer of right calf with necrosis of muscle** CC
L97.214 **Non-pressure chronic ulcer of right calf with necrosis of bone** CC
L97.219 **Non-pressure chronic ulcer of right calf with unspecified severity** CC
L97.22 **Non-pressure chronic ulcer of left calf**
L97.221 **Non-pressure chronic ulcer of left calf limited to breakdown of skin** CC
L97.222 **Non-pressure chronic ulcer of left calf with fat layer exposed** CC
L97.223 **Non-pressure chronic ulcer of left calf with necrosis of muscle** CC
L97.224 **Non-pressure chronic ulcer of left calf with necrosis of bone** CC
L97.229 **Non-pressure chronic ulcer of left calf with unspecified severity** CC

L97.3 **Non-pressure chronic ulcer of ankle**
L97.30 **Non-pressure chronic ulcer of unspecified ankle**
L97.301 **Non-pressure chronic ulcer of unspecified ankle limited to breakdown of skin** CC
L97.302 **Non-pressure chronic ulcer of unspecified ankle with fat layer exposed** CC
L97.303 **Non-pressure chronic ulcer of unspecified ankle with necrosis of muscle** CC
L97.304 **Non-pressure chronic ulcer of unspecified ankle with necrosis of bone** CC
L97.309 **Non-pressure chronic ulcer of unspecified ankle with unspecified severity** CC
L97.31 **Non-pressure chronic ulcer of right ankle**
L97.311 **Non-pressure chronic ulcer of right ankle limited to breakdown of skin** CC
L97.312 **Non-pressure chronic ulcer of right ankle with fat layer exposed** CC
L97.313 **Non-pressure chronic ulcer of right ankle with necrosis of muscle** CC
L97.314 **Non-pressure chronic ulcer of right ankle with necrosis of bone** CC

Unacceptable principal diagnosis symbol per Medicare code edits · Code exempt from diagnosis present on admission requirement
Questionable admission · CC Complication or comorbidity · CC/MCC exclusion · MCC Major complication or comorbidity
Principal diagnosis as its own CC · Principal diagnosis as its own MCC · Z code as first-listed diagnosis

L97.319 Non-pressure chronic ulcer of right ankle with unspecified severity

L97.32 Non-pressure chronic ulcer of left ankle

L97.321 Non-pressure chronic ulcer of left ankle limited to breakdown of skin

L97.322 Non-pressure chronic ulcer of left ankle with fat layer exposed

L97.323 Non-pressure chronic ulcer of left ankle with necrosis of muscle

L97.324 Non-pressure chronic ulcer of left ankle with necrosis of bone

L97.329 Non-pressure chronic ulcer of left ankle with unspecified severity

L97.4 Non-pressure chronic ulcer of heel and midfoot

Non-pressure chronic ulcer of plantar surface of midfoot

L97.40 Non-pressure chronic ulcer of unspecified heel and midfoot

L97.401 Non-pressure chronic ulcer of unspecified heel and midfoot limited to breakdown of skin

L97.402 Non-pressure chronic ulcer of unspecified heel and midfoot with fat layer exposed

L97.403 Non-pressure chronic ulcer of unspecified heel and midfoot with necrosis of muscle

L97.404 Non-pressure chronic ulcer of unspecified heel and midfoot with necrosis of bone

L97.409 Non-pressure chronic ulcer of unspecified heel and midfoot with unspecified severity

L97.41 Non-pressure chronic ulcer of right heel and midfoot

L97.411 Non-pressure chronic ulcer of right heel and midfoot limited to breakdown of skin

L97.412 Non-pressure chronic ulcer of right heel and midfoot with fat layer exposed

L97.413 Non-pressure chronic ulcer of right heel and midfoot with necrosis of muscle

L97.414 Non-pressure chronic ulcer of right heel and midfoot with necrosis of bone

L97.419 Non-pressure chronic ulcer of right heel and midfoot with unspecified severity

L97.42 Non-pressure chronic ulcer of left heel and midfoot

L97.421 Non-pressure chronic ulcer of left heel and midfoot limited to breakdown of skin

AHA: Q1, 2016

L97.422 Non-pressure chronic ulcer of left heel and midfoot with fat layer exposed

L97.423 Non-pressure chronic ulcer of left heel and midfoot with necrosis of muscle

L97.424 Non-pressure chronic ulcer of left heel and midfoot with necrosis of bone

L97.429 Non-pressure chronic ulcer of left heel and midfoot with unspecified severity

L97.5 Non-pressure chronic ulcer of other part of foot

Non-pressure chronic ulcer of toe

L97.50 Non-pressure chronic ulcer of other part of unspecified foot

L97.501 Non-pressure chronic ulcer of other part of unspecified foot limited to breakdown of skin

L97.502 Non-pressure chronic ulcer of other part of unspecified foot with fat layer exposed

L97.503 Non-pressure chronic ulcer of other part of unspecified foot with necrosis of muscle

L97.504 Non-pressure chronic ulcer of other part of unspecified foot with necrosis of bone

L97.509 Non-pressure chronic ulcer of other part of unspecified foot with unspecified severity

L97.51 Non-pressure chronic ulcer of other part of right foot

L97.511 Non-pressure chronic ulcer of other part of right foot limited to breakdown of skin

L97.512 Non-pressure chronic ulcer of other part of right foot with fat layer exposed

L97.513 Non-pressure chronic ulcer of other part of right foot with necrosis of muscle

L97.514 Non-pressure chronic ulcer of other part of right foot with necrosis of bone

L97.519 Non-pressure chronic ulcer of other part of right foot with unspecified severity

L97.52 Non-pressure chronic ulcer of other part of left foot

L97.521 Non-pressure chronic ulcer of other part of left foot limited to breakdown of skin

L97.522 Non-pressure chronic ulcer of other part of left foot with fat layer exposed

L97.523 Non-pressure chronic ulcer of other part of left foot with necrosis of muscle

L97.524 Non-pressure chronic ulcer of other part of left foot with necrosis of bone

L97.529 Non-pressure chronic ulcer of other part of left foot with unspecified severity

L97.8 Non-pressure chronic ulcer of other part of lower leg

L97.80 Non-pressure chronic ulcer of other part of unspecified lower leg

L97.801 Non-pressure chronic ulcer of other part of unspecified lower leg limited to breakdown of skin

L97.802 Non-pressure chronic ulcer of other part of unspecified lower leg with fat layer exposed

L97.803 Non-pressure chronic ulcer of other part of unspecified lower leg with necrosis of muscle

L97.804 Non-pressure chronic ulcer of other part of unspecified lower leg with necrosis of bone

L97.809 Non-pressure chronic ulcer of other part of unspecified lower leg with unspecified severity

L97.81 Non-pressure chronic ulcer of other part of right lower leg

L97.811 Non-pressure chronic ulcer of other part of right lower leg limited to breakdown of skin

L97.812 Non-pressure chronic ulcer of other part of right lower leg with fat layer exposed

L97.813 Non-pressure chronic ulcer of other part of right lower leg with necrosis of muscle

L97.814 Non-pressure chronic ulcer of other part of right lower leg with necrosis of bone

L97.819 Non-pressure chronic ulcer of other part of right lower leg with unspecified severity

L97.82 Non-pressure chronic ulcer of other part of left lower leg

L97.821 Non-pressure chronic ulcer of other part of left lower leg limited to breakdown of skin

L97.822 Non-pressure chronic ulcer of other part of left lower leg with fat layer exposed

L97.823 Non-pressure chronic ulcer of other part of left lower leg with necrosis of muscle

L97.824 Non-pressure chronic ulcer of other part of left lower leg with necrosis of bone

L97.829 Non-pressure chronic ulcer of other part of left lower leg with unspecified severity

L97.9 Non-pressure chronic ulcer of unspecified part of lower leg

L97.90 Non-pressure chronic ulcer of unspecified part of unspecified lower leg

L97.901 Non-pressure chronic ulcer of unspecified part of unspecified lower leg limited to breakdown of skin

L97.902 Non-pressure chronic ulcer of unspecified part of unspecified lower leg with fat layer exposed

L97.903 Non-pressure chronic ulcer of unspecified part of unspecified lower leg with necrosis of muscle CC

L97.904 Non-pressure chronic ulcer of unspecified part of unspecified lower leg with necrosis of bone CC

L97.909 Non-pressure chronic ulcer of unspecified part of unspecified lower leg with unspecified severity CC

L97.91 Non-pressure chronic ulcer of unspecified part of right lower leg

L97.911 Non-pressure chronic ulcer of unspecified part of right lower leg limited to breakdown of skin CC

L97.912 Non-pressure chronic ulcer of unspecified part of right lower leg with fat layer exposed CC

L97.913 Non-pressure chronic ulcer of unspecified part of right lower leg with necrosis of muscle CC

L97.914 Non-pressure chronic ulcer of unspecified part of right lower leg with necrosis of bone CC

L97.919 Non-pressure chronic ulcer of unspecified part of right lower leg with unspecified severity CC

L97.92 Non-pressure chronic ulcer of unspecified part of left lower leg

L97.921 Non-pressure chronic ulcer of unspecified part of left lower leg limited to breakdown of skin CC

L97.922 Non-pressure chronic ulcer of unspecified part of left lower leg with fat layer exposed CC

L97.923 Non-pressure chronic ulcer of unspecified part of left lower leg with necrosis of muscle CC

L97.924 Non-pressure chronic ulcer of unspecified part of left lower leg with necrosis of bone CC

L97.929 Non-pressure chronic ulcer of unspecified part of left lower leg with unspecified severity CC

L98 Other disorders of skin and subcutaneous tissue, not elsewhere classified

L98.0 Pyogenic granuloma

EXCLUDES2 *pyogenic granuloma of gingiva (K06.8)*
pyogenic granuloma of maxillary alveolar ridge (K04.5)
pyogenic granuloma of oral mucosa (K13.4)

L98.1 Factitial dermatitis

Neurotic excoriation

EXCLUDES1 *Excoriation (skin-picking) disorder (F42.4)*

L98.2 Febrile neutrophilic dermatosis [Sweet]

L98.3 Eosinophilic cellulitis [Wells] CC

L98.4 Non-pressure chronic ulcer of skin, not elsewhere classified

Chronic ulcer of skin NOS
Tropical ulcer NOS
Ulcer of skin NOS

EXCLUDES2 *pressure ulcer (pressure area) (L89.-)*
gangrene (I96)
skin infections (L00-L08)
specific infections classified to A00-B99
ulcer of lower limb NEC (L97.-)
varicose ulcer (I83.0-I82.2)

L98.41 Non-pressure chronic ulcer of buttock

L98.411 Non-pressure chronic ulcer of buttock limited to breakdown of skin

L98.412 Non-pressure chronic ulcer of buttock with fat layer exposed

L98.413 Non-pressure chronic ulcer of buttock with necrosis of muscle

L98.414 Non-pressure chronic ulcer of buttock with necrosis of bone

L98.419 Non-pressure chronic ulcer of buttock with unspecified severity

L98.42 Non-pressure chronic ulcer of back

L98.421 Non-pressure chronic ulcer of back limited to breakdown of skin

L98.422 Non-pressure chronic ulcer of back with fat layer exposed

L98.423 Non-pressure chronic ulcer of back with necrosis of muscle

L98.424 Non-pressure chronic ulcer of back with necrosis of bone

L98.429 Non-pressure chronic ulcer of back with unspecified severity

L98.49 Non-pressure chronic ulcer of skin of other sites

Non-pressure chronic ulcer of skin NOS

L98.491 Non-pressure chronic ulcer of skin of other sites limited to breakdown of skin

L98.492 Non-pressure chronic ulcer of skin of other sites with fat layer exposed

L98.493 Non-pressure chronic ulcer of skin of other sites with necrosis of muscle

L98.494 Non-pressure chronic ulcer of skin of other sites with necrosis of bone

L98.499 Non-pressure chronic ulcer of skin of other sites with unspecified severity

L98.5 Mucinosis of the skin

Focal mucinosis
Lichen myxedematosus
Reticular erythematous mucinosis

EXCLUDES1 *focal oral mucinosis (K13.79)*
myxedema (E03.9)

L98.6 Other infiltrative disorders of the skin and subcutaneous tissue

EXCLUDES1 *hyalinosis cutis et mucosae (E78.89)*

● L98.7 Excessive and redundant skin and subcutaneous tissue CC/MCC Exc

Loose or sagging skin following bariatric surgery weight loss
Loose or sagging skin following dietary weight loss
Loose or sagging skin, NOS

EXCLUDES2 *acquired excess or redundant skin of eyelid (H02.3-)*
congenital excess or redundant skin of eyelid (Q10.3)
skin changes due to chronic exposure to nonionizing radiation (L57.-)

L98.8 Other specified disorders of the skin and subcutaneous tissue

L98.9 Disorder of the skin and subcutaneous tissue, unspecified

L99 Other disorders of skin and subcutaneous tissue in diseases classified elsewhere

Code first underlying disease, such as:
amyloidosis (E85.-)

EXCLUDES1 *skin disorders in diabetes (E08-E13 with .62)*
skin disorders in gonorrhea (A54.89)
skin disorders in syphilis (A51.31, A52.79)

PDx Unacceptable principal diagnosis symbol per Medicare code edits | POA Code exempt from diagnosis present on admission requirement | ? Questionable admission | CC Complication or comorbidity | CC/MCC Exc CC/MCC exclusion | MCC Major complication or comorbidity | PDx CC Principal diagnosis as its own CC | PDx MCC Principal diagnosis as its own MCC | Z1 Z code as first-listed diagnosis

Chapter 13: Diseases of the Musculoskeletal System and Connective Tissue (M00-M99)

Guidelines for Assigning Codes From This Chapter

When you need to report a joint or spine disorder, a musculoskeletal deformity, or a pathologic fracture, you're likely to find your code in Chapter 13.

List of Sections

- M00-M25 Arthropathies
- M26-M27 Dentofacial anomalies [including malocclusion] and other disorders of jaw
- M30-M36 Systemic connective tissue disorders
- M40-M54 Dorsopathies
- M60-M79 Soft tissue disorders
- M80-M94 Osteopathies and chondropathies
- M95 Other disorders of the musculoskeletal system and connective tissue
- M96 Intraoperative and postprocedural complications and disorders of musculoskeletal system, not elsewhere classified
- M99 Biomechanical lesions, not elsewhere classified

Highlights From the ICD-10-CM Official Guidelines for Coding and Reporting

For Chapter 13, the ICD-10-CM Official Guidelines for Coding and Reporting concentrate on proper coding of site and laterality, acute traumatic versus chronic or recurrent musculoskeletal conditions, coding of pathologic fractures, and osteoporosis. The information below is from Section I.C.13 of the 2017 Official Guidelines.

Specificity is Key

- Select the code that designates the specific bone, joint or muscle involved and the side of the body.
- Use the "multiple sites" code, if one is available, instead of coding each site separately.
- Code the bone, not the joint, if a condition, such as avascular necrosis or osteoporosis, affects the end of the bone and includes the joint.

Acute Traumatic vs Chronic or Recurrent

Before choosing between acute traumatic and chronic or recurrent codes, remember that a condition can be the result of previous injury or trauma or a recurrent condition. You'll find bone, joint, or muscle conditions that are the result of a healed injury in chapter 13, as well as recurrent conditions. Remember to code acute injuries from Chapter 19.

Use the 7th Character for Pathologic Fractures

A pathologic fracture is a break in a weakened bone caused by disease, such as a tumor, rather than trauma or stress. Coding varies based on the stage of the treatment.

Active treatment: To report a pathologic fracture receiving active treatment, you use a code from Chapter 13 range M84.4- to M84.6- (Pathological fracture…) ending in 7th character A. According to the guidelines, "Examples of active treatment are surgical treatment, emergency department encounter, evaluation and continuing treatment by the same or a different physician." Remember that it doesn't matter if the provider is seeing the patient for the first time.

Aftercare: Select a code with 7th character D for encounters after the patient has completed active treatment. You'll find other 7th character options listed under each subcategory in the Tabular List to identify subsequent encounters for treatment of problems associated with healing, such as malunions, nonunions, and sequelae.

If complications arise after surgical treatment, use the appropriate complication codes.

Bone up on Osteoporosis Coding

Osteoporosis is a systemic condition, affecting the whole body, so you won't find site codes in category M81 (*Osteoporosis without current pathological fracture, os*). If an osteoporosis patient sustains a fracture, choose a code from M80 (*Osteoporosis with current pathological fracture*) to identify the site of the fracture, not the osteoporosis.

Without current fracture: Use category M81 for patients without a current fracture, even if they have had a fracture due to osteoporosis in the past. For those patients, assign status code Z87.310 (*Personal history of [healed] osteoporosis fracture*) after M81.

With current fracture: Select a code from M80 based on fracture site. Never use a traumatic fracture code for a patient with known osteoporosis.

Anatomy of the Musculoskeletal System

Introduction

Osteology (Osteo: bone; logy: study) is the branch of anatomy that deals with the detailed analysis of structure, function and diseases of the skeletal elements. It constitutes the bony framework of the body. The human bony skeleton is composed of the below mentioned components (and is derived from the mesoderm, which is the primary germ cell layer).

Skeletal Region	Body Structure	Quantity of bones
Axial Skeleton (The trunk)	Skull	22
	Hyoid Bone	1
	Ribs & Sternum	25
	Vertebral Column	26
Appendicular Skeleton (The limbs)	Upper Extremities	64
	Lower Extremities	62
Auditory Ossicles		6

1. **Structure of a Normal Human Bone:** Bone is comprised of a rigid structure, which is based on dense connective tissue. A normal human bone is made up of the following essential macro and micro elements:
   a) Periosteum
   b) Medullary Membrane
   c) Marrow
   d) Blood Vessels and Nerves of Bone
   e) Haversian Canals (Canals of Havers)
   f) Lamellae
   g) Lacunae
   h) Canaliculi
   i) Perichondrium
   j) Osteoblasts
   k) Osteoclasts
   l) Medullary spaces
   m) Epiphysis
   n) Diaphysis
   o) Metaphysis
2. **The Vertebral Column**
   a) Anatomical Detail: The vertebral column is composed of a continuous series of compact bones that articulate with each other via intervertebral discs, and are called vertebrae. The structure forms the dorsal aspect of the trunk. The vertebral column is also called spine. The spinal cord traverses through the spinal canal of the vertebral column. The individual vertebrae remain connected together by intervertebral discs. The cervical, thoracic, and lumbar vertebrae are termed true vertebrae. However, sacral and coccygeal ones are false vertebrae. The concept behind considering them as true or false is based on mobility of the individual vertebrae through intervertebral discs. Cervical, thoracic and lumbar vertebrae are moveable to some extent and therefore termed as true vertebral bodies. In contrast, the sacral-coccygeal section is rather fixed and thus not categorized as true vertebrae. Each vertebral segment is associated with a portion of spinal cord, which travels the entire vertebral column, and each spinal cord segment has specific physiology and functions. The vertebral bodies communicate with each other through the pads of elastic fibro-cartilage. These flexible pads constitute the intervertebral discs, which help in the movement of vertebral bodies and provide protection from trauma or shocks. However, the length of the adult vertebral column ranges from 60-70 cm. The entire vertebral column is based on a total of 33 vertebrae that are categorized (below) in accordance with the occupied region.
      i) neck or the cervical region is composed of seven cervical vertebrae.
      ii) back or thorax region contains 12 thoracic vertebrae.
      iii) loin or lumbar region is based on five lumbar vertebrae.
      iv) sacrum forms five (fused) sacral vertebrae.
      v) coccyx (tail) has usually four (fused) coccygeal vertebrae.

   b) Cervical Vertebrae

      These are small and delicate bones, which are marked by the existence of a foramen in every transverse process. The cervical region is based on the seven cervical bones (C1-C7). However, the first cervical vertebra is known as Atlas and the second one is Axis.

   c) Thoracic Vertebrae

      Thoracic vertebrae are 12 in quantity (T1–T12), and communicate with the head (tubercles) of ribs in the thoracic region through articular facets of the transverse processes. Their body structure is similar to the shape of the heart, with nearly circular vertebral foramina.

   d) Lumbar Vertebrae

      These are five vertebrae (L1-L5), with kidney shaped bodies. Lumbar vertebrae are in fact the most toughest and robust in configuration. These are enlarged in size and marked by the absence of a transverse process foramen and vertebral facets. They are true vertebrae, thereby allowing flexion and extension movements via flexible intervertebral discs. Their broad lamellae, large bodies, long transverse processes, and strong pedicles make them suitable to support additional body weight as compared to other similar vertebrae.

   e) Sacral Vertebrae

      These are five vertebral bodies (S1-S5), which constitute a portion of the pelvic cavity. Sacral vertebral bodies consist of five separate segments that get fused together at maturity. As a matter of fact, these vertebrae lack intervertebral discs, which restrict their mobility and put them into the category of false vertebrae.

   f) Coccygeal Vertebrae

      The four coccygeal vertebrae constitute the human vestigial tail bone, in which vertebral bodies are fused together without the existence of any intervertebral disc. Movement of the individual vertebral bodies is restricted due to their interfusion. Hence, these are considered as false vertebrae. The number of bones in the coccygeal region may rarely vary between three to five vertebrae, in few individuals.
3. **Thorax; Anatomical Detail**
   The part of the trunk situated between the neck and abdomen constitutes the thorax. The thoracic cavity is bounded by ribs, sternum, costal cartilages, and the thoracic vertebrae. The thorax is also known as the chest region. The osseocartilaginous cage of the thorax covers and protects the prime organs of circulation and respiration. Furthermore, this osseocartilaginous cage is composed mainly of the ribcage, shoulder girdle, and spine.

   The 12 thoracic vertebrae and certain component of the ribs constitute the posterior (back) wall of the thoracic cavity. However, the anterior (front) region is composed of sternum and the costal cartilages. The entire human chest (thorax) region contains multiple organs, muscles, bones, vasculature, internal and external structures. These contents include heart, lungs, thymus, pectoral muscles, scapula, sternum, ribs, aorta, trachea, diaphragm, and mammary glands etc.
4. **Sternum (Chest or Breast Bone)**
   a) Sternum: It is a flat and long bone situated in the center of the thorax and forms the midline of the anterior thoracic cage. It articulates with both clavicles (collar bones) through its upper ends. It is composed of the following three (interfused) components:
      i) manubrium
      ii) body (gladiolus/corpus sterni)
      iii) xiphoid process (processus xiphoideus/ensiform or xiphoid appendix) ribs.

   b) Ribs are the elongated, flattened, lightweight, resilient, and twisted bones that are the essential constituent of the thoracic skeleton. The total number of ribs in the human body is 24 (12 on each side). The ribs can be classified as follows:
      i) True Ribs-These are also called vertebrosternal ribs. True ribs comprise the first seven ribs that communicate (to the dorsum) with the vertebral column as well as sternum (in front) via costal cartilages.
      ii) False Ribs-These are also called vertebrochondral ribs. False ribs comprise the eighth, ninth, and tenth ribs that are indirectly attached to the sternum through costal cartilages. The individual cartilages of each of these ribs are connected to the cartilage of the rib lying just above them.
      iii) Floating Ribs-These are also termed vertebral ribs. These ribs include the 11th and 12th ribs that are free at their anterior extremities (without any attachment with the sternum) and are connected to the vertebral bodies on their dorsal ends.

5. **The Skull**
   The human skull is based on the skeleton of the head. Several bones of the skull integrate together to form the cranium (or the skull). The skull can be categorized as follows:
   a) The Brain Box or Brain Case (The Calvaria). It constitutes the upper cranium and contains the brain.
   b) The Facial Skeleton comprises the portion of skull (other than the brain box) and includes the mandible bone of the face.

The Composition of Human Skull

The Calvaria	
Paired Bones	Unpaired Bones
i) Parietal	i) Frontal
ii) Temporal	ii) Occipital
	iii) Sphenoid
	iv) Ethmoid
The Facial Skeleton	
Paired Bones	Unpaired Bones
iii) Maxilla	v) Mandible
iv) Zygomatic	vi) Vomer
v) Nasal	
vi) Lacrimal	
vii) Palatine	
viii) Inferior Nasal Concha	

   c. The Facial Bones- The facial skeleton comprises the lower and anterior portion of the human skull and includes the following bones:
      i) nasal bones
      ii) maxillae (upper jaw)
      iii) lacrimal bone
      iv) zygomatic bone
      v) palatine bone
      vi) inferior nasal concha
      vii) vomer
      viii) mandible (lower jaw)
      ix) hyoid bone
6. **The Bones of the Upper Extremity**
   a. Clavicle
      The clavicle is also called the collar bone that forms the anterior portion of the shoulder girdle. The clavicles are two in number and called the right and left clavicles.
   b. Scapula
      The scapula is also called the shoulder blade and constitutes the back portion of the shoulder girdle. It is a flat bone that articulates with the clavicle and humerus. It also contains a triangular process that projects laterally and is called the acromion. Additionally, the upper part of the neck of the scapula contains a curved process, which is known as the coracoid process. The scapulae are two in number (right and left scapula).
   c. Humerus
      The humerus is the long bone of the arm that begins from the shoulder and ends up at the elbow. It is the largest bone of the upper extremity and consists of the following major components:
      i) greater tubercle (greater tuberosity)
      ii) lesser tubercle (lesser tuberosity)
      iii) body or shaft (corpus humeri)
      iv) anterior, lateral, and medial borders
      v) medial and lateral epicondyles
      vi) radial sulcus (musculospiral groove)
      vii) lateral and medial supracondylar ridges
      viii) deltoid tuberosity.
   d. Ulna
      The ulna is one of the two long and prismatic bones of the forearm that extends parallel with the radius. The ulna possesses a body and two extremities. The proximal or upper extremity contains olecranon and coronoid processes, and the semilunar and radial notches respectively. The body or shaft of the ulna is also known as the corpus ulnae. The lower or distal extremity is comprised of an articular eminence (the head of the ulna) and a nonarticular eminence (the styloid process).
   e. Radius
      The radius is one of the two long bones of the forearm that extends laterally with the ulna. Its lower end participates in the formation of the wrist joint and upper end helps to create the elbow joint. The upper or proximal extremity consists of a head, neck, and tuberosity. The body or shaft is also known as the corpus radii. The lateral surface of the lower extremity contains a conical projection, which is known as the styloid process.
   f. Carpus
      The carpus region of the hand contains the carpal bones, which consist of a total of eight bones positioned in proximal and distal rows to facilitate uninterrupted movement of the wrist joint. The carpal bones of the proximal row are: navicular, lunate, triangular, and pisiform. The bones of the distal row are: greater multangular, lesser multangular, capitate, and hamate.
   g. Metacarpus
      The metacarpus region of hand is based on cylindrical (metacarpal) bones that are five in number and constitute the intermediary portion of the bony skeleton of hand. The first through fifth metacarpal bones belong to the thumb, index, middle, ring and little fingers respectively.
   h. Phalanges of the Hand
      The phalanges (finger bones) of the hand constitute the fingers. These are 14 in number. Each finger consists of three phalanges. However, the thumb consists of only two phalanges. A single finger bone has a body, with two extremities. The finger bones serve to facilitate the basic functions of the hand, like-effective grasping of objects and writing, etc.
7. **The Bones of the Lower Extremity**
   a. Hip Bone
      The hip bone is also known as the coxal bone. It's based on three components: ilium, ischium, and pubis. The ilium holds the flank. It is the broad portion situated on top of the large cup-shaped articular cavity, the acetabulum. The ischium forms the lower back part of the hip bone that facilitates sitting. It's located downward from the acetabulum and is the strongest component of the hip bone, containing an enlarged opening, the obturator foramen. The pubis is the lower frontal portion of the hip bone, which is located medially below the acetabulum. It supports the internal organs of reproduction. The angle across the pubic symphysis is known as the pubic arch.
   b. Pelvis
      The pelvis consists of a bony ring that provides a connecting medium between the vertebral column and femurs. It is based on the following 4 bones:
      i) The hip bones are two in number.
      ii) The sacrum-The fused vertebrae that are five in number and connected to the hip bones.
      iii) The coccyx-The fused vertebrae that are four in number and constitute the tailbone.

      The space surrounded by the pelvic girdle is known as the pelvic cavity. The pelvic girdle bears the entire weight of the trunk and upper body while sitting and transfers this weight to the lower limbs during standing, walking, or running.
   c. Femur
      The femur is one of the two largest, longest, and strongest bones in the human skeleton that bears the load of the upper body via the pelvis in standing, walking, or running. It also participates in the formation of the hip and knee joints. The components of a normal femur bone are as follows:

      The Upper (Proximal) Extremity consists of the following elements:
      i) Head
      ii) Neck
      iii) Greater Trochanter
      iv) Lesser Trochanter

      The Body or Shaft-The body is cylindrical in shape, lies between the upper and lower extremities and is also known as corpus femoris.

      The Lower (Distal) Extremity -The distal extremity is based on two projections (the lateral and medial condyles). These projections (condyles) are separated in front by an articular depression, known as the patellar surface. The same condyles are further interrupted from behind by a deep pit, which is termed as the intercondyloid fossa.

d. Patella

The knee cap (patella) is a flat, thick, circular-triangular, and dense cancellous articular bone that is situated on the frontal portion of the knee joint. The superior border is thick and forms the base of patella. The patella is further marked by medial and lateral borders. The apex of patella is a pointed region that provides attachment to the patellar ligament. The patella articulates with the femur through the patellofemoral joint.

e. Tibia

The tibia (shin bone) is located medially in the lower leg and is regarded as the largest and strongest bone of the skeleton after the femur. It also participates in the formation of the knee and ankle joints. The tibia is composed of the following elements:

i) upper (proximal) end – The proximal extremity is composed of the projections, which are known as the medial and lateral condyles. The condylar surfaces further merge to form an eminence on the frontal side, which is known as the tibial tuberosity.

ii) body or shaft of tibia – The shaft of the tibia is also known as corpus tibiae and contains the anterior crest (or border), the medial border, and the interosseous crest (or lateral border).

iii) lower (distal) end – The distal extremity contains the inferior articular surface, the anterior surface, the posterior surface, the lateral surface, and the medial surface. However, the medial surface extends medially to form a pyramidal process, which is termed as the medial malleolus.

f. Fibula

The fibula (calf bone) is located laterally in the lower leg and runs laterally with the adjacent shin bone (tibia). It's a thin and slender bone which is composed of a body with upper and lower extremities. The lower or distal extremity constitutes the lateral malleolus, which is also known as the external malleolus or malleolus lateralis.

g. Tarsus

The tarsus region of foot is based on the following seven tarsal bones:

i) calcaneus

ii) talus

iii) cuboid

iv) navicular

v) three cuneiforms

h. Phalanges of the Foot

The phalanges of the foot constitute the region of forefoot. These are also known as the toe bones. The great toe (hallux) contains two phalanges (proximal and distal). The proximal and distal phalangeal bones of the great toe articulate with each other to form the first interphalangeal joint. The proximal phalanges of the other toes articulate with their respective metatarsal heads to form the metatarsophalangeal joints.

8. Syndesmology (The Articulations or Joints)

Syndesmology is defined as the branch of anatomy that deals with the joints and their components (including ligaments). The junctions of bones, where multiple parts of the individual bones connect together, are called articulations or joints. These articulations are further supported by sheets of tough fibrous tissue that connect the joint bones together and are termed ligaments. Various components of the joints are listed below:

a) Bones

b) Cartilages

The cartilages are flexible nonvascular structures composed of connective tissue and found mainly in joints. A cartilage can be categorized into the following elements:

c) Hyaline cartilage

d) White fibrocartilage

The white fibrocartilage can further be categorized into four subcategories:

i) interarticular fibrocartilage

ii) connecting fibrocartilage

iii) circumferential fibrocartilage

iv) stratiform fibrocartilage

e) Yellow or elastic fibrocartilage

f) Articular Capsule

The articular capsule is also known as the joint capsule that completely covers and protects the freely movable (synovial) joints.

g) Mucous Sheaths

The mucous sheaths cover a part of the fibroosseous canals and surface of the tendons that glide upon these canals to facilitate the movement of these tendons on their respective canals.

9. Classification of Joints

The joints can be classified into the following three classes:

a) Synarthroses (Immovable Joints)

b) Amphiarthroses (Slightly Movable Joints)

c) Diarthroses (Freely Movable Joints)

10. Joints of the Trunk

a) Joints between Vertebral Bodies

The articulations between the individual vertebral bodies are based on the amphiarthrodial (slightly movable) intervertebral joints that possess only a very slight degree of mobility.

b) Joints between Vertebral Arches

The articulations between the individual vertebral arches are carried out through the two pairs of articular processes. The articular processes of a typical vertebral arch connect together with the articular processes of the adjacent vertebral arch to form true diarthrosis of arthrodial variety.

c) Joints of the Atlas with the Axis

The atlas forms three diarthroses with the axis. Moreover, the articulations of the axis with the atlas are known as the Atlantoaxial articulations.

d) Joints of the Vertebral Column with the Cranium

The atlas forms two articulations (known as diarthrosis) with the occipital bone. The occipital condyles interact with the articular surfaces of the atlas to constitute diarthroses. The synovial stratum covers the articular capsules around the condyles of the occipital bone.

e) Joints of the Mandible

The temporomandibular articulation forms an arthrodial diarthrosis. The temporal mandibular fossa and mandibular condyle interact together to constitute the temporomandibular articulation.

f) Joints of the Ribs with the Vertebrae

The head and tubercle of a typical rib articulates with the vertebral column to form a costovertebral articulation.

g) Joints of the Vertebral Column with the Pelvis

The fifth lumbar vertebra connects with the sacrum to form the lumbosacral articulation. The inner lip of the iliac crest connects with the transverse processes of the fifth lumbar vertebra through iliolumbar ligament.

h) Joints of the Pelvis

The articulations of the pelvis are mainly based on the following types of joints:

i) symphysis pubis

The two pubic bones articulate with each other to constitute a joint, which is known as the symphysis pubis.

ii) sacroiliac articulation

The auricular surfaces of sacrum and ilium connect with each other to form an amphiarthrodial joint, which is termed as the sacroiliac articulation.

iii) sacrococcygeal symphysis

The apex of the sacrum and base of the coccyx articulate with each other to form an amphiarthrodial joint, which is known as the sacrococcygeal symphysis.

11. Joints of Upper Extremity

a) The Acromioclavicular Joint

The medial aspect of the acromion (of the scapula) connects with the acromial end of the clavicle to constitute the acromioclavicular articulation. However, this type of joint is categorized as an arthrodial diarthrosis.

b) The Shoulder Joint

The humeral articulation constitutes the shoulder joint, which is an enarthrodial (ball and socket) joint and considered as the largest joint of the upper limb. The shoulder joint offers an extended range of movement and is composed of the articular head of humerus and the shallow glenoid cavity of the scapula. The ligaments of the shoulder joint include the articular capsule (capsular ligament), glenoid labrum (glenoid ligament) as well as the glenohumeral, coracohumeral, and transverse humeral ligaments.

c) The Elbow Joint

The elbow articulation falls under the category of hinge joint (ginglymus diarthrosis). The elbow joint performs the flexion and extension movements around a transversely placed single axis. The elbow joint consists of the humerus, ulna, and radius bones. An elbow joint is formed when the trochlea of humerus connects with the semilunar notch of ulna and the capitulum of humerus interacts with the cup (shallow-depression or fovea) on the proximal aspect of the head of the radius. The articular surfaces of the elbow joint are enclosed by and interact with each other through a well defined articular capsule.

d) The Radioulnar Joint

The radioulnar joint is based on two articulations positioned at the proximal and distal ends of the radius and ulna. These articulations facilitate the rotational movements of the radius around its longitudinal axis to constitute a uniaxial diarthrosis, which is known as lateral ginglymus.

e) The Radiocarpal Joint

The radiocarpal articulation is also known as the wrist joint, which is a type of condyloid articulation. The distal (lower) end of radius, discus articularis (the articular disc), and the proximal articular surfaces of navicular, lunate and triquetral bones (including their interosseous ligaments) together constitute the wrist articulation. Moreover, the wrist joint is completely encapsulated by the articular capsule.

f) The Intercarpal Joint

The carpal joints are based on the articulations between the carpal bones with limited range of movement. These joints consist of the arthrodial diarthroses and are therefore known as the gliding joints. The carpal bone articulations are characterized as follows:

i) Proximal Row (Carpal) Joint
ii) Distal Row (Carpal) Joint
iii) Transverse (Carpal) Joint

g) The Carpometacarpal joint

The Carpometacarpal (CMC) joints are based on the interaction between the carpal and metacarpal bones. However, the carpometacarpal articulation of the thumb region differs from the articulations of the other four metacarpal bones with the carpus. Therefore, the carpometacarpal articulations can be categorized as follows:

h) The Joints of the other Four Metacarpal Bones with the Carpus

These types of carpometacarpal articulations are formed by the connections between the bases of the second, third, fourth, and fifth medial metacarpal bones and the four bones of the distal carpal row.

i) The Intermetacarpal Joints

The four medial metacarpal bones articulate with each other to form the arthrodial diarthroses, which are known as the intermetacarpal joints.

j) The Metacarpophalangeal Joints

With the exception of the thumb, the spherical head of each metacarpal bone articulates with the shallow oval cavity on the base of the first phalanx to constitute the metacarpophalangeal joints. The metacarpophalangeal articulations facilitate flexion, extension, adduction, abduction, and circumduction type of joint movements.

k) The Joints of the Digits

The interphalangeal joints are categorized as hinge joints that are two in number for each finger and only one for the thumb. The interphalangeal joints can perform movements like flexion and extension.

12. Joints of the Lower Extremity

a) The Hip Joint

The coxal articulation constitutes the hip joint, which is a type of enarthrodial diarthrosis (ball and socket joint). The articular surfaces of the hip joint consist of the head of the femur and a cup shaped cavity (acetabulum) that connect together to constitute the coxal articulation. The hip joint can perform multi-axial movements like rotation, flexion, extension, abduction, and adduction. The hip joint cavity is completely encapsulated by an articular capsule or the capsular ligament. Other ligaments of the hip joint are described below:

i) iliofemoral ligament (ligamentum iliofemorale/Y-ligament/ligament of Bigelow)
ii) pubocapsular ligament (ligamentum pubocapsulare/pubofemoral ligament)
iii) ischiocapsular ligament (ligamentum ischiocapsulare/ischiocapsular band/ligament of Bertin)
iv) ligamentum teres femoris
v) glenoidal labrum (labrum glenoidale/cotyloid ligament)
vi) transverse acetabular ligament (ligamentum transversum acetabuli/ transverse ligament)

b) The Knee Joint

The knee articulation/joint is considered as the largest articulation in the human body and related to the ginglymus (hinge) variety of diarthroses. However, its structure is more elaborate and complicated. The articular surfaces of the knee joint pertain to specific portions of the femur, tibia and patella bones. The ligaments associated with the knee joint are as follows:

i) articular capsule (capsula articularis/capsular ligament)
ii) ligamentum patellae (anterior ligament)
iii) oblique popliteal ligament (ligamentum popliteum obliquum/ posterior ligament)
iv) tibial collateral ligament (ligamentum collaterale tibiale/internal lateral ligament)
v) fibular collateral ligament (ligamentum collaterale fibulare/external lateral or long external lateral ligament)
vi) anterior cruciate ligament (ligamentum cruciatum anterius/external crucial ligament)
vii) posterior cruciate ligament (ligamentum cruciatum posterius/ internal crucial ligament)
viii) medial meniscus (meniscus medialis/internal semilunar fibrocartilage)
ix) lateral meniscus (meniscus lateralis/external semilunar fibrocartilage)
x) transverse ligament (ligamentum transversum genu)
xi) coronary ligaments
xii) synovial membrane encapsulates the upper border of the patella and the lower portion of the front of the femur. The movements associated with the knee joint are flexion, extension, internal, and external rotation.

c) The Joints between Tibia and Fibula

The articulations between the tibia and fibula constitute the tibiofibular joints. The fibula articulates with the tibia through its proximal and distal ends. The proximal tibiofibular joint is an arthrodial articulation between head of the fibula and lateral condyle of the tibia. The interosseous membrane acts as an accessory ligament to bind the shafts of tibia and fibula together. However, the tibiofibular syndesmosis constitutes the distal tibiofibular joint, which presents a series of ligaments that are accessory to the ankle joint.

d) The Talocrural Joint

The talocrural articulation constitutes the ankle joint, which is a ginglymus variety of diarthrosis. In other words, the ankle joint is a type of hinge joint. The ankle joint facilitates the movements like dorsiflexion and extension.

e) The Intertarsal Joints

The intertarsal articulations (joints) are diarthroses that facilitate the gliding movements of the foot. These joints can be categorized in the following manner:

i) talocalcaneal joint
ii) talocalcaneonavicular joint
iii) calcaneocuboid joint
iv) cuneonavicular joint
v) cuboideonavicular joint
vi) intercuneiform and cuneocuboid joint

f) The Tarsometatarsal Joint

The tarsometatarsal joints include the articular surfaces of the cuneiform, the cuboid, and the metatarsal bones. The articular facets of the three cuneiform and cuboid bones connect with the bases of the five metatarsal bones to constitute the tarsometatarsal articulations.

g) The Intermetatarsal Joint

The articular facets on the bases of the four metatarsal bones connect with each other via dorsal, plantar, and interosseous ligaments to form the intermetatarsal joints. However, no ligament acts to connect the first metatarsal base with the second one.

h) The Metatarsophalangeal Joint

The metatarsophalangeal joints are types of modified ball and socket articulations, wherein globular heads of metatarsal bones articulate with the shallow cups upon the bases of the first phalanges via plantar and collateral ligaments. These joints are encapsulated by an articular capsule.

i) The Joints of the Digits

The articulations between the digits constitute the interphalangeal joints. The phalanges of the toes connect with each other to form the interphalangeal articulations. The great toe possesses only one interphalangeal joint. However, every other toe (except great toe) comprises of two interphalangeal joints.

13. The Muscular System
Introduction

The muscle cells of the human body facilitate the movements of various body parts through their special function of contraction in response to a requisite external or internal stimulus. These muscle cells can be characterized under the below mentioned three different classes:

a) Striated Muscle Cells

The striated muscle cells are those voluntary muscle cells that constitute the skeletal muscular system.

b) Non Striated Muscle Cells

The nonstriated muscle cells are those involuntary muscle cells that occur in the vessel walls and hollow viscera.

c) Cardiac Muscle Cells

The cardiac muscle cells consist of those striated cells that constitute the substance of the heart. However, these muscle cells are involuntary in nature.

14. The Muscles of the Trunk
The muscles of the back are based on the following group of muscles:

a) Splenius

The splenius muscles constitute the superficial layer of the intrinsic back muscles that occupy the back of neck and upper portion of the thoracic region. The splenius muscles overlap the vertical muscles like a bandage and have the following two types:

i) splenius capitis

ii) splenius cervicis

b) Sacrospinalis (Erector Spinae)

The erector spinae muscles are positioned in a groove between the angle of the ribs and spinal processes on each side of the vertebral column. The erector spinae is divided into the following three muscle columns:

c) Iliocostalis

The lateral column is further divided into the following muscle components:

i) iliocostalis lumborum (iliocostalis/sacrolumbalis muscle)

ii) iliocostalis dorsi (musculus accessorius)

iii) iliocostalis cervicis (cervicalis ascendens)

d) Longissimus

i) longissimus dorsi

ii) longissimus cervicis (transversalis cervicis)

iii) longissimus capitis (trachelomastoid muscle)

e) Spinalis

i) spinalis dorsi

ii) spinalis cervicis (spinalis coli)

iii) spinalis capitis (biventer cervicis)

f) Semispinalis

The semispinalis constitute the deeper layer of intrinsic back muscles. These muscles originate from half of the vertebral column and are categorized into three distinct parts:

i) semispinalis dorsi

ii) semispinalis cervicis (semispinalis colli)

iii) semispinalis capitis (complexus)

g) Multifidus (Multifidus Spinae)

The multifidus consists of short triangular muscular bundles that remain apparent from sacrum to the axis.

h) Rotatores (Rotatores Spinae)

It remains confined in the thoracic region.

i) Interspinales and Intertransversarii (Intertransversales) are best developed and most distinct in the cervical region and considered as the smallest of the deep back muscles.

15. The Muscles of the Pelvis
The muscles of the pelvis include the following:

a) Obturator Internus

b) Piriformis

c) Levator Ani (Pubococcygeus and Iliococcygeus)

d) Coccygeus (Ischiococcygeus)

16. The Muscles of the Upper Extremity

a) The muscles that connect the upper extremity to the vertebral column are defined below:

i) trapezius

ii) rhomboideus major

iii) latissimus dorsi

iv) rhomboideus minor

v) levator scapulae

b) The Muscles Connecting the Upper Extremity to the Anterior and Lateral Thoracic Walls

i) pectoralis major

ii) subclavius

iii) pectoralis minor

iv) serratus anterior

c) The Muscles of the Shoulder

i) Deltoid muscle originates from the lateral third portion of clavicle, the acromion, and the spine of scapula. However, it gets inserted into the deltoid tuberosity of humerus. This muscle facilitates the abduction and medial and lateral rotation of the arm.

ii) Subscapularis muscle originates from the subscapular fossa that forms the ventral surface of scapula. However, it gets inserted into the lesser tubercle of humerus. The subscapularis helps to medially rotate and adduct the arm and fixes the humeral head in the glenoid cavity (of the scapula).

iii) Supraspinatus muscle originates from the supraspinatous fossa of scapula and gets inserted into the superior facet of greater tubercle of humerus. This muscle assists the deltoid in the abduction of the arm.

iv) Infraspinatus muscle arises from the infraspinatous fossa of scapula and gets inserted into the middle facet of the greater tubercle of humerus. This muscle helps in the lateral rotation of the arm and fixes the head of humerus into the glenoid cavity of scapula.

v) Teres Minor muscle originates from the middle portion of lateral border of scapula and gets inserted into the inferior facet of greater tubercle of humerus. Like infraspinatus, teres minor muscle also helps in the lateral rotation of the arm and fixes the head of humerus into the glenoid cavity of scapula.

vi) Teres Major muscle arises from the posterior surface of the inferior angle of scapula and gets inserted into the medial lip of the intertubercular groove of humerus. This muscle facilitates the adduction and medial rotation of the arm.

d) The Muscles of the Arm

i) coracobrachialis

ii) biceps brachii

iii) brachialis

iv) triceps brachii

e) The Muscles of the Forearm: muscles of the Anterior Compartment of Forearm

The Muscles of the Superficial (First) Layer

i) pronator teres

ii) flexor carpi radialis

iii) the palmaris longus

iv) flexor carpi ulnaris

f) The Muscle of the Intermediate (Second) Layer

i) flexor digitorum superficialis

The Muscles of the Deep (Third) Layer

i) flexor digitorum profundus

ii) flexor pollicis longus

iii) pronator quadrates

g) Muscles of the Posterior Compartment of Forearm of the Superficial Layer

i) brachioradialis

ii) extensor carpi radialis longus

iii) extensor carpii radialis brevis

iv) extensor digitorum
v) extensor digiti minimi
vi) extensor carpi ulnaris

h) The Muscles of the Deep Layer
i) supinator
ii) abductor pollicis longus
iii) extensor pollicis longus
iv) extensor pollicis brevis
v) extensor indicis

i) The Muscles of the Hand: Thenar Muscles
i) opponens pollicis
ii) abductor pollicis brevis
iii) flexor pollicis brevis
iv) adductor pollicis

Hypothenar muscles
i) abductor digiti minimi
ii) flexor digiti minimi Brevis
iii) opponens digiti minimi

j) The Short Muscles
i) Lumbricals
ii) Dorsal Interossei
iii) Palmar Interossei

17. The Muscles of the Thigh: Anterior Thigh Muscles

a) The below mentioned anterior thigh muscles are based on the anterior compartment of thigh:
i) pectineus
ii) iliopsoas
iii) psoas major
iv) iliacus
v) femoris
vi) vastus lateralis
vii) vastus intermedius
viii) vastus medialis

b) Medial Thigh Muscles
i) adductor longus
ii) adductor brevis
iii) adductor magnus
iv) gracilis
v) obturator externus

c) Gluteal Region Muscles
i) gluteus maximus
ii) gluteus medius
iii) gluteus minimus
iv) tensor fasciae latae
v) piriformis
vi) obturator internus
vii) superior and inferior gemelli
viii) quadratus femoris

d) Posterior Thigh Muscles
i) semitendinosus
ii) semimembranosus
iii) biceps femoris (long head)

e) The Muscles of the Leg: The Anterior Compartment Muscles
i) tibialis anterior
ii) extensor hallucis longus
iii) extensor digitorum longus
iv) fibularis tertius

f) The Lateral Compartment Muscles
i) fibularis longus
ii) fibularis brevis

g) The Posterior Compartment Muscles: Superficial Muscle Group
i) gastrocnemius
ii) soleus
iii) plantaris

h) The Deep Muscle Group
i) Popliteus
ii) Flexor Hallucis Longus
iii) Flexor Digitorum Longus
iv) Tibialis Posterior

i) The Muscles of the Foot: First Layer Muscles
i) abductor hallucis
ii) flexor digitorum brevis
iii) abductor digiti minimi

j) Second Layer Muscles
i) quadratus plantae
ii) lumbricals

k) The Third Layer Muscles
i) flexor hallucis brevis
ii) adductor hallucis
iii) flexor digiti minimi brevis

l) The Fourth Layer Muscles
i) plantar interossei (three muscles)
ii) dorsal interossei (four muscles)

m) Muscles of Dorsum of Foot
i) extensor digitorum brevis
ii) extensor hallucis brevis

Common Pathologies

Rotator Cuff Tendinitis

Rotator cuff tendinitis, often with inflammation of the subacromial bursa overlying it, is the most common cause of shoulder pain other than trauma. In rotator cuff tendinitis, also known as impingement syndrome, the rotator cuff degenerates from rubbing against the acromion and/or the acromioclavicular joint. This results in irritation of the tendons and inflammation of the normally smooth bursa that line the tendons. Symptoms include pain, swelling, and tenderness at the front of the shoulder.

Frozen Shoulder

Frozen shoulder, also called adhesive capsulitis, causes pain and stiffness in the shoulder. It is characterized by progressive pain and global loss of motion in the shoulder. Movement of the shoulder is severely restricted. Pain is usually constant, worse at night. Inflammation of the capsule restricts movement of the bones in the shoulder joint. The pathophysiology of frozen shoulder is still unclear. As the condition progresses, the stiffness may continue to the point where range of motion can be severely limited.

De Quervain's Tenosynovitis

De Quervain's tenosynovitis is a painful condition affecting the tendons on the thumb side of wrist. Tendons include the extensor pollicis brevis and the abductor pollicis longus tendons. When the tendons swell, they rub against the walls of the narrow canal they pass through. Pain at the base of the thumb and in the lower arm results from the ongoing irritation. Pain is reproduced by stretching the tendons with the thumb inside a closed fist.

Carpal Tunnel Syndrome

Carpal tunnel syndrome is caused by compression of the median nerve at the wrist. Carpal tunnel is a narrow passageway of ligament and bones at the base of your hand. It contains nerve and tendons. Carpal tunnel syndrome results in a feeling of intermittent numbness of the thumb, index, and long fingers and the radial side of the ring finger. Symptoms are often worse at night or after use of vibrating tools or great force.

Dupuytren Contracture

Dupuytren's contracture refers to a thickening of the underlying fibrous tissue beneath the skin of the palm of the hand and of the fingers. It involves the palmar fascia of the hand. The finger affected by contracture cannot be straightened completely, which can complicate everyday activities. The ring finger is affected most often.

Osteoarthrosis

Osteoarthrosis is a noninflammatory degenerative join disease. The cause of osteoarthritis is unknown. Symptoms may include degeneration of the articular cartilage, hypertrophy of bone at the margins, changes in the synovial membrane, tenderness, stiffness, locking and sometimes an effusion. It can occur in multiple joints, but the symptoms will likely only be noticeable in just one or two joints. Primary symptoms of osteoarthritis include joint pain, stiffness upon arising, and locking of the joint with continued immobility.

Stages of Rheumatoid Arthritis

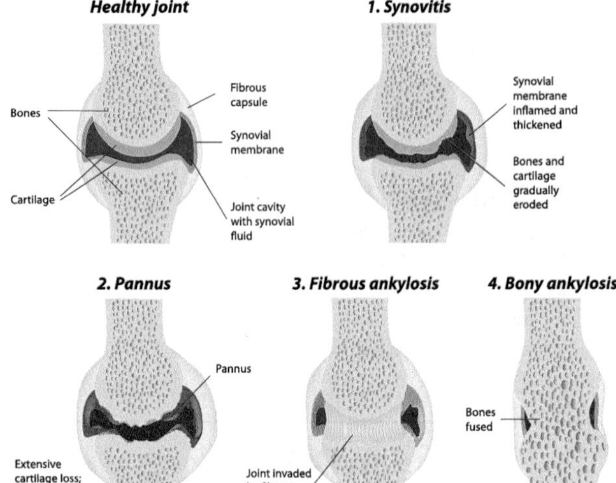

Rheumatoid arthritis

Rheumatoid arthritis is a chronic autoimmune disease that progresses over time, resulting in disability. It is characterized by pain, swelling, and inflammation in the joints and surrounding tissues. It can also affect other organs in the body. The cause of rheumatoid arthritis is not known. It can affect any joint but is common in the wrist and fingers. It can be a disabling and painful condition, which can lead to substantial loss of functioning and mobility.

Common types of Arthritis

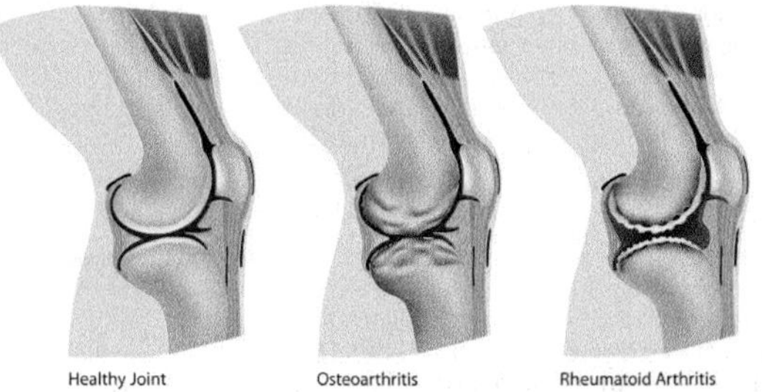

Osteoporosis

Osteoporosis is a systemic bone disease characterized as the diminishment of bone mass and damage of bone micro-structure. It is a silent disease. It causes bones to become weak and brittle. Its risk factors include aging, being female, low body weight, low sex hormones or menopause, smoking, and some medications. Hip, wrist, and spine fractures commonly result from osteoporosis.

Osteoporosis

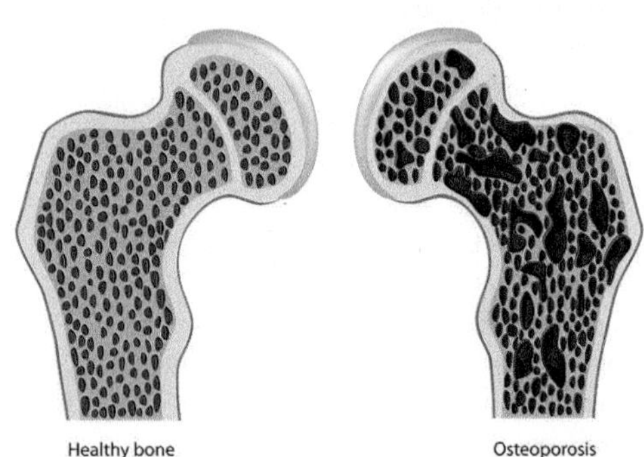

Septic Arthritis

Septic arthritis is the purulent invasion of a joint by an infectious agent which produces arthritis. Septic arthritis develops when bacteria or other tiny disease-causing microorganisms spread through the bloodstream to a joint. This inflammatory process, which is considered sterile because the skin remains unbroken, usually results from a bacterial infection in a location elsewhere in the body.

Meralgia Paresthetica

Meralgia paresthetica is a condition characterized by tingling, numbness and burning pain in the outer part of your thigh. Pain in the outer thigh is caused by injury to lateral cutaneous nerve of thigh. The nerve passes through the inguinal ligament, at its lateral end, at the level of the anterosuperior iliac spine, and becomes entrapped. It typically occurs in isolation

Diseases of the musculoskeletal system and connective tissue (M00-M99)

NOTES Use an external cause code following the code for the musculoskeletal condition, if applicable, to identify the cause of the musculoskeletal condition

EXCLUDES2 *arthropathic psoriasis (L40.5-)*
certain conditions originating in the perinatal period (P04-P96)
certain infectious and parasitic diseases (A00-B99)
compartment syndrome (traumatic) (T79.A-)
complications of pregnancy, childbirth and the puerperium (O00-O9A)
congenital malformations, deformations, and chromosomal abnormalities (Q00-Q99)
endocrine, nutritional and metabolic diseases (E00-E88)
injury, poisoning and certain other consequences of external causes (S00-T88)
neoplasms (C00-D49)
symptoms, signs and abnormal clinical and laboratory findings, not elsewhere classified (R00-R94)

This chapter contains the following blocks:

- **M00-M02** Infectious arthropathies
- **M04** Autoinflammatory syndromes
- **M05-M14** Inflammatory polyarthropathies
- **M15-M19** Osteoarthritis
- **M20-M25** Other joint disorders
- **M26-M27** Dentofacial anomalies [including malocclusion] and other disorders of jaw
- **M30-M36** Systemic connective tissue disorders
- **M40-M43** Deforming dorsopathies
- **M45-M49** Spondylopathies
- **M50-M54** Other dorsopathies
- **M60-M63** Disorders of muscles
- **M65-M67** Disorders of synovium and tendon
- **M70-M79** Other soft tissue disorders
- **M80-M85** Disorders of bone density and structure
- **M86-M90** Other osteopathies
- **M91-M94** Chondropathies
- **M95** Other disorders of the musculoskeletal system and connective tissue
- **M96** Intraoperative and postprocedural complications and disorders of musculoskeletal system, not elsewhere classified
- **M97** Periprosthetic fracture around internal prosthetic joint
- **M99** Biomechanical lesions, not elsewhere classified

Arthropathies (M00-M25)

INCLUDES *Disorders affecting predominantly peripheral (limb) joints*

Infectious arthropathies (M00-M02)

NOTES This block comprises arthropathies due to microbiological agents. Distinction is made between the following types of etiological relationship:
a) direct infection of joint, where organisms invade synovial tissue and microbial antigen is present in the joint;
b) indirect infection, which may be of two types: a reactive arthropathy, where microbial infection of the body is established but neither organisms nor antigens can be identified in the joint, and a postinfective arthropathy, where microbial antigen is present but recovery of an organism is inconstant and evidence of local multiplication is lacking.

(4) **M00 Pyogenic arthritis**

(5) **M00.0 Staphylococcal arthritis and polyarthritis**
Use additional code (B95.61-B95.8) to identify bacterial agent
EXCLUDES2 *infection and inflammatory reaction due to internal joint prosthesis (T84.5-)*

M00.00 Staphylococcal arthritis, unspecified joint
(6) **M00.01** Staphylococcal arthritis, shoulder
M00.011 Staphylococcal arthritis, right shoulder
M00.012 Staphylococcal arthritis, left shoulder
M00.019 Staphylococcal arthritis, unspecified shoulder
(6) **M00.02** Staphylococcal arthritis, elbow
M00.021 Staphylococcal arthritis, right elbow
M00.022 Staphylococcal arthritis, left elbow
M00.029 Staphylococcal arthritis, unspecified elbow
(6) **M00.03** Staphylococcal arthritis, wrist
Staphylococcal arthritis of carpal bones
M00.031 Staphylococcal arthritis, right wrist
M00.032 Staphylococcal arthritis, left wrist
M00.039 Staphylococcal arthritis, unspecified wrist
(6) **M00.04** Staphylococcal arthritis, hand
Staphylococcal arthritis of metacarpus and phalanges
M00.041 Staphylococcal arthritis, right hand
M00.042 Staphylococcal arthritis, left hand
M00.049 Staphylococcal arthritis, unspecified hand
(6) **M00.05** Staphylococcal arthritis, hip
M00.051 Staphylococcal arthritis, right hip
M00.052 Staphylococcal arthritis, left hip
M00.059 Staphylococcal arthritis, unspecified hip
(6) **M00.06** Staphylococcal arthritis, knee
M00.061 Staphylococcal arthritis, right knee
M00.062 Staphylococcal arthritis, left knee
M00.069 Staphylococcal arthritis, unspecified knee
(6) **M00.07** Staphylococcal arthritis, ankle and foot
Staphylococcal arthritis, tarsus, metatarsus and phalanges
M00.071 Staphylococcal arthritis, right ankle and foot
M00.072 Staphylococcal arthritis, left ankle and foot
M00.079 Staphylococcal arthritis, unspecified ankle and foot
M00.08 Staphylococcal arthritis, vertebrae
M00.09 Staphylococcal polyarthritis

(5) **M00.1 Pneumococcal arthritis and polyarthritis**
M00.10 Pneumococcal arthritis, unspecified joint
(6) **M00.11** Pneumococcal arthritis, shoulder
M00.111 Pneumococcal arthritis, right shoulder
M00.112 Pneumococcal arthritis, left shoulder
M00.119 Pneumococcal arthritis, unspecified shoulder
(6) **M00.12** Pneumococcal arthritis, elbow
M00.121 Pneumococcal arthritis, right elbow
M00.122 Pneumococcal arthritis, left elbow
M00.129 Pneumococcal arthritis, unspecified elbow
(6) **M00.13** Pneumococcal arthritis, wrist
Pneumococcal arthritis of carpal bones
M00.131 Pneumococcal arthritis, right wrist
M00.132 Pneumococcal arthritis, left wrist
M00.139 Pneumococcal arthritis, unspecified wrist
(6) **M00.14** Pneumococcal arthritis, hand
Pneumococcal arthritis of metacarpus and phalanges
M00.141 Pneumococcal arthritis, right hand
M00.142 Pneumococcal arthritis, left hand
M00.149 Pneumococcal arthritis, unspecified hand
(6) **M00.15** Pneumococcal arthritis, hip
M00.151 Pneumococcal arthritis, right hip
M00.152 Pneumococcal arthritis, left hip
M00.159 Pneumococcal arthritis, unspecified hip
(6) **M00.16** Pneumococcal arthritis, knee
M00.161 Pneumococcal arthritis, right knee
M00.162 Pneumococcal arthritis, left knee
M00.169 Pneumococcal arthritis, unspecified knee
(6) **M00.17** Pneumococcal arthritis, ankle and foot
Pneumococcal arthritis, tarsus, metatarsus and phalanges
M00.171 Pneumococcal arthritis, right ankle and foot

Unspecified Code Other Specified Code Manifestation Code N Newborn P Pediatric M Maternity A Adult ♂ Male ♀ Female
● New Code ▲ Revised Code Title ►◄ Revised Text NOTES INCLUDES EXCLUDES1 Not coded here EXCLUDES2 Not included here
(4) 4th character required (5) 5th character required (6) 6th character required (7) 7th character required
(7) Extension 'X' Alert HAC Hospital-acquired condition (HAC) alert AHA AHA Coding Clinic©

M00.172 Pneumococcal arthritis, left ankle and foot
M00.179 Pneumococcal arthritis, unspecified ankle and foot
M00.18 Pneumococcal arthritis, vertebrae
M00.19 Pneumococcal polyarthritis

M00.2 Other streptococcal arthritis and polyarthritis
Use additional code (B95.0-B95.2, B95.4-B95.5) to identify bacterial agent
M00.20 Other streptococcal arthritis, unspecified joint
M00.21 Other streptococcal arthritis, shoulder
M00.211 Other streptococcal arthritis, right shoulder
M00.212 Other streptococcal arthritis, left shoulder
M00.219 Other streptococcal arthritis, unspecified shoulder
M00.22 Other streptococcal arthritis, elbow
M00.221 Other streptococcal arthritis, right elbow
M00.222 Other streptococcal arthritis, left elbow
M00.229 Other streptococcal arthritis, unspecified elbow
M00.23 Other streptococcal arthritis, wrist
Other streptococcal arthritis of carpal bones
M00.231 Other streptococcal arthritis, right wrist
M00.232 Other streptococcal arthritis, left wrist
M00.239 Other streptococcal arthritis, unspecified wrist
M00.24 Other streptococcal arthritis, hand
Other streptococcal arthritis metacarpus and phalanges
M00.241 Other streptococcal arthritis, right hand
M00.242 Other streptococcal arthritis, left hand
M00.249 Other streptococcal arthritis, unspecified hand
M00.25 Other streptococcal arthritis, hip
M00.251 Other streptococcal arthritis, right hip
M00.252 Other streptococcal arthritis, left hip
M00.259 Other streptococcal arthritis, unspecified hip
M00.26 Other streptococcal arthritis, knee
M00.261 Other streptococcal arthritis, right knee
M00.262 Other streptococcal arthritis, left knee
M00.269 Other streptococcal arthritis, unspecified knee
M00.27 Other streptococcal arthritis, ankle and foot
Other streptococcal arthritis, tarsus, metatarsus and phalanges
M00.271 Other streptococcal arthritis, right ankle and foot
M00.272 Other streptococcal arthritis, left ankle and foot
M00.279 Other streptococcal arthritis, unspecified ankle and foot
M00.28 Other streptococcal arthritis, vertebrae
M00.29 Other streptococcal polyarthritis

M00.8 Arthritis and polyarthritis due to other bacteria
Use additional code (B96) to identify bacteria
M00.80 Arthritis due to other bacteria, unspecified joint
M00.81 Arthritis due to other bacteria, shoulder
M00.811 Arthritis due to other bacteria, right shoulder
M00.812 Arthritis due to other bacteria, left shoulder
M00.819 Arthritis due to other bacteria, unspecified shoulder
M00.82 Arthritis due to other bacteria, elbow
M00.821 Arthritis due to other bacteria, right elbow
M00.822 Arthritis due to other bacteria, left elbow
M00.829 Arthritis due to other bacteria, unspecified elbow
M00.83 Arthritis due to other bacteria, wrist
Arthritis due to other bacteria, carpal bones
M00.831 Arthritis due to other bacteria, right wrist
M00.832 Arthritis due to other bacteria, left wrist
M00.839 Arthritis due to other bacteria, unspecified wrist
M00.84 Arthritis due to other bacteria, hand
Arthritis due to other bacteria, metacarpus and phalanges
M00.841 Arthritis due to other bacteria, right hand
M00.842 Arthritis due to other bacteria, left hand
M00.849 Arthritis due to other bacteria, unspecified hand
M00.85 Arthritis due to other bacteria, hip
M00.851 Arthritis due to other bacteria, right hip
M00.852 Arthritis due to other bacteria, left hip
M00.859 Arthritis due to other bacteria, unspecified hip
M00.86 Arthritis due to other bacteria, knee
M00.861 Arthritis due to other bacteria, right knee
M00.862 Arthritis due to other bacteria, left knee
M00.869 Arthritis due to other bacteria, unspecified knee
M00.87 Arthritis due to other bacteria, ankle and foot
Arthritis due to other bacteria, tarsus, metatarsus, and phalanges
M00.871 Arthritis due to other bacteria, right ankle and foot
M00.872 Arthritis due to other bacteria, left ankle and foot
M00.879 Arthritis due to other bacteria, unspecified ankle and foot
M00.88 Arthritis due to other bacteria, vertebrae
M00.89 Polyarthritis due to other bacteria
M00.9 Pyogenic arthritis, unspecified
Infective arthritis NOS

M01 Direct infections of joint in infectious and parasitic diseases classified elsewhere
Code first underlying disease, such as:
leprosy [Hansen's disease] (A30.-)
mycoses (B35-B49)
O'nyong-nyong fever (A92.1)
paratyphoid fever (A01.1-A01.4)

EXCLUDES1 *arthropathy in Lyme disease (A69.23)*
gonococcal arthritis (A54.42)
meningococcal arthritis (A39.83)
mumps arthritis (B26.85)
postinfective arthropathy (M02.-)
postmeningococcal arthritis (A39.84)
reactive arthritis (M02.3)
rubella arthritis (B06.82)
sarcoidosis arthritis (D86.86)
typhoid fever arthritis (A01.04)
tuberculosis arthritis (A18.01-A18.02)

M01.X Direct infection of joint in infectious and parasitic diseases classified elsewhere
M01.X0 Direct infection of unspecified joint in infectious and parasitic diseases classified elsewhere
M01.X1 Direct infection of shoulder joint in infectious and parasitic diseases classified elsewhere
M01.X11 Direct infection of right shoulder in infectious and parasitic diseases classified elsewhere
M01.X12 Direct infection of left shoulder in infectious and parasitic diseases classified elsewhere

Unacceptable principal diagnosis symbol per Medicare code edits — Code exempt from diagnosis present on admission requirement
Questionable admission — Complication or comorbidity — CC/MCC exclusion — Major complication or comorbidity
Principal diagnosis as its own CC — Principal diagnosis as its own MCC — Z code as first-listed diagnosis

When symbols appear on a code that requires a 7th character extension, refer to Appendix D to identify applicable 7th character codes.

M01.X19 Direct infection of unspecified shoulder in infectious and parasitic diseases classified elsewhere

M01.X2 Direct infection of elbow in infectious and parasitic diseases classified elsewhere

M01.X21 Direct infection of right elbow in infectious and parasitic diseases classified elsewhere

M01.X22 Direct infection of left elbow in infectious and parasitic diseases classified elsewhere

M01.X29 Direct infection of unspecified elbow in infectious and parasitic diseases classified elsewhere

M01.X3 Direct infection of wrist in infectious and parasitic diseases classified elsewhere

Direct infection of carpal bones in infectious and parasitic diseases classified elsewhere

M01.X31 Direct infection of right wrist in infectious and parasitic diseases classified elsewhere

M01.X32 Direct infection of left wrist in infectious and parasitic diseases classified elsewhere

M01.X39 Direct infection of unspecified wrist in infectious and parasitic diseases classified elsewhere

M01.X4 Direct infection of hand in infectious and parasitic diseases classified elsewhere

Direct infection of metacarpus and phalanges in infectious and parasitic diseases classified elsewhere

M01.X41 Direct infection of right hand in infectious and parasitic diseases classified elsewhere

M01.X42 Direct infection of left hand in infectious and parasitic diseases classified elsewhere

M01.X49 Direct infection of unspecified hand in infectious and parasitic diseases classified elsewhere

M01.X5 Direct infection of hip in infectious and parasitic diseases classified elsewhere

M01.X51 Direct infection of right hip in infectious and parasitic diseases classified elsewhere

M01.X52 Direct infection of left hip in infectious and parasitic diseases classified elsewhere

M01.X59 Direct infection of unspecified hip in infectious and parasitic diseases classified elsewhere

M01.X6 Direct infection of knee in infectious and parasitic diseases classified elsewhere

M01.X61 Direct infection of right knee in infectious and parasitic diseases classified elsewhere

M01.X62 Direct infection of left knee in infectious and parasitic diseases classified elsewhere

M01.X69 Direct infection of unspecified knee in infectious and parasitic diseases classified elsewhere

M01.X7 Direct infection of ankle and foot in infectious and parasitic diseases classified elsewhere

Direct infection of tarsus, metatarsus and phalanges in infectious and parasitic diseases classified elsewhere

M01.X71 Direct infection of right ankle and foot in infectious and parasitic diseases classified elsewhere

M01.X72 Direct infection of left ankle and foot in infectious and parasitic diseases classified elsewhere

M01.X79 Direct infection of unspecified ankle and foot in infectious and parasitic diseases classified elsewhere

M01.X8 Direct infection of vertebrae in infectious and parasitic diseases classified elsewhere

M01.X9 Direct infection of multiple joints in infectious and parasitic diseases classified elsewhere

M02 Postinfective and reactive arthropathies

Code first underlying disease, such as:
congenital syphilis [Clutton's joints] (A50.5)
enteritis due to Yersinia enterocolitica (A04.6)
infective endocarditis (I33.0)
viral hepatitis (B15-B19)

EXCLUDES1 *Behçet's disease (M35.2)*
direct infections of joint in infectious and parasitic diseases classified elsewhere (M01.-)
postmeningococcal arthritis (A39.84)
mumps arthritis (B26.85)
rubella arthritis (B06.82)
syphilis arthritis (late) (A52.77)
rheumatic fever (I00)
tabetic arthropathy [Charcôt's] (A52.16)

M02.0 Arthropathy following intestinal bypass

M02.00 Arthropathy following intestinal bypass, unspecified site

M02.01 Arthropathy following intestinal bypass, shoulder

M02.011 Arthropathy following intestinal bypass, right shoulder

M02.012 Arthropathy following intestinal bypass, left shoulder

M02.019 Arthropathy following intestinal bypass, unspecified shoulder

M02.02 Arthropathy following intestinal bypass, elbow

M02.021 Arthropathy following intestinal bypass, right elbow

M02.022 Arthropathy following intestinal bypass, left elbow

M02.029 Arthropathy following intestinal bypass, unspecified elbow

M02.03 Arthropathy following intestinal bypass, wrist

Arthropathy following intestinal bypass, carpal bones

M02.031 Arthropathy following intestinal bypass, right wrist

M02.032 Arthropathy following intestinal bypass, left wrist

M02.039 Arthropathy following intestinal bypass, unspecified wrist

M02.04 Arthropathy following intestinal bypass, hand

Arthropathy following intestinal bypass, metacarpals and phalanges

M02.041 Arthropathy following intestinal bypass, right hand

M02.042 Arthropathy following intestinal bypass, left hand

M02.049 Arthropathy following intestinal bypass, unspecified hand

M02.05 Arthropathy following intestinal bypass, hip

M02.051 Arthropathy following intestinal bypass, right hip

M02.052 Arthropathy following intestinal bypass, left hip

M02.059 Arthropathy following intestinal bypass, unspecified hip

M02.06 Arthropathy following intestinal bypass, knee

M02.061 Arthropathy following intestinal bypass, right knee

M02.062 Arthropathy following intestinal bypass, left knee

M02.069 Arthropathy following intestinal bypass, unspecified knee

M02.07 Arthropathy following intestinal bypass, ankle and foot

Arthropathy following intestinal bypass, tarsus, metatarsus and phalanges

M02.071 Arthropathy following intestinal bypass, right ankle and foot

Unspecified Code Other Specified Code Manifestation Code N Newborn P Pediatric M Maternity A Adult ♂ Male ♀ Female
● New Code ▲ Revised Code Title ►◄ Revised Text NOTES INCLUDES EXCLUDES1 Not coded here EXCLUDES2 Not included here
4th character required 5th character required 6th character required 7th character required
Extension 'X' Alert HAC Hospital-acquired condition (HAC) alert AHA AHA Coding Clinic©

M02.072 Arthropathy following intestinal bypass, left ankle and foot
M02.079 Arthropathy following intestinal bypass, unspecified ankle and foot
M02.08 Arthropathy following intestinal bypass, vertebrae
M02.09 Arthropathy following intestinal bypass, multiple sites

M02.1 Postdysenteric arthropathy
M02.10 Postdysenteric arthropathy, unspecified site
M02.11 Postdysenteric arthropathy, shoulder
M02.111 Postdysenteric arthropathy, right shoulder
M02.112 Postdysenteric arthropathy, left shoulder
M02.119 Postdysenteric arthropathy, unspecified shoulder
M02.12 Postdysenteric arthropathy, elbow
M02.121 Postdysenteric arthropathy, right elbow
M02.122 Postdysenteric arthropathy, left elbow
M02.129 Postdysenteric arthropathy, unspecified elbow
M02.13 Postdysenteric arthropathy, wrist
Postdysenteric arthropathy, carpal bones
M02.131 Postdysenteric arthropathy, right wrist
M02.132 Postdysenteric arthropathy, left wrist
M02.139 Postdysenteric arthropathy, unspecified wrist
M02.14 Postdysenteric arthropathy, hand
Postdysenteric arthropathy, metacarpus and phalanges
M02.141 Postdysenteric arthropathy, right hand
M02.142 Postdysenteric arthropathy, left hand
M02.149 Postdysenteric arthropathy, unspecified hand
M02.15 Postdysenteric arthropathy, hip
M02.151 Postdysenteric arthropathy, right hip
M02.152 Postdysenteric arthropathy, left hip
M02.159 Postdysenteric arthropathy, unspecified hip
M02.16 Postdysenteric arthropathy, knee
M02.161 Postdysenteric arthropathy, right knee
M02.162 Postdysenteric arthropathy, left knee
M02.169 Postdysenteric arthropathy, unspecified knee
M02.17 Postdysenteric arthropathy, ankle and foot
Postdysenteric arthropathy, tarsus, metatarsus and phalanges
M02.171 Postdysenteric arthropathy, right ankle and foot
M02.172 Postdysenteric arthropathy, left ankle and foot
M02.179 Postdysenteric arthropathy, unspecified ankle and foot
M02.18 Postdysenteric arthropathy, vertebrae
M02.19 Postdysenteric arthropathy, multiple sites

M02.2 Postimmunization arthropathy
M02.20 Postimmunization arthropathy, unspecified site
M02.21 Postimmunization arthropathy, shoulder
M02.211 Postimmunization arthropathy, right shoulder
M02.212 Postimmunization arthropathy, left shoulder
M02.219 Postimmunization arthropathy, unspecified shoulder
M02.22 Postimmunization arthropathy, elbow
M02.221 Postimmunization arthropathy, right elbow
M02.222 Postimmunization arthropathy, left elbow
M02.229 Postimmunization arthropathy, unspecified elbow
M02.23 Postimmunization arthropathy, wrist
Postimmunization arthropathy, carpal bones
M02.231 Postimmunization arthropathy, right wrist
M02.232 Postimmunization arthropathy, left wrist
M02.239 Postimmunization arthropathy, unspecified wrist
M02.24 Postimmunization arthropathy, hand
Postimmunization arthropathy, metacarpus and phalanges
M02.241 Postimmunization arthropathy, right hand
M02.242 Postimmunization arthropathy, left hand
M02.249 Postimmunization arthropathy, unspecified hand
M02.25 Postimmunization arthropathy, hip
M02.251 Postimmunization arthropathy, right hip
M02.252 Postimmunization arthropathy, left hip
M02.259 Postimmunization arthropathy, unspecified hip
M02.26 Postimmunization arthropathy, knee
M02.261 Postimmunization arthropathy, right knee
M02.262 Postimmunization arthropathy, left knee
M02.269 Postimmunization arthropathy, unspecified knee
M02.27 Postimmunization arthropathy, ankle and foot
Postimmunization arthropathy, tarsus, metatarsus and phalanges
M02.271 Postimmunization arthropathy, right ankle and foot
M02.272 Postimmunization arthropathy, left ankle and foot
M02.279 Postimmunization arthropathy, unspecified ankle and foot
M02.28 Postimmunization arthropathy, vertebrae
M02.29 Postimmunization arthropathy, multiple sites

M02.3 Reiter's disease
Reactive arthritis
M02.30 Reiter's disease, unspecified site
M02.31 Reiter's disease, shoulder
M02.311 Reiter's disease, right shoulder
M02.312 Reiter's disease, left shoulder
M02.319 Reiter's disease, unspecified shoulder
M02.32 Reiter's disease, elbow
M02.321 Reiter's disease, right elbow
M02.322 Reiter's disease, left elbow
M02.329 Reiter's disease, unspecified elbow
M02.33 Reiter's disease, wrist
Reiter's disease, carpal bones
M02.331 Reiter's disease, right wrist
M02.332 Reiter's disease, left wrist
M02.339 Reiter's disease, unspecified wrist
M02.34 Reiter's disease, hand
Reiter's disease, metacarpus and phalanges
M02.341 Reiter's disease, right hand
M02.342 Reiter's disease, left hand
M02.349 Reiter's disease, unspecified hand
M02.35 Reiter's disease, hip
M02.351 Reiter's disease, right hip
M02.352 Reiter's disease, left hip
M02.359 Reiter's disease, unspecified hip
M02.36 Reiter's disease, knee
M02.361 Reiter's disease, right knee
M02.362 Reiter's disease, left knee
M02.369 Reiter's disease, unspecified knee
M02.37 Reiter's disease, ankle and foot
Reiter's disease, tarsus, metatarsus and phalanges
M02.371 Reiter's disease, right ankle and foot
M02.372 Reiter's disease, left ankle and foot
M02.379 Reiter's disease, unspecified ankle and foot
M02.38 Reiter's disease, vertebrae
M02.39 Reiter's disease, multiple sites

M02.8 Other reactive arthropathies
M02.80 Other reactive arthropathies, unspecified site
M02.81 Other reactive arthropathies, shoulder
M02.811 Other reactive arthropathies, right shoulder

Unacceptable principal diagnosis symbol per Medicare code edits · Code exempt from diagnosis present on admission requirement
Questionable admission · Complication or comorbidity · CC/MCC exclusion · Major complication or comorbidity
Principal diagnosis as its own CC · Principal diagnosis as its own MCC · Z code as first-listed diagnosis

M02.812 Other reactive arthropathies, left shoulder CC
M02.819 Other reactive arthropathies, unspecified shoulder CC
M02.82 Other reactive arthropathies, elbow
M02.821 Other reactive arthropathies, right elbow CC
M02.822 Other reactive arthropathies, left elbow CC
M02.829 Other reactive arthropathies, unspecified elbow CC
M02.83 Other reactive arthropathies, wrist
Other reactive arthropathies, carpal bones
M02.831 Other reactive arthropathies, right wrist CC
M02.832 Other reactive arthropathies, left wrist CC
M02.839 Other reactive arthropathies, unspecified wrist CC
M02.84 Other reactive arthropathies, hand
Other reactive arthropathies, metacarpus and phalanges
M02.841 Other reactive arthropathies, right hand CC
M02.842 Other reactive arthropathies, left hand CC
M02.849 Other reactive arthropathies, unspecified hand CC
M02.85 Other reactive arthropathies, hip
M02.851 Other reactive arthropathies, right hip CC
M02.852 Other reactive arthropathies, left hip CC
M02.859 Other reactive arthropathies, unspecified hip CC
M02.86 Other reactive arthropathies, knee
M02.861 Other reactive arthropathies, right knee CC
M02.862 Other reactive arthropathies, left knee CC
M02.869 Other reactive arthropathies, unspecified knee CC
M02.87 Other reactive arthropathies, ankle and foot
Other reactive arthropathies, tarsus, metatarsus and phalanges
M02.871 Other reactive arthropathies, right ankle and foot CC
M02.872 Other reactive arthropathies, left ankle and foot CC
M02.879 Other reactive arthropathies, unspecified ankle and foot CC
M02.88 Other reactive arthropathies, vertebrae CC
M02.89 Other reactive arthropathies, multiple sites CC
M02.9 Reactive arthropathy, unspecified

Autoinflammatory syndromes (M04)

● M04 Autoinflammatory syndromes
EXCLUDES2 Crohn's disease (K50.-)
● M04.1 Periodic fever syndromes
Familial Mediterranean fever
Hyperimmunoglobin D syndrome
Mevalonate kinase deficiency
Tumor necrosis factor receptor associated periodic syndrome [TRAPS]
● M04.2 Cryopyrin-associated periodic syndromes
Chronic infantile neurological, cutaneous and articular syndrome [CINCA]
Familial cold autoinflammatory syndrome
Familial cold urticaria
Muckle-Wells syndrome
Neonatal onset multisystemic inflammatory disorder [NOMID]
● M04.8 Other autoinflammatory syndromes
Blau syndrome
Deficiency of interleukin 1 receptor antagonist [DIRA]
Majeed syndrome
Periodic fever, aphthous stomatitis, pharyngitis, and adenopathy syndrome [PFAPA]
Pyogenic arthritis, pyoderma gangrenosum, and acne syndrome [PAPA]
● M04.9 Autoinflammatory syndrome, unspecified

Inflammatory polyarthropathies (M05-M14)

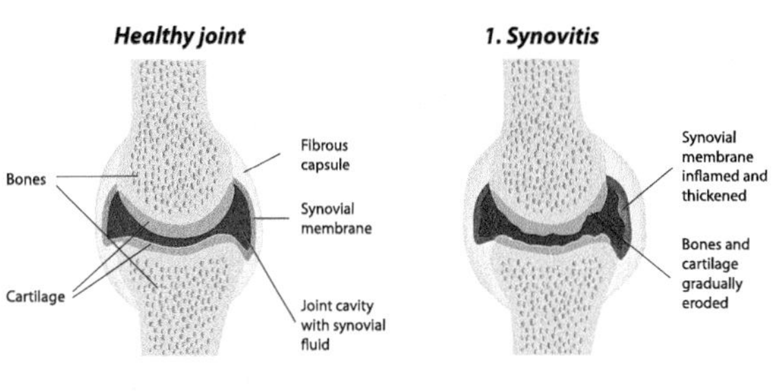

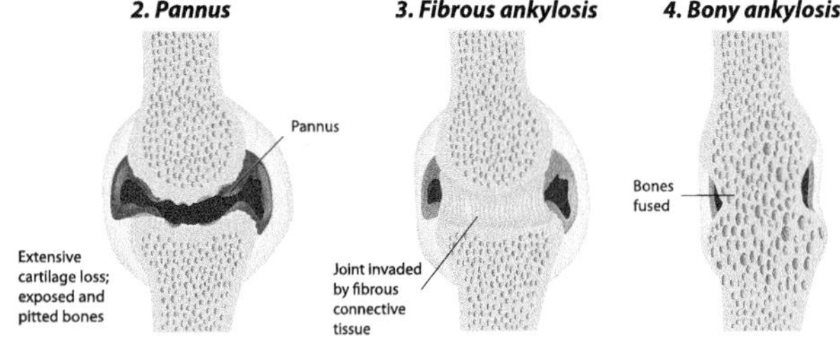

Figure 13.1 Stages of rheumatoid athritis

M05 Rheumatoid arthritis with rheumatoid factor
EXCLUDES1 *rheumatic fever (I00)*
juvenile rheumatoid arthritis (M08.-)
rheumatoid arthritis of spine (M45.-)
M05.0 Felty's syndrome
Rheumatoid arthritis with splenoadenomegaly and leukopenia
M05.00 Felty's syndrome, unspecified site
M05.01 Felty's syndrome, shoulder
M05.011 Felty's syndrome, right shoulder
M05.012 Felty's syndrome, left shoulder
M05.019 Felty's syndrome, unspecified shoulder
M05.02 Felty's syndrome, elbow
M05.021 Felty's syndrome, right elbow
M05.022 Felty's syndrome, left elbow
M05.029 Felty's syndrome, unspecified elbow
M05.03 Felty's syndrome, wrist
Felty's syndrome, carpal bones
M05.031 Felty's syndrome, right wrist
M05.032 Felty's syndrome, left wrist
M05.039 Felty's syndrome, unspecified wrist
M05.04 Felty's syndrome, hand
Felty's syndrome, metacarpus and phalanges
M05.041 Felty's syndrome, right hand
M05.042 Felty's syndrome, left hand
M05.049 Felty's syndrome, unspecified hand
M05.05 Felty's syndrome, hip
M05.051 Felty's syndrome, right hip
M05.052 Felty's syndrome, left hip
M05.059 Felty's syndrome, unspecified hip
M05.06 Felty's syndrome, knee
M05.061 Felty's syndrome, right knee
M05.062 Felty's syndrome, left knee
M05.069 Felty's syndrome, unspecified knee
M05.07 Felty's syndrome, ankle and foot
Felty's syndrome, tarsus, metatarsus and phalanges
M05.071 Felty's syndrome, right ankle and foot
M05.072 Felty's syndrome, left ankle and foot
M05.079 Felty's syndrome, unspecified ankle and foot
M05.09 Felty's syndrome, multiple sites
M05.1 Rheumatoid lung disease with rheumatoid arthritis

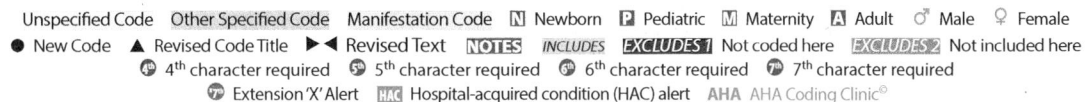

Unspecified Code Other Specified Code Manifestation Code N Newborn P Pediatric M Maternity A Adult ♂ Male ♀ Female
● New Code ▲ Revised Code Title ►◄ Revised Text NOTES INCLUDES EXCLUDES1 Not coded here EXCLUDES2 Not included here
4th character required 5th character required 6th character required 7th character required
Extension 'X' Alert HAC Hospital-acquired condition (HAC) alert AHA AHA Coding Clinic©

M05.10 Rheumatoid lung disease with rheumatoid arthritis of unspecified site

M05.11 Rheumatoid lung disease with rheumatoid arthritis of shoulder
- M05.111 Rheumatoid lung disease with rheumatoid arthritis of right shoulder
- M05.112 Rheumatoid lung disease with rheumatoid arthritis of left shoulder
- M05.119 Rheumatoid lung disease with rheumatoid arthritis of unspecified shoulder

M05.12 Rheumatoid lung disease with rheumatoid arthritis of elbow
- M05.121 Rheumatoid lung disease with rheumatoid arthritis of right elbow
- M05.122 Rheumatoid lung disease with rheumatoid arthritis of left elbow
- M05.129 Rheumatoid lung disease with rheumatoid arthritis of unspecified elbow

M05.13 Rheumatoid lung disease with rheumatoid arthritis of wrist

Rheumatoid lung disease with rheumatoid arthritis, carpal bones
- M05.131 Rheumatoid lung disease with rheumatoid arthritis of right wrist
- M05.132 Rheumatoid lung disease with rheumatoid arthritis of left wrist
- M05.139 Rheumatoid lung disease with rheumatoid arthritis of unspecified wrist

M05.14 Rheumatoid lung disease with rheumatoid arthritis of hand

Rheumatoid lung disease with rheumatoid arthritis, metacarpus and phalanges
- M05.141 Rheumatoid lung disease with rheumatoid arthritis of right hand
- M05.142 Rheumatoid lung disease with rheumatoid arthritis of left hand
- M05.149 Rheumatoid lung disease with rheumatoid arthritis of unspecified hand

M05.15 Rheumatoid lung disease with rheumatoid arthritis of hip
- M05.151 Rheumatoid lung disease with rheumatoid arthritis of right hip
- M05.152 Rheumatoid lung disease with rheumatoid arthritis of left hip
- M05.159 Rheumatoid lung disease with rheumatoid arthritis of unspecified hip

M05.16 Rheumatoid lung disease with rheumatoid arthritis of knee
- M05.161 Rheumatoid lung disease with rheumatoid arthritis of right knee
- M05.162 Rheumatoid lung disease with rheumatoid arthritis of left knee
- M05.169 Rheumatoid lung disease with rheumatoid arthritis of unspecified knee

M05.17 Rheumatoid lung disease with rheumatoid arthritis of ankle and foot

Rheumatoid lung disease with rheumatoid arthritis, tarsus, metatarsus and phalanges
- M05.171 Rheumatoid lung disease with rheumatoid arthritis of right ankle and foot
- M05.172 Rheumatoid lung disease with rheumatoid arthritis of left ankle and foot
- M05.179 Rheumatoid lung disease with rheumatoid arthritis of unspecified ankle and foot

M05.19 Rheumatoid lung disease with rheumatoid arthritis of multiple sites

M05.2 Rheumatoid vasculitis with rheumatoid arthritis

M05.20 Rheumatoid vasculitis with rheumatoid arthritis of unspecified site

M05.21 Rheumatoid vasculitis with rheumatoid arthritis of shoulder
- M05.211 Rheumatoid vasculitis with rheumatoid arthritis of right shoulder
- M05.212 Rheumatoid vasculitis with rheumatoid arthritis of left shoulder
- M05.219 Rheumatoid vasculitis with rheumatoid arthritis of unspecified shoulder

M05.22 Rheumatoid vasculitis with rheumatoid arthritis of elbow
- M05.221 Rheumatoid vasculitis with rheumatoid arthritis of right elbow
- M05.222 Rheumatoid vasculitis with rheumatoid arthritis of left elbow
- M05.229 Rheumatoid vasculitis with rheumatoid arthritis of unspecified elbow

M05.23 Rheumatoid vasculitis with rheumatoid arthritis of wrist

Rheumatoid vasculitis with rheumatoid arthritis, carpal bones
- M05.231 Rheumatoid vasculitis with rheumatoid arthritis of right wrist
- M05.232 Rheumatoid vasculitis with rheumatoid arthritis of left wrist
- M05.239 Rheumatoid vasculitis with rheumatoid arthritis of unspecified wrist

M05.24 Rheumatoid vasculitis with rheumatoid arthritis of hand

Rheumatoid vasculitis with rheumatoid arthritis, metacarpus and phalanges
- M05.241 Rheumatoid vasculitis with rheumatoid arthritis of right hand
- M05.242 Rheumatoid vasculitis with rheumatoid arthritis of left hand
- M05.249 Rheumatoid vasculitis with rheumatoid arthritis of unspecified hand

M05.25 Rheumatoid vasculitis with rheumatoid arthritis of hip
- M05.251 Rheumatoid vasculitis with rheumatoid arthritis of right hip
- M05.252 Rheumatoid vasculitis with rheumatoid arthritis of left hip
- M05.259 Rheumatoid vasculitis with rheumatoid arthritis of unspecified hip

M05.26 Rheumatoid vasculitis with rheumatoid arthritis of knee
- M05.261 Rheumatoid vasculitis with rheumatoid arthritis of right knee
- M05.262 Rheumatoid vasculitis with rheumatoid arthritis of left knee
- M05.269 Rheumatoid vasculitis with rheumatoid arthritis of unspecified knee

M05.27 Rheumatoid vasculitis with rheumatoid arthritis of ankle and foot

Rheumatoid vasculitis with rheumatoid arthritis, tarsus, metatarsus and phalanges
- M05.271 Rheumatoid vasculitis with rheumatoid arthritis of right ankle and foot
- M05.272 Rheumatoid vasculitis with rheumatoid arthritis of left ankle and foot
- M05.279 Rheumatoid vasculitis with rheumatoid arthritis of unspecified ankle and foot

M05.29 Rheumatoid vasculitis with rheumatoid arthritis of multiple sites

M05.3 Rheumatoid heart disease with rheumatoid arthritis

Rheumatoid carditis
Rheumatoid endocarditis
Rheumatoid myocarditis
Rheumatoid pericarditis

M05.30 Rheumatoid heart disease with rheumatoid arthritis of unspecified site

M05.31 Rheumatoid heart disease with rheumatoid arthritis of shoulder
- M05.311 Rheumatoid heart disease with rheumatoid arthritis of right shoulder
- M05.312 Rheumatoid heart disease with rheumatoid arthritis of left shoulder
- M05.319 Rheumatoid heart disease with rheumatoid arthritis of unspecified shoulder

Unacceptable principal diagnosis symbol per Medicare code edits · Code exempt from diagnosis present on admission requirement · Questionable admission · Complication or comorbidity · CC/MCC exclusion · Major complication or comorbidity · Principal diagnosis as its own CC · Principal diagnosis as its own MCC · Z code as first-listed diagnosis

When symbols appear on a code that requires a 7th character extension, refer to Appendix D to identify applicable 7th character codes.

M05.32 Rheumatoid heart disease with rheumatoid arthritis of elbow
M05.321 Rheumatoid heart disease with rheumatoid arthritis of right elbow
M05.322 Rheumatoid heart disease with rheumatoid arthritis of left elbow
M05.329 Rheumatoid heart disease with rheumatoid arthritis of unspecified elbow

M05.33 Rheumatoid heart disease with rheumatoid arthritis of wrist
Rheumatoid heart disease with rheumatoid arthritis, carpal bones
M05.331 Rheumatoid heart disease with rheumatoid arthritis of right wrist
M05.332 Rheumatoid heart disease with rheumatoid arthritis of left wrist
M05.339 Rheumatoid heart disease with rheumatoid arthritis of unspecified wrist

M05.34 Rheumatoid heart disease with rheumatoid arthritis of hand
Rheumatoid heart disease with rheumatoid arthritis, metacarpus and phalanges
M05.341 Rheumatoid heart disease with rheumatoid arthritis of right hand
M05.342 Rheumatoid heart disease with rheumatoid arthritis of left hand
M05.349 Rheumatoid heart disease with rheumatoid arthritis of unspecified hand

M05.35 Rheumatoid heart disease with rheumatoid arthritis of hip
M05.351 Rheumatoid heart disease with rheumatoid arthritis of right hip
M05.352 Rheumatoid heart disease with rheumatoid arthritis of left hip
M05.359 Rheumatoid heart disease with rheumatoid arthritis of unspecified hip

M05.36 Rheumatoid heart disease with rheumatoid arthritis of knee
M05.361 Rheumatoid heart disease with rheumatoid arthritis of right knee
M05.362 Rheumatoid heart disease with rheumatoid arthritis of left knee
M05.369 Rheumatoid heart disease with rheumatoid arthritis of unspecified knee

M05.37 Rheumatoid heart disease with rheumatoid arthritis of ankle and foot
Rheumatoid heart disease with rheumatoid arthritis, tarsus, metatarsus and phalanges
M05.371 Rheumatoid heart disease with rheumatoid arthritis of right ankle and foot
M05.372 Rheumatoid heart disease with rheumatoid arthritis of left ankle and foot
M05.379 Rheumatoid heart disease with rheumatoid arthritis of unspecified ankle and foot

M05.39 Rheumatoid heart disease with rheumatoid arthritis of multiple sites

M05.4 Rheumatoid myopathy with rheumatoid arthritis
M05.40 Rheumatoid myopathy with rheumatoid arthritis of unspecified site

M05.41 Rheumatoid myopathy with rheumatoid arthritis of shoulder
M05.411 Rheumatoid myopathy with rheumatoid arthritis of right shoulder
M05.412 Rheumatoid myopathy with rheumatoid arthritis of left shoulder
M05.419 Rheumatoid myopathy with rheumatoid arthritis of unspecified shoulder

M05.42 Rheumatoid myopathy with rheumatoid arthritis of elbow
M05.421 Rheumatoid myopathy with rheumatoid arthritis of right elbow
M05.422 Rheumatoid myopathy with rheumatoid arthritis of left elbow
M05.429 Rheumatoid myopathy with rheumatoid arthritis of unspecified elbow

M05.43 Rheumatoid myopathy with rheumatoid arthritis of wrist
Rheumatoid myopathy with rheumatoid arthritis, carpal bones
M05.431 Rheumatoid myopathy with rheumatoid arthritis of right wrist
M05.432 Rheumatoid myopathy with rheumatoid arthritis of left wrist
M05.439 Rheumatoid myopathy with rheumatoid arthritis of unspecified wrist

M05.44 Rheumatoid myopathy with rheumatoid arthritis of hand
Rheumatoid myopathy with rheumatoid arthritis, metacarpus and phalanges
M05.441 Rheumatoid myopathy with rheumatoid arthritis of right hand
M05.442 Rheumatoid myopathy with rheumatoid arthritis of left hand
M05.449 Rheumatoid myopathy with rheumatoid arthritis of unspecified hand

M05.45 Rheumatoid myopathy with rheumatoid arthritis of hip
M05.451 Rheumatoid myopathy with rheumatoid arthritis of right hip
M05.452 Rheumatoid myopathy with rheumatoid arthritis of left hip
M05.459 Rheumatoid myopathy with rheumatoid arthritis of unspecified hip

M05.46 Rheumatoid myopathy with rheumatoid arthritis of knee
M05.461 Rheumatoid myopathy with rheumatoid arthritis of right knee
M05.462 Rheumatoid myopathy with rheumatoid arthritis of left knee
M05.469 Rheumatoid myopathy with rheumatoid arthritis of unspecified knee

M05.47 Rheumatoid myopathy with rheumatoid arthritis of ankle and foot
Rheumatoid myopathy with rheumatoid arthritis, tarsus, metatarsus and phalanges
M05.471 Rheumatoid myopathy with rheumatoid arthritis of right ankle and foot
M05.472 Rheumatoid myopathy with rheumatoid arthritis of left ankle and foot
M05.479 Rheumatoid myopathy with rheumatoid arthritis of unspecified ankle and foot

M05.49 Rheumatoid myopathy with rheumatoid arthritis of multiple sites

M05.5 Rheumatoid polyneuropathy with rheumatoid arthritis
M05.50 Rheumatoid polyneuropathy with rheumatoid arthritis of unspecified site

M05.51 Rheumatoid polyneuropathy with rheumatoid arthritis of shoulder
M05.511 Rheumatoid polyneuropathy with rheumatoid arthritis of right shoulder
M05.512 Rheumatoid polyneuropathy with rheumatoid arthritis of left shoulder
M05.519 Rheumatoid polyneuropathy with rheumatoid arthritis of unspecified shoulder

M05.52 Rheumatoid polyneuropathy with rheumatoid arthritis of elbow
M05.521 Rheumatoid polyneuropathy with rheumatoid arthritis of right elbow
M05.522 Rheumatoid polyneuropathy with rheumatoid arthritis of left elbow
M05.529 Rheumatoid polyneuropathy with rheumatoid arthritis of unspecified elbow

M05.53 Rheumatoid polyneuropathy with rheumatoid arthritis of wrist
Rheumatoid polyneuropathy with rheumatoid arthritis, carpal bones
M05.531 Rheumatoid polyneuropathy with rheumatoid arthritis of right wrist
M05.532 Rheumatoid polyneuropathy with rheumatoid arthritis of left wrist

Unspecified Code Other Specified Code Manifestation Code N Newborn P Pediatric M Maternity A Adult ♂ Male ♀ Female
● New Code ▲ Revised Code Title ►◄ Revised Text NOTES INCLUDES EXCLUDES1 Not coded here EXCLUDES2 Not included here
4th character required 5th character required 6th character required 7th character required
Extension 'X' Alert HAC Hospital-acquired condition (HAC) alert AHA AHA Coding Clinic©

M05.539 Rheumatoid polyneuropathy with rheumatoid arthritis of unspecified wrist

M05.54 Rheumatoid polyneuropathy with rheumatoid arthritis of hand
Rheumatoid polyneuropathy with rheumatoid arthritis, metacarpus and phalanges
M05.541 Rheumatoid polyneuropathy with rheumatoid arthritis of right hand
M05.542 Rheumatoid polyneuropathy with rheumatoid arthritis of left hand
M05.549 Rheumatoid polyneuropathy with rheumatoid arthritis of unspecified hand

M05.55 Rheumatoid polyneuropathy with rheumatoid arthritis of hip
M05.551 Rheumatoid polyneuropathy with rheumatoid arthritis of right hip
M05.552 Rheumatoid polyneuropathy with rheumatoid arthritis of left hip
M05.559 Rheumatoid polyneuropathy with rheumatoid arthritis of unspecified hip

M05.56 Rheumatoid polyneuropathy with rheumatoid arthritis of knee
M05.561 Rheumatoid polyneuropathy with rheumatoid arthritis of right knee
M05.562 Rheumatoid polyneuropathy with rheumatoid arthritis of left knee
M05.569 Rheumatoid polyneuropathy with rheumatoid arthritis of unspecified knee

M05.57 Rheumatoid polyneuropathy with rheumatoid arthritis of ankle and foot
Rheumatoid polyneuropathy with rheumatoid arthritis, tarsus, metatarsus and phalanges
M05.571 Rheumatoid polyneuropathy with rheumatoid arthritis of right ankle and foot
M05.572 Rheumatoid polyneuropathy with rheumatoid arthritis of left ankle and foot
M05.579 Rheumatoid polyneuropathy with rheumatoid arthritis of unspecified ankle and foot

M05.59 Rheumatoid polyneuropathy with rheumatoid arthritis of multiple sites

M05.6 Rheumatoid arthritis with involvement of other organs and systems

M05.60 Rheumatoid arthritis of unspecified site with involvement of other organs and systems

M05.61 Rheumatoid arthritis of shoulder with involvement of other organs and systems
M05.611 Rheumatoid arthritis of right shoulder with involvement of other organs and systems
M05.612 Rheumatoid arthritis of left shoulder with involvement of other organs and systems
M05.619 Rheumatoid arthritis of unspecified shoulder with involvement of other organs and systems

M05.62 Rheumatoid arthritis of elbow with involvement of other organs and systems
M05.621 Rheumatoid arthritis of right elbow with involvement of other organs and systems
M05.622 Rheumatoid arthritis of left elbow with involvement of other organs and systems
M05.629 Rheumatoid arthritis of unspecified elbow with involvement of other organs and systems

M05.63 Rheumatoid arthritis of wrist with involvement of other organs and systems
Rheumatoid arthritis of carpal bones with involvement of other organs and systems
M05.631 Rheumatoid arthritis of right wrist with involvement of other organs and systems
M05.632 Rheumatoid arthritis of left wrist with involvement of other organs and systems
M05.639 Rheumatoid arthritis of unspecified wrist with involvement of other organs and systems

M05.64 Rheumatoid arthritis of hand with involvement of other organs and systems
Rheumatoid arthritis of metacarpus and phalanges with involvement of other organs and systems
M05.641 Rheumatoid arthritis of right hand with involvement of other organs and systems
M05.642 Rheumatoid arthritis of left hand with involvement of other organs and systems
M05.649 Rheumatoid arthritis of unspecified hand with involvement of other organs and systems

M05.65 Rheumatoid arthritis of hip with involvement of other organs and systems
M05.651 Rheumatoid arthritis of right hip with involvement of other organs and systems
M05.652 Rheumatoid arthritis of left hip with involvement of other organs and systems
M05.659 Rheumatoid arthritis of unspecified hip with involvement of other organs and systems

M05.66 Rheumatoid arthritis of knee with involvement of other organs and systems
M05.661 Rheumatoid arthritis of right knee with involvement of other organs and systems
M05.662 Rheumatoid arthritis of left knee with involvement of other organs and systems
M05.669 Rheumatoid arthritis of unspecified knee with involvement of other organs and systems

M05.67 Rheumatoid arthritis of ankle and foot with involvement of other organs and systems
Rheumatoid arthritis of tarsus, metatarsus and phalanges with involvement of other organs and systems
M05.671 Rheumatoid arthritis of right ankle and foot with involvement of other organs and systems
M05.672 Rheumatoid arthritis of left ankle and foot with involvement of other organs and systems
M05.679 Rheumatoid arthritis of unspecified ankle and foot with involvement of other organs and systems

M05.69 Rheumatoid arthritis of multiple sites with involvement of other organs and systems

M05.7 Rheumatoid arthritis with rheumatoid factor without organ or systems involvement

M05.70 Rheumatoid arthritis with rheumatoid factor of unspecified site without organ or systems involvement

M05.71 Rheumatoid arthritis with rheumatoid factor of shoulder without organ or systems involvement
M05.711 Rheumatoid arthritis with rheumatoid factor of right shoulder without organ or systems involvement
M05.712 Rheumatoid arthritis with rheumatoid factor of left shoulder without organ or systems involvement
M05.719 Rheumatoid arthritis with rheumatoid factor of unspecified shoulder without organ or systems involvement

M05.72 Rheumatoid arthritis with rheumatoid factor of elbow without organ or systems involvement
M05.721 Rheumatoid arthritis with rheumatoid factor of right elbow without organ or systems involvement
M05.722 Rheumatoid arthritis with rheumatoid factor of left elbow without organ or systems involvement
M05.729 Rheumatoid arthritis with rheumatoid factor of unspecified elbow without organ or systems involvement

M05.73 Rheumatoid arthritis with rheumatoid factor of wrist without organ or systems involvement
M05.731 Rheumatoid arthritis with rheumatoid factor of right wrist without organ or systems involvement

Unacceptable principal diagnosis symbol per Medicare code edits · Code exempt from diagnosis present on admission requirement
Questionable admission · Complication or comorbidity · CC/MCC exclusion · Major complication or comorbidity
Principal diagnosis as its own CC · Principal diagnosis as its own MCC · Z code as first-listed diagnosis

When symbols appear on a code that requires a 7th character extension, refer to Appendix D to identify applicable 7th character codes.

M05.732 Rheumatoid arthritis with rheumatoid factor of left wrist without organ or systems involvement
M05.739 Rheumatoid arthritis with rheumatoid factor of unspecified wrist without organ or systems involvement
M05.74 Rheumatoid arthritis with rheumatoid factor of hand without organ or systems involvement
M05.741 Rheumatoid arthritis with rheumatoid factor of right hand without organ or systems involvement
M05.742 Rheumatoid arthritis with rheumatoid factor of left hand without organ or systems involvement
M05.749 Rheumatoid arthritis with rheumatoid factor of unspecified hand without organ or systems involvement
M05.75 Rheumatoid arthritis with rheumatoid factor of hip without organ or systems involvement
M05.751 Rheumatoid arthritis with rheumatoid factor of right hip without organ or systems involvement
M05.752 Rheumatoid arthritis with rheumatoid factor of left hip without organ or systems involvement
M05.759 Rheumatoid arthritis with rheumatoid factor of unspecified hip without organ or systems involvement
M05.76 Rheumatoid arthritis with rheumatoid factor of knee without organ or systems involvement
M05.761 Rheumatoid arthritis with rheumatoid factor of right knee without organ or systems involvement
M05.762 Rheumatoid arthritis with rheumatoid factor of left knee without organ or systems involvement
M05.769 Rheumatoid arthritis with rheumatoid factor of unspecified knee without organ or systems involvement
M05.77 Rheumatoid arthritis with rheumatoid factor of ankle and foot without organ or systems involvement
M05.771 Rheumatoid arthritis with rheumatoid factor of right ankle and foot without organ or systems involvement
M05.772 Rheumatoid arthritis with rheumatoid factor of left ankle and foot without organ or systems involvement
M05.779 Rheumatoid arthritis with rheumatoid factor of unspecified ankle and foot without organ or systems involvement
M05.79 Rheumatoid arthritis with rheumatoid factor of multiple sites without organ or systems involvement
M05.8 Other rheumatoid arthritis with rheumatoid factor
M05.80 Other rheumatoid arthritis with rheumatoid factor of unspecified site
M05.81 Other rheumatoid arthritis with rheumatoid factor of shoulder
M05.811 Other rheumatoid arthritis with rheumatoid factor of right shoulder
M05.812 Other rheumatoid arthritis with rheumatoid factor of left shoulder
M05.819 Other rheumatoid arthritis with rheumatoid factor of unspecified shoulder
M05.82 Other rheumatoid arthritis with rheumatoid factor of elbow
M05.821 Other rheumatoid arthritis with rheumatoid factor of right elbow
M05.822 Other rheumatoid arthritis with rheumatoid factor of left elbow
M05.829 Other rheumatoid arthritis with rheumatoid factor of unspecified elbow
M05.83 Other rheumatoid arthritis with rheumatoid factor of wrist
M05.831 Other rheumatoid arthritis with rheumatoid factor of right wrist
M05.832 Other rheumatoid arthritis with rheumatoid factor of left wrist
M05.839 Other rheumatoid arthritis with rheumatoid factor of unspecified wrist
M05.84 Other rheumatoid arthritis with rheumatoid factor of hand
M05.841 Other rheumatoid arthritis with rheumatoid factor of right hand
M05.842 Other rheumatoid arthritis with rheumatoid factor of left hand
M05.849 Other rheumatoid arthritis with rheumatoid factor of unspecified hand
M05.85 Other rheumatoid arthritis with rheumatoid factor of hip
M05.851 Other rheumatoid arthritis with rheumatoid factor of right hip
M05.852 Other rheumatoid arthritis with rheumatoid factor of left hip
M05.859 Other rheumatoid arthritis with rheumatoid factor of unspecified hip
M05.86 Other rheumatoid arthritis with rheumatoid factor of knee
M05.861 Other rheumatoid arthritis with rheumatoid factor of right knee
M05.862 Other rheumatoid arthritis with rheumatoid factor of left knee
M05.869 Other rheumatoid arthritis with rheumatoid factor of unspecified knee
M05.87 Other rheumatoid arthritis with rheumatoid factor of ankle and foot
M05.871 Other rheumatoid arthritis with rheumatoid factor of right ankle and foot
M05.872 Other rheumatoid arthritis with rheumatoid factor of left ankle and foot
M05.879 Other rheumatoid arthritis with rheumatoid factor of unspecified ankle and foot
M05.89 Other rheumatoid arthritis with rheumatoid factor of multiple sites
M05.9 Rheumatoid arthritis with rheumatoid factor, unspecified
M06 Other rheumatoid arthritis
M06.0 Rheumatoid arthritis without rheumatoid factor
M06.00 Rheumatoid arthritis without rheumatoid factor, unspecified site
M06.01 Rheumatoid arthritis without rheumatoid factor, shoulder
M06.011 Rheumatoid arthritis without rheumatoid factor, right shoulder
M06.012 Rheumatoid arthritis without rheumatoid factor, left shoulder
M06.019 Rheumatoid arthritis without rheumatoid factor, unspecified shoulder
M06.02 Rheumatoid arthritis without rheumatoid factor, elbow
M06.021 Rheumatoid arthritis without rheumatoid factor, right elbow
M06.022 Rheumatoid arthritis without rheumatoid factor, left elbow
M06.029 Rheumatoid arthritis without rheumatoid factor, unspecified elbow
M06.03 Rheumatoid arthritis without rheumatoid factor, wrist
M06.031 Rheumatoid arthritis without rheumatoid factor, right wrist
M06.032 Rheumatoid arthritis without rheumatoid factor, left wrist
M06.039 Rheumatoid arthritis without rheumatoid factor, unspecified wrist
M06.04 Rheumatoid arthritis without rheumatoid factor, hand
M06.041 Rheumatoid arthritis without rheumatoid factor, right hand
M06.042 Rheumatoid arthritis without rheumatoid factor, left hand
M06.049 Rheumatoid arthritis without rheumatoid factor, unspecified hand

Unspecified Code Other Specified Code Manifestation Code N Newborn P Pediatric M Maternity A Adult ♂ Male ♀ Female
● New Code ▲ Revised Code Title ►◄ Revised Text NOTES INCLUDES EXCLUDES1 Not coded here EXCLUDES2 Not included here
4th character required 5th character required 6th character required 7th character required
Extension 'X' Alert HAC Hospital-acquired condition (HAC) alert AHA AHA Coding Clinic©

M06.05 Rheumatoid arthritis without rheumatoid factor, hip
M06.051 Rheumatoid arthritis without rheumatoid factor, right hip
M06.052 Rheumatoid arthritis without rheumatoid factor, left hip
M06.059 Rheumatoid arthritis without rheumatoid factor, unspecified hip
M06.06 Rheumatoid arthritis without rheumatoid factor, knee
M06.061 Rheumatoid arthritis without rheumatoid factor, right knee
M06.062 Rheumatoid arthritis without rheumatoid factor, left knee
M06.069 Rheumatoid arthritis without rheumatoid factor, unspecified knee
M06.07 Rheumatoid arthritis without rheumatoid factor, ankle and foot
M06.071 Rheumatoid arthritis without rheumatoid factor, right ankle and foot
M06.072 Rheumatoid arthritis without rheumatoid factor, left ankle and foot
M06.079 Rheumatoid arthritis without rheumatoid factor, unspecified ankle and foot
M06.08 Rheumatoid arthritis without rheumatoid factor, vertebrae
M06.09 Rheumatoid arthritis without rheumatoid factor, multiple sites
M06.1 Adult-onset Still's disease A
EXCLUDES1 *Still's disease NOS (M08.2-)*
M06.2 Rheumatoid bursitis
M06.20 Rheumatoid bursitis, unspecified site
M06.21 Rheumatoid bursitis, shoulder
M06.211 Rheumatoid bursitis, right shoulder
M06.212 Rheumatoid bursitis, left shoulder
M06.219 Rheumatoid bursitis, unspecified shoulder
M06.22 Rheumatoid bursitis, elbow
M06.221 Rheumatoid bursitis, right elbow
M06.222 Rheumatoid bursitis, left elbow
M06.229 Rheumatoid bursitis, unspecified elbow
M06.23 Rheumatoid bursitis, wrist
M06.231 Rheumatoid bursitis, right wrist
M06.232 Rheumatoid bursitis, left wrist
M06.239 Rheumatoid bursitis, unspecified wrist
M06.24 Rheumatoid bursitis, hand
M06.241 Rheumatoid bursitis, right hand
M06.242 Rheumatoid bursitis, left hand
M06.249 Rheumatoid bursitis, unspecified hand
M06.25 Rheumatoid bursitis, hip
M06.251 Rheumatoid bursitis, right hip
M06.252 Rheumatoid bursitis, left hip
M06.259 Rheumatoid bursitis, unspecified hip
M06.26 Rheumatoid bursitis, knee
M06.261 Rheumatoid bursitis, right knee
M06.262 Rheumatoid bursitis, left knee
M06.269 Rheumatoid bursitis, unspecified knee
M06.27 Rheumatoid bursitis, ankle and foot
M06.271 Rheumatoid bursitis, right ankle and foot
M06.272 Rheumatoid bursitis, left ankle and foot
M06.279 Rheumatoid bursitis, unspecified ankle and foot
M06.28 Rheumatoid bursitis, vertebrae
M06.29 Rheumatoid bursitis, multiple sites
M06.3 Rheumatoid nodule
M06.30 Rheumatoid nodule, unspecified site
M06.31 Rheumatoid nodule, shoulder
M06.311 Rheumatoid nodule, right shoulder
M06.312 Rheumatoid nodule, left shoulder
M06.319 Rheumatoid nodule, unspecified shoulder
M06.32 Rheumatoid nodule, elbow
M06.321 Rheumatoid nodule, right elbow
M06.322 Rheumatoid nodule, left elbow
M06.329 Rheumatoid nodule, unspecified elbow
M06.33 Rheumatoid nodule, wrist
M06.331 Rheumatoid nodule, right wrist
M06.332 Rheumatoid nodule, left wrist
M06.339 Rheumatoid nodule, unspecified wrist
M06.34 Rheumatoid nodule, hand
M06.341 Rheumatoid nodule, right hand
M06.342 Rheumatoid nodule, left hand
M06.349 Rheumatoid nodule, unspecified hand
M06.35 Rheumatoid nodule, hip
M06.351 Rheumatoid nodule, right hip
M06.352 Rheumatoid nodule, left hip
M06.359 Rheumatoid nodule, unspecified hip
M06.36 Rheumatoid nodule, knee
M06.361 Rheumatoid nodule, right knee
M06.362 Rheumatoid nodule, left knee
M06.369 Rheumatoid nodule, unspecified knee
M06.37 Rheumatoid nodule, ankle and foot
M06.371 Rheumatoid nodule, right ankle and foot
M06.372 Rheumatoid nodule, left ankle and foot
M06.379 Rheumatoid nodule, unspecified ankle and foot
M06.38 Rheumatoid nodule, vertebrae
M06.39 Rheumatoid nodule, multiple sites
M06.4 Inflammatory polyarthropathy
EXCLUDES1 *polyarthritis NOS (M13.0)*
M06.8 Other specified rheumatoid arthritis
M06.80 Other specified rheumatoid arthritis, unspecified site
M06.81 Other specified rheumatoid arthritis, shoulder
M06.811 Other specified rheumatoid arthritis, right shoulder
M06.812 Other specified rheumatoid arthritis, left shoulder
M06.819 Other specified rheumatoid arthritis, unspecified shoulder
M06.82 Other specified rheumatoid arthritis, elbow
M06.821 Other specified rheumatoid arthritis, right elbow
M06.822 Other specified rheumatoid arthritis, left elbow
M06.829 Other specified rheumatoid arthritis, unspecified elbow
M06.83 Other specified rheumatoid arthritis, wrist
M06.831 Other specified rheumatoid arthritis, right wrist
M06.832 Other specified rheumatoid arthritis, left wrist
M06.839 Other specified rheumatoid arthritis, unspecified wrist
M06.84 Other specified rheumatoid arthritis, hand
M06.841 Other specified rheumatoid arthritis, right hand
M06.842 Other specified rheumatoid arthritis, left hand
M06.849 Other specified rheumatoid arthritis, unspecified hand
M06.85 Other specified rheumatoid arthritis, hip
M06.851 Other specified rheumatoid arthritis, right hip
M06.852 Other specified rheumatoid arthritis, left hip
M06.859 Other specified rheumatoid arthritis, unspecified hip
M06.86 Other specified rheumatoid arthritis, knee
M06.861 Other specified rheumatoid arthritis, right knee
M06.862 Other specified rheumatoid arthritis, left knee
M06.869 Other specified rheumatoid arthritis, unspecified knee
M06.87 Other specified rheumatoid arthritis, ankle and foot
M06.871 Other specified rheumatoid arthritis, right ankle and foot
M06.872 Other specified rheumatoid arthritis, left ankle and foot

Unacceptable principal diagnosis symbol per Medicare code edits — Code exempt from diagnosis present on admission requirement
Questionable admission — Complication or comorbidity — CC/MCC exclusion — Major complication or comorbidity
Principal diagnosis as its own CC — Principal diagnosis as its own MCC — Z code as first-listed diagnosis

 When symbols appear on a code that requires a 7th character extension, refer to Appendix D to identify applicable 7th character codes.

M06.879 Other specified rheumatoid arthritis, unspecified ankle and foot
M06.88 Other specified rheumatoid arthritis, vertebrae
M06.89 Other specified rheumatoid arthritis, multiple sites
M06.9 Rheumatoid arthritis, unspecified

M07 Enteropathic arthropathies
Code also associated enteropathy, such as:
regional enteritis [Crohn's disease] (K50.-)
ulcerative colitis (K51.-)
EXCLUDES1 *psoriatic arthropathies (L40.5-)*

M07.6 Enteropathic arthropathies
M07.60 Enteropathic arthropathies, unspecified site
M07.61 Enteropathic arthropathies, shoulder
M07.611 Enteropathic arthropathies, right shoulder
M07.612 Enteropathic arthropathies, left shoulder
M07.619 Enteropathic arthropathies, unspecified shoulder
M07.62 Enteropathic arthropathies, elbow
M07.621 Enteropathic arthropathies, right elbow
M07.622 Enteropathic arthropathies, left elbow
M07.629 Enteropathic arthropathies, unspecified elbow
M07.63 Enteropathic arthropathies, wrist
M07.631 Enteropathic arthropathies, right wrist
M07.632 Enteropathic arthropathies, left wrist
M07.639 Enteropathic arthropathies, unspecified wrist
M07.64 Enteropathic arthropathies, hand
M07.641 Enteropathic arthropathies, right hand
M07.642 Enteropathic arthropathies, left hand
M07.649 Enteropathic arthropathies, unspecified hand
M07.65 Enteropathic arthropathies, hip
M07.651 Enteropathic arthropathies, right hip
M07.652 Enteropathic arthropathies, left hip
M07.659 Enteropathic arthropathies, unspecified hip
M07.66 Enteropathic arthropathies, knee
M07.661 Enteropathic arthropathies, right knee
M07.662 Enteropathic arthropathies, left knee
M07.669 Enteropathic arthropathies, unspecified knee
M07.67 Enteropathic arthropathies, ankle and foot
M07.671 Enteropathic arthropathies, right ankle and foot
M07.672 Enteropathic arthropathies, left ankle and foot
M07.679 Enteropathic arthropathies, unspecified ankle and foot
M07.68 Enteropathic arthropathies, vertebrae
M07.69 Enteropathic arthropathies, multiple sites

M08 Juvenile arthritis
Code also any associated underlying condition, such as:
regional enteritis [Crohn's disease] (K50.-)
ulcerative colitis (K51.-)
EXCLUDES1 *arthropathy in Whipple's disease (M14.8)*
Felty's syndrome (M05.0)
juvenile dermatomyositis (M33.0-)
psoriatic juvenile arthropathy (L40.54)

M08.0 Unspecified juvenile rheumatoid arthritis
Juvenile rheumatoid arthritis with or without rheumatoid factor
M08.00 Unspecified juvenile rheumatoid arthritis of unspecified site
M08.01 Unspecified juvenile rheumatoid arthritis, shoulder
M08.011 Unspecified juvenile rheumatoid arthritis, right shoulder
M08.012 Unspecified juvenile rheumatoid arthritis, left shoulder
M08.019 Unspecified juvenile rheumatoid arthritis, unspecified shoulder
M08.02 Unspecified juvenile rheumatoid arthritis of elbow
M08.021 Unspecified juvenile rheumatoid arthritis, right elbow
M08.022 Unspecified juvenile rheumatoid arthritis, left elbow
M08.029 Unspecified juvenile rheumatoid arthritis, unspecified elbow
M08.03 Unspecified juvenile rheumatoid arthritis, wrist
M08.031 Unspecified juvenile rheumatoid arthritis, right wrist
M08.032 Unspecified juvenile rheumatoid arthritis, left wrist
M08.039 Unspecified juvenile rheumatoid arthritis, unspecified wrist
M08.04 Unspecified juvenile rheumatoid arthritis, hand
M08.041 Unspecified juvenile rheumatoid arthritis, right hand
M08.042 Unspecified juvenile rheumatoid arthritis, left hand
M08.049 Unspecified juvenile rheumatoid arthritis, unspecified hand
M08.05 Unspecified juvenile rheumatoid arthritis, hip
M08.051 Unspecified juvenile rheumatoid arthritis, right hip
M08.052 Unspecified juvenile rheumatoid arthritis, left hip
M08.059 Unspecified juvenile rheumatoid arthritis, unspecified hip
M08.06 Unspecified juvenile rheumatoid arthritis, knee
M08.061 Unspecified juvenile rheumatoid arthritis, right knee
M08.062 Unspecified juvenile rheumatoid arthritis, left knee
M08.069 Unspecified juvenile rheumatoid arthritis, unspecified knee
M08.07 Unspecified juvenile rheumatoid arthritis, ankle and foot
M08.071 Unspecified juvenile rheumatoid arthritis, right ankle and foot
M08.072 Unspecified juvenile rheumatoid arthritis, left ankle and foot
M08.079 Unspecified juvenile rheumatoid arthritis, unspecified ankle and foot
M08.08 Unspecified juvenile rheumatoid arthritis, vertebrae
M08.09 Unspecified juvenile rheumatoid arthritis, multiple sites

M08.1 Juvenile ankylosing spondylitis
EXCLUDES1 *ankylosing spondylitis in adults (M45.0-)*

M08.2 Juvenile rheumatoid arthritis with systemic onset
Still's disease NOS
EXCLUDES1 *adult-onset Still's disease (M06.1-)*
M08.20 Juvenile rheumatoid arthritis with systemic onset, unspecified site
M08.21 Juvenile rheumatoid arthritis with systemic onset, shoulder
M08.211 Juvenile rheumatoid arthritis with systemic onset, right shoulder
M08.212 Juvenile rheumatoid arthritis with systemic onset, left shoulder
M08.219 Juvenile rheumatoid arthritis with systemic onset, unspecified shoulder
M08.22 Juvenile rheumatoid arthritis with systemic onset, elbow
M08.221 Juvenile rheumatoid arthritis with systemic onset, right elbow
M08.222 Juvenile rheumatoid arthritis with systemic onset, left elbow
M08.229 Juvenile rheumatoid arthritis with systemic onset, unspecified elbow
M08.23 Juvenile rheumatoid arthritis with systemic onset, wrist
M08.231 Juvenile rheumatoid arthritis with systemic onset, right wrist
M08.232 Juvenile rheumatoid arthritis with systemic onset, left wrist
M08.239 Juvenile rheumatoid arthritis with systemic onset, unspecified wrist

Unspecified Code Other Specified Code Manifestation Code N Newborn P Pediatric M Maternity A Adult ♂ Male ♀ Female
● New Code ▲ Revised Code Title ►◄ Revised Text NOTES INCLUDES EXCLUDES1 Not coded here EXCLUDES2 Not included here
4th character required 5th character required 6th character required 7th character required
Extension 'X' Alert HAC Hospital-acquired condition (HAC) alert AHA AHA Coding Clinic©

M08.24 Juvenile rheumatoid arthritis with systemic onset, hand
M08.241 Juvenile rheumatoid arthritis with systemic onset, right hand
M08.242 Juvenile rheumatoid arthritis with systemic onset, left hand
M08.249 Juvenile rheumatoid arthritis with systemic onset, unspecified hand
M08.25 Juvenile rheumatoid arthritis with systemic onset, hip
M08.251 Juvenile rheumatoid arthritis with systemic onset, right hip
M08.252 Juvenile rheumatoid arthritis with systemic onset, left hip
M08.259 Juvenile rheumatoid arthritis with systemic onset, unspecified hip
M08.26 Juvenile rheumatoid arthritis with systemic onset, knee
M08.261 Juvenile rheumatoid arthritis with systemic onset, right knee
M08.262 Juvenile rheumatoid arthritis with systemic onset, left knee
M08.269 Juvenile rheumatoid arthritis with systemic onset, unspecified knee
M08.27 Juvenile rheumatoid arthritis with systemic onset, ankle and foot
M08.271 Juvenile rheumatoid arthritis with systemic onset, right ankle and foot
M08.272 Juvenile rheumatoid arthritis with systemic onset, left ankle and foot
M08.279 Juvenile rheumatoid arthritis with systemic onset, unspecified ankle and foot
M08.28 Juvenile rheumatoid arthritis with systemic onset, vertebrae
M08.29 Juvenile rheumatoid arthritis with systemic onset, multiple sites
M08.3 Juvenile rheumatoid polyarthritis (seronegative)
M08.4 Pauciarticular juvenile rheumatoid arthritis
M08.40 Pauciarticular juvenile rheumatoid arthritis, unspecified site
M08.41 Pauciarticular juvenile rheumatoid arthritis, shoulder
M08.411 Pauciarticular juvenile rheumatoid arthritis, right shoulder
M08.412 Pauciarticular juvenile rheumatoid arthritis, left shoulder
M08.419 Pauciarticular juvenile rheumatoid arthritis, unspecified shoulder
M08.42 Pauciarticular juvenile rheumatoid arthritis, elbow
M08.421 Pauciarticular juvenile rheumatoid arthritis, right elbow
M08.422 Pauciarticular juvenile rheumatoid arthritis, left elbow
M08.429 Pauciarticular juvenile rheumatoid arthritis, unspecified elbow
M08.43 Pauciarticular juvenile rheumatoid arthritis, wrist
M08.431 Pauciarticular juvenile rheumatoid arthritis, right wrist
M08.432 Pauciarticular juvenile rheumatoid arthritis, left wrist
M08.439 Pauciarticular juvenile rheumatoid arthritis, unspecified wrist
M08.44 Pauciarticular juvenile rheumatoid arthritis, hand
M08.441 Pauciarticular juvenile rheumatoid arthritis, right hand
M08.442 Pauciarticular juvenile rheumatoid arthritis, left hand
M08.449 Pauciarticular juvenile rheumatoid arthritis, unspecified hand
M08.45 Pauciarticular juvenile rheumatoid arthritis, hip
M08.451 Pauciarticular juvenile rheumatoid arthritis, right hip
M08.452 Pauciarticular juvenile rheumatoid arthritis, left hip
M08.459 Pauciarticular juvenile rheumatoid arthritis, unspecified hip
M08.46 Pauciarticular juvenile rheumatoid arthritis, knee
M08.461 Pauciarticular juvenile rheumatoid arthritis, right knee
M08.462 Pauciarticular juvenile rheumatoid arthritis, left knee
M08.469 Pauciarticular juvenile rheumatoid arthritis, unspecified knee
M08.47 Pauciarticular juvenile rheumatoid arthritis, ankle and foot
M08.471 Pauciarticular juvenile rheumatoid arthritis, right ankle and foot
M08.472 Pauciarticular juvenile rheumatoid arthritis, left ankle and foot
M08.479 Pauciarticular juvenile rheumatoid arthritis, unspecified ankle and foot
M08.48 Pauciarticular juvenile rheumatoid arthritis, vertebrae
M08.8 Other juvenile arthritis
M08.80 Other juvenile arthritis, unspecified site
M08.81 Other juvenile arthritis, shoulder
M08.811 Other juvenile arthritis, right shoulder
M08.812 Other juvenile arthritis, left shoulder
M08.819 Other juvenile arthritis, unspecified shoulder
M08.82 Other juvenile arthritis, elbow
M08.821 Other juvenile arthritis, right elbow
M08.822 Other juvenile arthritis, left elbow
M08.829 Other juvenile arthritis, unspecified elbow
M08.83 Other juvenile arthritis, wrist
M08.831 Other juvenile arthritis, right wrist
M08.832 Other juvenile arthritis, left wrist
M08.839 Other juvenile arthritis, unspecified wrist
M08.84 Other juvenile arthritis, hand
M08.841 Other juvenile arthritis, right hand
M08.842 Other juvenile arthritis, left hand
M08.849 Other juvenile arthritis, unspecified hand
M08.85 Other juvenile arthritis, hip
M08.851 Other juvenile arthritis, right hip
M08.852 Other juvenile arthritis, left hip
M08.859 Other juvenile arthritis, unspecified hip
M08.86 Other juvenile arthritis, knee
M08.861 Other juvenile arthritis, right knee
M08.862 Other juvenile arthritis, left knee
M08.869 Other juvenile arthritis, unspecified knee
M08.87 Other juvenile arthritis, ankle and foot
M08.871 Other juvenile arthritis, right ankle and foot
M08.872 Other juvenile arthritis, left ankle and foot
M08.879 Other juvenile arthritis, unspecified ankle and foot
M08.88 Other juvenile arthritis, other specified site
Other juvenile arthritis, vertebrae
M08.89 Other juvenile arthritis, multiple sites
M08.9 Juvenile arthritis, unspecified
EXCLUDES1 *juvenile rheumatoid arthritis, unspecified (M08.0-)*
M08.90 Juvenile arthritis, unspecified, unspecified site
M08.91 Juvenile arthritis, unspecified, shoulder
M08.911 Juvenile arthritis, unspecified, right shoulder
M08.912 Juvenile arthritis, unspecified, left shoulder
M08.919 Juvenile arthritis, unspecified, unspecified shoulder
M08.92 Juvenile arthritis, unspecified, elbow
M08.921 Juvenile arthritis, unspecified, right elbow
M08.922 Juvenile arthritis, unspecified, left elbow
M08.929 Juvenile arthritis, unspecified, unspecified elbow
M08.93 Juvenile arthritis, unspecified, wrist
M08.931 Juvenile arthritis, unspecified, right wrist
M08.932 Juvenile arthritis, unspecified, left wrist

Unacceptable principal diagnosis symbol per Medicare code edits · Code exempt from diagnosis present on admission requirement
Questionable admission · Complication or comorbidity · CC/MCC exclusion · Major complication or comorbidity
Principal diagnosis as its own CC · Principal diagnosis as its own MCC · Z code as first-listed diagnosis

M08.939 Juvenile arthritis, unspecified, unspecified wrist
M08.94 Juvenile arthritis, unspecified, hand
M08.941 Juvenile arthritis, unspecified, right hand
M08.942 Juvenile arthritis, unspecified, left hand
M08.949 Juvenile arthritis, unspecified, unspecified hand
M08.95 Juvenile arthritis, unspecified, hip
M08.951 Juvenile arthritis, unspecified, right hip
M08.952 Juvenile arthritis, unspecified, left hip
M08.959 Juvenile arthritis, unspecified, unspecified hip
M08.96 Juvenile arthritis, unspecified, knee
M08.961 Juvenile arthritis, unspecified, right knee
M08.962 Juvenile arthritis, unspecified, left knee
M08.969 Juvenile arthritis, unspecified, unspecified knee
M08.97 Juvenile arthritis, unspecified, ankle and foot
M08.971 Juvenile arthritis, unspecified, right ankle and foot
M08.972 Juvenile arthritis, unspecified, left ankle and foot
M08.979 Juvenile arthritis, unspecified, unspecified ankle and foot
M08.98 Juvenile arthritis, unspecified, vertebrae
M08.99 Juvenile arthritis, unspecified, multiple sites

M1A Chronic gout

Use additional code to identify:
Autonomic neuropathy in diseases classified elsewhere (G99.0)
Calculus of urinary tract in diseases classified elsewhere (N22)
Cardiomyopathy in diseases classified elsewhere (I43)
Disorders of external ear in diseases classified elsewhere (H61.1-, H62.8-)
Disorders of iris and ciliary body in diseases classified elsewhere (H22)
Glomerular disorders in diseases classified elsewhere (N08)

EXCLUDES1 *gout NOS (M10.-)*

EXCLUDES2 *acute gout (M10.-)*

The appropriate 7th character is to be added to each code from category M1A
0 = without tophus (tophi)
1 = with tophus (tophi)

M1A.0 Idiopathic chronic gout
Chronic gouty bursitis
Primary chronic gout
M1A.00 Idiopathic chronic gout, unspecified site
M1A.01 Idiopathic chronic gout, shoulder
M1A.011 Idiopathic chronic gout, right shoulder
M1A.012 Idiopathic chronic gout, left shoulder
M1A.019 Idiopathic chronic gout, unspecified shoulder
M1A.02 Idiopathic chronic gout, elbow
M1A.021 Idiopathic chronic gout, right elbow
M1A.022 Idiopathic chronic gout, left elbow
M1A.029 Idiopathic chronic gout, unspecified elbow
M1A.03 Idiopathic chronic gout, wrist
M1A.031 Idiopathic chronic gout, right wrist
M1A.032 Idiopathic chronic gout, left wrist
M1A.039 Idiopathic chronic gout, unspecified wrist
M1A.04 Idiopathic chronic gout, hand
M1A.041 Idiopathic chronic gout, right hand
M1A.042 Idiopathic chronic gout, left hand
M1A.049 Idiopathic chronic gout, unspecified hand
M1A.05 Idiopathic chronic gout, hip
M1A.051 Idiopathic chronic gout, right hip
M1A.052 Idiopathic chronic gout, left hip
M1A.059 Idiopathic chronic gout, unspecified hip
M1A.06 Idiopathic chronic gout, knee
M1A.061 Idiopathic chronic gout, right knee
M1A.062 Idiopathic chronic gout, left knee
M1A.069 Idiopathic chronic gout, unspecified knee
M1A.07 Idiopathic chronic gout, ankle and foot
M1A.071 Idiopathic chronic gout, right ankle and foot
M1A.072 Idiopathic chronic gout, left ankle and foot
M1A.079 Idiopathic chronic gout, unspecified ankle and foot
M1A.08 Idiopathic chronic gout, vertebrae
M1A.09 Idiopathic chronic gout, multiple sites

M1A.1 Lead-induced chronic gout
Code first toxic effects of lead and its compounds (T56.0-)
M1A.10 Lead-induced chronic gout, unspecified site
M1A.11 Lead-induced chronic gout, shoulder
M1A.111 Lead-induced chronic gout, right shoulder
M1A.112 Lead-induced chronic gout, left shoulder
M1A.119 Lead-induced chronic gout, unspecified shoulder
M1A.12 Lead-induced chronic gout, elbow
M1A.121 Lead-induced chronic gout, right elbow
M1A.122 Lead-induced chronic gout, left elbow
M1A.129 Lead-induced chronic gout, unspecified elbow
M1A.13 Lead-induced chronic gout, wrist
M1A.131 Lead-induced chronic gout, right wrist
M1A.132 Lead-induced chronic gout, left wrist
M1A.139 Lead-induced chronic gout, unspecified wrist
M1A.14 Lead-induced chronic gout, hand
M1A.141 Lead-induced chronic gout, right hand
M1A.142 Lead-induced chronic gout, left hand
M1A.149 Lead-induced chronic gout, unspecified hand
M1A.15 Lead-induced chronic gout, hip
M1A.151 Lead-induced chronic gout, right hip
M1A.152 Lead-induced chronic gout, left hip
M1A.159 Lead-induced chronic gout, unspecified hip
M1A.16 Lead-induced chronic gout, knee
M1A.161 Lead-induced chronic gout, right knee
M1A.162 Lead-induced chronic gout, left knee
M1A.169 Lead-induced chronic gout, unspecified knee
M1A.17 Lead-induced chronic gout, ankle and foot
M1A.171 Lead-induced chronic gout, right ankle and foot
M1A.172 Lead-induced chronic gout, left ankle and foot
M1A.179 Lead-induced chronic gout, unspecified ankle and foot
M1A.18 Lead-induced chronic gout, vertebrae
M1A.19 Lead-induced chronic gout, multiple sites

M1A.2 Drug-induced chronic gout
Use additional code for adverse effect, if applicable, to identify drug (T36-T50 with fifth or sixth character 5)
M1A.20 Drug-induced chronic gout, unspecified site
M1A.21 Drug-induced chronic gout, shoulder
M1A.211 Drug-induced chronic gout, right shoulder
M1A.212 Drug-induced chronic gout, left shoulder
M1A.219 Drug-induced chronic gout, unspecified shoulder
M1A.22 Drug-induced chronic gout, elbow
M1A.221 Drug-induced chronic gout, right elbow
M1A.222 Drug-induced chronic gout, left elbow
M1A.229 Drug-induced chronic gout, unspecified elbow
M1A.23 Drug-induced chronic gout, wrist
M1A.231 Drug-induced chronic gout, right wrist
M1A.232 Drug-induced chronic gout, left wrist
M1A.239 Drug-induced chronic gout, unspecified wrist
M1A.24 Drug-induced chronic gout, hand
M1A.241 Drug-induced chronic gout, right hand
M1A.242 Drug-induced chronic gout, left hand

Unspecified Code · Other Specified Code · Manifestation Code · N Newborn · P Pediatric · M Maternity · A Adult · ♂ Male · ♀ Female
● New Code · ▲ Revised Code Title · ►◄ Revised Text · NOTES · INCLUDES · EXCLUDES1 Not coded here · EXCLUDES2 Not included here
4th character required · 5th character required · 6th character required · 7th character required
Extension 'X' Alert · HAC Hospital-acquired condition (HAC) alert · AHA AHA Coding Clinic©

 When symbols appear on a code that requires a 7th character extension, refer to Appendix D to identify applicable 7th character codes.

M1A.249 Drug-induced chronic gout, unspecified hand
M1A.25 Drug-induced chronic gout, hip
M1A.251 Drug-induced chronic gout, right hip
M1A.252 Drug-induced chronic gout, left hip
M1A.259 Drug-induced chronic gout, unspecified hip
M1A.26 Drug-induced chronic gout, knee
M1A.261 Drug-induced chronic gout, right knee
M1A.262 Drug-induced chronic gout, left knee
M1A.269 Drug-induced chronic gout, unspecified knee
M1A.27 Drug-induced chronic gout, ankle and foot
M1A.271 Drug-induced chronic gout, right ankle and foot
M1A.272 Drug-induced chronic gout, left ankle and foot
M1A.279 Drug-induced chronic gout, unspecified ankle and foot
M1A.28 Drug-induced chronic gout, vertebrae
M1A.29 Drug-induced chronic gout, multiple sites
M1A.3 Chronic gout due to renal impairment
Code first associated renal disease
M1A.30 Chronic gout due to renal impairment, unspecified site
M1A.31 Chronic gout due to renal impairment, shoulder
M1A.311 Chronic gout due to renal impairment, right shoulder
M1A.312 Chronic gout due to renal impairment, left shoulder
M1A.319 Chronic gout due to renal impairment, unspecified shoulder
M1A.32 Chronic gout due to renal impairment, elbow
M1A.321 Chronic gout due to renal impairment, right elbow
M1A.322 Chronic gout due to renal impairment, left elbow
M1A.329 Chronic gout due to renal impairment, unspecified elbow
M1A.33 Chronic gout due to renal impairment, wrist
M1A.331 Chronic gout due to renal impairment, right wrist
M1A.332 Chronic gout due to renal impairment, left wrist
M1A.339 Chronic gout due to renal impairment, unspecified wrist
M1A.34 Chronic gout due to renal impairment, hand
M1A.341 Chronic gout due to renal impairment, right hand
M1A.342 Chronic gout due to renal impairment, left hand
M1A.349 Chronic gout due to renal impairment, unspecified hand
M1A.35 Chronic gout due to renal impairment, hip
M1A.351 Chronic gout due to renal impairment, right hip
M1A.352 Chronic gout due to renal impairment, left hip
M1A.359 Chronic gout due to renal impairment, unspecified hip
M1A.36 Chronic gout due to renal impairment, knee
M1A.361 Chronic gout due to renal impairment, right knee
M1A.362 Chronic gout due to renal impairment, left knee
M1A.369 Chronic gout due to renal impairment, unspecified knee
M1A.37 Chronic gout due to renal impairment, ankle and foot
M1A.371 Chronic gout due to renal impairment, right ankle and foot
M1A.372 Chronic gout due to renal impairment, left ankle and foot
M1A.379 Chronic gout due to renal impairment, unspecified ankle and foot
M1A.38 Chronic gout due to renal impairment, vertebrae
M1A.39 Chronic gout due to renal impairment, multiple sites
M1A.4 Other secondary chronic gout
Code first associated condition
M1A.40 Other secondary chronic gout, unspecified site
M1A.41 Other secondary chronic gout, shoulder
M1A.411 Other secondary chronic gout, right shoulder
M1A.412 Other secondary chronic gout, left shoulder
M1A.419 Other secondary chronic gout, unspecified shoulder
M1A.42 Other secondary chronic gout, elbow
M1A.421 Other secondary chronic gout, right elbow
M1A.422 Other secondary chronic gout, left elbow
M1A.429 Other secondary chronic gout, unspecified elbow
M1A.43 Other secondary chronic gout, wrist
M1A.431 Other secondary chronic gout, right wrist
M1A.432 Other secondary chronic gout, left wrist
M1A.439 Other secondary chronic gout, unspecified wrist
M1A.44 Other secondary chronic gout, hand
M1A.441 Other secondary chronic gout, right hand
M1A.442 Other secondary chronic gout, left hand
M1A.449 Other secondary chronic gout, unspecified hand
M1A.45 Other secondary chronic gout, hip
M1A.451 Other secondary chronic gout, right hip
M1A.452 Other secondary chronic gout, left hip
M1A.459 Other secondary chronic gout, unspecified hip
M1A.46 Other secondary chronic gout, knee
M1A.461 Other secondary chronic gout, right knee
M1A.462 Other secondary chronic gout, left knee
M1A.469 Other secondary chronic gout, unspecified knee
M1A.47 Other secondary chronic gout, ankle and foot
M1A.471 Other secondary chronic gout, right ankle and foot
M1A.472 Other secondary chronic gout, left ankle and foot
M1A.479 Other secondary chronic gout, unspecified ankle and foot
M1A.48 Other secondary chronic gout, vertebrae
M1A.49 Other secondary chronic gout, multiple sites
M1A.9 Chronic gout, unspecified

M10 Gout
Acute gout
Gout attack
Gout flare
Podagra
Use additional code to identify:
Autonomic neuropathy in diseases classified elsewhere (G99.0)
Calculus of urinary tract in diseases classified elsewhere (N22)
Cardiomyopathy in diseases classified elsewhere (I43)
Disorders of external ear in diseases classified elsewhere (H61.1-, H62.8-)
Disorders of iris and ciliary body in diseases classified elsewhere (H22)
Glomerular disorders in diseases classified elsewhere (N08)
EXCLUDES2 *chronic gout (M1A.-)*
M10.0 Idiopathic gout
Gouty bursitis
Primary gout
M10.00 Idiopathic gout, unspecified site
M10.01 Idiopathic gout, shoulder
M10.011 Idiopathic gout, right shoulder
M10.012 Idiopathic gout, left shoulder
M10.019 Idiopathic gout, unspecified shoulder
M10.02 Idiopathic gout, elbow
M10.021 Idiopathic gout, right elbow
M10.022 Idiopathic gout, left elbow

Unacceptable principal diagnosis symbol per Medicare code edits · Code exempt from diagnosis present on admission requirement · Questionable admission · Complication or comorbidity · CC/MCC exclusion · Major complication or comorbidity · Principal diagnosis as its own CC · Principal diagnosis as its own MCC · Z code as first-listed diagnosis

M10.029 Idiopathic gout, unspecified elbow
M10.03 Idiopathic gout, wrist
M10.031 Idiopathic gout, right wrist
M10.032 Idiopathic gout, left wrist
M10.039 Idiopathic gout, unspecified wrist
M10.04 Idiopathic gout, hand
M10.041 Idiopathic gout, right hand
M10.042 Idiopathic gout, left hand
M10.049 Idiopathic gout, unspecified hand
M10.05 Idiopathic gout, hip
M10.051 Idiopathic gout, right hip
M10.052 Idiopathic gout, left hip
M10.059 Idiopathic gout, unspecified hip
M10.06 Idiopathic gout, knee
M10.061 Idiopathic gout, right knee
M10.062 Idiopathic gout, left knee
M10.069 Idiopathic gout, unspecified knee
M10.07 Idiopathic gout, ankle and foot
M10.071 Idiopathic gout, right ankle and foot
M10.072 Idiopathic gout, left ankle and foot
M10.079 Idiopathic gout, unspecified ankle and foot
M10.08 Idiopathic gout, vertebrae
M10.09 Idiopathic gout, multiple sites
M10.1 Lead-induced gout
Code first toxic effects of lead and its compounds (T56.0-)
M10.10 Lead-induced gout, unspecified site
M10.11 Lead-induced gout, shoulder
M10.111 Lead-induced gout, right shoulder
M10.112 Lead-induced gout, left shoulder
M10.119 Lead-induced gout, unspecified shoulder
M10.12 Lead-induced gout, elbow
M10.121 Lead-induced gout, right elbow
M10.122 Lead-induced gout, left elbow
M10.129 Lead-induced gout, unspecified elbow
M10.13 Lead-induced gout, wrist
M10.131 Lead-induced gout, right wrist
M10.132 Lead-induced gout, left wrist
M10.139 Lead-induced gout, unspecified wrist
M10.14 Lead-induced gout, hand
M10.141 Lead-induced gout, right hand
M10.142 Lead-induced gout, left hand
M10.149 Lead-induced gout, unspecified hand
M10.15 Lead-induced gout, hip
M10.151 Lead-induced gout, right hip
M10.152 Lead-induced gout, left hip
M10.159 Lead-induced gout, unspecified hip
M10.16 Lead-induced gout, knee
M10.161 Lead-induced gout, right knee
M10.162 Lead-induced gout, left knee
M10.169 Lead-induced gout, unspecified knee
M10.17 Lead-induced gout, ankle and foot
M10.171 Lead-induced gout, right ankle and foot
M10.172 Lead-induced gout, left ankle and foot
M10.179 Lead-induced gout, unspecified ankle and foot
M10.18 Lead-induced gout, vertebrae
M10.19 Lead-induced gout, multiple sites
M10.2 Drug-induced gout
Use additional code for adverse effect, if applicable, to identify drug (T36-T50 with fifth or sixth character 5)
M10.20 Drug-induced gout, unspecified site
M10.21 Drug-induced gout, shoulder
M10.211 Drug-induced gout, right shoulder
M10.212 Drug-induced gout, left shoulder
M10.219 Drug-induced gout, unspecified shoulder
M10.22 Drug-induced gout, elbow
M10.221 Drug-induced gout, right elbow
M10.222 Drug-induced gout, left elbow
M10.229 Drug-induced gout, unspecified elbow
M10.23 Drug-induced gout, wrist
M10.231 Drug-induced gout, right wrist
M10.232 Drug-induced gout, left wrist
M10.239 Drug-induced gout, unspecified wrist
M10.24 Drug-induced gout, hand
M10.241 Drug-induced gout, right hand
M10.242 Drug-induced gout, left hand
M10.249 Drug-induced gout, unspecified hand
M10.25 Drug-induced gout, hip
M10.251 Drug-induced gout, right hip
M10.252 Drug-induced gout, left hip
M10.259 Drug-induced gout, unspecified hip
M10.26 Drug-induced gout, knee
M10.261 Drug-induced gout, right knee
M10.262 Drug-induced gout, left knee
M10.269 Drug-induced gout, unspecified knee
M10.27 Drug-induced gout, ankle and foot
M10.271 Drug-induced gout, right ankle and foot
M10.272 Drug-induced gout, left ankle and foot
M10.279 Drug-induced gout, unspecified ankle and foot
M10.28 Drug-induced gout, vertebrae
M10.29 Drug-induced gout, multiple sites
M10.3 Gout due to renal impairment
Code first associated renal disease
M10.30 Gout due to renal impairment, unspecified site
M10.31 Gout due to renal impairment, shoulder
M10.311 Gout due to renal impairment, right shoulder
M10.312 Gout due to renal impairment, left shoulder
M10.319 Gout due to renal impairment, unspecified shoulder
M10.32 Gout due to renal impairment, elbow
M10.321 Gout due to renal impairment, right elbow
M10.322 Gout due to renal impairment, left elbow
M10.329 Gout due to renal impairment, unspecified elbow
M10.33 Gout due to renal impairment, wrist
M10.331 Gout due to renal impairment, right wrist
M10.332 Gout due to renal impairment, left wrist
M10.339 Gout due to renal impairment, unspecified wrist
M10.34 Gout due to renal impairment, hand
M10.341 Gout due to renal impairment, right hand
M10.342 Gout due to renal impairment, left hand
M10.349 Gout due to renal impairment, unspecified hand
M10.35 Gout due to renal impairment, hip
M10.351 Gout due to renal impairment, right hip
M10.352 Gout due to renal impairment, left hip
M10.359 Gout due to renal impairment, unspecified hip
M10.36 Gout due to renal impairment, knee
M10.361 Gout due to renal impairment, right knee
M10.362 Gout due to renal impairment, left knee
M10.369 Gout due to renal impairment, unspecified knee
M10.37 Gout due to renal impairment, ankle and foot
M10.371 Gout due to renal impairment, right ankle and foot
M10.372 Gout due to renal impairment, left ankle and foot
M10.379 Gout due to renal impairment, unspecified ankle and foot
M10.38 Gout due to renal impairment, vertebrae
M10.39 Gout due to renal impairment, multiple sites
M10.4 Other secondary gout
Code first associated condition
M10.40 Other secondary gout, unspecified site
M10.41 Other secondary gout, shoulder
M10.411 Other secondary gout, right shoulder
M10.412 Other secondary gout, left shoulder
M10.419 Other secondary gout, unspecified shoulder

M10.42 Other secondary gout, elbow
M10.421 Other secondary gout, right elbow
M10.422 Other secondary gout, left elbow
M10.429 Other secondary gout, unspecified elbow
M10.43 Other secondary gout, wrist
M10.431 Other secondary gout, right wrist
M10.432 Other secondary gout, left wrist
M10.439 Other secondary gout, unspecified wrist
M10.44 Other secondary gout, hand
M10.441 Other secondary gout, right hand
M10.442 Other secondary gout, left hand
M10.449 Other secondary gout, unspecified hand
M10.45 Other secondary gout, hip
M10.451 Other secondary gout, right hip
M10.452 Other secondary gout, left hip
M10.459 Other secondary gout, unspecified hip
M10.46 Other secondary gout, knee
M10.461 Other secondary gout, right knee
M10.462 Other secondary gout, left knee
M10.469 Other secondary gout, unspecified knee
M10.47 Other secondary gout, ankle and foot
M10.471 Other secondary gout, right ankle and foot
M10.472 Other secondary gout, left ankle and foot
M10.479 Other secondary gout, unspecified ankle and foot
M10.48 Other secondary gout, vertebrae
M10.49 Other secondary gout, multiple sites
M10.9 Gout, unspecified
Gout NOS
M11 Other crystal arthropathies
M11.0 Hydroxyapatite deposition disease
M11.00 Hydroxyapatite deposition disease, unspecified site
M11.01 Hydroxyapatite deposition disease, shoulder
M11.011 Hydroxyapatite deposition disease, right shoulder
M11.012 Hydroxyapatite deposition disease, left shoulder
M11.019 Hydroxyapatite deposition disease, unspecified shoulder
M11.02 Hydroxyapatite deposition disease, elbow
M11.021 Hydroxyapatite deposition disease, right elbow
M11.022 Hydroxyapatite deposition disease, left elbow
M11.029 Hydroxyapatite deposition disease, unspecified elbow
M11.03 Hydroxyapatite deposition disease, wrist
M11.031 Hydroxyapatite deposition disease, right wrist
M11.032 Hydroxyapatite deposition disease, left wrist
M11.039 Hydroxyapatite deposition disease, unspecified wrist
M11.04 Hydroxyapatite deposition disease, hand
M11.041 Hydroxyapatite deposition disease, right hand
M11.042 Hydroxyapatite deposition disease, left hand
M11.049 Hydroxyapatite deposition disease, unspecified hand
M11.05 Hydroxyapatite deposition disease, hip
M11.051 Hydroxyapatite deposition disease, right hip
M11.052 Hydroxyapatite deposition disease, left hip
M11.059 Hydroxyapatite deposition disease, unspecified hip
M11.06 Hydroxyapatite deposition disease, knee
M11.061 Hydroxyapatite deposition disease, right knee
M11.062 Hydroxyapatite deposition disease, left knee
M11.069 Hydroxyapatite deposition disease, unspecified knee
M11.07 Hydroxyapatite deposition disease, ankle and foot
M11.071 Hydroxyapatite deposition disease, right ankle and foot
M11.072 Hydroxyapatite deposition disease, left ankle and foot
M11.079 Hydroxyapatite deposition disease, unspecified ankle and foot
M11.08 Hydroxyapatite deposition disease, vertebrae
M11.09 Hydroxyapatite deposition disease, multiple sites
M11.1 Familial chondrocalcinosis
M11.10 Familial chondrocalcinosis, unspecified site
M11.11 Familial chondrocalcinosis, shoulder
M11.111 Familial chondrocalcinosis, right shoulder
M11.112 Familial chondrocalcinosis, left shoulder
M11.119 Familial chondrocalcinosis, unspecified shoulder
M11.12 Familial chondrocalcinosis, elbow
M11.121 Familial chondrocalcinosis, right elbow
M11.122 Familial chondrocalcinosis, left elbow
M11.129 Familial chondrocalcinosis, unspecified elbow
M11.13 Familial chondrocalcinosis, wrist
M11.131 Familial chondrocalcinosis, right wrist
M11.132 Familial chondrocalcinosis, left wrist
M11.139 Familial chondrocalcinosis, unspecified wrist
M11.14 Familial chondrocalcinosis, hand
M11.141 Familial chondrocalcinosis, right hand
M11.142 Familial chondrocalcinosis, left hand
M11.149 Familial chondrocalcinosis, unspecified hand
M11.15 Familial chondrocalcinosis, hip
M11.151 Familial chondrocalcinosis, right hip
M11.152 Familial chondrocalcinosis, left hip
M11.159 Familial chondrocalcinosis, unspecified hip
M11.16 Familial chondrocalcinosis, knee
M11.161 Familial chondrocalcinosis, right knee
M11.162 Familial chondrocalcinosis, left knee
M11.169 Familial chondrocalcinosis, unspecified knee
M11.17 Familial chondrocalcinosis, ankle and foot
M11.171 Familial chondrocalcinosis, right ankle and foot
M11.172 Familial chondrocalcinosis, left ankle and foot
M11.179 Familial chondrocalcinosis, unspecified ankle and foot
M11.18 Familial chondrocalcinosis, vertebrae
M11.19 Familial chondrocalcinosis, multiple sites
M11.2 Other chondrocalcinosis
Chondrocalcinosis NOS
M11.20 Other chondrocalcinosis, unspecified site
M11.21 Other chondrocalcinosis, shoulder
M11.211 Other chondrocalcinosis, right shoulder
M11.212 Other chondrocalcinosis, left shoulder
M11.219 Other chondrocalcinosis, unspecified shoulder
M11.22 Other chondrocalcinosis, elbow
M11.221 Other chondrocalcinosis, right elbow
M11.222 Other chondrocalcinosis, left elbow
M11.229 Other chondrocalcinosis, unspecified elbow
M11.23 Other chondrocalcinosis, wrist
M11.231 Other chondrocalcinosis, right wrist
M11.232 Other chondrocalcinosis, left wrist
M11.239 Other chondrocalcinosis, unspecified wrist
M11.24 Other chondrocalcinosis, hand
M11.241 Other chondrocalcinosis, right hand
M11.242 Other chondrocalcinosis, left hand

Unacceptable principal diagnosis symbol per Medicare code edits · Code exempt from diagnosis present on admission requirement
Questionable admission · Complication or comorbidity · CC/MCC exclusion · Major complication or comorbidity
Principal diagnosis as its own CC · Principal diagnosis as its own MCC · Z code as first-listed diagnosis

When symbols appear on a code that requires a 7th character extension, refer to Appendix D to identify applicable 7th character codes.

M11.249 Other chondrocalcinosis, unspecified hand
M11.25 Other chondrocalcinosis, hip
M11.251 Other chondrocalcinosis, right hip
M11.252 Other chondrocalcinosis, left hip
M11.259 Other chondrocalcinosis, unspecified hip
M11.26 Other chondrocalcinosis, knee
M11.261 Other chondrocalcinosis, right knee
M11.262 Other chondrocalcinosis, left knee
M11.269 Other chondrocalcinosis, unspecified knee
M11.27 Other chondrocalcinosis, ankle and foot
M11.271 Other chondrocalcinosis, right ankle and foot
M11.272 Other chondrocalcinosis, left ankle and foot
M11.279 Other chondrocalcinosis, unspecified ankle and foot
M11.28 Other chondrocalcinosis, vertebrae
M11.29 Other chondrocalcinosis, multiple sites
M11.8 Other specified crystal arthropathies
M11.80 Other specified crystal arthropathies, unspecified site
M11.81 Other specified crystal arthropathies, shoulder
M11.811 Other specified crystal arthropathies, right shoulder
M11.812 Other specified crystal arthropathies, left shoulder
M11.819 Other specified crystal arthropathies, unspecified shoulder
M11.82 Other specified crystal arthropathies, elbow
M11.821 Other specified crystal arthropathies, right elbow
M11.822 Other specified crystal arthropathies, left elbow
M11.829 Other specified crystal arthropathies, unspecified elbow
M11.83 Other specified crystal arthropathies, wrist
M11.831 Other specified crystal arthropathies, right wrist
M11.832 Other specified crystal arthropathies, left wrist
M11.839 Other specified crystal arthropathies, unspecified wrist
M11.84 Other specified crystal arthropathies, hand
M11.841 Other specified crystal arthropathies, right hand
M11.842 Other specified crystal arthropathies, left hand
M11.849 Other specified crystal arthropathies, unspecified hand
M11.85 Other specified crystal arthropathies, hip
M11.851 Other specified crystal arthropathies, right hip
M11.852 Other specified crystal arthropathies, left hip
M11.859 Other specified crystal arthropathies, unspecified hip
M11.86 Other specified crystal arthropathies, knee
M11.861 Other specified crystal arthropathies, right knee
M11.862 Other specified crystal arthropathies, left knee
M11.869 Other specified crystal arthropathies, unspecified knee
M11.87 Other specified crystal arthropathies, ankle and foot
M11.871 Other specified crystal arthropathies, right ankle and foot
M11.872 Other specified crystal arthropathies, left ankle and foot
M11.879 Other specified crystal arthropathies, unspecified ankle and foot
M11.88 Other specified crystal arthropathies, vertebrae
M11.89 Other specified crystal arthropathies, multiple sites
M11.9 Crystal arthropathy, unspecified

M12 Other and unspecified arthropathy
EXCLUDES1 *arthrosis (M15-M19)*
cricoarytenoid arthropathy (J38.7)
M12.0 Chronic postrheumatic arthropathy [Jaccoud]
M12.00 Chronic postrheumatic arthropathy [Jaccoud], unspecified site
M12.01 Chronic postrheumatic arthropathy [Jaccoud], shoulder
M12.011 Chronic postrheumatic arthropathy [Jaccoud], right shoulder
M12.012 Chronic postrheumatic arthropathy [Jaccoud], left shoulder
M12.019 Chronic postrheumatic arthropathy [Jaccoud], unspecified shoulder
M12.02 Chronic postrheumatic arthropathy [Jaccoud], elbow
M12.021 Chronic postrheumatic arthropathy [Jaccoud], right elbow
M12.022 Chronic postrheumatic arthropathy [Jaccoud], left elbow
M12.029 Chronic postrheumatic arthropathy [Jaccoud], unspecified elbow
M12.03 Chronic postrheumatic arthropathy [Jaccoud], wrist
M12.031 Chronic postrheumatic arthropathy [Jaccoud], right wrist
M12.032 Chronic postrheumatic arthropathy [Jaccoud], left wrist
M12.039 Chronic postrheumatic arthropathy [Jaccoud], unspecified wrist
M12.04 Chronic postrheumatic arthropathy [Jaccoud], hand
M12.041 Chronic postrheumatic arthropathy [Jaccoud], right hand
M12.042 Chronic postrheumatic arthropathy [Jaccoud], left hand
M12.049 Chronic postrheumatic arthropathy [Jaccoud], unspecified hand
M12.05 Chronic postrheumatic arthropathy [Jaccoud], hip
M12.051 Chronic postrheumatic arthropathy [Jaccoud], right hip
M12.052 Chronic postrheumatic arthropathy [Jaccoud], left hip
M12.059 Chronic postrheumatic arthropathy [Jaccoud], unspecified hip
M12.06 Chronic postrheumatic arthropathy [Jaccoud], knee
M12.061 Chronic postrheumatic arthropathy [Jaccoud], right knee
M12.062 Chronic postrheumatic arthropathy [Jaccoud], left knee
M12.069 Chronic postrheumatic arthropathy [Jaccoud], unspecified knee
M12.07 Chronic postrheumatic arthropathy [Jaccoud], ankle and foot
M12.071 Chronic postrheumatic arthropathy [Jaccoud], right ankle and foot
M12.072 Chronic postrheumatic arthropathy [Jaccoud], left ankle and foot
M12.079 Chronic postrheumatic arthropathy [Jaccoud], unspecified ankle and foot
M12.08 Chronic postrheumatic arthropathy [Jaccoud], other specified site
Chronic postrheumatic arthropathy [Jaccoud], vertebrae
M12.09 Chronic postrheumatic arthropathy [Jaccoud], multiple sites
M12.1 Kaschin-Beck disease
Osteochondroarthrosis deformans endemica
M12.10 Kaschin-Beck disease, unspecified site
M12.11 Kaschin-Beck disease, shoulder
M12.111 Kaschin-Beck disease, right shoulder
M12.112 Kaschin-Beck disease, left shoulder
M12.119 Kaschin-Beck disease, unspecified shoulder
M12.12 Kaschin-Beck disease, elbow
M12.121 Kaschin-Beck disease, right elbow
M12.122 Kaschin-Beck disease, left elbow
M12.129 Kaschin-Beck disease, unspecified elbow

Unspecified Code | Other Specified Code | Manifestation Code | N Newborn | P Pediatric | M Maternity | A Adult | ♂ Male | ♀ Female
● New Code | ▲ Revised Code Title | ►◄ Revised Text | NOTES | INCLUDES | EXCLUDES1 Not coded here | EXCLUDES2 Not included here
4th character required | 5th character required | 6th character required | 7th character required
Extension 'X' Alert | HAC Hospital-acquired condition (HAC) alert | AHA AHA Coding Clinic©

M12.13 Kaschin-Beck disease, wrist
M12.131 Kaschin-Beck disease, right wrist
M12.132 Kaschin-Beck disease, left wrist
M12.139 Kaschin-Beck disease, unspecified wrist
M12.14 Kaschin-Beck disease, hand
M12.141 Kaschin-Beck disease, right hand
M12.142 Kaschin-Beck disease, left hand
M12.149 Kaschin-Beck disease, unspecified hand
M12.15 Kaschin-Beck disease, hip
M12.151 Kaschin-Beck disease, right hip
M12.152 Kaschin-Beck disease, left hip
M12.159 Kaschin-Beck disease, unspecified hip
M12.16 Kaschin-Beck disease, knee
M12.161 Kaschin-Beck disease, right knee
M12.162 Kaschin-Beck disease, left knee
M12.169 Kaschin-Beck disease, unspecified knee
M12.17 Kaschin-Beck disease, ankle and foot
M12.171 Kaschin-Beck disease, right ankle and foot
M12.172 Kaschin-Beck disease, left ankle and foot
M12.179 Kaschin-Beck disease, unspecified ankle and foot
M12.18 Kaschin-Beck disease, vertebrae
M12.19 Kaschin-Beck disease, multiple sites
M12.2 Villonodular synovitis (pigmented)
M12.20 Villonodular synovitis (pigmented), unspecified site
M12.21 Villonodular synovitis (pigmented), shoulder
M12.211 Villonodular synovitis (pigmented), right shoulder
M12.212 Villonodular synovitis (pigmented), left shoulder
M12.219 Villonodular synovitis (pigmented), unspecified shoulder
M12.22 Villonodular synovitis (pigmented), elbow
M12.221 Villonodular synovitis (pigmented), right elbow
M12.222 Villonodular synovitis (pigmented), left elbow
M12.229 Villonodular synovitis (pigmented), unspecified elbow
M12.23 Villonodular synovitis (pigmented), wrist
M12.231 Villonodular synovitis (pigmented), right wrist
M12.232 Villonodular synovitis (pigmented), left wrist
M12.239 Villonodular synovitis (pigmented), unspecified wrist
M12.24 Villonodular synovitis (pigmented), hand
M12.241 Villonodular synovitis (pigmented), right hand
M12.242 Villonodular synovitis (pigmented), left hand
M12.249 Villonodular synovitis (pigmented), unspecified hand
M12.25 Villonodular synovitis (pigmented), hip
M12.251 Villonodular synovitis (pigmented), right hip
M12.252 Villonodular synovitis (pigmented), left hip
M12.259 Villonodular synovitis (pigmented), unspecified hip
M12.26 Villonodular synovitis (pigmented), knee
M12.261 Villonodular synovitis (pigmented), right knee
M12.262 Villonodular synovitis (pigmented), left knee
M12.269 Villonodular synovitis (pigmented), unspecified knee
M12.27 Villonodular synovitis (pigmented), ankle and foot
M12.271 Villonodular synovitis (pigmented), right ankle and foot
M12.272 Villonodular synovitis (pigmented), left ankle and foot
M12.279 Villonodular synovitis (pigmented), unspecified ankle and foot
M12.28 Villonodular synovitis (pigmented), other specified site
Villonodular synovitis (pigmented), vertebrae
M12.29 Villonodular synovitis (pigmented), multiple sites
M12.3 Palindromic rheumatism
M12.30 Palindromic rheumatism, unspecified site
M12.31 Palindromic rheumatism, shoulder
M12.311 Palindromic rheumatism, right shoulder
M12.312 Palindromic rheumatism, left shoulder
M12.319 Palindromic rheumatism, unspecified shoulder
M12.32 Palindromic rheumatism, elbow
M12.321 Palindromic rheumatism, right elbow
M12.322 Palindromic rheumatism, left elbow
M12.329 Palindromic rheumatism, unspecified elbow
M12.33 Palindromic rheumatism, wrist
M12.331 Palindromic rheumatism, right wrist
M12.332 Palindromic rheumatism, left wrist
M12.339 Palindromic rheumatism, unspecified wrist
M12.34 Palindromic rheumatism, hand
M12.341 Palindromic rheumatism, right hand
M12.342 Palindromic rheumatism, left hand
M12.349 Palindromic rheumatism, unspecified hand
M12.35 Palindromic rheumatism, hip
M12.351 Palindromic rheumatism, right hip
M12.352 Palindromic rheumatism, left hip
M12.359 Palindromic rheumatism, unspecified hip
M12.36 Palindromic rheumatism, knee
M12.361 Palindromic rheumatism, right knee
M12.362 Palindromic rheumatism, left knee
M12.369 Palindromic rheumatism, unspecified knee
M12.37 Palindromic rheumatism, ankle and foot
M12.371 Palindromic rheumatism, right ankle and foot
M12.372 Palindromic rheumatism, left ankle and foot
M12.379 Palindromic rheumatism, unspecified ankle and foot
M12.38 Palindromic rheumatism, other specified site
Palindromic rheumatism, vertebrae
M12.39 Palindromic rheumatism, multiple sites
M12.4 Intermittent hydrarthrosis
M12.40 Intermittent hydrarthrosis, unspecified site
M12.41 Intermittent hydrarthrosis, shoulder
M12.411 Intermittent hydrarthrosis, right shoulder
M12.412 Intermittent hydrarthrosis, left shoulder
M12.419 Intermittent hydrarthrosis, unspecified shoulder
M12.42 Intermittent hydrarthrosis, elbow
M12.421 Intermittent hydrarthrosis, right elbow
M12.422 Intermittent hydrarthrosis, left elbow
M12.429 Intermittent hydrarthrosis, unspecified elbow
M12.43 Intermittent hydrarthrosis, wrist
M12.431 Intermittent hydrarthrosis, right wrist
M12.432 Intermittent hydrarthrosis, left wrist
M12.439 Intermittent hydrarthrosis, unspecified wrist
M12.44 Intermittent hydrarthrosis, hand
M12.441 Intermittent hydrarthrosis, right hand
M12.442 Intermittent hydrarthrosis, left hand
M12.449 Intermittent hydrarthrosis, unspecified hand
M12.45 Intermittent hydrarthrosis, hip
M12.451 Intermittent hydrarthrosis, right hip
M12.452 Intermittent hydrarthrosis, left hip
M12.459 Intermittent hydrarthrosis, unspecified hip
M12.46 Intermittent hydrarthrosis, knee
M12.461 Intermittent hydrarthrosis, right knee

Unacceptable principal diagnosis symbol per Medicare code edits | Code exempt from diagnosis present on admission requirement
Questionable admission | Complication or comorbidity | CC/MCC exclusion | Major complication or comorbidity
Principal diagnosis as its own CC | Principal diagnosis as its own MCC | Z code as first-listed diagnosis

When symbols appear on a code that requires a 7th character extension, refer to Appendix D to identify applicable 7th character codes.

M12.462 Intermittent hydrarthrosis, left knee
M12.469 Intermittent hydrarthrosis, unspecified knee
M12.47 Intermittent hydrarthrosis, ankle and foot
M12.471 Intermittent hydrarthrosis, right ankle and foot
M12.472 Intermittent hydrarthrosis, left ankle and foot
M12.479 Intermittent hydrarthrosis, unspecified ankle and foot
M12.48 Intermittent hydrarthrosis, other site
M12.49 Intermittent hydrarthrosis, multiple sites
M12.5 Traumatic arthropathy
EXCLUDES1 *current injury-see Alphabetic Index*
post-traumatic osteoarthritis of first carpometacarpal joint (M18.2-M18.3)
post-traumatic osteoarthritis of hip (M16.4-M16.5)
post-traumatic osteoarthritis of knee (M17.2-M17.3)
post-traumatic osteoarthritis NOS (M19.1-)
post-traumatic osteoarthritis of other single joints (M19.1-)
M12.50 Traumatic arthropathy, unspecified site
M12.51 Traumatic arthropathy, shoulder
M12.511 Traumatic arthropathy, right shoulder
M12.512 Traumatic arthropathy, left shoulder
M12.519 Traumatic arthropathy, unspecified shoulder
M12.52 Traumatic arthropathy, elbow
M12.521 Traumatic arthropathy, right elbow
M12.522 Traumatic arthropathy, left elbow
M12.529 Traumatic arthropathy, unspecified elbow
M12.53 Traumatic arthropathy, wrist
M12.531 Traumatic arthropathy, right wrist
M12.532 Traumatic arthropathy, left wrist
M12.539 Traumatic arthropathy, unspecified wrist
M12.54 Traumatic arthropathy, hand
M12.541 Traumatic arthropathy, right hand
M12.542 Traumatic arthropathy, left hand
M12.549 Traumatic arthropathy, unspecified hand
M12.55 Traumatic arthropathy, hip
M12.551 Traumatic arthropathy, right hip
M12.552 Traumatic arthropathy, left hip
AHA: Q1, 2015
M12.559 Traumatic arthropathy, unspecified hip
M12.56 Traumatic arthropathy, knee
M12.561 Traumatic arthropathy, right knee
M12.562 Traumatic arthropathy, left knee
M12.569 Traumatic arthropathy, unspecified knee
M12.57 Traumatic arthropathy, ankle and foot
M12.571 Traumatic arthropathy, right ankle and foot
M12.572 Traumatic arthropathy, left ankle and foot
M12.579 Traumatic arthropathy, unspecified ankle and foot
M12.58 Traumatic arthropathy, other specified site
Traumatic arthropathy, vertebrae
M12.59 Traumatic arthropathy, multiple sites
M12.8 Other specific arthropathies, not elsewhere classified
Transient arthropathy
M12.80 Other specific arthropathies, not elsewhere classified, unspecified site
M12.81 Other specific arthropathies, not elsewhere classified, shoulder
M12.811 Other specific arthropathies, not elsewhere classified, right shoulder
M12.812 Other specific arthropathies, not elsewhere classified, left shoulder
M12.819 Other specific arthropathies, not elsewhere classified, unspecified shoulder
M12.82 Other specific arthropathies, not elsewhere classified, elbow
M12.821 Other specific arthropathies, not elsewhere classified, right elbow
M12.822 Other specific arthropathies, not elsewhere classified, left elbow
M12.829 Other specific arthropathies, not elsewhere classified, unspecified elbow
M12.83 Other specific arthropathies, not elsewhere classified, wrist
M12.831 Other specific arthropathies, not elsewhere classified, right wrist
M12.832 Other specific arthropathies, not elsewhere classified, left wrist
M12.839 Other specific arthropathies, not elsewhere classified, unspecified wrist
M12.84 Other specific arthropathies, not elsewhere classified, hand
M12.841 Other specific arthropathies, not elsewhere classified, right hand
M12.842 Other specific arthropathies, not elsewhere classified, left hand
M12.849 Other specific arthropathies, not elsewhere classified, unspecified hand
M12.85 Other specific arthropathies, not elsewhere classified, hip
M12.851 Other specific arthropathies, not elsewhere classified, right hip
M12.852 Other specific arthropathies, not elsewhere classified, left hip
M12.859 Other specific arthropathies, not elsewhere classified, unspecified hip
M12.86 Other specific arthropathies, not elsewhere classified, knee
M12.861 Other specific arthropathies, not elsewhere classified, right knee
M12.862 Other specific arthropathies, not elsewhere classified, left knee
M12.869 Other specific arthropathies, not elsewhere classified, unspecified knee
M12.87 Other specific arthropathies, not elsewhere classified, ankle and foot
M12.871 Other specific arthropathies, not elsewhere classified, right ankle and foot
M12.872 Other specific arthropathies, not elsewhere classified, left ankle and foot
M12.879 Other specific arthropathies, not elsewhere classified, unspecified ankle and foot
M12.88 Other specific arthropathies, not elsewhere classified, other specified site
Other specific arthropathies, not elsewhere classified, vertebrae
M12.89 Other specific arthropathies, not elsewhere classified, multiple sites
M12.9 Arthropathy, unspecified
M13 Other arthritis
EXCLUDES1 *arthrosis (M15-M19)*
osteoarthritis (M15-M19)
M13.0 Polyarthritis, unspecified
M13.1 Monoarthritis , not elsewhere classified
M13.10 Monoarthritis, not elsewhere classified, unspecified site
M13.11 Monoarthritis, not elsewhere classified, shoulder
M13.111 Monoarthritis, not elsewhere classified, right shoulder
M13.112 Monoarthritis, not elsewhere classified, left shoulder
M13.119 Monoarthritis, not elsewhere classified, unspecified shoulder
M13.12 Monoarthritis, not elsewhere classified, elbow
M13.121 Monoarthritis, not elsewhere classified, right elbow
M13.122 Monoarthritis, not elsewhere classified, left elbow
M13.129 Monoarthritis, not elsewhere classified, unspecified elbow
M13.13 Monoarthritis, not elsewhere classified, wrist
M13.131 Monoarthritis, not elsewhere classified, right wrist

Unspecified Code Other Specified Code Manifestation Code N Newborn P Pediatric M Maternity A Adult ♂ Male ♀ Female
● New Code ▲ Revised Code Title ▶◀ Revised Text NOTES INCLUDES EXCLUDES1 Not coded here EXCLUDES2 Not included here
4th character required 5th character required 6th character required 7th character required
Extension 'X' Alert HAC Hospital-acquired condition (HAC) alert AHA AHA Coding Clinic©

- M13.132 Monoarthritis, not elsewhere classified, left wrist
- M13.139 Monoarthritis, not elsewhere classified, unspecified wrist
- M13.14 Monoarthritis, not elsewhere classified, hand
  - M13.141 Monoarthritis, not elsewhere classified, right hand
  - M13.142 Monoarthritis, not elsewhere classified, left hand
  - M13.149 Monoarthritis, not elsewhere classified, unspecified hand
- M13.15 Monoarthritis, not elsewhere classified, hip
  - M13.151 Monoarthritis, not elsewhere classified, right hip
  - M13.152 Monoarthritis, not elsewhere classified, left hip
  - M13.159 Monoarthritis, not elsewhere classified, unspecified hip
- M13.16 Monoarthritis, not elsewhere classified, knee
  - M13.161 Monoarthritis, not elsewhere classified, right knee
  - M13.162 Monoarthritis, not elsewhere classified, left knee
  - M13.169 Monoarthritis, not elsewhere classified, unspecified knee
- M13.17 Monoarthritis, not elsewhere classified, ankle and foot
  - M13.171 Monoarthritis, not elsewhere classified, right ankle and foot
  - M13.172 Monoarthritis, not elsewhere classified, left ankle and foot
  - M13.179 Monoarthritis, not elsewhere classified, unspecified ankle and foot

M13.8 Other specified arthritis
Allergic arthritis
EXCLUDES1 *osteoarthritis (M15-M19)*

- M13.80 Other specified arthritis, unspecified site
- M13.81 Other specified arthritis, shoulder
  - M13.811 Other specified arthritis, right shoulder
  - M13.812 Other specified arthritis, left shoulder
  - M13.819 Other specified arthritis, unspecified shoulder
- M13.82 Other specified arthritis, elbow
  - M13.821 Other specified arthritis, right elbow
  - M13.822 Other specified arthritis, left elbow
  - M13.829 Other specified arthritis, unspecified elbow
- M13.83 Other specified arthritis, wrist
  - M13.831 Other specified arthritis, right wrist
  - M13.832 Other specified arthritis, left wrist
  - M13.839 Other specified arthritis, unspecified wrist
- M13.84 Other specified arthritis, hand
  - M13.841 Other specified arthritis, right hand
  - M13.842 Other specified arthritis, left hand
  - M13.849 Other specified arthritis, unspecified hand
- M13.85 Other specified arthritis, hip
  - M13.851 Other specified arthritis, right hip
  - M13.852 Other specified arthritis, left hip
  - M13.859 Other specified arthritis, unspecified hip
- M13.86 Other specified arthritis, knee
  - M13.861 Other specified arthritis, right knee
  - M13.862 Other specified arthritis, left knee
  - M13.869 Other specified arthritis, unspecified knee
- M13.87 Other specified arthritis, ankle and foot
  - M13.871 Other specified arthritis, right ankle and foot
  - M13.872 Other specified arthritis, left ankle and foot
  - M13.879 Other specified arthritis, unspecified ankle and foot
- M13.88 Other specified arthritis, other site
- M13.89 Other specified arthritis, multiple sites

M14 Arthropathies in other diseases classified elsewhere

EXCLUDES1 *arthropathy in:*
diabetes mellitus (E08-E13 with .61-)
hematological disorders (M36.2-M36.3)
hypersensitivity reactions (M36.4)
neoplastic disease (M36.1)
neurosyphilis (A52.16)
sarcoidosis (D86.86)
enteropathic arthropathies (M07.-)
juvenile psoriatic arthropathy (L40.54)
lipoid dermatoarthritis (E78.81)

M14.6 Charcôt's joint
Neuropathic arthropathy
EXCLUDES1 *Charcôt's joint in diabetes mellitus (E08-E13 with .610)*
Charcôt's joint in tabes dorsalis (A52.16)

- M14.60 Charcôt's joint, unspecified site
- M14.61 Charcôt's joint, shoulder
  - M14.611 Charcôt's joint, right shoulder
  - M14.612 Charcôt's joint, left shoulder
  - M14.619 Charcôt's joint, unspecified shoulder
- M14.62 Charcôt's joint, elbow
  - M14.621 Charcôt's joint, right elbow
  - M14.622 Charcôt's joint, left elbow
  - M14.629 Charcôt's joint, unspecified elbow
- M14.63 Charcôt's joint, wrist
  - M14.631 Charcôt's joint, right wrist
  - M14.632 Charcôt's joint, left wrist
  - M14.639 Charcôt's joint, unspecified wrist
- M14.64 Charcôt's joint, hand
  - M14.641 Charcôt's joint, right hand
  - M14.642 Charcôt's joint, left hand
  - M14.649 Charcôt's joint, unspecified hand
- M14.65 Charcôt's joint, hip
  - M14.651 Charcôt's joint, right hip
  - M14.652 Charcôt's joint, left hip
  - M14.659 Charcôt's joint, unspecified hip
- M14.66 Charcôt's joint, knee
  - M14.661 Charcôt's joint, right knee
  - M14.662 Charcôt's joint, left knee
  - M14.669 Charcôt's joint, unspecified knee
- M14.67 Charcôt's joint, ankle and foot
  - M14.671 Charcôt's joint, right ankle and foot
  - M14.672 Charcôt's joint, left ankle and foot
  - M14.679 Charcôt's joint, unspecified ankle and foot
- M14.68 Charcôt's joint, vertebrae
- M14.69 Charcôt's joint, multiple sites

M14.8 Arthropathies in other specified diseases classified elsewhere
Code first underlying disease, such as:
amyloidosis (E85.-)
erythema multiforme (L51.-)
erythema nodosum (L52)
hemochromatosis (E83.11-)
hyperparathyroidism (E21.-)
hypothyroidism (E00-E03)
sickle-cell disorders (D57.-)
thyrotoxicosis [hyperthyroidism] (E05.-)
Whipple's disease (K90.81)

- M14.80 Arthropathies in other specified diseases classified elsewhere, unspecified site
- M14.81 Arthropathies in other specified diseases classified elsewhere, shoulder
  - M14.811 Arthropathies in other specified diseases classified elsewhere, right shoulder
  - M14.812 Arthropathies in other specified diseases classified elsewhere, left shoulder
  - M14.819 Arthropathies in other specified diseases classified elsewhere, unspecified shoulder
- M14.82 Arthropathies in other specified diseases classified elsewhere, elbow
  - M14.821 Arthropathies in other specified diseases classified elsewhere, right elbow
  - M14.822 Arthropathies in other specified diseases classified elsewhere, left elbow

Unacceptable principal diagnosis symbol per Medicare code edits · Code exempt from diagnosis present on admission requirement
Questionable admission · Complication or comorbidity · CC/MCC exclusion · Major complication or comorbidity
Principal diagnosis as its own CC · Principal diagnosis as its own MCC · Z code as first-listed diagnosis

M14.829 Arthropathies in other specified diseases classified elsewhere, unspecified elbow
M14.83 Arthropathies in other specified diseases classified elsewhere, wrist
M14.831 Arthropathies in other specified diseases classified elsewhere, right wrist
M14.832 Arthropathies in other specified diseases classified elsewhere, left wrist
M14.839 Arthropathies in other specified diseases classified elsewhere, unspecified wrist
M14.84 Arthropathies in other specified diseases classified elsewhere, hand
M14.841 Arthropathies in other specified diseases classified elsewhere, right hand
M14.842 Arthropathies in other specified diseases classified elsewhere, left hand
M14.849 Arthropathies in other specified diseases classified elsewhere, unspecified hand
M14.85 Arthropathies in other specified diseases classified elsewhere, hip
M14.851 Arthropathies in other specified diseases classified elsewhere, right hip
M14.852 Arthropathies in other specified diseases classified elsewhere, left hip
M14.859 Arthropathies in other specified diseases classified elsewhere, unspecified hip
M14.86 Arthropathies in other specified diseases classified elsewhere, knee
M14.861 Arthropathies in other specified diseases classified elsewhere, right knee
M14.862 Arthropathies in other specified diseases classified elsewhere, left knee
M14.869 Arthropathies in other specified diseases classified elsewhere, unspecified knee
M14.87 Arthropathies in other specified diseases classified elsewhere, ankle and foot
M14.871 Arthropathies in other specified diseases classified elsewhere, right ankle and foot
M14.872 Arthropathies in other specified diseases classified elsewhere, left ankle and foot
M14.879 Arthropathies in other specified diseases classified elsewhere, unspecified ankle and foot
M14.88 Arthropathies in other specified diseases classified elsewhere, vertebrae
M14.89 Arthropathies in other specified diseases classified elsewhere, multiple sites

Osteoarthritis (M15-M19)

EXCLUDES2 *osteoarthritis of spine (M47.-)*

M15 Polyosteoarthritis
INCLUDES *arthritis of multiple sites*
EXCLUDES1 *bilateral involvement of single joint (M16-M19)*
M15.0 Primary generalized (osteo)arthritis
M15.1 Heberden's nodes (with arthropathy)
Interphalangeal distal osteoarthritis
M15.2 Bouchard's nodes (with arthropathy)
Juxtaphalangeal distal osteoarthritis
M15.3 Secondary multiple arthritis
Post-traumatic polyosteoarthritis
M15.4 Erosive (osteo)arthritis
M15.8 Other polyosteoarthritis
M15.9 Polyosteoarthritis, unspecified
Generalized osteoarthritis NOS

M16 Osteoarthritis of hip
M16.0 Bilateral primary osteoarthritis of hip
M16.1 Unilateral primary osteoarthritis of hip
Primary osteoarthritis of hip NOS
M16.10 Unilateral primary osteoarthritis, unspecified hip
M16.11 Unilateral primary osteoarthritis, right hip
M16.12 Unilateral primary osteoarthritis, left hip
M16.2 Bilateral osteoarthritis resulting from hip dysplasia
M16.3 Unilateral osteoarthritis resulting from hip dysplasia
Dysplastic osteoarthritis of hip NOS
M16.30 Unilateral osteoarthritis resulting from hip dysplasia, unspecified hip
M16.31 Unilateral osteoarthritis resulting from hip dysplasia, right hip
M16.32 Unilateral osteoarthritis resulting from hip dysplasia, left hip
M16.4 Bilateral post-traumatic osteoarthritis of hip
M16.5 Unilateral post-traumatic osteoarthritis of hip
Post-traumatic osteoarthritis of hip NOS
M16.50 Unilateral post-traumatic osteoarthritis, unspecified hip
M16.51 Unilateral post-traumatic osteoarthritis, right hip
M16.52 Unilateral post-traumatic osteoarthritis, left hip
M16.6 Other bilateral secondary osteoarthritis of hip
M16.7 Other unilateral secondary osteoarthritis of hip
Secondary osteoarthritis of hip NOS
M16.9 Osteoarthritis of hip, unspecified

M17 Osteoarthritis of knee
M17.0 Bilateral primary osteoarthritis of knee
M17.1 Unilateral primary osteoarthritis of knee
Primary osteoarthritis of knee NOS
M17.10 Unilateral primary osteoarthritis, unspecified knee
M17.11 Unilateral primary osteoarthritis, right knee
M17.12 Unilateral primary osteoarthritis, left knee
M17.2 Bilateral post-traumatic osteoarthritis of knee
M17.3 Unilateral post-traumatic osteoarthritis of knee
Post-traumatic osteoarthritis of knee NOS
M17.30 Unilateral post-traumatic osteoarthritis, unspecified knee
M17.31 Unilateral post-traumatic osteoarthritis, right knee
M17.32 Unilateral post-traumatic osteoarthritis, left knee
M17.4 Other bilateral secondary osteoarthritis of knee
M17.5 Other unilateral secondary osteoarthritis of knee
Secondary osteoarthritis of knee NOS
M17.9 Osteoarthritis of knee, unspecified

M18 Osteoarthritis of first carpometacarpal joint
M18.0 Bilateral primary osteoarthritis of first carpometacarpal joints
M18.1 Unilateral primary osteoarthritis of first carpometacarpal joint
Primary osteoarthritis of first carpometacarpal joint NOS
M18.10 Unilateral primary osteoarthritis of first carpometacarpal joint, unspecified hand
M18.11 Unilateral primary osteoarthritis of first carpometacarpal joint, right hand
M18.12 Unilateral primary osteoarthritis of first carpometacarpal joint, left hand
M18.2 Bilateral post-traumatic osteoarthritis of first carpometacarpal joints
M18.3 Unilateral post-traumatic osteoarthritis of first carpometacarpal joint
Post-traumatic osteoarthritis of first carpometacarpal joint NOS
M18.30 Unilateral post-traumatic osteoarthritis of first carpometacarpal joint, unspecified hand
M18.31 Unilateral post-traumatic osteoarthritis of first carpometacarpal joint, right hand
M18.32 Unilateral post-traumatic osteoarthritis of first carpometacarpal joint, left hand
M18.4 Other bilateral secondary osteoarthritis of first carpometacarpal joints
M18.5 Other unilateral secondary osteoarthritis of first carpometacarpal joint
Secondary osteoarthritis of first carpometacarpal joint NOS
M18.50 Other unilateral secondary osteoarthritis of first carpometacarpal joint, unspecified hand
M18.51 Other unilateral secondary osteoarthritis of first carpometacarpal joint, right hand
M18.52 Other unilateral secondary osteoarthritis of first carpometacarpal joint, left hand
M18.9 Osteoarthritis of first carpometacarpal joint, unspecified

M19 Other and unspecified osteoarthritis
EXCLUDES1 *polyarthritis (M15.-)*
EXCLUDES2 *arthrosis of spine (M47.-)*
hallux rigidus (M20.2)
osteoarthritis of spine (M47.-)

Unspecified Code | Other Specified Code | Manifestation Code | N Newborn | P Pediatric | M Maternity | A Adult | ♂ Male | ♀ Female
● New Code ▲ Revised Code Title ►◄ Revised Text NOTES INCLUDES EXCLUDES1 Not coded here EXCLUDES2 Not included here
4th character required | 5th character required | 6th character required | 7th character required
Extension 'X' Alert | HAC Hospital-acquired condition (HAC) alert | AHA AHA Coding Clinic©

M19.0 Primary osteoarthritis of other joints
M19.01 Primary osteoarthritis, shoulder
M19.011 Primary osteoarthritis, right shoulder
M19.012 Primary osteoarthritis, left shoulder
M19.019 Primary osteoarthritis, unspecified shoulder
M19.02 Primary osteoarthritis, elbow
M19.021 Primary osteoarthritis, right elbow
M19.022 Primary osteoarthritis, left elbow
M19.029 Primary osteoarthritis, unspecified elbow
M19.03 Primary osteoarthritis, wrist
M19.031 Primary osteoarthritis, right wrist
M19.032 Primary osteoarthritis, left wrist
M19.039 Primary osteoarthritis, unspecified wrist
M19.04 Primary osteoarthritis, hand
EXCLUDES2 *primary osteoarthritis of first carpometacarpal joint (M18.0-, M18.1-)*
M19.041 Primary osteoarthritis, right hand
M19.042 Primary osteoarthritis, left hand
M19.049 Primary osteoarthritis, unspecified hand
M19.07 Primary osteoarthritis ankle and foot
M19.071 Primary osteoarthritis, right ankle and foot
M19.072 Primary osteoarthritis, left ankle and foot
M19.079 Primary osteoarthritis, unspecified ankle and foot
M19.1 Post-traumatic osteoarthritis of other joints
M19.11 Post-traumatic osteoarthritis, shoulder
M19.111 Post-traumatic osteoarthritis, right shoulder
M19.112 Post-traumatic osteoarthritis, left shoulder
M19.119 Post-traumatic osteoarthritis, unspecified shoulder
M19.12 Post-traumatic osteoarthritis, elbow
M19.121 Post-traumatic osteoarthritis, right elbow
M19.122 Post-traumatic osteoarthritis, left elbow
M19.129 Post-traumatic osteoarthritis, unspecified elbow
M19.13 Post-traumatic osteoarthritis, wrist
M19.131 Post-traumatic osteoarthritis, right wrist
M19.132 Post-traumatic osteoarthritis, left wrist
M19.139 Post-traumatic osteoarthritis, unspecified wrist
M19.14 Post-traumatic osteoarthritis, hand
EXCLUDES2 *post-traumatic osteoarthritis of first carpometacarpal joint (M18.2-, M18.3-)*
M19.141 Post-traumatic osteoarthritis, right hand
M19.142 Post-traumatic osteoarthritis, left hand
M19.149 Post-traumatic osteoarthritis, unspecified hand
M19.17 Post-traumatic osteoarthritis, ankle and foot
M19.171 Post-traumatic osteoarthritis, right ankle and foot
M19.172 Post-traumatic osteoarthritis, left ankle and foot
M19.179 Post-traumatic osteoarthritis, unspecified ankle and foot
M19.2 Secondary osteoarthritis of other joints
M19.21 Secondary osteoarthritis, shoulder
M19.211 Secondary osteoarthritis, right shoulder
M19.212 Secondary osteoarthritis, left shoulder
M19.219 Secondary osteoarthritis, unspecified shoulder
M19.22 Secondary osteoarthritis, elbow
M19.221 Secondary osteoarthritis, right elbow
M19.222 Secondary osteoarthritis, left elbow
M19.229 Secondary osteoarthritis, unspecified elbow
M19.23 Secondary osteoarthritis, wrist
M19.231 Secondary osteoarthritis, right wrist
M19.232 Secondary osteoarthritis, left wrist
M19.239 Secondary osteoarthritis, unspecified wrist
M19.24 Secondary osteoarthritis, hand
M19.241 Secondary osteoarthritis, right hand
M19.242 Secondary osteoarthritis, left hand
M19.249 Secondary osteoarthritis, unspecified hand
M19.27 Secondary osteoarthritis, ankle and foot
M19.271 Secondary osteoarthritis, right ankle and foot
M19.272 Secondary osteoarthritis, left ankle and foot
M19.279 Secondary osteoarthritis, unspecified ankle and foot
M19.9 Osteoarthritis, unspecified site
M19.90 Unspecified osteoarthritis, unspecified site
Arthrosis NOS
Arthritis NOS
Osteoarthritis NOS
M19.91 Primary osteoarthritis, unspecified site
Primary osteoarthritis NOS
M19.92 Post-traumatic osteoarthritis, unspecified site
Post-traumatic osteoarthritis NOS
M19.93 Secondary osteoarthritis, unspecified site
Secondary osteoarthritis NOS

Other joint disorders (M20-M25)

EXCLUDES2 *joints of the spine (M40-M54)*

M20 Acquired deformities of fingers and toes
EXCLUDES1 *acquired absence of fingers and toes (Z89.-)*
congenital absence of fingers and toes (Q71.3-, Q72.3-)
congenital deformities and malformations of fingers and toes (Q66.-, Q68-Q70, Q74.-)
M20.0 Deformity of finger(s)
EXCLUDES1 *clubbing of fingers (R68.3)*
palmar fascial fibromatosis [Dupuytren] (M72.0)
trigger finger (M65.3)
M20.00 Unspecified deformity of finger(s)
M20.001 Unspecified deformity of right finger(s)
M20.002 Unspecified deformity of left finger(s)
M20.009 Unspecified deformity of unspecified finger(s)
M20.01 Mallet finger
M20.011 Mallet finger of right finger(s)
M20.012 Mallet finger of left finger(s)
M20.019 Mallet finger of unspecified finger(s)
M20.02 Boutonnière deformity
M20.021 Boutonnière deformity of right finger(s)
M20.022 Boutonnière deformity of left finger(s)
M20.029 Boutonnière deformity of unspecified finger(s)
M20.03 Swan-neck deformity
M20.031 Swan-neck deformity of right finger(s)
M20.032 Swan-neck deformity of left finger(s)
M20.039 Swan-neck deformity of unspecified finger(s)
M20.09 Other deformity of finger(s)
M20.091 Other deformity of right finger(s)
M20.092 Other deformity of left finger(s)
M20.099 Other deformity of finger(s), unspecified finger(s)

Unacceptable principal diagnosis symbol per Medicare code edits; Code exempt from diagnosis present on admission requirement
Questionable admission; Complication or comorbidity; CC/MCC exclusion; Major complication or comorbidity
Principal diagnosis as its own CC; Principal diagnosis as its own MCC; Z code as first-listed diagnosis

 When symbols appear on a code that requires a 7th character extension, refer to Appendix D to identify applicable 7th character codes.

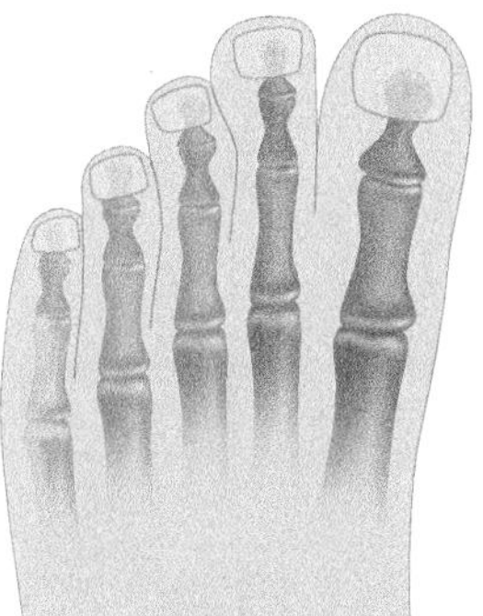

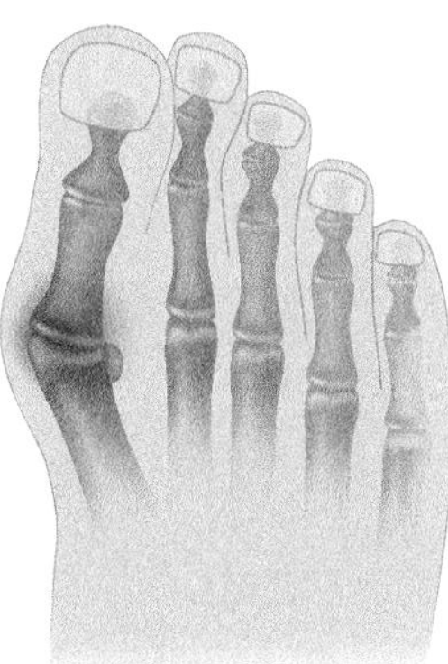

Figure 13.2 Bunion

M20.1 Hallux valgus (acquired)
EXCLUDES2 *bunion (M21.6-)*
M20.10 Hallux valgus (acquired), unspecified foot
M20.11 Hallux valgus (acquired), right foot
M20.12 Hallux valgus (acquired), left foot
M20.2 Hallux rigidus
M20.20 Hallux rigidus, unspecified foot
M20.21 Hallux rigidus, right foot
M20.22 Hallux rigidus, left foot
M20.3 Hallux varus (acquired)
M20.30 Hallux varus (acquired), unspecified foot
M20.31 Hallux varus (acquired), right foot
M20.32 Hallux varus (acquired), left foot
M20.4 Other hammer toe(s) (acquired)
M20.40 Other hammer toe(s) (acquired), unspecified foot
M20.41 Other hammer toe(s) (acquired), right foot
M20.42 Other hammer toe(s) (acquired), left foot
M20.5 Other deformities of toe(s) (acquired)
M20.5X Other deformities of toe(s) (acquired)
M20.5X1 Other deformities of toe(s) (acquired), right foot
M20.5X2 Other deformities of toe(s) (acquired), left foot
M20.5X9 Other deformities of toe(s) (acquired), unspecified foot
M20.6 Acquired deformities of toe(s), unspecified
M20.60 Acquired deformities of toe(s), unspecified, unspecified foot
M20.61 Acquired deformities of toe(s), unspecified, right foot
M20.62 Acquired deformities of toe(s), unspecified, left foot
M21 Other acquired deformities of limbs
EXCLUDES1 *acquired absence of limb (Z89.-)*
congenital absence of limbs (Q71-Q73)
congenital deformities and malformations of limbs (Q65-Q66, Q68-Q74)
EXCLUDES2 *acquired deformities of fingers or toes (M20.-)*
coxa plana (M91.2)
M21.0 Valgus deformity, not elsewhere classified
EXCLUDES1 *metatarsus valgus (Q66.6)*
talipes calcaneovalgus (Q66.4)
M21.00 Valgus deformity, not elsewhere classified, unspecified site
M21.02 Valgus deformity, not elsewhere classified, elbow
Cubitus valgus
M21.021 Valgus deformity, not elsewhere classified, right elbow
M21.022 Valgus deformity, not elsewhere classified, left elbow
M21.029 Valgus deformity, not elsewhere classified, unspecified elbow
M21.05 Valgus deformity, not elsewhere classified, hip
M21.051 Valgus deformity, not elsewhere classified, right hip
M21.052 Valgus deformity, not elsewhere classified, left hip
M21.059 Valgus deformity, not elsewhere classified, unspecified hip
M21.06 Valgus deformity, not elsewhere classified, knee
Genu valgum
Knock knee
M21.061 Valgus deformity, not elsewhere classified, right knee
M21.062 Valgus deformity, not elsewhere classified, left knee
M21.069 Valgus deformity, not elsewhere classified, unspecified knee
M21.07 Valgus deformity, not elsewhere classified, ankle
M21.071 Valgus deformity, not elsewhere classified, right ankle
M21.072 Valgus deformity, not elsewhere classified, left ankle
M21.079 Valgus deformity, not elsewhere classified, unspecified ankle
M21.1 Varus deformity, not elsewhere classified
EXCLUDES1 *metatarsus varus ▶(Q66.22)◀*
tibia vara (M92.5)
M21.10 Varus deformity, not elsewhere classified, unspecified site
M21.12 Varus deformity, not elsewhere classified, elbow
Cubitus varus, elbow
M21.121 Varus deformity, not elsewhere classified, right elbow
M21.122 Varus deformity, not elsewhere classified, left elbow
M21.129 Varus deformity, not elsewhere classified, unspecified elbow
M21.15 Varus deformity, not elsewhere classified, hip
M21.151 Varus deformity, not elsewhere classified, right hip
M21.152 Varus deformity, not elsewhere classified, left hip
M21.159 Varus deformity, not elsewhere classified, unspecified
M21.16 Varus deformity, not elsewhere classified, knee
Bow leg
Genu varum
M21.161 Varus deformity, not elsewhere classified, right knee
M21.162 Varus deformity, not elsewhere classified, left knee
M21.169 Varus deformity, not elsewhere classified, unspecified knee
M21.17 Varus deformity, not elsewhere classified, ankle
M21.171 Varus deformity, not elsewhere classified, right ankle
M21.172 Varus deformity, not elsewhere classified, left ankle
M21.179 Varus deformity, not elsewhere classified, unspecified ankle
M21.2 Flexion deformity
M21.20 Flexion deformity, unspecified site
M21.21 Flexion deformity, shoulder
M21.211 Flexion deformity, right shoulder
M21.212 Flexion deformity, left shoulder
M21.219 Flexion deformity, unspecified shoulder
M21.22 Flexion deformity, elbow
M21.221 Flexion deformity, right elbow
M21.222 Flexion deformity, left elbow
M21.229 Flexion deformity, unspecified elbow
M21.23 Flexion deformity, wrist
M21.231 Flexion deformity, right wrist
M21.232 Flexion deformity, left wrist
M21.239 Flexion deformity, unspecified wrist
M21.24 Flexion deformity, finger joints
M21.241 Flexion deformity, right finger joints

Unspecified Code | Other Specified Code | Manifestation Code | N Newborn | P Pediatric | M Maternity | A Adult | ♂ Male | ♀ Female
● New Code | ▲ Revised Code Title | ▶◀ Revised Text | NOTES | INCLUDES | EXCLUDES1 Not coded here | EXCLUDES2 Not included here
4th character required | 5th character required | 6th character required | 7th character required
Extension 'X' Alert | HAC Hospital-acquired condition (HAC) alert | AHA AHA Coding Clinic©

M21.242 Flexion deformity, left finger joints
M21.249 Flexion deformity, unspecified finger joints
M21.25 Flexion deformity, hip
M21.251 Flexion deformity, right hip
M21.252 Flexion deformity, left hip
M21.259 Flexion deformity, unspecified hip
M21.26 Flexion deformity, knee
M21.261 Flexion deformity, right knee
M21.262 Flexion deformity, left knee
M21.269 Flexion deformity, unspecified knee
M21.27 Flexion deformity, ankle and toes
M21.271 Flexion deformity, right ankle and toes
M21.272 Flexion deformity, left ankle and toes
M21.279 Flexion deformity, unspecified ankle and toes
M21.3 Wrist or foot drop (acquired)
M21.33 Wrist drop (acquired)
M21.331 Wrist drop, right wrist
M21.332 Wrist drop, left wrist
M21.339 Wrist drop, unspecified wrist
M21.37 Foot drop (acquired)
M21.371 Foot drop, right foot
M21.372 Foot drop, left foot
M21.379 Foot drop, unspecified foot

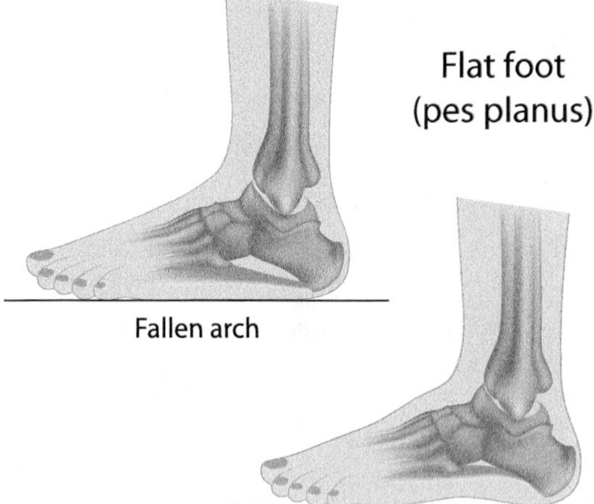

Figure 13.3 Illustration showing normal and flat foot

M21.4 Flat foot [pes planus] (acquired)
EXCLUDES1 *congenital pes planus (Q66.5-)*
M21.40 Flat foot [pes planus] (acquired), unspecified foot
M21.41 Flat foot [pes planus] (acquired), right foot
M21.42 Flat foot [pes planus] (acquired), left foot
M21.5 Acquired clawhand, clubhand, clawfoot and clubfoot
EXCLUDES1 *clubfoot, not specified as acquired (Q66.89)*
M21.51 Acquired clawhand
M21.511 Acquired clawhand, right hand
M21.512 Acquired clawhand, left hand
M21.519 Acquired clawhand, unspecified hand
M21.52 Acquired clubhand
M21.521 Acquired clubhand, right hand
M21.522 Acquired clubhand, left hand
M21.529 Acquired clubhand, unspecified hand
M21.53 Acquired clawfoot
M21.531 Acquired clawfoot, right foot
M21.532 Acquired clawfoot, left foot
M21.539 Acquired clawfoot, unspecified foot
M21.54 Acquired clubfoot
M21.541 Acquired clubfoot, right foot
M21.542 Acquired clubfoot, left foot
M21.549 Acquired clubfoot, unspecified foot

M21.6 Other acquired deformities of foot
EXCLUDES2 *deformities of toe (acquired) ▶(M20.1-M20.6-)◀*
● M21.61 Bunion
● M21.611 Bunion of right foot
● M21.612 Bunion of left foot
● M21.619 Bunion of unspecified foot
● M21.62 Bunionette
● M21.621 Bunionette of right foot
● M21.622 Bunionette of left foot
● M21.629 Bunionette of unspecified foot
M21.6X Other acquired deformities of foot
M21.6X1 Other acquired deformities of right foot
M21.6X2 Other acquired deformities of left foot
M21.6X9 Other acquired deformities of unspecified foot
M21.7 Unequal limb length (acquired)
NOTES The site used should correspond to the shorter limb
M21.70 Unequal limb length (acquired), unspecified site
M21.72 Unequal limb length (acquired), humerus
M21.721 Unequal limb length (acquired), right humerus
M21.722 Unequal limb length (acquired), left humerus
M21.729 Unequal limb length (acquired), unspecified humerus
M21.73 Unequal limb length (acquired), ulna and radius
M21.731 Unequal limb length (acquired), right ulna
M21.732 Unequal limb length (acquired), left ulna
M21.733 Unequal limb length (acquired), right radius
M21.734 Unequal limb length (acquired), left radius
M21.739 Unequal limb length (acquired), unspecified ulna and radius
M21.75 Unequal limb length (acquired), femur
M21.751 Unequal limb length (acquired), right femur
M21.752 Unequal limb length (acquired), left femur
M21.759 Unequal limb length (acquired), unspecified femur
M21.76 Unequal limb length (acquired), tibia and fibula
M21.761 Unequal limb length (acquired), right tibia
M21.762 Unequal limb length (acquired), left tibia
M21.763 Unequal limb length (acquired), right fibula
M21.764 Unequal limb length (acquired), left fibula
M21.769 Unequal limb length (acquired), unspecified tibia and fibula
M21.8 Other specified acquired deformities of limbs
EXCLUDES2 *coxa plana (M91.2)*
M21.80 Other specified acquired deformities of unspecified limb
M21.82 Other specified acquired deformities of upper arm
M21.821 Other specified acquired deformities of right upper arm
M21.822 Other specified acquired deformities of left upper arm
M21.829 Other specified acquired deformities of unspecified upper arm
M21.83 Other specified acquired deformities of forearm
M21.831 Other specified acquired deformities of right forearm
M21.832 Other specified acquired deformities of left forearm
M21.839 Other specified acquired deformities of unspecified forearm
M21.85 Other specified acquired deformities of thigh
M21.851 Other specified acquired deformities of right thigh
M21.852 Other specified acquired deformities of left thigh
M21.859 Other specified acquired deformities of unspecified thigh
M21.86 Other specified acquired deformities of lower leg

Unacceptable principal diagnosis symbol per Medicare code edits; Code exempt from diagnosis present on admission requirement; Questionable admission; Complication or comorbidity; CC/MCC exclusion; Major complication or comorbidity; Principal diagnosis as its own CC; Principal diagnosis as its own MCC; Z code as first-listed diagnosis

M21.861 Other specified acquired deformities of right lower leg
M21.862 Other specified acquired deformities of left lower leg
M21.869 Other specified acquired deformities of unspecified lower leg
M21.9 Unspecified acquired deformity of limb and hand
M21.90 Unspecified acquired deformity of unspecified limb
M21.92 Unspecified acquired deformity of upper arm
M21.921 Unspecified acquired deformity of right upper arm
M21.922 Unspecified acquired deformity of left upper arm
M21.929 Unspecified acquired deformity of unspecified upper arm
M21.93 Unspecified acquired deformity of forearm
M21.931 Unspecified acquired deformity of right forearm
M21.932 Unspecified acquired deformity of left forearm
M21.939 Unspecified acquired deformity of unspecified forearm
M21.94 Unspecified acquired deformity of hand
M21.941 Unspecified acquired deformity of hand, right hand
M21.942 Unspecified acquired deformity of hand, left hand
M21.949 Unspecified acquired deformity of hand, unspecified hand
M21.95 Unspecified acquired deformity of thigh
M21.951 Unspecified acquired deformity of right thigh
M21.952 Unspecified acquired deformity of left thigh
M21.959 Unspecified acquired deformity of unspecified thigh
M21.96 Unspecified acquired deformity of lower leg
M21.961 Unspecified acquired deformity of right lower leg
M21.962 Unspecified acquired deformity of left lower leg
M21.969 Unspecified acquired deformity of unspecified lower leg

M22 Disorder of patella
EXCLUDES1 *traumatic dislocation of patella (S83.0-)*
M22.0 Recurrent dislocation of patella
M22.00 Recurrent dislocation of patella, unspecified knee
M22.01 Recurrent dislocation of patella, right knee
M22.02 Recurrent dislocation of patella, left knee
M22.1 Recurrent subluxation of patella
Incomplete dislocation of patella
M22.10 Recurrent subluxation of patella, unspecified knee
M22.11 Recurrent subluxation of patella, right knee
M22.12 Recurrent subluxation of patella, left knee
M22.2 Patellofemoral disorders
M22.2X Patellofemoral disorders
M22.2X1 Patellofemoral disorders, right knee
M22.2X2 Patellofemoral disorders, left knee
M22.2X9 Patellofemoral disorders, unspecified knee
M22.3 Other derangements of patella
M22.3X Other derangements of patella
M22.3X1 Other derangements of patella, right knee
M22.3X2 Other derangements of patella, left knee
M22.3X9 Other derangements of patella, unspecified knee
M22.4 Chondromalacia patellae
M22.40 Chondromalacia patellae, unspecified knee
M22.41 Chondromalacia patellae, right knee
M22.42 Chondromalacia patellae, left knee
M22.8 Other disorders of patella
M22.8X Other disorders of patella
M22.8X1 Other disorders of patella, right knee
M22.8X2 Other disorders of patella, left knee
M22.8X9 Other disorders of patella, unspecified knee
M22.9 Unspecified disorder of patella
M22.90 Unspecified disorder of patella, unspecified knee
M22.91 Unspecified disorder of patella, right knee
M22.92 Unspecified disorder of patella, left knee

M23 Internal derangement of knee
EXCLUDES1 *ankylosis (M24.66)*
current injury - see injury of knee and lower leg (S80-S89)
deformity of knee (M21.-)
osteochondritis dissecans (M93.2)
recurrent dislocation or subluxation of joints (M24.4)
recurrent dislocation or subluxation of patella (M22.0-M22.1)
M23.0 Cystic meniscus
M23.00 Cystic meniscus, unspecified meniscus
Cystic meniscus, unspecified lateral meniscus
Cystic meniscus, unspecified medial meniscus
M23.000 Cystic meniscus, unspecified lateral meniscus, right knee
M23.001 Cystic meniscus, unspecified lateral meniscus, left knee
M23.002 Cystic meniscus, unspecified lateral meniscus, unspecified knee
M23.003 Cystic meniscus, unspecified medial meniscus, right knee
M23.004 Cystic meniscus, unspecified medial meniscus, left knee
M23.005 Cystic meniscus, unspecified medial meniscus, unspecified knee
M23.006 Cystic meniscus, unspecified meniscus, right knee
M23.007 Cystic meniscus, unspecified meniscus, left knee
M23.009 Cystic meniscus, unspecified meniscus, unspecified knee
M23.01 Cystic meniscus, anterior horn of medial meniscus
M23.011 Cystic meniscus, anterior horn of medial meniscus, right knee
M23.012 Cystic meniscus, anterior horn of medial meniscus, left knee
M23.019 Cystic meniscus, anterior horn of medial meniscus, unspecified knee
M23.02 Cystic meniscus, posterior horn of medial meniscus
M23.021 Cystic meniscus, posterior horn of medial meniscus, right knee
M23.022 Cystic meniscus, posterior horn of medial meniscus, left knee
M23.029 Cystic meniscus, posterior horn of medial meniscus, unspecified knee
M23.03 Cystic meniscus, other medial meniscus
M23.031 Cystic meniscus, other medial meniscus, right knee
M23.032 Cystic meniscus, other medial meniscus, left knee
M23.039 Cystic meniscus, other medial meniscus, unspecified knee
M23.04 Cystic meniscus, anterior horn of lateral meniscus
M23.041 Cystic meniscus, anterior horn of lateral meniscus, right knee
M23.042 Cystic meniscus, anterior horn of lateral meniscus, left knee
M23.049 Cystic meniscus, anterior horn of lateral meniscus, unspecified knee
M23.05 Cystic meniscus, posterior horn of lateral meniscus
M23.051 Cystic meniscus, posterior horn of lateral meniscus, right knee
M23.052 Cystic meniscus, posterior horn of lateral meniscus, left knee
M23.059 Cystic meniscus, posterior horn of lateral meniscus, unspecified knee
M23.06 Cystic meniscus, other lateral meniscus
M23.061 Cystic meniscus, other lateral meniscus, right knee
M23.062 Cystic meniscus, other lateral meniscus, left knee

Unspecified Code | Other Specified Code | Manifestation Code | N Newborn | P Pediatric | M Maternity | A Adult | ♂ Male | ♀ Female
● New Code | ▲ Revised Code Title | ►◄ Revised Text | NOTES | INCLUDES | EXCLUDES1 Not coded here | EXCLUDES2 Not included here
4th character required | 5th character required | 6th character required | 7th character required
Extension 'X' Alert | HAC Hospital-acquired condition (HAC) alert | AHA AHA Coding Clinic©

When symbols appear on a code that requires a 7th character extension, refer to Appendix D to identify applicable 7th character codes.

M23.069 Cystic meniscus, other lateral meniscus, unspecified knee

M23.2 Derangement of meniscus due to old tear or injury
Old bucket-handle tear

M23.20 Derangement of unspecified meniscus due to old tear or injury
Derangement of unspecified lateral meniscus due to old tear or injury
Derangement of unspecified medial meniscus due to old tear or injury

M23.200 Derangement of unspecified lateral meniscus due to old tear or injury, right knee
M23.201 Derangement of unspecified lateral meniscus due to old tear or injury, left knee
M23.202 Derangement of unspecified lateral meniscus due to old tear or injury, unspecified knee
M23.203 Derangement of unspecified medial meniscus due to old tear or injury, right knee
M23.204 Derangement of unspecified medial meniscus due to old tear or injury, left knee
M23.205 Derangement of unspecified medial meniscus due to old tear or injury, unspecified knee
M23.206 Derangement of unspecified meniscus due to old tear or injury, right knee
M23.207 Derangement of unspecified meniscus due to old tear or injury, left knee
M23.209 Derangement of unspecified meniscus due to old tear or injury, unspecified knee

M23.21 Derangement of anterior horn of medial meniscus due to old tear or injury
M23.211 Derangement of anterior horn of medial meniscus due to old tear or injury, right knee
M23.212 Derangement of anterior horn of medial meniscus due to old tear or injury, left knee
M23.219 Derangement of anterior horn of medial meniscus due to old tear or injury, unspecified knee

M23.22 Derangement of posterior horn of medial meniscus due to old tear or injury
M23.221 Derangement of posterior horn of medial meniscus due to old tear or injury, right knee
M23.222 Derangement of posterior horn of medial meniscus due to old tear or injury, left knee
M23.229 Derangement of posterior horn of medial meniscus due to old tear or injury, unspecified knee

M23.23 Derangement of other medial meniscus due to old tear or injury
M23.231 Derangement of other medial meniscus due to old tear or injury, right knee
M23.232 Derangement of other medial meniscus due to old tear or injury, left knee
M23.239 Derangement of other medial meniscus due to old tear or injury, unspecified knee

M23.24 Derangement of anterior horn of lateral meniscus due to old tear or injury
M23.241 Derangement of anterior horn of lateral meniscus due to old tear or injury, right knee
M23.242 Derangement of anterior horn of lateral meniscus due to old tear or injury, left knee
M23.249 Derangement of anterior horn of lateral meniscus due to old tear or injury, unspecified knee

M23.25 Derangement of posterior horn of lateral meniscus due to old tear or injury
M23.251 Derangement of posterior horn of lateral meniscus due to old tear or injury, right knee
M23.252 Derangement of posterior horn of lateral meniscus due to old tear or injury, left knee
M23.259 Derangement of posterior horn of lateral meniscus due to old tear or injury, unspecified knee

M23.26 Derangement of other lateral meniscus due to old tear or injury
M23.261 Derangement of other lateral meniscus due to old tear or injury, right knee
M23.262 Derangement of other lateral meniscus due to old tear or injury, left knee
M23.269 Derangement of other lateral meniscus due to old tear or injury, unspecified knee

M23.3 Other meniscus derangements
Degenerate meniscus
Detached meniscus
Retained meniscus

M23.30 Other meniscus derangements, unspecified meniscus
Other meniscus derangements, unspecified lateral meniscus
Other meniscus derangements, unspecified medial meniscus

M23.300 Other meniscus derangements, unspecified lateral meniscus, right knee
M23.301 Other meniscus derangements, unspecified lateral meniscus, left knee
M23.302 Other meniscus derangements, unspecified lateral meniscus, unspecified knee
M23.303 Other meniscus derangements, unspecified medial meniscus, right knee
M23.304 Other meniscus derangements, unspecified medial meniscus, left knee
M23.305 Other meniscus derangements, unspecified medial meniscus, unspecified knee
M23.306 Other meniscus derangements, unspecified meniscus, right knee
M23.307 Other meniscus derangements, unspecified meniscus, left knee
M23.309 Other meniscus derangements, unspecified meniscus, unspecified knee

M23.31 Other meniscus derangements, anterior horn of medial meniscus
M23.311 Other meniscus derangements, anterior horn of medial meniscus, right knee
M23.312 Other meniscus derangements, anterior horn of medial meniscus, left knee
M23.319 Other meniscus derangements, anterior horn of medial meniscus, unspecified knee

M23.32 Other meniscus derangements, posterior horn of medial meniscus
M23.321 Other meniscus derangements, posterior horn of medial meniscus, right knee
M23.322 Other meniscus derangements, posterior horn of medial meniscus, left knee
M23.329 Other meniscus derangements, posterior horn of medial meniscus, unspecified knee

M23.33 Other meniscus derangements, other medial meniscus
M23.331 Other meniscus derangements, other medial meniscus, right knee
M23.332 Other meniscus derangements, other medial meniscus, left knee
M23.339 Other meniscus derangements, other medial meniscus, unspecified knee

M23.34 Other meniscus derangements, anterior horn of lateral meniscus
M23.341 Other meniscus derangements, anterior horn of lateral meniscus, right knee

Unacceptable principal diagnosis symbol per Medicare code edits; Code exempt from diagnosis present on admission requirement; Questionable admission; Complication or comorbidity; CC/MCC exclusion; Major complication or comorbidity; Principal diagnosis as its own CC; Principal diagnosis as its own MCC; Z code as first-listed diagnosis

M23.342 Other meniscus derangements, anterior horn of lateral meniscus, left knee
M23.349 Other meniscus derangements, anterior horn of lateral meniscus, unspecified knee
M23.35 Other meniscus derangements, posterior horn of lateral meniscus
M23.351 Other meniscus derangements, posterior horn of lateral meniscus, right knee
M23.352 Other meniscus derangements, posterior horn of lateral meniscus, left knee
M23.359 Other meniscus derangements, posterior horn of lateral meniscus, unspecified knee
M23.36 Other meniscus derangements, other lateral meniscus
M23.361 Other meniscus derangements, other lateral meniscus, right knee
M23.362 Other meniscus derangements, other lateral meniscus, left knee
M23.369 Other meniscus derangements, other lateral meniscus, unspecified knee
M23.4 Loose body in knee
M23.40 Loose body in knee, unspecified knee
M23.41 Loose body in knee, right knee
M23.42 Loose body in knee, left knee
M23.5 Chronic instability of knee
M23.50 Chronic instability of knee, unspecified knee
M23.51 Chronic instability of knee, right knee
M23.52 Chronic instability of knee, left knee
M23.6 Other spontaneous disruption of ligament(s) of knee
M23.60 Other spontaneous disruption of unspecified ligament of knee
M23.601 Other spontaneous disruption of unspecified ligament of right knee
M23.602 Other spontaneous disruption of unspecified ligament of left knee
M23.609 Other spontaneous disruption of unspecified ligament of unspecified knee
M23.61 Other spontaneous disruption of anterior cruciate ligament of knee
M23.611 Other spontaneous disruption of anterior cruciate ligament of right knee
M23.612 Other spontaneous disruption of anterior cruciate ligament of left knee
M23.619 Other spontaneous disruption of anterior cruciate ligament of unspecified knee
M23.62 Other spontaneous disruption of posterior cruciate ligament of knee
M23.621 Other spontaneous disruption of posterior cruciate ligament of right knee
M23.622 Other spontaneous disruption of posterior cruciate ligament of left knee
M23.629 Other spontaneous disruption of posterior cruciate ligament of unspecified knee
M23.63 Other spontaneous disruption of medial collateral ligament of knee
M23.631 Other spontaneous disruption of medial collateral ligament of right knee
M23.632 Other spontaneous disruption of medial collateral ligament of left knee
M23.639 Other spontaneous disruption of medial collateral ligament of unspecified knee
M23.64 Other spontaneous disruption of lateral collateral ligament of knee
M23.641 Other spontaneous disruption of lateral collateral ligament of right knee
M23.642 Other spontaneous disruption of lateral collateral ligament of left knee
M23.649 Other spontaneous disruption of lateral collateral ligament of unspecified knee
M23.67 Other spontaneous disruption of capsular ligament of knee
M23.671 Other spontaneous disruption of capsular ligament of right knee
M23.672 Other spontaneous disruption of capsular ligament of left knee
M23.679 Other spontaneous disruption of capsular ligament of unspecified knee
M23.8 Other internal derangements of knee
Laxity of ligament of knee
Snapping knee
M23.8X Other internal derangements of knee
M23.8X1 Other internal derangements of right knee
M23.8X2 Other internal derangements of left knee
M23.8X9 Other internal derangements of unspecified knee
M23.9 Unspecified internal derangement of knee
M23.90 Unspecified internal derangement of unspecified knee
M23.91 Unspecified internal derangement of right knee
M23.92 Unspecified internal derangement of left knee

M24 Other specific joint derangements
EXCLUDES1 *current injury - see injury of joint by body region*
EXCLUDES2 *ganglion (M67.4)*
snapping knee (M23.8-)
temporomandibular joint disorders (M26.6-)
M24.0 Loose body in joint
EXCLUDES2 *loose body in knee (M23.4)*
M24.00 Loose body in unspecified joint
M24.01 Loose body in shoulder
M24.011 Loose body in right shoulder
M24.012 Loose body in left shoulder
M24.019 Loose body in unspecified shoulder
M24.02 Loose body in elbow
M24.021 Loose body in right elbow
M24.022 Loose body in left elbow
M24.029 Loose body in unspecified elbow
M24.03 Loose body in wrist
M24.031 Loose body in right wrist
M24.032 Loose body in left wrist
M24.039 Loose body in unspecified wrist
M24.04 Loose body in finger joints
M24.041 Loose body in right finger joint(s)
M24.042 Loose body in left finger joint(s)
M24.049 Loose body in unspecified finger joint(s)
M24.05 Loose body in hip
M24.051 Loose body in right hip
M24.052 Loose body in left hip
M24.059 Loose body in unspecified hip
M24.07 Loose body in ankle and toe joints
M24.071 Loose body in right ankle
M24.072 Loose body in left ankle
M24.073 Loose body in unspecified ankle
M24.074 Loose body in right toe joint(s)
M24.075 Loose body in left toe joint(s)
M24.076 Loose body in unspecified toe joints
M24.08 Loose body, other site
M24.1 Other articular cartilage disorders
EXCLUDES2 *chondrocalcinosis (M11.1, M11.2-)*
internal derangement of knee (M23.-)
metastatic calcification (E83.5)
ochronosis (E70.2)
M24.10 Other articular cartilage disorders, unspecified site
M24.11 Other articular cartilage disorders, shoulder
M24.111 Other articular cartilage disorders, right shoulder
M24.112 Other articular cartilage disorders, left shoulder
M24.119 Other articular cartilage disorders, unspecified shoulder
M24.12 Other articular cartilage disorders, elbow
M24.121 Other articular cartilage disorders, right elbow
M24.122 Other articular cartilage disorders, left elbow
M24.129 Other articular cartilage disorders, unspecified elbow

Unspecified Code | Other Specified Code | Manifestation Code | N Newborn | P Pediatric | M Maternity | A Adult | ♂ Male | ♀ Female
● New Code | ▲ Revised Code Title | ►◄ Revised Text | NOTES | INCLUDES | EXCLUDES1 Not coded here | EXCLUDES2 Not included here
4th character required | 5th character required | 6th character required | 7th character required
Extension 'X' Alert | HAC Hospital-acquired condition (HAC) alert | AHA AHA Coding Clinic©

M24.13 Other articular cartilage disorders, wrist
M24.131 Other articular cartilage disorders, right wrist
M24.132 Other articular cartilage disorders, left wrist
M24.139 Other articular cartilage disorders, unspecified wrist
M24.14 Other articular cartilage disorders, hand
M24.141 Other articular cartilage disorders, right hand
M24.142 Other articular cartilage disorders, left hand
M24.149 Other articular cartilage disorders, unspecified hand
M24.15 Other articular cartilage disorders, hip
M24.151 Other articular cartilage disorders, right hip
M24.152 Other articular cartilage disorders, left hip
M24.159 Other articular cartilage disorders, unspecified hip
M24.17 Other articular cartilage disorders, ankle and foot
M24.171 Other articular cartilage disorders, right ankle
M24.172 Other articular cartilage disorders, left ankle
M24.173 Other articular cartilage disorders, unspecified ankle
M24.174 Other articular cartilage disorders, right foot
M24.175 Other articular cartilage disorders, left foot
M24.176 Other articular cartilage disorders, unspecified foot

M24.2 Disorder of ligament
Instability secondary to old ligament injury
Ligamentous laxity NOS
EXCLUDES1 *familial ligamentous laxity (M35.7)*
EXCLUDES2 *internal derangement of knee (M23.5-M23.89)*
M24.20 Disorder of ligament, unspecified site
M24.21 Disorder of ligament, shoulder
M24.211 Disorder of ligament, right shoulder
M24.212 Disorder of ligament, left shoulder
M24.219 Disorder of ligament, unspecified shoulder
M24.22 Disorder of ligament, elbow
M24.221 Disorder of ligament, right elbow
M24.222 Disorder of ligament, left elbow
M24.229 Disorder of ligament, unspecified elbow
M24.23 Disorder of ligament, wrist
M24.231 Disorder of ligament, right wrist
M24.232 Disorder of ligament, left wrist
M24.239 Disorder of ligament, unspecified wrist
M24.24 Disorder of ligament, hand
M24.241 Disorder of ligament, right hand
M24.242 Disorder of ligament, left hand
M24.249 Disorder of ligament, unspecified hand
M24.25 Disorder of ligament, hip
M24.251 Disorder of ligament, right hip
M24.252 Disorder of ligament, left hip
M24.259 Disorder of ligament, unspecified hip
M24.27 Disorder of ligament, ankle and foot
M24.271 Disorder of ligament, right ankle
M24.272 Disorder of ligament, left ankle
M24.273 Disorder of ligament, unspecified ankle
M24.274 Disorder of ligament, right foot
M24.275 Disorder of ligament, left foot
M24.276 Disorder of ligament, unspecified foot
M24.28 Disorder of ligament, vertebrae

M24.3 Pathological dislocation of joint, not elsewhere classified
EXCLUDES1 *congenital dislocation or displacement of joint- see congenital malformations and deformations of the musculoskeletal system (Q65-Q79)*
current injury - see injury of joints and ligaments by body region
recurrent dislocation of joint (M24.4-)
M24.30 Pathological dislocation of unspecified joint, not elsewhere classified
M24.31 Pathological dislocation of shoulder, not elsewhere classified
M24.311 Pathological dislocation of right shoulder, not elsewhere classified
M24.312 Pathological dislocation of left shoulder, not elsewhere classified
M24.319 Pathological dislocation of unspecified shoulder, not elsewhere classified
M24.32 Pathological dislocation of elbow, not elsewhere classified
M24.321 Pathological dislocation of right elbow, not elsewhere classified
M24.322 Pathological dislocation of left elbow, not elsewhere classified
M24.329 Pathological dislocation of unspecified elbow, not elsewhere classified
M24.33 Pathological dislocation of wrist, not elsewhere classified
M24.331 Pathological dislocation of right wrist, not elsewhere classified
M24.332 Pathological dislocation of left wrist, not elsewhere classified
M24.339 Pathological dislocation of unspecified wrist, not elsewhere classified
M24.34 Pathological dislocation of hand, not elsewhere classified
M24.341 Pathological dislocation of right hand, not elsewhere classified
M24.342 Pathological dislocation of left hand, not elsewhere classified
M24.349 Pathological dislocation of unspecified hand, not elsewhere classified
M24.35 Pathological dislocation of hip, not elsewhere classified
M24.351 Pathological dislocation of right hip, not elsewhere classified
M24.352 Pathological dislocation of left hip, not elsewhere classified
M24.359 Pathological dislocation of unspecified hip, not elsewhere classified
M24.36 Pathological dislocation of knee, not elsewhere classified
M24.361 Pathological dislocation of right knee, not elsewhere classified
M24.362 Pathological dislocation of left knee, not elsewhere classified
M24.369 Pathological dislocation of unspecified knee, not elsewhere classified
M24.37 Pathological dislocation of ankle and foot, not elsewhere classified
M24.371 Pathological dislocation of right ankle, not elsewhere classified
M24.372 Pathological dislocation of left ankle, not elsewhere classified
M24.373 Pathological dislocation of unspecified ankle, not elsewhere classified
M24.374 Pathological dislocation of right foot, not elsewhere classified
M24.375 Pathological dislocation of left foot, not elsewhere classified
M24.376 Pathological dislocation of unspecified foot, not elsewhere classified

M24.4 Recurrent dislocation of joint
Recurrent subluxation of joint
EXCLUDES2 *recurrent dislocation of patella (M22.0-M22.1)*
recurrent vertebral dislocation (M43.3-, M43.4, M43.5-)
M24.40 Recurrent dislocation, unspecified joint
M24.41 Recurrent dislocation, shoulder
M24.411 Recurrent dislocation, right shoulder
M24.412 Recurrent dislocation, left shoulder
M24.419 Recurrent dislocation, unspecified shoulder
M24.42 Recurrent dislocation, elbow

Unacceptable principal diagnosis symbol per Medicare code edits; Code exempt from diagnosis present on admission requirement
Questionable admission; Complication or comorbidity; CC/MCC exclusion; Major complication or comorbidity
Principal diagnosis as its own CC; Principal diagnosis as its own MCC; Z code as first-listed diagnosis

When symbols appear on a code that requires a 7th character extension, refer to Appendix D to identify applicable 7th character codes.

M24.421 Recurrent dislocation, right elbow
M24.422 Recurrent dislocation, left elbow
M24.429 Recurrent dislocation, unspecified elbow
M24.43 Recurrent dislocation, wrist
M24.431 Recurrent dislocation, right wrist
M24.432 Recurrent dislocation, left wrist
M24.439 Recurrent dislocation, unspecified wrist
M24.44 Recurrent dislocation, hand and finger(s)
M24.441 Recurrent dislocation, right hand
M24.442 Recurrent dislocation, left hand
M24.443 Recurrent dislocation, unspecified hand
M24.444 Recurrent dislocation, right finger
M24.445 Recurrent dislocation, left finger
M24.446 Recurrent dislocation, unspecified finger
M24.45 Recurrent dislocation, hip
M24.451 Recurrent dislocation, right hip
M24.452 Recurrent dislocation, left hip
M24.459 Recurrent dislocation, unspecified hip
M24.46 Recurrent dislocation, knee
M24.461 Recurrent dislocation, right knee
M24.462 Recurrent dislocation, left knee
M24.469 Recurrent dislocation, unspecified knee
M24.47 Recurrent dislocation, ankle, foot and toes
M24.471 Recurrent dislocation, right ankle
M24.472 Recurrent dislocation, left ankle
M24.473 Recurrent dislocation, unspecified ankle
M24.474 Recurrent dislocation, right foot
M24.475 Recurrent dislocation, left foot
M24.476 Recurrent dislocation, unspecified foot
M24.477 Recurrent dislocation, right toe(s)
M24.478 Recurrent dislocation, left toe(s)
M24.479 Recurrent dislocation, unspecified toe(s)

M24.5 Contracture of joint

EXCLUDES1 *contracture of muscle without contracture of joint (M62.4-)*
contracture of tendon (sheath) without contracture of joint (M62.4-)
Dupuytren's contracture (M72.0)

EXCLUDES2 *acquired deformities of limbs (M20-M21)*

M24.50 Contracture, unspecified joint
M24.51 Contracture, shoulder
M24.511 Contracture, right shoulder
M24.512 Contracture, left shoulder
M24.519 Contracture, unspecified shoulder
M24.52 Contracture, elbow
M24.521 Contracture, right elbow
M24.522 Contracture, left elbow
M24.529 Contracture, unspecified elbow
M24.53 Contracture, wrist
M24.531 Contracture, right wrist
M24.532 Contracture, left wrist
M24.539 Contracture, unspecified wrist
M24.54 Contracture, hand
M24.541 Contracture, right hand
M24.542 Contracture, left hand
M24.549 Contracture, unspecified hand
M24.55 Contracture, hip
M24.551 Contracture, right hip
AHA: Q2, 2016
M24.552 Contracture, left hip
AHA: Q2, 2016
M24.559 Contracture, unspecified hip
M24.56 Contracture, knee
M24.561 Contracture, right knee
AHA: Q2, 2016
M24.562 Contracture, left knee
AHA: Q2, 2016
M24.569 Contracture, unspecified knee
M24.57 Contracture, ankle and foot
M24.571 Contracture, right ankle
M24.572 Contracture, left ankle
M24.573 Contracture, unspecified ankle
M24.574 Contracture, right foot
M24.575 Contracture, left foot
M24.576 Contracture, unspecified foot

M24.6 Ankylosis of joint

EXCLUDES1 *stiffness of joint without ankylosis (M25.6-)*

EXCLUDES2 *spine (M43.2-)*

M24.60 Ankylosis, unspecified joint
M24.61 Ankylosis, shoulder
M24.611 Ankylosis, right shoulder
M24.612 Ankylosis, left shoulder
M24.619 Ankylosis, unspecified shoulder
M24.62 Ankylosis, elbow
M24.621 Ankylosis, right elbow
M24.622 Ankylosis, left elbow
M24.629 Ankylosis, unspecified elbow
M24.63 Ankylosis, wrist
M24.631 Ankylosis, right wrist
M24.632 Ankylosis, left wrist
M24.639 Ankylosis, unspecified wrist
M24.64 Ankylosis, hand
M24.641 Ankylosis, right hand
M24.642 Ankylosis, left hand
M24.649 Ankylosis, unspecified hand
M24.65 Ankylosis, hip
M24.651 Ankylosis, right hip
M24.652 Ankylosis, left hip
M24.659 Ankylosis, unspecified hip
M24.66 Ankylosis, knee
M24.661 Ankylosis, right knee
M24.662 Ankylosis, left knee
M24.669 Ankylosis, unspecified knee
M24.67 Ankylosis, ankle and foot
M24.671 Ankylosis, right ankle
M24.672 Ankylosis, left ankle
M24.673 Ankylosis, unspecified ankle
M24.674 Ankylosis, right foot
M24.675 Ankylosis, left foot
M24.676 Ankylosis, unspecified foot

M24.7 Protrusio acetabuli

M24.8 Other specific joint derangements, not elsewhere classified

EXCLUDES2 *iliotibial band syndrome (M76.3)*

M24.80 Other specific joint derangements of unspecified joint, not elsewhere classified
M24.81 Other specific joint derangements of shoulder , not elsewhere classified
M24.811 Other specific joint derangements of right shoulder, not elsewhere classified
M24.812 Other specific joint derangements of left shoulder, not elsewhere classified
M24.819 Other specific joint derangements of unspecified shoulder, not elsewhere classified
M24.82 Other specific joint derangements of elbow , not elsewhere classified
M24.821 Other specific joint derangements of right elbow, not elsewhere classified
M24.822 Other specific joint derangements of left elbow, not elsewhere classified
M24.829 Other specific joint derangements of unspecified elbow, not elsewhere classified
M24.83 Other specific joint derangements of wrist , not elsewhere classified
M24.831 Other specific joint derangements of right wrist, not elsewhere classified
M24.832 Other specific joint derangements of left wrist, not elsewhere classified
M24.839 Other specific joint derangements of unspecified wrist, not elsewhere classified
M24.84 Other specific joint derangements of hand , not elsewhere classified
M24.841 Other specific joint derangements of right hand, not elsewhere classified

Unspecified Code Other Specified Code Manifestation Code N Newborn P Pediatric M Maternity A Adult ♂ Male ♀ Female
● New Code ▲ Revised Code Title ►◄ Revised Text NOTES INCLUDES EXCLUDES1 Not coded here EXCLUDES2 Not included here
4th character required 5th character required 6th character required 7th character required
Extension 'X' Alert HAC Hospital-acquired condition (HAC) alert AHA AHA Coding Clinic©

M24.842 Other specific joint derangements of left hand, not elsewhere classified
M24.849 Other specific joint derangements of unspecified hand, not elsewhere classified
M24.85 Other specific joint derangements of hip, not elsewhere classified
Irritable hip
M24.851 Other specific joint derangements of right hip, not elsewhere classified
M24.852 Other specific joint derangements of left hip, not elsewhere classified
M24.859 Other specific joint derangements of unspecified hip, not elsewhere classified
M24.87 Other specific joint derangements of ankle and foot, not elsewhere classified
M24.871 Other specific joint derangements of right ankle, not elsewhere classified
M24.872 Other specific joint derangements of left ankle, not elsewhere classified
M24.873 Other specific joint derangements of unspecified ankle, not elsewhere classified
M24.874 Other specific joint derangements of right foot, not elsewhere classified
M24.875 Other specific joint derangements left foot, not elsewhere classified
M24.876 Other specific joint derangements of unspecified foot, not elsewhere classified
M24.9 Joint derangement, unspecified
M25 Other joint disorder, not elsewhere classified
EXCLUDES2 *abnormality of gait and mobility (R26.-)*
acquired deformities of limb (M20-M21)
calcification of bursa (M71.4-)
calcification of shoulder (joint) (M75.3)
calcification of tendon (M65.2-)
difficulty in walking (R26.2)
temporomandibular joint disorder (M26.6-)
M25.0 Hemarthrosis
EXCLUDES1 *current injury - see injury of joint by body region*
hemophilic arthropathy (M36.2)
M25.00 Hemarthrosis, unspecified joint CC
M25.01 Hemarthrosis, shoulder
M25.011 Hemarthrosis, right shoulder CC
M25.012 Hemarthrosis, left shoulder CC
M25.019 Hemarthrosis, unspecified shoulder CC
M25.02 Hemarthrosis, elbow
M25.021 Hemarthrosis, right elbow CC
M25.022 Hemarthrosis, left elbow CC
M25.029 Hemarthrosis, unspecified elbow CC
M25.03 Hemarthrosis, wrist
M25.031 Hemarthrosis, right wrist CC
M25.032 Hemarthrosis, left wrist CC
M25.039 Hemarthrosis, unspecified wrist CC
M25.04 Hemarthrosis, hand
M25.041 Hemarthrosis, right hand CC
M25.042 Hemarthrosis, left hand CC
M25.049 Hemarthrosis, unspecified hand CC
M25.05 Hemarthrosis, hip
M25.051 Hemarthrosis, right hip CC
M25.052 Hemarthrosis, left hip CC
M25.059 Hemarthrosis, unspecified hip CC
M25.06 Hemarthrosis, knee
M25.061 Hemarthrosis, right knee CC
M25.062 Hemarthrosis, left knee CC
M25.069 Hemarthrosis, unspecified knee CC
M25.07 Hemarthrosis, ankle and foot
M25.071 Hemarthrosis, right ankle CC
M25.072 Hemarthrosis, left ankle CC
M25.073 Hemarthrosis, unspecified ankle CC
M25.074 Hemarthrosis, right foot CC
M25.075 Hemarthrosis, left foot CC
M25.076 Hemarthrosis, unspecified foot CC
M25.08 Hemarthrosis, other specified site CC
Hemarthrosis, vertebrae
M25.1 Fistula of joint
M25.10 Fistula, unspecified joint
M25.11 Fistula, shoulder
M25.111 Fistula, right shoulder
M25.112 Fistula, left shoulder
M25.119 Fistula, unspecified shoulder
M25.12 Fistula, elbow
M25.121 Fistula, right elbow
M25.122 Fistula, left elbow
M25.129 Fistula, unspecified elbow
M25.13 Fistula, wrist
M25.131 Fistula, right wrist
M25.132 Fistula, left wrist
M25.139 Fistula, unspecified wrist
M25.14 Fistula, hand
M25.141 Fistula, right hand
M25.142 Fistula, left hand
M25.149 Fistula, unspecified hand
M25.15 Fistula, hip
M25.151 Fistula, right hip
M25.152 Fistula, left hip
M25.159 Fistula, unspecified hip
M25.16 Fistula, knee
M25.161 Fistula, right knee
M25.162 Fistula, left knee
M25.169 Fistula, unspecified knee
M25.17 Fistula, ankle and foot
M25.171 Fistula, right ankle
M25.172 Fistula, left ankle
M25.173 Fistula, unspecified ankle
M25.174 Fistula, right foot
M25.175 Fistula, left foot
M25.176 Fistula, unspecified foot
M25.18 Fistula, other specified site
Fistula, vertebrae
M25.2 Flail joint
M25.20 Flail joint, unspecified joint
M25.21 Flail joint, shoulder
M25.211 Flail joint, right shoulder
M25.212 Flail joint, left shoulder
M25.219 Flail joint, unspecified shoulder
M25.22 Flail joint, elbow
M25.221 Flail joint, right elbow
M25.222 Flail joint, left elbow
M25.229 Flail joint, unspecified elbow
M25.23 Flail joint, wrist
M25.231 Flail joint, right wrist
M25.232 Flail joint, left wrist
M25.239 Flail joint, unspecified wrist
M25.24 Flail joint, hand
M25.241 Flail joint, right hand
M25.242 Flail joint, left hand
M25.249 Flail joint, unspecified hand
M25.25 Flail joint, hip
M25.251 Flail joint, right hip
M25.252 Flail joint, left hip
M25.259 Flail joint, unspecified hip
M25.26 Flail joint, knee
M25.261 Flail joint, right knee
M25.262 Flail joint, left knee
M25.269 Flail joint, unspecified knee
M25.27 Flail joint, ankle and foot
M25.271 Flail joint, right ankle and foot
M25.272 Flail joint, left ankle and foot
M25.279 Flail joint, unspecified ankle and foot
M25.28 Flail joint, other site
M25.3 Other instability of joint
EXCLUDES1 *instability of joint secondary to old ligament injury (M24.2-)*
instability of joint secondary to removal of joint prosthesis (M96.8-)

PDx Unacceptable principal diagnosis symbol per Medicare code edits POA Code exempt from diagnosis present on admission requirement
? Questionable admission CC Complication or comorbidity CC/MCC Exc CC/MCC exclusion MCC Major complication or comorbidity
PDx CC Principal diagnosis as its own CC PDx MCC Principal diagnosis as its own MCC Z1 Z code as first-listed diagnosis

EXCLUDES2 *spinal instabilities (M53.2-)*
M25.30 Other instability, unspecified joint
M25.31 Other instability, shoulder
M25.311 Other instability, right shoulder
M25.312 Other instability, left shoulder
M25.319 Other instability, unspecified shoulder
M25.32 Other instability, elbow
M25.321 Other instability, right elbow
M25.322 Other instability, left elbow
M25.329 Other instability, unspecified elbow
M25.33 Other instability, wrist
M25.331 Other instability, right wrist
M25.332 Other instability, left wrist
M25.339 Other instability, unspecified wrist
M25.34 Other instability, hand
M25.341 Other instability, right hand
M25.342 Other instability, left hand
M25.349 Other instability, unspecified hand
M25.35 Other instability, hip
M25.351 Other instability, right hip
M25.352 Other instability, left hip
M25.359 Other instability, unspecified hip
M25.36 Other instability, knee
M25.361 Other instability, right knee
M25.362 Other instability, left knee
M25.369 Other instability, unspecified knee
M25.37 Other instability, ankle and foot
M25.371 Other instability, right ankle
M25.372 Other instability, left ankle
M25.373 Other instability, unspecified ankle
M25.374 Other instability, right foot
M25.375 Other instability, left foot
M25.376 Other instability, unspecified foot
M25.4 Effusion of joint
EXCLUDES1 *hydrarthrosis in yaws (A66.6)*
intermittent hydrarthrosis (M12.4-)
other infective (teno)synovitis (M65.1-)
M25.40 Effusion, unspecified joint
M25.41 Effusion, shoulder
M25.411 Effusion, right shoulder
M25.412 Effusion, left shoulder
M25.419 Effusion, unspecified shoulder
M25.42 Effusion, elbow
M25.421 Effusion, right elbow
M25.422 Effusion, left elbow
M25.429 Effusion, unspecified elbow
M25.43 Effusion, wrist
M25.431 Effusion, right wrist
M25.432 Effusion, left wrist
M25.439 Effusion, unspecified wrist
M25.44 Effusion, hand
M25.441 Effusion, right hand
M25.442 Effusion, left hand
M25.449 Effusion, unspecified hand
M25.45 Effusion, hip
M25.451 Effusion, right hip
M25.452 Effusion, left hip
M25.459 Effusion, unspecified hip
M25.46 Effusion, knee
M25.461 Effusion, right knee
M25.462 Effusion, left knee
M25.469 Effusion, unspecified knee
M25.47 Effusion, ankle and foot
M25.471 Effusion, right ankle
M25.472 Effusion, left ankle
M25.473 Effusion, unspecified ankle
M25.474 Effusion, right foot
M25.475 Effusion, left foot
M25.476 Effusion, unspecified foot
M25.48 Effusion, other site
M25.5 Pain in joint
EXCLUDES2 *pain in hand (M79.64-)*
pain in fingers (M79.64-)
pain in foot (M79.67-)
pain in limb (M79.6-)
pain in toes (M79.67-)
M25.50 Pain in unspecified joint
M25.51 Pain in shoulder
M25.511 Pain in right shoulder
M25.512 Pain in left shoulder
M25.519 Pain in unspecified shoulder
M25.52 Pain in elbow
M25.521 Pain in right elbow
M25.522 Pain in left elbow
M25.529 Pain in unspecified elbow
M25.53 Pain in wrist
M25.531 Pain in right wrist
M25.532 Pain in left wrist
M25.539 Pain in unspecified wrist
● M25.54 Pain in joints of hand
● M25.541 Pain in joints of right hand CC/MCC Exc
● M25.542 Pain in joints of left hand CC/MCC Exc
● M25.549 Pain in joints of unspecified hand CC/MCC Exc
Pain in joints of hand NOS
M25.55 Pain in hip
M25.551 Pain in right hip
M25.552 Pain in left hip
M25.559 Pain in unspecified hip
M25.56 Pain in knee
M25.561 Pain in right knee
M25.562 Pain in left knee
M25.569 Pain in unspecified knee
M25.57 Pain in ankle and joints of foot
M25.571 Pain in right ankle and joints of right foot
M25.572 Pain in left ankle and joints of left foot
M25.579 Pain in unspecified ankle and joints of unspecified foot
M25.6 Stiffness of joint, not elsewhere classified
EXCLUDES1 *ankylosis of joint (M24.6-)*
contracture of joint (M24.5-)
M25.60 Stiffness of unspecified joint, not elsewhere classified
M25.61 Stiffness of shoulder, not elsewhere classified
M25.611 Stiffness of right shoulder, not elsewhere classified
M25.612 Stiffness of left shoulder, not elsewhere classified
M25.619 Stiffness of unspecified shoulder, not elsewhere classified
M25.62 Stiffness of elbow, not elsewhere classified
M25.621 Stiffness of right elbow, not elsewhere classified
M25.622 Stiffness of left elbow, not elsewhere classified
M25.629 Stiffness of unspecified elbow, not elsewhere classified
M25.63 Stiffness of wrist, not elsewhere classified
M25.631 Stiffness of right wrist, not elsewhere classified
M25.632 Stiffness of left wrist, not elsewhere classified
M25.639 Stiffness of unspecified wrist, not elsewhere classified
M25.64 Stiffness of hand, not elsewhere classified
M25.641 Stiffness of right hand, not elsewhere classified
M25.642 Stiffness of left hand, not elsewhere classified
M25.649 Stiffness of unspecified hand, not elsewhere classified
M25.65 Stiffness of hip, not elsewhere classified
M25.651 Stiffness of right hip, not elsewhere classified
M25.652 Stiffness of left hip, not elsewhere classified

Unspecified Code Other Specified Code Manifestation Code N Newborn P Pediatric M Maternity A Adult ♂ Male ♀ Female
● New Code ▲ Revised Code Title ►◄ Revised Text NOTES INCLUDES EXCLUDES1 Not coded here EXCLUDES2 Not included here
4th character required 5th character required 6th character required 7th character required
Extension 'X' Alert HAC Hospital-acquired condition (HAC) alert AHA AHA Coding Clinic©

M25.659 Stiffness of unspecified hip, not elsewhere classified
M25.66 Stiffness of knee, not elsewhere classified
M25.661 Stiffness of right knee, not elsewhere classified
M25.662 Stiffness of left knee, not elsewhere classified
M25.669 Stiffness of unspecified knee, not elsewhere classified
M25.67 Stiffness of ankle and foot, not elsewhere classified
M25.671 Stiffness of right ankle, not elsewhere classified
M25.672 Stiffness of left ankle, not elsewhere classified
M25.673 Stiffness of unspecified ankle, not elsewhere classified
M25.674 Stiffness of right foot, not elsewhere classified
M25.675 Stiffness of left foot, not elsewhere classified
M25.676 Stiffness of unspecified foot, not elsewhere classified
M25.7 Osteophyte
M25.70 Osteophyte, unspecified joint
M25.71 Osteophyte, shoulder
M25.711 Osteophyte, right shoulder
M25.712 Osteophyte, left shoulder
M25.719 Osteophyte, unspecified shoulder
M25.72 Osteophyte, elbow
M25.721 Osteophyte, right elbow
M25.722 Osteophyte, left elbow
M25.729 Osteophyte, unspecified elbow
M25.73 Osteophyte, wrist
M25.731 Osteophyte, right wrist
M25.732 Osteophyte, left wrist
M25.739 Osteophyte, unspecified wrist
M25.74 Osteophyte, hand
M25.741 Osteophyte, right hand
M25.742 Osteophyte, left hand
M25.749 Osteophyte, unspecified hand
M25.75 Osteophyte, hip
M25.751 Osteophyte, right hip
M25.752 Osteophyte, left hip
M25.759 Osteophyte, unspecified hip
M25.76 Osteophyte, knee
M25.761 Osteophyte, right knee
M25.762 Osteophyte, left knee
M25.769 Osteophyte, unspecified knee
M25.77 Osteophyte, ankle and foot
M25.771 Osteophyte, right ankle
M25.772 Osteophyte, left ankle
M25.773 Osteophyte, unspecified ankle
M25.774 Osteophyte, right foot
M25.775 Osteophyte, left foot
M25.776 Osteophyte, unspecified foot
M25.78 Osteophyte, vertebrae
M25.8 Other specified joint disorders
M25.80 Other specified joint disorders, unspecified joint
M25.81 Other specified joint disorders, shoulder
M25.811 Other specified joint disorders, right shoulder
M25.812 Other specified joint disorders, left shoulder
M25.819 Other specified joint disorders, unspecified shoulder
M25.82 Other specified joint disorders, elbow
M25.821 Other specified joint disorders, right elbow
M25.822 Other specified joint disorders, left elbow
M25.829 Other specified joint disorders, unspecified elbow
M25.83 Other specified joint disorders, wrist
M25.831 Other specified joint disorders, right wrist
M25.832 Other specified joint disorders, left wrist
M25.839 Other specified joint disorders, unspecified wrist
M25.84 Other specified joint disorders, hand
M25.841 Other specified joint disorders, right hand
M25.842 Other specified joint disorders, left hand
M25.849 Other specified joint disorders, unspecified hand
M25.85 Other specified joint disorders, hip
M25.851 Other specified joint disorders, right hip
M25.852 Other specified joint disorders, left hip
M25.859 Other specified joint disorders, unspecified hip
M25.86 Other specified joint disorders, knee
M25.861 Other specified joint disorders, right knee
M25.862 Other specified joint disorders, left knee
M25.869 Other specified joint disorders, unspecified knee
M25.87 Other specified joint disorders, ankle and foot
M25.871 Other specified joint disorders, right ankle and foot
M25.872 Other specified joint disorders, left ankle and foot
M25.879 Other specified joint disorders, unspecified ankle and foot
M25.9 Joint disorder, unspecified

Dentofacial anomalies [including malocclusion] and other disorders of jaw (M26-M27)

EXCLUDES1 *hemifacial atrophy or hypertrophy (Q67.4)*
unilateral condylar hyperplasia or hypoplasia (M27.8)

M26 Dentofacial anomalies [including malocclusion]
M26.0 Major anomalies of jaw size
EXCLUDES1 *acromegaly (E22.0)*
Robin's syndrome (Q87.0)
M26.00 Unspecified anomaly of jaw size
M26.01 Maxillary hyperplasia
M26.02 Maxillary hypoplasia
M26.03 Mandibular hyperplasia
M26.04 Mandibular hypoplasia
M26.05 Macrogenia
M26.06 Microgenia
M26.07 Excessive tuberosity of jaw
Entire maxillary tuberosity
M26.09 Other specified anomalies of jaw size
M26.1 Anomalies of jaw-cranial base relationship
M26.10 Unspecified anomaly of jaw-cranial base relationship
M26.11 Maxillary asymmetry
M26.12 Other jaw asymmetry
M26.19 Other specified anomalies of jaw-cranial base relationship
M26.2 Anomalies of dental arch relationship
M26.20 Unspecified anomaly of dental arch relationship
M26.21 Malocclusion, Angle's class
M26.211 Malocclusion, Angle's class I
Neutro-occlusion
M26.212 Malocclusion, Angle's class II
Disto-occlusion Division I
Disto-occlusion Division II
M26.213 Malocclusion, Angle's class III
Mesio-occlusion
M26.219 Malocclusion, Angle's class, unspecified
M26.22 Open occlusal relationship
M26.220 Open anterior occlusal relationship
Anterior openbite
M26.221 Open posterior occlusal relationship
Posterior openbite
M26.23 Excessive horizontal overlap
Excessive horizontal overjet
M26.24 Reverse articulation
Crossbite (anterior) (posterior)
M26.25 Anomalies of interarch distance
M26.29 Other anomalies of dental arch relationship

Unacceptable principal diagnosis symbol per Medicare code edits · Code exempt from diagnosis present on admission requirement
Questionable admission · Complication or comorbidity · CC/MCC exclusion · Major complication or comorbidity
Principal diagnosis as its own CC · Principal diagnosis as its own MCC · Z code as first-listed diagnosis

Midline deviation of dental arch
Overbite (excessive) deep
Overbite (excessive) horizontal
Overbite (excessive) vertical
Posterior lingual occlusion of mandibular teeth

M26.3 Anomalies of tooth position of fully erupted tooth or teeth
EXCLUDES2 *embedded and impacted teeth (K01.-)*

M26.30 Unspecified anomaly of tooth position of fully erupted tooth or teeth
Abnormal spacing of fully erupted tooth or teeth NOS
Displacement of fully erupted tooth or teeth NOS
Transposition of fully erupted tooth or teeth NOS

M26.31 Crowding of fully erupted teeth

M26.32 Excessive spacing of fully erupted teeth
Diastema of fully erupted tooth or teeth NOS

M26.33 Horizontal displacement of fully erupted tooth or teeth
Tipped tooth or teeth
Tipping of fully erupted tooth

M26.34 Vertical displacement of fully erupted tooth or teeth
Extruded tooth
Infraeruption of tooth or teeth
Supraeruption of tooth or teeth

M26.35 Rotation of fully erupted tooth or teeth

M26.36 Insufficient interocclusal distance of fully erupted teeth (ridge)
Lack of adequate intermaxillary vertical dimension of fully erupted teeth

M26.37 Excessive interocclusal distance of fully erupted teeth
Excessive intermaxillary vertical dimension of fully erupted teeth
Loss of occlusal vertical dimension of fully erupted teeth

M26.39 Other anomalies of tooth position of fully erupted tooth or teeth

M26.4 Malocclusion, unspecified

M26.5 Dentofacial functional abnormalities
EXCLUDES1 *bruxism (F45.8)*
teeth-grinding NOS (F45.8)

M26.50 Dentofacial functional abnormalities, unspecified

M26.51 Abnormal jaw closure

M26.52 Limited mandibular range of motion

M26.53 Deviation in opening and closing of the mandible

M26.54 Insufficient anterior guidance
Insufficient anterior occlusal guidance

M26.55 Centric occlusion maximum intercuspation discrepancy
EXCLUDES1 *centric occlusion NOS (M26.59)*

M26.56 Non-working side interference
Balancing side interference

M26.57 Lack of posterior occlusal support

M26.59 Other dentofacial functional abnormalities
Centric occlusion (of teeth) NOS
Malocclusion due to abnormal swallowing
Malocclusion due to mouth breathing
Malocclusion due to tongue, lip or finger habits

M26.6 Temporomandibular joint disorders
EXCLUDES2 *current temporomandibular joint dislocation (S03.0)*
current temporomandibular joint sprain (S03.4)

M26.60 Temporomandibular joint disorder, unspecified

● **M26.601 Right temporomandibular joint disorder, unspecified** CC/MCC Exc

● **M26.602 Left temporomandibular joint disorder, unspecified** CC/MCC Exc

● **M26.603 Bilateral temporomandibular joint disorder, unspecified** CC/MCC Exc

● **M26.609 Unspecified temporomandibular joint disorder, unspecified side** CC/MCC Exc
Temporomandibular joint disorder NOS

M26.61 Adhesions and ankylosis of temporomandibular joint

● **M26.611 Adhesions and ankylosis of right temporomandibular joint** CC/MCC Exc

● **M26.612 Adhesions and ankylosis of left temporomandibular joint** CC/MCC Exc

● **M26.613 Adhesions and ankylosis of bilateral temporomandibular joint** CC/MCC Exc

● **M26.619 Adhesions and ankylosis of temporomandibular joint, unspecified side** CC/MCC Exc

M26.62 Arthralgia of temporomandibular joint

● **M26.621 Arthralgia of right temporomandibular joint** CC/MCC Exc

● **M26.622 Arthralgia of left temporomandibular joint** CC/MCC Exc

● **M26.623 Arthralgia of bilateral temporomandibular joint** CC/MCC Exc

● **M26.629 Arthralgia of temporomandibular joint, unspecified side** CC/MCC Exc

M26.63 Articular disc disorder of temporomandibular joint

● **M26.631 Articular disc disorder of right temporomandibular joint** CC/MCC Exc

● **M26.632 Articular disc disorder of left temporomandibular joint** CC/MCC Exc

● **M26.633 Articular disc disorder of bilateral temporomandibular joint** CC/MCC Exc

● **M26.639 Articular disc disorder of temporomandibular joint, unspecified side** CC/MCC Exc

M26.69 Other specified disorders of temporomandibular joint

M26.7 Dental alveolar anomalies

M26.70 Unspecified alveolar anomaly

M26.71 Alveolar maxillary hyperplasia

M26.72 Alveolar mandibular hyperplasia

M26.73 Alveolar maxillary hypoplasia

M26.74 Alveolar mandibular hypoplasia

M26.79 Other specified alveolar anomalies

M26.8 Other dentofacial anomalies

M26.81 Anterior soft tissue impingement
Anterior soft tissue impingement on teeth

M26.82 Posterior soft tissue impingement
Posterior soft tissue impingement on teeth

M26.89 Other dentofacial anomalies

M26.9 Dentofacial anomaly, unspecified

M27 Other diseases of jaws

M27.0 Developmental disorders of jaws
Latent bone cyst of jaw
Stafne's cyst
Torus mandibularis
Torus palatinus

M27.1 Giant cell granuloma, central
Giant cell granuloma NOS
EXCLUDES1 *peripheral giant cell granuloma (K06.8)*

M27.2 Inflammatory conditions of jaws
Osteitis of jaw(s)
Osteomyelitis (neonatal) jaw(s)
Osteoradionecrosis jaw(s)
Periostitis jaw(s)
Sequestrum of jaw bone
Use additional code (W88-W90, X39.0) to identify radiation, if radiation-induced
EXCLUDES2 *osteonecrosis of jaw due to drug (M87.180)*

M27.3 Alveolitis of jaws
Alveolar osteitis
Dry socket

M27.4 Other and unspecified cysts of jaw
EXCLUDES1 *cysts of oral region (K09.-)*
latent bone cyst of jaw (M27.0)
Stafne's cyst (M27.0)

M27.40 Unspecified cyst of jaw
Cyst of jaw NOS

M27.49 Other cysts of jaw
Aneurysmal cyst of jaw
Hemorrhagic cyst of jaw
Traumatic cyst of jaw

M27.5 Periradicular pathology associated with previous endodontic treatment

M27.51 Perforation of root canal space due to endodontic treatment

Unspecified Code | Other Specified Code | Manifestation Code | N Newborn | P Pediatric | M Maternity | A Adult | ♂ Male | ♀ Female
● New Code | ▲ Revised Code Title | ►◄ Revised Text | NOTES | INCLUDES | EXCLUDES1 Not coded here | EXCLUDES2 Not included here
4th character required | 5th character required | 6th character required | 7th character required
Extension 'X' Alert | HAC Hospital-acquired condition (HAC) alert | AHA AHA Coding Clinic©

When symbols appear on a code that requires a 7th character extension, refer to Appendix D to identify applicable 7th character codes.

M27.52 **Endodontic overfill**
M27.53 **Endodontic underfill**
M27.59 **Other periradicular pathology associated with previous endodontic treatment**

M27.6 **Endosseous dental implant failure**
M27.61 **Osseointegration failure of dental implant**
Hemorrhagic complications of dental implant placement
Iatrogenic osseointegration failure of dental implant
Osseointegration failure of dental implant due to complications of systemic disease
Osseointegration failure of dental implant due to poor bone quality
Pre-integration failure of dental implant NOS
Pre-osseointegration failure of dental implant
M27.62 **Post-osseointegration biological failure of dental implant**
Failure of dental implant due to lack of attached gingiva
Failure of dental implant due to occlusal trauma (caused by poor prosthetic design)
Failure of dental implant due to parafunctional habits
Failure of dental implant due to periodontal infection (peri-implantitis)
Failure of dental implant due to poor oral hygiene
Iatrogenic post-osseointegration failure of dental implant
Post-osseointegration failure of dental implant due to complications of systemic disease
M27.63 **Post-osseointegration mechanical failure of dental implant**
Failure of dental prosthesis causing loss of dental implant
Fracture of dental implant
EXCLUDES2 *cracked tooth (K03.81)*
fractured dental restorative material with loss of material (K08.531)
fractured dental restorative material without loss of material (K08.530)
fractured tooth (S02.5)
M27.69 **Other endosseous dental implant failure**
Dental implant failure NOS

M27.8 **Other specified diseases of jaws**
Cherubism
Exostosis
Fibrous dysplasia
Unilateral condylar hyperplasia
Unilateral condylar hypoplasia
EXCLUDES1 *jaw pain (R68.84)*
M27.9 **Disease of jaws, unspecified**

Systemic connective tissue disorders (M30-M36)

INCLUDES *autoimmune disease NOS*
collagen (vascular) disease NOS
systemic autoimmune disease
systemic collagen (vascular) disease
EXCLUDES1 *autoimmune disease, single organ or single cell-type -code to relevant condition category*

M30 **Polyarteritis nodosa and related conditions**
EXCLUDES1 *microscopic polyarteritis (M31.7)*
M30.0 **Polyarteritis nodosa** CC
M30.1 **Polyarteritis with lung involvement [Churg-Strauss]** CC
Allergic granulomatous angiitis
M30.2 **Juvenile polyarteritis** CC
M30.3 **Mucocutaneous lymph node syndrome [Kawasaki]** CC
M30.8 **Other conditions related to polyarteritis nodosa** CC
Polyangiitis overlap syndrome

M31 **Other necrotizing vasculopathies**
M31.0 **Hypersensitivity angiitis** CC
Goodpasture's syndrome
M31.1 **Thrombotic microangiopathy** MCC
Thrombotic thrombocytopenic purpura
M31.2 **Lethal midline granuloma** CC
M31.3 **Wegener's granulomatosis**
Necrotizing respiratory granulomatosis
M31.30 **Wegener's granulomatosis without renal involvement** CC
Wegener's granulomatosis NOS
M31.31 **Wegener's granulomatosis with renal involvement** CC
M31.4 **Aortic arch syndrome [Takayasu]** CC
M31.5 **Giant cell arteritis with polymyalgia rheumatica**
M31.6 **Other giant cell arteritis**
M31.7 **Microscopic polyangiitis** CC
Microscopic polyarteritis
EXCLUDES1 *polyarteritis nodosa (M30.0)*
M31.8 **Other specified necrotizing vasculopathies** CC
Hypocomplementemic vasculitis
Septic vasculitis
M31.9 **Necrotizing vasculopathy, unspecified** CC

M32 **Systemic lupus erythematosus (SLE)**
EXCLUDES1 *lupus erythematosus (discoid) (NOS) (L93.0)*
M32.0 **Drug-induced systemic lupus erythematosus**
Use additional code for adverse effect, if applicable, to identify drug (T36-T50 with fifth or sixth character 5)
M32.1 **Systemic lupus erythematosus with organ or system involvement**
M32.10 **Systemic lupus erythematosus, organ or system involvement unspecified**
M32.11 **Endocarditis in systemic lupus erythematosus** CC PDx
Libman-Sacks disease
M32.12 **Pericarditis in systemic lupus erythematosus** CC PDx
Lupus pericarditis
M32.13 **Lung involvement in systemic lupus erythematosus**
Pleural effusion due to systemic lupus erythematosus
M32.14 **Glomerular disease in systemic lupus erythematosus**
Lupus renal disease NOS
AHA: Q4, 2013
M32.15 **Tubulo-interstitial nephropathy in systemic lupus erythematosus**
M32.19 **Other organ or system involvement in systemic lupus erythematosus**
M32.8 **Other forms of systemic lupus erythematosus**
M32.9 **Systemic lupus erythematosus, unspecified**
SLE NOS
Systemic lupus erythematosus NOS
Systemic lupus erythematosus without organ involvement

M33 **Dermatopolymyositis**
M33.0 **Juvenile dermatopolymyositis**
M33.00 **Juvenile dermatopolymyositis, organ involvement unspecified** CC
M33.01 **Juvenile dermatopolymyositis with respiratory involvement** CC
M33.02 **Juvenile dermatopolymyositis with myopathy** CC PDx
M33.09 **Juvenile dermatopolymyositis with other organ involvement** CC
M33.1 **Other dermatopolymyositis**
M33.10 **Other dermatopolymyositis, organ involvement unspecified** CC
M33.11 **Other dermatopolymyositis with respiratory involvement** CC
M33.12 **Other dermatopolymyositis with myopathy** CC PDx
M33.19 **Other dermatopolymyositis with other organ involvement** CC
M33.2 **Polymyositis**
M33.20 **Polymyositis, organ involvement unspecified** CC
M33.21 **Polymyositis with respiratory involvement** CC
M33.22 **Polymyositis with myopathy** CC PDx
M33.29 **Polymyositis with other organ involvement** CC
M33.9 **Dermatopolymyositis, unspecified**
M33.90 **Dermatopolymyositis, unspecified, organ involvement unspecified** CC
M33.91 **Dermatopolymyositis, unspecified with respiratory involvement** CC
M33.92 **Dermatopolymyositis, unspecified with myopathy** CC PDx
M33.99 **Dermatopolymyositis, unspecified with other organ involvement** CC

M34 **Systemic sclerosis [scleroderma]**
EXCLUDES1 *circumscribed scleroderma (L94.0)*

PDx Unacceptable principal diagnosis symbol per Medicare code edits — POA Code exempt from diagnosis present on admission requirement
Q Questionable admission — CC Complication or comorbidity — CC/MCC Exc CC/MCC exclusion — MCC Major complication or comorbidity
PDx CC Principal diagnosis as its own CC — PDx MCC Principal diagnosis as its own MCC — Z Z code as first-listed diagnosis

neonatal scleroderma (P83.8)
M34.0 Progressive systemic sclerosis
M34.1 CR(E)ST syndrome
Combination of calcinosis, Raynaud's phenomenon, esophageal dysfunction, sclerodactyly, telangiectasia
M34.2 Systemic sclerosis induced by drug and chemical
Code first poisoning due to drug or toxin, if applicable (T36-T65 with fifth or sixth character 1-4 or 6)
Use additional code for adverse effect, if applicable, to identify drug (T36-T50 with fifth or sixth character 5)
M34.8 Other forms of systemic sclerosis
M34.81 Systemic sclerosis with lung involvement
M34.82 Systemic sclerosis with myopathy
M34.83 Systemic sclerosis with polyneuropathy
M34.89 Other systemic sclerosis
M34.9 Systemic sclerosis, unspecified
M35 Other systemic involvement of connective tissue
EXCLUDES1 *reactive perforating collagenosis (L87.1)*
M35.0 Sicca syndrome [Sjögren]
M35.00 Sicca syndrome, unspecified
M35.01 Sicca syndrome with keratoconjunctivitis
M35.02 Sicca syndrome with lung involvement
M35.03 Sicca syndrome with myopathy
M35.04 Sicca syndrome with tubulo-interstitial nephropathy
Renal tubular acidosis in sicca syndrome
M35.09 Sicca syndrome with other organ involvement
M35.1 Other overlap syndromes
Mixed connective tissue disease
EXCLUDES1 *polyangiitis overlap syndrome (M30.8)*
M35.2 Behçet's disease
M35.3 Polymyalgia rheumatica
EXCLUDES1 *polymyalgia rheumatica with giant cell arteritis (M31.5)*
M35.4 Diffuse (eosinophilic) fasciitis
M35.5 Multifocal fibrosclerosis
M35.6 Relapsing panniculitis [Weber-Christian]
EXCLUDES1 *lupus panniculitis (L93.2)*
panniculitis NOS (M79.3-)
M35.7 Hypermobility syndrome
Familial ligamentous laxity
EXCLUDES1 *Ehlers-Danlos syndrome (Q79.6)*
ligamentous laxity, NOS (M24.2-)
M35.8 Other specified systemic involvement of connective tissue
M35.9 Systemic involvement of connective tissue, unspecified
Autoimmune disease (systemic) NOS
Collagen (vascular) disease NOS
M36 Systemic disorders of connective tissue in diseases classified elsewhere
EXCLUDES2 *arthropathies in diseases classified elsewhere (M14.-)*
M36.0 Dermato(poly)myositis in neoplastic disease
Code first underlying neoplasm (C00-D49)
M36.1 Arthropathy in neoplastic disease
Code first underlying neoplasm, such as:
leukemia (C91-C95)
malignant histiocytosis (C96.A)
multiple myeloma (C90.0)
M36.2 Hemophilic arthropathy
Hemarthrosis in hemophilic arthropathy
Code first underlying disease, such as:
factor VIII deficiency (D66)
with vascular defect (D68.0)
factor IX deficiency (D67)
hemophilia (classical) (D66)
hemophilia B (D67)
hemophilia C (D68.1)
M36.3 Arthropathy in other blood disorders
M36.4 Arthropathy in hypersensitivity reactions classified elsewhere
Code first underlying disease, such as:
Henoch (-Schönlein) purpura (D69.0)
serum sickness (T80.6-)
M36.8 Systemic disorders of connective tissue in other diseases classified elsewhere
Code first underlying disease, such as:
alkaptonuria (E70.2)
hypogammaglobulinemia (D80.-)
ochronosis (E70.2)

Dorsopathies (M40-M54)

Deforming dorsopathies (M40-M43)

M40 Kyphosis and lordosis
EXCLUDES1 *congenital kyphosis and lordosis (Q76.4)*
kyphoscoliosis (M41.-)
postprocedural kyphosis and lordosis (M96.-)
M40.0 Postural kyphosis
EXCLUDES1 *osteochondrosis of spine (M42.-)*
M40.00 Postural kyphosis, site unspecified
M40.03 Postural kyphosis, cervicothoracic region
M40.04 Postural kyphosis, thoracic region
M40.05 Postural kyphosis, thoracolumbar region
M40.1 Other secondary kyphosis
M40.10 Other secondary kyphosis, site unspecified
M40.12 Other secondary kyphosis, cervical region
M40.13 Other secondary kyphosis, cervicothoracic region
M40.14 Other secondary kyphosis, thoracic region
M40.15 Other secondary kyphosis, thoracolumbar region
M40.2 Other and unspecified kyphosis
M40.20 Unspecified kyphosis
M40.202 Unspecified kyphosis, cervical region
M40.203 Unspecified kyphosis, cervicothoracic region
M40.204 Unspecified kyphosis, thoracic region
M40.205 Unspecified kyphosis, thoracolumbar region
M40.209 Unspecified kyphosis, site unspecified
M40.29 Other kyphosis
M40.292 Other kyphosis, cervical region
M40.293 Other kyphosis, cervicothoracic region
M40.294 Other kyphosis, thoracic region
M40.295 Other kyphosis, thoracolumbar region
M40.299 Other kyphosis, site unspecified
M40.3 Flatback syndrome
M40.30 Flatback syndrome, site unspecified
M40.35 Flatback syndrome, thoracolumbar region
M40.36 Flatback syndrome, lumbar region
M40.37 Flatback syndrome, lumbosacral region
M40.4 Postural lordosis
Acquired lordosis
M40.40 Postural lordosis, site unspecified
M40.45 Postural lordosis, thoracolumbar region
M40.46 Postural lordosis, lumbar region
M40.47 Postural lordosis, lumbosacral region
M40.5 Lordosis, unspecified
M40.50 Lordosis, unspecified, site unspecified
M40.55 Lordosis, unspecified, thoracolumbar region
M40.56 Lordosis, unspecified, lumbar region
M40.57 Lordosis, unspecified, lumbosacral region
M41 Scoliosis
INCLUDES *kyphoscoliosis*
EXCLUDES1 *congenital scoliosis NOS (Q67.5)*
congenital scoliosis due to bony malformation (Q76.3)
postural congenital scoliosis (Q67.5)
kyphoscoliotic heart disease (I27.1)
postprocedural scoliosis (M96.-)
M41.0 Infantile idiopathic scoliosis
M41.00 Infantile idiopathic scoliosis, site unspecified
M41.02 Infantile idiopathic scoliosis, cervical region
M41.03 Infantile idiopathic scoliosis, cervicothoracic region
M41.04 Infantile idiopathic scoliosis, thoracic region
M41.05 Infantile idiopathic scoliosis, thoracolumbar region
M41.06 Infantile idiopathic scoliosis, lumbar region
M41.07 Infantile idiopathic scoliosis, lumbosacral region

Unspecified Code Other Specified Code Manifestation Code N Newborn P Pediatric M Maternity A Adult ♂ Male ♀ Female
● New Code ▲ Revised Code Title ►◄ Revised Text NOTES INCLUDES EXCLUDES1 Not coded here EXCLUDES2 Not included here
4th character required 5th character required 6th character required 7th character required
Extension 'X' Alert HAC Hospital-acquired condition (HAC) alert AHA AHA Coding Clinic©

M41.08 Infantile idiopathic scoliosis, sacral and sacrococcygeal region

M41.1 Juvenile and adolescent idiopathic scoliosis

M41.11 Juvenile idiopathic scoliosis

M41.112 Juvenile idiopathic scoliosis, cervical region
M41.113 Juvenile idiopathic scoliosis, cervicothoracic region
M41.114 Juvenile idiopathic scoliosis, thoracic region
M41.115 Juvenile idiopathic scoliosis, thoracolumbar region
M41.116 Juvenile idiopathic scoliosis, lumbar region
M41.117 Juvenile idiopathic scoliosis, lumbosacral region
M41.119 Juvenile idiopathic scoliosis, site unspecified

M41.12 Adolescent scoliosis

M41.122 Adolescent idiopathic scoliosis, cervical region
M41.123 Adolescent idiopathic scoliosis, cervicothoracic region
M41.124 Adolescent idiopathic scoliosis, thoracic region
M41.125 Adolescent idiopathic scoliosis, thoracolumbar region
M41.126 Adolescent idiopathic scoliosis, lumbar region
M41.127 Adolescent idiopathic scoliosis, lumbosacral region
M41.129 Adolescent idiopathic scoliosis, site unspecified

M41.2 Other idiopathic scoliosis

M41.20 Other idiopathic scoliosis, site unspecified
M41.22 Other idiopathic scoliosis, cervical region
M41.23 Other idiopathic scoliosis, cervicothoracic region
M41.24 Other idiopathic scoliosis, thoracic region
M41.25 Other idiopathic scoliosis, thoracolumbar region
M41.26 Other idiopathic scoliosis, lumbar region
M41.27 Other idiopathic scoliosis, lumbosacral region

M41.3 Thoracogenic scoliosis

M41.30 Thoracogenic scoliosis, site unspecified
M41.34 Thoracogenic scoliosis, thoracic region
M41.35 Thoracogenic scoliosis, thoracolumbar region

M41.4 Neuromuscular scoliosis

Scoliosis secondary to cerebral palsy, Friedreich's ataxia, poliomyelitis and other neuromuscular disorders
Code also underlying condition

M41.40 Neuromuscular scoliosis, site unspecified
M41.41 Neuromuscular scoliosis, occipito-atlanto-axial region
M41.42 Neuromuscular scoliosis, cervical region
M41.43 Neuromuscular scoliosis, cervicothoracic region
M41.44 Neuromuscular scoliosis, thoracic region
M41.45 Neuromuscular scoliosis, thoracolumbar region
M41.46 Neuromuscular scoliosis, lumbar region
M41.47 Neuromuscular scoliosis, lumbosacral region

M41.5 Other secondary scoliosis

M41.50 Other secondary scoliosis, site unspecified
M41.52 Other secondary scoliosis, cervical region
M41.53 Other secondary scoliosis, cervicothoracic region
M41.54 Other secondary scoliosis, thoracic region
M41.55 Other secondary scoliosis, thoracolumbar region
M41.56 Other secondary scoliosis, lumbar region
M41.57 Other secondary scoliosis, lumbosacral region

M41.8 Other forms of scoliosis

M41.80 Other forms of scoliosis, site unspecified
M41.82 Other forms of scoliosis, cervical region
M41.83 Other forms of scoliosis, cervicothoracic region
M41.84 Other forms of scoliosis, thoracic region
M41.85 Other forms of scoliosis, thoracolumbar region
M41.86 Other forms of scoliosis, lumbar region
M41.87 Other forms of scoliosis, lumbosacral region

M41.9 Scoliosis, unspecified

M42 Spinal osteochondrosis

M42.0 Juvenile osteochondrosis of spine

Calvé's disease
Scheuermann's disease
EXCLUDES1 *postural kyphosis (M40.0)*

M42.00 Juvenile osteochondrosis of spine, site unspecified
M42.01 Juvenile osteochondrosis of spine, occipito-atlanto-axial region
M42.02 Juvenile osteochondrosis of spine, cervical region
M42.03 Juvenile osteochondrosis of spine, cervicothoracic region
M42.04 Juvenile osteochondrosis of spine, thoracic region
M42.05 Juvenile osteochondrosis of spine, thoracolumbar region
M42.06 Juvenile osteochondrosis of spine, lumbar region
M42.07 Juvenile osteochondrosis of spine, lumbosacral region
M42.08 Juvenile osteochondrosis of spine, sacral and sacrococcygeal region
M42.09 Juvenile osteochondrosis of spine, multiple sites in spine

M42.1 Adult osteochondrosis of spine

M42.10 Adult osteochondrosis of spine, site unspecified A
M42.11 Adult osteochondrosis of spine, occipito-atlanto-axial region A
M42.12 Adult osteochondrosis of spine, cervical region A
M42.13 Adult osteochondrosis of spine, cervicothoracic region A
M42.14 Adult osteochondrosis of spine, thoracic region A
M42.15 Adult osteochondrosis of spine, thoracolumbar region A
M42.16 Adult osteochondrosis of spine, lumbar region A
M42.17 Adult osteochondrosis of spine, lumbosacral region A
M42.18 Adult osteochondrosis of spine, sacral and sacrococcygeal region A
M42.19 Adult osteochondrosis of spine, multiple sites in spine A

M42.9 Spinal osteochondrosis, unspecified

M43 Other deforming dorsopathies

EXCLUDES1 *congenital spondylolysis and spondylolisthesis (Q76.2)*
hemivertebra (Q76.3-Q76.4)
Klippel-Feil syndrome (Q76.1)
lumbarization and sacralization (Q76.4)
platyspondylisis (Q76.4)
spina bifida occulta (Q76.0)
spinal curvature in osteoporosis (M80.-)
spinal curvature in Paget's disease of bone [osteitis deformans] (M88.-)

M43.0 Spondylolysis

EXCLUDES1 *congenital spondylolysis (Q76.2)*
spondylolisthesis (M43.1)

M43.00 Spondylolysis, site unspecified
M43.01 Spondylolysis, occipito-atlanto-axial region
M43.02 Spondylolysis, cervical region
M43.03 Spondylolysis, cervicothoracic region
M43.04 Spondylolysis, thoracic region
M43.05 Spondylolysis, thoracolumbar region
M43.06 Spondylolysis, lumbar region
M43.07 Spondylolysis, lumbosacral region
M43.08 Spondylolysis, sacral and sacrococcygeal region
M43.09 Spondylolysis, multiple sites in spine

M43.1 Spondylolisthesis

EXCLUDES1 *acute traumatic of lumbosacral region (S33.1)*
acute traumatic of sites other than lumbosacral- code to Fracture, vertebra, by region
congenital spondylolisthesis (Q76.2)

M43.10 Spondylolisthesis, site unspecified
M43.11 Spondylolisthesis, occipito-atlanto-axial region
M43.12 Spondylolisthesis, cervical region
M43.13 Spondylolisthesis, cervicothoracic region

Unacceptable principal diagnosis symbol per Medicare code edits | Code exempt from diagnosis present on admission requirement
Questionable admission | Complication or comorbidity | CC/MCC exclusion | Major complication or comorbidity
Principal diagnosis as its own CC | Principal diagnosis as its own MCC | Z code as first-listed diagnosis

M43.14 **Spondylolisthesis, thoracic region**
M43.15 **Spondylolisthesis, thoracolumbar region**
M43.16 **Spondylolisthesis, lumbar region**
M43.17 **Spondylolisthesis, lumbosacral region**
M43.18 **Spondylolisthesis, sacral and sacrococcygeal region**
M43.19 **Spondylolisthesis, multiple sites in spine**

(5) M43.2 **Fusion of spine**
Ankylosis of spinal joint
EXCLUDES1 *ankylosing spondylitis (M45.0-)*
congenital fusion of spine (Q76.4)
EXCLUDES2 *arthrodesis status (Z98.1)*
pseudoarthrosis after fusion or arthrodesis (M96.0)
M43.20 **Fusion of spine, site unspecified**
M43.21 **Fusion of spine, occipito-atlanto-axial region**
M43.22 **Fusion of spine, cervical region**
M43.23 **Fusion of spine, cervicothoracic region**
M43.24 **Fusion of spine, thoracic region**
M43.25 **Fusion of spine, thoracolumbar region**
M43.26 **Fusion of spine, lumbar region**
M43.27 **Fusion of spine, lumbosacral region**
M43.28 **Fusion of spine, sacral and sacrococcygeal region**

M43.3 **Recurrent atlantoaxial dislocation with myelopathy**
M43.4 **Other recurrent atlantoaxial dislocation**

(5) M43.5 **Other recurrent vertebral dislocation**
EXCLUDES1 *biomechanical lesions NEC (M99.-)*
(6) M43.5X **Other recurrent vertebral dislocation**
M43.5X2 **Other recurrent vertebral dislocation, cervical region**
M43.5X3 **Other recurrent vertebral dislocation, cervicothoracic region**
M43.5X4 **Other recurrent vertebral dislocation, thoracic region**
M43.5X5 **Other recurrent vertebral dislocation, thoracolumbar region**
M43.5X6 **Other recurrent vertebral dislocation, lumbar region**
M43.5X7 **Other recurrent vertebral dislocation, lumbosacral region**
M43.5X8 **Other recurrent vertebral dislocation, sacral and sacrococcygeal region**
M43.5X9 **Other recurrent vertebral dislocation, site unspecified**

M43.6 **Torticollis**
EXCLUDES1 *congenital (sternomastoid) torticollis (Q68.0)*
current injury - see Injury, of spine, by body region
ocular torticollis (R29.891)
psychogenic torticollis (F45.8)
spasmodic torticollis (G24.3)
torticollis due to birth injury (P15.2)

(5) M43.8 **Other specified deforming dorsopathies**
EXCLUDES2 *kyphosis and lordosis (M40.-)*
scoliosis (M41.-)
(6) M43.8X **Other specified deforming dorsopathies**
M43.8X1 **Other specified deforming dorsopathies, occipito-atlanto-axial region**
M43.8X2 **Other specified deforming dorsopathies, cervical region**
M43.8X3 **Other specified deforming dorsopathies, cervicothoracic region**
M43.8X4 **Other specified deforming dorsopathies, thoracic region**
M43.8X5 **Other specified deforming dorsopathies, thoracolumbar region**
M43.8X6 **Other specified deforming dorsopathies, lumbar region**
M43.8X7 **Other specified deforming dorsopathies, lumbosacral region**
M43.8X8 **Other specified deforming dorsopathies, sacral and sacrococcygeal region**
M43.8X9 **Other specified deforming dorsopathies, site unspecified**

M43.9 **Deforming dorsopathy, unspecified**
Curvature of spine NOS

Spondylopathies (M45-M49)

Healthy spine — Ankylosing spondylitis
Body of vertebra
Disc
Inflammation of joints
Fusion of bones "bamboo spine"

Figure 13.4 Healthy spine changing in to ankylosing spondylitis

(4) M45 **Ankylosing spondylitis**
Rheumatoid arthritis of spine
EXCLUDES1 *arthropathy in Reiter's disease (M02.3-)*
juvenile (ankylosing) spondylitis (M08.1)
EXCLUDES2 *Behçet's disease (M35.2)*
M45.0 **Ankylosing spondylitis of multiple sites in spine**
M45.1 **Ankylosing spondylitis of occipito-atlanto-axial region**
M45.2 **Ankylosing spondylitis of cervical region**
M45.3 **Ankylosing spondylitis of cervicothoracic region**
M45.4 **Ankylosing spondylitis of thoracic region**
M45.5 **Ankylosing spondylitis of thoracolumbar region**
M45.6 **Ankylosing spondylitis lumbar region**
M45.7 **Ankylosing spondylitis of lumbosacral region**
M45.8 **Ankylosing spondylitis sacral and sacrococcygeal region**
M45.9 **Ankylosing spondylitis of unspecified sites in spine**

(4) M46 **Other inflammatory spondylopathies**
(5) M46.0 **Spinal enthesopathy**
Disorder of ligamentous or muscular attachments of spine
M46.00 **Spinal enthesopathy, site unspecified**
M46.01 **Spinal enthesopathy, occipito-atlanto-axial region**
M46.02 **Spinal enthesopathy, cervical region**
M46.03 **Spinal enthesopathy, cervicothoracic region**
M46.04 **Spinal enthesopathy, thoracic region**
M46.05 **Spinal enthesopathy, thoracolumbar region**
M46.06 **Spinal enthesopathy, lumbar region**
M46.07 **Spinal enthesopathy, lumbosacral region**
M46.08 **Spinal enthesopathy, sacral and sacrococcygeal region**
M46.09 **Spinal enthesopathy, multiple sites in spine**
M46.1 **Sacroiliitis, not elsewhere classified**
(5) M46.2 **Osteomyelitis of vertebra**
M46.20 **Osteomyelitis of vertebra, site unspecified** CC
M46.21 **Osteomyelitis of vertebra, occipito-atlanto-axial region** CC
M46.22 **Osteomyelitis of vertebra, cervical region** CC
M46.23 **Osteomyelitis of vertebra, cervicothoracic region** CC
M46.24 **Osteomyelitis of vertebra, thoracic region** CC
M46.25 **Osteomyelitis of vertebra, thoracolumbar region** CC
M46.26 **Osteomyelitis of vertebra, lumbar region** CC
M46.27 **Osteomyelitis of vertebra, lumbosacral region** CC
M46.28 **Osteomyelitis of vertebra, sacral and sacrococcygeal region** CC
(5) M46.3 **Infection of intervertebral disc (pyogenic)**
Use additional code (B95-B97) to identify infectious agent.
M46.30 **Infection of intervertebral disc (pyogenic), site unspecified** CC
M46.31 **Infection of intervertebral disc (pyogenic), occipito-atlanto-axial region** CC
M46.32 **Infection of intervertebral disc (pyogenic), cervical region** CC
M46.33 **Infection of intervertebral disc (pyogenic), cervicothoracic region** CC
M46.34 **Infection of intervertebral disc (pyogenic), thoracic region** CC

Unspecified Code | Other Specified Code | Manifestation Code | N Newborn | P Pediatric | M Maternity | A Adult | ♂ Male | ♀ Female
● New Code | ▲ Revised Code Title | ►◄ Revised Text | NOTES | INCLUDES | EXCLUDES1 Not coded here | EXCLUDES2 Not included here
(4) 4th character required | (5) 5th character required | (6) 6th character required | (7) 7th character required
(X) Extension 'X' Alert | HAC Hospital-acquired condition (HAC) alert | AHA AHA Coding Clinic©

M46.35 Infection of intervertebral disc (pyogenic), thoracolumbar region CC
M46.36 Infection of intervertebral disc (pyogenic), lumbar region CC
M46.37 Infection of intervertebral disc (pyogenic), lumbosacral region CC
M46.38 Infection of intervertebral disc (pyogenic), sacral and sacrococcygeal region CC
M46.39 Infection of intervertebral disc (pyogenic), multiple sites in spine CC

M46.4 Discitis, unspecified
M46.40 Discitis, unspecified, site unspecified
M46.41 Discitis, unspecified, occipito-atlanto-axial region
M46.42 Discitis, unspecified, cervical region
M46.43 Discitis, unspecified, cervicothoracic region
M46.44 Discitis, unspecified, thoracic region
M46.45 Discitis, unspecified, thoracolumbar region
M46.46 Discitis, unspecified, lumbar region
M46.47 Discitis, unspecified, lumbosacral region
M46.48 Discitis, unspecified, sacral and sacrococcygeal region
M46.49 Discitis, unspecified, multiple sites in spine

M46.5 Other infective spondylopathies
M46.50 Other infective spondylopathies, site unspecified
M46.51 Other infective spondylopathies, occipito-atlanto-axial region
M46.52 Other infective spondylopathies, cervical region
M46.53 Other infective spondylopathies, cervicothoracic region
M46.54 Other infective spondylopathies, thoracic region
M46.55 Other infective spondylopathies, thoracolumbar region
M46.56 Other infective spondylopathies, lumbar region
M46.57 Other infective spondylopathies, lumbosacral region
M46.58 Other infective spondylopathies, sacral and sacrococcygeal region
M46.59 Other infective spondylopathies, multiple sites in spine

M46.8 Other specified inflammatory spondylopathies
M46.80 Other specified inflammatory spondylopathies, site unspecified
M46.81 Other specified inflammatory spondylopathies, occipito-atlanto-axial region
M46.82 Other specified inflammatory spondylopathies, cervical region
M46.83 Other specified inflammatory spondylopathies, cervicothoracic region
M46.84 Other specified inflammatory spondylopathies, thoracic region
M46.85 Other specified inflammatory spondylopathies, thoracolumbar region
M46.86 Other specified inflammatory spondylopathies, lumbar region
M46.87 Other specified inflammatory spondylopathies, lumbosacral region
M46.88 Other specified inflammatory spondylopathies, sacral and sacrococcygeal region
M46.89 Other specified inflammatory spondylopathies, multiple sites in spine

M46.9 Unspecified inflammatory spondylopathy
M46.90 Unspecified inflammatory spondylopathy, site unspecified
M46.91 Unspecified inflammatory spondylopathy, occipito-atlanto-axial region
M46.92 Unspecified inflammatory spondylopathy, cervical region
M46.93 Unspecified inflammatory spondylopathy, cervicothoracic region
M46.94 Unspecified inflammatory spondylopathy, thoracic region
M46.95 Unspecified inflammatory spondylopathy, thoracolumbar region
M46.96 Unspecified inflammatory spondylopathy, lumbar region
M46.97 Unspecified inflammatory spondylopathy, lumbosacral region
M46.98 Unspecified inflammatory spondylopathy, sacral and sacrococcygeal region
M46.99 Unspecified inflammatory spondylopathy, multiple sites in spine

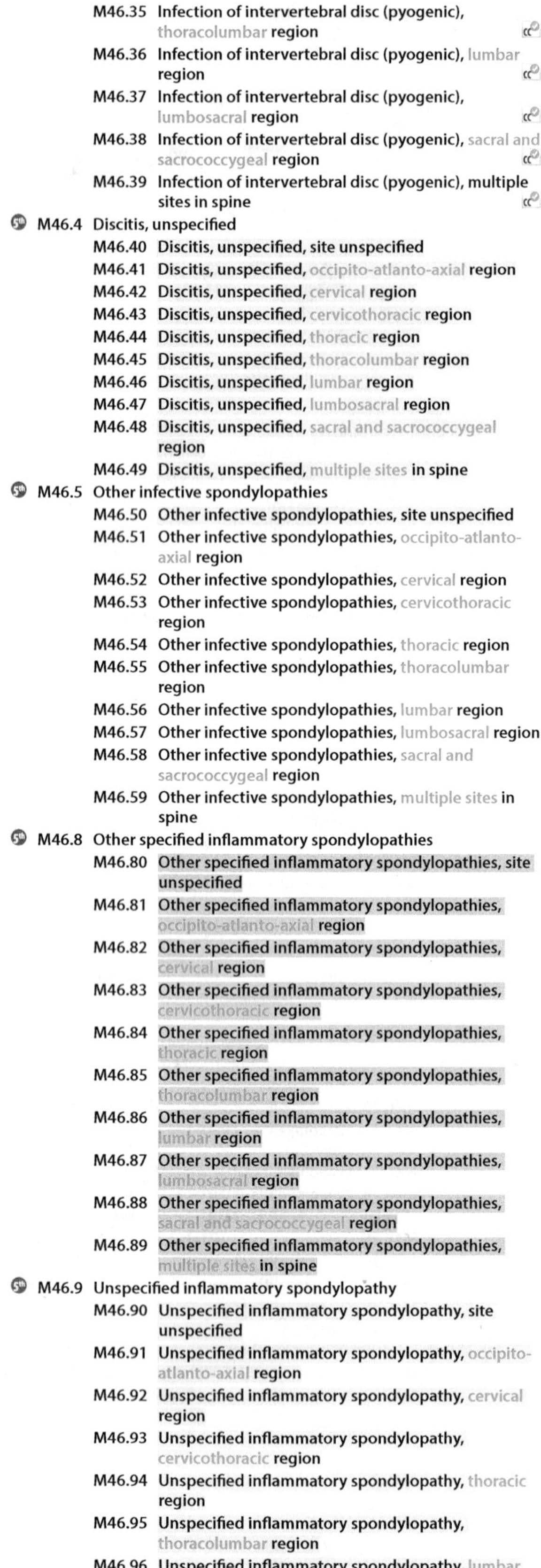

Figure 13.5 Remarkable changes in healthy and osteoarthritic spine

M47 Spondylosis
INCLUDES *arthrosis or osteoarthritis of spine*
degeneration of facet joints

M47.0 Anterior spinal and vertebral artery compression syndromes
M47.01 Anterior spinal artery compression syndromes
M47.011 Anterior spinal artery compression syndromes, occipito-atlanto-axial region CC
M47.012 Anterior spinal artery compression syndromes, cervical region CC
M47.013 Anterior spinal artery compression syndromes, cervicothoracic region CC
M47.014 Anterior spinal artery compression syndromes, thoracic region CC
M47.015 Anterior spinal artery compression syndromes, thoracolumbar region CC
M47.016 Anterior spinal artery compression syndromes, lumbar region CC
M47.019 Anterior spinal artery compression syndromes, site unspecified CC
M47.02 Vertebral artery compression syndromes
M47.021 Vertebral artery compression syndromes, occipito-atlanto-axial region CC
M47.022 Vertebral artery compression syndromes, cervical region CC
M47.029 Vertebral artery compression syndromes, site unspecified CC

M47.1 Other spondylosis with myelopathy
Spondylogenic compression of spinal cord
EXCLUDES1 *vertebral subluxation (M43.3-M43.59)*
M47.10 Other spondylosis with myelopathy, site unspecified CC
M47.11 Other spondylosis with myelopathy, occipito-atlanto-axial region CC
M47.12 Other spondylosis with myelopathy, cervical region CC
M47.13 Other spondylosis with myelopathy, cervicothoracic region CC

Unacceptable principal diagnosis symbol per Medicare code edits; Code exempt from diagnosis present on admission requirement; Questionable admission; CC Complication or comorbidity; CC/MCC exclusion; MCC Major complication or comorbidity; Principal diagnosis as its own CC; Principal diagnosis as its own MCC; Z code as first-listed diagnosis

M47.14 Other spondylosis with myelopathy, thoracic region
M47.15 Other spondylosis with myelopathy, thoracolumbar region
M47.16 Other spondylosis with myelopathy, lumbar region
M47.2 Other spondylosis with radiculopathy
M47.20 Other spondylosis with radiculopathy, site unspecified
M47.21 Other spondylosis with radiculopathy, occipito-atlanto-axial region
M47.22 Other spondylosis with radiculopathy, cervical region
M47.23 Other spondylosis with radiculopathy, cervicothoracic region
M47.24 Other spondylosis with radiculopathy, thoracic region
M47.25 Other spondylosis with radiculopathy, thoracolumbar region
M47.26 Other spondylosis with radiculopathy, lumbar region
M47.27 Other spondylosis with radiculopathy, lumbosacral region
M47.28 Other spondylosis with radiculopathy, sacral and sacrococcygeal region
M47.8 Other spondylosis
M47.81 Spondylosis without myelopathy or radiculopathy
M47.811 Spondylosis without myelopathy or radiculopathy, occipito-atlanto-axial region
M47.812 Spondylosis without myelopathy or radiculopathy, cervical region
M47.813 Spondylosis without myelopathy or radiculopathy, cervicothoracic region
M47.814 Spondylosis without myelopathy or radiculopathy, thoracic region
M47.815 Spondylosis without myelopathy or radiculopathy, thoracolumbar region
M47.816 Spondylosis without myelopathy or radiculopathy, lumbar region
M47.817 Spondylosis without myelopathy or radiculopathy, lumbosacral region
M47.818 Spondylosis without myelopathy or radiculopathy, sacral and sacrococcygeal region
M47.819 Spondylosis without myelopathy or radiculopathy, site unspecified
M47.89 Other spondylosis
M47.891 Other spondylosis, occipito-atlanto-axial region
M47.892 Other spondylosis, cervical region
M47.893 Other spondylosis, cervicothoracic region
M47.894 Other spondylosis, thoracic region
M47.895 Other spondylosis, thoracolumbar region
M47.896 Other spondylosis, lumbar region
M47.897 Other spondylosis, lumbosacral region
M47.898 Other spondylosis, sacral and sacrococcygeal region
M47.899 Other spondylosis, site unspecified
M47.9 Spondylosis, unspecified
M48 Other spondylopathies
M48.0 Spinal stenosis
Caudal stenosis
M48.00 Spinal stenosis, site unspecified
M48.01 Spinal stenosis, occipito-atlanto-axial region
M48.02 Spinal stenosis, cervical region
M48.03 Spinal stenosis, cervicothoracic region
M48.04 Spinal stenosis, thoracic region
M48.05 Spinal stenosis, thoracolumbar region
M48.06 Spinal stenosis, lumbar region
M48.07 Spinal stenosis, lumbosacral region
M48.08 Spinal stenosis, sacral and sacrococcygeal region
M48.1 Ankylosing hyperostosis [Forestier]
Diffuse idiopathic skeletal hyperostosis [DISH]
M48.10 Ankylosing hyperostosis [Forestier], site unspecified
M48.11 Ankylosing hyperostosis [Forestier], occipito-atlanto-axial region
M48.12 Ankylosing hyperostosis [Forestier], cervical region
M48.13 Ankylosing hyperostosis [Forestier], cervicothoracic region
M48.14 Ankylosing hyperostosis [Forestier], thoracic region
M48.15 Ankylosing hyperostosis [Forestier], thoracolumbar region
M48.16 Ankylosing hyperostosis [Forestier], lumbar region
M48.17 Ankylosing hyperostosis [Forestier], lumbosacral region
M48.18 Ankylosing hyperostosis [Forestier], sacral and sacrococcygeal region
M48.19 Ankylosing hyperostosis [Forestier], multiple sites in spine
M48.2 Kissing spine
M48.20 Kissing spine, site unspecified
M48.21 Kissing spine, occipito-atlanto-axial region
M48.22 Kissing spine, cervical region
M48.23 Kissing spine, cervicothoracic region
M48.24 Kissing spine, thoracic region
M48.25 Kissing spine, thoracolumbar region
M48.26 Kissing spine, lumbar region
M48.27 Kissing spine, lumbosacral region
M48.3 Traumatic spondylopathy
M48.30 Traumatic spondylopathy, site unspecified
M48.31 Traumatic spondylopathy, occipito-atlanto-axial region
M48.32 Traumatic spondylopathy, cervical region
M48.33 Traumatic spondylopathy, cervicothoracic region
M48.34 Traumatic spondylopathy, thoracic region
M48.35 Traumatic spondylopathy, thoracolumbar region
M48.36 Traumatic spondylopathy, lumbar region
M48.37 Traumatic spondylopathy, lumbosacral region
M48.38 Traumatic spondylopathy, sacral and sacrococcygeal region
M48.4 Fatigue fracture of vertebra
Stress fracture of vertebra
EXCLUDES1 *pathological fracture NOS (M84.4-)*
pathological fracture of vertebra due to neoplasm (M84.58)
pathological fracture of vertebra due to other diagnosis (M84.68)
pathological fracture of vertebra due to osteoporosis (M80.-)
traumatic fracture of vertebrae (S12.0-S12.3-, S22.0-, S32.0-)

The appropriate 7th character is to be added to each code from subcategory M48.4:
A = initial encounter for fracture
D = subsequent encounter for fracture with routine healing
G = subsequent encounter for fracture with delayed healing
S = sequela of fracture

M48.40 Fatigue fracture of vertebra, site unspecified
M48.41 Fatigue fracture of vertebra, occipito-atlanto-axial region
M48.42 Fatigue fracture of vertebra, cervical region
M48.43 Fatigue fracture of vertebra, cervicothoracic region
M48.44 Fatigue fracture of vertebra, thoracic region
M48.45 Fatigue fracture of vertebra, thoracolumbar region
M48.46 Fatigue fracture of vertebra, lumbar region
M48.47 Fatigue fracture of vertebra, lumbosacral region
M48.48 Fatigue fracture of vertebra, sacral and sacrococcygeal region
M48.5 Collapsed vertebra, not elsewhere classified
Collapsed vertebra NOS
Compression fracture of vertebra NOS
Wedging of vertebra NOS
EXCLUDES1 *current injury - see Injury of spine, by body region*
fatigue fracture of vertebra (M48.4)
pathological fracture of vertebra due to neoplasm (M84.58)

Unspecified Code | Other Specified Code | Manifestation Code | N Newborn | P Pediatric | M Maternity | A Adult | ♂ Male | ♀ Female
● New Code | ▲ Revised Code Title | ►◄ Revised Text | NOTES | INCLUDES | EXCLUDES1 Not coded here | EXCLUDES2 Not included here
4th character required | 5th character required | 6th character required | 7th character required
Extension 'X' Alert | HAC Hospital-acquired condition (HAC) alert | AHA AHA Coding Clinic©

pathological fracture of vertebra due to other diagnosis (M84.68)
pathological fracture of vertebra due to osteoporosis (M80.-)
pathological fracture NOS (M84.4-)
stress fracture of vertebra (M48.4-)
traumatic fracture of vertebra (S12.-, S22.-, S32.-)

The appropriate 7th character is to be added to each code from subcategory M48.5:
A = initial encounter for fracture
D = subsequent encounter for fracture with routine healing
G = subsequent encounter for fracture with delayed healing
S = sequela of fracture

M48.50 Collapsed vertebra, not elsewhere classified, site unspecified
M48.51 Collapsed vertebra, not elsewhere classified, occipito-atlanto-axial region
M48.52 Collapsed vertebra, not elsewhere classified, cervical region
M48.53 Collapsed vertebra, not elsewhere classified, cervicothoracic region
M48.54 Collapsed vertebra, not elsewhere classified, thoracic region
M48.55 Collapsed vertebra, not elsewhere classified, thoracolumbar region
M48.56 Collapsed vertebra, not elsewhere classified, lumbar region
M48.57 Collapsed vertebra, not elsewhere classified, lumbosacral region
M48.58 Collapsed vertebra, not elsewhere classified, sacral and sacrococcygeal region

M48.8 Other specified spondylopathies
Ossification of posterior longitudinal ligament

M48.8X Other specified spondylopathies
M48.8X1 Other specified spondylopathies, occipito-atlanto-axial region
M48.8X2 Other specified spondylopathies, cervical region
M48.8X3 Other specified spondylopathies, cervicothoracic region
M48.8X4 Other specified spondylopathies, thoracic region
M48.8X5 Other specified spondylopathies, thoracolumbar region
M48.8X6 Other specified spondylopathies, lumbar region
M48.8X7 Other specified spondylopathies, lumbosacral region
M48.8X8 Other specified spondylopathies, sacral and sacrococcygeal region
M48.8X9 Other specified spondylopathies, site unspecified

M48.9 Spondylopathy, unspecified

M49 Spondylopathies in diseases classified elsewhere
INCLUDES *curvature of spine in diseases classified elsewhere*
deformity of spine in diseases classified elsewhere
kyphosis in diseases classified elsewhere
scoliosis in diseases classified elsewhere
spondylopathy in diseases classified elsewhere

Code first underlying disease, such as:
brucellosis (A23.-)
Charcot-Marie-Tooth disease (G60.0)
enterobacterial infections (A01-A04)
osteitis fibrosa cystica (E21.0)

EXCLUDES1 *curvature of spine in tuberculosis [Pott's] (A18.01)*
enteropathic arthropathies (M07.-)
gonococcal spondylitis (A54.41)
neuropathic [tabes dorsalis] spondylitis (A52.11)
neuropathic spondylopathy in syringomyelia (G95.0)
neuropathic spondylopathy in tabes dorsalis (A52.11)
nonsyphilitic neuropathic spondylopathy NEC (G98.0)
spondylitis in syphilis (acquired) (A52.77)
tuberculous spondylitis (A18.01)
typhoid fever spondylitis (A01.05)

M49.8 Spondylopathy in diseases classified elsewhere
M49.80 Spondylopathy in diseases classified elsewhere, site unspecified
M49.81 Spondylopathy in diseases classified elsewhere, occipito-atlanto-axial region
M49.82 Spondylopathy in diseases classified elsewhere, cervical region
M49.83 Spondylopathy in diseases classified elsewhere, cervicothoracic region
M49.84 Spondylopathy in diseases classified elsewhere, thoracic region
M49.85 Spondylopathy in diseases classified elsewhere, thoracolumbar region
M49.86 Spondylopathy in diseases classified elsewhere, lumbar region
M49.87 Spondylopathy in diseases classified elsewhere, lumbosacral region
M49.88 Spondylopathy in diseases classified elsewhere, sacral and sacrococcygeal region
M49.89 Spondylopathy in diseases classified elsewhere, multiple sites in spine

Other dorsopathies (M50-M54)

EXCLUDES1 *current injury - see injury of spine by body region*
discitis NOS (M46.4-)

M50 Cervical disc disorders
NOTES code to the most superior level of disorder
INCLUDES *cervicothoracic disc disorders with cervicalgia*
cervicothoracic disc disorders
AHA: Q1, 2016

M50.0 Cervical disc disorder with myelopathy
AHA: Q1, 2016
M50.00 Cervical disc disorder with myelopathy, unspecified cervical region
M50.01 Cervical disc disorder with myelopathy, high cervical region
C2-C3 disc disorder with myelopathy
C3-C4 disc disorder with myelopathy
AHA: Q1, 2016

M50.02 Cervical disc disorder with myelopathy, mid-cervical region
● M50.020 Cervical disc disorder with myelopathy, mid-cervical region, unspecified level
● M50.021 Cervical disc disorder at C4-C5 level with myelopathy
C4-C5 disc disorder with myelopathy
● M50.022 Cervical disc disorder at C5-C6 level with myelopathy
C5-C6 disc disorder with myelopathy
● M50.023 Cervical disc disorder at C6-C7 level with myelopathy
C6-C7 disc disorder with myelopathy

M50.03 Cervical disc disorder with myelopathy, cervicothoracic region
C7-T1 disc disorder with myelopathy

M50.1 Cervical disc disorder with radiculopathy
EXCLUDES2 *brachial radiculitis NOS (M54.13)*
M50.10 Cervical disc disorder with radiculopathy, unspecified cervical region
M50.11 Cervical disc disorder with radiculopathy, high cervical region
C2-C3 disc disorder with radiculopathy
C3 radiculopathy due to disc disorder
C3-C4 disc disorder with radiculopathy
C4 radiculopathy due to disc disorder

M50.12 Cervical disc disorder with radiculopathy, mid-cervical region
● M50.120 Mid-cervical disc disorder, unspecified
● M50.121 Cervical disc disorder at C4-C5 level with radiculopathy
C4-C5 disc disorder with radiculopathy
C5 radiculopathy due to disc disorder
● M50.122 Cervical disc disorder at C5-C6 level with radiculopathy

Unacceptable principal diagnosis symbol per Medicare code edits | Code exempt from diagnosis present on admission requirement | Questionable admission | Complication or comorbidity | CC/MCC exclusion | Major complication or comorbidity | Principal diagnosis as its own CC | Principal diagnosis as its own MCC | Z code as first-listed diagnosis

C5-C6 disc disorder with radiculopathy
C6 radiculopathy due to disc disorder
● **M50.123 Cervical disc disorder at C6-C7 level with radiculopathy**
C6-C7 disc disorder with radiculopathy
C7 radiculopathy due to disc disorder
M50.13 Cervical disc disorder with radiculopathy, cervicothoracic region
C7-T1 disc disorder with radiculopathy
C8 radiculopathy due to disc disorder
M50.2 Other cervical disc displacement
M50.20 Other cervical disc displacement, unspecified cervical region
M50.21 Other cervical disc displacement, high cervical region
Other C2-C3 cervical disc displacement
Other C3-C4 cervical disc displacement
M50.22 Other cervical disc displacement, mid-cervical region
● **M50.220 Other cervical disc displacement, mid-cervical region, unspecified level** CC/MCC Exc
● **M50.221 Other cervical disc displacement at C4-C5 level** CC/MCC Exc
Other C4-C5 cervical disc displacement
● **M50.222 Other cervical disc displacement at C5-C6 level** CC/MCC Exc
Other C5-C6 cervical disc displacement
● **M50.223 Other cervical disc displacement at C6-C7 level** CC/MCC Exc
Other C6-C7 cervical disc displacement
M50.23 Other cervical disc displacement, cervicothoracic region
Other C7-T1 cervical disc displacement
M50.3 Other cervical disc degeneration
M50.30 Other cervical disc degeneration, unspecified cervical region
M50.31 Other cervical disc degeneration, high cervical region
Other C2-C3 cervical disc degeneration
Other C3-C4 cervical disc degeneration
M50.32 Other cervical disc degeneration, mid-cervical region
● **M50.320 Other cervical disc degeneration, mid-cervical region, unspecified level**
● **M50.321 Other cervical disc degeneration at C4-C5 level**
Other C4-C5 cervical disc degeneration
● **M50.322 Other cervical disc degeneration at C5-C6 level**
Other C5-C6 cervical disc degeneration
● **M50.323 Other cervical disc degeneration at C6-C7 level**
Other C6-C7 cervical disc degeneration
M50.33 Other cervical disc degeneration, cervicothoracic region
Other C7-T1 cervical disc degeneration
M50.8 Other cervical disc disorders
M50.80 Other cervical disc disorders, unspecified cervical region
M50.81 Other cervical disc disorders, high cervical region
Other C2-C3 cervical disc disorders
Other C3-C4 cervical disc disorders
M50.82 Other cervical disc disorders, mid-cervical region
● **M50.820 Other cervical disc disorders, mid-cervical region, unspecified level**
● **M50.821 Other cervical disc disorders at C4-C5 level**
Other C4-C5 cervical disc disorders
● **M50.822 Other cervical disc disorders at C5-C6 level**
Other C5-C6 cervical disc disorders
● **M50.823 Other cervical disc disorders at C6-C7 level**
Other C6-C7 cervical disc disorders
M50.83 Other cervical disc disorders, cervicothoracic region
Other C7-T1 cervical disc disorders
M50.9 Cervical disc disorder, unspecified
M50.90 Cervical disc disorder, unspecified, unspecified cervical region
M50.91 Cervical disc disorder, unspecified, high cervical region
C2-C3 cervical disc disorder, unspecified
C3-C4 cervical disc disorder, unspecified
M50.92 Cervical disc disorder, unspecified, mid-cervical region
● **M50.920 Unspecified cervical disc disorder, mid-cervical region, unspecified level**
● **M50.921 Unspecified cervical disc disorder at C4-C5 level**
Unspecified C4-C5 cervical disc disorder
● **M50.922 Unspecified cervical disc disorder at C5-C6 level**
Unspecified C5-C6 cervical disc disorder
● **M50.923 Unspecified cervical disc disorder at C6-C7 level**
Unspecified C6-C7 cervical disc disorder
M50.93 Cervical disc disorder, unspecified, cervicothoracic region
C7-T1 cervical disc disorder, unspecified

M51 Thoracic, thoracolumbar, and lumbosacral intervertebral disc disorders
EXCLUDES2 *cervical and cervicothoracic disc disorders (M50.-)*
sacral and sacrococcygeal disorders (M53.3)
M51.0 Thoracic, thoracolumbar and lumbosacral intervertebral disc disorders with myelopathy
M51.04 Intervertebral disc disorders with myelopathy, thoracic region CC
M51.05 Intervertebral disc disorders with myelopathy, thoracolumbar region CC
M51.06 Intervertebral disc disorders with myelopathy, lumbar region CC
M51.1 Thoracic, thoracolumbar and lumbosacral intervertebral disc disorders with radiculopathy
Sciatica due to intervertebral disc disorder
EXCLUDES1 *lumbar radiculitis NOS (M54.16)*
sciatica NOS (M54.3)
M51.14 Intervertebral disc disorders with radiculopathy, thoracic region
M51.15 Intervertebral disc disorders with radiculopathy, thoracolumbar region
M51.16 Intervertebral disc disorders with radiculopathy, lumbar region
M51.17 Intervertebral disc disorders with radiculopathy, lumbosacral region
M51.2 Other thoracic, thoracolumbar and lumbosacral intervertebral disc displacement
Lumbago due to displacement of intervertebral disc
M51.24 Other intervertebral disc displacement, thoracic region
M51.25 Other intervertebral disc displacement, thoracolumbar region
M51.26 Other intervertebral disc displacement, lumbar region
M51.27 Other intervertebral disc displacement, lumbosacral region
M51.3 Other thoracic, thoracolumbar and lumbosacral intervertebral disc degeneration
AHA: Q3, 2013
M51.34 Other intervertebral disc degeneration, thoracic region
M51.35 Other intervertebral disc degeneration, thoracolumbar region
M51.36 Other intervertebral disc degeneration, lumbar region
M51.37 Other intervertebral disc degeneration, lumbosacral region
M51.4 Schmorl's nodes
M51.44 Schmorl's nodes, thoracic region
M51.45 Schmorl's nodes, thoracolumbar region
M51.46 Schmorl's nodes, lumbar region
M51.47 Schmorl's nodes, lumbosacral region
M51.8 Other thoracic, thoracolumbar and lumbosacral intervertebral disc disorders

Unspecified Code | Other Specified Code | Manifestation Code | N Newborn | P Pediatric | M Maternity | A Adult | ♂ Male | ♀ Female
● New Code ▲ Revised Code Title ►◄ Revised Text NOTES INCLUDES EXCLUDES1 Not coded here EXCLUDES2 Not included here
4th character required 5th character required 6th character required 7th character required
Extension 'X' Alert HAC Hospital-acquired condition (HAC) alert AHA AHA Coding Clinic©

M51.84 Other intervertebral disc disorders, thoracic region
M51.85 Other intervertebral disc disorders, thoracolumbar region
M51.86 Other intervertebral disc disorders, lumbar region
M51.87 Other intervertebral disc disorders, lumbosacral region
M51.9 Unspecified thoracic, thoracolumbar and lumbosacral intervertebral disc disorder

M53 Other and unspecified dorsopathies, not elsewhere classified
M53.0 Cervicocranial syndrome
Posterior cervical sympathetic syndrome
M53.1 Cervicobrachial syndrome
EXCLUDES2 *cervical disc disorder (M50.-)*
thoracic outlet syndrome (G54.0)
M53.2 Spinal instabilities
M53.2X Spinal instabilities
M53.2X1 Spinal instabilities, occipito-atlanto-axial region
M53.2X2 Spinal instabilities, cervical region
M53.2X3 Spinal instabilities, cervicothoracic region
M53.2X4 Spinal instabilities, thoracic region
M53.2X5 Spinal instabilities, thoracolumbar region
M53.2X6 Spinal instabilities, lumbar region
M53.2X7 Spinal instabilities, lumbosacral region
M53.2X8 Spinal instabilities, sacral and sacrococcygeal region
M53.2X9 Spinal instabilities, site unspecified
M53.3 Sacrococcygeal disorders, not elsewhere classified
Coccygodynia
M53.8 Other specified dorsopathies
M53.80 Other specified dorsopathies, site unspecified
M53.81 Other specified dorsopathies, occipito-atlanto-axial region
M53.82 Other specified dorsopathies, cervical region
M53.83 Other specified dorsopathies, cervicothoracic region
M53.84 Other specified dorsopathies, thoracic region
M53.85 Other specified dorsopathies, thoracolumbar region
M53.86 Other specified dorsopathies, lumbar region
M53.87 Other specified dorsopathies, lumbosacral region
M53.88 Other specified dorsopathies, sacral and sacrococcygeal region
M53.9 Dorsopathy, unspecified

M54 Dorsalgia
EXCLUDES1 *psychogenic dorsalgia (F45.41)*
M54.0 Panniculitis affecting regions of neck and back
EXCLUDES1 *lupus panniculitis (L93.2)*
panniculitis NOS (M79.3)
relapsing [Weber-Christian] panniculitis (M35.6)
M54.00 Panniculitis affecting regions of neck and back, site unspecified
M54.01 Panniculitis affecting regions of neck and back, occipito-atlanto-axial region
M54.02 Panniculitis affecting regions of neck and back, cervical region
M54.03 Panniculitis affecting regions of neck and back, cervicothoracic region
M54.04 Panniculitis affecting regions of neck and back, thoracic region
M54.05 Panniculitis affecting regions of neck and back, thoracolumbar region
M54.06 Panniculitis affecting regions of neck and back, lumbar region
M54.07 Panniculitis affecting regions of neck and back, lumbosacral region
M54.08 Panniculitis affecting regions of neck and back, sacral and sacrococcygeal region
M54.09 Panniculitis affecting regions, neck and back, multiple sites in spine
M54.1 Radiculopathy
Brachial neuritis or radiculitis NOS
Lumbar neuritis or radiculitis NOS
Lumbosacral neuritis or radiculitis NOS
Thoracic neuritis or radiculitis NOS
Radiculitis NOS
EXCLUDES1 *neuralgia and neuritis NOS (M79.2)*
radiculopathy with cervical disc disorder (M50.1)
radiculopathy with lumbar and other intervertebral disc disorder (M51.1-)
radiculopathy with spondylosis (M47.2-)
M54.10 Radiculopathy, site unspecified
M54.11 Radiculopathy, occipito-atlanto-axial region
M54.12 Radiculopathy, cervical region
M54.13 Radiculopathy, cervicothoracic region
M54.14 Radiculopathy, thoracic region
M54.15 Radiculopathy, thoracolumbar region
M54.16 Radiculopathy, lumbar region
M54.17 Radiculopathy, lumbosacral region
M54.18 Radiculopathy, sacral and sacrococcygeal region
M54.2 Cervicalgia
EXCLUDES1 *cervicalgia due to intervertebral cervical disc disorder (M50.-)*
M54.3 Sciatica
EXCLUDES1 *lesion of sciatic nerve (G57.0)*
sciatica due to intervertebral disc disorder (M51.1-)
sciatica with lumbago (M54.4-)
M54.30 Sciatica, unspecified side
M54.31 Sciatica, right side
M54.32 Sciatica, left side
M54.4 Lumbago with sciatica
EXCLUDES1 *lumbago with sciatica due to intervertebral disc disorder (M51.1-)*
M54.40 Lumbago with sciatica, unspecified side
M54.41 Lumbago with sciatica, right side
M54.42 Lumbago with sciatica, left side
AHA: Q2, 2016
M54.5 Low back pain
Loin pain
Lumbago NOS
EXCLUDES1 *low back strain (S39.012)*
lumbago due to intervertebral disc displacement (M51.2-)
lumbago with sciatica (M54.4-)
M54.6 Pain in thoracic spine
EXCLUDES1 *pain in thoracic spine due to intervertebral disc disorder (M51.-)*
M54.8 Other dorsalgia
EXCLUDES1 *dorsalgia in thoracic region (M54.6)*
low back pain (M54.5)
M54.81 Occipital neuralgia
M54.89 Other dorsalgia
M54.9 Dorsalgia, unspecified
Backache NOS
Back pain NOS

Soft tissue disorders (M60-M79)

Disorders of muscles (M60-M63)

EXCLUDES1 *dermatopolymyositis (M33.-)*
muscular dystrophies and myopathies (G71-G72)
myopathy in amyloidosis (E85.-)
myopathy in polyarteritis nodosa (M30.0)
myopathy in rheumatoid arthritis (M05.32)
myopathy in scleroderma (M34.-)
myopathy in Sjögren's syndrome (M35.03)
myopathy in systemic lupus erythematosus (M32.-)

M60 Myositis
EXCLUDES2 *inclusion body myositis [IBM] (G72.41)*
M60.0 Infective myositis
Tropical pyomyositis
Use additional code (B95-B97) to identify infectious agent
M60.00 Infective myositis, unspecified site
M60.000 Infective myositis, unspecified right arm CC

Unacceptable principal diagnosis symbol per Medicare code edits · Code exempt from diagnosis present on admission requirement
Questionable admission · Complication or comorbidity · CC/MCC exclusion · Major complication or comorbidity
Principal diagnosis as its own CC · Principal diagnosis as its own MCC · Z code as first-listed diagnosis

 When symbols appear on a code that requires a 7th character extension, refer to Appendix D to identify applicable 7th character codes.

Infective myositis, right upper limb NOS
M60.001 Infective myositis, unspecified left arm
Infective myositis, left upper limb NOS
M60.002 Infective myositis, unspecified arm
Infective myositis, upper limb NOS
M60.003 Infective myositis, unspecified right leg
Infective myositis, right lower limb NOS
M60.004 Infective myositis, unspecified left leg
Infective myositis, left lower limb NOS
M60.005 Infective myositis, unspecified leg
Infective myositis, lower limb NOS
M60.009 Infective myositis, unspecified site
M60.01 Infective myositis, shoulder
M60.011 Infective myositis, right shoulder
M60.012 Infective myositis, left shoulder
M60.019 Infective myositis, unspecified shoulder
M60.02 Infective myositis, upper arm
M60.021 Infective myositis, right upper arm
M60.022 Infective myositis, left upper arm
M60.029 Infective myositis, unspecified upper arm
M60.03 Infective myositis, forearm
M60.031 Infective myositis, right forearm
M60.032 Infective myositis, left forearm
M60.039 Infective myositis, unspecified forearm
M60.04 Infective myositis, hand and fingers
M60.041 Infective myositis, right hand
M60.042 Infective myositis, left hand
M60.043 Infective myositis, unspecified hand
M60.044 Infective myositis, right finger(s)
M60.045 Infective myositis, left finger(s)
M60.046 Infective myositis, unspecified finger(s)
M60.05 Infective myositis, thigh
M60.051 Infective myositis, right thigh
M60.052 Infective myositis, left thigh
M60.059 Infective myositis, unspecified thigh
M60.06 Infective myositis, lower leg
M60.061 Infective myositis, right lower leg
M60.062 Infective myositis, left lower leg
M60.069 Infective myositis, unspecified lower leg
M60.07 Infective myositis, ankle , foot and toes
M60.070 Infective myositis, right ankle
M60.071 Infective myositis, left ankle
M60.072 Infective myositis, unspecified ankle
M60.073 Infective myositis, right foot
M60.074 Infective myositis, left foot
M60.075 Infective myositis, unspecified foot
M60.076 Infective myositis, right toe(s)
M60.077 Infective myositis, left toe(s)
M60.078 Infective myositis, unspecified toe(s)
M60.08 Infective myositis, other site
M60.09 Infective myositis, multiple sites
M60.1 Interstitial myositis
M60.10 Interstitial myositis of unspecified site
M60.11 Interstitial myositis, shoulder
M60.111 Interstitial myositis, right shoulder
M60.112 Interstitial myositis, left shoulder
M60.119 Interstitial myositis, unspecified shoulder
M60.12 Interstitial myositis, upper arm
M60.121 Interstitial myositis, right upper arm
M60.122 Interstitial myositis, left upper arm
M60.129 Interstitial myositis, unspecified upper arm
M60.13 Interstitial myositis, forearm
M60.131 Interstitial myositis, right forearm
M60.132 Interstitial myositis, left forearm
M60.139 Interstitial myositis, unspecified forearm
M60.14 Interstitial myositis, hand
M60.141 Interstitial myositis, right hand
M60.142 Interstitial myositis, left hand
M60.149 Interstitial myositis, unspecified hand
M60.15 Interstitial myositis, thigh
M60.151 Interstitial myositis, right thigh
M60.152 Interstitial myositis, left thigh
M60.159 Interstitial myositis, unspecified thigh
M60.16 Interstitial myositis, lower leg
M60.161 Interstitial myositis, right lower leg
M60.162 Interstitial myositis, left lower leg
M60.169 Interstitial myositis, unspecified lower leg
M60.17 Interstitial myositis, ankle and foot
M60.171 Interstitial myositis, right ankle and foot
M60.172 Interstitial myositis, left ankle and foot
M60.179 Interstitial myositis, unspecified ankle and foot
M60.18 Interstitial myositis, other site
M60.19 Interstitial myositis, multiple sites
M60.2 Foreign body granuloma of soft tissue, not elsewhere classified
Use additional code to identify the type of retained foreign body (Z18.-)
EXCLUDES1 *foreign body granuloma of skin and subcutaneous tissue (L92.3)*
M60.20 Foreign body granuloma of soft tissue, not elsewhere classified, unspecified site
M60.21 Foreign body granuloma of soft tissue, not elsewhere classified, shoulder
M60.211 Foreign body granuloma of soft tissue, not elsewhere classified, right shoulder
M60.212 Foreign body granuloma of soft tissue, not elsewhere classified, left shoulder
M60.219 Foreign body granuloma of soft tissue, not elsewhere classified, unspecified shoulder
M60.22 Foreign body granuloma of soft tissue, not elsewhere classified, upper arm
M60.221 Foreign body granuloma of soft tissue, not elsewhere classified, right upper arm
M60.222 Foreign body granuloma of soft tissue, not elsewhere classified, left upper arm
M60.229 Foreign body granuloma of soft tissue, not elsewhere classified, unspecified upper arm
M60.23 Foreign body granuloma of soft tissue, not elsewhere classified, forearm
M60.231 Foreign body granuloma of soft tissue, not elsewhere classified, right forearm
M60.232 Foreign body granuloma of soft tissue, not elsewhere classified, left forearm
M60.239 Foreign body granuloma of soft tissue, not elsewhere classified, unspecified forearm
M60.24 Foreign body granuloma of soft tissue, not elsewhere classified, hand
M60.241 Foreign body granuloma of soft tissue, not elsewhere classified, right hand
M60.242 Foreign body granuloma of soft tissue, not elsewhere classified, left hand
M60.249 Foreign body granuloma of soft tissue, not elsewhere classified, unspecified hand
M60.25 Foreign body granuloma of soft tissue, not elsewhere classified, thigh
M60.251 Foreign body granuloma of soft tissue, not elsewhere classified, right thigh
M60.252 Foreign body granuloma of soft tissue, not elsewhere classified, left thigh
M60.259 Foreign body granuloma of soft tissue, not elsewhere classified, unspecified thigh
M60.26 Foreign body granuloma of soft tissue, not elsewhere classified, lower leg
M60.261 Foreign body granuloma of soft tissue, not elsewhere classified, right lower leg
M60.262 Foreign body granuloma of soft tissue, not elsewhere classified, left lower leg
M60.269 Foreign body granuloma of soft tissue, not elsewhere classified, unspecified lower leg

Unspecified Code Other Specified Code Manifestation Code N Newborn P Pediatric M Maternity A Adult ♂ Male ♀ Female
● New Code ▲ Revised Code Title ►◄ Revised Text NOTES INCLUDES EXCLUDES1 Not coded here EXCLUDES2 Not included here
4th character required 5th character required 6th character required 7th character required
Extension 'X' Alert HAC Hospital-acquired condition (HAC) alert AHA AHA Coding Clinic©

M60.27 Foreign body granuloma of soft tissue, not elsewhere classified, ankle and foot
M60.271 Foreign body granuloma of soft tissue, not elsewhere classified, right ankle and foot
M60.272 Foreign body granuloma of soft tissue, not elsewhere classified, left ankle and foot
M60.279 Foreign body granuloma of soft tissue, not elsewhere classified, unspecified ankle and foot
M60.28 Foreign body granuloma of soft tissue, not elsewhere classified, other site
M60.8 Other myositis
M60.80 Other myositis, unspecified site
M60.81 Other myositis shoulder
M60.811 Other myositis, right shoulder
M60.812 Other myositis, left shoulder
M60.819 Other myositis, unspecified shoulder
M60.82 Other myositis, upper arm
M60.821 Other myositis, right upper arm
M60.822 Other myositis, left upper arm
M60.829 Other myositis, unspecified upper arm
M60.83 Other myositis, forearm
M60.831 Other myositis, right forearm
M60.832 Other myositis, left forearm
M60.839 Other myositis, unspecified forearm
M60.84 Other myositis, hand
M60.841 Other myositis, right hand
M60.842 Other myositis, left hand
M60.849 Other myositis, unspecified hand
M60.85 Other myositis, thigh
M60.851 Other myositis, right thigh
M60.852 Other myositis, left thigh
M60.859 Other myositis, unspecified thigh
M60.86 Other myositis, lower leg
M60.861 Other myositis, right lower leg
M60.862 Other myositis, left lower leg
M60.869 Other myositis, unspecified lower leg
M60.87 Other myositis, ankle and foot
M60.871 Other myositis, right ankle and foot
M60.872 Other myositis, left ankle and foot
M60.879 Other myositis, unspecified ankle and foot
M60.88 Other myositis, other site
M60.89 Other myositis, multiple sites
M60.9 Myositis, unspecified
M61 Calcification and ossification of muscle
M61.0 Myositis ossificans traumatica
M61.00 Myositis ossificans traumatica, unspecified site
M61.01 Myositis ossificans traumatica, shoulder
M61.011 Myositis ossificans traumatica, right shoulder
M61.012 Myositis ossificans traumatica, left shoulder
M61.019 Myositis ossificans traumatica, unspecified shoulder
M61.02 Myositis ossificans traumatica, upper arm
M61.021 Myositis ossificans traumatica, right upper arm
M61.022 Myositis ossificans traumatica, left upper arm
M61.029 Myositis ossificans traumatica, unspecified upper arm
M61.03 Myositis ossificans traumatica, forearm
M61.031 Myositis ossificans traumatica, right forearm
M61.032 Myositis ossificans traumatica, left forearm
M61.039 Myositis ossificans traumatica, unspecified forearm
M61.04 Myositis ossificans traumatica, hand
M61.041 Myositis ossificans traumatica, right hand
M61.042 Myositis ossificans traumatica, left hand
M61.049 Myositis ossificans traumatica, unspecified hand
M61.05 Myositis ossificans traumatica, thigh
M61.051 Myositis ossificans traumatica, right thigh
M61.052 Myositis ossificans traumatica, left thigh
M61.059 Myositis ossificans traumatica, unspecified thigh
M61.06 Myositis ossificans traumatica, lower leg
M61.061 Myositis ossificans traumatica, right lower leg
M61.062 Myositis ossificans traumatica, left lower leg
M61.069 Myositis ossificans traumatica, unspecified lower leg
M61.07 Myositis ossificans traumatica, ankle and foot
M61.071 Myositis ossificans traumatica, right ankle and foot
M61.072 Myositis ossificans traumatica, left ankle and foot
M61.079 Myositis ossificans traumatica, unspecified ankle and foot
M61.08 Myositis ossificans traumatica, other site
M61.09 Myositis ossificans traumatica, multiple sites
M61.1 Myositis ossificans progressiva
Fibrodysplasia ossificans progressiva
M61.10 Myositis ossificans progressiva, unspecified site
M61.11 Myositis ossificans progressiva, shoulder
M61.111 Myositis ossificans progressiva, right shoulder
M61.112 Myositis ossificans progressiva, left shoulder
M61.119 Myositis ossificans progressiva, unspecified shoulder
M61.12 Myositis ossificans progressiva, upper arm
M61.121 Myositis ossificans progressiva, right upper arm
M61.122 Myositis ossificans progressiva, left upper arm
M61.129 Myositis ossificans progressiva, unspecified arm
M61.13 Myositis ossificans progressiva, forearm
M61.131 Myositis ossificans progressiva, right forearm
M61.132 Myositis ossificans progressiva, left forearm
M61.139 Myositis ossificans progressiva, unspecified forearm
M61.14 Myositis ossificans progressiva, hand and finger (s)
M61.141 Myositis ossificans progressiva, right hand
M61.142 Myositis ossificans progressiva, left hand
M61.143 Myositis ossificans progressiva, unspecified hand
M61.144 Myositis ossificans progressiva, right finger(s)
M61.145 Myositis ossificans progressiva, left finger(s)
M61.146 Myositis ossificans progressiva, unspecified finger(s)
M61.15 Myositis ossificans progressiva, thigh
M61.151 Myositis ossificans progressiva, right thigh
M61.152 Myositis ossificans progressiva, left thigh
M61.159 Myositis ossificans progressiva, unspecified thigh
M61.16 Myositis ossificans progressiva, lower leg
M61.161 Myositis ossificans progressiva, right lower leg
M61.162 Myositis ossificans progressiva, left lower leg
M61.169 Myositis ossificans progressiva, unspecified lower leg
M61.17 Myositis ossificans progressiva, ankle, foot and toe(s)
M61.171 Myositis ossificans progressiva, right ankle
M61.172 Myositis ossificans progressiva, left ankle

Unacceptable principal diagnosis symbol per Medicare code edits · Code exempt from diagnosis present on admission requirement
Questionable admission · Complication or comorbidity · CC/MCC exclusion · Major complication or comorbidity
Principal diagnosis as its own CC · Principal diagnosis as its own MCC · Z code as first-listed diagnosis

M61.173 Myositis ossificans progressiva, unspecified ankle
M61.174 Myositis ossificans progressiva, right foot
M61.175 Myositis ossificans progressiva, left foot
M61.176 Myositis ossificans progressiva, unspecified foot
M61.177 Myositis ossificans progressiva, right toe(s)
M61.178 Myositis ossificans progressiva, left toe(s)
M61.179 Myositis ossificans progressiva, unspecified toe(s)
M61.18 Myositis ossificans progressiva, other site
M61.19 Myositis ossificans progressiva, multiple sites
M61.2 Paralytic calcification and ossification of muscle
Myositis ossificans associated with quadriplegia or paraplegia
M61.20 Paralytic calcification and ossification of muscle, unspecified site
M61.21 Paralytic calcification and ossification of muscle, shoulder
M61.211 Paralytic calcification and ossification of muscle, right shoulder
M61.212 Paralytic calcification and ossification of muscle, left shoulder
M61.219 Paralytic calcification and ossification of muscle, unspecified shoulder
M61.22 Paralytic calcification and ossification of muscle, upper arm
M61.221 Paralytic calcification and ossification of muscle, right upper arm
M61.222 Paralytic calcification and ossification of muscle, left upper arm
M61.229 Paralytic calcification and ossification of muscle, unspecified upper arm
M61.23 Paralytic calcification and ossification of muscle, forearm
M61.231 Paralytic calcification and ossification of muscle, right forearm
M61.232 Paralytic calcification and ossification of muscle, left forearm
M61.239 Paralytic calcification and ossification of muscle, unspecified forearm
M61.24 Paralytic calcification and ossification of muscle, hand
M61.241 Paralytic calcification and ossification of muscle, right hand
M61.242 Paralytic calcification and ossification of muscle, left hand
M61.249 Paralytic calcification and ossification of muscle, unspecified hand
M61.25 Paralytic calcification and ossification of muscle, thigh
M61.251 Paralytic calcification and ossification of muscle, right thigh
M61.252 Paralytic calcification and ossification of muscle, left thigh
M61.259 Paralytic calcification and ossification of muscle, unspecified thigh
M61.26 Paralytic calcification and ossification of muscle, lower leg
M61.261 Paralytic calcification and ossification of muscle, right lower leg
M61.262 Paralytic calcification and ossification of muscle, left lower leg
M61.269 Paralytic calcification and ossification of muscle, unspecified lower leg
M61.27 Paralytic calcification and ossification of muscle, ankle and foot
M61.271 Paralytic calcification and ossification of muscle, right ankle and foot
M61.272 Paralytic calcification and ossification of muscle, left ankle and foot
M61.279 Paralytic calcification and ossification of muscle, unspecified ankle and foot
M61.28 Paralytic calcification and ossification of muscle, other site
M61.29 Paralytic calcification and ossification of muscle, multiple sites
M61.3 Calcification and ossification of muscles associated with burns
Myositis ossificans associated with burns
M61.30 Calcification and ossification of muscles associated with burns, unspecified site
M61.31 Calcification and ossification of muscles associated with burns, shoulder
M61.311 Calcification and ossification of muscles associated with burns, right shoulder
M61.312 Calcification and ossification of muscles associated with burns, left shoulder
M61.319 Calcification and ossification of muscles associated with burns, unspecified shoulder
M61.32 Calcification and ossification of muscles associated with burns, upper arm
M61.321 Calcification and ossification of muscles associated with burns, right upper arm
M61.322 Calcification and ossification of muscles associated with burns, left upper arm
M61.329 Calcification and ossification of muscles associated with burns, unspecified upper arm
M61.33 Calcification and ossification of muscles associated with burns, forearm
M61.331 Calcification and ossification of muscles associated with burns, right forearm
M61.332 Calcification and ossification of muscles associated with burns, left forearm
M61.339 Calcification and ossification of muscles associated with burns, unspecified forearm
M61.34 Calcification and ossification of muscles associated with burns, hand
M61.341 Calcification and ossification of muscles associated with burns, right hand
M61.342 Calcification and ossification of muscles associated with burns, left hand
M61.349 Calcification and ossification of muscles associated with burns, unspecified hand
M61.35 Calcification and ossification of muscles associated with burns, thigh
M61.351 Calcification and ossification of muscles associated with burns, right thigh
M61.352 Calcification and ossification of muscles associated with burns, left thigh
M61.359 Calcification and ossification of muscles associated with burns, unspecified thigh
M61.36 Calcification and ossification of muscles associated with burns, lower leg
M61.361 Calcification and ossification of muscles associated with burns, right lower leg
M61.362 Calcification and ossification of muscles associated with burns, left lower leg
M61.369 Calcification and ossification of muscles associated with burns, unspecified lower leg
M61.37 Calcification and ossification of muscles associated with burns, ankle and foot
M61.371 Calcification and ossification of muscles associated with burns, right ankle and foot
M61.372 Calcification and ossification of muscles associated with burns, left ankle and foot
M61.379 Calcification and ossification of muscles associated with burns, unspecified ankle and foot
M61.38 Calcification and ossification of muscles associated with burns, other site
M61.39 Calcification and ossification of muscles associated with burns, multiple sites
M61.4 Other calcification of muscle
EXCLUDES1 *calcific tendinitis NOS (M65.2-)*
calcific tendinitis of shoulder (M75.3)
M61.40 Other calcification of muscle, unspecified site
M61.41 Other calcification of muscle, shoulder

Unspecified Code Other Specified Code Manifestation Code N Newborn P Pediatric M Maternity A Adult ♂ Male ♀ Female
● New Code ▲ Revised Code Title ►◄ Revised Text NOTES INCLUDES EXCLUDES1 Not coded here EXCLUDES2 Not included here
4th character required 5th character required 6th character required 7th character required
Extension 'X' Alert HAC Hospital-acquired condition (HAC) alert AHA AHA Coding Clinic©

M61.411 Other calcification of muscle, right shoulder
M61.412 Other calcification of muscle, left shoulder
M61.419 Other calcification of muscle, unspecified shoulder
M61.42 Other calcification of muscle, upper arm
M61.421 Other calcification of muscle, right upper arm
M61.422 Other calcification of muscle, left upper arm
M61.429 Other calcification of muscle, unspecified upper arm
M61.43 Other calcification of muscle, forearm
M61.431 Other calcification of muscle, right forearm
M61.432 Other calcification of muscle, left forearm
M61.439 Other calcification of muscle, unspecified forearm
M61.44 Other calcification of muscle, hand
M61.441 Other calcification of muscle, right hand
M61.442 Other calcification of muscle, left hand
M61.449 Other calcification of muscle, unspecified hand
M61.45 Other calcification of muscle, thigh
M61.451 Other calcification of muscle, right thigh
M61.452 Other calcification of muscle, left thigh
M61.459 Other calcification of muscle, unspecified thigh
M61.46 Other calcification of muscle, lower leg
M61.461 Other calcification of muscle, right lower leg
M61.462 Other calcification of muscle, left lower leg
M61.469 Other calcification of muscle, unspecified lower leg
M61.47 Other calcification of muscle, ankle and foot
M61.471 Other calcification of muscle, right ankle and foot
M61.472 Other calcification of muscle, left ankle and foot
M61.479 Other calcification of muscle, unspecified ankle and foot
M61.48 Other calcification of muscle, other site
M61.49 Other calcification of muscle, multiple sites
M61.5 Other ossification of muscle
M61.50 Other ossification of muscle, unspecified site
M61.51 Other ossification of muscle, shoulder
M61.511 Other ossification of muscle, right shoulder
M61.512 Other ossification of muscle, left shoulder
M61.519 Other ossification of muscle, unspecified shoulder
M61.52 Other ossification of muscle, upper arm
M61.521 Other ossification of muscle, right upper arm
M61.522 Other ossification of muscle, left upper arm
M61.529 Other ossification of muscle, unspecified upper arm
M61.53 Other ossification of muscle, forearm
M61.531 Other ossification of muscle, right forearm
M61.532 Other ossification of muscle, left forearm
M61.539 Other ossification of muscle, unspecified forearm
M61.54 Other ossification of muscle, hand
M61.541 Other ossification of muscle, right hand
M61.542 Other ossification of muscle, left hand
M61.549 Other ossification of muscle, unspecified hand
M61.55 Other ossification of muscle, thigh
M61.551 Other ossification of muscle, right thigh
M61.552 Other ossification of muscle, left thigh
M61.559 Other ossification of muscle, unspecified thigh
M61.56 Other ossification of muscle, lower leg
M61.561 Other ossification of muscle, right lower leg
M61.562 Other ossification of muscle, left lower leg
M61.569 Other ossification of muscle, unspecified lower leg
M61.57 Other ossification of muscle, ankle and foot
M61.571 Other ossification of muscle, right ankle and foot
M61.572 Other ossification of muscle, left ankle and foot
M61.579 Other ossification of muscle, unspecified ankle and foot
M61.58 Other ossification of muscle, other site
M61.59 Other ossification of muscle, multiple sites
M61.9 Calcification and ossification of muscle, unspecified

M62 Other disorders of muscle
EXCLUDES1 *alcoholic myopathy (G72.1)*
cramp and spasm (R25.2)
drug-induced myopathy (G72.0)
myalgia (M79.1)
stiff-man syndrome (G25.82)
EXCLUDES2 *nontraumatic hematoma of muscle (M79.81)*

M62.0 Separation of muscle (nontraumatic)
Diastasis of muscle
EXCLUDES1 *diastasis recti complicating pregnancy, labor and delivery (O71.8)*
traumatic separation of muscle- see strain of muscle by body region
M62.00 Separation of muscle (nontraumatic), unspecified site
M62.01 Separation of muscle (nontraumatic), shoulder
M62.011 Separation of muscle (nontraumatic), right shoulder
M62.012 Separation of muscle (nontraumatic), left shoulder
M62.019 Separation of muscle (nontraumatic), unspecified shoulder
M62.02 Separation of muscle (nontraumatic), upper arm
M62.021 Separation of muscle (nontraumatic), right upper arm
M62.022 Separation of muscle (nontraumatic), left upper arm
M62.029 Separation of muscle (nontraumatic), unspecified upper arm
M62.03 Separation of muscle (nontraumatic), forearm
M62.031 Separation of muscle (nontraumatic), right forearm
M62.032 Separation of muscle (nontraumatic), left forearm
M62.039 Separation of muscle (nontraumatic), unspecified forearm
M62.04 Separation of muscle (nontraumatic), hand
M62.041 Separation of muscle (nontraumatic), right hand
M62.042 Separation of muscle (nontraumatic), left hand
M62.049 Separation of muscle (nontraumatic), unspecified hand
M62.05 Separation of muscle (nontraumatic), thigh
M62.051 Separation of muscle (nontraumatic), right thigh
M62.052 Separation of muscle (nontraumatic), left thigh
M62.059 Separation of muscle (nontraumatic), unspecified thigh
M62.06 Separation of muscle (nontraumatic), lower leg
M62.061 Separation of muscle (nontraumatic), right lower leg
M62.062 Separation of muscle (nontraumatic), left lower leg
M62.069 Separation of muscle (nontraumatic), unspecified lower leg
M62.07 Separation of muscle (nontraumatic), ankle and foot

Unacceptable principal diagnosis symbol per Medicare code edits · Code exempt from diagnosis present on admission requirement
Questionable admission · Complication or comorbidity · CC/MCC exclusion · Major complication or comorbidity
Principal diagnosis as its own CC · Principal diagnosis as its own MCC · Z code as first-listed diagnosis

M62.071 Separation of muscle (nontraumatic), right ankle and foot
M62.072 Separation of muscle (nontraumatic), left ankle and foot
M62.079 Separation of muscle (nontraumatic), unspecified ankle and foot
M62.08 Separation of muscle (nontraumatic), other site
M62.1 Other rupture of muscle (nontraumatic)
EXCLUDES1 *traumatic rupture of muscle - see strain of muscle by body region*
EXCLUDES2 *rupture of tendon (M66.-)*
M62.10 Other rupture of muscle (nontraumatic), unspecified site
M62.11 Other rupture of muscle (nontraumatic), shoulder
M62.111 Other rupture of muscle (nontraumatic), right shoulder
M62.112 Other rupture of muscle (nontraumatic), left shoulder
M62.119 Other rupture of muscle (nontraumatic), unspecified shoulder
M62.12 Other rupture of muscle (nontraumatic), upper arm
M62.121 Other rupture of muscle (nontraumatic), right upper arm
M62.122 Other rupture of muscle (nontraumatic), left upper arm
M62.129 Other rupture of muscle (nontraumatic), unspecified upper arm
M62.13 Other rupture of muscle (nontraumatic), forearm
M62.131 Other rupture of muscle (nontraumatic), right forearm
M62.132 Other rupture of muscle (nontraumatic), left forearm
M62.139 Other rupture of muscle (nontraumatic), unspecified forearm
M62.14 Other rupture of muscle (nontraumatic), hand
M62.141 Other rupture of muscle (nontraumatic), right hand
M62.142 Other rupture of muscle (nontraumatic), left hand
M62.149 Other rupture of muscle (nontraumatic), unspecified hand
M62.15 Other rupture of muscle (nontraumatic), thigh
M62.151 Other rupture of muscle (nontraumatic), right thigh
M62.152 Other rupture of muscle (nontraumatic), left thigh
M62.159 Other rupture of muscle (nontraumatic), unspecified thigh
M62.16 Other rupture of muscle (nontraumatic), lower leg
M62.161 Other rupture of muscle (nontraumatic), right lower leg
M62.162 Other rupture of muscle (nontraumatic), left lower leg
M62.169 Other rupture of muscle (nontraumatic), unspecified lower leg
M62.17 Other rupture of muscle (nontraumatic), ankle and foot
M62.171 Other rupture of muscle (nontraumatic), right ankle and foot
M62.172 Other rupture of muscle (nontraumatic), left ankle and foot
M62.179 Other rupture of muscle (nontraumatic), unspecified ankle and foot
M62.18 Other rupture of muscle (nontraumatic), other site
M62.2 Nontraumatic ischemic infarction of muscle
EXCLUDES1 *compartment syndrome (traumatic) (T79.A-)*
nontraumatic compartment syndrome (M79.A-)
traumatic ischemia of muscle (T79.6)
rhabdomyolysis (M62.82)
Volkmann's ischemic contracture (T79.6)
M62.20 Nontraumatic ischemic infarction of muscle, unspecified site
M62.21 Nontraumatic ischemic infarction of muscle, shoulder
M62.211 Nontraumatic ischemic infarction of muscle, right shoulder
M62.212 Nontraumatic ischemic infarction of muscle, left shoulder
M62.219 Nontraumatic ischemic infarction of muscle, unspecified shoulder
M62.22 Nontraumatic ischemic infarction of muscle, upper arm
M62.221 Nontraumatic ischemic infarction of muscle, right upper arm
M62.222 Nontraumatic ischemic infarction of muscle, left upper arm
M62.229 Nontraumatic ischemic infarction of muscle, unspecified upper arm
M62.23 Nontraumatic ischemic infarction of muscle, forearm
M62.231 Nontraumatic ischemic infarction of muscle, right forearm
M62.232 Nontraumatic ischemic infarction of muscle, left forearm
M62.239 Nontraumatic ischemic infarction of muscle, unspecified forearm
M62.24 Nontraumatic ischemic infarction of muscle, hand
M62.241 Nontraumatic ischemic infarction of muscle, right hand
M62.242 Nontraumatic ischemic infarction of muscle, left hand
M62.249 Nontraumatic ischemic infarction of muscle, unspecified hand
M62.25 Nontraumatic ischemic infarction of muscle, thigh
M62.251 Nontraumatic ischemic infarction of muscle, right thigh
M62.252 Nontraumatic ischemic infarction of muscle, left thigh
M62.259 Nontraumatic ischemic infarction of muscle, unspecified thigh
M62.26 Nontraumatic ischemic infarction of muscle, lower leg
M62.261 Nontraumatic ischemic infarction of muscle, right lower leg
M62.262 Nontraumatic ischemic infarction of muscle, left lower leg
M62.269 Nontraumatic ischemic infarction of muscle, unspecified lower leg
M62.27 Nontraumatic ischemic infarction of muscle, ankle and foot
M62.271 Nontraumatic ischemic infarction of muscle, right ankle and foot
M62.272 Nontraumatic ischemic infarction of muscle, left ankle and foot
M62.279 Nontraumatic ischemic infarction of muscle, unspecified ankle and foot
M62.28 Nontraumatic ischemic infarction of muscle, other site
M62.3 Immobility syndrome (paraplegic)
M62.4 Contracture of muscle
Contracture of tendon (sheath)
EXCLUDES1 *contracture of joint (M24.5-)*
M62.40 Contracture of muscle, unspecified site
M62.41 Contracture of muscle, shoulder
M62.411 Contracture of muscle, right shoulder
M62.412 Contracture of muscle, left shoulder
M62.419 Contracture of muscle, unspecified shoulder
M62.42 Contracture of muscle, upper arm
M62.421 Contracture of muscle, right upper arm
M62.422 Contracture of muscle, left upper arm
M62.429 Contracture of muscle, unspecified upper arm
M62.43 Contracture of muscle, forearm
M62.431 Contracture of muscle, right forearm
M62.432 Contracture of muscle, left forearm
M62.439 Contracture of muscle, unspecified forearm
M62.44 Contracture of muscle, hand
M62.441 Contracture of muscle, right hand

Unspecified Code | Other Specified Code | Manifestation Code | N Newborn | P Pediatric | M Maternity | A Adult | ♂ Male | ♀ Female
● New Code | ▲ Revised Code Title | ►◄ Revised Text | NOTES | INCLUDES | EXCLUDES1 Not coded here | EXCLUDES2 Not included here
4th character required | 5th character required | 6th character required | 7th character required
Extension 'X' Alert | HAC Hospital-acquired condition (HAC) alert | AHA AHA Coding Clinic©

M62.442 Contracture of muscle, left hand
M62.449 Contracture of muscle, unspecified hand
M62.45 Contracture of muscle, thigh
M62.451 Contracture of muscle, right thigh
M62.452 Contracture of muscle, left thigh
M62.459 Contracture of muscle, unspecified thigh
M62.46 Contracture of muscle, lower leg
M62.461 Contracture of muscle, right lower leg
M62.462 Contracture of muscle, left lower leg
M62.469 Contracture of muscle, unspecified lower leg
M62.47 Contracture of muscle, ankle and foot
M62.471 Contracture of muscle, right ankle and foot
M62.472 Contracture of muscle, left ankle and foot
M62.479 Contracture of muscle, unspecified ankle and foot
M62.48 Contracture of muscle, other site
M62.49 Contracture of muscle, multiple sites
M62.5 Muscle wasting and atrophy, not elsewhere classified
Disuse atrophy NEC
EXCLUDES1 *neuralgic amyotrophy (G54.5)*
progressive muscular atrophy (G12.29)
sarcopenia (M62.84)
EXCLUDES2 *pelvic muscle wasting (N81.84)*
M62.50 Muscle wasting and atrophy, not elsewhere classified, unspecified site
M62.51 Muscle wasting and atrophy, not elsewhere classified, shoulder
M62.511 Muscle wasting and atrophy, not elsewhere classified, right shoulder
M62.512 Muscle wasting and atrophy, not elsewhere classified, left shoulder
M62.519 Muscle wasting and atrophy, not elsewhere classified, unspecified shoulder
M62.52 Muscle wasting and atrophy, not elsewhere classified, upper arm
M62.521 Muscle wasting and atrophy, not elsewhere classified, right upper arm
M62.522 Muscle wasting and atrophy, not elsewhere classified, left upper arm
M62.529 Muscle wasting and atrophy, not elsewhere classified, unspecified upper arm
M62.53 Muscle wasting and atrophy, not elsewhere classified, forearm
M62.531 Muscle wasting and atrophy, not elsewhere classified, right forearm
M62.532 Muscle wasting and atrophy, not elsewhere classified, left forearm
M62.539 Muscle wasting and atrophy, not elsewhere classified, unspecified forearm
M62.54 Muscle wasting and atrophy, not elsewhere classified, hand
M62.541 Muscle wasting and atrophy, not elsewhere classified, right hand
M62.542 Muscle wasting and atrophy, not elsewhere classified, left hand
M62.549 Muscle wasting and atrophy, not elsewhere classified, unspecified hand
M62.55 Muscle wasting and atrophy, not elsewhere classified, thigh
M62.551 Muscle wasting and atrophy, not elsewhere classified, right thigh
M62.552 Muscle wasting and atrophy, not elsewhere classified, left thigh
M62.559 Muscle wasting and atrophy, not elsewhere classified, unspecified thigh
M62.56 Muscle wasting and atrophy, not elsewhere classified, lower leg
M62.561 Muscle wasting and atrophy, not elsewhere classified, right lower leg
M62.562 Muscle wasting and atrophy, not elsewhere classified, left lower leg
M62.569 Muscle wasting and atrophy, not elsewhere classified, unspecified lower leg
M62.57 Muscle wasting and atrophy, not elsewhere classified, ankle and foot
M62.571 Muscle wasting and atrophy, not elsewhere classified, right ankle and foot
M62.572 Muscle wasting and atrophy, not elsewhere classified, left ankle and foot
M62.579 Muscle wasting and atrophy, not elsewhere classified, unspecified ankle and foot
M62.58 Muscle wasting and atrophy, not elsewhere classified, other site
M62.59 Muscle wasting and atrophy, not elsewhere classified, multiple sites
M62.8 Other specified disorders of muscle
EXCLUDES2 *nontraumatic hematoma of muscle (M79.81)*
M62.81 Muscle weakness (generalized)
EXCLUDES1 *muscle weakness in sarcopenia (M62.84)*
M62.82 Rhabdomyolysis
EXCLUDES1 *traumatic rhabdomyolysis (T79.6)*
M62.83 Muscle spasm
M62.830 Muscle spasm of back
M62.831 Muscle spasm of calf
Charley-horse
M62.838 Other muscle spasm
● M62.84 Sarcopenia
Age-related sarcopenia
Code first underlying disease, if applicable, such as:
disorders of myoneural junction and muscle disease in diseases classified elsewhere (G73.-)
other and unspecified myopathies (G72.-)
primary disorders of muscles (G71.-)
M62.89 Other specified disorders of muscle
Muscle (sheath) hernia
M62.9 Disorder of muscle, unspecified
M63 Disorders of muscle in diseases classified elsewhere
Code first underlying disease, such as:
leprosy (A30.-)
neoplasm (C49.-, C79.89, D21.-, D48.1)
schistosomiasis (B65.-)
trichinellosis (B75)
EXCLUDES1 *myopathy in cysticercosis (B69.81)*
myopathy in endocrine diseases (G73.7)
myopathy in metabolic diseases (G73.7)
myopathy in sarcoidosis (D86.87)
myopathy in secondary syphilis (A51.49)
myopathy in syphilis (late) (A52.78)
myopathy in toxoplasmosis (B58.82)
myopathy in tuberculosis (A18.09)
M63.8 Disorders of muscle in diseases classified elsewhere
M63.80 Disorders of muscle in diseases classified elsewhere, unspecified site
M63.81 Disorders of muscle in diseases classified elsewhere, shoulder
M63.811 Disorders of muscle in diseases classified elsewhere, right shoulder
M63.812 Disorders of muscle in diseases classified elsewhere, left shoulder
M63.819 Disorders of muscle in diseases classified elsewhere, unspecified shoulder
M63.82 Disorders of muscle in diseases classified elsewhere, upper arm
M63.821 Disorders of muscle in diseases classified elsewhere, right upper arm
M63.822 Disorders of muscle in diseases classified elsewhere, left upper arm
M63.829 Disorders of muscle in diseases classified elsewhere, unspecified upper arm
M63.83 Disorders of muscle in diseases classified elsewhere, forearm
M63.831 Disorders of muscle in diseases classified elsewhere, right forearm

Unacceptable principal diagnosis symbol per Medicare code edits · Code exempt from diagnosis present on admission requirement · Questionable admission · Complication or comorbidity · CC/MCC exclusion · Major complication or comorbidity · Principal diagnosis as its own CC · Principal diagnosis as its own MCC · Z code as first-listed diagnosis

When symbols appear on a code that requires a 7th character extension, refer to Appendix D to identify applicable 7th character codes.

M63.832 Disorders of muscle in diseases classified elsewhere, left forearm
M63.839 Disorders of muscle in diseases classified elsewhere, unspecified forearm
M63.84 Disorders of muscle in diseases classified elsewhere, hand
M63.841 Disorders of muscle in diseases classified elsewhere, right hand
M63.842 Disorders of muscle in diseases classified elsewhere, left hand
M63.849 Disorders of muscle in diseases classified elsewhere, unspecified hand
M63.85 Disorders of muscle in diseases classified elsewhere, thigh
M63.851 Disorders of muscle in diseases classified elsewhere, right thigh
M63.852 Disorders of muscle in diseases classified elsewhere, left thigh
M63.859 Disorders of muscle in diseases classified elsewhere, unspecified thigh
M63.86 Disorders of muscle in diseases classified elsewhere, lower leg
M63.861 Disorders of muscle in diseases classified elsewhere, right lower leg
M63.862 Disorders of muscle in diseases classified elsewhere, left lower leg
M63.869 Disorders of muscle in diseases classified elsewhere, unspecified lower leg
M63.87 Disorders of muscle in diseases classified elsewhere, ankle and foot
M63.871 Disorders of muscle in diseases classified elsewhere, right ankle and foot
M63.872 Disorders of muscle in diseases classified elsewhere, left ankle and foot
M63.879 Disorders of muscle in diseases classified elsewhere, unspecified ankle and foot
M63.88 Disorders of muscle in diseases classified elsewhere, other site
M63.89 Disorders of muscle in diseases classified elsewhere, multiple sites

Disorders of synovium and tendon (M65-M67)

M65 Synovitis and tenosynovitis

EXCLUDES1 *chronic crepitant synovitis of hand and wrist (M70.0-)*
current injury - see injury of ligament or tendon by body region
soft tissue disorders related to use, overuse and pressure (M70.-)

M65.0 Abscess of tendon sheath
Use additional code (B95-B96) to identify bacterial agent.
M65.00 Abscess of tendon sheath, unspecified site
M65.01 Abscess of tendon sheath, shoulder
M65.011 Abscess of tendon sheath, right shoulder
M65.012 Abscess of tendon sheath, left shoulder
M65.019 Abscess of tendon sheath, unspecified shoulder
M65.02 Abscess of tendon sheath, upper arm
M65.021 Abscess of tendon sheath, right upper arm
M65.022 Abscess of tendon sheath, left upper arm
M65.029 Abscess of tendon sheath, unspecified upper arm
M65.03 Abscess of tendon sheath, forearm
M65.031 Abscess of tendon sheath, right forearm
M65.032 Abscess of tendon sheath, left forearm
M65.039 Abscess of tendon sheath, unspecified forearm
M65.04 Abscess of tendon sheath, hand
M65.041 Abscess of tendon sheath, right hand
M65.042 Abscess of tendon sheath, left hand
M65.049 Abscess of tendon sheath, unspecified hand
M65.05 Abscess of tendon sheath, thigh
M65.051 Abscess of tendon sheath, right thigh
M65.052 Abscess of tendon sheath, left thigh
M65.059 Abscess of tendon sheath, unspecified thigh
M65.06 Abscess of tendon sheath, lower leg
M65.061 Abscess of tendon sheath, right lower leg
M65.062 Abscess of tendon sheath, left lower leg
M65.069 Abscess of tendon sheath, unspecified lower leg
M65.07 Abscess of tendon sheath, ankle and foot
M65.071 Abscess of tendon sheath, right ankle and foot
M65.072 Abscess of tendon sheath, left ankle and foot
M65.079 Abscess of tendon sheath, unspecified ankle and foot
M65.08 Abscess of tendon sheath, other site

M65.1 Other infective (teno)synovitis
M65.10 Other infective (teno)synovitis, unspecified site
M65.11 Other infective (teno)synovitis, shoulder
M65.111 Other infective (teno)synovitis, right shoulder
M65.112 Other infective (teno)synovitis, left shoulder
M65.119 Other infective (teno)synovitis, unspecified shoulder
M65.12 Other infective (teno)synovitis, elbow
M65.121 Other infective (teno)synovitis, right elbow
M65.122 Other infective (teno)synovitis, left elbow
M65.129 Other infective (teno)synovitis, unspecified elbow
M65.13 Other infective (teno)synovitis, wrist
M65.131 Other infective (teno)synovitis, right wrist
M65.132 Other infective (teno)synovitis, left wrist
M65.139 Other infective (teno)synovitis, unspecified wrist
M65.14 Other infective (teno)synovitis, hand
M65.141 Other infective (teno)synovitis, right hand
M65.142 Other infective (teno)synovitis, left hand
M65.149 Other infective (teno)synovitis, unspecified hand
M65.15 Other infective (teno)synovitis, hip
M65.151 Other infective (teno)synovitis, right hip
M65.152 Other infective (teno)synovitis, left hip
M65.159 Other infective (teno)synovitis, unspecified hip
M65.16 Other infective (teno)synovitis, knee
M65.161 Other infective (teno)synovitis, right knee
M65.162 Other infective (teno)synovitis, left knee
M65.169 Other infective (teno)synovitis, unspecified knee
M65.17 Other infective (teno)synovitis, ankle and foot
M65.171 Other infective (teno)synovitis, right ankle and foot
M65.172 Other infective (teno)synovitis, left ankle and foot
M65.179 Other infective (teno)synovitis, unspecified ankle and foot
M65.18 Other infective (teno)synovitis, other site
M65.19 Other infective (teno)synovitis, multiple sites

M65.2 Calcific tendinitis

EXCLUDES1 *tendinitis as classified in M75-M77*
calcified tendinitis of shoulder (M75.3)

M65.20 Calcific tendinitis, unspecified site
M65.22 Calcific tendinitis, upper arm
M65.221 Calcific tendinitis, right upper arm
M65.222 Calcific tendinitis, left upper arm
M65.229 Calcific tendinitis, unspecified upper arm
M65.23 Calcific tendinitis, forearm
M65.231 Calcific tendinitis, right forearm
M65.232 Calcific tendinitis, left forearm
M65.239 Calcific tendinitis, unspecified forearm
M65.24 Calcific tendinitis, hand
M65.241 Calcific tendinitis, right hand
M65.242 Calcific tendinitis, left hand

Unspecified Code Other Specified Code Manifestation Code N Newborn P Pediatric M Maternity A Adult ♂ Male ♀ Female
● New Code ▲ Revised Code Title ►◄ Revised Text NOTES INCLUDES EXCLUDES1 Not coded here EXCLUDES2 Not included here
4th character required 5th character required 6th character required 7th character required
Extension 'X' Alert HAC Hospital-acquired condition (HAC) alert AHA AHA Coding Clinic©

M65.249 Calcific tendinitis, unspecified hand
M65.25 Calcific tendinitis, thigh
M65.251 Calcific tendinitis, right thigh
M65.252 Calcific tendinitis, left thigh
M65.259 Calcific tendinitis, unspecified thigh
M65.26 Calcific tendinitis, lower leg
M65.261 Calcific tendinitis, right lower leg
M65.262 Calcific tendinitis, left lower leg
M65.269 Calcific tendinitis, unspecified lower leg
M65.27 Calcific tendinitis, ankle and foot
M65.271 Calcific tendinitis, right ankle and foot
M65.272 Calcific tendinitis, left ankle and foot
M65.279 Calcific tendinitis, unspecified ankle and foot
M65.28 Calcific tendinitis, other site
M65.29 Calcific tendinitis, multiple sites
M65.3 Trigger finger
Nodular tendinous disease
M65.30 Trigger finger, unspecified finger
M65.31 Trigger thumb
M65.311 Trigger thumb, right thumb
M65.312 Trigger thumb, left thumb
M65.319 Trigger thumb, unspecified thumb
M65.32 Trigger finger, index finger
M65.321 Trigger finger, right index finger
M65.322 Trigger finger, left index finger
M65.329 Trigger finger, unspecified index finger
M65.33 Trigger finger, middle finger
M65.331 Trigger finger, right middle finger
M65.332 Trigger finger, left middle finger
M65.339 Trigger finger, unspecified middle finger
M65.34 Trigger finger, ring finger
M65.341 Trigger finger, right ring finger
M65.342 Trigger finger, left ring finger
M65.349 Trigger finger, unspecified ring finger
M65.35 Trigger finger, little finger
M65.351 Trigger finger, right little finger
M65.352 Trigger finger, left little finger
M65.359 Trigger finger, unspecified little finger
M65.4 Radial styloid tenosynovitis [de Quervain]
M65.8 Other synovitis and tenosynovitis
M65.80 Other synovitis and tenosynovitis, unspecified site
M65.81 Other synovitis and tenosynovitis, shoulder
M65.811 Other synovitis and tenosynovitis, right shoulder
M65.812 Other synovitis and tenosynovitis, left shoulder
M65.819 Other synovitis and tenosynovitis, unspecified shoulder
M65.82 Other synovitis and tenosynovitis, upper arm
M65.821 Other synovitis and tenosynovitis, right upper arm
M65.822 Other synovitis and tenosynovitis, left upper arm
M65.829 Other synovitis and tenosynovitis, unspecified upper arm
M65.83 Other synovitis and tenosynovitis, forearm
M65.831 Other synovitis and tenosynovitis, right forearm
M65.832 Other synovitis and tenosynovitis, left forearm
M65.839 Other synovitis and tenosynovitis, unspecified forearm
M65.84 Other synovitis and tenosynovitis, hand
M65.841 Other synovitis and tenosynovitis, right hand
M65.842 Other synovitis and tenosynovitis, left hand
M65.849 Other synovitis and tenosynovitis, unspecified hand
M65.85 Other synovitis and tenosynovitis, thigh
M65.851 Other synovitis and tenosynovitis, right thigh
M65.852 Other synovitis and tenosynovitis, left thigh
M65.859 Other synovitis and tenosynovitis, unspecified thigh
M65.86 Other synovitis and tenosynovitis, lower leg
M65.861 Other synovitis and tenosynovitis, right lower leg
M65.862 Other synovitis and tenosynovitis, left lower leg
M65.869 Other synovitis and tenosynovitis, unspecified lower leg
M65.87 Other synovitis and tenosynovitis, ankle and foot
M65.871 Other synovitis and tenosynovitis, right ankle and foot
M65.872 Other synovitis and tenosynovitis, left ankle and foot
M65.879 Other synovitis and tenosynovitis, unspecified ankle and foot
M65.88 Other synovitis and tenosynovitis, other site
M65.89 Other synovitis and tenosynovitis, multiple sites
M65.9 Synovitis and tenosynovitis, unspecified
M66 Spontaneous rupture of synovium and tendon
INCLUDES *rupture that occurs when a normal force is applied to tissues that are inferred to have less than normal strength*
EXCLUDES2 *rotator cuff syndrome (M75.1-)*
rupture where an abnormal force is applied to normal tissue - see injury of tendon by body region
M66.0 Rupture of popliteal cyst
M66.1 Rupture of synovium
Rupture of synovial cyst
EXCLUDES2 *rupture of popliteal cyst (M66.0)*
M66.10 Rupture of synovium, unspecified joint
M66.11 Rupture of synovium, shoulder
M66.111 Rupture of synovium, right shoulder
M66.112 Rupture of synovium, left shoulder
M66.119 Rupture of synovium, unspecified shoulder
M66.12 Rupture of synovium, elbow
M66.121 Rupture of synovium, right elbow
M66.122 Rupture of synovium, left elbow
M66.129 Rupture of synovium, unspecified elbow
M66.13 Rupture of synovium, wrist
M66.131 Rupture of synovium, right wrist
M66.132 Rupture of synovium, left wrist
M66.139 Rupture of synovium, unspecified wrist
M66.14 Rupture of synovium, hand and fingers
M66.141 Rupture of synovium, right hand
M66.142 Rupture of synovium, left hand
M66.143 Rupture of synovium, unspecified hand
M66.144 Rupture of synovium, right finger(s)
M66.145 Rupture of synovium, left finger(s)
M66.146 Rupture of synovium, unspecified finger(s)
M66.15 Rupture of synovium, hip
M66.151 Rupture of synovium, right hip
M66.152 Rupture of synovium, left hip
M66.159 Rupture of synovium, unspecified hip
M66.17 Rupture of synovium, ankle, foot and toes
M66.171 Rupture of synovium, right ankle
M66.172 Rupture of synovium, left ankle
M66.173 Rupture of synovium, unspecified ankle
M66.174 Rupture of synovium, right foot
M66.175 Rupture of synovium, left foot
M66.176 Rupture of synovium, unspecified foot
M66.177 Rupture of synovium, right toe(s)
M66.178 Rupture of synovium, left toe(s)
M66.179 Rupture of synovium, unspecified toe(s)
M66.18 Rupture of synovium, other site
M66.2 Spontaneous rupture of extensor tendons
M66.20 Spontaneous rupture of extensor tendons, unspecified site
M66.21 Spontaneous rupture of extensor tendons, shoulder

PDx Unacceptable principal diagnosis symbol per Medicare code edits; POA Code exempt from diagnosis present on admission requirement
Q Questionable admission; CC Complication or comorbidity; CC/MCC Exc CC/MCC exclusion; MCC Major complication or comorbidity
PDx CC Principal diagnosis as its own CC; PDx MCC Principal diagnosis as its own MCC; Z1 Z code as first-listed diagnosis

 When symbols appear on a code that requires a 7th character extension, refer to Appendix D to identify applicable 7th character codes.

M66.211 Spontaneous rupture of extensor tendons, right shoulder
M66.212 Spontaneous rupture of extensor tendons, left shoulder
M66.219 Spontaneous rupture of extensor tendons, unspecified shoulder
M66.22 Spontaneous rupture of extensor tendons, upper arm
M66.221 Spontaneous rupture of extensor tendons, right upper arm
M66.222 Spontaneous rupture of extensor tendons, left upper arm
M66.229 Spontaneous rupture of extensor tendons, unspecified upper arm
M66.23 Spontaneous rupture of extensor tendons, forearm
M66.231 Spontaneous rupture of extensor tendons, right forearm
M66.232 Spontaneous rupture of extensor tendons, left forearm
M66.239 Spontaneous rupture of extensor tendons, unspecified forearm
M66.24 Spontaneous rupture of extensor tendons, hand
M66.241 Spontaneous rupture of extensor tendons, right hand
M66.242 Spontaneous rupture of extensor tendons, left hand
M66.249 Spontaneous rupture of extensor tendons, unspecified hand
M66.25 Spontaneous rupture of extensor tendons, thigh
M66.251 Spontaneous rupture of extensor tendons, right thigh
M66.252 Spontaneous rupture of extensor tendons, left thigh
M66.259 Spontaneous rupture of extensor tendons, unspecified thigh
M66.26 Spontaneous rupture of extensor tendons, lower leg
M66.261 Spontaneous rupture of extensor tendons, right lower leg
M66.262 Spontaneous rupture of extensor tendons, left lower leg
M66.269 Spontaneous rupture of extensor tendons, unspecified lower leg
M66.27 Spontaneous rupture of extensor tendons, ankle and foot
M66.271 Spontaneous rupture of extensor tendons, right ankle and foot
M66.272 Spontaneous rupture of extensor tendons, left ankle and foot
M66.279 Spontaneous rupture of extensor tendons, unspecified ankle and foot
M66.28 Spontaneous rupture of extensor tendons, other site
M66.29 Spontaneous rupture of extensor tendons, multiple sites
M66.3 Spontaneous rupture of flexor tendons
M66.30 Spontaneous rupture of flexor tendons, unspecified site
M66.31 Spontaneous rupture of flexor tendons, shoulder
M66.311 Spontaneous rupture of flexor tendons, right shoulder
M66.312 Spontaneous rupture of flexor tendons, left shoulder
M66.319 Spontaneous rupture of flexor tendons, unspecified shoulder
M66.32 Spontaneous rupture of flexor tendons, upper arm
M66.321 Spontaneous rupture of flexor tendons, right upper arm
M66.322 Spontaneous rupture of flexor tendons, left upper arm
M66.329 Spontaneous rupture of flexor tendons, unspecified upper arm
M66.33 Spontaneous rupture of flexor tendons, forearm
M66.331 Spontaneous rupture of flexor tendons, right forearm
M66.332 Spontaneous rupture of flexor tendons, left forearm
M66.339 Spontaneous rupture of flexor tendons, unspecified forearm
M66.34 Spontaneous rupture of flexor tendons, hand
M66.341 Spontaneous rupture of flexor tendons, right hand
M66.342 Spontaneous rupture of flexor tendons, left hand
M66.349 Spontaneous rupture of flexor tendons, unspecified hand
M66.35 Spontaneous rupture of flexor tendons, thigh
M66.351 Spontaneous rupture of flexor tendons, right thigh
M66.352 Spontaneous rupture of flexor tendons, left thigh
M66.359 Spontaneous rupture of flexor tendons, unspecified thigh
M66.36 Spontaneous rupture of flexor tendons, lower leg
M66.361 Spontaneous rupture of flexor tendons, right lower leg
M66.362 Spontaneous rupture of flexor tendons, left lower leg
M66.369 Spontaneous rupture of flexor tendons, unspecified lower leg
M66.37 Spontaneous rupture of flexor tendons, ankle and foot
M66.371 Spontaneous rupture of flexor tendons, right ankle and foot
M66.372 Spontaneous rupture of flexor tendons, left ankle and foot
M66.379 Spontaneous rupture of flexor tendons, unspecified ankle and foot
M66.38 Spontaneous rupture of flexor tendons, other site
M66.39 Spontaneous rupture of flexor tendons, multiple sites
M66.8 Spontaneous rupture of other tendons
M66.80 Spontaneous rupture of other tendons, unspecified site
M66.81 Spontaneous rupture of other tendons, shoulder
M66.811 Spontaneous rupture of other tendons, right shoulder
M66.812 Spontaneous rupture of other tendons, left shoulder
M66.819 Spontaneous rupture of other tendons, unspecified shoulder
M66.82 Spontaneous rupture of other tendons, upper arm
M66.821 Spontaneous rupture of other tendons, right upper arm
M66.822 Spontaneous rupture of other tendons, left upper arm
M66.829 Spontaneous rupture of other tendons, unspecified upper arm
M66.83 Spontaneous rupture of other tendons, forearm
M66.831 Spontaneous rupture of other tendons, right forearm
M66.832 Spontaneous rupture of other tendons, left forearm
M66.839 Spontaneous rupture of other tendons, unspecified forearm
M66.84 Spontaneous rupture of other tendons, hand
M66.841 Spontaneous rupture of other tendons, right hand
M66.842 Spontaneous rupture of other tendons, left hand
M66.849 Spontaneous rupture of other tendons, unspecified hand
M66.85 Spontaneous rupture of other tendons, thigh
M66.851 Spontaneous rupture of other tendons, right thigh
M66.852 Spontaneous rupture of other tendons, left thigh
M66.859 Spontaneous rupture of other tendons, unspecified thigh
M66.86 Spontaneous rupture of other tendons, lower leg
M66.861 Spontaneous rupture of other tendons, right lower leg

Unspecified Code Other Specified Code Manifestation Code N Newborn P Pediatric M Maternity A Adult ♂ Male ♀ Female
● New Code ▲ Revised Code Title ►◄ Revised Text NOTES INCLUDES EXCLUDES1 Not coded here EXCLUDES2 Not included here
4th character required 5th character required 6th character required 7th character required
Extension 'X' Alert HAC Hospital-acquired condition (HAC) alert AHA AHA Coding Clinic©

M66.862 Spontaneous rupture of other tendons, left lower leg
M66.869 Spontaneous rupture of other tendons, unspecified lower leg
M66.87 Spontaneous rupture of other tendons, ankle and foot
M66.871 Spontaneous rupture of other tendons, right ankle and foot
M66.872 Spontaneous rupture of other tendons, left ankle and foot
M66.879 Spontaneous rupture of other tendons, unspecified ankle and foot
M66.88 Spontaneous rupture of other tendons, other
M66.89 Spontaneous rupture of other tendons, multiple sites
M66.9 Spontaneous rupture of unspecified tendon
Rupture at musculotendinous junction, nontraumatic
M67 Other disorders of synovium and tendon
EXCLUDES1 *palmar fascial fibromatosis [Dupuytren] (M72.0)*
tendinitis NOS (M77.9-)
xanthomatosis localized to tendons (E78.2)
M67.0 Short Achilles tendon (acquired)
M67.00 Short Achilles tendon (acquired), unspecified ankle
M67.01 Short Achilles tendon (acquired), right ankle
M67.02 Short Achilles tendon (acquired), left ankle
M67.2 Synovial hypertrophy, not elsewhere classified
EXCLUDES1 *villonodular synovitis (pigmented) (M12.2-)*
M67.20 Synovial hypertrophy, not elsewhere classified, unspecified site
M67.21 Synovial hypertrophy, not elsewhere classified, shoulder
M67.211 Synovial hypertrophy, not elsewhere classified, right shoulder
M67.212 Synovial hypertrophy, not elsewhere classified, left shoulder
M67.219 Synovial hypertrophy, not elsewhere classified, unspecified shoulder
M67.22 Synovial hypertrophy, not elsewhere classified, upper arm
M67.221 Synovial hypertrophy, not elsewhere classified, right upper arm
M67.222 Synovial hypertrophy, not elsewhere classified, left upper arm
M67.229 Synovial hypertrophy, not elsewhere classified, unspecified upper arm
M67.23 Synovial hypertrophy, not elsewhere classified, forearm
M67.231 Synovial hypertrophy, not elsewhere classified, right forearm
M67.232 Synovial hypertrophy, not elsewhere classified, left forearm
M67.239 Synovial hypertrophy, not elsewhere classified, unspecified forearm
M67.24 Synovial hypertrophy, not elsewhere classified, hand
M67.241 Synovial hypertrophy, not elsewhere classified, right hand
M67.242 Synovial hypertrophy, not elsewhere classified, left hand
M67.249 Synovial hypertrophy, not elsewhere classified, unspecified hand
M67.25 Synovial hypertrophy, not elsewhere classified, thigh
M67.251 Synovial hypertrophy, not elsewhere classified, right thigh
M67.252 Synovial hypertrophy, not elsewhere classified, left thigh
M67.259 Synovial hypertrophy, not elsewhere classified, unspecified thigh
M67.26 Synovial hypertrophy, not elsewhere classified, lower leg
M67.261 Synovial hypertrophy, not elsewhere classified, right lower leg
M67.262 Synovial hypertrophy, not elsewhere classified, left lower leg
M67.269 Synovial hypertrophy, not elsewhere classified, unspecified lower leg
M67.27 Synovial hypertrophy, not elsewhere classified, ankle and foot
M67.271 Synovial hypertrophy, not elsewhere classified, right ankle and foot
M67.272 Synovial hypertrophy, not elsewhere classified, left ankle and foot
M67.279 Synovial hypertrophy, not elsewhere classified, unspecified ankle and foot
M67.28 Synovial hypertrophy, not elsewhere classified, other site
M67.29 Synovial hypertrophy, not elsewhere classified, multiple sites
M67.3 Transient synovitis
Toxic synovitis
EXCLUDES1 *palindromic rheumatism (M12.3-)*
M67.30 Transient synovitis, unspecified site
M67.31 Transient synovitis, shoulder
M67.311 Transient synovitis, right shoulder
M67.312 Transient synovitis, left shoulder
M67.319 Transient synovitis, unspecified shoulder
M67.32 Transient synovitis, elbow
M67.321 Transient synovitis, right elbow
M67.322 Transient synovitis, left elbow
M67.329 Transient synovitis, unspecified elbow
M67.33 Transient synovitis, wrist
M67.331 Transient synovitis, right wrist
M67.332 Transient synovitis, left wrist
M67.339 Transient synovitis, unspecified wrist
M67.34 Transient synovitis, hand
M67.341 Transient synovitis, right hand
M67.342 Transient synovitis, left hand
M67.349 Transient synovitis, unspecified hand
M67.35 Transient synovitis, hip
M67.351 Transient synovitis, right hip
M67.352 Transient synovitis, left hip
M67.359 Transient synovitis, unspecified hip
M67.36 Transient synovitis, knee
M67.361 Transient synovitis, right knee
M67.362 Transient synovitis, left knee
M67.369 Transient synovitis, unspecified knee
M67.37 Transient synovitis, ankle and foot
M67.371 Transient synovitis, right ankle and foot
M67.372 Transient synovitis, left ankle and foot
M67.379 Transient synovitis, unspecified ankle and foot
M67.38 Transient synovitis, other site
M67.39 Transient synovitis, multiple sites
M67.4 Ganglion
Ganglion of joint or tendon (sheath)
EXCLUDES1 *ganglion in yaws (A66.6)*
EXCLUDES2 *cyst of bursa (M71.2-M71.3)*
cyst of synovium (M71.2-M71.3)
M67.40 Ganglion, unspecified site
M67.41 Ganglion, shoulder
M67.411 Ganglion, right shoulder
M67.412 Ganglion, left shoulder
M67.419 Ganglion, unspecified shoulder
M67.42 Ganglion, elbow
M67.421 Ganglion, right elbow
M67.422 Ganglion, left elbow
M67.429 Ganglion, unspecified elbow
M67.43 Ganglion, wrist
M67.431 Ganglion, right wrist
M67.432 Ganglion, left wrist
M67.439 Ganglion, unspecified wrist
M67.44 Ganglion, hand
M67.441 Ganglion, right hand
M67.442 Ganglion, left hand
M67.449 Ganglion, unspecified hand
M67.45 Ganglion, hip
M67.451 Ganglion, right hip
M67.452 Ganglion, left hip
M67.459 Ganglion, unspecified hip

Unacceptable principal diagnosis symbol per Medicare code edits · Code exempt from diagnosis present on admission requirement
Questionable admission · Complication or comorbidity · CC/MCC exclusion · Major complication or comorbidity
Principal diagnosis as its own CC · Principal diagnosis as its own MCC · Z code as first-listed diagnosis

M67.46 Ganglion, knee
M67.461 Ganglion, right knee
M67.462 Ganglion, left knee
M67.469 Ganglion, unspecified knee
M67.47 Ganglion, ankle and foot
M67.471 Ganglion, right ankle and foot
M67.472 Ganglion, left ankle and foot
M67.479 Ganglion, unspecified ankle and foot
M67.48 Ganglion, other site
M67.49 Ganglion, multiple sites
M67.5 Plica syndrome
Plica knee
M67.50 Plica syndrome, unspecified knee
M67.51 Plica syndrome, right knee
M67.52 Plica syndrome, left knee
M67.8 Other specified disorders of synovium and tendon
M67.80 Other specified disorders of synovium and tendon, unspecified site
M67.81 Other specified disorders of synovium and tendon, shoulder
M67.811 Other specified disorders of synovium, right shoulder
M67.812 Other specified disorders of synovium, left shoulder
M67.813 Other specified disorders of tendon, right shoulder
M67.814 Other specified disorders of tendon, left shoulder
M67.819 Other specified disorders of synovium and tendon, unspecified shoulder
M67.82 Other specified disorders of synovium and tendon, elbow
M67.821 Other specified disorders of synovium, right elbow
M67.822 Other specified disorders of synovium, left elbow
M67.823 Other specified disorders of tendon, right elbow
M67.824 Other specified disorders of tendon, left elbow
M67.829 Other specified disorders of synovium and tendon, unspecified elbow
M67.83 Other specified disorders of synovium and tendon, wrist
M67.831 Other specified disorders of synovium, right wrist
M67.832 Other specified disorders of synovium, left wrist
M67.833 Other specified disorders of tendon, right wrist
M67.834 Other specified disorders of tendon, left wrist
M67.839 Other specified disorders of synovium and tendon, unspecified forearm
M67.84 Other specified disorders of synovium and tendon, hand
M67.841 Other specified disorders of synovium, right hand
M67.842 Other specified disorders of synovium, left hand
M67.843 Other specified disorders of tendon, right hand
M67.844 Other specified disorders of tendon, left hand
M67.849 Other specified disorders of synovium and tendon, unspecified hand
M67.85 Other specified disorders of synovium and tendon, hip
M67.851 Other specified disorders of synovium, right hip
M67.852 Other specified disorders of synovium, left hip
M67.853 Other specified disorders of tendon, right hip
M67.854 Other specified disorders of tendon, left hip
M67.859 Other specified disorders of synovium and tendon, unspecified hip
M67.86 Other specified disorders of synovium and tendon, knee
M67.861 Other specified disorders of synovium, right knee
M67.862 Other specified disorders of synovium, left knee
M67.863 Other specified disorders of tendon, right knee
M67.864 Other specified disorders of tendon, left knee
M67.869 Other specified disorders of synovium and tendon, unspecified knee
M67.87 Other specified disorders of synovium and tendon, ankle and foot
M67.871 Other specified disorders of synovium, right ankle and foot
M67.872 Other specified disorders of synovium, left ankle and foot
M67.873 Other specified disorders of tendon, right ankle and foot
M67.874 Other specified disorders of tendon, left ankle and foot
M67.879 Other specified disorders of synovium and tendon, unspecified ankle and foot
M67.88 Other specified disorders of synovium and tendon, other site
M67.89 Other specified disorders of synovium and tendon, multiple sites
M67.9 Unspecified disorder of synovium and tendon
M67.90 Unspecified disorder of synovium and tendon, unspecified site
M67.91 Unspecified disorder of synovium and tendon, shoulder
M67.911 Unspecified disorder of synovium and tendon, right shoulder
M67.912 Unspecified disorder of synovium and tendon, left shoulder
M67.919 Unspecified disorder of synovium and tendon, unspecified shoulder
M67.92 Unspecified disorder of synovium and tendon, upper arm
M67.921 Unspecified disorder of synovium and tendon, right upper arm
M67.922 Unspecified disorder of synovium and tendon, left upper arm
M67.929 Unspecified disorder of synovium and tendon, unspecified upper arm
M67.93 Unspecified disorder of synovium and tendon, forearm
M67.931 Unspecified disorder of synovium and tendon, right forearm
M67.932 Unspecified disorder of synovium and tendon, left forearm
M67.939 Unspecified disorder of synovium and tendon, unspecified forearm
M67.94 Unspecified disorder of synovium and tendon, hand
M67.941 Unspecified disorder of synovium and tendon, right hand
M67.942 Unspecified disorder of synovium and tendon, left hand
M67.949 Unspecified disorder of synovium and tendon, unspecified hand
M67.95 Unspecified disorder of synovium and tendon, thigh
M67.951 Unspecified disorder of synovium and tendon, right thigh
M67.952 Unspecified disorder of synovium and tendon, left thigh
M67.959 Unspecified disorder of synovium and tendon, unspecified thigh
M67.96 Unspecified disorder of synovium and tendon, lower leg

Unspecified Code | Other Specified Code | Manifestation Code | N Newborn | P Pediatric | M Maternity | A Adult | ♂ Male | ♀ Female
● New Code | ▲ Revised Code Title | ►◄ Revised Text | NOTES | INCLUDES | EXCLUDES1 Not coded here | EXCLUDES2 Not included here
4th character required | 5th character required | 6th character required | 7th character required
Extension 'X' Alert | HAC Hospital-acquired condition (HAC) alert | AHA AHA Coding Clinic©

M67.961 Unspecified disorder of synovium and tendon, right lower leg
M67.962 Unspecified disorder of synovium and tendon, left lower leg
M67.969 Unspecified disorder of synovium and tendon, unspecified lower leg
M67.97 Unspecified disorder of synovium and tendon, ankle and foot
M67.971 Unspecified disorder of synovium and tendon, right ankle and foot
M67.972 Unspecified disorder of synovium and tendon, left ankle and foot
M67.979 Unspecified disorder of synovium and tendon, unspecified ankle and foot
M67.98 Unspecified disorder of synovium and tendon, other site
M67.99 Unspecified disorder of synovium and tendon, multiple sites

Other soft tissue disorders (M70-M79)

M70 Soft tissue disorders related to use, overuse and pressure
INCLUDES *soft tissue disorders of occupational origin*
Use additional external cause code to identify activity causing disorder (Y93.-)
EXCLUDES1 *bursitis NOS (M71.9-)*
EXCLUDES2 *bursitis of shoulder (M75.5)*
enthesopathies (M76-M77)
pressure ulcer (pressure area) (L89.-)

M70.0 Crepitant synovitis (acute) (chronic) of hand and wrist
M70.03 Crepitant synovitis (acute) (chronic), wrist
M70.031 Crepitant synovitis (acute) (chronic), right wrist
M70.032 Crepitant synovitis (acute) (chronic), left wrist
M70.039 Crepitant synovitis (acute) (chronic), unspecified wrist
M70.04 Crepitant synovitis (acute) (chronic), hand
M70.041 Crepitant synovitis (acute) (chronic), right hand
M70.042 Crepitant synovitis (acute) (chronic), left hand
M70.049 Crepitant synovitis (acute) (chronic), unspecified hand
M70.1 Bursitis of hand
M70.10 Bursitis, unspecified hand
M70.11 Bursitis, right hand
M70.12 Bursitis, left hand
M70.2 Olecranon bursitis
M70.20 Olecranon bursitis, unspecified elbow
M70.21 Olecranon bursitis, right elbow
M70.22 Olecranon bursitis, left elbow
M70.3 Other bursitis of elbow
M70.30 Other bursitis of elbow, unspecified elbow
M70.31 Other bursitis of elbow, right elbow
M70.32 Other bursitis of elbow, left elbow
M70.4 Prepatellar bursitis
M70.40 Prepatellar bursitis, unspecified knee
M70.41 Prepatellar bursitis, right knee
M70.42 Prepatellar bursitis, left knee
M70.5 Other bursitis of knee
M70.50 Other bursitis of knee, unspecified knee
M70.51 Other bursitis of knee, right knee
M70.52 Other bursitis of knee, left knee
M70.6 Trochanteric bursitis
Trochanteric tendinitis
M70.60 Trochanteric bursitis, unspecified hip
M70.61 Trochanteric bursitis, right hip
M70.62 Trochanteric bursitis, left hip
M70.7 Other bursitis of hip
Ischial bursitis
M70.70 Other bursitis of hip, unspecified hip
M70.71 Other bursitis of hip, right hip
M70.72 Other bursitis of hip, left hip

M70.8 Other soft tissue disorders related to use, overuse and pressure
M70.80 Other soft tissue disorders related to use, overuse and pressure of unspecified site
M70.81 Other soft tissue disorders related to use, overuse and pressure of shoulder
M70.811 Other soft tissue disorders related to use, overuse and pressure, right shoulder
M70.812 Other soft tissue disorders related to use, overuse and pressure, left shoulder
M70.819 Other soft tissue disorders related to use, overuse and pressure, unspecified shoulder
M70.82 Other soft tissue disorders related to use, overuse and pressure of upper arm
M70.821 Other soft tissue disorders related to use, overuse and pressure, right upper arm
M70.822 Other soft tissue disorders related to use, overuse and pressure, left upper arm
M70.829 Other soft tissue disorders related to use, overuse and pressure, unspecified upper arms
M70.83 Other soft tissue disorders related to use, overuse and pressure of forearm
M70.831 Other soft tissue disorders related to use, overuse and pressure, right forearm
M70.832 Other soft tissue disorders related to use, overuse and pressure, left forearm
M70.839 Other soft tissue disorders related to use, overuse and pressure, unspecified forearm
M70.84 Other soft tissue disorders related to use, overuse and pressure of hand
M70.841 Other soft tissue disorders related to use, overuse and pressure, right hand
M70.842 Other soft tissue disorders related to use, overuse and pressure, left hand
M70.849 Other soft tissue disorders related to use, overuse and pressure, unspecified hand
M70.85 Other soft tissue disorders related to use, overuse and pressure of thigh
M70.851 Other soft tissue disorders related to use, overuse and pressure, right thigh
M70.852 Other soft tissue disorders related to use, overuse and pressure, left thigh
M70.859 Other soft tissue disorders related to use, overuse and pressure, unspecified thigh
M70.86 Other soft tissue disorders related to use, overuse and pressure lower leg
M70.861 Other soft tissue disorders related to use, overuse and pressure, right lower leg
M70.862 Other soft tissue disorders related to use, overuse and pressure, left lower leg
M70.869 Other soft tissue disorders related to use, overuse and pressure, unspecified leg
M70.87 Other soft tissue disorders related to use, overuse and pressure of ankle and foot
M70.871 Other soft tissue disorders related to use, overuse and pressure, right ankle and foot
M70.872 Other soft tissue disorders related to use, overuse and pressure, left ankle and foot
M70.879 Other soft tissue disorders related to use, overuse and pressure, unspecified ankle and foot
M70.88 Other soft tissue disorders related to use, overuse and pressure other site
M70.89 Other soft tissue disorders related to use, overuse and pressure multiple sites
M70.9 Unspecified soft tissue disorder related to use, overuse and pressure
M70.90 Unspecified soft tissue disorder related to use, overuse and pressure of unspecified site
M70.91 Unspecified soft tissue disorder related to use, overuse and pressure of shoulder
M70.911 Unspecified soft tissue disorder related to use, overuse and pressure, right shoulder

Unacceptable principal diagnosis symbol per Medicare code edits · Code exempt from diagnosis present on admission requirement
Questionable admission · Complication or comorbidity · CC/MCC exclusion · Major complication or comorbidity
Principal diagnosis as its own CC · Principal diagnosis as its own MCC · Z code as first-listed diagnosis

M70.912 Unspecified soft tissue disorder related to use, overuse and pressure, left shoulder
M70.919 Unspecified soft tissue disorder related to use, overuse and pressure, unspecified shoulder
M70.92 Unspecified soft tissue disorder related to use, overuse and pressure of upper arm
M70.921 Unspecified soft tissue disorder related to use, overuse and pressure, right upper arm
M70.922 Unspecified soft tissue disorder related to use, overuse and pressure, left upper arm
M70.929 Unspecified soft tissue disorder related to use, overuse and pressure, unspecified upper arm
M70.93 Unspecified soft tissue disorder related to use, overuse and pressure of forearm
M70.931 Unspecified soft tissue disorder related to use, overuse and pressure, right forearm
M70.932 Unspecified soft tissue disorder related to use, overuse and pressure, left forearm
M70.939 Unspecified soft tissue disorder related to use, overuse and pressure, unspecified forearm
M70.94 Unspecified soft tissue disorder related to use, overuse and pressure of hand
M70.941 Unspecified soft tissue disorder related to use, overuse and pressure, right hand
M70.942 Unspecified soft tissue disorder related to use, overuse and pressure, left hand
M70.949 Unspecified soft tissue disorder related to use, overuse and pressure, unspecified hand
M70.95 Unspecified soft tissue disorder related to use, overuse and pressure of thigh
M70.951 Unspecified soft tissue disorder related to use, overuse and pressure, right thigh
M70.952 Unspecified soft tissue disorder related to use, overuse and pressure, left thigh
M70.959 Unspecified soft tissue disorder related to use, overuse and pressure, unspecified thigh
M70.96 Unspecified soft tissue disorder related to use, overuse and pressure lower leg
M70.961 Unspecified soft tissue disorder related to use, overuse and pressure, right lower leg
M70.962 Unspecified soft tissue disorder related to use, overuse and pressure, left lower leg
M70.969 Unspecified soft tissue disorder related to use, overuse and pressure, unspecified lower leg
M70.97 Unspecified soft tissue disorder related to use, overuse and pressure of ankle and foot
M70.971 Unspecified soft tissue disorder related to use, overuse and pressure, right ankle and foot
M70.972 Unspecified soft tissue disorder related to use, overuse and pressure, left ankle and foot
M70.979 Unspecified soft tissue disorder related to use, overuse and pressure, unspecified ankle and foot
M70.98 Unspecified soft tissue disorder related to use, overuse and pressure other
M70.99 Unspecified soft tissue disorder related to use, overuse and pressure multiple sites

M71 Other bursopathies
EXCLUDES1 *bunion (M20.1)*
bursitis related to use, overuse or pressure (M70.-)
enthesopathies (M76-M77)

M71.0 Abscess of bursa
Use additional code (B95.-, B96.-) to identify causative organism
M71.00 Abscess of bursa, unspecified site
M71.01 Abscess of bursa, shoulder
M71.011 Abscess of bursa, right shoulder
M71.012 Abscess of bursa, left shoulder
M71.019 Abscess of bursa, unspecified shoulder
M71.02 Abscess of bursa, elbow
M71.021 Abscess of bursa, right elbow
M71.022 Abscess of bursa, left elbow
M71.029 Abscess of bursa, unspecified elbow
M71.03 Abscess of bursa, wrist
M71.031 Abscess of bursa, right wrist
M71.032 Abscess of bursa, left wrist
M71.039 Abscess of bursa, unspecified wrist
M71.04 Abscess of bursa, hand
M71.041 Abscess of bursa, right hand
M71.042 Abscess of bursa, left hand
M71.049 Abscess of bursa, unspecified hand
M71.05 Abscess of bursa, hip
M71.051 Abscess of bursa, right hip
M71.052 Abscess of bursa, left hip
M71.059 Abscess of bursa, unspecified hip
M71.06 Abscess of bursa, knee
M71.061 Abscess of bursa, right knee
M71.062 Abscess of bursa, left knee
M71.069 Abscess of bursa, unspecified knee
M71.07 Abscess of bursa, ankle and foot
M71.071 Abscess of bursa, right ankle and foot
M71.072 Abscess of bursa, left ankle and foot
M71.079 Abscess of bursa, unspecified ankle and foot
M71.08 Abscess of bursa, other site
M71.09 Abscess of bursa, multiple sites

M71.1 Other infective bursitis
Use additional code (B95.-, B96.-) to identify causative organism
M71.10 Other infective bursitis, unspecified site
M71.11 Other infective bursitis, shoulder
M71.111 Other infective bursitis, right shoulder
M71.112 Other infective bursitis, left shoulder
M71.119 Other infective bursitis, unspecified shoulder
M71.12 Other infective bursitis, elbow
M71.121 Other infective bursitis, right elbow
M71.122 Other infective bursitis, left elbow
M71.129 Other infective bursitis, unspecified elbow
M71.13 Other infective bursitis, wrist
M71.131 Other infective bursitis, right wrist
M71.132 Other infective bursitis, left wrist
M71.139 Other infective bursitis, unspecified wrist
M71.14 Other infective bursitis, hand
M71.141 Other infective bursitis, right hand
M71.142 Other infective bursitis, left hand
M71.149 Other infective bursitis, unspecified hand
M71.15 Other infective bursitis, hip
M71.151 Other infective bursitis, right hip
M71.152 Other infective bursitis, left hip
M71.159 Other infective bursitis, unspecified hip
M71.16 Other infective bursitis, knee
M71.161 Other infective bursitis, right knee
M71.162 Other infective bursitis, left knee
M71.169 Other infective bursitis, unspecified knee
M71.17 Other infective bursitis, ankle and foot
M71.171 Other infective bursitis, right ankle and foot
M71.172 Other infective bursitis, left ankle and foot
M71.179 Other infective bursitis, unspecified ankle and foot
M71.18 Other infective bursitis, other site
M71.19 Other infective bursitis, multiple sites

M71.2 Synovial cyst of popliteal space [Baker]
EXCLUDES1 *synovial cyst of popliteal space with rupture (M66.0)*
M71.20 Synovial cyst of popliteal space [Baker], unspecified knee
M71.21 Synovial cyst of popliteal space [Baker], right knee
M71.22 Synovial cyst of popliteal space [Baker], left knee

M71.3 Other bursal cyst

Unspecified Code Other Specified Code Manifestation Code N Newborn P Pediatric M Maternity A Adult ♂ Male ♀ Female
● New Code ▲ Revised Code Title ►◄ Revised Text NOTES INCLUDES EXCLUDES1 Not coded here EXCLUDES2 Not included here
4th character required 5th character required 6th character required 7th character required
Extension 'X' Alert HAC Hospital-acquired condition (HAC) alert AHA AHA Coding Clinic©

Synovial cyst NOS
EXCLUDES1 *synovial cyst with rupture (M66.1-)*
M71.30 Other bursal cyst, unspecified site
M71.31 Other bursal cyst, shoulder
M71.311 Other bursal cyst, right shoulder
M71.312 Other bursal cyst, left shoulder
M71.319 Other bursal cyst, unspecified shoulder
M71.32 Other bursal cyst, elbow
M71.321 Other bursal cyst, right elbow
M71.322 Other bursal cyst, left elbow
M71.329 Other bursal cyst, unspecified elbow
M71.33 Other bursal cyst, wrist
M71.331 Other bursal cyst, right wrist
M71.332 Other bursal cyst, left wrist
M71.339 Other bursal cyst, unspecified wrist
M71.34 Other bursal cyst, hand
M71.341 Other bursal cyst, right hand
M71.342 Other bursal cyst, left hand
M71.349 Other bursal cyst, unspecified hand
M71.35 Other bursal cyst, hip
M71.351 Other bursal cyst, right hip
M71.352 Other bursal cyst, left hip
M71.359 Other bursal cyst, unspecified hip
M71.37 Other bursal cyst, ankle and foot
M71.371 Other bursal cyst, right ankle and foot
M71.372 Other bursal cyst, left ankle and foot
M71.379 Other bursal cyst, unspecified ankle and foot
M71.38 Other bursal cyst, other site
M71.39 Other bursal cyst, multiple sites

M71.4 Calcium deposit in bursa
EXCLUDES2 *calcium deposit in bursa of shoulder (M75.3)*
M71.40 Calcium deposit in bursa, unspecified site
M71.42 Calcium deposit in bursa, elbow
M71.421 Calcium deposit in bursa, right elbow
M71.422 Calcium deposit in bursa, left elbow
M71.429 Calcium deposit in bursa, unspecified elbow
M71.43 Calcium deposit in bursa, wrist
M71.431 Calcium deposit in bursa, right wrist
M71.432 Calcium deposit in bursa, left wrist
M71.439 Calcium deposit in bursa, unspecified wrist
M71.44 Calcium deposit in bursa, hand
M71.441 Calcium deposit in bursa, right hand
M71.442 Calcium deposit in bursa, left hand
M71.449 Calcium deposit in bursa, unspecified hand
M71.45 Calcium deposit in bursa, hip
M71.451 Calcium deposit in bursa, right hip
M71.452 Calcium deposit in bursa, left hip
M71.459 Calcium deposit in bursa, unspecified hip
M71.46 Calcium deposit in bursa, knee
M71.461 Calcium deposit in bursa, right knee
M71.462 Calcium deposit in bursa, left knee
M71.469 Calcium deposit in bursa, unspecified knee
M71.47 Calcium deposit in bursa, ankle and foot
M71.471 Calcium deposit in bursa, right ankle and foot
M71.472 Calcium deposit in bursa, left ankle and foot
M71.479 Calcium deposit in bursa, unspecified ankle and foot
M71.48 Calcium deposit in bursa, other site
M71.49 Calcium deposit in bursa, multiple sites

M71.5 Other bursitis, not elsewhere classified
EXCLUDES1 *bursitis NOS (M71.9-)*
EXCLUDES2 *bursitis of shoulder (M75.5)*
bursitis of tibial collateral [Pellegrini-Stieda] ►(M76.4-)◄
M71.50 Other bursitis, not elsewhere classified, unspecified site
M71.52 Other bursitis, not elsewhere classified, elbow
M71.521 Other bursitis, not elsewhere classified, right elbow
M71.522 Other bursitis, not elsewhere classified, left elbow
M71.529 Other bursitis, not elsewhere classified, unspecified elbow
M71.53 Other bursitis, not elsewhere classified, wrist
M71.531 Other bursitis, not elsewhere classified, right wrist
M71.532 Other bursitis, not elsewhere classified, left wrist
M71.539 Other bursitis, not elsewhere classified, unspecified wrist
M71.54 Other bursitis, not elsewhere classified, hand
M71.541 Other bursitis, not elsewhere classified, right hand
M71.542 Other bursitis, not elsewhere classified, left hand
M71.549 Other bursitis, not elsewhere classified, unspecified hand
M71.55 Other bursitis, not elsewhere classified, hip
M71.551 Other bursitis, not elsewhere classified, right hip
M71.552 Other bursitis, not elsewhere classified, left hip
M71.559 Other bursitis, not elsewhere classified, unspecified hip
M71.56 Other bursitis, not elsewhere classified, knee
M71.561 Other bursitis, not elsewhere classified, right knee
M71.562 Other bursitis, not elsewhere classified, left knee
M71.569 Other bursitis, not elsewhere classified, unspecified knee
M71.57 Other bursitis, not elsewhere classified, ankle and foot
M71.571 Other bursitis, not elsewhere classified, right ankle and foot
M71.572 Other bursitis, not elsewhere classified, left ankle and foot
M71.579 Other bursitis, not elsewhere classified, unspecified ankle and foot
M71.58 Other bursitis, not elsewhere classified, other site

M71.8 Other specified bursopathies
M71.80 Other specified bursopathies, unspecified site
M71.81 Other specified bursopathies, shoulder
M71.811 Other specified bursopathies, right shoulder
M71.812 Other specified bursopathies, left shoulder
M71.819 Other specified bursopathies, unspecified shoulder
M71.82 Other specified bursopathies, elbow
M71.821 Other specified bursopathies, right elbow
M71.822 Other specified bursopathies, left elbow
M71.829 Other specified bursopathies, unspecified elbow
M71.83 Other specified bursopathies, wrist
M71.831 Other specified bursopathies, right wrist
M71.832 Other specified bursopathies, left wrist
M71.839 Other specified bursopathies, unspecified wrist
M71.84 Other specified bursopathies, hand
M71.841 Other specified bursopathies, right hand
M71.842 Other specified bursopathies, left hand
M71.849 Other specified bursopathies, unspecified hand

Unacceptable principal diagnosis symbol per Medicare code edits | Code exempt from diagnosis present on admission requirement
Questionable admission | Complication or comorbidity | CC/MCC exclusion | Major complication or comorbidity
Principal diagnosis as its own CC | Principal diagnosis as its own MCC | Z code as first-listed diagnosis

M71.85 Other specified bursopathies, hip
M71.851 Other specified bursopathies, right hip
M71.852 Other specified bursopathies, left hip
M71.859 Other specified bursopathies, unspecified hip
M71.86 Other specified bursopathies, knee
M71.861 Other specified bursopathies, right knee
M71.862 Other specified bursopathies, left knee
M71.869 Other specified bursopathies, unspecified knee
M71.87 Other specified bursopathies, ankle and foot
M71.871 Other specified bursopathies, right ankle and foot
M71.872 Other specified bursopathies, left ankle and foot
M71.879 Other specified bursopathies, unspecified ankle and foot
M71.88 Other specified bursopathies, other site
M71.89 Other specified bursopathies, multiple sites
M71.9 Bursopathy, unspecified
Bursitis NOS

M72 Fibroblastic disorders
EXCLUDES2 *retroperitoneal fibromatosis (D48.3)*
M72.0 Palmar fascial fibromatosis [Dupuytren] A
M72.1 Knuckle pads
M72.2 Plantar fascial fibromatosis
Plantar fasciitis
M72.4 Pseudosarcomatous fibromatosis
Nodular fasciitis
M72.6 Necrotizing fasciitis MCC
Use additional code (B95.-, B96.-) to identify causative organism
M72.8 Other fibroblastic disorders
Abscess of fascia
Fasciitis NEC
Other infective fasciitis
Use additional code to (B95.-, B96.-) identify causative organism
EXCLUDES1 *diffuse (eosinophilic) fasciitis (M35.4)*
necrotizing fasciitis (M72.6)
nodular fasciitis (M72.4)
perirenal fasciitis NOS (N13.5)
perirenal fasciitis with infection (N13.6)
plantar fasciitis (M72.2)
M72.9 Fibroblastic disorder, unspecified
Fasciitis NOS
Fibromatosis NOS

M75 Shoulder lesions
EXCLUDES2 *shoulder-hand syndrome (M89.0-)*
M75.0 Adhesive capsulitis of shoulder
Frozen shoulder
Periarthritis of shoulder
M75.00 Adhesive capsulitis of unspecified shoulder
M75.01 Adhesive capsulitis of right shoulder
M75.02 Adhesive capsulitis of left shoulder
M75.1 Rotator cuff tear or rupture, not specified as traumatic
Rotator cuff syndrome
Supraspinatus tear or rupture, not specified as traumatic
Supraspinatus syndrome
EXCLUDES1 *tear of rotator cuff, traumatic (S46.01-)*
M75.10 Unspecified rotator cuff tear or rupture, not specified as traumatic
M75.100 Unspecified rotator cuff tear or rupture of unspecified shoulder, not specified as traumatic
M75.101 Unspecified rotator cuff tear or rupture of right shoulder, not specified as traumatic
M75.102 Unspecified rotator cuff tear or rupture of left shoulder, not specified as traumatic
M75.11 Incomplete rotator cuff tear or rupture not specified as traumatic
M75.110 Incomplete rotator cuff tear or rupture of unspecified shoulder, not specified as traumatic
M75.111 Incomplete rotator cuff tear or rupture of right shoulder, not specified as traumatic
M75.112 Incomplete rotator cuff tear or rupture of left shoulder, not specified as traumatic
M75.12 Complete rotator cuff tear or rupture not specified as traumatic
M75.120 Complete rotator cuff tear or rupture of unspecified shoulder, not specified as traumatic
M75.121 Complete rotator cuff tear or rupture of right shoulder, not specified as traumatic
M75.122 Complete rotator cuff tear or rupture of left shoulder, not specified as traumatic
M75.2 Bicipital tendinitis
M75.20 Bicipital tendinitis, unspecified shoulder
M75.21 Bicipital tendinitis, right shoulder
M75.22 Bicipital tendinitis, left shoulder
M75.3 Calcific tendinitis of shoulder
Calcified bursa of shoulder
M75.30 Calcific tendinitis of unspecified shoulder
M75.31 Calcific tendinitis of right shoulder
M75.32 Calcific tendinitis of left shoulder
M75.4 Impingement syndrome of shoulder
M75.40 Impingement syndrome of unspecified shoulder
M75.41 Impingement syndrome of right shoulder
M75.42 Impingement syndrome of left shoulder
M75.5 Bursitis of shoulder
M75.50 Bursitis of unspecified shoulder
M75.51 Bursitis of right shoulder
M75.52 Bursitis of left shoulder
M75.8 Other shoulder lesions
M75.80 Other shoulder lesions, unspecified shoulder
M75.81 Other shoulder lesions, right shoulder
M75.82 Other shoulder lesions, left shoulder
M75.9 Shoulder lesion, unspecified
M75.90 Shoulder lesion, unspecified, unspecified shoulder
M75.91 Shoulder lesion, unspecified, right shoulder
M75.92 Shoulder lesion, unspecified, left shoulder

M76 Enthesopathies, lower limb, excluding foot
EXCLUDES2 *bursitis due to use, overuse and pressure (M70.-)*
enthesopathies of ankle and foot (M77.5-)
M76.0 Gluteal tendinitis
M76.00 Gluteal tendinitis, unspecified hip
M76.01 Gluteal tendinitis, right hip
M76.02 Gluteal tendinitis, left hip
M76.1 Psoas tendinitis
M76.10 Psoas tendinitis, unspecified hip
M76.11 Psoas tendinitis, right hip
M76.12 Psoas tendinitis, left hip
M76.2 Iliac crest spur
M76.20 Iliac crest spur, unspecified hip
M76.21 Iliac crest spur, right hip
M76.22 Iliac crest spur, left hip
M76.3 Iliotibial band syndrome
M76.30 Iliotibial band syndrome, unspecified leg
M76.31 Iliotibial band syndrome, right leg
M76.32 Iliotibial band syndrome, left leg
M76.4 Tibial collateral bursitis [Pellegrini-Stieda]
M76.40 Tibial collateral bursitis [Pellegrini-Stieda], unspecified leg
M76.41 Tibial collateral bursitis [Pellegrini-Stieda], right leg
M76.42 Tibial collateral bursitis [Pellegrini-Stieda], left leg
M76.5 Patellar tendinitis
M76.50 Patellar tendinitis, unspecified knee
M76.51 Patellar tendinitis, right knee
M76.52 Patellar tendiitis, left knee

Unspecified Code | Other Specified Code | Manifestation Code | N Newborn | P Pediatric | M Maternity | A Adult | ♂ Male | ♀ Female
● New Code | ▲ Revised Code Title | ►◄ Revised Text | NOTES | INCLUDES | EXCLUDES1 Not coded here | EXCLUDES2 Not included here
4th character required | 5th character required | 6th character required | 7th character required
Extension 'X' Alert | HAC Hospital-acquired condition (HAC) alert | AHA AHA Coding Clinic©

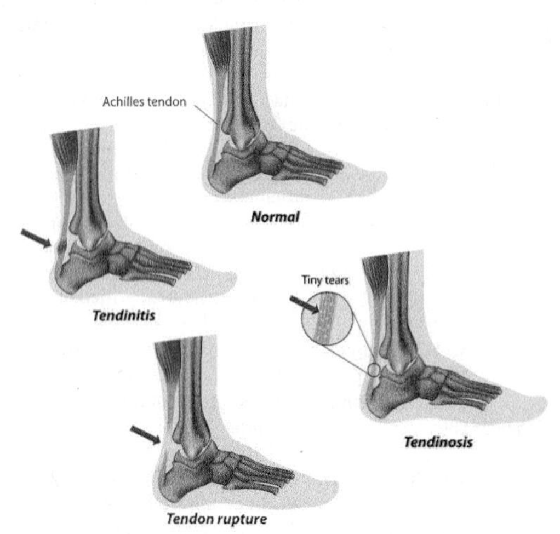

Figure 13.6 Achilles tendon problems

M76.6 Achilles tendinitis
Achilles bursitis
M76.60 Achilles tendinitis, unspecified leg
M76.61 Achilles tendinitis, right leg
M76.62 Achilles tendinitis, left leg
M76.7 Peroneal tendinitis
M76.70 Peroneal tendinitis, unspecified leg
M76.71 Peroneal tendinitis, right leg
M76.72 Peroneal tendinitis, left leg
M76.8 Other specified enthesopathies of lower limb, excluding foot
M76.81 Anterior tibial syndrome
M76.811 Anterior tibial syndrome, right leg
M76.812 Anterior tibial syndrome, left leg
M76.819 Anterior tibial syndrome, unspecified leg
M76.82 Posterior tibial tendinitis
M76.821 Posterior tibial tendinitis, right leg
M76.822 Posterior tibial tendinitis, left leg
M76.829 Posterior tibial tendinitis, unspecified leg
M76.89 Other specified enthesopathies of lower limb, excluding foot
M76.891 Other specified enthesopathies of right lower limb, excluding foot
M76.892 Other specified enthesopathies of left lower limb, excluding foot
M76.899 Other specified enthesopathies of unspecified lower limb, excluding foot
M76.9 Unspecified enthesopathy, lower limb, excluding foot
M77 Other enthesopathies
EXCLUDES1 *bursitis NOS (M71.9-)*
EXCLUDES2 *bursitis due to use, overuse and pressure (M70.-)*
osteophyte (M25.7)
spinal enthesopathy (M46.0-)
M77.0 Medial epicondylitis
M77.00 Medial epicondylitis, unspecified elbow
M77.01 Medial epicondylitis, right elbow
M77.02 Medial epicondylitis, left elbow
M77.1 Lateral epicondylitis
Tennis elbow
M77.10 Lateral epicondylitis, unspecified elbow
M77.11 Lateral epicondylitis, right elbow
M77.12 Lateral epicondylitis, left elbow
M77.2 Periarthritis of wrist
M77.20 Periarthritis, unspecified wrist
M77.21 Periarthritis, right wrist
M77.22 Periarthritis, left wrist
M77.3 Calcaneal spur
M77.30 Calcaneal spur, unspecified foot
M77.31 Calcaneal spur, right foot
M77.32 Calcaneal spur, left foot
M77.4 Metatarsalgia
EXCLUDES1 *Morton's metatarsalgia (G57.6)*
M77.40 Metatarsalgia, unspecified foot
M77.41 Metatarsalgia, right foot
M77.42 Metatarsalgia, left foot
M77.5 Other enthesopathy of foot
M77.50 Other enthesopathy of unspecified foot
M77.51 Other enthesopathy of right foot
M77.52 Other enthesopathy of left foot
M77.8 Other enthesopathies, not elsewhere classified
M77.9 Enthesopathy, unspecified
Bone spur NOS
Capsulitis NOS
Periarthritis NOS
Tendinitis NOS
M79 Other and unspecified soft tissue disorders, not elsewhere classified
EXCLUDES1 *psychogenic rheumatism (F45.8)*
soft tissue pain, psychogenic (F45.41)
M79.0 Rheumatism, unspecified
EXCLUDES1 *fibromyalgia (M79.7)*
palindromic rheumatism (M12.3-)
M79.1 Myalgia
Myofascial pain syndrome
EXCLUDES1 *fibromyalgia (M79.7)*
myositis (M60.-)
M79.2 Neuralgia and neuritis, unspecified
EXCLUDES1 *brachial radiculitis NOS (M54.1)*
lumbosacral radiculitis NOS (M54.1)
mononeuropathies (G56-G58)
radiculitis NOS (M54.1)
sciatica (M54.3-M54.4)
M79.3 Panniculitis, unspecified
EXCLUDES1 *lupus panniculitis (L93.2)*
neck and back panniculitis (M54.0-)
relapsing [Weber-Christian] panniculitis (M35.6)
M79.4 Hypertrophy of (infrapatellar) fat pad
M79.5 Residual foreign body in soft tissue
EXCLUDES1 *foreign body granuloma of skin and subcutaneous tissue (L92.3)*
foreign body granuloma of soft tissue (M60.2-)
M79.6 Pain in limb, hand, foot, fingers and toes
EXCLUDES2 *pain in joint (M25.5-)*
M79.60 Pain in limb, unspecified
M79.601 Pain in right arm
Pain in right upper limb NOS
M79.602 Pain in left arm
Pain in left upper limb NOS
M79.603 Pain in arm, unspecified
Pain in upper limb NOS
M79.604 Pain in right leg
Pain in right lower limb NOS
M79.605 Pain in left leg
Pain in left lower limb NOS
M79.606 Pain in leg, unspecified
Pain in lower limb NOS
M79.609 Pain in unspecified limb
Pain in limb NOS
M79.62 Pain in upper arm
Pain in axillary region
M79.621 Pain in right upper arm
M79.622 Pain in left upper arm
M79.629 Pain in unspecified upper arm
M79.63 Pain in forearm
M79.631 Pain in right forearm
M79.632 Pain in left forearm
M79.639 Pain in unspecified forearm
M79.64 Pain in hand and fingers
M79.641 Pain in right hand
M79.642 Pain in left hand
M79.643 Pain in unspecified hand
M79.644 Pain in right finger(s)

Unacceptable principal diagnosis symbol per Medicare code edits | Code exempt from diagnosis present on admission requirement | Questionable admission | Complication or comorbidity | CC/MCC exclusion | Major complication or comorbidity | Principal diagnosis as its own CC | Principal diagnosis as its own MCC | Z code as first-listed diagnosis

M79.645 Pain in left finger(s)
M79.646 Pain in unspecified finger(s)
M79.65 Pain in thigh
M79.651 Pain in right thigh
M79.652 Pain in left thigh
M79.659 Pain in unspecified thigh
M79.66 Pain in lower leg
M79.661 Pain in right lower leg
M79.662 Pain in left lower leg
M79.669 Pain in unspecified lower leg
M79.67 Pain in foot and toes
M79.671 Pain in right foot
M79.672 Pain in left foot
M79.673 Pain in unspecified foot
M79.674 Pain in right toe(s)
M79.675 Pain in left toe(s)
M79.676 Pain in unspecified toe(s)
M79.7 Fibromyalgia
Fibromyositis
Fibrositis
Myofibrositis
M79.A Nontraumatic compartment syndrome
Code first , if applicable, associated postprocedural complication
EXCLUDES1 *compartment syndrome NOS (T79.A-)*
fibromyalgia (M79.7)
nontraumatic ischemic infarction of muscle (M62.2-)
traumatic compartment syndrome (T79.A-)
M79.A1 Nontraumatic compartment syndrome of upper extremity
Nontraumatic compartment syndrome of shoulder, arm, forearm, wrist, hand, and fingers
M79.A11 Nontraumatic compartment syndrome of right upper extremity
M79.A12 Nontraumatic compartment syndrome of left upper extremity
M79.A19 Nontraumatic compartment syndrome of unspecified upper extremity
M79.A2 Nontraumatic compartment syndrome of lower extremity
Nontraumatic compartment syndrome of hip, buttock, thigh, leg, foot, and toes
M79.A21 Nontraumatic compartment syndrome of right lower extremity
M79.A22 Nontraumatic compartment syndrome of left lower extremity
M79.A29 Nontraumatic compartment syndrome of unspecified lower extremity
M79.A3 Nontraumatic compartment syndrome of abdomen
M79.A9 Nontraumatic compartment syndrome of other sites
M79.8 Other specified soft tissue disorders
M79.81 Nontraumatic hematoma of soft tissue
Nontraumatic hematoma of muscle
Nontraumatic seroma of muscle and soft tissue
M79.89 Other specified soft tissue disorders
Polyalgia
M79.9 Soft tissue disorder, unspecified

Osteopathies and chondropathies (M80-M94)

Disorders of bone density and structure (M80-M85)

Osteoporosis

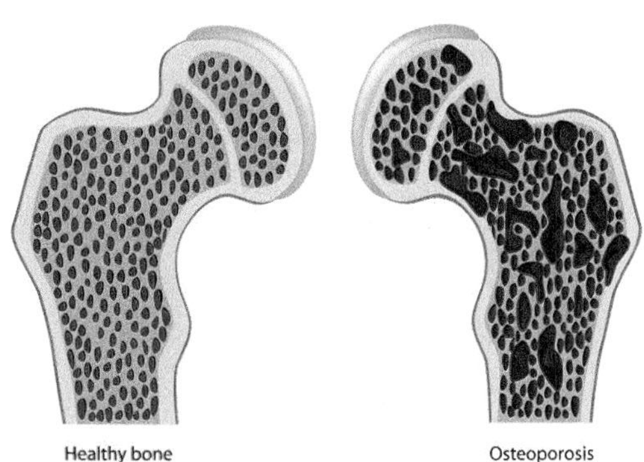

Figure 13.7 Reduced bone matrix in osteoporosis

M80 Osteoporosis with current pathological fracture
INCLUDES *osteoporosis with current fragility fracture*
Use additional code to identify major osseous defect, if applicable (M89.7-)
EXCLUDES1 *collapsed vertebra NOS (M48.5)*
pathological fracture NOS (M84.4)
wedging of vertebra NOS (M48.5)
EXCLUDES2 *personal history of (healed) osteoporosis fracture (Z87.310)*
The appropriate 7th character is to be added to each code from category M80:
A = initial encounter for fracture
D = subsequent encounter for fracture with routine healing
G = subsequent encounter for fracture with delayed healing
K = subsequent encounter for fracture with nonunion
P = subsequent encounter for fracture with malunion
S = sequela
M80.0 Age-related osteoporosis with current pathological fracture
Involutional osteoporosis with current pathological fracture
Osteoporosis NOS with current pathological fracture
Postmenopausal osteoporosis with current pathological fracture
Senile osteoporosis with current pathological fracture
M80.00 Age-related osteoporosis with current pathological fracture, unspecified site A
M80.01 Age-related osteoporosis with current pathological fracture, shoulder
M80.011 Age-related osteoporosis with current pathological fracture, right shoulder A
M80.012 Age-related osteoporosis with current pathological fracture, left shoulder A
M80.019 Age-related osteoporosis with current pathological fracture, unspecified shoulder A
M80.02 Age-related osteoporosis with current pathological fracture, humerus
M80.021 Age-related osteoporosis with current pathological fracture, right humerus A
M80.022 Age-related osteoporosis with current pathological fracture, left humerus A
M80.029 Age-related osteoporosis with current pathological fracture, unspecified humerus A
M80.03 Age-related osteoporosis with current pathological fracture, forearm
Age-related osteoporosis with current pathological fracture of wrist
M80.031 Age-related osteoporosis with current pathological fracture, right forearm A

M80.032 Age-related osteoporosis with current pathological fracture, left forearm

M80.039 Age-related osteoporosis with current pathological fracture, unspecified forearm

M80.04 Age-related osteoporosis with current pathological fracture, hand

M80.041 Age-related osteoporosis with current pathological fracture, right hand

M80.042 Age-related osteoporosis with current pathological fracture, left hand

M80.049 Age-related osteoporosis with current pathological fracture, unspecified hand

M80.05 Age-related osteoporosis with current pathological fracture, femur

Age-related osteoporosis with current pathological fracture of hip

M80.051 Age-related osteoporosis with current pathological fracture, right femur

M80.052 Age-related osteoporosis with current pathological fracture, left femur

M80.059 Age-related osteoporosis with current pathological fracture, unspecified femur

M80.06 Age-related osteoporosis with current pathological fracture, lower leg

M80.061 Age-related osteoporosis with current pathological fracture, right lower leg

M80.062 Age-related osteoporosis with current pathological fracture, left lower leg

M80.069 Age-related osteoporosis with current pathological fracture, unspecified lower leg

M80.07 Age-related osteoporosis with current pathological fracture, ankle and foot

M80.071 Age-related osteoporosis with current pathological fracture, right ankle and foot

M80.072 Age-related osteoporosis with current pathological fracture, left ankle and foot

M80.079 Age-related osteoporosis with current pathological fracture, unspecified ankle and foot

M80.08 Age-related osteoporosis with current pathological fracture, vertebra(e)

M80.8 Other osteoporosis with current pathological fracture

Drug-induced osteoporosis with current pathological fracture
Idiopathic osteoporosis with current pathological fracture
Osteoporosis of disuse with current pathological fracture
Postoophorectomy osteoporosis with current pathological fracture
Postsurgical malabsorption osteoporosis with current pathological fracture
Post-traumatic osteoporosis with current pathological fracture
Use additional code for adverse effect, if applicable, to identify drug (T36-T50 with fifth or sixth character 5)

M80.80 Other osteoporosis with current pathological fracture, unspecified site

M80.81 Other osteoporosis with pathological fracture, shoulder

M80.811 Other osteoporosis with current pathological fracture, right shoulder

M80.812 Other osteoporosis with current pathological fracture, left shoulder

M80.819 Other osteoporosis with current pathological fracture, unspecified shoulder

M80.82 Other osteoporosis with current pathological fracture, humerus

M80.821 Other osteoporosis with current pathological fracture, right humerus

M80.822 Other osteoporosis with current pathological fracture, left humerus

M80.829 Other osteoporosis with current pathological fracture, unspecified humerus

M80.83 Other osteoporosis with current pathological fracture, forearm

Other osteoporosis with current pathological fracture of wrist

M80.831 Other osteoporosis with current pathological fracture, right forearm

M80.832 Other osteoporosis with current pathological fracture, left forearm

M80.839 Other osteoporosis with current pathological fracture, unspecified forearm

M80.84 Other osteoporosis with current pathological fracture, hand

M80.841 Other osteoporosis with current pathological fracture, right hand

M80.842 Other osteoporosis with current pathological fracture, left hand

M80.849 Other osteoporosis with current pathological fracture, unspecified hand

M80.85 Other osteoporosis with current pathological fracture, femur

Other osteoporosis with current pathological fracture of hip

M80.851 Other osteoporosis with current pathological fracture, right femur

M80.852 Other osteoporosis with current pathological fracture, left femur

M80.859 Other osteoporosis with current pathological fracture, unspecified femur

M80.86 Other osteoporosis with current pathological fracture, lower leg

M80.861 Other osteoporosis with current pathological fracture, right lower leg

M80.862 Other osteoporosis with current pathological fracture, left lower leg

M80.869 Other osteoporosis with current pathological fracture, unspecified lower leg

M80.87 Other osteoporosis with current pathological fracture, ankle and foot

M80.871 Other osteoporosis with current pathological fracture, right ankle and foot

M80.872 Other osteoporosis with current pathological fracture, left ankle and foot

M80.879 Other osteoporosis with current pathological fracture, unspecified ankle and foot

M80.88 Other osteoporosis with current pathological fracture, vertebra(e)

M81 Osteoporosis without current pathological fracture

Use additional code to identify:
major osseous defect, if applicable (M89.7-)
personal history of (healed) osteoporosis fracture, if applicable (Z87.310)

EXCLUDES1 *osteoporosis with current pathological fracture (M80.-)*
Sudeck's atrophy (M89.0)

M81.0 Age-related osteoporosis without current pathological fracture

Involutional osteoporosis without current pathological fracture
Osteoporosis NOS
Postmenopausal osteoporosis without current pathological fracture
Senile osteoporosis without current pathological fracture

M81.6 Localized osteoporosis [Lequesne]

EXCLUDES1 *Sudeck's atrophy (M89.0)*

M81.8 Other osteoporosis without current pathological fracture

Drug-induced osteoporosis without current pathological fracture
Idiopathic osteoporosis without current pathological fracture
Osteoporosis of disuse without current pathological fracture
Postoophorectomy osteoporosis without current pathological fracture
Postsurgical malabsorption osteoporosis without current pathological fracture
Post-traumatic osteoporosis without current pathological fracture
Use additional code for adverse effect, if applicable, to identify drug (T36-T50 with fifth or sixth character 5)

Unacceptable principal diagnosis symbol per Medicare code edits · Code exempt from diagnosis present on admission requirement
Questionable admission · Complication or comorbidity · CC/MCC exclusion · Major complication or comorbidity
Principal diagnosis as its own CC · Principal diagnosis as its own MCC · Z code as first-listed diagnosis

M83 Adult osteomalacia
EXCLUDES1 *infantile and juvenile osteomalacia (E55.0)*
renal osteodystrophy (N25.0)
rickets (active) (E55.0)
rickets (active) sequelae (E64.3)
vitamin D-resistant osteomalacia (E83.3)
vitamin D-resistant rickets (active) (E83.3)

M83.0 Puerperal osteomalacia M ♀
M83.1 Senile osteomalacia A
M83.2 Adult osteomalacia due to malabsorption A
Postsurgical malabsorption osteomalacia in adults
M83.3 Adult osteomalacia due to malnutrition A
M83.4 Aluminum bone disease
M83.5 Other drug-induced osteomalacia in adults A
Use additional code for adverse effect, if applicable, to identify drug (T36-T50 with fifth or sixth character 5)
M83.8 Other adult osteomalacia A
M83.9 Adult osteomalacia, unspecified A

M84 Disorder of continuity of bone
EXCLUDES2 *traumatic fracture of bone-see fracture, by site*

M84.3 Stress fracture
Fatigue fracture
March fracture
Stress fracture NOS
Stress reaction
Use additional external cause code(s) to identify the cause of the stress fracture
EXCLUDES1 *pathological fracture NOS (M84.4.-)*
pathological fracture due to osteoporosis (M80.-)
traumatic fracture (S12.-, S22.-, S32.-, S42.-, S52.-, S62.-, S72.-, S82.-, S92.-)
EXCLUDES2 *personal history of (healed) stress (fatigue) fracture (Z87.312)*
stress fracture of vertebra (M48.4-)

The appropriate 7th character is to be added to each code from subcategory M84.3:
A = initial encounter for fracture
D = subsequent encounter for fracture with routine healing
G = subsequent encounter for fracture with delayed healing
K = subsequent encounter for fracture with nonunion
P = subsequent encounter for fracture with malunion
S = sequela

M84.30 Stress fracture, unspecified site CC
M84.31 Stress fracture, shoulder
M84.311 Stress fracture, right shoulder CC
M84.312 Stress fracture, left shoulder CC
M84.319 Stress fracture, unspecified shoulder CC
M84.32 Stress fracture, humerus
M84.321 Stress fracture, right humerus CC
M84.322 Stress fracture, left humerus CC
M84.329 Stress fracture, unspecified humerus CC
M84.33 Stress fracture, ulna and radius
M84.331 Stress fracture, right ulna CC
M84.332 Stress fracture, left ulna CC
M84.333 Stress fracture, right radius CC
M84.334 Stress fracture, left radius CC
M84.339 Stress fracture, unspecified ulna and radius CC
M84.34 Stress fracture, hand and fingers
M84.341 Stress fracture, right hand CC
M84.342 Stress fracture, left hand CC
M84.343 Stress fracture, unspecified hand CC
M84.344 Stress fracture, right finger(s) CC
M84.345 Stress fracture, left finger(s) CC
M84.346 Stress fracture, unspecified finger(s) CC
M84.35 Stress fracture, pelvis and femur
Stress fracture, hip
M84.350 Stress fracture, pelvis CC
M84.351 Stress fracture, right femur CC
M84.352 Stress fracture, left femur CC
M84.353 Stress fracture, unspecified femur CC
M84.359 Stress fracture, hip, unspecified CC
M84.36 Stress fracture, tibia and fibula
M84.361 Stress fracture, right tibia CC
M84.362 Stress fracture, left tibia CC
M84.363 Stress fracture, right fibula CC
M84.364 Stress fracture, left fibula CC
M84.369 Stress fracture, unspecified tibia and fibula CC
M84.37 Stress fracture, ankle, foot and toes
M84.371 Stress fracture, right ankle CC
M84.372 Stress fracture, left ankle CC
M84.373 Stress fracture, unspecified ankle CC
M84.374 Stress fracture, right foot CC
M84.375 Stress fracture, left foot CC
M84.376 Stress fracture, unspecified foot CC
M84.377 Stress fracture, right toe(s) CC
M84.378 Stress fracture, left toe(s) CC
M84.379 Stress fracture, unspecified toe(s) CC
M84.38 Stress fracture, other site CC
EXCLUDES2 *stress fracture of vertebra (M48.4-)*

M84.4 Pathological fracture, not elsewhere classified
Chronic fracture
Pathological fracture NOS
EXCLUDES1 *collapsed vertebra NEC (M48.5)*
pathological fracture in neoplastic disease (M84.5-)
pathological fracture in osteoporosis (M80.-)
pathological fracture in other disease (M84.6-)
stress fracture (M84.3-)
traumatic fracture (S12.-, S22.-, S32.-, S42.-, S52.-, S62.-, S72.-, S82.-, S92.-)
EXCLUDES2 *personal history of (healed) pathological fracture (Z87.311)*

The appropriate 7th character is to be added to each code from subcategory M84.4:
A = initial encounter for fracture
D = subsequent encounter for fracture with routine healing
G = subsequent encounter for fracture with delayed healing
K = subsequent encounter for fracture with nonunion
P = subsequent encounter for fracture with malunion
S = sequela

M84.40 Pathological fracture, unspecified site CC
M84.41 Pathological fracture, shoulder
M84.411 Pathological fracture, right shoulder CC
M84.412 Pathological fracture, left shoulder CC
M84.419 Pathological fracture, unspecified shoulder CC
M84.42 Pathological fracture, humerus
M84.421 Pathological fracture, right humerus CC
M84.422 Pathological fracture, left humerus CC
M84.429 Pathological fracture, unspecified humerus CC
M84.43 Pathological fracture, ulna and radius
M84.431 Pathological fracture, right ulna CC
M84.432 Pathological fracture, left ulna CC
M84.433 Pathological fracture, right radius CC
M84.434 Pathological fracture, left radius CC
M84.439 Pathological fracture, unspecified ulna and radius CC
M84.44 Pathological fracture, hand and fingers
M84.441 Pathological fracture, right hand CC
M84.442 Pathological fracture, left hand CC
M84.443 Pathological fracture, unspecified hand CC
M84.444 Pathological fracture, right finger(s) CC
M84.445 Pathological fracture, left finger(s) CC
M84.446 Pathological fracture, unspecified finger(s) CC
M84.45 Pathological fracture, femur and pelvis
M84.451 Pathological fracture, right femur CC
M84.452 Pathological fracture, left femur CC

Unspecified Code | Other Specified Code | Manifestation Code | N Newborn | P Pediatric | M Maternity | A Adult | ♂ Male | ♀ Female
● New Code | ▲ Revised Code Title | ►◄ Revised Text | NOTES | INCLUDES | EXCLUDES1 Not coded here | EXCLUDES2 Not included here
4th character required | 5th character required | 6th character required | 7th character required
Extension 'X' Alert | HAC Hospital-acquired condition (HAC) alert | AHA AHA Coding Clinic©

M84.453 Pathological fracture, unspecified femur
M84.454 Pathological fracture, pelvis
M84.459 Pathological fracture, hip, unspecified
M84.46 Pathological fracture, tibia and fibula
M84.461 Pathological fracture, right tibia
M84.462 Pathological fracture, left tibia
M84.463 Pathological fracture, right fibula
M84.464 Pathological fracture, left fibula
M84.469 Pathological fracture, unspecified tibia and fibula
M84.47 Pathological fracture, ankle , foot and toes
M84.471 Pathological fracture, right ankle
M84.472 Pathological fracture, left ankle
M84.473 Pathological fracture, unspecified ankle
M84.474 Pathological fracture, right foot
M84.475 Pathological fracture, left foot
M84.476 Pathological fracture, unspecified foot
M84.477 Pathological fracture, right toe(s)
M84.478 Pathological fracture, left toe(s)
M84.479 Pathological fracture, unspecified toe(s)
M84.48 Pathological fracture, other site

M84.5 Pathological fracture in neoplastic disease
Code also underlying neoplasm
The appropriate 7th character is to be added to each code from subcategory M84.5:
A = initial encounter for fracture
D = subsequent encounter for fracture with routine healing
G = subsequent encounter for fracture with delayed healing
K = subsequent encounter for fracture with nonunion
P = subsequent encounter for fracture with malunion
S = sequela

M84.50 Pathological fracture in neoplastic disease, unspecified site
M84.51 Pathological fracture in neoplastic disease, shoulder
M84.511 Pathological fracture in neoplastic disease, right shoulder
M84.512 Pathological fracture in neoplastic disease, left shoulder
M84.519 Pathological fracture in neoplastic disease, unspecified shoulder
M84.52 Pathological fracture in neoplastic disease, humerus
M84.521 Pathological fracture in neoplastic disease, right humerus
M84.522 Pathological fracture in neoplastic disease, left humerus
M84.529 Pathological fracture in neoplastic disease, unspecified humerus
M84.53 Pathological fracture in neoplastic disease, ulna and radius
M84.531 Pathological fracture in neoplastic disease, right ulna
M84.532 Pathological fracture in neoplastic disease, left ulna
M84.533 Pathological fracture in neoplastic disease, right radius
M84.534 Pathological fracture in neoplastic disease, left radius
M84.539 Pathological fracture in neoplastic disease, unspecified ulna and radius
M84.54 Pathological fracture in neoplastic disease, hand
M84.541 Pathological fracture in neoplastic disease, right hand
M84.542 Pathological fracture in neoplastic disease, left hand
M84.549 Pathological fracture in neoplastic disease, unspecified hand
M84.55 Pathological fracture in neoplastic disease, pelvis and femur
M84.550 Pathological fracture in neoplastic disease, pelvis
M84.551 Pathological fracture in neoplastic disease, right femur
M84.552 Pathological fracture in neoplastic disease, left femur
M84.553 Pathological fracture in neoplastic disease, unspecified femur
M84.559 Pathological fracture in neoplastic disease, hip, unspecified
M84.56 Pathological fracture in neoplastic disease, tibia and fibula
M84.561 Pathological fracture in neoplastic disease, right tibia
M84.562 Pathological fracture in neoplastic disease, left tibia
M84.563 Pathological fracture in neoplastic disease, right fibula
M84.564 Pathological fracture in neoplastic disease, left fibula
M84.569 Pathological fracture in neoplastic disease, unspecified tibia and fibula
M84.57 Pathological fracture in neoplastic disease, ankle and foot
M84.571 Pathological fracture in neoplastic disease, right ankle
M84.572 Pathological fracture in neoplastic disease, left ankle
M84.573 Pathological fracture in neoplastic disease, unspecified ankle
M84.574 Pathological fracture in neoplastic disease, right foot
M84.575 Pathological fracture in neoplastic disease, left foot
M84.576 Pathological fracture in neoplastic disease, unspecified foot
M84.58 Pathological fracture in neoplastic disease, other specified site
Pathological fracture in neoplastic disease, vertebrae

M84.6 Pathological fracture in other disease
Code also underlying condition
EXCLUDES1 *pathological fracture in osteoporosis (M80.-)*
The appropriate 7th character is to be added to each code from subcategory M84.6:
A = initial encounter for fracture
D = subsequent encounter for fracture with routine healing
G = subsequent encounter for fracture with delayed healing
K = subsequent encounter for fracture with nonunion
P = subsequent encounter for fracture with malunion
S = sequela

M84.60 Pathological fracture in other disease, unspecified site
M84.61 Pathological fracture in other disease, shoulder
M84.611 Pathological fracture in other disease, right shoulder
M84.612 Pathological fracture in other disease, left shoulder
M84.619 Pathological fracture in other disease, unspecified shoulder
M84.62 Pathological fracture in other disease, humerus
M84.621 Pathological fracture in other disease, right humerus
M84.622 Pathological fracture in other disease, left humerus
M84.629 Pathological fracture in other disease, unspecified humerus
M84.63 Pathological fracture in other disease, ulna and radius
M84.631 Pathological fracture in other disease, right ulna
M84.632 Pathological fracture in other disease, left ulna
M84.633 Pathological fracture in other disease, right radius
M84.634 Pathological fracture in other disease, left radius

Unacceptable principal diagnosis symbol per Medicare code edits · Code exempt from diagnosis present on admission requirement
Questionable admission · Complication or comorbidity · CC/MCC exclusion · Major complication or comorbidity
Principal diagnosis as its own CC · Principal diagnosis as its own MCC · Z code as first-listed diagnosis

When symbols appear on a code that requires a 7th character extension, refer to Appendix D to identify applicable 7th character codes.

M84.639 Pathological fracture in other disease, unspecified ulna and radius CC
M84.64 Pathological fracture in other disease, hand
M84.641 Pathological fracture in other disease, right hand CC
M84.642 Pathological fracture in other disease, left hand CC
M84.649 Pathological fracture in other disease, unspecified hand CC
M84.65 Pathological fracture in other disease, pelvis and femur
M84.650 Pathological fracture in other disease, pelvis CC
M84.651 Pathological fracture in other disease, right femur CC
M84.652 Pathological fracture in other disease, left femur CC
M84.653 Pathological fracture in other disease, unspecified femur CC
M84.659 Pathological fracture in other disease, hip, unspecified CC
M84.66 Pathological fracture in other disease, tibia and fibula
M84.661 Pathological fracture in other disease, right tibia CC
M84.662 Pathological fracture in other disease, left tibia CC
M84.663 Pathological fracture in other disease, right fibula CC
M84.664 Pathological fracture in other disease, left fibula CC
M84.669 Pathological fracture in other disease, unspecified tibia and fibula CC
M84.67 Pathological fracture in other disease, ankle and foot
M84.671 Pathological fracture in other disease, right ankle CC
M84.672 Pathological fracture in other disease, left ankle CC
M84.673 Pathological fracture in other disease, unspecified ankle CC
M84.674 Pathological fracture in other disease, right foot CC
M84.675 Pathological fracture in other disease, left foot CC
M84.676 Pathological fracture in other disease, unspecified foot CC
M84.68 Pathological fracture in other disease, other site CC
● M84.7 Nontraumatic fracture, not elsewhere classified
● M84.75 Atypical femoral fracture

The appropriate 7th character is to be added to each code from M84.75:

A = initial encounter for fracture
D = subsequent encounter for fracture with routine healing
G = subsequent encounter for fracture with delayed healing
K = subsequent encounter for fracture with nonunion
P = subsequent encounter for fracture with malunion
S = sequela

● M84.750 Atypical femoral fracture, unspecified CC CC/MCC Exc
● M84.751 Incomplete atypical femoral fracture, right leg CC CC/MCC Exc
● M84.752 Incomplete atypical femoral fracture, left leg CC CC/MCC Exc
● M84.753 Incomplete atypical femoral fracture, unspecified leg CC CC/MCC Exc
● M84.754 Complete transverse atypical femoral fracture, right leg CC CC/MCC Exc
● M84.755 Complete transverse atypical femoral fracture, left leg CC CC/MCC Exc
● M84.756 Complete transverse atypical femoral fracture, unspecified leg CC CC/MCC Exc
● M84.757 Complete oblique atypical femoral fracture, right leg CC CC/MCC Exc
● M84.758 Complete oblique atypical femoral fracture, left leg CC CC/MCC Exc
● M84.759 Complete oblique atypical femoral fracture, unspecified leg CC CC/MCC Exc
M84.8 Other disorders of continuity of bone
M84.80 Other disorders of continuity of bone, unspecified site
M84.81 Other disorders of continuity of bone, shoulder
M84.811 Other disorders of continuity of bone, right shoulder
M84.812 Other disorders of continuity of bone, left shoulder
M84.819 Other disorders of continuity of bone, unspecified shoulder
M84.82 Other disorders of continuity of bone, humerus
M84.821 Other disorders of continuity of bone, right humerus
M84.822 Other disorders of continuity of bone, left humerus
M84.829 Other disorders of continuity of bone, unspecified humerus
M84.83 Other disorders of continuity of bone, ulna and radius
M84.831 Other disorders of continuity of bone, right ulna
M84.832 Other disorders of continuity of bone, left ulna
M84.833 Other disorders of continuity of bone, right radius
M84.834 Other disorders of continuity of bone, left radius
M84.839 Other disorders of continuity of bone, unspecified ulna and radius
M84.84 Other disorders of continuity of bone, hand
M84.841 Other disorders of continuity of bone, right hand
M84.842 Other disorders of continuity of bone, left hand
M84.849 Other disorders of continuity of bone, unspecified hand
M84.85 Other disorders of continuity of bone, pelvic region and thigh
M84.851 Other disorders of continuity of bone, right pelvic region and thigh
M84.852 Other disorders of continuity of bone, left pelvic region and thigh
M84.859 Other disorders of continuity of bone, unspecified pelvic region and thigh
M84.86 Other disorders of continuity of bone, tibia and fibula
M84.861 Other disorders of continuity of bone, right tibia
M84.862 Other disorders of continuity of bone, left tibia
M84.863 Other disorders of continuity of bone, right fibula
M84.864 Other disorders of continuity of bone, left fibula
M84.869 Other disorders of continuity of bone, unspecified tibia and fibula
M84.87 Other disorders of continuity of bone, ankle and foot
M84.871 Other disorders of continuity of bone, right ankle and foot
M84.872 Other disorders of continuity of bone, left ankle and foot
M84.879 Other disorders of continuity of bone, unspecified ankle and foot
M84.88 Other disorders of continuity of bone, other site
M84.9 Disorder of continuity of bone, unspecified
M85 Other disorders of bone density and structure

EXCLUDES1 *osteogenesis imperfecta (Q78.0)*
osteopetrosis (Q78.2)
osteopoikilosis (Q78.8)
polyostotic fibrous dysplasia (Q78.1)

Unspecified Code Other Specified Code Manifestation Code N Newborn P Pediatric M Maternity A Adult ♂ Male ♀ Female
● New Code ▲ Revised Code Title ►◄ Revised Text NOTES INCLUDES EXCLUDES1 Not coded here EXCLUDES2 Not included here
4th character required 5th character required 6th character required 7th character required
Extension 'X' Alert HAC Hospital-acquired condition (HAC) alert AHA AHA Coding Clinic©

M85.0 Fibrous dysplasia (monostotic)
EXCLUDES2 *fibrous dysplasia of jaw (M27.8)*
M85.00 Fibrous dysplasia (monostotic), unspecified site
M85.01 Fibrous dysplasia (monostotic), shoulder
M85.011 Fibrous dysplasia (monostotic), right shoulder
M85.012 Fibrous dysplasia (monostotic), left shoulder
M85.019 Fibrous dysplasia (monostotic), unspecified shoulder
M85.02 Fibrous dysplasia (monostotic), upper arm
M85.021 Fibrous dysplasia (monostotic), right upper arm
M85.022 Fibrous dysplasia (monostotic), left upper arm
M85.029 Fibrous dysplasia (monostotic), unspecified upper arm
M85.03 Fibrous dysplasia (monostotic), forearm
M85.031 Fibrous dysplasia (monostotic), right forearm
M85.032 Fibrous dysplasia (monostotic), left forearm
M85.039 Fibrous dysplasia (monostotic), unspecified forearm
M85.04 Fibrous dysplasia (monostotic), hand
M85.041 Fibrous dysplasia (monostotic), right hand
M85.042 Fibrous dysplasia (monostotic), left hand
M85.049 Fibrous dysplasia (monostotic), unspecified hand
M85.05 Fibrous dysplasia (monostotic), thigh
M85.051 Fibrous dysplasia (monostotic), right thigh
M85.052 Fibrous dysplasia (monostotic), left thigh
M85.059 Fibrous dysplasia (monostotic), unspecified thigh
M85.06 Fibrous dysplasia (monostotic), lower leg
M85.061 Fibrous dysplasia (monostotic), right lower leg
M85.062 Fibrous dysplasia (monostotic), left lower leg
M85.069 Fibrous dysplasia (monostotic), unspecified lower leg
M85.07 Fibrous dysplasia (monostotic), ankle and foot
M85.071 Fibrous dysplasia (monostotic), right ankle and foot
M85.072 Fibrous dysplasia (monostotic), left ankle and foot
M85.079 Fibrous dysplasia (monostotic), unspecified ankle and foot
M85.08 Fibrous dysplasia (monostotic), other site
M85.09 Fibrous dysplasia (monostotic), multiple sites
M85.1 Skeletal fluorosis
M85.10 Skeletal fluorosis, unspecified site
M85.11 Skeletal fluorosis, shoulder
M85.111 Skeletal fluorosis, right shoulder
M85.112 Skeletal fluorosis, left shoulder
M85.119 Skeletal fluorosis, unspecified shoulder
M85.12 Skeletal fluorosis, upper arm
M85.121 Skeletal fluorosis, right upper arm
M85.122 Skeletal fluorosis, left upper arm
M85.129 Skeletal fluorosis, unspecified upper arm
M85.13 Skeletal fluorosis, forearm
M85.131 Skeletal fluorosis, right forearm
M85.132 Skeletal fluorosis, left forearm
M85.139 Skeletal fluorosis, unspecified forearm
M85.14 Skeletal fluorosis, hand
M85.141 Skeletal fluorosis, right hand
M85.142 Skeletal fluorosis, left hand
M85.149 Skeletal fluorosis, unspecified hand
M85.15 Skeletal fluorosis, thigh
M85.151 Skeletal fluorosis, right thigh
M85.152 Skeletal fluorosis, left thigh
M85.159 Skeletal fluorosis, unspecified thigh
M85.16 Skeletal fluorosis, lower leg
M85.161 Skeletal fluorosis, right lower leg
M85.162 Skeletal fluorosis, left lower leg
M85.169 Skeletal fluorosis, unspecified lower leg
M85.17 Skeletal fluorosis, ankle and foot
M85.171 Skeletal fluorosis, right ankle and foot
M85.172 Skeletal fluorosis, left ankle and foot
M85.179 Skeletal fluorosis, unspecified ankle and foot
M85.18 Skeletal fluorosis, other site
M85.19 Skeletal fluorosis, multiple sites
M85.2 Hyperostosis of skull
M85.3 Osteitis condensans
M85.30 Osteitis condensans, unspecified site
M85.31 Osteitis condensans, shoulder
M85.311 Osteitis condensans, right shoulder
M85.312 Osteitis condensans, left shoulder
M85.319 Osteitis condensans, unspecified shoulder
M85.32 Osteitis condensans, upper arm
M85.321 Osteitis condensans, right upper arm
M85.322 Osteitis condensans, left upper arm
M85.329 Osteitis condensans, unspecified upper arm
M85.33 Osteitis condensans, forearm
M85.331 Osteitis condensans, right forearm
M85.332 Osteitis condensans, left forearm
M85.339 Osteitis condensans, unspecified forearm
M85.34 Osteitis condensans, hand
M85.341 Osteitis condensans, right hand
M85.342 Osteitis condensans, left hand
M85.349 Osteitis condensans, unspecified hand
M85.35 Osteitis condensans, thigh
M85.351 Osteitis condensans, right thigh
M85.352 Osteitis condensans, left thigh
M85.359 Osteitis condensans, unspecified thigh
M85.36 Osteitis condensans, lower leg
M85.361 Osteitis condensans, right lower leg
M85.362 Osteitis condensans, left lower leg
M85.369 Osteitis condensans, unspecified lower leg
M85.37 Osteitis condensans, ankle and foot
M85.371 Osteitis condensans, right ankle and foot
M85.372 Osteitis condensans, left ankle and foot
M85.379 Osteitis condensans, unspecified ankle and foot
M85.38 Osteitis condensans, other site
M85.39 Osteitis condensans, multiple sites
M85.4 Solitary bone cyst
EXCLUDES2 *solitary cyst of jaw (M27.4)*
M85.40 Solitary bone cyst, unspecified site
M85.41 Solitary bone cyst, shoulder
M85.411 Solitary bone cyst, right shoulder
M85.412 Solitary bone cyst, left shoulder
M85.419 Solitary bone cyst, unspecified shoulder
M85.42 Solitary bone cyst, humerus
M85.421 Solitary bone cyst, right humerus
M85.422 Solitary bone cyst, left humerus
M85.429 Solitary bone cyst, unspecified humerus
M85.43 Solitary bone cyst, ulna and radius
M85.431 Solitary bone cyst, right ulna and radius
M85.432 Solitary bone cyst, left ulna and radius
M85.439 Solitary bone cyst, unspecified ulna and radius
M85.44 Solitary bone cyst, hand
M85.441 Solitary bone cyst, right hand
M85.442 Solitary bone cyst, left hand
M85.449 Solitary bone cyst, unspecified hand
M85.45 Solitary bone cyst, pelvis
M85.451 Solitary bone cyst, right pelvis
M85.452 Solitary bone cyst, left pelvis
M85.459 Solitary bone cyst, unspecified pelvis
M85.46 Solitary bone cyst, tibia and fibula
M85.461 Solitary bone cyst, right tibia and fibula

Unacceptable principal diagnosis symbol per Medicare code edits · Code exempt from diagnosis present on admission requirement
Questionable admission · Complication or comorbidity · CC/MCC exclusion · Major complication or comorbidity
Principal diagnosis as its own CC · Principal diagnosis as its own MCC · Z code as first-listed diagnosis

M85.462 Solitary bone cyst, left tibia and fibula
M85.469 Solitary bone cyst, unspecified tibia and fibula
M85.47 Solitary bone cyst, ankle and foot
M85.471 Solitary bone cyst, right ankle and foot
M85.472 Solitary bone cyst, left ankle and foot
M85.479 Solitary bone cyst, unspecified ankle and foot
M85.48 Solitary bone cyst, other site
M85.5 Aneurysmal bone cyst
EXCLUDES2 *aneurysmal cyst of jaw (M27.4)*
M85.50 Aneurysmal bone cyst, unspecified site
M85.51 Aneurysmal bone cyst, shoulder
M85.511 Aneurysmal bone cyst, right shoulder
M85.512 Aneurysmal bone cyst, left shoulder
M85.519 Aneurysmal bone cyst, unspecified shoulder
M85.52 Aneurysmal bone cyst, upper arm
M85.521 Aneurysmal bone cyst, right upper arm
M85.522 Aneurysmal bone cyst, left upper arm
M85.529 Aneurysmal bone cyst, unspecified upper arm
M85.53 Aneurysmal bone cyst, forearm
M85.531 Aneurysmal bone cyst, right forearm
M85.532 Aneurysmal bone cyst, left forearm
M85.539 Aneurysmal bone cyst, unspecified forearm
M85.54 Aneurysmal bone cyst, hand
M85.541 Aneurysmal bone cyst, right hand
M85.542 Aneurysmal bone cyst, left hand
M85.549 Aneurysmal bone cyst, unspecified hand
M85.55 Aneurysmal bone cyst, thigh
M85.551 Aneurysmal bone cyst, right thigh
M85.552 Aneurysmal bone cyst, left thigh
M85.559 Aneurysmal bone cyst, unspecified thigh
M85.56 Aneurysmal bone cyst, lower leg
M85.561 Aneurysmal bone cyst, right lower leg
M85.562 Aneurysmal bone cyst, left lower leg
M85.569 Aneurysmal bone cyst, unspecified lower leg
M85.57 Aneurysmal bone cyst, ankle and foot
M85.571 Aneurysmal bone cyst, right ankle and foot
M85.572 Aneurysmal bone cyst, left ankle and foot
M85.579 Aneurysmal bone cyst, unspecified ankle and foot
M85.58 Aneurysmal bone cyst, other site
M85.59 Aneurysmal bone cyst, multiple sites
M85.6 Other cyst of bone
EXCLUDES1 *cyst of jaw NEC (M27.4)*
osteitis fibrosa cystica generalisata [von Recklinghausen's disease of bone] (E21.0)
M85.60 Other cyst of bone, unspecified site
M85.61 Other cyst of bone, shoulder
M85.611 Other cyst of bone, right shoulder
M85.612 Other cyst of bone, left shoulder
M85.619 Other cyst of bone, unspecified shoulder
M85.62 Other cyst of bone, upper arm
M85.621 Other cyst of bone, right upper arm
M85.622 Other cyst of bone, left upper arm
M85.629 Other cyst of bone, unspecified upper arm
M85.63 Other cyst of bone, forearm
M85.631 Other cyst of bone, right forearm
M85.632 Other cyst of bone, left forearm
M85.639 Other cyst of bone, unspecified forearm
M85.64 Other cyst of bone, hand
M85.641 Other cyst of bone, right hand
M85.642 Other cyst of bone, left hand
M85.649 Other cyst of bone, unspecified hand
M85.65 Other cyst of bone, thigh
M85.651 Other cyst of bone, right thigh
M85.652 Other cyst of bone, left thigh
M85.659 Other cyst of bone, unspecified thigh
M85.66 Other cyst of bone, lower leg
M85.661 Other cyst of bone, right lower leg
M85.662 Other cyst of bone, left lower leg
M85.669 Other cyst of bone, unspecified lower leg
M85.67 Other cyst of bone, ankle and foot
M85.671 Other cyst of bone, right ankle and foot
M85.672 Other cyst of bone, left ankle and foot
M85.679 Other cyst of bone, unspecified ankle and foot
M85.68 Other cyst of bone, other site
M85.69 Other cyst of bone, multiple sites
M85.8 Other specified disorders of bone density and structure
Hyperostosis of bones, except skull
Osteosclerosis, acquired
EXCLUDES1 *diffuse idiopathic skeletal hyperostosis [DISH] (M48.1)*
osteosclerosis congenita (Q77.4)
osteosclerosis fragilitas (generalista) (Q78.2)
osteosclerosis myelofibrosis (D75.81)
M85.80 Other specified disorders of bone density and structure, unspecified site
M85.81 Other specified disorders of bone density and structure, shoulder
M85.811 Other specified disorders of bone density and structure, right shoulder
M85.812 Other specified disorders of bone density and structure, left shoulder
M85.819 Other specified disorders of bone density and structure, unspecified shoulder
M85.82 Other specified disorders of bone density and structure, upper arm
M85.821 Other specified disorders of bone density and structure, right upper arm
M85.822 Other specified disorders of bone density and structure, left upper arm
M85.829 Other specified disorders of bone density and structure, unspecified upper arm
M85.83 Other specified disorders of bone density and structure, forearm
M85.831 Other specified disorders of bone density and structure, right forearm
M85.832 Other specified disorders of bone density and structure, left forearm
M85.839 Other specified disorders of bone density and structure, unspecified forearm
M85.84 Other specified disorders of bone density and structure, hand
M85.841 Other specified disorders of bone density and structure, right hand
M85.842 Other specified disorders of bone density and structure, left hand
M85.849 Other specified disorders of bone density and structure, unspecified hand
M85.85 Other specified disorders of bone density and structure, thigh
M85.851 Other specified disorders of bone density and structure, right thigh
M85.852 Other specified disorders of bone density and structure, left thigh
M85.859 Other specified disorders of bone density and structure, unspecified thigh
M85.86 Other specified disorders of bone density and structure, lower leg
M85.861 Other specified disorders of bone density and structure, right lower leg
M85.862 Other specified disorders of bone density and structure, left lower leg
M85.869 Other specified disorders of bone density and structure, unspecified lower leg
M85.87 Other specified disorders of bone density and structure, ankle and foot
M85.871 Other specified disorders of bone density and structure, right ankle and foot
M85.872 Other specified disorders of bone density and structure, left ankle and foot

Unspecified Code Other Specified Code Manifestation Code N Newborn P Pediatric M Maternity A Adult ♂ Male ♀ Female
● New Code ▲ Revised Code Title ►◄ Revised Text NOTES INCLUDES EXCLUDES1 Not coded here EXCLUDES2 Not included here
4th character required 5th character required 6th character required 7th character required
Extension 'X' Alert HAC Hospital-acquired condition (HAC) alert AHA AHA Coding Clinic©

M85.879 Other specified disorders of bone density and structure, unspecified ankle and foot
M85.88 Other specified disorders of bone density and structure, other site
M85.89 Other specified disorders of bone density and structure, multiple sites
M85.9 Disorder of bone density and structure, unspecified

Other osteopathies (M86-M90)

EXCLUDES1 *postprocedural osteopathies ►(M96.-)◄*

M86 Osteomyelitis
Use additional code (B95-B97) to identify infectious agent
Use additional code to identify major osseous defect, if applicable (M89.7-)

EXCLUDES1 *osteomyelitis due to:*
echinococcus (B67.2)
gonococcus (A54.43)
salmonella (A02.24)

EXCLUDES2 *osteomyelitis of:*
orbit (H05.0-)
petrous bone (H70.2-)
vertebra (M46.2-)

M86.0 Acute hematogenous osteomyelitis
M86.00 Acute hematogenous osteomyelitis, unspecified site CC
M86.01 Acute hematogenous osteomyelitis, shoulder
M86.011 Acute hematogenous osteomyelitis, right shoulder CC
M86.012 Acute hematogenous osteomyelitis, left shoulder CC
M86.019 Acute hematogenous osteomyelitis, unspecified shoulder CC
M86.02 Acute hematogenous osteomyelitis, humerus
M86.021 Acute hematogenous osteomyelitis, right humerus CC
M86.022 Acute hematogenous osteomyelitis, left humerus CC
M86.029 Acute hematogenous osteomyelitis, unspecified humerus CC
M86.03 Acute hematogenous osteomyelitis, radius and ulna
M86.031 Acute hematogenous osteomyelitis, right radius and ulna CC
M86.032 Acute hematogenous osteomyelitis, left radius and ulna CC
M86.039 Acute hematogenous osteomyelitis, unspecified radius and ulna CC
M86.04 Acute hematogenous osteomyelitis, hand
M86.041 Acute hematogenous osteomyelitis, right hand CC
M86.042 Acute hematogenous osteomyelitis, left hand CC
M86.049 Acute hematogenous osteomyelitis, unspecified hand CC
M86.05 Acute hematogenous osteomyelitis, femur
M86.051 Acute hematogenous osteomyelitis, right femur CC
M86.052 Acute hematogenous osteomyelitis, left femur CC
M86.059 Acute hematogenous osteomyelitis, unspecified femur CC
M86.06 Acute hematogenous osteomyelitis, tibia and fibula
M86.061 Acute hematogenous osteomyelitis, right tibia and fibula CC
M86.062 Acute hematogenous osteomyelitis, left tibia and fibula CC
M86.069 Acute hematogenous osteomyelitis, unspecified tibia and fibula CC
M86.07 Acute hematogenous osteomyelitis, ankle and foot
M86.071 Acute hematogenous osteomyelitis, right ankle and foot CC
M86.072 Acute hematogenous osteomyelitis, left ankle and foot CC
M86.079 Acute hematogenous osteomyelitis, unspecified ankle and foot CC
M86.08 Acute hematogenous osteomyelitis, other sites CC
M86.09 Acute hematogenous osteomyelitis, multiple sites CC

M86.1 Other acute osteomyelitis
M86.10 Other acute osteomyelitis, unspecified site CC
M86.11 Other acute osteomyelitis, shoulder
M86.111 Other acute osteomyelitis, right shoulder CC
M86.112 Other acute osteomyelitis, left shoulder CC
M86.119 Other acute osteomyelitis, unspecified shoulder CC
M86.12 Other acute osteomyelitis, humerus
M86.121 Other acute osteomyelitis, right humerus CC
M86.122 Other acute osteomyelitis, left humerus CC
M86.129 Other acute osteomyelitis, unspecified humerus CC
M86.13 Other acute osteomyelitis, radius and ulna
M86.131 Other acute osteomyelitis, right radius and ulna CC
M86.132 Other acute osteomyelitis, left radius and ulna CC
M86.139 Other acute osteomyelitis, unspecified radius and ulna CC
M86.14 Other acute osteomyelitis, hand
M86.141 Other acute osteomyelitis, right hand CC
M86.142 Other acute osteomyelitis, left hand CC
M86.149 Other acute osteomyelitis, unspecified hand CC
M86.15 Other acute osteomyelitis, femur
M86.151 Other acute osteomyelitis, right femur CC
M86.152 Other acute osteomyelitis, left femur CC
M86.159 Other acute osteomyelitis, unspecified femur CC
M86.16 Other acute osteomyelitis, tibia and fibula
M86.161 Other acute osteomyelitis, right tibia and fibula CC
M86.162 Other acute osteomyelitis, left tibia and fibula CC
M86.169 Other acute osteomyelitis, unspecified tibia and fibula CC
M86.17 Other acute osteomyelitis, ankle and foot
M86.171 Other acute osteomyelitis, right ankle and foot CC
M86.172 Other acute osteomyelitis, left ankle and foot CC
M86.179 Other acute osteomyelitis, unspecified ankle and foot CC
M86.18 Other acute osteomyelitis, other site CC
M86.19 Other acute osteomyelitis, multiple sites CC

M86.2 Subacute osteomyelitis
M86.20 Subacute osteomyelitis, unspecified site CC
M86.21 Subacute osteomyelitis, shoulder
M86.211 Subacute osteomyelitis, right shoulder CC
M86.212 Subacute osteomyelitis, left shoulder CC
M86.219 Subacute osteomyelitis, unspecified shoulder CC
M86.22 Subacute osteomyelitis, humerus
M86.221 Subacute osteomyelitis, right humerus CC
M86.222 Subacute osteomyelitis, left humerus CC
M86.229 Subacute osteomyelitis, unspecified humerus CC
M86.23 Subacute osteomyelitis, radius and ulna
M86.231 Subacute osteomyelitis, right radius and ulna CC
M86.232 Subacute osteomyelitis, left radius and ulna CC
M86.239 Subacute osteomyelitis, unspecified radius and ulna CC
M86.24 Subacute osteomyelitis, hand
M86.241 Subacute osteomyelitis, right hand CC
M86.242 Subacute osteomyelitis, left hand CC

Unacceptable principal diagnosis symbol per Medicare code edits · Code exempt from diagnosis present on admission requirement
Questionable admission · Complication or comorbidity · CC/MCC exclusion · Major complication or comorbidity
Principal diagnosis as its own CC · Principal diagnosis as its own MCC · Z code as first-listed diagnosis

When symbols appear on a code that requires a 7th character extension, refer to Appendix D to identify applicable 7th character codes.

M86.249 Subacute osteomyelitis, unspecified hand
M86.25 Subacute osteomyelitis, femur
M86.251 Subacute osteomyelitis, right femur
M86.252 Subacute osteomyelitis, left femur
M86.259 Subacute osteomyelitis, unspecified femur
M86.26 Subacute osteomyelitis, tibia and fibula
M86.261 Subacute osteomyelitis, right tibia and fibula
M86.262 Subacute osteomyelitis, left tibia and fibula
M86.269 Subacute osteomyelitis, unspecified tibia and fibula
M86.27 Subacute osteomyelitis, ankle and foot
M86.271 Subacute osteomyelitis, right ankle and foot
M86.272 Subacute osteomyelitis, left ankle and foot
M86.279 Subacute osteomyelitis, unspecified ankle and foot
M86.28 Subacute osteomyelitis, other site
M86.29 Subacute osteomyelitis, multiple sites
M86.3 Chronic multifocal osteomyelitis
M86.30 Chronic multifocal osteomyelitis, unspecified site
M86.31 Chronic multifocal osteomyelitis, shoulder
M86.311 Chronic multifocal osteomyelitis, right shoulder
M86.312 Chronic multifocal osteomyelitis, left shoulder
M86.319 Chronic multifocal osteomyelitis, unspecified shoulder
M86.32 Chronic multifocal osteomyelitis, humerus
M86.321 Chronic multifocal osteomyelitis, right humerus
M86.322 Chronic multifocal osteomyelitis, left humerus
M86.329 Chronic multifocal osteomyelitis, unspecified humerus
M86.33 Chronic multifocal osteomyelitis, radius and ulna
M86.331 Chronic multifocal osteomyelitis, right radius and ulna
M86.332 Chronic multifocal osteomyelitis, left radius and ulna
M86.339 Chronic multifocal osteomyelitis, unspecified radius and ulna
M86.34 Chronic multifocal osteomyelitis, hand
M86.341 Chronic multifocal osteomyelitis, right hand
M86.342 Chronic multifocal osteomyelitis, left hand
M86.349 Chronic multifocal osteomyelitis, unspecified hand
M86.35 Chronic multifocal osteomyelitis, femur
M86.351 Chronic multifocal osteomyelitis, right femur
M86.352 Chronic multifocal osteomyelitis, left femur
M86.359 Chronic multifocal osteomyelitis, unspecified femur
M86.36 Chronic multifocal osteomyelitis, tibia and fibula
M86.361 Chronic multifocal osteomyelitis, right tibia and fibula
M86.362 Chronic multifocal osteomyelitis, left tibia and fibula
M86.369 Chronic multifocal osteomyelitis, unspecified tibia and fibula
M86.37 Chronic multifocal osteomyelitis, ankle and foot
M86.371 Chronic multifocal osteomyelitis, right ankle and foot
M86.372 Chronic multifocal osteomyelitis, left ankle and foot
M86.379 Chronic multifocal osteomyelitis, unspecified ankle and foot
M86.38 Chronic multifocal osteomyelitis, other site
M86.39 Chronic multifocal osteomyelitis, multiple sites
M86.4 Chronic osteomyelitis with draining sinus
M86.40 Chronic osteomyelitis with draining sinus, unspecified site
M86.41 Chronic osteomyelitis with draining sinus, shoulder
M86.411 Chronic osteomyelitis with draining sinus, right shoulder
M86.412 Chronic osteomyelitis with draining sinus, left shoulder
M86.419 Chronic osteomyelitis with draining sinus, unspecified shoulder
M86.42 Chronic osteomyelitis with draining sinus, humerus
M86.421 Chronic osteomyelitis with draining sinus, right humerus
M86.422 Chronic osteomyelitis with draining sinus, left humerus
M86.429 Chronic osteomyelitis with draining sinus, unspecified humerus
M86.43 Chronic osteomyelitis with draining sinus, radius and ulna
M86.431 Chronic osteomyelitis with draining sinus, right radius and ulna
M86.432 Chronic osteomyelitis with draining sinus, left radius and ulna
M86.439 Chronic osteomyelitis with draining sinus, unspecified radius and ulna
M86.44 Chronic osteomyelitis with draining sinus, hand
M86.441 Chronic osteomyelitis with draining sinus, right hand
M86.442 Chronic osteomyelitis with draining sinus, left hand
M86.449 Chronic osteomyelitis with draining sinus, unspecified hand
M86.45 Chronic osteomyelitis with draining sinus, femur
M86.451 Chronic osteomyelitis with draining sinus, right femur
M86.452 Chronic osteomyelitis with draining sinus, left femur
M86.459 Chronic osteomyelitis with draining sinus, unspecified femur
M86.46 Chronic osteomyelitis with draining sinus, tibia and fibula
M86.461 Chronic osteomyelitis with draining sinus, right tibia and fibula
M86.462 Chronic osteomyelitis with draining sinus, left tibia and fibula
M86.469 Chronic osteomyelitis with draining sinus, unspecified tibia and fibula
M86.47 Chronic osteomyelitis with draining sinus, ankle and foot
M86.471 Chronic osteomyelitis with draining sinus, right ankle and foot
M86.472 Chronic osteomyelitis with draining sinus, left ankle and foot
M86.479 Chronic osteomyelitis with draining sinus, unspecified ankle and foot
M86.48 Chronic osteomyelitis with draining sinus, other site
M86.49 Chronic osteomyelitis with draining sinus, multiple sites
M86.5 Other chronic hematogenous osteomyelitis
M86.50 Other chronic hematogenous osteomyelitis, unspecified site
M86.51 Other chronic hematogenous osteomyelitis, shoulder
M86.511 Other chronic hematogenous osteomyelitis, right shoulder
M86.512 Other chronic hematogenous osteomyelitis, left shoulder
M86.519 Other chronic hematogenous osteomyelitis, unspecified shoulder
M86.52 Other chronic hematogenous osteomyelitis, humerus
M86.521 Other chronic hematogenous osteomyelitis, right humerus

Unspecified Code · Other Specified Code · Manifestation Code · N Newborn · P Pediatric · M Maternity · A Adult · ♂ Male · ♀ Female
● New Code · ▲ Revised Code Title · ►◄ Revised Text · NOTES · INCLUDES · EXCLUDES 1 Not coded here · EXCLUDES 2 Not included here
4th character required · 5th character required · 6th character required · 7th character required
Extension 'X' Alert · HAC Hospital-acquired condition (HAC) alert · AHA AHA Coding Clinic©

M86.522 Other chronic hematogenous osteomyelitis, left humerus
M86.529 Other chronic hematogenous osteomyelitis, unspecified humerus
M86.53 Other chronic hematogenous osteomyelitis, radius and ulna
M86.531 Other chronic hematogenous osteomyelitis, right radius and ulna
M86.532 Other chronic hematogenous osteomyelitis, left radius and ulna
M86.539 Other chronic hematogenous osteomyelitis, unspecified radius and ulna
M86.54 Other chronic hematogenous osteomyelitis, hand
M86.541 Other chronic hematogenous osteomyelitis, right hand
M86.542 Other chronic hematogenous osteomyelitis, left hand
M86.549 Other chronic hematogenous osteomyelitis, unspecified hand
M86.55 Other chronic hematogenous osteomyelitis, femur
M86.551 Other chronic hematogenous osteomyelitis, right femur
M86.552 Other chronic hematogenous osteomyelitis, left femur
M86.559 Other chronic hematogenous osteomyelitis, unspecified femur
M86.56 Other chronic hematogenous osteomyelitis, tibia and fibula
M86.561 Other chronic hematogenous osteomyelitis, right tibia and fibula
M86.562 Other chronic hematogenous osteomyelitis, left tibia and fibula
M86.569 Other chronic hematogenous osteomyelitis, unspecified tibia and fibula
M86.57 Other chronic hematogenous osteomyelitis, ankle and foot
M86.571 Other chronic hematogenous osteomyelitis, right ankle and foot
M86.572 Other chronic hematogenous osteomyelitis, left ankle and foot
M86.579 Other chronic hematogenous osteomyelitis, unspecified ankle and foot
M86.58 Other chronic hematogenous osteomyelitis, other site
M86.59 Other chronic hematogenous osteomyelitis, multiple sites
M86.6 Other chronic osteomyelitis
M86.60 Other chronic osteomyelitis, unspecified site
M86.61 Other chronic osteomyelitis, shoulder
M86.611 Other chronic osteomyelitis, right shoulder
M86.612 Other chronic osteomyelitis, left shoulder
M86.619 Other chronic osteomyelitis, unspecified shoulder
M86.62 Other chronic osteomyelitis, humerus
M86.621 Other chronic osteomyelitis, right humerus
M86.622 Other chronic osteomyelitis, left humerus
M86.629 Other chronic osteomyelitis, unspecified humerus
M86.63 Other chronic osteomyelitis, radius and ulna
M86.631 Other chronic osteomyelitis, right radius and ulna
M86.632 Other chronic osteomyelitis, left radius and ulna
M86.639 Other chronic osteomyelitis, unspecified radius and ulna
M86.64 Other chronic osteomyelitis, hand
M86.641 Other chronic osteomyelitis, right hand
M86.642 Other chronic osteomyelitis, left hand
M86.649 Other chronic osteomyelitis, unspecified hand
M86.65 Other chronic osteomyelitis, thigh
M86.651 Other chronic osteomyelitis, right thigh
M86.652 Other chronic osteomyelitis, left thigh
M86.659 Other chronic osteomyelitis, unspecified thigh
M86.66 Other chronic osteomyelitis, tibia and fibula
M86.661 Other chronic osteomyelitis, right tibia and fibula
M86.662 Other chronic osteomyelitis, left tibia and fibula
M86.669 Other chronic osteomyelitis, unspecified tibia and fibula
M86.67 Other chronic osteomyelitis, ankle and foot
M86.671 Other chronic osteomyelitis, right ankle and foot
AHA: Q1, 2016
M86.672 Other chronic osteomyelitis, left ankle and foot
M86.679 Other chronic osteomyelitis, unspecified ankle and foot
M86.68 Other chronic osteomyelitis, other site
M86.69 Other chronic osteomyelitis, multiple sites
M86.8 Other osteomyelitis
Brodie's abscess
M86.8X Other osteomyelitis
M86.8X0 Other osteomyelitis, multiple sites
M86.8X1 Other osteomyelitis, shoulder
M86.8X2 Other osteomyelitis, upper arm
M86.8X3 Other osteomyelitis, forearm
M86.8X4 Other osteomyelitis, hand
M86.8X5 Other osteomyelitis, thigh
M86.8X6 Other osteomyelitis, lower leg
M86.8X7 Other osteomyelitis, ankle and foot
M86.8X8 Other osteomyelitis, other site
M86.8X9 Other osteomyelitis, unspecified sites
M86.9 Osteomyelitis, unspecified
Infection of bone NOS
Periostitis without osteomyelitis
M87 Osteonecrosis
INCLUDES *avascular necrosis of bone*
Use additional code to identify major osseous defect, if applicable (M89.7-)
EXCLUDES1 *juvenile osteonecrosis (M91-M92)*
osteochondropathies (M90-M93)
M87.0 Idiopathic aseptic necrosis of bone
M87.00 Idiopathic aseptic necrosis of unspecified bone
M87.01 Idiopathic aseptic necrosis of shoulder
Idiopathic aseptic necrosis of clavicle and scapula
M87.011 Idiopathic aseptic necrosis of right shoulder
M87.012 Idiopathic aseptic necrosis of left shoulder
M87.019 Idiopathic aseptic necrosis of unspecified shoulder
M87.02 Idiopathic aseptic necrosis of humerus
M87.021 Idiopathic aseptic necrosis of right humerus
M87.022 Idiopathic aseptic necrosis of left humerus
M87.029 Idiopathic aseptic necrosis of unspecified humerus
M87.03 Idiopathic aseptic necrosis of radius, ulna and carpus
M87.031 Idiopathic aseptic necrosis of right radius
M87.032 Idiopathic aseptic necrosis of left radius
M87.033 Idiopathic aseptic necrosis of unspecified radius
M87.034 Idiopathic aseptic necrosis of right ulna
M87.035 Idiopathic aseptic necrosis of left ulna

Unacceptable principal diagnosis symbol per Medicare code edits | Code exempt from diagnosis present on admission requirement
Questionable admission | Complication or comorbidity | CC/MCC exclusion | Major complication or comorbidity
Principal diagnosis as its own CC | Principal diagnosis as its own MCC | Z code as first-listed diagnosis

M87.036 Idiopathic aseptic necrosis of unspecified ulna CC
M87.037 Idiopathic aseptic necrosis of right carpus CC
M87.038 Idiopathic aseptic necrosis of left carpus CC
M87.039 Idiopathic aseptic necrosis of unspecified carpus CC
M87.04 Idiopathic aseptic necrosis of hand and fingers
Idiopathic aseptic necrosis of metacarpals and phalanges of hands
M87.041 Idiopathic aseptic necrosis of right hand CC
M87.042 Idiopathic aseptic necrosis of left hand CC
M87.043 Idiopathic aseptic necrosis of unspecified hand CC
M87.044 Idiopathic aseptic necrosis of right finger(s) CC
M87.045 Idiopathic aseptic necrosis of left finger(s) CC
M87.046 Idiopathic aseptic necrosis of unspecified finger(s) CC
M87.05 Idiopathic aseptic necrosis of pelvis and femur
M87.050 Idiopathic aseptic necrosis of pelvis CC
M87.051 Idiopathic aseptic necrosis of right femur CC
M87.052 Idiopathic aseptic necrosis of left femur CC
M87.059 Idiopathic aseptic necrosis of unspecified femur CC
Idiopathic aseptic necrosis of hip NOS
M87.06 Idiopathic aseptic necrosis of tibia and fibula
M87.061 Idiopathic aseptic necrosis of right tibia CC
M87.062 Idiopathic aseptic necrosis of left tibia CC
M87.063 Idiopathic aseptic necrosis of unspecified tibia CC
M87.064 Idiopathic aseptic necrosis of right fibula CC
M87.065 Idiopathic aseptic necrosis of left fibula CC
M87.066 Idiopathic aseptic necrosis of unspecified fibula CC
M87.07 Idiopathic aseptic necrosis of ankle, foot and toes
Idiopathic aseptic necrosis of metatarsus, tarsus, and phalanges of toes
M87.071 Idiopathic aseptic necrosis of right ankle CC
M87.072 Idiopathic aseptic necrosis of left ankle CC
M87.073 Idiopathic aseptic necrosis of unspecified ankle CC
M87.074 Idiopathic aseptic necrosis of right foot CC
M87.075 Idiopathic aseptic necrosis of left foot CC
M87.076 Idiopathic aseptic necrosis of unspecified foot CC
M87.077 Idiopathic aseptic necrosis of right toe(s) CC
M87.078 Idiopathic aseptic necrosis of left toe(s) CC
M87.079 Idiopathic aseptic necrosis of unspecified toe(s) CC
M87.08 Idiopathic aseptic necrosis of bone, other site CC
M87.09 Idiopathic aseptic necrosis of bone, multiple sites CC
M87.1 Osteonecrosis due to drugs
Use additional code for adverse effect, if applicable, to identify drug (T36-T50 with fifth or sixth character 5)
M87.10 Osteonecrosis due to drugs, unspecified bone CC
M87.11 Osteonecrosis due to drugs, shoulder
M87.111 Osteonecrosis due to drugs, right shoulder CC
M87.112 Osteonecrosis due to drugs, left shoulder CC
M87.119 Osteonecrosis due to drugs, unspecified shoulder CC
M87.12 Osteonecrosis due to drugs, humerus
M87.121 Osteonecrosis due to drugs, right humerus CC
M87.122 Osteonecrosis due to drugs, left humerus CC
M87.129 Osteonecrosis due to drugs, unspecified humerus CC
M87.13 Osteonecrosis due to drugs of radius, ulna and carpus
M87.131 Osteonecrosis due to drugs of right radius CC
M87.132 Osteonecrosis due to drugs of left radius CC
M87.133 Osteonecrosis due to drugs of unspecified radius CC
M87.134 Osteonecrosis due to drugs of right ulna CC
M87.135 Osteonecrosis due to drugs of left ulna CC
M87.136 Osteonecrosis due to drugs of unspecified ulna CC
M87.137 Osteonecrosis due to drugs of right carpus CC
M87.138 Osteonecrosis due to drugs of left carpus CC
M87.139 Osteonecrosis due to drugs of unspecified carpus CC
M87.14 Osteonecrosis due to drugs, hand and fingers
M87.141 Osteonecrosis due to drugs, right hand CC
M87.142 Osteonecrosis due to drugs, left hand CC
M87.143 Osteonecrosis due to drugs, unspecified hand CC
M87.144 Osteonecrosis due to drugs, right f inger(s) CC
M87.145 Osteonecrosis due to drugs, left finger(s) CC
M87.146 Osteonecrosis due to drugs, unspecified finger(s) CC
M87.15 Osteonecrosis due to drugs, pelvis and femur
M87.150 Osteonecrosis due to drugs, pelvis CC
M87.151 Osteonecrosis due to drugs, right femur CC
M87.152 Osteonecrosis due to drugs, left femur CC
M87.159 Osteonecrosis due to drugs, unspecified femur CC
M87.16 Osteonecrosis due to drugs, tibia and fibula
M87.161 Osteonecrosis due to drugs, right tibia CC
M87.162 Osteonecrosis due to drugs, left tibia CC
M87.163 Osteonecrosis due to drugs, unspecified tibia CC
M87.164 Osteonecrosis due to drugs, right fibula CC
M87.165 Osteonecrosis due to drugs, left fibula CC
M87.166 Osteonecrosis due to drugs, unspecified fibula CC
M87.17 Osteonecrosis due to drugs, ankle, foot and toes
M87.171 Osteonecrosis due to drugs, right ankle CC
M87.172 Osteonecrosis due to drugs, left ankle CC
M87.173 Osteonecrosis due to drugs, unspecified ankle CC
M87.174 Osteonecrosis due to drugs, right foot CC
M87.175 Osteonecrosis due to drugs, left foot CC
M87.176 Osteonecrosis due to drugs, unspecified foot CC
M87.177 Osteonecrosis due to drugs, right toe(s) CC
M87.178 Osteonecrosis due to drugs, left toe(s) CC
M87.179 Osteonecrosis due to drugs, unspecified toe(s) CC
M87.18 Osteonecrosis due to drugs, other site
M87.180 Osteonecrosis due to drugs, jaw CC
M87.188 Osteonecrosis due to drugs, other site CC
M87.19 Osteonecrosis due to drugs, multiple sites CC
M87.2 Osteonecrosis due to previous trauma
M87.20 Osteonecrosis due to previous trauma, unspecified bone CC
M87.21 Osteonecrosis due to previous trauma, shoulder
M87.211 Osteonecrosis due to previous trauma, right shoulder CC

Unspecified Code Other Specified Code Manifestation Code N Newborn P Pediatric M Maternity A Adult ♂ Male ♀ Female
● New Code ▲ Revised Code Title ►◄ Revised Text NOTES INCLUDES EXCLUDES 1 Not coded here EXCLUDES 2 Not included here
4th character required 5th character required 6th character required 7th character required
Extension 'X' Alert HAC Hospital-acquired condition (HAC) alert AHA AHA Coding Clinic®

M87.212 Osteonecrosis due to previous trauma, left shoulder CC
M87.219 Osteonecrosis due to previous trauma, unspecified shoulder CC
M87.22 Osteonecrosis due to previous trauma, humerus
M87.221 Osteonecrosis due to previous trauma, right humerus CC
M87.222 Osteonecrosis due to previous trauma, left humerus CC
M87.229 Osteonecrosis due to previous trauma, unspecified humerus CC
M87.23 Osteonecrosis due to previous trauma of radius, ulna and carpus
M87.231 Osteonecrosis due to previous trauma of right radius CC
M87.232 Osteonecrosis due to previous trauma of left radius CC
M87.233 Osteonecrosis due to previous trauma of unspecified radius CC
M87.234 Osteonecrosis due to previous trauma of right ulna CC
M87.235 Osteonecrosis due to previous trauma of left ulna CC
M87.236 Osteonecrosis due to previous trauma of unspecified ulna CC
M87.237 Osteonecrosis due to previous trauma of right carpus CC
M87.238 Osteonecrosis due to previous trauma of left carpus CC
M87.239 Osteonecrosis due to previous trauma of unspecified carpus CC
M87.24 Osteonecrosis due to previous trauma, hand and fingers
M87.241 Osteonecrosis due to previous trauma, right hand CC
M87.242 Osteonecrosis due to previous trauma, left hand CC
M87.243 Osteonecrosis due to previous trauma, unspecified hand CC
M87.244 Osteonecrosis due to previous trauma, right finger(s) CC
M87.245 Osteonecrosis due to previous trauma, left finger(s) CC
M87.246 Osteonecrosis due to previous trauma, unspecified finger(s) CC
M87.25 Osteonecrosis due to previous trauma, pelvis and femur
M87.250 Osteonecrosis due to previous trauma, pelvis CC
M87.251 Osteonecrosis due to previous trauma, right femur CC
M87.252 Osteonecrosis due to previous trauma, left femur CC
M87.256 Osteonecrosis due to previous trauma, unspecified femur CC
M87.26 Osteonecrosis due to previous trauma, tibia and fibula
M87.261 Osteonecrosis due to previous trauma, right tibia CC
M87.262 Osteonecrosis due to previous trauma, left tibia CC
M87.263 Osteonecrosis due to previous trauma, unspecified tibia CC
M87.264 Osteonecrosis due to previous trauma, right fibula CC
M87.265 Osteonecrosis due to previous trauma, left fibula CC
M87.266 Osteonecrosis due to previous trauma, unspecified fibula CC
M87.27 Osteonecrosis due to previous trauma, ankle, foot and toes
M87.271 Osteonecrosis due to previous trauma, right ankle CC
M87.272 Osteonecrosis due to previous trauma, left ankle CC
M87.273 Osteonecrosis due to previous trauma, unspecified ankle CC
M87.274 Osteonecrosis due to previous trauma, right foot CC
M87.275 Osteonecrosis due to previous trauma, left foot CC
M87.276 Osteonecrosis due to previous trauma, unspecified foot CC
M87.277 Osteonecrosis due to previous trauma, right toe(s) CC
M87.278 Osteonecrosis due to previous trauma, left toe(s) CC
M87.279 Osteonecrosis due to previous trauma, unspecified toe(s) CC
M87.28 Osteonecrosis due to previous trauma, other site CC
M87.29 Osteonecrosis due to previous trauma, multiple sites CC
M87.3 Other secondary osteonecrosis
M87.30 Other secondary osteonecrosis, unspecified bone CC
M87.31 Other secondary osteonecrosis, shoulder
M87.311 Other secondary osteonecrosis, right shoulder CC
M87.312 Other secondary osteonecrosis, left shoulder CC
M87.319 Other secondary osteonecrosis, unspecified shoulder CC
M87.32 Other secondary osteonecrosis, humerus
M87.321 Other secondary osteonecrosis, right humerus CC
M87.322 Other secondary osteonecrosis, left humerus CC
M87.329 Other secondary osteonecrosis, unspecified humerus CC
M87.33 Other secondary osteonecrosis of radius, ulna and carpus
M87.331 Other secondary osteonecrosis of right radius CC
M87.332 Other secondary osteonecrosis of left radius CC
M87.333 Other secondary osteonecrosis of unspecified radius CC
M87.334 Other secondary osteonecrosis of right ulna CC
M87.335 Other secondary osteonecrosis of left ulna CC
M87.336 Other secondary osteonecrosis of unspecified ulna CC
M87.337 Other secondary osteonecrosis of right carpus CC
M87.338 Other secondary osteonecrosis of left carpus CC
M87.339 Other secondary osteonecrosis of unspecified carpus CC
M87.34 Other secondary osteonecrosis, hand and fingers
M87.341 Other secondary osteonecrosis, right hand CC
M87.342 Other secondary osteonecrosis, left hand CC
M87.343 Other secondary osteonecrosis, unspecified hand CC
M87.344 Other secondary osteonecrosis, right finger(s) CC
M87.345 Other secondary osteonecrosis, left finger(s) CC
M87.346 Other secondary osteonecrosis, unspecified finger(s) CC
M87.35 Other secondary osteonecrosis, pelvis and femur
M87.350 Other secondary osteonecrosis, pelvis CC
M87.351 Other secondary osteonecrosis, right femur CC
M87.352 Other secondary osteonecrosis, left femur CC
M87.353 Other secondary osteonecrosis, unspecified femur CC
M87.36 Other secondary osteonecrosis, tibia and fibula

PDx Unacceptable principal diagnosis symbol per Medicare code edits; POA Code exempt from diagnosis present on admission requirement
Q Questionable admission; CC Complication or comorbidity; CC/MCC Exc CC/MCC exclusion; MCC Major complication or comorbidity
PDx CC Principal diagnosis as its own CC; PDx MCC Principal diagnosis as its own MCC; Z1 Z code as first-listed diagnosis

M87.361 Other secondary osteonecrosis, right tibia
M87.362 Other secondary osteonecrosis, left tibia
M87.363 Other secondary osteonecrosis, unspecified tibia
M87.364 Other secondary osteonecrosis, right fibula
M87.365 Other secondary osteonecrosis, left fibula
M87.366 Other secondary osteonecrosis, unspecified fibula
M87.37 Other secondary osteonecrosis, ankle and foot
M87.371 Other secondary osteonecrosis, right ankle
M87.372 Other secondary osteonecrosis, left ankle
M87.373 Other secondary osteonecrosis, unspecified ankle
M87.374 Other secondary osteonecrosis, right foot
M87.375 Other secondary osteonecrosis, left foot
M87.376 Other secondary osteonecrosis, unspecified foot
M87.377 Other secondary osteonecrosis, right toe(s)
M87.378 Other secondary osteonecrosis, left toe(s)
M87.379 Other secondary osteonecrosis, unspecified toe(s)
M87.38 Other secondary osteonecrosis, other site
M87.39 Other secondary osteonecrosis, multiple sites
M87.8 Other osteonecrosis
M87.80 Other osteonecrosis, unspecified bone
M87.81 Other osteonecrosis, shoulder
M87.811 Other osteonecrosis, right shoulder
M87.812 Other osteonecrosis, left shoulder
M87.819 Other osteonecrosis, unspecified shoulder
M87.82 Other osteonecrosis, humerus
M87.821 Other osteonecrosis, right humerus
M87.822 Other osteonecrosis, left humerus
M87.829 Other osteonecrosis, unspecified humerus
M87.83 Other osteonecrosis of radius, ulna and carpus
M87.831 Other osteonecrosis of right radius
M87.832 Other osteonecrosis of left radius
M87.833 Other osteonecrosis of unspecified radius
M87.834 Other osteonecrosis of right ulna
M87.835 Other osteonecrosis of left ulna
M87.836 Other osteonecrosis of unspecified ulna
M87.837 Other osteonecrosis of right carpus
M87.838 Other osteonecrosis of left carpus
M87.839 Other osteonecrosis of unspecified carpus
M87.84 Other osteonecrosis, hand and fingers
M87.841 Other osteonecrosis, right hand
M87.842 Other osteonecrosis, left hand
M87.843 Other osteonecrosis, unspecified hand
M87.844 Other osteonecrosis, right finger(s)
M87.845 Other osteonecrosis, left finger(s)
M87.849 Other osteonecrosis, unspecified finger(s)
M87.85 Other osteonecrosis, pelvis and femur
M87.850 Other osteonecrosis, pelvis
M87.851 Other osteonecrosis, right femur
M87.852 Other osteonecrosis, left femur
M87.859 Other osteonecrosis, unspecified femur
M87.86 Other osteonecrosis, tibia and fibula
M87.861 Other osteonecrosis, right tibia
M87.862 Other osteonecrosis, left tibia
M87.863 Other osteonecrosis, unspecified tibia
M87.864 Other osteonecrosis, right fibula
M87.865 Other osteonecrosis, left fibula
M87.869 Other osteonecrosis, unspecified fibula
M87.87 Other osteonecrosis, ankle, foot and toes
M87.871 Other osteonecrosis, right ankle
M87.872 Other osteonecrosis, left ankle
M87.873 Other osteonecrosis, unspecified ankle
M87.874 Other osteonecrosis, right foot
M87.875 Other osteonecrosis, left foot
M87.876 Other osteonecrosis, unspecified foot
M87.877 Other osteonecrosis, right toe(s)
M87.878 Other osteonecrosis, left toe(s)
M87.879 Other osteonecrosis, unspecified toe(s)
M87.88 Other osteonecrosis, other site
M87.89 Other osteonecrosis, multiple sites
M87.9 Osteonecrosis, unspecified
Necrosis of bone NOS
M88 Osteitis deformans [Paget's disease of bone]
EXCLUDES1 *osteitis deformans in neoplastic disease (M90.6)*
M88.0 Osteitis deformans of skull
M88.1 Osteitis deformans of vertebrae
M88.8 Osteitis deformans of other bones
M88.81 Osteitis deformans of shoulder
M88.811 Osteitis deformans of right shoulder
M88.812 Osteitis deformans of left shoulder
M88.819 Osteitis deformans of unspecified shoulder
M88.82 Osteitis deformans of upper arm
M88.821 Osteitis deformans of right upper arm
M88.822 Osteitis deformans of left upper arm
M88.829 Osteitis deformans of unspecified upper arm
M88.83 Osteitis deformans of forearm
M88.831 Osteitis deformans of right forearm
M88.832 Osteitis deformans of left forearm
M88.839 Osteitis deformans of unspecified forearm
M88.84 Osteitis deformans of hand
M88.841 Osteitis deformans of right hand
M88.842 Osteitis deformans of left hand
M88.849 Osteitis deformans of unspecified hand
M88.85 Osteitis deformans of thigh
M88.851 Osteitis deformans of right thigh
M88.852 Osteitis deformans of left thigh
M88.859 Osteitis deformans of unspecified thigh
M88.86 Osteitis deformans of lower leg
M88.861 Osteitis deformans of right lower leg
M88.862 Osteitis deformans of left lower leg
M88.869 Osteitis deformans of unspecified lower leg
M88.87 Osteitis deformans of ankle and foot
M88.871 Osteitis deformans of right ankle and foot
M88.872 Osteitis deformans of left ankle and foot
M88.879 Osteitis deformans of unspecified ankle and foot
M88.88 Osteitis deformans of other bones
EXCLUDES2 *osteitis deformans of skull (M88.0)*
osteitis deformans of vertebrae (M88.1)
M88.89 Osteitis deformans of multiple sites
M88.9 Osteitis deformans of unspecified bone
M89 Other disorders of bone
M89.0 Algoneurodystrophy
Shoulder-hand syndrome
Sudeck's atrophy
EXCLUDES1 *causalgia, lower limb (G57.7-)*
causalgia, upper limb (G56.4-)
complex regional pain syndrome II, lower limb (G57.7-)
complex regional pain syndrome II, upper limb (G56.4-)
reflex sympathetic dystrophy (G90.5-)
M89.00 Algoneurodystrophy, unspecified site
M89.01 Algoneurodystrophy, shoulder
M89.011 Algoneurodystrophy, right shoulder
M89.012 Algoneurodystrophy, left shoulder

M89.019 Algoneurodystrophy, unspecified shoulder
M89.02 Algoneurodystrophy, upper arm
M89.021 Algoneurodystrophy, right upper arm
M89.022 Algoneurodystrophy, left upper arm
M89.029 Algoneurodystrophy, unspecified upper arm
M89.03 Algoneurodystrophy, forearm
M89.031 Algoneurodystrophy, right forearm
M89.032 Algoneurodystrophy, left forearm
M89.039 Algoneurodystrophy, unspecified forearm
M89.04 Algoneurodystrophy, hand
M89.041 Algoneurodystrophy, right hand
M89.042 Algoneurodystrophy, left hand
M89.049 Algoneurodystrophy, unspecified hand
M89.05 Algoneurodystrophy, thigh
M89.051 Algoneurodystrophy, right thigh
M89.052 Algoneurodystrophy, left thigh
M89.059 Algoneurodystrophy, unspecified thigh
M89.06 Algoneurodystrophy, lower leg
M89.061 Algoneurodystrophy, right lower leg
M89.062 Algoneurodystrophy, left lower leg
M89.069 Algoneurodystrophy, unspecified lower leg
M89.07 Algoneurodystrophy, ankle and foot
M89.071 Algoneurodystrophy, right ankle and foot
M89.072 Algoneurodystrophy, left ankle and foot
M89.079 Algoneurodystrophy, unspecified ankle and foot
M89.08 Algoneurodystrophy, other site
M89.09 Algoneurodystrophy, multiple sites
M89.1 Physeal arrest
Arrest of growth plate
Epiphyseal arrest
Growth plate arrest
M89.12 Physeal arrest, humerus
M89.121 Complete physeal arrest, right proximal humerus
M89.122 Complete physeal arrest, left proximal humerus
M89.123 Partial physeal arrest, right proximal humerus
M89.124 Partial physeal arrest, left proximal humerus
M89.125 Complete physeal arrest, right distal humerus
M89.126 Complete physeal arrest, left distal humerus
M89.127 Partial physeal arrest, right distal humerus
M89.128 Partial physeal arrest, left distal humerus
M89.129 Physeal arrest, humerus, unspecified
M89.13 Physeal arrest, forearm
M89.131 Complete physeal arrest, right distal radius
M89.132 Complete physeal arrest, left distal radius
M89.133 Partial physeal arrest, right distal radius
M89.134 Partial physeal arrest, left distal radius
M89.138 Other physeal arrest of forearm
M89.139 Physeal arrest, forearm, unspecified
M89.15 Physeal arrest, femur
M89.151 Complete physeal arrest, right proximal femur
M89.152 Complete physeal arrest, left proximal femur
M89.153 Partial physeal arrest, right proximal femur
M89.154 Partial physeal arrest, left proximal femur
M89.155 Complete physeal arrest, right distal femur
M89.156 Complete physeal arrest, left distal femur
M89.157 Partial physeal arrest, right distal femur
M89.158 Partial physeal arrest, left distal femur
M89.159 Physeal arrest, femur, unspecified
M89.16 Physeal arrest, lower leg
M89.160 Complete physeal arrest, right proximal tibia
M89.161 Complete physeal arrest, left proximal tibia
M89.162 Partial physeal arrest, right proximal tibia
M89.163 Partial physeal arrest, left proximal tibia
M89.164 Complete physeal arrest, right distal tibia
M89.165 Complete physeal arrest, left distal tibia
M89.166 Partial physeal arrest, right distal tibia
M89.167 Partial physeal arrest, left distal tibia
M89.168 Other physeal arrest of lower leg
M89.169 Physeal arrest, lower leg, unspecified
M89.18 Physeal arrest, other site
M89.2 Other disorders of bone development and growth
M89.20 Other disorders of bone development and growth, unspecified site
M89.21 Other disorders of bone development and growth, shoulder
M89.211 Other disorders of bone development and growth, right shoulder
M89.212 Other disorders of bone development and growth, left shoulder
M89.219 Other disorders of bone development and growth, unspecified shoulder
M89.22 Other disorders of bone development and growth, humerus
M89.221 Other disorders of bone development and growth, right humerus
M89.222 Other disorders of bone development and growth, left humerus
M89.229 Other disorders of bone development and growth, unspecified humerus
M89.23 Other disorders of bone development and growth, ulna and radius
M89.231 Other disorders of bone development and growth, right ulna
M89.232 Other disorders of bone development and growth, left ulna
M89.233 Other disorders of bone development and growth, right radius
M89.234 Other disorders of bone development and growth, left radius
M89.239 Other disorders of bone development and growth, unspecified ulna and radius
M89.24 Other disorders of bone development and growth, hand
M89.241 Other disorders of bone development and growth, right hand
M89.242 Other disorders of bone development and growth, left hand
M89.249 Other disorders of bone development and growth, unspecified hand
M89.25 Other disorders of bone development and growth, femur
M89.251 Other disorders of bone development and growth, right femur
M89.252 Other disorders of bone development and growth, left femur
M89.259 Other disorders of bone development and growth, unspecified femur
M89.26 Other disorders of bone development and growth, tibia and fibula
M89.261 Other disorders of bone development and growth, right tibia
M89.262 Other disorders of bone development and growth, left tibia
M89.263 Other disorders of bone development and growth, right fibula
M89.264 Other disorders of bone development and growth, left fibula
M89.269 Other disorders of bone development and growth, unspecified lower leg
M89.27 Other disorders of bone development and growth, ankle and foot
M89.271 Other disorders of bone development and growth, right ankle and foot

Unacceptable principal diagnosis symbol per Medicare code edits | Code exempt from diagnosis present on admission requirement
Questionable admission | Complication or comorbidity | CC/MCC exclusion | Major complication or comorbidity
Principal diagnosis as its own CC | Principal diagnosis as its own MCC | Z code as first-listed diagnosis

M89.272 Other disorders of bone development and growth, left ankle and foot
M89.279 Other disorders of bone development and growth, unspecified ankle and foot
M89.28 Other disorders of bone development and growth, other site
M89.29 Other disorders of bone development and growth, multiple sites
M89.3 Hypertrophy of bone
M89.30 Hypertrophy of bone, unspecified site
M89.31 Hypertrophy of bone, shoulder
M89.311 Hypertrophy of bone, right shoulder
M89.312 Hypertrophy of bone, left shoulder
M89.319 Hypertrophy of bone, unspecified shoulder
M89.32 Hypertrophy of bone, humerus
M89.321 Hypertrophy of bone, right humerus
M89.322 Hypertrophy of bone, left humerus
M89.329 Hypertrophy of bone, unspecified humerus
M89.33 Hypertrophy of bone, ulna and radius
M89.331 Hypertrophy of bone, right ulna
M89.332 Hypertrophy of bone, left ulna
M89.333 Hypertrophy of bone, right radius
M89.334 Hypertrophy of bone, left radius
M89.339 Hypertrophy of bone, unspecified ulna and radius
M89.34 Hypertrophy of bone, hand
M89.341 Hypertrophy of bone, right hand
M89.342 Hypertrophy of bone, left hand
M89.349 Hypertrophy of bone, unspecified hand
M89.35 Hypertrophy of bone, femur
M89.351 Hypertrophy of bone, right femur
M89.352 Hypertrophy of bone, left femur
M89.359 Hypertrophy of bone, unspecified femur
M89.36 Hypertrophy of bone, tibia and fibula
M89.361 Hypertrophy of bone, right tibia
M89.362 Hypertrophy of bone, left tibia
M89.363 Hypertrophy of bone, right fibula
M89.364 Hypertrophy of bone, left fibula
M89.369 Hypertrophy of bone, unspecified tibia and fibula
M89.37 Hypertrophy of bone, ankle and foot
M89.371 Hypertrophy of bone, right ankle and foot
M89.372 Hypertrophy of bone, left ankle and foot
M89.379 Hypertrophy of bone, unspecified ankle and foot
M89.38 Hypertrophy of bone, other site
M89.39 Hypertrophy of bone, multiple sites
M89.4 Other hypertrophic osteoarthropathy
Marie-Bamberger disease
Pachydermoperiostosis
M89.40 Other hypertrophic osteoarthropathy, unspecified site
M89.41 Other hypertrophic osteoarthropathy, shoulder
M89.411 Other hypertrophic osteoarthropathy, right shoulder
M89.412 Other hypertrophic osteoarthropathy, left shoulder
M89.419 Other hypertrophic osteoarthropathy, unspecified shoulder
M89.42 Other hypertrophic osteoarthropathy, upper arm
M89.421 Other hypertrophic osteoarthropathy, right upper arm
M89.422 Other hypertrophic osteoarthropathy, left upper arm
M89.429 Other hypertrophic osteoarthropathy, unspecified upper arm
M89.43 Other hypertrophic osteoarthropathy, forearm
M89.431 Other hypertrophic osteoarthropathy, right forearm
M89.432 Other hypertrophic osteoarthropathy, left forearm
M89.439 Other hypertrophic osteoarthropathy, unspecified forearm
M89.44 Other hypertrophic osteoarthropathy, hand
M89.441 Other hypertrophic osteoarthropathy, right hand
M89.442 Other hypertrophic osteoarthropathy, left hand
M89.449 Other hypertrophic osteoarthropathy, unspecified hand
M89.45 Other hypertrophic osteoarthropathy, thigh
M89.451 Other hypertrophic osteoarthropathy, right thigh
M89.452 Other hypertrophic osteoarthropathy, left thigh
M89.459 Other hypertrophic osteoarthropathy, unspecified thigh
M89.46 Other hypertrophic osteoarthropathy, lower leg
M89.461 Other hypertrophic osteoarthropathy, right lower leg
M89.462 Other hypertrophic osteoarthropathy, left lower leg
M89.469 Other hypertrophic osteoarthropathy, unspecified lower leg
M89.47 Other hypertrophic osteoarthropathy, ankle and foot
M89.471 Other hypertrophic osteoarthropathy, right ankle and foot
M89.472 Other hypertrophic osteoarthropathy, left ankle and foot
M89.479 Other hypertrophic osteoarthropathy, unspecified ankle and foot
M89.48 Other hypertrophic osteoarthropathy, other site
M89.49 Other hypertrophic osteoarthropathy, multiple sites
M89.5 Osteolysis
Use additional code to identify major osseous defect, if applicable (M89.7-)
EXCLUDES2 *periprosthetic osteolysis of internal prosthetic joint (T84.05-)*
M89.50 Osteolysis, unspecified site
M89.51 Osteolysis, shoulder
M89.511 Osteolysis, right shoulder
M89.512 Osteolysis, left shoulder
M89.519 Osteolysis, unspecified shoulder
M89.52 Osteolysis, upper arm
M89.521 Osteolysis, right upper arm
M89.522 Osteolysis, left upper arm
M89.529 Osteolysis, unspecified upper arm
M89.53 Osteolysis, forearm
M89.531 Osteolysis, right forearm
M89.532 Osteolysis, left forearm
M89.539 Osteolysis, unspecified forearm
M89.54 Osteolysis, hand
M89.541 Osteolysis, right hand
M89.542 Osteolysis, left hand
M89.549 Osteolysis, unspecified hand
M89.55 Osteolysis, thigh
M89.551 Osteolysis, right thigh
M89.552 Osteolysis, left thigh
M89.559 Osteolysis, unspecified thigh
M89.56 Osteolysis, lower leg
M89.561 Osteolysis, right lower leg
M89.562 Osteolysis, left lower leg
M89.569 Osteolysis, unspecified lower leg
M89.57 Osteolysis, ankle and foot
M89.571 Osteolysis, right ankle and foot
M89.572 Osteolysis, left ankle and foot
M89.579 Osteolysis, unspecified ankle and foot
M89.58 Osteolysis, other site
M89.59 Osteolysis, multiple sites
M89.6 Osteopathy after poliomyelitis
Use additional code (B91) to identify previous poliomyelitis
EXCLUDES1 *postpolio syndrome (G14)*
M89.60 Osteopathy after poliomyelitis, unspecified site
M89.61 Osteopathy after poliomyelitis, shoulder

Unspecified Code Other Specified Code Manifestation Code N Newborn P Pediatric M Maternity A Adult ♂ Male ♀ Female
● New Code ▲ Revised Code Title ►◄ Revised Text NOTES INCLUDES EXCLUDES1 Not coded here EXCLUDES2 Not included here
4th character required 5th character required 6th character required 7th character required
Extension 'X' Alert HAC Hospital-acquired condition (HAC) alert AHA AHA Coding Clinic©

M89.611 Osteopathy after poliomyelitis, right shoulder
M89.612 Osteopathy after poliomyelitis, left shoulder
M89.619 Osteopathy after poliomyelitis, unspecified shoulder
M89.62 Osteopathy after poliomyelitis, upper arm
M89.621 Osteopathy after poliomyelitis, right upper arm
M89.622 Osteopathy after poliomyelitis, left upper arm
M89.629 Osteopathy after poliomyelitis, unspecified upper arm
M89.63 Osteopathy after poliomyelitis, forearm
M89.631 Osteopathy after poliomyelitis, right forearm
M89.632 Osteopathy after poliomyelitis, left forearm
M89.639 Osteopathy after poliomyelitis, unspecified forearm
M89.64 Osteopathy after poliomyelitis, hand
M89.641 Osteopathy after poliomyelitis, right hand
M89.642 Osteopathy after poliomyelitis, left hand
M89.649 Osteopathy after poliomyelitis, unspecified hand
M89.65 Osteopathy after poliomyelitis, thigh
M89.651 Osteopathy after poliomyelitis, right thigh
M89.652 Osteopathy after poliomyelitis, left thigh
M89.659 Osteopathy after poliomyelitis, unspecified thigh
M89.66 Osteopathy after poliomyelitis, lower leg
M89.661 Osteopathy after poliomyelitis, right lower leg
M89.662 Osteopathy after poliomyelitis, left lower leg
M89.669 Osteopathy after poliomyelitis, unspecified lower leg
M89.67 Osteopathy after poliomyelitis, ankle and foot
M89.671 Osteopathy after poliomyelitis, right ankle and foot
M89.672 Osteopathy after poliomyelitis, left ankle and foot
M89.679 Osteopathy after poliomyelitis, unspecified ankle and foot
M89.68 Osteopathy after poliomyelitis, other site
M89.69 Osteopathy after poliomyelitis, multiple sites
M89.7 Major osseous defect
Code first underlying disease, if known, such as:
aseptic necrosis of bone (M87.-)
malignant neoplasm of bone (C40.-)
osteolysis (M89.5)
osteomyelitis (M86.-)
osteonecrosis (M87.-)
osteoporosis (M80.-, M81.-)
periprosthetic osteolysis (T84.05-)
M89.70 Major osseous defect, unspecified site
M89.71 Major osseous defect, shoulder region
Major osseous defect clavicle or scapula
M89.711 Major osseous defect, right shoulder region
M89.712 Major osseous defect, left shoulder region
M89.719 Major osseous defect, unspecified shoulder region
M89.72 Major osseous defect, humerus
M89.721 Major osseous defect, right humerus
M89.722 Major osseous defect, left humerus
M89.729 Major osseous defect, unspecified humerus
M89.73 Major osseous defect, forearm
Major osseous defect of radius and ulna
M89.731 Major osseous defect, right forearm
M89.732 Major osseous defect, left forearm
M89.739 Major osseous defect, unspecified forearm
M89.74 Major osseous defect, hand
Major osseous defect of carpus, fingers, metacarpus
M89.741 Major osseous defect, right hand
M89.742 Major osseous defect, left hand
M89.749 Major osseous defect, unspecified hand
M89.75 Major osseous defect, pelvic region and thigh
Major osseous defect of femur and pelvis
M89.751 Major osseous defect, right pelvic region and thigh
M89.752 Major osseous defect, left pelvic region and thigh
M89.759 Major osseous defect, unspecified pelvic region and thigh
M89.76 Major osseous defect, lower leg
Major osseous defect of fibula and tibia
M89.761 Major osseous defect, right lower leg
M89.762 Major osseous defect, left lower leg
M89.769 Major osseous defect, unspecified lower leg
M89.77 Major osseous defect, ankle and foot
Major osseous defect of metatarsus, tarsus, toes
M89.771 Major osseous defect, right ankle and foot
M89.772 Major osseous defect, left ankle and foot
M89.779 Major osseous defect, unspecified ankle and foot
M89.78 Major osseous defect, other site
M89.79 Major osseous defect, multiple sites
M89.8 Other specified disorders of bone
Infantile cortical hyperostoses
Post-traumatic subperiosteal ossification
M89.8X Other specified disorders of bone
M89.8X0 Other specified disorders of bone, multiple sites
M89.8X1 Other specified disorders of bone, shoulder
M89.8X2 Other specified disorders of bone, upper arm
M89.8X3 Other specified disorders of bone, forearm
M89.8X4 Other specified disorders of bone, hand
M89.8X5 Other specified disorders of bone, thigh
M89.8X6 Other specified disorders of bone, lower leg
M89.8X7 Other specified disorders of bone, ankle and foot
M89.8X8 Other specified disorders of bone, other site
M89.8X9 Other specified disorders of bone, unspecified site
M89.9 Disorder of bone, unspecified
M90 Osteopathies in diseases classified elsewhere
EXCLUDES1 *osteochondritis, osteomyelitis, and osteopathy (in):*
cryptococcosis (B45.3)
diabetes mellitus (E08-E13 with .69-)
gonococcal (A54.43)
neurogenic syphilis (A52.11)
renal osteodystrophy (N25.0)
salmonellosis (A02.24)
secondary syphilis (A51.46)
syphilis (late) (A52.77)
M90.5 Osteonecrosis in diseases classified elsewhere
Code first underlying disease, such as:
caisson disease (T70.3)
hemoglobinopathy (D50-D64)
M90.50 Osteonecrosis in diseases classified elsewhere, unspecified site
M90.51 Osteonecrosis in diseases classified elsewhere, shoulder
M90.511 Osteonecrosis in diseases classified elsewhere, right shoulder
M90.512 Osteonecrosis in diseases classified elsewhere, left shoulder
M90.519 Osteonecrosis in diseases classified elsewhere, unspecified shoulder

Unacceptable principal diagnosis symbol per Medicare code edits | Code exempt from diagnosis present on admission requirement
Questionable admission | Complication or comorbidity | CC/MCC exclusion | Major complication or comorbidity
Principal diagnosis as its own CC | Principal diagnosis as its own MCC | Z code as first-listed diagnosis

M90.52 Osteonecrosis in diseases classified elsewhere, upper arm
- M90.521 Osteonecrosis in diseases classified elsewhere, right upper arm
- M90.522 Osteonecrosis in diseases classified elsewhere, left upper arm
- M90.529 Osteonecrosis in diseases classified elsewhere, unspecified upper arm

M90.53 Osteonecrosis in diseases classified elsewhere, forearm
- M90.531 Osteonecrosis in diseases classified elsewhere, right forearm
- M90.532 Osteonecrosis in diseases classified elsewhere, left forearm
- M90.539 Osteonecrosis in diseases classified elsewhere, unspecified forearm

M90.54 Osteonecrosis in diseases classified elsewhere, hand
- M90.541 Osteonecrosis in diseases classified elsewhere, right hand
- M90.542 Osteonecrosis in diseases classified elsewhere, left hand
- M90.549 Osteonecrosis in diseases classified elsewhere, unspecified hand

M90.55 Osteonecrosis in diseases classified elsewhere, thigh
- M90.551 Osteonecrosis in diseases classified elsewhere, right thigh
- M90.552 Osteonecrosis in diseases classified elsewhere, left thigh
- M90.559 Osteonecrosis in diseases classified elsewhere, unspecified thigh

M90.56 Osteonecrosis in diseases classified elsewhere, lower leg
- M90.561 Osteonecrosis in diseases classified elsewhere, right lower leg
- M90.562 Osteonecrosis in diseases classified elsewhere, left lower leg
- M90.569 Osteonecrosis in diseases classified elsewhere, unspecified lower leg

M90.57 Osteonecrosis in diseases classified elsewhere, ankle and foot
- M90.571 Osteonecrosis in diseases classified elsewhere, right ankle and foot
- M90.572 Osteonecrosis in diseases classified elsewhere, left ankle and foot
- M90.579 Osteonecrosis in diseases classified elsewhere, unspecified ankle and foot

M90.58 Osteonecrosis in diseases classified elsewhere, other site

M90.59 Osteonecrosis in diseases classified elsewhere, multiple sites

M90.6 Osteitis deformans in neoplastic diseases

Osteitis deformans in malignant neoplasm of bone

Code first the neoplasm (C40.-, C41.-)

EXCLUDES1 *osteitis deformans [Paget's disease of bone] (M88.-)*

M90.60 Osteitis deformans in neoplastic diseases, unspecified site

M90.61 Osteitis deformans in neoplastic diseases, shoulder
- M90.611 Osteitis deformans in neoplastic diseases, right shoulder
- M90.612 Osteitis deformans in neoplastic diseases, left shoulder
- M90.619 Osteitis deformans in neoplastic diseases, unspecified shoulder

M90.62 Osteitis deformans in neoplastic diseases, upper arm
- M90.621 Osteitis deformans in neoplastic diseases, right upper arm
- M90.622 Osteitis deformans in neoplastic diseases, left upper arm
- M90.629 Osteitis deformans in neoplastic diseases, unspecified upper arm

M90.63 Osteitis deformans in neoplastic diseases, forearm
- M90.631 Osteitis deformans in neoplastic diseases, right forearm
- M90.632 Osteitis deformans in neoplastic diseases, left forearm
- M90.639 Osteitis deformans in neoplastic diseases, unspecified forearm

M90.64 Osteitis deformans in neoplastic diseases, hand
- M90.641 Osteitis deformans in neoplastic diseases, right hand
- M90.642 Osteitis deformans in neoplastic diseases, left hand
- M90.649 Osteitis deformans in neoplastic diseases, unspecified hand

M90.65 Osteitis deformans in neoplastic diseases, thigh
- M90.651 Osteitis deformans in neoplastic diseases, right thigh
- M90.652 Osteitis deformans in neoplastic diseases, left thigh
- M90.659 Osteitis deformans in neoplastic diseases, unspecified thigh

M90.66 Osteitis deformans in neoplastic diseases, lower leg
- M90.661 Osteitis deformans in neoplastic diseases, right lower leg
- M90.662 Osteitis deformans in neoplastic diseases, left lower leg
- M90.669 Osteitis deformans in neoplastic diseases, unspecified lower leg

M90.67 Osteitis deformans in neoplastic diseases, ankle and foot
- M90.671 Osteitis deformans in neoplastic diseases, right ankle and foot
- M90.672 Osteitis deformans in neoplastic diseases, left ankle and foot
- M90.679 Osteitis deformans in neoplastic diseases, unspecified ankle and foot

M90.68 Osteitis deformans in neoplastic diseases, other site

M90.69 Osteitis deformans in neoplastic diseases, multiple sites

M90.8 Osteopathy in diseases classified elsewhere

Code first underlying disease, such as:

rickets (E55.0)

vitamin-D-resistant rickets (E83.3)

M90.80 Osteopathy in diseases classified elsewhere, unspecified site

M90.81 Osteopathy in diseases classified elsewhere, shoulder
- M90.811 Osteopathy in diseases classified elsewhere, right shoulder
- M90.812 Osteopathy in diseases classified elsewhere, left shoulder
- M90.819 Osteopathy in diseases classified elsewhere, unspecified shoulder

M90.82 Osteopathy in diseases classified elsewhere, upper arm
- M90.821 Osteopathy in diseases classified elsewhere, right upper arm
- M90.822 Osteopathy in diseases classified elsewhere, left upper arm
- M90.829 Osteopathy in diseases classified elsewhere, unspecified upper arm

M90.83 Osteopathy in diseases classified elsewhere, forearm
- M90.831 Osteopathy in diseases classified elsewhere, right forearm
- M90.832 Osteopathy in diseases classified elsewhere, left forearm
- M90.839 Osteopathy in diseases classified elsewhere, unspecified forearm

M90.84 Osteopathy in diseases classified elsewhere, hand
- M90.841 Osteopathy in diseases classified elsewhere, right hand
- M90.842 Osteopathy in diseases classified elsewhere, left hand
- M90.849 Osteopathy in diseases classified elsewhere, unspecified hand

M90.85 Osteopathy in diseases classified elsewhere, thigh
- M90.851 Osteopathy in diseases classified elsewhere, right thigh
- M90.852 Osteopathy in diseases classified elsewhere, left thigh

Unspecified Code | Other Specified Code | Manifestation Code | N Newborn | P Pediatric | M Maternity | A Adult | ♂ Male | ♀ Female
● New Code | ▲ Revised Code Title | ►◄ Revised Text | NOTES | INCLUDES | EXCLUDES1 Not coded here | EXCLUDES2 Not included here
4th character required | 5th character required | 6th character required | 7th character required
Extension 'X' Alert | HAC Hospital-acquired condition (HAC) alert | AHA AHA Coding Clinic©

M90.859 Osteopathy in diseases classified elsewhere, unspecified thigh

M90.86 Osteopathy in diseases classified elsewhere, lower leg
- M90.861 Osteopathy in diseases classified elsewhere, right lower leg
- M90.862 Osteopathy in diseases classified elsewhere, left lower leg
- M90.869 Osteopathy in diseases classified elsewhere, unspecified lower leg

M90.87 Osteopathy in diseases classified elsewhere, ankle and foot
- M90.871 Osteopathy in diseases classified elsewhere, right ankle and foot
- M90.872 Osteopathy in diseases classified elsewhere, left ankle and foot
- M90.879 Osteopathy in diseases classified elsewhere, unspecified ankle and foot

M90.88 Osteopathy in diseases classified elsewhere, other site

M90.89 Osteopathy in diseases classified elsewhere, multiple sites

Chondropathies (M91-M94)

EXCLUDES1 *postprocedural chondropathies (M96.-)*

M91 Juvenile osteochondrosis of hip and pelvis

EXCLUDES1 *slipped upper femoral epiphysis (nontraumatic) (M93.0)*

M91.0 Juvenile osteochondrosis of pelvis
Osteochondrosis (juvenile) of acetabulum
Osteochondrosis (juvenile) of iliac crest [Buchanan]
Osteochondrosis (juvenile) of ischiopubic synchondrosis [van Neck]
Osteochondrosis (juvenile) of symphysis pubis [Pierson]

M91.1 Juvenile osteochondrosis of head of femur [Legg-Calvé-Perthes]
- M91.10 Juvenile osteochondrosis of head of femur [Legg-Calvé-Perthes], unspecified leg
- M91.11 Juvenile osteochondrosis of head of femur [Legg-Calvé-Perthes], right leg
- M91.12 Juvenile osteochondrosis of head of femur [Legg-Calvé-Perthes], left leg

M91.2 Coxa plana
Hip deformity due to previous juvenile osteochondrosis
- M91.20 Coxa plana, unspecified hip
- M91.21 Coxa plana, right hip
- M91.22 Coxa plana, left hip

M91.3 Pseudocoxalgia
- M91.30 Pseudocoxalgia, unspecified hip
- M91.31 Pseudocoxalgia, right hip
- M91.32 Pseudocoxalgia, left hip

M91.4 Coxa magna
- M91.40 Coxa magna, unspecified hip
- M91.41 Coxa magna, right hip
- M91.42 Coxa magna, left hip

M91.8 Other juvenile osteochondrosis of hip and pelvis
Juvenile osteochondrosis after reduction of congenital dislocation of hip
- M91.80 Other juvenile osteochondrosis of hip and pelvis, unspecified leg
- M91.81 Other juvenile osteochondrosis of hip and pelvis, right leg
- M91.82 Other juvenile osteochondrosis of hip and pelvis, left leg

M91.9 Juvenile osteochondrosis of hip and pelvis, unspecified
- M91.90 Juvenile osteochondrosis of hip and pelvis, unspecified, unspecified leg
- M91.91 Juvenile osteochondrosis of hip and pelvis, unspecified, right leg
- M91.92 Juvenile osteochondrosis of hip and pelvis, unspecified, left leg

M92 Other juvenile osteochondrosis

M92.0 Juvenile osteochondrosis of humerus
Osteochondrosis (juvenile) of capitulum of humerus [Panner]
Osteochondrosis (juvenile) of head of humerus [Haas]
- M92.00 Juvenile osteochondrosis of humerus, unspecified arm
- M92.01 Juvenile osteochondrosis of humerus, right arm
- M92.02 Juvenile osteochondrosis of humerus, left arm

M92.1 Juvenile osteochondrosis of radius and ulna
Osteochondrosis (juvenile) of lower ulna [Burns]
Osteochondrosis (juvenile) of radial head [Brailsford]
- M92.10 Juvenile osteochondrosis of radius and ulna, unspecified arm
- M92.11 Juvenile osteochondrosis of radius and ulna, right arm
- M92.12 Juvenile osteochondrosis of radius and ulna, left arm

M92.2 Juvenile osteochondrosis, hand

M92.20 Unspecified juvenile osteochondrosis, hand
- M92.201 Unspecified juvenile osteochondrosis, right hand
- M92.202 Unspecified juvenile osteochondrosis, left hand
- M92.209 Unspecified juvenile osteochondrosis, unspecified hand

M92.21 Osteochondrosis (juvenile) of carpal lunate [Kienböck]
- M92.211 Osteochondrosis (juvenile) of carpal lunate [Kienböck], right hand
- M92.212 Osteochondrosis (juvenile) of carpal lunate [Kienböck], left hand
- M92.219 Osteochondrosis (juvenile) of carpal lunate [Kienböck], unspecified hand

M92.22 Osteochondrosis (juvenile) of metacarpal heads [Mauclaire]
- M92.221 Osteochondrosis (juvenile) of metacarpal heads [Mauclaire], right hand
- M92.222 Osteochondrosis (juvenile) of metacarpal heads [Mauclaire], left hand
- M92.229 Osteochondrosis (juvenile) of metacarpal heads [Mauclaire], unspecified hand

M92.29 Other juvenile osteochondrosis, hand
- M92.291 Other juvenile osteochondrosis, right hand
- M92.292 Other juvenile osteochondrosis, left hand
- M92.299 Other juvenile osteochondrosis, unspecified hand

M92.3 Other juvenile osteochondrosis, upper limb
- M92.30 Other juvenile osteochondrosis, unspecified upper limb
- M92.31 Other juvenile osteochondrosis, right upper limb
- M92.32 Other juvenile osteochondrosis, left upper limb

M92.4 Juvenile osteochondrosis of patella
Osteochondrosis (juvenile) of primary patellar center [Köhler]
Osteochondrosis (juvenile) of secondary patellar centre [Sinding Larsen]
- M92.40 Juvenile osteochondrosis of patella, unspecified knee
- M92.41 Juvenile osteochondrosis of patella, right knee
- M92.42 Juvenile osteochondrosis of patella, left knee

M92.5 Juvenile osteochondrosis of tibia and fibula
Osteochondrosis (juvenile) of proximal tibia [Blount]
Osteochondrosis (juvenile) of tibial tubercle [Osgood-Schlatter]
Tibia vara
- M92.50 Juvenile osteochondrosis of tibia and fibula, unspecified leg
- M92.51 Juvenile osteochondrosis of tibia and fibula, right leg
- M92.52 Juvenile osteochondrosis of tibia and fibula, left leg

M92.6 Juvenile osteochondrosis of tarsus
Osteochondrosis (juvenile) of calcaneum [Sever]
Osteochondrosis (juvenile) of os tibiale externum [Haglund]
Osteochondrosis (juvenile) of talus [Diaz]
Osteochondrosis (juvenile) of tarsal navicular [Köhler]
- M92.60 Juvenile osteochondrosis of tarsus, unspecified ankle
- M92.61 Juvenile osteochondrosis of tarsus, right ankle
- M92.62 Juvenile osteochondrosis of tarsus, left ankle

M92.7 Juvenile osteochondrosis of metatarsus
Osteochondrosis (juvenile) of fifth metatarsus [Iselin]
Osteochondrosis (juvenile) of second metatarsus [Freiberg]

Unacceptable principal diagnosis symbol per Medicare code edits · Code exempt from diagnosis present on admission requirement · Questionable admission · Complication or comorbidity · CC/MCC exclusion · Major complication or comorbidity · Principal diagnosis as its own CC · Principal diagnosis as its own MCC · Z code as first-listed diagnosis

M92.70 Juvenile osteochondrosis of metatarsus, unspecified foot
M92.71 Juvenile osteochondrosis of metatarsus, right foot
M92.72 Juvenile osteochondrosis of metatarsus, left foot

M92.8 Other specified juvenile osteochondrosis
Calcaneal apophysitis

M92.9 Juvenile osteochondrosis, unspecified
Juvenile apophysitis NOS
Juvenile epiphysitis NOS
Juvenile osteochondritis NOS
Juvenile osteochondrosis NOS

M93 Other osteochondropathies
EXCLUDES2 *osteochondrosis of spine (M42.-)*

M93.0 Slipped upper femoral epiphysis (nontraumatic)
Use additional code for associated chondrolysis (M94.3)

M93.00 Unspecified slipped upper femoral epiphysis (nontraumatic)
M93.001 Unspecified slipped upper femoral epiphysis (nontraumatic), right hip
M93.002 Unspecified slipped upper femoral epiphysis (nontraumatic), left hip
M93.003 Unspecified slipped upper femoral epiphysis (nontraumatic), unspecified hip

M93.01 Acute slipped upper femoral epiphysis (nontraumatic)
M93.011 Acute slipped upper femoral epiphysis (nontraumatic), right hip
M93.012 Acute slipped upper femoral epiphysis (nontraumatic), left hip
M93.013 Acute slipped upper femoral epiphysis (nontraumatic), unspecified hip

M93.02 Chronic slipped upper femoral epiphysis (nontraumatic)
M93.021 Chronic slipped upper femoral epiphysis (nontraumatic), right hip
M93.022 Chronic slipped upper femoral epiphysis (nontraumatic), left hip
M93.023 Chronic slipped upper femoral epiphysis (nontraumatic), unspecified hip

M93.03 Acute on chronic slipped upper femoral epiphysis (nontraumatic)
M93.031 Acute on chronic slipped upper femoral epiphysis (nontraumatic), right hip
M93.032 Acute on chronic slipped upper femoral epiphysis (nontraumatic), left hip
M93.033 Acute on chronic slipped upper femoral epiphysis (nontraumatic), unspecified hip

M93.1 Kienböck's disease of adults A
Adult osteochondrosis of carpal lunates

M93.2 Osteochondritis dissecans
M93.20 Osteochondritis dissecans of unspecified site

M93.21 Osteochondritis dissecans of shoulder
M93.211 Osteochondritis dissecans, right shoulder
M93.212 Osteochondritis dissecans, left shoulder
M93.219 Osteochondritis dissecans, unspecified shoulder

M93.22 Osteochondritis dissecans of elbow
M93.221 Osteochondritis dissecans, right elbow
M93.222 Osteochondritis dissecans, left elbow
M93.229 Osteochondritis dissecans, unspecified elbow

M93.23 Osteochondritis dissecans of wrist
M93.231 Osteochondritis dissecans, right wrist
M93.232 Osteochondritis dissecans, left wrist
M93.239 Osteochondritis dissecans, unspecified wrist

M93.24 Osteochondritis dissecans of joints of hand
M93.241 Osteochondritis dissecans, joints of right hand
M93.242 Osteochondritis dissecans, joints of left hand
M93.249 Osteochondritis dissecans, joints of unspecified hand

M93.25 Osteochondritis dissecans of hip
M93.251 Osteochondritis dissecans, right hip
M93.252 Osteochondritis dissecans, left hip
M93.259 Osteochondritis dissecans, unspecified hip

M93.26 Osteochondritis dissecans knee
M93.261 Osteochondritis dissecans, right knee
M93.262 Osteochondritis dissecans, left knee
M93.269 Osteochondritis dissecans, unspecified knee

M93.27 Osteochondritis dissecans of ankle and joints of foot
M93.271 Osteochondritis dissecans, right ankle and joints of right foot
M93.272 Osteochondritis dissecans, left ankle and joints of left foot
M93.279 Osteochondritis dissecans, unspecified ankle and joints of foot

M93.28 Osteochondritis dissecans other site
M93.29 Osteochondritis dissecans multiple sites

M93.8 Other specified osteochondropathies
M93.80 Other specified osteochondropathies of unspecified site

M93.81 Other specified osteochondropathies of shoulder
M93.811 Other specified osteochondropathies, right shoulder
M93.812 Other specified osteochondropathies, left shoulder
M93.819 Other specified osteochondropathies, unspecified shoulder

M93.82 Other specified osteochondropathies of upper arm
M93.821 Other specified osteochondropathies, right upper arm
M93.822 Other specified osteochondropathies, left upper arm
M93.829 Other specified osteochondropathies, unspecified upper arm

M93.83 Other specified osteochondropathies of forearm
M93.831 Other specified osteochondropathies, right forearm
M93.832 Other specified osteochondropathies, left forearm
M93.839 Other specified osteochondropathies, unspecified forearm

M93.84 Other specified osteochondropathies of hand
M93.841 Other specified osteochondropathies, right hand
M93.842 Other specified osteochondropathies, left hand
M93.849 Other specified osteochondropathies, unspecified hand

M93.85 Other specified osteochondropathies of thigh
M93.851 Other specified osteochondropathies, right thigh
M93.852 Other specified osteochondropathies, left thigh
M93.859 Other specified osteochondropathies, unspecified thigh

M93.86 Other specified osteochondropathies lower leg
M93.861 Other specified osteochondropathies, right lower leg
M93.862 Other specified osteochondropathies, left lower leg
M93.869 Other specified osteochondropathies, unspecified lower leg

M93.87 Other specified osteochondropathies of ankle and foot
M93.871 Other specified osteochondropathies, right ankle and foot
M93.872 Other specified osteochondropathies, left ankle and foot
M93.879 Other specified osteochondropathies, unspecified ankle and foot

M93.88 Other specified osteochondropathies other
M93.89 Other specified osteochondropathies multiple sites

M93.9 Osteochondropathy, unspecified
Apophysitis NOS
Epiphysitis NOS

Unspecified Code Other Specified Code Manifestation Code N Newborn P Pediatric M Maternity A Adult ♂ Male ♀ Female
● New Code ▲ Revised Code Title ►◄ Revised Text NOTES INCLUDES EXCLUDES1 Not coded here EXCLUDES2 Not included here
4th character required 5th character required 6th character required 7th character required
Extension 'X' Alert HAC Hospital-acquired condition (HAC) alert AHA AHA Coding Clinic©

Osteochondritis NOS
Osteochondrosis NOS
M93.90 Osteochondropathy, unspecified of unspecified site
M93.91 Osteochondropathy, unspecified of shoulder
M93.911 Osteochondropathy, unspecified, right shoulder
M93.912 Osteochondropathy, unspecified, left shoulder
M93.919 Osteochondropathy, unspecified, unspecified shoulder
M93.92 Osteochondropathy, unspecified of upper arm
M93.921 Osteochondropathy, unspecified, right upper arm
M93.922 Osteochondropathy, unspecified, left upper arm
M93.929 Osteochondropathy, unspecified, unspecified upper arm
M93.93 Osteochondropathy, unspecified of forearm
M93.931 Osteochondropathy, unspecified, right forearm
M93.932 Osteochondropathy, unspecified, left forearm
M93.939 Osteochondropathy, unspecified, unspecified forearm
M93.94 Osteochondropathy, unspecified of hand
M93.941 Osteochondropathy, unspecified, right hand
M93.942 Osteochondropathy, unspecified, left hand
M93.949 Osteochondropathy, unspecified, unspecified hand
M93.95 Osteochondropathy, unspecified of thigh
M93.951 Osteochondropathy, unspecified, right thigh
M93.952 Osteochondropathy, unspecified, left thigh
M93.959 Osteochondropathy, unspecified, unspecified thigh
M93.96 Osteochondropathy, unspecified lower leg
M93.961 Osteochondropathy, unspecified, right lower leg
M93.962 Osteochondropathy, unspecified, left lower leg
M93.969 Osteochondropathy, unspecified, unspecified lower leg
M93.97 Osteochondropathy, unspecified of ankle and foot
M93.971 Osteochondropathy, unspecified, right ankle and foot
M93.972 Osteochondropathy, unspecified, left ankle and foot
M93.979 Osteochondropathy, unspecified, unspecified ankle and foot
M93.98 Osteochondropathy, unspecified other
M93.99 Osteochondropathy, unspecified multiple sites
M94 Other disorders of cartilage
M94.0 Chondrocostal junction syndrome [Tietze]
Costochondritis
M94.1 Relapsing polychondritis
M94.2 Chondromalacia
EXCLUDES1 *chondromalacia patellae (M22.4)*
M94.20 Chondromalacia, unspecified site
M94.21 Chondromalacia, shoulder
M94.211 Chondromalacia, right shoulder
M94.212 Chondromalacia, left shoulder
M94.219 Chondromalacia, unspecified shoulder
M94.22 Chondromalacia, elbow
M94.221 Chondromalacia, right elbow
M94.222 Chondromalacia, left elbow
M94.229 Chondromalacia, unspecified elbow
M94.23 Chondromalacia, wrist
M94.231 Chondromalacia, right wrist
M94.232 Chondromalacia, left wrist
M94.239 Chondromalacia, unspecified wrist
M94.24 Chondromalacia, joints of hand
M94.241 Chondromalacia, joints of right hand
M94.242 Chondromalacia, joints of left hand
M94.249 Chondromalacia, joints of unspecified hand
M94.25 Chondromalacia, hip
M94.251 Chondromalacia, right hip
M94.252 Chondromalacia, left hip
M94.259 Chondromalacia, unspecified hip
M94.26 Chondromalacia, knee
M94.261 Chondromalacia, right knee
M94.262 Chondromalacia, left knee
M94.269 Chondromalacia, unspecified knee
M94.27 Chondromalacia, ankle and joints of foot
M94.271 Chondromalacia, right ankle and joints of right foot
M94.272 Chondromalacia, left ankle and joints of left foot
M94.279 Chondromalacia, unspecified ankle and joints of foot
M94.28 Chondromalacia, other site
M94.29 Chondromalacia, multiple sites
M94.3 Chondrolysis
Code first any associated slipped upper femoral epiphysis (nontraumatic) (M93.0-)
M94.35 Chondrolysis, hip
M94.351 Chondrolysis, right hip
M94.352 Chondrolysis, left hip
M94.359 Chondrolysis, unspecified hip
M94.8 Other specified disorders of cartilage
M94.8X Other specified disorders of cartilage
M94.8X0 Other specified disorders of cartilage, multiple sites
M94.8X1 Other specified disorders of cartilage, shoulder
M94.8X2 Other specified disorders of cartilage, upper arm
M94.8X3 Other specified disorders of cartilage, forearm
M94.8X4 Other specified disorders of cartilage, hand
M94.8X5 Other specified disorders of cartilage, thigh
M94.8X6 Other specified disorders of cartilage, lower leg
M94.8X7 Other specified disorders of cartilage, ankle and foot
M94.8X8 Other specified disorders of cartilage, other site
M94.8X9 Other specified disorders of cartilage, unspecified sites
M94.9 Disorder of cartilage, unspecified

Other disorders of the musculoskeletal system and connective tissue (M95)

M95 Other acquired deformities of musculoskeletal system and connective tissue
EXCLUDES2 *acquired absence of limbs and organs (Z89-Z90)*
acquired deformities of limbs (M20-M21)
congenital malformations and deformations of the musculoskeletal system (Q65-Q79)
deforming dorsopathies (M40-M43)
dentofacial anomalies [including malocclusion] (M26.-)
postprocedural musculoskeletal disorders (M96.-)
M95.0 Acquired deformity of nose
EXCLUDES2 *deviated nasal septum (J34.2)*
M95.1 Cauliflower ear
EXCLUDES2 *other acquired deformities of ear (H61.1)*
M95.10 Cauliflower ear, unspecified ear
M95.11 Cauliflower ear, right ear
M95.12 Cauliflower ear, left ear
M95.2 Other acquired deformity of head
M95.3 Acquired deformity of neck
M95.4 Acquired deformity of chest and rib
M95.5 Acquired deformity of pelvis

Unacceptable principal diagnosis symbol per Medicare code edits; Code exempt from diagnosis present on admission requirement
Questionable admission; Complication or comorbidity; CC/MCC exclusion; Major complication or comorbidity
Principal diagnosis as its own CC; Principal diagnosis as its own MCC; Z code as first-listed diagnosis

When symbols appear on a code that requires a 7th character extension, refer to Appendix D to identify applicable 7th character codes.

EXCLUDES1 *maternal care for known or suspected disproportion (O33.-)*

M95.8 Other specified acquired deformities of musculoskeletal system

M95.9 Acquired deformity of musculoskeletal system, unspecified

Intraoperative and postprocedural complications and disorders of musculoskeletal system, not elsewhere classified (M96)

M96 Intraoperative and postprocedural complications and disorders of musculoskeletal system, not elsewhere classified

EXCLUDES2 *arthropathy following intestinal bypass (M02.0-)*
complications of internal orthopedic prosthetic devices, implants and grafts (T84.-)
disorders associated with osteoporosis (M80)
periprosthetic fracture around internal prosthetic joint (M97.-)
presence of functional implants and other devices (Z96-Z97)

M96.0 Pseudarthrosis after fusion or arthrodesis CC

M96.1 Postlaminectomy syndrome, not elsewhere classified

M96.2 Postradiation kyphosis

M96.3 Postlaminectomy kyphosis

M96.4 Postsurgical lordosis

M96.5 Postradiation scoliosis

M96.6 Fracture of bone following insertion of orthopedic implant, joint prosthesis, or bone plate

Intraoperative fracture of bone during insertion of orthopedic implant, joint prosthesis, or bone plate

EXCLUDES2 *complication of internal orthopedic devices, implants or grafts (T84.-)*

M96.62 Fracture of humerus following insertion of orthopedic implant, joint prosthesis, or bone plate

M96.621 Fracture of humerus following insertion of orthopedic implant, joint prosthesis, or bone plate, right arm CC

M96.622 Fracture of humerus following insertion of orthopedic implant, joint prosthesis, or bone plate, left arm CC

M96.629 Fracture of humerus following insertion of orthopedic implant, joint prosthesis, or bone plate, unspecified arm CC

M96.63 Fracture of radius or ulna following insertion of orthopedic implant, joint prosthesis, or bone plate

M96.631 Fracture of radius or ulna following insertion of orthopedic implant, joint prosthesis, or bone plate, right arm CC

M96.632 Fracture of radius or ulna following insertion of orthopedic implant, joint prosthesis, or bone plate, left arm CC

M96.639 Fracture of radius or ulna following insertion of orthopedic implant, joint prosthesis, or bone plate, unspecified arm CC

M96.65 Fracture of pelvis following insertion of orthopedic implant, joint prosthesis, or bone plate CC

M96.66 Fracture of femur following insertion of orthopedic implant, joint prosthesis, or bone plate

M96.661 Fracture of femur following insertion of orthopedic implant, joint prosthesis, or bone plate, right leg CC

M96.662 Fracture of femur following insertion of orthopedic implant, joint prosthesis, or bone plate, left leg CC

M96.669 Fracture of femur following insertion of orthopedic implant, joint prosthesis, or bone plate, unspecified leg CC

M96.67 Fracture of tibia or fibula following insertion of orthopedic implant, joint prosthesis, or bone plate

M96.671 Fracture of tibia or fibula following insertion of orthopedic implant, joint prosthesis, or bone plate, right leg CC

M96.672 Fracture of tibia or fibula following insertion of orthopedic implant, joint prosthesis, or bone plate, left leg CC

M96.679 Fracture of tibia or fibula following insertion of orthopedic implant, joint prosthesis, or bone plate, unspecified leg CC

M96.69 Fracture of other bone following insertion of orthopedic implant, joint prosthesis, or bone plate CC

M96.8 Other intraoperative and postprocedural complications and disorders of musculoskeletal system, not elsewhere classified

M96.81 Intraoperative hemorrhage and hematoma of a musculoskeletal structure complicating a procedure

EXCLUDES1 *intraoperative hemorrhage and hematoma of a musculoskeletal structure due to accidental puncture and laceration during a procedure (M96.82-)*

M96.810 Intraoperative hemorrhage and hematoma of a musculoskeletal structure complicating a musculoskeletal system procedure CC

M96.811 Intraoperative hemorrhage and hematoma of a musculoskeletal structure complicating other procedure CC

M96.82 Accidental puncture and laceration of a musculoskeletal structure during a procedure

M96.820 Accidental puncture and laceration of a musculoskeletal structure during a musculoskeletal system procedure CC

M96.821 Accidental puncture and laceration of a musculoskeletal structure during other procedure CC

▲ M96.83 Postprocedural ▶hemorrhage of◀ a musculoskeletal structure following a procedure

▲ M96.830 Postprocedural ▶hemorrhage of◀ a musculoskeletal structure following a musculoskeletal system procedure CC

▲ M96.831 Postprocedural ▶hemorrhage of◀ a musculoskeletal structure following other procedure CC

● M96.84 Postprocedural hematoma and seroma of a musculoskeletal structure following a procedure

● M96.840 Postprocedural hematoma of a musculoskeletal structure following a musculoskeletal system procedure CC CC/MCC Exc

● M96.841 Postprocedural hematoma of a musculoskeletal structure following other procedure CC CC/MCC Exc

● M96.842 Postprocedural seroma of a musculoskeletal structure following a musculoskeletal system procedure

● M96.843 Postprocedural seroma of a musculoskeletal structure following other procedure

M96.89 Other intraoperative and postprocedural complications and disorders of the musculoskeletal system CC

Instability of joint secondary to removal of joint prosthesis

Use additional code, if applicable, to further specify disorder

Periprosthetic fracture around internal prosthetic joint (M97)

● M97 Periprosthetic fracture around internal prosthetic joint
EXCLUDES2 *fracture of bone following insertion of orthopedic implant, joint prosthesis or bone plate (M96.6-)*
breakage (fracture) of prosthetic joint (T84.01-)
The appropriate 7th character is to be added to each code from category M97
A = initial encounter
D = subsequent encounter
S = sequela
● M97.0 Periprosthetic fracture around internal prosthetic hip joint
● M97.01 Periprosthetic fracture around internal prosthetic right hip joint CC CC/MCC Exc
● M97.02 Periprosthetic fracture around internal prosthetic left hip joint CC CC/MCC Exc
● M97.1 Periprosthetic fracture around internal prosthetic knee joint
● M97.11 Periprosthetic fracture around internal prosthetic right knee joint CC CC/MCC Exc
● M97.12 Periprosthetic fracture around internal prosthetic left knee joint CC CC/MCC Exc
● M97.2 Periprosthetic fracture around internal prosthetic ankle joint
● M97.21 Periprosthetic fracture around internal prosthetic right ankle joint CC CC/MCC Exc
● M97.22 Periprosthetic fracture around internal prosthetic left ankle joint CC CC/MCC Exc
● M97.3 Periprosthetic fracture around internal prosthetic shoulder joint
● M97.31 Periprosthetic fracture around internal prosthetic right shoulder joint CC CC/MCC Exc
● M97.32 Periprosthetic fracture around internal prosthetic left shoulder joint CC CC/MCC Exc
● M97.4 Periprosthetic fracture around internal prosthetic elbow joint
● M97.41 Periprosthetic fracture around internal prosthetic right elbow joint CC CC/MCC Exc
● M97.42 Periprosthetic fracture around internal prosthetic left elbow joint CC CC/MCC Exc
● M97.8 Periprosthetic fracture around other internal prosthetic joint CC CC/MCC Exc
Periprosthetic fracture around internal prosthetic finger joint
Periprosthetic fracture around internal prosthetic spinal joint
Periprosthetic fracture around internal prosthetic toe joint
Periprosthetic fracture around internal prosthetic wrist joint
Use additional code to identify the joint (Z96.6-)
● M97.9 Periprosthetic fracture around unspecified internal prosthetic joint CC CC/MCC Exc

Biomechanical lesions, not elsewhere classified (M99)

M99 Biomechanical lesions, not elsewhere classified
NOTES This category should not be used if the condition can be classified elsewhere.
M99.0 Segmental and somatic dysfunction
M99.00 Segmental and somatic dysfunction of head region
M99.01 Segmental and somatic dysfunction of cervical region
M99.02 Segmental and somatic dysfunction of thoracic region
M99.03 Segmental and somatic dysfunction of lumbar region
M99.04 Segmental and somatic dysfunction of sacral region
M99.05 Segmental and somatic dysfunction of pelvic region
M99.06 Segmental and somatic dysfunction of lower extremity
M99.07 Segmental and somatic dysfunction of upper extremity
M99.08 Segmental and somatic dysfunction of rib cage
M99.09 Segmental and somatic dysfunction of abdomen and other regions
M99.1 Subluxation complex (vertebral)
M99.10 Subluxation complex (vertebral) of head region CC HAC
M99.11 Subluxation complex (vertebral) of cervical region CC HAC
M99.12 Subluxation complex (vertebral) of thoracic region
M99.13 Subluxation complex (vertebral) of lumbar region
M99.14 Subluxation complex (vertebral) of sacral region
M99.15 Subluxation complex (vertebral) of pelvic region
M99.16 Subluxation complex (vertebral) of lower extremity
M99.17 Subluxation complex (vertebral) of upper extremity
M99.18 Subluxation complex (vertebral) of rib cage CC HAC
M99.19 Subluxation complex (vertebral) of abdomen and other regions
M99.2 Subluxation stenosis of neural canal
M99.20 Subluxation stenosis of neural canal of head region
M99.21 Subluxation stenosis of neural canal of cervical region
M99.22 Subluxation stenosis of neural canal of thoracic region
M99.23 Subluxation stenosis of neural canal of lumbar region
M99.24 Subluxation stenosis of neural canal of sacral region
M99.25 Subluxation stenosis of neural canal of pelvic region
M99.26 Subluxation stenosis of neural canal of lower extremity
M99.27 Subluxation stenosis of neural canal of upper extremity
M99.28 Subluxation stenosis of neural canal of rib cage
M99.29 Subluxation stenosis of neural canal of abdomen and other regions
M99.3 Osseous stenosis of neural canal
M99.30 Osseous stenosis of neural canal of head region
M99.31 Osseous stenosis of neural canal of cervical region
M99.32 Osseous stenosis of neural canal of thoracic region
M99.33 Osseous stenosis of neural canal of lumbar region
M99.34 Osseous stenosis of neural canal of sacral region
M99.35 Osseous stenosis of neural canal of pelvic region
M99.36 Osseous stenosis of neural canal of lower extremity
M99.37 Osseous stenosis of neural canal of upper extremity
M99.38 Osseous stenosis of neural canal of rib cage
M99.39 Osseous stenosis of neural canal of abdomen and other regions
M99.4 Connective tissue stenosis of neural canal
M99.40 Connective tissue stenosis of neural canal of head region
M99.41 Connective tissue stenosis of neural canal of cervical region
M99.42 Connective tissue stenosis of neural canal of thoracic region
M99.43 Connective tissue stenosis of neural canal of lumbar region
M99.44 Connective tissue stenosis of neural canal of sacral region
M99.45 Connective tissue stenosis of neural canal of pelvic region
M99.46 Connective tissue stenosis of neural canal of lower extremity
M99.47 Connective tissue stenosis of neural canal of upper extremity
M99.48 Connective tissue stenosis of neural canal of rib cage
M99.49 Connective tissue stenosis of neural canal of abdomen and other regions
M99.5 Intervertebral disc stenosis of neural canal
M99.50 Intervertebral disc stenosis of neural canal of head region
M99.51 Intervertebral disc stenosis of neural canal of cervical region
M99.52 Intervertebral disc stenosis of neural canal of thoracic region
M99.53 Intervertebral disc stenosis of neural canal of lumbar region
M99.54 Intervertebral disc stenosis of neural canal of sacral region
M99.55 Intervertebral disc stenosis of neural canal of pelvic region
M99.56 Intervertebral disc stenosis of neural canal of lower extremity
M99.57 Intervertebral disc stenosis of neural canal of upper extremity

Unacceptable principal diagnosis symbol per Medicare code edits · Code exempt from diagnosis present on admission requirement · Questionable admission · CC Complication or comorbidity · CC/MCC Exc CC/MCC exclusion · MCC Major complication or comorbidity · Principal diagnosis as its own CC · Principal diagnosis as its own MCC · Z code as first-listed diagnosis

M99.58 Intervertebral disc stenosis of neural canal of rib cage
M99.59 Intervertebral disc stenosis of neural canal of abdomen and other regions

M99.6 Osseous and subluxation stenosis of intervertebral foramina
M99.60 Osseous and subluxation stenosis of intervertebral foramina of head region
M99.61 Osseous and subluxation stenosis of intervertebral foramina of cervical region
M99.62 Osseous and subluxation stenosis of intervertebral foramina of thoracic region
M99.63 Osseous and subluxation stenosis of intervertebral foramina of lumbar region
M99.64 Osseous and subluxation stenosis of intervertebral foramina of sacral region
M99.65 Osseous and subluxation stenosis of intervertebral foramina of pelvic region
M99.66 Osseous and subluxation stenosis of intervertebral foramina of lower extremity
M99.67 Osseous and subluxation stenosis of intervertebral foramina of upper extremity
M99.68 Osseous and subluxation stenosis of intervertebral foramina of rib cage
M99.69 Osseous and subluxation stenosis of intervertebral foramina of abdomen and other regions

M99.7 Connective tissue and disc stenosis of intervertebral foramina
M99.70 Connective tissue and disc stenosis of intervertebral foramina of head region
M99.71 Connective tissue and disc stenosis of intervertebral foramina of cervical region
M99.72 Connective tissue and disc stenosis of intervertebral foramina of thoracic region
M99.73 Connective tissue and disc stenosis of intervertebral foramina of lumbar region
M99.74 Connective tissue and disc stenosis of intervertebral foramina of sacral region
M99.75 Connective tissue and disc stenosis of intervertebral foramina of pelvic region
M99.76 Connective tissue and disc stenosis of intervertebral foramina of lower extremity
M99.77 Connective tissue and disc stenosis of intervertebral foramina of upper extremity
M99.78 Connective tissue and disc stenosis of intervertebral foramina of rib cage
M99.79 Connective tissue and disc stenosis of intervertebral foramina of abdomen and other regions

M99.8 Other biomechanical lesions
M99.80 Other biomechanical lesions of head region
M99.81 Other biomechanical lesions of cervical region
M99.82 Other biomechanical lesions of thoracic region
M99.83 Other biomechanical lesions of lumbar region
M99.84 Other biomechanical lesions of sacral region
M99.85 Other biomechanical lesions of pelvic region
M99.86 Other biomechanical lesions of lower extremity
M99.87 Other biomechanical lesions of upper extremity
M99.88 Other biomechanical lesions of rib cage
M99.89 Other biomechanical lesions of abdomen and other regions

M99.9 Biomechanical lesion, unspecified

This page intentionally left blank

Chapter 14: Diseases of the Genitourinary System (N00-N99)

Guidelines for Assigning Codes From This Chapter

The genitourinary system, which Chapter 14 covers, includes both the reproductive organs and the urinary organs. You'll find codes related to the kidneys and urinary tract; the male genital organs, including the prostate and infertility issues; the breasts; female pelvic organs; and the female genital tract, including diagnoses such as endometriosis and menopause.

List of Sections

- N00-N08: Glomerular diseases
- N10-N16: Renal tubulo-interstitial diseases
- N17-N19: Acute kidney failure and chronic kidney disease
- N20-N23: Urolithiasis
- N25-N29: Other disorders of kidney and ureter
- N30-N39: Other diseases of the urinary system
- N40-N53: Diseases of male genital organs
- N60-N65: Disorders of breast
- N70-N77: Inflammatory diseases of female pelvic organs
- N80-N98: Noninflammatory disorders of female genital tract
- N99: Intraoperative and postprocedural complications and disorders of genitourinary system, not elsewhere classified

Highlights From the ICD-10-CM Official Guidelines for Coding and Reporting

Although there are a variety of diagnoses in Chapter 14, the ICD-10-CM Official Guidelines for Coding and Reporting focus on proper coding of chronic kidney disease. The information below is from Section I.C.14 of the 2017 Official Guidelines.

Capture All the Information for Chronic Kidney Disease Coding

An important element of coding chronic kidney disease (CKD) is reporting the stage, from 1-5. For instance, you report stage 1 using N18.1 (*Chronic kidney disease, stage 1*) and stage 2 using N18.2 (*Chronic kidney disease, stage 2 [mild]*). Stage 3 (N18.3) is considered moderate and stage 4 (N18.4) severe. The codes for stage 1 and stage 5 (N18.5) have not been classified according to severity.

There's also a distinct code for end stage renal disease (ESRD), N18.6 (*End stage renal disease*). When documentation shows both a stage and ESRD, you should report only ESRD code N18.6 and not the code for the stage.

Transplant: When a patient who has had a kidney transplant has CKD, you should report the appropriate code for the CKD stage and Z94.0 (*Kidney transplant status*). Note that CKD following kidney transplant does not qualify as a complication, so you should not code it as such. When the documentation isn't clear about whether or not the CKD is a complication, ask the provider for clarification. See section g in Chapter 19 of the Official Guidelines for codes for transplant failure or rejection.

Other conditions: When the patient has another condition in addition to CKD, such as diabetes mellitus (Chapter 4) or hypertension (Chapter 9), be sure to review each condition's code for rules on proper sequencing and reporting.

Check Chapter 1 for Urosepsis Rule

You won't find every relevant guideline for Chapter 14 in the Chapter 14 section of the Official Guidelines. You'll find one important example in the Chapter 1 guidelines for Infectious and Parasitic Diseases.

In Section I.C.1.d, you'll find a note explaining that the term urosepsis has no clinical meaning, and it has no default code in the Alphabetic Index. If a provider documents urosepsis, you must ask for clarification. If he identifies a urinary tract infection, you would select the code based on the location of the infection. You should also report a code for the infecting organism if known.

Anatomy of the Male Reproductive System

1. **The male reproductive system includes the following:**
   a) The primary sex organs (or the Testes/Male Gonads) that produce sperms and the male sex hormones.
   b) The accessory organs (or the scrotum and ducts) that support the testes and transport the sperm.
   c) The accessory glands that produce secretions for constituting the semen.
   d) The penis, which acts as a transporting and supporting structure of the male reproductive system
2. **The anatomy of structures/components of the male reproductive system is further described below:**
   a) Scrotum
      i) It is an extension from the abdominal wall that supports the testes.
      ii) It is divided into two lateral pouches via a septum, and each pouch contains a single testis.
      iii) The scrotal sac serves to provide protection to the sperms from the changes in the external environment.
   b) The Testes
      i) The testes are covered by a capsule of connective tissue, which is known as the tunica albuginea.
      ii) The tunica albuginea travels inwards to constitute a series of compartments, which are known as lobules.
      iii) A single lobule carries convoluted seminiferous tubules for spermatogenesis.
      iv) Male sex hormone (testosterone) is produced by the interstitial cells of Leydig that remain located in the individual lobules.
   c) The Spermatozoa (or Mature Sperm Cell)
      i) A typical sperm cell is composed of a head, a middle piece, and a tail (or flagellum)
      ii) Spermatozoa can survive up to a period of 48 hours in the female reproductive tract. Approximately three hundred million spermatozoa are produced on a daily basis in a male.
   d) The Ducts of the Male Reproductive System
      i) Convoluted seminiferous tubules of the testis contain the mature sperm cells.
      ii) A tightly coiled structure (or epididymis) is positioned on the posterior border of the testis.
      iii) The straightened epididymis is known as the ductus deferens (or vas deferens).
      iv) The spermatic cord is a sheath that contains the vas deferens and empties into the ejaculatory duct.
      v) The urethra is regarded as the terminal duct of the male reproductive system. The ejaculatory duct ejects the spermatozoa into the urethra. Moreover, the urethra provides a common passage for both sperm and urine.
      vi) The urethra traverses through the prostate gland, urogenital diaphragm, and penis.
   e) The Accessory Glands
      i) Paired seminal vesicles generate the alkaline viscous part of the semen and transfer it to the ejaculatory duct.
      ii) The prostate gland produces the semen that provides a medium to the sperm cells for swimming.
      iii) Bulbourethral glands (or Cowper's glands) generate the viscous mucus that acts as a lubricant for sexual intercourse.
   f) Semen
      i) Semen is a milky fluid, which is a mixture of the matured sperm cells and secretions of the accessory glands.
      ii) It provides a transport medium for the sperm.
   g) The Penis
      i) It acts to transport the matured sperms to the female reproductive tract.
      ii) It is composed of a shaft, and the terminal point of the shaft is known as the glans penis (or head). The head of the penis is covered with loose skin, which is called the prepuce or foreskin.

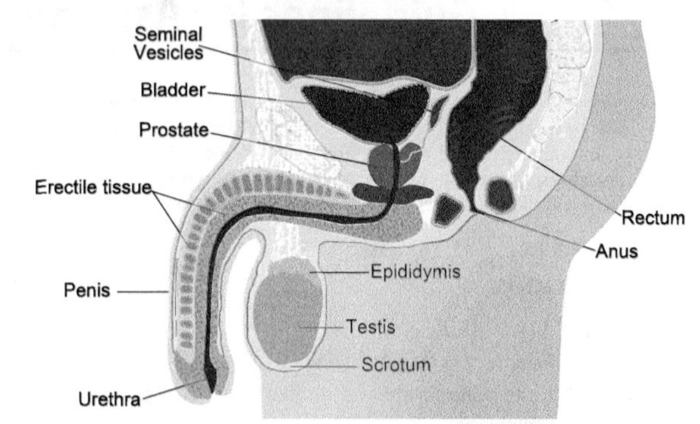

Common Pathologies

Benign Prostate Hyperplasia
Benign prostate hyperplasia (BPH) is a noncancerous enlargement of the prostate gland, typically in older males. It compresses the urethra and makes urination difficult. BPH symptoms are also known as lower urinary tract symptoms, or LUTS.

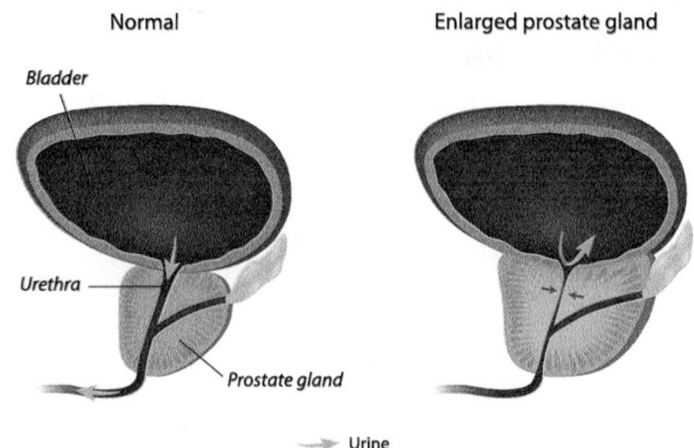

Gynecomastia
Gynecomastia refers to enlargement of the male breast, common in adolescents and the elderly, which is due to an imbalance of sex hormones.

Hypospadias
Hypospadias is a medical condition present from birth in some males in which the opening of the urethra is on the underside of the penis instead of at its tip.

Orchitis
Orchitis, an inflammation of the testicles, results from infection with bacteria or the mumps virus. It can affect one or both testes.

Torsion of Testis
Testicular torsion is a painful condition in which the spermatic cord, which supplies blood to a testicle, twists and obstructs blood flow.

Hydrocele
Hydrocele refers to an abnormal accumulation of fluid in a sac-type structure, such as a testicle.

Phimosis
Phimosis is a painful condition in which the foreskin, or prepuce, cannot be retracted from the head, or glans, of the penis due to scarring or stricture.

Balanitis
Balanitis causes redness, swelling, and pain of the foreskin, or prepuce, due to inflammation or bacterial infection.

Anatomy of the Urinary System

1. **An Outline of the Urinary System**
   a) Two Kidneys
   b) Two Ureters
   c) The Urinary Bladder
   d) The Urethra
   e) The urinary system maintains the state of homeostasis by regulating water and solutes in the human body.
   f) Kidneys produce the urine and function as the major filtering organs of the urinary system.
   g) Urine is composed of components like urea, water, ions, and toxic wastes that need to be regulated in the human body by the entire urinary system.
2. **The Functions of Kidneys**
   a) Excretion
   b) Maintenance of blood volume and concentration
   c) pH regulation
   d) Maintenance of blood pressure
   e) Maintenance of erythrocyte concentration
   f) The conversion of vitamin D to its active form (or calciferol).
3. **The Anatomy of Kidneys**
   a) Kidneys are situated between the parietal peritoneum and posterior wall of abdomen.
   b) There is a notch (known as hilum) located in the concave center of each kidney. The ureter exits the kidney, and blood vessels, lymph vessels and nerves enter and leave the kidney through the hilum.
   c) The kidney is surrounded by the following three layers:
      i) The innermost layer of the kidney is known as the renal capsule. It acts as a barrier against trauma and infection.
      ii) Adipose capsule is the middle layer of the kidney. It is made up of fatty tissue and protects the kidney from blows.
      iii) The renal fascia is the outermost layer of the kidney. It serves to attach the kidney to the abdominal wall.
   d) Cortex is the outer region of the kidney.
   e) Medulla is the inner area of the kidney.
   f) Renal pyramids are striated triangular structures that are found within the medulla. The bases of these pyramids face toward the cortex. However, their tips point to the center of the kidney and are known as the renal papillae.
   g) The renal columns constitute the cortical material that extends between the pyramids.
   h) The parenchyma of the kidney is formed by the cortex and renal pyramids.
   i) The parenchyma is further composed of the microscopic units or nephrons, which are the structural and functional units of the kidneys.
   j) The minor calyx is a funnel-shaped structure that surrounds the tip of each renal pyramid. The function of this minor calyx is to collect the urine from the ducts of the renal pyramids. The minor calyces integrate to constitute the major calyces.
   k) The renal pelvis is the large collecting funnel that is formed by a bunch of major calyces. The renal pelvis is further narrowed and extended to constitute the ureter.
4. **The Ureter**
   a) It is the extension of the renal pelvis of the kidney and communicates with the urinary bladder.
   b) They are two in number and carry urine from the renal pelvis to the urinary bladder.
   c) Urine is expelled from the bladder by the act of micturition.
5. **The Urethra**
   a) It is a thin walled tube that connects the floor of the urinary bladder to the genitals for the expulsion of fluids (urine, semen, etc.) out of the body.
   b) It is located in the wall of the vagina and above the vaginal opening in females. The female urethral orifice is the opening of the urethra and situated between the vaginal opening and clitoris.
   c) It lies below the bladder in males and travels through the prostate gland and penis.
   d) The opening at the tip of the male penis is known as the male urethral orifice.
   e) The external urethral sphincter is a striated muscle and provides voluntary control of urination.

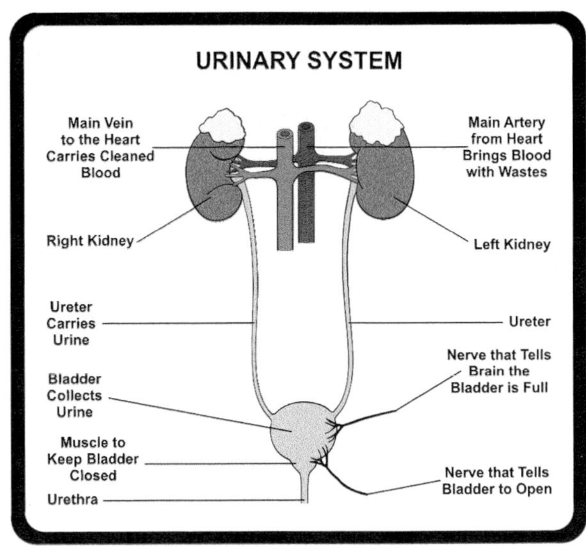

Common Pathologies

Glomerulonephritis
Glomerulonephritis, also known as nephritic syndrome, is a disease of the kidney, characterized by inflammation of the glomeruli, small structures through which the kidney filters urine. Inflammation of the glomeruli prevents the kidneys from being able to filter the urine. Fluid and toxins then build up in the body and can lead to chronic renal failure, also known as chronic kidney failure (CKD).

Acute Renal Failure
Acute renal failure refers to the inability of the kidneys to filter waste products, resulting in the buildup of toxic substances in the blood.

Chronic Kidney Disease
Chronic kidney disease, or CKD, is a condition of gradual loss of kidney function, described in five stages, with stage 1 being the least severe and stage 5 being end stage renal disease, requiring dialysis or kidney transplant for treatment.

Bladder Cancer
Bladder cancer is an abnormal growth of cells in the bladder, typically beginning in the lining of the bladder and then spreading throughout the bladder and to adjacent organs.

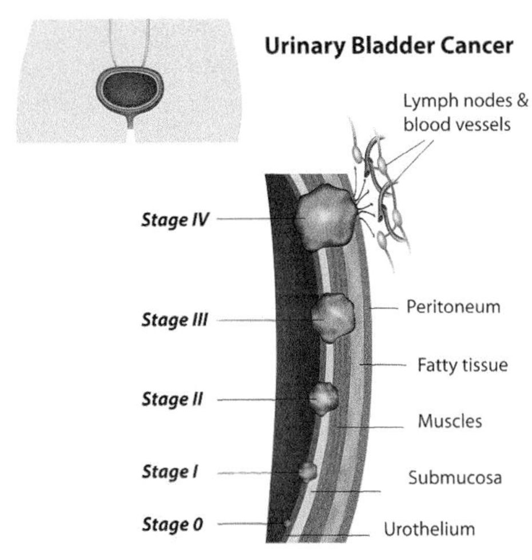

Interstitial Cystitis

Interstitial cystitis is an inflammatory condition of the bladder that results in ongoing pain and feeling the need to urinate urgently and frequently.

Cystocele

Cystocele is a condition that occurs when the tough fibrous wall between a woman's bladder and her vagina weakens, allowing the bladder to droop into the vagina.

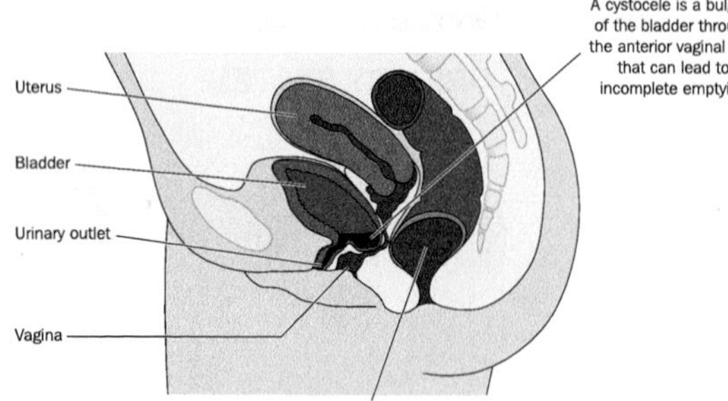
A cystocele is a bulging of the bladder through the anterior vaginal wall that can lead to incomplete emptying
Uterus
Bladder
Urinary outlet
Vagina

UTI

A urinary tract infection, or UTI, is a bacterial infection of one or more structures in the urinary tract, typically involving the bladder or urethra.

Kidney Stones

A kidney stone, also known as a calculus, results from a buildup of mineral salts or other such material in the kidney. Kidney stones vary in size. Larger stones can block the flow of urine, resulting in severe pain and blood in the urine.

Diseases of the genitourinary system (N00-N99)

EXCLUDES2 *certain conditions originating in the perinatal period (P04-P96)*
certain infectious and parasitic diseases (A00-B99)
complications of pregnancy, childbirth and the puerperium (O00-O9A)
congenital malformations, deformations and chromosomal abnormalities (Q00-Q99)
endocrine, nutritional and metabolic diseases (E00-E88)
injury, poisoning and certain other consequences of external causes (S00-T88)
neoplasms (C00-D49)
symptoms, signs and abnormal clinical and laboratory findings, not elsewhere classified (R00-R94)

This chapter contains the following blocks:

N00-N08	Glomerular diseases
N10-N16	Renal tubulo-interstitial diseases
N17-N19	Acute kidney failure and chronic kidney disease
N20-N23	Urolithiasis
N25-N29	Other disorders of kidney and ureter
N30-N39	Other diseases of the urinary system
N40-N53	Diseases of male genital organs
N60-N65	Disorders of breast
N70-N77	Inflammatory diseases of female pelvic organs
N80-N98	Noninflammatory disorders of female genital tract
N99	Intraoperative and postprocedural complications and disorders of genitourinary system, not elsewhere classified

Glomerular diseases (N00-N08)

Code also any associated kidney failure (N17-N19).

EXCLUDES1 *hypertensive chronic kidney disease (I12.-)*

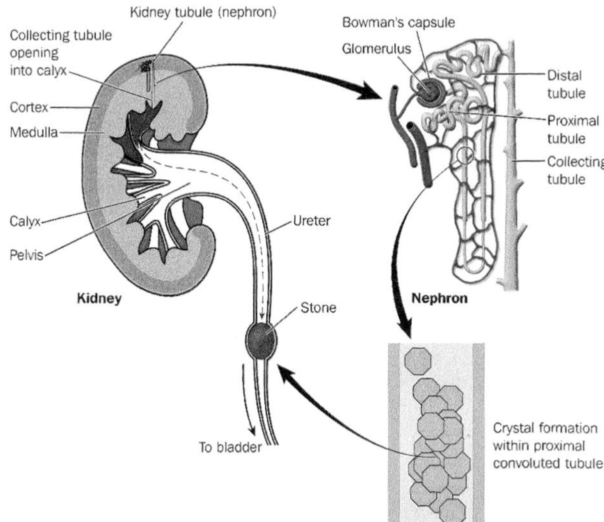

Figure 14.1 Kidney and nephron showing calculus (stone) formation

N00 Acute nephritic syndrome (4th character required)

INCLUDES *acute glomerular disease*
acute glomerulonephritis
acute nephritis

EXCLUDES1 *acute tubulo-interstitial nephritis (N10)*
nephritic syndrome NOS (N05.-)

N00.0 Acute nephritic syndrome with minor glomerular abnormality MCC
Acute nephritic syndrome with minimal change lesion

N00.1 Acute nephritic syndrome with focal and segmental glomerular lesions MCC
Acute nephritic syndrome with focal and segmental hyalinosis
Acute nephritic syndrome with focal and segmental sclerosis
Acute nephritic syndrome with focal glomerulonephritis

N00.2 Acute nephritic syndrome with diffuse membranous glomerulonephritis MCC

N00.3 Acute nephritic syndrome with diffuse mesangial proliferative glomerulonephritis MCC

N00.4 Acute nephritic syndrome with diffuse endocapillary proliferative glomerulonephritis MCC

N00.5 Acute nephritic syndrome with diffuse mesangiocapillary glomerulonephritis MCC
Acute nephritic syndrome with membranoproliferative glomerulonephritis, types 1 and 3, or NOS

N00.6 Acute nephritic syndrome with dense deposit disease MCC
Acute nephritic syndrome with membranoproliferative glomerulonephritis, type 2

N00.7 Acute nephritic syndrome with diffuse crescentic glomerulonephritis MCC
Acute nephritic syndrome with extracapillary glomerulonephritis

N00.8 Acute nephritic syndrome with other morphologic changes MCC
Acute nephritic syndrome with proliferative glomerulonephritis NOS

N00.9 Acute nephritic syndrome with unspecified morphologic changes MCC

N01 Rapidly progressive **nephritic syndrome** (4th character required)

INCLUDES *rapidly progressive glomerular disease*
rapidly progressive glomerulonephritis
rapidly progressive nephritis

EXCLUDES1 *nephritic syndrome NOS (N05.-)*

N01.0 Rapidly progressive nephritic syndrome with minor glomerular abnormality MCC
Rapidly progressive nephritic syndrome with minimal change lesion

N01.1 Rapidly progressive nephritic syndrome with focal and segmental glomerular lesions MCC
Rapidly progressive nephritic syndrome with focal and segmental hyalinosis
Rapidly progressive nephritic syndrome with focal and segmental sclerosis
Rapidly progressive nephritic syndrome with focal glomerulonephritis

N01.2 Rapidly progressive nephritic syndrome with diffuse membranous glomerulonephritis MCC

N01.3 Rapidly progressive nephritic syndrome with diffuse mesangial proliferative glomerulonephritis MCC

N01.4 Rapidly progressive nephritic syndrome with diffuse endocapillary proliferative glomerulonephritis MCC

N01.5 Rapidly progressive nephritic syndrome with diffuse mesangiocapillary glomerulonephritis MCC
Rapidly progressive nephritic syndrome with membranoproliferative glomerulonephritis, types 1 and 3, or NOS

N01.6 Rapidly progressive nephritic syndrome with dense deposit disease MCC
Rapidly progressive nephritic syndrome with membranoproliferative glomerulonephritis, type 2

N01.7 Rapidly progressive nephritic syndrome with diffuse crescentic glomerulonephritis MCC
Rapidly progressive nephritic syndrome with extracapillary glomerulonephritis

N01.8 Rapidly progressive nephritic syndrome with other morphologic changes MCC
Rapidly progressive nephritic syndrome with proliferative glomerulonephritis NOS

N01.9 Rapidly progressive nephritic syndrome with unspecified morphologic changes MCC

N02 Recurrent and persistent hematuria (4th character required)

EXCLUDES1 *acute cystitis with hematuria (N30.01)*
hematuria NOS (R31.9)
hematuria not associated with specified morphologic lesions (R31.-)

N02.0 Recurrent and persistent hematuria with minor glomerular abnormality CC
Recurrent and persistent hematuria with minimal change lesion

Unspecified Code Other Specified Code Manifestation Code N Newborn P Pediatric M Maternity A Adult ♂ Male ♀ Female
● New Code ▲ Revised Code Title ►◄ Revised Text NOTES INCLUDES EXCLUDES1 Not coded here EXCLUDES2 Not included here
4th character required 5th character required 6th character required 7th character required
Extension 'X' Alert HAC Hospital-acquired condition (HAC) alert AHA AHA Coding Clinic®

N02.1 **Recurrent and persistent hematuria** with focal and segmental glomerular lesions
Recurrent and persistent hematuria with focal and segmental hyalinosis
Recurrent and persistent hematuria with focal and segmental sclerosis
Recurrent and persistent hematuria with focal glomerulonephritis

N02.2 **Recurrent and persistent hematuria** with diffuse membranous glomerulonephritis

N02.3 **Recurrent and persistent hematuria** with diffuse mesangial proliferative glomerulonephritis

N02.4 **Recurrent and persistent hematuria** with diffuse endocapillary proliferative glomerulonephritis

N02.5 **Recurrent and persistent hematuria** with diffuse mesangiocapillary glomerulonephritis
Recurrent and persistent hematuria with membranoproliferative glomerulonephritis, types 1 and 3, or NOS

N02.6 **Recurrent and persistent hematuria** with dense deposit disease
Recurrent and persistent hematuria with membranoproliferative glomerulonephritis, type 2

N02.7 **Recurrent and persistent hematuria** with diffuse crescentic glomerulonephritis
Recurrent and persistent hematuria with extracapillary glomerulonephritis

N02.8 **Recurrent and persistent hematuria with other morphologic changes**
Recurrent and persistent hematuria with proliferative glomerulonephritis NOS

N02.9 **Recurrent and persistent hematuria with unspecified morphologic changes**

N03 Chronic **nephritic syndrome**

INCLUDES *chronic glomerular disease*
chronic glomerulonephritis
chronic nephritis

EXCLUDES1 *chronic tubulo-interstitial nephritis (N11.-)*
diffuse sclerosing glomerulonephritis (N05.8-)
nephritic syndrome NOS (N05.-)

N03.0 **Chronic nephritic syndrome** with minor glomerular abnormality
Chronic nephritic syndrome with minimal change lesion

N03.1 **Chronic nephritic syndrome** with focal and segmental glomerular lesions
Chronic nephritic syndrome with focal and segmental hyalinosis
Chronic nephritic syndrome with focal and segmental sclerosis
Chronic nephritic syndrome with focal glomerulonephritis

N03.2 **Chronic nephritic syndrome** with diffuse membranous glomerulonephritis

N03.3 **Chronic nephritic syndrome** with diffuse mesangial proliferative glomerulonephritis

N03.4 **Chronic nephritic syndrome** with diffuse endocapillary proliferative glomerulonephritis

N03.5 **Chronic nephritic syndrome** with diffuse mesangiocapillary glomerulonephritis
Chronic nephritic syndrome with membranoproliferative glomerulonephritis, types 1 and 3, or NOS

N03.6 **Chronic nephritic syndrome** with dense deposit disease
Chronic nephritic syndrome with membranoproliferative glomerulonephritis, type 2

N03.7 **Chronic nephritic syndrome with diffuse crescentic glomerulonephritis**
Chronic nephritic syndrome with extracapillary glomerulonephritis

N03.8 **Chronic nephritic syndrome with other morphologic changes**
Chronic nephritic syndrome with proliferative glomerulonephritis NOS

N03.9 **Chronic nephritic syndrome with unspecified morphologic changes**

N04 Nephrotic syndrome

INCLUDES *congenital nephrotic syndrome*
lipoid nephrosis

N04.0 **Nephrotic syndrome** with minor glomerular abnormality
Nephrotic syndrome with minimal change lesion

N04.1 **Nephrotic syndrome** with focal and segmental glomerular lesions
Nephrotic syndrome with focal and segmental hyalinosis
Nephrotic syndrome with focal and segmental sclerosis
Nephrotic syndrome with focal glomerulonephritis

N04.2 **Nephrotic syndrome** with diffuse membranous glomerulonephritis

N04.3 **Nephrotic syndrome** with diffuse mesangial proliferative glomerulonephritis

N04.4 **Nephrotic syndrome** with diffuse endocapillary proliferative glomerulonephritis

N04.5 **Nephrotic syndrome** with diffuse mesangiocapillary glomerulonephritis
Nephrotic syndrome with membranoproliferative glomerulonephritis, types 1 and 3, or NOS

N04.6 **Nephrotic syndrome** with dense deposit disease
Nephrotic syndrome with membranoproliferative glomerulonephritis, type 2

N04.7 **Nephrotic syndrome** with diffuse crescentic glomerulonephritis
Nephrotic syndrome with extracapillary glomerulonephritis

N04.8 **Nephrotic syndrome with other morphologic changes**
Nephrotic syndrome with proliferative glomerulonephritis NOS

N04.9 **Nephrotic syndrome with unspecified morphologic changes**

N05 Unspecified nephritic syndrome

INCLUDES *glomerular disease NOS*
glomerulonephritis NOS
nephritis NOS
nephropathy NOS and renal disease NOS with morphological lesion specified in .0-.8

EXCLUDES1 *nephropathy NOS with no stated morphological lesion (N28.9)*
renal disease NOS with no stated morphological lesion (N28.9)
tubulo-interstitial nephritis NOS (N12)

N05.0 **Unspecified nephritic syndrome** with minor glomerular abnormality
Unspecified nephritic syndrome with minimal change lesion

N05.1 **Unspecified nephritic syndrome** with focal and segmental glomerular lesions
Unspecified nephritic syndrome with focal and segmental hyalinosis
Unspecified nephritic syndrome with focal and segmental sclerosis
Unspecified nephritic syndrome with focal glomerulonephritis

N05.2 **Unspecified nephritic syndrome** with diffuse membranous glomerulonephritis

N05.3 **Unspecified nephritic syndrome** with diffuse mesangial proliferative glomerulonephritis

N05.4 **Unspecified nephritic syndrome** with diffuse endocapillary proliferative glomerulonephritis

N05.5 **Unspecified nephritic syndrome** with diffuse mesangiocapillary glomerulonephritis
Unspecified nephritic syndrome with membranoproliferative glomerulonephritis, types 1 and 3, or NOS

N05.6 **Unspecified nephritic syndrome** with dense deposit disease
Unspecified nephritic syndrome with membranoproliferative glomerulonephritis, type 2

N05.7 **Unspecified nephritic syndrome** with diffuse crescentic glomerulonephritis
Unspecified nephritic syndrome with extracapillary glomerulonephritis

N05.8 **Unspecified nephritic syndrome** with other morphologic changes
Unspecified nephritic syndrome with proliferative glomerulonephritis NOS

N05.9 **Unspecified nephritic syndrome** with unspecified morphologic changes

N06 Isolated proteinuria with specified morphological lesion

EXCLUDES1 *Proteinuria not associated with specific morphologic lesions (R80.0)*

N06.0 **Isolated proteinuria** with minor glomerular abnormality
Isolated proteinuria with minimal change lesion

Unacceptable principal diagnosis symbol per Medicare code edits · Code exempt from diagnosis present on admission requirement
Questionable admission · Complication or comorbidity · CC/MCC exclusion · Major complication or comorbidity
Principal diagnosis as its own CC · Principal diagnosis as its own MCC · Z code as first-listed diagnosis

When symbols appear on a code that requires a 7th character extension, refer to Appendix D to identify applicable 7th character codes.

N06.1 **Isolated proteinuria** with focal and segmental glomerular lesions
Isolated proteinuria with focal and segmental hyalinosis
Isolated proteinuria with focal and segmental sclerosis
Isolated proteinuria with focal glomerulonephritis

N06.2 **Isolated proteinuria** with diffuse membranous glomerulonephritis

N06.3 **Isolated proteinuria** with diffuse mesangial proliferative glomerulonephritis

N06.4 **Isolated proteinuria** with diffuse endocapillary proliferative glomerulonephritis

N06.5 **Isolated proteinuria** with diffuse mesangiocapillary glomerulonephritis
Isolated proteinuria with membranoproliferative glomerulonephritis, types 1 and 3, or NOS

N06.6 **Isolated proteinuria** with dense deposit disease
Isolated proteinuria with membranoproliferative glomerulonephritis, type 2

N06.7 **Isolated proteinuria** with diffuse crescentic glomerulonephritis
Isolated proteinuria with extracapillary glomerulonephritis

N06.8 **Isolated proteinuria with other morphologic lesion**
Isolated proteinuria with proliferative glomerulonephritis NOS

N06.9 **Isolated proteinuria with unspecified morphologic lesion**

N07 **Hereditary nephropathy, not elsewhere classified**
EXCLUDES2 *Alport's syndrome (Q87.81-)*
hereditary amyloid nephropathy (E85.-)
nail patella syndrome (Q87.2)
non-neuropathic heredofamilial amyloidosis (E85.-)

N07.0 **Hereditary nephropathy, not elsewhere classified** with minor glomerular abnormality
Hereditary nephropathy, not elsewhere classified with minimal change lesion

N07.1 **Hereditary nephropathy, not elsewhere classified** with focal and segmental glomerular lesions
Hereditary nephropathy, not elsewhere classified with focal and segmental hyalinosis
Hereditary nephropathy, not elsewhere classified with focal and segmental sclerosis
Hereditary nephropathy, not elsewhere classified with focal glomerulonephritis

N07.2 **Hereditary nephropathy, not elsewhere classified** with diffuse membranous glomerulonephritis

N07.3 **Hereditary nephropathy, not elsewhere classified** with diffuse mesangial proliferative glomerulonephritis

N07.4 **Hereditary nephropathy, not elsewhere classified** with diffuse endocapillary proliferative glomerulonephritis

N07.5 **Hereditary nephropathy, not elsewhere classified** with diffuse mesangiocapillary glomerulonephritis
Hereditary nephropathy, not elsewhere classified with membranoproliferative glomerulonephritis, types 1 and 3, or NOS

N07.6 **Hereditary nephropathy, not elsewhere classified** with dense deposit disease
Hereditary nephropathy, not elsewhere classified with membranoproliferative glomerulonephritis, type 2

N07.7 **Hereditary nephropathy, not elsewhere classified** with diffuse crescentic glomerulonephritis
Hereditary nephropathy, not elsewhere classified with extracapillary glomerulonephritis

N07.8 **Hereditary nephropathy, not elsewhere classified with other morphologic lesions**
Hereditary nephropathy, not elsewhere classified with proliferative glomerulonephritis NOS

N07.9 **Hereditary nephropathy, not elsewhere classified with unspecified morphologic lesions**

N08 **Glomerular disorders in diseases classified elsewhere**
Glomerulonephritis
Nephritis
Nephropathy
Code first underlying disease, such as:
amyloidosis (E85.-)
congenital syphilis (A50.5)
cryoglobulinemia (D89.1)
disseminated intravascular coagulation (D65)
gout (M1A.-, M10.-)
microscopic polyangiitis (M31.7)
multiple myeloma (C90.0-)
sepsis (A40.0-A41.9)
sickle-cell disease (D57.0-D57.8)
EXCLUDES1 *glomerulonephritis, nephritis and nephropathy (in):*
antiglomerular basement membrane disease (M31.0)
diabetes (E08-E13 with .21)
gonococcal (A54.21)
Goodpasture's syndrome (M31.0)
hemolytic-uremic syndrome (D59.3)
lupus (M32.14)
mumps (B26.83)
syphilis (A52.75)
systemic lupus erythematosus (M32.14)
Wegener's granulomatosis (M31.31)
pyelonephritis in diseases classified elsewhere (N16)
renal tubulo-interstitial disorders classified elsewhere (N16)

Renal tubulo-interstitial diseases (N10-N16)

INCLUDES *pyelonephritis*
EXCLUDES1 *pyeloureteritis cystica (N28.85)*

▲ N10 **Acute ►pyelonephritis◄**
Acute infectious interstitial nephritis
Acute pyelitis
Acute ►tubulo-interstitial nephritis◄
Hemoglobin nephrosis
Myoglobin nephrosis
Use additional code (B95-B97), to identify infectious agent.

N11 **Chronic tubulo-interstitial nephritis**
INCLUDES *chronic infectious interstitial nephritis*
chronic pyelitis
chronic pyelonephritis
Use additional code (B95-B97), to identify infectious agent.

N11.0 **Nonobstructive reflux-associated chronic pyelonephritis**
Pyelonephritis (chronic) associated with (vesicoureteral) reflux
EXCLUDES1 *vesicoureteral reflux NOS (N13.70)*

N11.1 **Chronic obstructive pyelonephritis**
Pyelonephritis (chronic) associated with anomaly of pelviureteric junction
Pyelonephritis (chronic) associated with anomaly of pyeloureteric junction
Pyelonephritis (chronic) associated with crossing of vessel
Pyelonephritis (chronic) associated with kinking of ureter
Pyelonephritis (chronic) associated with obstruction of ureter
Pyelonephritis (chronic) associated with stricture of pelviureteric junction
Pyelonephritis (chronic) associated with stricture of ureter
EXCLUDES1 *calculous pyelonephritis (N20.9)*
obstructive uropathy (N13.-)

N11.8 **Other chronic tubulo-interstitial nephritis**
Nonobstructive chronic pyelonephritis NOS

N11.9 **Chronic tubulo-interstitial nephritis, unspecified**
Chronic interstitial nephritis NOS
Chronic pyelitis NOS
Chronic pyelonephritis NOS

N12 **Tubulo-interstitial nephritis, not specified as acute or chronic**
Interstitial nephritis NOS
Pyelitis NOS
Pyelonephritis NOS
EXCLUDES1 *calculous pyelonephritis (N20.9)*

N13 **Obstructive and reflux uropathy**
EXCLUDES2 *calculus of kidney and ureter without hydronephrosis (N20.-)*
congenital obstructive defects of renal pelvis and ureter (Q62.0-Q62.3)
hydronephrosis with ureteropelvic junction obstruction (Q62.1)
obstructive pyelonephritis (N11.1)

● N13.0 Hydronephrosis with ureteropelvic junction **obstruction**
Hydronephrosis due to acquired occlusion of ureteropelvic junction
EXCLUDES2 *Hydronephrosis with ureteropelvic junction obstruction due to calculus (N13.2)*

Unspecified Code Other Specified Code Manifestation Code N Newborn P Pediatric M Maternity A Adult ♂ Male ♀ Female
● New Code ▲ Revised Code Title ►◄ Revised Text NOTES INCLUDES EXCLUDES1 Not coded here EXCLUDES2 Not included here
4th character required 5th character required 6th character required 7th character required
Extension 'X' Alert HAC Hospital-acquired condition (HAC) alert AHA AHA Coding Clinic©

N13.1 **Hydronephrosis with ureteral stricture, not elsewhere classified**

EXCLUDES1 *Hydronephrosis with ureteral stricture with infection (N13.6)*

N13.2 **Hydronephrosis with renal and ureteral calculous obstruction**

EXCLUDES1 *Hydronephrosis with renal and ureteral calculous obstruction with infection (N13.6)*

N13.3 **Other and unspecified hydronephrosis**

EXCLUDES1 *hydronephrosis with infection (N13.6)*

N13.30 **Unspecified hydronephrosis**

N13.39 **Other hydronephrosis**

N13.4 **Hydroureter**

EXCLUDES1 *congenital hydroureter (Q62.3-)*
hydroureter with infection (N13.6)
vesicoureteral-reflux with hydroureter (N13.73-)

N13.5 **Crossing vessel and stricture of ureter without hydronephrosis**

Kinking and stricture of ureter without hydronephrosis

EXCLUDES1 *Crossing vessel and stricture of ureter without hydronephrosis with infection (N13.6)*

N13.6 **Pyonephrosis**

Conditions in ▶N13.0-N13.5◀ with infection
Obstructive uropathy with infection
Use additional code (B95-B97), to identify infectious agent.

N13.7 **Vesicoureteral-reflux**

EXCLUDES1 *reflux-associated pyelonephritis (N11.0)*

N13.70 **Vesicoureteral-reflux, unspecified**

Vesicoureteral-reflux NOS

N13.71 **Vesicoureteral-reflux** without reflux nephropathy

N13.72 **Vesicoureteral-reflux** with reflux nephropathy without hydroureter

N13.721 **Vesicoureteral-reflux with reflux nephropathy without hydroureter,** unilateral

N13.722 **Vesicoureteral-reflux with reflux nephropathy without hydroureter,** bilateral

N13.729 **Vesicoureteral-reflux with reflux nephropathy without hydroureter, unspecified**

N13.73 **Vesicoureteral-reflux** with reflux nephropathy with hydroureter

N13.731 **Vesicoureteral-reflux with reflux nephropathy with hydroureter,** unilateral

N13.732 **Vesicoureteral-reflux with reflux nephropathy with hydroureter,** bilateral

N13.739 **Vesicoureteral-reflux with reflux nephropathy with hydroureter, unspecified**

N13.8 **Other obstructive and reflux uropathy**

Urinary tract obstruction due to specified cause
Code first , if applicable, any causal condition, such as:
enlarged prostate (N40.1)

N13.9 **Obstructive and reflux uropathy, unspecified**

Urinary tract obstruction NOS

N14 **Drug- and heavy-metal-induced tubulo-interstitial and tubular conditions**

Code first poisoning due to drug or toxin, if applicable (T36-T65 with fifth or sixth character 1-4 or 6)
Use additional code for adverse effect, if applicable, to identify drug (T36-T50 with fifth or sixth character 5)

N14.0 **Analgesic nephropathy**

N14.1 **Nephropathy induced by other drugs, medicaments and biological substances**

N14.2 **Nephropathy induced by unspecified drug, medicament or biological substance**

N14.3 **Nephropathy induced by heavy metals**

N14.4 **Toxic nephropathy, not elsewhere classified**

N15 **Other renal tubulo-interstitial diseases**

N15.0 **Balkan nephropathy**

Balkan endemic nephropathy

N15.1 **Renal and perinephric abscess**

N15.8 **Other specified renal tubulo-interstitial diseases**

N15.9 **Renal tubulo-interstitial disease, unspecified**

Infection of kidney NOS

EXCLUDES1 *urinary tract infection NOS (N39.0)*

N16 **Renal tubulo-interstitial disorders in diseases classified elsewhere**

Pyelonephritis
Tubulo-interstitial nephritis
Code first underlying disease, such as:
brucellosis (A23.0-A23.9)
cryoglobulinemia (D89.1)
glycogen storage disease (E74.0)
leukemia (C91-C95)
lymphoma (C81.0-C85.9, C96.0-C96.9)
multiple myeloma (C90.0-)
sepsis (A40.0-A41.9)
Wilson's disease (E83.0)

EXCLUDES1 *diphtheritic pyelonephritis and tubulo-interstitial nephritis (A36.84)*
pyelonephritis and tubulo-interstitial nephritis in candidiasis (B37.49)
pyelonephritis and tubulo-interstitial nephritis in cystinosis (E72.04)
pyelonephritis and tubulo-interstitial nephritis in salmonella infection (A02.25)
pyelonephritis and tubulo-interstitial nephritis in sarcoidosis (D86.84)
pyelonephritis and tubulo-interstitial nephritis in sicca syndrome [Sjogren's] (M35.04)
pyelonephritis and tubulo-interstitial nephritis in systemic lupus erythematosus (M32.15)
pyelonephritis and tubulo-interstitial nephritis in toxoplasmosis (B58.83)
renal tubular degeneration in diabetes (E08-E13 with .29)
syphilitic pyelonephritis and tubulo-interstitial nephritis (A52.75)

Acute kidney failure and chronic kidney disease (N17-N19)

EXCLUDES2 *congenital renal failure (P96.0)*
drug- and heavy-metal-induced tubulo-interstitial and tubular conditions (N14.-)
extrarenal uremia (R39.2)
hemolytic-uremic syndrome (D59.3)
hepatorenal syndrome (K76.7)
postpartum hepatorenal syndrome (O90.4)
posttraumatic renal failure (T79.5)
prerenal uremia (R39.2)
renal failure complicating abortion or ectopic or molar pregnancy (O00-O07, O08.4)
renal failure following labor and delivery (O90.4)
renal failure postprocedural (N99.0)

N17 Acute **kidney failure**

Code also associated underlying condition

EXCLUDES1 *posttraumatic renal failure (T79.5)*

N17.0 **Acute kidney failure** with tubular necrosis

Acute tubular necrosis
Renal tubular necrosis
Tubular necrosis NOS

N17.1 **Acute kidney failure** with acute cortical necrosis

Acute cortical necrosis
Cortical necrosis NOS
Renal cortical necrosis

N17.2 **Acute kidney failure** with medullary necrosis

Medullary [papillary] necrosis NOS
Acute medullary [papillary] necrosis
Renal medullary [papillary] necrosis

N17.8 **Other acute kidney failure**

N17.9 **Acute kidney failure, unspecified**

Acute kidney injury (nontraumatic)

EXCLUDES2 *traumatic kidney injury (S37.0-)*

Unacceptable principal diagnosis symbol per Medicare code edits · Code exempt from diagnosis present on admission requirement · Questionable admission · Complication or comorbidity · CC/MCC exclusion · Major complication or comorbidity · Principal diagnosis as its own CC · Principal diagnosis as its own MCC · Z code as first-listed diagnosis

N18 Chronic kidney disease (CKD)
Code first any associated:
diabetic chronic kidney disease (E08.22, E09.22, E10.22, E11.22, E13.22)
hypertensive chronic kidney disease (I12.-, I13.-)
Use additional code to identify kidney transplant status, if applicable, (Z94.0)

N18.1 Chronic kidney disease, stage 1

N18.2 Chronic kidney disease, stage 2 (mild)

N18.3 Chronic kidney disease, stage 3 (moderate)

N18.4 Chronic kidney disease, stage 4 (severe) CC
AHA: Q1, 2013

N18.5 Chronic kidney disease, stage 5 CC
EXCLUDES1 *chronic kidney disease, stage 5 requiring chronic dialysis (N18.6)*

N18.6 End stage renal disease MCC
Chronic kidney disease requiring chronic dialysis
Use additional code to identify dialysis status (Z99.2)
AHA: Q4, 2013

N18.9 Chronic kidney disease, unspecified
Chronic renal disease
Chronic renal failure NOS
Chronic renal insufficiency
Chronic uremia

N19 Unspecified kidney failure
Uremia NOS
EXCLUDES1 *acute kidney failure (N17.-)*
chronic kidney disease (N18.-)
chronic uremia (N18.9)
extrarenal uremia (R39.2)
prerenal uremia (R39.2)
renal insufficiency (acute) (N28.9)
uremia of newborn (P96.0)

Urolithiasis (N20-N23)

N20 Calculus of kidney and ureter
Calculous pyelonephritis
EXCLUDES1 *nephrocalcinosis (E83.5)*
that with hydronephrosis (N13.2)

N20.0 Calculus of kidney
Nephrolithiasis NOS
Renal calculus
Renal stone
Staghorn calculus
Stone in kidney

N20.1 Calculus of ureter CC
Ureteric stone

N20.2 Calculus of kidney with calculus of ureter CC

N20.9 Urinary calculus, unspecified

N21 Calculus of lower urinary tract
INCLUDES *calculus of lower urinary tract with cystitis and urethritis*

N21.0 Calculus in bladder
Calculus in diverticulum of bladder
Urinary bladder stone
EXCLUDES2 *staghorn calculus (N20.0)*

N21.1 Calculus in urethra
EXCLUDES2 *calculus of prostate (N42.0)*

N21.8 Other lower urinary tract calculus

N21.9 Calculus of lower urinary tract, unspecified
EXCLUDES1 *calculus of urinary tract NOS (N20.9)*

N22 Calculus of urinary tract in diseases classified elsewhere
Code first underlying disease, such as:
gout (M1A.-, M10.-)
schistosomiasis (B65.0-B65.9)

N23 Unspecified renal colic

Other disorders of kidney and ureter (N25-N29)

EXCLUDES2 *disorders of kidney and ureter with urolithiasis (N20-N23)*

N25 Disorders resulting from impaired renal tubular function
EXCLUDES1 *metabolic disorders classifiable to E70-E88*

N25.0 Renal osteodystrophy
Azotemic osteodystrophy
Phosphate-losing tubular disorders
Renal rickets
Renal short stature

N25.1 Nephrogenic diabetes insipidus CC
EXCLUDES1 *diabetes insipidus NOS (E23.2)*

N25.8 Other disorders resulting from impaired renal tubular function

N25.81 Secondary hyperparathyroidism of renal origin CC
EXCLUDES1 *secondary hyperparathyroidism, non-renal (E21.1)*

N25.89 Other disorders resulting from impaired renal tubular function
Hypokalemic nephropathy
Lightwood-Albright syndrome
Renal tubular acidosis NOS

N25.9 Disorder resulting from impaired renal tubular function, unspecified

N26 Unspecified contracted kidney
EXCLUDES1 *contracted kidney due to hypertension (I12.-)*
diffuse sclerosing glomerulonephritis (N05.8.-)
hypertensive nephrosclerosis (arteriolar) (arteriosclerotic) (I12.-)
small kidney of unknown cause (N27.-)

N26.1 Atrophy of kidney (terminal)

N26.2 Page kidney

N26.9 Renal sclerosis, unspecified

N27 Small kidney of unknown cause
INCLUDES *oligonephronia*

N27.0 Small kidney, unilateral

N27.1 Small kidney, bilateral

N27.9 Small kidney, unspecified

N28 Other disorders of kidney and ureter, not elsewhere classified

N28.0 Ischemia and infarction of kidney CC
Renal artery embolism
Renal artery obstruction
Renal artery occlusion
Renal artery thrombosis
Renal infarct
EXCLUDES1 *atherosclerosis of renal artery (extrarenal part) (I70.1)*
congenital stenosis of renal artery (Q27.1)
Goldblatt's kidney (I70.1)

N28.1 Cyst of kidney, acquired
Cyst (multiple)(solitary) of kidney, acquired
EXCLUDES1 *cystic kidney disease (congenital) (Q61.-)*

N28.8 Other specified disorders of kidney and ureter
EXCLUDES1 *hydroureter (N13.4)*
ureteric stricture with hydronephrosis (N13.1)
ureteric stricture without hydronephrosis (N13.5)

N28.81 Hypertrophy of kidney

N28.82 Megaloureter

N28.83 Nephroptosis

N28.84 Pyelitis cystica CC

N28.85 Pyeloureteritis cystica CC

N28.86 Ureteritis cystica CC

N28.89 Other specified disorders of kidney and ureter

N28.9 Disorder of kidney and ureter, unspecified
Nephropathy NOS
Renal disease (acute) NOS
Renal insufficiency (acute)
EXCLUDES1 *chronic renal insufficiency (N18.9)*
unspecified nephritic syndrome (N05.-)
AHA: Q1, 2016

Unspecified Code | Other Specified Code | Manifestation Code | N Newborn | P Pediatric | M Maternity | A Adult | ♂ Male | ♀ Female
● New Code | ▲ Revised Code Title | ►◄ Revised Text | NOTES | INCLUDES | EXCLUDES1 Not coded here | EXCLUDES2 Not included here
4th character required | 5th character required | 6th character required | 7th character required
Extension 'X' Alert | HAC Hospital-acquired condition (HAC) alert | AHA AHA Coding Clinic©

When symbols appear on a code that requires a 7th character extension, refer to Appendix D to identify applicable 7th character codes.

N29 **Other disorders of kidney and ureter in diseases classified elsewhere**
Code first underlying disease, such as:
amyloidosis (E85.-)
nephrocalcinosis (E83.5)
schistosomiasis (B65.0-B65.9)
EXCLUDES1 *disorders of kidney and ureter in:*
cystinosis (E72.0)
gonorrhea (A54.21)
syphilis (A52.75)
tuberculosis (A18.11)

Other diseases of the urinary system (N30-N39)

EXCLUDES1 *urinary infection (complicating):*
abortion or ectopic or molar pregnancy (O00-O07, O08.8)
pregnancy, childbirth and the puerperium (O23.-, O75.3, O86.2-)

N30 **Cystitis**
Use additional code to identify infectious agent (B95-B97)
EXCLUDES1 *prostatocystitis (N41.3)*

N30.0 **Acute cystitis**
EXCLUDES1 *irradiation cystitis (N30.4-)*
trigonitis (N30.3-)
N30.00 **Acute cystitis without hematuria** CC
N30.01 **Acute cystitis with hematuria** CC

N30.1 **Interstitial cystitis (chronic)**
N30.10 **Interstitial cystitis (chronic) without hematuria**
N30.11 **Interstitial cystitis (chronic) with hematuria**

N30.2 **Other chronic cystitis**
N30.20 **Other chronic cystitis without hematuria**
N30.21 **Other chronic cystitis with hematuria**

N30.3 **Trigonitis**
Urethrotrigonitis
N30.30 **Trigonitis without hematuria**
N30.31 **Trigonitis with hematuria**

N30.4 **Irradiation cystitis**
N30.40 **Irradiation cystitis without hematuria** CC
N30.41 **Irradiation cystitis with hematuria** CC

N30.8 **Other cystitis**
Abscess of bladder
N30.80 **Other cystitis without hematuria**
N30.81 **Other cystitis with hematuria**

N30.9 **Cystitis, unspecified**
N30.90 **Cystitis, unspecified without hematuria**
N30.91 **Cystitis, unspecified with hematuria**

N31 **Neuromuscular dysfunction of bladder, not elsewhere classified**
Use additional code to identify any associated urinary incontinence (N39.3-N39.4-)
EXCLUDES1 *cord bladder NOS (G95.89)*
neurogenic bladder due to cauda equina syndrome (G83.4)
neuromuscular dysfunction due to spinal cord lesion (G95.89)

N31.0 **Uninhibited neuropathic bladder, not elsewhere classified**
N31.1 **Reflex neuropathic bladder, not elsewhere classified**
N31.2 **Flaccid neuropathic bladder, not elsewhere classified**
Atonic (motor) (sensory) neuropathic bladder
Autonomous neuropathic bladder
Nonreflex neuropathic bladder
N31.8 **Other neuromuscular dysfunction of bladder**
N31.9 **Neuromuscular dysfunction of bladder, unspecified**
Neurogenic bladder dysfunction NOS

N32 **Other disorders of bladder**
EXCLUDES2 *calculus of bladder (N21.0)*
cystocele (N81.1-)
hernia or prolapse of bladder, female (N81.1-)

N32.0 **Bladder-neck obstruction**
Bladder-neck stenosis (acquired)
EXCLUDES1 *congenital bladder-neck obstruction (Q64.3-)*
N32.1 **Vesicointestinal fistula** CC
Vesicorectal fistula
N32.2 **Vesical fistula, not elsewhere classified** CC
EXCLUDES1 *fistula between bladder and female genital tract (N82.0-N82.1)*
N32.3 **Diverticulum of bladder**
EXCLUDES1 *congenital diverticulum of bladder (Q64.6)*
diverticulitis of bladder (N30.8-)

N32.8 **Other specified disorders of bladder**
N32.81 **Overactive bladder**
Detrusor muscle hyperactivity
EXCLUDES1 *frequent urination due to specified bladder condition- code to condition*
N32.89 **Other specified disorders of bladder**
Bladder hemorrhage
Bladder hypertrophy
Calcified bladder
Contracted bladder
N32.9 **Bladder disorder, unspecified**

N33 **Bladder disorders in diseases classified elsewhere**
Code first underlying disease, such as:
schistosomiasis (B65.0-B65.9)
EXCLUDES1 *bladder disorder in syphilis (A52.76)*
bladder disorder in tuberculosis (A18.12)
candidal cystitis (B37.41)
chlamydial cystitis (A56.01)
cystitis in gonorrhea (A54.01)
cystitis in neurogenic bladder (N31.-)
diphtheritic cystitis (A36.85)
syphilitic cystitis (A52.76)
trichomonal cystitis (A59.03)

N34 **Urethritis and urethral syndrome**
Use additional code (B95-B97), to identify infectious agent.
EXCLUDES2 *Reiter's disease (M02.3-)*
urethritis in diseases with a predominantly sexual mode of transmission (A50-A64)
urethrotrigonitis (N30.3-)

N34.0 **Urethral abscess** CC
Abscess (of) Cowper's gland
Abscess (of) Littré's gland
Abscess (of) urethral (gland)
Periurethral abscess
EXCLUDES1 *urethral caruncle (N36.2)*
N34.1 **Nonspecific urethritis**
Nongonococcal urethritis
Nonvenereal urethritis
N34.2 **Other urethritis**
Meatitis, urethral
Postmenopausal urethritis
Ulcer of urethra (meatus)
Urethritis NOS
N34.3 **Urethral syndrome, unspecified**

N35 **Urethral stricture**
EXCLUDES1 *congenital urethral stricture (Q64.3-)*
postprocedural urethral stricture (N99.1-)

N35.0 **Post-traumatic urethral stricture**
Urethral stricture due to injury
EXCLUDES1 *postprocedural urethral stricture (N99.1-)*
N35.01 **Post-traumatic urethral stricture, male**
N35.010 **Post-traumatic urethral stricture, male, meatal** ♂
N35.011 **Post-traumatic bulbous urethral stricture**
N35.012 **Post-traumatic membranous urethral stricture**
N35.013 **Post-traumatic anterior urethral stricture**
N35.014 **Post-traumatic urethral stricture, male, unspecified** ♂
N35.02 **Post-traumatic urethral stricture, female**
N35.021 **Urethral stricture due to childbirth** ♀
N35.028 **Other post-traumatic urethral stricture, female** ♀

N35.1 **Postinfective urethral stricture, not elsewhere classified**
EXCLUDES1 *urethral stricture associated with schistosomiasis (B65.-, N29)*
gonococcal urethral stricture (A54.01)
syphilitic urethral stricture (A52.76)
N35.11 **Postinfective urethral stricture, not elsewhere classified, male**

PDx Unacceptable principal diagnosis symbol per Medicare code edits · POA Code exempt from diagnosis present on admission requirement
Q Questionable admission · CC Complication or comorbidity · CC/MCC Exc CC/MCC exclusion · MCC Major complication or comorbidity
Principal diagnosis as its own CC · Principal diagnosis as its own MCC · Z code as first-listed diagnosis

 When symbols appear on a code that requires a 7th character extension, refer to Appendix D to identify applicable 7th character codes.

N35.111 **Postinfective urethral stricture, not elsewhere classified, male, meatal** ♂

N35.112 **Postinfective bulbous urethral stricture, not elsewhere classified**

N35.113 **Postinfective membranous urethral stricture, not elsewhere classified**

N35.114 **Postinfective anterior urethral stricture, not elsewhere classified**

N35.119 **Postinfective urethral stricture, not elsewhere classified, male, unspecified** ♂

N35.12 **Postinfective urethral stricture, not elsewhere classified, female** ♀

N35.8 **Other urethral stricture**

EXCLUDES1 *postprocedural urethral stricture (N99.1-)*

N35.9 **Urethral stricture, unspecified**

4th N36 **Other disorders of urethra**

N36.0 **Urethral fistula** cc

Urethroperineal fistula
Urethrorectal fistula
Urinary fistula NOS

EXCLUDES1 *urethroscrotal fistula ▶(N50.89)◀*
urethrovaginal fistula (N82.1)
urethrovesicovaginal fistula (N82.1)

N36.1 **Urethral diverticulum**

N36.2 **Urethral caruncle**

5th N36.4 **Urethral functional and muscular disorders**

Use additional code to identify associated urinary stress incontinence (N39.3)

N36.41 **Hypermobility of urethra**

N36.42 **Intrinsic sphincter deficiency (ISD)**

N36.43 **Combined hypermobility of urethra and intrinsic sphincter deficiency**

N36.44 **Muscular disorders of urethra**

Bladder sphincter dyssynergy

N36.5 **Urethral false passage**

N36.8 **Other specified disorders of urethra**

EXCLUDES1 *congenital urethrocele (Q64.7)*
female urethrocele (N81.0)

N36.9 **Urethral disorder, unspecified**

N37 **Urethral disorders in diseases classified elsewhere**

Code first underlying disease

EXCLUDES1 *urethritis (in):*
candidal infection (B37.41)
chlamydial (A56.01)
gonorrhea (A54.01)
syphilis (A52.76)
trichomonal infection (A59.03)
tuberculosis (A18.13)

4th N39 **Other disorders of urinary system**

EXCLUDES2 *hematuria NOS (R31.-)*
recurrent or persistent hematuria (N02.-)
recurrent or persistent hematuria with specified morphological lesion (N02.-)
proteinuria NOS (R80.-)

N39.0 **Urinary tract infection, site not specified** cc

Use additional code (B95-B97), to identify infectious agent.

EXCLUDES1 *candidiasis of urinary tract (B37.4-)*
neonatal urinary tract infection (P39.3)
urinary tract infection of specified site, such as:
cystitis (N30.-)
urethritis (N34.-)

N39.3 **Stress incontinence (female) (male)**

Code also any associated overactive bladder (N32.81)

EXCLUDES1 *mixed incontinence (N39.46)*

5th N39.4 **Other specified urinary incontinence**

Code also any associated overactive bladder (N32.81)

EXCLUDES1 *enuresis NOS (R32)*
functional urinary incontinence (R39.81)
urinary incontinence associated with cognitive impairment (R39.81)
urinary incontinence NOS (R32)
urinary incontinence of nonorganic origin (F98.0)

N39.41 **Urge incontinence**

EXCLUDES1 *mixed incontinence (N39.46)*

N39.42 **Incontinence without sensory awareness**

Insensible (urinary) incontinence

N39.43 **Post-void dribbling**

N39.44 **Nocturnal enuresis**

N39.45 **Continuous leakage**

N39.46 **Mixed incontinence**

Urge and stress incontinence

6th N39.49 **Other specified urinary incontinence**

N39.490 **Overflow incontinence**

● N39.491 **Coital incontinence**

● N39.492 **Postural (urinary) incontinence**

N39.498 **Other specified urinary incontinence**

Reflex incontinence
Total incontinence

N39.8 **Other specified disorders of urinary system**

N39.9 **Disorder of urinary system, unspecified**

Diseases of male genital organs (N40-N53)

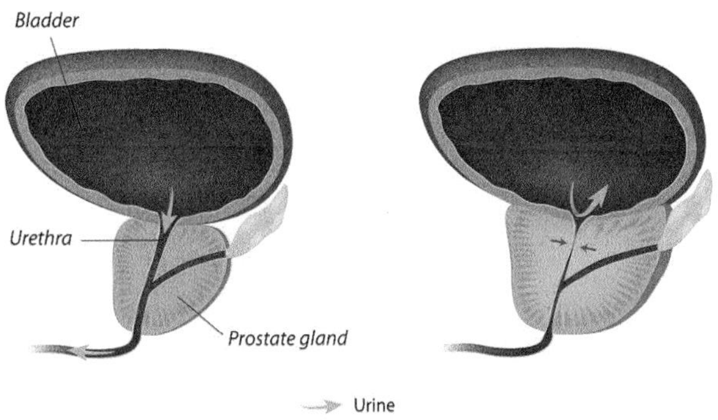

Normal — Enlarged prostate gland

Bladder
Urethra
Prostate gland
Urine

Figure 14.2 Benign prostatic hyperplasia

▲ 4th N40 ▶**Benign prostatic hyperplasia**◀

INCLUDES *adenofibromatous hypertrophy of prostate*
benign hypertrophy of the prostate
benign prostatic hypertrophy
BPH
enlarged prostate
nodular prostate
polyp of prostate

EXCLUDES1 *benign neoplasms of prostate (adenoma, benign) (fibroadenoma) (fibroma) (myoma) (D29.1)*

EXCLUDES2 *malignant neoplasm of prostate (C61)*

▲ N40.0 ▶**Benign prostatic hyperplasia**◀ **without lower urinary tract symptoms** A ♂

Enlarged prostate without LUTS
Enlarged prostate NOS

▲ N40.1 ▶**Benign prostatic hyperplasia**◀ **with lower urinary tract symptoms** A ♂

Enlarged prostate with LUTS

Use additional code for associated symptoms, when specified:
incomplete bladder emptying (R39.14)
nocturia (R35.1)
straining on urination (R39.16)
urinary frequency (R35.0)
urinary hesitancy (R39.11)
urinary incontinence (N39.4-)
urinary obstruction (N13.8)
urinary retention (R33.8)
urinary urgency (R39.15)
weak urinary stream (R39.12)

N40.2 **Nodular prostate without lower urinary tract symptoms** A ♂

Nodular prostate without LUTS

N40.3 Nodular prostate with lower urinary tract symptoms A ♂
Use additional code for associated symptoms, when specified:
incomplete bladder emptying (R39.14)
nocturia (R35.1)
straining on urination (R39.16)
urinary frequency (R35.0)
urinary hesitancy (R39.11)
urinary incontinence (N39.4-)
urinary obstruction (N13.8)
urinary retention (R33.8)
urinary urgency (R39.15)
weak urinary stream (R39.12)

N41 Inflammatory diseases of prostate
Use additional code (B95-B97), to identify infectious agent.
N41.0 Acute prostatitis A CC ♂
N41.1 Chronic prostatitis A ♂
N41.2 Abscess of prostate A CC ♂
N41.3 Prostatocystitis A ♂
N41.4 Granulomatous prostatitis A ♂
N41.8 Other inflammatory diseases of prostate A ♂
N41.9 Inflammatory disease of prostate, unspecified A ♂
Prostatitis NOS

N42 Other and unspecified disorders of prostate
N42.0 Calculus of prostate A ♂
Prostatic stone
N42.1 Congestion and hemorrhage of prostate A ♂
EXCLUDES1 *enlarged prostate (N40.-)*
hematuria (R31.-)
hyperplasia of prostate (N40.-)
inflammatory diseases of prostate (N41.-)
N42.3 Dysplasia of prostate
● N42.30 Unspecified dysplasia of prostate CC/MCC Exc
● N42.31 Prostatic intraepithelial neoplasia CC/MCC Exc
PIN
Prostatic intraepithelial neoplasia I (PIN I)
Prostatic intraepithelial neoplasia II (PIN II)
EXCLUDES1 *prostatic intraepithelial neoplasia III (PIN III) (D07.5)*
● N42.32 Atypical small acinar proliferation of prostate CC/MCC Exc
● N42.39 Other dysplasia of prostate CC/MCC Exc
N42.8 Other specified disorders of prostate
N42.81 Prostatodynia syndrome A ♂
Painful prostate syndrome
N42.82 Prostatosis syndrome A ♂
N42.83 Cyst of prostate A ♂
N42.89 Other specified disorders of prostate A ♂
N42.9 Disorder of prostate, unspecified A ♂

N43 Hydrocele and spermatocele
INCLUDES *hydrocele of spermatic cord, testis or tunica vaginalis*
EXCLUDES1 *congenital hydrocele (P83.5)*
N43.0 Encysted hydrocele ♂
N43.1 Infected hydrocele CC ♂
Use additional code (B95-B97), to identify infectious agent
N43.2 Other hydrocele ♂
N43.3 Hydrocele, unspecified ♂
N43.4 Spermatocele of epididymis
Spermatic cyst
N43.40 Spermatocele of epididymis, unspecified ♂
N43.41 Spermatocele of epididymis, single ♂
N43.42 Spermatocele of epididymis, multiple ♂

N44 Noninflammatory disorders of testis
N44.0 Torsion of testis
N44.00 Torsion of testis, unspecified CC ♂
N44.01 Extravaginal torsion of spermatic cord CC ♂
N44.02 Intravaginal torsion of spermatic cord CC ♂
Torsion of spermatic cord NOS
N44.03 Torsion of appendix testis CC ♂
N44.04 Torsion of appendix epididymis CC ♂
N44.1 Cyst of tunica albuginea testis ♂
N44.2 Benign cyst of testis ♂
N44.8 Other noninflammatory disorders of the testis ♂

N45 Orchitis and epididymitis
Use additional code (B95-B97), to identify infectious agent.
N45.1 Epididymitis ♂
N45.2 Orchitis ♂
N45.3 Epididymo-orchitis ♂
N45.4 Abscess of epididymis or testis CC ♂

N46 Male infertility
EXCLUDES1 *vasectomy status (Z98.52)*
N46.0 Azoospermia
Absolute male infertility
Male infertility due to germinal (cell) aplasia
Male infertility due to spermatogenic arrest (complete)
N46.01 Organic azoospermia A ♂
Azoospermia NOS
N46.02 Azoospermia due to extratesticular causes
Code also associated cause
N46.021 Azoospermia due to drug therapy A ♂
N46.022 Azoospermia due to infection A ♂
N46.023 Azoospermia due to obstruction of efferent ducts A ♂
N46.024 Azoospermia due to radiation A ♂
N46.025 Azoospermia due to systemic disease A ♂
N46.029 Azoospermia due to other extratesticular causes A ♂
N46.1 Oligospermia
Male infertility due to germinal cell desquamation
Male infertility due to hypospermatogenesis
Male infertility due to incomplete spermatogenic arrest
N46.11 Organic oligospermia A ♂
Oligospermia NOS
N46.12 Oligospermia due to extratesticular causes
Code also associated cause
N46.121 Oligospermia due to drug therapy A ♂
N46.122 Oligospermia due to infection A ♂
N46.123 Oligospermia due to obstruction of efferent ducts A ♂
N46.124 Oligospermia due to radiation A ♂
N46.125 Oligospermia due to systemic disease A ♂
N46.129 Oligospermia due to other extratesticular causes A ♂
N46.8 Other male infertility A ♂
N46.9 Male infertility, unspecified A ♂

N47 Disorders of prepuce
N47.0 Adherent prepuce, newborn N ♂
N47.1 Phimosis ♂
N47.2 Paraphimosis ♂
N47.3 Deficient foreskin ♂
N47.4 Benign cyst of prepuce ♂
N47.5 Adhesions of prepuce and glans penis ♂
N47.6 Balanoposthitis ♂
Use additional code (B95-B97), to identify infectious agent.
EXCLUDES1 *balanitis (N48.1)*
N47.7 Other inflammatory diseases of prepuce ♂
Use additional code (B95-B97), to identify infectious agent.
N47.8 Other disorders of prepuce ♂

N48 Other disorders of penis
N48.0 Leukoplakia of penis ♂
Balanitis xerotica obliterans
Kraurosis of penis
Lichen sclerosus of external male genital organs
EXCLUDES1 *carcinoma in situ of penis (D07.4)*
N48.1 Balanitis ♂
Use additional code (B95-B97), to identify infectious agent
EXCLUDES1 *amebic balanitis (A06.8)*
balanitis xerotica obliterans (N48.0)
candidal balanitis (B37.42)
gonococcal balanitis (A54.23)
herpesviral [herpes simplex] balanitis (A60.01)

PDx Unacceptable principal diagnosis symbol per Medicare code edits · POA Code exempt from diagnosis present on admission requirement
Q Questionable admission · CC Complication or comorbidity · CC/MCC Exc CC/MCC exclusion · MCC Major complication or comorbidity
PDx CC Principal diagnosis as its own CC · PDx MCC Principal diagnosis as its own MCC · Z1 Z code as first-listed diagnosis

When symbols appear on a code that requires a 7th character extension, refer to Appendix D to identify applicable 7th character codes.

N48.2 Other inflammatory disorders of penis
Use additional code (B95-B97), to identify infectious agent.
EXCLUDES1 *balanitis (N48.1)*
balanitis xerotica obliterans (N48.0)
balanoposthitis (N47.6)
N48.21 Abscess of corpus cavernosum and penis ♂
N48.22 Cellulitis of corpus cavernosum and penis ♂
N48.29 Other inflammatory disorders of penis ♂

N48.3 Priapism
Painful erection
Code first underlying cause
N48.30 Priapism, unspecified ♂
N48.31 Priapism due to trauma ♂
N48.32 Priapism due to disease classified elsewhere ♂
N48.33 Priapism, drug-induced ♂
N48.39 Other priapism ♂

N48.5 Ulcer of penis ♂
N48.6 Induration penis plastica ♂
Peyronie's disease
Plastic induration of penis

N48.8 Other specified disorders of penis
N48.81 Thrombosis of superficial vein of penis ♂
N48.82 Acquired torsion of penis ♂
Acquired torsion of penis NOS
EXCLUDES1 *congenital torsion of penis (Q55.63)*
N48.83 Acquired buried penis ♂
EXCLUDES1 *congenital hidden penis (Q55.64)*
N48.89 Other specified disorders of penis ♂

N48.9 Disorder of penis, unspecified ♂

N49 Inflammatory disorders of male genital organs, not elsewhere classified
Use additional code (B95-B97), to identify infectious agent
EXCLUDES1 *inflammation of penis (N48.1, N48.2-)*
orchitis and epididymitis (N45.-)
N49.0 Inflammatory disorders of seminal vesicle ♂
Vesiculitis NOS
N49.1 Inflammatory disorders of spermatic cord, tunica vaginalis and vas deferens ♂
Vasitis
N49.2 Inflammatory disorders of scrotum ♂
N49.3 Fournier gangrene ♂
N49.8 Inflammatory disorders of other specified male genital organs ♂
Inflammation of multiple sites in male genital organs
N49.9 Inflammatory disorder of unspecified male genital organ ♂
Abscess of unspecified male genital organ
Boil of unspecified male genital organ
Carbuncle of unspecified male genital organ
Cellulitis of unspecified male genital organ

N50 Other and unspecified disorders of male genital organs
EXCLUDES2 *torsion of testis (N44.0-)*
N50.0 Atrophy of testis ♂
N50.1 Vascular disorders of male genital organs ♂
Hematocele, NOS, of male genital organs
Hemorrhage of male genital organs
Thrombosis of male genital organs
N50.3 Cyst of epididymis ♂
N50.8 Other specified disorders of male genital organs
● N50.81 Testicular pain
● N50.811 Right testicular pain CC/MCC Exc
● N50.812 Left testicular pain CC/MCC Exc
● N50.819 Testicular pain, unspecified CC/MCC Exc
● N50.82 Scrotal pain CC/MCC Exc
● N50.89 Other specified disorders of the male genital organs CC/MCC Exc
Atrophy of scrotum, seminal vesicle, spermatic cord, tunica vaginalis and vas deferens
Chylocele, tunica vaginalis (nonfilarial) NOS
Edema of scrotum, seminal vesicle, spermatic cord, tunica vaginalis and vas deferens
Hypertrophy of scrotum, seminal vesicle, spermatic cord, tunica vaginalis and vas deferens
Stricture of spermatic cord, tunica vaginalis, and vas deferens
Ulcer of scrotum, seminal vesicle, spermatic cord, testis, tunica vaginalis and vas deferens
Urethroscrotal fistula
N50.9 Disorder of male genital organs, unspecified ♂

N51 Disorders of male genital organs in diseases classified elsewhere ♂
Code first underlying disease, such as:
filariasis (B74.0-B74.9)
EXCLUDES1 *amebic balanitis (A06.8)*
candidal balanitis (B37.42)
gonococcal balanitis (A54.23)
gonococcal prostatitis (A54.22)
herpesviral [herpes simplex] balanitis (A60.01)
trichomonal prostatitis (A59.02)
tuberculous prostatitis (A18.14)

N52 Male erectile dysfunction
EXCLUDES1 *psychogenic impotence (F52.21)*
N52.0 Vasculogenic erectile dysfunction
N52.01 Erectile dysfunction due to arterial insufficiency A ♂
N52.02 Corporo-venous occlusive erectile dysfunction A ♂
N52.03 Combined arterial insufficiency and corporo-venous occlusive erectile dysfunction A ♂
N52.1 Erectile dysfunction due to diseases classified elsewhere A ♂
Code first underlying disease
N52.2 Drug-induced erectile dysfunction A ♂
▲ N52.3 ▶Postprocedural◀ erectile dysfunction
N52.31 Erectile dysfunction following radical prostatectomy A ♂
N52.32 Erectile dysfunction following radical cystectomy A ♂
N52.33 Erectile dysfunction following urethral surgery A ♂
N52.34 Erectile dysfunction following simple prostatectomy A ♂
● N52.35 Erectile dysfunction following radiation therapy CC/MCC Exc
● N52.36 Erectile dysfunction following interstitial seed therapy CC/MCC Exc
● N52.37 Erectile dysfunction following prostate ablative therapy CC/MCC Exc
Erectile dysfunction following cryotherapy
Erectile dysfunction following other prostate ablative therapies
Erectile dysfunction following ultrasound ablative therapies
▲ N52.39 Other ▶and unspecified postprocedural◀ erectile dysfunction A ♂
N52.8 Other male erectile dysfunction A ♂
N52.9 Male erectile dysfunction, unspecified A ♂
Impotence NOS

N53 Other male sexual dysfunction
EXCLUDES1 *psychogenic sexual dysfunction (F52.-)*
N53.1 Ejaculatory dysfunction
EXCLUDES1 *premature ejaculation (F52.4)*
N53.11 Retarded ejaculation ♂
N53.12 Painful ejaculation ♂
N53.13 Anejaculatory orgasm ♂
N53.14 Retrograde ejaculation ♂
N53.19 Other ejaculatory dysfunction ♂
Ejaculatory dysfunction NOS
N53.8 Other male sexual dysfunction ♂
N53.9 Unspecified male sexual dysfunction ♂

Disorders of breast (N60-N65)

EXCLUDES1 *disorders of breast associated with childbirth (O91-O92)*

N60 Benign mammary dysplasia
INCLUDES *fibrocystic mastopathy*
N60.0 Solitary cyst of breast
Cyst of breast
N60.01 Solitary cyst of right breast
N60.02 Solitary cyst of left breast

Unspecified Code Other Specified Code Manifestation Code N Newborn P Pediatric M Maternity A Adult ♂ Male ♀ Female
● New Code ▲ Revised Code Title ▶◀ Revised Text NOTES INCLUDES EXCLUDES1 Not coded here EXCLUDES2 Not included here
4th character required 5th character required 6th character required 7th character required
Extension 'X' Alert HAC Hospital-acquired condition (HAC) alert AHA AHA Coding Clinic©

N60.09 Solitary cyst of unspecified breast

N60.1 Diffuse cystic mastopathy
Cystic breast
Fibrocystic disease of breast
EXCLUDES1 *diffuse cystic mastopathy with epithelial proliferation (N60.3-)*

N60.11 Diffuse cystic mastopathy of right breast

N60.12 Diffuse cystic mastopathy of left breast

N60.19 Diffuse cystic mastopathy of unspecified breast

N60.2 Fibroadenosis of breast
Adenofibrosis of breast
EXCLUDES2 *fibroadenoma of breast (D24.-)*

N60.21 Fibroadenosis of right breast

N60.22 Fibroadenosis of left breast

N60.29 Fibroadenosis of unspecified breast

N60.3 Fibrosclerosis of breast
Cystic mastopathy with epithelial proliferation

N60.31 Fibrosclerosis of right breast

N60.32 Fibrosclerosis of left breast

N60.39 Fibrosclerosis of unspecified breast

N60.4 Mammary duct ectasia

N60.41 Mammary duct ectasia of right breast

N60.42 Mammary duct ectasia of left breast

N60.49 Mammary duct ectasia of unspecified breast

N60.8 Other benign mammary dysplasias

N60.81 Other benign mammary dysplasias of right breast

N60.82 Other benign mammary dysplasias of left breast

N60.89 Other benign mammary dysplasias of unspecified breast

N60.9 Unspecified benign mammary dysplasia

N60.91 Unspecified benign mammary dysplasia of right breast

N60.92 Unspecified benign mammary dysplasia of left breast

N60.99 Unspecified benign mammary dysplasia of unspecified breast

N61 Inflammatory disorders of breast
EXCLUDES1 *inflammatory carcinoma of breast (C50.9)*
inflammatory disorder of breast associated with childbirth (O91.-)
neonatal infective mastitis (P39.0)
thrombophlebitis of breast [Mondor's disease] (I80.8)

● N61.0 Mastitis without abscess
Infective mastitis (acute) (nonpuerperal) (subacute)
Mastitis (acute) (nonpuerperal) (subacute) NOS
Cellulitis (acute) (nonpuerperal) (subacute) of breast NOS
Cellulitis (acute) (nonpuerperal) (subacute) of nipple NOS

● N61.1 Abscess of the breast and nipple
Abscess (acute) (chronic) (nonpuerperal) of areola
Abscess (acute) (chronic) (nonpuerperal) of breast
Carbuncle of breast
Mastitis with abscess

N62 Hypertrophy of breast
Gynecomastia
Hypertrophy of breast NOS
Massive pubertal hypertrophy of breast
EXCLUDES1 *breast engorgement of newborn (P83.4)*
disproportion of reconstructed breast (N65.1)

N63 Unspecified lump in breast
Nodule(s) NOS in breast

N64 Other disorders of breast
EXCLUDES2 *mechanical complication of breast prosthesis and implant (T85.4-)*

N64.0 Fissure and fistula of nipple

N64.1 Fat necrosis of breast
Fat necrosis (segmental) of breast
Code first breast necrosis due to breast graft ▶(T85.898)◀

N64.2 Atrophy of breast

N64.3 Galactorrhea not associated with childbirth

N64.4 Mastodynia

N64.5 Other signs and symptoms in breast
EXCLUDES2 *abnormal findings on diagnostic imaging of breast (R92.-)*

N64.51 Induration of breast

N64.52 Nipple discharge
EXCLUDES1 *abnormal findings in nipple discharge (R89.-)*

N64.53 Retraction of nipple

N64.59 Other signs and symptoms in breast

N64.8 Other specified disorders of breast

N64.81 Ptosis of breast
EXCLUDES1 *ptosis of native breast in relation to reconstructed breast (N65.1)*

N64.82 Hypoplasia of breast
Micromastia
EXCLUDES1 *congenital absence of breast (Q83.0)*
hypoplasia of native breast in relation to reconstructed breast (N65.1)

N64.89 Other specified disorders of breast
Galactocele
Subinvolution of breast (postlactational)

N64.9 Disorder of breast, unspecified

N65 Deformity and disproportion of reconstructed breast

N65.0 Deformity of reconstructed breast
Contour irregularity in reconstructed breast
Excess tissue in reconstructed breast
Misshapen reconstructed breast

N65.1 Disproportion of reconstructed breast
Breast asymmetry between native breast and reconstructed breast
Disproportion between native breast and reconstructed breast

Inflammatory diseases of female pelvic organs (N70-N77)

EXCLUDES1 *inflammatory diseases of female pelvic organs complicating:*
abortion or ectopic or molar pregnancy (O00-O07, O08.0)
pregnancy, childbirth and the puerperium (O23.-, O75.3, O85, O86.-)

N70 Salpingitis and oophoritis
INCLUDES *abscess (of) fallopian tube*
abscess (of) ovary
pyosalpinx
salpingo-oophoritis
tubo-ovarian abscess
tubo-ovarian inflammatory disease
Use additional code (B95-B97), to identify infectious agent
EXCLUDES1 *gonococcal infection (A54.24)*
tuberculous infection (A18.17)

N70.0 Acute salpingitis and oophoritis

N70.01 Acute salpingitis

N70.02 Acute oophoritis

N70.03 Acute salpingitis and oophoritis

N70.1 Chronic salpingitis and oophoritis
Hydrosalpinx

N70.11 Chronic salpingitis

N70.12 Chronic oophoritis

N70.13 Chronic salpingitis and oophoritis

N70.9 Salpingitis and oophoritis, unspecified

N70.91 Salpingitis, unspecified

N70.92 Oophoritis, unspecified

N70.93 Salpingitis and oophoritis, unspecified

N71 Inflammatory disease of uterus, except cervix
INCLUDES *endo (myo) metritis*
metritis
myometritis
pyometra
uterine abscess
Use additional code (B95-B97), to identify infectious agent
EXCLUDES1 *hyperplastic endometritis (N85.0-)*
infection of uterus following delivery (O85, O86.-)

N71.0 Acute inflammatory disease of uterus

N71.1 Chronic inflammatory disease of uterus

N71.9 Inflammatory disease of uterus, unspecified

N72 Inflammatory disease of cervix uteri
INCLUDES *cervicitis (with or without erosion or ectropion)*
endocervicitis (with or without erosion or ectropion)
exocervicitis (with or without erosion or ectropion)
Use additional code (B95-B97), to identify infectious agent
EXCLUDES1 *erosion and ectropion of cervix without cervicitis (N86)*

Unacceptable principal diagnosis symbol per Medicare code edits; Code exempt from diagnosis present on admission requirement
Questionable admission; Complication or comorbidity; CC/MCC exclusion; Major complication or comorbidity
Principal diagnosis as its own CC; Principal diagnosis as its own MCC; Z code as first-listed diagnosis

When symbols appear on a code that requires a 7th character extension, refer to Appendix D to identify applicable 7th character codes.

CHAPTER 14: DISEASES OF THE GENITOURINARY SYSTEM (N00-N99)

N73 Other female pelvic inflammatory diseases
Use additional code (B95-B97), to identify infectious agent.
N73.0 Acute parametritis and pelvic cellulitis
Abscess of broad ligament
Abscess of parametrium
Pelvic cellulitis, female
N73.1 Chronic parametritis and pelvic cellulitis
Any condition in N73.0 specified as chronic
EXCLUDES1 *tuberculous parametritis and pelvic cellultis (A18.17)*
N73.2 Unspecified parametritis and pelvic cellulitis
Any condition in N73.0 unspecified whether acute or chronic
N73.3 Female acute pelvic peritonitis
N73.4 Female chronic pelvic peritonitis
EXCLUDES1 *tuberculous pelvic (female) peritonitis (A18.17)*
N73.5 Female pelvic peritonitis, unspecified
N73.6 Female pelvic peritoneal adhesions (postinfective)
EXCLUDES2 *postprocedural pelvic peritoneal adhesions (N99.4)*
N73.8 Other specified female pelvic inflammatory diseases
N73.9 Female pelvic inflammatory disease, unspecified
Female pelvic infection or inflammation NOS

N74 Female pelvic inflammatory disorders in diseases classified elsewhere
Code first underlying disease
EXCLUDES1 *chlamydial cervicitis (A56.02)*
chlamydial pelvic inflammatory disease (A56.11)
gonococcal cervicitis (A54.03)
gonococcal pelvic inflammatory disease (A54.24)
herpesviral [herpes simplex] cervicitis (A60.03)
herpesviral [herpes simplex] pelvic inflammatory disease (A60.09)
syphilitic cervicitis (A52.76)
syphilitic pelvic inflammatory disease (A52.76)
trichomonal cervicitis (A59.09)
tuberculous cervicitis (A18.16)
tuberculous pelvic inflammatory disease (A18.17)

N75 Diseases of Bartholin's gland
N75.0 Cyst of Bartholin's gland
N75.1 Abscess of Bartholin's gland
N75.8 Other diseases of Bartholin's gland
Bartholinitis
N75.9 Disease of Bartholin's gland, unspecified

N76 Other inflammation of vagina and vulva
Use additional code (B95-B97), to identify infectious agent
EXCLUDES2 *senile (atrophic) vaginitis (N95.2)*
vulvar vestibulitis (N94.810)
N76.0 Acute vaginitis
Acute vulvovaginitis
Vaginitis NOS
Vulvovaginitis NOS
N76.1 Subacute and chronic vaginitis
Chronic vulvovaginitis
Subacute vulvovaginitis
N76.2 Acute vulvitis
Vulvitis NOS
N76.3 Subacute and chronic vulvitis
N76.4 Abscess of vulva
Furuncle of vulva
N76.5 Ulceration of vagina
N76.6 Ulceration of vulva
N76.8 Other specified inflammation of vagina and vulva
N76.81 Mucositis (ulcerative) of vagina and vulva
Code also type of associated therapy, such as:
antineoplastic and immunosuppressive drugs (T45.1X-)
radiological procedure and radiotherapy (Y84.2)
EXCLUDES2 *gastrointestinal mucositis (ulcerative) (K92.81)*
nasal mucositis (ulcerative) (J34.81)
oral mucositis (ulcerative) (K12.3-)
N76.89 Other specified inflammation of vagina and vulva

N77 Vulvovaginal ulceration and inflammation in diseases classified elsewhere
N77.0 Ulceration of vulva in diseases classified elsewhere
Code first underlying disease, such as:
Behçet's disease (M35.2)
EXCLUDES1 *ulceration of vulva in gonococcal infection (A54.02)*
ulceration of vulva in herpesviral [herpes simplex] infection (A60.04)
ulceration of vulva in syphilis (A51.0)
ulceration of vulva in tuberculosis (A18.18)
N77.1 Vaginitis, vulvitis and vulvovaginitis in diseases classified elsewhere
Code first underlying disease, such as:
pinworm (B80)
EXCLUDES1 *candidal vulvovaginitis (B37.3)*
chlamydial vulvovaginitis (A56.02)
gonococcal vulvovaginitis (A54.02)
herpesviral [herpes simplex] vulvovaginitis (A60.04)
trichomonal vulvovaginitis (A59.01)
tuberculous vulvovaginitis (A18.18)
vulvovaginitis in early syphilis (A51.0)
vulvovaginitis in late syphilis (A52.76)

Noninflammatory disorders of female genital tract (N80-N98)

N80 Endometriosis
N80.0 Endometriosis of uterus
Adenomyosis
EXCLUDES1 *stromal endometriosis (D39.0)*
N80.1 Endometriosis of ovary
N80.2 Endometriosis of fallopian tube
N80.3 Endometriosis of pelvic peritoneum
N80.4 Endometriosis of rectovaginal septum and vagina
N80.5 Endometriosis of intestine
N80.6 Endometriosis in cutaneous scar
N80.8 Other endometriosis
N80.9 Endometriosis, unspecified

N81 Female genital prolapse
EXCLUDES1 *genital prolapse complicating pregnancy, labor or delivery (O34.5-)*
prolapse and hernia of ovary and fallopian tube ►(N83.4-)◄
prolapse of vaginal vault after hysterectomy (N99.3)
N81.0 Urethrocele
EXCLUDES1 *urethrocele with cystocele (N81.1-)*
urethrocele with prolapse of uterus (N81.2-N81.4)
N81.1 Cystocele
Cystocele with urethrocele
Cystourethrocele
EXCLUDES1 *cystocele with prolapse of uterus (N81.2-N81.4)*
N81.10 Cystocele, unspecified
Prolapse of (anterior) vaginal wall NOS
N81.11 Cystocele, midline
N81.12 Cystocele, lateral
Paravaginal cystocele
N81.2 Incomplete uterovaginal prolapse
First degree uterine prolapse
Prolapse of cervix NOS
Second degree uterine prolapse
EXCLUDES1 *cervical stump prolapse (N81.85)*
N81.3 Complete uterovaginal prolapse
Procidentia (uteri) NOS
Third degree uterine prolapse
N81.4 Uterovaginal prolapse, unspecified
Prolapse of uterus NOS
N81.5 Vaginal enterocele
EXCLUDES1 *enterocele with prolapse of uterus (N81.2-N81.4)*
N81.6 Rectocele
Prolapse of posterior vaginal wall
Use additional code for any associated fecal incontinence, if applicable (R15.-)
EXCLUDES2 *perineocele (N81.81)*
rectal prolapse (K62.3)
rectocele with prolapse of uterus (N81.2-N81.4)

Unspecified Code Other Specified Code Manifestation Code N Newborn P Pediatric M Maternity A Adult ♂ Male ♀ Female
● New Code ▲ Revised Code Title ►◄ Revised Text NOTES INCLUDES EXCLUDES1 Not coded here EXCLUDES2 Not included here
4th character required 5th character required 6th character required 7th character required
Extension 'X' Alert HAC Hospital-acquired condition (HAC) alert AHA AHA Coding Clinic©

N81.8 Other female genital prolapse
- N81.81 Perineocele ♀
- N81.82 Incompetence or weakening of pubocervical tissue ♀
- N81.83 Incompetence or weakening of rectovaginal tissue ♀
- N81.84 Pelvic muscle wasting ♀
  Disuse atrophy of pelvic muscles and anal sphincter
- N81.85 Cervical stump prolapse ♀
- N81.89 Other female genital prolapse ♀
  Deficient perineum
  Old laceration of muscles of pelvic floor

N81.9 Female genital prolapse, unspecified ♀

N82 Fistulae involving female genital tract

EXCLUDES1 *vesicointestinal fistulae (N32.1)*

- N82.0 Vesicovaginal fistula CC ♀
- N82.1 Other female urinary-genital tract fistulae CC ♀
  Cervicovesical fistula
  Ureterovaginal fistula
  Urethrovaginal fistula
  Uteroureteric fistula
  Uterovesical fistula
- N82.2 Fistula of vagina to small intestine CC ♀
- N82.3 Fistula of vagina to large intestine CC ♀
  Rectovaginal fistula
- N82.4 Other female intestinal-genital tract fistulae CC ♀
  Intestinouterine fistula
- N82.5 Female genital tract-skin fistulae CC ♀
  Uterus to abdominal wall fistula
  Vaginoperineal fistula
- N82.8 Other female genital tract fistulae CC ♀
- N82.9 Female genital tract fistula, unspecified CC ♀

N83 Noninflammatory disorders of ovary, fallopian tube and broad ligament

EXCLUDES2 *hydrosalpinx (N70.1-)*

N83.0 Follicular cyst of ovary
  Cyst of graafian follicle
  Hemorrhagic follicular cyst (of ovary)
- ● N83.00 Follicular cyst of ovary, unspecified side CC/MCC Exc ♀
- ● N83.01 Follicular cyst of right ovary CC/MCC Exc ♀
- ● N83.02 Follicular cyst of left ovary CC/MCC Exc ♀

N83.1 Corpus luteum cyst
  Hemorrhagic corpus luteum cyst
- ● N83.10 Corpus luteum cyst of ovary, unspecified side CC/MCC Exc ♀
- ● N83.11 Corpus luteum cyst of right ovary CC/MCC Exc ♀
- ● N83.12 Corpus luteum cyst of left ovary CC/MCC Exc ♀

N83.2 Other and unspecified ovarian cysts
  EXCLUDES1 *developmental ovarian cyst (Q50.1)*
  neoplastic ovarian cyst (D27.-)
  polycystic ovarian syndrome (E28.2)
  Stein-Leventhal syndrome (E28.2)
- N83.20 Unspecified ovarian cysts
  - ● N83.201 Unspecified ovarian cyst, right side CC/MCC Exc ♀
  - ● N83.202 Unspecified ovarian cyst, left side CC/MCC Exc ♀
  - ● N83.209 Unspecified ovarian cyst, unspecified side CC/MCC Exc ♀
    Ovarian cyst, NOS
- N83.29 Other ovarian cysts
  Retention cyst of ovary
  Simple cyst of ovary
  - ● N83.291 Other ovarian cyst, right side CC/MCC Exc ♀
  - ● N83.292 Other ovarian cyst, left side CC/MCC Exc ♀
  - ● N83.299 Other ovarian cyst, unspecified side CC/MCC Exc ♀

N83.3 Acquired atrophy of ovary and fallopian tube
- N83.31 Acquired atrophy of ovary
  - ● N83.311 Acquired atrophy of right ovary CC/MCC Exc ♀
  - ● N83.312 Acquired atrophy of left ovary CC/MCC Exc ♀
  - ● N83.319 Acquired atrophy of ovary, unspecified side CC/MCC Exc ♀
    Acquired atrophy of ovary, NOS
- N83.32 Acquired atrophy of fallopian tube
  - ● N83.321 Acquired atrophy of right fallopian tube CC/MCC Exc ♀
  - ● N83.322 Acquired atrophy of left fallopian tube CC/MCC Exc ♀
  - ● N83.329 Acquired atrophy of fallopian tube, unspecified side CC/MCC Exc ♀
    Acquired atrophy of fallopian tube, NOS
- N83.33 Acquired atrophy of ovary and fallopian tube
  - ● N83.331 Acquired atrophy of right ovary and fallopian tube CC/MCC Exc ♀
  - ● N83.332 Acquired atrophy of left ovary and fallopian tube CC/MCC Exc ♀
  - ● N83.339 Acquired atrophy of ovary and fallopian tube, unspecified side CC/MCC Exc ♀
    Acquired atrophy of ovary and fallopian tube, NOS

N83.4 Prolapse and hernia of ovary and fallopian tube
- ● N83.40 Prolapse and hernia of ovary and fallopian tube, unspecified side CC/MCC Exc ♀
  Prolapse and hernia of ovary and fallopian tube, NOS
- ● N83.41 Prolapse and hernia of right ovary and fallopian tube CC/MCC Exc ♀
- ● N83.42 Prolapse and hernia of left ovary and fallopian tube CC/MCC Exc ♀

N83.5 Torsion of ovary, ovarian pedicle and fallopian tube
  Torsion of accessory tube
- N83.51 Torsion of ovary and ovarian pedicle
  - ● N83.511 Torsion of right ovary and ovarian pedicle CC CC/MCC Exc ♀
  - ● N83.512 Torsion of left ovary and ovarian pedicle CC CC/MCC Exc ♀
  - ● N83.519 Torsion of ovary and ovarian pedicle, unspecified side CC CC/MCC Exc ♀
    Torsion of ovary and ovarian pedicle, NOS
- N83.52 Torsion of fallopian tube
  Torsion of hydatid of Morgagni
  - ● N83.521 Torsion of right fallopian tube CC CC/MCC Exc ♀
  - ● N83.522 Torsion of left fallopian tube CC CC/MCC Exc ♀
  - ● N83.529 Torsion of fallopian tube, unspecified side CC CC/MCC Exc ♀
    Torsion of fallopian tube, NOS
- N83.53 Torsion of ovary, ovarian pedicle and fallopian tube CC ♀

N83.6 Hematosalpinx ♀
  EXCLUDES1 *hematosalpinx (with) (in):*
  hematocolpos (N89.7)
  hematometra (N85.7)
  tubal pregnancy ▶(O00.1-)◀

N83.7 Hematoma of broad ligament ♀

N83.8 Other noninflammatory disorders of ovary, fallopian tube and broad ligament ♀
  Broad ligament laceration syndrome [Allen-Masters]

N83.9 Noninflammatory disorder of ovary, fallopian tube and broad ligament, unspecified ♀

N84 Polyp of female genital tract

EXCLUDES1 *adenomatous polyp (D28.-)*
placental polyp (O90.89)

- N84.0 Polyp of corpus uteri ♀
  Polyp of endometrium
  Polyp of uterus NOS
  EXCLUDES1 *polypoid endometrial hyperplasia (N85.0-)*
- N84.1 Polyp of cervix uteri ♀
  Mucous polyp of cervix
- N84.2 Polyp of vagina ♀
- N84.3 Polyp of vulva ♀
  Polyp of labia
- N84.8 Polyp of other parts of female genital tract ♀
- N84.9 Polyp of female genital tract, unspecified ♀

N85 Other noninflammatory disorders of uterus, except cervix

EXCLUDES1 *endometriosis (N80.-)*
inflammatory diseases of uterus (N71.-)
noninflammatory disorders of cervix, except malposition (N86-N88)
polyp of corpus uteri (N84.0)
uterine prolapse (N81.-)

PDx Unacceptable principal diagnosis symbol per Medicare code edits; POA Code exempt from diagnosis present on admission requirement; ? Questionable admission; CC Complication or comorbidity; CC/MCC Exc CC/MCC exclusion; MCC Major complication or comorbidity; PDx CC Principal diagnosis as its own CC; PDx MCC Principal diagnosis as its own MCC; Z1 Z code as first-listed diagnosis

N85.0 Endometrial hyperplasia

N85.00 **Endometrial hyperplasia, unspecified** ♀
Hyperplasia (adenomatous) (cystic) (glandular) of endometrium
Hyperplastic endometritis

N85.01 Benign **endometrial hyperplasia** ♀
Endometrial hyperplasia (complex) (simple) without atypia

N85.02 Endometrial intraepithelial neoplasia [EIN] ♀
Endometrial hyperplasia with atypia
EXCLUDES1 *malignant neoplasm of endometrium (with endometrial intraepithelial neoplasia [EIN]) (C54.1)*

N85.2 Hypertrophy **of uterus** ♀
Bulky or enlarged uterus
EXCLUDES1 *puerperal hypertrophy of uterus (O90.89)*

N85.3 Subinvolution **of uterus** ♀
EXCLUDES1 *puerperal subinvolution of uterus (O90.89)*

N85.4 Malposition **of uterus** ♀
Anteversion of uterus
Retroflexion of uterus
Retroversion of uterus
EXCLUDES1 *malposition of uterus complicating pregnancy, labor or delivery (O34.5-, O65.5)*

N85.5 Inversion **of uterus** ♀
EXCLUDES1 *current obstetric trauma (O71.2)*
postpartum inversion of uterus (O71.2)

N85.6 Intrauterine synechiae ♀

N85.7 Hematometra ♀
Hematosalpinx with hematometra
EXCLUDES1 *hematometra with hematocolpos (N89.7)*

N85.8 **Other specified noninflammatory disorders of uterus** ♀
Atrophy of uterus, acquired
Fibrosis of uterus NOS

N85.9 **Noninflammatory disorder of uterus, unspecified** ♀
Disorder of uterus NOS

N86 **Erosion and ectropion of cervix uteri** ♀
Decubitus (trophic) ulcer of cervix
Eversion of cervix
EXCLUDES1 *erosion and ectropion of cervix with cervicitis (N72)*

N87 Dysplasia **of cervix uteri**
EXCLUDES1 *abnormal results from cervical cytologic examination without histologic confirmation (R87.61-)*
carcinoma in situ of cervix uteri (D06.-)
cervical intraepithelial neoplasia III [CIN III] (D06.-)
HGSIL of cervix (R87.613)
severe dysplasia of cervix uteri (D06.-)

N87.0 Mild **cervical dysplasia** ♀
Cervical intraepithelial neoplasia I [CIN I]

N87.1 Moderate **cervical dysplasia** ♀
Cervical intraepithelial neoplasia II [CIN II]

N87.9 **Dysplasia of cervix uteri, unspecified** ♀
Anaplasia of cervix
Cervical atypism
Cervical dysplasia NOS

N88 Other **noninflammatory disorders of cervix uteri**
EXCLUDES2 *inflammatory disease of cervix (N72)*
polyp of cervix (N84.1)

N88.0 **Leukoplakia of cervix uteri** ♀

N88.1 **Old laceration of cervix uteri** ♀
Adhesions of cervix
EXCLUDES1 *current obstetric trauma (O71.3)*

N88.2 **Stricture and stenosis of cervix uteri** ♀
EXCLUDES1 *stricture and stenosis of cervix uteri complicating labor (O65.5)*

N88.3 **Incompetence of cervix uteri** ♀
Investigation and management of (suspected) cervical incompetence in a nonpregnant woman
EXCLUDES1 *cervical incompetence complicating pregnancy (O34.3-)*

N88.4 **Hypertrophic elongation of cervix uteri** ♀

N88.8 **Other specified noninflammatory disorders of cervix uteri** ♀
EXCLUDES1 *current obstetric trauma (O71.3)*

N88.9 **Noninflammatory disorder of cervix uteri, unspecified** ♀

N89 Other **noninflammatory disorders of vagina**
EXCLUDES1 *abnormal results from vaginal cytologic examination without histologic confirmation (R87.62-)*
carcinoma in situ of vagina (D07.2)
HGSIL of vagina (R87.623)
inflammation of vagina (N76.-)
senile (atrophic) vaginitis (N95.2)
severe dysplasia of vagina (D07.2)
trichomonal leukorrhea (A59.00)
vaginal intraepithelial neoplasia [VAIN], grade III (D07.2)

N89.0 Mild **vaginal dysplasia** ♀
Vaginal intraepithelial neoplasia [VAIN], grade I

N89.1 Moderate **vaginal dysplasia** ♀
Vaginal intraepithelial neoplasia [VAIN], grade II

N89.3 **Dysplasia of vagina, unspecified** ♀

N89.4 **Leukoplakia of vagina** ♀

N89.5 **Stricture and atresia of vagina** ♀
Vaginal adhesions
Vaginal stenosis
EXCLUDES1 *congenital atresia or stricture (Q52.4)*
postprocedural adhesions of vagina (N99.2)

N89.6 **Tight hymenal ring** ♀
Rigid hymen
Tight introitus
EXCLUDES1 *imperforate hymen (Q52.3)*

N89.7 **Hematocolpos** ♀
Hematocolpos with hematometra or hematosalpinx

N89.8 **Other specified noninflammatory disorders of vagina** ♀
Leukorrhea NOS
Old vaginal laceration
Pessary ulcer of vagina
EXCLUDES1 *current obstetric trauma (O70.-, O71.4, O71.7-O71.8)*
old laceration involving muscles of pelvic floor (N81.8)

N89.9 **Noninflammatory disorder of vagina, unspecified** ♀

N90 **Other noninflammatory disorders of vulva and perineum**
EXCLUDES1 *anogenital (venereal) warts (A63.0)*
carcinoma in situ of vulva (D07.1)
condyloma acuminatum (A63.0)
current obstetric trauma (O70.-, O71.7-O71.8)
inflammation of vulva (N76.-)
severe dysplasia of vulva (D07.1)
vulvar intraepithelial neoplasm III [VIN III] (D07.1)

N90.0 **Mild vulvar dysplasia** ♀
Vulvar intraepithelial neoplasia [VIN], grade I

N90.1 **Moderate vulvar dysplasia** ♀
Vulvar intraepithelial neoplasia [VIN], grade II

N90.3 **Dysplasia of vulva, unspecified** ♀

N90.4 **Leukoplakia of vulva** ♀
Dystrophy of vulva
Kraurosis of vulva
Lichen sclerosus of external female genital organs

N90.5 **Atrophy of vulva** ♀
Stenosis of vulva

N90.6 **Hypertrophy of vulva**

● N90.60 Unspecified **hypertrophy of vulva** CC/MCC Exc
Unspecified hypertrophy of labia

● N90.61 Childhood asymmetric labium majus enlargement CC/MCC Exc
CALME

● N90.69 Other specified **hypertrophy of vulva** CC/MCC Exc
Other specified hypertrophy of labia

N90.7 **Vulvar cyst** ♀

N90.8 Other specified **noninflammatory disorders of vulva and perineum**

N90.81 **Female genital mutilation status**
Female genital cutting status

N90.810 **Female genital mutilation status, unspecified** ♀
Female genital cutting status, unspecified
Female genital mutilation status NOS

N90.811 **Female genital mutilation** Type I **status** ♀
Clitorectomy status
Female genital cutting Type I status

Unspecified Code | Other Specified Code | Manifestation Code | N Newborn | P Pediatric | M Maternity | A Adult | ♂ Male | ♀ Female
● New Code | ▲ Revised Code Title | ►◄ Revised Text | NOTES | INCLUDES | EXCLUDES1 Not coded here | EXCLUDES2 Not included here
4th character required | 5th character required | 6th character required | 7th character required
Extension 'X' Alert | HAC Hospital-acquired condition (HAC) alert | AHA AHA Coding Clinic©

When symbols appear on a code that requires a 7th character extension, refer to Appendix D to identify applicable 7th character codes.

N90.812 **Female genital mutilation Type II status** ♀
Clitorectomy with excision of labia minora status
Female genital cutting Type II status
N90.813 **Female genital mutilation Type III status** ♀
Female genital cutting Type III status
Infibulation status
N90.818 **Other female genital mutilation status** ♀
Female genital cutting Type IV status
Female genital mutilation Type IV status
Other female genital cutting status
N90.89 **Other specified noninflammatory disorders of vulva and perineum** ♀
Adhesions of vulva
Hypertrophy of clitoris
N90.9 **Noninflammatory disorder of vulva and perineum, unspecified** ♀

N91 **Absent, scanty and rare menstruation**
EXCLUDES1 *ovarian dysfunction (E28.-)*
N91.0 **Primary amenorrhea** ♀
N91.1 **Secondary amenorrhea** ♀
N91.2 **Amenorrhea, unspecified** ♀
N91.3 **Primary oligomenorrhea** ♀
N91.4 **Secondary oligomenorrhea** ♀
N91.5 **Oligomenorrhea, unspecified** ♀
Hypomenorrhea NOS

N92 **Excessive, frequent and irregular menstruation**
EXCLUDES1 *postmenopausal bleeding (N95.0)*
precocious puberty (menstruation) (E30.1)
N92.0 **Excessive and frequent menstruation with regular cycle** ♀
Heavy periods NOS
Menorrhagia NOS
Polymenorrhea
N92.1 **Excessive and frequent menstruation with irregular cycle** ♀
Irregular intermenstrual bleeding
Irregular, shortened intervals between menstrual bleeding
Menometrorrhagia
Metrorrhagia
N92.2 **Excessive menstruation at puberty** ♀
Excessive bleeding associated with onset of menstrual periods
Pubertal menorrhagia
Puberty bleeding
N92.3 **Ovulation bleeding** ♀
Regular intermenstrual bleeding
N92.4 **Excessive bleeding in the premenopausal period** ♀
Climacteric menorrhagia or metrorrhagia
Menopausal menorrhagia or metrorrhagia
Preclimacteric menorrhagia or metrorrhagia
Premenopausal menorrhagia or metrorrhagia
N92.5 **Other specified irregular menstruation** ♀
N92.6 **Irregular menstruation, unspecified** ♀
Irregular bleeding NOS
Irregular periods NOS
EXCLUDES1 *irregular menstruation with:*
lengthened intervals or scanty bleeding (N91.3-N91.5)
shortened intervals or excessive bleeding (N92.1)

N93 **Other abnormal uterine and vaginal bleeding**
EXCLUDES1 *neonatal vaginal hemorrhage (P54.6)*
precocious puberty (menstruation) (E30.1)
pseudomenses (P54.6)
N93.0 **Postcoital and contact bleeding** ♀
● N93.1 **Pre-pubertal vaginal bleeding**
N93.8 **Other specified abnormal uterine and vaginal bleeding** ♀
Dysfunctional or functional uterine or vaginal bleeding NOS
N93.9 **Abnormal uterine and vaginal bleeding, unspecified** ♀

N94 **Pain and other conditions associated with female genital organs and menstrual cycle**
N94.0 **Mittelschmerz** ♀
N94.1 **Dyspareunia**
EXCLUDES1 *psychogenic dyspareunia (F52.6)*
● N94.10 **Unspecified dyspareunia**
● N94.11 **Superficial (introital) dyspareunia**
● N94.12 **Deep dyspareunia**
● N94.19 **Other specified dyspareunia**
N94.2 **Vaginismus** ♀
EXCLUDES1 *psychogenic vaginismus (F52.5)*
N94.3 **Premenstrual tension syndrome** ♀
Premenstrual dysphoric disorder
Code also associated menstrual migraine (G43.82-, G43.83-)
EXCLUDES1 *Premenstrual dysphoric disorder (F32.81)*
N94.4 **Primary dysmenorrhea** ♀
N94.5 **Secondary dysmenorrhea** ♀
N94.6 **Dysmenorrhea, unspecified** ♀
EXCLUDES1 *psychogenic dysmenorrhea (F45.8)*
N94.8 **Other specified conditions associated with female genital organs and menstrual cycle**
N94.81 **Vulvodynia**
N94.810 **Vulvar vestibulitis** ♀
N94.818 **Other vulvodynia** ♀
N94.819 **Vulvodynia, unspecified** ♀
Vulvodynia NOS
N94.89 **Other specified conditions associated with female genital organs and menstrual cycle** ♀
N94.9 **Unspecified condition associated with female genital organs and menstrual cycle** ♀

N95 **Menopausal and other perimenopausal disorders**
Menopausal and other perimenopausal disorders due to naturally occurring (age-related) menopause and perimenopause
EXCLUDES1 *excessive bleeding in the premenopausal period (N92.4)*
menopausal and perimenopausal disorders due to artificial or premature menopause (E89.4-, E28.31-)
premature menopause (E28.31-)
EXCLUDES2 *postmenopausal osteoporosis (M81.0-)*
postmenopausal osteoporosis with current pathological fracture (M80.0-)
postmenopausal urethritis (N34.2)
N95.0 **Postmenopausal bleeding** ♀
N95.1 **Menopausal and female climacteric states** ♀
Symptoms such as flushing, sleeplessness, headache, lack of concentration, associated with natural (age-related) menopause
Use additional code for associated symptoms
EXCLUDES1 *asymptomatic menopausal state (Z78.0)*
symptoms associated with artificial menopause (E89.41)
symptoms associated with premature menopause (E28.310)
N95.2 **Postmenopausal atrophic vaginitis** ♀
Senile (atrophic) vaginitis
N95.8 **Other specified menopausal and perimenopausal disorders** ♀
N95.9 **Unspecified menopausal and perimenopausal disorder** ♀

N96 **Recurrent pregnancy loss** ♀
Investigation or care in a nonpregnant woman with history of recurrent pregnancy loss
EXCLUDES1 *recurrent pregancy loss with current pregnancy (O26.2-)*

N97 **Female infertility**
INCLUDES *inability to achieve a pregnancy*
sterility, female NOS
EXCLUDES1 *female infertility associated with:*
hypopituitarism (E23.0)
Stein-Leventhal syndrome (E28.2)
EXCLUDES2 *incompetence of cervix uteri (N88.3)*
N97.0 **Female infertility associated with anovulation** ♀
N97.1 **Female infertility of tubal origin** ♀
Female infertility associated with congenital anomaly of tube
Female infertility due to tubal block
Female infertility due to tubal occlusion
Female infertility due to tubal stenosis
N97.2 **Female infertility of uterine origin** ♀
Female infertility associated with congenital anomaly of uterus
Female infertility due to nonimplantation of ovum
N97.8 **Female infertility of other origin** ♀
N97.9 **Female infertility, unspecified** ♀

N98 **Complications associated with artificial fertilization**
N98.0 **Infection associated with artificial insemination** CC ♀
N98.1 **Hyperstimulation of ovaries** CC ♀
Hyperstimulation of ovaries NOS
Hyperstimulation of ovaries associated with induced ovulation

PDx Unacceptable principal diagnosis symbol per Medicare code edits · POA Code exempt from diagnosis present on admission requirement · Q Questionable admission · CC Complication or comorbidity · CC/MCC Excl CC/MCC exclusion · MCC Major complication or comorbidity · Principal diagnosis as its own CC · Principal diagnosis as its own MCC · Z Z code as first-listed diagnosis

N98.2 Complications of attempted introduction of fertilized ovum following in vitro fertilization CC ♀
N98.3 Complications of attempted introduction of embryo in embryo transfer CC ♀
N98.8 Other complications associated with artificial fertilization CC ♀
N98.9 Complication associated with artificial fertilization, unspecified CC ♀

Intraoperative and postprocedural complications and disorders of genitourinary system, not elsewhere classified (N99)

N99 Intraoperative and postprocedural complications and disorders of genitourinary system, not elsewhere classified

EXCLUDES2 *irradiation cystitis (N30.4-)*
postoophorectomy osteoporosis with current pathological fracture (M80.8-)
postoophorectomy osteoporosis without current pathological fracture (M81.8)

N99.0 Postprocedural (acute) (chronic) kidney failure
Use additional code to type of kidney disease

N99.1 Postprocedural urethral stricture
Postcatheterization urethral stricture

N99.11 Postprocedural urethral stricture, male
N99.110 Postprocedural urethral stricture, male, meatal ♂
N99.111 Postprocedural bulbous urethral stricture
N99.112 Postprocedural membranous urethral stricture
▲ N99.113 Postprocedural anterior ▶bulbous◀ urethral stricture
N99.114 Postprocedural urethral stricture, male, unspecified ♂
● N99.115 Postprocedural fossa navicularis urethral stricture CC/MCC Exc

N99.12 Postprocedural urethral stricture, female ♀

N99.2 Postprocedural adhesions of vagina ♀
N99.3 Prolapse of vaginal vault after hysterectomy ♀
N99.4 Postprocedural pelvic peritoneal adhesions

EXCLUDES2 *pelvic peritoneal adhesions NOS (N73.6)*
postinfective pelvic peritoneal adhesions (N73.6)

N99.5 Complications of stoma of urinary tract

EXCLUDES2 *mechanical complication of ▶urinary catheter◀ (T83.0-)*

N99.51 Complication of cystostomy
N99.510 Cystostomy hemorrhage CC
N99.511 Cystostomy infection CC
N99.512 Cystostomy malfunction CC
N99.518 Other cystostomy complication CC

▲ N99.52 Complication of ▶incontinent◀ external stoma of urinary tract
▲ N99.520 Hemorrhage of ▶incontinent◀ external stoma of urinary tract
▲ N99.521 Infection of ▶incontinent◀ external stoma of urinary tract
▲ N99.522 Malfunction of ▶incontinent◀ external stoma of urinary tract
● N99.523 Herniation of incontinent stoma of urinary tract
● N99.524 Stenosis of incontinent stoma of urinary tract
▲ N99.528 Other complication of ▶incontinent◀ external stoma of urinary tract

▲ N99.53 Complication of ▶continent◀ stoma of urinary tract
▲ N99.530 Hemorrhage of ▶continent◀ stoma of urinary tract
▲ N99.531 Infection of ▶continent◀ stoma of urinary tract
▲ N99.532 Malfunction of ▶continent◀ stoma of urinary tract
● N99.533 Herniation of continent stoma of urinary tract
● N99.534 Stenosis of continent stoma of urinary tract
▲ N99.538 Other complication of ▶continent◀ stoma of urinary tract

N99.6 Intraoperative hemorrhage and hematoma of a genitourinary system organ or structure complicating a procedure

EXCLUDES1 *intraoperative hemorrhage and hematoma of a genitourinary system organ or structure due to accidental puncture or laceration during a procedure (N99.7-)*

N99.61 Intraoperative hemorrhage and hematoma of a genitourinary system organ or structure complicating a genitourinary system procedure CC
N99.62 Intraoperative hemorrhage and hematoma of a genitourinary system organ or structure complicating other procedure CC

N99.7 Accidental puncture and laceration of a genitourinary system organ or structure during a procedure

N99.71 Accidental puncture and laceration of a genitourinary system organ or structure during a genitourinary system procedure CC
N99.72 Accidental puncture and laceration of a genitourinary system organ or structure during other procedure CC

N99.8 Other intraoperative and postprocedural complications and disorders of genitourinary system

N99.81 Other intraoperative complications of genitourinary system
▲ N99.82 Postprocedural ▶hemorrhage of◀ a genitourinary system organ or structure following a procedure
▲ N99.820 Postprocedural ▶hemorrhage of◀ a genitourinary system organ or structure following a genitourinary system procedure CC
▲ N99.821 Postprocedural ▶hemorrhage of◀ a genitourinary system organ or structure following other procedure CC
N99.83 Residual ovary syndrome ♀
● N99.84 Postprocedural hematoma and seroma of a genitourinary system organ or structure following a procedure
● N99.840 Postprocedural hematoma of a genitourinary system organ or structure following a genitourinary system procedure
● N99.841 Postprocedural hematoma of a genitourinary system organ or structure following other procedure
● N99.842 Postprocedural seroma of a genitourinary system organ or structure following a genitourinary system procedure
● N99.843 Postprocedural seroma of a genitourinary system organ or structure following other procedure
N99.89 Other postprocedural complications and disorders of genitourinary system

Unspecified Code Other Specified Code Manifestation Code N Newborn P Pediatric M Maternity A Adult ♂ Male ♀ Female
● New Code ▲ Revised Code Title ▶◀ Revised Text NOTES INCLUDES EXCLUDES1 Not coded here EXCLUDES2 Not included here
4th character required 5th character required 6th character required 7th character required
Extension 'X' Alert HAC Hospital-acquired condition (HAC) alert AHA AHA Coding Clinic©

This page intentionally left blank

Chapter 15: Pregnancy, Childbirth and the Puerperium (O00-O9A)

Guidelines for Assigning Codes From This Chapter

As Chapter 15's name indicates, you'll find codes here for diagnoses related to pregnancy, childbirth, and the puerperium (the weeks immediately after the birth). This chapter primarily includes codes for complications, but it also includes codes for normal delivery.

List of Sections

- O00-O08: Pregnancy with abortive outcome
- O09: Supervision of high risk pregnancy
- O10-O16: Edema, proteinuria and hypertensive disorders in pregnancy, childbirth and the puerperium
- -O29: Other maternal disorders predominantly related to pregnancy
- O30-O48: Maternal care related to the fetus and amniotic cavity and possible delivery problems
- O60-O77: Complications of labor and delivery
- O80-O82: Encounter for delivery
- O85-O92: Complications predominantly related to the puerperium
- O94-O9A: Other obstetric conditions, not elsewhere classified

Highlights From the ICD-10-CM Official Guidelines for Coding and Reporting

The Official Guidelines for Chapter 15 cover a variety of topics, including when to look outside the chapter for the proper codes. One important rule for this chapter is that generally these codes trump codes from other chapters. Also important is that these codes belong on claims for the mother, not for the newborn. You can read the complete guidelines for this chapter in Section I.C.15 of the 2017 Official Guidelines.

Keep in Mind That Z Codes May Apply Instead

Note that when a patient presents for an encounter and the pregnancy is incidental, meaning that the reason for the encounter is not the pregnancy, you should report Z33.1 (*Pregnant state, incidental*), instead of a code from Chapter 15. The provider's documentation should clearly state that the reason for the visit is not the pregnancy.

Also, if a patient presents for routine prenatal visits and no codes from Chapter 15 apply because there are no pregnancy complications, you should assign Z34.0 (*Encounter for supervision of normal first pregnancy*) or Z34.8 (*Encounter for supervision of other normal pregnancy*), or Z34.9 (*Encounter for supervision of normal pregnancy, unspecified*) as the diagnosis. To clarify, do not use these codes with codes from Chapter 15.

Code High-Risk Supervision as Primary Diagnosis

Assign a code from category O09 (**Supervision of high-risk pregnancy**) as the first-listed diagnosis. Other chapter 15 codes may also be reported when appropriate.

Identify the Trimester with a Final Character

Most of the codes in Chapter 15 require a final character to indicate which trimester the complication occurs in. Here are the time frames for each trimester:

- First trimester Less than 14 weeks, 0 days
- Second trimester 14 weeks, 0 days through 27 weeks and 6 days
- Third trimester 28 weeks through delivery

Certain conditions always occurs in a specific trimester, and sometimes, the trimester of pregnancy is simply not applicable to the condition. Some conditions may occur in more than one trimester but not in every trimester. You must check the documentation and the index to determine whether a final character is needed for certain codes. The final character is based on the trimester at the time of admission or encounter, whether the condition is pre-existing or occurred during the pregnancy.

In childbirth option. Whenever you have an "in childbirth" option a complication that occurs during delivery, use that code.

Unspecified trimester. Although a final character exists for an unspecified trimester, you should not assign that code unless the record fails to document the trimester and it is impossible to get the record clarified.

Overlapping trimesters. Assign the final character based on which trimester the patient was in at the time of admission/encounter for the complication, even if the complication developed prior to admission or is a pre-existing condition. Do not assign the character for the trimester at the time of discharge.

Identify Fetus with 7th Character in Multiple Gestation Complications

Certain categories of complication diagnoses codes (O31, O32, O33.3 - O33.6, O35, O36, O40, O41, O60.1, O60.2, O64, and O69) require that you assign a seventh character to identify the fetus affected. Use a 0 as the seventh character for:

- Single gestations
- Insufficient documentation to determine the affected fetus and clarification is not possible.
- When the affected fetus cannot be clinically determined.

If the pregnancy is a multiple-gestation pregnancy, fetuses one through five are identified with corresponding seventh characters of 1-5. A seventh character of 9 identifies "other."

Delivery May Affect Complication Coding

No delivery: For an encounter where delivery doesn't happen, choose the complication that led to the encounter as the principal diagnosis. If there's more than one complication, you may report any one of them first.

Delivery: When reporting the delivery encounter, your principal diagnosis needs to represent the "main circumstances or complication of the delivery" if the delivery is complicated. If the patient has a cesarean section (C-section), choose the code responsible for admission as the principal code, even if it's unrelated to the condition that led to the C-section. Also be sure to include a code for outcome of the delivery (Z37) in the maternal record.

Focus on Maternal Impact of Fetal Conditions

Heed the code descriptors before you use codes from O35 (*Maternal care for known or suspected fetal abnormality and damage*) or O36 (*Maternal care for other fetal problems*). As the definitions specify, those codes are appropriate only when the condition is one "affecting the management of the mother," such as a condition that leads to additional tests or performing in utero surgery. The mere existence of the fetal condition is insufficient reason to assign one of these codes if it doesn't affect the mother's care.

In utero surgery. In utero surgery on a fetus should be reported as an obstetric encounter. A diagnosis code from category O35 to identify the fetal condition is appropriate along with the appropriate procedure code. Never use perinatal codes from Chapter 16 on the mother's record.

Remember Sequencing for Pregnant Patients With HIV or Diabetes

HIV: Choose O98.7- (*Human immunodeficiency [HIV] disease complicating pregnancy, childbirth and the puerperium*) as the principal diagnosis for a patient who is admitted because of an HIV-related illness and who is pregnant or recently gave birth. Then, depending on the patient's HIV status, add B20 (*Human immunodeficiency virus [HIV] disease*) — which includes AIDS, AIDS-related complex, and symptomatic HIV infection — or Z21 (*Asymptomatic human immunodeficiency virus [HIV] infection status*), which includes HIV positive, NOS.

Diabetes: Code first one of the codes from the category O24 (*Diabetes mellitus in pregnancy, childbirth, and the puerperium*). Then, add an appropriate diabetes code from Chapter 4 code(s) (E08-E13).

For pre-existing diabetes mellitus in pregnancy, you have two codes to choose from O24.01 (type 1) and O24.11 (type 2). Add an additional character 1-3 for the first through third trimesters and 9 for unspecified trimester. You have other codes in this same category for diabetes mellitus in childbirth and puerperium.

For gestational diabetes in pregnancy, choose from the subcategory O24.41, adding additional characters for diet controlled (0), insulin controlled (4), and unspecified control (9). This category does not specify the trimester. Do not use any other code from category O24 when you report this code.

If the patient is receiving insulin to control the diabetes, you should also add Z79.4 (*Long-term [current] use of insulin*).

If the patient is diagnosed with abnormal glucose tolerance but not diabetes mellitus, you should assign a code from subcategory O99.81 (*Abnormal glucose complicating pregnancy, childbirth, and the puerperium*).

Don't Overlook Other Complications

Sepsis and septic shock. If you assign a code from chapter 15 for a complication of sepsis during pregnancy, delivery, abortion, or the puerperium, assign an additional code to identify the specific type of infective agent, if known. In addition, look to the subcategory R65.2- (*Severe sepsis*) if severe sepsis is present, with additional code(s) to identify affected organs, if appropriate.

For example, if you assign code O85 (*Puerperal sepsis*) caused by a bacteria, you would add a code from categories B95-B96 (*Bacterial infections in conditions classified elsewhere*) to identify the cause of the infection. Do not use codes from category A40.- (*Streptococcal sepsis*) or A41.- (*Other sepsis*) when you assign O85 for puerperal sepsis.

Alcohol. Assign a code from subcategory O99.31 (*Alcohol use complicating pregnancy, childbirth, and the puerperium*) when a pregnant patient uses alcohol during the pregnancy or postpartum period. Classify manifestations of alcohol use with an additional code from category F10 (*Alcohol-related disorders*).

Tobacco. When a pregnant patient uses any tobacco product during pregnancy or the postpartum period, report it with codes in subcategory O99.33 (*Smoking [tobacco] complicating pregnancy, childbirth, and the puerperium*) along with a code from category F17 (*Nicotine dependence*) to identify the type of nicotine dependence.

Other adverse events and effects. If a pregnant patient suffers a complication due to poisoning, toxicity from a drug or other substance, underdosing of a drug, or other adverse effect, chose a code from subcategory O9A.2 (*Injury, poisoning and certain other consequences of external causes complicating pregnancy, childbirth, and the puerperium*) as a primary diagnosis. Follow it with additional code(s) that to specify the cause of the complication. See Chapter 19, Adverse effects, poisoning, underdosing, and toxic effects.

Factor Complication's Time Frame Into Coding Choice

Resolved before delivery: Although you shouldn't report O80 (*Normal delivery*) when a complication code from Chapter 15 applies, you may report 080 if the patient had a previous complication that resolved by the time of the delivery admission. You can report diagnosis codes from other chapters if they are not complicating the pregnancy or delivery.

Remember to assign Z37.0 (*Single live birth*) for the outcome of delivery with O80; no other outcome of delivery code is acceptable with O80.

Complications after delivery: The Official Guidelines define postpartum as the 6 weeks after delivery. But you may report Chapter 15 codes even after this time if the provider documents the condition is pregnancy-related. Peripartum is the last month of pregnancy and five months after delivery. Chapter 15 codes can even be assigned after the peripartum period provided the documentation supports a pregnancy-related complication, such as pregnancy-associated cardiomyopathy.

Pregnancy-associated cardiomyopathy. When a patient who does not have pre-existing heart disease develops cardiomyopathy as a result of her pregnancy, assign code O90.3 (*Peripartum cardiomyopathy*). Although it may be diagnosed in the third trimester, pregnancy-related cardiomyopathy can continue for months after delivery — therefore, the diagnosis *peripartum cardiomyopathy*. You can only use this code, however, for a pregnant patient without pre-existing heart disease.

Sequelae of pregnancy-related complications. If a patient develops a condition resulting from a complication (a sequela) and requires care or treatment after the complication has resolved, code the condition (sequela) first and then code O94 (Sequelae of complication of pregnancy, childbirth, and the puerperium).

Don't Get Thrown by Delivery Outside Hospital

When a patient presents for routine care after delivering outside of the hospital, report **Z39.0** (*Encounter for care and examination of mother immediately after delivery*). If the patient presents with complications after delivering outside the hospital, choose codes based on those complications. You can use this code anytime after the postpartum period.

Watch Definitions and Circumstances for Accurate Abortion Coding

Definitions: Abortion simply means premature termination of pregnancy. You may be familiar with the term miscarriage, which in medical language is a spontaneous abortion. An induced abortion is an elective termination of pregnancy, regardless of the reason. You may see the words *incomplete abortion* referring to retained products of conception (fetus and/or placenta) following either a spontaneous or elective abortion.

Fetus liveborn: When the fetus is liveborn during an attempted pregnancy termination, you should report Z33.2 (*Encounter for elective termination of pregnancy*) and a code from category Z37 (*Outcome of Delivery*).

Post-abortion retained products of conception. If a patient retains tissue from the placenta or fetus after an elective termination of pregnancy, you would assign a code from codes O07.4 (*Failed attempted termination of pregnancy without complication*) and Z33.2 (*Encounter for elective termination of pregnancy*). If the retained products followed a spontaneous abortion, you would assign a code from category O03 (*Spontaneous abortion*). These codes can be appropriate even when the patient had a discharge diagnosis of complete abortion.

Complications: Other codes from Chapter 15 that identify documented complications of the pregnancy can be used in combination with codes from categories O07 (*Failed attempted termination of pregnancy*) and O08 (*Complications following ectopic and molar pregnancy*).

Don't Overlook Codes for Abuse in a Pregnant Patient

Sequence codes for suspected or confirmed abuse first before assigning appropriate codes to report the specific injury or sexual abuse, or codes to identify the abuser. Subcategories to report abuse include:

- O9A.3 — *Physical abuse complicating pregnancy, childbirth, and the puerperium*
- O9A.4 — *Sexual abuse complicating pregnancy, childbirth, and the puerperium*
- O9A.5 — *Psychological abuse complicating pregnancy, childbirth, and the puerperium*

See Chapter 19, Adult and child abuse, neglect and other maltreatment for additional codes.

Anatomy of the Female Reproductive System

1. **The female reproductive system includes the following:**
   a) The ovaries or female gonads are the primary sex organs of the female reproductive system.
   b) The uterine (or fallopian) tubes, uterus, vagina and external genitalia serve as the accessory organs of the female reproductive system.
   c) The accessory glands act to produce the mucus for providing lubrication during sexual intercourse.
2. **The anatomy of structures/components of the female reproductive system is further described below:**
   a) The Ovaries
      i) Ovaries are the paired glands in the upper pelvic cavity and remain located on each side of the uterus.
      ii) Capsule of the ovary is termed as the tunica albuginea. The outer region of the ovarian capsule is known as the cortex, which contains the ovarian follicles (or eggs).
      iii) Ovaries facilitate the discharge of eggs in ovulation and secrete the female sex hormones estrogen and progesterone.
   b) The Uterine (or Fallopian) Tubes
      i) Fallopian tubes are two in number and serve to transport the ova from the ovaries to the uterus.
      ii) The open end of the fallopian tube is of the shape of a funnel and is known as the infundibulum. The infundibulum is surrounded by the fimbriae, which form a fringe of fingerlike projections.
   c) The Uterus
      i) The uterus is known as the site of menstruation and fetal development.
      ii) The uterus is a pear shaped organ. The dome shaped part of the uterus above the uterine tubes is known as the fundus. The major tapering portion of the uterus is called the body. However, the narrow inferior part of the uterus is known as the cervix (or cervix uteri/neck of uterus).
      iii) The uterine cavity forms the interior of the body of uterus. The interior portion of the cervix is known as the cervical canal.
      iv) The internal os is the opening between the uterine wall and the cervical canal. The external os is the opening between the cervical canal and the vagina.
      v) The endometrium is the innermost layer of the uterine wall and forms the site of implantation of the fertilized egg.
      vi) The myometrium is the middle layer of the wall of uterus and composed of the smooth muscle.
      vii) The perimetrium (or visceral peritoneum) is the outermost layer of the uterine wall.
   d) The Vagina
      i) Its provides a passage for the menstrual flow. It is the lower part of the birth canal and serves as a receptacle for the penis during sexual intercourse.
      ii) Its attachment to the cervix is surrounded by a recess, which is known as the fornix.
   e) The External Genitalia of the Female
      i) The external genitalia of the female are known as the vulva (or pudendum).
      ii) The mons pubis (or veneris) is a rounded eminence of adipose or fatty tissue upon the pubic symphysis.
      iii) The outer fatty folds of the vulva that extend from the mons pubis are known as the labia majora.
      iv) Inner and highly vascular connective tissue folds of the vulva are known as the labia minora. These folds lack hairs and are also known as the nymphae.
      v) The small mass of erectile tissue at the anterior junction of labia minora is known as the clitoris. The clitoris remains covered with a skin layer, which is known as the prepuce. The glans is the exposed part of the clitoris.
      vi) The vestibule is an opening between the folds of the labia minora. This opening contains a thin fold of tissue (or the hymen) that gets ruptured at the time of the first sexual intercourse.
      vii) The vestibule is further linked to the vaginal and urethral orifices.
      viii) Lesser vestibular or Skene's glands secrete mucus, and the openings of their ducts lie on each side of the urethral orifice.
      ix) Bartholin's or greater vestibular glands generate mucus to facilitate the process of sexual intercourse. The openings of these glands lie on each side of the vaginal orifice.
   f) The Perineum
      i) The perineum is a region between the thighs and buttocks of both males and females. This area marks the boundary of the pelvic outlet and provides passage to the urogenital ducts and rectum.
      ii) The perineum is further divided into an anterior urogenital triangle containing the external genitalia, and a posterior anal triangle containing the anus.
   g) The Menstrual Cycle
      i) The menstrual cycle is also known by the names of menstruation or menses.
      ii) The menstrual cycle is divided into the menstrual, proliferative, and secretory phases.
      iii) The shedding of the endometrial lining of uterus, blood, and tissue fluid occurs during the menstrual phase of the menstrual cycle.
      iv) The proliferative phase of the menstrual cycle is also known as the follicular phase. The lining of the uterus grows and proliferates during this phase. The process of ovulation also starts in the follicular phase, wherein the egg ruptures from the Graafian follicle and the rising estrogen levels cause the endometrial lining of the uterus to thicken. The follicle eventually collapses and gets transformed to the corpus luteum.
      v) The estrogen and progesterone hormones are secreted during the secretory phase of the menstrual cycle. The fertilization and implantation process can occur in this stage after the hymen rupture during the first sexual intercourse. The corpus luteum degenerates and gets transformed to corpus albicans if the fertilization and implantation processes do not occur during this phase.
      vi) Following fertilization, the development of placenta is started. The placenta facilitates the secretion of estrogen and progesterone hormones to support the pregnancy and breast development for the production of milk inside the mammary glands.
   h) The Mammary Glands
      i) They serve to produce milk in females and are found in both males and females.
      ii) The mammary ducts expand into milk storage sinuses (or ampullae) near the nipple.
      iii) The areola is a circular pigmented area around the nipple.
      iv) They facilitate the process of lactation (which includes milk production and its ejection from the nipple).
   i) Pregnancy and Embryonic Development
      i) Pregnancy is initiated with the formation of a viable zygote (or fertilized egg) by the union of the male sperm and the female ovum (or fertilization).
      ii) Fertilization occurs in the outer third portion of the fallopian tube.
      iii) The zygote travels down the uterine tube and forms the blastocyst or blastula through mitotic division.
      iv) The zygote eventually gets transformed to the chorionic vesicle in the uterine cavity. This chorionic vesicle secretes the chorionic gonadotropin hormone that gets embedded in the endometrial lining and maintains it via hormones.
      v) The ectoderm forms the outer layer of the germ cells and develops into skin and nervous system.
      vi) The endoderm initially consists of the flattened cells that form the epithelial linings of the internal organs.
      vii) The mesoderm induces the formation of coelom (or the fluid-filled cavity within the mesoderm) and gives rise to muscles, bones, cartilages, connective tissues, and other structures.
      viii) The chorionic villi are the projections of the trophoblast (or the fluid-filled sphere of the blastocyst). These chorionic villi communicate with the uterine tissue to form the placenta.
      ix) The amnion is the fluid filled sac that surrounds and protects the embryo as the placenta is formed.
      x) The umbilical cord or birth cord is the stalk that connects the fetus (or embryo) to the placenta.
      xi) The placenta serves to exchange oxygen, nutrients, and wastes between the embryo and the mother.

xii) With the ongoing pregnancy, the uterus expands in the abdominal cavity for accommodating the growing fetus.

xiii) Childbirth (or parturition) is induced by uterine contractions, and this process is termed as the labor.

xiv) The dilation stage involves the complete dilation of the cervix by the head of the fetus. The amniotic fluid (or bag of waters) is also released during the rupture of the amnion.

xv) The child moves out through the cervix and vagina during the expulsion stage.

xvi) The placental stage (or afterbirth) is marked by the detachment of the placenta from the uterus following the birth.

Common Pathologies

Dysfunctional uterine bleeding (DUB)
Dysfunctional uterine bleeding, or DUB, refers to bleeding originating from the uterus due to changes in hormone levels, common in adolescents and women nearing menopause.

Endometriosis
Endometriosis is a condition in which the tissue that lines the inside of the uterus, known as the endometrium, grows outside of the uterus, including on other organs in the pelvis.

Fibroids
Fibroids, also known as myomas or leiomyomas, are solid, benign tumors made of fibrous tissue that develop and grow in the muscular walls of the uterus. They tend to form during a woman's childbearing years and may grow fast or slow. Symptoms include heavy or prolonged menstrual bleeding, pelvic pain, and urinary symptoms due to pressure on the bladder. There are four types of fibroids: intramural, subserosal, submucosal, and cervical.

Intramural
These are located in the wall of the uterus. These are the most common types of fibroids.

Subserosal
These are located outside the wall of the uterus. They may grow in the form stalks, called pedunculated fibroids. Subserosal fibroids can become quite large.

Submucosal
These are located in the muscle beneath the lining of the uterus wall.

Cervical
These are located in the neck of the womb (the cervix).

Uterine fibroids

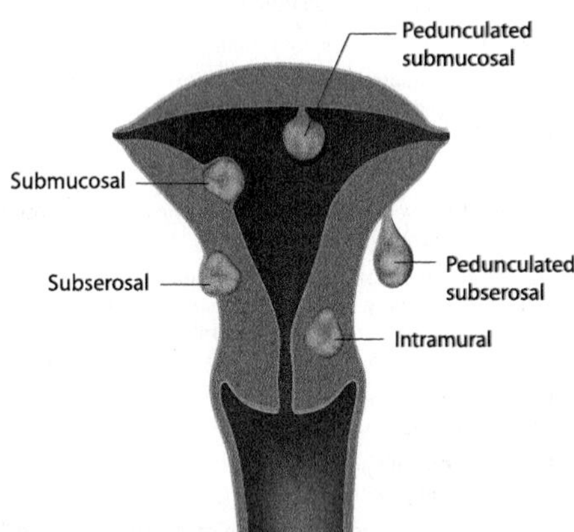

Gonorrhea
Gonorrhea is a sexually transmitted disease, or STD, that results from infection with the bacterium Neisseria gonorrhoeae. It damages the reproductive system and can be passed from mother to baby during delivery.

Urinary Incontinence
Urinary incontinence refers to the inability to hold urine. It is often caused by weakness of the external sphincter muscle of the urethra, the duct through which urine exits the body. It is more common in women.

Polycystic Ovarian Syndrome (PCOS)
Polycystic ovarian syndrome, or PCOS, is characterized by small cysts on the ovaries and is associated with a hormone imbalance that results in a variety of symptoms, which may include infertility. PCOS is also known as Stein-Leventhal syndrome.

Pregnancy, childbirth and the puerperium (O00-O9A)

NOTES CODES FROM THIS CHAPTER ARE FOR USE ONLY ON MATERNAL RECORDS, NEVER ON NEWBORN RECORDS
Codes from this chapter are for use for conditions related to or aggravated by the pregnancy, childbirth, or by the puerperium (maternal causes or obstetric causes)
Trimesters are counted from the first day of the last menstrual period. They are defined as follows:
1st trimester- less than 14 weeks 0 days
2nd trimester- 14 weeks 0 days to less than 28 weeks 0 days
3rd trimester- 28 weeks 0 days until delivery

Use additional code from category Z3A, Weeks of gestation, to identify the specific week of the pregnancy, ►if known◄.

EXCLUDES1 *supervision of normal pregnancy (Z34.-)*

EXCLUDES2 *mental and behavioral disorders associated with the puerperium (F53)*
obstetrical tetanus (A34)
postpartum necrosis of pituitary gland (E23.0)
puerperal osteomalacia (M83.0)

This chapter contains the following blocks:

Pregnancy with abortive outcome (O00-O08)

EXCLUDES1 *continuing pregnancy in multiple gestation after abortion of one fetus or more (O31.1-, O31.3-)*

④ **O00 Ectopic pregnancy**
INCLUDES *ruptured ectopic pregnancy*
Use additional code from category O08 to identify any associated complication

⑤ **O00.0** Abdominal **pregnancy**
EXCLUDES1 *maternal care for viable fetus in abdominal pregnancy (O36.7-)*

● **O00.00 Abdominal pregnancy** without intrauterine pregnancy CC CC/MCC Exc
Abdominal pregnancy NOS

● **O00.01 Abdominal pregnancy** with intrauterine pregnancy CC CC/MCC Exc

⑤ **O00.1** Tubal **pregnancy**
Fallopian pregnancy
Rupture of (fallopian) tube due to pregnancy
Tubal abortion

● **O00.10 Tubal pregnancy** without intrauterine pregnancy CC CC/MCC Exc
Tubal pregnancy NOS

● **O00.11 Tubal pregnancy** with intrauterine pregnancy CC CC/MCC Exc

⑤ **O00.2** Ovarian **pregnancy**

● **O00.20 Ovarian pregnancy** without intrauterine pregnancy CC CC/MCC Exc
Ovarian pregnancy NOS

● **O00.21 Ovarian pregnancy** with intrauterine pregnancy CC CC/MCC Exc

⑤ **O00.8 Other ectopic pregnancy**
Cervical pregnancy
Cornual pregnancy
Intraligamentous pregnancy
Mural pregnancy

● **O00.80 Other ectopic pregnancy** without intrauterine pregnancy CC CC/MCC Exc
Other ectopic pregnancy NOS

● **O00.81 Other ectopic pregnancy** with intrauterine pregnancy CC CC/MCC Exc

⑤ **O00.9 Ectopic pregnancy, unspecified**

● **O00.90 Unspecified ectopic pregnancy** without intrauterine pregnancy CC CC/MCC Exc
Ectopic pregnancy NOS

● **O00.91 Unspecified ectopic pregnancy** with intrauterine pregnancy CC CC/MCC Exc

④ **O01 Hydatidiform mole**
Use additional code from category O08 to identify any associated complication.
EXCLUDES1 *chorioadenoma (destruens) (D39.2)*
malignant hydatidiform mole (D39.2)

O01.0 Classical **hydatidiform mole** M ♀
Complete hydatidiform mole

O01.1 Incomplete and partial **hydatidiform mole** M ♀

O01.9 Hydatidiform mole, unspecified M ♀
Trophoblastic disease NOS
Vesicular mole NOS

④ **O02 Other abnormal products of conception**
Use additional code from category O08 to identify any associated complication.
EXCLUDES1 *papyraceous fetus (O31.0-)*

O02.0 Blighted ovum and nonhydatidiform mole M ♀
Carneous mole
Fleshy mole
Intrauterine mole NOS
Molar pregnancy NEC
Pathological ovum

O02.1 Missed abortion M ♀
Early fetal death, before completion of 20 weeks of gestation, with retention of dead fetus
EXCLUDES1 *failed induced abortion (O07.-)*
fetal death (intrauterine) (late) (O36.4)
missed abortion with blighted ovum (O02.0)
missed abortion with hydatidiform mole (O01.-)
missed abortion with nonhydatidiform (O02.0)
missed abortion with other abnormal products of conception (O02.8-)
missed delivery (O36.4)
stillbirth (P95)

⑤ **O02.8 Other specified abnormal products of conception**
EXCLUDES1 *abnormal products of conception with blighted ovum (O02.0)*
abnormal products of conception with hydatidiform mole (O01.-)
abnormal products of conception with nonhydatidiform mole (O02.0)

O02.81 Inappropriate change in quantitative human chorionic gonadotropin (hCG) in early pregnancy M ♀
Biochemical pregnancy
Chemical pregnancy
Inappropriate level of quantitative human chorionic gonadotropin (hCG) for gestational age in early pregnancy

O02.89 Other abnormal products of conception M ♀

O02.9 Abnormal product of conception, unspecified M ♀

④ **O03 Spontaneous abortion**
NOTES Incomplete abortion includes retained products of conception following spontaneous abortion
INCLUDES *miscarriage*

O03.0 Genital tract and pelvic infection **following** incomplete **spontaneous abortion** M CC ♀
Endometritis following incomplete spontaneous abortion
Oophoritis following incomplete spontaneous abortion
Parametritis following incomplete spontaneous abortion
Pelvic peritonitis following incomplete spontaneous abortion
Salpingitis following incomplete spontaneous abortion
Salpingo-oophoritis following incomplete spontaneous abortion
EXCLUDES1 *sepsis following incomplete spontaneous abortion (O03.37)*
urinary tract infection following incomplete spontaneous abortion (O03.38)

Unspecified Code | Other Specified Code | Manifestation Code | N Newborn | P Pediatric | M Maternity | A Adult | ♂ Male | ♀ Female
● New Code | ▲ Revised Code Title | ►◄ Revised Text | NOTES | INCLUDES | EXCLUDES1 Not coded here | EXCLUDES2 Not included here
④ 4th character required | ⑤ 5th character required | ⑥ 6th character required | ⑦ 7th character required
Extension 'X' Alert | HAC Hospital-acquired condition (HAC) alert | AHA AHA Coding Clinic©

O03.1 Delayed or excessive hemorrhage following incomplete spontaneous abortion M ♀
Afibrinogenemia following incomplete spontaneous abortion
Defibrination syndrome following incomplete spontaneous abortion
Hemolysis following incomplete spontaneous abortion
Intravascular coagulation following incomplete spontaneous abortion

O03.2 Embolism following incomplete spontaneous abortion M MCC ♀
Air embolism following incomplete spontaneous abortion
Amniotic fluid embolism following incomplete spontaneous abortion
Blood-clot embolism following incomplete spontaneous abortion
Embolism NOS following incomplete spontaneous abortion
Fat embolism following incomplete spontaneous abortion
Pulmonary embolism following incomplete spontaneous abortion
Pyemic embolism following incomplete spontaneous abortion
Septic or septicopyemic embolism following incomplete spontaneous abortion
Soap embolism following incomplete spontaneous abortion

O03.3 Other and unspecified complications following incomplete spontaneous abortion

O03.30 Unspecified complication following incomplete spontaneous abortion M CC ♀

O03.31 Shock following incomplete spontaneous abortion M MCC ♀
Circulatory collapse following incomplete spontaneous abortion
Shock (postprocedural) following incomplete spontaneous abortion
EXCLUDES1 *shock due to infection following incomplete spontaneous abortion (O03.37)*

O03.32 Renal failure following incomplete spontaneous abortion M MCC ♀
Kidney failure (acute) following incomplete spontaneous abortion
Oliguria following incomplete spontaneous abortion
Renal shutdown following incomplete spontaneous abortion
Renal tubular necrosis following incomplete spontaneous abortion
Uremia following incomplete spontaneous abortion

O03.33 Metabolic disorder following incomplete spontaneous abortion M CC ♀

O03.34 Damage to pelvic organs following incomplete spontaneous abortion M CC ♀
Laceration, perforation, tear or chemical damage of bladder following incomplete spontaneous abortion
Laceration, perforation, tear or chemical damage of bowel following incomplete spontaneous abortion
Laceration, perforation, tear or chemical damage of broad ligament following incomplete spontaneous abortion
Laceration, perforation, tear or chemical damage of cervix following incomplete spontaneous abortion
Laceration, perforation, tear or chemical damage of periurethral tissue following incomplete spontaneous abortion
Laceration, perforation, tear or chemical damage of uterus following incomplete spontaneous abortion
Laceration, perforation, tear or chemical damage of vagina following incomplete spontaneous abortion

O03.35 Other venous complications following incomplete spontaneous abortion M CC ♀

O03.36 Cardiac arrest following incomplete spontaneous abortion M CC ♀

O03.37 Sepsis following incomplete spontaneous abortion M CC ♀
Use additional code to identify infectious agent (B95-B97)
Use additional code to identify severe sepsis, if applicable (R65.2-)
EXCLUDES1 *septic or septicopyemic embolism following incomplete spontaneous abortion (O03.2)*

O03.38 Urinary tract infection following incomplete spontaneous abortion M CC ♀
Cystitis following incomplete spontaneous abortion

O03.39 Incomplete spontaneous abortion with other complications M CC ♀

O03.4 Incomplete spontaneous abortion without complication M ♀

O03.5 Genital tract and pelvic infection following complete or unspecified spontaneous abortion M CC ♀
Endometritis following complete or unspecified spontaneous abortion
Oophoritis following complete or unspecified spontaneous abortion
Parametritis following complete or unspecified spontaneous abortion
Pelvic peritonitis following complete or unspecified spontaneous abortion
Salpingitis following complete or unspecified spontaneous abortion
Salpingo-oophoritis following complete or unspecified spontaneous abortion
EXCLUDES1 *sepsis following complete or unspecified spontaneous abortion (O03.87)*
urinary tract infection following complete or unspecified spontaneous abortion (O03.88)

O03.6 Delayed or excessive hemorrhage following complete or unspecified spontaneous abortion M ♀
Afibrinogenemia following complete or unspecified spontaneous abortion
Defibrination syndrome following complete or unspecified spontaneous abortion
Hemolysis following complete or unspecified spontaneous abortion
Intravascular coagulation following complete or unspecified spontaneous abortion

O03.7 Embolism following complete or unspecified spontaneous abortion M CC ♀
Air embolism following complete or unspecified spontaneous abortion
Amniotic fluid embolism following complete or unspecified spontaneous abortion
Blood-clot embolism following complete or unspecified spontaneous abortion
Embolism NOS following complete or unspecified spontaneous abortion
Fat embolism following complete or unspecified spontaneous abortion
Pulmonary embolism following complete or unspecified spontaneous abortion
Pyemic embolism following complete or unspecified spontaneous abortion
Septic or septicopyemic embolism following complete or unspecified spontaneous abortion
Soap embolism following complete or unspecified spontaneous abortion

O03.8 Other and unspecified complications following complete or unspecified spontaneous abortion

O03.80 Unspecified complication following complete or unspecified spontaneous abortion M CC ♀

O03.81 Shock following complete or unspecified spontaneous abortion M MCC ♀
Circulatory collapse following complete or unspecified spontaneous abortion
Shock (postprocedural) following complete or unspecified spontaneous abortion
EXCLUDES1 *shock due to infection following complete or unspecified spontaneous abortion (O03.87)*

O03.82 Renal failure following complete or unspecified spontaneous abortion M MCC ♀
Kidney failure (acute) following complete or unspecified spontaneous abortion
Oliguria following complete or unspecified spontaneous abortion
Renal shutdown following complete or unspecified spontaneous abortion
Renal tubular necrosis following complete or unspecified spontaneous abortion
Uremia following complete or unspecified spontaneous abortion

O03.83 Metabolic disorder following complete or unspecified spontaneous abortion M CC ♀

O03.84 Damage to pelvic organs following complete or unspecified spontaneous abortion M CC ♀

Unacceptable principal diagnosis symbol per Medicare code edits · Code exempt from diagnosis present on admission requirement
Questionable admission · Complication or comorbidity · CC/MCC exclusion · Major complication or comorbidity
Principal diagnosis as its own CC · Principal diagnosis as its own MCC · Z code as first-listed diagnosis

Laceration, perforation, tear or chemical damage of bladder following complete or unspecified spontaneous abortion
Laceration, perforation, tear or chemical damage of bowel following complete or unspecified spontaneous abortion
Laceration, perforation, tear or chemical damage of broad ligament following complete or unspecified spontaneous abortion
Laceration, perforation, tear or chemical damage of cervix following complete or unspecified spontaneous abortion
Laceration, perforation, tear or chemical damage of periurethral tissue following complete or unspecified spontaneous abortion
Laceration, perforation, tear or chemical damage of uterus following complete or unspecified spontaneous abortion
Laceration, perforation, tear or chemical damage of vagina following complete or unspecified spontaneous abortion

O03.85 Other venous complications following complete or unspecified spontaneous abortion M cc ♀

O03.86 Cardiac arrest following complete or unspecified spontaneous abortion M cc ♀

O03.87 Sepsis following complete or unspecified spontaneous abortion M cc ♀
Use additional code to identify infectious agent (B95-B97)
Use additional code to identify severe sepsis, if applicable (R65.2-)
EXCLUDES1 *septic or septicopyemic embolism following complete or unspecified spontaneous abortion (O03.7)*

O03.88 Urinary tract infection following complete or unspecified spontaneous abortion M cc ♀
Cystitis following complete or unspecified spontaneous abortion

O03.89 Complete or unspecified spontaneous abortion with other complications M cc ♀

O03.9 Complete or unspecified spontaneous abortion without complication M ♀
Miscarriage NOS
Spontaneous abortion NOS

O04 Complications following (induced) termination of pregnancy (4th character required)
INCLUDES *complications following (induced) termination of pregnancy*
EXCLUDES1 *encounter for elective termination of pregnancy, uncomplicated (Z33.2)*
failed attempted termination of pregnancy (O07.-)

O04.5 Genital tract and pelvic infection following (induced) termination of pregnancy M cc ♀
Endometritis following (induced) termination of pregnancy
Oophoritis following (induced) termination of pregnancy
Parametritis following (induced) termination of pregnancy
Pelvic peritonitis following (induced) termination of pregnancy
Salpingitis following (induced) termination of pregnancy
Salpingo-oophoritis following (induced) termination of pregnancy
EXCLUDES1 *sepsis following (induced) termination of pregnancy (O04.87)*
urinary tract infection following (induced) termination of pregnancy (O04.88)

O04.6 Delayed or excessive hemorrhage following (induced) termination of pregnancy M ♀
Afibrinogenemia following (induced) termination of pregnancy
Defibrination syndrome following (induced) termination of pregnancy
Hemolysis following (induced) termination of pregnancy
Intravascular coagulation following (induced) termination of pregnancy

O04.7 Embolism following (induced) termination of pregnancy M MCC ♀
Air embolism following (induced) termination of pregnancy
Amniotic fluid embolism following (induced) termination of pregnancy
Blood-clot embolism following (induced) termination of pregnancy
Embolism NOS following (induced) termination of pregnancy
Fat embolism following (induced) termination of pregnancy
Pulmonary embolism following (induced) termination of pregnancy
Pyemic embolism following (induced) termination of pregnancy
Septic or septicopyemic embolism following (induced) termination of pregnancy
Soap embolism following (induced) termination of pregnancy

O04.8 (Induced) termination of pregnancy with other and unspecified complications (5th character required)

O04.80 (Induced) termination of pregnancy with unspecified complications M cc ♀

O04.81 Shock following (induced) termination of pregnancy M MCC ♀
Circulatory collapse following (induced) termination of pregnancy
Shock (postprocedural) following (induced) termination of pregnancy
EXCLUDES1 *shock due to infection following (induced) termination of pregnancy (O04.87)*

O04.82 Renal failure following (induced) termination of pregnancy M MCC ♀
Kidney failure (acute) following (induced) termination of pregnancy
Oliguria following (induced) termination of pregnancy
Renal shutdown following (induced) termination of pregnancy
Renal tubular necrosis following (induced) termination of pregnancy
Uremia following (induced) termination of pregnancy

O04.83 Metabolic disorder following (induced) termination of pregnancy M cc ♀

O04.84 Damage to pelvic organs following (induced) termination of pregnancy M cc ♀
Laceration, perforation, tear or chemical damage of bladder following (induced) termination of pregnancy
Laceration, perforation, tear or chemical damage of bowel following (induced) termination of pregnancy
Laceration, perforation, tear or chemical damage of broad ligament following (induced) termination of pregnancy
Laceration, perforation, tear or chemical damage of cervix following (induced) termination of pregnancy
Laceration, perforation, tear or chemical damage of periurethral tissue following (induced) termination of pregnancy
Laceration, perforation, tear or chemical damage of uterus following (induced) termination of pregnancy
Laceration, perforation, tear or chemical damage of vagina following (induced) termination of pregnancy

O04.85 Other venous complications following (induced) termination of pregnancy M cc ♀

O04.86 Cardiac arrest following (induced) termination of pregnancy M cc ♀

O04.87 Sepsis following (induced) termination of pregnancy M cc ♀
Use additional code to identify infectious agent (B95-B97)
Use additional code to identify severe sepsis, if applicable (R65.2-)
EXCLUDES1 *septic or septicopyemic embolism following (induced) termination of pregnancy (O04.7)*

O04.88 Urinary tract infection following (induced) termination of pregnancy M cc ♀
Cystitis following (induced) termination of pregnancy

O04.89 (Induced) termination of pregnancy with other complications M cc ♀

O07 Failed attempted termination of pregnancy (4th character required)
INCLUDES *failure of attempted induction of termination of pregnancy*
incomplete elective abortion
EXCLUDES1 *incomplete spontaneous abortion (O03.0-)*

O07.0 Genital tract and pelvic infection following failed attempted termination of pregnancy M cc ♀
Endometritis following failed attempted termination of pregnancy
Oophoritis following failed attempted termination of pregnancy
Parametritis following failed attempted termination of pregnancy

Pelvic peritonitis following failed attempted termination of pregnancy
Salpingitis following failed attempted termination of pregnancy
Salpingo-oophoritis following failed attempted termination of pregnancy

EXCLUDES1 *sepsis following failed attempted termination of pregnancy (O07.37)*
urinary tract infection following failed attempted termination of pregnancy (O07.38)

O07.1 **Delayed or excessive hemorrhage following failed attempted termination of pregnancy** M cc ♀
Afibrinogenemia following failed attempted termination of pregnancy
Defibrination syndrome following failed attempted termination of pregnancy
Hemolysis following failed attempted termination of pregnancy
Intravascular coagulation following failed attempted termination of pregnancy

O07.2 **Embolism following failed attempted termination of pregnancy** M MCC ♀
Air embolism following failed attempted termination of pregnancy
Amniotic fluid embolism following failed attempted termination of pregnancy
Blood-clot embolism following failed attempted termination of pregnancy
Embolism NOS following failed attempted termination of pregnancy
Fat embolism following failed attempted termination of pregnancy
Pulmonary embolism following failed attempted termination of pregnancy
Pyemic embolism following failed attempted termination of pregnancy
Septic or septicopyemic embolism following failed attempted termination of pregnancy
Soap embolism following failed attempted termination of pregnancy

5th O07.3 **Failed attempted termination of pregnancy with other and unspecified complications**

O07.30 **Failed attempted termination of pregnancy with unspecified complications** M cc ♀

O07.31 **Shock following failed attempted termination of pregnancy** M MCC ♀
Circulatory collapse following failed attempted termination of pregnancy
Shock (postprocedural) following failed attempted termination of pregnancy

EXCLUDES1 *shock due to infection following failed attempted termination of pregnancy (O07.37)*

O07.32 **Renal failure following failed attempted termination of pregnancy** M MCC ♀
Kidney failure (acute) following failed attempted termination of pregnancy
Oliguria following failed attempted termination of pregnancy
Renal shutdown following failed attempted termination of pregnancy
Renal tubular necrosis following failed attempted termination of pregnancy
Uremia following failed attempted termination of pregnancy

O07.33 **Metabolic disorder following failed attempted termination of pregnancy** M cc ♀

O07.34 **Damage to pelvic organs following failed attempted termination of pregnancy** M cc ♀
Laceration, perforation, tear or chemical damage of bladder following failed attempted termination of pregnancy
Laceration, perforation, tear or chemical damage of bowel following failed attempted termination of pregnancy
Laceration, perforation, tear or chemical damage of broad ligament following failed attempted termination of pregnancy
Laceration, perforation, tear or chemical damage of cervix following failed attempted termination of pregnancy
Laceration, perforation, tear or chemical damage of periurethral tissue following failed attempted termination of pregnancy
Laceration, perforation, tear or chemical damage of uterus following failed attempted termination of pregnancy
Laceration, perforation, tear or chemical damage of vagina following failed attempted termination of pregnancy

O07.35 **Other venous complications following failed attempted termination of pregnancy** M cc ♀

O07.36 **Cardiac arrest following failed attempted termination of pregnancy** M cc ♀

O07.37 **Sepsis following failed attempted termination of pregnancy** M cc ♀
Use additional code (B95-B97), to identify infectious agent
Use additional code (R65.2-) to identify severe sepsis, if applicable

EXCLUDES1 *septic or septicopyemic embolism following failed attempted termination of pregnancy (O07.2)*

O07.38 **Urinary tract infection following failed attempted termination of pregnancy** M cc ♀
Cystitis following failed attempted termination of pregnancy

O07.39 **Failed attempted termination of pregnancy with other complications** M cc ♀

O07.4 **Failed attempted termination of pregnancy without complication** M ♀

4th O08 **Complications following ectopic and molar pregnancy**
This category is for use with categories O00-O02 to identify any associated complications

O08.0 **Genital tract and pelvic infection following ectopic and molar pregnancy** M cc ♀
Endometritis following ectopic and molar pregnancy
Oophoritis following ectopic and molar pregnancy
Parametritis following ectopic and molar pregnancy
Pelvic peritonitis following ectopic and molar pregnancy
Salpingitis following ectopic and molar pregnancy
Salpingo-oophoritis following ectopic and molar pregnancy

EXCLUDES1 *sepsis following ectopic and molar pregnancy (O08.82)*
urinary tract infection (O08.83)

O08.1 **Delayed or excessive hemorrhage following ectopic and molar pregnancy** M cc ♀
Afibrinogenemia following ectopic and molar pregnancy
Defibrination syndrome following ectopic and molar pregnancy
Hemolysis following ectopic and molar pregnancy
Intravascular coagulation following ectopic and molar pregnancy

EXCLUDES1 *delayed or excessive hemorrhage due to incomplete abortion (O03.1)*

O08.2 **Embolism following ectopic and molar pregnancy** M MCC ♀
Air embolism following ectopic and molar pregnancy
Amniotic fluid embolism following ectopic and molar pregnancy
Blood-clot embolism following ectopic and molar pregnancy
Embolism NOS following ectopic and molar pregnancy
Fat embolism following ectopic and molar pregnancy
Pulmonary embolism following ectopic and molar pregnancy
Pyemic embolism following ectopic and molar pregnancy
Septic or septicopyemic embolism following ectopic and molar pregnancy
Soap embolism following ectopic and molar pregnancy

O08.3 **Shock following ectopic and molar pregnancy** M MCC ♀
Circulatory collapse following ectopic and molar pregnancy
Shock (postprocedural) following ectopic and molar pregnancy

EXCLUDES1 *shock due to infection following ectopic and molar pregnancy (O08.82)*

O08.4 **Renal failure following ectopic and molar pregnancy** M MCC ♀
Kidney failure (acute) following ectopic and molar pregnancy
Oliguria following ectopic and molar pregnancy
Renal shutdown following ectopic and molar pregnancy
Renal tubular necrosis following ectopic and molar pregnancy
Uremia following ectopic and molar pregnancy

O08.5 **Metabolic disorders following an ectopic and molar pregnancy** M cc ♀

1st 1st trimester 2nd 2nd trimester 3rd 3rd trimester PDx Unacceptable principal diagnosis symbol per Medicare code edits
POA Code exempt from diagnosis present on admission requirement ? Questionable admission CC Complication or comorbidity
CC/MCC Excl CC/MCC exclusion MCC Major complication or comorbidity PDx CC Principal diagnosis as its own CC
PDx MCC Principal diagnosis as its own MCC Z-1 Z code as first-listed diagnosis

O08.6 Damage to pelvic organs and tissues following an ectopic and molar pregnancy
Laceration, perforation, tear or chemical damage of bladder following an ectopic and molar pregnancy
Laceration, perforation, tear or chemical damage of bowel following an ectopic and molar pregnancy
Laceration, perforation, tear or chemical damage of broad ligament following an ectopic and molar pregnancy
Laceration, perforation, tear or chemical damage of cervix following an ectopic and molar pregnancy
Laceration, perforation, tear or chemical damage of periurethral tissue following an ectopic and molar pregnancy
Laceration, perforation, tear or chemical damage of uterus following an ectopic and molar pregnancy
Laceration, perforation, tear or chemical damage of vagina following an ectopic and molar pregnancy

O08.7 Other venous complications following an ectopic and molar pregnancy

O08.8 Other complications following an ectopic and molar pregnancy

O08.81 Cardiac arrest following an ectopic and molar pregnancy

O08.82 Sepsis following ectopic and molar pregnancy
Use additional code (B95-B97), to identify infectious agent
Use additional code (R65.2-) to identify severe sepsis, if applicable
EXCLUDES1 *septic or septicopyemic embolism following ectopic and molar pregnancy (O08.2)*

O08.83 Urinary tract infection following an ectopic and molar pregnancy
Cystitis following an ectopic and molar pregnancy

O08.89 Other complications following an ectopic and molar pregnancy

O08.9 Unspecified complication following an ectopic and molar pregnancy

Supervision of high risk pregnancy (O09)

O09 Supervision of high risk pregnancy

O09.0 Supervision of pregnancy with history of infertility

O09.00 Supervision of pregnancy with history of infertility, unspecified trimester

O09.01 Supervision of pregnancy with history of infertility, first trimester

O09.02 Supervision of pregnancy with history of infertility, second trimester

O09.03 Supervision of pregnancy with history of infertility, third trimester

▲ O09.1 Supervision of pregnancy with history of ▶ectopic pregnancy◀

▲ O09.10 Supervision of pregnancy with history of ▶ectopic pregnancy◀, unspecified trimester

▲ O09.11 Supervision of pregnancy with history of ▶ectopic pregnancy◀, first trimester

▲ O09.12 Supervision of pregnancy with history of ▶ectopic pregnancy◀, second trimester

▲ O09.13 Supervision of pregnancy with history of ▶ectopic pregnancy◀, third trimester

● O09.A Supervision of pregnancy with history of molar pregnancy

● O09.A0 Supervision of pregnancy with history of molar pregnancy, unspecified trimester

● O09.A1 Supervision of pregnancy with history of molar pregnancy, first trimester

● O09.A2 Supervision of pregnancy with history of molar pregnancy, second trimester

● O09.A3 Supervision of pregnancy with history of molar pregnancy, third trimester

O09.2 Supervision of pregnancy with other poor reproductive or obstetric history
EXCLUDES2 *pregnancy care for patient with history of recurrent pregnancy loss (O26.2-)*

O09.21 Supervision of pregnancy with history of pre-term labor

O09.211 Supervision of pregnancy with history of pre-term labor, first trimeter

O09.212 Supervision of pregnancy with history of pre-term labor, second trimester

O09.213 Supervision of pregnancy with history of pre-term labor, third trimester

O09.219 Supervision of pregnancy with history of pre-term labor, unspecified t rimester

O09.29 Supervision of pregnancy with other poor reproductive or obstetric history
Supervision of pregnancy with history of neonatal death
Supervision of pregnancy with history of stillbirth

O09.291 Supervision of pregnancy with other poor reproductive or obstetric history, first trimester

O09.292 Supervision of pregnancy with other poor reproductive or obstetric history, second trimester

O09.293 Supervision of pregnancy with other poor reproductive or obstetric history, third trimester

O09.299 Supervision of pregnancy with other poor reproductive or obstetric history, unspecified trimester

O09.3 Supervision of pregnancy with insufficient antenatal care
Supervision of concealed pregnancy
Supervision of hidden pregnancy

O09.30 Supervision of pregnancy with insufficient antenatal care, unspecified trimester

O09.31 Supervision of pregnancy with insufficient antenatal care, first trimester

O09.32 Supervision of pregnancy with insufficient antenatal care, second trimester

O09.33 Supervision of pregnancy with insufficient antenatal care, third trimester

O09.4 Supervision of pregnancy with grand multiparity

O09.40 Supervision of pregnancy with grand multiparity, unspecified trimester

O09.41 Supervision of pregnancy with grand multiparity, first trimester

O09.42 Supervision of pregnancy with grand multiparity, second trimester

O09.43 Supervision of pregnancy with grand multiparity, third trimester

O09.5 Supervision of elderly primigravida and multigravida
Pregnancy for a female 35 years and older at expected date of delivery

O09.51 Supervision of elderly primigravida

O09.511 Supervision of elderly primigravida, first trimester

O09.512 Supervision of elderly primigravida, second trimester

O09.513 Supervision of elderly primigravida, third trimester

O09.519 Supervision of elderly primigravida, unspecified trimester

O09.52 Supervision of elderly multigravida

O09.521 Supervision of elderly multigravida, first trimester

O09.522 Supervision of elderly multigravida, second trimester

O09.523 Supervision of elderly multigravida, third trimester

O09.529 Supervision of elderly multigravida, unspecified trimester

O09.6 Supervision of young primigravida and multigravida
Supervision of pregnancy for a female less than 16 years old at expected date of delivery

O09.61 Supervision of young primigravida

O09.611 Supervision of young primigravida, first trimester

Unspecified Code Other Specified Code Manifestation Code N Newborn P Pediatric M Maternity A Adult ♂ Male ♀ Female
● New Code ▲ Revised Code Title ▶◀ Revised Text NOTES INCLUDES EXCLUDES1 Not coded here EXCLUDES2 Not included here
4th character required 5th character required 6th character required 7th character required
Extension 'X' Alert HAC Hospital-acquired condition (HAC) alert AHA AHA Coding Clinic©

O09.612 Supervision of young primigravida, second trimester
O09.613 Supervision of young primigravida, third trimester
O09.619 Supervision of young primigravida, unspecified trimester
O09.62 Supervision of young multigravida
O09.621 Supervision of young multigravida, first trimester
O09.622 Supervision of young multigravida, second trimester
O09.623 Supervision of young multigravida, third trimester
O09.629 Supervision of young multigravida, unspecified trimester
O09.7 Supervision of high risk pregnancy due to social problems
O09.70 Supervision of high risk pregnancy due to social problems, unspecified trimester
O09.71 Supervision of high risk pregnancy due to social problems, first trimester
O09.72 Supervision of high risk pregnancy due to social problems, second trimester
O09.73 Supervision of high risk pregnancy due to social problems, third trimester
O09.8 Supervision of other high risk pregnancies
O09.81 Supervision of pregnancy resulting from assisted reproductive technology

Supervision of pregnancy resulting from in-vitro fertilization

EXCLUDES2 *gestational carrier status (Z33.3)*

O09.811 Supervision of pregnancy resulting from assisted reproductive technology, first trimester
O09.812 Supervision of pregnancy resulting from assisted reproductive technology, second trimester
O09.813 Supervision of pregnancy resulting from assisted reproductive technology, third trimester
O09.819 Supervision of pregnancy resulting from assisted reproductive technology, unspecified trimester
O09.82 Supervision of pregnancy with history of in utero procedure during previous pregnancy
O09.821 Supervision of pregnancy with history of in utero procedure during previous pregnancy, first trimester
O09.822 Supervision of pregnancy with history of in utero procedure during previous pregnancy, second trimester
O09.823 Supervision of pregnancy with history of in utero procedure during previous pregnancy, third trimester
O09.829 Supervision of pregnancy with history of in utero procedure during previous pregnancy, unspecified trimester

EXCLUDES1 *supervision of pregnancy affected by in utero procedure during current pregnancy (O35.7)*

O09.89 Supervision of other high risk pregnancies
O09.891 Supervision of other high risk pregnancies, first trimester
O09.892 Supervision of other high risk pregnancies, second trimester
O09.893 Supervision of other high risk pregnancies, third trimester
O09.899 Supervision of other high risk pregnancies, unspecified trimester
O09.9 Supervision of high risk pregnancy, unspecified
O09.90 Supervision of high risk pregnancy, unspecified, unspecified trimester
O09.91 Supervision of high risk pregnancy, unspecified, first trimester
O09.92 Supervision of high risk pregnancy, unspecified, second trimester
O09.93 Supervision of high risk pregnancy, unspecified, third trimester

Edema, proteinuria and hypertensive disorders in pregnancy, childbirth and the puerperium (O10-O16)

O10 Pre-existing hypertension complicating pregnancy, childbirth and the puerperium

INCLUDES *pre-existing hypertension with pre-existing proteinuria complicating pregnancy, childbirth and the puerperium*

EXCLUDES2 *pre-existing hypertension with superimposed pre-eclampsia complicating pregnancy, childbirth and the puerperium (O11.-)*

O10.0 Pre-existing essential hypertension complicating pregnancy, childbirth and the puerperium

Any condition in I10 specified as a reason for obstetric care during pregnancy, childbirth or the puerperium

O10.01 Pre-existing essential hypertension complicating pregnancy,
O10.011 Pre-existing essential hypertension complicating pregnancy, first trimester
O10.012 Pre-existing essential hypertension complicating pregnancy, second trimester
O10.013 Pre-existing essential hypertension complicating pregnancy, third trimester
O10.019 Pre-existing essential hypertension complicating pregnancy, unspecified trimester
O10.02 Pre-existing essential hypertension complicating childbirth
O10.03 Pre-existing essential hypertension complicating the puerperium
O10.1 Pre-existing hypertensive heart disease complicating pregnancy, childbirth and the puerperium

Any condition in I11 specified as a reason for obstetric care during pregnancy, childbirth or the puerperium

Use additional code from I11 to identify the type of hypertensive heart disease

O10.11 Pre-existing hypertensive heart disease complicating pregnancy
O10.111 Pre-existing hypertensive heart disease complicating pregnancy, first trimester
O10.112 Pre-existing hypertensive heart disease complicating pregnancy, second trimester
O10.113 Pre-existing hypertensive heart disease complicating pregnancy, third trimester
O10.119 Pre-existing hypertensive heart disease complicating pregnancy, unspecified trimester
O10.12 Pre-existing hypertensive heart disease complicating childbirth
O10.13 Pre-existing hypertensive heart disease complicating the puerperium
O10.2 Pre-existing hypertensive chronic kidney disease complicating pregnancy, childbirth and the puerperium

Any condition in I12 specified as a reason for obstetric care during pregnancy, childbirth or the puerperium

Use additional code from I12 to identify the type of hypertensive chronic kidney disease

O10.21 Pre-existing hypertensive chronic kidney disease complicating pregnancy
O10.211 Pre-existing hypertensive chronic kidney disease complicating pregnancy, first trimester
O10.212 Pre-existing hypertensive chronic kidney disease complicating pregnancy, second trimester
O10.213 Pre-existing hypertensive chronic kidney disease complicating pregnancy, third trimester

1st 1st trimester 2nd 2nd trimester 3rd 3rd trimester PDx Unacceptable principal diagnosis symbol per Medicare code edits
POA Code exempt from diagnosis present on admission requirement ? Questionable admission CC Complication or comorbidity
CC/MCC Exc CC/MCC exclusion MCC Major complication or comorbidity PDx Principal diagnosis as its own CC
PDx Principal diagnosis as its own MCC Z1 Z code as first-listed diagnosis

O10.219 Pre-existing hypertensive chronic kidney disease complicating pregnancy, unspecified trimester

O10.22 Pre-existing hypertensive chronic kidney disease complicating childbirth

O10.23 Pre-existing hypertensive chronic kidney disease complicating the puerperium

O10.3 Pre-existing hypertensive heart and chronic kidney disease complicating pregnancy, childbirth and the puerperium
Any condition in I13 specified as a reason for obstetric care during pregnancy, childbirth or the puerperium
Use additional code from I13 to identify the type of hypertensive heart and chronic kidney disease

O10.31 Pre-existing hypertensive heart and chronic kidney disease complicating pregnancy

O10.311 Pre-existing hypertensive heart and chronic kidney disease complicating pregnancy, first trimester

O10.312 Pre-existing hypertensive heart and chronic kidney disease complicating pregnancy, second trimester

O10.313 Pre-existing hypertensive heart and chronic kidney disease complicating pregnancy, third trimester

O10.319 Pre-existing hypertensive heart and chronic kidney disease complicating pregnancy, unspecified trimester

O10.32 Pre-existing hypertensive heart and chronic kidney disease complicating childbirth

O10.33 Pre-existing hypertensive heart and chronic kidney disease complicating the puerperium

O10.4 Pre-existing secondary hypertension complicating pregnancy, childbirth and the puerperium
Any condition in I15 specified as a reason for obstetric care during pregnancy, childbirth or the puerperium
Use additional code from I15 to identify the type of secondary hypertension

O10.41 Pre-existing secondary hypertension complicating pregnancy

O10.411 Pre-existing secondary hypertension complicating pregnancy, first trimester

O10.412 Pre-existing secondary hypertension complicating pregnancy, second trimester

O10.413 Pre-existing secondary hypertension complicating pregnancy, third trimester

O10.419 Pre-existing secondary hypertension complicating pregnancy, unspecified trimester

O10.42 Pre-existing secondary hypertension complicating childbirth

O10.43 Pre-existing secondary hypertension complicating the puerperium

O10.9 Unspecified pre-existing hypertension complicating pregnancy, childbirth and the puerperium

O10.91 Unspecified pre-existing hypertension complicating pregnancy

O10.911 Unspecified pre-existing hypertension complicating pregnancy, first trimester

O10.912 Unspecified pre-existing hypertension complicating pregnancy, second trimester

O10.913 Unspecified pre-existing hypertension complicating pregnancy, third trimester

O10.919 Unspecified pre-existing hypertension complicating pregnancy, unspecified trimester

O10.92 Unspecified pre-existing hypertension complicating childbirth

O10.93 Unspecified pre-existing hypertension complicating the puerperium

O11 Pre-existing hypertension with pre-eclampsia
INCLUDES *conditions in O10 complicated by pre-eclampsia*
pre-eclampsia superimposed pre-existing hypertension
Use additional code from O10 to identify the type of hypertension

O11.1 Pre-existing hypertension with pre-eclampsia, first trimester

O11.2 Pre-existing hypertension with pre-eclampsia, second trimester

O11.3 Pre-existing hypertension with pre-eclampsia, third trimester

● O11.4 Pre-existing hypertension with pre-eclampsia, complicating childbirth

● O11.5 Pre-existing hypertension with pre-eclampsia, complicating the puerperium

O11.9 Pre-existing hypertension with pre-eclampsia, unspecified trimester

O12 Gestational [pregnancy-induced] edema and proteinuria without hypertension

O12.0 Gestational edema

O12.00 Gestational edema, unspecified trimester

O12.01 Gestational edema, first trimester

O12.02 Gestational edema, second trimester

O12.03 Gestational edema, third trimester

● O12.04 Gestational edema, complicating childbirth

● O12.05 Gestational edema, complicating the puerperium

O12.1 Gestational proteinuria

O12.10 Gestational proteinuria, unspecified trimester

O12.11 Gestational proteinuria, first trimester

O12.12 Gestational proteinuria, second trimester

O12.13 Gestational proteinuria, third trimester

● O12.14 Gestational proteinuria, complicating childbirth

● O12.15 Gestational proteinuria, complicating the puerperium

O12.2 Gestational edema with proteinuria

O12.20 Gestational edema with proteinuria, unspecified trimester

O12.21 Gestational edema with proteinuria, first trimester

O12.22 Gestational edema with proteinuria, second trimester

O12.23 Gestational edema with proteinuria, third trimester

● O12.24 Gestational edema with proteinuria, complicating childbirth

● O12.25 Gestational edema with proteinuria, complicating the puerperium

O13 Gestational [pregnancy-induced] hypertension without significant proteinuria
INCLUDES *gestational hypertension NOS*
transient hypertension of pregnancy

O13.1 Gestational [pregnancy-induced] hypertension without significant proteinuria, first trimester

O13.2 Gestational [pregnancy-induced] hypertension without significant proteinuria, second trimester

O13.3 Gestational [pregnancy-induced] hypertension without significant proteinuria, third trimester

● O13.4 Gestational [pregnancy-induced] hypertension without significant proteinuria, complicating childbirth

● O13.5 Gestational [pregnancy-induced] hypertension without significant proteinuria, complicating the puerperium

O13.9 Gestational [pregnancy-induced] hypertension without significant proteinuria, unspecified trimester

O14 Pre-eclampsia
EXCLUDES1 *pre-existing hypertension with pre-eclampsia (O11)*

O14.0 Mild to moderate pre-eclampsia

O14.00 Mild to moderate pre-eclampsia, unspecified trimester

O14.02 Mild to moderate pre-eclampsia, second trimester

O14.03 Mild to moderate pre-eclampsia, third trimester

Unspecified Code Other Specified Code Manifestation Code N Newborn P Pediatric M Maternity A Adult ♂ Male ♀ Female
● New Code ▲ Revised Code Title ►◄ Revised Text NOTES INCLUDES EXCLUDES1 Not coded here EXCLUDES2 Not included here
4th character required 5th character required 6th character required 7th character required
Extension 'X' Alert HAC Hospital-acquired condition (HAC) alert AHA AHA Coding Clinic©

- O14.04 Mild to moderate pre-eclampsia, complicating childbirth
- O14.05 Mild to moderate pre-eclampsia, complicating the puerperium

O14.1 Severe pre-eclampsia
EXCLUDES1 *HELLP syndrome (O14.2-)*
- O14.10 Severe pre-eclampsia, unspecified trimester
- O14.12 Severe pre-eclampsia, second trimester
- O14.13 Severe pre-eclampsia, third trimester
- O14.14 Severe pre-eclampsia complicating childbirth
- O14.15 Severe pre-eclampsia, complicating the puerperium

O14.2 HELLP syndrome
Severe pre-eclampsia with hemolysis, elevated liver enzymes and low platelet count (HELLP)
- O14.20 HELLP syndrome (HELLP), unspecified trimester
- O14.22 HELLP syndrome (HELLP), second trimester
- O14.23 HELLP syndrome (HELLP), third trimester
- O14.24 HELLP syndrome, complicating childbirth
- O14.25 HELLP syndrome, complicating the puerperium

O14.9 Unspecified pre-eclampsia
- O14.90 Unspecified pre-eclampsia, unspecifiedtrimester
- O14.92 Unspecified pre-eclampsia, second trimester
- O14.93 Unspecified pre-eclampsia, third trimester
- O14.94 Unspecified pre-eclampsia, complicating childbirth
- O14.95 Unspecified pre-eclampsia, complicating the puerperium

O15 Eclampsia
INCLUDES *convulsions following conditions in O10-O14 and O16*

▲ O15.0 Eclampsia ▶complicating◀ pregnancy
- ▲ O15.00 Eclampsia ▶complicating◀ pregnancy, unspecified trimester
- ▲ O15.02 Eclampsia ▶complicating◀ pregnancy, second trimester
- ▲ O15.03 Eclampsia ▶complicating◀ pregnancy, third trimester

▲ O15.1 Eclampsia ▶complicating◀ labor
▲ O15.2 Eclampsia ▶complicating◀ the puerperium
O15.9 Eclampsia, unspecified as to time period
Eclampsia NOS

O16 Unspecified maternal hypertension
- O16.1 Unspecified maternal hypertension, first trimester
- O16.2 Unspecified maternal hypertension, second trimester
- O16.3 Unspecified maternal hypertension, third trimester
- O16.4 Unspecified maternal hypertension, complicating childbirth
- O16.5 Unspecified maternal hypertension, complicating the puerperium
- O16.9 Unspecified maternal hypertension, unspecified trimester

Other maternal disorders predominantly related to pregnancy (O20-O29)

EXCLUDES2 *maternal care related to the fetus and amniotic cavity and possible delivery problems (O30-O48)*
maternal diseases classifiable elsewhere but complicating pregnancy, labor and delivery, and the puerperium (O98-O99)

O20 Hemorrhage in early pregnancy
INCLUDES *hemorrhage before completion of 20 weeks gestation*
EXCLUDES1 *pregnancy with abortive outcome (O00-O08)*
- O20.0 Threatened abortion
  Hemorrhage specified as due to threatened abortion
- O20.8 Other hemorrhage in early pregnancy
- O20.9 Hemorrhage in early pregnancy, unspecified

O21 Excessive vomiting in pregnancy
- O21.0 Mild hyperemesis gravidarum
  Hyperemesis gravidarum, mild or unspecified, starting before the end of the 20th week of gestation
- O21.1 Hyperemesis gravidarum with metabolic disturbance
  Hyperemesis gravidarum, starting before the end of the 20th week of gestation, with metabolic disturbance such as carbohydrate depletion
  Hyperemesis gravidarum, starting before the end of the 20th week of gestation, with metabolic disturbance such as dehydration
  Hyperemesis gravidarum, starting before the end of the 20th week of gestation, with metabolic disturbance such as electrolyte imbalance
- O21.2 Late vomiting of pregnancy
  Excessive vomiting starting after 20 completed weeks of gestation
- O21.8 Other vomiting complicating pregnancy
  Vomiting due to diseases classified elsewhere, complicating pregnancy
  Use additional code, to identify cause.
- O21.9 Vomiting of pregnancy, unspecified

O22 Venous complications and hemorrhoids in pregnancy
EXCLUDES1 *venous complications of:*
abortion NOS (O03.9)
ectopic or molar pregnancy (O08.7)
failed attempted abortion (O07.35)
induced abortion (O04.85)
spontaneous abortion (O03.89)
EXCLUDES2 *obstetric pulmonary embolism (O88.-)*
venous complications and hemorrhoids of childbirth and the puerperium (O87.-)

O22.0 Varicose veins of lower extremity in pregnancy
Varicose veins NOS in pregnancy
- O22.00 Varicose veins of lower extremity in pregnancy, unspecified trimester
- O22.01 Varicose veins of lower extremity in pregnancy, first trimester
- O22.02 Varicose veins of lower extremity in pregnancy, second trimester
- O22.03 Varicose veins of lower extremity in pregnancy, third trimester

O22.1 Genital varices in pregnancy
Perineal varices in pregnancy
Vaginal varices in pregnancy
Vulval varices in pregnancy
- O22.10 Genital varices in pregnancy, unspecifiedtrimester
- O22.11 Genital varices in pregnancy, first trimester
- O22.12 Genital varices in pregnancy, second trimester
- O22.13 Genital varices in pregnancy, third trimester

O22.2 Superficial thrombophlebitis in pregnancy
Phlebitis in pregnancy NOS
Thrombophlebitis of legs in pregnancy
Thrombosis in pregnancy NOS
Use additional code to identify the superficial thrombophlebitis (I80.0-)
- O22.20 Superficial thrombophlebitis in pregnancy, unspecified trimester
- O22.21 Superficial thrombophlebitis in pregnancy, first trimester
- O22.22 Superficial thrombophlebitis in pregnancy, second trimester
- O22.23 Superficial thrombophlebitis in pregnancy, third trimester

O22.3 Deep phlebothrombosis in pregnancy
Deep vein thrombosis, antepartum
Use additional code to identify the deep vein thrombosis (I82.4-, I82.5-, I82.62-. I82.72-)
Use additional code, if applicable, for associated long-term (current) use of anticoagulants (Z79.01)
- O22.30 Deep phlebothrombosis in pregnancy, unspecified trimester
- O22.31 Deep phlebothrombosis in pregnancy, first trimester
- O22.32 Deep phlebothrombosis in pregnancy, second trimester

1st 1st trimester 2nd 2nd trimester 3rd 3rd trimester Unacceptable principal diagnosis symbol per Medicare code edits
Code exempt from diagnosis present on admission requirement ? Questionable admission CC Complication or comorbidity
CC/MCC Exc CC/MCC exclusion MCC Major complication or comorbidity Principal diagnosis as its own CC
Principal diagnosis as its own MCC Z code as first-listed diagnosis

O22.33 Deep phlebothrombosis in pregnancy, third trimester
O22.4 Hemorrhoids in pregnancy
O22.40 Hemorrhoids in pregnancy, unspecified trimester
O22.41 Hemorrhoids in pregnancy, first trimester
O22.42 Hemorrhoids in pregnancy, second trimester
O22.43 Hemorrhoids in pregnancy, third trimester
O22.5 Cerebral venous thrombosis in pregnancy
Cerebrovenous sinus thrombosis in pregnancy
O22.50 Cerebral venous thrombosis in pregnancy, unspecified trimester
O22.51 Cerebral venous thrombosis in pregnancy, first trimester
O22.52 Cerebral venous thrombosis in pregnancy, second trimester
O22.53 Cerebral venous thrombosis in pregnancy, third trimester
O22.8 Other venous complications in pregnancy
O22.8X Other venous complications in pregnancy
O22.8X1 Other venous complications in pregnancy, first trimester
O22.8X2 Other venous complications in pregnancy, second trimester
O22.8X3 Other venous complications in pregnancy, third trimester
O22.8X9 Other venous complications in pregnancy, unspecified trimester
O22.9 Venous complication in pregnancy, unspecified
Gestational phlebitis NOS
Gestational phlebopathy NOS
Gestational thrombosis NOS
O22.90 Venous complication in pregnancy, unspecified, unspecified trimester
O22.91 Venous complication in pregnancy, unspecified, first trimester
O22.92 Venous complication in pregnancy, unspecified, second trimester
O22.93 Venous complication in pregnancy, unspecified, third trimester

O23 Infections of genitourinary tract in pregnancy
Use additional code to identify organism (B95.-, B96.-)
EXCLUDES2 *gonococcal infections complicating pregnancy, childbirth and the puerperium (O98.2)*
infections with a predominantly sexual mode of transmission NOS complicating pregnancy, childbirth and the puerperium (O98.3)
syphilis complicating pregnancy, childbirth and the puerperium (O98.1)
tuberculosis of genitourinary system complicating pregnancy, childbirth and the puerperium (O98.0)
venereal disease NOS complicating pregnancy, childbirth and the puerperium (O98.3)
O23.0 Infections of kidney in pregnancy
Pyelonephritis in pregnancy
O23.00 Infections of kidney in pregnancy, unspecified trimester
O23.01 Infections of kidney in pregnancy, first trimester
O23.02 Infections of kidney in pregnancy, second trimester
O23.03 Infections of kidney in pregnancy, third trimester
O23.1 Infections of bladder in pregnancy
O23.10 Infections of bladder in pregnancy, unspecified trimester
O23.11 Infections of bladder in pregnancy, first trimester
O23.12 Infections of bladder in pregnancy, second trimester
O23.13 Infections of bladder in pregnancy, third trimester
O23.2 Infections of urethra in pregnancy
O23.20 Infections of urethra in pregnancy, unspecified trimester
O23.21 Infections of urethra in pregnancy, first trimester
O23.22 Infections of urethra in pregnancy, second trimester
O23.23 Infections of urethra in pregnancy, third trimester
O23.3 Infections of other parts of urinary tract in pregnancy
O23.30 Infections of other parts of urinary tract in pregnancy, unspecified trimester
O23.31 Infections of other parts of urinary tract in pregnancy, first trimester
O23.32 Infections of other parts of urinary tract in pregnancy, second trimester
O23.33 Infections of other parts of urinary tract in pregnancy, third trimester
O23.4 Unspecified infection of urinary tract in pregnancy
O23.40 Unspecified infection of urinary tract in pregnancy, unspecified trimester
O23.41 Unspecified infection of urinary tract in pregnancy, first trimester
O23.42 Unspecified infection of urinary tract in pregnancy, second trimester
O23.43 Unspecified infection of urinary tract in pregnancy, third trimester
O23.5 Infections of the genital tract in pregnancy
O23.51 Infection of cervix in pregnancy
O23.511 Infections of cervix in pregnancy, first trimester
O23.512 Infections of cervix in pregnancy, second trimester
O23.513 Infections of cervix in pregnancy, third trimester
O23.519 Infections of cervix in pregnancy, unspecified trimester
O23.52 Salpingo-oophoritis in pregnancy
Oophoritis in pregnancy
Salpingitis in pregnancy
O23.521 Salpingo-oophoritis in pregnancy, first trimester
O23.522 Salpingo-oophoritis in pregnancy, second trimester
O23.523 Salpingo-oophoritis in pregnancy, third trimester
O23.529 Salpingo-oophoritis in pregnancy, unspecified trimester
O23.59 Infection of other part of genital tract in pregnancy
O23.591 Infection of other part of genital tract in pregnancy, first trimester
O23.592 Infection of other part of genital tract in pregnancy, second trimester
O23.593 Infection of other part of genital tract in pregnancy, third trimester
O23.599 Infection of other part of genital tract in pregnancy, unspecified trimester
O23.9 Unspecified genitourinary tract infection in pregnancy
Genitourinary tract infection in pregnancy NOS
O23.90 Unspecified genitourinary tract infection in pregnancy, unspecified trimester
O23.91 Unspecified genitourinary tract infection in pregnancy, first trimester
O23.92 Unspecified genitourinary tract infection in pregnancy, second trimester
O23.93 Unspecified genitourinary tract infection in pregnancy, third trimester

O24 Diabetes mellitus in pregnancy, childbirth, and the puerperium
▲ O24.0 Pre-existing ▶type 1 diabetes mellitus◀, in pregnancy, childbirth and the puerperium
Juvenile onset diabetes mellitus, in pregnancy, childbirth and the puerperium
Ketosis-prone diabetes mellitus in pregnancy, childbirth and the puerperium
Use additional code from category E10 to further identify any manifestations

Unspecified Code | Other Specified Code | Manifestation Code | N Newborn | P Pediatric | M Maternity | A Adult | ♂ Male | ♀ Female
● New Code | ▲ Revised Code Title | ▶◀ Revised Text | NOTES | INCLUDES | EXCLUDES1 Not coded here | EXCLUDES2 Not included here
4th character required | 5th character required | 6th character required | 7th character required
Extension 'X' Alert | HAC Hospital-acquired condition (HAC) alert | AHA AHA Coding Clinic©

O22.33 - O24.0
CHAPTER 15: PREGNANCY, CHILDBIRTH AND THE PUERPERIUM (O00-O9A)

▲ O24.01 Pre-existing ▶type 1 diabetes mellitus◀, in pregnancy
- ▲ O24.011 Pre-existing ▶type 1 diabetes mellitus◀, in pregnancy, first trimester
- ▲ O24.012 Pre-existing ▶type 1 diabetes mellitus◀, in pregnancy, second trimester
- ▲ O24.013 Pre-existing ▶type 1 diabetes mellitus◀, in pregnancy, third trimester
- ▲ O24.019 Pre-existing ▶type 1 diabetes mellitus◀, in pregnancy, unspecified trimester

▲ O24.02 Pre-existing ▶type 1 diabetes mellitus◀, in childbirth

▲ O24.03 Pre-existing ▶type 1 diabetes mellitus◀, in the puerperium

▲ O24.1 Pre-existing ▶type 2 diabetes mellitus◀, in pregnancy, childbirth and the puerperium

Insulin-resistant diabetes mellitus in pregnancy, childbirth and the puerperium

Use additional code (for):

from category E11 to further identify any manifestations

long-term (current) use of insulin (Z79.4)

▲ O24.11 Pre-existing ▶type 2 diabetes mellitus◀, in pregnancy
- ▲ O24.111 Pre-existing ▶type 2 diabetes mellitus◀, in pregnancy, first trimester
- ▲ O24.112 Pre-existing ▶type 2 diabetes mellitus◀, in pregnancy, second trimester
- ▲ O24.113 Pre-existing ▶type 2 diabetes mellitus◀, in pregnancy, third trimester
- ▲ O24.119 Pre-existing ▶type 2 diabetes mellitus◀, in pregnancy, unspecified trimester

▲ O24.12 Pre-existing ▶type 2 diabetes mellitus◀, in childbirth

▲ O24.13 Pre-existing ▶type 2 diabetes mellitus◀, in the puerperium

O24.3 Unspecified pre-existing diabetes mellitus in pregnancy, childbirth and the puerperium

Use additional code (for):

from category E11 to further identify any manifestation

long-term (current) use of insulin (Z79.4)

O24.31 Unspecified pre-existing diabetes mellitus in pregnancy
- O24.311 Unspecified pre-existing diabetes mellitus in pregnancy, first trimester
- O24.312 Unspecified pre-existing diabetes mellitus in pregnancy, second trimester
- O24.313 Unspecified pre-existing diabetes mellitus in pregnancy, third trimester
- O24.319 Unspecified pre-existing diabetes mellitus in pregnancy, unspecifiedtrimester

O24.32 Unspecified pre-existing diabetes mellitus in childbirth

O24.33 Unspecified pre-existing diabetes mellitus in the puerperium

O24.4 Gestational diabetes mellitus

Diabetes mellitus arising in pregnancy

Gestational diabetes mellitus NOS

O24.41 Gestational diabetes mellitus in pregnancy
- O24.410 Gestational diabetes mellitus in pregnancy, diet controlled
- O24.414 Gestational diabetes mellitus in pregnancy, insulin controlled
- ● O24.415 Gestational diabetes mellitus in pregnancy, controlled by oral hypoglycemic drugs
  Gestational diabetes mellitus in pregnancy, controlled by oral antidiabetic drugs
- O24.419 Gestational diabetes mellitus in pregnancy, unspecified control
  AHA: Q4, 2015

O24.42 Gestational diabetes mellitus in childbirth
- O24.420 Gestational diabetes mellitus in childbirth, diet controlled
- O24.424 Gestational diabetes mellitus in childbirth, insulin controlled
- ● O24.425 Gestational diabetes mellitus in childbirth, controlled by oral hypoglycemic drugs
  Gestational diabetes mellitus in childbirth, controlled by oral antidiabetic drugs
- O24.429 Gestational diabetes mellitus in childbirth, unspecified control

O24.43 Gestational diabetes mellitus in the puerperium
- O24.430 Gestational diabetes mellitus in the puerperium, diet controlled
- O24.434 Gestational diabetes mellitus in the puerperium, insulin controlled
- ● O24.435 Gestational diabetes mellitus in puerperium, controlled by oral hypoglycemic drugs
  Gestational diabetes mellitus in puerperium, controlled by oral antidiabetic drugs
- O24.439 Gestational diabetes mellitus in the puerperium, unspecified control

O24.8 Other pre-existing diabetes mellitus in pregnancy, childbirth, and the puerperium

Use additional code (for):

from categories E08, E09 and E13 to further identify any manifestation

long-term (current) use of insulin (Z79.4)

O24.81 Other pre-existing diabetes mellitus in pregnancy
- O24.811 Other pre-existing diabetes mellitus in pregnancy, first trimester
- O24.812 Other pre-existing diabetes mellitus in pregnancy, second trimester
- O24.813 Other pre-existing diabetes mellitus in pregnancy, third trimester
- O24.819 Other pre-existing diabetes mellitus in pregnancy, unspecified trimester

O24.82 Other pre-existing diabetes mellitus in childbirth

O24.83 Other pre-existing diabetes mellitus in the puerperium

O24.9 Unspecified diabetes mellitus in pregnancy, childbirth and the puerperium

Use additional code for long-term (current) use of insulin (Z79.4)

O24.91 Unspecified diabetes mellitus in pregnancy
- O24.911 Unspecified diabetes mellitus in pregnancy, first trimester
- O24.912 Unspecified diabetes mellitus in pregnancy, second trimester
- O24.913 Unspecified diabetes mellitus in pregnancy, third trimester
- O24.919 Unspecified diabetes mellitus in pregnancy, unspecified trimester

O24.92 Unspecified diabetes mellitus in childbirth

O24.93 Unspecified diabetes mellitus in the puerperium

O25 Malnutrition in pregnancy, childbirth and the puerperium

O25.1 Malnutrition in pregnancy
- O25.10 Malnutrition in pregnancy, unspecifiedtrimester
- O25.11 Malnutrition in pregnancy, first trimester
- O25.12 Malnutrition in pregnancy, second trimester
- O25.13 Malnutrition in pregnancy, third trimester

O25.2 Malnutrition in childbirth

O25.3 Malnutrition in the puerperium

O26 Maternal care for other conditions predominantly related to pregnancy

O26.0 Excessive weight gain in pregnancy

EXCLUDES2 *gestational edema (O12.0, O12.2)*
- O26.00 Excessive weight gain in pregnancy, unspecified trimester
- O26.01 Excessive weight gain in pregnancy, first trimester
- O26.02 Excessive weight gain in pregnancy, second trimester
- O26.03 Excessive weight gain in pregnancy, third trimester

1st 1st trimester 2nd 2nd trimester 3rd 3rd trimester Unacceptable principal diagnosis symbol per Medicare code edits
Code exempt from diagnosis present on admission requirement Questionable admission Complication or comorbidity
CC/MCC exclusion Major complication or comorbidity Principal diagnosis as its own CC
Principal diagnosis as its own MCC Z code as first-listed diagnosis

O26.1 Low weight gain in pregnancy
- O26.10 Low weight gain in pregnancy, unspecified trimester
- O26.11 Low weight gain in pregnancy, first trimester
- O26.12 Low weight gain in pregnancy, second trimester
- O26.13 Low weight gain in pregnancy, third trimester

O26.2 Pregnancy care for patient with recurrent pregnancy loss
- O26.20 Pregnancy care for patient with recurrent pregnancy loss, unspecified trimester
- O26.21 Pregnancy care for patient with recurrent pregnancy loss, first trimester
- O26.22 Pregnancy care for patient with recurrent pregnancy loss, second trimester
- O26.23 Pregnancy care for patient with recurrent pregnancy loss, third trimester

O26.3 Retained intrauterine contraceptive device in pregnancy
- O26.30 Retained intrauterine contraceptive device in pregnancy, unspecified trimester
- O26.31 Retained intrauterine contraceptive device in pregnancy, first trimester
- O26.32 Retained intrauterine contraceptive device in pregnancy, second trimester
- O26.33 Retained intrauterine contraceptive device in pregnancy, third trimester

O26.4 Herpes gestationis
- O26.40 Herpes gestationis, unspecified trimester
- O26.41 Herpes gestationis, first trimester
- O26.42 Herpes gestationis, second trimester
- O26.43 Herpes gestationis, third trimester

O26.5 Maternal hypotension syndrome

Supine hypotensive syndrome
- O26.50 Maternal hypotension syndrome, unspecified trimester
- O26.51 Maternal hypotension syndrome, first trimester
- O26.52 Maternal hypotension syndrome, second trimester
- O26.53 Maternal hypotension syndrome, third trimester

O26.6 Liver and biliary tract disorders in pregnancy, childbirth and the puerperium

Use additional code to identify the specific disorder

EXCLUDES2 *hepatorenal syndrome following labor and delivery (O90.4)*

- O26.61 Liver and biliary tract disorders in pregnancy
  - O26.611 Liver and biliary tract disorders in pregnancy, first trimester
  - O26.612 Liver and biliary tract disorders in pregnancy, second trimester
  - O26.613 Liver and biliary tract disorders in pregnancy, third trimester
  - O26.619 Liver and biliary tract disorders in pregnancy, unspecified trimester
- O26.62 Liver and biliary tract disorders in childbirth
- O26.63 Liver and biliary tract disorders in the puerperium

O26.7 Subluxation of symphysis (pubis) in pregnancy, childbirth and the puerperium

EXCLUDES1 *traumatic separation of symphysis (pubis) during childbirth (O71.6)*

- O26.71 Subluxation of symphysis (pubis) in pregnancy
  - O26.711 Subluxation of symphysis (pubis) in pregnancy, first trimester
  - O26.712 Subluxation of symphysis (pubis) in pregnancy, second trimester
  - O26.713 Subluxation of symphysis (pubis) in pregnancy, third trimester
  - O26.719 Subluxation of symphysis (pubis) in pregnancy, unspecified trimester
- O26.72 Subluxation of symphysis (pubis) in childbirth
- O26.73 Subluxation of symphysis (pubis) in the puerperium

O26.8 Other specified pregnancy related conditions

- O26.81 Pregnancy related exhaustion and fatigue
  - O26.811 Pregnancy related exhaustion and fatigue, first trimester
  - O26.812 Pregnancy related exhaustion and fatigue, second trimester
  - O26.813 Pregnancy related exhaustion and fatigue, third trimester
  - O26.819 Pregnancy related exhaustion and fatigue, unspecified trimester
- O26.82 Pregnancy related peripheral neuritis
  - O26.821 Pregnancy related peripheral neuritis, first trimester
  - O26.822 Pregnancy related peripheral neuritis, second trimester
  - O26.823 Pregnancy related peripheral neuritis, third trimester
  - O26.829 Pregnancy related peripheral neuritis, unspecified trimester
- O26.83 Pregnancy related renal disease

  Use additional code to identify the specific disorder
  - O26.831 Pregnancy related renal disease, first trimester
  - O26.832 Pregnancy related renal disease, second trimester
  - O26.833 Pregnancy related renal disease, third trimester
  - O26.839 Pregnancy related renal disease, unspecified trimester
- O26.84 Uterine size-date discrepancy complicating pregnancy

  EXCLUDES1 *encounter for suspected problem with fetal growth ruled out (Z03.74)*
  - O26.841 Uterine size-date discrepancy, first trimester
  - O26.842 Uterine size-date discrepancy, second trimester
  - O26.843 Uterine size-date discrepancy, third trimester
  - O26.849 Uterine size-date discrepancy, unspecified trimester
- O26.85 Spotting complicating pregnancy
  - O26.851 Spotting complicating pregnancy, first trimester
  - O26.852 Spotting complicating pregnancy, second trimester
  - O26.853 Spotting complicating pregnancy, third trimester
  - O26.859 Spotting complicating pregnancy, unspecified trimester
- O26.86 Pruritic urticarial papules and plaques of pregnancy (PUPPP)

  Polymorphic eruption of pregnancy
- O26.87 Cervical shortening

  EXCLUDES1 *encounter for suspected cervical shortening ruled out (Z03.75)*
  - O26.872 Cervical shortening, second trimester
  - O26.873 Cervical shortening, third trimester
  - O26.879 Cervical shortening, unspecified trimester
- O26.89 Other specified pregnancy related conditions
  - O26.891 Other specified pregnancy related conditions, first trimester
  - O26.892 Other specified pregnancy related conditions, second trimester
  - O26.893 Other specified pregnancy related conditions, third trimester

    AHA: Q3, 2015
  - O26.899 Other specified pregnancy related conditions, unspecified trimester

O26.9 Pregnancy related conditions, unspecified
- O26.90 Pregnancy related conditions, unspecified, unspecified trimester

Unspecified Code | Other Specified Code | Manifestation Code | N Newborn | P Pediatric | M Maternity | A Adult | ♂ Male | ♀ Female
● New Code | ▲ Revised Code Title | ►◄ Revised Text | NOTES | INCLUDES | EXCLUDES1 Not coded here | EXCLUDES2 Not included here
4th character required | 5th character required | 6th character required | 7th character required
Extension 'X' Alert | HAC Hospital-acquired condition (HAC) alert | AHA AHA Coding Clinic©

O26.91 Pregnancy related conditions, unspecified, first trimester 1st M ♀
O26.92 Pregnancy related conditions, unspecified, second trimester 2nd M ♀
O26.93 Pregnancy related conditions, unspecified, third trimester 3rd M ♀

4th O28 Abnormal findings on antenatal screening of mother
EXCLUDES1 *diagnostic findings classified elsewhere - see Alphabetical Index*
O28.0 Abnormal hematological finding on antenatal screening of mother M ♀
O28.1 Abnormal biochemical finding on antenatal screening of mother M ♀
O28.2 Abnormal cytological finding on antenatal screening of mother M ♀
O28.3 Abnormal ultrasonic finding on antenatal screening of mother M ♀
O28.4 Abnormal radiological finding on antenatal screening of mother M ♀
O28.5 Abnormal chromosomal and genetic finding on antenatal screening of mother M ♀
O28.8 Other abnormal findings on antenatal screening of mother M ♀
O28.9 Unspecified abnormal findings on antenatal screening of mother M ♀

4th O29 Complications of anesthesia during pregnancy
INCLUDES *maternal complications arising from the administration of a general, regional or local anesthetic, analgesic or other sedation during pregnancy*
Use additional code, if necessary, to identify the complication
EXCLUDES2 *complications of anesthesia during labor and delivery (O74.-)*
complications of anesthesia during the puerperium (O89.-)

5th O29.0 Pulmonary complications of anesthesia during pregnancy
6th O29.01 Aspiration pneumonitis due to anesthesia during pregnancy
Inhalation of stomach contents or secretions NOS due to anesthesia during pregnancy
Mendelson's syndrome due to anesthesia during pregnancy
O29.011 Aspiration pneumonitis due to anesthesia during pregnancy, first trimester 1st M ♀
O29.012 Aspiration pneumonitis due to anesthesia during pregnancy, second trimester 2nd M ♀
O29.013 Aspiration pneumonitis due to anesthesia during pregnancy, third trimester 3rd M ♀
O29.019 Aspiration pneumonitis due to anesthesia during pregnancy, unspecified trimester M ♀
6th O29.02 Pressure collapse of lung due to anesthesia during pregnancy
O29.021 Pressure collapse of lung due to anesthesia during pregnancy, first trimester 1st M ♀
O29.022 Pressure collapse of lung due to anesthesia during pregnancy, second trimester 2nd M ♀
O29.023 Pressure collapse of lung due to anesthesia during pregnancy, third trimester 3rd M ♀
O29.029 Pressure collapse of lung due to anesthesia during pregnancy, unspecified trimester M ♀
6th O29.09 Other pulmonary complications of anesthesia during pregnancy
O29.091 Other pulmonary complications of anesthesia during pregnancy, first trimester 1st M ♀
O29.092 Other pulmonary complications of anesthesia during pregnancy, second trimester 2nd M ♀
O29.093 Other pulmonary complications of anesthesia during pregnancy, third trimester 3rd M ♀
O29.099 Other pulmonary complications of anesthesia during pregnancy, unspecified trimester M ♀

5th O29.1 Cardiac complications of anesthesia during pregnancy
6th O29.11 Cardiac arrest due to anesthesia during pregnancy
O29.111 Cardiac arrest due to anesthesia during pregnancy, first trimester 1st M ♀
O29.112 Cardiac arrest due to anesthesia during pregnancy, second trimester 2nd M ♀
O29.113 Cardiac arrest due to anesthesia during pregnancy, third trimester 3rd M ♀
O29.119 Cardiac arrest due to anesthesia during pregnancy, unspecified trimester M ♀
6th O29.12 Cardiac failure due to anesthesia during pregnancy
O29.121 Cardiac failure due to anesthesia during pregnancy, first trimester 1st M ♀
O29.122 Cardiac failure due to anesthesia during pregnancy, second trimester 2nd M ♀
O29.123 Cardiac failure due to anesthesia during pregnancy, third trimester 3rd M ♀
O29.129 Cardiac failure due to anesthesia during pregnancy, unspecified trimester M ♀
6th O29.19 Other cardiac complications of anesthesia during pregnancy
O29.191 Other cardiac complications of anesthesia during pregnancy, first trimester 1st M ♀
O29.192 Other cardiac complications of anesthesia during pregnancy, second trimester 2nd M ♀
O29.193 Other cardiac complications of anesthesia during pregnancy, third trimester 3rd M ♀
O29.199 Other cardiac complications of anesthesia during pregnancy, unspecified trimester M ♀

5th O29.2 Central nervous system complications of anesthesia during pregnancy
6th O29.21 Cerebral anoxia due to anesthesia during pregnancy
O29.211 Cerebral anoxia due to anesthesia during pregnancy, first trimester 1st M ♀
O29.212 Cerebral anoxia due to anesthesia during pregnancy, second trimester 2nd M ♀
O29.213 Cerebral anoxia due to anesthesia during pregnancy, third trimester 3rd M ♀
O29.219 Cerebral anoxia due to anesthesia during pregnancy, unspecified trimester M ♀
6th O29.29 Other central nervous system complications of anesthesia during pregnancy
O29.291 Other central nervous system complications of anesthesia during pregnancy, first trimester 1st M ♀
O29.292 Other central nervous system complications of anesthesia during pregnancy, second trimester 2nd M ♀
O29.293 Other central nervous system complications of anesthesia during pregnancy, third trimester 3rd M ♀
O29.299 Other central nervous system complications of anesthesia during pregnancy, unspecified trimester M ♀

5th O29.3 Toxic reaction to local anesthesia during pregnancy
6th O29.3X Toxic reaction to local anesthesia during pregnancy
O29.3X1 Toxic reaction to local anesthesia during pregnancy, first trimester 1st M ♀
O29.3X2 Toxic reaction to local anesthesia during pregnancy, second trimester 2nd M ♀
O29.3X3 Toxic reaction to local anesthesia during pregnancy, third trimester 3rd M ♀
O29.3X9 Toxic reaction to local anesthesia during pregnancy, unspecified trimester M ♀

5th O29.4 Spinal and epidural anesthesia induced headache during pregnancy
O29.40 Spinal and epidural anesthesia induced headache during pregnancy, unspecified trimester M ♀
O29.41 Spinal and epidural anesthesia induced headache during pregnancy, first trimester 1st M ♀
O29.42 Spinal and epidural anesthesia induced headache during pregnancy, second trimester 2nd M ♀

1st 1st trimester 2nd 2nd trimester 3rd 3rd trimester PDx Unacceptable principal diagnosis symbol per Medicare code edits
POA Code exempt from diagnosis present on admission requirement ? Questionable admission CC Complication or comorbidity
CC/MCC Exc CC/MCC exclusion MCC Major complication or comorbidity PDx CC Principal diagnosis as its own CC
PDx MCC Principal diagnosis as its own MCC Z1 Z code as first-listed diagnosis

O29.43 Spinal and epidural anesthesia induced headache during pregnancy, third trimester

O29.5 Other complications of spinal and epidural anesthesia during pregnancy

O29.5X Other complications of spinal and epidural anesthesia during pregnancy

O29.5X1 Other complications of spinal and epidural anesthesia during pregnancy, first trimester

O29.5X2 Other complications of spinal and epidural anesthesia during pregnancy, second trimester

O29.5X3 Other complications of spinal and epidural anesthesia during pregnancy, third trimester

O29.5X9 Other complications of spinal and epidural anesthesia during pregnancy, unspecified trimester

O29.6 Failed or difficult intubation for anesthesia during pregnancy

O29.60 Failed or difficult intubation for anesthesia during pregnancy, unspecified trimester

O29.61 Failed or difficult intubation for anesthesia during pregnancy, first trimester

O29.62 Failed or difficult intubation for anesthesia during pregnancy, second trimester

O29.63 Failed or difficult intubation for anesthesia during pregnancy, third trimester

O29.8 Other complications of anesthesia during pregnancy

O29.8X Other complications of anesthesia during pregnancy

O29.8X1 Other complications of anesthesia during pregnancy, first trimester

O29.8X2 Other complications of anesthesia during pregnancy, second trimester

O29.8X3 Other complications of anesthesia during pregnancy, third trimester

O29.8X9 Other complications of anesthesia during pregnancy, unspecified trimester

O29.9 Unspecified complication of anesthesia during pregnancy

O29.90 Unspecified complication of anesthesia during pregnancy, unspecified trimester

O29.91 Unspecified complication of anesthesia during pregnancy, first trimester

O29.92 Unspecified complication of anesthesia during pregnancy, second trimester

O29.93 Unspecified complication of anesthesia during pregnancy, third trimester

Maternal care related to the fetus and amniotic cavity and possible delivery problems (O30-O48)

O30 Multiple gestation

Code also any complications specific to multiple gestation

O30.0 Twin pregnancy

O30.00 Twin pregnancy, unspecified number of placenta and unspecified number of amniotic sacs

O30.001 Twin pregnancy, unspecified number of placenta and unspecified number of amniotic sacs, first trimester

O30.002 Twin pregnancy, unspecified number of placenta and unspecified number of amniotic sacs, second trimester

O30.003 Twin pregnancy, unspecified number of placenta and unspecified number of amniotic sacs, third trimester

O30.009 Twin pregnancy, unspecified number of placenta and unspecified number of amniotic sacs, unspecified trimester

O30.01 Twin pregnancy, monochorionic/monoamniotic

Twin pregnancy, one placenta, one amniotic sac

EXCLUDES1 *conjoined twins (O30.02-)*

O30.011 Twin pregnancy, monochorionic/monoamniotic, first trimester

O30.012 Twin pregnancy, monochorionic/monoamniotic, second trimester

O30.013 Twin pregnancy, monochorionic/monoamniotic, third trimester

O30.019 Twin pregnancy, monochorionic/monoamniotic, unspecified trimester

O30.02 Conjoined twin pregnancy

O30.021 Conjoined twin pregnancy, first trimester

O30.022 Conjoined twin pregnancy, second trimester

O30.023 Conjoined twin pregnancy, third trimester

O30.029 Conjoined twin pregnancy, unspecified trimester

O30.03 Twin pregnancy, monochorionic/diamniotic

Twin pregnancy, one placenta, two amniotic sacs

O30.031 Twin pregnancy, monochorionic/diamniotic, first trimester

O30.032 Twin pregnancy, monochorionic/diamniotic, second trimester

O30.033 Twin pregnancy, monochorionic/diamniotic, third trimester

O30.039 Twin pregnancy, monochorionic/diamniotic, unspecified trimester

O30.04 Twin pregnancy, dichorionic/diamniotic

Twin pregnancy, two placentae, two amniotic sacs

O30.041 Twin pregnancy, dichorionic/diamniotic, first trimester

O30.042 Twin pregnancy, dichorionic/diamniotic, second trimester

O30.043 Twin pregnancy, dichorionic/diamniotic, third trimester

O30.049 Twin pregnancy, dichorionic/diamniotic, unspecified trimester

O30.09 Twin pregnancy, unable to determine number of placenta and number of amniotic sacs

O30.091 Twin pregnancy, unable to determine number of placenta and number of amniotic sacs, first trimester

O30.092 Twin pregnancy, unable to determine number of placenta and number of amniotic sacs, second trimester

O30.093 Twin pregnancy, unable to determine number of placenta and number of amniotic sacs, third trimester

O30.099 Twin pregnancy, unable to determine number of placenta and number of amniotic sacs, unspecified trimester

O30.1 Triplet pregnancy

O30.10 Triplet pregnancy, unspecified number of placenta and unspecified number of amniotic sacs

O30.101 Triplet pregnancy, unspecified number of placenta and unspecified number of amniotic sacs, first trimester

O30.102 Triplet pregnancy, unspecified number of placenta and unspecified number of amniotic sacs, second trimester

O30.103 Triplet pregnancy, unspecified number of placenta and unspecified number of amniotic sacs, third trimester

AHA: Q2, 2016

O30.109 Triplet pregnancy, unspecified number of placenta and unspecified number of amniotic sacs, unspecified trimester

O30.11 Triplet pregnancy with two or more monochorionic fetuses

O30.111 Triplet pregnancy with two or more monochorionic fetuses, first trimester

Unspecified Code Other Specified Code Manifestation Code N Newborn P Pediatric M Maternity A Adult ♂ Male ♀ Female
● New Code ▲ Revised Code Title ►◄ Revised Text NOTES INCLUDES EXCLUDES1 Not coded here EXCLUDES2 Not included here
4th character required 5th character required 6th character required 7th character required
Extension 'X' Alert HAC Hospital-acquired condition (HAC) alert AHA AHA Coding Clinic©

O30.112 Triplet pregnancy with two or more monochorionic fetuses, second trimester 2nd M CC ♀ PDx

O30.113 Triplet pregnancy with two or more monochorionic fetuses, third trimester 3rd M CC ♀ PDx

O30.119 Triplet pregnancy with two or more monochorionic fetuses, unspecified trimester M ♀ PDx

6th O30.12 Triplet pregnancy with two or more monoamniotic fetuses

O30.121 Triplet pregnancy with two or more monoamniotic fetuses, first trimester 1st M CC ♀ PDx

O30.122 Triplet pregnancy with two or more monoamniotic fetuses, second trimester 2nd M CC ♀ PDx

O30.123 Triplet pregnancy with two or more monoamniotic fetuses, third trimester 3rd M CC ♀ PDx

O30.129 Triplet pregnancy with two or more monoamniotic fetuses, unspecified trimester M ♀ PDx

6th O30.19 Triplet pregnancy, unable to determine number of placenta and number of amniotic sacs

O30.191 Triplet pregnancy, unable to determine number of placenta and number of amniotic sacs, first trimester 1st M CC ♀ PDx

O30.192 Triplet pregnancy, unable to determine number of placenta and number of amniotic sacs, second trimester 2nd M CC ♀ PDx

O30.193 Triplet pregnancy, unable to determine number of placenta and number of amniotic sacs, third trimester 3rd M CC ♀ PDx

O30.199 Triplet pregnancy, unable to determine number of placenta and number of amniotic sacs, unspecified trimester M ♀ PDx

5th O30.2 Quadruplet pregnancy

6th O30.20 Quadruplet pregnancy, unspecified number of placenta and unspecified number of amniotic sacs

O30.201 Quadruplet pregnancy, unspecified number of placenta and unspecified number of amniotic sacs, first trimester 1st M CC ♀ PDx

O30.202 Quadruplet pregnancy, unspecified number of placenta and unspecified number of amniotic sacs, second trimester 2nd M CC ♀ PDx

O30.203 Quadruplet pregnancy, unspecified number of placenta and unspecified number of amniotic sacs, third trimester 3rd M CC ♀ PDx

O30.209 Quadruplet pregnancy, unspecified number of placenta and unspecified number of amniotic sacs, unspecified trimester M ♀ PDx

6th O30.21 Quadruplet pregnancy with two or more monochorionic fetuses

O30.211 Quadruplet pregnancy with two or more monochorionic fetuses, first trimester 1st M CC ♀ PDx

O30.212 Quadruplet pregnancy with two or more monochorionic fetuses, second trimester 2nd M CC ♀ PDx

O30.213 Quadruplet pregnancy with two or more monochorionic fetuses, third trimester 3rd M CC ♀ PDx

O30.219 Quadruplet pregnancy with two or more monochorionic fetuses, unspecified trimester M ♀ PDx

6th O30.22 Quadruplet pregnancy with two or more monoamniotic fetuses

O30.221 Quadruplet pregnancy with two or more monoamniotic fetuses, first trimester 1st M CC ♀ PDx

O30.222 Quadruplet pregnancy with two or more monoamniotic fetuses, second trimester 2nd M CC ♀ PDx

O30.223 Quadruplet pregnancy with two or more monoamniotic fetuses, third trimester 3rd M CC ♀ PDx

O30.229 Quadruplet pregnancy with two or more monoamniotic fetuses, unspecified trimester M ♀ PDx

6th O30.29 Quadruplet pregnancy, unable to determine number of placenta and number of amniotic sacs

O30.291 Quadruplet pregnancy, unable to determine number of placenta and number of amniotic sacs, first trimester 1st M CC ♀ PDx

O30.292 Quadruplet pregnancy, unable to determine number of placenta and number of amniotic sacs, second trimester 2nd M CC ♀ PDx

O30.293 Quadruplet pregnancy, unable to determine number of placenta and number of amniotic sacs, third trimester 3rd M CC ♀ PDx

O30.299 Quadruplet pregnancy, unable to determine number of placenta and number of amniotic sacs, unspecified trimester M ♀ PDx

5th O30.8 Other specified multiple gestation

Multiple gestation pregnancy greater then quadruplets

6th O30.80 Other specified multiple gestation, unspecified number of placenta and unspecified number of amniotic sacs

O30.801 Other specified multiple gestation, unspecified number of placenta and unspecified number of amniotic sacs, first trimester 1st M CC ♀ PDx

O30.802 Other specified multiple gestation, unspecified number of placenta and unspecified number of amniotic sacs, second trimester 2nd M CC ♀ PDx

O30.803 Other specified multiple gestation, unspecified number of placenta and unspecified number of amniotic sacs, third trimester 3rd M CC ♀ PDx

O30.809 Other specified multiple gestation, unspecified number of placenta and unspecified number of amniotic sacs, unspecified trimester M ♀ PDx

6th O30.81 Other specified multiple gestation with two or more monochorionic fetuses

O30.811 Other specified multiple gestation with two or more monochorionic fetuses, first trimester 1st M CC ♀ PDx

O30.812 Other specified multiple gestation with two or more monochorionic fetuses, second trimester 2nd M CC ♀ PDx

O30.813 Other specified multiple gestation with two or more monochorionic fetuses, third trimester 3rd M CC ♀ PDx

O30.819 Other specified multiple gestation with two or more monochorionic fetuses, unspecified trimester M ♀ PDx

6th O30.82 Other specified multiple gestation with two or more monoamniotic fetuses

O30.821 Other specified multiple gestation with two or more monoamniotic fetuses, first trimester 1st M CC ♀ PDx

O30.822 Other specified multiple gestation with two or more monoamniotic fetuses, second trimester 2nd M CC ♀ PDx

O30.823 Other specified multiple gestation with two or more monoamniotic fetuses, third trimester 3rd M CC ♀ PDx

O30.829 Other specified multiple gestation with two or more monoamniotic fetuses, unspecified trimester M ♀ PDx

6th O30.89 Other specified multiple gestation, unable to determine number of placenta and number of amniotic sacs

1st 1st trimester 2nd 2nd trimester 3rd 3rd trimester PDx Unacceptable principal diagnosis symbol per Medicare code edits
POA Code exempt from diagnosis present on admission requirement ? Questionable admission CC Complication or comorbidity
CC/MCC Exc CC/MCC exclusion MCC Major complication or comorbidity PDx CC Principal diagnosis as its own CC
PDx MCC Principal diagnosis as its own MCC Z1 Z code as first-listed diagnosis

O30.891 Other specified multiple gestation, unable to determine number of placenta and number of amniotic sacs, first trimester 1st M ♀ PDx

O30.892 Other specified multiple gestation, unable to determine number of placenta and number of amniotic sacs, second trimester 2nd M ♀ PDx

O30.893 Other specified multiple gestation, unable to determine number of placenta and number of amniotic sacs, third trimester 3rd M ♀ PDx

O30.899 Other specified multiple gestation, unable to determine number of placenta and number of amniotic sacs, unspecified trimester M ♀ PDx

O30.9 Multiple gestation, unspecified
Multiple pregnancy NOS

O30.90 Multiple gestation, unspecified, unspecified trimester M ♀

O30.91 Multiple gestation, unspecified, first trimester 1st M ♀

O30.92 Multiple gestation, unspecified, second trimester 2nd M ♀

O30.93 Multiple gestation, unspecified, third trimester 3rd M ♀

O31 Complications specific to multiple gestation

EXCLUDES2 *delayed delivery of second twin, triplet, etc. (O63.2)*
malpresentation of one fetus or more (O32.9)
placental transfusion syndromes (O43.0-)

One of the following 7th characters is to be assigned to each code under category O31. 7th character 0 is for single gestations and multiple gestations where the fetus is unspecified. 7th characters 1 through 9 are for cases of multiple gestations to identify the fetus for which the code applies. The appropriate code from category O30, Multiple gestation, must also be assigned when assigning a code from category O31 that has a 7th character of 1 through 9.

0 = not applicable or unspecified
1 = fetus 1
2 = fetus 2
3 = fetus 3
4 = fetus 4
5 = fetus 5
9 = other fetus

AHA: Q4, 2012

O31.0 Papyraceous fetus
Fetus compressus

O31.00 Papyraceous fetus, unspecified trimester M ♀

O31.01 Papyraceous fetus, first trimester 1st M ♀

O31.02 Papyraceous fetus, second trimester 2nd M ♀

O31.03 Papyraceous fetus, third trimester 3rd M ♀

O31.1 Continuing pregnancy after spontaneous abortion of one fetus or more

O31.10 Continuing pregnancy after spontaneous abortion of one fetus or more, unspecified trimester M ♀

O31.11 Continuing pregnancy after spontaneous abortion of one fetus or more, first trimester 1st M ♀

O31.12 Continuing pregnancy after spontaneous abortion of one fetus or more, second trimester 2nd M ♀

O31.13 Continuing pregnancy after spontaneous abortion of one fetus or more, third trimester 3rd M ♀

O31.2 Continuing pregnancy after intrauterine death of one fetus or more

O31.20 Continuing pregnancy after intrauterine death of one fetus or more, unspecified trimester M ♀

O31.21 Continuing pregnancy after intrauterine death of one fetus or more, first trimester 1st M ♀

O31.22 Continuing pregnancy after intrauterine death of one fetus or more, second trimester 2nd M ♀

O31.23 Continuing pregnancy after intrauterine death of one fetus or more, third trimester 3rd M ♀

O31.3 Continuing pregnancy after elective fetal reduction of one fetus or more
Continuing pregnancy after selective termination of one fetus or more

O31.30 Continuing pregnancy after elective fetal reduction of one fetus or more, unspecified trimester M ♀

O31.31 Continuing pregnancy after elective fetal reduction of one fetus or more, first trimester 1st M ♀

O31.32 Continuing pregnancy after elective fetal reduction of one fetus or more, second trimester 2nd M ♀

O31.33 Continuing pregnancy after elective fetal reduction of one fetus or more, third trimester 3rd M ♀

O31.8 Other complications specific to multiple gestation

O31.8X Other complications specific to multiple gestation

O31.8X1 Other complications specific to multiple gestation, first trimester 1st M ♀

O31.8X2 Other complications specific to multiple gestation, second trimester 2nd M ♀

O31.8X3 Other complications specific to multiple gestation, third trimester 3rd M ♀

O31.8X9 Other complications specific to multiple gestation, unspecified trimester M ♀

O32 Maternal care for malpresentation of fetus

INCLUDES *the listed conditions as a reason for observation, hospitalization or other obstetric care of the mother, or for cesarean delivery before onset of labor*

EXCLUDES1 *malpresentation of fetus with obstructed labor (O64.-)*

One of the following 7th characters is to be assigned to each code under category O32. 7th character 0 is for single gestations and multiple gestations where the fetus is unspecified. 7th characters 1 through 9 are for cases of multiple gestations to identify the fetus for which the code applies. The appropriate code from category O30, Multiple gestation, must also be assigned when assigning a code from category O32 that has a 7th character of 1 through 9.

0 = not applicable or unspecified
1 = fetus 1
2 = fetus 2
3 = fetus 3
4 = fetus 4
5 = fetus 5
9 = other fetus

AHA: Q4, 2012

O32.0 Maternal care for unstable lie M ♀

O32.1 Maternal care for breech presentation M ♀
Maternal care for buttocks presentation
Maternal care for complete breech
Maternal care for frank breech

EXCLUDES1 *footling presentation (O32.8)*
incomplete breech (O32.8)

O32.2 Maternal care for transverse and oblique lie M ♀
Maternal care for oblique presentation
Maternal care for transverse presentation

O32.3 Maternal care for face, brow and chin presentation M ♀

O32.4 Maternal care for high head at term M ♀
Maternal care for failure of head to enter pelvic brim

O32.6 Maternal care for compound presentation M ♀

O32.8 Maternal care for other malpresentation of fetus M ♀
Maternal care for footling presentation
Maternal care for incomplete breech

O32.9 Maternal care for malpresentation of fetus, unspecified M ♀

O33 Maternal care for disproportion

INCLUDES *the listed conditions as a reason for observation, hospitalization or other obstetric care of the mother, or for cesarean delivery before onset of labor*

EXCLUDES1 *disproportion with obstructed labor (O65-O66)*

O33.0 Maternal care for disproportion due to deformity of maternal pelvic bones M ♀
Maternal care for disproportion due to pelvic deformity causing disproportion NOS

O33.1 Maternal care for disproportion due to generally contracted pelvis M ♀
Maternal care for disproportion due to contracted pelvis NOS causing disproportion

O33.2 Maternal care for disproportion due to inlet contraction of pelvis M ♀
Maternal care for disproportion due to inlet contraction (pelvis) causing disproportion

Unspecified Code Other Specified Code Manifestation Code N Newborn P Pediatric M Maternity A Adult ♂ Male ♀ Female
● New Code ▲ Revised Code Title ►◄ Revised Text NOTES INCLUDES EXCLUDES1 Not coded here EXCLUDES2 Not included here
4th character required 5th character required 6th character required 7th character required
Extension 'X' Alert HAC Hospital-acquired condition (HAC) alert AHA AHA Coding Clinic©

O33.3 **Maternal care for disproportion due to outlet contraction of pelvis**
Maternal care for disproportion due to mid-cavity contraction (pelvis)
Maternal care for disproportion due to outlet contraction (pelvis)
One of the following 7th characters is to be assigned to code O33.3. 7th character 0 is for single gestations and multiple gestations where the fetus is unspecified. 7th characters 1 through 9 are for cases of multiple gestations to identify the fetus for which the code applies. The appropriate code from category O30, Multiple gestation, must also be assigned when assigning code O33.3 with a 7th character of 1 through 9.
0 = not applicable or unspecified
1 = fetus 1
2 = fetus 2
3 = fetus 3
4 = fetus 4
5 = fetus 5
9 = other fetus

O33.4 **Maternal care for disproportion of mixed maternal and fetal origin**
One of the following 7th characters is to be assigned to code O33.4. 7th character 0 is for single gestations and multiple gestations where the fetus is unspecified. 7th characters 1 through 9 are for cases of multiple gestations to identify the fetus for which the code applies. The appropriate code from category O30, Multiple gestation, must also be assigned when assigning code O33.4 with a 7th character of 1 through 9.
0 = not applicable or unspecified
1 = fetus 1
2 = fetus 2
3 = fetus 3
4 = fetus 4
5 = fetus 5
9 = other fetus

O33.5 **Maternal care for disproportion due to unusually large fetus**
Maternal care for disproportion due to disproportion of fetal origin with normally formed fetus
Maternal care for disproportion due to fetal disproportion NOS
One of the following 7th characters is to be assigned to code O33.5. 7th character 0 is for single gestations and multiple gestations where the fetus is unspecified. 7th characters 1 through 9 are for cases of multiple gestations to identify the fetus for which the code applies. The appropriate code from category O30, Multiple gestation, must also be assigned when assigning code O33.5 with a 7th character of 1 through 9.
0 = not applicable or unspecified
1 = fetus 1
2 = fetus 2
3 = fetus 3
4 = fetus 4
5 = fetus 5
9 = other fetus

O33.6 **Maternal care for disproportion due to hydrocephalic fetus**
One of the following 7th characters is to be assigned to code O33.6. 7th character 0 is for single gestations and multiple gestations where the fetus is unspecified. 7th characters 1 through 9 are for cases of multiple gestations to identify the fetus for which the code applies. The appropriate code from category O30, Multiple gestation, must also be assigned when assigning code O33.6 with a 7th character of 1 through 9.
0 = not applicable or unspecified
1 = fetus 1
2 = fetus 2
3 = fetus 3
4 = fetus 4
5 = fetus 5
9 = other fetus

O33.7 **Maternal care for disproportion due to other fetal deformities**
Maternal care for disproportion due to fetal ascites
Maternal care for disproportion due to fetal hydrops
Maternal care for disproportion due to fetal meningomyelocele
Maternal care for disproportion due to fetal sacral teratoma
Maternal care for disproportion due to fetal tumor
One of the following 7th characters is to be assigned to code O33.7. 7th character 0 is for single gestations and multiple gestations where the fetus is unspecified. 7th characters 1 through 9 are for cases of multiple gestations to identify the fetus for which the code applies. The appropriate code from category O30, Multiple gestation, must also be assigned when assigning code O33.7 with a 7th character of 1 through 9.
0 = not applicable or unspecified
1 = fetus 1
2 = fetus 2
3 = fetus 3
4 = fetus 4
5 = fetus 5
9 = other fetus

EXCLUDES1 *obstructed labor due to other fetal deformities (O66.3)*

O33.8 **Maternal care for disproportion of other origin**

O33.9 **Maternal care for disproportion, unspecified**
Maternal care for disproportion due to cephalopelvic disproportion NOS
Maternal care for disproportion due to fetopelvic disproportion NOS

O34 **Maternal care for abnormality of pelvic organs**
INCLUDES *the listed conditions as a reason for hospitalization or other obstetric care of the mother, or for cesarean delivery before onset of labor*
Code first any associated obstructed labor (O65.5)
Use additional code for specific condition

O34.0 **Maternal care for congenital malformation of uterus**
Maternal care for double uterus
Maternal care for uterus bicornis
O34.00 **Maternal care for unspecified congenital malformation of uterus, unspecified trimester**
O34.01 **Maternal care for unspecified congenital malformation of uterus, first trimester**
O34.02 **Maternal care for unspecified congenital malformation of uterus, second trimester**
O34.03 **Maternal care for unspecified congenital malformation of uterus, third trimester**

O34.1 **Maternal care for benign tumor of corpus uteri**
EXCLUDES2 *maternal care for benign tumor of cervix (O34.4-)*
maternal care for malignant neoplasm of uterus (O9A.1-)
O34.10 **Maternal care for benign tumor of corpus uteri, unspecified trimester**
O34.11 **Maternal care for benign tumor of corpus uteri, first trimester**
O34.12 **Maternal care for benign tumor of corpus uteri, second trimester**
O34.13 **Maternal care for benign tumor of corpus uteri, third trimester**

O34.2 **Maternal care due to uterine scar from previous surgery**
O34.21 **Maternal care for scar from previous cesarean delivery**
● O34.211 **Maternal care for low transverse scar from previous cesarean delivery**
● O34.212 **Maternal care for vertical scar from previous cesarean delivery**
Maternal care for classical scar from previous cesarean delivery
● O34.219 **Maternal care for unspecified type scar from previous cesarean delivery**
O34.29 **Maternal care due to uterine scar from other previous surgery**
Maternal care due to uterine scar from other transmural uterine incision

O34.3 **Maternal care for cervical incompetence**
Maternal care for cerclage with or without cervical incompetence
Maternal care for Shirodkar suture with or without cervical incompetence
O34.30 **Maternal care for cervical incompetence, unspecified trimester**
O34.31 **Maternal care for cervical incompetence, first trimester**

1st 1st trimester 2nd 2nd trimester 3rd 3rd trimester Unacceptable principal diagnosis symbol per Medicare code edits
Code exempt from diagnosis present on admission requirement ? Questionable admission CC Complication or comorbidity
CC/MCC exclusion MCC Major complication or comorbidity Principal diagnosis as its own CC
Principal diagnosis as its own MCC Z1 Z code as first-listed diagnosis

When symbols appear on a code that requires a 7th character extension, refer to Appendix D to identify applicable 7th character codes.

O34.32 Maternal care for cervical incompetence, second trimester 2nd M MCC ♀
O34.33 Maternal care for cervical incompetence, third trimester 3rd M MCC ♀
O34.4 Maternal care for other abnormalities of cervix
O34.40 Maternal care for other abnormalities of cervix, unspecified trimester M ♀
O34.41 Maternal care for other abnormalities of cervix, first trimester 1st M ♀
O34.42 Maternal care for other abnormalities of cervix, second trimester 2nd M ♀
O34.43 Maternal care for other abnormalities of cervix, third trimester 3rd M ♀
O34.5 Maternal care for other abnormalities of gravid uterus
O34.51 Maternal care for incarceration of gravid uterus
O34.511 Maternal care for incarceration of gravid uterus, first trimester 1st M ♀
O34.512 Maternal care for incarceration of gravid uterus, secondtrimester 2nd M ♀
O34.513 Maternal care for incarceration of gravid uterus, third trimester 3rd M ♀
O34.519 Maternal care for incarceration of gravid uterus, unspecified trimester M ♀
O34.52 Maternal care for prolapse of gravid uterus
O34.521 Maternal care for prolapse of gravid uterus, first trimester 1st M ♀
O34.522 Maternal care for prolapse of gravid uterus, second trimester 2nd M ♀
O34.523 Maternal care for prolapse of gravid uterus, third trimester 3rd M ♀
O34.529 Maternal care for prolapse of gravid uterus, unspecified trimester M ♀
O34.53 Maternal care for retroversion of gravid uterus
O34.531 Maternal care for retroversion of gravid uterus, first trimester 1st M ♀
O34.532 Maternal care for retroversion of gravid uterus, second trimester 2nd M ♀
O34.533 Maternal care for retroversion of gravid uterus, third trimester 3rd M ♀
O34.539 Maternal care for retroversion of gravid uterus, unspecified trimester M ♀
O34.59 Maternal care for other abnormalities of gravid uterus
O34.591 Maternal care for other abnormalities of gravid uterus, first trimester 1st M ♀
O34.592 Maternal care for other abnormalities of gravid uterus, second trimester 2nd M ♀
O34.593 Maternal care for other abnormalities of gravid uterus, third trimester 3rd M ♀
O34.599 Maternal care for other abnormalities of gravid uterus, unspecified trimester M ♀
O34.6 Maternal care for abnormality of vagina
EXCLUDES2 *maternal care for vaginal varices in pregnancy (O22.1-)*
O34.60 Maternal care for abnormality of vagina, unspecified trimester M ♀
O34.61 Maternal care for abnormality of vagina, first trimester 1st M ♀
O34.62 Maternal care for abnormality of vagina, second trimester 2nd M ♀
O34.63 Maternal care for abnormality of vagina, third trimester 3rd M ♀
O34.7 Maternal care for abnormality of vulva and perineum
EXCLUDES2 *maternal care for perineal and vulval varices in pregnancy (O22.1-)*
O34.70 Maternal care for abnormality of vulva and perineum, unspecified trimester M ♀
O34.71 Maternal care for abnormality of vulva and perineum, first trimester 1st M ♀
O34.72 Maternal care for abnormality of vulva and perineum, second trimester 2nd M ♀
O34.73 Maternal care for abnormality of vulva and perineum, third trimester 3rd M ♀
O34.8 Maternal care for other abnormalities of pelvic organs
O34.80 Maternal care for other abnormalities of pelvic organs, unspecified trimester M ♀
O34.81 Maternal care for other abnormalities of pelvic organs, first trimester 1st M ♀
O34.82 Maternal care for other abnormalities of pelvic organs, second trimester 2nd M ♀
O34.83 Maternal care for other abnormalities of pelvic organs, third trimester 3rd M ♀
O34.9 Maternal care for abnormality of pelvic organ, unspecified
O34.90 Maternal care for abnormality of pelvic organ, unspecified, unspecified trimester M ♀
O34.91 Maternal care for abnormality of pelvic organ, unspecified, first trimester 1st M ♀
O34.92 Maternal care for abnormality of pelvic organ, unspecified, second trimester 2nd M ♀
O34.93 Maternal care for abnormality of pelvic organ, unspecified, third trimester 3rd M ♀

O35 Maternal care for known or suspected fetal abnormality and damage
INCLUDES *the listed conditions in the fetus as a reason for hospitalization or other obstetric care to the mother, or for termination of pregnancy*
Code also any associated maternal condition
EXCLUDES1 *encounter for suspected maternal and fetal conditions ruled out (Z03.7-)*

One of the following 7th characters is to be assigned to each code under category O35. 7th character 0 is for single gestations and multiple gestations where the fetus is unspecified. 7th characters 1 through 9 are for cases of multiple gestations to identify the fetus for which the code applies. The appropriate code from category O30, Multiple gestation, must also be assigned when assigning a code from category O35 that has a 7th character of 1 through 9.
0 = not applicable or unspecified
1 = fetus 1
2 = fetus 2
3 = fetus 3
4 = fetus 4
5 = fetus 5
9 = other fetus

O35.0 Maternal care for (suspected) central nervous system malformation in fetus M ♀
Maternal care for fetal anencephaly
Maternal care for fetal hydrocephalus
Maternal care for fetal spina bifida
EXCLUDES2 *chromosomal abnormality in fetus (O35.1)*
O35.1 Maternal care for (suspected) chromosomal abnormality in fetus M ♀
O35.2 Maternal care for (suspected) hereditary disease in fetus M ♀
EXCLUDES2 *chromosomal abnormality in fetus (O35.1)*
O35.3 Maternal care for (suspected) damage to fetus from viral disease in mother M ♀
Maternal care for damage to fetus from maternal cytomegalovirus infection
Maternal care for damage to fetus from maternal rubella
O35.4 Maternal care for (suspected) damage to fetus from alcohol M ♀
O35.5 Maternal care for (suspected) damage to fetus by drugs M ♀
Maternal care for damage to fetus from drug addiction
O35.6 Maternal care for (suspected) damage to fetus by radiation M ♀
O35.7 Maternal care for (suspected) damage to fetus by other medical procedures M ♀
Maternal care for damage to fetus by amniocentesis
Maternal care for damage to fetus by biopsy procedures
Maternal care for damage to fetus by hematological investigation
Maternal care for damage to fetus by intrauterine contraceptive device
Maternal care for damage to fetus by intrauterine surgery
O35.8 Maternal care for other (suspected) fetal abnormality and damage M ♀
Maternal care for damage to fetus from maternal listeriosis
Maternal care for damage to fetus from maternal toxoplasmosis
O35.9 Maternal care for (suspected) fetal abnormality and damage, unspecified M ♀

Unspecified Code | Other Specified Code | Manifestation Code | N Newborn | P Pediatric | M Maternity | A Adult | ♂ Male | ♀ Female
● New Code ▲ Revised Code Title ►◄ Revised Text NOTES INCLUDES EXCLUDES1 Not coded here EXCLUDES2 Not included here
4th character required | 5th character required | 6th character required | 7th character required
Extension 'X' Alert | HAC Hospital-acquired condition (HAC) alert | AHA AHA Coding Clinic©

O36 Maternal care for other fetal problems

INCLUDES *the listed conditions in the fetus as a reason for hospitalization or other obstetric care of the mother, or for termination of pregnancy*

EXCLUDES1 *encounter for suspected maternal and fetal conditions ruled out (Z03.7-)*

placental transfusion syndromes (O43.0-)

EXCLUDES2 *labor and delivery complicated by fetal stress (O77.-)*

One of the following 7th characters is to be assigned to each code under category O36. 7th character 0 is for single gestations and multiple gestations where the fetus is unspecified. 7th characters 1 through 9 are for cases of multiple gestations to identify the fetus for which the code applies. The appropriate code from category O30, Multiple gestation, must also be assigned when assigning a code from category O36 that has a 7th character of 1 through 9.

- 0 = not applicable or unspecified
- 1 = fetus 1
- 2 = fetus 2
- 3 = fetus 3
- 4 = fetus 4
- 5 = fetus 5
- 9 = other fetus

AHA: Q3, 2015

O36.0 Maternal care for rhesus isoimmunization
Maternal care for Rh incompatibility (with hydrops fetalis)

O36.01 Maternal care for anti-D [Rh] antibodies

O36.011 Maternal care for anti-D [Rh] antibodies, first trimester 1st CC M ♀

O36.012 Maternal care for anti-D [Rh] antibodies, second trimester 2nd CC M ♀

O36.013 Maternal care for anti-D [Rh] antibodies, third trimester 3rd CC M ♀

O36.019 Maternal care for anti-D [Rh] antibodies, unspecified trimester M ♀

O36.09 Maternal care for other rhesus isoimmunization

O36.091 Maternal care for other rhesus isoimmunization, first trimester 1st CC M ♀

O36.092 Maternal care for other rhesus isoimmunization, second trimester 2nd CC M ♀

O36.093 Maternal care for other rhesus isoimmunization, third trimester 3rd CC M ♀

O36.099 Maternal care for other rhesus isoimmunization, unspecified trimester M ♀

O36.1 Maternal care for other isoimmunization
Maternal care for ABO isoimmunization

O36.11 Maternal care for Anti-A sensitization
Maternal care for isoimmunization NOS (with hydrops fetalis)

O36.111 Maternal care for Anti-A sensitization, first trimester 1st M ♀

O36.112 Maternal care for Anti-A sensitization, second trimester 2nd M ♀

O36.113 Maternal care for Anti-A sensitization, third trimester 3rd M ♀

O36.119 Maternal care for Anti-A sensitization, unspecified trimester M ♀

O36.19 Maternal care for other isoimmunization
Maternal care for Anti-B sensitization

O36.191 Maternal care for other isoimmunization, first trimester 1st M ♀

O36.192 Maternal care for other isoimmunization, second trimester 2nd M ♀

O36.193 Maternal care for other isoimmunization, third trimester 3rd M ♀

O36.199 Maternal care for other isoimmunization, unspecified trimester M ♀

O36.2 Maternal care for hydrops fetalis
Maternal care for hydrops fetalis NOS
Maternal care for hydrops fetalis not associated with isoimmunization

EXCLUDES1 *hydrops fetalis associated with ABO isoimmunization (O36.1-)*

hydrops fetalis associated with rhesus isoimmunization (O36.0-)

O36.20 Maternal care for hydrops fetalis, unspecified trimester M ♀

O36.21 Maternal care for hydrops fetalis, first trimester 1st M ♀

O36.22 Maternal care for hydrops fetalis, second trimester 2nd M ♀

O36.23 Maternal care for hydrops fetalis, third trimester 3rd M ♀

O36.4 Maternal care for intrauterine death CC M ♀
Maternal care for intrauterine fetal death NOS
Maternal care for intrauterine fetal death after completion of 20 weeks of gestation
Maternal care for late fetal death
Maternal care for missed delivery

EXCLUDES1 *missed abortion (O02.1)*

stillbirth (P95)

O36.5 Maternal care for known or suspected poor fetal growth

O36.51 Maternal care for known or suspected placental insufficiency

O36.511 Maternal care for known or suspected placental insufficiency, first trimester 1st M ♀

O36.512 Maternal care for known or suspected placental insufficiency, second trimester 2nd M ♀

O36.513 Maternal care for known or suspected placental insufficiency, third trimester 3rd M ♀

O36.519 Maternal care for known or suspected placental insufficiency, unspecified trimester M ♀

O36.59 Maternal care for other known or suspected poor fetal growth
Maternal care for known or suspected light-for-dates NOS
Maternal care for known or suspected small-for-dates NOS

O36.591 Maternal care for other known or suspected poor fetal growth, first trimester 1st M ♀

O36.592 Maternal care for other known or suspected poor fetal growth, second trimester 2nd M ♀

O36.593 Maternal care for other known or suspected poor fetal growth, third trimester 3rd M ♀

O36.599 Maternal care for other known or suspected poor fetal growth, unspecified trimester M ♀

O36.6 Maternal care for excessive fetal growth
Maternal care for known or suspected large-for-dates

O36.60 Maternal care for excessive fetal growth, unspecified trimester M ♀

O36.61 Maternal care for excessive fetal growth, first trimester 1st M ♀

O36.62 Maternal care for excessive fetal growth, second trimester 2nd M ♀

O36.63 Maternal care for excessive fetal growth, third trimester 3rd M ♀

O36.7 Maternal care for viable fetus in abdominal pregnancy

O36.70 Maternal care for viable fetus in abdominal pregnancy, unspecified trimester M ♀

O36.71 Maternal care for viable fetus in abdominal pregnancy, first trimester 1st M ♀

O36.72 Maternal care for viable fetus in abdominal pregnancy, second trimester 2nd M ♀

O36.73 Maternal care for viable fetus in abdominal pregnancy, third trimester 3rd M ♀

O36.8 Maternal care for other specified fetal problems

O36.80 Pregnancy with inconclusive fetal viability
Encounter to determine fetal viability of pregnancy PDx M ♀

1st 1st trimester 2nd 2nd trimester 3rd 3rd trimester PDx Unacceptable principal diagnosis symbol per Medicare code edits
POA Code exempt from diagnosis present on admission requirement ? Questionable admission CC Complication or comorbidity
CC/MCC Excl CC/MCC exclusion MCC Major complication or comorbidity PDx Principal diagnosis as its own CC
PDx Principal diagnosis as its own MCC Z1 Z code as first-listed diagnosis

O36.81 Decreased fetal movements
- O36.812 Decreased fetal movements, second trimester 2nd M ♀
- O36.813 Decreased fetal movements, third trimester 3rd M ♀
- O36.819 Decreased fetal movements, unspecified trimester M ♀

O36.82 Fetal anemia and thrombocytopenia
- O36.821 Fetal anemia and thrombocytopenia, first trimester 1st M ♀
- O36.822 Fetal anemia and thrombocytopenia, second trimester 2nd M ♀
- O36.823 Fetal anemia and thrombocytopenia, third trimester 3rd M ♀
- O36.829 Fetal anemia and thrombocytopenia, unspecified trimester M ♀

O36.89 Maternal care for other specified fetal problems
- O36.891 Maternal care for other specified fetal problems, first trimester 1st M ♀
- O36.892 Maternal care for other specified fetal problems, second trimester 2nd M ♀
- O36.893 Maternal care for other specified fetal problems, third trimester 3rd M ♀
- O36.899 Maternal care for other specified fetal problems, unspecified trimester M ♀

O36.9 Maternal care for fetal problem, unspecified
- O36.90 Maternal care for fetal problem, unspecified, unspecified trimester M ♀
- O36.91 Maternal care for fetal problem, unspecified, first trimester 1st M ♀
- O36.92 Maternal care for fetal problem, unspecified, second trimester 2nd M ♀
- O36.93 Maternal care for fetal problem, unspecified, third trimester 3rd M ♀

O40 Polyhydramnios

INCLUDES *hydramnios*

EXCLUDES1 *encounter for suspected maternal and fetal conditions ruled out (Z03.7-)*

One of the following 7th characters is to be assigned to each code under category O40. 7th character 0 is for single gestations and multiple gestations where the fetus is unspecified. 7th characters 1 through 9 are for cases of multiple gestations to identify the fetus for which the code applies. The appropriate code from category O30, Multiple gestation, must also be assigned when assigning a code from category O40 that has a 7th character of 1 through 9.

- 0 = not applicable or unspecified
- 1 = fetus 1
- 2 = fetus 2
- 3 = fetus 3
- 4 = fetus 4
- 5 = fetus 5
- 9 = other fetus

- O40.1 Polyhydramnios, first trimester 1st M ♀
- O40.2 Polyhydramnios, second trimester 2nd M ♀
- O40.3 Polyhydramnios, third trimester 3rd M ♀
- O40.9 Polyhydramnios, unspecified trimester M ♀

O41 Other disorders of amniotic fluid and membranes

EXCLUDES1 *encounter for suspected maternal and fetal conditions ruled out (Z03.7-)*

One of the following 7th characters is to be assigned to each code under category O41. 7th character 0 is for single gestations and multiple gestations where the fetus is unspecified. 7th characters 1 through 9 are for cases of multiple gestations to identify the fetus for which the code applies. The appropriate code from category O30, Multiple gestation, must also be assigned when assigning a code from category O41 that has a 7th character of 1 through 9.

- 0 = not applicable or unspecified
- 1 = fetus 1
- 2 = fetus 2
- 3 = fetus 3
- 4 = fetus 4
- 5 = fetus 5
- 9 = other fetus

O41.0 Oligohydramnios

Oligohydramnios without rupture of membranes
- O41.00 Oligohydramnios, unspecified trimester M ♀
- O41.01 Oligohydramnios, first trimester 1st CC M ♀
- O41.02 Oligohydramnios, second trimester 2nd CC M ♀
- O41.03 Oligohydramnios, third trimester 3rd CC M ♀

O41.1 Infection of amniotic sac and membranes

O41.10 Infection of amniotic sac and membranes, unspecified
- O41.101 Infection of amniotic sac and membranes, unspecified, first trimester 1st MCC M ♀
- O41.102 Infection of amniotic sac and membranes, unspecified, second trimester 2nd MCC M ♀
- O41.103 Infection of amniotic sac and membranes, unspecified, third trimester 3rd MCC M ♀
- O41.109 Infection of amniotic sac and membranes, unspecified, unspecified trimester M ♀

O41.12 Chorioamnionitis
- O41.121 Chorioamnionitis, first trimester 1st MCC M ♀
- O41.122 Chorioamnionitis, second trimester 2nd MCC M ♀
- O41.123 Chorioamnionitis, third trimester 3rd MCC M ♀
- O41.129 Chorioamnionitis, unspecified trimester M ♀

O41.14 Placentitis
- O41.141 Placentitis, first trimester 1st MCC M ♀
- O41.142 Placentitis, second trimester 2nd MCC M ♀
- O41.143 Placentitis, third trimester 3rd MCC M ♀
- O41.149 Placentitis, unspecified trimester M ♀

O41.8 Other specified disorders of amniotic fluid and membranes

O41.8X Other specified disorders of amniotic fluid and membranes
- O41.8X1 Other specified disorders of amniotic fluid and membranes, first trimester 1st M ♀
- O41.8X2 Other specified disorders of amniotic fluid and membranes, second trimester 2nd M ♀
- O41.8X3 Other specified disorders of amniotic fluid and membranes, third trimester 3rd M ♀
- O41.8X9 Other specified disorders of amniotic fluid and membranes, unspecified trimester M ♀

O41.9 Disorder of amniotic fluid and membranes, unspecified
- O41.90 Disorder of amniotic fluid and membranes, unspecified, unspecified trimester M ♀
- O41.91 Disorder of amniotic fluid and membranes, unspecified, first trimester 1st M ♀
- O41.92 Disorder of amniotic fluid and membranes, unspecified, second trimester 2nd M ♀
- O41.93 Disorder of amniotic fluid and membranes, unspecified, third trimester 3rd M ♀

O42 Premature rupture of membranes

O42.0 Premature rupture of membranes, onset of labor within 24 hours of rupture
- O42.00 Premature rupture of membranes, onset of labor within 24 hours of rupture, unspecified weeks of gestation M ♀

O42.01 Preterm premature rupture of membranes, onset of labor within 24 hours of rupture

Premature rupture of membranes before 37 completed weeks of gestation
- O42.011 Preterm premature rupture of membranes, onset of labor within 24 hours of rupture, first trimester 1st M ♀
- O42.012 Preterm premature rupture of membranes, onset of labor within 24 hours of rupture, second trimester 2nd M ♀
- O42.013 Preterm premature rupture of membranes, onset of labor within 24 hours of rupture, third trimester 3rd M ♀

Unspecified Code | Other Specified Code | Manifestation Code | N Newborn | P Pediatric | M Maternity | A Adult | ♂ Male | ♀ Female
● New Code | ▲ Revised Code Title | ►◄ Revised Text | NOTES | INCLUDES | EXCLUDES1 Not coded here | EXCLUDES2 Not included here
4th character required | 5th character required | 6th character required | 7th character required
Extension 'X' Alert | HAC Hospital-acquired condition (HAC) alert | AHA AHA Coding Clinic©

O42.019 Preterm premature rupture of membranes, onset of labor within 24 hours of rupture, unspecified trimester M ♀

O42.02 Full-term premature rupture of membranes, onset of labor within 24 hours of rupture 3rd M ♀
Premature rupture of membranes ▶at or after 37 completed weeks of gestation, onset of labor within 24 hours of rupture◀

5th O42.1 Premature rupture of membranes, onset of labor more than 24 hours following rupture

O42.10 Premature rupture of membranes, onset of labor more than 24 hours following rupture, unspecified weeks of gestation M ♀

6th O42.11 Preterm premature rupture of membranes, onset of labor more than 24 hours following rupture
Premature rupture of membranes before 37 completed weeks of gestation

O42.111 Preterm premature rupture of membranes, onset of labor more than 24 hours following rupture, first trimester 1st M ♀

O42.112 Preterm premature rupture of membranes, onset of labor more than 24 hours following rupture, second trimester 2nd M ♀

O42.113 Preterm premature rupture of membranes, onset of labor more than 24 hours following rupture, third trimester 3rd M ♀

O42.119 Preterm premature rupture of membranes, onset of labor more than 24 hours following rupture, unspecified trimester M ♀

O42.12 Full-term premature rupture of membranes, onset of labor more than 24 hours following rupture 3rd M ♀
Premature rupture of membranes ▶at or after 37 completed weeks of gestation, onset of labor more than 24 hours following rupture◀

5th O42.9 Premature rupture of membranes, unspecified as to length of time between rupture and onset of labor

O42.90 Premature rupture of membranes, unspecified as to length of time between rupture and onset of labor, unspecified weeks of gestation M ♀

6th O42.91 Preterm premature rupture of membranes, unspecified as to length of time between rupture and onset of labor
Premature rupture of membranes before 37 completed weeks of gestation

O42.911 Preterm premature rupture of membranes, unspecified as to length of time between rupture and onset of labor, first trimester 1st M ♀

O42.912 Preterm premature rupture of membranes, unspecified as to length of time between rupture and onset of labor, second trimester 2nd M ♀

O42.913 Preterm premature rupture of membranes, unspecified as to length of time between rupture and onset of labor, third trimester 3rd M ♀

O42.919 Preterm premature rupture of membranes, unspecified as to length of time between rupture and onset of labor, unspecified trimester M ♀

O42.92 Full-term premature rupture of membranes, unspecified as to length of time between rupture and onset of labor 3rd M ♀
Premature rupture of membranes ▶at or after 37 completed weeks of gestation, unspecified as to length of time between rupture and onset of labor◀

4th O43 Placental disorders

EXCLUDES2 *maternal care for poor fetal growth due to placental insufficiency (O36.5-)*
placenta previa (O44.-)
placental polyp (O90.89)
placentitis (O41.14-)
premature separation of placenta [abruptio placentae] (O45.-)

5th O43.0 Placental transfusion syndromes

6th O43.01 Fetomaternal placental transfusion syndrome
Maternofetal placental transfusion syndrome

O43.011 Fetomaternal placental transfusion syndrome, first trimester 1st M ♀

O43.012 Fetomaternal placental transfusion syndrome, second trimester 2nd M ♀

O43.013 Fetomaternal placental transfusion syndrome, third trimester 3rd M ♀

O43.019 Fetomaternal placental transfusion syndrome, unspecified trimester M ♀

6th O43.02 Fetus-to-fetus placental transfusion syndrome

O43.021 Fetus-to-fetus placental transfusion syndrome, first trimester 1st M ♀

O43.022 Fetus-to-fetus placental transfusion syndrome, second trimester 2nd M ♀

O43.023 Fetus-to-fetus placental transfusion syndrome, third trimester 3rd M ♀

O43.029 Fetus-to-fetus placental transfusion syndrome, unspecified trimester M ♀

5th O43.1 Malformation of placenta

6th O43.10 Malformation of placenta, unspecified
Abnormal placenta NOS

O43.101 Malformation of placenta, unspecified, first trimester 1st M ♀

O43.102 Malformation of placenta, unspecified, second trimester 2nd M ♀

O43.103 Malformation of placenta, unspecified, third trimester 3rd M ♀

O43.109 Malformation of placenta, unspecified, unspecified trimester M ♀

6th O43.11 Circumvallate placenta

O43.111 Circumvallate placenta, first trimester 1st M ♀

O43.112 Circumvallate placenta, second trimester 2nd M ♀

O43.113 Circumvallate placenta, third trimester 3rd M ♀

O43.119 Circumvallate placenta, unspecified trimester M ♀

6th O43.12 Velamentous insertion of umbilical cord

O43.121 Velamentous insertion of umbilical cord, first trimester 1st M ♀

O43.122 Velamentous insertion of umbilical cord, second trimester 2nd M ♀

O43.123 Velamentous insertion of umbilical cord, third trimester 3rd M ♀

O43.129 Velamentous insertion of umbilical cord, unspecified trimester M ♀

6th O43.19 Other malformation of placenta

O43.191 Other malformation of placenta, first trimester 1st M ♀

O43.192 Other malformation of placenta, second trimester 2nd M ♀

O43.193 Other malformation of placenta, third trimester 3rd M ♀

O43.199 Other malformation of placenta, unspecified trimester M ♀

5th O43.2 Morbidly adherent placenta
Code also associated third stage postpartum hemorrhage, if applicable (O72.0)

EXCLUDES1 *retained placenta (O73.-)*

6th O43.21 Placenta accreta

O43.211 Placenta accreta, first trimester 1st M ♀

O43.212 Placenta accreta, second trimester 2nd M ♀

O43.213 Placenta accreta, third trimester 3rd M ♀

O43.219 Placenta accreta, unspecified trimester M ♀

6th O43.22 Placenta increta

O43.221 Placenta increta, first trimester 1st M ♀

O43.222 Placenta increta, second trimester 2nd M ♀

O43.223 Placenta increta, third trimester 3rd M ♀

O43.229 Placenta increta, unspecified trimester M ♀

6th O43.23 Placenta percreta

1st 1st trimester 2nd 2nd trimester 3rd 3rd trimester Unacceptable principal diagnosis symbol per Medicare code edits
Code exempt from diagnosis present on admission requirement ? Questionable admission CC Complication or comorbidity
CC/MCC exclusion MCC Major complication or comorbidity Principal diagnosis as its own CC
Principal diagnosis as its own MCC Z1 Z code as first-listed diagnosis

O43.231 Placenta percreta, first trimester 1st M ♀
O43.232 Placenta percreta, second trimester 2nd M ♀
O43.233 Placenta percreta, third trimester 3rd M ♀
O43.239 Placenta percreta, unspecified trimester M ♀

⑤ O43.8 Other placental disorders
⑥ O43.81 Placental infarction
O43.811 Placental infarction, first trimester 1st M ♀
O43.812 Placental infarction, second trimester 2nd M ♀
O43.813 Placental infarction, third trimester 3rd M ♀
O43.819 Placental infarction, unspecified trimester M ♀
⑥ O43.89 Other placental disorders
Placental dysfunction
O43.891 Other placental disorders, first trimester 1st M ♀
O43.892 Other placental disorders, second trimester 2nd M ♀
O43.893 Other placental disorders, third trimester 3rd M ♀
O43.899 Other placental disorders, unspecified trimester M ♀

⑤ O43.9 Unspecified placental disorder
O43.90 Unspecified placental disorder, unspecified trimester M ♀
O43.91 Unspecified placental disorder, first trimester 1st M ♀
O43.92 Unspecified placental disorder, second trimester 2nd M ♀
O43.93 Unspecified placental disorder, third trimester 3rd M ♀

④ O44 Placenta previa
▲ ⑤ O44.0 ▶Complete placenta previa NOS or◀ without hemorrhage
Placenta previa NOS
▲ O44.00 ▶Complete placenta previa NOS or◀ without hemorrhage, unspecified trimester M ♀
▲ O44.01 ▶Complete placenta previa NOS or◀ without hemorrhage, first trimester 1st M CC ♀
▲ O44.02 ▶Complete placenta previa NOS or◀ without hemorrhage, second trimester 2nd M CC ♀
▲ O44.03 ▶Complete placenta previa NOS or◀ without hemorrhage, third trimester 3rd M CC ♀
▲ ⑤ O44.1 ▶Complete◀ placenta previa with hemorrhage
EXCLUDES1 *labor and delivery complicated by hemorrhage from vasa previa (O69.4)*
▲ O44.10 ▶Complete◀ placenta previa with hemorrhage, unspecified trimester M ♀
▲ O44.11 ▶Complete◀ placenta previa with hemorrhage, first trimester 1st M MCC ♀
▲ O44.12 ▶Complete◀ placenta previa with hemorrhage, second trimester 2nd M MCC ♀
▲ O44.13 ▶Complete◀ placenta previa with hemorrhage, third trimester 3rd M MCC ♀
● ⑤ O44.2 Partial placenta previa without hemorrhage
Marginal placenta previa, NOS or without hemorrhage
● O44.20 Partial placenta previa NOS or without hemorrhage, unspecified trimester CC/MCC Exc
● O44.21 Partial placenta previa NOS or without hemorrhage, first trimester 1st CC CC/MCC Exc
● O44.22 Partial placenta previa NOS or without hemorrhage, second trimester 2nd CC CC/MCC Exc
● O44.23 Partial placenta previa NOS or without hemorrhage, third trimester 3rd CC CC/MCC Exc
● ⑤ O44.3 Partial placenta previa with hemorrhage
Marginal placenta previa with hemorrhage
● O44.30 Partial placenta previa with hemorrhage, unspecified trimester CC/MCC Exc
● O44.31 Partial placenta previa with hemorrhage, first trimester 1st CC/MCC Exc MCC
● O44.32 Partial placenta previa with hemorrhage, second trimester 2nd CC/MCC Exc MCC
● O44.33 Partial placenta previa with hemorrhage, third trimester 3rd CC/MCC Exc MCC
● ⑤ O44.4 Low lying placenta NOS or without hemorrhage
Low implantation of placenta NOS or without hemorrhage
● O44.40 Low lying placenta NOS or without hemorrhage, unspecified trimester CC/MCC Exc
● O44.41 Low lying placenta NOS or without hemorrhage, first trimester 1st CC CC/MCC Exc
● O44.42 Low lying placenta NOS or without hemorrhage, second trimester 2nd CC CC/MCC Exc
● O44.43 Low lying placenta NOS or without hemorrhage, third trimester 3rd CC CC/MCC Exc
● ⑤ O44.5 Low lying placenta with hemorrhage
Low implantation of placenta with hemorrhage
● O44.50 Low lying placenta with hemorrhage, unspecified trimester CC/MCC Exc
● O44.51 Low lying placenta with hemorrhage, first trimester 1st CC/MCC Exc MCC
● O44.52 Low lying placenta with hemorrhage, second trimester 2nd CC/MCC Exc MCC
● O44.53 Low lying placenta with hemorrhage, third trimester 3rd CC/MCC Exc MCC

④ O45 Premature separation of placenta [abruptio placentae]
⑤ O45.0 Premature separation of placenta with coagulation defect
⑥ O45.00 Premature separation of placenta with coagulation defect, unspecified
O45.001 Premature separation of placenta with coagulation defect, unspecified, first trimester 1st M MCC ♀
O45.002 Premature separation of placenta with coagulation defect, unspecified, second trimester 2nd M MCC ♀
O45.003 Premature separation of placenta with coagulation defect, unspecified, third trimester 3rd M MCC ♀
O45.009 Premature separation of placenta with coagulation defect, unspecified, unspecified trimester M ♀
⑥ O45.01 Premature separation of placenta with afibrinogenemia
Premature separation of placenta with hypofibrinogenemia
O45.011 Premature separation of placenta with afibrinogenemia, first trimester 1st M MCC ♀
O45.012 Premature separation of placenta with afibrinogenemia, second trimester 2nd M MCC ♀
O45.013 Premature separation of placenta with afibrinogenemia, third trimester 3rd M MCC ♀
O45.019 Premature separation of placenta with afibrinogenemia, unspecified trimester M ♀
⑥ O45.02 Premature separation of placenta with disseminated intravascular coagulation
O45.021 Premature separation of placenta with disseminated intravascular coagulation, first trimester 1st M MCC ♀
O45.022 Premature separation of placenta with disseminated intravascular coagulation, second trimester 2nd M MCC ♀
O45.023 Premature separation of placenta with disseminated intravascular coagulation, third trimester 3rd M MCC ♀
O45.029 Premature separation of placenta with disseminated intravascular coagulation, unspecified trimester M ♀
⑥ O45.09 Premature separation of placenta with other coagulation defect
O45.091 Premature separation of placenta with other coagulation defect, first trimester 1st M MCC ♀
O45.092 Premature separation of placenta with other coagulation defect, second trimester 2nd M MCC ♀

Unspecified Code Other Specified Code Manifestation Code N Newborn P Pediatric M Maternity A Adult ♂ Male ♀ Female
● New Code ▲ Revised Code Title ▶◀ Revised Text NOTES INCLUDES EXCLUDES1 Not coded here EXCLUDES2 Not included here
④ 4th character required ⑤ 5th character required ⑥ 6th character required ⑦ 7th character required
Extension 'X' Alert HAC Hospital-acquired condition (HAC) alert AHA AHA Coding Clinic®

O45.093 Premature separation of placenta with other coagulation defect, third trimester

O45.099 Premature separation of placenta with other coagulation defect, unspecified trimester

O45.8 Other premature separation of placenta

O45.8X Other premature separation of placenta

O45.8X1 Other premature separation of placenta, first trimester

O45.8X2 Other premature separation of placenta, second trimester

O45.8X3 Other premature separation of placenta, third trimester

O45.8X9 Other premature separation of placenta, unspecified trimester

O45.9 Premature separation of placenta, unspecified

Abruptio placentae NOS

O45.90 Premature separation of placenta, unspecified, unspecified trimester

O45.91 Premature separation of placenta, unspecified, first trimester

O45.92 Premature separation of placenta, unspecified, second trimester

O45.93 Premature separation of placenta, unspecified, third trimester

O46 Antepartum hemorrhage, not elsewhere classified

EXCLUDES1 *hemorrhage in early pregnancy (O20.-)*
intrapartum hemorrhage NEC (O67.-)
placenta previa (O44.-)
premature separation of placenta [abruptio placentae] (O45.-)

O46.0 Antepartum hemorrhage with coagulation defect

O46.00 Antepartum hemorrhage with coagulation defect, unspecified

O46.001 Antepartum hemorrhage with coagulation defect, unspecified, first trimester

O46.002 Antepartum hemorrhage with coagulation defect, unspecified, second trimester

O46.003 Antepartum hemorrhage with coagulation defect, unspecified, third trimester

O46.009 Antepartum hemorrhage with coagulation defect, unspecified, unspecified trimester

O46.01 Antepartum hemorrhage with afibrinogenemia

Antepartum hemorrhage with hypofibrinogenemia

O46.011 Antepartum hemorrhage with afibrinogenemia, first trimester

O46.012 Antepartum hemorrhage with afibrinogenemia, second trimester

O46.013 Antepartum hemorrhage with afibrinogenemia, third trimester

O46.019 Antepartum hemorrhage with afibrinogenemia, unspecified trimester

O46.02 Antepartum hemorrhage with disseminated intravascular coagulation

O46.021 Antepartum hemorrhage with disseminated intravascular coagulation, first trimester

O46.022 Antepartum hemorrhage with disseminated intravascular coagulation, second trimester

O46.023 Antepartum hemorrhage with disseminated intravascular coagulation, third trimester

O46.029 Antepartum hemorrhage with disseminated intravascular coagulation, unspecified trimester

O46.09 Antepartum hemorrhage with other coagulation defect

O46.091 Antepartum hemorrhage with other coagulation defect, first trimester

O46.092 Antepartum hemorrhage with other coagulation defect, second trimester

O46.093 Antepartum hemorrhage with other coagulation defect, third trimester

O46.099 Antepartum hemorrhage with other coagulation defect, unspecified trimester

O46.8 Other antepartum hemorrhage

O46.8X Other antepartum hemorrhage

O46.8X1 Other antepartum hemorrhage, first trimester

O46.8X2 Other antepartum hemorrhage, second trimester

O46.8X3 Other antepartum hemorrhage, third trimester

O46.8X9 Other antepartum hemorrhage, unspecified trimester

O46.9 Antepartum hemorrhage, unspecified

O46.90 Antepartum hemorrhage, unspecified, unspecified trimester

O46.91 Antepartum hemorrhage, unspecified, first trimester

O46.92 Antepartum hemorrhage, unspecified, second trimester

O46.93 Antepartum hemorrhage, unspecified, third trimester

O47 False labor

INCLUDES *Braxton Hicks contractions*
threatened labor

EXCLUDES1 *preterm labor (O60.-)*

O47.0 False labor before 37 completed weeks of gestation

O47.00 False labor before 37 completed weeks of gestation, unspecified trimester

O47.02 False labor before 37 completed weeks of gestation, second trimester

O47.03 False labor before 37 completed weeks of gestation, third trimester

O47.1 False labor at or after 37 completed weeks of gestation

O47.9 False labor, unspecified

O48 Late pregnancy

O48.0 Post-term pregnancy

Pregnancy over 40 completed weeks to 42 completed weeks gestation

O48.1 Prolonged pregnancy

Pregnancy which has advanced beyond 42 completed weeks gestation

Complications of labor and delivery (O60-O77)

O60 Preterm labor

INCLUDES *onset (spontaneous) of labor before 37 completed weeks of gestation*

EXCLUDES1 *false labor (O47.0-)*
threatened labor NOS (O47.0-)

O60.0 Preterm labor without delivery

O60.00 Preterm labor without delivery, unspecified trimester

O60.02 Preterm labor without delivery, second trimester

O60.03 Preterm labor without delivery, third trimester

O60.1 Preterm labor with preterm delivery

One of the following 7th characters is to be assigned to each code under subcategory O60.1. 7th character 0 is for single gestations and multiple gestations where the fetus is unspecified. 7th characters 1 through 9 are for cases of multiple gestations to identify the fetus for which the code applies. The appropriate code from category O30, Multiple

1st 1st trimester 2nd 2nd trimester 3rd 3rd trimester Unacceptable principal diagnosis symbol per Medicare code edits
Code exempt from diagnosis present on admission requirement Questionable admission CC Complication or comorbidity
CC/MCC exclusion MCC Major complication or comorbidity Principal diagnosis as its own CC
Principal diagnosis as its own MCC Z code as first-listed diagnosis

gestation, must also be assigned when assigning a code from subcategory O60.1 that has a 7th character of 1 through 9.

0 = not applicable or unspecified
1 = fetus 1
2 = fetus 2
3 = fetus 3
4 = fetus 4
5 = fetus 5
9 = other fetus

O60.10 Preterm labor with preterm delivery, unspecified trimester CC M ♀
Preterm labor with delivery NOS
O60.12 Preterm labor second trimester with preterm delivery second trimester 2nd MCC M ♀
O60.13 Preterm labor second trimester with preterm delivery third trimester 2nd 3rd MCC M ♀
O60.14 Preterm labor third trimester with preterm delivery third trimester 3rd MCC M ♀
AHA: Q2, 2016

O60.2 Term delivery with preterm labor
One of the following 7th characters is to be assigned to each code under subcategory O60.2. 7th character 0 is for single gestations and multiple gestations where the fetus is unspecified. 7th characters 1 through 9 are for cases of multiple gestations to identify the fetus for which the code applies. The appropriate code from category O30, Multiple gestation, must also be assigned when assigning a code from subcategory O60.2 that has a 7th character of 1 through 9.

0 = not applicable or unspecified
1 = fetus 1
2 = fetus 2
3 = fetus 3
4 = fetus 4
5 = fetus 5
9 = other fetus

O60.20 Term delivery with preterm labor, unspecified trimester CC M ♀
O60.22 Term delivery with preterm labor, second trimester 2nd MCC M ♀
O60.23 Term delivery with preterm labor, third trimester 3rd MCC M ♀

O61 Failed induction of labor
O61.0 Failed medical induction of labor M ♀
Failed induction (of labor) by oxytocin
Failed induction (of labor) by prostaglandins
O61.1 Failed instrumental induction of labor M ♀
Failed mechanical induction (of labor)
Failed surgical induction (of labor)
O61.8 Other failed induction of labor M ♀
O61.9 Failed induction of labor, unspecified M ♀

O62 Abnormalities of forces of labor
O62.0 Primary inadequate contractions M ♀
Failure of cervical dilatation
Primary hypotonic uterine dysfunction
Uterine inertia during latent phase of labor
O62.1 Secondary uterine inertia M ♀
Arrested active phase of labor
Secondary hypotonic uterine dysfunction
O62.2 Other uterine inertia M ♀
Atony of uterus without hemorrhage
Atony of uterus NOS
Desultory labor
Hypotonic uterine dysfunction NOS
Irregular labor
Poor contractions
Slow slope active phase of labor
Uterine inertia NOS
EXCLUDES1 *atony of uterus with hemorrhage (postpartum) (O72.1)*
postpartum atony of uterus without hemorrhage (O75.89)
O62.3 Precipitate labor M ♀
O62.4 Hypertonic, incoordinate, and prolonged uterine contractions M ♀
Cervical spasm
Contraction ring dystocia
Dyscoordinate labor
Hour-glass contraction of uterus
Hypertonic uterine dysfunction
Incoordinate uterine action
Tetanic contractions
Uterine dystocia NOS
Uterine spasm
EXCLUDES1 *dystocia (fetal) (maternal) NOS (O66.9)*
O62.8 Other abnormalities of forces of labor M ♀
O62.9 Abnormality of forces of labor, unspecified M ♀

O63 Long labor
O63.0 Prolonged first stage (of labor) M ♀
O63.1 Prolonged second stage (of labor) M ♀
O63.2 Delayed delivery of second twin, triplet, etc. M ♀
O63.9 Long labor, unspecified M CC ♀
Prolonged labor NOS

O64 Obstructed labor due to malposition and malpresentation of fetus
One of the following 7th characters is to be assigned to each code under category O64. 7th character 0 is for single gestations and multiple gestations where the fetus is unspecified. 7th characters 1 through 9 are for cases of multiple gestations to identify the fetus for which the code applies. The appropriate code from category O30, Multiple gestation, must also be assigned when assigning a code from category O64 that has a 7th character of 1 through 9.

0 = not applicable or unspecified
1 = fetus 1
2 = fetus 2
3 = fetus 3
4 = fetus 4
5 = fetus 5
9 = other fetus

O64.0 Obstructed labor due to incomplete rotation of fetal head M ♀
Deep transverse arrest
Obstructed labor due to persistent occipitoiliac (position)
Obstructed labor due to persistent occipitoposterior (position)
Obstructed labor due to persistent occipitosacral (position)
Obstructed labor due to persistent occipitotransverse (position)
O64.1 Obstructed labor due to breech presentation M ♀
Obstructed labor due to buttocks presentation
Obstructed labor due to complete breech presentation
Obstructed labor due to frank breech presentation
O64.2 Obstructed labor due to face presentation M ♀
Obstructed labor due to chin presentation
O64.3 Obstructed labor due to brow presentation M ♀
O64.4 Obstructed labor due to shoulder presentation M ♀
Prolapsed arm
EXCLUDES1 *impacted shoulders (O66.0)*
shoulder dystocia (O66.0)
O64.5 Obstructed labor due to compound presentation M ♀
O64.8 Obstructed labor due to other malposition and malpresentation M ♀
Obstructed labor due to footling presentation
Obstructed labor due to incomplete breech presentation
O64.9 Obstructed labor due to malposition and malpresentation, unspecified M ♀

O65 Obstructed labor due to maternal pelvic abnormality
O65.0 Obstructed labor due to deformed pelvis M ♀
O65.1 Obstructed labor due to generally contracted pelvis M ♀
O65.2 Obstructed labor due to pelvic inlet contraction M ♀
O65.3 Obstructed labor due to pelvic outlet and mid-cavity contraction M ♀
O65.4 Obstructed labor due to fetopelvic disproportion, unspecified M ♀
EXCLUDES1 *dystocia due to abnormality of fetus (O66.2-O66.3)*
O65.5 Obstructed labor due to abnormality of maternal pelvic organs M ♀
Obstructed labor due to conditions listed in O34.-
Use additional code to identify abnormality of pelvic organs O34.-
O65.8 Obstructed labor due to other maternal pelvic abnormalities M ♀
O65.9 Obstructed labor due to maternal pelvic abnormality, unspecified M ♀

Unspecified Code | Other Specified Code | Manifestation Code | N Newborn | P Pediatric | M Maternity | A Adult | ♂ Male | ♀ Female
● New Code ▲ Revised Code Title ►◄ Revised Text NOTES INCLUDES EXCLUDES1 Not coded here EXCLUDES2 Not included here
4th character required | 5th character required | 6th character required | 7th character required
Extension 'X' Alert | HAC Hospital-acquired condition (HAC) alert | AHA AHA Coding Clinic©

O66 Other obstructed labor

O66.0 Obstructed labor due to shoulder dystocia M ♀
Impacted shoulders

O66.1 Obstructed labor due to locked twins M ♀

O66.2 Obstructed labor due to unusually large fetus M ♀

O66.3 Obstructed labor due to other abnormalities of fetus M ♀
Dystocia due to fetal ascites
Dystocia due to fetal hydrops
Dystocia due to fetal meningomyelocele
Dystocia due to fetal sacral teratoma
Dystocia due to fetal tumor
Dystocia due to hydrocephalic fetus
Use additional code to identify cause of obstruction

O66.4 Failed trial of labor

O66.40 Failed trial of labor, unspecified M ♀

O66.41 Failed attempted vaginal birth after previous cesarean delivery M ♀
Code first rupture of uterus, if applicable (O71.0-, O71.1)

O66.5 Attempted application of vacuum extractor and forceps M POA ♀
Attempted application of vacuum or forceps, with subsequent delivery by forceps or cesarean delivery

O66.6 Obstructed labor due to other multiple fetuses M ♀

O66.8 Other specified obstructed labor M ♀
Use additional code to identify cause of obstruction

O66.9 Obstructed labor, unspecified M ♀
Dystocia NOS
Fetal dystocia NOS
Maternal dystocia NOS

O67 Labor and delivery complicated by intrapartum hemorrhage, not elsewhere classified

EXCLUDES1 *antepartum hemorrhage NEC (O46.-)*
placenta previa (O44.-)
premature separation of placenta [abruptio placentae] (O45.-)

EXCLUDES2 *postpartum hemorrhage (O72.-)*

O67.0 Intrapartum hemorrhage with coagulation defect M MCC ♀
Intrapartum hemorrhage (excessive) associated with afibrinogenemia
Intrapartum hemorrhage (excessive) associated with disseminated intravascular coagulation
Intrapartum hemorrhage (excessive) associated with hyperfibrinolysis
Intrapartum hemorrhage (excessive) associated with hypofibrinogenemia

O67.8 Other intrapartum hemorrhage M ♀
Excessive intrapartum hemorrhage

O67.9 Intrapartum hemorrhage, unspecified M ♀

O68 Labor and delivery complicated by abnormality of fetal acid-base balance M CC ♀
Fetal acidemia complicating labor and delivery
Fetal acidosis complicating labor and delivery
Fetal alkalosis complicating labor and delivery
Fetal metabolic acidemia complicating labor and delivery

EXCLUDES1 *fetal stress NOS (O77.9)*
labor and delivery complicated by electrocardiographic evidence of fetal stress (O77.8)
labor and delivery complicated by ultrasonic evidence of fetal stress (O77.8)

EXCLUDES2 *abnormality in fetal heart rate or rhythm (O76)*
labor and delivery complicated by meconium in amniotic fluid (O77.0)

O69 Labor and delivery complicated by umbilical cord complications

One of the following 7th characters is to be assigned to each code under category O69. 7th character 0 is for single gestations and multiple gestations where the fetus is unspecified. 7th characters 1 through 9 are for cases of multiple gestations to identify the fetus for which the code applies. The appropriate code from category O30, Multiple gestation, must also be assigned when assigning a code from category O69 that has a 7th character of 1 through 9.

0 = not applicable or unspecified
1 = fetus 1
2 = fetus 2
3 = fetus 3
4 = fetus 4
5 = fetus 5
9 = other fetus

O69.0 Labor and delivery complicated by prolapse of cord M ♀

O69.1 Labor and delivery complicated by cord around neck, with compression M ♀

EXCLUDES1 *labor and delivery complicated by cord around neck, without compression (O69.81)*

O69.2 Labor and delivery complicated by other cord entanglement, with compression M ♀
Labor and delivery complicated by compression of cord NOS
Labor and delivery complicated by entanglement of cords of twins in monoamniotic sac
Labor and delivery complicated by knot in cord

EXCLUDES1 *labor and delivery complicated by other cord entanglement, without compression (O69.82)*

O69.3 Labor and delivery complicated by short cord M ♀

O69.4 Labor and delivery complicated by vasa previa M ♀
Labor and delivery complicated by hemorrhage from vasa previa

O69.5 Labor and delivery complicated by vascular lesion of cord M ♀
Labor and delivery complicated by cord bruising
Labor and delivery complicated by cord hematoma
Labor and delivery complicated by thrombosis of umbilical vessels

O69.8 Labor and delivery complicated by other cord complications

O69.81 Labor and delivery complicated by cord around neck, without compression M ♀

O69.82 Labor and delivery complicated by other cord entanglement, without compression M ♀

O69.89 Labor and delivery complicated by other cord complications M ♀

O69.9 Labor and delivery complicated by cord complication, unspecified M ♀

O70 Perineal laceration during delivery

INCLUDES *episiotomy extended by laceration*

EXCLUDES1 *obstetric high vaginal laceration alone (O71.4)*

O70.0 First degree perineal laceration during delivery M ♀
Perineal laceration, rupture or tear involving fourchette during delivery
Perineal laceration, rupture or tear involving labia during delivery
Perineal laceration, rupture or tear involving skin during delivery
Perineal laceration, rupture or tear involving vagina during delivery
Perineal laceration, rupture or tear involving vulva during delivery
Slight perineal laceration, rupture or tear during delivery

O70.1 Second degree perineal laceration during delivery M ♀
Perineal laceration, rupture or tear during delivery as in O70.0, also involving pelvic floor
Perineal laceration, rupture or tear during delivery as in O70.0, also involving perineal muscles
Perineal laceration, rupture or tear during delivery as in O70.0, also involving vaginal muscles

EXCLUDES1 *perineal laceration involving anal sphincter (O70.2)*

AHA: Q2, 2016

O70.2 Third degree perineal laceration during delivery
Perineal laceration, rupture or tear during delivery as in O70.1, also involving anal sphincter
Perineal laceration, rupture or tear during delivery as in O70.1, also involving rectovaginal septum
Perineal laceration, rupture or tear during delivery as in O70.1, also involving sphincter NOS

EXCLUDES1 *anal sphincter tear during delivery without third degree perineal laceration (O70.4)*
perineal laceration involving anal or rectal mucosa (O70.3)

● **O70.20 Third degree perineal laceration during delivery, unspecified** CC CC/MCC Exc

● **O70.21 Third degree perineal laceration during delivery, IIIa** CC CC/MCC Exc
Third degree perineal laceration during delivery with less than 50% of external anal sphincter (EAS) thickness torn

1st 1st trimester 2nd 2nd trimester 3rd 3rd trimester PDx Unacceptable principal diagnosis symbol per Medicare code edits
POA Code exempt from diagnosis present on admission requirement ? Questionable admission CC Complication or comorbidity
CC/MCC Exc CC/MCC exclusion MCC Major complication or comorbidity PDx CC Principal diagnosis as its own CC
PDx MCC Principal diagnosis as its own MCC Z1 Z code as first-listed diagnosis

● O70.22 **Third degree perineal laceration during delivery,** IIIb
Third degree perineal laceration during delivery with more than 50% external anal sphincter (EAS) thickness torn

● O70.23 **Third degree perineal laceration during delivery,** IIIc
Third degree perineal laceration during delivery with both external anal sphincter (EAS) and internal anal sphincter (IAS) torn

O70.3 Fourth degree **perineal laceration during delivery** M ♀
Perineal laceration, rupture or tear during delivery as in O70.2, also involving anal mucosa
Perineal laceration, rupture or tear during delivery as in O70.2, also involving rectal mucosa

O70.4 Anal sphincter tear **complicating delivery, not associated with third degree laceration** M ♀
EXCLUDES1 *anal sphincter tear with third degree perineal laceration (O70.2)*

O70.9 **Perineal laceration during delivery, unspecified** M ♀

O71 Other obstetric trauma
INCLUDES *obstetric damage from instruments*

O71.0 **Rupture of uterus (spontaneous)** before onset of labor
EXCLUDES1 *disruption of (current) cesarean delivery wound (O90.0)*
laceration of uterus, NEC (O71.81)

O71.00 **Rupture of uterus before onset of labor, unspecified trimester** M ♀

O71.02 **Rupture of uterus before onset of labor,** second trimester 2nd M ♀

O71.03 **Rupture of uterus before onset of labor,** third trimester 3rd M ♀

O71.1 **Rupture of uterus** during labor M ♀
Rupture of uterus not stated as occurring before onset of labor
EXCLUDES1 *disruption of cesarean delivery wound (O90.0)*
laceration of uterus, NEC (O71.81)

O71.2 **Postpartum** inversion of uterus M ♀

O71.3 **Obstetric** laceration of cervix M ♀
Annular detachment of cervix

O71.4 **Obstetric** high vaginal laceration **alone** M ♀
Laceration of vaginal wall without perineal laceration
EXCLUDES1 *obstetric high vaginal laceration with perineal laceration (O70.-)*

O71.5 **Other obstetric injury to pelvic organs** M ♀
Obstetric injury to bladder
Obstetric injury to urethra
EXCLUDES2 *obstetric periurethral trauma (O71.82)*

O71.6 **Obstetric damage to** pelvic joints and ligaments M ♀
Obstetric avulsion of inner symphyseal cartilage
Obstetric damage to coccyx
Obstetric traumatic separation of symphysis (pubis)

O71.7 **Obstetric** hematoma of pelvis M ♀
Obstetric hematoma of perineum
Obstetric hematoma of vagina
Obstetric hematoma of vulva

O71.8 **Other specified obstetric trauma**

O71.81 **Laceration of uterus, not elsewhere classified** M ♀

O71.82 **Other specified trauma to perineum and vulva** M ♀
Obstetric periurethral trauma

O71.89 **Other specified obstetric trauma** M ♀

O71.9 **Obstetric trauma, unspecified** M ♀

O72 Postpartum hemorrhage
INCLUDES *hemorrhage after delivery of fetus or infant*

O72.0 Third-stage **hemorrhage** M ♀
Hemorrhage associated with retained, trapped or adherent placenta
Retained placenta NOS
Code also type of adherent placenta (O43.2-)

O72.1 Other immediate **postpartum hemorrhage** M ♀
Hemorrhage following delivery of placenta
Postpartum hemorrhage (atonic) NOS
Uterine atony with hemorrhage
EXCLUDES1 *uterine atony NOS (O62.2)*
uterine atony without hemorrhage (O62.2)
postpartum atony of uterus without hemorrhage (O75.89)

O72.2 Delayed and secondary **postpartum hemorrhage** M ♀
Hemorrhage associated with retained portions of placenta or membranes after the first 24 hours following delivery of placenta
Retained products of conception NOS, following delivery

O72.3 **Postpartum** coagulation defects M ♀
Postpartum afibrinogenemia
Postpartum fibrinolysis

O73 Retained placenta and membranes, without hemorrhage
EXCLUDES1 *placenta accreta (O43.21-)*
placenta increta (O43.22-)
placenta percreta (O43.23-)

O73.0 **Retained** placenta **without hemorrhage** M ♀
Adherent placenta, without hemorrhage
Trapped placenta without hemorrhage

O73.1 **Retained** portions of placenta and membranes**, without hemorrhage** M ♀
Retained products of conception following delivery, without hemorrhage

O74 Complications of anesthesia during labor and delivery
INCLUDES *maternal complications arising from the administration of a general, regional or local anesthetic, analgesic or other sedation during labor and delivery*
Use additional code, if applicable, to identify specific complication

O74.0 Aspiration pneumonitis **due to anesthesia during labor and delivery** M ♀
Inhalation of stomach contents or secretions NOS due to anesthesia during labor and delivery
Mendelson's syndrome due to anesthesia during labor and delivery

O74.1 Other pulmonary complications **of anesthesia during labor and delivery** M ♀

O74.2 Cardiac complications **of anesthesia during labor and delivery** M ♀

O74.3 Central nervous system complications **of anesthesia during labor and delivery** M ♀

O74.4 Toxic reaction **to local anesthesia during labor and delivery** M ♀

O74.5 Spinal and epidural anesthesia-induced headache **during labor and delivery** M ♀

O74.6 **Other complications of** spinal and epidural anesthesia **during labor and delivery** M ♀

O74.7 Failed or difficult intubation **for anesthesia during labor and delivery** M ♀

O74.8 **Other complications of anesthesia during labor and delivery** M ♀

O74.9 **Complication of anesthesia during labor and delivery, unspecified** M ♀

O75 Other complications of labor and delivery, not elsewhere classified
EXCLUDES2 *puerperal (postpartum) infection (O86.-)*
puerperal (postpartum) sepsis (O85)

O75.0 **Maternal distress during labor and delivery** M ♀

O75.1 **Shock during or following labor and delivery** M ♀
Obstetric shock following labor and delivery

O75.2 **Pyrexia during labor, not elsewhere classified** M ♀

O75.3 **Other infection during labor** M ♀
Sepsis during labor
Use additional code (B95-B97), to identify infectious agent

O75.4 **Other complications of obstetric surgery and procedures** M ♀
Cardiac arrest following obstetric surgery or procedures
Cardiac failure following obstetric surgery or procedures
Cerebral anoxia following obstetric surgery or procedures
Pulmonary edema following obstetric surgery or procedures
Use additional code to identify specific complication
EXCLUDES2 *complications of anesthesia during labor and delivery (O74.-)*
disruption of obstetrical (surgical) wound (O90.0-O90.1)
hematoma of obstetrical (surgical) wound (O90.2)
infection of obstetrical (surgical) wound (O86.0)

O75.5 **Delayed delivery after artificial rupture of membranes** M ♀

O75.8 Other specified **complications of labor and delivery**

Unspecified Code | Other Specified Code | Manifestation Code | N Newborn | P Pediatric | M Maternity | A Adult | ♂ Male | ♀ Female
● New Code | ▲ Revised Code Title | ►◄ Revised Text | NOTES | INCLUDES | EXCLUDES1 Not coded here | EXCLUDES2 Not included here
4th character required | 5th character required | 6th character required | 7th character required
Extension 'X' Alert | HAC Hospital-acquired condition (HAC) alert | AHA AHA Coding Clinic©

O75.81 **Maternal exhaustion complicating labor and delivery**

O75.82 **Onset (spontaneous) of labor after 37 completed weeks of gestation but before 39 completed weeks gestation, with delivery by (planned) cesarean section**
Delivery by (planned) cesarean section occurring after 37 completed weeks of gestation but before 39 completed weeks gestation due to (spontaneous) onset of labor
Code first to specify reason for planned cesarean section such as:
cephalopelvic disproportion (normally formed fetus) (O33.9)
previous cesarean delivery (O34.21)

O75.89 **Other specified complications of labor and delivery**

O75.9 **Complication of labor and delivery, unspecified**

O76 **Abnormality in fetal heart rate and rhythm complicating labor and delivery**
Depressed fetal heart rate tones complicating labor and delivery
Fetal bradycardia complicating labor and delivery
Fetal heart rate decelerations complicating labor and delivery
Fetal heart rate irregularity complicating labor and delivery
Fetal heart rate abnormal variability complicating labor and delivery
Fetal tachycardia complicating labor and delivery
Non-reassuring fetal heart rate or rhythm complicating labor and delivery
EXCLUDES1 *fetal stress NOS (O77.9)*
labor and delivery complicated by electrocardiographic evidence of fetal stress (O77.8)
labor and delivery complicated by ultrasonic evidence of fetal stress (O77.8)
EXCLUDES2 *fetal metabolic acidemia (O68)*
other fetal stress (O77.0-O77.1)
AHA: Q4, 2013

O77 **Other fetal stress complicating labor and delivery**
AHA: Q4, 2013

O77.0 **Labor and delivery complicated by meconium in amniotic fluid**
AHA: Q4, 2013

O77.1 **Fetal stress in labor or delivery due to drug administration**

O77.8 **Labor and delivery complicated by other evidence of fetal stress**
Labor and delivery complicated by electrocardiographic evidence of fetal stress
Labor and delivery complicated by ultrasonic evidence of fetal stress
EXCLUDES1 *abnormality of fetal acid-base balance (O68)*
abnormality in fetal heart rate or rhythm (O76)
fetal metabolic acidemia (O68)

O77.9 **Labor and delivery complicated by fetal stress, unspecified**
EXCLUDES1 *abnormality of fetal acid-base balance (O68)*
abnormality in fetal heart rate or rhythm (O76)
fetal metabolic acidemia (O68)

Encounter for delivery (O80-O82)

O80 **Encounter for full-term uncomplicated delivery**
Delivery requiring minimal or no assistance, with or without episiotomy, without fetal manipulation [e.g., rotation version] or instrumentation [forceps] of a spontaneous, cephalic, vaginal, full-term, single, live-born infant. This code is for use as a single diagnosis code and is not to be used with any other code from chapter 15.
Use additional code to indicate outcome of delivery (Z37.0)

O82 **Encounter for cesarean delivery without indication**
Use additional code to indicate outcome of delivery (Z37.0)

Complications predominantly related to the puerperium (O85-O92)

EXCLUDES2 *mental and behavioral disorders associated with the puerperium (F53)*
obstetrical tetanus (A34)
puerperal osteomalacia (M83.0)

O85 **Puerperal sepsis**
Postpartum sepsis
Puerperal peritonitis
Puerperal pyemia
Use additional code (B95-B97), to identify infectious agent
Use additional code (R65.2-) to identify severe sepsis, if applicable
EXCLUDES1 *fever of unknown origin following delivery (O86.4)*
genital tract infection following delivery (O86.1-)
obstetric pyemic and septic embolism (O88.3-)
puerperal septic thrombophlebitis (O86.81)
urinary tract infection following delivery (O86.2-)
EXCLUDES2 *sepsis during labor (O75.3)*

O86 **Other puerperal infections**
Use additional code (B95-B97), to identify infectious agent
EXCLUDES2 *infection during labor (O75.3)*
obstetrical tetanus (A34)

O86.0 **Infection of obstetric surgical wound**
Infected cesarean delivery wound following delivery
Infected perineal repair following delivery

O86.1 **Other infection of genital tract following delivery**

O86.11 **Cervicitis following delivery**

O86.12 **Endometritis following delivery**

O86.13 **Vaginitis following delivery**

O86.19 **Other infection of genital tract following delivery**

O86.2 **Urinary tract infection following delivery**

O86.20 **Urinary tract infection following delivery, unspecified**
Puerperal urinary tract infection NOS

O86.21 **Infection of kidney following delivery**

O86.22 **Infection of bladder following delivery**
Infection of urethra following delivery

O86.29 **Other urinary tract infection following delivery**

O86.4 **Pyrexia of unknown origin following delivery**
Puerperal infection NOS following delivery
Puerperal pyrexia NOS following delivery
EXCLUDES2 *pyrexia during labor (O75.2)*

O86.8 **Other specified puerperal infections**

O86.81 **Puerperal septic thrombophlebitis**

O86.89 **Other specified puerperal infections**

O87 **Venous complications and hemorrhoids in the puerperium**
INCLUDES *venous complications in labor, delivery and the puerperium*
EXCLUDES2 *obstetric embolism (O88.-)*
puerperal septic thrombophlebitis (O86.81)
venous complications in pregnancy (O22.-)

O87.0 **Superficial thrombophlebitis in the puerperium**
Puerperal phlebitis NOS
Puerperal thrombosis NOS

O87.1 **Deep phlebothrombosis in the puerperium**
Deep vein thrombosis, postpartum
Pelvic thrombophlebitis, postpartum
Use additional code to identify the deep vein thrombosis (I82.4-, I82.5-, I82.62-. I82.72-)
Use additional code, if applicable, for associated long-term (current) use of anticoagulants (Z79.01)

O87.2 **Hemorrhoids in the puerperium**

O87.3 **Cerebral venous thrombosis in the puerperium**
Cerebrovenous sinus thrombosis in the puerperium

O87.4 **Varicose veins of lower extremity in the puerperium**

O87.8 **Other venous complications in the puerperium**
Genital varices in the puerperium

O87.9 **Venous complication in the puerperium, unspecified**
Puerperal phlebopathy NOS

O88 **Obstetric embolism**
EXCLUDES1 *embolism complicating abortion NOS (O03.2)*
embolism complicating ectopic or molar pregnancy (O08.2)
embolism complicating failed attempted abortion (O07.2)
embolism complicating induced abortion (O04.7)
embolism complicating spontaneous abortion (O03.2, O03.7)

1st 1st trimester · 2nd 2nd trimester · 3rd 3rd trimester · Unacceptable principal diagnosis symbol per Medicare code edits · Code exempt from diagnosis present on admission requirement · Questionable admission · Complication or comorbidity · CC/MCC exclusion · Major complication or comorbidity · Principal diagnosis as its own CC · Principal diagnosis as its own MCC · Z code as first-listed diagnosis

O88.0 Obstetric air embolism
O88.01 Obstetric air embolism in pregnancy
O88.011 Air embolism in pregnancy, first trimester
O88.012 Air embolism in pregnancy, second trimester
O88.013 Air embolism in pregnancy, third trimester
O88.019 Air embolism in pregnancy, unspecified trimester
O88.02 Air embolism in childbirth
O88.03 Air embolism in the puerperium
O88.1 Amniotic fluid embolism
Anaphylactoid syndrome in pregnancy
O88.11 Amniotic fluid embolism in pregnancy
O88.111 Amniotic fluid embolism in pregnancy, first trimester
O88.112 Amniotic fluid embolism in pregnancy, second trimester
O88.113 Amniotic fluid embolism in pregnancy, third trimester
O88.119 Amniotic fluid embolism in pregnancy, unspecified trimester
O88.12 Amniotic fluid embolism in childbirth
O88.13 Amniotic fluid embolism in the puerperium
O88.2 Obstetric thromboembolism
O88.21 Thromboembolism in pregnancy
Obstetric (pulmonary) embolism NOS
O88.211 Thromboembolism in pregnancy, first trimester
O88.212 Thromboembolism in pregnancy, second trimester
O88.213 Thromboembolism in pregnancy, third trimester
O88.219 Thromboembolism in pregnancy, unspecified trimester
O88.22 Thromboembolism in childbirth
O88.23 Thromboembolism in the puerperium
Puerperal (pulmonary) embolism NOS
O88.3 Obstetric pyemic and septic embolism
O88.31 Pyemic and septic embolism in pregnancy
O88.311 Pyemic and septic embolism in pregnancy, first trimester
O88.312 Pyemic and septic embolism in pregnancy, second trimester
O88.313 Pyemic and septic embolism in pregnancy, third trimester
O88.319 Pyemic and septic embolism in pregnancy, unspecified trimester
O88.32 Pyemic and septic embolism in childbirth
O88.33 Pyemic and septic embolism in the puerperium
O88.8 Other obstetric embolism
Obstetric fat embolism
O88.81 Other embolism in pregnancy
O88.811 Other embolism in pregnancy, first trimester
O88.812 Other embolism in pregnancy, second trimester
O88.813 Other embolism in pregnancy, third trimester
O88.819 Other embolism in pregnancy, unspecified trimester
O88.82 Other embolism in childbirth
O88.83 Other embolism in the puerperium
O89 Complications of anesthesia during the puerperium
INCLUDES *maternal complications arising from the administration of a general, regional or local anesthetic, analgesic or other sedation during the puerperium*
Use additional code, if applicable, to identify specific complication
O89.0 Pulmonary complications of anesthesia during the puerperium
O89.01 Aspiration pneumonitis due to anesthesia during the puerperium
Inhalation of stomach contents or secretions NOS due to anesthesia during the puerperium
Mendelson's syndrome due to anesthesia during the puerperium
O89.09 Other pulmonary complications of anesthesia during the puerperium
O89.1 Cardiac complications of anesthesia during the puerperium
O89.2 Central nervous system complications of anesthesia during the puerperium
O89.3 Toxic reaction to local anesthesia during the puerperium
O89.4 Spinal and epidural anesthesia-induced headache during the puerperium
O89.5 Other complications of spinal and epidural anesthesia during the puerperium
O89.6 Failed or difficult intubation for anesthesia during the puerperium
O89.8 Other complications of anesthesia during the puerperium
O89.9 Complication of anesthesia during the puerperium, unspecified
O90 Complications of the puerperium, not elsewhere classified
O90.0 Disruption of cesarean delivery wound
Dehiscence of cesarean delivery wound
EXCLUDES1 *rupture of uterus (spontaneous) before onset of labor (O71.0-)*
rupture of uterus during labor (O71.1)
O90.1 Disruption of perineal obstetric wound
Disruption of wound of episiotomy
Disruption of wound of perineal laceration
Secondary perineal tear
O90.2 Hematoma of obstetric wound
O90.3 Peripartum cardiomyopathy
Conditions in I42.- arising during pregnancy and the puerperium
EXCLUDES1 *pre-existing heart disease complicating pregnancy and the puerperium (O99.4-)*
O90.4 Postpartum acute kidney failure
Hepatorenal syndrome following labor and delivery
O90.5 Postpartum thyroiditis
O90.6 Postpartum mood disturbance
Postpartum blues
Postpartum dysphoria
Postpartum sadness
EXCLUDES1 *postpartum depression (F53)*
puerperal psychosis (F53)
O90.8 Other complications of the puerperium, not elsewhere classified
O90.81 Anemia of the puerperium
Postpartum anemia NOS
EXCLUDES1 *pre-existing anemia complicating the puerperium (O99.03)*
O90.89 Other complications of the puerperium, not elsewhere classified
Placental polyp
O90.9 Complication of the puerperium, unspecified
O91 Infections of breast associated with pregnancy, the puerperium and lactation
Use additional code to identify infection
O91.0 Infection of nipple associated with pregnancy, the puerperium and lactation
O91.01 Infection of nipple associated with pregnancy
Gestational abscess of nipple
O91.011 Infection of nipple associated with pregnancy, first trimester
O91.012 Infection of nipple associated with pregnancy, second trimester
O91.013 Infection of nipple associated with pregnancy, third trimester
O91.019 Infection of nipple associated with pregnancy, unspecified trimester
O91.02 Infection of nipple associated with the puerperium
Puerperal abscess of nipple
O91.03 Infection of nipple associated with lactation
Abscess of nipple associated with lactation

Unspecified Code Other Specified Code Manifestation Code N Newborn P Pediatric M Maternity A Adult ♂ Male ♀ Female
● New Code ▲ Revised Code Title ►◄ Revised Text NOTES INCLUDES EXCLUDES1 Not coded here EXCLUDES2 Not included here
4th character required 5th character required 6th character required 7th character required
Extension 'X' Alert HAC Hospital-acquired condition (HAC) alert AHA AHA Coding Clinic®

O91.1 Abscess of breast associated with pregnancy, the puerperium and lactation
O91.11 Abscess of breast associated with pregnancy
Gestational mammary abscess
Gestational purulent mastitis
Gestational subareolar abscess
O91.111 Abscess of breast associated with pregnancy, first trimester
O91.112 Abscess of breast associated with pregnancy, second trimester
O91.113 Abscess of breast associated with pregnancy, third trimester
O91.119 Abscess of breast associated with pregnancy, unspecified trimester
O91.12 Abscess of breast associated with the puerperium
Puerperal mammary abscess
Puerperal purulent mastitis
Puerperal subareolar abscess
O91.13 Abscess of breast associated with lactation
Mammary abscess associated with lactation
Purulent mastitis associated with lactation
Subareolar abscess associated with lactation
O91.2 Nonpurulent mastitis associated with pregnancy, the puerperium and lactation
O91.21 Nonpurulent mastitis associated with pregnancy
Gestational interstitial mastitis
Gestational lymphangitis of breast
Gestational mastitis NOS
Gestational parenchymatous mastitis
O91.211 Nonpurulent mastitis associated with pregnancy, first trimester
O91.212 Nonpurulent mastitis associated with pregnancy, second trimester
O91.213 Nonpurulent mastitis associated with pregnancy, third trimester
O91.219 Nonpurulent mastitis associated with pregnancy, unspecified trimester
O91.22 Nonpurulent mastitis associated with the puerperium
Puerperal interstitial mastitis
Puerperal lymphangitis of breast
Puerperal mastitis NOS
Puerperal parenchymatous mastitis
O91.23 Nonpurulent mastitis associated with lactation
Interstitial mastitis associated with lactation
Lymphangitis of breast associated with lactation
Mastitis NOS associated with lactation
Parenchymatous mastitis associated with lactation

O92 Other disorders of breast and disorders of lactation associated with pregnancy and the puerperium
O92.0 Retracted nipple associated with pregnancy, the puerperium, and lactation
O92.01 Retracted nipple associated with pregnancy
O92.011 Retracted nipple associated with pregnancy, first trimester
O92.012 Retracted nipple associated with pregnancy, second trimester
O92.013 Retracted nipple associated with pregnancy, third trimester
O92.019 Retracted nipple associated with pregnancy, unspecified trimester
O92.02 Retracted nipple associated with the puerperium
O92.03 Retracted nipple associated with lactation
O92.1 Cracked nipple associated with pregnancy, the puerperium, and lactation
Fissure of nipple, gestational or puerperal
O92.11 Cracked nipple associated with pregnancy
O92.111 Cracked nipple associated with pregnancy, first trimester
O92.112 Cracked nipple associated with pregnancy, second trimester
O92.113 Cracked nipple associated with pregnancy, third trimester
O92.119 Cracked nipple associated with pregnancy, unspecified trimester
O92.12 Cracked nipple associated with the puerperium
O92.13 Cracked nipple associated with lactation
O92.2 Other and unspecified disorders of breast associated with pregnancy and the puerperium
O92.20 Unspecified disorder of breast associated with pregnancy and the puerperium
O92.29 Other disorders of breast associated with pregnancy and the puerperium
O92.3 Agalactia
Primary agalactia
EXCLUDES1 *Elective agalactia (O92.5)*
Secondary agalactia (O92.5)
Therapeutic agalactia (O92.5)
O92.4 Hypogalactia
O92.5 Suppressed lactation
Elective agalactia
Secondary agalactia
Therapeutic agalactia
EXCLUDES1 *primary agalactia (O92.3)*
O92.6 Galactorrhea
O92.7 Other and unspecified disorders of lactation
O92.70 Unspecified disorders of lactation
O92.79 Other disorders of lactation
Puerperal galactocele

Other obstetric conditions, not elsewhere classified (O94-O9A)

O94 Sequelae of complication of pregnancy, childbirth, and the puerperium
NOTES This category is to be used to indicate conditions in O00-O77.-, O85-O94 and O98-O9A.- as the cause of late effects. The sequelae include conditions specified as such, or as late effects, which may occur at any time after the puerperium
Code first condition resulting from (sequela) of complication of pregnancy, childbirth, and the puerperium

O98 Maternal infectious and parasitic diseases classifiable elsewhere but complicating pregnancy, childbirth and the puerperium
INCLUDES *the listed conditions when complicating the pregnant state, when aggravated by the pregnancy, or as a reason for obstetric care*
Use additional code (Chapter 1), to identify specific infectious or parasitic disease
EXCLUDES2 *herpes gestationis (O26.4-)*
infectious carrier state (O99.82-, O99.83-)
obstetrical tetanus (A34)
puerperal infection (O86.-)
puerperal sepsis (O85)
when the reason for maternal care is that the disease is known or suspected to have affected the fetus (O35-O36)
O98.0 Tuberculosis complicating pregnancy, childbirth and the puerperium
Conditions in A15-A19
O98.01 Tuberculosis complicating pregnancy
O98.011 Tuberculosis complicating pregnancy, first trimester
O98.012 Tuberculosis complicating pregnancy, second trimester
O98.013 Tuberculosis complicating pregnancy, third trimester
O98.019 Tuberculosis complicating pregnancy, unspecified trimester
O98.02 Tuberculosis complicating childbirth
O98.03 Tuberculosis complicating the puerperium
O98.1 Syphilis complicating pregnancy, childbirth and the puerperium
Conditions in A50-A53
O98.11 Syphilis complicating pregnancy
O98.111 Syphilis complicating pregnancy, first trimester
O98.112 Syphilis complicating pregnancy, second trimester

1st trimester 2nd trimester 3rd trimester Unacceptable principal diagnosis symbol per Medicare code edits
Code exempt from diagnosis present on admission requirement Questionable admission Complication or comorbidity
CC/MCC exclusion Major complication or comorbidity Principal diagnosis as its own CC
Principal diagnosis as its own MCC Z code as first-listed diagnosis

O98.113 Syphilis complicating pregnancy, third trimester
O98.119 Syphilis complicating pregnancy, unspecified trimester
O98.12 Syphilis complicating childbirth
O98.13 Syphilis complicating the puerperium

O98.2 Gonorrhea complicating pregnancy, childbirth and the puerperium
Conditions in A54.-
O98.21 Gonorrhea complicating pregnancy
O98.211 Gonorrhea complicating pregnancy, first trimester
O98.212 Gonorrhea complicating pregnancy, second trimester
O98.213 Gonorrhea complicating pregnancy, third trimester
O98.219 Gonorrhea complicating pregnancy, unspecified trimester
O98.22 Gonorrhea complicating childbirth
O98.23 Gonorrhea complicating the puerperium

O98.3 Other infections with a predominantly sexual mode of transmission complicating pregnancy, childbirth and the puerperium
Conditions in A55-A64
O98.31 Other infections with a predominantly sexual mode of transmission complicating pregnancy
O98.311 Other infections with a predominantly sexual mode of transmission complicating pregnancy, first trimester
O98.312 Other infections with a predominantly sexual mode of transmission complicating pregnancy, second trimester
O98.313 Other infections with a predominantly sexual mode of transmission complicating pregnancy, third trimester
O98.319 Other infections with a predominantly sexual mode of transmission complicating pregnancy, unspecified trimester
O98.32 Other infections with a predominantly sexual mode of transmission complicating childbirth
O98.33 Other infections with a predominantly sexual mode of transmission complicating the puerperium

O98.4 Viral hepatitis complicating pregnancy, childbirth and the puerperium
Conditions in B15-B19
O98.41 Viral hepatitis complicating pregnancy
O98.411 Viral hepatitis complicating pregnancy, first trimester
O98.412 Viral hepatitis complicating pregnancy, second trimester
O98.413 Viral hepatitis complicating pregnancy, third trimester
O98.419 Viral hepatitis complicating pregnancy, unspecified trimester
O98.42 Viral hepatitis complicating childbirth
O98.43 Viral hepatitis complicating the puerperium

O98.5 Other viral diseases complicating pregnancy, childbirth and the puerperium
Conditions in A80-B09, B25-B34, R87.81-, R87.82-
EXCLUDES1 *human immunodeficiency virus [HIV] disease complicating pregnancy, childbirth and the puerperium (O98.7-)*
O98.51 Other viral diseases complicating pregnancy
O98.511 Other viral diseases complicating pregnancy, first trimester
O98.512 Other viral diseases complicating pregnancy, second trimester
O98.513 Other viral diseases complicating pregnancy, third trimester
O98.519 Other viral diseases complicating pregnancy, unspecified trimester
O98.52 Other viral diseases complicating childbirth
O98.53 Other viral diseases complicating the puerperium

O98.6 Protozoal diseases complicating pregnancy, childbirth and the puerperium
Conditions in B50-B64
O98.61 Protozoal diseases complicating pregnancy
O98.611 Protozoal diseases complicating pregnancy, first trimester
O98.612 Protozoal diseases complicating pregnancy, second trimester
O98.613 Protozoal diseases complicating pregnancy, third trimester
O98.619 Protozoal diseases complicating pregnancy, unspecified trimester
O98.62 Protozoal diseases complicating childbirth
O98.63 Protozoal diseases complicating the puerperium

O98.7 Human immunodeficiency virus [HIV] disease complicating pregnancy, childbirth and the puerperium
Use additional code to identify the type of HIV disease:
Acquired immune deficiency syndrome (AIDS) (B20)
Asymptomatic HIV status (Z21)
HIV positive NOS (Z21)
Symptomatic HIV disease (B20)
O98.71 Human immunodeficiency virus [HIV] disease complicating pregnancy
O98.711 Human immunodeficiency virus [HIV] disease complicating pregnancy, first trimester
O98.712 Human immunodeficiency virus [HIV] disease complicating pregnancy, second trimester
O98.713 Human immunodeficiency virus [HIV] disease complicating pregnancy, third trimester
O98.719 Human immunodeficiency virus [HIV] disease complicating pregnancy, unspecified trimester
O98.72 Human immunodeficiency virus [HIV] disease complicating childbirth
O98.73 Human immunodeficiency virus [HIV] disease complicating the puerperium

O98.8 Other maternal infectious and parasitic diseases complicating pregnancy, childbirth and the puerperium
O98.81 Other maternal infectious and parasitic diseases complicating pregnancy
O98.811 Other maternal infectious and parasitic diseases complicating pregnancy, first trimester
O98.812 Other maternal infectious and parasitic diseases complicating pregnancy, second trimester
O98.813 Other maternal infectious and parasitic diseases complicating pregnancy, third trimester
O98.819 Other maternal infectious and parasitic diseases complicating pregnancy, unspecified trimester
O98.82 Other maternal infectious and parasitic diseases complicating childbirth
O98.83 Other maternal infectious and parasitic diseases complicating the puerperium

O98.9 Unspecified maternal infectious and parasitic disease complicating pregnancy, childbirth and the puerperium
O98.91 Unspecified maternal infectious and parasitic disease complicating pregnancy
O98.911 Unspecified maternal infectious and parasitic disease complicating pregnancy, first trimester
O98.912 Unspecified maternal infectious and parasitic disease complicating pregnancy, second trimester
O98.913 Unspecified maternal infectious and parasitic disease complicating pregnancy, third trimester
O98.919 Unspecified maternal infectious and parasitic disease complicating pregnancy, unspecified trimester

Unspecified Code | Other Specified Code | Manifestation Code | N Newborn | P Pediatric | M Maternity | A Adult | ♂ Male | ♀ Female
● New Code | ▲ Revised Code Title | ►◄ Revised Text | NOTES | INCLUDES | EXCLUDES1 Not coded here | EXCLUDES2 Not included here
4th character required | 5th character required | 6th character required | 7th character required
Extension 'X' Alert | HAC Hospital-acquired condition (HAC) alert | AHA AHA Coding Clinic©

O98.92 **Unspecified maternal infectious and parasitic disease complicating childbirth** M CC ♀

O98.93 **Unspecified maternal infectious and parasitic disease complicating the puerperium** M CC ♀

(4th) **O99 Other maternal diseases classifiable elsewhere but complicating pregnancy, childbirth and the puerperium**

INCLUDES *conditions which complicate the pregnant state, are aggravated by the pregnancy or are a main reason for obstetric care*

Use additional code to identify specific condition

EXCLUDES2 *when the reason for maternal care is that the condition is known or suspected to have affected the fetus (O35-O36)*

(5th) O99.0 **Anemia complicating pregnancy, childbirth and the puerperium**

Conditions in D50-D64

EXCLUDES1 *anemia arising in the puerperium (O90.81)*
postpartum anemia NOS (O90.81)

(6th) O99.01 **Anemia complicating pregnancy**

O99.011 **Anemia complicating pregnancy, first trimester** 1st M ♀

O99.012 **Anemia complicating pregnancy, second trimester** 2nd M ♀

O99.013 **Anemia complicating pregnancy, third trimester** 3rd M ♀

O99.019 **Anemia complicating pregnancy, unspecified trimester** M ♀

O99.02 **Anemia complicating childbirth** M ♀

O99.03 **Anemia complicating the puerperium** M ♀

EXCLUDES1 *postpartum anemia not pre-existing prior to delivery (O90.81)*

(5th) O99.1 **Other diseases of the blood and blood-forming organs and certain disorders involving the immune mechanism complicating pregnancy, childbirth and the puerperium**

Conditions in D65-D89

EXCLUDES2 *hemorrhage with coagulation defects (O45.-, O46.0-, O67.0, O72.3)*

(6th) O99.11 **Other diseases of the blood and blood-forming organs and certain disorders involving the immune mechanism complicating pregnancy**

O99.111 **Other diseases of the blood and blood-forming organs and certain disorders involving the immune mechanism complicating pregnancy, first trimester** 1st M CC ♀

O99.112 **Other diseases of the blood and blood-forming organs and certain disorders involving the immune mechanism complicating pregnancy, second trimester** 2nd M CC ♀

O99.113 **Other diseases of the blood and blood-forming organs and certain disorders involving the immune mechanism complicating pregnancy, third trimester** 3rd M CC ♀

O99.119 **Other diseases of the blood and blood-forming organs and certain disorders involving the immune mechanism complicating pregnancy, unspecified trimester** M CC ♀

O99.12 **Other diseases of the blood and blood-forming organs and certain disorders involving the immune mechanism complicating childbirth** M CC ♀

O99.13 **Other diseases of the blood and blood-forming organs and certain disorders involving the immune mechanism complicating the puerperium** M CC ♀

(5th) O99.2 **Endocrine, nutritional and metabolic diseases complicating pregnancy, childbirth and the puerperium**

Conditions in E00-E88

EXCLUDES2 *diabetes mellitus (O24.-)*
malnutrition (O25.-)
postpartum thyroiditis (O90.5)

(6th) O99.21 **Obesity complicating pregnancy, childbirth, and the puerperium**

Use additional code to identify the type of obesity (E66.-)

O99.210 **Obesity complicating pregnancy, unspecified trimester** M ♀

O99.211 **Obesity complicating pregnancy, first trimester** 1st M ♀

O99.212 **Obesity complicating pregnancy, second trimester** 2nd M ♀

O99.213 **Obesity complicating pregnancy, third trimester** 3rd M ♀

O99.214 **Obesity complicating childbirth** M ♀

O99.215 **Obesity complicating the puerperium** M ♀

(6th) O99.28 **Other endocrine, nutritional and metabolic diseases complicating pregnancy, childbirth and the puerperium**

O99.280 **Endocrine, nutritional and metabolic diseases complicating pregnancy, unspecified trimester** M ♀

O99.281 **Endocrine, nutritional and metabolic diseases complicating pregnancy, first trimester** 1st M ♀

O99.282 **Endocrine, nutritional and metabolic diseases complicating pregnancy, second trimester** 2nd M ♀

O99.283 **Endocrine, nutritional and metabolic diseases complicating pregnancy, third trimester** 3rd M ♀

O99.284 **Endocrine, nutritional and metabolic diseases complicating childbirth** M ♀

O99.285 **Endocrine, nutritional and metabolic diseases complicating the puerperium** M ♀

(5th) O99.3 **Mental disorders and diseases of the nervous system complicating pregnancy, childbirth and the puerperium**

(6th) O99.31 **Alcohol use complicating pregnancy, childbirth, and the puerperium**

Use additional code(s) from F10 to identify manifestations of the alcohol use

O99.310 **Alcohol use complicating pregnancy, unspecified trimester** M ♀

O99.311 **Alcohol use complicating pregnancy, first trimester** 1st M ♀

O99.312 **Alcohol use complicating pregnancy, second trimester** 2nd M ♀

O99.313 **Alcohol use complicating pregnancy, third trimester** 3rd M ♀

O99.314 **Alcohol use complicating childbirth** M ♀

O99.315 **Alcohol use complicating the puerperium** M ♀

(6th) O99.32 **Drug use complicating pregnancy, childbirth, and the puerperium**

Use additional code(s) from F11-F16 and F18-F19 to identify manifestations of the drug use

O99.320 **Drug use complicating pregnancy, unspecified trimester** M ♀

O99.321 **Drug use complicating pregnancy, first trimester** 1st M CC ♀

O99.322 **Drug use complicating pregnancy, second trimester** 2nd M CC ♀

O99.323 **Drug use complicating pregnancy, third trimester** 3rd M CC ♀

O99.324 **Drug use complicating childbirth** M CC ♀

O99.325 **Drug use complicating the puerperium** M CC ♀

▲ (6th) O99.33 **►Tobacco use disorder◄ complicating pregnancy, childbirth, and the puerperium**

Smoking complicating pregnancy, childbirth, and the puerperium

Use additional code from category F17 to identify type of tobacco nicotine dependence

O99.330 **Smoking (tobacco) complicating pregnancy, unspecified trimester** M ♀

O99.331 **Smoking (tobacco) complicating pregnancy, first trimester** 1st M ♀

O99.332 **Smoking (tobacco) complicating pregnancy, second trimester** 2nd M ♀

O99.333 **Smoking (tobacco) complicating pregnancy, third trimester** 3rd M ♀

O99.334 **Smoking (tobacco) complicating childbirth** M ♀

O99.335 **Smoking (tobacco) complicating the puerperium** M ♀

1st 1st trimester 2nd 2nd trimester 3rd 3rd trimester PDx Unacceptable principal diagnosis symbol per Medicare code edits
POA Code exempt from diagnosis present on admission requirement ? Questionable admission CC Complication or comorbidity
CC/MCC Excl CC/MCC exclusion MCC Major complication or comorbidity PDx CC Principal diagnosis as its own CC
PDx MCC Principal diagnosis as its own MCC Z1 Z code as first-listed diagnosis

When symbols appear on a code that requires a 7th character extension, refer to Appendix D to identify applicable 7th character codes.

O99.34 Other mental disorders complicating pregnancy, childbirth, and the puerperium
Conditions in F01-F09 and F20-F99
EXCLUDES2 *postpartum mood disturbance (O90.6)*
postnatal psychosis (F53)
puerperal psychosis (F53)
O99.340 Other mental disorders complicating pregnancy, unspecified trimester M ♀
O99.341 Other mental disorders complicating pregnancy, first trimester 1st M ♀
O99.342 Other mental disorders complicating pregnancy, second trimester 2nd M ♀
O99.343 Other mental disorders complicating pregnancy, third trimester 3rd M ♀
O99.344 Other mental disorders complicating childbirth M ♀
O99.345 Other mental disorders complicating the puerperium M ♀
O99.35 Diseases of the nervous system complicating pregnancy, childbirth, and the puerperium
Conditions in G00-G99
EXCLUDES2 *pregnancy related peripheral neuritis (O26.8-)*
O99.350 Diseases of the nervous system complicating pregnancy, unspecified trimester M ♀
O99.351 Diseases of the nervous system complicating pregnancy, first trimester 1st M ♀
O99.352 Diseases of the nervous system complicating pregnancy, second trimester 2nd M ♀
O99.353 Diseases of the nervous system complicating pregnancy, third trimester 3rd M ♀
O99.354 Diseases of the nervous system complicating childbirth M CC ♀
O99.355 Diseases of the nervous system complicating the puerperium M CC ♀
O99.4 Diseases of the circulatory system complicating pregnancy, childbirth and the puerperium
Conditions in I00-I99
EXCLUDES1 *peripartum cardiomyopathy (O90.3)*
EXCLUDES2 *hypertensive disorders (O10-O16)*
obstetric embolism (O88.-)
venous complications and cerebrovenous sinus thrombosis in labor, childbirth and the puerperium (O87.-)
venous complications and cerebrovenous sinus thrombosis in pregnancy (O22.-)
O99.41 Diseases of the circulatory system complicating pregnancy
O99.411 Diseases of the circulatory system complicating pregnancy, first trimester 1st M CC ♀
O99.412 Diseases of the circulatory system complicating pregnancy, second trimester 2nd M CC ♀
O99.413 Diseases of the circulatory system complicating pregnancy, third trimester 3rd M CC ♀
O99.419 Diseases of the circulatory system complicating pregnancy, unspecified trimester M ♀
O99.42 Diseases of the circulatory system complicating childbirth M MCC ♀
O99.43 Diseases of the circulatory system complicating the puerperium M CC ♀
O99.5 Diseases of the respiratory system complicating pregnancy, childbirth and the puerperium
Conditions in J00-J99
O99.51 Diseases of the respiratory system complicating pregnancy
O99.511 Diseases of the respiratory system complicating pregnancy, first trimester 1st M ♀
O99.512 Diseases of the respiratory system complicating pregnancy, second trimester 2nd M ♀
O99.513 Diseases of the respiratory system complicating pregnancy, third trimester 3rd M ♀
O99.519 Diseases of the respiratory system complicating pregnancy, unspecified trimester M ♀
O99.52 Diseases of the respiratory system complicating childbirth M ♀
O99.53 Diseases of the respiratory system complicating the puerperium M ♀
O99.6 Diseases of the digestive system complicating pregnancy, childbirth and the puerperium
Conditions in K00-K93
EXCLUDES2 *hemorrhoids in pregnancy (O22.4-)*
liver and biliary tract disorders in pregnancy, childbirth and the puerperium (O26.6-)
O99.61 Diseases of the digestive system complicating pregnancy
O99.611 Diseases of the digestive system complicating pregnancy, first trimester 1st M ♀
O99.612 Diseases of the digestive system complicating pregnancy, second trimester 2nd M ♀
O99.613 Diseases of the digestive system complicating pregnancy, third trimester 3rd M ♀
O99.619 Diseases of the digestive system complicating pregnancy, unspecified trimester M ♀
O99.62 Diseases of the digestive system complicating childbirth M ♀
O99.63 Diseases of the digestive system complicating the puerperium M ♀
O99.7 Diseases of the skin and subcutaneous tissue complicating pregnancy, childbirth and the puerperium
Conditions in L00-L99
EXCLUDES2 *herpes gestationis (O26.4)*
pruritic urticarial papules and plaques of pregnancy (PUPPP) (O26.86)
O99.71 Diseases of the skin and subcutaneous tissue complicating pregnancy
O99.711 Diseases of the skin and subcutaneous tissue complicating pregnancy, first trimester 1st M ♀
O99.712 Diseases of the skin and subcutaneous tissue complicating pregnancy, second trimester 2nd M ♀
O99.713 Diseases of the skin and subcutaneous tissue complicating pregnancy, third trimester 3rd M ♀
O99.719 Diseases of the skin and subcutaneous tissue complicating pregnancy, unspecified trimester M ♀
O99.72 Diseases of the skin and subcutaneous tissue complicating childbirth M ♀
O99.73 Diseases of the skin and subcutaneous tissue complicating the puerperium M ♀
O99.8 Other specified diseases and conditions complicating pregnancy, childbirth and the puerperium
Conditions in D00-D48, H00-H95, M00-N99, and Q00-Q99
Use additional code to identify condition
EXCLUDES2 *genitourinary infections in pregnancy (O23.-)*
infection of genitourinary tract following delivery (O86.1-O86.3)
malignant neoplasm complicating pregnancy, childbirth and the puerperium (O9A.1-)
maternal care for known or suspected abnormality of maternal pelvic organs (O34.-)
postpartum acute kidney failure (O90.4)
traumatic injuries in pregnancy (O9A.2-)
O99.81 Abnormal glucose complicating pregnancy, childbirth and the puerperium
EXCLUDES1 *gestational diabetes (O24.4-)*

O99.810 Abnormal glucose complicating pregnancy M ♀
O99.814 Abnormal glucose complicating childbirth M ♀
O99.815 Abnormal glucose complicating the puerperium M ♀

O99.82 Streptococcus B carrier state complicating pregnancy, childbirth and the puerperium

EXCLUDES1 *Carrier of streptococcus group B (GBS) in a nonpregnant woman (Z22.330)*

O99.820 Streptococcus B carrier state complicating pregnancy M ♀ PDx
O99.824 Streptococcus B carrier state complicating childbirth M ♀
O99.825 Streptococcus B carrier state complicating the puerperium M ♀ PDx

O99.83 Other infection carrier state complicating pregnancy, childbirth and the puerperium
Use additional code to identify the carrier state (Z22.-)

O99.830 Other infection carrier state complicating pregnancy M cc ♀
O99.834 Other infection carrier state complicating childbirth M cc ♀
O99.835 Other infection carrier state complicating the puerperium M cc ♀

O99.84 Bariatric surgery status complicating pregnancy, childbirth and the puerperium
Gastric banding status complicating pregnancy, childbirth and the puerperium
Gastric bypass status for obesity complicating pregnancy, childbirth and the puerperium
Obesity surgery status complicating pregnancy, childbirth and the puerperium

O99.840 Bariatric surgery status complicating pregnancy, unspecified trimester M ♀
O99.841 Bariatric surgery status complicating pregnancy, first trimester 1st M ♀
O99.842 Bariatric surgery status complicating pregnancy, second trimester 2nd M ♀
O99.843 Bariatric surgery status complicating pregnancy, third trimester 3rd M ♀
O99.844 Bariatric surgery status complicating childbirth M ♀
O99.845 Bariatric surgery status complicating the puerperium M ♀

O99.89 Other specified diseases and conditions complicating pregnancy, childbirth and the puerperium M ♀

O9A Maternal malignant neoplasms, traumatic injuries and abuse classifiable elsewhere but complicating pregnancy, childbirth and the puerperium

O9A.1 Malignant neoplasm complicating pregnancy, childbirth and the puerperium
Conditions in C00-C96
Use additional code to identify neoplasm

EXCLUDES2 *maternal care for benign tumor of corpus uteri (O34.1-)*
maternal care for benign tumor of cervix (O34.4-)

O9A.11 Malignant neoplasm complicating pregnancy

O9A.111 Malignant neoplasm complicating pregnancy, first trimester 1st M ♀
O9A.112 Malignant neoplasm complicating pregnancy, second trimester 2nd M ♀
O9A.113 Malignant neoplasm complicating pregnancy, third trimester 3rd M ♀
O9A.119 Malignant neoplasm complicating pregnancy, unspecified trimester M ♀

O9A.12 Malignant neoplasm complicating childbirth M ♀
O9A.13 Malignant neoplasm complicating the puerperium M ♀
AHA: Q3, 2015

O9A.2 Injury, poisoning and certain other consequences of external causes complicating pregnancy, childbirth and the puerperium
Conditions in S00-T88, except T74 and T76
Use additional code(s) to identify the injury or poisoning

EXCLUDES2 *physical, sexual and psychological abuse complicating pregnancy, childbirth and the puerperium (O9A.3-, O9A.4-, O9A.5-)*

O9A.21 Injury, poisoning and certain other consequences of external causes complicating pregnancy

O9A.211 Injury, poisoning and certain other consequences of external causes complicating pregnancy, first trimester 1st M ♀
O9A.212 Injury, poisoning and certain other consequences of external causes complicating pregnancy, second trimester 2nd M ♀
O9A.213 Injury, poisoning and certain other consequences of external causes complicating pregnancy, third trimester 3rd M ♀
O9A.219 Injury, poisoning and certain other consequences of external causes complicating pregnancy, unspecified trimester M ♀

O9A.22 Injury, poisoning and certain other consequences of external causes complicating childbirth M ♀
O9A.23 Injury, poisoning and certain other consequences of external causes complicating the puerperium M ♀

O9A.3 Physical abuse complicating pregnancy, childbirth and the puerperium
Conditions in T74.11 or T76.11
Use additional code (if applicable):
to identify any associated current injury due to physical abuse
to identify the perpetrator of abuse (Y07.-)

EXCLUDES2 *sexual abuse complicating pregnancy, childbirth and the puerperium (O9A.4)*

O9A.31 Physical abuse complicating pregnancy

O9A.311 Physical abuse complicating pregnancy, first trimester 1st M ♀
O9A.312 Physical abuse complicating pregnancy, second trimester 2nd M ♀
O9A.313 Physical abuse complicating pregnancy, third trimester 3rd M ♀
O9A.319 Physical abuse complicating pregnancy, unspecified trimester M ♀

O9A.32 Physical abuse complicating childbirth M ♀
O9A.33 Physical abuse complicating the puerperium M ♀

O9A.4 Sexual abuse complicating pregnancy, childbirth and the puerperium
Conditions in T74.21 or T76.21
Use additional code (if applicable):
to identify any associated current injury due to sexual abuse
to identify the perpetrator of abuse (Y07.-)

O9A.41 Sexual abuse complicating pregnancy

O9A.411 Sexual abuse complicating pregnancy, first trimester 1st M ♀
O9A.412 Sexual abuse complicating pregnancy, second trimester 2nd M ♀
O9A.413 Sexual abuse complicating pregnancy, third trimester 3rd M ♀
O9A.419 Sexual abuse complicating pregnancy, unspecified trimester M ♀

O9A.42 Sexual abuse complicating childbirth M ♀
O9A.43 Sexual abuse complicating the puerperium M ♀

O9A.5 Psychological abuse complicating pregnancy, childbirth and the puerperium
Conditions in T74.31 or T76.31
Use additional code to identify the perpetrator of abuse (Y07.-)

O9A.51 Psychological abuse complicating pregnancy

O9A.511 Psychological abuse complicating pregnancy, first trimester 1st M ♀
O9A.512 Psychological abuse complicating pregnancy, second trimester 2nd M ♀
O9A.513 Psychological abuse complicating pregnancy, third trimester 3rd M ♀
O9A.519 Psychological abuse complicating pregnancy, unspecified trimester M ♀

O9A.52 Psychological abuse complicating childbirth M ♀
O9A.53 Psychological abuse complicating the puerperium M ♀

1st 1st trimester 2nd 2nd trimester 3rd 3rd trimester PDx Unacceptable principal diagnosis symbol per Medicare code edits
POA Code exempt from diagnosis present on admission requirement ? Questionable admission cc Complication or comorbidity
CC/MCC Exc CC/MCC exclusion MCC Major complication or comorbidity PDx CC Principal diagnosis as its own CC
PDx MCC Principal diagnosis as its own MCC Z1 Z code as first-listed diagnosis

 When symbols appear on a code that requires a 7th character extension, refer to Appendix D to identify applicable 7th character codes.

Chapter 16: Certain Conditions Originating in the Perinatal Period (P00-P96)

Guidelines for Assigning Codes From This Chapter

Chapter 16's title refers to the perinatal period, which includes the period before birth as well as 28 days after birth. But the key to properly applying these codes is understanding that you never use them on the maternal record. Use these for the specific patient (whether an infant or older) who has a condition with origins just before the patient was born or in the first four weeks of life.

List of Categories

- P00-P04: Newborn affected by maternal factors and by complications of pregnancy, labor, and delivery
- P05-P08: Disorders of newborn related to length of gestation and fetal growth
- P09: Abnormal findings on neonatal screening
- P10-P15: Birth trauma
- P19-P29: Respiratory and cardiovascular disorders specific to the perinatal period
- P35-P39: Infections specific to the perinatal period
- P50-P61: Hemorrhagic and hematological disorders of newborn
- P70-P74: Transitory endocrine and metabolic disorders specific to newborn
- P76-P78: Digestive system disorders of newborn
- P80-P83: Conditions involving the integument and temperature regulation of newborn
- P84: Other problems with newborn
- P90-P96: Other disorders originating in the perinatal period

Highlights From the ICD-10-CM Official Guidelines for Coding and Reporting

The Chapter 16 ICD-10-CM Official Guidelines for Coding and Reporting help you with assigning codes for conditions arising before birth and in the 28 days after. The information below is from Section I.C.16 of the 2017 Official Guidelines.

Factor In These 6 General Rules

The guidelines start with general rules for Chapter 16 coding:

1. You should never use Chapter 16 codes or codes from category Z38 (*Liveborn infants according to place of birth and type of delivery*) on the maternal record nor should you use Chapter 15 codes on a newborn record.
2. Code P95 (*Stillbirth*) is used only in facilities that record stillbirths separately. Do not use any other code with P95, and do not include it on the mother's record.
3. If a condition present at birth continues throughout the patient's life, Chapter 16 codes still apply.
4. On a newborn record, the delivering hospital reports the appropriate liveborn code from category Z38 (*Liveborn infants according to place of birth and type of delivery*). Then the hospital reports the appropriate Chapter 16 code followed by any relevant codes from other chapters that provide more details. Should the baby be transferred to another hospital, the receiving hospital should not assign Z38.- codes.
5. Chapter 16 includes codes for conditions caused by the birth process, not for community-acquired conditions. But if a condition could be either and the record doesn't specify, you should use a Chapter 16 code.
6. The Chapter 16 guidelines instruct you to report all clinically significant conditions noted on the routine newborn exam. In relation to the newborn exam, a condition is clinically significant if it requires any of the following:

- Clinical evaluation
- Therapy
- Diagnostic services
- An extended hospital stay
- Higher than normal nursing care and/or monitoring
- Watching because of the implications on the patient's future health.

Keep in mind that this last bullet in particular applies to coding the newborn exam, and you shouldn't assume it applies to coding in other areas.

Use Caution When Assigning Premature, Slow Fetal Growth, Malnutrition, and Low Birth Weight Codes

Note that the guidelines indicate that because providers have different definitions of prematurity, you should assign a prematurity code only when the provider documents prematurity.

Carefully check the documentation before you assign codes from categories P05 (*Disorders of newborn related to slow fetal growth and fetal malnutrition*) and P07 (*Disorders of newborn related to short gestation and low birth weight, not elsewhere classified*). Go by the documented birth weight and estimated gestational age. Keep these points in mind:

- Do not assign codes from the P05 category in combination with codes from P07.
- Code birth weight before gestational age, if both are documented, with appropriate codes from the P07 category.
- Codes from category P07 can be used for adults if their current health is impacted by those conditions.

See also Chapter 21 for more codes for other factors influencing health status..

Start With This Chapter for Newborn Sepsis

For newborn sepsis, you should report a code from category P36 (*Bacterial sepsis of newborn, includes congenital sepsis*), rather than codes from Chapter 1, Certain Infectious and Parasitic Diseases. If the documentation doesn't indicate whether the sepsis is congenital or community-acquired, the default is congenital, and you should assign a code from the P36 category. Most of the P36 code descriptors include the causative organism. However, if you have to use a code that does not identify the organism, you should add a code from category B95 (Streptococcus, Staphylococcus, and Enterococcus as the cause of diseases classified elsewhere) or B96 (Other bacterial agents as the cause of diseases classified elsewhere). If appropriate, you can use additional codes from R65.2- (*Severe sepsis*) to report severe sepsis and associated organ dysfunction.

Certain conditions originating in the perinatal period (P00-P96)

NOTES Codes from this chapter are for use on newborn records only, never on maternal records

INCLUDES *conditions that have their origin in the fetal or perinatal period (before birth through the first 28 days after birth) even if morbidity occurs later*

EXCLUDES2 *congenital malformations, deformations and chromosomal abnormalities (Q00-Q99)*
endocrine, nutritional and metabolic diseases (E00-E88)
injury, poisoning and certain other consequences of external causes (S00-T88)
neoplasms (C00-D49)
tetanus neonatorum (A33)

This chapter contains the following blocks:

P00-P04	Newborn affected by maternal factors and by complications of pregnancy, labor, and delivery
P05-P08	Disorders of newborn related to length of gestation and fetal growth
P09	Abnormal findings on neonatal screening
P10-P15	Birth trauma
P19-P29	Respiratory and cardiovascular disorders specific to the perinatal period
P35-P39	Infections specific to the perinatal period
P50-P61	Hemorrhagic and hematological disorders of newborn
P70-P74	Transitory endocrine and metabolic disorders specific to newborn
P76-P78	Digestive system disorders of newborn
P80-P83	Conditions involving the integument and temperature regulation of newborn
P84	Other problems with newborn
P90-P96	Other disorders originating in the perinatal period

Newborn affected by maternal factors and by complications of pregnancy, labor, and delivery (P00-P04)

NOTES ▶These codes are for use when the listed maternal conditions are specified as the cause of confirmed morbidity or potential morbidity which have their origin in the perinatal period (before birth through the first 28 days after birth).◀

▲ 4th **P00 ▶Newborn affected◀ by maternal conditions that may be unrelated to present pregnancy**
Code first any current condition in newborn
EXCLUDES2 *encounter for observation of newborn for suspected diseases and conditions ruled out (Z05.-)*
newborn affected by maternal complications of pregnancy (P01.-)
newborn affected by maternal endocrine and metabolic disorders (P70-P74)
newborn affected by noxious substances transmitted via placenta or breast milk (P04.-)

▲ P00.0 **▶Newborn affected◀ by maternal hypertensive disorders** N POA
▶Newborn affected◀ by maternal conditions classifiable to O10-O11, O13-O16

▲ P00.1 **▶Newborn affected◀ by maternal renal and urinary tract diseases** N POA
▶Newborn affected◀ by maternal conditions classifiable to N00-N39

▲ P00.2 **▶Newborn affected◀ by maternal infectious and parasitic diseases** N POA
▶Newborn affected◀ by maternal infectious disease classifiable to A00-B99, J09 and J10
EXCLUDES1 *infections specific to the perinatal period (P35-P39)*
maternal genital tract or other localized infections (P00.8)
AHA: Q3, 2015

▲ P00.3 **▶Newborn affected◀ by other maternal circulatory and respiratory diseases** N POA
▶Newborn affected◀ by maternal conditions classifiable to I00-I99, J00-J99, Q20-Q34 and not included in P00.0, P00.2

▲ P00.4 **▶Newborn affected◀ by maternal nutritional disorders** N POA
▶Newborn affected◀ by maternal disorders classifiable to E40-E64
Maternal malnutrition NOS

▲ P00.5 **▶Newborn affected◀ by maternal injury** N POA
▶Newborn affected◀ by maternal conditions classifiable to O9A.2-

▲ P00.6 **▶Newborn affected◀ by surgical procedure on mother** N POA
▶Newborn affected◀ by amniocentesis
EXCLUDES1 *Cesarean delivery for present delivery (P03.4)*
damage to placenta from amniocentesis, Cesarean delivery or surgical induction (P02.1)
previous surgery to uterus or pelvic organs (P03.89)
EXCLUDES2 *newborn affected by complication of (fetal) intrauterine procedure (P96.5)*

▲ P00.7 **▶Newborn affected◀ by other medical procedures on mother, not elsewhere classified** N POA
▶Newborn affected◀ by radiation to mother
EXCLUDES1 *damage to placenta from amniocentesis, cesarean delivery or surgical induction (P02.1)*
newborn affected by other complications of labor and delivery (P03.-)

▲ 5th P00.8 **▶Newborn affected◀ by other maternal conditions**

▲ P00.81 **▶Newborn affected◀ by periodontal disease in mother** N POA

▲ P00.89 **▶Newborn affected◀ by other maternal conditions** N POA
▶Newborn affected◀ by conditions classifiable to T80-T88
▶Newborn affected◀ by maternal genital tract or other localized infections
▶Newborn affected◀ by maternal systemic lupus erythematosus

▲ P00.9 **▶Newborn affected◀ by unspecified maternal condition** N POA

▲ 4th **P01 ▶Newborn affected◀ by maternal complications of pregnancy**
Code first any current condition in newborn
EXCLUDES2 *encounter for observation of newborn for suspected diseases and conditions ruled out (Z05.-)*

▲ P01.0 **▶Newborn affected◀ by incompetent cervix** N

▲ P01.1 **▶Newborn affected◀ by premature rupture of membranes** N

▲ P01.2 **▶Newborn affected◀ by oligohydramnios** N
EXCLUDES1 *oligohydramnios due to premature rupture of membranes (P01.1)*

▲ P01.3 **▶Newborn affected◀ by polyhydramnios** N
▶Newborn affected◀ by hydramnios

▲ P01.4 **▶Newborn affected◀ by ectopic pregnancy** N
▶Newborn affected◀ by abdominal pregnancy

▲ P01.5 **▶Newborn affected◀ by multiple pregnancy** N
▶Newborn affected◀ by triplet (pregnancy)
▶Newborn affected◀ by twin (pregnancy)

▲ P01.6 **▶Newborn affected◀ by maternal death** N

▲ P01.7 **▶Newborn affected◀ by malpresentation before labor** N
▶Newborn affected◀ by breech presentation before labor
▶Newborn affected◀ by external version before labor
▶Newborn affected◀ by face presentation before labor
▶Newborn affected◀ by transverse lie before labor
▶Newborn affected◀ by unstable lie before labor

▲ P01.8 **▶Newborn affected◀ by other maternal complications of pregnancy** N

▲ P01.9 **▶Newborn affected◀ by maternal complication of pregnancy, unspecified** N

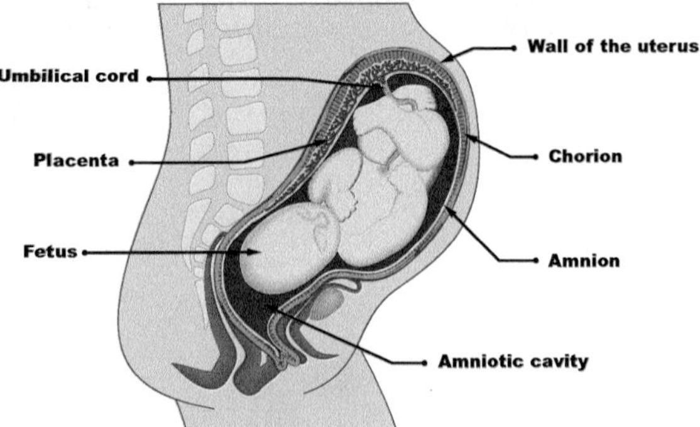

Figure 16.1 Uterine cavity

▲ P02 ▶Newborn affected◀ by complications of placenta, cord and membranes
Code first any current condition in newborn
EXCLUDES2 *encounter for observation of newborn for suspected diseases and conditions ruled out (Z05.-)*

▲ P02.0 ▶Newborn affected◀ by placenta previa N

▲ P02.1 ▶Newborn affected◀ by other forms of placental separation and hemorrhage N
▶Newborn affected◀ by abruptio placenta
▶Newborn affected◀ by accidental hemorrhage
▶Newborn affected◀ by antepartum hemorrhage
▶Newborn affected◀ by damage to placenta from amniocentesis, cesarean delivery or surgical induction
▶Newborn affected◀ by maternal blood loss
▶Newborn affected◀ by premature separation of placenta

▲ P02.2 ▶Newborn affected◀ by other and unspecified morphological and functional abnormalities of placenta

▲ P02.20 ▶Newborn affected◀ by unspecified morphological and functional abnormalities of placenta N

▲ P02.29 ▶Newborn affected◀ by other morphological and functional abnormalities of placenta N
▶Newborn affected◀ by placental dysfunction
▶Newborn affected◀ by placental infarction
▶Newborn affected◀ by placental insufficiency

▲ P02.3 ▶Newborn affected◀ by placental transfusion syndromes N
▶Newborn affected◀ by placental and cord abnormalities resulting in twin-to-twin or other transplacental transfusion

▲ P02.4 ▶Newborn affected◀ by prolapsed cord N

▲ P02.5 ▶Newborn affected◀ by other compression of umbilical cord N
▶Newborn affected◀ by umbilical cord (tightly) around neck
▶Newborn affected◀ by entanglement of umbilical cord
▶Newborn affected◀ by knot in umbilical cord

▲ P02.6 ▶Newborn affected◀ by other and unspecified conditions of umbilical cord

▲ P02.60 ▶Newborn affected◀ by unspecified conditions of umbilical cord N

▲ P02.69 ▶Newborn affected◀ by other conditions of umbilical cord N
▶Newborn affected◀ by short umbilical cord
▶Newborn affected◀ by vasa previa
EXCLUDES1 *newborn affected by single umbilical artery (Q27.0)*

▲ P02.7 ▶Newborn affected◀ by chorioamnionitis N
▶Newborn affected◀ by amnionitis
▶Newborn affected◀ by membranitis
▶Newborn affected◀ by placentitis

▲ P02.8 ▶Newborn affected◀ by other abnormalities of membranes N

▲ P02.9 ▶Newborn affected◀ by abnormality of membranes, unspecified N

▲ P03 ▶Newborn affected◀ by other complications of labor and delivery
Code first any current condition in newborn
EXCLUDES2 *encounter for observation of newborn for suspected diseases and conditions ruled out (Z05.-)*

▲ P03.0 ▶Newborn affected◀ by breech delivery and extraction N

▲ P03.1 ▶Newborn affected◀ by other malpresentation, malposition and disproportion during labor and delivery N
▶Newborn affected◀ by contracted pelvis
▶Newborn affected◀ by conditions classifiable to O64-O66
▶Newborn affected◀ by persistent occipitoposterior
▶Newborn affected◀ by transverse lie

▲ P03.2 ▶Newborn affected◀ by forceps delivery N

▲ P03.3 ▶Newborn affected◀ by delivery by vacuum extractor [ventouse] N

▲ P03.4 ▶Newborn affected◀ by Cesarean delivery N

▲ P03.5 ▶Newborn affected◀ by precipitate delivery N
▶Newborn affected◀ by rapid second stage

▲ P03.6 ▶Newborn affected◀ by abnormal uterine contractions N
▶Newborn affected◀ by conditions classifiable to O62.-, except O62.3
▶Newborn affected◀ by hypertonic labor
▶Newborn affected◀ by uterine inertia

▲ P03.8 ▶Newborn affected◀ by other specified complications of labor and delivery

▲ P03.81 ▶Newborn affected◀ by abnormality in fetal (intrauterine) heart rate or rhythm
EXCLUDES1 *neonatal cardiac dysrhythmia (P29.1-)*

▲ P03.810 ▶Newborn affected◀ by abnormality in fetal (intrauterine) heart rate or rhythm before the onset of labor N

▲ P03.811 ▶Newborn affected◀ by abnormality in fetal (intrauterine) heart rate or rhythm during labor N

▲ P03.819 ▶Newborn affected◀ by abnormality in fetal (intrauterine) heart rate or rhythm, unspecified as to time of onset N

P03.82 Meconium passage during delivery N
EXCLUDES1 *meconium aspiration (P24.00, P24.01)*
meconium staining (P96.83)

▲ P03.89 ▶Newborn affected◀ by other specified complications of labor and delivery N
▶Newborn affected◀ by abnormality of maternal soft tissues
▶Newborn affected◀ by conditions classifiable to O60-O75 and by procedures used in labor and delivery not included in P02.- and P03.0-P03.6
▶Newborn affected◀ by induction of labor

▲ P03.9 ▶Newborn affected◀ by complication of labor and delivery, unspecified N

▲ P04 ▶Newborn affected◀ by noxious substances transmitted via placenta or breast milk
INCLUDES *nonteratogenic effects of substances transmitted via placenta*
EXCLUDES2 *congenital malformations (Q00-Q99)*
encounter for observation of newborn for suspected diseases and conditions ruled out (Z05.-)
neonatal jaundice from excessive hemolysis due to drugs or toxins transmitted from mother (P58.4)
newborn in contact with and (suspected) exposures hazardous to health not transmitted via placenta or breast milk (Z77.-)

▲ P04.0 ▶Newborn affected◀ by maternal anesthesia and analgesia in pregnancy, labor and delivery N
▶Newborn affected◀ by reactions and intoxications from maternal opiates and tranquilizers administered during labor and delivery

▲ P04.1 ▶Newborn affected◀ by other maternal medication N
▶Newborn affected◀ by cancer chemotherapy
▶Newborn affected◀ by cytotoxic drugs
EXCLUDES1 *dysmorphism due to warfarin (Q86.2)*
fetal hydantoin syndrome (Q86.1)
maternal use of drugs of addiction (P04.4-)

▲ P04.2 ▶Newborn affected◀ by maternal use of tobacco N
▶Newborn affected◀ by exposure in utero to tobacco smoke
EXCLUDES2 *newborn exposure to environmental tobacco smoke (P96.81)*

▲ P04.3 ▶Newborn affected◀ by maternal use of alcohol N
EXCLUDES1 *fetal alcohol syndrome (Q86.0)*

▲ P04.4 Newborn affected by maternal use of drugs of addiction

▲ P04.41 ▶Newborn affected◀ by maternal use of cocaine N
'Crack baby'

▲ P04.49 ▶Newborn affected◀ by maternal use of other drugs of addiction N
EXCLUDES2 *▶Newborn affected◀ by maternal anesthesia and analgesia (P04.0)*
withdrawal symptoms from maternal use of drugs of addiction (P96.1)

▲ P04.5 ▶Newborn affected◀ by maternal use of nutritional chemical substances N

▲ P04.6 ▶Newborn affected◀ by maternal exposure to environmental chemical substances N

▲ P04.8 ▶Newborn affected◀ by other maternal noxious substances N

▲ P04.9 ▶Newborn affected◀ by maternal noxious substance, unspecified N

Disorders of newborn related to length of gestation and fetal growth (P05-P08)

P05 Disorders of newborn related to slow fetal growth and fetal malnutrition

P05.0 Newborn light for gestational age
Newborn light-for-dates
Weight below but length above 10th percentile for gestational age

Unspecified Code Other Specified Code Manifestation Code N Newborn P Pediatric M Maternity A Adult ♂ Male ♀ Female
● New Code ▲ Revised Code Title ▶◀ Revised Text NOTES INCLUDES EXCLUDES1 Not coded here EXCLUDES2 Not included here
4th character required 5th character required 6th character required 7th character required
Extension 'X' Alert HAC Hospital-acquired condition (HAC) alert AHA AHA Coding Clinic©

P05.00 **Newborn light for gestational age, unspecified weight** N
P05.01 **Newborn light for gestational age,** less than 500 grams N
P05.02 **Newborn light for gestational age,** 500-749 grams N
P05.03 **Newborn light for gestational age,** 750-999 grams N
P05.04 **Newborn light for gestational age,** 1000-1249 grams N
P05.05 **Newborn light for gestational age,** 1250-1499 grams N
P05.06 **Newborn light for gestational age,** 1500-1749 grams N
P05.07 **Newborn light for gestational age,** 1750-1999 grams N
P05.08 **Newborn light for gestational age,** 2000-2499 grams N
● P05.09 **Newborn light for gestational age,** 2500 grams and over
Newborn light for gestational age, other

P05.1 **Newborn small for gestational age**
Newborn small-and-light-for-dates
Newborn small-for-dates
Weight and length below 10th percentile for gestational age
P05.10 **Newborn small for gestational age, unspecified weight** N
P05.11 **Newborn small for gestational age,** less than 500 grams N
P05.12 **Newborn small for gestational age,** 500-749 grams N
P05.13 **Newborn small for gestational age,** 750-999 grams N
P05.14 **Newborn small for gestational age,** 1000-1249 grams N
P05.15 **Newborn small for gestational age,** 1250-1499 grams N
P05.16 **Newborn small for gestational age,** 1500-1749 grams N
P05.17 **Newborn small for gestational age,** 1750-1999 grams N
P05.18 **Newborn small for gestational age,** 2000-2499 grams N
● P05.19 **Newborn small for gestational age, other**
Newborn small for gestational age, 2500 grams and over

P05.2 **Newborn affected by fetal (intrauterine) malnutrition not light or small for gestational age** N
Infant, not light or small for gestational age, showing signs of fetal malnutrition, such as dry, peeling skin and loss of subcutaneous tissue
EXCLUDES1 *newborn affected by fetal malnutrition with light for gestational age (P05.0-)*
newborn affected by fetal malnutrition with small for gestational age (P05.1-)

P05.9 **Newborn affected by slow intrauterine growth, unspecified** N
Newborn affected by fetal growth retardation NOS

P07 **Disorders of newborn related to short gestation and low birth weight, not elsewhere classified**
NOTES When both birth weight and gestational age of the newborn are available, both should be coded with birth weight sequenced before gestational age
INCLUDES *the listed conditions, without further specification, as the cause of morbidity or additional care, in newborn*

P07.0 Extremely low **birth weight newborn**
Newborn birth weight 999 g. or less
EXCLUDES1 *low birth weight due to slow fetal growth and fetal malnutrition (P05.-)*
P07.00 **Extremely low birth weight newborn, unspecified weight** N
P07.01 **Extremely low birth weight newborn,** less than 500 grams N
P07.02 **Extremely low birth weight newborn,** 500-749 grams N
P07.03 **Extremely low birth weight newborn,** 750-999 grams N

P07.1 Other low **birth weight newborn**
Newborn birth weight 1000-2499 g.
EXCLUDES1 *low birth weight due to slow fetal growth and fetal malnutrition (P05.-)*
P07.10 **Other low birth weight newborn, unspecified weight** N
P07.14 **Other low birth weight newborn,** 1000-1249 grams N
P07.15 **Other low birth weight newborn,** 1250-1499 grams N
P07.16 **Other low birth weight newborn,** 1500-1749 grams N
P07.17 **Other low birth weight newborn,** 1750-1999 grams N
P07.18 **Other low birth weight newborn,** 2000-2499 grams N

P07.2 Extreme immaturity **of newborn**
Less than 28 completed weeks (less than 196 completed days) of gestation.
P07.20 **Extreme immaturity of newborn, unspecified weeks of gestation** N
Gestational age less than 28 completed weeks NOS
P07.21 **Extreme immaturity of newborn, gestational age** less than 23 completed weeks N
Extreme immaturity of newborn, gestational age less than 23 weeks, 0 days
P07.22 **Extreme immaturity of newborn, gestational age** 23 completed weeks N
Extreme immaturity of newborn, gestational age 23 weeks, 0 days through 23 weeks, 6 days
P07.23 **Extreme immaturity of newborn, gestational age** 24 completed weeks N
Extreme immaturity of newborn, gestational age 24 weeks, 0 days through 24 weeks, 6 days
P07.24 **Extreme immaturity of newborn, gestational age** 25 completed weeks N
Extreme immaturity of newborn, gestational age 25 weeks, 0 days through 25 weeks, 6 days
P07.25 **Extreme immaturity of newborn, gestational age** 26 completed weeks N
Extreme immaturity of newborn, gestational age 26 weeks, 0 days through 26 weeks, 6 days
P07.26 **Extreme immaturity of newborn, gestational age** 27 completed weeks N
Extreme immaturity of newborn, gestational age 27 weeks, 0 days through 27 weeks, 6 days

P07.3 Preterm **[premature] newborn [other]**
28 completed weeks or more but less than 37 completed weeks (196 completed days but less than 259 completed days) of gestation.
Prematurity NOS
P07.30 **Preterm newborn, unspecified weeks of gestation** N
P07.31 **Preterm newborn, gestational age** 28 completed weeks N
Preterm newborn, gestational age 28 weeks, 0 days through 28 weeks, 6 days
P07.32 **Preterm newborn, gestational age** 29 completed weeks N
Preterm newborn, gestational age 29 weeks, 0 days through 29 weeks, 6 days
P07.33 **Preterm newborn, gestational age** 30 completed weeks N
Preterm newborn, gestational age 30 weeks, 0 days through 30 weeks, 6 days
P07.34 **Preterm newborn, gestational age** 31 completed weeks N
Preterm newborn, gestational age 31 weeks, 0 days through 31 weeks, 6 days
P07.35 **Preterm newborn, gestational age** 32 completed weeks N
Preterm newborn, gestational age 32 weeks, 0 days through 32 weeks, 6 days
P07.36 **Preterm newborn, gestational age** 33 completed weeks N
Preterm newborn, gestational age 33 weeks, 0 days through 33 weeks, 6 days
P07.37 **Preterm newborn, gestational age** 34 completed weeks N
Preterm newborn, gestational age 34 weeks, 0 days through 34 weeks, 6 days

Unacceptable principal diagnosis symbol per Medicare code edits · Code exempt from diagnosis present on admission requirement
Questionable admission · Complication or comorbidity · CC/MCC exclusion · Major complication or comorbidity
Principal diagnosis as its own CC · Principal diagnosis as its own MCC · Z code as first-listed diagnosis

P07.38 **Preterm newborn, gestational age 35 completed weeks** N
Preterm newborn, gestational age 35 weeks, 0 days through 35 weeks, 6 days

P07.39 **Preterm newborn, gestational age 36 completed weeks** N
Preterm newborn, gestational age 36 weeks, 0 days through 36 weeks, 6 days

P08 Disorders of newborn related to long gestation and high birth weight

NOTES When both birth weight and gestational age of the newborn are available, priority of assignment should be given to birth weight

INCLUDES *the listed conditions, without further specification, as causes of morbidity or additional care, in newborn*

P08.0 **Exceptionally large newborn baby** N
Usually implies a birth weight of 4500 g. or more
EXCLUDES1 *syndrome of infant of diabetic mother (P70.1)*
syndrome of infant of mother with gestational diabetes (P70.0)

P08.1 **Other heavy for gestational age newborn** N
Other newborn heavy- or large-for-dates regardless of period of gestation
Usually implies a birth weight of 4000 g. to 4499 g.
EXCLUDES1 *newborn with a birth weight of 4500 or more (P08.0)*
syndrome of infant of diabetic mother (P70.1)
syndrome of infant of mother with gestational diabetes (P70.0).

P08.2 **Late newborn, not heavy for gestational age**

P08.21 **Post-term newborn** N
Newborn with gestation period over 40 completed weeks to 42 completed weeks

P08.22 **Prolonged gestation of newborn** N
Newborn with gestation period over 42 completed weeks (294 days or more), not heavy- or large-for-dates.
Postmaturity NOS

Abnormal findings on neonatal screening (P09)

P09 **Abnormal findings on neonatal screening** N
Use additional code to identify signs, symptoms and conditions associated with the screening
EXCLUDES2 *nonspecific serologic evidence of human immunodeficiency virus [HIV] (R75)*

Birth trauma (P10-P15)

P10 Intracranial laceration and hemorrhage due to birth injury
EXCLUDES1 *intracranial hemorrhage of newborn NOS (P52.9)*
intracranial hemorrhage of newborn due to anoxia or hypoxia (P52.-)
nontraumatic intracranial hemorrhage of newborn (P52.-)

P10.0 **Subdural hemorrhage due to birth injury** N MCC
Subdural hematoma (localized) due to birth injury
EXCLUDES1 *subdural hemorrhage accompanying tentorial tear (P10.4)*

P10.1 **Cerebral hemorrhage due to birth injury** N MCC

P10.2 **Intraventricular hemorrhage due to birth injury** N CC

P10.3 **Subarachnoid hemorrhage due to birth injury** N MCC

P10.4 **Tentorial tear due to birth injury** N MCC

P10.8 **Other intracranial lacerations and hemorrhages due to birth injury** N MCC

P10.9 **Unspecified intracranial laceration and hemorrhage due to birth injury** N MCC

P11 Other birth injuries to central nervous system

P11.0 **Cerebral edema due to birth injury** N MCC

P11.1 **Other specified brain damage due to birth injury** N

P11.2 **Unspecified brain damage due to birth injury** N MCC

P11.3 **Birth injury to facial nerve** N
Facial palsy due to birth injury

P11.4 **Birth injury to other cranial nerves** N

P11.5 **Birth injury to spine and spinal cord** N
Fracture of spine due to birth injury

P11.9 **Birth injury to central nervous system, unspecified** N MCC

P12 Birth injury to scalp

P12.0 **Cephalhematoma due to birth injury** N

P12.1 **Chignon (from vacuum extraction) due to birth injury** N

P12.2 **Epicranial subaponeurotic hemorrhage due to birth injury** N CC
Subgaleal hemorrhage

P12.3 **Bruising of scalp due to birth injury** N

P12.4 **Injury of scalp of newborn due to monitoring equipment** N
Sampling incision of scalp of newborn
Scalp clip (electrode) injury of newborn

P12.8 **Other birth injuries to scalp**

P12.81 **Caput succedaneum** N

P12.89 **Other birth injuries to scalp** N

P12.9 **Birth injury to scalp, unspecified** N

P13 Birth injury to skeleton
EXCLUDES2 *birth injury to spine (P11.5)*

P13.0 **Fracture of skull due to birth injury** N

P13.1 **Other birth injuries to skull** N
EXCLUDES1 *cephalhematoma (P12.0)*

P13.2 **Birth injury to femur** N

P13.3 **Birth injury to other long bones** N

P13.4 **Fracture of clavicle due to birth injury** N

P13.8 **Birth injuries to other parts of skeleton** N

P13.9 **Birth injury to skeleton, unspecified** N

P14 Birth injury to peripheral nervous system

P14.0 **Erb's paralysis due to birth injury** N

P14.1 **Klumpke's paralysis due to birth injury** N

P14.2 **Phrenic nerve paralysis due to birth injury** N

P14.3 **Other brachial plexus birth injuries** N

P14.8 **Birth injuries to other parts of peripheral nervous system** N

P14.9 **Birth injury to peripheral nervous system, unspecified** N

P15 Other birth injuries

P15.0 **Birth injury to liver** N
Rupture of liver due to birth injury

P15.1 **Birth injury to spleen** N
Rupture of spleen due to birth injury

P15.2 **Sternomastoid injury due to birth injury** N

P15.3 **Birth injury to eye** N
Subconjunctival hemorrhage due to birth injury
Traumatic glaucoma due to birth injury

P15.4 **Birth injury to face** N
Facial congestion due to birth injury

P15.5 **Birth injury to external genitalia** N

P15.6 **Subcutaneous fat necrosis due to birth injury** N

P15.8 **Other specified birth injuries** N

P15.9 **Birth injury, unspecified** N

Respiratory and cardiovascular disorders specific to the perinatal period (P19-P29)

P19 Metabolic acidemia in newborn
INCLUDES *metabolic acidemia in newborn*

P19.0 **Metabolic acidemia in newborn first noted before onset of labor** N

P19.1 **Metabolic acidemia in newborn first noted during labor** N

P19.2 **Metabolic acidemia noted at birth** N

P19.9 **Metabolic acidemia, unspecified** N

P22 Respiratory distress of newborn
EXCLUDES1 *respiratory arrest of newborn (P28.81)*
respiratory failure of newborn NOS (P28.5)

P22.0 **Respiratory distress syndrome of newborn** N MCC
Cardiorespiratory distress syndrome of newborn
Hyaline membrane disease
Idiopathic respiratory distress syndrome [IRDS or RDS] of newborn
Pulmonary hypoperfusion syndrome
Respiratory distress syndrome, type I

P22.1 **Transient tachypnea of newborn** N
Idiopathic tachypnea of newborn
Respiratory distress syndrome, type II
Wet lung syndrome

Unspecified Code Other Specified Code Manifestation Code N Newborn P Pediatric M Maternity A Adult ♂ Male ♀ Female
● New Code ▲ Revised Code Title ►◄ Revised Text NOTES INCLUDES EXCLUDES1 Not coded here EXCLUDES2 Not included here
4th character required 5th character required 6th character required 7th character required
Extension 'X' Alert HAC Hospital-acquired condition (HAC) alert AHA AHA Coding Clinic©

P22.8 Other respiratory distress of newborn N
P22.9 **Respiratory distress of newborn, unspecified** N

P23 Congenital pneumonia
INCLUDES *infective pneumonia acquired in utero or during birth*
EXCLUDES1 *neonatal pneumonia resulting from aspiration (P24.-)*
P23.0 Congenital pneumonia due to viral agent N MCC
Use additional code (B97) to identify organism
EXCLUDES1 *congenital rubella pneumonitis (P35.0)*
P23.1 Congenital pneumonia due to Chlamydia N MCC
P23.2 Congenital pneumonia due to staphylococcus N MCC
P23.3 Congenital pneumonia due to streptococcus, group B N MCC
P23.4 Congenital pneumonia due to Escherichia coli N MCC
P23.5 Congenital pneumonia due to Pseudomonas N MCC
P23.6 Congenital pneumonia due to other bacterial agents N MCC
Congenital pneumonia due to Hemophilus influenzae
Congenital pneumonia due to Klebsiella pneumoniae
Congenital pneumonia due to Mycoplasma
Congenital pneumonia due to Streptococcus, except group B
Use additional code (B95-B96) to identify organism
P23.8 Congenital pneumonia due to other organisms N MCC
P23.9 **Congenital pneumonia, unspecified** N MCC

P24 Neonatal aspiration
INCLUDES *aspiration in utero and during delivery*
P24.0 Meconium aspiration
EXCLUDES1 *meconium passage (without aspiration) during delivery (P03.82)*
meconium staining (P96.83)
P24.00 Meconium aspiration without respiratory symptoms N
Meconium aspiration NOS
P24.01 Meconium aspiration with respiratory symptoms N MCC
Meconium aspiration pneumonia
Meconium aspiration pneumonitis
Meconium aspiration syndrome NOS
Use additional code to identify any secondary pulmonary hypertension, if applicable (I27.2)
P24.1 Neonatal aspiration of (clear) amniotic fluid and mucus
Neonatal aspiration of liquor (amnii)
P24.10 Neonatal aspiration of (clear) amniotic fluid and mucus without respiratory symptoms N
Neonatal aspiration of amniotic fluid and mucus NOS
P24.11 Neonatal aspiration of (clear) amniotic fluid and mucus with respiratory symptoms N MCC
Neonatal aspiration of amniotic fluid and mucus with pneumonia
Neonatal aspiration of amniotic fluid and mucus with pneumonitis
Use additional code to identify any secondary pulmonary hypertension, if applicable (I27.2)
P24.2 Neonatal aspiration of blood
P24.20 Neonatal aspiration of blood without respiratory symptoms N
Neonatal aspiration of blood NOS
P24.21 Neonatal aspiration of blood with respiratory symptoms N MCC
Neonatal aspiration of blood with pneumonia
Neonatal aspiration of blood with pneumonitis
Use additional code to identify any secondary pulmonary hypertension, if applicable (I27.2)
P24.3 Neonatal aspiration of milk and regurgitated food
Neonatal aspiration of stomach contents
P24.30 Neonatal aspiration of milk and regurgitated food without respiratory symptoms N
Neonatal aspiration of milk and regurgitated food NOS
P24.31 Neonatal aspiration of milk and regurgitated food with respiratory symptoms N MCC
Neonatal aspiration of milk and regurgitated food with pneumonia
Neonatal aspiration of milk and regurgitated food with pneumonitis
Use additional code to identify any secondary pulmonary hypertension, if applicable (I27.2)
P24.8 Other neonatal aspiration
P24.80 Other neonatal aspiration without respiratory symptoms N
Neonatal aspiration NEC
P24.81 Other neonatal aspiration with respiratory symptoms N MCC
Neonatal aspiration pneumonia NEC
Neonatal aspiration with pneumonitis NEC
Neonatal aspiration with pneumonia NOS
Neonatal aspiration with pneumonitis NOS
Use additional code to identify any secondary pulmonary hypertension, if applicable (I27.2)
P24.9 **Neonatal aspiration, unspecified** N

P25 Interstitial emphysema and related conditions originating in the perinatal period
P25.0 Interstitial emphysema originating in the perinatal period N MCC
P25.1 Pneumothorax originating in the perinatal period N MCC
P25.2 Pneumomediastinum originating in the perinatal period N MCC
P25.3 Pneumopericardium originating in the perinatal period N MCC
P25.8 Other conditions related to interstitial emphysema originating in the perinatal period N MCC

P26 Pulmonary hemorrhage originating in the perinatal period
EXCLUDES1 *acute idiopathic hemorrhage in infants over 28 days old (R04.81)*
P26.0 Tracheobronchial hemorrhage originating in the perinatal period N MCC
P26.1 Massive pulmonary hemorrhage originating in the perinatal period N MCC
P26.8 Other pulmonary hemorrhages originating in the perinatal period N MCC
P26.9 **Unspecified pulmonary hemorrhage originating in the perinatal period** N MCC

P27 Chronic respiratory disease originating in the perinatal period
EXCLUDES1 *respiratory distress of newborn (P22.0-P22.9)*
P27.0 Wilson-Mikity syndrome MCC
Pulmonary dysmaturity
P27.1 Bronchopulmonary dysplasia originating in the perinatal period MCC
P27.8 Other chronic respiratory diseases originating in the perinatal period MCC
Congenital pulmonary fibrosis
Ventilator lung in newborn
P27.9 **Unspecified chronic respiratory disease originating in the perinatal period** MCC

P28 Other respiratory conditions originating in the perinatal period
EXCLUDES1 *congenital malformations of the respiratory system (Q30-Q34)*
P28.0 Primary atelectasis of newborn N CC
Primary failure to expand terminal respiratory units
Pulmonary hypoplasia associated with short gestation
Pulmonary immaturity NOS
P28.1 Other and unspecified atelectasis of newborn
P28.10 **Unspecified atelectasis of newborn** N CC
Atelectasis of newborn NOS
P28.11 Resorption atelectasis without respiratory distress syndrome N CC
EXCLUDES1 *resorption atelectasis with respiratory distress syndrome (P22.0)*
P28.19 Other atelectasis of newborn N CC
Partial atelectasis of newborn
Secondary atelectasis of newborn
P28.2 Cyanotic attacks of newborn N CC
EXCLUDES1 *apnea of newborn (P28.3-P28.4)*
P28.3 Primary sleep apnea of newborn N CC
Central sleep apnea of newborn
Obstructive sleep apnea of newborn
Sleep apnea of newborn NOS
P28.4 Other apnea of newborn N CC
Apnea of prematurity
Obstructive apnea of newborn
EXCLUDES1 *obstructive sleep apnea of newborn (P28.3)*
P28.5 Respiratory failure of newborn N MCC
EXCLUDES1 *respiratory arrest of newborn (P28.81)*
respiratory distress of newborn (P22.0-)

Unacceptable principal diagnosis symbol per Medicare code edits · Code exempt from diagnosis present on admission requirement
Questionable admission · CC Complication or comorbidity · CC/MCC exclusion · MCC Major complication or comorbidity
Principal diagnosis as its own CC · Principal diagnosis as its own MCC · Z code as first-listed diagnosis

P28.8 Other specified respiratory conditions of newborn
- P28.81 Respiratory arrest of newborn
- P28.89 Other specified respiratory conditions of newborn
  - Congenital laryngeal stridor
  - Sniffles in newborn
  - Snuffles in newborn
  - EXCLUDES1 *early congenital syphilitic rhinitis (A50.05)*

P28.9 Respiratory condition of newborn, unspecified
- Respiratory depression in newborn

P29 Cardiovascular disorders originating in the perinatal period
- EXCLUDES1 *congenital malformations of the circulatory system (Q20-Q28)*

P29.0 Neonatal cardiac failure

P29.1 Neonatal cardiac dysrhythmia
- P29.11 Neonatal tachycardia
- P29.12 Neonatal bradycardia

P29.2 Neonatal hypertension

P29.3 Persistent fetal circulation
- Delayed closure of ductus arteriosus
- (Persistent) pulmonary hypertension of newborn

P29.4 Transient myocardial ischemia in newborn

P29.8 Other cardiovascular disorders originating in the perinatal period
- P29.81 Cardiac arrest of newborn
- P29.89 Other cardiovascular disorders originating in the perinatal period

P29.9 Cardiovascular disorder originating in the perinatal period, unspecified

Infections specific to the perinatal period (P35-P39)

Infections acquired in utero, during birth via the umbilicus, or during the first 28 days after birth

EXCLUDES2 *asymptomatic human immunodeficiency virus [HIV] infection status (Z21)*
congenital gonococcal infection (A54.-)
congenital pneumonia (P23.-)
congenital syphilis (A50.-)
human immunodeficiency virus [HIV] disease (B20)
infant botulism (A48.51)
infectious diseases not specific to the perinatal period (A00-B99, J09, J10.-)
intestinal infectious disease (A00-A09)
laboratory evidence of human immunodeficiency virus [HIV] (R75)
tetanus neonatorum (A33)

P35 Congenital viral diseases
- INCLUDES *infections acquired in utero or during birth*

P35.0 Congenital rubella syndrome
- Congenital rubella pneumonitis

P35.1 Congenital cytomegalovirus infection

P35.2 Congenital herpesviral [herpes simplex] infection

P35.3 Congenital viral hepatitis

P35.8 Other congenital viral diseases
- Congenital varicella [chickenpox]

P35.9 Congenital viral disease, unspecified

P36 Bacterial sepsis of newborn
- INCLUDES *congenital sepsis*
- Use additional code(s), if applicable, to identify severe sepsis (R65.2-) and associated acute organ dysfunction(s)

P36.0 Sepsis of newborn due to streptococcus, group B

P36.1 Sepsis of newborn due to other and unspecified streptococci
- P36.10 Sepsis of newborn due to unspecified streptococci
- P36.19 Sepsis of newborn due to other streptococci

P36.2 Sepsis of newborn due to Staphylococcus aureus

P36.3 Sepsis of newborn due to other and unspecified staphylococci
- P36.30 Sepsis of newborn due to unspecified staphylococci
- P36.39 Sepsis of newborn due to other staphylococci

P36.4 Sepsis of newborn due to Escherichia coli

P36.5 Sepsis of newborn due to anaerobes

P36.8 Other bacterial sepsis of newborn
- Use additional code from category B96 to identify organism

P36.9 Bacterial sepsis of newborn, unspecified

P37 Other congenital infectious and parasitic diseases
- EXCLUDES2 *congenital syphilis (A50.-)*
  infectious neonatal diarrhea (A00-A09)
  necrotizing enterocolitis in newborn (P77.-)
  noninfectious neonatal diarrhea (P78.3)
  ophthalmia neonatorum due to gonococcus (A54.31)
  tetanus neonatorum (A33)

P37.0 Congenital tuberculosis

P37.1 Congenital toxoplasmosis
- Hydrocephalus due to congenital toxoplasmosis

P37.2 Neonatal (disseminated) listeriosis

P37.3 Congenital falciparum malaria

P37.4 Other congenital malaria

P37.5 Neonatal candidiasis

P37.8 Other specified congenital infectious and parasitic diseases

P37.9 Congenital infectious or parasitic disease, unspecified

P38 Omphalitis of newborn
- EXCLUDES1 *omphalitis not of newborn (L08.82)*
  tetanus omphalitis (A33)
  umbilical hemorrhage of newborn (P51.-)

P38.1 Omphalitis with mild hemorrhage

P38.9 Omphalitis without hemorrhage
- Omphalitis of newborn NOS

P39 Other infections specific to the perinatal period
- Use additional code to identify organism or specific infection

P39.0 Neonatal infective mastitis
- EXCLUDES1 *breast engorgement of newborn (P83.4)*
  noninfective mastitis of newborn (P83.4)

P39.1 Neonatal conjunctivitis and dacryocystitis
- Neonatal chlamydial conjunctivitis
- Ophthalmia neonatorum NOS
- EXCLUDES1 *gonococcal conjunctivitis (A54.31)*

P39.2 Intra-amniotic infection affecting newborn, not elsewhere classified

P39.3 Neonatal urinary tract infection

P39.4 Neonatal skin infection
- Neonatal pyoderma
- EXCLUDES1 *pemphigus neonatorum (L00)*
  staphylococcal scalded skin syndrome (L00)

P39.8 Other specified infections specific to the perinatal period

P39.9 Infection specific to the perinatal period, unspecified

Hemorrhagic and hematological disorders of newborn (P50-P61)

EXCLUDES1 *congenital stenosis and stricture of bile ducts (Q44.3)*
Crigler-Najjar syndrome (E80.5)
Dubin-Johnson syndrome (E80.6)
Gilbert syndrome (E80.4)
hereditary hemolytic anemias (D55-D58)

P50 Newborn affected by intrauterine (fetal) blood loss
- EXCLUDES1 *congenital anemia from intrauterine (fetal) blood loss (P61.3)*

P50.0 Newborn affected by intrauterine (fetal) blood loss from vasa previa

P50.1 Newborn affected by intrauterine (fetal) blood loss from ruptured cord

P50.2 Newborn affected by intrauterine (fetal) blood loss from placenta

P50.3 Newborn affected by hemorrhage into co-twin

P50.4 Newborn affected by hemorrhage into maternal circulation

P50.5 Newborn affected by intrauterine (fetal) blood loss from cut end of co-twin's cord

Unspecified Code | Other Specified Code | Manifestation Code | N Newborn | P Pediatric | M Maternity | A Adult | ♂ Male | ♀ Female
● New Code | ▲ Revised Code Title | ►◄ Revised Text | NOTES | INCLUDES | EXCLUDES1 Not coded here | EXCLUDES2 Not included here
4th character required | 5th character required | 6th character required | 7th character required
Extension 'X' Alert | HAC Hospital-acquired condition (HAC) alert | AHA AHA Coding Clinic©

P50.8 Newborn affected by other intrauterine (fetal) blood loss N
P50.9 Newborn affected by intrauterine (fetal) blood loss, unspecified N
Newborn affected by fetal hemorrhage NOS

P51 Umbilical hemorrhage of newborn
EXCLUDES1 *omphalitis with mild hemorrhage (P38.1)*
umbilical hemorrhage from cut end of co-twins cord (P50.5)
P51.0 Massive umbilical hemorrhage of newborn N
P51.8 Other umbilical hemorrhages of newborn N
Slipped umbilical ligature NOS
P51.9 Umbilical hemorrhage of newborn, unspecified N

P52 Intracranial nontraumatic hemorrhage of newborn
INCLUDES *intracranial hemorrhage due to anoxia or hypoxia*
EXCLUDES1 *intracranial hemorrhage due to birth injury (P10.-)*
intracranial hemorrhage due to other injury (S06.-)
P52.0 Intraventricular (nontraumatic) hemorrhage, grade 1, of newborn N CC
Subependymal hemorrhage (without intraventricular extension)
Bleeding into germinal matrix
P52.1 Intraventricular (nontraumatic) hemorrhage, grade 2, of newborn N CC
Subependymal hemorrhage with intraventricular extension
Bleeding into ventricle
P52.2 Intraventricular (nontraumatic) hemorrhage, grade 3 and grade 4, of newborn
P52.21 Intraventricular (nontraumatic) hemorrhage, grade 3, of newborn N MCC
Subependymal hemorrhage with intraventricular extension with enlargement of ventricle
P52.22 Intraventricular (nontraumatic) hemorrhage, grade 4, of newborn N MCC
Bleeding into cerebral cortex
Subependymal hemorrhage with intracerebral extension
P52.3 Unspecified intraventricular (nontraumatic) hemorrhage of newborn N CC
P52.4 Intracerebral (nontraumatic) hemorrhage of newborn N MCC
P52.5 Subarachnoid (nontraumatic) hemorrhage of newborn N MCC
P52.6 Cerebellar (nontraumatic) and posterior fossa hemorrhage of newborn N MCC
P52.8 Other intracranial (nontraumatic) hemorrhages of newborn N MCC
P52.9 Intracranial (nontraumatic) hemorrhage of newborn, unspecified N MCC

P53 Hemorrhagic disease of newborn N CC
Vitamin K deficiency of newborn
AHA: Q4, 2004

P54 Other neonatal hemorrhages
EXCLUDES1 *newborn affected by (intrauterine) blood loss (P50.-)*
pulmonary hemorrhage originating in the perinatal period (P26.-)
P54.0 Neonatal hematemesis N
EXCLUDES1 *neonatal hematemesis due to swallowed maternal blood (P78.2)*
P54.1 Neonatal melena N MCC
EXCLUDES1 *neonatal melena due to swallowed maternal blood (P78.2)*
P54.2 Neonatal rectal hemorrhage N MCC
P54.3 Other neonatal gastrointestinal hemorrhage N MCC
P54.4 Neonatal adrenal hemorrhage N CC
P54.5 Neonatal cutaneous hemorrhage N
Neonatal bruising
Neonatal ecchymoses
Neonatal petechiae
Neonatal superficial hematomata
EXCLUDES2 *bruising of scalp due to birth injury (P12.3)*
cephalhematoma due to birth injury (P12.0)
P54.6 Neonatal vaginal hemorrhage N ♀
Neonatal pseudomenses
P54.8 Other specified neonatal hemorrhages N
P54.9 Neonatal hemorrhage, unspecified N

P55 Hemolytic disease of newborn
P55.0 Rh isoimmunization of newborn N
P55.1 ABO isoimmunization of newborn N
AHA: Q3, 2015
P55.8 Other hemolytic diseases of newborn N
P55.9 Hemolytic disease of newborn, unspecified N

P56 Hydrops fetalis due to hemolytic disease
EXCLUDES1 *hydrops fetalis NOS (P83.2)*
P56.0 Hydrops fetalis due to isoimmunization N MCC
P56.9 Hydrops fetalis due to other and unspecified hemolytic disease
P56.90 Hydrops fetalis due to unspecified hemolytic disease N MCC
P56.99 Hydrops fetalis due to other hemolytic disease N MCC

P57 Kernicterus
P57.0 Kernicterus due to isoimmunization N MCC
P57.8 Other specified kernicterus N MCC
EXCLUDES1 *Crigler-Najjar syndrome (E80.5)*
P57.9 Kernicterus, unspecified N MCC

P58 Neonatal jaundice due to other excessive hemolysis
EXCLUDES1 *jaundice due to isoimmunization (P55-P57)*
P58.0 Neonatal jaundice due to bruising N
P58.1 Neonatal jaundice due to bleeding N
P58.2 Neonatal jaundice due to infection N
P58.3 Neonatal jaundice due to polycythemia N
P58.4 Neonatal jaundice due to drugs or toxins transmitted from mother or given to newborn
Code first poisoning due to drug or toxin, if applicable (T36-T65 with fifth or sixth character 1-4 or 6)
Use additional code for adverse effect, if applicable, to identify drug (T36-T50 with fifth or sixth character 5)
P58.41 Neonatal jaundice due to drugs or toxins transmitted from mother N
P58.42 Neonatal jaundice due to drugs or toxins given to newborn N
P58.5 Neonatal jaundice due to swallowed maternal blood N
P58.8 Neonatal jaundice due to other specified excessive hemolysis N
P58.9 Neonatal jaundice due to excessive hemolysis, unspecified N

P59 Neonatal jaundice from other and unspecified causes
EXCLUDES1 *jaundice due to inborn errors of metabolism (E70-E88)*
kernicterus (P57.-)
P59.0 Neonatal jaundice associated with preterm delivery N
Hyperbilirubinemia of prematurity
Jaundice due to delayed conjugation associated with preterm delivery
P59.1 Inspissated bile syndrome N MCC
P59.2 Neonatal jaundice from other and unspecified hepatocellular damage
EXCLUDES1 *congenital viral hepatitis (P35.3)*
P59.20 Neonatal jaundice from unspecified hepatocellular damage N MCC
P59.29 Neonatal jaundice from other hepatocellular damage N MCC
Neonatal giant cell hepatitis
Neonatal (idiopathic) hepatitis
P59.3 Neonatal jaundice from breast milk inhibitor N
P59.8 Neonatal jaundice from other specified causes N
P59.9 Neonatal jaundice, unspecified N
Neonatal physiological jaundice (intense)(prolonged) NOS
AHA: Q3, 2015

P60 Disseminated intravascular coagulation of newborn N MCC
Defibrination syndrome of newborn

P61 Other perinatal hematological disorders
EXCLUDES1 *transient hypogammaglobulinemia of infancy (D80.7)*
P61.0 Transient neonatal thrombocytopenia N MCC
Neonatal thrombocytopenia due to exchange transfusion
Neonatal thrombocytopenia due to idiopathic maternal thrombocytopenia
Neonatal thrombocytopenia due to isoimmunization
P61.1 Polycythemia neonatorum N
P61.2 Anemia of prematurity N CC
P61.3 Congenital anemia from fetal blood loss N CC

Unacceptable principal diagnosis symbol per Medicare code edits · Code exempt from diagnosis present on admission requirement · Questionable admission · CC Complication or comorbidity · CC/MCC exclusion · MCC Major complication or comorbidity · Principal diagnosis as its own CC · Principal diagnosis as its own MCC · Z code as first-listed diagnosis

 When symbols appear on a code that requires a 7th character extension, refer to Appendix D to identify applicable 7th character codes.

P61.4 **Other congenital anemias, not elsewhere classified** N CC
Congenital anemia NOS
P61.5 **Transient neonatal neutropenia** N MCC
EXCLUDES1 *congenital neutropenia (nontransient) (D70.0)*
P61.6 **Other transient neonatal disorders of coagulation** N CC
P61.8 **Other specified perinatal hematological disorders** N
P61.9 **Perinatal hematological disorder, unspecified** N

Transitory endocrine and metabolic disorders specific to newborn (P70-P74)

INCLUDES *transitory endocrine and metabolic disturbances caused by the infant's response to maternal endocrine and metabolic factors, or its adjustment to extrauterine environment*

P70 **Transitory disorders of carbohydrate metabolism specific to newborn**
P70.0 **Syndrome of infant of mother with gestational diabetes** N
Newborn (with hypoglycemia) affected by maternal gestational diabetes
EXCLUDES1 *newborn (with hypoglycemia) affected by maternal (pre-existing) diabetes mellitus (P70.1)*
syndrome of infant of a diabetic mother (P70.1)
P70.1 **Syndrome of infant of a diabetic mother** N
Newborn (with hypoglycemia) affected by maternal (pre-existing) diabetes mellitus
EXCLUDES1 *newborn (with hypoglycemia) affected by maternal gestational diabetes (P70.0)*
syndrome of infant of mother with gestational diabetes (P70.0)
P70.2 **Neonatal diabetes mellitus** N CC
P70.3 **Iatrogenic neonatal hypoglycemia** N
P70.4 **Other neonatal hypoglycemia** N
Transitory neonatal hypoglycemia
P70.8 **Other transitory disorders of carbohydrate metabolism of newborn** N CC
P70.9 **Transitory disorder of carbohydrate metabolism of newborn, unspecified** N

P71 **Transitory neonatal disorders of calcium and magnesium metabolism**
P71.0 **Cow's milk hypocalcemia in newborn** N CC
P71.1 **Other neonatal hypocalcemia** N CC
EXCLUDES1 *neonatal hypoparathyroidism (P71.4)*
P71.2 **Neonatal hypomagnesemia** N CC
P71.3 **Neonatal tetany without calcium or magnesium deficiency** N CC
Neonatal tetany NOS
P71.4 **Transitory neonatal hypoparathyroidism** N CC
P71.8 **Other transitory neonatal disorders of calcium and magnesium metabolism** N CC
P71.9 **Transitory neonatal disorder of calcium and magnesium metabolism, unspecified** N CC

P72 **Other transitory neonatal endocrine disorders**
EXCLUDES1 *congenital hypothyroidism with or without goiter (E03.0-E03.1)*
dyshormogenetic goiter (E07.1)
Pendred's syndrome (E07.1)
P72.0 **Neonatal goiter, not elsewhere classified** N CC
Transitory congenital goiter with normal functioning
P72.1 **Transitory neonatal hyperthyroidism** N CC
Neonatal thyrotoxicosis
P72.2 **Other transitory neonatal disorders of thyroid function, not elsewhere classified** N CC
Transitory neonatal hypothyroidism
P72.8 **Other specified transitory neonatal endocrine disorders** N CC
P72.9 **Transitory neonatal endocrine disorder, unspecified** N

P74 **Other transitory neonatal electrolyte and metabolic disturbances**
P74.0 **Late metabolic acidosis of newborn** N MCC
EXCLUDES1 *(fetal) metabolic acidosis of newborn (P19)*
P74.1 **Dehydration of newborn** N
P74.2 **Disturbances of sodium balance of newborn** N
P74.3 **Disturbances of potassium balance of newborn** N
P74.4 **Other transitory electrolyte disturbances of newborn** N
P74.5 **Transitory tyrosinemia of newborn** N CC
P74.6 **Transitory hyperammonemia of newborn** N CC
P74.8 **Other transitory metabolic disturbances of newborn** N CC
Amino-acid metabolic disorders described as transitory
P74.9 **Transitory metabolic disturbance of newborn, unspecified** N

Digestive system disorders of newborn (P76-P78)

P76 **Other intestinal obstruction of newborn**
P76.0 **Meconium plug syndrome** N
Meconium ileus NOS
EXCLUDES1 *meconium ileus in cystic fibrosis (E84.11)*
P76.1 **Transitory ileus of newborn** N CC
EXCLUDES1 *Hirschsprung's disease (Q43.1)*
P76.2 **Intestinal obstruction due to inspissated milk** N
P76.8 **Other specified intestinal obstruction of newborn** N
EXCLUDES1 *intestinal obstruction classifiable to K56.-*
P76.9 **Intestinal obstruction of newborn, unspecified** N

P77 **Necrotizing enterocolitis of newborn**
P77.1 **Stage 1 necrotizing enterocolitis in newborn** N MCC
Necrotizing enterocolitis without pneumatosis, without perforation
P77.2 **Stage 2 necrotizing enterocolitis in newborn** N MCC
Necrotizing enterocolitis with pneumatosis, without perforation
P77.3 **Stage 3 necrotizing enterocolitis in newborn** N MCC
Necrotizing enterocolitis with perforation
Necrotizing enterocolitis with pneumatosis and perforation
P77.9 **Necrotizing enterocolitis in newborn, unspecified** N MCC
Necrotizing enterocolitis in newborn, NOS

P78 **Other perinatal digestive system disorders**
EXCLUDES1 *cystic fibrosis (E84.0-E84.9)*
neonatal gastrointestinal hemorrhages (P54.0-P54.3)
P78.0 **Perinatal intestinal perforation** N MCC
Meconium peritonitis
P78.1 **Other neonatal peritonitis** N
Neonatal peritonitis NOS
P78.2 **Neonatal hematemesis and melena due to swallowed maternal blood** N
P78.3 **Noninfective neonatal diarrhea** N
Neonatal diarrhea NOS
P78.8 **Other specified perinatal digestive system disorders**
P78.81 **Congenital cirrhosis (of liver)** N
P78.82 **Peptic ulcer of newborn** N
P78.83 **Newborn esophageal reflux** N
Neonatal esophageal reflux
P78.89 **Other specified perinatal digestive system disorders** N
P78.9 **Perinatal digestive system disorder, unspecified** N

Conditions involving the integument and temperature regulation of newborn (P80-P83)

P80 **Hypothermia of newborn**
P80.0 **Cold injury syndrome** N
Severe and usually chronic hypothermia associated with a pink flushed appearance, edema and neurological and biochemical abnormalities.
EXCLUDES1 *mild hypothermia of newborn (P80.8)*
P80.8 **Other hypothermia of newborn** N
Mild hypothermia of newborn
P80.9 **Hypothermia of newborn, unspecified** N

P81 **Other disturbances of temperature regulation of newborn**
P81.0 **Environmental hyperthermia of newborn** N
P81.8 **Other specified disturbances of temperature regulation of newborn** N
P81.9 **Disturbance of temperature regulation of newborn, unspecified** N
Fever of newborn NOS

P83 **Other conditions of integument specific to newborn**
EXCLUDES1 *congenital malformations of skin and integument (Q80-Q84)*
hydrops fetalis due to hemolytic disease (P56.-)
neonatal skin infection (P39.4)

Unspecified Code Other Specified Code Manifestation Code N Newborn P Pediatric M Maternity A Adult ♂ Male ♀ Female
● New Code ▲ Revised Code Title ►◄ Revised Text NOTES INCLUDES EXCLUDES1 Not coded here EXCLUDES2 Not included here
4th character required 5th character required 6th character required 7th character required
Extension 'X' Alert HAC Hospital-acquired condition (HAC) alert AHA AHA Coding Clinic©

staphylococcal scalded skin syndrome (L00)
EXCLUDES2 cradle cap (L21.0)
diaper [napkin] dermatitis (L22)

P83.0 **Sclerema neonatorum**
P83.1 **Neonatal erythema toxicum**
P83.2 **Hydrops fetalis not due to hemolytic disease**
Hydrops fetalis NOS
P83.3 **Other and unspecified edema specific to newborn**
P83.30 **Unspecified edema specific to newborn**
P83.39 **Other edema specific to newborn**
P83.4 **Breast engorgement of newborn**
Noninfective mastitis of newborn
P83.5 **Congenital hydrocele**
P83.6 **Umbilical polyp of newborn**
P83.8 **Other specified conditions of integument specific to newborn**
Bronze baby syndrome
Neonatal scleroderma
Urticaria neonatorum
P83.9 **Condition of the integument specific to newborn, unspecified**

Other problems with newborn (P84)

P84 **Other problems with newborn**
Acidemia of newborn
Acidosis of newborn
Anoxia of newborn NOS
Asphyxia of newborn NOS
Hypercapnia of newborn
Hypoxemia of newborn
Hypoxia of newborn NOS
Mixed metabolic and respiratory acidosis of newborn
EXCLUDES1 *intracranial hemorrhage due to anoxia or hypoxia (P52.-)*
hypoxic ischemic encephalopathy [HIE] (P91.6-)
late metabolic acidosis of newborn (P74.0)

Other disorders originating in the perinatal period (P90-P96)

P90 **Convulsions of newborn**
EXCLUDES1 *benign myoclonic epilepsy in infancy (G40.3-)*
benign neonatal convulsions (familial) (G40.3-)
P91 **Other disturbances of cerebral status of newborn**
P91.0 **Neonatal cerebral ischemia**
P91.1 **Acquired periventricular cysts of newborn**
P91.2 **Neonatal cerebral leukomalacia**
Periventricular leukomalacia
P91.3 **Neonatal cerebral irritability**
P91.4 **Neonatal cerebral depression**
P91.5 **Neonatal coma**
P91.6 **Hypoxic ischemic encephalopathy [HIE]**
P91.60 **Hypoxic ischemic encephalopathy [HIE], unspecified**
P91.61 **Mild hypoxic ischemic encephalopathy [HIE]**
P91.62 **Moderate hypoxic ischemic encephalopathy [HIE]**
P91.63 **Severe hypoxic ischemic encephalopathy [HIE]**
P91.8 **Other specified disturbances of cerebral status of newborn**
P91.9 **Disturbance of cerebral status of newborn, unspecified**
P92 **Feeding problems of newborn**
EXCLUDES1 *feeding problems in child over 28 days old (R63.3)*
P92.0 **Vomiting of newborn**
EXCLUDES1 *vomiting of child over 28 days old (R11.-)*
P92.01 **Bilious vomiting of newborn**
EXCLUDES1 *bilious vomiting in child over 28 days old (R11.14)*
P92.09 **Other vomiting of newborn**
EXCLUDES1 *regurgitation of food in newborn (P92.1)*
P92.1 **Regurgitation and rumination of newborn**
P92.2 **Slow feeding of newborn**
P92.3 **Underfeeding of newborn**
P92.4 **Overfeeding of newborn**
P92.5 **Neonatal difficulty in feeding at breast**
P92.6 **Failure to thrive in newborn**
EXCLUDES1 *failure to thrive in child over 28 days old (R62.51)*
P92.8 **Other feeding problems of newborn**
P92.9 **Feeding problem of newborn, unspecified**
P93 **Reactions and intoxications due to drugs administered to newborn**
INCLUDES *reactions and intoxications due to drugs administered to fetus affecting newborn*
EXCLUDES1 *jaundice due to drugs or toxins transmitted from mother or given to newborn (P58.4-)*
reactions and intoxications from maternal opiates, tranquilizers and other medication (P04.0-P04.1, P04.4)
withdrawal symptoms from maternal use of drugs of addiction (P96.1)
withdrawal symptoms from therapeutic use of drugs in newborn (P96.2)
P93.0 **Grey baby syndrome**
Grey syndrome from chloramphenicol administration in newborn
P93.8 **Other reactions and intoxications due to drugs administered to newborn**
Use additional code for adverse effect, if applicable, to identify drug (T36-T50 with fifth or sixth character 5)
P94 **Disorders of muscle tone of newborn**
P94.0 **Transient neonatal myasthenia gravis**
EXCLUDES1 *myasthenia gravis (G70.0)*
P94.1 **Congenital hypertonia**
P94.2 **Congenital hypotonia**
Floppy baby syndrome, unspecified
P94.8 **Other disorders of muscle tone of newborn**
P94.9 **Disorder of muscle tone of newborn, unspecified**
P95 **Stillbirth**
Deadborn fetus NOS
Fetal death of unspecified cause
Stillbirth NOS
EXCLUDES1 *maternal care for intrauterine death (O36.4)*
missed abortion (O02.1)
outcome of delivery, stillbirth (Z37.1, Z37.3, Z37.4, Z37.7)
P96 **Other conditions originating in the perinatal period**
P96.0 **Congenital renal failure**
Uremia of newborn
P96.1 **Neonatal withdrawal symptoms from maternal use of drugs of addiction**
Drug withdrawal syndrome in infant of dependent mother
Neonatal abstinence syndrome
EXCLUDES1 *reactions and intoxications from maternal opiates and tranquilizers administered during labor and delivery (P04.0)*
P96.2 **Withdrawal symptoms from therapeutic use of drugs in newborn**
P96.3 **Wide cranial sutures of newborn**
Neonatal craniotabes
P96.5 **Complication to newborn due to (fetal) intrauterine procedure**
EXCLUDES2 *►newborn affected◄ by amniocentesis (P00.6)*
P96.8 **Other specified conditions originating in the perinatal period**
P96.81 **Exposure to (parental) (environmental) tobacco smoke in the perinatal period**
EXCLUDES2 *newborn affected by in utero exposure to tobacco (P04.2)*
exposure to environmental tobacco smoke after the perinatal period (Z77.22)
P96.82 **Delayed separation of umbilical cord**
P96.83 **Meconium staining**
EXCLUDES1 *meconium aspiration (P24.00, P24.01)*
meconium passage during delivery (P03.82)
P96.89 **Other specified conditions originating in the perinatal period**
Use additional code to specify condition
P96.9 **Condition originating in the perinatal period, unspecified**
Congenital debility NOS

Unacceptable principal diagnosis symbol per Medicare code edits; Code exempt from diagnosis present on admission requirement
Questionable admission; Complication or comorbidity; CC/MCC exclusion; Major complication or comorbidity
Principal diagnosis as its own CC; Principal diagnosis as its own MCC; Z code as first-listed diagnosis

Chapter 17: Congenital Malformations, Deformations, and Chromosomal Abnormalities (Q00-Q99)

Guidelines for Assigning Codes From This Chapter

To report a condition present from birth, you should use a code from Chapter 17. Examples of conditions you'll find here include spina bifida, ventricular septal defect, patent ductus arteriosus, and congenital hip deformities.

List of Categories

- Q00-Q07: Congenital malformations of the nervous system
- Q10-Q18: Congenital malformations of eye, ear, face and neck
- Q20-Q28: Congenital malformations of the circulatory system
- Q30-Q34: Congenital malformations of the respiratory system
- Q35-Q37: Cleft lip and cleft palate
- Q38-Q45: Other congenital malformations of the digestive system
- Q50-Q56: Congenital malformations of genital organs
- Q60-Q64: Congenital malformations of the urinary system
- Q65-Q79: Congenital malformations and deformations of the musculoskeletal system
- Q80-Q89: Other congenital malformations
- Q90-Q99: Chromosomal abnormalities, not elsewhere classified

Highlights From the ICD-10-CM Official Guidelines for Coding and Reporting

The ICD-10-CM Official Guidelines for Coding and Reporting for Chapter 17 supply helpful information for reporting congenital anomalies, which you may report as either primary or secondary diagnoses. The information below is from Section I.C.17 of the 2017 Official Guidelines.

Keep Your Manifestation Coding in Line With the Rules

In some cases, an anomaly may not have a unique code, but you may report codes for manifestations of the anomaly.

But when there is a unique code for the anomaly, you shouldn't report codes for typical manifestations of that anomaly.

Don't Limit Code Use Based on Age

Although congenital means present from birth, that doesn't put an age restriction on the patients these codes apply to. You may report a congenital anomaly code for a patient of any age. In fact, providers may not identify some types of congenital anomalies until years after the patient's birth.

When the provider identifies the anomaly at birth, the guidelines offer specific rules for coding the birth. You should report the appropriate liveborn infant code from **category Z38** (*Liveborn infants according to place of birth and type of delivery*), followed by the code for the anomaly.

Caution: If the congenital anomaly is documented as corrected, you should report a personal history code for that anomaly.

Congenital malformations, deformations and chromosomal abnormalities (Q00-Q99)

NOTES Codes from this chapter are not for use on maternal or fetal records

EXCLUDES2 *inborn errors of metabolism (E70-E88)*

This chapter contains the following blocks:

Q00-Q07 Congenital malformations of the nervous system
Q10-Q18 Congenital malformations of eye, ear, face and neck
Q20-Q28 Congenital malformations of the circulatory system
Q30-Q34 Congenital malformations of the respiratory system
Q35-Q37 Cleft lip and cleft palate
Q38-Q45 Other congenital malformations of the digestive system
Q50-Q56 Congenital malformations of genital organs
Q60-Q64 Congenital malformations of the urinary system
Q65-Q79 Congenital malformations and deformations of the musculoskeletal system
Q80-Q89 Other congenital malformations
Q90-Q99 Chromosomal abnormalities, not elsewhere classified

Congenital malformations of the nervous system (Q00-Q07)

Q00 Anencephaly and similar malformations

Q00.0 Anencephaly POA MCC
Acephaly
Acrania
Amyelencephaly
Hemianencephaly
Hemicephaly

Q00.1 Craniorachischisis POA MCC

Q00.2 Iniencephaly POA MCC

Q01 Encephalocele

INCLUDES *Arnold-Chiari syndrome, type III*
encephalocystocele
encephalomyelocele
hydroencephalocele
hydromeningocele, cranial
meningocele, cerebral
meningoencephalocele

EXCLUDES1 *Meckel-Gruber syndrome (Q61.9)*

Q01.0 Frontal **encephalocele** CC POA

Q01.1 Nasofrontal **encephalocele** CC POA

Q01.2 Occipital **encephalocele** CC POA

Q01.8 Encephalocele of other sites CC POA

Q01.9 Encephalocele, unspecified CC POA

Q02 Microcephaly POA

INCLUDES *hydromicrocephaly*
micrencephalon

EXCLUDES1 *Meckel-Gruber syndrome (Q61.9)*

Q03 Congenital hydrocephalus

INCLUDES *hydrocephalus in newborn*

EXCLUDES1 *Arnold-Chiari syndrome, type II (Q07.0-)*
acquired hydrocephalus (G91.-)
hydrocephalus due to congenital toxoplasmosis (P37.1)
hydrocephalus with spina bifida (Q05.0-Q05.4)

Q03.0 Malformations of aqueduct of Sylvius POA
Anomaly of aqueduct of Sylvius
Obstruction of aqueduct of Sylvius, congenital
Stenosis of aqueduct of Sylvius

Q03.1 Atresia of foramina of Magendie and Luschka POA
Dandy-Walker syndrome

Q03.8 Other congenital hydrocephalus POA

Q03.9 Congenital hydrocephalus, unspecified POA

Q04 Other congenital malformations of brain

EXCLUDES1 *cyclopia (Q87.0)*
macrocephaly (Q75.3)

Q04.0 Congenital malformations of corpus callosum POA MCC
Agenesis of corpus callosum

Q04.1 Arhinencephaly POA MCC

Q04.2 Holoprosencephaly POA MCC

Q04.3 Other reduction deformities **of brain** POA MCC
Absence of part of brain
Agenesis of part of brain
Agyria
Aplasia of part of brain
Hydranencephaly
Hypoplasia of part of brain
Lissencephaly
Microgyria
Pachygyria

EXCLUDES1 *congenital malformations of corpus callosum (Q04.0)*

Q04.4 Septo-optic dysplasia **of brain** CC POA

Q04.5 Megalencephaly CC POA

Q04.6 Congenital cerebral cysts CC POA
Porencephaly
Schizencephaly

EXCLUDES1 *acquired porencephalic cyst (G93.0)*

Q04.8 Other specified **congenital malformations of brain** CC POA
Arnold-Chiari syndrome, type IV
Macrogyria

Q04.9 Congenital malformation **of brain, unspecified** POA
Congenital anomaly NOS of brain
Congenital deformity NOS of brain
Congenital disease or lesion NOS of brain
Multiple anomalies NOS of brain, congenital

Q05 Spina bifida

INCLUDES *hydromeningocele (spinal)*
meningocele (spinal)
meningomyelocele
myelocele
myelomeningocele
rachischisis
spina bifida (aperta)(cystica)
syringomyelocele

Use additional code for any associated paraplegia (paraparesis) (G82.2-)

EXCLUDES1 *Arnold-Chiari syndrome, type II (Q07.0-)*
spina bifida occulta (Q76.0)

Q05.0 Cervical **spina bifida** with hydrocephalus CC POA

Q05.1 Thoracic **spina bifida** with hydrocephalus CC POA
Dorsal spina bifida with hydrocephalus
Thoracolumbar spina bifida with hydrocephalus

Q05.2 Lumbar **spina bifida** with hydrocephalus CC POA
Lumbosacral spina bifida with hydrocephalus

Q05.3 Sacral **spina bifida** with hydrocephalus CC POA

Q05.4 Unspecified spina bifida with hydrocephalus CC POA

Q05.5 Cervical **spina bifida** without hydrocephalus POA

Q05.6 Thoracic **spina bifida** without hydrocephalus POA
Dorsal spina bifida NOS
Thoracolumbar spina bifida NOS

Q05.7 Lumbar **spina bifida** without hydrocephalus POA
Lumbosacral spina bifida NOS

Q05.8 Sacral **spina bifida** without hydrocephalus POA

Q05.9 Spina bifida, unspecified POA

Q06 Other **congenital malformations of** spinal cord

Q06.0 Amyelia POA

Q06.1 Hypoplasia and dysplasia of spinal cord POA
Atelomyelia
Myelatelia
Myelodysplasia of spinal cord

Q06.2 Diastematomyelia POA

Q06.3 Other congenital cauda equina malformations POA

Q06.4 Hydromyelia POA
Hydrorachis

Q06.8 Other specified congenital malformations of spinal cord POA

Q06.9 Congenital malformation of spinal cord, unspecified POA
Congenital anomaly NOS of spinal cord
Congenital deformity NOS of spinal cord
Congenital disease or lesion NOS of spinal cord

Q07 Other **congenital malformations of** nervous system

EXCLUDES2 *congenital central alveolar hypoventilation syndrome (G47.35)*
familial dysautonomia [Riley-Day] (G90.1)
neurofibromatosis (nonmalignant) (Q85.0-)

PDx Unacceptable principal diagnosis symbol per Medicare code edits | POA Code exempt from diagnosis present on admission requirement
Questionable admission | CC Complication or comorbidity | CC/MCC Exc CC/MCC exclusion | MCC Major complication or comorbidity
PDx CC Principal diagnosis as its own CC | PDx MCC Principal diagnosis as its own MCC | Z1 Z code as first-listed diagnosis

When symbols appear on a code that requires a 7th character extension, refer to Appendix D to identify applicable 7th character codes.

Q07.0 Arnold-Chiari syndrome
Arnold-Chiari syndrome, type II
EXCLUDES1 *Arnold-Chiari syndrome, type III (Q01.-)*
Arnold-Chiari syndrome, type IV (Q04.8)
Q07.00 Arnold-Chiari syndrome without spina bifida or hydrocephalus
Q07.01 Arnold-Chiari syndrome with spina bifida
Q07.02 Arnold-Chiari syndrome with hydrocephalus
Q07.03 Arnold-Chiari syndrome with spina bifida and hydrocephalus
Q07.8 Other specified congenital malformations of nervous system
Agenesis of nerve
Displacement of brachial plexus
Jaw-winking syndrome
Marcus Gunn's syndrome
Q07.9 Congenital malformation of nervous system, unspecified
Congenital anomaly NOS of nervous system
Congenital deformity NOS of nervous system
Congenital disease or lesion NOS of nervous system

Congenital malformations of eye, ear, face and neck (Q10-Q18)

EXCLUDES2 *cleft lip and cleft palate (Q35-Q37)*
congenital malformation of cervical spine (Q05.0, Q05.5, Q67.5, Q76.0-Q76.4)
congenital malformation of larynx (Q31.-)
congenital malformation of lip NEC (Q38.0)
congenital malformation of nose (Q30.-)
congenital malformation of parathyroid gland (Q89.2)
congenital malformation of thyroid gland (Q89.2)

Q10 Congenital malformations of eyelid, lacrimal apparatus and orbit
EXCLUDES1 *cryptophthalmos NOS (Q11.2)*
cryptophthalmos syndrome (Q87.0)
Q10.0 Congenital ptosis
Q10.1 Congenital ectropion
Q10.2 Congenital entropion
Q10.3 Other congenital malformations of eyelid
Ablepharon
Blepharophimosis, congenital
Coloboma of eyelid
Congenital absence or agenesis of cilia
Congenital absence or agenesis of eyelid
Congenital accessory eyelid
Congenital accessory eye muscle
Congenital malformation of eyelid NOS
Q10.4 Absence and agenesis of lacrimal apparatus
Congenital absence of punctum lacrimale
Q10.5 Congenital stenosis and stricture of lacrimal duct
Q10.6 Other congenital malformations of lacrimal apparatus
Congenital malformation of lacrimal apparatus NOS
Q10.7 Congenital malformation of orbit

Q11 Anophthalmos, microphthalmos and macrophthalmos
Q11.0 Cystic eyeball
Q11.1 Other anophthalmos
Anophthalmos NOS
Agenesis of eye
Aplasia of eye
Q11.2 Microphthalmos
Cryptophthalmos NOS
Dysplasia of eye
Hypoplasia of eye
Rudimentary eye
EXCLUDES1 *cryptophthalmos syndrome (Q87.0)*
AHA: Q4, 2004
Q11.3 Macrophthalmos
EXCLUDES1 *macrophthalmos in congenital glaucoma (Q15.0)*

Q12 Congenital lens malformations
Q12.0 Congenital cataract
Q12.1 Congenital displaced lens
Q12.2 Coloboma of lens
Q12.3 Congenital aphakia
Q12.4 Spherophakia
Q12.8 Other congenital lens malformations
Microphakia
Q12.9 Congenital lens malformation, unspecified

Q13 Congenital malformations of anterior segment of eye
Q13.0 Coloboma of iris
Coloboma NOS
Q13.1 Absence of iris
Aniridia
Use additional code for associated glaucoma (H42)
Q13.2 Other congenital malformations of iris
Anisocoria, congenital
Atresia of pupil
Congenital malformation of iris NOS
Corectopia
Q13.3 Congenital corneal opacity
Q13.4 Other congenital corneal malformations
Congenital malformation of cornea NOS
Microcornea
Peter's anomaly
Q13.5 Blue sclera
Q13.8 Other congenital malformations of anterior segment of eye
Q13.81 Rieger's anomaly
Use additional code for associated glaucoma (H42)
Q13.89 Other congenital malformations of anterior segment of eye
Q13.9 Congenital malformation of anterior segment of eye, unspecified

Q14 Congenital malformations of posterior segment of eye
EXCLUDES2 *optic nerve hypoplasia (H47.03-)*
Q14.0 Congenital malformation of vitreous humor
Congenital vitreous opacity
Q14.1 Congenital malformation of retina
Congenital retinal aneurysm
Q14.2 Congenital malformation of optic disc
Coloboma of optic disc
Q14.3 Congenital malformation of choroid
Q14.8 Other congenital malformations of posterior segment of eye
Coloboma of the fundus
Q14.9 Congenital malformation of posterior segment of eye, unspecified

Q15 Other congenital malformations of eye
EXCLUDES1 *congenital nystagmus (H55.01)*
ocular albinism (E70.31-)
optic nerve hypoplasia (H47.03-)
retinitis pigmentosa (H35.52)
Q15.0 Congenital glaucoma
Axenfeld's anomaly
Buphthalmos
Glaucoma of childhood
Glaucoma of newborn
Hydrophthalmos
Keratoglobus, congenital, with glaucoma
Macrocornea with glaucoma
Macrophthalmos in congenital glaucoma
Megalocornea with glaucoma
Q15.8 Other specified congenital malformations of eye
Q15.9 Congenital malformation of eye, unspecified
Congenital anomaly of eye
Congenital deformity of eye

Q16 Congenital malformations of ear causing impairment of hearing
EXCLUDES1 *congenital deafness (H90.-)*
Q16.0 Congenital absence of (ear) auricle
Q16.1 Congenital absence, atresia and stricture of auditory canal (external)
Congenital atresia or stricture of osseous meatus
Q16.2 Absence of eustachian tube
Q16.3 Congenital malformation of ear ossicles
Congenital fusion of ear ossicles
Q16.4 Other congenital malformations of middle ear
Congenital malformation of middle ear NOS
Q16.5 Congenital malformation of inner ear
Congenital anomaly of membranous labyrinth
Congenital anomaly of organ of Corti

Unspecified Code Other Specified Code Manifestation Code N Newborn P Pediatric M Maternity A Adult ♂ Male ♀ Female
● New Code ▲ Revised Code Title ►◄ Revised Text NOTES INCLUDES EXCLUDES1 Not coded here EXCLUDES2 Not included here
4th character required 5th character required 6th character required 7th character required
Extension 'X' Alert HAC Hospital-acquired condition (HAC) alert AHA AHA Coding Clinic®

Q16.9 **Congenital malformation of ear causing impairment of hearing, unspecified** POA
Congenital absence of ear NOS

Q17 Other **congenital malformations of** ear
EXCLUDES1 *congenital malformations of ear with impairment of hearing (Q16.0-Q16.9)*
preauricular sinus (Q18.1)

Q17.0 **Accessory auricle** POA
Accessory tragus
Polyotia
Preauricular appendage or tag
Supernumerary ear
Supernumerary lobule

Q17.1 **Macrotia** POA

Q17.2 **Microtia** POA

Q17.3 **Other misshapen ear** POA
Pointed ear

Q17.4 **Misplaced ear** POA
Low-set ears
EXCLUDES1 *cervical auricle (Q18.2)*

Q17.5 **Prominent ear** POA
Bat ear

Q17.8 **Other specified congenital malformations of ear** POA
Congenital absence of lobe of ear

Q17.9 **Congenital malformation of ear, unspecified** POA
Congenital anomaly of ear NOS

Q18 Other **congenital malformations of** face and neck
EXCLUDES1 *cleft lip and cleft palate (Q35-Q37)*
conditions classified to Q67.0-Q67.4
congenital malformations of skull and face bones (Q75.-)
cyclopia (Q87.0)
dentofacial anomalies [including malocclusion] (M26.-)
malformation syndromes affecting facial appearance (Q87.0)
persistent thyroglossal duct (Q89.2)

Q18.0 **Sinus, fistula and cyst of branchial cleft** POA
Branchial vestige

Q18.1 **Preauricular sinus and cyst** POA
Fistula of auricle, congenital
Cervicoaural fistula

Q18.2 **Other branchial cleft malformations** POA
Branchial cleft malformation NOS
Cervical auricle
Otocephaly

Q18.3 **Webbing of neck** POA
Pterygium colli

Q18.4 **Macrostomia** POA

Q18.5 **Microstomia** POA

Q18.6 **Macrocheilia** POA
Hypertrophy of lip, congenital

Q18.7 **Microcheilia** POA

Q18.8 **Other specified congenital malformations of face and neck** POA
Medial cyst of face and neck
Medial fistula of face and neck
Medial sinus of face and neck

Q18.9 **Congenital malformation of face and neck, unspecified** POA
Congenital anomaly NOS of face and neck

Congenital malformations of the circulatory system (Q20-Q28)

Q20 **Congenital malformations of** cardiac chambers and connections
EXCLUDES1 *dextrocardia with situs inversus (Q89.3)*
mirror-image atrial arrangement with situs inversus (Q89.3)

Q20.0 **Common arterial trunk** POA MCC
Persistent truncus arteriosus
EXCLUDES1 *aortic septal defect (Q21.4)*

Q20.1 **Double** outlet right **ventricle** POA MCC
Taussig-Bing syndrome

Q20.2 **Double** outlet left **ventricle** POA MCC

Q20.3 **Discordant ventriculoarterial connection** POA MCC
Dextrotransposition of aorta
Transposition of great vessels (complete)

Q20.4 **Double** inlet **ventricle** POA MCC
Common ventricle
Cor triloculare biatriatum
Single ventricle

Q20.5 **Discordant** atrioventricular **connection** CC POA
Corrected transposition
Levotransposition
Ventricular inversion

Q20.6 **Isomerism of atrial appendages** POA
Isomerism of atrial appendages with asplenia or polysplenia

Q20.8 **Other congenital malformations of cardiac chambers and connections** POA
Cor binoculare

Q20.9 **Congenital malformation of cardiac chambers and connections, unspecified** POA

Q21 **Congenital malformations of** cardiac septa
EXCLUDES1 *acquired cardiac septal defect (I51.0)*

Q21.0 Ventricular **septal defect** CC POA
Roger's disease

Q21.1 Atrial **septal defect** CC POA
Coronary sinus defect
Patent or persistent foramen ovale
Patent or persistent ostium secundum defect (type II)
Patent or persistent sinus venosus defect

Q21.2 Atrioventricular **septal defect** CC POA
Common atrioventricular canal
Endocardial cushion defect
Ostium primum atrial septal defect (type I)

Q21.3 **Tetralogy of Fallot** POA MCC
Ventricular septal defect with pulmonary stenosis or atresia, dextroposition of aorta and hypertrophy of right ventricle.

Q21.4 Aortopulmonary **septal defect** POA
Aortic septal defect
Aortopulmonary window

Q21.8 **Other congenital malformations of cardiac septa** POA
Eisenmenger's defect
Pentalogy of Fallot
EXCLUDES1 *Eisenmenger's complex (I27.8)*
Eisenmenger's syndrome (I27.8)

Q21.9 **Congenital malformation of cardiac septum, unspecified** POA
Septal (heart) defect NOS

Q22 **Congenital malformations of** pulmonary and tricuspid valves

Q22.0 **Pulmonary** valve atresia POA MCC

Q22.1 **Congenital pulmonary valve** stenosis CC POA

Q22.2 **Congenital pulmonary valve** insufficiency CC POA
Congenital pulmonary valve regurgitation

Q22.3 **Other congenital malformations of pulmonary valve** CC POA
Congenital malformation of pulmonary valve NOS
Supernumerary cusps of pulmonary valve

Q22.4 **Congenital** tricuspid stenosis POA MCC
Congenital tricuspid atresia

Q22.5 **Ebstein's anomaly** POA MCC

Q22.6 **Hypoplastic** right heart **syndrome** POA MCC

Q22.8 **Other congenital malformations of tricuspid valve** POA MCC

Q22.9 **Congenital malformation of tricuspid valve, unspecified** POA MCC

Q23 **Congenital malformations of** aortic and mitral valves

Q23.0 **Congenital** stenosis **of aortic valve** CC POA
Congenital aortic atresia
Congenital aortic stenosis NOS
EXCLUDES1 *congenital stenosis of aortic valve in hypoplastic left heart syndrome (Q23.4)*
congenital subaortic stenosis (Q24.4)
supravalvular aortic stenosis (congenital) (Q25.3)

Q23.1 **Congenital** insufficiency **of aortic valve** CC POA
Bicuspid aortic valve
Congenital aortic insufficiency

Q23.2 **Congenital** mitral stenosis CC POA
Congenital mitral atresia

Q23.3 **Congenital** mitral insufficiency CC POA

Q23.4 **Hypoplastic** left heart syndrome POA MCC

Q23.8 **Other congenital malformations of aortic and mitral valves** POA

Q23.9 **Congenital malformation of aortic and mitral valves, unspecified** POA

Q24 Other **congenital malformations of** heart
EXCLUDES1 *endocardial fibroelastosis (I42.4)*

PDx Unacceptable principal diagnosis symbol per Medicare code edits; POA Code exempt from diagnosis present on admission requirement; ? Questionable admission; CC Complication or comorbidity; CC/MCC Exc CC/MCC exclusion; MCC Major complication or comorbidity; PDx CC Principal diagnosis as its own CC; PDx MCC Principal diagnosis as its own MCC; Z1 Z code as first-listed diagnosis

Q24.0 Dextrocardia
EXCLUDES1 *dextrocardia with situs inversus (Q89.3)*
isomerism of atrial appendages (with asplenia or polysplenia) (Q20.6)
mirror-image atrial arrangement with situs inversus (Q89.3)

Q24.1 Levocardia

Q24.2 Cor triatriatum

Q24.3 Pulmonary infundibular stenosis
Subvalvular pulmonic stenosis

Q24.4 Congenital subaortic stenosis

Q24.5 Malformation of coronary vessels
Congenital coronary (artery) aneurysm

Q24.6 Congenital heart block

Q24.8 Other specified congenital malformations of heart
Congenital diverticulum of left ventricle
Congenital malformation of myocardium
Congenital malformation of pericardium
Malposition of heart
Uhl's disease

Q24.9 Congenital malformation of heart, unspecified
Congenital anomaly of heart
Congenital disease of heart

Q25 Congenital malformations of great arteries

Q25.0 Patent ductus arteriosus
Patent ductus Botallo
Persistent ductus arteriosus

Q25.1 Coarctation of aorta
Coarctation of aorta (preductal) (postductal)
Stenosis of aorta

Q25.2 Atresia of aorta

● **Q25.21 Interruption of aortic arch**
Atresia of aortic arch

● **Q25.29 Other atresia of aorta**
Atresia of aorta

Q25.3 Supravalvular aortic stenosis
EXCLUDES1 *congenital aortic stenosis NOS (Q23.0)*
congenital stenosis of aortic valve (Q23.0)

Q25.4 Other congenital malformations of aorta
EXCLUDES1 *hypoplasia of aorta in hypoplastic left heart syndrome (Q23.4)*

● **Q25.40 Congenital malformation of aorta unspecified**

● **Q25.41 Absence and aplasia of aorta**

● **Q25.42 Hypoplasia of aorta**

● **Q25.43 Congenital aneurysm of aorta**
Congenital aneurysm of aortic root
Congenital aneurysm of aortic sinus

● **Q25.44 Congenital dilation of aorta**

● **Q25.45 Double aortic arch**
Vascular ring of aorta

● **Q25.46 Tortuous aortic arch**
Persistent convolutions of aortic arch

● **Q25.47 Right aortic arch**
Persistent right aortic arch

● **Q25.48 Anomalous origin of subclavian artery**

● **Q25.49 Other congenital malformations of aorta**

Q25.5 Atresia of pulmonary artery

Q25.6 Stenosis of pulmonary artery
Supravalvular pulmonary stenosis

Q25.7 Other congenital malformations of pulmonary artery

Q25.71 Coarctation of pulmonary artery

Q25.72 Congenital pulmonary arteriovenous malformation
Congenital pulmonary arteriovenous aneurysm

Q25.79 Other congenital malformations of pulmonary artery
Aberrant pulmonary artery
Agenesis of pulmonary artery
Congenital aneurysm of pulmonary artery
Congenital anomaly of pulmonary artery
Hypoplasia of pulmonary artery

Q25.8 Other congenital malformations of other great arteries

Q25.9 Congenital malformation of great arteries, unspecified

Q26 Congenital malformations of great veins

Q26.0 Congenital stenosis of vena cava
Congenital stenosis of vena cava (inferior)(superior)

Q26.1 Persistent left superior vena cava

Q26.2 Total anomalous pulmonary venous connection
Total anomalous pulmonary venous return [TAPVR], subdiaphragmatic
Total anomalous pulmonary venous return [TAPVR], supradiaphragmatic

Q26.3 Partial anomalous pulmonary venous connection
Partial anomalous pulmonary venous return

Q26.4 Anomalous pulmonary venous connection, unspecified

Q26.5 Anomalous portal venous connection

Q26.6 Portal vein-hepatic artery fistula

Q26.8 Other congenital malformations of great veins
Absence of vena cava (inferior) (superior)
Azygos continuation of inferior vena cava
Persistent left posterior cardinal vein
Scimitar syndrome

Q26.9 Congenital malformation of great vein, unspecified
Congenital anomaly of vena cava (inferior) (superior) NOS

Q27 Other congenital malformations of peripheral vascular system
EXCLUDES2 *anomalies of cerebral and precerebral vessels (Q28.0-Q28.3)*
anomalies of coronary vessels (Q24.5)
anomalies of pulmonary artery (Q25.5-Q25.7)
congenital retinal aneurysm (Q14.1)
hemangioma and lymphangioma (D18.-)

Q27.0 Congenital absence and hypoplasia of umbilical artery
Single umbilical artery

Q27.1 Congenital renal artery stenosis

Q27.2 Other congenital malformations of renal artery
Congenital malformation of renal artery NOS
Multiple renal arteries

Q27.3 Arteriovenous malformation (peripheral)
Arteriovenous aneurysm
EXCLUDES1 *acquired arteriovenous aneurysm (I77.0)*
EXCLUDES2 *arteriovenous malformation of cerebral vessels (Q28.2)*
arteriovenous malformation of precerebral vessels (Q28.0)

Q27.30 Arteriovenous malformation, site unspecified

Q27.31 Arteriovenous malformation of vessel of upper limb

Q27.32 Arteriovenous malformation of vessel of lower limb

Q27.33 Arteriovenous malformation of digestive system vessel

Q27.34 Arteriovenous malformation of renal vessel

Q27.39 Arteriovenous malformation, other site

Q27.4 Congenital phlebectasia

Q27.8 Other specified congenital malformations of peripheral vascular system
Absence of peripheral vascular system
Atresia of peripheral vascular system
Congenital aneurysm (peripheral)
Congenital stricture, artery
Congenital varix
EXCLUDES1 *arteriovenous malformation (Q27.3-)*

Q27.9 Congenital malformation of peripheral vascular system, unspecified
Anomaly of artery or vein NOS

Q28 Other congenital malformations of circulatory system
EXCLUDES1 *congenital aneurysm NOS (Q27.8)*
congenital coronary aneurysm (Q24.5)
ruptured cerebral arteriovenous malformation (I60.8)
ruptured malformation of precerebral vessels (I72.0)
EXCLUDES2 *congenital peripheral aneurysm (Q27.8)*
congenital pulmonary aneurysm (Q25.79)
congenital retinal aneurysm (Q14.1)

Q28.0 Arteriovenous malformation of precerebral vessels
Congenital arteriovenous precerebral aneurysm (nonruptured)

Unspecified Code | Other Specified Code | Manifestation Code | N Newborn | P Pediatric | M Maternity | A Adult | ♂ Male | ♀ Female
● New Code | ▲ Revised Code Title | ►◄ Revised Text | NOTES | INCLUDES | EXCLUDES1 Not coded here | EXCLUDES2 Not included here
4th character required | 5th character required | 6th character required | 7th character required
Extension 'X' Alert | HAC Hospital-acquired condition (HAC) alert | AHA AHA Coding Clinic®

Q28.1 Other malformations of precerebral vessels
Congenital malformation of precerebral vessels NOS
Congenital precerebral aneurysm (nonruptured)

Q28.2 Arteriovenous malformation of cerebral vessels
Arteriovenous malformation of brain NOS
Congenital arteriovenous cerebral aneurysm (nonruptured)

Q28.3 Other malformations of cerebral vessels
Congenital cerebral aneurysm (nonruptured)
Congenital malformation of cerebral vessels NOS
Developmental venous anomaly

Q28.8 Other specified congenital malformations of circulatory system
Congenital aneurysm, specified site NEC
Spinal vessel anomaly

Q28.9 Congenital malformation of circulatory system, unspecified

Congenital malformations of the respiratory system (Q30-Q34)

Q30 Congenital malformations of nose
EXCLUDES1 *congenital deviation of nasal septum (Q67.4)*

Q30.0 Choanal atresia
Atresia of nares (anterior) (posterior)
Congenital stenosis of nares (anterior) (posterior)

Q30.1 Agenesis and underdevelopment of nose
Congenital absent of nose

Q30.2 Fissured, notched and cleft nose

Q30.3 Congenital perforated nasal septum

Q30.8 Other congenital malformations of nose
Accessory nose
Congenital anomaly of nasal sinus wall

Q30.9 Congenital malformation of nose, unspecified

Q31 Congenital malformations of larynx
EXCLUDES1 *congenital laryngeal stridor NOS (P28.89)*

Q31.0 Web of larynx
Glottic web of larynx
Subglottic web of larynx
Web of larynx NOS

Q31.1 Congenital subglottic stenosis

Q31.2 Laryngeal hypoplasia

Q31.3 Laryngocele

Q31.5 Congenital laryngomalacia

Q31.8 Other congenital malformations of larynx
Absence of larynx
Agenesis of larynx
Atresia of larynx
Congenital cleft thyroid cartilage
Congenital fissure of epiglottis
Congenital stenosis of larynx NEC
Posterior cleft of cricoid cartilage

Q31.9 Congenital malformation of larynx, unspecified

Q32 Congenital malformations of trachea and bronchus
EXCLUDES1 *congenital bronchiectasis (Q33.4)*

Q32.0 Congenital tracheomalacia

Q32.1 Other congenital malformations of trachea
Atresia of trachea
Congenital anomaly of tracheal cartilage
Congenital dilatation of trachea
Congenital malformation of trachea
Congenital stenosis of trachea
Congenital tracheocele

Q32.2 Congenital bronchomalacia

Q32.3 Congenital stenosis of bronchus

Q32.4 Other congenital malformations of bronchus
Absence of bronchus
Agenesis of bronchus
Atresia of bronchus
Congenital diverticulum of bronchus
Congenital malformation of bronchus NOS

Q33 Congenital malformations of lung

Q33.0 Congenital cystic lung
Congenital cystic lung disease
Congenital honeycomb lung
Congenital polycystic lung disease
EXCLUDES1 *cystic fibrosis (E84.0)*
cystic lung disease, acquired or unspecified (J98.4)

Q33.1 Accessory lobe of lung
Azygos lobe (fissured), lung

Q33.2 Sequestration of lung

Q33.3 Agenesis of lung
Congenital absence of lung (lobe)

Q33.4 Congenital bronchiectasis

Q33.5 Ectopic tissue in lung

Q33.6 Congenital hypoplasia and dysplasia of lung
EXCLUDES1 *pulmonary hypoplasia associated with short gestation (P28.0)*

Q33.8 Other congenital malformations of lung

Q33.9 Congenital malformation of lung, unspecified

Q34 Other congenital malformations of respiratory system
EXCLUDES2 *congenital central alveolar hypoventilation syndrome (G47.35)*

Q34.0 Anomaly of pleura

Q34.1 Congenital cyst of mediastinum

Q34.8 Other specified congenital malformations of respiratory system
Atresia of nasopharynx

Q34.9 Congenital malformation of respiratory system, unspecified
Congenital absence of respiratory system
Congenital anomaly of respiratory system NOS

Cleft lip and cleft palate (Q35-Q37)

Use additional code to identify associated malformation of the nose (Q30.2)

EXCLUDES1 *Robin's syndrome (Q87.0)*

Q35 Cleft palate
INCLUDES *fissure of palate*
palatoschisis
EXCLUDES1 *cleft palate with cleft lip (Q37.-)*

Q35.1 Cleft hard palate

Q35.3 Cleft soft palate

Q35.5 Cleft hard palate with cleft soft palate

Q35.7 Cleft uvula

Q35.9 Cleft palate, unspecified
Cleft palate NOS

Q36 Cleft lip
INCLUDES *cheiloschisis*
congenital fissure of lip
harelip
labium leporinum
EXCLUDES1 *cleft lip with cleft palate (Q37.-)*

Q36.0 Cleft lip, bilateral

Q36.1 Cleft lip, median

Q36.9 Cleft lip, unilateral
Cleft lip NOS

Q37 Cleft palate with cleft lip
INCLUDES *cheilopalatoschisis*

Q37.0 Cleft hard palate with bilateral cleft lip

Q37.1 Cleft hard palate with unilateral cleft lip
Cleft hard palate with cleft lip NOS

Q37.2 Cleft soft palate with bilateral cleft lip

Q37.3 Cleft soft palate with unilateral cleft lip
Cleft soft palate with cleft lip NOS

Q37.4 Cleft hard and soft palate with bilateral cleft lip

Q37.5 Cleft hard and soft palate with unilateral cleft lip
Cleft hard and soft palate with cleft lip NOS

Q37.8 Unspecified cleft palate with bilateral cleft lip

Q37.9 Unspecified cleft palate with unilateral cleft lip
Cleft palate with cleft lip NOS

Unacceptable principal diagnosis symbol per Medicare code edits · Code exempt from diagnosis present on admission requirement
Questionable admission · Complication or comorbidity · CC/MCC exclusion · Major complication or comorbidity
Principal diagnosis as its own CC · Principal diagnosis as its own MCC · Z code as first-listed diagnosis

Other congenital malformations of the digestive system (Q38-Q45)

Q38 Other congenital malformations of tongue, mouth and pharynx
EXCLUDES1 *dentofacial anomalies (M26.-)*
macrostomia (Q18.4)
microstomia (Q18.5)

Q38.0 Congenital malformations of lips, not elsewhere classified
Congenital fistula of lip
Congenital malformation of lip NOS
Van der Woude's syndrome
EXCLUDES1 *cleft lip (Q36.-)*
cleft lip with cleft palate (Q37.-)
macrocheilia (Q18.6)
microcheilia (Q18.7)

Q38.1 Ankyloglossia
Tongue tie

Q38.2 Macroglossia
Congenital hypertrophy of tongue

Q38.3 Other congenital malformations of tongue
Aglossia
Bifid tongue
Congenital adhesion of tongue
Congenital fissure of tongue
Congenital malformation of tongue NOS
Double tongue
Hypoglossia
Hypoplasia of tongue
Microglossia

Q38.4 Congenital malformations of salivary glands and ducts
Atresia of salivary glands and ducts
Congenital absence of salivary glands and ducts
Congenital accessory salivary glands and ducts
Congenital fistula of salivary gland

Q38.5 Congenital malformations of palate, not elsewhere classified
Congenital absence of uvula
Congenital malformation of palate NOS
Congenital high arched palate
EXCLUDES1 *cleft palate (Q35.-)*
cleft palate with cleft lip (Q37.-)

Q38.6 Other congenital malformations of mouth
Congenital malformation of mouth NOS

Q38.7 Congenital pharyngeal pouch
Congenital diverticulum of pharynx
EXCLUDES1 *pharyngeal pouch syndrome (D82.1)*

Q38.8 Other congenital malformations of pharynx
Congenital malformation of pharynx NOS
Imperforate pharynx

Q39 Congenital malformations of esophagus

Q39.0 Atresia of esophagus without fistula
Atresia of esophagus NOS

Q39.1 Atresia of esophagus with tracheo-esophageal fistula
Atresia of esophagus with broncho-esophageal fistula

Q39.2 Congenital tracheo-esophageal fistula without atresia
Congenital tracheo-esophageal fistula NOS

Q39.3 Congenital stenosis and stricture of esophagus

Q39.4 Esophageal web

Q39.5 Congenital dilatation of esophagus
Congenital cardiospasm

Q39.6 Congenital diverticulum of esophagus
Congenital esophageal pouch

Q39.8 Other congenital malformations of esophagus
Congenital absence of esophagus
Congenital displacement of esophagus
Congenital duplication of esophagus

Q39.9 Congenital malformation of esophagus, unspecified

Q40 Other congenital malformations of upper alimentary tract

Q40.0 Congenital hypertrophic pyloric stenosis
Congenital or infantile constriction
Congenital or infantile hypertrophy
Congenital or infantile spasm
Congenital or infantile stenosis
Congenital or infantile stricture

Q40.1 Congenital hiatus hernia
Congenital displacement of cardia through esophageal hiatus
EXCLUDES1 *congenital diaphragmatic hernia (Q79.0)*

Q40.2 Other specified congenital malformations of stomach
Congenital displacement of stomach
Congenital diverticulum of stomach
Congenital hourglass stomach
Congenital duplication of stomach
Megalogastria
Microgastria

Q40.3 Congenital malformation of stomach, unspecified

Q40.8 Other specified congenital malformations of upper alimentary tract

Q40.9 Congenital malformation of upper alimentary tract, unspecified
Congenital anomaly of upper alimentary tract
Congenital deformity of upper alimentary tract

Q41 Congenital absence, atresia and stenosis of small intestine
INCLUDES *congenital obstruction, occlusion or stricture of small intestine or intestine NOS*
EXCLUDES1 *cystic fibrosis with intestinal manifestation (E84.11)*
meconium ileus NOS (without cystic fibrosis) (P76.0)

Q41.0 Congenital absence, atresia and stenosis of duodenum

Q41.1 Congenital absence, atresia and stenosis of jejunum
Apple peel syndrome
Imperforate jejunum

Q41.2 Congenital absence, atresia and stenosis of ileum

Q41.8 Congenital absence, atresia and stenosis of other specified parts of small intestine

Q41.9 Congenital absence, atresia and stenosis of small intestine, part unspecified
Congenital absence, atresia and stenosis of intestine NOS

Q42 Congenital absence, atresia and stenosis of large intestine
INCLUDES *congenital obstruction, occlusion and stricture of large intestine*

Q42.0 Congenital absence, atresia and stenosis of rectum with fistula

Q42.1 Congenital absence, atresia and stenosis of rectum without fistula
Imperforate rectum

Q42.2 Congenital absence, atresia and stenosis of anus with fistula

Q42.3 Congenital absence, atresia and stenosis of anus without fistula
Imperforate anus

Q42.8 Congenital absence, atresia and stenosis of other parts of large intestine

Q42.9 Congenital absence, atresia and stenosis of large intestine, part unspecified

Q43 Other congenital malformations of intestine

Q43.0 Meckel's diverticulum (displaced) (hypertrophic)
Persistent omphalomesenteric duct
Persistent vitelline duct

Q43.1 Hirschsprung's disease
Aganglionosis
Congenital (aganglionic) megacolon

Q43.2 Other congenital functional disorders of colon
Congenital dilatation of colon

Q43.3 Congenital malformations of intestinal fixation
Congenital omental, anomalous adhesions [bands]
Congenital peritoneal adhesions [bands]
Incomplete rotation of cecum and colon
Insufficient rotation of cecum and colon
Jackson's membrane
Malrotation of colon
Rotation failure of cecum and colon
Universal mesentery

Q43.4 Duplication of intestine

Q43.5 Ectopic anus

Q43.6 Congenital fistula of rectum and anus
EXCLUDES1 *congenital fistula of anus with absence, atresia and stenosis (Q42.2)*
congenital fistula of rectum with absence, atresia and stenosis (Q42.0)

Unspecified Code | Other Specified Code | Manifestation Code | N Newborn | P Pediatric | M Maternity | A Adult | ♂ Male | ♀ Female
● New Code ▲ Revised Code Title ►◄ Revised Text NOTES INCLUDES EXCLUDES1 Not coded here EXCLUDES2 Not included here
4th character required 5th character required 6th character required 7th character required
Extension 'X' Alert HAC Hospital-acquired condition (HAC) alert AHA AHA Coding Clinic©

congenital rectovaginal fistula (Q52.2)
congenital urethrorectal fistula (Q64.73)
pilonidal fistula or sinus (L05.-)

Q43.7 **Persistent cloaca**
Cloaca NOS

Q43.8 **Other specified congenital malformations of intestine**
Congenital blind loop syndrome
Congenital diverticulitis, colon
Congenital diverticulum, intestine
Dolichocolon
Megaloappendix
Megaloduodenum
Microcolon
Transposition of appendix
Transposition of colon
Transposition of intestine

Q43.9 **Congenital malformation of intestine, unspecified**

Q44 **Congenital malformations of gallbladder, bile ducts and liver**

Q44.0 **Agenesis, aplasia and hypoplasia of gallbladder**
Congenital absence of gallbladder

Q44.1 **Other congenital malformations of gallbladder**
Congenital malformation of gallbladder NOS
Intrahepatic gallbladder

Q44.2 **Atresia of bile ducts**

Q44.3 **Congenital stenosis and stricture of bile ducts**

Q44.4 **Choledochal cyst**

Q44.5 **Other congenital malformations of bile ducts**
Accessory hepatic duct
Biliary duct duplication
Congenital malformation of bile duct NOS
Cystic duct duplication

Q44.6 **Cystic disease of liver**
Fibrocystic disease of liver

Q44.7 **Other congenital malformations of liver**
Accessory liver
Alagille's syndrome
Congenital absence of liver
Congenital hepatomegaly
Congenital malformation of liver NOS

Q45 **Other congenital malformations of digestive system**

EXCLUDES2 *congenital diaphragmatic hernia (Q79.0)*
congenital hiatus hernia (Q40.1)

Q45.0 **Agenesis, aplasia and hypoplasia of pancreas**
Congenital absence of pancreas

Q45.1 **Annular pancreas**

Q45.2 **Congenital pancreatic cyst**

Q45.3 **Other congenital malformations of pancreas and pancreatic duct**
Accessory pancreas
Congenital malformation of pancreas or pancreatic duct NOS

EXCLUDES1 *congenital diabetes mellitus (E10.-)*
cystic fibrosis (E84.0-E84.9)
fibrocystic disease of pancreas (E84.-)
neonatal diabetes mellitus (P70.2)

Q45.8 **Other specified congenital malformations of digestive system**
Absence (complete) (partial) of alimentary tract NOS
Duplication of digestive system
Malposition, congenital of digestive system

Q45.9 **Congenital malformation of digestive system, unspecified**
Congenital anomaly of digestive system
Congenital deformity of digestive system

Congenital malformations of genital organs (Q50-Q56)

EXCLUDES1 *androgen insensitivity syndrome (E34.5-)*
syndromes associated with anomalies in the number and form of chromosomes (Q90-Q99)

Q50 **Congenital malformations of ovaries, fallopian tubes and broad ligaments**

Q50.0 **Congenital absence of ovary**

EXCLUDES1 *Turner's syndrome (Q96.-)*

Q50.01 **Congenital absence of ovary, unilateral**

Q50.02 **Congenital absence of ovary, bilateral**

Q50.1 **Developmental ovarian cyst**

Q50.2 **Congenital torsion of ovary**

Q50.3 **Other congenital malformations of ovary**

Q50.31 **Accessory ovary**

Q50.32 **Ovarian streak**
46, XX with streak gonads

Q50.39 **Other congenital malformation of ovary**
Congenital malformation of ovary NOS

Q50.4 **Embryonic cyst of fallopian tube**
Fimbrial cyst

Q50.5 **Embryonic cyst of broad ligament**
Epoophoron cyst
Parovarian cyst

Q50.6 **Other congenital malformations of fallopian tube and broad ligament**
Absence of fallopian tube and broad ligament
Accessory fallopian tube and broad ligament
Atresia of fallopian tube and broad ligament
Congenital malformation of fallopian tube or broad ligament NOS

Q51 **Congenital malformations of uterus and cervix**

Q51.0 **Agenesis and aplasia of uterus**
Congenital absence of uterus

Q51.1 **Doubling of uterus with doubling of cervix and vagina**

Q51.10 **Doubling of uterus with doubling of cervix and vagina without obstruction**
Doubling of uterus with doubling of cervix and vagina NOS

Q51.11 **Doubling of uterus with doubling of cervix and vagina with obstruction**

Q51.2 **Other doubling of uterus**
Doubling of uterus NOS
Septate uterus, complete or partial

Q51.3 **Bicornate uterus**
Bicornate uterus, complete or partial

Q51.4 **Unicornate uterus**
Unicornate uterus with or without a separate uterine horn
Uterus with only one functioning horn

Q51.5 **Agenesis and aplasia of cervix**
Congenital absence of cervix

Q51.6 **Embryonic cyst of cervix**

Q51.7 **Congenital fistulae between uterus and digestive and urinary tracts**

Q51.8 **Other congenital malformations of uterus and cervix**

Q51.81 **Other congenital malformations of uterus**

Q51.810 **Arcuate uterus**
Arcuatus uterus

Q51.811 **Hypoplasia of uterus**

Q51.818 **Other congenital malformations of uterus**
Müllerian anomaly of uterus NEC

Q51.82 **Other congenital malformations of cervix**

Q51.820 **Cervical duplication**

Q51.821 **Hypoplasia of cervix**

Q51.828 **Other congenital malformations of cervix**

Q51.9 **Congenital malformation of uterus and cervix, unspecified**

Q52 **Other congenital malformations of female genitalia**

Q52.0 **Congenital absence of vagina**
Vaginal agenesis, total or partial

Q52.1 **Doubling of vagina**

EXCLUDES1 *doubling of vagina with doubling of uterus and cervix (Q51.1-)*

Q52.10 **Doubling of vagina, unspecified**
Septate vagina NOS

Q52.11 **Transverse vaginal septum**

Q52.12 **Longitudinal vaginal septum**

● Q52.120 **Longitudinal vaginal septum, nonobstructing**

● Q52.121 **Longitudinal vaginal septum, obstructing, right side**

● Q52.122 **Longitudinal vaginal septum, obstructing, left side**

● Q52.123 **Longitudinal vaginal septum, microperforate, right side**

Unacceptable principal diagnosis symbol per Medicare code edits · Code exempt from diagnosis present on admission requirement · Questionable admission · Complication or comorbidity · CC/MCC exclusion · Major complication or comorbidity · Principal diagnosis as its own CC · Principal diagnosis as its own MCC · Z code as first-listed diagnosis

● Q52.124 Longitudinal vaginal septum, microperforate, left side
● Q52.129 Other and unspecified longitudinal vaginal septum
Q52.2 Congenital rectovaginal fistula POA ♀
EXCLUDES1 *cloaca (Q43.7)*
Q52.3 Imperforate hymen POA ♀
Q52.4 Other congenital malformations of vagina POA ♀
Canal of Nuck cyst, congenital
Congenital malformation of vagina NOS
Embryonic vaginal cyst
Gartner's duct cyst
Q52.5 Fusion of labia POA ♀
Q52.6 Congenital malformation of clitoris POA ♀
⑤ Q52.7 Other and unspecified congenital malformations of vulva
Q52.70 Unspecified congenital malformations of vulva POA ♀
Congenital malformation of vulva NOS
Q52.71 Congenital absence of vulva POA ♀
Q52.79 Other congenital malformations of vulva POA ♀
Congenital cyst of vulva
Q52.8 Other specified congenital malformations of female genitalia POA ♀
Q52.9 Congenital malformation of female genitalia, unspecified POA ♀

④ Q53 Undescended and ectopic testicle
⑤ Q53.0 Ectopic testis
Q53.00 Ectopic testis, unspecified POA ♂
Q53.01 Ectopic testis, unilateral POA ♂
Q53.02 Ectopic testes, bilateral POA ♂
⑤ Q53.1 Undescended testicle, unilateral
Q53.10 Unspecified undescended testicle, unilateral POA ♂
Q53.11 Abdominal testis, unilateral POA ♂
Q53.12 Ectopic perineal testis, unilateral POA ♂
⑤ Q53.2 Undescended testicle, bilateral
Q53.20 Undescended testicle, unspecified, bilateral POA ♂
Q53.21 Abdominal testis, bilateral POA ♂
Q53.22 Ectopic perineal testis, bilateral POA ♂
Q53.9 Undescended testicle, unspecified POA ♂
Cryptorchism NOS

④ Q54 Hypospadias
EXCLUDES1 *epispadias (Q64.0)*
Q54.0 Hypospadias, balanic POA ♂
Hypospadias, coronal
Hypospadias, glandular
Q54.1 Hypospadias, penile POA ♂
Q54.2 Hypospadias, penoscrotal POA ♂
Q54.3 Hypospadias, perineal POA ♂
Q54.4 Congenital chordee POA ♂
Chordee without hypospadias
Q54.8 Other hypospadias POA ♂
Hypospadias with intersex state
Q54.9 Hypospadias, unspecified POA ♂

④ Q55 Other congenital malformations of male genital organs
EXCLUDES1 *congenital hydrocele (P83.5)*
hypospadias (Q54.-)
Q55.0 Absence and aplasia of testis POA ♂
Monorchism
Q55.1 Hypoplasia of testis and scrotum POA ♂
Fusion of testes
⑤ Q55.2 Other and unspecified congenital malformations of testis and scrotum
Q55.20 Unspecified congenital malformations of testis and scrotum POA ♂
Congenital malformation of testis or scrotum NOS
Q55.21 Polyorchism POA ♂
Q55.22 Retractile testis POA ♂
Q55.23 Scrotal transposition POA ♂
Q55.29 Other congenital malformations of testis and scrotum POA ♂
Q55.3 Atresia of vas deferens POA ♂
Code first any associated cystic fibrosis (E84.-)
Q55.4 Other congenital malformations of vas deferens, epididymis, seminal vesicles and prostate POA ♂
Absence or aplasia of prostate
Absence or aplasia of spermatic cord
Congenital malformation of vas deferens, epididymis, seminal vesicles or prostate NOS
Q55.5 Congenital absence and aplasia of penis POA ♂
⑤ Q55.6 Other congenital malformations of penis
Q55.61 Curvature of penis (lateral) POA ♂
Q55.62 Hypoplasia of penis POA ♂
Micropenis
Q55.63 Congenital torsion of penis POA ♂
EXCLUDES1 *acquired torsion of penis (N48.82)*
Q55.64 Hidden penis POA ♂
Buried penis
Concealed penis
EXCLUDES1 *acquired buried penis (N48.83)*
Q55.69 Other congenital malformation of penis POA ♂
Congenital malformation of penis NOS
Q55.7 Congenital vasocutaneous fistula POA ♂
Q55.8 Other specified congenital malformations of male genital organs POA ♂
Q55.9 Congenital malformation of male genital organ, unspecified POA ♂
Congenital anomaly of male genital organ
Congenital deformity of male genital organ

④ Q56 Indeterminate sex and pseudohermaphroditism
EXCLUDES1 *46,XX true hermaphrodite (Q99.1)*
androgen insensitivity syndrome (E34.5-)
chimera 46,XX/46,XY true hermaphrodite (Q99.0)
female pseudohermaphroditism with adrenocortical disorder (E25.-)
pseudohermaphroditism with specified chromosomal anomaly (Q96-Q99)
pure gonadal dysgenesis (Q99.1)
Q56.0 Hermaphroditism, not elsewhere classified POA
Ovotestis
Q56.1 Male pseudohermaphroditism, not elsewhere classified POA ♂
46, XY with streak gonads
Male pseudohermaphroditism NOS
Q56.2 Female pseudohermaphroditism, not elsewhere classified POA ♀
Female pseudohermaphroditism NOS
Q56.3 Pseudohermaphroditism, unspecified POA
Q56.4 Indeterminate sex, unspecified POA
Ambiguous genitalia

Congenital malformations of the urinary system (Q60-Q64)

④ Q60 Renal agenesis and other reduction defects of kidney
INCLUDES *congenital absence of kidney*
congenital atrophy of kidney
infantile atrophy of kidney
Q60.0 Renal agenesis, unilateral CC POA
Q60.1 Renal agenesis, bilateral CC POA
Q60.2 Renal agenesis, unspecified CC POA
Q60.3 Renal hypoplasia, unilateral CC POA
Q60.4 Renal hypoplasia, bilateral CC POA
Q60.5 Renal hypoplasia, unspecified CC POA
Q60.6 Potter's syndrome CC POA

④ Q61 Cystic kidney disease
EXCLUDES1 *acquired cyst of kidney (N28.1)*
Potter's syndrome (Q60.6)
⑤ Q61.0 Congenital renal cyst
Q61.00 Congenital renal cyst, unspecified CC POA
Cyst of kidney NOS (congenital)
Q61.01 Congenital single renal cyst CC POA
Q61.02 Congenital multiple renal cysts CC POA
⑤ Q61.1 Polycystic kidney, infantile type
Polycystic kidney, autosomal recessive
Q61.11 Cystic dilatation of collecting ducts CC POA
Q61.19 Other polycystic kidney, infantile type CC POA
Q61.2 Polycystic kidney, adult type CC POA
Polycystic kidney, autosomal dominant

Unspecified Code Other Specified Code Manifestation Code N Newborn P Pediatric M Maternity A Adult ♂ Male ♀ Female
● New Code ▲ Revised Code Title ►◄ Revised Text NOTES INCLUDES EXCLUDES1 Not coded here EXCLUDES2 Not included here
④ 4th character required ⑤ 5th character required ⑥ 6th character required ⑦ 7th character required
⑦ Extension 'X' Alert HAC Hospital-acquired condition (HAC) alert AHA AHA Coding Clinic©

Q61.3 **Polycystic kidney, unspecified**
Q61.4 **Renal dysplasia**
Multicystic dysplastic kidney
Multicystic kidney (development)
Multicystic kidney disease
Multicystic renal dysplasia
EXCLUDES1 *polycystic kidney disease (Q61.11-Q61.3)*
Q61.5 **Medullary cystic kidney**
Nephronopthisis
Sponge kidney NOS
Q61.8 **Other cystic kidney diseases**
Fibrocystic kidney
Fibrocystic renal degeneration or disease
Q61.9 **Cystic kidney disease, unspecified**
Meckel-Gruber syndrome

Q62 **Congenital obstructive defects of renal pelvis and congenital malformations of ureter**
Q62.0 **Congenital hydronephrosis**
Q62.1 **Congenital occlusion of ureter**
Atresia and stenosis of ureter
Q62.10 **Congenital occlusion of ureter, unspecified**
Q62.11 **Congenital occlusion of ureteropelvic junction**
Q62.12 **Congenital occlusion of ureterovesical orifice**
Q62.2 **Congenital megaureter**
Congenital dilatation of ureter
Q62.3 **Other obstructive defects of renal pelvis and ureter**
Q62.31 **Congenital ureterocele, orthotopic**
Q62.32 **Cecoureterocele**
Ectopic ureterocele
Q62.39 **Other obstructive defects of renal pelvis and ureter**
Ureteropelvic junction obstruction NOS
Q62.4 **Agenesis of ureter**
Congenital absence ureter
Q62.5 **Duplication of ureter**
Accessory ureter
Double ureter
Q62.6 **Malposition of ureter**
Q62.60 **Malposition of ureter, unspecified**
Q62.61 **Deviation of ureter**
Q62.62 **Displacement of ureter**
Q62.63 **Anomalous implantation of ureter**
Ectopia of ureter
Ectopic ureter
Q62.69 **Other malposition of ureter**
Q62.7 **Congenital vesico-uretero-renal reflux**
Q62.8 **Other congenital malformations of ureter**
Anomaly of ureter NOS

Q63 **Other congenital malformations of kidney**
EXCLUDES1 *congenital nephrotic syndrome (N04.-)*
Q63.0 **Accessory kidney**
Q63.1 **Lobulated, fused and horseshoe kidney**
Q63.2 **Ectopic kidney**
Congenital displaced kidney
Malrotation of kidney
Q63.3 **Hyperplastic and giant kidney**
Compensatory hypertrophy of kidney
Q63.8 **Other specified congenital malformations of kidney**
Congenital renal calculi
Q63.9 **Congenital malformation of kidney, unspecified**

Q64 **Other congenital malformations of urinary system**
Q64.0 **Epispadias**
EXCLUDES1 *hypospadias (Q54.-)*
Q64.1 **Exstrophy of urinary bladder**
Q64.10 **Exstrophy of urinary bladder, unspecified**
Ectopia vesicae
Q64.11 **Supravesical fissure of urinary bladder**
Q64.12 **Cloacal extrophy of urinary bladder**
Q64.19 **Other exstrophy of urinary bladder**
Extroversion of bladder
Q64.2 **Congenital posterior urethral valves**
Q64.3 **Other atresia and stenosis of urethra and bladder neck**
Q64.31 **Congenital bladder neck obstruction**
Congenital obstruction of vesicourethral orifice
Q64.32 **Congenital stricture of urethra**
Q64.33 **Congenital stricture of urinary meatus**
Q64.39 **Other atresia and stenosis of urethra and bladder neck**
Atresia and stenosis of urethra and bladder neck NOS
Q64.4 **Malformation of urachus**
Cyst of urachus
Patent urachus
Prolapse of urachus
Q64.5 **Congenital absence of bladder and urethra**
Q64.6 **Congenital diverticulum of bladder**
Q64.7 **Other and unspecified congenital malformations of bladder and urethra**
EXCLUDES1 *congenital prolapse of bladder (mucosa) (Q79.4)*
Q64.70 **Unspecified congenital malformation of bladder and urethra**
Malformation of bladder or urethra NOS
Q64.71 **Congenital prolapse of urethra**
Q64.72 **Congenital prolapse of urinary meatus**
Q64.73 **Congenital urethrorectal fistula**
Q64.74 **Double urethra**
Q64.75 **Double urinary meatus**
Q64.79 **Other congenital malformations of bladder and urethra**
Q64.8 **Other specified congenital malformations of urinary system**
Q64.9 **Congenital malformation of urinary system, unspecified**
Congenital anomaly NOS of urinary system
Congenital deformity NOS of urinary system

Congenital malformations and deformations of the musculoskeletal system (Q65-Q79)

Q65 **Congenital deformities of hip**
EXCLUDES1 *clicking hip (R29.4)*
Q65.0 **Congenital dislocation of hip, unilateral**
Q65.00 **Congenital dislocation of unspecified hip, unilateral**
Q65.01 **Congenital dislocation of right hip, unilateral**
Q65.02 **Congenital dislocation of left hip, unilateral**
Q65.1 **Congenital dislocation of hip, bilateral**
Q65.2 **Congenital dislocation of hip, unspecified**
Q65.3 **Congenital partial dislocation of hip, unilateral**
Q65.30 **Congenital partial dislocation of unspecified hip, unilateral**
Q65.31 **Congenital partial dislocation of right hip, unilateral**
Q65.32 **Congenital partial dislocation of left hip, unilateral**
Q65.4 **Congenital partial dislocation of hip, bilateral**
Q65.5 **Congenital partial dislocation of hip, unspecified**
Q65.6 **Congenital unstable hip**
Congenital dislocatable hip
Q65.8 **Other congenital deformities of hip**
Q65.81 **Congenital coxa valga**
Q65.82 **Congenital coxa vara**
Q65.89 **Other specified congenital deformities of hip**
Anteversion of femoral neck
Congenital acetabular dysplasia
Q65.9 **Congenital deformity of hip, unspecified**

Q66 **Congenital deformities of feet**
EXCLUDES1 *reduction defects of feet (Q72.-)*
valgus deformities (acquired) (M21.0-)
varus deformities (acquired) (M21.1-)
Q66.0 **Congenital talipes equinovarus**
Q66.1 **Congenital talipes calcaneovarus**
Q66.2 **Congenital metatarsus (primus) varus**
● Q66.21 **Congenital metatarsus primus varus**
● Q66.22 **Congenital metatarsus adductus**
Congenital metatarsus varus
Q66.3 **Other congenital varus deformities of feet**
Hallux varus, congenital

Unacceptable principal diagnosis symbol per Medicare code edits; Code exempt from diagnosis present on admission requirement; Questionable admission; Complication or comorbidity; CC/MCC exclusion; Major complication or comorbidity; Principal diagnosis as its own CC; Principal diagnosis as its own MCC; Z code as first-listed diagnosis

When symbols appear on a code that requires a 7th character extension, refer to Appendix D to identify applicable 7th character codes.

Q66.4 Congenital talipes calcaneovalgus POA
Q66.5 Congenital pes planus
Congenital flat foot
Congenital rigid flat foot
Congenital spastic (everted) flat foot
EXCLUDES1 *pes planus, acquired (M21.4)*
Q66.50 **Congenital pes planus, unspecified foot** POA
Q66.51 **Congenital pes planus, right foot** POA
Q66.52 **Congenital pes planus, left foot** POA
Q66.6 **Other congenital valgus deformities of feet** POA
Congenital metatarsus valgus
Q66.7 Congenital pes cavus POA
Q66.8 Other congenital deformities of feet
Q66.80 **Congenital vertical talus deformity, unspecified foot** POA
Q66.81 **Congenital vertical talus deformity, right foot** POA
Q66.82 **Congenital vertical talus deformity, left foot** POA
Q66.89 **Other specified congenital deformities of feet** POA
Congenital asymmetric talipes
Congenital clubfoot NOS
Congenital talipes NOS
Congenital tarsal coalition
Hammer toe, congenital
Q66.9 **Congenital deformity of feet, unspecified** POA
Q67 **Congenital musculoskeletal deformities of head, face, spine and chest**
EXCLUDES1 *congenital malformation syndromes classified to Q87.-*
Potter's syndrome (Q60.6)
Q67.0 Congenital facial asymmetry POA
Q67.1 Congenital compression facies POA
Q67.2 Dolichocephaly POA
Q67.3 Plagiocephaly POA
Q67.4 **Other congenital deformities of skull, face and jaw** POA
Congenital depressions in skull
Congenital hemifacial atrophy or hypertrophy
Deviation of nasal septum, congenital
Squashed or bent nose, congenital
EXCLUDES1 *dentofacial anomalies [including malocclusion] (M26.-)*
syphilitic saddle nose (A50.5)
Q67.5 **Congenital deformity of spine** CC POA
Congenital postural scoliosis
Congenital scoliosis NOS
EXCLUDES1 *infantile idiopathic scoliosis (M41.0)*
scoliosis due to congenital bony malformation (Q76.3)
Q67.6 Pectus excavatum POA
Congenital funnel chest
Q67.7 Pectus carinatum POA
Congenital pigeon chest
Q67.8 **Other congenital deformities of chest** CC POA
Congenital deformity of chest wall NOS
Q68 Other congenital musculoskeletal deformities
EXCLUDES1 *reduction defects of limb(s) (Q71-Q73)*
EXCLUDES2 *congenital myotonic chondrodystrophy (G71.13)*
Q68.0 **Congenital deformity of sternocleidomastoid muscle** POA
Congenital contracture of sternocleidomastoid (muscle)
Congenital (sternomastoid) torticollis
Sternomastoid tumor (congenital)
Q68.1 **Congenital deformity of finger(s) and hand** CC POA
Congenital clubfinger
Spade-like hand (congenital)
Q68.2 **Congenital deformity of knee** POA
Congenital dislocation of knee
Congenital genu recurvatum
Q68.3 **Congenital bowing of femur** POA
EXCLUDES1 *anteversion of femur (neck) (Q65.89)*
Q68.4 **Congenital bowing of tibia and fibula** POA
Q68.5 **Congenital bowing of long bones of leg, unspecified** POA
Q68.6 Discoid meniscus POA
Q68.8 **Other specified congenital musculoskeletal deformities** POA
Congenital deformity of clavicle
Congenital deformity of elbow
Congenital deformity of forearm
Congenital deformity of scapula
Congenital deformity of wrist
Congenital dislocation of elbow
Congenital dislocation of shoulder
Congenital dislocation of wrist
Q69 **Polydactyly**
Q69.0 Accessory finger(s) POA
Q69.1 Accessory thumb(s) POA
Q69.2 Accessory toe(s) POA
Accessory hallux
Q69.9 **Polydactyly, unspecified** POA
Supernumerary digit(s) NOS
Q70 **Syndactyly**
Q70.0 Fused fingers
Complex syndactyly of fingers with synostosis
Q70.00 **Fused fingers, unspecified hand** POA
Q70.01 **Fused fingers, right hand** POA
Q70.02 **Fused fingers, left hand** POA
Q70.03 **Fused fingers, bilateral** POA
Q70.1 Webbed fingers
Simple syndactyly of fingers without synostosis
Q70.10 **Webbed fingers, unspecified hand** POA
Q70.11 **Webbed fingers, right hand** POA
Q70.12 **Webbed fingers, left hand** POA
Q70.13 **Webbed fingers, bilateral** POA
Q70.2 Fused toes
Complex syndactyly of toes with synostosis
Q70.20 **Fused toes, unspecified foot** POA
Q70.21 **Fused toes, right foot** POA
Q70.22 **Fused toes, left foot** POA
Q70.23 **Fused toes, bilateral** POA
Q70.3 Webbed toes
Simple syndactyly of toes without synostosis
Q70.30 **Webbed toes, unspecified foot** POA
Q70.31 **Webbed toes, right foot** POA
Q70.32 **Webbed toes, left foot** POA
Q70.33 **Webbed toes, bilateral** POA
Q70.4 **Polysyndactyly, unspecified** POA
EXCLUDES1 *specified syndactyly of hand and feet - code to specified conditions (Q70.0- -Q70.3-)*
Q70.9 **Syndactyly, unspecified** POA
Symphalangy NOS
Q71 **Reduction defects of upper limb**
Q71.0 **Congenital complete absence of upper limb**
Q71.00 **Congenital complete absence of unspecified upper limb** POA
Q71.01 **Congenital complete absence of right upper limb** POA
Q71.02 **Congenital complete absence of left upper limb** POA
Q71.03 **Congenital complete absence of upper limb, bilateral** POA
Q71.1 **Congenital absence of upper arm and forearm with hand present**
Q71.10 **Congenital absence of unspecified upper arm and forearm with hand present** POA
Q71.11 **Congenital absence of right upper arm and forearm with hand present** POA
Q71.12 **Congenital absence of left upper arm and forearm with hand present** POA
Q71.13 **Congenital absence of upper arm and forearm with hand present, bilateral** POA
Q71.2 **Congenital absence of both forearm and hand**
Q71.20 **Congenital absence of both forearm and hand, unspecified upper limb** POA
Q71.21 **Congenital absence of both forearm and hand, right upper limb** POA
Q71.22 **Congenital absence of both forearm and hand, left upper limb** POA
Q71.23 **Congenital absence of both forearm and hand, bilateral** POA
Q71.3 **Congenital absence of hand and finger**
Q71.30 **Congenital absence of unspecified hand and finger** POA
Q71.31 **Congenital absence of right hand and finger** POA

Unspecified Code Other Specified Code Manifestation Code N Newborn P Pediatric M Maternity A Adult ♂ Male ♀ Female
● New Code ▲ Revised Code Title ►◄ Revised Text NOTES INCLUDES EXCLUDES1 Not coded here EXCLUDES2 Not included here
4th character required 5th character required 6th character required 7th character required
Extension 'X' Alert HAC Hospital-acquired condition (HAC) alert AHA AHA Coding Clinic©

Q71.32 Congenital absence of left hand and finger
Q71.33 Congenital absence of hand and finger, bilateral
Q71.4 Longitudinal reduction defect of radius
Clubhand (congenital)
Radial clubhand
Q71.40 Longitudinal reduction defect of unspecified radius
Q71.41 Longitudinal reduction defect of right radius
Q71.42 Longitudinal reduction defect of left radius
Q71.43 Longitudinal reduction defect of radius, bilateral
Q71.5 Longitudinal reduction defect of ulna
Q71.50 Longitudinal reduction defect of unspecified ulna
Q71.51 Longitudinal reduction defect of right ulna
Q71.52 Longitudinal reduction defect of left ulna
Q71.53 Longitudinal reduction defect of ulna, bilateral
Q71.6 Lobster-claw hand
Q71.60 Lobster-claw hand, unspecified hand
Q71.61 Lobster-claw right hand
Q71.62 Lobster-claw left hand
Q71.63 Lobster-claw hand, bilateral
Q71.8 Other reduction defects of upper limb
Q71.81 Congenital shortening of upper limb
Q71.811 Congenital shortening of right upper limb
Q71.812 Congenital shortening of left upper limb
Q71.813 Congenital shortening of upper limb, bilateral
Q71.819 Congenital shortening of unspecified upper limb
Q71.89 Other reduction defects of upper limb
Q71.891 Other reduction defects of right upper limb
Q71.892 Other reduction defects of left upper limb
Q71.893 Other reduction defects of upper limb, bilateral
Q71.899 Other reduction defects of unspecified upper limb
Q71.9 Unspecified reduction defect of upper limb
Q71.90 Unspecified reduction defect of unspecified upper limb
Q71.91 Unspecified reduction defect of right upper limb
Q71.92 Unspecified reduction defect of left upper limb
Q71.93 Unspecified reduction defect of upper limb, bilateral

Q72 Reduction defects of lower limb
Q72.0 Congenital complete absence of lower limb
Q72.00 Congenital complete absence of unspecified lower limb
Q72.01 Congenital complete absence of right lower limb
Q72.02 Congenital complete absence of left lower limb
Q72.03 Congenital complete absence of lower limb, bilateral
Q72.1 Congenital absence of thigh and lower leg with foot present
Q72.10 Congenital absence of unspecified thigh and lower leg with foot present
Q72.11 Congenital absence of right thigh and lower leg with foot present
Q72.12 Congenital absence of left thigh and lower leg with foot present
Q72.13 Congenital absence of thigh and lower leg with foot present, bilateral
Q72.2 Congenital absence of both lower leg and foot
Q72.20 Congenital absence of both lower leg and foot, unspecified lower limb
Q72.21 Congenital absence of both lower leg and foot, right lower limb
Q72.22 Congenital absence of both lower leg and foot, left lower limb
Q72.23 Congenital absence of both lower leg and foot, bilateral
Q72.3 Congenital absence of foot and toe(s)
Q72.30 Congenital absence of unspecified foot and toe(s)
Q72.31 Congenital absence of right foot and toe(s)
Q72.32 Congenital absence of left foot and toe(s)
Q72.33 Congenital absence of foot and toe(s), bilateral
Q72.4 Longitudinal reduction defect of femur
Proximal femoral focal deficiency
Q72.40 Longitudinal reduction defect of unspecified femur
Q72.41 Longitudinal reduction defect of right femur
Q72.42 Longitudinal reduction defect of left femur
Q72.43 Longitudinal reduction defect of femur, bilateral
Q72.5 Longitudinal reduction defect of tibia
Q72.50 Longitudinal reduction defect of unspecified tibia
Q72.51 Longitudinal reduction defect of right tibia
Q72.52 Longitudinal reduction defect of left tibia
Q72.53 Longitudinal reduction defect of tibia, bilateral
Q72.6 Longitudinal reduction defect of fibula
Q72.60 Longitudinal reduction defect of unspecified fibula
Q72.61 Longitudinal reduction defect of right fibula
Q72.62 Longitudinal reduction defect of left fibula
Q72.63 Longitudinal reduction defect of fibula, bilateral
Q72.7 Split foot
Q72.70 Split foot, unspecified lower limb
Q72.71 Split foot, right lower limb
Q72.72 Split foot, left lower limb
Q72.73 Split foot, bilateral
Q72.8 Other reduction defects of lower limb
Q72.81 Congenital shortening of lower limb
Q72.811 Congenital shortening of right lower limb
Q72.812 Congenital shortening of left lower limb
Q72.813 Congenital shortening of lower limb, bilateral
Q72.819 Congenital shortening of unspecified lower limb
Q72.89 Other reduction defects of lower limb
Q72.891 Other reduction defects of right lower limb
Q72.892 Other reduction defects of left lower limb
Q72.893 Other reduction defects of lower limb, bilateral
Q72.899 Other reduction defects of unspecified lower limb
Q72.9 Unspecified reduction defect of lower limb
Q72.90 Unspecified reduction defect of unspecified lower limb
Q72.91 Unspecified reduction defect of right lower limb
Q72.92 Unspecified reduction defect of left lower limb
Q72.93 Unspecified reduction defect of lower limb, bilateral

Q73 Reduction defects of unspecified limb
Q73.0 Congenital absence of unspecified limb(s)
Amelia NOS
Q73.1 Phocomelia, unspecified limb(s)
Phocomelia NOS
Q73.8 Other reduction defects of unspecified limb(s)
Longitudinal reduction deformity of unspecified limb(s)
Ectromelia of limb NOS
Hemimelia of limb NOS
Reduction defect of limb NOS

Q74 Other congenital malformations of limb(s)
EXCLUDES1 *polydactyly (Q69.-)*
reduction defect of limb (Q71-Q73)
syndactyly (Q70.-)
Q74.0 Other congenital malformations of upper limb(s), including shoulder girdle
Accessory carpal bones
Cleidocranial dysostosis
Congenital pseudarthrosis of clavicle

Unacceptable principal diagnosis symbol per Medicare code edits; Code exempt from diagnosis present on admission requirement; Questionable admission; Complication or comorbidity; CC/MCC exclusion; Major complication or comorbidity; Principal diagnosis as its own CC; Principal diagnosis as its own MCC; Z code as first-listed diagnosis

Macrodactylia (fingers)
Madelung's deformity
Radioulnar synostosis
Sprengel's deformity
Triphalangeal thumb

Q74.1 Congenital malformation of knee
Congenital absence of patella
Congenital dislocation of patella
Congenital genu valgum
Congenital genu varum
Rudimentary patella
EXCLUDES1 *congenital dislocation of knee (Q68.2)*
congenital genu recurvatum (Q68.2)
nail patella syndrome (Q87.2)

Q74.2 Other congenital malformations of lower limb(s), including pelvic girdle
Congenital fusion of sacroiliac joint
Congenital malformation of ankle joint
Congenital malformation of sacroiliac joint
EXCLUDES1 *anteversion of femur (neck) (Q65.89)*

Q74.3 Arthrogryposis multiplex congenita

Q74.8 Other specified congenital malformations of limb(s)

Q74.9 Unspecified congenital malformation of limb(s)
Congenital anomaly of limb(s) NOS

Q75 Other congenital malformations of skull and face bones
EXCLUDES1 *congenital malformation of face NOS (Q18.-)*
congenital malformation syndromes classified to Q87.-
dentofacial anomalies [including malocclusion] (M26.-)
musculoskeletal deformities of head and face (Q67.0-Q67.4)
skull defects associated with congenital anomalies of brain such as:
anencephaly (Q00.0)
encephalocele (Q01.-)
hydrocephalus (Q03.-)
microcephaly (Q02)

Q75.0 Craniosynostosis
Acrocephaly
Imperfect fusion of skull
Oxycephaly
Trigonocephaly

Q75.1 Craniofacial dysostosis
Crouzon's disease

Q75.2 Hypertelorism

Q75.3 Macrocephaly

Q75.4 Mandibulofacial dysostosis
Franceschetti syndrome
Treacher Collins syndrome

Q75.5 Oculomandibular dysostosis

Q75.8 Other specified congenital malformations of skull and face bones
Absence of skull bone, congenital
Congenital deformity of forehead
Platybasia

Q75.9 Congenital malformation of skull and face bones, unspecified
Congenital anomaly of face bones NOS
Congenital anomaly of skull NOS

Q76 Congenital malformations of spine and bony thorax
EXCLUDES1 *congenital musculoskeletal deformities of spine and chest (Q67.5-Q67.8)*

Q76.0 Spina bifida occulta
EXCLUDES1 *meningocele (spinal) (Q05.-)*
spina bifida (aperta) (cystica) (Q05.-)

Q76.1 Klippel-Feil syndrome
Cervical fusion syndrome

Q76.2 Congenital spondylolisthesis
Congenital spondylolysis
EXCLUDES1 *spondylolisthesis (acquired) (M43.1-)*
spondylolysis (acquired) (M43.0-)

Q76.3 Congenital scoliosis due to congenital bony malformation
Hemivertebra fusion or failure of segmentation with scoliosis

Q76.4 Other congenital malformations of spine, not associated with scoliosis

Q76.41 Congenital kyphosis

Q76.411 Congenital kyphosis, occipito-atlanto-axial region

Q76.412 Congenital kyphosis, cervical region

Q76.413 Congenital kyphosis, cervicothoracic region

Q76.414 Congenital kyphosis, thoracic region

Q76.415 Congenital kyphosis, thoracolumbar region

Q76.419 Congenital kyphosis, unspecified region

Q76.42 Congenital lordosis

Q76.425 Congenital lordosis, thoracolumbar region

Q76.426 Congenital lordosis, lumbar region

Q76.427 Congenital lordosis, lumbosacral region

Q76.428 Congenital lordosis, sacral and sacrococcygeal region

Q76.429 Congenital lordosis, unspecified region

Q76.49 Other congenital malformations of spine, not associated with scoliosis
Congenital absence of vertebra NOS
Congenital fusion of spine NOS
Congenital malformation of lumbosacral (joint) (region) NOS
Congenital malformation of spine NOS
Hemivertebra NOS
Malformation of spine NOS
Platyspondylisis NOS
Supernumerary vertebra NOS

Q76.5 Cervical rib
Supernumerary rib in cervical region

Q76.6 Other congenital malformations of ribs
Accessory rib
Congenital absence of rib
Congenital fusion of ribs
Congenital malformation of ribs NOS
EXCLUDES1 *short rib syndrome (Q77.2)*

Q76.7 Congenital malformation of sternum
Congenital absence of sternum
Sternum bifidum

Q76.8 Other congenital malformations of bony thorax

Q76.9 Congenital malformation of bony thorax, unspecified

Q77 Osteochondrodysplasia with defects of growth of tubular bones and spine
EXCLUDES1 *mucopolysaccharidosis (E76.0-E76.3)*
EXCLUDES2 *congenital myotonic chondrodystrophy (G71.13)*

Q77.0 Achondrogenesis
Hypochondrogenesis

Q77.1 Thanatophoric short stature

Q77.2 Short rib syndrome
Asphyxiating thoracic dysplasia [Jeune]

Q77.3 Chondrodysplasia punctata
EXCLUDES1 *Rhizomelic chondrodysplasia punctata (E71.43)*

Q77.4 Achondroplasia
Hypochondroplasia
Osteosclerosis congenita

Q77.5 Diastrophic dysplasia

Q77.6 Chondroectodermal dysplasia
Ellis-van Creveld syndrome

Q77.7 Spondyloepiphyseal dysplasia

Q77.8 Other osteochondrodysplasia with defects of growth of tubular bones and spine

Q77.9 Osteochondrodysplasia with defects of growth of tubular bones and spine, unspecified

Q78 Other osteochondrodysplasias
EXCLUDES2 *congenital myotonic chondrodystrophy (G71.13)*

Q78.0 Osteogenesis imperfecta
Fragilitas ossium
Osteopsathyrosis

Q78.1 Polyostotic fibrous dysplasia
Albright(-McCune)(-Sternberg) syndrome

Unspecified Code | Other Specified Code | Manifestation Code | N Newborn | P Pediatric | M Maternity | A Adult | ♂ Male | ♀ Female
● New Code | ▲ Revised Code Title | ►◄ Revised Text | NOTES | INCLUDES | EXCLUDES1 Not coded here | EXCLUDES2 Not included here
4th character required | 5th character required | 6th character required | 7th character required
Extension 'X' Alert | HAC Hospital-acquired condition (HAC) alert | AHA AHA Coding Clinic®

Q78.2 **Osteopetrosis**
Albers-Schönberg syndrome
Osteosclerosis NOS
Q78.3 **Progressive diaphyseal dysplasia**
Camurati-Engelmann syndrome
Q78.4 **Enchondromatosis**
Maffucci's syndrome
Ollier's disease
Q78.5 **Metaphyseal dysplasia**
Pyle's syndrome
Q78.6 **Multiple congenital exostoses**
Diaphyseal aclasis
Q78.8 **Other specified osteochondrodysplasias**
Osteopoikilosis
Q78.9 **Osteochondrodysplasia, unspecified**
Chondrodystrophy NOS
Osteodystrophy NOS

Q79 **Congenital malformations of musculoskeletal system, not elsewhere classified**
EXCLUDES2 *congenital (sternomastoid) torticollis (Q68.0)*
Q79.0 **Congenital diaphragmatic hernia**
EXCLUDES1 *congenital hiatus hernia (Q40.1)*
Q79.1 **Other congenital malformations of diaphragm**
Absence of diaphragm
Congenital malformation of diaphragm NOS
Eventration of diaphragm
Q79.2 **Exomphalos**
Omphalocele
EXCLUDES1 *umbilical hernia (K42.-)*
Q79.3 **Gastroschisis**
Q79.4 **Prune belly syndrome**
Congenital prolapse of bladder mucosa
Eagle-Barrett syndrome
Q79.5 **Other congenital malformations of abdominal wall**
EXCLUDES1 *umbilical hernia (K42.-)*
Q79.51 **Congenital hernia of bladder**
Q79.59 **Other congenital malformations of abdominal wall**
Q79.6 **Ehlers-Danlos syndrome**
Q79.8 **Other congenital malformations of musculoskeletal system**
Absence of muscle
Absence of tendon
Accessory muscle
Amyotrophia congenita
Congenital constricting bands
Congenital shortening of tendon
Poland syndrome
Q79.9 **Congenital malformation of musculoskeletal system, unspecified**
Congenital anomaly of musculoskeletal system NOS
Congenital deformity of musculoskeletal system NOS

Other congenital malformations (Q80-Q89)

Q80 **Congenital ichthyosis**
EXCLUDES1 *Refsum's disease (G60.1)*
Q80.0 **Ichthyosis vulgaris**
Q80.1 **X-linked ichthyosis**
Q80.2 **Lamellar ichthyosis**
Collodion baby
Q80.3 **Congenital bullous ichthyosiform erythroderma**
Q80.4 **Harlequin fetus**
Q80.8 **Other congenital ichthyosis**
Q80.9 **Congenital ichthyosis, unspecified**

Q81 **Epidermolysis bullosa**
Q81.0 **Epidermolysis bullosa simplex**
EXCLUDES1 *Cockayne's syndrome (Q87.1)*
Q81.1 **Epidermolysis bullosa letalis**
Herlitz' syndrome
Q81.2 **Epidermolysis bullosa dystrophica**
Q81.8 **Other epidermolysis bullosa**
Q81.9 **Epidermolysis bullosa, unspecified**

Q82 **Other congenital malformations of skin**
EXCLUDES1 *acrodermatitis enteropathica (E83.2)*
congenital erythropoietic porphyria (E80.0)
pilonidal cyst or sinus (L05.-)
Sturge-Weber (-Dimitri) syndrome (Q85.8)
Q82.0 **Hereditary lymphedema**
Q82.1 **Xeroderma pigmentosum**
Q82.2 **Mastocytosis**
Urticaria pigmentosa
EXCLUDES1 *malignant mastocytosis (C96.2)*
Q82.3 **Incontinentia pigmenti**
Q82.4 **Ectodermal dysplasia (anhidrotic)**
EXCLUDES1 *Ellis-van Creveld syndrome (Q77.6)*
Q82.5 **Congenital non-neoplastic nevus**
Birthmark NOS
Flammeus Nevus
Portwine Nevus
Sanguineous Nevus
Strawberry Nevus
Vascular Nevus NOS
Verrucous Nevus
EXCLUDES2 *Café au lait spots (L81.3)*
lentigo (L81.4)
nevus NOS (D22.-)
araneus nevus (I78.1)
melanocytic nevus (D22.-)
pigmented nevus (D22.-)
spider nevus (I78.1)
stellar nevus (I78.1)
● Q82.6 **Congenital sacral dimple**
Parasacral dimple
EXCLUDES2 *pilonidal cyst with abscess (L05.01)*
pilonidal cyst without abscess (L05.91)
Q82.8 **Other specified congenital malformations of skin**
Abnormal palmar creases
Accessory skin tags
Benign familial pemphigus [Hailey-Hailey]
Congenital poikiloderma
Cutis laxa (hyperelastica)
Dermatoglyphic anomalies
Inherited keratosis palmaris et plantaris
Keratosis follicularis [Darier-White]
EXCLUDES1 *Ehlers-Danlos syndrome (Q79.6)*
AHA: Q1, 2016
Q82.9 **Congenital malformation of skin, unspecified**

Q83 **Congenital malformations of breast**
EXCLUDES2 *absence of pectoral muscle (Q79.8)*
hypoplasia of breast (N64.82)
micromastia (N64.82)
Q83.0 **Congenital absence of breast with absent nipple**
Q83.1 **Accessory breast**
Supernumerary breast
Q83.2 **Absent nipple**
Q83.3 **Accessory nipple**
Supernumerary nipple
Q83.8 **Other congenital malformations of breast**
Q83.9 **Congenital malformation of breast, unspecified**

Q84 **Other congenital malformations of integument**
Q84.0 **Congenital alopecia**
Congenital atrichosis
Q84.1 **Congenital morphological disturbances of hair, not elsewhere classified**
Beaded hair
Monilethrix
Pili annulati
EXCLUDES1 *Menkes' kinky hair syndrome (E83.0)*
Q84.2 **Other congenital malformations of hair**
Congenital hypertrichosis
Congenital malformation of hair NOS
Persistent lanugo
Q84.3 **Anonychia**
EXCLUDES1 *nail patella syndrome (Q87.2)*
Q84.4 **Congenital leukonychia**
Q84.5 **Enlarged and hypertrophic nails**
Congenital onychauxis
Pachyonychia

Unacceptable principal diagnosis symbol per Medicare code edits · Code exempt from diagnosis present on admission requirement
Questionable admission · Complication or comorbidity · CC/MCC exclusion · Major complication or comorbidity
Principal diagnosis as its own CC · Principal diagnosis as its own MCC · Z code as first-listed diagnosis

Q84.6 **Other congenital malformations of nails**
Congenital clubnail
Congenital koilonychia
Congenital malformation of nail NOS
Q84.8 **Other specified congenital malformations of integument**
Aplasia cutis congenita
Q84.9 **Congenital malformation of integument, unspecified**
Congenital anomaly of integument NOS
Congenital deformity of integument NOS

Q85 **Phakomatoses, not elsewhere classified**
EXCLUDES1 *ataxia telangiectasia [Louis-Bar] (G11.3)*
familial dysautonomia [Riley-Day] (G90.1)
Q85.0 **Neurofibromatosis (nonmalignant)**
Q85.00 **Neurofibromatosis, unspecified**
Q85.01 **Neurofibromatosis, type 1**
Von Recklinghausen disease
Q85.02 **Neurofibromatosis, type 2**
Acoustic neurofibromatosis
Q85.03 **Schwannomatosis**
Q85.09 **Other neurofibromatosis**
Q85.1 **Tuberous sclerosis**
Bourneville's disease
Epiloia
Q85.8 **Other phakomatoses, not elsewhere classified**
Peutz-Jeghers Syndrome
Sturge-Weber(-Dimitri) syndrome
von Hippel-Lindau syndrome
EXCLUDES1 *Meckel-Gruber syndrome (Q61.9)*
Q85.9 **Phakomatosis, unspecified**
Hamartosis NOS

Q86 **Congenital malformation syndromes due to known exogenous causes , not elsewhere classified**
EXCLUDES2 *iodine-deficiency-related hypothyroidism (E00-E02)*
nonteratogenic effects of substances transmitted via placenta or breast milk (P04.-)
Q86.0 **Fetal alcohol syndrome (dysmorphic)**
Q86.1 **Fetal hydantoin syndrome**
Meadow's syndrome
Q86.2 **Dysmorphism due to warfarin**
Q86.8 **Other congenital malformation syndromes due to known exogenous causes**

Q87 **Other specified congenital malformation syndromes affecting multiple systems**
Use additional code(s) to identify all associated manifestations
Q87.0 **Congenital malformation syndromes predominantly affecting facial appearance**
Acrocephalopolysyndactyly
Acrocephalosyndactyly [Apert]
Cryptophthalmos syndrome
Cyclopia
Goldenhar syndrome
Moebius syndrome
Oro-facial-digital syndrome
Robin syndrome
Whistling face
Q87.1 **Congenital malformation syndromes predominantly associated with short stature**
Aarskog syndrome
Cockayne syndrome
De Lange syndrome
Dubowitz syndrome
Noonan syndrome
Prader-Willi syndrome
Robinow-Silverman-Smith syndrome
Russell-Silver syndrome
Seckel syndrome
EXCLUDES1 *Ellis-van Creveld syndrome (Q77.6)*
Smith-Lemli-Opitz syndrome (E78.72)
Q87.2 **Congenital malformation syndromes predominantly involving limbs**
Holt-Oram syndrome
Klippel-Trenaunay-Weber syndrome
Nail patella syndrome
Rubinstein-Taybi syndrome
Sirenomelia syndrome
Thrombocytopenia with absent radius [TAR] syndrome
VATER syndrome
Q87.3 **Congenital malformation syndromes involving early overgrowth**
Beckwith-Wiedemann syndrome
Sotos syndrome
Weaver syndrome
Q87.4 **Marfan's syndrome**
Q87.40 **Marfan's syndrome, unspecified**
Q87.41 **Marfan's syndrome with cardiovascular manifestations**
Q87.410 **Marfan's syndrome with aortic dilation**
Q87.418 **Marfan's syndrome with other cardiovascular manifestations**
Q87.42 **Marfan's syndrome with ocular manifestations**
Q87.43 **Marfan's syndrome with skeletal manifestation**
Q87.5 **Other congenital malformation syndromes with other skeletal changes**
Q87.8 **Other specified congenital malformation syndromes, not elsewhere classified**
EXCLUDES1 *Zellweger syndrome (E71.510)*
Q87.81 **Alport syndrome**
Use additional code to identify stage of chronic kidney disease (N18.1-N18.6)
● Q87.82 **Arterial tortuosity syndrome**
Q87.89 **Other specified congenital malformation syndromes, not elsewhere classified**
Laurence-Moon (-Bardet)-Biedl syndrome

Q89 **Other congenital malformations, not elsewhere classified**
Q89.0 **Congenital absence and malformations of spleen**
EXCLUDES1 *isomerism of atrial appendages (with asplenia or polysplenia) (Q20.6)*
Q89.01 **Asplenia (congenital)**
Q89.09 **Congenital malformations of spleen**
Congenital splenomegaly
Q89.1 **Congenital malformations of adrenal gland**
EXCLUDES1 *adrenogenital disorders (E25.-)*
congenital adrenal hyperplasia (E25.0)
Q89.2 **Congenital malformations of other endocrine glands**
Congenital malformation of parathyroid or thyroid gland
Persistent thyroglossal duct
Thyroglossal cyst
EXCLUDES1 *congenital goiter (E03.0)*
congenital hypothyroidism (E03.1)
Q89.3 **Situs inversus**
Dextrocardia with situs inversus
Mirror-image atrial arrangement with situs inversus
Situs inversus or transversus abdominalis
Situs inversus or transversus thoracis
Transposition of abdominal viscera
Transposition of thoracic viscera
EXCLUDES1 *dextrocardia NOS (Q24.0)*
Q89.4 **Conjoined twins**
Craniopagus
Dicephaly
Pygopagus
Thoracopagus
Q89.7 **Multiple congenital malformations, not elsewhere classified**
Multiple congenital anomalies NOS
Multiple congenital deformities NOS
EXCLUDES1 *congenital malformation syndromes affecting multiple systems (Q87.-)*
Q89.8 **Other specified congenital malformations**
Use additional code(s) to identify all associated manifestations
Q89.9 **Congenital malformation, unspecified**
Congenital anomaly NOS
Congenital deformity NOS

Unspecified Code · Other Specified Code · Manifestation Code · N Newborn · P Pediatric · M Maternity · A Adult · ♂ Male · ♀ Female
● New Code · ▲ Revised Code Title · ►◄ Revised Text · NOTES · INCLUDES · EXCLUDES1 Not coded here · EXCLUDES2 Not included here
4th character required · 5th character required · 6th character required · 7th character required
Extension 'X' Alert · HAC Hospital-acquired condition (HAC) alert · AHA AHA Coding Clinic©

Chromosomal abnormalities, not elsewhere classified (Q90-Q99)

EXCLUDES2 *mitochondrial metabolic disorders (E88.4-)*

Q90 Down syndrome
Use additional code(s) to identify any associated physical conditions and degree of intellectual disabilities (F70-F79)
- Q90.0 **Trisomy 21, nonmosaicism (meiotic nondisjunction)**
- Q90.1 **Trisomy 21, mosaicism (mitotic nondisjunction)**
- Q90.2 **Trisomy 21, translocation**
- Q90.9 **Down syndrome, unspecified**
  Trisomy 21 NOS

Q91 Trisomy 18 and Trisomy 13
- Q91.0 **Trisomy 18, nonmosaicism (meiotic nondisjunction)**
- Q91.1 **Trisomy 18, mosaicism (mitotic nondisjunction)**
- Q91.2 **Trisomy 18, translocation**
- Q91.3 **Trisomy 18, unspecified**
- Q91.4 **Trisomy 13, nonmosaicism (meiotic nondisjunction)**
- Q91.5 **Trisomy 13, mosaicism (mitotic nondisjunction)**
- Q91.6 **Trisomy 13, translocation**
- Q91.7 **Trisomy 13, unspecified**

Q92 Other trisomies and partial trisomies of the autosomes, not elsewhere classified
INCLUDES *unbalanced translocations and insertions*
EXCLUDES1 *trisomies of chromosomes 13, 18, 21 (Q90-Q91)*
- Q92.0 **Whole chromosome trisomy, nonmosaicism (meiotic nondisjunction)**
- Q92.1 **Whole chromosome trisomy, mosaicism (mitotic nondisjunction)**
- Q92.2 **Partial trisomy**
  Less than whole arm duplicated
  Whole arm or more duplicated
  EXCLUDES1 *partial trisomy due to unbalanced translocation (Q92.5)*
- Q92.5 **Duplications with other complex rearrangements**
  Partial trisomy due to unbalanced translocations
  Code also any associated deletions due to unbalanced translocations, inversions and insertions (Q93.7)
- Q92.6 **Marker chromosomes**
  Trisomies due to dicentrics
  Trisomies due to extra rings
  Trisomies due to isochromosomes
  Individual with marker heterochromatin
  - Q92.61 **Marker chromosomes in normal individual**
  - Q92.62 **Marker chromosomes in abnormal individual**
- Q92.7 **Triploidy and polyploidy**
- Q92.8 **Other specified trisomies and partial trisomies of autosomes**
  Duplications identified by fluorescence in situ hybridization (FISH)
  Duplications identified by in situ hybridization (ISH)
  Duplications seen only at prometaphase
- Q92.9 **Trisomy and partial trisomy of autosomes, unspecified**

Q93 Monosomies and deletions from the autosomes, not elsewhere classified
- Q93.0 **Whole chromosome monosomy, nonmosaicism (meiotic nondisjunction)**
- Q93.1 **Whole chromosome monosomy, mosaicism (mitotic nondisjunction)**
- Q93.2 **Chromosome replaced with ring, dicentric or isochromosome**
- Q93.3 **Deletion of short arm of chromosome 4**
  Wolff-Hirschorn syndrome
- Q93.4 **Deletion of short arm of chromosome 5**
  Cri-du-chat syndrome
- Q93.5 **Other deletions of part of a chromosome**
  Angelman syndrome
- Q93.7 **Deletions with other complex rearrangements**
  Deletions due to unbalanced translocations, inversions and insertions
  Code also any associated duplications due to unbalanced translocations, inversions and insertions (Q92.5)
- Q93.8 **Other deletions from the autosomes**
  - Q93.81 **Velo-cardio-facial syndrome**
    Deletion 22q11.2
  - Q93.88 **Other microdeletions**
    Miller-Dieker syndrome
    Smith-Magenis syndrome
  - Q93.89 **Other deletions from the autosomes**
    Deletions identified by fluorescence in situ hybridization (FISH)
    Deletions identified by in situ hybridization (ISH)
    Deletions seen only at prometaphase
- Q93.9 **Deletion from autosomes, unspecified**

Q95 Balanced rearrangements and structural markers, not elsewhere classified
INCLUDES *Robertsonian and balanced reciprocal translocations and insertions*
- Q95.0 **Balanced translocation and insertion in normal individual**
- Q95.1 **Chromosome inversion in normal individual**
- Q95.2 **Balanced autosomal rearrangement in abnormal individual**
- Q95.3 **Balanced sex/autosomal rearrangement in abnormal individual**
- Q95.5 **Individual with autosomal fragile site**
- Q95.8 **Other balanced rearrangements and structural markers**
- Q95.9 **Balanced rearrangement and structural marker, unspecified**

Q96 Turner's syndrome
EXCLUDES1 *Noonan syndrome (Q87.1)*
- Q96.0 **Karyotype 45, X**
- Q96.1 **Karyotype 46, X iso (Xq)**
  Karyotype 46, isochromosome Xq
- Q96.2 **Karyotype 46, X with abnormal sex chromosome, except iso (Xq)**
  Karyotype 46, X with abnormal sex chromosome, except isochromosome Xq
- Q96.3 **Mosaicism, 45, X/46, XX or XY**
- Q96.4 **Mosaicism, 45, X/other cell line(s) with abnormal sex chromosome**
- Q96.8 **Other variants of Turner's syndrome**
- Q96.9 **Turner's syndrome, unspecified**

Q97 Other sex chromosome abnormalities, female phenotype, not elsewhere classified
EXCLUDES1 *Turner's syndrome (Q96.-)*
- Q97.0 **Karyotype 47, XXX**
- Q97.1 **Female with more than three X chromosomes**
- Q97.2 **Mosaicism, lines with various numbers of X chromosomes**
- Q97.3 **Female with 46, XY karyotype**
- Q97.8 **Other specified sex chromosome abnormalities, female phenotype**
- Q97.9 **Sex chromosome abnormality, female phenotype, unspecified**

Q98 Other sex chromosome abnormalities, male phenotype, not elsewhere classified
- Q98.0 **Klinefelter syndrome karyotype 47, XXY**
- Q98.1 **Klinefelter syndrome, male with more than two X chromosomes**
- Q98.3 **Other male with 46, XX karyotype**
- Q98.4 **Klinefelter syndrome, unspecified**
- Q98.5 **Karyotype 47, XYY**
- Q98.6 **Male with structurally abnormal sex chromosome**
- Q98.7 **Male with sex chromosome mosaicism**
- Q98.8 **Other specified sex chromosome abnormalities, male phenotype**
- Q98.9 **Sex chromosome abnormality, male phenotype, unspecified**

Q99 Other chromosome abnormalities, not elsewhere classified
- Q99.0 **Chimera 46, XX/46, XY**
  Chimera 46, XX/46, XY true hermaphrodite
- Q99.1 **46, XX true hermaphrodite**
  46, XX with streak gonads
  46, XY with streak gonads
  Pure gonadal dysgenesis
- Q99.2 **Fragile X chromosome**
  Fragile X syndrome
- Q99.8 **Other specified chromosome abnormalities**
- Q99.9 **Chromosomal abnormality, unspecified**

Unacceptable principal diagnosis symbol per Medicare code edits — Code exempt from diagnosis present on admission requirement
Questionable admission — Complication or comorbidity — CC/MCC exclusion — Major complication or comorbidity
Principal diagnosis as its own CC — Principal diagnosis as its own MCC — Z code as first-listed diagnosis

Chapter 18: Symptoms, Signs, and Abnormal Clinical and Laboratory Findings, Not Elsewhere Classified (R00-R99)

Guidelines for Assigning Codes From This Chapter

Chapter 18 is your go-to chapter for codes when the documentation doesn't include a definitive diagnosis, but documentation does include the signs or symptoms that triggered the visit. You'll also find the codes you'll use when the results of a test, such as an electrocardiogram or urinalysis, are abnormal.

Caution: You may find codes for signs and symptoms associated with specific diagnoses in other chapters, as well.

List of Sections

- R00-R09: Symptoms and signs involving the circulatory and respiratory systems
- R10-R19: Symptoms and signs involving the digestive system and abdomen
- R20-R23: Symptoms and signs involving the skin and subcutaneous tissue
- R25-R29: Symptoms and signs involving the nervous and musculoskeletal systems
- R30-R39: Symptoms and signs involving the genitourinary system
- R40-R46: Symptoms and signs involving cognition, perception, emotional state and behavior
- R47-R49: Symptoms and signs involving speech and voice
- R50-R69: General symptoms and signs
- R70-R79: Abnormal findings on examination of blood, without diagnosis
- R80-R82: Abnormal findings on examination of urine, without diagnosis
- R83-R89: Abnormal findings on examination of other body fluids, substances and tissues, without diagnosis
- R90-R94: Abnormal findings on diagnostic imaging and in function studies, without diagnosis
- R97: Abnormal tumor markers
- R99: Ill-defined and unknown cause of mortality

Highlights From the ICD-10-CM Official Guidelines for Coding and Reporting

The Chapter 18 ICD-10-CM Official Guidelines for Coding and Reporting help you with assigning codes for when a diagnosis has not yet been determined or when a patient has symptoms or manifestations unrelated to the diagnosis. The information below is from Section I.C.18 of the 2017 Official Guidelines.

Apply These General Guidelines from Chapter 18

The Chapter Guidelines include these instructions:

- You may use the signs and symptoms codes when the provider hasn't confirmed a definitive diagnosis.
- You should not report signs and symptoms if they're a usual part of the disease process for the confirmed diagnosis you're reporting or if the diagnosis code is a combination code that includes the symptoms in the descriptor.
- You may report signs and symptoms not usually associated with the confirmed diagnosis you're reporting, but code the primary diagnosis first.

Heed the Rules for These Specific Circumstances

Repeated falls. When a patient presents for a workup to investigate the reason for recent falls, use code R29.6 (*Repeated falls*). When a patient presents for a different problem but is at risk for repeated falls due to a history of falling, Z91.81 (*History of falling*) should be assigned. Sometimes, you can use both codes for the same encounter, for example, if the patient had fallen in the past followed by an interval without falls and then starts having repeated falls again.

Coma scale. When a patient presents with loss of consciousness or reduced alertness after a traumatic brain injury or cerebrovascular accident (stroke), the provider generally performs a neurological examination to determine the patient's level of conscious. He follows specific guidelines that have associated scores, which are added up to determine the coma score. EMTs and ER nurses may report coma scores when the patient presents initially, but some facilities may capture a coma score at intervals throughout the patient's stay. Regardless of R40.221 who assigns the score, the initial score documented in the medical record should always be assigned a code.

When assigning coma scale codes, remember these guidelines:

1. Sequence the coma scale codes after the diagnosis code(s).
2. Choose one code from each subcategory: R40.21 (Coma scale, eyes open), R40.22 (... best verbal response), R40.23 (... best motor response) to get a complete scale.
3. Add a 7th character to indicate when the scale took place; you should use the same 7th character for all three codes.
4. If only the total score is documented, choose code R40.24- (Glasgow coma scale, total score).

Used principally by trauma registries, R40.2 codes for coma may also be employed in any facility where this information is collected.

Functional quadriplegia. Functional quadriplegia is the inability to use one's arms or legs due to some cause other than a neurological deficit. Do not assign code R53.2 (*functional quadriplegia*) when a patient is documented to have quadriplegia as a result of brain or spinal cord injury or disease (see code categories G80.8, G82.5, and I63). Report R53.2 only when the medical records specifically documents functional quadriplegia.

SIRS due to noninfectious process. Patients can develop systemic inflammatory response syndrome (SIRS) as a result of trauma, pancreatitis, malignant neoplasm, or other noninfectious processes. When the medical record documents such a condition in conjunction with SIRS and no infection is documented, you should code first the primary diagnosis. Then, code R65.10 (*Systemic inflammatory response syndrome [SIRS] of noninfectious origin without acute organ dysfunction*), or R65.11 (*... with acute organ dysfunction*) if acute organ dysfunction resulting from the SIRS is documented. In the latter case, report a separate code for the specific type of organ dysfunction(s). If the record documents acute organ dysfunction but does not connect it to the primary diagnosis or SIRS, query the provider.

Death NOS. Use code R99 (*Ill-defined and unknown cause of mortality*) only when a patient is pronounced dead upon arrival. Do not use this code for the discharge disposition of death.

Remember These Additional Rules from the General Guidelines

Check Chapter 1 rule for HIV test. The guidelines for Chapter 1, Infectious and Parasitic Diseases, will help keep you on track when reporting an encounter for HIV testing. You should report an HIV code only for confirmed cases of HIV, so when a patient with signs and symptoms presents for HIV testing, you should report the signs and symptoms rather than HIV (Section I.C.1.a.2.h).

Remember different rules for 'probable' diagnoses: Section IV.I, which relates to coding outpatient encounters, includes a rule every coder should know: "Do not code diagnoses documented as 'probable,' 'suspected,' 'questionable,' 'rule out,' or 'working diagnosis' or other similar terms indicating uncertainty. Rather, code the condition(s) to the highest degree of certainty for that encounter/visit, such as symptoms, signs, abnormal test results, or other reason for the visit."

Caution: As Section IV.I also explains, the above rule "differs from the coding practices used by short-term, acute care, long-term care and psychiatric hospitals." Section II.H explains that those inpatient hospitals may report uncertain diagnoses as established diagnoses.

Symptoms, signs and abnormal clinical and laboratory findings, not elsewhere classified (R00-R99)

NOTES This chapter includes symptoms, signs, abnormal results of clinical or other investigative procedures, and ill-defined conditions regarding which no diagnosis classifiable elsewhere is recorded. Signs and symptoms that point rather definitely to a given diagnosis have been assigned to a category in other chapters of the classification. In general, categories in this chapter include the less well-defined conditions and symptoms that, without the necessary study of the case to establish a final diagnosis, point perhaps equally to two or more diseases or to two or more systems of the body. Practically all categories in the chapter could be designated 'not otherwise specified', 'unknown etiology' or 'transient'. The Alphabetical Index should be consulted to determine which symptoms and signs are to be allocated here and which to other chapters. The residual subcategories, numbered .8, are generally provided for other relevant symptoms that cannot be allocated elsewhere in the classification.
The conditions and signs or symptoms included in categories R00-R94 consist of:
(a) cases for which no more specific diagnosis can be made even after all the facts bearing on the case have been investigated;
(b) signs or symptoms existing at the time of initial encounter that proved to be transient and whose causes could not be determined;
(c) provisional diagnosis in a patient who failed to return for further investigation or care;
(d) cases referred elsewhere for investigation or treatment before the diagnosis was made;
(e) cases in which a more precise diagnosis was not available for any other reason;
(f) certain symptoms, for which supplementary information is provided, that represent important problems in medical care in their own right.

EXCLUDES2 *abnormal findings on antenatal screening of mother (O28.-)*
certain conditions originating in the perinatal period (P04-P96)
signs and symptoms classified in the body system chapters
signs and symptoms of breast (N63, N64.5)

This chapter contains the following blocks:

R00-R09	Symptoms and signs involving the circulatory and respiratory systems
R10-R19	Symptoms and signs involving the digestive system and abdomen
R20-R23	Symptoms and signs involving the skin and subcutaneous tissue
R25-R29	Symptoms and signs involving the nervous and musculoskeletal systems
R30-R39	Symptoms and signs involving the genitourinary system
R40-R46	Symptoms and signs involving cognition, perception, emotional state and behavior
R47-R49	Symptoms and signs involving speech and voice
R50-R69	General symptoms and signs
R70-R79	Abnormal findings on examination of blood, without diagnosis
R80-R82	Abnormal findings on examination of urine, without diagnosis
R83-R89	Abnormal findings on examination of other body fluids, substances and tissues, without diagnosis
R90-R94	Abnormal findings on diagnostic imaging and in function studies, without diagnosis
R97	Abnormal tumor markers
R99	Ill-defined and unknown cause of mortality

Symptoms and signs involving the circulatory and respiratory systems (R00-R09)

4th **R00 Abnormalities of heart beat**
EXCLUDES1 *abnormalities originating in the perinatal period (P29.1-)*
EXCLUDES2 *specified arrhythmias (I47-I49)*
R00.0 **Tachycardia, unspecified**
Rapid heart beat
Sinoauricular tachycardia NOS
Sinus [sinusal] tachycardia NOS
EXCLUDES1 *neonatal tachycardia (P29.11)*
paroxysmal tachycardia (I47.-)
R00.1 **Bradycardia, unspecified**
Sinoatrial bradycardia
Sinus bradycardia
Slow heart beat
Vagal bradycardia
Use additional code for adverse effect, if applicable, to identify drug (T36-T50 with fifth or sixth character 5)
EXCLUDES1 *neonatal bradycardia (P29.12)*
R00.2 **Palpitations**
Awareness of heart beat
R00.8 **Other abnormalities of heart beat**
R00.9 **Unspecified abnormalities of heart beat**

4th **R01 Cardiac murmurs and other cardiac sounds**
EXCLUDES1 *cardiac murmurs and sounds originating in the perinatal period (P29.8)*
R01.0 **Benign and innocent cardiac murmurs**
Functional cardiac murmur
R01.1 **Cardiac murmur, unspecified**
Cardiac bruit NOS
Heart murmur NOS
Systolic murmur NOS
R01.2 **Other cardiac sounds**
Cardiac dullness, increased or decreased
Precordial friction

4th **R03 Abnormal blood-pressure reading, without diagnosis**
R03.0 **Elevated blood-pressure reading, without diagnosis of hypertension** Q
NOTES This category is to be used to record an episode of elevated blood pressure in a patient in whom no formal diagnosis of hypertension has been made, or as an isolated incidental finding.
R03.1 **Nonspecific low blood-pressure reading**
EXCLUDES1 *hypotension (I95.-)*
maternal hypotension syndrome (O26.5-)
neurogenic orthostatic hypotension (G90.3)

4th **R04 Hemorrhage from respiratory passages**
R04.0 **Epistaxis**
Hemorrhage from nose
Nosebleed
R04.1 **Hemorrhage from throat**
EXCLUDES2 *hemoptysis (R04.2)*
R04.2 **Hemoptysis** CC
Blood-stained sputum
Cough with hemorrhage
AHA: Q4, 2013
5th R04.8 **Hemorrhage from other sites in respiratory passages**
R04.81 **Acute idiopathic pulmonary hemorrhage in infants** P CC
AIPHI
Acute idiopathic hemorrhage in infants over 28 days old
EXCLUDES1 *perinatal pulmonary hemorrhage (P26.-)*
von Willebrand's disease (D68.0)
R04.89 **Hemorrhage from other sites in respiratory passages** CC
Pulmonary hemorrhage NOS
R04.9 **Hemorrhage from respiratory passages, unspecified** CC

R05 Cough
EXCLUDES1 *cough with hemorrhage (R04.2)*
smoker's cough (J41.0)
AHA: Q2, 2016

4th **R06 Abnormalities of breathing**
EXCLUDES1 *acute respiratory distress syndrome (J80)*
respiratory arrest (R09.2)
respiratory arrest of newborn (P28.81)
respiratory distress syndrome of newborn (P22.-)
respiratory failure (J96.-)
respiratory failure of newborn (P28.5)
5th R06.0 **Dyspnea**
EXCLUDES1 *tachypnea NOS (R06.82)*
transient tachypnea of newborn (P22.1)
R06.00 **Dyspnea, unspecified**
R06.01 **Orthopnea**
R06.02 **Shortness of breath**

PDx Unacceptable principal diagnosis symbol per Medicare code edits · POA Code exempt from diagnosis present on admission requirement
Q Questionable admission · CC Complication or comorbidity · CC/MCC Excl CC/MCC exclusion · MCC Major complication or comorbidity
Principal diagnosis as its own CC · Principal diagnosis as its own MCC · Z code as first-listed diagnosis

R06.09 Other forms of dyspnea
R06.1 **Stridor**
EXCLUDES1 *congenital laryngeal stridor (P28.89)*
laryngismus (stridulus) (J38.5)
R06.2 **Wheezing**
AHA: Q2, 2016
EXCLUDES1 *Asthma (J45.-)*
R06.3 **Periodic breathing**
Cheyne-Stokes breathing
R06.4 **Hyperventilation**
EXCLUDES1 *psychogenic hyperventilation (F45.8)*
R06.5 **Mouth breathing**
EXCLUDES2 *dry mouth NOS (R68.2)*
R06.6 **Hiccough**
EXCLUDES1 *psychogenic hiccough (F45.8)*
R06.7 **Sneezing**
R06.8 **Other abnormalities of breathing**
R06.81 **Apnea, not elsewhere classified**
Apnea NOS
EXCLUDES1 *apnea (of) newborn (P28.4)*
sleep apnea (G47.3-)
sleep apnea of newborn (primary) (P28.3)
R06.82 **Tachypnea, not elsewhere classified**
Tachypnea NOS
EXCLUDES1 *transitory tachypnea of newborn (P22.1)*
R06.83 **Snoring**
R06.89 **Other abnormalities of breathing**
Breath-holding (spells)
Sighing
R06.9 **Unspecified abnormalities of breathing**
R07 **Pain in throat and chest**
EXCLUDES1 *epidemic myalgia (B33.0)*
EXCLUDES2 *jaw pain R68.84*
pain in breast (N64.4)
R07.0 **Pain in throat**
EXCLUDES1 *chronic sore throat (J31.2)*
sore throat (acute) NOS (J02.9)
EXCLUDES2 *dysphagia (R13.1-)*
pain in neck (M54.2)
R07.1 **Chest pain on breathing**
Painful respiration
R07.2 **Precordial pain**
R07.8 **Other chest pain**
R07.81 **Pleurodynia**
Pleurodynia NOS
EXCLUDES1 *epidemic pleurodynia (B33.0)*
R07.82 **Intercostal pain**
R07.89 **Other chest pain**
Anterior chest-wall pain NOS
R07.9 **Chest pain, unspecified**
R09 **Other symptoms and signs involving the circulatory and respiratory system**
EXCLUDES1 *acute respiratory distress syndrome (J80)*
respiratory arrest of newborn (P28.81)
respiratory distress syndrome of newborn (P22.0)
respiratory failure (J96.-)
respiratory failure of newborn (P28.5)
R09.0 **Asphyxia and hypoxemia**
EXCLUDES1 *asphyxia due to carbon monoxide (T58.-)*
asphyxia due to foreign body in respiratory tract (T17.-)
birth (intrauterine) asphyxia (P84)
hypercapnia (R06.4)
hyperventilation (R06.4)
traumatic asphyxia (T71.-)
R09.01 **Asphyxia**
R09.02 **Hypoxemia**
R09.1 **Pleurisy**
EXCLUDES1 *pleurisy with effusion (J90)*
R09.2 **Respiratory arrest**
Cardiorespiratory failure
EXCLUDES1 *cardiac arrest (I46.-)*
respiratory arrest of newborn (P28.81)
respiratory distress of newborn (P22.0)
respiratory failure (J96.-)
respiratory failure of newborn (P28.5)
respiratory insufficiency (R06.89)
respiratory insufficiency of newborn (P28.5)
R09.3 **Abnormal sputum**
Abnormal amount of sputum
Abnormal color of sputum
Abnormal odor of sputum
Excessive sputum
EXCLUDES1 *blood-stained sputum (R04.2)*
R09.8 **Other specified symptoms and signs involving the circulatory and respiratory systems**
R09.81 **Nasal congestion**
R09.82 **Postnasal drip**
R09.89 **Other specified symptoms and signs involving the circulatory and respiratory systems**
Bruit (arterial)
Abnormal chest percussion
Feeling of foreign body in throat
Friction sounds in chest
Chest tympany
Choking sensation
Rales
Weak pulse
EXCLUDES2 *foreign body in throat (T17.2-)*
wheezing (R06.2)

Symptoms and signs involving the digestive system and abdomen (R10-R19)

EXCLUDES2 *congenital or infantile pylorospasm (Q40.0)*
gastrointestinal hemorrhage (K92.0-K92.2)
intestinal obstruction (K56.-)
newborn gastrointestinal hemorrhage (P54.0-P54.3)
newborn intestinal obstruction (P76.-)
pylorospasm (K31.3)
signs and symptoms involving the urinary system (R30-R39)
symptoms referable to female genital organs (N94.-)
symptoms referable to male genital organs (N48-N50)

R10 **Abdominal and pelvic pain**
EXCLUDES1 *renal colic (N23)*
EXCLUDES2 *dorsalgia (M54.-)*
flatulence and related conditions (R14.-)
R10.0 **Acute abdomen**
Severe abdominal pain (generalized) (with abdominal rigidity)
EXCLUDES1 *abdominal rigidity NOS (R19.3)*
generalized abdominal pain NOS (R10.84)
localized abdominal pain (R10.1-R10.3-)
R10.1 **Pain localized to upper abdomen**
R10.10 **Upper abdominal pain, unspecified**
R10.11 **Right upper quadrant pain**
R10.12 **Left upper quadrant pain**
R10.13 **Epigastric pain**
Dyspepsia
EXCLUDES1 *functional dyspepsia (K30)*
R10.2 **Pelvic and perineal pain**
EXCLUDES1 *vulvodynia (N94.81)*
R10.3 **Pain localized to other parts of lower abdomen**
R10.30 **Lower abdominal pain, unspecified**
R10.31 **Right lower quadrant pain**
R10.32 **Left lower quadrant pain**
R10.33 **Periumbilical pain**
R10.8 **Other abdominal pain**
R10.81 **Abdominal tenderness**
Abdominal tenderness NOS
R10.811 **Right upper quadrant abdominal tenderness**

Unspecified Code · Other Specified Code · Manifestation Code · N Newborn · P Pediatric · M Maternity · A Adult · ♂ Male · ♀ Female
● New Code · ▲ Revised Code Title · ►◄ Revised Text · NOTES · INCLUDES · EXCLUDES1 Not coded here · EXCLUDES2 Not included here
4th character required · 5th character required · 6th character required · 7th character required
Extension 'X' Alert · HAC Hospital-acquired condition (HAC) alert · AHA AHA Coding Clinic®

R10.812 Left upper quadrant abdominal tenderness
R10.813 Right lower quadrant abdominal tenderness
R10.814 Left lower quadrant abdominal tenderness
R10.815 Periumbilic abdominal tenderness
R10.816 Epigastric abdominal tenderness
R10.817 Generalized abdominal tenderness
R10.819 Abdominal tenderness, unspecified site

R10.82 Rebound abdominal tenderness
R10.821 Right upper quadrant rebound abdominal tenderness
R10.822 Left upper quadrant rebound abdominal tenderness
R10.823 Right lower quadrant rebound abdominal tenderness
R10.824 Left lower quadrant rebound abdominal tenderness
R10.825 Periumbilic rebound abdominal tenderness
R10.826 Epigastric rebound abdominal tenderness
R10.827 Generalized rebound abdominal tenderness
R10.829 Rebound abdominal tenderness, unspecified site

R10.83 Colic
Colic NOS
Infantile colic
EXCLUDES1 *colic in adult and child over 12 months old (R10.84)*

R10.84 Generalized abdominal pain
EXCLUDES1 *generalized abdominal pain associated with acute abdomen (R10.0)*

R10.9 Unspecified abdominal pain

R11 Nausea and vomiting
EXCLUDES1 *cyclical vomiting associated with migraine (G43.A-)*
excessive vomiting in pregnancy (O21.-)
hematemesis (K92.0)
neonatal hematemesis (P54.0)
newborn vomiting (P92.0-)
psychogenic vomiting ►(F50.89)◄
vomiting associated with bulimia nervosa (F50.2)
vomiting following gastrointestinal surgery (K91.0)

R11.0 Nausea
Nausea NOS
Nausea without vomiting

R11.1 Vomiting
R11.10 Vomiting, unspecified
Vomiting NOS
R11.11 Vomiting without nausea
R11.12 Projectile vomiting
R11.13 Vomiting of fecal matter
R11.14 Bilious vomiting
Bilious emesis

R11.2 Nausea with vomiting, unspecified
Persistent nausea with vomiting NOS

R12 Heartburn
EXCLUDES1 *dyspepsia NOS (R10.13)*
functional dyspepsia (K30)

R13 Aphagia and dysphagia
R13.0 Aphagia
Inability to swallow
EXCLUDES1 *psychogenic aphagia (F50.9)*

R13.1 Dysphagia
Code first, if applicable, dysphagia following cerebrovascular disease (I69. with final characters -91)
EXCLUDES1 *psychogenic dysphagia (F45.8)*
R13.10 Dysphagia, unspecified
Difficulty in swallowing NOS
R13.11 Dysphagia, oral phase
R13.12 Dysphagia, oropharyngeal phase
R13.13 Dysphagia, pharyngeal phase
R13.14 Dysphagia, pharyngoesophageal phase
R13.19 Other dysphagia
Cervical dysphagia
Neurogenic dysphagia

R14 Flatulence and related conditions
EXCLUDES1 *psychogenic aerophagy (F45.8)*
R14.0 Abdominal distension (gaseous)
Bloating
Tympanites (abdominal) (intestinal)
R14.1 Gas pain
R14.2 Eructation
R14.3 Flatulence

R15 Fecal incontinence
INCLUDES *encopresis NOS*
EXCLUDES1 *fecal incontinence of nonorganic origin (F98.1)*
R15.0 Incomplete defecation
EXCLUDES1 *constipation (K59.0-)*
fecal impaction (K56.41)
R15.1 Fecal smearing
Fecal soiling
R15.2 Fecal urgency
R15.9 Full incontinence of feces
Fecal incontinence NOS

R16 Hepatomegaly and splenomegaly, not elsewhere classified
R16.0 Hepatomegaly, not elsewhere classified
Hepatomegaly NOS
R16.1 Splenomegaly, not elsewhere classified
Splenomegaly NOS
R16.2 Hepatomegaly with splenomegaly, not elsewhere classified
Hepatosplenomegaly NOS

R17 Unspecified jaundice
EXCLUDES1 *neonatal jaundice (P55, P57-P59)*

R18 Ascites
INCLUDES *fluid in peritoneal cavity*
EXCLUDES1 *ascites in alcoholic cirrhosis (K70.31)*
ascites in alcoholic hepatitis (K70.11)
ascites in toxic liver disease with chronic active hepatitis (K71.51)
R18.0 Malignant ascites
Code first malignancy, such as:
malignant neoplasm of ovary (C56.-)
secondary malignant neoplasm of retroperitoneum and peritoneum (C78.6)
R18.8 Other ascites
Ascites NOS
Peritoneal effusion (chronic)

R19 Other symptoms and signs involving the digestive system and abdomen
EXCLUDES1 *acute abdomen (R10.0)*

R19.0 Intra-abdominal and pelvic swelling, mass and lump
EXCLUDES1 *abdominal distension (gaseous) (R14.-)*
ascites (R18.-)
R19.00 Intra-abdominal and pelvic swelling, mass and lump, unspecified site
R19.01 Right upper quadrant abdominal swelling, mass and lump
R19.02 Left upper quadrant abdominal swelling, mass and lump
R19.03 Right lower quadrant abdominal swelling, mass and lump
R19.04 Left lower quadrant abdominal swelling, mass and lump
R19.05 Periumbilic swelling, mass or lump
Diffuse or generalized umbilical swelling or mass
R19.06 Epigastric swelling, mass or lump
R19.07 Generalized intra-abdominal and pelvic swelling, mass and lump
Diffuse or generalized intra-abdominal swelling or mass NOS
Diffuse or generalized pelvic swelling or mass NOS
R19.09 Other intra-abdominal and pelvic swelling, mass and lump

Unacceptable principal diagnosis symbol per Medicare code edits; Code exempt from diagnosis present on admission requirement
Questionable admission; Complication or comorbidity; CC/MCC exclusion; Major complication or comorbidity
Principal diagnosis as its own CC; Principal diagnosis as its own MCC; Z code as first-listed diagnosis

 When symbols appear on a code that requires a 7th character extension, refer to Appendix D to identify applicable 7th character codes.

R19.1 Abnormal bowel sounds
R19.11 Absent bowel sounds
R19.12 Hyperactive bowel sounds
R19.15 Other abnormal bowel sounds
Abnormal bowel sounds NOS
R19.2 Visible peristalsis
Hyperperistalsis
R19.3 Abdominal rigidity
EXCLUDES1 *abdominal rigidity with severe abdominal pain (R10.0)*
R19.30 Abdominal rigidity, unspecified site
R19.31 Right upper quadrant abdominal rigidity
R19.32 Left upper quadrant abdominal rigidity
R19.33 Right lower quadrant abdominal rigidity
R19.34 Left lower quadrant abdominal rigidity
R19.35 Periumbilic abdominal rigidity
R19.36 Epigastric abdominal rigidity
R19.37 Generalized abdominal rigidity
R19.4 Change in bowel habit
EXCLUDES1 *constipation (K59.0-)*
functional diarrhea (K59.1)
R19.5 Other fecal abnormalities
Abnormal stool color
Bulky stools
Mucus in stools
Occult blood in feces
Occult blood in stools
EXCLUDES1 *melena (K92.1)*
neonatal melena (P54.1)
R19.6 Halitosis
R19.7 Diarrhea, unspecified
Diarrhea NOS
EXCLUDES1 *functional diarrhea (K59.1)*
neonatal diarrhea (P78.3)
psychogenic diarrhea (F45.8)
R19.8 Other specified symptoms and signs involving the digestive system and abdomen

Symptoms and signs involving the skin and subcutaneous tissue (R20-R23)

EXCLUDES2 *symptoms relating to breast (N64.4-N64.5)*
R20 Disturbances of skin sensation
EXCLUDES1 *dissociative anesthesia and sensory loss (F44.6)*
psychogenic disturbances (F45.8)
R20.0 Anesthesia of skin
R20.1 Hypoesthesia of skin
R20.2 Paresthesia of skin
Formication
Pins and needles
Tingling skin
EXCLUDES1 *acroparesthesia (I73.8)*
R20.3 Hyperesthesia
R20.8 Other disturbances of skin sensation
R20.9 Unspecified disturbances of skin sensation
R21 Rash and other nonspecific skin eruption
INCLUDES *rash NOS*
EXCLUDES1 *specified type of rash- code to condition*
vesicular eruption (R23.8)
R22 Localized swelling, mass and lump of skin and subcutaneous tissue
INCLUDES *subcutaneous nodules (localized)(superficial)*
EXCLUDES1 *abnormal findings on diagnostic imaging (R90-R93)*
edema (R60.-)
enlarged lymph nodes (R59.-)
localized adiposity (E65)
swelling of joint (M25.4-)
R22.0 Localized swelling, mass and lump, head
R22.1 Localized swelling, mass and lump, neck
R22.2 Localized swelling, mass and lump, trunk
EXCLUDES1 *intra-abdominal or pelvic mass and lump (R19.0-)*
intra-abdominal or pelvic swelling (R19.0-)
EXCLUDES2 *breast mass and lump (N63)*
R22.3 Localized swelling, mass and lump, upper limb
R22.30 Localized swelling, mass and lump, unspecified upper limb
R22.31 Localized swelling, mass and lump, right upper limb
R22.32 Localized swelling, mass and lump, left upper limb
R22.33 Localized swelling, mass and lump, upper limb, bilateral
R22.4 Localized swelling, mass and lump, lower limb
R22.40 Localized swelling, mass and lump, unspecified lower limb
R22.41 Localized swelling, mass and lump, right lower limb
R22.42 Localized swelling, mass and lump, left lower limb
R22.43 Localized swelling, mass and lump, lower limb, bilateral
R22.9 Localized swelling, mass and lump, unspecified
R23 Other skin changes
R23.0 Cyanosis
EXCLUDES1 *acrocyanosis (I73.8)*
cyanotic attacks of newborn (P28.2)
R23.1 Pallor
Clammy skin
R23.2 Flushing
Excessive blushing
Code first , if applicable, menopausal and female climacteric states (N95.1)
R23.3 Spontaneous ecchymoses
Petechiae
EXCLUDES1 *ecchymoses of newborn (P54.5)*
purpura (D69.-)
R23.4 Changes in skin texture
Desquamation of skin
Induration of skin
Scaling of skin
EXCLUDES1 *epidermal thickening NOS (L85.9)*
R23.8 Other skin changes
R23.9 Unspecified skin changes

Symptoms and signs involving the nervous and musculoskeletal systems (R25-R29)

R25 Abnormal involuntary movements
EXCLUDES1 *specific movement disorders (G20-G26)*
stereotyped movement disorders (F98.4)
tic disorders (F95.-)
R25.0 Abnormal head movements
R25.1 Tremor, unspecified
EXCLUDES1 *chorea NOS (G25.5)*
essential tremor (G25.0)
hysterical tremor (F44.4)
intention tremor (G25.2)
R25.2 Cramp and spasm
EXCLUDES2 *carpopedal spasm (R29.0)*
charley-horse (M62.831)
infantile spasms (G40.4-)
muscle spasm of back (M62.830)
muscle spasm of calf (M62.831)
R25.3 Fasciculation
Twitching NOS
R25.8 Other abnormal involuntary movements
R25.9 Unspecified abnormal involuntary movements
R26 Abnormalities of gait and mobility
EXCLUDES1 *ataxia NOS (R27.0)*
hereditary ataxia (G11.-)
locomotor (syphilitic) ataxia (A52.11)
immobility syndrome (paraplegic) (M62.3)
R26.0 Ataxic gait
Staggering gait
R26.1 Paralytic gait
Spastic gait

R26.2 Difficulty in walking, not elsewhere classified
EXCLUDES1 *falling (R29.6)*
unsteadiness on feet (R26.81)
AHA: Q2, 2016
R26.8 Other abnormalities of gait and mobility
R26.81 Unsteadiness on feet
R26.89 Other abnormalities of gait and mobility
R26.9 Unspecified abnormalities of gait and mobility

R27 Other lack of coordination
EXCLUDES1 *ataxic gait (R26.0)*
hereditary ataxia (G11.-)
vertigo NOS (R42)
R27.0 Ataxia, unspecified
EXCLUDES1 *ataxia following cerebrovascular disease (I69. with final characters -93)*
R27.8 Other lack of coordination
R27.9 Unspecified lack of coordination

R29 Other symptoms and signs involving the nervous and musculoskeletal systems
R29.0 Tetany
Carpopedal spasm
EXCLUDES1 *hysterical tetany (F44.5)*
neonatal tetany (P71.3)
parathyroid tetany (E20.9)
post-thyroidectomy tetany (E89.2)
R29.1 Meningismus
R29.2 Abnormal reflex
EXCLUDES2 *abnormal pupillary reflex (H57.0)*
hyperactive gag reflex (J39.2)
vasovagal reaction or syncope (R55)
R29.3 Abnormal posture
R29.4 Clicking hip
EXCLUDES1 *congenital deformities of hip (Q65.-)*
R29.5 Transient paralysis
Code first any associated spinal cord injury (S14.0, S14.1-, S24.0, S24.1-, S34.0-, S34.1-)
EXCLUDES1 *transient ischemic attack (G45.9)*
R29.6 Repeated falls
Falling
Tendency to fall
EXCLUDES2 *at risk for falling (Z91.81)*
history of falling (Z91.81)
AHA: Q2, 2016
● R29.7 National Institutes of Health Stroke Scale (NIHSS) score
Code first the type of cerebral infarction (I63-)
● R29.70 NIHSS score 0-9
● R29.700 NIHSS score 0
● R29.701 NIHSS score 1
● R29.702 NIHSS score 2
● R29.703 NIHSS score 3
● R29.704 NIHSS score 4
● R29.705 NIHSS score 5
● R29.706 NIHSS score 6
● R29.707 NIHSS score 7
● R29.708 NIHSS score 8
● R29.709 NIHSS score 9
● R29.71 NIHSS score 10-19
● R29.710 NIHSS score 10
● R29.711 NIHSS score 11
● R29.712 NIHSS score 12
● R29.713 NIHSS score 13
● R29.714 NIHSS score 14
● R29.715 NIHSS score 15
● R29.716 NIHSS score 16
● R29.717 NIHSS score 17
● R29.718 NIHSS score 18
● R29.719 NIHSS score 19
● R29.72 NIHSS score 20-29
● R29.720 NIHSS score 20
● R29.721 NIHSS score 21
● R29.722 NIHSS score 22
● R29.723 NIHSS score 23
● R29.724 NIHSS score 24
● R29.725 NIHSS score 25
● R29.726 NIHSS score 26
● R29.727 NIHSS score 27
● R29.728 NIHSS score 28
● R29.729 NIHSS score 29
● R29.73 NIHSS score 30-39
● R29.730 NIHSS score 30
● R29.731 NIHSS score 31
● R29.732 NIHSS score 32
● R29.733 NIHSS score 33
● R29.734 NIHSS score 34
● R29.735 NIHSS score 35
● R29.736 NIHSS score 36
● R29.737 NIHSS score 37
● R29.738 NIHSS score 38
● R29.739 NIHSS score 39
● R29.74 NIHSS score 40-42
● R29.740 NIHSS score 40
● R29.741 NIHSS score 41
● R29.742 NIHSS score 42
R29.8 Other symptoms and signs involving the nervous and musculoskeletal systems
R29.81 Other symptoms and signs involving the nervous system
R29.810 Facial weakness
Facial droop
EXCLUDES1 *Bell's palsy (G51.0)*
facial weakness following cerebrovascular disease (I69. with final characters -92)
R29.818 Other symptoms and signs involving the nervous system
R29.89 Other symptoms and signs involving the musculoskeletal system
EXCLUDES2 *pain in limb (M79.6-)*
R29.890 Loss of height
EXCLUDES1 *osteoporosis (M80-M81)*
R29.891 Ocular torticollis
EXCLUDES1 *congenital (sternomastoid) torticollis Q68.0*
psychogenic torticollis (F45.8)
spasmodic torticollis (G24.3)
torticollis due to birth injury (P15.8)
torticollis NOS M43.6
R29.898 Other symptoms and signs involving the musculoskeletal system
R29.9 Unspecified symptoms and signs involving the nervous and musculoskeletal systems
R29.90 Unspecified symptoms and signs involving the nervous system
R29.91 Unspecified symptoms and signs involving the musculoskeletal system

Symptoms and signs involving the genitourinary system (R30-R39)

R30 Pain associated with micturition
EXCLUDES1 *psychogenic pain associated with micturition (F45.8)*
R30.0 Dysuria
Strangury
R30.1 Vesical tenesmus
R30.9 Painful micturition, unspecified
Painful urination NOS

R31 Hematuria
EXCLUDES1 *hematuria included with underlying conditions, such as:*
acute cystitis with hematuria (N30.01)
recurrent and persistent hematuria in glomerular diseases (N02.-)
R31.0 Gross hematuria
R31.1 Benign essential microscopic hematuria

Unacceptable principal diagnosis symbol per Medicare code edits — Code exempt from diagnosis present on admission requirement
Questionable admission — Complication or comorbidity — CC/MCC exclusion — Major complication or comorbidity
Principal diagnosis as its own CC — Principal diagnosis as its own MCC — Z code as first-listed diagnosis

R31.2 Other microscopic hematuria
- ● R31.21 Asymptomatic microscopic hematuria CC/MCC Exc
  AMH
- ● R31.29 Other microscopic hematuria CC/MCC Exc

R31.9 Hematuria, unspecified

R32 Unspecified urinary incontinence
Enuresis NOS
EXCLUDES1 *functional urinary incontinence (R39.81)*
nonorganic enuresis (F98.0)
stress incontinence and other specified urinary incontinence (N39.3-N39.4-)
urinary incontinence associated with cognitive impairment (R39.81)

R33 Retention of urine
EXCLUDES1 *psychogenic retention of urine (F45.8)*

R33.0 Drug induced retention of urine
Use additional code for adverse effect, if applicable, to identify drug (T36-T50 with fifth or sixth character 5)

R33.8 Other retention of urine
Code first, if applicable, any causal condition, such as:
enlarged prostate (N40.1)

R33.9 Retention of urine, unspecified

R34 Anuria and oliguria
EXCLUDES1 *anuria and oliguria complicating abortion or ectopic or molar pregnancy (O00-O07, O08.4)*
anuria and oliguria complicating pregnancy (O26.83-)
anuria and oliguria complicating the puerperium (O90.4)

R35 Polyuria
Code first, if applicable, any causal condition, such as:
enlarged prostate (N40.1)
EXCLUDES1 *psychogenic polyuria (F45.8)*

R35.0 Frequency of micturition

R35.1 Nocturia

R35.8 Other polyuria
Polyuria NOS

R36 Urethral discharge

R36.0 Urethral discharge without blood

R36.1 Hematospermia ♂

R36.9 Urethral discharge, unspecified
Penile discharge NOS
Urethrorrhea

R37 Sexual dysfunction, unspecified

R39 Other and unspecified symptoms and signs involving the genitourinary system

R39.0 Extravasation of urine CC

R39.1 Other difficulties with micturition
Code first, if applicable, any causal condition, such as:
enlarged prostate (N40.1)
- R39.11 Hesitancy of micturition
- R39.12 Poor urinary stream
  Weak urinary steam
- R39.13 Splitting of urinary stream
- R39.14 Feeling of incomplete bladder emptying
- R39.15 Urgency of urination
  EXCLUDES1 *urge incontinence (N39.41, N39.46)*
- R39.16 Straining to void
- R39.19 Other difficulties with micturition
  - ● R39.191 Need to immediately re-void
  - ● R39.192 Position dependent micturition
  - ● R39.198 Other difficulties with micturition

R39.2 Extrarenal uremia
Prerenal uremia
EXCLUDES1 *uremia NOS (N19)*

R39.8 Other symptoms and signs involving the genitourinary system
- R39.81 Functional urinary incontinence
  Urinary incontinence due to cognitive impairment, or severe physical disability or immobility
  EXCLUDES1 *stress incontinence and other specified urinary incontinence (N39.3-N39.4-)*
  urinary incontinence NOS (R32)
- ● R39.82 Chronic bladder pain CC/MCC Exc
- R39.89 Other symptoms and signs involving the genitourinary system

R39.9 Unspecified symptoms and signs involving the genitourinary system

Symptoms and signs involving cognition, perception, emotional state and behavior (R40-R46)

EXCLUDES2 *symptoms and signs constituting part of a pattern of mental disorder (F01-F99)*

R40 Somnolence, stupor and coma
EXCLUDES1 *neonatal coma (P91.5)*
somnolence, stupor and coma in diabetes (E08-E13)
somnolence, stupor and coma in hepatic failure (K72.-)
somnolence, stupor and coma in hypoglycemia (nondiabetic) (E15)

R40.0 Somnolence
Drowsiness
EXCLUDES1 *coma (R40.2-)*

R40.1 Stupor
Catatonic stupor
Semicoma
EXCLUDES1 *catatonic schizophrenia (F20.2)*
coma (R40.2-)
depressive stupor (F31-F33)
dissociative stupor (F44.2)
manic stupor (F30.2)

R40.2 Coma
Code first any associated:
fracture of skull (S02.-)
intracranial injury (S06.-)
NOTES One code from ▶each subcategory◀, R40.21-R40.23, is required to complete the coma scale

- R40.20 Unspecified coma MCC
  Coma NOS
  Unconsciousness NOS
- R40.21 Coma scale, eyes open
  The following appropriate 7th character is to be added to subcategory R40.21-:
  0 = unspecified time
  1 = in the field [EMT or ambulance]
  2 = at arrival to emergency department
  3 = at hospital admission
  4 = 24 hours or more after hospital admission
  - R40.211 Coma scale, eyes open, never MCC
  - R40.212 Coma scale, eyes open, to pain MCC
  - R40.213 Coma scale, eyes open, to sound
  - R40.214 Coma scale, eyes open, spontaneous
- R40.22 Coma scale, best verbal response
  The following appropriate 7th character is to be added to subcategory R40.22-:
  0 = unspecified time
  1 = in the field [EMT or ambulance]
  2 = at arrival to emergency department
  3 = at hospital admission
  4 = 24 hours or more after hospital admission
  - R40.221 Coma scale, best verbal response, none MCC
  - R40.222 Coma scale, best verbal response, incomprehensible words MCC
  - R40.223 Coma scale, best verbal response, inappropriate words
  - R40.224 Coma scale, best verbal response, confused conversation
  - R40.225 Coma scale, best verbal response, oriented
- R40.23 Coma scale, best motor response
  The following appropriate 7th character is to be added to subcategory R40.23-:
  0 = unspecified time
  1 = in the field [EMT or ambulance]
  2 = at arrival to emergency department
  3 = at hospital admission
  4 = 24 hours or more after hospital admission

Unspecified Code | Other Specified Code | Manifestation Code | N Newborn | P Pediatric | M Maternity | A Adult | ♂ Male | ♀ Female
● New Code | ▲ Revised Code Title | ▶◀ Revised Text | NOTES | INCLUDES | EXCLUDES1 Not coded here | EXCLUDES2 Not included here
4th character required | 5th character required | 6th character required | 7th character required
Extension 'X' Alert | HAC Hospital-acquired condition (HAC) alert | AHA AHA Coding Clinic©

R40.231 Coma scale, best motor response, none
R40.232 Coma scale, best motor response, extension
R40.233 Coma scale, best motor response, abnormal
R40.234 Coma scale, best motor response, flexion withdrawal
R40.235 Coma scale, best motor response, localizes pain
R40.236 Coma scale, best motor response, obeys commands

R40.24 Glasgow coma scale, total score
NOTES Assign a code from subcategory R40.24, when only the total coma score is documented
The following appropriate 7th character is to be added to subcategory R40.24-:
0 = unspecified time
1 = in the field [EMT or ambulance]
2 = at arrival to emergency department
3 = at hospital admission
4 = 24 hours or more after hospital admission

R40.241 Glasgow coma scale score 13-15
R40.242 Glasgow coma scale score 9-12
R40.243 Glasgow coma scale score 3-8
R40.244 Other coma, without documented Glasgow coma scale score, or with partial score reported

R40.3 Persistent vegetative state
R40.4 Transient alteration of awareness

R41 Other symptoms and signs involving cognitive functions and awareness
EXCLUDES1 *dissociative [conversion] disorders (F44.-)*
mild cognitive impairment, so stated (G31.84)

R41.0 Disorientation, unspecified
Confusion NOS
Delirium NOS
R41.1 Anterograde amnesia
R41.2 Retrograde amnesia
R41.3 Other amnesia
Amnesia NOS
Memory loss NOS
EXCLUDES1 *amnestic disorder due to known physiologic condition (F04)*
amnestic syndrome due to psychoactive substance use (F10-F19 with 5th character .6)
mild memory disturbance due to known physiological condition (F06.8)
transient global amnesia (G45.4)
R41.4 Neurologic neglect syndrome
Asomatognosia
Hemi-akinesia
Hemi-inattention
Hemispatial neglect
Left-sided neglect
Sensory neglect
Visuospatial neglect
EXCLUDES1 *visuospatial deficit (R41.842)*

R41.8 Other symptoms and signs involving cognitive functions and awareness
R41.81 Age-related cognitive decline
Senility NOS
R41.82 Altered mental status, unspecified
Change in mental status NOS
EXCLUDES1 *altered level of consciousness (R40.-)*
altered mental status due to known condition - code to condition
delirium NOS (R41.0)
R41.83 Borderline intellectual functioning
IQ level 71 to 84
EXCLUDES1 *intellectual disabilities (F70-F79)*
R41.84 Other specified cognitive deficit
EXCLUDES1 *cognitive deficits as sequelae of cerebrovascular disease (I69.01-, I69.11-, I69.21-, I69.31-, I69.81-, I69.91-)*
R41.840 Attention and concentration deficit
EXCLUDES1 *attention-deficit hyperactivity disorders (F90.-)*
R41.841 Cognitive communication deficit
R41.842 Visuospatial deficit
R41.843 Psychomotor deficit
R41.844 Frontal lobe and executive function deficit
R41.89 Other symptoms and signs involving cognitive functions and awareness
Anosognosia
R41.9 Unspecified symptoms and signs involving cognitive functions and awareness

R42 Dizziness and giddiness
Light-headedness
Vertigo NOS
EXCLUDES1 *vertiginous syndromes (H81.-)*
vertigo from infrasound (T75.23)
AHA: Q4, 2015

R43 Disturbances of smell and taste
R43.0 Anosmia
R43.1 Parosmia
R43.2 Parageusia
R43.8 Other disturbances of smell and taste
Mixed disturbance of smell and taste
R43.9 Unspecified disturbances of smell and taste

R44 Other symptoms and signs involving general sensations and perceptions
EXCLUDES1 *alcoholic hallucinations (F1.5)*
hallucinations in drug psychosis (F11-F19 with .5)
hallucinations in mood disorders with psychotic symptoms (F30.2, F31.5, F32.3, F33.3)
hallucinations in schizophrenia, schizotypal and delusional disorders (F20-F29)
EXCLUDES2 *disturbances of skin sensation (R20.-)*
R44.0 Auditory hallucinations
R44.1 Visual hallucinations
R44.2 Other hallucinations
R44.3 Hallucinations, unspecified
R44.8 Other symptoms and signs involving general sensations and perceptions
R44.9 Unspecified symptoms and signs involving general sensations and perceptions

R45 Symptoms and signs involving emotional state
R45.0 Nervousness
Nervous tension
R45.1 Restlessness and agitation
R45.2 Unhappiness
R45.3 Demoralization and apathy
EXCLUDES1 *anhedonia (R45.84)*
R45.4 Irritability and anger
R45.5 Hostility
R45.6 Violent behavior
R45.7 State of emotional shock and stress, unspecified
R45.8 Other symptoms and signs involving emotional state
R45.81 Low self-esteem
R45.82 Worries
R45.83 Excessive crying of child, adolescent or adult
EXCLUDES1 *excessive crying of infant (baby) R68.11*
R45.84 Anhedonia
R45.85 Homicidal and suicidal ideations
EXCLUDES1 *suicide attempt (T14.91)*
R45.850 Homicidal ideations
R45.851 Suicidal ideations
R45.86 Emotional lability
R45.87 Impulsiveness
R45.89 Other symptoms and signs involving emotional state

Unacceptable principal diagnosis symbol per Medicare code edits | Code exempt from diagnosis present on admission requirement
Questionable admission | Complication or comorbidity | CC/MCC exclusion | Major complication or comorbidity
Principal diagnosis as its own CC | Principal diagnosis as its own MCC | Z code as first-listed diagnosis

 When symbols appear on a code that requires a 7th character extension, refer to Appendix D to identify applicable 7th character codes.

R46 Symptoms and signs involving appearance and behavior
EXCLUDES1 *appearance and behavior in schizophrenia, schizotypal and delusional disorders (F20-F29)*
mental and behavioral disorders (F01-F99)
R46.0 Very low level of personal hygiene
R46.1 Bizarre personal appearance
R46.2 Strange and inexplicable behavior
R46.3 Overactivity
R46.4 Slowness and poor responsiveness
EXCLUDES1 *stupor (R40.1)*
R46.5 Suspiciousness and marked evasiveness
R46.6 Undue concern and preoccupation with stressful events
R46.7 Verbosity and circumstantial detail obscuring reason for contact
R46.8 Other symptoms and signs involving appearance and behavior
R46.81 Obsessive-compulsive behavior PDx
EXCLUDES1 *obsessive-compulsive disorder ▶(F42.-)◀*
R46.89 Other symptoms and signs involving appearance and behavior PDx

Symptoms and signs involving speech and voice (R47-R49)

R47 Speech disturbances, not elsewhere classified
EXCLUDES1 *autism (F84.0)*
cluttering (F80.81)
specific developmental disorders of speech and language (F80.-)
stuttering (F80.81)
R47.0 Dysphasia and aphasia
R47.01 Aphasia CC
EXCLUDES1 *aphasia following cerebrovascular disease (I69. with final characters -20)*
progressive isolated aphasia (G31.01)
R47.02 Dysphasia
EXCLUDES1 *dysphasia following cerebrovascular disease (I69. with final characters -21)*
R47.1 Dysarthria and anarthria
EXCLUDES1 *dysarthria following cerebrovascular disease (I69. with final characters -22)*
R47.8 Other speech disturbances
EXCLUDES1 *dysarthria following cerebrovascular disease (I69. with final characters -28)*
R47.81 Slurred speech
R47.82 Fluency disorder in conditions classified elsewhere
Stuttering in conditions classified elsewhere
Code first underlying disease or condition, such as:
Parkinson's disease (G20)
EXCLUDES1 *adult onset fluency disorder (F98.5)*
childhood onset fluency disorder (F80.81)
fluency disorder (stuttering) following cerebrovascular disease (I69. with final characters -23)
R47.89 Other speech disturbances
R47.9 Unspecified speech disturbances
R48 Dyslexia and other symbolic dysfunctions, not elsewhere classified
EXCLUDES1 *specific developmental disorders of scholastic skills (F81.-)*
R48.0 Dyslexia and alexia
R48.1 Agnosia
Astereognosia (astereognosis)
Autotopagnosia
EXCLUDES1 *visual object agnosia (R48.3)*
R48.2 Apraxia
EXCLUDES1 *apraxia following cerebrovascular disease (I69. with final characters -90)*
R48.3 Visual agnosia
Prosopagnosia
Simultanagnosia (asimultagnosia)
R48.8 Other symbolic dysfunctions
Acalculia
Agraphia
R48.9 Unspecified symbolic dysfunctions
R49 Voice and resonance disorders
EXCLUDES1 *psychogenic voice and resonance disorders (F44.4)*
R49.0 Dysphonia
Hoarseness
R49.1 Aphonia
Loss of voice
R49.2 Hypernasality and hyponasality
R49.21 Hypernasality
R49.22 Hyponasality
R49.8 Other voice and resonance disorders
R49.9 Unspecified voice and resonance disorder
Change in voice NOS
Resonance disorder NOS

General symptoms and signs (R50-R69)

R50 Fever of other and unknown origin
EXCLUDES1 *chills without fever (R68.83)*
febrile convulsions (R56.0-)
fever of unknown origin during labor (O75.2)
fever of unknown origin in newborn (P81.9)
hypothermia due to illness (R68.0)
malignant hyperthermia due to anesthesia (T88.3)
puerperal pyrexia NOS (O86.4)
R50.2 Drug induced fever
Use additional code for adverse effect, if applicable, to identify drug (T36-T50 with fifth or sixth character 5)
EXCLUDES1 *postvaccination (postimmunization) fever (R50.83)*
R50.8 Other specified fever
R50.81 Fever presenting with conditions classified elsewhere
Code first underlying condition when associated fever is present, such as with:
leukemia (C91-C95)
neutropenia (D70.-)
sickle-cell disease (D57.-)
R50.82 Postprocedural fever
EXCLUDES1 *postprocedural infection ▶(T81.4-)◀*
posttransfusion fever (R50.84)
postvaccination (postimmunization) fever (R50.83)
R50.83 Postvaccination fever
Postimmunization fever
R50.84 Febrile nonhemolytic transfusion reaction
FNHTR
Posttransfusion fever
R50.9 Fever, unspecified
Fever NOS
Fever of unknown origin [FUO]
Fever with chills
Fever with rigors
Hyperpyrexia NOS
Persistent fever
Pyrexia NOS
R51 Headache
Facial pain NOS
EXCLUDES1 *atypical face pain (G50.1)*
migraine and other headache syndromes (G43-G44)
trigeminal neuralgia (G50.0)
R52 Pain, unspecified
Acute pain NOS
Generalized pain NOS
Pain NOS
EXCLUDES1 *acute and chronic pain, not elsewhere classified (G89.-)*
localized pain, unspecified type - code to pain by site, such as:
abdomen pain (R10.-)
back pain (M54.9)
breast pain (N64.4)
chest pain (R07.1-R07.9)
ear pain (H92.0-)
eye pain (H57.1)
headache (R51)

joint pain (M25.5-)
limb pain (M79.6-)
lumbar region pain (M54.5)
pelvic and perineal pain (R10.2)
shoulder pain (M25.51-)
spine pain (M54.-)
throat pain (R07.0)
tongue pain (K14.6)
tooth pain (K08.8)
renal colic (N23)
pain disorders exclusively related to psychological factors (F45.41)

R53 Malaise and fatigue

R53.0 Neoplastic (malignant) related fatigue
Code first associated neoplasm

R53.1 Weakness
Asthenia NOS
EXCLUDES1 *age-related weakness (R54)*
muscle weakness (M62.8-)
sarcopenia (M62.84)
senile asthenia (R54)

R53.2 Functional quadriplegia MCC
Complete immobility due to severe physical disability or frailty
EXCLUDES1 *frailty NOS (R54)*
hysterical paralysis (F44.4)
immobility syndrome (M62.3)
neurologic quadriplegia (G82.5-)
quadriplegia (G82.50)
AHA: Q2, 2016

R53.8 Other malaise and fatigue
EXCLUDES1 *combat exhaustion and fatigue (F43.0)*
congenital debility (P96.9)
exhaustion and fatigue due to depressive episode (F32.-)
exhaustion and fatigue due to excessive exertion (T73.3)
exhaustion and fatigue due to exposure (T73.2)
exhaustion and fatigue due to heat (T67.-)
exhaustion and fatigue due to pregnancy (O26.8-)
exhaustion and fatigue due to recurrent depressive episode (F33)
exhaustion and fatigue due to senile debility (R54)

R53.81 Other malaise
Chronic debility
Debility NOS
General physical deterioration
Malaise NOS
Nervous debility
EXCLUDES1 *age-related physical debility (R54)*

R53.82 Chronic fatigue, unspecified
Chronic fatigue syndrome NOS
EXCLUDES1 *postviral fatigue syndrome (G93.3)*

R53.83 Other fatigue
Fatigue NOS
Lack of energy
Lethargy
Tiredness

R54 Age-related physical debility A
Frailty
Old age
Senescence
Senile asthenia
Senile debility
EXCLUDES1 *age-related cognitive decline (R41.81)*
sarcopenia (M62.84)
senile psychosis (F03)
senility NOS (R41.81)

R55 Syncope and collapse
Blackout
Fainting
Vasovagal attack
EXCLUDES1 *cardiogenic shock (R57.0)*
carotid sinus syncope (G90.01)
heat syncope (T67.1)
neurocirculatory asthenia (F45.8)
neurogenic orthostatic hypotension (G90.3)
orthostatic hypotension (I95.1)
postprocedural shock (T81.1-)
psychogenic syncope (F48.8)
shock NOS (R57.9)
shock complicating or following abortion or ectopic or molar pregnancy (O00-O07, O08.3)
shock complicating or following labor and delivery (O75.1)
Stokes-Adams attack (I45.9)
unconsciousness NOS (R40.2-)

R56 Convulsions, not elsewhere classified
EXCLUDES1 *dissociative convulsions and seizures (F44.5)*
epileptic convulsions and seizures (G40.-)
newborn convulsions and seizures (P90)

R56.0 Febrile convulsions

R56.00 Simple febrile convulsions CC
Febrile convulsion NOS
Febrile seizure NOS

R56.01 Complex febrile convulsions CC
Atypical febrile seizure
Complex febrile seizure
Complicated febrile seizure
EXCLUDES1 *status epilepticus (G40.901)*

R56.1 Post traumatic seizures CC
EXCLUDES1 *post traumatic epilepsy (G40.-)*

R56.9 Unspecified convulsions
Convulsion disorder
Fit NOS
Recurrent convulsions
Seizure(s) (convulsive) NOS

R57 Shock, not elsewhere classified
EXCLUDES1 *anaphylactic shock NOS (T78.2)*
anaphylactic reaction or shock due to adverse food reaction (T78.0-)
anaphylactic shock due to adverse effect of correct drug or medicament properly administered (T88.6)
anaphylactic shock due to serum (T80.5-)
anesthetic shock (T88.3)
electric shock (T75.4)
obstetric shock (O75.1)
postprocedural shock (T81.1-)
psychic shock (F43.0)
septic shock (R65.21)
shock complicating or following ectopic or molar pregnancy (O00-O07, O08.3)
shock due to lightning (T75.01)
traumatic shock (T79.4)
toxic shock syndrome (A48.3)

R57.0 Cardiogenic shock MCC
R57.1 Hypovolemic shock MCC
R57.8 Other shock MCC
R57.9 Shock, unspecified CC
Failure of peripheral circulation NOS

R58 Hemorrhage, not elsewhere classified
Hemorrhage NOS
EXCLUDES1 *hemorrhage included with underlying conditions, such as:*
acute duodenal ulcer with hemorrhage (K26.0)
acute gastritis with bleeding (K29.01)
ulcerative enterocolitis with rectal bleeding (K51.01)

R59 Enlarged lymph nodes
INCLUDES *swollen glands*
EXCLUDES1 *lymphadenitis NOS (I88.9)*
acute lymphadenitis (L04.-)
chronic lymphadenitis (I88.1)
mesenteric (acute) (chronic) lymphadenitis (I88.0)

Unacceptable principal diagnosis symbol per Medicare code edits | Code exempt from diagnosis present on admission requirement | Questionable admission | CC Complication or comorbidity | CC/MCC exclusion | MCC Major complication or comorbidity | Principal diagnosis as its own CC | Principal diagnosis as its own MCC | Z code as first-listed diagnosis

R59.0 Localized enlarged lymph nodes
R59.1 Generalized enlarged lymph nodes
Lymphadenopathy NOS
R59.9 Enlarged lymph nodes, unspecified

R60 Edema, not elsewhere classified
EXCLUDES1 *angioneurotic edema (T78.3)*
ascites (R18.-)
cerebral edema (G93.6)
cerebral edema due to birth injury (P11.0)
edema of larynx (J38.4)
edema of nasopharynx (J39.2)
edema of pharynx (J39.2)
gestational edema (O12.0-)
hereditary edema (Q82.0)
hydrops fetalis NOS (P83.2)
hydrothorax (J94.8)
nutritional edema (E40-E46)
hydrops fetalis NOS (P83.2)
newborn edema (P83.3)
pulmonary edema (J81.-)
R60.0 Localized edema
R60.1 Generalized edema
R60.9 Edema, unspecified
Fluid retention NOS

R61 Generalized hyperhidrosis
Excessive sweating
Night sweats
Secondary hyperhidrosis
Code first , if applicable, menopausal and female climacteric states (N95.1)
EXCLUDES1 *focal (primary) (secondary) hyperhidrosis (L74.5-)*
Frey's syndrome (L74.52)
localized (primary) (secondary) hyperhidrosis (L74.5-)

R62 Lack of expected normal physiological development in childhood and adults
EXCLUDES1 *delayed puberty (E30.0)*
gonadal dysgenesis (Q99.1)
hypopituitarism (E23.0)
R62.0 Delayed milestone in childhood P
Delayed attainment of expected physiological developmental stage
Late talker
Late walker
R62.5 Other and unspecified lack of expected normal physiological development in childhood
EXCLUDES1 *HIV disease resulting in failure to thrive (B20)*
physical retardation due to malnutrition (E45)
R62.50 Unspecified lack of expected normal physiological development in childhood P
Infantilism NOS
R62.51 Failure to thrive (child) P
Failure to gain weight
EXCLUDES1 *failure to thrive in child under 28 days old (P92.6)*
R62.52 Short stature (child) P
Lack of growth
Physical retardation
Short stature NOS
EXCLUDES1 *short stature due to endocrine disorder (E34.3)*
R62.59 Other lack of expected normal physiological development in childhood P
R62.7 Adult failure to thrive A

R63 Symptoms and signs concerning food and fluid intake
EXCLUDES1 *bulimia NOS (F50.2)*
eating disorders of nonorganic origin (F50.-)
malnutrition (E40-E46)
R63.0 Anorexia
Loss of appetite
EXCLUDES1 *anorexia nervosa (F50.0-)*
loss of appetite of nonorganic origin ▶(F50.89)◀
R63.1 Polydipsia
Excessive thirst
R63.2 Polyphagia
Excessive eating
Hyperalimentation NOS
R63.3 Feeding difficulties
Feeding problem (elderly) (infant) NOS
EXCLUDES1 *feeding problems of newborn (P92.-)*
infant feeding disorder of nonorganic origin (F98.2-)
R63.4 Abnormal weight loss
R63.5 Abnormal weight gain
EXCLUDES1 *excessive weight gain in pregnancy (O26.0-)*
obesity (E66.-)
R63.6 Underweight
Use additional code to identify body mass index (BMI), if known (Z68.-)
EXCLUDES1 *abnormal weight loss (R63.4)*
anorexia nervosa (F50.0-)
malnutrition (E40-E46)
R63.8 Other symptoms and signs concerning food and fluid intake

R64 Cachexia CC
Wasting syndrome
Code first underlying condition, if known
EXCLUDES1 *abnormal weight loss (R63.4)*
nutritional marasmus (E41)

R65 Symptoms and signs specifically associated with systemic inflammation and infection
R65.1 Systemic inflammatory response syndrome (SIRS) of non-infectious origin
Code first underlying condition, such as:
heatstroke (T67.0)
injury and trauma (S00-T88)
EXCLUDES1 *sepsis- code to infection*
severe sepsis (R65.2)
R65.10 Systemic inflammatory response syndrome (SIRS) of non-infectious origin without acute organ dysfunction CC
Systemic inflammatory response syndrome (SIRS) NOS
R65.11 Systemic inflammatory response syndrome (SIRS) of non-infectious origin with acute organ dysfunction MCC
Use additional code to identify specific acute organ dysfunction, such as:
acute kidney failure (N17.-)
acute respiratory failure (J96.0-)
critical illness myopathy (G72.81)
critical illness polyneuropathy (G62.81)
disseminated intravascular coagulopathy [DIC] (D65)
encephalopathy (metabolic) (septic) (G93.41)
hepatic failure (K72.0-)
R65.2 Severe sepsis
Infection with associated acute organ dysfunction
Sepsis with acute organ dysfunction
Sepsis with multiple organ dysfunction
Systemic inflammatory response syndrome due to infectious process with acute organ dysfunction
Code first underlying infection, such as:
infection following a procedure ▶(T81.4-)◀
infections following infusion, transfusion and therapeutic injection (T80.2-)
puerperal sepsis (O85)
sepsis following complete or unspecified spontaneous abortion (O03.87)
sepsis following ectopic and molar pregnancy (O08.82)
sepsis following incomplete spontaneous abortion (O03.37)
sepsis following (induced) termination of pregnancy (O04.87)
sepsis NOS (A41.9)
Use additional code to identify specific acute organ dysfunction, such as:
acute kidney failure (N17.-)
acute respiratory failure (J96.0-)
critical illness myopathy (G72.81)
critical illness polyneuropathy (G62.81)
disseminated intravascular coagulopathy [DIC] (D65)
encephalopathy (metabolic) (septic) (G93.41)
hepatic failure (K72.0-)

Unspecified Code Other Specified Code Manifestation Code N Newborn P Pediatric M Maternity A Adult ♂ Male ♀ Female
● New Code ▲ Revised Code Title ▶◀ Revised Text NOTES INCLUDES EXCLUDES1 Not coded here EXCLUDES2 Not included here
4th character required 5th character required 6th character required 7th character required
Extension 'X' Alert HAC Hospital-acquired condition (HAC) alert AHA AHA Coding Clinic©

R65.20 **Severe sepsis** without septic shock MCC
Severe sepsis NOS
AHA: Q4, 2013

R65.21 **Severe sepsis** with septic shock MCC PDx MCC

R68 **Other general symptoms and signs**

R68.0 **Hypothermia, not associated with low environmental temperature**
EXCLUDES1 *hypothermia NOS (accidental) (T68)*
hypothermia due to anesthesia (T88.51)
hypothermia due to low environmental temperature (T68)
newborn hypothermia (P80.-)

R68.1 **Nonspecific symptoms peculiar to infancy**
EXCLUDES1 *colic, infantile (R10.83)*
neonatal cerebral irritability (P91.3)
teething syndrome (K00.7)

R68.11 **Excessive crying of infant (baby)** P
EXCLUDES1 *excessive crying of child, adolescent, or adult (R45.83)*

R68.12 **Fussy infant (baby)** P
Irritable infant

R68.13 **Apparent life threatening event in infant (ALTE)** P
Apparent life threatening event in newborn
Code first confirmed diagnosis, if known
Use additional code(s) for associated signs and symptoms if no confirmed diagnosis established, or if signs and symptoms are not associated routinely with confirmed diagnosis, or provide additional information for cause of ALTE

R68.19 **Other nonspecific symptoms peculiar to infancy** P

R68.2 **Dry mouth, unspecified**
EXCLUDES1 *dry mouth due to dehydration (E86.0)*
dry mouth due to sicca syndrome [Sjögren] (M35.0-)
salivary gland hyposecretion (K11.7)

R68.3 **Clubbing of fingers**
Clubbing of nails
EXCLUDES1 *congenital clubfinger (Q68.1)*

R68.8 **Other general symptoms and signs**

R68.81 **Early satiety**

R68.82 **Decreased libido** A
Decreased sexual desire

R68.83 **Chills (without fever)**
Chills NOS
EXCLUDES1 *chills with fever (R50.9)*

R68.84 **Jaw pain**
Mandibular pain
Maxilla pain
EXCLUDES1 *temporomandibular joint arthralgia ►(M26.62-)◄*

R68.89 **Other general symptoms and signs**

R69 **Illness, unspecified**
Unknown and unspecified cases of morbidity

Abnormal findings on examination of blood, without diagnosis (R70-R79)

EXCLUDES2 *abnormal findings on antenatal screening of mother (O28.-)*
abnormalities of lipids (E78.-)
abnormalities of platelets and thrombocytes (D69.-)
abnormalities of white blood cells classified elsewhere (D70-D72)
coagulation hemorrhagic disorders (D65-D68)
diagnostic abnormal findings classified elsewhere - see Alphabetical Index
hemorrhagic and hematological disorders of newborn (P50-P61)

R70 **Elevated erythrocyte sedimentation rate and abnormality of plasma viscosity**

R70.0 **Elevated erythrocyte sedimentation rate**

R70.1 **Abnormal plasma viscosity**

R71 **Abnormality of red blood cells**
EXCLUDES1 *anemias (D50-D64)*
anemia of premature infant (P61.2)
benign (familial) polycythemia (D75.0)
congenital anemias (P61.2-P61.4)
newborn anemia due to isoimmunization (P55.-)
polycythemia neonatorum (P61.1)
polycythemia NOS (D75.1)
polycythemia vera (D45)
secondary polycythemia (D75.1)

R71.0 **Precipitous drop in hematocrit** CC
Drop (precipitous) in hemoglobin
Drop in hematocrit

R71.8 **Other abnormality of red blood cells**
Abnormal red-cell morphology NOS
Abnormal red-cell volume NOS
Anisocytosis
Poikilocytosis

R73 **Elevated blood glucose level**
EXCLUDES1 *diabetes mellitus (E08-E13)*
diabetes mellitus in pregnancy, childbirth and the puerperium (O24.-)
neonatal disorders (P70.0-P70.2)
postsurgical hypoinsulinemia (E89.1)

R73.0 **Abnormal glucose**
EXCLUDES1 *abnormal glucose in pregnancy (O99.81-)*
diabetes mellitus (E08-E13)
dysmetabolic syndrome X (E88.81)
gestational diabetes (O24.4-)
glycosuria (R81)
hypoglycemia (E16.2)

R73.01 **Impaired fasting glucose**
Elevated fasting glucose

R73.02 **Impaired glucose tolerance (oral)**
Elevated glucose tolerance

● R73.03 Prediabetes
Latent diabetes

R73.09 **Other abnormal glucose**
Abnormal glucose NOS
Abnormal non-fasting glucose tolerance

R73.9 **Hyperglycemia, unspecified**

R74 **Abnormal serum enzyme levels**

R74.0 **Nonspecific elevation of levels of transaminase and lactic acid dehydrogenase [LDH]**

R74.8 **Abnormal levels of other serum enzymes**
Abnormal level of acid phosphatase
Abnormal level of alkaline phosphatase
Abnormal level of amylase
Abnormal level of lipase [triacylglycerol lipase]

R74.9 **Abnormal serum enzyme level, unspecified**

R75 **Inconclusive laboratory evidence of human immunodeficiency virus [HIV]**
Nonconclusive HIV-test finding in infants
EXCLUDES1 *asymptomatic human immunodeficiency virus [HIV] infection status (Z21)*
human immunodeficiency virus [HIV] disease (B20)

R76 Other **abnormal immunological findings in serum**

R76.0 **Raised antibody titer**
EXCLUDES1 *isoimmunization in pregnancy (O36.0-O36.1)*
isoimmunization affecting newborn (P55.-)

R76.1 **Nonspecific reaction to test for tuberculosis**

R76.11 **Nonspecific reaction to** tuberculin skin test without active tuberculosis
Abnormal result of Mantoux test
PPD positive
Tuberculin (skin test) positive
Tuberculin (skin test) reactor
EXCLUDES1 *nonspecific reaction to cell mediated immunity measurement of gamma interferon antigen response without active tuberculosis (R76.12)*

R76.12 **Nonspecific reaction to** cell mediated immunity measurement of gamma interferon antigen response without active tuberculosis
Nonspecific reaction to QuantiFERON-TB test (QFT) without active tuberculosis
EXCLUDES1 *nonspecific reaction to tuberculin skin test without active tuberculosis (R76.11)*
positive tuberculin skin test (R76.11)

PDx Unacceptable principal diagnosis symbol per Medicare code edits · POA Code exempt from diagnosis present on admission requirement
Q Questionable admission · CC Complication or comorbidity · CC/MCC Excl CC/MCC exclusion · MCC Major complication or comorbidity
PDx CC Principal diagnosis as its own CC · PDx MCC Principal diagnosis as its own MCC · Z Z code as first-listed diagnosis

 When symbols appear on a code that requires a 7th character extension, refer to Appendix D to identify applicable 7th character codes.

R76.8 Other specified abnormal immunological findings in serum
Raised level of immunoglobulins NOS
R76.9 Abnormal immunological finding in serum, unspecified

R77 Other abnormalities of plasma proteins
EXCLUDES1 *disorders of plasma-protein metabolism (E88.0)*
R77.0 Abnormality of albumin
R77.1 Abnormality of globulin
Hyperglobulinemia NOS
R77.2 Abnormality of alpha fetoprotein
R77.8 Other specified abnormalities of plasma proteins
R77.9 Abnormality of plasma protein, unspecified

R78 Findings of drugs and other substances, not normally found in blood
Use additional code to identify the any retained foreign body, if applicable (Z18.-)
EXCLUDES1 *mental or behavioral disorders due to psychoactive substance use (F10-F19)*
R78.0 Finding of alcohol in blood
Use additional external cause code (Y90.-), for detail regarding alcohol level.
R78.1 Finding of opiate drug in blood
R78.2 Finding of cocaine in blood
R78.3 Finding of hallucinogen in blood
R78.4 Finding of other drugs of addictive potential in blood
R78.5 Finding of other psychotropic drug in blood
R78.6 Finding of steroid agent in blood
R78.7 Finding of abnormal level of heavy metals in blood
R78.71 Abnormal lead level in blood
EXCLUDES1 *lead poisoning (T56.0-)*
R78.79 Finding of abnormal level of heavy metals in blood
R78.8 Finding of other specified substances, not normally found in blood
R78.81 Bacteremia
EXCLUDES1 *sepsis-code to specified ►infection◄*
R78.89 Finding of other specified substances, not normally found in blood
Finding of abnormal level of lithium in blood
R78.9 Finding of unspecified substance, not normally found in blood

R79 Other abnormal findings of blood chemistry
Use additional code to identify any retained foreign body, if applicable (Z18.-)
EXCLUDES1 *abnormality of fluid, electrolyte or acid-base balance (E86-E87)*
asymptomatic hyperuricemia (E79.0)
hyperglycemia NOS (R73.9)
hypoglycemia NOS (E16.2)
neonatal hypoglycemia (P70.3-P70.4)
specific findings indicating disorder of amino-acid metabolism (E70-E72)
specific findings indicating disorder of carbohydrate metabolism (E73-E74)
specific findings indicating disorder of lipid metabolism (E75.-)
R79.0 Abnormal level of blood mineral
Abnormal blood level of cobalt
Abnormal blood level of copper
Abnormal blood level of iron
Abnormal blood level of magnesium
Abnormal blood level of mineral NEC
Abnormal blood level of zinc
EXCLUDES1 *abnormal level of lithium (R78.89)*
disorders of mineral metabolism (E83.-)
neonatal hypomagnesemia (P71.2)
nutritional mineral deficiency (E58-E61)
R79.1 Abnormal coagulation profile
Abnormal or prolonged bleeding time
Abnormal or prolonged coagulation time
Abnormal or prolonged partial thromboplastin time [PTT]
Abnormal or prolonged prothrombin time [PT]
EXCLUDES1 *coagulation defects (D68.-)*
R79.8 Other specified abnormal findings of blood chemistry
R79.81 Abnormal blood-gas level
R79.82 Elevated C-reactive protein (CRP)
R79.89 Other specified abnormal findings of blood chemistry
R79.9 Abnormal finding of blood chemistry, unspecified

Abnormal findings on examination of urine, without diagnosis (R80-R82)

EXCLUDES1 *abnormal findings on antenatal screening of mother (O28.-)*
diagnostic abnormal findings classified elsewhere - see Alphabetical Index
specific findings indicating disorder of amino-acid metabolism (E70-E72)
specific findings indicating disorder of carbohydrate metabolism (E73-E74)

R80 Proteinuria
EXCLUDES1 *gestational proteinuria (O12.1-)*
R80.0 Isolated proteinuria
Idiopathic proteinuria
EXCLUDES1 *isolated proteinuria with specific morphological lesion (N06.-)*
R80.1 Persistent proteinuria, unspecified
R80.2 Orthostatic proteinuria, unspecified
Postural proteinuria
R80.3 Bence Jones proteinuria
R80.8 Other proteinuria
R80.9 Proteinuria, unspecified
Albuminuria NOS

R81 Glycosuria
EXCLUDES1 *renal glycosuria (E74.8)*

R82 Other and unspecified abnormal findings in urine
INCLUDES *chromoabnormalities in urine*
Use additional code to identify any retained foreign body, if applicable (Z18.-)
EXCLUDES2 *hematuria (R31.-)*
R82.0 Chyluria
EXCLUDES1 *filarial chyluria (B74.-)*
R82.1 Myoglobinuria
R82.2 Biliuria
R82.3 Hemoglobinuria
EXCLUDES1 *hemoglobinuria due to hemolysis from external causes NEC (D59.6)*
hemoglobinuria due to paroxysmal nocturnal [Marchiafava-Micheli] (D59.5)
R82.4 Acetonuria
Ketonuria
R82.5 Elevated urine levels of drugs, medicaments and biological substances
Elevated urine levels of catecholamines
Elevated urine levels of indoleacetic acid
Elevated urine levels of 17-ketosteroids
Elevated urine levels of steroids
R82.6 Abnormal urine levels of substances chiefly nonmedicinal as to source
Abnormal urine level of heavy metals
R82.7 Abnormal findings on microbiological examination of urine
EXCLUDES1 *colonization status (Z22.-)*
● R82.71 Bacteriuria CC/MCC Exc
● R82.79 Other abnormal findings on microbiological examination of urine CC/MCC Exc
Positive culture findings of urine
R82.8 Abnormal findings on cytological and histological examination of urine
R82.9 Other and unspecified abnormal findings in urine
R82.90 Unspecified abnormal findings in urine
R82.91 Other chromoabnormalities of urine
Chromoconversion (dipstick)
Idiopathic dipstick converts positive for blood with no cellular forms in sediment
EXCLUDES1 *hemoglobinuria (R82.3)*
myoglobinuria (R82.1)
R82.99 Other abnormal findings in urine
Cells and casts in urine
Crystalluria
Melanuria

Unspecified Code | Other Specified Code | Manifestation Code | N Newborn | P Pediatric | M Maternity | A Adult | ♂ Male | ♀ Female
● New Code | ▲ Revised Code Title | ►◄ Revised Text | NOTES | INCLUDES | EXCLUDES1 Not coded here | EXCLUDES2 Not included here
4th character required | 5th character required | 6th character required | 7th character required
Extension 'X' Alert | HAC Hospital-acquired condition (HAC) alert | AHA AHA Coding Clinic©

Abnormal findings on examination of other body fluids, substances and tissues, without diagnosis (R83-R89)

EXCLUDES1 *abnormal findings on antenatal screening of mother (O28.-)*
diagnostic abnormal findings classified elsewhere - see Alphabetical Index

EXCLUDES2 *abnormal findings on examination of blood, without diagnosis (R70-R79)*
abnormal findings on examination of urine, without diagnosis (R80-R82)
abnormal tumor markers (R97.-)

R83 Abnormal findings in cerebrospinal fluid

R83.0 Abnormal level of enzymes in cerebrospinal fluid

R83.1 Abnormal level of hormones in cerebrospinal fluid

R83.2 Abnormal level of other drugs, medicaments and biological substances in cerebrospinal fluid

R83.3 Abnormal level of substances chiefly nonmedicinal as to source in cerebrospinal fluid

R83.4 Abnormal immunological findings in cerebrospinal fluid

R83.5 Abnormal microbiological findings in cerebrospinal fluid
Positive culture findings in cerebrospinal fluid
EXCLUDES1 *colonization status (Z22.-)*

R83.6 Abnormal cytological findings in cerebrospinal fluid

R83.8 Other abnormal findings in cerebrospinal fluid
Abnormal chromosomal findings in cerebrospinal fluid

R83.9 Unspecified abnormal finding in cerebrospinal fluid

R84 Abnormal findings in specimens from respiratory organs and thorax

INCLUDES *abnormal findings in bronchial washings*
abnormal findings in nasal secretions
abnormal findings in pleural fluid
abnormal findings in sputum
abnormal findings in throat scrapings

EXCLUDES1 *blood-stained sputum (R04.2)*

R84.0 Abnormal level of enzymes in specimens from respiratory organs and thorax

R84.1 Abnormal level of hormones in specimens from respiratory organs and thorax

R84.2 Abnormal level of other drugs, medicaments and biological substances in specimens from respiratory organs and thorax

R84.3 Abnormal level of substances chiefly nonmedicinal as to source in specimens from respiratory organs and thorax

R84.4 Abnormal immunological findings in specimens from respiratory organs and thorax

R84.5 Abnormal microbiological findings in specimens from respiratory organs and thorax
Positive culture findings in specimens from respiratory organs and thorax
EXCLUDES1 *colonization status (Z22.-)*

R84.6 Abnormal cytological findings in specimens from respiratory organs and thorax

R84.7 Abnormal histological findings in specimens from respiratory organs and thorax

R84.8 Other abnormal findings in specimens from respiratory organs and thorax
Abnormal chromosomal findings in specimens from respiratory organs and thorax

R84.9 Unspecified abnormal finding in specimens from respiratory organs and thorax

R85 Abnormal findings in specimens from digestive organs and abdominal cavity

INCLUDES *abnormal findings in peritoneal fluid*
abnormal findings in saliva

EXCLUDES1 *cloudy peritoneal dialysis effluent (R88.0)*
fecal abnormalities (R19.5)

R85.0 Abnormal level of enzymes in specimens from digestive organs and abdominal cavity

R85.1 Abnormal level of hormones in specimens from digestive organs and abdominal cavity

R85.2 Abnormal level of other drugs, medicaments and biological substances in specimens from digestive organs and abdominal cavity

R85.3 Abnormal level of substances chiefly nonmedicinal as to source in specimens from digestive organs and abdominal cavity

R85.4 Abnormal immunological findings in specimens from digestive organs and abdominal cavity

R85.5 Abnormal microbiological findings in specimens from digestive organs and abdominal cavity
Positive culture findings in specimens from digestive organs and abdominal cavity
EXCLUDES1 *colonization status (Z22.-)*

R85.6 Abnormal cytological findings in specimens from digestive organs and abdominal cavity

R85.61 Abnormal cytologic smear of anus

EXCLUDES1 *abnormal cytological findings in specimens from other digestive organs and abdominal cavity (R85.69)*
carcinoma in situ of anus (histologically confirmed) (D01.3)
anal intraepithelial neoplasia I [AIN I] (K62.82)
anal intraepithelial neoplasia II [AIN II] (K62.82)
anal intraepithelial neoplasia III [AIN III] (D01.3)
dysplasia (mild) (moderate) of anus (histologically confirmed) (K62.82)
severe dysplasia of anus (histologically confirmed) (D01.3)

EXCLUDES2 *anal high risk human papillomavirus (HPV) DNA test positive (R85.81)*
anal low risk human papillomavirus (HPV) DNA test positive (R85.82)

R85.610 Atypical squamous cells of undetermined significance on cytologic smear of anus (ASC-US)

R85.611 Atypical squamous cells cannot exclude high grade squamous intraepithelial lesion on cytologic smear of anus (ASC-H)

R85.612 Low grade squamous intraepithelial lesion on cytologic smear of anus (LGSIL)

R85.613 High grade squamous intraepithelial lesion on cytologic smear of anus (HGSIL)

R85.614 Cytologic evidence of malignancy on smear of anus

R85.615 Unsatisfactory cytologic smear of anus
Inadequate sample of cytologic smear of anus

R85.616 Satisfactory anal smear but lacking transformation zone

R85.618 Other abnormal cytological findings on specimens from anus

R85.619 Unspecified abnormal cytological findings in specimens from anus
Abnormal anal cytology NOS
Atypical glandular cells of anus NOS

R85.69 Abnormal cytological findings in specimens from other digestive organs and abdominal cavity

R85.7 Abnormal histological findings in specimens from digestive organs and abdominal cavity

R85.8 Other abnormal findings in specimens from digestive organs and abdominal cavity

R85.81 Anal high risk human papillomavirus (HPV) DNA test positive
EXCLUDES1 *anogenital warts due to human papillomavirus (HPV) (A63.0)*
condyloma acuminatum (A63.0)

R85.82 Anal low risk human papillomavirus (HPV) DNA test positive
Use additional code for associated human papillomavirus (B97.7)

R85.89 Other abnormal findings in specimens from digestive organs and abdominal cavity
Abnormal chromosomal findings in specimens from digestive organs and abdominal cavity

R85.9 Unspecified abnormal finding in specimens from digestive organs and abdominal cavity

Unacceptable principal diagnosis symbol per Medicare code edits · Code exempt from diagnosis present on admission requirement
Questionable admission · Complication or comorbidity · CC/MCC exclusion · Major complication or comorbidity
Principal diagnosis as its own CC · Principal diagnosis as its own MCC · Z code as first-listed diagnosis

R86 Abnormal findings in specimens from male genital organs

INCLUDES *abnormal findings in prostatic secretions*
abnormal findings in semen, seminal fluid
abnormal spermatozoa

EXCLUDES1 *azoospermia (N46.0-)*
oligospermia (N46.1-)

R86.0 Abnormal level of enzymes in specimens from male genital organs ♂

R86.1 Abnormal level of hormones in specimens from male genital organs ♂

R86.2 Abnormal level of other drugs, medicaments and biological substances in specimens from male genital organs ♂

R86.3 Abnormal level of substances chiefly nonmedicinal as to source in specimens from male genital organs ♂

R86.4 Abnormal immunological findings in specimens from male genital organs ♂

R86.5 Abnormal microbiological findings in specimens from male genital organs ♂

Positive culture findings in specimens from male genital organs

EXCLUDES1 *colonization status (Z22.-)*

R86.6 Abnormal cytological findings in specimens from male genital organs ♂

R86.7 Abnormal histological findings in specimens from male genital organs ♂

R86.8 Other abnormal findings in specimens from male genital organs ♂

Abnormal chromosomal findings in specimens from male genital organs

R86.9 Unspecified abnormal finding in specimens from male genital organs ♂

R87 Abnormal findings in specimens from female genital organs

INCLUDES *abnormal findings in secretion and smears from cervix uteri*
abnormal findings in secretion and smears from vagina
abnormal findings in secretion and smears from vulva

R87.0 Abnormal level of enzymes in specimens from female genital organs ♀

R87.1 Abnormal level of hormones in specimens from female genital organs ♀

R87.2 Abnormal level of other drugs, medicaments and biological substances in specimens from female genital organs ♀

R87.3 Abnormal level of substances chiefly nonmedicinal as to source in specimens from female genital organs ♀

R87.4 Abnormal immunological findings in specimens from female genital organs ♀

R87.5 Abnormal microbiological findings in specimens from female genital organs ♀

Positive culture findings in specimens from female genital organs

EXCLUDES1 *colonization status (Z22.-)*

R87.6 Abnormal cytological findings in specimens from female genital organs

R87.61 Abnormal cytological findings in specimens from cervix uteri

EXCLUDES1 *abnormal cytological findings in specimens from other female genital organs (R87.69)*
abnormal cytological findings in specimens from vagina (R87.62-)
carcinoma in situ of cervix uteri (histologically confirmed) (D06.-)
cervical intraepithelial neoplasia I [CIN I] (N87.0)
cervical intraepithelial neoplasia II [CIN II] (N87.1)
cervical intraepithelial neoplasia III [CIN III] (D06.-)
dysplasia (mild) (moderate) of cervix uteri (histologically confirmed) (N87.-)
severe dysplasia of cervix uteri (histologically confirmed) (D06.-)

EXCLUDES2 *cervical high risk human papillomavirus (HPV) DNA test positive (R87.810)*
cervical low risk human papillomavirus (HPV) DNA test positive (R87.820)

R87.610 Atypical squamous cells of undetermined significance on cytologic smear of cervix (ASC-US) ♀

R87.611 Atypical squamous cells cannot exclude high grade squamous intraepithelial lesion on cytologic smear of cervix (ASC-H) ♀

R87.612 Low grade squamous intraepithelial lesion on cytologic smear of cervix (LGSIL) ♀

R87.613 High grade squamous intraepithelial lesion on cytologic smear of cervix (HGSIL) ♀

R87.614 Cytologic evidence of malignancy on smear of cervix ♀

R87.615 Unsatisfactory cytologic smear of cervix ♀

Inadequate sample of cytologic smear of cervix

R87.616 Satisfactory cervical smear but lacking transformation zone ♀

R87.618 Other abnormal cytological findings on specimens from cervix uteri ♀

R87.619 Unspecified abnormal cytological findings in specimens from cervix uteri ♀

Abnormal cervical cytology NOS
Abnormal Papanicolaou smear of cervix NOS
Abnormal thin preparation smear of cervix NOS
Atypical endocervical cells of cervix NOS
Atypical endometrial cells of cervix NOS
Atypical glandular cells of cervix NOS

R87.62 Abnormal cytological findings in specimens from vagina

Use additional code to identify acquired absence of uterus and cervix, if applicable (Z90.71-)

EXCLUDES1 *abnormal cytological findings in specimens from cervix uteri (R87.61-)*
abnormal cytological findings in specimens from other female genital organs (R87.69)
carcinoma in situ of vagina (histologically confirmed) (D07.2)
vaginal intraepithelial neoplasia I [VAIN I] (N89.0)
vaginal intraepithelial neoplasia II [VAIN II] (N89.1)
vaginal intraepithelial neoplasia III [VAIN III] (D07.2)
dysplasia (mild) (moderate) of vagina (histologically confirmed) (N89.-)
severe dysplasia of vagina (histologically confirmed) (D07.2)

EXCLUDES2 *vaginal high risk human papillomavirus (HPV) DNA test positive (R87.811)*
vaginal low risk human papillomavirus (HPV) DNA test positive (R87.821)

R87.620 Atypical squamous cells of undetermined significance on cytologic smear of vagina (ASC-US) ♀

R87.621 Atypical squamous cells cannot exclude high grade squamous intraepithelial lesion on cytologic smear of vagina (ASC-H) ♀

R87.622 Low grade squamous intraepithelial lesion on cytologic smear of vagina (LGSIL) ♀

R87.623 High grade squamous intraepithelial lesion on cytologic smear of vagina (HGSIL) ♀

R87.624 Cytologic evidence of malignancy on smear of vagina ♀

R87.625 Unsatisfactory cytologic smear of vagina ♀

Inadequate sample of cytologic smear of vagina

Unspecified Code Other Specified Code Manifestation Code N Newborn P Pediatric M Maternity A Adult ♂ Male ♀ Female
● New Code ▲ Revised Code Title ►◄ Revised Text NOTES INCLUDES EXCLUDES1 Not coded here EXCLUDES2 Not included here
4th character required 5th character required 6th character required 7th character required
Extension 'X' Alert HAC Hospital-acquired condition (HAC) alert AHA AHA Coding Clinic©

R87.628 **Other abnormal cytological findings on specimens from vagina** ♀

R87.629 **Unspecified abnormal cytological findings in specimens from vagina** ♀
Abnormal Papanicolaou smear of vagina NOS
Abnormal thin preparation smear of vagina NOS
Abnormal vaginal cytology NOS
Atypical endocervical cells of vagina NOS
Atypical endometrial cells of vagina NOS
Atypical glandular cells of vagina NOS

R87.69 **Abnormal cytological findings in specimens from other female genital organs** ♀
Abnormal cytological findings in specimens from female genital organs NOS
EXCLUDES1 *dysplasia of vulva (histologically confirmed) (N90.0-N90.3)*

R87.7 **Abnormal histological findings in specimens from female genital organs** ♀
EXCLUDES1 *carcinoma in situ (histologically confirmed) of female genital organs (D06-D07.3)*
cervical intraepithelial neoplasia I [CIN I] (N87.0)
cervical intraepithelial neoplasia II [CIN II] (N87.1)
cervical intraepithelial neoplasia III [CIN III] (D06.-)
dysplasia (mild) (moderate) of cervix uteri (histologically confirmed) (N87.-)
dysplasia (mild) (moderate) of vagina (histologically confirmed) (N89.-)
vaginal intraepithelial neoplasia I [VAIN I] (N89.0)
vaginal intraepithelial neoplasia II [VAIN II] (N89.1)
vaginal intraepithelial neoplasia III [VAIN III] (D07.2)
severe dysplasia of cervix uteri (histologically confirmed) (D06.-)
severe dysplasia of vagina (histologically confirmed) (D07.2)

R87.8 **Other abnormal findings in specimens from female genital organs**

R87.81 **High risk human papillomavirus (HPV) DNA test positive from female genital organs**
EXCLUDES1 *anogenital warts due to human papillomavirus (HPV) (A63.0)*
condyloma acuminatum (A63.0)

R87.810 **Cervical high risk human papillomavirus (HPV) DNA test positive** ♀

R87.811 **Vaginal high risk human papillomavirus (HPV) DNA test positive** ♀

R87.82 **Low risk human papillomavirus (HPV) DNA test positive from female genital organs**
Use additional code for associated human papillomavirus (B97.7)

R87.820 **Cervical low risk human papillomavirus (HPV) DNA test positive** ♀

R87.821 **Vaginal low risk human papillomavirus (HPV) DNA test positive** ♀

R87.89 **Other abnormal findings in specimens from female genital organs** ♀
Abnormal chromosomal findings in specimens from female genital organs

R87.9 **Unspecified abnormal finding in specimens from female genital organs** ♀

R88 **Abnormal findings in other body fluids and substances**

R88.0 **Cloudy (hemodialysis) (peritoneal) dialysis effluent**

R88.8 **Abnormal findings in other body fluids and substances**

R89 **Abnormal findings in specimens from other organs, systems and tissues**
INCLUDES *abnormal findings in nipple discharge*
abnormal findings in synovial fluid
abnormal findings in wound secretions

R89.0 **Abnormal level of enzymes in specimens from other organs, systems and tissues**

R89.1 **Abnormal level of hormones in specimens from other organs, systems and tissues**

R89.2 **Abnormal level of other drugs, medicaments and biological substances in specimens from other organs, systems and tissues**

R89.3 **Abnormal level of substances chiefly nonmedicinal as to source in specimens from other organs, systems and tissues**

R89.4 **Abnormal immunological findings in specimens from other organs, systems and tissues**

R89.5 **Abnormal microbiological findings in specimens from other organs, systems and tissues**
Positive culture findings in specimens from other organs, systems and tissues
EXCLUDES1 *colonization status (Z22.-)*

R89.6 **Abnormal cytological findings in specimens from other organs, systems and tissues**

R89.7 **Abnormal histological findings in specimens from other organs, systems and tissues**

R89.8 **Other abnormal findings in specimens from other organs, systems and tissues**
Abnormal chromosomal findings in specimens from other organs, systems and tissues

R89.9 **Unspecified abnormal finding in specimens from other organs, systems and tissues**

Abnormal findings on diagnostic imaging and in function studies, without diagnosis (R90-R94)

INCLUDES *nonspecific abnormal findings on diagnostic imaging by computerized axial tomography [CAT scan]*
nonspecific abnormal findings on diagnostic imaging by magnetic resonance imaging [MRI][NMR]
nonspecific abnormal findings on diagnostic imaging by positron emission tomography [PET scan]
nonspecific abnormal findings on diagnostic imaging by thermography
nonspecific abnormal findings on diagnostic imaging by ultrasound [echogram]
nonspecific abnormal findings on diagnostic imaging by X-ray examination

EXCLUDES1 *abnormal findings on antenatal screening of mother (O28.-)*
diagnostic abnormal findings classified elsewhere - see Alphabetical Index

R90 **Abnormal findings on diagnostic imaging of central nervous system**

R90.0 **Intracranial space-occupying lesion found on diagnostic imaging of central nervous system**

R90.8 **Other abnormal findings on diagnostic imaging of central nervous system**

R90.81 **Abnormal echoencephalogram**

R90.82 **White matter disease, unspecified**

R90.89 **Other abnormal findings on diagnostic imaging of central nervous system**
Other cerebrovascular abnormality found on diagnostic imaging of central nervous system

R91 **Abnormal findings on diagnostic imaging of lung**

R91.1 **Solitary pulmonary nodule**
Coin lesion lung
Solitary pulmonary nodule, subsegmental branch of the bronchial tree

R91.8 **Other nonspecific abnormal finding of lung field**
Lung mass NOS found on diagnostic imaging of lung
Pulmonary infiltrate NOS
Shadow, lung

R92 **Abnormal and inconclusive findings on diagnostic imaging of breast**

R92.0 **Mammographic microcalcification found on diagnostic imaging of breast**
EXCLUDES2 *mammographic calcification (calculus) found on diagnostic imaging of breast (R92.1)*

R92.1 **Mammographic calcification found on diagnostic imaging of breast**
Mammographic calculus found on diagnostic imaging of breast

R92.2 **Inconclusive mammogram**
Dense breasts NOS
Inconclusive mammogram NEC
Inconclusive mammography due to dense breasts
Inconclusive mammography NEC
AHA: Q1, 2015

Unacceptable principal diagnosis symbol per Medicare code edits · Code exempt from diagnosis present on admission requirement
Questionable admission · Complication or comorbidity · CC/MCC exclusion · Major complication or comorbidity
Principal diagnosis as its own CC · Principal diagnosis as its own MCC · Z code as first-listed diagnosis

R92.8 **Other abnormal and inconclusive findings on diagnostic imaging of breast**

R93 **Abnormal findings on diagnostic imaging of other body structures**

R93.0 **Abnormal findings on diagnostic imaging of skull and head, not elsewhere classified**

EXCLUDES1 *intracranial space-occupying lesion found on diagnostic imaging (R90.0)*

R93.1 **Abnormal findings on diagnostic imaging of heart and coronary circulation**

Abnormal echocardiogram NOS
Abnormal heart shadow

R93.2 **Abnormal findings on diagnostic imaging of liver and biliary tract**

Nonvisualization of gallbladder

R93.3 **Abnormal findings on diagnostic imaging of other parts of digestive tract**

R93.4 **Abnormal findings on diagnostic imaging of urinary organs**

EXCLUDES2 *hypertrophy of kidney (N28.81)*

● R93.41 **Abnormal radiologic findings on diagnostic imaging of renal pelvis, ureter, or bladder**

Filling defect of bladder found on diagnostic imaging
Filling defect of renal pelvis found on diagnostic imaging
Filling defect of ureter found on diagnostic imaging

● R93.42 **Abnormal radiologic findings on diagnostic imaging of kidney**

● R93.421 **Abnormal radiologic findings on diagnostic imaging of right kidney**

● R93.422 **Abnormal radiologic findings on diagnostic imaging of left kidney**

● R93.429 **Abnormal radiologic findings on diagnostic imaging of unspecified kidney**

● R93.49 **Abnormal radiologic findings on diagnostic imaging of other urinary organs**

R93.5 **Abnormal findings on diagnostic imaging of other abdominal regions, including retroperitoneum**

R93.6 **Abnormal findings on diagnostic imaging of limbs**

EXCLUDES2 *abnormal finding in skin and subcutaneous tissue (R93.8)*

R93.7 **Abnormal findings on diagnostic imaging of other parts of musculoskeletal system**

EXCLUDES2 *abnormal findings on diagnostic imaging of skull (R93.0)*

R93.8 **Abnormal findings on diagnostic imaging of other specified body structures**

Abnormal finding by radioisotope localization of placenta
Abnormal radiological finding in skin and subcutaneous tissue
Mediastinal shift

R93.9 **Diagnostic imaging inconclusive due to excess body fat of patient**

R94 **Abnormal results of function studies**

INCLUDES *abnormal results of radionuclide [radioisotope] uptake studies*
abnormal results of scintigraphy

R94.0 **Abnormal results of function studies of central nervous system**

R94.01 **Abnormal electroencephalogram [EEG]**

R94.02 **Abnormal brain scan**

R94.09 **Abnormal results of other function studies of central nervous system**

R94.1 **Abnormal results of function studies of peripheral nervous system and special senses**

R94.11 **Abnormal results of function studies of eye**

R94.110 **Abnormal electro-oculogram [EOG]**

R94.111 **Abnormal electroretinogram [ERG]**

Abnormal retinal function study

R94.112 **Abnormal visually evoked potential [VEP]**

R94.113 **Abnormal oculomotor study**

R94.118 **Abnormal results of other function studies of eye**

R94.12 **Abnormal results of function studies of ear and other special senses**

R94.120 **Abnormal auditory function study**

R94.121 **Abnormal vestibular function study**

R94.128 **Abnormal results of other function studies of ear and other special senses**

R94.13 **Abnormal results of function studies of peripheral nervous system**

R94.130 **Abnormal response to nerve stimulation, unspecified**

R94.131 **Abnormal electromyogram [EMG]**

EXCLUDES1 *electromyogram of eye (R94.113)*

R94.138 **Abnormal results of other function studies of peripheral nervous system**

R94.2 **Abnormal results of pulmonary function studies**

Reduced ventilatory capacity
Reduced vital capacity

R94.3 **Abnormal results of cardiovascular function studies**

R94.30 **Abnormal result of cardiovascular function study, unspecified**

R94.31 **Abnormal electrocardiogram [ECG] [EKG]**

EXCLUDES1 *long QT syndrome (I45.81)*

R94.39 **Abnormal result of other cardiovascular function study**

Abnormal electrophysiological intracardiac studies
Abnormal phonocardiogram
Abnormal vectorcardiogram

R94.4 **Abnormal results of kidney function studies**

Abnormal renal function test

R94.5 **Abnormal results of liver function studies**

R94.6 **Abnormal results of thyroid function studies**

R94.7 **Abnormal results of other endocrine function studies**

EXCLUDES2 *abnormal glucose (R73.0-)*

R94.8 **Abnormal results of function studies of other organs and systems**

Abnormal basal metabolic rate [BMR]
Abnormal bladder function test
Abnormal splenic function test

Abnormal tumor markers (R97)

R97 **Abnormal tumor markers**

Elevated tumor associated antigens [TAA]
Elevated tumor specific antigens [TSA]

R97.0 **Elevated carcinoembryonic antigen [CEA]**

R97.1 **Elevated cancer antigen 125 [CA 125]** ♀

R97.2 **Elevated prostate specific antigen [PSA]**

● R97.20 **Elevated prostate specific antigen [PSA]** CC/MCC Exc

● R97.21 **Rising PSA following treatment for malignant neoplasm of prostate** CC/MCC Exc

R97.8 **Other abnormal tumor markers**

Ill-defined and unknown cause of mortality (R99)

R99 **Ill-defined and unknown cause of mortality**

Death (unexplained) NOS
Unspecified cause of mortality

Unspecified Code Other Specified Code Manifestation Code N Newborn P Pediatric M Maternity A Adult ♂ Male ♀ Female
● New Code ▲ Revised Code Title ►◄ Revised Text NOTES INCLUDES EXCLUDES1 Not coded here EXCLUDES2 Not included here
4th character required 5th character required 6th character required 7th character required
Extension 'X' Alert HAC Hospital-acquired condition (HAC) alert AHA AHA Coding Clinic©

When symbols appear on a code that requires a 7th character extension, refer to Appendix D to identify applicable 7th character codes.

This page intentionally left blank

Chapter 19: Injury, Poisoning, and Certain other Consequences of External Causes (S00-T88)

Guidelines for Assigning Codes From This Chapter

Chapter 19 covers a wide variety of injuries, complications, and types of toxin exposure. Burns, contusions, fractures, and poisonings are just a few of the conditions you'll find in this chapter. You'll also use codes in this chapter to report late effects of injuries, poisonings, and other similar conditions. Be sure to read the instructions ICD-10-CM includes at the beginning of this chapter in the coding manual. You may be surprised to learn that when a code title includes more than one injury site, the use of "and" means "either or both sites." "With" is the term that shows the code requires both sites.

List of Sections

- S00-S09: Injuries to the head
- S10-S19: Injuries to the neck
- S20-S29: Injuries to the thorax
- S30-S39: Injuries to the abdomen, lower back, lumbar spine, pelvis and external genitals
- S40-S49: Injuries to the shoulder and upper arm
- S50-S59: Injuries to the elbow and forearm
- S60-S69: Injuries to the wrist, hand and fingers
- S70-S79: Injuries to the hip and thigh
- S80-S89: Injuries to the knee and lower leg
- S90-S99: Injuries to the ankle and foot
- T07-T88: Injury, poisoning and certain other consequences of external causes

Highlights From the ICD-10-CM Official Guidelines for Coding and Reporting

The ICD-10-CM Official Guidelines for Coding and Reporting for Chapter 19 supply important guidance on everything from the application of 7th characters to coding the complications of care. The information below is from Section I.C.19 of the 2017 Official Guidelines.

Get to Know 7th Character Options

You'll find 7th characters throughout chapter 19. Except for fractures, choose A for an *initial encounter*, D for a *subsequent encounter*, and S for *sequela* (late effect). Here are some tips to help you choose:

- The initial encounter (A) means active treatment—not the first time the provider sees the patient. Examples include surgery, emergency department visit, and evaluation and continuing treatment by the same or a different physician.
- Active treatment for complication codes must be treatment for the condition described by the code
- Choose subsequent encounter (D) for routine care after the initial encounter. Examples include cast change or removal, an X-ray to check healing status of a fracture, removal of an external or internal fixation device, medication adjustment, and other follow-up visits.
- When a 7th character is available to identify subsequent care, don't use aftercare Z codes.
- Code both the injury and a late effect, or sequela, but remember to append the S to the injury code—not the sequela code.

Keep These Fundamentals in Mind for Trauma Cases

- Report each injury separately unless ICD-10-CM offers a combination code for the specific injuries
- Sequence first the injury the provider states is most serious
- Don't report abrasions and contusions associated with a more serious injury, but you should report minor injuries to peripheral nerves and blood vessels as secondary codes after reporting the larger associated injury.

Watch for Expanded 7th Character Options for Traumatic Fractures

In addition to initial encounter, subsequent encounter, and sequela codes, you'll choose a 7th character to describe aspects of the fracture.

- **Nonunion vs malunion.** For subsequent care, choose K, M, or N for nonunion and P, Q, or R for malunion.
- **Open vs closed.** Code as closed if the provider doesn't specify open or closed.
- **Displaced or nondisplaced.** Code as displaced if the provider doesn't specify.

For aftercare, assign an acute fracture code with the appropriate 7th character—not a Z code.

Don't choose a traumatic fracture code when a fracture is due to osteoporosis. Look to category M80 in chapter 13.

Sequencing. When a patient has more than one fracture, your first code should be the most severe fracture.

Watch These Areas When Reporting Burns and Corrosion

ICD-10-CM distinguishes between thermal burns (from a heat source) and corrosion (a chemical burn). Classify current burns (T20-T25) by depth, extent and by agent (X code) as first degree (erythema), second degree (blistering), and third degree (full-thickness involvement). Classify burns of the eye and internal organs (T26-T28) by site, not by degree.

Classify burns of the same local site (three-character category level, T20-T28) but of different degrees to the subcategory identifying the highest degree recorded in the diagnosis.

Sequencing: When a patient has more than one burn, your first code should be for the highest degree of burn. If those burns of different degrees are at the same site, based on the three-digit categories, report only the code for the highest degree.

A patient may have both internal and external burns, or the patient may have burns as well as related conditions. In those cases, your first code should reflect the reason for admission.

Nonhealing burns: Use an acute burn code for nonhealing burns.

Infection: For infected burn sites, use an additional code for the infection.

Separate sites: Assign a separate code for each burn site. Avoid using unspecified category T30.

Rule of nines: Proper use of codes in categories T31 (burns) and T32 (corrosion) depends on understanding the "rule of nines":

- Head and neck: 9 percent
- Each arm: 9 percent
- Each leg: 18 percent
- Anterior trunk: 18 percent
- Posterior trunk: 18 percent
- Genitalia: 1 percent.

The above list shows the basic body surface estimate, but providers may vary from this list for children, whose heads are proportionately larger than adults', and for patients who have large buttocks, thighs, or abdomens with burns.

Sequelae. When the patient presents for treatment of late effects of a burn or corrosion, such as scars or joint contracture, report the burn or corrosion code with 7th character S.

Keep in mind that burns and corrosions don't heal at the same rate, and you can report sequela codes alongside current burn codes.

External cause. Don't forget to assign a code to identify the source of a burn, its intent, and the place where it occurred.

Check Additional Code Requirements for Adverse Effects, Poisonings, and Toxic Effects

Codes in categories T36-T65 are combination codes that combine the substance taken and the intent. Don't report an external cause code. Here are the basics:

- Don't code from the Table of Drugs and Chemicals. Always code from the tabular

- Use as many codes as necessary to describe all ingested substances.
- Assign a code only once if the same code describes the causative agent for more than one adverse reaction.
- Code each substance individually unless a combination code is available.

Adverse effect: When the patient presents with an adverse effect from a correctly prescribed and administered drug, first report the effect and then report a code from T36-T50, Poisoning by, adverse effects of and underdosing of drugs, medicaments and biological substances.

Poisoning: Poisoning codes (T36-T50) apply in cases of:

- Error in drug prescription or administration
- Intentional overdose
- Interaction of a nonprescribed agent with a properly prescribed and administered agent
- Interaction of alcohol and a drug.

You should report the poisoning code first followed by a code for the manifestation. You may report a drug abuse or dependence code as well when appropriate.

Underdosing: When the patient takes less medication than prescribed, assign a code from categories T36-T50, with a fifth or sixth character of "6." Never assign an underdosing code as the principal or first listed code. If underdosing causes a relapse or exacerbation of a medical condition, code the condition. Code the intent, if known, with a noncompliance or complication of care code.

Toxic effect: When reporting a toxic effect (T51-T65), use the appropriate Z code to indicate whether the intent was accidental, intentional self-harm, assault, or undetermined.

Report Abuse, Neglect and Other Maltreatment First

When reporting abuse, neglect, and maltreatment, sequence first the code from categories T74.- or T76.- for abuse, neglect and other maltreatment, followed by any accompanying mental health or injury code(s).

If the documentation in the medical record states abuse or neglect is suspected, code from T76-. Report a code from T74- only if the document specifies abuse or neglect is confirmed.

If there are physical injuries, choose an external cause code from the assault section (X92-Y08). If the perpetrator is known, code Y07 unless the documentation says abuse is only "suspected."

If a suspected case of abuse, neglect, mistreatment or alleged rape or sexual abuse is ruled out during an encounter, code Z04.71, Z04.41, or Z04.42, not a code from T76.

Apply Special Rules for Medical Device and Transplant Complications

Basics: After reporting a code from T80-T88, Complications of Surgical and Medical Care, Not Elsewhere Classified, you have to decide whether to report an additional code to identify the complication. Only report an additional code if it adds specificity to the code you've reported.

Pain due to medical devices: You'll find specific codes for pain due to medical devices in the T code section of the ICD-10-CM. Use additional code(s) from category G89 to identify acute or chronic pain due to presence of the device, implant or graft (G89.18 or G89.28).

Non-kidney transplant: Before reporting a code from T86 (*Complications of transplanted organs and tissues for a complication related to a nonkidney organ transplant*), remember that you shouldn't assign the code unless the complication affects the function of the organ.

Kidney transplant: Chronic kidney disease (CKD) following kidney transplant does not qualify as a complication, so you should not code it as such. Use T86.1- (*Complications of kidney transplant*), for complications such as failure or rejection. Use an additional code to report the specific complication. See Chapter 14 to report CKD.

Complication of care codes: Some of the complications of care codes include the nature of the complication as well as the type of procedure that caused the complication. You won't report an additional external cause code for the procedure.

Sequence intraoperative and postprocedural complication codes found in body system chapters first. Then code any specific complications.

Injury, poisoning and certain other consequences of external causes (S00-T88)

NOTES Use secondary code(s) from Chapter 20, External causes of morbidity, to indicate cause of injury. Codes within the T section that include the external cause do not require an additional external cause code

Use additional code to identify any retained foreign body, if applicable (Z18.-)

EXCLUDES1 *birth trauma (P10-P15)*
obstetric trauma (O70-O71)

This chapter contains the following blocks:

- S00-S09 Injuries to the head
- S10-S19 Injuries to the neck
- S20-S29 Injuries to the thorax
- S30-S39 Injuries to the abdomen, lower back, lumbar spine, pelvis and external genitals
- S40-S49 Injuries to the shoulder and upper arm
- S50-S59 Injuries to the elbow and forearm
- S60-S69 Injuries to the wrist, hand and fingers
- S70-S79 Injuries to the hip and thigh
- S80-S89 Injuries to the knee and lower leg
- S90-S99 Injuries to the ankle and foot
- T07 Injuries involving multiple body regions
- T14 Injury of unspecified body region
- T15-T19 Effects of foreign body entering through natural orifice
- T20-T32 Burns and corrosions
- T20-T25 Burns and corrosions of external body surface, specified by site
- T26-T28 Burns and corrosions confined to eye and internal organs
- T30-T32 Burns and corrosions of multiple and unspecified body regions
- T33-T34 Frostbite
- T36-T50 Poisoning by, adverse effect of and underdosing of drugs, medicaments and biological substances
- T51-T65 Toxic effects of substances chiefly nonmedicinal as to source
- T66-T78 Other and unspecified effects of external causes
- T79 Certain early complications of trauma
- T80-T88 Complications of surgical and medical care, not elsewhere classified

NOTES The chapter uses the S-section for coding different types of injuries related to single body regions and the T-section to cover injuries to unspecified body regions as well as poisoning and certain other consequences of external causes.

Injuries to the head (S00-S09)

INCLUDES *injuries of ear*
injuries of eye
injuries of face [any part]
injuries of gum
injuries of jaw
injuries of oral cavity
injuries of palate
injuries of periocular area
injuries of scalp
injuries of temporomandibular joint area
injuries of tongue
injuries of tooth

Code also for any associated infection

EXCLUDES2 *burns and corrosions (T20-T32)*
effects of foreign body in ear (T16)
effects of foreign body in larynx (T17.3)
effects of foreign body in mouth NOS (T18.0)
effects of foreign body in nose (T17.0-T17.1)
effects of foreign body in pharynx (T17.2)
effects of foreign body on external eye (T15.-)
frostbite (T33-T34)
insect bite or sting, venomous (T63.4)

S00 Superficial injury of head

EXCLUDES1 *diffuse cerebral contusion (S06.2-)*
focal cerebral contusion (S06.3-)
injury of eye and orbit (S05.-)
open wound of head (S01.-)

The appropriate 7th character is to be added to each code from category S00
A = initial encounter
D = subsequent encounter
S = sequela

S00.0 Superficial injury of scalp
- S00.00 Unspecified superficial injury of scalp
- S00.01 Abrasion of scalp
- S00.02 Blister (nonthermal) of scalp
- S00.03 Contusion of scalp
  Bruise of scalp
  Hematoma of scalp
- S00.04 External constriction of part of scalp
- S00.05 Superficial foreign body of scalp
  Splinter in the scalp
- S00.06 Insect bite (nonvenomous) of scalp
- S00.07 Other superficial bite of scalp
  EXCLUDES1 *open bite of scalp (S01.05)*

S00.1 Contusion of eyelid and periocular area
Black eye
EXCLUDES2 *contusion of eyeball and orbital tissues (S05.1)*
- S00.10 Contusion of unspecified eyelid and periocular area
- S00.11 Contusion of right eyelid and periocular area
- S00.12 Contusion of left eyelid and periocular area

S00.2 Other and unspecified superficial injuries of eyelid and periocular area
EXCLUDES2 *superficial injury of conjunctiva and cornea (S05.0-)*
- S00.20 Unspecified superficial injury of eyelid and periocular area
  - S00.201 Unspecified superficial injury of right eyelid and periocular area
  - S00.202 Unspecified superficial injury of left eyelid and periocular area
  - S00.209 Unspecified superficial injury of unspecified eyelid and periocular area
- S00.21 Abrasion of eyelid and periocular area
  - S00.211 Abrasion of right eyelid and periocular area
  - S00.212 Abrasion of left eyelid and periocular area
  - S00.219 Abrasion of unspecified eyelid and periocular area
- S00.22 Blister (nonthermal) of eyelid and periocular area
  - S00.221 Blister (nonthermal) of right eyelid and periocular area
  - S00.222 Blister (nonthermal) of left eyelid and periocular area
  - S00.229 Blister (nonthermal) of unspecified eyelid and periocular area
- S00.24 External constriction of eyelid and periocular area
  - S00.241 External constriction of right eyelid and periocular area
  - S00.242 External constriction of left eyelid and periocular area
  - S00.249 External constriction of unspecified eyelid and periocular area
- S00.25 Superficial foreign body of eyelid and periocular area
  Splinter of eyelid and periocular area
  EXCLUDES2 *retained foreign body in eyelid (H02.81-)*
  - S00.251 Superficial foreign body of right eyelid and periocular area
  - S00.252 Superficial foreign body of left eyelid and periocular area
  - S00.259 Superficial foreign body of unspecified eyelid and periocular area
- S00.26 Insect bite (nonvenomous) of eyelid and periocular area
  - S00.261 Insect bite (nonvenomous) of right eyelid and periocular area
  - S00.262 Insect bite (nonvenomous) of left eyelid and periocular area

Unspecified Code | Other Specified Code | Manifestation Code | N Newborn | P Pediatric | M Maternity | A Adult | ♂ Male | ♀ Female
● New Code | ▲ Revised Code Title | ►◄ Revised Text | NOTES | INCLUDES | EXCLUDES1 Not coded here | EXCLUDES2 Not included here
4th character required | 5th character required | 6th character required | 7th character required
Extension 'X' Alert | HAC Hospital-acquired condition (HAC) alert | AHA AHA Coding Clinic©

S00.269 Insect bite (nonvenomous) of unspecified eyelid and periocular area

S00.27 Other superficial bite of eyelid and periocular area

EXCLUDES1 *open bite of eyelid and periocular area (S01.15)*

S00.271 Other superficial bite of right eyelid and periocular area

S00.272 Other superficial bite of left eyelid and periocular area

S00.279 Other superficial bite of unspecified eyelid and periocular area

S00.3 Superficial injury of nose

S00.30 Unspecified superficial injury of nose

S00.31 Abrasion of nose

S00.32 Blister (nonthermal) of nose

S00.33 Contusion of nose
Bruise of nose
Hematoma of nose

S00.34 External constriction of nose

S00.35 Superficial foreign body of nose
Splinter in the nose

S00.36 Insect bite (nonvenomous) of nose

S00.37 Other superficial bite of nose

EXCLUDES1 *open bite of nose (S01.25)*

S00.4 Superficial injury of ear

S00.40 Unspecified superficial injury of ear

S00.401 Unspecified superficial injury of right ear

S00.402 Unspecified superficial injury of left ear

S00.409 Unspecified superficial injury of unspecified ear

S00.41 Abrasion of ear

S00.411 Abrasion of right ear

S00.412 Abrasion of left ear

S00.419 Abrasion of unspecified ear

S00.42 Blister (nonthermal) of ear

S00.421 Blister (nonthermal) of right ear

S00.422 Blister (nonthermal) of left ear

S00.429 Blister (nonthermal) of unspecified ear

S00.43 Contusion of ear
Bruise of ear
Hematoma of ear

S00.431 Contusion of right ear

S00.432 Contusion of left ear

S00.439 Contusion of unspecified ear

S00.44 External constriction of ear

S00.441 External constriction of right ear

S00.442 External constriction of left ear

S00.449 External constriction of unspecified ear

S00.45 Superficial foreign body of ear
Splinter in the ear

S00.451 Superficial foreign body of right ear

S00.452 Superficial foreign body of left ear

S00.459 Superficial foreign body of unspecified ear

S00.46 Insect bite (nonvenomous) of ear

S00.461 Insect bite (nonvenomous) of right ear

S00.462 Insect bite (nonvenomous) of left ear

S00.469 Insect bite (nonvenomous) of unspecified ear

S00.47 Other superficial bite of ear

EXCLUDES1 *open bite of ear (S01.35)*

S00.471 Other superficial bite of right ear

S00.472 Other superficial bite of left ear

S00.479 Other superficial bite of unspecified ear

S00.5 Superficial injury of lip and oral cavity

S00.50 Unspecified superficial injury of lip and oral cavity

S00.501 Unspecified superficial injury of lip

S00.502 Unspecified superficial injury of oral cavity

S00.51 Abrasion of lip and oral cavity

S00.511 Abrasion of lip

S00.512 Abrasion of oral cavity

S00.52 Blister (nonthermal) of lip and oral cavity

S00.521 Blister (nonthermal) of lip

S00.522 Blister (nonthermal) of oral cavity

S00.53 Contusion of lip and oral cavity

S00.531 Contusion of lip
Bruise of lip
Hematoma of oral cavity

S00.532 Contusion of oral cavity
Bruise of lip
Hematoma of oral cavity

S00.54 External constriction of lip and oral cavity

S00.541 External constriction of lip

S00.542 External constriction of oral cavity

S00.55 Superficial foreign body of lip and oral cavity

S00.551 Superficial foreign body of lip
Splinter of lip and oral cavity

S00.552 Superficial foreign body of oral cavity
Splinter of lip and oral cavity

S00.56 Insect bite (nonvenomous) of lip and oral cavity

S00.561 Insect bite (nonvenomous) of lip

S00.562 Insect bite (nonvenomous) of oral cavity

S00.57 Other superficial bite of lip and oral cavity

S00.571 Other superficial bite of lip

EXCLUDES1 *open bite of lip (S01.551)*

S00.572 Other superficial bite of oral cavity

EXCLUDES1 *open bite of oral cavity (S01.552)*

S00.8 Superficial injury of other parts of head
Superficial injuries of face [any part]

S00.80 Unspecified superficial injury of other part of head

S00.81 Abrasion of other part of head

S00.82 Blister (nonthermal) of other part of head

S00.83 Contusion of other part of head
Bruise of other part of head
Hematoma of other part of head

S00.84 External constriction of other part of head

S00.85 Superficial foreign body of other part of head
Splinter in other part of head

S00.86 Insect bite (nonvenomous) of other part of head

S00.87 Other superficial bite of other part of head

EXCLUDES1 *open bite of other part of head (S01.85)*

S00.9 Superficial injury of unspecified part of head

S00.90 Unspecified superficial injury of unspecified part of head

S00.91 Abrasion of unspecified part of head

S00.92 Blister (nonthermal) of unspecified part of head

S00.93 Contusion of unspecified part of head
Bruise of head
Hematoma of head

S00.94 External constriction of unspecified part of head

S00.95 Superficial foreign body of unspecified part of head
Splinter of head

S00.96 Insect bite (nonvenomous) of unspecified part of head

S00.97 Other superficial bite of unspecified part of head

EXCLUDES1 *open bite of head (S01.95)*

S01 Open wound of head

Code also any associated:
injury of cranial nerve (S04.-)
injury of muscle and tendon of head (S09.1-)
intracranial injury (S06.-)
wound infection

EXCLUDES1 *open skull fracture (S02.- with 7th character B)*

EXCLUDES2 *injury of eye and orbit (S05.-)*
traumatic amputation of part of head (S08.-)

The appropriate 7th character is to be added to each code from category S01
A = initial encounter
D = subsequent encounter
S = sequela

S01.0 Open wound of scalp

EXCLUDES1 *avulsion of scalp (S08.0)*

S01.00 Unspecified open wound of scalp

S01.01 Laceration without foreign body of scalp

Unacceptable principal diagnosis symbol per Medicare code edits | Code exempt from diagnosis present on admission requirement | Questionable admission | Complication or comorbidity | CC/MCC exclusion | Major complication or comorbidity | Principal diagnosis as its own CC | Principal diagnosis as its own MCC | Z code as first-listed diagnosis

- S01.02 Laceration with foreign body of scalp
  AHA: Q1, 2015
- S01.03 Puncture wound without foreign body of scalp
- S01.04 Puncture wound with foreign body of scalp
- S01.05 Open bite of scalp
  Bite of scalp NOS
  EXCLUDES1 *superficial bite of scalp (S00.06, S00.07-)*

S01.1 Open wound of eyelid and periocular area
Open wound of eyelid and periocular area with or without involvement of lacrimal passages

- S01.10 Unspecified open wound of eyelid and periocular area
  - S01.101 Unspecified open wound of right eyelid and periocular area
  - S01.102 Unspecified open wound of left eyelid and periocular area
  - S01.109 Unspecified open wound of unspecified eyelid and periocular area
- S01.11 Laceration without foreign body of eyelid and periocular area
  - S01.111 Laceration without foreign body of right eyelid and periocular area
  - S01.112 Laceration without foreign body of left eyelid and periocular area
  - S01.119 Laceration without foreign body of unspecified eyelid and periocular area
- S01.12 Laceration with foreign body of eyelid and periocular area
  - S01.121 Laceration with foreign body of right eyelid and periocular area
  - S01.122 Laceration with foreign body of left eyelid and periocular area
  - S01.129 Laceration with foreign body of unspecified eyelid and periocular area
- S01.13 Puncture wound without foreign body of eyelid and periocular area
  - S01.131 Puncture wound without foreign body of right eyelid and periocular area
  - S01.132 Puncture wound without foreign body of left eyelid and periocular area
  - S01.139 Puncture wound without foreign body of unspecified eyelid and periocular area
- S01.14 Puncture wound with foreign body of eyelid and periocular area
  - S01.141 Puncture wound with foreign body of right eyelid and periocular area
  - S01.142 Puncture wound with foreign body of left eyelid and periocular area
  - S01.149 Puncture wound with foreign body of unspecified eyelid and periocular area
- S01.15 Open bite of eyelid and periocular area
  Bite of eyelid and periocular area NOS
  EXCLUDES1 *superficial bite of eyelid and periocular area (S00.26, S00.27)*
  - S01.151 Open bite of right eyelid and periocular area
  - S01.152 Open bite of left eyelid and periocular area
  - S01.159 Open bite of unspecified eyelid and periocular area

S01.2 Open wound of nose

- S01.20 Unspecified open wound of nose
- S01.21 Laceration without foreign body of nose
  AHA: Q1, 2015
- S01.22 Laceration with foreign body of nose
- S01.23 Puncture wound without foreign body of nose
- S01.24 Puncture wound with foreign body of nose
- S01.25 Open bite of nose
  Bite of nose NOS
  EXCLUDES1 *superficial bite of nose (S00.36, S00.37)*

S01.3 Open wound of ear

- S01.30 Unspecified open wound of ear
  - S01.301 Unspecified open wound of right ear
  - S01.302 Unspecified open wound of left ear
  - S01.309 Unspecified open wound of unspecified ear
- S01.31 Laceration without foreign body of ear
  - S01.311 Laceration without foreign body of right ear
  - S01.312 Laceration without foreign body of left ear
  - S01.319 Laceration without foreign body of unspecified ear
- S01.32 Laceration with foreign body of ear
  - S01.321 Laceration with foreign body of right ear
  - S01.322 Laceration with foreign body of left ear
  - S01.329 Laceration with foreign body of unspecified ear
- S01.33 Puncture wound without foreign body of ear
  - S01.331 Puncture wound without foreign body of right ear
  - S01.332 Puncture wound without foreign body of left ear
  - S01.339 Puncture wound without foreign body of unspecified ear
- S01.34 Puncture wound with foreign body of ear
  - S01.341 Puncture wound with foreign body of right ear
  - S01.342 Puncture wound with foreign body of left ear
  - S01.349 Puncture wound with foreign body of unspecified ear
- S01.35 Open bite of ear
  Bite of ear NOS
  EXCLUDES1 *superficial bite of ear (S00.46, S00.47)*
  - S01.351 Open bite of right ear
  - S01.352 Open bite of left ear
  - S01.359 Open bite of unspecified ear

S01.4 Open wound of cheek and temporomandibular area

- S01.40 Unspecified open wound of cheek and temporomandibular area
  - S01.401 Unspecified open wound of right cheek and temporomandibular area
  - S01.402 Unspecified open wound of left cheek and temporomandibular area
  - S01.409 Unspecified open wound of unspecified cheek and temporomandibular area
- S01.41 Laceration without foreign body of cheek and temporomandibular area
  - S01.411 Laceration without foreign body of right cheek and temporomandibular area
    AHA: Q1, 2015
  - S01.412 Laceration without foreign body of left cheek and temporomandibular area
  - S01.419 Laceration without foreign body of unspecified cheek and temporomandibular area
- S01.42 Laceration with foreign body of cheek and temporomandibular area
  - S01.421 Laceration with foreign body of right cheek and temporomandibular area
  - S01.422 Laceration with foreign body of left cheek and temporomandibular area
  - S01.429 Laceration with foreign body of unspecified cheek and temporomandibular area
- S01.43 Puncture wound without foreign body of cheek and temporomandibular area
  - S01.431 Puncture wound without foreign body of right cheek and temporomandibular area
  - S01.432 Puncture wound without foreign body of left cheek and temporomandibular area
  - S01.439 Puncture wound without foreign body of unspecified cheek and temporomandibular area
- S01.44 Puncture wound with foreign body of cheek and temporomandibular area
  - S01.441 Puncture wound with foreign body of right cheek and temporomandibular area

S01.442 Puncture wound with foreign body of left cheek and temporomandibular area
S01.449 Puncture wound with foreign body of unspecified cheek and temporomandibular area
S01.45 Open bite of cheek and temporomandibular area
Bite of cheek and temporomandibular area NOS
EXCLUDES2 *superficial bite of cheek and temporomandibular area (S00.86, S00.87)*
S01.451 Open bite of right cheek and temporomandibular area
S01.452 Open bite of left cheek and temporomandibular area
S01.459 Open bite of unspecified cheek and temporomandibular area
S01.5 Open wound of lip and oral cavity
EXCLUDES2 *tooth dislocation (S03.2)*
tooth fracture (S02.5)
S01.50 Unspecified open wound of lip and oral cavity
S01.501 Unspecified open wound of lip
S01.502 Unspecified open wound of oral cavity
S01.51 Laceration of lip and oral cavity without foreign body
S01.511 Laceration without foreign body of lip
S01.512 Laceration without foreign body of oral cavity
S01.52 Laceration of lip and oral cavity with foreign body
S01.521 Laceration with foreign body of lip
S01.522 Laceration with foreign body of oral cavity
S01.53 Puncture wound of lip and oral cavity without foreign body
S01.531 Puncture wound without foreign body of lip
S01.532 Puncture wound without foreign body of oral cavity
S01.54 Puncture wound of lip and oral cavity with foreign body
S01.541 Puncture wound with foreign body of lip
S01.542 Puncture wound with foreign body of oral cavity
S01.55 Open bite of lip and oral cavity
S01.551 Open bite of lip
Bite of lip NOS
EXCLUDES1 *superficial bite of lip (S00.571)*
S01.552 Open bite of oral cavity
Bite of oral cavity NOS
EXCLUDES1 *superficial bite of oral cavity (S00.572)*
S01.8 Open wound of other parts of head
S01.80 Unspecified open wound of other part of head
S01.81 Laceration without foreign body of other part of head
S01.82 Laceration with foreign body of other part of head
S01.83 Puncture wound without foreign body of other part of head
S01.84 Puncture wound with foreign body of other part of head
S01.85 Open bite of other part of head
Bite of other part of head NOS
EXCLUDES1 *superficial bite of other part of head (S00.85)*
S01.9 Open wound of unspecified part of head
S01.90 Unspecified open wound of unspecified part of head
S01.91 Laceration without foreign body of unspecified part of head
S01.92 Laceration with foreign body of unspecified part of head
S01.93 Puncture wound without foreign body of unspecified part of head
S01.94 Puncture wound with foreign body of unspecified part of head
S01.95 Open bite of unspecified part of head
Bite of head NOS
EXCLUDES1 *superficial bite of head NOS (S00.97)*

S02 Fracture of skull and facial bones
NOTES A fracture not indicated as open or closed should be coded to closed
Code also any associated intracranial injury (S06.-)
The appropriate 7th character is to be added to each code from category S02
A = initial encounter for closed fracture
B = initial encounter for open fracture
D = subsequent encounter for fracture with routine healing
G = subsequent encounter for fracture with delayed healing
K = subsequent encounter for fracture with nonunion
S = sequela
S02.0 Fracture of vault of skull CC HAC MCC
Fracture of frontal bone
Fracture of parietal bone
S02.1 Fracture of base of skull
EXCLUDES1 *orbit NOS (S02.8)*
EXCLUDES2 *orbital floor (S02.3-)*
S02.10 Unspecified fracture of base of skull
● S02.101 Fracture of base of skull, right side CC CC/MCC Exc MCC
● S02.102 Fracture of base of skull, left side CC CC/MCC Exc MCC
● S02.109 Fracture of base of skull, unspecified side CC CC/MCC Exc MCC
S02.11 Fracture of occiput
▲ S02.110 Type I occipital condyle fracture, ►unspecified side◄ CC HAC MCC
▲ S02.111 Type II occipital condyle fracture, ►unspecified side◄ CC HAC MCC
▲ S02.112 Type III occipital condyle fracture, ►unspecified side◄ CC HAC MCC
S02.113 Unspecified occipital condyle fracture CC HAC MCC
▲ S02.118 Other fracture of occiput, ►unspecified side◄ CC HAC MCC
S02.119 Unspecified fracture of occiput CC HAC MCC
● S02.11A Type I occipital condyle fracture, right side CC CC/MCC Exc MCC
● S02.11B Type I occipital condyle fracture, left side CC CC/MCC Exc MCC
● S02.11C Type II occipital condyle fracture, right side CC CC/MCC Exc MCC
● S02.11D Type II occipital condyle fracture, left side CC CC/MCC Exc MCC
● S02.11E Type III occipital condyle fracture, right side CC CC/MCC Exc MCC
● S02.11F Type III occipital condyle fracture, left side CC CC/MCC Exc MCC
● S02.11G Other fracture of occiput, right side CC CC/MCC Exc MCC
● S02.11H Other fracture of occiput, left side CC CC/MCC Exc MCC
S02.19 Other fracture of base of skull CC HAC MCC
Fracture of anterior fossa of base of skull
Fracture of ethmoid sinus
Fracture of frontal sinus
Fracture of middle fossa of base of skull
Fracture of orbital roof
Fracture of posterior fossa of base of skull
Fracture of sphenoid
Fracture of temporal bone
S02.2 Fracture of nasal bones CC HAC
S02.3 Fracture of orbital floor
EXCLUDES1 *orbit NOS (S02.8)*
EXCLUDES2 *orbital roof (S02.1-)*
● S02.30 Fracture of orbital floor, unspecified side CC CC/MCC Exc
● S02.31 Fracture of orbital floor, right side CC CC/MCC Exc
● S02.32 Fracture of orbital floor, left side CC CC/MCC Exc
S02.4 Fracture of malar, maxillary and zygoma bones
Fracture of superior maxilla
Fracture of upper jaw (bone)
Fracture of zygomatic process of temporal bone
S02.40 Fracture of malar, maxillary and zygoma bones, unspecified

Unacceptable principal diagnosis symbol per Medicare code edits | Code exempt from diagnosis present on admission requirement
Questionable admission | CC Complication or comorbidity | CC/MCC Exc CC/MCC exclusion | MCC Major complication or comorbidity
Principal diagnosis as its own CC | Principal diagnosis as its own MCC | Z code as first-listed diagnosis

 When symbols appear on a code that requires a 7th character extension, refer to Appendix D to identify applicable 7th character codes.

▲ S02.400 Malar fracture, ▶unspecified side◀ CC HAC
▲ S02.401 Maxillary fracture, unspecified ▶side◀ CC HAC
▲ S02.402 Zygomatic fracture, unspecified ▶side◀ CC HAC
● S02.40A Malar fracture, right side CC CC/MCC Exc
● S02.40B Malar fracture, left side CC CC/MCC Exc
● S02.40C Maxillary fracture, right side CC CC/MCC Exc
● S02.40D Maxillary fracture, left side CC CC/MCC Exc
● S02.40E Zygomatic fracture, right side CC CC/MCC Exc
● S02.40F Zygomatic fracture, left side CC CC/MCC Exc

S02.41 LeFort fracture
S02.411 LeFort I fracture CC HAC
S02.412 LeFort II fracture CC HAC
S02.413 LeFort III fracture CC HAC

S02.42 Fracture of alveolus of maxilla CC HAC

S02.5 Fracture of tooth (traumatic) CC
Broken tooth
EXCLUDES1 *cracked tooth (nontraumatic) (K03.81)*

S02.6 Fracture of mandible
Fracture of lower jaw (bone)

S02.60 Fracture of mandible, unspecified
▲ S02.600 Fracture of unspecified part of body of mandible, ▶unspecified side◀ CC HAC
● S02.601 Fracture of unspecified part of body of right mandible CC CC/MCC Exc
● S02.602 Fracture of unspecified part of body of left mandible CC CC/MCC Exc
S02.609 Fracture of mandible, unspecified CC HAC

S02.61 Fracture of condylar process of mandible
● S02.610 Fracture of condylar process of mandible, unspecified side CC CC/MCC Exc
● S02.611 Fracture of condylar process of right mandible CC CC/MCC Exc
● S02.612 Fracture of condylar process of left mandible CC CC/MCC Exc

S02.62 Fracture of subcondylar process of mandible
● S02.620 Fracture of subcondylar process of mandible, unspecified side CC CC/MCC Exc
● S02.621 Fracture of subcondylar process of right mandible CC CC/MCC Exc
● S02.622 Fracture of subcondylar process of left mandible CC CC/MCC Exc

S02.63 Fracture of coronoid process of mandible CC HAC
● S02.630 Fracture of coronoid process of mandible, unspecified side CC CC/MCC Exc
● S02.631 Fracture of coronoid process of right mandible CC CC/MCC Exc
● S02.632 Fracture of coronoid process of left mandible CC CC/MCC Exc

S02.64 Fracture of ramus of mandible
● S02.640 Fracture of ramus of mandible, unspecified side CC CC/MCC Exc
● S02.641 Fracture of ramus of right mandible CC CC/MCC Exc
● S02.642 Fracture of ramus of left mandible CC CC/MCC Exc

S02.65 Fracture of angle of mandible
● S02.650 Fracture of angle of mandible, unspecified side CC CC/MCC Exc
● S02.651 Fracture of angle of right mandible CC CC/MCC Exc
● S02.652 Fracture of angle of left mandible CC CC/MCC Exc

S02.66 Fracture of symphysis of mandible CC HAC

S02.67 Fracture of alveolus of mandible
● S02.670 Fracture of alveolus of mandible, unspecified side CC CC/MCC Exc
● S02.671 Fracture of alveolus of right mandible CC CC/MCC Exc
● S02.672 Fracture of alveolus of left mandible CC CC/MCC Exc

S02.69 Fracture of mandible of other specified site CC HAC

S02.8 Fractures of other specified skull and facial bones
Fracture of orbit NOS
Fracture of palate
EXCLUDES1 *fracture of orbital floor (S02.3-)*
fracture of orbital roof (S02.1-)
● S02.80 Fracture of other specified skull and facial bones, unspecified side CC CC/MCC Exc
● S02.81 Fracture of other specified skull and facial bones, right side CC CC/MCC Exc
● S02.82 Fracture of other specified skull and facial bones, left side CC CC/MCC Exc

S02.9 Fracture of unspecified skull and facial bones
S02.91 Unspecified fracture of skull CC HAC MCC
S02.92 Unspecified fracture of facial bones CC HAC

S03 Dislocation and sprain of joints and ligaments of head

INCLUDES *avulsion of joint (capsule) or ligament of head*
laceration of cartilage, joint (capsule) or ligament of head
sprain of cartilage, joint (capsule) or ligament of head
traumatic hemarthrosis of joint or ligament of head
traumatic rupture of joint or ligament of head
traumatic subluxation of joint or ligament of head
traumatic tear of joint or ligament of head

Code also any associated open wound
EXCLUDES2 *Strain of muscle or tendon of head (S09.1)*

The appropriate 7th character is to be added to each code from category S03
A = initial encounter
D = subsequent encounter
S = sequela

S03.0 Dislocation of jaw
Dislocation of jaw (cartilage) (meniscus)
Dislocation of mandible
Dislocation of temporomandibular (joint)
● S03.00 Dislocation of jaw, unspecified side CC/MCC Exc
● S03.01 Dislocation of jaw, right side CC/MCC Exc
● S03.02 Dislocation of jaw, left side CC/MCC Exc
● S03.03 Dislocation of jaw, bilateral CC/MCC Exc

S03.1 Dislocation of septal cartilage of nose
S03.2 Dislocation of tooth
S03.4 Sprain of jaw
Sprain of temporomandibular (joint) (ligament)
● S03.40 Sprain of jaw, unspecified side
● S03.41 Sprain of jaw, right side
● S03.42 Sprain of jaw, left side
● S03.43 Sprain of jaw, bilateral
S03.8 Sprain of joints and ligaments of other parts of head
S03.9 Sprain of joints and ligaments of unspecified parts of head

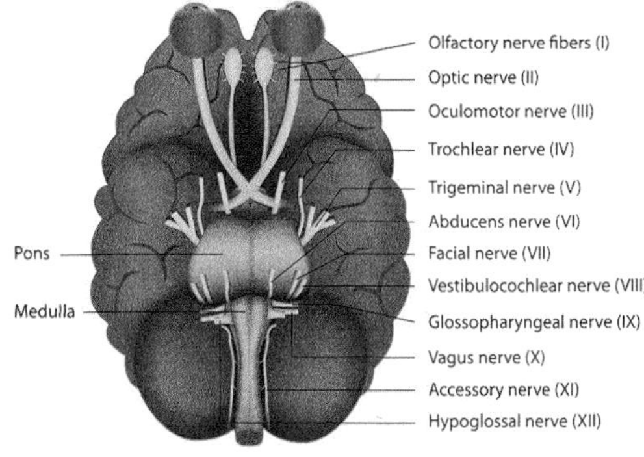

Figure 15.1 Cranial nerves

S04 Injury of cranial nerve

The selection of side should be based on the side of the body being affected
Code first any associated intracranial injury (S06.-)
Code also any associated:
open wound of head (S01.-)
skull fracture (S02.-)

Unspecified Code | Other Specified Code | Manifestation Code | N Newborn | P Pediatric | M Maternity | A Adult | ♂ Male | ♀ Female
● New Code | ▲ Revised Code Title | ▶◀ Revised Text | NOTES | INCLUDES | EXCLUDES1 Not coded here | EXCLUDES2 Not included here
4th character required | 5th character required | 6th character required | 7th character required
Extension 'X' Alert | HAC Hospital-acquired condition (HAC) alert | AHA AHA Coding Clinic©

The appropriate 7th character is to be added to each code from category S04

- A = initial encounter
- D = subsequent encounter
- S = sequela

S04.0 Injury of optic nerve and pathways

Use additional code to identify any visual field defect or blindness (H53.4-, H54)

S04.01 Injury of optic nerve

Injury of 2nd cranial nerve

- **S04.011 Injury of optic nerve, right eye** CC
- **S04.012 Injury of optic nerve, left eye** CC
- **S04.019 Injury of optic nerve, unspecified eye** CC
  Injury of optic nerve NOS

S04.02 Injury of optic chiasm CC

S04.03 Injury of optic tract and pathways

Injury of optic radiation

- **S04.031 Injury of optic tract and pathways, right eye** CC
- **S04.032 Injury of optic tract and pathways, left eye** CC
- **S04.039 Injury of optic tract and pathways, unspecified eye** CC
  Injury of optic tract and pathways NOS

S04.04 Injury of visual cortex

- **S04.041 Injury of visual cortex, right eye** CC
- **S04.042 Injury of visual cortex, left eye** CC
- **S04.049 Injury of visual cortex, unspecified eye** CC
  Injury of visual cortex NOS

S04.1 Injury of oculomotor nerve

Injury of 3rd cranial nerve

- **S04.10 Injury of oculomotor nerve, unspecified side** CC
- **S04.11 Injury of oculomotor nerve, right side** CC
- **S04.12 Injury of oculomotor nerve, left side** CC

S04.2 Injury of trochlear nerve

Injury of 4th cranial nerve

- **S04.20 Injury of trochlear nerve, unspecified side** CC
- **S04.21 Injury of trochlear nerve, right side** CC
- **S04.22 Injury of trochlear nerve, left side** CC

S04.3 Injury of trigeminal nerve

Injury of 5th cranial nerve

- **S04.30 Injury of trigeminal nerve, unspecified side** CC
- **S04.31 Injury of trigeminal nerve, right side** CC
- **S04.32 Injury of trigeminal nerve, left side** CC

S04.4 Injury of abducent nerve

Injury of 6th cranial nerve

- **S04.40 Injury of abducent nerve, unspecified side** CC
- **S04.41 Injury of abducent nerve, right side** CC
- **S04.42 Injury of abducent nerve, left side** CC

S04.5 Injury of facial nerve

Injury of 7th cranial nerve

- **S04.50 Injury of facial nerve, unspecified side** CC
- **S04.51 Injury of facial nerve, right side** CC
- **S04.52 Injury of facial nerve, left side** CC

S04.6 Injury of acoustic nerve

Injury of auditory nerve
Injury of 8th cranial nerve

- **S04.60 Injury of acoustic nerve, unspecified side** CC
- **S04.61 Injury of acoustic nerve, right side** CC
- **S04.62 Injury of acoustic nerve, left side** CC

S04.7 Injury of accessory nerve

Injury of 11th cranial nerve

- **S04.70 Injury of accessory nerve, unspecified side** CC
- **S04.71 Injury of accessory nerve, right side** CC
- **S04.72 Injury of accessory nerve, left side** CC

S04.8 Injury of other cranial nerves

S04.81 Injury of olfactory [1st] nerve

- **S04.811 Injury of olfactory [1st] nerve, right side** CC
- **S04.812 Injury of olfactory [1st] nerve, left side** CC
- **S04.819 Injury of olfactory [1st] nerve, unspecified side** CC

S04.89 Injury of other cranial nerves

Injury of vagus [10th] nerve

- **S04.891 Injury of other cranial nerves, right side** CC
- **S04.892 Injury of other cranial nerves, left side** CC
- **S04.899 Injury of other cranial nerves, unspecified side** CC

S04.9 Injury of unspecified cranial nerve CC

S05 Injury of eye and orbit

INCLUDES *open wound of eye and orbit*

EXCLUDES2 *2nd cranial [optic] nerve injury (S04.0-)*
3rd cranial [oculomotor] nerve injury (S04.1-)
open wound of eyelid and periocular area (S01.1-)
orbital bone fracture (S02.1-, S02.3-, S02.8-)
superficial injury of eyelid (S00.1-S00.2)

The appropriate 7th character is to be added to each code from category S05

- A = initial encounter
- D = subsequent encounter
- S = sequela

S05.0 Injury of conjunctiva and corneal abrasion without foreign body

EXCLUDES1 *foreign body in conjunctival sac (T15.1)*
foreign body in cornea (T15.0)

- **S05.00 Injury of conjunctiva and corneal abrasion without foreign body, unspecified eye**
- **S05.01 Injury of conjunctiva and corneal abrasion without foreign body, right eye**
- **S05.02 Injury of conjunctiva and corneal abrasion without foreign body, left eye**

S05.1 Contusion of eyeball and orbital tissues

Traumatic hyphema

EXCLUDES2 *black eye NOS (S00.1)*
contusion of eyelid and periocular area (S00.1)

- **S05.10 Contusion of eyeball and orbital tissues, unspecified eye**
- **S05.11 Contusion of eyeball and orbital tissues, right eye**
- **S05.12 Contusion of eyeball and orbital tissues, left eye**

S05.2 Ocular laceration and rupture with prolapse or loss of intraocular tissue

- **S05.20 Ocular laceration and rupture with prolapse or loss of intraocular tissue, unspecified eye** CC
- **S05.21 Ocular laceration and rupture with prolapse or loss of intraocular tissue, right eye** CC
- **S05.22 Ocular laceration and rupture with prolapse or loss of intraocular tissue, left eye** CC

S05.3 Ocular laceration without prolapse or loss of intraocular tissue

Laceration of eye NOS

- **S05.30 Ocular laceration without prolapse or loss of intraocular tissue, unspecified eye** CC
- **S05.31 Ocular laceration without prolapse or loss of intraocular tissue, right eye** CC
- **S05.32 Ocular laceration without prolapse or loss of intraocular tissue, left eye** CC

S05.4 Penetrating wound of orbit with or without foreign body

EXCLUDES2 *retained (old) foreign body following penetrating wound in orbit (H05.5-)*

- **S05.40 Penetrating wound of orbit with or without foreign body, unspecified eye** CC
- **S05.41 Penetrating wound of orbit with or without foreign body, right eye** CC
- **S05.42 Penetrating wound of orbit with or without foreign body, left eye** CC

S05.5 Penetrating wound with foreign body of eyeball

EXCLUDES2 *retained (old) intraocular foreign body (H44.6-, H44.7)*

- **S05.50 Penetrating wound with foreign body of unspecified eyeball** CC
- **S05.51 Penetrating wound with foreign body of right eyeball** CC
- **S05.52 Penetrating wound with foreign body of left eyeball** CC

S05.6 Penetrating wound without foreign body of eyeball

Ocular penetration NOS

- **S05.60 Penetrating wound without foreign body of unspecified eyeball**

Unacceptable principal diagnosis symbol per Medicare code edits · Code exempt from diagnosis present on admission requirement · Questionable admission · CC Complication or comorbidity · CC/MCC exclusion · MCC Major complication or comorbidity · Principal diagnosis as its own CC · Principal diagnosis as its own MCC · Z code as first-listed diagnosis

S05.61 Penetrating wound without foreign body of right eyeball
S05.62 Penetrating wound without foreign body of left eyeball
S05.7 Avulsion of eye
Traumatic enucleation
S05.70 Avulsion of unspecified eye CC
S05.71 Avulsion of right eye CC
S05.72 Avulsion of left eye CC
S05.8 Other injuries of eye and orbit
Lacrimal duct injury
S05.8X Other injuries of eye and orbit
S05.8X1 Other injuries of right eye and orbit CC
S05.8X2 Other injuries of left eye and orbit CC
S05.8X9 Other injuries of unspecified eye and orbit CC
S05.9 Unspecified injury of eye and orbit
Injury of eye NOS
S05.90 Unspecified injury of unspecified eye and orbit
S05.91 Unspecified injury of right eye and orbit CC
S05.92 Unspecified injury of left eye and orbit CC
S06 Intracranial injury
INCLUDES *traumatic brain injury*
Code also any associated:
open wound of head (S01.-)
skull fracture (S02.-)
EXCLUDES1 *head injury NOS (S09.90)*
The appropriate 7th character is to be added to each code from category S06
A = initial encounter
D = subsequent encounter
S = sequela
S06.0 Concussion
Commotio cerebri
EXCLUDES1 *concussion with other intracranial injuries classified in ►subcategories S06.1- to S06.6-, S06.81- and S06.82-◄ code to specified intracranial injury*
S06.0X Concussion
S06.0X0 Concussion without loss of consciousness
S06.0X1 Concussion with loss of consciousness of 30 minutes or less CC HAC
S06.0X9 Concussion with loss of consciousness of unspecified duration CC HAC
Concussion NOS
S06.1 Traumatic cerebral edema
Diffuse traumatic cerebral edema
Focal traumatic cerebral edema
S06.1X Traumatic cerebral edema
S06.1X0 Traumatic cerebral edema without loss of consciousness MCC PDx MCC
AHA: Q1, 2015
S06.1X1 Traumatic cerebral edema with loss of consciousness of 30 minutes or less HAC MCC PDx MCC
S06.1X2 Traumatic cerebral edema with loss of consciousness of 31 minutes to 59 minutes HAC MCC PDx MCC
S06.1X3 Traumatic cerebral edema with loss of consciousness of 1 hour to 5 hours 59 minutes HAC MCC PDx MCC
S06.1X4 Traumatic cerebral edema with loss of consciousness of 6 hours to 24 hours HAC MCC PDx MCC
S06.1X5 Traumatic cerebral edema with loss of consciousness greater than 24 hours with return to pre-existing conscious level HAC MCC PDx MCC
S06.1X6 Traumatic cerebral edema with loss of consciousness greater than 24 hours without return to pre-existing conscious level with patient surviving HAC MCC PDx MCC
S06.1X7 Traumatic cerebral edema with loss of consciousness of any duration with death due to brain injury prior to regaining consciousness HAC MCC PDx MCC
S06.1X8 Traumatic cerebral edema with loss of consciousness of any duration with death due to other cause prior to regaining consciousness HAC MCC PDx MCC
S06.1X9 Traumatic cerebral edema with loss of consciousness of unspecified duration HAC MCC PDx MCC
Traumatic cerebral edema NOS
S06.2 Diffuse traumatic brain injury
Diffuse axonal brain injury
EXCLUDES1 *traumatic diffuse cerebral edema (S06.1X-)*
S06.2X Diffuse traumatic brain injury
S06.2X0 Diffuse traumatic brain injury without loss of consciousness
S06.2X1 Diffuse traumatic brain injury with loss of consciousness of 30 minutes or less CC HAC
S06.2X2 Diffuse traumatic brain injury with loss of consciousness of 31 minutes to 59 minutes CC HAC
S06.2X3 Diffuse traumatic brain injury with loss of consciousness of 1 hour to 5 hours 59 minutes CC HAC
S06.2X4 Diffuse traumatic brain injury with loss of consciousness of 6 hours to 24 hours CC HAC
S06.2X5 Diffuse traumatic brain injury with loss of consciousness greater than 24 hours with return to pre-existing conscious levels CC HAC
S06.2X6 Diffuse traumatic brain injury with loss of consciousness greater than 24 hours without return to pre-existing conscious level with patient surviving HAC MCC
S06.2X7 Diffuse traumatic brain injury with loss of consciousness of any duration with death due to brain injury prior to regaining consciousness HAC MCC
S06.2X8 Diffuse traumatic brain injury with loss of consciousness of any duration with death due to other cause prior to regaining consciousness HAC MCC
S06.2X9 Diffuse traumatic brain injury with loss of consciousness of unspecified duration CC HAC
Diffuse traumatic brain injury NOS
S06.3 Focal traumatic brain injury
EXCLUDES1 *any condition classifiable to S06.4-S06.6*
focal cerebral edema (S06.1)
S06.30 Unspecified focal traumatic brain injury
S06.300 Unspecified focal traumatic brain injury without loss of consciousness
S06.301 Unspecified focal traumatic brain injury with loss of consciousness of 30 minutes or less CC HAC
S06.302 Unspecified focal traumatic brain injury with loss of consciousness of 31 minutes to 59 minutes CC HAC
S06.303 Unspecified focal traumatic brain injury with loss of consciousness of 1 hour to 5 hours 59 minutes CC HAC
S06.304 Unspecified focal traumatic brain injury with loss of consciousness of 6 hours to 24 hours CC HAC
S06.305 Unspecified focal traumatic brain injury with loss of consciousness greater than 24 hours with return to pre-existing conscious level CC HAC
S06.306 Unspecified focal traumatic brain injury with loss of consciousness greater than 24 hours without return to pre-existing conscious level with patient surviving HAC MCC
S06.307 Unspecified focal traumatic brain injury with loss of consciousness of any duration with death due to brain injury prior to regaining consciousness HAC MCC

Unspecified Code Other Specified Code Manifestation Code N Newborn P Pediatric M Maternity A Adult ♂ Male ♀ Female
● New Code ▲ Revised Code Title ►◄ Revised Text NOTES INCLUDES EXCLUDES1 Not coded here EXCLUDES2 Not included here
4th character required 5th character required 6th character required 7th character required
Extension 'X' Alert HAC Hospital-acquired condition (HAC) alert AHA AHA Coding Clinic®

S06.308 Unspecified focal traumatic brain injury with loss of consciousness of any duration with death due to other cause prior to regaining consciousness HAC MCC

S06.309 Unspecified focal traumatic brain injury with loss of consciousness of unspecified duration CC HAC

Unspecified focal traumatic brain injury NOS

S06.31 Contusion and laceration of right cerebrum

S06.310 Contusion and laceration of right cerebrum without loss of consciousness HAC MCC

S06.311 Contusion and laceration of right cerebrum with loss of consciousness of 30 minutes or less HAC MCC

S06.312 Contusion and laceration of right cerebrum with loss of consciousness of 31 minutes to 59 minutes HAC MCC

S06.313 Contusion and laceration of right cerebrum with loss of consciousness of 1 hour to 5 hours 59 minutes HAC MCC

S06.314 Contusion and laceration of right cerebrum with loss of consciousness of 6 hours to 24 hours HAC MCC

S06.315 Contusion and laceration of right cerebrum with loss of consciousness greater than 24 hours with return to pre-existing conscious level HAC MCC

S06.316 Contusion and laceration of right cerebrum with loss of consciousness greater than 24 hours without return to pre-existing conscious level with patient surviving HAC MCC

S06.317 Contusion and laceration of right cerebrum with loss of consciousness of any duration with death due to brain injury prior to regaining consciousness HAC MCC

S06.318 Contusion and laceration of right cerebrum with loss of consciousness of any duration with death due to other cause prior to regaining consciousness HAC MCC

S06.319 Contusion and laceration of right cerebrum with loss of consciousness of unspecified duration HAC MCC

Contusion and laceration of right cerebrum NOS

S06.32 Contusion and laceration of left cerebrum

S06.320 Contusion and laceration of left cerebrum without loss of consciousness HAC MCC

S06.321 Contusion and laceration of left cerebrum with loss of consciousness of 30 minutes or less HAC MCC

S06.322 Contusion and laceration of left cerebrum with loss of consciousness of 31 minutes to 59 minutes HAC MCC

S06.323 Contusion and laceration of left cerebrum with loss of consciousness of 1 hour to 5 hours 59 minutes HAC MCC

S06.324 Contusion and laceration of left cerebrum with loss of consciousness of 6 hours to 24 hours HAC MCC

S06.325 Contusion and laceration of left cerebrum with loss of consciousness greater than 24 hours with return to pre-existing conscious level HAC MCC

S06.326 Contusion and laceration of left cerebrum with loss of consciousness greater than 24 hours without return to pre-existing conscious level with patient surviving HAC MCC

S06.327 Contusion and laceration of left cerebrum with loss of consciousness of any duration with death due to brain injury prior to regaining consciousness HAC MCC

S06.328 Contusion and laceration of left cerebrum with loss of consciousness of any duration with death due to other cause prior to regaining consciousness HAC MCC

S06.329 Contusion and laceration of left cerebrum with loss of consciousness of unspecified duration HAC MCC

Contusion and laceration of left cerebrum NOS

S06.33 Contusion and laceration of cerebrum, unspecified

S06.330 Contusion and laceration of cerebrum, unspecified, without loss of consciousness HAC MCC

S06.331 Contusion and laceration of cerebrum, unspecified, with loss of consciousness of 30 minutes or less HAC MCC

S06.332 Contusion and laceration of cerebrum, unspecified, with loss of consciousness of 31 minutes to 59 minutes HAC MCC

S06.333 Contusion and laceration of cerebrum, unspecified, with loss of consciousness of 1 hour to 5 hours 59 minutes HAC MCC

S06.334 Contusion and laceration of cerebrum, unspecified, with loss of consciousness of 6 hours to 24 hours HAC MCC

S06.335 Contusion and laceration of cerebrum, unspecified, with loss of consciousness greater than 24 hours with return to pre-existing conscious level HAC MCC

S06.336 Contusion and laceration of cerebrum, unspecified, with loss of consciousness greater than 24 hours without return to pre-existing conscious level with patient surviving HAC MCC

S06.337 Contusion and laceration of cerebrum, unspecified, with loss of consciousness of any duration with death due to brain injury prior to regaining consciousness HAC MCC

S06.338 Contusion and laceration of cerebrum, unspecified, with loss of consciousness of any duration with death due to other cause prior to regaining consciousness HAC MCC

S06.339 Contusion and laceration of cerebrum, unspecified, with loss of consciousness of unspecified duration HAC MCC

Contusion and laceration of cerebrum NOS

S06.34 Traumatic hemorrhage of right cerebrum

Traumatic intracerebral hemorrhage and hematoma of right cerebrum

S06.340 Traumatic hemorrhage of right cerebrum without loss of consciousness HAC MCC

AHA: Q1, 2015

S06.341 Traumatic hemorrhage of right cerebrum with loss of consciousness of 30 minutes or less HAC MCC

S06.342 Traumatic hemorrhage of right cerebrum with loss of consciousness of 31 minutes to 59 minutes HAC MCC

S06.343 Traumatic hemorrhage of right cerebrum with loss of consciousness of 1 hours to 5 hours 59 minutes HAC MCC

S06.344 Traumatic hemorrhage of right cerebrum with loss of consciousness of 6 hours to 24 hours HAC MCC

S06.345 Traumatic hemorrhage of right cerebrum with loss of consciousness greater than 24 hours with return to pre-existing conscious level HAC MCC

S06.346 Traumatic hemorrhage of right cerebrum with loss of consciousness greater than 24 hours without return to pre-existing conscious level with patient surviving HAC MCC

S06.347 Traumatic hemorrhage of right cerebrum with loss of consciousness of any duration

Unacceptable principal diagnosis symbol per Medicare code edits; Code exempt from diagnosis present on admission requirement; Questionable admission; Complication or comorbidity; CC/MCC exclusion; Major complication or comorbidity; Principal diagnosis as its own CC; Principal diagnosis as its own MCC; Z code as first-listed diagnosis

When symbols appear on a code that requires a 7th character extension, refer to Appendix D to identify applicable 7th character codes.

with death due to brain injury prior to regaining consciousness HAC MCC

S06.348 Traumatic hemorrhage of right cerebrum with loss of consciousness of any duration with death due to other cause prior to regaining consciousness HAC MCC

S06.349 Traumatic hemorrhage of right cerebrum with loss of consciousness of unspecified duration HAC MCC
Traumatic hemorrhage of right cerebrum NOS

S06.35 Traumatic hemorrhage of left cerebrum
Traumatic intracerebral hemorrhage and hematoma of left cerebrum

S06.350 Traumatic hemorrhage of left cerebrum without loss of consciousness HAC MCC

S06.351 Traumatic hemorrhage of left cerebrum with loss of consciousness of 30 minutes or less HAC MCC

S06.352 Traumatic hemorrhage of left cerebrum with loss of consciousness of 31 minutes to 59 minutes HAC MCC

S06.353 Traumatic hemorrhage of left cerebrum with loss of consciousness of 1 hours to 5 hours 59 minutes HAC MCC

S06.354 Traumatic hemorrhage of left cerebrum with loss of consciousness of 6 hours to 24 hours HAC MCC

S06.355 Traumatic hemorrhage of left cerebrum with loss of consciousness greater than 24 hours with return to pre-existing conscious level HAC MCC

S06.356 Traumatic hemorrhage of left cerebrum with loss of consciousness greater than 24 hours without return to pre-existing conscious level with patient surviving HAC MCC

S06.357 Traumatic hemorrhage of left cerebrum with loss of consciousness of any duration with death due to brain injury prior to regaining consciousness HAC MCC

S06.358 Traumatic hemorrhage of left cerebrum with loss of consciousness of any duration with death due to other cause prior to regaining consciousness HAC MCC

S06.359 Traumatic hemorrhage of left cerebrum with loss of consciousness of unspecified duration HAC MCC
Traumatic hemorrhage of left cerebrum NOS

S06.36 Traumatic hemorrhage of cerebrum, unspecified
Traumatic intracerebral hemorrhage and hematoma, unspecified

S06.360 Traumatic hemorrhage of cerebrum, unspecified, without loss of consciousness HAC MCC

S06.361 Traumatic hemorrhage of cerebrum, unspecified, with loss of consciousness of 30 minutes or less HAC MCC

S06.362 Traumatic hemorrhage of cerebrum, unspecified, with loss of consciousness of 31 minutes to 59 minutes HAC MCC

S06.363 Traumatic hemorrhage of cerebrum, unspecified, with loss of consciousness of 1 hours to 5 hours 59 minutes HAC MCC

S06.364 Traumatic hemorrhage of cerebrum, unspecified, with loss of consciousness of 6 hours to 24 hours HAC MCC

S06.365 Traumatic hemorrhage of cerebrum, unspecified, with loss of consciousness greater than 24 hours with return to pre-existing conscious level HAC MCC

S06.366 Traumatic hemorrhage of cerebrum, unspecified, with loss of consciousness greater than 24 hours without return to pre-existing conscious level with patient surviving HAC MCC

S06.367 Traumatic hemorrhage of cerebrum, unspecified, with loss of consciousness of any duration with death due to brain injury prior to regaining consciousness HAC MCC

S06.368 Traumatic hemorrhage of cerebrum, unspecified, with loss of consciousness of any duration with death due to other cause prior to regaining consciousness HAC MCC

S06.369 Traumatic hemorrhage of cerebrum, unspecified, with loss of consciousness of unspecified duration HAC MCC
Traumatic hemorrhage of cerebrum NOS

S06.37 Contusion, laceration, and hemorrhage of cerebellum

S06.370 Contusion, laceration, and hemorrhage of cerebellum without loss of consciousness HAC MCC

S06.371 Contusion, laceration, and hemorrhage of cerebellum with loss of consciousness of 30 minutes or less CC HAC

S06.372 Contusion, laceration, and hemorrhage of cerebellum with loss of consciousness of 31 minutes to 59 minutes CC HAC

S06.373 Contusion, laceration, and hemorrhage of cerebellum with loss of consciousness of 1 hour to 5 hours 59 minutes CC HAC

S06.374 Contusion, laceration, and hemorrhage of cerebellum with loss of consciousness of 6 hours to 24 hours CC HAC

S06.375 Contusion, laceration, and hemorrhage of cerebellum with loss of consciousness greater than 24 hours with return to pre-existing conscious level CC HAC

S06.376 Contusion, laceration, and hemorrhage of cerebellum with loss of consciousness greater than 24 hours without return to pre-existing conscious level with patient surviving HAC MCC

S06.377 Contusion, laceration, and hemorrhage of cerebellum with loss of consciousness of any duration with death due to brain injury prior to regaining consciousness HAC MCC

S06.378 Contusion, laceration, and hemorrhage of cerebellum with loss of consciousness of any duration with death due to other cause prior to regaining consciousness HAC MCC

S06.379 Contusion, laceration, and hemorrhage of cerebellum with loss of consciousness of unspecified duration CC HAC
Contusion, laceration, and hemorrhage of cerebellum NOS

S06.38 Contusion, laceration, and hemorrhage of brainstem

S06.380 Contusion, laceration, and hemorrhage of brainstem without loss of consciousness HAC MCC

S06.381 Contusion, laceration, and hemorrhage of brainstem with loss of consciousness of 30 minutes or less CC HAC

S06.382 Contusion, laceration, and hemorrhage of brainstem with loss of consciousness of 31 minutes to 59 minutes CC HAC

S06.383 Contusion, laceration, and hemorrhage of brainstem with loss of consciousness of 1 hour to 5 hours 59 minutes CC HAC

S06.384 Contusion, laceration, and hemorrhage of brainstem with loss of consciousness of 6 hours to 24 hours CC HAC

S06.385 Contusion, laceration, and hemorrhage of brainstem with loss of consciousness greater than 24 hours with return to pre-existing conscious level CC HAC

S06.386 Contusion, laceration, and hemorrhage of brainstem with loss of consciousness greater than 24 hours without return to

Unspecified Code Other Specified Code Manifestation Code N Newborn P Pediatric M Maternity A Adult ♂ Male ♀ Female
● New Code ▲ Revised Code Title ►◄ Revised Text NOTES INCLUDES EXCLUDES1 Not coded here EXCLUDES2 Not included here
4th character required 5th character required 6th character required 7th character required
Extension 'X' Alert HAC Hospital-acquired condition (HAC) alert AHA AHA Coding Clinic®

pre-existing conscious level with patient surviving HAC MCC

S06.387 Contusion, laceration, and hemorrhage of brainstem with loss of consciousness of any duration with death due to brain injury prior to regaining consciousness HAC MCC

S06.388 Contusion, laceration, and hemorrhage of brainstem with loss of consciousness of any duration with death due to other cause prior to regaining consciousness HAC MCC

S06.389 Contusion, laceration, and hemorrhage of brainstem with loss of consciousness of unspecified duration CC HAC

Contusion, laceration, and hemorrhage of brainstem NOS

S06.4 Epidural hemorrhage

Extradural hemorrhage NOS

Extradural hemorrhage (traumatic)

S06.4X Epidural hemorrhage

S06.4X0 Epidural hemorrhage without loss of consciousness HAC MCC

S06.4X1 Epidural hemorrhage with loss of consciousness of 30 minutes or less HAC MCC

S06.4X2 Epidural hemorrhage with loss of consciousness of 31 minutes to 59 minutes HAC MCC

S06.4X3 Epidural hemorrhage with loss of consciousness of 1 hour to 5 hours 59 minutes HAC MCC

S06.4X4 Epidural hemorrhage with loss of consciousness of 6 hours to 24 hours HAC MCC

S06.4X5 Epidural hemorrhage with loss of consciousness greater than 24 hours with return to pre-existing conscious level HAC MCC

S06.4X6 Epidural hemorrhage with loss of consciousness greater than 24 hours without return to pre-existing conscious level with patient surviving HAC MCC

S06.4X7 Epidural hemorrhage with loss of consciousness of any duration with death due to brain injury prior to regaining consciousness HAC MCC

S06.4X8 Epidural hemorrhage with loss of consciousness of any duration with death due to other causes prior to regaining consciousness HAC MCC

S06.4X9 Epidural hemorrhage with loss of consciousness of unspecified duration HAC MCC

Epidural hemorrhage NOS

S06.5 Traumatic subdural hemorrhage

S06.5X Traumatic subdural hemorrhage

S06.5X0 Traumatic subdural hemorrhage without loss of consciousness HAC MCC

AHA: Q3, 2015

S06.5X1 Traumatic subdural hemorrhage with loss of consciousness of 30 minutes or less HAC MCC

S06.5X2 Traumatic subdural hemorrhage with loss of consciousness of 31 minutes to 59 minutes HAC MCC

S06.5X3 Traumatic subdural hemorrhage with loss of consciousness of 1 hour to 5 hours 59 minutes HAC MCC

S06.5X4 Traumatic subdural hemorrhage with loss of consciousness of 6 hours to 24 hours HAC MCC

S06.5X5 Traumatic subdural hemorrhage with loss of consciousness greater than 24 hours with return to pre-existing conscious level HAC MCC

S06.5X6 Traumatic subdural hemorrhage with loss of consciousness greater than 24 hours without return to pre-existing conscious level with patient surviving HAC MCC

S06.5X7 Traumatic subdural hemorrhage with loss of consciousness of any duration with death due to brain injury before regaining consciousness HAC MCC

S06.5X8 Traumatic subdural hemorrhage with loss of consciousness of any duration with death due to other cause before regaining consciousness HAC MCC

S06.5X9 Traumatic subdural hemorrhage with loss of consciousness of unspecified duration HAC MCC

Traumatic subdural hemorrhage NOS

S06.6 Traumatic subarachnoid hemorrhage

S06.6X Traumatic subarachnoid hemorrhage

S06.6X0 Traumatic subarachnoid hemorrhage without loss of consciousness HAC MCC

AHA: Q3, 2015

S06.6X1 Traumatic subarachnoid hemorrhage with loss of consciousness of 30 minutes or less HAC MCC

S06.6X2 Traumatic subarachnoid hemorrhage with loss of consciousness of 31 minutes to 59 minutes HAC MCC

S06.6X3 Traumatic subarachnoid hemorrhage with loss of consciousness of 1 hour to 5 hours 59 minutes HAC MCC

S06.6X4 Traumatic subarachnoid hemorrhage with loss of consciousness of 6 hours to 24 hours HAC MCC

S06.6X5 Traumatic subarachnoid hemorrhage with loss of consciousness greater than 24 hours with return to pre-existing conscious level HAC MCC

S06.6X6 Traumatic subarachnoid hemorrhage with loss of consciousness greater than 24 hours without return to pre-existing conscious level with patient surviving HAC MCC

S06.6X7 Traumatic subarachnoid hemorrhage with loss of consciousness of any duration with death due to brain injury prior to regaining consciousness HAC MCC

S06.6X8 Traumatic subarachnoid hemorrhage with loss of consciousness of any duration with death due to other cause prior to regaining consciousness HAC MCC

S06.6X9 Traumatic subarachnoid hemorrhage with loss of consciousness of unspecified duration HAC MCC

Traumatic subarachnoid hemorrhage NOS

S06.8 Other specified intracranial injuries

S06.81 Injury of right internal carotid artery, intracranial portion, not elsewhere classified

S06.810 Injury of right internal carotid artery, intracranial portion, not elsewhere classified without loss of consciousness

S06.811 Injury of right internal carotid artery, intracranial portion, not elsewhere classified with loss of consciousness of 30 minutes or less CC HAC

S06.812 Injury of right internal carotid artery, intracranial portion, not elsewhere classified with loss of consciousness of 31 minutes to 59 minutes CC HAC

S06.813 Injury of right internal carotid artery, intracranial portion, not elsewhere classified with loss of consciousness of 1 hour to 5 hours 59 minutes CC HAC

S06.814 Injury of right internal carotid artery, intracranial portion, not elsewhere classified with loss of consciousness of 6 hours to 24 hours CC HAC

S06.815 Injury of right internal carotid artery, intracranial portion, not elsewhere classified with loss of consciousness

PDx Unacceptable principal diagnosis symbol per Medicare code edits · POA Code exempt from diagnosis present on admission requirement · Q Questionable admission · CC Complication or comorbidity · CC/MCC Excl CC/MCC exclusion · MCC Major complication or comorbidity · PDx CC Principal diagnosis as its own CC · PDx MCC Principal diagnosis as its own MCC · Z1 Z code as first-listed diagnosis

greater than 24 hours with return to pre-existing conscious level CC HAC

S06.816 Injury of right internal carotid artery, intracranial portion, not elsewhere classified with loss of consciousness greater than 24 hours without return to pre-existing conscious level with patient surviving HAC MCC

S06.817 Injury of right internal carotid artery, intracranial portion, not elsewhere classified with loss of consciousness of any duration with death due to brain injury prior to regaining consciousness HAC MCC

S06.818 Injury of right internal carotid artery, intracranial portion, not elsewhere classified with loss of consciousness of any duration with death due to other cause prior to regaining consciousness HAC MCC

S06.819 Injury of right internal carotid artery, intracranial portion, not elsewhere classified with loss of consciousness of unspecified duration CC HAC

Injury of right internal carotid artery, intracranial portion, not elsewhere classified NOS

S06.82 Injury of left internal carotid artery, intracranial portion, not elsewhere classified

S06.820 Injury of left internal carotid artery, intracranial portion, not elsewhere classified without loss of consciousness

S06.821 Injury of left internal carotid artery, intracranial portion, not elsewhere classified with loss of consciousness of 30 minutes or less CC HAC

S06.822 Injury of left internal carotid artery, intracranial portion, not elsewhere classified with loss of consciousness of 31 minutes to 59 minutes CC HAC

S06.823 Injury of left internal carotid artery, intracranial portion, not elsewhere classified with loss of consciousness of 1 hour to 5 hours 59 minutes CC HAC

S06.824 Injury of left internal carotid artery, intracranial portion, not elsewhere classified with loss of consciousness of 6 hours to 24 hours CC HAC

S06.825 Injury of left internal carotid artery, intracranial portion, not elsewhere classified with loss of consciousness greater than 24 hours with return to pre-existing conscious level CC HAC

S06.826 Injury of left internal carotid artery, intracranial portion, not elsewhere classified with loss of consciousness greater than 24 hours without return to pre-existing conscious level with patient surviving HAC MCC

S06.827 Injury of left internal carotid artery, intracranial portion, not elsewhere classified with loss of consciousness of any duration with death due to brain injury prior to regaining consciousness HAC MCC

S06.828 Injury of left internal carotid artery, intracranial portion, not elsewhere classified with loss of consciousness of any duration with death due to other cause prior to regaining consciousness HAC MCC

S06.829 Injury of left internal carotid artery, intracranial portion, not elsewhere classified with loss of consciousness of unspecified duration CC HAC

Injury of left internal carotid artery, intracranial portion, not elsewhere classified NOS

S06.89 Other specified intracranial injury

EXCLUDES1 *concussion (S06.0X-)*

S06.890 Other specified intracranial injury without loss of consciousness

S06.891 Other specified intracranial injury with loss of consciousness of 30 minutes or less CC HAC

S06.892 Other specified intracranial injury with loss of consciousness of 31 minutes to 59 minutes CC HAC

S06.893 Other specified intracranial injury with loss of consciousness of 1 hour to 5 hours 59 minutes CC HAC

S06.894 Other specified intracranial injury with loss of consciousness of 6 hours to 24 hours CC HAC

S06.895 Other specified intracranial injury with loss of consciousness greater than 24 hours with return to pre-existing conscious level CC HAC

S06.896 Other specified intracranial injury with loss of consciousness greater than 24 hours without return to pre-existing conscious level with patient surviving HAC MCC

S06.897 Other specified intracranial injury with loss of consciousness of any duration with death due to brain injury prior to regaining consciousness HAC MCC

S06.898 Other specified intracranial injury with loss of consciousness of any duration with death due to other cause prior to regaining consciousness HAC MCC

S06.899 Other specified intracranial injury with loss of consciousness of unspecified duration CC HAC

S06.9 Unspecified intracranial injury

Brain injury NOS
Head injury NOS with loss of consciousness
Traumatic brain injury NOS

EXCLUDES1 *conditions classifiable to S06.0- to S06.8-code to specified intracranial injury*
head injury NOS (S09.90)

S06.9X Unspecified intracranial injury

S06.9X0 Unspecified intracranial injury without loss of consciousness

S06.9X1 Unspecified intracranial injury with loss of consciousness of 30 minutes or less CC HAC

S06.9X2 Unspecified intracranial injury with loss of consciousness of 31 minutes to 59 minutes CC HAC

S06.9X3 Unspecified intracranial injury with loss of consciousness of 1 hour to 5 hours 59 minutes CC HAC

S06.9X4 Unspecified intracranial injury with loss of consciousness of 6 hours to 24 hours CC HAC

S06.9X5 Unspecified intracranial injury with loss of consciousness greater than 24 hours with return to pre-existing conscious level CC HAC

S06.9X6 Unspecified intracranial injury with loss of consciousness greater than 24 hours without return to pre-existing conscious level with patient surviving HAC MCC

S06.9X7 Unspecified intracranial injury with loss of consciousness of any duration with death due to brain injury prior to regaining consciousness HAC MCC

S06.9X8 Unspecified intracranial injury with loss of consciousness of any duration with death due to other cause prior to regaining consciousness HAC MCC

S06.9X9 Unspecified intracranial injury with loss of consciousness of unspecified duration CC HAC

S07 Crushing injury of head

Use additional code for all associated injuries, such as:

intracranial injuries (S06.-)
skull fractures (S02.-)

The appropriate 7th character is to be added to each code from category S07
A = initial encounter
D = subsequent encounter
S = sequela

S07.0 Crushing injury of face
S07.1 Crushing injury of skull
S07.8 Crushing injury of other parts of head
S07.9 Crushing injury of head, part unspecified

S08 Avulsion and traumatic amputation of part of head
An amputation not identified as partial or complete should be coded to complete

The appropriate 7th character is to be added to each code from category S08
A = initial encounter
D = subsequent encounter
S = sequela

S08.0 Avulsion of scalp
S08.1 Traumatic amputation of ear
S08.11 Complete traumatic amputation of ear
S08.111 Complete traumatic amputation of right ear
S08.112 Complete traumatic amputation of left ear
S08.119 Complete traumatic amputation of unspecified ear
S08.12 Partial traumatic amputation of ear
S08.121 Partial traumatic amputation of right ear
S08.122 Partial traumatic amputation of left ear
S08.129 Partial traumatic amputation of unspecified ear
S08.8 Traumatic amputation of other parts of head
S08.81 Traumatic amputation of nose
S08.811 Complete traumatic amputation of nose
S08.812 Partial traumatic amputation of nose
S08.89 Traumatic amputation of other parts of head

S09 Other and unspecified injuries of head

The appropriate 7th character is to be added to each code from category S09
A = initial encounter
D = subsequent encounter
S = sequela

S09.0 Injury of blood vessels of head, not elsewhere classified
EXCLUDES1 *injury of cerebral blood vessels (S06.-)*
injury of precerebral blood vessels (S15.-)
S09.1 Injury of muscle and tendon of head
Code also any associated open wound (S01.-)
EXCLUDES2 *sprain to joints and ligament of head (S03.9)*
S09.10 Unspecified injury of muscle and tendon of head
Injury of muscle and tendon of head NOS
S09.11 Strain of muscle and tendon of head
S09.12 Laceration of muscle and tendon of head
S09.19 Other specified injury of muscle and tendon of head
S09.2 Traumatic rupture of ear drum
EXCLUDES1 *traumatic rupture of ear drum due to blast injury (S09.31-)*
S09.20 Traumatic rupture of unspecified ear drum
S09.21 Traumatic rupture of right ear drum
S09.22 Traumatic rupture of left ear drum
S09.3 Other specified and unspecified injury of middle and inner ear
EXCLUDES1 *injury to ear NOS (S09.91-)*
EXCLUDES2 *injury to external ear (S00.4-, S01.3-, S08.1-)*
S09.30 Unspecified injury of middle and inner ear
S09.301 Unspecified injury of right middle and inner ear
S09.302 Unspecified injury of left middle and inner ear
S09.309 Unspecified injury of unspecified middle and inner ear
S09.31 Primary blast injury of ear
Blast injury of ear NOS
S09.311 Primary blast injury of right ear
S09.312 Primary blast injury of left ear
S09.313 Primary blast injury of ear, bilateral
S09.319 Primary blast injury of unspecified ear
S09.39 Other specified injury of middle and inner ear
Secondary blast injury to ear
S09.391 Other specified injury of right middle and inner ear
S09.392 Other specified injury of left middle and inner ear
S09.399 Other specified injury of unspecified middle and inner ear
S09.8 Other specified injuries of head
S09.9 Unspecified injury of face and head
S09.90 Unspecified injury of head
Head injury NOS
EXCLUDES1 *brain injury NOS (S06.9-)*
head injury NOS with loss of consciousness (S06.9-)
intracranial injury NOS (S06.9-)
S09.91 Unspecified injury of ear
Injury of ear NOS
S09.92 Unspecified injury of nose
Injury of nose NOS
S09.93 Unspecified injury of face
Injury of face NOS

Injuries to the neck (S10-S19)

INCLUDES *injuries of nape*
injuries of supraclavicular region
injuries of throat
EXCLUDES2 *burns and corrosions (T20-T32)*
effects of foreign body in esophagus (T18.1)
effects of foreign body in larynx (T17.3)
effects of foreign body in pharynx (T17.2)
effects of foreign body in trachea (T17.4)
frostbite (T33-T34)
insect bite or sting, venomous (T63.4)

S10 Superficial injury of neck

The appropriate 7th character is to be added to each code from category S10
A = initial encounter
D = subsequent encounter
S = sequela

S10.0 Contusion of throat
Contusion of cervical esophagus
Contusion of larynx
Contusion of pharynx
Contusion of trachea
S10.1 Other and unspecified superficial injuries of throat
S10.10 Unspecified superficial injuries of throat
S10.11 Abrasion of throat
S10.12 Blister (nonthermal) of throat
S10.14 External constriction of part of throat
S10.15 Superficial foreign body of throat
Splinter in the throat
S10.16 Insect bite (nonvenomous) of throat
S10.17 Other superficial bite of throat
EXCLUDES1 *open bite of throat (S11.85)*
S10.8 Superficial injury of other specified parts of neck
S10.80 Unspecified superficial injury of other specified part of neck
S10.81 Abrasion of other specified part of neck
S10.82 Blister (nonthermal) of other specified part of neck
S10.83 Contusion of other specified part of neck
S10.84 External constriction of other specified part of neck
S10.85 Superficial foreign body of other specified part of neck
Splinter in other specified part of neck
S10.86 Insect bite of other specified part of neck
S10.87 Other superficial bite of other specified part of neck

Unacceptable principal diagnosis symbol per Medicare code edits · Code exempt from diagnosis present on admission requirement
Questionable admission · Complication or comorbidity · CC/MCC exclusion · Major complication or comorbidity
Principal diagnosis as its own CC · Principal diagnosis as its own MCC · Z code as first-listed diagnosis

EXCLUDES1 *open bite of other specified parts of neck (S11.85)*

S10.9 Superficial injury of unspecified part of neck
- S10.90 Unspecified superficial injury of unspecified part of neck
- S10.91 Abrasion of unspecified part of neck
- S10.92 Blister (nonthermal) of unspecified part of neck
- S10.93 Contusion of unspecified part of neck
- S10.94 External constriction of unspecified part of neck
- S10.95 Superficial foreign body of unspecified part of neck
- S10.96 Insect bite of unspecified part of neck
- S10.97 Other superficial bite of unspecified part of neck

S11 Open wound of neck

Code also any associated:
- spinal cord injury (S14.0, S14.1-)
- wound infection

EXCLUDES2 *open fracture of vertebra (S12.- with 7th character B)*

The appropriate 7th character is to be added to each code from category S11
- A = initial encounter
- D = subsequent encounter
- S = sequela

S11.0 Open wound of larynx and trachea
- S11.01 Open wound of larynx
  - EXCLUDES2 *open wound of vocal cord (S11.03)*
  - S11.011 Laceration without foreign body of larynx MCC
  - S11.012 Laceration with foreign body of larynx MCC
  - S11.013 Puncture wound without foreign body of larynx MCC
  - S11.014 Puncture wound with foreign body of larynx MCC
  - S11.015 Open bite of larynx MCC
    - Bite of larynx NOS
  - S11.019 Unspecified open wound of larynx MCC
- S11.02 Open wound of trachea
  - Open wound of cervical trachea
  - Open wound of trachea NOS
  - EXCLUDES2 *open wound of thoracic trachea (S27.5-)*
  - S11.021 Laceration without foreign body of trachea MCC
  - S11.022 Laceration with foreign body of trachea MCC
  - S11.023 Puncture wound without foreign body of trachea MCC
  - S11.024 Puncture wound with foreign body of trachea MCC
  - S11.025 Open bite of trachea MCC
    - Bite of trachea NOS
  - S11.029 Unspecified open wound of trachea MCC
- S11.03 Open wound of vocal cord
  - S11.031 Laceration without foreign body of vocal cord MCC
  - S11.032 Laceration with foreign body of vocal cord MCC
  - S11.033 Puncture wound without foreign body of vocal cord MCC
  - S11.034 Puncture wound with foreign body of vocal cord MCC
  - S11.035 Open bite of vocal cord MCC
    - Bite of vocal cord NOS
  - S11.039 Unspecified open wound of vocal cord MCC

S11.1 Open wound of thyroid gland
- S11.10 Unspecified open wound of thyroid gland CC
- S11.11 Laceration without foreign body of thyroid gland CC
- S11.12 Laceration with foreign body of thyroid gland CC
- S11.13 Puncture wound without foreign body of thyroid gland CC
- S11.14 Puncture wound with foreign body of thyroid gland CC
- S11.15 Open bite of thyroid gland CC
  - Bite of thyroid gland NOS

S11.2 Open wound of pharynx and cervical esophagus

EXCLUDES1 *open wound of esophagus NOS (S27.8-)*
- S11.20 Unspecified open wound of pharynx and cervical esophagus CC
- S11.21 Laceration without foreign body of pharynx and cervical esophagus CC
- S11.22 Laceration with foreign body of pharynx and cervical esophagus CC
- S11.23 Puncture wound without foreign body of pharynx and cervical esophagus CC
- S11.24 Puncture wound with foreign body of pharynx and cervical esophagus CC
- S11.25 Open bite of pharynx and cervical esophagus CC
  - Bite of pharynx and cervical esophagus NOS

S11.8 Open wound of other specified parts of neck
- S11.80 Unspecified open wound of other specified part of neck
- S11.81 Laceration without foreign body of other specified part of neck
- S11.82 Laceration with foreign body of other specified part of neck
- S11.83 Puncture wound without foreign body of other specified part of neck
- S11.84 Puncture wound with foreign body of other specified part of neck
- S11.85 Open bite of other specified part of neck
  - Bite of other specified part of neck NOS
  - EXCLUDES1 *superficial bite of other specified part of neck (S10.87)*
- S11.89 Other open wound of other specified part of neck

S11.9 Open wound of unspecified part of neck
- S11.90 Unspecified open wound of unspecified part of neck
- S11.91 Laceration without foreign body of unspecified part of neck
- S11.92 Laceration with foreign body of unspecified part of neck
- S11.93 Puncture wound without foreign body of unspecified part of neck
- S11.94 Puncture wound with foreign body of unspecified part of neck
- S11.95 Open bite of unspecified part of neck
  - Bite of neck NOS
  - EXCLUDES1 *superficial bite of neck (S10.97)*

S12 Fracture of cervical vertebra and other parts of neck

NOTES A fracture not indicated as displaced or nondisplaced should be coded to displaced

A fracture not indicated as open or closed should be coded to closed

INCLUDES *fracture of cervical neural arch*
fracture of cervical spine
fracture of cervical spinous process
fracture of cervical transverse process
fracture of cervical vertebral arch
fracture of neck

Code first any associated cervical spinal cord injury (S14.0, S14.1-)

The appropriate 7th character is to be added to all codes from subcategories S12.0-S12.6
- A = initial encounter for closed fracture
- B = initial encounter for open fracture
- D = subsequent encounter for fracture with routine healing
- G = subsequent encounter for fracture with delayed healing
- K = subsequent encounter for fracture with nonunion
- S = sequela

S12.0 Fracture of first cervical vertebra

Atlas
- S12.00 Unspecified fracture of first cervical vertebra
  - S12.000 Unspecified displaced fracture of first cervical vertebra CC HAC MCC
  - S12.001 Unspecified nondisplaced fracture of first cervical vertebra CC HAC MCC
- S12.01 Stable burst fracture of first cervical vertebra CC HAC MCC
- S12.02 Unstable burst fracture of first cervical vertebra CC HAC MCC
- S12.03 Posterior arch fracture of first cervical vertebra
  - S12.030 Displaced posterior arch fracture of first cervical vertebra CC HAC MCC

Unspecified Code | Other Specified Code | Manifestation Code | N Newborn | P Pediatric | M Maternity | A Adult | ♂ Male | ♀ Female
● New Code | ▲ Revised Code Title | ►◄ Revised Text | NOTES | INCLUDES | EXCLUDES1 Not coded here | EXCLUDES2 Not included here
4th character required | 5th character required | 6th character required | 7th character required
Extension 'X' Alert | HAC Hospital-acquired condition (HAC) alert | AHA AHA Coding Clinic©

When symbols appear on a code that requires a 7th character extension, refer to Appendix D to identify applicable 7th character codes.

S12.031 Nondisplaced posterior arch fracture of first cervical vertebra CC HAC MCC
S12.04 Lateral mass fracture of first cervical vertebra
S12.040 Displaced lateral mass fracture of first cervical vertebra CC HAC MCC
S12.041 Nondisplaced lateral mass fracture of first cervical vertebra CC HAC MCC
S12.09 Other fracture of first cervical vertebra
S12.090 Other displaced fracture of first cervical vertebra CC HAC MCC
S12.091 Other nondisplaced fracture of first cervical vertebra CC HAC MCC
S12.1 Fracture of second cervical vertebra
Axis
S12.10 Unspecified fracture of second cervical vertebra
S12.100 Unspecified displaced fracture of second cervical vertebra CC HAC MCC
S12.101 Unspecified nondisplaced fracture of second cervical vertebra CC HAC MCC
S12.11 Type II dens fracture
S12.110 Anterior displaced Type II dens fracture CC HAC MCC
S12.111 Posterior displaced Type II dens fracture CC HAC MCC
S12.112 Nondisplaced Type II dens fracture CC HAC MCC
S12.12 Other dens fracture
S12.120 Other displaced dens fracture CC HAC MCC
S12.121 Other nondisplaced dens fracture CC HAC MCC
S12.13 Unspecified traumatic spondylolisthesis of second cervical vertebra
S12.130 Unspecified traumatic displaced spondylolisthesis of second cervical vertebra CC HAC MCC
S12.131 Unspecified traumatic nondisplaced spondylolisthesis of second cervical vertebra CC HAC MCC
S12.14 Type III traumatic spondylolisthesis of second cervical vertebra CC HAC MCC
S12.15 Other traumatic spondylolisthesis of second cervical vertebra
S12.150 Other traumatic displaced spondylolisthesis of second cervical vertebra CC HAC MCC
S12.151 Other traumatic nondisplaced spondylolisthesis of second cervical vertebra CC HAC MCC
S12.19 Other fracture of second cervical vertebra
S12.190 Other displaced fracture of second cervical vertebra CC HAC MCC
S12.191 Other nondisplaced fracture of second cervical vertebra CC HAC MCC
S12.2 Fracture of third cervical vertebra
S12.20 Unspecified fracture of third cervical vertebra
S12.200 Unspecified displaced fracture of third cervical vertebra CC HAC MCC
S12.201 Unspecified nondisplaced fracture of third cervical vertebra CC HAC MCC
S12.23 Unspecified traumatic spondylolisthesis of third cervical vertebra
S12.230 Unspecified traumatic displaced spondylolisthesis of third cervical vertebra CC HAC MCC
S12.231 Unspecified traumatic nondisplaced spondylolisthesis of third cervical vertebra CC HAC MCC
S12.24 Type III traumatic spondylolisthesis of third cervical vertebra CC HAC MCC
S12.25 Other traumatic spondylolisthesis of third cervical vertebra
S12.250 Other traumatic displaced spondylolisthesis of third cervical vertebra CC HAC MCC
S12.251 Other traumatic nondisplaced spondylolisthesis of third cervical vertebra CC HAC MCC
S12.29 Other fracture of third cervical vertebra
S12.290 Other displaced fracture of third cervical vertebra CC HAC MCC
S12.291 Other nondisplaced fracture of third cervical vertebra CC HAC MCC
S12.3 Fracture of fourth cervical vertebra
S12.30 Unspecified fracture of fourth cervical vertebra
S12.300 Unspecified displaced fracture of fourth cervical vertebra CC HAC MCC
S12.301 Unspecified nondisplaced fracture of fourth cervical vertebra CC HAC MCC
S12.33 Unspecified traumatic spondylolisthesis of fourth cervical vertebra
S12.330 Unspecified traumatic displaced spondylolisthesis of fourth cervical vertebra CC HAC MCC
S12.331 Unspecified traumatic nondisplaced spondylolisthesis of fourth cervical vertebra CC HAC MCC
S12.34 Type III traumatic spondylolisthesis of fourth cervical vertebra CC HAC MCC
S12.35 Other traumatic spondylolisthesis of fourth cervical vertebra
S12.350 Other traumatic displaced spondylolisthesis of fourth cervical vertebra CC HAC MCC
S12.351 Other traumatic nondisplaced spondylolisthesis of fourth cervical vertebra CC HAC MCC
S12.39 Other fracture of fourth cervical vertebra
S12.390 Other displaced fracture of fourth cervical vertebra CC HAC MCC
S12.391 Other nondisplaced fracture of fourth cervical vertebra CC HAC MCC
S12.4 Fracture of fifth cervical vertebra
S12.40 Unspecified fracture of fifth cervical vertebra
S12.400 Unspecified displaced fracture of fifth cervical vertebra CC HAC MCC
S12.401 Unspecified nondisplaced fracture of fifth cervical vertebra CC HAC MCC
S12.43 Unspecified traumatic spondylolisthesis of fifth cervical vertebra
S12.430 Unspecified traumatic displaced spondylolisthesis of fifth cervical vertebra CC HAC MCC
S12.431 Unspecified traumatic nondisplaced spondylolisthesis of fifth cervical vertebra CC HAC MCC
S12.44 Type III traumatic spondylolisthesis of fifth cervical vertebra CC HAC MCC
S12.45 Other traumatic spondylolisthesis of fifth cervical vertebra
S12.450 Other traumatic displaced spondylolisthesis of fifth cervical vertebra CC HAC MCC
S12.451 Other traumatic nondisplaced spondylolisthesis of fifth cervical vertebra CC HAC MCC
S12.49 Other fracture of fifth cervical vertebra
S12.490 Other displaced fracture of fifth cervical vertebra CC HAC MCC
S12.491 Other nondisplaced fracture of fifth cervical vertebra CC HAC MCC
S12.5 Fracture of sixth cervical vertebra
S12.50 Unspecified fracture of sixth cervical vertebra
S12.500 Unspecified displaced fracture of sixth cervical vertebra CC HAC MCC
S12.501 Unspecified nondisplaced fracture of sixth cervical vertebra CC HAC MCC
S12.53 Unspecified traumatic spondylolisthesis of sixth cervical vertebra

PDx Unacceptable principal diagnosis symbol per Medicare code edits; POA Code exempt from diagnosis present on admission requirement
? Questionable admission; CC Complication or comorbidity; CC/MCC Exc CC/MCC exclusion; MCC Major complication or comorbidity
PDx CC Principal diagnosis as its own CC; PDx MCC Principal diagnosis as its own MCC; Z1 Z code as first-listed diagnosis

S12.530 Unspecified traumatic displaced spondylolisthesis of sixth cervical vertebra CC HAC MCC
S12.531 Unspecified traumatic nondisplaced spondylolisthesis of sixth cervical vertebra CC HAC MCC
S12.54 Type III traumatic spondylolisthesis of sixth cervical vertebra CC HAC MCC
S12.55 Other traumatic spondylolisthesis of sixth cervical vertebra
S12.550 Other traumatic displaced spondylolisthesis of sixth cervical vertebra CC HAC MCC
S12.551 Other traumatic nondisplaced spondylolisthesis of sixth cervical vertebra CC HAC MCC
S12.59 Other fracture of sixth cervical vertebra
S12.590 Other displaced fracture of sixth cervical vertebra CC HAC MCC
S12.591 Other nondisplaced fracture of sixth cervical vertebra CC HAC MCC
S12.6 Fracture of seventh cervical vertebra
S12.60 Unspecified fracture of seventh cervical vertebra
S12.600 Unspecified displaced fracture of seventh cervical vertebra CC HAC MCC
S12.601 Unspecified nondisplaced fracture of seventh cervical vertebra CC HAC MCC
S12.63 Unspecified traumatic spondylolisthesis of seventh cervical vertebra
S12.630 Unspecified traumatic displaced spondylolisthesis of seventh cervical vertebra CC HAC MCC
S12.631 Unspecified traumatic nondisplaced spondylolisthesis of seventh cervical vertebra CC HAC MCC
S12.64 Type III traumatic spondylolisthesis of seventh cervical vertebra CC HAC MCC
S12.65 Other traumatic spondylolisthesis of seventh cervical vertebra
S12.650 Other traumatic displaced spondylolisthesis of seventh cervical vertebra CC HAC MCC
S12.651 Other traumatic nondisplaced spondylolisthesis of seventh cervical vertebra CC HAC MCC
S12.69 Other fracture of seventh cervical vertebra
S12.690 Other displaced fracture of seventh cervical vertebra CC HAC MCC
S12.691 Other nondisplaced fracture of seventh cervical vertebra CC HAC MCC
S12.8 Fracture of other parts of neck HAC MCC
Hyoid bone
Larynx
Thyroid cartilage
Trachea
The appropriate 7th character is to be added to code S12.8
A = initial encounter
D = subsequent encounter
S = sequela
S12.9 Fracture of neck, unspecified CC HAC
Fracture of neck NOS
Fracture of cervical spine NOS
Fracture of cervical vertebra NOS
The appropriate 7th character is to be added to code S12.9
A = initial encounter
D = subsequent encounter
S = sequela
S13 Dislocation and sprain of joints and ligaments at neck level
INCLUDES *avulsion of joint or ligament at neck level*
laceration of cartilage, joint or ligament at neck level
sprain of cartilage, joint or ligament at neck level
traumatic hemarthrosis of joint or ligament at neck level
traumatic rupture of joint or ligament at neck level
traumatic subluxation of joint or ligament at neck level
traumatic tear of joint or ligament at neck level
Code also any associated open wound
EXCLUDES2 *strain of muscle or tendon at neck level (S16.1)*
The appropriate 7th character is to be added to each code from category S13
A = initial encounter
D = subsequent encounter
S = sequela
S13.0 Traumatic rupture of cervical intervertebral disc CC HAC
EXCLUDES1 *rupture or displacement (nontraumatic) of cervical intervertebral disc NOS (M50.-)*
S13.1 Subluxation and dislocation of cervical vertebrae
Code also any associated:
open wound of neck (S11.-)
spinal cord injury (S14.1-)
EXCLUDES2 *fracture of cervical vertebrae (S12.0-S12.3-)*
S13.10 Subluxation and dislocation of unspecified cervical vertebrae
S13.100 Subluxation of unspecified cervical vertebrae CC HAC
S13.101 Dislocation of unspecified cervical vertebrae CC HAC
S13.11 Subluxation and dislocation of C0/C1 cervical vertebrae
Subluxation and dislocation of atlantooccipital joint
Subluxation and dislocation of atloidooccipital joint
Subluxation and dislocation of occipitoatloid joint
S13.110 Subluxation of C0/C1 cervical vertebrae CC HAC
S13.111 Dislocation of C0/C1 cervical vertebrae CC HAC
S13.12 Subluxation and dislocation of C1/C2 cervical vertebrae
Subluxation and dislocation of atlantoaxial joint
S13.120 Subluxation of C1/C2 cervical vertebrae CC HAC
S13.121 Dislocation of C1/C2 cervical vertebrae CC HAC
S13.13 Subluxation and dislocation of C2/C3 cervical vertebrae
S13.130 Subluxation of C2/C3 cervical vertebrae CC HAC
S13.131 Dislocation of C2/C3 cervical vertebrae CC HAC
S13.14 Subluxation and dislocation of C3/C4 cervical vertebrae
S13.140 Subluxation of C3/C4 cervical vertebrae CC HAC
S13.141 Dislocation of C3/C4 cervical vertebrae CC HAC
S13.15 Subluxation and dislocation of C4/C5 cervical vertebrae
S13.150 Subluxation of C4/C5 cervical vertebrae CC HAC
S13.151 Dislocation of C4/C5 cervical vertebrae CC HAC
S13.16 Subluxation and dislocation of C5/C6 cervical vertebrae
S13.160 Subluxation of C5/C6 cervical vertebrae CC HAC
S13.161 Dislocation of C5/C6 cervical vertebrae CC HAC
S13.17 Subluxation and dislocation of C6/C7 cervical vertebrae
S13.170 Subluxation of C6/C7 cervical vertebrae CC HAC
S13.171 Dislocation of C6/C7 cervical vertebrae CC HAC
S13.18 Subluxation and dislocation of C7/T1 cervical vertebrae
S13.180 Subluxation of C7/T1 cervical vertebrae CC HAC
S13.181 Dislocation of C7/T1 cervical vertebrae CC HAC
S13.2 Dislocation of other and unspecified parts of neck
S13.20 Dislocation of unspecified parts of neck CC HAC

Unspecified Code Other Specified Code Manifestation Code N Newborn P Pediatric M Maternity A Adult ♂ Male ♀ Female
● New Code ▲ Revised Code Title ►◄ Revised Text NOTES INCLUDES EXCLUDES1 Not coded here EXCLUDES2 Not included here
4th character required 5th character required 6th character required 7th character required
Extension 'X' Alert HAC Hospital-acquired condition (HAC) alert AHA AHA Coding Clinic©

S13.29 Dislocation of other parts of neck CC HAC

S13.4 Sprain of ligaments of cervical spine
- Sprain of anterior longitudinal (ligament), cervical
- Sprain of atlanto-axial (joints)
- Sprain of atlanto-occipital (joints)
- Whiplash injury of cervical spine

S13.5 Sprain of thyroid region
- Sprain of cricoarytenoid (joint) (ligament)
- Sprain of cricothyroid (joint) (ligament)
- Sprain of thyroid cartilage

S13.8 Sprain of joints and ligaments of other parts of neck

S13.9 Sprain of joints and ligaments of unspecified parts of neck

S14 Injury of nerves and spinal cord at neck level

NOTES Code to highest level of cervical cord injury

Code also any associated:
- fracture of cervical vertebra (S12.0--S12.6.-)
- open wound of neck (S11.-)
- transient paralysis (R29.5)

The appropriate 7th character is to be added to each code from category S14
- A = initial encounter
- D = subsequent encounter
- S = sequela

S14.0 Concussion and edema of cervical spinal cord MCC

S14.1 Other and unspecified injuries of cervical spinal cord

S14.10 Unspecified injury of cervical spinal cord
- S14.101 Unspecified injury at C1 level of cervical spinal cord HAC MCC
- S14.102 Unspecified injury at C2 level of cervical spinal cord HAC MCC
- S14.103 Unspecified injury at C3 level of cervical spinal cord HAC MCC
- S14.104 Unspecified injury at C4 level of cervical spinal cord HAC MCC
- S14.105 Unspecified injury at C5 level of cervical spinal cord HAC MCC
- S14.106 Unspecified injury at C6 level of cervical spinal cord HAC MCC
- S14.107 Unspecified injury at C7 level of cervical spinal cord HAC MCC
- S14.108 Unspecified injury at C8 level of cervical spinal cord MCC
- S14.109 Unspecified injury at unspecified level of cervical spinal cord HAC
  - Injury of cervical spinal cord NOS

S14.11 Complete lesion of cervical spinal cord
- S14.111 Complete lesion at C1 level of cervical spinal cord HAC MCC
- S14.112 Complete lesion at C2 level of cervical spinal cord HAC MCC
- S14.113 Complete lesion at C3 level of cervical spinal cord HAC MCC
- S14.114 Complete lesion at C4 level of cervical spinal cord HAC MCC
- S14.115 Complete lesion at C5 level of cervical spinal cord HAC MCC
- S14.116 Complete lesion at C6 level of cervical spinal cord HAC MCC
- S14.117 Complete lesion at C7 level of cervical spinal cord HAC MCC
- S14.118 Complete lesion at C8 level of cervical spinal cord MCC
- S14.119 Complete lesion at unspecified level of cervical spinal cord

S14.12 Central cord syndrome of cervical spinal cord
- S14.121 Central cord syndrome at C1 level of cervical spinal cord HAC MCC
- S14.122 Central cord syndrome at C2 level of cervical spinal cord HAC MCC
- S14.123 Central cord syndrome at C3 level of cervical spinal cord HAC MCC
- S14.124 Central cord syndrome at C4 level of cervical spinal cord HAC MCC
- S14.125 Central cord syndrome at C5 level of cervical spinal cord HAC MCC
- S14.126 Central cord syndrome at C6 level of cervical spinal cord HAC MCC
- S14.127 Central cord syndrome at C7 level of cervical spinal cord HAC MCC
- S14.128 Central cord syndrome at C8 level of cervical spinal cord MCC
- S14.129 Central cord syndrome at unspecified level of cervical spinal cord

S14.13 Anterior cord syndrome of cervical spinal cord
- S14.131 Anterior cord syndrome at C1 level of cervical spinal cord HAC MCC
- S14.132 Anterior cord syndrome at C2 level of cervical spinal cord HAC MCC
- S14.133 Anterior cord syndrome at C3 level of cervical spinal cord HAC MCC
- S14.134 Anterior cord syndrome at C4 level of cervical spinal cord HAC MCC
- S14.135 Anterior cord syndrome at C5 level of cervical spinal cord HAC MCC
- S14.136 Anterior cord syndrome at C6 level of cervical spinal cord HAC MCC
- S14.137 Anterior cord syndrome at C7 level of cervical spinal cord HAC MCC
- S14.138 Anterior cord syndrome at C8 level of cervical spinal cord MCC
- S14.139 Anterior cord syndrome at unspecified level of cervical spinal cord

S14.14 Brown-Séquard syndrome of cervical spinal cord
- S14.141 Brown-Séquard syndrome at C1 level of cervical spinal cord MCC
- S14.142 Brown-Séquard syndrome at C2 level of cervical spinal cord MCC
- S14.143 Brown-Séquard syndrome at C3 level of cervical spinal cord MCC
- S14.144 Brown-Séquard syndrome at C4 level of cervical spinal cord MCC
- S14.145 Brown-Séquard syndrome at C5 level of cervical spinal cord MCC
- S14.146 Brown-Séquard syndrome at C6 level of cervical spinal cord MCC
- S14.147 Brown-Séquard syndrome at C7 level of cervical spinal cord MCC
- S14.148 Brown-Séquard syndrome at C8 level of cervical spinal cord MCC
- S14.149 Brown-Séquard syndrome at unspecified level of cervical spinal cord

S14.15 Other incomplete lesions of cervical spinal cord
- Incomplete lesion of cervical spinal cord NOS
- Posterior cord syndrome of cervical spinal cord
- S14.151 Other incomplete lesion at C1 level of cervical spinal cord HAC MCC
- S14.152 Other incomplete lesion at C2 level of cervical spinal cord HAC MCC
- S14.153 Other incomplete lesion at C3 level of cervical spinal cord HAC MCC
- S14.154 Other incomplete lesion at C4 level of cervical spinal cord HAC MCC
- S14.155 Other incomplete lesion at C5 level of cervical spinal cord HAC MCC
- S14.156 Other incomplete lesion at C6 level of cervical spinal cord HAC MCC
- S14.157 Other incomplete lesion at C7 level of cervical spinal cord HAC MCC
- S14.158 Other incomplete lesion at C8 level of cervical spinal cord MCC
- S14.159 Other incomplete lesion at unspecified level of cervical spinal cord

S14.2 Injury of nerve root of cervical spine

S14.3 Injury of brachial plexus

S14.4 Injury of peripheral nerves of neck

S14.5 Injury of cervical sympathetic nerves

S14.8 Injury of other specified nerves of neck

S14.9 Injury of unspecified nerves of neck

S15 Injury of blood vessels at neck level

Code also any associated open wound (S11.-)

PDx Unacceptable principal diagnosis symbol per Medicare code edits · POA Code exempt from diagnosis present on admission requirement
? Questionable admission · CC Complication or comorbidity · CC/MCC Exc CC/MCC exclusion · MCC Major complication or comorbidity
PDx CC Principal diagnosis as its own CC · PDx MCC Principal diagnosis as its own MCC · Z1 Z code as first-listed diagnosis

 When symbols appear on a code that requires a 7th character extension, refer to Appendix D to identify applicable 7th character codes.

The appropriate 7th character is to be added to each code from category S15
A = initial encounter
D = subsequent encounter
S = sequela

S15.0 Injury of carotid artery of neck
Injury of carotid artery (common) (external) (internal, extracranial portion)
Injury of carotid artery NOS
EXCLUDES1 *injury of internal carotid artery, intracranial portion (S06.8)*
S15.00 Unspecified injury of carotid artery
S15.001 Unspecified injury of right carotid artery
S15.002 Unspecified injury of left carotid artery
S15.009 Unspecified injury of unspecified carotid artery
S15.01 Minor laceration of carotid artery
Incomplete transection of carotid artery
Laceration of carotid artery NOS
Superficial laceration of carotid artery
S15.011 Minor laceration of right carotid artery
S15.012 Minor laceration of left carotid artery
S15.019 Minor laceration of unspecified carotid artery
S15.02 Major laceration of carotid artery
Complete transection of carotid artery
Traumatic rupture of carotid artery
S15.021 Major laceration of right carotid artery
S15.022 Major laceration of left carotid artery
S15.029 Major laceration of unspecified carotid artery
S15.09 Other specified injury of carotid artery
S15.091 Other specified injury of right carotid artery
S15.092 Other specified injury of left carotid artery
S15.099 Other specified injury of unspecified carotid artery

S15.1 Injury of vertebral artery
S15.10 Unspecified injury of vertebral artery
S15.101 Unspecified injury of right vertebral artery
S15.102 Unspecified injury of left vertebral artery
S15.109 Unspecified injury of unspecified vertebral artery
S15.11 Minor laceration of vertebral artery
Incomplete transection of vertebral artery
Laceration of vertebral artery NOS
Superficial laceration of vertebral artery
S15.111 Minor laceration of right vertebral artery
S15.112 Minor laceration of left vertebral artery
S15.119 Minor laceration of unspecified vertebral artery
S15.12 Major laceration of vertebral artery
Complete transection of vertebral artery
Traumatic rupture of vertebral artery
S15.121 Major laceration of right vertebral artery
S15.122 Major laceration of left vertebral artery
S15.129 Major laceration of unspecified vertebral artery
S15.19 Other specified injury of vertebral artery
S15.191 Other specified injury of right vertebral artery
S15.192 Other specified injury of left vertebral artery
S15.199 Other specified injury of unspecified vertebral artery

S15.2 Injury of external jugular vein
S15.20 Unspecified injury of external jugular vein
S15.201 Unspecified injury of right external jugular vein
S15.202 Unspecified injury of left external jugular vein
S15.209 Unspecified injury of unspecified external jugular vein
S15.21 Minor laceration of external jugular vein
Incomplete transection of external jugular vein
Laceration of external jugular vein NOS
Superficial laceration of external jugular vein
S15.211 Minor laceration of right external jugular vein
S15.212 Minor laceration of left external jugular vein
S15.219 Minor laceration of unspecified external jugular vein
S15.22 Major laceration of external jugular vein
Complete transection of external jugular vein
Traumatic rupture of external jugular vein
S15.221 Major laceration of right external jugular vein
S15.222 Major laceration of left external jugular vein
S15.229 Major laceration of unspecified external jugular vein
S15.29 Other specified injury of external jugular vein
S15.291 Other specified injury of right external jugular vein
S15.292 Other specified injury of left external jugular vein
S15.299 Other specified injury of unspecified external jugular vein

S15.3 Injury of internal jugular vein
S15.30 Unspecified injury of internal jugular vein
S15.301 Unspecified injury of right internal jugular vein
S15.302 Unspecified injury of left internal jugular vein
S15.309 Unspecified injury of unspecified internal jugular vein
S15.31 Minor laceration of internal jugular vein
Incomplete transection of internal jugular vein
Laceration of internal jugular vein NOS
Superficial laceration of internal jugular vein
S15.311 Minor laceration of right internal jugular vein
S15.312 Minor laceration of left internal jugular vein
S15.319 Minor laceration of unspecified internal jugular vein
S15.32 Major laceration of internal jugular vein
Complete transection of internal jugular vein
Traumatic rupture of internal jugular vein
S15.321 Major laceration of right internal jugular vein
S15.322 Major laceration of left internal jugular vein
S15.329 Major laceration of unspecified internal jugular vein
S15.39 Other specified injury of internal jugular vein
S15.391 Other specified injury of right internal jugular vein
S15.392 Other specified injury of left internal jugular vein
S15.399 Other specified injury of unspecified internal jugular vein

S15.8 Injury of other specified blood vessels at neck level
S15.9 Injury of unspecified blood vessel at neck level

S16 Injury of muscle, fascia and tendon at neck level
Code also any associated open wound (S11.-)
EXCLUDES2 *sprain of joint or ligament at neck level (S13.9)*
The appropriate 7th character is to be added to each code from category S16
A = initial encounter
D = subsequent encounter
S = sequela
S16.1 Strain of muscle, fascia and tendon at neck level
S16.2 Laceration of muscle, fascia and tendon at neck level

Unspecified Code | Other Specified Code | Manifestation Code | N Newborn | P Pediatric | M Maternity | A Adult | ♂ Male | ♀ Female
● New Code | ▲ Revised Code Title | ►◄ Revised Text | NOTES | INCLUDES | EXCLUDES1 Not coded here | EXCLUDES2 Not included here
4th character required | 5th character required | 6th character required | 7th character required
Extension 'X' Alert | HAC Hospital-acquired condition (HAC) alert | AHA AHA Coding Clinic®

When symbols appear on a code that requires a 7th character extension, refer to Appendix D to identify applicable 7th character codes.

S16.8 Other specified injury of muscle, fascia and tendon at neck level
S16.9 Unspecified injury of muscle, fascia and tendon at neck level

S17 Crushing injury of neck
Use additional code for all associated injuries, such as:
injury of blood vessels (S15.-)
open wound of neck (S11.-)
spinal cord injury (S14.0, S14.1-)
vertebral fracture (S12.0--S12.3-)
The appropriate 7th character is to be added to each code from category S17
A = initial encounter
D = subsequent encounter
S = sequela
S17.0 Crushing injury of larynx and trachea CC HAC
S17.8 Crushing injury of other specified parts of neck CC HAC
S17.9 Crushing injury of neck, part unspecified CC HAC

S19 Other specified and unspecified injuries of neck
The appropriate 7th character is to be added to each code from category S19
A = initial encounter
D = subsequent encounter
S = sequela
S19.8 Other specified injuries of neck
S19.80 Other specified injuries of unspecified part of neck
S19.81 Other specified injuries of larynx
S19.82 Other specified injuries of cervical trachea
EXCLUDES2 *other specified injury of thoracic trachea (S27.5-)*
S19.83 Other specified injuries of vocal cord
S19.84 Other specified injuries of thyroid gland
S19.85 Other specified injuries of pharynx and cervical esophagus
S19.89 Other specified injuries of other specified part of neck
S19.9 Unspecified injury of neck

Injuries to the thorax (S20-S29)

INCLUDES *injuries of breast*
injuries of chest (wall)
injuries of interscapular area
EXCLUDES2 *burns and corrosions (T20-T32)*
effects of foreign body in bronchus (T17.5)
effects of foreign body in esophagus (T18.1)
effects of foreign body in lung (T17.8)
effects of foreign body in trachea (T17.4)
frostbite (T33-T34)
injuries of axilla
injuries of clavicle
injuries of scapular region
injuries of shoulder
insect bite or sting, venomous (T63.4)

S20 Superficial injury of thorax
The appropriate 7th character is to be added to each code from category S20
A = initial encounter
D = subsequent encounter
S = sequela
S20.0 Contusion of breast
S20.00 Contusion of breast, unspecified breast
S20.01 Contusion of right breast
S20.02 Contusion of left breast
S20.1 Other and unspecified superficial injuries of breast
S20.10 Unspecified superficial injuries of breast
S20.101 Unspecified superficial injuries of breast, right breast
S20.102 Unspecified superficial injuries of breast, left breast
S20.109 Unspecified superficial injuries of breast, unspecified breast
S20.11 Abrasion of breast
S20.111 Abrasion of breast, right breast
S20.112 Abrasion of breast, left breast
S20.119 Abrasion of breast, unspecified breast
S20.12 Blister (nonthermal) of breast
S20.121 Blister (nonthermal) of breast, right breast
S20.122 Blister (nonthermal) of breast, left breast
S20.129 Blister (nonthermal) of breast, unspecified breast
S20.14 External constriction of part of breast
S20.141 External constriction of part of breast, right breast
S20.142 External constriction of part of breast, left breast
S20.149 External constriction of part of breast, unspecified breast
S20.15 Superficial foreign body of breast
Splinter in the breast
S20.151 Superficial foreign body of breast, right breast
S20.152 Superficial foreign body of breast, left breast
S20.159 Superficial foreign body of breast, unspecified breast
S20.16 Insect bite (nonvenomous) of breast
S20.161 Insect bite (nonvenomous) of breast, right breast
S20.162 Insect bite (nonvenomous) of breast, left breast
S20.169 Insect bite (nonvenomous) of breast, unspecified breast
S20.17 Other superficial bite of breast
EXCLUDES1 *open bite of breast (S21.05-)*
S20.171 Other superficial bite of breast, right breast
S20.172 Other superficial bite of breast, left breast
S20.179 Other superficial bite of breast, unspecified breast
S20.2 Contusion of thorax
S20.20 Contusion of thorax, unspecified
S20.21 Contusion of front wall of thorax
S20.211 Contusion of right front wall of thorax
S20.212 Contusion of left front wall of thorax
S20.219 Contusion of unspecified front wall of thorax
S20.22 Contusion of back wall of thorax
S20.221 Contusion of right back wall of thorax
S20.222 Contusion of left back wall of thorax
S20.229 Contusion of unspecified back wall of thorax
S20.3 Other and unspecified superficial injuries of front wall of thorax
S20.30 Unspecified superficial injuries of front wall of thorax
S20.301 Unspecified superficial injuries of right front wall of thorax
S20.302 Unspecified superficial injuries of left front wall of thorax
S20.309 Unspecified superficial injuries of unspecified front wall of thorax
S20.31 Abrasion of front wall of thorax
S20.311 Abrasion of right front wall of thorax
S20.312 Abrasion of left front wall of thorax
S20.319 Abrasion of unspecified front wall of thorax
S20.32 Blister (nonthermal) of front wall of thorax
S20.321 Blister (nonthermal) of right front wall of thorax
S20.322 Blister (nonthermal) of left front wall of thorax
S20.329 Blister (nonthermal) of unspecified front wall of thorax
S20.34 External constriction of front wall of thorax
S20.341 External constriction of right front wall of thorax

Unacceptable principal diagnosis symbol per Medicare code edits | Code exempt from diagnosis present on admission requirement
Questionable admission | Complication or comorbidity | CC/MCC exclusion | Major complication or comorbidity
Principal diagnosis as its own CC | Principal diagnosis as its own MCC | Z code as first-listed diagnosis

S20.342 External constriction of left front wall of thorax
S20.349 External constriction of unspecified front wall of thorax
S20.35 Superficial foreign body of front wall of thorax
Splinter in front wall of thorax
S20.351 Superficial foreign body of right front wall of thorax
S20.352 Superficial foreign body of left front wall of thorax
S20.359 Superficial foreign body of unspecified front wall of thorax
S20.36 Insect bite (nonvenomous) of front wall of thorax
S20.361 Insect bite (nonvenomous) of right front wall of thorax
S20.362 Insect bite (nonvenomous) of left front wall of thorax
S20.369 Insect bite (nonvenomous) of unspecified front wall of thorax
S20.37 Other superficial bite of front wall of thorax
EXCLUDES1 *open bite of front wall of thorax (S21.14)*
S20.371 Other superficial bite of right front wall of thorax
S20.372 Other superficial bite of left front wall of thorax
S20.379 Other superficial bite of unspecified front wall of thorax
S20.4 Other and unspecified superficial injuries of back wall of thorax
S20.40 Unspecified superficial injuries of back wall of thorax
S20.401 Unspecified superficial injuries of right back wall of thorax
S20.402 Unspecified superficial injuries of left back wall of thorax
S20.409 Unspecified superficial injuries of unspecified back wall of thorax
S20.41 Abrasion of back wall of thorax
S20.411 Abrasion of right back wall of thorax
S20.412 Abrasion of left back wall of thorax
S20.419 Abrasion of unspecified back wall of thorax
S20.42 Blister (nonthermal) of back wall of thorax
S20.421 Blister (nonthermal) of right back wall of thorax
S20.422 Blister (nonthermal) of left back wall of thorax
S20.429 Blister (nonthermal) of unspecified back wall of thorax
S20.44 External constriction of back wall of thorax
S20.441 External constriction of right back wall of thorax
S20.442 External constriction of left back wall of thorax
S20.449 External constriction of unspecified back wall of thorax
S20.45 Superficial foreign body of back wall of thorax
Splinter of back wall of thorax
S20.451 Superficial foreign body of right back wall of thorax
S20.452 Superficial foreign body of left back wall of thorax
S20.459 Superficial foreign body of unspecified back wall of thorax
S20.46 Insect bite (nonvenomous) of back wall of thorax
S20.461 Insect bite (nonvenomous) of right back wall of thorax
S20.462 Insect bite (nonvenomous) of left back wall of thorax
S20.469 Insect bite (nonvenomous) of unspecified back wall of thorax
S20.47 Other superficial bite of back wall of thorax
EXCLUDES1 *open bite of back wall of thorax (S21.24)*
S20.471 Other superficial bite of right back wall of thorax
S20.472 Other superficial bite of left back wall of thorax
S20.479 Other superficial bite of unspecified back wall of thorax
S20.9 Superficial injury of unspecified parts of thorax
EXCLUDES1 *contusion of thorax NOS (S20.20)*
S20.90 Unspecified superficial injury of unspecified parts of thorax
Superficial injury of thoracic wall NOS
S20.91 Abrasion of unspecified parts of thorax
S20.92 Blister (nonthermal) of unspecified parts of thorax
S20.94 External constriction of unspecified parts of thorax
S20.95 Superficial foreign body of unspecified parts of thorax
Splinter in thorax NOS
S20.96 Insect bite (nonvenomous) of unspecified parts of thorax
S20.97 Other superficial bite of unspecified parts of thorax
EXCLUDES1 *open bite of thorax NOS (S21.95)*

S21 Open wound of thorax
Code also any associated injury, such as:
- injury of heart (S26.-)
- injury of intrathoracic organs (S27.-)
- rib fracture (S22.3-, S22.4-)
- spinal cord injury (S24.0-, S24.1-)
- traumatic hemopneumothorax (S27.3)
- traumatic hemothorax (S27.1)
- traumatic pneumothorax (S27.0)
- wound infection

EXCLUDES1 *traumatic amputation (partial) of thorax (S28.1)*

The appropriate 7th character is to be added to each code from category S21
A = initial encounter
D = subsequent encounter
S = sequela

S21.0 Open wound of breast
S21.00 Unspecified open wound of breast
S21.001 Unspecified open wound of right breast
S21.002 Unspecified open wound of left breast
S21.009 Unspecified open wound of unspecified breast
S21.01 Laceration without foreign body of breast
S21.011 Laceration without foreign body of right breast
S21.012 Laceration without foreign body of left breast
S21.019 Laceration without foreign body of unspecified breast
S21.02 Laceration with foreign body of breast
S21.021 Laceration with foreign body of right breast
S21.022 Laceration with foreign body of left breast
S21.029 Laceration with foreign body of unspecified breast
S21.03 Puncture wound without foreign body of breast
S21.031 Puncture wound without foreign body of right breast
S21.032 Puncture wound without foreign body of left breast
S21.039 Puncture wound without foreign body of unspecified breast
S21.04 Puncture wound with foreign body of breast
S21.041 Puncture wound with foreign body of right breast
S21.042 Puncture wound with foreign body of left breast
S21.049 Puncture wound with foreign body of unspecified breast
S21.05 Open bite of breast
Bite of breast NOS
EXCLUDES1 *superficial bite of breast (S20.17)*
S21.051 Open bite of right breast
S21.052 Open bite of left breast
S21.059 Open bite of unspecified breast

S21.1 Open wound of front wall of thorax without penetration into thoracic cavity
Open wound of chest without penetration into thoracic cavity
S21.10 Unspecified open wound of front wall of thorax without penetration into thoracic cavity
S21.101 Unspecified open wound of right front wall of thorax without penetration into thoracic cavity CC
S21.102 Unspecified open wound of left front wall of thorax without penetration into thoracic cavity CC
S21.109 Unspecified open wound of unspecified front wall of thorax without penetration into thoracic cavity CC
S21.11 Laceration without foreign body of front wall of thorax without penetration into thoracic cavity
S21.111 Laceration without foreign body of right front wall of thorax without penetration into thoracic cavity CC
S21.112 Laceration without foreign body of left front wall of thorax without penetration into thoracic cavity CC
S21.119 Laceration without foreign body of unspecified front wall of thorax without penetration into thoracic cavity CC
S21.12 Laceration with foreign body of front wall of thorax without penetration into thoracic cavity
S21.121 Laceration with foreign body of right front wall of thorax without penetration into thoracic cavity CC
S21.122 Laceration with foreign body of left front wall of thorax without penetration into thoracic cavity CC
S21.129 Laceration with foreign body of unspecified front wall of thorax without penetration into thoracic cavity CC
S21.13 Puncture wound without foreign body of front wall of thorax without penetration into thoracic cavity
S21.131 Puncture wound without foreign body of right front wall of thorax without penetration into thoracic cavity CC
S21.132 Puncture wound without foreign body of left front wall of thorax without penetration into thoracic cavity CC
S21.139 Puncture wound without foreign body of unspecified front wall of thorax without penetration into thoracic cavity CC
S21.14 Puncture wound with foreign body of front wall of thorax without penetration into thoracic cavity
S21.141 Puncture wound with foreign body of right front wall of thorax without penetration into thoracic cavity CC
S21.142 Puncture wound with foreign body of left front wall of thorax without penetration into thoracic cavity CC
S21.149 Puncture wound with foreign body of unspecified front wall of thorax without penetration into thoracic cavity CC
S21.15 Open bite of front wall of thorax without penetration into thoracic cavity
Bite of front wall of thorax NOS
EXCLUDES1 *superficial bite of front wall of thorax (S20.37)*
S21.151 Open bite of right front wall of thorax without penetration into thoracic cavity CC
S21.152 Open bite of left front wall of thorax without penetration into thoracic cavity CC
S21.159 Open bite of unspecified front wall of thorax without penetration into thoracic cavity CC
S21.2 Open wound of back wall of thorax without penetration into thoracic cavity
S21.20 Unspecified open wound of back wall of thorax without penetration into thoracic cavity
S21.201 Unspecified open wound of right back wall of thorax without penetration into thoracic cavity
S21.202 Unspecified open wound of left back wall of thorax without penetration into thoracic cavity
S21.209 Unspecified open wound of unspecified back wall of thorax without penetration into thoracic cavity
S21.21 Laceration without foreign body of back wall of thorax without penetration into thoracic cavity
S21.211 Laceration without foreign body of right back wall of thorax without penetration into thoracic cavity
S21.212 Laceration without foreign body of left back wall of thorax without penetration into thoracic cavity
S21.219 Laceration without foreign body of unspecified back wall of thorax without penetration into thoracic cavity
S21.22 Laceration with foreign body of back wall of thorax without penetration into thoracic cavity
S21.221 Laceration with foreign body of right back wall of thorax without penetration into thoracic cavity
S21.222 Laceration with foreign body of left back wall of thorax without penetration into thoracic cavity
S21.229 Laceration with foreign body of unspecified back wall of thorax without penetration into thoracic cavity
S21.23 Puncture wound without foreign body of back wall of thorax without penetration into thoracic cavity
S21.231 Puncture wound without foreign body of right back wall of thorax without penetration into thoracic cavity
S21.232 Puncture wound without foreign body of left back wall of thorax without penetration into thoracic cavity
S21.239 Puncture wound without foreign body of unspecified back wall of thorax without penetration into thoracic cavity
S21.24 Puncture wound with foreign body of back wall of thorax without penetration into thoracic cavity
S21.241 Puncture wound with foreign body of right back wall of thorax without penetration into thoracic cavity
S21.242 Puncture wound with foreign body of left back wall of thorax without penetration into thoracic cavity
S21.249 Puncture wound with foreign body of unspecified back wall of thorax without penetration into thoracic cavity
S21.25 Open bite of back wall of thorax without penetration into thoracic cavity
Bite of back wall of thorax NOS
EXCLUDES1 *superficial bite of back wall of thorax (S20.47)*
S21.251 Open bite of right back wall of thorax without penetration into thoracic cavity
S21.252 Open bite of left back wall of thorax without penetration into thoracic cavity
S21.259 Open bite of unspecified back wall of thorax without penetration into thoracic cavity
S21.3 Open wound of front wall of thorax with penetration into thoracic cavity
Open wound of chest with penetration into thoracic cavity
S21.30 Unspecified open wound of front wall of thorax with penetration into thoracic cavity
S21.301 Unspecified open wound of right front wall of thorax with penetration into thoracic cavity MCC
S21.302 Unspecified open wound of left front wall of thorax with penetration into thoracic cavity MCC

Unacceptable principal diagnosis symbol per Medicare code edits · Code exempt from diagnosis present on admission requirement
Questionable admission · CC Complication or comorbidity · CC/MCC exclusion · MCC Major complication or comorbidity
Principal diagnosis as its own CC · Principal diagnosis as its own MCC · Z code as first-listed diagnosis

S21.309 Unspecified open wound of unspecified front wall of thorax with penetration into thoracic cavity MCC

S21.31 Laceration without foreign body of front wall of thorax with penetration into thoracic cavity

S21.311 Laceration without foreign body of right front wall of thorax with penetration into thoracic cavity MCC

S21.312 Laceration without foreign body of left front wall of thorax with penetration into thoracic cavity MCC

S21.319 Laceration without foreign body of unspecified front wall of thorax with penetration into thoracic cavity MCC

S21.32 Laceration with foreign body of front wall of thorax with penetration into thoracic cavity

S21.321 Laceration with foreign body of right front wall of thorax with penetration into thoracic cavity MCC

S21.322 Laceration with foreign body of left front wall of thorax with penetration into thoracic cavity MCC

S21.329 Laceration with foreign body of unspecified front wall of thorax with penetration into thoracic cavity MCC

S21.33 Puncture wound without foreign body of front wall of thorax with penetration into thoracic cavity

S21.331 Puncture wound without foreign body of right front wall of thorax with penetration into thoracic cavity MCC

S21.332 Puncture wound without foreign body of left front wall of thorax with penetration into thoracic cavity MCC

S21.339 Puncture wound without foreign body of unspecified front wall of thorax with penetration into thoracic cavity MCC

S21.34 Puncture wound with foreign body of front wall of thorax with penetration into thoracic cavity

S21.341 Puncture wound with foreign body of right front wall of thorax with penetration into thoracic cavity MCC

S21.342 Puncture wound with foreign body of left front wall of thorax with penetration into thoracic cavity MCC

S21.349 Puncture wound with foreign body of unspecified front wall of thorax with penetration into thoracic cavity MCC

S21.35 Open bite of front wall of thorax with penetration into thoracic cavity

EXCLUDES1 *superficial bite of front wall of thorax (S20.37)*

S21.351 Open bite of right front wall of thorax with penetration into thoracic cavity MCC

S21.352 Open bite of left front wall of thorax with penetration into thoracic cavity MCC

S21.359 Open bite of unspecified front wall of thorax with penetration into thoracic cavity MCC

S21.4 Open wound of back wall of thorax with penetration into thoracic cavity

S21.40 Unspecified open wound of back wall of thorax with penetration into thoracic cavity

S21.401 Unspecified open wound of right back wall of thorax with penetration into thoracic cavity MCC

S21.402 Unspecified open wound of left back wall of thorax with penetration into thoracic cavity MCC

S21.409 Unspecified open wound of unspecified back wall of thorax with penetration into thoracic cavity MCC

S21.41 Laceration without foreign body of back wall of thorax with penetration into thoracic cavity

S21.411 Laceration without foreign body of right back wall of thorax with penetration into thoracic cavity MCC

S21.412 Laceration without foreign body of left back wall of thorax with penetration into thoracic cavity MCC

S21.419 Laceration without foreign body of unspecified back wall of thorax with penetration into thoracic cavity MCC

S21.42 Laceration with foreign body of back wall of thorax with penetration into thoracic cavity

S21.421 Laceration with foreign body of right back wall of thorax with penetration into thoracic cavity MCC

S21.422 Laceration with foreign body of left back wall of thorax with penetration into thoracic cavity MCC

S21.429 Laceration with foreign body of unspecified back wall of thorax with penetration into thoracic cavity MCC

S21.43 Puncture wound without foreign body of back wall of thorax with penetration into thoracic cavity

S21.431 Puncture wound without foreign body of right back wall of thorax with penetration into thoracic cavity MCC

S21.432 Puncture wound without foreign body of left back wall of thorax with penetration into thoracic cavity MCC

S21.439 Puncture wound without foreign body of unspecified back wall of thorax with penetration into thoracic cavity MCC

S21.44 Puncture wound with foreign body of back wall of thorax with penetration into thoracic cavity

S21.441 Puncture wound with foreign body of right back wall of thorax with penetration into thoracic cavity MCC

S21.442 Puncture wound with foreign body of left back wall of thorax with penetration into thoracic cavity MCC

S21.449 Puncture wound with foreign body of unspecified back wall of thorax with penetration into thoracic cavity MCC

S21.45 Open bite of back wall of thorax with penetration into thoracic cavity

Bite of back wall of thorax NOS

EXCLUDES1 *superficial bite of back wall of thorax (S20.47)*

S21.451 Open bite of right back wall of thorax with penetration into thoracic cavity MCC

S21.452 Open bite of left back wall of thorax with penetration into thoracic cavity MCC

S21.459 Open bite of unspecified back wall of thorax with penetration into thoracic cavity MCC

S21.9 Open wound of unspecified part of thorax

Open wound of thoracic wall NOS

S21.90 Unspecified open wound of unspecified part of thorax CC

S21.91 Laceration without foreign body of unspecified part of thorax CC

S21.92 Laceration with foreign body of unspecified part of thorax CC

S21.93 Puncture wound without foreign body of unspecified part of thorax CC

S21.94 Puncture wound with foreign body of unspecified part of thorax CC

S21.95 Open bite of unspecified part of thorax CC

EXCLUDES1 *superficial bite of thorax (S20.97)*

S22 Fracture of rib(s), sternum and thoracic spine

NOTES A fracture not indicated as displaced or nondisplaced should be coded to displaced

A fracture not indicated as open or closed should be coded to closed

INCLUDES *fracture of thoracic neural arch*

fracture of thoracic spinous process

fracture of thoracic transverse process

fracture of thoracic vertebra

fracture of thoracic vertebral arch

Code first any associated:

injury of intrathoracic organ (S27.-)

spinal cord injury (S24.0-, S24.1-)

Unspecified Code Other Specified Code Manifestation Code N Newborn P Pediatric M Maternity A Adult ♂ Male ♀ Female
● New Code ▲ Revised Code Title ►◄ Revised Text NOTES INCLUDES EXCLUDES1 Not coded here EXCLUDES2 Not included here
4th character required 5th character required 6th character required 7th character required
Extension 'X' Alert HAC Hospital-acquired condition (HAC) alert AHA AHA Coding Clinic®

EXCLUDES1 *transection of thorax (S28.1)*
EXCLUDES2 *fracture of clavicle (S42.0-)*
fracture of scapula (S42.1-)

The appropriate 7th character is to be added to each code from category S22
A = initial encounter for closed fracture
B = initial encounter for open fracture
D = subsequent encounter for fracture with routine healing
G = subsequent encounter for fracture with delayed healing
K = subsequent encounter for fracture with nonunion
S = sequela

S22.0 Fracture of thoracic vertebra
S22.00 Fracture of unspecified thoracic vertebra
S22.000 Wedge compression fracture of unspecified thoracic vertebra CC HAC MCC
S22.001 Stable burst fracture of unspecified thoracic vertebra CC HAC MCC
S22.002 Unstable burst fracture of unspecified thoracic vertebra CC HAC MCC
S22.008 Other fracture of unspecified thoracic vertebra CC HAC MCC
S22.009 Unspecified fracture of unspecified thoracic vertebra CC HAC MCC
S22.01 Fracture of first thoracic vertebra
S22.010 Wedge compression fracture of first thoracic vertebra CC HAC MCC
S22.011 Stable burst fracture of first thoracic vertebra CC HAC MCC
S22.012 Unstable burst fracture of first thoracic vertebra CC HAC MCC
S22.018 Other fracture of first thoracic vertebra CC HAC MCC
S22.019 Unspecified fracture of first thoracic vertebra CC HAC MCC
S22.02 Fracture of second thoracic vertebra
S22.020 Wedge compression fracture of second thoracic vertebra CC HAC MCC
S22.021 Stable burst fracture of second thoracic vertebra CC HAC MCC
S22.022 Unstable burst fracture of second thoracic vertebra CC HAC MCC
S22.028 Other fracture of second thoracic vertebra CC HAC MCC
S22.029 Unspecified fracture of second thoracic vertebra CC HAC MCC
S22.03 Fracture of third thoracic vertebra
S22.030 Wedge compression fracture of third thoracic vertebra CC HAC MCC
S22.031 Stable burst fracture of third thoracic vertebra CC HAC MCC
S22.032 Unstable burst fracture of third thoracic vertebra CC HAC MCC
S22.038 Other fracture of third thoracic vertebra CC HAC MCC
S22.039 Unspecified fracture of third thoracic vertebra CC HAC MCC
S22.04 Fracture of fourth thoracic vertebra
S22.040 Wedge compression fracture of fourth thoracic vertebra CC HAC MCC
S22.041 Stable burst fracture of fourth thoracic vertebra CC HAC MCC
S22.042 Unstable burst fracture of fourth thoracic vertebra CC HAC MCC
S22.048 Other fracture of fourth thoracic vertebra CC HAC MCC
S22.049 Unspecified fracture of fourth thoracic vertebra CC HAC MCC
S22.05 Fracture of T5-T6 vertebra
S22.050 Wedge compression fracture of T5-T6 vertebra CC HAC MCC
S22.051 Stable burst fracture of T5-T6 vertebra CC HAC MCC
S22.052 Unstable burst fracture of T5-T6 vertebra CC HAC MCC
S22.058 Other fracture of T5-T6 vertebra CC HAC MCC
S22.059 Unspecified fracture of T5-T6 vertebra CC HAC MCC
S22.06 Fracture of T7-T8 vertebra
S22.060 Wedge compression fracture of T7-T8 vertebra CC HAC MCC
S22.061 Stable burst fracture of T7-T8 vertebra CC HAC MCC
S22.062 Unstable burst fracture of T7-T8 vertebra CC HAC MCC
S22.068 Other fracture of T7-T8 thoracic vertebra CC HAC MCC
S22.069 Unspecified fracture of T7-T8 vertebra CC HAC MCC
S22.07 Fracture of T9-T10 vertebra
S22.070 Wedge compression fracture of T9-T10 vertebra CC HAC MCC
S22.071 Stable burst fracture of T9-T10 vertebra CC HAC MCC
S22.072 Unstable burst fracture of T9-T10 vertebra CC HAC MCC
S22.078 Other fracture of T9-T10 vertebra CC HAC MCC
S22.079 Unspecified fracture of T9-T10 vertebra CC HAC MCC
S22.08 Fracture of T11-T12 vertebra
S22.080 Wedge compression fracture of T11-T12 vertebra CC HAC MCC
S22.081 Stable burst fracture of T11-T12 vertebra CC HAC MCC
S22.082 Unstable burst fracture of T11-T12 vertebra CC HAC MCC
S22.088 Other fracture of T11-T12 vertebra CC HAC MCC
S22.089 Unspecified fracture of T11-T12 vertebra CC HAC MCC

S22.2 Fracture of sternum
S22.20 Unspecified fracture of sternum CC HAC MCC
S22.21 Fracture of manubrium CC HAC MCC
S22.22 Fracture of body of sternum CC HAC MCC
S22.23 Sternal manubrial dissociation CC HAC MCC
S22.24 Fracture of xiphoid process CC HAC MCC

S22.3 Fracture of one rib
S22.31 Fracture of one rib, right side CC HAC MCC
S22.32 Fracture of one rib, left side CC HAC MCC
S22.39 Fracture of one rib, unspecified side CC HAC MCC

S22.4 Multiple fractures of ribs
Fractures of two or more ribs
EXCLUDES1 *flail chest (S22.5-)*
S22.41 Multiple fractures of ribs, right side CC HAC MCC
S22.42 Multiple fractures of ribs, left side CC HAC MCC
S22.43 Multiple fractures of ribs, bilateral CC HAC MCC
S22.49 Multiple fractures of ribs, unspecified side CC HAC MCC

S22.5 Flail chest CC HAC MCC
S22.9 Fracture of bony thorax, part unspecified CC HAC MCC

S23 Dislocation and sprain of joints and ligaments of thorax
INCLUDES *avulsion of joint or ligament of thorax*
laceration of cartilage, joint or ligament of thorax
sprain of cartilage, joint or ligament of thorax
traumatic hemarthrosis of joint or ligament of thorax
traumatic rupture of joint or ligament of thorax
traumatic subluxation of joint or ligament of thorax
traumatic tear of joint or ligament of thorax
Code also any associated open wound
EXCLUDES2 *dislocation, sprain of sternoclavicular joint (S43.2, S43.6)*
strain of muscle or tendon of thorax (S29.01-)

The appropriate 7th character is to be added to each code from category S23
A = initial encounter
D = subsequent encounter
S = sequela

S23.0 Traumatic rupture of thoracic intervertebral disc
EXCLUDES1 *rupture or displacement (nontraumatic) of thoracic intervertebral disc NOS (M51.- with fifth character 4)*

PDx Unacceptable principal diagnosis symbol per Medicare code edits; POA Code exempt from diagnosis present on admission requirement
Q Questionable admission; CC Complication or comorbidity; CC/MCC Exc CC/MCC exclusion; MCC Major complication or comorbidity
PDx CC Principal diagnosis as its own CC; PDx MCC Principal diagnosis as its own MCC; Z1 Z code as first-listed diagnosis

S23.1 Subluxation and dislocation of thoracic vertebra
Code also any associated
open wound of thorax (S21.-)
spinal cord injury (S24.0-, S24.1-)
EXCLUDES2 *fracture of thoracic vertebrae (S22.0-)*
S23.10 Subluxation and dislocation of unspecified thoracic vertebra
S23.100 Subluxation of unspecified thoracic vertebra
S23.101 Dislocation of unspecified thoracic vertebra
S23.11 Subluxation and dislocation of T1/T2 thoracic vertebra
S23.110 Subluxation of T1/T2 thoracic vertebra
S23.111 Dislocation of T1/T2 thoracic vertebra
S23.12 Subluxation and dislocation of T2/T3-T3/T4 thoracic vertebra
S23.120 Subluxation of T2/T3 thoracic vertebra
S23.121 Dislocation of T2/T3 thoracic vertebra
S23.122 Subluxation of T3/T4 thoracic vertebra
S23.123 Dislocation of T3/T4 thoracic vertebra
S23.13 Subluxation and dislocation of T4/T5-T5/T6 thoracic vertebra
S23.130 Subluxation of T4/T5 thoracic vertebra
S23.131 Dislocation of T4/T5 thoracic vertebra
S23.132 Subluxation of T5/T6 thoracic vertebra
S23.133 Dislocation of T5/T6 thoracic vertebra
S23.14 Subluxation and dislocation of T6/T7-T7/T8 thoracic vertebra
S23.140 Subluxation of T6/T7 thoracic vertebra
S23.141 Dislocation of T6/T7 thoracic vertebra
S23.142 Subluxation of T7/T8 thoracic vertebra
S23.143 Dislocation of T7/T8 thoracic vertebra
S23.15 Subluxation and dislocation of T8/T9-T9/T10 thoracic vertebra
S23.150 Subluxation of T8/T9 thoracic vertebra
S23.151 Dislocation of T8/T9 thoracic vertebra
S23.152 Subluxation of T9/T10 thoracic vertebra
S23.153 Dislocation of T9/T10 thoracic vertebra
S23.16 Subluxation and dislocation of T10/T11-T11/T12 thoracic vertebra
S23.160 Subluxation of T10/T11 thoracic vertebra
S23.161 Dislocation of T10/T11 thoracic vertebra
S23.162 Subluxation of T11/T12 thoracic vertebra
S23.163 Dislocation of T11/T12 thoracic vertebra
S23.17 Subluxation and dislocation of T12/L1 thoracic vertebra
S23.170 Subluxation of T12/L1 thoracic vertebra
S23.171 Dislocation of T12/L1 thoracic vertebra
S23.2 Dislocation of other and unspecified parts of thorax
S23.20 Dislocation of unspecified part of thorax
S23.29 Dislocation of other parts of thorax
S23.3 Sprain of ligaments of thoracic spine
S23.4 Sprain of ribs and sternum
S23.41 Sprain of ribs
S23.42 Sprain of sternum
S23.420 Sprain of sternoclavicular (joint) (ligament)
S23.421 Sprain of chondrosternal joint
S23.428 Other sprain of sternum
S23.429 Unspecified sprain of sternum
S23.8 Sprain of other specified parts of thorax
S23.9 Sprain of unspecified parts of thorax
S24 Injury of nerves and spinal cord at thorax level
NOTES Code to highest level of thoracic spinal cord injury
Injuries to the spinal cord (S24.0 and S24.1) refer to the cord level and not bone level injury, and can affect nerve roots at and below the level given.
Code also any associated:
fracture of thoracic vertebra (S22.0-)
open wound of thorax (S21.-)
transient paralysis (R29.5)
EXCLUDES2 *injury of brachial plexus (S14.3)*

The appropriate 7th character is to be added to each code from category S24
A = initial encounter
D = subsequent encounter
S = sequela
S24.0 Concussion and edema of thoracic spinal cord MCC
S24.1 Other and unspecified injuries of thoracic spinal cord
S24.10 Unspecified injury of thoracic spinal cord
S24.101 Unspecified injury at T1 level of thoracic spinal cord HAC MCC
S24.102 Unspecified injury at T2-T6 level of thoracic spinal cord HAC MCC
S24.103 Unspecified injury at T7-T10 level of thoracic spinal cord HAC MCC
S24.104 Unspecified injury at T11-T12 level of thoracic spinal cord HAC MCC
S24.109 Unspecified injury at unspecified level of thoracic spinal cord HAC
Injury of thoracic spinal cord NOS
S24.11 Complete lesion of thoracic spinal cord
S24.111 Complete lesion at T1 level of thoracic spinal cord HAC MCC
S24.112 Complete lesion at T2-T6 level of thoracic spinal cord HAC MCC
S24.113 Complete lesion at T7-T10 level of thoracic spinal cord HAC MCC
S24.114 Complete lesion at T11-T12 level of thoracic spinal cord HAC MCC
S24.119 Complete lesion at unspecified level of thoracic spinal cord
S24.13 Anterior cord syndrome of thoracic spinal cord
S24.131 Anterior cord syndrome at T1 level of thoracic spinal cord HAC MCC
S24.132 Anterior cord syndrome at T2-T6 level of thoracic spinal cord HAC MCC
S24.133 Anterior cord syndrome at T7-T10 level of thoracic spinal cord HAC MCC
S24.134 Anterior cord syndrome at T11-T12 level of thoracic spinal cord HAC MCC
S24.139 Anterior cord syndrome at unspecified level of thoracic spinal cord
S24.14 Brown-Séquard syndrome of thoracic spinal cord
S24.141 Brown-Séquard syndrome at T1 level of thoracic spinal cord MCC
S24.142 Brown-Séquard syndrome at T2-T6 level of thoracic spinal cord MCC
S24.143 Brown-Séquard syndrome at T7-T10 level of thoracic spinal cord MCC
S24.144 Brown-Séquard syndrome at T11-T12 level of thoracic spinal cord MCC
S24.149 Brown-Séquard syndrome at unspecified level of thoracic spinal cord
S24.15 Other incomplete lesions of thoracic spinal cord
Incomplete lesion of thoracic spinal cord NOS
Posterior cord syndrome of thoracic spinal cord
S24.151 Other incomplete lesion at T1 level of thoracic spinal cord HAC MCC
S24.152 Other incomplete lesion at T2-T6 level of thoracic spinal cord HAC MCC
S24.153 Other incomplete lesion at T7-T10 level of thoracic spinal cord HAC MCC
S24.154 Other incomplete lesion at T11-T12 level of thoracic spinal cord HAC MCC
S24.159 Other incomplete lesion at unspecified level of thoracic spinal cord
S24.2 Injury of nerve root of thoracic spine
S24.3 Injury of peripheral nerves of thorax
S24.4 Injury of thoracic sympathetic nervous system
Injury of cardiac plexus
Injury of esophageal plexus
Injury of pulmonary plexus
Injury of stellate ganglion
Injury of thoracic sympathetic ganglion
S24.8 Injury of other specified nerves of thorax
S24.9 Injury of unspecified nerve of thorax
S25 Injury of blood vessels of thorax

Unspecified Code Other Specified Code Manifestation Code N Newborn P Pediatric M Maternity A Adult ♂ Male ♀ Female
● New Code ▲ Revised Code Title ►◄ Revised Text NOTES INCLUDES EXCLUDES1 Not coded here EXCLUDES2 Not included here
4th character required 5th character required 6th character required 7th character required
Extension 'X' Alert HAC Hospital-acquired condition (HAC) alert AHA AHA Coding Clinic®

Code also any associated open wound (S21.-)

The appropriate 7th character is to be added to each code from category S25

A = initial encounter
D = subsequent encounter
S = sequela

S25.0 Injury of thoracic aorta
Injury of aorta NOS
S25.00 Unspecified injury of thoracic aorta MCC
S25.01 Minor laceration of thoracic aorta MCC
Incomplete transection of thoracic aorta
Laceration of thoracic aorta NOS
Superficial laceration of thoracic aorta
S25.02 Major laceration of thoracic aorta MCC
Complete transection of thoracic aorta
Traumatic rupture of thoracic aorta
S25.09 Other specified injury of thoracic aorta MCC

S25.1 Injury of innominate or subclavian artery
S25.10 Unspecified injury of innominate or subclavian artery
S25.101 Unspecified injury of right innominate or subclavian artery MCC
S25.102 Unspecified injury of left innominate or subclavian artery MCC
S25.109 Unspecified injury of unspecified innominate or subclavian artery MCC
S25.11 Minor laceration of innominate or subclavian artery
Incomplete transection of innominate or subclavian artery
Laceration of innominate or subclavian artery NOS
Superficial laceration of innominate or subclavian artery
S25.111 Minor laceration of right innominate or subclavian artery MCC
S25.112 Minor laceration of left innominate or subclavian artery MCC
S25.119 Minor laceration of unspecified innominate or subclavian artery MCC
S25.12 Major laceration of innominate or subclavian artery
Complete transection of innominate or subclavian artery
Traumatic rupture of innominate or subclavian artery
S25.121 Major laceration of right innominate or subclavian artery MCC
S25.122 Major laceration of left innominate or subclavian artery MCC
S25.129 Major laceration of unspecified innominate or subclavian artery MCC
S25.19 Other specified injury of innominate or subclavian artery
S25.191 Other specified injury of right innominate or subclavian artery MCC
S25.192 Other specified injury of left innominate or subclavian artery MCC
S25.199 Other specified injury of unspecified innominate or subclavian artery MCC

S25.2 Injury of superior vena cava
Injury of vena cava NOS
S25.20 Unspecified injury of superior vena cava MCC
S25.21 Minor laceration of superior vena cava MCC
Incomplete transection of superior vena cava
Laceration of superior vena cava NOS
Superficial laceration of superior vena cava
S25.22 Major laceration of superior vena cava MCC
Complete transection of superior vena cava
Traumatic rupture of superior vena cava
S25.29 Other specified injury of superior vena cava MCC

S25.3 Injury of innominate or subclavian vein
S25.30 Unspecified injury of innominate or subclavian vein
S25.301 Unspecified injury of right innominate or subclavian vein MCC
S25.302 Unspecified injury of left innominate or subclavian vein MCC
S25.309 Unspecified injury of unspecified innominate or subclavian vein MCC
S25.31 Minor laceration of innominate or subclavian vein
Incomplete transection of innominate or subclavian vein
Laceration of innominate or subclavian vein NOS
Superficial laceration of innominate or subclavian vein
S25.311 Minor laceration of right innominate or subclavian vein MCC
S25.312 Minor laceration of left innominate or subclavian vein MCC
S25.319 Minor laceration of unspecified innominate or subclavian vein MCC
S25.32 Major laceration of innominate or subclavian vein
Complete transection of innominate or subclavian vein
Traumatic rupture of innominate or subclavian vein
S25.321 Major laceration of right innominate or subclavian vein MCC
S25.322 Major laceration of left innominate or subclavian vein MCC
S25.329 Major laceration of unspecified innominate or subclavian vein MCC
S25.39 Other specified injury of innominate or subclavian vein
S25.391 Other specified injury of right innominate or subclavian vein MCC
S25.392 Other specified injury of left innominate or subclavian vein MCC
S25.399 Other specified injury of unspecified innominate or subclavian vein MCC

S25.4 Injury of pulmonary blood vessels
S25.40 Unspecified injury of pulmonary blood vessels
S25.401 Unspecified injury of right pulmonary blood vessels MCC
S25.402 Unspecified injury of left pulmonary blood vessels MCC
S25.409 Unspecified injury of unspecified pulmonary blood vessels MCC
S25.41 Minor laceration of pulmonary blood vessels
Incomplete transection of pulmonary blood vessels
Laceration of pulmonary blood vessels NOS
Superficial laceration of pulmonary blood vessels
S25.411 Minor laceration of right pulmonary blood vessels MCC
S25.412 Minor laceration of left pulmonary blood vessels MCC
S25.419 Minor laceration of unspecified pulmonary blood vessels MCC
S25.42 Major laceration of pulmonary blood vessels
Complete transection of pulmonary blood vessels
Traumatic rupture of pulmonary blood vessels
S25.421 Major laceration of right pulmonary blood vessels MCC
S25.422 Major laceration of left pulmonary blood vessels MCC
S25.429 Major laceration of unspecified pulmonary blood vessels MCC
S25.49 Other specified injury of pulmonary blood vessels
S25.491 Other specified injury of right pulmonary blood vessels MCC
S25.492 Other specified injury of left pulmonary blood vessels MCC
S25.499 Other specified injury of unspecified pulmonary blood vessels MCC

S25.5 Injury of intercostal blood vessels
S25.50 Unspecified injury of intercostal blood vessels
S25.501 Unspecified injury of intercostal blood vessels, right side CC
S25.502 Unspecified injury of intercostal blood vessels, left side CC
S25.509 Unspecified injury of intercostal blood vessels, unspecified side CC
S25.51 Laceration of intercostal blood vessels
S25.511 Laceration of intercostal blood vessels, right side CC
S25.512 Laceration of intercostal blood vessels, left side CC

Unacceptable principal diagnosis symbol per Medicare code edits — Code exempt from diagnosis present on admission requirement
Questionable admission — Complication or comorbidity — CC/MCC exclusion — Major complication or comorbidity
Principal diagnosis as its own CC — Principal diagnosis as its own MCC — Z code as first-listed diagnosis

S25.519 Laceration of intercostal blood vessels, unspecified side CC
S25.59 Other specified injury of intercostal blood vessels
S25.591 Other specified injury of intercostal blood vessels, right side CC
S25.592 Other specified injury of intercostal blood vessels, left side CC
S25.599 Other specified injury of intercostal blood vessels, unspecified side CC
S25.8 Injury of other blood vessels of thorax
Injury of azygos vein
Injury of mammary artery or vein
S25.80 Unspecified injury of other blood vessels of thorax
S25.801 Unspecified injury of other blood vessels of thorax, right side CC
S25.802 Unspecified injury of other blood vessels of thorax, left side CC
S25.809 Unspecified injury of other blood vessels of thorax, unspecified side CC
S25.81 Laceration of other blood vessels of thorax
S25.811 Laceration of other blood vessels of thorax, right side CC
S25.812 Laceration of other blood vessels of thorax, left side CC
S25.819 Laceration of other blood vessels of thorax, unspecified side CC
S25.89 Other specified injury of other blood vessels of thorax
S25.891 Other specified injury of other blood vessels of thorax, right side CC
S25.892 Other specified injury of other blood vessels of thorax, left side CC
S25.899 Other specified injury of other blood vessels of thorax, unspecified side CC
S25.9 Injury of unspecified blood vessel of thorax
S25.90 Unspecified injury of unspecified blood vessel of thorax CC
S25.91 Laceration of unspecified blood vessel of thorax CC
S25.99 Other specified injury of unspecified blood vessel of thorax CC
S26 Injury of heart
Code also any associated:
open wound of thorax (S21.-)
traumatic hemopneumothorax (S27.2)
traumatic hemothorax (S27.1)
traumatic pneumothorax (S27.0)
The appropriate 7th character is to be added to each code from category S26
A = initial encounter
D = subsequent encounter
S = sequela
S26.0 Injury of heart with hemopericardium
S26.00 Unspecified injury of heart with hemopericardium CC
S26.01 Contusion of heart with hemopericardium CC
S26.02 Laceration of heart with hemopericardium
S26.020 Mild laceration of heart with hemopericardium MCC
Laceration of heart without penetration of heart chamber
S26.021 Moderate laceration of heart with hemopericardium MCC
Laceration of heart with penetration of heart chamber
S26.022 Major laceration of heart with hemopericardium MCC
Laceration of heart with penetration of multiple heart chambers
S26.09 Other injury of heart with hemopericardium CC
S26.1 Injury of heart without hemopericardium
S26.10 Unspecified injury of heart without hemopericardium CC
S26.11 Contusion of heart without hemopericardium CC
S26.12 Laceration of heart without hemopericardium MCC
S26.19 Other injury of heart without hemopericardium CC
S26.9 Injury of heart, unspecified with or without hemopericardium
S26.90 Unspecified injury of heart, unspecified with or without hemopericardium CC
S26.91 Contusion of heart, unspecified with or without hemopericardium CC
S26.92 Laceration of heart, unspecified with or without hemopericardium MCC
Laceration of heart NOS
S26.99 Other injury of heart, unspecified with or without hemopericardium CC
S27 Injury of other and unspecified intrathoracic organs
Code also any associated open wound of thorax (S21.-)
EXCLUDES2 *injury of cervical esophagus (S10-S19)*
injury of trachea (cervical) (S10-S19)
The appropriate 7th character is to be added to each code from category S27
A = initial encounter
D = subsequent encounter
S = sequela
S27.0 Traumatic pneumothorax CC
EXCLUDES1 *spontaneous pneumothorax (J93.-)*
S27.1 Traumatic hemothorax MCC
S27.2 Traumatic hemopneumothorax MCC
S27.3 Other and unspecified injuries of lung
S27.30 Unspecified injury of lung
S27.301 Unspecified injury of lung, unilateral CC
S27.302 Unspecified injury of lung, bilateral CC
S27.309 Unspecified injury of lung, unspecified CC
S27.31 Primary blast injury of lung
Blast injury of lung NOS
S27.311 Primary blast injury of lung, unilateral CC
S27.312 Primary blast injury of lung, bilateral CC
S27.319 Primary blast injury of lung, unspecified CC
S27.32 Contusion of lung
S27.321 Contusion of lung, unilateral CC
S27.322 Contusion of lung, bilateral CC
S27.329 Contusion of lung, unspecified CC
S27.33 Laceration of lung
S27.331 Laceration of lung, unilateral MCC
S27.332 Laceration of lung, bilateral MCC
S27.339 Laceration of lung, unspecified MCC
S27.39 Other injuries of lung
Secondary blast injury of lung
S27.391 Other injuries of lung, unilateral CC
S27.392 Other injuries of lung, bilateral CC
S27.399 Other injuries of lung, unspecified CC
S27.4 Injury of bronchus
S27.40 Unspecified injury of bronchus
S27.401 Unspecified injury of bronchus, unilateral MCC
S27.402 Unspecified injury of bronchus, bilateral MCC
S27.409 Unspecified injury of bronchus, unspecified MCC
S27.41 Primary blast injury of bronchus
Blast injury of bronchus NOS
S27.411 Primary blast injury of bronchus, unilateral MCC
S27.412 Primary blast injury of bronchus, bilateral MCC
S27.419 Primary blast injury of bronchus, unspecified MCC
S27.42 Contusion of bronchus
S27.421 Contusion of bronchus, unilateral MCC
S27.422 Contusion of bronchus, bilateral MCC
S27.429 Contusion of bronchus, unspecified MCC
S27.43 Laceration of bronchus
S27.431 Laceration of bronchus, unilateral MCC
S27.432 Laceration of bronchus, bilateral MCC
S27.439 Laceration of bronchus, unspecified MCC
S27.49 Other injury of bronchus
Secondary blast injury of bronchus
S27.491 Other injury of bronchus, unilateral MCC

Unspecified Code Other Specified Code Manifestation Code N Newborn P Pediatric M Maternity A Adult ♂ Male ♀ Female
● New Code ▲ Revised Code Title ►◄ Revised Text NOTES INCLUDES EXCLUDES1 Not coded here EXCLUDES2 Not included here
4th character required 5th character required 6th character required 7th character required
Extension 'X' Alert HAC Hospital-acquired condition (HAC) alert AHA AHA Coding Clinic©

S27.492 Other injury of bronchus, bilateral
S27.499 Other injury of bronchus, unspecified
S27.5 Injury of thoracic trachea
S27.50 Unspecified injury of thoracic trachea
S27.51 Primary blast injury of thoracic trachea
Blast injury of thoracic trachea NOS
S27.52 Contusion of thoracic trachea
S27.53 Laceration of thoracic trachea
S27.59 Other injury of thoracic trachea
Secondary blast injury of thoracic trachea
S27.6 Injury of pleura
S27.60 Unspecified injury of pleura
S27.63 Laceration of pleura
S27.69 Other injury of pleura
S27.8 Injury of other specified intrathoracic organs
S27.80 Injury of diaphragm
S27.802 Contusion of diaphragm
S27.803 Laceration of diaphragm
S27.808 Other injury of diaphragm
S27.809 Unspecified injury of diaphragm
S27.81 Injury of esophagus (thoracic part)
S27.812 Contusion of esophagus (thoracic part)
S27.813 Laceration of esophagus (thoracic part)
S27.818 Other injury of esophagus (thoracic part)
S27.819 Unspecified injury of esophagus (thoracic part)
S27.89 Injury of other specified intrathoracic organs
Injury of lymphatic thoracic duct
Injury of thymus gland
S27.892 Contusion of other specified intrathoracic organs
S27.893 Laceration of other specified intrathoracic organs
S27.898 Other injury of other specified intrathoracic organs
S27.899 Unspecified injury of other specified intrathoracic organs
S27.9 Injury of unspecified intrathoracic organ
S28 Crushing injury of thorax, and traumatic amputation of part of thorax
The appropriate 7th character is to be added to each code from category S28
A = initial encounter
D = subsequent encounter
S = sequela
S28.0 Crushed chest
Use additional code for all associated injuries
EXCLUDES1 *flail chest (S22.5)*
S28.1 Traumatic amputation (partial) of part of thorax, except breast
S28.2 Traumatic amputation of breast
S28.21 Complete traumatic amputation of breast
Traumatic amputation of breast NOS
S28.211 Complete traumatic amputation of right breast
S28.212 Complete traumatic amputation of left breast
S28.219 Complete traumatic amputation of unspecified breast
S28.22 Partial traumatic amputation of breast
S28.221 Partial traumatic amputation of right breast
S28.222 Partial traumatic amputation of left breast
S28.229 Partial traumatic amputation of unspecified breast
S29 Other and unspecified injuries of thorax
Code also any associated open wound (S21.-)
The appropriate 7th character is to be added to each code from category S29
A = initial encounter
D = subsequent encounter
S = sequela
S29.0 Injury of muscle and tendon at thorax level
S29.00 Unspecified injury of muscle and tendon of thorax
S29.001 Unspecified injury of muscle and tendon of front wall of thorax
S29.002 Unspecified injury of muscle and tendon of back wall of thorax
S29.009 Unspecified injury of muscle and tendon of unspecified wall of thorax
S29.01 Strain of muscle and tendon of thorax
S29.011 Strain of muscle and tendon of front wall of thorax
S29.012 Strain of muscle and tendon of back wall of thorax
S29.019 Strain of muscle and tendon of unspecified wall of thorax
S29.02 Laceration of muscle and tendon of thorax
S29.021 Laceration of muscle and tendon of front wall of thorax
S29.022 Laceration of muscle and tendon of back wall of thorax
S29.029 Laceration of muscle and tendon of unspecified wall of thorax
S29.09 Other injury of muscle and tendon of thorax
S29.091 Other injury of muscle and tendon of front wall of thorax
S29.092 Other injury of muscle and tendon of back wall of thorax
S29.099 Other injury of muscle and tendon of unspecified wall of thorax
S29.8 Other specified injuries of thorax
S29.9 Unspecified injury of thorax

Injuries to the abdomen, lower back, lumbar spine, pelvis and external genitals (S30-S39)

INCLUDES *injuries to the abdominal wall*
injuries to the anus
injuries to the buttock
injuries to the external genitalia
injuries to the flank
injuries to the groin

EXCLUDES2 *burns and corrosions (T20-T32)*
effects of foreign body in anus and rectum (T18.5)
effects of foreign body in genitourinary tract (T19.-)
effects of foreign body in stomach, small intestine and colon (T18.2-T18.4)
frostbite (T33-T34)
insect bite or sting, venomous (T63.4)

S30 Superficial injury of abdomen, lower back, pelvis and external genitals
EXCLUDES2 *superficial injury of hip (S70.-)*
The appropriate 7th character is to be added to each code from category S30
A = initial encounter
D = subsequent encounter
S = sequela
S30.0 Contusion of lower back and pelvis
Contusion of buttock
S30.1 Contusion of abdominal wall
Contusion of flank
Contusion of groin
S30.2 Contusion of external genital organs
S30.20 Contusion of unspecified external genital organ
S30.201 Contusion of unspecified external genital organ, male ♂
S30.202 Contusion of unspecified external genital organ, female ♀
S30.21 Contusion of penis ♂
S30.22 Contusion of scrotum and testes ♂
S30.23 Contusion of vagina and vulva ♀
S30.3 Contusion of anus
S30.8 Other superficial injuries of abdomen, lower back, pelvis and external genitals

Unacceptable principal diagnosis symbol per Medicare code edits; Code exempt from diagnosis present on admission requirement; Questionable admission; CC Complication or comorbidity; CC/MCC exclusion; MCC Major complication or comorbidity; Principal diagnosis as its own CC; Principal diagnosis as its own MCC; Z code as first-listed diagnosis

 When symbols appear on a code that requires a 7th character extension, refer to Appendix D to identify applicable 7th character codes.

S30.81 Abrasion of abdomen, lower back, pelvis and external genitals
S30.810 Abrasion of lower back and pelvis
S30.811 Abrasion of abdominal wall
S30.812 Abrasion of penis ♂
S30.813 Abrasion of scrotum and testes ♂
S30.814 Abrasion of vagina and vulva ♀
S30.815 Abrasion of unspecified external genital organs, male ♂
S30.816 Abrasion of unspecified external genital organs, female ♀
S30.817 Abrasion of anus
S30.82 Blister (nonthermal) of abdomen, lower back, pelvis and external genitals
S30.820 Blister (nonthermal) of lower back and pelvis
S30.821 Blister (nonthermal) of abdominal wall
S30.822 Blister (nonthermal) of penis ♂
S30.823 Blister (nonthermal) of scrotum and testes ♂
S30.824 Blister (nonthermal) of vagina and vulva ♀
S30.825 Blister (nonthermal) of unspecified external genital organs, male ♂
S30.826 Blister (nonthermal) of unspecified external genital organs, female ♀
S30.827 Blister (nonthermal) of anus
S30.84 External constriction of abdomen, lower back, pelvis and external genitals
S30.840 External constriction of lower back and pelvis
S30.841 External constriction of abdominal wall
S30.842 External constriction of penis ♂
Hair tourniquet syndrome of penis
Use additional cause code to identify the constricting item (W49.0-)
S30.843 External constriction of scrotum and testes ♂
S30.844 External constriction of vagina and vulva ♀
S30.845 External constriction of unspecified external genital organs, male ♂
S30.846 External constriction of unspecified external genital organs, female ♀
S30.85 Superficial foreign body of abdomen, lower back, pelvis and external genitals
Splinter in the abdomen, lower back, pelvis and external genitals
S30.850 Superficial foreign body of lower back and pelvis
S30.851 Superficial foreign body of abdominal wall
S30.852 Superficial foreign body of penis ♂
S30.853 Superficial foreign body of scrotum and testes ♂
S30.854 Superficial foreign body of vagina and vulva ♀
S30.855 Superficial foreign body of unspecified external genital organs, male ♂
S30.856 Superficial foreign body of unspecified external genital organs, female ♀
S30.857 Superficial foreign body of anus
S30.86 Insect bite (nonvenomous) of abdomen, lower back, pelvis and external genitals
S30.860 Insect bite (nonvenomous) of lower back and pelvis
S30.861 Insect bite (nonvenomous) of abdominal wall
S30.862 Insect bite (nonvenomous) of penis ♂
S30.863 Insect bite (nonvenomous) of scrotum and testes ♂
S30.864 Insect bite (nonvenomous) of vagina and vulva ♀
S30.865 Insect bite (nonvenomous) of unspecified external genital organs, male ♂
S30.866 Insect bite (nonvenomous) of unspecified external genital organs, female ♀
S30.867 Insect bite (nonvenomous) of anus
S30.87 Other superficial bite of abdomen, lower back, pelvis and external genitals
EXCLUDES1 *open bite of abdomen, lower back, pelvis and external genitals (S31.05, S31.15, S31.25, S31.35, S31.45, S31.55)*
S30.870 Other superficial bite of lower back and pelvis
S30.871 Other superficial bite of abdominal wall
S30.872 Other superficial bite of penis ♂
S30.873 Other superficial bite of scrotum and testes ♂
S30.874 Other superficial bite of vagina and vulva ♀
S30.875 Other superficial bite of unspecified external genital organs, male ♂
S30.876 Other superficial bite of unspecified external genital organs, female ♀
S30.877 Other superficial bite of anus
S30.9 Unspecified superficial injury of abdomen, lower back, pelvis and external genitals
S30.91 Unspecified superficial injury of lower back and pelvis
S30.92 Unspecified superficial injury of abdominal wall
S30.93 Unspecified superficial injury of penis ♂
S30.94 Unspecified superficial injury of scrotum and testes ♂
S30.95 Unspecified superficial injury of vagina and vulva ♀
S30.96 Unspecified superficial injury of unspecified external genital organs, male ♂
S30.97 Unspecified superficial injury of unspecified external genital organs, female ♀
S30.98 Unspecified superficial injury of anus

S31 Open wound of abdomen, lower back, pelvis and external genitals
Code also any associated:
spinal cord injury (S24.0, S24.1-, S34.0-, S34.1-)
wound infection
EXCLUDES1 *traumatic amputation of part of abdomen, lower back and pelvis (S38.2-, S38.3)*
EXCLUDES2 *open wound of hip (S71.00-S71.02)*
open fracture of pelvis (S32.1--S32.9 with 7th character B)
The appropriate 7th character is to be added to each code from category S31
A = initial encounter
D = subsequent encounter
S = sequela
S31.0 Open wound of lower back and pelvis
S31.00 Unspecified open wound of lower back and pelvis
S31.000 Unspecified open wound of lower back and pelvis without penetration into retroperitoneum
Unspecified open wound of lower back and pelvis NOS
S31.001 Unspecified open wound of lower back and pelvis with penetration into retroperitoneum MCC
S31.01 Laceration without foreign body of lower back and pelvis
S31.010 Laceration without foreign body of lower back and pelvis without penetration into retroperitoneum
Laceration without foreign body of lower back and pelvis NOS
S31.011 Laceration without foreign body of lower back and pelvis with penetration into retroperitoneum MCC
S31.02 Laceration with foreign body of lower back and pelvis
S31.020 Laceration with foreign body of lower back and pelvis without penetration into retroperitoneum
Laceration with foreign body of lower back and pelvis NOS

Unspecified Code Other Specified Code Manifestation Code N Newborn P Pediatric M Maternity A Adult ♂ Male ♀ Female
● New Code ▲ Revised Code Title ►◄ Revised Text NOTES INCLUDES EXCLUDES1 Not coded here EXCLUDES2 Not included here
4th character required 5th character required 6th character required 7th character required
Extension 'X' Alert HAC Hospital-acquired condition (HAC) alert AHA AHA Coding Clinic©

S31.021 Laceration with foreign body of lower back and pelvis with penetration into retroperitoneum MCC

S31.03 Puncture wound without foreign body of lower back and pelvis

S31.030 Puncture wound without foreign body of lower back and pelvis without penetration into retroperitoneum
Puncture wound without foreign body of lower back and pelvis NOS

S31.031 Puncture wound without foreign body of lower back and pelvis with penetration into retroperitoneum MCC

S31.04 Puncture wound with foreign body of lower back and pelvis

S31.040 Puncture wound with foreign body of lower back and pelvis without penetration into retroperitoneum
Puncture wound with foreign body of lower back and pelvis NOS

S31.041 Puncture wound with foreign body of lower back and pelvis with penetration into retroperitoneum MCC

S31.05 Open bite of lower back and pelvis
Bite of lower back and pelvis NOS
EXCLUDES1 *superficial bite of lower back and pelvis (S30.860, S30.870)*

S31.050 Open bite of lower back and pelvis without penetration into retroperitoneum
Open bite of lower back and pelvis NOS

S31.051 Open bite of lower back and pelvis with penetration into retroperitoneum MCC

S31.1 Open wound of abdominal wall without penetration into peritoneal cavity
Open wound of abdominal wall NOS
EXCLUDES2 *open wound of abdominal wall with penetration into peritoneal cavity (S31.6-)*

S31.10 Unspecified open wound of abdominal wall without penetration into peritoneal cavity

S31.100 Unspecified open wound of abdominal wall, right upper quadrant without penetration into peritoneal cavity

S31.101 Unspecified open wound of abdominal wall, left upper quadrant without penetration into peritoneal cavity

S31.102 Unspecified open wound of abdominal wall, epigastric region without penetration into peritoneal cavity

S31.103 Unspecified open wound of abdominal wall, right lower quadrant without penetration into peritoneal cavity

S31.104 Unspecified open wound of abdominal wall, left lower quadrant without penetration into peritoneal cavity

S31.105 Unspecified open wound of abdominal wall, periumbilic region without penetration into peritoneal cavity

S31.109 Unspecified open wound of abdominal wall, unspecified quadrant without penetration into peritoneal cavity
Unspecified open wound of abdominal wall NOS

S31.11 Laceration without foreign body of abdominal wall without penetration into peritoneal cavity

S31.110 Laceration without foreign body of abdominal wall, right upper quadrant without penetration into peritoneal cavity

S31.111 Laceration without foreign body of abdominal wall, left upper quadrant without penetration into peritoneal cavity

S31.112 Laceration without foreign body of abdominal wall, epigastric region without penetration into peritoneal cavity

S31.113 Laceration without foreign body of abdominal wall, right lower quadrant without penetration into peritoneal cavity

S31.114 Laceration without foreign body of abdominal wall, left lower quadrant without penetration into peritoneal cavity

S31.115 Laceration without foreign body of abdominal wall, periumbilic region without penetration into peritoneal cavity

S31.119 Laceration without foreign body of abdominal wall, unspecified quadrant without penetration into peritoneal cavity

S31.12 Laceration with foreign body of abdominal wall without penetration into peritoneal cavity

S31.120 Laceration of abdominal wall with foreign body, right upper quadrant without penetration into peritoneal cavity

S31.121 Laceration of abdominal wall with foreign body, left upper quadrant without penetration into peritoneal cavity

S31.122 Laceration of abdominal wall with foreign body, epigastric region without penetration into peritoneal cavity

S31.123 Laceration of abdominal wall with foreign body, right lower quadrant without penetration into peritoneal cavity

S31.124 Laceration of abdominal wall with foreign body, left lower quadrant without penetration into peritoneal cavity

S31.125 Laceration of abdominal wall with foreign body, periumbilic region without penetration into peritoneal cavity

S31.129 Laceration of abdominal wall with foreign body, unspecified quadrant without penetration into peritoneal cavity

S31.13 Puncture wound of abdominal wall without foreign body without penetration into peritoneal cavity

S31.130 Puncture wound of abdominal wall without foreign body, right upper quadrant without penetration into peritoneal cavity

S31.131 Puncture wound of abdominal wall without foreign body, left upper quadrant without penetration into peritoneal cavity

S31.132 Puncture wound of abdominal wall without foreign body, epigastric region without penetration into peritoneal cavity

S31.133 Puncture wound of abdominal wall without foreign body, right lower quadrant without penetration into peritoneal cavity

S31.134 Puncture wound of abdominal wall without foreign body, left lower quadrant without penetration into peritoneal cavity

S31.135 Puncture wound of abdominal wall without foreign body, periumbilic region without penetration into peritoneal cavity

S31.139 Puncture wound of abdominal wall without foreign body, unspecified quadrant without penetration into peritoneal cavity

S31.14 Puncture wound of abdominal wall with foreign body without penetration into peritoneal cavity

S31.140 Puncture wound of abdominal wall with foreign body, right upper quadrant without penetration into peritoneal cavity

S31.141 Puncture wound of abdominal wall with foreign body, left upper quadrant without penetration into peritoneal cavity

S31.142 Puncture wound of abdominal wall with foreign body, epigastric region without penetration into peritoneal cavity

S31.143 Puncture wound of abdominal wall with foreign body, right lower quadrant without penetration into peritoneal cavity

S31.144 Puncture wound of abdominal wall with foreign body, left lower quadrant without penetration into peritoneal cavity

S31.145 Puncture wound of abdominal wall with foreign body, periumbilic region without penetration into peritoneal cavity

Unacceptable principal diagnosis symbol per Medicare code edits | Code exempt from diagnosis present on admission requirement | Questionable admission | Complication or comorbidity | CC/MCC exclusion | Major complication or comorbidity | Principal diagnosis as its own CC | Principal diagnosis as its own MCC | Z code as first-listed diagnosis

When symbols appear on a code that requires a 7th character extension, refer to Appendix D to identify applicable 7th character codes.

S31.149 Puncture wound of abdominal wall with foreign body, unspecified quadrant without penetration into peritoneal cavity

S31.15 Open bite of abdominal wall without penetration into peritoneal cavity
Bite of abdominal wall NOS
EXCLUDES1 *superficial bite of abdominal wall (S30.871)*

S31.150 Open bite of abdominal wall, right upper quadrant without penetration into peritoneal cavity
S31.151 Open bite of abdominal wall, left upper quadrant without penetration into peritoneal cavity
S31.152 Open bite of abdominal wall, epigastric region without penetration into peritoneal cavity
S31.153 Open bite of abdominal wall, right lower quadrant without penetration into peritoneal cavity
S31.154 Open bite of abdominal wall, left lower quadrant without penetration into peritoneal cavity
S31.155 Open bite of abdominal wall, periumbilic region without penetration into peritoneal cavity
S31.159 Open bite of abdominal wall, unspecified quadrant without penetration into peritoneal cavity

S31.2 Open wound of penis
S31.20 Unspecified open wound of penis ♂
S31.21 Laceration without foreign body of penis ♂
S31.22 Laceration with foreign body of penis ♂
S31.23 Puncture wound without foreign body of penis ♂
S31.24 Puncture wound with foreign body of penis ♂
S31.25 Open bite of penis ♂
Bite of penis NOS
EXCLUDES1 *superficial bite of penis (S30.862, S30.872)*

S31.3 Open wound of scrotum and testes
S31.30 Unspecified open wound of scrotum and testes ♂
S31.31 Laceration without foreign body of scrotum and testes ♂
S31.32 Laceration with foreign body of scrotum and testes ♂
S31.33 Puncture wound without foreign body of scrotum and testes ♂
S31.34 Puncture wound with foreign body of scrotum and testes ♂
S31.35 Open bite of scrotum and testes ♂
Bite of scrotum and testes NOS
EXCLUDES1 *superficial bite of scrotum and testes (S30.863, S30.873)*

S31.4 Open wound of vagina and vulva
EXCLUDES1 *injury to vagina and vulva during delivery (O70.-, O71.4)*
S31.40 Unspecified open wound of vagina and vulva ♀
S31.41 Laceration without foreign body of vagina and vulva ♀
S31.42 Laceration with foreign body of vagina and vulva ♀
S31.43 Puncture wound without foreign body of vagina and vulva ♀
S31.44 Puncture wound with foreign body of vagina and vulva ♀
S31.45 Open bite of vagina and vulva ♀
Bite of vagina and vulva NOS
EXCLUDES1 *superficial bite of vagina and vulva (S30.864, S30.874)*

S31.5 Open wound of unspecified external genital organs
EXCLUDES1 *traumatic amputation of external genital organs (S38.21, S38.22)*

S31.50 Unspecified open wound of unspecified external genital organs
S31.501 Unspecified open wound of unspecified external genital organs, male ♂
S31.502 Unspecified open wound of unspecified external genital organs, female ♀

S31.51 Laceration without foreign body of unspecified external genital organs
S31.511 Laceration without foreign body of unspecified external genital organs, male ♂
S31.512 Laceration without foreign body of unspecified external genital organs, female ♀

S31.52 Laceration with foreign body of unspecified external genital organs
S31.521 Laceration with foreign body of unspecified external genital organs, male ♂
S31.522 Laceration with foreign body of unspecified external genital organs, female ♀

S31.53 Puncture wound without foreign body of unspecified external genital organs
S31.531 Puncture wound without foreign body of unspecified external genital organs, male ♂
S31.532 Puncture wound without foreign body of unspecified external genital organs, female ♀

S31.54 Puncture wound with foreign body of unspecified external genital organs
S31.541 Puncture wound with foreign body of unspecified external genital organs, male ♂
S31.542 Puncture wound with foreign body of unspecified external genital organs, female ♀

S31.55 Open bite of unspecified external genital organs
Bite of unspecified external genital organs NOS
EXCLUDES1 *superficial bite of unspecified external genital organs (S30.865, S30.866, S30.875, S30.876)*
S31.551 Open bite of unspecified external genital organs, male ♂
S31.552 Open bite of unspecified external genital organs, female ♀

S31.6 Open wound of abdominal wall with penetration into peritoneal cavity

S31.60 Unspecified open wound of abdominal wall with penetration into peritoneal cavity
S31.600 Unspecified open wound of abdominal wall, right upper quadrant with penetration into peritoneal cavity MCC
S31.601 Unspecified open wound of abdominal wall, left upper quadrant with penetration into peritoneal cavity MCC
S31.602 Unspecified open wound of abdominal wall, epigastric region with penetration into peritoneal cavity MCC
S31.603 Unspecified open wound of abdominal wall, right lower quadrant with penetration into peritoneal cavity MCC
S31.604 Unspecified open wound of abdominal wall, left lower quadrant with penetration into peritoneal cavity MCC
S31.605 Unspecified open wound of abdominal wall, periumbilic region with penetration into peritoneal cavity MCC
S31.609 Unspecified open wound of abdominal wall, unspecified quadrant with penetration into peritoneal cavity MCC

S31.61 Laceration without foreign body of abdominal wall with penetration into peritoneal cavity
S31.610 Laceration without foreign body of abdominal wall, right upper quadrant with penetration into peritoneal cavity MCC
S31.611 Laceration without foreign body of abdominal wall, left upper quadrant with penetration into peritoneal cavity MCC
S31.612 Laceration without foreign body of abdominal wall, epigastric region with penetration into peritoneal cavity MCC

Unspecified Code Other Specified Code Manifestation Code N Newborn P Pediatric M Maternity A Adult ♂ Male ♀ Female
● New Code ▲ Revised Code Title ►◄ Revised Text NOTES INCLUDES EXCLUDES1 Not coded here EXCLUDES2 Not included here
4th character required 5th character required 6th character required 7th character required
Extension 'X' Alert HAC Hospital-acquired condition (HAC) alert AHA AHA Coding Clinic©

S31.613 Laceration without foreign body of abdominal wall, right lower quadrant with penetration into peritoneal cavity MCC
AHA: Q4, 2015

S31.614 Laceration without foreign body of abdominal wall, left lower quadrant with penetration into peritoneal cavity MCC

S31.615 Laceration without foreign body of abdominal wall, periumbilic region with penetration into peritoneal cavity MCC

S31.619 Laceration without foreign body of abdominal wall, unspecified quadrant with penetration into peritoneal cavity MCC

S31.62 Laceration with foreign body of abdominal wall with penetration into peritoneal cavity

S31.620 Laceration with foreign body of abdominal wall, right upper quadrant with penetration into peritoneal cavity MCC

S31.621 Laceration with foreign body of abdominal wall, left upper quadrant with penetration into peritoneal cavity MCC

S31.622 Laceration with foreign body of abdominal wall, epigastric region with penetration into peritoneal cavity MCC

S31.623 Laceration with foreign body of abdominal wall, right lower quadrant with penetration into peritoneal cavity MCC

S31.624 Laceration with foreign body of abdominal wall, left lower quadrant with penetration into peritoneal cavity MCC

S31.625 Laceration with foreign body of abdominal wall, periumbilic region with penetration into peritoneal cavity MCC

S31.629 Laceration with foreign body of abdominal wall, unspecified quadrant with penetration into peritoneal cavity MCC

S31.63 Puncture wound without foreign body of abdominal wall with penetration into peritoneal cavity

S31.630 Puncture wound without foreign body of abdominal wall, right upper quadrant with penetration into peritoneal cavity MCC

S31.631 Puncture wound without foreign body of abdominal wall, left upper quadrant with penetration into peritoneal cavity MCC

S31.632 Puncture wound without foreign body of abdominal wall, epigastric region with penetration into peritoneal cavity MCC

S31.633 Puncture wound without foreign body of abdominal wall, right lower quadrant with penetration into peritoneal cavity MCC

S31.634 Puncture wound without foreign body of abdominal wall, left lower quadrant with penetration into peritoneal cavity MCC

S31.635 Puncture wound without foreign body of abdominal wall, periumbilic region with penetration into peritoneal cavity MCC

S31.639 Puncture wound without foreign body of abdominal wall, unspecified quadrant with penetration into peritoneal cavity MCC

S31.64 Puncture wound with foreign body of abdominal wall with penetration into peritoneal cavity

S31.640 Puncture wound with foreign body of abdominal wall, right upper quadrant with penetration into peritoneal cavity MCC

S31.641 Puncture wound with foreign body of abdominal wall, left upper quadrant with penetration into peritoneal cavity MCC

S31.642 Puncture wound with foreign body of abdominal wall, epigastric region with penetration into peritoneal cavity MCC

S31.643 Puncture wound with foreign body of abdominal wall, right lower quadrant with penetration into peritoneal cavity MCC

S31.644 Puncture wound with foreign body of abdominal wall, left lower quadrant with penetration into peritoneal cavity MCC

S31.645 Puncture wound with foreign body of abdominal wall, periumbilic region with penetration into peritoneal cavity MCC

S31.649 Puncture wound with foreign body of abdominal wall, unspecified quadrant with penetration into peritoneal cavity MCC

S31.65 Open bite of abdominal wall with penetration into peritoneal cavity

EXCLUDES1 *superficial bite of abdominal wall (S30.861, S30.871)*

S31.650 Open bite of abdominal wall, right upper quadrant with penetration into peritoneal cavity MCC

S31.651 Open bite of abdominal wall, left upper quadrant with penetration into peritoneal cavity MCC

S31.652 Open bite of abdominal wall, epigastric region with penetration into peritoneal cavity MCC

S31.653 Open bite of abdominal wall, right lower quadrant with penetration into peritoneal cavity MCC

S31.654 Open bite of abdominal wall, left lower quadrant with penetration into peritoneal cavity MCC

S31.655 Open bite of abdominal wall, periumbilic region with penetration into peritoneal cavity MCC

S31.659 Open bite of abdominal wall, unspecified quadrant with penetration into peritoneal cavity MCC

S31.8 Open wound of other parts of abdomen, lower back and pelvis

S31.80 Open wound of unspecified buttock

S31.801 Laceration without foreign body of unspecified buttock

S31.802 Laceration with foreign body of unspecified buttock

S31.803 Puncture wound without foreign body of unspecified buttock

S31.804 Puncture wound with foreign body of unspecified buttock

S31.805 Open bite of unspecified buttock
Bite of buttock NOS
EXCLUDES1 *superficial bite of buttock (S30.870)*

S31.809 Unspecified open wound of unspecified buttock

S31.81 Open wound of right buttock

S31.811 Laceration without foreign body of right buttock

S31.812 Laceration with foreign body of right buttock

S31.813 Puncture wound without foreign body of right buttock

S31.814 Puncture wound with foreign body of right buttock

S31.815 Open bite of right buttock
Bite of right buttock NOS
EXCLUDES1 *superficial bite of buttock (S30.870)*

S31.819 Unspecified open wound of right buttock

S31.82 Open wound of left buttock

S31.821 Laceration without foreign body of left buttock

S31.822 Laceration with foreign body of left buttock

S31.823 Puncture wound without foreign body of left buttock

S31.824 Puncture wound with foreign body of left buttock

S31.825 Open bite of left buttock
Bite of left buttock NOS
EXCLUDES1 *superficial bite of buttock (S30.870)*

S31.829 Unspecified open wound of left buttock

PDx Unacceptable principal diagnosis symbol per Medicare code edits · POA Code exempt from diagnosis present on admission requirement
? Questionable admission · CC Complication or comorbidity · CC/MCC Exc CC/MCC exclusion · MCC Major complication or comorbidity
PDx CC Principal diagnosis as its own CC · PDx MCC Principal diagnosis as its own MCC · Z Z code as first-listed diagnosis

S31.83 Open wound of anus
- S31.831 Laceration without foreign body of anus
- S31.832 Laceration with foreign body of anus
- S31.833 Puncture wound without foreign body of anus
- S31.834 Puncture wound with foreign body of anus
- S31.835 Open bite of anus
  Bite of anus NOS
  EXCLUDES1 *superficial bite of anus (S30.877)*
- S31.839 Unspecified open wound of anus

S32 Fracture of lumbar spine and pelvis

NOTES A fracture not indicated as displaced or nondisplaced should be coded to displaced
A fracture not indicated as opened or closed should be coded to closed

INCLUDES *fracture of lumbosacral neural arch*
fracture of lumbosacral spinous process
fracture of lumbosacral transverse process
fracture of lumbosacral vertebra
fracture of lumbosacral vertebral arch

Code first any associated spinal cord and spinal nerve injury (S34.-)

EXCLUDES1 *transection of abdomen (S38.3)*

EXCLUDES2 *fracture of hip NOS (S72.0-)*

The appropriate 7th character is to be added to each code from category S32
- A = initial encounter for closed fracture
- B = initial encounter for open fracture
- D = subsequent encounter for fracture with routine healing
- G = subsequent encounter for fracture with delayed healing
- K = subsequent encounter for fracture with nonunion
- S = sequela

S32.0 Fracture of lumbar vertebra
Fracture of lumbar spine NOS

S32.00 Fracture of unspecified lumbar vertebra
- S32.000 Wedge compression fracture of unspecified lumbar vertebra CC HAC MCC
- S32.001 Stable burst fracture of unspecified lumbar vertebra CC HAC MCC
- S32.002 Unstable burst fracture of unspecified lumbar vertebra CC HAC MCC
- S32.008 Other fracture of unspecified lumbar vertebra CC HAC MCC
- S32.009 Unspecified fracture of unspecified lumbar vertebra CC HAC MCC

S32.01 Fracture of first lumbar vertebra
- S32.010 Wedge compression fracture of first lumbar vertebra CC HAC MCC
- S32.011 Stable burst fracture of first lumbar vertebra CC HAC MCC
- S32.012 Unstable burst fracture of first lumbar vertebra CC HAC MCC
- S32.018 Other fracture of first lumbar vertebra CC HAC MCC
- S32.019 Unspecified fracture of first lumbar vertebra CC HAC MCC

S32.02 Fracture of second lumbar vertebra
- S32.020 Wedge compression fracture of second lumbar vertebra CC HAC MCC
- S32.021 Stable burst fracture of second lumbar vertebra CC HAC MCC
- S32.022 Unstable burst fracture of second lumbar vertebra CC HAC MCC
- S32.028 Other fracture of second lumbar vertebra CC HAC MCC
- S32.029 Unspecified fracture of second lumbar vertebra CC HAC MCC

S32.03 Fracture of third lumbar vertebra
- S32.030 Wedge compression fracture of third lumbar vertebra CC HAC MCC
- S32.031 Stable burst fracture of third lumbar vertebra CC HAC MCC
- S32.032 Unstable burst fracture of third lumbar vertebra CC HAC MCC
- S32.038 Other fracture of third lumbar vertebra CC HAC MCC
- S32.039 Unspecified fracture of third lumbar vertebra CC HAC MCC

S32.04 Fracture of fourth lumbar vertebra
- S32.040 Wedge compression fracture of fourth lumbar vertebra CC HAC MCC
- S32.041 Stable burst fracture of fourth lumbar vertebra CC HAC MCC
- S32.042 Unstable burst fracture of fourth lumbar vertebra CC HAC MCC
- S32.048 Other fracture of fourth lumbar vertebra CC HAC MCC
- S32.049 Unspecified fracture of fourth lumbar vertebra CC HAC MCC

S32.05 Fracture of fifth lumbar vertebra
- S32.050 Wedge compression fracture of fifth lumbar vertebra CC HAC MCC
- S32.051 Stable burst fracture of fifth lumbar vertebra CC HAC MCC
- S32.052 Unstable burst fracture of fifth lumbar vertebra CC HAC MCC
- S32.058 Other fracture of fifth lumbar vertebra CC HAC MCC
- S32.059 Unspecified fracture of fifth lumbar vertebra CC HAC MCC

S32.1 Fracture of sacrum
For vertical fractures, code to most medial fracture extension
Use two codes if both a vertical and transverse fracture are present
Code also any associated fracture of pelvic ring (S32.8-)

- S32.10 Unspecified fracture of sacrum CC HAC MCC

S32.11 Zone I fracture of sacrum
Vertical sacral ala fracture of sacrum
- S32.110 Nondisplaced Zone I fracture of sacrum CC HAC MCC
- S32.111 Minimally displaced Zone I fracture of sacrum CC HAC MCC
- S32.112 Severely displaced Zone I fracture of sacrum CC HAC MCC
- S32.119 Unspecified Zone I fracture of sacrum CC HAC MCC

S32.12 Zone II fracture of sacrum
Vertical foraminal region fracture of sacrum
- S32.120 Nondisplaced Zone II fracture of sacrum CC HAC MCC
- S32.121 Minimally displaced Zone II fracture of sacrum CC HAC MCC
- S32.122 Severely displaced Zone II fracture of sacrum CC HAC MCC
- S32.129 Unspecified Zone II fracture of sacrum CC HAC MCC

S32.13 Zone III fracture of sacrum
Vertical fracture into spinal canal region of sacrum
- S32.130 Nondisplaced Zone III fracture of sacrum CC HAC MCC
- S32.131 Minimally displaced Zone III fracture of sacrum CC HAC MCC
- S32.132 Severely displaced Zone III fracture of sacrum CC HAC MCC
- S32.139 Unspecified Zone III fracture of sacrum CC HAC MCC

- S32.14 Type 1 fracture of sacrum CC HAC MCC
  Transverse flexion fracture of sacrum without displacement
- S32.15 Type 2 fracture of sacrum CC HAC MCC
  Transverse flexion fracture of sacrum with posterior displacement
- S32.16 Type 3 fracture of sacrum CC HAC MCC
  Transverse extension fracture of sacrum with anterior displacement
- S32.17 Type 4 fracture of sacrum CC HAC MCC
  Transverse segmental comminution of upper sacrum
- S32.19 Other fracture of sacrum CC HAC MCC

S32.2 Fracture of coccyx CC HAC MCC

S32.3 Fracture of ilium

Unspecified Code | Other Specified Code | Manifestation Code | N Newborn | P Pediatric | M Maternity | A Adult | ♂ Male | ♀ Female
● New Code ▲ Revised Code Title ►◄ Revised Text NOTES INCLUDES EXCLUDES1 Not coded here EXCLUDES2 Not included here
4th character required 5th character required 6th character required 7th character required
Extension 'X' Alert HAC Hospital-acquired condition (HAC) alert AHA AHA Coding Clinic®

When symbols appear on a code that requires a 7th character extension, refer to Appendix D to identify applicable 7th character codes.

EXCLUDES1 *fracture of ilium with associated disruption of pelvic ring (S32.8-)*

S32.30 Unspecified fracture of ilium
- S32.301 Unspecified fracture of right ilium CC HAC MCC
- S32.302 Unspecified fracture of left ilium CC HAC MCC
- S32.309 Unspecified fracture of unspecified ilium CC HAC MCC

S32.31 Avulsion fracture of ilium
- S32.311 Displaced avulsion fracture of right ilium CC HAC MCC
- S32.312 Displaced avulsion fracture of left ilium CC HAC MCC
- S32.313 Displaced avulsion fracture of unspecified ilium CC HAC MCC
- S32.314 Nondisplaced avulsion fracture of right ilium CC HAC MCC
- S32.315 Nondisplaced avulsion fracture of left ilium CC HAC MCC
- S32.316 Nondisplaced avulsion fracture of unspecified ilium CC HAC MCC

S32.39 Other fracture of ilium
- S32.391 Other fracture of right ilium CC HAC MCC
- S32.392 Other fracture of left ilium CC HAC MCC
- S32.399 Other fracture of unspecified ilium CC HAC MCC

S32.4 Fracture of acetabulum

Code also any associated fracture of pelvic ring (S32.8-)

S32.40 Unspecified fracture of acetabulum
- S32.401 Unspecified fracture of right acetabulum CC HAC MCC
- S32.402 Unspecified fracture of left acetabulum CC HAC MCC
- S32.409 Unspecified fracture of unspecified acetabulum CC HAC MCC

S32.41 Fracture of anterior wall of acetabulum
- S32.411 Displaced fracture of anterior wall of right acetabulum CC HAC MCC
- S32.412 Displaced fracture of anterior wall of left acetabulum CC HAC MCC
- S32.413 Displaced fracture of anterior wall of unspecified acetabulum CC HAC MCC
- S32.414 Nondisplaced fracture of anterior wall of right acetabulum CC HAC MCC
- S32.415 Nondisplaced fracture of anterior wall of left acetabulum CC HAC MCC
- S32.416 Nondisplaced fracture of anterior wall of unspecified acetabulum CC HAC MCC

S32.42 Fracture of posterior wall of acetabulum
- S32.421 Displaced fracture of posterior wall of right acetabulum CC HAC MCC
- S32.422 Displaced fracture of posterior wall of left acetabulum CC HAC MCC
- S32.423 Displaced fracture of posterior wall of unspecified acetabulum CC HAC MCC
- S32.424 Nondisplaced fracture of posterior wall of right acetabulum CC HAC MCC
- S32.425 Nondisplaced fracture of posterior wall of left acetabulum CC HAC MCC
- S32.426 Nondisplaced fracture of posterior wall of unspecified acetabulum CC HAC MCC

S32.43 Fracture of anterior column [iliopubic] of acetabulum
- S32.431 Displaced fracture of anterior column [iliopubic] of right acetabulum CC HAC MCC
- S32.432 Displaced fracture of anterior column [iliopubic] of left acetabulum CC HAC MCC
- S32.433 Displaced fracture of anterior column [iliopubic] of unspecified acetabulum CC HAC MCC
- S32.434 Nondisplaced fracture of anterior column [iliopubic] of right acetabulum CC HAC MCC
- S32.435 Nondisplaced fracture of anterior column [iliopubic] of left acetabulum CC HAC MCC
- S32.436 Nondisplaced fracture of anterior column [iliopubic] of unspecified acetabulum CC HAC MCC

S32.44 Fracture of posterior column [ilioischial] of acetabulum
- S32.441 Displaced fracture of posterior column [ilioischial] of right acetabulum CC HAC MCC
- S32.442 Displaced fracture of posterior column [ilioischial] of left acetabulum CC HAC MCC
- S32.443 Displaced fracture of posterior column [ilioischial] of unspecified acetabulum CC HAC MCC
- S32.444 Nondisplaced fracture of posterior column [ilioischial] of right acetabulum CC HAC MCC
- S32.445 Nondisplaced fracture of posterior column [ilioischial] of left acetabulum CC HAC MCC
- S32.446 Nondisplaced fracture of posterior column [ilioischial] of unspecified acetabulum CC HAC MCC

S32.45 Transverse fracture of acetabulum
- S32.451 Displaced transverse fracture of right acetabulum CC HAC MCC
- S32.452 Displaced transverse fracture of left acetabulum CC HAC MCC
- S32.453 Displaced transverse fracture of unspecified acetabulum CC HAC MCC
- S32.454 Nondisplaced transverse fracture of right acetabulum CC HAC MCC
- S32.455 Nondisplaced transverse fracture of left acetabulum CC HAC MCC
- S32.456 Nondisplaced transverse fracture of unspecified acetabulum CC HAC MCC

S32.46 Associated transverse-posterior fracture of acetabulum
- S32.461 Displaced associated transverse-posterior fracture of right acetabulum CC HAC MCC
- S32.462 Displaced associated transverse-posterior fracture of left acetabulum CC HAC MCC
- S32.463 Displaced associated transverse-posterior fracture of unspecified acetabulum CC HAC MCC
- S32.464 Nondisplaced associated transverse-posterior fracture of right acetabulum CC HAC MCC
- S32.465 Nondisplaced associated transverse-posterior fracture of left acetabulum CC HAC MCC
- S32.466 Nondisplaced associated transverse-posterior fracture of unspecified acetabulum CC HAC MCC

S32.47 Fracture of medial wall of acetabulum
- S32.471 Displaced fracture of medial wall of right acetabulum CC HAC MCC
- S32.472 Displaced fracture of medial wall of left acetabulum CC HAC MCC
- S32.473 Displaced fracture of medial wall of unspecified acetabulum CC HAC MCC
- S32.474 Nondisplaced fracture of medial wall of right acetabulum CC HAC MCC
- S32.475 Nondisplaced fracture of medial wall of left acetabulum CC HAC MCC
- S32.476 Nondisplaced fracture of medial wall of unspecified acetabulum CC HAC MCC

S32.48 Dome fracture of acetabulum
- S32.481 Displaced dome fracture of right acetabulum CC HAC MCC
- S32.482 Displaced dome fracture of left acetabulum CC HAC MCC
- S32.483 Displaced dome fracture of unspecified acetabulum CC HAC MCC
- S32.484 Nondisplaced dome fracture of right acetabulum CC HAC MCC
- S32.485 Nondisplaced dome fracture of left acetabulum CC HAC MCC

Unacceptable principal diagnosis symbol per Medicare code edits · Code exempt from diagnosis present on admission requirement · Questionable admission · CC Complication or comorbidity · CC/MCC Exclusion · MCC Major complication or comorbidity · Principal diagnosis as its own CC · Principal diagnosis as its own MCC · Z code as first-listed diagnosis

When symbols appear on a code that requires a 7th character extension, refer to Appendix D to identify applicable 7th character codes.

S32.486 Nondisplaced dome fracture of unspecified acetabulum CC HAC MCC

S32.49 Other specified fracture of acetabulum
S32.491 Other specified fracture of right acetabulum CC HAC MCC
S32.492 Other specified fracture of left acetabulum CC HAC MCC
S32.499 Other specified fracture of unspecified acetabulum CC HAC MCC

S32.5 Fracture of pubis
EXCLUDES1 *fracture of pubis with associated disruption of pelvic ring (S32.8-)*

S32.50 Unspecified fracture of pubis
S32.501 Unspecified fracture of right pubis CC HAC MCC
S32.502 Unspecified fracture of left pubis CC HAC MCC
S32.509 Unspecified fracture of unspecified pubis CC HAC MCC

S32.51 Fracture of superior rim of pubis
S32.511 Fracture of superior rim of right pubis CC HAC MCC
S32.512 Fracture of superior rim of left pubis CC HAC MCC
S32.519 Fracture of superior rim of unspecified pubis CC HAC MCC

S32.59 Other specified fracture of pubis
S32.591 Other specified fracture of right pubis CC HAC MCC
S32.592 Other specified fracture of left pubis CC HAC MCC
S32.599 Other specified fracture of unspecified pubis CC HAC MCC

S32.6 Fracture of ischium
EXCLUDES1 *fracture of ischium with associated disruption of pelvic ring (S32.8-)*

S32.60 Unspecified fracture of ischium
S32.601 Unspecified fracture of right ischium CC HAC MCC
S32.602 Unspecified fracture of left ischium CC HAC MCC
S32.609 Unspecified fracture of unspecified ischium CC HAC MCC

S32.61 Avulsion fracture of ischium
S32.611 Displaced avulsion fracture of right ischium CC HAC MCC
S32.612 Displaced avulsion fracture of left ischium CC HAC MCC
S32.613 Displaced avulsion fracture of unspecified ischium CC HAC MCC
S32.614 Nondisplaced avulsion fracture of right ischium CC HAC MCC
S32.615 Nondisplaced avulsion fracture of left ischium CC HAC MCC
S32.616 Nondisplaced avulsion fracture of unspecified ischium CC HAC MCC

S32.69 Other specified fracture of ischium
S32.691 Other specified fracture of right ischium CC HAC MCC
S32.692 Other specified fracture of left ischium CC HAC MCC
S32.699 Other specified fracture of unspecified ischium CC HAC MCC

S32.8 Fracture of other parts of pelvis
Code also any associated:
fracture of acetabulum (S32.4-)
sacral fracture (S32.1-)

S32.81 Multiple fractures of pelvis with disruption of pelvic ring
Multiple pelvic fractures with disruption of pelvic circle
S32.810 Multiple fractures of pelvis with stable disruption of pelvic ring CC HAC MCC
S32.811 Multiple fractures of pelvis with unstable disruption of pelvic ring CC HAC MCC

S32.82 Multiple fractures of pelvis without disruption of pelvic ring CC HAC MCC
Multiple pelvic fractures without disruption of pelvic circle
S32.89 Fracture of other parts of pelvis CC HAC MCC

S32.9 Fracture of unspecified parts of lumbosacral spine and pelvis CC HAC MCC
Fracture of lumbosacral spine NOS
Fracture of pelvis NOS

S33 Dislocation and sprain of joints and ligaments of lumbar spine and pelvis
INCLUDES *avulsion of joint or ligament of lumbar spine and pelvis*
laceration of cartilage, joint or ligament of lumbar spine and pelvis
sprain of cartilage, joint or ligament of lumbar spine and pelvis
traumatic hemarthrosis of joint or ligament of lumbar spine and pelvis
traumatic rupture of joint or ligament of lumbar spine and pelvis
traumatic subluxation of joint or ligament of lumbar spine and pelvis
traumatic tear of joint or ligament of lumbar spine and pelvis
Code also any associated open wound
EXCLUDES1 *nontraumatic rupture or displacement of lumbar intervertebral disc NOS (M51.-)*
obstetric damage to pelvic joints and ligaments (O71.6)
EXCLUDES2 *dislocation and sprain of joints and ligaments of hip (S73.-)*
strain of muscle of lower back and pelvis (S39.01-)

The appropriate 7th character is to be added to each code from category S33
A = initial encounter
D = subsequent encounter
S = sequela

S33.0 Traumatic rupture of lumbar intervertebral disc
EXCLUDES1 *rupture or displacement (nontraumatic) of lumbar intervertebral disc NOS (M51.- with fifth character 6)*

S33.1 Subluxation and dislocation of lumbar vertebra
Code also any associated:
open wound of abdomen, lower back and pelvis (S31)
spinal cord injury (S24.0, S24.1-, S34.0-, S34.1-)
EXCLUDES2 *fracture of lumbar vertebrae (S32.0-)*

S33.10 Subluxation and dislocation of unspecified lumbar vertebra
S33.100 Subluxation of unspecified lumbar vertebra
S33.101 Dislocation of unspecified lumbar vertebra

S33.11 Subluxation and dislocation of L1/L2 lumbar vertebra
S33.110 Subluxation of L1/L2 lumbar vertebra
S33.111 Dislocation of L1/L2 lumbar vertebra

S33.12 Subluxation and dislocation of L2/L3 lumbar vertebra
S33.120 Subluxation of L2/L3 lumbar vertebra
S33.121 Dislocation of L2/L3 lumbar vertebra

S33.13 Subluxation and dislocation of L3/L4 lumbar vertebra
S33.130 Subluxation of L3/L4 lumbar vertebra
S33.131 Dislocation of L3/L4 lumbar vertebra

S33.14 Subluxation and dislocation of L4/L5 lumbar vertebra
S33.140 Subluxation of L4/L5 lumbar vertebra
S33.141 Dislocation of L4/L5 lumbar vertebra

S33.2 Dislocation of sacroiliac and sacrococcygeal joint

S33.3 Dislocation of other and unspecified parts of lumbar spine and pelvis
S33.30 Dislocation of unspecified parts of lumbar spine and pelvis
S33.39 Dislocation of other parts of lumbar spine and pelvis

S33.4 Traumatic rupture of symphysis pubis
S33.5 Sprain of ligaments of lumbar spine
S33.6 Sprain of sacroiliac joint
S33.8 Sprain of other parts of lumbar spine and pelvis

Unspecified Code | Other Specified Code | Manifestation Code | N Newborn | P Pediatric | M Maternity | A Adult | ♂ Male | ♀ Female
● New Code | ▲ Revised Code Title | ►◄ Revised Text | NOTES | INCLUDES | EXCLUDES1 Not coded here | EXCLUDES2 Not included here
4th character required | 5th character required | 6th character required | 7th character required
Extension 'X' Alert | HAC Hospital-acquired condition (HAC) alert | AHA AHA Coding Clinic©

When symbols appear on a code that requires a 7th character extension, refer to Appendix D to identify applicable 7th character codes.

S33.9 Sprain of unspecified parts of lumbar spine and pelvis

S34 Injury of lumbar and sacral spinal cord and nerves at abdomen, lower back and pelvis level

NOTES Code to highest level of lumbar cord injury
Injuries to the spinal cord (S34.0 and S34.1) refer to the cord level and not bone level injury, and can affect nerve roots at and below the level given.

Code also any associated:
fracture of vertebra (S22.0-, S32.0-)
open wound of abdomen, lower back and pelvis (S31.-)
transient paralysis (R29.5)

The appropriate 7th character is to be added to each code from category S34
A = initial encounter
D = subsequent encounter
S = sequela

S34.0 Concussion and edema of lumbar and sacral spinal cord
S34.01 Concussion and edema of lumbar spinal cord MCC
S34.02 Concussion and edema of sacral spinal cord MCC
Concussion and edema of conus medullaris

S34.1 Other and unspecified injury of lumbar and sacral spinal cord
S34.10 Unspecified injury to lumbar spinal cord
S34.101 Unspecified injury to L1 level of lumbar spinal cord HAC MCC
Unspecified injury to lumbar spinal cord level 1
S34.102 Unspecified injury to L2 level of lumbar spinal cord HAC MCC
Unspecified injury to lumbar spinal cord level 2
S34.103 Unspecified injury to L3 level of lumbar spinal cord HAC MCC
Unspecified injury to lumbar spinal cord level 3
S34.104 Unspecified injury to L4 level of lumbar spinal cord HAC MCC
Unspecified injury to lumbar spinal cord level 4
S34.105 Unspecified injury to L5 level of lumbar spinal cord HAC MCC
Unspecified injury to lumbar spinal cord level 5
S34.109 Unspecified injury to unspecified level of lumbar spinal cord HAC MCC

S34.11 Complete lesion of lumbar spinal cord
S34.111 Complete lesion of L1 level of lumbar spinal cord HAC MCC
Complete lesion of lumbar spinal cord level 1
S34.112 Complete lesion of L2 level of lumbar spinal cord HAC MCC
Complete lesion of lumbar spinal cord level 2
S34.113 Complete lesion of L3 level of lumbar spinal cord HAC MCC
Complete lesion of lumbar spinal cord level 3
S34.114 Complete lesion of L4 level of lumbar spinal cord HAC MCC
Complete lesion of lumbar spinal cord level 4
S34.115 Complete lesion of L5 level of lumbar spinal cord HAC MCC
Complete lesion of lumbar spinal cord level 5
S34.119 Complete lesion of unspecified level of lumbar spinal cord HAC MCC

S34.12 Incomplete lesion of lumbar spinal cord
S34.121 Incomplete lesion of L1 level of lumbar spinal cord HAC MCC
Incomplete lesion of lumbar spinal cord level 1
S34.122 Incomplete lesion of L2 level of lumbar spinal cord HAC MCC
Incomplete lesion of lumbar spinal cord level 2
S34.123 Incomplete lesion of L3 level of lumbar spinal cord HAC MCC
Incomplete lesion of lumbar spinal cord level 3
S34.124 Incomplete lesion of L4 level of lumbar spinal cord HAC MCC
Incomplete lesion of lumbar spinal cord level 4
S34.125 Incomplete lesion of L5 level of lumbar spinal cord HAC MCC
Incomplete lesion of lumbar spinal cord level 5
S34.129 Incomplete lesion of unspecified level of lumbar spinal cord HAC MCC

S34.13 Other and unspecified injury to sacral spinal cord
Other injury to conus medullaris
S34.131 Complete lesion of sacral spinal cord HAC MCC
Complete lesion of conus medullaris
S34.132 Incomplete lesion of sacral spinal cord HAC MCC
Incomplete lesion of conus medullaris
S34.139 Unspecified injury to sacral spinal cord HAC MCC
Unspecified injury of conus medullaris

S34.2 Injury of nerve root of lumbar and sacral spine
S34.21 Injury of nerve root of lumbar spine
S34.22 Injury of nerve root of sacral spine

S34.3 Injury of cauda equina HAC MCC

S34.4 Injury of lumbosacral plexus

S34.5 Injury of lumbar, sacral and pelvic sympathetic nerves
Injury of celiac ganglion or plexus
Injury of hypogastric plexus
Injury of mesenteric plexus (inferior) (superior)
Injury of splanchnic nerve

S34.6 Injury of peripheral nerve(s) at abdomen, lower back and pelvis level

S34.8 Injury of other nerves at abdomen, lower back and pelvis level

S34.9 Injury of unspecified nerves at abdomen, lower back and pelvis level

S35 Injury of blood vessels at abdomen, lower back and pelvis level

Code also any associated open wound (S31.-)

The appropriate 7th character is to be added to each code from category S35
A = initial encounter
D = subsequent encounter
S = sequela

S35.0 Injury of abdominal aorta
EXCLUDES1 *injury of aorta NOS (S25.0)*
S35.00 Unspecified injury of abdominal aorta MCC
S35.01 Minor laceration of abdominal aorta MCC
Incomplete transection of abdominal aorta
Laceration of abdominal aorta NOS
Superficial laceration of abdominal aorta
S35.02 Major laceration of abdominal aorta MCC
Complete transection of abdominal aorta
Traumatic rupture of abdominal aorta
S35.09 Other injury of abdominal aorta MCC

S35.1 Injury of inferior vena cava
Injury of hepatic vein
EXCLUDES1 *injury of vena cava NOS (S25.2)*
S35.10 Unspecified injury of inferior vena cava MCC
S35.11 Minor laceration of inferior vena cava MCC
Incomplete transection of inferior vena cava
Laceration of inferior vena cava NOS
Superficial laceration of inferior vena cava
S35.12 Major laceration of inferior vena cava MCC
Complete transection of inferior vena cava
Traumatic rupture of inferior vena cava
S35.19 Other injury of inferior vena cava MCC

S35.2 Injury of celiac or mesenteric artery and branches
S35.21 Injury of celiac artery
S35.211 Minor laceration of celiac artery MCC
Incomplete transection of celiac artery
Laceration of celiac artery NOS

PDx Unacceptable principal diagnosis symbol per Medicare code edits | POA Code exempt from diagnosis present on admission requirement
? Questionable admission | CC Complication or comorbidity | CC/MCC Exc CC/MCC exclusion | MCC Major complication or comorbidity
PDx CC Principal diagnosis as its own CC | PDx MCC Principal diagnosis as its own MCC | Z1 Z code as first-listed diagnosis

Superficial laceration of celiac artery
S35.212 Major laceration of celiac artery MCC
Complete transection of celiac artery
Traumatic rupture of celiac artery
S35.218 Other injury of celiac artery MCC
S35.219 Unspecified injury of celiac artery MCC
S35.22 Injury of superior mesenteric artery
S35.221 Minor laceration of superior mesenteric artery MCC
Incomplete transection of superior mesenteric artery
Laceration of superior mesenteric artery NOS
Superficial laceration of superior mesenteric artery
S35.222 Major laceration of superior mesenteric artery MCC
Complete transection of superior mesenteric artery
Traumatic rupture of superior mesenteric artery
S35.228 Other injury of superior mesenteric artery MCC
S35.229 Unspecified injury of superior mesenteric artery MCC
S35.23 Injury of inferior mesenteric artery
S35.231 Minor laceration of inferior mesenteric artery MCC
Incomplete transection of inferior mesenteric artery
Laceration of inferior mesenteric artery NOS
Superficial laceration of inferior mesenteric artery
S35.232 Major laceration of inferior mesenteric artery MCC
Complete transection of inferior mesenteric artery
Traumatic rupture of inferior mesenteric artery
S35.238 Other injury of inferior mesenteric a rtery MCC
S35.239 Unspecified injury of inferior mesenteric artery MCC
S35.29 Injury of branches of celiac and mesenteric artery
Injury of gastric artery
Injury of gastroduodenal artery
Injury of hepatic artery
Injury of splenic artery
S35.291 Minor laceration of branches of celiac and mesenteric artery MCC
Incomplete transection of branches of celiac and mesenteric artery
Laceration of branches of celiac and mesenteric artery NOS
Superficial laceration of branches of celiac and mesenteric artery
S35.292 Major laceration of branches of celiac and mesenteric artery MCC
Complete transection of branches of celiac and mesenteric artery
Traumatic rupture of branches of celiac and mesenteric artery
S35.298 Other injury of branches of celiac and mesenteric artery MCC
S35.299 Unspecified injury of branches of celiac and mesenteric artery MCC
S35.3 Injury of portal or splenic vein and branches
S35.31 Injury of portal vein
S35.311 Laceration of portal vein MCC
S35.318 Other specified injury of portal vein MCC
S35.319 Unspecified injury of portal vein MCC
S35.32 Injury of splenic vein
S35.321 Laceration of splenic vein MCC
S35.328 Other specified injury of splenic vein MCC
S35.329 Unspecified injury of splenic vein MCC
S35.33 Injury of superior mesenteric vein
S35.331 Laceration of superior mesenteric vein MCC
S35.338 Other specified injury of superior mesenteric vein MCC
S35.339 Unspecified injury of superior mesenteric vein MCC
S35.34 Injury of inferior mesenteric vein
S35.341 Laceration of inferior mesenteric vein MCC
S35.348 Other specified injury of inferior mesenteric vein MCC
S35.349 Unspecified injury of inferior mesenteric vein MCC
S35.4 Injury of renal blood vessels
S35.40 Unspecified injury of renal blood vessel
S35.401 Unspecified injury of right renal artery MCC
S35.402 Unspecified injury of left renal artery MCC
S35.403 Unspecified injury of unspecified renal artery MCC
S35.404 Unspecified injury of right renal vein MCC
S35.405 Unspecified injury of left renal vein MCC
S35.406 Unspecified injury of unspecified renal vein MCC
S35.41 Laceration of renal blood vessel
S35.411 Laceration of right renal artery MCC
S35.412 Laceration of left renal artery MCC
S35.413 Laceration of unspecified renal artery MCC
S35.414 Laceration of right renal vein MCC
S35.415 Laceration of left renal vein MCC
S35.416 Laceration of unspecified renal vein MCC
S35.49 Other specified injury of renal blood vessel
S35.491 Other specified injury of right renal artery MCC
S35.492 Other specified injury of left renal artery MCC
S35.493 Other specified injury of unspecified renal artery MCC
S35.494 Other specified injury of right renal vein MCC
S35.495 Other specified injury of left renal vein MCC
S35.496 Other specified injury of unspecified renal vein MCC
S35.5 Injury of iliac blood vessels
S35.50 Injury of unspecified iliac blood vessel(s) MCC
S35.51 Injury of iliac artery or vein
Injury of hypogastric artery or vein
S35.511 Injury of right iliac artery MCC
S35.512 Injury of left iliac artery MCC
S35.513 Injury of unspecified iliac artery MCC
S35.514 Injury of right iliac vein MCC
S35.515 Injury of left iliac vein MCC
S35.516 Injury of unspecified iliac vein MCC
S35.53 Injury of uterine artery or vein
S35.531 Injury of right uterine artery CC ♀
S35.532 Injury of left uterine artery CC ♀
S35.533 Injury of unspecified uterine artery CC ♀
S35.534 Injury of right uterine vein CC ♀
S35.535 Injury of left uterine vein CC ♀
S35.536 Injury of unspecified uterine vein CC ♀
S35.59 Injury of other iliac blood vessels MCC
S35.8 Injury of other blood vessels at abdomen, lower back and pelvis level
Injury of ovarian artery or vein
S35.8X Injury of other blood vessels at abdomen, lower back and pelvis level
S35.8X1 Laceration of other blood vessels at abdomen, lower back and pelvis level CC
S35.8X8 Other specified injury of other blood vessels at abdomen, lower back and pelvis level CC
S35.8X9 Unspecified injury of other blood vessels at abdomen, lower back and pelvis level CC
S35.9 Injury of unspecified blood vessel at abdomen, lower back and pelvis level
S35.90 Unspecified injury of unspecified blood vessel at abdomen, lower back and pelvis level CC

Unspecified Code Other Specified Code Manifestation Code N Newborn P Pediatric M Maternity A Adult ♂ Male ♀ Female
● New Code ▲ Revised Code Title ►◄ Revised Text NOTES INCLUDES EXCLUDES1 Not coded here EXCLUDES2 Not included here
4th character required 5th character required 6th character required 7th character required
Extension 'X' Alert HAC Hospital-acquired condition (HAC) alert AHA AHA Coding Clinic©

S35.91 Laceration of unspecified blood vessel at abdomen, lower back and pelvis level CC
S35.99 Other specified injury of unspecified blood vessel at abdomen, lower back and pelvis level CC

S36 Injury of intra-abdominal organs
Code also any associated open wound (S31.-)
The appropriate 7th character is to be added to each code from category S36
A = initial encounter
D = subsequent encounter
S = sequela

S36.0 Injury of spleen
- S36.00 Unspecified injury of spleen CC
- S36.02 Contusion of spleen
  - S36.020 Minor contusion of spleen CC
    Contusion of spleen less than 2 cm
  - S36.021 Major contusion of spleen CC
    Contusion of spleen greater than 2 cm
  - S36.029 Unspecified contusion of spleen CC
    AHA: Q1, 2015
- S36.03 Laceration of spleen
  - S36.030 Superficial (capsular) laceration of spleen CC
    Laceration of spleen less than 1 cm
    Minor laceration of spleen
  - S36.031 Moderate laceration of spleen MCC
    Laceration of spleen 1 to 3 cm
  - S36.032 Major laceration of spleen MCC
    Avulsion of spleen
    Laceration of spleen greater than 3 cm
    Massive laceration of spleen
    Multiple moderate lacerations of spleen
    Stellate laceration of spleen
  - S36.039 Unspecified laceration of spleen CC
- S36.09 Other injury of spleen CC

S36.1 Injury of liver and gallbladder and bile duct
- S36.11 Injury of liver
  - S36.112 Contusion of liver CC
  - S36.113 Laceration of liver, unspecified degree CC
  - S36.114 Minor laceration of liver CC
    Laceration involving capsule only, or, without significant involvement of hepatic parenchyma [i.e., less than 1 cm deep]
  - S36.115 Moderate laceration of liver MCC
    Laceration involving parenchyma but without major disruption of parenchyma [i.e., less than 10 cm long and less than 3 cm deep]
  - S36.116 Major laceration of liver MCC
    Laceration with significant disruption of hepatic parenchyma [i.e., greater than 10 cm long and 3 cm deep]
    Multiple moderate lacerations, with or without hematoma
    Stellate laceration of liver
  - S36.118 Other injury of liver CC
  - S36.119 Unspecified injury of liver CC
- S36.12 Injury of gallbladder
  - S36.122 Contusion of gallbladder CC
  - S36.123 Laceration of gallbladder CC
  - S36.128 Other injury of gallbladder CC
  - S36.129 Unspecified injury of gallbladder CC
- S36.13 Injury of bile duct CC

S36.2 Injury of pancreas
- S36.20 Unspecified injury of pancreas
  - S36.200 Unspecified injury of head of pancreas CC
  - S36.201 Unspecified injury of body of pancreas CC
  - S36.202 Unspecified injury of tail of pancreas CC
  - S36.209 Unspecified injury of unspecified part of pancreas CC
- S36.22 Contusion of pancreas
  - S36.220 Contusion of head of pancreas CC
  - S36.221 Contusion of body of pancreas CC
  - S36.222 Contusion of tail of pancreas CC
  - S36.229 Contusion of unspecified part of pancreas CC
- S36.23 Laceration of pancreas, unspecified degree
  - S36.230 Laceration of head of pancreas, unspecified degree CC
  - S36.231 Laceration of body of pancreas, unspecified degree CC
  - S36.232 Laceration of tail of pancreas, unspecified degree CC
  - S36.239 Laceration of unspecified part of pancreas, unspecified degree CC
- S36.24 Minor laceration of pancreas
  - S36.240 Minor laceration of head of pancreas CC
  - S36.241 Minor laceration of body of pancreas CC
  - S36.242 Minor laceration of tail of pancreas CC
  - S36.249 Minor laceration of unspecified part of pancreas CC
- S36.25 Moderate laceration of pancreas
  - S36.250 Moderate laceration of head of pancreas CC
  - S36.251 Moderate laceration of body of pancreas CC
  - S36.252 Moderate laceration of tail of pancreas CC
  - S36.259 Moderate laceration of unspecified part of pancreas CC
- S36.26 Major laceration of pancreas
  - S36.260 Major laceration of head of pancreas CC
  - S36.261 Major laceration of body of pancreas CC
  - S36.262 Major laceration of tail of pancreas CC
  - S36.269 Major laceration of unspecified part of pancreas CC
- S36.29 Other injury of pancreas
  - S36.290 Other injury of head of pancreas CC
  - S36.291 Other injury of body of pancreas CC
  - S36.292 Other injury of tail of pancreas CC
  - S36.299 Other injury of unspecified part of pancreas CC

S36.3 Injury of stomach
- S36.30 Unspecified injury of stomach CC
- S36.32 Contusion of stomach CC
- S36.33 Laceration of stomach CC
- S36.39 Other injury of stomach CC

S36.4 Injury of small intestine
- S36.40 Unspecified injury of small intestine
  - S36.400 Unspecified injury of duodenum CC
  - S36.408 Unspecified injury of other part of small intestine CC
  - S36.409 Unspecified injury of unspecified part of small intestine CC
- S36.41 Primary blast injury of small intestine
  Blast injury of small intestine NOS
  - S36.410 Primary blast injury of duodenum CC
  - S36.418 Primary blast injury of other part of small intestine CC
  - S36.419 Primary blast injury of unspecified part of small intestine CC
- S36.42 Contusion of small intestine
  - S36.420 Contusion of duodenum CC
  - S36.428 Contusion of other part of small intestine CC
  - S36.429 Contusion of unspecified part of small intestine CC
- S36.43 Laceration of small intestine
  - S36.430 Laceration of duodenum CC
  - S36.438 Laceration of other part of small intestine CC
  - S36.439 Laceration of unspecified part of small intestine CC
- S36.49 Other injury of small intestine
  - S36.490 Other injury of duodenum CC
  - S36.498 Other injury of other part of small intestine CC
  - S36.499 Other injury of unspecified part of small intestine CC

Unacceptable principal diagnosis symbol per Medicare code edits | Code exempt from diagnosis present on admission requirement
Questionable admission | Complication or comorbidity | CC/MCC exclusion | Major complication or comorbidity
Principal diagnosis as its own CC | Principal diagnosis as its own MCC | Z code as first-listed diagnosis

S36.5 Injury of colon
EXCLUDES2 injury of rectum (S36.6-)
S36.50 Unspecified injury of colon
S36.500 Unspecified injury of ascending [right] colon
S36.501 Unspecified injury of transverse colon
S36.502 Unspecified injury of descending [left] colon
S36.503 Unspecified injury of sigmoid colon
S36.508 Unspecified injury of other part of colon
S36.509 Unspecified injury of unspecified part of colon
S36.51 Primary blast injury of colon
Blast injury of colon NOS
S36.510 Primary blast injury of ascending [right] colon
S36.511 Primary blast injury of transverse colon
S36.512 Primary blast injury of descending [left] colon
S36.513 Primary blast injury of sigmoid colon
S36.518 Primary blast injury of other part of colon
S36.519 Primary blast injury of unspecified part of colon
S36.52 Contusion of colon
S36.520 Contusion of ascending [right] colon
S36.521 Contusion of transverse colon
S36.522 Contusion of descending [left] colon
S36.523 Contusion of sigmoid colon
S36.528 Contusion of other part of colon
S36.529 Contusion of unspecified part of colon
S36.53 Laceration of colon
S36.530 Laceration of ascending [right] colon
S36.531 Laceration of transverse colon
S36.532 Laceration of descending [left] colon
S36.533 Laceration of sigmoid colon
S36.538 Laceration of other part of colon
S36.539 Laceration of unspecified part of colon
S36.59 Other injury of colon
Secondary blast injury of colon
S36.590 Other injury of ascending [right] colon
S36.591 Other injury of transverse colon
S36.592 Other injury of descending [left] colon
S36.593 Other injury of sigmoid colon
S36.598 Other injury of other part of colon
S36.599 Other injury of unspecified part of colon
S36.6 Injury of rectum
S36.60 Unspecified injury of rectum
S36.61 Primary blast injury of rectum
Blast injury of rectum NOS
S36.62 Contusion of rectum
S36.63 Laceration of rectum
S36.69 Other injury of rectum
Secondary blast injury of rectum
S36.8 Injury of other intra-abdominal organs
S36.81 Injury of peritoneum
S36.89 Injury of other intra-abdominal organs
Injury of retroperitoneum
S36.892 Contusion of other intra-abdominal organs
S36.893 Laceration of other intra-abdominal organs
S36.898 Other injury of other intra-abdominal organs
S36.899 Unspecified injury of other intra-abdominal organs
S36.9 Injury of unspecified intra-abdominal organ
S36.90 Unspecified injury of unspecified intra-abdominal organ
S36.92 Contusion of unspecified intra-abdominal organ
S36.93 Laceration of unspecified intra-abdominal organ
S36.99 Other injury of unspecified intra-abdominal organ

S37 Injury of urinary and pelvic organs
Code also any associated open wound (S31.-)
EXCLUDES1 obstetric trauma to pelvic organs (O71.-)
EXCLUDES2 injury of peritoneum (S36.81)
injury of retroperitoneum (S36.89-)
The appropriate 7th character is to be added to each code from category S37
A = initial encounter
D = subsequent encounter
S = sequela
S37.0 Injury of kidney
EXCLUDES2 acute kidney injury (nontraumatic) (N17.9)
S37.00 Unspecified injury of kidney
S37.001 Unspecified injury of right kidney
S37.002 Unspecified injury of left kidney
S37.009 Unspecified injury of unspecified kidney
S37.01 Minor contusion of kidney
Contusion of kidney less than 2 cm
Contusion of kidney NOS
S37.011 Minor contusion of right kidney
S37.012 Minor contusion of left kidney
S37.019 Minor contusion of unspecified kidney
S37.02 Major contusion of kidney
Contusion of kidney greater than 2 cm
S37.021 Major contusion of right kidney
S37.022 Major contusion of left kidney
S37.029 Major contusion of unspecified kidney
S37.03 Laceration of kidney, unspecified degree
S37.031 Laceration of right kidney, unspecified degree
S37.032 Laceration of left kidney, unspecified degree
S37.039 Laceration of unspecified kidney, unspecified degree
S37.04 Minor laceration of kidney
Laceration of kidney less than 1 cm
S37.041 Minor laceration of right kidney
S37.042 Minor laceration of left kidney
S37.049 Minor laceration of unspecified kidney
S37.05 Moderate laceration of kidney
Laceration of kidney 1 to 3 cm
S37.051 Moderate laceration of right kidney
S37.052 Moderate laceration of left kidney
S37.059 Moderate laceration of unspecified kidney
S37.06 Major laceration of kidney
Avulsion of kidney
Laceration of kidney greater than 3 cm
Massive laceration of kidney
Multiple moderate lacerations of kidney
Stellate laceration of kidney
S37.061 Major laceration of right kidney MCC
S37.062 Major laceration of left kidney MCC
S37.069 Major laceration of unspecified kidney MCC
S37.09 Other injury of kidney
S37.091 Other injury of right kidney MCC
S37.092 Other injury of left kidney MCC
S37.099 Other injury of unspecified kidney MCC
S37.1 Injury of ureter
S37.10 Unspecified injury of ureter
S37.12 Contusion of ureter
S37.13 Laceration of ureter
S37.19 Other injury of ureter
S37.2 Injury of bladder
S37.20 Unspecified injury of bladder
S37.22 Contusion of bladder
S37.23 Laceration of bladder
S37.29 Other injury of bladder
S37.3 Injury of urethra
S37.30 Unspecified injury of urethra
S37.32 Contusion of urethra
S37.33 Laceration of urethra

Unspecified Code Other Specified Code Manifestation Code N Newborn P Pediatric M Maternity A Adult ♂ Male ♀ Female
● New Code ▲ Revised Code Title ►◄ Revised Text NOTES INCLUDES EXCLUDES1 Not coded here EXCLUDES2 Not included here
4th character required 5th character required 6th character required 7th character required
Extension 'X' Alert HAC Hospital-acquired condition (HAC) alert AHA AHA Coding Clinic©

S37.39 Other injury of urethra

S37.4 Injury of ovary

S37.40 Unspecified injury of ovary

S37.401 Unspecified injury of ovary, unilateral ♀

S37.402 Unspecified injury of ovary, bilateral ♀

S37.409 Unspecified injury of ovary, unspecified ♀

S37.42 Contusion of ovary

S37.421 Contusion of ovary, unilateral ♀

S37.422 Contusion of ovary, bilateral ♀

S37.429 Contusion of ovary, unspecified ♀

S37.43 Laceration of ovary

S37.431 Laceration of ovary, unilateral ♀

S37.432 Laceration of ovary, bilateral ♀

S37.439 Laceration of ovary, unspecified ♀

S37.49 Other injury of ovary

S37.491 Other injury of ovary, unilateral ♀

S37.492 Other injury of ovary, bilateral ♀

S37.499 Other injury of ovary, unspecified ♀

S37.5 Injury of fallopian tube

S37.50 Unspecified injury of fallopian tube

S37.501 Unspecified injury of fallopian tube, unilateral ♀

S37.502 Unspecified injury of fallopian tube, bilateral ♀

S37.509 Unspecified injury of fallopian tube, unspecified ♀

S37.51 Primary blast injury of fallopian tube

Blast injury of fallopian tube NOS

S37.511 Primary blast injury of fallopian tube, unilateral ♀

S37.512 Primary blast injury of fallopian tube, bilateral ♀

S37.519 Primary blast injury of fallopian tube, unspecified ♀

S37.52 Contusion of fallopian tube

S37.521 Contusion of fallopian tube, unilateral ♀

S37.522 Contusion of fallopian tube, bilateral ♀

S37.529 Contusion of fallopian tube, unspecified ♀

S37.53 Laceration of fallopian tube

S37.531 Laceration of fallopian tube, unilateral ♀

S37.532 Laceration of fallopian tube, bilateral ♀

S37.539 Laceration of fallopian tube, unspecified ♀

S37.59 Other injury of fallopian tube

Secondary blast injury of fallopian tube

S37.591 Other injury of fallopian tube, unilateral ♀

S37.592 Other injury of fallopian tube, bilateral ♀

S37.599 Other injury of fallopian tube, unspecified ♀

S37.6 Injury of uterus

EXCLUDES1 *injury to gravid uterus (O9A.2-)*

injury to uterus during delivery (O71.-)

S37.60 Unspecified injury of uterus ♀

S37.62 Contusion of uterus ♀

S37.63 Laceration of uterus ♀

S37.69 Other injury of uterus ♀

S37.8 Injury of other urinary and pelvic organs

S37.81 Injury of adrenal gland

S37.812 Contusion of adrenal gland

S37.813 Laceration of adrenal gland

S37.818 Other injury of adrenal gland

S37.819 Unspecified injury of adrenal gland

S37.82 Injury of prostate

S37.822 Contusion of prostate ♂

S37.823 Laceration of prostate ♂

S37.828 Other injury of prostate ♂

S37.829 Unspecified injury of prostate ♂

S37.89 Injury of other urinary and pelvic organ

S37.892 Contusion of other urinary and pelvic organ

S37.893 Laceration of other urinary and pelvic organ

S37.898 Other injury of other urinary and pelvic organ

S37.899 Unspecified injury of other urinary and pelvic organ

S37.9 Injury of unspecified urinary and pelvic organ

S37.90 Unspecified injury of unspecified urinary and pelvic organ

S37.92 Contusion of unspecified urinary and pelvic organ

S37.93 Laceration of unspecified urinary and pelvic organ

S37.99 Other injury of unspecified urinary and pelvic organ

S38 Crushing injury and traumatic amputation of abdomen, lower back, pelvis and external genitals

An amputation not identified as partial or complete should be coded to complete

The appropriate 7th character is to be added to each code from category S38

A = initial encounter

D = subsequent encounter

S = sequela

S38.0 Crushing injury of external genital organs

Use additional code for any associated injuries

S38.00 Crushing injury of unspecified external genital organs

S38.001 Crushing injury of unspecified external genital organs, male ♂

S38.002 Crushing injury of unspecified external genital organs, female ♀

S38.01 Crushing injury of penis ♂

S38.02 Crushing injury of scrotum and testis ♂

S38.03 Crushing injury of vulva ♀

S38.1 Crushing injury of abdomen, lower back, and pelvis

Use additional code for all associated injuries, such as:

fracture of thoracic or lumbar spine and pelvis (S22.0-, S32.-)

injury to intra-abdominal organs (S36.-)

injury to urinary and pelvic organs (S37.-)

open wound of abdominal wall (S31.-)

spinal cord injury (S34.0, S34.1-)

EXCLUDES2 *crushing injury of external genital organs (S38.0-)*

S38.2 Traumatic amputation of external genital organs

S38.21 Traumatic amputation of female external genital organs

Traumatic amputation of clitoris

Traumatic amputation of labium (majus) (minus)

Traumatic amputation of vulva

S38.211 Complete traumatic amputation of female external genital organs ♀

S38.212 Partial traumatic amputation of female external genital organs ♀

S38.22 Traumatic amputation of penis

S38.221 Complete traumatic amputation of penis ♂

S38.222 Partial traumatic amputation of penis ♂

S38.23 Traumatic amputation of scrotum and testis

S38.231 Complete traumatic amputation of scrotum and testis ♂

S38.232 Partial traumatic amputation of scrotum and testis ♂

S38.3 Transection (partial) of abdomen

S39 Other and unspecified injuries of abdomen, lower back, pelvis and external genitals

Code also any associated open wound (S31.-)

EXCLUDES2 *sprain of joints and ligaments of lumbar spine and pelvis (S33.-)*

The appropriate 7th character is to be added to each code from category S39

A = initial encounter

D = subsequent encounter

S = sequela

S39.0 Injury of muscle, fascia and tendon of abdomen, lower back and pelvis

S39.00 Unspecified injury of muscle, fascia and tendon of abdomen, lower back and pelvis

S39.001 Unspecified injury of muscle, fascia and tendon of abdomen

Unacceptable principal diagnosis symbol per Medicare code edits — Code exempt from diagnosis present on admission requirement — Questionable admission — Complication or comorbidity — CC/MCC exclusion — Major complication or comorbidity — Principal diagnosis as its own CC — Principal diagnosis as its own MCC — Z code as first-listed diagnosis

 When symbols appear on a code that requires a 7th character extension, refer to Appendix D to identify applicable 7th character codes.

S39.002 Unspecified injury of muscle, fascia and tendon of lower back
S39.003 Unspecified injury of muscle, fascia and tendon of pelvis
S39.01 Strain of muscle, fascia and tendon of abdomen, lower back and pelvis
S39.011 Strain of muscle, fascia and tendon of abdomen
S39.012 Strain of muscle, fascia and tendon of lower back
S39.013 Strain of muscle, fascia and tendon of pelvis
S39.02 Laceration of muscle, fascia and tendon of abdomen, lower back and pelvis
S39.021 Laceration of muscle, fascia and tendon of abdomen
S39.022 Laceration of muscle, fascia and tendon of lower back
S39.023 Laceration of muscle, fascia and tendon of pelvis
S39.09 Other injury of muscle, fascia and tendon of abdomen, lower back and pelvis
S39.091 Other injury of muscle, fascia and tendon of abdomen
S39.092 Other injury of muscle, fascia and tendon of lower back
S39.093 Other injury of muscle, fascia and tendon of pelvis
S39.8 Other specified injuries of abdomen, lower back, pelvis and external genitals
S39.81 Other specified injuries of abdomen
S39.82 Other specified injuries of lower back
S39.83 Other specified injuries of pelvis
S39.84 Other specified injuries of external genitals
S39.840 Fracture of corpus cavernosum penis ♂
S39.848 Other specified injuries of external genitals
S39.9 Unspecified injury of abdomen, lower back, pelvis and external genitals
S39.91 Unspecified injury of abdomen
S39.92 Unspecified injury of lower back
S39.93 Unspecified injury of pelvis
S39.94 Unspecified injury of external genitals

Injuries to the shoulder and upper arm (S40-S49)

INCLUDES *injuries of axilla*
injuries of scapular region

EXCLUDES2 *burns and corrosions (T20-T32)*
frostbite (T33-T34)
injuries of elbow (S50-S59)
insect bite or sting, venomous (T63.4)

S40 Superficial injury of shoulder and upper arm
The appropriate 7th character is to be added to each code from category S40
A = initial encounter
D = subsequent encounter
S = sequela
S40.0 Contusion of shoulder and upper arm
S40.01 Contusion of shoulder
S40.011 Contusion of right shoulder
S40.012 Contusion of left shoulder
S40.019 Contusion of unspecified shoulder
S40.02 Contusion of upper arm
S40.021 Contusion of right upper arm
S40.022 Contusion of left upper arm
S40.029 Contusion of unspecified upper arm
S40.2 Other superficial injuries of shoulder
S40.21 Abrasion of shoulder
S40.211 Abrasion of right shoulder
S40.212 Abrasion of left shoulder
S40.219 Abrasion of unspecified shoulder
S40.22 Blister (nonthermal) of shoulder
S40.221 Blister (nonthermal) of right shoulder
S40.222 Blister (nonthermal) of left shoulder
S40.229 Blister (nonthermal) of unspecified shoulder
S40.24 External constriction of shoulder
S40.241 External constriction of right shoulder
S40.242 External constriction of left shoulder
S40.249 External constriction of unspecified shoulder
S40.25 Superficial foreign body of shoulder
Splinter in the shoulder
S40.251 Superficial foreign body of right shoulder
S40.252 Superficial foreign body of left shoulder
S40.259 Superficial foreign body of unspecified shoulder
S40.26 Insect bite (nonvenomous) of shoulder
S40.261 Insect bite (nonvenomous) of right shoulder
S40.262 Insect bite (nonvenomous) of left shoulder
S40.269 Insect bite (nonvenomous) of unspecified shoulder
S40.27 Other superficial bite of shoulder
EXCLUDES1 *open bite of shoulder (S41.05)*
S40.271 Other superficial bite of right shoulder
S40.272 Other superficial bite of left shoulder
S40.279 Other superficial bite of unspecified shoulder
S40.8 Other superficial injuries of upper arm
S40.81 Abrasion of upper arm
S40.811 Abrasion of right upper arm
S40.812 Abrasion of left upper arm
S40.819 Abrasion of unspecified upper arm
S40.82 Blister (nonthermal) of upper arm
S40.821 Blister (nonthermal) of right upper arm
S40.822 Blister (nonthermal) of left upper arm
S40.829 Blister (nonthermal) of unspecified upper arm
S40.84 External constriction of upper arm
S40.841 External constriction of right upper arm
S40.842 External constriction of left upper arm
S40.849 External constriction of unspecified upper arm
S40.85 Superficial foreign body of upper arm
Splinter in the upper arm
S40.851 Superficial foreign body of right upper arm
S40.852 Superficial foreign body of left upper arm
S40.859 Superficial foreign body of unspecified upper arm
S40.86 Insect bite (nonvenomous) of upper arm
S40.861 Insect bite (nonvenomous) of right upper arm
S40.862 Insect bite (nonvenomous) of left upper arm
S40.869 Insect bite (nonvenomous) of unspecified upper arm
S40.87 Other superficial bite of upper arm
EXCLUDES1 *open bite of upper arm (S41.14)*
EXCLUDES2 *other superficial bite of shoulder (S40.27-)*
S40.871 Other superficial bite of right upper arm
S40.872 Other superficial bite of left upper arm
S40.879 Other superficial bite of unspecified upper arm
S40.9 Unspecified superficial injury of shoulder and upper arm
S40.91 Unspecified superficial injury of shoulder
S40.911 Unspecified superficial injury of right shoulder
S40.912 Unspecified superficial injury of left shoulder
S40.919 Unspecified superficial injury of unspecified shoulder
S40.92 Unspecified superficial injury of upper arm

Unspecified Code Other Specified Code Manifestation Code N Newborn P Pediatric M Maternity A Adult ♂ Male ♀ Female
● New Code ▲ Revised Code Title ►◄ Revised Text NOTES INCLUDES EXCLUDES1 Not coded here EXCLUDES2 Not included here
4th character required 5th character required 6th character required 7th character required
Extension 'X' Alert HAC Hospital-acquired condition (HAC) alert AHA AHA Coding Clinic©

S40.921 Unspecified superficial injury of right upper arm
S40.922 Unspecified superficial injury of left upper arm
S40.929 Unspecified superficial injury of unspecified upper arm

S41 Open wound of shoulder and upper arm
Code also any associated wound infection
EXCLUDES1 *traumatic amputation of shoulder and upper arm (S48.-)*
EXCLUDES2 *open fracture of shoulder and upper arm (S42.- with 7th character B or C)*
The appropriate 7th character is to be added to each code from category S41
A = initial encounter
D = subsequent encounter
S = sequela

S41.0 Open wound of shoulder
S41.00 Unspecified open wound of shoulder
S41.001 Unspecified open wound of right shoulder
S41.002 Unspecified open wound of left shoulder
S41.009 Unspecified open wound of unspecified shoulder
S41.01 Laceration without foreign body of shoulder
S41.011 Laceration without foreign body of right shoulder
S41.012 Laceration without foreign body of left shoulder
S41.019 Laceration without foreign body of unspecified shoulder
S41.02 Laceration with foreign body of shoulder
S41.021 Laceration with foreign body of right shoulder
S41.022 Laceration with foreign body of left shoulder
S41.029 Laceration with foreign body of unspecified shoulder
S41.03 Puncture wound without foreign body of shoulder
S41.031 Puncture wound without foreign body of right shoulder
S41.032 Puncture wound without foreign body of left shoulder
S41.039 Puncture wound without foreign body of unspecified shoulder
S41.04 Puncture wound with foreign body of shoulder
S41.041 Puncture wound with foreign body of right shoulder
S41.042 Puncture wound with foreign body of left shoulder
S41.049 Puncture wound with foreign body of unspecified shoulder
S41.05 Open bite of shoulder
Bite of shoulder NOS
EXCLUDES1 *superficial bite of shoulder (S40.27)*
S41.051 Open bite of right shoulder
S41.052 Open bite of left shoulder
S41.059 Open bite of unspecified shoulder

S41.1 Open wound of upper arm
S41.10 Unspecified open wound of upper arm
S41.101 Unspecified open wound of right upper arm
S41.102 Unspecified open wound of left upper arm
S41.109 Unspecified open wound of unspecified upper arm
S41.11 Laceration without foreign body of upper arm
S41.111 Laceration without foreign body of right upper arm
S41.112 Laceration without foreign body of left upper arm
S41.119 Laceration without foreign body of unspecified upper arm
S41.12 Laceration with foreign body of upper arm
S41.121 Laceration with foreign body of right upper arm
S41.122 Laceration with foreign body of left upper arm
S41.129 Laceration with foreign body of unspecified upper arm
S41.13 Puncture wound without foreign body of upper arm
S41.131 Puncture wound without foreign body of right upper arm
S41.132 Puncture wound without foreign body of left upper arm
S41.139 Puncture wound without foreign body of unspecified upper arm
S41.14 Puncture wound with foreign body of upper arm
S41.141 Puncture wound with foreign body of right upper arm
S41.142 Puncture wound with foreign body of left upper arm
S41.149 Puncture wound with foreign body of unspecified upper arm
S41.15 Open bite of upper arm
Bite of upper arm NOS
EXCLUDES1 *superficial bite of upper arm (S40.87)*
S41.151 Open bite of right upper arm
S41.152 Open bite of left upper arm
S41.159 Open bite of unspecified upper arm

S42 Fracture of shoulder and upper arm
NOTES A fracture not indicated as displaced or nondisplaced should be coded to displaced
A fracture not indicated as open or closed should be coded to closed
EXCLUDES1 *traumatic amputation of shoulder and upper arm (S48.-)*
The appropriate 7th character is to be added to all codes from category S42
A = initial encounter for closed fracture
B = initial encounter for open fracture
D = subsequent encounter for fracture with routine healing
G = subsequent encounter for fracture with delayed healing
K = subsequent encounter for fracture with nonunion
P = subsequent encounter for fracture with malunion
S = sequela

S42.0 Fracture of clavicle
S42.00 Fracture of unspecified part of clavicle
S42.001 Fracture of unspecified part of right clavicle CC HAC
S42.002 Fracture of unspecified part of left clavicle CC HAC
S42.009 Fracture of unspecified part of unspecified clavicle CC HAC
S42.01 Fracture of sternal end of clavicle
S42.011 Anterior displaced fracture of sternal end of right clavicle CC HAC
S42.012 Anterior displaced fracture of sternal end of left clavicle CC HAC
S42.013 Anterior displaced fracture of sternal end of unspecified clavicle CC HAC
Displaced fracture of sternal end of clavicle NOS
S42.014 Posterior displaced fracture of sternal end of right clavicle CC HAC
S42.015 Posterior displaced fracture of sternal end of left clavicle CC HAC
S42.016 Posterior displaced fracture of sternal end of unspecified clavicle CC HAC
S42.017 Nondisplaced fracture of sternal end of right clavicle CC HAC
S42.018 Nondisplaced fracture of sternal end of left clavicle CC HAC
S42.019 Nondisplaced fracture of sternal end of unspecified clavicle CC HAC
S42.02 Fracture of shaft of clavicle
S42.021 Displaced fracture of shaft of right clavicle CC HAC
S42.022 Displaced fracture of shaft of left clavicle CC HAC
S42.023 Displaced fracture of shaft of unspecified clavicle CC HAC

Unacceptable principal diagnosis symbol per Medicare code edits — Code exempt from diagnosis present on admission requirement
Questionable admission — Complication or comorbidity — CC/MCC exclusion — Major complication or comorbidity
Principal diagnosis as its own CC — Principal diagnosis as its own MCC — Z code as first-listed diagnosis

S42.024 Nondisplaced fracture of shaft of right clavicle
S42.025 Nondisplaced fracture of shaft of left clavicle
S42.026 Nondisplaced fracture of shaft of unspecified clavicle

S42.03 Fracture of lateral end of clavicle
Fracture of acromial end of clavicle
S42.031 Displaced fracture of lateral end of right clavicle
S42.032 Displaced fracture of lateral end of left clavicle
S42.033 Displaced fracture of lateral end of unspecified clavicle
S42.034 Nondisplaced fracture of lateral end of right clavicle
S42.035 Nondisplaced fracture of lateral end of left clavicle
S42.036 Nondisplaced fracture of lateral end of unspecified clavicle

S42.1 Fracture of scapula

S42.10 Fracture of unspecified part of scapula
S42.101 Fracture of unspecified part of scapula, right shoulder
S42.102 Fracture of unspecified part of scapula, left shoulder
S42.109 Fracture of unspecified part of scapula, unspecified shoulder

S42.11 Fracture of body of scapula
S42.111 Displaced fracture of body of scapula, right shoulder
S42.112 Displaced fracture of body of scapula, left shoulder
S42.113 Displaced fracture of body of scapula, unspecified shoulder
S42.114 Nondisplaced fracture of body of scapula, right shoulder
S42.115 Nondisplaced fracture of body of scapula, left shoulder
S42.116 Nondisplaced fracture of body of scapula, unspecified shoulder

S42.12 Fracture of acromial process
S42.121 Displaced fracture of acromial process, right shoulder
S42.122 Displaced fracture of acromial process, left shoulder
S42.123 Displaced fracture of acromial process, unspecified shoulder
S42.124 Nondisplaced fracture of acromial process, right shoulder
S42.125 Nondisplaced fracture of acromial process, left shoulder
S42.126 Nondisplaced fracture of acromial process, unspecified shoulder

S42.13 Fracture of coracoid process
S42.131 Displaced fracture of coracoid process, right shoulder
S42.132 Displaced fracture of coracoid process, left shoulder
S42.133 Displaced fracture of coracoid process, unspecified shoulder
S42.134 Nondisplaced fracture of coracoid process, right shoulder
S42.135 Nondisplaced fracture of coracoid process, left shoulder
S42.136 Nondisplaced fracture of coracoid process, unspecified shoulder

S42.14 Fracture of glenoid cavity of scapula
S42.141 Displaced fracture of glenoid cavity of scapula, right shoulder
S42.142 Displaced fracture of glenoid cavity of scapula, left shoulder
S42.143 Displaced fracture of glenoid cavity of scapula, unspecified shoulder
S42.144 Nondisplaced fracture of glenoid cavity of scapula, right shoulder
S42.145 Nondisplaced fracture of glenoid cavity of scapula, left shoulder
S42.146 Nondisplaced fracture of glenoid cavity of scapula, unspecified shoulder

S42.15 Fracture of neck of scapula
S42.151 Displaced fracture of neck of scapula, right shoulder
S42.152 Displaced fracture of neck of scapula, left shoulder
S42.153 Displaced fracture of neck of scapula, unspecified shoulder
S42.154 Nondisplaced fracture of neck of scapula, right shoulder
S42.155 Nondisplaced fracture of neck of scapula, left shoulder
S42.156 Nondisplaced fracture of neck of scapula, unspecified shoulder

S42.19 Fracture of other part of scapula
S42.191 Fracture of other part of scapula, right shoulder
S42.192 Fracture of other part of scapula, left shoulder
S42.199 Fracture of other part of scapula, unspecified shoulder

S42.2 Fracture of upper end of humerus
Fracture of proximal end of humerus
EXCLUDES2 *fracture of shaft of humerus (S42.3-)*
physeal fracture of upper end of humerus (S49.0-)

S42.20 Unspecified fracture of upper end of humerus
S42.201 Unspecified fracture of upper end of right humerus
S42.202 Unspecified fracture of upper end of left humerus
S42.209 Unspecified fracture of upper end of unspecified humerus

S42.21 Unspecified fracture of surgical neck of humerus
Fracture of neck of humerus NOS
S42.211 Unspecified displaced fracture of surgical neck of right humerus
S42.212 Unspecified displaced fracture of surgical neck of left humerus
S42.213 Unspecified displaced fracture of surgical neck of unspecified humerus
S42.214 Unspecified nondisplaced fracture of surgical neck of right humerus
S42.215 Unspecified nondisplaced fracture of surgical neck of left humerus
S42.216 Unspecified nondisplaced fracture of surgical neck of unspecified humerus

S42.22 2-part fracture of surgical neck of humerus
S42.221 2-part displaced fracture of surgical neck of right humerus
S42.222 2-part displaced fracture of surgical neck of left humerus
S42.223 2-part displaced fracture of surgical neck of unspecified humerus
S42.224 2-part nondisplaced fracture of surgical neck of right humerus
S42.225 2-part nondisplaced fracture of surgical neck of left humerus
S42.226 2-part nondisplaced fracture of surgical neck of unspecified humerus

S42.23 3-part fracture of surgical neck of humerus
S42.231 3-part fracture of surgical neck of right humerus
S42.232 3-part fracture of surgical neck of left humerus
S42.239 3-part fracture of surgical neck of unspecified humerus

S42.24 4-part fracture of surgical neck of humerus
S42.241 4-part fracture of surgical neck of right humerus
S42.242 4-part fracture of surgical neck of left humerus

Unspecified Code Other Specified Code Manifestation Code N Newborn P Pediatric M Maternity A Adult ♂ Male ♀ Female
● New Code ▲ Revised Code Title ►◄ Revised Text NOTES INCLUDES EXCLUDES1 Not coded here EXCLUDES2 Not included here
4th character required 5th character required 6th character required 7th character required
Extension 'X' Alert HAC Hospital-acquired condition (HAC) alert AHA AHA Coding Clinic®

S42.249 4-part fracture of surgical neck of unspecified humerus CC HAC MCC

S42.25 Fracture of greater tuberosity of humerus

S42.251 Displaced fracture of greater tuberosity of right humerus CC HAC MCC

S42.252 Displaced fracture of greater tuberosity of left humerus CC HAC MCC

S42.253 Displaced fracture of greater tuberosity of unspecified humerus CC HAC MCC

S42.254 Nondisplaced fracture of greater tuberosity of right humerus CC HAC MCC

S42.255 Nondisplaced fracture of greater tuberosity of left humerus CC HAC MCC

S42.256 Nondisplaced fracture of greater tuberosity of unspecified humerus CC HAC MCC

S42.26 Fracture of lesser tuberosity of humerus

S42.261 Displaced fracture of lesser tuberosity of right humerus CC HAC MCC

S42.262 Displaced fracture of lesser tuberosity of left humerus CC HAC MCC

S42.263 Displaced fracture of lesser tuberosity of unspecified humerus CC HAC MCC

S42.264 Nondisplaced fracture of lesser tuberosity of right humerus CC HAC MCC

S42.265 Nondisplaced fracture of lesser tuberosity of left humerus CC HAC MCC

S42.266 Nondisplaced fracture of lesser tuberosity of unspecified humerus CC HAC MCC

S42.27 Torus fracture of upper end of humerus

The appropriate 7th character is to be added to all codes in subcategory S42.27

A = initial encounter for closed fracture
D = subsequent encounter for fracture with routine healing
G = subsequent encounter for fracture with delayed healing
K = subsequent encounter for fracture with nonunion
P = subsequent encounter for fracture with malunion
S = sequela

S42.271 Torus fracture of upper end of right humerus CC HAC

S42.272 Torus fracture of upper end of left humerus CC HAC

S42.279 Torus fracture of upper end of unspecified humerus CC HAC

S42.29 Other fracture of upper end of humerus

Fracture of anatomical neck of humerus
Fracture of articular head of humerus

S42.291 Other displaced fracture of upper end of right humerus CC HAC MCC

S42.292 Other displaced fracture of upper end of left humerus CC HAC MCC

S42.293 Other displaced fracture of upper end of unspecified humerus CC HAC MCC

S42.294 Other nondisplaced fracture of upper end of right humerus CC HAC MCC

S42.295 Other nondisplaced fracture of upper end of left humerus CC HAC MCC

S42.296 Other nondisplaced fracture of upper end of unspecified humerus CC HAC MCC

S42.3 Fracture of shaft of humerus

Fracture of humerus NOS
Fracture of upper arm NOS

EXCLUDES2 *physeal fractures of upper end of humerus (S49.0-)*
physeal fractures of lower end of humerus (S49.1-)

S42.30 Unspecified fracture of shaft of humerus

S42.301 Unspecified fracture of shaft of humerus, right arm CC HAC MCC

S42.302 Unspecified fracture of shaft of humerus, left arm CC HAC MCC

S42.309 Unspecified fracture of shaft of humerus, unspecified arm CC HAC MCC

S42.31 Greenstick fracture of shaft of humerus

The appropriate 7th character is to be added to all codes in subcategory S42.31

A = initial encounter for closed fracture
D = subsequent encounter for fracture with routine healing
G = subsequent encounter for fracture with delayed healing
K = subsequent encounter for fracture with nonunion
P = subsequent encounter for fracture with malunion
S = sequela

S42.311 Greenstick fracture of shaft of humerus, right arm CC HAC

S42.312 Greenstick fracture of shaft of humerus, left arm CC HAC

S42.319 Greenstick fracture of shaft of humerus, unspecified arm CC HAC

S42.32 Transverse fracture of shaft of humerus

S42.321 Displaced transverse fracture of shaft of humerus, right arm CC HAC MCC

S42.322 Displaced transverse fracture of shaft of humerus, left arm CC HAC MCC

S42.323 Displaced transverse fracture of shaft of humerus, unspecified arm CC HAC MCC

S42.324 Nondisplaced transverse fracture of shaft of humerus, right arm CC HAC MCC

S42.325 Nondisplaced transverse fracture of shaft of humerus, left arm CC HAC MCC

S42.326 Nondisplaced transverse fracture of shaft of humerus, unspecified arm CC HAC MCC

S42.33 Oblique fracture of shaft of humerus

S42.331 Displaced oblique fracture of shaft of humerus, right arm CC HAC MCC

S42.332 Displaced oblique fracture of shaft of humerus, left arm CC HAC MCC

S42.333 Displaced oblique fracture of shaft of humerus, unspecified arm CC HAC MCC

S42.334 Nondisplaced oblique fracture of shaft of humerus, right arm CC HAC MCC

S42.335 Nondisplaced oblique fracture of shaft of humerus, left arm CC HAC MCC

S42.336 Nondisplaced oblique fracture of shaft of humerus, unspecified arm CC HAC MCC

S42.34 Spiral fracture of shaft of humerus

S42.341 Displaced spiral fracture of shaft of humerus, right arm CC HAC MCC

S42.342 Displaced spiral fracture of shaft of humerus, left arm CC HAC MCC

S42.343 Displaced spiral fracture of shaft of humerus, unspecified arm CC HAC MCC

S42.344 Nondisplaced spiral fracture of shaft of humerus, right arm CC HAC MCC

S42.345 Nondisplaced spiral fracture of shaft of humerus, left arm CC HAC MCC

S42.346 Nondisplaced spiral fracture of shaft of humerus, unspecified arm CC HAC MCC

S42.35 Comminuted fracture of shaft of humerus

S42.351 Displaced comminuted fracture of shaft of humerus, right arm CC HAC MCC

S42.352 Displaced comminuted fracture of shaft of humerus, left arm CC HAC MCC

S42.353 Displaced comminuted fracture of shaft of humerus, unspecified arm CC HAC MCC

S42.354 Nondisplaced comminuted fracture of shaft of humerus, right arm CC HAC MCC

S42.355 Nondisplaced comminuted fracture of shaft of humerus, left arm CC HAC MCC

S42.356 Nondisplaced comminuted fracture of shaft of humerus, unspecified arm CC HAC MCC

S42.36 Segmental fracture of shaft of humerus

S42.361 Displaced segmental fracture of shaft of humerus, right arm CC HAC MCC

S42.362 Displaced segmental fracture of shaft of humerus, left arm CC HAC MCC

Unacceptable principal diagnosis symbol per Medicare code edits — Code exempt from diagnosis present on admission requirement
Questionable admission — Complication or comorbidity — CC/MCC exclusion — Major complication or comorbidity
Principal diagnosis as its own CC — Principal diagnosis as its own MCC — Z code as first-listed diagnosis

S42.363 Displaced segmental fracture of shaft of humerus, unspecified arm
S42.364 Nondisplaced segmental fracture of shaft of humerus, right arm
S42.365 Nondisplaced segmental fracture of shaft of humerus, left arm
S42.366 Nondisplaced segmental fracture of shaft of humerus, unspecified arm
S42.39 Other fracture of shaft of humerus
S42.391 Other fracture of shaft of right humerus
S42.392 Other fracture of shaft of left humerus
S42.399 Other fracture of shaft of unspecified humerus
S42.4 Fracture of lower end of humerus
Fracture of distal end of humerus
EXCLUDES2 *fracture of shaft of humerus (S42.3-)*
physeal fracture of lower end of humerus (S49.1-)
S42.40 Unspecified fracture of lower end of humerus
Fracture of elbow NOS
S42.401 Unspecified fracture of lower end of right humerus
S42.402 Unspecified fracture of lower end of left humerus
S42.409 Unspecified fracture of lower end of unspecified humerus
S42.41 Simple supracondylar fracture without intercondylar fracture of humerus
S42.411 Displaced simple supracondylar fracture without intercondylar fracture of right humerus
S42.412 Displaced simple supracondylar fracture without intercondylar fracture of left humerus
S42.413 Displaced simple supracondylar fracture without intercondylar fracture of unspecified humerus
S42.414 Nondisplaced simple supracondylar fracture without intercondylar fracture of right humerus
S42.415 Nondisplaced simple supracondylar fracture without intercondylar fracture of left humerus
S42.416 Nondisplaced simple supracondylar fracture without intercondylar fracture of unspecified humerus
S42.42 Comminuted supracondylar fracture without intercondylar fracture of humerus
S42.421 Displaced comminuted supracondylar fracture without intercondylar fracture of right humerus
S42.422 Displaced comminuted supracondylar fracture without intercondylar fracture of left humerus
S42.423 Displaced comminuted supracondylar fracture without intercondylar fracture of unspecified humerus
S42.424 Nondisplaced comminuted supracondylar fracture without intercondylar fracture of right humerus
S42.425 Nondisplaced comminuted supracondylar fracture without intercondylar fracture of left humerus
S42.426 Nondisplaced comminuted supracondylar fracture without intercondylar fracture of unspecified humerus
S42.43 Fracture (avulsion) of lateral epicondyle of humerus
S42.431 Displaced fracture (avulsion) of lateral epicondyle of right humerus
S42.432 Displaced fracture (avulsion) of lateral epicondyle of left humerus
S42.433 Displaced fracture (avulsion) of lateral epicondyle of unspecified humerus
S42.434 Nondisplaced fracture (avulsion) of lateral epicondyle of right humerus
S42.435 Nondisplaced fracture (avulsion) of lateral epicondyle of left humerus
S42.436 Nondisplaced fracture (avulsion) of lateral epicondyle of unspecified humerus
S42.44 Fracture (avulsion) of medial epicondyle of humerus
S42.441 Displaced fracture (avulsion) of medial epicondyle of right humerus
S42.442 Displaced fracture (avulsion) of medial epicondyle of left humerus
S42.443 Displaced fracture (avulsion) of medial epicondyle of unspecified humerus
S42.444 Nondisplaced fracture (avulsion) of medial epicondyle of right humerus
S42.445 Nondisplaced fracture (avulsion) of medial epicondyle of left humerus
S42.446 Nondisplaced fracture (avulsion) of medial epicondyle of unspecified humerus
S42.447 Incarcerated fracture (avulsion) of medial epicondyle of right humerus
S42.448 Incarcerated fracture (avulsion) of medial epicondyle of left humerus
S42.449 Incarcerated fracture (avulsion) of medial epicondyle of unspecified humerus
S42.45 Fracture of lateral condyle of humerus
Fracture of capitellum of humerus
S42.451 Displaced fracture of lateral condyle of right humerus
S42.452 Displaced fracture of lateral condyle of left humerus
S42.453 Displaced fracture of lateral condyle of unspecified humerus
S42.454 Nondisplaced fracture of lateral condyle of right humerus
S42.455 Nondisplaced fracture of lateral condyle of left humerus
S42.456 Nondisplaced fracture of lateral condyle of unspecified humerus
S42.46 Fracture of medial condyle of humerus
Trochlea fracture of humerus
S42.461 Displaced fracture of medial condyle of right humerus
S42.462 Displaced fracture of medial condyle of left humerus
S42.463 Displaced fracture of medial condyle of unspecified humerus
S42.464 Nondisplaced fracture of medial condyle of right humerus
S42.465 Nondisplaced fracture of medial condyle of left humerus
S42.466 Nondisplaced fracture of medial condyle of unspecified humerus
S42.47 Transcondylar fracture of humerus
S42.471 Displaced transcondylar fracture of right humerus
S42.472 Displaced transcondylar fracture of left humerus
S42.473 Displaced transcondylar fracture of unspecified humerus
S42.474 Nondisplaced transcondylar fracture of right humerus
S42.475 Nondisplaced transcondylar fracture of left humerus
S42.476 Nondisplaced transcondylar fracture of unspecified humerus
S42.48 Torus fracture of lower end of humerus
The appropriate 7th character is to be added to all codes in subcategory S42.48
A = initial encounter for closed fracture
D = subsequent encounter for fracture with routine healing

Unspecified Code Other Specified Code Manifestation Code N Newborn P Pediatric M Maternity A Adult ♂ Male ♀ Female
● New Code ▲ Revised Code Title ►◄ Revised Text NOTES INCLUDES EXCLUDES1 Not coded here EXCLUDES2 Not included here
4th character required 5th character required 6th character required 7th character required
Extension 'X' Alert HAC Hospital-acquired condition (HAC) alert AHA AHA Coding Clinic©

G = subsequent encounter for fracture with delayed healing
K = subsequent encounter for fracture with nonunion
P = subsequent encounter for fracture with malunion
S = sequela

- S42.481 Torus fracture of lower end of right humerus CC HAC
- S42.482 Torus fracture of lower end of left humerus CC HAC
- S42.489 Torus fracture of lower end of unspecified humerus CC HAC

S42.49 Other fracture of lower end of humerus
- S42.491 Other displaced fracture of lower end of right humerus CC HAC MCC
- S42.492 Other displaced fracture of lower end of left humerus CC HAC MCC
- S42.493 Other displaced fracture of lower end of unspecified humerus CC HAC MCC
- S42.494 Other nondisplaced fracture of lower end of right humerus CC HAC MCC
- S42.495 Other nondisplaced fracture of lower end of left humerus CC HAC MCC
- S42.496 Other nondisplaced fracture of lower end of unspecified humerus CC HAC MCC

S42.9 Fracture of shoulder girdle, part unspecified
Fracture of shoulder NOS
- S42.90 Fracture of unspecified shoulder girdle, part unspecified CC HAC MCC
- S42.91 Fracture of right shoulder girdle, part unspecified CC HAC MCC
- S42.92 Fracture of left shoulder girdle, part unspecified CC HAC MCC

S43 Dislocation and sprain of joints and ligaments of shoulder girdle

INCLUDES *avulsion of joint or ligament of shoulder girdle*
laceration of cartilage, joint or ligament of shoulder girdle
sprain of cartilage, joint or ligament of shoulder girdle
traumatic hemarthrosis of joint or ligament of shoulder girdle
traumatic rupture of joint or ligament of shoulder girdle
traumatic subluxation of joint or ligament of shoulder girdle
traumatic tear of joint or ligament of shoulder girdle

Code also any associated open wound

EXCLUDES2 *strain of muscle, fascia and tendon of shoulder and upper arm (S46.-)*

The appropriate 7th character is to be added to each code from category S43
A = initial encounter
D = subsequent encounter
S = sequela

S43.0 Subluxation and dislocation of shoulder joint
Dislocation of glenohumeral joint
Subluxation of glenohumeral joint

S43.00 Unspecified subluxation and dislocation of shoulder joint
Dislocation of humerus NOS
Subluxation of humerus NOS
- S43.001 Unspecified subluxation of right shoulder joint
- S43.002 Unspecified subluxation of left shoulder joint
- S43.003 Unspecified subluxation of unspecified shoulder joint
- S43.004 Unspecified dislocation of right shoulder joint
- S43.005 Unspecified dislocation of left shoulder joint
- S43.006 Unspecified dislocation of unspecified shoulder joint

S43.01 Anterior subluxation and dislocation of humerus
- S43.011 Anterior subluxation of right humerus
- S43.012 Anterior subluxation of left humerus
- S43.013 Anterior subluxation of unspecified humerus
- S43.014 Anterior dislocation of right humerus
- S43.015 Anterior dislocation of left humerus
- S43.016 Anterior dislocation of unspecified humerus

S43.02 Posterior subluxation and dislocation of humerus
- S43.021 Posterior subluxation of right humerus
- S43.022 Posterior subluxation of left humerus
- S43.023 Posterior subluxation of unspecified humerus
- S43.024 Posterior dislocation of right humerus
- S43.025 Posterior dislocation of left humerus
- S43.026 Posterior dislocation of unspecified humerus

S43.03 Inferior subluxation and dislocation of humerus
- S43.031 Inferior subluxation of right humerus
- S43.032 Inferior subluxation of left humerus
- S43.033 Inferior subluxation of unspecified humerus
- S43.034 Inferior dislocation of right humerus
- S43.035 Inferior dislocation of left humerus
- S43.036 Inferior dislocation of unspecified humerus

S43.08 Other subluxation and dislocation of shoulder joint
- S43.081 Other subluxation of right shoulder joint
- S43.082 Other subluxation of left shoulder joint
- S43.083 Other subluxation of unspecified shoulder joint
- S43.084 Other dislocation of right shoulder joint
- S43.085 Other dislocation of left shoulder joint
- S43.086 Other dislocation of unspecified shoulder joint

S43.1 Subluxation and dislocation of acromioclavicular joint

S43.10 Unspecified dislocation of acromioclavicular joint
- S43.101 Unspecified dislocation of right acromioclavicular joint
- S43.102 Unspecified dislocation of left acromioclavicular joint
- S43.109 Unspecified dislocation of unspecified acromioclavicular joint

S43.11 Subluxation of acromioclavicular joint
- S43.111 Subluxation of right acromioclavicular joint
- S43.112 Subluxation of left acromioclavicular joint
- S43.119 Subluxation of unspecified acromioclavicular joint

S43.12 Dislocation of acromioclavicular joint, 100%-200% displacement
- S43.121 Dislocation of right acromioclavicular joint, 100%-200% displacement
- S43.122 Dislocation of left acromioclavicular joint, 100%-200% displacement
- S43.129 Dislocation of unspecified acromioclavicular joint, 100%-200% displacement

S43.13 Dislocation of acromioclavicular joint, greater than 200% displacement
- S43.131 Dislocation of right acromioclavicular joint, greater than 200% displacement
- S43.132 Dislocation of left acromioclavicular joint, greater than 200% displacement
- S43.139 Dislocation of unspecified acromioclavicular joint, greater than 200% displacement

S43.14 Inferior dislocation of acromioclavicular joint
- S43.141 Inferior dislocation of right acromioclavicular joint
- S43.142 Inferior dislocation of left acromioclavicular joint
- S43.149 Inferior dislocation of unspecified acromioclavicular joint

S43.15 Posterior dislocation of acromioclavicular joint
- S43.151 Posterior dislocation of right acromioclavicular joint
- S43.152 Posterior dislocation of left acromioclavicular joint

Unacceptable principal diagnosis symbol per Medicare code edits; Code exempt from diagnosis present on admission requirement
Questionable admission; Complication or comorbidity; CC/MCC exclusion; Major complication or comorbidity
Principal diagnosis as its own CC; Principal diagnosis as its own MCC; Z code as first-listed diagnosis

S43.159 Posterior dislocation of unspecified acromioclavicular joint

S43.2 Subluxation and dislocation of sternoclavicular joint

S43.20 Unspecified subluxation and dislocation of sternoclavicular joint

S43.201 Unspecified subluxation of right sternoclavicular joint HAC

S43.202 Unspecified subluxation of left sternoclavicular joint HAC

S43.203 Unspecified subluxation of unspecified sternoclavicular joint HAC

S43.204 Unspecified dislocation of right sternoclavicular joint HAC

S43.205 Unspecified dislocation of left sternoclavicular joint HAC

S43.206 Unspecified dislocation of unspecified sternoclavicular joint HAC

S43.21 Anterior subluxation and dislocation of sternoclavicular joint

S43.211 Anterior subluxation of right sternoclavicular joint HAC

S43.212 Anterior subluxation of left sternoclavicular joint HAC

S43.213 Anterior subluxation of unspecified sternoclavicular joint HAC

S43.214 Anterior dislocation of right sternoclavicular joint HAC

S43.215 Anterior dislocation of left sternoclavicular joint HAC

S43.216 Anterior dislocation of unspecified sternoclavicular joint HAC

S43.22 Posterior subluxation and dislocation of sternoclavicular joint

S43.221 Posterior subluxation of right sternoclavicular joint HAC

S43.222 Posterior subluxation of left sternoclavicular joint HAC

S43.223 Posterior subluxation of unspecified sternoclavicular joint HAC

S43.224 Posterior dislocation of right sternoclavicular joint HAC

S43.225 Posterior dislocation of left sternoclavicular joint HAC

S43.226 Posterior dislocation of unspecified sternoclavicular joint HAC

S43.3 Subluxation and dislocation of other and unspecified parts of shoulder girdle

S43.30 Subluxation and dislocation of unspecified parts of shoulder girdle
Dislocation of shoulder girdle NOS
Subluxation of shoulder girdle NOS

S43.301 Subluxation of unspecified parts of right shoulder girdle

S43.302 Subluxation of unspecified parts of left shoulder girdle

S43.303 Subluxation of unspecified parts of unspecified shoulder girdle

S43.304 Dislocation of unspecified parts of right shoulder girdle

S43.305 Dislocation of unspecified parts of left shoulder girdle

S43.306 Dislocation of unspecified parts of unspecified shoulder girdle

S43.31 Subluxation and dislocation of scapula

S43.311 Subluxation of right scapula

S43.312 Subluxation of left scapula

S43.313 Subluxation of unspecified scapula

S43.314 Dislocation of right scapula

S43.315 Dislocation of left scapula

S43.316 Dislocation of unspecified scapula

S43.39 Subluxation and dislocation of other parts of shoulder girdle

S43.391 Subluxation of other parts of right shoulder girdle

S43.392 Subluxation of other parts of left shoulder girdle

S43.393 Subluxation of other parts of unspecified shoulder girdle

S43.394 Dislocation of other parts of right shoulder girdle

S43.395 Dislocation of other parts of left shoulder girdle

S43.396 Dislocation of other parts of unspecified shoulder girdle

S43.4 Sprain of shoulder joint

S43.40 Unspecified sprain of shoulder joint

S43.401 Unspecified sprain of right shoulder joint

S43.402 Unspecified sprain of left shoulder joint

S43.409 Unspecified sprain of unspecified shoulder joint

S43.41 Sprain of coracohumeral (ligament)

S43.411 Sprain of right coracohumeral (ligament)

S43.412 Sprain of left coracohumeral (ligament)

S43.419 Sprain of unspecified coracohumeral (ligament)

S43.42 Sprain of rotator cuff capsule

EXCLUDES1 *rotator cuff syndrome (complete) (incomplete), not specified as traumatic (M75.1-)*

EXCLUDES2 *injury of tendon of rotator cuff (S46.0-)*

S43.421 Sprain of right rotator cuff capsule

S43.422 Sprain of left rotator cuff capsule

S43.429 Sprain of unspecified rotator cuff capsule

S43.43 Superior glenoid labrum lesion
SLAP lesion

S43.431 Superior glenoid labrum lesion of right shoulder

S43.432 Superior glenoid labrum lesion of left shoulder

S43.439 Superior glenoid labrum lesion of unspecified shoulder

S43.49 Other sprain of shoulder joint

S43.491 Other sprain of right shoulder joint

S43.492 Other sprain of left shoulder joint

S43.499 Other sprain of unspecified shoulder joint

S43.5 Sprain of acromioclavicular joint
Sprain of acromioclavicular ligament

S43.50 Sprain of unspecified acromioclavicular joint

S43.51 Sprain of right acromioclavicular joint

S43.52 Sprain of left acromioclavicular joint

S43.6 Sprain of sternoclavicular joint

S43.60 Sprain of unspecified sternoclavicular joint

S43.61 Sprain of right sternoclavicular joint

S43.62 Sprain of left sternoclavicular joint

S43.8 Sprain of other specified parts of shoulder girdle

S43.80 Sprain of other specified parts of unspecified shoulder girdle

S43.81 Sprain of other specified parts of right shoulder girdle

S43.82 Sprain of other specified parts of left shoulder girdle

S43.9 Sprain of unspecified parts of shoulder girdle

S43.90 Sprain of unspecified parts of unspecified shoulder girdle
Sprain of shoulder girdle NOS

S43.91 Sprain of unspecified parts of right shoulder girdle

S43.92 Sprain of unspecified parts of left shoulder girdle

S44 Injury of nerves at shoulder and upper arm level
Code also any associated open wound (S41.-)

EXCLUDES2 *injury of brachial plexus (S14.3-)*

The appropriate 7th character is to be added to each code from category S44
A = initial encounter
D = subsequent encounter
S = sequela

S44.0 Injury of ulnar nerve at upper arm level

EXCLUDES1 *ulnar nerve NOS (S54.0)*

S44.00 Injury of ulnar nerve at upper arm level, unspecified arm

S44.01 Injury of ulnar nerve at upper arm level, right arm

S44.02 Injury of ulnar nerve at upper arm level, left arm

Unspecified Code Other Specified Code Manifestation Code N Newborn P Pediatric M Maternity A Adult ♂ Male ♀ Female
● New Code ▲ Revised Code Title ▶◀ Revised Text NOTES INCLUDES EXCLUDES1 Not coded here EXCLUDES2 Not included here
4th character required 5th character required 6th character required 7th character required
Extension 'X' Alert HAC Hospital-acquired condition (HAC) alert AHA AHA Coding Clinic©

S44.1 Injury of median nerve at upper arm level
EXCLUDES1 *median nerve NOS (S54.1)*
S44.10 Injury of median nerve at upper arm level, unspecified arm
S44.11 Injury of median nerve at upper arm level, right arm
S44.12 Injury of median nerve at upper arm level, left arm
S44.2 Injury of radial nerve at upper arm level
EXCLUDES1 *radial nerve NOS (S54.2)*
S44.20 Injury of radial nerve at upper arm level, unspecified arm
S44.21 Injury of radial nerve at upper arm level, right arm
S44.22 Injury of radial nerve at upper arm level, left arm
S44.3 Injury of axillary nerve
S44.30 Injury of axillary nerve, unspecified arm
S44.31 Injury of axillary nerve, right arm
S44.32 Injury of axillary nerve, left arm
S44.4 Injury of musculocutaneous nerve
S44.40 Injury of musculocutaneous nerve, unspecified arm
S44.41 Injury of musculocutaneous nerve, right arm
S44.42 Injury of musculocutaneous nerve, left arm
S44.5 Injury of cutaneous sensory nerve at shoulder and upper arm level
S44.50 Injury of cutaneous sensory nerve at shoulder and upper arm level, unspecified arm
S44.51 Injury of cutaneous sensory nerve at shoulder and upper arm level, right arm
S44.52 Injury of cutaneous sensory nerve at shoulder and upper arm level, left arm
S44.8 Injury of other nerves at shoulder and upper arm level
S44.8X Injury of other nerves at shoulder and upper arm level
S44.8X1 Injury of other nerves at shoulder and upper arm level, right arm
S44.8X2 Injury of other nerves at shoulder and upper arm level, left arm
S44.8X9 Injury of other nerves at shoulder and upper arm level, unspecified arm
S44.9 Injury of unspecified nerve at shoulder and upper arm level
S44.90 Injury of unspecified nerve at shoulder and upper arm level, unspecified arm
S44.91 Injury of unspecified nerve at shoulder and upper arm level, right arm
S44.92 Injury of unspecified nerve at shoulder and upper arm level, left arm

S45 Injury of blood vessels at shoulder and upper arm level
Code also any associated open wound (S41.-)
EXCLUDES2 *injury of subclavian artery (S25.1)*
injury of subclavian vein (S25.3)
The appropriate 7th character is to be added to each code from category S45
A = initial encounter
D = subsequent encounter
S = sequela
S45.0 Injury of axillary artery
S45.00 Unspecified injury of axillary artery
S45.001 Unspecified injury of axillary artery, right side MCC
S45.002 Unspecified injury of axillary artery, left side MCC
S45.009 Unspecified injury of axillary artery, unspecified side MCC
S45.01 Laceration of axillary artery
S45.011 Laceration of axillary artery, right side MCC
S45.012 Laceration of axillary artery, left side MCC
S45.019 Laceration of axillary artery, unspecified side MCC
S45.09 Other specified injury of axillary artery
S45.091 Other specified injury of axillary artery, right side MCC
S45.092 Other specified injury of axillary artery, left side MCC
S45.099 Other specified injury of axillary artery, unspecified side MCC
S45.1 Injury of brachial artery
S45.10 Unspecified injury of brachial artery
S45.101 Unspecified injury of brachial artery, right side CC
S45.102 Unspecified injury of brachial artery, left side CC
S45.109 Unspecified injury of brachial artery, unspecified side CC
S45.11 Laceration of brachial artery
S45.111 Laceration of brachial artery, right side CC
S45.112 Laceration of brachial artery, left side CC
S45.119 Laceration of brachial artery, unspecified side CC
S45.19 Other specified injury of brachial artery
S45.191 Other specified injury of brachial artery, right side CC
S45.192 Other specified injury of brachial artery, left side CC
S45.199 Other specified injury of brachial artery, unspecified side CC
S45.2 Injury of axillary or brachial vein
S45.20 Unspecified injury of axillary or brachial vein
S45.201 Unspecified injury of axillary or brachial vein, right side CC
S45.202 Unspecified injury of axillary or brachial vein, left side CC
S45.209 Unspecified injury of axillary or brachial vein, unspecified side CC
S45.21 Laceration of axillary or brachial vein
S45.211 Laceration of axillary or brachial vein, right side CC
S45.212 Laceration of axillary or brachial vein, left side CC
S45.219 Laceration of axillary or brachial vein, unspecified side CC
S45.29 Other specified injury of axillary or brachial vein
S45.291 Other specified injury of axillary or brachial vein, right side CC
S45.292 Other specified injury of axillary or brachial vein, left side CC
S45.299 Other specified injury of axillary or brachial vein, unspecified side CC
S45.3 Injury of superficial vein at shoulder and upper arm level
S45.30 Unspecified injury of superficial vein at shoulder and upper arm level
S45.301 Unspecified injury of superficial vein at shoulder and upper arm level, right arm CC
S45.302 Unspecified injury of superficial vein at shoulder and upper arm level, left arm CC
S45.309 Unspecified injury of superficial vein at shoulder and upper arm level, unspecified arm CC
S45.31 Laceration of superficial vein at shoulder and upper arm level
S45.311 Laceration of superficial vein at shoulder and upper arm level, right arm CC
S45.312 Laceration of superficial vein at shoulder and upper arm level, left arm CC
S45.319 Laceration of superficial vein at shoulder and upper arm level, unspecified arm CC
S45.39 Other specified injury of superficial vein at shoulder and upper arm level
S45.391 Other specified injury of superficial vein at shoulder and upper arm level, right arm CC
S45.392 Other specified injury of superficial vein at shoulder and upper arm level, left arm CC
S45.399 Other specified injury of superficial vein at shoulder and upper arm level, unspecified arm CC
S45.8 Injury of other specified blood vessels at shoulder and upper arm level
S45.80 Unspecified injury of other specified blood vessels at shoulder and upper arm level

Unacceptable principal diagnosis symbol per Medicare code edits | Code exempt from diagnosis present on admission requirement
Questionable admission | CC Complication or comorbidity | CC/MCC exclusion | MCC Major complication or comorbidity
Principal diagnosis as its own CC | Principal diagnosis as its own MCC | Z code as first-listed diagnosis

When symbols appear on a code that requires a 7th character extension, refer to Appendix D to identify applicable 7th character codes.

S45.801 Unspecified injury of other specified blood vessels at shoulder and upper arm level, right arm
S45.802 Unspecified injury of other specified blood vessels at shoulder and upper arm level, left arm
S45.809 Unspecified injury of other specified blood vessels at shoulder and upper arm level, unspecified arm
S45.81 Laceration of other specified blood vessels at shoulder and upper arm level
S45.811 Laceration of other specified blood vessels at shoulder and upper arm level, right arm
S45.812 Laceration of other specified blood vessels at shoulder and upper arm level, left arm
S45.819 Laceration of other specified blood vessels at shoulder and upper arm level, unspecified arm
S45.89 Other specified injury of other specified blood vessels at shoulder and upper arm level
S45.891 Other specified injury of other specified blood vessels at shoulder and upper arm level, right arm
S45.892 Other specified injury of other specified blood vessels at shoulder and upper arm level, left arm
S45.899 Other specified injury of other specified blood vessels at shoulder and upper arm level, unspecified arm
S45.9 Injury of unspecified blood vessel at shoulder and upper arm level
S45.90 Unspecified injury of unspecified blood vessel at shoulder and upper arm level
S45.901 Unspecified injury of unspecified blood vessel at shoulder and upper arm level, right arm
S45.902 Unspecified injury of unspecified blood vessel at shoulder and upper arm level, left arm
S45.909 Unspecified injury of unspecified blood vessel at shoulder and upper arm level, unspecified arm
S45.91 Laceration of unspecified blood vessel at shoulder and upper arm level
S45.911 Laceration of unspecified blood vessel at shoulder and upper arm level, right arm
S45.912 Laceration of unspecified blood vessel at shoulder and upper arm level, left arm
S45.919 Laceration of unspecified blood vessel at shoulder and upper arm level, unspecified arm
S45.99 Other specified injury of unspecified blood vessel at shoulder and upper arm level
S45.991 Other specified injury of unspecified blood vessel at shoulder and upper arm level, right arm
S45.992 Other specified injury of unspecified blood vessel at shoulder and upper arm level, left arm
S45.999 Other specified injury of unspecified blood vessel at shoulder and upper arm level, unspecified arm

S46 Injury of muscle, fascia and tendon at shoulder and upper arm level
Code also any associated open wound (S41.-)
EXCLUDES2 *injury of muscle, fascia and tendon at elbow (S56.-)*
sprain of joints and ligaments of shoulder girdle (S43.9)
The appropriate 7th character is to be added to each code from category S46
A = initial encounter
D = subsequent encounter
S = sequela

S46.0 Injury of muscle(s) and tendon(s) of the rotator cuff of shoulder
S46.00 Unspecified injury of muscle(s) and tendon(s) of the rotator cuff of shoulder
S46.001 Unspecified injury of muscle(s) and tendon(s) of the rotator cuff of right shoulder
S46.002 Unspecified injury of muscle(s) and tendon(s) of the rotator cuff of left shoulder
S46.009 Unspecified injury of muscle(s) and tendon(s) of the rotator cuff of unspecified shoulder
S46.01 Strain of muscle(s) and tendon(s) of the rotator cuff of shoulder
S46.011 Strain of muscle(s) and tendon(s) of the rotator cuff of right shoulder
S46.012 Strain of muscle(s) and tendon(s) of the rotator cuff of left shoulder
S46.019 Strain of muscle(s) and tendon(s) of the rotator cuff of unspecified shoulder
S46.02 Laceration of muscle(s) and tendon(s) of the rotator cuff of shoulder
S46.021 Laceration of muscle(s) and tendon(s) of the rotator cuff of right shoulder
S46.022 Laceration of muscle(s) and tendon(s) of the rotator cuff of left shoulder
S46.029 Laceration of muscle(s) and tendon(s) of the rotator cuff of unspecified shoulder
S46.09 Other injury of muscle(s) and tendon(s) of the rotator cuff of shoulder
S46.091 Other injury of muscle(s) and tendon(s) of the rotator cuff of right shoulder
S46.092 Other injury of muscle(s) and tendon(s) of the rotator cuff of left shoulder
S46.099 Other injury of muscle(s) and tendon(s) of the rotator cuff of unspecified shoulder
S46.1 Injury of muscle, fascia and tendon of long head of biceps
S46.10 Unspecified injury of muscle, fascia and tendon of long head of biceps
S46.101 Unspecified injury of muscle, fascia and tendon of long head of biceps, right arm
S46.102 Unspecified injury of muscle, fascia and tendon of long head of biceps, left arm
S46.109 Unspecified injury of muscle, fascia and tendon of long head of biceps, unspecified arm
S46.11 Strain of muscle, fascia and tendon of long head of biceps
S46.111 Strain of muscle, fascia and tendon of long head of biceps, right arm
S46.112 Strain of muscle, fascia and tendon of long head of biceps, left arm
S46.119 Strain of muscle, fascia and tendon of long head of biceps, unspecified arm
S46.12 Laceration of muscle, fascia and tendon of long head of biceps
S46.121 Laceration of muscle, fascia and tendon of long head of biceps, right arm
S46.122 Laceration of muscle, fascia and tendon of long head of biceps, left arm
S46.129 Laceration of muscle, fascia and tendon of long head of biceps, unspecified arm
S46.19 Other injury of muscle, fascia and tendon of long head of biceps
S46.191 Other injury of muscle, fascia and tendon of long head of biceps, right arm
S46.192 Other injury of muscle, fascia and tendon of long head of biceps, left arm
S46.199 Other injury of muscle, fascia and tendon of long head of biceps, unspecified arm
S46.2 Injury of muscle, fascia and tendon of other parts of biceps
S46.20 Unspecified injury of muscle, fascia and tendon of other parts of biceps
S46.201 Unspecified injury of muscle, fascia and tendon of other parts of biceps, right arm
S46.202 Unspecified injury of muscle, fascia and tendon of other parts of biceps, left arm

Unspecified Code Other Specified Code Manifestation Code N Newborn P Pediatric M Maternity A Adult ♂ Male ♀ Female
● New Code ▲ Revised Code Title ►◄ Revised Text NOTES INCLUDES EXCLUDES1 Not coded here EXCLUDES2 Not included here
4th character required 5th character required 6th character required 7th character required
Extension 'X' Alert HAC Hospital-acquired condition (HAC) alert AHA AHA Coding Clinic©

- S46.209 Unspecified injury of muscle, fascia and tendon of other parts of biceps, unspecified arm
- S46.21 Strain of muscle, fascia and tendon of other parts of biceps
  - S46.211 Strain of muscle, fascia and tendon of other parts of biceps, right arm
  - S46.212 Strain of muscle, fascia and tendon of other parts of biceps, left arm
  - S46.219 Strain of muscle, fascia and tendon of other parts of biceps, unspecified arm
- S46.22 Laceration of muscle, fascia and tendon of other parts of biceps
  - S46.221 Laceration of muscle, fascia and tendon of other parts of biceps, right arm CC
  - S46.222 Laceration of muscle, fascia and tendon of other parts of biceps, left arm CC
  - S46.229 Laceration of muscle, fascia and tendon of other parts of biceps, unspecified arm CC
- S46.29 Other injury of muscle, fascia and tendon of other parts of biceps
  - S46.291 Other injury of muscle, fascia and tendon of other parts of biceps, right arm
  - S46.292 Other injury of muscle, fascia and tendon of other parts of biceps, left arm
  - S46.299 Other injury of muscle, fascia and tendon of other parts of biceps, unspecified arm

S46.3 Injury of muscle, fascia and tendon of triceps
- S46.30 Unspecified injury of muscle, fascia and tendon of triceps
  - S46.301 Unspecified injury of muscle, fascia and tendon of triceps, right arm
  - S46.302 Unspecified injury of muscle, fascia and tendon of triceps, left arm
  - S46.309 Unspecified injury of muscle, fascia and tendon of triceps, unspecified arm
- S46.31 Strain of muscle, fascia and tendon of triceps
  - S46.311 Strain of muscle, fascia and tendon of triceps, right arm
  - S46.312 Strain of muscle, fascia and tendon of triceps, left arm
  - S46.319 Strain of muscle, fascia and tendon of triceps, unspecified arm
- S46.32 Laceration of muscle, fascia and tendon of triceps
  - S46.321 Laceration of muscle, fascia and tendon of triceps, right arm CC
  - S46.322 Laceration of muscle, fascia and tendon of triceps, left arm CC
  - S46.329 Laceration of muscle, fascia and tendon of triceps, unspecified arm CC
- S46.39 Other injury of muscle, fascia and tendon of triceps
  - S46.391 Other injury of muscle, fascia and tendon of triceps, right arm
  - S46.392 Other injury of muscle, fascia and tendon of triceps, left arm
  - S46.399 Other injury of muscle, fascia and tendon of triceps, unspecified arm

S46.8 Injury of other muscles, fascia and tendons at shoulder and upper arm level
- S46.80 Unspecified injury of other muscles, fascia and tendons at shoulder and upper arm level
  - S46.801 Unspecified injury of other muscles, fascia and tendons at shoulder and upper arm level, right arm
  - S46.802 Unspecified injury of other muscles, fascia and tendons at shoulder and upper arm level, left arm
  - S46.809 Unspecified injury of other muscles, fascia and tendons at shoulder and upper arm level, unspecified arm
- S46.81 Strain of other muscles, fascia and tendons at shoulder and upper arm level
  - S46.811 Strain of other muscles, fascia and tendons at shoulder and upper arm level, right arm
  - S46.812 Strain of other muscles, fascia and tendons at shoulder and upper arm level, left arm
  - S46.819 Strain of other muscles, fascia and tendons at shoulder and upper arm level, unspecified arm
- S46.82 Laceration of other muscles, fascia and tendons at shoulder and upper arm level
  - S46.821 Laceration of other muscles, fascia and tendons at shoulder and upper arm level, right arm CC
  - S46.822 Laceration of other muscles, fascia and tendons at shoulder and upper arm level, left arm CC
  - S46.829 Laceration of other muscles, fascia and tendons at shoulder and upper arm level, unspecified arm CC
- S46.89 Other injury of other muscles, fascia and tendons at shoulder and upper arm level
  - S46.891 Other injury of other muscles, fascia and tendons at shoulder and upper arm level, right arm
  - S46.892 Other injury of other muscles, fascia and tendons at shoulder and upper arm level, left arm
  - S46.899 Other injury of other muscles, fascia and tendons at shoulder and upper arm level, unspecified arm

S46.9 Injury of unspecified muscle, fascia and tendon at shoulder and upper arm level
- S46.90 Unspecified injury of unspecified muscle, fascia and tendon at shoulder and upper arm level
  - S46.901 Unspecified injury of unspecified muscle, fascia and tendon at shoulder and upper arm level, right arm
  - S46.902 Unspecified injury of unspecified muscle, fascia and tendon at shoulder and upper arm level, left arm
  - S46.909 Unspecified injury of unspecified muscle, fascia and tendon at shoulder and upper arm level, unspecified arm
- S46.91 Strain of unspecified muscle, fascia and tendon at shoulder and upper arm level
  - S46.911 Strain of unspecified muscle, fascia and tendon at shoulder and upper arm level, right arm
  - S46.912 Strain of unspecified muscle, fascia and tendon at shoulder and upper arm level, left arm
  - S46.919 Strain of unspecified muscle, fascia and tendon at shoulder and upper arm level, unspecified arm
- S46.92 Laceration of unspecified muscle, fascia and tendon at shoulder and upper arm level
  - S46.921 Laceration of unspecified muscle, fascia and tendon at shoulder and upper arm level, right arm CC
  - S46.922 Laceration of unspecified muscle, fascia and tendon at shoulder and upper arm level, left arm CC
  - S46.929 Laceration of unspecified muscle, fascia and tendon at shoulder and upper arm level, unspecified arm CC
- S46.99 Other injury of unspecified muscle, fascia and tendon at shoulder and upper arm level
  - S46.991 Other injury of unspecified muscle, fascia and tendon at shoulder and upper arm level, right arm
  - S46.992 Other injury of unspecified muscle, fascia and tendon at shoulder and upper arm level, left arm
  - S46.999 Other injury of unspecified muscle, fascia and tendon at shoulder and upper arm level, unspecified arm

S47 Crushing injury of shoulder and upper arm

Use additional code for all associated injuries

EXCLUDES2 *crushing injury of elbow (S57.0-)*

PDx Unacceptable principal diagnosis symbol per Medicare code edits · POA Code exempt from diagnosis present on admission requirement · Q Questionable admission · CC Complication or comorbidity · CC/MCC Exc CC/MCC exclusion · MCC Major complication or comorbidity · PDx CC Principal diagnosis as its own CC · PDx MCC Principal diagnosis as its own MCC · Z1 Z code as first-listed diagnosis

 When symbols appear on a code that requires a 7th character extension, refer to Appendix D to identify applicable 7th character codes.

The appropriate 7th character is to be added to each code from category S47
A = initial encounter
D = subsequent encounter
S = sequela

S47.1 Crushing injury of right shoulder and upper arm
S47.2 Crushing injury of left shoulder and upper arm
S47.9 Crushing injury of shoulder and upper arm, unspecified arm

S48 Traumatic amputation of shoulder and upper arm
An amputation not identified as partial or complete should be coded to complete
EXCLUDES1 *traumatic amputation at elbow level (S58.0)*
The appropriate 7th character is to be added to each code from category S48
A = initial encounter
D = subsequent encounter
S = sequela

S48.0 Traumatic amputation at shoulder joint
S48.01 Complete traumatic amputation at shoulder joint
S48.011 Complete traumatic amputation at right shoulder joint
S48.012 Complete traumatic amputation at left shoulder joint
S48.019 Complete traumatic amputation at unspecified shoulder joint
S48.02 Partial traumatic amputation at shoulder joint
S48.021 Partial traumatic amputation at right shoulder joint
S48.022 Partial traumatic amputation at left shoulder joint
S48.029 Partial traumatic amputation at unspecified shoulder joint
S48.1 Traumatic amputation at level between shoulder and elbow
S48.11 Complete traumatic amputation at level between shoulder and elbow
S48.111 Complete traumatic amputation at level between right shoulder and elbow
S48.112 Complete traumatic amputation at level between left shoulder and elbow
S48.119 Complete traumatic amputation at level between unspecified shoulder and elbow
S48.12 Partial traumatic amputation at level between shoulder and elbow
S48.121 Partial traumatic amputation at level between right shoulder and elbow
S48.122 Partial traumatic amputation at level between left shoulder and elbow
S48.129 Partial traumatic amputation at level between unspecified shoulder and elbow
S48.9 Traumatic amputation of shoulder and upper arm, level unspecified
S48.91 Complete traumatic amputation of shoulder and upper arm, level unspecified
S48.911 Complete traumatic amputation of right shoulder and upper arm, level unspecified
S48.912 Complete traumatic amputation of left shoulder and upper arm, level unspecified
S48.919 Complete traumatic amputation of unspecified shoulder and upper arm, level unspecified
S48.92 Partial traumatic amputation of shoulder and upper arm, level unspecified
S48.921 Partial traumatic amputation of right shoulder and upper arm, level unspecified
S48.922 Partial traumatic amputation of left shoulder and upper arm, level unspecified
S48.929 Partial traumatic amputation of unspecified shoulder and upper arm, level unspecified

S49 Other and unspecified injuries of shoulder and upper arm
The appropriate 7th character is to be added to each code from subcategories S49.0 and S49.1
A = initial encounter for closed fracture
D = subsequent encounter for fracture with routine healing
G = subsequent encounter for fracture with delayed healing
K = subsequent encounter for fracture with nonunion
P = subsequent encounter for fracture with malunion
S = sequela

S49.0 Physeal fracture of upper end of humerus
S49.00 Unspecified physeal fracture of upper end of humerus
S49.001 Unspecified physeal fracture of upper end of humerus, right arm HAC
S49.002 Unspecified physeal fracture of upper end of humerus, left arm HAC
S49.009 Unspecified physeal fracture of upper end of humerus, unspecified arm HAC
S49.01 Salter-Harris Type I physeal fracture of upper end of humerus
S49.011 Salter-Harris Type I physeal fracture of upper end of humerus, right arm HAC
S49.012 Salter-Harris Type I physeal fracture of upper end of humerus, left arm HAC
S49.019 Salter-Harris Type I physeal fracture of upper end of humerus, unspecified arm HAC
S49.02 Salter-Harris Type II physeal fracture of upper end of humerus
S49.021 Salter-Harris Type II physeal fracture of upper end of humerus, right arm HAC
S49.022 Salter-Harris Type II physeal fracture of upper end of humerus, left arm HAC
S49.029 Salter-Harris Type II physeal fracture of upper end of humerus, unspecified arm HAC
S49.03 Salter-Harris Type III physeal fracture of upper end of humerus
▲ S49.031 ▶Salter-Harris◀ Type III physeal fracture of upper end of humerus, right arm HAC
▲ S49.032 ▶Salter-Harris◀ Type III physeal fracture of upper end of humerus, left arm HAC
▲ S49.039 ▶Salter-Harris◀ Type III physeal fracture of upper end of humerus, unspecified arm HAC
S49.04 Salter-Harris Type IV physeal fracture of upper end of humerus
S49.041 Salter-Harris Type IV physeal fracture of upper end of humerus, right arm HAC
S49.042 Salter-Harris Type IV physeal fracture of upper end of humerus, left arm HAC
S49.049 Salter-Harris Type IV physeal fracture of upper end of humerus, unspecified arm HAC
S49.09 Other physeal fracture of upper end of humerus
S49.091 Other physeal fracture of upper end of humerus, right arm HAC
S49.092 Other physeal fracture of upper end of humerus, left arm HAC
S49.099 Other physeal fracture of upper end of humerus, unspecified arm HAC
S49.1 Physeal fracture of lower end of humerus
S49.10 Unspecified physeal fracture of lower end of humerus
S49.101 Unspecified physeal fracture of lower end of humerus, right arm HAC
S49.102 Unspecified physeal fracture of lower end of humerus, left arm HAC
S49.109 Unspecified physeal fracture of lower end of humerus, unspecified arm HAC
S49.11 Salter-Harris Type I physeal fracture of lower end of humerus
S49.111 Salter-Harris Type I physeal fracture of lower end of humerus, right arm HAC
S49.112 Salter-Harris Type I physeal fracture of lower end of humerus, left arm HAC

Unspecified Code Other Specified Code Manifestation Code N Newborn P Pediatric M Maternity A Adult ♂ Male ♀ Female
● New Code ▲ Revised Code Title ▶◀ Revised Text NOTES INCLUDES EXCLUDES1 Not coded here EXCLUDES2 Not included here
4th character required 5th character required 6th character required 7th character required
Extension 'X' Alert HAC Hospital-acquired condition (HAC) alert AHA AHA Coding Clinic©

S49.119 Salter-Harris Type I physeal fracture of lower end of humerus, unspecified arm CC HAC

S49.12 Salter-Harris Type II physeal fracture of lower end of humerus

S49.121 Salter-Harris Type II physeal fracture of lower end of humerus, right arm CC HAC

S49.122 Salter-Harris Type II physeal fracture of lower end of humerus, left arm CC HAC

S49.129 Salter-Harris Type II physeal fracture of lower end of humerus, unspecified arm CC HAC

▲ S49.13 ▶Salter-Harris◀ Type III physeal fracture of lower end of humerus

▲ S49.131 ▶Salter-Harris◀ Type III physeal fracture of lower end of humerus, right arm CC HAC

▲ S49.132 ▶Salter-Harris◀ Type III physeal fracture of lower end of humerus, left arm CC HAC

▲ S49.139 ▶Salter-Harris◀ Type III physeal fracture of lower end of humerus, unspecified arm CC HAC

S49.14 Salter-Harris Type IV physeal fracture of lower end of humerus

S49.141 Salter-Harris Type IV physeal fracture of lower end of humerus, right arm CC HAC

S49.142 Salter-Harris Type IV physeal fracture of lower end of humerus, left arm CC HAC

S49.149 Salter-Harris Type IV physeal fracture of lower end of humerus, unspecified arm CC HAC

S49.19 Other physeal fracture of lower end of humerus

S49.191 Other physeal fracture of lower end of humerus, right arm CC HAC

S49.192 Other physeal fracture of lower end of humerus, left arm CC HAC

S49.199 Other physeal fracture of lower end of humerus, unspecified arm CC HAC

S49.8 Other specified injuries of shoulder and upper arm

The appropriate 7th character is to be added to each code in subcategory S49.8
A = initial encounter
D = subsequent encounter
S = sequela

S49.80 Other specified injuries of shoulder and upper arm, unspecified arm

S49.81 Other specified injuries of right shoulder and upper arm

S49.82 Other specified injuries of left shoulder and upper arm

S49.9 Unspecified injury of shoulder and upper arm

The appropriate 7th character is to be added to each code in subcategory S49.9
A = initial encounter
D = subsequent encounter
S = sequela

S49.90 Unspecified injury of shoulder and upper arm, unspecified arm

S49.91 Unspecified injury of right shoulder and upper arm

S49.92 Unspecified injury of left shoulder and upper arm

Injuries to the elbow and forearm (S50-S59)

EXCLUDES2 *burns and corrosions (T20-T32)*
frostbite (T33-T34)
injuries of wrist and hand (S60-S69)
insect bite or sting, venomous (T63.4)

S50 Superficial injury of elbow and forearm

EXCLUDES2 *superficial injury of wrist and hand (S60.-)*

The appropriate 7th character is to be added to each code from category S50
A = initial encounter
D = subsequent encounter
S = sequela

S50.0 Contusion of elbow

S50.00 Contusion of unspecified elbow

S50.01 Contusion of right elbow

S50.02 Contusion of left elbow

S50.1 Contusion of forearm

S50.10 Contusion of unspecified forearm

S50.11 Contusion of right forearm

S50.12 Contusion of left forearm

S50.3 Other superficial injuries of elbow

S50.31 Abrasion of elbow

S50.311 Abrasion of right elbow

S50.312 Abrasion of left elbow

S50.319 Abrasion of unspecified elbow

S50.32 Blister (nonthermal) of elbow

S50.321 Blister (nonthermal) of right elbow

S50.322 Blister (nonthermal) of left elbow

S50.329 Blister (nonthermal) of unspecified elbow

S50.34 External constriction of elbow

S50.341 External constriction of right elbow

S50.342 External constriction of left elbow

S50.349 External constriction of unspecified elbow

S50.35 Superficial foreign body of elbow

Splinter in the elbow

S50.351 Superficial foreign body of right elbow

S50.352 Superficial foreign body of left elbow

S50.359 Superficial foreign body of unspecified elbow

S50.36 Insect bite (nonvenomous) of elbow

S50.361 Insect bite (nonvenomous) of right elbow

S50.362 Insect bite (nonvenomous) of left elbow

S50.369 Insect bite (nonvenomous) of unspecified elbow

S50.37 Other superficial bite of elbow

EXCLUDES1 *open bite of elbow (S51.04)*

S50.371 Other superficial bite of right elbow

S50.372 Other superficial bite of left elbow

S50.379 Other superficial bite of unspecified elbow

S50.8 Other superficial injuries of forearm

S50.81 Abrasion of forearm

S50.811 Abrasion of right forearm

S50.812 Abrasion of left forearm

S50.819 Abrasion of unspecified forearm

S50.82 Blister (nonthermal) of forearm

S50.821 Blister (nonthermal) of right forearm

S50.822 Blister (nonthermal) of left forearm

S50.829 Blister (nonthermal) of unspecified forearm

S50.84 External constriction of forearm

S50.841 External constriction of right forearm

S50.842 External constriction of left forearm

S50.849 External constriction of unspecified forearm

S50.85 Superficial foreign body of forearm

Splinter in the forearm

S50.851 Superficial foreign body of right forearm

S50.852 Superficial foreign body of left forearm

S50.859 Superficial foreign body of unspecified forearm

S50.86 Insect bite (nonvenomous) of forearm

S50.861 Insect bite (nonvenomous) of right forearm

S50.862 Insect bite (nonvenomous) of left forearm

S50.869 Insect bite (nonvenomous) of unspecified forearm

S50.87 Other superficial bite of forearm

EXCLUDES1 *open bite of forearm (S51.84)*

S50.871 Other superficial bite of right forearm

S50.872 Other superficial bite of left forearm

S50.879 Other superficial bite of unspecified forearm

S50.9 Unspecified superficial injury of elbow and forearm

S50.90 Unspecified superficial injury of elbow

PDx Unacceptable principal diagnosis symbol per Medicare code edits · POA Code exempt from diagnosis present on admission requirement
Q Questionable admission · CC Complication or comorbidity · CC/MCC Exc CC/MCC exclusion · MCC Major complication or comorbidity
PDx CC Principal diagnosis as its own CC · PDx MCC Principal diagnosis as its own MCC · Z1 Z code as first-listed diagnosis

S50.901 Unspecified superficial injury of right elbow
S50.902 Unspecified superficial injury of left elbow
S50.909 Unspecified superficial injury of unspecified elbow
S50.91 Unspecified superficial injury of forearm
S50.911 Unspecified superficial injury of right forearm
S50.912 Unspecified superficial injury of left forearm
S50.919 Unspecified superficial injury of unspecified forearm

S51 Open wound of elbow and forearm
Code also any associated wound infection
EXCLUDES1 *open fracture of elbow and forearm (S52.- with open fracture 7th character)*
traumatic amputation of elbow and forearm (S58.-)
EXCLUDES2 *open wound of wrist and hand (S61.-)*
The appropriate 7th character is to be added to each code from category S51
A = initial encounter
D = subsequent encounter
S = sequela

S51.0 Open wound of elbow
S51.00 Unspecified open wound of elbow
S51.001 Unspecified open wound of right elbow
AHA: Q4, 2012
S51.002 Unspecified open wound of left elbow
S51.009 Unspecified open wound of unspecified elbow
Open wound of elbow NOS
S51.01 Laceration without foreign body of elbow
S51.011 Laceration without foreign body of right elbow
S51.012 Laceration without foreign body of left elbow
S51.019 Laceration without foreign body of unspecified elbow
S51.02 Laceration with foreign body of elbow
S51.021 Laceration with foreign body of right elbow
S51.022 Laceration with foreign body of left elbow
S51.029 Laceration with foreign body of unspecified elbow
S51.03 Puncture wound without foreign body of elbow
S51.031 Puncture wound without foreign body of right elbow
S51.032 Puncture wound without foreign body of left elbow
S51.039 Puncture wound without foreign body of unspecified elbow
S51.04 Puncture wound with foreign body of elbow
S51.041 Puncture wound with foreign body of right elbow
S51.042 Puncture wound with foreign body of left elbow
S51.049 Puncture wound with foreign body of unspecified elbow
S51.05 Open bite of elbow
Bite of elbow NOS
EXCLUDES1 *superficial bite of elbow (S50.36, S50.37)*
S51.051 Open bite, right elbow
S51.052 Open bite, left elbow
S51.059 Open bite, unspecified elbow

S51.8 Open wound of forearm
EXCLUDES2 *open wound of elbow (S51.0-)*
S51.80 Unspecified open wound of forearm
S51.801 Unspecified open wound of right forearm
S51.802 Unspecified open wound of left forearm
S51.809 Unspecified open wound of unspecified forearm
Open wound of forearm NOS
S51.81 Laceration without foreign body of forearm
S51.811 Laceration without foreign body of right forearm
S51.812 Laceration without foreign body of left forearm
S51.819 Laceration without foreign body of unspecified forearm
S51.82 Laceration with foreign body of forearm
S51.821 Laceration with foreign body of right forearm
S51.822 Laceration with foreign body of left forearm
S51.829 Laceration with foreign body of unspecified forearm
S51.83 Puncture wound without foreign body of forearm
S51.831 Puncture wound without foreign body of right forearm
S51.832 Puncture wound without foreign body of left forearm
S51.839 Puncture wound without foreign body of unspecified forearm
S51.84 Puncture wound with foreign body of forearm
S51.841 Puncture wound with foreign body of right forearm
S51.842 Puncture wound with foreign body of left forearm
S51.849 Puncture wound with foreign body of unspecified forearm
S51.85 Open bite of forearm
Bite of forearm NOS
EXCLUDES1 *superficial bite of forearm (S50.86, S50.87)*
S51.851 Open bite of right forearm
S51.852 Open bite of left forearm
S51.859 Open bite of unspecified forearm

S52 Fracture of forearm
NOTES A fracture not indicated as displaced or nondisplaced should be coded to displaced
A fracture not indicated as open or closed should be coded to closed
The open fracture designations are based on the Gustilo open fracture classification
EXCLUDES1 *traumatic amputation of forearm (S58.-)*
EXCLUDES2 *fracture at wrist and hand level (S62.-)*
The appropriate 7th character is to be added to all codes from category S52
A = initial encounter for closed fracture
B = initial encounter for open fracture type I or II initial encounter for open fracture NOS
C = initial encounter for open fracture type IIIA, IIIB, or IIIC
D = subsequent encounter for closed fracture with routine healing
E = subsequent encounter for open fracture type I or II with routine healing
F = subsequent encounter for open fracture type IIIA, IIIB, or IIIC with routine healing
G = subsequent encounter for closed fracture with delayed healing
H = subsequent encounter for open fracture type I or II with delayed healing
J = subsequent encounter for open fracture type IIIA, IIIB, or IIIC with delayed healing
K = subsequent encounter for closed fracture with nonunion
M = subsequent encounter for open fracture type I or II with nonunion
N = subsequent encounter for open fracture type IIIA, IIIB, or IIIC with nonunion
P = subsequent encounter for closed fracture with malunion
Q = subsequent encounter for open fracture type I or II with malunion
R = subsequent encounter for open fracture type IIIA, IIIB, or IIIC with malunion
S = sequela

S52.0 Fracture of upper end of ulna
Fracture of proximal end of ulna
EXCLUDES2 *fracture of elbow NOS (S42.40-)*
fractures of shaft of ulna (S52.2-)

Unspecified Code Other Specified Code Manifestation Code N Newborn P Pediatric M Maternity A Adult ♂ Male ♀ Female
● New Code ▲ Revised Code Title ►◄ Revised Text NOTES INCLUDES EXCLUDES1 Not coded here EXCLUDES2 Not included here
4th character required 5th character required 6th character required 7th character required
Extension 'X' Alert HAC Hospital-acquired condition (HAC) alert AHA AHA Coding Clinic©

S52.00 Unspecified fracture of upper end of ulna
- S52.001 Unspecified fracture of upper end of right ulna
- S52.002 Unspecified fracture of upper end of left ulna
- S52.009 Unspecified fracture of upper end of unspecified ulna

S52.01 Torus fracture of upper end of ulna

The appropriate 7th character is to be added to all codes in subcategory S52.01
- A = initial encounter for closed fracture
- D = subsequent encounter for fracture with routine healing
- G = subsequent encounter for fracture with delayed healing
- K = subsequent encounter for fracture with nonunion
- P = subsequent encounter for fracture with malunion
- S = sequela

- S52.011 Torus fracture of upper end of right ulna
- S52.012 Torus fracture of upper end of left ulna
- S52.019 Torus fracture of upper end of unspecified ulna

S52.02 Fracture of olecranon process without intraarticular extension of ulna
- S52.021 Displaced fracture of olecranon process without intraarticular extension of right ulna
- S52.022 Displaced fracture of olecranon process without intraarticular extension of left ulna
- S52.023 Displaced fracture of olecranon process without intraarticular extension of unspecified ulna
- S52.024 Nondisplaced fracture of olecranon process without intraarticular extension of right ulna
- S52.025 Nondisplaced fracture of olecranon process without intraarticular extension of left ulna
- S52.026 Nondisplaced fracture of olecranon process without intraarticular extension of unspecified ulna

S52.03 Fracture of olecranon process with intraarticular extension of ulna
- S52.031 Displaced fracture of olecranon process with intraarticular extension of right ulna
- S52.032 Displaced fracture of olecranon process with intraarticular extension of left ulna
- S52.033 Displaced fracture of olecranon process with intraarticular extension of unspecified ulna
- S52.034 Nondisplaced fracture of olecranon process with intraarticular extension of right ulna
- S52.035 Nondisplaced fracture of olecranon process with intraarticular extension of left ulna
- S52.036 Nondisplaced fracture of olecranon process with intraarticular extension of unspecified ulna

S52.04 Fracture of coronoid process of ulna
- S52.041 Displaced fracture of coronoid process of right ulna
- S52.042 Displaced fracture of coronoid process of left ulna
- S52.043 Displaced fracture of coronoid process of unspecified ulna
- S52.044 Nondisplaced fracture of coronoid process of right ulna
- S52.045 Nondisplaced fracture of coronoid process of left ulna
- S52.046 Nondisplaced fracture of coronoid process of unspecified ulna

S52.09 Other fracture of upper end of ulna
- S52.091 Other fracture of upper end of right ulna
- S52.092 Other fracture of upper end of left ulna
- S52.099 Other fracture of upper end of unspecified ulna

S52.1 Fracture of upper end of radius

Fracture of proximal end of radius

EXCLUDES2 *physeal fractures of upper end of radius (S59.2-)*
fracture of shaft of radius (S52.3-)

S52.10 Unspecified fracture of upper end of radius
- S52.101 Unspecified fracture of upper end of right radius
- S52.102 Unspecified fracture of upper end of left radius
- S52.109 Unspecified fracture of upper end of unspecified radius

S52.11 Torus fracture of upper end of radius

The appropriate 7th character is to be added to all codes in subcategory S52.11
- A = initial encounter for closed fracture
- D = subsequent encounter for fracture with routine healing
- G = subsequent encounter for fracture with delayed healing
- K = subsequent encounter for fracture with nonunion
- P = subsequent encounter for fracture with malunion
- S = sequela

- S52.111 Torus fracture of upper end of right radius
- S52.112 Torus fracture of upper end of left radius
- S52.119 Torus fracture of upper end of unspecified radius

S52.12 Fracture of head of radius
- S52.121 Displaced fracture of head of right radius
- S52.122 Displaced fracture of head of left radius
- S52.123 Displaced fracture of head of unspecified radius
- S52.124 Nondisplaced fracture of head of right radius
- S52.125 Nondisplaced fracture of head of left radius
- S52.126 Nondisplaced fracture of head of unspecified radius

S52.13 Fracture of neck of radius
- S52.131 Displaced fracture of neck of right radius
- S52.132 Displaced fracture of neck of left radius
- S52.133 Displaced fracture of neck of unspecified radius
- S52.134 Nondisplaced fracture of neck of right radius
- S52.135 Nondisplaced fracture of neck of left radius
- S52.136 Nondisplaced fracture of neck of unspecified radius

S52.18 Other fracture of upper end of radius
- S52.181 Other fracture of upper end of right radius
- S52.182 Other fracture of upper end of left radius
- S52.189 Other fracture of upper end of unspecified radius

S52.2 Fracture of shaft of ulna

S52.20 Unspecified fracture of shaft of ulna

Fracture of ulna NOS

Unacceptable principal diagnosis symbol per Medicare code edits | Code exempt from diagnosis present on admission requirement | Questionable admission | Complication or comorbidity | CC/MCC exclusion | Major complication or comorbidity | Principal diagnosis as its own CC | Principal diagnosis as its own MCC | Z code as first-listed diagnosis

 When symbols appear on a code that requires a 7th character extension, refer to Appendix D to identify applicable 7th character codes.

- S52.201 Unspecified fracture of shaft of right ulna CC HAC MCC
- S52.202 Unspecified fracture of shaft of left ulna CC HAC MCC
- S52.209 Unspecified fracture of shaft of unspecified ulna CC HAC MCC

S52.21 Greenstick fracture of shaft of ulna

The appropriate 7th character is to be added to all codes in subcategory S52.21
- A = initial encounter for closed fracture
- D = subsequent encounter for fracture with routine healing
- G = subsequent encounter for fracture with delayed healing
- K = subsequent encounter for fracture with nonunion
- P = subsequent encounter for fracture with malunion
- S = sequela

- S52.211 Greenstick fracture of shaft of right ulna CC HAC
- S52.212 Greenstick fracture of shaft of left ulna CC HAC
- S52.219 Greenstick fracture of shaft of unspecified ulna CC HAC

S52.22 Transverse fracture of shaft of ulna
- S52.221 Displaced transverse fracture of shaft of right ulna CC HAC MCC
- S52.222 Displaced transverse fracture of shaft of left ulna CC HAC MCC
- S52.223 Displaced transverse fracture of shaft of unspecified ulna CC HAC MCC
- S52.224 Nondisplaced transverse fracture of shaft of right ulna CC HAC MCC
- S52.225 Nondisplaced transverse fracture of shaft of left ulna CC HAC MCC
- S52.226 Nondisplaced transverse fracture of shaft of unspecified ulna CC HAC MCC

S52.23 Oblique fracture of shaft of ulna
- S52.231 Displaced oblique fracture of shaft of right ulna CC HAC MCC
- S52.232 Displaced oblique fracture of shaft of left ulna CC HAC MCC
- S52.233 Displaced oblique fracture of shaft of unspecified ulna CC HAC MCC
- S52.234 Nondisplaced oblique fracture of shaft of right ulna CC HAC MCC
- S52.235 Nondisplaced oblique fracture of shaft of left ulna CC HAC MCC
- S52.236 Nondisplaced oblique fracture of shaft of unspecified ulna CC HAC MCC

S52.24 Spiral fracture of shaft of ulna
- S52.241 Displaced spiral fracture of shaft of ulna, right arm CC HAC MCC
- S52.242 Displaced spiral fracture of shaft of ulna, left arm CC HAC MCC
- S52.243 Displaced spiral fracture of shaft of ulna, unspecified arm CC HAC MCC
- S52.244 Nondisplaced spiral fracture of shaft of ulna, right arm CC HAC MCC
- S52.245 Nondisplaced spiral fracture of shaft of ulna, left arm CC HAC MCC
- S52.246 Nondisplaced spiral fracture of shaft of ulna, unspecified arm CC HAC MCC

S52.25 Comminuted fracture of shaft of ulna
- S52.251 Displaced comminuted fracture of shaft of ulna, right arm CC HAC MCC
- S52.252 Displaced comminuted fracture of shaft of ulna, left arm CC HAC MCC
- S52.253 Displaced comminuted fracture of shaft of ulna, unspecified arm CC HAC MCC
- S52.254 Nondisplaced comminuted fracture of shaft of ulna, right arm CC HAC MCC
- S52.255 Nondisplaced comminuted fracture of shaft of ulna, left arm CC HAC MCC
- S52.256 Nondisplaced comminuted fracture of shaft of ulna, unspecified arm CC HAC MCC

S52.26 Segmental fracture of shaft of ulna
- S52.261 Displaced segmental fracture of shaft of ulna, right arm CC HAC MCC
- S52.262 Displaced segmental fracture of shaft of ulna, left arm CC HAC MCC
- S52.263 Displaced segmental fracture of shaft of ulna, unspecified arm CC HAC MCC
- S52.264 Nondisplaced segmental fracture of shaft of ulna, right arm CC HAC MCC
- S52.265 Nondisplaced segmental fracture of shaft of ulna, left arm CC HAC MCC
- S52.266 Nondisplaced segmental fracture of shaft of ulna, unspecified arm CC HAC MCC

S52.27 Monteggia's fracture of ulna

Fracture of upper shaft of ulna with dislocation of radial head
- S52.271 Monteggia's fracture of right ulna CC MCC
- S52.272 Monteggia's fracture of left ulna CC MCC
- S52.279 Monteggia's fracture of unspecified ulna CC MCC

S52.28 Bent bone of ulna
- S52.281 Bent bone of right ulna CC HAC MCC
- S52.282 Bent bone of left ulna CC HAC MCC
- S52.283 Bent bone of unspecified ulna CC HAC MCC

S52.29 Other fracture of shaft of ulna
- S52.291 Other fracture of shaft of right ulna CC HAC MCC
- S52.292 Other fracture of shaft of left ulna CC HAC MCC
- S52.299 Other fracture of shaft of unspecified ulna CC HAC MCC

S52.3 Fracture of shaft of radius

S52.30 Unspecified fracture of shaft of radius
- S52.301 Unspecified fracture of shaft of right radius CC HAC MCC
- S52.302 Unspecified fracture of shaft of left radius CC HAC MCC
- S52.309 Unspecified fracture of shaft of unspecified radius CC HAC MCC

S52.31 Greenstick fracture of shaft of radius

The appropriate 7th character is to be added to all codes in subcategory S52.31
- A = initial encounter for closed fracture
- D = subsequent encounter for fracture with routine healing
- G = subsequent encounter for fracture with delayed healing
- K = subsequent encounter for fracture with nonunion
- P = subsequent encounter for fracture with malunion
- S = sequela

- S52.311 Greenstick fracture of shaft of radius, right arm CC HAC
- S52.312 Greenstick fracture of shaft of radius, left arm CC HAC
- S52.319 Greenstick fracture of shaft of radius, unspecified arm CC HAC

S52.32 Transverse fracture of shaft of radius
- S52.321 Displaced transverse fracture of shaft of right radius CC HAC MCC
- S52.322 Displaced transverse fracture of shaft of left radius CC HAC MCC
- S52.323 Displaced transverse fracture of shaft of unspecified radius CC HAC MCC
- S52.324 Nondisplaced transverse fracture of shaft of right radius CC HAC MCC
- S52.325 Nondisplaced transverse fracture of shaft of left radius CC HAC MCC
- S52.326 Nondisplaced transverse fracture of shaft of unspecified radius CC HAC MCC

S52.33 Oblique fracture of shaft of radius

Unspecified Code Other Specified Code Manifestation Code N Newborn P Pediatric M Maternity A Adult ♂ Male ♀ Female
● New Code ▲ Revised Code Title ►◄ Revised Text NOTES INCLUDES EXCLUDES1 Not coded here EXCLUDES2 Not included here
4th character required 5th character required 6th character required 7th character required
Extension 'X' Alert HAC Hospital-acquired condition (HAC) alert AHA AHA Coding Clinic®

S52.331 Displaced oblique fracture of shaft of right radius CC HAC MCC
S52.332 Displaced oblique fracture of shaft of left radius CC HAC MCC
S52.333 Displaced oblique fracture of shaft of unspecified radius CC HAC MCC
S52.334 Nondisplaced oblique fracture of shaft of right radius CC HAC MCC
S52.335 Nondisplaced oblique fracture of shaft of left radius CC HAC MCC
S52.336 Nondisplaced oblique fracture of shaft of unspecified radius CC HAC MCC

S52.34 Spiral fracture of shaft of radius
S52.341 Displaced spiral fracture of shaft of radius, right arm CC HAC MCC
S52.342 Displaced spiral fracture of shaft of radius, left arm CC HAC MCC
S52.343 Displaced spiral fracture of shaft of radius, unspecified arm CC HAC MCC
S52.344 Nondisplaced spiral fracture of shaft of radius, right arm CC HAC MCC
S52.345 Nondisplaced spiral fracture of shaft of radius, left arm CC HAC MCC
S52.346 Nondisplaced spiral fracture of shaft of radius, unspecified arm CC HAC MCC

S52.35 Comminuted fracture of shaft of radius
S52.351 Displaced comminuted fracture of shaft of radius, right arm CC HAC MCC
S52.352 Displaced comminuted fracture of shaft of radius, left arm CC HAC MCC
S52.353 Displaced comminuted fracture of shaft of radius, unspecified arm CC HAC MCC
S52.354 Nondisplaced comminuted fracture of shaft of radius, right arm CC HAC MCC
S52.355 Nondisplaced comminuted fracture of shaft of radius, left arm CC HAC MCC
S52.356 Nondisplaced comminuted fracture of shaft of radius, unspecified arm CC HAC MCC

S52.36 Segmental fracture of shaft of radius
S52.361 Displaced segmental fracture of shaft of radius, right arm CC HAC MCC
S52.362 Displaced segmental fracture of shaft of radius, left arm CC HAC MCC
S52.363 Displaced segmental fracture of shaft of radius, unspecified arm CC HAC MCC
S52.364 Nondisplaced segmental fracture of shaft of radius, right arm CC HAC MCC
S52.365 Nondisplaced segmental fracture of shaft of radius, left arm CC HAC MCC
S52.366 Nondisplaced segmental fracture of shaft of radius, unspecified arm CC HAC MCC

S52.37 Galeazzi's fracture
Fracture of lower shaft of radius with radioulnar joint dislocation
S52.371 Galeazzi's fracture of right radius CC MCC
S52.372 Galeazzi's fracture of left radius CC MCC
S52.379 Galeazzi's fracture of unspecified radius CC MCC

S52.38 Bent bone of radius
S52.381 Bent bone of right radius CC HAC MCC
S52.382 Bent bone of left radius CC HAC MCC
S52.389 Bent bone of unspecified radius CC HAC MCC

S52.39 Other fracture of shaft of radius
S52.391 Other fracture of shaft of radius, right arm CC HAC MCC
S52.392 Other fracture of shaft of radius, left arm CC HAC MCC
S52.399 Other fracture of shaft of radius, unspecified arm CC HAC MCC

S52.5 Fracture of lower end of radius
Fracture of distal end of radius
EXCLUDES2 *physeal fractures of lower end of radius (S59.2-)*

S52.50 Unspecified fracture of the lower end of radius
S52.501 Unspecified fracture of the lower end of right radius CC HAC MCC
S52.502 Unspecified fracture of the lower end of left radius CC HAC MCC
S52.509 Unspecified fracture of the lower end of unspecified radius CC HAC MCC

S52.51 Fracture of radial styloid process
S52.511 Displaced fracture of right radial styloid process CC HAC MCC
S52.512 Displaced fracture of left radial styloid process CC HAC MCC
S52.513 Displaced fracture of unspecified radial styloid process CC HAC MCC
S52.514 Nondisplaced fracture of right radial styloid process CC HAC MCC
S52.515 Nondisplaced fracture of left radial styloid process CC HAC MCC
S52.516 Nondisplaced fracture of unspecified radial styloid process CC HAC MCC

S52.52 Torus fracture of lower end of radius
The appropriate 7th character is to be added to all codes in subcategory S52.52
A = initial encounter for closed fracture
D = subsequent encounter for fracture with routine healing
G = subsequent encounter for fracture with delayed healing
K = subsequent encounter for fracture with nonunion
P = subsequent encounter for fracture with malunion
S = sequela
S52.521 Torus fracture of lower end of right r adius CC HAC
S52.522 Torus fracture of lower end of left radius CC HAC
S52.529 Torus fracture of lower end of unspecified radius CC HAC

S52.53 Colles' fracture
S52.531 Colles' fracture of right radius CC HAC MCC
S52.532 Colles' fracture of left radius CC HAC MCC
AHA: Q2, 2016
S52.539 Colles' fracture of unspecified radius CC HAC MCC

S52.54 Smith's fracture
S52.541 Smith's fracture of right radius CC HAC MCC
S52.542 Smith's fracture of left radius CC HAC MCC
S52.549 Smith's fracture of unspecified radius CC HAC MCC

S52.55 Other extraarticular fracture of lower end of radius
S52.551 Other extraarticular fracture of lower end of right radius CC HAC MCC
S52.552 Other extraarticular fracture of lower end of left radius CC HAC MCC
S52.559 Other extraarticular fracture of lower end of unspecified radius CC HAC MCC

S52.56 Barton's fracture
S52.561 Barton's fracture of right radius CC HAC MCC
S52.562 Barton's fracture of left radius CC HAC MCC
S52.569 Barton's fracture of unspecified radius CC HAC MCC

S52.57 Other intraarticular fracture of lower end of radius
S52.571 Other intraarticular fracture of lower end of right radius CC HAC MCC
S52.572 Other intraarticular fracture of lower end of left radius CC HAC MCC
S52.579 Other intraarticular fracture of lower end of unspecified radius CC HAC MCC

S52.59 Other fractures of lower end of radius
S52.591 Other fractures of lower end of right radius CC HAC MCC
S52.592 Other fractures of lower end of left radius CC HAC MCC
S52.599 Other fractures of lower end of unspecified radius CC HAC MCC

S52.6 Fracture of lower end of ulna
S52.60 Unspecified fracture of lower end of ulna

PDx Unacceptable principal diagnosis symbol per Medicare code edits · POA Code exempt from diagnosis present on admission requirement
? Questionable admission · CC Complication or comorbidity · CC/MCC Excl CC/MCC exclusion · MCC Major complication or comorbidity
PDx Principal diagnosis as its own CC · PDx Principal diagnosis as its own MCC · Z Z code as first-listed diagnosis

S52.601 Unspecified fracture of lower end of right ulna CC HAC MCC
S52.602 Unspecified fracture of lower end of left ulna CC HAC MCC
S52.609 Unspecified fracture of lower end of unspecified ulna CC HAC MCC
S52.61 Fracture of ulna styloid process
S52.611 Displaced fracture of right ulna styloid process CC HAC MCC
S52.612 Displaced fracture of left ulna styloid process CC HAC MCC
S52.613 Displaced fracture of unspecified ulna styloid process CC HAC MCC
S52.614 Nondisplaced fracture of right ulna styloid process CC HAC MCC
S52.615 Nondisplaced fracture of left ulna styloid process CC HAC MCC
S52.616 Nondisplaced fracture of unspecified ulna styloid process CC HAC MCC
S52.62 Torus fracture of lower end of ulna
The appropriate 7th character is to be added to all codes in subcategory S52.62
A = initial encounter for closed fracture
D = subsequent encounter for fracture with routine healing
G = subsequent encounter for fracture with delayed healing
K = subsequent encounter for fracture with nonunion
P = subsequent encounter for fracture with malunion
S = sequela
S52.621 Torus fracture of lower end of right ulna CC HAC
S52.622 Torus fracture of lower end of left ulna CC HAC
S52.629 Torus fracture of lower end of unspecified ulna CC HAC
S52.69 Other fracture of lower end of ulna
S52.691 Other fracture of lower end of right ulna CC HAC MCC
S52.692 Other fracture of lower end of left ulna CC HAC MCC
S52.699 Other fracture of lower end of unspecified ulna CC HAC MCC
S52.9 Unspecified fracture of forearm
S52.90 Unspecified fracture of unspecified forearm CC HAC MCC
S52.91 Unspecified fracture of right forearm CC HAC MCC
S52.92 Unspecified fracture of left forearm CC HAC MCC
S53 Dislocation and sprain of joints and ligaments of elbow
INCLUDES *avulsion of joint or ligament of elbow*
laceration of cartilage, joint or ligament of elbow
sprain of cartilage, joint or ligament of elbow
traumatic hemarthrosis of joint or ligament of elbow
traumatic rupture of joint or ligament of elbow
traumatic subluxation of joint or ligament of elbow
traumatic tear of joint or ligament of elbow
Code also any associated open wound
EXCLUDES2 *strain of muscle, fascia and tendon at forearm level (S56.-)*
The appropriate 7th character is to be added to each code from category S53
A = initial encounter
D = subsequent encounter
S = sequela
S53.0 Subluxation and dislocation of radial head
Dislocation of radiohumeral joint
Subluxation of radiohumeral joint
EXCLUDES1 *Monteggia's fracture-dislocation (S52.27-)*
S53.00 Unspecified subluxation and dislocation of radial head
S53.001 Unspecified subluxation of right radial head
S53.002 Unspecified subluxation of left radial head
S53.003 Unspecified subluxation of unspecified radial head
S53.004 Unspecified dislocation of right radial head
S53.005 Unspecified dislocation of left radial head
S53.006 Unspecified dislocation of unspecified radial head
S53.01 Anterior subluxation and dislocation of radial head
Anteromedial subluxation and dislocation of radial head
S53.011 Anterior subluxation of right radial head
S53.012 Anterior subluxation of left radial head
S53.013 Anterior subluxation of unspecified radial head
S53.014 Anterior dislocation of right radial head
S53.015 Anterior dislocation of left radial head
S53.016 Anterior dislocation of unspecified radial head
S53.02 Posterior subluxation and dislocation of radial head
Posterolateral subluxation and dislocation of radial head
S53.021 Posterior subluxation of right radial head
S53.022 Posterior subluxation of left radial head
S53.023 Posterior subluxation of unspecified radial head
S53.024 Posterior dislocation of right radial head
S53.025 Posterior dislocation of left radial head
S53.026 Posterior dislocation of unspecified radial head
S53.03 Nursemaid's elbow
S53.031 Nursemaid's elbow, right elbow
AHA: Q1, 2015
S53.032 Nursemaid's elbow, left elbow
S53.033 Nursemaid's elbow, unspecified elbow
S53.09 Other subluxation and dislocation of radial head
S53.091 Other subluxation of right radial head
S53.092 Other subluxation of left radial head
S53.093 Other subluxation of unspecified radial head
S53.094 Other dislocation of right radial head
S53.095 Other dislocation of left radial head
S53.096 Other dislocation of unspecified radial head
S53.1 Subluxation and dislocation of ulnohumeral joint
Subluxation and dislocation of elbow NOS
EXCLUDES1 *dislocation of radial head alone (S53.0-)*
S53.10 Unspecified subluxation and dislocation of ulnohumeral joint
S53.101 Unspecified subluxation of right ulnohumeral joint
S53.102 Unspecified subluxation of left ulnohumeral joint
S53.103 Unspecified subluxation of unspecified ulnohumeral joint
S53.104 Unspecified dislocation of right ulnohumeral joint
S53.105 Unspecified dislocation of left ulnohumeral joint
S53.106 Unspecified dislocation of unspecified ulnohumeral joint
S53.11 Anterior subluxation and dislocation of ulnohumeral joint
S53.111 Anterior subluxation of right ulnohumeral joint
S53.112 Anterior subluxation of left ulnohumeral joint
S53.113 Anterior subluxation of unspecified ulnohumeral joint
S53.114 Anterior dislocation of right ulnohumeral joint
AHA: Q4, 2012
S53.115 Anterior dislocation of left ulnohumeral joint

Unspecified Code Other Specified Code Manifestation Code N Newborn P Pediatric M Maternity A Adult ♂ Male ♀ Female
● New Code ▲ Revised Code Title ►◄ Revised Text NOTES INCLUDES EXCLUDES1 Not coded here EXCLUDES2 Not included here
4th character required 5th character required 6th character required 7th character required
Extension 'X' Alert HAC Hospital-acquired condition (HAC) alert AHA AHA Coding Clinic®

S53.116 Anterior dislocation of unspecified ulnohumeral joint

S53.12 Posterior subluxation and dislocation of ulnohumeral joint

S53.121 Posterior subluxation of right ulnohumeral joint

S53.122 Posterior subluxation of left ulnohumeral joint

S53.123 Posterior subluxation of unspecified ulnohumeral joint

S53.124 Posterior dislocation of right ulnohumeral joint

S53.125 Posterior dislocation of left ulnohumeral joint

S53.126 Posterior dislocation of unspecified ulnohumeral joint

S53.13 Medial subluxation and dislocation of ulnohumeral joint

S53.131 Medial subluxation of right ulnohumeral joint

S53.132 Medial subluxation of left ulnohumeral joint

S53.133 Medial subluxation of unspecified ulnohumeral joint

S53.134 Medial dislocation of right ulnohumeral joint

S53.135 Medial dislocation of left ulnohumeral joint

S53.136 Medial dislocation of unspecified ulnohumeral joint

S53.14 Lateral subluxation and dislocation of ulnohumeral joint

S53.141 Lateral subluxation of right ulnohumeral joint

S53.142 Lateral subluxation of left ulnohumeral joint

S53.143 Lateral subluxation of unspecified ulnohumeral joint

S53.144 Lateral dislocation of right ulnohumeral joint

S53.145 Lateral dislocation of left ulnohumeral joint

S53.146 Lateral dislocation of unspecified ulnohumeral joint

S53.19 Other subluxation and dislocation of ulnohumeral joint

S53.191 Other subluxation of right ulnohumeral joint

S53.192 Other subluxation of left ulnohumeral joint

S53.193 Other subluxation of unspecified ulnohumeral joint

S53.194 Other dislocation of right ulnohumeral joint

S53.195 Other dislocation of left ulnohumeral joint

S53.196 Other dislocation of unspecified ulnohumeral joint

S53.2 Traumatic rupture of radial collateral ligament

EXCLUDES1 *sprain of radial collateral ligament NOS (S53.43-)*

S53.20 Traumatic rupture of unspecified radial collateral ligament

S53.21 Traumatic rupture of right radial collateral ligament

S53.22 Traumatic rupture of left radial collateral ligament

S53.3 Traumatic rupture of ulnar collateral ligament

EXCLUDES1 *sprain of ulnar collateral ligament (S53.44-)*

S53.30 Traumatic rupture of unspecified ulnar collateral ligament

S53.31 Traumatic rupture of right ulnar collateral ligament

S53.32 Traumatic rupture of left ulnar collateral ligament

S53.4 Sprain of elbow

EXCLUDES2 *traumatic rupture of radial collateral ligament (S53.2-)*
traumatic rupture of ulnar collateral ligament (S53.3-)

S53.40 Unspecified sprain of elbow

S53.401 Unspecified sprain of right elbow

S53.402 Unspecified sprain of left elbow

S53.409 Unspecified sprain of unspecified elbow
Sprain of elbow NOS

S53.41 Radiohumeral (joint) sprain

S53.411 Radiohumeral (joint) sprain of right elbow

S53.412 Radiohumeral (joint) sprain of left elbow

S53.419 Radiohumeral (joint) sprain of unspecified elbow

S53.42 Ulnohumeral (joint) sprain

S53.421 Ulnohumeral (joint) sprain of right elbow

S53.422 Ulnohumeral (joint) sprain of left elbow

S53.429 Ulnohumeral (joint) sprain of unspecified elbow

S53.43 Radial collateral ligament sprain

S53.431 Radial collateral ligament sprain of right elbow

S53.432 Radial collateral ligament sprain of left elbow

S53.439 Radial collateral ligament sprain of unspecified elbow

S53.44 Ulnar collateral ligament sprain

S53.441 Ulnar collateral ligament sprain of right elbow

S53.442 Ulnar collateral ligament sprain of left elbow

S53.449 Ulnar collateral ligament sprain of unspecified elbow

S53.49 Other sprain of elbow

S53.491 Other sprain of right elbow

S53.492 Other sprain of left elbow

S53.499 Other sprain of unspecified elbow

S54 Injury of nerves at forearm level

Code also any associated open wound (S51.-)

EXCLUDES2 *injury of nerves at wrist and hand level (S64.-)*

The appropriate 7th character is to be added to each code from category S54

A = initial encounter
D = subsequent encounter
S = sequela

S54.0 Injury of ulnar nerve at forearm level
Injury of ulnar nerve NOS

S54.00 Injury of ulnar nerve at forearm level, unspecified arm

S54.01 Injury of ulnar nerve at forearm level, right arm

S54.02 Injury of ulnar nerve at forearm level, left arm

S54.1 Injury of median nerve at forearm level
Injury of median nerve NOS

S54.10 Injury of median nerve at forearm level, unspecified arm

S54.11 Injury of median nerve at forearm level, right arm

S54.12 Injury of median nerve at forearm level, left arm

S54.2 Injury of radial nerve at forearm level
Injury of radial nerve NOS

S54.20 Injury of radial nerve at forearm level, unspecified arm

S54.21 Injury of radial nerve at forearm level, right arm

S54.22 Injury of radial nerve at forearm level, left arm

S54.3 Injury of cutaneous sensory nerve at forearm level

S54.30 Injury of cutaneous sensory nerve at forearm level, unspecified arm

S54.31 Injury of cutaneous sensory nerve at forearm level, right arm

S54.32 Injury of cutaneous sensory nerve at forearm level, left arm

S54.8 Injury of other nerves at forearm level

▲ S54.8X ►Injury◄ of other nerves at forearm level

▲ S54.8X1 ►Injury◄ of other nerves at forearm level, right arm

▲ S54.8X2 ►Injury◄ of other nerves at forearm level, left arm

▲ S54.8X9 ►Injury◄ of other nerves at forearm level, unspecified arm

S54.9 Injury of unspecified nerve at forearm level

Unacceptable principal diagnosis symbol per Medicare code edits · Code exempt from diagnosis present on admission requirement
Questionable admission · Complication or comorbidity · CC/MCC exclusion · Major complication or comorbidity
Principal diagnosis as its own CC · Principal diagnosis as its own MCC · Z code as first-listed diagnosis

S54.90 Injury of unspecified nerve at forearm level, unspecified arm
S54.91 Injury of unspecified nerve at forearm level, right arm
S54.92 Injury of unspecified nerve at forearm level, left arm

S55 Injury of blood vessels at forearm level
Code also any associated open wound (S51.-)
EXCLUDES2 *injury of blood vessels at wrist and hand level (S65.-)*
injury of brachial vessels (S45.1-S45.2)
The appropriate 7th character is to be added to each code from category S55
A = initial encounter
D = subsequent encounter
S = sequela

S55.0 Injury of ulnar artery at forearm level
S55.00 Unspecified injury of ulnar artery at forearm level
S55.001 Unspecified injury of ulnar artery at forearm level, right arm
S55.002 Unspecified injury of ulnar artery at forearm level, left arm
S55.009 Unspecified injury of ulnar artery at forearm level, unspecified arm
S55.01 Laceration of ulnar artery at forearm level
S55.011 Laceration of ulnar artery at forearm level, right arm
S55.012 Laceration of ulnar artery at forearm level, left arm
S55.019 Laceration of ulnar artery at forearm level, unspecified arm
S55.09 Other specified injury of ulnar artery at forearm level
S55.091 Other specified injury of ulnar artery at forearm level, right arm
S55.092 Other specified injury of ulnar artery at forearm level, left arm
S55.099 Other specified injury of ulnar artery at forearm level, unspecified arm

S55.1 Injury of radial artery at forearm level
S55.10 Unspecified injury of radial artery at forearm level
S55.101 Unspecified injury of radial artery at forearm level, right arm
S55.102 Unspecified injury of radial artery at forearm level, left arm
S55.109 Unspecified injury of radial artery at forearm level, unspecified arm
S55.11 Laceration of radial artery at forearm level
S55.111 Laceration of radial artery at forearm level, right arm
S55.112 Laceration of radial artery at forearm level, left arm
S55.119 Laceration of radial artery at forearm level, unspecified arm
S55.19 Other specified injury of radial artery at forearm level
S55.191 Other specified injury of radial artery at forearm level, right arm
S55.192 Other specified injury of radial artery at forearm level, left arm
S55.199 Other specified injury of radial artery at forearm level, unspecified arm

S55.2 Injury of vein at forearm level
S55.20 Unspecified injury of vein at forearm level
S55.201 Unspecified injury of vein at forearm level, right arm
S55.202 Unspecified injury of vein at forearm level, left arm
S55.209 Unspecified injury of vein at forearm level, unspecified arm
S55.21 Laceration of vein at forearm level
S55.211 Laceration of vein at forearm level, right arm
S55.212 Laceration of vein at forearm level, left arm
S55.219 Laceration of vein at forearm level, unspecified arm
S55.29 Other specified injury of vein at forearm level
S55.291 Other specified injury of vein at forearm level, right arm
S55.292 Other specified injury of vein at forearm level, left arm
S55.299 Other specified injury of vein at forearm level, unspecified arm

S55.8 Injury of other blood vessels at forearm level
S55.80 Unspecified injury of other blood vessels at forearm level
S55.801 Unspecified injury of other blood vessels at forearm level, right arm
S55.802 Unspecified injury of other blood vessels at forearm level, left arm
S55.809 Unspecified injury of other blood vessels at forearm level, unspecified arm
S55.81 Laceration of other blood vessels at forearm level
S55.811 Laceration of other blood vessels at forearm level, right arm
S55.812 Laceration of other blood vessels at forearm level, left arm
S55.819 Laceration of other blood vessels at forearm level, unspecified arm
S55.89 Other specified injury of other blood vessels at forearm level
S55.891 Other specified injury of other blood vessels at forearm level, right arm
S55.892 Other specified injury of other blood vessels at forearm level, left arm
S55.899 Other specified injury of other blood vessels at forearm level, unspecified arm

S55.9 Injury of unspecified blood vessel at forearm level
S55.90 Unspecified injury of unspecified blood vessel at forearm level
S55.901 Unspecified injury of unspecified blood vessel at forearm level, right arm
S55.902 Unspecified injury of unspecified blood vessel at forearm level, left arm
S55.909 Unspecified injury of unspecified blood vessel at forearm level, unspecified arm
S55.91 Laceration of unspecified blood vessel at forearm level
S55.911 Laceration of unspecified blood vessel at forearm level, right arm
S55.912 Laceration of unspecified blood vessel at forearm level, left arm
S55.919 Laceration of unspecified blood vessel at forearm level, unspecified arm
S55.99 Other specified injury of unspecified blood vessel at forearm level
S55.991 Other specified injury of unspecified blood vessel at forearm level, right arm
S55.992 Other specified injury of unspecified blood vessel at forearm level, left arm
S55.999 Other specified injury of unspecified blood vessel at forearm level, unspecified arm

S56 Injury of muscle, fascia and tendon at forearm level
Code also any associated open wound (S51.-)
EXCLUDES2 *injury of muscle, fascia and tendon at or below wrist (S66.-)*
sprain of joints and ligaments of elbow (S53.4-)
The appropriate 7th character is to be added to each code from category S56
A = initial encounter
D = subsequent encounter
S = sequela

S56.0 Injury of flexor muscle, fascia and tendon of thumb at forearm level
S56.00 Unspecified injury of flexor muscle, fascia and tendon of thumb at forearm level
S56.001 Unspecified injury of flexor muscle, fascia and tendon of right thumb at forearm level
S56.002 Unspecified injury of flexor muscle, fascia and tendon of left thumb at forearm level

Unspecified Code Other Specified Code Manifestation Code N Newborn P Pediatric M Maternity A Adult ♂ Male ♀ Female
● New Code ▲ Revised Code Title ►◄ Revised Text NOTES INCLUDES EXCLUDES1 Not coded here EXCLUDES2 Not included here
4th character required 5th character required 6th character required 7th character required
Extension 'X' Alert HAC Hospital-acquired condition (HAC) alert AHA AHA Coding Clinic©

S56.009 Unspecified injury of flexor muscle, fascia and tendon of unspecified thumb at forearm level

S56.01 Strain of flexor muscle, fascia and tendon of thumb at forearm level

S56.011 Strain of flexor muscle, fascia and tendon of right thumb at forearm level

S56.012 Strain of flexor muscle, fascia and tendon of left thumb at forearm level

S56.019 Strain of flexor muscle, fascia and tendon of unspecified thumb at forearm level

S56.02 Laceration of flexor muscle, fascia and tendon of thumb at forearm level

S56.021 Laceration of flexor muscle, fascia and tendon of right thumb at forearm level CC

S56.022 Laceration of flexor muscle, fascia and tendon of left thumb at forearm level CC

S56.029 Laceration of flexor muscle, fascia and tendon of unspecified thumb at forearm level CC

S56.09 Other injury of flexor muscle, fascia and tendon of thumb at forearm level

S56.091 Other injury of flexor muscle, fascia and tendon of right thumb at forearm level

S56.092 Other injury of flexor muscle, fascia and tendon of left thumb at forearm level

S56.099 Other injury of flexor muscle, fascia and tendon of unspecified thumb at forearm level

S56.1 Injury of flexor muscle, fascia and tendon of other and unspecified finger at forearm level

S56.10 Unspecified injury of flexor muscle, fascia and tendon of other and unspecified finger at forearm level

S56.101 Unspecified injury of flexor muscle, fascia and tendon of right index finger at forearm level

S56.102 Unspecified injury of flexor muscle, fascia and tendon of left index finger at forearm level

S56.103 Unspecified injury of flexor muscle, fascia and tendon of right middle finger at forearm level

S56.104 Unspecified injury of flexor muscle, fascia and tendon of left middle finger at forearm level

S56.105 Unspecified injury of flexor muscle, fascia and tendon of right ring finger at forearm level

S56.106 Unspecified injury of flexor muscle, fascia and tendon of left ring finger at forearm level

S56.107 Unspecified injury of flexor muscle, fascia and tendon of right little finger at forearm level

S56.108 Unspecified injury of flexor muscle, fascia and tendon of left little finger at forearm level

S56.109 Unspecified injury of flexor muscle, fascia and tendon of unspecified finger at forearm level

S56.11 Strain of flexor muscle, fascia and tendon of other and unspecified finger at forearm level

S56.111 Strain of flexor muscle, fascia and tendon of right index finger at forearm level

S56.112 Strain of flexor muscle, fascia and tendon of left index finger at forearm level

S56.113 Strain of flexor muscle, fascia and tendon of right middle finger at forearm level

S56.114 Strain of flexor muscle, fascia and tendon of left middle finger at forearm level

S56.115 Strain of flexor muscle, fascia and tendon of right ring finger at forearm level

S56.116 Strain of flexor muscle, fascia and tendon of left ring finger at forearm level

S56.117 Strain of flexor muscle, fascia and tendon of right little finger at forearm level

S56.118 Strain of flexor muscle, fascia and tendon of left little finger at forearm level

S56.119 Strain of flexor muscle, fascia and tendon of finger of unspecified finger at forearm level

S56.12 Laceration of flexor muscle, fascia and tendon of other and unspecified finger at forearm level

S56.121 Laceration of flexor muscle, fascia and tendon of right index finger at forearm level CC

S56.122 Laceration of flexor muscle, fascia and tendon of left index finger at forearm level CC

S56.123 Laceration of flexor muscle, fascia and tendon of right middle finger at forearm level CC

S56.124 Laceration of flexor muscle, fascia and tendon of left middle finger at forearm level CC

S56.125 Laceration of flexor muscle, fascia and tendon of right ring finger at forearm level CC

S56.126 Laceration of flexor muscle, fascia and tendon of left ring finger at forearm level CC

S56.127 Laceration of flexor muscle, fascia and tendon of right little finger at forearm level CC

S56.128 Laceration of flexor muscle, fascia and tendon of left little finger at forearm level CC

S56.129 Laceration of flexor muscle, fascia and tendon of unspecified finger at forearm level CC

S56.19 Other injury of flexor muscle, fascia and tendon of other and unspecified finger at forearm level

S56.191 Other injury of flexor muscle, fascia and tendon of right index finger at forearm level

S56.192 Other injury of flexor muscle, fascia and tendon of left index finger at forearm level

S56.193 Other injury of flexor muscle, fascia and tendon of right middle finger at forearm level

S56.194 Other injury of flexor muscle, fascia and tendon of left middle finger at forearm level

S56.195 Other injury of flexor muscle, fascia and tendon of right ring finger at forearm level

S56.196 Other injury of flexor muscle, fascia and tendon of left ring finger at forearm level

S56.197 Other injury of flexor muscle, fascia and tendon of right little finger at forearm level

S56.198 Other injury of flexor muscle, fascia and tendon of left little finger at forearm level

S56.199 Other injury of flexor muscle, fascia and tendon of unspecified finger at forearm level

S56.2 Injury of other flexor muscle, fascia and tendon at forearm level

S56.20 Unspecified injury of other flexor muscle, fascia and tendon at forearm level

S56.201 Unspecified injury of other flexor muscle, fascia and tendon at forearm level, right arm

S56.202 Unspecified injury of other flexor muscle, fascia and tendon at forearm level, left arm

S56.209 Unspecified injury of other flexor muscle, fascia and tendon at forearm level, unspecified arm

S56.21 Strain of other flexor muscle, fascia and tendon at forearm level

Unacceptable principal diagnosis symbol per Medicare code edits | Code exempt from diagnosis present on admission requirement
Questionable admission | Complication or comorbidity | CC/MCC exclusion | Major complication or comorbidity
Principal diagnosis as its own CC | Principal diagnosis as its own MCC | Z code as first-listed diagnosis

S56.211 Strain of other flexor muscle, fascia and tendon at forearm level, right arm
S56.212 Strain of other flexor muscle, fascia and tendon at forearm level, left arm
S56.219 Strain of other flexor muscle, fascia and tendon at forearm level, unspecified arm
S56.22 Laceration of other flexor muscle, fascia and tendon at forearm level
S56.221 Laceration of other flexor muscle, fascia and tendon at forearm level, right arm
S56.222 Laceration of other flexor muscle, fascia and tendon at forearm level, left arm
S56.229 Laceration of other flexor muscle, fascia and tendon at forearm level, unspecified arm
S56.29 Other injury of other flexor muscle, fascia and tendon at forearm level
S56.291 Other injury of other flexor muscle, fascia and tendon at forearm level, right arm
S56.292 Other injury of other flexor muscle, fascia and tendon at forearm level, left arm
S56.299 Other injury of other flexor muscle, fascia and tendon at forearm level, unspecified arm
S56.3 Injury of extensor or abductor muscles, fascia and tendons of thumb at forearm level
S56.30 Unspecified injury of extensor or abductor muscles, fascia and tendons of thumb at forearm level
S56.301 Unspecified injury of extensor or abductor muscles, fascia and tendons of right thumb at forearm level
S56.302 Unspecified injury of extensor or abductor muscles, fascia and tendons of left thumb at forearm level
S56.309 Unspecified injury of extensor or abductor muscles, fascia and tendons of unspecified thumb at forearm level
S56.31 Strain of extensor or abductor muscles, fascia and tendons of thumb at forearm level
S56.311 Strain of extensor or abductor muscles, fascia and tendons of right thumb at forearm level
S56.312 Strain of extensor or abductor muscles, fascia and tendons of left thumb at forearm level
S56.319 Strain of extensor or abductor muscles, fascia and tendons of unspecified thumb at forearm level
S56.32 Laceration of extensor or abductor muscles, fascia and tendons of thumb at forearm level
S56.321 Laceration of extensor or abductor muscles, fascia and tendons of right thumb at forearm level
S56.322 Laceration of extensor or abductor muscles, fascia and tendons of left thumb at forearm level
S56.329 Laceration of extensor or abductor muscles, fascia and tendons of unspecified thumb at forearm level
S56.39 Other injury of extensor or abductor muscles, fascia and tendons of thumb at forearm level
S56.391 Other injury of extensor or abductor muscles, fascia and tendons of right thumb at forearm level
S56.392 Other injury of extensor or abductor muscles, fascia and tendons of left thumb at forearm level
S56.399 Other injury of extensor or abductor muscles, fascia and tendons of unspecified thumb at forearm level
S56.4 Injury of extensor muscle, fascia and tendon of other and unspecified finger at forearm level
S56.40 Unspecified injury of extensor muscle, fascia and tendon of other and unspecified finger at forearm level
S56.401 Unspecified injury of extensor muscle, fascia and tendon of right index finger at forearm level
S56.402 Unspecified injury of extensor muscle, fascia and tendon of left index finger at forearm level
S56.403 Unspecified injury of extensor muscle, fascia and tendon of right middle finger at forearm level
S56.404 Unspecified injury of extensor muscle, fascia and tendon of left middle finger at forearm level
S56.405 Unspecified injury of extensor muscle, fascia and tendon of right ring finger at forearm level
S56.406 Unspecified injury of extensor muscle, fascia and tendon of left ring finger at forearm level
S56.407 Unspecified injury of extensor muscle, fascia and tendon of right little finger at forearm level
S56.408 Unspecified injury of extensor muscle, fascia and tendon of left little finger at forearm level
S56.409 Unspecified injury of extensor muscle, fascia and tendon of unspecified finger at forearm level
S56.41 Strain of extensor muscle, fascia and tendon of other and unspecified finger at forearm level
S56.411 Strain of extensor muscle, fascia and tendon of right index finger at forearm level
S56.412 Strain of extensor muscle, fascia and tendon of left index finger at forearm level
S56.413 Strain of extensor muscle, fascia and tendon of right middle finger at forearm level
S56.414 Strain of extensor muscle, fascia and tendon of left middle finger at forearm level
S56.415 Strain of extensor muscle, fascia and tendon of right ring finger at forearm level
S56.416 Strain of extensor muscle, fascia and tendon of left ring finger at forearm level
S56.417 Strain of extensor muscle, fascia and tendon of right little finger at forearm level
S56.418 Strain of extensor muscle, fascia and tendon of left little finger at forearm level
S56.419 Strain of extensor muscle, fascia and tendon of finger, unspecified finger at forearm level
S56.42 Laceration of extensor muscle, fascia and tendon of other and unspecified finger at forearm level
S56.421 Laceration of extensor muscle, fascia and tendon of right index finger at forearm level
S56.422 Laceration of extensor muscle, fascia and tendon of left index finger at forearm level
S56.423 Laceration of extensor muscle, fascia and tendon of right middle finger at forearm level
S56.424 Laceration of extensor muscle, fascia and tendon of left middle finger at forearm level
S56.425 Laceration of extensor muscle, fascia and tendon of right ring finger at forearm level
S56.426 Laceration of extensor muscle, fascia and tendon of left ring finger at forearm level
S56.427 Laceration of extensor muscle, fascia and tendon of right little finger at forearm level

Unspecified Code Other Specified Code Manifestation Code N Newborn P Pediatric M Maternity A Adult ♂ Male ♀ Female
● New Code ▲ Revised Code Title ►◄ Revised Text NOTES INCLUDES EXCLUDES1 Not coded here EXCLUDES2 Not included here
4th character required 5th character required 6th character required 7th character required
Extension 'X' Alert HAC Hospital-acquired condition (HAC) alert AHA AHA Coding Clinic©

S56.428 Laceration of extensor muscle, fascia and tendon of left little finger at forearm level
S56.429 Laceration of extensor muscle, fascia and tendon of unspecified finger at forearm level
S56.49 Other injury of extensor muscle, fascia and tendon of other and unspecified finger at forearm level
S56.491 Other injury of extensor muscle, fascia and tendon of right index finger at forearm level
S56.492 Other injury of extensor muscle, fascia and tendon of left index finger at forearm level
S56.493 Other injury of extensor muscle, fascia and tendon of right middle finger at forearm level
S56.494 Other injury of extensor muscle, fascia and tendon of left middle finger at forearm level
S56.495 Other injury of extensor muscle, fascia and tendon of right ring finger at forearm level
S56.496 Other injury of extensor muscle, fascia and tendon of left ring finger at forearm level
S56.497 Other injury of extensor muscle, fascia and tendon of right little finger at forearm level
S56.498 Other injury of extensor muscle, fascia and tendon of left little finger at forearm level
S56.499 Other injury of extensor muscle, fascia and tendon of unspecified finger at forearm level
S56.5 Injury of other extensor muscle, fascia and tendon at forearm level
S56.50 Unspecified injury of other extensor muscle, fascia and tendon at forearm level
S56.501 Unspecified injury of other extensor muscle, fascia and tendon at forearm level, right arm
S56.502 Unspecified injury of other extensor muscle, fascia and tendon at forearm level, left arm
S56.509 Unspecified injury of other extensor muscle, fascia and tendon at forearm level, unspecified arm
S56.51 Strain of other extensor muscle, fascia and tendon at forearm level
S56.511 Strain of other extensor muscle, fascia and tendon at forearm level, right arm
S56.512 Strain of other extensor muscle, fascia and tendon at forearm level, left arm
S56.519 Strain of other extensor muscle, fascia and tendon at forearm level, unspecified arm
S56.52 Laceration of other extensor muscle, fascia and tendon at forearm level
S56.521 Laceration of other extensor muscle, fascia and tendon at forearm level, right arm
S56.522 Laceration of other extensor muscle, fascia and tendon at forearm level, left arm
S56.529 Laceration of other extensor muscle, fascia and tendon at forearm level, unspecified arm
S56.59 Other injury of other extensor muscle, fascia and tendon at forearm level
S56.591 Other injury of other extensor muscle, fascia and tendon at forearm level, right arm
S56.592 Other injury of other extensor muscle, fascia and tendon at forearm level, left arm
S56.599 Other injury of other extensor muscle, fascia and tendon at forearm level, unspecified arm
S56.8 Injury of other muscles, fascia and tendons at forearm level
S56.80 Unspecified injury of other muscles, fascia and tendons at forearm level
S56.801 Unspecified injury of other muscles, fascia and tendons at forearm level, right arm
S56.802 Unspecified injury of other muscles, fascia and tendons at forearm level, left arm
S56.809 Unspecified injury of other muscles, fascia and tendons at forearm level, unspecified arm
S56.81 Strain of other muscles, fascia and tendons at forearm level
S56.811 Strain of other muscles, fascia and tendons at forearm level, right arm
S56.812 Strain of other muscles, fascia and tendons at forearm level, left arm
S56.819 Strain of other muscles, fascia and tendons at forearm level, unspecified arm
S56.82 Laceration of other muscles, fascia and tendons at forearm level
S56.821 Laceration of other muscles, fascia and tendons at forearm level, right arm
S56.822 Laceration of other muscles, fascia and tendons at forearm level, left arm
S56.829 Laceration of other muscles, fascia and tendons at forearm level, unspecified arm
S56.89 Other injury of other muscles, fascia and tendons at forearm level
S56.891 Other injury of other muscles, fascia and tendons at forearm level, right arm
S56.892 Other injury of other muscles, fascia and tendons at forearm level, left arm
S56.899 Other injury of other muscles, fascia and tendons at forearm level, unspecified arm
S56.9 Injury of unspecified muscles, fascia and tendons at forearm level
S56.90 Unspecified injury of unspecified muscles, fascia and tendons at forearm level
S56.901 Unspecified injury of unspecified muscles, fascia and tendons at forearm level, right arm
S56.902 Unspecified injury of unspecified muscles, fascia and tendons at forearm level, left arm
S56.909 Unspecified injury of unspecified muscles, fascia and tendons at forearm level, unspecified arm
S56.91 Strain of unspecified muscles, fascia and tendons at forearm level
S56.911 Strain of unspecified muscles, fascia and tendons at forearm level, right arm
S56.912 Strain of unspecified muscles, fascia and tendons at forearm level, left arm
S56.919 Strain of unspecified muscles, fascia and tendons at forearm level, unspecified arm
S56.92 Laceration of unspecified muscles, fascia and tendons at forearm level
S56.921 Laceration of unspecified muscles, fascia and tendons at forearm level, right arm
S56.922 Laceration of unspecified muscles, fascia and tendons at forearm level, left arm
S56.929 Laceration of unspecified muscles, fascia and tendons at forearm level, unspecified arm
S56.99 Other injury of unspecified muscles, fascia and tendons at forearm level
S56.991 Other injury of unspecified muscles, fascia and tendons at forearm level, right arm
S56.992 Other injury of unspecified muscles, fascia and tendons at forearm level, left arm
S56.999 Other injury of unspecified muscles, fascia and tendons at forearm level, unspecified arm

Unacceptable principal diagnosis symbol per Medicare code edits — Code exempt from diagnosis present on admission requirement
Questionable admission — Complication or comorbidity — CC/MCC exclusion — Major complication or comorbidity
Principal diagnosis as its own CC — Principal diagnosis as its own MCC — Z code as first-listed diagnosis

S57 Crushing injury of elbow and forearm
Use additional code(s) for all associated injuries
EXCLUDES2 *crushing injury of wrist and hand (S67.-)*
The appropriate 7th character is to be added to each code from category S57
A = initial encounter
D = subsequent encounter
S = sequela

S57.0 Crushing injury of elbow
- S57.00 Crushing injury of unspecified elbow
- S57.01 Crushing injury of right elbow
- S57.02 Crushing injury of left elbow

S57.8 Crushing injury of forearm
- S57.80 Crushing injury of unspecified forearm
- S57.81 Crushing injury of right forearm
- S57.82 Crushing injury of left forearm

S58 Traumatic amputation of elbow and forearm
An amputation not identified as partial or complete should be coded to complete
EXCLUDES1 *traumatic amputation of wrist and hand (S68.-)*
The appropriate 7th character is to be added to each code from category S58
A = initial encounter
D = subsequent encounter
S = sequela

S58.0 Traumatic amputation at elbow level
- S58.01 Complete traumatic amputation at elbow level
  - S58.011 Complete traumatic amputation at elbow level, right arm
  - S58.012 Complete traumatic amputation at elbow level, left arm
  - S58.019 Complete traumatic amputation at elbow level, unspecified arm
- S58.02 Partial traumatic amputation at elbow level
  - S58.021 Partial traumatic amputation at elbow level, right arm
  - S58.022 Partial traumatic amputation at elbow level, left arm
  - S58.029 Partial traumatic amputation at elbow level, unspecified arm

S58.1 Traumatic amputation at level between elbow and wrist
- S58.11 Complete traumatic amputation at level between elbow and wrist
  - S58.111 Complete traumatic amputation at level between elbow and wrist, right arm
  - S58.112 Complete traumatic amputation at level between elbow and wrist, left arm
  - S58.119 Complete traumatic amputation at level between elbow and wrist, unspecified arm
- S58.12 Partial traumatic amputation at level between elbow and wrist
  - S58.121 Partial traumatic amputation at level between elbow and wrist, right arm
  - S58.122 Partial traumatic amputation at level between elbow and wrist, left arm
  - S58.129 Partial traumatic amputation at level between elbow and wrist, unspecified arm

S58.9 Traumatic amputation of forearm, level unspecified
EXCLUDES1 *traumatic amputation of wrist (S68.-)*
- S58.91 Complete traumatic amputation of forearm, level unspecified
  - S58.911 Complete traumatic amputation of right forearm, level unspecified
  - S58.912 Complete traumatic amputation of left forearm, level unspecified
  - S58.919 Complete traumatic amputation of unspecified forearm, level unspecified
- S58.92 Partial traumatic amputation of forearm, level unspecified
  - S58.921 Partial traumatic amputation of right forearm, level unspecified
  - S58.922 Partial traumatic amputation of left forearm, level unspecified
  - S58.929 Partial traumatic amputation of unspecified forearm, level unspecified

S59 Other and unspecified injuries of elbow and forearm
EXCLUDES2 *other and unspecified injuries of wrist and hand (S69.-)*
The appropriate 7th character is to be added to each code from subcategories S59.0, S59.1, and S59.2
A = initial encounter for closed fracture
D = subsequent encounter for fracture with routine healing
G = subsequent encounter for fracture with delayed healing
K = subsequent encounter for fracture with nonunion
P = subsequent encounter for fracture with malunion
S = sequela

S59.0 Physeal fracture of lower end of ulna
- S59.00 Unspecified physeal fracture of lower end of ulna
  - S59.001 Unspecified physeal fracture of lower end of ulna, right arm HAC
  - S59.002 Unspecified physeal fracture of lower end of ulna, left arm HAC
  - S59.009 Unspecified physeal fracture of lower end of ulna, unspecified arm HAC
- S59.01 Salter-Harris Type I physeal fracture of lower end of ulna
  - S59.011 Salter-Harris Type I physeal fracture of lower end of ulna, right arm HAC
  - S59.012 Salter-Harris Type I physeal fracture of lower end of ulna, left arm HAC
  - S59.019 Salter-Harris Type I physeal fracture of lower end of ulna, unspecified arm HAC
- S59.02 Salter-Harris Type II physeal fracture of lower end of ulna
  - S59.021 Salter-Harris Type II physeal fracture of lower end of ulna, right arm HAC
  - S59.022 Salter-Harris Type II physeal fracture of lower end of ulna, left arm HAC
  - S59.029 Salter-Harris Type II physeal fracture of lower end of ulna, unspecified arm HAC
- S59.03 Salter-Harris Type III physeal fracture of lower end of ulna
  - S59.031 Salter-Harris Type III physeal fracture of lower end of ulna, right arm HAC
  - S59.032 Salter-Harris Type III physeal fracture of lower end of ulna, left arm HAC
  - S59.039 Salter-Harris Type III physeal fracture of lower end of ulna, unspecified arm HAC
- S59.04 Salter-Harris Type IV physeal fracture of lower end of ulna
  - S59.041 Salter-Harris Type IV physeal fracture of lower end of ulna, right arm HAC
  - S59.042 Salter-Harris Type IV physeal fracture of lower end of ulna, left arm HAC
  - S59.049 Salter-Harris Type IV physeal fracture of lower end of ulna, unspecified arm HAC
- S59.09 Other physeal fracture of lower end of ulna
  - S59.091 Other physeal fracture of lower end of ulna, right arm HAC
  - S59.092 Other physeal fracture of lower end of ulna, left arm HAC
  - S59.099 Other physeal fracture of lower end of ulna, unspecified arm HAC

S59.1 Physeal fracture of upper end of radius
- S59.10 Unspecified physeal fracture of upper end of radius
  - S59.101 Unspecified physeal fracture of upper end of radius, right arm
  - S59.102 Unspecified physeal fracture of upper end of radius, left arm
  - S59.109 Unspecified physeal fracture of upper end of radius, unspecified arm
- S59.11 Salter-Harris Type I physeal fracture of upper end of radius
  - S59.111 Salter-Harris Type I physeal fracture of upper end of radius, right arm
  - S59.112 Salter-Harris Type I physeal fracture of upper end of radius, left arm
  - S59.119 Salter-Harris Type I physeal fracture of upper end of radius, unspecified arm

Unspecified Code Other Specified Code Manifestation Code N Newborn P Pediatric M Maternity A Adult ♂ Male ♀ Female
● New Code ▲ Revised Code Title ►◄ Revised Text NOTES INCLUDES EXCLUDES1 Not coded here EXCLUDES2 Not included here
4th character required 5th character required 6th character required 7th character required
Extension 'X' Alert HAC Hospital-acquired condition (HAC) alert AHA AHA Coding Clinic®

S59.12 Salter-Harris Type II physeal fracture of upper end of radius
S59.121 Salter-Harris Type II physeal fracture of upper end of radius, right arm
S59.122 Salter-Harris Type II physeal fracture of upper end of radius, left arm
S59.129 Salter-Harris Type II physeal fracture of upper end of radius, unspecified arm
S59.13 Salter-Harris Type III physeal fracture of upper end of radius
S59.131 Salter-Harris Type III physeal fracture of upper end of radius, right arm
S59.132 Salter-Harris Type III physeal fracture of upper end of radius, left arm
S59.139 Salter-Harris Type III physeal fracture of upper end of radius, unspecified arm
S59.14 Salter-Harris Type IV physeal fracture of upper end of radius
S59.141 Salter-Harris Type IV physeal fracture of upper end of radius, right arm
S59.142 Salter-Harris Type IV physeal fracture of upper end of radius, left arm
S59.149 Salter-Harris Type IV physeal fracture of upper end of radius, unspecified arm
S59.19 Other physeal fracture of upper end of radius
S59.191 Other physeal fracture of upper end of radius, right arm
S59.192 Other physeal fracture of upper end of radius, left arm
S59.199 Other physeal fracture of upper end of radius, unspecified arm
S59.2 Physeal fracture of lower end of radius
S59.20 Unspecified physeal fracture of lower end of radius
S59.201 Unspecified physeal fracture of lower end of radius, right arm HAC
S59.202 Unspecified physeal fracture of lower end of radius, left arm HAC
S59.209 Unspecified physeal fracture of lower end of radius, unspecified arm HAC
S59.21 Salter-Harris Type I physeal fracture of lower end of radius
S59.211 Salter-Harris Type I physeal fracture of lower end of radius, right arm HAC
S59.212 Salter-Harris Type I physeal fracture of lower end of radius, left arm HAC
S59.219 Salter-Harris Type I physeal fracture of lower end of radius, unspecified arm HAC
S59.22 Salter-Harris Type II physeal fracture of lower end of radius
S59.221 Salter-Harris Type II physeal fracture of lower end of radius, right arm HAC
S59.222 Salter-Harris Type II physeal fracture of lower end of radius, left arm HAC
S59.229 Salter-Harris Type II physeal fracture of lower end of radius, unspecified arm HAC
S59.23 Salter-Harris Type III physeal fracture of lower end of radius
S59.231 Salter-Harris Type III physeal fracture of lower end of radius, right arm HAC
S59.232 Salter-Harris Type III physeal fracture of lower end of radius, left arm HAC
S59.239 Salter-Harris Type III physeal fracture of lower end of radius, unspecified arm HAC
S59.24 Salter-Harris Type IV physeal fracture of lower end of radius
S59.241 Salter-Harris Type IV physeal fracture of lower end of radius, right arm HAC
S59.242 Salter-Harris Type IV physeal fracture of lower end of radius, left arm HAC
S59.249 Salter-Harris Type IV physeal fracture of lower end of radius, unspecified arm HAC
S59.29 Other physeal fracture of lower end of radius
S59.291 Other physeal fracture of lower end of radius, right arm HAC
S59.292 Other physeal fracture of lower end of radius, left arm HAC
S59.299 Other physeal fracture of lower end of radius, unspecified arm HAC
S59.8 Other specified injuries of elbow and forearm
The appropriate 7th character is to be added to each code in subcategory S59.8
A = initial encounter
D = subsequent encounter
S = sequela
S59.80 Other specified injuries of elbow
S59.801 Other specified injuries of right elbow
S59.802 Other specified injuries of left elbow
S59.809 Other specified injuries of unspecified elbow
S59.81 Other specified injuries of forearm
S59.811 Other specified injuries right forearm
S59.812 Other specified injuries left forearm
S59.819 Other specified injuries unspecified forearm
S59.9 Unspecified injury of elbow and forearm
The appropriate 7th character is to be added to each code in subcategory S59.9
A = initial encounter
D = subsequent encounter
S = sequela
S59.90 Unspecified injury of elbow
S59.901 Unspecified injury of right elbow
S59.902 Unspecified injury of left elbow
S59.909 Unspecified injury of unspecified elbow
S59.91 Unspecified injury of forearm
S59.911 Unspecified injury of right forearm
S59.912 Unspecified injury of left forearm
S59.919 Unspecified injury of unspecified forearm

Unacceptable principal diagnosis symbol per Medicare code edits | Code exempt from diagnosis present on admission requirement | Questionable admission | Complication or comorbidity | CC/MCC exclusion | Major complication or comorbidity | Principal diagnosis as its own CC | Principal diagnosis as its own MCC | Z code as first-listed diagnosis

Injuries to the wrist, hand and fingers (S60-S69)

EXCLUDES2 *burns and corrosions (T20-T32)*
frostbite (T33-T34)
insect bite or sting, venomous (T63.4)

S60 Superficial injury of wrist, hand and fingers
The appropriate 7th character is to be added to each code from category S60
A = initial encounter
D = subsequent encounter
S = sequela

S60.0 Contusion of finger without damage to nail
EXCLUDES1 *contusion involving nail (matrix) (S60.1)*
S60.00 Contusion of unspecified finger without damage to nail
Contusion of finger(s) NOS
S60.01 Contusion of thumb without damage to nail
S60.011 Contusion of right thumb without damage to nail
S60.012 Contusion of left thumb without damage to nail
S60.019 Contusion of unspecified thumb without damage to nail
S60.02 Contusion of index finger without damage to nail
S60.021 Contusion of right index finger without damage to nail
S60.022 Contusion of left index finger without damage to nail
S60.029 Contusion of unspecified index finger without damage to nail
S60.03 Contusion of middle finger without damage to nail
S60.031 Contusion of right middle finger without damage to nail
S60.032 Contusion of left middle finger without damage to nail
S60.039 Contusion of unspecified middle finger without damage to nail
S60.04 Contusion of ring finger without damage to nail
S60.041 Contusion of right ring finger without damage to nail
S60.042 Contusion of left ring finger without damage to nail
S60.049 Contusion of unspecified ring finger without damage to nail
S60.05 Contusion of little finger without damage to nail
S60.051 Contusion of right little finger without damage to nail
S60.052 Contusion of left little finger without damage to nail
S60.059 Contusion of unspecified little finger without damage to nail

S60.1 Contusion of finger with damage to nail
S60.10 Contusion of unspecified finger with damage to nail
S60.11 Contusion of thumb with damage to nail
S60.111 Contusion of right thumb with damage to nail
S60.112 Contusion of left thumb with damage to nail
S60.119 Contusion of unspecified thumb with damage to nail
S60.12 Contusion of index finger with damage to nail
S60.121 Contusion of right index finger with damage to nail
S60.122 Contusion of left index finger with damage to nail
S60.129 Contusion of unspecified index finger with damage to nail
S60.13 Contusion of middle finger with damage to nail
S60.131 Contusion of right middle finger with damage to nail
S60.132 Contusion of left middle finger with damage to nail
S60.139 Contusion of unspecified middle finger with damage to nail
S60.14 Contusion of ring finger with damage to nail
S60.141 Contusion of right ring finger with damage to nail
S60.142 Contusion of left ring finger with damage to nail
S60.149 Contusion of unspecified ring finger with damage to nail
S60.15 Contusion of little finger with damage to nail
S60.151 Contusion of right little finger with damage to nail
S60.152 Contusion of left little finger with damage to nail
S60.159 Contusion of unspecified little finger with damage to nail

S60.2 Contusion of wrist and hand
EXCLUDES2 *contusion of fingers (S60.0-, S60.1-)*
S60.21 Contusion of wrist
S60.211 Contusion of right wrist
S60.212 Contusion of left wrist
S60.219 Contusion of unspecified wrist
S60.22 Contusion of hand
S60.221 Contusion of right hand
S60.222 Contusion of left hand
S60.229 Contusion of unspecified hand

S60.3 Other superficial injuries of thumb
S60.31 Abrasion of thumb
S60.311 Abrasion of right thumb
S60.312 Abrasion of left thumb
S60.319 Abrasion of unspecified thumb
S60.32 Blister (nonthermal) of thumb
S60.321 Blister (nonthermal) of right thumb
S60.322 Blister (nonthermal) of left thumb
S60.329 Blister (nonthermal) of unspecified thumb
S60.34 External constriction of thumb
Hair tourniquet syndrome of thumb
Use additional cause code to identify the constricting item (W49.0-)
S60.341 External constriction of right thumb
S60.342 External constriction of left thumb
S60.349 External constriction of unspecified thumb
S60.35 Superficial foreign body of thumb
Splinter in the thumb
S60.351 Superficial foreign body of right thumb
S60.352 Superficial foreign body of left thumb
S60.359 Superficial foreign body of unspecified thumb
S60.36 Insect bite (nonvenomous) of thumb
S60.361 Insect bite (nonvenomous) of right thumb
S60.362 Insect bite (nonvenomous) of left thumb
S60.369 Insect bite (nonvenomous) of unspecified thumb
S60.37 Other superficial bite of thumb
EXCLUDES1 *open bite of thumb (S61.05-, S61.15-)*
S60.371 Other superficial bite of right thumb
S60.372 Other superficial bite of left thumb
S60.379 Other superficial bite of unspecified thumb
S60.39 Other superficial injuries of thumb
S60.391 Other superficial injuries of right thumb
S60.392 Other superficial injuries of left thumb
S60.399 Other superficial injuries of unspecified thumb

S60.4 Other superficial injuries of other fingers
S60.41 Abrasion of fingers
S60.410 Abrasion of right index finger
S60.411 Abrasion of left index finger
S60.412 Abrasion of right middle finger
S60.413 Abrasion of left middle finger
S60.414 Abrasion of right ring finger
S60.415 Abrasion of left ring finger
S60.416 Abrasion of right little finger
S60.417 Abrasion of left little finger
S60.418 Abrasion of other finger

Unspecified Code Other Specified Code Manifestation Code N Newborn P Pediatric M Maternity A Adult ♂ Male ♀ Female
● New Code ▲ Revised Code Title ►◄ Revised Text NOTES INCLUDES EXCLUDES1 Not coded here EXCLUDES2 Not included here
4th character required 5th character required 6th character required 7th character required
Extension 'X' Alert HAC Hospital-acquired condition (HAC) alert AHA AHA Coding Clinic©

Abrasion of specified finger with unspecified laterality

S60.419 Abrasion of unspecified finger

S60.42 Blister (nonthermal) of fingers

S60.420 Blister (nonthermal) of right index finger

S60.421 Blister (nonthermal) of left index finger

S60.422 Blister (nonthermal) of right middle finger

S60.423 Blister (nonthermal) of left middle finger

S60.424 Blister (nonthermal) of right ring finger

S60.425 Blister (nonthermal) of left ring finger

S60.426 Blister (nonthermal) of right little finger

S60.427 Blister (nonthermal) of left little finger

S60.428 Blister (nonthermal) of other finger

Blister (nonthermal) of specified finger with unspecified laterality

S60.429 Blister (nonthermal) of unspecified finger

S60.44 External constriction of fingers

Hair tourniquet syndrome of finger

Use additional cause code to identify the constricting item (W49.0-)

S60.440 External constriction of right index finger

S60.441 External constriction of left index finger

S60.442 External constriction of right middle finger

S60.443 External constriction of left middle finger

S60.444 External constriction of right ring finger

S60.445 External constriction of left ring finger

S60.446 External constriction of right little finger

S60.447 External constriction of left little finger

S60.448 External constriction of other finger

External constriction of specified finger with unspecified laterality

S60.449 External constriction of unspecified finger

S60.45 Superficial foreign body of fingers

Splinter in the finger(s)

S60.450 Superficial foreign body of right index finger

S60.451 Superficial foreign body of left index finger

S60.452 Superficial foreign body of right middle finger

S60.453 Superficial foreign body of left middle finger

S60.454 Superficial foreign body of right ring finger

S60.455 Superficial foreign body of left ring finger

S60.456 Superficial foreign body of right little finger

S60.457 Superficial foreign body of left little finger

S60.458 Superficial foreign body of other finger

Superficial foreign body of specified finger with unspecified laterality

S60.459 Superficial foreign body of unspecified finger

S60.46 Insect bite (nonvenomous) of fingers

S60.460 Insect bite (nonvenomous) of right index finger

S60.461 Insect bite (nonvenomous) of left index finger

S60.462 Insect bite (nonvenomous) of right middle finger

S60.463 Insect bite (nonvenomous) of left middle finger

S60.464 Insect bite (nonvenomous) of right ring finger

S60.465 Insect bite (nonvenomous) of left ring finger

S60.466 Insect bite (nonvenomous) of right little finger

S60.467 Insect bite (nonvenomous) of left little finger

S60.468 Insect bite (nonvenomous) of other finger

Insect bite (nonvenomous) of specified finger with unspecified laterality

S60.469 Insect bite (nonvenomous) of unspecified finger

S60.47 Other superficial bite of fingers

EXCLUDES1 *open bite of fingers (S61.25-, S61.35-)*

S60.470 Other superficial bite of right index finger

S60.471 Other superficial bite of left index finger

S60.472 Other superficial bite of right middle finger

S60.473 Other superficial bite of left middle finger

S60.474 Other superficial bite of right ring finger

S60.475 Other superficial bite of left ring finger

S60.476 Other superficial bite of right little finger

S60.477 Other superficial bite of left little finger

S60.478 Other superficial bite of other finger

Other superficial bite of specified finger with unspecified laterality

S60.479 Other superficial bite of unspecified finger

S60.5 Other superficial injuries of hand

EXCLUDES2 *superficial injuries of fingers (S60.3-, S60.4-)*

S60.51 Abrasion of hand

S60.511 Abrasion of right hand

S60.512 Abrasion of left hand

S60.519 Abrasion of unspecified hand

S60.52 Blister (nonthermal) of hand

S60.521 Blister (nonthermal) of right hand

S60.522 Blister (nonthermal) of left hand

S60.529 Blister (nonthermal) of unspecified hand

S60.54 External constriction of hand

S60.541 External constriction of right hand

S60.542 External constriction of left hand

S60.549 External constriction of unspecified hand

S60.55 Superficial foreign body of hand

Splinter in the hand

S60.551 Superficial foreign body of right hand

S60.552 Superficial foreign body of left hand

S60.559 Superficial foreign body of unspecified hand

S60.56 Insect bite (nonvenomous) of hand

S60.561 Insect bite (nonvenomous) of right hand

S60.562 Insect bite (nonvenomous) of left hand

S60.569 Insect bite (nonvenomous) of unspecified hand

S60.57 Other superficial bite of hand

EXCLUDES1 *open bite of hand (S61.45-)*

S60.571 Other superficial bite of hand of right hand

S60.572 Other superficial bite of hand of left hand

S60.579 Other superficial bite of hand of unspecified hand

S60.8 Other superficial injuries of wrist

S60.81 Abrasion of wrist

S60.811 Abrasion of right wrist

S60.812 Abrasion of left wrist

S60.819 Abrasion of unspecified wrist

S60.82 Blister (nonthermal) of wrist

S60.821 Blister (nonthermal) of right wrist

S60.822 Blister (nonthermal) of left wrist

S60.829 Blister (nonthermal) of unspecified wrist

S60.84 External constriction of wrist

S60.841 External constriction of right wrist

S60.842 External constriction of left wrist

S60.849 External constriction of unspecified wrist

S60.85 Superficial foreign body of wrist

Splinter in the wrist

S60.851 Superficial foreign body of right wrist

S60.852 Superficial foreign body of left wrist

S60.859 Superficial foreign body of unspecified wrist

S60.86 Insect bite (nonvenomous) of wrist

S60.861 Insect bite (nonvenomous) of right wrist

S60.862 Insect bite (nonvenomous) of left wrist

S60.869 Insect bite (nonvenomous) of unspecified wrist

Unacceptable principal diagnosis symbol per Medicare code edits | Code exempt from diagnosis present on admission requirement
Questionable admission | Complication or comorbidity | CC/MCC exclusion | Major complication or comorbidity
Principal diagnosis as its own CC | Principal diagnosis as its own MCC | Z code as first-listed diagnosis

S60.87 Other superficial bite of wrist
EXCLUDES1 *open bite of wrist (S61.55)*
S60.871 Other superficial bite of right wrist
S60.872 Other superficial bite of left wrist
S60.879 Other superficial bite of unspecified wrist
S60.9 Unspecified superficial injury of wrist, hand and fingers
S60.91 Unspecified superficial injury of wrist
S60.911 Unspecified superficial injury of right wrist
S60.912 Unspecified superficial injury of left wrist
S60.919 Unspecified superficial injury of unspecified wrist
S60.92 Unspecified superficial injury of hand
S60.921 Unspecified superficial injury of right hand
S60.922 Unspecified superficial injury of left hand
S60.929 Unspecified superficial injury of unspecified hand
S60.93 Unspecified superficial injury of thumb
S60.931 Unspecified superficial injury of right thumb
S60.932 Unspecified superficial injury of left thumb
S60.939 Unspecified superficial injury of unspecified thumb
S60.94 Unspecified superficial injury of other fingers
S60.940 Unspecified superficial injury of right index finger
S60.941 Unspecified superficial injury of left index finger
S60.942 Unspecified superficial injury of right middle finger
S60.943 Unspecified superficial injury of left middle finger
S60.944 Unspecified superficial injury of right ring finger
S60.945 Unspecified superficial injury of left ring finger
S60.946 Unspecified superficial injury of right little finger
S60.947 Unspecified superficial injury of left little finger
S60.948 Unspecified superficial injury of other finger
Unspecified superficial injury of specified finger with unspecified laterality
S60.949 Unspecified superficial injury of unspecified finger

S61 Open wound of wrist, hand and fingers
Code also any associated wound infection
EXCLUDES1 *open fracture of wrist, hand and finger (S62.- with 7th character B)*
traumatic amputation of wrist and hand (S68.-)
The appropriate 7th character is to be added to each code from category S61
A = initial encounter
D = subsequent encounter
S = sequela
S61.0 Open wound of thumb without damage to nail
EXCLUDES1 *open wound of thumb with damage to nail (S61.1-)*
S61.00 Unspecified open wound of thumb without damage to nail
S61.001 Unspecified open wound of right thumb without damage to nail
S61.002 Unspecified open wound of left thumb without damage to nail
S61.009 Unspecified open wound of unspecified thumb without damage to nail
S61.01 Laceration without foreign body of thumb without damage to nail
S61.011 Laceration without foreign body of right thumb without damage to nail
S61.012 Laceration without foreign body of left thumb without damage to nail
S61.019 Laceration without foreign body of unspecified thumb without damage to nail
S61.02 Laceration with foreign body of thumb without damage to nail
S61.021 Laceration with foreign body of right thumb without damage to nail
S61.022 Laceration with foreign body of left thumb without damage to nail
S61.029 Laceration with foreign body of unspecified thumb without damage to nail
S61.03 Puncture wound without foreign body of thumb without damage to nail
S61.031 Puncture wound without foreign body of right thumb without damage to nail
S61.032 Puncture wound without foreign body of left thumb without damage to nail
S61.039 Puncture wound without foreign body of unspecified thumb without damage to nail
S61.04 Puncture wound with foreign body of thumb without damage to nail
S61.041 Puncture wound with foreign body of right thumb without damage to nail
S61.042 Puncture wound with foreign body of left thumb without damage to nail
S61.049 Puncture wound with foreign body of unspecified thumb without damage to nail
S61.05 Open bite of thumb without damage to nail
Bite of thumb NOS
EXCLUDES1 *superficial bite of thumb (S60.36-, S60.37-)*
S61.051 Open bite of right thumb without damage to nail
S61.052 Open bite of left thumb without damage to nail
S61.059 Open bite of unspecified thumb without damage to nail
S61.1 Open wound of thumb with damage to nail
S61.10 Unspecified open wound of thumb with damage to nail
S61.101 Unspecified open wound of right thumb with damage to nail
S61.102 Unspecified open wound of left thumb with damage to nail
S61.109 Unspecified open wound of unspecified thumb with damage to nail
S61.11 Laceration without foreign body of thumb with damage to nail
S61.111 Laceration without foreign body of right thumb with damage to nail
S61.112 Laceration without foreign body of left thumb with damage to nail
S61.119 Laceration without foreign body of unspecified thumb with damage to nail
S61.12 Laceration with foreign body of thumb with damage to nail
S61.121 Laceration with foreign body of right thumb with damage to nail
S61.122 Laceration with foreign body of left thumb with damage to nail
S61.129 Laceration with foreign body of unspecified thumb with damage to nail
S61.13 Puncture wound without foreign body of thumb with damage to nail
S61.131 Puncture wound without foreign body of right thumb with damage to nail
S61.132 Puncture wound without foreign body of left thumb with damage to nail
S61.139 Puncture wound without foreign body of unspecified thumb with damage to nail
S61.14 Puncture wound with foreign body of thumb with damage to nail
S61.141 Puncture wound with foreign body of right thumb with damage to nail

Unspecified Code Other Specified Code Manifestation Code N Newborn P Pediatric M Maternity A Adult ♂ Male ♀ Female
● New Code ▲ Revised Code Title ►◄ Revised Text NOTES INCLUDES EXCLUDES1 Not coded here EXCLUDES2 Not included here
4th character required 5th character required 6th character required 7th character required
Extension 'X' Alert HAC Hospital-acquired condition (HAC) alert AHA AHA Coding Clinic©

S61.142 Puncture wound with foreign body of left thumb with damage to nail
S61.149 Puncture wound with foreign body of unspecified thumb with damage to nail
S61.15 Open bite of thumb with damage to nail
Bite of thumb with damage to nail NOS
EXCLUDES1 *superficial bite of thumb (S60.36-, S60.37-)*
S61.151 Open bite of right thumb with damage to nail
S61.152 Open bite of left thumb with damage to nail
S61.159 Open bite of unspecified thumb with damage to nail
S61.2 Open wound of other finger without damage to nail
EXCLUDES1 *open wound of finger involving nail (matrix) (S61.3-)*
EXCLUDES2 *open wound of thumb without damage to nail (S61.0-)*
S61.20 Unspecified open wound of other finger without damage to nail
S61.200 Unspecified open wound of right index finger without damage to nail
S61.201 Unspecified open wound of left index finger without damage to nail
S61.202 Unspecified open wound of right middle finger without damage to nail
S61.203 Unspecified open wound of left middle finger without damage to nail
S61.204 Unspecified open wound of right ring finger without damage to nail
S61.205 Unspecified open wound of left ring finger without damage to nail
S61.206 Unspecified open wound of right little finger without damage to nail
S61.207 Unspecified open wound of left little finger without damage to nail
S61.208 Unspecified open wound of other finger without damage to nail
Unspecified open wound of specified finger with unspecified laterality without damage to nail
S61.209 Unspecified open wound of unspecified finger without damage to nail
S61.21 Laceration without foreign body of finger without damage to nail
S61.210 Laceration without foreign body of right index finger without damage to nail
S61.211 Laceration without foreign body of left index finger without damage to nail
S61.212 Laceration without foreign body of right middle finger without damage to nail
S61.213 Laceration without foreign body of left middle finger without damage to nail
S61.214 Laceration without foreign body of right ring finger without damage to nail
S61.215 Laceration without foreign body of left ring finger without damage to nail
S61.216 Laceration without foreign body of right little finger without damage to nail
S61.217 Laceration without foreign body of left little finger without damage to nail
S61.218 Laceration without foreign body of other finger without damage to nail
Laceration without foreign body of specified finger with unspecified laterality without damage to nail
S61.219 Laceration without foreign body of unspecified finger without damage to nail
S61.22 Laceration with foreign body of finger without damage to nail
S61.220 Laceration with foreign body of right index finger without damage to nail
S61.221 Laceration with foreign body of left index finger without damage to nail
S61.222 Laceration with foreign body of right middle finger without damage to nail
S61.223 Laceration with foreign body of left middle finger without damage to nail
S61.224 Laceration with foreign body of right ring finger without damage to nail
S61.225 Laceration with foreign body of left ring finger without damage to nail
S61.226 Laceration with foreign body of right little finger without damage to nail
S61.227 Laceration with foreign body of left little finger without damage to nail
S61.228 Laceration with foreign body of other finger without damage to nail
Laceration with foreign body of specified finger with unspecified laterality without damage to nail
S61.229 Laceration with foreign body of unspecified finger without damage to nail
S61.23 Puncture wound without foreign body of finger without damage to nail
S61.230 Puncture wound without foreign body of right index finger without damage to nail
S61.231 Puncture wound without foreign body of left index finger without damage to nail
S61.232 Puncture wound without foreign body of right middle finger without damage to nail
S61.233 Puncture wound without foreign body of left middle finger without damage to nail
S61.234 Puncture wound without foreign body of right ring finger without damage to nail
S61.235 Puncture wound without foreign body of left ring finger without damage to nail
S61.236 Puncture wound without foreign body of right little finger without damage to nail
S61.237 Puncture wound without foreign body of left little finger without damage to nail
S61.238 Puncture wound without foreign body of other finger without damage to nail
Puncture wound without foreign body of specified finger with unspecified laterality without damage to nail
S61.239 Puncture wound without foreign body of unspecified finger without damage to nail
S61.24 Puncture wound with foreign body of finger without damage to nail
S61.240 Puncture wound with foreign body of right index finger without damage to nail
S61.241 Puncture wound with foreign body of left index finger without damage to nail
S61.242 Puncture wound with foreign body of right middle finger without damage to nail
S61.243 Puncture wound with foreign body of left middle finger without damage to nail
S61.244 Puncture wound with foreign body of right ring finger without damage to nail
S61.245 Puncture wound with foreign body of left ring finger without damage to nail
S61.246 Puncture wound with foreign body of right little finger without damage to nail
S61.247 Puncture wound with foreign body of left little finger without damage to nail
S61.248 Puncture wound with foreign body of other finger without damage to nail
Puncture wound with foreign body of specified finger with unspecified laterality without damage to nail
S61.249 Puncture wound with foreign body of unspecified finger without damage to nail
S61.25 Open bite of finger without damage to nail
Bite of finger without damage to nail NOS
EXCLUDES1 *superficial bite of finger (S60.46-, S60.47-)*
S61.250 Open bite of right index finger without damage to nail
S61.251 Open bite of left index finger without damage to nail
S61.252 Open bite of right middle finger without damage to nail

Unacceptable principal diagnosis symbol per Medicare code edits · Code exempt from diagnosis present on admission requirement
Questionable admission · Complication or comorbidity · CC/MCC exclusion · Major complication or comorbidity
Principal diagnosis as its own CC · Principal diagnosis as its own MCC · Z code as first-listed diagnosis

S61.253 Open bite of left middle finger without damage to nail
S61.254 Open bite of right ring finger without damage to nail
S61.255 Open bite of left ring finger without damage to nail
S61.256 Open bite of right little finger without damage to nail
S61.257 Open bite of left little finger without damage to nail
S61.258 Open bite of other finger without damage to nail
Open bite of specified finger with unspecified laterality without damage to nail
S61.259 Open bite of unspecified finger without damage to nail

S61.3 Open wound of other finger with damage to nail

S61.30 Unspecified open wound of finger with damage to nail
S61.300 Unspecified open wound of right index finger with damage to nail
S61.301 Unspecified open wound of left index finger with damage to nail
S61.302 Unspecified open wound of right middle finger with damage to nail
S61.303 Unspecified open wound of left middle finger with damage to nail
S61.304 Unspecified open wound of right ring finger with damage to nail
S61.305 Unspecified open wound of left ring finger with damage to nail
S61.306 Unspecified open wound of right little finger with damage to nail
S61.307 Unspecified open wound of left little finger with damage to nail
S61.308 Unspecified open wound of other finger with damage to nail
Unspecified open wound of specified finger with unspecified laterality with damage to nail
S61.309 Unspecified open wound of unspecified finger with damage to nail

S61.31 Laceration without foreign body of finger with damage to nail
S61.310 Laceration without foreign body of right index finger with damage to nail
S61.311 Laceration without foreign body of left index finger with damage to nail
S61.312 Laceration without foreign body of right middle finger with damage to nail
S61.313 Laceration without foreign body of left middle finger with damage to nail
S61.314 Laceration without foreign body of right ring finger with damage to nail
S61.315 Laceration without foreign body of left ring finger with damage to nail
S61.316 Laceration without foreign body of right little finger with damage to nail
S61.317 Laceration without foreign body of left little finger with damage to nail
S61.318 Laceration without foreign body of other finger with damage to nail
Laceration without foreign body of specified finger with unspecified laterality with damage to nail
S61.319 Laceration without foreign body of unspecified finger with damage to nail

S61.32 Laceration with foreign body of finger with damage to nail
S61.320 Laceration with foreign body of right index finger with damage to nail
S61.321 Laceration with foreign body of left index finger with damage to nail
S61.322 Laceration with foreign body of right middle finger with damage to nail
S61.323 Laceration with foreign body of left middle finger with damage to nail
S61.324 Laceration with foreign body of right ring finger with damage to nail
S61.325 Laceration with foreign body of left ring finger with damage to nail
S61.326 Laceration with foreign body of right little finger with damage to nail
S61.327 Laceration with foreign body of left little finger with damage to nail
S61.328 Laceration with foreign body of other finger with damage to nail
Laceration with foreign body of specified finger with unspecified laterality with damage to nail
S61.329 Laceration with foreign body of unspecified finger with damage to nail

S61.33 Puncture wound without foreign body of finger with damage to nail
S61.330 Puncture wound without foreign body of right index finger with damage to nail
S61.331 Puncture wound without foreign body of left index finger with damage to nail
S61.332 Puncture wound without foreign body of right middle finger with damage to nail
S61.333 Puncture wound without foreign body of left middle finger with damage to nail
S61.334 Puncture wound without foreign body of right ring finger with damage to nail
S61.335 Puncture wound without foreign body of left ring finger with damage to nail
S61.336 Puncture wound without foreign body of right little finger with damage to nail
S61.337 Puncture wound without foreign body of left little finger with damage to nail
S61.338 Puncture wound without foreign body of other finger with damage to nail
Puncture wound without foreign body of specified finger with unspecified laterality with damage to nail
S61.339 Puncture wound without foreign body of unspecified finger with damage to nail

S61.34 Puncture wound with foreign body of finger with damage to nail
S61.340 Puncture wound with foreign body of right index finger with damage to nail
S61.341 Puncture wound with foreign body of left index finger with damage to nail
S61.342 Puncture wound with foreign body of right middle finger with damage to nail
S61.343 Puncture wound with foreign body of left middle finger with damage to nail
S61.344 Puncture wound with foreign body of right ring finger with damage to nail
S61.345 Puncture wound with foreign body of left ring finger with damage to nail
S61.346 Puncture wound with foreign body of right little finger with damage to nail
S61.347 Puncture wound with foreign body of left little finger with damage to nail
S61.348 Puncture wound with foreign body of other finger with damage to nail
Puncture wound with foreign body of specified finger with unspecified laterality with damage to nail
S61.349 Puncture wound with foreign body of unspecified finger with damage to nail

S61.35 Open bite of finger with damage to nail
Bite of finger with damage to nail NOS
EXCLUDES1 *superficial bite of finger (S60.46-, S60.47-)*
S61.350 Open bite of right index finger with damage to nail
S61.351 Open bite of left index finger with damage to nail
S61.352 Open bite of right middle finger with damage to nail

Unspecified Code Other Specified Code Manifestation Code N Newborn P Pediatric M Maternity A Adult ♂ Male ♀ Female
● New Code ▲ Revised Code Title ►◄ Revised Text NOTES INCLUDES EXCLUDES1 Not coded here EXCLUDES2 Not included here
4th character required 5th character required 6th character required 7th character required
Extension 'X' Alert HAC Hospital-acquired condition (HAC) alert AHA AHA Coding Clinic©

S61.353 Open bite of left middle finger with damage to nail
S61.354 Open bite of right ring finger with damage to nail
S61.355 Open bite of left ring finger with damage to nail
S61.356 Open bite of right little finger with damage to nail
S61.357 Open bite of left little finger with damage to nail
S61.358 Open bite of other finger with damage to nail
Open bite of specified finger with unspecified laterality with damage to nail
S61.359 Open bite of unspecified finger with damage to nail

S61.4 Open wound of hand
S61.40 Unspecified open wound of hand
S61.401 Unspecified open wound of right hand
S61.402 Unspecified open wound of left hand
S61.409 Unspecified open wound of unspecified hand
S61.41 Laceration without foreign body of hand
S61.411 Laceration without foreign body of right hand
S61.412 Laceration without foreign body of left hand
S61.419 Laceration without foreign body of unspecified hand
S61.42 Laceration with foreign body of hand
S61.421 Laceration with foreign body of right hand
S61.422 Laceration with foreign body of left hand
S61.429 Laceration with foreign body of unspecified hand
S61.43 Puncture wound without foreign body of hand
S61.431 Puncture wound without foreign body of right hand
S61.432 Puncture wound without foreign body of left hand
S61.439 Puncture wound without foreign body of unspecified hand
S61.44 Puncture wound with foreign body of hand
S61.441 Puncture wound with foreign body of right hand
S61.442 Puncture wound with foreign body of left hand
S61.449 Puncture wound with foreign body of unspecified hand
S61.45 Open bite of hand
Bite of hand NOS
EXCLUDES1 *superficial bite of hand (S60.56-, S60.57-)*
S61.451 Open bite of right hand
S61.452 Open bite of left hand
S61.459 Open bite of unspecified hand

S61.5 Open wound of wrist
S61.50 Unspecified open wound of wrist
S61.501 Unspecified open wound of right wrist
S61.502 Unspecified open wound of left wrist
S61.509 Unspecified open wound of unspecified wrist
S61.51 Laceration without foreign body of wrist
S61.511 Laceration without foreign body of right wrist
S61.512 Laceration without foreign body of left wrist
S61.519 Laceration without foreign body of unspecified wrist
S61.52 Laceration with foreign body of wrist
S61.521 Laceration with foreign body of right wrist
S61.522 Laceration with foreign body of left wrist
S61.529 Laceration with foreign body of unspecified wrist
S61.53 Puncture wound without foreign body of wrist
S61.531 Puncture wound without foreign body of right wrist
S61.532 Puncture wound without foreign body of left wrist
S61.539 Puncture wound without foreign body of unspecified wrist
S61.54 Puncture wound with foreign body of wrist
S61.541 Puncture wound with foreign body of right wrist
S61.542 Puncture wound with foreign body of left wrist
S61.549 Puncture wound with foreign body of unspecified wrist
S61.55 Open bite of wrist
Bite of wrist NOS
EXCLUDES1 *superficial bite of wrist (S60.86-, S60.87-)*
S61.551 Open bite of right wrist
S61.552 Open bite of left wrist
S61.559 Open bite of unspecified wrist

S62 Fracture at wrist and hand level
NOTES A fracture not indicated as displaced or nondisplaced should be coded to displaced
A fracture not indicated as open or closed should be coded to closed
EXCLUDES1 *traumatic amputation of wrist and hand (S68.-)*
EXCLUDES2 *fracture of distal parts of ulna and radius (S52.-)*

The appropriate 7th character is to be added to each code from category S62
A = initial encounter for closed fracture
B = initial encounter for open fracture
D = subsequent encounter for fracture with routine healing
G = subsequent encounter for fracture with delayed healing
K = subsequent encounter for fracture with nonunion
P = subsequent encounter for fracture with malunion
S = sequela

S62.0 Fracture of navicular [scaphoid] bone of wrist
S62.00 Unspecified fracture of navicular [scaphoid] bone of wrist
S62.001 Unspecified fracture of navicular [scaphoid] bone of right wrist CC HAC
S62.002 Unspecified fracture of navicular [scaphoid] bone of left wrist CC HAC
AHA: Q4, 2012
S62.009 Unspecified fracture of navicular [scaphoid] bone of unspecified wrist CC HAC
S62.01 Fracture of distal pole of navicular [scaphoid] bone of wrist
Fracture of volar tuberosity of navicular [scaphoid] bone of wrist
S62.011 Displaced fracture of distal pole of navicular [scaphoid] bone of right wrist CC HAC
S62.012 Displaced fracture of distal pole of navicular [scaphoid] bone of left wrist CC HAC
S62.013 Displaced fracture of distal pole of navicular [scaphoid] bone of unspecified wrist CC HAC
S62.014 Nondisplaced fracture of distal pole of navicular [scaphoid] bone of right wrist CC HAC
S62.015 Nondisplaced fracture of distal pole of navicular [scaphoid] bone of left wrist CC HAC
S62.016 Nondisplaced fracture of distal pole of navicular [scaphoid] bone of unspecified wrist CC HAC
S62.02 Fracture of middle third of navicular [scaphoid] bone of wrist
S62.021 Displaced fracture of middle third of navicular [scaphoid] bone of right wrist CC HAC
S62.022 Displaced fracture of middle third of navicular [scaphoid] bone of left wrist CC HAC

Unacceptable principal diagnosis symbol per Medicare code edits · Code exempt from diagnosis present on admission requirement
Questionable admission · Complication or comorbidity · CC/MCC exclusion · Major complication or comorbidity
Principal diagnosis as its own CC · Principal diagnosis as its own MCC · Z code as first-listed diagnosis

S62.023 Displaced fracture of middle third of navicular [scaphoid] bone of unspecified wrist HAC
S62.024 Nondisplaced fracture of middle third of navicular [scaphoid] bone of right wrist HAC
S62.025 Nondisplaced fracture of middle third of navicular [scaphoid] bone of left wrist HAC
S62.026 Nondisplaced fracture of middle third of navicular [scaphoid] bone of unspecified wrist HAC
S62.03 Fracture of proximal third of navicular [scaphoid] bone of wrist
S62.031 Displaced fracture of proximal third of navicular [scaphoid] bone of right wrist HAC
S62.032 Displaced fracture of proximal third of navicular [scaphoid] bone of left wrist HAC
S62.033 Displaced fracture of proximal third of navicular [scaphoid] bone of unspecified wrist HAC
S62.034 Nondisplaced fracture of proximal third of navicular [scaphoid] bone of right wrist HAC
S62.035 Nondisplaced fracture of proximal third of navicular [scaphoid] bone of left wrist HAC
S62.036 Nondisplaced fracture of proximal third of navicular [scaphoid] bone of unspecified wrist HAC

S62.1 Fracture of other and unspecified carpal bone(s)
EXCLUDES2 *fracture of scaphoid of wrist (S62.0-)*

S62.10 Fracture of unspecified carpal bone
Fracture of wrist NOS
S62.101 Fracture of unspecified carpal bone, right wrist HAC
S62.102 Fracture of unspecified carpal bone, left wrist HAC
AHA: Q4, 2012
S62.109 Fracture of unspecified carpal bone, unspecified wrist HAC

S62.11 Fracture of triquetrum [cuneiform] bone of wrist
S62.111 Displaced fracture of triquetrum [cuneiform] bone, right wrist HAC
S62.112 Displaced fracture of triquetrum [cuneiform] bone, left wrist HAC
S62.113 Displaced fracture of triquetrum [cuneiform] bone, unspecified wrist HAC
S62.114 Nondisplaced fracture of triquetrum [cuneiform] bone, right wrist HAC
S62.115 Nondisplaced fracture of triquetrum [cuneiform] bone, left wrist HAC
S62.116 Nondisplaced fracture of triquetrum [cuneiform] bone, unspecified wrist HAC

S62.12 Fracture of lunate [semilunar]
S62.121 Displaced fracture of lunate [semilunar], right wrist HAC
S62.122 Displaced fracture of lunate [semilunar], left wrist HAC
S62.123 Displaced fracture of lunate [semilunar], unspecified wrist HAC
S62.124 Nondisplaced fracture of lunate [semilunar], right wrist HAC
S62.125 Nondisplaced fracture of lunate [semilunar], left wrist HAC
S62.126 Nondisplaced fracture of lunate [semilunar], unspecified wrist HAC

S62.13 Fracture of capitate [os magnum] bone
S62.131 Displaced fracture of capitate [os magnum] bone, right wrist HAC
S62.132 Displaced fracture of capitate [os magnum] bone, left wrist HAC
S62.133 Displaced fracture of capitate [os magnum] bone, unspecified wrist HAC
S62.134 Nondisplaced fracture of capitate [os magnum] bone, right wrist HAC
S62.135 Nondisplaced fracture of capitate [os magnum] bone, left wrist HAC
S62.136 Nondisplaced fracture of capitate [os magnum] bone, unspecified wrist HAC

S62.14 Fracture of body of hamate [unciform] bone
Fracture of hamate [unciform] bone NOS
S62.141 Displaced fracture of body of hamate [unciform] bone, right wrist HAC
S62.142 Displaced fracture of body of hamate [unciform] bone, left wrist HAC
S62.143 Displaced fracture of body of hamate [unciform] bone, unspecified wrist HAC
S62.144 Nondisplaced fracture of body of hamate [unciform] bone, right wrist HAC
S62.145 Nondisplaced fracture of body of hamate [unciform] bone, left wrist HAC
S62.146 Nondisplaced fracture of body of hamate [unciform] bone, unspecified wrist HAC

S62.15 Fracture of hook process of hamate [unciform] bone
Fracture of unciform process of hamate [unciform] bone
S62.151 Displaced fracture of hook process of hamate [unciform] bone, right wrist HAC
S62.152 Displaced fracture of hook process of hamate [unciform] bone, left wrist HAC
S62.153 Displaced fracture of hook process of hamate [unciform] bone, unspecified wrist HAC
S62.154 Nondisplaced fracture of hook process of hamate [unciform] bone, right wrist HAC
S62.155 Nondisplaced fracture of hook process of hamate [unciform] bone, left wrist HAC
S62.156 Nondisplaced fracture of hook process of hamate [unciform] bone, unspecified wrist HAC

S62.16 Fracture of pisiform
S62.161 Displaced fracture of pisiform, right wrist HAC
S62.162 Displaced fracture of pisiform, left wrist HAC
S62.163 Displaced fracture of pisiform, unspecified wrist HAC
S62.164 Nondisplaced fracture of pisiform, right wrist HAC
S62.165 Nondisplaced fracture of pisiform, left wrist HAC
S62.166 Nondisplaced fracture of pisiform, unspecified wrist HAC

S62.17 Fracture of trapezium [larger multangular]
S62.171 Displaced fracture of trapezium [larger multangular], right wrist HAC
S62.172 Displaced fracture of trapezium [larger multangular], left wrist HAC
S62.173 Displaced fracture of trapezium [larger multangular], unspecified wrist HAC
S62.174 Nondisplaced fracture of trapezium [larger multangular], right wrist HAC
S62.175 Nondisplaced fracture of trapezium [larger multangular], left wrist HAC
S62.176 Nondisplaced fracture of trapezium [larger multangular], unspecified wrist HAC

S62.18 Fracture of trapezoid [smaller multangular]
S62.181 Displaced fracture of trapezoid [smaller multangular], right wrist HAC

Unspecified Code Other Specified Code Manifestation Code N Newborn P Pediatric M Maternity A Adult ♂ Male ♀ Female
● New Code ▲ Revised Code Title ►◄ Revised Text NOTES INCLUDES EXCLUDES1 Not coded here EXCLUDES2 Not included here
4th character required 5th character required 6th character required 7th character required
Extension 'X' Alert HAC Hospital-acquired condition (HAC) alert AHA AHA Coding Clinic©

S62.182 Displaced fracture of trapezoid [smaller multangular], left wrist CC HAC
S62.183 Displaced fracture of trapezoid [smaller multangular], unspecified wrist CC HAC
S62.184 Nondisplaced fracture of trapezoid [smaller multangular], right wrist CC HAC
S62.185 Nondisplaced fracture of trapezoid [smaller multangular], left wrist CC HAC
S62.186 Nondisplaced fracture of trapezoid [smaller multangular], unspecified wrist CC HAC

S62.2 Fracture of first metacarpal bone
S62.20 Unspecified fracture of first metacarpal bone
S62.201 Unspecified fracture of first metacarpal bone, right hand CC HAC
S62.202 Unspecified fracture of first metacarpal bone, left hand CC HAC
S62.209 Unspecified fracture of first metacarpal bone, unspecified hand CC HAC
S62.21 Bennett's fracture
S62.211 Bennett's fracture, right hand CC
S62.212 Bennett's fracture, left hand CC
S62.213 Bennett's fracture, unspecified hand CC
S62.22 Rolando's fracture
S62.221 Displaced Rolando's fracture, right hand CC
S62.222 Displaced Rolando's fracture, left hand CC
S62.223 Displaced Rolando's fracture, unspecified hand CC
S62.224 Nondisplaced Rolando's fracture, right hand CC
S62.225 Nondisplaced Rolando's fracture, left hand CC
S62.226 Nondisplaced Rolando's fracture, unspecified hand CC
S62.23 Other fracture of base of first metacarpal bone
S62.231 Other displaced fracture of base of first metacarpal bone, right hand CC HAC
S62.232 Other displaced fracture of base of first metacarpal bone, left hand CC HAC
S62.233 Other displaced fracture of base of first metacarpal bone, unspecified hand CC HAC
S62.234 Other nondisplaced fracture of base of first metacarpal bone, right hand CC HAC
S62.235 Other nondisplaced fracture of base of first metacarpal bone, left hand CC HAC
S62.236 Other nondisplaced fracture of base of first metacarpal bone, unspecified hand CC HAC
S62.24 Fracture of shaft of first metacarpal bone
S62.241 Displaced fracture of shaft of first metacarpal bone, right hand CC HAC
S62.242 Displaced fracture of shaft of first metacarpal bone, left hand CC HAC
S62.243 Displaced fracture of shaft of first metacarpal bone, unspecified hand CC HAC
S62.244 Nondisplaced fracture of shaft of first metacarpal bone, right hand CC HAC
S62.245 Nondisplaced fracture of shaft of first metacarpal bone, left hand CC HAC
S62.246 Nondisplaced fracture of shaft of first metacarpal bone, unspecified hand CC HAC
S62.25 Fracture of neck of first metacarpal bone
S62.251 Displaced fracture of neck of first metacarpal bone, right hand CC HAC
S62.252 Displaced fracture of neck of first metacarpal bone, left hand CC HAC
S62.253 Displaced fracture of neck of first metacarpal bone, unspecified hand CC HAC
S62.254 Nondisplaced fracture of neck of first metacarpal bone, right hand CC HAC
S62.255 Nondisplaced fracture of neck of first metacarpal bone, left hand CC HAC
S62.256 Nondisplaced fracture of neck of first metacarpal bone, unspecified hand CC HAC
S62.29 Other fracture of first metacarpal bone
S62.291 Other fracture of first metacarpal bone, right hand CC HAC
S62.292 Other fracture of first metacarpal bone, left hand CC HAC
S62.299 Other fracture of first metacarpal bone, unspecified hand CC HAC

S62.3 Fracture of other and unspecified metacarpal bone
EXCLUDES2 *fracture of first metacarpal bone (S62.2-)*
S62.30 Unspecified fracture of other metacarpal bone
S62.300 Unspecified fracture of second metacarpal bone, right hand CC HAC
S62.301 Unspecified fracture of second metacarpal bone, left hand CC HAC
S62.302 Unspecified fracture of third metacarpal bone, right hand CC HAC
S62.303 Unspecified fracture of third metacarpal bone, left hand CC HAC
S62.304 Unspecified fracture of fourth metacarpal bone, right hand CC HAC
S62.305 Unspecified fracture of fourth metacarpal bone, left hand CC HAC
S62.306 Unspecified fracture of fifth metacarpal bone, right hand CC HAC
S62.307 Unspecified fracture of fifth metacarpal bone, left hand CC HAC
S62.308 Unspecified fracture of other metacarpal bone CC HAC
Unspecified fracture of specified metacarpal bone with unspecified laterality
S62.309 Unspecified fracture of unspecified metacarpal bone CC HAC
S62.31 Displaced fracture of base of other metacarpal bone
S62.310 Displaced fracture of base of second metacarpal bone, right hand CC HAC
S62.311 Displaced fracture of base of second metacarpal bone. left hand CC HAC
S62.312 Displaced fracture of base of third metacarpal bone, right hand CC HAC
S62.313 Displaced fracture of base of third metacarpal bone, left hand CC HAC
S62.314 Displaced fracture of base of fourth metacarpal bone, right hand CC HAC
S62.315 Displaced fracture of base of fourth metacarpal bone, left hand CC HAC
S62.316 Displaced fracture of base of fifth metacarpal bone, right hand CC HAC
S62.317 Displaced fracture of base of fifth metacarpal bone. left hand CC HAC
S62.318 Displaced fracture of base of other metacarpal bone CC HAC
Displaced fracture of base of specified metacarpal bone with unspecified laterality
S62.319 Displaced fracture of base of unspecified metacarpal bone CC HAC
S62.32 Displaced fracture of shaft of other metacarpal bone
S62.320 Displaced fracture of shaft of second metacarpal bone, right hand CC HAC
S62.321 Displaced fracture of shaft of second metacarpal bone, left hand CC HAC

PDx Unacceptable principal diagnosis symbol per Medicare code edits · POA Code exempt from diagnosis present on admission requirement
? Questionable admission · CC Complication or comorbidity · CC/MCC Exc CC/MCC exclusion · MCC Major complication or comorbidity
PDx CC Principal diagnosis as its own CC · PDx MCC Principal diagnosis as its own MCC · Z Z code as first-listed diagnosis

When symbols appear on a code that requires a 7th character extension, refer to Appendix D to identify applicable 7th character codes.

S62.322 Displaced fracture of shaft of third metacarpal bone, right hand
S62.323 Displaced fracture of shaft of third metacarpal bone, left hand
S62.324 Displaced fracture of shaft of fourth metacarpal bone, right hand
S62.325 Displaced fracture of shaft of fourth metacarpal bone, left hand
S62.326 Displaced fracture of shaft of fifth metacarpal bone, right hand
S62.327 Displaced fracture of shaft of fifth metacarpal bone, left hand
S62.328 Displaced fracture of shaft of other metacarpal bone
Displaced fracture of shaft of specified metacarpal bone with unspecified laterality
S62.329 Displaced fracture of shaft of unspecified metacarpal bone

S62.33 Displaced fracture of neck of other metacarpal bone
S62.330 Displaced fracture of neck of second metacarpal bone, right hand
S62.331 Displaced fracture of neck of second metacarpal bone, left hand
S62.332 Displaced fracture of neck of third metacarpal bone, right hand
S62.333 Displaced fracture of neck of third metacarpal bone, left hand
S62.334 Displaced fracture of neck of fourth metacarpal bone, right hand
S62.335 Displaced fracture of neck of fourth metacarpal bone, left hand
S62.336 Displaced fracture of neck of fifth metacarpal bone, right hand
S62.337 Displaced fracture of neck of fifth metacarpal bone, left hand
S62.338 Displaced fracture of neck of other metacarpal bone
Displaced fracture of neck of specified metacarpal bone with unspecified laterality
S62.339 Displaced fracture of neck of unspecified metacarpal bone

S62.34 Nondisplaced fracture of base of other metacarpal bone
S62.340 Nondisplaced fracture of base of second metacarpal bone, right hand
S62.341 Nondisplaced fracture of base of second metacarpal bone. left hand
S62.342 Nondisplaced fracture of base of third metacarpal bone, right hand
S62.343 Nondisplaced fracture of base of third metacarpal bone, left hand
S62.344 Nondisplaced fracture of base of fourth metacarpal bone, right hand
S62.345 Nondisplaced fracture of base of fourth metacarpal bone, left hand
S62.346 Nondisplaced fracture of base of fifth metacarpal bone, right hand
S62.347 Nondisplaced fracture of base of fifth metacarpal bone. left hand
S62.348 Nondisplaced fracture of base of other metacarpal bone
Nondisplaced fracture of base of specified metacarpal bone with unspecified laterality
S62.349 Nondisplaced fracture of base of unspecified metacarpal bone

S62.35 Nondisplaced fracture of shaft of other metacarpal bone
S62.350 Nondisplaced fracture of shaft of second metacarpal bone, right hand
S62.351 Nondisplaced fracture of shaft of second metacarpal bone, left hand
S62.352 Nondisplaced fracture of shaft of third metacarpal bone, right hand
S62.353 Nondisplaced fracture of shaft of third metacarpal bone, left hand
S62.354 Nondisplaced fracture of shaft of fourth metacarpal bone, right hand
S62.355 Nondisplaced fracture of shaft of fourth metacarpal bone, left hand
S62.356 Nondisplaced fracture of shaft of fifth metacarpal bone, right hand
S62.357 Nondisplaced fracture of shaft of fifth metacarpal bone, left hand
S62.358 Nondisplaced fracture of shaft of other metacarpal bone
Nondisplaced fracture of shaft of specified metacarpal bone with unspecified laterality
S62.359 Nondisplaced fracture of shaft of unspecified metacarpal bone

S62.36 Nondisplaced fracture of neck of other metacarpal bone
S62.360 Nondisplaced fracture of neck of second metacarpal bone, right hand
S62.361 Nondisplaced fracture of neck of second metacarpal bone, left hand
S62.362 Nondisplaced fracture of neck of third metacarpal bone, right hand
S62.363 Nondisplaced fracture of neck of third metacarpal bone, left hand
S62.364 Nondisplaced fracture of neck of fourth metacarpal bone, right hand
S62.365 Nondisplaced fracture of neck of fourth metacarpal bone, left hand
S62.366 Nondisplaced fracture of neck of fifth metacarpal bone, right hand
S62.367 Nondisplaced fracture of neck of fifth metacarpal bone, left hand
S62.368 Nondisplaced fracture of neck of other metacarpal bone
Nondisplaced fracture of neck of specified metacarpal bone with unspecified laterality
S62.369 Nondisplaced fracture of neck of unspecified metacarpal bone

S62.39 Other fracture of other metacarpal bone
S62.390 Other fracture of second metacarpal bone, right hand
S62.391 Other fracture of second metacarpal bone, left hand
S62.392 Other fracture of third metacarpal bone, right hand
S62.393 Other fracture of third metacarpal bone, left hand
S62.394 Other fracture of fourth metacarpal bone, right hand
S62.395 Other fracture of fourth metacarpal bone, left hand
S62.396 Other fracture of fifth metacarpal bone, right hand
S62.397 Other fracture of fifth metacarpal bone, left hand
S62.398 Other fracture of other metacarpal bone

Unspecified Code | Other Specified Code | Manifestation Code | N Newborn | P Pediatric | M Maternity | A Adult | ♂ Male | ♀ Female
● New Code | ▲ Revised Code Title | ►◄ Revised Text | NOTES | INCLUDES | EXCLUDES1 Not coded here | EXCLUDES2 Not included here
4th character required | 5th character required | 6th character required | 7th character required
Extension 'X' Alert | HAC Hospital-acquired condition (HAC) alert | AHA AHA Coding Clinic®

Other fracture of specified metacarpal bone with unspecified laterality

S62.399 Other fracture of unspecified metacarpal bone

S62.5 Fracture of thumb

S62.50 Fracture of unspecified phalanx of thumb

S62.501 Fracture of unspecified phalanx of right thumb

S62.502 Fracture of unspecified phalanx of left thumb

S62.509 Fracture of unspecified phalanx of unspecified thumb

S62.51 Fracture of proximal phalanx of thumb

S62.511 Displaced fracture of proximal phalanx of right thumb

S62.512 Displaced fracture of proximal phalanx of left thumb

S62.513 Displaced fracture of proximal phalanx of unspecified thumb

S62.514 Nondisplaced fracture of proximal phalanx of right thumb

S62.515 Nondisplaced fracture of proximal phalanx of left thumb

S62.516 Nondisplaced fracture of proximal phalanx of unspecified thumb

S62.52 Fracture of distal phalanx of thumb

S62.521 Displaced fracture of distal phalanx of right thumb

S62.522 Displaced fracture of distal phalanx of left thumb

S62.523 Displaced fracture of distal phalanx of unspecified thumb

S62.524 Nondisplaced fracture of distal phalanx of right thumb

S62.525 Nondisplaced fracture of distal phalanx of left thumb

S62.526 Nondisplaced fracture of distal phalanx of unspecified thumb

S62.6 Fracture of other and unspecified finger(s)

EXCLUDES2 *fracture of thumb (S62.5-)*

S62.60 Fracture of unspecified phalanx of finger

S62.600 Fracture of unspecified phalanx of right index finger

S62.601 Fracture of unspecified phalanx of left index finger

S62.602 Fracture of unspecified phalanx of right middle finger

S62.603 Fracture of unspecified phalanx of left middle finger

S62.604 Fracture of unspecified phalanx of right ring finger

S62.605 Fracture of unspecified phalanx of left ring finger

S62.606 Fracture of unspecified phalanx of right little finger

S62.607 Fracture of unspecified phalanx of left little finger

S62.608 Fracture of unspecified phalanx of other finger

Fracture of unspecified phalanx of specified finger with unspecified laterality

S62.609 Fracture of unspecified phalanx of unspecified finger

S62.61 Displaced fracture of proximal phalanx of finger

S62.610 Displaced fracture of proximal phalanx of right index finger

S62.611 Displaced fracture of proximal phalanx of left index finger

S62.612 Displaced fracture of proximal phalanx of right middle finger

S62.613 Displaced fracture of proximal phalanx of left middle finger

S62.614 Displaced fracture of proximal phalanx of right ring finger

S62.615 Displaced fracture of proximal phalanx of left ring finger

S62.616 Displaced fracture of proximal phalanx of right little finger

S62.617 Displaced fracture of proximal phalanx of left little finger

S62.618 Displaced fracture of proximal phalanx of other finger

Displaced fracture of proximal phalanx of specified finger with unspecified laterality

S62.619 Displaced fracture of proximal phalanx of unspecified finger

S62.62 Displaced fracture of medial phalanx of finger

S62.620 Displaced fracture of medial phalanx of right index finger

S62.621 Displaced fracture of medial phalanx of left index finger

S62.622 Displaced fracture of medial phalanx of right middle finger

S62.623 Displaced fracture of medial phalanx of left middle finger

S62.624 Displaced fracture of medial phalanx of right ring finger

S62.625 Displaced fracture of medial phalanx of left ring finger

S62.626 Displaced fracture of medial phalanx of right little finger

S62.627 Displaced fracture of medial phalanx of left little finger

S62.628 Displaced fracture of medial phalanx of other finger

Displaced fracture of medial phalanx of specified finger with unspecified laterality

S62.629 Displaced fracture of medial phalanx of unspecified finger

S62.63 Displaced fracture of distal phalanx of finger

S62.630 Displaced fracture of distal phalanx of right index finger

S62.631 Displaced fracture of distal phalanx of left index finger

S62.632 Displaced fracture of distal phalanx of right middle finger

S62.633 Displaced fracture of distal phalanx of left middle finger

S62.634 Displaced fracture of distal phalanx of right ring finger

S62.635 Displaced fracture of distal phalanx of left ring finger

S62.636 Displaced fracture of distal phalanx of right little finger

S62.637 Displaced fracture of distal phalanx of left little finger

S62.638 Displaced fracture of distal phalanx of other finger

Displaced fracture of distal phalanx of specified finger with unspecified laterality

S62.639 Displaced fracture of distal phalanx of unspecified finger

S62.64 Nondisplaced fracture of proximal phalanx of finger

S62.640 Nondisplaced fracture of proximal phalanx of right index finger

S62.641 Nondisplaced fracture of proximal phalanx of left index finger

S62.642 Nondisplaced fracture of proximal phalanx of right middle finger

S62.643 Nondisplaced fracture of proximal phalanx of left middle finger

S62.644 Nondisplaced fracture of proximal phalanx of right ring finger

S62.645 Nondisplaced fracture of proximal phalanx of left ring finger

S62.646 Nondisplaced fracture of proximal phalanx of right little finger

S62.647 Nondisplaced fracture of proximal phalanx of left little finger

S62.648 Nondisplaced fracture of proximal phalanx of other finger

Unacceptable principal diagnosis symbol per Medicare code edits — Code exempt from diagnosis present on admission requirement — Questionable admission — Complication or comorbidity — CC/MCC exclusion — Major complication or comorbidity — Principal diagnosis as its own CC — Principal diagnosis as its own MCC — Z code as first-listed diagnosis

Nondisplaced fracture of proximal phalanx of specified finger with unspecified laterality

S62.649 Nondisplaced fracture of proximal phalanx of unspecified finger HAC

S62.65 Nondisplaced fracture of medial phalanx of finger

S62.650 Nondisplaced fracture of medial phalanx of right index finger HAC

S62.651 Nondisplaced fracture of medial phalanx of left index finger HAC

S62.652 Nondisplaced fracture of medial phalanx of right middle finger HAC

S62.653 Nondisplaced fracture of medial phalanx of left middle finger HAC

S62.654 Nondisplaced fracture of medial phalanx of right ring finger HAC

S62.655 Nondisplaced fracture of medial phalanx of left ring finger HAC

S62.656 Nondisplaced fracture of medial phalanx of right little finger HAC

S62.657 Nondisplaced fracture of medial phalanx of left little finger HAC

S62.658 Nondisplaced fracture of medial phalanx of other finger HAC

Nondisplaced fracture of medial phalanx of specified finger with unspecified laterality

S62.659 Nondisplaced fracture of medial phalanx of unspecified finger HAC

S62.66 Nondisplaced fracture of distal phalanx of finger

S62.660 Nondisplaced fracture of distal phalanx of right index finger HAC

S62.661 Nondisplaced fracture of distal phalanx of left index finger HAC

S62.662 Nondisplaced fracture of distal phalanx of right middle finger HAC

S62.663 Nondisplaced fracture of distal phalanx of left middle finger HAC

S62.664 Nondisplaced fracture of distal phalanx of right ring finger HAC

S62.665 Nondisplaced fracture of distal phalanx of left ring finger HAC

S62.666 Nondisplaced fracture of distal phalanx of right little finger HAC

S62.667 Nondisplaced fracture of distal phalanx of left little finger HAC

S62.668 Nondisplaced fracture of distal phalanx of other finger HAC

Nondisplaced fracture of distal phalanx of specified finger with unspecified laterality

S62.669 Nondisplaced fracture of distal phalanx of unspecified finger HAC

S62.9 Unspecified fracture of wrist and hand

S62.90 Unspecified fracture of unspecified wrist and hand HAC

S62.91 Unspecified fracture of right wrist and hand HAC

S62.92 Unspecified fracture of left wrist and hand HAC

S63 Dislocation and sprain of joints and ligaments at wrist and hand level

INCLUDES *avulsion of joint or ligament at wrist and hand level*
laceration of cartilage, joint or ligament at wrist and hand level
sprain of cartilage, joint or ligament at wrist and hand level
traumatic hemarthrosis of joint or ligament at wrist and hand level
traumatic rupture of joint or ligament at wrist and hand level
traumatic subluxation of joint or ligament at wrist and hand level
traumatic tear of joint or ligament at wrist and hand level

Code also any associated open wound

EXCLUDES2 *strain of muscle, fascia and tendon of wrist and hand (S66.-)*

The appropriate 7th character is to be added to each code from category S63
A = initial encounter
D = subsequent encounter
S = sequela

S63.0 Subluxation and dislocation of wrist and hand joints

S63.00 Unspecified subluxation and dislocation of wrist and hand

Dislocation of carpal bone NOS
Dislocation of distal end of radius NOS
Subluxation of carpal bone NOS
Subluxation of distal end of radius NOS

S63.001 Unspecified subluxation of right wrist and hand

S63.002 Unspecified subluxation of left wrist and hand

S63.003 Unspecified subluxation of unspecified wrist and hand

S63.004 Unspecified dislocation of right wrist and hand

S63.005 Unspecified dislocation of left wrist and hand

S63.006 Unspecified dislocation of unspecified wrist and hand

S63.01 Subluxation and dislocation of distal radioulnar joint

S63.011 Subluxation of distal radioulnar joint of right wrist

S63.012 Subluxation of distal radioulnar joint of left wrist

S63.013 Subluxation of distal radioulnar joint of unspecified wrist

S63.014 Dislocation of distal radioulnar joint of right wrist

S63.015 Dislocation of distal radioulnar joint of left wrist

S63.016 Dislocation of distal radioulnar joint of unspecified wrist

S63.02 Subluxation and dislocation of radiocarpal joint

S63.021 Subluxation of radiocarpal joint of right wrist

S63.022 Subluxation of radiocarpal joint of left wrist

S63.023 Subluxation of radiocarpal joint of unspecified wrist

S63.024 Dislocation of radiocarpal joint of right wrist

S63.025 Dislocation of radiocarpal joint of left wrist

S63.026 Dislocation of radiocarpal joint of unspecified wrist

S63.03 Subluxation and dislocation of midcarpal joint

S63.031 Subluxation of midcarpal joint of right wrist

S63.032 Subluxation of midcarpal joint of left wrist

S63.033 Subluxation of midcarpal joint of unspecified wrist

S63.034 Dislocation of midcarpal joint of right wrist

S63.035 Dislocation of midcarpal joint of left wrist

S63.036 Dislocation of midcarpal joint of unspecified wrist

S63.04 Subluxation and dislocation of carpometacarpal joint of thumb

EXCLUDES2 *interphalangeal subluxation and dislocation of thumb (S63.1-)*

S63.041 Subluxation of carpometacarpal joint of right thumb

S63.042 Subluxation of carpometacarpal joint of left thumb

S63.043 Subluxation of carpometacarpal joint of unspecified thumb

S63.044 Dislocation of carpometacarpal joint of right thumb

S63.045 Dislocation of carpometacarpal joint of left thumb

S63.046 Dislocation of carpometacarpal joint of unspecified thumb

S63.05 Subluxation and dislocation of other carpometacarpal joint

EXCLUDES2 *subluxation and dislocation of carpometacarpal joint of thumb (S63.04-)*

Unspecified Code | Other Specified Code | Manifestation Code | N Newborn | P Pediatric | M Maternity | A Adult | ♂ Male | ♀ Female
● New Code | ▲ Revised Code Title | ►◄ Revised Text | NOTES | INCLUDES | EXCLUDES1 Not coded here | EXCLUDES2 Not included here
4th character required | 5th character required | 6th character required | 7th character required
Extension 'X' Alert | HAC Hospital-acquired condition (HAC) alert | AHA AHA Coding Clinic©

S63.051 Subluxation of other carpometacarpal joint of right hand
S63.052 Subluxation of other carpometacarpal joint of left hand
S63.053 Subluxation of other carpometacarpal joint of unspecified hand
S63.054 Dislocation of other carpometacarpal joint of right hand
S63.055 Dislocation of other carpometacarpal joint of left hand
S63.056 Dislocation of other carpometacarpal joint of unspecified hand

S63.06 Subluxation and dislocation of metacarpal (bone), proximal end
S63.061 Subluxation of metacarpal (bone), proximal end of right hand
S63.062 Subluxation of metacarpal (bone), proximal end of left hand
S63.063 Subluxation of metacarpal (bone), proximal end of unspecified hand
S63.064 Dislocation of metacarpal (bone), proximal end of right hand
S63.065 Dislocation of metacarpal (bone), proximal end of left hand
S63.066 Dislocation of metacarpal (bone), proximal end of unspecified hand

S63.07 Subluxation and dislocation of distal end of ulna
S63.071 Subluxation of distal end of right ulna
S63.072 Subluxation of distal end of left ulna
S63.073 Subluxation of distal end of unspecified ulna
S63.074 Dislocation of distal end of right ulna
S63.075 Dislocation of distal end of left ulna
S63.076 Dislocation of distal end of unspecified ulna

S63.09 Other subluxation and dislocation of wrist and hand
S63.091 Other subluxation of right wrist and hand
S63.092 Other subluxation of left wrist and hand
S63.093 Other subluxation of unspecified wrist and hand
S63.094 Other dislocation of right wrist and hand
S63.095 Other dislocation of left wrist and hand
S63.096 Other dislocation of unspecified wrist and hand

S63.1 Subluxation and dislocation of thumb

S63.10 Unspecified subluxation and dislocation of thumb
S63.101 Unspecified subluxation of right thumb
S63.102 Unspecified subluxation of left thumb
S63.103 Unspecified subluxation of unspecified thumb
S63.104 Unspecified dislocation of right thumb
S63.105 Unspecified dislocation of left thumb
S63.106 Unspecified dislocation of unspecified thumb

S63.11 Subluxation and dislocation of metacarpophalangeal joint of thumb
S63.111 Subluxation of metacarpophalangeal joint of right thumb
S63.112 Subluxation of metacarpophalangeal joint of left thumb
S63.113 Subluxation of metacarpophalangeal joint of unspecified thumb
S63.114 Dislocation of metacarpophalangeal joint of right thumb
S63.115 Dislocation of metacarpophalangeal joint of left thumb
S63.116 Dislocation of metacarpophalangeal joint of unspecified thumb

S63.12 Subluxation and dislocation of unspecified interphalangeal joint of thumb
S63.121 Subluxation of unspecified interphalangeal joint of right thumb
S63.122 Subluxation of unspecified interphalangeal joint of left thumb
S63.123 Subluxation of unspecified interphalangeal joint of unspecified thumb
S63.124 Dislocation of unspecified interphalangeal joint of right thumb
S63.125 Dislocation of unspecified interphalangeal joint of left thumb
S63.126 Dislocation of unspecified interphalangeal joint of unspecified thumb

S63.13 Subluxation and dislocation of proximal interphalangeal joint of thumb
S63.131 Subluxation of proximal interphalangeal joint of right thumb
S63.132 Subluxation of proximal interphalangeal joint of left thumb
S63.133 Subluxation of proximal interphalangeal joint of unspecified thumb
S63.134 Dislocation of proximal interphalangeal joint of right thumb
S63.135 Dislocation of proximal interphalangeal joint of left thumb
S63.136 Dislocation of proximal interphalangeal joint of unspecified thumb

S63.14 Subluxation and dislocation of distal interphalangeal joint of thumb
S63.141 Subluxation of distal interphalangeal joint of right thumb
S63.142 Subluxation of distal interphalangeal joint of left thumb
S63.143 Subluxation of distal interphalangeal joint of unspecified thumb
S63.144 Dislocation of distal interphalangeal joint of right thumb
S63.145 Dislocation of distal interphalangeal joint of left thumb
S63.146 Dislocation of distal interphalangeal joint of unspecified thumb

S63.2 Subluxation and dislocation of other finger(s)
EXCLUDES2 *subluxation and dislocation of thumb (S63.1-)*

S63.20 Unspecified subluxation of other finger
S63.200 Unspecified subluxation of right index finger
S63.201 Unspecified subluxation of left index finger
S63.202 Unspecified subluxation of right middle finger
S63.203 Unspecified subluxation of left middle finger
S63.204 Unspecified subluxation of right ring finger
S63.205 Unspecified subluxation of left ring finger
S63.206 Unspecified subluxation of right little finger
S63.207 Unspecified subluxation of left little finger
S63.208 Unspecified subluxation of other finger
Unspecified subluxation of specified finger with unspecified laterality
S63.209 Unspecified subluxation of unspecified finger

S63.21 Subluxation of metacarpophalangeal joint of finger
S63.210 Subluxation of metacarpophalangeal joint of right index finger
S63.211 Subluxation of metacarpophalangeal joint of left index finger
S63.212 Subluxation of metacarpophalangeal joint of right middle finger
S63.213 Subluxation of metacarpophalangeal joint of left middle finger
S63.214 Subluxation of metacarpophalangeal joint of right ring finger
S63.215 Subluxation of metacarpophalangeal joint of left ring finger
S63.216 Subluxation of metacarpophalangeal joint of right little finger

Unacceptable principal diagnosis symbol per Medicare code edits · Code exempt from diagnosis present on admission requirement · Questionable admission · Complication or comorbidity · CC/MCC exclusion · Major complication or comorbidity · Principal diagnosis as its own CC · Principal diagnosis as its own MCC · Z code as first-listed diagnosis

S63.217 Subluxation of metacarpophalangeal joint of left little finger
S63.218 Subluxation of metacarpophalangeal joint of other finger
Subluxation of metacarpophalangeal joint of specified finger with unspecified laterality
S63.219 Subluxation of metacarpophalangeal joint of unspecified finger
S63.22 Subluxation of unspecified interphalangeal joint of finger
S63.220 Subluxation of unspecified interphalangeal joint of right index finger
S63.221 Subluxation of unspecified interphalangeal joint of left index finger
S63.222 Subluxation of unspecified interphalangeal joint of right middle finger
S63.223 Subluxation of unspecified interphalangeal joint of left middle finger
S63.224 Subluxation of unspecified interphalangeal joint of right ring finger
S63.225 Subluxation of unspecified interphalangeal joint of left ring finger
S63.226 Subluxation of unspecified interphalangeal joint of right little finger
S63.227 Subluxation of unspecified interphalangeal joint of left little finger
S63.228 Subluxation of unspecified interphalangeal joint of other finger
Subluxation of unspecified interphalangeal joint of specified finger with unspecified laterality
S63.229 Subluxation of unspecified interphalangeal joint of unspecified finger
S63.23 Subluxation of proximal interphalangeal joint of finger
S63.230 Subluxation of proximal interphalangeal joint of right index finger
S63.231 Subluxation of proximal interphalangeal joint of left index finger
S63.232 Subluxation of proximal interphalangeal joint of right middle finger
S63.233 Subluxation of proximal interphalangeal joint of left middle finger
S63.234 Subluxation of proximal interphalangeal joint of right ring finger
S63.235 Subluxation of proximal interphalangeal joint of left ring finger
S63.236 Subluxation of proximal interphalangeal joint of right little finger
S63.237 Subluxation of proximal interphalangeal joint of left little finger
S63.238 Subluxation of proximal interphalangeal joint of other finger
Subluxation of proximal interphalangeal joint of specified finger with unspecified laterality
S63.239 Subluxation of proximal interphalangeal joint of unspecified finger
S63.24 Subluxation of distal interphalangeal joint of finger
S63.240 Subluxation of distal interphalangeal joint of right index finger
S63.241 Subluxation of distal interphalangeal joint of left index finger
S63.242 Subluxation of distal interphalangeal joint of right middle finger
S63.243 Subluxation of distal interphalangeal joint of left middle finger
S63.244 Subluxation of distal interphalangeal joint of right ring finger
S63.245 Subluxation of distal interphalangeal joint of left ring finger
S63.246 Subluxation of distal interphalangeal joint of right little finger
S63.247 Subluxation of distal interphalangeal joint of left little finger
S63.248 Subluxation of distal interphalangeal joint of other finger
Subluxation of distal interphalangeal joint of specified finger with unspecified laterality
S63.249 Subluxation of distal interphalangeal joint of unspecified finger
S63.25 Unspecified dislocation of other finger
S63.250 Unspecified dislocation of right index finger
S63.251 Unspecified dislocation of left index finger
S63.252 Unspecified dislocation of right middle finger
S63.253 Unspecified dislocation of left middle finger
S63.254 Unspecified dislocation of right ring finger
S63.255 Unspecified dislocation of left ring finger
S63.256 Unspecified dislocation of right little finger
S63.257 Unspecified dislocation of left little finger
S63.258 Unspecified dislocation of other finger
Unspecified dislocation of specified finger with unspecified laterality
S63.259 Unspecified dislocation of unspecified finger
Unspecified dislocation of specified finger with unspecified laterality
S63.26 Dislocation of metacarpophalangeal joint of finger
S63.260 Dislocation of metacarpophalangeal joint of right index finger
S63.261 Dislocation of metacarpophalangeal joint of left index finger
S63.262 Dislocation of metacarpophalangeal joint of right middle finger
S63.263 Dislocation of metacarpophalangeal joint of left middle finger
S63.264 Dislocation of metacarpophalangeal joint of right ring finger
S63.265 Dislocation of metacarpophalangeal joint of left ring finger
S63.266 Dislocation of metacarpophalangeal joint of right little finger
S63.267 Dislocation of metacarpophalangeal joint of left little finger
S63.268 Dislocation of metacarpophalangeal joint of other finger
Dislocation of metacarpophalangeal joint of specified finger with unspecified laterality
S63.269 Dislocation of metacarpophalangeal joint of unspecified finger
S63.27 Dislocation of unspecified interphalangeal joint of finger
S63.270 Dislocation of unspecified interphalangeal joint of right index finger
S63.271 Dislocation of unspecified interphalangeal joint of left index finger
S63.272 Dislocation of unspecified interphalangeal joint of right middle finger
S63.273 Dislocation of unspecified interphalangeal joint of left middle finger
S63.274 Dislocation of unspecified interphalangeal joint of right ring finger
S63.275 Dislocation of unspecified interphalangeal joint of left ring finger
S63.276 Dislocation of unspecified interphalangeal joint of right little finger
S63.277 Dislocation of unspecified interphalangeal joint of left little finger
S63.278 Dislocation of unspecified interphalangeal joint of other finger
Dislocation of unspecified interphalangeal joint of specified finger with unspecified laterality

Unspecified Code Other Specified Code Manifestation Code N Newborn P Pediatric M Maternity A Adult ♂ Male ♀ Female
● New Code ▲ Revised Code Title ►◄ Revised Text NOTES INCLUDES EXCLUDES1 Not coded here EXCLUDES2 Not included here
4th character required 5th character required 6th character required 7th character required
Extension 'X' Alert HAC Hospital-acquired condition (HAC) alert AHA AHA Coding Clinic©

S63.279 Dislocation of unspecified interphalangeal joint of unspecified finger
Dislocation of unspecified interphalangeal joint of specified finger without specified laterality

S63.28 Dislocation of proximal interphalangeal joint of finger
S63.280 Dislocation of proximal interphalangeal joint of right index finger
S63.281 Dislocation of proximal interphalangeal joint of left index finger
S63.282 Dislocation of proximal interphalangeal joint of right middle finger
S63.283 Dislocation of proximal interphalangeal joint of left middle finger
S63.284 Dislocation of proximal interphalangeal joint of right ring finger
S63.285 Dislocation of proximal interphalangeal joint of left ring finger
S63.286 Dislocation of proximal interphalangeal joint of right little finger
S63.287 Dislocation of proximal interphalangeal joint of left little finger
S63.288 Dislocation of proximal interphalangeal joint of other finger
Dislocation of proximal interphalangeal joint of specified finger with unspecified laterality
S63.289 Dislocation of proximal interphalangeal joint of unspecified finger

S63.29 Dislocation of distal interphalangeal joint of finger
S63.290 Dislocation of distal interphalangeal joint of right index finger
S63.291 Dislocation of distal interphalangeal joint of left index finger
S63.292 Dislocation of distal interphalangeal joint of right middle finger
S63.293 Dislocation of distal interphalangeal joint of left middle finger
S63.294 Dislocation of distal interphalangeal joint of right ring finger
S63.295 Dislocation of distal interphalangeal joint of left ring finger
S63.296 Dislocation of distal interphalangeal joint of right little finger
S63.297 Dislocation of distal interphalangeal joint of left little finger
S63.298 Dislocation of distal interphalangeal joint of other finger
Dislocation of distal interphalangeal joint of specified finger with unspecified laterality
S63.299 Dislocation of distal interphalangeal joint of unspecified finger

S63.3 Traumatic rupture of ligament of wrist
S63.30 Traumatic rupture of unspecified ligament of wrist
S63.301 Traumatic rupture of unspecified ligament of right wrist
S63.302 Traumatic rupture of unspecified ligament of left wrist
S63.309 Traumatic rupture of unspecified ligament of unspecified wrist

S63.31 Traumatic rupture of collateral ligament of wrist
S63.311 Traumatic rupture of collateral ligament of right wrist
S63.312 Traumatic rupture of collateral ligament of left wrist
S63.319 Traumatic rupture of collateral ligament of unspecified wrist

S63.32 Traumatic rupture of radiocarpal ligament
S63.321 Traumatic rupture of right radiocarpal ligament
S63.322 Traumatic rupture of left radiocarpal ligament
S63.329 Traumatic rupture of unspecified radiocarpal ligament

S63.33 Traumatic rupture of ulnocarpal (palmar) ligament
S63.331 Traumatic rupture of right ulnocarpal (palmar) ligament
S63.332 Traumatic rupture of left ulnocarpal (palmar) ligament
S63.339 Traumatic rupture of unspecified ulnocarpal (palmar) ligament

S63.39 Traumatic rupture of other ligament of wrist
S63.391 Traumatic rupture of other ligament of right wrist
S63.392 Traumatic rupture of other ligament of left wrist
S63.399 Traumatic rupture of other ligament of unspecified wrist

S63.4 Traumatic rupture of ligament of finger at metacarpophalangeal and interphalangeal joint(s)
S63.40 Traumatic rupture of unspecified ligament of finger at metacarpophalangeal and interphalangeal joint
S63.400 Traumatic rupture of unspecified ligament of right index finger at metacarpophalangeal and interphalangeal joint
S63.401 Traumatic rupture of unspecified ligament of left index finger at metacarpophalangeal and interphalangeal joint
S63.402 Traumatic rupture of unspecified ligament of right middle finger at metacarpophalangeal and interphalangeal joint
S63.403 Traumatic rupture of unspecified ligament of left middle finger at metacarpophalangeal and interphalangeal joint
S63.404 Traumatic rupture of unspecified ligament of right ring finger at metacarpophalangeal and interphalangeal joint
S63.405 Traumatic rupture of unspecified ligament of left ring finger at metacarpophalangeal and interphalangeal joint
S63.406 Traumatic rupture of unspecified ligament of right little finger at metacarpophalangeal and interphalangeal joint
S63.407 Traumatic rupture of unspecified ligament of left little finger at metacarpophalangeal and interphalangeal joint
S63.408 Traumatic rupture of unspecified ligament of other finger at metacarpophalangeal and interphalangeal joint
Traumatic rupture of unspecified ligament of specified finger with unspecified laterality at metacarpophalangeal and interphalangeal joint
S63.409 Traumatic rupture of unspecified ligament of unspecified finger at metacarpophalangeal and interphalangeal joint

S63.41 Traumatic rupture of collateral ligament of finger at metacarpophalangeal and interphalangeal joint
S63.410 Traumatic rupture of collateral ligament of right index finger at metacarpophalangeal and interphalangeal joint
S63.411 Traumatic rupture of collateral ligament of left index finger at metacarpophalangeal and interphalangeal joint
S63.412 Traumatic rupture of collateral ligament of right middle finger at metacarpophalangeal and interphalangeal joint
S63.413 Traumatic rupture of collateral ligament of left middle finger at metacarpophalangeal and interphalangeal joint

Unacceptable principal diagnosis symbol per Medicare code edits · Code exempt from diagnosis present on admission requirement
Questionable admission · Complication or comorbidity · CC/MCC exclusion · Major complication or comorbidity
Principal diagnosis as its own CC · Principal diagnosis as its own MCC · Z code as first-listed diagnosis

S63.414 Traumatic rupture of collateral ligament of right ring finger at metacarpophalangeal and interphalangeal joint
S63.415 Traumatic rupture of collateral ligament of left ring finger at metacarpophalangeal and interphalangeal joint
S63.416 Traumatic rupture of collateral ligament of right little finger at metacarpophalangeal and interphalangeal joint
S63.417 Traumatic rupture of collateral ligament of left little finger at metacarpophalangeal and interphalangeal joint
S63.418 Traumatic rupture of collateral ligament of other finger at metacarpophalangeal and interphalangeal joint
Traumatic rupture of collateral ligament of specified finger with unspecified laterality at metacarpophalangeal and interphalangeal joint
S63.419 Traumatic rupture of collateral ligament of unspecified finger at metacarpophalangeal and interphalangeal joint

S63.42 Traumatic rupture of palmar ligament of finger at metacarpophalangeal and interphalangeal joint
S63.420 Traumatic rupture of palmar ligament of right index finger at metacarpophalangeal and interphalangeal joint
S63.421 Traumatic rupture of palmar ligament of left index finger at metacarpophalangeal and interphalangeal joint
S63.422 Traumatic rupture of palmar ligament of right middle finger at metacarpophalangeal and interphalangeal joint
S63.423 Traumatic rupture of palmar ligament of left middle finger at metacarpophalangeal and interphalangeal joint
S63.424 Traumatic rupture of palmar ligament of right ring finger at metacarpophalangeal and interphalangeal joint
S63.425 Traumatic rupture of palmar ligament of left ring finger at metacarpophalangeal and interphalangeal joint
S63.426 Traumatic rupture of palmar ligament of right little finger at metacarpophalangeal and interphalangeal joint
S63.427 Traumatic rupture of palmar ligament of left little finger at metacarpophalangeal and interphalangeal joint
S63.428 Traumatic rupture of palmar ligament of other finger at metacarpophalangeal and interphalangeal joint
Traumatic rupture of palmar ligament of specified finger with unspecified laterality at metacarpophalangeal and interphalangeal joint
S63.429 Traumatic rupture of palmar ligament of unspecified finger at metacarpophalangeal and interphalangeal joint

S63.43 Traumatic rupture of volar plate of finger at metacarpophalangeal and interphalangeal joint
S63.430 Traumatic rupture of volar plate of right index finger at metacarpophalangeal and interphalangeal joint
S63.431 Traumatic rupture of volar plate of left index finger at metacarpophalangeal and interphalangeal joint
S63.432 Traumatic rupture of volar plate of right middle finger at metacarpophalangeal and interphalangeal joint
S63.433 Traumatic rupture of volar plate of left middle finger at metacarpophalangeal and interphalangeal joint
S63.434 Traumatic rupture of volar plate of right ring finger at metacarpophalangeal and interphalangeal joint
S63.435 Traumatic rupture of volar plate of left ring finger at metacarpophalangeal and interphalangeal joint
S63.436 Traumatic rupture of volar plate of right little finger at metacarpophalangeal and interphalangeal joint
S63.437 Traumatic rupture of volar plate of left little finger at metacarpophalangeal and interphalangeal joint
S63.438 Traumatic rupture of volar plate of other finger at metacarpophalangeal and interphalangeal joint
Traumatic rupture of volar plate of specified finger with unspecified laterality at metacarpophalangeal and interphalangeal joint
S63.439 Traumatic rupture of volar plate of unspecified finger at metacarpophalangeal and interphalangeal joint

S63.49 Traumatic rupture of other ligament of finger at metacarpophalangeal and interphalangeal joint
S63.490 Traumatic rupture of other ligament of right index finger at metacarpophalangeal and interphalangeal joint
S63.491 Traumatic rupture of other ligament of left index finger at metacarpophalangeal and interphalangeal joint
S63.492 Traumatic rupture of other ligament of right middle finger at metacarpophalangeal and interphalangeal joint
S63.493 Traumatic rupture of other ligament of left middle finger at metacarpophalangeal and interphalangeal joint
S63.494 Traumatic rupture of other ligament of right ring finger at metacarpophalangeal and interphalangeal joint
S63.495 Traumatic rupture of other ligament of left ring finger at metacarpophalangeal and interphalangeal joint
S63.496 Traumatic rupture of other ligament of right little finger at metacarpophalangeal and interphalangeal joint
S63.497 Traumatic rupture of other ligament of left little finger at metacarpophalangeal and interphalangeal joint
S63.498 Traumatic rupture of other ligament of other finger at metacarpophalangeal and interphalangeal joint
Traumatic rupture of ligament of specified finger with unspecified laterality at metacarpophalangeal and interphalangeal joint
S63.499 Traumatic rupture of other ligament of unspecified finger at metacarpophalangeal and interphalangeal joint

S63.5 Other and unspecified sprain of wrist
S63.50 Unspecified sprain of wrist
S63.501 Unspecified sprain of right wrist
S63.502 Unspecified sprain of left wrist
S63.509 Unspecified sprain of unspecified wrist
S63.51 Sprain of carpal (joint)
S63.511 Sprain of carpal joint of right wrist
S63.512 Sprain of carpal joint of left wrist
S63.519 Sprain of carpal joint of unspecified wrist
S63.52 Sprain of radiocarpal joint
EXCLUDES1 *traumatic rupture of radiocarpal ligament (S63.32-)*
S63.521 Sprain of radiocarpal joint of right wrist
S63.522 Sprain of radiocarpal joint of left wrist
S63.529 Sprain of radiocarpal joint of unspecified wrist
S63.59 Other specified sprain of wrist
S63.591 Other specified sprain of right wrist
S63.592 Other specified sprain of left wrist

Unspecified Code Other Specified Code Manifestation Code N Newborn P Pediatric M Maternity A Adult ♂ Male ♀ Female
● New Code ▲ Revised Code Title ►◄ Revised Text NOTES INCLUDES EXCLUDES1 Not coded here EXCLUDES2 Not included here
4th character required 5th character required 6th character required 7th character required
Extension 'X' Alert HAC Hospital-acquired condition (HAC) alert AHA AHA Coding Clinic©

S63.599 Other specified sprain of unspecified wrist
S63.6 Other and unspecified sprain of finger(s)
EXCLUDES1 *traumatic rupture of ligament of finger at metacarpophalangeal and interphalangeal joint(s) (S63.4-)*
S63.60 Unspecified sprain of thumb
S63.601 Unspecified sprain of right thumb
S63.602 Unspecified sprain of left thumb
S63.609 Unspecified sprain of unspecified thumb
S63.61 Unspecified sprain of other and unspecified finger(s)
S63.610 Unspecified sprain of right index finger
S63.611 Unspecified sprain of left index finger
S63.612 Unspecified sprain of right middle finger
S63.613 Unspecified sprain of left middle finger
S63.614 Unspecified sprain of right ring finger
S63.615 Unspecified sprain of left ring finger
S63.616 Unspecified sprain of right little finger
S63.617 Unspecified sprain of left little finger
S63.618 Unspecified sprain of other finger
Unspecified sprain of specified finger with unspecified laterality
S63.619 Unspecified sprain of unspecified finger
S63.62 Sprain of interphalangeal joint of thumb
S63.621 Sprain of interphalangeal joint of right thumb
S63.622 Sprain of interphalangeal joint of left thumb
S63.629 Sprain of interphalangeal joint of unspecified thumb
S63.63 Sprain of interphalangeal joint of other and unspecified finger(s)
S63.630 Sprain of interphalangeal joint of right index finger
S63.631 Sprain of interphalangeal joint of left index finger
S63.632 Sprain of interphalangeal joint of right middle finger
S63.633 Sprain of interphalangeal joint of left middle finger
S63.634 Sprain of interphalangeal joint of right ring finger
S63.635 Sprain of interphalangeal joint of left ring finger
S63.636 Sprain of interphalangeal joint of right little finger
S63.637 Sprain of interphalangeal joint of left little finger
S63.638 Sprain of interphalangeal joint of other finger
S63.639 Sprain of interphalangeal joint of unspecified finger
S63.64 Sprain of metacarpophalangeal joint of thumb
S63.641 Sprain of metacarpophalangeal joint of right thumb
S63.642 Sprain of metacarpophalangeal joint of left thumb
S63.649 Sprain of metacarpophalangeal joint of unspecified thumb
S63.65 Sprain of metacarpophalangeal joint of other and unspecified finger(s)
S63.650 Sprain of metacarpophalangeal joint of right index finger
S63.651 Sprain of metacarpophalangeal joint of left index finger
S63.652 Sprain of metacarpophalangeal joint of right middle finger
S63.653 Sprain of metacarpophalangeal joint of left middle finger
S63.654 Sprain of metacarpophalangeal joint of right ring finger
S63.655 Sprain of metacarpophalangeal joint of left ring finger
S63.656 Sprain of metacarpophalangeal joint of right little finger
S63.657 Sprain of metacarpophalangeal joint of left little finger
S63.658 Sprain of metacarpophalangeal joint of other finger
Sprain of metacarpophalangeal joint of specified finger with unspecified laterality
S63.659 Sprain of metacarpophalangeal joint of unspecified finger
S63.68 Other sprain of thumb
S63.681 Other sprain of right thumb
S63.682 Other sprain of left thumb
S63.689 Other sprain of unspecified thumb
S63.69 Other sprain of other and unspecified finger(s)
S63.690 Other sprain of right index finger
S63.691 Other sprain of left index finger
S63.692 Other sprain of right middle finger
S63.693 Other sprain of left middle finger
S63.694 Other sprain of right ring finger
S63.695 Other sprain of left ring finger
S63.696 Other sprain of right little finger
S63.697 Other sprain of left little finger
S63.698 Other sprain of other finger
Other sprain of specified finger with unspecified laterality
S63.699 Other sprain of unspecified finger
S63.8 Sprain of other part of wrist and hand
S63.8X Sprain of other part of wrist and hand
S63.8X1 Sprain of other part of right wrist and hand
S63.8X2 Sprain of other part of left wrist and hand
S63.8X9 Sprain of other part of unspecified wrist and hand
S63.9 Sprain of unspecified part of wrist and hand
S63.90 Sprain of unspecified part of unspecified wrist and hand
S63.91 Sprain of unspecified part of right wrist and hand
S63.92 Sprain of unspecified part of left wrist and hand
S64 Injury of nerves at wrist and hand level
Code also any associated open wound (S61.-)
The appropriate 7th character is to be added to each code from category S64
A = initial encounter
D = subsequent encounter
S = sequela
S64.0 Injury of ulnar nerve at wrist and hand level
S64.00 Injury of ulnar nerve at wrist and hand level of unspecified arm
S64.01 Injury of ulnar nerve at wrist and hand level of right arm
S64.02 Injury of ulnar nerve at wrist and hand level of left arm
S64.1 Injury of median nerve at wrist and hand level
S64.10 Injury of median nerve at wrist and hand level of unspecified arm
S64.11 Injury of median nerve at wrist and hand level of right arm
S64.12 Injury of median nerve at wrist and hand level of left arm
S64.2 Injury of radial nerve at wrist and hand level
S64.20 Injury of radial nerve at wrist and hand level of unspecified arm
S64.21 Injury of radial nerve at wrist and hand level of right arm
S64.22 Injury of radial nerve at wrist and hand level of left arm
S64.3 Injury of digital nerve of thumb
S64.30 Injury of digital nerve of unspecified thumb
S64.31 Injury of digital nerve of right thumb
S64.32 Injury of digital nerve of left thumb
S64.4 Injury of digital nerve of other and unspecified finger
S64.40 Injury of digital nerve of unspecified finger
S64.49 Injury of digital nerve of other finger
S64.490 Injury of digital nerve of right index finger
S64.491 Injury of digital nerve of left index finger

Unacceptable principal diagnosis symbol per Medicare code edits · Code exempt from diagnosis present on admission requirement
Questionable admission · Complication or comorbidity · CC/MCC exclusion · Major complication or comorbidity
Principal diagnosis as its own CC · Principal diagnosis as its own MCC · Z code as first-listed diagnosis

S64.492 Injury of digital nerve of right middle finger
S64.493 Injury of digital nerve of left middle finger
S64.494 Injury of digital nerve of right ring finger
S64.495 Injury of digital nerve of left ring finger
S64.496 Injury of digital nerve of right little finger
S64.497 Injury of digital nerve of left little finger
S64.498 Injury of digital nerve of other finger
Injury of digital nerve of specified finger with unspecified laterality
S64.8 Injury of other nerves at wrist and hand level
S64.8X Injury of other nerves at wrist and hand level
S64.8X1 Injury of other nerves at wrist and hand level of right arm
S64.8X2 Injury of other nerves at wrist and hand level of left arm
S64.8X9 Injury of other nerves at wrist and hand level of unspecified arm
S64.9 Injury of unspecified nerve at wrist and hand level
S64.90 Injury of unspecified nerve at wrist and hand level of unspecified arm
S64.91 Injury of unspecified nerve at wrist and hand level of right arm
S64.92 Injury of unspecified nerve at wrist and hand level of left arm
S65 Injury of blood vessels at wrist and hand level
Code also any associated open wound (S61.-)
The appropriate 7th character is to be added to each code from category S65
A = initial encounter
D = subsequent encounter
S = sequela
S65.0 Injury of ulnar artery at wrist and hand level
S65.00 Unspecified injury of ulnar artery at wrist and hand level
S65.001 Unspecified injury of ulnar artery at wrist and hand level of right arm
S65.002 Unspecified injury of ulnar artery at wrist and hand level of left arm
S65.009 Unspecified injury of ulnar artery at wrist and hand level of unspecified arm
S65.01 Laceration of ulnar artery at wrist and hand level
S65.011 Laceration of ulnar artery at wrist and hand level of right arm
S65.012 Laceration of ulnar artery at wrist and hand level of left arm
S65.019 Laceration of ulnar artery at wrist and hand level of unspecified arm
S65.09 Other specified injury of ulnar artery at wrist and hand level
S65.091 Other specified injury of ulnar artery at wrist and hand level of right arm
S65.092 Other specified injury of ulnar artery at wrist and hand level of left arm
S65.099 Other specified injury of ulnar artery at wrist and hand level of unspecified arm
S65.1 Injury of radial artery at wrist and hand level
S65.10 Unspecified injury of radial artery at wrist and hand level
S65.101 Unspecified injury of radial artery at wrist and hand level of right arm
S65.102 Unspecified injury of radial artery at wrist and hand level of left arm
S65.109 Unspecified injury of radial artery at wrist and hand level of unspecified arm
S65.11 Laceration of radial artery at wrist and hand level
S65.111 Laceration of radial artery at wrist and hand level of right arm
S65.112 Laceration of radial artery at wrist and hand level of left arm
S65.119 Laceration of radial artery at wrist and hand level of unspecified arm
S65.19 Other specified injury of radial artery at wrist and hand level
S65.191 Other specified injury of radial artery at wrist and hand level of right arm
S65.192 Other specified injury of radial artery at wrist and hand level of left arm
S65.199 Other specified injury of radial artery at wrist and hand level of unspecified arm
S65.2 Injury of superficial palmar arch
S65.20 Unspecified injury of superficial palmar arch
S65.201 Unspecified injury of superficial palmar arch of right hand
S65.202 Unspecified injury of superficial palmar arch of left hand
S65.209 Unspecified injury of superficial palmar arch of unspecified hand
S65.21 Laceration of superficial palmar arch
S65.211 Laceration of superficial palmar arch of right hand
S65.212 Laceration of superficial palmar arch of left hand
S65.219 Laceration of superficial palmar arch of unspecified hand
S65.29 Other specified injury of superficial palmar arch
S65.291 Other specified injury of superficial palmar arch of right hand
S65.292 Other specified injury of superficial palmar arch of left hand
S65.299 Other specified injury of superficial palmar arch of unspecified hand
S65.3 Injury of deep palmar arch
S65.30 Unspecified injury of deep palmar arch
S65.301 Unspecified injury of deep palmar arch of right hand
S65.302 Unspecified injury of deep palmar arch of left hand
S65.309 Unspecified injury of deep palmar arch of unspecified hand
S65.31 Laceration of deep palmar arch
S65.311 Laceration of deep palmar arch of right hand
S65.312 Laceration of deep palmar arch of left hand
S65.319 Laceration of deep palmar arch of unspecified hand
S65.39 Other specified injury of deep palmar arch
S65.391 Other specified injury of deep palmar arch of right hand
S65.392 Other specified injury of deep palmar arch of left hand
S65.399 Other specified injury of deep palmar arch of unspecified hand
S65.4 Injury of blood vessel of thumb
S65.40 Unspecified injury of blood vessel of thumb
S65.401 Unspecified injury of blood vessel of right thumb
S65.402 Unspecified injury of blood vessel of left thumb
S65.409 Unspecified injury of blood vessel of unspecified thumb
S65.41 Laceration of blood vessel of thumb
S65.411 Laceration of blood vessel of right thumb
S65.412 Laceration of blood vessel of left thumb
S65.419 Laceration of blood vessel of unspecified thumb
S65.49 Other specified injury of blood vessel of thumb
S65.491 Other specified injury of blood vessel of right thumb
S65.492 Other specified injury of blood vessel of left thumb
S65.499 Other specified injury of blood vessel of unspecified thumb
S65.5 Injury of blood vessel of other and unspecified finger
S65.50 Unspecified injury of blood vessel of other and unspecified finger

Unspecified Code | Other Specified Code | Manifestation Code | N Newborn | P Pediatric | M Maternity | A Adult | ♂ Male | ♀ Female
● New Code | ▲ Revised Code Title | ►◄ Revised Text | NOTES | INCLUDES | EXCLUDES 1 Not coded here | EXCLUDES 2 Not included here
4th character required | 5th character required | 6th character required | 7th character required
Extension 'X' Alert | HAC Hospital-acquired condition (HAC) alert | AHA AHA Coding Clinic®

S65.500 Unspecified injury of blood vessel of right index finger
S65.501 Unspecified injury of blood vessel of left index finger
S65.502 Unspecified injury of blood vessel of right middle finger
S65.503 Unspecified injury of blood vessel of left middle finger
S65.504 Unspecified injury of blood vessel of right ring finger
S65.505 Unspecified injury of blood vessel of left ring finger
S65.506 Unspecified injury of blood vessel of right little finger
S65.507 Unspecified injury of blood vessel of left little finger
S65.508 Unspecified injury of blood vessel of other finger
Unspecified injury of blood vessel of specified finger with unspecified laterality
S65.509 Unspecified injury of blood vessel of unspecified finger

S65.51 Laceration of blood vessel of other and unspecified finger
S65.510 Laceration of blood vessel of right index finger
S65.511 Laceration of blood vessel of left index finger
S65.512 Laceration of blood vessel of right middle finger
S65.513 Laceration of blood vessel of left middle finger
S65.514 Laceration of blood vessel of right ring finger
S65.515 Laceration of blood vessel of left ring finger
S65.516 Laceration of blood vessel of right little finger
S65.517 Laceration of blood vessel of left little finger
S65.518 Laceration of blood vessel of other finger
Laceration of blood vessel of specified finger with unspecified laterality
S65.519 Laceration of blood vessel of unspecified finger

S65.59 Other specified injury of blood vessel of other and unspecified finger
S65.590 Other specified injury of blood vessel of right index finger
S65.591 Other specified injury of blood vessel of left index finger
S65.592 Other specified injury of blood vessel of right middle finger
S65.593 Other specified injury of blood vessel of left middle finger
S65.594 Other specified injury of blood vessel of right ring finger
S65.595 Other specified injury of blood vessel of left ring finger
S65.596 Other specified injury of blood vessel of right little finger
S65.597 Other specified injury of blood vessel of left little finger
S65.598 Other specified injury of blood vessel of other finger
Other specified injury of blood vessel of specified finger with unspecified laterality
S65.599 Other specified injury of blood vessel of unspecified finger

S65.8 Injury of other blood vessels at wrist and hand level
S65.80 Unspecified injury of other blood vessels at wrist and hand level
S65.801 Unspecified injury of other blood vessels at wrist and hand level of right arm
S65.802 Unspecified injury of other blood vessels at wrist and hand level of left arm
S65.809 Unspecified injury of other blood vessels at wrist and hand level of unspecified arm

S65.81 Laceration of other blood vessels at wrist and hand level
S65.811 Laceration of other blood vessels at wrist and hand level of right arm
S65.812 Laceration of other blood vessels at wrist and hand level of left arm
S65.819 Laceration of other blood vessels at wrist and hand level of unspecified arm

S65.89 Other specified injury of other blood vessels at wrist and hand level
S65.891 Other specified injury of other blood vessels at wrist and hand level of right arm
S65.892 Other specified injury of other blood vessels at wrist and hand level of left arm
S65.899 Other specified injury of other blood vessels at wrist and hand level of unspecified arm

S65.9 Injury of unspecified blood vessel at wrist and hand level
S65.90 Unspecified injury of unspecified blood vessel at wrist and hand level
S65.901 Unspecified injury of unspecified blood vessel at wrist and hand level of right arm
S65.902 Unspecified injury of unspecified blood vessel at wrist and hand level of left arm
S65.909 Unspecified injury of unspecified blood vessel at wrist and hand level of unspecified arm

S65.91 Laceration of unspecified blood vessel at wrist and hand level
S65.911 Laceration of unspecified blood vessel at wrist and hand level of right arm
S65.912 Laceration of unspecified blood vessel at wrist and hand level of left arm
S65.919 Laceration of unspecified blood vessel at wrist and hand level of unspecified arm

S65.99 Other specified injury of unspecified blood vessel at wrist and hand level
S65.991 Other specified injury of unspecified blood vessel at wrist and hand of right arm
S65.992 Other specified injury of unspecified blood vessel at wrist and hand of left arm
S65.999 Other specified injury of unspecified blood vessel at wrist and hand of unspecified arm

S66 Injury of muscle, fascia and tendon at wrist and hand level
Code also any associated open wound (S61.-)
EXCLUDES2 *sprain of joints and ligaments of wrist and hand (S63.-)*
The appropriate 7th character is to be added to each code from category S66
A = initial encounter
D = subsequent encounter
S = sequela

S66.0 Injury of long flexor muscle, fascia and tendon of thumb at wrist and hand level
S66.00 Unspecified injury of long flexor muscle, fascia and tendon of thumb at wrist and hand level
S66.001 Unspecified injury of long flexor muscle, fascia and tendon of right thumb at wrist and hand level
S66.002 Unspecified injury of long flexor muscle, fascia and tendon of left thumb at wrist and hand level
S66.009 Unspecified injury of long flexor muscle, fascia and tendon of unspecified thumb at wrist and hand level

Unacceptable principal diagnosis symbol per Medicare code edits | Code exempt from diagnosis present on admission requirement
Questionable admission | Complication or comorbidity | CC/MCC exclusion | Major complication or comorbidity
Principal diagnosis as its own CC | Principal diagnosis as its own MCC | Z code as first-listed diagnosis

S66.01 Strain of long flexor muscle, fascia and tendon of thumb at wrist and hand level

S66.011 Strain of long flexor muscle, fascia and tendon of right thumb at wrist and hand level

S66.012 Strain of long flexor muscle, fascia and tendon of left thumb at wrist and hand level

S66.019 Strain of long flexor muscle, fascia and tendon of unspecified thumb at wrist and hand level

S66.02 Laceration of long flexor muscle, fascia and tendon of thumb at wrist and hand level

S66.021 Laceration of long flexor muscle, fascia and tendon of right thumb at wrist and hand level

S66.022 Laceration of long flexor muscle, fascia and tendon of left thumb at wrist and hand level

S66.029 Laceration of long flexor muscle, fascia and tendon of unspecified thumb at wrist and hand level

S66.09 Other specified injury of long flexor muscle, fascia and tendon of thumb at wrist and hand level

S66.091 Other specified injury of long flexor muscle, fascia and tendon of right thumb at wrist and hand level

S66.092 Other specified injury of long flexor muscle, fascia and tendon of left thumb at wrist and hand level

S66.099 Other specified injury of long flexor muscle, fascia and tendon of unspecified thumb at wrist and hand level

S66.1 Injury of flexor muscle, fascia and tendon of other and unspecified finger at wrist and hand level

EXCLUDES2 *Injury of long flexor muscle, fascia and tendon of thumb at wrist and hand level (S66.0-)*

S66.10 Unspecified injury of flexor muscle, fascia and tendon of other and unspecified finger at wrist and hand level

S66.100 Unspecified injury of flexor muscle, fascia and tendon of right index finger at wrist and hand level

S66.101 Unspecified injury of flexor muscle, fascia and tendon of left index finger at wrist and hand level

S66.102 Unspecified injury of flexor muscle, fascia and tendon of right middle finger at wrist and hand level

S66.103 Unspecified injury of flexor muscle, fascia and tendon of left middle finger at wrist and hand level

S66.104 Unspecified injury of flexor muscle, fascia and tendon of right ring finger at wrist and hand level

S66.105 Unspecified injury of flexor muscle, fascia and tendon of left ring finger at wrist and hand level

S66.106 Unspecified injury of flexor muscle, fascia and tendon of right little finger at wrist and hand level

S66.107 Unspecified injury of flexor muscle, fascia and tendon of left little finger at wrist and hand level

S66.108 Unspecified injury of flexor muscle, fascia and tendon of other finger at wrist and hand level

Unspecified injury of flexor muscle, fascia and tendon of specified finger with unspecified laterality at wrist and hand level

S66.109 Unspecified injury of flexor muscle, fascia and tendon of unspecified finger at wrist and hand level

S66.11 Strain of flexor muscle, fascia and tendon of other and unspecified finger at wrist and hand level

S66.110 Strain of flexor muscle, fascia and tendon of right index finger at wrist and hand level

S66.111 Strain of flexor muscle, fascia and tendon of left index finger at wrist and hand level

S66.112 Strain of flexor muscle, fascia and tendon of right middle finger at wrist and hand level

S66.113 Strain of flexor muscle, fascia and tendon of left middle finger at wrist and hand level

S66.114 Strain of flexor muscle, fascia and tendon of right ring finger at wrist and hand level

S66.115 Strain of flexor muscle, fascia and tendon of left ring finger at wrist and hand level

S66.116 Strain of flexor muscle, fascia and tendon of right little finger at wrist and hand level

S66.117 Strain of flexor muscle, fascia and tendon of left little finger at wrist and hand level

S66.118 Strain of flexor muscle, fascia and tendon of other finger at wrist and hand level

Strain of flexor muscle, fascia and tendon of specified finger with unspecified laterality at wrist and hand level

S66.119 Strain of flexor muscle, fascia and tendon of unspecified finger at wrist and hand level

S66.12 Laceration of flexor muscle, fascia and tendon of other and unspecified finger at wrist and hand level

S66.120 Laceration of flexor muscle, fascia and tendon of right index finger at wrist and hand level

S66.121 Laceration of flexor muscle, fascia and tendon of left index finger at wrist and hand level

S66.122 Laceration of flexor muscle, fascia and tendon of right middle finger at wrist and hand level

S66.123 Laceration of flexor muscle, fascia and tendon of left middle finger at wrist and hand level

S66.124 Laceration of flexor muscle, fascia and tendon of right ring finger at wrist and hand level

S66.125 Laceration of flexor muscle, fascia and tendon of left ring finger at wrist and hand level

S66.126 Laceration of flexor muscle, fascia and tendon of right little finger at wrist and hand level

S66.127 Laceration of flexor muscle, fascia and tendon of left little finger at wrist and hand level

S66.128 Laceration of flexor muscle, fascia and tendon of other finger at wrist and hand level

Laceration of flexor muscle, fascia and tendon of specified finger with unspecified laterality at wrist and hand level

S66.129 Laceration of flexor muscle, fascia and tendon of unspecified finger at wrist and hand level

S66.19 Other injury of flexor muscle, fascia and tendon of other and unspecified finger at wrist and hand level

S66.190 Other injury of flexor muscle, fascia and tendon of right index finger at wrist and hand level

S66.191 Other injury of flexor muscle, fascia and tendon of left index finger at wrist and hand level

S66.192 Other injury of flexor muscle, fascia and tendon of right middle finger at wrist and hand level

S66.193 Other injury of flexor muscle, fascia and tendon of left middle finger at wrist and hand level

Unspecified Code Other Specified Code Manifestation Code N Newborn P Pediatric M Maternity A Adult ♂ Male ♀ Female
● New Code ▲ Revised Code Title ►◄ Revised Text NOTES INCLUDES EXCLUDES1 Not coded here EXCLUDES2 Not included here
4th character required 5th character required 6th character required 7th character required
Extension 'X' Alert HAC Hospital-acquired condition (HAC) alert AHA AHA Coding Clinic®

S66.194 Other injury of flexor muscle, fascia and tendon of right ring finger at wrist and hand level
S66.195 Other injury of flexor muscle, fascia and tendon of left ring finger at wrist and hand level
S66.196 Other injury of flexor muscle, fascia and tendon of right little finger at wrist and hand level
S66.197 Other injury of flexor muscle, fascia and tendon of left little finger at wrist and hand level
S66.198 Other injury of flexor muscle, fascia and tendon of other finger at wrist and hand level
Other injury of flexor muscle, fascia and tendon of specified finger with unspecified laterality at wrist and hand level
S66.199 Other injury of flexor muscle, fascia and tendon of unspecified finger at wrist and hand level

S66.2 Injury of extensor muscle, fascia and tendon of thumb at wrist and hand level
S66.20 Unspecified injury of extensor muscle, fascia and tendon of thumb at wrist and hand level
S66.201 Unspecified injury of extensor muscle, fascia and tendon of right thumb at wrist and hand level
S66.202 Unspecified injury of extensor muscle, fascia and tendon of left thumb at wrist and hand level
S66.209 Unspecified injury of extensor muscle, fascia and tendon of unspecified thumb at wrist and hand level
S66.21 Strain of extensor muscle, fascia and tendon of thumb at wrist and hand level
S66.211 Strain of extensor muscle, fascia and tendon of right thumb at wrist and hand level
S66.212 Strain of extensor muscle, fascia and tendon of left thumb at wrist and hand level
S66.219 Strain of extensor muscle, fascia and tendon of unspecified thumb at wrist and hand level
S66.22 Laceration of extensor muscle, fascia and tendon of thumb at wrist and hand level
S66.221 Laceration of extensor muscle, fascia and tendon of right thumb at wrist and hand level CC
S66.222 Laceration of extensor muscle, fascia and tendon of left thumb at wrist and hand level CC
S66.229 Laceration of extensor muscle, fascia and tendon of unspecified thumb at wrist and hand level CC
S66.29 Other specified injury of extensor muscle, fascia and tendon of thumb at wrist and hand level
S66.291 Other specified injury of extensor muscle, fascia and tendon of right thumb at wrist and hand level
S66.292 Other specified injury of extensor muscle, fascia and tendon of left thumb at wrist and hand level
S66.299 Other specified injury of extensor muscle, fascia and tendon of unspecified thumb at wrist and hand level

S66.3 Injury of extensor muscle, fascia and tendon of other and unspecified finger at wrist and hand level
EXCLUDES2 *Injury of extensor muscle, fascia and tendon of thumb at wrist and hand level (S66.2-)*
S66.30 Unspecified injury of extensor muscle, fascia and tendon of other and unspecified finger at wrist and hand level
S66.300 Unspecified injury of extensor muscle, fascia and tendon of right index finger at wrist and hand level
S66.301 Unspecified injury of extensor muscle, fascia and tendon of left index finger at wrist and hand level
S66.302 Unspecified injury of extensor muscle, fascia and tendon of right middle finger at wrist and hand level
S66.303 Unspecified injury of extensor muscle, fascia and tendon of left middle finger at wrist and hand level
S66.304 Unspecified injury of extensor muscle, fascia and tendon of right ring finger at wrist and hand level
S66.305 Unspecified injury of extensor muscle, fascia and tendon of left ring finger at wrist and hand level
S66.306 Unspecified injury of extensor muscle, fascia and tendon of right little finger at wrist and hand level
S66.307 Unspecified injury of extensor muscle, fascia and tendon of left little finger at wrist and hand level
S66.308 Unspecified injury of extensor muscle, fascia and tendon of other finger at wrist and hand level
Unspecified injury of extensor muscle, fascia and tendon of specified finger with unspecified laterality at wrist and hand level
S66.309 Unspecified injury of extensor muscle, fascia and tendon of unspecified finger at wrist and hand level
S66.31 Strain of extensor muscle, fascia and tendon of other and unspecified finger at wrist and hand level
S66.310 Strain of extensor muscle, fascia and tendon of right index finger at wrist and hand level
S66.311 Strain of extensor muscle, fascia and tendon of left index finger at wrist and hand level
S66.312 Strain of extensor muscle, fascia and tendon of right middle finger at wrist and hand level
S66.313 Strain of extensor muscle, fascia and tendon of left middle finger at wrist and hand level
S66.314 Strain of extensor muscle, fascia and tendon of right ring finger at wrist and hand level
S66.315 Strain of extensor muscle, fascia and tendon of left ring finger at wrist and hand level
S66.316 Strain of extensor muscle, fascia and tendon of right little finger at wrist and hand level
S66.317 Strain of extensor muscle, fascia and tendon of left little finger at wrist and hand level
S66.318 Strain of extensor muscle, fascia and tendon of other finger at wrist and hand level
Strain of extensor muscle, fascia and tendon of specified finger with unspecified laterality at wrist and hand level
S66.319 Strain of extensor muscle, fascia and tendon of unspecified finger at wrist and hand level
S66.32 Laceration of extensor muscle, fascia and tendon of other and unspecified finger at wrist and hand level
S66.320 Laceration of extensor muscle, fascia and tendon of right index finger at wrist and hand level CC
S66.321 Laceration of extensor muscle, fascia and tendon of left index finger at wrist and hand level CC
S66.322 Laceration of extensor muscle, fascia and tendon of right middle finger at wrist and hand level CC

PDx Unacceptable principal diagnosis symbol per Medicare code edits · POA Code exempt from diagnosis present on admission requirement
? Questionable admission · CC Complication or comorbidity · CC/MCC Excl CC/MCC exclusion · MCC Major complication or comorbidity
PDx CC Principal diagnosis as its own CC · PDx MCC Principal diagnosis as its own MCC · Z Z code as first-listed diagnosis

S66.323 Laceration of extensor muscle, fascia and tendon of left middle finger at wrist and hand level

S66.324 Laceration of extensor muscle, fascia and tendon of right ring finger at wrist and hand level

S66.325 Laceration of extensor muscle, fascia and tendon of left ring finger at wrist and hand level

S66.326 Laceration of extensor muscle, fascia and tendon of right little finger at wrist and hand level

S66.327 Laceration of extensor muscle, fascia and tendon of left little finger at wrist and hand level

S66.328 Laceration of extensor muscle, fascia and tendon of other finger at wrist and hand level

Laceration of extensor muscle, fascia and tendon of specified finger with unspecified laterality at wrist and hand level

S66.329 Laceration of extensor muscle, fascia and tendon of unspecified finger at wrist and hand level

S66.39 Other injury of extensor muscle, fascia and tendon of other and unspecified finger at wrist and hand level

S66.390 Other injury of extensor muscle, fascia and tendon of right index finger at wrist and hand level

S66.391 Other injury of extensor muscle, fascia and tendon of left index finger at wrist and hand level

S66.392 Other injury of extensor muscle, fascia and tendon of right middle finger at wrist and hand level

S66.393 Other injury of extensor muscle, fascia and tendon of left middle finger at wrist and hand level

S66.394 Other injury of extensor muscle, fascia and tendon of right ring finger at wrist and hand level

S66.395 Other injury of extensor muscle, fascia and tendon of left ring finger at wrist and hand level

S66.396 Other injury of extensor muscle, fascia and tendon of right little finger at wrist and hand level

S66.397 Other injury of extensor muscle, fascia and tendon of left little finger at wrist and hand level

S66.398 Other injury of extensor muscle, fascia and tendon of other finger at wrist and hand level

Other injury of extensor muscle, fascia and tendon of specified finger with unspecified laterality at wrist and hand level

S66.399 Other injury of extensor muscle, fascia and tendon of unspecified finger at wrist and hand level

S66.4 Injury of intrinsic muscle, fascia and tendon of thumb at wrist and hand level

S66.40 Unspecified injury of intrinsic muscle, fascia and tendon of thumb at wrist and hand level

S66.401 Unspecified injury of intrinsic muscle, fascia and tendon of right thumb at wrist and hand level

S66.402 Unspecified injury of intrinsic muscle, fascia and tendon of left thumb at wrist and hand level

S66.409 Unspecified injury of intrinsic muscle, fascia and tendon of unspecified thumb at wrist and hand level

S66.41 Strain of intrinsic muscle, fascia and tendon of thumb at wrist and hand level

S66.411 Strain of intrinsic muscle, fascia and tendon of right thumb at wrist and hand level

S66.412 Strain of intrinsic muscle, fascia and tendon of left thumb at wrist and hand level

S66.419 Strain of intrinsic muscle, fascia and tendon of unspecified thumb at wrist and hand level

S66.42 Laceration of intrinsic muscle, fascia and tendon of thumb at wrist and hand level

S66.421 Laceration of intrinsic muscle, fascia and tendon of right thumb at wrist and hand level

S66.422 Laceration of intrinsic muscle, fascia and tendon of left thumb at wrist and hand level

S66.429 Laceration of intrinsic muscle, fascia and tendon of unspecified thumb at wrist and hand level

S66.49 Other specified injury of intrinsic muscle, fascia and tendon of thumb at wrist and hand level

S66.491 Other specified injury of intrinsic muscle, fascia and tendon of right thumb at wrist and hand level

S66.492 Other specified injury of intrinsic muscle, fascia and tendon of left thumb at wrist and hand level

S66.499 Other specified injury of intrinsic muscle, fascia and tendon of unspecified thumb at wrist and hand level

S66.5 Injury of intrinsic muscle , fascia and tendon of other and unspecified finger at wrist and hand level

EXCLUDES2 *injury of intrinsic muscle, fascia and tendon of thumb at wrist and hand level (S66.4-)*

S66.50 Unspecified injury of intrinsic muscle, fascia and tendon of other and unspecified finger at wrist and hand level

S66.500 Unspecified injury of intrinsic muscle, fascia and tendon of right index finger at wrist and hand level

S66.501 Unspecified injury of intrinsic muscle, fascia and tendon of left index finger at wrist and hand level

S66.502 Unspecified injury of intrinsic muscle, fascia and tendon of right middle finger at wrist and hand level

S66.503 Unspecified injury of intrinsic muscle, fascia and tendon of left middle finger at wrist and hand level

S66.504 Unspecified injury of intrinsic muscle, fascia and tendon of right ring finger at wrist and hand level

S66.505 Unspecified injury of intrinsic muscle, fascia and tendon of left ring finger at wrist and hand level

S66.506 Unspecified injury of intrinsic muscle, fascia and tendon of right little finger at wrist and hand level

S66.507 Unspecified injury of intrinsic muscle, fascia and tendon of left little finger at wrist and hand level

S66.508 Unspecified injury of intrinsic muscle, fascia and tendon of other finger at wrist and hand level

Unspecified injury of intrinsic muscle, fascia and tendon of specified finger with unspecified laterality at wrist and hand level

S66.509 Unspecified injury of intrinsic muscle, fascia and tendon of unspecified finger at wrist and hand level

S66.51 Strain of intrinsic muscle, fascia and tendon of other and unspecified finger at wrist and hand level

S66.510 Strain of intrinsic muscle, fascia and tendon of right index finger at wrist and hand level

S66.511 Strain of intrinsic muscle, fascia and tendon of left index finger at wrist and hand level

Unspecified Code Other Specified Code Manifestation Code N Newborn P Pediatric M Maternity A Adult ♂ Male ♀ Female
● New Code ▲ Revised Code Title ►◄ Revised Text NOTES INCLUDES EXCLUDES1 Not coded here EXCLUDES2 Not included here
4th character required 5th character required 6th character required 7th character required
Extension 'X' Alert HAC Hospital-acquired condition (HAC) alert AHA AHA Coding Clinic©

S66.512 Strain of intrinsic muscle, fascia and tendon of right middle finger at wrist and hand level
S66.513 Strain of intrinsic muscle, fascia and tendon of left middle finger at wrist and hand level
S66.514 Strain of intrinsic muscle, fascia and tendon of right ring finger at wrist and hand level
S66.515 Strain of intrinsic muscle, fascia and tendon of left ring finger at wrist and hand level
S66.516 Strain of intrinsic muscle, fascia and tendon of right little finger at wrist and hand level
S66.517 Strain of intrinsic muscle, fascia and tendon of left little finger at wrist and hand level
S66.518 Strain of intrinsic muscle, fascia and tendon of other finger at wrist and hand level
Strain of intrinsic muscle, fascia and tendon of specified finger with unspecified laterality at wrist and hand level
S66.519 Strain of intrinsic muscle, fascia and tendon of unspecified finger at wrist and hand level

S66.52 Laceration of intrinsic muscle, fascia and tendon of other and unspecified finger at wrist and hand level
S66.520 Laceration of intrinsic muscle, fascia and tendon of right index finger at wrist and hand level CC
S66.521 Laceration of intrinsic muscle, fascia and tendon of left index finger at wrist and hand level CC
S66.522 Laceration of intrinsic muscle, fascia and tendon of right middle finger at wrist and hand level CC
S66.523 Laceration of intrinsic muscle, fascia and tendon of left middle finger at wrist and hand level CC
S66.524 Laceration of intrinsic muscle, fascia and tendon of right ring finger at wrist and hand level CC
S66.525 Laceration of intrinsic muscle, fascia and tendon of left ring finger at wrist and hand level CC
S66.526 Laceration of intrinsic muscle, fascia and tendon of right little finger at wrist and hand level CC
S66.527 Laceration of intrinsic muscle, fascia and tendon of left little finger at wrist and hand level CC
S66.528 Laceration of intrinsic muscle, fascia and tendon of other finger at wrist and hand level CC
Laceration of intrinsic muscle, fascia and tendon of specified finger with unspecified laterality at wrist and hand level
S66.529 Laceration of intrinsic muscle, fascia and tendon of unspecified finger at wrist and hand level CC

S66.59 Other injury of intrinsic muscle, fascia and tendon of other and unspecified finger at wrist and hand level
S66.590 Other injury of intrinsic muscle, fascia and tendon of right index finger at wrist and hand level
S66.591 Other injury of intrinsic muscle, fascia and tendon of left index finger at wrist and hand level
S66.592 Other injury of intrinsic muscle, fascia and tendon of right middle finger at wrist and hand level
S66.593 Other injury of intrinsic muscle, fascia and tendon of left middle finger at wrist and hand level
S66.594 Other injury of intrinsic muscle, fascia and tendon of right ring finger at wrist and hand level
S66.595 Other injury of intrinsic muscle, fascia and tendon of left ring finger at wrist and hand level
S66.596 Other injury of intrinsic muscle, fascia and tendon of right little finger at wrist and hand level
S66.597 Other injury of intrinsic muscle, fascia and tendon of left little finger at wrist and hand level
S66.598 Other injury of intrinsic muscle, fascia and tendon of other finger at wrist and hand level
Other injury of intrinsic muscle, fascia and tendon of specified finger with unspecified laterality at wrist and hand level
S66.599 Other injury of intrinsic muscle, fascia and tendon of unspecified finger at wrist and hand level

S66.8 Injury of other specified muscles, fascia and tendons at wrist and hand level

S66.80 Unspecified injury of other specified muscles, fascia and tendons at wrist and hand level
S66.801 Unspecified injury of other specified muscles, fascia and tendons at wrist and hand level, right hand
S66.802 Unspecified injury of other specified muscles, fascia and tendons at wrist and hand level, left hand
S66.809 Unspecified injury of other specified muscles, fascia and tendons at wrist and hand level, unspecified hand

S66.81 Strain of other specified muscles, fascia and tendons at wrist and hand level
S66.811 Strain of other specified muscles, fascia and tendons at wrist and hand level, right hand
S66.812 Strain of other specified muscles, fascia and tendons at wrist and hand level, left hand
S66.819 Strain of other specified muscles, fascia and tendons at wrist and hand level, unspecified hand

S66.82 Laceration of other specified muscles, fascia and tendons at wrist and hand level
S66.821 Laceration of other specified muscles, fascia and tendons at wrist and hand level, right hand CC
S66.822 Laceration of other specified muscles, fascia and tendons at wrist and hand level, left hand CC
S66.829 Laceration of other specified muscles, fascia and tendons at wrist and hand level, unspecified hand CC

S66.89 Other injury of other specified muscles, fascia and tendons at wrist and hand level
S66.891 Other injury of other specified muscles, fascia and tendons at wrist and hand level, right hand
S66.892 Other injury of other specified muscles, fascia and tendons at wrist and hand level, left hand
S66.899 Other injury of other specified muscles, fascia and tendons at wrist and hand level, unspecified hand

S66.9 Injury of unspecified muscle, fascia and tendon at wrist and hand level

S66.90 Unspecified injury of unspecified muscle, fascia and tendon at wrist and hand level
S66.901 Unspecified injury of unspecified muscle, fascia and tendon at wrist and hand level, right hand
S66.902 Unspecified injury of unspecified muscle, fascia and tendon at wrist and hand level, left hand

Unacceptable principal diagnosis symbol per Medicare code edits — Code exempt from diagnosis present on admission requirement
Questionable admission — CC Complication or comorbidity — CC/MCC exclusion — MCC Major complication or comorbidity
Principal diagnosis as its own CC — Principal diagnosis as its own MCC — Z code as first-listed diagnosis

S66.909 Unspecified injury of unspecified muscle, fascia and tendon at wrist and hand level, unspecified hand
S66.91 Strain of unspecified muscle, fascia and tendon at wrist and hand level
S66.911 Strain of unspecified muscle, fascia and tendon at wrist and hand level, right hand
S66.912 Strain of unspecified muscle, fascia and tendon at wrist and hand level, left hand
S66.919 Strain of unspecified muscle, fascia and tendon at wrist and hand level, unspecified hand
S66.92 Laceration of unspecified muscle, fascia and tendon at wrist and hand level
S66.921 Laceration of unspecified muscle, fascia and tendon at wrist and hand level, right hand
S66.922 Laceration of unspecified muscle, fascia and tendon at wrist and hand level, left hand
S66.929 Laceration of unspecified muscle, fascia and tendon at wrist and hand level, unspecified hand
S66.99 Other injury of unspecified muscle, fascia and tendon at wrist and hand level
S66.991 Other injury of unspecified muscle, fascia and tendon at wrist and hand level, right hand
S66.992 Other injury of unspecified muscle, fascia and tendon at wrist and hand level, left hand
S66.999 Other injury of unspecified muscle, fascia and tendon at wrist and hand level, unspecified hand

S67 Crushing injury of wrist, hand and fingers
Use additional code for all associated injuries, such as:
fracture of wrist and hand (S62.-)
open wound of wrist and hand (S61.-)
The appropriate 7th character is to be added to each code from category S67
A = initial encounter
D = subsequent encounter
S = sequela

S67.0 Crushing injury of thumb
S67.00 Crushing injury of unspecified thumb
S67.01 Crushing injury of right thumb
S67.02 Crushing injury of left thumb
S67.1 Crushing injury of other and unspecified finger(s)
EXCLUDES2 *crushing injury of thumb (S67.0-)*
S67.10 Crushing injury of unspecified finger(s)
S67.19 Crushing injury of other finger(s)
S67.190 Crushing injury of right index finger
S67.191 Crushing injury of left index finger
S67.192 Crushing injury of right middle finger
S67.193 Crushing injury of left middle finger
S67.194 Crushing injury of right ring finger
S67.195 Crushing injury of left ring finger
S67.196 Crushing injury of right little finger
S67.197 Crushing injury of left little finger
S67.198 Crushing injury of other finger
Crushing injury of specified finger with unspecified laterality
S67.2 Crushing injury of hand
EXCLUDES2 *crushing injury of fingers (S67.1-)*
crushing injury of thumb (S67.0-)
S67.20 Crushing injury of unspecified hand
S67.21 Crushing injury of right hand
S67.22 Crushing injury of left hand
S67.3 Crushing injury of wrist
S67.30 Crushing injury of unspecified wrist
S67.31 Crushing injury of right wrist
S67.32 Crushing injury of left wrist
S67.4 Crushing injury of wrist and hand
EXCLUDES1 *crushing injury of hand alone (S67.2-)*
crushing injury of wrist alone (S67.3-)
EXCLUDES2 *crushing injury of fingers (S67.1-)*
crushing injury of thumb (S67.0-)
S67.40 Crushing injury of unspecified wrist and hand
S67.41 Crushing injury of right wrist and hand
S67.42 Crushing injury of left wrist and hand
S67.9 Crushing injury of unspecified part(s) of wrist, hand and fingers
S67.90 Crushing injury of unspecified part(s) of unspecified wrist, hand and fingers
S67.91 Crushing injury of unspecified part(s) of right wrist, hand and fingers
S67.92 Crushing injury of unspecified part(s) of left wrist, hand and fingers

S68 Traumatic amputation of wrist, hand and fingers
An amputation not identified as partial or complete should be coded to complete
The appropriate 7th character is to be added to each code from category S68
A = initial encounter
D = subsequent encounter
S = sequela

S68.0 Traumatic metacarpophalangeal amputation of thumb
Traumatic amputation of thumb NOS
S68.01 Complete traumatic metacarpophalangeal amputation of thumb
S68.011 Complete traumatic metacarpophalangeal amputation of right thumb
S68.012 Complete traumatic metacarpophalangeal amputation of left thumb
S68.019 Complete traumatic metacarpophalangeal amputation of unspecified thumb
S68.02 Partial traumatic metacarpophalangeal amputation of thumb
S68.021 Partial traumatic metacarpophalangeal amputation of right thumb
S68.022 Partial traumatic metacarpophalangeal amputation of left thumb
S68.029 Partial traumatic metacarpophalangeal amputation of unspecified thumb
S68.1 Traumatic metacarpophalangeal amputation of other and unspecified finger
Traumatic amputation of finger NOS
EXCLUDES2 *traumatic metacarpophalangeal amputation of thumb (S68.0-)*
S68.11 Complete traumatic metacarpophalangeal amputation of other and unspecified finger
S68.110 Complete traumatic metacarpophalangeal amputation of right index finger
S68.111 Complete traumatic metacarpophalangeal amputation of left index finger
S68.112 Complete traumatic metacarpophalangeal amputation of right middle finger
S68.113 Complete traumatic metacarpophalangeal amputation of left middle finger
S68.114 Complete traumatic metacarpophalangeal amputation of right ring finger
S68.115 Complete traumatic metacarpophalangeal amputation of left ring finger
S68.116 Complete traumatic metacarpophalangeal amputation of right little finger
S68.117 Complete traumatic metacarpophalangeal amputation of left little finger

S68.118 Complete traumatic metacarpophalangeal amputation of other finger
Complete traumatic metacarpophalangeal amputation of specified finger with unspecified laterality
S68.119 Complete traumatic metacarpophalangeal amputation of unspecified finger
S68.12 Partial traumatic metacarpophalangeal amputation of other and unspecified finger
S68.120 Partial traumatic metacarpophalangeal amputation of right index finger
S68.121 Partial traumatic metacarpophalangeal amputation of left index finger
S68.122 Partial traumatic metacarpophalangeal amputation of right middle finger
S68.123 Partial traumatic metacarpophalangeal amputation of left middle finger
S68.124 Partial traumatic metacarpophalangeal amputation of right ring finger
S68.125 Partial traumatic metacarpophalangeal amputation of left ring finger
S68.126 Partial traumatic metacarpophalangeal amputation of right little finger
S68.127 Partial traumatic metacarpophalangeal amputation of left little finger
S68.128 Partial traumatic metacarpophalangeal amputation of other finger
Partial traumatic metacarpophalangeal amputation of specified finger with unspecified laterality
S68.129 Partial traumatic metacarpophalangeal amputation of unspecified finger
S68.4 Traumatic amputation of hand at wrist level
Traumatic amputation of hand NOS
Traumatic amputation of wrist
S68.41 Complete traumatic amputation of hand at wrist level
S68.411 Complete traumatic amputation of right hand at wrist level CC
S68.412 Complete traumatic amputation of left hand at wrist level CC
S68.419 Complete traumatic amputation of unspecified hand at wrist level CC
S68.42 Partial traumatic amputation of hand at wrist level
S68.421 Partial traumatic amputation of right hand at wrist level CC
S68.422 Partial traumatic amputation of left hand at wrist level CC
S68.429 Partial traumatic amputation of unspecified hand at wrist level CC
S68.5 Traumatic transphalangeal amputation of thumb
Traumatic interphalangeal joint amputation of thumb
S68.51 Complete traumatic transphalangeal amputation of thumb
S68.511 Complete traumatic transphalangeal amputation of right thumb
S68.512 Complete traumatic transphalangeal amputation of left thumb
S68.519 Complete traumatic transphalangeal amputation of unspecified thumb
S68.52 Partial traumatic transphalangeal amputation of thumb
S68.521 Partial traumatic transphalangeal amputation of right thumb
S68.522 Partial traumatic transphalangeal amputation of left thumb
S68.529 Partial traumatic transphalangeal amputation of unspecified thumb
S68.6 Traumatic transphalangeal amputation of other and unspecified finger
S68.61 Complete traumatic transphalangeal amputation of other and unspecified finger(s)
S68.610 Complete traumatic transphalangeal amputation of right index finger
S68.611 Complete traumatic transphalangeal amputation of left index finger
S68.612 Complete traumatic transphalangeal amputation of right middle finger
S68.613 Complete traumatic transphalangeal amputation of left middle finger
S68.614 Complete traumatic transphalangeal amputation of right ring finger
S68.615 Complete traumatic transphalangeal amputation of left ring finger
S68.616 Complete traumatic transphalangeal amputation of right little finger
S68.617 Complete traumatic transphalangeal amputation of left little finger
S68.618 Complete traumatic transphalangeal amputation of other finger
Complete traumatic transphalangeal amputation of specified finger with unspecified laterality
S68.619 Complete traumatic transphalangeal amputation of unspecified finger
S68.62 Partial traumatic transphalangeal amputation of other and unspecified finger
S68.620 Partial traumatic transphalangeal amputation of right index finger
S68.621 Partial traumatic transphalangeal amputation of left index finger
S68.622 Partial traumatic transphalangeal amputation of right middle finger
S68.623 Partial traumatic transphalangeal amputation of left middle finger
S68.624 Partial traumatic transphalangeal amputation of right ring finger
S68.625 Partial traumatic transphalangeal amputation of left ring finger
S68.626 Partial traumatic transphalangeal amputation of right little finger
S68.627 Partial traumatic transphalangeal amputation of left little finger
S68.628 Partial traumatic transphalangeal amputation of other finger
Partial traumatic transphalangeal amputation of specified finger with unspecified laterality
S68.629 Partial traumatic transphalangeal amputation of unspecified finger
S68.7 Traumatic transmetacarpal amputation of hand
S68.71 Complete traumatic transmetacarpal amputation of hand
S68.711 Complete traumatic transmetacarpal amputation of right hand CC
S68.712 Complete traumatic transmetacarpal amputation of left hand CC
S68.719 Complete traumatic transmetacarpal amputation of unspecified hand CC
S68.72 Partial traumatic transmetacarpal amputation of hand
S68.721 Partial traumatic transmetacarpal amputation of right hand CC
S68.722 Partial traumatic transmetacarpal amputation of left hand CC
S68.729 Partial traumatic transmetacarpal amputation of unspecified hand CC
S69 Other and unspecified injuries of wrist, hand and finger(s)
The appropriate 7th character is to be added to each code from category S69
A = initial encounter
D = subsequent encounter
S = sequela
S69.8 Other specified injuries of wrist, hand and finger(s)
S69.80 Other specified injuries of unspecified wrist, hand and finger(s)
S69.81 Other specified injuries of right wrist, hand and finger(s)
S69.82 Other specified injuries of left wrist, hand and finger(s)

PDx Unacceptable principal diagnosis symbol per Medicare code edits POA Code exempt from diagnosis present on admission requirement
Q Questionable admission CC Complication or comorbidity CC/MCC Exc CC/MCC exclusion MCC Major complication or comorbidity
PDx CC Principal diagnosis as its own CC PDx MCC Principal diagnosis as its own MCC Z1 Z code as first-listed diagnosis

S69.9 Unspecified injury of wrist, hand and finger(s)
- S69.90 Unspecified injury of unspecified wrist, hand and finger(s)
- S69.91 Unspecified injury of right wrist, hand and finger(s)
- S69.92 Unspecified injury of left wrist, hand and finger(s)

Injuries to the hip and thigh (S70-S79)

EXCLUDES2 *burns and corrosions (T20-T32)*
frostbite (T33-T34)
snake bite (T63.0-)
venomous insect bite or sting (T63.4-)

S70 Superficial injury of hip and thigh

The appropriate 7th character is to be added to each code from category S70
A = initial encounter
D = subsequent encounter
S = sequela

S70.0 Contusion of hip
- S70.00 Contusion of unspecified hip
- S70.01 Contusion of right hip
- S70.02 Contusion of left hip

S70.1 Contusion of thigh
- S70.10 Contusion of unspecified thigh
- S70.11 Contusion of right thigh
- S70.12 Contusion of left thigh

S70.2 Other superficial injuries of hip
- S70.21 Abrasion of hip
  - S70.211 Abrasion, right hip
  - S70.212 Abrasion, left hip
  - S70.219 Abrasion, unspecified hip
- S70.22 Blister (nonthermal) of hip
  - S70.221 Blister (nonthermal), right hip
  - S70.222 Blister (nonthermal), left hip
  - S70.229 Blister (nonthermal), unspecified hip
- S70.24 External constriction of hip
  - S70.241 External constriction, right hip
  - S70.242 External constriction, left hip
  - S70.249 External constriction, unspecified hip
- S70.25 Superficial foreign body of hip
  Splinter in the hip
  - S70.251 Superficial foreign body, right hip
  - S70.252 Superficial foreign body, left hip
  - S70.259 Superficial foreign body, unspecified hip
- S70.26 Insect bite (nonvenomous) of hip
  - S70.261 Insect bite (nonvenomous), right hip
  - S70.262 Insect bite (nonvenomous), left hip
  - S70.269 Insect bite (nonvenomous), unspecified hip
- S70.27 Other superficial bite of hip
  EXCLUDES1 *open bite of hip (S71.05-)*
  - S70.271 Other superficial bite of hip, right hip
  - S70.272 Other superficial bite of hip, left hip
  - S70.279 Other superficial bite of hip, unspecified hip

S70.3 Other superficial injuries of thigh
- S70.31 Abrasion of thigh
  - S70.311 Abrasion, right thigh
  - S70.312 Abrasion, left thigh
  - S70.319 Abrasion, unspecified thigh
- S70.32 Blister (nonthermal) of thigh
  - S70.321 Blister (nonthermal), right thigh
  - S70.322 Blister (nonthermal), left thigh
  - S70.329 Blister (nonthermal), unspecified thigh
- S70.34 External constriction of thigh
  - S70.341 External constriction, right thigh
  - S70.342 External constriction, left thigh
  - S70.349 External constriction, unspecified thigh
- S70.35 Superficial foreign body of thigh
  Splinter in the thigh
  - S70.351 Superficial foreign body, right thigh
  - S70.352 Superficial foreign body, left thigh
  - S70.359 Superficial foreign body, unspecified thigh
- S70.36 Insect bite (nonvenomous) of thigh
  - S70.361 Insect bite (nonvenomous), right thigh
  - S70.362 Insect bite (nonvenomous), left thigh
  - S70.369 Insect bite (nonvenomous), unspecified thigh
- S70.37 Other superficial bite of thigh
  EXCLUDES1 *open bite of thigh (S71.15)*
  - S70.371 Other superficial bite of right thigh
  - S70.372 Other superficial bite of left thigh
  - S70.379 Other superficial bite of unspecified thigh

S70.9 Unspecified superficial injury of hip and thigh
- S70.91 Unspecified superficial injury of hip
  - S70.911 Unspecified superficial injury of right hip
  - S70.912 Unspecified superficial injury of left hip
  - S70.919 Unspecified superficial injury of unspecified hip
- S70.92 Unspecified superficial injury of thigh
  - S70.921 Unspecified superficial injury of right thigh
  - S70.922 Unspecified superficial injury of left thigh
  - S70.929 Unspecified superficial injury of unspecified thigh

S71 Open wound of hip and thigh

Code also any associated wound infection

EXCLUDES1 *open fracture of hip and thigh (S72.-)*
traumatic amputation of hip and thigh (S78.-)

EXCLUDES2 *bite of venomous animal (T63.-)*
open wound of ankle, foot and toes (S91.-)
open wound of knee and lower leg (S81.-)

The appropriate 7th character is to be added to each code from category S71
A = initial encounter
D = subsequent encounter
S = sequela

S71.0 Open wound of hip
- S71.00 Unspecified open wound of hip
  - S71.001 Unspecified open wound, right hip
  - S71.002 Unspecified open wound, left hip
  - S71.009 Unspecified open wound, unspecified hip
- S71.01 Laceration without foreign body of hip
  - S71.011 Laceration without foreign body, right hip
  - S71.012 Laceration without foreign body, left hip
  - S71.019 Laceration without foreign body, unspecified hip
- S71.02 Laceration with foreign body of hip
  - S71.021 Laceration with foreign body, right hip
  - S71.022 Laceration with foreign body, left hip
  - S71.029 Laceration with foreign body, unspecified hip
- S71.03 Puncture wound without foreign body of hip
  - S71.031 Puncture wound without foreign body, right hip
  - S71.032 Puncture wound without foreign body, left hip
  - S71.039 Puncture wound without foreign body, unspecified hip
- S71.04 Puncture wound with foreign body of hip
  - S71.041 Puncture wound with foreign body, right hip
  - S71.042 Puncture wound with foreign body, left hip
  - S71.049 Puncture wound with foreign body, unspecified hip
- S71.05 Open bite of hip
  Bite of hip NOS
  EXCLUDES1 *superficial bite of hip (S70.26, S70.27)*
  - S71.051 Open bite, right hip
  - S71.052 Open bite, left hip
  - S71.059 Open bite, unspecified hip

S71.1 Open wound of thigh
- S71.10 Unspecified open wound of thigh

Unspecified Code | Other Specified Code | Manifestation Code | N Newborn | P Pediatric | M Maternity | A Adult | ♂ Male | ♀ Female
● New Code | ▲ Revised Code Title | ►◄ Revised Text | NOTES | INCLUDES | EXCLUDES1 Not coded here | EXCLUDES2 Not included here
4th character required | 5th character required | 6th character required | 7th character required
Extension 'X' Alert | HAC Hospital-acquired condition (HAC) alert | AHA AHA Coding Clinic©

S71.101 Unspecified open wound, right thigh
S71.102 Unspecified open wound, left thigh
S71.109 Unspecified open wound, unspecified thigh

S71.11 Laceration without foreign body of thigh
S71.111 Laceration without foreign body, right thigh
S71.112 Laceration without foreign body, left thigh
S71.119 Laceration without foreign body, unspecified thigh

S71.12 Laceration with foreign body of thigh
S71.121 Laceration with foreign body, right thigh
S71.122 Laceration with foreign body, left thigh
S71.129 Laceration with foreign body, unspecified thigh

S71.13 Puncture wound without foreign body of thigh
S71.131 Puncture wound without foreign body, right thigh
S71.132 Puncture wound without foreign body, left thigh
S71.139 Puncture wound without foreign body, unspecified thigh

S71.14 Puncture wound with foreign body of thigh
S71.141 Puncture wound with foreign body, right thigh
S71.142 Puncture wound with foreign body, left thigh
S71.149 Puncture wound with foreign body, unspecified thigh

S71.15 Open bite of thigh
Bite of thigh NOS
EXCLUDES1 *superficial bite of thigh (S70.37-)*
S71.151 Open bite, right thigh
S71.152 Open bite, left thigh
S71.159 Open bite, unspecified thigh

S72 Fracture of femur
NOTES A fracture not indicated as displaced or nondisplaced should be coded to displaced
A fracture not indicated as open or closed should be coded to closed
The open fracture designations are based on the Gustilo open fracture classification
EXCLUDES1 *traumatic amputation of hip and thigh (S78.-)*
EXCLUDES2 *fracture of lower leg and ankle (S82.-)*
fracture of foot (S92.-)
periprosthetic fracture of prosthetic implant of hip (T84.040, T84.041)

The appropriate 7th character is to be added to all codes from category S72
A = initial encounter for closed fracture
B = initial encounter for open fracture type I or II initial encounter for open fracture NOS
C = initial encounter for open fracture type IIIA, IIIB, or IIIC
D = subsequent encounter for closed fracture with routine healing
E = subsequent encounter for open fracture type I or II with routine healing
F = subsequent encounter for open fracture type IIIA, IIIB, or IIIC with routine healing
G = subsequent encounter for closed fracture with delayed healing
H = subsequent encounter for open fracture type I or II with delayed healing
J = subsequent encounter for open fracture type IIIA, IIIB, or IIIC with delayed healing
K = subsequent encounter for closed fracture with nonunion
M = subsequent encounter for open fracture type I or II with nonunion
N = subsequent encounter for open fracture type IIIA, IIIB, or IIIC with nonunion
P = subsequent encounter for closed fracture with malunion
Q = subsequent encounter for open fracture type I or II with malunion
R = subsequent encounter for open fracture type IIIA, IIIB, or IIIC with malunion
S = sequela

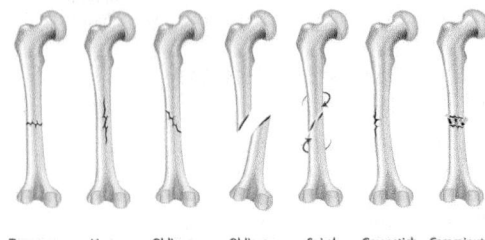

Figure 16.1 Types of bone fractures

S72.0 Fracture of head and neck of femur
EXCLUDES2 *physeal fracture of upper end of femur (S79.0-)*

S72.00 Fracture of unspecified part of neck of femur
Fracture of hip NOS
Fracture of neck of femur NOS
S72.001 Fracture of unspecified part of neck of right femur CC HAC MCC
S72.002 Fracture of unspecified part of neck of left femur CC HAC MCC
AHA: Q4, 2015
S72.009 Fracture of unspecified part of neck of unspecified femur CC HAC MCC

S72.01 Unspecified intracapsular fracture of femur
Subcapital fracture of femur
S72.011 Unspecified intracapsular fracture of right femur CC HAC MCC
S72.012 Unspecified intracapsular fracture of left femur CC HAC MCC
S72.019 Unspecified intracapsular fracture of unspecified femur CC HAC MCC

S72.02 Fracture of epiphysis (separation) (upper) of femur
Transepiphyseal fracture of femur
EXCLUDES1 *capital femoral epiphyseal fracture (pediatric) of femur (S79.01-)*
Salter-Harris Type I physeal fracture of upper end of femur (S79.01-)
S72.021 Displaced fracture of epiphysis (separation) (upper) of right femur CC HAC MCC
S72.022 Displaced fracture of epiphysis (separation) (upper) of left femur CC HAC MCC
S72.023 Displaced fracture of epiphysis (separation) (upper) of unspecified femur CC HAC MCC
S72.024 Nondisplaced fracture of epiphysis (separation) (upper) of right femur CC HAC MCC
S72.025 Nondisplaced fracture of epiphysis (separation) (upper) of left femur CC HAC MCC
S72.026 Nondisplaced fracture of epiphysis (separation) (upper) of unspecified femur CC HAC MCC

S72.03 Midcervical fracture of femur
Transcervical fracture of femur NOS
S72.031 Displaced midcervical fracture of right femur CC HAC MCC
S72.032 Displaced midcervical fracture of left femur CC HAC MCC
S72.033 Displaced midcervical fracture of unspecified femur CC HAC MCC
S72.034 Nondisplaced midcervical fracture of right femur CC HAC MCC
S72.035 Nondisplaced midcervical fracture of left femur CC HAC MCC

Unacceptable principal diagnosis symbol per Medicare code edits; Code exempt from diagnosis present on admission requirement
Questionable admission; CC Complication or comorbidity; CC/MCC exclusion; MCC Major complication or comorbidity
Principal diagnosis as its own CC; Principal diagnosis as its own MCC; Z code as first-listed diagnosis

 When symbols appear on a code that requires a 7th character extension, refer to Appendix D to identify applicable 7th character codes.

S72.036 Nondisplaced midcervical fracture of unspecified femur CC HAC MCC

S72.04 Fracture of base of neck of femur
Cervicotrochanteric fracture of femur

S72.041 Displaced fracture of base of neck of right femur CC HAC MCC

S72.042 Displaced fracture of base of neck of left femur CC HAC MCC

S72.043 Displaced fracture of base of neck of unspecified femur CC HAC MCC

S72.044 Nondisplaced fracture of base of neck of right femur CC HAC MCC

S72.045 Nondisplaced fracture of base of neck of left femur CC HAC MCC

S72.046 Nondisplaced fracture of base of neck of unspecified femur CC HAC MCC

S72.05 Unspecified fracture of head of femur
Fracture of head of femur NOS

S72.051 Unspecified fracture of head of right femur CC HAC MCC

S72.052 Unspecified fracture of head of left femur CC HAC MCC

S72.059 Unspecified fracture of head of unspecified femur CC HAC MCC

S72.06 Articular fracture of head of femur

S72.061 Displaced articular fracture of head of right femur CC HAC MCC

S72.062 Displaced articular fracture of head of left femur CC HAC MCC

S72.063 Displaced articular fracture of head of unspecified femur CC HAC MCC

S72.064 Nondisplaced articular fracture of head of right femur CC HAC MCC

S72.065 Nondisplaced articular fracture of head of left femur CC HAC MCC

S72.066 Nondisplaced articular fracture of head of unspecified femur CC HAC MCC

S72.09 Other fracture of head and neck of femur

S72.091 Other fracture of head and neck of right femur CC HAC MCC

S72.092 Other fracture of head and neck of left femur CC HAC MCC

S72.099 Other fracture of head and neck of unspecified femur CC HAC MCC

S72.1 Pertrochanteric fracture

S72.10 Unspecified trochanteric fracture of femur
Fracture of trochanter NOS

S72.101 Unspecified trochanteric fracture of right femur CC HAC MCC

S72.102 Unspecified trochanteric fracture of left femur CC HAC MCC

S72.109 Unspecified trochanteric fracture of unspecified femur CC HAC MCC

S72.11 Fracture of greater trochanter of femur

S72.111 Displaced fracture of greater trochanter of right femur CC HAC MCC

S72.112 Displaced fracture of greater trochanter of left femur CC HAC MCC

S72.113 Displaced fracture of greater trochanter of unspecified femur CC HAC MCC

S72.114 Nondisplaced fracture of greater trochanter of right femur CC HAC MCC

S72.115 Nondisplaced fracture of greater trochanter of left femur CC HAC MCC

S72.116 Nondisplaced fracture of greater trochanter of unspecified femur CC HAC MCC

S72.12 Fracture of lesser trochanter of femur

S72.121 Displaced fracture of lesser trochanter of right femur CC HAC MCC

S72.122 Displaced fracture of lesser trochanter of left femur CC HAC MCC

S72.123 Displaced fracture of lesser trochanter of unspecified femur CC HAC MCC

S72.124 Nondisplaced fracture of lesser trochanter of right femur CC HAC MCC

S72.125 Nondisplaced fracture of lesser trochanter of left femur CC HAC MCC

S72.126 Nondisplaced fracture of lesser trochanter of unspecified femur CC HAC MCC

S72.13 Apophyseal fracture of femur
EXCLUDES1 *chronic (nontraumatic) slipped upper femoral epiphysis (M93.0-)*

S72.131 Displaced apophyseal fracture of right femur CC HAC MCC

S72.132 Displaced apophyseal fracture of left femur CC HAC MCC

S72.133 Displaced apophyseal fracture of unspecified femur CC HAC MCC

S72.134 Nondisplaced apophyseal fracture of right femur CC HAC MCC

S72.135 Nondisplaced apophyseal fracture of left femur CC HAC MCC

S72.136 Nondisplaced apophyseal fracture of unspecified femur CC HAC MCC

S72.14 Intertrochanteric fracture of femur

S72.141 Displaced intertrochanteric fracture of right femur CC HAC MCC
AHA: Q4, 2013

S72.142 Displaced intertrochanteric fracture of left femur CC HAC MCC

S72.143 Displaced intertrochanteric fracture of unspecified femur CC HAC MCC

S72.144 Nondisplaced intertrochanteric fracture of right femur CC HAC MCC

S72.145 Nondisplaced intertrochanteric fracture of left femur CC HAC MCC

S72.146 Nondisplaced intertrochanteric fracture of unspecified femur CC HAC MCC

S72.2 Subtrochanteric fracture of femur

S72.21 Displaced subtrochanteric fracture of right femur CC HAC MCC

S72.22 Displaced subtrochanteric fracture of left femur CC HAC MCC

S72.23 Displaced subtrochanteric fracture of unspecified femur CC HAC MCC

S72.24 Nondisplaced subtrochanteric fracture of right femur CC HAC MCC

S72.25 Nondisplaced subtrochanteric fracture of left femur CC HAC MCC

S72.26 Nondisplaced subtrochanteric fracture of unspecified femur CC HAC MCC

S72.3 Fracture of shaft of femur

S72.30 Unspecified fracture of shaft of femur

S72.301 Unspecified fracture of shaft of right femur CC HAC MCC

S72.302 Unspecified fracture of shaft of left femur CC HAC MCC

S72.309 Unspecified fracture of shaft of unspecified femur CC HAC MCC

S72.32 Transverse fracture of shaft of femur

S72.321 Displaced transverse fracture of shaft of right femur CC HAC MCC

S72.322 Displaced transverse fracture of shaft of left femur CC HAC MCC

S72.323 Displaced transverse fracture of shaft of unspecified femur CC HAC MCC

S72.324 Nondisplaced transverse fracture of shaft of right femur CC HAC MCC

S72.325 Nondisplaced transverse fracture of shaft of left femur CC HAC MCC

S72.326 Nondisplaced transverse fracture of shaft of unspecified femur CC HAC MCC

S72.33 Oblique fracture of shaft of femur

S72.331 Displaced oblique fracture of shaft of right femur CC HAC MCC

S72.332 Displaced oblique fracture of shaft of left femur CC HAC MCC

Unspecified Code | Other Specified Code | Manifestation Code | N Newborn | P Pediatric | M Maternity | A Adult | ♂ Male | ♀ Female
● New Code | ▲ Revised Code Title | ►◄ Revised Text | NOTES | INCLUDES | EXCLUDES1 Not coded here | EXCLUDES2 Not included here
4th character required | 5th character required | 6th character required | 7th character required
Extension 'X' Alert | HAC Hospital-acquired condition (HAC) alert | AHA AHA Coding Clinic®

S72.333 Displaced oblique fracture of shaft of unspecified femur CC HAC MCC
S72.334 Nondisplaced oblique fracture of shaft of right femur CC HAC MCC
S72.335 Nondisplaced oblique fracture of shaft of left femur CC HAC MCC
S72.336 Nondisplaced oblique fracture of shaft of unspecified femur CC HAC MCC

S72.34 Spiral fracture of shaft of femur
S72.341 Displaced spiral fracture of shaft of right femur CC HAC MCC
S72.342 Displaced spiral fracture of shaft of left femur CC HAC MCC
S72.343 Displaced spiral fracture of shaft of unspecified femur CC HAC MCC
S72.344 Nondisplaced spiral fracture of shaft of right femur CC HAC MCC
S72.345 Nondisplaced spiral fracture of shaft of left femur CC HAC MCC
S72.346 Nondisplaced spiral fracture of shaft of unspecified femur CC HAC MCC

S72.35 Comminuted fracture of shaft of femur
S72.351 Displaced comminuted fracture of shaft of right femur CC HAC MCC
S72.352 Displaced comminuted fracture of shaft of left femur CC HAC MCC
S72.353 Displaced comminuted fracture of shaft of unspecified femur CC HAC MCC
S72.354 Nondisplaced comminuted fracture of shaft of right femur CC HAC MCC
S72.355 Nondisplaced comminuted fracture of shaft of left femur CC HAC MCC
S72.356 Nondisplaced comminuted fracture of shaft of unspecified femur CC HAC MCC

S72.36 Segmental fracture of shaft of femur
S72.361 Displaced segmental fracture of shaft of right femur CC HAC MCC
S72.362 Displaced segmental fracture of shaft of left femur CC HAC MCC
S72.363 Displaced segmental fracture of shaft of unspecified femur CC HAC MCC
S72.364 Nondisplaced segmental fracture of shaft of right femur CC HAC MCC
S72.365 Nondisplaced segmental fracture of shaft of left femur CC HAC MCC
S72.366 Nondisplaced segmental fracture of shaft of unspecified femur CC HAC MCC

S72.39 Other fracture of shaft of femur
S72.391 Other fracture of shaft of right femur CC HAC MCC
S72.392 Other fracture of shaft of left femur CC HAC MCC
S72.399 Other fracture of shaft of unspecified femur CC HAC MCC

S72.4 Fracture of lower end of femur
Fracture of distal end of femur
EXCLUDES2 *fracture of shaft of femur (S72.3-)*
physeal fracture of lower end of femur (S79.1-)

S72.40 Unspecified fracture of lower end of femur
S72.401 Unspecified fracture of lower end of right femur CC HAC MCC
S72.402 Unspecified fracture of lower end of left femur CC HAC MCC
S72.409 Unspecified fracture of lower end of unspecified femur CC HAC MCC

S72.41 Unspecified condyle fracture of lower end of femur
Condyle fracture of femur NOS
S72.411 Displaced unspecified condyle fracture of lower end of right femur CC HAC MCC
S72.412 Displaced unspecified condyle fracture of lower end of left femur CC HAC MCC
S72.413 Displaced unspecified condyle fracture of lower end of unspecified femur CC HAC MCC
S72.414 Nondisplaced unspecified condyle fracture of lower end of right femur CC HAC MCC
S72.415 Nondisplaced unspecified condyle fracture of lower end of left femur CC HAC MCC
S72.416 Nondisplaced unspecified condyle fracture of lower end of unspecified femur CC HAC MCC

S72.42 Fracture of lateral condyle of femur
S72.421 Displaced fracture of lateral condyle of right femur CC HAC MCC
S72.422 Displaced fracture of lateral condyle of left femur CC HAC MCC
S72.423 Displaced fracture of lateral condyle of unspecified femur CC HAC MCC
S72.424 Nondisplaced fracture of lateral condyle of right femur CC HAC MCC
S72.425 Nondisplaced fracture of lateral condyle of left femur CC HAC MCC
S72.426 Nondisplaced fracture of lateral condyle of unspecified femur CC HAC MCC

S72.43 Fracture of medial condyle of femur
S72.431 Displaced fracture of medial condyle of right femur CC HAC MCC
S72.432 Displaced fracture of medial condyle of left femur CC HAC MCC
S72.433 Displaced fracture of medial condyle of unspecified femur CC HAC MCC
S72.434 Nondisplaced fracture of medial condyle of right femur CC HAC MCC
S72.435 Nondisplaced fracture of medial condyle of left femur CC HAC MCC
S72.436 Nondisplaced fracture of medial condyle of unspecified femur CC HAC MCC

S72.44 Fracture of lower epiphysis (separation) of femur
EXCLUDES1 *Salter-Harris Type I physeal fracture of lower end of femur (S79.11-)*
S72.441 Displaced fracture of lower epiphysis (separation) of right femur CC HAC MCC
S72.442 Displaced fracture of lower epiphysis (separation) of left femur CC HAC MCC
S72.443 Displaced fracture of lower epiphysis (separation) of unspecified femur CC HAC MCC
S72.444 Nondisplaced fracture of lower epiphysis (separation) of right femur CC HAC MCC
S72.445 Nondisplaced fracture of lower epiphysis (separation) of left femur CC HAC MCC
S72.446 Nondisplaced fracture of lower epiphysis (separation) of unspecified femur CC HAC MCC

S72.45 Supracondylar fracture without intracondylar extension of lower end of femur
Supracondylar fracture of lower end of femur NOS
EXCLUDES1 *supracondylar fracture with intracondylar extension of lower end of femur (S72.46-)*
S72.451 Displaced supracondylar fracture without intracondylar extension of lower end of right femur CC HAC MCC
S72.452 Displaced supracondylar fracture without intracondylar extension of lower end of left femur CC HAC MCC
S72.453 Displaced supracondylar fracture without intracondylar extension of lower end of unspecified femur CC HAC MCC
S72.454 Nondisplaced supracondylar fracture without intracondylar extension of lower end of right femur CC HAC MCC

Unacceptable principal diagnosis symbol per Medicare code edits; Code exempt from diagnosis present on admission requirement; Questionable admission; Complication or comorbidity; CC/MCC exclusion; Major complication or comorbidity; Principal diagnosis as its own CC; Principal diagnosis as its own MCC; Z code as first-listed diagnosis

S72.455 Nondisplaced supracondylar fracture without intracondylar extension of lower end of left femur CC HAC MCC
S72.456 Nondisplaced supracondylar fracture without intracondylar extension of lower end of unspecified femur CC HAC MCC

S72.46 Supracondylar fracture with intracondylar extension of lower end of femur
EXCLUDES1 *supracondylar fracture without intracondylar extension of lower end of femur (S72.45-)*
S72.461 Displaced supracondylar fracture with intracondylar extension of lower end of right femur CC HAC MCC
S72.462 Displaced supracondylar fracture with intracondylar extension of lower end of left femur CC HAC MCC
S72.463 Displaced supracondylar fracture with intracondylar extension of lower end of unspecified femur CC HAC MCC
S72.464 Nondisplaced supracondylar fracture with intracondylar extension of lower end of right femur CC HAC MCC
S72.465 Nondisplaced supracondylar fracture with intracondylar extension of lower end of left femur CC HAC MCC
S72.466 Nondisplaced supracondylar fracture with intracondylar extension of lower end of unspecified femur CC HAC MCC

S72.47 Torus fracture of lower end of femur
The appropriate 7th character is to be added to all codes in subcategory S72.47
A = initial encounter for closed fracture
D = subsequent encounter for fracture with routine healing
G = subsequent encounter for fracture with delayed healing
K = subsequent encounter for fracture with nonunion
P = subsequent encounter for fracture with malunion
S = sequela
S72.471 Torus fracture of lower end of right femur CC HAC
S72.472 Torus fracture of lower end of left femur CC HAC
S72.479 Torus fracture of lower end of unspecified femur CC HAC

S72.49 Other fracture of lower end of femur
S72.491 Other fracture of lower end of right femur CC HAC MCC
S72.492 Other fracture of lower end of left femur CC HAC MCC
S72.499 Other fracture of lower end of unspecified femur CC HAC MCC

S72.8 Other fracture of femur
S72.8X Other fracture of femur
S72.8X1 Other fracture of right femur CC HAC MCC
S72.8X2 Other fracture of left femur CC HAC MCC
S72.8X9 Other fracture of unspecified femur CC HAC MCC

S72.9 Unspecified fracture of femur
Fracture of thigh NOS
Fracture of upper leg NOS
EXCLUDES1 *fracture of hip NOS (S72.00-, S72.01-)*
S72.90 Unspecified fracture of unspecified femur CC HAC MCC
S72.91 Unspecified fracture of right femur CC HAC MCC
S72.92 Unspecified fracture of left femur CC HAC MCC

S73 Dislocation and sprain of joint and ligaments of hip
INCLUDES *avulsion of joint or ligament of hip*
laceration of cartilage, joint or ligament of hip
sprain of cartilage, joint or ligament of hip
traumatic hemarthrosis of joint or ligament of hip
traumatic rupture of joint or ligament of hip
traumatic subluxation of joint or ligament of hip
traumatic tear of joint or ligament of hip
Code also any associated open wound
EXCLUDES2 *strain of muscle, fascia and tendon of hip and thigh (S76.-)*
The appropriate 7th character is to be added to each code from category S73
A = initial encounter
D = subsequent encounter
S = sequela

S73.0 Subluxation and dislocation of hip
EXCLUDES2 *dislocation and subluxation of hip prosthesis (T84.020, T84.021)*

S73.00 Unspecified subluxation and dislocation of hip
Dislocation of hip NOS
Subluxation of hip NOS
S73.001 Unspecified subluxation of right hip CC HAC
S73.002 Unspecified subluxation of left hip CC HAC
S73.003 Unspecified subluxation of unspecified hip CC HAC
S73.004 Unspecified dislocation of right hip CC HAC
S73.005 Unspecified dislocation of left hip CC HAC
S73.006 Unspecified dislocation of unspecified hip CC HAC

S73.01 Posterior subluxation and dislocation of hip
S73.011 Posterior subluxation of right hip CC HAC
S73.012 Posterior subluxation of left hip CC HAC
S73.013 Posterior subluxation of unspecified hip CC HAC
S73.014 Posterior dislocation of right hip CC HAC
S73.015 Posterior dislocation of left hip CC HAC
S73.016 Posterior dislocation of unspecified hip CC HAC

S73.02 Obturator subluxation and dislocation of hip
S73.021 Obturator subluxation of right hip CC HAC
S73.022 Obturator subluxation of left hip CC HAC
S73.023 Obturator subluxation of unspecified hip CC HAC
S73.024 Obturator dislocation of right hip CC HAC
S73.025 Obturator dislocation of left hip CC HAC
S73.026 Obturator dislocation of unspecified hip CC HAC

S73.03 Other anterior dislocation of hip
S73.031 Other anterior subluxation of right hip CC HAC
S73.032 Other anterior subluxation of left hip CC HAC
S73.033 Other anterior subluxation of unspecified hip CC HAC
S73.034 Other anterior dislocation of right hip CC HAC
S73.035 Other anterior dislocation of left hip CC HAC
S73.036 Other anterior dislocation of unspecified hip CC HAC

S73.04 Central dislocation of hip
S73.041 Central subluxation of right hip CC HAC
S73.042 Central subluxation of left hip CC HAC

Unspecified Code Other Specified Code Manifestation Code N Newborn P Pediatric M Maternity A Adult ♂ Male ♀ Female
● New Code ▲ Revised Code Title ►◄ Revised Text NOTES INCLUDES EXCLUDES1 Not coded here EXCLUDES2 Not included here
4th character required 5th character required 6th character required 7th character required
Extension 'X' Alert HAC Hospital-acquired condition (HAC) alert AHA AHA Coding Clinic©

S73.043 Central subluxation of unspecified hip CC HAC
S73.044 Central dislocation of right hip CC HAC
S73.045 Central dislocation of left hip CC HAC
S73.046 Central dislocation of unspecified hip CC HAC

S73.1 Sprain of hip
S73.10 Unspecified sprain of hip
S73.101 Unspecified sprain of right hip
S73.102 Unspecified sprain of left hip
S73.109 Unspecified sprain of unspecified hip
S73.11 Iliofemoral ligament sprain of hip
S73.111 Iliofemoral ligament sprain of right hip
S73.112 Iliofemoral ligament sprain of left hip
S73.119 Iliofemoral ligament sprain of unspecified hip
S73.12 Ischiocapsular (ligament) sprain of hip
S73.121 Ischiocapsular ligament sprain of right hip
S73.122 Ischiocapsular ligament sprain of left hip
S73.129 Ischiocapsular ligament sprain of unspecified hip
S73.19 Other sprain of hip
S73.191 Other sprain of right hip
S73.192 Other sprain of left hip
S73.199 Other sprain of unspecified hip

S74 Injury of nerves at hip and thigh level

Code also any associated open wound (S71.-)

EXCLUDES2 *injury of nerves at ankle and foot level (S94.-)*
injury of nerves at lower leg level (S84.-)

The appropriate 7th character is to be added to each code from category S74
A = initial encounter
D = subsequent encounter
S = sequela

S74.0 Injury of sciatic nerve at hip and thigh level
S74.00 Injury of sciatic nerve at hip and thigh level, unspecified leg
S74.01 Injury of sciatic nerve at hip and thigh level, right leg
S74.02 Injury of sciatic nerve at hip and thigh level, left leg
S74.1 Injury of femoral nerve at hip and thigh level
S74.10 Injury of femoral nerve at hip and thigh level, unspecified leg
S74.11 Injury of femoral nerve at hip and thigh level, right leg
S74.12 Injury of femoral nerve at hip and thigh level, left leg
S74.2 Injury of cutaneous sensory nerve at hip and thigh level
S74.20 Injury of cutaneous sensory nerve at hip and thigh level, unspecified leg
S74.21 Injury of cutaneous sensory nerve at hip and high level, right leg
S74.22 Injury of cutaneous sensory nerve at hip and thigh level, left leg
S74.8 Injury of other nerves at hip and thigh level
S74.8X Injury of other nerves at hip and thigh level
S74.8X1 Injury of other nerves at hip and thigh level, right leg
S74.8X2 Injury of other nerves at hip and thigh level, left leg
S74.8X9 Injury of other nerves at hip and thigh level, unspecified leg
S74.9 Injury of unspecified nerve at hip and thigh level
S74.90 Injury of unspecified nerve at hip and thigh level, unspecified leg
S74.91 Injury of unspecified nerve at hip and thigh level, right leg
S74.92 Injury of unspecified nerve at hip and thigh level, left leg

S75 Injury of blood vessels at hip and thigh level

Code also any associated open wound (S71.-)

EXCLUDES2 *injury of blood vessels at lower leg level (S85.-)*
injury of popliteal artery (S85.0)

The appropriate 7th character is to be added to each code from category S75
A = initial encounter
D = subsequent encounter
S = sequela

S75.0 Injury of femoral artery
S75.00 Unspecified injury of femoral artery
S75.001 Unspecified injury of femoral artery, right leg MCC
S75.002 Unspecified injury of femoral artery, left leg MCC
S75.009 Unspecified injury of femoral artery, unspecified leg MCC
S75.01 Minor laceration of femoral artery
Incomplete transection of femoral artery
Laceration of femoral artery NOS
Superficial laceration of femoral artery
S75.011 Minor laceration of femoral artery, right leg MCC
S75.012 Minor laceration of femoral artery, left leg MCC
S75.019 Minor laceration of femoral artery, unspecified leg MCC
S75.02 Major laceration of femoral artery
Complete transection of femoral artery
Traumatic rupture of femoral artery
S75.021 Major laceration of femoral artery, right leg MCC
S75.022 Major laceration of femoral artery, left leg MCC
S75.029 Major laceration of femoral artery, unspecified leg MCC
S75.09 Other specified injury of femoral artery
S75.091 Other specified injury of femoral artery, right leg MCC
S75.092 Other specified injury of femoral artery, left leg MCC
S75.099 Other specified injury of femoral artery, unspecified leg MCC
S75.1 Injury of femoral vein at hip and thigh level
S75.10 Unspecified injury of femoral vein at hip and thigh level
S75.101 Unspecified injury of femoral vein at hip and thigh level, right leg MCC
S75.102 Unspecified injury of femoral vein at hip and thigh level, left leg MCC
S75.109 Unspecified injury of femoral vein at hip and thigh level, unspecified leg MCC
S75.11 Minor laceration of femoral vein at hip and thigh level
Incomplete transection of femoral vein at hip and thigh level
Laceration of femoral vein at hip and thigh level NOS
Superficial laceration of femoral vein at hip and thigh level
S75.111 Minor laceration of femoral vein at hip and thigh level, right leg MCC
S75.112 Minor laceration of femoral vein at hip and thigh level, left leg MCC
S75.119 Minor laceration of femoral vein at hip and thigh level, unspecified leg MCC
S75.12 Major laceration of femoral vein at hip and thigh level
Complete transection of femoral vein at hip and thigh level
Traumatic rupture of femoral vein at hip and thigh level
S75.121 Major laceration of femoral vein at hip and thigh level, right leg MCC
S75.122 Major laceration of femoral vein at hip and thigh level, left leg MCC
S75.129 Major laceration of femoral vein at hip and thigh level, unspecified leg MCC
S75.19 Other specified injury of femoral vein at hip and thigh level

PDx Unacceptable principal diagnosis symbol per Medicare code edits   POA Code exempt from diagnosis present on admission requirement
Q Questionable admission   CC Complication or comorbidity   CC/MCC Exc CC/MCC exclusion   MCC Major complication or comorbidity
PDx CC Principal diagnosis as its own CC   PDx MCC Principal diagnosis as its own MCC   Z1 Z code as first-listed diagnosis

S75.191 Other specified injury of femoral vein at hip and thigh level, right leg MCC
S75.192 Other specified injury of femoral vein at hip and thigh level, left leg MCC
S75.199 Other specified injury of femoral vein at hip and thigh level, unspecified leg MCC

S75.2 Injury of greater saphenous vein at hip and thigh level
EXCLUDES1 *greater saphenous vein NOS (S85.3)*

S75.20 Unspecified injury of greater saphenous vein at hip and thigh level
S75.201 Unspecified injury of greater saphenous vein at hip and thigh level, right leg CC
S75.202 Unspecified injury of greater saphenous vein at hip and thigh level, left leg CC
S75.209 Unspecified injury of greater saphenous vein at hip and thigh level, unspecified leg CC

S75.21 Minor laceration of greater saphenous vein at hip and thigh level
Incomplete transection of greater saphenous vein at hip and thigh level
Laceration of greater saphenous vein at hip and thigh level NOS
Superficial laceration of greater saphenous vein at hip and thigh level
S75.211 Minor laceration of greater saphenous vein at hip and thigh level, right leg CC
S75.212 Minor laceration of greater saphenous vein at hip and thigh level, left leg CC
S75.219 Minor laceration of greater saphenous vein at hip and thigh level, unspecified leg CC

S75.22 Major laceration of greater saphenous vein at hip and thigh level
Complete transection of greater saphenous vein at hip and thigh level
Traumatic rupture of greater saphenous vein at hip and thigh level
S75.221 Major laceration of greater saphenous vein at hip and thigh level, right leg CC
S75.222 Major laceration of greater saphenous vein at hip and thigh level, left leg CC
S75.229 Major laceration of greater saphenous vein at hip and thigh level, unspecified leg CC

S75.29 Other specified injury of greater saphenous vein at hip and thigh level
S75.291 Other specified injury of greater saphenous vein at hip and thigh level, right leg CC
S75.292 Other specified injury of greater saphenous vein at hip and thigh level, left leg CC
S75.299 Other specified injury of greater saphenous vein at hip and thigh level, unspecified leg CC

S75.8 Injury of other blood vessels at hip and thigh level

S75.80 Unspecified injury of other blood vessels at hip and thigh level
S75.801 Unspecified injury of other blood vessels at hip and thigh level, right leg CC
S75.802 Unspecified injury of other blood vessels at hip and thigh level, left leg CC
S75.809 Unspecified injury of other blood vessels at hip and thigh level, unspecified leg CC

S75.81 Laceration of other blood vessels at hip and thigh level
S75.811 Laceration of other blood vessels at hip and thigh level, right leg CC
S75.812 Laceration of other blood vessels at hip and thigh level, left leg CC
S75.819 Laceration of other blood vessels at hip and thigh level, unspecified leg CC

S75.89 Other specified injury of other blood vessels at hip and thigh level
S75.891 Other specified injury of other blood vessels at hip and thigh level, right leg CC
S75.892 Other specified injury of other blood vessels at hip and thigh level, left leg CC
S75.899 Other specified injury of other blood vessels at hip and thigh level, unspecified leg CC

S75.9 Injury of unspecified blood vessel at hip and thigh level

S75.90 Unspecified injury of unspecified blood vessel at hip and thigh level
S75.901 Unspecified injury of unspecified blood vessel at hip and thigh level, right leg CC
S75.902 Unspecified injury of unspecified blood vessel at hip and thigh level, left leg CC
S75.909 Unspecified injury of unspecified blood vessel at hip and thigh level, unspecified leg CC

S75.91 Laceration of unspecified blood vessel at hip and thigh level
S75.911 Laceration of unspecified blood vessel at hip and thigh level, right leg CC
S75.912 Laceration of unspecified blood vessel at hip and thigh level, left leg CC
S75.919 Laceration of unspecified blood vessel at hip and thigh level, unspecified leg CC

S75.99 Other specified injury of unspecified blood vessel at hip and thigh level
S75.991 Other specified injury of unspecified blood vessel at hip and thigh level, right leg CC
S75.992 Other specified injury of unspecified blood vessel at hip and thigh level, left leg CC
S75.999 Other specified injury of unspecified blood vessel at hip and thigh level, unspecified leg CC

S76 Injury of muscle, fascia and tendon at hip and thigh level
Code also any associated open wound (S71.-)
EXCLUDES2 *injury of muscle, fascia and tendon at lower leg level (S86)*
sprain of joint and ligament of hip (S73.1)

The appropriate 7th character is to be added to each code from category S76
A = initial encounter
D = subsequent encounter
S = sequela

S76.0 Injury of muscle, fascia and tendon of hip

S76.00 Unspecified injury of muscle, fascia and tendon of hip
S76.001 Unspecified injury of muscle, fascia and tendon of right hip
S76.002 Unspecified injury of muscle, fascia and tendon of left hip
S76.009 Unspecified injury of muscle, fascia and tendon of unspecified hip

S76.01 Strain of muscle, fascia and tendon of hip
S76.011 Strain of muscle, fascia and tendon of right hip
S76.012 Strain of muscle, fascia and tendon of left hip
S76.019 Strain of muscle, fascia and tendon of unspecified hip

S76.02 Laceration of muscle, fascia and tendon of hip
S76.021 Laceration of muscle, fascia and tendon of right hip CC
S76.022 Laceration of muscle, fascia and tendon of left hip CC
S76.029 Laceration of muscle, fascia and tendon of unspecified hip CC

S76.09 Other specified injury of muscle, fascia and tendon of hip
S76.091 Other specified injury of muscle, fascia and tendon of right hip
S76.092 Other specified injury of muscle, fascia and tendon of left hip
S76.099 Other specified injury of muscle, fascia and tendon of unspecified hip

Unspecified Code Other Specified Code Manifestation Code N Newborn P Pediatric M Maternity A Adult ♂ Male ♀ Female
● New Code ▲ Revised Code Title ►◄ Revised Text NOTES INCLUDES EXCLUDES1 Not coded here EXCLUDES2 Not included here
4th character required 5th character required 6th character required 7th character required
Extension 'X' Alert HAC Hospital-acquired condition (HAC) alert AHA AHA Coding Clinic©

S76.1 Injury of quadriceps muscle, fascia and tendon
Injury of patellar ligament (tendon)
- S76.10 Unspecified injury of quadriceps muscle, fascia and tendon
  - S76.101 Unspecified injury of right quadriceps muscle, fascia and tendon
  - S76.102 Unspecified injury of left quadriceps muscle, fascia and tendon
  - S76.109 Unspecified injury of unspecified quadriceps muscle, fascia and tendon
- S76.11 Strain of quadriceps muscle, fascia and tendon
  - S76.111 Strain of right quadriceps muscle, fascia and tendon
  - S76.112 Strain of left quadriceps muscle, fascia and tendon
  - S76.119 Strain of unspecified quadriceps muscle, fascia and tendon
- S76.12 Laceration of quadriceps muscle, fascia and tendon
  - S76.121 Laceration of right quadriceps muscle, fascia and tendon CC
  - S76.122 Laceration of left quadriceps muscle, fascia and tendon CC
  - S76.129 Laceration of unspecified quadriceps muscle, fascia and tendon CC
- S76.19 Other specified injury of quadriceps muscle, fascia and tendon
  - S76.191 Other specified injury of right quadriceps muscle, fascia and tendon
  - S76.192 Other specified injury of left quadriceps muscle, fascia and tendon
  - S76.199 Other specified injury of unspecified quadriceps muscle, fascia and tendon

S76.2 Injury of adductor muscle, fascia and tendon of thigh
- S76.20 Unspecified injury of adductor muscle, fascia and tendon of thigh
  - S76.201 Unspecified injury of adductor muscle, fascia and tendon of right thigh
  - S76.202 Unspecified injury of adductor muscle, fascia and tendon of left thigh
  - S76.209 Unspecified injury of adductor muscle, fascia and tendon of unspecified thigh
- S76.21 Strain of adductor muscle, fascia and tendon of thigh
  - S76.211 Strain of adductor muscle, fascia and tendon of right thigh
  - S76.212 Strain of adductor muscle, fascia and tendon of left thigh
  - S76.219 Strain of adductor muscle, fascia and tendon of unspecified thigh
- S76.22 Laceration of adductor muscle, fascia and tendon of thigh
  - S76.221 Laceration of adductor muscle, fascia and tendon of right thigh CC
  - S76.222 Laceration of adductor muscle, fascia and tendon of left thigh CC
  - S76.229 Laceration of adductor muscle, fascia and tendon of unspecified thigh CC
- S76.29 Other injury of adductor muscle, fascia and tendon of thigh
  - S76.291 Other injury of adductor muscle, fascia and tendon of right thigh
  - S76.292 Other injury of adductor muscle, fascia and tendon of left thigh
  - S76.299 Other injury of adductor muscle, fascia and tendon of unspecified thigh

S76.3 Injury of muscle, fascia and tendon of the posterior muscle group at thigh level
- S76.30 Unspecified injury of muscle, fascia and tendon of the posterior muscle group at thigh level
  - S76.301 Unspecified injury of muscle, fascia and tendon of the posterior muscle group at thigh level, right thigh
  - S76.302 Unspecified injury of muscle, fascia and tendon of the posterior muscle group at thigh level, left thigh
  - S76.309 Unspecified injury of muscle, fascia and tendon of the posterior muscle group at thigh level, unspecified thigh
- S76.31 Strain of muscle, fascia and tendon of the posterior muscle group at thigh level
  - S76.311 Strain of muscle, fascia and tendon of the posterior muscle group at thigh level, right thigh
  - S76.312 Strain of muscle, fascia and tendon of the posterior muscle group at thigh level, left thigh
  - S76.319 Strain of muscle, fascia and tendon of the posterior muscle group at thigh level, unspecified thigh
- S76.32 Laceration of muscle, fascia and tendon of the posterior muscle group at thigh level
  - S76.321 Laceration of muscle, fascia and tendon of the posterior muscle group at thigh level, right thigh CC
  - S76.322 Laceration of muscle, fascia and tendon of the posterior muscle group at thigh level, left thigh CC
  - S76.329 Laceration of muscle, fascia and tendon of the posterior muscle group at thigh level, unspecified thigh CC
- S76.39 Other specified injury of muscle, fascia and tendon of the posterior muscle group at thigh level
  - S76.391 Other specified injury of muscle, fascia and tendon of the posterior muscle group at thigh level, right thigh
  - S76.392 Other specified injury of muscle, fascia and tendon of the posterior muscle group at thigh level, left thigh
  - S76.399 Other specified injury of muscle, fascia and tendon of the posterior muscle group at thigh level, unspecified thigh

S76.8 Injury of other specified muscles, fascia and tendons at thigh level
- S76.80 Unspecified injury of other specified muscles, fascia and tendons at thigh level
  - S76.801 Unspecified injury of other specified muscles, fascia and tendons at thigh level, right thigh
  - S76.802 Unspecified injury of other specified muscles, fascia and tendons at thigh level, left thigh
  - S76.809 Unspecified injury of other specified muscles, fascia and tendons at thigh level, unspecified thigh
- S76.81 Strain of other specified muscles, fascia and tendons at thigh level
  - S76.811 Strain of other specified muscles, fascia and tendons at thigh level, right thigh
  - S76.812 Strain of other specified muscles, fascia and tendons at thigh level, left thigh
  - S76.819 Strain of other specified muscles, fascia and tendons at thigh level, unspecified thigh
- S76.82 Laceration of other specified muscles, fascia and tendons at thigh level
  - S76.821 Laceration of other specified muscles, fascia and tendons at thigh level, right thigh CC
  - S76.822 Laceration of other specified muscles, fascia and tendons at thigh level, left thigh CC
  - S76.829 Laceration of other specified muscles, fascia and tendons at thigh level, unspecified thigh CC
- S76.89 Other injury of other specified muscles, fascia and tendons at thigh level
  - S76.891 Other injury of other specified muscles, fascia and tendons at thigh level, right thigh
  - S76.892 Other injury of other specified muscles, fascia and tendons at thigh level, left thigh

PDx Unacceptable principal diagnosis symbol per Medicare code edits · POA Code exempt from diagnosis present on admission requirement
? Questionable admission · CC Complication or comorbidity · CC/MCC Exc CC/MCC exclusion · MCC Major complication or comorbidity
PDx CC Principal diagnosis as its own CC · PDx MCC Principal diagnosis as its own MCC · Z Z code as first-listed diagnosis

S76.899 Other injury of other specified muscles, fascia and tendons at thigh level, unspecified thigh

S76.9 Injury of unspecified muscles, fascia and tendons at thigh level

S76.90 Unspecified injury of unspecified muscles, fascia and tendons at thigh level

S76.901 Unspecified injury of unspecified muscles, fascia and tendons at thigh level, right thigh

S76.902 Unspecified injury of unspecified muscles, fascia and tendons at thigh level, left thigh

S76.909 Unspecified injury of unspecified muscles, fascia and tendons at thigh level, unspecified thigh

S76.91 Strain of unspecified muscles, fascia and tendons at thigh level

S76.911 Strain of unspecified muscles, fascia and tendons at thigh level, right thigh

S76.912 Strain of unspecified muscles, fascia and tendons at thigh level, left thigh

S76.919 Strain of unspecified muscles, fascia and tendons at thigh level, unspecified thigh

S76.92 Laceration of unspecified muscles, fascia and tendons at thigh level

S76.921 Laceration of unspecified muscles, fascia and tendons at thigh level, right thigh CC

S76.922 Laceration of unspecified muscles, fascia and tendons at thigh level, left thigh CC

S76.929 Laceration of unspecified muscles, fascia and tendons at thigh level, unspecified thigh CC

S76.99 Other specified injury of unspecified muscles, fascia and tendons at thigh level

S76.991 Other specified injury of unspecified muscles, fascia and tendons at thigh level, right thigh

S76.992 Other specified injury of unspecified muscles, fascia and tendons at thigh level, left thigh

S76.999 Other specified injury of unspecified muscles, fascia and tendons at thigh level, unspecified thigh

S77 Crushing injury of hip and thigh

Use additional code(s) for all associated injuries

EXCLUDES2 *crushing injury of ankle and foot (S97.-)*
crushing injury of lower leg (S87.-)

The appropriate 7th character is to be added to each code from category S77

A = initial encounter
D = subsequent encounter
S = sequela

S77.0 Crushing injury of hip

S77.00 Crushing injury of unspecified hip CC HAC

S77.01 Crushing injury of right hip CC HAC

S77.02 Crushing injury of left hip CC HAC

S77.1 Crushing injury of thigh

S77.10 Crushing injury of unspecified thigh CC HAC

S77.11 Crushing injury of right thigh CC HAC

S77.12 Crushing injury of left thigh CC HAC

S77.2 Crushing injury of hip with thigh

S77.20 Crushing injury of unspecified hip with thigh

S77.21 Crushing injury of right hip with thigh

S77.22 Crushing injury of left hip with thigh

S78 Traumatic amputation of hip and thigh

An amputation not identified as partial or complete should be coded to complete

EXCLUDES1 *traumatic amputation of knee (S88.0-)*

The appropriate 7th character is to be added to each code from category S78

A = initial encounter
D = subsequent encounter
S = sequela

S78.0 Traumatic amputation at hip joint

S78.01 Complete traumatic amputation at hip joint

S78.011 Complete traumatic amputation at right hip joint CC

S78.012 Complete traumatic amputation at left hip joint CC

S78.019 Complete traumatic amputation at unspecified hip joint CC

S78.02 Partial traumatic amputation at hip joint

S78.021 Partial traumatic amputation at right hip joint CC

S78.022 Partial traumatic amputation at left hip joint CC

S78.029 Partial traumatic amputation at unspecified hip joint CC

S78.1 Traumatic amputation at level between hip and knee

EXCLUDES1 *traumatic amputation of knee (S88.0-)*

S78.11 Complete traumatic amputation at level between hip and knee

S78.111 Complete traumatic amputation at level between right hip and knee CC

S78.112 Complete traumatic amputation at level between left hip and knee CC

S78.119 Complete traumatic amputation at level between unspecified hip and knee CC

S78.12 Partial traumatic amputation at level between hip and knee

S78.121 Partial traumatic amputation at level between right hip and knee CC

S78.122 Partial traumatic amputation at level between left hip and knee CC

S78.129 Partial traumatic amputation at level between unspecified hip and knee CC

S78.9 Traumatic amputation of hip and thigh, level unspecified

S78.91 Complete traumatic amputation of hip and thigh, level unspecified

S78.911 Complete traumatic amputation of right hip and thigh, level unspecified CC

S78.912 Complete traumatic amputation of left hip and thigh, level unspecified CC

S78.919 Complete traumatic amputation of unspecified hip and thigh, level unspecified CC

S78.92 Partial traumatic amputation of hip and thigh, level unspecified

S78.921 Partial traumatic amputation of right hip and thigh, level unspecified CC

S78.922 Partial traumatic amputation of left hip and thigh, level unspecified CC

S78.929 Partial traumatic amputation of unspecified hip and thigh, level unspecified CC

S79 Other and unspecified injuries of hip and thigh

NOTES A fracture not indicated as open or closed should be coded to closed

The appropriate 7th character is to be added to each code from subcategories S79.0 and S79.1

A = initial encounter for closed fracture
D = subsequent encounter for fracture with routine healing
G = subsequent encounter for fracture with delayed healing
K = subsequent encounter for fracture with nonunion
P = subsequent encounter for fracture with malunion
S = sequela

S79.0 Physeal fracture of upper end of femur

EXCLUDES1 *apophyseal fracture of upper end of femur (S72.13-)*
nontraumatic slipped upper femoral epiphysis (M93.0-)

S79.00 Unspecified physeal fracture of upper end of femur

S79.001 Unspecified physeal fracture of upper end of right femur CC HAC MCC

S79.002 Unspecified physeal fracture of upper end of left femur CC HAC MCC

S79.009 Unspecified physeal fracture of upper end of unspecified femur CC HAC MCC

Unspecified Code Other Specified Code Manifestation Code N Newborn P Pediatric M Maternity A Adult ♂ Male ♀ Female
● New Code ▲ Revised Code Title ►◄ Revised Text NOTES INCLUDES EXCLUDES1 Not coded here EXCLUDES2 Not included here
4th character required 5th character required 6th character required 7th character required
Extension 'X' Alert HAC Hospital-acquired condition (HAC) alert AHA AHA Coding Clinic©

S79.01 Salter-Harris Type I physeal fracture of upper end of femur
Acute on chronic slipped capital femoral epiphysis (traumatic)
Acute slipped capital femoral epiphysis (traumatic)
Capital femoral epiphyseal fracture
EXCLUDES1 *chronic slipped upper femoral epiphysis (nontraumatic) (M93.02-)*
S79.011 Salter-Harris Type I physeal fracture of upper end of right femur CC HAC MCC
S79.012 Salter-Harris Type I physeal fracture of upper end of left femur CC HAC MCC
S79.019 Salter-Harris Type I physeal fracture of upper end of unspecified femur CC HAC MCC
S79.09 Other physeal fracture of upper end of femur
S79.091 Other physeal fracture of upper end of right femur CC HAC MCC
S79.092 Other physeal fracture of upper end of left femur CC HAC MCC
S79.099 Other physeal fracture of upper end of unspecified femur CC HAC MCC
S79.1 Physeal fracture of lower end of femur
S79.10 Unspecified physeal fracture of lower end of femur
S79.101 Unspecified physeal fracture of lower end of right femur CC HAC
S79.102 Unspecified physeal fracture of lower end of left femur CC HAC
S79.109 Unspecified physeal fracture of lower end of unspecified femur CC HAC
S79.11 Salter-Harris Type I physeal fracture of lower end of femur
S79.111 Salter-Harris Type I physeal fracture of lower end of right femur CC HAC
S79.112 Salter-Harris Type I physeal fracture of lower end of left femur CC HAC
S79.119 Salter-Harris Type I physeal fracture of lower end of unspecified femur CC HAC
S79.12 Salter-Harris Type II physeal fracture of lower end of femur
S79.121 Salter-Harris Type II physeal fracture of lower end of right femur CC HAC
S79.122 Salter-Harris Type II physeal fracture of lower end of left femur CC HAC
S79.129 Salter-Harris Type II physeal fracture of lower end of unspecified femur CC HAC
S79.13 Salter-Harris Type III physeal fracture of lower end of femur
S79.131 Salter-Harris Type III physeal fracture of lower end of right femur CC HAC
S79.132 Salter-Harris Type III physeal fracture of lower end of left femur CC HAC
S79.139 Salter-Harris Type III physeal fracture of lower end of unspecified femur CC HAC
S79.14 Salter-Harris Type IV physeal fracture of lower end of femur
S79.141 Salter-Harris Type IV physeal fracture of lower end of right femur CC HAC
S79.142 Salter-Harris Type IV physeal fracture of lower end of left femur CC HAC
S79.149 Salter-Harris Type IV physeal fracture of lower end of unspecified femur CC HAC
S79.19 Other physeal fracture of lower end of femur
S79.191 Other physeal fracture of lower end of right femur CC HAC
S79.192 Other physeal fracture of lower end of left femur CC HAC
S79.199 Other physeal fracture of lower end of unspecified femur CC HAC
S79.8 Other specified injuries of hip and thigh
The appropriate 7th character is to be added to each code in subcategory S79.8
A = initial encounter
D = subsequent encounter
S = sequela
S79.81 Other specified injuries of hip
S79.811 Other specified injuries of right hip
S79.812 Other specified injuries of left hip
S79.819 Other specified injuries of unspecified hip
S79.82 Other specified injuries of thigh
S79.821 Other specified injuries of right thigh
S79.822 Other specified injuries of left thigh
S79.829 Other specified injuries of unspecified thigh
S79.9 Unspecified injury of hip and thigh
The appropriate 7th character is to be added to each code in subcategory S79.9
A = initial encounter
D = subsequent encounter
S = sequela
S79.91 Unspecified injury of hip
S79.911 Unspecified injury of right hip
S79.912 Unspecified injury of left hip
S79.919 Unspecified injury of unspecified hip
S79.92 Unspecified injury of thigh
S79.921 Unspecified injury of right thigh
S79.922 Unspecified injury of left thigh
S79.929 Unspecified injury of unspecified thigh

Injuries to the knee and lower leg (S80-S89)

EXCLUDES2 *burns and corrosions (T20-T32)*
frostbite (T33-T34)
injuries of ankle and foot, except fracture of ankle and malleolus (S90-S99)
insect bite or sting, venomous (T63.4)

S80 Superficial injury of knee and lower leg
EXCLUDES2 *superficial injury of ankle and foot (S90.-)*
The appropriate 7th character is to be added to each code from category S80
A = initial encounter
D = subsequent encounter
S = sequela
S80.0 Contusion of knee
S80.00 Contusion of unspecified knee
S80.01 Contusion of right knee
S80.02 Contusion of left knee
S80.1 Contusion of lower leg
S80.10 Contusion of unspecified lower leg
S80.11 Contusion of right lower leg
S80.12 Contusion of left lower leg
S80.2 Other superficial injuries of knee
S80.21 Abrasion of knee
S80.211 Abrasion, right knee
S80.212 Abrasion, left knee
S80.219 Abrasion, unspecified knee
S80.22 Blister (nonthermal) of knee
S80.221 Blister (nonthermal), right knee
S80.222 Blister (nonthermal), left knee
S80.229 Blister (nonthermal), unspecified knee
S80.24 External constriction of knee
S80.241 External constriction, right knee
S80.242 External constriction, left knee
S80.249 External constriction, unspecified knee
S80.25 Superficial foreign body of knee
Splinter in the knee
S80.251 Superficial foreign body, right knee
S80.252 Superficial foreign body, left knee
S80.259 Superficial foreign body, unspecified knee
S80.26 Insect bite (nonvenomous) of knee
S80.261 Insect bite (nonvenomous), right knee
S80.262 Insect bite (nonvenomous), left knee
S80.269 Insect bite (nonvenomous), unspecified knee

Unacceptable principal diagnosis symbol per Medicare code edits · Code exempt from diagnosis present on admission requirement
Questionable admission · CC Complication or comorbidity · CC/MCC exclusion · MCC Major complication or comorbidity
Principal diagnosis as its own CC · Principal diagnosis as its own MCC · Z code as first-listed diagnosis

S80.27 Other superficial bite of knee
EXCLUDES1 *open bite of knee (S81.05-)*
S80.271 Other superficial bite of right knee
S80.272 Other superficial bite of left knee
S80.279 Other superficial bite of unspecified knee
S80.8 Other superficial injuries of lower leg
S80.81 Abrasion of lower leg
S80.811 Abrasion, right lower leg
S80.812 Abrasion, left lower leg
S80.819 Abrasion, unspecified lower leg
S80.82 Blister (nonthermal) of lower leg
S80.821 Blister (nonthermal), right lower leg
S80.822 Blister (nonthermal), left lower leg
S80.829 Blister (nonthermal), unspecified lower leg
S80.84 External constriction of lower leg
S80.841 External constriction, right lower leg
S80.842 External constriction, left lower leg
S80.849 External constriction, unspecified lower leg
S80.85 Superficial foreign body of lower leg
Splinter in the lower leg
S80.851 Superficial foreign body, right lower leg
S80.852 Superficial foreign body, left lower leg
S80.859 Superficial foreign body, unspecified lower leg
S80.86 Insect bite (nonvenomous) of lower leg
S80.861 Insect bite (nonvenomous), right lower leg
S80.862 Insect bite (nonvenomous), left lower leg
S80.869 Insect bite (nonvenomous), unspecified lower leg
S80.87 Other superficial bite of lower leg
EXCLUDES1 *open bite of lower leg (S81.85-)*
S80.871 Other superficial bite, right lower leg
S80.872 Other superficial bite, left lower leg
S80.879 Other superficial bite, unspecified lower leg
S80.9 Unspecified superficial injury of knee and lower leg
S80.91 Unspecified superficial injury of knee
S80.911 Unspecified superficial injury of right knee
S80.912 Unspecified superficial injury of left knee
S80.919 Unspecified superficial injury of unspecified knee
S80.92 Unspecified superficial injury of lower leg
S80.921 Unspecified superficial injury of right lower leg
S80.922 Unspecified superficial injury of left lower leg
S80.929 Unspecified superficial injury of unspecified lower leg

S81 Open wound of knee and lower leg
Code also any associated wound infection
EXCLUDES1 *open fracture of knee and lower leg (S82.-)*
traumatic amputation of lower leg (S88.-)
EXCLUDES2 *open wound of ankle and foot (S91.-)*
The appropriate 7th character is to be added to each code from category S81
A = initial encounter
D = subsequent encounter
S = sequela
S81.0 Open wound of knee
S81.00 Unspecified open wound of knee
S81.001 Unspecified open wound, right knee
S81.002 Unspecified open wound, left knee
S81.009 Unspecified open wound, unspecified knee
S81.01 Laceration without foreign body of knee
S81.011 Laceration without foreign body, right knee
S81.012 Laceration without foreign body, left knee
S81.019 Laceration without foreign body, unspecified knee
S81.02 Laceration with foreign body of knee
S81.021 Laceration with foreign body, right knee
S81.022 Laceration with foreign body, left knee
S81.029 Laceration with foreign body, unspecified knee
S81.03 Puncture wound without foreign body of knee
S81.031 Puncture wound without foreign body, right knee
S81.032 Puncture wound without foreign body, left knee
S81.039 Puncture wound without foreign body, unspecified knee
S81.04 Puncture wound with foreign body of knee
S81.041 Puncture wound with foreign body, right knee
S81.042 Puncture wound with foreign body, left knee
S81.049 Puncture wound with foreign body, unspecified knee
S81.05 Open bite of knee
Bite of knee NOS
EXCLUDES1 *superficial bite of knee (S80.27-)*
S81.051 Open bite, right knee
S81.052 Open bite, left knee
S81.059 Open bite, unspecified knee
S81.8 Open wound of lower leg
S81.80 Unspecified open wound of lower leg
S81.801 Unspecified open wound, right lower leg
S81.802 Unspecified open wound, left lower leg
S81.809 Unspecified open wound, unspecified lower leg
S81.81 Laceration without foreign body of lower leg
S81.811 Laceration without foreign body, right lower leg
S81.812 Laceration without foreign body, left lower leg
S81.819 Laceration without foreign body, unspecified lower leg
S81.82 Laceration with foreign body of lower leg
S81.821 Laceration with foreign body, right lower leg
S81.822 Laceration with foreign body, left lower leg
S81.829 Laceration with foreign body, unspecified lower leg
S81.83 Puncture wound without foreign body of lower leg
S81.831 Puncture wound without foreign body, right lower leg
S81.832 Puncture wound without foreign body, left lower leg
S81.839 Puncture wound without foreign body, unspecified lower leg
S81.84 Puncture wound with foreign body of lower leg
S81.841 Puncture wound with foreign body, right lower leg
S81.842 Puncture wound with foreign body, left lower leg
S81.849 Puncture wound with foreign body, unspecified lower leg
S81.85 Open bite of lower leg
Bite of lower leg NOS
EXCLUDES1 *superficial bite of lower leg (S80.86-, S80.87-)*
S81.851 Open bite, right lower leg
S81.852 Open bite, left lower leg
S81.859 Open bite, unspecified lower leg

S82 Fracture of lower leg, including ankle
NOTES A fracture not indicated as displaced or nondisplaced should be coded to displaced
A fracture not indicated as open or closed should be coded to closed
The open fracture designations are based on the Gustilo open fracture classification
INCLUDES *fracture of malleolus*

EXCLUDES1 *traumatic amputation of lower leg (S88.-)*
EXCLUDES2 *fracture of foot, except ankle (S92.-)*
periprosthetic fracture of prosthetic implant of knee (T84.042, T84.043)

The appropriate 7th character is to be added to all codes from category S82
- A = initial encounter for closed fracture
- B = initial encounter for open fracture type I or II
  initial encounter for open fracture NOS
- C = initial encounter for open fracture type IIIA, IIIB, or IIIC
- D = subsequent encounter for closed fracture with routine healing
- E = subsequent encounter for open fracture type I or II with routine healing
- F = subsequent encounter for open fracture type IIIA, IIIB, or IIIC with routine healing
- G = subsequent encounter for closed fracture with delayed healing
- H = subsequent encounter for open fracture type I or II with delayed healing
- J = subsequent encounter for open fracture type IIIA, IIIB, or IIIC with delayed healing
- K = subsequent encounter for closed fracture with nonunion
- M = subsequent encounter for open fracture type I or II with nonunion
- N = subsequent encounter for open fracture type IIIA, IIIB, or IIIC with nonunion
- P = subsequent encounter for closed fracture with malunion
- Q = subsequent encounter for open fracture type I or II with malunion
- R = subsequent encounter for open fracture type IIIA, IIIB, or IIIC with malunion
- S = sequela

5th **S82.0** Fracture of patella
Knee cap

6th **S82.00** Unspecified fracture of patella
- 7th S82.001 Unspecified fracture of right patella CC HAC
- 7th S82.002 Unspecified fracture of left patella CC HAC
- 7th S82.009 Unspecified fracture of unspecified patella CC HAC

6th **S82.01** Osteochondral fracture of patella
- 7th S82.011 Displaced osteochondral fracture of right patella CC HAC
- 7th S82.012 Displaced osteochondral fracture of left patella CC HAC
- 7th S82.013 Displaced osteochondral fracture of unspecified patella CC HAC
- 7th S82.014 Nondisplaced osteochondral fracture of right patella CC HAC
- 7th S82.015 Nondisplaced osteochondral fracture of left patella CC HAC
- 7th S82.016 Nondisplaced osteochondral fracture of unspecified patella CC HAC

6th **S82.02** Longitudinal fracture of patella
- 7th S82.021 Displaced longitudinal fracture of right patella CC HAC
- 7th S82.022 Displaced longitudinal fracture of left patella CC HAC
- 7th S82.023 Displaced longitudinal fracture of unspecified patella CC HAC
- 7th S82.024 Nondisplaced longitudinal fracture of right patella CC HAC
- 7th S82.025 Nondisplaced longitudinal fracture of left patella CC HAC
- 7th S82.026 Nondisplaced longitudinal fracture of unspecified patella CC HAC

6th **S82.03** Transverse fracture of patella
- 7th S82.031 Displaced transverse fracture of right patella CC HAC
- 7th S82.032 Displaced transverse fracture of left patella CC HAC
- 7th S82.033 Displaced transverse fracture of unspecified patella CC HAC
- 7th S82.034 Nondisplaced transverse fracture of right patella CC HAC
- 7th S82.035 Nondisplaced transverse fracture of left patella CC HAC
- 7th S82.036 Nondisplaced transverse fracture of unspecified patella CC HAC

6th **S82.04** Comminuted fracture of patella
- 7th S82.041 Displaced comminuted fracture of right patella CC HAC
- 7th S82.042 Displaced comminuted fracture of left patella CC HAC
- 7th S82.043 Displaced comminuted fracture of unspecified patella CC HAC
- 7th S82.044 Nondisplaced comminuted fracture of right patella CC HAC
- 7th S82.045 Nondisplaced comminuted fracture of left patella CC HAC
- 7th S82.046 Nondisplaced comminuted fracture of unspecified patella CC HAC

6th **S82.09** Other fracture of patella
- 7th S82.091 Other fracture of right patella CC HAC
- 7th S82.092 Other fracture of left patella CC HAC
- 7th S82.099 Other fracture of unspecified patella CC HAC

5th **S82.1** Fracture of upper end of tibia
Fracture of proximal end of tibia
EXCLUDES2 *fracture of shaft of tibia (S82.2-)*
physeal fracture of upper end of tibia (S89.0-)

6th **S82.10** Unspecified fracture of upper end of tibia
- 7th S82.101 Unspecified fracture of upper end of right tibia CC HAC MCC
- 7th S82.102 Unspecified fracture of upper end of left tibia CC HAC MCC
- 7th S82.109 Unspecified fracture of upper end of unspecified tibia CC HAC MCC

6th **S82.11** Fracture of tibial spine
- 7th S82.111 Displaced fracture of right tibial spine CC HAC MCC
- 7th S82.112 Displaced fracture of left tibial spine CC HAC MCC
- 7th S82.113 Displaced fracture of unspecified tibial spine CC HAC MCC
- 7th S82.114 Nondisplaced fracture of right tibial spine CC HAC MCC
- 7th S82.115 Nondisplaced fracture of left tibial spine CC HAC MCC
- 7th S82.116 Nondisplaced fracture of unspecified tibial spine CC HAC MCC

6th **S82.12** Fracture of lateral condyle of tibia
- 7th S82.121 Displaced fracture of lateral condyle of right tibia CC HAC MCC
- 7th S82.122 Displaced fracture of lateral condyle of left tibia CC HAC MCC
- 7th S82.123 Displaced fracture of lateral condyle of unspecified tibia CC HAC MCC
- 7th S82.124 Nondisplaced fracture of lateral condyle of right tibia CC HAC MCC
- 7th S82.125 Nondisplaced fracture of lateral condyle of left tibia CC HAC MCC
- 7th S82.126 Nondisplaced fracture of lateral condyle of unspecified tibia CC HAC MCC

6th **S82.13** Fracture of medial condyle of tibia
- 7th S82.131 Displaced fracture of medial condyle of right tibia CC HAC MCC
- 7th S82.132 Displaced fracture of medial condyle of left tibia CC HAC MCC
- 7th S82.133 Displaced fracture of medial condyle of unspecified tibia CC HAC MCC
- 7th S82.134 Nondisplaced fracture of medial condyle of right tibia CC HAC MCC
- 7th S82.135 Nondisplaced fracture of medial condyle of left tibia CC HAC MCC
- 7th S82.136 Nondisplaced fracture of medial condyle of unspecified tibia CC HAC MCC

PDx Unacceptable principal diagnosis symbol per Medicare code edits · POA Code exempt from diagnosis present on admission requirement
? Questionable admission · CC Complication or comorbidity · CC/MCC Exc CC/MCC exclusion · MCC Major complication or comorbidity
PDx CC Principal diagnosis as its own CC · PDx MCC Principal diagnosis as its own MCC · Z1 Z code as first-listed diagnosis

S82.14 Bicondylar fracture of tibia
Fracture of tibial plateau NOS
S82.141 Displaced bicondylar fracture of right tibia CC HAC MCC
S82.142 Displaced bicondylar fracture of left tibia CC HAC MCC
S82.143 Displaced bicondylar fracture of unspecified tibia CC HAC MCC
S82.144 Nondisplaced bicondylar fracture of right tibia CC HAC MCC
S82.145 Nondisplaced bicondylar fracture of left tibia CC HAC MCC
S82.146 Nondisplaced bicondylar fracture of unspecified tibia CC HAC MCC
S82.15 Fracture of tibial tuberosity
S82.151 Displaced fracture of right tibial tuberosity CC HAC MCC
S82.152 Displaced fracture of left tibial tuberosity CC HAC MCC
S82.153 Displaced fracture of unspecified tibial tuberosity CC HAC MCC
S82.154 Nondisplaced fracture of right tibial tuberosity CC HAC MCC
S82.155 Nondisplaced fracture of left tibial tuberosity CC HAC MCC
S82.156 Nondisplaced fracture of unspecified tibial tuberosity CC HAC MCC
S82.16 Torus fracture of upper end of tibia
The appropriate 7th character is to be added to all codes in subcategory S82.16
A = initial encounter for closed fracture
D = subsequent encounter for fracture with routine healing
G = subsequent encounter for fracture with delayed healing
K = subsequent encounter for fracture with nonunion
P = subsequent encounter for fracture with malunion
S = sequela
S82.161 Torus fracture of upper end of right tibia CC HAC
S82.162 Torus fracture of upper end of left tibia CC HAC
S82.169 Torus fracture of upper end of unspecified tibia CC HAC
S82.19 Other fracture of upper end of tibia
S82.191 Other fracture of upper end of right tibia CC HAC MCC
S82.192 Other fracture of upper end of left tibia CC HAC MCC
S82.199 Other fracture of upper end of unspecified tibia CC HAC MCC
S82.2 Fracture of shaft of tibia
S82.20 Unspecified fracture of shaft of tibia
Fracture of tibia NOS
S82.201 Unspecified fracture of shaft of right tibia CC HAC MCC
S82.202 Unspecified fracture of shaft of left tibia CC HAC MCC
S82.209 Unspecified fracture of shaft of unspecified tibia CC HAC MCC
S82.22 Transverse fracture of shaft of tibia
S82.221 Displaced transverse fracture of shaft of right tibia CC HAC MCC
S82.222 Displaced transverse fracture of shaft of left tibia CC HAC MCC
S82.223 Displaced transverse fracture of shaft of unspecified tibia CC HAC MCC
S82.224 Nondisplaced transverse fracture of shaft of right tibia CC HAC MCC
S82.225 Nondisplaced transverse fracture of shaft of left tibia CC HAC MCC
S82.226 Nondisplaced transverse fracture of shaft of unspecified tibia CC HAC MCC
S82.23 Oblique fracture of shaft of tibia
S82.231 Displaced oblique fracture of shaft of right tibia CC HAC MCC
S82.232 Displaced oblique fracture of shaft of left tibia CC HAC MCC
S82.233 Displaced oblique fracture of shaft of unspecified tibia CC HAC MCC
S82.234 Nondisplaced oblique fracture of shaft of right tibia CC HAC MCC
AHA: Q1, 2015
S82.235 Nondisplaced oblique fracture of shaft of left tibia CC HAC MCC
S82.236 Nondisplaced oblique fracture of shaft of unspecified tibia CC HAC MCC
S82.24 Spiral fracture of shaft of tibia
Toddler fracture
S82.241 Displaced spiral fracture of shaft of right tibia CC HAC MCC
S82.242 Displaced spiral fracture of shaft of left tibia CC HAC MCC
S82.243 Displaced spiral fracture of shaft of unspecified tibia CC HAC MCC
S82.244 Nondisplaced spiral fracture of shaft of right tibia CC HAC MCC
S82.245 Nondisplaced spiral fracture of shaft of left tibia CC HAC MCC
S82.246 Nondisplaced spiral fracture of shaft of unspecified tibia CC HAC MCC
S82.25 Comminuted fracture of shaft of tibia
S82.251 Displaced comminuted fracture of shaft of right tibia CC HAC MCC
S82.252 Displaced comminuted fracture of shaft of left tibia CC HAC MCC
S82.253 Displaced comminuted fracture of shaft of unspecified tibia CC HAC MCC
S82.254 Nondisplaced comminuted fracture of shaft of right tibia CC HAC MCC
S82.255 Nondisplaced comminuted fracture of shaft of left tibia CC HAC MCC
S82.256 Nondisplaced comminuted fracture of shaft of unspecified tibia CC HAC MCC
S82.26 Segmental fracture of shaft of tibia
S82.261 Displaced segmental fracture of shaft of right tibia CC HAC MCC
S82.262 Displaced segmental fracture of shaft of left tibia CC HAC MCC
S82.263 Displaced segmental fracture of shaft of unspecified tibia CC HAC MCC
S82.264 Nondisplaced segmental fracture of shaft of right tibia CC HAC MCC
S82.265 Nondisplaced segmental fracture of shaft of left tibia CC HAC MCC
S82.266 Nondisplaced segmental fracture of shaft of unspecified tibia CC HAC MCC
S82.29 Other fracture of shaft of tibia
S82.291 Other fracture of shaft of right tibia CC HAC MCC
S82.292 Other fracture of shaft of left tibia CC HAC MCC
S82.299 Other fracture of shaft of unspecified tibia CC HAC MCC
S82.3 Fracture of lower end of tibia
EXCLUDES1 *bimalleolar fracture of lower leg (S82.84-)*
fracture of medial malleolus alone (S82.5-)
Maisonneuve's fracture (S82.86-)
pilon fracture of distal tibia (S82.87-)
trimalleolar fractures of lower leg (S82.85-)
S82.30 Unspecified fracture of lower end of tibia
S82.301 Unspecified fracture of lower end of right tibia CC HAC
S82.302 Unspecified fracture of lower end of left tibia CC HAC
S82.309 Unspecified fracture of lower end of unspecified tibia CC HAC

Unspecified Code Other Specified Code Manifestation Code N Newborn P Pediatric M Maternity A Adult ♂ Male ♀ Female
● New Code ▲ Revised Code Title ►◄ Revised Text NOTES INCLUDES EXCLUDES1 Not coded here EXCLUDES2 Not included here
4th character required 5th character required 6th character required 7th character required
Extension 'X' Alert HAC Hospital-acquired condition (HAC) alert AHA AHA Coding Clinic©

S82.31 Torus fracture of lower end of tibia
The appropriate 7th character is to be added to all codes in subcategory S82.31
A = initial encounter for closed fracture
D = subsequent encounter for fracture with routine healing
G = subsequent encounter for fracture with delayed healing
K = subsequent encounter for fracture with nonunion
P = subsequent encounter for fracture with malunion
S = sequela
S82.311 Torus fracture of lower end of right tibia CC HAC
S82.312 Torus fracture of lower end of left tibia CC HAC
S82.319 Torus fracture of lower end of unspecified tibia CC HAC
S82.39 Other fracture of lower end of tibia
S82.391 Other fracture of lower end of right tibia CC HAC
S82.392 Other fracture of lower end of left tibia CC HAC
AHA: Q1, 2015
S82.399 Other fracture of lower end of unspecified tibia CC HAC
S82.4 Fracture of shaft of fibula
EXCLUDES2 *fracture of lateral malleolus alone (S82.6-)*
S82.40 Unspecified fracture of shaft of fibula
S82.401 Unspecified fracture of shaft of right fibula CC HAC MCC
S82.402 Unspecified fracture of shaft of left fibula CC HAC MCC
S82.409 Unspecified fracture of shaft of unspecified fibula CC HAC MCC
S82.42 Transverse fracture of shaft of fibula
S82.421 Displaced transverse fracture of shaft of right fibula CC HAC MCC
S82.422 Displaced transverse fracture of shaft of left fibula CC HAC MCC
S82.423 Displaced transverse fracture of shaft of unspecified fibula CC HAC MCC
S82.424 Nondisplaced transverse fracture of shaft of right fibula CC HAC MCC
S82.425 Nondisplaced transverse fracture of shaft of left fibula CC HAC MCC
S82.426 Nondisplaced transverse fracture of shaft of unspecified fibula CC HAC MCC
S82.43 Oblique fracture of shaft of fibula
S82.431 Displaced oblique fracture of shaft of right fibula CC HAC MCC
S82.432 Displaced oblique fracture of shaft of left fibula CC HAC MCC
S82.433 Displaced oblique fracture of shaft of unspecified fibula CC HAC MCC
S82.434 Nondisplaced oblique fracture of shaft of right fibula CC HAC MCC
S82.435 Nondisplaced oblique fracture of shaft of left fibula CC HAC MCC
S82.436 Nondisplaced oblique fracture of shaft of unspecified fibula CC HAC MCC
S82.44 Spiral fracture of shaft of fibula
S82.441 Displaced spiral fracture of shaft of right fibula CC HAC MCC
S82.442 Displaced spiral fracture of shaft of left fibula CC HAC MCC
S82.443 Displaced spiral fracture of shaft of unspecified fibula CC HAC MCC
S82.444 Nondisplaced spiral fracture of shaft of right fibula CC HAC MCC
S82.445 Nondisplaced spiral fracture of shaft of left fibula CC HAC MCC
S82.446 Nondisplaced spiral fracture of shaft of unspecified fibula CC HAC MCC
S82.45 Comminuted fracture of shaft of fibula
S82.451 Displaced comminuted fracture of shaft of right fibula CC HAC MCC
S82.452 Displaced comminuted fracture of shaft of left fibula CC HAC MCC
S82.453 Displaced comminuted fracture of shaft of unspecified fibula CC HAC MCC
S82.454 Nondisplaced comminuted fracture of shaft of right fibula CC HAC MCC
S82.455 Nondisplaced comminuted fracture of shaft of left fibula CC HAC MCC
S82.456 Nondisplaced comminuted fracture of shaft of unspecified fibula CC HAC MCC
S82.46 Segmental fracture of shaft of fibula
S82.461 Displaced segmental fracture of shaft of right fibula CC HAC MCC
S82.462 Displaced segmental fracture of shaft of left fibula CC HAC MCC
S82.463 Displaced segmental fracture of shaft of unspecified fibula CC HAC MCC
S82.464 Nondisplaced segmental fracture of shaft of right fibula CC HAC MCC
S82.465 Nondisplaced segmental fracture of shaft of left fibula CC HAC MCC
S82.466 Nondisplaced segmental fracture of shaft of unspecified fibula CC HAC MCC
S82.49 Other fracture of shaft of fibula
S82.491 Other fracture of shaft of right fibula CC HAC MCC
S82.492 Other fracture of shaft of left fibula CC HAC MCC
S82.499 Other fracture of shaft of unspecified fibula CC HAC MCC
S82.5 Fracture of medial malleolus
EXCLUDES1 *pilon fracture of distal tibia (S82.87-)*
Salter-Harris type III of lower end of tibia (S89.13-)
Salter-Harris type IV of lower end of tibia (S89.14-)
S82.51 Displaced fracture of medial malleolus of right tibia CC HAC
S82.52 Displaced fracture of medial malleolus of left tibia CC HAC
S82.53 Displaced fracture of medial malleolus of unspecified tibia CC HAC
S82.54 Nondisplaced fracture of medial malleolus of right tibia CC HAC
S82.55 Nondisplaced fracture of medial malleolus of left tibia CC HAC
S82.56 Nondisplaced fracture of medial malleolus of unspecified tibia CC HAC
S82.6 Fracture of lateral malleolus
EXCLUDES1 *pilon fracture of distal tibia (S82.87-)*
S82.61 Displaced fracture of lateral malleolus of right fibula CC HAC
S82.62 Displaced fracture of lateral malleolus of left fibula CC HAC
S82.63 Displaced fracture of lateral malleolus of unspecified fibula CC HAC
S82.64 Nondisplaced fracture of lateral malleolus of right fibula CC HAC
S82.65 Nondisplaced fracture of lateral malleolus of left fibula CC HAC
S82.66 Nondisplaced fracture of lateral malleolus of unspecified fibula CC HAC
S82.8 Other fractures of lower leg
S82.81 Torus fracture of upper end of fibula
The appropriate 7th character is to be added to all codes in subcategory S82.81
A = initial encounter for closed fracture
D = subsequent encounter for fracture with routine healing
G = subsequent encounter for fracture with delayed healing
K = subsequent encounter for fracture with nonunion
P = subsequent encounter for fracture with malunion
S = sequela

PDx Unacceptable principal diagnosis symbol per Medicare code edits · POA Code exempt from diagnosis present on admission requirement
? Questionable admission · CC Complication or comorbidity · CC/MCC Exc CC/MCC exclusion · MCC Major complication or comorbidity
PDx Principal diagnosis as its own CC · PDx Principal diagnosis as its own MCC · Z Z code as first-listed diagnosis

S82.811 Torus fracture of upper end of right fibula
S82.812 Torus fracture of upper end of left fibula
S82.819 Torus fracture of upper end of unspecified fibula
S82.82 Torus fracture of lower end of fibula
The appropriate 7th character is to be added to all codes in subcategory S82.82
A = initial encounter for closed fracture
D = subsequent encounter for fracture with routine healing
G = subsequent encounter for fracture with delayed healing
K = subsequent encounter for fracture with nonunion
P = subsequent encounter for fracture with malunion
S = sequela
S82.821 Torus fracture of lower end of right fibula
S82.822 Torus fracture of lower end of left fibula
S82.829 Torus fracture of lower end of unspecified fibula
S82.83 Other fracture of upper and lower end of fibula
S82.831 Other fracture of upper and lower end of right fibula HAC
S82.832 Other fracture of upper and lower end of left fibula HAC
S82.839 Other fracture of upper and lower end of unspecified fibula HAC
S82.84 Bimalleolar fracture of lower leg
S82.841 Displaced bimalleolar fracture of right lower leg HAC
S82.842 Displaced bimalleolar fracture of left lower leg HAC
S82.843 Displaced bimalleolar fracture of unspecified lower leg HAC
S82.844 Nondisplaced bimalleolar fracture of right lower leg HAC
S82.845 Nondisplaced bimalleolar fracture of left lower leg HAC
S82.846 Nondisplaced bimalleolar fracture of unspecified lower leg HAC
S82.85 Trimalleolar fracture of lower leg
S82.851 Displaced trimalleolar fracture of right lower leg HAC
S82.852 Displaced trimalleolar fracture of left lower leg HAC
S82.853 Displaced trimalleolar fracture of unspecified lower leg HAC
S82.854 Nondisplaced trimalleolar fracture of right lower leg HAC
S82.855 Nondisplaced trimalleolar fracture of left lower leg HAC
S82.856 Nondisplaced trimalleolar fracture of unspecified lower leg HAC
S82.86 Maisonneuve's fracture
S82.861 Displaced Maisonneuve's fracture of right leg
S82.862 Displaced Maisonneuve's fracture of left leg
S82.863 Displaced Maisonneuve's fracture of unspecified leg
S82.864 Nondisplaced Maisonneuve's fracture of right leg
S82.865 Nondisplaced Maisonneuve's fracture of left leg
S82.866 Nondisplaced Maisonneuve's fracture of unspecified leg
S82.87 Pilon fracture of tibia
S82.871 Displaced pilon fracture of right tibia HAC
S82.872 Displaced pilon fracture of left tibia HAC
S82.873 Displaced pilon fracture of unspecified tibia HAC
S82.874 Nondisplaced pilon fracture of right tibia HAC
S82.875 Nondisplaced pilon fracture of left tibia HAC
S82.876 Nondisplaced pilon fracture of unspecified tibia HAC
S82.89 Other fractures of lower leg
Fracture of ankle NOS
S82.891 Other fracture of right lower leg HAC
S82.892 Other fracture of left lower leg HAC
S82.899 Other fracture of unspecified lower leg HAC
S82.9 Unspecified fracture of lower leg
S82.90 Unspecified fracture of unspecified lower leg HAC
S82.91 Unspecified fracture of right lower leg HAC
S82.92 Unspecified fracture of left lower leg HAC
S83 Dislocation and sprain of joints and ligaments of knee
INCLUDES *avulsion of joint or ligament of knee*
laceration of cartilage, joint or ligament of knee
sprain of cartilage, joint or ligament of knee
traumatic hemarthrosis of joint or ligament of knee
traumatic rupture of joint or ligament of knee
traumatic subluxation of joint or ligament of knee
traumatic tear of joint or ligament of knee
Code also any associated open wound
EXCLUDES1 *derangement of patella (M22.0-M22.3)*
injury of patellar ligament (tendon) (S76.1-)
internal derangement of knee (M23.-)
old dislocation of knee (M24.36)
pathological dislocation of knee (M24.36)
recurrent dislocation of knee (M22.0)
EXCLUDES2 *strain of muscle, fascia and tendon of lower leg (S86.-)*
The appropriate 7th character is to be added to each code from category S83
A = initial encounter
D = subsequent encounter
S = sequela
S83.0 Subluxation and dislocation of patella
S83.00 Unspecified subluxation and dislocation of patella
S83.001 Unspecified subluxation of right patella
S83.002 Unspecified subluxation of left patella
S83.003 Unspecified subluxation of unspecified patella
S83.004 Unspecified dislocation of right patella
S83.005 Unspecified dislocation of left patella
S83.006 Unspecified dislocation of unspecified patella
S83.01 Lateral subluxation and dislocation of patella
S83.011 Lateral subluxation of right patella
S83.012 Lateral subluxation of left patella
S83.013 Lateral subluxation of unspecified patella
S83.014 Lateral dislocation of right patella
S83.015 Lateral dislocation of left patella
S83.016 Lateral dislocation of unspecified patella
S83.09 Other subluxation and dislocation of patella
S83.091 Other subluxation of right patella
S83.092 Other subluxation of left patella
S83.093 Other subluxation of unspecified patella
S83.094 Other dislocation of right patella
S83.095 Other dislocation of left patella
S83.096 Other dislocation of unspecified patella
S83.1 Subluxation and dislocation of knee
EXCLUDES2 *instability of knee prosthesis (T84.022, T84.023)*
S83.10 Unspecified subluxation and dislocation of knee
S83.101 Unspecified subluxation of right knee
S83.102 Unspecified subluxation of left knee
S83.103 Unspecified subluxation of unspecified knee
S83.104 Unspecified dislocation of right knee
S83.105 Unspecified dislocation of left knee

Unspecified Code Other Specified Code Manifestation Code N Newborn P Pediatric M Maternity A Adult ♂ Male ♀ Female
● New Code ▲ Revised Code Title ►◄ Revised Text NOTES INCLUDES EXCLUDES1 Not coded here EXCLUDES2 Not included here
4th character required 5th character required 6th character required 7th character required
Extension 'X' Alert HAC Hospital-acquired condition (HAC) alert AHA AHA Coding Clinic®

S83.106 Unspecified dislocation of unspecified knee

S83.11 Anterior subluxation and dislocation of proximal end of tibia
Posterior subluxation and dislocation of distal end of femur
- S83.111 Anterior subluxation of proximal end of tibia, right knee
- S83.112 Anterior subluxation of proximal end of tibia, left knee
- S83.113 Anterior subluxation of proximal end of tibia, unspecified knee
- S83.114 Anterior dislocation of proximal end of tibia, right knee
- S83.115 Anterior dislocation of proximal end of tibia, left knee
- S83.116 Anterior dislocation of proximal end of tibia, unspecified knee

S83.12 Posterior subluxation and dislocation of proximal end of tibia
Anterior dislocation of distal end of femur
- S83.121 Posterior subluxation of proximal end of tibia, right knee
- S83.122 Posterior subluxation of proximal end of tibia, left knee
- S83.123 Posterior subluxation of proximal end of tibia, unspecified knee
- S83.124 Posterior dislocation of proximal end of tibia, right knee
- S83.125 Posterior dislocation of proximal end of tibia, left knee
- S83.126 Posterior dislocation of proximal end of tibia, unspecified knee

S83.13 Medial subluxation and dislocation of proximal end of tibia
- S83.131 Medial subluxation of proximal end of tibia, right knee
- S83.132 Medial subluxation of proximal end of tibia, left knee
- S83.133 Medial subluxation of proximal end of tibia, unspecified knee
- S83.134 Medial dislocation of proximal end of tibia, right knee
- S83.135 Medial dislocation of proximal end of tibia, left knee
- S83.136 Medial dislocation of proximal end of tibia, unspecified knee

S83.14 Lateral subluxation and dislocation of proximal end of tibia
- S83.141 Lateral subluxation of proximal end of tibia, right knee
- S83.142 Lateral subluxation of proximal end of tibia, left knee
- S83.143 Lateral subluxation of proximal end of tibia, unspecified knee
- S83.144 Lateral dislocation of proximal end of tibia, right knee
- S83.145 Lateral dislocation of proximal end of tibia, left knee
- S83.146 Lateral dislocation of proximal end of tibia, unspecified knee

S83.19 Other subluxation and dislocation of knee
- S83.191 Other subluxation of right knee
- S83.192 Other subluxation of left knee
- S83.193 Other subluxation of unspecified knee
- S83.194 Other dislocation of right knee
- S83.195 Other dislocation of left knee
- S83.196 Other dislocation of unspecified knee

S83.2 Tear of meniscus, current injury
EXCLUDES1 *old bucket-handle tear (M23.2)*

S83.20 Tear of unspecified meniscus, current injury
Tear of meniscus of knee NOS
- S83.200 Bucket-handle tear of unspecified meniscus, current injury, right knee
- S83.201 Bucket-handle tear of unspecified meniscus, current injury, left knee
- S83.202 Bucket-handle tear of unspecified meniscus, current injury, unspecified knee
- S83.203 Other tear of unspecified meniscus, current injury, right knee
- S83.204 Other tear of unspecified meniscus, current injury, left knee
- S83.205 Other tear of unspecified meniscus, current injury, unspecified knee
- S83.206 Unspecified tear of unspecified meniscus, current injury, right knee
- S83.207 Unspecified tear of unspecified meniscus, current injury, left knee
- S83.209 Unspecified tear of unspecified meniscus, current injury, unspecified knee

S83.21 Bucket-handle tear of medial meniscus, current injury
- S83.211 Bucket-handle tear of medial meniscus, current injury, right knee
- S83.212 Bucket-handle tear of medial meniscus, current injury, left knee
- S83.219 Bucket-handle tear of medial meniscus, current injury, unspecified knee

S83.22 Peripheral tear of medial meniscus, current injury
- S83.221 Peripheral tear of medial meniscus, current injury, right knee
- S83.222 Peripheral tear of medial meniscus, current injury, left knee
- S83.229 Peripheral tear of medial meniscus, current injury, unspecified knee

S83.23 Complex tear of medial meniscus, current injury
- S83.231 Complex tear of medial meniscus, current injury, right knee
- S83.232 Complex tear of medial meniscus, current injury, left knee
- S83.239 Complex tear of medial meniscus, current injury, unspecified knee

S83.24 Other tear of medial meniscus, current injury
- S83.241 Other tear of medial meniscus, current injury, right knee
- S83.242 Other tear of medial meniscus, current injury, left knee
- S83.249 Other tear of medial meniscus, current injury, unspecified knee

S83.25 Bucket-handle tear of lateral meniscus, current injury
- S83.251 Bucket-handle tear of lateral meniscus, current injury, right knee
- S83.252 Bucket-handle tear of lateral meniscus, current injury, left knee
- S83.259 Bucket-handle tear of lateral meniscus, current injury, unspecified knee

S83.26 Peripheral tear of lateral meniscus, current injury
- S83.261 Peripheral tear of lateral meniscus, current injury, right knee
- S83.262 Peripheral tear of lateral meniscus, current injury, left knee
- S83.269 Peripheral tear of lateral meniscus, current injury, unspecified knee

S83.27 Complex tear of lateral meniscus, current injury
- S83.271 Complex tear of lateral meniscus, current injury, right knee
- S83.272 Complex tear of lateral meniscus, current injury, left knee
- S83.279 Complex tear of lateral meniscus, current injury, unspecified knee

S83.28 Other tear of lateral meniscus, current injury
- S83.281 Other tear of lateral meniscus, current injury, right knee
- S83.282 Other tear of lateral meniscus, current injury, left knee
- S83.289 Other tear of lateral meniscus, current injury, unspecified knee

S83.3 Tear of articular cartilage of knee, current
- S83.30 Tear of articular cartilage of unspecified knee, current
- S83.31 Tear of articular cartilage of right knee, current

Unacceptable principal diagnosis symbol per Medicare code edits
Code exempt from diagnosis present on admission requirement
Questionable admission
Complication or comorbidity
CC/MCC exclusion
Major complication or comorbidity
Principal diagnosis as its own CC
Principal diagnosis as its own MCC
Z code as first-listed diagnosis

S83.32 Tear of articular cartilage of left knee, current
S83.4 Sprain of collateral ligament of knee
S83.40 Sprain of unspecified collateral ligament of knee
S83.401 Sprain of unspecified collateral ligament of right knee
S83.402 Sprain of unspecified collateral ligament of left knee
S83.409 Sprain of unspecified collateral ligament of unspecified knee
S83.41 Sprain of medial collateral ligament of knee
Sprain of tibial collateral ligament
S83.411 Sprain of medial collateral ligament of right knee
S83.412 Sprain of medial collateral ligament of left knee
S83.419 Sprain of medial collateral ligament of unspecified knee
S83.42 Sprain of lateral collateral ligament of knee
Sprain of fibular collateral ligament
S83.421 Sprain of lateral collateral ligament of right knee
S83.422 Sprain of lateral collateral ligament of left knee
S83.429 Sprain of lateral collateral ligament of unspecified knee
S83.5 Sprain of cruciate ligament of knee
S83.50 Sprain of unspecified cruciate ligament of knee
S83.501 Sprain of unspecified cruciate ligament of right knee
S83.502 Sprain of unspecified cruciate ligament of left knee
S83.509 Sprain of unspecified cruciate ligament of unspecified knee
S83.51 Sprain of anterior cruciate ligament of knee
S83.511 Sprain of anterior cruciate ligament of right knee
AHA: Q2, 2016
S83.512 Sprain of anterior cruciate ligament of left knee
S83.519 Sprain of anterior cruciate ligament of unspecified knee
S83.52 Sprain of posterior cruciate ligament of knee
S83.521 Sprain of posterior cruciate ligament of right knee
S83.522 Sprain of posterior cruciate ligament of left knee
S83.529 Sprain of posterior cruciate ligament of unspecified knee
S83.6 Sprain of the superior tibiofibular joint and ligament
S83.60 Sprain of the superior tibiofibular joint and ligament, unspecified knee
S83.61 Sprain of the superior tibiofibular joint and ligament, right knee
S83.62 Sprain of the superior tibiofibular joint and ligament, left knee
S83.8 Sprain of other specified parts of knee
S83.8X Sprain of other specified parts of knee
S83.8X1 Sprain of other specified parts of right knee
S83.8X2 Sprain of other specified parts of left knee
S83.8X9 Sprain of other specified parts of unspecified knee
S83.9 Sprain of unspecified site of knee
S83.90 Sprain of unspecified site of unspecified knee
S83.91 Sprain of unspecified site of right knee
S83.92 Sprain of unspecified site of left knee
S84 Injury of nerves at lower leg level
Code also any associated open wound (S81.-)
EXCLUDES2 *injury of nerves at ankle and foot level (S94.-)*
The appropriate 7th character is to be added to each code from category S84
A = initial encounter
D = subsequent encounter
S = sequela
S84.0 Injury of tibial nerve at lower leg level
S84.00 Injury of tibial nerve at lower leg level, unspecified leg
S84.01 Injury of tibial nerve at lower leg level, right leg
S84.02 Injury of tibial nerve at lower leg level, left leg
S84.1 Injury of peroneal nerve at lower leg level
S84.10 Injury of peroneal nerve at lower leg level, unspecified leg
S84.11 Injury of peroneal nerve at lower leg level, right leg
S84.12 Injury of peroneal nerve at lower leg level, left leg
S84.2 Injury of cutaneous sensory nerve at lower leg level
S84.20 Injury of cutaneous sensory nerve at lower leg level, unspecified leg
S84.21 Injury of cutaneous sensory nerve at lower leg level, right leg
S84.22 Injury of cutaneous sensory nerve at lower leg level, left leg
S84.8 Injury of other nerves at lower leg level
S84.80 Injury of other nerves at lower leg level
S84.801 Injury of other nerves at lower leg level, right leg
S84.802 Injury of other nerves at lower leg level, left leg
S84.809 Injury of other nerves at lower leg level, unspecified leg
S84.9 Injury of unspecified nerve at lower leg level
S84.90 Injury of unspecified nerve at lower leg level, unspecified leg
S84.91 Injury of unspecified nerve at lower leg level, right leg
S84.92 Injury of unspecified nerve at lower leg level, left leg
S85 Injury of blood vessels at lower leg level
Code also any associated open wound (S81.-)
EXCLUDES2 *injury of blood vessels at ankle and foot level (S95.-)*
The appropriate 7th character is to be added to each code from category S85
A = initial encounter
D = subsequent encounter
S = sequela
S85.0 Injury of popliteal artery
S85.00 Unspecified injury of popliteal artery
S85.001 Unspecified injury of popliteal artery, right leg MCC
S85.002 Unspecified injury of popliteal artery, left leg MCC
S85.009 Unspecified injury of popliteal artery, unspecified leg MCC
S85.01 Laceration of popliteal artery
S85.011 Laceration of popliteal artery, right leg MCC
S85.012 Laceration of popliteal artery, left leg MCC
S85.019 Laceration of popliteal artery, unspecified leg MCC
S85.09 Other specified injury of popliteal artery
S85.091 Other specified injury of popliteal artery, right leg MCC
S85.092 Other specified injury of popliteal artery, left leg MCC
S85.099 Other specified injury of popliteal artery, unspecified leg MCC
S85.1 Injury of tibial artery
S85.10 Unspecified injury of unspecified tibial artery
Injury of tibial artery NOS
S85.101 Unspecified injury of unspecified tibial artery, right leg CC
S85.102 Unspecified injury of unspecified tibial artery, left leg CC
S85.109 Unspecified injury of unspecified tibial artery, unspecified leg CC
S85.11 Laceration of unspecified tibial artery
S85.111 Laceration of unspecified tibial artery, right leg CC
S85.112 Laceration of unspecified tibial artery, left leg CC
S85.119 Laceration of unspecified tibial artery, unspecified leg CC
S85.12 Other specified injury of unspecified tibial artery

Unspecified Code Other Specified Code Manifestation Code N Newborn P Pediatric M Maternity A Adult ♂ Male ♀ Female
● New Code ▲ Revised Code Title ►◄ Revised Text NOTES INCLUDES EXCLUDES1 Not coded here EXCLUDES2 Not included here
4th character required 5th character required 6th character required 7th character required
Extension 'X' Alert HAC Hospital-acquired condition (HAC) alert AHA AHA Coding Clinic©

- S85.121 Other specified injury of unspecified tibial artery, right leg CC
- S85.122 Other specified injury of unspecified tibial artery, left leg CC
- S85.129 Other specified injury of unspecified tibial artery, unspecified leg CC

S85.13 Unspecified injury of anterior tibial artery
- S85.131 Unspecified injury of anterior tibial artery, right leg CC
- S85.132 Unspecified injury of anterior tibial artery, left leg CC
- S85.139 Unspecified injury of anterior tibial artery, unspecified leg CC

S85.14 Laceration of anterior tibial artery
- S85.141 Laceration of anterior tibial artery, right leg CC
- S85.142 Laceration of anterior tibial artery, left leg CC
- S85.149 Laceration of anterior tibial artery, unspecified leg CC

S85.15 Other specified injury of anterior tibial artery
- S85.151 Other specified injury of anterior tibial artery, right leg CC
- S85.152 Other specified injury of anterior tibial artery, left leg CC
- S85.159 Other specified injury of anterior tibial artery, unspecified leg CC

S85.16 Unspecified injury of posterior tibial artery
- S85.161 Unspecified injury of posterior tibial artery, right leg CC
- S85.162 Unspecified injury of posterior tibial artery, left leg CC
- S85.169 Unspecified injury of posterior tibial artery, unspecified leg CC

S85.17 Laceration of posterior tibial artery
- S85.171 Laceration of posterior tibial artery, right leg CC
- S85.172 Laceration of posterior tibial artery, left leg CC
- S85.179 Laceration of posterior tibial artery, unspecified leg CC

S85.18 Other specified injury of posterior tibial artery
- S85.181 Other specified injury of posterior tibial artery, right leg CC
- S85.182 Other specified injury of posterior tibial artery, left leg CC
- S85.189 Other specified injury of posterior tibial artery, unspecified leg CC

S85.2 Injury of peroneal artery

S85.20 Unspecified injury of peroneal artery
- S85.201 Unspecified injury of peroneal artery, right leg CC
- S85.202 Unspecified injury of peroneal artery, left leg CC
- S85.209 Unspecified injury of peroneal artery, unspecified leg CC

S85.21 Laceration of peroneal artery
- S85.211 Laceration of peroneal artery, right leg CC
- S85.212 Laceration of peroneal artery, left leg CC
- S85.219 Laceration of peroneal artery, unspecified leg CC

S85.29 Other specified injury of peroneal artery
- S85.291 Other specified injury of peroneal artery, right leg CC
- S85.292 Other specified injury of peroneal artery, left leg CC
- S85.299 Other specified injury of peroneal artery, unspecified leg CC

S85.3 Injury of greater saphenous vein at lower leg level
Injury of greater saphenous vein NOS
Injury of saphenous vein NOS

S85.30 Unspecified injury of greater saphenous vein at lower leg level
- S85.301 Unspecified injury of greater saphenous vein at lower leg level, right leg CC
- S85.302 Unspecified injury of greater saphenous vein at lower leg level, left leg CC
- S85.309 Unspecified injury of greater saphenous vein at lower leg level, unspecified leg CC

S85.31 Laceration of greater saphenous vein at lower leg level
- S85.311 Laceration of greater saphenous vein at lower leg level, right leg CC
- S85.312 Laceration of greater saphenous vein at lower leg level, left leg CC
- S85.319 Laceration of greater saphenous vein at lower leg level, unspecified leg CC

S85.39 Other specified injury of greater saphenous vein at lower leg level
- S85.391 Other specified injury of greater saphenous vein at lower leg level, right leg CC
- S85.392 Other specified injury of greater saphenous vein at lower leg level, left leg CC
- S85.399 Other specified injury of greater saphenous vein at lower leg level, unspecified leg CC

S85.4 Injury of lesser saphenous vein at lower leg level

S85.40 Unspecified injury of lesser saphenous vein at lower leg level
- S85.401 Unspecified injury of lesser saphenous vein at lower leg level, right leg CC
- S85.402 Unspecified injury of lesser saphenous vein at lower leg level, left leg CC
- S85.409 Unspecified injury of lesser saphenous vein at lower leg level, unspecified leg CC

S85.41 Laceration of lesser saphenous vein at lower leg level
- S85.411 Laceration of lesser saphenous vein at lower leg level, right leg CC
- S85.412 Laceration of lesser saphenous vein at lower leg level, left leg CC
- S85.419 Laceration of lesser saphenous vein at lower leg level, unspecified leg CC

S85.49 Other specified injury of lesser saphenous vein at lower leg level
- S85.491 Other specified injury of lesser saphenous vein at lower leg level, right leg CC
- S85.492 Other specified injury of lesser saphenous vein at lower leg level, left leg CC
- S85.499 Other specified injury of lesser saphenous vein at lower leg level, unspecified leg CC

S85.5 Injury of popliteal vein

S85.50 Unspecified injury of popliteal vein
- S85.501 Unspecified injury of popliteal vein, right leg MCC
- S85.502 Unspecified injury of popliteal vein, left leg MCC
- S85.509 Unspecified injury of popliteal vein, unspecified leg MCC

S85.51 Laceration of popliteal vein
- S85.511 Laceration of popliteal vein, right leg MCC
- S85.512 Laceration of popliteal vein, left leg MCC
- S85.519 Laceration of popliteal vein, unspecified leg MCC

S85.59 Other specified injury of popliteal vein
- S85.591 Other specified injury of popliteal vein, right leg MCC
- S85.592 Other specified injury of popliteal vein, left leg MCC
- S85.599 Other specified injury of popliteal vein, unspecified leg MCC

S85.8 Injury of other blood vessels at lower leg level

S85.80 Unspecified injury of other blood vessels at lower leg level
- S85.801 Unspecified injury of other blood vessels at lower leg level, right leg CC
- S85.802 Unspecified injury of other blood vessels at lower leg level, left leg CC

Unacceptable principal diagnosis symbol per Medicare code edits · Code exempt from diagnosis present on admission requirement
Questionable admission · CC Complication or comorbidity · CC/MCC exclusion · MCC Major complication or comorbidity
Principal diagnosis as its own CC · Principal diagnosis as its own MCC · Z code as first-listed diagnosis

S85.809 Unspecified injury of other blood vessels at lower leg level, unspecified leg

S85.81 Laceration of other blood vessels at lower leg level
S85.811 Laceration of other blood vessels at lower leg level, right leg
S85.812 Laceration of other blood vessels at lower leg level, left leg
S85.819 Laceration of other blood vessels at lower leg level, unspecified leg

S85.89 Other specified injury of other blood vessels at lower leg level
S85.891 Other specified injury of other blood vessels at lower leg level, right leg
S85.892 Other specified injury of other blood vessels at lower leg level, left leg
S85.899 Other specified injury of other blood vessels at lower leg level, unspecified leg

S85.9 Injury of unspecified blood vessel at lower leg level

S85.90 Unspecified injury of unspecified blood vessel at lower leg level
S85.901 Unspecified injury of unspecified blood vessel at lower leg level, right leg
S85.902 Unspecified injury of unspecified blood vessel at lower leg level, left leg
S85.909 Unspecified injury of unspecified blood vessel at lower leg level, unspecified leg

S85.91 Laceration of unspecified blood vessel at lower leg level
S85.911 Laceration of unspecified blood vessel at lower leg level, right leg
S85.912 Laceration of unspecified blood vessel at lower leg level, left leg
S85.919 Laceration of unspecified blood vessel at lower leg level, unspecified leg

S85.99 Other specified injury of unspecified blood vessel at lower leg level
S85.991 Other specified injury of unspecified blood vessel at lower leg level, right leg
S85.992 Other specified injury of unspecified blood vessel at lower leg level, left leg
S85.999 Other specified injury of unspecified blood vessel at lower leg level, unspecified leg

S86 Injury of muscle, fascia and tendon at lower leg level

Code also any associated open wound (S81.-)

EXCLUDES2 *injury of muscle, fascia and tendon at ankle (S96.-)*
injury of patellar ligament (tendon) (S76.1-)
sprain of joints and ligaments of knee (S83.-)

The appropriate 7th character is to be added to each code from category S86
A = initial encounter
D = subsequent encounter
S = sequela

S86.0 Injury of Achilles tendon

S86.00 Unspecified injury of Achilles tendon
S86.001 Unspecified injury of right Achilles tendon
S86.002 Unspecified injury of left Achilles tendon
S86.009 Unspecified injury of unspecified Achilles tendon

S86.01 Strain of Achilles tendon
S86.011 Strain of right Achilles tendon
S86.012 Strain of left Achilles tendon
S86.019 Strain of unspecified Achilles tendon

S86.02 Laceration of Achilles tendon
S86.021 Laceration of right Achilles tendon
S86.022 Laceration of left Achilles tendon
S86.029 Laceration of unspecified Achilles tendon

S86.09 Other specified injury of Achilles tendon
S86.091 Other specified injury of right Achilles tendon
S86.092 Other specified injury of left Achilles tendon
S86.099 Other specified injury of unspecified Achilles tendon

S86.1 Injury of other muscle(s) and tendon(s) of posterior muscle group at lower leg level

S86.10 Unspecified injury of other muscle(s) and tendon(s) of posterior muscle group at lower leg level
S86.101 Unspecified injury of other muscle(s) and tendon(s) of posterior muscle group at lower leg level, right leg
S86.102 Unspecified injury of other muscle(s) and tendon(s) of posterior muscle group at lower leg level, left leg
S86.109 Unspecified injury of other muscle(s) and tendon(s) of posterior muscle group at lower leg level, unspecified leg

S86.11 Strain of other muscle(s) and tendon(s) of posterior muscle group at lower leg level
S86.111 Strain of other muscle(s) and tendon(s) of posterior muscle group at lower leg level, right leg
S86.112 Strain of other muscle(s) and tendon(s) of posterior muscle group at lower leg level, left leg
S86.119 Strain of other muscle(s) and tendon(s) of posterior muscle group at lower leg level, unspecified leg

S86.12 Laceration of other muscle(s) and tendon(s) of posterior muscle group at lower leg level
S86.121 Laceration of other muscle(s) and tendon(s) of posterior muscle group at lower leg level, right leg
S86.122 Laceration of other muscle(s) and tendon(s) of posterior muscle group at lower leg level, left leg
S86.129 Laceration of other muscle(s) and tendon(s) of posterior muscle group at lower leg level, unspecified leg

S86.19 Other injury of other muscle(s) and tendon(s) of posterior muscle group at lower leg level
S86.191 Other injury of other muscle(s) and tendon(s) of posterior muscle group at lower leg level, right leg
S86.192 Other injury of other muscle(s) and tendon(s) of posterior muscle group at lower leg level, left leg
S86.199 Other injury of other muscle(s) and tendon(s) of posterior muscle group at lower leg level, unspecified leg

S86.2 Injury of muscle(s) and tendon(s) of anterior muscle group at lower leg level

S86.20 Unspecified injury of muscle(s) and tendon(s) of anterior muscle group at lower leg level
S86.201 Unspecified injury of muscle(s) and tendon(s) of anterior muscle group at lower leg level, right leg
S86.202 Unspecified injury of muscle(s) and tendon(s) of anterior muscle group at lower leg level, left leg
S86.209 Unspecified injury of muscle(s) and tendon(s) of anterior muscle group at lower leg level, unspecified leg

S86.21 Strain of muscle(s) and tendon(s) of anterior muscle group at lower leg level
S86.211 Strain of muscle(s) and tendon(s) of anterior muscle group at lower leg level, right leg
S86.212 Strain of muscle(s) and tendon(s) of anterior muscle group at lower leg level, left leg
S86.219 Strain of muscle(s) and tendon(s) of anterior muscle group at lower leg level, unspecified leg

S86.22 Laceration of muscle(s) and tendon(s) of anterior muscle group at lower leg level
S86.221 Laceration of muscle(s) and tendon(s) of anterior muscle group at lower leg level, right leg

Unspecified Code | Other Specified Code | Manifestation Code | N Newborn | P Pediatric | M Maternity | A Adult | ♂ Male | ♀ Female
● New Code | ▲ Revised Code Title | ►◄ Revised Text | NOTES | INCLUDES | EXCLUDES1 Not coded here | EXCLUDES2 Not included here
4th character required | 5th character required | 6th character required | 7th character required
Extension 'X' Alert | HAC Hospital-acquired condition (HAC) alert | AHA AHA Coding Clinic©

S86.222 Laceration of muscle(s) and tendon(s) of anterior muscle group at lower leg level, left leg CC
S86.229 Laceration of muscle(s) and tendon(s) of anterior muscle group at lower leg level, unspecified leg CC
S86.29 Other injury of muscle(s) and tendon(s) of anterior muscle group at lower leg level
S86.291 Other injury of muscle(s) and tendon(s) of anterior muscle group at lower leg level, right leg
S86.292 Other injury of muscle(s) and tendon(s) of anterior muscle group at lower leg level, left leg
S86.299 Other injury of muscle(s) and tendon(s) of anterior muscle group at lower leg level, unspecified leg
S86.3 Injury of muscle(s) and tendon(s) of peroneal muscle group at lower leg level
S86.30 Unspecified injury of muscle(s) and tendon(s) of peroneal muscle group at lower leg level
S86.301 Unspecified injury of muscle(s) and tendon(s) of peroneal muscle group at lower leg level, right leg
S86.302 Unspecified injury of muscle(s) and tendon(s) of peroneal muscle group at lower leg level, left leg
S86.309 Unspecified injury of muscle(s) and tendon(s) of peroneal muscle group at lower leg level, unspecified leg
S86.31 Strain of muscle(s) and tendon(s) of peroneal muscle group at lower leg level
S86.311 Strain of muscle(s) and tendon(s) of peroneal muscle group at lower leg level, right leg
S86.312 Strain of muscle(s) and tendon(s) of peroneal muscle group at lower leg level, left leg
S86.319 Strain of muscle(s) and tendon(s) of peroneal muscle group at lower leg level, unspecified leg
S86.32 Laceration of muscle(s) and tendon(s) of peroneal muscle group at lower leg level
S86.321 Laceration of muscle(s) and tendon(s) of peroneal muscle group at lower leg level, right leg CC
S86.322 Laceration of muscle(s) and tendon(s) of peroneal muscle group at lower leg level, left leg CC
S86.329 Laceration of muscle(s) and tendon(s) of peroneal muscle group at lower leg level, unspecified leg CC
S86.39 Other injury of muscle(s) and tendon(s) of peroneal muscle group at lower leg level
S86.391 Other injury of muscle(s) and tendon(s) of peroneal muscle group at lower leg level, right leg
S86.392 Other injury of muscle(s) and tendon(s) of peroneal muscle group at lower leg level, left leg
S86.399 Other injury of muscle(s) and tendon(s) of peroneal muscle group at lower leg level, unspecified leg
S86.8 Injury of other muscles and tendons at lower leg level
S86.80 Unspecified injury of other muscles and tendons at lower leg level
S86.801 Unspecified injury of other muscle(s) and tendon(s) at lower leg level, right leg
S86.802 Unspecified injury of other muscle(s) and tendon(s) at lower leg level, left leg
S86.809 Unspecified injury of other muscle(s) and tendon(s) at lower leg level, unspecified leg
S86.81 Strain of other muscles and tendons at lower leg level
S86.811 Strain of other muscle(s) and tendon(s) at lower leg level, right leg
S86.812 Strain of other muscle(s) and tendon(s) at lower leg level, left leg
S86.819 Strain of other muscle(s) and tendon(s) at lower leg level, unspecified leg
S86.82 Laceration of other muscles and tendons at lower leg level
S86.821 Laceration of other muscle(s) and tendon(s) at lower leg level, right leg CC
S86.822 Laceration of other muscle(s) and tendon(s) at lower leg level, left leg CC
S86.829 Laceration of other muscle(s) and tendon(s) at lower leg level, unspecified leg CC
S86.89 Other injury of other muscles and tendons at lower leg level
S86.891 Other injury of other muscle(s) and tendon(s) at lower leg level, right leg
S86.892 Other injury of other muscle(s) and tendon(s) at lower leg level, left leg
S86.899 Other injury of other muscle(s) and tendon(s) at lower leg level, unspecified leg
S86.9 Injury of unspecified muscle and tendon at lower leg level
S86.90 Unspecified injury of unspecified muscle and tendon at lower leg level
S86.901 Unspecified injury of unspecified muscle(s) and tendon(s) at lower leg level, right leg
S86.902 Unspecified injury of unspecified muscle(s) and tendon(s) at lower leg level, left leg
S86.909 Unspecified injury of unspecified muscle(s) and tendon(s) at lower leg level, unspecified leg
S86.91 Strain of unspecified muscle and tendon at lower leg level
S86.911 Strain of unspecified muscle(s) and tendon(s) at lower leg level, right leg
S86.912 Strain of unspecified muscle(s) and tendon(s) at lower leg level, left leg
S86.919 Strain of unspecified muscle(s) and tendon(s) at lower leg level, unspecified leg
S86.92 Laceration of unspecified muscle and tendon at lower leg level
S86.921 Laceration of unspecified muscle(s) and tendon(s) at lower leg level, right leg CC
S86.922 Laceration of unspecified muscle(s) and tendon(s) at lower leg level, left leg CC
S86.929 Laceration of unspecified muscle(s) and tendon(s) at lower leg level, unspecified leg CC
S86.99 Other injury of unspecified muscle and tendon at lower leg level
S86.991 Other injury of unspecified muscle(s) and tendon(s) at lower leg level, right leg
S86.992 Other injury of unspecified muscle(s) and tendon(s) at lower leg level, left leg
S86.999 Other injury of unspecified muscle(s) and tendon(s) at lower leg level, unspecified leg

S87 Crushing injury of lower leg
Use additional code(s) for all associated injuries
EXCLUDES2 *crushing injury of ankle and foot (S97.-)*
The appropriate 7th character is to be added to each code from category S87
A = initial encounter
D = subsequent encounter
S = sequela
S87.0 Crushing injury of knee
S87.00 Crushing injury of unspecified knee
S87.01 Crushing injury of right knee
S87.02 Crushing injury of left knee
S87.8 Crushing injury of lower leg

PDx Unacceptable principal diagnosis symbol per Medicare code edits · POA Code exempt from diagnosis present on admission requirement · ? Questionable admission · CC Complication or comorbidity · CC/MCC Exc CC/MCC exclusion · MCC Major complication or comorbidity · PDx CC Principal diagnosis as its own CC · PDx MCC Principal diagnosis as its own MCC · Z1 Z code as first-listed diagnosis

S87.80 Crushing injury of unspecified lower leg
S87.81 Crushing injury of right lower leg
S87.82 Crushing injury of left lower leg

S88 Traumatic amputation of lower leg
An amputation not identified as partial or complete should be coded to complete
EXCLUDES1 *traumatic amputation of ankle and foot (S98.-)*
The appropriate 7th character is to be added to each code from category S88
A = initial encounter
D = subsequent encounter
S = sequela

S88.0 Traumatic amputation at knee level
S88.01 Complete traumatic amputation at knee level
S88.011 Complete traumatic amputation at knee level, right lower leg
S88.012 Complete traumatic amputation at knee level, left lower leg
S88.019 Complete traumatic amputation at knee level, unspecified lower leg
S88.02 Partial traumatic amputation at knee level
S88.021 Partial traumatic amputation at knee level, right lower leg
S88.022 Partial traumatic amputation at knee level, left lower leg
S88.029 Partial traumatic amputation at knee level, unspecified lower leg

S88.1 Traumatic amputation at level between knee and ankle
S88.11 Complete traumatic amputation at level between knee and ankle
S88.111 Complete traumatic amputation at level between knee and ankle, right lower leg
S88.112 Complete traumatic amputation at level between knee and ankle, left lower leg
S88.119 Complete traumatic amputation at level between knee and ankle, unspecified lower leg
S88.12 Partial traumatic amputation at level between knee and ankle
S88.121 Partial traumatic amputation at level between knee and ankle, right lower leg
S88.122 Partial traumatic amputation at level between knee and ankle, left lower leg
S88.129 Partial traumatic amputation at level between knee and ankle, unspecified lower leg

S88.9 Traumatic amputation of lower leg, level unspecified
S88.91 Complete traumatic amputation of lower leg, level unspecified
S88.911 Complete traumatic amputation of right lower leg, level unspecified
S88.912 Complete traumatic amputation of left lower leg, level unspecified
S88.919 Complete traumatic amputation of unspecified lower leg, level unspecified
S88.92 Partial traumatic amputation of lower leg, level unspecified
S88.921 Partial traumatic amputation of right lower leg, level unspecified
S88.922 Partial traumatic amputation of left lower leg, level unspecified
S88.929 Partial traumatic amputation of unspecified lower leg, level unspecified

S89 Other and unspecified injuries of lower leg
NOTES A fracture not indicated as open or closed should be coded to closed
EXCLUDES2 *other and unspecified injuries of ankle and foot (S99.-)*
The appropriate 7th character is to be added to each code from subcategories S89.0, S89.1, S89.2, and S89.3
A = initial encounter for closed fracture
D = subsequent encounter for fracture with routine healing
G = subsequent encounter for fracture with delayed healing
K = subsequent encounter for fracture with nonunion
P = subsequent encounter for fracture with malunion
S = sequela

S89.0 Physeal fracture of upper end of tibia
S89.00 Unspecified physeal fracture of upper end of tibia
S89.001 Unspecified physeal fracture of upper end of right tibia HAC
S89.002 Unspecified physeal fracture of upper end of left tibia HAC
S89.009 Unspecified physeal fracture of upper end of unspecified tibia HAC
S89.01 Salter-Harris Type I physeal fracture of upper end of tibia
S89.011 Salter-Harris Type I physeal fracture of upper end of right tibia HAC
S89.012 Salter-Harris Type I physeal fracture of upper end of left tibia HAC
S89.019 Salter-Harris Type I physeal fracture of upper end of unspecified tibia HAC
S89.02 Salter-Harris Type II physeal fracture of upper end of tibia
S89.021 Salter-Harris Type II physeal fracture of upper end of right tibia HAC
S89.022 Salter-Harris Type II physeal fracture of upper end of left tibia HAC
S89.029 Salter-Harris Type II physeal fracture of upper end of unspecified tibia HAC
S89.03 Salter-Harris Type III physeal fracture of upper end of tibia
S89.031 Salter-Harris Type III physeal fracture of upper end of right tibia HAC
S89.032 Salter-Harris Type III physeal fracture of upper end of left tibia HAC
S89.039 Salter-Harris Type III physeal fracture of upper end of unspecified tibia HAC
S89.04 Salter-Harris Type IV physeal fracture of upper end of tibia
S89.041 Salter-Harris Type IV physeal fracture of upper end of right tibia HAC
S89.042 Salter-Harris Type IV physeal fracture of upper end of left tibia HAC
S89.049 Salter-Harris Type IV physeal fracture of upper end of unspecified tibia HAC
S89.09 Other physeal fracture of upper end of tibia
S89.091 Other physeal fracture of upper end of right tibia HAC
S89.092 Other physeal fracture of upper end of left tibia HAC
S89.099 Other physeal fracture of upper end of unspecified tibia HAC

S89.1 Physeal fracture of lower end of tibia
S89.10 Unspecified physeal fracture of lower end of tibia
S89.101 Unspecified physeal fracture of lower end of right tibia
S89.102 Unspecified physeal fracture of lower end of left tibia
S89.109 Unspecified physeal fracture of lower end of unspecified tibia
S89.11 Salter-Harris Type I physeal fracture of lower end of tibia
S89.111 Salter-Harris Type I physeal fracture of lower end of right tibia
S89.112 Salter-Harris Type I physeal fracture of lower end of left tibia
S89.119 Salter-Harris Type I physeal fracture of lower end of unspecified tibia
S89.12 Salter-Harris Type II physeal fracture of lower end of tibia
S89.121 Salter-Harris Type II physeal fracture of lower end of right tibia
S89.122 Salter-Harris Type II physeal fracture of lower end of left tibia

Unspecified Code Other Specified Code Manifestation Code N Newborn P Pediatric M Maternity A Adult ♂ Male ♀ Female
● New Code ▲ Revised Code Title ►◄ Revised Text NOTES INCLUDES EXCLUDES1 Not coded here EXCLUDES2 Not included here
4th character required 5th character required 6th character required 7th character required
Extension 'X' Alert HAC Hospital-acquired condition (HAC) alert AHA AHA Coding Clinic©

S89.129 Salter-Harris Type II physeal fracture of lower end of unspecified tibia

S89.13 Salter-Harris Type III physeal fracture of lower end of tibia

EXCLUDES1 *fracture of medial malleolus (adult) (S82.5-)*

S89.131 Salter-Harris Type III physeal fracture of lower end of right tibia

S89.132 Salter-Harris Type III physeal fracture of lower end of left tibia

S89.139 Salter-Harris Type III physeal fracture of lower end of unspecified tibia

S89.14 Salter-Harris Type IV physeal fracture of lower end of tibia

EXCLUDES1 *fracture of medial malleolus (adult) (S82.5-)*

S89.141 Salter-Harris Type IV physeal fracture of lower end of right tibia

S89.142 Salter-Harris Type IV physeal fracture of lower end of left tibia

S89.149 Salter-Harris Type IV physeal fracture of lower end of unspecified tibia

S89.19 Other physeal fracture of lower end of tibia

S89.191 Other physeal fracture of lower end of right tibia

S89.192 Other physeal fracture of lower end of left tibia

S89.199 Other physeal fracture of lower end of unspecified tibia

S89.2 Physeal fracture of upper end of fibula

S89.20 Unspecified physeal fracture of upper end of fibula

S89.201 Unspecified physeal fracture of upper end of right fibula

S89.202 Unspecified physeal fracture of upper end of left fibula

S89.209 Unspecified physeal fracture of upper end of unspecified fibula

S89.21 Salter-Harris Type I physeal fracture of upper end of fibula

S89.211 Salter-Harris Type I physeal fracture of upper end of right fibula

S89.212 Salter-Harris Type I physeal fracture of upper end of left fibula

S89.219 Salter-Harris Type I physeal fracture of upper end of unspecified fibula

S89.22 Salter-Harris Type II physeal fracture of upper end of fibula

S89.221 Salter-Harris Type II physeal fracture of upper end of right fibula

S89.222 Salter-Harris Type II physeal fracture of upper end of left fibula

S89.229 Salter-Harris Type II physeal fracture of upper end of unspecified fibula

S89.29 Other physeal fracture of upper end of fibula

S89.291 Other physeal fracture of upper end of right fibula

S89.292 Other physeal fracture of upper end of left fibula

S89.299 Other physeal fracture of upper end of unspecified fibula

S89.3 Physeal fracture of lower end of fibula

S89.30 Unspecified physeal fracture of lower end of fibula

S89.301 Unspecified physeal fracture of lower end of right fibula

S89.302 Unspecified physeal fracture of lower end of left fibula

S89.309 Unspecified physeal fracture of lower end of unspecified fibula

S89.31 Salter-Harris Type I physeal fracture of lower end of fibula

S89.311 Salter-Harris Type I physeal fracture of lower end of right fibula

S89.312 Salter-Harris Type I physeal fracture of lower end of left fibula

S89.319 Salter-Harris Type I physeal fracture of lower end of unspecified fibula

S89.32 Salter-Harris Type II physeal fracture of lower end of fibula

S89.321 Salter-Harris Type II physeal fracture of lower end of right fibula

S89.322 Salter-Harris Type II physeal fracture of lower end of left fibula

S89.329 Salter-Harris Type II physeal fracture of lower end of unspecified fibula

S89.39 Other physeal fracture of lower end of fibula

S89.391 Other physeal fracture of lower end of right fibula

S89.392 Other physeal fracture of lower end of left fibula

S89.399 Other physeal fracture of lower end of unspecified fibula

S89.8 Other specified injuries of lower leg

The appropriate 7th character is to be added to each code in subcategory S89.8

A = initial encounter
D = subsequent encounter
S = sequela

S89.80 Other specified injuries of unspecified lower leg

S89.81 Other specified injuries of right lower leg

S89.82 Other specified injuries of left lower leg

S89.9 Unspecified injury of lower leg

The appropriate 7th character is to be added to each code in subcategory S89.9

A = initial encounter
D = subsequent encounter
S = sequela

S89.90 Unspecified injury of unspecified lower leg

S89.91 Unspecified injury of right lower leg

S89.92 Unspecified injury of left lower leg

Injuries to the ankle and foot (S90-S99)

EXCLUDES2 *burns and corrosions (T20-T32)*
fracture of ankle and malleolus (S82.-)
frostbite (T33-T34)
insect bite or sting, venomous (T63.4)

S90 Superficial injury of ankle, foot and toes

The appropriate 7th character is to be added to each code from category S90

A = initial encounter
D = subsequent encounter
S = sequela

S90.0 Contusion of ankle

S90.00 Contusion of unspecified ankle

S90.01 Contusion of right ankle

S90.02 Contusion of left ankle

S90.1 Contusion of toe without damage to nail

S90.11 Contusion of great toe without damage to nail

S90.111 Contusion of right great toe without damage to nail

S90.112 Contusion of left great toe without damage to nail

S90.119 Contusion of unspecified great toe without damage to nail

S90.12 Contusion of lesser toe without damage to nail

S90.121 Contusion of right lesser toe(s) without damage to nail

S90.122 Contusion of left lesser toe(s) without damage to nail

S90.129 Contusion of unspecified lesser toe(s) without damage to nail

Contusion of toe NOS

S90.2 Contusion of toe with damage to nail

S90.21 Contusion of great toe with damage to nail

S90.211 Contusion of right great toe with damage to nail

S90.212 Contusion of left great toe with damage to nail

S90.219 Contusion of unspecified great toe with damage to nail

Unacceptable principal diagnosis symbol per Medicare code edits — Code exempt from diagnosis present on admission requirement — Questionable admission — Complication or comorbidity — CC/MCC exclusion — Major complication or comorbidity — Principal diagnosis as its own CC — Principal diagnosis as its own MCC — Z code as first-listed diagnosis

S90.22 Contusion of lesser toe with damage to nail
S90.221 Contusion of right lesser toe(s) with damage to nail
S90.222 Contusion of left lesser toe(s) with damage to nail
S90.229 Contusion of unspecified lesser toe(s) with damage to nail
S90.3 Contusion of foot
EXCLUDES2 *contusion of toes (S90.1-, S90.2-)*
S90.30 Contusion of unspecified foot
Contusion of foot NOS
S90.31 Contusion of right foot
S90.32 Contusion of left foot
S90.4 Other superficial injuries of toe
S90.41 Abrasion of toe
S90.411 Abrasion, right great toe
S90.412 Abrasion, left great toe
S90.413 Abrasion, unspecified great toe
S90.414 Abrasion, right lesser toe(s)
S90.415 Abrasion, left lesser toe(s)
S90.416 Abrasion, unspecified lesser toe(s)
S90.42 Blister (nonthermal) of toe
S90.421 Blister (nonthermal), right great toe
S90.422 Blister (nonthermal), left great toe
S90.423 Blister (nonthermal), unspecified great toe
S90.424 Blister (nonthermal), right lesser toe(s)
S90.425 Blister (nonthermal), left lesser toe(s)
S90.426 Blister (nonthermal), unspecified lesser toe(s)
S90.44 External constriction of toe
Hair tourniquet syndrome of toe
S90.441 External constriction, right great toe
S90.442 External constriction, left great toe
S90.443 External constriction, unspecified great toe
S90.444 External constriction, right lesser toe(s)
S90.445 External constriction, left lesser toe(s)
S90.446 External constriction, unspecified lesser toe(s)
S90.45 Superficial foreign body of toe
Splinter in the toe
S90.451 Superficial foreign body, right great toe
S90.452 Superficial foreign body, left great toe
S90.453 Superficial foreign body, unspecified great toe
S90.454 Superficial foreign body, right lesser toe(s)
S90.455 Superficial foreign body, left lesser toe(s)
S90.456 Superficial foreign body, unspecified lesser toe(s)
S90.46 Insect bite (nonvenomous) of toe
S90.461 Insect bite (nonvenomous), right great toe
S90.462 Insect bite (nonvenomous), left great toe
S90.463 Insect bite (nonvenomous), unspecified great toe
S90.464 Insect bite (nonvenomous), right lesser toe(s)
S90.465 Insect bite (nonvenomous), left lesser toe(s)
S90.466 Insect bite (nonvenomous), unspecified lesser toe(s)
S90.47 Other superficial bite of toe
EXCLUDES1 *open bite of toe (S91.15-, S91.25-)*
S90.471 Other superficial bite of right great toe
S90.472 Other superficial bite of left great toe
S90.473 Other superficial bite of unspecified great toe
S90.474 Other superficial bite of right lesser toe(s)
S90.475 Other superficial bite of left lesser toe(s)
S90.476 Other superficial bite of unspecified lesser toe(s)
S90.5 Other superficial injuries of ankle
S90.51 Abrasion of ankle
S90.511 Abrasion, right ankle
S90.512 Abrasion, left ankle
S90.519 Abrasion, unspecified ankle
S90.52 Blister (nonthermal) of ankle
S90.521 Blister (nonthermal), right ankle
S90.522 Blister (nonthermal), left ankle
S90.529 Blister (nonthermal), unspecified ankle
S90.54 External constriction of ankle
S90.541 External constriction, right ankle
S90.542 External constriction, left ankle
S90.549 External constriction, unspecified ankle
S90.55 Superficial foreign body of ankle
Splinter in the ankle
S90.551 Superficial foreign body, right ankle
S90.552 Superficial foreign body, left ankle
S90.559 Superficial foreign body, unspecified ankle
S90.56 Insect bite (nonvenomous) of ankle
S90.561 Insect bite (nonvenomous), right ankle
S90.562 Insect bite (nonvenomous), left ankle
S90.569 Insect bite (nonvenomous), unspecified ankle
S90.57 Other superficial bite of ankle
EXCLUDES1 *open bite of ankle (S91.05-)*
S90.571 Other superficial bite of ankle, right ankle
S90.572 Other superficial bite of ankle, left ankle
S90.579 Other superficial bite of ankle, unspecified ankle
S90.8 Other superficial injuries of foot
S90.81 Abrasion of foot
S90.811 Abrasion, right foot
S90.812 Abrasion, left foot
S90.819 Abrasion, unspecified foot
S90.82 Blister (nonthermal) of foot
S90.821 Blister (nonthermal), right foot
S90.822 Blister (nonthermal), left foot
S90.829 Blister (nonthermal), unspecified foot
S90.84 External constriction of foot
S90.841 External constriction, right foot
S90.842 External constriction, left foot
S90.849 External constriction, unspecified foot
S90.85 Superficial foreign body of foot
Splinter in the foot
S90.851 Superficial foreign body, right foot
S90.852 Superficial foreign body, left foot
S90.859 Superficial foreign body, unspecified foot
S90.86 Insect bite (nonvenomous) of foot
S90.861 Insect bite (nonvenomous), right foot
S90.862 Insect bite (nonvenomous), left foot
S90.869 Insect bite (nonvenomous), unspecified foot
S90.87 Other superficial bite of foot
EXCLUDES1 *open bite of foot (S91.35-)*
S90.871 Other superficial bite of right foot
S90.872 Other superficial bite of left foot
S90.879 Other superficial bite of unspecified foot
S90.9 Unspecified superficial injury of ankle, foot and toe
S90.91 Unspecified superficial injury of ankle
S90.911 Unspecified superficial injury of right ankle
S90.912 Unspecified superficial injury of left ankle
S90.919 Unspecified superficial injury of unspecified ankle
S90.92 Unspecified superficial injury of foot
S90.921 Unspecified superficial injury of right foot
S90.922 Unspecified superficial injury of left foot
S90.929 Unspecified superficial injury of unspecified foot
S90.93 Unspecified superficial injury of toes
S90.931 Unspecified superficial injury of right great toe
S90.932 Unspecified superficial injury of left great toe
S90.933 Unspecified superficial injury of unspecified great toe

Unspecified Code Other Specified Code Manifestation Code N Newborn P Pediatric M Maternity A Adult ♂ Male ♀ Female
● New Code ▲ Revised Code Title ►◄ Revised Text NOTES INCLUDES EXCLUDES1 Not coded here EXCLUDES2 Not included here
4th character required 5th character required 6th character required 7th character required
Extension 'X' Alert HAC Hospital-acquired condition (HAC) alert AHA AHA Coding Clinic©

S90.934 Unspecified superficial injury of right lesser toe(s)
S90.935 Unspecified superficial injury of left lesser toe(s)
S90.936 Unspecified superficial injury of unspecified lesser toe(s)

S91 Open wound of ankle, foot and toes
Code also any associated wound infection
EXCLUDES1 *open fracture of ankle, foot and toes (S92.-with 7th character B)*
traumatic amputation of ankle and foot (S98.-)
The appropriate 7th character is to be added to each code from category S91
A = initial encounter
D = subsequent encounter
S = sequela

S91.0 Open wound of ankle
S91.00 Unspecified open wound of ankle
S91.001 Unspecified open wound, right ankle
S91.002 Unspecified open wound, left ankle
S91.009 Unspecified open wound, unspecified ankle
S91.01 Laceration without foreign body of ankle
S91.011 Laceration without foreign body, right ankle
S91.012 Laceration without foreign body, left ankle
S91.019 Laceration without foreign body, unspecified ankle
S91.02 Laceration with foreign body of ankle
S91.021 Laceration with foreign body, right ankle
S91.022 Laceration with foreign body, left ankle
S91.029 Laceration with foreign body, unspecified ankle
S91.03 Puncture wound without foreign body of ankle
S91.031 Puncture wound without foreign body, right ankle
S91.032 Puncture wound without foreign body, left ankle
S91.039 Puncture wound without foreign body, unspecified ankle
S91.04 Puncture wound with foreign body of ankle
S91.041 Puncture wound with foreign body, right ankle
S91.042 Puncture wound with foreign body, left ankle
S91.049 Puncture wound with foreign body, unspecified ankle
S91.05 Open bite of ankle
EXCLUDES1 *superficial bite of ankle (S90.56-, S90.57-)*
S91.051 Open bite, right ankle
S91.052 Open bite, left ankle
S91.059 Open bite, unspecified ankle

S91.1 Open wound of toe without damage to nail
S91.10 Unspecified open wound of toe without damage to nail
S91.101 Unspecified open wound of right great toe without damage to nail
S91.102 Unspecified open wound of left great toe without damage to nail
S91.103 Unspecified open wound of unspecified great toe without damage to nail
S91.104 Unspecified open wound of right lesser toe(s) without damage to nail
S91.105 Unspecified open wound of left lesser toe(s) without damage to nail
S91.106 Unspecified open wound of unspecified lesser toe(s) without damage to nail
S91.109 Unspecified open wound of unspecified toe(s) without damage to nail
S91.11 Laceration without foreign body of toe without damage to nail
S91.111 Laceration without foreign body of right great toe without damage to nail
S91.112 Laceration without foreign body of left great toe without damage to nail
S91.113 Laceration without foreign body of unspecified great toe without damage to nail
S91.114 Laceration without foreign body of right lesser toe(s) without damage to nail
S91.115 Laceration without foreign body of left lesser toe(s) without damage to nail
S91.116 Laceration without foreign body of unspecified lesser toe(s) without damage to nail
S91.119 Laceration without foreign body of unspecified toe without damage to nail
S91.12 Laceration with foreign body of toe without damage to nail
S91.121 Laceration with foreign body of right great toe without damage to nail
S91.122 Laceration with foreign body of left great toe without damage to nail
S91.123 Laceration with foreign body of unspecified great toe without damage to nail
S91.124 Laceration with foreign body of right lesser toe(s) without damage to nail
S91.125 Laceration with foreign body of left lesser toe(s) without damage to nail
S91.126 Laceration with foreign body of unspecified lesser toe(s) without damage to nail
S91.129 Laceration with foreign body of unspecified toe(s) without damage to nail
S91.13 Puncture wound without foreign body of toe without damage to nail
S91.131 Puncture wound without foreign body of right great toe without damage to nail
S91.132 Puncture wound without foreign body of left great toe without damage to nail
S91.133 Puncture wound without foreign body of unspecified great toe without damage to nail
S91.134 Puncture wound without foreign body of right lesser toe(s) without damage to nail
S91.135 Puncture wound without foreign body of left lesser toe(s) without damage to nail
S91.136 Puncture wound without foreign body of unspecified lesser toe(s) without damage to nail
S91.139 Puncture wound without foreign body of unspecified toe(s) without damage to nail
S91.14 Puncture wound with foreign body of toe without damage to nail
S91.141 Puncture wound with foreign body of right great toe without damage to nail
S91.142 Puncture wound with foreign body of left great toe without damage to nail
S91.143 Puncture wound with foreign body of unspecified great toe without damage to nail
S91.144 Puncture wound with foreign body of right lesser toe(s) without damage to nail
S91.145 Puncture wound with foreign body of left lesser toe(s) without damage to nail
S91.146 Puncture wound with foreign body of unspecified lesser toe(s) without damage to nail
S91.149 Puncture wound with foreign body of unspecified toe(s) without damage to nail
S91.15 Open bite of toe without damage to nail
Bite of toe NOS
EXCLUDES1 *superficial bite of toe (S90.46-, S90.47-)*
S91.151 Open bite of right great toe without damage to nail
S91.152 Open bite of left great toe without damage to nail

Unacceptable principal diagnosis symbol per Medicare code edits | Code exempt from diagnosis present on admission requirement
Questionable admission | Complication or comorbidity | CC/MCC exclusion | Major complication or comorbidity
Principal diagnosis as its own CC | Principal diagnosis as its own MCC | Z code as first-listed diagnosis

S91.153 Open bite of unspecified great toe without damage to nail
S91.154 Open bite of right lesser toe(s) without damage to nail
S91.155 Open bite of left lesser toe(s) without damage to nail
S91.156 Open bite of unspecified lesser toe(s) without damage to nail
S91.159 Open bite of unspecified toe(s) without damage to nail

S91.2 Open wound of toe with damage to nail

S91.20 Unspecified open wound of toe with damage to nail
S91.201 Unspecified open wound of right great toe with damage to nail
S91.202 Unspecified open wound of left great toe with damage to nail
S91.203 Unspecified open wound of unspecified great toe with damage to nail
S91.204 Unspecified open wound of right lesser toe(s) with damage to nail
S91.205 Unspecified open wound of left lesser toe(s) with damage to nail
S91.206 Unspecified open wound of unspecified lesser toe(s) with damage to nail
S91.209 Unspecified open wound of unspecified toe(s) with damage to nail

S91.21 Laceration without foreign body of toe with damage to nail
S91.211 Laceration without foreign body of right great toe with damage to nail
S91.212 Laceration without foreign body of left great toe with damage to nail
S91.213 Laceration without foreign body of unspecified great toe with damage to nail
S91.214 Laceration without foreign body of right lesser toe(s) with damage to nail
S91.215 Laceration without foreign body of left lesser toe(s) with damage to nail
S91.216 Laceration without foreign body of unspecified lesser toe(s) with damage to nail
S91.219 Laceration without foreign body of unspecified toe(s) with damage to nail

S91.22 Laceration with foreign body of toe with damage to nail
S91.221 Laceration with foreign body of right great toe with damage to nail
S91.222 Laceration with foreign body of left great toe with damage to nail
S91.223 Laceration with foreign body of unspecified great toe with damage to nail
S91.224 Laceration with foreign body of right lesser toe(s) with damage to nail
S91.225 Laceration with foreign body of left lesser toe(s) with damage to nail
S91.226 Laceration with foreign body of unspecified lesser toe(s) with damage to nail
S91.229 Laceration with foreign body of unspecified toe(s) with damage to nail

S91.23 Puncture wound without foreign body of toe with damage to nail
S91.231 Puncture wound without foreign body of right great toe with damage to nail
S91.232 Puncture wound without foreign body of left great toe with damage to nail
S91.233 Puncture wound without foreign body of unspecified great toe with damage to nail
S91.234 Puncture wound without foreign body of right lesser toe(s) with damage to nail
S91.235 Puncture wound without foreign body of left lesser toe(s) with damage to nail
S91.236 Puncture wound without foreign body of unspecified lesser toe(s) with damage to nail
S91.239 Puncture wound without foreign body of unspecified toe(s) with damage to nail

S91.24 Puncture wound with foreign body of toe with damage to nail
S91.241 Puncture wound with foreign body of right great toe with damage to nail
S91.242 Puncture wound with foreign body of left great toe with damage to nail
S91.243 Puncture wound with foreign body of unspecified great toe with damage to nail
S91.244 Puncture wound with foreign body of right lesser toe(s) with damage to nail
S91.245 Puncture wound with foreign body of left lesser toe(s) with damage to nail
S91.246 Puncture wound with foreign body of unspecified lesser toe(s) with damage to nail
S91.249 Puncture wound with foreign body of unspecified toe(s) with damage to nail

S91.25 Open bite of toe with damage to nail
Bite of toe with damage to nail NOS
EXCLUDES1 *superficial bite of toe (S90.46-, S90.47-)*
S91.251 Open bite of right great toe with damage to nail
S91.252 Open bite of left great toe with damage to nail
S91.253 Open bite of unspecified great toe with damage to nail
S91.254 Open bite of right lesser toe(s) with damage to nail
S91.255 Open bite of left lesser toe(s) with damage to nail
S91.256 Open bite of unspecified lesser toe(s) with damage to nail
S91.259 Open bite of unspecified toe(s) with damage to nail

S91.3 Open wound of foot

S91.30 Unspecified open wound of foot
S91.301 Unspecified open wound, right foot
S91.302 Unspecified open wound, left foot
S91.309 Unspecified open wound, unspecified foot

S91.31 Laceration without foreign body of foot
S91.311 Laceration without foreign body, right foot
S91.312 Laceration without foreign body, left foot
S91.319 Laceration without foreign body, unspecified foot

S91.32 Laceration with foreign body of foot
S91.321 Laceration with foreign body, right foot
S91.322 Laceration with foreign body, left foot
S91.329 Laceration with foreign body, unspecified foot

S91.33 Puncture wound without foreign body of foot
S91.331 Puncture wound without foreign body, right foot
S91.332 Puncture wound without foreign body, left foot
S91.339 Puncture wound without foreign body, unspecified foot

S91.34 Puncture wound with foreign body of foot
S91.341 Puncture wound with foreign body, right foot
S91.342 Puncture wound with foreign body, left foot
S91.349 Puncture wound with foreign body, unspecified foot

S91.35 Open bite of foot
EXCLUDES1 *superficial bite of foot (S90.86-, S90.87-)*
S91.351 Open bite, right foot
S91.352 Open bite, left foot
S91.359 Open bite, unspecified foot

Unspecified Code | Other Specified Code | Manifestation Code | N Newborn | P Pediatric | M Maternity | A Adult | ♂ Male | ♀ Female
● New Code | ▲ Revised Code Title | ►◄ Revised Text | NOTES | INCLUDES | EXCLUDES1 Not coded here | EXCLUDES2 Not included here
4th character required | 5th character required | 6th character required | 7th character required
Extension 'X' Alert | HAC Hospital-acquired condition (HAC) alert | AHA AHA Coding Clinic®

S92 Fracture of foot and toe, except ankle

NOTES A fracture not indicated as displaced or nondisplaced should be coded to displaced
A fracture not indicated as open or closed should be coded to closed

EXCLUDES1 *traumatic amputation of ankle and foot (S98.-)*

EXCLUDES2 *fracture of ankle (S82.-)*
fracture of malleolus (S82.-)

The appropriate 7th character is to be added to each code from category S92
A = initial encounter for closed fracture
B = initial encounter for open fracture
D = subsequent encounter for fracture with routine healing
G = subsequent encounter for fracture with delayed healing
K = subsequent encounter for fracture with nonunion
P = subsequent encounter for fracture with malunion
S = sequela

S92.0 Fracture of calcaneus
Heel bone
Os calcis
EXCLUDES2 *Physeal fracture of calcaneus (S99.0-)*

S92.00 Unspecified fracture of calcaneus
S92.001 Unspecified fracture of right calcaneus CC HAC
S92.002 Unspecified fracture of left calcaneus CC HAC
S92.009 Unspecified fracture of unspecified calcaneus CC HAC

S92.01 Fracture of body of calcaneus
S92.011 Displaced fracture of body of right calcaneus CC HAC
S92.012 Displaced fracture of body of left calcaneus CC HAC
S92.013 Displaced fracture of body of unspecified calcaneus CC HAC
S92.014 Nondisplaced fracture of body of right calcaneus CC HAC
S92.015 Nondisplaced fracture of body of left calcaneus CC HAC
S92.016 Nondisplaced fracture of body of unspecified calcaneus CC HAC

S92.02 Fracture of anterior process of calcaneus
S92.021 Displaced fracture of anterior process of right calcaneus CC HAC
S92.022 Displaced fracture of anterior process of left calcaneus CC HAC
S92.023 Displaced fracture of anterior process of unspecified calcaneus CC HAC
S92.024 Nondisplaced fracture of anterior process of right calcaneus CC HAC
S92.025 Nondisplaced fracture of anterior process of left calcaneus CC HAC
S92.026 Nondisplaced fracture of anterior process of unspecified calcaneus CC HAC

S92.03 Avulsion fracture of tuberosity of calcaneus
S92.031 Displaced avulsion fracture of tuberosity of right calcaneus CC HAC
S92.032 Displaced avulsion fracture of tuberosity of left calcaneus CC HAC
S92.033 Displaced avulsion fracture of tuberosity of unspecified calcaneus CC HAC
S92.034 Nondisplaced avulsion fracture of tuberosity of right calcaneus CC HAC
S92.035 Nondisplaced avulsion fracture of tuberosity of left calcaneus CC HAC
S92.036 Nondisplaced avulsion fracture of tuberosity of unspecified calcaneus CC HAC

S92.04 Other fracture of tuberosity of calcaneus
S92.041 Displaced other fracture of tuberosity of right calcaneus CC HAC
S92.042 Displaced other fracture of tuberosity of left calcaneus CC HAC
S92.043 Displaced other fracture of tuberosity of unspecified calcaneus CC HAC
S92.044 Nondisplaced other fracture of tuberosity of right calcaneus CC HAC
S92.045 Nondisplaced other fracture of tuberosity of left calcaneus CC HAC
S92.046 Nondisplaced other fracture of tuberosity of unspecified calcaneus CC HAC

S92.05 Other extraarticular fracture of calcaneus
S92.051 Displaced other extraarticular fracture of right calcaneus CC HAC
S92.052 Displaced other extraarticular fracture of left calcaneus CC HAC
S92.053 Displaced other extraarticular fracture of unspecified calcaneus CC HAC
S92.054 Nondisplaced other extraarticular fracture of right calcaneus CC HAC
S92.055 Nondisplaced other extraarticular fracture of left calcaneus CC HAC
S92.056 Nondisplaced other extraarticular fracture of unspecified calcaneus CC HAC

S92.06 Intraarticular fracture of calcaneus
S92.061 Displaced intraarticular fracture of right calcaneus CC HAC
S92.062 Displaced intraarticular fracture of left calcaneus CC HAC
S92.063 Displaced intraarticular fracture of unspecified calcaneus CC HAC
S92.064 Nondisplaced intraarticular fracture of right calcaneus CC HAC
S92.065 Nondisplaced intraarticular fracture of left calcaneus CC HAC
S92.066 Nondisplaced intraarticular fracture of unspecified calcaneus CC HAC

S92.1 Fracture of talus
Astragalus

S92.10 Unspecified fracture of talus
S92.101 Unspecified fracture of right talus CC HAC
S92.102 Unspecified fracture of left talus CC HAC
S92.109 Unspecified fracture of unspecified talus CC HAC

S92.11 Fracture of neck of talus
S92.111 Displaced fracture of neck of right talus CC HAC
S92.112 Displaced fracture of neck of left talus CC HAC
S92.113 Displaced fracture of neck of unspecified talus CC HAC
S92.114 Nondisplaced fracture of neck of right talus CC HAC
S92.115 Nondisplaced fracture of neck of left talus CC HAC
S92.116 Nondisplaced fracture of neck of unspecified talus CC HAC

S92.12 Fracture of body of talus
S92.121 Displaced fracture of body of right talus CC HAC
S92.122 Displaced fracture of body of left talus CC HAC
S92.123 Displaced fracture of body of unspecified talus CC HAC
S92.124 Nondisplaced fracture of body of right talus CC HAC
S92.125 Nondisplaced fracture of body of left talus CC HAC
S92.126 Nondisplaced fracture of body of unspecified talus CC HAC

S92.13 Fracture of posterior process of talus

Unacceptable principal diagnosis symbol per Medicare code edits · Code exempt from diagnosis present on admission requirement
Questionable admission · Complication or comorbidity · CC/MCC exclusion · Major complication or comorbidity
Principal diagnosis as its own CC · Principal diagnosis as its own MCC · Z code as first-listed diagnosis

S92.131 Displaced fracture of posterior process of right talus HAC
S92.132 Displaced fracture of posterior process of left talus HAC
S92.133 Displaced fracture of posterior process of unspecified talus HAC
S92.134 Nondisplaced fracture of posterior process of right talus HAC
S92.135 Nondisplaced fracture of posterior process of left talus HAC
S92.136 Nondisplaced fracture of posterior process of unspecified talus HAC

S92.14 Dome fracture of talus
EXCLUDES1 *osteochondritis dissecans (M93.2)*
S92.141 Displaced dome fracture of right talus HAC
S92.142 Displaced dome fracture of left talus HAC
S92.143 Displaced dome fracture of unspecified talus HAC
S92.144 Nondisplaced dome fracture of right talus HAC
S92.145 Nondisplaced dome fracture of left talus HAC
S92.146 Nondisplaced dome fracture of unspecified talus HAC

S92.15 Avulsion fracture (chip fracture) of talus
S92.151 Displaced avulsion fracture (chip fracture) of right talus HAC
S92.152 Displaced avulsion fracture (chip fracture) of left talus HAC
S92.153 Displaced avulsion fracture (chip fracture) of unspecified talus HAC
S92.154 Nondisplaced avulsion fracture (chip fracture) of right talus HAC
S92.155 Nondisplaced avulsion fracture (chip fracture) of left talus HAC
S92.156 Nondisplaced avulsion fracture (chip fracture) of unspecified talus HAC

S92.19 Other fracture of talus
S92.191 Other fracture of right talus HAC
S92.192 Other fracture of left talus HAC
S92.199 Other fracture of unspecified talus HAC

S92.2 Fracture of other and unspecified tarsal bone(s)
S92.20 Fracture of unspecified tarsal bone(s)
S92.201 Fracture of unspecified tarsal bone(s) of right foot HAC
S92.202 Fracture of unspecified tarsal bone(s) of left foot HAC
S92.209 Fracture of unspecified tarsal bone(s) of unspecified foot HAC

S92.21 Fracture of cuboid bone
S92.211 Displaced fracture of cuboid bone of right foot HAC
S92.212 Displaced fracture of cuboid bone of left foot HAC
S92.213 Displaced fracture of cuboid bone of unspecified foot HAC
S92.214 Nondisplaced fracture of cuboid bone of right foot HAC
S92.215 Nondisplaced fracture of cuboid bone of left foot HAC
S92.216 Nondisplaced fracture of cuboid bone of unspecified foot HAC

S92.22 Fracture of lateral cuneiform
S92.221 Displaced fracture of lateral cuneiform of right foot HAC
S92.222 Displaced fracture of lateral cuneiform of left foot HAC
S92.223 Displaced fracture of lateral cuneiform of unspecified foot HAC
S92.224 Nondisplaced fracture of lateral cuneiform of right foot HAC
S92.225 Nondisplaced fracture of lateral cuneiform of left foot HAC
S92.226 Nondisplaced fracture of lateral cuneiform of unspecified foot HAC

S92.23 Fracture of intermediate cuneiform
S92.231 Displaced fracture of intermediate cuneiform of right foot HAC
S92.232 Displaced fracture of intermediate cuneiform of left foot HAC
S92.233 Displaced fracture of intermediate cuneiform of unspecified foot HAC
S92.234 Nondisplaced fracture of intermediate cuneiform of right foot HAC
S92.235 Nondisplaced fracture of intermediate cuneiform of left foot HAC
S92.236 Nondisplaced fracture of intermediate cuneiform of unspecified foot HAC

S92.24 Fracture of medial cuneiform
S92.241 Displaced fracture of medial cuneiform of right foot HAC
S92.242 Displaced fracture of medial cuneiform of left foot HAC
S92.243 Displaced fracture of medial cuneiform of unspecified foot HAC
S92.244 Nondisplaced fracture of medial cuneiform of right foot HAC
S92.245 Nondisplaced fracture of medial cuneiform of left foot HAC
S92.246 Nondisplaced fracture of medial cuneiform of unspecified foot HAC

S92.25 Fracture of navicular [scaphoid] of foot
S92.251 Displaced fracture of navicular [scaphoid] of right foot HAC
S92.252 Displaced fracture of navicular [scaphoid] of left foot HAC
S92.253 Displaced fracture of navicular [scaphoid] of unspecified foot HAC
S92.254 Nondisplaced fracture of navicular [scaphoid] of right foot HAC
S92.255 Nondisplaced fracture of navicular [scaphoid] of left foot HAC
S92.256 Nondisplaced fracture of navicular [scaphoid] of unspecified foot HAC

S92.3 Fracture of metatarsal bone(s)
EXCLUDES2 *Physeal fracture of metatarsal (S99.1-)*

S92.30 Fracture of unspecified metatarsal bone(s)
S92.301 Fracture of unspecified metatarsal bone(s), right foot HAC
S92.302 Fracture of unspecified metatarsal bone(s), left foot HAC
S92.309 Fracture of unspecified metatarsal bone(s), unspecified foot HAC

S92.31 Fracture of first metatarsal bone
S92.311 Displaced fracture of first metatarsal bone, right foot HAC
S92.312 Displaced fracture of first metatarsal bone, left foot HAC
S92.313 Displaced fracture of first metatarsal bone, unspecified foot HAC
S92.314 Nondisplaced fracture of first metatarsal bone, right foot HAC
S92.315 Nondisplaced fracture of first metatarsal bone, left foot HAC
S92.316 Nondisplaced fracture of first metatarsal bone, unspecified foot HAC

S92.32 Fracture of second metatarsal bone
S92.321 Displaced fracture of second metatarsal bone, right foot HAC
S92.322 Displaced fracture of second metatarsal bone, left foot HAC
S92.323 Displaced fracture of second metatarsal bone, unspecified foot HAC
S92.324 Nondisplaced fracture of second metatarsal bone, right foot HAC
S92.325 Nondisplaced fracture of second metatarsal bone, left foot HAC

Unspecified Code | Other Specified Code | Manifestation Code | N Newborn | P Pediatric | M Maternity | A Adult | ♂ Male | ♀ Female
● New Code | ▲ Revised Code Title | ►◄ Revised Text | NOTES | INCLUDES | EXCLUDES1 Not coded here | EXCLUDES2 Not included here
4th character required | 5th character required | 6th character required | 7th character required
Extension 'X' Alert | HAC Hospital-acquired condition (HAC) alert | AHA AHA Coding Clinic©

- S92.326 Nondisplaced fracture of second metatarsal bone, unspecified foot CC HAC
- S92.33 Fracture of third metatarsal bone
  - S92.331 Displaced fracture of third metatarsal bone, right foot CC HAC
  - S92.332 Displaced fracture of third metatarsal bone, left foot CC HAC
  - S92.333 Displaced fracture of third metatarsal bone, unspecified foot CC HAC
  - S92.334 Nondisplaced fracture of third metatarsal bone, right foot CC HAC
  - S92.335 Nondisplaced fracture of third metatarsal bone, left foot CC HAC
  - S92.336 Nondisplaced fracture of third metatarsal bone, unspecified foot CC HAC
- S92.34 Fracture of fourth metatarsal bone
  - S92.341 Displaced fracture of fourth metatarsal bone, right foot CC HAC
  - S92.342 Displaced fracture of fourth metatarsal bone, left foot CC HAC
  - S92.343 Displaced fracture of fourth metatarsal bone, unspecified foot CC HAC
  - S92.344 Nondisplaced fracture of fourth metatarsal bone, right foot CC HAC
  - S92.345 Nondisplaced fracture of fourth metatarsal bone, left foot CC HAC
  - S92.346 Nondisplaced fracture of fourth metatarsal bone, unspecified foot CC HAC
- S92.35 Fracture of fifth metatarsal bone
  - S92.351 Displaced fracture of fifth metatarsal bone, right foot CC HAC
  - S92.352 Displaced fracture of fifth metatarsal bone, left foot CC HAC
  - S92.353 Displaced fracture of fifth metatarsal bone, unspecified foot CC HAC
  - S92.354 Nondisplaced fracture of fifth metatarsal bone, right foot CC HAC
  - S92.355 Nondisplaced fracture of fifth metatarsal bone, left foot CC HAC
  - S92.356 Nondisplaced fracture of fifth metatarsal bone, unspecified foot CC HAC

S92.4 Fracture of great toe

EXCLUDES2 *Physeal fracture of phalanx of toe (S99.2-)*

- S92.40 Unspecified fracture of great toe
  - S92.401 Displaced unspecified fracture of right great toe CC
  - S92.402 Displaced unspecified fracture of left great toe CC
  - S92.403 Displaced unspecified fracture of unspecified great toe CC
  - S92.404 Nondisplaced unspecified fracture of right great toe CC
  - S92.405 Nondisplaced unspecified fracture of left great toe CC
  - S92.406 Nondisplaced unspecified fracture of unspecified great toe CC
- S92.41 Fracture of proximal phalanx of great toe
  - S92.411 Displaced fracture of proximal phalanx of right great toe CC
  - S92.412 Displaced fracture of proximal phalanx of left great toe CC
  - S92.413 Displaced fracture of proximal phalanx of unspecified great toe CC
  - S92.414 Nondisplaced fracture of proximal phalanx of right great toe CC
  - S92.415 Nondisplaced fracture of proximal phalanx of left great toe CC
  - S92.416 Nondisplaced fracture of proximal phalanx of unspecified great toe CC
- S92.42 Fracture of distal phalanx of great toe
  - S92.421 Displaced fracture of distal phalanx of right great toe CC
  - S92.422 Displaced fracture of distal phalanx of left great toe CC
  - S92.423 Displaced fracture of distal phalanx of unspecified great toe CC
  - S92.424 Nondisplaced fracture of distal phalanx of right great toe CC
  - S92.425 Nondisplaced fracture of distal phalanx of left great toe CC
  - S92.426 Nondisplaced fracture of distal phalanx of unspecified great toe CC
- S92.49 Other fracture of great toe
  - S92.491 Other fracture of right great toe CC
  - S92.492 Other fracture of left great toe CC
  - S92.499 Other fracture of unspecified great toe CC

S92.5 Fracture of lesser toe(s)

EXCLUDES2 *Physeal fracture of phalanx of toe (S99.2-)*

- S92.50 Unspecified fracture of lesser toe(s)
  - S92.501 Displaced unspecified fracture of right lesser toe(s) CC
  - S92.502 Displaced unspecified fracture of left lesser toe(s) CC
  - S92.503 Displaced unspecified fracture of unspecified lesser toe(s) CC
  - S92.504 Nondisplaced unspecified fracture of right lesser toe(s) CC
  - S92.505 Nondisplaced unspecified fracture of left lesser toe(s) CC
  - S92.506 Nondisplaced unspecified fracture of unspecified lesser toe(s) CC
- S92.51 Fracture of proximal phalanx of lesser toe(s)
  - S92.511 Displaced fracture of proximal phalanx of right lesser toe(s) CC
  - S92.512 Displaced fracture of proximal phalanx of left lesser toe(s) CC
  - S92.513 Displaced fracture of proximal phalanx of unspecified lesser toe(s) CC
  - S92.514 Nondisplaced fracture of proximal phalanx of right lesser toe(s) CC
  - S92.515 Nondisplaced fracture of proximal phalanx of left lesser toe(s) CC
  - S92.516 Nondisplaced fracture of proximal phalanx of unspecified lesser toe(s) CC
- S92.52 Fracture of medial phalanx of lesser toe(s)
  - S92.521 Displaced fracture of medial phalanx of right lesser toe(s) CC
  - S92.522 Displaced fracture of medial phalanx of left lesser toe(s) CC
  - S92.523 Displaced fracture of medial phalanx of unspecified lesser toe(s) CC
  - S92.524 Nondisplaced fracture of medial phalanx of right lesser toe(s) CC
  - S92.525 Nondisplaced fracture of medial phalanx of left lesser toe(s) CC
  - S92.526 Nondisplaced fracture of medial phalanx of unspecified lesser toe(s) CC
- S92.53 Fracture of distal phalanx of lesser toe(s)
  - S92.531 Displaced fracture of distal phalanx of right lesser toe(s) CC
  - S92.532 Displaced fracture of distal phalanx of left lesser toe(s) CC
  - S92.533 Displaced fracture of distal phalanx of unspecified lesser toe(s) CC
  - S92.534 Nondisplaced fracture of distal phalanx of right lesser toe(s) CC
  - S92.535 Nondisplaced fracture of distal phalanx of left lesser toe(s) CC
  - S92.536 Nondisplaced fracture of distal phalanx of unspecified lesser toe(s) CC
- S92.59 Other fracture of lesser toe(s)

Unacceptable principal diagnosis symbol per Medicare code edits · Code exempt from diagnosis present on admission requirement · Questionable admission · Complication or comorbidity · CC/MCC exclusion · Major complication or comorbidity · Principal diagnosis as its own CC · Principal diagnosis as its own MCC · Z code as first-listed diagnosis

When symbols appear on a code that requires a 7th character extension, refer to Appendix D to identify applicable 7th character codes.

S92.591 Other fracture of right lesser toe(s)
S92.592 Other fracture of left lesser toe(s)
S92.599 Other fracture of unspecified lesser toe(s)

● S92.8 Other fracture of foot, except ankle

● S92.81 Other fracture of foot
Sesamoid fracture of foot

● S92.811 Other fracture of right foot
● S92.812 Other fracture of left foot
● S92.819 Other fracture of unspecified foot

S92.9 Unspecified fracture of foot and toe

S92.90 Unspecified fracture of foot

S92.901 Unspecified fracture of right foot HAC
S92.902 Unspecified fracture of left foot HAC
S92.909 Unspecified fracture of unspecified foot HAC

S92.91 Unspecified fracture of toe

S92.911 Unspecified fracture of right toe(s)
S92.912 Unspecified fracture of left toe(s)
S92.919 Unspecified fracture of unspecified toe(s)

S93 Dislocation and sprain of joints and ligaments at ankle, foot and toe level

INCLUDES *avulsion of joint or ligament of ankle, foot and toe*
laceration of cartilage, joint or ligament of ankle, foot and toe
sprain of cartilage, joint or ligament of ankle, foot and toe
traumatic hemarthrosis of joint or ligament of ankle, foot and toe
traumatic rupture of joint or ligament of ankle, foot and toe
traumatic subluxation of joint or ligament of ankle, foot and toe
traumatic tear of joint or ligament of ankle, foot and toe

Code also any associated open wound

EXCLUDES2 *strain of muscle and tendon of ankle and foot (S96.-)*

The appropriate 7th character is to be added to each code from category S93
A = initial encounter
D = subsequent encounter
S = sequela

S93.0 Subluxation and dislocation of ankle joint
Subluxation and dislocation of astragalus
Subluxation and dislocation of fibula, lower end
Subluxation and dislocation of talus
Subluxation and dislocation of tibia, lower end

S93.01 Subluxation of right ankle joint
S93.02 Subluxation of left ankle joint
S93.03 Subluxation of unspecified ankle joint
S93.04 Dislocation of right ankle joint
S93.05 Dislocation of left ankle joint
S93.06 Dislocation of unspecified ankle joint

S93.1 Subluxation and dislocation of toe

S93.10 Unspecified subluxation and dislocation of toe
Dislocation of toe NOS
Subluxation of toe NOS

S93.101 Unspecified subluxation of right toe(s)
S93.102 Unspecified subluxation of left toe(s)
S93.103 Unspecified subluxation of unspecified toe(s)
S93.104 Unspecified dislocation of right toe(s)
S93.105 Unspecified dislocation of left toe(s)
S93.106 Unspecified dislocation of unspecified toe(s)

S93.11 Dislocation of interphalangeal joint

S93.111 Dislocation of interphalangeal joint of right great toe
S93.112 Dislocation of interphalangeal joint of left great toe
S93.113 Dislocation of interphalangeal joint of unspecified great toe
S93.114 Dislocation of interphalangeal joint of right lesser toe(s)
S93.115 Dislocation of interphalangeal joint of left lesser toe(s)
S93.116 Dislocation of interphalangeal joint of unspecified lesser toe(s)
S93.119 Dislocation of interphalangeal joint of unspecified toe(s)

S93.12 Dislocation of metatarsophalangeal joint

S93.121 Dislocation of metatarsophalangeal joint of right great toe
S93.122 Dislocation of metatarsophalangeal joint of left great toe
S93.123 Dislocation of metatarsophalangeal joint of unspecified great toe
S93.124 Dislocation of metatarsophalangeal joint of right lesser toe(s)
S93.125 Dislocation of metatarsophalangeal joint of left lesser toe(s)
S93.126 Dislocation of metatarsophalangeal joint of unspecified lesser toe(s)
S93.129 Dislocation of metatarsophalangeal joint of unspecified toe(s)

S93.13 Subluxation of interphalangeal joint

S93.131 Subluxation of interphalangeal joint of right great toe
S93.132 Subluxation of interphalangeal joint of left great toe
S93.133 Subluxation of interphalangeal joint of unspecified great toe
S93.134 Subluxation of interphalangeal joint of right lesser toe(s)
S93.135 Subluxation of interphalangeal joint of left lesser toe(s)
S93.136 Subluxation of interphalangeal joint of unspecified lesser toe(s)
S93.139 Subluxation of interphalangeal joint of unspecified toe(s)

S93.14 Subluxation of metatarsophalangeal joint

S93.141 Subluxation of metatarsophalangeal joint of right great toe
S93.142 Subluxation of metatarsophalangeal joint of left great toe
S93.143 Subluxation of metatarsophalangeal joint of unspecified great toe
S93.144 Subluxation of metatarsophalangeal joint of right lesser toe(s)
S93.145 Subluxation of metatarsophalangeal joint of left lesser toe(s)
S93.146 Subluxation of metatarsophalangeal joint of unspecified lesser toe(s)
S93.149 Subluxation of metatarsophalangeal joint of unspecified toe(s)

S93.3 Subluxation and dislocation of foot

EXCLUDES2 *dislocation of toe (S93.1-)*

S93.30 Unspecified subluxation and dislocation of foot
Dislocation of foot NOS
Subluxation of foot NOS

S93.301 Unspecified subluxation of right foot
S93.302 Unspecified subluxation of left foot
S93.303 Unspecified subluxation of unspecified foot
S93.304 Unspecified dislocation of right foot
S93.305 Unspecified dislocation of left foot
S93.306 Unspecified dislocation of unspecified foot

S93.31 Subluxation and dislocation of tarsal joint

S93.311 Subluxation of tarsal joint of right foot
S93.312 Subluxation of tarsal joint of left foot
S93.313 Subluxation of tarsal joint of unspecified foot
S93.314 Dislocation of tarsal joint of right foot
S93.315 Dislocation of tarsal joint of left foot
S93.316 Dislocation of tarsal joint of unspecified foot

S93.32 Subluxation and dislocation of tarsometatarsal joint

Unspecified Code | Other Specified Code | Manifestation Code | N Newborn | P Pediatric | M Maternity | A Adult | ♂ Male | ♀ Female
● New Code ▲ Revised Code Title ▶◀ Revised Text NOTES INCLUDES EXCLUDES1 Not coded here EXCLUDES2 Not included here
4th character required 5th character required 6th character required 7th character required
Extension 'X' Alert HAC Hospital-acquired condition (HAC) alert AHA AHA Coding Clinic©

S93.321 Subluxation of tarsometatarsal joint of right foot
S93.322 Subluxation of tarsometatarsal joint of left foot
S93.323 Subluxation of tarsometatarsal joint of unspecified foot
S93.324 Dislocation of tarsometatarsal joint of right foot
S93.325 Dislocation of tarsometatarsal joint of left foot
S93.326 Dislocation of tarsometatarsal joint of unspecified foot

S93.33 Other subluxation and dislocation of foot
S93.331 Other subluxation of right foot
S93.332 Other subluxation of left foot
S93.333 Other subluxation of unspecified foot
S93.334 Other dislocation of right foot
S93.335 Other dislocation of left foot
S93.336 Other dislocation of unspecified foot

S93.4 Sprain of ankle
EXCLUDES2 *injury of Achilles tendon (S86.0-)*

S93.40 Sprain of unspecified ligament of ankle
Sprain of ankle NOS
Sprained ankle NOS
S93.401 Sprain of unspecified ligament of right ankle
S93.402 Sprain of unspecified ligament of left ankle
S93.409 Sprain of unspecified ligament of unspecified ankle

S93.41 Sprain of calcaneofibular ligament
S93.411 Sprain of calcaneofibular ligament of right ankle
S93.412 Sprain of calcaneofibular ligament of left ankle
S93.419 Sprain of calcaneofibular ligament of unspecified ankle

S93.42 Sprain of deltoid ligament
S93.421 Sprain of deltoid ligament of right ankle
S93.422 Sprain of deltoid ligament of left ankle
S93.429 Sprain of deltoid ligament of unspecified ankle

S93.43 Sprain of tibiofibular ligament
S93.431 Sprain of tibiofibular ligament of right ankle
S93.432 Sprain of tibiofibular ligament of left ankle
S93.439 Sprain of tibiofibular ligament of unspecified ankle

S93.49 Sprain of other ligament of ankle
Sprain of internal collateral ligament
Sprain of talofibular ligament
S93.491 Sprain of other ligament of right ankle
S93.492 Sprain of other ligament of left ankle
S93.499 Sprain of other ligament of unspecified ankle

S93.5 Sprain of toe

S93.50 Unspecified sprain of toe
S93.501 Unspecified sprain of right great toe
S93.502 Unspecified sprain of left great toe
S93.503 Unspecified sprain of unspecified great toe
S93.504 Unspecified sprain of right lesser toe(s)
S93.505 Unspecified sprain of left lesser toe(s)
S93.506 Unspecified sprain of unspecified lesser toe(s)
S93.509 Unspecified sprain of unspecified toe(s)

S93.51 Sprain of interphalangeal joint of toe
S93.511 Sprain of interphalangeal joint of right great toe
S93.512 Sprain of interphalangeal joint of left great toe
S93.513 Sprain of interphalangeal joint of unspecified great toe
S93.514 Sprain of interphalangeal joint of right lesser toe(s)
S93.515 Sprain of interphalangeal joint of left lesser toe(s)
S93.516 Sprain of interphalangeal joint of unspecified lesser toe(s)
S93.519 Sprain of interphalangeal joint of unspecified toe(s)

S93.52 Sprain of metatarsophalangeal joint of toe
S93.521 Sprain of metatarsophalangeal joint of right great toe
S93.522 Sprain of metatarsophalangeal joint of left great toe
S93.523 Sprain of metatarsophalangeal joint of unspecified great toe
S93.524 Sprain of metatarsophalangeal joint of right lesser toe(s)
S93.525 Sprain of metatarsophalangeal joint of left lesser toe(s)
S93.526 Sprain of metatarsophalangeal joint of unspecified lesser toe(s)
S93.529 Sprain of metatarsophalangeal joint of unspecified toe(s)

S93.6 Sprain of foot
EXCLUDES2 *sprain of metatarsophalangeal joint of toe (S93.52-)*
sprain of toe (S93.5-)

S93.60 Unspecified sprain of foot
S93.601 Unspecified sprain of right foot
S93.602 Unspecified sprain of left foot
S93.609 Unspecified sprain of unspecified foot

S93.61 Sprain of tarsal ligament of foot
S93.611 Sprain of tarsal ligament of right foot
S93.612 Sprain of tarsal ligament of left foot
S93.619 Sprain of tarsal ligament of unspecified foot

S93.62 Sprain of tarsometatarsal ligament of foot
S93.621 Sprain of tarsometatarsal ligament of right foot
S93.622 Sprain of tarsometatarsal ligament of left foot
S93.629 Sprain of tarsometatarsal ligament of unspecified foot

S93.69 Other sprain of foot
S93.691 Other sprain of right foot
S93.692 Other sprain of left foot
S93.699 Other sprain of unspecified foot

S94 Injury of nerves at ankle and foot level
Code also any associated open wound (S91.-)
The appropriate 7th character is to be added to each code from category S94
A = initial encounter
D = subsequent encounter
S = sequela

S94.0 Injury of lateral plantar nerve
S94.00 Injury of lateral plantar nerve, unspecified leg
S94.01 Injury of lateral plantar nerve, right leg
S94.02 Injury of lateral plantar nerve, left leg

S94.1 Injury of medial plantar nerve
S94.10 Injury of medial plantar nerve, unspecified leg
S94.11 Injury of medial plantar nerve, right leg
S94.12 Injury of medial plantar nerve, left leg

S94.2 Injury of deep peroneal nerve at ankle and foot level
Injury of terminal, lateral branch of deep peroneal nerve
S94.20 Injury of deep peroneal nerve at ankle and foot level, unspecified leg
S94.21 Injury of deep peroneal nerve at ankle and foot level, right leg
S94.22 Injury of deep peroneal nerve at ankle and foot level, left leg

S94.3 Injury of cutaneous sensory nerve at ankle and foot level
S94.30 Injury of cutaneous sensory nerve at ankle and foot level, unspecified leg
S94.31 Injury of cutaneous sensory nerve at ankle and foot level, right leg

Unacceptable principal diagnosis symbol per Medicare code edits; Code exempt from diagnosis present on admission requirement
Questionable admission; Complication or comorbidity; CC/MCC exclusion; Major complication or comorbidity
Principal diagnosis as its own CC; Principal diagnosis as its own MCC; Z code as first-listed diagnosis

S94.32 Injury of cutaneous sensory nerve at ankle and foot level, left leg
S94.8 Injury of other nerves at ankle and foot level
S94.8X Injury of other nerves at ankle and foot level
S94.8X1 Injury of other nerves at ankle and foot level, right leg
S94.8X2 Injury of other nerves at ankle and foot level, left leg
S94.8X9 Injury of other nerves at ankle and foot level, unspecified leg
S94.9 Injury of unspecified nerve at ankle and foot level
S94.90 Injury of unspecified nerve at ankle and foot level, unspecified leg
S94.91 Injury of unspecified nerve at ankle and foot level, right leg
S94.92 Injury of unspecified nerve at ankle and foot level, left leg

S95 Injury of blood vessels at ankle and foot level
Code also any associated open wound (S91.-)
EXCLUDES2 *injury of posterior tibial artery and vein (S85.1-, S85.8-)*
The appropriate 7th character is to be added to each code from category S95
A = initial encounter
D = subsequent encounter
S = sequela

S95.0 Injury of dorsal artery of foot
S95.00 Unspecified injury of dorsal artery of foot
S95.001 Unspecified injury of dorsal artery of right foot
S95.002 Unspecified injury of dorsal artery of left foot
S95.009 Unspecified injury of dorsal artery of unspecified foot
S95.01 Laceration of dorsal artery of foot
S95.011 Laceration of dorsal artery of right foot
S95.012 Laceration of dorsal artery of left foot
S95.019 Laceration of dorsal artery of unspecified foot
S95.09 Other specified injury of dorsal artery of foot
S95.091 Other specified injury of dorsal artery of right foot
S95.092 Other specified injury of dorsal artery of left foot
S95.099 Other specified injury of dorsal artery of unspecified foot
S95.1 Injury of plantar artery of foot
S95.10 Unspecified injury of plantar artery of foot
S95.101 Unspecified injury of plantar artery of right foot
S95.102 Unspecified injury of plantar artery of left foot
S95.109 Unspecified injury of plantar artery of unspecified foot
S95.11 Laceration of plantar artery of foot
S95.111 Laceration of plantar artery of right foot
S95.112 Laceration of plantar artery of left foot
S95.119 Laceration of plantar artery of unspecified foot
S95.19 Other specified injury of plantar artery of foot
S95.191 Other specified injury of plantar artery of right foot
S95.192 Other specified injury of plantar artery of left foot
S95.199 Other specified injury of plantar artery of unspecified foot
S95.2 Injury of dorsal vein of foot
S95.20 Unspecified injury of dorsal vein of foot
S95.201 Unspecified injury of dorsal vein of right foot
S95.202 Unspecified injury of dorsal vein of left foot
S95.209 Unspecified injury of dorsal vein of unspecified foot
S95.21 Laceration of dorsal vein of foot
S95.211 Laceration of dorsal vein of right foot
S95.212 Laceration of dorsal vein of left foot
S95.219 Laceration of dorsal vein of unspecified foot
S95.29 Other specified injury of dorsal vein of foot
S95.291 Other specified injury of dorsal vein of right foot
S95.292 Other specified injury of dorsal vein of left foot
S95.299 Other specified injury of dorsal vein of unspecified foot
S95.8 Injury of other blood vessels at ankle and foot level
S95.80 Unspecified injury of other blood vessels at ankle and foot level
S95.801 Unspecified injury of other blood vessels at ankle and foot level, right leg
S95.802 Unspecified injury of other blood vessels at ankle and foot level, left leg
S95.809 Unspecified injury of other blood vessels at ankle and foot level, unspecified leg
S95.81 Laceration of other blood vessels at ankle and foot level
S95.811 Laceration of other blood vessels at ankle and foot level, right leg
S95.812 Laceration of other blood vessels at ankle and foot level, left leg
S95.819 Laceration of other blood vessels at ankle and foot level, unspecified leg
S95.89 Other specified injury of other blood vessels at ankle and foot level
S95.891 Other specified injury of other blood vessels at ankle and foot level, right leg
S95.892 Other specified injury of other blood vessels at ankle and foot level, left leg
S95.899 Other specified injury of other blood vessels at ankle and foot level, unspecified leg
S95.9 Injury of unspecified blood vessel at ankle and foot level
S95.90 Unspecified injury of unspecified blood vessel at ankle and foot level
S95.901 Unspecified injury of unspecified blood vessel at ankle and foot level, right leg
S95.902 Unspecified injury of unspecified blood vessel at ankle and foot level, left leg
S95.909 Unspecified injury of unspecified blood vessel at ankle and foot level, unspecified leg
S95.91 Laceration of unspecified blood vessel at ankle and foot level
S95.911 Laceration of unspecified blood vessel at ankle and foot level, right leg
S95.912 Laceration of unspecified blood vessel at ankle and foot level, left leg
S95.919 Laceration of unspecified blood vessel at ankle and foot level, unspecified leg
S95.99 Other specified injury of unspecified blood vessel at ankle and foot level
S95.991 Other specified injury of unspecified blood vessel at ankle and foot level, right leg
S95.992 Other specified injury of unspecified blood vessel at ankle and foot level, left leg
S95.999 Other specified injury of unspecified blood vessel at ankle and foot level, unspecified leg

S96 Injury of muscle and tendon at ankle and foot level
Code also any associated open wound (S91.-)
EXCLUDES2 *injury of Achilles tendon (S86.0-)*
sprain of joints and ligaments of ankle and foot (S93.-)
The appropriate 7th character is to be added to each code from category S96
A = initial encounter
D = subsequent encounter
S = sequela

Unspecified Code Other Specified Code Manifestation Code N Newborn P Pediatric M Maternity A Adult ♂ Male ♀ Female
● New Code ▲ Revised Code Title ►◄ Revised Text NOTES INCLUDES EXCLUDES1 Not coded here EXCLUDES2 Not included here
4th character required 5th character required 6th character required 7th character required
Extension 'X' Alert HAC Hospital-acquired condition (HAC) alert AHA AHA Coding Clinic©

S96.0 Injury of muscle and tendon of long flexor muscle of toe at ankle and foot level
S96.00 Unspecified injury of muscle and tendon of long flexor muscle of toe at ankle and foot level
S96.001 Unspecified injury of muscle and tendon of long flexor muscle of toe at ankle and foot level, right foot
S96.002 Unspecified injury of muscle and tendon of long flexor muscle of toe at ankle and foot level, left foot
S96.009 Unspecified injury of muscle and tendon of long flexor muscle of toe at ankle and foot level, unspecified foot
S96.01 Strain of muscle and tendon of long flexor muscle of toe at ankle and foot level
S96.011 Strain of muscle and tendon of long flexor muscle of toe at ankle and foot level, right foot
S96.012 Strain of muscle and tendon of long flexor muscle of toe at ankle and foot level, left foot
S96.019 Strain of muscle and tendon of long flexor muscle of toe at ankle and foot level, unspecified foot
S96.02 Laceration of muscle and tendon of long flexor muscle of toe at ankle and foot level
S96.021 Laceration of muscle and tendon of long flexor muscle of toe at ankle and foot level, right foot CC
S96.022 Laceration of muscle and tendon of long flexor muscle of toe at ankle and foot level, left foot CC
S96.029 Laceration of muscle and tendon of long flexor muscle of toe at ankle and foot level, unspecified foot CC
S96.09 Other injury of muscle and tendon of long flexor muscle of toe at ankle and foot level
S96.091 Other injury of muscle and tendon of long flexor muscle of toe at ankle and foot level, right foot
S96.092 Other injury of muscle and tendon of long flexor muscle of toe at ankle and foot level, left foot
S96.099 Other injury of muscle and tendon of long flexor muscle of toe at ankle and foot level, unspecified foot
S96.1 Injury of muscle and tendon of long extensor muscle of toe at ankle and foot level
S96.10 Unspecified injury of muscle and tendon of long extensor muscle of toe at ankle and foot level
S96.101 Unspecified injury of muscle and tendon of long extensor muscle of toe at ankle and foot level, right foot
S96.102 Unspecified injury of muscle and tendon of long extensor muscle of toe at ankle and foot level, left foot
S96.109 Unspecified injury of muscle and tendon of long extensor muscle of toe at ankle and foot level, unspecified foot
S96.11 Strain of muscle and tendon of long extensor muscle of toe at ankle and foot level
S96.111 Strain of muscle and tendon of long extensor muscle of toe at ankle and foot level, right foot
S96.112 Strain of muscle and tendon of long extensor muscle of toe at ankle and foot level, left foot
S96.119 Strain of muscle and tendon of long extensor muscle of toe at ankle and foot level, unspecified foot
S96.12 Laceration of muscle and tendon of long extensor muscle of toe at ankle and foot level
S96.121 Laceration of muscle and tendon of long extensor muscle of toe at ankle and foot level, right foot CC
S96.122 Laceration of muscle and tendon of long extensor muscle of toe at ankle and foot level, left foot CC
S96.129 Laceration of muscle and tendon of long extensor muscle of toe at ankle and foot level, unspecified foot CC
S96.19 Other specified injury of muscle and tendon of long extensor muscle of toe at ankle and foot level
S96.191 Other specified injury of muscle and tendon of long extensor muscle of toe at ankle and foot level, right foot
S96.192 Other specified injury of muscle and tendon of long extensor muscle of toe at ankle and foot level, left foot
S96.199 Other specified injury of muscle and tendon of long extensor muscle of toe at ankle and foot level, unspecified foot
S96.2 Injury of intrinsic muscle and tendon at ankle and foot level
S96.20 Unspecified injury of intrinsic muscle and tendon at ankle and foot level
S96.201 Unspecified injury of intrinsic muscle and tendon at ankle and foot level, right foot
S96.202 Unspecified injury of intrinsic muscle and tendon at ankle and foot level, left foot
S96.209 Unspecified injury of intrinsic muscle and tendon at ankle and foot level, unspecified foot
S96.21 Strain of intrinsic muscle and tendon at ankle and foot level
S96.211 Strain of intrinsic muscle and tendon at ankle and foot level, right foot
S96.212 Strain of intrinsic muscle and tendon at ankle and foot level, left foot
S96.219 Strain of intrinsic muscle and tendon at ankle and foot level, unspecified foot
S96.22 Laceration of intrinsic muscle and tendon at ankle and foot level
S96.221 Laceration of intrinsic muscle and tendon at ankle and foot level, right foot CC
S96.222 Laceration of intrinsic muscle and tendon at ankle and foot level, left foot CC
S96.229 Laceration of intrinsic muscle and tendon at ankle and foot level, unspecified foot CC
S96.29 Other specified injury of intrinsic muscle and tendon at ankle and foot level
S96.291 Other specified injury of intrinsic muscle and tendon at ankle and foot level, right foot
S96.292 Other specified injury of intrinsic muscle and tendon at ankle and foot level, left foot
S96.299 Other specified injury of intrinsic muscle and tendon at ankle and foot level, unspecified foot
S96.8 Injury of other specified muscles and tendons at ankle and foot level
S96.80 Unspecified injury of other specified muscles and tendons at ankle and foot level
S96.801 Unspecified injury of other specified muscles and tendons at ankle and foot level, right foot
S96.802 Unspecified injury of other specified muscles and tendons at ankle and foot level, left foot
S96.809 Unspecified injury of other specified muscles and tendons at ankle and foot level, unspecified foot
S96.81 Strain of other specified muscles and tendons at ankle and foot level
S96.811 Strain of other specified muscles and tendons at ankle and foot level, right foot
S96.812 Strain of other specified muscles and tendons at ankle and foot level, left foot
S96.819 Strain of other specified muscles and tendons at ankle and foot level, unspecified foot

Unacceptable principal diagnosis symbol per Medicare code edits · Code exempt from diagnosis present on admission requirement
Questionable admission · Complication or comorbidity · CC/MCC exclusion · Major complication or comorbidity
Principal diagnosis as its own CC · Principal diagnosis as its own MCC · Z code as first-listed diagnosis

S96.82 Laceration of other specified muscles and tendons at ankle and foot level
S96.821 Laceration of other specified muscles and tendons at ankle and foot level, right foot
S96.822 Laceration of other specified muscles and tendons at ankle and foot level, left foot
S96.829 Laceration of other specified muscles and tendons at ankle and foot level, unspecified foot
S96.89 Other specified injury of other specified muscles and tendons at ankle and foot level
S96.891 Other specified injury of other specified muscles and tendons at ankle and foot level, right foot
S96.892 Other specified injury of other specified muscles and tendons at ankle and foot level, left foot
S96.899 Other specified injury of other specified muscles and tendons at ankle and foot level, unspecified foot
S96.9 Injury of unspecified muscle and tendon at ankle and foot level
S96.90 Unspecified injury of unspecified muscle and tendon at ankle and foot level
S96.901 Unspecified injury of unspecified muscle and tendon at ankle and foot level, right foot
S96.902 Unspecified injury of unspecified muscle and tendon at ankle and foot level, left foot
S96.909 Unspecified injury of unspecified muscle and tendon at ankle and foot level, unspecified foot
S96.91 Strain of unspecified muscle and tendon at ankle and foot level
S96.911 Strain of unspecified muscle and tendon at ankle and foot level, right foot
S96.912 Strain of unspecified muscle and tendon at ankle and foot level, left foot
S96.919 Strain of unspecified muscle and tendon at ankle and foot level, unspecified foot
S96.92 Laceration of unspecified muscle and tendon at ankle and foot level
S96.921 Laceration of unspecified muscle and tendon at ankle and foot level, right foot
S96.922 Laceration of unspecified muscle and tendon at ankle and foot level, left foot
S96.929 Laceration of unspecified muscle and tendon at ankle and foot level, unspecified foot
S96.99 Other specified injury of unspecified muscle and tendon at ankle and foot level
S96.991 Other specified injury of unspecified muscle and tendon at ankle and foot level, right foot
S96.992 Other specified injury of unspecified muscle and tendon at ankle and foot level, left foot
S96.999 Other specified injury of unspecified muscle and tendon at ankle and foot level, unspecified foot

S97 Crushing injury of ankle and foot
Use additional code(s) for all associated injuries
The appropriate 7th character is to be added to each code from category S97
A = initial encounter
D = subsequent encounter
S = sequela
S97.0 Crushing injury of ankle
S97.00 Crushing injury of unspecified ankle
S97.01 Crushing injury of right ankle
S97.02 Crushing injury of left ankle
S97.1 Crushing injury of toe
S97.10 Crushing injury of unspecified toe(s)
S97.101 Crushing injury of unspecified right toe(s)
S97.102 Crushing injury of unspecified left toe(s)
S97.109 Crushing injury of unspecified toe(s)
Crushing injury of toe NOS
S97.11 Crushing injury of great toe
S97.111 Crushing injury of right great toe
S97.112 Crushing injury of left great toe
S97.119 Crushing injury of unspecified great toe
S97.12 Crushing injury of lesser toe(s)
S97.121 Crushing injury of right lesser toe(s)
S97.122 Crushing injury of left lesser toe(s)
S97.129 Crushing injury of unspecified lesser toe(s)
S97.8 Crushing injury of foot
S97.80 Crushing injury of unspecified foot
Crushing injury of foot NOS
S97.81 Crushing injury of right foot
S97.82 Crushing injury of left foot

S98 Traumatic amputation of ankle and foot
An amputation not identified as partial or complete should be coded to complete
The appropriate 7th character is to be added to each code from category S98
A = initial encounter
D = subsequent encounter
S = sequela
S98.0 Traumatic amputation of foot at ankle level
S98.01 Complete traumatic amputation of foot at ankle level
S98.011 Complete traumatic amputation of right foot at ankle level
S98.012 Complete traumatic amputation of left foot at ankle level
S98.019 Complete traumatic amputation of unspecified foot at ankle level
S98.02 Partial traumatic amputation of foot at ankle level
S98.021 Partial traumatic amputation of right foot at ankle level
S98.022 Partial traumatic amputation of left foot at ankle level
S98.029 Partial traumatic amputation of unspecified foot at ankle level
S98.1 Traumatic amputation of one toe
S98.11 Complete traumatic amputation of great toe
S98.111 Complete traumatic amputation of right great toe
S98.112 Complete traumatic amputation of left great toe
S98.119 Complete traumatic amputation of unspecified great toe
S98.12 Partial traumatic amputation of great toe
S98.121 Partial traumatic amputation of right great toe
S98.122 Partial traumatic amputation of left great toe
S98.129 Partial traumatic amputation of unspecified great toe
S98.13 Complete traumatic amputation of one lesser toe
Traumatic amputation of toe NOS
S98.131 Complete traumatic amputation of one right lesser toe
S98.132 Complete traumatic amputation of one left lesser toe
S98.139 Complete traumatic amputation of one unspecified lesser toe
S98.14 Partial traumatic amputation of one lesser toe
S98.141 Partial traumatic amputation of one right lesser toe
S98.142 Partial traumatic amputation of one left lesser toe
S98.149 Partial traumatic amputation of one unspecified lesser toe
S98.2 Traumatic amputation of two or more lesser toes

Unspecified Code Other Specified Code Manifestation Code N Newborn P Pediatric M Maternity A Adult ♂ Male ♀ Female
● New Code ▲ Revised Code Title ►◄ Revised Text NOTES INCLUDES EXCLUDES1 Not coded here EXCLUDES2 Not included here
4th character required 5th character required 6th character required 7th character required
Extension 'X' Alert HAC Hospital-acquired condition (HAC) alert AHA AHA Coding Clinic®

S98.21 Complete traumatic amputation of two or more lesser toes
S98.211 Complete traumatic amputation of two or more right lesser toes
S98.212 Complete traumatic amputation of two or more left lesser toes
S98.219 Complete traumatic amputation of two or more unspecified lesser toes
S98.22 Partial traumatic amputation of two or more lesser toes
S98.221 Partial traumatic amputation of two or more right lesser toes
S98.222 Partial traumatic amputation of two or more left lesser toes
S98.229 Partial traumatic amputation of two or more unspecified lesser toes
S98.3 Traumatic amputation of midfoot
S98.31 Complete traumatic amputation of midfoot
S98.311 Complete traumatic amputation of right midfoot
S98.312 Complete traumatic amputation of left midfoot
S98.319 Complete traumatic amputation of unspecified midfoot
S98.32 Partial traumatic amputation of midfoot
S98.321 Partial traumatic amputation of right midfoot
S98.322 Partial traumatic amputation of left midfoot
S98.329 Partial traumatic amputation of unspecified midfoot
S98.9 Traumatic amputation of foot, level unspecified
S98.91 Complete traumatic amputation of foot, level unspecified
S98.911 Complete traumatic amputation of right foot, level unspecified
S98.912 Complete traumatic amputation of left foot, level unspecified
S98.919 Complete traumatic amputation of unspecified foot, level unspecified
S98.92 Partial traumatic amputation of foot, level unspecified
S98.921 Partial traumatic amputation of right foot, level unspecified
S98.922 Partial traumatic amputation of left foot, level unspecified
S98.929 Partial traumatic amputation of unspecified foot, level unspecified
S99 Other and unspecified injuries of ankle and foot
● S99.0 Physeal fracture of calcaneus

The appropriate 7th character is to be added to each code from subcategories S99.0

A = initial encounter for closed fracture
B = initial encounter for open fracture
D = subsequent encounter for fracture with routine healing
G = subsequent encounter for fracture with delayed healing
K = subsequent encounter for fracture with nonunion
P = subsequent encounter for fracture with malunion
S = sequela

● S99.00 Unspecified physeal fracture of calcaneus
● S99.001 Unspecified physeal fracture of right calcaneus
● S99.002 Unspecified physeal fracture of left calcaneus
● S99.009 Unspecified physeal fracture of unspecified calcaneus
● S99.01 Salter-Harris Type I physeal fracture of calcaneus
● S99.011 Salter-Harris Type I physeal fracture of right calcaneus
● S99.012 Salter-Harris Type I physeal fracture of left calcaneus
● S99.019 Salter-Harris Type I physeal fracture of unspecified calcaneus
● S99.02 Salter-Harris Type II physeal fracture of calcaneus
● S99.021 Salter-Harris Type II physeal fracture of right calcaneus
● S99.022 Salter-Harris Type II physeal fracture of left calcaneus
● S99.029 Salter-Harris Type II physeal fracture of unspecified calcaneus
● S99.03 Salter-Harris Type III physeal fracture of calcaneus
● S99.031 Salter-Harris Type III physeal fracture of right calcaneus
● S99.032 Salter-Harris Type III physeal fracture of left calcaneus
● S99.039 Salter-Harris Type III physeal fracture of unspecified calcaneus
● S99.04 Salter-Harris Type IV physeal fracture of calcaneus
● S99.041 Salter-Harris Type IV physeal fracture of right calcaneus
● S99.042 Salter-Harris Type IV physeal fracture of left calcaneus
● S99.049 Salter-Harris Type IV physeal fracture of unspecified calcaneus
● S99.09 Other physeal fracture of calcaneus
● S99.091 Other physeal fracture of right calcaneus
● S99.092 Other physeal fracture of left calcaneus
● S99.099 Other physeal fracture of unspecified calcaneus
● S99.1 Physeal fracture of metatarsal

The appropriate 7th character is to be added to each code from subcategories S99.1

A = initial encounter for closed fracture
B = initial encounter for open fracture
D = subsequent encounter for fracture with routine healing
G = subsequent encounter for fracture with delayed healing
K = subsequent encounter for fracture with nonunion
P = subsequent encounter for fracture with malunion
S = sequela

● S99.10 Unspecified physeal fracture of metatarsal
● S99.101 Unspecified physeal fracture of right metatarsal
● S99.102 Unspecified physeal fracture of left metatarsal
● S99.109 Unspecified physeal fracture of unspecified metatarsal
● S99.11 Salter-Harris Type I physeal fracture of metatarsal
● S99.111 Salter-Harris Type I physeal fracture of right metatarsal
● S99.112 Salter-Harris Type I physeal fracture of left metatarsal
● S99.119 Salter-Harris Type I physeal fracture of unspecified metatarsal
● S99.12 Salter-Harris Type II physeal fracture of metatarsal
● S99.121 Salter-Harris Type II physeal fracture of right metatarsal
● S99.122 Salter-Harris Type II physeal fracture of left metatarsal
● S99.129 Salter-Harris Type II physeal fracture of unspecified metatarsal
● S99.13 Salter-Harris Type III physeal fracture of metatarsal
● S99.131 Salter-Harris Type III physeal fracture of right metatarsal
● S99.132 Salter-Harris Type III physeal fracture of left metatarsal
● S99.139 Salter-Harris Type III physeal fracture of unspecified metatarsal
● S99.14 Salter-Harris Type IV physeal fracture of metatarsal
● S99.141 Salter-Harris Type IV physeal fracture of right metatarsal
● S99.142 Salter-Harris Type IV physeal fracture of left metatarsal
● S99.149 Salter-Harris Type IV physeal fracture of unspecified metatarsal
● S99.19 Other physeal fracture of metatarsal
● S99.191 Other physeal fracture of right metatarsal
● S99.192 Other physeal fracture of left metatarsal

Unacceptable principal diagnosis symbol per Medicare code edits; Code exempt from diagnosis present on admission requirement; Questionable admission; Complication or comorbidity; CC/MCC exclusion; Major complication or comorbidity; Principal diagnosis as its own CC; Principal diagnosis as its own MCC; Z code as first-listed diagnosis

 When symbols appear on a code that requires a 7th character extension, refer to Appendix D to identify applicable 7th character codes.

● S99.199 Other physeal fracture of unspecified metatarsal

● S99.2 Physeal fracture of phalanx of toe

The appropriate 7th character is to be added to each code from subcategories S99.2
A = initial encounter for closed fracture
B = initial encounter for open fracture
D = subsequent encounter for fracture with routine healing
G = subsequent encounter for fracture with delayed healing
K = subsequent encounter for fracture with nonunion
P = subsequent encounter for fracture with malunion
S = sequela

● S99.20 Unspecified physeal fracture of phalanx of toe
● S99.201 Unspecified physeal fracture of phalanx of right toe
● S99.202 Unspecified physeal fracture of phalanx of left toe
● S99.209 Unspecified physeal fracture of phalanx of unspecified toe

● S99.21 Salter-Harris Type I physeal fracture of phalanx of toe
● S99.211 Salter-Harris Type I physeal fracture of phalanx of right toe
● S99.212 Salter-Harris Type I physeal fracture of phalanx of left toe
● S99.219 Salter-Harris Type I physeal fracture of phalanx of unspecified toe

● S99.22 Salter-Harris Type II physeal fracture of phalanx of toe
● S99.221 Salter-Harris Type II physeal fracture of phalanx of right toe
● S99.222 Salter-Harris Type II physeal fracture of phalanx of left toe
● S99.229 Salter-Harris Type II physeal fracture of phalanx of unspecified toe

● S99.23 Salter-Harris Type III physeal fracture of phalanx of toe
● S99.231 Salter-Harris Type III physeal fracture of phalanx of right toe
● S99.232 Salter-Harris Type III physeal fracture of phalanx of left toe
● S99.239 Salter-Harris Type III physeal fracture of phalanx of unspecified toe

● S99.24 Salter-Harris Type IV physeal fracture of phalanx of toe
● S99.241 Salter-Harris Type IV physeal fracture of phalanx of right toe
● S99.242 Salter-Harris Type IV physeal fracture of phalanx of left toe
● S99.249 Salter-Harris Type IV physeal fracture of phalanx of unspecified toe

● S99.29 Other physeal fracture of phalanx of toe
● S99.291 Other physeal fracture of phalanx of right toe
● S99.292 Other physeal fracture of phalanx of left toe
● S99.299 Other physeal fracture of phalanx of unspecified toe

S99.8 Other specified injuries of ankle and foot

The appropriate 7th character is to be added to each code from subcategory S99.8
A = initial encounter
D = subsequent encounter
S = sequela

S99.81 Other specified injuries of ankle
S99.811 Other specified injuries of right ankle
S99.812 Other specified injuries of left ankle
S99.819 Other specified injuries of unspecified ankle

S99.82 Other specified injuries of foot
S99.821 Other specified injuries of right foot
S99.822 Other specified injuries of left foot
S99.829 Other specified injuries of unspecified foot

S99.9 Unspecified injury of ankle and foot

The appropriate 7th character is to be added to each code from subcategory S99.9
A = initial encounter
D = subsequent encounter
S = sequela

S99.91 Unspecified injury of ankle
S99.911 Unspecified injury of right ankle
S99.912 Unspecified injury of left ankle
S99.919 Unspecified injury of unspecified ankle

S99.92 Unspecified injury of foot
S99.921 Unspecified injury of right foot
S99.922 Unspecified injury of left foot
S99.929 Unspecified injury of unspecified foot

Injury, poisoning and certain other consequences of external causes (T07-T88)

Injuries involving multiple body regions (T07)

EXCLUDES1 *burns and corrosions (T20-T32)*
frostbite (T33-T34)
insect bite or sting, venomous (T63.4)
sunburn (L55.-)

T07 Unspecified multiple injuries
EXCLUDES1 *injury NOS (T14)*

Injury of unspecified body region (T14)

T14 Injury of unspecified body region
EXCLUDES1 *multiple unspecified injuries (T07)*

T14.8 Other injury of unspecified body region
Abrasion NOS
Contusion NOS
Crush injury NOS
Fracture NOS
Skin injury NOS
Vascular injury NOS

T14.9 Unspecified injury
T14.90 Injury, unspecified
Injury NOS
T14.91 Suicide attempt
Attempted suicide NOS

Effects of foreign body entering through natural orifice (T15-T19)

EXCLUDES2 *foreign body accidentally left in operation wound (T81.5-)*
foreign body in penetrating wound - See open wound by body region
residual foreign body in soft tissue (M79.5)
splinter, without open wound - See superficial injury by body region

T15 Foreign body on external eye
EXCLUDES2 *foreign body in penetrating wound of orbit and eye ball (S05.4-, S05.5-)*
open wound of eyelid and periocular area (S01.1-)
retained foreign body in eyelid (H02.8-)
retained (old) foreign body in penetrating wound of orbit and eye ball (H05.5-, H44.6-, H44.7-)
superficial foreign body of eyelid and periocular area (S00.25-)

The appropriate 7th character is to be added to each code from category T15
A = initial encounter
D = subsequent encounter
S = sequela

T15.0 Foreign body in cornea
T15.00 Foreign body in cornea, unspecified eye
T15.01 Foreign body in cornea, right eye
T15.02 Foreign body in cornea, left eye

Unspecified Code Other Specified Code Manifestation Code N Newborn P Pediatric M Maternity A Adult ♂ Male ♀ Female
● New Code ▲ Revised Code Title ►◄ Revised Text NOTES INCLUDES EXCLUDES1 Not coded here EXCLUDES2 Not included here
4th character required 5th character required 6th character required 7th character required
Extension 'X' Alert HAC Hospital-acquired condition (HAC) alert AHA AHA Coding Clinic©

T15.1 Foreign body in conjunctival sac
T15.10 Foreign body in conjunctival sac, unspecified eye
T15.11 Foreign body in conjunctival sac, right eye
T15.12 Foreign body in conjunctival sac, left eye
T15.8 Foreign body in other and multiple parts of external eye
Foreign body in lacrimal punctum
T15.80 Foreign body in other and multiple parts of external eye, unspecified eye
T15.81 Foreign body in other and multiple parts of external eye, right eye
T15.82 Foreign body in other and multiple parts of external eye, left eye
T15.9 Foreign body on external eye, part unspecified
T15.90 Foreign body on external eye, part unspecified, unspecified eye
T15.91 Foreign body on external eye, part unspecified, right eye
T15.92 Foreign body on external eye, part unspecified, left eye
T16 Foreign body in ear
INCLUDES *foreign body in auditory canal*
The appropriate 7th character is to be added to each code from category T16
A = initial encounter
D = subsequent encounter
S = sequela
T16.1 Foreign body in right ear
T16.2 Foreign body in left ear
T16.9 Foreign body in ear, unspecified ear
T17 Foreign body in respiratory tract
The appropriate 7th character is to be added to each code from category T17
A = initial encounter
D = subsequent encounter
S = sequela
T17.0 Foreign body in nasal sinus
T17.1 Foreign body in nostril
Foreign body in nose NOS
T17.2 Foreign body in pharynx
Foreign body in nasopharynx
Foreign body in throat NOS
T17.20 Unspecified foreign body in pharynx
T17.200 Unspecified foreign body in pharynx causing asphyxiation
T17.208 Unspecified foreign body in pharynx causing other injury
T17.21 Gastric contents in pharynx
Aspiration of gastric contents into pharynx
Vomitus in pharynx
T17.210 Gastric contents in pharynx causing asphyxiation
T17.218 Gastric contents in pharynx causing other injury
T17.22 Food in pharynx
Bones in pharynx
Seeds in pharynx
T17.220 Food in pharynx causing asphyxiation
T17.228 Food in pharynx causing other injury
T17.29 Other foreign object in pharynx
T17.290 Other foreign object in pharynx causing asphyxiation
T17.298 Other foreign object in pharynx causing other injury
T17.3 Foreign body in larynx
T17.30 Unspecified foreign body in larynx
T17.300 Unspecified foreign body in larynx causing asphyxiation
T17.308 Unspecified foreign body in larynx causing other injury
T17.31 Gastric contents in larynx
Aspiration of gastric contents into larynx
Vomitus in larynx
T17.310 Gastric contents in larynx causing asphyxiation
T17.318 Gastric contents in larynx causing other injury
T17.32 Food in larynx
►Bones◄ in larynx
Seeds in larynx
T17.320 Food in larynx causing asphyxiation
T17.328 Food in larynx causing other injury
T17.39 Other foreign object in larynx
T17.390 Other foreign object in larynx causing asphyxiation
T17.398 Other foreign object in larynx causing other injury
T17.4 Foreign body in trachea
T17.40 Unspecified foreign body in trachea
T17.400 Unspecified foreign body in trachea causing asphyxiation CC
T17.408 Unspecified foreign body in trachea causing other injury CC
T17.41 Gastric contents in trachea
Aspiration of gastric contents into trachea
Vomitus in trachea
T17.410 Gastric contents in trachea causing asphyxiation CC
T17.418 Gastric contents in trachea causing other injury CC
T17.42 Food in trachea
Bones in trachea
Seeds in trachea
T17.420 Food in trachea causing asphyxiation CC
T17.428 Food in trachea causing other injury CC
T17.49 Other foreign object in trachea
T17.490 Other foreign object in trachea causing asphyxiation CC
T17.498 Other foreign object in trachea causing other injury CC
T17.5 Foreign body in bronchus
T17.50 Unspecified foreign body in bronchus
T17.500 Unspecified foreign body in bronchus causing asphyxiation CC
T17.508 Unspecified foreign body in bronchus causing other injury CC
T17.51 Gastric contents in bronchus
Aspiration of gastric contents into bronchus
Vomitus in bronchus
T17.510 Gastric contents in bronchus causing asphyxiation CC
T17.518 Gastric contents in bronchus causing other injury CC
T17.52 Food in bronchus
Bones in bronchus
Seeds in bronchus
T17.520 Food in bronchus causing asphyxiation CC
T17.528 Food in bronchus causing other injury CC
T17.59 Other foreign object in bronchus
T17.590 Other foreign object in bronchus causing asphyxiation CC
T17.598 Other foreign object in bronchus causing other injury CC
T17.8 Foreign body in other parts of respiratory tract
Foreign body in bronchioles
Foreign body in lung
T17.80 Unspecified foreign body in other parts of respiratory tract
T17.800 Unspecified foreign body in other parts of respiratory tract causing asphyxiation CC
T17.808 Unspecified foreign body in other parts of respiratory tract causing other injury CC
T17.81 Gastric contents in other parts of respiratory tract
Aspiration of gastric contents into other parts of respiratory tract
Vomitus in other parts of respiratory tract
T17.810 Gastric contents in other parts of respiratory tract causing asphyxiation CC
T17.818 Gastric contents in other parts of respiratory tract causing other injury CC

Unacceptable principal diagnosis symbol per Medicare code edits | Code exempt from diagnosis present on admission requirement
Questionable admission | Complication or comorbidity | CC/MCC exclusion | Major complication or comorbidity
Principal diagnosis as its own CC | Principal diagnosis as its own MCC | Z code as first-listed diagnosis

T17.82 Food in other parts of respiratory tract
Bones in other parts of respiratory tract
Seeds in other parts of respiratory tract
T17.820 Food in other parts of respiratory tract causing asphyxiation
T17.828 Food in other parts of respiratory tract causing other injury
T17.89 Other foreign object in other parts of respiratory tract
T17.890 Other foreign object in other parts of respiratory tract causing asphyxiation
T17.898 Other foreign object in other parts of respiratory tract causing other injury
T17.9 Foreign body in respiratory tract, part unspecified
T17.90 Unspecified foreign body in respiratory tract, part unspecified
T17.900 Unspecified foreign body in respiratory tract, part unspecified causing asphyxiation
T17.908 Unspecified foreign body in respiratory tract, part unspecified causing other injury
T17.91 Gastric contents in respiratory tract, part unspecified
Aspiration of gastric contents into respiratory tract, part unspecified
Vomitus in trachea respiratory tract, part unspecified
T17.910 Gastric contents in respiratory tract, part unspecified causing asphyxiation
T17.918 Gastric contents in respiratory tract, part unspecified causing other injury
T17.92 Food in respiratory tract, part unspecified
Bones in respiratory tract, part unspecified
Seeds in respiratory tract, part unspecified
T17.920 Food in respiratory tract, part unspecified causing asphyxiation
T17.928 Food in respiratory tract, part unspecified causing other injury
T17.99 Other foreign object in respiratory tract, part unspecified
T17.990 Other foreign object in respiratory tract, part unspecified in causing asphyxiation
T17.998 Other foreign object in respiratory tract, part unspecified causing other injury

T18 Foreign body in alimentary tract
EXCLUDES2 *foreign body in pharynx (T17.2-)*
The appropriate 7th character is to be added to each code from category T18
A = initial encounter
D = subsequent encounter
S = sequela
T18.0 Foreign body in mouth
T18.1 Foreign body in esophagus
EXCLUDES2 *foreign body in respiratory tract (T17.-)*
T18.10 Unspecified foreign body in esophagus
T18.100 Unspecified foreign body in esophagus causing compression of trachea
Unspecified foreign body in esophagus causing obstruction of respiration
T18.108 Unspecified foreign body in esophagus causing other injury
T18.11 Gastric contents in esophagus
Vomitus in esophagus
T18.110 Gastric contents in esophagus causing compression of trachea
Gastric contents in esophagus causing obstruction of respiration
T18.118 Gastric contents in esophagus causing other injury
T18.12 Food in esophagus
Bones in esophagus
Seeds in esophagus
T18.120 Food in esophagus causing compression of trachea
Food in esophagus causing obstruction of respiration
T18.128 Food in esophagus causing other injury
T18.19 Other foreign object in esophagus
T18.190 Other foreign object in esophagus causing compression of trachea
Other foreign body in esophagus causing obstruction of respiration
T18.198 Other foreign object in esophagus causing other injury
T18.2 Foreign body in stomach
T18.3 Foreign body in small intestine
T18.4 Foreign body in colon
T18.5 Foreign body in anus and rectum
Foreign body in rectosigmoid (junction)
T18.8 Foreign body in other parts of alimentary tract
T18.9 Foreign body of alimentary tract, part unspecified
Foreign body in digestive system NOS
Swallowed foreign body NOS

T19 Foreign body in genitourinary tract
EXCLUDES2 *complications due to implanted mesh (T83.7-)*
mechanical complications of contraceptive device (intrauterine) (vaginal) (T83.3-)
presence of contraceptive device (intrauterine) (vaginal) (Z97.5)
The appropriate 7th character is to be added to each code from category T19
A = initial encounter
D = subsequent encounter
S = sequela
T19.0 Foreign body in urethra
T19.1 Foreign body in bladder
T19.2 Foreign body in vulva and vagina ♀
T19.3 Foreign body in uterus ♀
T19.4 Foreign body in penis ♂
T19.8 Foreign body in other parts of genitourinary tract
T19.9 Foreign body in genitourinary tract, part unspecified

Burns and corrosions (T20-T32)

INCLUDES *burns (thermal) from electrical heating appliances*
burns (thermal) from electricity
burns (thermal) from flame
burns (thermal) from friction
burns (thermal) from hot air and hot gases
burns (thermal) from hot objects
burns (thermal) from lightning
burns (thermal) from radiation
chemical burn [corrosion] (external) (internal)
scalds
EXCLUDES2 *erythema [dermatitis] ab igne (L59.0)*
radiation-related disorders of the skin and subcutaneous tissue (L55-L59)
sunburn (L55.-)

Unspecified Code Other Specified Code Manifestation Code N Newborn P Pediatric M Maternity A Adult ♂ Male ♀ Female
● New Code ▲ Revised Code Title ►◄ Revised Text NOTES INCLUDES EXCLUDES1 Not coded here EXCLUDES2 Not included here
4th character required 5th character required 6th character required 7th character required
Extension 'X' Alert HAC Hospital-acquired condition (HAC) alert AHA AHA Coding Clinic©

Burns and corrosions of external body surface, specified by site (T20-T25)

INCLUDES *burns and corrosions of first degree [erythema]*
burns and corrosions of second degree [blisters][epidermal loss]
burns and corrosions of third degree [deep necrosis of underlying tissue] [full- thickness skin loss]

Use additional code from category T31 or T32 to identify extent of body surface involved

T20 Burn and corrosion of head, face, and neck
EXCLUDES2 *burn and corrosion of ear drum (T28.41, T28.91)*
burn and corrosion of eye and adnexa (T26.-)
burn and corrosion of mouth and pharynx (T28.0)

The appropriate 7th character is to be added to each code from category T20
A = initial encounter
D = subsequent encounter
S = sequela

T20.0 Burn of unspecified degree of head, face, and neck
Use additional external cause code to identify the source, place and intent of the burn (X00-X19, X75-X77, X96-X98, Y92)
T20.00 Burn of unspecified degree of head, face, and neck, unspecified site
T20.01 Burn of unspecified degree of ear [any part, except ear drum]
EXCLUDES2 *burn of ear drum (T28.41-)*
T20.011 Burn of unspecified degree of right ear [any part, except ear drum]
T20.012 Burn of unspecified degree of left ear [any part, except ear drum]
T20.019 Burn of unspecified degree of unspecified ear [any part, except ear drum]
T20.02 Burn of unspecified degree of lip(s)
T20.03 Burn of unspecified degree of chin
T20.04 Burn of unspecified degree of nose (septum)
T20.05 Burn of unspecified degree of scalp [any part]
T20.06 Burn of unspecified degree of forehead and cheek
T20.07 Burn of unspecified degree of neck
T20.09 Burn of unspecified degree of multiple sites of head, face, and neck

T20.1 Burn of first degree of head, face, and neck
Use additional external cause code to identify the source, place and intent of the burn (X00-X19, X75-X77, X96-X98, Y92)
T20.10 Burn of first degree of head, face, and neck, unspecified site
T20.11 Burn of first degree of ear [any part, except ear drum]
EXCLUDES2 *burn of ear drum (T28.41-)*
T20.111 Burn of first degree of right ear [any part, except ear drum]
T20.112 Burn of first degree of left ear [any part, except ear drum]
T20.119 Burn of first degree of unspecified ear [any part, except ear drum]
T20.12 Burn of first degree of lip(s)
T20.13 Burn of first degree of chin
T20.14 Burn of first degree of nose (septum)
T20.15 Burn of first degree of scalp [any part]
T20.16 Burn of first degree of forehead and cheek
T20.17 Burn of first degree of neck
T20.19 Burn of first degree of multiple sites of head, face, and neck

T20.2 Burn of second degree of head, face, and neck
Use additional external cause code to identify the source, place and intent of the burn (X00-X19, X75-X77, X96-X98, Y92)
T20.20 Burn of second degree of head, face, and neck, unspecified site
T20.21 Burn of second degree of ear [any part, except ear drum]
EXCLUDES2 *burn of ear drum (T28.41-)*
T20.211 Burn of second degree of right ear [any part, except ear drum]
T20.212 Burn of second degree of left ear [any part, except ear drum]
T20.219 Burn of second degree of unspecified ear [any part, except ear drum]
T20.22 Burn of second degree of lip(s)
T20.23 Burn of second degree of chin
T20.24 Burn of second degree of nose (septum)
T20.25 Burn of second degree of scalp [any part]
AHA: Q1, 2015
T20.26 Burn of second degree of forehead and cheek
T20.27 Burn of second degree of neck
T20.29 Burn of second degree of multiple sites of head, face, and neck

T20.3 Burn of third degree of head, face, and neck
Use additional external cause code to identify the source, place and intent of the burn (X00-X19, X75-X77, X96-X98, Y92)
T20.30 Burn of third degree of head, face, and neck, unspecified site CC HAC
T20.31 Burn of third degree of ear [any part, except ear drum]
EXCLUDES2 *burn of ear drum (T28.41-)*
T20.311 Burn of third degree of right ear [any part, except ear drum] CC HAC
T20.312 Burn of third degree of left ear [any part, except ear drum] CC HAC
AHA: Q1, 2015
T20.319 Burn of third degree of unspecified ear [any part, except ear drum] CC HAC
T20.32 Burn of third degree of lip(s) CC HAC
T20.33 Burn of third degree of chin CC HAC
T20.34 Burn of third degree of nose (septum) CC HAC
T20.35 Burn of third degree of scalp [any part] CC HAC
T20.36 Burn of third degree of forehead and cheek CC HAC
T20.37 Burn of third degree of neck CC HAC
T20.39 Burn of third degree of multiple sites of head, face, and neck CC HAC

T20.4 Corrosion of unspecified degree of head, face, and neck
Code first (T51-T65) to identify chemical and intent
Use additional external cause code to identify place (Y92)
T20.40 Corrosion of unspecified degree of head, face, and neck, unspecified site
T20.41 Corrosion of unspecified degree of ear [any part, except ear drum]
EXCLUDES2 *corrosion of ear drum (T28.91-)*
T20.411 Corrosion of unspecified degree of right ear [any part, except ear drum]
T20.412 Corrosion of unspecified degree of left ear [any part, except ear drum]
T20.419 Corrosion of unspecified degree of unspecified ear [any part, except ear drum]
T20.42 Corrosion of unspecified degree of lip(s)
T20.43 Corrosion of unspecified degree of chin
T20.44 Corrosion of unspecified degree of nose (septum)
T20.45 Corrosion of unspecified degree of scalp [any part]
T20.46 Corrosion of unspecified degree of forehead and cheek
T20.47 Corrosion of unspecified degree of neck
T20.49 Corrosion of unspecified degree of multiple sites of head, face, and neck

T20.5 Corrosion of first degree of head, face, and neck
Code first (T51-T65) to identify chemical and intent
Use additional external cause code to identify place (Y92)
T20.50 Corrosion of first degree of head, face, and neck, unspecified site
T20.51 Corrosion of first degree of ear [any part, except ear drum]
EXCLUDES2 *corrosion of ear drum (T28.91-)*
T20.511 Corrosion of first degree of right ear [any part, except ear drum]

Unacceptable principal diagnosis symbol per Medicare code edits | Code exempt from diagnosis present on admission requirement
Questionable admission | Complication or comorbidity | CC/MCC exclusion | Major complication or comorbidity
Principal diagnosis as its own CC | Principal diagnosis as its own MCC | Z code as first-listed diagnosis

When symbols appear on a code that requires a 7th character extension, refer to Appendix D to identify applicable 7th character codes.

T20.512 Corrosion of first degree of left ear [any part, except ear drum]
T20.519 Corrosion of first degree of unspecified ear [any part, except ear drum]
T20.52 Corrosion of first degree of lip(s)
T20.53 Corrosion of first degree of chin
T20.54 Corrosion of first degree of nose (septum)
T20.55 Corrosion of first degree of scalp [any part]
T20.56 Corrosion of first degree of forehead and cheek
T20.57 Corrosion of first degree of neck
T20.59 Corrosion of first degree of multiple sites of head, face, and neck

T20.6 Corrosion of second degree of head, face, and neck
Code first (T51-T65) to identify chemical and intent
Use additional external cause code to identify place (Y92)
T20.60 Corrosion of second degree of head, face, and neck, unspecified site
T20.61 Corrosion of second degree of ear [any part, except ear drum]
EXCLUDES2 *corrosion of ear drum (T28.91-)*
T20.611 Corrosion of second degree of right ear [any part, except ear drum]
T20.612 Corrosion of second degree of left ear [any part, except ear drum]
T20.619 Corrosion of second degree of unspecified ear [any part, except ear drum]
T20.62 Corrosion of second degree of lip(s)
T20.63 Corrosion of second degree of chin
T20.64 Corrosion of second degree of nose (septum)
T20.65 Corrosion of second degree of scalp [any part]
T20.66 Corrosion of second degree of forehead and cheek
T20.67 Corrosion of second degree of neck
T20.69 Corrosion of second degree of multiple sites of head, face, and neck

T20.7 Corrosion of third degree of head, face, and neck
Code first (T51-T65) to identify chemical and intent
Use additional external cause code to identify place (Y92)
T20.70 Corrosion of third degree of head, face, and neck, unspecified site CC HAC
T20.71 Corrosion of third degree of ear [any part, except ear drum]
EXCLUDES2 *corrosion of ear drum (T28.91-)*
T20.711 Corrosion of third degree of right ear [any part, except ear drum] CC HAC
T20.712 Corrosion of third degree of left ear [any part, except ear drum] CC HAC
T20.719 Corrosion of third degree of unspecified ear [any part, except ear drum] CC HAC
T20.72 Corrosion of third degree of lip(s) CC HAC
T20.73 Corrosion of third degree of chin CC HAC
T20.74 Corrosion of third degree of nose (septum) CC HAC
T20.75 Corrosion of third degree of scalp [any part] CC HAC
T20.76 Corrosion of third degree of forehead and cheek CC HAC
T20.77 Corrosion of third degree of neck CC HAC
T20.79 Corrosion of third degree of multiple sites of head, face, and neck CC HAC

T21 Burn and corrosion of trunk
INCLUDES *burns and corrosion of hip region*
EXCLUDES2 *burns and corrosion of axilla (T22.- with fifth character 4)*
burns and corrosion of scapular region (T22.- with fifth character 6)
burns and corrosion of shoulder (T22.- with fifth character 5)

The appropriate 7th character is to be added to each code from category T21
A = initial encounter
D = subsequent encounter
S = sequela

T21.0 Burn of unspecified degree of trunk
Use additional external cause code to identify the source, place and intent of the burn (X00-X19, X75-X77, X96-X98, Y92)
T21.00 Burn of unspecified degree of trunk, unspecified site
T21.01 Burn of unspecified degree of chest wall
Burn of unspecified degree of breast
T21.02 Burn of unspecified degree of abdominal wall
Burn of unspecified degree of flank
Burn of unspecified degree of groin
T21.03 Burn of unspecified degree of upper back
Burn of unspecified degree of interscapular region
T21.04 Burn of unspecified degree of lower back
T21.05 Burn of unspecified degree of buttock
Burn of unspecified degree of anus
T21.06 Burn of unspecified degree of male genital region ♂
Burn of unspecified degree of penis
Burn of unspecified degree of scrotum
Burn of unspecified degree of testis
T21.07 Burn of unspecified degree of female genital region ♀
Burn of unspecified degree of labium (majus) (minus)
Burn of unspecified degree of perineum
Burn of unspecified degree of vulva
EXCLUDES2 *burn of vagina (T28.3)*
T21.09 Burn of unspecified degree of other site of trunk

T21.1 Burn of first degree of trunk
Use additional external cause code to identify the source, place and intent of the burn (X00-X19, X75-X77, X96-X98, Y92)
T21.10 Burn of first degree of trunk, unspecified site
T21.11 Burn of first degree of chest wall
Burn of first degree of breast
T21.12 Burn of first degree of abdominal wall
Burn of first degree of flank
Burn of first degree of groin
T21.13 Burn of first degree of upper back
Burn of first degree of interscapular region
T21.14 Burn of first degree of lower back
T21.15 Burn of first degree of buttock
Burn of first degree of anus
T21.16 Burn of first degree of male genital region ♂
Burn of first degree of penis
Burn of first degree of scrotum
Burn of first degree of testis
T21.17 Burn of first degree of female genital region ♀
Burn of first degree of labium (majus) (minus)
Burn of first degree of perineum
Burn of first degree of vulva
EXCLUDES2 *burn of vagina (T28.3)*
T21.19 Burn of first degree of other site of trunk

T21.2 Burn of second degree of trunk
Use additional external cause code to identify the source, place and intent of the burn (X00-X19, X75-X77, X96-X98, Y92)
T21.20 Burn of second degree of trunk, unspecified site
T21.21 Burn of second degree of chest wall
Burn of second degree of breast
T21.22 Burn of second degree of abdominal wall
Burn of second degree of flank
Burn of second degree of groin
T21.23 Burn of second degree of upper back
Burn of second degree of interscapular region
T21.24 Burn of second degree of lower back
T21.25 Burn of second degree of buttock
Burn of second degree of anus
T21.26 Burn of second degree of male genital region ♂
Burn of second degree of penis
Burn of second degree of scrotum
Burn of second degree of testis
T21.27 Burn of second degree of female genital region ♀
Burn of second degree of labium (majus) (minus)
Burn of second degree of perineum
Burn of second degree of vulva
EXCLUDES2 *burn of vagina (T28.3)*
T21.29 Burn of second degree of other site of trunk

T21.3 Burn of third degree of trunk
Use additional external cause code to identify the source, place and intent of the burn (X00-X19, X75-X77, X96-X98, Y92)

Unspecified Code | Other Specified Code | Manifestation Code | N Newborn | P Pediatric | M Maternity | A Adult | ♂ Male | ♀ Female
● New Code | ▲ Revised Code Title | ►◄ Revised Text | NOTES | INCLUDES | EXCLUDES1 Not coded here | EXCLUDES2 Not included here
4th character required | 5th character required | 6th character required | 7th character required
Extension 'X' Alert | HAC Hospital-acquired condition (HAC) alert | AHA AHA Coding Clinic©

T21.30 **Burn of third degree of trunk, unspecified site** CC HAC

T21.31 **Burn of third degree of chest wall** CC HAC
Burn of third degree of breast
AHA: Q2, 2016

T21.32 **Burn of third degree of abdominal wall** CC HAC
Burn of third degree of flank
Burn of third degree of groin

T21.33 **Burn of third degree of upper back** CC HAC
Burn of third degree of interscapular region

T21.34 **Burn of third degree of lower back** CC HAC

T21.35 **Burn of third degree of buttock** CC HAC
Burn of third degree of anus

T21.36 **Burn of third degree of male genital region** CC HAC ♂
Burn of third degree of penis
Burn of third degree of scrotum
Burn of third degree of testis

T21.37 **Burn of third degree of female genital region** CC HAC ♀
Burn of third degree of labium (majus) (minus)
Burn of third degree of perineum
Burn of third degree of vulva
EXCLUDES2 *burn of vagina (T28.3)*

T21.39 **Burn of third degree of other site of trunk** CC HAC

T21.4 **Corrosion of unspecified degree of trunk**
Code first (T51-T65) to identify chemical and intent
Use additional external cause code to identify place (Y92)

T21.40 **Corrosion of unspecified degree of trunk, unspecified site**

T21.41 **Corrosion of unspecified degree of chest wall**
Corrosion of unspecified degree of breast

T21.42 **Corrosion of unspecified degree of abdominal wall**
Corrosion of unspecified degree of flank
Corrosion of unspecified degree of groin

T21.43 **Corrosion of unspecified degree of upper back**
Corrosion of unspecified degree of interscapular region

T21.44 **Corrosion of unspecified degree of lower back**

T21.45 **Corrosion of unspecified degree of buttock**
Corrosion of unspecified degree of anus

T21.46 **Corrosion of unspecified degree of male genital region** ♂
Corrosion of unspecified degree of penis
Corrosion of unspecified degree of scrotum
Corrosion of unspecified degree of testis

T21.47 **Corrosion of unspecified degree of female genital region** ♀
Corrosion of unspecified degree of labium (majus) (minus)
Corrosion of unspecified degree of perineum
Corrosion of unspecified degree of vulva
EXCLUDES2 *corrosion of vagina (T28.8)*

T21.49 **Corrosion of unspecified degree of other site of trunk**

T21.5 **Corrosion of first degree of trunk**
Code first (T51-T65) to identify chemical and intent
Use additional external cause code to identify place (Y92)

T21.50 **Corrosion of first degree of trunk, unspecified site**

T21.51 **Corrosion of first degree of chest wall**
Corrosion of first degree of breast

T21.52 **Corrosion of first degree of abdominal wall**
Corrosion of first degree of flank
Corrosion of first degree of groin

T21.53 **Corrosion of first degree of upper back**
Corrosion of first degree of interscapular region

T21.54 **Corrosion of first degree of lower back**

T21.55 **Corrosion of first degree of buttock**
Corrosion of first degree of anus

T21.56 **Corrosion of first degree of male genital region** ♂
Corrosion of first degree of penis
Corrosion of first degree of scrotum
Corrosion of first degree of testis

T21.57 **Corrosion of first degree of female genital region** ♀
Corrosion of first degree of labium (majus) (minus)
Corrosion of first degree of perineum
Corrosion of first degree of vulva
EXCLUDES2 *corrosion of vagina (T28.8)*

T21.59 **Corrosion of first degree of other site of trunk**

T21.6 **Corrosion of second degree of trunk**
Code first (T51-T65) to identify chemical and intent
Use additional external cause code to identify place (Y92)

T21.60 **Corrosion of second degree of trunk, unspecified site**

T21.61 **Corrosion of second degree of chest wall**
Corrosion of second degree of breast

T21.62 **Corrosion of second degree of abdominal wall**
Corrosion of second degree of flank
Corrosion of second degree of groin

T21.63 **Corrosion of second degree of upper back**
Corrosion of second degree of interscapular region

T21.64 **Corrosion of second degree of lower back**

T21.65 **Corrosion of second degree of buttock**
Corrosion of second degree of anus

T21.66 **Corrosion of second degree of male genital region** ♂
Corrosion of second degree of penis
Corrosion of second degree of scrotum
Corrosion of second degree of testis

T21.67 **Corrosion of second degree of female genital region** ♀
Corrosion of second degree of labium (majus) (minus)
Corrosion of second degree of perineum
Corrosion of second degree of vulva
EXCLUDES2 *corrosion of vagina (T28.8)*

T21.69 **Corrosion of second degree of other site of trunk**

T21.7 **Corrosion of third degree of trunk**
Code first (T51-T65) to identify chemical and intent
Use additional external cause code to identify place (Y92)

T21.70 **Corrosion of third degree of trunk, unspecified site** CC HAC

T21.71 **Corrosion of third degree of chest wall** CC HAC
Corrosion of third degree of breast

T21.72 **Corrosion of third degree of abdominal wall** CC HAC
Corrosion of third degree of flank
Corrosion of third degree of groin

T21.73 **Corrosion of third degree of upper back** CC HAC
Corrosion of third degree of interscapular region

T21.74 **Corrosion of third degree of lower back** CC HAC

T21.75 **Corrosion of third degree of buttock** CC HAC
Corrosion of third degree of anus

T21.76 **Corrosion of third degree of male genital region** CC HAC ♂
Corrosion of third degree of penis
Corrosion of third degree of scrotum
Corrosion of third degree of testis

T21.77 **Corrosion of third degree of female genital region** CC HAC ♀
Corrosion of third degree of labium (majus) (minus)
Corrosion of third degree of perineum
Corrosion of third degree of vulva
EXCLUDES2 *corrosion of vagina (T28.8)*

T21.79 **Corrosion of third degree of other site of trunk** CC HAC

T22 **Burn and corrosion of shoulder and upper limb, except wrist and hand**
EXCLUDES2 *burn and corrosion of interscapular region (T21.-)*
burn and corrosion of wrist and hand (T23.-)

The appropriate 7th character is to be added to each code from category T22
A = initial encounter
D = subsequent encounter
S = sequela

T22.0 **Burn of unspecified degree of shoulder and upper limb, except wrist and hand**
Use additional external cause code to identify the source, place and intent of the burn (X00-X19, X75-X77, X96-X98, Y92)

T22.00 **Burn of unspecified degree of shoulder and upper limb, except wrist and hand, unspecified site**

T22.01 **Burn of unspecified degree of forearm**

T22.011 **Burn of unspecified degree of right forearm**

Unacceptable principal diagnosis symbol per Medicare code edits | Code exempt from diagnosis present on admission requirement
Questionable admission | Complication or comorbidity | CC/MCC exclusion | Major complication or comorbidity
Principal diagnosis as its own CC | Principal diagnosis as its own MCC | Z code as first-listed diagnosis

T22.012 Burn of unspecified degree of left forearm
T22.019 Burn of unspecified degree of unspecified forearm
T22.02 Burn of unspecified degree of elbow
T22.021 Burn of unspecified degree of right elbow
T22.022 Burn of unspecified degree of left elbow
T22.029 Burn of unspecified degree of unspecified elbow
T22.03 Burn of unspecified degree of upper arm
T22.031 Burn of unspecified degree of right upper arm
T22.032 Burn of unspecified degree of left upper arm
T22.039 Burn of unspecified degree of unspecified upper arm
T22.04 Burn of unspecified degree of axilla
T22.041 Burn of unspecified degree of right axilla
T22.042 Burn of unspecified degree of left axilla
T22.049 Burn of unspecified degree of unspecified axilla
T22.05 Burn of unspecified degree of shoulder
T22.051 Burn of unspecified degree of right shoulder
T22.052 Burn of unspecified degree of left shoulder
T22.059 Burn of unspecified degree of unspecified shoulder
T22.06 Burn of unspecified degree of scapular region
T22.061 Burn of unspecified degree of right scapular region
T22.062 Burn of unspecified degree of left scapular region
T22.069 Burn of unspecified degree of unspecified scapular region
T22.09 Burn of unspecified degree of multiple sites of shoulder and upper limb, except wrist and hand
T22.091 Burn of unspecified degree of multiple sites of right shoulder and upper limb, except wrist and hand
T22.092 Burn of unspecified degree of multiple sites of left shoulder and upper limb, except wrist and hand
T22.099 Burn of unspecified degree of multiple sites of unspecified shoulder and upper limb, except wrist and hand
T22.1 Burn of first degree of shoulder and upper limb, except wrist and hand
Use additional external cause code to identify the source, place and intent of the burn (X00-X19, X75-X77, X96-X98, Y92)
T22.10 Burn of first degree of shoulder and upper limb, except wrist and hand, unspecified site
T22.11 Burn of first degree of forearm
T22.111 Burn of first degree of right forearm
T22.112 Burn of first degree of left forearm
T22.119 Burn of first degree of unspecified forearm
T22.12 Burn of first degree of elbow
T22.121 Burn of first degree of right elbow
T22.122 Burn of first degree of left elbow
T22.129 Burn of first degree of unspecified elbow
T22.13 Burn of first degree of upper arm
T22.131 Burn of first degree of right upper arm
T22.132 Burn of first degree of left upper arm
T22.139 Burn of first degree of unspecified upper arm
T22.14 Burn of first degree of axilla
T22.141 Burn of first degree of right axilla
T22.142 Burn of first degree of left axilla
T22.149 Burn of first degree of unspecified axilla
T22.15 Burn of first degree of shoulder
T22.151 Burn of first degree of right shoulder
T22.152 Burn of first degree of left shoulder
T22.159 Burn of first degree of unspecified shoulder
T22.16 Burn of first degree of scapular region
T22.161 Burn of first degree of right scapular region
T22.162 Burn of first degree of left scapular region
T22.169 Burn of first degree of unspecified scapular region
T22.19 Burn of first degree of multiple sites of shoulder and upper limb, except wrist and hand
T22.191 Burn of first degree of multiple sites of right shoulder and upper limb, except wrist and hand
T22.192 Burn of first degree of multiple sites of left shoulder and upper limb, except wrist and hand
T22.199 Burn of first degree of multiple sites of unspecified shoulder and upper limb, except wrist and hand
T22.2 Burn of second degree of shoulder and upper limb, except wrist and hand
Use additional external cause code to identify the source, place and intent of the burn (X00-X19, X75-X77, X96-X98, Y92)
T22.20 Burn of second degree of shoulder and upper limb, except wrist and hand, unspecified site
T22.21 Burn of second degree of forearm
T22.211 Burn of second degree of right forearm
T22.212 Burn of second degree of left forearm
T22.219 Burn of second degree of unspecified forearm
T22.22 Burn of second degree of elbow
T22.221 Burn of second degree of right elbow
T22.222 Burn of second degree of left elbow
T22.229 Burn of second degree of unspecified elbow
T22.23 Burn of second degree of upper arm
T22.231 Burn of second degree of right upper arm
T22.232 Burn of second degree of left upper arm
T22.239 Burn of second degree of unspecified upper arm
T22.24 Burn of second degree of axilla
T22.241 Burn of second degree of right axilla
T22.242 Burn of second degree of left axilla
T22.249 Burn of second degree of unspecified axilla
T22.25 Burn of second degree of shoulder
T22.251 Burn of second degree of right shoulder
T22.252 Burn of second degree of left shoulder
T22.259 Burn of second degree of unspecified shoulder
T22.26 Burn of second degree of scapular region
T22.261 Burn of second degree of right scapular region
T22.262 Burn of second degree of left scapular region
T22.269 Burn of second degree of unspecified scapular region
T22.29 Burn of second degree of multiple sites of shoulder and upper limb, except wrist and hand
T22.291 Burn of second degree of multiple sites of right shoulder and upper limb, except wrist and hand
T22.292 Burn of second degree of multiple sites of left shoulder and upper limb, except wrist and hand
T22.299 Burn of second degree of multiple sites of unspecified shoulder and upper limb, except wrist and hand
T22.3 Burn of third degree of shoulder and upper limb, except wrist and hand
Use additional external cause code to identify the source, place and intent of the burn (X00-X19, X75-X77, X96-X98, Y92)
T22.30 Burn of third degree of shoulder and upper limb, except wrist and hand, unspecified site CC HAC
T22.31 Burn of third degree of forearm

Unspecified Code Other Specified Code Manifestation Code N Newborn P Pediatric M Maternity A Adult ♂ Male ♀ Female
● New Code ▲ Revised Code Title ►◄ Revised Text NOTES INCLUDES EXCLUDES1 Not coded here EXCLUDES2 Not included here
4th character required 5th character required 6th character required 7th character required
Extension 'X' Alert HAC Hospital-acquired condition (HAC) alert AHA AHA Coding Clinic©

- T22.311 Burn of third degree of right forearm CC HAC
- T22.312 Burn of third degree of left forearm CC HAC
- T22.319 Burn of third degree of unspecified forearm CC HAC

T22.32 Burn of third degree of elbow
- T22.321 Burn of third degree of right elbow CC HAC
- T22.322 Burn of third degree of left elbow CC HAC
- T22.329 Burn of third degree of unspecified elbow CC HAC

T22.33 Burn of third degree of upper arm
- T22.331 Burn of third degree of right upper arm CC HAC
- T22.332 Burn of third degree of left upper arm CC HAC
- T22.339 Burn of third degree of unspecified upper arm CC HAC

T22.34 Burn of third degree of axilla
- T22.341 Burn of third degree of right axilla CC HAC
- T22.342 Burn of third degree of left axilla CC HAC
- T22.349 Burn of third degree of unspecified axilla CC HAC

T22.35 Burn of third degree of shoulder
- T22.351 Burn of third degree of right shoulder CC HAC
- T22.352 Burn of third degree of left shoulder CC HAC
- T22.359 Burn of third degree of unspecified shoulder CC HAC

T22.36 Burn of third degree of scapular region
- T22.361 Burn of third degree of right scapular region CC HAC
- T22.362 Burn of third degree of left scapular region CC HAC
- T22.369 Burn of third degree of unspecified scapular region CC HAC

T22.39 Burn of third degree of multiple sites of shoulder and upper limb, except wrist and hand
- T22.391 Burn of third degree of multiple sites of right shoulder and upper limb, except wrist and hand CC HAC
- T22.392 Burn of third degree of multiple sites of left shoulder and upper limb, except wrist and hand CC HAC
- T22.399 Burn of third degree of multiple sites of unspecified shoulder and upper limb, except wrist and hand CC HAC

T22.4 Corrosion of unspecified degree of shoulder and upper limb, except wrist and hand

Code first (T51-T65) to identify chemical and intent

Use additional external cause code to identify place (Y92)

T22.40 Corrosion of unspecified degree of shoulder and upper limb, except wrist and hand, unspecified site

T22.41 Corrosion of unspecified degree of forearm
- T22.411 Corrosion of unspecified degree of right forearm
- T22.412 Corrosion of unspecified degree of left forearm
- T22.419 Corrosion of unspecified degree of unspecified forearm

T22.42 Corrosion of unspecified degree of elbow
- T22.421 Corrosion of unspecified degree of right elbow
- T22.422 Corrosion of unspecified degree of left elbow
- T22.429 Corrosion of unspecified degree of unspecified elbow

T22.43 Corrosion of unspecified degree of upper arm
- T22.431 Corrosion of unspecified degree of right upper arm
- T22.432 Corrosion of unspecified degree of left upper arm
- T22.439 Corrosion of unspecified degree of unspecified upper arm

T22.44 Corrosion of unspecified degree of axilla
- T22.441 Corrosion of unspecified degree of right axilla
- T22.442 Corrosion of unspecified degree of left axilla
- T22.449 Corrosion of unspecified degree of unspecified axilla

T22.45 Corrosion of unspecified degree of shoulder
- T22.451 Corrosion of unspecified degree of right shoulder
- T22.452 Corrosion of unspecified degree of left shoulder
- T22.459 Corrosion of unspecified degree of unspecified shoulder

T22.46 Corrosion of unspecified degree of scapular region
- T22.461 Corrosion of unspecified degree of right scapular region
- T22.462 Corrosion of unspecified degree of left scapular region
- T22.469 Corrosion of unspecified degree of unspecified scapular region

T22.49 Corrosion of unspecified degree of multiple sites of shoulder and upper limb, except wrist and hand
- T22.491 Corrosion of unspecified degree of multiple sites of right shoulder and upper limb, except wrist and hand
- T22.492 Corrosion of unspecified degree of multiple sites of left shoulder and upper limb, except wrist and hand
- T22.499 Corrosion of unspecified degree of multiple sites of unspecified shoulder and upper limb, except wrist and hand

T22.5 Corrosion of first degree of shoulder and upper limb, except wrist and hand

Code first (T51-T65) to identify chemical and intent

Use additional external cause code to identify place (Y92)

T22.50 Corrosion of first degree of shoulder and upper limb, except wrist and hand unspecified site

T22.51 Corrosion of first degree of forearm
- T22.511 Corrosion of first degree of right forearm
- T22.512 Corrosion of first degree of left forearm
- T22.519 Corrosion of first degree of unspecified forearm

T22.52 Corrosion of first degree of elbow
- T22.521 Corrosion of first degree of right elbow
- T22.522 Corrosion of first degree of left elbow
- T22.529 Corrosion of first degree of unspecified elbow

T22.53 Corrosion of first degree of upper arm
- T22.531 Corrosion of first degree of right upper arm
- T22.532 Corrosion of first degree of left upper arm
- T22.539 Corrosion of first degree of unspecified upper arm

T22.54 Corrosion of first degree of axilla
- T22.541 Corrosion of first degree of right axilla
- T22.542 Corrosion of first degree of left axilla
- T22.549 Corrosion of first degree of unspecified axilla

T22.55 Corrosion of first degree of shoulder
- T22.551 Corrosion of first degree of right shoulder
- T22.552 Corrosion of first degree of left shoulder
- T22.559 Corrosion of first degree of unspecified shoulder

T22.56 Corrosion of first degree of scapular region
- T22.561 Corrosion of first degree of right scapular region
- T22.562 Corrosion of first degree of left scapular region
- T22.569 Corrosion of first degree of unspecified scapular region

Unacceptable principal diagnosis symbol per Medicare code edits · Code exempt from diagnosis present on admission requirement
Questionable admission · CC Complication or comorbidity · CC/MCC exclusion · MCC Major complication or comorbidity
Principal diagnosis as its own CC · Principal diagnosis as its own MCC · Z code as first-listed diagnosis

T22.59 Corrosion of first degree of multiple sites of shoulder and upper limb, except wrist and hand
T22.591 Corrosion of first degree of multiple sites of right shoulder and upper limb, except wrist and hand
T22.592 Corrosion of first degree of multiple sites of left shoulder and upper limb, except wrist and hand
T22.599 Corrosion of first degree of multiple sites of unspecified shoulder and upper limb, except wrist and hand
T22.6 Corrosion of second degree of shoulder and upper limb, except wrist and hand
Code first (T51-T65) to identify chemical and intent
Use additional external cause code to identify place (Y92)
T22.60 Corrosion of second degree of shoulder and upper limb, except wrist and hand, unspecified site
T22.61 Corrosion of second degree of forearm
T22.611 Corrosion of second degree of right forearm
T22.612 Corrosion of second degree of left forearm
T22.619 Corrosion of second degree of unspecified forearm
T22.62 Corrosion of second degree of elbow
T22.621 Corrosion of second degree of right elbow
T22.622 Corrosion of second degree of left elbow
T22.629 Corrosion of second degree of unspecified elbow
T22.63 Corrosion of second degree of upper arm
T22.631 Corrosion of second degree of right upper arm
T22.632 Corrosion of second degree of left upper arm
T22.639 Corrosion of second degree of unspecified upper arm
T22.64 Corrosion of second degree of axilla
T22.641 Corrosion of second degree of right axilla
T22.642 Corrosion of second degree of left axilla
T22.649 Corrosion of second degree of unspecified axilla
T22.65 Corrosion of second degree of shoulder
T22.651 Corrosion of second degree of right shoulder
T22.652 Corrosion of second degree of left shoulder
T22.659 Corrosion of second degree of unspecified shoulder
T22.66 Corrosion of second degree of scapular region
T22.661 Corrosion of second degree of right scapular region
T22.662 Corrosion of second degree of left scapular region
T22.669 Corrosion of second degree of unspecified scapular region
T22.69 Corrosion of second degree of multiple sites of shoulder and upper limb, except wrist and hand
T22.691 Corrosion of second degree of multiple sites of right shoulder and upper limb, except wrist and hand
T22.692 Corrosion of second degree of multiple sites of left shoulder and upper limb, except wrist and hand
T22.699 Corrosion of second degree of multiple sites of unspecified shoulder and upper limb, except wrist and hand
T22.7 Corrosion of third degree of shoulder and upper limb, except wrist and hand
Code first (T51-T65) to identify chemical and intent
Use additional external cause code to identify place (Y92)
T22.70 Corrosion of third degree of shoulder and upper limb, except wrist and hand, unspecified site HAC
T22.71 Corrosion of third degree of forearm
T22.711 Corrosion of third degree of right forearm HAC
T22.712 Corrosion of third degree of left forearm HAC
T22.719 Corrosion of third degree of unspecified forearm HAC
T22.72 Corrosion of third degree of elbow
T22.721 Corrosion of third degree of right elbow HAC
T22.722 Corrosion of third degree of left elbow HAC
T22.729 Corrosion of third degree of unspecified elbow HAC
T22.73 Corrosion of third degree of upper arm
T22.731 Corrosion of third degree of right upper arm HAC
T22.732 Corrosion of third degree of left upper arm HAC
T22.739 Corrosion of third degree of unspecified upper arm HAC
T22.74 Corrosion of third degree of axilla
T22.741 Corrosion of third degree of right axilla HAC
T22.742 Corrosion of third degree of left axilla HAC
T22.749 Corrosion of third degree of unspecified axilla HAC
T22.75 Corrosion of third degree of shoulder
T22.751 Corrosion of third degree of right shoulder HAC
T22.752 Corrosion of third degree of left shoulder HAC
T22.759 Corrosion of third degree of unspecified shoulder HAC
T22.76 Corrosion of third degree of scapular region
T22.761 Corrosion of third degree of right scapular region HAC
T22.762 Corrosion of third degree of left scapular region HAC
T22.769 Corrosion of third degree of unspecified scapular region HAC
T22.79 Corrosion of third degree of multiple sites of shoulder and upper limb, except wrist and hand
T22.791 Corrosion of third degree of multiple sites of right shoulder and upper limb, except wrist and hand HAC
T22.792 Corrosion of third degree of multiple sites of left shoulder and upper limb, except wrist and hand HAC
T22.799 Corrosion of third degree of multiple sites of unspecified shoulder and upper limb, except wrist and hand HAC

T23 Burn and corrosion of wrist and hand
The appropriate 7th character is to be added to each code from category T23
A = initial encounter
D = subsequent encounter
S = sequela
T23.0 Burn of unspecified degree of wrist and hand
Use additional external cause code to identify the source, place and intent of the burn (X00-X19, X75-X77, X96-X98, Y92)
T23.00 Burn of unspecified degree of hand, unspecified site
T23.001 Burn of unspecified degree of right hand, unspecified site
T23.002 Burn of unspecified degree of left hand, unspecified site
T23.009 Burn of unspecified degree of unspecified hand, unspecified site
T23.01 Burn of unspecified degree of thumb (nail)
T23.011 Burn of unspecified degree of right thumb (nail)
T23.012 Burn of unspecified degree of left thumb (nail)
T23.019 Burn of unspecified degree of unspecified thumb (nail)

Unspecified Code Other Specified Code Manifestation Code N Newborn P Pediatric M Maternity A Adult ♂ Male ♀ Female
● New Code ▲ Revised Code Title ►◄ Revised Text NOTES INCLUDES EXCLUDES1 Not coded here EXCLUDES2 Not included here
4th character required 5th character required 6th character required 7th character required
Extension 'X' Alert HAC Hospital-acquired condition (HAC) alert AHA AHA Coding Clinic®

T23.02 Burn of unspecified degree of single finger (nail) except thumb
T23.021 Burn of unspecified degree of single right finger (nail) except thumb
T23.022 Burn of unspecified degree of single left finger (nail) except thumb
T23.029 Burn of unspecified degree of unspecified single finger (nail) except thumb
T23.03 Burn of unspecified degree of multiple fingers (nail), not including thumb
T23.031 Burn of unspecified degree of multiple right fingers (nail), not including thumb
T23.032 Burn of unspecified degree of multiple left fingers (nail), not including thumb
T23.039 Burn of unspecified degree of unspecified multiple fingers (nail), not including thumb
T23.04 Burn of unspecified degree of multiple fingers (nail), including thumb
T23.041 Burn of unspecified degree of multiple right fingers (nail), including thumb
T23.042 Burn of unspecified degree of multiple left fingers (nail), including thumb
T23.049 Burn of unspecified degree of unspecified multiple fingers (nail), including thumb
T23.05 Burn of unspecified degree of palm
T23.051 Burn of unspecified degree of right palm
T23.052 Burn of unspecified degree of left palm
T23.059 Burn of unspecified degree of unspecified palm
T23.06 Burn of unspecified degree of back of hand
T23.061 Burn of unspecified degree of back of right hand
T23.062 Burn of unspecified degree of back of left hand
T23.069 Burn of unspecified degree of back of unspecified hand
T23.07 Burn of unspecified degree of wrist
T23.071 Burn of unspecified degree of right wrist
T23.072 Burn of unspecified degree of left wrist
T23.079 Burn of unspecified degree of unspecified wrist
T23.09 Burn of unspecified degree of multiple sites of wrist and hand
T23.091 Burn of unspecified degree of multiple sites of right wrist and hand
T23.092 Burn of unspecified degree of multiple sites of left wrist and hand
T23.099 Burn of unspecified degree of multiple sites of unspecified wrist and hand
T23.1 Burn of first degree of wrist and hand
Use additional external cause code to identify the source, place and intent of the burn (X00-X19, X75-X77, X96-X98, Y92)
T23.10 Burn of first degree of hand, unspecified site
T23.101 Burn of first degree of right hand, unspecified site
T23.102 Burn of first degree of left hand, unspecified site
T23.109 Burn of first degree of unspecified hand, unspecified site
T23.11 Burn of first degree of thumb (nail)
T23.111 Burn of first degree of right thumb (nail)
T23.112 Burn of first degree of left thumb (nail)
T23.119 Burn of first degree of unspecified thumb (nail)
T23.12 Burn of first degree of single finger (nail) except thumb
T23.121 Burn of first degree of single right finger (nail) except thumb
T23.122 Burn of first degree of single left finger (nail) except thumb
T23.129 Burn of first degree of unspecified single finger (nail) except thumb
T23.13 Burn of first degree of multiple fingers (nail), not including thumb
T23.131 Burn of first degree of multiple right fingers (nail), not including thumb
T23.132 Burn of first degree of multiple left fingers (nail), not including thumb
T23.139 Burn of first degree of unspecified multiple fingers (nail), not including thumb
T23.14 Burn of first degree of multiple fingers (nail), including thumb
T23.141 Burn of first degree of multiple right fingers (nail), including thumb
T23.142 Burn of first degree of multiple left fingers (nail), including thumb
T23.149 Burn of first degree of unspecified multiple fingers (nail), including thumb
T23.15 Burn of first degree of palm
T23.151 Burn of first degree of right palm
T23.152 Burn of first degree of left palm
T23.159 Burn of first degree of unspecified palm
T23.16 Burn of first degree of back of hand
T23.161 Burn of first degree of back of right hand
T23.162 Burn of first degree of back of left hand
T23.169 Burn of first degree of back of unspecified hand
T23.17 Burn of first degree of wrist
T23.171 Burn of first degree of right wrist
T23.172 Burn of first degree of left wrist
T23.179 Burn of first degree of unspecified wrist
T23.19 Burn of first degree of multiple sites of wrist and hand
T23.191 Burn of first degree of multiple sites of right wrist and hand
T23.192 Burn of first degree of multiple sites of left wrist and hand
T23.199 Burn of first degree of multiple sites of unspecified wrist and hand
T23.2 Burn of second degree of wrist and hand
Use additional external cause code to identify the source, place and intent of the burn (X00-X19, X75-X77, X96-X98, Y92)
T23.20 Burn of second degree of hand, unspecified site
T23.201 Burn of second degree of right hand, unspecified site
T23.202 Burn of second degree of left hand, unspecified site
T23.209 Burn of second degree of unspecified hand, unspecified site
T23.21 Burn of second degree of thumb (nail)
T23.211 Burn of second degree of right thumb (nail)
T23.212 Burn of second degree of left thumb (nail)
T23.219 Burn of second degree of unspecified thumb (nail)
T23.22 Burn of second degree of single finger (nail) except thumb
T23.221 Burn of second degree of single right finger (nail) except thumb
T23.222 Burn of second degree of single left finger (nail) except thumb
T23.229 Burn of second degree of unspecified single finger (nail) except thumb
T23.23 Burn of second degree of multiple fingers (nail), not including thumb
T23.231 Burn of second degree of multiple right fingers (nail), not including thumb
T23.232 Burn of second degree of multiple left fingers (nail), not including thumb
T23.239 Burn of second degree of unspecified multiple fingers (nail), not including thumb
T23.24 Burn of second degree of multiple fingers (nail), including thumb
T23.241 Burn of second degree of multiple right fingers (nail), including thumb

Unacceptable principal diagnosis symbol per Medicare code edits · Code exempt from diagnosis present on admission requirement
Questionable admission · Complication or comorbidity · CC/MCC exclusion · Major complication or comorbidity
Principal diagnosis as its own CC · Principal diagnosis as its own MCC · Z code as first-listed diagnosis

 When symbols appear on a code that requires a 7th character extension, refer to Appendix D to identify applicable 7th character codes.

T23.242 Burn of second degree of multiple left fingers (nail), including thumb
T23.249 Burn of second degree of unspecified multiple fingers (nail), including thumb
T23.25 Burn of second degree of palm
T23.251 Burn of second degree of right palm
T23.252 Burn of second degree of left palm
T23.259 Burn of second degree of unspecified palm
T23.26 Burn of second degree of back of hand
T23.261 Burn of second degree of back of right hand
T23.262 Burn of second degree of back of left hand
T23.269 Burn of second degree of back of unspecified hand
T23.27 Burn of second degree of wrist
T23.271 Burn of second degree of right wrist
T23.272 Burn of second degree of left wrist
T23.279 Burn of second degree of unspecified wrist
T23.29 Burn of second degree of multiple sites of wrist and hand
T23.291 Burn of second degree of multiple sites of right wrist and hand
T23.292 Burn of second degree of multiple sites of left wrist and hand
T23.299 Burn of second degree of multiple sites of unspecified wrist and hand

T23.3 Burn of third degree of wrist and hand
Use additional external cause code to identify the source, place and intent of the burn (X00-X19, X75-X77, X96-X98, Y92)
T23.30 Burn of third degree of hand, unspecified site
T23.301 Burn of third degree of right hand, unspecified site HAC
AHA: Q1, 2015
T23.302 Burn of third degree of left hand, unspecified site HAC
AHA: Q2, 2016
T23.309 Burn of third degree of unspecified hand, unspecified site HAC
T23.31 Burn of third degree of thumb (nail)
T23.311 Burn of third degree of right thumb (nail) HAC
T23.312 Burn of third degree of left thumb (nail) HAC
T23.319 Burn of third degree of unspecified thumb (nail) HAC
T23.32 Burn of third degree of single finger (nail) except thumb
T23.321 Burn of third degree of single right finger (nail) except thumb HAC
T23.322 Burn of third degree of single left finger (nail) except thumb HAC
T23.329 Burn of third degree of unspecified single finger (nail) except thumb HAC
T23.33 Burn of third degree of multiple fingers (nail), not including thumb
T23.331 Burn of third degree of multiple right fingers (nail), not including thumb HAC
T23.332 Burn of third degree of multiple left fingers (nail), not including thumb HAC
T23.339 Burn of third degree of unspecified multiple fingers (nail), not including thumb HAC
T23.34 Burn of third degree of multiple fingers (nail), including thumb
T23.341 Burn of third degree of multiple right fingers (nail), including thumb HAC
T23.342 Burn of third degree of multiple left fingers (nail), including thumb HAC
T23.349 Burn of third degree of unspecified multiple fingers (nail), including thumb HAC
T23.35 Burn of third degree of palm
T23.351 Burn of third degree of right palm HAC
T23.352 Burn of third degree of left palm HAC
T23.359 Burn of third degree of unspecified palm HAC
T23.36 Burn of third degree of back of hand
T23.361 Burn of third degree of back of right hand HAC
T23.362 Burn of third degree of back of left hand HAC
T23.369 Burn of third degree of back of unspecified hand HAC
T23.37 Burn of third degree of wrist
T23.371 Burn of third degree of right wrist HAC
T23.372 Burn of third degree of left wrist HAC
T23.379 Burn of third degree of unspecified wrist HAC
T23.39 Burn of third degree of multiple sites of wrist and hand
T23.391 Burn of third degree of multiple sites of right wrist and hand HAC
T23.392 Burn of third degree of multiple sites of left wrist and hand HAC
T23.399 Burn of third degree of multiple sites of unspecified wrist and hand HAC

T23.4 Corrosion of unspecified degree of wrist and hand
Code first (T51-T65) to identify chemical and intent
Use additional external cause code to identify place (Y92)
T23.40 Corrosion of unspecified degree of hand, unspecified site
T23.401 Corrosion of unspecified degree of right hand, unspecified site
T23.402 Corrosion of unspecified degree of left hand, unspecified site
T23.409 Corrosion of unspecified degree of unspecified hand, unspecified site
T23.41 Corrosion of unspecified degree of thumb (nail)
T23.411 Corrosion of unspecified degree of right thumb (nail)
T23.412 Corrosion of unspecified degree of left thumb (nail)
T23.419 Corrosion of unspecified degree of unspecified thumb (nail)
T23.42 Corrosion of unspecified degree of single finger (nail) except thumb
T23.421 Corrosion of unspecified degree of single right finger (nail) except thumb
T23.422 Corrosion of unspecified degree of single left finger (nail) except thumb
T23.429 Corrosion of unspecified degree of unspecified single finger (nail) except thumb
T23.43 Corrosion of unspecified degree of multiple fingers (nail), not including thumb
T23.431 Corrosion of unspecified degree of multiple right fingers (nail), not including thumb
T23.432 Corrosion of unspecified degree of multiple left fingers (nail), not including thumb
T23.439 Corrosion of unspecified degree of unspecified multiple fingers (nail), not including thumb
T23.44 Corrosion of unspecified degree of multiple fingers (nail), including thumb
T23.441 Corrosion of unspecified degree of multiple right fingers (nail), including thumb
T23.442 Corrosion of unspecified degree of multiple left fingers (nail), including thumb

Unspecified Code | Other Specified Code | Manifestation Code | N Newborn | P Pediatric | M Maternity | A Adult | ♂ Male | ♀ Female
● New Code | ▲ Revised Code Title | ►◄ Revised Text | NOTES | INCLUDES | EXCLUDES 1 Not coded here | EXCLUDES 2 Not included here
4th character required | 5th character required | 6th character required | 7th character required
Extension 'X' Alert | HAC Hospital-acquired condition (HAC) alert | AHA AHA Coding Clinic©

T23.449 Corrosion of unspecified degree of unspecified multiple fingers (nail), including thumb
T23.45 Corrosion of unspecified degree of palm
T23.451 Corrosion of unspecified degree of right palm
T23.452 Corrosion of unspecified degree of left palm
T23.459 Corrosion of unspecified degree of unspecified palm
T23.46 Corrosion of unspecified degree of back of hand
T23.461 Corrosion of unspecified degree of back of right hand
T23.462 Corrosion of unspecified degree of back of left hand
T23.469 Corrosion of unspecified degree of back of unspecified hand
T23.47 Corrosion of unspecified degree of wrist
T23.471 Corrosion of unspecified degree of right wrist
T23.472 Corrosion of unspecified degree of left wrist
T23.479 Corrosion of unspecified degree of unspecified wrist
T23.49 Corrosion of unspecified degree of multiple sites of wrist and hand
T23.491 Corrosion of unspecified degree of multiple sites of right wrist and hand
T23.492 Corrosion of unspecified degree of multiple sites of left wrist and hand
T23.499 Corrosion of unspecified degree of multiple sites of unspecified wrist and hand
T23.5 Corrosion of first degree of wrist and hand
Code first (T51-T65) to identify chemical and intent
Use additional external cause code to identify place (Y92)
T23.50 Corrosion of first degree of hand, unspecified site
T23.501 Corrosion of first degree of right hand, unspecified site
T23.502 Corrosion of first degree of left hand, unspecified site
T23.509 Corrosion of first degree of unspecified hand, unspecified site
T23.51 Corrosion of first degree of thumb (nail)
T23.511 Corrosion of first degree of right thumb (nail)
T23.512 Corrosion of first degree of left thumb (nail)
T23.519 Corrosion of first degree of unspecified thumb (nail)
T23.52 Corrosion of first degree of single finger (nail) except thumb
T23.521 Corrosion of first degree of single right finger (nail) except thumb
T23.522 Corrosion of first degree of single left finger (nail) except thumb
T23.529 Corrosion of first degree of unspecified single finger (nail) except thumb
T23.53 Corrosion of first degree of multiple fingers (nail), not including thumb
T23.531 Corrosion of first degree of multiple right fingers (nail), not including thumb
T23.532 Corrosion of first degree of multiple left fingers (nail), not including thumb
T23.539 Corrosion of first degree of unspecified multiple fingers (nail), not including thumb
T23.54 Corrosion of first degree of multiple fingers (nail), including thumb
T23.541 Corrosion of first degree of multiple right fingers (nail), including thumb
T23.542 Corrosion of first degree of multiple left fingers (nail), including thumb
T23.549 Corrosion of first degree of unspecified multiple fingers (nail), including thumb
T23.55 Corrosion of first degree of palm
T23.551 Corrosion of first degree of right palm
T23.552 Corrosion of first degree of left palm
T23.559 Corrosion of first degree of unspecified palm
T23.56 Corrosion of first degree of back of hand
T23.561 Corrosion of first degree of back of right hand
T23.562 Corrosion of first degree of back of left hand
T23.569 Corrosion of first degree of back of unspecified hand
T23.57 Corrosion of first degree of wrist
T23.571 Corrosion of first degree of right wrist
T23.572 Corrosion of first degree of left wrist
T23.579 Corrosion of first degree of unspecified wrist
T23.59 Corrosion of first degree of multiple sites of wrist and hand
T23.591 Corrosion of first degree of multiple sites of right wrist and hand
T23.592 Corrosion of first degree of multiple sites of left wrist and hand
T23.599 Corrosion of first degree of multiple sites of unspecified wrist and hand
T23.6 Corrosion of second degree of wrist and hand
Code first (T51-T65) to identify chemical and intent
Use additional external cause code to identify place (Y92)
T23.60 Corrosion of second degree of hand, unspecified site
T23.601 Corrosion of second degree of right hand, unspecified site
T23.602 Corrosion of second degree of left hand, unspecified site
T23.609 Corrosion of second degree of unspecified hand, unspecified site
T23.61 Corrosion of second degree of thumb (nail)
T23.611 Corrosion of second degree of right thumb (nail)
T23.612 Corrosion of second degree of left thumb (nail)
T23.619 Corrosion of second degree of unspecified thumb (nail)
T23.62 Corrosion of second degree of single finger (nail) except thumb
T23.621 Corrosion of second degree of single right finger (nail) except thumb
T23.622 Corrosion of second degree of single left finger (nail) except thumb
T23.629 Corrosion of second degree of unspecified single finger (nail) except thumb
T23.63 Corrosion of second degree of multiple fingers (nail), not including thumb
T23.631 Corrosion of second degree of multiple right fingers (nail), not including thumb
T23.632 Corrosion of second degree of multiple left fingers (nail), not including thumb
T23.639 Corrosion of second degree of unspecified multiple fingers (nail), not including thumb
T23.64 Corrosion of second degree of multiple fingers (nail), including thumb
T23.641 Corrosion of second degree of multiple right fingers (nail), including thumb
T23.642 Corrosion of second degree of multiple left fingers (nail), including thumb
T23.649 Corrosion of second degree of unspecified multiple fingers (nail), including thumb
T23.65 Corrosion of second degree of palm
T23.651 Corrosion of second degree of right palm
T23.652 Corrosion of second degree of left palm
T23.659 Corrosion of second degree of unspecified palm
T23.66 Corrosion of second degree of back of hand
T23.661 Corrosion of second degree back of right hand

Unacceptable principal diagnosis symbol per Medicare code edits — Code exempt from diagnosis present on admission requirement
Questionable admission — Complication or comorbidity — CC/MCC exclusion — Major complication or comorbidity
Principal diagnosis as its own CC — Principal diagnosis as its own MCC — Z code as first-listed diagnosis

T23.662 Corrosion of second degree back of left hand
T23.669 Corrosion of second degree back of unspecified hand
T23.67 Corrosion of second degree of wrist
T23.671 Corrosion of second degree of right wrist
T23.672 Corrosion of second degree of left wrist
T23.679 Corrosion of second degree of unspecified wrist
T23.69 Corrosion of second degree of multiple sites of wrist and hand
T23.691 Corrosion of second degree of multiple sites of right wrist and hand
T23.692 Corrosion of second degree of multiple sites of left wrist and hand
T23.699 Corrosion of second degree of multiple sites of unspecified wrist and hand
T23.7 Corrosion of third degree of wrist and hand
Code first (T51-T65) to identify chemical and intent
Use additional external cause code to identify place (Y92)
T23.70 Corrosion of third degree of hand, unspecified site
T23.701 Corrosion of third degree of right hand, unspecified site CC HAC
T23.702 Corrosion of third degree of left hand, unspecified site CC HAC
T23.709 Corrosion of third degree of unspecified hand, unspecified site CC HAC
T23.71 Corrosion of third degree of thumb (nail)
T23.711 Corrosion of third degree of right thumb (nail) CC HAC
T23.712 Corrosion of third degree of left thumb (nail) CC HAC
T23.719 Corrosion of third degree of unspecified thumb (nail) CC HAC
T23.72 Corrosion of third degree of single finger (nail) except thumb
T23.721 Corrosion of third degree of single right finger (nail) except thumb CC HAC
T23.722 Corrosion of third degree of single left finger (nail) except thumb CC HAC
T23.729 Corrosion of third degree of unspecified single finger (nail) except thumb CC HAC
T23.73 Corrosion of third degree of multiple fingers (nail), not including thumb
T23.731 Corrosion of third degree of multiple right fingers (nail), not including thumb CC HAC
T23.732 Corrosion of third degree of multiple left fingers (nail), not including thumb CC HAC
T23.739 Corrosion of third degree of unspecified multiple fingers (nail), not including thumb CC HAC
T23.74 Corrosion of third degree of multiple fingers (nail), including thumb
T23.741 Corrosion of third degree of multiple right fingers (nail), including thumb CC HAC
T23.742 Corrosion of third degree of multiple left fingers (nail), including thumb CC HAC
T23.749 Corrosion of third degree of unspecified multiple fingers (nail), including thumb CC HAC
T23.75 Corrosion of third degree of palm
T23.751 Corrosion of third degree of right palm CC HAC
T23.752 Corrosion of third degree of left palm CC HAC
T23.759 Corrosion of third degree of unspecified palm CC HAC
T23.76 Corrosion of third degree of back of hand
T23.761 Corrosion of third degree of back of right hand CC HAC
T23.762 Corrosion of third degree of back of left hand CC HAC
T23.769 Corrosion of third degree back of unspecified hand CC HAC
T23.77 Corrosion of third degree of wrist
T23.771 Corrosion of third degree of right wrist CC HAC
T23.772 Corrosion of third degree of left wrist CC HAC
T23.779 Corrosion of third degree of unspecified wrist CC HAC
T23.79 Corrosion of third degree of multiple sites of wrist and hand
T23.791 Corrosion of third degree of multiple sites of right wrist and hand CC HAC
T23.792 Corrosion of third degree of multiple sites of left wrist and hand CC HAC
T23.799 Corrosion of third degree of multiple sites of unspecified wrist and hand CC HAC

T24 Burn and corrosion of lower limb, except ankle and foot
EXCLUDES2 *burn and corrosion of ankle and foot (T25.-)*
burn and corrosion of hip region (T21.-)
The appropriate 7th character is to be added to each code from category T24
A = initial encounter
D = subsequent encounter
S = sequela
T24.0 Burn of unspecified degree of lower limb, except ankle and foot
Use additional external cause code to identify the source, place and intent of the burn (X00-X19, X75-X77, X96-X98, Y92)
T24.00 Burn of unspecified degree of unspecified site of lower limb, except ankle and foot
T24.001 Burn of unspecified degree of unspecified site of right lower limb, except ankle and foot
T24.002 Burn of unspecified degree of unspecified site of left lower limb, except ankle and foot
T24.009 Burn of unspecified degree of unspecified site of unspecified lower limb, except ankle and foot
T24.01 Burn of unspecified degree of thigh
T24.011 Burn of unspecified degree of right thigh
T24.012 Burn of unspecified degree of left thigh
T24.019 Burn of unspecified degree of unspecified thigh
T24.02 Burn of unspecified degree of knee
T24.021 Burn of unspecified degree of right knee
T24.022 Burn of unspecified degree of left knee
T24.029 Burn of unspecified degree of unspecified knee
T24.03 Burn of unspecified degree of lower leg
T24.031 Burn of unspecified degree of right lower leg
T24.032 Burn of unspecified degree of left lower leg
T24.039 Burn of unspecified degree of unspecified lower leg
T24.09 Burn of unspecified degree of multiple sites of lower limb, except ankle and foot
T24.091 Burn of unspecified degree of multiple sites of right lower limb, except ankle and foot
T24.092 Burn of unspecified degree of multiple sites of left lower limb, except ankle and foot
T24.099 Burn of unspecified degree of multiple sites of unspecified lower limb, except ankle and foot
T24.1 Burn of first degree of lower limb, except ankle and foot
Use additional external cause code to identify the source, place and intent of the burn (X00-X19, X75-X77, X96-X98, Y92)
T24.10 Burn of first degree of unspecified site of lower limb, except ankle and foot
T24.101 Burn of first degree of unspecified site of right lower limb, except ankle and foot

Unspecified Code | Other Specified Code | Manifestation Code | N Newborn | P Pediatric | M Maternity | A Adult | ♂ Male | ♀ Female
● New Code ▲ Revised Code Title ►◄ Revised Text NOTES INCLUDES EXCLUDES1 Not coded here EXCLUDES2 Not included here
4th character required 5th character required 6th character required 7th character required
Extension 'X' Alert HAC Hospital-acquired condition (HAC) alert AHA AHA Coding Clinic©

T24.102 Burn of first degree of unspecified site of left lower limb, except ankle and foot
T24.109 Burn of first degree of unspecified site of unspecified lower limb, except ankle and foot
T24.11 Burn of first degree of thigh
T24.111 Burn of first degree of right thigh
T24.112 Burn of first degree of left thigh
T24.119 Burn of first degree of unspecified thigh
T24.12 Burn of first degree of knee
T24.121 Burn of first degree of right knee
T24.122 Burn of first degree of left knee
T24.129 Burn of first degree of unspecified knee
T24.13 Burn of first degree of lower leg
T24.131 Burn of first degree of right lower leg
T24.132 Burn of first degree of left lower leg
T24.139 Burn of first degree of unspecified lower leg
T24.19 Burn of first degree of multiple sites of lower limb, except ankle and foot
T24.191 Burn of first degree of multiple sites of right lower limb, except ankle and foot
T24.192 Burn of first degree of multiple sites of left lower limb, except ankle and foot
T24.199 Burn of first degree of multiple sites of unspecified lower limb, except ankle and foot

T24.2 Burn of second degree of lower limb, except ankle and foot
Use additional external cause code to identify the source, place and intent of the burn (X00-X19, X75-X77, X96-X98, Y92)
T24.20 Burn of second degree of unspecified site of lower limb, except ankle and foot
T24.201 Burn of second degree of unspecified site of right lower limb, except ankle and foot
T24.202 Burn of second degree of unspecified site of left lower limb, except ankle and foot
T24.209 Burn of second degree of unspecified site of unspecified lower limb, except ankle and foot
T24.21 Burn of second degree of thigh
T24.211 Burn of second degree of right thigh
T24.212 Burn of second degree of left thigh
T24.219 Burn of second degree of unspecified thigh
T24.22 Burn of second degree of knee
T24.221 Burn of second degree of right knee
T24.222 Burn of second degree of left knee
T24.229 Burn of second degree of unspecified knee
T24.23 Burn of second degree of lower leg
T24.231 Burn of second degree of right lower leg
T24.232 Burn of second degree of left lower leg
T24.239 Burn of second degree of unspecified lower leg
T24.29 Burn of second degree of multiple sites of lower limb, except ankle and foot
T24.291 Burn of second degree of multiple sites of right lower limb, except ankle and foot
T24.292 Burn of second degree of multiple sites of left lower limb, except ankle and foot
T24.299 Burn of second degree of multiple sites of unspecified lower limb, except ankle and foot

T24.3 Burn of third degree of lower limb, except ankle and foot
Use additional external cause code to identify the source, place and intent of the burn (X00-X19, X75-X77, X96-X98, Y92)
T24.30 Burn of third degree of unspecified site of lower limb, except ankle and foot
T24.301 Burn of third degree of unspecified site of right lower limb, except ankle and foot CC HAC
T24.302 Burn of third degree of unspecified site of left lower limb, except ankle and foot CC HAC
T24.309 Burn of third degree of unspecified site of unspecified lower limb, except ankle and foot CC HAC
T24.31 Burn of third degree of thigh
T24.311 Burn of third degree of right thigh CC HAC
T24.312 Burn of third degree of left thigh CC HAC
T24.319 Burn of third degree of unspecified thigh CC HAC
T24.32 Burn of third degree of knee
T24.321 Burn of third degree of right knee CC HAC
T24.322 Burn of third degree of left knee CC HAC
T24.329 Burn of third degree of unspecified knee CC HAC
T24.33 Burn of third degree of lower leg
T24.331 Burn of third degree of right lower leg CC HAC
T24.332 Burn of third degree of left lower leg CC HAC
T24.339 Burn of third degree of unspecified lower leg CC HAC
T24.39 Burn of third degree of multiple sites of lower limb, except ankle and foot
T24.391 Burn of third degree of multiple sites of right lower limb, except ankle and foot CC HAC
AHA: Q2, 2016
T24.392 Burn of third degree of multiple sites of left lower limb, except ankle and foot CC HAC
AHA: Q2, 2016
T24.399 Burn of third degree of multiple sites of unspecified lower limb, except ankle and foot CC HAC

T24.4 Corrosion of unspecified degree of lower limb, except ankle and foot
Code first (T51-T65) to identify chemical and intent
Use additional external cause code to identify place (Y92)
T24.40 Corrosion of unspecified degree of unspecified site of lower limb, except ankle and foot
T24.401 Corrosion of unspecified degree of unspecified site of right lower limb, except ankle and foot
T24.402 Corrosion of unspecified degree of unspecified site of left lower limb, except ankle and foot
T24.409 Corrosion of unspecified degree of unspecified site of unspecified lower limb, except ankle and foot
T24.41 Corrosion of unspecified degree of thigh
T24.411 Corrosion of unspecified degree of right thigh
T24.412 Corrosion of unspecified degree of left thigh
T24.419 Corrosion of unspecified degree of unspecified thigh
T24.42 Corrosion of unspecified degree of knee
T24.421 Corrosion of unspecified degree of right knee
T24.422 Corrosion of unspecified degree of left knee
T24.429 Corrosion of unspecified degree of unspecified knee
T24.43 Corrosion of unspecified degree of lower leg
T24.431 Corrosion of unspecified degree of right lower leg
T24.432 Corrosion of unspecified degree of left lower leg
T24.439 Corrosion of unspecified degree of unspecified lower leg
T24.49 Corrosion of unspecified degree of multiple sites of lower limb, except ankle and foot

Unacceptable principal diagnosis symbol per Medicare code edits · Code exempt from diagnosis present on admission requirement
Questionable admission · CC Complication or comorbidity · CC/MCC Excl CC/MCC exclusion · MCC Major complication or comorbidity
PDx Principal diagnosis as its own CC · PDx Principal diagnosis as its own MCC · Z code as first-listed diagnosis

T24.491 Corrosion of unspecified degree of multiple sites of right lower limb, except ankle and foot
T24.492 Corrosion of unspecified degree of multiple sites of left lower limb, except ankle and foot
T24.499 Corrosion of unspecified degree of multiple sites of unspecified lower limb, except ankle and foot

T24.5 Corrosion of first degree of lower limb, except ankle and foot
Code first (T51-T65) to identify chemical and intent
Use additional external cause code to identify place (Y92)
T24.50 Corrosion of first degree of unspecified site of lower limb, except ankle and foot
T24.501 Corrosion of first degree of unspecified site of right lower limb, except ankle and foot
T24.502 Corrosion of first degree of unspecified site of left lower limb, except ankle and foot
T24.509 Corrosion of first degree of unspecified site of unspecified lower limb, except ankle and foot
T24.51 Corrosion of first degree of thigh
T24.511 Corrosion of first degree of right thigh
T24.512 Corrosion of first degree of left thigh
T24.519 Corrosion of first degree of unspecified thigh
T24.52 Corrosion of first degree of knee
T24.521 Corrosion of first degree of right knee
T24.522 Corrosion of first degree of left knee
T24.529 Corrosion of first degree of unspecified knee
T24.53 Corrosion of first degree of lower leg
T24.531 Corrosion of first degree of right lower leg
T24.532 Corrosion of first degree of left lower leg
T24.539 Corrosion of first degree of unspecified lower leg
T24.59 Corrosion of first degree of multiple sites of lower limb, except ankle and foot
T24.591 Corrosion of first degree of multiple sites of right lower limb, except ankle and foot
T24.592 Corrosion of first degree of multiple sites of left lower limb, except ankle and foot
T24.599 Corrosion of first degree of multiple sites of unspecified lower limb, except ankle and foot

T24.6 Corrosion of second degree of lower limb, except ankle and foot
Code first (T51-T65) to identify chemical and intent
Use additional external cause code to identify place (Y92)
T24.60 Corrosion of second degree of unspecified site of lower limb, except ankle and foot
T24.601 Corrosion of second degree of unspecified site of right lower limb, except ankle and foot
T24.602 Corrosion of second degree of unspecified site of left lower limb, except ankle and foot
T24.609 Corrosion of second degree of unspecified site of unspecified lower limb, except ankle and foot
T24.61 Corrosion of second degree of thigh
T24.611 Corrosion of second degree of right thigh
T24.612 Corrosion of second degree of left thigh
T24.619 Corrosion of second degree of unspecified thigh
T24.62 Corrosion of second degree of knee
T24.621 Corrosion of second degree of right knee
T24.622 Corrosion of second degree of left knee
T24.629 Corrosion of second degree of unspecified knee
T24.63 Corrosion of second degree of lower leg
T24.631 Corrosion of second degree of right lower leg
T24.632 Corrosion of second degree of left lower leg
T24.639 Corrosion of second degree of unspecified lower leg
T24.69 Corrosion of second degree of multiple site s of lower limb, except ankle and foot
T24.691 Corrosion of second degree of multiple sites of right lower limb, except ankle and foot
T24.692 Corrosion of second degree of multiple sites of left lower limb, except ankle and foot
T24.699 Corrosion of second degree of multiple sites of unspecified lower limb, except ankle and foot

T24.7 Corrosion of third degree of lower limb, except ankle and foot
Code first (T51-T65) to identify chemical and intent
Use additional external cause code to identify place (Y92)
T24.70 Corrosion of third degree of unspecified site of lower limb, except ankle and foot
T24.701 Corrosion of third degree of unspecified site of right lower limb, except ankle and foot HAC
T24.702 Corrosion of third degree of unspecified site of left lower limb, except ankle and foot HAC
T24.709 Corrosion of third degree of unspecified site of unspecified lower limb, except ankle and foot HAC
T24.71 Corrosion of third degree of thigh
T24.711 Corrosion of third degree of right thigh HAC
T24.712 Corrosion of third degree of left thigh HAC
T24.719 Corrosion of third degree of unspecified thigh HAC
T24.72 Corrosion of third degree of knee
T24.721 Corrosion of third degree of right knee HAC
T24.722 Corrosion of third degree of left knee HAC
T24.729 Corrosion of third degree of unspecified knee HAC
T24.73 Corrosion of third degree of lower leg
T24.731 Corrosion of third degree of right lower leg HAC
T24.732 Corrosion of third degree of left lower leg HAC
T24.739 Corrosion of third degree of unspecified lower leg HAC
T24.79 Corrosion of third degree of multiple sites of lower limb, except ankle and foot
T24.791 Corrosion of third degree of multiple sites of right lower limb, except ankle and foot HAC
T24.792 Corrosion of third degree of multiple sites of left lower limb, except ankle and foot HAC
T24.799 Corrosion of third degree of multiple sites of unspecified lower limb, except ankle and foot HAC

T25 Burn and corrosion of ankle and foot
The appropriate 7th character is to be added to each code from category T25
A = initial encounter
D = subsequent encounter
S = sequela
T25.0 Burn of unspecified degree of ankle and foot
Use additional external cause code to identify the source, place and intent of the burn (X00-X19, X75-X77, X96-X98, Y92)
T25.01 Burn of unspecified degree of ankle
T25.011 Burn of unspecified degree of right ankle
T25.012 Burn of unspecified degree of left ankle
T25.019 Burn of unspecified degree of unspecified ankle

Unspecified Code | Other Specified Code | Manifestation Code | N Newborn | P Pediatric | M Maternity | A Adult | ♂ Male | ♀ Female
● New Code ▲ Revised Code Title ►◄ Revised Text NOTES INCLUDES EXCLUDES1 Not coded here EXCLUDES2 Not included here
4th character required 5th character required 6th character required 7th character required
Extension 'X' Alert HAC Hospital-acquired condition (HAC) alert AHA AHA Coding Clinic®

T25.02 Burn of unspecified degree of foot
EXCLUDES2 burn of unspecified degree of toe(s) (nail) (T25.03-)
T25.021 Burn of unspecified degree of right foot
T25.022 Burn of unspecified degree of left foot
T25.029 Burn of unspecified degree of unspecified foot
T25.03 Burn of unspecified degree of toe(s) (nail)
T25.031 Burn of unspecified degree of right toe(s) (nail)
T25.032 Burn of unspecified degree of left toe(s) (nail)
T25.039 Burn of unspecified degree of unspecified toe(s) (nail)
T25.09 Burn of unspecified degree of multiple sites of ankle and foot
T25.091 Burn of unspecified degree of multiple sites of right ankle and foot
T25.092 Burn of unspecified degree of multiple sites of left ankle and foot
T25.099 Burn of unspecified degree of multiple sites of unspecified ankle and foot

T25.1 Burn of first degree of ankle and foot
Use additional external cause code to identify the source, place and intent of the burn (X00-X19, X75-X77, X96-X98, Y92)
T25.11 Burn of first degree of ankle
T25.111 Burn of first degree of right ankle
T25.112 Burn of first degree of left ankle
T25.119 Burn of first degree of unspecified ankle
T25.12 Burn of first degree of foot
EXCLUDES2 burn of first degree of toe(s) (nail) (T25.13-)
T25.121 Burn of first degree of right foot
T25.122 Burn of first degree of left foot
T25.129 Burn of first degree of unspecified foot
T25.13 Burn of first degree of toe(s) (nail)
T25.131 Burn of first degree of right toe(s) (nail)
T25.132 Burn of first degree of left toe(s) (nail)
T25.139 Burn of first degree of unspecified toe(s) (nail)
T25.19 Burn of first degree of multiple sites of ankle and foot
T25.191 Burn of first degree of multiple sites of right ankle and foot
T25.192 Burn of first degree of multiple sites of left ankle and foot
T25.199 Burn of first degree of multiple sites of unspecified ankle and foot

T25.2 Burn of second degree of ankle and foot
Use additional external cause code to identify the source, place and intent of the burn (X00-X19, X75-X77, X96-X98, Y92)
T25.21 Burn of second degree of ankle
T25.211 Burn of second degree of right ankle
T25.212 Burn of second degree of left ankle
T25.219 Burn of second degree of unspecified ankle
T25.22 Burn of second degree of foot
EXCLUDES2 burn of second degree of toe(s) (nail) (T25.23-)
T25.221 Burn of second degree of right foot
T25.222 Burn of second degree of left foot
T25.229 Burn of second degree of unspecified foot
T25.23 Burn of second degree of toe(s) (nail)
T25.231 Burn of second degree of right toe(s) (nail)
T25.232 Burn of second degree of left toe(s) (nail)
T25.239 Burn of second degree of unspecified toe(s) (nail)
T25.29 Burn of second degree of multiple sites of ankle and foot
T25.291 Burn of second degree of multiple sites of right ankle and foot
T25.292 Burn of second degree of multiple sites of left ankle and foot
T25.299 Burn of second degree of multiple sites of unspecified ankle and foot

T25.3 Burn of third degree of ankle and foot
Use additional external cause code to identify the source, place and intent of the burn (X00-X19, X75-X77, X96-X98, Y92)
T25.31 Burn of third degree of ankle
T25.311 Burn of third degree of right ankle CC HAC
T25.312 Burn of third degree of left ankle CC HAC
T25.319 Burn of third degree of unspecified ankle CC HAC
T25.32 Burn of third degree of foot
EXCLUDES2 burn of third degree of toe(s) (nail) (T25.33-)
T25.321 Burn of third degree of right foot CC HAC
T25.322 Burn of third degree of left foot CC HAC
T25.329 Burn of third degree of unspecified foot CC HAC
T25.33 Burn of third degree of toe(s) (nail)
T25.331 Burn of third degree of right toe(s) (nail) CC HAC
T25.332 Burn of third degree of left toe(s) (nail) CC HAC
T25.339 Burn of third degree of unspecified toe(s) (nail) CC HAC
T25.39 Burn of third degree of multiple sites of ankle and foot
T25.391 Burn of third degree of multiple sites of right ankle and foot CC HAC
T25.392 Burn of third degree of multiple sites of left ankle and foot CC HAC
T25.399 Burn of third degree of multiple sites of unspecified ankle and foot CC HAC

T25.4 Corrosion of unspecified degree of ankle and foot
Code first (T51-T65) to identify chemical and intent
Use additional external cause code to identify place (Y92)
T25.41 Corrosion of unspecified degree of ankle
T25.411 Corrosion of unspecified degree of right ankle
T25.412 Corrosion of unspecified degree of left ankle
T25.419 Corrosion of unspecified degree of unspecified ankle
T25.42 Corrosion of unspecified degree of foot
EXCLUDES2 corrosion of unspecified degree of toe(s) (nail) (T25.43-)
T25.421 Corrosion of unspecified degree of right foot
T25.422 Corrosion of unspecified degree of left foot
T25.429 Corrosion of unspecified degree of unspecified foot
T25.43 Corrosion of unspecified degree of toe(s) (nail)
T25.431 Corrosion of unspecified degree of right toe(s) (nail)
T25.432 Corrosion of unspecified degree of left toe(s) (nail)
T25.439 Corrosion of unspecified degree of unspecified toe(s) (nail)
T25.49 Corrosion of unspecified degree of multiple sites of ankle and foot
T25.491 Corrosion of unspecified degree of multiple sites of right ankle and foot
T25.492 Corrosion of unspecified degree of multiple sites of left ankle and foot
T25.499 Corrosion of unspecified degree of multiple sites of unspecified ankle and foot

T25.5 Corrosion of first degree of ankle and foot
Code first (T51-T65) to identify chemical and intent
Use additional external cause code to identify place (Y92)
T25.51 Corrosion of first degree of ankle
T25.511 Corrosion of first degree of right ankle
T25.512 Corrosion of first degree of left ankle
T25.519 Corrosion of first degree of unspecified ankle
T25.52 Corrosion of first degree of foot
EXCLUDES2 corrosion of first degree of toe(s) (nail) (T25.53-)

PDx Unacceptable principal diagnosis symbol per Medicare code edits; POA Code exempt from diagnosis present on admission requirement
Q Questionable admission; CC Complication or comorbidity; CC/MCC Excl CC/MCC exclusion; MCC Major complication or comorbidity
PDx CC Principal diagnosis as its own CC; PDx MCC Principal diagnosis as its own MCC; Z1 Z code as first-listed diagnosis

When symbols appear on a code that requires a 7th character extension, refer to Appendix D to identify applicable 7th character codes.

T25.521 Corrosion of first degree of right foot
T25.522 Corrosion of first degree of left foot
T25.529 Corrosion of first degree of unspecified foot
T25.53 Corrosion of first degree of toe(s) (nail)
T25.531 Corrosion of first degree of right toe(s) (nail)
T25.532 Corrosion of first degree of left toe(s) (nail)
T25.539 Corrosion of first degree of unspecified toe(s) (nail)
T25.59 Corrosion of first degree of multiple site s of ankle and foot
T25.591 Corrosion of first degree of multiple sites of right ankle and foot
T25.592 Corrosion of first degree of multiple sites of left ankle and foot
T25.599 Corrosion of first degree of multiple sites of unspecified ankle and foot
T25.6 Corrosion of second degree of ankle and foot
Code first (T51-T65) to identify chemical and intent
Use additional external cause code to identify place (Y92)
T25.61 Corrosion of second degree of ankle
T25.611 Corrosion of second degree of right ankle
T25.612 Corrosion of second degree of left ankle
T25.619 Corrosion of second degree of unspecified ankle
T25.62 Corrosion of second degree of foot
EXCLUDES2 *corrosion of second degree of toe(s) (nail) (T25.63-)*
T25.621 Corrosion of second degree of right foot
T25.622 Corrosion of second degree of left foot
T25.629 Corrosion of second degree of unspecified foot
T25.63 Corrosion of second degree of toe(s) (nail)
T25.631 Corrosion of second degree of right toe(s) (nail)
T25.632 Corrosion of second degree of left toe(s) (nail)
T25.639 Corrosion of second degree of unspecified toe(s) (nail)
T25.69 Corrosion of second degree of multiple sites of ankle and foot
T25.691 Corrosion of second degree of right ankle and foot
T25.692 Corrosion of second degree of left ankle and foot
T25.699 Corrosion of second degree of unspecified ankle and foot
T25.7 Corrosion of third degree of ankle and foot
Code first (T51-T65) to identify chemical and intent
Use additional external cause code to identify place (Y92)
T25.71 Corrosion of third degree of ankle
T25.711 Corrosion of third degree of right ankle CC HAC
T25.712 Corrosion of third degree of left ankle CC HAC
T25.719 Corrosion of third degree of unspecified ankle CC HAC
T25.72 Corrosion of third degree of foot
EXCLUDES2 *corrosion of third degree of toe(s) (nail) (T25.73-)*
T25.721 Corrosion of third degree of right foot CC HAC
T25.722 Corrosion of third degree of left foot CC HAC
T25.729 Corrosion of third degree of unspecified foot CC HAC
T25.73 Corrosion of third degree of toe(s) (nail)
T25.731 Corrosion of third degree of right toe(s) (nail) CC HAC
T25.732 Corrosion of third degree of left toe(s) (nail) CC HAC
T25.739 Corrosion of third degree of unspecified toe(s) (nail) CC HAC
T25.79 Corrosion of third degree of multiple sites of ankle and foot
T25.791 Corrosion of third degree of multiple sites of right ankle and foot CC HAC
T25.792 Corrosion of third degree of multiple sites of left ankle and foot CC HAC
T25.799 Corrosion of third degree of multiple sites of unspecified ankle and foot CC HAC

Burns and corrosions confined to eye and internal organs (T26-T28)

T26 Burn and corrosion confined to eye and adnexa
The appropriate 7th character is to be added to each code from category T26
A = initial encounter
D = subsequent encounter
S = sequela
T26.0 Burn of eyelid and periocular area
Use additional external cause code to identify the source, place and intent of the burn (X00-X19, X75-X77, X96-X98, Y92)
T26.00 Burn of unspecified eyelid and periocular area
T26.01 Burn of right eyelid and periocular area
T26.02 Burn of left eyelid and periocular area
T26.1 Burn of cornea and conjunctival sac
Use additional external cause code to identify the source, place and intent of the burn (X00-X19, X75-X77, X96-X98, Y92)
T26.10 Burn of cornea and conjunctival sac, unspecified eye
T26.11 Burn of cornea and conjunctival sac, right eye
T26.12 Burn of cornea and conjunctival sac, left eye
T26.2 Burn with resulting rupture and destruction of eyeball
Use additional external cause code to identify the source, place and intent of the burn (X00-X19, X75-X77, X96-X98, Y92)
T26.20 Burn with resulting rupture and destruction of unspecified eyeball CC HAC
T26.21 Burn with resulting rupture and destruction of right eyeball CC HAC
T26.22 Burn with resulting rupture and destruction of left eyeball CC HAC
T26.3 Burns of other specified parts of eye and adnexa
Use additional external cause code to identify the source, place and intent of the burn (X00-X19, X75-X77, X96-X98, Y92)
T26.30 Burns of other specified parts of unspecified eye and adnexa
T26.31 Burns of other specified parts of right eye and adnexa
T26.32 Burns of other specified parts of left eye and adnexa
T26.4 Burn of eye and adnexa, part unspecified
Use additional external cause code to identify the source, place and intent of the burn (X00-X19, X75-X77, X96-X98, Y92)
T26.40 Burn of unspecified eye and adnexa, part unspecified
T26.41 Burn of right eye and adnexa, part unspecified
T26.42 Burn of left eye and adnexa, part unspecified
T26.5 Corrosion of eyelid and periocular area
Code first (T51-T65) to identify chemical and intent
Use additional external cause code to identify place (Y92)
T26.50 Corrosion of unspecified eyelid and periocular area
T26.51 Corrosion of right eyelid and periocular area
T26.52 Corrosion of left eyelid and periocular area
T26.6 Corrosion of cornea and conjunctival sac
Code first (T51-T65) to identify chemical and intent
Use additional external cause code to identify place (Y92)
T26.60 Corrosion of cornea and conjunctival sac, unspecified eye
T26.61 Corrosion of cornea and conjunctival sac, right eye
T26.62 Corrosion of cornea and conjunctival sac, left eye
T26.7 Corrosion with resulting rupture and destruction of eyeball

Unspecified Code | Other Specified Code | Manifestation Code | N Newborn | P Pediatric | M Maternity | A Adult | ♂ Male | ♀ Female
● New Code | ▲ Revised Code Title | ►◄ Revised Text | NOTES | INCLUDES | EXCLUDES1 Not coded here | EXCLUDES2 Not included here
4th character required | 5th character required | 6th character required | 7th character required
Extension 'X' Alert | HAC Hospital-acquired condition (HAC) alert | AHA AHA Coding Clinic©

Code first (T51-T65) to identify chemical and intent
Use additional external cause code to identify place (Y92)

- T26.70 **Corrosion with resulting rupture and destruction of unspecified eyeball** CC HAC
- T26.71 **Corrosion with resulting rupture and destruction of right eyeball** CC HAC
- T26.72 **Corrosion with resulting rupture and destruction of left eyeball** CC HAC

T26.8 **Corrosions of other specified parts of eye and adnexa**
Code first (T51-T65) to identify chemical and intent
Use additional external cause code to identify place (Y92)

- T26.80 **Corrosions of other specified parts of unspecified eye and adnexa**
- T26.81 **Corrosions of other specified parts of right eye and adnexa**
- T26.82 **Corrosions of other specified parts of left eye and adnexa**

T26.9 **Corrosion of eye and adnexa, part unspecified**
Code first (T51-T65) to identify chemical and intent
Use additional external cause code to identify place (Y92)

- T26.90 **Corrosion of unspecified eye and adnexa, part unspecified**
- T26.91 **Corrosion of right eye and adnexa, part unspecified**
- T26.92 **Corrosion of left eye and adnexa, part unspecified**

T27 **Burn and corrosion of respiratory tract**
Use additional external cause code to identify the source and intent of the burn (X00-X19, X75-X77, X96-X98)
Use additional external cause code to identify place (Y92)
The appropriate 7th character is to be added to each code from category T27
A = initial encounter
D = subsequent encounter
S = sequela

- T27.0 **Burn of larynx and trachea** CC HAC
- T27.1 **Burn involving larynx and trachea with lung** CC HAC
- T27.2 **Burn of other parts of respiratory tract** CC HAC
  Burn of thoracic cavity
- T27.3 **Burn of respiratory tract, part unspecified** CC HAC
  Code first (T51-T65) to identify chemical and intent for codes T27.4-T27.7
- T27.4 **Corrosion of larynx and trachea** CC HAC
- T27.5 **Corrosion involving larynx and trachea with lung** CC HAC
- T27.6 **Corrosion of other parts of respiratory tract** CC HAC
- T27.7 **Corrosion of respiratory tract, part unspecified** CC HAC

T28 **Burn and corrosion of other internal organs**
Use additional external cause code to identify the source and intent of the burn (X00-X19, X75-X77, X96-X98)
Use additional external cause code to identify place (Y92)
The appropriate 7th character is to be added to each code from category T28
A = initial encounter
D = subsequent encounter
S = sequela

- T28.0 **Burn of mouth and pharynx**
- T28.1 **Burn of esophagus** CC HAC
- T28.2 **Burn of other parts of alimentary tract** CC HAC
- T28.3 **Burn of internal genitourinary organs**
- T28.4 **Burns of other and unspecified internal organs**
  - T28.40 **Burn of unspecified internal organ**
  - T28.41 **Burn of ear drum**
    - T28.411 **Burn of right ear drum**
    - T28.412 **Burn of left ear drum**
    - T28.419 **Burn of unspecified ear drum**
  - T28.49 **Burn of other internal organ**
    Code first (T51-T65) to identify chemical and intent for T28.5-T28.9-
- T28.5 **Corrosion of mouth and pharynx**
- T28.6 **Corrosion of esophagus** CC HAC
- T28.7 **Corrosion of other parts of alimentary tract** CC HAC
- T28.8 **Corrosion of internal genitourinary organs**
- T28.9 **Corrosions of other and unspecified internal organs**
  - T28.90 **Corrosions of unspecified internal organs**
  - T28.91 **Corrosions of ear drum**
    - T28.911 **Corrosions of right ear drum**
    - T28.912 **Corrosions of left ear drum**
    - T28.919 **Corrosions of unspecified ear drum**
  - T28.99 **Corrosions of other internal organs**

Burns and corrosions of multiple and unspecified body regions (T30-T32)

T30 **Burn and corrosion, body region unspecified**

- T30.0 **Burn of unspecified body region, unspecified degree**
  This code is not for inpatient use. Code to specified site and degree of burns
  Burn NOS
  Multiple burns NOS
- T30.4 **Corrosion of unspecified body region, unspecified degree**
  This code is not for inpatient use. Code to specified site and degree of corrosion
  Corrosion NOS
  Multiple corrosion NOS

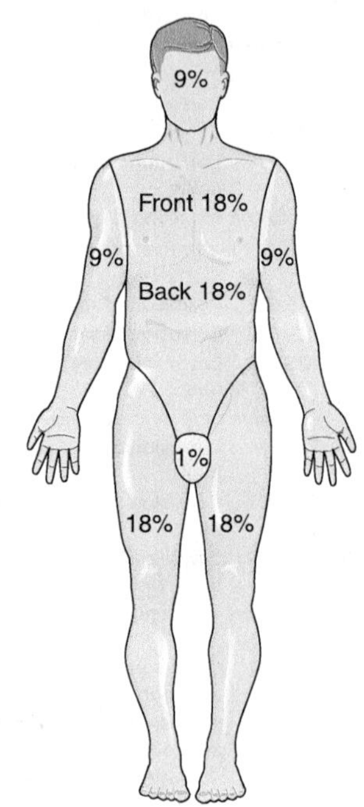

Figure 17.1 Rule of Nine: Percentage of burn areas

T31 **Burns classified according to extent of body surface involved**
NOTES This category is to be used as the primary code only when the site of the burn is unspecified. It should be used as a supplementary code with categories T20-T25 when the site is specified.

- T31.0 **Burns involving less than 10% of body surface**
- T31.1 **Burns involving 10-19% of body surface**
  - T31.10 **Burns involving 10-19% of body surface with 0% to 9% third degree burns** CC HAC
    Burns involving 10-19% of body surface NOS
  - T31.11 **Burns involving 10-19% of body surface with 10-19% third degree burns** CC HAC
- T31.2 **Burns involving 20-29% of body surface**
  - T31.20 **Burns involving 20-29% of body surface with 0% to 9% third degree burns** CC HAC
    Burns involving 20-29% of body surface NOS
  - T31.21 **Burns involving 20-29% of body surface with 10-19% third degree burns** HAC MCC
  - T31.22 **Burns involving 20-29% of body surface with 20-29% third degree burns** HAC MCC
- T31.3 **Burns involving 30-39% of body surface**
  - T31.30 **Burns involving 30-39% of body surface with 0% to 9% third degree burns** CC HAC
    Burns involving 30-39% of body surface NOS

Unacceptable principal diagnosis symbol per Medicare code edits; Code exempt from diagnosis present on admission requirement; Questionable admission; CC Complication or comorbidity; CC/MCC exclusion; MCC Major complication or comorbidity; Principal diagnosis as its own CC; Principal diagnosis as its own MCC; Z code as first-listed diagnosis

T31.31 Burns involving 30-39% of body surface with 10-19% third degree burns HAC MCC
T31.32 Burns involving 30-39% of body surface with 20-29% third degree burns HAC MCC
T31.33 Burns involving 30-39% of body surface with 30-39% third degree burns HAC MCC

T31.4 Burns involving 40-49% of body surface
T31.40 Burns involving 40-49% of body surface with 0% to 9% third degree burns CC HAC
Burns involving 40-49% of body surface NOS
T31.41 Burns involving 40-49% of body surface with 10-19% third degree burns HAC MCC
T31.42 Burns involving 40-49% of body surface with 20-29% third degree burns HAC MCC
T31.43 Burns involving 40-49% of body surface with 30-39% third degree burns HAC MCC
T31.44 Burns involving 40-49% of body surface with 40-49% third degree burns HAC MCC

T31.5 Burns involving 50-59% of body surface
T31.50 Burns involving 50-59% of body surface with 0% to 9% third degree burns CC HAC
Burns involving 50-59% of body surface NOS
T31.51 Burns involving 50-59% of body surface with 10-19% third degree burns HAC MCC
T31.52 Burns involving 50-59% of body surface with 20-29% third degree burns HAC MCC
T31.53 Burns involving 50-59% of body surface with 30-39% third degree burns HAC MCC
T31.54 Burns involving 50-59% of body surface with 40-49% third degree burns HAC MCC
T31.55 Burns involving 50-59% of body surface with 50-59% third degree burns HAC MCC

T31.6 Burns involving 60-69% of body surface
T31.60 Burns involving 60-69% of body surface with 0% to 9% third degree burns CC HAC
Burns involving 60-69% of body surface NOS
T31.61 Burns involving 60-69% of body surface with 10-19% third degree burns HAC MCC
T31.62 Burns involving 60-69% of body surface with 20-29% third degree burns HAC MCC
T31.63 Burns involving 60-69% of body surface with 30-39% third degree burns HAC MCC
T31.64 Burns involving 60-69% of body surface with 40-49% third degree burns HAC MCC
T31.65 Burns involving 60-69% of body surface with 50-59% third degree burns HAC MCC
T31.66 Burns involving 60-69% of body surface with 60-69% third degree burns HAC MCC

T31.7 Burns involving 70-79% of body surface
T31.70 Burns involving 70-79% of body surface with 0% to 9% third degree burns CC HAC
Burns involving 70-79% of body surface NOS
T31.71 Burns involving 70-79% of body surface with 10-19% third degree burns HAC MCC
T31.72 Burns involving 70-79% of body surface with 20-29% third degree burns HAC MCC
T31.73 Burns involving 70-79% of body surface with 30-39% third degree burns HAC MCC
T31.74 Burns involving 70-79% of body surface with 40-49% third degree burns HAC MCC
T31.75 Burns involving 70-79% of body surface with 50-59% third degree burns HAC MCC
T31.76 Burns involving 70-79% of body surface with 60-69% third degree burns HAC MCC
T31.77 Burns involving 70-79% of body surface with 70-79% third degree burns HAC MCC

T31.8 Burns involving 80-89% of body surface
T31.80 Burns involving 80-89% of body surface with 0% to 9% third degree burns CC HAC
Burns involving 80-89% of body surface NOS
T31.81 Burns involving 80-89% of body surface with 10-19% third degree burns HAC MCC
T31.82 Burns involving 80-89% of body surface with 20-29% third degree burns HAC MCC
T31.83 Burns involving 80-89% of body surface with 30-39% third degree burns HAC MCC
T31.84 Burns involving 80-89% of body surface with 40-49% third degree burns HAC MCC
T31.85 Burns involving 80-89% of body surface with 50-59% third degree burns HAC MCC
T31.86 Burns involving 80-89% of body surface with 60-69% third degree burns HAC MCC
T31.87 Burns involving 80-89% of body surface with 70-79% third degree burns HAC MCC
T31.88 Burns involving 80-89% of body surface with 80-89% third degree burns HAC MCC

T31.9 Burns involving 90% or more of body surface
T31.90 Burns involving 90% or more of body surface with 0% to 9% third degree burns CC HAC
Burns involving 90% or more of body surface NOS
T31.91 Burns involving 90% or more of body surface with 10-19% third degree burns HAC MCC
T31.92 Burns involving 90% or more of body surface with 20-29% third degree burns HAC MCC
T31.93 Burns involving 90% or more of body surface with 30-39% third degree burns HAC MCC
T31.94 Burns involving 90% or more of body surface with 40-49% third degree burns HAC MCC
T31.95 Burns involving 90% or more of body surface with 50-59% third degree burns HAC MCC
T31.96 Burns involving 90% or more of body surface with 60-69% third degree burns HAC MCC
T31.97 Burns involving 90% or more of body surface with 70-79% third degree burns HAC MCC
T31.98 Burns involving 90% or more of body surface with 80-89% third degree burns HAC MCC
T31.99 Burns involving 90% or more of body surface with 90% or more third degree burns HAC MCC

T32 Corrosions classified according to extent of body surface involved

NOTES This category is to be used as the primary code only when the site of the corrosion is unspecified. It may be used as a supplementary code with categories T20-T25 when the site is specified.

T32.0 Corrosions involving less than 10% of body surface

T32.1 Corrosions involving 10-19% of body surface
T32.10 Corrosions involving 10-19% of body surface with 0% to 9% third degree corrosion CC HAC
Corrosions involving 10-19% of body surface NOS
T32.11 Corrosions involving 10-19% of body surface with 10-19% third degree corrosion CC HAC

T32.2 Corrosions involving 20-29% of body surface
T32.20 Corrosions involving 20-29% of body surface with 0% to 9% third degree corrosion CC HAC
T32.21 Corrosions involving 20-29% of body surface with 10-19% third degree corrosion HAC MCC
T32.22 Corrosions involving 20-29% of body surface with 20-29% third degree corrosion HAC MCC

T32.3 Corrosions involving 30-39% of body surface
T32.30 Corrosions involving 30-39% of body surface with 0% to 9% third degree corrosion CC HAC
T32.31 Corrosions involving 30-39% of body surface with 10-19% third degree corrosion HAC MCC
T32.32 Corrosions involving 30-39% of body surface with 20-29% third degree corrosion HAC MCC
T32.33 Corrosions involving 30-39% of body surface with 30-39% third degree corrosion HAC MCC

T32.4 Corrosions involving 40-49% of body surface
T32.40 Corrosions involving 40-49% of body surface with 0% to 9% third degree corrosion CC HAC
T32.41 Corrosions involving 40-49% of body surface with 10-19% third degree corrosion HAC MCC
T32.42 Corrosions involving 40-49% of body surface with 20-29% third degree corrosion HAC MCC
T32.43 Corrosions involving 40-49% of body surface with 30-39% third degree corrosion HAC MCC
T32.44 Corrosions involving 40-49% of body surface with 40-49% third degree corrosion HAC MCC

T32.5 Corrosions involving 50-59% of body surface
T32.50 Corrosions involving 50-59% of body surface with 0% to 9% third degree corrosion CC HAC
T32.51 Corrosions involving 50-59% of body surface with 10-19% third degree corrosion HAC MCC

Unspecified Code Other Specified Code Manifestation Code N Newborn P Pediatric M Maternity A Adult ♂ Male ♀ Female
● New Code ▲ Revised Code Title ►◄ Revised Text NOTES INCLUDES EXCLUDES1 Not coded here EXCLUDES2 Not included here
4th character required 5th character required 6th character required 7th character required
Extension 'X' Alert HAC Hospital-acquired condition (HAC) alert AHA AHA Coding Clinic©

T32.52 Corrosions involving 50-59% of body surface with 20-29% third degree corrosion HAC MCC
T32.53 Corrosions involving 50-59% of body surface with 30-39% third degree corrosion HAC MCC
T32.54 Corrosions involving 50-59% of body surface with 40-49% third degree corrosion HAC MCC
T32.55 Corrosions involving 50-59% of body surface with 50-59% third degree corrosion HAC MCC

T32.6 Corrosions involving 60-69% of body surface
T32.60 Corrosions involving 60-69% of body surface with 0% to 9% third degree corrosion CC HAC
T32.61 Corrosions involving 60-69% of body surface with 10-19% third degree corrosion HAC MCC
T32.62 Corrosions involving 60-69% of body surface with 20-29% third degree corrosion HAC MCC
T32.63 Corrosions involving 60-69% of body surface with 30-39% third degree corrosion HAC MCC
T32.64 Corrosions involving 60-69% of body surface with 40-49% third degree corrosion HAC MCC
T32.65 Corrosions involving 60-69% of body surface with 50-59% third degree corrosion HAC MCC
T32.66 Corrosions involving 60-69% of body surface with 60-69% third degree corrosion HAC MCC

T32.7 Corrosions involving 70-79% of body surface
T32.70 Corrosions involving 70-79% of body surface with 0% to 9% third degree corrosion CC HAC
T32.71 Corrosions involving 70-79% of body surface with 10-19% third degree corrosion HAC MCC
T32.72 Corrosions involving 70-79% of body surface with 20-29% third degree corrosion HAC MCC
T32.73 Corrosions involving 70-79% of body surface with 30-39% third degree corrosion HAC MCC
T32.74 Corrosions involving 70-79% of body surface with 40-49% third degree corrosion HAC MCC
T32.75 Corrosions involving 70-79% of body surface with 50-59% third degree corrosion HAC MCC
T32.76 Corrosions involving 70-79% of body surface with 60-69% third degree corrosion HAC MCC
T32.77 Corrosions involving 70-79% of body surface with 70-79% third degree corrosion HAC MCC

T32.8 Corrosions involving 80-89% of body surface
T32.80 Corrosions involving 80-89% of body surface with 0% to 9% third degree corrosion CC HAC
T32.81 Corrosions involving 80-89% of body surface with 10-19% third degree corrosion HAC MCC
T32.82 Corrosions involving 80-89% of body surface with 20-29% third degree corrosion HAC MCC
T32.83 Corrosions involving 80-89% of body surface with 30-39% third degree corrosion HAC MCC
T32.84 Corrosions involving 80-89% of body surface with 40-49% third degree corrosion HAC MCC
T32.85 Corrosions involving 80-89% of body surface with 50-59% third degree corrosion HAC MCC
T32.86 Corrosions involving 80-89% of body surface with 60-69% third degree corrosion HAC MCC
T32.87 Corrosions involving 80-89% of body surface with 70-79% third degree corrosion HAC MCC
T32.88 Corrosions involving 80-89% of body surface with 80-89% third degree corrosion HAC MCC

T32.9 Corrosions involving 90% or more of body surface
T32.90 Corrosions involving 90% or more of body surface with 0% to 9% third degree corrosion CC HAC
T32.91 Corrosions involving 90% or more of body surface with 10-19% third degree corrosion HAC MCC
T32.92 Corrosions involving 90% or more of body surface with 20-29% third degree corrosion HAC MCC
T32.93 Corrosions involving 90% or more of body surface with 30-39% third degree corrosion HAC MCC
T32.94 Corrosions involving 90% or more of body surface with 40-49% third degree corrosion HAC MCC
T32.95 Corrosions involving 90% or more of body surface with 50-59% third degree corrosion HAC MCC
T32.96 Corrosions involving 90% or more of body surface with 60-69% third degree corrosion HAC MCC
T32.97 Corrosions involving 90% or more of body surface with 70-79% third degree corrosion HAC MCC
T32.98 Corrosions involving 90% or more of body surface with 80-89% third degree corrosion HAC MCC
T32.99 Corrosions involving 90% or more of body surface with 90% or more third degree corrosion HAC MCC

Frostbite (T33-T34)

EXCLUDES2 *hypothermia and other effects of reduced temperature (T68, T69.-)*

T33 Superficial frostbite

INCLUDES *frostbite with partial thickness skin loss*

The appropriate 7th character is to be added to each code from category T33
A = initial encounter
D = subsequent encounter
S = sequela

T33.0 Superficial frostbite of head
T33.01 Superficial frostbite of ear
T33.011 Superficial frostbite of right ear CC HAC
T33.012 Superficial frostbite of left ear CC HAC
T33.019 Superficial frostbite of unspecified ear CC HAC
T33.02 Superficial frostbite of nose CC HAC
T33.09 Superficial frostbite of other part of head CC HAC
T33.1 Superficial frostbite of neck CC HAC
T33.2 Superficial frostbite of thorax CC HAC
T33.3 Superficial frostbite of abdominal wall, lower back and pelvis CC HAC
T33.4 Superficial frostbite of arm

EXCLUDES2 *superficial frostbite of wrist and hand (T33.5-)*

T33.40 Superficial frostbite of unspecified arm CC HAC
T33.41 Superficial frostbite of right arm CC HAC
T33.42 Superficial frostbite of left arm CC HAC
T33.5 Superficial frostbite of wrist, hand, and fingers
T33.51 Superficial frostbite of wrist
T33.511 Superficial frostbite of right wrist CC HAC
T33.512 Superficial frostbite of left wrist CC HAC
T33.519 Superficial frostbite of unspecified wrist CC HAC
T33.52 Superficial frostbite of hand

EXCLUDES2 *superficial frostbite of fingers (T33.53-)*

T33.521 Superficial frostbite of right hand CC HAC
T33.522 Superficial frostbite of left hand CC HAC
T33.529 Superficial frostbite of unspecified hand CC HAC
T33.53 Superficial frostbite of finger(s)
T33.531 Superficial frostbite of right finger(s) CC HAC
T33.532 Superficial frostbite of left finger(s) CC HAC
T33.539 Superficial frostbite of unspecified finger(s) CC HAC
T33.6 Superficial frostbite of hip and thigh
T33.60 Superficial frostbite of unspecified hip and thigh CC HAC
T33.61 Superficial frostbite of right hip and thigh CC HAC
T33.62 Superficial frostbite of left hip and thigh CC HAC
T33.7 Superficial frostbite of knee and lower leg

EXCLUDES2 *superficial frostbite of ankle and foot (T33.8-)*

T33.70 Superficial frostbite of unspecified knee and lower leg CC HAC
T33.71 Superficial frostbite of right knee and lower leg CC HAC
T33.72 Superficial frostbite of left knee and lower leg CC HAC
T33.8 Superficial frostbite of ankle, foot, and toe(s)

PDx Unacceptable principal diagnosis symbol per Medicare code edits; POA Code exempt from diagnosis present on admission requirement
Q Questionable admission; CC Complication or comorbidity; CC/MCC Exc CC/MCC exclusion; MCC Major complication or comorbidity
PDx CC Principal diagnosis as its own CC; PDx MCC Principal diagnosis as its own MCC; Z1 Z code as first-listed diagnosis

T33.81 Superficial frostbite of ankle
T33.811 Superficial frostbite of right ankle
T33.812 Superficial frostbite of left ankle
T33.819 Superficial frostbite of unspecified ankle
T33.82 Superficial frostbite of foot
T33.821 Superficial frostbite of right foot
T33.822 Superficial frostbite of left foot
T33.829 Superficial frostbite of unspecified foot
T33.83 Superficial frostbite of toe(s)
T33.831 Superficial frostbite of right toe(s)
T33.832 Superficial frostbite of left toe(s)
T33.839 Superficial frostbite of unspecified toe(s)
T33.9 Superficial frostbite of other and unspecified sites
T33.90 Superficial frostbite of unspecified sites
Superficial frostbite NOS
T33.99 Superficial frostbite of other sites
Superficial frostbite of leg NOS
Superficial frostbite of trunk NOS

T34 Frostbite with tissue necrosis
The appropriate 7th character is to be added to each code from category T34
A = initial encounter
D = subsequent encounter
S = sequela
T34.0 Frostbite with tissue necrosis of head
T34.01 Frostbite with tissue necrosis of ear
T34.011 Frostbite with tissue necrosis of right ear
T34.012 Frostbite with tissue necrosis of left ear
T34.019 Frostbite with tissue necrosis of unspecified ear
T34.02 Frostbite with tissue necrosis of nose
T34.09 Frostbite with tissue necrosis of other part of head
T34.1 Frostbite with tissue necrosis of neck
T34.2 Frostbite with tissue necrosis of thorax
T34.3 Frostbite with tissue necrosis of abdominal wall, lower back and pelvis
T34.4 Frostbite with tissue necrosis of arm
EXCLUDES2 *frostbite with tissue necrosis of wrist and hand (T34.5-)*
T34.40 Frostbite with tissue necrosis of unspecified arm
T34.41 Frostbite with tissue necrosis of right arm
T34.42 Frostbite with tissue necrosis of left arm
T34.5 Frostbite with tissue necrosis of wrist, hand, and finger(s)
T34.51 Frostbite with tissue necrosis of wrist
T34.511 Frostbite with tissue necrosis of right wrist
T34.512 Frostbite with tissue necrosis of left wrist
T34.519 Frostbite with tissue necrosis of unspecified wrist
T34.52 Frostbite with tissue necrosis of hand
EXCLUDES2 *frostbite with tissue necrosis of finger(s) (T34.53-)*
T34.521 Frostbite with tissue necrosis of right hand
T34.522 Frostbite with tissue necrosis of left hand
T34.529 Frostbite with tissue necrosis of unspecified hand
T34.53 Frostbite with tissue necrosis of finger(s)
T34.531 Frostbite with tissue necrosis of right finger(s)
T34.532 Frostbite with tissue necrosis of left finger(s)
T34.539 Frostbite with tissue necrosis of unspecified finger(s)
T34.6 Frostbite with tissue necrosis of hip and thigh
T34.60 Frostbite with tissue necrosis of unspecified hip and thigh
T34.61 Frostbite with tissue necrosis of right hip and thigh
T34.62 Frostbite with tissue necrosis of left hip and thigh
T34.7 Frostbite with tissue necrosis of knee and lower leg
EXCLUDES2 *frostbite with tissue necrosis of ankle and foot (T34.8-)*
T34.70 Frostbite with tissue necrosis of unspecified knee and lower leg
T34.71 Frostbite with tissue necrosis of right knee and lower leg
T34.72 Frostbite with tissue necrosis of left knee and lower leg
T34.8 Frostbite with tissue necrosis of ankle, foot, and toe(s)
T34.81 Frostbite with tissue necrosis of ankle
T34.811 Frostbite with tissue necrosis of right ankle
T34.812 Frostbite with tissue necrosis of left ankle
T34.819 Frostbite with tissue necrosis of unspecified ankle
T34.82 Frostbite with tissue necrosis of foot
T34.821 Frostbite with tissue necrosis of right foot
T34.822 Frostbite with tissue necrosis of left foot
T34.829 Frostbite with tissue necrosis of unspecified foot
T34.83 Frostbite with tissue necrosis of toe(s)
T34.831 Frostbite with tissue necrosis of right toe(s)
T34.832 Frostbite with tissue necrosis of left toe(s)
T34.839 Frostbite with tissue necrosis of unspecified toe(s)
T34.9 Frostbite with tissue necrosis of other and unspecified sites
T34.90 Frostbite with tissue necrosis of unspecified sites
Frostbite with tissue necrosis NOS
T34.99 Frostbite with tissue necrosis of other sites
Frostbite with tissue necrosis of leg NOS
Frostbite with tissue necrosis of trunk NOS

Poisoning by, adverse effects of and underdosing of drugs, medicaments and biological substances (T36-T50)

INCLUDES *adverse effect of correct substance properly administered*
poisoning by overdose of substance
poisoning by wrong substance given or taken in error
underdosing by (inadvertently) (deliberately) taking less substance than prescribed or instructed

Code first , for adverse effects, the nature of the adverse effect, such as:
adverse effect NOS (T88.7)
aspirin gastritis (K29.-)
blood disorders (D56-D76)
contact dermatitis (L23-L25)
dermatitis due to substances taken internally (L27.-)
nephropathy (N14.0-N14.2)

NOTES The drug giving rise to the adverse effect should be identified by use of codes from categories T36-T50 with fifth or sixth character 5.

Use additional code(s) to specify:
manifestations of poisoning
underdosing or failure in dosage during medical and surgical care (Y63.6, Y63.8-Y63.9)
underdosing of medication regimen (Z91.12-, Z91.13-)

EXCLUDES1 *toxic reaction to local anesthesia in pregnancy (O29.3-)*

EXCLUDES2 *abuse and dependence of psychoactive substances (F10-F19)*
abuse of non-dependence-producing substances (F55.-)
drug reaction and poisoning affecting newborn (P00-P96)
pathological drug intoxication (inebriation) (F10-F19)

T36 Poisoning by, adverse effect of and underdosing of systemic antibiotics

EXCLUDES1 *antineoplastic antibiotics (T45.1-)*
locally applied antibiotic NEC (T49.0)
topically used antibiotic for ear, nose and throat (T49.6)
topically used antibiotic for eye (T49.5)

The appropriate 7th character is to be added to each code from category T36
A = initial encounter
D = subsequent encounter
S = sequela

T36.0 **Poisoning by, adverse effect of and underdosing of penicillins**
T36.0X **Poisoning by, adverse effect of and underdosing of penicillins**
T36.0X1 **Poisoning by penicillins, accidental (unintentional)**
Poisoning by penicillins NOS
T36.0X2 **Poisoning by penicillins, intentional self-harm**
T36.0X3 **Poisoning by penicillins, assault**
T36.0X4 **Poisoning by penicillins, undetermined**
T36.0X5 **Adverse effect of penicillins**
T36.0X6 **Underdosing of penicillins**

T36.1 **Poisoning by, adverse effect of and underdosing of cephalosporins and other beta-lactam antibiotics**
T36.1X **Poisoning by, adverse effect of and underdosing of cephalosporins and other beta-lactam antibiotics**
T36.1X1 **Poisoning by cephalosporins and other beta-lactam antibiotics, accidental (unintentional)**
Poisoning by cephalosporins and other beta-lactam antibiotics NOS
T36.1X2 **Poisoning by cephalosporins and other beta-lactam antibiotics, intentional self-harm**
T36.1X3 **Poisoning by cephalosporins and other beta-lactam antibiotics, assault**
T36.1X4 **Poisoning by cephalosporins and other beta-lactam antibiotics, undetermined**
T36.1X5 **Adverse effect of cephalosporins and other beta-lactam antibiotics**
T36.1X6 **Underdosing of cephalosporins and other beta-lactam antibiotics**

T36.2 **Poisoning by, adverse effect of and underdosing of chloramphenicol group**
T36.2X **Poisoning by, adverse effect of and underdosing of chloramphenicol group**
T36.2X1 **Poisoning by chloramphenicol group, accidental (unintentional)**
Poisoning by chloramphenicol group NOS
T36.2X2 **Poisoning by chloramphenicol group, intentional self-harm**
T36.2X3 **Poisoning by chloramphenicol group, assault**
T36.2X4 **Poisoning by chloramphenicol group, undetermined**
T36.2X5 **Adverse effect of chloramphenicol group**
T36.2X6 **Underdosing of chloramphenicol group**

T36.3 **Poisoning by, adverse effect of and underdosing of macrolides**
T36.3X **Poisoning by, adverse effect of and underdosing of macrolides**
T36.3X1 **Poisoning by macrolides, accidental (unintentional)**
Poisoning by macrolides NOS
T36.3X2 **Poisoning by macrolides, intentional self-harm**
T36.3X3 **Poisoning by macrolides, assault**
T36.3X4 **Poisoning by macrolides, undetermined**
T36.3X5 **Adverse effect of macrolides**
T36.3X6 **Underdosing of macrolides**

T36.4 **Poisoning by, adverse effect of and underdosing of tetracyclines**
T36.4X **Poisoning by, adverse effect of and underdosing of tetracyclines**
T36.4X1 **Poisoning by tetracyclines, accidental (unintentional)**
Poisoning by tetracyclines NOS
T36.4X2 **Poisoning by tetracyclines, intentional self-harm**
T36.4X3 **Poisoning by tetracyclines, assault**
T36.4X4 **Poisoning by tetracyclines, undetermined**
T36.4X5 **Adverse effect of tetracyclines**
T36.4X6 **Underdosing of tetracyclines**

T36.5 **Poisoning by, adverse effect of and underdosing of aminoglycosides**
Poisoning by, adverse effect of and underdosing of streptomycin
T36.5X **Poisoning by, adverse effect of and underdosing of aminoglycosides**
T36.5X1 **Poisoning by aminoglycosides, accidental (unintentional)**
Poisoning by aminoglycosides NOS
T36.5X2 **Poisoning by aminoglycosides, intentional self-harm**
T36.5X3 **Poisoning by aminoglycosides, assault**
T36.5X4 **Poisoning by aminoglycosides, undetermined**
T36.5X5 **Adverse effect of aminoglycosides**
T36.5X6 **Underdosing of aminoglycosides**

T36.6 **Poisoning by, adverse effect of and underdosing of rifampicins**
T36.6X **Poisoning by, adverse effect of and underdosing of rifampicins**
T36.6X1 **Poisoning by rifampicins, accidental (unintentional)**
Poisoning by rifampicins NOS
T36.6X2 **Poisoning by rifampicins, intentional self-harm**
T36.6X3 **Poisoning by rifampicins, assault**
T36.6X4 **Poisoning by rifampicins, undetermined**
T36.6X5 **Adverse effect of rifampicins**
T36.6X6 **Underdosing of rifampicins**

T36.7 **Poisoning by, adverse effect of and underdosing of antifungal antibiotics, systemically used**
T36.7X **Poisoning by, adverse effect of and underdosing of antifungal antibiotics , systemically used**
T36.7X1 **Poisoning by antifungal antibiotics, systemically used, accidental (unintentional)**
Poisoning by antifungal antibiotics, systemically used NOS
T36.7X2 **Poisoning by antifungal antibiotics, systemically used, intentional self-harm**
T36.7X3 **Poisoning by antifungal antibiotics, systemically used, assault**
T36.7X4 **Poisoning by antifungal antibiotics, systemically used, undetermined**
T36.7X5 **Adverse effect of antifungal antibiotics, systemically used**
T36.7X6 **Underdosing of antifungal antibiotics, systemically used**

T36.8 **Poisoning by, adverse effect of and underdosing of other systemic antibiotics**
T36.8X **Poisoning by, adverse effect of and underdosing of other systemic antibiotics**
T36.8X1 **Poisoning by other systemic antibiotics, accidental (unintentional)**
Poisoning by other systemic antibiotics NOS
T36.8X2 **Poisoning by other systemic antibiotics, intentional self-harm**
T36.8X3 **Poisoning by other systemic antibiotics, assault**
T36.8X4 **Poisoning by other systemic antibiotics, undetermined**
T36.8X5 **Adverse effect of other systemic antibiotics**
T36.8X6 **Underdosing of other systemic antibiotics**

T36.9 **Poisoning by, adverse effect of and underdosing of unspecified systemic antibiotic**
T36.91 **Poisoning by unspecified systemic antibiotic, accidental (unintentional)**
Poisoning by systemic antibiotic NOS

Unacceptable principal diagnosis symbol per Medicare code edits — Code exempt from diagnosis present on admission requirement
Questionable admission — Complication or comorbidity — CC/MCC exclusion — Major complication or comorbidity
Principal diagnosis as its own CC — Principal diagnosis as its own MCC — Z code as first-listed diagnosis

T36.92 Poisoning by unspecified systemic antibiotic, intentional self-harm
T36.93 Poisoning by unspecified systemic antibiotic, assault
T36.94 Poisoning by unspecified systemic antibiotic, undetermined
T36.95 Adverse effect of unspecified systemic antibiotic
T36.96 Underdosing of unspecified systemic antibiotic

T37 Poisoning by, adverse effect of and underdosing of other systemic anti- infectives and antiparasitics

EXCLUDES1 *anti-infectives topically used for ear, nose and throat (T49.6-)*
anti-infectives topically used for eye (T49.5-)
locally applied anti-infectives NEC (T49.0-)

The appropriate 7th character is to be added to each code from category T37
A = initial encounter
D = subsequent encounter
S = sequela

T37.0 Poisoning by, adverse effect of and underdosing of sulfonamides
T37.0X Poisoning by, adverse effect of and underdosing of sulfonamides
T37.0X1 Poisoning by sulfonamides, accidental (unintentional)
Poisoning by sulfonamides NOS
T37.0X2 Poisoning by sulfonamides, intentional self-harm
T37.0X3 Poisoning by sulfonamides, assault
T37.0X4 Poisoning by sulfonamides, undetermined
T37.0X5 Adverse effect of sulfonamides
T37.0X6 Underdosing of sulfonamides

T37.1 Poisoning by, adverse effect of and underdosing of antimycobacterial drugs
EXCLUDES1 *rifampicins (T36.6-)*
streptomycin (T36.5-)
T37.1X Poisoning by, adverse effect of and underdosing of antimycobacterial drugs
T37.1X1 Poisoning by antimycobacterial drugs, accidental (unintentional)
Poisoning by antimycobacterial drugs NOS
T37.1X2 Poisoning by antimycobacterial drugs, intentional self-harm
T37.1X3 Poisoning by antimycobacterial drugs, assault
T37.1X4 Poisoning by antimycobacterial drugs, undetermined
T37.1X5 Adverse effect of antimycobacterial drugs
T37.1X6 Underdosing of antimycobacterial drugs

T37.2 Poisoning by, adverse effect of and underdosing of antimalarials and drugs acting on other blood protozoa
EXCLUDES1 *hydroxyquinoline derivatives (T37.8-)*
T37.2X Poisoning by, adverse effect of and underdosing of antimalarials and drugs acting on other blood protozoa
T37.2X1 Poisoning by antimalarials and drugs acting on other blood protozoa, accidental (unintentional)
Poisoning by antimalarials and drugs acting on other blood protozoa NOS
T37.2X2 Poisoning by antimalarials and drugs acting on other blood protozoa, intentional self-harm
T37.2X3 Poisoning by antimalarials and drugs acting on other blood protozoa, assault
T37.2X4 Poisoning by antimalarials and drugs acting on other blood protozoa, undetermined
T37.2X5 Adverse effect of antimalarials and drugs acting on other blood protozoa
T37.2X6 Underdosing of antimalarials and drugs acting on other blood protozoa

T37.3 Poisoning by, adverse effect of and underdosing of other antiprotozoal drugs
T37.3X Poisoning by, adverse effect of and underdosing of other antiprotozoal drugs
T37.3X1 Poisoning by other antiprotozoal drugs, accidental (unintentional)
Poisoning by other antiprotozoal drugs NOS
T37.3X2 Poisoning by other antiprotozoal drugs, intentional self-harm
T37.3X3 Poisoning by other antiprotozoal drugs, assault
T37.3X4 Poisoning by other antiprotozoal drugs, undetermined
T37.3X5 Adverse effect of other antiprotozoal drugs
T37.3X6 Underdosing of other antiprotozoal drugs

T37.4 Poisoning by, adverse effect of and underdosing of anthelminthics
T37.4X Poisoning by, adverse effect of and underdosing of anthelminthics
T37.4X1 Poisoning by anthelminthics, accidental (unintentional)
Poisoning by anthelminthics NOS
T37.4X2 Poisoning by anthelminthics, intentional self-harm
T37.4X3 Poisoning by anthelminthics, assault
T37.4X4 Poisoning by anthelminthics, undetermined
T37.4X5 Adverse effect of anthelminthics
T37.4X6 Underdosing of anthelminthics

T37.5 Poisoning by, adverse effect of and underdosing of antiviral drugs
EXCLUDES1 *amantadine (T42.8-)*
cytarabine (T45.1-)
T37.5X Poisoning by, adverse effect of and underdosing of antiviral drugs
T37.5X1 Poisoning by antiviral drugs, accidental (unintentional)
Poisoning by antiviral drugs NOS
T37.5X2 Poisoning by antiviral drugs, intentional self-harm
T37.5X3 Poisoning by antiviral drugs, assault
T37.5X4 Poisoning by antiviral drugs, undetermined
T37.5X5 Adverse effect of antiviral drugs
T37.5X6 Underdosing of antiviral drugs

T37.8 Poisoning by, adverse effect of and underdosing of other specified systemic anti-infectives and antiparasitics
Poisoning by, adverse effect of and underdosing of hydroxyquinoline derivatives
EXCLUDES1 *antimalarial drugs (T37.2-)*
T37.8X Poisoning by, adverse effect of and underdosing of other specified systemic anti-infectives and antiparasitics
T37.8X1 Poisoning by other specified systemic anti-infectives and antiparasitics, accidental (unintentional)
Poisoning by other specified systemic anti-infectives and antiparasitics NOS
T37.8X2 Poisoning by other specified systemic anti-infectives and antiparasitics, intentional self-harm
T37.8X3 Poisoning by other specified systemic anti-infectives and antiparasitics, assault
T37.8X4 Poisoning by other specified systemic anti-infectives and antiparasitics, undetermined
T37.8X5 Adverse effect of other specified systemic anti-infectives and antiparasitics
T37.8X6 Underdosing of other specified systemic anti-infectives and antiparasitics

T37.9 Poisoning by, adverse effect of and underdosing of unspecified systemic anti-infective and antiparasitics
T37.91 Poisoning by unspecified systemic anti-infective and antiparasitics, accidental (unintentional)
Poisoning by, adverse effect of and underdosing of systemic anti-infective and antiparasitics NOS
T37.92 Poisoning by unspecified systemic anti-infective and antiparasitics, intentional self-harm

Unspecified Code | Other Specified Code | Manifestation Code | N Newborn | P Pediatric | M Maternity | A Adult | ♂ Male | ♀ Female
● New Code ▲ Revised Code Title ►◄ Revised Text NOTES INCLUDES EXCLUDES1 Not coded here EXCLUDES2 Not included here
4th character required 5th character required 6th character required 7th character required
Extension 'X' Alert HAC Hospital-acquired condition (HAC) alert AHA AHA Coding Clinic®

T37.93 Poisoning by unspecified systemic anti-infective and antiparasitics, assault

T37.94 Poisoning by unspecified systemic anti-infective and antiparasitics, undetermined

T37.95 Adverse effect of unspecified systemic anti-infective and antiparasitic

T37.96 Underdosing of unspecified systemic anti-infectives and antiparasitics

T38 Poisoning by, adverse effect of and underdosing of hormones and their synthetic substitutes and antagonists, not elsewhere classified

EXCLUDES1 *mineralocorticoids and their antagonists (T50.0-)*
oxytocic hormones (T48.0-)
parathyroid hormones and derivatives (T50.9-)

The appropriate 7th character is to be added to each code from category T38

A = initial encounter
D = subsequent encounter
S = sequela

T38.0 Poisoning by, adverse effect of and underdosing of glucocorticoids and synthetic analogues

EXCLUDES1 *glucocorticoids, topically used (T49.-)*

T38.0X Poisoning by, adverse effect of and underdosing of glucocorticoids and synthetic analogues

T38.0X1 Poisoning by glucocorticoids and synthetic analogues, accidental (unintentional)
Poisoning by glucocorticoids and synthetic analogues NOS

T38.0X2 Poisoning by glucocorticoids and synthetic analogues, intentional self-harm

T38.0X3 Poisoning by glucocorticoids and synthetic analogues, assault

T38.0X4 Poisoning by glucocorticoids and synthetic analogues, undetermined

T38.0X5 Adverse effect of glucocorticoids and synthetic analogues

T38.0X6 Underdosing of glucocorticoids and synthetic analogues

T38.1 Poisoning by, adverse effect of and underdosing of thyroid hormones and substitutes

T38.1X Poisoning by, adverse effect of and underdosing of thyroid hormones and substitutes

T38.1X1 Poisoning by thyroid hormones and substitutes, accidental (unintentional)
Poisoning by thyroid hormones and substitutes NOS

T38.1X2 Poisoning by thyroid hormones and substitutes, intentional self-harm

T38.1X3 Poisoning by thyroid hormones and substitutes, assault

T38.1X4 Poisoning by thyroid hormones and substitutes, undetermined

T38.1X5 Adverse effect of thyroid hormones and substitutes

T38.1X6 Underdosing of thyroid hormones and substitutes

T38.2 Poisoning by, adverse effect of and underdosing of antithyroid drugs

T38.2X Poisoning by, adverse effect of and underdosing of antithyroid drugs

T38.2X1 Poisoning by antithyroid drugs, accidental (unintentional)
Poisoning by antithyroid drugs NOS

T38.2X2 Poisoning by antithyroid drugs, intentional self-harm

T38.2X3 Poisoning by antithyroid drugs, assault

T38.2X4 Poisoning by antithyroid drugs, undetermined

T38.2X5 Adverse effect of antithyroid drugs

T38.2X6 Underdosing of antithyroid drugs

T38.3 Poisoning by, adverse effect of and underdosing of insulin and oral hypoglycemic [antidiabetic] drugs

T38.3X Poisoning by, adverse effect of and underdosing of insulin and oral hypoglycemic [antidiabetic] drugs

T38.3X1 Poisoning by insulin and oral hypoglycemic [antidiabetic] drugs, accidental (unintentional)
Poisoning by insulin and oral hypoglycemic [antidiabetic] drugs NOS

T38.3X2 Poisoning by insulin and oral hypoglycemic [antidiabetic] drugs, intentional self-harm

T38.3X3 Poisoning by insulin and oral hypoglycemic [antidiabetic] drugs, assault

T38.3X4 Poisoning by insulin and oral hypoglycemic [antidiabetic] drugs, undetermined

T38.3X5 Adverse effect of insulin and oral hypoglycemic [antidiabetic] drugs

T38.3X6 Underdosing of insulin and oral hypoglycemic [antidiabetic] drugs

T38.4 Poisoning by, adverse effect of and underdosing of oral contraceptives
Poisoning by, adverse effect of and underdosing of multiple- and single-ingredient oral contraceptive preparations

T38.4X Poisoning by, adverse effect of and underdosing of oral contraceptives

T38.4X1 Poisoning by oral contraceptives, accidental (unintentional)
Poisoning by oral contraceptives NOS

T38.4X2 Poisoning by oral contraceptives, intentional self-harm

T38.4X3 Poisoning by oral contraceptives, assault

T38.4X4 Poisoning by oral contraceptives, undetermined

T38.4X5 Adverse effect of oral contraceptives

T38.4X6 Underdosing of oral contraceptives

T38.5 Poisoning by, adverse effect of and underdosing of other estrogens and progestogens
Poisoning by, adverse effect of and underdosing of estrogens and progestogens mixtures and substitutes

T38.5X Poisoning by, adverse effect of and underdosing of other estrogens and progestogens

T38.5X1 Poisoning by other estrogens and progestogens, accidental (unintentional)
Poisoning by other estrogens and progestogens NOS

T38.5X2 Poisoning by other estrogens and progestogens, intentional self-harm

T38.5X3 Poisoning by other estrogens and progestogens, assault

T38.5X4 Poisoning by other estrogens and progestogens, undetermined

T38.5X5 Adverse effect of other estrogens and progestogens

T38.5X6 Underdosing of other estrogens and progestogens

T38.6 Poisoning by, adverse effect of and underdosing of antigonadotrophins, antiestrogens, antiandrogens, not elsewhere classified
Poisoning by, adverse effect of and underdosing of tamoxifen

T38.6X Poisoning by, adverse effect of and underdosing of antigonadotrophins, antiestrogens, antiandrogens, not elsewhere classified

T38.6X1 Poisoning by antigonadotrophins, antiestrogens, antiandrogens, not elsewhere classified, accidental (unintentional)
Poisoning by antigonadotrophins, antiestrogens, antiandrogens, not elsewhere classified NOS

T38.6X2 Poisoning by antigonadotrophins, antiestrogens, antiandrogens, not elsewhere classified, intentional self-harm

T38.6X3 Poisoning by antigonadotrophins, antiestrogens, antiandrogens, not elsewhere classified, assault

T38.6X4 Poisoning by antigonadotrophins, antiestrogens, antiandrogens, not elsewhere classified, undetermined

Unacceptable principal diagnosis symbol per Medicare code edits | Code exempt from diagnosis present on admission requirement | Questionable admission | Complication or comorbidity | CC/MCC exclusion | Major complication or comorbidity | Principal diagnosis as its own CC | Principal diagnosis as its own MCC | Z code as first-listed diagnosis

T38.6X5 Adverse effect of antigonadotrophins, antiestrogens, antiandrogens, not elsewhere classified
T38.6X6 Underdosing of antigonadotrophins, antiestrogens, antiandrogens, not elsewhere classified

T38.7 Poisoning by, adverse effect of and underdosing of androgens and anabolic congeners
T38.7X Poisoning by, adverse effect of and underdosing of androgens and anabolic congeners
T38.7X1 Poisoning by androgens and anabolic congeners, accidental (unintentional)
Poisoning by androgens and anabolic congeners NOS
T38.7X2 Poisoning by androgens and anabolic congeners, intentional self-harm
T38.7X3 Poisoning by androgens and anabolic congeners, assault
T38.7X4 Poisoning by androgens and anabolic congeners, undetermined
T38.7X5 Adverse effect of androgens and anabolic congeners
T38.7X6 Underdosing of androgens and anabolic congeners

T38.8 Poisoning by, adverse effect of and underdosing of other and unspecified hormones and synthetic substitutes
T38.80 Poisoning by, adverse effect of and underdosing of unspecified hormones and synthetic substitutes
T38.801 Poisoning by unspecified hormones and synthetic substitutes, accidental (unintentional)
Poisoning by unspecified hormones and synthetic substitutes NOS
T38.802 Poisoning by unspecified hormones and synthetic substitutes, intentional self-harm
T38.803 Poisoning by unspecified hormones and synthetic substitutes, assault
T38.804 Poisoning by unspecified hormones and synthetic substitutes, undetermined
T38.805 Adverse effect of unspecified hormones and synthetic substitutes
T38.806 Underdosing of unspecified hormones and synthetic substitutes
T38.81 Poisoning by, adverse effect of and underdosing of anterior pituitary [adenohypophyseal] hormones
T38.811 Poisoning by anterior pituitary [adenohypophyseal] hormones, accidental (unintentional)
Poisoning by anterior pituitary [adenohypophyseal] hormones NOS
T38.812 Poisoning by anterior pituitary [adenohypophyseal] hormones, intentional self-harm
T38.813 Poisoning by anterior pituitary [adenohypophyseal] hormones, assault
T38.814 Poisoning by anterior pituitary [adenohypophyseal] hormones, undetermined
T38.815 Adverse effect of anterior pituitary [adenohypophyseal] hormones
T38.816 Underdosing of anterior pituitary [adenohypophyseal] hormones
T38.89 Poisoning by, adverse effect of and underdosing of other hormones and synthetic substitutes
T38.891 Poisoning by other hormones and synthetic substitutes, accidental (unintentional)
Poisoning by other hormones and synthetic substitutes NOS
T38.892 Poisoning by other hormones and synthetic substitutes, intentional self-harm
T38.893 Poisoning by other hormones and synthetic substitutes, assault
T38.894 Poisoning by other hormones and synthetic substitutes, undetermined
T38.895 Adverse effect of other hormones and synthetic substitutes
T38.896 Underdosing of other hormones and synthetic substitutes

T38.9 Poisoning by, adverse effect of and underdosing of other and unspecified hormone antagonists
T38.90 Poisoning by, adverse effect of and underdosing of unspecified hormone antagonists
T38.901 Poisoning by unspecified hormone antagonists, accidental (unintentional)
Poisoning by unspecified hormone antagonists NOS
T38.902 Poisoning by unspecified hormone antagonists, intentional self-harm
T38.903 Poisoning by unspecified hormone antagonists, assault
T38.904 Poisoning by unspecified hormone antagonists, undetermined
T38.905 Adverse effect of unspecified hormone antagonists
T38.906 Underdosing of unspecified hormone antagonists
T38.99 Poisoning by, adverse effect of and underdosing of other hormone antagonists
T38.991 Poisoning by other hormone antagonists, accidental (unintentional)
Poisoning by other hormone antagonists NOS
T38.992 Poisoning by other hormone antagonists, intentional self-harm
T38.993 Poisoning by other hormone antagonists, assault
T38.994 Poisoning by other hormone antagonists, undetermined
T38.995 Adverse effect of other hormone antagonists
T38.996 Underdosing of other hormone antagonists

T39 Poisoning by, adverse effect of and underdosing of nonopioid analgesics, antipyretics and antirheumatics

The appropriate 7th character is to be added to each code from category T39
A = initial encounter
D = subsequent encounter
S = sequela

T39.0 Poisoning by, adverse effect of and underdosing of salicylates
T39.01 Poisoning by, adverse effect of and underdosing of aspirin
Poisoning by, adverse effect of and underdosing of acetylsalicylic acid
T39.011 Poisoning by aspirin, accidental (unintentional)
T39.012 Poisoning by aspirin, intentional self-harm
T39.013 Poisoning by aspirin, assault
T39.014 Poisoning by aspirin, undetermined
T39.015 Adverse effect of aspirin
AHA: Q1, 2016
T39.016 Underdosing of aspirin
T39.09 Poisoning by, adverse effect of and underdosing of other salicylates
T39.091 Poisoning by salicylates, accidental (unintentional)
Poisoning by salicylates NOS
T39.092 Poisoning by salicylates, intentional self-harm
T39.093 Poisoning by salicylates, assault
T39.094 Poisoning by salicylates, undetermined
T39.095 Adverse effect of salicylates
T39.096 Underdosing of salicylates

T39.1 Poisoning by, adverse effect of and underdosing of 4-Aminophenol derivatives
T39.1X Poisoning by, adverse effect of and underdosing of 4-Aminophenol derivative s
T39.1X1 Poisoning by 4-Aminophenol derivatives, accidental (unintentional)

Unspecified Code Other Specified Code Manifestation Code N Newborn P Pediatric M Maternity A Adult ♂ Male ♀ Female
● New Code ▲ Revised Code Title ►◄ Revised Text NOTES INCLUDES EXCLUDES 1 Not coded here EXCLUDES 2 Not included here
4th character required 5th character required 6th character required 7th character required
Extension 'X' Alert HAC Hospital-acquired condition (HAC) alert AHA AHA Coding Clinic©

Poisoning by 4-Aminophenol derivatives NOS

- T39.1X2 **Poisoning by 4-Aminophenol derivatives, intentional self-harm**
- T39.1X3 **Poisoning by 4-Aminophenol derivatives, assault**
- T39.1X4 **Poisoning by 4-Aminophenol derivatives, undetermined**
- T39.1X5 **Adverse effect of 4-Aminophenol derivatives**
- T39.1X6 **Underdosing of 4-Aminophenol derivatives**

T39.2 **Poisoning by, adverse effect of and underdosing of pyrazolone derivatives**

T39.2X **Poisoning by, adverse effect of and underdosing of pyrazolone derivatives**

- T39.2X1 **Poisoning by pyrazolone derivatives, accidental (unintentional)**
  Poisoning by pyrazolone derivatives NOS
- T39.2X2 **Poisoning by pyrazolone derivatives, intentional self-harm**
- T39.2X3 **Poisoning by pyrazolone derivatives, assault**
- T39.2X4 **Poisoning by pyrazolone derivatives, undetermined**
- T39.2X5 **Adverse effect of pyrazolone derivatives**
- T39.2X6 **Underdosing of pyrazolone derivatives**

T39.3 **Poisoning by, adverse effect of and underdosing of other nonsteroidal anti-inflammatory drugs [NSAID]**

T39.31 **Poisoning by, adverse effect of and underdosing of propionic acid derivatives**

Poisoning by, adverse effect of and underdosing of fenoprofen
Poisoning by, adverse effect of and underdosing of flurbiprofen
Poisoning by, adverse effect of and underdosing of ibuprofen
Poisoning by, adverse effect of and underdosing of ketoprofen
Poisoning by, adverse effect of and underdosing of naproxen
Poisoning by, adverse effect of and underdosing of oxaprozin

- T39.311 **Poisoning by propionic acid derivatives, accidental (unintentional)**
- T39.312 **Poisoning by propionic acid derivatives, intentional self-harm**
- T39.313 **Poisoning by propionic acid derivatives, assault**
- T39.314 **Poisoning by propionic acid derivatives, undetermined**
- T39.315 **Adverse effect of propionic acid derivatives**
- T39.316 **Underdosing of propionic acid derivatives**

T39.39 **Poisoning by, adverse effect of and underdosing of other nonsteroidal anti-inflammatory drugs [NSAID]**

- T39.391 **Poisoning by other nonsteroidal anti-inflammatory drugs [NSAID], accidental (unintentional)**
  Poisoning by other nonsteroidal anti-inflammatory drugs NOS
- T39.392 **Poisoning by other nonsteroidal anti-inflammatory drugs [NSAID], intentional self-harm**
- T39.393 **Poisoning by other nonsteroidal anti-inflammatory drugs [NSAID], assault**
- T39.394 **Poisoning by other nonsteroidal anti-inflammatory drugs [NSAID], undetermined**
- T39.395 **Adverse effect of other nonsteroidal anti-inflammatory drugs [NSAID]**
- T39.396 **Underdosing of other nonsteroidal anti-inflammatory drugs [NSAID]**

T39.4 **Poisoning by, adverse effect of and underdosing of antirheumatics, not elsewhere classified**

EXCLUDES1 *poisoning by, adverse effect of and underdosing of glucocorticoids (T38.0-)*
poisoning by, adverse effect of and underdosing of salicylates (T39.0-)

T39.4X **Poisoning by, adverse effect of and underdosing of antirheumatics, not elsewhere classified**

- T39.4X1 **Poisoning by antirheumatics, not elsewhere classified, accidental (unintentional)**
  Poisoning by antirheumatics, not elsewhere classified NOS
- T39.4X2 **Poisoning by antirheumatics, not elsewhere classified, intentional self-harm**
- T39.4X3 **Poisoning by antirheumatics, not elsewhere classified, assault**
- T39.4X4 **Poisoning by antirheumatics, not elsewhere classified, undetermined**
- T39.4X5 **Adverse effect of antirheumatics, not elsewhere classified**
- T39.4X6 **Underdosing of antirheumatics, not elsewhere classified**

T39.8 **Poisoning by, adverse effect of and underdosing of other nonopioid analgesics and antipyretics, not elsewhere classified**

T39.8X **Poisoning by, adverse effect of and underdosing of other nonopioid analgesics and antipyretics, not elsewhere classified**

- T39.8X1 **Poisoning by other nonopioid analgesics and antipyretics, not elsewhere classified, accidental (unintentional)**
  Poisoning by other nonopioid analgesics and antipyretics, not elsewhere classified NOS
- T39.8X2 **Poisoning by other nonopioid analgesics and antipyretics, not elsewhere classified, intentional self-harm**
- T39.8X3 **Poisoning by other nonopioid analgesics and antipyretics, not elsewhere classified, assault**
- T39.8X4 **Poisoning by other nonopioid analgesics and antipyretics, not elsewhere classified, undetermined**
- T39.8X5 **Adverse effect of other nonopioid analgesics and antipyretics, not elsewhere classified**
- T39.8X6 **Underdosing of other nonopioid analgesics and antipyretics, not elsewhere classified**

T39.9 **Poisoning by, adverse effect of and underdosing of unspecified nonopioid analgesic, antipyretic and antirheumatic**

- T39.91 **Poisoning by unspecified nonopioid analgesic, antipyretic and antirheumatic, accidental (unintentional)**
  Poisoning by nonopioid analgesic, antipyretic and antirheumatic NOS
- T39.92 **Poisoning by unspecified nonopioid analgesic, antipyretic and antirheumatic, intentional self-harm**
- T39.93 **Poisoning by unspecified nonopioid analgesic, antipyretic and antirheumatic, assault**
- T39.94 **Poisoning by unspecified nonopioid analgesic, antipyretic and antirheumatic, undetermined**
- T39.95 **Adverse effect of unspecified nonopioid analgesic, antipyretic and antirheumatic**
- T39.96 **Underdosing of unspecified nonopioid analgesic, antipyretic and antirheumatic**

T40 **Poisoning by, adverse effect of and underdosing of narcotics and psychodysleptics [hallucinogens]**

EXCLUDES2 *drug dependence and related mental and behavioral disorders due to psychoactive substance use (F10.-F19.-)*

The appropriate 7th character is to be added to each code from category T40

A = initial encounter
D = subsequent encounter
S = sequela

T40.0 **Poisoning by, adverse effect of and underdosing of opium**

T40.0X **Poisoning by, adverse effect of and underdosing of opium**

Unacceptable principal diagnosis symbol per Medicare code edits — Code exempt from diagnosis present on admission requirement
Questionable admission — Complication or comorbidity — CC/MCC exclusion — Major complication or comorbidity
Principal diagnosis as its own CC — Principal diagnosis as its own MCC — Z code as first-listed diagnosis

T40.0X1 Poisoning by opium, accidental (unintentional)
Poisoning by opium NOS
T40.0X2 Poisoning by opium, intentional self-harm
T40.0X3 Poisoning by opium, assault
T40.0X4 Poisoning by opium, undetermined
T40.0X5 Adverse effect of opium
T40.0X6 Underdosing of opium
T40.1 Poisoning by and adverse effect of heroin
T40.1X Poisoning by and adverse effect of heroin
T40.1X1 Poisoning by heroin, accidental (unintentional)
Poisoning by heroin NOS
T40.1X2 Poisoning by heroin, intentional self-harm
T40.1X3 Poisoning by heroin, assault
T40.1X4 Poisoning by heroin, undetermined
T40.2 Poisoning by, adverse effect of and underdosing of other opioids
T40.2X Poisoning by, adverse effect of and underdosing of other opioids
T40.2X1 Poisoning by other opioids, accidental (unintentional)
Poisoning by other opioids NOS
T40.2X2 Poisoning by other opioids, intentional self-harm
T40.2X3 Poisoning by other opioids, assault
T40.2X4 Poisoning by other opioids, undetermined
T40.2X5 Adverse effect of other opioids
T40.2X6 Underdosing of other opioids
T40.3 Poisoning by, adverse effect of and underdosing of methadone
T40.3X Poisoning by, adverse effect of and underdosing of methadone
T40.3X1 Poisoning by methadone, accidental (unintentional)
Poisoning by methadone NOS
T40.3X2 Poisoning by methadone, intentional self-harm
T40.3X3 Poisoning by methadone, assault
T40.3X4 Poisoning by methadone, undetermined
T40.3X5 Adverse effect of methadone
T40.3X6 Underdosing of methadone
T40.4 Poisoning by, adverse effect of and underdosing of other synthetic narcotics
T40.4X Poisoning by, adverse effect of and underdosing of other synthetic narcotics
T40.4X1 Poisoning by other synthetic narcotics, accidental (unintentional)
Poisoning by other synthetic narcotics NOS
T40.4X2 Poisoning by other synthetic narcotics, intentional self-harm
T40.4X3 Poisoning by other synthetic narcotics, assault
T40.4X4 Poisoning by other synthetic narcotics, undetermined
T40.4X5 Adverse effect of other synthetic narcotics
T40.4X6 Underdosing of other synthetic narcotics
T40.5 Poisoning by, adverse effect of and underdosing of cocaine
T40.5X Poisoning by, adverse effect of and underdosing of cocaine
T40.5X1 Poisoning by cocaine, accidental (unintentional)
Poisoning by cocaine NOS
AHA: Q2, 2016
T40.5X2 Poisoning by cocaine, intentional self-harm
T40.5X3 Poisoning by cocaine, assault
T40.5X4 Poisoning by cocaine, undetermined
T40.5X5 Adverse effect of cocaine
T40.5X6 Underdosing of cocaine
T40.6 Poisoning by, adverse effect of and underdosing of other and unspecified narcotics
T40.60 Poisoning by, adverse effect of and underdosing of unspecified narcotics
T40.601 Poisoning by unspecified narcotics, accidental (unintentional)
Poisoning by narcotics NOS
T40.602 Poisoning by unspecified narcotics, intentional self-harm
T40.603 Poisoning by unspecified narcotics, assault
T40.604 Poisoning by unspecified narcotics, undetermined
T40.605 Adverse effect of unspecified narcotics
T40.606 Underdosing of unspecified narcotics
T40.69 Poisoning by, adverse effect of and underdosing of other narcotics
T40.691 Poisoning by other narcotics, accidental (unintentional)
Poisoning by other narcotics NOS
T40.692 Poisoning by other narcotics, intentional self-harm
T40.693 Poisoning by other narcotics, assault
T40.694 Poisoning by other narcotics, undetermined
T40.695 Adverse effect of other narcotics
T40.696 Underdosing of other narcotics
T40.7 Poisoning by, adverse effect of and underdosing of cannabis (derivatives)
T40.7X Poisoning by, adverse effect of and underdosing of cannabis (derivatives)
T40.7X1 Poisoning by cannabis (derivatives), accidental (unintentional)
Poisoning by cannabis NOS
T40.7X2 Poisoning by cannabis (derivatives), intentional self-harm
T40.7X3 Poisoning by cannabis (derivatives), assault
T40.7X4 Poisoning by cannabis (derivatives), undetermined
T40.7X5 Adverse effect of cannabis (derivatives)
T40.7X6 Underdosing of cannabis (derivatives)
T40.8 Poisoning by and adverse effect of lysergide [LSD]
T40.8X Poisoning by and adverse effect of lysergide [LSD]
T40.8X1 Poisoning by lysergide [LSD], accidental (unintentional)
Poisoning by lysergide [LSD]NOS
T40.8X2 Poisoning by lysergide [LSD], intentional self-harm
T40.8X3 Poisoning by lysergide [LSD], assault
T40.8X4 Poisoning by lysergide [LSD], undetermined
T40.9 Poisoning by, adverse effect of and underdosing of other and unspecified psychodysleptics [hallucinogens]
T40.90 Poisoning by, adverse effect of and underdosing of unspecified psychodysleptics [hallucinogens]
T40.901 Poisoning by unspecified psychodysleptics [hallucinogens], accidental (unintentional)
T40.902 Poisoning by unspecified psychodysleptics [hallucinogens], intentional self-harm
T40.903 Poisoning by unspecified psychodysleptics [hallucinogens], assault
T40.904 Poisoning by unspecified psychodysleptics [hallucinogens], undetermined
T40.905 Adverse effect of unspecified psychodysleptics [hallucinogens]
T40.906 Underdosing of unspecified psychodysleptics
T40.99 Poisoning by, adverse effect of and underdosing of other psychodysleptics [hallucinogens]
T40.991 Poisoning by other psychodysleptics [hallucinogens], accidental (unintentional)
Poisoning by other psychodysleptics [hallucinogens] NOS
T40.992 Poisoning by other psychodysleptics [hallucinogens], intentional self-harm

Unspecified Code Other Specified Code Manifestation Code N Newborn P Pediatric M Maternity A Adult ♂ Male ♀ Female
● New Code ▲ Revised Code Title ►◄ Revised Text NOTES INCLUDES EXCLUDES1 Not coded here EXCLUDES2 Not included here
4th character required 5th character required 6th character required 7th character required
Extension 'X' Alert HAC Hospital-acquired condition (HAC) alert AHA AHA Coding Clinic©

T40.993 Poisoning by other psychodysleptics [hallucinogens], assault
T40.994 Poisoning by other psychodysleptics [hallucinogens], undetermined
T40.995 Adverse effect of other psychodysleptics [hallucinogens]
T40.996 Underdosing of other psychodysleptics

T41 Poisoning by, adverse effect of and underdosing of anesthetics and therapeutic gases

EXCLUDES1 *benzodiazepines (T42.4-)*
cocaine (T40.5-)
complications of anesthesia during pregnancy (O29.-)
complications of anesthesia during labor and delivery (O74.-)
complications of anesthesia during the puerperium (O89.-)
opioids (T40.0-T40.2-)

The appropriate 7th character is to be added to each code from category T41
A = initial encounter
D = subsequent encounter
S = sequela

T41.0 Poisoning by, adverse effect of and underdosing of inhaled anesthetics
EXCLUDES1 *oxygen (T41.5-)*

T41.0X Poisoning by, adverse effect of and underdosing of inhaled anesthetics
T41.0X1 Poisoning by inhaled anesthetics, accidental (unintentional)
Poisoning by inhaled anesthetics NOS
T41.0X2 Poisoning by inhaled anesthetics, intentional self-harm
T41.0X3 Poisoning by inhaled anesthetics, assault
T41.0X4 Poisoning by inhaled anesthetics, undetermined
T41.0X5 Adverse effect of inhaled anesthetics
T41.0X6 Underdosing of inhaled anesthetics

T41.1 Poisoning by, adverse effect of and underdosing of intravenous anesthetics
Poisoning by, adverse effect of and underdosing of thiobarbiturates

T41.1X Poisoning by, adverse effect of and underdosing of intravenous anesthetics
T41.1X1 Poisoning by intravenous anesthetics, accidental (unintentional)
Poisoning by intravenous anesthetics NOS
T41.1X2 Poisoning by intravenous anesthetics, intentional self-harm
T41.1X3 Poisoning by intravenous anesthetics, assault
T41.1X4 Poisoning by intravenous anesthetics, undetermined
T41.1X5 Adverse effect of intravenous anesthetics
T41.1X6 Underdosing of intravenous anesthetics

T41.2 Poisoning by, adverse effect of and underdosing of other and unspecified general anesthetics

T41.20 Poisoning by, adverse effect of and underdosing of unspecified general anesthetics
T41.201 Poisoning by unspecified general anesthetics, accidental (unintentional)
Poisoning by general anesthetics NOS
T41.202 Poisoning by unspecified general anesthetics, intentional self-harm
T41.203 Poisoning by unspecified general anesthetics, assault
T41.204 Poisoning by unspecified general anesthetics, undetermined
T41.205 Adverse effect of unspecified general anesthetics
T41.206 Underdosing of unspecified general anesthetics

T41.29 Poisoning by, adverse effect of and underdosing of other general anesthetics
T41.291 Poisoning by other general anesthetics, accidental (unintentional)
Poisoning by other general anesthetics NOS
T41.292 Poisoning by other general anesthetics, intentional self-harm
T41.293 Poisoning by other general anesthetics, assault
T41.294 Poisoning by other general anesthetics, undetermined
T41.295 Adverse effect of other general anesthetics
T41.296 Underdosing of other general anesthetics

T41.3 Poisoning by, adverse effect of and underdosing of local anesthetics
Cocaine (topical)
EXCLUDES2 *poisoning by cocaine used as a central nervous system stimulant (T40.5X1-T40.5X4)*

T41.3X Poisoning by, adverse effect of and underdosing of local anesthetics
T41.3X1 Poisoning by local anesthetics, accidental (unintentional)
Poisoning by local anesthetics NOS
T41.3X2 Poisoning by local anesthetics, intentional self-harm
T41.3X3 Poisoning by local anesthetics, assault
T41.3X4 Poisoning by local anesthetics, undetermined
T41.3X5 Adverse effect of local anesthetics
T41.3X6 Underdosing of local anesthetics

T41.4 Poisoning by, adverse effect of and underdosing of unspecified anesthetic
T41.41 Poisoning by unspecified anesthetic, accidental (unintentional)
Poisoning by anesthetic NOS
T41.42 Poisoning by unspecified anesthetic, intentional self-harm
T41.43 Poisoning by unspecified anesthetic, assault
T41.44 Poisoning by unspecified anesthetic, undetermined
T41.45 Adverse effect of unspecified anesthetic
T41.46 Underdosing of unspecified anesthetics

T41.5 Poisoning by, adverse effect of and underdosing of therapeutic gases

T41.5X Poisoning by, adverse effect of and underdosing of therapeutic gases
T41.5X1 Poisoning by therapeutic gases, accidental (unintentional)
Poisoning by therapeutic gases NOS
T41.5X2 Poisoning by therapeutic gases, intentional self-harm
T41.5X3 Poisoning by therapeutic gases, assault
T41.5X4 Poisoning by therapeutic gases, undetermined
T41.5X5 Adverse effect of therapeutic gases
T41.5X6 Underdosing of therapeutic gases

T42 Poisoning by, adverse effect of and underdosing of antiepileptic, sedative- hypnotic and antiparkinsonism drugs

EXCLUDES2 *drug dependence and related mental and behavioral disorders due to psychoactive substance use (F10.--F19.-)*

The appropriate 7th character is to be added to each code from category T42
A = initial encounter
D = subsequent encounter
S = sequela

T42.0 Poisoning by, adverse effect of and underdosing of hydantoin derivatives

T42.0X Poisoning by, adverse effect of and underdosing of hydantoin derivatives
T42.0X1 Poisoning by hydantoin derivatives, accidental (unintentional)
Poisoning by hydantoin derivatives NOS
T42.0X2 Poisoning by hydantoin derivatives, intentional self-harm
T42.0X3 Poisoning by hydantoin derivatives, assault
T42.0X4 Poisoning by hydantoin derivatives, undetermined
T42.0X5 Adverse effect of hydantoin derivatives
T42.0X6 Underdosing of hydantoin derivatives

Unacceptable principal diagnosis symbol per Medicare code edits | Code exempt from diagnosis present on admission requirement
Questionable admission | Complication or comorbidity | CC/MCC exclusion | Major complication or comorbidity
Principal diagnosis as its own CC | Principal diagnosis as its own MCC | Z code as first-listed diagnosis

T42.1 Poisoning by, adverse effect of and underdosing of iminostilbenes
Poisoning by, adverse effect of and underdosing of carbamazepine

T42.1X Poisoning by, adverse effect of and underdosing of iminostilbenes

T42.1X1 Poisoning by iminostilbenes, accidental (unintentional)
Poisoning by iminostilbenes NOS

T42.1X2 Poisoning by iminostilbenes, intentional self-harm

T42.1X3 Poisoning by iminostilbenes, assault

T42.1X4 Poisoning by iminostilbenes, undetermined

T42.1X5 Adverse effect of iminostilbenes

T42.1X6 Underdosing of iminostilbenes

T42.2 Poisoning by, adverse effect of and underdosing of succinimides and oxazolidinediones

T42.2X Poisoning by, adverse effect of and underdosing of succinimides and oxazolidinediones

T42.2X1 Poisoning by succinimides and oxazolidinediones, accidental (unintentional)
Poisoning by succinimides and oxazolidinediones NOS

T42.2X2 Poisoning by succinimides and oxazolidinediones, intentional self-harm

T42.2X3 Poisoning by succinimides and oxazolidinediones, assault

T42.2X4 Poisoning by succinimides and oxazolidinediones, undetermined

T42.2X5 Adverse effect of succinimides and oxazolidinediones

T42.2X6 Underdosing of succinimides and oxazolidinediones

T42.3 Poisoning by, adverse effect of and underdosing of barbiturates
EXCLUDES1 *poisoning by, adverse effect of and underdosing of thiobarbiturates (T41.1-)*

T42.3X Poisoning by, adverse effect of and underdosing of barbiturates

T42.3X1 Poisoning by barbiturates, accidental (unintentional)
Poisoning by barbiturates NOS

T42.3X2 Poisoning by barbiturates, intentional self-harm

T42.3X3 Poisoning by barbiturates, assault

T42.3X4 Poisoning by barbiturates, undetermined

T42.3X5 Adverse effect of barbiturates

T42.3X6 Underdosing of barbiturates

T42.4 Poisoning by, adverse effect of and underdosing of benzodiazepines

T42.4X Poisoning by, adverse effect of and underdosing of benzodiazepines

T42.4X1 Poisoning by benzodiazepines, accidental (unintentional)
Poisoning by benzodiazepines NOS

T42.4X2 Poisoning by benzodiazepines, intentional self-harm

T42.4X3 Poisoning by benzodiazepines, assault

T42.4X4 Poisoning by benzodiazepines, undetermined

T42.4X5 Adverse effect of benzodiazepines

T42.4X6 Underdosing of benzodiazepines

T42.5 Poisoning by, adverse effect of and underdosing of mixed antiepileptics

T42.5X Poisoning by, adverse effect of and underdosing of antiepileptics

T42.5X1 Poisoning by mixed antiepileptics, accidental (unintentional)
Poisoning by mixed antiepileptics NOS

T42.5X2 Poisoning by mixed antiepileptics, intentional self-harm

T42.5X3 Poisoning by mixed antiepileptics, assault

T42.5X4 Poisoning by mixed antiepileptics, undetermined

T42.5X5 Adverse effect of mixed antiepileptics

T42.5X6 Underdosing of mixed antiepileptics

T42.6 Poisoning by, adverse effect of and underdosing of other antiepileptic and sedative-hypnotic drugs
Poisoning by, adverse effect of and underdosing of methaqualone
Poisoning by, adverse effect of and underdosing of valproic acid
EXCLUDES1 *poisoning by, adverse effect of and underdosing of carbamazepine (T42.1-)*

T42.6X Poisoning by, adverse effect of and underdosing of other antiepileptic and sedative-hypnotic drugs

T42.6X1 Poisoning by other antiepileptic and sedative-hypnotic drugs, accidental (unintentional)
Poisoning by other antiepileptic and sedative-hypnotic drugs NOS

T42.6X2 Poisoning by other antiepileptic and sedative-hypnotic drugs, intentional self-harm

T42.6X3 Poisoning by other antiepileptic and sedative-hypnotic drugs, assault

T42.6X4 Poisoning by other antiepileptic and sedative-hypnotic drugs, undetermined

T42.6X5 Adverse effect of other antiepileptic and sedative-hypnotic drugs

T42.6X6 Underdosing of other antiepileptic and sedative-hypnotic drugs

T42.7 Poisoning by, adverse effect of and underdosing of unspecified antiepileptic and sedative-hypnotic drugs

T42.71 Poisoning by unspecified antiepileptic and sedative-hypnotic drugs, accidental (unintentional)
Poisoning by antiepileptic and sedative-hypnotic drugs NOS

T42.72 Poisoning by unspecified antiepileptic and sedative-hypnotic drugs, intentional self-harm

T42.73 Poisoning by unspecified antiepileptic and sedative-hypnotic drugs, assault

T42.74 Poisoning by unspecified antiepileptic and sedative-hypnotic drugs, undetermined

T42.75 Adverse effect of unspecified antiepileptic and sedative-hypnotic drugs

T42.76 Underdosing of unspecified antiepileptic and sedative-hypnotic drugs

T42.8 Poisoning by, adverse effect of and underdosing of antiparkinsonism drugs and other central muscle-tone depressants
Poisoning by, adverse effect of and underdosing of amantadine

T42.8X Poisoning by, adverse effect of and underdosing of antiparkinsonism drugs and other central muscle-tone depressants

T42.8X1 Poisoning by antiparkinsonism drugs and other central muscle-tone depressants, accidental (unintentional)
Poisoning by antiparkinsonism drugs and other central muscle-tone depressants NOS

T42.8X2 Poisoning by antiparkinsonism drugs and other central muscle-tone depressants, intentional self-harm

T42.8X3 Poisoning by antiparkinsonism drugs and other central muscle-tone depressants, assault

T42.8X4 Poisoning by antiparkinsonism drugs and other central muscle-tone depressants, undetermined

T42.8X5 Adverse effect of antiparkinsonism drugs and other central muscle-tone depressants

T42.8X6 Underdosing of antiparkinsonism drugs and other central muscle-tone depressants

T43 Poisoning by, adverse effect of and underdosing of psychotropic drugs, not elsewhere classified
EXCLUDES1 *appetite depressants (T50.5-)*
barbiturates (T42.3-)
benzodiazepines (T42.4-)
methaqualone (T42.6-)

Unspecified Code Other Specified Code Manifestation Code N Newborn P Pediatric M Maternity A Adult ♂ Male ♀ Female
● New Code ▲ Revised Code Title ►◄ Revised Text NOTES INCLUDES EXCLUDES1 Not coded here EXCLUDES2 Not included here
4th character required 5th character required 6th character required 7th character required
Extension 'X' Alert HAC Hospital-acquired condition (HAC) alert AHA AHA Coding Clinic©

psychodysleptics [hallucinogens] (T40.7-T40.9-)

EXCLUDES2 *drug dependence and related mental and behavioral disorders due to psychoactive substance use (F10.- -F19.-)*

The appropriate 7th character is to be added to each code from category T43

A = initial encounter

D = subsequent encounter

S = sequela

T43.0 Poisoning by, adverse effect of and underdosing of tricyclic and tetracyclic antidepressants

T43.01 Poisoning by, adverse effect of and underdosing of tricyclic antidepressants

T43.011 Poisoning by tricyclic antidepressants, accidental (unintentional)

Poisoning by tricyclic antidepressants NOS

T43.012 Poisoning by tricyclic antidepressants, intentional self-harm

T43.013 Poisoning by tricyclic antidepressants, assault

T43.014 Poisoning by tricyclic antidepressants, undetermined

T43.015 Adverse effect of tricyclic antidepressants

T43.016 Underdosing of tricyclic antidepressants

T43.02 Poisoning by, adverse effect of and underdosing of tetracyclic antidepressants

T43.021 Poisoning by tetracyclic antidepressants, accidental (unintentional)

Poisoning by tetracyclic antidepressants NOS

T43.022 Poisoning by tetracyclic antidepressants, intentional self-harm

T43.023 Poisoning by tetracyclic antidepressants, assault

T43.024 Poisoning by tetracyclic antidepressants, undetermined

T43.025 Adverse effect of tetracyclic antidepressants

T43.026 Underdosing of tetracyclic antidepressants

T43.1 Poisoning by, adverse effect of and underdosing of monoamine-oxidase-inhibitor antidepressants

T43.1X Poisoning by, adverse effect of and underdosing of monoamine-oxidase-inhibitor antidepressants

T43.1X1 Poisoning by monoamine-oxidase-inhibitor antidepressants, accidental (unintentional)

Poisoning by monoamine-oxidase-inhibitor antidepressants NOS

T43.1X2 Poisoning by monoamine-oxidase-inhibitor antidepressants, intentional self-harm

T43.1X3 Poisoning by monoamine-oxidase-inhibitor antidepressants, assault

T43.1X4 Poisoning by monoamine-oxidase-inhibitor antidepressants, undetermined

T43.1X5 Adverse effect of monoamine-oxidase-inhibitor antidepressants

T43.1X6 Underdosing of monoamine-oxidase-inhibitor antidepressants

T43.2 Poisoning by, adverse effect of and underdosing of other and unspecified antidepressants

T43.20 Poisoning by, adverse effect of and underdosing of unspecified antidepressants

T43.201 Poisoning by unspecified antidepressants, accidental (unintentional)

Poisoning by antidepressants NOS

T43.202 Poisoning by unspecified antidepressants, intentional self-harm

T43.203 Poisoning by unspecified antidepressants, assault

T43.204 Poisoning by unspecified antidepressants, undetermined

T43.205 Adverse effect of unspecified antidepressants

T43.206 Underdosing of unspecified antidepressants

T43.21 Poisoning by, adverse effect of and underdosing of selective serotonin and norepinephrine reuptake inhibitors

Poisoning by, adverse effect of and underdosing of SSNRI antidepressants

T43.211 Poisoning by selective serotonin and norepinephrine reuptake inhibitors, accidental (unintentional)

T43.212 Poisoning by selective serotonin and norepinephrine reuptake inhibitors, intentional self-harm

T43.213 Poisoning by selective serotonin and norepinephrine reuptake inhibitors, assault

T43.214 Poisoning by selective serotonin and norepinephrine reuptake inhibitors, undetermined

T43.215 Adverse effect of selective serotonin and norepinephrine reuptake inhibitors

T43.216 Underdosing of selective serotonin and norepinephrine reuptake inhibitors

T43.22 Poisoning by, adverse effect of and underdosing of selective serotonin reuptake inhibitors

Poisoning by, adverse effect of and underdosing of SSRI antidepressants

T43.221 Poisoning by selective serotonin reuptake inhibitors, accidental (unintentional)

T43.222 Poisoning by selective serotonin reuptake inhibitors, intentional self-harm

T43.223 Poisoning by selective serotonin reuptake inhibitors, assault

T43.224 Poisoning by selective serotonin reuptake inhibitors, undetermined

T43.225 Adverse effect of selective serotonin reuptake inhibitors

T43.226 Underdosing of selective serotonin reuptake inhibitors

T43.29 Poisoning by, adverse effect of and underdosing of other antidepressants

T43.291 Poisoning by other antidepressants, accidental (unintentional)

Poisoning by other antidepressants NOS

T43.292 Poisoning by other antidepressants, intentional self-harm

T43.293 Poisoning by other antidepressants, assault

T43.294 Poisoning by other antidepressants, undetermined

T43.295 Adverse effect of other antidepressants

T43.296 Underdosing of other antidepressants

T43.3 Poisoning by, adverse effect of and underdosing of phenothiazine antipsychotics and neuroleptics

T43.3X Poisoning by, adverse effect of and underdosing of phenothiazine antipsychotics and neuroleptics

T43.3X1 Poisoning by phenothiazine antipsychotics and neuroleptics, accidental (unintentional)

Poisoning by phenothiazine antipsychotics and neuroleptics NOS

T43.3X2 Poisoning by phenothiazine antipsychotics and neuroleptics, intentional self-harm

T43.3X3 Poisoning by phenothiazine antipsychotics and neuroleptics, assault

T43.3X4 Poisoning by phenothiazine antipsychotics and neuroleptics, undetermined

T43.3X5 Adverse effect of phenothiazine antipsychotics and neuroleptics

T43.3X6 Underdosing of phenothiazine antipsychotics and neuroleptics

T43.4 Poisoning by, adverse effect of and underdosing of butyrophenone and thiothixene neuroleptics

T43.4X Poisoning by, adverse effect of and underdosing of butyrophenone and thiothixene neuroleptics

Unacceptable principal diagnosis symbol per Medicare code edits · Code exempt from diagnosis present on admission requirement · Questionable admission · Complication or comorbidity · CC/MCC exclusion · Major complication or comorbidity · Principal diagnosis as its own CC · Principal diagnosis as its own MCC · Z code as first-listed diagnosis

T43.4X1 Poisoning by butyrophenone and thiothixene neuroleptics, accidental (unintentional)
Poisoning by butyrophenone and thiothixene neuroleptics NOS
T43.4X2 Poisoning by butyrophenone and thiothixene neuroleptics, intentional self-harm
T43.4X3 Poisoning by butyrophenone and thiothixene neuroleptics, assault
T43.4X4 Poisoning by butyrophenone and thiothixene neuroleptics, undetermined
T43.4X5 Adverse effect of butyrophenone and thiothixene neuroleptics
T43.4X6 Underdosing of butyrophenone and thiothixene neuroleptics

T43.5 Poisoning by, adverse effect of and underdosing of other and unspecified antipsychotics and neuroleptics
EXCLUDES1 *poisoning by, adverse effect of and underdosing of rauwolfia (T46.5-)*

T43.50 Poisoning by, adverse effect of and underdosing of unspecified antipsychotics and neuroleptics
T43.501 Poisoning by unspecified antipsychotics and neuroleptics, accidental (unintentional)
Poisoning by antipsychotics and neuroleptics NOS
T43.502 Poisoning by unspecified antipsychotics and neuroleptics, intentional self-harm
T43.503 Poisoning by unspecified antipsychotics and neuroleptics, assault
T43.504 Poisoning by unspecified antipsychotics and neuroleptics, undetermined
T43.505 Adverse effect of unspecified antipsychotics and neuroleptics
T43.506 Underdosing of unspecified antipsychotics and neuroleptics

T43.59 Poisoning by, adverse effect of and underdosing of other antipsychotics and neuroleptics
T43.591 Poisoning by other antipsychotics and neuroleptics, accidental (unintentional)
Poisoning by other antipsychotics and neuroleptics NOS
T43.592 Poisoning by other antipsychotics and neuroleptics, intentional self-harm
T43.593 Poisoning by other antipsychotics and neuroleptics, assault
T43.594 Poisoning by other antipsychotics and neuroleptics, undetermined
T43.595 Adverse effect of other antipsychotics and neuroleptics
T43.596 Underdosing of other antipsychotics and neuroleptics

T43.6 Poisoning by, adverse effect of and underdosing of psychostimulants
EXCLUDES1 *poisoning by, adverse effect of and underdosing of cocaine (T40.5-)*

T43.60 Poisoning by, adverse effect of and underdosing of unspecified psychostimulant
T43.601 Poisoning by unspecified psychostimulants, accidental (unintentional)
Poisoning by psychostimulants NOS
T43.602 Poisoning by unspecified psychostimulants, intentional self-harm
T43.603 Poisoning by unspecified psychostimulants, assault
T43.604 Poisoning by unspecified psychostimulants, undetermined
T43.605 Adverse effect of unspecified psychostimulants
T43.606 Underdosing of unspecified psychostimulants

T43.61 Poisoning by, adverse effect of and underdosing of caffeine
T43.611 Poisoning by caffeine, accidental (unintentional)
Poisoning by caffeine NOS
T43.612 Poisoning by caffeine, intentional self-harm
T43.613 Poisoning by caffeine, assault
T43.614 Poisoning by caffeine, undetermined
T43.615 Adverse effect of caffeine
T43.616 Underdosing of caffeine

T43.62 Poisoning by, adverse effect of and underdosing of amphetamines
Poisoning by, adverse effect of and underdosing of methamphetamines
T43.621 Poisoning by amphetamines, accidental (unintentional)
Poisoning by amphetamines NOS
T43.622 Poisoning by amphetamines, intentional self-harm
T43.623 Poisoning by amphetamines, assault
T43.624 Poisoning by amphetamines, undetermined
T43.625 Adverse effect of amphetamines
T43.626 Underdosing of amphetamines

T43.63 Poisoning by, adverse effect of and underdosing of methylphenidate
T43.631 Poisoning by methylphenidate, accidental (unintentional)
Poisoning by methylphenidate NOS
T43.632 Poisoning by methylphenidate, intentional self-harm
T43.633 Poisoning by methylphenidate, assault
T43.634 Poisoning by methylphenidate, undetermined
T43.635 Adverse effect of methylphenidate
T43.636 Underdosing of methylphenidate

T43.69 Poisoning by, adverse effect of and underdosing of other psychostimulants
T43.691 Poisoning by other psychostimulants, accidental (unintentional)
Poisoning by other psychostimulants NOS
T43.692 Poisoning by other psychostimulants, intentional self-harm
T43.693 Poisoning by other psychostimulants, assault
T43.694 Poisoning by other psychostimulants, undetermined
T43.695 Adverse effect of other psychostimulants
T43.696 Underdosing of other psychostimulants

T43.8 Poisoning by, adverse effect of and underdosing of other psychotropic drugs
T43.8X Poisoning by, adverse effect of and underdosing of other psychotropic drugs
T43.8X1 Poisoning by other psychotropic drugs, accidental (unintentional)
Poisoning by other psychotropic drugs NOS
T43.8X2 Poisoning by other psychotropic drugs, intentional self-harm
T43.8X3 Poisoning by other psychotropic drugs, assault
T43.8X4 Poisoning by other psychotropic drugs, undetermined
T43.8X5 Adverse effect of other psychotropic drugs
T43.8X6 Underdosing of other psychotropic drugs

T43.9 Poisoning by, adverse effect of and underdosing of unspecified psychotropic drug
T43.91 Poisoning by unspecified psychotropic drug, accidental (unintentional)
Poisoning by psychotropic drug NOS
T43.92 Poisoning by unspecified psychotropic drug, intentional self-harm
T43.93 Poisoning by unspecified psychotropic drug, assault
T43.94 Poisoning by unspecified psychotropic drug, undetermined
T43.95 Adverse effect of unspecified psychotropic drug
T43.96 Underdosing of unspecified psychotropic drug

T44 Poisoning by, adverse effect of and underdosing of drugs primarily affecting the autonomic nervous system

Unspecified Code | Other Specified Code | Manifestation Code | N Newborn | P Pediatric | M Maternity | A Adult | ♂ Male | ♀ Female
● New Code ▲ Revised Code Title ►◄ Revised Text NOTES INCLUDES EXCLUDES1 Not coded here EXCLUDES2 Not included here
4th character required 5th character required 6th character required 7th character required
Extension 'X' Alert HAC Hospital-acquired condition (HAC) alert AHA AHA Coding Clinic©

The appropriate 7th character is to be added to each code from category T44
A = initial encounter
D = subsequent encounter
S = sequela

T44.0 Poisoning by, adverse effect of and underdosing of anticholinesterase agents
- **T44.0X** Poisoning by, adverse effect of and underdosing of anticholinesterase agents
  - **T44.0X1** Poisoning by anticholinesterase agents, accidental (unintentional)
    Poisoning by anticholinesterase agents NOS
  - **T44.0X2** Poisoning by anticholinesterase agents, intentional self-harm
  - **T44.0X3** Poisoning by anticholinesterase agents, assault
  - **T44.0X4** Poisoning by anticholinesterase agents, undetermined
  - **T44.0X5** Adverse effect of anticholinesterase agents
  - **T44.0X6** Underdosing of anticholinesterase agents

T44.1 Poisoning by, adverse effect of and underdosing of other parasympathomimetics [cholinergics]
- **T44.1X** Poisoning by, adverse effect of and underdosing of other parasympathomimetics [cholinergics]
  - **T44.1X1** Poisoning by other parasympathomimetics [cholinergics], accidental (unintentional)
    Poisoning by other parasympathomimetics [cholinergics] NOS
  - **T44.1X2** Poisoning by other parasympathomimetics [cholinergics], intentional self-harm
  - **T44.1X3** Poisoning by other parasympathomimetics [cholinergics], assault
  - **T44.1X4** Poisoning by other parasympathomimetics [cholinergics], undetermined
  - **T44.1X5** Adverse effect of other parasympathomimetics [cholinergics]
  - **T44.1X6** Underdosing of other parasympathomimetics

T44.2 Poisoning by, adverse effect of and underdosing of ganglionic blocking drugs
- **T44.2X** Poisoning by, adverse effect of and underdosing of ganglionic blocking drugs
  - **T44.2X1** Poisoning by ganglionic blocking drugs, accidental (unintentional)
    Poisoning by ganglionic blocking drugs NOS
  - **T44.2X2** Poisoning by ganglionic blocking drugs, intentional self-harm
  - **T44.2X3** Poisoning by ganglionic blocking drugs, assault
  - **T44.2X4** Poisoning by ganglionic blocking drugs, undetermined
  - **T44.2X5** Adverse effect of ganglionic blocking drugs
  - **T44.2X6** Underdosing of ganglionic blocking drugs

T44.3 Poisoning by, adverse effect of and underdosing of other parasympatholytics [anticholinergics and antimuscarinics] and spasmolytics
Poisoning by, adverse effect of and underdosing of papaverine
- **T44.3X** Poisoning by, adverse effect of and underdosing of other parasympatholytics [anticholinergics and antimuscarinics] and spasmolytics
  - **T44.3X1** Poisoning by other parasympatholytics [anticholinergics and antimuscarinics] and spasmolytics, accidental (unintentional)
    Poisoning by other parasympatholytics [anticholinergics and antimuscarinics] and spasmolytics NOS
  - **T44.3X2** Poisoning by other parasympatholytics [anticholinergics and antimuscarinics] and spasmolytics, intentional self-harm
  - **T44.3X3** Poisoning by other parasympatholytics [anticholinergics and antimuscarinics] and spasmolytics, assault
  - **T44.3X4** Poisoning by other parasympatholytics [anticholinergics and antimuscarinics] and spasmolytics, undetermined
  - **T44.3X5** Adverse effect of other parasympatholytics [anticholinergics and antimuscarinics] and spasmolytics
  - **T44.3X6** Underdosing of other parasympatholytics [anticholinergics and antimuscarinics] and spasmolytics

T44.4 Poisoning by, adverse effect of and underdosing of predominantly alpha-adrenoreceptor agonists
Poisoning by, adverse effect of and underdosing of metaraminol
- **T44.4X** Poisoning by, adverse effect of and underdosing of predominantly alpha-adrenoreceptor agonists
  - **T44.4X1** Poisoning by predominantly alpha-adrenoreceptor agonists, accidental (unintentional)
    Poisoning by predominantly alpha-adrenoreceptor agonists NOS
  - **T44.4X2** Poisoning by predominantly alpha-adrenoreceptor agonists, intentional self-harm
  - **T44.4X3** Poisoning by predominantly alpha-adrenoreceptor agonists, assault
  - **T44.4X4** Poisoning by predominantly alpha-adrenoreceptor agonists, undetermined
  - **T44.4X5** Adverse effect of predominantly alpha-adrenoreceptor agonists
  - **T44.4X6** Underdosing of predominantly alpha-adrenoreceptor agonists

T44.5 Poisoning by, adverse effect of and underdosing of predominantly beta-adrenoreceptor agonists
EXCLUDES1 *poisoning by, adverse effect of and underdosing of beta-adrenoreceptor agonists used in asthma therapy (T48.6-)*
- **T44.5X** Poisoning by, adverse effect of and underdosing of predominantly beta-adrenoreceptor agonists
  - **T44.5X1** Poisoning by predominantly beta-adrenoreceptor agonists, accidental (unintentional)
    Poisoning by predominantly beta-adrenoreceptor agonists NOS
  - **T44.5X2** Poisoning by predominantly beta-adrenoreceptor agonists, intentional self-harm
  - **T44.5X3** Poisoning by predominantly beta-adrenoreceptor agonists, assault
  - **T44.5X4** Poisoning by predominantly beta-adrenoreceptor agonists, undetermined
  - **T44.5X5** Adverse effect of predominantly beta-adrenoreceptor agonists
  - **T44.5X6** Underdosing of predominantly beta-adrenoreceptor agonists

T44.6 Poisoning by, adverse effect of and underdosing of alpha-adrenoreceptor antagonists
EXCLUDES1 *poisoning by, adverse effect of and underdosing of ergot alkaloids (T48.0)*
- **T44.6X** Poisoning by, adverse effect of and underdosing of alpha-adrenoreceptor antagonists
  - **T44.6X1** Poisoning by alpha-adrenoreceptor antagonists, accidental (unintentional)
    Poisoning by alpha-adrenoreceptor antagonists NOS
  - **T44.6X2** Poisoning by alpha-adrenoreceptor antagonists, intentional self-harm
  - **T44.6X3** Poisoning by alpha-adrenoreceptor antagonists, assault
  - **T44.6X4** Poisoning by alpha-adrenoreceptor antagonists, undetermined
  - **T44.6X5** Adverse effect of alpha-adrenoreceptor antagonists
  - **T44.6X6** Underdosing of alpha-adrenoreceptor antagonists

Unacceptable principal diagnosis symbol per Medicare code edits · Code exempt from diagnosis present on admission requirement · Questionable admission · Complication or comorbidity · CC/MCC exclusion · Major complication or comorbidity · Principal diagnosis as its own CC · Principal diagnosis as its own MCC · Z code as first-listed diagnosis

T44.7 Poisoning by, adverse effect of and underdosing of beta-adrenoreceptor antagonists

T44.7X Poisoning by, adverse effect of and underdosing of beta-adrenoreceptor antagonists

T44.7X1 Poisoning by beta-adrenoreceptor antagonists, accidental (unintentional)
Poisoning by beta-adrenoreceptor antagonists NOS

T44.7X2 Poisoning by beta-adrenoreceptor antagonists, intentional self-harm

T44.7X3 Poisoning by beta-adrenoreceptor antagonists, assault

T44.7X4 Poisoning by beta-adrenoreceptor antagonists, undetermined

T44.7X5 Adverse effect of beta-adrenoreceptor antagonists

T44.7X6 Underdosing of beta-adrenoreceptor antagonists

T44.8 Poisoning by, adverse effect of and underdosing of centrally-acting and adrenergic-neuron- blocking agents

EXCLUDES1 *poisoning by, adverse effect of and underdosing of clonidine (T46.5)*
poisoning by, adverse effect of and underdosing of guanethidine (T46.5)

T44.8X Poisoning by, adverse effect of and underdosing of centrally-acting and adrenergic- neuron-blocking agents

T44.8X1 Poisoning by centrally-acting and adrenergic-neuron-blocking agents, accidental (unintentional)
Poisoning by centrally-acting and adrenergic-neuron-blocking agents NOS

T44.8X2 Poisoning by centrally-acting and adrenergic-neuron-blocking agents, intentional self-harm

T44.8X3 Poisoning by centrally-acting and adrenergic-neuron-blocking agents, assault

T44.8X4 Poisoning by centrally-acting and adrenergic-neuron-blocking agents, undetermined

T44.8X5 Adverse effect of centrally-acting and adrenergic-neuron-blocking agents

T44.8X6 Underdosing of centrally-acting and adrenergic-neuron-blocking agents

T44.9 Poisoning by, adverse effect of and underdosing of other and unspecified drugs primarily affecting the autonomic nervous system
Poisoning by, adverse effect of and underdosing of drug stimulating both alpha and beta-adrenoreceptors

T44.90 Poisoning by, adverse effect of and underdosing of unspecified drugs primarily affecting the autonomic nervous system

T44.901 Poisoning by unspecified drugs primarily affecting the autonomic nervous system, accidental (unintentional)
Poisoning by unspecified drugs primarily affecting the autonomic nervous system NOS

T44.902 Poisoning by unspecified drugs primarily affecting the autonomic nervous system, intentional self-harm

T44.903 Poisoning by unspecified drugs primarily affecting the autonomic nervous system, assault

T44.904 Poisoning by unspecified drugs primarily affecting the autonomic nervous system, undetermined

T44.905 Adverse effect of unspecified drugs primarily affecting the autonomic nervous system

T44.906 Underdosing of unspecified drugs primarily affecting the autonomic nervous system

T44.99 Poisoning by, adverse effect of and underdosing of other drugs primarily affecting the autonomic nervous system

T44.991 Poisoning by other drug primarily affecting the autonomic nervous system, accidental (unintentional)
Poisoning by other drugs primarily affecting the autonomic nervous system NOS

T44.992 Poisoning by other drug primarily affecting the autonomic nervous system, intentional self-harm

T44.993 Poisoning by other drug primarily affecting the autonomic nervous system, assault

T44.994 Poisoning by other drug primarily affecting the autonomic nervous system, undetermined

T44.995 Adverse effect of other drug primarily affecting the autonomic nervous system

T44.996 Underdosing of other drug primarily affecting the autonomic nervous system

T45 Poisoning by, adverse effect of and underdosing of primarily systemic and hematological agents, not elsewhere classified

The appropriate 7th character is to be added to each code from category T45
A = initial encounter
D = subsequent encounter
S = sequela

T45.0 Poisoning by, adverse effect of and underdosing of antiallergic and antiemetic drugs

EXCLUDES1 *poisoning by, adverse effect of and underdosing of phenothiazine-based neuroleptics (T43.3)*

T45.0X Poisoning by, adverse effect of and underdosing of antiallergic and antiemetic drugs

T45.0X1 Poisoning by antiallergic and antiemetic drugs, accidental (unintentional)
Poisoning by antiallergic and antiemetic drugs NOS

T45.0X2 Poisoning by antiallergic and antiemetic drugs, intentional self-harm

T45.0X3 Poisoning by antiallergic and antiemetic drugs, assault

T45.0X4 Poisoning by antiallergic and antiemetic drugs, undetermined

T45.0X5 Adverse effect of antiallergic and antiemetic drugs

T45.0X6 Underdosing of antiallergic and antiemetic drugs

T45.1 Poisoning by, adverse effect of and underdosing of antineoplastic and immunosuppressive drugs

EXCLUDES1 *poisoning by, adverse effect of and underdosing of tamoxifen (T38.6)*

T45.1X Poisoning by, adverse effect of and underdosing of antineoplastic and immunosuppressive drugs

T45.1X1 Poisoning by antineoplastic and immunosuppressive drugs, accidental (unintentional)
Poisoning by antineoplastic and immunosuppressive drugs NOS

T45.1X2 Poisoning by antineoplastic and immunosuppressive drugs, intentional self-harm

T45.1X3 Poisoning by antineoplastic and immunosuppressive drugs, assault

T45.1X4 Poisoning by antineoplastic and immunosuppressive drugs, undetermined

T45.1X5 Adverse effect of antineoplastic and immunosuppressive drugs

T45.1X6 Underdosing of antineoplastic and immunosuppressive drugs

T45.2 Poisoning by, adverse effect of and underdosing of vitamins

EXCLUDES2 *poisoning by, adverse effect of and underdosing of nicotinic acid (derivatives) (T46.7)*
poisoning by, adverse effect of and underdosing of iron (T45.4)
poisoning by, adverse effect of and underdosing of vitamin K (T45.7)

Unspecified Code Other Specified Code Manifestation Code N Newborn P Pediatric M Maternity A Adult ♂ Male ♀ Female
● New Code ▲ Revised Code Title ►◄ Revised Text NOTES INCLUDES EXCLUDES1 Not coded here EXCLUDES2 Not included here
4th character required 5th character required 6th character required 7th character required
Extension 'X' Alert HAC Hospital-acquired condition (HAC) alert AHA AHA Coding Clinic©

T45.2X Poisoning by, adverse effect of and underdosing of vitamins
- T45.2X1 Poisoning by vitamins, accidental (unintentional)
  Poisoning by vitamins NOS
- T45.2X2 Poisoning by vitamins, intentional self-harm
- T45.2X3 Poisoning by vitamins, assault
- T45.2X4 Poisoning by vitamins, undetermined
- T45.2X5 Adverse effect of vitamins
- T45.2X6 Underdosing of vitamins
  EXCLUDES1 *vitamin deficiencies (E50-E56)*

T45.3 Poisoning by, adverse effect of and underdosing of enzymes

T45.3X Poisoning by, adverse effect of and underdosing of enzymes
- T45.3X1 Poisoning by enzymes, accidental (unintentional)
  Poisoning by enzymes NOS
- T45.3X2 Poisoning by enzymes, intentional self-harm
- T45.3X3 Poisoning by enzymes, assault
- T45.3X4 Poisoning by enzymes, undetermined
- T45.3X5 Adverse effect of enzymes
- T45.3X6 Underdosing of enzymes

T45.4 Poisoning by, adverse effect of and underdosing of iron and its compounds

T45.4X Poisoning by, adverse effect of and underdosing of iron and its compounds
- T45.4X1 Poisoning by iron and its compounds, accidental (unintentional)
  Poisoning by iron and its compounds NOS
- T45.4X2 Poisoning by iron and its compounds, intentional self-harm
- T45.4X3 Poisoning by iron and its compounds, assault
- T45.4X4 Poisoning by iron and its compounds, undetermined
- T45.4X5 Adverse effect of iron and its compounds
- T45.4X6 Underdosing of iron and its compounds
  EXCLUDES1 *iron deficiency (E61.1)*

T45.5 Poisoning by, adverse effect of and underdosing of anticoagulants and antithrombotic drugs

T45.51 Poisoning by, adverse effect of and underdosing of anticoagulants
- T45.511 Poisoning by anticoagulants, accidental (unintentional)
  Poisoning by anticoagulants NOS
- T45.512 Poisoning by anticoagulants, intentional self-harm
- T45.513 Poisoning by anticoagulants, assault
- T45.514 Poisoning by anticoagulants, undetermined
- T45.515 Adverse effect of anticoagulants
  AHA: Q1, 2016
- T45.516 Underdosing of anticoagulants

T45.52 Poisoning by, adverse effect of and underdosing of antithrombotic drugs
Poisoning by, adverse effect of and underdosing of antiplatelet drugs
EXCLUDES2 *poisoning by, adverse effect of and underdosing of aspirin (T39.01-)*
poisoning by, adverse effect of and underdosing of acetylsalicylic acid (T39.01-)
- T45.521 Poisoning by antithrombotic drugs, accidental (unintentional)
  Poisoning by antithrombotic drug NOS
- T45.522 Poisoning by antithrombotic drugs, intentional self-harm
- T45.523 Poisoning by antithrombotic drugs, assault
- T45.524 Poisoning by antithrombotic drugs, undetermined
- T45.525 Adverse effect of antithrombotic drugs
  AHA: Q1, 2016
- T45.526 Underdosing of antithrombotic drugs

T45.6 Poisoning by, adverse effect of and underdosing of fibrinolysis-affecting drugs

T45.60 Poisoning by, adverse effect of and underdosing of unspecified fibrinolysis-affecting drugs
- T45.601 Poisoning by unspecified fibrinolysis-affecting drugs, accidental (unintentional)
  Poisoning by fibrinolysis-affecting drug NOS
- T45.602 Poisoning by unspecified fibrinolysis-affecting drugs, intentional self-harm
- T45.603 Poisoning by unspecified fibrinolysis-affecting drugs, assault
- T45.604 Poisoning by unspecified fibrinolysis-affecting drugs, undetermined
- T45.605 Adverse effect of unspecified fibrinolysis-affecting drugs
- T45.606 Underdosing of unspecified fibrinolysis-affecting drugs

T45.61 Poisoning by, adverse effect of and underdosing of thrombolytic drugs
- T45.611 Poisoning by thrombolytic drug, accidental (unintentional)
  Poisoning by thrombolytic drug NOS
- T45.612 Poisoning by thrombolytic drug, intentional self-harm
- T45.613 Poisoning by thrombolytic drug, assault
- T45.614 Poisoning by thrombolytic drug, undetermined
- T45.615 Adverse effect of thrombolytic drugs
- T45.616 Underdosing of thrombolytic drugs

T45.62 Poisoning by, adverse effect of and underdosing of hemostatic drugs
- T45.621 Poisoning by hemostatic drug, accidental (unintentional)
  Poisoning by hemostatic drug NOS
- T45.622 Poisoning by hemostatic drug, intentional self-harm
- T45.623 Poisoning by hemostatic drug, assault
- T45.624 Poisoning by hemostatic drug, undetermined
- T45.625 Adverse effect of hemostatic drug
- T45.626 Underdosing of hemostatic drugs

T45.69 Poisoning by, adverse effect of and underdosing of other fibrinolysis-affecting drugs
- T45.691 Poisoning by other fibrinolysis-affecting drugs, accidental (unintentional)
  Poisoning by other fibrinolysis-affecting drug NOS
- T45.692 Poisoning by other fibrinolysis-affecting drugs, intentional self-harm
- T45.693 Poisoning by other fibrinolysis-affecting drugs, assault
- T45.694 Poisoning by other fibrinolysis-affecting drugs, undetermined
- T45.695 Adverse effect of other fibrinolysis-affecting drugs
- T45.696 Underdosing of other fibrinolysis-affecting drugs

T45.7 Poisoning by, adverse effect of and underdosing of anticoagulant antagonists, vitamin K and other coagulants

T45.7X Poisoning by, adverse effect of and underdosing of anticoagulant antagonists, vitamin K and other coagulants
- T45.7X1 Poisoning by anticoagulant antagonists, vitamin K and other coagulants, accidental (unintentional)
  Poisoning by anticoagulant antagonists, vitamin K and other coagulants NOS
- T45.7X2 Poisoning by anticoagulant antagonists, vitamin K and other coagulants, intentional self-harm
- T45.7X3 Poisoning by anticoagulant antagonists, vitamin K and other coagulants, assault
- T45.7X4 Poisoning by anticoagulant antagonists, vitamin K and other coagulants, undetermined

Unacceptable principal diagnosis symbol per Medicare code edits · Code exempt from diagnosis present on admission requirement
Questionable admission · Complication or comorbidity · CC/MCC exclusion · Major complication or comorbidity
Principal diagnosis as its own CC · Principal diagnosis as its own MCC · Z code as first-listed diagnosis

T45.7X5 Adverse effect of anticoagulant antagonists, vitamin K and other coagulants

T45.7X6 Underdosing of anticoagulant antagonist, vitamin K and other coagulants

EXCLUDES1 *vitamin K deficiency (E56.1)*

T45.8 Poisoning by, adverse effect of and underdosing of other primarily systemic and hematological agents

Poisoning by, adverse effect of and underdosing of liver preparations and other antianemic agents

Poisoning by, adverse effect of and underdosing of natural blood and blood products

Poisoning by, adverse effect of and underdosing of plasma substitute

EXCLUDES2 *poisoning by, adverse effect of and underdosing of immunoglobulin (T50.Z1)*

poisoning by, adverse effect of and underdosing of iron (T45.4)

transfusion reactions (T80.-)

T45.8X Poisoning by, adverse effect of and underdosing of other primarily systemic and hematological agents

T45.8X1 Poisoning by other primarily systemic and hematological agents, accidental (unintentional)

Poisoning by other primarily systemic and hematological agents NOS

T45.8X2 Poisoning by other primarily systemic and hematological agents, intentional self-harm

T45.8X3 Poisoning by other primarily systemic and hematological agents, assault

T45.8X4 Poisoning by other primarily systemic and hematological agents, undetermined

T45.8X5 Adverse effect of other primarily systemic and hematological agents

T45.8X6 Underdosing of other primarily systemic and hematological agents

T45.9 Poisoning by, adverse effect of and underdosing of unspecified primarily systemic and hematological agent

T45.91 Poisoning by unspecified primarily systemic and hematological agent, accidental (unintentional)

Poisoning by primarily systemic and hematological agent NOS

T45.92 Poisoning by unspecified primarily systemic and hematological agent, intentional self-harm

T45.93 Poisoning by unspecified primarily systemic and hematological agent, assault

T45.94 Poisoning by unspecified primarily systemic and hematological agent, undetermined

T45.95 Adverse effect of unspecified primarily systemic and hematological agent

T45.96 Underdosing of unspecified primarily systemic and hematological agent

T46 Poisoning by, adverse effect of and underdosing of agents primarily affecting the cardiovascular system

EXCLUDES1 *poisoning by, adverse effect of and underdosing of metaraminol (T44.4)*

The appropriate 7th character is to be added to each code from category T46

A = initial encounter
D = subsequent encounter
S = sequela

T46.0 Poisoning by, adverse effect of and underdosing of cardiac-stimulant glycosides and drugs of similar action

T46.0X Poisoning by, adverse effect of and underdosing of cardiac-stimulant glycosides and drugs of similar action

T46.0X1 Poisoning by cardiac-stimulant glycosides and drugs of similar action, accidental (unintentional)

Poisoning by cardiac-stimulant glycosides and drugs of similar action NOS

T46.0X2 Poisoning by cardiac-stimulant glycosides and drugs of similar action, intentional self-harm

T46.0X3 Poisoning by cardiac-stimulant glycosides and drugs of similar action, assault

T46.0X4 Poisoning by cardiac-stimulant glycosides and drugs of similar action, undetermined

T46.0X5 Adverse effect of cardiac-stimulant glycosides and drugs of similar action

T46.0X6 Underdosing of cardiac-stimulant glycosides and drugs of similar action

T46.1 Poisoning by, adverse effect of and underdosing of calcium-channel blockers

T46.1X Poisoning by, adverse effect of and underdosing of calcium-channel blockers

T46.1X1 Poisoning by calcium-channel blockers, accidental (unintentional)

Poisoning by calcium-channel blockers NOS

T46.1X2 Poisoning by calcium-channel blockers, intentional self-harm

T46.1X3 Poisoning by calcium-channel blockers, assault

T46.1X4 Poisoning by calcium-channel blockers, undetermined

T46.1X5 Adverse effect of calcium-channel blockers

T46.1X6 Underdosing of calcium-channel blockers

T46.2 Poisoning by, adverse effect of and underdosing of other antidysrhythmic drugs, not elsewhere classified

EXCLUDES1 *poisoning by, adverse effect of and underdosing of beta-adrenoreceptor antagonists (T44.7-)*

T46.2X Poisoning by, adverse effect of and underdosing of other antidysrhythmic drugs

T46.2X1 Poisoning by other antidysrhythmic drugs, accidental (unintentional)

Poisoning by other antidysrhythmic drugs NOS

T46.2X2 Poisoning by other antidysrhythmic drugs, intentional self-harm

T46.2X3 Poisoning by other antidysrhythmic drugs, assault

T46.2X4 Poisoning by other antidysrhythmic drugs, undetermined

T46.2X5 Adverse effect of other antidysrhythmic drugs

T46.2X6 Underdosing of other antidysrhythmic drugs

T46.3 Poisoning by, adverse effect of and underdosing of coronary vasodilators

Poisoning by, adverse effect of and underdosing of dipyridamole

EXCLUDES1 *poisoning by, adverse effect of and underdosing of calcium-channel blockers (T46.1)*

T46.3X Poisoning by, adverse effect of and underdosing of coronary vasodilators

T46.3X1 Poisoning by coronary vasodilators, accidental (unintentional)

Poisoning by coronary vasodilators NOS

T46.3X2 Poisoning by coronary vasodilators, intentional self-harm

T46.3X3 Poisoning by coronary vasodilators, assault

T46.3X4 Poisoning by coronary vasodilators, undetermined

T46.3X5 Adverse effect of coronary vasodilators

T46.3X6 Underdosing of coronary vasodilators

T46.4 Poisoning by, adverse effect of and underdosing of angiotensin-converting-enzyme inhibitors

T46.4X Poisoning by, adverse effect of and underdosing of angiotensin-converting-enzyme inhibitors

T46.4X1 Poisoning by angiotensin-converting-enzyme inhibitors, accidental (unintentional)

Poisoning by angiotensin-converting-enzyme inhibitors NOS

T46.4X2 Poisoning by angiotensin-converting-enzyme inhibitors, intentional self-harm

T46.4X3 Poisoning by angiotensin-converting-enzyme inhibitors, assault

T46.4X4 Poisoning by angiotensin-converting-enzyme inhibitors, undetermined
T46.4X5 Adverse effect of angiotensin-converting-enzyme inhibitors
T46.4X6 Underdosing of angiotensin-converting-enzyme inhibitors

T46.5 Poisoning by, adverse effect of and underdosing of other antihypertensive drugs
EXCLUDES2 *poisoning by, adverse effect of and underdosing of beta-adrenoreceptor antagonists (T44.7)*
poisoning by, adverse effect of and underdosing of calcium-channel blockers (T46.1)
poisoning by, adverse effect of and underdosing of diuretics (T50.0-T50.2)

T46.5X Poisoning by, adverse effect of and underdosing of other antihypertensive drugs
T46.5X1 Poisoning by other antihypertensive drugs, accidental (unintentional)
Poisoning by other antihypertensive drugs NOS
T46.5X2 Poisoning by other antihypertensive drugs, intentional self-harm
T46.5X3 Poisoning by other antihypertensive drugs, assault
T46.5X4 Poisoning by other antihypertensive drugs, undetermined
T46.5X5 Adverse effect of other antihypertensive drugs
T46.5X6 Underdosing of other antihypertensive drugs

T46.6 Poisoning by, adverse effect of and underdosing of antihyperlipidemic and antiarteriosclerotic drugs
T46.6X Poisoning by, adverse effect of and underdosing of antihyperlipidemic and antiarteriosclerotic drugs
T46.6X1 Poisoning by antihyperlipidemic and antiarteriosclerotic drugs, accidental (unintentional)
Poisoning by antihyperlipidemic and antiarteriosclerotic drugs NOS
T46.6X2 Poisoning by antihyperlipidemic and antiarteriosclerotic drugs, intentional self-harm
T46.6X3 Poisoning by antihyperlipidemic and antiarteriosclerotic drugs, assault
T46.6X4 Poisoning by antihyperlipidemic and antiarteriosclerotic drugs, undetermined
T46.6X5 Adverse effect of antihyperlipidemic and antiarteriosclerotic drugs
T46.6X6 Underdosing of antihyperlipidemic and antiarteriosclerotic drugs

T46.7 Poisoning by, adverse effect of and underdosing of peripheral vasodilators
Poisoning by, adverse effect of and underdosing of nicotinic acid (derivatives)
EXCLUDES1 *poisoning by, adverse effect of and underdosing of papaverine (T44.3)*
T46.7X Poisoning by, adverse effect of and underdosing of peripheral vasodilators
T46.7X1 Poisoning by peripheral vasodilators, accidental (unintentional)
Poisoning by peripheral vasodilators NOS
T46.7X2 Poisoning by peripheral vasodilators, intentional self-harm
T46.7X3 Poisoning by peripheral vasodilators, assault
T46.7X4 Poisoning by peripheral vasodilators, undetermined
T46.7X5 Adverse effect of peripheral vasodilators
T46.7X6 Underdosing of peripheral vasodilators

T46.8 Poisoning by, adverse effect of and underdosing of antivaricose drugs, including sclerosing agents
T46.8X Poisoning by, adverse effect of and underdosing of antivaricose drugs, including sclerosing agents
T46.8X1 Poisoning by antivaricose drugs, including sclerosing agents, accidental (unintentional)
Poisoning by antivaricose drugs, including sclerosing agents NOS
T46.8X2 Poisoning by antivaricose drugs, including sclerosing agents, intentional self-harm
T46.8X3 Poisoning by antivaricose drugs, including sclerosing agents, assault
T46.8X4 Poisoning by antivaricose drugs, including sclerosing agents, undetermined
T46.8X5 Adverse effect of antivaricose drugs, including sclerosing agents
T46.8X6 Underdosing of antivaricose drugs, including sclerosing agents

T46.9 Poisoning by, adverse effect of and underdosing of other and unspecified agents primarily affecting the cardiovascular system
T46.90 Poisoning by, adverse effect of and underdosing of unspecified agents primarily affecting the cardiovascular system
T46.901 Poisoning by unspecified agents primarily affecting the cardiovascular system, accidental (unintentional)
T46.902 Poisoning by unspecified agents primarily affecting the cardiovascular system, intentional self-harm
T46.903 Poisoning by unspecified agents primarily affecting the cardiovascular system, assault
T46.904 Poisoning by unspecified agents primarily affecting the cardiovascular system, undetermined
T46.905 Adverse effect of unspecified agents primarily affecting the cardiovascular system
T46.906 Underdosing of unspecified agents primarily affecting the cardiovascular system
T46.99 Poisoning by, adverse effect of and underdosing of other agents primarily affecting the cardiovascular system
T46.991 Poisoning by other agents primarily affecting the cardiovascular system, accidental (unintentional)
T46.992 Poisoning by other agents primarily affecting the cardiovascular system, intentional self-harm
T46.993 Poisoning by other agents primarily affecting the cardiovascular system, assault
T46.994 Poisoning by other agents primarily affecting the cardiovascular system, undetermined
T46.995 Adverse effect of other agents primarily affecting the cardiovascular system
T46.996 Underdosing of other agents primarily affecting the cardiovascular system

T47 Poisoning by, adverse effect of and underdosing of agents primarily affecting the gastrointestinal system
The appropriate 7th character is to be added to each code from category T47
A = initial encounter
D = subsequent encounter
S = sequela

T47.0 Poisoning by, adverse effect of and underdosing of histamine H2-receptor blockers
T47.0X Poisoning by, adverse effect of and underdosing of histamine H2-receptor blockers
T47.0X1 Poisoning by histamine H2-receptor blockers, accidental (unintentional)
Poisoning by histamine H2-receptor blockers NOS
T47.0X2 Poisoning by histamine H2-receptor blockers, intentional self-harm
T47.0X3 Poisoning by histamine H2-receptor blockers, assault
T47.0X4 Poisoning by histamine H2-receptor blockers, undetermined

Unacceptable principal diagnosis symbol per Medicare code edits | Code exempt from diagnosis present on admission requirement
Questionable admission | Complication or comorbidity | CC/MCC exclusion | Major complication or comorbidity
Principal diagnosis as its own CC | Principal diagnosis as its own MCC | Z code as first-listed diagnosis

T47.0X5 Adverse effect of histamine H2-receptor blockers
T47.0X6 Underdosing of histamine H2-receptor blockers

T47.1 Poisoning by, adverse effect of and underdosing of other antacids and anti-gastric-secretion drugs
T47.1X Poisoning by, adverse effect of and underdosing of other antacids and anti-gastric-secretion drugs
T47.1X1 Poisoning by other antacids and anti-gastric-secretion drugs, accidental (unintentional)
Poisoning by other antacids and anti-gastric-secretion drugs NOS
T47.1X2 Poisoning by other antacids and anti-gastric-secretion drugs, intentional self-harm
T47.1X3 Poisoning by other antacids and anti-gastric-secretion drugs, assault
T47.1X4 Poisoning by other antacids and anti-gastric-secretion drugs, undetermined
T47.1X5 Adverse effect of other antacids and anti-gastric-secretion drugs
T47.1X6 Underdosing of other antacids and anti-gastric-secretion drugs

T47.2 Poisoning by, adverse effect of and underdosing of stimulant laxatives
T47.2X Poisoning by, adverse effect of and underdosing of stimulant laxatives
T47.2X1 Poisoning by stimulant laxatives, accidental (unintentional)
Poisoning by stimulant laxatives NOS
T47.2X2 Poisoning by stimulant laxatives, intentional self-harm
T47.2X3 Poisoning by stimulant laxatives, assault
T47.2X4 Poisoning by stimulant laxatives, undetermined
T47.2X5 Adverse effect of stimulant laxatives
T47.2X6 Underdosing of stimulant laxatives

T47.3 Poisoning by, adverse effect of and underdosing of saline and osmotic laxatives
T47.3X Poisoning by and adverse effect of saline and osmotic laxatives
T47.3X1 Poisoning by saline and osmotic laxatives, accidental (unintentional)
Poisoning by saline and osmotic laxatives NOS
T47.3X2 Poisoning by saline and osmotic laxatives, intentional self-harm
T47.3X3 Poisoning by saline and osmotic laxatives, assault
T47.3X4 Poisoning by saline and osmotic laxatives, undetermined
T47.3X5 Adverse effect of saline and osmotic laxatives
T47.3X6 Underdosing of saline and osmotic laxatives

T47.4 Poisoning by, adverse effect of and underdosing of other laxatives
T47.4X Poisoning by, adverse effect of and underdosing of other laxatives
T47.4X1 Poisoning by other laxatives, accidental (unintentional)
Poisoning by other laxatives NOS
T47.4X2 Poisoning by other laxatives, intentional self-harm
T47.4X3 Poisoning by other laxatives, assault
T47.4X4 Poisoning by other laxatives, undetermined
T47.4X5 Adverse effect of other laxatives
T47.4X6 Underdosing of other laxatives

T47.5 Poisoning by, adverse effect of and underdosing of digestants
T47.5X Poisoning by, adverse effect of and underdosing of digestants
T47.5X1 Poisoning by digestants, accidental (unintentional)
Poisoning by digestants NOS
T47.5X2 Poisoning by digestants, intentional self-harm
T47.5X3 Poisoning by digestants, assault
T47.5X4 Poisoning by digestants, undetermined
T47.5X5 Adverse effect of digestants
T47.5X6 Underdosing of digestants

T47.6 Poisoning by, adverse effect of and underdosing of antidiarrheal drugs
EXCLUDES2 *poisoning by, adverse effect of and underdosing of systemic antibiotics and other anti-infectives (T36-T37)*
T47.6X Poisoning by, adverse effect of and underdosing of antidiarrheal drugs
T47.6X1 Poisoning by antidiarrheal drugs, accidental (unintentional)
Poisoning by antidiarrheal drugs NOS
T47.6X2 Poisoning by antidiarrheal drugs, intentional self-harm
T47.6X3 Poisoning by antidiarrheal drugs, assault
T47.6X4 Poisoning by antidiarrheal drugs, undetermined
T47.6X5 Adverse effect of antidiarrheal drugs
T47.6X6 Underdosing of antidiarrheal drugs

T47.7 Poisoning by, adverse effect of and underdosing of emetics
T47.7X Poisoning by, adverse effect of and underdosing of emetics
T47.7X1 Poisoning by emetics, accidental (unintentional)
Poisoning by emetics NOS
T47.7X2 Poisoning by emetics, intentional self-harm
T47.7X3 Poisoning by emetics, assault
T47.7X4 Poisoning by emetics, undetermined
T47.7X5 Adverse effect of emetics
T47.7X6 Underdosing of emetics

T47.8 Poisoning by, adverse effect of and underdosing of other agents primarily affecting gastrointestinal system
T47.8X Poisoning by, adverse effect of and underdosing of other agents primarily affecting gastrointestinal system
T47.8X1 Poisoning by other agents primarily affecting gastrointestinal system, accidental (unintentional)
Poisoning by other agents primarily affecting gastrointestinal system NOS
T47.8X2 Poisoning by other agents primarily affecting gastrointestinal system, intentional self-harm
T47.8X3 Poisoning by other agents primarily affecting gastrointestinal system, assault
T47.8X4 Poisoning by other agents primarily affecting gastrointestinal system, undetermined
T47.8X5 Adverse effect of other agents primarily affecting gastrointestinal system
T47.8X6 Underdosing of other agents primarily affecting gastrointestinal system

T47.9 Poisoning by, adverse effect of and underdosing of unspecified agents primarily affecting the gastrointestinal system
T47.91 Poisoning by unspecified agents primarily affecting the gastrointestinal system, accidental (unintentional)
Poisoning by agents primarily affecting the gastrointestinal system NOS
T47.92 Poisoning by unspecified agents primarily affecting the gastrointestinal system, intentional self-harm
T47.93 Poisoning by unspecified agents primarily affecting the gastrointestinal system, assault
T47.94 Poisoning by unspecified agents primarily affecting the gastrointestinal system, undetermined
T47.95 Adverse effect of unspecified agents primarily affecting the gastrointestinal system
T47.96 Underdosing of unspecified agents primarily affecting the gastrointestinal system

Unspecified Code Other Specified Code Manifestation Code N Newborn P Pediatric M Maternity A Adult ♂ Male ♀ Female
● New Code ▲ Revised Code Title ►◄ Revised Text NOTES INCLUDES EXCLUDES1 Not coded here EXCLUDES2 Not included here
4th character required 5th character required 6th character required 7th character required
Extension 'X' Alert HAC Hospital-acquired condition (HAC) alert AHA AHA Coding Clinic©

T48 Poisoning by, adverse effect of and underdosing of agents primarily acting on smooth and skeletal muscles and the respiratory system

The appropriate 7th character is to be added to each code from category T48

A = initial encounter

D = subsequent encounter

S = sequela

T48.0 Poisoning by, adverse effect of and underdosing of oxytocic drugs

EXCLUDES1 *poisoning by, adverse effect of and underdosing of estrogens, progestogens and antagonists (T38.4-T38.6)*

T48.0X Poisoning by, adverse effect of and underdosing of oxytocic drugs

T48.0X1 Poisoning by oxytocic drugs, accidental (unintentional)

Poisoning by oxytocic drugs NOS

T48.0X2 Poisoning by oxytocic drugs, intentional self-harm

T48.0X3 Poisoning by oxytocic drugs, assault

T48.0X4 Poisoning by oxytocic drugs, undetermined

T48.0X5 Adverse effect of oxytocic drugs

T48.0X6 Underdosing of oxytocic drugs

T48.1 Poisoning by, adverse effect of and underdosing of skeletal muscle relaxants [neuromuscular blocking agents]

T48.1X Poisoning by, adverse effect of and underdosing of skeletal muscle relaxants [neuromuscular blocking agents]

T48.1X1 Poisoning by skeletal muscle relaxants [neuromuscular blocking agents], accidental (unintentional)

Poisoning by skeletal muscle relaxants [neuromuscular blocking agents] NOS

T48.1X2 Poisoning by skeletal muscle relaxants [neuromuscular blocking agents], intentional self-harm

T48.1X3 Poisoning by skeletal muscle relaxants [neuromuscular blocking agents], assault

T48.1X4 Poisoning by skeletal muscle relaxants [neuromuscular blocking agents], undetermined

T48.1X5 Adverse effect of skeletal muscle relaxants [neuromuscular blocking agents]

T48.1X6 Underdosing of skeletal muscle relaxants [neuromuscular blocking agents]

T48.2 Poisoning by, adverse effect of and underdosing of other and unspecified drugs acting on muscles

T48.20 Poisoning by, adverse effect of and underdosing of unspecified drugs acting on muscles

T48.201 Poisoning by unspecified drugs acting on muscles, accidental (unintentional)

Poisoning by unspecified drugs acting on muscles NOS

T48.202 Poisoning by unspecified drugs acting on muscles, intentional self-harm

T48.203 Poisoning by unspecified drugs acting on muscles, assault

T48.204 Poisoning by unspecified drugs acting on muscles, undetermined

T48.205 Adverse effect of unspecified drugs acting on muscles

T48.206 Underdosing of unspecified drugs acting on muscles

T48.29 Poisoning by, adverse effect of and underdosing of other drugs acting on muscles

T48.291 Poisoning by other drugs acting on muscles, accidental (unintentional)

Poisoning by other drugs acting on muscles NOS

T48.292 Poisoning by other drugs acting on muscles, intentional self-harm

T48.293 Poisoning by other drugs acting on muscles, assault

T48.294 Poisoning by other drugs acting on muscles, undetermined

T48.295 Adverse effect of other drugs acting on muscles

T48.296 Underdosing of other drugs acting on muscles

T48.3 Poisoning by, adverse effect of and underdosing of antitussives

T48.3X Poisoning by, adverse effect of and underdosing of antitussives

T48.3X1 Poisoning by antitussives, accidental (unintentional)

Poisoning by antitussives NOS

T48.3X2 Poisoning by antitussives, intentional self-harm

T48.3X3 Poisoning by antitussives, assault

T48.3X4 Poisoning by antitussives, undetermined

T48.3X5 Adverse effect of antitussives

T48.3X6 Underdosing of antitussives

T48.4 Poisoning by, adverse effect of and underdosing of expectorants

T48.4X Poisoning by, adverse effect of and underdosing of expectorants

T48.4X1 Poisoning by expectorants, accidental (unintentional)

Poisoning by expectorants NOS

T48.4X2 Poisoning by expectorants, intentional self-harm

T48.4X3 Poisoning by expectorants, assault

T48.4X4 Poisoning by expectorants, undetermined

T48.4X5 Adverse effect of expectorants

T48.4X6 Underdosing of expectorants

T48.5 Poisoning by, adverse effect of and underdosing of other anti-common-cold drugs

Poisoning by, adverse effect of and underdosing of decongestants

EXCLUDES2 *poisoning by, adverse effect of and underdosing of antipyretics, NEC (T39.9-)*

poisoning by, adverse effect of and underdosing of non-steroidal antiinflammatory drugs (T39.3-)

poisoning by, adverse effect of and underdosing of salicylates (T39.0-)

T48.5X Poisoning by, adverse effect of and underdosing of other anti-common-cold drugs

T48.5X1 Poisoning by other anti-common-cold drugs, accidental (unintentional)

Poisoning by other anti-common-cold drugs NOS

T48.5X2 Poisoning by other anti-common-cold drugs, intentional self-harm

T48.5X3 Poisoning by other anti-common-cold drugs, assault

T48.5X4 Poisoning by other anti-common-cold drugs, undetermined

T48.5X5 Adverse effect of other anti-common-cold drugs

T48.5X6 Underdosing of other anti-common-cold drugs

T48.6 Poisoning by, adverse effect of and underdosing of antiasthmatics, not elsewhere classified

Poisoning by, adverse effect of and underdosing of beta-adrenoreceptor agonists used in asthma therapy

EXCLUDES1 *poisoning by, adverse effect of and underdosing of beta-adrenoreceptor agonists not used in asthma therapy (T44.5)*

poisoning by, adverse effect of and underdosing of anterior pituitary [adenohypophyseal] hormones (T38.8)

T48.6X Poisoning by, adverse effect of and underdosing of antiasthmatics

T48.6X1 Poisoning by antiasthmatics, accidental (unintentional)

Poisoning by antiasthmatics NOS

T48.6X2 Poisoning by antiasthmatics, intentional self-harm

T48.6X3 Poisoning by antiasthmatics, assault

T48.6X4 Poisoning by antiasthmatics, undetermined

Unacceptable principal diagnosis symbol per Medicare code edits · Code exempt from diagnosis present on admission requirement
Questionable admission · Complication or comorbidity · CC/MCC exclusion · Major complication or comorbidity
Principal diagnosis as its own CC · Principal diagnosis as its own MCC · Z code as first-listed diagnosis

T48.6X5 Adverse effect of antiasthmatics
T48.6X6 Underdosing of antiasthmatics

T48.9 Poisoning by, adverse effect of and underdosing of other and unspecified agents primarily acting on the respiratory system

T48.90 Poisoning by, adverse effect of and underdosing of unspecified agents primarily acting on the respiratory system
T48.901 Poisoning by unspecified agents primarily acting on the respiratory system, accidental (unintentional)
T48.902 Poisoning by unspecified agents primarily acting on the respiratory system, intentional self-harm
T48.903 Poisoning by unspecified agents primarily acting on the respiratory system, assault
T48.904 Poisoning by unspecified agents primarily acting on the respiratory system, undetermined
T48.905 Adverse effect of unspecified agents primarily acting on the respiratory system
T48.906 Underdosing of unspecified agents primarily acting on the respiratory system

T48.99 Poisoning by, adverse effect of and underdosing of other agents primarily acting on the respiratory system
T48.991 Poisoning by other agents primarily acting on the respiratory system, accidental (unintentional)
T48.992 Poisoning by other agents primarily acting on the respiratory system, intentional self-harm
T48.993 Poisoning by other agents primarily acting on the respiratory system, assault
T48.994 Poisoning by other agents primarily acting on the respiratory system, undetermined
T48.995 Adverse effect of other agents primarily acting on the respiratory system
T48.996 Underdosing of other agents primarily acting on the respiratory system

T49 Poisoning by, adverse effect of and underdosing of topical agents primarily affecting skin and mucous membrane and by ophthalmological, otorhinorlaryngological and dental drugs

INCLUDES *poisoning by, adverse effect of and underdosing of glucocorticoids, topically used*

The appropriate 7th character is to be added to each code from category T49
A = initial encounter
D = subsequent encounter
S = sequela

T49.0 Poisoning by, adverse effect of and underdosing of local antifungal, anti-infective and anti-inflammatory drugs

T49.0X Poisoning by, adverse effect of and underdosing of local antifungal, anti-infective and anti-inflammatory drugs
T49.0X1 Poisoning by local antifungal, anti-infective and anti-inflammatory drugs, accidental (unintentional)
Poisoning by local antifungal, anti-infective and anti-inflammatory drugs NOS
T49.0X2 Poisoning by local antifungal, anti-infective and anti-inflammatory drugs, intentional self-harm
T49.0X3 Poisoning by local antifungal, anti-infective and anti-inflammatory drugs, assault
T49.0X4 Poisoning by local antifungal, anti-infective and anti-inflammatory drugs, undetermined
T49.0X5 Adverse effect of local antifungal, anti-infective and anti-inflammatory drugs
T49.0X6 Underdosing of local antifungal, anti-infective and anti-inflammatory drugs

T49.1 Poisoning by, adverse effect of and underdosing of antipruritics

T49.1X Poisoning by, adverse effect of and underdosing of antipruritics
T49.1X1 Poisoning by antipruritics, accidental (unintentional)
Poisoning by antipruritics NOS
T49.1X2 Poisoning by antipruritics, intentional self-harm
T49.1X3 Poisoning by antipruritics, assault
T49.1X4 Poisoning by antipruritics, undetermined
T49.1X5 Adverse effect of antipruritics
T49.1X6 Underdosing of antipruritics

T49.2 Poisoning by, adverse effect of and underdosing of local astringents and local detergents

T49.2X Poisoning by, adverse effect of and underdosing of local astringents and local detergents
T49.2X1 Poisoning by local astringents and local detergents, accidental (unintentional)
Poisoning by local astringents and local detergents NOS
T49.2X2 Poisoning by local astringents and local detergents, intentional self-harm
T49.2X3 Poisoning by local astringents and local detergents, assault
T49.2X4 Poisoning by local astringents and local detergents, undetermined
T49.2X5 Adverse effect of local astringents and local detergents
T49.2X6 Underdosing of local astringents and local detergents

T49.3 Poisoning by, adverse effect of and underdosing of emollients, demulcents and protectants

T49.3X Poisoning by, adverse effect of and underdosing of emollients, demulcents and protectants
T49.3X1 Poisoning by emollients, demulcents and protectants, accidental (unintentional)
Poisoning by emollients, demulcents and protectants NOS
T49.3X2 Poisoning by emollients, demulcents and protectants, intentional self-harm
T49.3X3 Poisoning by emollients, demulcents and protectants, assault
T49.3X4 Poisoning by emollients, demulcents and protectants, undetermined
T49.3X5 Adverse effect of emollients, demulcents and protectants
T49.3X6 Underdosing of emollients, demulcents and protectants

T49.4 Poisoning by, adverse effect of and underdosing of keratolytics, keratoplastics, and other hair treatment drugs and preparations

T49.4X Poisoning by, adverse effect of and underdosing of keratolytics, keratoplastics, and other hair treatment drugs and preparations
T49.4X1 Poisoning by keratolytics, keratoplastics, and other hair treatment drugs and preparations, accidental (unintentional)
Poisoning by keratolytics, keratoplastics, and other hair treatment drugs and preparations NOS
T49.4X2 Poisoning by keratolytics, keratoplastics, and other hair treatment drugs and preparations, intentional self-harm
T49.4X3 Poisoning by keratolytics, keratoplastics, and other hair treatment drugs and preparations, assault
T49.4X4 Poisoning by keratolytics, keratoplastics, and other hair treatment drugs and preparations, undetermined
T49.4X5 Adverse effect of keratolytics, keratoplastics, and other hair treatment drugs and preparations
T49.4X6 Underdosing of keratolytics, keratoplastics, and other hair treatment drugs and preparations

T49.5 Poisoning by, adverse effect of and underdosing of ophthalmological drugs and preparations

T49.5X Poisoning by, adverse effect of and underdosing of ophthalmological drugs and preparations

Unspecified Code Other Specified Code Manifestation Code N Newborn P Pediatric M Maternity A Adult ♂ Male ♀ Female
● New Code ▲ Revised Code Title ►◄ Revised Text NOTES INCLUDES EXCLUDES1 Not coded here EXCLUDES2 Not included here
4th character required 5th character required 6th character required 7th character required
Extension 'X' Alert HAC Hospital-acquired condition (HAC) alert AHA AHA Coding Clinic©

T49.5X1 Poisoning by ophthalmological drugs and preparations, accidental (unintentional)
Poisoning by ophthalmological drugs and preparations NOS
T49.5X2 Poisoning by ophthalmological drugs and preparations, intentional self-harm
T49.5X3 Poisoning by ophthalmological drugs and preparations, assault
T49.5X4 Poisoning by ophthalmological drugs and preparations, undetermined
T49.5X5 Adverse effect of ophthalmological drugs and preparations
T49.5X6 Underdosing of ophthalmological drugs and preparations

T49.6 Poisoning by, adverse effect of and underdosing of otorhinolaryngological drugs and preparations
T49.6X Poisoning by, adverse effect of and underdosing of otorhinolaryngological drugs and preparations
T49.6X1 Poisoning by otorhinolaryngological drugs and preparations, accidental (unintentional)
Poisoning by otorhinolaryngological drugs and preparations NOS
T49.6X2 Poisoning by otorhinolaryngological drugs and preparations, intentional self-harm
T49.6X3 Poisoning by otorhinolaryngological drugs and preparations, assault
T49.6X4 Poisoning by otorhinolaryngological drugs and preparations, undetermined
T49.6X5 Adverse effect of otorhinolaryngological drugs and preparations
T49.6X6 Underdosing of otorhinolaryngological drugs and preparations

T49.7 Poisoning by, adverse effect of and underdosing of dental drugs, topically applied
T49.7X Poisoning by, adverse effect of and underdosing of dental drugs, topically applied
T49.7X1 Poisoning by dental drugs, topically applied, accidental (unintentional)
Poisoning by dental drugs, topically applied NOS
T49.7X2 Poisoning by dental drugs, topically applied, intentional self-harm
T49.7X3 Poisoning by dental drugs, topically applied, assault
T49.7X4 Poisoning by dental drugs, topically applied, undetermined
T49.7X5 Adverse effect of dental drugs, topically applied
T49.7X6 Underdosing of dental drugs, topically applied

T49.8 Poisoning by, adverse effect of and underdosing of other topical agents
Poisoning by, adverse effect of and underdosing of spermicides
T49.8X Poisoning by, adverse effect of and underdosing of other topical agents
T49.8X1 Poisoning by other topical agents, accidental (unintentional)
Poisoning by other topical agents NOS
T49.8X2 Poisoning by other topical agents, intentional self-harm
T49.8X3 Poisoning by other topical agents, assault
T49.8X4 Poisoning by other topical agents, undetermined
T49.8X5 Adverse effect of other topical agents
T49.8X6 Underdosing of other topical agents

T49.9 Poisoning by, adverse effect of and underdosing of unspecified topical agent
T49.91 Poisoning by unspecified topical agent, accidental (unintentional)
T49.92 Poisoning by unspecified topical agent, intentional self-harm
T49.93 Poisoning by unspecified topical agent, assault
T49.94 Poisoning by unspecified topical agent, undetermined
T49.95 Adverse effect of unspecified topical agent
T49.96 Underdosing of unspecified topical agent

T50 Poisoning by, adverse effect of and underdosing of diuretics and other and unspecified drugs, medicaments and biological substances
The appropriate 7th character is to be added to each code from category T50
A = initial encounter
D = subsequent encounter
S = sequela

T50.0 Poisoning by, adverse effect of and underdosing of mineralocorticoids and their antagonists
T50.0X Poisoning by, adverse effect of and underdosing of mineralocorticoids and their antagonists
T50.0X1 Poisoning by mineralocorticoids and their antagonists, accidental (unintentional)
Poisoning by mineralocorticoids and their antagonists NOS
T50.0X2 Poisoning by mineralocorticoids and their antagonists, intentional self-harm
T50.0X3 Poisoning by mineralocorticoids and their antagonists, assault
T50.0X4 Poisoning by mineralocorticoids and their antagonists, undetermined
T50.0X5 Adverse effect of mineralocorticoids and their antagonists
T50.0X6 Underdosing of mineralocorticoids and their antagonists

T50.1 Poisoning by, adverse effect of and underdosing of loop [high-ceiling] diuretics
T50.1X Poisoning by, adverse effect of and underdosing of loop [high-ceiling] diuretics
T50.1X1 Poisoning by loop [high-ceiling] diuretics, accidental (unintentional)
Poisoning by loop [high-ceiling] diuretics NOS
T50.1X2 Poisoning by loop [high-ceiling] diuretics, intentional self-harm
T50.1X3 Poisoning by loop [high-ceiling] diuretics, assault
T50.1X4 Poisoning by loop [high-ceiling] diuretics, undetermined
T50.1X5 Adverse effect of loop [high-ceiling] diuretics
T50.1X6 Underdosing of loop [high-ceiling] diuretics

T50.2 Poisoning by, adverse effect of and underdosing of carbonic-anhydrase inhibitors, benzothiadiazides and other diuretics
Poisoning by, adverse effect of and underdosing of acetazolamide
T50.2X Poisoning by, adverse effect of and underdosing of carbonic-anhydrase inhibitors, benzothiadiazides and other diuretics
T50.2X1 Poisoning by carbonic-anhydrase inhibitors, benzothiadiazides and other diuretics, accidental (unintentional)
Poisoning by carbonic-anhydrase inhibitors, benzothiadiazides and other diuretics NOS
T50.2X2 Poisoning by carbonic-anhydrase inhibitors, benzothiadiazides and other diuretics, intentional self-harm
T50.2X3 Poisoning by carbonic-anhydrase inhibitors, benzothiadiazides and other diuretics, assault
T50.2X4 Poisoning by carbonic-anhydrase inhibitors, benzothiadiazides and other diuretics, undetermined
T50.2X5 Adverse effect of carbonic-anhydrase inhibitors, benzothiadiazides and other diuretics
T50.2X6 Underdosing of carbonic-anhydrase inhibitors, benzothiadiazides and other diuretics

T50.3 Poisoning by, adverse effect of and underdosing of electrolytic, caloric and water-balance agents
Poisoning by, adverse effect of and underdosing of oral rehydration salts

Unacceptable principal diagnosis symbol per Medicare code edits · Code exempt from diagnosis present on admission requirement
Questionable admission · Complication or comorbidity · CC/MCC exclusion · Major complication or comorbidity
Principal diagnosis as its own CC · Principal diagnosis as its own MCC · Z code as first-listed diagnosis

When symbols appear on a code that requires a 7th character extension, refer to Appendix D to identify applicable 7th character codes.

T50.3X Poisoning by, adverse effect of and underdosing of electrolytic, caloric and water-balance agents
- T50.3X1 Poisoning by electrolytic, caloric and water-balance agents, accidental (unintentional)
  Poisoning by electrolytic, caloric and water-balance agents NOS
- T50.3X2 Poisoning by electrolytic, caloric and water-balance agents, intentional self-harm
- T50.3X3 Poisoning by electrolytic, caloric and water-balance agents, assault
- T50.3X4 Poisoning by electrolytic, caloric and water-balance agents, undetermined
- T50.3X5 Adverse effect of electrolytic, caloric and water-balance agents
- T50.3X6 Underdosing of electrolytic, caloric and water-balance agents

T50.4 Poisoning by, adverse effect of and underdosing of drugs affecting uric acid metabolism

T50.4X Poisoning by, adverse effect of and underdosing of drugs affecting uric acid metabolism
- T50.4X1 Poisoning by drugs affecting uric acid metabolism, accidental (unintentional)
  Poisoning by drugs affecting uric acid metabolism NOS
- T50.4X2 Poisoning by drugs affecting uric acid metabolism, intentional self-harm
- T50.4X3 Poisoning by drugs affecting uric acid metabolism, assault
- T50.4X4 Poisoning by drugs affecting uric acid metabolism, undetermined
- T50.4X5 Adverse effect of drugs affecting uric acid metabolism
- T50.4X6 Underdosing of drugs affecting uric acid metabolism

T50.5 Poisoning by, adverse effect of and underdosing of appetite depressants

T50.5X Poisoning by, adverse effect of and underdosing of appetite depressants
- T50.5X1 Poisoning by appetite depressants, accidental (unintentional)
  Poisoning by appetite depressants NOS
- T50.5X2 Poisoning by appetite depressants, intentional self-harm
- T50.5X3 Poisoning by appetite depressants, assault
- T50.5X4 Poisoning by appetite depressants, undetermined
- T50.5X5 Adverse effect of appetite depressants
- T50.5X6 Underdosing of appetite depressants

T50.6 Poisoning by, adverse effect of and underdosing of antidotes and chelating agents

Poisoning by, adverse effect of and underdosing of alcohol deterrents

T50.6X Poisoning by, adverse effect of and underdosing of antidotes and chelating agents
- T50.6X1 Poisoning by antidotes and chelating agents, accidental (unintentional)
  Poisoning by antidotes and chelating agents NOS
- T50.6X2 Poisoning by antidotes and chelating agents, intentional self-harm
- T50.6X3 Poisoning by antidotes and chelating agents, assault
- T50.6X4 Poisoning by antidotes and chelating agents, undetermined
- T50.6X5 Adverse effect of antidotes and chelating agents
- T50.6X6 Underdosing of antidotes and chelating agents

T50.7 Poisoning by, adverse effect of and underdosing of analeptics and opioid receptor antagonists

T50.7X Poisoning by, adverse effect of and underdosing of analeptics and opioid receptor antagonists
- T50.7X1 Poisoning by analeptics and opioid receptor antagonists, accidental (unintentional)
  Poisoning by analeptics and opioid receptor antagonists NOS
- T50.7X2 Poisoning by analeptics and opioid receptor antagonists, intentional self-harm
- T50.7X3 Poisoning by analeptics and opioid receptor antagonists, assault
- T50.7X4 Poisoning by analeptics and opioid receptor antagonists, undetermined
- T50.7X5 Adverse effect of analeptics and opioid receptor antagonists
- T50.7X6 Underdosing of analeptics and opioid receptor antagonists

T50.8 Poisoning by, adverse effect of and underdosing of diagnostic agents

T50.8X Poisoning by, adverse effect of and underdosing of diagnostic agents
- T50.8X1 Poisoning by diagnostic agents, accidental (unintentional)
  Poisoning by diagnostic agents NOS
- T50.8X2 Poisoning by diagnostic agents, intentional self-harm
- T50.8X3 Poisoning by diagnostic agents, assault
- T50.8X4 Poisoning by diagnostic agents, undetermined
- T50.8X5 Adverse effect of diagnostic agents
- T50.8X6 Underdosing of diagnostic agents

T50.A Poisoning by, adverse effect of and underdosing of bacterial vaccines

T50.A1 Poisoning by, adverse effect of and underdosing of pertussis vaccine , including combinations with a pertussis component
- T50.A11 Poisoning by pertussis vaccine, including combinations with a pertussis component, accidental (unintentional)
- T50.A12 Poisoning by pertussis vaccine, including combinations with a pertussis component, intentional self-harm
- T50.A13 Poisoning by pertussis vaccine, including combinations with a pertussis component, assault
- T50.A14 Poisoning by pertussis vaccine, including combinations with a pertussis component, undetermined
- T50.A15 Adverse effect of pertussis vaccine, including combinations with a pertussis component
- T50.A16 Underdosing of pertussis vaccine, including combinations with a pertussis component

T50.A2 Poisoning by, adverse effect of and underdosing of mixed bacterial vaccines without a pertussis component
- T50.A21 Poisoning by mixed bacterial vaccines without a pertussis component, accidental (unintentional)
- T50.A22 Poisoning by mixed bacterial vaccines without a pertussis component, intentional self-harm
- T50.A23 Poisoning by mixed bacterial vaccines without a pertussis component, assault
- T50.A24 Poisoning by mixed bacterial vaccines without a pertussis component, undetermined
- T50.A25 Adverse effect of mixed bacterial vaccines without a pertussis component
- T50.A26 Underdosing of mixed bacterial vaccines without a pertussis component

T50.A9 Poisoning by, adverse effect of and underdosing of other bacterial vaccines
- T50.A91 Poisoning by other bacterial vaccines, accidental (unintentional)
- T50.A92 Poisoning by other bacterial vaccines, intentional self-harm

T50.A93 Poisoning by other bacterial vaccines, assault
T50.A94 Poisoning by other bacterial vaccines, undetermined
T50.A95 Adverse effect of other bacterial vaccines
T50.A96 Underdosing of other bacterial vaccines

T50.B Poisoning by, adverse effect of and underdosing of viral vaccines

T50.B1 Poisoning by, adverse effect of and underdosing of smallpox vaccines
T50.B11 Poisoning by smallpox vaccines, accidental (unintentional)
T50.B12 Poisoning by smallpox vaccines, intentional self-harm
T50.B13 Poisoning by smallpox vaccines, assault
T50.B14 Poisoning by smallpox vaccines, undetermined
T50.B15 Adverse effect of smallpox vaccines
T50.B16 Underdosing of smallpox vaccines

T50.B9 Poisoning by, adverse effect of and underdosing of other viral vaccines
T50.B91 Poisoning by other viral vaccines, accidental (unintentional)
T50.B92 Poisoning by other viral vaccines, intentional self-harm
T50.B93 Poisoning by other viral vaccines, assault
T50.B94 Poisoning by other viral vaccines, undetermined
T50.B95 Adverse effect of other viral vaccines
T50.B96 Underdosing of other viral vaccines

T50.Z Poisoning by, adverse effect of and underdosing of other vaccines and biological substances

T50.Z1 Poisoning by, adverse effect of and underdosing of immunoglobulin
T50.Z11 Poisoning by immunoglobulin, accidental (unintentional)
T50.Z12 Poisoning by immunoglobulin, intentional self-harm
T50.Z13 Poisoning by immunoglobulin, assault
T50.Z14 Poisoning by immunoglobulin, undetermined
T50.Z15 Adverse effect of immunoglobulin
T50.Z16 Underdosing of immunoglobulin

T50.Z9 Poisoning by, adverse effect of and underdosing of other vaccines and biological substances
T50.Z91 Poisoning by other vaccines and biological substances, accidental (unintentional)
T50.Z92 Poisoning by other vaccines and biological substances, intentional self-harm
T50.Z93 Poisoning by other vaccines and biological substances, assault
T50.Z94 Poisoning by other vaccines and biological substances, undetermined
T50.Z95 Adverse effect of other vaccines and biological substances
T50.Z96 Underdosing of other vaccines and biological substances

T50.9 Poisoning by, adverse effect of and underdosing of other and unspecified drugs, medicaments and biological substances

T50.90 Poisoning by, adverse effect of and underdosing of unspecified drugs, medicaments and biological substances
T50.901 Poisoning by unspecified drugs, medicaments and biological substances, accidental (unintentional)
AHA: Q1, 2015
T50.902 Poisoning by unspecified drugs, medicaments and biological substances, intentional self-harm
T50.903 Poisoning by unspecified drugs, medicaments and biological substances, assault
T50.904 Poisoning by unspecified drugs, medicaments and biological substances, undetermined
T50.905 Adverse effect of unspecified drugs, medicaments and biological substances
T50.906 Underdosing of unspecified drugs, medicaments and biological substances

T50.99 Poisoning by, adverse effect of and underdosing of other drugs, medicaments and biological substances
T50.991 Poisoning by other drugs, medicaments and biological substances, accidental (unintentional)
T50.992 Poisoning by other drugs, medicaments and biological substances, intentional self-harm
T50.993 Poisoning by other drugs, medicaments and biological substances, assault
T50.994 Poisoning by other drugs, medicaments and biological substances, undetermined
T50.995 Adverse effect of other drugs, medicaments and biological substances
T50.996 Underdosing of other drugs, medicaments and biological substances

Toxic effects of substances chiefly nonmedicinal as to source (T51-T65)

NOTES When no intent is indicated code to accidental. Undetermined intent is only for use when there is specific documentation in the record that the intent of the toxic effect cannot be determined.

Use additional code(s):
for all associated manifestations of toxic effect, such as: respiratory conditions due to external agents (J60-J70)
personal history of foreign body fully removed (Z87.821)
to identify any retained foreign body, if applicable (Z18.-)

EXCLUDES1 *contact with and (suspected) exposure to toxic substances (Z77.-)*

T51 Toxic effect of alcohol

The appropriate 7th character is to be added to each code from category T51
A = initial encounter
D = subsequent encounter
S = sequela

T51.0 Toxic effect of ethanol
Toxic effect of ethyl alcohol
EXCLUDES2 *acute alcohol intoxication or 'hangover' effects (F10.129, F10.229, F10.929)*
drunkenness (F10.129, F10.229, F10.929)
pathological alcohol intoxication (F10.129, F10.229, F10.929)

T51.0X Toxic effect of ethanol
T51.0X1 Toxic effect of ethanol, accidental (unintentional)
Toxic effect of ethanol NOS
T51.0X2 Toxic effect of ethanol, intentional self-harm
T51.0X3 Toxic effect of ethanol, assault
T51.0X4 Toxic effect of ethanol, undetermined

T51.1 Toxic effect of methanol
Toxic effect of methyl alcohol

T51.1X Toxic effect of methanol
T51.1X1 Toxic effect of methanol, accidental (unintentional)
Toxic effect of methanol NOS
T51.1X2 Toxic effect of methanol, intentional self-harm
T51.1X3 Toxic effect of methanol, assault
T51.1X4 Toxic effect of methanol, undetermined

T51.2 Toxic effect of 2-Propanol
Toxic effect of isopropyl alcohol

T51.2X Toxic effect of 2-Propanol
T51.2X1 Toxic effect of 2-Propanol, accidental (unintentional)
Toxic effect of 2-Propanol NOS
T51.2X2 Toxic effect of 2-Propanol, intentional self-harm

Unacceptable principal diagnosis symbol per Medicare code edits · Code exempt from diagnosis present on admission requirement
Questionable admission · Complication or comorbidity · CC/MCC exclusion · Major complication or comorbidity
Principal diagnosis as its own CC · Principal diagnosis as its own MCC · Z code as first-listed diagnosis

T51.2X3 Toxic effect of 2-Propanol, assault
T51.2X4 Toxic effect of 2-Propanol, undetermined

T51.3 Toxic effect of fusel oil
Toxic effect of amyl alcohol
Toxic effect of butyl [1-butanol] alcohol
Toxic effect of propyl [1-propanol] alcohol
T51.3X Toxic effect of fusel oil
T51.3X1 Toxic effect of fusel oil, accidental (unintentional)
Toxic effect of fusel oil NOS
T51.3X2 Toxic effect of fusel oil, intentional self-harm
T51.3X3 Toxic effect of fusel oil, assault
T51.3X4 Toxic effect of fusel oil, undetermined

T51.8 Toxic effect of other alcohols
T51.8X Toxic effect of other alcohols
T51.8X1 Toxic effect of other alcohols, accidental (unintentional)
Toxic effect of other alcohols NOS
T51.8X2 Toxic effect of other alcohols, intentional self-harm
T51.8X3 Toxic effect of other alcohols, assault
T51.8X4 Toxic effect of other alcohols, undetermined

T51.9 Toxic effect of unspecified alcohol
T51.91 Toxic effect of unspecified alcohol, accidental (unintentional)
T51.92 Toxic effect of unspecified alcohol, intentional self-harm
T51.93 Toxic effect of unspecified alcohol, assault
T51.94 Toxic effect of unspecified alcohol, undetermined

T52 Toxic effect of organic solvents

EXCLUDES1 *halogen derivatives of aliphatic and aromatic hydrocarbons (T53.-)*

The appropriate 7th character is to be added to each code from category T52
A = initial encounter
D = subsequent encounter
S = sequela

T52.0 Toxic effects of petroleum products
Toxic effects of gasoline [petrol]
Toxic effects of kerosene [paraffin oil]
Toxic effects of paraffin wax
Toxic effects of ether petroleum
Toxic effects of naphtha petroleum
Toxic effects of spirit petroleum
T52.0X Toxic effects of petroleum products
T52.0X1 Toxic effect of petroleum products, accidental (unintentional)
Toxic effects of petroleum products NOS
T52.0X2 Toxic effect of petroleum products, intentional self-harm
T52.0X3 Toxic effect of petroleum products, assault
T52.0X4 Toxic effect of petroleum products, undetermined

T52.1 Toxic effects of benzene
EXCLUDES1 *homologues of benzene (T52.2)*
nitroderivatives and aminoderivatives of benzene and its homologues (T65.3)
T52.1X Toxic effects of benzene
T52.1X1 Toxic effect of benzene, accidental (unintentional)
Toxic effects of benzene NOS
T52.1X2 Toxic effect of benzene, intentional self-harm
T52.1X3 Toxic effect of benzene, assault
T52.1X4 Toxic effect of benzene, undetermined

T52.2 Toxic effects of homologues of benzene
Toxic effects of toluene [methylbenzene]
Toxic effects of xylene [dimethylbenzene]
T52.2X Toxic effects of homologues of benzene
T52.2X1 Toxic effect of homologues of benzene, accidental (unintentional)
Toxic effects of homologues of benzene NOS
T52.2X2 Toxic effect of homologues of benzene, intentional self-harm
T52.2X3 Toxic effect of homologues of benzene, assault
T52.2X4 Toxic effect of homologues of benzene, undetermined

T52.3 Toxic effects of glycols
T52.3X Toxic effects of glycols
T52.3X1 Toxic effect of glycols, accidental (unintentional)
Toxic effects of glycols NOS
T52.3X2 Toxic effect of glycols, intentional self-harm
T52.3X3 Toxic effect of glycols, assault
T52.3X4 Toxic effect of glycols, undetermined

T52.4 Toxic effects of ketones
T52.4X Toxic effects of ketones
T52.4X1 Toxic effect of ketones, accidental (unintentional)
Toxic effects of ketones NOS
T52.4X2 Toxic effect of ketones, intentional self-harm
T52.4X3 Toxic effect of ketones, assault
T52.4X4 Toxic effect of ketones, undetermined

T52.8 Toxic effects of other organic solvents
T52.8X Toxic effects of other organic solvents
T52.8X1 Toxic effect of other organic solvents, accidental (unintentional)
Toxic effects of other organic solvents NOS
T52.8X2 Toxic effect of other organic solvents, intentional self-harm
T52.8X3 Toxic effect of other organic solvents, assault
T52.8X4 Toxic effect of other organic solvents, undetermined

T52.9 Toxic effects of unspecified organic solvent
T52.91 Toxic effect of unspecified organic solvent, accidental (unintentional)
T52.92 Toxic effect of unspecified organic solvent, intentional self-harm
T52.93 Toxic effect of unspecified organic solvent, assault
T52.94 Toxic effect of unspecified organic solvent, undetermined

T53 Toxic effect of halogen derivatives of aliphatic and aromatic hydrocarbons

The appropriate 7th character is to be added to each code from category T53
A = initial encounter
D = subsequent encounter
S = sequela

T53.0 Toxic effects of carbon tetrachloride
Toxic effects of tetrachloromethane
T53.0X Toxic effects of carbon tetrachloride
T53.0X1 Toxic effect of carbon tetrachloride, accidental (unintentional)
Toxic effects of carbon tetrachloride NOS
T53.0X2 Toxic effect of carbon tetrachloride, intentional self-harm
T53.0X3 Toxic effect of carbon tetrachloride, assault
T53.0X4 Toxic effect of carbon tetrachloride, undetermined

T53.1 Toxic effects of chloroform
Toxic effects of trichloromethane
T53.1X Toxic effects of chloroform
T53.1X1 Toxic effect of chloroform, accidental (unintentional)
Toxic effects of chloroform NOS
T53.1X2 Toxic effect of chloroform, intentional self-harm
T53.1X3 Toxic effect of chloroform, assault
T53.1X4 Toxic effect of chloroform, undetermined

T53.2 Toxic effects of trichloroethylene

Toxic effects of trichloroethene

T53.2X Toxic effects of trichloroethylene

T53.2X1 Toxic effect of trichloroethylene, accidental (unintentional)
Toxic effects of trichloroethylene NOS

T53.2X2 Toxic effect of trichloroethylene, intentional self-harm

T53.2X3 Toxic effect of trichloroethylene, assault

T53.2X4 Toxic effect of trichloroethylene, undetermined

T53.3 Toxic effects of tetrachloroethylene
Toxic effects of perchloroethylene
Toxic effect of tetrachloroethene

T53.3X Toxic effects of tetrachloroethylene

T53.3X1 Toxic effect of tetrachloroethylene, accidental (unintentional)
Toxic effects of tetrachloroethylene NOS

T53.3X2 Toxic effect of tetrachloroethylene, intentional self-harm

T53.3X3 Toxic effect of tetrachloroethylene, assault

T53.3X4 Toxic effect of tetrachloroethylene, undetermined

T53.4 Toxic effects of dichloromethane
Toxic effects of methylene chloride

T53.4X Toxic effects of dichloromethane

T53.4X1 Toxic effect of dichloromethane, accidental (unintentional)
Toxic effects of dichloromethane NOS

T53.4X2 Toxic effect of dichloromethane, intentional self-harm

T53.4X3 Toxic effect of dichloromethane, assault

T53.4X4 Toxic effect of dichloromethane, undetermined

T53.5 Toxic effects of chlorofluorocarbons

T53.5X Toxic effects of chlorofluorocarbons

T53.5X1 Toxic effect of chlorofluorocarbons, accidental (unintentional)
Toxic effects of chlorofluorocarbons NOS

T53.5X2 Toxic effect of chlorofluorocarbons, intentional self-harm

T53.5X3 Toxic effect of chlorofluorocarbons, assault

T53.5X4 Toxic effect of chlorofluorocarbons, undetermined

T53.6 Toxic effects of other halogen derivatives of aliphatic hydrocarbons

T53.6X Toxic effects of other halogen derivatives of aliphatic hydrocarbons

T53.6X1 Toxic effect of other halogen derivatives of aliphatic hydrocarbons, accidental (unintentional)
Toxic effects of other halogen derivatives of aliphatic hydrocarbons NOS

T53.6X2 Toxic effect of other halogen derivatives of aliphatic hydrocarbons, intentional self-harm

T53.6X3 Toxic effect of other halogen derivatives of aliphatic hydrocarbons, assault

T53.6X4 Toxic effect of other halogen derivatives of aliphatic hydrocarbons, undetermined

T53.7 Toxic effects of other halogen derivatives of aromatic hydrocarbons

T53.7X Toxic effects of other halogen derivatives of aromatic hydrocarbons

T53.7X1 Toxic effect of other halogen derivatives of aromatic hydrocarbons, accidental (unintentional)
Toxic effects of other halogen derivatives of aromatic hydrocarbons NOS

T53.7X2 Toxic effect of other halogen derivatives of aromatic hydrocarbons, intentional self-harm

T53.7X3 Toxic effect of other halogen derivatives of aromatic hydrocarbons, assault

T53.7X4 Toxic effect of other halogen derivatives of aromatic hydrocarbons, undetermined

T53.9 Toxic effects of unspecified halogen derivatives of aliphatic and aromatic hydrocarbons

T53.91 Toxic effect of unspecified halogen derivatives of aliphatic and aromatic hydrocarbons, accidental (unintentional)

T53.92 Toxic effect of unspecified halogen derivatives of aliphatic and aromatic hydrocarbons, intentional self-harm

T53.93 Toxic effect of unspecified halogen derivatives of aliphatic and aromatic hydrocarbons, assault

T53.94 Toxic effect of unspecified halogen derivatives of aliphatic and aromatic hydrocarbons, undetermined

T54 Toxic effect of corrosive substances

The appropriate 7th character is to be added to each code from category T54
A = initial encounter
D = subsequent encounter
S = sequela

T54.0 Toxic effects of phenol and phenol homologues

T54.0X Toxic effects of phenol and phenol homologues

T54.0X1 Toxic effect of phenol and phenol homologues, accidental (unintentional)
Toxic effects of phenol and phenol homologues NOS

T54.0X2 Toxic effect of phenol and phenol homologues, intentional self-harm

T54.0X3 Toxic effect of phenol and phenol homologues, assault

T54.0X4 Toxic effect of phenol and phenol homologues, undetermined

T54.1 Toxic effects of other corrosive organic compounds

T54.1X Toxic effects of other corrosive organic compounds

T54.1X1 Toxic effect of other corrosive organic compounds, accidental (unintentional)
Toxic effects of other corrosive organic compounds NOS

T54.1X2 Toxic effect of other corrosive organic compounds, intentional self-harm

T54.1X3 Toxic effect of other corrosive organic compounds, assault

T54.1X4 Toxic effect of other corrosive organic compounds, undetermined

T54.2 Toxic effects of corrosive acids and acid-like substances
Toxic effects of hydrochloric acid
Toxic effects of sulfuric acid

T54.2X Toxic effects of corrosive acids and acid-like substances

T54.2X1 Toxic effect of corrosive acids and acid-like substances, accidental (unintentional)
Toxic effects of corrosive acids and acid-like substances NOS

T54.2X2 Toxic effect of corrosive acids and acid-like substances, intentional self-harm

T54.2X3 Toxic effect of corrosive acids and acid-like substances, assault

T54.2X4 Toxic effect of corrosive acids and acid-like substances, undetermined

T54.3 Toxic effects of corrosive alkalis and alkali-like substances
Toxic effects of potassium hydroxide
Toxic effects of sodium hydroxide

T54.3X Toxic effects of corrosive alkalis and alkali-like substances

T54.3X1 Toxic effect of corrosive alkalis and alkali-like substances, accidental (unintentional)
Toxic effects of corrosive alkalis and alkali-like substances NOS

T54.3X2 Toxic effect of corrosive alkalis and alkali-like substances, intentional self-harm

T54.3X3 Toxic effect of corrosive alkalis and alkali-like substances, assault

T54.3X4 Toxic effect of corrosive alkalis and alkali-like substances, undetermined

T54.9 Toxic effects of unspecified corrosive substance

T54.91 Toxic effect of unspecified corrosive substance, accidental (unintentional)

Unacceptable principal diagnosis symbol per Medicare code edits | Code exempt from diagnosis present on admission requirement
Questionable admission | Complication or comorbidity | CC/MCC exclusion | Major complication or comorbidity
Principal diagnosis as its own CC | Principal diagnosis as its own MCC | Z code as first-listed diagnosis

T54.92 Toxic effect of unspecified corrosive substance, intentional self-harm
T54.93 Toxic effect of unspecified corrosive substance, assault
T54.94 Toxic effect of unspecified corrosive substance, undetermined

T55 Toxic effect of soaps and detergents
The appropriate 7th character is to be added to each code from category T55
A = initial encounter
D = subsequent encounter
S = sequela
T55.0 Toxic effect of soaps
T55.0X Toxic effect of soaps
T55.0X1 Toxic effect of soaps, accidental (unintentional)
Toxic effect of soaps NOS
T55.0X2 Toxic effect of soaps, intentional self-harm
T55.0X3 Toxic effect of soaps, assault
T55.0X4 Toxic effect of soaps, undetermined
T55.1 Toxic effect of detergents
T55.1X Toxic effect of detergents
T55.1X1 Toxic effect of detergents, accidental (unintentional)
Toxic effect of detergents NOS
T55.1X2 Toxic effect of detergents, intentional self-harm
T55.1X3 Toxic effect of detergents, assault
T55.1X4 Toxic effect of detergents, undetermined

T56 Toxic effect of metals
INCLUDES *toxic effects of fumes and vapors of metals*
toxic effects of metals from all sources, except medicinal substances
Use additional code to identify any retained metal foreign body, if applicable (Z18.0-, T18.1-)
EXCLUDES1 *arsenic and its compounds (T57.0)*
manganese and its compounds (T57.2)
The appropriate 7th character is to be added to each code from category T56
A = initial encounter
D = subsequent encounter
S = sequela
T56.0 Toxic effects of lead and its compounds
T56.0X Toxic effects of lead and its compounds
T56.0X1 Toxic effect of lead and its compounds, accidental (unintentional)
Toxic effects of lead and its compounds NOS
T56.0X2 Toxic effect of lead and its compounds, intentional self-harm
T56.0X3 Toxic effect of lead and its compounds, assault
T56.0X4 Toxic effect of lead and its compounds, undetermined
T56.1 Toxic effects of mercury and its compounds
T56.1X Toxic effects of mercury and its compounds
T56.1X1 Toxic effect of mercury and its compounds, accidental (unintentional)
Toxic effects of mercury and its compounds NOS
T56.1X2 Toxic effect of mercury and its compounds, intentional self-harm
T56.1X3 Toxic effect of mercury and its compounds, assault
T56.1X4 Toxic effect of mercury and its compounds, undetermined
T56.2 Toxic effects of chromium and its compounds
T56.2X Toxic effects of chromium and its compounds
T56.2X1 Toxic effect of chromium and its compounds, accidental (unintentional)
Toxic effects of chromium and its compounds NOS
T56.2X2 Toxic effect of chromium and its compounds, intentional self-harm
T56.2X3 Toxic effect of chromium and its compounds, assault
T56.2X4 Toxic effect of chromium and its compounds, undetermined
T56.3 Toxic effects of cadmium and its compounds
T56.3X Toxic effects of cadmium and its compounds
T56.3X1 Toxic effect of cadmium and its compounds, accidental (unintentional)
Toxic effects of cadmium and its compounds NOS
T56.3X2 Toxic effect of cadmium and its compounds, intentional self-harm
T56.3X3 Toxic effect of cadmium and its compounds, assault
T56.3X4 Toxic effect of cadmium and its compounds, undetermined
T56.4 Toxic effects of copper and its compounds
T56.4X Toxic effects of copper and its compounds
T56.4X1 Toxic effect of copper and its compounds, accidental (unintentional)
Toxic effects of copper and its compounds NOS
T56.4X2 Toxic effect of copper and its compounds, intentional self-harm
T56.4X3 Toxic effect of copper and its compounds, assault
T56.4X4 Toxic effect of copper and its compounds, undetermined
T56.5 Toxic effects of zinc and its compounds
T56.5X Toxic effects of zinc and its compounds
T56.5X1 Toxic effect of zinc and its compounds, accidental (unintentional)
Toxic effects of zinc and its compounds NOS
T56.5X2 Toxic effect of zinc and its compounds, intentional self-harm
T56.5X3 Toxic effect of zinc and its compounds, assault
T56.5X4 Toxic effect of zinc and its compounds, undetermined
T56.6 Toxic effects of tin and its compounds
T56.6X Toxic effects of tin and its compounds
T56.6X1 Toxic effect of tin and its compounds, accidental (unintentional)
Toxic effects of tin and its compounds NOS
T56.6X2 Toxic effect of tin and its compounds, intentional self-harm
T56.6X3 Toxic effect of tin and its compounds, assault
T56.6X4 Toxic effect of tin and its compounds, undetermined
T56.7 Toxic effects of beryllium and its compounds
T56.7X Toxic effects of beryllium and its compounds
T56.7X1 Toxic effect of beryllium and its compounds, accidental (unintentional)
Toxic effects of beryllium and its compounds NOS
T56.7X2 Toxic effect of beryllium and its compounds, intentional self-harm
T56.7X3 Toxic effect of beryllium and its compounds, assault
T56.7X4 Toxic effect of beryllium and its compounds, undetermined
T56.8 Toxic effects of other metals
T56.81 Toxic effect of thallium
T56.811 Toxic effect of thallium, accidental (unintentional)
Toxic effect of thallium NOS
T56.812 Toxic effect of thallium, intentional self-harm
T56.813 Toxic effect of thallium, assault
T56.814 Toxic effect of thallium, undetermined
T56.89 Toxic effects of other metals
T56.891 Toxic effect of other metals, accidental (unintentional)
Toxic effects of other metals NOS

Unspecified Code Other Specified Code Manifestation Code N Newborn P Pediatric M Maternity A Adult ♂ Male ♀ Female
● New Code ▲ Revised Code Title ►◄ Revised Text NOTES INCLUDES EXCLUDES1 Not coded here EXCLUDES2 Not included here
4th character required 5th character required 6th character required 7th character required
Extension 'X' Alert HAC Hospital-acquired condition (HAC) alert AHA AHA Coding Clinic©

T56.892 Toxic effect of other metals, intentional self-harm
T56.893 Toxic effect of other metals, assault
T56.894 Toxic effect of other metals, undetermined
T56.9 Toxic effects of unspecified metal
T56.91 Toxic effect of unspecified metal, accidental (unintentional)
T56.92 Toxic effect of unspecified metal, intentional self-harm
T56.93 Toxic effect of unspecified metal, assault
T56.94 Toxic effect of unspecified metal, undetermined

T57 Toxic effect of other inorganic substances
The appropriate 7th character is to be added to each code from category T57
A = initial encounter
D = subsequent encounter
S = sequela

T57.0 Toxic effect of arsenic and its compounds
T57.0X Toxic effect of arsenic and its compounds
T57.0X1 Toxic effect of arsenic and its compounds, accidental (unintentional)
Toxic effect of arsenic and its compounds NOS
T57.0X2 Toxic effect of arsenic and its compounds, intentional self-harm
T57.0X3 Toxic effect of arsenic and its compounds, assault
T57.0X4 Toxic effect of arsenic and its compounds, undetermined
T57.1 Toxic effect of phosphorus and its compounds
EXCLUDES1 *organophosphate insecticides (T60.0)*
T57.1X Toxic effect of phosphorus and its compounds
T57.1X1 Toxic effect of phosphorus and its compounds, accidental (unintentional)
Toxic effect of phosphorus and its compounds NOS
T57.1X2 Toxic effect of phosphorus and its compounds, intentional self-harm
T57.1X3 Toxic effect of phosphorus and its compounds, assault
T57.1X4 Toxic effect of phosphorus and its compounds, undetermined
T57.2 Toxic effect of manganese and its compounds
T57.2X Toxic effect of manganese and its compounds
T57.2X1 Toxic effect of manganese and its compounds, accidental (unintentional)
Toxic effect of manganese and its compounds NOS
T57.2X2 Toxic effect of manganese and its compounds, intentional self-harm
T57.2X3 Toxic effect of manganese and its compounds, assault
T57.2X4 Toxic effect of manganese and its compounds, undetermined
T57.3 Toxic effect of hydrogen cyanide
T57.3X Toxic effect of hydrogen cyanide
T57.3X1 Toxic effect of hydrogen cyanide, accidental (unintentional)
Toxic effect of hydrogen cyanide NOS
T57.3X2 Toxic effect of hydrogen cyanide, intentional self-harm
T57.3X3 Toxic effect of hydrogen cyanide, assault
T57.3X4 Toxic effect of hydrogen cyanide, undetermined
T57.8 Toxic effect of other specified inorganic substances
T57.8X Toxic effect of other specified inorganic substances
T57.8X1 Toxic effect of other specified inorganic substances, accidental (unintentional)
Toxic effect of other specified inorganic substances NOS
T57.8X2 Toxic effect of other specified inorganic substances, intentional self-harm
T57.8X3 Toxic effect of other specified inorganic substances, assault
T57.8X4 Toxic effect of other specified inorganic substances, undetermined
T57.9 Toxic effect of unspecified inorganic substance
T57.91 Toxic effect of unspecified inorganic substance, accidental (unintentional)
T57.92 Toxic effect of unspecified inorganic substance, intentional self-harm
T57.93 Toxic effect of unspecified inorganic substance, assault
T57.94 Toxic effect of unspecified inorganic substance, undetermined

T58 Toxic effect of carbon monoxide
INCLUDES *asphyxiation from carbon monoxide*
toxic effect of carbon monoxide from all sources
The appropriate 7th character is to be added to each code from category T58
A = initial encounter
D = subsequent encounter
S = sequela

T58.0 Toxic effect of carbon monoxide from motor vehicle exhaust
Toxic effect of exhaust gas from gas engine
Toxic effect of exhaust gas from motor pump
T58.01 Toxic effect of carbon monoxide from motor vehicle exhaust, accidental (unintentional)
T58.02 Toxic effect of carbon monoxide from motor vehicle exhaust, intentional self-harm
T58.03 Toxic effect of carbon monoxide from motor vehicle exhaust, assault
T58.04 Toxic effect of carbon monoxide from motor vehicle exhaust, undetermined
T58.1 Toxic effect of carbon monoxide from utility gas
Toxic effect of acetylene
Toxic effect of gas NOS used for lighting, heating, cooking
Toxic effect of water gas
T58.11 Toxic effect of carbon monoxide from utility gas, accidental (unintentional)
T58.12 Toxic effect of carbon monoxide from utility gas, intentional self-harm
T58.13 Toxic effect of carbon monoxide from utility gas, assault
T58.14 Toxic effect of carbon monoxide from utility gas, undetermined
T58.2 Toxic effect of carbon monoxide from incomplete combustion of other domestic fuels
Toxic effect of carbon monoxide from incomplete combustion of coal, coke, kerosene, wood
T58.2X Toxic effect of carbon monoxide from incomplete combustion of other domestic fuels
T58.2X1 Toxic effect of carbon monoxide from incomplete combustion of other domestic fuels, accidental (unintentional)
T58.2X2 Toxic effect of carbon monoxide from incomplete combustion of other domestic fuels, intentional self-harm
T58.2X3 Toxic effect of carbon monoxide from incomplete combustion of other domestic fuels, assault
T58.2X4 Toxic effect of carbon monoxide from incomplete combustion of other domestic fuels, undetermined
T58.8 Toxic effect of carbon monoxide from other source
Toxic effect of carbon monoxide from blast furnace gas
Toxic effect of carbon monoxide from fuels in industrial use
Toxic effect of carbon monoxide from kiln vapor
T58.8X Toxic effect of carbon monoxide from other source
T58.8X1 Toxic effect of carbon monoxide from other source, accidental (unintentional)
T58.8X2 Toxic effect of carbon monoxide from other source, intentional self-harm
T58.8X3 Toxic effect of carbon monoxide from other source, assault
T58.8X4 Toxic effect of carbon monoxide from other source, undetermined
T58.9 Toxic effect of carbon monoxide from unspecified source
T58.91 Toxic effect of carbon monoxide from unspecified source, accidental (unintentional)

Unacceptable principal diagnosis symbol per Medicare code edits · Code exempt from diagnosis present on admission requirement
Questionable admission · Complication or comorbidity · CC/MCC exclusion · Major complication or comorbidity
Principal diagnosis as its own CC · Principal diagnosis as its own MCC · Z code as first-listed diagnosis

T58.92 Toxic effect of carbon monoxide from unspecified source, intentional self-harm
T58.93 Toxic effect of carbon monoxide from unspecified source, assault
T58.94 Toxic effect of carbon monoxide from unspecified source, undetermined

T59 Toxic effect of other gases, fumes and vapors
INCLUDES *aerosol propellants*
EXCLUDES1 *chlorofluorocarbons (T53.5)*
The appropriate 7th character is to be added to each code from category T59
A = initial encounter
D = subsequent encounter
S = sequela

T59.0 Toxic effect of nitrogen oxides
T59.0X Toxic effect of nitrogen oxides
T59.0X1 Toxic effect of nitrogen oxides, accidental (unintentional)
Toxic effect of nitrogen oxides NOS
T59.0X2 Toxic effect of nitrogen oxides, intentional self-harm
T59.0X3 Toxic effect of nitrogen oxides, assault
T59.0X4 Toxic effect of nitrogen oxides, undetermined

T59.1 Toxic effect of sulfur dioxide
T59.1X Toxic effect of sulfur dioxide
T59.1X1 Toxic effect of sulfur dioxide, accidental (unintentional)
Toxic effect of sulfur dioxide NOS
T59.1X2 Toxic effect of sulfur dioxide, intentional self-harm
T59.1X3 Toxic effect of sulfur dioxide, assault
T59.1X4 Toxic effect of sulfur dioxide, undetermined

T59.2 Toxic effect of formaldehyde
T59.2X Toxic effect of formaldehyde
T59.2X1 Toxic effect of formaldehyde, accidental (unintentional)
Toxic effect of formaldehyde NOS
T59.2X2 Toxic effect of formaldehyde, intentional self-harm
T59.2X3 Toxic effect of formaldehyde, assault
T59.2X4 Toxic effect of formaldehyde, undetermined

T59.3 Toxic effect of lacrimogenic gas
Toxic effect of tear gas
T59.3X Toxic effect of lacrimogenic gas
T59.3X1 Toxic effect of lacrimogenic gas, accidental (unintentional)
Toxic effect of lacrimogenic gas NOS
T59.3X2 Toxic effect of lacrimogenic gas, intentional self-harm
T59.3X3 Toxic effect of lacrimogenic gas, assault
T59.3X4 Toxic effect of lacrimogenic gas, undetermined

T59.4 Toxic effect of chlorine gas
T59.4X Toxic effect of chlorine gas
T59.4X1 Toxic effect of chlorine gas, accidental (unintentional)
Toxic effect of chlorine gas NOS
T59.4X2 Toxic effect of chlorine gas, intentional self-harm
T59.4X3 Toxic effect of chlorine gas, assault
T59.4X4 Toxic effect of chlorine gas, undetermined

T59.5 Toxic effect of fluorine gas and hydrogen fluoride
T59.5X Toxic effect of fluorine gas and hydrogen fluoride
T59.5X1 Toxic effect of fluorine gas and hydrogen fluoride, accidental (unintentional)
Toxic effect of fluorine gas and hydrogen fluoride NOS
T59.5X2 Toxic effect of fluorine gas and hydrogen fluoride, intentional self-harm
T59.5X3 Toxic effect of fluorine gas and hydrogen fluoride, assault
T59.5X4 Toxic effect of fluorine gas and hydrogen fluoride, undetermined

T59.6 Toxic effect of hydrogen sulfide
T59.6X Toxic effect of hydrogen sulfide
T59.6X1 Toxic effect of hydrogen sulfide, accidental (unintentional)
Toxic effect of hydrogen sulfide NOS
T59.6X2 Toxic effect of hydrogen sulfide, intentional self-harm
T59.6X3 Toxic effect of hydrogen sulfide, assault
T59.6X4 Toxic effect of hydrogen sulfide, undetermined

T59.7 Toxic effect of carbon dioxide
T59.7X Toxic effect of carbon dioxide
T59.7X1 Toxic effect of carbon dioxide, accidental (unintentional)
Toxic effect of carbon dioxide NOS
T59.7X2 Toxic effect of carbon dioxide, intentional self-harm
T59.7X3 Toxic effect of carbon dioxide, assault
T59.7X4 Toxic effect of carbon dioxide, undetermined

T59.8 Toxic effect of other specified gases, fumes and vapors
T59.81 Toxic effect of smoke
Smoke inhalation
EXCLUDES2 *toxic effect of cigarette (tobacco) smoke (T65.22-)*
T59.811 Toxic effect of smoke, accidental (unintentional)
Toxic effect of smoke NOS
AHA: Q4, 2013
T59.812 Toxic effect of smoke, intentional self-harm
T59.813 Toxic effect of smoke, assault
T59.814 Toxic effect of smoke, undetermined
T59.89 Toxic effect of other specified gases, fumes and vapors
T59.891 Toxic effect of other specified gases, fumes and vapors, accidental (unintentional)
T59.892 Toxic effect of other specified gases, fumes and vapors, intentional self-harm
T59.893 Toxic effect of other specified gases, fumes and vapors, assault
T59.894 Toxic effect of other specified gases, fumes and vapors, undetermined

T59.9 Toxic effect of unspecified gases, fumes and vapors
T59.91 Toxic effect of unspecified gases, fumes and vapors, accidental (unintentional)
T59.92 Toxic effect of unspecified gases, fumes and vapors, intentional self-harm
T59.93 Toxic effect of unspecified gases, fumes and vapors, assault
T59.94 Toxic effect of unspecified gases, fumes and vapors, undetermined

T60 Toxic effect of pesticides
INCLUDES *toxic effect of wood preservatives*
The appropriate 7th character is to be added to each code from category T60
A = initial encounter
D = subsequent encounter
S = sequela

T60.0 Toxic effect of organophosphate and carbamate insecticides
T60.0X Toxic effect of organophosphate and carbamate insecticides
T60.0X1 Toxic effect of organophosphate and carbamate insecticides, accidental (unintentional)
Toxic effect of organophosphate and carbamate insecticides NOS
T60.0X2 Toxic effect of organophosphate and carbamate insecticides, intentional self-harm
T60.0X3 Toxic effect of organophosphate and carbamate insecticides, assault

Unspecified Code Other Specified Code Manifestation Code N Newborn P Pediatric M Maternity A Adult ♂ Male ♀ Female
● New Code ▲ Revised Code Title ►◄ Revised Text NOTES INCLUDES EXCLUDES1 Not coded here EXCLUDES2 Not included here
4th character required 5th character required 6th character required 7th character required
Extension 'X' Alert HAC Hospital-acquired condition (HAC) alert AHA AHA Coding Clinic©

T60.0X4 Toxic effect of organophosphate and carbamate insecticides, undetermined

T60.1 Toxic effect of halogenated insecticides

EXCLUDES1 *chlorinated hydrocarbon (T53.-)*

T60.1X Toxic effect of halogenated insecticides

T60.1X1 Toxic effect of halogenated insecticides, accidental (unintentional)
Toxic effect of halogenated insecticides NOS

T60.1X2 Toxic effect of halogenated insecticides, intentional self-harm

T60.1X3 Toxic effect of halogenated insecticides, assault

T60.1X4 Toxic effect of halogenated insecticides, undetermined

T60.2 Toxic effect of other insecticides

T60.2X Toxic effect of other insecticides

T60.2X1 Toxic effect of other insecticides, accidental (unintentional)
Toxic effect of other insecticides NOS

T60.2X2 Toxic effect of other insecticides, intentional self-harm

T60.2X3 Toxic effect of other insecticides, assault

T60.2X4 Toxic effect of other insecticides, undetermined

T60.3 Toxic effect of herbicides and fungicides

T60.3X Toxic effect of herbicides and fungicides

T60.3X1 Toxic effect of herbicides and fungicides, accidental (unintentional)
Toxic effect of herbicides and fungicides NOS

T60.3X2 Toxic effect of herbicides and fungicides, intentional self-harm

T60.3X3 Toxic effect of herbicides and fungicides, assault

T60.3X4 Toxic effect of herbicides and fungicides, undetermined

T60.4 Toxic effect of rodenticides

EXCLUDES1 *strychnine and its salts (T65.1)*
thallium (T56.81-)

T60.4X Toxic effect of rodenticides

T60.4X1 Toxic effect of rodenticides, accidental (unintentional)
Toxic effect of rodenticides NOS

T60.4X2 Toxic effect of rodenticides, intentional self-harm

T60.4X3 Toxic effect of rodenticides, assault

T60.4X4 Toxic effect of rodenticides, undetermined

T60.8 Toxic effect of other pesticides

T60.8X Toxic effect of other pesticides

T60.8X1 Toxic effect of other pesticides, accidental (unintentional)
Toxic effect of other pesticides NOS

T60.8X2 Toxic effect of other pesticides, intentional self-harm

T60.8X3 Toxic effect of other pesticides, assault

T60.8X4 Toxic effect of other pesticides, undetermined

T60.9 Toxic effect of unspecified pesticide

T60.91 Toxic effect of unspecified pesticide, accidental (unintentional)

T60.92 Toxic effect of unspecified pesticide, intentional self-harm

T60.93 Toxic effect of unspecified pesticide, assault

T60.94 Toxic effect of unspecified pesticide, undetermined

T61 Toxic effect of noxious substances eaten as seafood

EXCLUDES1 *allergic reaction to food, such as:*
anaphylactic reaction or shock due to adverse food reaction (T78.0-)
bacterial foodborne intoxications (A05.-)
dermatitis (L23.6, L25.4, L27.2)
food protein-induced enterocolitis syndrome (K52.21)
food protein-induced enteropathy (K52.22)
gastroenteritis (noninfective) (K52.29)
toxic effect of aflatoxin and other mycotoxins (T64)
toxic effect of cyanides (T65.0-)
toxic effect of harmful algae bloom (T65.82-)
toxic effect of hydrogen cyanide (T57.3-)
toxic effect of mercury (T56.1-)
toxic effect of red tide (T65.82-)

The appropriate 7th character is to be added to each code from category T61
A = initial encounter
D = subsequent encounter
S = sequela

T61.0 Ciguatera fish poisoning

T61.01 Ciguatera fish poisoning, accidental (unintentional)

T61.02 Ciguatera fish poisoning, intentional self-harm

T61.03 Ciguatera fish poisoning, assault

T61.04 Ciguatera fish poisoning, undetermined

T61.1 Scombroid fish poisoning
Histamine-like syndrome

T61.11 Scombroid fish poisoning, accidental (unintentional)

T61.12 Scombroid fish poisoning, intentional self-harm

T61.13 Scombroid fish poisoning, assault

T61.14 Scombroid fish poisoning, undetermined

T61.7 Other fish and shellfish poisoning

T61.77 Other fish poisoning

T61.771 Other fish poisoning, accidental (unintentional)

T61.772 Other fish poisoning, intentional self-harm

T61.773 Other fish poisoning, assault

T61.774 Other fish poisoning, undetermined

T61.78 Other shellfish poisoning

T61.781 Other shellfish poisoning, accidental (unintentional)

T61.782 Other shellfish poisoning, intentional self-harm

T61.783 Other shellfish poisoning, assault

T61.784 Other shellfish poisoning, undetermined

T61.8 Toxic effect of other seafood

T61.8X Toxic effect of other seafood

T61.8X1 Toxic effect of other seafood, accidental (unintentional)

T61.8X2 Toxic effect of other seafood, intentional self-harm

T61.8X3 Toxic effect of other seafood, assault

T61.8X4 Toxic effect of other seafood, undetermined

T61.9 Toxic effect of unspecified seafood

T61.91 Toxic effect of unspecified seafood, accidental (unintentional)

T61.92 Toxic effect of unspecified seafood, intentional self-harm

T61.93 Toxic effect of unspecified seafood, assault

T61.94 Toxic effect of unspecified seafood, undetermined

T62 Toxic effect of other noxious substances eaten as food

EXCLUDES1 *allergic reaction to food, such as:*
anaphylactic shock (reaction) due to adverse food reaction (T78.0-)
bacterial food borne intoxications (A05.-)
dermatitis (L23.6, L25.4, L27.2)
food protein-induced enterocolitis syndrome (K52.21)
food protein-induced enteropathy (K52.22)
gastroenteritis (noninfective) (K52.29)
toxic effect of aflatoxin and other mycotoxins (T64)
toxic effect of cyanides (T65.0-)
toxic effect of hydrogen cyanide (T57.3-)
toxic effect of mercury (T56.1-)

The appropriate 7th character is to be added to each code from category T62
A = initial encounter
D = subsequent encounter
S = sequela

T62.0 Toxic effect of ingested mushrooms

Unacceptable principal diagnosis symbol per Medicare code edits; Code exempt from diagnosis present on admission requirement; Questionable admission; Complication or comorbidity; CC/MCC exclusion; Major complication or comorbidity; Principal diagnosis as its own CC; Principal diagnosis as its own MCC; Z code as first-listed diagnosis

T62.0X Toxic effect of ingested mushrooms
- T62.0X1 Toxic effect of ingested mushrooms, accidental (unintentional)
  Toxic effect of ingested mushrooms NOS
- T62.0X2 Toxic effect of ingested mushrooms, intentional self-harm
- T62.0X3 Toxic effect of ingested mushrooms, assault
- T62.0X4 Toxic effect of ingested mushrooms, undetermined

T62.1 Toxic effect of ingested berries

T62.1X Toxic effect of ingested berries
- T62.1X1 Toxic effect of ingested berries, accidental (unintentional)
  Toxic effect of ingested berries NOS
- T62.1X2 Toxic effect of ingested berries, intentional self-harm
- T62.1X3 Toxic effect of ingested berries, assault
- T62.1X4 Toxic effect of ingested berries, undetermined

T62.2 Toxic effect of other ingested (parts of) plant(s)

T62.2X Toxic effect of other ingested (parts of) plant (s)
- T62.2X1 Toxic effect of other ingested (parts of) plant(s), accidental (unintentional)
  Toxic effect of other ingested (parts of) plant(s) NOS
- T62.2X2 Toxic effect of other ingested (parts of) plant(s), intentional self-harm
- T62.2X3 Toxic effect of other ingested (parts of) plant(s), assault
- T62.2X4 Toxic effect of other ingested (parts of) plant(s), undetermined

T62.8 Toxic effect of other specified noxious substances eaten as food

T62.8X Toxic effect of other specified noxious substances eaten as food
- T62.8X1 Toxic effect of other specified noxious substances eaten as food, accidental (unintentional)
  Toxic effect of other specified noxious substances eaten as food NOS
- T62.8X2 Toxic effect of other specified noxious substances eaten as food, intentional self-harm
- T62.8X3 Toxic effect of other specified noxious substances eaten as food, assault
- T62.8X4 Toxic effect of other specified noxious substances eaten as food, undetermined

T62.9 Toxic effect of unspecified noxious substance eaten as food
- T62.91 Toxic effect of unspecified noxious substance eaten as food, accidental (unintentional)
  Toxic effect of unspecified noxious substance eaten as food NOS
- T62.92 Toxic effect of unspecified noxious substance eaten as food, intentional self-harm
- T62.93 Toxic effect of unspecified noxious substance eaten as food, assault
- T62.94 Toxic effect of unspecified noxious substance eaten as food, undetermined

T63 Toxic effect of contact with venomous animals and plants

INCLUDES *bite or touch of venomous animal*
pricked or stuck by thorn or leaf

EXCLUDES2 *ingestion of toxic animal or plant (T61.-, T62.-)*

The appropriate 7th character is to be added to each code from category T63
- A = initial encounter
- D = subsequent encounter
- S = sequela

T63.0 Toxic effect of snake venom

T63.00 Toxic effect of unspecified snake venom
- T63.001 Toxic effect of unspecified snake venom, accidental (unintentional)
  Toxic effect of unspecified snake venom NOS
- T63.002 Toxic effect of unspecified snake venom, intentional self-harm
- T63.003 Toxic effect of unspecified snake venom, assault
- T63.004 Toxic effect of unspecified snake venom, undetermined

T63.01 Toxic effect of rattlesnake venom
- T63.011 Toxic effect of rattlesnake venom, accidental (unintentional)
  Toxic effect of rattlesnake venom NOS
- T63.012 Toxic effect of rattlesnake venom, intentional self-harm
- T63.013 Toxic effect of rattlesnake venom, assault
- T63.014 Toxic effect of rattlesnake venom, undetermined

T63.02 Toxic effect of coral snake venom
- T63.021 Toxic effect of coral snake venom, accidental (unintentional)
  Toxic effect of coral snake venom NOS
- T63.022 Toxic effect of coral snake venom, intentional self-harm
- T63.023 Toxic effect of coral snake venom, assault
- T63.024 Toxic effect of coral snake venom, undetermined

T63.03 Toxic effect of taipan venom
- T63.031 Toxic effect of taipan venom, accidental (unintentional)
  Toxic effect of taipan venom NOS
- T63.032 Toxic effect of taipan venom, intentional self-harm
- T63.033 Toxic effect of taipan venom, assault
- T63.034 Toxic effect of taipan venom, undetermined

T63.04 Toxic effect of cobra venom
- T63.041 Toxic effect of cobra venom, accidental (unintentional)
  Toxic effect of cobra venom NOS
- T63.042 Toxic effect of cobra venom, intentional self-harm
- T63.043 Toxic effect of cobra venom, assault
- T63.044 Toxic effect of cobra venom, undetermined

T63.06 Toxic effect of venom of other North and South American snake
- T63.061 Toxic effect of venom of other North and South American snake, accidental (unintentional)
  Toxic effect of venom of other North and South American snake NOS
- T63.062 Toxic effect of venom of other North and South American snake, intentional self-harm
- T63.063 Toxic effect of venom of other North and South American snake, assault
- T63.064 Toxic effect of venom of other North and South American snake, undetermined

T63.07 Toxic effect of venom of other Australian snake
- T63.071 Toxic effect of venom of other Australian snake, accidental (unintentional)
  Toxic effect of venom of other Australian snake NOS
- T63.072 Toxic effect of venom of other Australian snake, intentional self-harm
- T63.073 Toxic effect of venom of other Australian snake, assault
- T63.074 Toxic effect of venom of other Australian snake, undetermined

T63.08 Toxic effect of venom of other African and Asian snake
- T63.081 Toxic effect of venom of other African and Asian snake, accidental (unintentional)
  Toxic effect of venom of other African and Asian snake NOS
- T63.082 Toxic effect of venom of other African and Asian snake, intentional self-harm
- T63.083 Toxic effect of venom of other African and Asian snake, assault

- T63.084 Toxic effect of venom of other African and Asian snake, undetermined
- T63.09 Toxic effect of venom of other snake
  - T63.091 Toxic effect of venom of other snake, accidental (unintentional)
    Toxic effect of venom of other snake NOS
  - T63.092 Toxic effect of venom of other snake, intentional self-harm
  - T63.093 Toxic effect of venom of other snake, assault
  - T63.094 Toxic effect of venom of other snake, undetermined
- T63.1 Toxic effect of venom of other reptiles
  - T63.11 Toxic effect of venom of gila monster
    - T63.111 Toxic effect of venom of gila monster, accidental (unintentional)
      Toxic effect of venom of gila monster NOS
    - T63.112 Toxic effect of venom of gila monster, intentional self-harm
    - T63.113 Toxic effect of venom of gila monster, assault
    - T63.114 Toxic effect of venom of gila monster, undetermined
  - T63.12 Toxic effect of venom of other venomous lizard
    - T63.121 Toxic effect of venom of other venomous lizard, accidental (unintentional)
      Toxic effect of venom of other venomous lizard NOS
    - T63.122 Toxic effect of venom of other venomous lizard, intentional self-harm
    - T63.123 Toxic effect of venom of other venomous lizard, assault
    - T63.124 Toxic effect of venom of other venomous lizard, undetermined
  - T63.19 Toxic effect of venom of other reptiles
    - T63.191 Toxic effect of venom of other reptiles, accidental (unintentional)
      Toxic effect of venom of other reptiles NOS
    - T63.192 Toxic effect of venom of other reptiles, intentional self-harm
    - T63.193 Toxic effect of venom of other reptiles, assault
    - T63.194 Toxic effect of venom of other reptiles, undetermined
- T63.2 Toxic effect of venom of scorpion
  - T63.2X Toxic effect of venom of scorpion
    - T63.2X1 Toxic effect of venom of scorpion, accidental (unintentional)
      Toxic effect of venom of scorpion NOS
    - T63.2X2 Toxic effect of venom of scorpion, intentional self-harm
    - T63.2X3 Toxic effect of venom of scorpion, assault
    - T63.2X4 Toxic effect of venom of scorpion, undetermined
- T63.3 Toxic effect of venom of spider
  - T63.30 Toxic effect of unspecified spider venom
    - T63.301 Toxic effect of unspecified spider venom, accidental (unintentional)
    - T63.302 Toxic effect of unspecified spider venom, intentional self-harm
    - T63.303 Toxic effect of unspecified spider venom, assault
    - T63.304 Toxic effect of unspecified spider venom, undetermined
  - T63.31 Toxic effect of venom of black widow spider
    - T63.311 Toxic effect of venom of black widow spider, accidental (unintentional)
    - T63.312 Toxic effect of venom of black widow spider, intentional self-harm
    - T63.313 Toxic effect of venom of black widow spider, assault
    - T63.314 Toxic effect of venom of black widow spider, undetermined
  - T63.32 Toxic effect of venom of tarantula
    - T63.321 Toxic effect of venom of tarantula, accidental (unintentional)
    - T63.322 Toxic effect of venom of tarantula, intentional self-harm
    - T63.323 Toxic effect of venom of tarantula, assault
    - T63.324 Toxic effect of venom of tarantula, undetermined
  - T63.33 Toxic effect of venom of brown recluse spider
    - T63.331 Toxic effect of venom of brown recluse spider, accidental (unintentional)
    - T63.332 Toxic effect of venom of brown recluse spider, intentional self-harm
    - T63.333 Toxic effect of venom of brown recluse spider, assault
    - T63.334 Toxic effect of venom of brown recluse spider, undetermined
  - T63.39 Toxic effect of venom of other spider
    - T63.391 Toxic effect of venom of other spider, accidental (unintentional)
    - T63.392 Toxic effect of venom of other spider, intentional self-harm
    - T63.393 Toxic effect of venom of other spider, assault
    - T63.394 Toxic effect of venom of other spider, undetermined
- T63.4 Toxic effect of venom of other arthropods
  - T63.41 Toxic effect of venom of centipedes and venomous millipedes
    - T63.411 Toxic effect of venom of centipedes and venomous millipedes, accidental (unintentional)
    - T63.412 Toxic effect of venom of centipedes and venomous millipedes, intentional self-harm
    - T63.413 Toxic effect of venom of centipedes and venomous millipedes, assault
    - T63.414 Toxic effect of venom of centipedes and venomous millipedes, undetermined
  - T63.42 Toxic effect of venom of ants
    - T63.421 Toxic effect of venom of ants, accidental (unintentional)
    - T63.422 Toxic effect of venom of ants, intentional self-harm
    - T63.423 Toxic effect of venom of ants, assault
    - T63.424 Toxic effect of venom of ants, undetermined
  - T63.43 Toxic effect of venom of caterpillars
    - T63.431 Toxic effect of venom of caterpillars, accidental (unintentional)
    - T63.432 Toxic effect of venom of caterpillars, intentional self-harm
    - T63.433 Toxic effect of venom of caterpillars, assault
    - T63.434 Toxic effect of venom of caterpillars, undetermined
  - T63.44 Toxic effect of venom of bees
    - T63.441 Toxic effect of venom of bees, accidental (unintentional)
    - T63.442 Toxic effect of venom of bees, intentional self-harm
    - T63.443 Toxic effect of venom of bees, assault
    - T63.444 Toxic effect of venom of bees, undetermined
  - T63.45 Toxic effect of venom of hornets
    - T63.451 Toxic effect of venom of hornets, accidental (unintentional)
    - T63.452 Toxic effect of venom of hornets, intentional self-harm
    - T63.453 Toxic effect of venom of hornets, assault
    - T63.454 Toxic effect of venom of hornets, undetermined
  - T63.46 Toxic effect of venom of wasps
    Toxic effect of yellow jacket
    - T63.461 Toxic effect of venom of wasps, accidental (unintentional)
    - T63.462 Toxic effect of venom of wasps, intentional self-harm
    - T63.463 Toxic effect of venom of wasps, assault

Unacceptable principal diagnosis symbol per Medicare code edits | Code exempt from diagnosis present on admission requirement
Questionable admission | Complication or comorbidity | CC/MCC exclusion | Major complication or comorbidity
Principal diagnosis as its own CC | Principal diagnosis as its own MCC | Z code as first-listed diagnosis

T63.464 Toxic effect of venom of wasps, undetermined
T63.48 Toxic effect of venom of other arthropod
T63.481 Toxic effect of venom of other arthropod, accidental (unintentional)
T63.482 Toxic effect of venom of other arthropod, intentional self-harm
T63.483 Toxic effect of venom of other arthropod, assault
T63.484 Toxic effect of venom of other arthropod, undetermined
T63.5 Toxic effect of contact with venomous fish
EXCLUDES2 *poisoning by ingestion of fish (T61.-)*
T63.51 Toxic effect of contact with stingray
T63.511 Toxic effect of contact with stingray, accidental (unintentional)
T63.512 Toxic effect of contact with stingray, intentional self-harm
T63.513 Toxic effect of contact with stingray, assault
T63.514 Toxic effect of contact with stingray, undetermined
T63.59 Toxic effect of contact with other venomous fish
T63.591 Toxic effect of contact with other venomous fish, accidental (unintentional)
T63.592 Toxic effect of contact with other venomous fish, intentional self-harm
T63.593 Toxic effect of contact with other venomous fish, assault
T63.594 Toxic effect of contact with other venomous fish, undetermined
T63.6 Toxic effect of contact with other venomous marine animals
EXCLUDES1 *sea-snake venom (T63.09)*
EXCLUDES2 *poisoning by ingestion of shellfish (T61.78-)*
T63.61 Toxic effect of contact with Portuguese man-of-war
Toxic effect of contact with bluebottle
T63.611 Toxic effect of contact with Portuguese man-of-war, accidental (unintentional)
T63.612 Toxic effect of contact with Portuguese man-of-war, intentional self-harm
T63.613 Toxic effect of contact with Portuguese man-of-war, assault
T63.614 Toxic effect of contact with Portuguese man-of-war, undetermined
T63.62 Toxic effect of contact with other jellyfish
T63.621 Toxic effect of contact with other jellyfish, accidental (unintentional)
T63.622 Toxic effect of contact with other jellyfish, intentional self-harm
T63.623 Toxic effect of contact with other jellyfish, assault
T63.624 Toxic effect of contact with other jellyfish, undetermined
T63.63 Toxic effect of contact with sea anemone
T63.631 Toxic effect of contact with sea anemone, accidental (unintentional)
T63.632 Toxic effect of contact with sea anemone, intentional self-harm
T63.633 Toxic effect of contact with sea anemone, assault
T63.634 Toxic effect of contact with sea anemone, undetermined
T63.69 Toxic effect of contact with other venomous marine animals
T63.691 Toxic effect of contact with other venomous marine animals, accidental (unintentional)
T63.692 Toxic effect of contact with other venomous marine animals, intentional self-harm
T63.693 Toxic effect of contact with other venomous marine animals, assault
T63.694 Toxic effect of contact with other venomous marine animals, undetermined
T63.7 Toxic effect of contact with venomous plant
T63.71 Toxic effect of contact with venomous marine plant
T63.711 Toxic effect of contact with venomous marine plant, accidental (unintentional)
T63.712 Toxic effect of contact with venomous marine plant, intentional self-harm
T63.713 Toxic effect of contact with venomous marine plant, assault
T63.714 Toxic effect of contact with venomous marine plant, undetermined
T63.79 Toxic effect of contact with other venomous plant
T63.791 Toxic effect of contact with other venomous plant, accidental (unintentional)
T63.792 Toxic effect of contact with other venomous plant, intentional self-harm
T63.793 Toxic effect of contact with other venomous plant, assault
T63.794 Toxic effect of contact with other venomous plant, undetermined
T63.8 Toxic effect of contact with other venomous animals
T63.81 Toxic effect of contact with venomous frog
EXCLUDES1 *contact with nonvenomous frog (W62.0)*
T63.811 Toxic effect of contact with venomous frog, accidental (unintentional)
T63.812 Toxic effect of contact with venomous frog, intentional self-harm
T63.813 Toxic effect of contact with venomous frog, assault
T63.814 Toxic effect of contact with venomous frog, undetermined
T63.82 Toxic effect of contact with venomous toad
EXCLUDES1 *contact with nonvenomous toad (W62.1)*
T63.821 Toxic effect of contact with venomous toad, accidental (unintentional)
T63.822 Toxic effect of contact with venomous toad, intentional self-harm
T63.823 Toxic effect of contact with venomous toad, assault
T63.824 Toxic effect of contact with venomous toad, undetermined
T63.83 Toxic effect of contact with other venomous amphibian
EXCLUDES1 *contact with nonvenomous amphibian (W62.9)*
T63.831 Toxic effect of contact with other venomous amphibian, accidental (unintentional)
T63.832 Toxic effect of contact with other venomous amphibian, intentional self-harm
T63.833 Toxic effect of contact with other venomous amphibian, assault
T63.834 Toxic effect of contact with other venomous amphibian, undetermined
T63.89 Toxic effect of contact with other venomous animals
T63.891 Toxic effect of contact with other venomous animals, accidental (unintentional)
T63.892 Toxic effect of contact with other venomous animals, intentional self-harm
T63.893 Toxic effect of contact with other venomous animals, assault
T63.894 Toxic effect of contact with other venomous animals, undetermined
T63.9 Toxic effect of contact with unspecified venomous animal
T63.91 Toxic effect of contact with unspecified venomous animal, accidental (unintentional)
T63.92 Toxic effect of contact with unspecified venomous animal, intentional self-harm
T63.93 Toxic effect of contact with unspecified venomous animal, assault
T63.94 Toxic effect of contact with unspecified venomous animal, undetermined
T64 Toxic effect of aflatoxin and other mycotoxin food contaminants
The appropriate 7th character is to be added to each code from category T64

Unspecified Code Other Specified Code Manifestation Code N Newborn P Pediatric M Maternity A Adult ♂ Male ♀ Female
● New Code ▲ Revised Code Title ►◄ Revised Text NOTES INCLUDES EXCLUDES1 Not coded here EXCLUDES2 Not included here
4th character required 5th character required 6th character required 7th character required
Extension 'X' Alert HAC Hospital-acquired condition (HAC) alert AHA AHA Coding Clinic©

A = initial encounter
D = subsequent encounter
S = sequela

T64.0 Toxic effect of aflatoxin
- T64.01 Toxic effect of aflatoxin, accidental (unintentional)
- T64.02 Toxic effect of aflatoxin, intentional self-harm
- T64.03 Toxic effect of aflatoxin, assault
- T64.04 Toxic effect of aflatoxin, undetermined

T64.8 Toxic effect of other mycotoxin food contaminants
- T64.81 Toxic effect of other mycotoxin food contaminants, accidental (unintentional)
- T64.82 Toxic effect of other mycotoxin food contaminants, intentional self-harm
- T64.83 Toxic effect of other mycotoxin food contaminants, assault
- T64.84 Toxic effect of other mycotoxin food contaminants, undetermined

T65 Toxic effect of other and unspecified substances

The appropriate 7th character is to be added to each code from category T65
A = initial encounter
D = subsequent encounter
S = sequela

T65.0 Toxic effect of cyanides

EXCLUDES1 *hydrogen cyanide (T57.3-)*

T65.0X Toxic effect of cyanides
- T65.0X1 Toxic effect of cyanides, accidental (unintentional)
  Toxic effect of cyanides NOS
- T65.0X2 Toxic effect of cyanides, intentional self-harm
- T65.0X3 Toxic effect of cyanides, assault
- T65.0X4 Toxic effect of cyanides, undetermined

T65.1 Toxic effect of strychnine and its salts

T65.1X Toxic effect of strychnine and its salts
- T65.1X1 Toxic effect of strychnine and its salts, accidental (unintentional)
  Toxic effect of strychnine and its salts NOS
- T65.1X2 Toxic effect of strychnine and its salts, intentional self-harm
- T65.1X3 Toxic effect of strychnine and its salts, assault
- T65.1X4 Toxic effect of strychnine and its salts, undetermined

T65.2 Toxic effect of tobacco and nicotine

EXCLUDES2 *nicotine dependence (F17.-)*

T65.21 Toxic effect of chewing tobacco
- T65.211 Toxic effect of chewing tobacco, accidental (unintentional)
  Toxic effect of chewing tobacco NOS
- T65.212 Toxic effect of chewing tobacco, intentional self-harm
- T65.213 Toxic effect of chewing tobacco, assault
- T65.214 Toxic effect of chewing tobacco, undetermined

T65.22 Toxic effect of tobacco cigarettes
Toxic effect of tobacco smoke
Use additional code for exposure to second hand tobacco smoke (Z57.31, Z77.22)
- T65.221 Toxic effect of tobacco cigarettes, accidental (unintentional)
  Toxic effect of tobacco cigarettes NOS
- T65.222 Toxic effect of tobacco cigarettes, intentional self-harm
- T65.223 Toxic effect of tobacco cigarettes, assault
- T65.224 Toxic effect of tobacco cigarettes, undetermined

T65.29 Toxic effect of other tobacco and nicotine
- T65.291 Toxic effect of other tobacco and nicotine, accidental (unintentional)
  Toxic effect of other tobacco and nicotine NOS
- T65.292 Toxic effect of other tobacco and nicotine, intentional self-harm
- T65.293 Toxic effect of other tobacco and nicotine, assault
- T65.294 Toxic effect of other tobacco and nicotine, undetermined

T65.3 Toxic effect of nitroderivatives and aminoderivatives of benzene and its homologues
Toxic effect of anilin [benzenamine]
Toxic effect of nitrobenzene
Toxic effect of trinitrotoluene

T65.3X Toxic effect of nitroderivatives and aminoderivatives of benzene and its homologues
- T65.3X1 Toxic effect of nitroderivatives and aminoderivatives of benzene and its homologues, accidental (unintentional)
  Toxic effect of nitroderivatives and aminoderivatives of benzene and its homologues NOS
- T65.3X2 Toxic effect of nitroderivatives and aminoderivatives of benzene and its homologues, intentional self-harm
- T65.3X3 Toxic effect of nitroderivatives and aminoderivatives of benzene and its homologues, assault
- T65.3X4 Toxic effect of nitroderivatives and aminoderivatives of benzene and its homologues, undetermined

T65.4 Toxic effect of carbon disulfide

T65.4X Toxic effect of carbon disulfide
- T65.4X1 Toxic effect of carbon disulfide, accidental (unintentional)
  Toxic effect of carbon disulfide NOS
- T65.4X2 Toxic effect of carbon disulfide, intentional self-harm
- T65.4X3 Toxic effect of carbon disulfide, assault
- T65.4X4 Toxic effect of carbon disulfide, undetermined

T65.5 Toxic effect of nitroglycerin and other nitric acids and esters
Toxic effect of 1,2,3-Propanetriol trinitrate

T65.5X Toxic effect of nitroglycerin and other nitric acids and esters
- T65.5X1 Toxic effect of nitroglycerin and other nitric acids and esters, accidental (unintentional)
  Toxic effect of nitroglycerin and other nitric acids and esters NOS
- T65.5X2 Toxic effect of nitroglycerin and other nitric acids and esters, intentional self-harm
- T65.5X3 Toxic effect of nitroglycerin and other nitric acids and esters, assault
- T65.5X4 Toxic effect of nitroglycerin and other nitric acids and esters, undetermined

T65.6 Toxic effect of paints and dyes, not elsewhere classified

T65.6X Toxic effect of paints and dyes, not elsewhere classified
- T65.6X1 Toxic effect of paints and dyes, not elsewhere classified, accidental (unintentional)
  Toxic effect of paints and dyes NOS
- T65.6X2 Toxic effect of paints and dyes, not elsewhere classified, intentional self-harm
- T65.6X3 Toxic effect of paints and dyes, not elsewhere classified, assault
- T65.6X4 Toxic effect of paints and dyes, not elsewhere classified, undetermined

T65.8 Toxic effect of other specified substances

T65.81 Toxic effect of latex
- T65.811 Toxic effect of latex, accidental (unintentional)
  Toxic effect of latex NOS
- T65.812 Toxic effect of latex, intentional self-harm
- T65.813 Toxic effect of latex, assault
- T65.814 Toxic effect of latex, undetermined

T65.82 Toxic effect of harmful algae and algae toxins
Toxic effect of (harmful) algae bloom NOS
Toxic effect of blue-green algae bloom
Toxic effect of brown tide

Unacceptable principal diagnosis symbol per Medicare code edits · Code exempt from diagnosis present on admission requirement · Questionable admission · Complication or comorbidity · CC/MCC exclusion · Major complication or comorbidity · Principal diagnosis as its own CC · Principal diagnosis as its own MCC · Z code as first-listed diagnosis

Toxic effect of cyanobacteria bloom
Toxic effect of Florida red tide
Toxic effect of pfiesteria piscicida
Toxic effect of red tide

T65.821 **Toxic effect of harmful algae and algae toxins, accidental (unintentional)**
Toxic effect of harmful algae and algae toxins NOS

T65.822 **Toxic effect of harmful algae and algae toxins, intentional self-harm**

T65.823 **Toxic effect of harmful algae and algae toxins, assault**

T65.824 **Toxic effect of harmful algae and algae toxins, undetermined**

T65.83 Toxic effect of fiberglass

T65.831 **Toxic effect of fiberglass, accidental (unintentional)**
Toxic effect of fiberglass NOS

T65.832 **Toxic effect of fiberglass, intentional self-harm**

T65.833 **Toxic effect of fiberglass, assault**

T65.834 **Toxic effect of fiberglass, undetermined**

T65.89 Toxic effect of other specified substances

T65.891 **Toxic effect of other specified substances, accidental (unintentional)**
Toxic effect of other specified substances NOS

T65.892 **Toxic effect of other specified substances, intentional self-harm**

T65.893 **Toxic effect of other specified substances, assault**

T65.894 **Toxic effect of other specified substances, undetermined**

T65.9 Toxic effect of unspecified substance

T65.91 **Toxic effect of unspecified substance, accidental (unintentional)**
Poisoning NOS

T65.92 **Toxic effect of unspecified substance, intentional self-harm**

T65.93 **Toxic effect of unspecified substance, assault**

T65.94 **Toxic effect of unspecified substance, undetermined**

Other and unspecified effects of external causes (T66-T78)

T66 **Radiation sickness, unspecified**

EXCLUDES1 *specified adverse effects of radiation, such as:*
burns (T20-T31)
leukemia (C91-C95)
radiation gastroenteritis and colitis (K52.0)
radiation pneumonitis (J70.0)
radiation related disorders of the skin and subcutaneous tissue (L55-L59)
sunburn (L55.-)

The appropriate 7th character is to be added to code T66
A = initial encounter
D = subsequent encounter
S = sequela

T67 **Effects of heat and light**

EXCLUDES1 *erythema [dermatitis] ab igne (L59.0)*
malignant hyperpyrexia due to anesthesia (T88.3)
radiation-related disorders of the skin and subcutaneous tissue (L55-L59)

EXCLUDES2 *burns (T20-T31)*
sunburn (L55.-)
sweat disorder due to heat (L74-L75)

The appropriate 7th character is to be added to each code from category T67
A = initial encounter
D = subsequent encounter
S = sequela

T67.0 **Heatstroke and sunstroke** HAC
Heat apoplexy
Heat pyrexia
Siriasis
Thermoplegia
Use additional code(s) to identify any associated complications of heatstroke, such as:
coma and stupor (R40.-)
systemic inflammatory response syndrome (R65.1-)

T67.1 **Heat syncope**
Heat collapse

T67.2 **Heat cramp**

T67.3 **Heat exhaustion, anhydrotic**
Heat prostration due to water depletion
EXCLUDES1 *heat exhaustion due to salt depletion (T67.4)*

T67.4 **Heat exhaustion due to salt depletion**
Heat prostration due to salt (and water) depletion

T67.5 **Heat exhaustion, unspecified**
Heat prostration NOS

T67.6 **Heat fatigue, transient**

T67.7 **Heat edema**

T67.8 **Other effects of heat and light**

T67.9 **Effect of heat and light, unspecified**

T68 **Hypothermia**
Accidental hypothermia
Hypothermia NOS
Use additional code to identify source of exposure:
Exposure to excessive cold of man-made origin (W93)
Exposure to excessive cold of natural origin (X31)

EXCLUDES1 *hypothermia following anesthesia (T88.51)*
hypothermia not associated with low environmental temperature (R68.0)
hypothermia of newborn (P80.-)

EXCLUDES2 *frostbite (T33-T34)*

The appropriate 7th character is to be added to code T68
A = initial encounter
D = subsequent encounter
S = sequela

T69 **Other effects of reduced temperature**
Use additional code to identify source of exposure:
Exposure to excessive cold of man-made origin (W93)
Exposure to excessive cold of natural origin (X31)

EXCLUDES2 *frostbite (T33-T34)*

The appropriate 7th character is to be added to each code from category T69
A = initial encounter
D = subsequent encounter
S = sequela

T69.0 **Immersion hand and foot**

T69.01 **Immersion hand**

T69.011 **Immersion hand, right hand**

T69.012 **Immersion hand, left hand**

T69.019 **Immersion hand, unspecified hand**

T69.02 **Immersion foot**
Trench foot

T69.021 **Immersion foot, right foot** HAC

T69.022 **Immersion foot, left foot** HAC

T69.029 **Immersion foot, unspecified foot** HAC

T69.1 **Chilblains**

T69.8 **Other specified effects of reduced temperature**

T69.9 **Effect of reduced temperature, unspecified**

T70 **Effects of air pressure and water pressure**

The appropriate 7th character is to be added to each code from category T70
A = initial encounter
D = subsequent encounter
S = sequela

T70.0 **Otitic barotrauma**
Aero-otitis media
Effects of change in ambient atmospheric pressure or water pressure on ears

T70.1 **Sinus barotrauma**
Aerosinusitis
Effects of change in ambient atmospheric pressure on sinuses

T70.2 **Other and unspecified effects of high altitude**
EXCLUDES2 *polycythemia due to high altitude (D75.1)*

T70.20 **Unspecified effects of high altitude**

T70.29 **Other effects of high altitude**
Alpine sickness
Anoxia due to high altitude
Barotrauma NOS
Hypobaropathy
Mountain sickness

T70.3 **Caisson disease [decompression sickness]** CC HAC
Compressed-air disease
Diver's palsy or paralysis

T70.4 **Effects of high-pressure fluids**
Hydraulic jet injection (industrial)
Pneumatic jet injection (industrial)
Traumatic jet injection (industrial)

T70.8 **Other effects of air pressure and water pressure**

T70.9 **Effect of air pressure and water pressure, unspecified**

T71 **Asphyxiation**
Mechanical suffocation
Traumatic suffocation

EXCLUDES1 *acute respiratory distress (syndrome) (J80)*
anoxia due to high altitude (T70.2)
asphyxia NOS (R09.01)
asphyxia from carbon monoxide (T58.-)
asphyxia from inhalation of food or foreign body (T17.-)
asphyxia from other gases, fumes and vapors (T59.-)
respiratory distress (syndrome) in newborn (P22.-)

The appropriate 7th character is to be added to each code from category T71
A = initial encounter
D = subsequent encounter
S = sequela

T71.1 **Asphyxiation due to** mechanical threat to breathing
Suffocation due to mechanical threat to breathing

T71.11 **Asphyxiation due to** smothering under pillow

T71.111 **Asphyxiation due to smothering under pillow,** accidental CC HAC
Asphyxiation due to smothering under pillow NOS

T71.112 **Asphyxiation due to smothering under pillow,** intentional self-harm CC HAC

T71.113 **Asphyxiation due to smothering under pillow,** assault CC HAC

T71.114 **Asphyxiation due to smothering under pillow,** undetermined CC HAC

T71.12 **Asphyxiation due to** plastic bag

T71.121 **Asphyxiation due to plastic bag,** accidental CC HAC
Asphyxiation due to plastic bag NOS

T71.122 **Asphyxiation due to plastic bag,** intentional self-harm CC HAC

T71.123 **Asphyxiation due to plastic bag,** assault CC HAC

T71.124 **Asphyxiation due to plastic bag,** undetermined CC HAC

T71.13 **Asphyxiation due to being** trapped in bed linens

T71.131 **Asphyxiation due to being trapped in bed linens,** accidental CC HAC
Asphyxiation due to being trapped in bed linens NOS

T71.132 **Asphyxiation due to being trapped in bed linens,** intentional self-harm CC HAC

T71.133 **Asphyxiation due to being trapped in bed linens,** assault CC HAC

T71.134 **Asphyxiation due to being trapped in bed linens,** undetermined CC HAC

T71.14 **Asphyxiation due to smothering under another person's body (in bed)**

T71.141 **Asphyxiation due to smothering under another person's body (in bed),** accidental CC
Asphyxiation due to smothering under another person's body (in bed) NOS

T71.143 **Asphyxiation due to smothering under another person's body (in bed),** assault CC

T71.144 **Asphyxiation due to smothering under another person's body (in bed),** undetermined CC

T71.15 **Asphyxiation due to** smothering in furniture

T71.151 **Asphyxiation due to smothering in furniture,** accidental CC HAC
Asphyxiation due to smothering in furniture NOS

T71.152 **Asphyxiation due to smothering in furniture,** intentional self-harm CC HAC

T71.153 **Asphyxiation due to smothering in furniture,** assault CC HAC

T71.154 **Asphyxiation due to smothering in furniture,** undetermined CC HAC

T71.16 **Asphyxiation due to** hanging
Hanging by window shade cord
Use additional code for any associated injuries, such as:
crushing injury of neck (S17.-)
fracture of cervical vertebrae (S12.0-S12.2-)
open wound of neck (S11.-)

T71.161 **Asphyxiation due to hanging,** accidental CC HAC
Asphyxiation due to hanging NOS
Hanging NOS

T71.162 **Asphyxiation due to hanging,** intentional self-harm CC HAC

T71.163 **Asphyxiation due to hanging,** assault CC HAC

T71.164 **Asphyxiation due to hanging,** undetermined CC HAC

T71.19 **Asphyxiation due to mechanical threat to breathing** due to other causes

T71.191 **Asphyxiation due to mechanical threat to breathing due to other causes,** accidental CC HAC
Asphyxiation due to other causes NOS

T71.192 **Asphyxiation due to mechanical threat to breathing due to other causes,** intentional self-harm CC HAC

T71.193 **Asphyxiation due to mechanical threat to breathing due to other causes,** assault CC HAC

T71.194 **Asphyxiation due to mechanical threat to breathing due to other causes,** undetermined CC HAC

T71.2 **Asphyxiation due to** systemic oxygen deficiency due to low oxygen content in ambient air
Suffocation due to systemic oxygen deficiency due to low oxygen content in ambient air

T71.20 **Asphyxiation due to systemic oxygen deficiency due to low oxygen content in ambient air due to unspecified cause** CC HAC

T71.21 **Asphyxiation due to** cave-in or falling earth CC HAC
Use additional code for any associated cataclysm (X34-X38)

T71.22 **Asphyxiation due to** being trapped in a car trunk

T71.221 **Asphyxiation due to being trapped in a car trunk,** accidental CC

T71.222 **Asphyxiation due to being trapped in a car trunk,** intentional self-harm CC

T71.223 **Asphyxiation due to being trapped in a car trunk,** assault CC

T71.224 **Asphyxiation due to being trapped in a car trunk,** undetermined CC

T71.23 **Asphyxiation due to being** trapped in a **(discarded)** refrigerator

T71.231 **Asphyxiation due to being trapped in a (discarded) refrigerator,** accidental CC

T71.232 **Asphyxiation due to being trapped in a (discarded) refrigerator,** intentional self-harm CC

T71.233 **Asphyxiation due to being trapped in a (discarded) refrigerator,** assault CC

T71.234 **Asphyxiation due to being trapped in a (discarded) refrigerator,** undetermined CC

PDx Unacceptable principal diagnosis symbol per Medicare code edits; POA Code exempt from diagnosis present on admission requirement
? Questionable admission; CC Complication or comorbidity; CC/MCC Exc CC/MCC exclusion; MCC Major complication or comorbidity
PDx CC Principal diagnosis as its own CC; PDx MCC Principal diagnosis as its own MCC; Z-1 Z code as first-listed diagnosis

When symbols appear on a code that requires a 7th character extension, refer to Appendix D to identify applicable 7th character codes.

T71.29 Asphyxiation due to being trapped in other low oxygen environment CC HAC

T71.9 Asphyxiation due to unspecified cause CC HAC
Suffocation (by strangulation) due to unspecified cause
Suffocation NOS
Systemic oxygen deficiency due to low oxygen content in ambient air due to unspecified cause
Systemic oxygen deficiency due to mechanical threat to breathing due to unspecified cause
Traumatic asphyxia NOS

T73 Effects of other deprivation
The appropriate 7th character is to be added to each code from category T73
A = initial encounter
D = subsequent encounter
S = sequela

T73.0 Starvation
Deprivation of food
T73.1 Deprivation of water
T73.2 Exhaustion due to exposure
T73.3 Exhaustion due to excessive exertion
Exhaustion due to overexertion
T73.8 Other effects of deprivation
T73.9 Effect of deprivation, unspecified

T74 Adult and child abuse, neglect and other maltreatment, confirmed
Use additional code, if applicable, to identify any associated current injury
Use additional external cause code to identify perpetrator, if known (Y07.-)
EXCLUDES1 *abuse and maltreatment in pregnancy (O9A.3-, O9A.4-, O9A.5-)*
adult and child maltreatment, suspected (T76.-)
The appropriate 7th character is to be added to each code from category T74
A = initial encounter
D = subsequent encounter
S = sequela

T74.0 Neglect or abandonment, confirmed
T74.01 Adult neglect or abandonment, confirmed A CC
T74.02 Child neglect or abandonment, confirmed P CC
T74.1 Physical abuse, confirmed
EXCLUDES2 *sexual abuse (T74.2-)*
T74.11 Adult physical abuse, confirmed A CC
T74.12 Child physical abuse, confirmed P CC
EXCLUDES2 *shaken infant syndrome (T74.4)*
T74.2 Sexual abuse, confirmed
Rape, confirmed
Sexual assault, confirmed
T74.21 Adult sexual abuse, confirmed A CC
T74.22 Child sexual abuse, confirmed P CC
T74.3 Psychological abuse, confirmed
T74.31 Adult psychological abuse, confirmed A
T74.32 Child psychological abuse, confirmed P CC
T74.4 Shaken infant syndrome P CC
T74.9 Unspecified maltreatment, confirmed
T74.91 Unspecified adult maltreatment, confirmed A CC
T74.92 Unspecified child maltreatment, confirmed P CC

T75 Other and unspecified effects of other external causes
EXCLUDES1 *adverse effects NEC (T78.-)*
EXCLUDES2 *burns (electric) (T20-T31)*
The appropriate 7th character is to be added to each code from category T75
A = initial encounter
D = subsequent encounter
S = sequela

T75.0 Effects of lightning
Struck by lightning
T75.00 Unspecified effects of lightning
Struck by lightning NOS
T75.01 Shock due to being struck by lightning
T75.09 Other effects of lightning
Use additional code for other effects of lightning
T75.1 Unspecified effects of drowning and nonfatal submersion CC HAC
Immersion
EXCLUDES1 *specified effects of drowning- code to effects*
T75.2 Effects of vibration
T75.20 Unspecified effects of vibration
T75.21 Pneumatic hammer syndrome
T75.22 Traumatic vasospastic syndrome
T75.23 Vertigo from infrasound
EXCLUDES1 *vertigo NOS (R42)*
T75.29 Other effects of vibration
T75.3 Motion sickness
Airsickness
Seasickness
Travel sickness
Use additional external cause code to identify vehicle or type of motion (Y92.81-, Y93.5-)
T75.4 Electrocution
Shock from electric current
Shock from electroshock gun (taser)
T75.8 Other specified effects of external causes
T75.81 Effects of abnormal gravitation [G] forces
T75.82 Effects of weightlessness
T75.89 Other specified effects of external causes

T76 Adult and child abuse, neglect and other maltreatment, suspected
Use additional code, if applicable, to identify any associated current injury
EXCLUDES1 *adult and child maltreatment, confirmed (T74.-)*
suspected abuse and maltreatment in pregnancy (O9A.3-, O9A.4-, O9A.5-)
suspected adult physical abuse, ruled out (Z04.71)
suspected adult sexual abuse, ruled out (Z04.41)
suspected child physical abuse, ruled out (Z04.72)
suspected child sexual abuse, ruled out (Z04.42)
The appropriate 7th character is to be added to each code from category T76
A = initial encounter
D = subsequent encounter
S = sequela

T76.0 Neglect or abandonment, suspected
T76.01 Adult neglect or abandonment, suspected A CC
T76.02 Child neglect or abandonment, suspected P CC
T76.1 Physical abuse, suspected
T76.11 Adult physical abuse, suspected A CC
T76.12 Child physical abuse, suspected P CC
T76.2 Sexual abuse, suspected
Rape, suspected
Sexual abuse, suspected
EXCLUDES1 *alleged abuse, ruled out (Z04.7)*
T76.21 Adult sexual abuse, suspected A CC
T76.22 Child sexual abuse, suspected P CC
T76.3 Psychological abuse, suspected
T76.31 Adult psychological abuse, suspected A
T76.32 Child psychological abuse, suspected P CC
T76.9 Unspecified maltreatment, suspected
T76.91 Unspecified adult maltreatment, suspected A CC
T76.92 Unspecified child maltreatment, suspected P CC

T78 Adverse effects, not elsewhere classified
EXCLUDES2 *complications of surgical and medical care NEC (T80-T88)*
The appropriate 7th character is to be added to each code from category T78
A = initial encounter
D = subsequent encounter
S = sequela

T78.0 Anaphylactic reaction due to food
Anaphylactic reaction due to adverse food reaction
Anaphylactic shock or reaction due to nonpoisonous foods
Anaphylactoid reaction due to food

Unspecified Code | Other Specified Code | Manifestation Code | N Newborn | P Pediatric | M Maternity | A Adult | ♂ Male | ♀ Female
● New Code | ▲ Revised Code Title | ►◄ Revised Text | NOTES | INCLUDES | EXCLUDES1 Not coded here | EXCLUDES2 Not included here
4th character required | 5th character required | 6th character required | 7th character required
Extension 'X' Alert | HAC Hospital-acquired condition (HAC) alert | AHA AHA Coding Clinic®

T78.00 **Anaphylactic reaction due to unspecified food**
T78.01 **Anaphylactic reaction due to peanuts**
T78.02 **Anaphylactic reaction due to shellfish (crustaceans)**
T78.03 **Anaphylactic reaction due to other fish**
T78.04 **Anaphylactic reaction due to fruits and vegetables**
T78.05 **Anaphylactic reaction due to tree nuts and seeds**
EXCLUDES2 *anaphylactic reaction due to peanuts (T78.01)*
T78.06 **Anaphylactic reaction due to food additives**
T78.07 **Anaphylactic reaction due to milk and dairy products**
T78.08 **Anaphylactic reaction due to eggs**
T78.09 **Anaphylactic reaction due to other food products**

T78.1 **Other adverse food reactions, not elsewhere classified**
Use additional code to identify the type of reaction, ▶if applicable◀
EXCLUDES1 *anaphylactic reaction or shock due to adverse food reaction (T78.0-)*
anaphylactic reaction due to food (T78.0-)
bacterial food borne intoxications (A05.-)
EXCLUDES2 *allergic and dietetic gastroenteritis and colitis ▶(K52.29)◀*
allergic rhinitis due to food (J30.5)
dermatitis due to food in contact with skin (L23.6, L24.6, L25.4)
dermatitis due to ingested food (L27.2)
food protein-induced enterocolitis syndrome (K52.21)
food protein-induced enteropathy (K52.22)

T78.2 **Anaphylactic shock, unspecified**
Allergic shock
Anaphylactic reaction
Anaphylaxis
EXCLUDES1 *anaphylactic reaction or shock due to adverse effect of correct medicinal substance properly administered (T88.6)*
anaphylactic reaction or shock due to adverse food reaction (T78.0-)
anaphylactic reaction or shock due to serum (T80.5-)

T78.3 **Angioneurotic edema**
Allergic angioedema
Giant urticaria
Quincke's edema
EXCLUDES1 *serum urticaria (T80.6-)*
urticaria (L50.-)

T78.4 **Other and unspecified allergy**
EXCLUDES1 *specified types of allergic reaction such as:*
allergic diarrhea ▶(K52.29)◀
allergic gastroenteritis and colitis ▶(K52.29)◀
dermatitis (L23-L25, L27.-)
food protein-induced enterocolitis syndrome (K52.21)
food protein-induced enteropathy (K52.22)
hay fever (J30.1)
T78.40 **Allergy, unspecified**
Allergic reaction NOS
Hypersensitivity NOS
T78.41 **Arthus phenomenon**
Arthus reaction
T78.49 **Other allergy**

T78.8 **Other adverse effects, not elsewhere classified**

Certain early complications of trauma (T79)

T79 **Certain early complications of trauma, not elsewhere classified**
EXCLUDES2 *acute respiratory distress syndrome (J80)*
complications occurring during or following medical procedures (T80-T88)
complications of surgical and medical care NEC (T80-T88)
newborn respiratory distress syndrome (P22.0)
The appropriate 7th character is to be added to each code from category T79
A = initial encounter
D = subsequent encounter
S = sequela

T79.0 **Air embolism (traumatic)**
EXCLUDES1 *air embolism complicating abortion or ectopic or molar pregnancy (O00-O07, O08.2)*
air embolism complicating pregnancy, childbirth and the puerperium (O88.0)
air embolism following infusion, transfusion, and therapeutic injection (T80.0)
air embolism following procedure NEC (T81.7-)

T79.1 **Fat embolism (traumatic)**
EXCLUDES1 *fat embolism complicating:*
abortion or ectopic or molar pregnancy (O00-O07, O08.2)
pregnancy, childbirth and the puerperium (O88.8)

T79.2 **Traumatic secondary and recurrent hemorrhage and seroma**

T79.4 **Traumatic shock**
Shock (immediate) (delayed) following injury
EXCLUDES1 *anaphylactic shock due to adverse food reaction (T78.0-)*
anaphylactic shock due to correct medicinal substance properly administered (T88.6)
anaphylactic shock due to serum (T80.5-)
anaphylactic shock NOS (T78.2)
anesthetic shock (T88.2)
electric shock (T75.4)
nontraumatic shock NEC (R57.-)
obstetric shock (O75.1)
postprocedural shock (T81.1-)
septic shock (R65.21)
shock complicating abortion or ectopic or molar pregnancy (O00-O07, O08.3)
shock due to lightning (T75.01)
shock NOS (R57.9)

T79.5 **Traumatic anuria**
Crush syndrome
Renal failure following crushing

T79.6 **Traumatic ischemia of muscle**
Traumatic rhabdomyolysis
Volkmann's ischemic contracture
EXCLUDES2 *anterior tibial syndrome (M76.8)*
compartment syndrome (traumatic) (T79.A-)
nontraumatic ischemia of muscle (M62.2-)

T79.7 **Traumatic subcutaneous emphysema**
EXCLUDES1 *emphysema NOS (J43)*
emphysema (subcutaneous) resulting from a procedure (T81.82)

T79.A **Traumatic compartment syndrome**
EXCLUDES1 *fibromyalgia (M79.7)*
nontraumatic compartment syndrome (M79.A-)
traumatic ischemic infarction of muscle (T79.6)
T79.A0 **Compartment syndrome, unspecified**
Compartment syndrome NOS
T79.A1 **Traumatic compartment syndrome of upper extremity**
Traumatic compartment syndrome of shoulder, arm, forearm, wrist, hand, and fingers
T79.A11 **Traumatic compartment syndrome of right upper extremity**
T79.A12 **Traumatic compartment syndrome of left upper extremity**
T79.A19 **Traumatic compartment syndrome of unspecified upper extremity**
T79.A2 **Traumatic compartment syndrome of lower extremity**
Traumatic compartment syndrome of hip, buttock, thigh, leg, foot, and toes
T79.A21 **Traumatic compartment syndrome of right lower extremity**

Unacceptable principal diagnosis symbol per Medicare code edits | Code exempt from diagnosis present on admission requirement | Questionable admission | Complication or comorbidity | CC/MCC exclusion | Major complication or comorbidity | Principal diagnosis as its own CC | Principal diagnosis as its own MCC | Z code as first-listed diagnosis

When symbols appear on a code that requires a 7th character extension, refer to Appendix D to identify applicable 7th character codes.

T79.A22 Traumatic compartment syndrome of left lower extremity

T79.A29 Traumatic compartment syndrome of unspecified lower extremity

T79.A3 Traumatic compartment syndrome of abdomen

T79.A9 Traumatic compartment syndrome of other sites

T79.8 Other early complications of trauma

T79.9 Unspecified early complication of trauma

Complications of surgical and medical care, not elsewhere classified (T80-T88)

Use additional code for adverse effect, if applicable, to identify drug (T36-T50 with fifth or sixth character 5)

Use additional code(s) to identify the specified condition resulting from the complication

Use additional code to identify devices involved and details of circumstances (Y62-Y82)

EXCLUDES2 *any encounters with medical care for postprocedural conditions in which no complications are present, such as:*
artificial opening status (Z93.-)
closure of external stoma (Z43.-)
fitting and adjustment of external prosthetic device (Z44.-)
burns and corrosions from local applications and irradiation (T20-T32)
complications of surgical procedures during pregnancy, childbirth and the puerperium (O00-O9A)
mechanical complication of respirator [ventilator] (J95.850)
poisoning and toxic effects of drugs and chemicals (T36-T65 with fifth or sixth character 1-4 or 6)
postprocedural fever (R50.82)
specified complications classified elsewhere, such as:
cerebrospinal fluid leak from spinal puncture (G97.0)
colostomy malfunction (K94.0-)
disorders of fluid and electrolyte imbalance (E86-E87)
functional disturbances following cardiac surgery (I97.0-I97.1)
intraoperative and postprocedural complications of specified body systems (D78.-, E36.-, E89.-, G97.3-, G97.4, H59.3-, H59.-, H95.2-, H95.3, I97.4-, I97.5, J95.6-, J95.7, K91.6-, L76.-, M96.-, N99.-)
ostomy complications (J95.0-, K94.-, N99.5-)
postgastric surgery syndromes (K91.1)
postlaminectomy syndrome NEC (M96.1)
postmastectomy lymphedema syndrome (I97.2)
postsurgical blind-loop syndrome (K91.2)
ventilator associated pneumonia (J95.851)

T80 Complications following infusion, transfusion and therapeutic injection

INCLUDES *complications following perfusion*

EXCLUDES2 *bone marrow transplant rejection (T86.01)*
febrile nonhemolytic transfusion reaction (R50.84)
fluid overload due to transfusion (E87.71)
posttransfusion purpura (D69.51)
transfusion associated circulatory overload (TACO) (E87.71)
transfusion (red blood cell) associated hemochromatosis (E83.111)
transfusion related acute lung injury (TRALI) (J95.84)

The appropriate 7th character is to be added to each code from category T80
A = initial encounter
D = subsequent encounter
S = sequela

T80.0 Air embolism following infusion, transfusion and therapeutic injection HAC MCC

T80.1 Vascular complications following infusion, transfusion and therapeutic injection

Use additional code to identify the vascular complication

EXCLUDES2 *extravasation of vesicant agent (T80.81-)*
infiltration of vesicant agent (T80.81-)
vascular complications specified as due to prosthetic devices, implants and grafts (T82.8-, ▶T83.8-, T84.8-, T85.8-◀)
postprocedural vascular complications (T81.7-)

T80.2 Infections following infusion, transfusion and therapeutic injection

Use additional code to identify the specific infection, such as: sepsis (A41.9)

Use additional code (R65.2-) to identify severe sepsis, if applicable

EXCLUDES2 *infections specified as due to prosthetic devices, implants and grafts (T82.6-T82.7, T83.5-T83.6, T84.5-T84.7, T85.7)*
postprocedural infections ▶(T81.4-)◀

T80.21 Infection due to central venous catheter

Infection due to pulmonary artery catheter (Swan-Ganz catheter)

T80.211 Bloodstream infection due to central venous catheter HAC
Catheter-related bloodstream infection (CRBSI) NOS
Central line-associated bloodstream infection (CLABSI)
Bloodstream infection due to Hickman catheter
Bloodstream infection due to peripherally inserted central catheter (PICC)
Bloodstream infection due to portacath (Port-a-Cath®)
Bloodstream infection due to pulmonary artery catheter
Bloodstream infection due to triple lumen catheter
Bloodstream infection due to umbilical venous catheter

T80.212 Local infection due to central venous catheter HAC
Exit or insertion site infection
Local infection due to Hickman catheter
Local infection due to peripherally inserted central catheter (PICC)
Local infection due to portacath (Port-a-Cath®)
Local infection due to pulmonary artery catheter
Local infection due to triple lumen catheter
Local infection due to umbilical venous catheter
Port or reservoir infection
Tunnel infection

T80.218 Other infection due to central venous catheter HAC
Other central line-associated infection
Other infection due to Hickman catheter
Other infection due to peripherally inserted central catheter (PICC)
Other infection due to portacath (Port-a-Cath®)
Other infection due to pulmonary artery catheter
Other infection due to triple lumen catheter
Other infection due to umbilical venous catheter

T80.219 Unspecified infection due to central venous catheter HAC
Central line-associated infection NOS
Unspecified infection due to Hickman catheter
Unspecified infection due to peripherally inserted central catheter (PICC)
Unspecified infection due to portacath (Port-a-Cath®)
Unspecified infection due to pulmonary artery catheter
Unspecified infection due to triple lumen catheter
Unspecified infection due to umbilical venous catheter

Unspecified Code Other Specified Code Manifestation Code N Newborn P Pediatric M Maternity A Adult ♂ Male ♀ Female
● New Code ▲ Revised Code Title ►◄ Revised Text NOTES INCLUDES EXCLUDES1 Not coded here EXCLUDES2 Not included here
4th character required 5th character required 6th character required 7th character required
Extension 'X' Alert HAC Hospital-acquired condition (HAC) alert AHA AHA Coding Clinic®

T80.22 **Acute infection following transfusion, infusion, or injection of blood and blood products**

T80.29 **Infection following other infusion, transfusion and therapeutic injection**

T80.3 ABO incompatibility **reaction due to transfusion of blood or blood products**

EXCLUDES1 *minor blood group antigens reactions (Duffy) (E) (K(ell)) (Kidd) (Lewis) (M) (N) (P) (S) (T80.A)*

T80.30 **ABO incompatibility reaction due to transfusion of blood or blood products, unspecified** HAC

ABO incompatibility blood transfusion NOS
Reaction to ABO incompatibility from transfusion NOS

T80.31 **ABO incompatibility** with hemolytic transfusion reaction

T80.310 **ABO incompatibility with** acute **hemolytic transfusion reaction** HAC

ABO incompatibility with hemolytic transfusion reaction less than 24 hours after transfusion
Acute hemolytic transfusion reaction (AHTR) due to ABO incompatibility

T80.311 **ABO incompatibility with** delayed **hemolytic transfusion reaction** HAC

ABO incompatibility with hemolytic transfusion reaction 24 hours or more after transfusion
Delayed hemolytic transfusion reaction (DHTR) due to ABO incompatibility

T80.319 **ABO incompatibility with hemolytic transfusion reaction, unspecified** HAC

ABO incompatibility with hemolytic transfusion reaction at unspecified time after transfusion
Hemolytic transfusion reaction (HTR) due to ABO incompatibility NOS

T80.39 **Other ABO incompatibility reaction due to transfusion of blood or blood products** HAC

Delayed serologic transfusion reaction (DSTR) from ABO incompatibility
Other ABO incompatible blood transfusion
Other reaction to ABO incompatible blood transfusion

T80.4 Rh incompatibility **reaction due to transfusion of blood or blood products**

Reaction due to incompatibility of Rh antigens (C) (c) (D) (E) (e)

T80.40 **Rh incompatibility reaction due to transfusion of blood or blood products, unspecified**

Reaction due to Rh factor in transfusion NOS
Rh incompatible blood transfusion NOS

T80.41 **Rh incompatibility** with hemolytic transfusion reaction

T80.410 **Rh incompatibility with** acute **hemolytic transfusion reaction**

Acute hemolytic transfusion reaction (AHTR) due to Rh incompatibility
Rh incompatibility with hemolytic transfusion reaction less than 24 hours after transfusion

T80.411 **Rh incompatibility with** delayed **hemolytic transfusion reaction**

Delayed hemolytic transfusion reaction (DHTR) due to Rh incompatibility
Rh incompatibility with hemolytic transfusion reaction 24 hours or more after transfusion

T80.419 **Rh incompatibility with hemolytic transfusion reaction, unspecified**

Rh incompatibility with hemolytic transfusion reaction at unspecified time after transfusion
Hemolytic transfusion reaction (HTR) due to Rh incompatibility NOS

T80.49 **Other Rh incompatibility reaction due to transfusion of blood or blood products**

Delayed serologic transfusion reaction (DSTR) from Rh incompatibility
Other reaction to Rh incompatible blood transfusion

T80.A Non-ABO incompatibility **reaction due to transfusion of blood or blood products**

Reaction due to incompatibility of minor antigens (Duffy) (Kell) (Kidd) (Lewis) (M) (N) (P) (S)

T80.A0 **Non-ABO incompatibility reaction due to transfusion of blood or blood products, unspecified**

Non-ABO antigen incompatibility reaction from transfusion NOS

T80.A1 **Non-ABO incompatibility** with hemolytic transfusion reaction

T80.A10 **Non-ABO incompatibility with** acute **hemolytic transfusion reaction**

Acute hemolytic transfusion reaction (AHTR) due to non-ABO incompatibility
Non-ABO incompatibility with hemolytic transfusion reaction less than 24 hours after transfusion

T80.A11 **Non-ABO incompatibility with** delayed **hemolytic transfusion reaction**

Delayed hemolytic transfusion reaction (DHTR) due to non-ABO incompatibility
Non-ABO incompatibility with hemolytic transfusion reaction 24 or more hours after transfusion

T80.A19 **Non-ABO incompatibility with hemolytic transfusion reaction, unspecified**

Hemolytic transfusion reaction (HTR) due to non-ABO incompatibility NOS
Non-ABO incompatibility with hemolytic transfusion reaction at unspecified time after transfusion

T80.A9 **Other non-ABO incompatibility reaction due to transfusion of blood or blood products**

Delayed serologic transfusion reaction (DSTR) from non-ABO incompatibility
Other reaction to non-ABO incompatible blood transfusion

T80.5 **Anaphylactic reaction due to serum**

Allergic shock due to serum
Anaphylactic shock due to serum
Anaphylactoid reaction due to serum
Anaphylaxis due to serum

EXCLUDES1 *ABO incompatibility reaction due to transfusion of blood or blood products (T80.3-)*
allergic reaction or shock NOS (T78.2)
anaphylactic reaction or shock NOS (T78.2)
anaphylactic reaction or shock due to adverse effect of correct medicinal substance properly administered (T88.6)
other serum reaction (T80.6-)

T80.51 **Anaphylactic reaction due to** administration of blood and blood products

T80.52 **Anaphylactic reaction due to** vaccination

T80.59 **Anaphylactic reaction due to other serum**

T80.6 **Other serum reactions**

Intoxication by serum
Protein sickness
Serum rash
Serum sickness
Serum urticaria

EXCLUDES2 *serum hepatitis ►(B16-B19)◄*

T80.61 **Other serum reaction** due to administration of blood and blood products

T80.62 **Other serum reaction** due to vaccination

T80.69 **Other** serum **reaction due to other** serum

T80.8 **Other complications following infusion, transfusion and therapeutic injection**

T80.81 **Extravasation of vesicant agent**

Infiltration of vesicant agent

T80.810 **Extravasation of vesicant antineoplastic chemotherapy**

Infiltration of vesicant antineoplastic chemotherapy

T80.818 **Extravasation of other vesicant agent**

Infiltration of other vesicant agent

T80.89 **Other complications following infusion, transfusion and therapeutic injection**

Delayed serologic transfusion reaction (DSTR), unspecified incompatibility

Unacceptable principal diagnosis symbol per Medicare code edits | Code exempt from diagnosis present on admission requirement
Questionable admission | Complication or comorbidity | CC/MCC exclusion | Major complication or comorbidity
Principal diagnosis as its own CC | Principal diagnosis as its own MCC | Z code as first-listed diagnosis

When symbols appear on a code that requires a 7th character extension, refer to Appendix D to identify applicable 7th character codes.

Use additional code to identify graft-versus-host reaction, if applicable, (D89.81-)

T80.9 Unspecified complication following infusion, transfusion and therapeutic injection

T80.90 Unspecified complication following infusion and therapeutic injection

T80.91 Hemolytic transfusion reaction, unspecified incompatibility

EXCLUDES1 *ABO incompatibility with hemolytic transfusion reaction (T80.31-)*

Non-ABO incompatibility with hemolytic transfusion reaction (T80.A1-)

Rh incompatibility with hemolytic transfusion reaction (T80.41-)

T80.910 Acute hemolytic transfusion reaction, unspecified incompatibility CC

T80.911 Delayed hemolytic transfusion reaction, unspecified incompatibility CC

T80.919 Hemolytic transfusion reaction, unspecified incompatibility, unspecified as acute or delayed CC

Hemolytic transfusion reaction NOS

T80.92 Unspecified transfusion reaction

Transfusion reaction NOS

T81 Complications of procedures, not elsewhere classified

Use additional code for adverse effect, if applicable, to identify drug (T36-T50 with fifth or sixth character 5)

EXCLUDES2 *complications following immunization (T88.0-T88.1)*

complications following infusion, transfusion and therapeutic injection (T80.-)

complications of transplanted organs and tissue (T86.-)

specified complications classified elsewhere, such as:

complication of prosthetic devices, implants and grafts (T82-T85)

dermatitis due to drugs and medicaments (L23.3, L24.4, L25.1, L27.0-L27.1)

endosseous dental implant failure (M27.6-)

floppy iris syndrome (IFIS) (intraoperative) H21.81

intraoperative and postprocedural complications of specific body system (D78.-, E36.-, E89.-, G97.3-, G97.4, H59.3-, H59.-, H95.2-, H95.3, I97.4-, I97.5, J95, K91.-, L76.-, M96.-, N99.-)

ostomy complications (J95.0-, K94.-, N99.5-)

plateau iris syndrome (post-iridectomy) (postprocedural) H21.82

poisoning and toxic effects of drugs and chemicals (T36-T65 with fifth or sixth character 1-4 or 6)

The appropriate 7th character is to be added to each code from category T81

A = initial encounter

D = subsequent encounter

S = sequela

T81.1 Postprocedural shock

Shock during or resulting from a procedure, not elsewhere classified

EXCLUDES1 *anaphylactic shock NOS (T78.2)*

anaphylactic shock due to correct substance properly administered (T88.6)

anaphylactic shock due to serum (T80.5-)

anesthetic shock (T88.2)

electric shock (T75.4)

obstetric shock (O75.1)

septic shock (R65.21)

shock following abortion or ectopic or molar pregnancy (O00-O07, O08.3)

traumatic shock (T79.4)

T81.10 Postprocedural shock unspecified CC

Collapse NOS during or resulting from a procedure, not elsewhere classified

Postprocedural failure of peripheral circulation

Postprocedural shock NOS

T81.11 Postprocedural cardiogenic shock MCC

T81.12 Postprocedural septic shock MCC PDx

Postprocedural endotoxic ▶shock resulting◀ from a procedure, not elsewhere classified

Postprocedural gram-negative ▶shock resulting◀ from a procedure, not elsewhere classified

Code first underlying infection

Use additional code, to identify any associated acute organ dysfunction, if applicable

T81.19 Other postprocedural shock MCC

Postprocedural hypovolemic shock

T81.3 Disruption of wound, not elsewhere classified

Disruption of any suture materials or other closure methods

EXCLUDES1 *breakdown (mechanical) of permanent sutures (T85.612)*

displacement of permanent sutures (T85.622)

disruption of cesarean delivery wound (O90.0)

disruption of perineal obstetric wound (O90.1)

mechanical complication of permanent sutures NEC (T85.692)

T81.30 Disruption of wound, unspecified CC

Disruption of wound NOS

T81.31 Disruption of external operation (surgical) wound, not elsewhere classified CC

Dehiscence of operation wound NOS

Disruption of operation wound NOS

Disruption or dehiscence of closure of cornea

Disruption or dehiscence of closure of mucosa

Disruption or dehiscence of closure of skin and subcutaneous tissue

Full-thickness skin disruption or dehiscence

Superficial disruption or dehiscence of operation wound

EXCLUDES1 *dehiscence of amputation stump (T87.81)*

AHA: Q1, 2015

T81.32 Disruption of internal operation (surgical) wound, not elsewhere classified CC

Deep disruption or dehiscence of operation wound NOS

Disruption or dehiscence of closure of internal organ or other internal tissue

Disruption or dehiscence of closure of muscle or muscle flap

Disruption or dehiscence of closure of ribs or rib cage

Disruption or dehiscence of closure of skull or craniotomy

Disruption or dehiscence of closure of sternum or sternotomy

Disruption or dehiscence of closure of tendon or ligament

Disruption or dehiscence of closure of superficial or muscular fascia

T81.33 Disruption of traumatic injury wound repair CC

Disruption or dehiscence of closure of traumatic laceration (external) (internal)

T81.4 Infection following a procedure CC HAC

Intra-abdominal abscess following a procedure

Postprocedural infection, not elsewhere classified

Sepsis following a procedure

Stitch abscess following a procedure

Subphrenic abscess following a procedure

Wound abscess following a procedure

Use additional code to identify infection

Use additional code (R65.2-) to identify severe sepsis, if applicable

EXCLUDES1 *obstetric surgical wound infection (O86.0)*

postprocedural fever NOS (R50.82)

postprocedural retroperitoneal abscess (K68.11)

EXCLUDES2 *bleb associated endophthalmitis (H59.4-)*

infection due to infusion, transfusion and therapeutic injection (T80.2-)

infection due to prosthetic devices, implants and grafts (T82.6-T82.7, T83.5-T83.6, T84.5-T84.7, T85.7)

AHA: Q4, 2015

T81.5 Complications of foreign body accidentally left in body following procedure

Unspecified Code Other Specified Code Manifestation Code N Newborn P Pediatric M Maternity A Adult ♂ Male ♀ Female
● New Code ▲ Revised Code Title ▶◀ Revised Text NOTES INCLUDES EXCLUDES1 Not coded here EXCLUDES2 Not included here
4th character required 5th character required 6th character required 7th character required
Extension 'X' Alert HAC Hospital-acquired condition (HAC) alert AHA AHA Coding Clinic©

T81.50 Unspecified complication of foreign body accidentally left in body following procedure

- T81.500 Unspecified complication of foreign body accidentally left in body following surgical operation CC HAC
- T81.501 Unspecified complication of foreign body accidentally left in body following infusion or transfusion CC HAC
- T81.502 Unspecified complication of foreign body accidentally left in body following kidney dialysis CC HAC
- T81.503 Unspecified complication of foreign body accidentally left in body following injection or immunization CC HAC
- T81.504 Unspecified complication of foreign body accidentally left in body following endoscopic examination CC HAC
- T81.505 Unspecified complication of foreign body accidentally left in body following heart catheterization CC HAC
- T81.506 Unspecified complication of foreign body accidentally left in body following aspiration, puncture or other catheterization CC HAC
- T81.507 Unspecified complication of foreign body accidentally left in body following removal of catheter or packing CC HAC
- T81.508 Unspecified complication of foreign body accidentally left in body following other procedure CC HAC
- T81.509 Unspecified complication of foreign body accidentally left in body following unspecified procedure CC HAC

T81.51 Adhesions due to foreign body accidentally left in body following procedure

- T81.510 Adhesions due to foreign body accidentally left in body following surgical operation CC HAC
- T81.511 Adhesions due to foreign body accidentally left in body following infusion or transfusion CC HAC
- T81.512 Adhesions due to foreign body accidentally left in body following kidney dialysis CC HAC
- T81.513 Adhesions due to foreign body accidentally left in body following injection or immunization CC HAC
- T81.514 Adhesions due to foreign body accidentally left in body following endoscopic examination CC HAC
- T81.515 Adhesions due to foreign body accidentally left in body following heart catheterization CC HAC
- T81.516 Adhesions due to foreign body accidentally left in body following aspiration, puncture or other catheterization CC HAC
- T81.517 Adhesions due to foreign body accidentally left in body following removal of catheter or packing CC HAC
- T81.518 Adhesions due to foreign body accidentally left in body following other procedure CC HAC
- T81.519 Adhesions due to foreign body accidentally left in body following unspecified procedure CC HAC

T81.52 Obstruction due to foreign body accidentally left in body following procedure

- T81.520 Obstruction due to foreign body accidentally left in body following surgical operation CC HAC
- T81.521 Obstruction due to foreign body accidentally left in body following infusion or transfusion CC HAC
- T81.522 Obstruction due to foreign body accidentally left in body following kidney dialysis CC HAC
- T81.523 Obstruction due to foreign body accidentally left in body following injection or immunization CC HAC
- T81.524 Obstruction due to foreign body accidentally left in body following endoscopic examination CC HAC
- T81.525 Obstruction due to foreign body accidentally left in body following heart catheterization CC HAC
- T81.526 Obstruction due to foreign body accidentally left in body following aspiration, puncture or other catheterization CC HAC
- T81.527 Obstruction due to foreign body accidentally left in body following removal of catheter or packing CC HAC
- T81.528 Obstruction due to foreign body accidentally left in body following other procedure CC HAC
- T81.529 Obstruction due to foreign body accidentally left in body following unspecified procedure CC HAC

T81.53 Perforation due to foreign body accidentally left in body following procedure

- T81.530 Perforation due to foreign body accidentally left in body following surgical operation CC HAC
- T81.531 Perforation due to foreign body accidentally left in body following infusion or transfusion CC HAC
- T81.532 Perforation due to foreign body accidentally left in body following kidney dialysis CC HAC
- T81.533 Perforation due to foreign body accidentally left in body following injection or immunization CC HAC
- T81.534 Perforation due to foreign body accidentally left in body following endoscopic examination CC HAC
- T81.535 Perforation due to foreign body accidentally left in body following heart catheterization CC HAC
- T81.536 Perforation due to foreign body accidentally left in body following aspiration, puncture or other catheterization CC HAC
- T81.537 Perforation due to foreign body accidentally left in body following removal of catheter or packing CC HAC
- T81.538 Perforation due to foreign body accidentally left in body following other procedure CC HAC
- T81.539 Perforation due to foreign body accidentally left in body following unspecified procedure CC HAC

T81.59 Other complications of foreign body accidentally left in body following procedure

EXCLUDES2 *obstruction or perforation due to prosthetic devices and implants intentionally left in body (T82.0-T82.5, T83.0-T83.4, T83.7, T84.0-T84.4, T85.0-T85.6)*

- T81.590 Other complications of foreign body accidentally left in body following surgical operation CC HAC
- T81.591 Other complications of foreign body accidentally left in body following infusion or transfusion CC HAC
- T81.592 Other complications of foreign body accidentally left in body following kidney dialysis CC HAC
- T81.593 Other complications of foreign body accidentally left in body following injection or immunization CC HAC

Unacceptable principal diagnosis symbol per Medicare code edits · Code exempt from diagnosis present on admission requirement
Questionable admission · Complication or comorbidity · CC/MCC exclusion · Major complication or comorbidity
Principal diagnosis as its own CC · Principal diagnosis as its own MCC · Z code as first-listed diagnosis

 When symbols appear on a code that requires a 7th character extension, refer to Appendix D to identify applicable 7th character codes.

T81.594 Other complications of foreign body accidentally left in body following endoscopic examination CC HAC
T81.595 Other complications of foreign body accidentally left in body following heart catheterization CC HAC
T81.596 Other complications of foreign body accidentally left in body following aspiration, puncture or other catheterization CC HAC
T81.597 Other complications of foreign body accidentally left in body following removal of catheter or packing CC HAC
T81.598 Other complications of foreign body accidentally left in body following other procedure CC HAC
T81.599 Other complications of foreign body accidentally left in body following unspecified procedure CC HAC

T81.6 Acute reaction to foreign substance accidentally left during a procedure
EXCLUDES2 *complications of foreign body accidentally left in body cavity or operation wound following procedure (T81.5-)*
T81.60 Unspecified acute reaction to foreign substance accidentally left during a procedure CC HAC
T81.61 Aseptic peritonitis due to foreign substance accidentally left during a procedure CC HAC
Chemical peritonitis
T81.69 Other acute reaction to foreign substance accidentally left during a procedure CC HAC

T81.7 Vascular complications following a procedure, not elsewhere classified
Air embolism following procedure NEC
Phlebitis or thrombophlebitis resulting from a procedure
EXCLUDES1 *embolism complicating abortion or ectopic or molar pregnancy (O00-O07, O08.2)*
embolism complicating pregnancy, childbirth and the puerperium (O88.-)
traumatic embolism (T79.0)
EXCLUDES2 *embolism due to prosthetic devices, implants and grafts (T82.8-, ▶T83.81, T84.8-, T85.81-◀)*
embolism following infusion, transfusion and therapeutic injection (T80.0)
T81.71 Complication of artery following a procedure, not elsewhere classified
T81.710 Complication of mesenteric artery following a procedure, not elsewhere classified CC
T81.711 Complication of renal artery following a procedure, not elsewhere classified CC
T81.718 Complication of other artery following a procedure, not elsewhere classified CC
T81.719 Complication of unspecified artery following a procedure, not elsewhere classified CC
T81.72 Complication of vein following a procedure, not elsewhere classified CC

T81.8 Other complications of procedures, not elsewhere classified
EXCLUDES2 *hypothermia following anesthesia (T88.51)*
malignant hyperpyrexia due to anesthesia (T88.3)
T81.81 Complication of inhalation therapy
T81.82 Emphysema (subcutaneous) resulting from a procedure
T81.83 Persistent postprocedural fistula CC
T81.89 Other complications of procedures, not elsewhere classified
Use additional code to specify complication, such as: postprocedural delirium (F05)
T81.9 Unspecified complication of procedure

T82 Complications of cardiac and vascular prosthetic devices, implants and grafts
EXCLUDES2 *failure and rejection of transplanted organs and tissue (T86.-)*
The appropriate 7th character is to be added to each code from category T82
A = initial encounter
D = subsequent encounter
S = sequela

T82.0 Mechanical complication of heart valve prosthesis
Mechanical complication of artificial heart valve
EXCLUDES1 *mechanical complication of biological heart valve graft (T82.22-)*
T82.01 Breakdown (mechanical) of heart valve prosthesis CC
T82.02 Displacement of heart valve prosthesis CC
Malposition of heart valve prosthesis
T82.03 Leakage of heart valve prosthesis CC
T82.09 Other mechanical complication of heart valve prosthesis CC
Obstruction (mechanical) of heart valve prosthesis
Perforation of heart valve prosthesis
Protrusion of heart valve prosthesis

T82.1 Mechanical complication of cardiac electronic device
T82.11 Breakdown (mechanical) of cardiac electronic device
T82.110 Breakdown (mechanical) of cardiac electrode CC
T82.111 Breakdown (mechanical) of cardiac pulse generator (battery) CC
T82.118 Breakdown (mechanical) of other cardiac electronic device CC
T82.119 Breakdown (mechanical) of unspecified cardiac electronic device CC
T82.12 Displacement of cardiac electronic device
Malposition of cardiac electronic device
T82.120 Displacement of cardiac electrode CC
T82.121 Displacement of cardiac pulse generator (battery) CC
T82.128 Displacement of other cardiac electronic device CC
T82.129 Displacement of unspecified cardiac electronic device CC
T82.19 Other mechanical complication of cardiac electronic device
Leakage of cardiac electronic device
Obstruction of cardiac electronic device
Perforation of cardiac electronic device
Protrusion of cardiac electronic device
T82.190 Other mechanical complication of cardiac electrode CC
T82.191 Other mechanical complication of cardiac pulse generator (battery) CC
T82.198 Other mechanical complication of other cardiac electronic device CC
T82.199 Other mechanical complication of unspecified cardiac device CC

T82.2 Mechanical complication of coronary artery bypass graft and biological heart valve graft
EXCLUDES1 *mechanical complication of artificial heart valve prosthesis (T82.0-)*
T82.21 Mechanical complication of coronary artery bypass graft
T82.211 Breakdown (mechanical) of coronary artery bypass graft CC
T82.212 Displacement of coronary artery bypass graft CC
Malposition of coronary artery bypass graft
T82.213 Leakage of coronary artery bypass graft CC
T82.218 Other mechanical complication of coronary artery bypass graft CC
Obstruction, mechanical of coronary artery bypass graft
Perforation of coronary artery bypass graft
Protrusion of coronary artery bypass graft
T82.22 Mechanical complication of biological heart valve graft
T82.221 Breakdown (mechanical) of biological heart valve graft CC
T82.222 Displacement of biological heart valve graft CC
Malposition of biological heart valve graft
T82.223 Leakage of biological heart valve graft CC

Unspecified Code Other Specified Code Manifestation Code N Newborn P Pediatric M Maternity A Adult ♂ Male ♀ Female
● New Code ▲ Revised Code Title ▶◀ Revised Text NOTES INCLUDES EXCLUDES1 Not coded here EXCLUDES2 Not included here
4th character required 5th character required 6th character required 7th character required
Extension 'X' Alert HAC Hospital-acquired condition (HAC) alert AHA AHA Coding Clinic©

T82.228 Other mechanical complication of biological heart valve graft
Obstruction of biological heart valve graft
Perforation of biological heart valve graft
Protrusion of biological heart valve graft

T82.3 Mechanical complication of other vascular grafts
T82.31 Breakdown (mechanical) of other vascular grafts
T82.310 Breakdown (mechanical) of aortic (bifurcation) graft (replacement)
T82.311 Breakdown (mechanical) of carotid arterial graft (bypass)
T82.312 Breakdown (mechanical) of femoral arterial graft (bypass)
T82.318 Breakdown (mechanical) of other vascular grafts
T82.319 Breakdown (mechanical) of unspecified vascular grafts
T82.32 Displacement of other vascular grafts
Malposition of other vascular grafts
T82.320 Displacement of aortic (bifurcation) graft (replacement)
T82.321 Displacement of carotid arterial graft (bypass)
T82.322 Displacement of femoral arterial graft (bypass)
T82.328 Displacement of other vascular grafts
T82.329 Displacement of unspecified vascular grafts
T82.33 Leakage of other vascular grafts
T82.330 Leakage of aortic (bifurcation) graft (replacement)
T82.331 Leakage of carotid arterial graft (bypass)
T82.332 Leakage of femoral arterial graft (bypass)
T82.338 Leakage of other vascular grafts
T82.339 Leakage of unspecified vascular graft
T82.39 Other mechanical complication of other vascular grafts
Obstruction (mechanical) of other vascular grafts
Perforation of other vascular grafts
Protrusion of other vascular grafts
T82.390 Other mechanical complication of aortic (bifurcation) graft (replacement)
T82.391 Other mechanical complication of carotid arterial graft (bypass)
T82.392 Other mechanical complication of femoral arterial graft (bypass)
T82.398 Other mechanical complication of other vascular grafts
T82.399 Other mechanical complication of unspecified vascular grafts

T82.4 Mechanical complication of vascular dialysis catheter
Mechanical complication of hemodialysis catheter
EXCLUDES1 *mechanical complication of intraperitoneal dialysis catheter (T85.62)*
T82.41 Breakdown (mechanical) of vascular dialysis catheter
T82.42 Displacement of vascular dialysis catheter
Malposition of vascular dialysis catheter
T82.43 Leakage of vascular dialysis catheter
T82.49 Other complication of vascular dialysis catheter
Obstruction (mechanical) of vascular dialysis catheter
Perforation of vascular dialysis catheter
Protrusion of vascular dialysis catheter

T82.5 Mechanical complication of other cardiac and vascular devices and implants
EXCLUDES2 *mechanical complication of epidural and subdural infusion catheter (T85.61)*
T82.51 Breakdown (mechanical) of other cardiac and vascular devices and implants
T82.510 Breakdown (mechanical) of surgically created arteriovenous fistula
T82.511 Breakdown (mechanical) of surgically created arteriovenous shunt
T82.512 Breakdown (mechanical) of artificial heart
T82.513 Breakdown (mechanical) of balloon (counterpulsation) device
T82.514 Breakdown (mechanical) of infusion catheter
T82.515 Breakdown (mechanical) of umbrella device
T82.518 Breakdown (mechanical) of other cardiac and vascular devices and implants
T82.519 Breakdown (mechanical) of unspecified cardiac and vascular devices and implants
T82.52 Displacement of other cardiac and vascular devices and implants
Malposition of other cardiac and vascular devices and implants
T82.520 Displacement of surgically created arteriovenous fistula
T82.521 Displacement of surgically created arteriovenous shunt
T82.522 Displacement of artificial heart
T82.523 Displacement of balloon (counterpulsation) device
T82.524 Displacement of infusion catheter
T82.525 Displacement of umbrella device
T82.528 Displacement of other cardiac and vascular devices and implants
T82.529 Displacement of unspecified cardiac and vascular devices and implants
T82.53 Leakage of other cardiac and vascular devices and implants
T82.530 Leakage of surgically created arteriovenous fistula
T82.531 Leakage of surgically created arteriovenous shunt
T82.532 Leakage of artificial heart
T82.533 Leakage of balloon (counterpulsation) device
T82.534 Leakage of infusion catheter
T82.535 Leakage of umbrella device
T82.538 Leakage of other cardiac and vascular devices and implants
T82.539 Leakage of unspecified cardiac and vascular devices and implants
T82.59 Other mechanical complication of other cardiac and vascular devices and implants
Obstruction (mechanical) of other cardiac and vascular devices and implants
Perforation of other cardiac and vascular devices and implants
Protrusion of other cardiac and vascular devices and implants
T82.590 Other mechanical complication of surgically created arteriovenous fistula
T82.591 Other mechanical complication of surgically created arteriovenous shunt
T82.592 Other mechanical complication of artificial heart
T82.593 Other mechanical complication of balloon (counterpulsation) device
T82.594 Other mechanical complication of infusion catheter
T82.595 Other mechanical complication of umbrella device
T82.598 Other mechanical complication of other cardiac and vascular devices and implants
T82.599 Other mechanical complication of unspecified cardiac and vascular devices and implants

T82.6 Infection and inflammatory reaction due to cardiac valve prosthesis HAC
Use additional code to identify infection

Unacceptable principal diagnosis symbol per Medicare code edits; Code exempt from diagnosis present on admission requirement; Questionable admission; Complication or comorbidity; CC/MCC exclusion; Major complication or comorbidity; Principal diagnosis as its own CC; Principal diagnosis as its own MCC; Z code as first-listed diagnosis

T82.7 Infection and inflammatory reaction due to other cardiac and vascular devices, implants and grafts CC HAC
Use additional code to identify infection
AHA: Q1, 2015

T82.8 **Other specified complications of cardiac and vascular prosthetic devices, implants and grafts**

▲ T82.81 Embolism ▶due to◀ cardiac and vascular prosthetic devices, implants and grafts
▲ T82.817 Embolism ▶due to◀ cardiac prosthetic devices, implants and grafts CC
▲ T82.818 Embolism ▶due to◀ vascular prosthetic devices, implants and grafts CC

▲ T82.82 Fibrosis ▶due to◀ cardiac and vascular prosthetic devices, implants and grafts
▲ T82.827 Fibrosis ▶due to◀ cardiac prosthetic devices, implants and grafts CC
▲ T82.828 Fibrosis ▶due to◀ vascular prosthetic devices, implants and grafts CC

▲ T82.83 Hemorrhage ▶due to◀ cardiac and vascular prosthetic devices, implants and grafts
▲ T82.837 Hemorrhage ▶due to◀ cardiac prosthetic devices, implants and grafts CC
▲ T82.838 Hemorrhage ▶due to◀ vascular prosthetic devices, implants and grafts CC

▲ T82.84 Pain ▶due to◀ cardiac and vascular prosthetic devices, implants and grafts
▲ T82.847 Pain ▶due to◀ cardiac prosthetic devices, implants and grafts CC
▲ T82.848 Pain ▶due to◀ vascular prosthetic devices, implants and grafts CC

▲ T82.85 Stenosis ▶due to◀ cardiac and vascular prosthetic devices, implants and grafts
● T82.855 Stenosis of coronary artery stent CC CC/MCC Exc
In-stent stenosis (restenosis) of coronary artery stent
Restenosis of coronary artery stent
● T82.856 Stenosis of peripheral vascular stent CC CC/MCC Exc
In-stent stenosis (restenosis) of peripheral vascular stent
Restenosis of peripheral vascular stent
▲ T82.857 Stenosis of ▶other◀ cardiac prosthetic devices, implants and grafts CC
▲ T82.858 Stenosis of ▶other◀ vascular prosthetic devices, implants and grafts CC

T82.86 Thrombosis of cardiac and vascular prosthetic devices, implants and grafts
▲ T82.867 Thrombosis ▶due to◀ cardiac prosthetic devices, implants and grafts CC
▲ T82.868 Thrombosis ▶due to◀ vascular prosthetic devices, implants and grafts CC

T82.89 Other specified complication of cardiac and vascular prosthetic devices, implants and grafts
T82.897 **Other specified complication of cardiac prosthetic devices, implants and grafts** CC
T82.898 **Other specified complication of vascular prosthetic devices, implants and grafts** CC

T82.9 Unspecified complication of cardiac and vascular prosthetic device, implant and graft CC

T83 Complications of genitourinary prosthetic devices, implants and grafts
EXCLUDES2 *failure and rejection of transplanted organs and tissue (T86.-)*
The appropriate 7th character is to be added to each code from category T83
A = initial encounter
D = subsequent encounter
S = sequela

▲ T83.0 Mechanical complication of ▶urinary catheter◀
EXCLUDES2 *complications of stoma of urinary tract (N99.5-)*

▲ T83.01 Breakdown (mechanical) of ▶urinary catheter◀
T83.010 Breakdown (mechanical) of cystostomy catheter CC
● T83.011 Breakdown (mechanical) of indwelling urethral catheter
● T83.012 Breakdown (mechanical) of nephrostomy catheter
▲ T83.018 Breakdown (mechanical) of other ▶urinary◀ catheter
Breakdown (mechanical) of Hopkins catheter
Breakdown (mechanical) of ileostomy catheter
Breakdown (mechanical) urostomy catheter

▲ T83.02 Displacement of ▶urinary catheter◀
Malposition of ▶urinary catheter◀
T83.020 Displacement of cystostomy catheter CC
● T83.021 Displacement of indwelling urethral catheter
● T83.022 Displacement of nephrostomy catheter
▲ T83.028 Displacement of other ▶urinary◀ catheter
Displacement of Hopkins catheter
Displacement of ileostomy catheter
Displacement of urostomy catheter

▲ T83.03 Leakage of ▶urinary catheter◀
T83.030 Leakage of cystostomy catheter CC
● T83.031 Leakage of indwelling urethral catheter
● T83.032 Leakage of nephrostomy catheter
▲ T83.038 Leakage of other ▶urinary◀ catheter
Leakage of Hopkins catheter
Leakage of ileostomy catheter
Leakage of urostomy catheter

▲ T83.09 Other mechanical complication of ▶urinary catheter◀
Obstruction (mechanical) of ▶urinary catheter◀
Perforation of ▶urinary catheter◀
Protrusion of ▶urinary catheter◀
T83.090 Other mechanical complication of cystostomy catheter CC
● T83.091 Other mechanical complication of indwelling urethral catheter
● T83.092 Other mechanical complication of nephrostomy catheter
▲ T83.098 Other mechanical complication of other ▶urinary◀ catheter
Other mechanical complication of Hopkins catheter
Other mechanical complication of ileostomy catheter
Other mechanical complication of urostomy catheter

T83.1 Mechanical complication of other urinary devices and implants

T83.11 Breakdown (mechanical) of other urinary devices and implants
T83.110 Breakdown (mechanical) of urinary electronic stimulator device CC
EXCLUDES2 *Breakdown (mechanical) of electrode (lead) for sacral nerve neurostimulator (T85.111)*
Breakdown (mechanical) of implanted electronic sacral neurostimulator, pulse generator or receiver (T85.113)
▲ T83.111 Breakdown (mechanical) of ▶implanted urinary sphincter◀ CC
▲ T83.112 Breakdown (mechanical) of ▶indwelling ureteral◀ stent CC
● T83.113 Breakdown (mechanical) of other urinary stents CC CC/MCC Exc
Breakdown (mechanical) of ileal conduit stent
Breakdown (mechanical) of nephroureteral stent
T83.118 Breakdown (mechanical) of other urinary devices and implants CC

T83.12 Displacement of other urinary devices and implants
Malposition of other urinary devices and implants
T83.120 Displacement of urinary electronic stimulator device CC

Unspecified Code **Other Specified Code** Manifestation Code N Newborn P Pediatric M Maternity A Adult ♂ Male ♀ Female
● New Code ▲ Revised Code Title ▶◀ Revised Text NOTES INCLUDES EXCLUDES1 Not coded here EXCLUDES2 Not included here
4th character required 5th character required 6th character required 7th character required
Extension 'X' Alert HAC Hospital-acquired condition (HAC) alert AHA AHA Coding Clinic©

EXCLUDES2 *Displacement of electrode (lead) for sacral nerve neurostimulator (T85.121)*

Displacement of implanted electronic sacral neurostimulator, pulse generator or receiver (T85.123)

▲ T83.121 **Displacement of ▶implanted urinary sphincter◀**

▲ T83.122 **Displacement of ▶indwelling ureteral◀ stent**

● T83.123 **Displacement of other urinary stents**

Displacement of ileal conduit stent
Displacement of nephroureteral stent

T83.128 **Displacement of other urinary devices and implants**

T83.19 **Other mechanical complication of other urinary devices and implants**

Leakage of other urinary devices and implants
Obstruction (mechanical) of other urinary devices and implants
Perforation of other urinary devices and implants
Protrusion of other urinary devices and implants

T83.190 **Other mechanical complication of urinary electronic stimulator device**

EXCLUDES2 *Other mechanical complication of electrode (lead) for sacral nerve neurostimulator (T85.191)*

Other mechanical complication of implanted electronic sacral neurostimulator, pulse generator or receiver (T85.193)

▲ T83.191 **Other mechanical complication of ▶implanted urinary◀ sphincter**

▲ T83.192 **Other mechanical complication of ▶indwelling ureteral◀ stent**

● T83.193 **Other mechanical complication of other urinary stent**

Other mechanical complication of ileal conduit stent
Other mechanical complication of nephroureteral stent

T83.198 **Other mechanical complication of other urinary devices and implants**

T83.2 **Mechanical complication of graft of urinary organ**

T83.21 **Breakdown (mechanical) of graft of urinary organ**

T83.22 **Displacement of graft of urinary organ**

Malposition of graft of urinary organ

T83.23 **Leakage of graft of urinary organ**

● T83.24 **Erosion of graft of urinary organ**

● T83.25 **Exposure of graft of urinary organ**

T83.29 **Other mechanical complication of graft of urinary organ**

Obstruction (mechanical) of graft of urinary organ
Perforation of graft of urinary organ
Protrusion of graft of urinary organ

T83.3 **Mechanical complication of intrauterine contraceptive device**

T83.31 **Breakdown (mechanical) of intrauterine contraceptive device** M ♀

T83.32 **Displacement of intrauterine contraceptive device** M ♀

Malposition of intrauterine contraceptive device
Missing string of intrauterine contraceptive device

T83.39 **Other mechanical complication of intrauterine contraceptive device** M ♀

Leakage of intrauterine contraceptive device
Obstruction (mechanical) of intrauterine contraceptive device
Perforation of intrauterine contraceptive device
Protrusion of intrauterine contraceptive device

T83.4 **Mechanical complication of other prosthetic devices, implants and grafts of genital tract**

T83.41 **Breakdown (mechanical) of other prosthetic devices, implants and grafts of genital tract**

▲ T83.410 **Breakdown (mechanical) of ▶implanted penile prosthesis◀** ♂

Breakdown (mechanical) of penile prosthesis cylinder
Breakdown (mechanical) of penile prosthesis pump
Breakdown (mechanical) of penile prosthesis reservoir

● T83.411 **Breakdown (mechanical) of implanted testicular prosthesis**

T83.418 **Breakdown (mechanical) of other prosthetic devices, implants and grafts of genital tract**

T83.42 **Displacement of other prosthetic devices, implants and grafts of genital tract**

Malposition of other prosthetic devices, implants and grafts of genital tract

▲ T83.420 **Displacement of ▶implanted penile prosthesis◀** ♂

Displacement of penile prosthesis cylinder
Displacement of penile prosthesis pump
Displacement of penile prosthesis reservoir

● T83.421 **Displacement of implanted testicular prosthesis**

T83.428 **Displacement of other prosthetic devices, implants and grafts of genital tract**

T83.49 **Other mechanical complication of other prosthetic devices, implants and grafts of genital tract**

Leakage of other prosthetic devices, implants and grafts of genital tract
Obstruction, mechanical of other prosthetic devices, implants and grafts of genital tract
Perforation of other prosthetic devices, implants and grafts of genital tract
Protrusion of other prosthetic devices, implants and grafts of genital tract

▲ T83.490 **Other mechanical complication of ▶implanted penile prosthesis◀** ♂

Other mechanical complication of penile prosthesis cylinder
Other mechanical complication of penile prosthesis pump
Other mechanical complication of penile prosthesis reservoir

● T83.491 **Other mechanical complication of implanted testicular prosthesis**

T83.498 **Other mechanical complication of other prosthetic devices, implants and grafts of genital tract**

T83.5 **Infection and inflammatory reaction due to prosthetic device, implant and graft in urinary system**

Use additional code to identify infection

▲ T83.51 **Infection and inflammatory reaction due to ▶urinary◀ catheter**

EXCLUDES2 *complications of stoma of urinary tract (N99.5-)*

● T83.510 **Infection and inflammatory reaction due to cystostomy catheter**

● T83.511 **Infection and inflammatory reaction due to indwelling urethral catheter**

● T83.512 **Infection and inflammatory reaction due to nephrostomy catheter**

● T83.518 **Infection and inflammatory reaction due to other urinary catheter**

Infection and inflammatory reaction due to Hopkins catheter
Infection and inflammatory reaction due to ileostomy catheter
Infection and inflammatory reaction due to urostomy catheter

T83.59 **Infection and inflammatory reaction due to prosthetic device, implant and graft in urinary system**

● T83.590 **Infection and inflammatory reaction due to implanted urinary neurostimulation device**

EXCLUDES2 *Infection and inflammatory reaction due to electrode lead*

Unacceptable principal diagnosis symbol per Medicare code edits; Code exempt from diagnosis present on admission requirement; Questionable admission; Complication or comorbidity; CC/MCC exclusion; Major complication or comorbidity; Principal diagnosis as its own CC; Principal diagnosis as its own MCC; Z code as first-listed diagnosis

of sacral nerve neurostimulator (T85.732)

Infection and inflammatory reaction due to pulse generator or receiver of sacral nerve neurostimulator (T85.734)

● **T83.591 Infection and inflammatory reaction due to implanted urinary sphincter**

● **T83.592 Infection and inflammatory reaction due to indwelling ureteral stent**

● **T83.593 Infection and inflammatory reaction due to other urinary stents**

Infection and inflammatory reaction due to ileal conduit stents

Infection and inflammatory reaction due to nephroureteral stent

● **T83.598 Infection and inflammatory reaction due to other prosthetic device, implant and graft in urinary system**

T83.6 Infection and inflammatory reaction due to prosthetic device, implant and graft in genital tract

Use additional code to identify infection

● **T83.61 Infection and inflammatory reaction due to implanted penile prosthesis**

Infection and inflammatory reaction due to penile prosthesis cylinder

Infection and inflammatory reaction due to penile prosthesis pump

Infection and inflammatory reaction due to penile prosthesis reservoir

● **T83.62 Infection and inflammatory reaction due to implanted testicular prosthesis**

● **T83.69 Infection and inflammatory reaction due to other prosthetic device, implant and graft in genital tract**

T83.7 Complications due to implanted mesh and other prosthetic materials

T83.71 Erosion of implanted mesh and other prosthetic materials to surrounding organ or tissue

▲ **T83.711 Erosion of implanted vaginal ▶mesh to◀ surrounding organ or tissue** ♀

Erosion of implanted vaginal ▶mesh into◀ pelvic floor muscles

● **T83.712 Erosion of implanted urethral mesh to surrounding organ or tissue**

Erosion of implanted female urethral sling

Erosion of implanted male urethral sling

Erosion of implanted urethral mesh into pelvic floor muscles

● **T83.713 Erosion of implanted urethral bulking agent to surrounding organ or tissue**

● **T83.714 Erosion of implanted ureteral bulking agent to surrounding organ or tissue**

▲ **T83.718 Erosion of other implanted ▶mesh to◀ organ or tissue**

● **T83.719 Erosion of other prosthetic materials to surrounding organ or tissue**

T83.72 Exposure of implanted mesh and other prosthetic materials into surrounding organ or tissue

Extrusion of implanted mesh

▲ **T83.721 Exposure of implanted vaginal mesh ▶into◀ vagina** ♀

Exposure of implanted vaginal ▶mesh through◀ vaginal wall

● **T83.722 Exposure of implanted urethral mesh into urethra**

Exposure of implanted female urethral sling

Exposure of implanted male urethral sling

Exposure of implanted urethral mesh through urethral wall

● **T83.723 Exposure of implanted urethral bulking agent into urethra**

● **T83.724 Exposure of implanted ureteral bulking agent into ureter**

▲ **T83.728 Exposure of other implanted mesh ▶into◀ organ or tissue**

● **T83.729 Exposure of other prosthetic materials into organ or tissue**

● **T83.79 Other specified complications due to other genitourinary prosthetic materials**

T83.8 Other specified complications of genitourinary prosthetic devices, implants and grafts

▲ **T83.81 Embolism ▶due to◀ genitourinary prosthetic devices, implants and grafts**

▲ **T83.82 Fibrosis ▶due◀ to genitourinary prosthetic devices, implants and grafts**

▲ **T83.83 Hemorrhage ▶due to◀ genitourinary prosthetic devices, implants and grafts**

▲ **T83.84 Pain ▶due to◀ genitourinary prosthetic devices, implants and grafts**

▲ **T83.85 Stenosis ▶due to◀ genitourinary prosthetic devices, implants and grafts**

▲ **T83.86 Thrombosis ▶due to◀ genitourinary prosthetic devices, implants and grafts**

T83.89 Other specified complication of genitourinary prosthetic devices, implants and grafts

T83.9 Unspecified complication of genitourinary prosthetic device, implant and graft

T84 Complications of internal orthopedic prosthetic devices, implants and grafts

EXCLUDES2 *failure and rejection of transplanted organs and tissues (T86.-)*

fracture of bone following insertion of orthopedic implant, joint prosthesis or bone plate (M96.6)

The appropriate 7th character is to be added to each code from category T84

A = initial encounter

D = subsequent encounter

S = sequela

T84.0 Mechanical complication of internal joint prosthesis

T84.01 Broken internal joint prosthesis

Breakage (fracture) of prosthetic joint

Broken prosthetic joint implant

EXCLUDES1 *periprosthetic joint implant fracture (T84.04)*

T84.010 Broken internal right hip prosthesis

T84.011 Broken internal left hip prosthesis

T84.012 Broken internal right knee prosthesis

T84.013 Broken internal left knee prosthesis

T84.018 Broken internal joint prosthesis, other site

Use additional code to identify the joint (Z96.6-)

T84.019 Broken internal joint prosthesis, unspecified site

T84.02 Dislocation of internal joint prosthesis

Instability of internal joint prosthesis

Subluxation of internal joint prosthesis

T84.020 Dislocation of internal right hip prosthesis

T84.021 Dislocation of internal left hip prosthesis

T84.022 Instability of internal right knee prosthesis

T84.023 Instability of internal left knee prosthesis

T84.028 Dislocation of other internal joint prosthesis

Use additional code to identify the joint (Z96.6-)

T84.029 Dislocation of unspecified internal joint prosthesis

T84.03 Mechanical loosening of internal prosthetic joint

Aseptic loosening of prosthetic joint

T84.030 Mechanical loosening of internal right hip prosthetic joint

T84.031 Mechanical loosening of internal left hip prosthetic joint

T84.032 Mechanical loosening of internal right knee prosthetic joint

T84.033 Mechanical loosening of internal left knee prosthetic joint
T84.038 Mechanical loosening of other internal prosthetic joint
Use additional code to identify the joint (Z96.6-)
T84.039 Mechanical loosening of unspecified internal prosthetic joint
T84.05 Periprosthetic osteolysis of internal prosthetic joint
Use additional code to identify major osseous defect, if applicable (M89.7-)
T84.050 Periprosthetic osteolysis of internal prosthetic right hip joint
T84.051 Periprosthetic osteolysis of internal prosthetic left hip joint
T84.052 Periprosthetic osteolysis of internal prosthetic right knee joint
T84.053 Periprosthetic osteolysis of internal prosthetic left knee joint
T84.058 Periprosthetic osteolysis of other internal prosthetic joint
Use additional code to identify the joint (Z96.6-)
T84.059 Periprosthetic osteolysis of unspecified internal prosthetic joint
T84.06 Wear of articular bearing surface of internal prosthetic joint
T84.060 Wear of articular bearing surface of internal prosthetic right hip joint
T84.061 Wear of articular bearing surface of internal prosthetic left hip joint
T84.062 Wear of articular bearing surface of internal prosthetic right knee joint
T84.063 Wear of articular bearing surface of internal prosthetic left knee joint
T84.068 Wear of articular bearing surface of other internal prosthetic joint
Use additional code to identify the joint (Z96.6-)
T84.069 Wear of articular bearing surface of unspecified internal prosthetic joint
T84.09 Other mechanical complication of internal joint prosthesis
Prosthetic joint implant failure NOS
T84.090 Other mechanical complication of internal right hip prosthesis
T84.091 Other mechanical complication of internal left hip prosthesis
T84.092 Other mechanical complication of internal right knee prosthesis
T84.093 Other mechanical complication of internal left knee prosthesis
T84.098 Other mechanical complication of other internal joint prosthesis
Use additional code to identify the joint (Z96.6-)
T84.099 Other mechanical complication of unspecified internal joint prosthesis
T84.1 Mechanical complication of internal fixation device of bones of limb
EXCLUDES2 *mechanical complication of internal fixation device of bones of feet (T84.2-)*
mechanical complication of internal fixation device of bones of fingers (T84.2-)
mechanical complication of internal fixation device of bones of hands (T84.2-)
mechanical complication of internal fixation device of bones of toes (T84.2-)
T84.11 Breakdown (mechanical) of internal fixation device of bones of limb
T84.110 Breakdown (mechanical) of internal fixation device of right humerus
T84.111 Breakdown (mechanical) of internal fixation device of left humerus
T84.112 Breakdown (mechanical) of internal fixation device of bone of right forearm
T84.113 Breakdown (mechanical) of internal fixation device of bone of left forearm
T84.114 Breakdown (mechanical) of internal fixation device of right femur
T84.115 Breakdown (mechanical) of internal fixation device of left femur
T84.116 Breakdown (mechanical) of internal fixation device of bone of right lower leg
T84.117 Breakdown (mechanical) of internal fixation device of bone of left lower leg
T84.119 Breakdown (mechanical) of internal fixation device of unspecified bone of limb
T84.12 Displacement of internal fixation device of bones of limb
Malposition of internal fixation device of bones of limb
T84.120 Displacement of internal fixation device of right humerus
T84.121 Displacement of internal fixation device of left humerus
T84.122 Displacement of internal fixation device of bone of right forearm
T84.123 Displacement of internal fixation device of bone of left forearm
T84.124 Displacement of internal fixation device of right femur
T84.125 Displacement of internal fixation device of left femur
T84.126 Displacement of internal fixation device of bone of right lower leg
T84.127 Displacement of internal fixation device of bone of left lower leg
T84.129 Displacement of internal fixation device of unspecified bone of limb
T84.19 Other mechanical complication of internal fixation device of bones of limb
Obstruction (mechanical) of internal fixation device of bones of limb
Perforation of internal fixation device of bones of limb
Protrusion of internal fixation device of bones of limb
T84.190 Other mechanical complication of internal fixation device of right humerus
T84.191 Other mechanical complication of internal fixation device of left humerus
T84.192 Other mechanical complication of internal fixation device of bone of right forearm
T84.193 Other mechanical complication of internal fixation device of bone of left forearm
T84.194 Other mechanical complication of internal fixation device of right femur
T84.195 Other mechanical complication of internal fixation device of left femur
T84.196 Other mechanical complication of internal fixation device of bone of right lower leg
T84.197 Other mechanical complication of internal fixation device of bone of left lower leg
T84.199 Other mechanical complication of internal fixation device of unspecified bone of limb
T84.2 Mechanical complication of internal fixation device of other bones
T84.21 Breakdown (mechanical) of internal fixation device of other bones
T84.210 Breakdown (mechanical) of internal fixation device of bones of hand and fingers
T84.213 Breakdown (mechanical) of internal fixation device of bones of foot and toes
T84.216 Breakdown (mechanical) of internal fixation device of vertebrae

Unacceptable principal diagnosis symbol per Medicare code edits; Code exempt from diagnosis present on admission requirement; Questionable admission; Complication or comorbidity; CC/MCC exclusion; Major complication or comorbidity; Principal diagnosis as its own CC; Principal diagnosis as its own MCC; Z code as first-listed diagnosis

T84.218 Breakdown (mechanical) of internal fixation device of other bones

T84.22 Displacement of internal fixation device of other bones
Malposition of internal fixation device of other bones

T84.220 Displacement of internal fixation device of bones of hand and fingers

T84.223 Displacement of internal fixation device of bones of foot and toes

T84.226 Displacement of internal fixation device of vertebrae

T84.228 Displacement of internal fixation device of other bones

T84.29 Other mechanical complication of internal fixation device of other bones
Obstruction (mechanical) of internal fixation device of other bones
Perforation of internal fixation device of other bones
Protrusion of internal fixation device of other bones

T84.290 Other mechanical complication of internal fixation device of bones of hand and fingers

T84.293 Other mechanical complication of internal fixation device of bones of foot and toes

T84.296 Other mechanical complication of internal fixation device of vertebrae

T84.298 Other mechanical complication of internal fixation device of other bones

T84.3 Mechanical complication of other bone devices, implants and grafts
EXCLUDES2 *other complications of bone graft (T86.83-)*

T84.31 Breakdown (mechanical) of other bone devices, implants and grafts

T84.310 Breakdown (mechanical) of electronic bone stimulator

T84.318 Breakdown (mechanical) of other bone devices, implants and grafts

T84.32 Displacement of other bone devices, implants and grafts
Malposition of other bone devices, implants and grafts

T84.320 Displacement of electronic bone stimulator

T84.328 Displacement of other bone devices, implants and grafts

T84.39 Other mechanical complication of other bone devices, implants and grafts
Obstruction (mechanical) of other bone devices, implants and grafts
Perforation of other bone devices, implants and grafts
Protrusion of other bone devices, implants and grafts

T84.390 Other mechanical complication of electronic bone stimulator

T84.398 Other mechanical complication of other bone devices, implants and grafts

T84.4 Mechanical complication of other internal orthopedic devices, implants and grafts

T84.41 Breakdown (mechanical) of other internal orthopedic devices, implants and grafts

T84.410 Breakdown (mechanical) of muscle and tendon graft

T84.418 Breakdown (mechanical) of other internal orthopedic devices, implants and grafts

T84.42 Displacement of other internal orthopedic devices, implants and grafts
Malposition of other internal orthopedic devices, implants and grafts

T84.420 Displacement of muscle and tendon graft

T84.428 Displacement of other internal orthopedic devices, implants and grafts

T84.49 Other mechanical complication of other internal orthopedic devices, implants and grafts
Mechanical complication of other internal orthopedic devices, implants and grafts NOS
Obstruction (mechanical) of other internal orthopedic devices, implants and grafts
Perforation of other internal orthopedic devices, implants and grafts
Protrusion of other internal orthopedic devices, implants and grafts

T84.490 Other mechanical complication of muscle and tendon graft

T84.498 Other mechanical complication of other internal orthopedic devices, implants and grafts

T84.5 Infection and inflammatory reaction due to internal joint prosthesis
Use additional code to identify infection

T84.50 Infection and inflammatory reaction due to unspecified internal joint prosthesis
AHA: Q1, 2015

T84.51 Infection and inflammatory reaction due to internal right hip prosthesis
AHA: Q4, 2015

T84.52 Infection and inflammatory reaction due to internal left hip prosthesis
AHA: Q1, 2015

T84.53 Infection and inflammatory reaction due to internal right knee prosthesis

T84.54 Infection and inflammatory reaction due to internal left knee prosthesis

T84.59 Infection and inflammatory reaction due to other internal joint prosthesis

T84.6 Infection and inflammatory reaction due to internal fixation device
Use additional code to identify infection

T84.60 Infection and inflammatory reaction due to internal fixation device of unspecified site HAC

T84.61 Infection and inflammatory reaction due to internal fixation device of arm

T84.610 Infection and inflammatory reaction due to internal fixation device of right humerus HAC

T84.611 Infection and inflammatory reaction due to internal fixation device of left humerus HAC

T84.612 Infection and inflammatory reaction due to internal fixation device of right radius HAC

T84.613 Infection and inflammatory reaction due to internal fixation device of left radius HAC

T84.614 Infection and inflammatory reaction due to internal fixation device of right ulna HAC

T84.615 Infection and inflammatory reaction due to internal fixation device of left ulna HAC

T84.619 Infection and inflammatory reaction due to internal fixation device of unspecified bone of arm HAC

T84.62 Infection and inflammatory reaction due to internal fixation device of leg

T84.620 Infection and inflammatory reaction due to internal fixation device of right femur

T84.621 Infection and inflammatory reaction due to internal fixation device of left femur

T84.622 Infection and inflammatory reaction due to internal fixation device of right tibia

T84.623 Infection and inflammatory reaction due to internal fixation device of left tibia

T84.624 Infection and inflammatory reaction due to internal fixation device of right fibula

T84.625 Infection and inflammatory reaction due to internal fixation device of left fibula

T84.629 Infection and inflammatory reaction due to internal fixation device of unspecified bone of leg

Unspecified Code | Other Specified Code | Manifestation Code | N Newborn | P Pediatric | M Maternity | A Adult | ♂ Male | ♀ Female
● New Code ▲ Revised Code Title ►◄ Revised Text NOTES INCLUDES EXCLUDES1 Not coded here EXCLUDES2 Not included here
4th character required 5th character required 6th character required 7th character required
Extension 'X' Alert HAC Hospital-acquired condition (HAC) alert AHA AHA Coding Clinic®

T84.63 **Infection and inflammatory reaction due to internal fixation device of spine** CC HAC

T84.69 **Infection and inflammatory reaction due to internal fixation device of other site** CC HAC

T84.7 Infection and inflammatory reaction due to other internal orthopedic prosthetic devices, implants and grafts CC HAC
Use additional code to identify infection

T84.8 Other specified complications of internal orthopedic prosthetic devices, implants and grafts

T84.81 **Embolism due to internal orthopedic prosthetic devices, implants and grafts** CC

T84.82 **Fibrosis due to internal orthopedic prosthetic devices, implants and grafts** CC

T84.83 **Hemorrhage due to internal orthopedic prosthetic devices, implants and grafts** CC

T84.84 **Pain due to internal orthopedic prosthetic devices, implants and grafts** CC

T84.85 **Stenosis due to internal orthopedic prosthetic devices, implants and grafts** CC

T84.86 **Thrombosis due to internal orthopedic prosthetic devices, implants and grafts** CC

T84.89 **Other specified complication of internal orthopedic prosthetic devices, implants and grafts** CC

T84.9 Unspecified complication of internal orthopedic prosthetic device, implant and graft CC

T85 Complications of other internal prosthetic devices, implants and grafts

EXCLUDES2 *failure and rejection of transplanted organs and tissue (T86.-)*

The appropriate 7th character is to be added to each code from category T85

A = initial encounter
D = subsequent encounter
S = sequela

T85.0 Mechanical complication of ventricular intracranial (communicating) shunt

T85.01 **Breakdown (mechanical) of ventricular intracranial (communicating) shunt** CC

T85.02 **Displacement of ventricular intracranial (communicating) shunt** CC
Malposition of ventricular intracranial (communicating) shunt

T85.03 **Leakage of ventricular intracranial (communicating) shunt** CC

T85.09 **Other mechanical complication of ventricular intracranial (communicating) shunt** CC
Obstruction (mechanical) of ventricular intracranial (communicating) shunt
Perforation of ventricular intracranial (communicating) shunt
Protrusion of ventricular intracranial (communicating) shunt

T85.1 Mechanical complication of implanted electronic stimulator of nervous system

T85.11 **Breakdown (mechanical) of implanted electronic stimulator of nervous system**

▲ T85.110 **Breakdown (mechanical) of implanted electronic neurostimulator ▶of brain electrode (lead)◀** CC

▲ T85.111 **Breakdown (mechanical) of implanted electronic neurostimulator ▶of peripheral nerve electrode (lead)◀** CC
Breakdown of electrode (lead) for cranial nerve neurostimulators
Breakdown of electrode (lead) for gastric neurostimulator
Breakdown of electrode (lead) for sacral nerve neurostimulator
Breakdown of electrode (lead) for vagal nerve neurostimulators

▲ T85.112 **Breakdown (mechanical) of implanted electronic neurostimulator ▶of spinal cord electrode (lead)◀** CC

● T85.113 **Breakdown (mechanical) of implanted electronic neurostimulator, generator** CC CC/MCC Exc
Breakdown (mechanical) of implanted electronic neurostimulator generator, brain, peripheral, gastric, spinal
Breakdown (mechanical) of implanted electronic sacral neurostimulator, pulse generator or receiver

T85.118 **Breakdown (mechanical) of other implanted electronic stimulator of nervous system** CC

T85.12 **Displacement of implanted electronic stimulator of nervous system**
Malposition of implanted electronic stimulator of nervous system

▲ T85.120 **Displacement of implanted electronic neurostimulator ▶of brain electrode (lead)◀** CC

▲ T85.121 **Displacement of implanted electronic neurostimulator ▶of peripheral nerve electrode (lead)◀** CC
Displacement of electrode (lead) for cranial nerve neurostimulators
Displacement of electrode (lead) for gastric neurostimulator
Displacement of electrode (lead) for sacral nerve neurostimulator
Displacement of electrode (lead) for vagal nerve neurostimulators

▲ T85.122 **Displacement of implanted electronic neurostimulator ▶of spinal cord electrode (lead)◀** CC

● ▲ T85.123 **Displacement of implanted electronic neurostimulator, generator** CC CC/MCC Exc
Displacement of implanted electronic neurostimulator generator, brain, peripheral, gastric, spinal
Displacement of implanted electronic sacral neurostimulator, pulse generator or receiver

T85.128 **Displacement of other implanted electronic stimulator of nervous system** CC

T85.19 **Other mechanical complication of implanted electronic stimulator of nervous system**
Leakage of implanted electronic stimulator of nervous system
Obstruction (mechanical) of implanted electronic stimulator of nervous system
Perforation of implanted electronic stimulator of nervous system
Protrusion of implanted electronic stimulator of nervous system

▲ T85.190 **Other mechanical complication of implanted electronic neurostimulator ▶of brain electrode (lead)◀** CC

▲ T85.191 **Other mechanical complication of implanted electronic neurostimulator ▶of peripheral nerve electrode (lead)◀** CC
Other mechanical complication of electrode (lead) for cranial nerve neurostimulators
Other mechanical complication of electrode (lead) for gastric neurostimulator
Other mechanical complication of electrode (lead) for sacral nerve neurostimulator
Other mechanical complication of electrode (lead) for vagal nerve neurostimulators

▲ T85.192 **Other mechanical complication of implanted electronic neurostimulator ▶of spinal cord electrode (lead)◀** CC

● T85.193 **Other mechanical complication of implanted electronic neurostimulator, generator** CC CC/MCC Exc
Other mechanical complication of implanted electronic neurostimulator generator, brain, peripheral, gastric, spinal
Other mechanical complication of implanted electronic sacral neurostimulator, pulse generator or receiver

PDx Unacceptable principal diagnosis symbol per Medicare code edits · POA Code exempt from diagnosis present on admission requirement
Q Questionable admission · CC Complication or comorbidity · CC/MCC Exc CC/MCC exclusion · MCC Major complication or comorbidity
PDx CC Principal diagnosis as its own CC · PDx MCC Principal diagnosis as its own MCC · Z1 Z code as first-listed diagnosis

T85.199 Other mechanical complication of other implanted electronic stimulator of nervous system

T85.2 Mechanical complication of intraocular lens

T85.21 Breakdown (mechanical) of intraocular lens

T85.22 Displacement of intraocular lens
Malposition of intraocular lens

T85.29 Other mechanical complication of intraocular lens
Obstruction (mechanical) of intraocular lens
Perforation of intraocular lens
Protrusion of intraocular lens

T85.3 Mechanical complication of other ocular prosthetic devices, implants and grafts
EXCLUDES2 *other complications of corneal graft (T86.84-)*

T85.31 Breakdown (mechanical) of other ocular prosthetic devices, implants and grafts

T85.310 Breakdown (mechanical) of prosthetic orbit of right eye

T85.311 Breakdown (mechanical) of prosthetic orbit of left eye

T85.318 Breakdown (mechanical) of other ocular prosthetic devices, implants and grafts

T85.32 Displacement of other ocular prosthetic devices, implants and grafts
Malposition of other ocular prosthetic devices, implants and grafts

T85.320 Displacement of prosthetic orbit of right eye

T85.321 Displacement of prosthetic orbit of left eye

T85.328 Displacement of other ocular prosthetic devices, implants and grafts

T85.39 Other mechanical complication of other ocular prosthetic devices, implants and grafts
Obstruction (mechanical) of other ocular prosthetic devices, implants and grafts
Perforation of other ocular prosthetic devices, implants and grafts
Protrusion of other ocular prosthetic devices, implants and grafts

T85.390 Other mechanical complication of prosthetic orbit of right eye

T85.391 Other mechanical complication of prosthetic orbit of left eye

T85.398 Other mechanical complication of other ocular prosthetic devices, implants and grafts

T85.4 Mechanical complication of breast prosthesis and implant

T85.41 Breakdown (mechanical) of breast prosthesis and implant

T85.42 Displacement of breast prosthesis and implant
Malposition of breast prosthesis and implant

T85.43 Leakage of breast prosthesis and implant

T85.44 Capsular contracture of breast implant

T85.49 Other mechanical complication of breast prosthesis and implant
Obstruction (mechanical) of breast prosthesis and implant
Perforation of breast prosthesis and implant
Protrusion of breast prosthesis and implant

T85.5 Mechanical complication of gastrointestinal prosthetic devices, implants and grafts

T85.51 Breakdown (mechanical) of gastrointestinal prosthetic devices, implants and grafts

T85.510 Breakdown (mechanical) of bile duct prosthesis

T85.511 Breakdown (mechanical) of esophageal anti-reflux device

T85.518 Breakdown (mechanical) of other gastrointestinal prosthetic devices, implants and grafts

T85.52 Displacement of gastrointestinal prosthetic devices, implants and grafts
Malposition of gastrointestinal prosthetic devices, implants and grafts

T85.520 Displacement of bile duct prosthesis

T85.521 Displacement of esophageal anti-reflux device

T85.528 Displacement of other gastrointestinal prosthetic devices, implants and grafts

T85.59 Other mechanical complication of gastrointestinal prosthetic devices, implants and grafts
Obstruction, mechanical of gastrointestinal prosthetic devices, implants and grafts
Perforation of gastrointestinal prosthetic devices, implants and grafts
Protrusion of gastrointestinal prosthetic devices, implants and grafts

T85.590 Other mechanical complication of bile duct prosthesis

T85.591 Other mechanical complication of esophageal anti-reflux device

T85.598 Other mechanical complication of other gastrointestinal prosthetic devices, implants and grafts

T85.6 Mechanical complication of other specified internal and external prosthetic devices, implants and grafts

T85.61 Breakdown (mechanical) of other specified internal prosthetic devices, implants and grafts

▲ T85.610 Breakdown (mechanical) of ▶cranial or spinal◀ infusion catheter
Breakdown (mechanical) of epidural infusion catheter
Breakdown (mechanical) of intrathecal infusion catheter
Breakdown (mechanical) of subarachnoid infusion catheter
Breakdown (mechanical) of subdural infusion catheter

T85.611 Breakdown (mechanical) of intraperitoneal dialysis catheter
EXCLUDES1 *mechanical complication of vascular dialysis catheter (T82.4-)*

T85.612 Breakdown (mechanical) of permanent sutures
EXCLUDES1 *mechanical complication of permanent (wire) suture used in bone repair (T84.1-T84.2)*

T85.613 Breakdown (mechanical) of artificial skin graft and decellularized allodermis
Failure of artificial skin graft and decellularized allodermis
Non-adherence of artificial skin graft and decellularized allodermis
Poor incorporation of artificial skin graft and decellularized allodermis
Shearing of artificial skin graft and decellularized allodermis

T85.614 Breakdown (mechanical) of insulin pump

● T85.615 Breakdown (mechanical) of other nervous system device, implant or graft
Breakdown (mechanical) of intrathecal infusion pump

T85.618 Breakdown (mechanical) of other specified internal prosthetic devices, implants and grafts

T85.62 Displacement of other specified internal prosthetic devices, implants and grafts
Malposition of other specified internal prosthetic devices, implants and grafts

▲ T85.620 Displacement of ▶cranial or spinal◀ infusion catheter
Displacement of epidural infusion catheter
Displacement of intrathecal infusion catheter
Displacement of subarachnoid infusion catheter
Displacement of subdural infusion catheter

T85.621 Displacement of intraperitoneal dialysis catheter
EXCLUDES1 *mechanical complication of vascular dialysis catheter (T82.4-)*

Unspecified Code | Other Specified Code | Manifestation Code | N Newborn | P Pediatric | M Maternity | A Adult | ♂ Male | ♀ Female
● New Code ▲ Revised Code Title ▶◀ Revised Text NOTES INCLUDES EXCLUDES1 Not coded here EXCLUDES2 Not included here
4th character required 5th character required 6th character required 7th character required
Extension 'X' Alert HAC Hospital-acquired condition (HAC) alert AHA AHA Coding Clinic©

T85.622 **Displacement of permanent sutures**
EXCLUDES1 *mechanical complication of permanent (wire) suture used in bone repair (T84.1-T84.2)*

T85.623 **Displacement of artificial skin graft and decellularized allodermis**
Dislodgement of artificial skin graft and decellularized allodermis
Displacement of artificial skin graft and decellularized allodermis

T85.624 **Displacement of insulin pump**

● T85.625 **Displacement of other nervous system device, implant or graft**
Displacement of intrathecal infusion pump

T85.628 **Displacement of other specified internal prosthetic devices, implants and grafts**
AHA: Q1, 2015

T85.63 **Leakage of other specified internal prosthetic devices, implants and grafts**

▲ T85.630 **Leakage of ►cranial or spinal◄ infusion catheter**
Leakage of epidural infusion catheter
Leakage of intrathecal infusion catheter infusion catheter
Leakage of subdural infusion catheter
Leakage of subarachnoid infusion catheter

T85.631 **Leakage of intraperitoneal dialysis catheter**
EXCLUDES1 *mechanical complication of vascular dialysis catheter (T82.4)*

T85.633 **Leakage of insulin pump**

● T85.635 **Leakage of other nervous system device, implant or graft**
Leakage of intrathecal infusion pump

T85.638 **Leakage of other specified internal prosthetic devices, implants and grafts**

T85.69 **Other mechanical complication of other specified internal prosthetic devices, implants and grafts**
Obstruction, mechanical of other specified internal prosthetic devices, implants and grafts
Perforation of other specified internal prosthetic devices, implants and grafts
Protrusion of other specified internal prosthetic devices, implants and grafts

▲ T85.690 **Other mechanical complication of ►cranial or spinal◄ infusion catheter**
Other mechanical complication of epidural infusion catheter
Other mechanical complication of intrathecal infusion catheter
Other mechanical complication of subarachnoid infusion catheter
Other mechanical complication of subdural infusion catheter

T85.691 **Other mechanical complication of intraperitoneal dialysis catheter**
EXCLUDES1 *mechanical complication of vascular dialysis catheter (T82.4)*

T85.692 **Other mechanical complication of permanent sutures**
EXCLUDES1 *mechanical complication of permanent (wire) suture used in bone repair (T84.1-T84.2)*

T85.693 **Other mechanical complication of artificial skin graft and decellularized allodermis**

T85.694 **Other mechanical complication of insulin pump**

● T85.695 **Other mechanical complication of other nervous system device, implant or graft**
Other mechanical complication of intrathecal infusion pump

T85.698 **Other mechanical complication of other specified internal prosthetic devices, implants and grafts**
Mechanical complication of nonabsorbable surgical material NOS

T85.7 **Infection and inflammatory reaction due to other internal prosthetic devices, implants and grafts**
Use additional code to identify infection

T85.71 **Infection and inflammatory reaction due to peritoneal dialysis catheter**

T85.72 **Infection and inflammatory reaction due to insulin pump**

● T85.73 **Infection and inflammatory reaction due to nervous system devices, implants and graft**

● T85.730 **Infection and inflammatory reaction due to ventricular intracranial (communicating) shunt**

● T85.731 **Infection and inflammatory reaction due to implanted electronic neurostimulator of brain, electrode (lead)**

● T85.732 **Infection and inflammatory reaction due to implanted electronic neurostimulator of peripheral nerve, electrode (lead)**
Infection and inflammatory reaction due to electrode (lead) for cranial nerve neurostimulators
Infection and inflammatory reaction due to electrode (lead) for gastric neurostimulator
Infection and inflammatory reaction due to electrode (lead) for sacral nerve neurostimulator
Infection and inflammatory reaction due to electrode (lead) for vagal nerve neurostimulators

● T85.733 **Infection and inflammatory reaction due to implanted electronic neurostimulator of spinal cord, electrode (lead)**

● T85.734 **Infection and inflammatory reaction due to implanted electronic neurostimulator, generator**
Generator pocket infection

● T85.735 **Infection and inflammatory reaction due to cranial or spinal infusion catheter**
Infection and inflammatory reaction due to epidural catheter
Infection and inflammatory reaction due to intrathecal infusion catheter
Infection and inflammatory reaction due to subarachnoid catheter
Infection and inflammatory reaction due to subdural catheter

● T85.738 **Infection and inflammatory reaction due to other nervous system device, implant or graft**
Infection and inflammatory reaction due to intrathecal infusion pump

T85.79 **Infection and inflammatory reaction due to other internal prosthetic devices, implants and grafts**

T85.8 **Other specified complications of internal prosthetic devices, implants and grafts, not elsewhere classified**

T85.81 **Embolism due to internal prosthetic devices, implants and grafts, not elsewhere classified**

● T85.810 **Embolism due to nervous system prosthetic devices, implants and grafts**

● T85.818 **Embolism due to other internal prosthetic devices, implants and grafts**

T85.82 **Fibrosis due to internal prosthetic devices, implants and grafts, not elsewhere classified**

● T85.820 **Fibrosis due to nervous system prosthetic devices, implants and grafts**

● T85.828 **Fibrosis due to other internal prosthetic devices, implants and grafts**

T85.83 **Hemorrhage due to internal prosthetic devices, implants and grafts, not elsewhere classified**

● T85.830 **Hemorrhage due to nervous system prosthetic devices, implants and grafts**

Unacceptable principal diagnosis symbol per Medicare code edits | Code exempt from diagnosis present on admission requirement
Questionable admission | Complication or comorbidity | CC/MCC exclusion | Major complication or comorbidity
Principal diagnosis as its own CC | Principal diagnosis as its own MCC | Z code as first-listed diagnosis

- ● T85.838 Hemorrhage due to other internal prosthetic devices, implants and grafts
- T85.84 Pain due to internal prosthetic devices, implants and grafts, not elsewhere classified
  - ● T85.840 Pain due to nervous system prosthetic devices, implants and grafts CC CC/MCC Exc
  - ● T85.848 Pain due to other internal prosthetic devices, implants and grafts
- T85.85 Stenosis due to internal prosthetic devices, implants and grafts, not elsewhere classified
  - ● T85.850 Stenosis due to nervous system prosthetic devices, implants and grafts CC CC/MCC Exc
  - ● T85.858 Stenosis due to other internal prosthetic devices, implants and grafts
- T85.86 Thrombosis due to internal prosthetic devices, implants and grafts, not elsewhere classified
  - ● T85.860 Thrombosis due to nervous system prosthetic devices, implants and grafts CC CC/MCC Exc
  - ● T85.868 Thrombosis due to other internal prosthetic devices, implants and grafts
- T85.89 Other specified complication of internal prosthetic devices, implants and grafts, not elsewhere classified
  Erosion or breakdown of subcutaneous device pocket
  - ● T85.890 Other specified complication of nervous system prosthetic devices, implants and grafts CC CC/MCC Exc
  - ● T85.898 Other specified complication of other internal prosthetic devices, implants and grafts

T85.9 Unspecified complication of internal prosthetic device, implant and graft
Complication of internal prosthetic device, implant and graft NOS

T86 Complications of transplanted organs and tissue

Use additional code to identify other transplant complications, such as:
graft-versus-host disease (D89.81-)
malignancy associated with organ transplant (C80.2)
post-transplant lymphoproliferative disorders (PTLD) (D47.Z1)

T86.0 Complications of bone marrow transplant
- T86.00 Unspecified complication of bone marrow transplant CC
- T86.01 Bone marrow transplant rejection CC
- T86.02 Bone marrow transplant failure CC
- T86.03 Bone marrow transplant infection CC
- T86.09 Other complications of bone marrow transplant CC

T86.1 Complications of kidney transplant
- T86.10 Unspecified complication of kidney transplant CC
- T86.11 Kidney transplant rejection CC
- T86.12 Kidney transplant failure CC
  AHA: Q1, 2013
- T86.13 Kidney transplant infection CC
  Use additional code to specify infection
- T86.19 Other complication of kidney transplant CC

T86.2 Complications of heart transplant
EXCLUDES1 *complication of:*
artificial heart device (T82.5)
heart-lung transplant (T86.3)
- T86.20 Unspecified complication of heart transplant CC
- T86.21 Heart transplant rejection CC
- T86.22 Heart transplant failure CC
- T86.23 Heart transplant infection CC
  Use additional code to specify infection
- T86.29 Other complications of heart transplant
  - T86.290 Cardiac allograft vasculopathy CC
    EXCLUDES1 *atherosclerosis of coronary arteries (I25.75-, I25.76-, I25.81-)*
  - T86.298 Other complications of heart transplant CC

T86.3 Complications of heart-lung transplant
- T86.30 Unspecified complication of heart-lung transplant CC PDx
- T86.31 Heart-lung transplant rejection CC PDx
- T86.32 Heart-lung transplant failure CC PDx
- T86.33 Heart-lung transplant infection CC PDx
  Use additional code to specify infection
- T86.39 Other complications of heart-lung transplant CC PDx

T86.4 Complications of liver transplant
- T86.40 Unspecified complication of liver transplant CC
- T86.41 Liver transplant rejection CC
- T86.42 Liver transplant failure CC
- T86.43 Liver transplant infection CC
  Use additional code to identify infection, such as:
  Cytomegalovirus (CMV) infection (B25.-)
- T86.49 Other complications of liver transplant CC

T86.5 Complications of stem cell transplant CC
Complications from stem cells from peripheral blood
Complications from stem cells from umbilical cord

T86.8 Complications of other transplanted organs and tissues
- T86.81 Complications of lung transplant
  EXCLUDES1 *complication of heart-lung transplant (T86.3-)*
  - T86.810 Lung transplant rejection CC
  - T86.811 Lung transplant failure CC
  - T86.812 Lung transplant infection CC
    Use additional code to specify infection
  - T86.818 Other complications of lung transplant CC
  - T86.819 Unspecified complication of lung transplant CC
- T86.82 Complications of skin graft (allograft) (autograft)
  EXCLUDES2 *complication of artificial skin graft (T85.693)*
  - T86.820 Skin graft (allograft) rejection CC
  - T86.821 Skin graft (allograft) (autograft) failure CC
  - T86.822 Skin graft (allograft) (autograft) infection CC
    Use additional code to specify infection
  - T86.828 Other complications of skin graft (allograft) (autograft) CC
  - T86.829 Unspecified complication of skin graft (allograft) (autograft) CC
- T86.83 Complications of bone graft
  EXCLUDES2 *mechanical complications of bone graft (T84.3-)*
  - T86.830 Bone graft rejection CC
  - T86.831 Bone graft failure CC
  - T86.832 Bone graft infection CC
    Use additional code to specify infection
  - T86.838 Other complications of bone graft CC
  - T86.839 Unspecified complication of bone graft CC
- T86.84 Complications of corneal transplant
  EXCLUDES2 *mechanical complications of corneal graft (T85.3-)*
  - T86.840 Corneal transplant rejection CC
  - T86.841 Corneal transplant failure CC
  - T86.842 Corneal transplant infection CC
    Use additional code to specify infection
  - T86.848 Other complications of corneal transplant CC
  - T86.849 Unspecified complication of corneal transplant CC
- T86.85 Complication of intestine transplant
  - T86.850 Intestine transplant rejection CC
  - T86.851 Intestine transplant failure CC
  - T86.852 Intestine transplant infection CC
    Use additional code to specify infection
  - T86.858 Other complications of intestine transplant CC
  - T86.859 Unspecified complication of intestine transplant CC
- T86.89 Complications of other transplanted tissue
  Transplant failure or rejection of pancreas
  - T86.890 Other transplanted tissue rejection CC
  - T86.891 Other transplanted tissue failure CC
  - T86.892 Other transplanted tissue infection CC
    Use additional code to specify infection
  - T86.898 Other complications of other transplanted tissue CC

T86.899 Unspecified complication of other transplanted tissue

T86.9 Complication of unspecified transplanted organ and tissue

T86.90 Unspecified complication of unspecified transplanted organ and tissue

T86.91 Unspecified transplanted organ and tissue rejection

T86.92 Unspecified transplanted organ and tissue failure

T86.93 Unspecified transplanted organ and tissue infection
Use additional code to specify infection

T86.99 Other complications of unspecified transplanted organ and tissue

T87 Complications peculiar to reattachment and amputation

T87.0 Complications of reattached (part of) upper extremity

T87.0X Complications of reattached (part of) upper extremity

T87.0X1 Complications of reattached (part of) right upper extremity

T87.0X2 Complications of reattached (part of) left upper extremity

T87.0X9 Complications of reattached (part of) unspecified upper extremity

T87.1 Complications of reattached (part of) lower extremity

T87.1X Complications of reattached (part of) lower extremity

T87.1X1 Complications of reattached (part of) right lower extremity

T87.1X2 Complications of reattached (part of) left lower extremity

T87.1X9 Complications of reattached (part of) unspecified lower extremity

T87.2 Complications of other reattached body part

T87.3 Neuroma of amputation stump

T87.30 Neuroma of amputation stump, unspecified extremity

T87.31 Neuroma of amputation stump, right upper extremity

T87.32 Neuroma of amputation stump, left upper extremity

T87.33 Neuroma of amputation stump, right lower extremity

T87.34 Neuroma of amputation stump, left lower extremity

T87.4 Infection of amputation stump

T87.40 Infection of amputation stump, unspecified extremity

T87.41 Infection of amputation stump, right upper extremity

T87.42 Infection of amputation stump, left upper extremity

T87.43 Infection of amputation stump, right lower extremity

T87.44 Infection of amputation stump, left lower extremity

T87.5 Necrosis of amputation stump

T87.50 Necrosis of amputation stump, unspecified extremity

T87.51 Necrosis of amputation stump, right upper extremity

T87.52 Necrosis of amputation stump, left upper extremity

T87.53 Necrosis of amputation stump, right lower extremity

T87.54 Necrosis of amputation stump, left lower extremity

T87.8 Other complications of amputation stump

T87.81 Dehiscence of amputation stump

T87.89 Other complications of amputation stump
Amputation stump contracture
Amputation stump contracture of next proximal joint
Amputation stump flexion
Amputation stump edema
Amputation stump hematoma
EXCLUDES2 *phantom limb syndrome (G54.6-G54.7)*

T87.9 Unspecified complications of amputation stump

T88 Other complications of surgical and medical care, not elsewhere classified

EXCLUDES2 *complication following infusion, transfusion and therapeutic injection (T80.-)*
complication following procedure NEC (T81.-)
complications of anesthesia in labor and delivery (O74.-)
complications of anesthesia in pregnancy (O29.-)
complications of anesthesia in puerperium (O89.-)
complications of devices, implants and grafts (T82-T85)
complications of obstetric surgery and procedure (O75.4)
dermatitis due to drugs and medicaments (L23.3, L24.4, L25.1, L27.0-L27.1)
poisoning and toxic effects of drugs and chemicals (T36-T65 with fifth or sixth character 1-4 or 6)
specified complications classified elsewhere

The appropriate 7th character is to be added to each code from category T88
A = initial encounter
D = subsequent encounter
S = sequela

T88.0 Infection following immunization
Sepsis following immunization

T88.1 Other complications following immunization, not elsewhere classified
Generalized vaccinia
Rash following immunization
EXCLUDES1 *vaccinia not from vaccine (B08.011)*
EXCLUDES2 *anaphylactic shock due to serum (T80.5-)*
other serum reactions (T80.6-)
postimmunization arthropathy (M02.2)
postimmunization encephalitis (G04.02)
postimmunization fever (R50.83)

T88.2 Shock due to anesthesia
Use additional code for adverse effect, if applicable, to identify drug (T41.- with fifth or sixth character 5)
EXCLUDES1 *complications of anesthesia (in):*
labor and delivery (O74.-)
pregnancy (O29.-)
puerperium (O89.-)
postprocedural shock NOS (T81.1-)

T88.3 Malignant hyperthermia due to anesthesia
Use additional code for adverse effect, if applicable, to identify drug (T41.- with fifth or sixth character 5)

T88.4 Failed or difficult intubation

T88.5 Other complications of anesthesia
Use additional code for adverse effect, if applicable, to identify drug (T41.- with fifth or sixth character 5)

T88.51 Hypothermia following anesthesia

T88.52 Failed moderate sedation during procedure
Failed conscious sedation during procedure
EXCLUDES2 *personal history of failed moderate sedation (Z92.83)*

● T88.53 Unintended awareness under general anesthesia during procedure
EXCLUDES2 *personal history of unintended awareness under general anesthesia (Z92.84)*

T88.59 Other complications of anesthesia

T88.6 Anaphylactic reaction due to adverse effect of correct drug or medicament properly administered
Anaphylactic shock due to adverse effect of correct drug or medicament properly administered
Anaphylactoid reaction NOS
Use additional code for adverse effect, if applicable, to identify drug (T36-T50 with fifth or sixth character 5)
EXCLUDES1 *anaphylactic reaction due to serum (T80.5-)*
anaphylactic shock or reaction due to adverse food reaction (T78.0-)

T88.7 Unspecified adverse effect of drug or medicament
Drug hypersensitivity NOS
Drug reaction NOS
Use additional code for adverse effect, if applicable, to identify drug (T36-T50 with fifth or sixth character 5)
EXCLUDES1 *specified adverse effects of drugs and medicaments (A00-R94 and T80-T88.6, T88.8)*

T88.8 Other specified complications of surgical and medical care, not elsewhere classified
Use additional code to identify the complication

T88.9 Complication of surgical and medical care, unspecified

Unacceptable principal diagnosis symbol per Medicare code edits · Code exempt from diagnosis present on admission requirement · Questionable admission · Complication or comorbidity · CC/MCC exclusion · Major complication or comorbidity · Principal diagnosis as its own CC · Principal diagnosis as its own MCC · Z code as first-listed diagnosis

When symbols appear on a code that requires a 7th character extension, refer to Appendix D to identify applicable 7th character codes.

Chapter 20: External Causes of Morbidity (V00-Y99)

Guidelines for Assigning Codes From This Chapter

Chapter 20's title refers to the cause of an injury or health condition, whether the intent behind the cause was intentional or unintentional/accidental (e.g., whether an injury was due to suicide or assault), the patient's location or activity at the time of the event, and whether the patient was a civilian or in the military.

The key to properly applying these codes is understanding that the purpose of these codes is for research — to provide data on the causes of injuries and other health conditions so that the government and healthcare agencies can come up with strategies to prevent them. There is no mandatory national requirement for reporting external causes of morbidity, but a state or individual payer may have such requirements. However, it is hoped that providers will voluntarily report these codes for the valuable data they provide, as noted above.

List of Sections

- V00-X58: Accidents
- X71-X83: Intentional self-harm
- X92-Y08: Assault
- Y21-Y33: Event of undetermined intent
- Y35-Y38: Legal intervention, operations of war, military operations, and terrorism
- Y62-Y84: Complications of medical and surgical care
- Y90-Y99: Supplementary factors related to causes of morbidity classified elsewhere

Highlights From the ICD-10-CM Official Guidelines for Coding and Reporting

The ICD-10-CM Official Guidelines for Coding and Reporting for Chapter 20 supply important guidance on everything from the application of 7th characters to sequencing codes in the correct order. The information below is from the 2017 Official Guidelines.

Know When to Apply an External Cause of Morbidity Code

The primary application for these codes is injuries. However, these codes may also apply to diseases, infections, and other health conditions that can be attributed to an external cause and that can be reported with a code in the range of A00.0-T88.9 or Z00-Z99. For example, if a stroke occurs during a boxing match or a player has a heart attack during a football game, it would be appropriate to apply an external cause code. *Never use a code from Chapter 20 as the principal or primary (first-listed) diagnosis code.*

Add a 7th Character for Each Encounter

Most of the codes in Chapter 20 require a 7th character (A, initial encounter; D, subsequent encounter; or S, Sequela) for each encounter while the patient is under treatment for an injury or condition. When the patient is seen by a new or different provider, match the 7th character to the encounter. That is, if a patient is seen in the emergency room for an injury, that's the initial encounter. If the patient is referred to a surgeon to repair a fracture, the encounter is still an initial encounter, because the patient is undergoing active treatment for the injury. Once the fracture has been repaired and is healing, follow-up visits would be coded as subsequent encounters. Sequela, of course, is used when the patient suffers a "late effect" or condition resulting from the trauma after the fracture has healed.

Note: Y92 is a notable exception to the 7th character code requirement.

Assign all external cause codes that apply. You may need multiple codes to fully explain the circumstances surrounding an injury or other condition. When not limited by the number you can record, add as many of these external cause codes as apply:

- Code cause of the injury or condition
- Code the intent — was it assault, self-inflicted, accidental, unknown?
- Code the location where the injury occurred.
- Code the activity the patient was involved in, if applicable
- Code the patient's status — driver, passenger, pedestrian; civilian or military; other

Get the Sequencing Right Every Time

Use the Alphabetic Index of External Causes to find the appropriate codes and watch Inclusion and Exclusion notes in the Tabular List to be sure you're applying the appropriate code(s). When you are applying external cause codes, keep these guidelines in mind:

1. External cause codes should be applied in the following order:

- Child and adult abuse
- Terrorism events
- Cataclysmic events
- Transport accidents

2. If you can record only one external cause code, use the one describing the cause most closely related to the primary diagnosis.
3. Separate injuries caused by separate events should be assigned a separate code for each cause.
4. If you can add more codes, cause and intent, including complications of surgery and medical care, always take precedence over codes for place, activity, or status.
5. Activity and status codes follow cause codes, if applicable, and if there is room on the form.

External cause codes aren't always necessary. Do not add an external cause code if the primary diagnosis code includes the cause, for example, many of the T poisoning codes in Chapter 19.

4. Sequence of events. When you choose a combination code that describes a sequence of events, the order of events should follow the same order in which the event happened. Try to choose a code that sequences the cause of the most serious injury first.

Place of occurrence, activity, and status. In general, Y92 (*Place of occurrence of the external cause*) codes, Y93 (*Activity codes*), and Y99 (External cause status) codes are assigned only for the initial encounter for treatment.

Rarely, a new injury, such as might occur during hospitalization, would require an the addition of a Y92 code to subsequent encounters. Seventh characters are not used with Y92 codes. The guidelines state, "Do not use place of occurrence code Y92.9 (*Unspecified place or not applicable*) if the place is not stated or is not applicable." As this statement appears to present a conflict, confirm the use of this code with your payer.

Add Y93 only if the activity is relevant to the diagnosis. Y93 codes do not apply to adverse effects, poisonings, or complications of surgery or medical care. The guidelines state, "Do not assign Y93.9 (*Activity, unspecified*) if the activity is not stated." This statement also appears to present a conflict, so confirm the use of this code with your payer.

Assign Y99 codes to indicate the work status of the person at the time of the causal event, whether military, nonmilitary, or student/volunteer in a nonwork activity. If there is no external cause code assigned, do not assign a Y99 code. Y99 codes are applicable to other external cause codes, such as transport accidents and falls but not to poisonings, adverse effects, injuries during surgery or medical care, or sequela. The guidelines also state, "Do not assign code Y99.9 (*Unspecified external cause status*) if the status is not stated." Again, confirm the use of this code with your payer to eliminate the conflict.

Look to X92-Y08 (Assault) for Child and Adult Abuse

Any of the assault codes may be applied to record the external cause of an injury due to confirmed abuse. When the person who inflicted the abuse or is responsible for neglect or maltreatment is known, add a code from Y07 (*Perpetrator of maltreatment and neglect*) to the assault code. See also Section I.C.19. Adult and child abuse, neglect and other maltreatment.

Know When to Use Undetermined Intent Category

Use an accidental intent code if the cause is not known or not specified. Use undetermined intent external cause codes only if the medical record specifies that the intent cannot be determined. All transport accident categories are assumed to be accidental.

No Need for Assault Code When Terrorism Code Applies

ICD-10-CM includes a specific definition for terrorism in an inclusion note with the category Y38 (*Terrorism*). When the cause of the patient's injury meets that terrorism definition, choose a code from the Y38 category. If there is more than one mechanism of injury, you can use an additional Y38 code to identify it. You should not report a separate assault code. Add an additional code from the Y92.- category for place of occurrence.

Don't use this category when the cause is "suspected" terrorism. Classify suspected cases of terrorism as assault.

Assign code Y38.9 (*Terrorism, secondary effects*) for injuries or conditions that occurred as a result of the terrorist event. Do not assign Y38.9 to injuries resulting from the initial terrorist act. You can report code Y38.9 with another Y38 code when an injury is sustained in both the initial terrorist event and as a result of subsequent related events.

Tabular List

External causes of morbidity (V00-Y99)

NOTES This chapter permits the classification of environmental events and circumstances as the cause of injury, and other adverse effects. Where a code from this section is applicable, it is intended that it shall be used secondary to a code from another chapter of the Classification indicating the nature of the condition. Most often, the condition will be classifiable to Chapter 19, Injury, poisoning and certain other consequences of external causes (S00-T88). Other conditions that may be stated to be due to external causes are classified in Chapters I to XVIII. For these conditions, codes from Chapter 20 should be used to provide additional information as to the cause of the condition.

This chapter contains the following blocks:

Accidents (V00-X58)

Transport accidents (V00-V99)

NOTES This section is structured in 12 groups. Those relating to land transport accidents (V00-V89) reflect the victim's mode of transport and are subdivided to identify the victim's 'counterpart' or the type of event. The vehicle of which the injured person is an occupant is identified in the first two characters since it is seen as the most important factor to identify for prevention purposes. A transport accident is one in which the vehicle involved must be moving or running or in use for transport purposes at the time of the accident.

Use additional code to identify:

Airbag injury (W22.1)

Type of street or road (Y92.4-)

Use of cellular telephone and other electronic equipment at the time of the transport accident (Y93.C-)

EXCLUDES1 *agricultural vehicles in stationary use or maintenance (W31.-)*

assault by crashing of motor vehicle (Y03.-)

automobile or motor cycle in stationary use or maintenance- code to type of accident

crashing of motor vehicle, undetermined intent (Y32)

intentional self-harm by crashing of motor vehicle (X82)

EXCLUDES2 *transport accidents due to cataclysm (X34-X38)*

NOTES Definitions ▶related to transport accidents◀:

(a) A transport accident ▶(V00-V99)◀ is any accident involving a device designed primarily for, or used at the time primarily for, conveying persons or good from one place to another.

(b) A public highway traffic way or street is the entire width between property lines (or other boundary lines) of land open to the public as a matter of right or custom for purposes of moving persons or property from one place to another. A roadway is that part of the public highway designed, improved and customarily used for vehicular traffic.

(c) A traffic accident is any vehicle accident occurring on the public highway [i.e. originating on, terminating on, or involving a vehicle partially on the highway]. A vehicle accident is assumed to have occurred on the public highway unless another place is specified, except in the case of accidents involving only off-road motor vehicles, which are classified as nontraffic accidents unless the contrary is stated.

(d) A nontraffic accident is any vehicle accident that occurs entirely in any place other than a public highway.

(e) A pedestrian is any person involved in an accident who was not at the time of the accident riding in or on a motor vehicle, railway train, streetcar or animal-drawn or other vehicle, or on a pedal cycle or animal. This includes, a person changing a tire, ▶working on a parked car, or a person on foot. It also includes the user of a pedestrian conveyance such as a baby stroller, ice-skates, skis, sled,◀ roller skates, a skateboard, nonmotorized or motorized wheelchair, motorized mobility scooter, or nonmotorized scooter.

(f) A driver is an occupant of a transport vehicle who is operating or intending to operate it.

(g) A passenger is any occupant of a transport vehicle other than the driver, except a person traveling on the outside of the vehicle.

(h) A person on the outside of a vehicle is any person being transported by a vehicle but not occupying the space normally reserved for the driver or passengers, or the space intended for the transport of property. This includes ▶a person travelling on the bodywork, bumper, fender, roof, running board or step of a vehicle, as well as, hanging on the outside of the◀ vehicle.

(i) A pedal cycle is any land transport vehicle operated solely by nonmotorized pedals including a bicycle or tricycle.

(j) A pedal cyclist is any person riding a pedal cycle or in a sidecar or trailer attached to a pedal cycle.
(k) A motorcycle is a two-wheeled motor vehicle with one or two riding saddles and sometimes with a third wheel for the support of a sidecar. The sidecar is considered part of the motorcycle. ▶This includes a moped, motor scooter, or motorized bicycle.◀
(l) A motorcycle rider is any person riding a motorcycle or in a sidecar or trailer attached to the motorcycle.
(m) A three-wheeled motor vehicle is a motorized tricycle designed primarily for on-road use. This includes a motor-driven tricycle, a motorized rickshaw, or a three-wheeled motor car.
(n) A car [automobile] is a four-wheeled motor vehicle designed primarily for carrying up to 7 persons. A trailer being towed by the car is considered part of the car. ▶It does not include a van or minivan - *see* definition (o)◀
(o) A pick-up truck or van is a four or six-wheeled motor vehicle designed for carrying passengers as well as property or cargo weighing less than the local limit for classification as a heavy goods vehicle, and not requiring a special driver's license. This includes a minivan and a sport-utility vehicle (SUV).
(p) A heavy transport vehicle is a motor vehicle designed primarily for carrying property, meeting local criteria for classification as a heavy goods vehicle in terms of weight and requiring a special driver's license.
(q) A bus (coach) is a motor vehicle designed or adapted primarily for carrying more than 10 passengers, and requiring a special driver's license.
(r) A railway train or railway vehicle is any device, with or without freight or passenger cars couple to it, designed for traffic on a railway track. This includes subterranean (subways) or elevated trains.
(s) A streetcar, is a device designed and used primarily for transporting passengers within a municipality, running on rails, usually subject to normal traffic control signals, and operated principally on a right-of-way that forms part of the roadway. This includes a tram or trolley that runs on rails. A trailer being towed by a streetcar is considered part of the streetcar.
(t) A special vehicle mainly used on industrial premises is a motor vehicle designed primarily for use within the buildings and premises of industrial or commercial establishments. This includes battery-powered ▶airport passenger vehicles or baggage/mail trucks,◀ forklifts, coal-cars in a coal mine, logging cars and trucks used in mines or quarries.
(u) A special vehicle mainly used in agriculture is a motor vehicle designed specifically for use in farming and agriculture (horticulture), to work the land, tend and harvest crops and transport materials on the farm. This includes harvesters, farm machinery and tractor and trailers.
(v) A special construction vehicle is a motor vehicle designed specifically for use on construction and demolition sites. This includes bulldozers, diggers, earth levellers, dump trucks. backhoes, front-end loaders, pavers, and mechanical shovels.
(w) A special all-terrain vehicle is a motor vehicle of special design to enable it to negotiate over rough or soft terrain , snow or sand. ▶Examples of special design are high construction, special wheels and tires, tracks, and support on a cushion of air.◀ This includes snow mobiles, All-terrain vehicles (ATV), and dune buggies. It does not include passenger vehicle designated as Sport Utility Vehicles. (SUV)
(x) A watercraft is any device designed for transporting passengers or goods on water. This includes motor or sail boats, ships, and hovercraft.
(y) An aircraft is any device for transporting passengers or goods in the air. This includes hot-air balloons, gliders, helicopters and airplanes.
(z) A military vehicle is any motorized vehicle operating on a public roadway owned by the military and being operated by a member of the military.

Pedestrian injured in transport accident (V00-V09)

INCLUDES *person changing tire on transport vehicle*
person examining engine of vehicle broken down in (on side of) road

EXCLUDES1 *fall due to non-transport collision with other person (W03)*
pedestrian on foot falling (slipping) on ice and snow (W00.-)
struck or bumped by another person (W51)

V00 Pedestrian conveyance accident
Use additional place of occurrence and activity external cause codes, if known (Y92.-, Y93.-)

EXCLUDES1 *collision with another person without fall (W51)*
fall due to person on foot colliding with another person on foot (W03)
fall from non-moving wheelchair, nonmotorized scooter and motorized mobility scooter without collision (W05.-)
pedestrian (conveyance) collision with other land transport vehicle (V01-V09)
pedestrian on foot falling (slipping) on ice and snow (W00.-)

The appropriate 7th character is to be added to each code from category V00
A = initial encounter
D = subsequent encounter
S = sequela

V00.0 Pedestrian on foot injured in collision with pedestrian conveyance
V00.01 Pedestrian on foot injured in collision with roller-skater
V00.02 Pedestrian on foot injured in collision with skateboarder
V00.09 Pedestrian on foot injured in collision with other pedestrian conveyance

V00.1 Rolling-type pedestrian conveyance accident
EXCLUDES1 *accident with baby stroller (V00.82-)*
accident with wheelchair (powered) (V00.81-)
accident with motorized mobility scooter (V00.83-)

V00.11 In-line roller-skate accident
V00.111 Fall from in-line roller-skates
V00.112 In-line roller-skater colliding with stationary object
V00.118 Other in-line roller-skate accident
EXCLUDES1 *roller-skater collision with other land transport vehicle (V01-V09 with 5th character 1)*

V00.12 Non-in- line roller-skate accident
V00.121 Fall from non-in-line roller-skates
V00.122 Non-in-line roller-skater colliding with stationary object
V00.128 Other non-in-line roller-skating accident
EXCLUDES1 *roller-skater collision with other land transport vehicle (V01-V09 with 5th character 1)*

V00.13 Skateboard accident
V00.131 Fall from skateboard
V00.132 Skateboarder colliding with stationary object
V00.138 Other skateboard accident
EXCLUDES1 *skateboarder collision with other land transport vehicle (V01-V09 with 5th character 2)*

V00.14 Scooter (nonmotorized) accident
EXCLUDES1 *motor scooter accident (V20-V29)*
V00.141 Fall from scooter (nonmotorized)
V00.142 Scooter (nonmotorized) colliding with stationary object

Unacceptable principal diagnosis symbol per Medicare code edits | Code exempt from diagnosis present on admission requirement
Questionable admission | Complication or comorbidity | CC/MCC exclusion | Major complication or comorbidity
Principal diagnosis as its own CC | Principal diagnosis as its own MCC | Z code as first-listed diagnosis

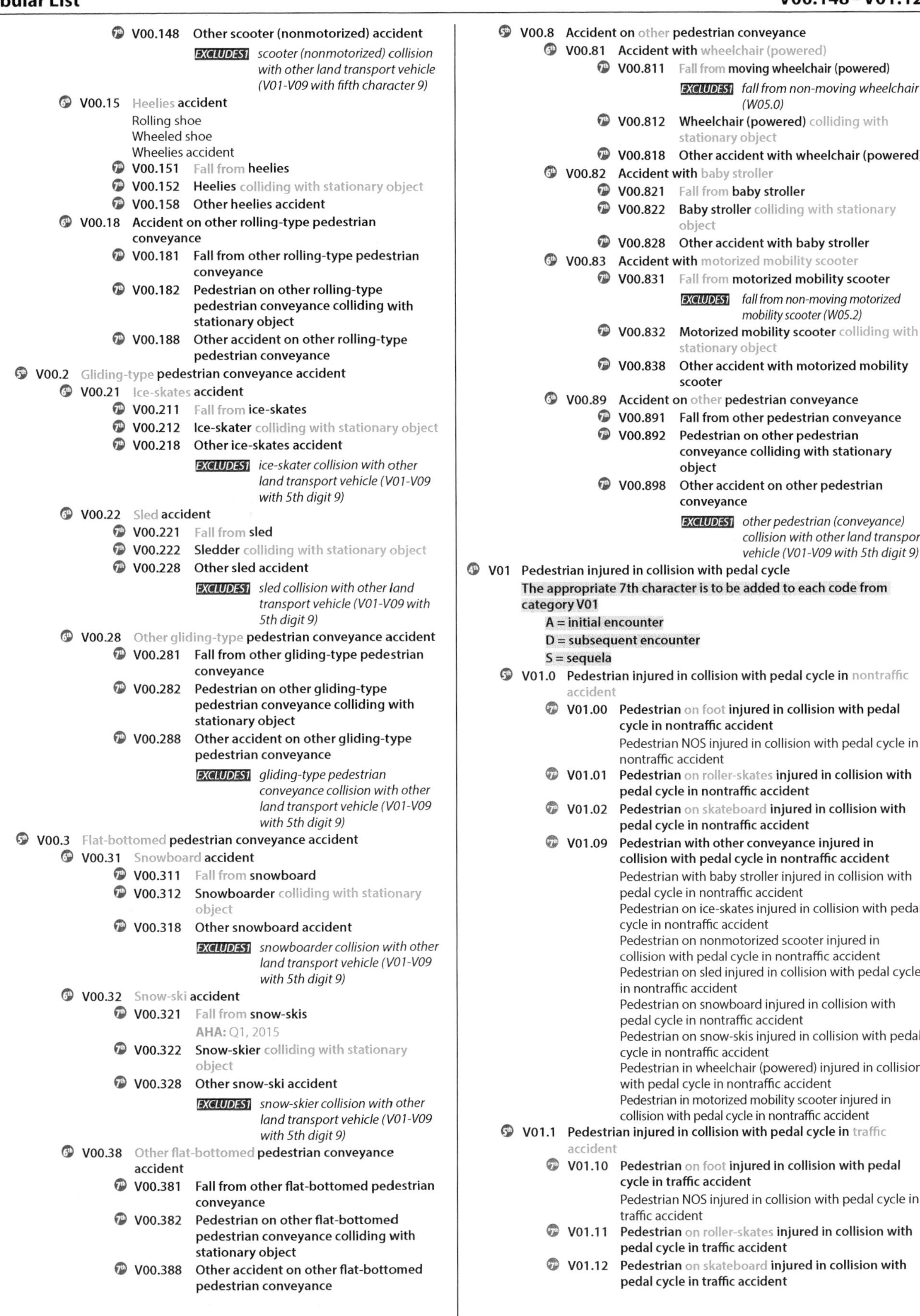

V00.148 Other scooter (nonmotorized) accident
EXCLUDES1 *scooter (nonmotorized) collision with other land transport vehicle (V01-V09 with fifth character 9)*

V00.15 Heelies accident
Rolling shoe
Wheeled shoe
Wheelies accident
V00.151 Fall from heelies
V00.152 Heelies colliding with stationary object
V00.158 Other heelies accident

V00.18 Accident on other rolling-type pedestrian conveyance
V00.181 Fall from other rolling-type pedestrian conveyance
V00.182 Pedestrian on other rolling-type pedestrian conveyance colliding with stationary object
V00.188 Other accident on other rolling-type pedestrian conveyance

V00.2 Gliding-type pedestrian conveyance accident
V00.21 Ice-skates accident
V00.211 Fall from ice-skates
V00.212 Ice-skater colliding with stationary object
V00.218 Other ice-skates accident
EXCLUDES1 *ice-skater collision with other land transport vehicle (V01-V09 with 5th digit 9)*

V00.22 Sled accident
V00.221 Fall from sled
V00.222 Sledder colliding with stationary object
V00.228 Other sled accident
EXCLUDES1 *sled collision with other land transport vehicle (V01-V09 with 5th digit 9)*

V00.28 Other gliding-type pedestrian conveyance accident
V00.281 Fall from other gliding-type pedestrian conveyance
V00.282 Pedestrian on other gliding-type pedestrian conveyance colliding with stationary object
V00.288 Other accident on other gliding-type pedestrian conveyance
EXCLUDES1 *gliding-type pedestrian conveyance collision with other land transport vehicle (V01-V09 with 5th digit 9)*

V00.3 Flat-bottomed pedestrian conveyance accident
V00.31 Snowboard accident
V00.311 Fall from snowboard
V00.312 Snowboarder colliding with stationary object
V00.318 Other snowboard accident
EXCLUDES1 *snowboarder collision with other land transport vehicle (V01-V09 with 5th digit 9)*

V00.32 Snow-ski accident
V00.321 Fall from snow-skis
AHA: Q1, 2015
V00.322 Snow-skier colliding with stationary object
V00.328 Other snow-ski accident
EXCLUDES1 *snow-skier collision with other land transport vehicle (V01-V09 with 5th digit 9)*

V00.38 Other flat-bottomed pedestrian conveyance accident
V00.381 Fall from other flat-bottomed pedestrian conveyance
V00.382 Pedestrian on other flat-bottomed pedestrian conveyance colliding with stationary object
V00.388 Other accident on other flat-bottomed pedestrian conveyance

V00.8 Accident on other pedestrian conveyance
V00.81 Accident with wheelchair (powered)
V00.811 Fall from moving wheelchair (powered)
EXCLUDES1 *fall from non-moving wheelchair (W05.0)*
V00.812 Wheelchair (powered) colliding with stationary object
V00.818 Other accident with wheelchair (powered)

V00.82 Accident with baby stroller
V00.821 Fall from baby stroller
V00.822 Baby stroller colliding with stationary object
V00.828 Other accident with baby stroller

V00.83 Accident with motorized mobility scooter
V00.831 Fall from motorized mobility scooter
EXCLUDES1 *fall from non-moving motorized mobility scooter (W05.2)*
V00.832 Motorized mobility scooter colliding with stationary object
V00.838 Other accident with motorized mobility scooter

V00.89 Accident on other pedestrian conveyance
V00.891 Fall from other pedestrian conveyance
V00.892 Pedestrian on other pedestrian conveyance colliding with stationary object
V00.898 Other accident on other pedestrian conveyance
EXCLUDES1 *other pedestrian (conveyance) collision with other land transport vehicle (V01-V09 with 5th digit 9)*

V01 Pedestrian injured in collision with pedal cycle
The appropriate 7th character is to be added to each code from category V01
A = initial encounter
D = subsequent encounter
S = sequela

V01.0 Pedestrian injured in collision with pedal cycle in nontraffic accident
V01.00 Pedestrian on foot injured in collision with pedal cycle in nontraffic accident
Pedestrian NOS injured in collision with pedal cycle in nontraffic accident
V01.01 Pedestrian on roller-skates injured in collision with pedal cycle in nontraffic accident
V01.02 Pedestrian on skateboard injured in collision with pedal cycle in nontraffic accident
V01.09 Pedestrian with other conveyance injured in collision with pedal cycle in nontraffic accident
Pedestrian with baby stroller injured in collision with pedal cycle in nontraffic accident
Pedestrian on ice-skates injured in collision with pedal cycle in nontraffic accident
Pedestrian on nonmotorized scooter injured in collision with pedal cycle in nontraffic accident
Pedestrian on sled injured in collision with pedal cycle in nontraffic accident
Pedestrian on snowboard injured in collision with pedal cycle in nontraffic accident
Pedestrian on snow-skis injured in collision with pedal cycle in nontraffic accident
Pedestrian in wheelchair (powered) injured in collision with pedal cycle in nontraffic accident
Pedestrian in motorized mobility scooter injured in collision with pedal cycle in nontraffic accident

V01.1 Pedestrian injured in collision with pedal cycle in traffic accident
V01.10 Pedestrian on foot injured in collision with pedal cycle in traffic accident
Pedestrian NOS injured in collision with pedal cycle in traffic accident
V01.11 Pedestrian on roller-skates injured in collision with pedal cycle in traffic accident
V01.12 Pedestrian on skateboard injured in collision with pedal cycle in traffic accident

Unspecified Code Other Specified Code Manifestation Code N Newborn P Pediatric M Maternity A Adult ♂ Male ♀ Female
● New Code ▲ Revised Code Title ►◄ Revised Text NOTES INCLUDES EXCLUDES1 Not coded here EXCLUDES2 Not included here
4th character required 5th character required 6th character required 7th character required
Extension 'X' Alert HAC Hospital-acquired condition (HAC) alert AHA AHA Coding Clinic©

V01.19 **Pedestrian with other conveyance injured in collision with pedal cycle in traffic accident**
Pedestrian with baby stroller injured in collision with pedal cycle in traffic accident
Pedestrian on ice-skates injured in collision with pedal cycle in traffic accident
Pedestrian on nonmotorized scooter injured in collision with pedal cycle in traffic accident
Pedestrian on sled injured in collision with pedal cycle in traffic accident
Pedestrian on snowboard injured in collision with pedal cycle in traffic accident
Pedestrian on snow-skis injured in collision with pedal cycle in traffic accident
Pedestrian in wheelchair (powered) injured in collision with pedal cycle in traffic accident
Pedestrian in motorized mobility scooter injured in collision with pedal cycle in traffic accident

V01.9 **Pedestrian injured in collision with pedal cycle,** unspecified whether traffic or nontraffic accident

V01.90 **Pedestrian on foot injured in collision with pedal cycle, unspecified whether traffic or nontraffic accident**
Pedestrian NOS injured in collision with pedal cycle, unspecified whether traffic or nontraffic accident

V01.91 **Pedestrian on roller-skates injured in collision with pedal cycle, unspecified whether traffic or nontraffic accident**

V01.92 **Pedestrian on skateboard injured in collision with pedal cycle, unspecified whether traffic or nontraffic accident**

V01.99 **Pedestrian with other conveyance injured in collision with pedal cycle, unspecified whether traffic or nontraffic accident**
Pedestrian with baby stroller injured in collision with pedal cycle, unspecified whether traffic or nontraffic accident
Pedestrian on ice-skates injured in collision with pedal cycle unspecified, whether traffic or nontraffic accident
Pedestrian on nonmotorized scooter injured in collision with pedal cycle, unspecified whether traffic or nontraffic accident
Pedestrian on sled injured in collision with pedal cycle unspecified, whether traffic or nontraffic accident
Pedestrian on snowboard injured in collision with pedal cycle, unspecified whether traffic or nontraffic accident
Pedestrian on snow-skis injured in collision with pedal cycle, unspecified whether traffic or nontraffic accident
Pedestrian in wheelchair (powered) injured in collision with pedal cycle, unspecified whether traffic or nontraffic accident
Pedestrian in motorized mobility scooter injured in collision with pedal cycle, unspecified whether traffic or nontraffic accident

V02 **Pedestrian injured in collision with** two- or three-wheeled motor vehicle

The appropriate 7th character is to be added to each code from category V02
A = initial encounter
D = subsequent encounter
S = sequela

V02.0 **Pedestrian injured** in **collision with two- or three-wheeled motor vehicle** in nontraffic accident

V02.00 **Pedestrian** on foot **injured in collision with two- or three-wheeled motor vehicle in nontraffic accident**
Pedestrian NOS injured in collision with two- or three-wheeled motor vehicle in nontraffic accident

V02.01 **Pedestrian** on roller-skates **injured in collision with two- or three-wheeled motor vehicle in nontraffic accident**

V02.02 **Pedestrian** on skateboard **injured in collision with two- or three-wheeled motor vehicle in nontraffic accident**

V02.09 **Pedestrian with other conveyance injured in collision with two- or three-wheeled motor vehicle in nontraffic accident**
Pedestrian with baby stroller injured in collision with two- or three-wheeled motor vehicle in nontraffic accident
Pedestrian on ice-skates injured in collision with two- or three-wheeled motor vehicle in nontraffic accident
Pedestrian on nonmotorized scooter injured in collision with two- or three-wheeled motor vehicle in nontraffic accident
Pedestrian on sled injured in collision with two- or three-wheeled motor vehicle in nontraffic accident
Pedestrian on snowboard injured in collision with two- or three-wheeled motor vehicle in nontraffic accident
Pedestrian on snow-skis injured in collision with two- or three-wheeled motor vehicle in nontraffic accident
Pedestrian in wheelchair (powered) injured in collision with two- or three-wheeled motor vehicle in nontraffic accident
Pedestrian in motorized mobility scooter injured in collision with two- or three-wheeled motor vehicle in nontraffic accident

V02.1 **Pedestrian injured in collision with two- or three-wheeled motor vehicle** in traffic accident

V02.10 **Pedestrian** on foot **injured in collision with two- or three-wheeled motor vehicle in traffic accident**
Pedestrian NOS injured in collision with two- or three-wheeled motor vehicle in traffic accident

V02.11 **Pedestrian** on roller-skates **injured in collision with two- or three-wheeled motor vehicle in traffic accident**

V02.12 **Pedestrian** on skateboard **injured in collision with two- or three-wheeled motor vehicle in traffic accident**

V02.19 **Pedestrian with other conveyance injured in collision with two- or three-wheeled motor vehicle in traffic accident**
Pedestrian with baby stroller injured in collision with two- or three-wheeled motor vehicle in traffic accident
Pedestrian on ice-skates injured in collision with two- or three-wheeled motor vehicle in traffic accident
Pedestrian on nonmotorized scooter injured in collision with two- or three-wheeled motor vehicle in traffic accident
Pedestrian on sled injured in collision with two- or three-wheeled motor vehicle in traffic accident
Pedestrian on snowboard injured in collision with two- or three-wheeled motor vehicle in traffic accident
Pedestrian on snow-skis injured in collision with two- or three-wheeled motor vehicle in traffic accident
Pedestrian in wheelchair (powered) injured in collision with two- or three-wheeled motor vehicle in traffic accident
Pedestrian in motorized mobility scooter injured in collision with two- or three-wheeled motor vehicle in traffic accident

V02.9 **Pedestrian injured in collision with two- or three-wheeled motor vehicle,** unspecified whether traffic or nontraffic accident

V02.90 **Pedestrian on foot injured in collision with two- or three-wheeled motor vehicle, unspecified whether traffic or nontraffic accident**
Pedestrian NOS injured in collision with two- or three-wheeled motor vehicle, unspecified whether traffic or nontraffic accident

V02.91 **Pedestrian on roller-skates injured in collision with two- or three-wheeled motor vehicle, unspecified whether traffic or nontraffic accident**

V02.92 **Pedestrian on skateboard injured in collision with two- or three-wheeled motor vehicle, unspecified whether traffic or nontraffic accident**

V02.99 **Pedestrian with other conveyance injured in collision with two- or three-wheeled motor vehicle, unspecified whether traffic or nontraffic accident**
Pedestrian with baby stroller injured in collision with two- or three-wheeled motor vehicle, unspecified whether traffic or nontraffic accident
Pedestrian on ice-skates injured in collision with two- or three-wheeled motor vehicle, unspecified whether traffic or nontraffic accident

Unacceptable principal diagnosis symbol per Medicare code edits · Code exempt from diagnosis present on admission requirement
Questionable admission · Complication or comorbidity · CC/MCC exclusion · Major complication or comorbidity
Principal diagnosis as its own CC · Principal diagnosis as its own MCC · Z code as first-listed diagnosis

Pedestrian on nonmotorized scooter injured in collision with two- or three-wheeled motor vehicle, unspecified whether traffic or nontraffic accident
Pedestrian on sled injured in collision with two- or three-wheeled motor vehicle, unspecified whether traffic or nontraffic accident
Pedestrian on snowboard injured in collision with two- or three-wheeled motor vehicle, unspecified whether traffic or nontraffic accident
Pedestrian on snow-skis injured in collision with two- or three-wheeled motor vehicle, unspecified whether traffic or nontraffic accident
Pedestrian in wheelchair (powered) injured in collision with two- or three-wheeled motor vehicle, unspecified whether traffic or nontraffic accident
Pedestrian in motorized mobility scooter injured in collision with two- or three-wheeled motor vehicle, unspecified whether traffic or nontraffic accident

V03 Pedestrian injured in collision with car, pick-up truck or van

The appropriate 7th character is to be added to each code from category V03
- **A = initial encounter**
- **D = subsequent encounter**
- **S = sequela**

V03.0 Pedestrian injured in collision with car, pick-up truck or van in nontraffic accident

V03.00 Pedestrian on foot **injured in collision with car, pick-up truck or van in nontraffic accident**
Pedestrian NOS injured in collision with car, pick-up truck or van in nontraffic accident

V03.01 Pedestrian on roller-skates **injured in collision with car, pick-up truck or van in nontraffic accident**

V03.02 Pedestrian on skateboard **injured in collision with car, pick-up truck or van in nontraffic accident**

V03.09 Pedestrian with other conveyance injured in collision with car, pick-up truck or van in nontraffic accident
Pedestrian with baby stroller injured in collision with car, pick-up truck or van in nontraffic accident
Pedestrian on ice-skates injured in collision with car, pick-up truck or van in nontraffic accident
Pedestrian on nonmotorized scooter injured in collision with car, pick-up truck or van in nontraffic accident
Pedestrian on sled injured in collision with car, pick-up truck or van in nontraffic accident
Pedestrian on snowboard injured in collision with car, pick-up truck or van in nontraffic accident
Pedestrian on snow-skis injured in collision with car, pick-up truck or van in nontraffic accident
Pedestrian in wheelchair (powered) injured in collision with car, pick-up truck or van in nontraffic accident
Pedestrian in motorized mobility scooter injured in collision with car, pick-up truck or van in nontraffic accident

V03.1 Pedestrian injured in collision with car, pick-up truck or van in traffic accident

V03.10 Pedestrian on foot **injured in collision with car, pick-up truck or van in traffic accident**
Pedestrian NOS injured in collision with car, pick-up truck or van in traffic accident

V03.11 Pedestrian on roller-skates **injured in collision with car, pick-up truck or van in traffic accident**

V03.12 Pedestrian on skateboard **injured in collision with car, pick-up truck or van in traffic accident**

V03.19 Pedestrian with other conveyance injured in collision with car, pick-up truck or van in traffic accident
Pedestrian with baby stroller injured in collision with car, pick-up truck or van in traffic accident
Pedestrian on ice-skates injured in collision with car, pick-up truck or van in traffic accident
Pedestrian on nonmotorized scooter injured in collision with car, pick-up truck or van in traffic accident
Pedestrian on sled injured in collision with car, pick-up truck or van in traffic accident
Pedestrian on snowboard injured in collision with car, pick-up truck or van in traffic accident
Pedestrian on snow-skis injured in collision with car, pick-up truck or van in traffic accident
Pedestrian in wheelchair (powered) injured in collision with car, pick-up truck or van in traffic accident
Pedestrian in motorized mobility scooter injured in collision with car, pick-up truck or van in traffic accident

V03.9 Pedestrian injured in collision with car, pick-up truck or van, unspecified whether traffic or nontraffic accident

V03.90 Pedestrian on foot injured in collision with car, pick-up truck or van, unspecified whether traffic or nontraffic accident
Pedestrian NOS injured in collision with car, pick-up truck or van, unspecified whether traffic or nontraffic accident

V03.91 Pedestrian on roller-skates injured in collision with car, pick-up truck or van, unspecified whether traffic or nontraffic accident

V03.92 Pedestrian on skateboard injured in collision with car, pick-up truck or van, unspecified whether traffic or nontraffic accident

V03.99 Pedestrian with other conveyance injured in collision with car, pick-up truck or van, unspecified whether traffic or nontraffic accident
Pedestrian with baby stroller injured in collision with car, pick-up truck or van, unspecified whether traffic or nontraffic accident
Pedestrian on ice-skates injured in collision with car, pick-up truck or van, unspecified whether traffic or nontraffic accident
Pedestrian on nonmotorized scooter injured in collision with car, pick-up truck or van, unspecified whether traffic or nontraffic accident
Pedestrian on sled injured in collision with car, pick-up truck or van in nontraffic accident
Pedestrian on snowboard injured in collision with car, pick-up truck or van, unspecified whether traffic or nontraffic accident
Pedestrian on snow-skis injured in collision with car, pick-up truck or van, unspecified whether traffic or nontraffic accident
Pedestrian in wheelchair (powered) injured in collision with car, pick-up truck or van, unspecified whether traffic or nontraffic accident
Pedestrian in motorized mobility scooter injured in collision with car, pick-up truck or van, unspecified whether traffic or nontraffic accident

V04 Pedestrian injured in collision with heavy transport vehicle or bus

EXCLUDES1 *pedestrian injured in collision with military vehicle (V09.01, V09.21)*

The appropriate 7th character is to be added to each code from category V04
- **A = initial encounter**
- **D = subsequent encounter**
- **S = sequela**

V04.0 Pedestrian injured in collision with heavy transport vehicle or bus in nontraffic accident

V04.00 Pedestrian on foot **injured in collision with heavy transport vehicle or bus in nontraffic accident**
Pedestrian NOS injured in collision with heavy transport vehicle or bus in nontraffic accident

V04.01 Pedestrian on roller-skates **injured in collision with heavy transport vehicle or bus in nontraffic accident**

V04.02 Pedestrian on skateboard **injured in collision with heavy transport vehicle or bus in nontraffic accident**

V04.09 Pedestrian with other conveyance injured in collision with heavy transport vehicle or bus in nontraffic accident
Pedestrian with baby stroller injured in collision with heavy transport vehicle or bus in nontraffic accident
Pedestrian on ice-skates injured in collision with heavy transport vehicle or bus in nontraffic accident
Pedestrian on nonmotorized scooter injured in collision with heavy transport vehicle or bus in nontraffic accident
Pedestrian on sled injured in collision with heavy transport vehicle or bus in nontraffic accident
Pedestrian on snowboard injured in collision with heavy transport vehicle or bus in nontraffic accident

Pedestrian on snow-skis injured in collision with heavy transport vehicle or bus in nontraffic accident
Pedestrian in wheelchair (powered) injured in collision with heavy transport vehicle or bus in nontraffic accident
Pedestrian in motorized mobility scooter injured in collision with heavy transport vehicle or bus in nontraffic accident

V04.1 Pedestrian injured in collision with heavy transport vehicle or bus in traffic accident

V04.10 Pedestrian on foot **injured in collision with heavy transport vehicle or bus in traffic accident**
Pedestrian NOS injured in collision with heavy transport vehicle or bus in traffic accident

V04.11 Pedestrian on roller-skates **injured in collision with heavy transport vehicle or bus in traffic accident**

V04.12 Pedestrian on skateboard **injured in collision with heavy transport vehicle or bus in traffic accident**

V04.19 Pedestrian with other conveyance injured in collision with heavy transport vehicle or bus in traffic accident
Pedestrian with baby stroller injured in collision with heavy transport vehicle or bus in traffic accident
Pedestrian on ice-skates injured in collision with heavy transport vehicle or bus in traffic accident
Pedestrian on nonmotorized scooter injured in collision with heavy transport vehicle or bus in traffic accident
Pedestrian on sled injured in collision with heavy transport vehicle or bus in traffic accident
Pedestrian on snowboard injured in collision with heavy transport vehicle or bus in traffic accident
Pedestrian on snow-skis injured in collision with heavy transport vehicle or bus in traffic accident
Pedestrian in wheelchair (powered) injured in collision with heavy transport vehicle or bus in traffic accident
Pedestrian in motorized mobility scooter injured in collision with heavy transport vehicle or bus in traffic accident

V04.9 Pedestrian injured in collision with heavy transport vehicle or bus, unspecified whether traffic or nontraffic accident

V04.90 Pedestrian on foot injured in collision with heavy transport vehicle or bus, unspecified whether traffic or nontraffic accident
Pedestrian NOS injured in collision with heavy transport vehicle or bus, unspecified whether traffic or nontraffic accident

V04.91 Pedestrian on roller-skates injured in collision with heavy transport vehicle or bus, unspecified whether traffic or nontraffic accident

V04.92 Pedestrian on skateboard injured in collision with heavy transport vehicle or bus, unspecified whether traffic or nontraffic accident

V04.99 Pedestrian with other conveyance injured in collision with heavy transport vehicle or bus, unspecified whether traffic or nontraffic accident
Pedestrian with baby stroller injured in collision with heavy transport vehicle or bus, unspecified whether traffic or nontraffic accident
Pedestrian on ice-skates injured in collision with heavy transport vehicle or bus, unspecified whether traffic or nontraffic accident
Pedestrian on nonmotorized scooter injured in collision with heavy transport vehicle or bus, unspecified whether traffic or nontraffic accident
Pedestrian on sled injured in collision with heavy transport vehicle or bus, unspecified whether traffic or nontraffic accident
Pedestrian on snowboard injured in collision with heavy transport vehicle or bus, unspecified whether traffic or nontraffic accident
Pedestrian on snow-skis injured in collision with heavy transport vehicle or bus, unspecified whether traffic or nontraffic accident
Pedestrian in wheelchair (powered) injured in collision with heavy transport vehicle or bus, unspecified whether traffic or nontraffic accident
Pedestrian in motorized mobility scooter injured in collision with heavy transport vehicle or bus, unspecified whether traffic or nontraffic accident

V05 Pedestrian injured in collision with railway train or railway vehicle

The appropriate 7th character is to be added to each code from category V05
A = initial encounter
D = subsequent encounter
S = sequela

V05.0 Pedestrian injured in collision with railway train or railway vehicle in nontraffic accident

V05.00 Pedestrian on foot **injured in collision with railway train or railway vehicle in nontraffic accident**
Pedestrian NOS injured in collision with railway train or railway vehicle in nontraffic accident

V05.01 Pedestrian on roller-skates **injured in collision with railway train or railway vehicle in nontraffic accident**

V05.02 Pedestrian on skateboard **injured in collision with railway train or railway vehicle in nontraffic accident**

V05.09 Pedestrian with other conveyance injured in collision with railway train or railway vehicle in nontraffic accident
Pedestrian with baby stroller injured in collision with railway train or railway vehicle in nontraffic accident
Pedestrian on ice-skates injured in collision with railway train or railway vehicle in nontraffic accident
Pedestrian on nonmotorized scooter injured in collision with railway train or railway vehicle in nontraffic accident
Pedestrian on sled injured in collision with railway train or railway vehicle in nontraffic accident
Pedestrian on snowboard injured in collision with railway train or railway vehicle in nontraffic accident
Pedestrian on snow-skis injured in collision with railway train or railway vehicle in nontraffic accident
Pedestrian in wheelchair (powered) injured in collision with railway train or railway vehicle in nontraffic accident
Pedestrian in motorized mobility scooter injured in collision with railway train or railway vehicle in nontraffic accident

V05.1 Pedestrian injured in collision with railway train or railway vehicle in traffic accident

V05.10 Pedestrian on foot **injured in collision with railway train or railway vehicle in traffic accident**
Pedestrian NOS injured in collision with railway train or railway vehicle in traffic accident

V05.11 Pedestrian on roller-skates **injured in collision with railway train or railway vehicle in traffic accident**

V05.12 Pedestrian on skateboard **injured in collision with railway train or railway vehicle in traffic accident**

V05.19 Pedestrian with other conveyance injured in collision with railway train or railway vehicle in traffic accident
Pedestrian with baby stroller injured in collision with railway train or railway vehicle in traffic accident
Pedestrian on ice-skates injured in collision with railway train or railway vehicle in traffic accident
Pedestrian on nonmotorized scooter injured in collision with railway train or railway vehicle in traffic accident
Pedestrian on sled injured in collision with railway train or railway vehicle in traffic accident
Pedestrian on snowboard injured in collision with railway train or railway vehicle in traffic accident
Pedestrian on snow-skis injured in collision with railway train or railway vehicle in traffic accident
Pedestrian in wheelchair (powered) injured in collision with railway train or railway vehicle in traffic accident
Pedestrian in motorized mobility scooter injured in collision with railway train or railway vehicle in traffic accident

V05.9 Pedestrian injured in collision with railway train or railway vehicle, unspecified whether traffic or nontraffic accident

V05.90 Pedestrian on foot injured in collision with railway train or railway vehicle, unspecified whether traffic or nontraffic accident
Pedestrian NOS injured in collision with railway train or railway vehicle, unspecified whether traffic or nontraffic accident

Unacceptable principal diagnosis symbol per Medicare code edits · Code exempt from diagnosis present on admission requirement
Questionable admission · Complication or comorbidity · CC/MCC exclusion · Major complication or comorbidity
Principal diagnosis as its own CC · Principal diagnosis as its own MCC · Z code as first-listed diagnosis

V05.91 **Pedestrian on roller-skates injured in collision with railway train or railway vehicle, unspecified whether traffic or nontraffic accident**

V05.92 **Pedestrian on skateboard injured in collision with railway train or railway vehicle, unspecified whether traffic or nontraffic accident**

V05.99 **Pedestrian with other conveyance injured in collision with railway train or railway vehicle, unspecified whether traffic or nontraffic accident**
Pedestrian with baby stroller injured in collision with railway train or railway vehicle, unspecified whether traffic or nontraffic
Pedestrian on ice-skates injured in collision with railway train or railway vehicle, unspecified whether traffic or nontraffic
Pedestrian on nonmotorized scooter injured in collision with railway train or railway vehicle, unspecified whether traffic or nontraffic
Pedestrian on sled injured in collision with railway train or railway vehicle, unspecified whether traffic or nontraffic
Pedestrian on snowboard injured in collision with railway train or railway vehicle, unspecified whether traffic or nontraffic
Pedestrian on snow-skis injured in collision with railway train or railway vehicle, unspecified whether traffic or nontraffic
Pedestrian in wheelchair (powered) injured in collision with railway train or railway vehicle, unspecified whether traffic or nontraffic
Pedestrian in motorized mobility scooter injured in collision with railway train or railway vehicle, unspecified whether traffic or nontraffic

V06 **Pedestrian injured in collision with other nonmotor vehicle**

INCLUDES *collision with animal-drawn vehicle, animal being ridden, nonpowered streetcar*

EXCLUDES1 *pedestrian injured in collision with pedestrian conveyance (V00.0-)*

The appropriate 7th character is to be added to each code from category V06
A = initial encounter
D = subsequent encounter
S = sequela

V06.0 **Pedestrian injured in collision with other nonmotor vehicle in nontraffic accident**

V06.00 **Pedestrian on foot injured in collision with other nonmotor vehicle in nontraffic accident**
Pedestrian NOS injured in collision with other nonmotor vehicle in nontraffic accident

V06.01 **Pedestrian on roller-skates injured in collision with other nonmotor vehicle in nontraffic accident**

V06.02 **Pedestrian on skateboard injured in collision with other nonmotor vehicle in nontraffic accident**

V06.09 **Pedestrian with other conveyance injured in collision with other nonmotor vehicle in nontraffic accident**
Pedestrian with baby stroller injured in collision with other nonmotor vehicle in nontraffic accident
Pedestrian on ice-skates injured in collision with other nonmotor vehicle in nontraffic accident
Pedestrian on nonmotorized scooter injured in collision with other nonmotor vehicle in nontraffic accident
Pedestrian on sled injured in collision with other nonmotor vehicle in nontraffic accident
Pedestrian on snowboard injured in collision with other nonmotor vehicle in nontraffic accident
Pedestrian on snow-skis injured in collision with other nonmotor vehicle in nontraffic accident
Pedestrian in wheelchair (powered) injured in collision with other nonmotor vehicle in nontraffic accident
Pedestrian in motorized mobility scooter injured in collision with other nonmotor vehicle in nontraffic accident

V06.1 **Pedestrian injured in collision with other nonmotor vehicle in traffic accident**

V06.10 **Pedestrian on foot injured in collision with other nonmotor vehicle in traffic accident**
Pedestrian NOS injured in collision with other nonmotor vehicle in traffic accident

V06.11 **Pedestrian on roller-skates injured in collision with other nonmotor vehicle in traffic accident**

V06.12 **Pedestrian on skateboard injured in collision with other nonmotor vehicle in traffic accident**

V06.19 **Pedestrian with other conveyance injured in collision with other nonmotor vehicle in traffic accident**
Pedestrian with baby stroller injured in collision with other nonmotor vehicle in nontraffic accident
Pedestrian on ice-skates injured in collision with other nonmotor vehicle in traffic accident
Pedestrian on nonmotorized scooter injured in collision with other nonmotor vehicle in traffic accident
Pedestrian on sled injured in collision with other nonmotor vehicle in traffic accident
Pedestrian on snowboard injured in collision with other nonmotor vehicle in traffic accident
Pedestrian on snow-skis injured in collision with other nonmotor vehicle in traffic accident
Pedestrian in wheelchair (powered) injured in collision with other nonmotor vehicle in traffic accident
Pedestrian in motorized mobility scooter injured in collision with other nonmotor vehicle in traffic accident

V06.9 **Pedestrian injured in collision with other nonmotor vehicle, unspecified whether traffic or nontraffic accident**

V06.90 **Pedestrian on foot injured in collision with other nonmotor vehicle, unspecified whether traffic or nontraffic accident**
Pedestrian NOS injured in collision with other nonmotor vehicle, unspecified whether traffic or nontraffic accident

V06.91 **Pedestrian on roller-skates injured in collision with other nonmotor vehicle, unspecified whether traffic or nontraffic accident**

V06.92 **Pedestrian on skateboard injured in collision with other nonmotor vehicle, unspecified whether traffic or nontraffic accident**

V06.99 **Pedestrian with other conveyance injured in collision with other nonmotor vehicle, unspecified whether traffic or nontraffic accident**
Pedestrian with baby stroller injured in collision with other nonmotor vehicle, unspecified whether traffic or nontraffic accident
Pedestrian on ice-skates injured in collision with other nonmotor vehicle, unspecified whether traffic or nontraffic accident
Pedestrian on nonmotorized scooter injured in collision with other nonmotor vehicle, unspecified whether traffic or nontraffic accident
Pedestrian on sled injured in collision with other nonmotor vehicle, unspecified whether traffic or nontraffic accident
Pedestrian on snowboard injured in collision with other nonmotor vehicle, unspecified whether traffic or nontraffic accident
Pedestrian on snow-skis injured in collision with other nonmotor vehicle, unspecified whether traffic or nontraffic accident
Pedestrian in wheelchair (powered) injured in collision with other nonmotor vehicle, unspecified whether traffic or nontraffic accident
Pedestrian in motorized mobility scooter injured in collision with other nonmotor vehicle, unspecified whether traffic or nontraffic accident

V09 **Pedestrian injured in other and unspecified transport accidents**

The appropriate 7th character is to be added to each code from category V09
A = initial encounter
D = subsequent encounter
S = sequela

V09.0 **Pedestrian injured in nontraffic accident involving other and unspecified motor vehicles**

V09.00 **Pedestrian injured in nontraffic accident involving unspecified motor vehicles**

V09.01 **Pedestrian injured in nontraffic accident involving military vehicle**

Unspecified Code Other Specified Code Manifestation Code N Newborn P Pediatric M Maternity A Adult ♂ Male ♀ Female
● New Code ▲ Revised Code Title ►◄ Revised Text NOTES INCLUDES EXCLUDES1 Not coded here EXCLUDES2 Not included here
4th character required 5th character required 6th character required 7th character required
Extension 'X' Alert HAC Hospital-acquired condition (HAC) alert AHA AHA Coding Clinic©

V09.09 Pedestrian injured in nontraffic accident involving other motor vehicles
Pedestrian injured in nontraffic accident by special vehicle
V09.1 Pedestrian injured in unspecified nontraffic accident
V09.2 Pedestrian injured in traffic accident involving other and unspecified motor vehicles
V09.20 Pedestrian injured in traffic accident involving unspecified motor vehicles
V09.21 Pedestrian injured in traffic accident involving military vehicle
V09.29 Pedestrian injured in traffic accident involving other motor vehicles
V09.3 Pedestrian injured in unspecified traffic accident
V09.9 Pedestrian injured in unspecified transport accident

Pedal cycle rider injured in transport accident (V10-V19)

INCLUDES *any non-motorized vehicle, excluding an animal-drawn vehicle, or a sidecar or trailer attached to the pedal cycle*

EXCLUDES2 *rupture of pedal cycle tire (W37.0)*

V10 Pedal cycle rider injured in collision with pedestrian or animal
EXCLUDES1 *pedal cycle rider collision with animal-drawn vehicle or animal being ridden (V16.-)*
The appropriate 7th character is to be added to each code from category V10
A = initial encounter
D = subsequent encounter
S = sequela
V10.0 Pedal cycle driver injured in collision with pedestrian or animal in nontraffic accident
V10.1 Pedal cycle passenger injured in collision with pedestrian or animal in nontraffic accident
V10.2 Unspecified pedal cyclist injured in collision with pedestrian or animal in nontraffic accident
V10.3 Person boarding or alighting a pedal cycle injured in collision with pedestrian or animal
V10.4 Pedal cycle driver injured in collision with pedestrian or animal in traffic accident
V10.5 Pedal cycle passenger injured in collision with pedestrian or animal in traffic accident
V10.9 Unspecified pedal cyclist injured in collision with pedestrian or animal in traffic accident
V11 Pedal cycle rider injured in collision with other pedal cycle
The appropriate 7th character is to be added to each code from category V11
A = initial encounter
D = subsequent encounter
S = sequela
V11.0 Pedal cycle driver injured in collision with other pedal cycle in nontraffic accident
V11.1 Pedal cycle passenger injured in collision with other pedal cycle in nontraffic accident
V11.2 Unspecified pedal cyclist injured in collision with other pedal cycle in nontraffic accident
V11.3 Person boarding or alighting a pedal cycle injured in collision with other pedal cycle
V11.4 Pedal cycle driver injured in collision with other pedal cycle in traffic accident
V11.5 Pedal cycle passenger injured in collision with other pedal cycle in traffic accident
V11.9 Unspecified pedal cyclist injured in collision with other pedal cycle in traffic accident
V12 Pedal cycle rider injured in collision with two- or three-wheeled motor vehicle
The appropriate 7th character is to be added to each code from category V12
A = initial encounter
D = subsequent encounter
S = sequela
V12.0 Pedal cycle driver injured in collision with two- or three-wheeled motor vehicle in nontraffic accident
V12.1 Pedal cycle passenger injured in collision with two- or three-wheeled motor vehicle in nontraffic accident
V12.2 Unspecified pedal cyclist injured in collision with two- or three-wheeled motor vehicle in nontraffic accident
V12.3 Person boarding or alighting a pedal cycle injured in collision with two- or three-wheeled motor vehicle
V12.4 Pedal cycle driver injured in collision with two- or three-wheeled motor vehicle in traffic accident
V12.5 Pedal cycle passenger injured in collision with two- or three-wheeled motor vehicle in traffic accident
V12.9 Unspecified pedal cyclist injured in collision with two- or three-wheeled motor vehicle in traffic accident
V13 Pedal cycle rider injured in collision with car, pick-up truck or van
The appropriate 7th character is to be added to each code from category V13
A = initial encounter
D = subsequent encounter
S = sequela
V13.0 Pedal cycle driver injured in collision with car, pick-up truck or van in nontraffic accident
V13.1 Pedal cycle passenger injured in collision with car, pick-up truck or van in nontraffic accident
V13.2 Unspecified pedal cyclist injured in collision with car, pick-up truck or van in nontraffic accident
V13.3 Person boarding or alighting a pedal cycle injured in collision with car, pick-up truck or van
V13.4 Pedal cycle driver injured in collision with car, pick-up truck or van in traffic accident
V13.5 Pedal cycle passenger injured in collision with car, pick-up truck or van in traffic accident
V13.9 Unspecified pedal cyclist injured in collision with car, pick-up truck or van in traffic accident
V14 Pedal cycle rider injured in collision with heavy transport vehicle or bus
EXCLUDES1 *pedal cycle rider injured in collision with military vehicle (V19.81)*
The appropriate 7th character is to be added to each code from category V14
A = initial encounter
D = subsequent encounter
S = sequela
V14.0 Pedal cycle driver injured in collision with heavy transport vehicle or bus in nontraffic accident
V14.1 Pedal cycle passenger injured in collision with heavy transport vehicle or bus in nontraffic accident
V14.2 Unspecified pedal cyclist injured in collision with heavy transport vehicle or bus in nontraffic accident
V14.3 Person boarding or alighting a pedal cycle injured in collision with heavy transport vehicle or bus
V14.4 Pedal cycle driver injured in collision with heavy transport vehicle or bus in traffic accident
V14.5 Pedal cycle passenger injured in collision with heavy transport vehicle or bus in traffic accident
V14.9 Unspecified pedal cyclist injured in collision with heavy transport vehicle or bus in traffic accident
V15 Pedal cycle rider injured in collision with railway train or railway vehicle
The appropriate 7th character is to be added to each code from category V15
A = initial encounter
D = subsequent encounter
S = sequela
V15.0 Pedal cycle driver injured in collision with railway train or railway vehicle in nontraffic accident
V15.1 Pedal cycle passenger injured in collision with railway train or railway vehicle in nontraffic accident
V15.2 Unspecified pedal cyclist injured in collision with railway train or railway vehicle in nontraffic accident
V15.3 Person boarding or alighting a pedal cycle injured in collision with railway train or railway vehicle
V15.4 Pedal cycle driver injured in collision with railway train or railway vehicle in traffic accident
V15.5 Pedal cycle passenger injured in collision with railway train or railway vehicle in traffic accident
V15.9 Unspecified pedal cyclist injured in collision with railway train or railway vehicle in traffic accident

Unacceptable principal diagnosis symbol per Medicare code edits | Code exempt from diagnosis present on admission requirement
Questionable admission | Complication or comorbidity | CC/MCC exclusion | Major complication or comorbidity
Principal diagnosis as its own CC | Principal diagnosis as its own MCC | Z code as first-listed diagnosis

V16 Pedal cycle rider injured in collision with other nonmotor vehicle
INCLUDES *collision with animal-drawn vehicle, animal being ridden, streetcar*
The appropriate 7th character is to be added to each code from category V16
A = initial encounter
D = subsequent encounter
S = sequela

V16.0 Pedal cycle driver injured in collision with other nonmotor vehicle in nontraffic accident
V16.1 Pedal cycle passenger injured in collision with other nonmotor vehicle in nontraffic accident
V16.2 Unspecified pedal cyclist injured in collision with other nonmotor vehicle in nontraffic accident
V16.3 Person boarding or alighting a pedal cycle injured in collision with other nonmotor vehicle in nontraffic accident
V16.4 Pedal cycle driver injured in collision with other nonmotor vehicle in traffic accident
V16.5 Pedal cycle passenger injured in collision with other nonmotor vehicle in traffic accident
V16.9 Unspecified pedal cyclist injured in collision with other nonmotor vehicle in traffic accident

V17 Pedal cycle rider injured in collision with fixed or stationary object
The appropriate 7th character is to be added to each code from category V17
A = initial encounter
D = subsequent encounter
S = sequela

V17.0 Pedal cycle driver injured in collision with fixed or stationary object in nontraffic accident
V17.1 Pedal cycle passenger injured in collision with fixed or stationary object in nontraffic accident
V17.2 Unspecified pedal cyclist injured in collision with fixed or stationary object in nontraffic accident
V17.3 Person boarding or alighting a pedal cycle injured in collision with fixed or stationary object
V17.4 Pedal cycle driver injured in collision with fixed or stationary object in traffic accident
V17.5 Pedal cycle passenger injured in collision with fixed or stationary object in traffic accident
V17.9 Unspecified pedal cyclist injured in collision with fixed or stationary object in traffic accident

V18 Pedal cycle rider injured in noncollision transport accident
INCLUDES *fall or thrown from pedal cycle (without antecedent collision)*
overturning pedal cycle NOS
overturning pedal cycle without collision
The appropriate 7th character is to be added to each code from category V18
A = initial encounter
D = subsequent encounter
S = sequela

V18.0 Pedal cycle driver injured in noncollision transport accident in nontraffic accident
V18.1 Pedal cycle passenger injured in noncollision transport accident in nontraffic accident
V18.2 Unspecified pedal cyclist injured in noncollision transport accident in nontraffic accident
V18.3 Person boarding or alighting a pedal cycle injured in noncollision transport accident
V18.4 Pedal cycle driver injured in noncollision transport accident in traffic accident
V18.5 Pedal cycle passenger injured in noncollision transport accident in traffic accident
V18.9 Unspecified pedal cyclist injured in noncollision transport accident in traffic accident

V19 Pedal cycle rider injured in other and unspecified transport accidents
The appropriate 7th character is to be added to each code from category V19
A = initial encounter
D = subsequent encounter
S = sequela

V19.0 Pedal cycle driver injured in collision with other and unspecified motor vehicles in nontraffic accident
V19.00 Pedal cycle driver injured in collision with unspecified motor vehicles in nontraffic accident
V19.09 Pedal cycle driver injured in collision with other motor vehicles in nontraffic accident
V19.1 Pedal cycle passenger injured in collision with other and unspecified motor vehicles in nontraffic accident
V19.10 Pedal cycle passenger injured in collision with unspecified motor vehicles in nontraffic accident
V19.19 Pedal cycle passenger injured in collision with other motor vehicles in nontraffic accident
V19.2 Unspecified pedal cyclist injured in collision with other and unspecified motor vehicles in nontraffic accident
V19.20 Unspecified pedal cyclist injured in collision with unspecified motor vehicles in nontraffic accident
Pedal cycle collision NOS, nontraffic
V19.29 Unspecified pedal cyclist injured in collision with other motor vehicles in nontraffic accident
V19.3 Pedal cyclist (driver) (passenger) injured in unspecified nontraffic accident
Pedal cycle accident NOS, nontraffic
Pedal cyclist injured in nontraffic accident NOS
V19.4 Pedal cycle driver injured in collision with other and unspecified motor vehicles in traffic accident
V19.40 Pedal cycle driver injured in collision with unspecified motor vehicles in traffic accident
V19.49 Pedal cycle driver injured in collision with other motor vehicles in traffic accident
V19.5 Pedal cycle passenger injured in collision with other and unspecified motor vehicles in traffic accident
V19.50 Pedal cycle passenger injured in collision with unspecified motor vehicles in traffic accident
V19.59 Pedal cycle passenger injured in collision with other motor vehicles in traffic accident
V19.6 Unspecified pedal cyclist injured in collision with other and unspecified motor vehicles in traffic accident
V19.60 Unspecified pedal cyclist injured in collision with unspecified motor vehicles in traffic accident
Pedal cycle collision NOS (traffic)
V19.69 Unspecified pedal cyclist injured in collision with other motor vehicles in traffic accident
V19.8 Pedal cyclist (driver) (passenger) injured in other specified transport accidents
V19.81 Pedal cyclist (driver) (passenger) injured in transport accident with military vehicle
V19.88 Pedal cyclist (driver) (passenger) injured in other specified transport accidents
V19.9 Pedal cyclist (driver) (passenger) injured in unspecified traffic accident
Pedal cycle accident NOS

Motorcycle rider injured in transport accident (V20-V29)

INCLUDES *moped*
motorcycle with sidecar
motorized bicycle
motor scooter
EXCLUDES1 *three-wheeled motor vehicle (V30-V39)*

V20 Motorcycle rider injured in collision with pedestrian or animal
EXCLUDES1 *motorcycle rider collision with animal-drawn vehicle or animal being ridden (V26.-)*
The appropriate 7th character is to be added to each code from category V20
A = initial encounter
D = subsequent encounter
S = sequela

V20.0 Motorcycle driver injured in collision with pedestrian or animal in nontraffic accident
V20.1 Motorcycle passenger injured in collision with pedestrian or animal in nontraffic accident
V20.2 Unspecified motorcycle rider injured in collision with pedestrian or animal in nontraffic accident
V20.3 Person boarding or alighting a motorcycle injured in collision with pedestrian or animal
V20.4 Motorcycle driver injured in collision with pedestrian or animal in traffic accident
V20.5 Motorcycle passenger injured in collision with pedestrian or animal in traffic accident

V20.9 Unspecified motorcycle rider injured in collision with pedestrian or animal in traffic accident

V21 Motorcycle rider injured in collision with pedal cycle

The appropriate 7th character is to be added to each code from category V21
A = initial encounter
D = subsequent encounter
S = sequela

V21.0 Motorcycle driver injured in collision with pedal cycle in nontraffic accident

V21.1 Motorcycle passenger injured in collision with pedal cycle in nontraffic accident

V21.2 Unspecified motorcycle rider injured in collision with pedal cycle in nontraffic accident

V21.3 Person boarding or alighting a motorcycle injured in collision with pedal cycle

V21.4 Motorcycle driver injured in collision with pedal cycle in traffic accident

V21.5 Motorcycle passenger injured in collision with pedal cycle in traffic accident

V21.9 Unspecified motorcycle rider injured in collision with pedal cycle in traffic accident

V22 Motorcycle rider injured in collision with two- or three-wheeled motor vehicle

The appropriate 7th character is to be added to each code from category V22
A = initial encounter
D = subsequent encounter
S = sequela

V22.0 Motorcycle driver injured in collision with two- or three-wheeled motor vehicle in nontraffic accident

V22.1 Motorcycle passenger injured in collision with two- or three-wheeled motor vehicle in nontraffic accident

V22.2 Unspecified motorcycle rider injured in collision with two- or three-wheeled motor vehicle in nontraffic accident

V22.3 Person boarding or alighting a motorcycle injured in collision with two- or three-wheeled motor vehicle

V22.4 Motorcycle driver injured in collision with two- or three-wheeled motor vehicle in traffic accident

V22.5 Motorcycle passenger injured in collision with two- or three-wheeled motor vehicle in traffic accident

V22.9 Unspecified motorcycle rider injured in collision with two- or three-wheeled motor vehicle in traffic accident

V23 Motorcycle rider injured in collision with car, pick-up truck or van

The appropriate 7th character is to be added to each code from category V23
A = initial encounter
D = subsequent encounter
S = sequela

V23.0 Motorcycle driver injured in collision with car, pick-up truck or van in nontraffic accident

V23.1 Motorcycle passenger injured in collision with car, pick-up truck or van in nontraffic accident

V23.2 Unspecified motorcycle rider injured in collision with car, pick-up truck or van in nontraffic accident

V23.3 Person boarding or alighting a motorcycle injured in collision with car, pick-up truck or van

V23.4 Motorcycle driver injured in collision with car, pick-up truck or van in traffic accident

V23.5 Motorcycle passenger injured in collision with car, pick-up truck or van in traffic accident

V23.9 Unspecified motorcycle rider injured in collision with car, pick-up truck or van in traffic accident

V24 Motorcycle rider injured in collision with heavy transport vehicle or bus

EXCLUDES1 *motorcycle rider injured in collision with military vehicle (V29.81)*

The appropriate 7th character is to be added to each code from category V24
A = initial encounter
D = subsequent encounter
S = sequela

V24.0 Motorcycle driver injured in collision with heavy transport vehicle or bus in nontraffic accident

V24.1 Motorcycle passenger injured in collision with heavy transport vehicle or bus in nontraffic accident

V24.2 Unspecified motorcycle rider injured in collision with heavy transport vehicle or bus in nontraffic accident

V24.3 Person boarding or alighting a motorcycle injured in collision with heavy transport vehicle or bus

V24.4 Motorcycle driver injured in collision with heavy transport vehicle or bus in traffic accident

V24.5 Motorcycle passenger injured in collision with heavy transport vehicle or bus in traffic accident

V24.9 Unspecified motorcycle rider injured in collision with heavy transport vehicle or bus in traffic accident

V25 Motorcycle rider injured in collision with railway train or railway vehicle

The appropriate 7th character is to be added to each code from category V25
A = initial encounter
D = subsequent encounter
S = sequela

V25.0 Motorcycle driver injured in collision with railway train or railway vehicle in nontraffic accident

V25.1 Motorcycle passenger injured in collision with railway train or railway vehicle in nontraffic accident

V25.2 Unspecified motorcycle rider injured in collision with railway train or railway vehicle in nontraffic accident

V25.3 Person boarding or alighting a motorcycle injured in collision with railway train or railway vehicle

V25.4 Motorcycle driver injured in collision with railway train or railway vehicle in traffic accident

V25.5 Motorcycle passenger injured in collision with railway train or railway vehicle in traffic accident

V25.9 Unspecified motorcycle rider injured in collision with railway train or railway vehicle in traffic accident

V26 Motorcycle rider injured in collision with other nonmotor vehicle

INCLUDES *collision with animal-drawn vehicle, animal being ridden, streetcar*

The appropriate 7th character is to be added to each code from category V26
A = initial encounter
D = subsequent encounter
S = sequela

V26.0 Motorcycle driver injured in collision with other nonmotor vehicle in nontraffic accident

V26.1 Motorcycle passenger injured in collision with other nonmotor vehicle in nontraffic accident

V26.2 Unspecified motorcycle rider injured in collision with other nonmotor vehicle in nontraffic accident

V26.3 Person boarding or alighting a motorcycle injured in collision with other nonmotor vehicle

V26.4 Motorcycle driver injured in collision with other nonmotor vehicle in traffic accident

V26.5 Motorcycle passenger injured in collision with other nonmotor vehicle in traffic accident

V26.9 Unspecified motorcycle rider injured in collision with other nonmotor vehicle in traffic accident

V27 Motorcycle rider injured in collision with fixed or stationary object

The appropriate 7th character is to be added to each code from category V27
A = initial encounter
D = subsequent encounter
S = sequela

V27.0 Motorcycle driver injured in collision with fixed or stationary object in nontraffic accident

V27.1 Motorcycle passenger injured in collision with fixed or stationary object in nontraffic accident

V27.2 Unspecified motorcycle rider injured in collision with fixed or stationary object in nontraffic accident

V27.3 Person boarding or alighting a motorcycle injured in collision with fixed or stationary object

V27.4 Motorcycle driver injured in collision with fixed or stationary object in traffic accident

V27.5 Motorcycle passenger injured in collision with fixed or stationary object in traffic accident

V27.9 Unspecified motorcycle rider injured in collision with fixed or stationary object in traffic accident

Unacceptable principal diagnosis symbol per Medicare code edits · Code exempt from diagnosis present on admission requirement
Questionable admission · Complication or comorbidity · CC/MCC exclusion · Major complication or comorbidity
Principal diagnosis as its own CC · Principal diagnosis as its own MCC · Z code as first-listed diagnosis

 When symbols appear on a code that requires a 7th character extension, refer to Appendix D to identify applicable 7th character codes.

V28 Motorcycle rider injured in noncollision transport accident

INCLUDES *fall or thrown from motorcycle (without antecedent collision)*
overturning motorcycle NOS
overturning motorcycle without collision

The appropriate 7th character is to be added to each code from category V28
A = initial encounter
D = subsequent encounter
S = sequela

V28.0 Motorcycle driver injured in noncollision transport accident in nontraffic accident
V28.1 Motorcycle passenger injured in noncollision transport accident in nontraffic accident
V28.2 Unspecified motorcycle rider injured in noncollision transport accident in nontraffic accident
V28.3 Person boarding or alighting a motorcycle injured in noncollision transport accident
V28.4 Motorcycle driver injured in noncollision transport accident in traffic accident
V28.5 Motorcycle passenger injured in noncollision transport accident in traffic accident
V28.9 Unspecified motorcycle rider injured in noncollision transport accident in traffic accident

V29 Motorcycle rider injured in other and unspecified transport accidents

The appropriate 7th character is to be added to each code from category V29
A = initial encounter
D = subsequent encounter
S = sequela

V29.0 Motorcycle driver injured in collision with other and unspecified motor vehicles in nontraffic accident
V29.00 Motorcycle driver injured in collision with unspecified motor vehicles in nontraffic accident
V29.09 Motorcycle driver injured in collision with other motor vehicles in nontraffic accident
V29.1 Motorcycle passenger injured in collision with other and unspecified motor vehicles in nontraffic accident
V29.10 Motorcycle passenger injured in collision with unspecified motor vehicles in nontraffic accident
V29.19 Motorcycle passenger injured in collision with other motor vehicles in nontraffic accident
V29.2 Unspecified motorcycle rider injured in collision with other and unspecified motor vehicles in nontraffic accident
V29.20 Unspecified motorcycle rider injured in collision with unspecified motor vehicles in nontraffic accident
Motorcycle collision NOS, nontraffic
V29.29 Unspecified motorcycle rider injured in collision with other motor vehicles in nontraffic accident
V29.3 Motorcycle rider (driver) (passenger) injured in unspecified nontraffic accident
Motorcycle accident NOS, nontraffic
Motorcycle rider injured in nontraffic accident NOS
V29.4 Motorcycle driver injured in collision with other and unspecified motor vehicles in traffic accident
V29.40 Motorcycle driver injured in collision with unspecified motor vehicles in traffic accident
V29.49 Motorcycle driver injured in collision with other motor vehicles in traffic accident
V29.5 Motorcycle passenger injured in collision with other and unspecified motor vehicles in traffic accident
V29.50 Motorcycle passenger injured in collision with unspecified motor vehicles in traffic accident
V29.59 Motorcycle passenger injured in collision with other motor vehicles in traffic accident
V29.6 Unspecified motorcycle rider injured in collision with other and unspecified motor vehicles in traffic accident
V29.60 Unspecified motorcycle rider injured in collision with unspecified motor vehicles in traffic accident
Motorcycle collision NOS (traffic)
V29.69 Unspecified motorcycle rider injured in collision with other motor vehicles in traffic accident
V29.8 Motorcycle rider (driver) (passenger) injured in other specified transport accidents
V29.81 Motorcycle rider (driver) (passenger) injured in transport accident with military vehicle
V29.88 Motorcycle rider (driver) (passenger) injured in other specified transport accidents
V29.9 Motorcycle rider (driver) (passenger) injured in unspecified traffic accident
Motorcycle accident NOS

Occupant of three-wheeled motor vehicle injured in transport accident (V30-V39)

INCLUDES *motorized tricycle*
motorized rickshaw
three-wheeled motor car

EXCLUDES1 *all-terrain vehicles (V86.-)*
motorcycle with sidecar (V20-V29)
vehicle designed primarily for off-road use (V86.-)

V30 Occupant of three-wheeled motor vehicle injured in collision with pedestrian or animal

EXCLUDES1 *three-wheeled motor vehicle collision with animal-drawn vehicle or animal being ridden (V36.-)*

The appropriate 7th character is to be added to each code from category V30
A = initial encounter
D = subsequent encounter
S = sequela

V30.0 Driver of three-wheeled motor vehicle injured in collision with pedestrian or animal in nontraffic accident
V30.1 Passenger in three-wheeled motor vehicle injured in collision with pedestrian or animal in nontraffic accident
V30.2 Person on outside of three-wheeled motor vehicle injured in collision with pedestrian or animal in nontraffic accident
V30.3 Unspecified occupant of three-wheeled motor vehicle injured in collision with pedestrian or animal in nontraffic accident
V30.4 Person boarding or alighting a three-wheeled motor vehicle injured in collision with pedestrian or animal
V30.5 Driver of three-wheeled motor vehicle injured in collision with pedestrian or animal in traffic accident
V30.6 Passenger in three-wheeled motor vehicle injured in collision with pedestrian or animal in traffic accident
V30.7 Person on outside of three-wheeled motor vehicle injured in collision with pedestrian or animal in traffic accident
V30.9 Unspecified occupant of three-wheeled motor vehicle injured in collision with pedestrian or animal in traffic accident

V31 Occupant of three-wheeled motor vehicle injured in collision with pedal cycle

The appropriate 7th character is to be added to each code from category V31
A = initial encounter
D = subsequent encounter
S = sequela

V31.0 Driver of three-wheeled motor vehicle injured in collision with pedal cycle in nontraffic accident
V31.1 Passenger in three-wheeled motor vehicle injured in collision with pedal cycle in nontraffic accident
V31.2 Person on outside of three-wheeled motor vehicle injured in collision with pedal cycle in nontraffic accident
V31.3 Unspecified occupant of three-wheeled motor vehicle injured in collision with pedal cycle in nontraffic accident
V31.4 Person boarding or alighting a three-wheeled motor vehicle injured in collision with pedal cycle
V31.5 Driver of three-wheeled motor vehicle injured in collision with pedal cycle in traffic accident
V31.6 Passenger in three-wheeled motor vehicle injured in collision with pedal cycle in traffic accident
V31.7 Person on outside of three-wheeled motor vehicle injured in collision with pedal cycle in traffic accident
V31.9 Unspecified occupant of three-wheeled motor vehicle injured in collision with pedal cycle in traffic accident

V32 Occupant of three-wheeled motor vehicle injured in collision with two- or three-wheeled motor vehicle

The appropriate 7th character is to be added to each code from category V32
A = initial encounter
D = subsequent encounter
S = sequela

Unspecified Code Other Specified Code Manifestation Code N Newborn P Pediatric M Maternity A Adult ♂ Male ♀ Female
● New Code ▲ Revised Code Title ►◄ Revised Text NOTES INCLUDES EXCLUDES1 Not coded here EXCLUDES2 Not included here
4th character required 5th character required 6th character required 7th character required
Extension 'X' Alert HAC Hospital-acquired condition (HAC) alert AHA AHA Coding Clinic©

V32.0 Driver of three-wheeled motor vehicle injured in collision with two- or three-wheeled motor vehicle in nontraffic accident
V32.1 Passenger in three-wheeled motor vehicle injured in collision with two- or three-wheeled motor vehicle in nontraffic accident
V32.2 Person on outside of three-wheeled motor vehicle injured in collision with two- or three-wheeled motor vehicle in nontraffic accident
V32.3 Unspecified occupant of three-wheeled motor vehicle injured in collision with two- or three-wheeled motor vehicle in nontraffic accident
V32.4 Person boarding or alighting a three-wheeled motor vehicle injured in collision with two- or three-wheeled motor vehicle
V32.5 Driver of three-wheeled motor vehicle injured in collision with two- or three-wheeled motor vehicle in traffic accident
V32.6 Passenger in three-wheeled motor vehicle injured in collision with two- or three-wheeled motor vehicle in traffic accident
V32.7 Person on outside of three-wheeled motor vehicle injured in collision with two- or three-wheeled motor vehicle in traffic accident
V32.9 Unspecified occupant of three-wheeled motor vehicle injured in collision with two- or three-wheeled motor vehicle in traffic accident

V33 Occupant of three-wheeled motor vehicle injured in collision with car, pick-up truck or van

The appropriate 7th character is to be added to each code from category V33
A = initial encounter
D = subsequent encounter
S = sequela

V33.0 Driver of three-wheeled motor vehicle injured in collision with car, pick-up truck or van in nontraffic accident
V33.1 Passenger in three-wheeled motor vehicle injured in collision with car, pick-up truck or van in nontraffic accident
V33.2 Person on outside of three-wheeled motor vehicle injured in collision with car, pick-up truck or van in nontraffic accident
V33.3 Unspecified occupant of three-wheeled motor vehicle injured in collision with car, pick-up truck or van in nontraffic accident
V33.4 Person boarding or alighting a three-wheeled motor vehicle injured in collision with car, pick-up truck or van
V33.5 Driver of three-wheeled motor vehicle injured in collision with car, pick-up truck or van in traffic accident
V33.6 Passenger in three-wheeled motor vehicle injured in collision with car, pick-up truck or van in traffic accident
V33.7 Person on outside of three-wheeled motor vehicle injured in collision with car, pick-up truck or van in traffic accident
V33.9 Unspecified occupant of three-wheeled motor vehicle injured in collision with car, pick-up truck or van in traffic accident

V34 Occupant of three-wheeled motor vehicle injured in collision with heavy transport vehicle or bus

EXCLUDES1 *occupant of three-wheeled motor vehicle injured in collision with military vehicle (V39.81)*

The appropriate 7th character is to be added to each code from category V34
A = initial encounter
D = subsequent encounter
S = sequela

V34.0 Driver of three-wheeled motor vehicle injured in collision with heavy transport vehicle or bus in nontraffic accident
V34.1 Passenger in three-wheeled motor vehicle injured in collision with heavy transport vehicle or bus in nontraffic accident
V34.2 Person on outside of three-wheeled motor vehicle injured in collision with heavy transport vehicle or bus in nontraffic accident
V34.3 Unspecified occupant of three-wheeled motor vehicle injured in collision with heavy transport vehicle or bus in nontraffic accident
V34.4 Person boarding or alighting a three-wheeled motor vehicle injured in collision with heavy transport vehicle or bus
V34.5 Driver of three-wheeled motor vehicle injured in collision with heavy transport vehicle or bus in traffic accident
V34.6 Passenger in three-wheeled motor vehicle injured in collision with heavy transport vehicle or bus in traffic accident
V34.7 Person on outside of three-wheeled motor vehicle injured in collision with heavy transport vehicle or bus in traffic accident
V34.9 Unspecified occupant of three-wheeled motor vehicle injured in collision with heavy transport vehicle or bus in traffic accident

V35 Occupant of three-wheeled motor vehicle injured in collision with railway train or railway vehicle

The appropriate 7th character is to be added to each code from category V35
A = initial encounter
D = subsequent encounter
S = sequela

V35.0 Driver of three-wheeled motor vehicle injured in collision with railway train or railway vehicle in nontraffic accident
V35.1 Passenger in three-wheeled motor vehicle injured in collision with railway train or railway vehicle in nontraffic accident
V35.2 Person on outside of three-wheeled motor vehicle injured in collision with railway train or railway vehicle in nontraffic accident
V35.3 Unspecified occupant of three-wheeled motor vehicle injured in collision with railway train or railway vehicle in nontraffic accident
V35.4 Person boarding or alighting a three-wheeled motor vehicle injured in collision with railway train or railway vehicle
V35.5 Driver of three-wheeled motor vehicle injured in collision with railway train or railway vehicle in traffic accident
V35.6 Passenger in three-wheeled motor vehicle injured in collision with railway train or railway vehicle in traffic accident
V35.7 Person on outside of three-wheeled motor vehicle injured in collision with railway train or railway vehicle in traffic accident
V35.9 Unspecified occupant of three-wheeled motor vehicle injured in collision with railway train or railway vehicle in traffic accident

V36 Occupant of three-wheeled motor vehicle injured in collision with other nonmotor vehicle

INCLUDES *collision with animal-drawn vehicle, animal being ridden, streetcar*

The appropriate 7th character is to be added to each code from category V36
A = initial encounter
D = subsequent encounter
S = sequela

V36.0 Driver of three-wheeled motor vehicle injured in collision with other nonmotor vehicle in nontraffic accident
V36.1 Passenger in three-wheeled motor vehicle injured in collision with other nonmotor vehicle in nontraffic accident
V36.2 Person on outside of three-wheeled motor vehicle injured in collision with other nonmotor vehicle in nontraffic accident
V36.3 Unspecified occupant of three-wheeled motor vehicle injured in collision with other nonmotor vehicle in nontraffic accident
V36.4 Person boarding or alighting a three-wheeled motor vehicle injured in collision with other nonmotor vehicle
V36.5 Driver of three-wheeled motor vehicle injured in collision with other nonmotor vehicle in traffic accident
V36.6 Passenger in three-wheeled motor vehicle injured in collision with other nonmotor vehicle in traffic accident
V36.7 Person on outside of three-wheeled motor vehicle injured in collision with other nonmotor vehicle in traffic accident
V36.9 Unspecified occupant of three-wheeled motor vehicle injured in collision with other nonmotor vehicle in traffic accident

V37 Occupant of three-wheeled motor vehicle injured in collision with fixed or stationary object

The appropriate 7th character is to be added to each code from category V37
A = initial encounter
D = subsequent encounter
S = sequela

V37.0 Driver of three-wheeled motor vehicle injured in collision with fixed or stationary object in nontraffic accident
V37.1 Passenger in three-wheeled motor vehicle injured in collision with fixed or stationary object in nontraffic accident
V37.2 Person on outside of three-wheeled motor vehicle injured in collision with fixed or stationary object in nontraffic accident

Unacceptable principal diagnosis symbol per Medicare code edits · Code exempt from diagnosis present on admission requirement
Questionable admission · Complication or comorbidity · CC/MCC exclusion · Major complication or comorbidity
Principal diagnosis as its own CC · Principal diagnosis as its own MCC · Z code as first-listed diagnosis

V37.3 Unspecified occupant of three-wheeled motor vehicle injured in collision with fixed or stationary object in nontraffic accident

V37.4 Person boarding or alighting a three-wheeled motor vehicle injured in collision with fixed or stationary object

V37.5 Driver of three-wheeled motor vehicle injured in collision with fixed or stationary object in traffic accident

V37.6 Passenger in three-wheeled motor vehicle injured in collision with fixed or stationary object in traffic accident

V37.7 Person on outside of three-wheeled motor vehicle injured in collision with fixed or stationary object in traffic accident

V37.9 Unspecified occupant of three-wheeled motor vehicle injured in collision with fixed or stationary object in traffic accident

V38 Occupant of three-wheeled motor vehicle injured in noncollision transport accident

INCLUDES *fall or thrown from three-wheeled motor vehicle*
overturning of three-wheeled motor vehicle NOS
overturning of three-wheeled motor vehicle without collision

The appropriate 7th character is to be added to each code from category V38
A = initial encounter
D = subsequent encounter
S = sequela

V38.0 Driver of three-wheeled motor vehicle injured in noncollision transport accident in nontraffic accident

V38.1 Passenger in three-wheeled motor vehicle injured in noncollision transport accident in nontraffic accident

V38.2 Person on outside of three-wheeled motor vehicle injured in noncollision transport accident in nontraffic accident

V38.3 Unspecified occupant of three-wheeled motor vehicle injured in noncollision transport accident in nontraffic accident

V38.4 Person boarding or alighting a three-wheeled motor vehicle injured in noncollision transport accident

V38.5 Driver of three-wheeled motor vehicle injured in noncollision transport accident in traffic accident

V38.6 Passenger in three-wheeled motor vehicle injured in noncollision transport accident in traffic accident

V38.7 Person on outside of three-wheeled motor vehicle injured in noncollision transport accident in traffic accident

V38.9 Unspecified occupant of three-wheeled motor vehicle injured in noncollision transport accident in traffic accident

V39 Occupant of three-wheeled motor vehicle injured in other and unspecified transport accidents

The appropriate 7th character is to be added to each code from category V39
A = initial encounter
D = subsequent encounter
S = sequela

V39.0 Driver of three-wheeled motor vehicle injured in collision with other and unspecified motor vehicles in nontraffic accident

V39.00 Driver of three-wheeled motor vehicle injured in collision with unspecified motor vehicles in nontraffic accident

V39.09 Driver of three-wheeled motor vehicle injured in collision with other motor vehicles in nontraffic accident

V39.1 Passenger in three-wheeled motor vehicle injured in collision with other and unspecified motor vehicles in nontraffic accident

V39.10 Passenger in three-wheeled motor vehicle injured in collision with unspecified motor vehicles in nontraffic accident

V39.19 Passenger in three-wheeled motor vehicle injured in collision with other motor vehicles in nontraffic accident

V39.2 Unspecified occupant of three-wheeled motor vehicle injured in collision with other and unspecified motor vehicles in nontraffic accident

V39.20 Unspecified occupant of three-wheeled motor vehicle injured in collision with unspecified motor vehicles in nontraffic accident
Collision NOS involving three-wheeled motor vehicle, nontraffic

V39.29 Unspecified occupant of three-wheeled motor vehicle injured in collision with other motor vehicles in nontraffic accident

V39.3 Occupant (driver) (passenger) of three-wheeled motor vehicle injured in unspecified nontraffic accident
Accident NOS involving three-wheeled motor vehicle, nontraffic
Occupant of three-wheeled motor vehicle injured in nontraffic accident NOS

V39.4 Driver of three-wheeled motor vehicle injured in collision with other and unspecified motor vehicles in traffic accident

V39.40 Driver of three-wheeled motor vehicle injured in collision with unspecified motor vehicles in traffic accident

V39.49 Driver of three-wheeled motor vehicle injured in collision with other motor vehicles in traffic accident

V39.5 Passenger in three-wheeled motor vehicle injured in collision with other and unspecified motor vehicles in traffic accident

V39.50 Passenger in three-wheeled motor vehicle injured in collision with unspecified motor vehicles in traffic accident

V39.59 Passenger in three-wheeled motor vehicle injured in collision with other motor vehicles in traffic accident

V39.6 Unspecified occupant of three-wheeled motor vehicle injured in collision with other and unspecified motor vehicles in traffic accident

V39.60 Unspecified occupant of three-wheeled motor vehicle injured in collision with unspecified motor vehicles in traffic accident
Collision NOS involving three-wheeled motor vehicle (traffic)

V39.69 Unspecified occupant of three-wheeled motor vehicle injured in collision with other motor vehicles in traffic accident

V39.8 Occupant (driver) (passenger) of three-wheeled motor vehicle injured in other specified transport accidents

V39.81 Occupant (driver) (passenger) of three-wheeled motor vehicle injured in transport accident with military vehicle

V39.89 Occupant (driver) (passenger) of three-wheeled motor vehicle injured in other specified transport accidents

V39.9 Occupant (driver) (passenger) of three-wheeled motor vehicle injured in unspecified traffic accident
Accident NOS involving three-wheeled motor vehicle

Car occupant injured in transport accident (V40-V49)

INCLUDES *a four-wheeled motor vehicle designed primarily for carrying passengers*
automobile (pulling a trailer or camper)

EXCLUDES1 *bus (V50-V59)*
minibus (V50-V59)
minivan (V50-V59)
motorcoach (V70-V79)
pick-up truck (V50-V59)
sport utility vehicle (SUV) (V50-V59)

V40 Car occupant injured in collision with pedestrian or animal

EXCLUDES1 *car collision with animal-drawn vehicle or animal being ridden (V46.-)*

The appropriate 7th character is to be added to each code from category V40
A = initial encounter
D = subsequent encounter
S = sequela

V40.0 Car driver injured in collision with pedestrian or animal in nontraffic accident

V40.1 Car passenger injured in collision with pedestrian or animal in nontraffic accident

V40.2 Person on outside of car injured in collision with pedestrian or animal in nontraffic accident

V40.3 Unspecified car occupant injured in collision with pedestrian or animal in nontraffic accident

V40.4 Person boarding or alighting a car injured in collision with pedestrian or animal

V40.5 Car driver injured in collision with pedestrian or animal in traffic accident

- V40.6 Car passenger injured in collision with pedestrian or animal in traffic accident
- V40.7 Person on outside of car injured in collision with pedestrian or animal in traffic accident
- V40.9 Unspecified car occupant injured in collision with pedestrian or animal in traffic accident

V41 Car occupant injured in collision with pedal cycle

The appropriate 7th character is to be added to each code from category V41
- A = initial encounter
- D = subsequent encounter
- S = sequela

- V41.0 Car driver injured in collision with pedal cycle in nontraffic accident
- V41.1 Car passenger injured in collision with pedal cycle in nontraffic accident
- V41.2 Person on outside of car injured in collision with pedal cycle in nontraffic accident
- V41.3 Unspecified car occupant injured in collision with pedal cycle in nontraffic accident
- V41.4 Person boarding or alighting a car injured in collision with pedal cycle
- V41.5 Car driver injured in collision with pedal cycle in traffic accident
- V41.6 Car passenger injured in collision with pedal cycle in traffic accident
- V41.7 Person on outside of car injured in collision with pedal cycle in traffic accident
- V41.9 Unspecified car occupant injured in collision with pedal cycle in traffic accident

V42 Car occupant injured in collision with two- or three-wheeled motor vehicle

The appropriate 7th character is to be added to each code from category V42
- A = initial encounter
- D = subsequent encounter
- S = sequela

- V42.0 Car driver injured in collision with two- or three-wheeled motor vehicle in nontraffic accident
- V42.1 Car passenger injured in collision with two- or three-wheeled motor vehicle in nontraffic accident
- V42.2 Person on outside of car injured in collision with two- or three-wheeled motor vehicle in nontraffic accident
- V42.3 Unspecified car occupant injured in collision with two- or three-wheeled motor vehicle in nontraffic accident
- V42.4 Person boarding or alighting a car injured in collision with two- or three-wheeled motor vehicle
- V42.5 Car driver injured in collision with two- or three-wheeled motor vehicle in traffic accident
- V42.6 Car passenger injured in collision with two- or three-wheeled motor vehicle in traffic accident
- V42.7 Person on outside of car injured in collision with two- or three-wheeled motor vehicle in traffic accident
- V42.9 Unspecified car occupant injured in collision with two- or three-wheeled motor vehicle in traffic accident

V43 Car occupant injured in collision with car, pick-up truck or van

The appropriate 7th character is to be added to each code from category V43
- A = initial encounter
- D = subsequent encounter
- S = sequela

- V43.0 Car driver injured in collision with car, pick-up truck or van in nontraffic accident
  - V43.01 Car driver injured in collision with sport utility vehicle in nontraffic accident
  - V43.02 Car driver injured in collision with other type car in nontraffic accident
  - V43.03 Car driver injured in collision with pick-up truck in nontraffic accident
  - V43.04 Car driver injured in collision with van in nontraffic accident
- V43.1 Car passenger injured in collision with car, pick-up truck or van in nontraffic accident
  - V43.11 Car passenger injured in collision with sport utility vehicle in nontraffic accident
  - V43.12 Car passenger injured in collision with other type car in nontraffic accident
  - V43.13 Car passenger injured in collision with pick-up in nontraffic accident
  - V43.14 Car passenger injured in collision with van in nontraffic accident
- V43.2 Person on outside of car injured in collision with car, pick-up truck or van in nontraffic accident
  - V43.21 Person on outside of car injured in collision with sport utility vehicle in nontraffic accident
  - V43.22 Person on outside of car injured in collision with other type car in nontraffic accident
  - V43.23 Person on outside of car injured in collision with pick-up truck in nontraffic accident
  - V43.24 Person on outside of car injured in collision with van in nontraffic accident
- V43.3 Unspecified car occupant injured in collision with car, pick-up truck or van in nontraffic accident
  - V43.31 Unspecified car occupant injured in collision with sport utility vehicle in nontraffic accident
  - V43.32 Unspecified car occupant injured in collision with other type car in nontraffic accident
  - V43.33 Unspecified car occupant injured in collision with pick-up truck in nontraffic accident
  - V43.34 Unspecified car occupant injured in collision with van in nontraffic accident
- V43.4 Person boarding or alighting a car injured in collision with car, pick-up truck or van
  - V43.41 Person boarding or alighting a car injured in collision with sport utility vehicle
  - V43.42 Person boarding or alighting a car injured in collision with other type car
  - V43.43 Person boarding or alighting a car injured in collision with pick-up truck
  - V43.44 Person boarding or alighting a car injured in collision with van
- V43.5 Car driver injured in collision with car, pick-up truck or van in traffic accident
  - V43.51 Car driver injured in collision with sport utility vehicle in traffic accident
  - V43.52 Car driver injured in collision with other type car in traffic accident
  - V43.53 Car driver injured in collision with pick-up truck in traffic accident
  - V43.54 Car driver injured in collision with van in traffic accident
- V43.6 Car passenger injured in collision with car, pick-up truck or van in traffic accident
  - V43.61 Car passenger injured in collision with sport utility vehicle in traffic accident
    AHA: Q1, 2015
  - V43.62 Car passenger injured in collision with other type car in traffic accident
  - V43.63 Car passenger injured in collision with pick-up truck in traffic accident
  - V43.64 Car passenger injured in collision with van in traffic accident
- V43.7 Person on outside of car injured in collision with car, pick-up truck or van in traffic accident
  - V43.71 Person on outside of car injured in collision with sport utility vehicle in traffic accident
  - V43.72 Person on outside of car injured in collision with other type car in traffic accident
  - V43.73 Person on outside of car injured in collision with pick-up truck in traffic accident
  - V43.74 Person on outside of car injured in collision with van in traffic accident
- V43.9 Unspecified car occupant injured in collision with car, pick-up truck or van in traffic accident
  - V43.91 Unspecified car occupant injured in collision with sport utility vehicle in traffic accident
  - V43.92 Unspecified car occupant injured in collision with other type car in traffic accident
  - V43.93 Unspecified car occupant injured in collision with pick-up truck in traffic accident

Unacceptable principal diagnosis symbol per Medicare code edits · Code exempt from diagnosis present on admission requirement · Questionable admission · Complication or comorbidity · CC/MCC exclusion · Major complication or comorbidity · Principal diagnosis as its own CC · Principal diagnosis as its own MCC · Z code as first-listed diagnosis

V43.94 Unspecified car occupant injured in collision with van in traffic accident

V44 Car occupant injured in collision with heavy transport vehicle or bus

EXCLUDES1 *car occupant injured in collision with military vehicle (V49.81)*

The appropriate 7th character is to be added to each code from category V44
A = initial encounter
D = subsequent encounter
S = sequela

V44.0 Car driver injured in collision with heavy transport vehicle or bus in nontraffic accident
V44.1 Car passenger injured in collision with heavy transport vehicle or bus in nontraffic accident
V44.2 Person on outside of car injured in collision with heavy transport vehicle or bus in nontraffic accident
V44.3 Unspecified car occupant injured in collision with heavy transport vehicle or bus in nontraffic accident
V44.4 Person boarding or alighting a car injured in collision with heavy transport vehicle or bus
V44.5 Car driver injured in collision with heavy transport vehicle or bus in traffic accident
V44.6 Car passenger injured in collision with heavy transport vehicle or bus in traffic accident
V44.7 Person on outside of car injured in collision with heavy transport vehicle or bus in traffic accident
V44.9 Unspecified car occupant injured in collision with heavy transport vehicle or bus in traffic accident

V45 Car occupant injured in collision with railway train or railway vehicle

The appropriate 7th character is to be added to each code from category V45
A = initial encounter
D = subsequent encounter
S = sequela

V45.0 Car driver injured in collision with railway train or railway vehicle in nontraffic accident
V45.1 Car passenger injured in collision with railway train or railway vehicle in nontraffic accident
V45.2 Person on outside of car injured in collision with railway train or railway vehicle in nontraffic accident
V45.3 Unspecified car occupant injured in collision with railway train or railway vehicle in nontraffic accident
V45.4 Person boarding or alighting a car injured in collision with railway train or railway vehicle
V45.5 Car driver injured in collision with railway train or railway vehicle in traffic accident
V45.6 Car passenger injured in collision with railway train or railway vehicle in traffic accident
V45.7 Person on outside of car injured in collision with railway train or railway vehicle in traffic accident
V45.9 Unspecified car occupant injured in collision with railway train or railway vehicle in traffic accident

V46 Car occupant injured in collision with other nonmotor vehicle

INCLUDES *collision with animal-drawn vehicle, animal being ridden, streetcar*

The appropriate 7th character is to be added to each code from category V46
A = initial encounter
D = subsequent encounter
S = sequela

V46.0 Car driver injured in collision with other nonmotor vehicle in nontraffic accident
V46.1 Car passenger injured in collision with other nonmotor vehicle in nontraffic accident
V46.2 Person on outside of car injured in collision with other nonmotor vehicle in nontraffic accident
V46.3 Unspecified car occupant injured in collision with other nonmotor vehicle in nontraffic accident
V46.4 Person boarding or alighting a car injured in collision with other nonmotor vehicle
V46.5 Car driver injured in collision with other nonmotor vehicle in traffic accident
V46.6 Car passenger injured in collision with other nonmotor vehicle in traffic accident
V46.7 Person on outside of car injured in collision with other nonmotor vehicle in traffic accident
V46.9 Unspecified car occupant injured in collision with other nonmotor vehicle in traffic accident

V47 Car occupant injured in collision with fixed or stationary object

The appropriate 7th character is to be added to each code from category V47
A = initial encounter
D = subsequent encounter
S = sequela

V47.0 Car driver injured in collision with fixed or stationary object in nontraffic accident
V47.1 Car passenger injured in collision with fixed or stationary object in nontraffic accident
V47.2 Person on outside of car injured in collision with fixed or stationary object in nontraffic accident
V47.3 Unspecified car occupant injured in collision with fixed or stationary object in nontraffic accident
V47.4 Person boarding or alighting a car injured in collision with fixed or stationary object
V47.5 Car driver injured in collision with fixed or stationary object in traffic accident
V47.6 Car passenger injured in collision with fixed or stationary object in traffic accident
V47.7 Person on outside of car injured in collision with fixed or stationary object in traffic accident
V47.9 Unspecified car occupant injured in collision with fixed or stationary object in traffic accident

V48 Car occupant injured in noncollision transport accident

INCLUDES *overturning car NOS*
overturning car without collision

The appropriate 7th character is to be added to each code from category V48
A = initial encounter
D = subsequent encounter
S = sequela

V48.0 Car driver injured in noncollision transport accident in nontraffic accident
V48.1 Car passenger injured in noncollision transport accident in nontraffic accident
V48.2 Person on outside of car injured in noncollision transport accident in nontraffic accident
V48.3 Unspecified car occupant injured in noncollision transport accident in nontraffic accident
V48.4 Person boarding or alighting a car injured in noncollision transport accident
V48.5 Car driver injured in noncollision transport accident in traffic accident
V48.6 Car passenger injured in noncollision transport accident in traffic accident
V48.7 Person on outside of car injured in noncollision transport accident in traffic accident
V48.9 Unspecified car occupant injured in noncollision transport accident in traffic accident

V49 Car occupant injured in other and unspecified transport accidents

The appropriate 7th character is to be added to each code from category V49
A = initial encounter
D = subsequent encounter
S = sequela

V49.0 Driver injured in collision with other and unspecified motor vehicles in nontraffic accident
V49.00 Driver injured in collision with unspecified motor vehicles in nontraffic accident
V49.09 Driver injured in collision with other motor vehicles in nontraffic accident
V49.1 Passenger injured in collision with other and unspecified motor vehicles in nontraffic accident
V49.10 Passenger injured in collision with unspecified motor vehicles in nontraffic accident
V49.19 Passenger injured in collision with other motor vehicles in nontraffic accident
V49.2 Unspecified car occupant injured in collision with other and unspecified motor vehicles in nontraffic accident
V49.20 Unspecified car occupant injured in collision with unspecified motor vehicles in nontraffic accident
Car collision NOS, nontraffic

Unspecified Code Other Specified Code Manifestation Code N Newborn P Pediatric M Maternity A Adult ♂ Male ♀ Female
● New Code ▲ Revised Code Title ►◄ Revised Text NOTES INCLUDES EXCLUDES1 Not coded here EXCLUDES2 Not included here
4th character required 5th character required 6th character required 7th character required
Extension 'X' Alert HAC Hospital-acquired condition (HAC) alert AHA AHA Coding Clinic©

- V49.29 Unspecified car occupant injured in collision with other motor vehicles in nontraffic accident
- V49.3 Car occupant (driver) (passenger) injured in unspecified nontraffic accident
  Car accident NOS, nontraffic
  Car occupant injured in nontraffic accident NOS
- V49.4 Driver injured in collision with other and unspecified motor vehicles in traffic accident
  - V49.40 Driver injured in collision with unspecified motor vehicles in traffic accident
  - V49.49 Driver injured in collision with other motor vehicles in traffic accident
- V49.5 Passenger injured in collision with other and unspecified motor vehicles in traffic accident
  - V49.50 Passenger injured in collision with unspecified motor vehicles in traffic accident
  - V49.59 Passenger injured in collision with other motor vehicles in traffic accident
- V49.6 Unspecified car occupant injured in collision with other and unspecified motor vehicles in traffic accident
  - V49.60 Unspecified car occupant injured in collision with unspecified motor vehicles in traffic accident
    Car collision NOS (traffic)
  - V49.69 Unspecified car occupant injured in collision with other motor vehicles in traffic accident
- V49.8 Car occupant (driver) (passenger) injured in other specified transport accidents
  - V49.81 Car occupant (driver) (passenger) injured in transport accident with military vehicle
  - V49.88 Car occupant (driver) (passenger) injured in other specified transport accidents
- V49.9 Car occupant (driver) (passenger) injured in unspecified traffic accident
  Car accident NOS

Occupant of pick-up truck or van injured in transport accident (V50-V59)

INCLUDES *a four or six wheel motor vehicle designed primarily for carrying passengers and property but weighing less than the local limit for classification as a heavy goods vehicle*
minibus
minivan
sport utility vehicle (SUV)
truck
van

EXCLUDES1 *heavy transport vehicle (V60-V69)*

V50 Occupant of pick-up truck or van injured in collision with pedestrian or animal

EXCLUDES1 *pick-up truck or van collision with animal-drawn vehicle or animal being ridden (V56.-)*

The appropriate 7th character is to be added to each code from category V50
A = initial encounter
D = subsequent encounter
S = sequela

- V50.0 Driver of pick-up truck or van injured in collision with pedestrian or animal in nontraffic accident
- V50.1 Passenger in pick-up truck or van injured in collision with pedestrian or animal in nontraffic accident
- V50.2 Person on outside of pick-up truck or van injured in collision with pedestrian or animal in nontraffic accident
- V50.3 Unspecified occupant of pick-up truck or van injured in collision with pedestrian or animal in nontraffic accident
- V50.4 Person boarding or alighting a pick-up truck or van injured in collision with pedestrian or animal
- V50.5 Driver of pick-up truck or van injured in collision with pedestrian or animal in traffic accident
- V50.6 Passenger in pick-up truck or van injured in collision with pedestrian or animal in traffic accident
- V50.7 Person on outside of pick-up truck or van injured in collision with pedestrian or animal in traffic accident
- V50.9 Unspecified occupant of pick-up truck or van injured in collision with pedestrian or animal in traffic accident

V51 Occupant of pick-up truck or van injured in collision with pedal cycle

The appropriate 7th character is to be added to each code from category V51
A = initial encounter
D = subsequent encounter
S = sequela

- V51.0 Driver of pick-up truck or van injured in collision with pedal cycle in nontraffic accident
- V51.1 Passenger in pick-up truck or van injured in collision with pedal cycle in nontraffic accident
- V51.2 Person on outside of pick-up truck or van injured in collision with pedal cycle in nontraffic accident
- V51.3 Unspecified occupant of pick-up truck or van injured in collision with pedal cycle in nontraffic accident
- V51.4 Person boarding or alighting a pick-up truck or van injured in collision with pedal cycle
- V51.5 Driver of pick-up truck or van injured in collision with pedal cycle in traffic accident
- V51.6 Passenger in pick-up truck or van injured in collision with pedal cycle in traffic accident
- V51.7 Person on outside of pick-up truck or van injured in collision with pedal cycle in traffic accident
- V51.9 Unspecified occupant of pick-up truck or van injured in collision with pedal cycle in traffic accident

V52 Occupant of pick-up truck or van injured in collision with two- or three-wheeled motor vehicle

The appropriate 7th character is to be added to each code from category V52
A = initial encounter
D = subsequent encounter
S = sequela

- V52.0 Driver of pick-up truck or van injured in collision with two- or three-wheeled motor vehicle in nontraffic accident
- V52.1 Passenger in pick-up truck or van injured in collision with two- or three-wheeled motor vehicle in nontraffic accident
- V52.2 Person on outside of pick-up truck or van injured in collision with two- or three-wheeled motor vehicle in nontraffic accident
- V52.3 Unspecified occupant of pick-up truck or van injured in collision with two- or three-wheeled motor vehicle in nontraffic accident
- V52.4 Person boarding or alighting a pick-up truck or van injured in collision with two- or three-wheeled motor vehicle
- V52.5 Driver of pick-up truck or van injured in collision with two- or three-wheeled motor vehicle in traffic accident
- V52.6 Passenger in pick-up truck or van injured in collision with two- or three-wheeled motor vehicle in traffic accident
- V52.7 Person on outside of pick-up truck or van injured in collision with two- or three-wheeled motor vehicle in traffic accident
- V52.9 Unspecified occupant of pick-up truck or van injured in collision with two- or three-wheeled motor vehicle in traffic accident

V53 Occupant of pick-up truck or van injured in collision with car, pick-up truck or van

The appropriate 7th character is to be added to each code from category V53
A = initial encounter
D = subsequent encounter
S = sequela

- V53.0 Driver of pick-up truck or van injured in collision with car, pick-up truck or van in nontraffic accident
- V53.1 Passenger in pick-up truck or van injured in collision with car, pick-up truck or van in nontraffic accident
- V53.2 Person on outside of pick-up truck or van injured in collision with car, pick-up truck or van in nontraffic accident
- V53.3 Unspecified occupant of pick-up truck or van injured in collision with car, pick-up truck or van in nontraffic accident
- V53.4 Person boarding or alighting a pick-up truck or van injured in collision with car, pick-up truck or van
- V53.5 Driver of pick-up truck or van injured in collision with car, pick-up truck or van in traffic accident
- V53.6 Passenger in pick-up truck or van injured in collision with car, pick-up truck or van in traffic accident
- V53.7 Person on outside of pick-up truck or van injured in collision with car, pick-up truck or van in traffic accident

Unacceptable principal diagnosis symbol per Medicare code edits · Code exempt from diagnosis present on admission requirement
Questionable admission · Complication or comorbidity · CC/MCC exclusion · Major complication or comorbidity
Principal diagnosis as its own CC · Principal diagnosis as its own MCC · Z code as first-listed diagnosis

V53.9 Unspecified occupant of pick-up truck or van injured in collision with car, pick-up truck or van in traffic accident

V54 Occupant of pick-up truck or van injured in collision with heavy transport vehicle or bus

EXCLUDES1 *occupant of pick-up truck or van injured in collision with military vehicle (V59.81)*

The appropriate 7th character is to be added to each code from category V54
A = initial encounter
D = subsequent encounter
S = sequela

V54.0 Driver of pick-up truck or van injured in collision with heavy transport vehicle or bus in nontraffic accident

V54.1 Passenger in pick-up truck or van injured in collision with heavy transport vehicle or bus in nontraffic accident

V54.2 Person on outside of pick-up truck or van injured in collision with heavy transport vehicle or bus in nontraffic accident

V54.3 Unspecified occupant of pick-up truck or van injured in collision with heavy transport vehicle or bus in nontraffic accident

V54.4 Person boarding or alighting a pick-up truck or van injured in collision with heavy transport vehicle or bus

V54.5 Driver of pick-up truck or van injured in collision with heavy transport vehicle or bus in traffic accident

V54.6 Passenger in pick-up truck or van injured in collision with heavy transport vehicle or bus in traffic accident

V54.7 Person on outside of pick-up truck or van injured in collision with heavy transport vehicle or bus in traffic accident

V54.9 Unspecified occupant of pick-up truck or van injured in collision with heavy transport vehicle or bus in traffic accident

V55 Occupant of pick-up truck or van injured in collision with railway train or railway vehicle

The appropriate 7th character is to be added to each code from category V55
A = initial encounter
D = subsequent encounter
S = sequela

V55.0 Driver of pick-up truck or van injured in collision with railway train or railway vehicle in nontraffic accident

V55.1 Passenger in pick-up truck or van injured in collision with railway train or railway vehicle in nontraffic accident

V55.2 Person on outside of pick-up truck or van injured in collision with railway train or railway vehicle in nontraffic accident

V55.3 Unspecified occupant of pick-up truck or van injured in collision with railway train or railway vehicle in nontraffic accident

V55.4 Person boarding or alighting a pick-up truck or van injured in collision with railway train or railway vehicle

V55.5 Driver of pick-up truck or van injured in collision with railway train or railway vehicle in traffic accident

V55.6 Passenger in pick-up truck or van injured in collision with railway train or railway vehicle in traffic accident

V55.7 Person on outside of pick-up truck or van injured in collision with railway train or railway vehicle in traffic accident

V55.9 Unspecified occupant of pick-up truck or van injured in collision with railway train or railway vehicle in traffic accident

V56 Occupant of pick-up truck or van injured in collision with other nonmotor vehicle

INCLUDES *collision with animal-drawn vehicle, animal being ridden, streetcar*

The appropriate 7th character is to be added to each code from category V56
A = initial encounter
D = subsequent encounter
S = sequela

V56.0 Driver of pick-up truck or van injured in collision with other nonmotor vehicle in nontraffic accident

V56.1 Passenger in pick-up truck or van injured in collision with other nonmotor vehicle in nontraffic accident

V56.2 Person on outside of pick-up truck or van injured in collision with other nonmotor vehicle in nontraffic accident

V56.3 Unspecified occupant of pick-up truck or van injured in collision with other nonmotor vehicle in nontraffic accident

V56.4 Person boarding or alighting a pick-up truck or van injured in collision with other nonmotor vehicle

V56.5 Driver of pick-up truck or van injured in collision with other nonmotor vehicle in traffic accident

V56.6 Passenger in pick-up truck or van injured in collision with other nonmotor vehicle in traffic accident

V56.7 Person on outside of pick-up truck or van injured in collision with other nonmotor vehicle in traffic accident

V56.9 Unspecified occupant of pick-up truck or van injured in collision with other nonmotor vehicle in traffic accident

V57 Occupant of pick-up truck or van injured in collision with fixed or stationary object

The appropriate 7th character is to be added to each code from category V57
A = initial encounter
D = subsequent encounter
S = sequela

V57.0 Driver of pick-up truck or van injured in collision with fixed or stationary object in nontraffic accident

V57.1 Passenger in pick-up truck or van injured in collision with fixed or stationary object in nontraffic accident

V57.2 Person on outside of pick-up truck or van injured in collision with fixed or stationary object in nontraffic accident

V57.3 Unspecified occupant of pick-up truck or van injured in collision with fixed or stationary object in nontraffic accident

V57.4 Person boarding or alighting a pick-up truck or van injured in collision with fixed or stationary object

V57.5 Driver of pick-up truck or van injured in collision with fixed or stationary object in traffic accident

V57.6 Passenger in pick-up truck or van injured in collision with fixed or stationary object in traffic accident

V57.7 Person on outside of pick-up truck or van injured in collision with fixed or stationary object in traffic accident

V57.9 Unspecified occupant of pick-up truck or van injured in collision with fixed or stationary object in traffic accident

V58 Occupant of pick-up truck or van injured in noncollision transport accident

INCLUDES *overturning pick-up truck or van NOS*
overturning pick-up truck or van without collision

The appropriate 7th character is to be added to each code from category V58
A = initial encounter
D = subsequent encounter
S = sequela

V58.0 Driver of pick-up truck or van injured in noncollision transport accident in nontraffic accident

V58.1 Passenger in pick-up truck or van injured in noncollision transport accident in nontraffic accident

V58.2 Person on outside of pick-up truck or van injured in noncollision transport accident in nontraffic accident

V58.3 Unspecified occupant of pick-up truck or van injured in noncollision transport accident in nontraffic accident

V58.4 Person boarding or alighting a pick-up truck or van injured in noncollision transport accident

V58.5 Driver of pick-up truck or van injured in noncollision transport accident in traffic accident

V58.6 Passenger in pick-up truck or van injured in noncollision transport accident in traffic accident

V58.7 Person on outside of pick-up truck or van injured in noncollision transport accident in traffic accident

V58.9 Unspecified occupant of pick-up truck or van injured in noncollision transport accident in traffic accident

V59 Occupant of pick-up truck or van injured in other and unspecified transport accidents

The appropriate 7th character is to be added to each code from category V59
A = initial encounter
D = subsequent encounter
S = sequela

V59.0 Driver of pick-up truck or van injured in collision with other and unspecified motor vehicles in nontraffic accident

V59.00 Driver of pick-up truck or van injured in collision with unspecified motor vehicles in nontraffic accident

Unspecified Code Other Specified Code Manifestation Code N Newborn P Pediatric M Maternity A Adult ♂ Male ♀ Female
● New Code ▲ Revised Code Title ►◄ Revised Text NOTES INCLUDES EXCLUDES1 Not coded here EXCLUDES2 Not included here
4th character required 5th character required 6th character required 7th character required
Extension 'X' Alert HAC Hospital-acquired condition (HAC) alert AHA AHA Coding Clinic©

V59.09 Driver of pick-up truck or van injured in collision with other motor vehicles in nontraffic accident

V59.1 Passenger in pick-up truck or van injured in collision with other and unspecified motor vehicles in nontraffic accident

V59.10 Passenger in pick-up truck or van injured in collision with unspecified motor vehicles in nontraffic accident

V59.19 Passenger in pick-up truck or van injured in collision with other motor vehicles in nontraffic accident

V59.2 Unspecified occupant of pick-up truck or van injured in collision with other and unspecified motor vehicles in nontraffic accident

V59.20 Unspecified occupant of pick-up truck or van injured in collision with unspecified motor vehicles in nontraffic accident
Collision NOS involving pick-up truck or van, nontraffic

V59.29 Unspecified occupant of pick-up truck or van injured in collision with other motor vehicles in nontraffic accident

V59.3 Occupant (driver) (passenger) of pick-up truck or van injured in unspecified nontraffic accident
Accident NOS involving pick-up truck or van, nontraffic
Occupant of pick-up truck or van injured in nontraffic accident NOS

V59.4 Driver of pick-up truck or van injured in collision with other and unspecified motor vehicles in traffic accident

V59.40 Driver of pick-up truck or van injured in collision with unspecified motor vehicles in traffic accident

V59.49 Driver of pick-up truck or van injured in collision with other motor vehicles in traffic accident

V59.5 Passenger in pick-up truck or van injured in collision with other and unspecified motor vehicles in traffic accident

V59.50 Passenger in pick-up truck or van injured in collision with unspecified motor vehicles in traffic accident

V59.59 Passenger in pick-up truck or van injured in collision with other motor vehicles in traffic accident

V59.6 Unspecified occupant of pick-up truck or van injured in collision with other and unspecified motor vehicles in traffic accident

V59.60 Unspecified occupant of pick-up truck or van injured in collision with unspecified motor vehicles in traffic accident
Collision NOS involving pick-up truck or van (traffic)

V59.69 Unspecified occupant of pick-up truck or van injured in collision with other motor vehicles in traffic accident

V59.8 Occupant (driver) (passenger) of pick-up truck or van injured in other specified transport accidents

V59.81 Occupant (driver) (passenger) of pick-up truck or van injured in transport accident with military vehicle

V59.88 Occupant (driver) (passenger) of pick-up truck or van injured in other specified transport accidents

V59.9 Occupant (driver) (passenger) of pick-up truck or van injured in unspecified traffic accident
Accident NOS involving pick-up truck or van

Occupant of heavy transport vehicle injured in transport accident (V60-V69)

INCLUDES *18 wheeler*
armored car
panel truck

EXCLUDES1 *bus*
motorcoach

V60 Occupant of heavy transport vehicle injured in collision with pedestrian or animal

EXCLUDES1 *heavy transport vehicle collision with animal-drawn vehicle or animal being ridden (V66.-)*

The appropriate 7th character is to be added to each code from category V60
A = initial encounter
D = subsequent encounter
S = sequela

V60.0 Driver of heavy transport vehicle injured in collision with pedestrian or animal in nontraffic accident

V60.1 Passenger in heavy transport vehicle injured in collision with pedestrian or animal in nontraffic accident

V60.2 Person on outside of heavy transport vehicle injured in collision with pedestrian or animal in nontraffic accident

V60.3 Unspecified occupant of heavy transport vehicle injured in collision with pedestrian or animal in nontraffic accident

V60.4 Person boarding or alighting a heavy transport vehicle injured in collision with pedestrian or animal

V60.5 Driver of heavy transport vehicle injured in collision with pedestrian or animal in traffic accident

V60.6 Passenger in heavy transport vehicle injured in collision with pedestrian or animal in traffic accident

V60.7 Person on outside of heavy transport vehicle injured in collision with pedestrian or animal in traffic accident

V60.9 Unspecified occupant of heavy transport vehicle injured in collision with pedestrian or animal in traffic accident

V61 Occupant of heavy transport vehicle injured in collision with pedal cycle

The appropriate 7th character is to be added to each code from category V61
A = initial encounter
D = subsequent encounter
S = sequela

V61.0 Driver of heavy transport vehicle injured in collision with pedal cycle in nontraffic accident

V61.1 Passenger in heavy transport vehicle injured in collision with pedal cycle in nontraffic accident

V61.2 Person on outside of heavy transport vehicle injured in collision with pedal cycle in nontraffic accident

V61.3 Unspecified occupant of heavy transport vehicle injured in collision with pedal cycle in nontraffic accident

V61.4 Person boarding or alighting a heavy transport vehicle injured in collision with pedal cycle while boarding or alighting

V61.5 Driver of heavy transport vehicle injured in collision with pedal cycle in traffic accident

V61.6 Passenger in heavy transport vehicle injured in collision with pedal cycle in traffic accident

V61.7 Person on outside of heavy transport vehicle injured in collision with pedal cycle in traffic accident

V61.9 Unspecified occupant of heavy transport vehicle injured in collision with pedal cycle in traffic accident

V62 Occupant of heavy transport vehicle injured in collision with two- or three-wheeled motor vehicle

The appropriate 7th character is to be added to each code from category V62
A = initial encounter
D = subsequent encounter
S = sequela

V62.0 Driver of heavy transport vehicle injured in collision with two- or three-wheeled motor vehicle in nontraffic accident

V62.1 Passenger in heavy transport vehicle injured in collision with two- or three-wheeled motor vehicle in nontraffic accident

V62.2 Person on outside of heavy transport vehicle injured in collision with two- or three-wheeled motor vehicle in nontraffic accident

V62.3 Unspecified occupant of heavy transport vehicle injured in collision with two- or three-wheeled motor vehicle in nontraffic accident

V62.4 Person boarding or alighting a heavy transport vehicle injured in collision with two- or three-wheeled motor vehicle

V62.5 Driver of heavy transport vehicle injured in collision with two- or three-wheeled motor vehicle in traffic accident

V62.6 Passenger in heavy transport vehicle injured in collision with two- or three-wheeled motor vehicle in traffic accident

V62.7 Person on outside of heavy transport vehicle injured in collision with two- or three-wheeled motor vehicle in traffic accident

V62.9 Unspecified occupant of heavy transport vehicle injured in collision with two- or three-wheeled motor vehicle in traffic accident

V63 Occupant of heavy transport vehicle injured in collision with car, pick-up truck or van

The appropriate 7th character is to be added to each code from category V63
A = initial encounter

Unacceptable principal diagnosis symbol per Medicare code edits — Code exempt from diagnosis present on admission requirement
Questionable admission — Complication or comorbidity — CC/MCC exclusion — Major complication or comorbidity
Principal diagnosis as its own CC — Principal diagnosis as its own MCC — Z code as first-listed diagnosis

D = subsequent encounter
S = sequela

- V63.0 Driver of heavy transport vehicle injured in collision with car, pick-up truck or van in nontraffic accident
- V63.1 Passenger in heavy transport vehicle injured in collision with car, pick-up truck or van in nontraffic accident
- V63.2 Person on outside of heavy transport vehicle injured in collision with car, pick-up truck or van in nontraffic accident
- V63.3 Unspecified occupant of heavy transport vehicle injured in collision with car, pick-up truck or van in nontraffic accident
- V63.4 Person boarding or alighting a heavy transport vehicle injured in collision with car, pick-up truck or van
- V63.5 Driver of heavy transport vehicle injured in collision with car, pick-up truck or van in traffic accident
- V63.6 Passenger in heavy transport vehicle injured in collision with car, pick-up truck or van in traffic accident
- V63.7 Person on outside of heavy transport vehicle injured in collision with car, pick-up truck or van in traffic accident
- V63.9 Unspecified occupant of heavy transport vehicle injured in collision with car, pick-up truck or van in traffic accident

V64 Occupant of heavy transport vehicle injured in collision with heavy transport vehicle or bus

EXCLUDES1 *occupant of heavy transport vehicle injured in collision with military vehicle (V69.81)*

The appropriate 7th character is to be added to each code from category V64
A = initial encounter
D = subsequent encounter
S = sequela

- V64.0 Driver of heavy transport vehicle injured in collision with heavy transport vehicle or bus in nontraffic accident
- V64.1 Passenger in heavy transport vehicle injured in collision with heavy transport vehicle or bus in nontraffic accident
- V64.2 Person on outside of heavy transport vehicle injured in collision with heavy transport vehicle or bus in nontraffic accident
- V64.3 Unspecified occupant of heavy transport vehicle injured in collision with heavy transport vehicle or bus in nontraffic accident
- V64.4 Person boarding or alighting a heavy transport vehicle injured in collision with heavy transport vehicle or bus while boarding or alighting
- V64.5 Driver of heavy transport vehicle injured in collision with heavy transport vehicle or bus in traffic accident
- V64.6 Passenger in heavy transport vehicle injured in collision with heavy transport vehicle or bus in traffic accident
- V64.7 Person on outside of heavy transport vehicle injured in collision with heavy transport vehicle or bus in traffic accident
- V64.9 Unspecified occupant of heavy transport vehicle injured in collision with heavy transport vehicle or bus in traffic accident

V65 Occupant of heavy transport vehicle injured in collision with railway train or railway vehicle

The appropriate 7th character is to be added to each code from category V65
A = initial encounter
D = subsequent encounter
S = sequela

- V65.0 Driver of heavy transport vehicle injured in collision with railway train or railway vehicle in nontraffic accident
- V65.1 Passenger in heavy transport vehicle injured in collision with railway train or railway vehicle in nontraffic accident
- V65.2 Person on outside of heavy transport vehicle injured in collision with railway train or railway vehicle in nontraffic accident
- V65.3 Unspecified occupant of heavy transport vehicle injured in collision with railway train or railway vehicle in nontraffic accident
- V65.4 Person boarding or alighting a heavy transport vehicle injured in collision with railway train or railway vehicle
- V65.5 Driver of heavy transport vehicle injured in collision with railway train or railway vehicle in traffic accident
- V65.6 Passenger in heavy transport vehicle injured in collision with railway train or railway vehicle in traffic accident
- V65.7 Person on outside of heavy transport vehicle injured in collision with railway train or railway vehicle in traffic accident
- V65.9 Unspecified occupant of heavy transport vehicle injured in collision with railway train or railway vehicle in traffic accident

V66 Occupant of heavy transport vehicle injured in collision with other nonmotor vehicle

INCLUDES *collision with animal-drawn vehicle, animal being ridden, streetcar*

The appropriate 7th character is to be added to each code from category V66
A = initial encounter
D = subsequent encounter
S = sequela

- V66.0 Driver of heavy transport vehicle injured in collision with other nonmotor vehicle in nontraffic accident
- V66.1 Passenger in heavy transport vehicle injured in collision with other nonmotor vehicle in nontraffic accident
- V66.2 Person on outside of heavy transport vehicle injured in collision with other nonmotor vehicle in nontraffic accident
- V66.3 Unspecified occupant of heavy transport vehicle injured in collision with other nonmotor vehicle in nontraffic accident
- V66.4 Person boarding or alighting a heavy transport vehicle injured in collision with other nonmotor vehicle
- V66.5 Driver of heavy transport vehicle injured in collision with other nonmotor vehicle in traffic accident
- V66.6 Passenger in heavy transport vehicle injured in collision with other nonmotor vehicle in traffic accident
- V66.7 Person on outside of heavy transport vehicle injured in collision with other nonmotor vehicle in traffic accident
- V66.9 Unspecified occupant of heavy transport vehicle injured in collision with other nonmotor vehicle in traffic accident

V67 Occupant of heavy transport vehicle injured in collision with fixed or stationary object

The appropriate 7th character is to be added to each code from category V67
A = initial encounter
D = subsequent encounter
S = sequela

- V67.0 Driver of heavy transport vehicle injured in collision with fixed or stationary object in nontraffic accident
- V67.1 Passenger in heavy transport vehicle injured in collision with fixed or stationary object in nontraffic accident
- V67.2 Person on outside of heavy transport vehicle injured in collision with fixed or stationary object in nontraffic accident
- V67.3 Unspecified occupant of heavy transport vehicle injured in collision with fixed or stationary object in nontraffic accident
- V67.4 Person boarding or alighting a heavy transport vehicle injured in collision with fixed or stationary object
- V67.5 Driver of heavy transport vehicle injured in collision with fixed or stationary object in traffic accident
- V67.6 Passenger in heavy transport vehicle injured in collision with fixed or stationary object in traffic accident
- V67.7 Person on outside of heavy transport vehicle injured in collision with fixed or stationary object in traffic accident
- V67.9 Unspecified occupant of heavy transport vehicle injured in collision with fixed or stationary object in traffic accident

V68 Occupant of heavy transport vehicle injured in noncollision transport accident

INCLUDES *overturning heavy transport vehicle NOS*
overturning heavy transport vehicle without collision

The appropriate 7th character is to be added to each code from category V68
A = initial encounter
D = subsequent encounter
S = sequela

- V68.0 Driver of heavy transport vehicle injured in noncollision transport accident in nontraffic accident
- V68.1 Passenger in heavy transport vehicle injured in noncollision transport accident in nontraffic accident
- V68.2 Person on outside of heavy transport vehicle injured in noncollision transport accident in nontraffic accident
- V68.3 Unspecified occupant of heavy transport vehicle injured in noncollision transport accident in nontraffic accident

Unspecified Code Other Specified Code Manifestation Code N Newborn P Pediatric M Maternity A Adult ♂ Male ♀ Female
● New Code ▲ Revised Code Title ►◄ Revised Text NOTES INCLUDES EXCLUDES1 Not coded here EXCLUDES2 Not included here
4th character required 5th character required 6th character required 7th character required
Extension 'X' Alert HAC Hospital-acquired condition (HAC) alert AHA AHA Coding Clinic®

V68.4 Person boarding or alighting a heavy transport vehicle injured in noncollision transport accident

V68.5 Driver of heavy transport vehicle injured in noncollision transport accident in traffic accident

V68.6 Passenger in heavy transport vehicle injured in noncollision transport accident in traffic accident

V68.7 Person on outside of heavy transport vehicle injured in noncollision transport accident in traffic accident

V68.9 Unspecified occupant of heavy transport vehicle injured in noncollision transport accident in traffic accident

V69 Occupant of heavy transport vehicle injured in other and unspecified transport accidents

The appropriate 7th character is to be added to each code from category V69
- A = initial encounter
- D = subsequent encounter
- S = sequela

V69.0 Driver of heavy transport vehicle injured in collision with other and unspecified motor vehicles in nontraffic accident

V69.00 Driver of heavy transport vehicle injured in collision with unspecified motor vehicles in nontraffic accident

V69.09 Driver of heavy transport vehicle injured in collision with other motor vehicles in nontraffic accident

V69.1 Passenger in heavy transport vehicle injured in collision with other and unspecified motor vehicles in nontraffic accident

V69.10 Passenger in heavy transport vehicle injured in collision with unspecified motor vehicles in nontraffic accident

V69.19 Passenger in heavy transport vehicle injured in collision with other motor vehicles in nontraffic accident

V69.2 Unspecified occupant of heavy transport vehicle injured in collision with other and unspecified motor vehicles in nontraffic accident

V69.20 Unspecified occupant of heavy transport vehicle injured in collision with unspecified motor vehicles in nontraffic accident

Collision NOS involving heavy transport vehicle, nontraffic

V69.29 Unspecified occupant of heavy transport vehicle injured in collision with other motor vehicles in nontraffic accident

V69.3 Occupant (driver) (passenger) of heavy transport vehicle injured in unspecified nontraffic accident

Accident NOS involving heavy transport vehicle, nontraffic
Occupant of heavy transport vehicle injured in nontraffic accident NOS

V69.4 Driver of heavy transport vehicle injured in collision with other and unspecified motor vehicles in traffic accident

V69.40 Driver of heavy transport vehicle injured in collision with unspecified motor vehicles in traffic accident

V69.49 Driver of heavy transport vehicle injured in collision with other motor vehicles in traffic accident

V69.5 Passenger in heavy transport vehicle injured in collision with other and unspecified motor vehicles in traffic accident

V69.50 Passenger in heavy transport vehicle injured in collision with unspecified motor vehicles in traffic accident

V69.59 Passenger in heavy transport vehicle injured in collision with other motor vehicles in traffic accident

V69.6 Unspecified occupant of heavy transport vehicle injured in collision with other and unspecified motor vehicles in traffic accident

V69.60 Unspecified occupant of heavy transport vehicle injured in collision with unspecified motor vehicles in traffic accident

Collision NOS involving heavy transport vehicle (traffic)

V69.69 Unspecified occupant of heavy transport vehicle injured in collision with other motor vehicles in traffic accident

V69.8 Occupant (driver) (passenger) of heavy transport vehicle injured in other specified transport accidents

V69.81 Occupant (driver) (passenger) of heavy transport vehicle injured in transport accidents with military vehicle

V69.88 Occupant (driver) (passenger) of heavy transport vehicle injured in other specified transport accidents

V69.9 Occupant (driver) (passenger) of heavy transport vehicle injured in unspecified traffic accident

Accident NOS involving heavy transport vehicle

Bus occupant injured in transport accident (V70-V79)

INCLUDES *motorcoach*

EXCLUDES1 *minibus (V50-V59)*

V70 Bus occupant injured in collision with pedestrian or animal

The appropriate 7th character is to be added to each code from category V70
- A = initial encounter
- D = subsequent encounter
- S = sequela

EXCLUDES1 *bus collision with animal-drawn vehicle or animal being ridden (V76.-)*

V70.0 Driver of bus injured in collision with pedestrian or animal in nontraffic accident

V70.1 Passenger on bus injured in collision with pedestrian or animal in nontraffic accident

V70.2 Person on outside of bus injured in collision with pedestrian or animal in nontraffic accident

V70.3 Unspecified occupant of bus injured in collision with pedestrian or animal in nontraffic accident

V70.4 Person boarding or alighting from bus injured in collision with pedestrian or animal

V70.5 Driver of bus injured in collision with pedestrian or animal in traffic accident

V70.6 Passenger on bus injured in collision with pedestrian or animal in traffic accident

V70.7 Person on outside of bus injured in collision with pedestrian or animal in traffic accident

V70.9 Unspecified occupant of bus injured in collision with pedestrian or animal in traffic accident

V71 Bus occupant injured in collision with pedal cycle

The appropriate 7th character is to be added to each code from category V71
- A = initial encounter
- D = subsequent encounter
- S = sequela

V71.0 Driver of bus injured in collision with pedal cycle in nontraffic accident

V71.1 Passenger on bus injured in collision with pedal cycle in nontraffic accident

V71.2 Person on outside of bus injured in collision with pedal cycle in nontraffic accident

V71.3 Unspecified occupant of bus injured in collision with pedal cycle in nontraffic accident

V71.4 Person boarding or alighting from bus injured in collision with pedal cycle

V71.5 Driver of bus injured in collision with pedal cycle in traffic accident

V71.6 Passenger on bus injured in collision with pedal cycle in traffic accident

V71.7 Person on outside of bus injured in collision with pedal cycle in traffic accident

V71.9 Unspecified occupant of bus injured in collision with pedal cycle in traffic accident

V72 Bus occupant injured in collision with two- or three-wheeled motor vehicle

The appropriate 7th character is to be added to each code from category V72
- A = initial encounter
- D = subsequent encounter
- S = sequela

V72.0 Driver of bus injured in collision with two- or three-wheeled motor vehicle in nontraffic accident

V72.1 Passenger on bus injured in collision with two- or three-wheeled motor vehicle in nontraffic accident

Unacceptable principal diagnosis symbol per Medicare code edits · Code exempt from diagnosis present on admission requirement · Questionable admission · Complication or comorbidity · CC/MCC exclusion · Major complication or comorbidity · Principal diagnosis as its own CC · Principal diagnosis as its own MCC · Z code as first-listed diagnosis

V72.2 Person on outside of bus injured in collision with two- or three-wheeled motor vehicle in nontraffic accident

V72.3 Unspecified occupant of bus injured in collision with two- or three-wheeled motor vehicle in nontraffic accident

V72.4 Person boarding or alighting from bus injured in collision with two- or three-wheeled motor vehicle

V72.5 Driver of bus injured in collision with two- or three-wheeled motor vehicle in traffic accident

V72.6 Passenger on bus injured in collision with two- or three-wheeled motor vehicle in traffic accident

V72.7 Person on outside of bus injured in collision with two- or three-wheeled motor vehicle in traffic accident

V72.9 Unspecified occupant of bus injured in collision with two- or three-wheeled motor vehicle in traffic accident

V73 Bus occupant injured in collision with car, pick-up truck or van

The appropriate 7th character is to be added to each code from category V73
- A = initial encounter
- D = subsequent encounter
- S = sequela

V73.0 Driver of bus injured in collision with car, pick-up truck or van in nontraffic accident

V73.1 Passenger on bus injured in collision with car, pick-up truck or van in nontraffic accident

V73.2 Person on outside of bus injured in collision with car, pick-up truck or van in nontraffic accident

V73.3 Unspecified occupant of bus injured in collision with car, pick-up truck or van in nontraffic accident

V73.4 Person boarding or alighting from bus injured in collision with car, pick-up truck or van

V73.5 Driver of bus injured in collision with car, pick-up truck or van in traffic accident

V73.6 Passenger on bus injured in collision with car, pick-up truck or van in traffic accident

V73.7 Person on outside of bus injured in collision with car, pick-up truck or van in traffic accident

V73.9 Unspecified occupant of bus injured in collision with car, pick-up truck or van in traffic accident

V74 Bus occupant injured in collision with heavy transport vehicle or bus

EXCLUDES1 *bus occupant injured in collision with military vehicle (V79.81)*

The appropriate 7th character is to be added to each code from category V74
- A = initial encounter
- D = subsequent encounter
- S = sequela

V74.0 Driver of bus injured in collision with heavy transport vehicle or bus in nontraffic accident

V74.1 Passenger on bus injured in collision with heavy transport vehicle or bus in nontraffic accident

V74.2 Person on outside of bus injured in collision with heavy transport vehicle or bus in nontraffic accident

V74.3 Unspecified occupant of bus injured in collision with heavy transport vehicle or bus in nontraffic accident

V74.4 Person boarding or alighting from bus injured in collision with heavy transport vehicle or bus

V74.5 Driver of bus injured in collision with heavy transport vehicle or bus in traffic accident

V74.6 Passenger on bus injured in collision with heavy transport vehicle or bus in traffic accident

V74.7 Person on outside of bus injured in collision with heavy transport vehicle or bus in traffic accident

V74.9 Unspecified occupant of bus injured in collision with heavy transport vehicle or bus in traffic accident

V75 Bus occupant injured in collision with railway train or railway vehicle

The appropriate 7th character is to be added to each code from category V75
- A = initial encounter
- D = subsequent encounter
- S = sequela

V75.0 Driver of bus injured in collision with railway train or railway vehicle in nontraffic accident

V75.1 Passenger on bus injured in collision with railway train or railway vehicle in nontraffic accident

V75.2 Person on outside of bus injured in collision with railway train or railway vehicle in nontraffic accident

V75.3 Unspecified occupant of bus injured in collision with railway train or railway vehicle in nontraffic accident

V75.4 Person boarding or alighting from bus injured in collision with railway train or railway vehicle

V75.5 Driver of bus injured in collision with railway train or railway vehicle in traffic accident

V75.6 Passenger on bus injured in collision with railway train or railway vehicle in traffic accident

V75.7 Person on outside of bus injured in collision with railway train or railway vehicle in traffic accident

V75.9 Unspecified occupant of bus injured in collision with railway train or railway vehicle in traffic accident

V76 Bus occupant injured in collision with other nonmotor vehicle

INCLUDES *collision with animal-drawn vehicle, animal being ridden, streetcar*

The appropriate 7th character is to be added to each code from category V76
- A = initial encounter
- D = subsequent encounter
- S = sequela

V76.0 Driver of bus injured in collision with other nonmotor vehicle in nontraffic accident

V76.1 Passenger on bus injured in collision with other nonmotor vehicle in nontraffic accident

V76.2 Person on outside of bus injured in collision with other nonmotor vehicle in nontraffic accident

V76.3 Unspecified occupant of bus injured in collision with other nonmotor vehicle in nontraffic accident

V76.4 Person boarding or alighting from bus injured in collision with other nonmotor vehicle

V76.5 Driver of bus injured in collision with other nonmotor vehicle in traffic accident

V76.6 Passenger on bus injured in collision with other nonmotor vehicle in traffic accident

V76.7 Person on outside of bus injured in collision with other nonmotor vehicle in traffic accident

V76.9 Unspecified occupant of bus injured in collision with other nonmotor vehicle in traffic accident

V77 Bus occupant injured in collision with fixed or stationary object

The appropriate 7th character is to be added to each code from category V77
- A = initial encounter
- D = subsequent encounter
- S = sequela

V77.0 Driver of bus injured in collision with fixed or stationary object in nontraffic accident

V77.1 Passenger on bus injured in collision with fixed or stationary object in nontraffic accident

V77.2 Person on outside of bus injured in collision with fixed or stationary object in nontraffic accident

V77.3 Unspecified occupant of bus injured in collision with fixed or stationary object in nontraffic accident

V77.4 Person boarding or alighting from bus injured in collision with fixed or stationary object

V77.5 Driver of bus injured in collision with fixed or stationary object in traffic accident

V77.6 Passenger on bus injured in collision with fixed or stationary object in traffic accident

V77.7 Person on outside of bus injured in collision with fixed or stationary object in traffic accident

V77.9 Unspecified occupant of bus injured in collision with fixed or stationary object in traffic accident

V78 Bus occupant injured in noncollision transport accident

INCLUDES *overturning bus NOS*
overturning bus without collision

The appropriate 7th character is to be added to each code from category V78
- A = initial encounter
- D = subsequent encounter
- S = sequela

V78.0 Driver of bus injured in noncollision transport accident in nontraffic accident

V78.1 Passenger on bus injured in noncollision transport accident in nontraffic accident

V78.2 Person on outside of bus injured in noncollision transport accident in nontraffic accident

Unspecified Code | Other Specified Code | Manifestation Code | N Newborn | P Pediatric | M Maternity | A Adult | ♂ Male | ♀ Female
● New Code ▲ Revised Code Title ►◄ Revised Text NOTES INCLUDES EXCLUDES1 Not coded here EXCLUDES2 Not included here
4th character required | 5th character required | 6th character required | 7th character required
Extension 'X' Alert | HAC Hospital-acquired condition (HAC) alert | AHA AHA Coding Clinic©

V78.3 Unspecified occupant of bus injured in noncollision transport accident in nontraffic accident

V78.4 Person boarding or alighting from bus injured in noncollision transport accident

V78.5 Driver of bus injured in noncollision transport accident in traffic accident

V78.6 Passenger on bus injured in noncollision transport accident in traffic accident

V78.7 Person on outside of bus injured in noncollision transport accident in traffic accident

V78.9 Unspecified occupant of bus injured in noncollision transport accident in traffic accident

V79 Bus occupant injured in other and unspecified transport accidents

The appropriate 7th character is to be added to each code from category V79

A = initial encounter
D = subsequent encounter
S = sequela

V79.0 Driver of bus injured in collision with other and unspecified motor vehicles in nontraffic accident

V79.00 Driver of bus injured in collision with unspecified motor vehicles in nontraffic accident

V79.09 Driver of bus injured in collision with other motor vehicles in nontraffic accident

V79.1 Passenger on bus injured in collision with other and unspecified motor vehicles in nontraffic accident

V79.10 Passenger on bus injured in collision with unspecified motor vehicles in nontraffic accident

V79.19 Passenger on bus injured in collision with other motor vehicles in nontraffic accident

V79.2 Unspecified bus occupant injured in collision with other and unspecified motor vehicles in nontraffic accident

V79.20 Unspecified bus occupant injured in collision with unspecified motor vehicles in nontraffic accident
Bus collision NOS, nontraffic

V79.29 Unspecified bus occupant injured in collision with other motor vehicles in nontraffic accident

V79.3 Bus occupant (driver) (passenger) injured in unspecified nontraffic accident
Bus accident NOS, nontraffic
Bus occupant injured in nontraffic accident NOS

V79.4 Driver of bus injured in collision with other and unspecified motor vehicles in traffic accident

V79.40 Driver of bus injured in collision with unspecified motor vehicles in traffic accident

V79.49 Driver of bus injured in collision with other motor vehicles in traffic accident

V79.5 Passenger on bus injured in collision with other and unspecified motor vehicles in traffic accident

V79.50 Passenger on bus injured in collision with unspecified motor vehicles in traffic accident

V79.59 Passenger on bus injured in collision with other motor vehicles in traffic accident

V79.6 Unspecified bus occupant injured in collision with other and unspecified motor vehicles in traffic accident

V79.60 Unspecified bus occupant injured in collision with unspecified motor vehicles in traffic accident
Bus collision NOS (traffic)

V79.69 Unspecified bus occupant injured in collision with other motor vehicles in traffic accident

V79.8 Bus occupant (driver) (passenger) injured in other specified transport accidents

V79.81 Bus occupant (driver) (passenger) injured in transport accidents with military vehicle

V79.88 Bus occupant (driver) (passenger) injured in other specified transport accidents

V79.9 Bus occupant (driver) (passenger) injured in unspecified traffic accident
Bus accident NOS

Other land transport accidents (V80-V89)

V80 Animal-rider or occupant of animal-drawn vehicle injured in transport accident

The appropriate 7th character is to be added to each code from category V80

A = initial encounter
D = subsequent encounter
S = sequela

V80.0 Animal-rider or occupant of animal drawn vehicle injured by fall from or being thrown from animal or animal-drawn vehicle in noncollision accident

V80.01 Animal-rider injured by fall from or being thrown from animal in noncollision accident

V80.010 Animal-rider injured by fall from or being thrown from horse in noncollision accident

V80.018 Animal-rider injured by fall from or being thrown from other animal in noncollision accident

V80.02 Occupant of animal-drawn vehicle injured by fall from or being thrown from animal-drawn vehicle in noncollision accident
Overturning animal-drawn vehicle NOS
Overturning animal-drawn vehicle without collision

V80.1 Animal-rider or occupant of animal-drawn vehicle injured in collision with pedestrian or animal

EXCLUDES1 *animal-rider or animal-drawn vehicle collision with animal-drawn vehicle or animal being ridden (V80.7)*

V80.11 Animal-rider injured in collision with pedestrian or animal

V80.12 Occupant of animal-drawn vehicle injured in collision with pedestrian or animal

V80.2 Animal-rider or occupant of animal-drawn vehicle injured in collision with pedal cycle

V80.21 Animal-rider injured in collision with pedal cycle

V80.22 Occupant of animal-drawn vehicle injured in collision with pedal cycle

V80.3 Animal-rider or occupant of animal-drawn vehicle injured in collision with two- or three-wheeled motor vehicle

V80.31 Animal-rider injured in collision with two- or three-wheeled motor vehicle

V80.32 Occupant of animal-drawn vehicle injured in collision with two- or three-wheeled motor vehicle

V80.4 Animal-rider or occupant of animal-drawn vehicle injured in collision with car, pick-up truck, van, heavy transport vehicle or bus

EXCLUDES1 *animal-rider injured in collision with military vehicle (V80.910)*
occupant of animal-drawn vehicle injured in collision with military vehicle (V80.920)

V80.41 Animal-rider injured in collision with car, pick-up truck, van, heavy transport vehicle or bus

V80.42 Occupant of animal-drawn vehicle injured in collision with car, pick-up truck, van, heavy transport vehicle or bus

V80.5 Animal-rider or occupant of animal-drawn vehicle injured in collision with other specified motor vehicle

V80.51 Animal-rider injured in collision with other specified motor vehicle

V80.52 Occupant of animal-drawn vehicle injured in collision with other specified motor vehicle

V80.6 Animal-rider or occupant of animal-drawn vehicle injured in collision with railway train or railway vehicle

V80.61 Animal-rider injured in collision with railway train or railway vehicle

V80.62 Occupant of animal-drawn vehicle injured in collision with railway train or railway vehicle

V80.7 Animal-rider or occupant of animal-drawn vehicle injured in collision with other nonmotor vehicles

V80.71 Animal-rider or occupant of animal-drawn vehicle injured in collision with animal being ridden

V80.710 Animal-rider injured in collision with other animal being ridden

V80.711 Occupant of animal-drawn vehicle injured in collision with animal being ridden

V80.72 Animal-rider or occupant of animal-drawn vehicle injured in collision with other animal-drawn vehicle

V80.720 Animal-rider injured in collision with animal-drawn vehicle

Unacceptable principal diagnosis symbol per Medicare code edits — Code exempt from diagnosis present on admission requirement — Questionable admission — Complication or comorbidity — CC/MCC exclusion — Major complication or comorbidity — Principal diagnosis as its own CC — Principal diagnosis as its own MCC — Z code as first-listed diagnosis

V80.721 Occupant of animal-drawn vehicle injured in collision with other animal-drawn vehicle

V80.73 Animal-rider or occupant of animal-drawn vehicle injured in collision with streetcar

V80.730 Animal-rider injured in collision with streetcar

V80.731 Occupant of animal-drawn vehicle injured in collision with streetcar

V80.79 Animal-rider or occupant of animal-drawn vehicle injured in collision with other nonmotor vehicles

V80.790 Animal-rider injured in collision with other nonmotor vehicles

V80.791 Occupant of animal-drawn vehicle injured in collision with other nonmotor vehicles

V80.8 Animal-rider or occupant of animal-drawn vehicle injured in collision with fixed or stationary object

V80.81 Animal-rider injured in collision with fixed or stationary object

V80.82 Occupant of animal-drawn vehicle injured in collision with fixed or stationary object

V80.9 Animal-rider or occupant of animal-drawn vehicle injured in other and unspecified transport accidents

V80.91 Animal-rider injured in other and unspecified transport accidents

V80.910 Animal-rider injured in transport accident with military vehicle

V80.918 Animal-rider injured in other transport accident

V80.919 Animal-rider injured in unspecified transport accident
Animal rider accident NOS

V80.92 Occupant of animal-drawn vehicle injured in other and unspecified transport accidents

V80.920 Occupant of animal-drawn vehicle injured in transport accident with military vehicle

V80.928 Occupant of animal-drawn vehicle injured in other transport accident

V80.929 Occupant of animal-drawn vehicle injured in unspecified transport accident
Animal-drawn vehicle accident NOS

V81 Occupant of railway train or railway vehicle injured in transport accident

INCLUDES *derailment of railway train or railway vehicle*
person on outside of train

EXCLUDES1 *streetcar (V82.-)*

The appropriate 7th character is to be added to each code from category V81
A = initial encounter
D = subsequent encounter
S = sequela

V81.0 Occupant of railway train or railway vehicle injured in collision with motor vehicle in nontraffic accident
EXCLUDES1 *Occupant of railway train or railway vehicle injured due to collision with military vehicle (V81.83)*

V81.1 Occupant of railway train or railway vehicle injured in collision with motor vehicle in traffic accident
EXCLUDES1 *Occupant of railway train or railway vehicle injured due to collision with military vehicle (V81.83)*

V81.2 Occupant of railway train or railway vehicle injured in collision with or hit by rolling stock

V81.3 Occupant of railway train or railway vehicle injured in collision with other object
Railway collision NOS

V81.4 Person injured while boarding or alighting from railway train or railway vehicle

V81.5 Occupant of railway train or railway vehicle injured by fall in railway train or railway vehicle

V81.6 Occupant of railway train or railway vehicle injured by fall from railway train or railway vehicle

V81.7 Occupant of railway train or railway vehicle injured in derailment without antecedent collision

V81.8 Occupant of railway train or railway vehicle injured in other specified railway accidents

V81.81 Occupant of railway train or railway vehicle injured due to explosion or fire on train

V81.82 Occupant of railway train or railway vehicle injured due to object falling onto train
Occupant of railway train or railway vehicle injured due to falling earth onto train
Occupant of railway train or railway vehicle injured due to falling rocks onto train
Occupant of railway train or railway vehicle injured due to falling snow onto train
Occupant of railway train or railway vehicle injured due to falling trees onto train

V81.83 Occupant of railway train or railway vehicle injured due to collision with military vehicle

V81.89 Occupant of railway train or railway vehicle injured due to other specified railway accident

V81.9 Occupant of railway train or railway vehicle injured in unspecified railway accident
Railway accident NOS

V82 Occupant of powered streetcar injured in transport accident

INCLUDES *interurban electric car*
person on outside of streetcar
tram (car)
trolley (car)

EXCLUDES1 *bus (V70-V79)*
motorcoach (V70-V79)
nonpowered streetcar (V76.-)
train (V81.-)

The appropriate 7th character is to be added to each code from category V82
A = initial encounter
D = subsequent encounter
S = sequela

V82.0 Occupant of streetcar injured in collision with motor vehicle in nontraffic accident

V82.1 Occupant of streetcar injured in collision with motor vehicle in traffic accident

V82.2 Occupant of streetcar injured in collision with or hit by rolling stock

V82.3 Occupant of streetcar injured in collision with other object
EXCLUDES1 *collision with animal-drawn vehicle or animal being ridden (V82.8)*

V82.4 Person injured while boarding or alighting from streetcar

V82.5 Occupant of streetcar injured by fall in streetcar
EXCLUDES1 *fall in streetcar:*
while boarding or alighting (V82.4)
with antecedent collision (V82.0-V82.3)

V82.6 Occupant of streetcar injured by fall from streetcar
EXCLUDES1 *fall from streetcar:*
while boarding or alighting (V82.4)
with antecedent collision (V82.0-V82.3)

V82.7 Occupant of streetcar injured in derailment without antecedent collision
EXCLUDES1 *occupant of streetcar injured in derailment with antecedent collision (V82.0-V82.3)*

V82.8 Occupant of streetcar injured in other specified transport accidents
Streetcar collision with military vehicle
Streetcar collision with train or nonmotor vehicles

V82.9 Occupant of streetcar injured in unspecified traffic accident
Streetcar accident NOS

V83 Occupant of special vehicle mainly used on industrial premises injured in transport accident

INCLUDES *battery-powered airport passenger vehicle*
battery-powered truck (baggage) (mail)
coal-car in mine
forklift (truck)
logging car
self-propelled industrial truck
station baggage truck (powered)
tram, truck, or tub (powered) in mine or quarry

EXCLUDES1 *special construction vehicles (V85.-)*
special industrial vehicle in stationary use or maintenance (W31.-)

Unspecified Code Other Specified Code Manifestation Code N Newborn P Pediatric M Maternity A Adult ♂ Male ♀ Female
● New Code ▲ Revised Code Title ►◄ Revised Text NOTES INCLUDES EXCLUDES1 Not coded here EXCLUDES2 Not included here
4th character required 5th character required 6th character required 7th character required
Extension 'X' Alert HAC Hospital-acquired condition (HAC) alert AHA AHA Coding Clinic©

The appropriate 7th character is to be added to each code from category V83
A = initial encounter
D = subsequent encounter
S = sequela

V83.0 Driver of special industrial vehicle injured in traffic accident
V83.1 Passenger of special industrial vehicle injured in traffic accident
V83.2 Person on outside of special industrial vehicle injured in traffic accident
V83.3 Unspecified occupant of special industrial vehicle injured in traffic accident
V83.4 Person injured while boarding or alighting from special industrial vehicle
V83.5 Driver of special industrial vehicle injured in nontraffic accident
V83.6 Passenger of special industrial vehicle injured in nontraffic accident
V83.7 Person on outside of special industrial vehicle injured in nontraffic accident
V83.9 Unspecified occupant of special industrial vehicle injured in nontraffic accident
Special-industrial-vehicle accident NOS

V84 Occupant of special vehicle mainly used in agriculture injured in transport accident
INCLUDES *self-propelled farm machinery*
tractor (and trailer)
EXCLUDES1 *animal-powered farm machinery accident (W30.8-)*
contact with combine harvester (W30.0)
special agricultural vehicle in stationary use or maintenance (W30.-)

The appropriate 7th character is to be added to each code from category V84
A = initial encounter
D = subsequent encounter
S = sequela

V84.0 Driver of special agricultural vehicle injured in traffic accident
V84.1 Passenger of special agricultural vehicle injured in traffic accident
V84.2 Person on outside of special agricultural vehicle injured in traffic accident
V84.3 Unspecified occupant of special agricultural vehicle injured in traffic accident
V84.4 Person injured while boarding or alighting from special agricultural vehicle
V84.5 Driver of special agricultural vehicle injured in nontraffic accident
V84.6 Passenger of special agricultural vehicle injured in nontraffic accident
V84.7 Person on outside of special agricultural vehicle injured in nontraffic accident
V84.9 Unspecified occupant of special agricultural vehicle injured in nontraffic accident
Special-agricultural vehicle accident NOS

V85 Occupant of special construction vehicle injured in transport accident
INCLUDES *bulldozer*
digger
dump truck
earth-leveller
mechanical shovel
road-roller
EXCLUDES1 *special industrial vehicle (V83.-)*
special construction vehicle in stationary use or maintenance (W31.-)

The appropriate 7th character is to be added to each code from category V85
A = initial encounter
D = subsequent encounter
S = sequela

V85.0 Driver of special construction vehicle injured in traffic accident
V85.1 Passenger of special construction vehicle injured in traffic accident
V85.2 Person on outside of special construction vehicle injured in traffic accident
V85.3 Unspecified occupant of special construction vehicle injured in traffic accident
V85.4 Person injured while boarding or alighting from special construction vehicle
V85.5 Driver of special construction vehicle injured in nontraffic accident
V85.6 Passenger of special construction vehicle injured in nontraffic accident
V85.7 Person on outside of special construction vehicle injured in nontraffic accident
V85.9 Unspecified occupant of special construction vehicle injured in nontraffic accident
Special-construction-vehicle accident NOS

V86 Occupant of special all-terrain or other off-road motor vehicle, injured in transport accident
EXCLUDES1 *special all-terrain vehicle in stationary use or maintenance (W31.-)*
sport-utility vehicle (V50-V59)
three-wheeled motor vehicle designed for on-road use (V30-V39)

The appropriate 7th character is to be added to each code from category V86
A = initial encounter
D = subsequent encounter
S = sequela

V86.0 Driver of special all-terrain or other off-road motor vehicle injured in traffic accident
V86.01 Driver of ambulance or fire engine injured in traffic accident
V86.02 Driver of snowmobile injured in traffic accident
V86.03 Driver of dune buggy injured in traffic accident
V86.04 Driver of military vehicle injured in traffic accident
V86.09 Driver of other special all-terrain or other off-road motor vehicle injured in traffic accident
Driver of dirt bike injured in traffic accident
Driver of go cart injured in traffic accident
Driver of golf cart injured in traffic accident
V86.1 Passenger of special all-terrain or other off-road motor vehicle injured in traffic accident
V86.11 Passenger of ambulance or fire engine injured in traffic accident
V86.12 Passenger of snowmobile injured in traffic accident
V86.13 Passenger of dune buggy injured in traffic accident
V86.14 Passenger of military vehicle injured in traffic accident
V86.19 Passenger of other special all-terrain or other off-road motor vehicle injured in traffic accident
Passenger of dirt bike injured in traffic accident
Passenger of go cart injured in traffic accident
Passenger of golf cart injured in traffic accident
V86.2 Person on outside of special all-terrain or other off-road motor vehicle injured in traffic accident
V86.21 Person on outside of ambulance or fire engine injured in traffic accident
V86.22 Person on outside of snowmobile injured in traffic accident
V86.23 Person on outside of dune buggy injured in traffic accident
V86.24 Person on outside of military vehicle injured in traffic accident
V86.29 Person on outside of other special all-terrain or other off-road motor vehicle injured in traffic accident
Person on outside of dirt bike injured in traffic accident
Person on outside of go cart in traffic accident
Person on outside of golf cart injured in traffic accident
V86.3 Unspecified occupant of special all-terrain or other off-road motor vehicle injured in traffic accident
V86.31 Unspecified occupant of ambulance or fire engine injured in traffic accident
V86.32 Unspecified occupant of snowmobile injured in traffic accident

Unacceptable principal diagnosis symbol per Medicare code edits | Code exempt from diagnosis present on admission requirement
Questionable admission | Complication or comorbidity | CC/MCC exclusion | Major complication or comorbidity
Principal diagnosis as its own CC | Principal diagnosis as its own MCC | Z code as first-listed diagnosis

V86.33 Unspecified occupant of dune buggy injured in traffic accident
V86.34 Unspecified occupant of military vehicle injured in traffic accident
V86.39 Unspecified occupant of other special all-terrain or other off-road motor vehicle injured in traffic accident
Unspecified occupant of dirt bike injured in traffic accident
Unspecified occupant of go cart injured in traffic accident
Unspecified occupant of golf cart injured in traffic accident

V86.4 Person injured while boarding or alighting from special all-terrain or other off-road motor vehicle
V86.41 Person injured while boarding or alighting from ambulance or fire engine
V86.42 Person injured while boarding or alighting from snowmobile
V86.43 Person injured while boarding or alighting from dune buggy
V86.44 Person injured while boarding or alighting from military vehicle
V86.49 Person injured while boarding or alighting from other special all-terrain or other off-road motor vehicle
Person injured while boarding or alighting from dirt bike
Person injured while boarding or alighting from go cart
Person injured while boarding or alighting from golf cart

V86.5 Driver of special all-terrain or other off-road motor vehicle injured in nontraffic accident
V86.51 Driver of ambulance or fire engine injured in nontraffic accident
V86.52 Driver of snowmobile injured in nontraffic accident
V86.53 Driver of dune buggy injured in nontraffic accident
V86.54 Driver of military vehicle injured in nontraffic accident
V86.59 Driver of other special all-terrain or other off-road motor vehicle injured in nontraffic accident
Driver of dirt bike injured in nontraffic accident
Driver of go cart injured in nontraffic accident
Driver of golf cart injured in nontraffic accident

V86.6 Passenger of special all-terrain or other off-road motor vehicle injured in nontraffic accident
V86.61 Passenger of ambulance or fire engine injured in nontraffic accident
V86.62 Passenger of snowmobile injured in nontraffic accident
V86.63 Passenger of dune buggy injured in nontraffic accident
V86.64 Passenger of military vehicle injured in nontraffic accident
V86.69 Passenger of other special all-terrain or other off-road motor vehicle injured in nontraffic accident
Passenger of dirt bike injured in nontraffic accident
Passenger of go cart injured in nontraffic accident
Passenger of golf cart injured in nontraffic accident

V86.7 Person on outside of special all-terrain or other off-road motor vehicle injured in nontraffic accident
V86.71 Person on outside of ambulance or fire engine injured in nontraffic accident
V86.72 Person on outside of snowmobile injured in nontraffic accident
V86.73 Person on outside of dune buggy injured in nontraffic accident
V86.74 Person on outside of military vehicle injured in nontraffic accident
V86.79 Person on outside of other special all-terrain or other off-road motor vehicles injured in nontraffic accident
Person on outside of dirt bike injured in nontraffic accident
Person on outside of go cart injured in nontraffic accident
Person on outside of golf cart injured in nontraffic accident

V86.9 Unspecified occupant of special all-terrain or other off-road motor vehicle injured in nontraffic accident
V86.91 Unspecified occupant of ambulance or fire engine injured in nontraffic accident
V86.92 Unspecified occupant of snowmobile injured in nontraffic accident
V86.93 Unspecified occupant of dune buggy injured in nontraffic accident
V86.94 Unspecified occupant of military vehicle injured in nontraffic accident
V86.99 Unspecified occupant of other special all-terrain or other off-road motor vehicle injured in nontraffic accident
All-terrain motor-vehicle accident NOS
Off-road motor-vehicle accident NOS
Other motor-vehicle accident NOS
Unspecified occupant of dirt bike injured in nontraffic accident
Unspecified occupant of go cart injured in nontraffic accident
Unspecified occupant of golf cart injured in nontraffic accident

V87 Traffic accident of specified type but victim's mode of transport unknown
EXCLUDES1 *collision involving:*
pedal cycle (V10-V19)
pedestrian (V01-V09)

The appropriate 7th character is to be added to each code from category V87
A = initial encounter
D = subsequent encounter
S = sequela

V87.0 Person injured in collision between car and two- or three-wheeled powered vehicle (traffic)
V87.1 Person injured in collision between other motor vehicle and two- or three-wheeled motor vehicle (traffic)
V87.2 Person injured in collision between car and pick-up truck or van (traffic)
V87.3 Person injured in collision between car and bus (traffic)
V87.4 Person injured in collision between car and heavy transport vehicle (traffic)
V87.5 Person injured in collision between heavy transport vehicle and bus (traffic)
V87.6 Person injured in collision between railway train or railway vehicle and car (traffic)
V87.7 Person injured in collision between other specified motor vehicles (traffic)
V87.8 Person injured in other specified noncollision transport accidents involving motor vehicle (traffic)
V87.9 Person injured in other specified (collision)(noncollision) transport accidents involving nonmotor vehicle (traffic)

V88 Nontraffic accident of specified type but victim's mode of transport unknown
EXCLUDES1 *collision involving:*
pedal cycle (V10-V19)
pedestrian (V01-V09)

The appropriate 7th character is to be added to each code from category V88
A = initial encounter
D = subsequent encounter
S = sequela

V88.0 Person injured in collision between car and two- or three-wheeled motor vehicle, nontraffic
V88.1 Person injured in collision between other motor vehicle and two- or three-wheeled motor vehicle, nontraffic
V88.2 Person injured in collision between car and pick-up truck or van , nontraffic
V88.3 Person injured in collision between car and bus , nontraffic
V88.4 Person injured in collision between car and heavy transport vehicle , nontraffic
V88.5 Person injured in collision between heavy transport vehicle and bus , nontraffic

Unspecified Code Other Specified Code Manifestation Code N Newborn P Pediatric M Maternity A Adult ♂ Male ♀ Female
● New Code ▲ Revised Code Title ►◄ Revised Text NOTES INCLUDES EXCLUDES1 Not coded here EXCLUDES2 Not included here
4th character required 5th character required 6th character required 7th character required
Extension 'X' Alert HAC Hospital-acquired condition (HAC) alert AHA AHA Coding Clinic©

V88.6 Person injured in collision between railway train or railway vehicle and car, nontraffic

V88.7 Person injured in collision between other specified motor vehicle, nontraffic

V88.8 Person injured in other specified noncollision transport accidents involving motor vehicle, nontraffic

V88.9 Person injured in other specified (collision)(noncollision) transport accidents involving nonmotor vehicle, nontraffic

V89 Motor- or nonmotor-vehicle accident, type of vehicle unspecified

The appropriate 7th character is to be added to each code from category V89
A = initial encounter
D = subsequent encounter
S = sequela

V89.0 Person injured in unspecified motor-vehicle accident, nontraffic
Motor-vehicle accident NOS, nontraffic

V89.1 Person injured in unspecified nonmotor-vehicle accident, nontraffic
Nonmotor-vehicle accident NOS (nontraffic)

V89.2 Person injured in unspecified motor-vehicle accident, traffic
Motor-vehicle accident [MVA] NOS
Road (traffic) accident [RTA] NOS

V89.3 Person injured in unspecified nonmotor-vehicle accident, traffic
Nonmotor-vehicle traffic accident NOS

V89.9 Person injured in unspecified vehicle accident
Collision NOS

Water transport accidents (V90-V94)

V90 Drowning and submersion due to accident to watercraft

EXCLUDES1 *civilian water transport accident involving military watercraft (V94.81-)*
fall into water not from watercraft (W16.-)
military watercraft accident in military or war operations (Y36.0-, Y37.0-)
water-transport-related drowning or submersion without accident to watercraft (V92.-)

The appropriate 7th character is to be added to each code from category V90
A = initial encounter
D = subsequent encounter
S = sequela

V90.0 Drowning and submersion due to watercraft overturning

V90.00 Drowning and submersion due to merchant ship overturning

V90.01 Drowning and submersion due to passenger ship overturning
Drowning and submersion due to Ferry-boat overturning
Drowning and submersion due to Liner overturning

V90.02 Drowning and submersion due to fishing boat overturning

V90.03 Drowning and submersion due to other powered watercraft overturning
Drowning and submersion due to Hovercraft (on open water) overturning
Drowning and submersion due to Jet ski overturning

V90.04 Drowning and submersion due to sailboat overturning

V90.05 Drowning and submersion due to canoe or kayak overturning

V90.06 Drowning and submersion due to (nonpowered) inflatable craft overturning

V90.08 Drowning and submersion due to other unpowered watercraft overturning
Drowning and submersion due to windsurfer overturning

V90.09 Drowning and submersion due to unspecified watercraft overturning
Drowning and submersion due to boat NOS overturning
Drowning and submersion due to ship NOS overturning
Drowning and submersion due to watercraft NOS overturning

V90.1 Drowning and submersion due to watercraft sinking

V90.10 Drowning and submersion due to merchant ship sinking

V90.11 Drowning and submersion due to passenger ship sinking
Drowning and submersion due to Ferry-boat sinking
Drowning and submersion due to Liner sinking

V90.12 Drowning and submersion due to fishing boat sinking

V90.13 Drowning and submersion due to other powered watercraft sinking
Drowning and submersion due to Hovercraft (on open water) sinking
Drowning and submersion due to Jet ski sinking

V90.14 Drowning and submersion due to sailboat sinking

V90.15 Drowning and submersion due to canoe or kayak sinking

V90.16 Drowning and submersion due to (nonpowered) inflatable craft sinking

V90.18 Drowning and submersion due to other unpowered watercraft sinking

V90.19 Drowning and submersion due to unspecified watercraft sinking
Drowning and submersion due to boat NOS sinking
Drowning and submersion due to ship NOS sinking
Drowning and submersion due to watercraft NOS sinking

V90.2 Drowning and submersion due to falling or jumping from burning watercraft

V90.20 Drowning and submersion due to falling or jumping from burning merchant ship

V90.21 Drowning and submersion due to falling or jumping from burning passenger ship
Drowning and submersion due to falling or jumping from burning Ferry-boat
Drowning and submersion due to falling or jumping from burning Liner

V90.22 Drowning and submersion due to falling or jumping from burning fishing boat

V90.23 Drowning and submersion due to falling or jumping from other burning powered watercraft
Drowning and submersion due to falling and jumping from burning Hovercraft (on open water)
Drowning and submersion due to falling and jumping from burning Jet ski

V90.24 Drowning and submersion due to falling or jumping from burning sailboat

V90.25 Drowning and submersion due to falling or jumping from burning canoe or kayak

V90.26 Drowning and submersion due to falling or jumping from burning (nonpowered) inflatable craft

V90.27 Drowning and submersion due to falling or jumping from burning water-skis

V90.28 Drowning and submersion due to falling or jumping from other burning unpowered watercraft
Drowning and submersion due to falling and jumping from burning surf-board
Drowning and submersion due to falling and jumping from burning windsurfer

V90.29 Drowning and submersion due to falling or jumping from unspecified burning watercraft
Drowning and submersion due to falling or jumping from burning boat NOS
Drowning and submersion due to falling or jumping from burning ship NOS
Drowning and submersion due to falling or jumping from burning watercraft NOS

V90.3 Drowning and submersion due to falling or jumping from crushed watercraft

V90.30 Drowning and submersion due to falling or jumping from crushed merchant ship

V90.31 Drowning and submersion due to falling or jumping from crushed passenger ship
Drowning and submersion due to falling and jumping from crushed Ferry boat

Unacceptable principal diagnosis symbol per Medicare code edits · Code exempt from diagnosis present on admission requirement
Questionable admission · Complication or comorbidity · CC/MCC exclusion · Major complication or comorbidity
Principal diagnosis as its own CC · Principal diagnosis as its own MCC · Z code as first-listed diagnosis

Drowning and submersion due to falling and jumping from crushed Liner

V90.32 **Drowning and submersion due to falling or jumping from crushed fishing boat**

V90.33 **Drowning and submersion due to falling or jumping from other crushed powered watercraft**
Drowning and submersion due to falling and jumping from crushed Hovercraft
Drowning and submersion due to falling and jumping from crushed Jet ski

V90.34 **Drowning and submersion due to falling or jumping from crushed sailboat**

V90.35 **Drowning and submersion due to falling or jumping from crushed canoe or kayak**

V90.36 **Drowning and submersion due to falling or jumping from crushed (nonpowered) inflatable craft**

V90.37 **Drowning and submersion due to falling or jumping from crushed water-skis**

V90.38 **Drowning and submersion due to falling or jumping from other crushed unpowered watercraft**
Drowning and submersion due to falling and jumping from crushed surf-board
Drowning and submersion due to falling and jumping from crushed windsurfer

V90.39 **Drowning and submersion due to falling or jumping from crushed unspecified watercraft**
Drowning and submersion due to falling and jumping from crushed boat NOS
Drowning and submersion due to falling and jumping from crushed ship NOS
Drowning and submersion due to falling and jumping from crushed watercraft NOS

V90.8 **Drowning and submersion due to other accident to watercraft**

V90.80 **Drowning and submersion due to other accident to merchant ship**

V90.81 **Drowning and submersion due to other accident to passenger ship**
Drowning and submersion due to other accident to Ferry-boat
Drowning and submersion due to other accident to Liner

V90.82 **Drowning and submersion due to other accident to fishing boat**

V90.83 **Drowning and submersion due to other accident to other powered watercraft**
Drowning and submersion due to other accident to Hovercraft (on open water)
Drowning and submersion due to other accident to Jet ski

V90.84 **Drowning and submersion due to other accident to sailboat**

V90.85 **Drowning and submersion due to other accident to canoe or kayak**

V90.86 **Drowning and submersion due to other accident to (nonpowered) inflatable craft**

V90.87 **Drowning and submersion due to other accident to water-skis**

V90.88 **Drowning and submersion due to other accident to other unpowered watercraft**
Drowning and submersion due to other accident to surf-board
Drowning and submersion due to other accident to windsurfer

V90.89 **Drowning and submersion due to other accident to unspecified watercraft**
Drowning and submersion due to other accident to boat NOS
Drowning and submersion due to other accident to ship NOS
Drowning and submersion due to other accident to watercraft NOS

V91 Other injury due to accident to watercraft

INCLUDES *any injury except drowning and submersion as a result of an accident to watercraft*

EXCLUDES1 *civilian water transport accident involving military watercraft (V94.81-)*
military watercraft accident in military or war operations (Y36, Y37.-)

EXCLUDES2 *drowning and submersion due to accident to watercraft (V90.-)*

The appropriate 7th character is to be added to each code from category V91
A = initial encounter
D = subsequent encounter
S = sequela

V91.0 **Burn due to watercraft on fire**

EXCLUDES1 *burn from localized fire or explosion on board ship without accident to watercraft (V93.-)*

V91.00 **Burn due to merchant ship on fire**

V91.01 **Burn due to passenger ship on fire**
Burn due to Ferry-boat on fire
Burn due to Liner on fire

V91.02 **Burn due to fishing boat on fire**

V91.03 **Burn due to other powered watercraft on fire**
Burn due to Hovercraft (on open water) on fire
Burn due to Jet ski on fire

V91.04 **Burn due to sailboat on fire**

V91.05 **Burn due to canoe or kayak on fire**

V91.06 **Burn due to (nonpowered) inflatable craft on fire**

V91.07 **Burn due to water-skis on fire**

V91.08 **Burn due to other unpowered watercraft on fire**

V91.09 **Burn due to unspecified watercraft on fire**
Burn due to boat NOS on fire
Burn due to ship NOS on fire
Burn due to watercraft NOS on fire

V91.1 **Crushed between watercraft and other watercraft or other object due to collision**
Crushed by lifeboat after abandoning ship in a collision

NOTES select the specified type of watercraft that the victim was on at the time of the collision

V91.10 **Crushed between merchant ship and other watercraft or other object due to collision**

V91.11 **Crushed between passenger ship and other watercraft or other object due to collision**
Crushed between Ferry-boat and other watercraft or other object due to collision
Crushed between Liner and other watercraft or other object due to collision

V91.12 **Crushed between fishing boat and other watercraft or other object due to collision**

V91.13 **Crushed between other powered watercraft and other watercraft or other object due to collision**
Crushed between Hovercraft (on open water) and other watercraft or other object due to collision
Crushed between Jet ski and other watercraft or other object due to collision

V91.14 **Crushed between sailboat and other watercraft or other object due to collision**

V91.15 **Crushed between canoe or kayak and other watercraft or other object due to collision**

V91.16 **Crushed between (nonpowered) inflatable craft and other watercraft or other object due to collision**

V91.18 **Crushed between other unpowered watercraft and other watercraft or other object due to collision**
Crushed between surfboard and other watercraft or other object due to collision
Crushed between windsurfer and other watercraft or other object due to collision

V91.19 **Crushed between unspecified watercraft and other watercraft or other object due to collision**
Crushed between boat NOS and other watercraft or other object due to collision
Crushed between ship NOS and other watercraft or other object due to collision
Crushed between watercraft NOS and other watercraft or other object due to collision

V91.2 **Fall due to collision between watercraft and other watercraft or other object**
Fall while remaining on watercraft after collision

NOTES select the specified type of watercraft that the victim was on at the time of the collision

EXCLUDES1 *crushed between watercraft and other watercraft and other object due to collision (V91.1-)*

Unspecified Code | Other Specified Code | Manifestation Code | N Newborn | P Pediatric | M Maternity | A Adult | ♂ Male | ♀ Female
● New Code | ▲ Revised Code Title | ►◄ Revised Text | NOTES | INCLUDES | EXCLUDES1 Not coded here | EXCLUDES2 Not included here
4th character required | 5th character required | 6th character required | 7th character required
Extension 'X' Alert | HAC Hospital-acquired condition (HAC) alert | AHA AHA Coding Clinic©

drowning and submersion due to falling from crushed watercraft (V90.3-)

V91.20 Fall due to collision between merchant ship and other watercraft or other object

V91.21 Fall due to collision between passenger ship and other watercraft or other object
Fall due to collision between Ferry-boat and other watercraft or other object
Fall due to collision between Liner and other watercraft or other object

V91.22 Fall due to collision between fishing boat and other watercraft or other object

V91.23 Fall due to collision between other powered watercraft and other watercraft or other object
Fall due to collision between Hovercraft (on open water) and other watercraft or other object
Fall due to collision between Jet ski and other watercraft or other object

V91.24 Fall due to collision between sailboat and other watercraft or other object

V91.25 Fall due to collision between canoe or kayak and other watercraft or other object

V91.26 Fall due to collision between (nonpowered) inflatable craft and other watercraft or other object

V91.29 Fall due to collision between unspecified watercraft and other watercraft or other object
Fall due to collision between boat NOS and other watercraft or other object
Fall due to collision between ship NOS and other watercraft or other object
Fall due to collision between watercraft NOS and other watercraft or other object

V91.3 Hit or struck by falling object due to accident to watercraft
Hit or struck by falling object (part of damaged watercraft or other object) after falling or jumping from damaged watercraft
EXCLUDES2 *drowning or submersion due to fall or jumping from damaged watercraft (V90.2-, V90.3-)*

V91.30 Hit or struck by falling object due to accident to merchant ship

V91.31 Hit or struck by falling object due to accident to passenger ship
Hit or struck by falling object due to accident to Ferry-boat
Hit or struck by falling object due to accident to Liner

V91.32 Hit or struck by falling object due to accident to fishing boat

V91.33 Hit or struck by falling object due to accident to other powered watercraft
Hit or struck by falling object due to accident to Hovercraft (on open water)
Hit or struck by falling object due to accident to Jet ski

V91.34 Hit or struck by falling object due to accident to sailboat

V91.35 Hit or struck by falling object due to accident to canoe or kayak

V91.36 Hit or struck by falling object due to accident to (nonpowered) inflatable craft

V91.37 Hit or struck by falling object due to accident to water-skis
Hit by water-skis after jumping off of water skis

V91.38 Hit or struck by falling object due to accident to other unpowered watercraft
Hit or struck by surf-board after falling off damaged surf-board
Hit or struck by object after falling off damaged windsurfer

V91.39 Hit or struck by falling object due to accident to unspecified watercraft
Hit or struck by falling object due to accident to boat NOS
Hit or struck by falling object due to accident to ship NOS
Hit or struck by falling object due to accident to watercraft NOS

V91.8 Other injury due to other accident to watercraft

V91.80 Other injury due to other accident to merchant ship

V91.81 Other injury due to other accident to passenger ship
Other injury due to other accident to Ferry-boat
Other injury due to other accident to Liner

V91.82 Other injury due to other accident to fishing boat

V91.83 Other injury due to other accident to other powered watercraft
Other injury due to other accident to Hovercraft (on open water)
Other injury due to other accident to Jet ski

V91.84 Other injury due to other accident to sailboat

V91.85 Other injury due to other accident to canoe or kayak

V91.86 Other injury due to other accident to (nonpowered) inflatable craft

V91.87 Other injury due to other accident to water-skis

V91.88 Other injury due to other accident to other unpowered watercraft
Other injury due to other accident to surf-board
Other injury due to other accident to windsurfer

V91.89 Other injury due to other accident to unspecified watercraft
Other injury due to other accident to boat NOS
Other injury due to other accident to ship NOS
Other injury due to other accident to watercraft NOS

V92 Drowning and submersion due to accident on board watercraft, without accident to watercraft

EXCLUDES1 *civilian water transport accident involving military watercraft (V94.81-)*
drowning or submersion due to accident to watercraft (V90-V91)
drowning or submersion of diver who voluntarily jumps from boat not involved in an accident (W16.711, W16.721)
fall into water without watercraft (W16.-)
military watercraft accident in military or war operations (Y36, Y37)

The appropriate 7th character is to be added to each code from category V92
A = initial encounter
D = subsequent encounter
S = sequela

V92.0 Drowning and submersion due to fall off watercraft
Drowning and submersion due to fall from gangplank of watercraft
Drowning and submersion due to fall overboard watercraft
EXCLUDES2 *hitting head on object or bottom of body of water due to fall from watercraft (V94.0-)*

V92.00 Drowning and submersion due to fall off merchant ship

V92.01 Drowning and submersion due to fall off passenger ship
Drowning and submersion due to fall off Ferry-boat
Drowning and submersion due to fall off Liner

V92.02 Drowning and submersion due to fall off fishing boat

V92.03 Drowning and submersion due to fall off other powered watercraft
Drowning and submersion due to fall off Hovercraft (on open water)
Drowning and submersion due to fall off Jet ski

V92.04 Drowning and submersion due to fall off sailboat

V92.05 Drowning and submersion due to fall off canoe or kayak

V92.06 Drowning and submersion due to fall off (nonpowered) inflatable craft

V92.07 Drowning and submersion due to fall off water-skis
EXCLUDES1 *drowning and submersion due to falling off burning water-skis (V90.27)*
drowning and submersion due to falling off crushed water-skis (V90.37)
hit by boat while water-skiing NOS (V94.X)

V92.08 Drowning and submersion due to fall off other unpowered watercraft
Drowning and submersion due to fall off surf-board
Drowning and submersion due to fall off windsurfer
EXCLUDES1 *drowning and submersion due to fall off burning unpowered watercraft (V90.28)*
drowning and submersion due to fall off crushed unpowered watercraft (V90.38)

Unacceptable principal diagnosis symbol per Medicare code edits; Code exempt from diagnosis present on admission requirement; Questionable admission; Complication or comorbidity; CC/MCC exclusion; Major complication or comorbidity; Principal diagnosis as its own CC; Principal diagnosis as its own MCC; Z code as first-listed diagnosis

drowning and submersion due to fall off damaged unpowered watercraft (V90.88)
drowning and submersion due to rider of nonpowered watercraft being hit by other watercraft (V94.-)
other injury due to rider of nonpowered watercraft being hit by other watercraft (V94.-)

V92.09 Drowning and submersion due to fall off unspecified watercraft
Drowning and submersion due to fall off boat NOS
Drowning and submersion due to fall off ship
Drowning and submersion due to fall off watercraft NOS

V92.1 Drowning and submersion due to being thrown overboard by motion of watercraft
EXCLUDES1 *drowning and submersion due to fall off surf-board (V92.08)*
drowning and submersion due to fall off water-skis (V92.07)
drowning and submersion due to fall off windsurfer (V92.08)

V92.10 Drowning and submersion due to being thrown overboard by motion of merchant ship

V92.11 Drowning and submersion due to being thrown overboard by motion of passenger ship
Drowning and submersion due to being thrown overboard by motion of Ferry-boat
Drowning and submersion due to being thrown overboard by motion of Liner

V92.12 Drowning and submersion due to being thrown overboard by motion of fishing boat

V92.13 Drowning and submersion due to being thrown overboard by motion of other powered watercraft
Drowning and submersion due to being thrown overboard by motion of Hovercraft

V92.14 Drowning and submersion due to being thrown overboard by motion of sailboat

V92.15 Drowning and submersion due to being thrown overboard by motion of canoe or kayak

V92.16 Drowning and submersion due to being thrown overboard by motion of (nonpowered) inflatable craft

V92.19 Drowning and submersion due to being thrown overboard by motion of unspecified watercraft
Drowning and submersion due to being thrown overboard by motion of boat NOS
Drowning and submersion due to being thrown overboard by motion of ship NOS
Drowning and submersion due to being thrown overboard by motion of watercraft NOS

V92.2 Drowning and submersion due to being washed overboard from watercraft
Code first any associated cataclysm (X37.0-)

V92.20 Drowning and submersion due to being washed overboard from merchant ship

V92.21 Drowning and submersion due to being washed overboard from passenger ship
Drowning and submersion due to being washed overboard from Ferry-boat
Drowning and submersion due to being washed overboard from Liner

V92.22 Drowning and submersion due to being washed overboard from fishing boat

V92.23 Drowning and submersion due to being washed overboard from other powered watercraft
Drowning and submersion due to being washed overboard from Hovercraft (on open water)
Drowning and submersion due to being washed overboard from Jet ski

V92.24 Drowning and submersion due to being washed overboard from sailboat

V92.25 Drowning and submersion due to being washed overboard from canoe or kayak

V92.26 Drowning and submersion due to being washed overboard from (nonpowered) inflatable craft

V92.27 Drowning and submersion due to being washed overboard from water-skis
EXCLUDES1 *drowning and submersion due to fall off water-skis (V92.07)*

V92.28 Drowning and submersion due to being washed overboard from other unpowered watercraft
Drowning and submersion due to being washed overboard from surf-board
Drowning and submersion due to being washed overboard from windsurfer

V92.29 Drowning and submersion due to being washed overboard from unspecified watercraft
Drowning and submersion due to being washed overboard from boat NOS
Drowning and submersion due to being washed overboard from ship NOS
Drowning and submersion due to being washed overboard from watercraft NOS

V93 Other injury due to accident on board watercraft, without accident to watercraft
EXCLUDES1 *civilian water transport accident involving military watercraft (V94.81-)*
other injury due to accident to watercraft (V91.-)
military watercraft accident in military or war operations (Y36, Y37.-)
EXCLUDES2 *drowning and submersion due to accident on board watercraft, without accident to watercraft (V92.-)*

The appropriate 7th character is to be added to each code from category V93
A = initial encounter
D = subsequent encounter
S = sequela

V93.0 Burn due to localized fire on board watercraft
EXCLUDES1 *burn due to watercraft on fire (V91.0-)*

V93.00 Burn due to localized fire on board merchant vessel

V93.01 Burn due to localized fire on board passenger vessel
Burn due to localized fire on board Ferry-boat
Burn due to localized fire on board Liner

V93.02 Burn due to localized fire on board fishing boat

V93.03 Burn due to localized fire on board other powered watercraft
Burn due to localized fire on board Hovercraft
Burn due to localized fire on board Jet ski

V93.04 Burn due to localized fire on board sailboat

V93.09 Burn due to localized fire on board unspecified watercraft
Burn due to localized fire on board boat NOS
Burn due to localized fire on board ship NOS
Burn due to localized fire on board watercraft NOS

V93.1 Other burn on board watercraft
Burn due to source other than fire on board watercraft
EXCLUDES1 *burn due to watercraft on fire (V91.0-)*

V93.10 Other burn on board merchant vessel

V93.11 Other burn on board passenger vessel
Other burn on board Ferry-boat
Other burn on board Liner

V93.12 Other burn on board fishing boat

V93.13 Other burn on board other powered watercraft
Other burn on board Hovercraft
Other burn on board Jet ski

V93.14 Other burn on board sailboat

V93.19 Other burn on board unspecified watercraft
Other burn on board boat NOS
Other burn on board ship NOS
Other burn on board watercraft NOS

V93.2 Heat exposure on board watercraft
EXCLUDES1 *exposure to man-made heat not aboard watercraft (W92)*
exposure to natural heat while on board watercraft (X30)
exposure to sunlight while on board watercraft (X32)
EXCLUDES2 *burn due to fire on board watercraft (V93.0-)*

V93.20 Heat exposure on board merchant ship

V93.21 Heat exposure on board passenger ship
Heat exposure on board Ferry-boat
Heat exposure on board Liner

Unspecified Code Other Specified Code Manifestation Code N Newborn P Pediatric M Maternity A Adult ♂ Male ♀ Female
● New Code ▲ Revised Code Title ►◄ Revised Text NOTES INCLUDES EXCLUDES1 Not coded here EXCLUDES2 Not included here
4th character required 5th character required 6th character required 7th character required
Extension 'X' Alert HAC Hospital-acquired condition (HAC) alert AHA AHA Coding Clinic©

V93.22 Heat exposure on board fishing boat
V93.23 Heat exposure on board other powered watercraft
Heat exposure on board hovercraft
V93.24 Heat exposure on board sailboat
V93.29 Heat exposure on board unspecified watercraft
Heat exposure on board boat NOS
Heat exposure on board ship NOS
Heat exposure on board watercraft NOS

V93.3 Fall on board watercraft
EXCLUDES1 *fall due to collision of watercraft (V91.2-)*
V93.30 Fall on board merchant ship
V93.31 Fall on board passenger ship
Fall on board Ferry-boat
Fall on board Liner
V93.32 Fall on board fishing boat
V93.33 Fall on board other powered watercraft
Fall on board Hovercraft (on open water)
Fall on board Jet ski
V93.34 Fall on board sailboat
V93.35 Fall on board canoe or kayak
V93.36 Fall on board (nonpowered) inflatable craft
V93.38 Fall on board other unpowered watercraft
V93.39 Fall on board unspecified watercraft
Fall on board boat NOS
Fall on board ship NOS
Fall on board watercraft NOS

V93.4 Struck by falling object on board watercraft
Hit by falling object on board watercraft
EXCLUDES1 *struck by falling object due to accident to watercraft (V91.3)*
V93.40 Struck by falling object on merchant ship
V93.41 Struck by falling object on passenger ship
Struck by falling object on Ferry-boat
Struck by falling object on Liner
V93.42 Struck by falling object on fishing boat
V93.43 Struck by falling object on other powered watercraft
Struck by falling object on Hovercraft
V93.44 Struck by falling object on sailboat
V93.48 Struck by falling object on other unpowered watercraft
V93.49 Struck by falling object on unspecified watercraft

V93.5 Explosion on board watercraft
Boiler explosion on steamship
EXCLUDES2 *fire on board watercraft (V93.0-)*
V93.50 Explosion on board merchant ship
V93.51 Explosion on board passenger ship
Explosion on board Ferry-boat
Explosion on board Liner
V93.52 Explosion on board fishing boat
V93.53 Explosion on board other powered watercraft
Explosion on board Hovercraft
Explosion on board Jet ski
V93.54 Explosion on board sailboat
V93.59 Explosion on board unspecified watercraft
Explosion on board boat NOS
Explosion on board ship NOS
Explosion on board watercraft NOS

V93.6 Machinery accident on board watercraft
EXCLUDES1 *machinery explosion on board watercraft (V93.4-)*
machinery fire on board watercraft (V93.0-)
V93.60 Machinery accident on board merchant ship
V93.61 Machinery accident on board passenger ship
Machinery accident on board Ferry-boat
Machinery accident on board Liner
V93.62 Machinery accident on board fishing boat
V93.63 Machinery accident on board other powered watercraft
Machinery accident on board Hovercraft
V93.64 Machinery accident on board sailboat
V93.69 Machinery accident on board unspecified watercraft
Machinery accident on board boat NOS
Machinery accident on board ship NOS
Machinery accident on board watercraft NOS

V93.8 Other injury due to other accident on board watercraft
Accidental poisoning by gases or fumes on watercraft
V93.80 Other injury due to other accident on board merchant ship
V93.81 Other injury due to other accident on board passenger ship
Other injury due to other accident on board Ferry-boat
Other injury due to other accident on board Liner
V93.82 Other injury due to other accident on board fishing boat
V93.83 Other injury due to other accident on board other powered watercraft
Other injury due to other accident on board Hovercraft
Other injury due to other accident on board Jet ski
V93.84 Other injury due to other accident on board sailboat
V93.85 Other injury due to other accident on board canoe or kayak
V93.86 Other injury due to other accident on board (nonpowered) inflatable craft
V93.87 Other injury due to other accident on board water-skis
Hit or struck by object while waterskiing
V93.88 Other injury due to other accident on board other unpowered watercraft
Hit or struck by object while surfing
Hit or struck by object while on board windsurfer
V93.89 Other injury due to other accident on board unspecified watercraft
Other injury due to other accident on board boat NOS
Other injury due to other accident on board ship NOS
Other injury due to other accident on board watercraft NOS

V94 Other and unspecified water transport accidents
EXCLUDES1 *military watercraft accidents in military or war operations (Y36, Y37)*

The appropriate 7th character is to be added to each code from category V94
A = initial encounter
D = subsequent encounter
S = sequela

V94.0 Hitting object or bottom of body of water due to fall from watercraft
EXCLUDES2 *drowning and submersion due to fall from watercraft (V92.0-)*

V94.1 Bather struck by watercraft
Swimmer hit by watercraft
V94.11 Bather struck by powered watercraft
V94.12 Bather struck by nonpowered watercraft

V94.2 Rider of nonpowered watercraft struck by other watercraft
V94.21 Rider of nonpowered watercraft struck by other nonpowered watercraft
Canoer hit by other nonpowered watercraft
Surfer hit by other nonpowered watercraft
Windsurfer hit by other nonpowered watercraft
V94.22 Rider of nonpowered watercraft struck by powered watercraft
Canoer hit by motorboat
Surfer hit by motorboat
Windsurfer hit by motorboat

V94.3 Injury to rider of (inflatable) watercraft being pulled behind other watercraft
V94.31 Injury to rider of (inflatable) recreational watercraft being pulled behind other watercraft
Injury to rider of inner-tube pulled behind motor boat
V94.32 Injury to rider of non-recreational watercraft being pulled behind other watercraft
Injury to occupant of dingy being pulled behind boat or ship
Injury to occupant of life-raft being pulled behind boat or ship

V94.4 Injury to barefoot water-skier
Injury to person being pulled behind boat or ship

V94.8 Other water transport accident
V94.81 Water transport accident involving military watercraft

Unacceptable principal diagnosis symbol per Medicare code edits | Code exempt from diagnosis present on admission requirement
Questionable admission | Complication or comorbidity | CC/MCC exclusion | Major complication or comorbidity
Principal diagnosis as its own CC | Principal diagnosis as its own MCC | Z code as first-listed diagnosis

V94.810 Civilian watercraft involved in water transport accident with military watercraft
Passenger on civilian watercraft injured due to accident with military watercraft
V94.811 Civilian in water injured by military watercraft
V94.818 Other water transport accident involving military watercraft
V94.89 Other water transport accident
V94.9 Unspecified water transport accident
Water transport accident NOS

Air and space transport accidents (V95-V97)

EXCLUDES1 *military aircraft accidents in military or war operations (Y36, Y37)*

V95 Accident to powered aircraft causing injury to occupant
The appropriate 7th character is to be added to each code from category V95
A = initial encounter
D = subsequent encounter
S = sequela

V95.0 Helicopter accident injuring occupant
V95.00 Unspecified helicopter accident injuring occupant
V95.01 Helicopter crash injuring occupant
V95.02 Forced landing of helicopter injuring occupant
V95.03 Helicopter collision injuring occupant
Helicopter collision with any object, fixed, movable or moving
V95.04 Helicopter fire injuring occupant
V95.05 Helicopter explosion injuring occupant
V95.09 Other helicopter accident injuring occupant

V95.1 Ultralight, microlight or powered-glider accident injuring occupant
V95.10 Unspecified ultralight, microlight or powered-glider accident injuring occupant
V95.11 Ultralight, microlight or powered-glider crash injuring occupant
V95.12 Forced landing of ultralight, microlight or powered-glider injuring occupant
V95.13 Ultralight, microlight or powered-glider collision injuring occupant
Ultralight, microlight or powered-glider collision with any object, fixed, movable or moving
V95.14 Ultralight, microlight or powered-glider fire injuring occupant
V95.15 Ultralight, microlight or powered-glider explosion injuring occupant
V95.19 Other ultralight, microlight or powered-glider accident injuring occupant

V95.2 Other private fixed-wing aircraft accident injuring occupant
V95.20 Unspecified accident to other private fixed-wing aircraft, injuring occupant
V95.21 Other private fixed-wing aircraft crash injuring occupant
V95.22 Forced landing of other private fixed-wing aircraft injuring occupant
V95.23 Other private fixed-wing aircraft collision injuring occupant
Other private fixed-wing aircraft collision with any object, fixed, movable or moving
V95.24 Other private fixed-wing aircraft fire injuring occupant
V95.25 Other private fixed-wing aircraft explosion injuring occupant
V95.29 Other accident to other private fixed-wing aircraft injuring occupant

V95.3 Commercial fixed-wing aircraft accident injuring occupant
V95.30 Unspecified accident to commercial fixed-wing aircraft injuring occupant
V95.31 Commercial fixed-wing aircraft crash injuring occupant
V95.32 Forced landing of commercial fixed-wing aircraft injuring occupant
V95.33 Commercial fixed-wing aircraft collision injuring occupant
Commercial fixed-wing aircraft collision with any object, fixed, movable or moving
V95.34 Commercial fixed-wing aircraft fire injuring occupant
V95.35 Commercial fixed-wing aircraft explosion injuring occupant
V95.39 Other accident to commercial fixed-wing aircraft injuring occupant

V95.4 Spacecraft accident injuring occupant
V95.40 Unspecified spacecraft accident injuring occupant
V95.41 Spacecraft crash injuring occupant
V95.42 Forced landing of spacecraft injuring occupant
V95.43 Spacecraft collision injuring occupant
Spacecraft collision with any object, fixed, moveable or moving
V95.44 Spacecraft fire injuring occupant
V95.45 Spacecraft explosion injuring occupant
V95.49 Other spacecraft accident injuring occupant
V95.8 Other powered aircraft accidents injuring occupant
V95.9 Unspecified aircraft accident injuring occupant
Aircraft accident NOS
Air transport accident NOS

V96 Accident to nonpowered aircraft causing injury to occupant
The appropriate 7th character is to be added to each code from category V96
A = initial encounter
D = subsequent encounter
S = sequela

V96.0 Balloon accident injuring occupant
V96.00 Unspecified balloon accident injuring occupant
V96.01 Balloon crash injuring occupant
V96.02 Forced landing of balloon injuring occupant
V96.03 Balloon collision injuring occupant
Balloon collision with any object, fixed, moveable or moving
V96.04 Balloon fire injuring occupant
V96.05 Balloon explosion injuring occupant
V96.09 Other balloon accident injuring occupant

V96.1 Hang-glider accident injuring occupant
V96.10 Unspecified hang-glider accident injuring occupant
V96.11 Hang-glider crash injuring occupant
V96.12 Forced landing of hang-glider injuring occupant
V96.13 Hang-glider collision injuring occupant
Hang-glider collision with any object, fixed, moveable or moving
V96.14 Hang-glider fire injuring occupant
V96.15 Hang-glider explosion injuring occupant
V96.19 Other hang-glider accident injuring occupant

V96.2 Glider (nonpowered) accident injuring occupant
V96.20 Unspecified glider (nonpowered) accident injuring occupant
V96.21 Glider (nonpowered) crash injuring occupant
V96.22 Forced landing of glider (nonpowered) injuring occupant
V96.23 Glider (nonpowered) collision injuring occupant
Glider (nonpowered) collision with any object, fixed, moveable or moving
V96.24 Glider (nonpowered) fire injuring occupant
V96.25 Glider (nonpowered) explosion injuring occupant
V96.29 Other glider (nonpowered) accident injuring occupant
V96.8 Other nonpowered-aircraft accidents injuring occupant
Kite carrying a person accident injuring occupant
V96.9 Unspecified nonpowered-aircraft accident injuring occupant
Nonpowered-aircraft accident NOS

V97 Other specified air transport accidents
The appropriate 7th character is to be added to each code from category V97
A = initial encounter
D = subsequent encounter
S = sequela
V97.0 Occupant of aircraft injured in other specified air transport accidents

Unspecified Code | Other Specified Code | Manifestation Code | N Newborn | P Pediatric | M Maternity | A Adult | ♂ Male | ♀ Female
● New Code | ▲ Revised Code Title | ►◄ Revised Text | NOTES | INCLUDES | EXCLUDES1 Not coded here | EXCLUDES2 Not included here
4th character required | 5th character required | 6th character required | 7th character required
Extension 'X' Alert | HAC Hospital-acquired condition (HAC) alert | AHA AHA Coding Clinic©

When symbols appear on a code that requires a 7th character extension, refer to Appendix D to identify applicable 7th character codes.

Fall in, on or from aircraft in air transport accident
EXCLUDES1 *accident while boarding or alighting aircraft (V97.1)*

V97.1 Person injured while boarding or alighting from aircraft

V97.2 Parachutist accident

V97.21 Parachutist entangled in object
Parachutist landing in tree

V97.22 Parachutist injured on landing

V97.29 Other parachutist accident

V97.3 Person on ground injured in air transport accident

V97.31 Hit by object falling from aircraft
Hit by crashing aircraft
Injured by aircraft hitting house
Injured by aircraft hitting car

V97.32 Injured by rotating propeller

V97.33 Sucked into jet engine

V97.39 Other injury to person on ground due to air transport accident

V97.8 Other air transport accidents, not elsewhere classified
EXCLUDES1 *aircraft accident NOS (V95.9)*
exposure to changes in air pressure during ascent or descent (W94.-)

V97.81 Air transport accident involving military aircraft

V97.810 Civilian aircraft involved in air transport accident with military aircraft
Passenger in civilian aircraft injured due to accident with military aircraft

V97.811 Civilian injured by military aircraft

V97.818 Other air transport accident involving military aircraft

V97.89 Other air transport accidents, not elsewhere classified
Injury from machinery on aircraft

Other and unspecified transport accidents (V98-V99)

EXCLUDES1 *vehicle accident, type of vehicle unspecified (V89.-)*

V98 Other specified transport accidents
The appropriate 7th character is to be added to each code from category V98
A = initial encounter
D = subsequent encounter
S = sequela

V98.0 Accident to, on or involving cable-car, not on rails
Caught or dragged by cable-car, not on rails
Fall or jump from cable-car, not on rails
Object thrown from or in cable-car, not on rails

V98.1 Accident to, on or involving land-yacht

V98.2 Accident to, on or involving ice yacht

V98.3 Accident to, on or involving ski lift
Accident to, on or involving ski chair-lift
Accident to, on or involving ski-lift with gondola

V98.8 Other specified transport accidents

V99 Unspecified transport accident
The appropriate 7th character is to be added to code V99
A = initial encounter
D = subsequent encounter
S = sequela

Other external causes of accidental injury (W00-X58)

Slipping, tripping, stumbling and falls (W00-W19)

EXCLUDES1 *assault involving a fall (Y01-Y02)*
fall from animal (V80.-)
fall (in) (from) machinery (in operation) (W28-W31)
fall (in) (from) transport vehicle (V01-V99)
intentional self-harm involving a fall (X80-X81)
EXCLUDES2 *at risk for fall (history of fall) Z91.81*
fall (in) (from) burning building (X00.-)
fall into fire (X00-X04, X08-X09)

W00 Fall due to ice and snow
INCLUDES *pedestrian on foot falling (slipping) on ice and snow*
EXCLUDES1 *fall on (from) ice and snow involving pedestrian conveyance (V00.-)*
fall from stairs and steps not due to ice and snow (W10.-)
The appropriate 7th character is to be added to each code from category W00
A = initial encounter
D = subsequent encounter
S = sequela

W00.0 Fall on same level due to ice and snow
AHA: Q2, 2016

W00.1 Fall from stairs and steps due to ice and snow

W00.2 Other fall from one level to another due to ice and snow

W00.9 Unspecified fall due to ice and snow

W01 Fall on same level from slipping, tripping and stumbling
INCLUDES *fall on moving sidewalk*
EXCLUDES1 *fall due to bumping (striking) against object (W18.0-)*
fall in shower or bathtub (W18.2-)
fall on same level NOS (W18.30)
fall on same level from slipping, tripping and stumbling due to ice or snow (W00.0)
fall off or from toilet (W18.1-)
slipping, tripping and stumbling NOS (W18.40)
slipping, tripping and stumbling without falling (W18.4-)
The appropriate 7th character is to be added to each code from category W01
A = initial encounter
D = subsequent encounter
S = sequela

W01.0 Fall on same level from slipping, tripping and stumbling without subsequent striking against object
Falling over animal

W01.1 Fall on same level from slipping, tripping and stumbling with subsequent striking against object

W01.10 Fall on same level from slipping, tripping and stumbling with subsequent striking against unspecified object

W01.11 Fall on same level from slipping, tripping and stumbling with subsequent striking against sharp object

W01.110 Fall on same level from slipping, tripping and stumbling with subsequent striking against sharp glass

W01.111 Fall on same level from slipping, tripping and stumbling with subsequent striking against power tool or machine

W01.118 Fall on same level from slipping, tripping and stumbling with subsequent striking against other sharp object

W01.119 Fall on same level from slipping, tripping and stumbling with subsequent striking against unspecified sharp object

W01.19 Fall on same level from slipping, tripping and stumbling with subsequent striking against other object

W01.190 Fall on same level from slipping, tripping and stumbling with subsequent striking against furniture

W01.198 Fall on same level from slipping, tripping and stumbling with subsequent striking against other object

W03 Other fall on same level due to collision with another person
Fall due to non-transport collision with other person
EXCLUDES1 *collision with another person without fall (W51)*
crushed or pushed by a crowd or human stampede (W52)
fall involving pedestrian conveyance (V00-V09)
fall due to ice or snow (W00)
fall on same level NOS (W18.30)
The appropriate 7th character is to be added to code W03
A = initial encounter
D = subsequent encounter

Unacceptable principal diagnosis symbol per Medicare code edits — Code exempt from diagnosis present on admission requirement — Questionable admission — CC Complication or comorbidity — CC/MCC exclusion — MCC Major complication or comorbidity — Principal diagnosis as its own CC — Principal diagnosis as its own MCC — Z code as first-listed diagnosis

 When symbols appear on a code that requires a 7th character extension, refer to Appendix D to identify applicable 7th character codes.

S = sequela
AHA: Q1, 2015

W04 Fall while being carried or supported by other persons
Accidentally dropped while being carried
The appropriate 7th character is to be added to code W04
A = initial encounter
D = subsequent encounter
S = sequela

W05 Fall from non-moving wheelchair, nonmotorized scooter and motorized mobility scooter
EXCLUDES1 *fall from moving wheelchair (powered) (V00.811)*
fall from moving motorized mobility scooter (V00.831)
fall from nonmotorized scooter (V00.141)
The appropriate 7th character is to be added to each code from category W05
A = initial encounter
D = subsequent encounter
S = sequela

W05.0 Fall from non-moving wheelchair
W05.1 Fall from non-moving nonmotorized scooter
W05.2 Fall from non-moving motorized mobility scooter

W06 Fall from bed
The appropriate 7th character is to be added to code W06
A = initial encounter
D = subsequent encounter
S = sequela

W07 Fall from chair
The appropriate 7th character is to be added to code W07
A = initial encounter
D = subsequent encounter
S = sequela

W08 Fall from other furniture
The appropriate 7th character is to be added to code W08
A = initial encounter
D = subsequent encounter
S = sequela

W09 Fall on and from playground equipment
EXCLUDES1 *fall involving recreational machinery (W31)*
The appropriate 7th character is to be added to each code from category W09
A = initial encounter
D = subsequent encounter
S = sequela

W09.0 Fall on or from playground slide
W09.1 Fall from playground swing
W09.2 Fall on or from jungle gym
W09.8 Fall on or from other playground equipment

W10 Fall on and from stairs and steps
EXCLUDES1 *Fall from stairs and steps due to ice and snow (W00.1)*
The appropriate 7th character is to be added to each code from category W10
A = initial encounter
D = subsequent encounter
S = sequela

W10.0 Fall (on)(from) escalator
W10.1 Fall (on)(from) sidewalk curb
W10.2 Fall (on)(from) incline
Fall (on) (from) ramp
W10.8 Fall (on) (from) other stairs and steps
W10.9 Fall (on) (from) unspecified stairs and steps

W11 Fall on and from ladder
The appropriate 7th character is to be added to code W11
A = initial encounter
D = subsequent encounter
S = sequela

W12 Fall on and from scaffolding
The appropriate 7th character is to be added to code W12
A = initial encounter
D = subsequent encounter
S = sequela

W13 Fall from, out of or through building or structure
The appropriate 7th character is to be added to each code from category W13
A = initial encounter
D = subsequent encounter
S = sequela

W13.0 Fall from, out of or through balcony
Fall from, out of or through railing
W13.1 Fall from, out of or through bridge
W13.2 Fall from, out of or through roof
W13.3 Fall through floor
W13.4 Fall from, out of or through window
EXCLUDES2 *fall with subsequent striking against sharp glass (W01.110)*
W13.8 Fall from, out of or through other building or structure
Fall from, out of or through viaduct
Fall from, out of or through wall
Fall from, out of or through flag-pole
W13.9 Fall from, out of or through building, not otherwise specified
EXCLUDES1 *collapse of a building or structure (W20.-)*
fall or jump from burning building or structure (X00.-)

W14 Fall from tree
The appropriate 7th character is to be added to code W14
A = initial encounter
D = subsequent encounter
S = sequela

W15 Fall from cliff
The appropriate 7th character is to be added to code W15
A = initial encounter
D = subsequent encounter
S = sequela

W16 Fall, jump or diving into water
EXCLUDES1 *accidental non-watercraft drowning and submersion not involving fall (W65-W74)*
effects of air pressure from diving (W94.-)
fall into water from watercraft (V90-V94)
hitting an object or against bottom when falling from watercraft (V94.0)
EXCLUDES2 *striking or hitting diving board (W21.4)*
The appropriate 7th character is to be added to each code from category W16
A = initial encounter
D = subsequent encounter
S = sequela

W16.0 Fall into swimming pool
Fall into swimming pool NOS
EXCLUDES1 *fall into empty swimming pool (W17.3)*
W16.01 Fall into swimming pool striking water surface
W16.011 Fall into swimming pool striking water surface causing drowning and submersion
EXCLUDES1 *drowning and submersion while in swimming pool without fall (W67)*
W16.012 Fall into swimming pool striking water surface causing other injury
W16.02 Fall into swimming pool striking bottom
W16.021 Fall into swimming pool striking bottom causing drowning and submersion
EXCLUDES1 *drowning and submersion while in swimming pool without fall (W67)*
W16.022 Fall into swimming pool striking bottom causing other injury
W16.03 Fall into swimming pool striking wall
W16.031 Fall into swimming pool striking wall causing drowning and submersion
EXCLUDES1 *drowning and submersion while in swimming pool without fall (W67)*
W16.032 Fall into swimming pool striking wall causing other injury
W16.1 Fall into natural body of water
Fall into lake
Fall into open sea

Unspecified Code Other Specified Code Manifestation Code N Newborn P Pediatric M Maternity A Adult ♂ Male ♀ Female
● New Code ▲ Revised Code Title ►◄ Revised Text NOTES INCLUDES EXCLUDES1 Not coded here EXCLUDES2 Not included here
4th character required 5th character required 6th character required 7th character required
Extension 'X' Alert HAC Hospital-acquired condition (HAC) alert AHA AHA Coding Clinic©

Fall into river
Fall into stream

W16.11 Fall into natural body of water striking water surface

W16.111 Fall into natural body of water striking water surface causing drowning and submersion

EXCLUDES1 *drowning and submersion while in natural body of water without fall (W69)*

W16.112 Fall into natural body of water striking water surface causing other injury

W16.12 Fall into natural body of water striking bottom

W16.121 Fall into natural body of water striking bottom causing drowning and submersion

EXCLUDES1 *drowning and submersion while in natural body of water without fall (W69)*

W16.122 Fall into natural body of water striking bottom causing other injury

W16.13 Fall into natural body of water striking side

W16.131 Fall into natural body of water striking side causing drowning and submersion

EXCLUDES1 *drowning and submersion while in natural body of water without fall (W69)*

W16.132 Fall into natural body of water striking side causing other injury

W16.2 Fall in (into) filled bathtub or bucket of water

W16.21 Fall in (into) filled bathtub

EXCLUDES1 *fall into empty bathtub (W18.2)*

W16.211 Fall in (into) filled bathtub causing drowning and submersion

EXCLUDES1 *drowning and submersion while in filled bathtub without fall (W65)*

W16.212 Fall in (into) filled bathtub causing other injury

W16.22 Fall in (into) bucket of water

W16.221 Fall in (into) bucket of water causing drowning and submersion

W16.222 Fall in (into) bucket of water causing other injury

W16.3 Fall into other water

Fall into fountain
Fall into reservoir

W16.31 Fall into other water striking water surface

W16.311 Fall into other water striking water surface causing drowning and submersion

EXCLUDES1 *drowning and submersion while in other water without fall (W73)*

W16.312 Fall into other water striking water surface causing other injury

W16.32 Fall into other water striking bottom

W16.321 Fall into other water striking bottom causing drowning and submersion

EXCLUDES1 *drowning and submersion while in other water without fall (W73)*

W16.322 Fall into other water striking bottom causing other injury

W16.33 Fall into other water striking wall

W16.331 Fall into other water striking wall causing drowning and submersion

EXCLUDES1 *drowning and submersion while in other water without fall (W73)*

W16.332 Fall into other water striking wall causing other injury

W16.4 Fall into unspecified water

W16.41 Fall into unspecified water causing drowning and submersion

W16.42 Fall into unspecified water causing other injury

W16.5 Jumping or diving into swimming pool

W16.51 Jumping or diving into swimming pool striking water surface

W16.511 Jumping or diving into swimming pool striking water surface causing drowning and submersion

EXCLUDES1 *drowning and submersion while in swimming pool without jumping or diving (W67)*

W16.512 Jumping or diving into swimming pool striking water surface causing other injury

W16.52 Jumping or diving into swimming pool striking bottom

W16.521 Jumping or diving into swimming pool striking bottom causing drowning and submersion

EXCLUDES1 *drowning and submersion while in swimming pool without jumping or diving (W67)*

W16.522 Jumping or diving into swimming pool striking bottom causing other injury

W16.53 Jumping or diving into swimming pool striking wall

W16.531 Jumping or diving into swimming pool striking wall causing drowning and submersion

EXCLUDES1 *drowning and submersion while in swimming pool without jumping or diving (W67)*

W16.532 Jumping or diving into swimming pool striking wall causing other injury

W16.6 Jumping or diving into natural body of water

Jumping or diving into lake
Jumping or diving into open sea
Jumping or diving into river
Jumping or diving into stream

W16.61 Jumping or diving into natural body of water striking water surface

W16.611 Jumping or diving into natural body of water striking water surface causing drowning and submersion

EXCLUDES1 *drowning and submersion while in natural body of water without jumping or diving (W69)*

W16.612 Jumping or diving into natural body of water striking water surface causing other injury

W16.62 Jumping or diving into natural body of water striking bottom

W16.621 Jumping or diving into natural body of water striking bottom causing drowning and submersion

EXCLUDES1 *drowning and submersion while in natural body of water without jumping or diving (W69)*

W16.622 Jumping or diving into natural body of water striking bottom causing other injury

W16.7 Jumping or diving from boat

EXCLUDES1 *Fall from boat into water -see watercraft accident (V90-V94)*

W16.71 Jumping or diving from boat striking water surface

W16.711 Jumping or diving from boat striking water surface causing drowning and submersion

W16.712 Jumping or diving from boat striking water surface causing other injury

W16.72 Jumping or diving from boat striking bottom

W16.721 Jumping or diving from boat striking bottom causing drowning and submersion

W16.722 Jumping or diving from boat striking bottom causing other injury

W16.8 Jumping or diving into other water

Jumping or diving into fountain
Jumping or diving into reservoir

W16.81 Jumping or diving into other water striking water surface

W16.811 Jumping or diving into other water striking water surface causing drowning and submersion

Unacceptable principal diagnosis symbol per Medicare code edits · Code exempt from diagnosis present on admission requirement · Questionable admission · Complication or comorbidity · CC/MCC exclusion · Major complication or comorbidity · Principal diagnosis as its own CC · Principal diagnosis as its own MCC · Z code as first-listed diagnosis

EXCLUDES1 *drowning and submersion while in other water without jumping or diving (W73)*

W16.812 Jumping or diving into other water striking water surface causing other injury

W16.82 Jumping or diving into other water striking bottom

W16.821 Jumping or diving into other water striking bottom causing drowning and submersion

EXCLUDES1 *drowning and submersion while in other water without jumping or diving (W73)*

W16.822 Jumping or diving into other water striking bottom causing other injury

W16.83 Jumping or diving into other water striking wall

W16.831 Jumping or diving into other water striking wall causing drowning and submersion

EXCLUDES1 *drowning and submersion while in other water without jumping or diving (W73)*

W16.832 Jumping or diving into other water striking wall causing other injury

W16.9 Jumping or diving into unspecified water

W16.91 Jumping or diving into unspecified water causing drowning and submersion

W16.92 Jumping or diving into unspecified water causing other injury

W17 Other fall from one level to another

The appropriate 7th character is to be added to each code from category W17

A = initial encounter
D = subsequent encounter
S = sequela

W17.0 Fall into well

W17.1 Fall into storm drain or manhole

W17.2 Fall into hole

Fall into pit

W17.3 Fall into empty swimming pool

EXCLUDES1 *fall into filled swimming pool (W16.0-)*

W17.4 Fall from dock

W17.8 Other fall from one level to another

W17.81 Fall down embankment (hill)

W17.82 Fall from (out of) grocery cart

Fall due to grocery cart tipping over

W17.89 Other fall from one level to another

Fall from cherry picker
Fall from lifting device
Fall from mobile elevated work platform [MEWP]
Fall from sky lift

W18 Other slipping, tripping and stumbling and falls

The appropriate 7th character is to be added to each code from category W18

A = initial encounter
D = subsequent encounter
S = sequela

W18.0 Fall due to bumping against object

Striking against object with subsequent fall

EXCLUDES1 *fall on same level due to slipping, tripping, or stumbling with subsequent striking against object (W01.1-)*

W18.00 Striking against unspecified object with subsequent fall

W18.01 Striking against sports equipment with subsequent fall

W18.02 Striking against glass with subsequent fall

W18.09 Striking against other object with subsequent fall

W18.1 Fall from or off toilet

W18.11 Fall from or off toilet without subsequent striking against object

Fall from (off) toilet NOS

W18.12 Fall from or off toilet with subsequent striking against object

W18.2 Fall in (into) shower or empty bathtub

EXCLUDES1 *fall in full bathtub causing drowning or submersion (W16.21-)*

W18.3 Other and unspecified fall on same level

W18.30 Fall on same level, unspecified

W18.31 Fall on same level due to stepping on an object

Fall on same level due to stepping on an animal

EXCLUDES1 *slipping, tripping and stumbling without fall due to stepping on animal (W18.41)*

W18.39 Other fall on same level

W18.4 Slipping, tripping and stumbling without falling

EXCLUDES1 *collision with another person without fall (W51)*

W18.40 Slipping, tripping and stumbling without falling, unspecified

W18.41 Slipping, tripping and stumbling without falling due to stepping on object

Slipping, tripping and stumbling without falling due to stepping on animal

EXCLUDES1 *slipping, tripping and stumbling with fall due to stepping on animal (W18.31)*

W18.42 Slipping, tripping and stumbling without falling due to stepping into hole or opening

W18.43 Slipping, tripping and stumbling without falling due to stepping from one level to another

W18.49 Other slipping, tripping and stumbling without falling

W19 Unspecified fall

Accidental fall NOS

The appropriate 7th character is to be added to code W19

A = initial encounter
D = subsequent encounter
S = sequela

AHA: Q4, 2012

Exposure to inanimate mechanical forces (W20-W49)

EXCLUDES1 *assault ▶(X92-Y09)◀*
contact or collision with animals or persons (W50-W64)
exposure to inanimate mechanical forces involving military or war operations (Y36.-, Y37.-)
intentional self-harm (X71-X83)

W20 Struck by thrown, projected or falling object

Code first any associated:
cataclysm (X34-X39)
lightning strike (T75.00)

EXCLUDES1 *falling object in machinery accident (W24, W28-W31)*
falling object in transport accident (V01-V99)
object set in motion by explosion (W35-W40)
object set in motion by firearm (W32-W34)
struck by thrown sports equipment (W21.-)

The appropriate 7th character is to be added to each code from category W20

A = initial encounter
D = subsequent encounter
S = sequela

W20.0 Struck by falling object in cave-in

EXCLUDES2 *asphyxiation due to cave-in (T71.21)*

W20.1 Struck by object due to collapse of building

EXCLUDES1 *struck by object due to collapse of burning building (X00.2, X02.2)*

W20.8 Other cause of strike by thrown, projected or falling object

EXCLUDES1 *struck by thrown sports equipment (W21.-)*

W21 Striking against or struck by sports equipment

EXCLUDES1 *assault with sports equipment (Y08.0-)*
striking against or struck by sports equipment with subsequent fall (W18.01)

The appropriate 7th character is to be added to each code from category W21

A = initial encounter
D = subsequent encounter
S = sequela

W21.0 Struck by hit or thrown ball

W21.00 Struck by hit or thrown ball, unspecified type

W21.01 Struck by football

W21.02 Struck by soccer ball

W21.03 Struck by baseball
W21.04 Struck by golf ball
W21.05 Struck by basketball
W21.06 Struck by volleyball
W21.07 Struck by softball
W21.09 Struck by other hit or thrown ball
W21.1 Struck by bat, racquet or club
W21.11 Struck by baseball bat
W21.12 Struck by tennis racquet
W21.13 Struck by golf club
W21.19 Struck by other bat, racquet or club
W21.2 Struck by hockey stick or puck
W21.21 Struck by hockey stick
W21.210 Struck by ice hockey stick
W21.211 Struck by field hockey stick
W21.22 Struck by hockey puck
W21.220 Struck by ice hockey puck
W21.221 Struck by field hockey puck
W21.3 Struck by sports foot wear
W21.31 Struck by shoe cleats
Stepped on by shoe cleats
W21.32 Struck by skate blades
Skated over by skate blades
W21.39 Struck by other sports foot wear
W21.4 Striking against diving board
Use additional code for subsequent falling into water, if applicable (W16.-)
W21.8 Striking against or struck by other sports equipment
W21.81 Striking against or struck by football helmet
W21.89 Striking against or struck by other sports equipment
W21.9 Striking against or struck by unspecified sports equipment

W22 Striking against or struck by other objects
EXCLUDES1 *striking against or struck by object with subsequent fall (W18.09)*
The appropriate 7th character is to be added to each code from category W22
A = initial encounter
D = subsequent encounter
S = sequela
W22.0 Striking against stationary object
EXCLUDES1 *striking against stationary sports equipment (W21.8)*
W22.01 Walked into wall
W22.02 Walked into lamppost
W22.03 Walked into furniture
W22.04 Striking against wall of swimming pool
W22.041 Striking against wall of swimming pool causing drowning and submersion
EXCLUDES1 *drowning and submersion while swimming without striking against wall (W67)*
W22.042 Striking against wall of swimming pool causing other injury
W22.09 Striking against other stationary object
W22.1 Striking against or struck by automobile airbag
W22.10 Striking against or struck by unspecified automobile airbag
W22.11 Striking against or struck by driver side automobile airbag
W22.12 Striking against or struck by front passenger side automobile airbag
W22.19 Striking against or struck by other automobile airbag
W22.8 Striking against or struck by other objects
Striking against or struck by object NOS
EXCLUDES1 *struck by thrown, projected or falling object (W20.-)*

W23 Caught, crushed, jammed or pinched in or between objects
EXCLUDES1 *injury caused by cutting or piercing instruments (W25-W27)*
injury caused by firearms malfunction (W32.1, W33.1-, W34.1-)
injury caused by lifting and transmission devices (W24.-)
injury caused by machinery (W28-W31)
injury caused by nonpowered hand tools (W27.-)
injury caused by transport vehicle being used as a means of transportation (V01-V99)
injury caused by struck by thrown, projected or falling object (W20.-)
The appropriate 7th character is to be added to each code from category W23
A = initial encounter
D = subsequent encounter
S = sequela
W23.0 Caught, crushed, jammed, or pinched between moving objects
W23.1 Caught, crushed, jammed, or pinched between stationary objects

W24 Contact with lifting and transmission devices, not elsewhere classified
EXCLUDES1 *transport accidents (V01-V99)*
The appropriate 7th character is to be added to each code from category W24
A = initial encounter
D = subsequent encounter
S = sequela
W24.0 Contact with lifting devices, not elsewhere classified
Contact with chain hoist
Contact with drive belt
Contact with pulley (block)
W24.1 Contact with transmission devices, not elsewhere classified
Contact with transmission belt or cable

W25 Contact with sharp glass
Code first any associated:
injury due to flying glass from explosion or firearm discharge (W32-W40)
transport accident (V00-V99)
EXCLUDES1 *fall on same level due to slipping, tripping and stumbling with subsequent striking against sharp glass (W01.10)*
striking against sharp glass with subsequent fall (W18.02)
EXCLUDES2 *glass embedded in skin (W45)*
The appropriate 7th character is to be added to code W25
A = initial encounter
D = subsequent encounter
S = sequela

▲ W26 Contact with ►other sharp objects◄
EXCLUDES2 *sharp object(s) embedded in skin (W45)*
The appropriate 7th character is to be added to each code from category W26
A = initial encounter
D = subsequent encounter
S = sequela
W26.0 Contact with knife
EXCLUDES1 *contact with electric knife (W29.1)*
W26.1 Contact with sword or dagger
● W26.2 Contact with edge of stiff paper
Paper cut
● W26.8 Contact with other sharp object(s), not elsewhere classified
Contact with tin can lid
● W26.9 Contact with unspecified sharp object(s)

W27 Contact with nonpowered hand tool
The appropriate 7th character is to be added to each code from category W27
A = initial encounter
D = subsequent encounter
S = sequela
W27.0 Contact with workbench tool
Contact with auger
Contact with axe
Contact with chisel
Contact with handsaw
Contact with screwdriver
W27.1 Contact with garden tool
Contact with hoe
Contact with nonpowered lawn mower
Contact with pitchfork
Contact with rake
W27.2 Contact with scissors

Unacceptable principal diagnosis symbol per Medicare code edits | Code exempt from diagnosis present on admission requirement
Questionable admission | Complication or comorbidity | CC/MCC exclusion | Major complication or comorbidity
Principal diagnosis as its own CC | Principal diagnosis as its own MCC | Z code as first-listed diagnosis

W27.3 Contact with needle (sewing)
EXCLUDES1 *contact with hypodermic needle (W46.-)*
W27.4 Contact with kitchen utensil
Contact with fork
Contact with ice-pick
Contact with can-opener NOS
W27.5 Contact with paper-cutter
W27.8 **Contact with nonpowered hand tool**
Contact with nonpowered sewing machine
Contact with shovel

W28 Contact with powered lawn mower
Powered lawn mower (commercial) (residential)
EXCLUDES1 *contact with nonpowered lawn mower (W27.1)*
EXCLUDES2 *exposure to electric current (W86.-)*
The appropriate 7th character is to be added to code W28
A = initial encounter
D = subsequent encounter
S = sequela

W29 Contact with other powered hand tools and household machinery
EXCLUDES1 *contact with commercial machinery (W31.82)*
contact with hot household appliance (X15)
contact with nonpowered hand tool (W27.-)
exposure to electric current (W86)
The appropriate 7th character is to be added to each code from category W29
A = initial encounter
D = subsequent encounter
S = sequela
W29.0 Contact with powered kitchen appliance
Contact with blender
Contact with can-opener
Contact with garbage disposal
Contact with mixer
W29.1 Contact with electric knife
W29.2 **Contact with other powered household machinery**
Contact with electric fan
Contact with powered dryer (clothes) (powered) (spin)
Contact with washing-machine
Contact with sewing machine
W29.3 Contact with powered garden and outdoor hand tools and machinery
Contact with chainsaw
Contact with edger
Contact with garden cultivator (tiller)
Contact with hedge trimmer
Contact with other powered garden tool
EXCLUDES1 *contact with powered lawn mower (W28)*
W29.4 Contact with nail gun
W29.8 **Contact with other powered hand tools and household machinery**
Contact with do-it-yourself tool NOS

W30 Contact with agricultural machinery
INCLUDES *animal-powered farm machine*
EXCLUDES1 *agricultural transport vehicle accident (V01-V99)*
explosion of grain store (W40.8)
exposure to electric current (W86.-)
The appropriate 7th character is to be added to each code from category W30
A = initial encounter
D = subsequent encounter
S = sequela
W30.0 Contact with combine harvester
Contact with reaper
Contact with thresher
W30.1 Contact with power take-off devices (PTO)
W30.2 Contact with hay derrick
W30.3 Contact with grain storage elevator
EXCLUDES1 *explosion of grain store (W40.8)*
W30.8 Contact with other specified agricultural machinery
W30.81 **Contact with agricultural transport vehicle in** stationary use
Contact with agricultural transport vehicle under repair, not on public roadway
EXCLUDES1 *agricultural transport vehicle accident (V01-V99)*
W30.89 **Contact with other specified agricultural machinery**
W30.9 **Contact with unspecified agricultural machinery**
Contact with farm machinery NOS

W31 Contact with other and unspecified **machinery**
EXCLUDES1 *contact with agricultural machinery (W30.-)*
contact with machinery in transport under own power or being towed by a vehicle (V01-V99)
exposure to electric current (W86)
The appropriate 7th character is to be added to each code from category W31
A = initial encounter
D = subsequent encounter
S = sequela
W31.0 Contact with mining and earth-drilling **machinery**
Contact with bore or drill (land) (seabed)
Contact with shaft hoist
Contact with shaft lift
Contact with undercutter
W31.1 Contact with metalworking **machines**
Contact with abrasive wheel
Contact with forging machine
Contact with lathe
Contact with mechanical shears
Contact with metal drilling machine
Contact with milling machine
Contact with power press
Contact with rolling-mill
Contact with metal sawing machine
W31.2 Contact with powered woodworking and forming **machines**
Contact with band saw
Contact with bench saw
Contact with circular saw
Contact with molding machine
Contact with overhead plane
Contact with powered saw
Contact with radial saw
Contact with sander
EXCLUDES1 *nonpowered woodworking tools (W27.0)*
W31.3 Contact with prime movers
Contact with gas turbine
Contact with internal combustion engine
Contact with steam engine
Contact with water driven turbine
W31.8 Contact with other specified **machinery**
W31.81 Contact with recreational **machinery**
Contact with roller coaster
W31.82 **Contact with other commercial machinery**
Contact with commercial electric fan
Contact with commercial kitchen appliances
Contact with commercial powered dryer (clothes) (powered) (spin)
Contact with commercial washing-machine
Contact with commercial sewing machine
EXCLUDES1 *contact with household machinery (W29.-)*
contact with powered lawn mower (W28)
W31.83 Contact with special construction vehicle in stationary use
Contact with special construction vehicle under repair, not on public roadway
EXCLUDES1 *special construction vehicle accident (V01-V99)*
W31.89 **Contact with other specified machinery**
W31.9 **Contact with unspecified machinery**
Contact with machinery NOS

W32 Accidental handgun **discharge and malfunction**
INCLUDES *accidental discharge and malfunction of gun for single hand use*
accidental discharge and malfunction of pistol
accidental discharge and malfunction of revolver
Handgun discharge and malfunction NOS
EXCLUDES1 *accidental airgun discharge and malfunction (W34.010, W34.110)*

Unspecified Code Other Specified Code Manifestation Code N Newborn P Pediatric M Maternity A Adult ♂ Male ♀ Female
● New Code ▲ Revised Code Title ►◄ Revised Text NOTES INCLUDES EXCLUDES1 Not coded here EXCLUDES2 Not included here
4th character required 5th character required 6th character required 7th character required
Extension 'X' Alert HAC Hospital-acquired condition (HAC) alert AHA AHA Coding Clinic®

accidental BB gun discharge and malfunction (W34.010, W34.110)
accidental pellet gun discharge and malfunction (W34.010, W34.110)
accidental shotgun discharge and malfunction (W33.01, W33.11)
assault by handgun discharge (X93)
handgun discharge involving legal intervention (Y35.0-)
handgun discharge involving military or war operations (Y36.4-)
intentional self-harm by handgun discharge (X72)
Very pistol discharge and malfunction (W34.09, W34.19)

The appropriate 7th character is to be added to each code from category W32
A = initial encounter
D = subsequent encounter
S = sequela

W32.0 Accidental handgun discharge
W32.1 Accidental handgun malfunction
Injury due to explosion of handgun (parts)
Injury due to malfunction of mechanism or component of handgun
Injury due to recoil of handgun
Powder burn from handgun

W33 Accidental rifle, shotgun and larger firearm discharge and malfunction
INCLUDES *rifle, shotgun and larger firearm discharge and malfunction NOS*
EXCLUDES1 *accidental airgun discharge and malfunction (W34.010, W34.110)*
accidental BB gun discharge and malfunction (W34.010, W34.110)
accidental handgun discharge and malfunction (W32.-)
accidental pellet gun discharge and malfunction (W34.010, W34.110)
assault by rifle, shotgun and larger firearm discharge (X94)
firearm discharge involving legal intervention (Y35.0-)
firearm discharge involving military or war operations (Y36.4-)
intentional self-harm by rifle, shotgun and larger firearm discharge (X73)

The appropriate 7th character is to be added to each code from category W33
A = initial encounter
D = subsequent encounter
S = sequela

W33.0 Accidental rifle, shotgun and larger firearm discharge
W33.00 Accidental discharge of unspecified larger firearm
Discharge of unspecified larger firearm NOS
W33.01 Accidental discharge of shotgun
Discharge of shotgun NOS
W33.02 Accidental discharge of hunting rifle
Discharge of hunting rifle NOS
W33.03 Accidental discharge of machine gun
Discharge of machine gun NOS
W33.09 Accidental discharge of other larger firearm
Discharge of other larger firearm NOS
W33.1 Accidental rifle, shotgun and larger firearm malfunction
Injury due to explosion of rifle, shotgun and larger firearm (parts)
Injury due to malfunction of mechanism or component of rifle, shotgun and larger firearm
Injury due to piercing, cutting, crushing or pinching due to (by) slide trigger mechanism, scope or other gun part
Injury due to recoil of rifle, shotgun and larger firearm
Powder burn from rifle, shotgun and larger firearm
W33.10 Accidental malfunction of unspecified larger firearm
Malfunction of unspecified larger firearm NOS
W33.11 Accidental malfunction of shotgun
Malfunction of shotgun NOS
W33.12 Accidental malfunction of hunting rifle
Malfunction of hunting rifle NOS
W33.13 Accidental malfunction of machine gun
Malfunction of machine gun NOS
W33.19 Accidental malfunction of other larger firearm
Malfunction of other larger firearm NOS

W34 Accidental discharge and malfunction from other and unspecified firearms and guns

The appropriate 7th character is to be added to each code from category W34
A = initial encounter
D = subsequent encounter
S = sequela
AHA: Q1, 2015

W34.0 Accidental discharge from other and unspecified firearms and guns
W34.00 Accidental discharge from unspecified firearms or gun
Discharge from firearm NOS
Gunshot wound NOS
Shot NOS
W34.01 Accidental discharge of gas, air or spring-operated guns
W34.010 Accidental discharge of airgun
Accidental discharge of BB gun
Accidental discharge of pellet gun
W34.011 Accidental discharge of paintball gun
Accidental injury due to paintball discharge
W34.018 Accidental discharge of other gas, air or spring-operated gun
W34.09 Accidental discharge from other specified firearms
Accidental discharge from Very pistol [flare]
W34.1 Accidental malfunction from other and unspecified firearms and guns
W34.10 Accidental malfunction from unspecified firearms or gun
Firearm malfunction NOS
W34.11 Accidental malfunction of gas, air or spring-operated guns
W34.110 Accidental malfunction of airgun
Accidental malfunction of BB gun
Accidental malfunction of pellet gun
W34.111 Accidental malfunction of paintball gun
Accidental injury due to paintball gun malfunction
W34.118 Accidental malfunction of other gas, air or spring-operated gun
W34.19 Accidental malfunction from other specified firearms
Accidental malfunction from Very pistol [flare]

W35 Explosion and rupture of boiler
EXCLUDES1 *explosion and rupture of boiler on watercraft (V93.4)*
The appropriate 7th character is to be added to code W35
A = initial encounter
D = subsequent encounter
S = sequela

W36 Explosion and rupture of gas cylinder
The appropriate 7th character is to be added to each code from category W36
A = initial encounter
D = subsequent encounter
S = sequela

W36.1 Explosion and rupture of aerosol can
W36.2 Explosion and rupture of air tank
W36.3 Explosion and rupture of pressurized-gas tank
W36.8 Explosion and rupture of other gas cylinder
W36.9 Explosion and rupture of unspecified gas cylinder

W37 Explosion and rupture of pressurized tire, pipe or hose
The appropriate 7th character is to be added to each code from category W37
A = initial encounter
D = subsequent encounter
S = sequela

W37.0 Explosion of bicycle tire
W37.8 Explosion and rupture of other pressurized tire, pipe or hose

W38 Explosion and rupture of other specified pressurized devices
The appropriate 7th character is to be added to code W38
A = initial encounter
D = subsequent encounter
S = sequela

W39 Discharge of firework
The appropriate 7th character is to be added to code W39
A = initial encounter

Unacceptable principal diagnosis symbol per Medicare code edits · Code exempt from diagnosis present on admission requirement
Questionable admission · Complication or comorbidity · CC/MCC exclusion · Major complication or comorbidity
Principal diagnosis as its own CC · Principal diagnosis as its own MCC · Z code as first-listed diagnosis

D = subsequent encounter
S = sequela

W40 Explosion of other materials
EXCLUDES1 assault by explosive material (X96)
explosion involving legal intervention (Y35.1-)
explosion involving military or war operations (Y36.0-, Y36.2-)
intentional self-harm by explosive material (X75)
The appropriate 7th character is to be added to each code from category W40
A = initial encounter
D = subsequent encounter
S = sequela

W40.0 Explosion of blasting material
Explosion of blasting cap
Explosion of detonator
Explosion of dynamite
Explosion of explosive (any) used in blasting operations

W40.1 Explosion of explosive gases
Explosion of acetylene
Explosion of butane
Explosion of coal gas
Explosion in mine NOS
Explosion of explosive gas
Explosion of fire damp
Explosion of gasoline fumes
Explosion of methane
Explosion of propane

W40.8 Explosion of other specified explosive materials
Explosion in dump NOS
Explosion in factory NOS
Explosion in grain store
Explosion in munitions
EXCLUDES1 explosion involving legal intervention (Y35.1-)
explosion involving military or war operations (Y36.0-, Y36.2-)

W40.9 Explosion of unspecified explosive materials
Explosion NOS

W42 Exposure to noise
The appropriate 7th character is to be added to each code from category W42
A = initial encounter
D = subsequent encounter
S = sequela

W42.0 Exposure to supersonic waves
W42.9 Exposure to other noise
Exposure to sound waves NOS

W45 Foreign body or object entering through skin
INCLUDES foreign body or object embedded in skin
nail embedded in skin
EXCLUDES2 contact with hand tools (nonpowered) (powered) (W27-W29)
contact with ▶other sharp object(s)◀ (W26.-)
contact with sharp glass (W25.-)
struck by objects (W20-W22)
The appropriate 7th character is to be added to each code from category W45
A = initial encounter
D = subsequent encounter
S = sequela

W45.0 Nail entering through skin
W45.8 Other foreign body or object entering through skin
Splinter in skin NOS

W46 Contact with hypodermic needle
The appropriate 7th character is to be added to each code from category W46
A = initial encounter
D = subsequent encounter
S = sequela

W46.0 Contact with hypodermic needle
Hypodermic needle stick NOS
W46.1 Contact with contaminated hypodermic needle

W49 Exposure to other inanimate mechanical forces
INCLUDES exposure to abnormal gravitational [G] forces
exposure to inanimate mechanical forces NEC
EXCLUDES1 exposure to inanimate mechanical forces involving military or war operations (Y36.-, Y37.-)
The appropriate 7th character is to be added to each code from category W49
A = initial encounter
D = subsequent encounter
S = sequela

W49.0 Item causing external constriction
W49.01 Hair causing external constriction
W49.02 String or thread causing external constriction
W49.03 Rubber band causing external constriction
W49.04 Ring or other jewelry causing external constriction
W49.09 Other specified item causing external constriction
W49.9 Exposure to other inanimate mechanical forces

Exposure to animate mechanical forces (W50-W64)

EXCLUDES1 Toxic effect of contact with venomous animals and plants (T63.-)

W50 Accidental hit, strike, kick, twist, bite or scratch by another person
INCLUDES hit, strike, kick, twist, bite, or scratch by another person NOS
EXCLUDES1 assault by bodily force (Y04)
struck by objects (W20-W22)
The appropriate 7th character is to be added to each code from category W50
A = initial encounter
D = subsequent encounter
S = sequela

W50.0 Accidental hit or strike by another person
Hit or strike by another person NOS
W50.1 Accidental kick by another person
Kick by another person NOS
W50.2 Accidental twist by another person
Twist by another person NOS
AHA: Q1, 2015
W50.3 Accidental bite by another person
Human bite
Bite by another person NOS
W50.4 Accidental scratch by another person
Scratch by another person NOS

W51 Accidental striking against or bumped into by another person
EXCLUDES1 assault by striking against or bumping into by another person (Y04.2)
fall due to collision with another person (W03)
The appropriate 7th character is to be added to code W51
A = initial encounter
D = subsequent encounter
S = sequela

W52 Crushed, pushed or stepped on by crowd or human stampede
Crushed, pushed or stepped on by crowd or human stampede with or without fall
The appropriate 7th character is to be added to code W52
A = initial encounter
D = subsequent encounter
S = sequela

W53 Contact with rodent
INCLUDES contact with saliva, feces or urine of rodent
The appropriate 7th character is to be added to each code from category W53
A = initial encounter
D = subsequent encounter
S = sequela

W53.0 Contact with mouse
W53.01 Bitten by mouse
W53.09 Other contact with mouse
W53.1 Contact with rat
W53.11 Bitten by rat
W53.19 Other contact with rat
W53.2 Contact with squirrel
W53.21 Bitten by squirrel
W53.29 Other contact with squirrel
W53.8 Contact with other rodent
W53.81 Bitten by other rodent
W53.89 Other contact with other rodent

Unspecified Code Other Specified Code Manifestation Code N Newborn P Pediatric M Maternity A Adult ♂ Male ♀ Female
● New Code ▲ Revised Code Title ▶◀ Revised Text NOTES INCLUDES EXCLUDES1 Not coded here EXCLUDES2 Not included here
4th character required 5th character required 6th character required 7th character required
Extension 'X' Alert HAC Hospital-acquired condition (HAC) alert AHA AHA Coding Clinic©

W54 Contact with dog

INCLUDES contact with saliva, feces or urine of dog

The appropriate 7th character is to be added to each code from category W54
A = initial encounter
D = subsequent encounter
S = sequela

W54.0 Bitten by dog
W54.1 Struck by dog
Knocked over by dog
W54.8 Other contact with dog

W55 Contact with other mammals

INCLUDES contact with saliva, feces or urine of mammal

EXCLUDES1 animal being ridden- see transport accidents
bitten or struck by dog (W54)
bitten or struck by rodent (W53.-)
contact with marine mammals (W56.-)

The appropriate 7th character is to be added to each code from category W55
A = initial encounter
D = subsequent encounter
S = sequela

W55.0 Contact with cat
W55.01 Bitten by cat
W55.03 Scratched by cat
W55.09 Other contact with cat
W55.1 Contact with horse
W55.11 Bitten by horse
W55.12 Struck by horse
W55.19 Other contact with horse
W55.2 Contact with cow
Contact with bull
W55.21 Bitten by cow
W55.22 Struck by cow
Gored by bull
W55.29 Other contact with cow
W55.3 Contact with other hoof stock
Contact with goats
Contact with sheep
W55.31 Bitten by other hoof stock
W55.32 Struck by other hoof stock
Gored by goat
Gored by ram
W55.39 Other contact with other hoof stock
W55.4 Contact with pig
W55.41 Bitten by pig
W55.42 Struck by pig
W55.49 Other contact with pig
W55.5 Contact with raccoon
W55.51 Bitten by raccoon
W55.52 Struck by raccoon
W55.59 Other contact with raccoon
W55.8 Contact with other mammals
W55.81 Bitten by other mammals
W55.82 Struck by other mammals
W55.89 Other contact with other mammals

W56 Contact with nonvenomous marine animal

EXCLUDES1 contact with venomous marine animal (T63.-)

The appropriate 7th character is to be added to each code from category W56
A = initial encounter
D = subsequent encounter
S = sequela

W56.0 Contact with dolphin
W56.01 Bitten by dolphin
W56.02 Struck by dolphin
W56.09 Other contact with dolphin
W56.1 Contact with sea lion
W56.11 Bitten by sea lion
W56.12 Struck by sea lion
W56.19 Other contact with sea lion
W56.2 Contact with orca
Contact with killer whale
W56.21 Bitten by orca
W56.22 Struck by orca
W56.29 Other contact with orca
W56.3 Contact with other marine mammals
W56.31 Bitten by other marine mammals
W56.32 Struck by other marine mammals
W56.39 Other contact with other marine mammals
W56.4 Contact with shark
W56.41 Bitten by shark
W56.42 Struck by shark
W56.49 Other contact with shark
W56.5 Contact with other fish
W56.51 Bitten by other fish
W56.52 Struck by other fish
W56.59 Other contact with other fish
W56.8 Contact with other nonvenomous marine animals
W56.81 Bitten by other nonvenomous marine animals
W56.82 Struck by other nonvenomous marine animals
W56.89 Other contact with other nonvenomous marine animals

W57 Bitten or stung by nonvenomous insect and other nonvenomous arthropods

EXCLUDES1 contact with venomous insects and arthropods (T63.2-, T63.3-, T63.4-)

The appropriate 7th character is to be added to code W57
A = initial encounter
D = subsequent encounter
S = sequela

W58 Contact with crocodile or alligator

The appropriate 7th character is to be added to each code from category W58
A = initial encounter
D = subsequent encounter
S = sequela

W58.0 Contact with alligator
W58.01 Bitten by alligator
W58.02 Struck by alligator
W58.03 Crushed by alligator
W58.09 Other contact with alligator
W58.1 Contact with crocodile
W58.11 Bitten by crocodile
W58.12 Struck by crocodile
W58.13 Crushed by crocodile
W58.19 Other contact with crocodile

W59 Contact with other nonvenomous reptiles

EXCLUDES1 contact with venomous reptile (T63.0-, T63.1-)

The appropriate 7th character is to be added to each code from category W59
A = initial encounter
D = subsequent encounter
S = sequela

W59.0 Contact with nonvenomous lizards
W59.01 Bitten by nonvenomous lizards
W59.02 Struck by nonvenomous lizards
W59.09 Other contact with nonvenomous lizards
Exposure to nonvenomous lizards
W59.1 Contact with nonvenomous snakes
W59.11 Bitten by nonvenomous snake
W59.12 Struck by nonvenomous snake
W59.13 Crushed by nonvenomous snake
W59.19 Other contact with nonvenomous snake
W59.2 Contact with turtles
EXCLUDES1 contact with tortoises (W59.8-)
W59.21 Bitten by turtle
W59.22 Struck by turtle
W59.29 Other contact with turtle
Exposure to turtles
W59.8 Contact with other nonvenomous reptiles
W59.81 Bitten by other nonvenomous reptiles
W59.82 Struck by other nonvenomous reptiles
W59.83 Crushed by other nonvenomous reptiles
W59.89 Other contact with other nonvenomous reptiles

W60 Contact with nonvenomous plant thorns and spines and sharp leaves

Unacceptable principal diagnosis symbol per Medicare code edits | Code exempt from diagnosis present on admission requirement
Questionable admission | Complication or comorbidity | CC/MCC exclusion | Major complication or comorbidity
Principal diagnosis as its own CC | Principal diagnosis as its own MCC | Z code as first-listed diagnosis

EXCLUDES1 *Contact with venomous plants (T63.7-)*

The appropriate 7th character is to be added to code W60
- A = initial encounter
- D = subsequent encounter
- S = sequela

W61 Contact with birds (domestic) (wild)

INCLUDES *contact with excreta of birds*

The appropriate 7th character is to be added to each code from category W61
- A = initial encounter
- D = subsequent encounter
- S = sequela

W61.0 Contact with parrot
- W61.01 Bitten by parrot
- W61.02 Struck by parrot
- W61.09 Other contact with parrot
  Exposure to parrots

W61.1 Contact with macaw
- W61.11 Bitten by macaw
- W61.12 Struck by macaw
- W61.19 Other contact with macaw
  Exposure to macaws

W61.2 Contact with other psittacines
- W61.21 Bitten by other psittacines
- W61.22 Struck by other psittacines
- W61.29 Other contact with other psittacines
  Exposure to other psittacines

W61.3 Contact with chicken
- W61.32 Struck by chicken
- W61.33 Pecked by chicken
- W61.39 Other contact with chicken
  Exposure to chickens

W61.4 Contact with turkey
- W61.42 Struck by turkey
- W61.43 Pecked by turkey
- W61.49 Other contact with turkey

W61.5 Contact with goose
- W61.51 Bitten by goose
- W61.52 Struck by goose
- W61.59 Other contact with goose

W61.6 Contact with duck
- W61.61 Bitten by duck
- W61.62 Struck by duck
- W61.69 Other contact with duck

W61.9 Contact with other birds
- W61.91 Bitten by other birds
- W61.92 Struck by other birds
- W61.99 Other contact with other birds
  Contact with bird NOS

W62 Contact with nonvenomous amphibians

EXCLUDES1 *contact with venomous amphibians (T63.81-R63.83)*

The appropriate 7th character is to be added to each code from category W62
- A = initial encounter
- D = subsequent encounter
- S = sequela

- W62.0 Contact with nonvenomous frogs
- W62.1 Contact with nonvenomous toads
- W62.9 Contact with other nonvenomous amphibians

W64 Exposure to other animate mechanical forces

INCLUDES *exposure to nonvenomous animal NOS*

EXCLUDES1 *contact with venomous animal (T63.-)*

The appropriate 7th character is to be added to code W64
- A = initial encounter
- D = subsequent encounter
- S = sequela

Accidental non-transport drowning and submersion (W65-W74)

EXCLUDES1 *accidental drowning and submersion due to fall into water (W16.-)*
accidental drowning and submersion due to water transport accident (V90.-, V92.-)

EXCLUDES2 *accidental drowning and submersion due to cataclysm (X34-X39)*

W65 Accidental drowning and submersion while in bath-tub

EXCLUDES1 *accidental drowning and submersion due to fall in (into) bathtub (W16.211)*

The appropriate 7th character is to be added to code W65
- A = initial encounter
- D = subsequent encounter
- S = sequela

W67 Accidental drowning and submersion while in swimming-pool

EXCLUDES1 *accidental drowning and submersion due to fall into swimming pool (W16.011, W16.021, W16.031)*
accidental drowning and submersion due to striking into wall of swimming pool (W22.041)

The appropriate 7th character is to be added to code W67
- A = initial encounter
- D = subsequent encounter
- S = sequela

W69 Accidental drowning and submersion while in natural water

Accidental drowning and submersion while in lake
Accidental drowning and submersion while in open sea
Accidental drowning and submersion while in river
Accidental drowning and submersion while in stream

EXCLUDES1 *accidental drowning and submersion due to fall into natural body of water (W16.111, W16.121, W16.131)*

The appropriate 7th character is to be added to code W69
- A = initial encounter
- D = subsequent encounter
- S = sequela

W73 Other specified cause of accidental non-transport drowning and submersion

Accidental drowning and submersion while in quenching tank
Accidental drowning and submersion while in reservoir

EXCLUDES1 *accidental drowning and submersion due to fall into other water (W16.311, W16.321, W16.331)*

The appropriate 7th character is to be added to code W73
- A = initial encounter
- D = subsequent encounter
- S = sequela

W74 Unspecified cause of accidental drowning and submersion

Drowning NOS

The appropriate 7th character is to be added to code W74
- A = initial encounter
- D = subsequent encounter
- S = sequela

Exposure to electric current, radiation and extreme ambient air temperature and pressure (W85-W99)

EXCLUDES1 *exposure to:*
failure in dosage of radiation or temperature during surgical and medical care (Y63.2-Y63.5)
lightning (T75.0-)
natural cold (X31)
natural heat (X30)
natural radiation NOS (X39)
radiological procedure and radiotherapy (Y84.2)
sunlight (X32)

W85 Exposure to electric transmission lines

Broken power line

The appropriate 7th character is to be added to code W85
- A = initial encounter
- D = subsequent encounter
- S = sequela

W86 Exposure to other specified electric current

The appropriate 7th character is to be added to each code from category W86
- A = initial encounter
- D = subsequent encounter
- S = sequela

- W86.0 Exposure to domestic wiring and appliances
- W86.1 Exposure to industrial wiring, appliances and electrical machinery

Exposure to conductors
Exposure to control apparatus
Exposure to electrical equipment and machinery
Exposure to transformers

W86.8 **Exposure to other electric current**
Exposure to wiring and appliances in or on farm (not farmhouse)
Exposure to wiring and appliances outdoors
Exposure to wiring and appliances in or on public building
Exposure to wiring and appliances in or on residential institutions
Exposure to wiring and appliances in or on schools

W88 **Exposure to ionizing radiation**
EXCLUDES1 *exposure to sunlight (X32)*
The appropriate 7th character is to be added to each code from category W88
A = initial encounter
D = subsequent encounter
S = sequela

W88.0 **Exposure to X-rays**
W88.1 **Exposure to radioactive isotopes**
W88.8 **Exposure to other ionizing radiation**

W89 **Exposure to man-made visible and ultraviolet light**
INCLUDES *exposure to welding light (arc)*
EXCLUDES1 *exposure to sunlight (X32)*
The appropriate 7th character is to be added to each code from category W89
A = initial encounter
D = subsequent encounter
S = sequela

W89.0 **Exposure to welding light (arc)**
W89.1 **Exposure to tanning bed**
W89.8 **Exposure to other man-made visible and ultraviolet light**
W89.9 **Exposure to unspecified man-made visible and ultraviolet light**

W90 **Exposure to other nonionizing radiation**
EXCLUDES1 *exposure to sunlight (X32)*
The appropriate 7th character is to be added to each code from category W90
A = initial encounter
D = subsequent encounter
S = sequela

W90.0 **Exposure to radiofrequency**
W90.1 **Exposure to infrared radiation**
W90.2 **Exposure to laser radiation**
W90.8 **Exposure to other nonionizing radiation**

W92 **Exposure to excessive heat of man-made origin**
The appropriate 7th character is to be added to code W92
A = initial encounter
D = subsequent encounter
S = sequela

W93 **Exposure to excessive cold of man-made origin**
The appropriate 7th character is to be added to each code from category W93
A = initial encounter
D = subsequent encounter
S = sequela

W93.0 **Contact with or inhalation of dry ice**
W93.01 **Contact with dry ice**
W93.02 **Inhalation of dry ice**

W93.1 **Contact with or inhalation of liquid air**
W93.11 **Contact with liquid air**
Contact with liquid hydrogen
Contact with liquid nitrogen
W93.12 **Inhalation of liquid air**
Inhalation of liquid hydrogen
Inhalation of liquid nitrogen

W93.2 **Prolonged exposure in deep freeze unit or refrigerator**
W93.8 **Exposure to other excessive cold of man-made origin**

W94 **Exposure to high and low air pressure and changes in air pressure**
The appropriate 7th character is to be added to each code from category W94
A = initial encounter
D = subsequent encounter
S = sequela

W94.0 **Exposure to prolonged high air pressure**
W94.1 **Exposure to prolonged low air pressure**
W94.11 **Exposure to residence or prolonged visit at high altitude**
W94.12 **Exposure to other prolonged low air pressure**
W94.2 **Exposure to rapid changes in air pressure during ascent**
W94.21 **Exposure to reduction in atmospheric pressure while surfacing from deep-water diving**
W94.22 **Exposure to reduction in atmospheric pressure while surfacing from underground**
W94.23 **Exposure to sudden change in air pressure in aircraft during ascent**
W94.29 **Exposure to other rapid changes in air pressure during ascent**
W94.3 **Exposure to rapid changes in air pressure during descent**
W94.31 **Exposure to sudden change in air pressure in aircraft during descent**
W94.32 **Exposure to high air pressure from rapid descent in water**
W94.39 **Exposure to other rapid changes in air pressure during descent**

W99 **Exposure to other man-made environmental factors**
The appropriate 7th character is to be added to code W99
A = initial encounter
D = subsequent encounter
S = sequela

Exposure to smoke, fire and flames (X00-X08)

EXCLUDES1 *arson (X97)*
EXCLUDES2 *explosions (W35-W40)*
lightning (T75.0-)
transport accident (V01-V99)

X00 **Exposure to uncontrolled fire in building or structure**
INCLUDES *conflagration in building or structure*
Code first any associated cataclysm
EXCLUDES2 *Exposure to ignition or melting of nightwear (X05)*
Exposure to ignition or melting of other clothing and apparel (X06.-)
Exposure to other specified smoke, fire and flames (X08.-)
The appropriate 7th character is to be added to each code from category X00
A = initial encounter
D = subsequent encounter
S = sequela

X00.0 **Exposure to flames in uncontrolled fire in building or structure**
AHA: Q2, 2016
X00.1 **Exposure to smoke in uncontrolled fire in building or structure**
X00.2 **Injury due to collapse of burning building or structure in uncontrolled fire**
EXCLUDES1 *injury due to collapse of building not on fire (W20.1)*
X00.3 **Fall from burning building or structure in uncontrolled fire**
X00.4 **Hit by object from burning building or structure in uncontrolled fire**
X00.5 **Jump from burning building or structure in uncontrolled fire**
X00.8 **Other exposure to uncontrolled fire in building or structure**

X01 **Exposure to uncontrolled fire, not in building or structure**
INCLUDES *exposure to forest fire*
The appropriate 7th character is to be added to each code from category X01
A = initial encounter
D = subsequent encounter
S = sequela

X01.0 **Exposure to flames in uncontrolled fire, not in building or structure**
X01.1 **Exposure to smoke in uncontrolled fire, not in building or structure**
X01.3 **Fall due to uncontrolled fire, not in building or structure**

Unacceptable principal diagnosis symbol per Medicare code edits; Code exempt from diagnosis present on admission requirement; Questionable admission; Complication or comorbidity; CC/MCC exclusion; Major complication or comorbidity; Principal diagnosis as its own CC; Principal diagnosis as its own MCC; Z code as first-listed diagnosis

X01.4 Hit by object due to uncontrolled fire, not in building or structure

X01.8 Other exposure to uncontrolled fire, not in building or structure

X02 Exposure to controlled fire in building or structure

INCLUDES *exposure to fire in fireplace*
exposure to fire in stove

The appropriate 7th character is to be added to each code from category X02
A = initial encounter
D = subsequent encounter
S = sequela

X02.0 Exposure to flames in controlled fire in building or structure

X02.1 Exposure to smoke in controlled fire in building or structure

X02.2 Injury due to collapse of burning building or structure in controlled fire

EXCLUDES1 *injury due to collapse of building not on fire (W20.1)*

X02.3 Fall from burning building or structure in controlled fire

X02.4 Hit by object from burning building or structure in controlled fire

X02.5 Jump from burning building or structure in controlled fire

X02.8 Other exposure to controlled fire in building or structure

X03 Exposure to controlled fire, not in building or structure

INCLUDES *exposure to bon fire*
exposure to camp-fire
exposure to trash fire

The appropriate 7th character is to be added to each code from category X03
A = initial encounter
D = subsequent encounter
S = sequela

X03.0 Exposure to flames in controlled fire, not in building or structure

X03.1 Exposure to smoke in controlled fire, not in building or structure

X03.3 Fall due to controlled fire, not in building or structure

X03.4 Hit by object due to controlled fire, not in building or structure

X03.8 Other exposure to controlled fire, not in building or structure

X04 Exposure to ignition of highly flammable material
Exposure to ignition of gasoline
Exposure to ignition of kerosene
Exposure to ignition of petrol

EXCLUDES2 *exposure to ignition or melting of nightwear (X05)*
exposure to ignition or melting of other clothing and apparel (X06)

The appropriate 7th character is to be added to code X04
A = initial encounter
D = subsequent encounter
S = sequela

AHA: Q2, 2016

X05 Exposure to ignition or melting of nightwear

EXCLUDES2 *exposure to uncontrolled fire in building or structure (X00.-)*
exposure to uncontrolled fire, not in building or structure (X01.-)
exposure to controlled fire in building or structure (X02.-)
exposure to controlled fire, not in building or structure (X03.-)
exposure to ignition of highly flammable materials (X04.-)

The appropriate 7th character is to be added to code X05
A = initial encounter
D = subsequent encounter
S = sequela

X06 Exposure to ignition or melting of other clothing and apparel

EXCLUDES2 *exposure to uncontrolled fire in building or structure (X00.-)*
exposure to uncontrolled fire, not in building or structure (X01.-)
exposure to controlled fire in building or structure (X02.-)
exposure to controlled fire, not in building or structure (X03.-)
exposure to ignition of highly flammable materials (X04.-)

The appropriate 7th character is to be added to each code from category X06
A = initial encounter
D = subsequent encounter
S = sequela

X06.0 Exposure to ignition of plastic jewelry

X06.1 Exposure to melting of plastic jewelry

X06.2 Exposure to ignition of other clothing and apparel

X06.3 Exposure to melting of other clothing and apparel

X08 Exposure to other specified smoke, fire and flames

The appropriate 7th character is to be added to each code from category X08
A = initial encounter
D = subsequent encounter
S = sequela

X08.0 Exposure to bed fire
Exposure to mattress fire

X08.00 Exposure to bed fire due to unspecified burning material

X08.01 Exposure to bed fire due to burning cigarette
AHA: Q1, 2015

X08.09 Exposure to bed fire due to other burning material

X08.1 Exposure to sofa fire

X08.10 Exposure to sofa fire due to unspecified burning material

X08.11 Exposure to sofa fire due to burning cigarette

X08.19 Exposure to sofa fire due to other burning material

X08.2 Exposure to other furniture fire

X08.20 Exposure to other furniture fire due to unspecified burning material

X08.21 Exposure to other furniture fire due to burning cigarette

X08.29 Exposure to other furniture fire due to other burning material

X08.8 Exposure to other specified smoke, fire and flames

Contact with heat and hot substances (X10-X19)

EXCLUDES1 *exposure to excessive natural heat (X30)*
exposure to fire and flames (X00-X09)

X10 Contact with hot drinks, food, fats and cooking oils

The appropriate 7th character is to be added to each code from category X10
A = initial encounter
D = subsequent encounter
S = sequela

X10.0 Contact with hot drinks

X10.1 Contact with hot food

X10.2 Contact with fats and cooking oils

X11 Contact with hot tap-water

INCLUDES *contact with boiling tap-water*
contact with boiling water NOS

EXCLUDES1 *contact with water heated on stove (X12)*

The appropriate 7th character is to be added to each code from category X11
A = initial encounter
D = subsequent encounter
S = sequela

X11.0 Contact with hot water in bath or tub

EXCLUDES1 *contact with running hot water in bath or tub (X11.1)*

X11.1 Contact with running hot water
Contact with hot water running out of hose
Contact with hot water running out of tap

X11.8 Contact with other hot tap-water
Contact with hot water in bucket
Contact with hot tap-water NOS

X12 Contact with other hot fluids
Contact with water heated on stove

EXCLUDES1 *hot (liquid) metals (X18)*

The appropriate 7th character is to be added to code X12
A = initial encounter
D = subsequent encounter
S = sequela

X13 Contact with steam and other hot vapors

The appropriate 7th character is to be added to each code from category X13
A = initial encounter
D = subsequent encounter
S = sequela

Unspecified Code Other Specified Code Manifestation Code N Newborn P Pediatric M Maternity A Adult ♂ Male ♀ Female
● New Code ▲ Revised Code Title ►◄ Revised Text NOTES INCLUDES EXCLUDES1 Not coded here EXCLUDES2 Not included here
4th character required 5th character required 6th character required 7th character required
Extension 'X' Alert HAC Hospital-acquired condition (HAC) alert AHA AHA Coding Clinic©

X13.0 Inhalation of steam and other hot vapors
X13.1 Other contact with steam and other hot vapors
X14 Contact with hot air and other hot gases
The appropriate 7th character is to be added to each code from category X14
A = initial encounter
D = subsequent encounter
S = sequela
X14.0 Inhalation of hot air and gases
X14.1 Other contact with hot air and other hot gases

X15 Contact with hot household appliances
EXCLUDES1 *contact with heating appliances (X16)*
contact with powered household appliances (W29.-)
exposure to controlled fire in building or structure due to household appliance (X02.8)
exposure to household appliances electrical current (W86.0)
The appropriate 7th character is to be added to each code from category X15
A = initial encounter
D = subsequent encounter
S = sequela
X15.0 Contact with hot stove (kitchen)
X15.1 Contact with hot toaster
X15.2 Contact with hotplate
X15.3 Contact with hot saucepan or skillet
X15.8 Contact with other hot household appliances
Contact with cooker
Contact with kettle
Contact with light bulbs
X16 Contact with hot heating appliances, radiators and pipes
EXCLUDES1 *contact with powered appliances (W29.-)*
exposure to controlled fire in building or structure due to appliance (X02.8)
exposure to industrial appliances electrical current (W86.1)
The appropriate 7th character is to be added to code X16
A = initial encounter
D = subsequent encounter
S = sequela
X17 Contact with hot engines, machinery and tools
EXCLUDES1 *contact with hot heating appliances, radiators and pipes (X16)*
contact with hot household appliances (X15)
The appropriate 7th character is to be added to code X17
A = initial encounter
D = subsequent encounter
S = sequela
X18 Contact with other hot metals
Contact with liquid metal
The appropriate 7th character is to be added to code X18
A = initial encounter
D = subsequent encounter
S = sequela
X19 Contact with other heat and hot substances
EXCLUDES1 *objects that are not normally hot, e.g., an object made hot by a house fire (X00-X09)*
The appropriate 7th character is to be added to code X19
A = initial encounter
D = subsequent encounter
S = sequela

Exposure to forces of nature (X30-X39)

X30 Exposure to excessive natural heat
Exposure to excessive heat as the cause of sunstroke
Exposure to heat NOS
EXCLUDES1 *excessive heat of man-made origin (W92)*
exposure to man-made radiation (W89)
exposure to sunlight (X32)
exposure to tanning bed (W89)
The appropriate 7th character is to be added to code X30
A = initial encounter
D = subsequent encounter
S = sequela

X31 Exposure to excessive natural cold
Excessive cold as the cause of chilblains NOS
Excessive cold as the cause of immersion foot or hand
Exposure to cold NOS
Exposure to weather conditions
EXCLUDES1 *cold of man-made origin (W93.-)*
contact with or inhalation of dry ice (W93.-)
contact with or inhalation of liquefied gas (W93.-)
The appropriate 7th character is to be added to code X31
A = initial encounter
D = subsequent encounter
S = sequela
X32 Exposure to sunlight
EXCLUDES1 *man-made radiation (tanning bed) (W89)*
The appropriate 7th character is to be added to code X32
A = initial encounter
D = subsequent encounter
S = sequela
X34 Earthquake
EXCLUDES2 *tidal wave (tsunami) due to earthquake (X37.41)*
The appropriate 7th character is to be added to code X34
A = initial encounter
D = subsequent encounter
S = sequela
X35 Volcanic eruption
EXCLUDES2 *tidal wave (tsunami) due to volcanic eruption (X37.41)*
The appropriate 7th character is to be added to code X35
A = initial encounter
D = subsequent encounter
S = sequela
X36 Avalanche, landslide and other earth movements
INCLUDES *victim of mudslide of cataclysmic nature*
EXCLUDES1 *earthquake (X34)*
EXCLUDES2 *transport accident involving collision with avalanche or landslide not in motion (V01-V99)*
The appropriate 7th character is to be added to each code from category X36
A = initial encounter
D = subsequent encounter
S = sequela
X36.0 Collapse of dam or man-made structure causing earth movement
X36.1 Avalanche, landslide, or mudslide
X37 Cataclysmic storm
The appropriate 7th character is to be added to each code from category X37
A = initial encounter
D = subsequent encounter
S = sequela
X37.0 Hurricane
Storm surge
Typhoon
X37.1 Tornado
Cyclone
Twister
X37.2 Blizzard (snow)(ice)
X37.3 Dust storm
X37.4 Tidal wave
X37.41 Tidal wave due to earthquake or volcanic eruption
Tidal wave NOS
Tsunami
X37.42 Tidal wave due to storm
X37.43 Tidal wave due to landslide
X37.8 Other cataclysmic storms
Cloudburst
Torrential rain
EXCLUDES2 *flood (X38)*
X37.9 Unspecified cataclysmic storm
Storm NOS
EXCLUDES1 *collapse of dam or man-made structure causing earth movement (X39.0)*

Unacceptable principal diagnosis symbol per Medicare code edits · Code exempt from diagnosis present on admission requirement
Questionable admission · Complication or comorbidity · CC/MCC exclusion · Major complication or comorbidity
Principal diagnosis as its own CC · Principal diagnosis as its own MCC · Z code as first-listed diagnosis

X38 Flood
Flood arising from remote storm
Flood of cataclysmic nature arising from melting snow
Flood resulting directly from storm
EXCLUDES1 *collapse of dam or man-made structure causing earth movement (X39.0)*
tidal wave NOS (X37.41)
tidal wave caused by storm (X37.2)
The appropriate 7th character is to be added to code X38
A = initial encounter
D = subsequent encounter
S = sequela

X39 **Exposure to** other forces of nature
The appropriate 7th character is to be added to each code from category X39
A = initial encounter
D = subsequent encounter
S = sequela

X39.0 **Exposure to** natural radiation
EXCLUDES1 *contact with and (suspected) exposure to radon and other naturally occurring radiation ►(Z77.123)◄*
exposure to man-made radiation (W88-W90)
exposure to sunlight (X32)

X39.01 **Exposure to** radon
X39.08 **Exposure to other natural radiation**
X39.8 **Other exposure to forces of nature**

Overexertion and strenuous or repetitive movements (X50)

● X50 **Overexertion and strenuous or repetitive movements**
The appropriate 7th character is to be added to each code from category X50
A = initial encounter
D = subsequent encounter
S = sequela

● X50.0 **Overexertion** from strenuous movement or load
Lifting heavy objects
Lifting weights

● X50.1 **Overexertion from** prolonged static or awkward postures
Prolonged bending
Prolonged kneeling
Prolonged reaching
Prolonged sitting
Prolonged standing
Prolonged twisting
Static bending
Static kneeling
Static reaching
Static sitting
Static standing
Static twisting

● X50.3 **Overexertion from** repetitive **movements**
Use of hand as hammer
EXCLUDES2 *Overuse from prolonged static or awkward postures (X50.1)*

● X50.9 Other and unspecified **overexertion or strenuous movements or** postures
Contact pressure
Contact stress

Accidental exposure to other specified factors (X52-X58)

X52 **Prolonged stay in weightless environment**
Weightlessness in spacecraft (simulator)
The appropriate 7th character is to be added to code X52
A = initial encounter
D = subsequent encounter
S = sequela

X58 **Exposure to other specified factors**
Accident NOS
Exposure NOS
The appropriate 7th character is to be added to code X58
A = initial encounter
D = subsequent encounter
S = sequela

Intentional self-harm (X71-X83)

Purposely self-inflicted injury
Suicide (attempted)

X71 **Intentional self-harm by** drowning and submersion
The appropriate 7th character is to be added to each code from category X71
A = initial encounter
D = subsequent encounter
S = sequela

X71.0 **Intentional self-harm by drowning and submersion** while in bathtub
X71.1 **Intentional self-harm by drowning and submersion** while in swimming pool
X71.2 **Intentional self-harm by drowning and submersion** after jump into swimming pool
X71.3 **Intentional self-harm by drowning and submersion in** natural water
X71.8 **Other intentional self-harm by drowning and submersion**
X71.9 **Intentional self-harm by drowning and submersion, unspecified**

X72 **Intentional self-harm by** handgun discharge
Intentional self-harm by gun for single hand use
Intentional self-harm by pistol
Intentional self-harm by revolver
EXCLUDES1 *Very pistol (X74.8)*
The appropriate 7th character is to be added to code X72
A = initial encounter
D = subsequent encounter
S = sequela

X73 **Intentional self-harm by rifle, shotgun and larger firearm discharge**
EXCLUDES1 *airgun (X74.01)*
The appropriate 7th character is to be added to each code from category X73
A = initial encounter
D = subsequent encounter
S = sequela

X73.0 **Intentional self-harm by** shotgun discharge
X73.1 **Intentional self-harm by** hunting rifle discharge
X73.2 **Intentional self-harm by** machine gun discharge
X73.8 **Intentional self-harm by other larger firearm discharge**
X73.9 **Intentional self-harm by unspecified larger firearm discharge**

X74 **Intentional self-harm by** other and unspecified **firearm and gun discharge**
The appropriate 7th character is to be added to each code from category X74
A = initial encounter
D = subsequent encounter
S = sequela

X74.0 **Intentional self-harm by** gas, air or spring-operated guns
X74.01 **Intentional self-harm by** airgun
Intentional self-harm by BB gun discharge
Intentional self-harm by pellet gun discharge
X74.02 **Intentional self-harm by** paintball gun
X74.09 **Intentional self-harm by other gas, air or spring-operated gun**
X74.8 **Intentional self-harm by other firearm discharge**
Intentional self-harm by Very pistol [flare] discharge
X74.9 **Intentional self-harm by unspecified firearm discharge**

X75 **Intentional self-harm by** explosive material
The appropriate 7th character is to be added to code X75
A = initial encounter
D = subsequent encounter
S = sequela

X76 **Intentional self-harm by** smoke, fire and flames
The appropriate 7th character is to be added to code X76
A = initial encounter
D = subsequent encounter
S = sequela

X77 **Intentional self-harm by** steam, hot vapors and hot objects
The appropriate 7th character is to be added to each code from category X77
A = initial encounter
D = subsequent encounter
S = sequela

X77.0 Intentional self-harm by steam or hot vapors
X77.1 Intentional self-harm by hot tap water
X77.2 Intentional self-harm by other hot fluids
X77.3 Intentional self-harm by hot household appliances
X77.8 Intentional self-harm by other hot objects
X77.9 Intentional self-harm by unspecified hot objects

X78 Intentional self-harm by sharp object
The appropriate 7th character is to be added to each code from category X78
A = initial encounter
D = subsequent encounter
S = sequela
X78.0 Intentional self-harm by sharp glass
X78.1 Intentional self-harm by knife
X78.2 Intentional self-harm by sword or dagger
X78.8 Intentional self-harm by other sharp object
X78.9 Intentional self-harm by unspecified sharp object

X79 Intentional self-harm by blunt object
The appropriate 7th character is to be added to code X79
A = initial encounter
D = subsequent encounter
S = sequela

X80 Intentional self-harm by jumping from a high place
Intentional fall from one level to another
The appropriate 7th character is to be added to code X80
A = initial encounter
D = subsequent encounter
S = sequela

X81 Intentional self-harm by jumping or lying in front of moving object
The appropriate 7th character is to be added to each code from category X81
A = initial encounter
D = subsequent encounter
S = sequela
X81.0 Intentional self-harm by jumping or lying in front of motor vehicle
X81.1 Intentional self-harm by jumping or lying in front of (subway) train
X81.8 Intentional self-harm by jumping or lying in front of other moving object

X82 Intentional self-harm by crashing of motor vehicle
The appropriate 7th character is to be added to each code from category X82
A = initial encounter
D = subsequent encounter
S = sequela
X82.0 Intentional collision of motor vehicle with other motor vehicle
X82.1 Intentional collision of motor vehicle with train
X82.2 Intentional collision of motor vehicle with tree
X82.8 Other intentional self-harm by crashing of motor vehicle

X83 Intentional self-harm by other specified means
EXCLUDES1 *intentional self-harm by poisoning or contact with toxic substance- See Table of Drugs and Chemicals*
The appropriate 7th character is to be added to each code from category X83
A = initial encounter
D = subsequent encounter
S = sequela
X83.0 Intentional self-harm by crashing of aircraft
X83.1 Intentional self-harm by electrocution
X83.2 Intentional self-harm by exposure to extremes of cold
X83.8 Intentional self-harm by other specified means

Assault (X92-Y09)

INCLUDES *homicide*
injuries inflicted by another person with intent to injure or kill, by any means

EXCLUDES1 *injuries due to legal intervention (Y35.-)*
injuries due to operations of war (Y36.-)
injuries due to terrorism (Y38.-)

X92 Assault by drowning and submersion
The appropriate 7th character is to be added to each code from category X92
A = initial encounter
D = subsequent encounter
S = sequela
X92.0 Assault by drowning and submersion while in bathtub
X92.1 Assault by drowning and submersion while in swimming pool
X92.2 Assault by drowning and submersion after push into swimming pool
X92.3 Assault by drowning and submersion in natural water
X92.8 Other assault by drowning and submersion
X92.9 Assault by drowning and submersion, unspecified

X93 Assault by handgun discharge
Assault by discharge of gun for single hand use
Assault by discharge of pistol
Assault by discharge of revolver
EXCLUDES1 *Very pistol (X95.8)*
The appropriate 7th character is to be added to code X93
A = initial encounter
D = subsequent encounter
S = sequela

X94 Assault by rifle, shotgun and larger firearm discharge
EXCLUDES1 *airgun (X95.01)*
The appropriate 7th character is to be added to each code from category X94
A = initial encounter
D = subsequent encounter
S = sequela
X94.0 Assault by shotgun
X94.1 Assault by hunting rifle
X94.2 Assault by machine gun
X94.8 Assault by other larger firearm discharge
X94.9 Assault by unspecified larger firearm discharge

X95 Assault by other and unspecified firearm and gun discharge
The appropriate 7th character is to be added to each code from category X95
A = initial encounter
D = subsequent encounter
S = sequela
X95.0 Assault by gas, air or spring-operated guns
X95.01 Assault by airgun discharge
Assault by BB gun discharge
Assault by pellet gun discharge
X95.02 Assault by paintball gun discharge
X95.09 Assault by other gas, air or spring-operated gun
X95.8 Assault by other firearm discharge
Assault by very pistol [flare] discharge
X95.9 Assault by unspecified firearm discharge

X96 Assault by explosive material
EXCLUDES1 *incendiary device (X97)*
terrorism involving explosive material (Y38.2-)
The appropriate 7th character is to be added to each code from category X96
A = initial encounter
D = subsequent encounter
S = sequela
X96.0 Assault by antipersonnel bomb
EXCLUDES1 *antipersonnel bomb use in military or war (Y36.2-)*
X96.1 Assault by gasoline bomb
X96.2 Assault by letter bomb
X96.3 Assault by fertilizer bomb
X96.4 Assault by pipe bomb
X96.8 Assault by other specified explosive
X96.9 Assault by unspecified explosive

X97 Assault by smoke, fire and flames
Assault by arson
Assault by cigarettes
Assault by incendiary device
The appropriate 7th character is to be added to code X97
A = initial encounter
D = subsequent encounter
S = sequela

Unacceptable principal diagnosis symbol per Medicare code edits · Code exempt from diagnosis present on admission requirement
Questionable admission · Complication or comorbidity · CC/MCC exclusion · Major complication or comorbidity
Principal diagnosis as its own CC · Principal diagnosis as its own MCC · Z code as first-listed diagnosis

X98 Assault by steam, hot vapors and hot objects
The appropriate 7th character is to be added to each code from category X98
A = initial encounter
D = subsequent encounter
S = sequela
X98.0 Assault by steam or hot vapors
X98.1 Assault by hot tap water
X98.2 Assault by hot fluids
X98.3 Assault by hot household appliances
X98.8 Assault by other hot objects
X98.9 Assault by unspecified hot objects

X99 Assault by sharp object
EXCLUDES1 *assault by strike by sports equipment (Y08.0-)*
The appropriate 7th character is to be added to each code from category X99
A = initial encounter
D = subsequent encounter
S = sequela
X99.0 Assault by sharp glass
X99.1 Assault by knife
X99.2 Assault by sword or dagger
X99.8 Assault by other sharp object
X99.9 Assault by unspecified sharp object
Assault by stabbing NOS

Y00 Assault by blunt object
EXCLUDES1 *assault by strike by sports equipment (Y08.0-)*
The appropriate 7th character is to be added to code Y00
A = initial encounter
D = subsequent encounter
S = sequela

Y01 Assault by pushing from high place
The appropriate 7th character is to be added to code Y01
A = initial encounter
D = subsequent encounter
S = sequela

Y02 Assault by pushing or placing victim in front of moving object
The appropriate 7th character is to be added to each code from category Y02
A = initial encounter
D = subsequent encounter
S = sequela
Y02.0 Assault by pushing or placing victim in front of motor vehicle
Y02.1 Assault by pushing or placing victim in front of (subway) train
Y02.8 Assault by pushing or placing victim in front of other moving object

Y03 Assault by crashing of motor vehicle
The appropriate 7th character is to be added to each code from category Y03
A = initial encounter
D = subsequent encounter
S = sequela
Y03.0 Assault by being hit or run over by motor vehicle
Y03.8 Other assault by crashing of motor vehicle

Y04 Assault by bodily force
EXCLUDES1 *assault by:*
submersion (X92.-)
use of weapon (X93-X95, X99, Y00)
The appropriate 7th character is to be added to each code from category Y04
A = initial encounter
D = subsequent encounter
S = sequela
Y04.0 Assault by unarmed brawl or fight
Y04.1 Assault by human bite
Y04.2 Assault by strike against or bumped into by another person
Y04.8 Assault by other bodily force
Assault by bodily force NOS

Y07 Perpetrator of assault, maltreatment and neglect
NOTES Codes from this category are for use only in cases of confirmed abuse (T74.-)
Selection of the correct perpetrator code is based on the relationship between the perpetrator and the victim
INCLUDES *perpetrator of abandonment*
perpetrator of emotional neglect
perpetrator of mental cruelty
perpetrator of physical abuse
perpetrator of physical neglect
perpetrator of sexual abuse
perpetrator of torture

Y07.0 Spouse or partner, perpetrator of maltreatment and neglect
Spouse or partner, perpetrator of maltreatment and neglect against spouse or partner
Y07.01 Husband, perpetrator of maltreatment and neglect
Y07.02 Wife, perpetrator of maltreatment and neglect
Y07.03 Male partner, perpetrator of maltreatment and neglect
Y07.04 Female partner, perpetrator of maltreatment and neglect

Y07.1 Parent (adoptive) (biological), perpetrator of maltreatment and neglect
Y07.11 Biological father, perpetrator of maltreatment and neglect
Y07.12 Biological mother, perpetrator of maltreatment and neglect
Y07.13 Adoptive father, perpetrator of maltreatment and neglect
Y07.14 Adoptive mother, perpetrator of maltreatment and neglect

Y07.4 Other family member, perpetrator of maltreatment and neglect
Y07.41 Sibling, perpetrator of maltreatment and neglect
EXCLUDES1 *stepsibling, perpetrator of maltreatment and neglect (Y07.435, Y07.436)*
Y07.410 Brother, perpetrator of maltreatment and neglect
Y07.411 Sister, perpetrator of maltreatment and neglect
Y07.42 Foster parent, perpetrator of maltreatment and neglect
Y07.420 Foster father, perpetrator of maltreatment and neglect
Y07.421 Foster mother, perpetrator of maltreatment and neglect
Y07.43 Stepparent or stepsibling, perpetrator of maltreatment and neglect
Y07.430 Stepfather, perpetrator of maltreatment and neglect
Y07.432 Male friend of parent (co-residing in household), perpetrator of maltreatment and neglect
Y07.433 Stepmother, perpetrator of maltreatment and neglect
Y07.434 Female friend of parent (co-residing in household), perpetrator of maltreatment and neglect
Y07.435 Stepbrother, perpetrator or maltreatment and neglect
Y07.436 Stepsister, perpetrator of maltreatment and neglect
Y07.49 Other family member, perpetrator of maltreatment and neglect
Y07.490 Male cousin, perpetrator of maltreatment and neglect
Y07.491 Female cousin, perpetrator of maltreatment and neglect
Y07.499 Other family member, perpetrator of maltreatment and neglect

Y07.5 Non-family member, perpetrator of maltreatment and neglect
Y07.50 Unspecified non-family member, perpetrator of maltreatment and neglect
Y07.51 Daycare provider, perpetrator of maltreatment and neglect
Y07.510 At-home childcare provider, perpetrator of maltreatment and neglect

Unspecified Code Other Specified Code Manifestation Code N Newborn P Pediatric M Maternity A Adult ♂ Male ♀ Female
● New Code ▲ Revised Code Title ►◄ Revised Text NOTES INCLUDES EXCLUDES1 Not coded here EXCLUDES2 Not included here
4th character required 5th character required 6th character required 7th character required
Extension 'X' Alert HAC Hospital-acquired condition (HAC) alert AHA AHA Coding Clinic©

Y07.511 Daycare center childcare provider, perpetrator of maltreatment and neglect
Y07.512 At-home adult care provider, perpetrator of maltreatment and neglect
Y07.513 Adult care center provider, perpetrator of maltreatment and neglect
Y07.519 Unspecified daycare provider, perpetrator of maltreatment and neglect
Y07.52 Healthcare provider, perpetrator of maltreatment and neglect
Y07.521 Mental health provider, perpetrator of maltreatment and neglect
Y07.528 Other therapist or healthcare provider, perpetrator of maltreatment and neglect
Nurse perpetrator of maltreatment and neglect
Occupational therapist perpetrator of maltreatment and neglect
Physical therapist perpetrator of maltreatment and neglect
Speech therapist perpetrator of maltreatment and neglect
Y07.529 Unspecified healthcare provider, perpetrator of maltreatment and neglect
Y07.53 Teacher or instructor, perpetrator of maltreatment and neglect
Coach, perpetrator of maltreatment and neglect
Y07.59 Other non-family member, perpetrator of maltreatment and neglect
Y07.9 Unspecified perpetrator of maltreatment and neglect

Y08 Assault by other specified means
The appropriate 7th character is to be added to each code from category Y08
A = initial encounter
D = subsequent encounter
S = sequela
Y08.0 Assault by strike by sport equipment
Y08.01 Assault by strike by hockey stick
Y08.02 Assault by strike by baseball bat
Y08.09 Assault by strike by other specified type of sport equipment
Y08.8 Assault by other specified means
Y08.81 Assault by crashing of aircraft
Y08.89 Assault by other specified means

Y09 Assault by unspecified means
Assassination (attempted) NOS
Homicide (attempted) NOS
Manslaughter (attempted) NOS
Murder (attempted) NOS

Event of undetermined intent (Y21-Y33)

Undetermined intent is only for use when there is specific documentation in the record that the intent of the injury cannot be determined. If no such documentation is present, code to accidental (unintentional)

Y21 Drowning and submersion, undetermined intent
The appropriate 7th character is to be added to each code from category Y21
A = initial encounter
D = subsequent encounter
S = sequela
Y21.0 Drowning and submersion while in bathtub, undetermined intent
Y21.1 Drowning and submersion after fall into bathtub, undetermined intent
Y21.2 Drowning and submersion while in swimming pool, undetermined intent
Y21.3 Drowning and submersion after fall into swimming pool, undetermined intent
Y21.4 Drowning and submersion in natural water, undetermined intent
Y21.8 Other drowning and submersion, undetermined intent
Y21.9 Unspecified drowning and submersion, undetermined intent

Y22 Handgun discharge, undetermined intent
Discharge of gun for single hand use, undetermined intent
Discharge of pistol, undetermined intent
Discharge of revolver, undetermined intent
EXCLUDES2 *very pistol (Y24.8)*
The appropriate 7th character is to be added to code Y22
A = initial encounter
D = subsequent encounter
S = sequela

Y23 Rifle, shotgun and larger firearm discharge, undetermined intent
EXCLUDES2 *airgun (Y24.0)*
The appropriate 7th character is to be added to each code from category Y23
A = initial encounter
D = subsequent encounter
S = sequela
Y23.0 Shotgun discharge, undetermined intent
Y23.1 Hunting rifle discharge, undetermined intent
Y23.2 Military firearm discharge, undetermined intent
Y23.3 Machine gun discharge, undetermined intent
Y23.8 Other larger firearm discharge, undetermined intent
Y23.9 Unspecified larger firearm discharge, undetermined intent

Y24 Other and unspecified firearm discharge, undetermined intent
The appropriate 7th character is to be added to each code from category Y24
A = initial encounter
D = subsequent encounter
S = sequela
Y24.0 Airgun discharge, undetermined intent
BB gun discharge, undetermined intent
Pellet gun discharge, undetermined intent
Y24.8 Other firearm discharge, undetermined intent
Paintball gun discharge, undetermined intent
Very pistol [flare] discharge, undetermined intent
Y24.9 Unspecified firearm discharge, undetermined intent

Y25 Contact with explosive material, undetermined intent
The appropriate 7th character is to be added to code Y25
A = initial encounter
D = subsequent encounter
S = sequela

Y26 Exposure to smoke, fire and flames, undetermined intent
The appropriate 7th character is to be added to code Y26
A = initial encounter
D = subsequent encounter
S = sequela

Y27 Contact with steam, hot vapors and hot objects, undetermined intent
The appropriate 7th character is to be added to each code from category Y27
A = initial encounter
D = subsequent encounter
S = sequela
Y27.0 Contact with steam and hot vapors, undetermined intent
Y27.1 Contact with hot tap water, undetermined intent
Y27.2 Contact with hot fluids, undetermined intent
Y27.3 Contact with hot household appliance, undetermined intent
Y27.8 Contact with other hot objects, undetermined intent
Y27.9 Contact with unspecified hot objects, undetermined intent

Y28 Contact with sharp object, undetermined intent
The appropriate 7th character is to be added to each code from category Y28
A = initial encounter
D = subsequent encounter
S = sequela
Y28.0 Contact with sharp glass, undetermined intent
Y28.1 Contact with knife, undetermined intent
Y28.2 Contact with sword or dagger, undetermined intent
Y28.8 Contact with other sharp object, undetermined intent
Y28.9 Contact with unspecified sharp object, undetermined intent

Y29 Contact with blunt object, undetermined intent
The appropriate 7th character is to be added to code Y29
A = initial encounter
D = subsequent encounter
S = sequela

Unacceptable principal diagnosis symbol per Medicare code edits · Code exempt from diagnosis present on admission requirement
Questionable admission · Complication or comorbidity · CC/MCC exclusion · Major complication or comorbidity
Principal diagnosis as its own CC · Principal diagnosis as its own MCC · Z code as first-listed diagnosis

Y30 Falling, jumping or pushed from a high place, undetermined intent
Victim falling from one level to another, undetermined intent
The appropriate 7th character is to be added to code Y30
A = initial encounter
D = subsequent encounter
S = sequela

Y31 Falling, lying or running before or into moving object, undetermined intent
The appropriate 7th character is to be added to code Y31
A = initial encounter
D = subsequent encounter
S = sequela

Y32 Crashing of motor vehicle, undetermined intent
The appropriate 7th character is to be added to code Y32
A = initial encounter
D = subsequent encounter
S = sequela

Y33 Other specified events, undetermined intent
The appropriate 7th character is to be added to code Y33
A = initial encounter
D = subsequent encounter
S = sequela

Legal intervention, operations of war, military operations, and terrorism (Y35-Y38)

Y35 Legal intervention
INCLUDES *any injury sustained as a result of an encounter with any law enforcement official, serving in any capacity at the time of the encounter, whether on-duty or off-duty. Includes: injury to law enforcement official, suspect and bystander*
The appropriate 7th character is to be added to each code from category Y35
A = initial encounter
D = subsequent encounter
S = sequela

Y35.0 Legal intervention involving firearm discharge
Y35.00 Legal intervention involving unspecified firearm discharge
Legal intervention involving gunshot wound
Legal intervention involving shot NOS
Y35.001 Legal intervention involving unspecified firearm discharge, law enforcement official injured
Y35.002 Legal intervention involving unspecified firearm discharge, bystander injured
Y35.003 Legal intervention involving unspecified firearm discharge, suspect injured
Y35.01 Legal intervention involving injury by machine gun
Y35.011 Legal intervention involving injury by machine gun, law enforcement official injured
Y35.012 Legal intervention involving injury by machine gun, bystander injured
Y35.013 Legal intervention involving injury by machine gun, suspect injured
Y35.02 Legal intervention involving injury by handgun
Y35.021 Legal intervention involving injury by handgun, law enforcement official injured
Y35.022 Legal intervention involving injury by handgun, bystander injured
Y35.023 Legal intervention involving injury by handgun, suspect injured
Y35.03 Legal intervention involving injury by rifle pellet
Y35.031 Legal intervention involving injury by rifle pellet, law enforcement official injured
Y35.032 Legal intervention involving injury by rifle pellet, bystander injured
Y35.033 Legal intervention involving injury by rifle pellet, suspect injured
Y35.04 Legal intervention involving injury by rubber bullet
Y35.041 Legal intervention involving injury by rubber bullet, law enforcement official injured
Y35.042 Legal intervention involving injury by rubber bullet, bystander injured
Y35.043 Legal intervention involving injury by rubber bullet, suspect injured
Y35.09 Legal intervention involving other firearm discharge
Y35.091 Legal intervention involving other firearm discharge, law enforcement official injured
Y35.092 Legal intervention involving other firearm discharge, bystander injured
Y35.093 Legal intervention involving other firearm discharge, suspect injured

Y35.1 Legal intervention involving explosives
Y35.10 Legal intervention involving unspecified explosives
Y35.101 Legal intervention involving unspecified explosives, law enforcement official injured
Y35.102 Legal intervention involving unspecified explosives, bystander injured
Y35.103 Legal intervention involving unspecified explosives, suspect injured
Y35.11 Legal intervention involving injury by dynamite
Y35.111 Legal intervention involving injury by dynamite, law enforcement official injured
Y35.112 Legal intervention involving injury by dynamite, bystander injured
Y35.113 Legal intervention involving injury by dynamite, suspect injured
Y35.12 Legal intervention involving injury by explosive shell
Y35.121 Legal intervention involving injury by explosive shell, law enforcement official injured
Y35.122 Legal intervention involving injury by explosive shell, bystander injured
Y35.123 Legal intervention involving injury by explosive shell, suspect injured
Y35.19 Legal intervention involving other explosives
Legal intervention involving injury by grenade
Legal intervention involving injury by mortar bomb
Y35.191 Legal intervention involving other explosives, law enforcement official injured
Y35.192 Legal intervention involving other explosives, bystander injured
Y35.193 Legal intervention involving other explosives, suspect injured

Y35.2 Legal intervention involving gas
Legal intervention involving asphyxiation by gas
Legal intervention involving poisoning by gas
Y35.20 Legal intervention involving unspecified gas
Y35.201 Legal intervention involving unspecified gas, law enforcement official injured
Y35.202 Legal intervention involving unspecified gas, bystander injured
Y35.203 Legal intervention involving unspecified gas, suspect injured
Y35.21 Legal intervention involving injury by tear gas
Y35.211 Legal intervention involving injury by tear gas, law enforcement official injured
Y35.212 Legal intervention involving injury by tear gas, bystander injured
Y35.213 Legal intervention involving injury by tear gas, suspect injured
Y35.29 Legal intervention involving other gas
Y35.291 Legal intervention involving other gas, law enforcement official injured
Y35.292 Legal intervention involving other gas, bystander injured
Y35.293 Legal intervention involving other gas, suspect injured

Y35.3 Legal intervention involving blunt objects
Legal intervention involving being hit or struck by blunt object

Unspecified Code Other Specified Code Manifestation Code N Newborn P Pediatric M Maternity A Adult ♂ Male ♀ Female
● New Code ▲ Revised Code Title ►◄ Revised Text NOTES INCLUDES EXCLUDES1 Not coded here EXCLUDES2 Not included here
4th character required 5th character required 6th character required 7th character required
Extension 'X' Alert HAC Hospital-acquired condition (HAC) alert AHA AHA Coding Clinic©

Y35.30 Legal intervention involving unspecified blunt objects
Y35.301 Legal intervention involving unspecified blunt objects, law enforcement official injured
Y35.302 Legal intervention involving unspecified blunt objects, bystander injured
Y35.303 Legal intervention involving unspecified blunt objects, suspect injured
Y35.31 Legal intervention involving baton
Y35.311 Legal intervention involving baton, law enforcement official injured
Y35.312 Legal intervention involving baton, bystander injured
Y35.313 Legal intervention involving baton, suspect injured
Y35.39 Legal intervention involving other blunt objects
Y35.391 Legal intervention involving other blunt objects, law enforcement official injured
Y35.392 Legal intervention involving other blunt objects, bystander injured
Y35.393 Legal intervention involving other blunt objects, suspect injured
Y35.4 Legal intervention involving sharp objects
Legal intervention involving being cut by sharp objects
Legal intervention involving being stabbed by sharp objects
Y35.40 Legal intervention involving unspecified sharp objects
Y35.401 Legal intervention involving unspecified sharp objects, law enforcement official injured
Y35.402 Legal intervention involving unspecified sharp objects, bystander injured
Y35.403 Legal intervention involving unspecified sharp objects, suspect injured
Y35.41 Legal intervention involving bayonet
Y35.411 Legal intervention involving bayonet, law enforcement official injured
Y35.412 Legal intervention involving bayonet, bystander injured
Y35.413 Legal intervention involving bayonet, suspect injured
Y35.49 Legal intervention involving other sharp objects
Y35.491 Legal intervention involving other sharp objects, law enforcement official injured
Y35.492 Legal intervention involving other sharp objects, bystander injured
Y35.493 Legal intervention involving other sharp objects, suspect injured
Y35.8 Legal intervention involving other specified means
Y35.81 Legal intervention involving manhandling
Y35.811 Legal intervention involving manhandling, law enforcement official injured
Y35.812 Legal intervention involving manhandling, bystander injured
Y35.813 Legal intervention involving manhandling, suspect injured
Y35.89 Legal intervention involving other specified means
Y35.891 Legal intervention involving other specified means, law enforcement official injured
Y35.892 Legal intervention involving other specified means, bystander injured
Y35.893 Legal intervention involving other specified means, suspect injured
Y35.9 Legal intervention, means unspecified
Y35.91 Legal intervention, means unspecified, law enforcement official injured
Y35.92 Legal intervention, means unspecified, bystander injured
Y35.93 Legal intervention, means unspecified, suspect injured
Y36 Operations of war
INCLUDES *injuries to military personnel and civilians caused by war, civil insurrection, and peacekeeping missions*
EXCLUDES1 *injury to military personnel occurring during peacetime military operations (Y37.-)*
military vehicles involved in transport accidents with non-military vehicle during peacetime (V09.01, V09.21, V19.81, V29.81, V39.81, V49.81, V59.81, V69.81, V79.81)

The appropriate 7th character is to be added to each code from category Y36
A = initial encounter
D = subsequent encounter
S = sequela

Y36.0 War operations involving explosion of marine weapons
Y36.00 War operations involving explosion of unspecified marine weapon
War operations involving underwater blast NOS
Y36.000 War operations involving explosion of unspecified marine weapon, military personnel
Y36.001 War operations involving explosion of unspecified marine weapon, civilian
Y36.01 War operations involving explosion of depth-charge
Y36.010 War operations involving explosion of depth-charge, military personnel
Y36.011 War operations involving explosion of depth-charge, civilian
Y36.02 War operations involving explosion of marine mine
War operations involving explosion of marine mine, at sea or in harbor
Y36.020 War operations involving explosion of marine mine, military personnel
Y36.021 War operations involving explosion of marine mine, civilian
Y36.03 War operations involving explosion of sea-based artillery shell
Y36.030 War operations involving explosion of sea-based artillery shell, military personnel
Y36.031 War operations involving explosion of sea-based artillery shell, civilian
Y36.04 War operations involving explosion of torpedo
Y36.040 War operations involving explosion of torpedo, military personnel
Y36.041 War operations involving explosion of torpedo, civilian
Y36.05 War operations involving accidental detonation of onboard marine weapons
Y36.050 War operations involving accidental detonation of onboard marine weapons, military personnel
Y36.051 War operations involving accidental detonation of onboard marine weapons, civilian
Y36.09 War operations involving explosion of other marine weapons
Y36.090 War operations involving explosion of other marine weapons, military personnel
Y36.091 War operations involving explosion of other marine weapons, civilian
Y36.1 War operations involving destruction of aircraft
Y36.10 War operations involving unspecified destruction of aircraft
Y36.100 War operations involving unspecified destruction of aircraft, military personnel
Y36.101 War operations involving unspecified destruction of aircraft, civilian
Y36.11 War operations involving destruction of aircraft due to enemy fire or explosives
War operations involving destruction of aircraft due to air to air missile
War operations involving destruction of aircraft due to explosive placed on aircraft
War operations involving destruction of aircraft due to rocket propelled grenade [RPG]
War operations involving destruction of aircraft due to small arms fire
War operations involving destruction of aircraft due to surface to air missile
Y36.110 War operations involving destruction of aircraft due to enemy fire or explosives, military personnel

Unacceptable principal diagnosis symbol per Medicare code edits | Code exempt from diagnosis present on admission requirement
Questionable admission | Complication or comorbidity | CC/MCC exclusion | Major complication or comorbidity
Principal diagnosis as its own CC | Principal diagnosis as its own MCC | Z code as first-listed diagnosis

Y36.111 War operations involving destruction of aircraft due to enemy fire or explosives, civilian

Y36.12 War operations involving destruction of aircraft due to collision with other aircraft

Y36.120 War operations involving destruction of aircraft due to collision with other aircraft, military personnel

Y36.121 War operations involving destruction of aircraft due to collision with other aircraft, civilian

Y36.13 War operations involving destruction of aircraft due to onboard fire

Y36.130 War operations involving destruction of aircraft due to onboard fire, military personnel

Y36.131 War operations involving destruction of aircraft due to onboard fire, civilian

Y36.14 War operations involving destruction of aircraft due to accidental detonation of onboard munitions and explosives

Y36.140 War operations involving destruction of aircraft due to accidental detonation of onboard munitions and explosives, military personnel

Y36.141 War operations involving destruction of aircraft due to accidental detonation of onboard munitions and explosives, civilian

Y36.19 War operations involving other destruction of aircraft

Y36.190 War operations involving other destruction of aircraft, military personnel

Y36.191 War operations involving other destruction of aircraft, civilian

Y36.2 War operations involving other explosions and fragments

EXCLUDES1 *war operations involving explosion of aircraft (Y36.1-)*
war operations involving explosion of marine weapons (Y36.0-)
war operations involving explosion of nuclear weapons (Y36.5-)
war operations involving explosion occurring after cessation of hostilities (Y36.8-)

Y36.20 War operations involving unspecified explosion and fragments

War operations involving air blast NOS
War operations involving blast NOS
War operations involving blast fragments NOS
War operations involving blast wave NOS
War operations involving blast wind NOS
War operations involving explosion NOS
War operations involving explosion of bomb NOS

Y36.200 War operations involving unspecified explosion and fragments, military personnel

Y36.201 War operations involving unspecified explosion and fragments, civilian

Y36.21 War operations involving explosion of aerial bomb

Y36.210 War operations involving explosion of aerial bomb, military personnel

Y36.211 War operations involving explosion of aerial bomb, civilian

Y36.22 War operations involving explosion of guided missile

Y36.220 War operations involving explosion of guided missile, military personnel

Y36.221 War operations involving explosion of guided missile, civilian

Y36.23 War operations involving explosion of improvised explosive device [IED]

War operations involving explosion of person-borne improvised explosive device [IED]
War operations involving explosion of vehicle-borne improvised explosive device [IED]
War operations involving explosion of roadside improvised explosive device [IED]

Y36.230 War operations involving explosion of improvised explosive device [IED], military personnel

Y36.231 War operations involving explosion of improvised explosive device [IED], civilian

Y36.24 War operations involving explosion due to accidental detonation and discharge of own munitions or munitions launch device

Y36.240 War operations involving explosion due to accidental detonation and discharge of own munitions or munitions launch device, military personnel

Y36.241 War operations involving explosion due to accidental detonation and discharge of own munitions or munitions launch device, civilian

Y36.25 War operations involving fragments from munitions

Y36.250 War operations involving fragments from munitions, military personnel

Y36.251 War operations involving fragments from munitions, civilian

Y36.26 War operations involving fragments of improvised explosive device [IED]

War operations involving fragments of person-borne improvised explosive device [IED]
War operations involving fragments of vehicle-borne improvised explosive device [IED]
War operations involving fragments of roadside improvised explosive device [IED]

Y36.260 War operations involving fragments of improvised explosive device [IED], military personnel

Y36.261 War operations involving fragments of improvised explosive device [IED], civilian

Y36.27 War operations involving fragments from weapons

Y36.270 War operations involving fragments from weapons, military personnel

Y36.271 War operations involving fragments from weapons, civilian

Y36.29 War operations involving other explosions and fragments

War operations involving explosion of grenade
War operations involving explosions of land mine
War operations involving shrapnel NOS

Y36.290 War operations involving other explosions and fragments, military personnel

Y36.291 War operations involving other explosions and fragments, civilian

Y36.3 War operations involving fires, conflagrations and hot substances

War operations involving smoke, fumes, and heat from fires, conflagrations and hot substances

EXCLUDES1 *war operations involving fires and conflagrations aboard military aircraft (Y36.1-)*
war operations involving fires and conflagrations aboard military watercraft (Y36.0-)
war operations involving fires and conflagrations caused indirectly by conventional weapons (Y36.2-)
war operations involving fires and thermal effects of nuclear weapons (Y36.53-)

Y36.30 War operations involving unspecified fire, conflagration and hot substance

Y36.300 War operations involving unspecified fire, conflagration and hot substance, military personnel

Y36.301 War operations involving unspecified fire, conflagration and hot substance, civilian

Y36.31 War operations involving gasoline bomb

War operations involving incendiary bomb
War operations involving petrol bomb

Y36.310 War operations involving gasoline bomb, military personnel

Y36.311 War operations involving gasoline bomb, civilian

Y36.32 War operations involving incendiary bullet

Y36.320 War operations involving incendiary bullet, military personnel

Unspecified Code Other Specified Code Manifestation Code N Newborn P Pediatric M Maternity A Adult ♂ Male ♀ Female
● New Code ▲ Revised Code Title ►◄ Revised Text NOTES INCLUDES EXCLUDES1 Not coded here EXCLUDES2 Not included here
4th character required 5th character required 6th character required 7th character required
Extension 'X' Alert HAC Hospital-acquired condition (HAC) alert AHA AHA Coding Clinic©

Y36.321 War operations involving incendiary bullet, civilian
Y36.33 War operations involving flamethrower
Y36.330 War operations involving flamethrower, military personnel
Y36.331 War operations involving flamethrower, civilian
Y36.39 War operations involving other fires, conflagrations and hot substances
Y36.390 War operations involving other fires, conflagrations and hot substances, military personnel
Y36.391 War operations involving other fires, conflagrations and hot substances, civilian
Y36.4 War operations involving firearm discharge and other forms of conventional warfare
Y36.41 War operations involving rubber bullets
Y36.410 War operations involving rubber bullets, military personnel
Y36.411 War operations involving rubber bullets, civilian
Y36.42 War operations involving firearms pellets
Y36.420 War operations involving firearms pellets, military personnel
Y36.421 War operations involving firearms pellets, civilian
Y36.43 War operations involving other firearms discharge
War operations involving bullets NOS
EXCLUDES1 *war operations involving munitions fragments (Y36.25-)*
war operations involving incendiary bullets (Y36.32-)
Y36.430 War operations involving other firearms discharge, military personnel
Y36.431 War operations involving other firearms discharge, civilian
Y36.44 War operations involving unarmed hand to hand combat
EXCLUDES1 *war operations involving combat using blunt or piercing object (Y36.45-)*
war operations involving intentional restriction of air and airway (Y36.46-)
war operations involving unintentional restriction of air and airway (Y36.47-)
Y36.440 War operations involving unarmed hand to hand combat, military personnel
Y36.441 War operations involving unarmed hand to hand combat, civilian
Y36.45 War operations involving combat using blunt or piercing object
Y36.450 War operations involving combat using blunt or piercing object, military personnel
Y36.451 War operations involving combat using blunt or piercing object, civilian
Y36.46 War operations involving intentional restriction of air and airway
Y36.460 War operations involving intentional restriction of air and airway, military personnel
Y36.461 War operations involving intentional restriction of air and airway, civilian
Y36.47 War operations involving unintentional restriction of air and airway
Y36.470 War operations involving unintentional restriction of air and airway, military personnel
Y36.471 War operations involving unintentional restriction of air and airway, civilian
Y36.49 War operations involving other forms of conventional warfare
Y36.490 War operations involving other forms of conventional warfare, military personnel
Y36.491 War operations involving other forms of conventional warfare, civilian
Y36.5 War operations involving nuclear weapons
War operations involving dirty bomb NOS
Y36.50 War operations involving unspecified effect of nuclear weapon
Y36.500 War operations involving unspecified effect of nuclear weapon, military personnel
Y36.501 War operations involving unspecified effect of nuclear weapon, civilian
Y36.51 War operations involving direct blast effect of nuclear weapon
War operations involving blast pressure of nuclear weapon
Y36.510 War operations involving direct blast effect of nuclear weapon, military personnel
Y36.511 War operations involving direct blast effect of nuclear weapon, civilian
Y36.52 War operations involving indirect blast effect of nuclear weapon
War operations involving being thrown by blast of nuclear weapon
War operations involving being struck or crushed by blast debris of nuclear weapon
Y36.520 War operations involving indirect blast effect of nuclear weapon, military personnel
Y36.521 War operations involving indirect blast effect of nuclear weapon, civilian
Y36.53 War operations involving thermal radiation effect of nuclear weapon
War operations involving direct heat from nuclear weapon
War operation involving fireball effects from nuclear weapon
Y36.530 War operations involving thermal radiation effect of nuclear weapon, military personnel
Y36.531 War operations involving thermal radiation effect of nuclear weapon, civilian
Y36.54 War operation involving nuclear radiation effects of nuclear weapon
War operation involving acute radiation exposure from nuclear weapon
War operation involving exposure to immediate ionizing radiation from nuclear weapon
War operation involving fallout exposure from nuclear weapon
War operation involving secondary effects of nuclear weapons
Y36.540 War operation involving nuclear radiation effects of nuclear weapon, military personnel.
Y36.541 War operation involving nuclear radiation effects of nuclear weapon, civilian
Y36.59 War operation involving other effects of nuclear weapons
Y36.590 War operation involving other effects of nuclear weapons, military personnel
Y36.591 War operation involving other effects of nuclear weapons, civilian
Y36.6 War operations involving biological weapons
Y36.6X War operations involving biological weapons
Y36.6X0 War operations involving biological weapons, military personnel
Y36.6X1 War operations involving biological weapons, civilian
Y36.7 War operations involving chemical weapons and other forms of unconventional warfare
EXCLUDES1 *war operations involving incendiary devices (Y36.3-, Y36.5-)*
Y36.7X War operations involving chemical weapons and other forms of unconventional warfare
Y36.7X0 War operations involving chemical weapons and other forms of unconventional warfare, military personnel

Unacceptable principal diagnosis symbol per Medicare code edits; Code exempt from diagnosis present on admission requirement; Questionable admission; Complication or comorbidity; CC/MCC exclusion; Major complication or comorbidity; Principal diagnosis as its own CC; Principal diagnosis as its own MCC; Z code as first-listed diagnosis

Y36.7X1 War operations involving chemical weapons and other forms of unconventional warfare, civilian

Y36.8 War operations occurring after cessation of hostilities
War operations classifiable to categories Y36.0-Y36.8 but occurring after cessation of hostilities

Y36.81 Explosion of mine placed during war operations but exploding after cessation of hostilities
Y36.810 Explosion of mine placed during war operations but exploding after cessation of hostilities, military personnel
Y36.811 Explosion of mine placed during war operations but exploding after cessation of hostilities, civilian

Y36.82 Explosion of bomb placed during war operations but exploding after cessation of hostilities
Y36.820 Explosion of bomb placed during war operations but exploding after cessation of hostilities, military personnel
Y36.821 Explosion of bomb placed during war operations but exploding after cessation of hostilities, civilian

Y36.88 Other war operations occurring after cessation of hostilities
Y36.880 Other war operations occurring after cessation of hostilities, military personnel
Y36.881 Other war operations occurring after cessation of hostilities, civilian

Y36.89 Unspecified war operations occurring after cessation of hostilities
Y36.890 Unspecified war operations occurring after cessation of hostilities, military personnel
Y36.891 Unspecified war operations occurring after cessation of hostilities, civilian

Y36.9 Other and unspecified war operations
Y36.90 War operations, unspecified
Y36.91 War operations involving unspecified weapon of mass destruction [WMD]
Y36.92 War operations involving friendly fire

Y37 Military operations

INCLUDES *injuries to military personnel and civilians occurring during peacetime on military property and during routine military exercises and operations*

EXCLUDES1 *military aircraft involved in aircraft accident with civilian aircraft (V97.81-)*
military vehicles involved in transport accident with civilian vehicle (V09.01, V09.21, V19.81, V29.81, V39.81, V49.81, V59.81, V69.81, V79.81)
military watercraft involved in water transport accident with civilian watercraft (V94.81-)
war operations (Y36.-)

The appropriate 7th character is to be added to each code from category Y37
A = initial encounter
D = subsequent encounter
S = sequela

Y37.0 Military operations involving explosion of marine weapons

Y37.00 Military operations involving explosion of unspecified marine weapon
Military operations involving underwater blast NOS
Y37.000 Military operations involving explosion of unspecified marine weapon, military personnel
Y37.001 Military operations involving explosion of unspecified marine weapon, civilian

Y37.01 Military operations involving explosion of depth-charge
Y37.010 Military operations involving explosion of depth-charge, military personnel
Y37.011 Military operations involving explosion of depth-charge, civilian

Y37.02 Military operations involving explosion of marine mine
Military operations involving explosion of marine mine, at sea or in harbor
Y37.020 Military operations involving explosion of marine mine, military personnel
Y37.021 Military operations involving explosion of marine mine, civilian

Y37.03 Military operations involving explosion of sea-based artillery shell
Y37.030 Military operations involving explosion of sea-based artillery shell, military personnel
Y37.031 Military operations involving explosion of sea-based artillery shell, civilian

Y37.04 Military operations involving explosion of torpedo
Y37.040 Military operations involving explosion of torpedo, military personnel
Y37.041 Military operations involving explosion of torpedo, civilian

Y37.05 Military operations involving accidental detonation of onboard marine weapons
Y37.050 Military operations involving accidental detonation of onboard marine weapons, military personnel
Y37.051 Military operations involving accidental detonation of onboard marine weapons, civilian

Y37.09 Military operations involving explosion of other marine weapons
Y37.090 Military operations involving explosion of other marine weapons, military personnel
Y37.091 Military operations involving explosion of other marine weapons, civilian

Y37.1 Military operations involving destruction of aircraft

Y37.10 Military operations involving unspecified destruction of aircraft
Y37.100 Military operations involving unspecified destruction of aircraft, military personnel
Y37.101 Military operations involving unspecified destruction of aircraft, civilian

Y37.11 Military operations involving destruction of aircraft due to enemy fire or explosives
Military operations involving destruction of aircraft due to air to air missile
Military operations involving destruction of aircraft due to explosive placed on aircraft
Military operations involving destruction of aircraft due to rocket propelled grenade [RPG]
Military operations involving destruction of aircraft due to small arms fire
Military operations involving destruction of aircraft due to surface to air missile
Y37.110 Military operations involving destruction of aircraft due to enemy fire or explosives, military personnel
Y37.111 Military operations involving destruction of aircraft due to enemy fire or explosives, civilian

Y37.12 Military operations involving destruction of aircraft due to collision with other aircraft
Y37.120 Military operations involving destruction of aircraft due to collision with other aircraft, military personnel
Y37.121 Military operations involving destruction of aircraft due to collision with other aircraft, civilian

Y37.13 Military operations involving destruction of aircraft due to onboard fire
Y37.130 Military operations involving destruction of aircraft due to onboard fire, military personnel
Y37.131 Military operations involving destruction of aircraft due to onboard fire, civilian

Y37.14 Military operations involving destruction of aircraft due to accidental detonation of onboard munitions and explosives
Y37.140 Military operations involving destruction of aircraft due to accidental detonation of onboard munitions and explosives, military personnel

Y37.141 **Military operations involving destruction of aircraft due to accidental detonation of onboard munitions and explosives, civilian**

Y37.19 **Military operations involving other destruction of aircraft**

Y37.190 **Military operations involving other destruction of aircraft, military personnel**

Y37.191 **Military operations involving other destruction of aircraft, civilian**

Y37.2 **Military operations involving other explosions and fragments**

EXCLUDES1 *military operations involving explosion of aircraft (Y37.1-)*
military operations involving explosion of marine weapons (Y37.0-)
military operations involving explosion of nuclear weapons (Y37.5-)

Y37.20 **Military operations involving unspecified explosion and fragments**

Military operations involving air blast NOS
Military operations involving blast NOS
Military operations involving blast fragments NOS
Military operations involving blast wave NOS
Military operations involving blast wind NOS
Military operations involving explosion NOS
Military operations involving explosion of bomb NOS

Y37.200 **Military operations involving unspecified explosion and fragments, military personnel**

Y37.201 **Military operations involving unspecified explosion and fragments, civilian**

Y37.21 **Military operations involving explosion of aerial bomb**

Y37.210 **Military operations involving explosion of aerial bomb, military personnel**

Y37.211 **Military operations involving explosion of aerial bomb, civilian**

Y37.22 **Military operations involving explosion of guided missile**

Y37.220 **Military operations involving explosion of guided missile, military personnel**

Y37.221 **Military operations involving explosion of guided missile, civilian**

Y37.23 **Military operations involving explosion of improvised explosive device [IED]**

Military operations involving explosion of person-borne improvised explosive device [IED]
Military operations involving explosion of vehicle-borne improvised explosive device [IED]
Military operations involving explosion of roadside improvised explosive device [IED]

Y37.230 **Military operations involving explosion of improvised explosive device [IED], military personnel**

Y37.231 **Military operations involving explosion of improvised explosive device [IED], civilian**

Y37.24 **Military operations involving explosion due to accidental detonation and discharge of own munitions or munitions launch device**

Y37.240 **Military operations involving explosion due to accidental detonation and discharge of own munitions or munitions launch device, military personnel**

Y37.241 **Military operations involving explosion due to accidental detonation and discharge of own munitions or munitions launch device, civilian**

Y37.25 **Military operations involving fragments from munitions**

Y37.250 **Military operations involving fragments from munitions, military personnel**

Y37.251 **Military operations involving fragments from munitions, civilian**

Y37.26 **Military operations involving fragments of improvised explosive device [IED]**

Military operations involving fragments of person-borne improvised explosive device [IED]
Military operations involving fragments of vehicle-borne improvised explosive device [IED]
Military operations involving fragments of roadside improvised explosive device [IED]

Y37.260 **Military operations involving fragments of improvised explosive device [IED], military personnel**

Y37.261 **Military operations involving fragments of improvised explosive device [IED], civilian**

Y37.27 **Military operations involving fragments from weapons**

Y37.270 **Military operations involving fragments from weapons, military personnel**

Y37.271 **Military operations involving fragments from weapons, civilian**

Y37.29 **Military operations involving other explosions and fragments**

Military operations involving explosion of grenade
Military operations involving explosions of land mine
Military operations involving shrapnel NOS

Y37.290 **Military operations involving other explosions and fragments, military personnel**

Y37.291 **Military operations involving other explosions and fragments, civilian**

Y37.3 **Military operations involving fires, conflagrations and hot substances**

Military operations involving smoke, fumes, and heat from fires, conflagrations and hot substances

EXCLUDES1 *military operations involving fires and conflagrations aboard military aircraft (Y37.1-)*
military operations involving fires and conflagrations aboard military watercraft (Y37.0-)
military operations involving fires and conflagrations caused indirectly by conventional weapons (Y37.2-)
military operations involving fires and thermal effects of nuclear weapons (Y36.53-)

Y37.30 **Military operations involving unspecified fire, conflagration and hot substance**

Y37.300 **Military operations involving unspecified fire, conflagration and hot substance, military personnel**

Y37.301 **Military operations involving unspecified fire, conflagration and hot substance, civilian**

Y37.31 **Military operations involving gasoline bomb**

Military operations involving incendiary bomb
Military operations involving petrol bomb

Y37.310 **Military operations involving gasoline bomb, military personnel**

Y37.311 **Military operations involving gasoline bomb, civilian**

Y37.32 **Military operations involving incendiary bullet**

Y37.320 **Military operations involving incendiary bullet, military personnel**

Y37.321 **Military operations involving incendiary bullet, civilian**

Y37.33 **Military operations involving flamethrower**

Y37.330 **Military operations involving flamethrower, military personnel**

Y37.331 **Military operations involving flamethrower, civilian**

Y37.39 **Military operations involving other fires, conflagrations and hot substances**

Y37.390 **Military operations involving other fires, conflagrations and hot substances, military personnel**

Y37.391 **Military operations involving other fires, conflagrations and hot substances, civilian**

Y37.4 **Military operations involving firearm discharge and other forms of conventional warfare**

Y37.41 **Military operations involving rubber bullets**

Y37.410 **Military operations involving rubber bullets, military personnel**

Y37.411 **Military operations involving rubber bullets, civilian**

Unacceptable principal diagnosis symbol per Medicare code edits; Code exempt from diagnosis present on admission requirement; Questionable admission; Complication or comorbidity; CC/MCC exclusion; Major complication or comorbidity; Principal diagnosis as its own CC; Principal diagnosis as its own MCC; Z code as first-listed diagnosis

Y37.42 Military operations involving firearms pellets
- Y37.420 Military operations involving firearms pellets, military personnel
- Y37.421 Military operations involving firearms pellets, civilian

Y37.43 Military operations involving other firearms discharge
Military operations involving bullets NOS
EXCLUDES1 *military operations involving munitions fragments (Y37.25-)*
military operations involving incendiary bullets (Y37.32-)
- Y37.430 Military operations involving other firearms discharge, military personnel
- Y37.431 Military operations involving other firearms discharge, civilian

Y37.44 Military operations involving unarmed hand to hand combat
EXCLUDES1 *military operations involving combat using blunt or piercing object (Y37.45-)*
military operations involving intentional restriction of air and airway (Y37.46-)
military operations involving unintentional restriction of air and airway (Y37.47-)
- Y37.440 Military operations involving unarmed hand to hand combat, military personnel
- Y37.441 Military operations involving unarmed hand to hand combat, civilian

Y37.45 Military operations involving combat using blunt or piercing object
- Y37.450 Military operations involving combat using blunt or piercing object, military personnel
- Y37.451 Military operations involving combat using blunt or piercing object, civilian

Y37.46 Military operations involving intentional restriction of air and airway
- Y37.460 Military operations involving intentional restriction of air and airway, military personnel
- Y37.461 Military operations involving intentional restriction of air and airway, civilian

Y37.47 Military operations involving unintentional restriction of air and airway
- Y37.470 Military operations involving unintentional restriction of air and airway, military personnel
- Y37.471 Military operations involving unintentional restriction of air and airway, civilian

Y37.49 Military operations involving other forms of conventional warfare
- Y37.490 Military operations involving other forms of conventional warfare, military personnel
- Y37.491 Military operations involving other forms of conventional warfare, civilian

Y37.5 Military operations involving nuclear weapons
Military operation involving dirty bomb NOS

Y37.50 Military operations involving unspecified effect of nuclear weapon
- Y37.500 Military operations involving unspecified effect of nuclear weapon, military personnel
- Y37.501 Military operations involving unspecified effect of nuclear weapon, civilian

Y37.51 Military operations involving direct blast effect of nuclear weapon
Military operations involving blast pressure of nuclear weapon
- Y37.510 Military operations involving direct blast effect of nuclear weapon, military personnel
- Y37.511 Military operations involving direct blast effect of nuclear weapon, civilian

Y37.52 Military operations involving indirect blast effect of nuclear weapon
Military operations involving being thrown by blast of nuclear weapon
Military operations involving being struck or crushed by blast debris of nuclear weapon
- Y37.520 Military operations involving indirect blast effect of nuclear weapon, military personnel
- Y37.521 Military operations involving indirect blast effect of nuclear weapon, civilian

Y37.53 Military operations involving thermal radiation effect of nuclear weapon
Military operations involving direct heat from nuclear weapon
Military operation involving fireball effects from nuclear weapon
- Y37.530 Military operations involving thermal radiation effect of nuclear weapon, military personnel
- Y37.531 Military operations involving thermal radiation effect of nuclear weapon, civilian

Y37.54 Military operation involving nuclear radiation effects of nuclear weapon
Military operation involving acute radiation exposure from nuclear weapon
Military operation involving exposure to immediate ionizing radiation from nuclear weapon
Military operation involving fallout exposure from nuclear weapon
Military operation involving secondary effects of nuclear weapons
- Y37.540 Military operation involving nuclear radiation effects of nuclear weapon, military personnel
- Y37.541 Military operation involving nuclear radiation effects of nuclear weapon, civilian

Y37.59 Military operation involving other effects of nuclear weapons
- Y37.590 Military operation involving other effects of nuclear weapons, military personnel
- Y37.591 Military operation involving other effects of nuclear weapons, civilian

Y37.6 Military operations involving biological weapons

Y37.6X Military operations involving biological weapons
- Y37.6X0 Military operations involving biological weapons, military personnel
- Y37.6X1 Military operations involving biological weapons, civilian

Y37.7 Military operations involving chemical weapons and other forms of unconventional warfare
EXCLUDES1 *military operations involving incendiary devices (Y36.3-, Y36.5-)*

Y37.7X Military operations involving chemical weapons and other forms of unconventional warfare
- Y37.7X0 Military operations involving chemical weapons and other forms of unconventional warfare, military personnel
- Y37.7X1 Military operations involving chemical weapons and other forms of unconventional warfare, civilian

Y37.9 Other and unspecified military operations
- Y37.90 Military operations, unspecified
- Y37.91 Military operations involving unspecified weapon of mass destruction [WMD]
- Y37.92 Military operations involving friendly fire

Y38 Terrorism
These codes are for use to identify injuries resulting from the unlawful use of force or violence against persons or property to intimidate or coerce a Government, the civilian population, or any segment thereof, in furtherance of political or social objective
Use additional code for place of occurrence (Y92.-)

Unspecified Code | Other Specified Code | Manifestation Code | N Newborn | P Pediatric | M Maternity | A Adult | ♂ Male | ♀ Female
● New Code | ▲ Revised Code Title | ►◄ Revised Text | NOTES | INCLUDES | EXCLUDES1 Not coded here | EXCLUDES2 Not included here
4th character required | 5th character required | 6th character required | 7th character required
Extension 'X' Alert | HAC Hospital-acquired condition (HAC) alert | AHA AHA Coding Clinic©

The appropriate 7th character is to be added to each code from category Y38

A = initial encounter

D = subsequent encounter

S = sequela

Y38.0 Terrorism involving explosion of marine weapons

Terrorism involving depth-charge
Terrorism involving marine mine
Terrorism involving mine NOS, at sea or in harbor
Terrorism involving sea-based artillery shell
Terrorism involving torpedo
Terrorism involving underwater blast

Y38.0X Terrorism involving explosion of marine weapons

Y38.0X1 Terrorism involving explosion of marine weapons, public safety official injured

Y38.0X2 Terrorism involving explosion of marine weapons, civilian injured

Y38.0X3 Terrorism involving explosion of marine weapons, terrorist injured

Y38.1 Terrorism involving destruction of aircraft

Terrorism involving aircraft burned
Terrorism involving aircraft exploded
Terrorism involving aircraft being shot down
Terrorism involving aircraft used as a weapon

Y38.1X Terrorism involving destruction of aircraft

Y38.1X1 Terrorism involving destruction of aircraft, public safety official injured

Y38.1X2 Terrorism involving destruction of aircraft, civilian injured

Y38.1X3 Terrorism involving destruction of aircraft, terrorist injured

Y38.2 Terrorism involving other explosions and fragments

Terrorism involving antipersonnel (fragments) bomb
Terrorism involving blast NOS
Terrorism involving explosion NOS
Terrorism involving explosion of breech block
Terrorism involving explosion of cannon block
Terrorism involving explosion (fragments) of artillery shell
Terrorism involving explosion (fragments) of bomb
Terrorism involving explosion (fragments) of grenade
Terrorism involving explosion (fragments) of guided missile
Terrorism involving explosion (fragments) of land mine
Terrorism involving explosion of mortar bomb
Terrorism involving explosion of munitions
Terrorism involving explosion (fragments) of rocket
Terrorism involving explosion (fragments) of shell
Terrorism involving shrapnel
Terrorism involving mine NOS, on land

EXCLUDES1 *terrorism involving explosion of nuclear weapon (Y38.5)*
terrorism involving suicide bomber (Y38.81)

Y38.2X Terrorism involving other explosions and fragments

Y38.2X1 Terrorism involving other explosions and fragments, public safety official injured

Y38.2X2 Terrorism involving other explosions and fragments, civilian injured

Y38.2X3 Terrorism involving other explosions and fragments, terrorist injured

Y38.3 Terrorism involving fires, conflagration and hot substances

Terrorism involving conflagration NOS
Terrorism involving fire NOS
Terrorism involving petrol bomb

EXCLUDES1 *terrorism involving fire or heat of nuclear weapon (Y38.5)*

Y38.3X Terrorism involving fires, conflagration and hot substances

Y38.3X1 Terrorism involving fires, conflagration and hot substances, public safety official injured

Y38.3X2 Terrorism involving fires, conflagration and hot substances, civilian injured

Y38.3X3 Terrorism involving fires, conflagration and hot substances, terrorist injured

Y38.4 Terrorism involving firearms

Terrorism involving carbine bullet
Terrorism involving machine gun bullet
Terrorism involving pellets (shotgun)
Terrorism involving pistol bullet
Terrorism involving rifle bullet
Terrorism involving rubber (rifle) bullet

Y38.4X Terrorism involving firearms

Y38.4X1 Terrorism involving firearms, public safety official injured

Y38.4X2 Terrorism involving firearms, civilian injured

Y38.4X3 Terrorism involving firearms, terrorist injured

Y38.5 Terrorism involving nuclear weapons

Terrorism involving blast effects of nuclear weapon
Terrorism involving exposure to ionizing radiation from nuclear weapon
Terrorism involving fireball effect of nuclear weapon
Terrorism involving heat from nuclear weapon

Y38.5X Terrorism involving nuclear weapons

Y38.5X1 Terrorism involving nuclear weapons, public safety official injured

Y38.5X2 Terrorism involving nuclear weapons, civilian injured

Y38.5X3 Terrorism involving nuclear weapons, terrorist injured

Y38.6 Terrorism involving biological weapons

Terrorism involving anthrax
Terrorism involving cholera
Terrorism involving smallpox

Y38.6X Terrorism involving biological weapons

Y38.6X1 Terrorism involving biological weapons, public safety official injured

Y38.6X2 Terrorism involving biological weapons, civilian injured

Y38.6X3 Terrorism involving biological weapons, terrorist injured

Y38.7 Terrorism involving chemical weapons

Terrorism involving gases, fumes, chemicals
Terrorism involving hydrogen cyanide
Terrorism involving phosgene
Terrorism involving sarin

Y38.7X Terrorism involving chemical weapons

Y38.7X1 Terrorism involving chemical weapons, public safety official injured

Y38.7X2 Terrorism involving chemical weapons, civilian injured

Y38.7X3 Terrorism involving chemical weapons, terrorist injured

Y38.8 Terrorism involving other and unspecified means

Y38.80 Terrorism involving unspecified means

Terrorism NOS

Y38.81 Terrorism involving suicide bomber

Y38.811 Terrorism involving suicide bomber, public safety official injured

Y38.812 Terrorism involving suicide bomber, civilian injured

Y38.89 Terrorism involving other **means**

Terrorism involving drowning and submersion
Terrorism involving lasers
Terrorism involving piercing or stabbing instruments

Y38.891 Terrorism involving other means, public safety official injured

Y38.892 Terrorism involving other means, civilian injured

Y38.893 Terrorism involving other means, terrorist injured

Y38.9 Terrorism, secondary effects

NOTES This code is for use to identify conditions occurring subsequent to a terrorist attack not those that are due to the initial terrorist attack

Y38.9X Terrorism, secondary effects

Y38.9X1 Terrorism, secondary effects, public safety official injured

Y38.9X2 Terrorism, secondary effects, civilian injured

Unacceptable principal diagnosis symbol per Medicare code edits | Code exempt from diagnosis present on admission requirement | Questionable admission | Complication or comorbidity | CC/MCC exclusion | Major complication or comorbidity | Principal diagnosis as its own CC | Principal diagnosis as its own MCC | Z code as first-listed diagnosis

Complications of medical and surgical care (Y62-Y84)

INCLUDES *complications of medical devices*
surgical and medical procedures as the cause of abnormal reaction of the patient, or of later complication, without mention of misadventure at the time of the procedure

Misadventures to patients during surgical and medical care (Y62-Y69)

EXCLUDES1 *surgical and medical procedures as the cause of abnormal reaction of the patient, without mention of misadventure at the time of the procedure (Y83-Y84)*
EXCLUDES2 *breakdown or malfunctioning of medical device (during procedure) (after implantation) (ongoing use) (Y70-Y82)*

Y62 Failure of sterile precautions during surgical and medical care
- **Y62.0 Failure of sterile precautions during surgical operation**
- **Y62.1 Failure of sterile precautions during infusion or transfusion**
- **Y62.2 Failure of sterile precautions during kidney dialysis and other perfusion**
- **Y62.3 Failure of sterile precautions during injection or immunization**
- **Y62.4 Failure of sterile precautions during endoscopic examination**
- **Y62.5 Failure of sterile precautions during heart catheterization**
- **Y62.6 Failure of sterile precautions during aspiration, puncture and other catheterization**
- **Y62.8 Failure of sterile precautions during other surgical and medical care**
- **Y62.9 Failure of sterile precautions during unspecified surgical and medical care**

Y63 Failure in dosage during surgical and medical care
EXCLUDES2 *accidental overdose of drug or wrong drug given in error (T36-T50)*
- **Y63.0 Excessive amount of blood or other fluid given during transfusion or infusion**
- **Y63.1 Incorrect dilution of fluid used during infusion**
- **Y63.2 Overdose of radiation given during therapy**
- **Y63.3 Inadvertent exposure of patient to radiation during medical care**
- **Y63.4 Failure in dosage in electroshock or insulin-shock therapy**
- **Y63.5 Inappropriate temperature in local application and packing**
- **Y63.6 Underdosing and nonadministration of necessary drug, medicament or biological substance**
- **Y63.8 Failure in dosage during other surgical and medical care**
- **Y63.9 Failure in dosage during unspecified surgical and medical care**

Y64 Contaminated medical or biological substances
- **Y64.0 Contaminated medical or biological substance, transfused or infused**
- **Y64.1 Contaminated medical or biological substance, injected or used for immunization**
- **Y64.8 Contaminated medical or biological substance administered by other means**
- **Y64.9 Contaminated medical or biological substance administered by unspecified means**
  Administered contaminated medical or biological substance NOS

Y65 Other misadventures during surgical and medical care
- **Y65.0 Mismatched blood in transfusion**
- **Y65.1 Wrong fluid used in infusion**
- **Y65.2 Failure in suture or ligature during surgical operation**
- **Y65.3 Endotracheal tube wrongly placed during anesthetic procedure**
- **Y65.4 Failure to introduce or to remove other tube or instrument**
- **Y65.5 Performance of wrong procedure (operation)**
  - **Y65.51 Performance of wrong procedure (operation) on correct patient**
    Wrong device implanted into correct surgical site
    EXCLUDES1 *performance of correct procedure (operation) on wrong side or body part (Y65.53)*
  - **Y65.52 Performance of procedure (operation) on patient not scheduled for surgery**
    Performance of procedure (operation) intended for another patient
    Performance of procedure (operation) on wrong patient
  - **Y65.53 Performance of correct procedure (operation) on wrong side or body part**
    Performance of correct procedure (operation) on wrong side
    Performance of correct procedure (operation) on wrong site
- **Y65.8 Other specified misadventures during surgical and medical care**

Y66 Nonadministration of surgical and medical care
Premature cessation of surgical and medical care
EXCLUDES1 *DNR status (Z66)*
palliative care (Z51.5)

Y69 Unspecified misadventure during surgical and medical care

Medical devices associated with adverse incidents in diagnostic and therapeutic use (Y70-Y82)

INCLUDES *breakdown or malfunction of medical devices (during use) (after implantation) (ongoing use)*
EXCLUDES2 *breakdown or malfunctioning of medical device (after implantation) (during procedure) (ongoing use) (Y70-Y82)*
later complications following use of medical devices without breakdown or malfunctioning of device (Y83-Y84)
misadventure to patients during surgical and medical care, classifiable to (Y62-Y69)
surgical and other medical procedures as the cause of abnormal reaction of the patient, or of later complication, without mention of misadventure at the time of the procedure (Y83-Y84)

Y70 Anesthesiology devices associated with adverse incidents
- **Y70.0 Diagnostic and monitoring anesthesiology devices associated with adverse incidents**
- **Y70.1 Therapeutic (nonsurgical) and rehabilitative anesthesiology devices associated with adverse incidents**
- **Y70.2 Prosthetic and other implants , materials and accessory anesthesiology devices associated with adverse incidents**
- **Y70.3 Surgical instruments , materials and anesthesiology devices (including sutures) associated with adverse incidents**
- **Y70.8 Miscellaneous anesthesiology devices associated with adverse incidents, not elsewhere classified**

Y71 Cardiovascular devices associated with adverse incidents
- **Y71.0 Diagnostic and monitoring cardiovascular devices associated with adverse incidents**
- **Y71.1 Therapeutic (nonsurgical) and rehabilitative cardiovascular devices associated with adverse incidents**
- **Y71.2 Prosthetic and other implants , materials and accessory cardiovascular devices associated with adverse incidents**
- **Y71.3 Surgical instruments , materials and cardiovascular devices (including sutures) associated with adverse incidents**
- **Y71.8 Miscellaneous cardiovascular devices associated with adverse incidents, not elsewhere classified**

Y72 Otorhinolaryngological devices associated with adverse incidents
- **Y72.0 Diagnostic and monitoring otorhinolaryngological devices associated with adverse incidents**
- **Y72.1 Therapeutic (nonsurgical) and rehabilitative otorhinolaryngological devices associated with adverse incidents**
- **Y72.2 Prosthetic and other implants , materials and accessory otorhinolaryngological devices associated with adverse incidents**
- **Y72.3 Surgical instruments , materials and otorhinolaryngological devices (including sutures) associated with adverse incidents**
- **Y72.8 Miscellaneous otorhinolaryngological devices associated with adverse incidents, not elsewhere classified**

Y73 Gastroenterology and urology devices associated with adverse incidents
- **Y73.0 Diagnostic and monitoring gastroenterology and urology devices associated with adverse incidents**
- **Y73.1 Therapeutic (nonsurgical) and rehabilitative gastroenterology and urology devices associated with adverse incidents**
- **Y73.2 Prosthetic and other implants , materials and accessory gastroenterology and urology devices associated with adverse incidents**
- **Y73.3 Surgical instruments, materials and gastroenterology and urology devices (including sutures) associated with adverse incidents**

Unspecified Code | Other Specified Code | Manifestation Code | N Newborn | P Pediatric | M Maternity | A Adult | ♂ Male | ♀ Female
● New Code | ▲ Revised Code Title | ►◄ Revised Text | NOTES | INCLUDES | EXCLUDES1 Not coded here | EXCLUDES2 Not included here
4th character required | 5th character required | 6th character required | 7th character required
Extension 'X' Alert | HAC Hospital-acquired condition (HAC) alert | AHA AHA Coding Clinic©

Y73.8 Miscellaneous gastroenterology and urology devices associated with adverse incidents, not elsewhere classified

Y74 General hospital and personal-use devices associated with adverse incidents

Y74.0 Diagnostic and monitoring general hospital and personal-use devices associated with adverse incidents

Y74.1 Therapeutic (nonsurgical) and rehabilitative general hospital and personal-use devices associated with adverse incidents

Y74.2 Prosthetic and other implants, materials and accessory general hospital and personal-use devices associated with adverse incidents

Y74.3 Surgical instruments, materials and general hospital and personal-use devices (including sutures) associated with adverse incidents

Y74.8 Miscellaneous general hospital and personal-use devices associated with adverse incidents, not elsewhere classified

Y75 Neurological devices associated with adverse incidents

Y75.0 Diagnostic and monitoring neurological devices associated with adverse incidents

Y75.1 Therapeutic (nonsurgical) and rehabilitative neurological devices associated with adverse incidents

Y75.2 Prosthetic and other implants, materials and neurological devices associated with adverse incidents

Y75.3 Surgical instruments, materials and neurological devices (including sutures) associated with adverse incidents

Y75.8 Miscellaneous neurological devices associated with adverse incidents, not elsewhere classified

Y76 Obstetric and gynecological devices associated with adverse incidents

Y76.0 Diagnostic and monitoring obstetric and gynecological devices associated with adverse incidents ♀

Y76.1 Therapeutic (nonsurgical) and rehabilitative obstetric and gynecological devices associated with adverse incidents ♀

Y76.2 Prosthetic and other implants, materials and accessory obstetric and gynecological devices associated with adverse incidents ♀

Y76.3 Surgical instruments, materials and obstetric and gynecological devices (including sutures) associated with adverse incidents ♀

Y76.8 Miscellaneous obstetric and gynecological devices associated with adverse incidents, not elsewhere classified ♀

Y77 Ophthalmic devices associated with adverse incidents

Y77.0 Diagnostic and monitoring ophthalmic devices associated with adverse incidents

Y77.1 Therapeutic (nonsurgical) and rehabilitative ophthalmic devices associated with adverse incidents

Y77.2 Prosthetic and other implants, materials and accessory ophthalmic devices associated with adverse incidents

Y77.3 Surgical instruments, materials and ophthalmic devices (including sutures) associated with adverse incidents

Y77.8 Miscellaneous ophthalmic devices associated with adverse incidents, not elsewhere classified

Y78 Radiological devices associated with adverse incidents

Y78.0 Diagnostic and monitoring radiological devices associated with adverse incidents

Y78.1 Therapeutic (nonsurgical) and rehabilitative radiological devices associated with adverse incidents

Y78.2 Prosthetic and other implants, materials and accessory radiological devices associated with adverse incidents

Y78.3 Surgical instruments, materials and radiological devices (including sutures) associated with adverse incidents

Y78.8 Miscellaneous radiological devices associated with adverse incidents, not elsewhere classified

Y79 Orthopedic devices associated with adverse incidents

Y79.0 Diagnostic and monitoring orthopedic devices associated with adverse incidents

Y79.1 Therapeutic (nonsurgical) and rehabilitative orthopedic devices associated with adverse incidents

Y79.2 Prosthetic and other implants, materials and accessory orthopedic devices associated with adverse incidents

Y79.3 Surgical instruments, materials and orthopedic devices (including sutures) associated with adverse incidents

Y79.8 Miscellaneous orthopedic devices associated with adverse incidents, not elsewhere classified

Y80 Physical medicine devices associated with adverse incidents

Y80.0 Diagnostic and monitoring physical medicine devices associated with adverse incidents

Y80.1 Therapeutic (nonsurgical) and rehabilitative physical medicine devices associated with adverse incidents

Y80.2 Prosthetic and other implants, materials and accessory physical medicine devices associated with adverse incidents

Y80.3 Surgical instruments, materials and physical medicine devices (including sutures) associated with adverse incidents

Y80.8 Miscellaneous physical medicine devices associated with adverse incidents, not elsewhere classified

Y81 General- and plastic-surgery devices associated with adverse incidents

Y81.0 Diagnostic and monitoring general- and plastic-surgery devices associated with adverse incidents

Y81.1 Therapeutic (nonsurgical) and rehabilitative general- and plastic-surgery devices associated with adverse incidents

Y81.2 Prosthetic and other implants, materials and accessory general- and plastic-surgery devices associated with adverse incidents

Y81.3 Surgical instruments, materials and general- and plastic-surgery devices (including sutures) associated with adverse incidents

Y81.8 Miscellaneous general- and plastic-surgery devices associated with adverse incidents, not elsewhere classified

Y82 Other and unspecified medical devices associated with adverse incidents

Y82.8 Other medical devices associated with adverse incidents

Y82.9 Unspecified medical devices associated with adverse incidents

Surgical and other medical procedures as the cause of abnormal reaction of the patient, or of later complication, without mention of misadventure at the time of the procedure (Y83-Y84)

EXCLUDES1 *misadventures to patients during surgical and medical care, classifiable to (Y62-Y69)*

EXCLUDES2 *breakdown or malfunctioning of medical device (after implantation) (during procedure) (ongoing use) (Y70-Y82)*

Y83 Surgical operation and other surgical procedures as the cause of abnormal reaction of the patient, or of later complication, without mention of misadventure at the time of the procedure

Y83.0 Surgical operation with transplant of whole organ as the cause of abnormal reaction of the patient, or of later complication, without mention of misadventure at the time of the procedure

Y83.1 Surgical operation with implant of artificial internal device as the cause of abnormal reaction of the patient, or of later complication, without mention of misadventure at the time of the procedure

Y83.2 Surgical operation with anastomosis, bypass or graft as the cause of abnormal reaction of the patient, or of later complication, without mention of misadventure at the time of the procedure

Y83.3 Surgical operation with formation of external stoma as the cause of abnormal reaction of the patient, or of later complication, without mention of misadventure at the time of the procedure

Y83.4 Other reconstructive surgery as the cause of abnormal reaction of the patient, or of later complication, without mention of misadventure at the time of the procedure

Y83.5 Amputation of limb(s) as the cause of abnormal reaction of the patient, or of later complication, without mention of misadventure at the time of the procedure

Y83.6 Removal of other organ (partial) (total) as the cause of abnormal reaction of the patient, or of later complication, without mention of misadventure at the time of the procedure

Y83.8 Other surgical procedures as the cause of abnormal reaction of the patient, or of later complication, without mention of misadventure at the time of the procedure

Y83.9 Surgical procedure, unspecified as the cause of abnormal reaction of the patient, or of later complication, without mention of misadventure at the time of the procedure

Unacceptable principal diagnosis symbol per Medicare code edits | Code exempt from diagnosis present on admission requirement
Questionable admission | Complication or comorbidity | CC/MCC exclusion | Major complication or comorbidity
Principal diagnosis as its own CC | Principal diagnosis as its own MCC | Z code as first-listed diagnosis

When symbols appear on a code that requires a 7th character extension, refer to Appendix D to identify applicable 7th character codes.

Y84 Other medical procedures as the cause of abnormal reaction of the patient, or of later complication, without mention of misadventure at the time of the procedure

Y84.0 Cardiac catheterization as the cause of abnormal reaction of the patient, or of later complication, without mention of misadventure at the time of the procedure

Y84.1 Kidney dialysis as the cause of abnormal reaction of the patient, or of later complication, without mention of misadventure at the time of the procedure

Y84.2 Radiological procedure and radiotherapy as the cause of abnormal reaction of the patient, or of later complication, without mention of misadventure at the time of the procedure

Y84.3 Shock therapy as the cause of abnormal reaction of the patient, or of later complication, without mention of misadventure at the time of the procedure

Y84.4 Aspiration of fluid as the cause of abnormal reaction of the patient, or of later complication, without mention of misadventure at the time of the procedure

Y84.5 Insertion of gastric or duodenal sound as the cause of abnormal reaction of the patient, or of later complication, without mention of misadventure at the time of the procedure

Y84.6 Urinary catheterization as the cause of abnormal reaction of the patient, or of later complication, without mention of misadventure at the time of the procedure

Y84.7 Blood-sampling as the cause of abnormal reaction of the patient, or of later complication, without mention of misadventure at the time of the procedure

Y84.8 Other medical procedures as the cause of abnormal reaction of the patient, or of later complication, without mention of misadventure at the time of the procedure

Y84.9 Medical procedure, unspecified as the cause of abnormal reaction of the patient, or of later complication, without mention of misadventure at the time of the procedure

Supplementary factors related to causes of morbidity classified elsewhere (Y90-Y99)

NOTES These categories may be used to provide supplementary information concerning causes of morbidity. They are not to be used for single-condition coding.

Y90 Evidence of alcohol involvement determined by blood alcohol level

Code first any associated alcohol related disorders (F10)

Y90.0 Blood alcohol level of less than 20 mg/100 ml

Y90.1 Blood alcohol level of 20-39 mg/100 ml

Y90.2 Blood alcohol level of 40-59 mg/100 ml

Y90.3 Blood alcohol level of 60-79 mg/100 ml

Y90.4 Blood alcohol level of 80-99 mg/100 ml

Y90.5 Blood alcohol level of 100-119 mg/100 ml

Y90.6 Blood alcohol level of 120-199 mg/100 ml

Y90.7 Blood alcohol level of 200-239 mg/100 ml

Y90.8 Blood alcohol level of 240 mg/100 ml or more

Y90.9 Presence of alcohol in blood, level not specified

Y92 Place of occurrence of the external cause

The following category is for use, when relevant, to identify the place of occurrence of the external cause. Use in conjunction with an activity code. Place of occurrence should be recorded only at the initial encounter for treatment

Y92.0 Non-institutional (private) residence as the place of occurrence of the external cause

EXCLUDES1 *abandoned or derelict house (Y92.89)*
home under construction but not yet occupied (Y92.6-)
institutional place of residence (Y92.1-)

Y92.00 Unspecified non-institutional (private) residence as the place of occurrence of the external cause

Y92.000 Kitchen of unspecified non-institutional (private) residence as the place of occurrence of the external cause POA

Y92.001 Dining room of unspecified non-institutional (private) residence as the place of occurrence of the external cause POA

Y92.002 Bathroom of unspecified non-institutional (private) residence single-family (private) house as the place of occurrence of the external cause POA

Y92.003 Bedroom of unspecified non-institutional (private) residence as the place of occurrence of the external cause POA

Y92.007 Garden or yard of unspecified non-institutional (private) residence as the place of occurrence of the external cause POA

Y92.008 Other place in unspecified non-institutional (private) residence as the place of occurrence of the external cause POA

Y92.009 Unspecified place in unspecified non-institutional (private) residence as the place of occurrence of the external cause POA

Home (NOS) as the place of occurrence of the external cause

Y92.01 Single-family non-institutional (private) house as the place of occurrence of the external cause

Farmhouse as the place of occurrence of the external cause

EXCLUDES1 *barn (Y92.71)*
chicken coop or hen house (Y92.72)
farm field (Y92.73)
orchard (Y92.74)
single family mobile home or trailer (Y92.02-)
slaughter house (Y92.86)

Y92.010 Kitchen of single-family (private) house as the place of occurrence of the external cause POA

Y92.011 Dining room of single-family (private) house as the place of occurrence of the external cause POA

Y92.012 Bathroom of single-family (private) house as the place of occurrence of the external cause POA

Y92.013 Bedroom of single-family (private) house as the place of occurrence of the external cause POA

Y92.014 Private driveway to single-family (private) house as the place of occurrence of the external cause POA

Y92.015 Private garage of single-family (private) house as the place of occurrence of the external cause POA

Y92.016 Swimming-pool in single-family (private) house or garden as the place of occurrence of the external cause POA

Y92.017 Garden or yard in single-family (private) house as the place of occurrence of the external cause POA

Y92.018 Other place in single-family (private) house as the place of occurrence of the external cause POA

Y92.019 Unspecified place in single-family (private) house as the place of occurrence of the external cause POA

Y92.02 Mobile home as the place of occurrence of the external cause

Y92.020 Kitchen in mobile home as the place of occurrence of the external cause POA

Y92.021 Dining room in mobile home as the place of occurrence of the external cause POA

Y92.022 Bathroom in mobile home as the place of occurrence of the external cause POA

Y92.023 Bedroom in mobile home as the place of occurrence of the external cause POA

Y92.024 Driveway of mobile home as the place of occurrence of the external cause POA

Y92.025 Garage of mobile home as the place of occurrence of the external cause POA

Y92.026 Swimming-pool of mobile home as the place of occurrence of the external cause POA

Y92.027 Garden or yard of mobile home as the place of occurrence of the external cause POA

Y92.028 Other place in mobile home as the place of occurrence of the external cause POA

Unspecified Code Other Specified Code Manifestation Code N Newborn P Pediatric M Maternity A Adult ♂ Male ♀ Female
● New Code ▲ Revised Code Title ►◄ Revised Text NOTES INCLUDES EXCLUDES1 Not coded here EXCLUDES2 Not included here
4th character required 5th character required 6th character required 7th character required
Extension 'X' Alert HAC Hospital-acquired condition (HAC) alert AHA AHA Coding Clinic©

Y92.029 Unspecified place in mobile home as the place of occurrence of the external cause

Y92.03 Apartment as the place of occurrence of the external cause
Condominium as the place of occurrence of the external cause
Co-op apartment as the place of occurrence of the external cause
Y92.030 Kitchen in apartment as the place of occurrence of the external cause
Y92.031 Bathroom in apartment as the place of occurrence of the external cause
Y92.032 Bedroom in apartment as the place of occurrence of the external cause
Y92.038 Other place in apartment as the place of occurrence of the external cause
Y92.039 Unspecified place in apartment as the place of occurrence of the external cause

Y92.04 Boarding-house as the place of occurrence of the external cause
Y92.040 Kitchen in boarding-house as the place of occurrence of the external cause
Y92.041 Bathroom in boarding-house as the place of occurrence of the external cause
Y92.042 Bedroom in boarding-house as the place of occurrence of the external cause
Y92.043 Driveway of boarding-house as the place of occurrence of the external cause
Y92.044 Garage of boarding-house as the place of occurrence of the external cause
Y92.045 Swimming-pool of boarding-house as the place of occurrence of the external cause
Y92.046 Garden or yard of boarding-house as the place of occurrence of the external cause
Y92.048 Other place in boarding-house as the place of occurrence of the external cause
Y92.049 Unspecified place in boarding-house as the place of occurrence of the external cause

Y92.09 Other non-institutional residence as the place of occurrence of the external cause
Y92.090 Kitchen in other non-institutional residence as the place of occurrence of the external cause
Y92.091 Bathroom in other non-institutional residence as the place of occurrence of the external cause
Y92.092 Bedroom in other non-institutional residence as the place of occurrence of the external cause
Y92.093 Driveway of other non-institutional residence as the place of occurrence of the external cause
Y92.094 Garage of other non-institutional residence as the place of occurrence of the external cause
Y92.095 Swimming-pool of other non-institutional residence as the place of occurrence of the external cause
Y92.096 Garden or yard of other non-institutional residence as the place of occurrence of the external cause
Y92.098 Other place in other non-institutional residence as the place of occurrence of the external cause
Y92.099 Unspecified place in other non-institutional residence as the place of occurrence of the external cause

Y92.1 Institutional (nonprivate) residence as the place of occurrence of the external cause
Y92.10 Unspecified residential institution as the place of occurrence of the external cause
Y92.11 Children's home and orphanage as the place of occurrence of the external cause
Y92.110 Kitchen in children's home and orphanage as the place of occurrence of the external cause
Y92.111 Bathroom in children's home and orphanage as the place of occurrence of the external cause
Y92.112 Bedroom in children's home and orphanage as the place of occurrence of the external cause
Y92.113 Driveway of children's home and orphanage as the place of occurrence of the external cause
Y92.114 Garage of children's home and orphanage as the place of occurrence of the external cause
Y92.115 Swimming-pool of children's home and orphanage as the place of occurrence of the external cause
Y92.116 Garden or yard of children's home and orphanage as the place of occurrence of the external cause
Y92.118 Other place in children's home and orphanage as the place of occurrence of the external cause
Y92.119 Unspecified place in children's home and orphanage as the place of occurrence of the external cause

Y92.12 Nursing home as the place of occurrence of the external cause
Home for the sick as the place of occurrence of the external cause
Hospice as the place of occurrence of the external cause
Y92.120 Kitchen in nursing home as the place of occurrence of the external cause
Y92.121 Bathroom in nursing home as the place of occurrence of the external cause
Y92.122 Bedroom in nursing home as the place of occurrence of the external cause
Y92.123 Driveway of nursing home as the place of occurrence of the external cause
Y92.124 Garage of nursing home as the place of occurrence of the external cause
Y92.125 Swimming-pool of nursing home as the place of occurrence of the external cause
Y92.126 Garden or yard of nursing home as the place of occurrence of the external cause
Y92.128 Other place in nursing home as the place of occurrence of the external cause
Y92.129 Unspecified place in nursing home as the place of occurrence of the external cause

Y92.13 Military base as the place of occurrence of the external cause
EXCLUDES1 *military training grounds (Y92.83)*
Y92.130 Kitchen on military base as the place of occurrence of the external cause
Y92.131 Mess hall on military base as the place of occurrence of the external cause
Y92.133 Barracks on military base as the place of occurrence of the external cause
Y92.135 Garage on military base as the place of occurrence of the external cause
Y92.136 Swimming-pool on military base as the place of occurrence of the external cause
Y92.137 Garden or yard on military base as the place of occurrence of the external cause
Y92.138 Other place on military base as the place of occurrence of the external cause
Y92.139 Unspecified place military base as the place of occurrence of the external cause

Y92.14 Prison as the place of occurrence of the external cause
Y92.140 Kitchen in prison as the place of occurrence of the external cause
Y92.141 Dining room in prison as the place of occurrence of the external cause

Unacceptable principal diagnosis symbol per Medicare code edits; Code exempt from diagnosis present on admission requirement; Questionable admission; Complication or comorbidity; CC/MCC exclusion; Major complication or comorbidity; Principal diagnosis as its own CC; Principal diagnosis as its own MCC; Z code as first-listed diagnosis

Y92.142 Bathroom in prison as the place of occurrence of the external cause POA
Y92.143 Cell of prison as the place of occurrence of the external cause POA
Y92.146 Swimming-pool of prison as the place of occurrence of the external cause POA
Y92.147 Courtyard of prison as the place of occurrence of the external cause POA
Y92.148 Other place in prison as the place of occurrence of the external cause POA
Y92.149 Unspecified place in prison as the place of occurrence of the external cause POA

Y92.15 Reform school as the place of occurrence of the external cause
Y92.150 Kitchen in reform school as the place of occurrence of the external cause POA
Y92.151 Dining room in reform school as the place of occurrence of the external cause POA
Y92.152 Bathroom in reform school as the place of occurrence of the external cause POA
Y92.153 Bedroom in reform school as the place of occurrence of the external cause POA
Y92.154 Driveway of reform school as the place of occurrence of the external cause POA
Y92.155 Garage of reform school as the place of occurrence of the external cause POA
Y92.156 Swimming-pool of reform school as the place of occurrence of the external cause POA
Y92.157 Garden or yard of reform school as the place of occurrence of the external cause POA
Y92.158 Other place in reform school as the place of occurrence of the external cause POA
Y92.159 Unspecified place in reform school as the place of occurrence of the external cause POA

Y92.16 School dormitory as the place of occurrence of the external cause
EXCLUDES1 *reform school as the place of occurrence of the external cause (Y92.15-)*
school buildings and grounds as the place of occurrence of the external cause (Y92.2-)
school sports and athletic areas as the place of occurrence of the external cause (Y92.3-)
Y92.160 Kitchen in school dormitory as the place of occurrence of the external cause POA
Y92.161 Dining room in school dormitory as the place of occurrence of the external cause POA
Y92.162 Bathroom in school dormitory as the place of occurrence of the external cause POA
Y92.163 Bedroom in school dormitory as the place of occurrence of the external cause POA
Y92.168 Other place in school dormitory as the place of occurrence of the external cause POA
Y92.169 Unspecified place in school dormitory as the place of occurrence of the external cause POA

Y92.19 Other specified residential institution as the place of occurrence of the external cause
Y92.190 Kitchen in other specified residential institution as the place of occurrence of the external cause POA
Y92.191 Dining room in other specified residential institution as the place of occurrence of the external cause POA
Y92.192 Bathroom in other specified residential institution as the place of occurrence of the external cause POA
Y92.193 Bedroom in other specified residential institution as the place of occurrence of the external cause POA
Y92.194 Driveway of other specified residential institution as the place of occurrence of the external cause POA
Y92.195 Garage of other specified residential institution as the place of occurrence of the external cause POA
Y92.196 Pool of other specified residential institution as the place of occurrence of the external cause POA
Y92.197 Garden or yard of other specified residential institution as the place of occurrence of the external cause POA
Y92.198 Other place in other specified residential institution as the place of occurrence of the external cause POA
Y92.199 Unspecified place in other specified residential institution as the place of occurrence of the external cause POA

Y92.2 School, other institution and public administrative area as the place of occurrence of the external cause
Building and adjacent grounds used by the general public or by a particular group of the public
EXCLUDES1 *building under construction as the place of occurrence of the external cause (Y92.6)*
residential institution as the place of occurrence of the external cause (Y92.1)
school dormitory as the place of occurrence of the external cause (Y92.16-)
sports and athletics area of schools as the place of occurrence of the external cause (Y92.3-)

Y92.21 School (private) (public) (state) as the place of occurrence of the external cause
Y92.210 Daycare center as the place of occurrence of the external cause POA
Y92.211 Elementary school as the place of occurrence of the external cause POA
Kindergarten as the place of occurrence of the external cause
Y92.212 Middle school as the place of occurrence of the external cause POA
Y92.213 High school as the place of occurrence of the external cause POA
AHA: Q4, 2012
Y92.214 College as the place of occurrence of the external cause POA
University as the place of occurrence of the external cause
Y92.215 Trade school as the place of occurrence of the external cause POA
Y92.218 Other school as the place of occurrence of the external cause POA
Y92.219 Unspecified school as the place of occurrence of the external cause POA

Y92.22 Religious institution as the place of occurrence of the external cause POA
Church as the place of occurrence of the external cause
Mosque as the place of occurrence of the external cause
Synagogue as the place of occurrence of the external cause

Y92.23 Hospital as the place of occurrence of the external cause
EXCLUDES1 *ambulatory (outpatient) health services establishments (Y92.53-)*
home for the sick as the place of occurrence of the external cause (Y92.12-)
hospice as the place of occurrence of the external cause (Y92.12-)
nursing home as the place of occurrence of the external cause (Y92.12-)
Y92.230 Patient room in hospital as the place of occurrence of the external cause POA
Y92.231 Patient bathroom in hospital as the place of occurrence of the external cause POA
Y92.232 Corridor of hospital as the place of occurrence of the external cause POA
Y92.233 Cafeteria of hospital as the place of occurrence of the external cause POA
Y92.234 Operating room of hospital as the place of occurrence of the external cause POA

Unspecified Code | Other Specified Code | Manifestation Code | N Newborn | P Pediatric | M Maternity | A Adult | ♂ Male | ♀ Female
● New Code ▲ Revised Code Title ►◄ Revised Text NOTES INCLUDES EXCLUDES1 Not coded here EXCLUDES2 Not included here
4th character required | 5th character required | 6th character required | 7th character required
Extension 'X' Alert | HAC Hospital-acquired condition (HAC) alert | AHA AHA Coding Clinic©

When symbols appear on a code that requires a 7th character extension, refer to Appendix D to identify applicable 7th character codes.

Y92.238 Other place in hospital as the place of occurrence of the external cause
Y92.239 Unspecified place in hospital as the place of occurrence of the external cause

Y92.24 Public administrative building as the place of occurrence of the external cause
Y92.240 Courthouse as the place of occurrence of the external cause
Y92.241 Library as the place of occurrence of the external cause
Y92.242 Post office as the place of occurrence of the external cause
Y92.243 City hall as the place of occurrence of the external cause
Y92.248 Other public administrative building as the place of occurrence of the external cause

Y92.25 Cultural building as the place of occurrence of the external cause
Y92.250 Art Gallery as the place of occurrence of the external cause
Y92.251 Museum as the place of occurrence of the external cause
Y92.252 Music hall as the place of occurrence of the external cause
Y92.253 Opera house as the place of occurrence of the external cause
Y92.254 Theater (live) as the place of occurrence of the external cause
Y92.258 Other cultural public building as the place of occurrence of the external cause

Y92.26 Movie house or cinema as the place of occurrence of the external cause

Y92.29 Other specified public building as the place of occurrence of the external cause
Assembly hall as the place of occurrence of the external cause
Clubhouse as the place of occurrence of the external cause

Y92.3 Sports and athletics area as the place of occurrence of the external cause

Y92.31 Athletic court as the place of occurrence of the external cause
EXCLUDES1 *tennis court in private home or garden (Y92.09)*
Y92.310 Basketball court as the place of occurrence of the external cause
Y92.311 Squash court as the place of occurrence of the external cause
Y92.312 Tennis court as the place of occurrence of the external cause
Y92.318 Other athletic court as the place of occurrence of the external cause

Y92.32 Athletic field as the place of occurrence of the external cause
Y92.320 Baseball field as the place of occurrence of the external cause
Y92.321 Football field as the place of occurrence of the external cause
Y92.322 Soccer field as the place of occurrence of the external cause
Y92.328 Other athletic field as the place of occurrence of the external cause
Cricket field as the place of occurrence of the external cause
Hockey field as the place of occurrence of the external cause

Y92.33 Skating rink as the place of occurrence of the external cause
Y92.330 Ice skating rink (indoor) (outdoor) as the place of occurrence of the external cause
Y92.331 Roller skating rink as the place of occurrence of the external cause

Y92.34 Swimming pool (public) as the place of occurrence of the external cause
EXCLUDES1 *swimming pool in private home or garden (Y92.016)*

Y92.39 Other specified sports and athletic area as the place of occurrence of the external cause
Golf-course as the place of occurrence of the external cause
Gymnasium as the place of occurrence of the external cause
Riding-school as the place of occurrence of the external cause
Stadium as the place of occurrence of the external cause

▲ Y92.4 ►Street, highway◄ and other paved roadways as the place of occurrence of the external cause
EXCLUDES1 *private driveway of residence (Y92.014, Y92.024, Y92.043, Y92.093, Y92.113, Y92.123, Y92.154, Y92.194)*

Y92.41 Street and highway as the place of occurrence of the external cause
Y92.410 Unspecified street and highway as the place of occurrence of the external cause
Road NOS as the place of occurrence of the external cause
Y92.411 Interstate highway as the place of occurrence of the external cause
Freeway as the place of occurrence of the external cause
Motorway as the place of occurrence of the external cause
Y92.412 Parkway as the place of occurrence of the external cause
Y92.413 State road as the place of occurrence of the external cause
Y92.414 Local residential or business street as the place of occurrence of the external cause
Y92.415 Exit ramp or entrance ramp of street or highway as the place of occurrence of the external cause

Y92.48 Other paved roadways as the place of occurrence of the external cause
Y92.480 Sidewalk as the place of occurrence of the external cause
Y92.481 Parking lot as the place of occurrence of the external cause
Y92.482 Bike path as the place of occurrence of the external cause
Y92.488 Other paved roadways as the place of occurrence of the external cause

Y92.5 Trade and service area as the place of occurrence of the external cause
EXCLUDES1 *garage in private home (Y92.015)*
schools and other public administration buildings (Y92.2-)

Y92.51 Private commercial establishments as the place of occurrence of the external cause
Y92.510 Bank as the place of occurrence of the external cause
Y92.511 Restaurant or café as the place of occurrence of the external cause
Y92.512 Supermarket, store or market as the place of occurrence of the external cause
Y92.513 Shop (commercial) as the place of occurrence of the external cause

Y92.52 Service areas as the place of occurrence of the external cause
Y92.520 Airport as the place of occurrence of the external cause
Y92.521 Bus station as the place of occurrence of the external cause
Y92.522 Railway station as the place of occurrence of the external cause
Y92.523 Highway rest stop as the place of occurrence of the external cause
Y92.524 Gas station as the place of occurrence of the external cause
Petroleum station as the place of occurrence of the external cause
Service station as the place of occurrence of the external cause

Unacceptable principal diagnosis symbol per Medicare code edits · Code exempt from diagnosis present on admission requirement
Questionable admission · Complication or comorbidity · CC/MCC exclusion · Major complication or comorbidity
Principal diagnosis as its own CC · Principal diagnosis as its own MCC · Z code as first-listed diagnosis

Y92.53 Ambulatory health services establishments as the place of occurrence of the external cause
- Y92.530 Ambulatory surgery center as the place of occurrence of the external cause POA
  - Outpatient surgery center, including that connected with a hospital as the place of occurrence of the external cause
  - Same day surgery center, including that connected with a hospital as the place of occurrence of the external cause
- Y92.531 Health care provider office as the place of occurrence of the external cause POA
  - Physician office as the place of occurrence of the external cause
- Y92.532 Urgent care center as the place of occurrence of the external cause POA
- Y92.538 Other ambulatory health services establishments as the place of occurrence of the external cause POA

Y92.59 Other trade areas as the place of occurrence of the external cause POA
- Office building as the place of occurrence of the external cause
- Casino as the place of occurrence of the external cause
- Garage (commercial) as the place of occurrence of the external cause
- Hotel as the place of occurrence of the external cause
- Radio or television station as the place of occurrence of the external cause
- Shopping mall as the place of occurrence of the external cause
- Warehouse as the place of occurrence of the external cause

Y92.6 Industrial and construction area as the place of occurrence of the external cause
- Y92.61 Building [any] under construction as the place of occurrence of the external cause POA
- Y92.62 Dock or shipyard as the place of occurrence of the external cause POA
  - Dockyard as the place of occurrence of the external cause
  - Dry dock as the place of occurrence of the external cause
  - Shipyard as the place of occurrence of the external cause
- Y92.63 Factory as the place of occurrence of the external cause POA
  - Factory building as the place of occurrence of the external cause
  - Factory premises as the place of occurrence of the external cause
  - Industrial yard as the place of occurrence of the external cause
- Y92.64 Mine or pit as the place of occurrence of the external cause POA
  - Mine as the place of occurrence of the external cause
- Y92.65 Oil rig as the place of occurrence of the external cause POA
  - Pit (coal) (gravel) (sand) as the place of occurrence of the external cause
- Y92.69 Other specified industrial and construction area as the place of occurrence of the external cause POA
  - Gasworks as the place of occurrence of the external cause
  - Power-station (coal) (nuclear) (oil) as the place of occurrence of the external cause
  - Tunnel under construction as the place of occurrence of the external cause
  - Workshop as the place of occurrence of the external cause

Y92.7 Farm as the place of occurrence of the external cause
- Ranch as the place of occurrence of the external cause
- EXCLUDES1 *farmhouse and home premises of farm (Y92.01-)*
- Y92.71 Barn as the place of occurrence of the external cause POA
- Y92.72 Chicken coop as the place of occurrence of the external cause POA
  - Hen house as the place of occurrence of the external cause
- Y92.73 Farm field as the place of occurrence of the external cause POA
- Y92.74 Orchard as the place of occurrence of the external cause POA
- Y92.79 Other farm location as the place of occurrence of the external cause POA

Y92.8 Other places as the place of occurrence of the external cause
- Y92.81 Transport vehicle as the place of occurrence of the external cause
  - EXCLUDES1 *transport accidents (V00-V99)*
  - Y92.810 Car as the place of occurrence of the external cause POA
  - Y92.811 Bus as the place of occurrence of the external cause POA
  - Y92.812 Truck as the place of occurrence of the external cause POA
  - Y92.813 Airplane as the place of occurrence of the external cause POA
  - Y92.814 Boat as the place of occurrence of the external cause POA
  - Y92.815 Train as the place of occurrence of the external cause POA
  - Y92.816 Subway car as the place of occurrence of the external cause POA
  - Y92.818 Other transport vehicle as the place of occurrence of the external cause POA
- Y92.82 Wilderness area
  - Y92.820 Desert as the place of occurrence of the external cause POA
  - Y92.821 Forest as the place of occurrence of the external cause POA
  - Y92.828 Other wilderness area as the place of occurrence of the external cause POA
    - Swamp as the place of occurrence of the external cause
    - Mountain as the place of occurrence of the external cause
    - Marsh as the place of occurrence of the external cause
    - Prairie as the place of occurrence of the external cause
- Y92.83 Recreation area as the place of occurrence of the external cause
  - Y92.830 Public park as the place of occurrence of the external cause POA
  - Y92.831 Amusement park as the place of occurrence of the external cause POA
  - Y92.832 Beach as the place of occurrence of the external cause POA
    - Seashore as the place of occurrence of the external cause
  - Y92.833 Campsite as the place of occurrence of the external cause POA
  - Y92.834 Zoological garden (Zoo) as the place of occurrence of the external cause POA
  - Y92.838 Other recreation area as the place of occurrence of the external cause POA
- Y92.84 Military training ground as the place of occurrence of the external cause POA
- Y92.85 Railroad track as the place of occurrence of the external cause POA
- Y92.86 Slaughter house as the place of occurrence of the external cause POA
- Y92.89 Other specified places as the place of occurrence of the external cause POA
  - Derelict house as the place of occurrence of the external cause

Y92.9 Unspecified place or not applicable POA

Unspecified Code | Other Specified Code | Manifestation Code | N Newborn | P Pediatric | M Maternity | A Adult | ♂ Male | ♀ Female
● New Code | ▲ Revised Code Title | ►◄ Revised Text | NOTES | INCLUDES | EXCLUDES1 Not coded here | EXCLUDES2 Not included here
4th character required | 5th character required | 6th character required | 7th character required
Extension 'X' Alert | HAC Hospital-acquired condition (HAC) alert | AHA AHA Coding Clinic®

Y93 Activity codes

NOTES Category Y93 is provided for use to indicate the activity of the person seeking healthcare for an injury or health condition, such as a heart attack while shoveling snow, which resulted from, or was contributed to, by the activity. These codes are appropriate for use for both acute injuries, such as those from chapter 19, and conditions that are due to the long-term, cumulative effects of an activity, such as those from chapter 13. They are also appropriate for use with external cause codes for cause and intent if identifying the activity provides additional information on the event. These codes should be used in conjunction with codes for external cause status (Y99) and place of occurrence (Y92).

This section contains the following broad activity categories:

Y93.0 Activities involving walking and running
Y93.1 Activities involving water and water craft
Y93.2 Activities involving ice and snow
Y93.3 Activities involving climbing, rappelling, and jumping off
Y93.4 Activities involving dancing and other rhythmic movement
Y93.5 Activities involving other sports and athletics played individually
Y93.6 Activities involving other sports and athletics played as a team or group
Y93.7 Activities involving other specified sports and athletics
Y93.A Activities involving other cardiorespiratory exercise
Y93.B Activities involving other muscle strengthening exercises
Y93.C Activities involving computer technology and electronic devices
Y93.D Activities involving arts and handcrafts
Y93.E Activities involving personal hygiene and interior property and clothing maintenance
Y93.F Activities involving caregiving
Y93.G Activities involving food preparation, cooking and grilling
Y93.H Activities involving exterior property and land maintenance, building and construction
Y93.I Activities involving roller coasters and other types of external motion
Y93.J Activities involving playing musical instrument
Y93.K Activities involving animal care
Y93.8 Activities, other specified
Y93.9 Activity, unspecified

Y93.0 Activities involving walking and running

EXCLUDES1 *activity, walking an animal (Y93.K1)*
activity, walking or running on a treadmill (Y93.A1)

Y93.01 Activity, walking, marching and hiking
Activity, walking, marching and hiking on level or elevated terrain
EXCLUDES1 *activity, mountain climbing (Y93.31)*

Y93.02 Activity, running

Y93.1 Activities involving water and water craft

EXCLUDES1 *activities involving ice (Y93.2-)*

Y93.11 Activity, swimming
Y93.12 Activity, springboard and platform diving
Y93.13 Activity, water polo
Y93.14 Activity, water aerobics and water exercise
Y93.15 Activity, underwater diving and snorkeling
Activity, SCUBA diving
Y93.16 Activity, rowing, canoeing, kayaking, rafting and tubing
Activity, canoeing, kayaking, rafting and tubing in calm and turbulent water
Y93.17 Activity, water skiing and wake boarding
Y93.18 Activity, surfing, windsurfing and boogie boarding
Activity, water sliding
Y93.19 Activity, other involving water and watercraft
Activity involving water NOS
Activity, parasailing
Activity, water survival training and testing

Y93.2 Activities involving ice and snow

EXCLUDES1 *activity, shoveling ice and snow (Y93.H1)*

Y93.21 Activity, ice skating
Activity, figure skating (singles) (pairs)
Activity, ice dancing
EXCLUDES1 *activity, ice hockey (Y93.22)*
Y93.22 Activity, ice hockey
Y93.23 Activity, snow (alpine) (downhill) skiing, snow boarding, sledding, tobogganing and snow tubing
EXCLUDES1 *activity, cross country skiing (Y93.24)*
Y93.24 Activity, cross country skiing
Activity, Nordic skiing
Y93.29 Activity, other involving ice and snow
Activity involving ice and snow NOS

Y93.3 Activities involving climbing, rappelling and jumping off

EXCLUDES1 *activity, hiking on level or elevated terrain (Y93.01)*
activity, jumping rope (Y93.56)
activity, trampoline jumping (Y93.44)

Y93.31 Activity, mountain climbing, rock climbing and wall climbing
Y93.32 Activity, rappelling
Y93.33 Activity, BASE jumping
Activity, Building, Antenna, Span, Earth jumping
Y93.34 Activity, bungee jumping
Y93.35 Activity, hang gliding
Y93.39 Activity, other involving climbing, rappelling and jumping off

Y93.4 Activities involving dancing and other rhythmic movement

EXCLUDES1 *activity, martial arts (Y93.75)*

Y93.41 Activity, dancing
AHA: Q4, 2012
Y93.42 Activity, yoga
Y93.43 Activity, gymnastics
Activity, rhythmic gymnastics
EXCLUDES1 *activity, trampolining (Y93.44)*
Y93.44 Activity, trampolining
Y93.45 Activity, cheerleading
Y93.49 Activity, other involving dancing and other rhythmic movements

Y93.5 Activities involving other sports and athletics played individually

EXCLUDES1 *activity, dancing (Y93.41)*
activity, gymnastic (Y93.43)
activity, trampolining (Y93.44)
activity, yoga (Y93.42)

Y93.51 Activity, roller skating (inline) and skateboarding
Y93.52 Activity, horseback riding
Y93.53 Activity, golf
Y93.54 Activity, bowling
Y93.55 Activity, bike riding
Y93.56 Activity, jumping rope
Y93.57 Activity, non-running track and field events
EXCLUDES1 *activity, running (any form) (Y93.02)*
Y93.59 Activity, other involving other sports and athletics played individually
EXCLUDES1 *activities involving climbing, rappelling, and jumping (Y93.3-)*
activities involving ice and snow (Y93.2-)
activities involving walking and running (Y93.0-)
activities involving water and watercraft (Y93.1-)

Y93.6 Activities involving other sports and athletics played as a team or group

EXCLUDES1 *activity, ice hockey (Y93.22)*
activity, water polo (Y93.13)

Y93.61 Activity, American tackle football
Activity, football NOS
Y93.62 Activity, American flag or touch football
Y93.63 Activity, rugby
Y93.64 Activity, baseball
Activity, softball
Y93.65 Activity, lacrosse and field hockey
AHA: Q1, 2015
Y93.66 Activity, soccer
Y93.67 Activity, basketball
Y93.68 Activity, volleyball (beach) (court)
Y93.6A Activity, physical games generally associated with school recess, summer camp and children
Activity, capture the flag
Activity, dodge ball
Activity, four square
Activity, kickball

Unacceptable principal diagnosis symbol per Medicare code edits; Code exempt from diagnosis present on admission requirement
Questionable admission; Complication or comorbidity; CC/MCC exclusion; Major complication or comorbidity
Principal diagnosis as its own CC; Principal diagnosis as its own MCC; Z code as first-listed diagnosis

Y93.69 **Activity, other involving other sports and athletics played as a team or group**
Activity, cricket

Y93.7 **Activities involving other specified sports and athletics**
Y93.71 **Activity, boxing**
Y93.72 **Activity, wrestling**
Y93.73 **Activity, racquet and hand sports**
Activity, handball
Activity, racquetball
Activity, squash
Activity, tennis
Y93.74 **Activity, frisbee**
Activity, ultimate frisbee
Y93.75 **Activity, martial arts**
Activity, combatives
Y93.79 **Activity, other specified sports and athletics**
EXCLUDES1 *sports and athletics activities specified in categories Y93.0-Y93.6*

Y93.A **Activities involving other cardiorespiratory exercise**
Activities involving physical training
Y93.A1 **Activity, exercise machines primarily for cardiorespiratory conditioning**
Activity, elliptical and stepper machines
Activity, stationary bike
Activity, treadmill
Y93.A2 **Activity, calisthenics**
Activity, jumping jacks
Activity, warm up and cool down
Y93.A3 **Activity, aerobic and step exercise**
Y93.A4 **Activity, circuit training**
Y93.A5 **Activity, obstacle course**
Activity, challenge course
Activity, confidence course
Y93.A6 **Activity, grass drills**
Activity, guerilla drills
Y93.A9 **Activity, other involving cardiorespiratory exercise**
EXCLUDES1 *activities involving cardiorespiratory exercise specified in categories Y93.0-Y93.7*

Y93.B **Activities involving other muscle strengthening exercises**
Y93.B1 **Activity, exercise machines primarily for muscle strengthening**
Y93.B2 **Activity, push-ups, pull-ups, sit-ups**
Y93.B3 **Activity, free weights**
Activity, barbells
Activity, dumbbells
Y93.B4 **Activity, Pilates**
Y93.B9 **Activity, other involving muscle strengthening exercises**
EXCLUDES1 *activities involving muscle strengthening specified in categories Y93.0-Y93.A*

Y93.C **Activities involving computer technology and electronic devices**
EXCLUDES1 *activity, electronic musical keyboard or instruments (Y93.J-)*
Y93.C1 **Activity, computer keyboarding**
Activity, electronic game playing using keyboard or other stationary device
Y93.C2 **Activity, hand held interactive electronic device**
Activity, cellular telephone and communication device
Activity, electronic game playing using interactive device
EXCLUDES1 *activity, electronic game playing using keyboard or other stationary device (Y93.C1)*
Y93.C9 **Activity, other involving computer technology and electronic devices**

Y93.D **Activities involving arts and handcrafts**
EXCLUDES1 *activities involving playing musical instrument (Y93.J-)*
Y93.D1 **Activity, knitting and crocheting**
Y93.D2 **Activity, sewing**
Y93.D3 **Activity, furniture building and finishing**
Activity, furniture repair
Y93.D9 **Activity, other involving arts and handcrafts**

Y93.E **Activities involving personal hygiene and interior property and clothing maintenance**
EXCLUDES1 *activities involving cooking and grilling (Y93.G-)*
activities involving exterior property and land maintenance, building and construction (Y93.H-)
activities involving caregiving (Y93.F-)
activity, dishwashing (Y93.G1)
activity, food preparation (Y93.G1)
activity, gardening (Y93.H2)
Y93.E1 **Activity, personal bathing and showering**
Y93.E2 **Activity, laundry**
Y93.E3 **Activity, vacuuming**
Y93.E4 **Activity, ironing**
Y93.E5 **Activity, floor mopping and cleaning**
Y93.E6 **Activity, residential relocation**
Activity, packing up and unpacking involved in moving to a new residence
Y93.E8 **Activity, other personal hygiene**
Y93.E9 **Activity, other interior property and clothing maintenance**

Y93.F **Activities involving caregiving**
Activity involving the provider of caregiving
Y93.F1 **Activity, caregiving, bathing**
Y93.F2 **Activity, caregiving, lifting**
Y93.F9 **Activity, other caregiving**

Y93.G **Activities involving food preparation, cooking and grilling**
Y93.G1 **Activity, food preparation and clean up**
Activity, dishwashing
Y93.G2 **Activity, grilling and smoking food**
Y93.G3 **Activity, cooking and baking**
Activity, use of stove, oven and microwave oven
Y93.G9 **Activity, other involving cooking and grilling**

Y93.H **Activities involving exterior property and land maintenance, building and construction**
Y93.H1 **Activity, digging, shoveling and raking**
Activity, dirt digging
Activity, raking leaves
Activity, snow shoveling
Y93.H2 **Activity, gardening and landscaping**
Activity, pruning, trimming shrubs, weeding
Y93.H3 **Activity, building and construction**
Y93.H9 **Activity, other involving exterior property and land maintenance, building and construction**

Y93.I **Activities involving roller coasters and other types of external motion**
Y93.I1 **Activity, roller coaster riding**
Y93.I9 **Activity, other involving external motion**

Y93.J **Activities involving playing musical instrument**
Activity involving playing electric musical instrument
Y93.J1 **Activity, piano playing**
Activity, musical keyboard (electronic) playing
Y93.J2 **Activity, drum and other percussion instrument playing**
Y93.J3 **Activity, string instrument playing**
Y93.J4 **Activity, winds and brass instrument playing**

Y93.K **Activities involving animal care**
EXCLUDES1 *activity, horseback riding (Y93.52)*
Y93.K1 **Activity, walking an animal**
Y93.K2 **Activity, milking an animal**
Y93.K3 **Activity, grooming and shearing an animal**
Y93.K9 **Activity, other involving animal care**

Y93.8 **Activities, other specified**
Y93.81 **Activity, refereeing a sports activity**
Y93.82 **Activity, spectator at an event**
Y93.83 **Activity, rough housing and horseplay**
AHA: Q1, 2015
Y93.84 **Activity, sleeping**
● Y93.85 **Activity, choking game**
Activity, blackout game
Activity, fainting game
Activity, pass out game
Y93.89 **Activity, other specified**

Y93.9 **Activity, unspecified**

Y95 **Nosocomial condition**
AHA: Q4, 2013

Unspecified Code | Other Specified Code | Manifestation Code | N Newborn | P Pediatric | M Maternity | A Adult | ♂ Male | ♀ Female
● New Code | ▲ Revised Code Title | ►◄ Revised Text | NOTES | INCLUDES | EXCLUDES1 Not coded here | EXCLUDES2 Not included here
4th character required | 5th character required | 6th character required | 7th character required
Extension 'X' Alert | HAC Hospital-acquired condition (HAC) alert | AHA AHA Coding Clinic©

Y99 External cause status

NOTES A single code from category Y99 should be used in conjunction with the external cause code(s) assigned to a record to indicate the status of the person at the time the event occurred.

Y99.0 Civilian activity done for income or pay

Civilian activity done for financial or other compensation

EXCLUDES1 *military activity (Y99.1)*
volunteer activity (Y99.2)

Y99.1 Military activity

EXCLUDES1 *activity of off duty military personnel (Y99.8)*

Y99.2 Volunteer activity

EXCLUDES1 *activity of child or other family member assisting in compensated work of other family member (Y99.8)*

Y99.8 Other external cause status

Activity NEC
Activity of child or other family member assisting in compensated work of other family member
Hobby not done for income
Leisure activity
Off-duty activity of military personnel
Recreation or sport not for income or while a student
Student activity

EXCLUDES1 *civilian activity done for income or compensation (Y99.0)*
military activity (Y99.1)

Y99.9 Unspecified external cause status

Unacceptable principal diagnosis symbol per Medicare code edits | Code exempt from diagnosis present on admission requirement
Questionable admission | Complication or comorbidity | CC/MCC exclusion | Major complication or comorbidity
Principal diagnosis as its own CC | Principal diagnosis as its own MCC | Z code as first-listed diagnosis

When symbols appear on a code that requires a 7th character extension, refer to Appendix D to identify applicable 7th character codes.

Chapter 21: Factors Influencing Health Status and Contact with Health Services (Z00-Z99)

Guidelines for Assigning Codes From This Chapter

Z codes are key to correct coding practices as both primary and secondary codes, giving information both about the nature of the encounter and the patient's circumstances.

List of Sections

- Z00-Z13: Persons encountering health services for examinations
- Z14-Z15: Genetic carrier and genetic susceptibility to disease
- Z16: Resistance to antimicrobial drugs
- Z17: Estrogen receptor status
- Z18: Retained foreign body fragments
- Z20-Z28: Persons with potential health hazards related to communicable diseases
- Z30-Z39: Persons encountering health services in circumstances related to reproduction
- Z40-Z53: Encounters for other specific health care
- Z55-Z65: Persons with potential health hazards related to socioeconomic and psychosocial circumstances
- Z66: Do not resuscitate status
- Z67: Blood type
- Z68: Body mass index [BMI]
- Z69-Z76: Persons encountering health services in other circumstances
- Z77-Z99: Persons with potential health hazards related to family and personal history and certain conditions influencing health status

Highlights From the ICD-10-CM Official Guidelines for Coding and Reporting

The ICD-10-CM Official Guidelines for Coding and Reporting cover a variety of rules to keep your Z code reporting on track. The information below summarizes the key points from Section I.C.21 of the 2017 Official Guideline.

4 Factors Trigger Z Code Use

The guidelines delineate the four main reasons you'll use Z codes:

- A healthy patient presenting for a specific encounter, such as organ donation, vaccination, or screenings
- Aftercare of an injury or disease
- Circumstances influencing health status or potential hazards to community health
- birth status

Other basic rules include that you may report Z codes in any healthcare setting, and that it's possible for Z codes to be primary or secondary codes, depending on the code and the circumstances.

Note: Z codes cannot be substituted for procedure codes; a procedure code must to be used in conjunction with a Z code to report the procedure performed.

Below are some of the main guidelines related to Z code categories.

Contact/Exposure Means No Signs/Symptoms

Use codes from category Z20 (*Contact with and [suspected] exposure to communicable diseases*) and Category Z77 (*Other contact with and [suspected] exposures hazardous to health*) for patients who have been exposed to the disease but who have no signs or symptoms of the disease. You can use them as primary codes for testing encounters or as secondary codes to supply information about risk.

Remember Z Codes for Inoculations and Vaccinations

Code Z23 represents inoculation and vaccination encounters. You may use code Z23 as a secondary code when the patient has the inoculation as part of a preventive healthcare visit. Use procedure codes to report the actual administration/injection and type of immunization.

Status Codes Add Information That May Affect Treatment

A status code offers information about the patient that may affect treatment, such as presence of a prosthetic. Don't confuse status codes with history codes, which you use when the patient doesn't have the condition anymore.

When you report a code from one of the body system chapters that includes the same information that's in the status code, don't report the status code. For example, do not report code Z94.1 (*Heart transplant status*) with a code from subcategory T86.2 (*Complications of heart transplant*). Z94.1 does not provide any additional information. But for encounters for weaning from a mechanical ventilator, you would assign a code from subcategory J96.1 (*Chronic respiratory failure*) followed by code Z99.11 (*Dependence on respirator [ventilator] status*), because the status code supplies more information about the patient's status.

For a full list of status codes/categories, see the Official Guidelines (Section I.C.21.c.3) in the beginning of this manual. Be sure to watch for the guidelines below in the list.

tPA status: In addition to the instructions ICD-10-CM includes with Z92.82 (*Status post administration of tPA [rtPA] in a different facility within the last 24 hours prior to admission to current facility*), you should know that only the receiving facility should report Z92.82 and the code applies even when the patient is still on tPA upon arrival at the receiving facility.

Drug use: Do not use codes from category Z79 (*Long-term [current] drug therapy*) for patients addicted to drugs or in detoxification/maintenance programs. Use drug dependence codes instead.

Genetic susceptibility: Assign codes from category Z15 (*Genetic susceptibility to disease*) only as a secondary code and if the patient has a gene that increases the patient's risk for that disease.

Apply History (of) Codes for Eradicated Conditions

The Z code section includes codes for both personal history and family history.

Personal history codes typically apply to conditions the patient used to have that have the potential to occur again. Family history codes represent conditions found in the patient's family, suggesting the patient may be at higher risk for the disease.

For a list of personal and family history codes and categories, see the Official Guidelines (Section I.C.21.c.4) in the beginning of this manual.

Hold Screening Codes for Patients With No Symptoms

Use the screening Z codes for tests on patients with no signs or symptoms of the disease being tested for. If a patient has a sign or symptom, then the test is diagnostic, and a screening code is not appropriate. Use the sign or symptom code for the test encounter instead.

You may use screening codes as either primary or secondary codes depending on the reason for the encounter. Note that when the screening is a usual part of an exam, such as a Pap smear during a routine pelvic exam, you do not need to report the screening code.

Screening Z code categories include the following:

- Z11 — Encounter for screening for infectious and parasitic diseases
- Z12 — Encounter for screening for malignant neoplasms
- Z13 — Encounter for screening for other diseases and disorders. Except: Z13.9, Encounter for screening, unspecified
- Z36 — Encounter for antenatal screening for mother

Think Twice Before Using These Observation Codes

You'll rarely use the observation Z codes because they apply only when the provider keeps a patient without signs or symptoms under observation for a suspected condition that the provider then rules out. Use observation codes only as the primary diagnosis code; other codes may be added only if they are unrelated to the reason for observation.

When a pregnant patient is seen for a suspected maternal or fetal condition that is ruled out during the encounter, you can assign a code from subcategory Z03.7 (*Encounter for suspected maternal and fetal conditions ruled out*). Do not use these conditions if the condition is confirmed.

Do not use if an illness or any signs or symptoms related to the suspected condition or problem are present. Use the appropriate diagnoses codes or signs or symptoms codes. It is acceptable to use additional codes with Z03.7 for conditions unrelated to the suspected condition.

Do not use codes from subcategory Z03.7 for antenatal screening encounters. See Section I.C.21. Screening.

Assign the appropriate code from categories O35, O36, O40 or O4 for encounters for suspected fetal condition that are inconclusive following testing and evaluation.

You'll find observation Z codes under the following:

- Z03 — *Encounter for medical observation for suspected diseases and conditions ruled out*
- Z04 — *Encounter for examination and observation for other reasons. Except: Z04.9 — Encounter for examination and observation for unspecified reason*

Aftercare Generally Applies to Recovering Patients

The guidelines categorize a variety of encounters as aftercare that you may not immediately think of as applying to patients in the healing or recovery phase after initial treatment is complete. The guidelines acknowledge this, pointing out that Z51.0 (*Encounter for antineoplastic radiation therapy*) and Z51.1 (*Encounter for antineoplastic chemotherapy and immunotherapy*) are exceptions to the definition of aftercare.

You typically use aftercare codes as the first-listed code, but these can also be additional codes in cases where the patient presents for treatment of another condition and aftercare also takes place. You may report other codes in addition to aftercare codes to provide additional information, such as status Z codes.

For a list of aftercare codes and categories, see the Official Guidelines (Section I.C.21.c.7) in the beginning of this manual.

Assign a Follow-Up for Encounters Related to Past Conditions

When the provider sees a patient to check on a condition that no longer exists following treatment, use a follow-up code. Note how these codes differ from aftercare, which typically refers to treatment for a healing condition or the consequences of that condition. You also would not use a follow-up code for injuries for which there are subsequent encounter codes with a 7th character.

To more fully explain the follow-up, you may report a history Z code as an additional code.

When a condition recurs, report the code for the condition rather than the follow-up code.

You'll find follow-up Z codes in these categories:

- Z08 — *Encounter for follow-up examination after completed treatment for malignant neoplasm*
- Z09 — *Encounter for follow-up examination after completed treatment for conditions other than malignant neoplasm*
- Z39 — *Encounter for maternal postpartum care and examination*

Use Donor Codes for Healthy Donors

Report a code from **category Z52** (*Donors of organs and tissues*) to identify an individual donating blood or body tissue. This code is not appropriate for self-donations, such as autografts, or cadaver donations.

Keep an Eye on Reason for Counseling

Use the counseling Z codes to identify encounters for counseling patients and/or families for specific conditions and circumstances. You don't need to report a counseling code with another diagnosis code when counseling is part of standard care.

For a list of counseling codes and categories, see the Official Guidelines (Section I.C.21.c.10) in the beginning of this manual.

Obstetrics and Related Conditions Have Strict Coding Rules

ICD-10-CM includes Z codes for pregnancy that you should use only when no code from the Obstetrics chapter applies, for example, category Z34 (*Encounter for supervision of normal pregnancy*).

You may assign codes from category Z3A (*Weeks of gestation*) to provide additional information about the pregnancy. When an admission extends beyond a single gestational week, use the date of the admission to determine weeks of gestation.

Be sure to include a code from Z37 (*Outcome of delivery*) on each maternity delivery record, but only as a secondary code.

For a list of obstetric-related codes and categories, see the Official Guidelines (Section I.C.21.c.11) in the beginning of this manual.

Track Down Newborn Guidelines in Other Sections

The guidelines direct you to see the Chapter 16 guidelines, as well as the observation code guidelines discussed above, for help with reporting newborn codes.

The categories include:

- Z76.1 — Encounter for health supervision and care of foundling
- Z00.1 — Encounter for routine child health examination
- Z38 — Liveborn infants according to place of birth and type of delivery

Routine and Administrative Exams Don't Involve Suspected Diagnoses

These codes for routine and administrative exams are not appropriate for exams related to diagnosing a suspected condition or for treatment. You'd use the related diagnosis code for those exams.

Note, however, that if the provider makes a diagnosis during a routine exam, you may report the routine exam followed by the confirmed diagnosis. Similarly, you may report additional codes for chronic or other conditions the patient already has.

You'll use these Z codes and categories for routine and administrative exams:

- Z00 — *Encounter for general examination without complaint, suspected or reported diagnosis*
- Z01 — *Encounter for other special examination without complaint, suspected or reported diagnosis*
- Z02 — *Encounter for administrative examination Except: Z02.9, Encounter for administrative examinations, unspecified*
- Z32.0- — *Encounter for pregnancy test*

Miscellaneous Z Codes Include Prophylactic Organ Removal

If a Z code doesn't fit into any of the other categories, you'll find it here. Examples include palliative care, elective surgery, and economic circumstances.

For a list of miscellaneous Z codes and categories, see the Official Guidelines (Section I.C.21.c.14) in the beginning of this manual.

Prophylactic organ removal: The guidelines give specific instructions for coding removal of organs to prevent disease. When a patient presents for removal of breasts, ovaries, or other organs because the patient has a genetic susceptibility to, or family history of, a specific cancer, you should report a code from category **Z40** (*Encounter for prophylactic surgery*). Then report another code for the genetic susceptibility or family history.

When a patient has cancer at one site and undergoes organ removal at another site to prevent cancer forming there, report the malignancy code in addition to a code from subcategory **Z40.0** (*Encounter for prophylactic surgery for risk factors related to malignant neoplasms*). But be sure to distinguish prophylactic removal from removal to treat a malignancy, "such as the removal of the testes for the treatment of prostate cancer," the guidelines warn.

Keep Nonspecific Z Codes as a Last Resort

ICD-10-CM offers nonspecific Z codes with the warning that their use should be very limited, particularly in the inpatient setting. One example of a nonspecific code is Z04.9 (*Encounter for examination and observation for unspecified reason*). Always try to find a more specific code describing the sign, symptom, or other reason for the encounter before choosing a nonspecific code.

For a list of nonspecific Z codes and categories, see the Official Guidelines (Section I.C.21.c.15) in the beginning of this manual.

Mark These Z Codes as Principal/First Listed Only

ICD-10-CM designates certain Z codes as reportable only as principal/first-listed diagnoses. The exception is that when more than one Z code meets the definition for principal/first-listed diagnosis, you may report these codes somewhere other than the primary spot.

For a list of Z codes you should report only as principal/first-listed codes, see the Official Guidelines (Section I.C.21.c.16) in the beginning of this or Appendix B, Z Codes as First-listed Diagnosis..

Factors influencing health status and contact with health services (Z00-Z99)

NOTES Z codes represent reasons for encounters. A corresponding procedure code must accompany a Z code if a procedure is performed. Categories Z00-Z99 are provided for occasions when circumstances other than a disease, injury or external cause classifiable to categories A00-Y89 are recorded as 'diagnoses' or 'problems'. This can arise in two main ways:
(a) When a person who may or may not be sick encounters the health services for some specific purpose, such as to receive limited care or service for a current condition, to donate an organ or tissue, to receive prophylactic vaccination (immunization), or to discuss a problem which is in itself not a disease or injury.
(b) When some circumstance or problem is present which influences the person's health status but is not in itself a current illness or injury.

This chapter contains the following blocks:

Z00-Z13	Persons encountering health services for examinations
Z14-Z15	Genetic carrier and genetic susceptibility to disease
Z16	Resistance to antimicrobial drugs
Z17	Estrogen receptor status
Z18	Retained foreign body fragments
Z19	Hormone sensitivity malignancy status
Z20-Z29	Persons with potential health hazards related to communicable diseases
Z30-Z39	Persons encountering health services in circumstances related to reproduction
Z40-Z53	Encounters for other specific health care
Z55-Z65	Persons with potential health hazards related to socioeconomic and psychosocial circumstances
Z66	Do not resuscitate status
Z67	Blood type
Z68	Body mass index (BMI)
Z69-Z76	Persons encountering health services in other circumstances
Z77-Z99	Persons with potential health hazards related to family and personal history and certain conditions influencing health status

Persons encountering health services for examinations (Z00-Z13)

NOTES Nonspecific abnormal findings disclosed at the time of these examinations are classified to categories R70-R94.

EXCLUDES1 *examinations related to pregnancy and reproduction (Z30-Z36, Z39.-)*

Z00 Encounter for general examination without complaint, suspected or reported diagnosis

EXCLUDES1 *encounter for examination for administrative purposes (Z02.-)*

EXCLUDES2 *encounter for pre-procedural examinations (Z01.81-)*

special screening examinations (Z11-Z13)

Z00.0 Encounter for general adult medical examination

Encounter for adult periodic examination (annual) (physical) and any associated laboratory and radiologic examinations

EXCLUDES1 *encounter for examination of sign or symptom- code to sign or symptom*

general health check-up of infant or child (Z00.12.-)

Z00.00 Encounter for general adult medical examination without abnormal findings A POA PDxIn Z1

Encounter for adult health check-up NOS

AHA: Q1, 2016

Z00.01 Encounter for general adult medical examination with abnormal findings A POA PDxIn Z1

Use additional code to identify abnormal findings

AHA: Q1, 2016

Z00.1 Encounter for newborn, infant and child health examinations

Z00.11 Newborn health examination

Health check for child under 29 days old

Use additional code to identify any abnormal findings

EXCLUDES1 *health check for child over 28 days old (Z00.12-)*

Z00.110 Health examination for newborn under 8 days old N POA PDxIn Z1

Health check for newborn under 8 days old

Z00.111 Health examination for newborn 8 to 28 days old N POA PDxIn Z1

Health check for newborn 8 to 28 days old

Newborn weight check

Z00.12 Encounter for routine child health examination

Encounter for development testing of infant or child

Health check (routine) for child over 28 days old

EXCLUDES1 *health check for child under 29 days old (Z00.11-)*

health supervision of foundling or other healthy infant or child (Z76.1-Z76.2)

newborn health examination (Z00.11-)

Z00.121 Encounter for routine child health examination with abnormal findings P POA PDxIn Z1

Use additional code to identify abnormal findings

AHA: Q1, 2016

Z00.129 Encounter for routine child health examination without abnormal findings P POA PDxIn Z1

Encounter for routine child health examination NOS

AHA: Q1, 2016

Z00.2 Encounter for examination for period of rapid growth in childhood P POA PDxIn Z1

Z00.3 Encounter for examination for adolescent development state P POA PDxIn Z1

Encounter for puberty development state

Z00.5 Encounter for examination of potential donor of organ and tissue POA PDxIn Z1

Z00.6 Encounter for examination for normal comparison and control in clinical research program POA

Examination of participant or control in clinical research program

Z00.7 Encounter for examination for period of delayed growth in childhood

Z00.70 Encounter for examination for period of delayed growth in childhood without abnormal findings P POA PDxIn Z1

Z00.71 Encounter for examination for period of delayed growth in childhood with abnormal findings P POA PDxIn Z1

Use additional code to identify abnormal findings

Z00.8 Encounter for other general examination POA PDxIn Z1

Encounter for health examination in population surveys

Z01 Encounter for other special examination without complaint, suspected or reported diagnosis

INCLUDES *routine examination of specific system*

NOTES Codes from category Z01 represent the reason for the encounter. A separate procedure code is required to identify any examinations or procedures performed

EXCLUDES1 *encounter for examination for administrative purposes (Z02.-)*

encounter for examination for suspected conditions, proven not to exist (Z03.-)

encounter for laboratory and radiologic examinations as a component of general medical examinations (Z00.0-)

encounter for laboratory, radiologic and imaging examinations for sign(s) and symptom(s) - code to the sign(s) or symptom(s)

EXCLUDES2 *screening examinations (Z11-Z13)*

Z01.0 Encounter for examination of eyes and vision

EXCLUDES1 *examination for driving license (Z02.4)*

Z01.00 Encounter for examination of eyes and vision without abnormal findings POA Z1

Encounter for examination of eyes and vision NOS

Z01.01 Encounter for examination of eyes and vision with abnormal findings POA Z1

Use additional code to identify abnormal findings

Z01.1 Encounter for examination of ears and hearing

Z01.10 Encounter for examination of ears and hearing without abnormal findings POA PDxIn Z1

Encounter for examination of ears and hearing NOS

Unspecified Code Other Specified Code Manifestation Code N Newborn P Pediatric M Maternity A Adult ♂ Male ♀ Female
● New Code ▲ Revised Code Title ►◄ Revised Text NOTES INCLUDES EXCLUDES1 Not coded here EXCLUDES2 Not included here
4th character required 5th character required 6th character required 7th character required
Extension 'X' Alert HAC Hospital-acquired condition (HAC) alert AHA AHA Coding Clinic©

Z01.11 Encounter for examination of ears and hearing with abnormal findings
Z01.110 Encounter for hearing examination following failed hearing screening
Z01.118 Encounter for examination of ears and hearing with other abnormal findings
Use additional code to identify abnormal findings
Z01.12 Encounter for hearing conservation and treatment
Z01.2 Encounter for dental examination and cleaning
Z01.20 Encounter for dental examination and cleaning without abnormal findings
Encounter for dental examination and cleaning NOS
Z01.21 Encounter for dental examination and cleaning with abnormal findings
Use additional code to identify abnormal findings
Z01.3 Encounter for examination of blood pressure
Z01.30 Encounter for examination of blood pressure without abnormal findings
Encounter for examination of blood pressure NOS
Z01.31 Encounter for examination of blood pressure with abnormal findings
Use additional code to identify abnormal findings
Z01.4 Encounter for gynecological examination
EXCLUDES2 *pregnancy examination or test (Z32.0-)*
routine examination for contraceptive maintenance (Z30.4-)
Z01.41 Encounter for routine gynecological examination
Encounter for general gynecological examination with or without cervical smear
Encounter for gynecological examination (general) (routine) NOS
Encounter for pelvic examination (annual) (periodic)
Use additional code:
for screening for human papillomavirus, if applicable, (Z11.51)
for screening vaginal pap smear, if applicable (Z12.72)
to identify acquired absence of uterus, if applicable (Z90.71-)
EXCLUDES1 *gynecologic examination status-post hysterectomy for malignant condition (Z08)*
screening cervical pap smear not a part of a routine gynecological examination (Z12.4)
Z01.411 Encounter for gynecological examination (general) (routine) with abnormal findings
Use additional code to identify abnormal findings
Z01.419 Encounter for gynecological examination (general) (routine) without abnormal findings
Z01.42 Encounter for cervical smear to confirm findings of recent normal smear following initial abnormal smear
Z01.8 Encounter for other specified special examinations
Z01.81 Encounter for preprocedural examinations
Encounter for preoperative examinations
Encounter for radiological and imaging examinations as part of preprocedural examination
Z01.810 Encounter for preprocedural cardiovascular examination
Z01.811 Encounter for preprocedural respiratory examination
Z01.812 Encounter for preprocedural laboratory examination
Blood and urine tests prior to treatment or procedure
Z01.818 Encounter for other preprocedural examination
Encounter for preprocedural examination NOS
Encounter for examinations prior to antineoplastic chemotherapy
Z01.82 Encounter for allergy testing
EXCLUDES1 *encounter for antibody response examination (Z01.84)*
Z01.83 Encounter for blood typing
Encounter for Rh typing
Z01.84 Encounter for antibody response examination
Encounter for immunity status testing
EXCLUDES1 *encounter for allergy testing (Z01.82)*
Z01.89 Encounter for other specified special examinations
Z02 Encounter for administrative examination
Z02.0 Encounter for examination for admission to educational institution
Encounter for examination for admission to preschool (education)
Encounter for examination for re-admission to school following illness or medical treatment
Z02.1 Encounter for pre-employment examination
Z02.2 Encounter for examination for admission to residential institution
EXCLUDES1 *examination for admission to prison (Z02.89)*
Z02.3 Encounter for examination for recruitment to armed forces
Z02.4 Encounter for examination for driving license
Z02.5 Encounter for examination for participation in sport
EXCLUDES1 *blood-alcohol and blood-drug test (Z02.83)*
Z02.6 Encounter for examination for insurance purposes
Z02.7 Encounter for issue of medical certificate
EXCLUDES1 *encounter for general medical examination (Z00-Z01, Z02.0-Z02.6, Z02.8-Z02.9,)*
Z02.71 Encounter for disability determination
Encounter for issue of medical certificate of incapacity
Encounter for issue of medical certificate of invalidity
Z02.79 Encounter for issue of other medical certificate
Z02.8 Encounter for other administrative examinations
Z02.81 Encounter for paternity testing
Z02.82 Encounter for adoption services
Z02.83 Encounter for blood-alcohol and blood-drug test
Use additional code for findings of alcohol or drugs in blood (R78.-)
Z02.89 Encounter for other administrative examinations
Encounter for examination for admission to prison
Encounter for examination for admission to summer camp
Encounter for immigration examination
Encounter for naturalization examination
Encounter for premarital examination
EXCLUDES1 *health supervision of foundling or other healthy infant or child (Z76.1-Z76.2)*
Z02.9 Encounter for administrative examinations, unspecified
Z03 Encounter for medical observation for suspected diseases and conditions ruled out
This category is to be used when a person without a diagnosis is suspected of having an abnormal condition, without signs or symptoms, which requires study, but after examination and observation, is ruled out. This category is also for use for administrative and legal observation status.
EXCLUDES1 *contact with and (suspected) exposures hazardous to health (Z77.-)*
newborn observation for suspected condition, ruled out (P00-P04)
person with feared complaint in whom no diagnosis is made (Z71.1)
signs or symptoms under study- code to signs or symptoms
Z03.6 Encounter for observation for suspected toxic effect from ingested substance ruled out
Encounter for observation for suspected adverse effect from drug
Encounter for observation for suspected poisoning

Unacceptable principal diagnosis symbol per Medicare code edits | Code exempt from diagnosis present on admission requirement
Questionable admission | Complication or comorbidity | CC/MCC exclusion | Major complication or comorbidity
Principal diagnosis as its own CC | Principal diagnosis as its own MCC | Z code as first-listed diagnosis

Z03.7 Encounter for suspected maternal and fetal conditions ruled out
Encounter for suspected maternal and fetal conditions not found
EXCLUDES1 *known or suspected fetal anomalies affecting management of mother, not ruled out (O26.-, O35.-, O36.-, O40.-, O41.-)*

Z03.71 Encounter for suspected problem with amniotic cavity and membrane ruled out
Encounter for suspected oligohydramnios ruled out
Encounter for suspected polyhydramnios ruled out

Z03.72 Encounter for suspected placental problem ruled out

Z03.73 Encounter for suspected fetal anomaly ruled out

Z03.74 Encounter for suspected problem with fetal growth ruled out

Z03.75 Encounter for suspected cervical shortening ruled out

Z03.79 Encounter for other suspected maternal and fetal conditions ruled out

Z03.8 Encounter for observation for other suspected diseases and conditions ruled out

Z03.81 Encounter for observation for suspected exposure to biological agents ruled out

Z03.810 Encounter for observation for suspected exposure to anthrax ruled out

Z03.818 Encounter for observation for suspected exposure to other biological agents ruled out

Z03.89 Encounter for observation for other suspected diseases and conditions ruled out

Z04 Encounter for examination and observation for other reasons
INCLUDES *encounter for examination for medicolegal reasons*
This category is to be used when a person without a diagnosis is suspected of having an abnormal condition, without signs or symptoms, which requires study, but after examination and observation, is ruled-out. This category is also for use for administrative and legal observation status.

Z04.1 Encounter for examination and observation following transport accident
EXCLUDES1 *encounter for examination and observation following work accident (Z04.2)*

Z04.2 Encounter for examination and observation following work accident

Z04.3 Encounter for examination and observation following other accident

Z04.4 Encounter for examination and observation following alleged rape
Encounter for examination and observation of victim following alleged rape
Encounter for examination and observation of victim following alleged sexual abuse

Z04.41 Encounter for examination and observation following alleged adult rape
Suspected adult rape, ruled out
Suspected adult sexual abuse, ruled out

Z04.42 Encounter for examination and observation following alleged child rape
Suspected child rape, ruled out
Suspected child sexual abuse, ruled out

Z04.6 Encounter for general psychiatric examination, requested by authority

Z04.7 Encounter for examination and observation following alleged physical abuse

Z04.71 Encounter for examination and observation following alleged adult physical abuse
Suspected adult physical abuse, ruled out
EXCLUDES1 *confirmed case of adult physical abuse (T74.-)*
encounter for examination and observation following alleged adult sexual abuse (Z04.41)
suspected case of adult physical abuse, not ruled out (T76.-)

Z04.72 Encounter for examination and observation following alleged child physical abuse
Suspected child physical abuse, ruled out
EXCLUDES1 *confirmed case of child physical abuse (T74.-)*
encounter for examination and observation following alleged child sexual abuse (Z04.42)
suspected case of child physical abuse, not ruled out (T76.-)

Z04.8 Encounter for examination and observation for other specified reasons
Encounter for examination and observation for request for expert evidence

Z04.9 Encounter for examination and observation for unspecified reason
Encounter for observation NOS

● Z05 Encounter for observation and evaluation of newborn for suspected diseases and conditions ruled out
This category is to be used for newborns, within the neonatal period (the first 28 days of life), who are suspected of having an abnormal condition unrelated to exposure from the mother or the birth process, but without signs or symptoms, and which, after examination and observation, is ruled out.
EXCLUDES2 *newborn observation for suspected condition, related to exposure from the mother or birth process (P00-P04)*

● Z05.0 Observation and evaluation of newborn for suspected cardiac condition ruled out

● Z05.1 Observation and evaluation of newborn for suspected infectious condition ruled out

● Z05.2 Observation and evaluation of newborn for suspected neurological condition ruled out

● Z05.3 Observation and evaluation of newborn for suspected respiratory condition ruled out

● Z05.4 Observation and evaluation of newborn for suspected genetic, metabolic or immunologic condition ruled out

● Z05.41 Observation and evaluation of newborn for suspected genetic condition ruled out

● Z05.42 Observation and evaluation of newborn for suspected metabolic condition ruled out

● Z05.43 Observation and evaluation of newborn for suspected immunologic condition ruled out

● Z05.5 Observation and evaluation of newborn for suspected gastrointestinal condition ruled out

● Z05.6 Observation and evaluation of newborn for suspected genitourinary condition ruled out

● Z05.7 Observation and evaluation of newborn for suspected skin, subcutaneous, musculoskeletal and connective tissue condition ruled out

● Z05.71 Observation and evaluation of newborn for suspected skin and subcutaneous tissue condition ruled out

● Z05.72 Observation and evaluation of newborn for suspected musculoskeletal condition ruled out

● Z05.73 Observation and evaluation of newborn for suspected connective tissue condition ruled out

● Z05.8 Observation and evaluation of newborn for other specified suspected condition ruled out

● Z05.9 Observation and evaluation of newborn for unspecified suspected condition ruled out

Z08 Encounter for follow-up examination after completed treatment for malignant neoplasm
Medical surveillance following completed treatment
Use additional code to identify any acquired absence of organs (Z90.-)
Use additional code to identify the personal history of malignant neoplasm (Z85.-)
EXCLUDES1 *aftercare following medical care (Z43-Z49, Z51)*

Z09 Encounter for follow-up examination after completed treatment for conditions other than malignant neoplasm
Medical surveillance following completed treatment
Use additional code to identify any applicable history of disease code (Z86.-, Z87.-)
EXCLUDES1 *aftercare following medical care (Z43-Z49, Z51)*
surveillance of contraception (Z30.4-)
surveillance of prosthetic and other medical devices (Z44-Z46)
AHA: Q1, 2015

Unspecified Code | Other Specified Code | Manifestation Code | N Newborn | P Pediatric | M Maternity | A Adult | ♂ Male | ♀ Female
● New Code | ▲ Revised Code Title | ►◄ Revised Text | NOTES | INCLUDES | EXCLUDES1 Not coded here | EXCLUDES2 Not included here
4th character required | 5th character required | 6th character required | 7th character required
Extension 'X' Alert | HAC Hospital-acquired condition (HAC) alert | AHA AHA Coding Clinic©

When symbols appear on a code that requires a 7th character extension, refer to Appendix D to identify applicable 7th character codes.

Z11 Encounter for screening for infectious and parasitic diseases
Screening is the testing for disease or disease precursors in asymptomatic individuals so that early detection and treatment can be provided for those who test positive for the disease.
EXCLUDES1 *encounter for diagnostic examination-code to sign or symptom*

Z11.0 Encounter for screening for intestinal infectious diseases

Z11.1 Encounter for screening for respiratory tuberculosis

Z11.2 Encounter for screening for other bacterial diseases

Z11.3 Encounter for screening for infections with a predominantly sexual mode of transmission
EXCLUDES2 *encounter for screening for human immunodeficiency virus [HIV] (Z11.4)*
encounter for screening for human papillomavirus (Z11.51)

Z11.4 Encounter for screening for human immunodeficiency virus [HIV]

Z11.5 Encounter for screening for other viral diseases
EXCLUDES2 *encounter for screening for viral intestinal disease (Z11.0)*

Z11.51 Encounter for screening for human papillomavirus (HPV)

Z11.59 Encounter for screening for other viral diseases

Z11.6 Encounter for screening for other protozoal diseases and helminthiases
EXCLUDES2 *encounter for screening for protozoal intestinal disease (Z11.0)*

Z11.8 Encounter for screening for other infectious and parasitic diseases
Encounter for screening for chlamydia
Encounter for screening for rickettsial
Encounter for screening for spirochetal
Encounter for screening for mycoses

Z11.9 Encounter for screening for infectious and parasitic diseases, unspecified

Z12 Encounter for screening for malignant neoplasms
Screening is the testing for disease or disease precursors in asymptomatic individuals so that early detection and treatment can be provided for those who test positive for the disease.
Use additional code to identify any family history of malignant neoplasm (Z80.-)
EXCLUDES1 *encounter for diagnostic examination-code to sign or symptom*

Z12.0 Encounter for screening for malignant neoplasm of stomach

Z12.1 Encounter for screening for malignant neoplasm of intestinal tract

Z12.10 Encounter for screening for malignant neoplasm of intestinal tract, unspecified

Z12.11 Encounter for screening for malignant neoplasm of colon
Encounter for screening colonoscopy NOS

Z12.12 Encounter for screening for malignant neoplasm of rectum

Z12.13 Encounter for screening for malignant neoplasm of small intestine

Z12.2 Encounter for screening for malignant neoplasm of respiratory organs

Z12.3 Encounter for screening for malignant neoplasm of breast

Z12.31 Encounter for screening mammogram for malignant neoplasm of breast
EXCLUDES1 *inconclusive mammogram (R92.2)*
AHA: Q1, 2015

Z12.39 Encounter for other screening for malignant neoplasm of breast

Z12.4 Encounter for screening for malignant neoplasm of cervix ♀
Encounter for screening pap smear for malignant neoplasm of cervix
EXCLUDES1 *when screening is part of general gynecological examination (Z01.4-)*
EXCLUDES2 *encounter for screening for human papillomavirus (Z11.51)*

Z12.5 Encounter for screening for malignant neoplasm of prostate ♂

Z12.6 Encounter for screening for malignant neoplasm of bladder

Z12.7 Encounter for screening for malignant neoplasm of other genitourinary organs

Z12.71 Encounter for screening for malignant neoplasm of testis ♂

Z12.72 Encounter for screening for malignant neoplasm of vagina ♀
Vaginal pap smear status-post hysterectomy for non-malignant condition
Use additional code to identify acquired absence of uterus (Z90.71-)
EXCLUDES1 *vaginal pap smear status-post hysterectomy for malignant conditions (Z08)*

Z12.73 Encounter for screening for malignant neoplasm of ovary ♀

Z12.79 Encounter for screening for malignant neoplasm of other genitourinary organs

Z12.8 Encounter for screening for malignant neoplasm of other sites

Z12.81 Encounter for screening for malignant neoplasm of oral cavity

Z12.82 Encounter for screening for malignant neoplasm of nervous system

Z12.83 Encounter for screening for malignant neoplasm of skin

Z12.89 Encounter for screening for malignant neoplasm of other sites

Z12.9 Encounter for screening for malignant neoplasm, site unspecified

Z13 Encounter for screening for other diseases and disorders
Screening is the testing for disease or disease precursors in asymptomatic individuals so that early detection and treatment can be provided for those who test positive for the disease.
EXCLUDES1 *encounter for diagnostic examination-code to sign or symptom*

Z13.0 Encounter for screening for diseases of the blood and blood-forming organs and certain disorders involving the immune mechanism

Z13.1 Encounter for screening for diabetes mellitus

Z13.2 Encounter for screening for nutritional, metabolic and other endocrine disorders

Z13.21 Encounter for screening for nutritional disorder

Z13.22 Encounter for screening for metabolic disorder

Z13.220 Encounter for screening for lipoid disorders
Encounter for screening for cholesterol level
Encounter for screening for hypercholesterolemia
Encounter for screening for hyperlipidemia

Z13.228 Encounter for screening for other metabolic disorders

Z13.29 Encounter for screening for other suspected endocrine disorder
EXCLUDES1 *encounter for screening for diabetes mellitus (Z13.1)*

Z13.4 Encounter for screening for certain developmental disorders in childhood
Encounter for screening for developmental handicaps in early childhood
EXCLUDES1 *routine development testing of infant or child (Z00.1-)*

Z13.5 Encounter for screening for eye and ear disorders
EXCLUDES2 *encounter for general hearing examination (Z01.1-)*
encounter for general vision examination (Z01.0-)

Z13.6 Encounter for screening for cardiovascular disorders

PDx Unacceptable principal diagnosis symbol per Medicare code edits · POA Code exempt from diagnosis present on admission requirement · Questionable admission · CC Complication or comorbidity · CC/MCC Exc CC/MCC exclusion · MCC Major complication or comorbidity · Principal diagnosis as its own CC · Principal diagnosis as its own MCC · Z code as first-listed diagnosis

Z13.7 Encounter for screening for genetic and chromosomal anomalies
EXCLUDES1 *genetic testing for procreative management (Z31.4-)*
Z13.71 Encounter for nonprocreative screening for genetic disease carrier status
Z13.79 Encounter for other screening for genetic and chromosomal anomalies
Z13.8 Encounter for screening for other specified diseases and disorders
EXCLUDES2 *screening for malignant neoplasms (Z12.-)*
Z13.81 Encounter for screening for digestive system disorders
Z13.810 Encounter for screening for upper gastrointestinal disorder
Z13.811 Encounter for screening for lower gastrointestinal disorder
EXCLUDES1 *encounter for screening for intestinal infectious disease (Z11.0)*
Z13.818 Encounter for screening for other digestive system disorders
Z13.82 Encounter for screening for musculoskeletal disorder
Z13.820 Encounter for screening for osteoporosis
Z13.828 Encounter for screening for other musculoskeletal disorder
Z13.83 Encounter for screening for respiratory disorder NEC
EXCLUDES1 *encounter for screening for respiratory tuberculosis (Z11.1)*
Z13.84 Encounter for screening for dental disorders
Z13.85 Encounter for screening for nervous system disorders
Z13.850 Encounter for screening for traumatic brain injury
Z13.858 Encounter for screening for other nervous system disorders
Z13.88 Encounter for screening for disorder due to exposure to contaminants
EXCLUDES1 *those exposed to contaminants without suspected disorders (Z57.-, Z77.-)*
Z13.89 Encounter for screening for other disorder
Encounter for screening for genitourinary disorders
Z13.9 Encounter for screening, unspecified

Genetic carrier and genetic susceptibility to disease (Z14-Z15)

Z14 Genetic carrier
Z14.0 Hemophilia A carrier
Z14.01 Asymptomatic hemophilia A carrier
Z14.02 Symptomatic hemophilia A carrier
Z14.1 Cystic fibrosis carrier
Z14.8 Genetic carrier of other disease
Z15 Genetic susceptibility to disease
INCLUDES *confirmed abnormal gene*
Use additional code, if applicable, for any associated family history of the disease (Z80-Z84)
EXCLUDES1 *chromosomal anomalies (Q90-Q99)*
Z15.0 Genetic susceptibility to malignant neoplasm
Code first , if applicable, any current malignant neoplasm (C00-C75, C81-C96)
Use additional code, if applicable, for any personal history of malignant neoplasm (Z85.-)
Z15.01 Genetic susceptibility to malignant neoplasm of breast
Z15.02 Genetic susceptibility to malignant neoplasm of ovary ♀
Z15.03 Genetic susceptibility to malignant neoplasm of prostate ♂
Z15.04 Genetic susceptibility to malignant neoplasm of endometrium ♀
Z15.09 Genetic susceptibility to other malignant neoplasm
Z15.8 Genetic susceptibility to other disease
Z15.81 Genetic susceptibility to multiple endocrine neoplasia [MEN]
EXCLUDES1 *multiple endocrine neoplasia [MEN] syndromes (E31.2-)*
Z15.89 Genetic susceptibility to other disease

Resistance to antimicrobial drugs (Z16)

Z16 Resistance to antimicrobial drugs
NOTES The codes in this category are provided for use as additional codes to identify the resistance and non-responsiveness of a condition to antimicrobial drugs.
Code first the infection
EXCLUDES1 *Methicillin resistant Staphylococcus aureus infection (A49.02)*
Methicillin resistant Staphylococcus aureus infection in diseases classified elsewhere (B95.62)
Methicillin resistant Staphylococcus aureus pneumonia (J15.212)
Sepsis due to Methicillin resistant Staphylococcus aureus (A41.02)
Z16.1 Resistance to beta lactam antibiotics
Z16.10 Resistance to unspecified beta lactam antibiotics
Z16.11 Resistance to penicillins
Resistance to amoxicillin
Resistance to ampicillin
Z16.12 Extended spectrum beta lactamase (ESBL) resistance
Z16.19 Resistance to other specified beta lactam antibiotics
Resistance to cephalosporins
Z16.2 Resistance to other antibiotics
Z16.20 Resistance to unspecified antibiotic
Resistance to antibiotics NOS
Z16.21 Resistance to vancomycin
Z16.22 Resistance to vancomycin related antibiotics
Z16.23 Resistance to quinolones and fluoroquinolones
Z16.24 Resistance to multiple antibiotics
Z16.29 Resistance to other single specified antibiotic
Resistance to aminoglycosides
Resistance to macrolides
Resistance to sulfonamides
Resistance to tetracyclines
Z16.3 Resistance to other antimicrobial drugs
EXCLUDES1 *resistance to antibiotics (Z16.1-, Z16.2-)*
Z16.30 Resistance to unspecified antimicrobial drugs
Drug resistance NOS
Z16.31 Resistance to antiparasitic drug(s)
Resistance to quinine and related compounds
Z16.32 Resistance to antifungal drug(s)
Z16.33 Resistance to antiviral drug(s)
Z16.34 Resistance to antimycobacterial drug(s)
Resistance to tuberculostatics
Z16.341 Resistance to single antimycobacterial drug
Resistance to antimycobacterial drug NOS
Z16.342 Resistance to multiple antimycobacterial drugs
Z16.35 Resistance to multiple antimicrobial drugs
EXCLUDES1 *Resistance to multiple antibiotics only (Z16.24)*
Z16.39 Resistance to other specified antimicrobial drug

Unspecified Code Other Specified Code Manifestation Code N Newborn P Pediatric M Maternity A Adult ♂ Male ♀ Female
● New Code ▲ Revised Code Title ►◄ Revised Text NOTES INCLUDES EXCLUDES1 Not coded here EXCLUDES2 Not included here
4th character required 5th character required 6th character required 7th character required
Extension 'X' Alert HAC Hospital-acquired condition (HAC) alert AHA AHA Coding Clinic©

Estrogen receptor status (Z17)

Z17 Estrogen receptor status
Code first malignant neoplasm of breast (C50.-)
- Z17.0 Estrogen receptor positive status [ER+]
- Z17.1 Estrogen receptor negative status [ER-]

Retained foreign body fragments (Z18)

Z18 Retained foreign body fragments

INCLUDES *embedded fragment (status)*
embedded splinter (status)
retained foreign body status

EXCLUDES1 *artificial joint prosthesis status (Z96.6-)*
foreign body accidentally left during a procedure (T81.5-)
foreign body entering through orifice (T15-T19)
in situ cardiac device (Z95.-)
organ or tissue replaced by means other than transplant (Z96.-, Z97.-)
organ or tissue replaced by transplant (Z94.-)
personal history of retained foreign body fully removed Z87.821
superficial foreign body (non-embedded splinter) - code to superficial foreign body, by site

- Z18.0 Retained radioactive fragments
  - Z18.01 Retained depleted uranium fragments
  - Z18.09 Other retained radioactive fragments
    Other retained depleted isotope fragments
    Retained nontherapeutic radioactive fragments
- Z18.1 Retained metal fragments
  EXCLUDES1 *retained radioactive metal fragments (Z18.01-Z18.09)*
  - Z18.10 Retained metal fragments, unspecified
    Retained metal fragment NOS
  - Z18.11 Retained magnetic metal fragments
  - Z18.12 Retained nonmagnetic metal fragments
- Z18.2 Retained plastic fragments
  Acrylics fragments
  Diethylhexylphthalates fragments
  Isocyanate fragments
- Z18.3 Retained organic fragments
  - Z18.31 Retained animal quills or spines
  - Z18.32 Retained tooth
  - Z18.33 Retained wood fragments
  - Z18.39 Other retained organic fragments
- Z18.8 Other specified retained foreign body
  - Z18.81 Retained glass fragments
  - Z18.83 Retained stone or crystalline fragments
    Retained concrete or cement fragments
  - Z18.89 Other specified retained foreign body fragments
- Z18.9 Retained foreign body fragments, unspecified material

Hormone sensitivity malignancy status (Z19)

● Z19 Hormone sensitivity malignancy status
Code first malignant neoplasm - see Table of Neoplasms, by site, malignant
- ● Z19.1 Hormone sensitive malignancy status
- ● Z19.2 Hormone resistant malignancy status
  Castrate resistant prostate malignancy status

Persons with potential health hazards related to communicable diseases (Z20-Z29)

Z20 Contact with and (suspected) exposure to communicable diseases

EXCLUDES1 *carrier of infectious disease (Z22.-)*
diagnosed current infectious or parasitic disease -see Alphabetic Index

EXCLUDES2 *personal history of infectious and parasitic diseases (Z86.1-)*

- Z20.0 Contact with and (suspected) exposure to intestinal infectious diseases
  - Z20.01 Contact with and (suspected) exposure to intestinal infectious diseases due to Escherichia coli (E. coli)
  - Z20.09 Contact with and (suspected) exposure to other intestinal infectious diseases
- Z20.1 Contact with and (suspected) exposure to tuberculosis
- Z20.2 Contact with and (suspected) exposure to infections with a predominantly sexual mode of transmission
- Z20.3 Contact with and (suspected) exposure to rabies
- Z20.4 Contact with and (suspected) exposure to rubella
- Z20.5 Contact with and (suspected) exposure to viral hepatitis
- Z20.6 Contact with and (suspected) exposure to human immunodeficiency virus [HIV]
  EXCLUDES1 *asymptomatic human immunodeficiency virus [HIV] HIV infection status (Z21)*
- Z20.7 Contact with and (suspected) exposure to pediculosis, acariasis and other infestations
- Z20.8 Contact with and (suspected) exposure to other communicable diseases
  - Z20.81 Contact with and (suspected) exposure to other bacterial communicable diseases
    - Z20.810 Contact with and (suspected) exposure to anthrax
    - Z20.811 Contact with and (suspected) exposure to meningococcus
    - Z20.818 Contact with and (suspected) exposure to other bacterial communicable diseases
  - Z20.82 Contact with and (suspected) exposure to other viral communicable diseases
    - Z20.820 Contact with and (suspected) exposure to varicella
    - Z20.828 Contact with and (suspected) exposure to other viral communicable diseases
  - Z20.89 Contact with and (suspected) exposure to other communicable diseases
- Z20.9 Contact with and (suspected) exposure to unspecified communicable disease

Z21 Asymptomatic human immunodeficiency virus [HIV] infection status
HIV positive NOS
Code first Human immunodeficiency virus [HIV] disease complicating pregnancy, childbirth and the puerperium, if applicable (O98.7-)

EXCLUDES1 *acquired immunodeficiency syndrome (B20)*
contact with human immunodeficiency virus [HIV] (Z20.6)
exposure to human immunodeficiency virus [HIV] (Z20.6)
human immunodeficiency virus [HIV] disease (B20)
inconclusive laboratory evidence of human immunodeficiency virus [HIV] (R75)

Z22 Carrier of infectious disease

INCLUDES *colonization status*
suspected carrier

EXCLUDES2 *carrier of viral hepatitis (B18.-)*

- Z22.0 Carrier of typhoid
- Z22.1 Carrier of other intestinal infectious diseases
- Z22.2 Carrier of diphtheria
- Z22.3 Carrier of other specified bacterial diseases
  - Z22.31 Carrier of bacterial disease due to meningococci
  - Z22.32 Carrier of bacterial disease due to staphylococci
    - Z22.321 Carrier or suspected carrier of Methicillin susceptible Staphylococcus aureus
      MSSA colonization
    - Z22.322 Carrier or suspected carrier of Methicillin resistant Staphylococcus aureus
      MRSA colonization
  - Z22.33 Carrier of bacterial disease due to streptococci
    - Z22.330 Carrier of Group B streptococcus
      EXCLUDES1 *Carrier of streptococcus group B (GBS) complicating pregnancy, childbirth and the puerperium (O99.82-)*
    - Z22.338 Carrier of other streptococcus
  - Z22.39 Carrier of other specified bacterial diseases

Unacceptable principal diagnosis symbol per Medicare code edits · Code exempt from diagnosis present on admission requirement
Questionable admission · Complication or comorbidity · CC/MCC exclusion · Major complication or comorbidity
Principal diagnosis as its own CC · Principal diagnosis as its own MCC · Z code as first-listed diagnosis

Z22.4 Carrier of infections with a predominantly sexual mode of transmission

Z22.6 Carrier of human T-lymphotropic virus type-1 [HTLV-1] infection

Z22.8 Carrier of other infectious diseases

Z22.9 Carrier of infectious disease, unspecified

Z23 Encounter for immunization

Code first any routine childhood examination

NOTES procedure codes are required to identify the types of immunizations given

Z28 Immunization not carried out and underimmunization status

INCLUDES *vaccination not carried out*

Z28.0 Immunization not carried out because of contraindication

Z28.01 Immunization not carried out because of acute illness of patient

Z28.02 Immunization not carried out because of chronic illness or condition of patient

Z28.03 Immunization not carried out because of immune compromised state of patient

Z28.04 Immunization not carried out because of patient allergy to vaccine or component

Z28.09 Immunization not carried out because of other contraindication

Z28.1 Immunization not carried out because of patient decision for reasons of belief or group pressure

Immunization not carried out because of religious belief

Z28.2 Immunization not carried out because of patient decision for other and unspecified reason

Z28.20 Immunization not carried out because of patient decision for unspecified reason

Z28.21 Immunization not carried out because of patient refusal

Z28.29 Immunization not carried out because of patient decision for other reason

Z28.3 Underimmunization status

Delinquent immunization status

Lapsed immunization schedule status

Z28.8 Immunization not carried out for other reason

Z28.81 Immunization not carried out due to patient having had the disease

Z28.82 Immunization not carried out because of caregiver refusal

Immunization not carried out because of guardian refusal

Immunization not carried out because of parent refusal

EXCLUDES1 *immunization not carried out because of caregiver refusal because of religious belief (Z28.1)*

Z28.89 Immunization not carried out for other reason

Z28.9 Immunization not carried out for unspecified reason

● Z29 Encounter for other prophylactic measures

EXCLUDES1 *desensitization to allergens (Z51.6)*
prophylactic surgery (Z40.-)

● Z29.1 Encounter for prophylactic immunotherapy

Encounter for administration of immunoglobulin

● Z29.11 Encounter for prophylactic immunotherapy for respiratory syncytial virus (RSV)

● Z29.12 Encounter for prophylactic antivenin

● Z29.13 Encounter for prophylactic Rho(D) immune globulin

● Z29.14 Encounter for prophylactic rabies immune globin

● Z29.3 Encounter for prophylactic fluoride administration

● Z29.8 Encounter for other specified prophylactic measures

● Z29.9 Encounter for prophylactic measures, unspecified

Persons encountering health services in circumstances related to reproduction (Z30-Z39)

Z30 Encounter for contraceptive management

Z30.0 Encounter for general counseling and advice on contraception

Z30.01 Encounter for initial prescription of contraceptives

EXCLUDES1 *encounter for surveillance of contraceptives (Z30.4-)*

Z30.011 Encounter for initial prescription of contraceptive pills

Z30.012 Encounter for prescription of emergency contraception

Encounter for postcoital contraception

Z30.013 Encounter for initial prescription of injectable contraceptive

Z30.014 Encounter for initial prescription of intrauterine contraceptive device

EXCLUDES1 *encounter for insertion of intrauterine contraceptive device (Z30.430, Z30.432)*

● Z30.015 Encounter for initial prescription of vaginal ring hormonal contraceptive

● Z30.016 Encounter for initial prescription of transdermal patch hormonal contraceptive device

● Z30.017 Encounter for initial prescription of implantable subdermal contraceptive

Z30.018 Encounter for initial prescription of other contraceptives

Encounter for initial prescription of barrier contraception

Encounter for initial prescription of diaphragm

Z30.019 Encounter for initial prescription of contraceptives, unspecified

Z30.02 Counseling and instruction in natural family planning to avoid pregnancy

Z30.09 Encounter for other general counseling and advice on contraception

Encounter for family planning advice NOS

Z30.2 Encounter for sterilization

Z30.4 Encounter for surveillance of contraceptives

Z30.40 Encounter for surveillance of contraceptives, unspecified

Z30.41 Encounter for surveillance of contraceptive pills

Encounter for repeat prescription for contraceptive pill

Z30.42 Encounter for surveillance of injectable contraceptive

Z30.43 Encounter for surveillance of intrauterine contraceptive device

Z30.430 Encounter for insertion of intrauterine contraceptive device

Z30.431 Encounter for routine checking of intrauterine contraceptive device

Z30.432 Encounter for removal of intrauterine contraceptive device

Z30.433 Encounter for removal and reinsertion of intrauterine contraceptive device

Encounter for replacement of intrauterine contraceptive device

● Z30.44 Encounter for surveillance of vaginal ring hormonal contraceptive device

● Z30.45 Encounter for surveillance of transdermal patch hormonal contraceptive device

● Z30.46 Encounter for surveillance of implantable subdermal contraceptive

Encounter for checking, reinsertion or removal of implantable subdermal contraceptive

Z30.49 Encounter for surveillance of other contraceptives

Encounter for surveillance of barrier contraception

Encounter for surveillance of diaphragm

Z30.8 Encounter for other contraceptive management

Encounter for postvasectomy sperm count

Encounter for routine examination for contraceptive maintenance

EXCLUDES1 *sperm count following sterilization reversal (Z31.42)*
sperm count for fertility testing (Z31.41)

Unspecified Code | Other Specified Code | Manifestation Code | N Newborn | P Pediatric | M Maternity | A Adult | ♂ Male | ♀ Female
● New Code | ▲ Revised Code Title | ►◄ Revised Text | NOTES | INCLUDES | EXCLUDES1 Not coded here | EXCLUDES2 Not included here
4th character required | 5th character required | 6th character required | 7th character required
Extension 'X' Alert | HAC Hospital-acquired condition (HAC) alert | AHA AHA Coding Clinic©

Z30.9 Encounter for contraceptive management, unspecified

Z31 Encounter for procreative management

EXCLUDES1 *complications associated with artificial fertilization (N98.-)*
female infertility (N97.-)
male infertility (N46.-)

Z31.0 Encounter for reversal of previous sterilization

Z31.4 Encounter for procreative investigation and testing

EXCLUDES1 *postvasectomy sperm count (Z30.8)*

Z31.41 Encounter for fertility testing
Encounter for fallopian tube patency testing
Encounter for sperm count for fertility testing

Z31.42 Aftercare following sterilization reversal
Sperm count following sterilization reversal

Z31.43 Encounter for genetic testing of female for procreative management
Use additional code for recurrent pregnancy loss, if applicable (N96, O26.2-)

EXCLUDES1 *nonprocreative genetic testing (Z13.7-)*

Z31.430 Encounter of female for testing for genetic disease carrier status for procreative management ♀

Z31.438 Encounter for other genetic testing of female for procreative management ♀

Z31.44 Encounter for genetic testing of male for procreative management

EXCLUDES1 *nonprocreative genetic testing (Z13.7-)*

Z31.440 Encounter of male for testing for genetic disease carrier status for procreative management ♂

Z31.441 Encounter for testing of male partner of patient with recurrent pregnancy loss A ♂

Z31.448 Encounter for other genetic testing of male for procreative management A ♂

Z31.49 Encounter for other procreative investigation and testing

Z31.5 Encounter for genetic counseling

Z31.6 Encounter for general counseling and advice on procreation

Z31.61 Procreative counseling and advice using natural family planning

Z31.62 Encounter for fertility preservation counseling
Encounter for fertility preservation counseling prior to cancer therapy
Encounter for fertility preservation counseling prior to surgical removal of gonads

Z31.69 Encounter for other general counseling and advice on procreation

● **Z31.7 Encounter for procreative management and counseling for gestational carrier**

EXCLUDES1 *pregnant state, gestational carrier (Z33.3)*

Z31.8 Encounter for other procreative management

Z31.81 Encounter for male factor infertility in female patient ♀

Z31.82 Encounter for Rh incompatibility status ♀
AHA: Q3, 2015

Z31.83 Encounter for assisted reproductive fertility procedure cycle ♀
Patient undergoing in vitro fertilization cycle
Use additional code to identify the type of infertility

EXCLUDES1 *pre-cycle diagnosis and testing - code to reason for encounter*

Z31.84 Encounter for fertility preservation procedure
Encounter for fertility preservation procedure prior to cancer therapy
Encounter for fertility preservation procedure prior to surgical removal of gonads

Z31.89 Encounter for other procreative management

Z31.9 Encounter for procreative management, unspecified

Z32 Encounter for pregnancy test and childbirth and childcare instruction

Z32.0 Encounter for pregnancy test

Z32.00 Encounter for pregnancy test, result unknown ♀
Encounter for pregnancy test NOS

Z32.01 Encounter for pregnancy test, result positive M ♀

Z32.02 Encounter for pregnancy test, result negative ♀

Z32.2 Encounter for childbirth instruction

Z32.3 Encounter for childcare instruction
Encounter for prenatal or postpartum childcare instruction

Z33 Pregnant state

Z33.1 Pregnant state, incidental M ♀
Pregnant state NOS

EXCLUDES1 *complications of pregnancy (O00-O9A)*
pregnant state, gestational carrier (Z33.3)

Z33.2 Encounter for elective termination of pregnancy M ♀

EXCLUDES1 *early fetal death with retention of dead fetus (O02.1)*
late fetal death (O36.4)
spontaneous abortion (O03)

● **Z33.3 Pregnant state, gestational carrier**

EXCLUDES1 *encounter for procreative management and counseling for gestational carrier (Z31.7)*

Z34 Encounter for supervision of normal pregnancy

EXCLUDES1 *any complication of pregnancy (O00-O9A)*
encounter for pregnancy test (Z32.0-)
encounter for supervision of high risk pregnancy (O09.-)

Z34.0 Encounter for supervision of normal first pregnancy

Z34.00 Encounter for supervision of normal first pregnancy, unspecified trimester M ♀

Z34.01 Encounter for supervision of normal first pregnancy, first trimester 1st M ♀

Z34.02 Encounter for supervision of normal first pregnancy, second trimester 2nd M ♀

Z34.03 Encounter for supervision of normal first pregnancy, third trimester 3rd M ♀

Z34.8 Encounter for supervision of other normal pregnancy

Z34.80 Encounter for supervision of other normal pregnancy, unspecified trimester M ♀

Z34.81 Encounter for supervision of other normal pregnancy, first trimester 1st M ♀

Z34.82 Encounter for supervision of other normal pregnancy, second trimester 2nd M ♀

Z34.83 Encounter for supervision of other normal pregnancy, third trimester 3rd M ♀

Z34.9 Encounter for supervision of normal pregnancy, unspecified

Z34.90 Encounter for supervision of normal pregnancy, unspecified, unspecified trimester M ♀

Z34.91 Encounter for supervision of normal pregnancy, unspecified, first trimester 1st M ♀

Z34.92 Encounter for supervision of normal pregnancy, unspecified, second trimester 2nd M ♀

Z34.93 Encounter for supervision of normal pregnancy, unspecified, third trimester 3rd M ♀

Z36 Encounter for antenatal screening of mother M ♀

EXCLUDES1 *abnormal findings on antenatal screening of mother (O28.-)*
diagnostic examination- code to sign or symptom
encounter for suspected maternal and fetal conditions ruled out (Z03.7-)
suspected fetal condition affecting management of pregnancy - code to condition in Chapter 15

EXCLUDES2 *genetic counseling and testing (Z31.43-, Z31.5)*
routine prenatal care (Z34)

Z3A Weeks of gestation

1st 1st trimester 2nd 2nd trimester 3rd 3rd trimester PDx Unacceptable principal diagnosis symbol per Medicare code edits
POA Code exempt from diagnosis present on admission requirement ? Questionable admission CC Complication or comorbidity
CC/MCC Excl CC/MCC exclusion MCC Major complication or comorbidity PDx CC Principal diagnosis as its own CC
PDx MCC Principal diagnosis as its own MCC Z1 Z code as first-listed diagnosis

NOTES Codes from category Z3A are for use, only on the maternal record, to indicate the weeks of gestation of the pregnancy, ▶if known.◀

Code first complications of pregnancy, childbirth and the puerperium (O00-O9A)

Z3A.0 Weeks of gestation of pregnancy, unspecified or less than 10 weeks
- Z3A.00 Weeks of gestation of pregnancy not specified
- Z3A.01 Less than 8 weeks gestation of pregnancy
- Z3A.08 8 weeks gestation of pregnancy
- Z3A.09 9 weeks gestation of pregnancy

Z3A.1 Weeks of gestation of pregnancy, weeks 10-19
- Z3A.10 10 weeks gestation of pregnancy
- Z3A.11 11 weeks gestation of pregnancy
- Z3A.12 12 weeks gestation of pregnancy
- Z3A.13 13 weeks gestation of pregnancy
- Z3A.14 14 weeks gestation of pregnancy
- Z3A.15 15 weeks gestation of pregnancy
- Z3A.16 16 weeks gestation of pregnancy
- Z3A.17 17 weeks gestation of pregnancy
- Z3A.18 18 weeks gestation of pregnancy
- Z3A.19 19 weeks gestation of pregnancy

Z3A.2 Weeks of gestation of pregnancy, weeks 20-29
- Z3A.20 20 weeks gestation of pregnancy
- Z3A.21 21 weeks gestation of pregnancy
- Z3A.22 22 weeks gestation of pregnancy
- Z3A.23 23 weeks gestation of pregnancy
- Z3A.24 24 weeks gestation of pregnancy
- Z3A.25 25 weeks gestation of pregnancy
- Z3A.26 26 weeks gestation of pregnancy
- Z3A.27 27 weeks gestation of pregnancy
- Z3A.28 28 weeks gestation of pregnancy
- Z3A.29 29 weeks gestation of pregnancy

Z3A.3 Weeks of gestation of pregnancy, weeks 30-39
- Z3A.30 30 weeks gestation of pregnancy
- Z3A.31 31 weeks gestation of pregnancy
- Z3A.32 32 weeks gestation of pregnancy
- Z3A.33 33 weeks gestation of pregnancy
- Z3A.34 34 weeks gestation of pregnancy
- Z3A.35 35 weeks gestation of pregnancy
- Z3A.36 36 weeks gestation of pregnancy
- Z3A.37 37 weeks gestation of pregnancy
- Z3A.38 38 weeks gestation of pregnancy
  AHA: Q2, 2016
- Z3A.39 39 weeks gestation of pregnancy

Z3A.4 Weeks of gestation of pregnancy, weeks 40 or greater
- Z3A.40 40 weeks gestation of pregnancy
- Z3A.41 41 weeks gestation of pregnancy
- Z3A.42 42 weeks gestation of pregnancy
- Z3A.49 Greater than 42 weeks gestation of pregnancy

Z37 Outcome of delivery

This category is intended for use as an additional code to identify the outcome of delivery on the mother's record. It is not for use on the newborn record.

EXCLUDES1 *stillbirth (P95)*

- Z37.0 Single live birth
  AHA: Q2, 2016
- Z37.1 Single stillbirth
- Z37.2 Twins, both liveborn
- Z37.3 Twins, one liveborn and one stillborn
- Z37.4 Twins, both stillborn
- Z37.5 Other multiple births, all liveborn
  - Z37.50 Multiple births, unspecified, all liveborn
  - Z37.51 Triplets, all liveborn
  - Z37.52 Quadruplets, all liveborn
  - Z37.53 Quintuplets, all liveborn
  - Z37.54 Sextuplets, all liveborn
  - Z37.59 Other multiple births, all liveborn
- Z37.6 Other multiple births, some liveborn
  - Z37.60 Multiple births, unspecified, some liveborn
  - Z37.61 Triplets, some liveborn
  - Z37.62 Quadruplets, some liveborn
  - Z37.63 Quintuplets, some liveborn
  - Z37.64 Sextuplets, some liveborn
  - Z37.69 Other multiple births, some liveborn
- Z37.7 Other multiple births, all stillborn
- Z37.9 Outcome of delivery, unspecified
  Multiple birth NOS
  Single birth NOS

Z38 Liveborn infants according to place of birth and type of delivery

This category is for use as the principal code on the initial record of a newborn baby. It is to be used for the initial birth record only. It is not to be used on the mother's record.

- Z38.0 Single liveborn infant, born in hospital
  Single liveborn infant, born in birthing center or other health care facility
  - Z38.00 Single liveborn infant, delivered vaginally
  - Z38.01 Single liveborn infant, delivered by cesarean
- Z38.1 Single liveborn infant, born outside hospital
- Z38.2 Single liveborn infant, unspecified as to place of birth
  Single liveborn infant NOS
- Z38.3 Twin liveborn infant, born in hospital
  - Z38.30 Twin liveborn infant, delivered vaginally
  - Z38.31 Twin liveborn infant, delivered by cesarean
- Z38.4 Twin liveborn infant, born outside hospital
- Z38.5 Twin liveborn infant, unspecified as to place of birth
- Z38.6 Other multiple liveborn infant, born in hospital
  - Z38.61 Triplet liveborn infant, delivered vaginally
  - Z38.62 Triplet liveborn infant, delivered by cesarean
  - Z38.63 Quadruplet liveborn infant, delivered vaginally
  - Z38.64 Quadruplet liveborn infant, delivered by cesarean
  - Z38.65 Quintuplet liveborn infant, delivered vaginally
  - Z38.66 Quintuplet liveborn infant, delivered by cesarean
  - Z38.68 Other multiple liveborn infant, delivered vaginally
  - Z38.69 Other multiple liveborn infant, delivered by cesarean
- Z38.7 Other multiple liveborn infant, born outside hospital
- Z38.8 Other multiple liveborn infant, unspecified as to place of birth

Z39 Encounter for maternal postpartum care and examination

- Z39.0 Encounter for care and examination of mother immediately after delivery
  Care and observation in uncomplicated cases when the delivery occurs outside a healthcare facility
  EXCLUDES1 *care for postpartum complication- see Alphabetic index*
- Z39.1 Encounter for care and examination of lactating mother
  Encounter for supervision of lactation
  EXCLUDES1 *disorders of lactation (O92.-)*
- Z39.2 Encounter for routine postpartum follow-up

Unspecified Code | Other Specified Code | Manifestation Code | N Newborn | P Pediatric | M Maternity | A Adult | ♂ Male | ♀ Female
● New Code | ▲ Revised Code Title | ▶◀ Revised Text | NOTES | INCLUDES | EXCLUDES1 Not coded here | EXCLUDES2 Not included here
4th character required | 5th character required | 6th character required | 7th character required
Extension 'X' Alert | HAC Hospital-acquired condition (HAC) alert | AHA AHA Coding Clinic®

When symbols appear on a code that requires a 7th character extension, refer to Appendix D to identify applicable 7th character codes.

Encounters for other specific health care (Z40-Z53)

Categories Z40-Z53 are intended for use to indicate a reason for care. They may be used for patients who have already been treated for a disease or injury, but who are receiving aftercare or prophylactic care, or care to consolidate the treatment, or to deal with a residual state

EXCLUDES2 *follow-up examination for medical surveillance after treatment (Z08-Z09)*

Z40 Encounter for prophylactic surgery

EXCLUDES1 *organ donations (Z52.-)*
therapeutic organ removal-code to condition

Z40.0 Encounter for prophylactic surgery for risk factors related to malignant neoplasms

Admission for prophylactic organ removal
Use additional code to identify risk factor

Z40.00 Encounter for prophylactic removal of unspecified organ
Z40.01 Encounter for prophylactic removal of breast
Z40.02 Encounter for prophylactic removal of ovary ♀
Z40.09 Encounter for prophylactic removal of other organ

Z40.8 Encounter for other prophylactic surgery PDx
Z40.9 Encounter for prophylactic surgery, unspecified PDx

Z41 Encounter for procedures for purposes other than remedying health state

Z41.1 Encounter for cosmetic surgery POA

Encounter for cosmetic breast implant
Encounter for cosmetic procedure

EXCLUDES1 *encounter for plastic and reconstructive surgery following medical procedure or healed injury (Z42.-)*
encounter for post-mastectomy breast implantation (Z42.1)

Z41.2 Encounter for routine and ritual male circumcision POA ♂
Z41.3 Encounter for ear piercing POA PDx
Z41.8 Encounter for other procedures for purposes other than remedying health state POA
Z41.9 Encounter for procedure for purposes other than remedying health state, unspecified POA PDx

Z42 Encounter for plastic and reconstructive surgery following medical procedure or healed injury

EXCLUDES1 *encounter for cosmetic plastic surgery (Z41.1)*
encounter for plastic surgery for treatment of current injury - code to relevant injury

Z42.1 Encounter for breast reconstruction following mastectomy A POA Z

EXCLUDES1 *deformity and disproportion of reconstructed breast (N65.1-)*

Z42.8 Encounter for other plastic and reconstructive surgery following medical procedure or healed injury POA Z

Z43 Encounter for attention to artificial openings

INCLUDES *closure of artificial openings*
passage of sounds or bougies through artificial openings
reforming artificial openings
removal of catheter from artificial openings
toilet or cleansing of artificial openings

EXCLUDES1 *artificial opening status only, without need for care (Z93.-)*
complications of external stoma (J95.0-, K94.-, N99.5-)

EXCLUDES2 *fitting and adjustment of prosthetic and other devices (Z44-Z46)*

Z43.0 Encounter for attention to tracheostomy POA
Z43.1 Encounter for attention to gastrostomy CC POA
Z43.2 Encounter for attention to ileostomy POA
Z43.3 Encounter for attention to colostomy POA
Z43.4 Encounter for attention to other artificial openings of digestive tract POA
Z43.5 Encounter for attention to cystostomy POA
Z43.6 Encounter for attention to other artificial openings of urinary tract POA

Encounter for attention to nephrostomy
Encounter for attention to ureterostomy
Encounter for attention to urethrostomy

Z43.7 Encounter for attention to artificial vagina POA
Z43.8 Encounter for attention to other artificial openings POA
Z43.9 Encounter for attention to unspecified artificial opening POA PDx

Z44 Encounter for fitting and adjustment of external prosthetic device

INCLUDES *removal or replacement of external prosthetic device*

EXCLUDES1 *malfunction or other complications of device - see Alphabetical Index*
presence of prosthetic device (Z97.-)

Z44.0 Encounter for fitting and adjustment of artificial arm

Z44.00 Encounter for fitting and adjustment of unspecified artificial arm

Z44.001 Encounter for fitting and adjustment of unspecified right artificial arm POA
Z44.002 Encounter for fitting and adjustment of unspecified left artificial arm POA
Z44.009 Encounter for fitting and adjustment of unspecified artificial arm, unspecified arm POA

Z44.01 Encounter for fitting and adjustment of complete artificial arm

Z44.011 Encounter for fitting and adjustment of complete right artificial arm POA
Z44.012 Encounter for fitting and adjustment of complete left artificial arm POA
Z44.019 Encounter for fitting and adjustment of complete artificial arm, unspecified arm POA

Z44.02 Encounter for fitting and adjustment of partial artificial arm

Z44.021 Encounter for fitting and adjustment of partial artificial right arm POA
Z44.022 Encounter for fitting and adjustment of partial artificial left arm POA
Z44.029 Encounter for fitting and adjustment of partial artificial arm, unspecified arm POA

Z44.1 Encounter for fitting and adjustment of artificial leg

Z44.10 Encounter for fitting and adjustment of unspecified artificial leg

Z44.101 Encounter for fitting and adjustment of unspecified right artificial leg POA
Z44.102 Encounter for fitting and adjustment of unspecified left artificial leg POA
Z44.109 Encounter for fitting and adjustment of unspecified artificial leg, unspecified leg POA

Z44.11 Encounter for fitting and adjustment of complete artificial leg

Z44.111 Encounter for fitting and adjustment of complete right artificial leg POA
Z44.112 Encounter for fitting and adjustment of complete left artificial leg POA
Z44.119 Encounter for fitting and adjustment of complete artificial leg, unspecified leg POA

Z44.12 Encounter for fitting and adjustment of partial artificial leg

Z44.121 Encounter for fitting and adjustment of partial artificial right leg POA
Z44.122 Encounter for fitting and adjustment of partial artificial left leg POA
Z44.129 Encounter for fitting and adjustment of partial artificial leg, unspecified leg POA

Z44.2 Encounter for fitting and adjustment of artificial eye

EXCLUDES1 *mechanical complication of ocular prosthesis (T85.3)*

Z44.20 Encounter for fitting and adjustment of artificial eye, unspecified POA
Z44.21 Encounter for fitting and adjustment of artificial right eye POA
Z44.22 Encounter for fitting and adjustment of artificial left eye POA

Z44.3 Encounter for fitting and adjustment of external breast prosthesis

EXCLUDES1 *complications of breast implant (T85.4-)*
encounter for adjustment or removal of breast implant (Z45.81-)
encounter for initial breast implant insertion for cosmetic breast augmentation (Z41.1)
encounter for breast reconstruction following mastectomy (Z42.1)

PDx Unacceptable principal diagnosis symbol per Medicare code edits — POA Code exempt from diagnosis present on admission requirement
? Questionable admission — CC Complication or comorbidity — CC/MCC Exc CC/MCC exclusion — MCC Major complication or comorbidity
PDx CC Principal diagnosis as its own CC — PDx MCC Principal diagnosis as its own MCC — Z Z code as first-listed diagnosis

Z44.30 Encounter for fitting and adjustment of external breast prosthesis, unspecified breast

Z44.31 Encounter for fitting and adjustment of external right breast prosthesis

Z44.32 Encounter for fitting and adjustment of external left breast prosthesis

Z44.8 Encounter for fitting and adjustment of other external prosthetic devices

Z44.9 Encounter for fitting and adjustment of unspecified external prosthetic device

Z45 Encounter for adjustment and management of implanted device

INCLUDES *removal or replacement of implanted device*

EXCLUDES1 *malfunction or other complications of device - see Alphabetical Index*

presence of prosthetic and other devices (Z95-Z97)

EXCLUDES2 *encounter for fitting and adjustment of non-implanted device (Z46.-)*

Z45.0 Encounter for adjustment and management of cardiac device

Z45.01 Encounter for adjustment and management of cardiac pacemaker

Encounter for adjustment and management of cardiac resynchronization therapy pacemaker (CRT-P)

EXCLUDES1 *encounter for adjustment and management of automatic implantable cardiac defibrillator with synchronous cardiac pacemaker (Z45.02)*

Z45.010 Encounter for checking and testing of cardiac pacemaker pulse generator [battery]

Encounter for replacing cardiac pacemaker pulse generator [battery]

Z45.018 Encounter for adjustment and management of other part of cardiac pacemaker

Z45.02 Encounter for adjustment and management of automatic implantable cardiac defibrillator

Encounter for adjustment and management of automatic implantable cardiac defibrillator with synchronous cardiac pacemaker

Encounter for adjustment and management of cardiac resynchronization therapy defibrillator (CRT-D)

Z45.09 Encounter for adjustment and management of other cardiac device

Z45.1 Encounter for adjustment and management of infusion pump

Z45.2 Encounter for adjustment and management of vascular access device

Encounter for adjustment and management of vascular catheters

EXCLUDES1 *encounter for adjustment and management of renal dialysis catheter (Z49.01)*

Z45.3 Encounter for adjustment and management of implanted devices of the special senses

Z45.31 Encounter for adjustment and management of implanted visual substitution device

Z45.32 Encounter for adjustment and management of implanted hearing device

EXCLUDES1 *Encounter for fitting and adjustment of hearing aide (Z46.1)*

Z45.320 Encounter for adjustment and management of bone conduction device

Z45.321 Encounter for adjustment and management of cochlear device

Z45.328 Encounter for adjustment and management of other implanted hearing device

Z45.4 Encounter for adjustment and management of implanted nervous system device

Z45.41 Encounter for adjustment and management of cerebrospinal fluid drainage device

Encounter for adjustment and management of cerebral ventricular (communicating) shunt

Z45.42 Encounter for adjustment and management of neuropacemaker (brain) (peripheral nerve) (spinal cord)

Z45.49 Encounter for adjustment and management of other implanted nervous system device

Z45.8 Encounter for adjustment and management of other implanted devices

Z45.81 Encounter for adjustment or removal of breast implant

Encounter for elective implant exchange (different material) (different size)

Encounter removal of tissue expander without synchronous insertion of permanent implant

EXCLUDES1 *complications of breast implant (T85.4-)*

encounter for initial breast implant insertion for cosmetic breast augmentation (Z41.1)

encounter for breast reconstruction following mastectomy (Z42.1)

Z45.811 Encounter for adjustment or removal of right breast implant

Z45.812 Encounter for adjustment or removal of left breast implant

Z45.819 Encounter for adjustment or removal of unspecified breast implant

Z45.82 Encounter for adjustment or removal of myringotomy device (stent) (tube)

Z45.89 Encounter for adjustment and management of other implanted devices

Z45.9 Encounter for adjustment and management of unspecified implanted device

Z46 Encounter for fitting and adjustment of other devices

INCLUDES *removal or replacement of other device*

EXCLUDES1 *malfunction or other complications of device - see Alphabetical Index*

EXCLUDES2 *encounter for fitting and management of implanted devices (Z45.-)*

issue of repeat prescription only (Z76.0)

presence of prosthetic and other devices (Z95-Z97)

Z46.0 Encounter for fitting and adjustment of spectacles and contact lenses

Z46.1 Encounter for fitting and adjustment of hearing aid

EXCLUDES1 *encounter for adjustment and management of implanted hearing device (Z45.32-)*

Z46.2 Encounter for fitting and adjustment of other devices related to nervous system and special senses

EXCLUDES2 *encounter for adjustment and management of implanted nervous system device (Z45.4-)*

encounter for adjustment and management of implanted visual substitution device (Z45.31)

Z46.3 Encounter for fitting and adjustment of dental prosthetic device

Encounter for fitting and adjustment of dentures

Z46.4 Encounter for fitting and adjustment of orthodontic device

Z46.5 Encounter for fitting and adjustment of other gastrointestinal appliance and device

EXCLUDES1 *encounter for attention to artificial openings of digestive tract (Z43.1-Z43.4)*

Z46.51 Encounter for fitting and adjustment of gastric lap band

Z46.59 Encounter for fitting and adjustment of other gastrointestinal appliance and device

Z46.6 Encounter for fitting and adjustment of urinary device

EXCLUDES2 *attention to artificial openings of urinary tract (Z43.5, Z43.6)*

Z46.8 Encounter for fitting and adjustment of other specified devices

Z46.81 Encounter for fitting and adjustment of insulin pump

Encounter for insulin pump instruction and training

Encounter for insulin pump titration

Z46.82 Encounter for fitting and adjustment of non-vascular catheter

Z46.89 Encounter for fitting and adjustment of other specified devices

Encounter for fitting and adjustment of wheelchair

Unspecified Code Other Specified Code Manifestation Code N Newborn P Pediatric M Maternity A Adult ♂ Male ♀ Female
● New Code ▲ Revised Code Title ►◄ Revised Text NOTES INCLUDES EXCLUDES1 Not coded here EXCLUDES2 Not included here
4th character required 5th character required 6th character required 7th character required
Extension 'X' Alert HAC Hospital-acquired condition (HAC) alert AHA AHA Coding Clinic©

Z46.9 **Encounter for fitting and adjustment of unspecified device**

Z47 Orthopedic aftercare

EXCLUDES1 *aftercare for healing fracture-code to fracture with 7th character D*

Z47.1 **Aftercare following joint replacement surgery**
Use additional code to identify the joint (Z96.6-)

Z47.2 **Encounter for removal of internal fixation device**

EXCLUDES1 *encounter for adjustment of internal fixation device for fracture treatment- code to fracture with appropriate 7th character*
encounter for removal of external fixation device- code to fracture with 7th character D
infection or inflammatory reaction to internal fixation device (T84.6-)
mechanical complication of internal fixation device (T84.1-)

Z47.3 **Aftercare following explantation of joint prosthesis**
Aftercare following explantation of joint prosthesis, staged procedure
Encounter for joint prosthesis insertion following prior explantation of joint prosthesis
AHA: Q1, 2015

Z47.31 **Aftercare following explantation of shoulder joint prosthesis**

EXCLUDES1 *acquired absence of shoulder joint following prior explantation of shoulder joint prosthesis (Z89.23-)*
shoulder joint prosthesis explantation status (Z89.23-)

Z47.32 **Aftercare following explantation of hip joint prosthesis**

EXCLUDES1 *acquired absence of hip joint following prior explantation of hip joint prosthesis (Z89.62-)*
hip joint prosthesis explantation status (Z89.62-)
AHA: Q1, 2015

Z47.33 **Aftercare following explantation of knee joint prosthesis**

EXCLUDES1 *acquired absence of knee joint following prior explantation of knee prosthesis (Z89.52-*
knee joint prosthesis explantation status (Z89.52-)

Z47.8 **Encounter for other orthopedic aftercare**

Z47.81 **Encounter for orthopedic aftercare following surgical amputation**
Use additional code to identify the limb amputated (Z89.-)

Z47.82 **Encounter for orthopedic aftercare following scoliosis surgery**

Z47.89 **Encounter for other orthopedic aftercare**
AHA: Q1, 2015

Z48 Encounter for other postprocedural aftercare

EXCLUDES1 *encounter for follow-up examination after completed treatment (Z08-Z09)*

EXCLUDES2 *encounter for attention to artificial openings (Z43.-)*
encounter for fitting and adjustment of prosthetic and other devices (Z44-Z46)

Z48.0 **Encounter for attention to dressings, sutures and drains**

EXCLUDES1 *encounter for planned postprocedural wound closure (Z48.1)*

Z48.00 **Encounter for change or removal of nonsurgical wound dressing**
Encounter for change or removal of wound dressing NOS

Z48.01 **Encounter for change or removal of surgical wound dressing**
AHA: Q4, 2015

Z48.02 **Encounter for removal of sutures**
Encounter for removal of staples
AHA: Q1, 2015

Z48.03 **Encounter for change or removal of drains**

Z48.1 **Encounter for planned postprocedural wound closure**

EXCLUDES1 *encounter for attention to dressings and sutures (Z48.0-)*

Z48.2 **Encounter for aftercare following organ transplant**

Z48.21 **Encounter for aftercare following heart transplant**

Z48.22 **Encounter for aftercare following kidney transplant**

Z48.23 **Encounter for aftercare following liver transplant**

Z48.24 **Encounter for aftercare following lung transplant**

Z48.28 **Encounter for aftercare following multiple organ transplant**

Z48.280 **Encounter for aftercare following heart-lung transplant**

Z48.288 **Encounter for aftercare following multiple organ transplant**

Z48.29 **Encounter for aftercare following other organ transplant**

Z48.290 **Encounter for aftercare following bone marrow transplant**

Z48.298 **Encounter for aftercare following other organ transplant**

Z48.3 **Aftercare following surgery for neoplasm**
Use additional code to identify the neoplasm

Z48.8 **Encounter for other specified postprocedural aftercare**

Z48.81 **Encounter for surgical aftercare following surgery on specified body systems**
These codes identify the body system requiring aftercare. They are for use in conjunction with other aftercare codes to fully explain the aftercare encounter. The condition treated should also be coded if still present.

EXCLUDES1 *aftercare for injury- code the injury with 7th character D*
aftercare following surgery for neoplasm (Z48.3)

EXCLUDES2 *aftercare following organ transplant (Z48.2-)*
orthopedic aftercare (Z47.-)

Z48.810 **Encounter for surgical aftercare following surgery on the sense organs**

Z48.811 **Encounter for surgical aftercare following surgery on the nervous system**

EXCLUDES2 *encounter for surgical aftercare following surgery on the sense organs (Z48.810)*

Z48.812 **Encounter for surgical aftercare following surgery on the circulatory system**
AHA: Q4, 2012

Z48.813 **Encounter for surgical aftercare following surgery on the respiratory system**

Z48.814 **Encounter for surgical aftercare following surgery on the teeth or oral cavity**

Z48.815 **Encounter for surgical aftercare following surgery on the digestive system**
AHA: Q4, 2015

Z48.816 **Encounter for surgical aftercare following surgery on the genitourinary system**

EXCLUDES1 *encounter for aftercare following sterilization reversal (Z31.42)*

Z48.817 **Encounter for surgical aftercare following surgery on the skin and subcutaneous tissue**
AHA: Q1, 2015

Z48.89 **Encounter for other specified surgical aftercare**

Z49 Encounter for care involving renal dialysis
Code also associated end stage renal disease (N18.6)

Z49.0 **Preparatory care for renal dialysis**
Encounter for dialysis instruction and training

Z49.01 **Encounter for fitting and adjustment of extracorporeal dialysis catheter**
Removal or replacement of renal dialysis catheter
Toilet or cleansing of renal dialysis catheter

Z49.02 **Encounter for fitting and adjustment of peritoneal dialysis catheter**

PDx Unacceptable principal diagnosis symbol per Medicare code edits — POA Code exempt from diagnosis present on admission requirement
Questionable admission — CC Complication or comorbidity — CC/MCC Exc CC/MCC exclusion — MCC Major complication or comorbidity
PDx CC Principal diagnosis as its own CC — PDx MCC Principal diagnosis as its own MCC — Z1 Z code as first-listed diagnosis

Z49.3 Encounter for adequacy testing for dialysis
Z49.31 Encounter for adequacy testing for hemodialysis
Z49.32 Encounter for adequacy testing for peritoneal dialysis
Encounter for peritoneal equilibration test

▲ Z51 Encounter for other aftercare ▶and medical care◀
Code also condition requiring care
EXCLUDES1 *follow-up examination after treatment (Z08-Z09)*
Z51.0 Encounter for antineoplastic radiation therapy
Z51.1 Encounter for antineoplastic chemotherapy and immunotherapy
EXCLUDES2 *encounter for chemotherapy and immunotherapy for nonneoplastic condition - code to condition*
Z51.11 Encounter for antineoplastic chemotherapy
AHA: Q3, 2015
Z51.12 Encounter for antineoplastic immunotherapy
Z51.5 Encounter for palliative care
● Z51.6 Encounter for desensitization to allergens
Z51.8 Encounter for other specified aftercare
EXCLUDES1 *holiday relief care (Z75.5)*
Z51.81 Encounter for therapeutic drug level monitoring
Code also any long-term (current) drug therapy (Z79.-)
EXCLUDES1 *encounter for blood-drug test for administrative or medicolegal reasons (Z02.83)*
Z51.89 Encounter for other specified aftercare
AHA: Q4, 2012

Z52 Donors of organs and tissues
INCLUDES *autologous and other living donors*
EXCLUDES1 *cadaveric donor - omit code*
examination of potential donor (Z00.5)
AHA: Q4, 2012
Z52.0 Blood donor
Z52.00 Unspecified blood donor
Z52.000 Unspecified donor, whole blood
Z52.001 Unspecified donor, stem cells
Z52.008 Unspecified donor, other blood
Z52.01 Autologous blood donor
Z52.010 Autologous donor, whole blood
Z52.011 Autologous donor, stem cells
Z52.018 Autologous donor, other blood
Z52.09 Other blood donor
Volunteer donor
Z52.090 Other blood donor, whole blood
Z52.091 Other blood donor, stem cells
Z52.098 Other blood donor, other blood
Z52.1 Skin donor
Z52.10 Skin donor, unspecified
Z52.11 Skin donor, autologous
Z52.19 Skin donor, other
Z52.2 Bone donor
Z52.20 Bone donor, unspecified
Z52.21 Bone donor, autologous
Z52.29 Bone donor, other
Z52.3 Bone marrow donor
Z52.4 Kidney donor
Z52.5 Cornea donor
Z52.6 Liver donor
AHA Q4, 2012
Z52.8 Donor of other specified organs or tissues
Z52.81 Egg (Oocyte) donor
Z52.810 Egg (Oocyte) donor under age 35, anonymous recipient
Egg donor under age 35 NOS
Z52.811 Egg (Oocyte) donor under age 35, designated recipient
Z52.812 Egg (Oocyte) donor age 35 and over, anonymous recipient
Egg donor age 35 and over NOS
Z52.813 Egg (Oocyte) donor age 35 and over, designated recipient
Z52.819 Egg (Oocyte) donor, unspecified
Z52.89 Donor of other specified organs or tissues
Z52.9 Donor of unspecified organ or tissue
Donor NOS

Z53 Persons encountering health services for specific procedures and treatment, not carried out
Z53.0 Procedure and treatment not carried out because of contraindication
Z53.01 Procedure and treatment not carried out due to patient smoking
Z53.09 Procedure and treatment not carried out because of other contraindication
Z53.1 Procedure and treatment not carried out because of patient's decision for reasons of belief and group pressure
Z53.2 Procedure and treatment not carried out because of patient's decision for other and unspecified reasons
Z53.20 Procedure and treatment not carried out because of patient's decision for unspecified reasons
Z53.21 Procedure and treatment not carried out due to patient leaving prior to being seen by health care provider
Z53.29 Procedure and treatment not carried out because of patient's decision for other reasons
● Z53.3 Procedure converted to open procedure
● Z53.31 Laparoscopic surgical procedure converted to open procedure
● Z53.32 Thoracoscopic surgical procedure converted to open procedure
● Z53.33 Arthroscopic surgical procedure converted to open procedure
● Z53.39 Other specified procedure converted to open procedure
Z53.8 Procedure and treatment not carried out for other reasons
Z53.9 Procedure and treatment not carried out, unspecified reason

Persons with potential health hazards related to socioeconomic and psychosocial circumstances (Z55-Z65)

Z55 Problems related to education and literacy
EXCLUDES1 *disorders of psychological development (F80-F89)*
Z55.0 Illiteracy and low-level literacy
Z55.1 Schooling unavailable and unattainable
Z55.2 Failed school examinations
Z55.3 Underachievement in school
Z55.4 Educational maladjustment and discord with teachers and classmates
Z55.8 Other problems related to education and literacy
Problems related to inadequate teaching
Z55.9 Problems related to education and literacy, unspecified
Academic problems NOS

Z56 Problems related to employment and unemployment
EXCLUDES2 *occupational exposure to risk factors (Z57.-)*
problems related to housing and economic circumstances (Z59.-)
Z56.0 Unemployment, unspecified
Z56.1 Change of job
Z56.2 Threat of job loss
Z56.3 Stressful work schedule
Z56.4 Discord with boss and workmates
Z56.5 Uncongenial work environment
Difficult conditions at work

Unspecified Code Other Specified Code Manifestation Code N Newborn P Pediatric M Maternity A Adult ♂ Male ♀ Female
● New Code ▲ Revised Code Title ▶◀ Revised Text NOTES INCLUDES EXCLUDES1 Not coded here EXCLUDES2 Not included here
4th character required 5th character required 6th character required 7th character required
Extension 'X' Alert HAC Hospital-acquired condition (HAC) alert AHA AHA Coding Clinic©

Z56.6 Other physical and mental strain related to work
Z56.8 Other problems related to employment
Z56.81 Sexual harassment on the job
Z56.82 Military deployment status
Individual (civilian or military) currently deployed in theater or in support of military war, peacekeeping and humanitarian operations
Z56.89 Other problems related to employment
Z56.9 Unspecified problems related to employment
Occupational problems NOS

Z57 Occupational exposure to risk factors
Z57.0 Occupational exposure to noise
Z57.1 Occupational exposure to radiation
Z57.2 Occupational exposure to dust
Z57.3 Occupational exposure to other air contaminants
Z57.31 Occupational exposure to environmental tobacco smoke
EXCLUDES2 *exposure to environmental tobacco smoke (Z77.22)*
Z57.39 Occupational exposure to other air contaminants
Z57.4 Occupational exposure to toxic agents in agriculture
Occupational exposure to solids, liquids, gases or vapors in agriculture
Z57.5 Occupational exposure to toxic agents in other industries
Occupational exposure to solids, liquids, gases or vapors in other industries
Z57.6 Occupational exposure to extreme temperature
Z57.7 Occupational exposure to vibration
Z57.8 Occupational exposure to other risk factors
Z57.9 Occupational exposure to unspecified risk factor

Z59 Problems related to housing and economic circumstances
EXCLUDES2 *problems related to upbringing (Z62.-)*
Z59.0 Homelessness
Z59.1 Inadequate housing
Lack of heating
Restriction of space
Technical defects in home preventing adequate care
Unsatisfactory surroundings
EXCLUDES1 *problems related to the natural and physical environment (Z77.1-)*
Z59.2 Discord with neighbors, lodgers and landlord
Z59.3 Problems related to living in residential institution
Boarding-school resident
EXCLUDES1 *institutional upbringing (Z62.2)*
Z59.4 Lack of adequate food and safe drinking water
Inadequate drinking water supply
EXCLUDES1 *effects of hunger (T73.0)*
inappropriate diet or eating habits (Z72.4)
malnutrition (E40-E46)
Z59.5 Extreme poverty
Z59.6 Low income
Z59.7 Insufficient social insurance and welfare support
Z59.8 Other problems related to housing and economic circumstances
Foreclosure on loan
Isolated dwelling
Problems with creditors
Z59.9 Problem related to housing and economic circumstances, unspecified

Z60 Problems related to social environment
Z60.0 Problems of adjustment to life-cycle transitions
Empty nest syndrome
Phase of life problem
Problem with adjustment to retirement [pension]
Z60.2 Problems related to living alone
Z60.3 Acculturation difficulty
Problem with migration
Problem with social transplantation
Z60.4 Social exclusion and rejection
Exclusion and rejection on the basis of personal characteristics, such as unusual physical appearance, illness or behavior.
EXCLUDES1 *target of adverse discrimination such as for racial or religious reasons (Z60.5)*
Z60.5 Target of (perceived) adverse discrimination and persecution
EXCLUDES1 *social exclusion and rejection (Z60.4)*
Z60.8 Other problems related to social environment
Z60.9 Problem related to social environment, unspecified

Z62 Problems related to upbringing
INCLUDES *current and past negative life events in childhood*
current and past problems of a child related to upbringing
EXCLUDES2 *maltreatment syndrome (T74.-)*
problems related to housing and economic circumstances (Z59.-)
Z62.0 Inadequate parental supervision and control
Z62.1 Parental overprotection
Z62.2 Upbringing away from parents
EXCLUDES1 *problems with boarding school (Z59.3)*
Z62.21 Child in welfare custody
Child in care of non-parental family member
Child in foster care
EXCLUDES2 *problem for parent due to child in welfare custody (Z63.5)*
Z62.22 Institutional upbringing
Child living in orphanage or group home
Z62.29 Other upbringing away from parents
Z62.3 Hostility towards and scapegoating of child
Z62.6 Inappropriate (excessive) parental pressure
Z62.8 Other specified problems related to upbringing
Z62.81 Personal history of abuse in childhood
Z62.810 Personal history of physical and sexual abuse in childhood
EXCLUDES1 *current child physical abuse (T74.12, T76.12)*
current child sexual abuse (T74.22, T76.22)
Z62.811 Personal history of psychological abuse in childhood
EXCLUDES1 *current child psychological abuse (T74.32, T76.32)*
Z62.812 Personal history of neglect in childhood
EXCLUDES1 *current child neglect (T74.02, T76.02)*
Z62.819 Personal history of unspecified abuse in childhood
EXCLUDES1 *current child abuse NOS (T74.92, T76.92)*
Z62.82 Parent-child conflict
Z62.820 Parent-biological child conflict
Parent-child problem NOS
Z62.821 Parent-adopted child conflict
Z62.822 Parent-foster child conflict
Z62.89 Other specified problems related to upbringing
Z62.890 Parent-child estrangement NEC
Z62.891 Sibling rivalry
Z62.898 Other specified problems related to upbringing
Z62.9 Problem related to upbringing, unspecified

Z63 Other problems related to primary support group, including family circumstances
EXCLUDES2 *maltreatment syndrome (T74.-, T76)*
parent-child problems (Z62.-)
problems related to negative life events in childhood (Z62.-)
problems related to upbringing (Z62.-)
Z63.0 Problems in relationship with spouse or partner
EXCLUDES1 *counseling for spousal or partner abuse problems (Z69.1)*
counseling related to sexual attitude, behavior, and orientation (Z70.-)
Z63.1 Problems in relationship with in-laws
Z63.3 Absence of family member
EXCLUDES1 *absence of family member due to disappearance and death (Z63.4)*

PDx Unacceptable principal diagnosis symbol per Medicare code edits; POA Code exempt from diagnosis present on admission requirement
Q Questionable admission; CC Complication or comorbidity; CC/MCC Exc CC/MCC exclusion; MCC Major complication or comorbidity
Principal diagnosis as its own CC; Principal diagnosis as its own MCC; Z1 Z code as first-listed diagnosis

absence of family member due to separation and divorce (Z63.5)

Z63.31 **Absence of family member due to military deployment**
Individual or family affected by other family member being on military deployment
EXCLUDES1 *family disruption due to return of family member from military deployment (Z63.71)*

Z63.32 **Other absence of family member**

Z63.4 **Disappearance and death of family member**
Assumed death of family member
Bereavement

Z63.5 **Disruption of family by separation and divorce**
Marital estrangement

Z63.6 **Dependent relative needing care at home**

Z63.7 **Other stressful life events affecting family and household**

Z63.71 **Stress on family due to return of family member from military deployment**
Individual or family affected by family member having returned from military deployment (current or past conflict)

Z63.72 **Alcoholism and drug addiction in family**

Z63.79 **Other stressful life events affecting family and household**
Anxiety (normal) about sick person in family
Health problems within family
Ill or disturbed family member
Isolated family

Z63.8 **Other specified problems related to primary support group**
Family discord NOS
Family estrangement NOS
High expressed emotional level within family
Inadequate family support NOS
Inadequate or distorted communication within family

Z63.9 **Problem related to primary support group, unspecified**
Relationship disorder NOS

Z64 **Problems related to certain psychosocial circumstances**

Z64.0 **Problems related to unwanted pregnancy**

Z64.1 **Problems related to multiparity**

Z64.4 **Discord with counselors**
Discord with probation officer
Discord with social worker

Z65 **Problems related to other psychosocial circumstances**

Z65.0 **Conviction in civil and criminal proceedings without imprisonment**

Z65.1 **Imprisonment and other incarceration**

Z65.2 **Problems related to release from prison**

Z65.3 **Problems related to other legal circumstances**
Arrest
Child custody or support proceedings
Litigation
Prosecution

Z65.4 **Victim of crime and terrorism**
Victim of torture

Z65.5 **Exposure to disaster, war and other hostilities**
EXCLUDES1 *target of perceived discrimination or persecution (Z60.5)*

Z65.8 **Other specified problems related to psychosocial circumstances**

Z65.9 **Problem related to unspecified psychosocial circumstances**

Do not resuscitate status (Z66)

Z66 **Do not resuscitate**
DNR status

Blood type (Z67)

Z67 **Blood type**
AHA: Q3, 2015

Z67.1 Type A **blood**

Z67.10 **Type A blood,** Rh positive

Z67.11 **Type A blood,** Rh negative

Z67.2 Type B **blood**

Z67.20 **Type B blood,** Rh positive

Z67.21 **Type B blood,** Rh negative

Z67.3 Type AB **blood**

Z67.30 **Type AB blood,** Rh positive

Z67.31 **Type AB blood,** Rh negative

Z67.4 Type O **blood**

Z67.40 **Type O blood,** Rh positive

Z67.41 **Type O blood,** Rh negative

Z67.9 Unspecified **blood type**

Z67.90 **Unspecified blood type,** Rh positive

Z67.91 **Unspecified blood type,** Rh negative
AHA: Q3, 2015

Body mass index [BMI] (Z68)

Z68 **Body mass index [BMI]**
Kilograms per meters squared
NOTES BMI adult codes are for use for persons 21 years of age or older
BMI pediatric codes are for use for persons 2-20 years of age. These percentiles are based on the growth charts published by the Centers for Disease Control and Prevention (CDC)

Z68.1 **Body mass index (BMI)** 19 or less**, adult**

Z68.2 **Body mass index (BMI)** 20-29**, adult**

Z68.20 **Body mass index (BMI)** 20.0-20.9**, adult**

Z68.21 **Body mass index (BMI)** 21.0-21.9**, adult**

Z68.22 **Body mass index (BMI)** 22.0-22.9**, adult**

Z68.23 **Body mass index (BMI)** 23.0-23.9**, adult**

Z68.24 **Body mass index (BMI)** 24.0-24.9**, adult**

Z68.25 **Body mass index (BMI)** 25.0-25.9**, adult**

Z68.26 **Body mass index (BMI)** 26.0-26.9**, adult**

Z68.27 **Body mass index (BMI)** 27.0-27.9**, adult**

Z68.28 **Body mass index (BMI)** 28.0-28.9**, adult**

Z68.29 **Body mass index (BMI)** 29.0-29.9**, adult**

Z68.3 **Body mass index (BMI)** 30-39**, adult**

Z68.30 **Body mass index (BMI)** 30.0-30.9**, adult**

Z68.31 **Body mass index (BMI)** 31.0-31.9**, adult**

Z68.32 **Body mass index (BMI)** 32.0-32.9**, adult**

Z68.33 **Body mass index (BMI)** 33.0-33.9**, adult**

Z68.34 **Body mass index (BMI)** 34.0-34.9**, adult**

Z68.35 **Body mass index (BMI)** 35.0-35.9**, adult**

Z68.36 **Body mass index (BMI)** 36.0-36.9**, adult**

Z68.37 **Body mass index (BMI)** 37.0-37.9**, adult**

Z68.38 **Body mass index (BMI)** 38.0-38.9**, adult**

Z68.39 **Body mass index (BMI)** 39.0-39.9**, adult**

Z68.4 **Body mass index (BMI)** 40 or greater**, adult**

Z68.41 **Body mass index (BMI)** 40.0-44.9**, adult**

Z68.42 **Body mass index (BMI)** 45.0-49.9**, adult**

Z68.43 **Body mass index (BMI)** 50-59.9 **, adult**

Z68.44 **Body mass index (BMI)** 60.0-69.9**, adult**

Z68.45 **Body mass index (BMI)** 70 or greater**, adult**

Z68.5 **Body mass index (BMI)** pediatric

Z68.51 **Body mass index (BMI) pediatric,** less than 5th percentile for age

Z68.52 **Body mass index (BMI) pediatric,** 5th percentile to less than 85th percentile for age

Z68.53 **Body mass index (BMI) pediatric,** 85th percentile to less than 95th percentile for age

Z68.54 **Body mass index (BMI) pediatric,** greater than or equal to 95th percentile for age

Persons encountering health services in other circumstances (Z69-Z76)

Z69 **Encounter for mental health services for victim and perpetrator of abuse**
INCLUDES *counseling for victims and perpetrators of abuse*

Z69.0 **Encounter for mental health services for** child **abuse problems**

Unspecified Code Other Specified Code Manifestation Code N Newborn P Pediatric M Maternity A Adult ♂ Male ♀ Female
● New Code ▲ Revised Code Title ►◄ Revised Text NOTES INCLUDES EXCLUDES1 Not coded here EXCLUDES2 Not included here
4th character required 5th character required 6th character required 7th character required
Extension 'X' Alert HAC Hospital-acquired condition (HAC) alert AHA AHA Coding Clinic©

Z69.01 Encounter for mental health services for parental child abuse
- Z69.010 Encounter for mental health services for victim of parental child abuse
- Z69.011 Encounter for mental health services for perpetrator of parental child abuse
  - EXCLUDES1 *encounter for mental health services for non-parental child abuse (Z69.02-)*

Z69.02 Encounter for mental health services for non-parental child abuse
- Z69.020 Encounter for mental health services for victim of non-parental child abuse
- Z69.021 Encounter for mental health services for perpetrator of non-parental child abuse

Z69.1 Encounter for mental health services for spousal or partner abuse problems
- Z69.11 Encounter for mental health services for victim of spousal or partner abuse
- Z69.12 Encounter for mental health services for perpetrator of spousal or partner abuse

Z69.8 Encounter for mental health services for victim or perpetrator of other abuse
- Z69.81 Encounter for mental health services for victim of other abuse
  - Encounter for rape victim counseling
- Z69.82 Encounter for mental health services for perpetrator of other abuse

Z70 Counseling related to sexual attitude, behavior and orientation

INCLUDES *encounter for mental health services for sexual attitude, behavior and orientation*

EXCLUDES2 *contraceptive or procreative counseling (Z30-Z31)*

- Z70.0 Counseling related to sexual attitude
- Z70.1 Counseling related to patient's sexual behavior and orientation
  - Patient concerned regarding impotence
  - Patient concerned regarding non-responsiveness
  - Patient concerned regarding promiscuity
  - Patient concerned regarding sexual orientation
- Z70.2 Counseling related to sexual behavior and orientation of third party
  - Advice sought regarding sexual behavior and orientation of child
  - Advice sought regarding sexual behavior and orientation of partner
  - Advice sought regarding sexual behavior and orientation of spouse
- Z70.3 Counseling related to combined concerns regarding sexual attitude, behavior and orientation
- Z70.8 Other sex counseling
  - Encounter for sex education
- Z70.9 Sex counseling, unspecified

Z71 Persons encountering health services for other counseling and medical advice, not elsewhere classified

EXCLUDES2 *contraceptive or procreation counseling (Z30-Z31)*
sex counseling (Z70.-)

- Z71.0 Person encountering health services to consult on behalf of another person
  - Person encountering health services to seek advice or treatment for non-attending third party
  - EXCLUDES2 *anxiety (normal) about sick person in family (Z63.7)*
    expectant (adoptive) parent(s) pre-birth pediatrician visit (Z76.81)
- Z71.1 Person with feared health complaint in whom no diagnosis is made
  - Person encountering health services with feared condition which was not demonstrated
  - Person encountering health services in which problem was normal state
  - 'Worried well'
  - EXCLUDES1 *medical observation for suspected diseases and conditions proven not to exist (Z03.-)*
- Z71.2 Person consulting for explanation of examination or test findings
- Z71.3 Dietary counseling and surveillance
  - Use additional code for any associated underlying medical condition
  - Use additional code to identify body mass index (BMI), if known (Z68.-)
- Z71.4 Alcohol abuse counseling and surveillance
  - Use additional code for alcohol abuse or dependence (F10.-)
  - Z71.41 Alcohol abuse counseling and surveillance of alcoholic
  - Z71.42 Counseling for family member of alcoholic
    - Counseling for significant other, partner, or friend of alcoholic
- Z71.5 Drug abuse counseling and surveillance
  - Use additional code for drug abuse or dependence (F11-F16, F18-F19)
  - Z71.51 Drug abuse counseling and surveillance of drug abuser
  - Z71.52 Counseling for family member of drug abuser
    - Counseling for significant other, partner, or friend of drug abuser
- Z71.6 Tobacco abuse counseling
  - Use additional code for nicotine dependence (F17.-)
- Z71.7 Human immunodeficiency virus [HIV] counseling
- Z71.8 Other specified counseling
  - EXCLUDES2 *counseling for contraception (Z30.0-)*
    counseling for genetics (Z31.5)
    counseling for procreative management (Z31.6-)
  - Z71.81 Spiritual or religious counseling
  - Z71.89 Other specified counseling
- Z71.9 Counseling, unspecified
  - Encounter for medical advice NOS

Z72 Problems related to lifestyle

EXCLUDES2 *problems related to life-management difficulty (Z73.-)*
problems related to socioeconomic and psychosocial circumstances (Z55-Z65)

- Z72.0 Tobacco use
  - Tobacco use NOS
  - EXCLUDES1 *history of tobacco dependence (Z87.891)*
    nicotine dependence (F17.2-)
    tobacco dependence (F17.2-)
    tobacco use during pregnancy (O99.33-)
- Z72.3 Lack of physical exercise
- Z72.4 Inappropriate diet and eating habits
  - EXCLUDES1 *behavioral eating disorders of infancy or childhood (F98.2.-F98.3)*
    eating disorders (F50.-)
    lack of adequate food (Z59.4)
    malnutrition and other nutritional deficiencies (E40-E64)
- Z72.5 High risk sexual behavior
  - Promiscuity
  - EXCLUDES1 *paraphilias (F65)*
  - Z72.51 High risk heterosexual behavior
  - Z72.52 High risk homosexual behavior
  - Z72.53 High risk bisexual behavior
- Z72.6 Gambling and betting
  - EXCLUDES1 *compulsive or pathological gambling (F63.0)*
- Z72.8 Other problems related to lifestyle
  - Z72.81 Antisocial behavior
    - EXCLUDES1 *conduct disorders (F91.-)*
    - Z72.810 Child and adolescent antisocial behavior
      - Antisocial behavior (child) (adolescent) without manifest psychiatric disorder
      - Delinquency NOS
      - Group delinquency
      - Offenses in the context of gang membership
      - Stealing in company with others
      - Truancy from school
    - Z72.811 Adult antisocial behavior
      - Adult antisocial behavior without manifest psychiatric disorder

Unacceptable principal diagnosis symbol per Medicare code edits | Code exempt from diagnosis present on admission requirement | Questionable admission | Complication or comorbidity | CC/MCC exclusion | Major complication or comorbidity | Principal diagnosis as its own CC | Principal diagnosis as its own MCC | Z code as first-listed diagnosis

Z72.82 Problems related to sleep
Z72.820 Sleep deprivation
Lack of adequate sleep
EXCLUDES1 *insomnia (G47.0-)*
Z72.821 Inadequate sleep hygiene
Bad sleep habits
Irregular sleep habits
Unhealthy sleep wake schedule
EXCLUDES1 *insomnia (F51.0-, G47.0-)*
Z72.89 Other problems related to lifestyle
Self-damaging behavior
Z72.9 Problem related to lifestyle, unspecified
Z73 Problems related to life management difficulty
EXCLUDES2 *problems related to socioeconomic and psychosocial circumstances (Z55-Z65)*
Z73.0 Burn-out
Z73.1 Type A behavior pattern
Z73.2 Lack of relaxation and leisure
Z73.3 Stress, not elsewhere classified
Physical and mental strain NOS
EXCLUDES1 *stress related to employment or unemployment (Z56.-)*
Z73.4 Inadequate social skills, not elsewhere classified
Z73.5 Social role conflict, not elsewhere classified
Z73.6 Limitation of activities due to disability
EXCLUDES1 *care-provider dependency (Z74.-)*
Z73.8 Other problems related to life management difficulty
Z73.81 Behavioral insomnia of childhood
Z73.810 Behavioral insomnia of childhood, sleep-onset association type
Z73.811 Behavioral insomnia of childhood, limit setting type
Z73.812 Behavioral insomnia of childhood, combined type
Z73.819 Behavioral insomnia of childhood, unspecified type
Z73.82 Dual sensory impairment
Z73.89 Other problems related to life management difficulty
Z73.9 Problem related to life management difficulty, unspecified
Z74 Problems related to care provider dependency
EXCLUDES2 *dependence on enabling machines or devices NEC (Z99.-)*
Z74.0 Reduced mobility
Z74.01 Bed confinement status
Bedridden
Z74.09 Other reduced mobility
Chair ridden
Reduced mobility NOS
EXCLUDES2 *wheelchair dependence (Z99.3)*
Z74.1 Need for assistance with personal care
Z74.2 Need for assistance at home and no other household member able to render care
Z74.3 Need for continuous supervision
Z74.8 Other problems related to care provider dependency
Z74.9 Problem related to care provider dependency, unspecified
Z75 Problems related to medical facilities and other health care
Z75.0 Medical services not available in home
EXCLUDES1 *no other household member able to render care (Z74.2)*
Z75.1 Person awaiting admission to adequate facility elsewhere
Z75.2 Other waiting period for investigation and treatment
Z75.3 Unavailability and inaccessibility of health-care facilities
EXCLUDES1 *bed unavailable (Z75.1)*
Z75.4 Unavailability and inaccessibility of other helping agencies
Z75.5 Holiday relief care
Z75.8 Other problems related to medical facilities and other health care
Z75.9 Unspecified problem related to medical facilities and other health care
Z76 Persons encountering health services in other circumstances
Z76.0 Encounter for issue of repeat prescription
Encounter for issue of repeat prescription for appliance
Encounter for issue of repeat prescription for medicaments
Encounter for issue of repeat prescription for spectacles
EXCLUDES2 *issue of medical certificate (Z02.7)*
repeat prescription for contraceptive (Z30.4-)
Z76.1 Encounter for health supervision and care of foundling
Z76.2 Encounter for health supervision and care of other healthy infant and child
Encounter for medical or nursing care or supervision of healthy infant under circumstances such as adverse socioeconomic conditions at home
Encounter for medical or nursing care or supervision of healthy infant under circumstances such as awaiting foster or adoptive placement
Encounter for medical or nursing care or supervision of healthy infant under circumstances such as maternal illness
Encounter for medical or nursing care or supervision of healthy infant under circumstances such as number of children at home preventing or interfering with normal care
Z76.3 Healthy person accompanying sick person
Z76.4 Other boarder to healthcare facility
EXCLUDES1 *homelessness (Z59.0)*
Z76.5 Malingerer [conscious simulation]
Person feigning illness (with obvious motivation)
EXCLUDES1 *factitious disorder (F68.1-)*
peregrinating patient (F68.1-)
Z76.8 Persons encountering health services in other specified circumstances
Z76.81 Expectant parent(s) prebirth pediatrician visit
Pre-adoption pediatrician visit for adoptive parent(s)
Z76.82 Awaiting organ transplant status
Patient waiting for organ availability
Z76.89 Persons encountering health services in other specified circumstances
Persons encountering health services NOS

Persons with potential health hazards related to family and personal history and certain conditions influencing health status (Z77-Z99)

Code also any follow-up examination (Z08-Z09)

Z77 Other contact with and (suspected) exposures hazardous to health
INCLUDES *contact with and (suspected) exposures to potential hazards to health*
EXCLUDES2 *contact with and (suspected) exposure to communicable diseases (Z20.-)*
exposure to (parental) (environmental) tobacco smoke in the perinatal period (P96.81)
►newborn affected◄ by noxious substances transmitted via placenta or breast milk (P04.-)
occupational exposure to risk factors (Z57.-)
retained foreign body (Z18.-)
retained foreign body fully removed (Z87.821)
toxic effects of substances chiefly nonmedicinal as to source (T51-T65)
Z77.0 Contact with and (suspected) exposure to hazardous, chiefly nonmedicinal, chemicals
Z77.01 Contact with and (suspected) exposure to hazardous metals
Z77.010 Contact with and (suspected) exposure to arsenic
Z77.011 Contact with and (suspected) exposure to lead
Z77.012 Contact with and (suspected) exposure to uranium
EXCLUDES1 *retained depleted uranium fragments (Z18.01)*
Z77.018 Contact with and (suspected) exposure to other hazardous metals
Contact with and (suspected) exposure to chromium compounds
Contact with and (suspected) exposure to nickel dust
Z77.02 Contact with and (suspected) exposure to hazardous aromatic compounds

Unspecified Code Other Specified Code Manifestation Code N Newborn P Pediatric M Maternity A Adult ♂ Male ♀ Female
● New Code ▲ Revised Code Title ►◄ Revised Text NOTES INCLUDES EXCLUDES1 Not coded here EXCLUDES2 Not included here
4th character required 5th character required 6th character required 7th character required
Extension 'X' Alert HAC Hospital-acquired condition (HAC) alert AHA AHA Coding Clinic©

Z77.020 Contact with and (suspected) exposure to aromatic amines

Z77.021 Contact with and (suspected) exposure to benzene

Z77.028 Contact with and (suspected) exposure to other hazardous aromatic compounds
Aromatic dyes NOS
Polycyclic aromatic hydrocarbons

Z77.09 Contact with and (suspected) exposure to other hazardous, chiefly nonmedicinal, chemicals

Z77.090 Contact with and (suspected) exposure to asbestos

Z77.098 Contact with and (suspected) exposure to other hazardous, chiefly nonmedicinal, chemicals
Dyes NOS

Z77.1 Contact with and (suspected) exposure to environmental pollution and hazards in the physical environment

Z77.11 Contact with and (suspected) exposure to environmental pollution

Z77.110 Contact with and (suspected) exposure to air pollution

Z77.111 Contact with and (suspected) exposure to water pollution

Z77.112 Contact with and (suspected) exposure to soil pollution

Z77.118 Contact with and (suspected) exposure to other environmental pollution

Z77.12 Contact with and (suspected) exposure to hazards in the physical environment

Z77.120 Contact with and (suspected) exposure to mold (toxic)

Z77.121 Contact with and (suspected) exposure to harmful algae and algae toxins
Contact with and (suspected) exposure to (harmful) algae bloom NOS
Contact with and (suspected) exposure to blue-green algae bloom
Contact with and (suspected) exposure to brown tide
Contact with and (suspected) exposure to cyanobacteria bloom
Contact with and (suspected) exposure to Florida red tide
Contact with and (suspected) exposure to pfiesteria piscicida
Contact with and (suspected) exposure to red tide

Z77.122 Contact with and (suspected) exposure to noise

Z77.123 Contact with and (suspected) exposure to radon and other naturally occuring radiation
EXCLUDES2 *radiation exposure as the cause of a confirmed condition (W88-W90, X39.0-)*
radiation sickness NOS (T66)

Z77.128 Contact with and (suspected) exposure to other hazards in the physical environment

Z77.2 Contact with and (suspected) exposure to other hazardous substances

Z77.21 Contact with and (suspected) exposure to potentially hazardous body fluids

Z77.22 Contact with and (suspected) exposure to environmental tobacco smoke (acute) (chronic)
Exposure to second hand tobacco smoke (acute) (chronic)
Passive smoking (acute) (chronic)
EXCLUDES1 *nicotine dependence (F17.-)*
tobacco use (Z72.0)
EXCLUDES2 *occupational exposure to environmental tobacco smoke (Z57.31)*

Z77.29 Contact with and (suspected) exposure to other hazardous substances
AHA: Q2 2016

Z77.9 Other contact with and (suspected) exposures hazardous to health

Z78 Other specified health status
EXCLUDES2 *asymptomatic human immunodeficiency virus [HIV] infection status (Z21)*
postprocedural status (Z93-Z99)
sex reassignment status (Z87.890)

Z78.0 Asymptomatic menopausal state
Menopausal state NOS
Postmenopausal status NOS
EXCLUDES2 *symptomatic menopausal state (N95.1)*

Z78.1 Physical restraint status
EXCLUDES1 *physical restraint due to a procedure - omit code*

Z78.9 Other specified health status

Z79 Long term (current) drug therapy
INCLUDES *long term (current) drug use for prophylactic purposes*
Code also any therapeutic drug level monitoring (Z51.81)
EXCLUDES2 *drug abuse and dependence (F11-F19)*
drug use complicating pregnancy, childbirth, and the puerperium (O99.32-)
long term (current) use of oral antidiabetic drugs (Z79.84)
long term (current) use of oral hypoglycemic drugs (Z79.84)

Z79.0 Long term (current) use of anticoagulants and antithrombotics/antiplatelets
EXCLUDES2 *long term (current) use of aspirin (Z79.82)*

Z79.01 Long term (current) use of anticoagulants

Z79.02 Long term (current) use of antithrombotics/antiplatelets

Z79.1 Long term (current) use of non-steroidal anti-inflammatories (NSAID)
EXCLUDES2 *long term (current) use of aspirin (Z79.82)*

Z79.2 Long term (current) use of antibiotics

Z79.3 Long term (current) use of hormonal contraceptives
Long term (current) use of birth control pill or patch

Z79.4 Long term (current) use of insulin

Z79.5 Long term (current) use of steroids

Z79.51 Long term (current) use of inhaled steroids

Z79.52 Long term (current) use of systemic steroids

Z79.8 Other long term (current) drug therapy

Z79.81 Long term (current) use of agents affecting estrogen receptors and estrogen levels
Code first , if applicable:
malignant neoplasm of breast (C50.-)
malignant neoplasm of prostate (C61)
Use additional code, if applicable, to identify:
estrogen receptor positive status (Z17.0)
family history of breast cancer (Z80.3)
genetic susceptibility to malignant neoplasm (cancer) (Z15.0-)
personal history of breast cancer (Z85.3)
personal history of prostate cancer (Z85.46)
postmenopausal status (Z78.0)
EXCLUDES1 *hormone replacement therapy (postmenopausal) (Z79.890)*

Z79.810 Long term (current) use of selective estrogen receptor modulators (SERMs)
Long term (current) use of raloxifene (Evista®)
Long term (current) use of tamoxifen (Nolvadex®)
Long term (current) use of toremifene (Fareston®)

Z79.811 Long term (current) use of aromatase inhibitors
Long term (current) use of anastrozole (Arimidex®)
Long term (current) use of exemestane (Aromasin®)
Long term (current) use of letrozole (Femara®)

Unacceptable principal diagnosis symbol per Medicare code edits · Code exempt from diagnosis present on admission requirement
Questionable admission · Complication or comorbidity · CC/MCC exclusion · Major complication or comorbidity
Principal diagnosis as its own CC · Principal diagnosis as its own MCC · Z code as first-listed diagnosis

Z79.818 Long term (current) use of other agents affecting estrogen receptors and estrogen levels POA PDx
Long term (current) use of estrogen receptor downregulators
Long term (current) use of fulvestrant (Faslodex®)
Long term (current) use of gonadotropin-releasing hormone (GnRH) agonist
Long term (current) use of goserelin acetate (Zoladex®)
Long term (current) use of leuprolide acetate (leuprorelin) (Lupron®)
Long term (current) use of megestrol acetate (Megace®)

Z79.82 Long term (current) use of aspirin POA

Z79.83 Long term (current) use of bisphosphonates POA PDx

● Z79.84 Long term (current) use of oral hypoglycemic drugs
Long term (current) use of oral antidiabetic drugs
EXCLUDES2 *long term (current) use of insulin (Z79.4)*

Z79.89 Other long term (current) drug therapy
Z79.890 Hormone replacement therapy (postmenopausal) POA ♀ PDx
Z79.891 Long term (current) use of opiate analgesic POA
Long term (current) use of methadone for pain management
EXCLUDES1 *methadone use NOS ►(F11.9-)◄*
use of methadone for treatment of heroin addiction (F11.2-)
Z79.899 Other long term (current) drug therapy POA
AHA Q3, 2015

Z80 Family history of primary malignant neoplasm

Z80.0 Family history of malignant neoplasm of digestive organs POA PDx
Conditions classifiable to C15-C26

Z80.1 Family history of malignant neoplasm of trachea, bronchus and lung POA PDx
Conditions classifiable to C33-C34

Z80.2 Family history of malignant neoplasm of other respiratory and intrathoracic organs POA PDx
Conditions classifiable to C30-C32, C37-C39

Z80.3 Family history of malignant neoplasm of breast POA PDx
Conditions classifiable to C50.-

Z80.4 Family history of malignant neoplasm of genital organs
Conditions classifiable to C51-C63
Z80.41 Family history of malignant neoplasm of ovary POA PDx
Z80.42 Family history of malignant neoplasm of prostate POA PDx
Z80.43 Family history of malignant neoplasm of testis POA PDx
Z80.49 Family history of malignant neoplasm of other genital organs POA PDx

Z80.5 Family history of malignant neoplasm of urinary tract
Conditions classifiable to C64-C68
Z80.51 Family history of malignant neoplasm of kidney POA PDx
Z80.52 Family history of malignant neoplasm of bladder POA PDx
Z80.59 Family history of malignant neoplasm of other urinary tract organ POA PDx

Z80.6 Family history of leukemia POA PDx
Conditions classifiable to C91-C95

Z80.7 Family history of other malignant neoplasms of lymphoid, hematopoietic and related tissues POA PDx
Conditions classifiable to C81-C90, C96.-

Z80.8 Family history of malignant neoplasm of other organs or systems POA PDx
Conditions classifiable to C00-C14, C40-C49, C69-C79

Z80.9 Family history of malignant neoplasm, unspecified POA PDx
Conditions classifiable to C80.1

Z81 Family history of mental and behavioral disorders

Z81.0 Family history of intellectual disabilities POA PDx
Conditions classifiable to F70-F79

Z81.1 Family history of alcohol abuse and dependence POA PDx
Conditions classifiable to F10.-

Z81.2 Family history of tobacco abuse and dependence POA PDx
Conditions classifiable to F17.-

Z81.3 Family history of other psychoactive substance abuse and dependence POA PDx
Conditions classifiable to F11-F16, F18-F19

Z81.4 Family history of other substance abuse and dependence POA PDx
Conditions classifiable to F55

Z81.8 Family history of other mental and behavioral disorders POA PDx
Conditions classifiable elsewhere in F01-F99

Z82 Family history of certain disabilities and chronic diseases (leading to disablement)

Z82.0 Family history of epilepsy and other diseases of the nervous system POA PDx
Conditions classifiable to G00-G99

Z82.1 Family history of blindness and visual loss POA PDx
Conditions classifiable to H54.-

Z82.2 Family history of deafness and hearing loss POA PDx
Conditions classifiable to H90-H91

Z82.3 Family history of stroke POA PDx
Conditions classifiable to I60-I64

Z82.4 Family history of ischemic heart disease and other diseases of the circulatory system
Conditions classifiable to I00-I52, I65-I99
Z82.41 Family history of sudden cardiac death POA PDx
Z82.49 Family history of ischemic heart disease and other diseases of the circulatory system POA PDx

Z82.5 Family history of asthma and other chronic lower respiratory diseases POA PDx
Conditions classifiable to J40-J47
EXCLUDES2 *family history of other diseases of the respiratory system (Z83.6)*

Z82.6 Family history of arthritis and other diseases of the musculoskeletal system and connective tissue
Conditions classifiable to M00-M99
Z82.61 Family history of arthritis POA PDx
Z82.62 Family history of osteoporosis POA PDx
Z82.69 Family history of other diseases of the musculoskeletal system and connective tissue POA PDx

Z82.7 Family history of congenital malformations, deformations and chromosomal abnormalities
Conditions classifiable to Q00-Q99
Z82.71 Family history of polycystic kidney POA PDx
Z82.79 Family history of other congenital malformations, deformations and chromosomal abnormalities POA PDx

Z82.8 Family history of other disabilities and chronic diseases leading to disablement, not elsewhere classified POA PDx

Z83 Family history of other specific disorders
EXCLUDES2 *contact with and (suspected) exposure to communicable disease in the family (Z20.-)*

Z83.0 Family history of human immunodeficiency virus [HIV] disease POA PDx
Conditions classifiable to B20

Z83.1 Family history of other infectious and parasitic diseases POA PDx
Conditions classifiable to A00-B19, B25-B94, B99

Z83.2 Family history of diseases of the blood and blood-forming organs and certain disorders involving the immune mechanism POA PDx
Conditions classifiable to D50-D89

Z83.3 Family history of diabetes mellitus POA PDx
Conditions classifiable to E08-E13

Z83.4 Family history of other endocrine, nutritional and metabolic diseases
Conditions classifiable to E00-E07, E15-E88
Z83.41 Family history of multiple endocrine neoplasia [MEN] syndrome POA PDx
● Z83.42 Family history of familial hypercholesterolemia
Z83.49 Family history of other endocrine, nutritional and metabolic diseases POA PDx

Z83.5 Family history of eye and ear disorders
Z83.51 Family history of eye disorders
Conditions classifiable to H00-H53, H55-H59
EXCLUDES2 *family history of blindness and visual loss (Z82.1)*

Unspecified Code | Other Specified Code | Manifestation Code | N Newborn | P Pediatric | M Maternity | A Adult | ♂ Male | ♀ Female
● New Code | ▲ Revised Code Title | ►◄ Revised Text | NOTES | INCLUDES | EXCLUDES1 Not coded here | EXCLUDES2 Not included here
4th character required | 5th character required | 6th character required | 7th character required
Extension 'X' Alert | HAC Hospital-acquired condition (HAC) alert | AHA AHA Coding Clinic©

Z83.511 Family history of glaucoma
Z83.518 Family history of other specified eye disorder
Z83.52 Family history of ear disorders
Conditions classifiable to H60-H83, H92-H95
EXCLUDES2 *family history of deafness and hearing loss (Z82.2)*
Z83.6 Family history of other diseases of the respiratory system
Conditions classifiable to J00-J39, J60-J99
EXCLUDES2 *family history of asthma and other chronic lower respiratory diseases (Z82.5)*
Z83.7 Family history of diseases of the digestive system
Conditions classifiable to K00-K93
Z83.71 Family history of colonic polyps
EXCLUDES1 *family history of malignant neoplasm of digestive organs (Z80.0)*
Z83.79 Family history of other diseases of the digestive system

Z84 Family history of other conditions
Z84.0 Family history of diseases of the skin and subcutaneous tissue
Conditions classifiable to L00-L99
Z84.1 Family history of disorders of kidney and ureter
Conditions classifiable to N00-N29
Z84.2 Family history of other diseases of the genitourinary system
Conditions classifiable to N30-N99
Z84.3 Family history of consanguinity
Z84.8 Family history of other specified conditions
Z84.81 Family history of carrier of genetic disease
● Z84.82 Family history of sudden infant death syndrome
Family history of SIDS
Z84.89 Family history of other specified conditions

Z85 Personal history of malignant neoplasm
Code first any follow-up examination after treatment of malignant neoplasm (Z08)
Use additional code to identify:
alcohol use and dependence (F10.-)
exposure to environmental tobacco smoke (Z77.22)
history of tobacco ▶dependence◀ (Z87.891)
occupational exposure to environmental tobacco smoke (Z57.31)
tobacco dependence (F17.-)
tobacco use (Z72.0)
EXCLUDES2 *personal history of benign neoplasm (Z86.01-)*
personal history of carcinoma-in-situ (Z86.00-)
Z85.0 Personal history of malignant neoplasm of digestive organs
Z85.00 Personal history of malignant neoplasm of unspecified digestive organ
Z85.01 Personal history of malignant neoplasm of esophagus
Conditions classifiable to C15
Z85.02 Personal history of malignant neoplasm of stomach
Z85.020 Personal history of malignant carcinoid tumor of stomach
Conditions classifiable to C7A.092
Z85.028 Personal history of other malignant neoplasm of stomach
Conditions classifiable to C16
Z85.03 Personal history of malignant neoplasm of large intestine
Z85.030 Personal history of malignant carcinoid tumor of large intestine
Conditions classifiable to C7A.022-C7A.025, C7A.029
Z85.038 Personal history of other malignant neoplasm of large intestine
Conditions classifiable to C18
Z85.04 Personal history of malignant neoplasm of rectum, rectosigmoid junction, and anus
Z85.040 Personal history of malignant carcinoid tumor of rectum
Conditions classifiable to C7A.026
Z85.048 Personal history of other malignant neoplasm of rectum, rectosigmoid junction, and anus
Conditions classifiable to C19-C21
Z85.05 Personal history of malignant neoplasm of liver
Conditions classifiable to C22
Z85.06 Personal history of malignant neoplasm of small intestine
Z85.060 Personal history of malignant carcinoid tumor of small intestine
Conditions classifiable to C7A.01-
Z85.068 Personal history of other malignant neoplasm of small intestine
Conditions classifiable to C17
Z85.07 Personal history of malignant neoplasm of pancreas
Conditions classifiable to C25
Z85.09 Personal history of malignant neoplasm of other digestive organs
Z85.1 Personal history of malignant neoplasm of trachea, bronchus and lung
Z85.11 Personal history of malignant neoplasm of bronchus and lung
Z85.110 Personal history of malignant carcinoid tumor of bronchus and lung
Conditions classifiable to C7A.090
Z85.118 Personal history of other malignant neoplasm of bronchus and lung
Conditions classifiable to C34
Z85.12 Personal history of malignant neoplasm of trachea
Conditions classifiable to C33
Z85.2 Personal history of malignant neoplasm of other respiratory and intrathoracic organs
Z85.20 Personal history of malignant neoplasm of unspecified respiratory organ
Z85.21 Personal history of malignant neoplasm of larynx
Conditions classifiable to C32
Z85.22 Personal history of malignant neoplasm of nasal cavities, middle ear, and accessory sinuses
Conditions classifiable to C30-C31
Z85.23 Personal history of malignant neoplasm of thymus
Z85.230 Personal history of malignant carcinoid tumor of thymus
Conditions classifiable to C7A.091
Z85.238 Personal history of other malignant neoplasm of thymus
Conditions classifiable to C37
Z85.29 Personal history of malignant neoplasm of other respiratory and intrathoracic organs
Z85.3 Personal history of malignant neoplasm of breast
Conditions classifiable to C50.-
Z85.4 Personal history of malignant neoplasm of genital organs
Conditions classifiable to C51-C63
Z85.40 Personal history of malignant neoplasm of unspecified female genital organ ♀
Z85.41 Personal history of malignant neoplasm of cervix uteri ♀
Z85.42 Personal history of malignant neoplasm of other parts of uterus ♀
Z85.43 Personal history of malignant neoplasm of ovary ♀
Z85.44 Personal history of malignant neoplasm of other female genital organs ♀
Z85.45 Personal history of malignant neoplasm of unspecified male genital organ ♂
Z85.46 Personal history of malignant neoplasm of prostate ♂
Z85.47 Personal history of malignant neoplasm of testis ♂
Z85.48 Personal history of malignant neoplasm of epididymis ♂

Unacceptable principal diagnosis symbol per Medicare code edits · Code exempt from diagnosis present on admission requirement · Questionable admission · Complication or comorbidity · CC/MCC exclusion · Major complication or comorbidity · Principal diagnosis as its own CC · Principal diagnosis as its own MCC · Z code as first-listed diagnosis

Z85.49 Personal history of malignant neoplasm of other male genital organs

Z85.5 Personal history of malignant neoplasm of urinary tract
Conditions classifiable to C64-C68

Z85.50 Personal history of malignant neoplasm of unspecified urinary tract organ

Z85.51 Personal history of malignant neoplasm of bladder

Z85.52 Personal history of malignant neoplasm of kidney
EXCLUDES1 *personal history of malignant neoplasm of renal pelvis (Z85.53)*

Z85.520 Personal history of malignant carcinoid tumor of kidney
Conditions classifiable to C7A.093

Z85.528 Personal history of other malignant neoplasm of kidney
Conditions classifiable to C64

Z85.53 Personal history of malignant neoplasm of renal pelvis

Z85.54 Personal history of malignant neoplasm of ureter

Z85.59 Personal history of malignant neoplasm of other urinary tract organ

Z85.6 Personal history of leukemia
Conditions classifiable to C91-C95
EXCLUDES1 *leukemia in remission C91.0-C95.9 with 5th character 1*

Z85.7 Personal history of other malignant neoplasms of lymphoid, hematopoietic and related tissues

Z85.71 Personal history of Hodgkin lymphoma
Conditions classifiable to C81

Z85.72 Personal history of non-Hodgkin lymphomas
Conditions classifiable to C82-C85

Z85.79 Personal history of other malignant neoplasms of lymphoid, hematopoietic and related tissues
Conditions classifiable to C88-C90, C96
EXCLUDES1 *multiple myeloma in remission (C90.01)*
plasma cell leukemia in remission (C90.11)
plasmacytoma in remission (C90.21)

Z85.8 Personal history of malignant neoplasms of other organs and systems
Conditions classifiable to C00-C14, C40-C49, ▶C69-C75, C7A.098, C76-C79◀

Z85.81 Personal history of malignant neoplasm of lip, oral cavity, and pharynx

Z85.810 Personal history of malignant neoplasm of tongue

Z85.818 Personal history of malignant neoplasm of other sites of lip, oral cavity, and pharynx

Z85.819 Personal history of malignant neoplasm of unspecified site of lip, oral cavity, and pharynx

Z85.82 Personal history of malignant neoplasm of skin

Z85.820 Personal history of malignant melanoma of skin
Conditions classifiable to C43

Z85.821 Personal history of Merkel cell carcinoma
Conditions classifiable to C4A

Z85.828 Personal history of other malignant neoplasm of skin
Conditions classifiable to C44

Z85.83 Personal history of malignant neoplasm of bone and soft tissue

Z85.830 Personal history of malignant neoplasm of bone

Z85.831 Personal history of malignant neoplasm of soft tissue
EXCLUDES2 *personal history of malignant neoplasm of skin (Z85.82-)*

Z85.84 Personal history of malignant neoplasm of eye and nervous tissue

Z85.840 Personal history of malignant neoplasm of eye

Z85.841 Personal history of malignant neoplasm of brain

Z85.848 Personal history of malignant neoplasm of other parts of nervous tissue

Z85.85 Personal history of malignant neoplasm of endocrine glands

Z85.850 Personal history of malignant neoplasm of thyroid

Z85.858 Personal history of malignant neoplasm of other endocrine glands

Z85.89 Personal history of malignant neoplasm of other organs and systems

Z85.9 Personal history of malignant neoplasm, unspecified
Conditions classifiable to C7A.00, C80.1

Z86 Personal history of certain other diseases
Code first any follow-up examination after treatment (Z09)

Z86.0 Personal history of in-situ and benign neoplasms and neoplasms of uncertain behavior
EXCLUDES2 *personal history of malignant neoplasms (Z85.-)*

Z86.00 Personal history of in-situ neoplasm
Conditions classifiable to D00-D09

Z86.000 Personal history of in-situ neoplasm of breast

Z86.001 Personal history of in-situ neoplasm of cervix uteri
Personal history of cervical intraepithelial neoplasia III [CIN III]

Z86.008 Personal history of in-situ neoplasm of other site
Personal history of vaginal intraepithelial neoplasia III [VAIN III]
Personal history of vulvar intraepithelial neoplasia III [VIN III]

Z86.01 Personal history of benign neoplasm

Z86.010 Personal history of colonic polyps

Z86.011 Personal history of benign neoplasm of the brain

Z86.012 Personal history of benign carcinoid tumor

Z86.018 Personal history of other benign neoplasm

Z86.03 Personal history of neoplasm of uncertain behavior

Z86.1 Personal history of infectious and parasitic diseases
Conditions classifiable to A00-B89, B99
EXCLUDES1 *personal history of infectious diseases specific to a body system*
sequelae of infectious and parasitic diseases (B90-B94)

Z86.11 Personal history of tuberculosis

Z86.12 Personal history of poliomyelitis

Z86.13 Personal history of malaria

Z86.14 Personal history of Methicillin resistant Staphylococcus aureus infection
Personal history of MRSA infection

Z86.19 Personal history of other infectious and parasitic diseases

Z86.2 Personal history of diseases of the blood and blood-forming organs and certain disorders involving the immune mechanism
Conditions classifiable to D50-D89

Z86.3 Personal history of endocrine, nutritional and metabolic diseases
Conditions classifiable to E00-E88

Z86.31 Personal history of diabetic foot ulcer
EXCLUDES2 *current diabetic foot ulcer (E08.621, E09.621, E10.621, E11.621, E13.621)*

Z86.32 Personal history of gestational diabetes
Personal history of conditions classifiable to O24.4-
EXCLUDES1 *gestational diabetes mellitus in current pregnancy (O24.4-)*

Z86.39 Personal history of other endocrine, nutritional and metabolic disease

Z86.5 Personal history of mental and behavioral disorders
Conditions classifiable to F40-F59
Z86.51 Personal history of combat and operational stress reaction
Z86.59 Personal history of other mental and behavioral disorders
Z86.6 Personal history of diseases of the nervous system and sense organs
Conditions classifiable to G00-G99, H00-H95
Z86.61 Personal history of infections of the central nervous system
Personal history of encephalitis
Personal history of meningitis
Z86.69 Personal history of other diseases of the nervous system and sense organs
Z86.7 Personal history of diseases of the circulatory system
Conditions classifiable to I00-I99
EXCLUDES2 *old myocardial infarction (I25.2)*
personal history of anaphylactic shock (Z87.892)
postmyocardial infarction syndrome (I24.1)
Z86.71 Personal history of venous thrombosis and embolism
Z86.711 Personal history of pulmonary embolism
Z86.718 Personal history of other venous thrombosis and embolism
Z86.72 Personal history of thrombophlebitis
Z86.73 Personal history of transient ischemic attack (TIA), and cerebral infarction without residual deficits
Personal history of prolonged reversible ischemic neurological deficit (PRIND)
Personal history of stroke NOS without residual deficits
EXCLUDES1 *personal history of traumatic brain injury (Z87.820)*
sequelae of cerebrovascular disease (I69.-)
Z86.74 Personal history of sudden cardiac arrest
Personal history of sudden cardiac death successfully resuscitated
Z86.79 Personal history of other diseases of the circulatory system
Z87 Personal history of other diseases and conditions
Code first any follow-up examination after treatment (Z09)
Z87.0 Personal history of diseases of the respiratory system
Conditions classifiable to J00-J99
Z87.01 Personal history of pneumonia (recurrent)
Z87.09 Personal history of other diseases of the respiratory system
Z87.1 Personal history of diseases of the digestive system
Conditions classifiable to K00-K93
Z87.11 Personal history of peptic ulcer disease
Z87.19 Personal history of other diseases of the digestive system
Z87.2 Personal history of diseases of the skin and subcutaneous tissue
Conditions classifiable to L00-L99
EXCLUDES2 *personal history of diabetic foot ulcer (Z86.31)*
Z87.3 Personal history of diseases of the musculoskeletal system and connective tissue
Conditions classifiable to M00-M99
EXCLUDES2 *personal history of (healed) traumatic fracture (Z87.81)*
Z87.31 Personal history of (healed) nontraumatic fracture
Z87.310 Personal history of (healed) osteoporosis fracture
Personal history of (healed) fragility fracture
Personal history of (healed) collapsed vertebra due to osteoporosis
Z87.311 Personal history of (healed) other pathological fracture
Personal history of (healed) collapsed vertebra NOS
EXCLUDES2 *personal history of osteoporosis fracture (Z87.310)*
Z87.312 Personal history of (healed) stress fracture
Personal history of (healed) fatigue fracture
Z87.39 Personal history of other diseases of the musculoskeletal system and connective tissue
Z87.4 Personal history of diseases of genitourinary system
Conditions classifiable to N00-N99
Z87.41 Personal history of dysplasia of the female genital tract
EXCLUDES1 *personal history of intraepithelial neoplasia III of female genital tract (Z87.001, Z87.008)*
personal history of malignant neoplasm of female genital tract (Z85.40-Z85.44)
Z87.410 Personal history of cervical dysplasia
Z87.411 Personal history of vaginal dysplasia
Z87.412 Personal history of vulvar dysplasia
Z87.42 Personal history of other diseases of the female genital tract
Z87.43 Personal history of diseases of male genital organs
Z87.430 Personal history of prostatic dysplasia
EXCLUDES1 *personal history of malignant neoplasm of prostate (Z85.46)*
Z87.438 Personal history of other diseases of male genital organs
Z87.44 Personal history of diseases of urinary system
EXCLUDES1 *personal history of malignant neoplasm of cervix uteri (Z85.41)*
Z87.440 Personal history of urinary (tract) infections
Z87.441 Personal history of nephrotic syndrome
Z87.442 Personal history of urinary calculi
Personal history of kidney stones
Z87.448 Personal history of other diseases of urinary system
Z87.5 Personal history of complications of pregnancy, childbirth and the puerperium
Conditions classifiable to O00-O9A
EXCLUDES2 *recurrent pregnancy loss (N96)*
Z87.51 Personal history of pre-term labor
EXCLUDES1 *current pregnancy with history of pre-term labor (O09.21-)*
Z87.59 Personal history of other complications of pregnancy, childbirth and the puerperium
Personal history of trophoblastic disease
Z87.7 Personal history of (corrected) congenital malformations
Conditions classifiable to Q00-Q89 that have been repaired or corrected
EXCLUDES1 *congenital malformations that have been partially corrected or repair but which still require medical treatment - code to condition*
EXCLUDES2 *other postprocedural states (Z98.-)*
personal history of medical treatment (Z92.-)
presence of cardiac and vascular implants and grafts (Z95.-)
presence of other devices (Z97.-)
presence of other functional implants (Z96.-)
transplanted organ and tissue status (Z94.-)
Z87.71 Personal history of (corrected) congenital malformations of genitourinary system
Z87.710 Personal history of (corrected) hypospadias
Z87.718 Personal history of other specified (corrected) congenital malformations of genitourinary system
Z87.72 Personal history of (corrected) congenital malformations of nervous system and sense organs
Z87.720 Personal history of (corrected) congenital malformations of eye

PDx Unacceptable principal diagnosis symbol per Medicare code edits; POA Code exempt from diagnosis present on admission requirement
Q Questionable admission; CC Complication or comorbidity; CC/MCC EXCL CC/MCC exclusion; MCC Major complication or comorbidity
PDx CC Principal diagnosis as its own CC; PDx MCC Principal diagnosis as its own MCC; Z1 Z code as first-listed diagnosis

Z87.721 Personal history of (corrected) congenital malformations of ear
Z87.728 Personal history of other specified (corrected) congenital malformations of nervous system and sense organs
Z87.73 Personal history of (corrected) congenital malformations of digestive system
Z87.730 Personal history of (corrected) cleft lip and palate
Z87.738 Personal history of other specified (corrected) congenital malformations of digestive system
Z87.74 Personal history of (corrected) congenital malformations of heart and circulatory system
Z87.75 Personal history of (corrected) congenital malformations of respiratory system
Z87.76 Personal history of (corrected) congenital malformations of integument, limbs and musculoskeletal system
Z87.79 Personal history of other (corrected) congenital malformations
Z87.790 Personal history of (corrected) congenital malformations of face and neck
Z87.798 Personal history of other (corrected) congenital malformations
Z87.8 Personal history of other specified conditions
EXCLUDES2 *personal history of self harm (Z91.5)*
Z87.81 Personal history of (healed) traumatic fracture
EXCLUDES2 *personal history of (healed) nontraumatic fracture (Z87.31-)*
Z87.82 Personal history of other (healed) physical injury and trauma
Conditions classifiable to S00-T88, except traumatic fractures
Z87.820 Personal history of traumatic brain injury
EXCLUDES1 *personal history of transient ischemic attack (TIA), and cerebral infarction without residual deficits (Z86.73)*
Z87.821 Personal history of retained foreign body fully removed
Z87.828 Personal history of other (healed) physical injury and trauma
Z87.89 Personal history of other specified conditions
Z87.890 Personal history of sex reassignment
Z87.891 Personal history of nicotine dependence
EXCLUDES1 *current nicotine dependence (F17.2-)*
Z87.892 Personal history of anaphylaxis
Code also allergy status such as:
allergy status to drugs, medicaments and biological substances (Z88.-)
allergy status, other than to drugs and biological substances (Z91.0-)
Z87.898 Personal history of other specified conditions
AHA: Q1, 2013
Z88 Allergy status to drugs, medicaments and biological substances
EXCLUDES2 *Allergy status, other than to drugs and biological substances (Z91.0-)*
Z88.0 Allergy status to penicillin
Z88.1 Allergy status to other antibiotic agents status
Z88.2 Allergy status to sulfonamides status
AHA: Q3, 2015
Z88.3 Allergy status to other anti-infective agents status
Z88.4 Allergy status to anesthetic agent status
Z88.5 Allergy status to narcotic agent status
Z88.6 Allergy status to analgesic agent status
Z88.7 Allergy status to serum and vaccine status
Z88.8 Allergy status to other drugs, medicaments and biological substances status
Z88.9 Allergy status to unspecified drugs, medicaments and biological substances status
Z89 Acquired absence of limb
INCLUDES *amputation status*
postprocedural loss of limb
post-traumatic loss of limb
EXCLUDES1 *acquired deformities of limbs (M20-M21)*
congenital absence of limbs (Q71-Q73)
Z89.0 Acquired absence of thumb and other finger(s)
Z89.01 Acquired absence of thumb
Z89.011 Acquired absence of right thumb
Z89.012 Acquired absence of left thumb
Z89.019 Acquired absence of unspecified thumb
Z89.02 Acquired absence of other finger(s)
EXCLUDES2 *acquired absence of thumb (Z89.01-)*
Z89.021 Acquired absence of right finger(s)
Z89.022 Acquired absence of left finger(s)
Z89.029 Acquired absence of unspecified finger(s)
Z89.1 Acquired absence of hand and wrist
Z89.11 Acquired absence of hand
Z89.111 Acquired absence of right hand
Z89.112 Acquired absence of left hand
Z89.119 Acquired absence of unspecified hand
Z89.12 Acquired absence of wrist
Disarticulation at wrist
Z89.121 Acquired absence of right wrist
Z89.122 Acquired absence of left wrist
Z89.129 Acquired absence of unspecified wrist
Z89.2 Acquired absence of upper limb above wrist
Z89.20 Acquired absence of upper limb, unspecified level
Z89.201 Acquired absence of right upper limb, unspecified level
Z89.202 Acquired absence of left upper limb, unspecified level
Z89.209 Acquired absence of unspecified upper limb, unspecified level
Acquired absence of arm NOS
Z89.21 Acquired absence of upper limb below elbow
Z89.211 Acquired absence of right upper limb below elbow
Z89.212 Acquired absence of left upper limb below elbow
Z89.219 Acquired absence of unspecified upper limb below elbow
Z89.22 Acquired absence of upper limb above elbow
Disarticulation at elbow
Z89.221 Acquired absence of right upper limb above elbow
Z89.222 Acquired absence of left upper limb above elbow
Z89.229 Acquired absence of unspecified upper limb above elbow
Z89.23 Acquired absence of shoulder
Acquired absence of shoulder joint following explantation of shoulder joint prosthesis, with or without presence of antibiotic-impregnated cement spacer
Z89.231 Acquired absence of right shoulder
Z89.232 Acquired absence of left shoulder
Z89.239 Acquired absence of unspecified shoulder
Z89.4 Acquired absence of toe(s), foot, and ankle
Z89.41 Acquired absence of great toe
Z89.411 Acquired absence of right great toe
Z89.412 Acquired absence of left great toe
Z89.419 Acquired absence of unspecified great toe

Unspecified Code | Other Specified Code | Manifestation Code | N Newborn | P Pediatric | M Maternity | A Adult | ♂ Male | ♀ Female
● New Code | ▲ Revised Code Title | ►◄ Revised Text | NOTES | INCLUDES | EXCLUDES1 Not coded here | EXCLUDES2 Not included here
4th character required | 5th character required | 6th character required | 7th character required
Extension 'X' Alert | HAC Hospital-acquired condition (HAC) alert | AHA AHA Coding Clinic©

Z89.42 Acquired absence of other toe(s)
EXCLUDES2 *acquired absence of great toe (Z89.41-)*
Z89.421 Acquired absence of other right toe(s)
Z89.422 Acquired absence of other left toe(s)
Z89.429 Acquired absence of other toe(s), unspecified side
Z89.43 Acquired absence of foot
Z89.431 Acquired absence of right foot
Z89.432 Acquired absence of left foot
Z89.439 Acquired absence of unspecified foot
Z89.44 Acquired absence of ankle
Disarticulation of ankle
Z89.441 Acquired absence of right ankle
Z89.442 Acquired absence of left ankle
Z89.449 Acquired absence of unspecified ankle
Z89.5 Acquired absence of leg below knee
Z89.51 Acquired absence of leg below knee
Z89.511 Acquired absence of right leg below knee
Z89.512 Acquired absence of left leg below knee
Z89.519 Acquired absence of unspecified leg below knee
Z89.52 Acquired absence of knee
Acquired absence of knee joint following explantation of knee joint prosthesis, with or without presence of antibiotic-impregnated cement spacer
Z89.521 Acquired absence of right knee
Z89.522 Acquired absence of left knee
Z89.529 Acquired absence of unspecified knee
Z89.6 Acquired absence of leg above knee
Z89.61 Acquired absence of leg above knee
Acquired absence of leg NOS
Disarticulation at knee
Z89.611 Acquired absence of right leg above knee
Z89.612 Acquired absence of left leg above knee
Z89.619 Acquired absence of unspecified leg above knee
Z89.62 Acquired absence of hip
Acquired absence of hip joint following explantation of hip joint prosthesis, with or without presence of antibiotic-impregnated cement spacer
Disarticulation at hip
Z89.621 Acquired absence of right hip joint
Z89.622 Acquired absence of left hip joint
Z89.629 Acquired absence of unspecified hip joint
Z89.9 Acquired absence of limb, unspecified
Z90 Acquired absence of organs, not elsewhere classified
INCLUDES *postprocedural or post-traumatic loss of body part NEC*
EXCLUDES1 *congenital absence - see Alphabetical Index*
EXCLUDES2 *postprocedural absence of endocrine glands (E89.-)*
Z90.0 Acquired absence of part of head and neck
Z90.01 Acquired absence of eye
Z90.02 Acquired absence of larynx
Z90.09 Acquired absence of other part of head and neck
Acquired absence of nose
EXCLUDES2 *teeth (K08.1)*
Z90.1 Acquired absence of breast and nipple
Z90.10 Acquired absence of unspecified breast and nipple
Z90.11 Acquired absence of right breast and nipple
Z90.12 Acquired absence of left breast and nipple
Z90.13 Acquired absence of bilateral breasts and nipples
Z90.2 Acquired absence of lung [part of]
Z90.3 Acquired absence of stomach [part of]
Z90.4 Acquired absence of other specified parts of digestive tract
Z90.41 Acquired absence of pancreas
Code also exocrine pancreatic insufficiency (K86.81)
Use additional code to identify any associated:
insulin use (Z79.4)
diabetes mellitus, postpancreatectomy (E13.-)
Z90.410 Acquired total absence of pancreas
Acquired absence of pancreas NOS
Z90.411 Acquired partial absence of pancreas
Z90.49 Acquired absence of other specified parts of digestive tract
Z90.5 Acquired absence of kidney
Z90.6 Acquired absence of other parts of urinary tract
Acquired absence of bladder
Z90.7 Acquired absence of genital organ(s)
EXCLUDES1 *personal history of sex reassignment (Z87.890)*
EXCLUDES2 *female genital mutilation status (N90.81-)*
Z90.71 Acquired absence of cervix and uterus
Z90.710 Acquired absence of both cervix and uterus
Acquired absence of uterus NOS
Status post total hysterectomy
Z90.711 Acquired absence of uterus with remaining cervical stump
Status post partial hysterectomy with remaining cervical stump
Z90.712 Acquired absence of cervix with remaining uterus
Z90.72 Acquired absence of ovaries
Z90.721 Acquired absence of ovaries, unilateral
Z90.722 Acquired absence of ovaries, bilateral
Z90.79 Acquired absence of other genital organ(s)
Z90.8 Acquired absence of other organs
Z90.81 Acquired absence of spleen
Z90.89 Acquired absence of other organs
Z91 Personal risk factors, not elsewhere classified
EXCLUDES2 *contact with and (suspected) exposures hazardous to health (Z77.-)*
exposure to pollution and other problems related to physical environment (Z77.1-)
personal history of physical injury and trauma (Z87.81, Z87.82-)
occupational exposure to risk factors (Z57.-)
Z91.0 Allergy status, other than to drugs and biological substances
EXCLUDES2 *Allergy status to drugs, medicaments, and biological substances (Z88.-)*
Z91.01 Food allergy status
EXCLUDES2 *food additives allergy status (Z91.02)*
Z91.010 Allergy to peanuts
Z91.011 Allergy to milk products
EXCLUDES1 *lactose intolerance (E73.-)*
Z91.012 Allergy to eggs
Z91.013 Allergy to seafood
Allergy to shellfish
Allergy to octopus or squid ink
Z91.018 Allergy to other foods
Allergy to nuts other than peanuts
Z91.02 Food additives allergy status
Z91.03 Insect allergy status
Z91.030 Bee allergy status
Z91.038 Other insect allergy status
Z91.04 Nonmedicinal substance allergy status
Z91.040 Latex allergy status
Latex sensitivity status
Z91.041 Radiographic dye allergy status
Allergy status to contrast media used for diagnostic X-ray procedure
Z91.048 Other nonmedicinal substance allergy status
Z91.09 Other allergy status, other than to drugs and biological substances
Z91.1 Patient's noncompliance with medical treatment and regimen
Z91.11 Patient's noncompliance with dietary regimen

Unacceptable principal diagnosis symbol per Medicare code edits — Code exempt from diagnosis present on admission requirement
Questionable admission — Complication or comorbidity — CC/MCC exclusion — Major complication or comorbidity
Principal diagnosis as its own CC — Principal diagnosis as its own MCC — Z code as first-listed diagnosis

Z91.12 Patient's intentional underdosing of medication regimen
Code first underdosing of medication (T36-T50) with fifth or sixth character 6
EXCLUDES1 *adverse effect of prescribed drug taken as directed- code to adverse effect*
poisoning (overdose) -code to poisoning
Z91.120 Patient's intentional underdosing of medication regimen due to financial hardship
Z91.128 Patient's intentional underdosing of medication regimen for other reason
Z91.13 Patient's unintentional underdosing of medication regimen
Code first underdosing of medication (T36-T50) with fifth or sixth character 6
EXCLUDES1 *adverse effect of prescribed drug taken as directed- code to adverse effect*
poisoning (overdose) -code to poisoning
Z91.130 Patient's unintentional underdosing of medication regimen due to age-related debility
Z91.138 Patient's unintentional underdosing of medication regimen for other reason
Z91.14 Patient's other noncompliance with medication regimen
Patient's underdosing of medication NOS
Z91.15 Patient's noncompliance with renal dialysis
Z91.19 Patient's noncompliance with other medical treatment and regimen
Z91.4 Personal history of psychological trauma, not elsewhere classified
Z91.41 Personal history of adult abuse
EXCLUDES2 *personal history of abuse in childhood (Z62.81-)*
Z91.410 Personal history of adult physical and sexual abuse
EXCLUDES1 *current adult physical abuse (T74.11, T76.11)*
current adult sexual abuse (T74.21, T76.11)
Z91.411 Personal history of adult psychological abuse
Z91.412 Personal history of adult neglect
EXCLUDES1 *current adult neglect (T74.01, T76.01)*
Z91.419 Personal history of unspecified adult abuse
Z91.49 Other personal history of psychological trauma, not elsewhere classified
Z91.5 Personal history of self-harm
Personal history of parasuicide
Personal history of self-poisoning
Personal history of suicide attempt
Z91.8 Other specified personal risk factors, not elsewhere classified
Z91.81 History of falling
At risk for falling
Z91.82 Personal history of military deployment
Individual (civilian or military) with past history of military war, peacekeeping and humanitarian deployment (current or past conflict)
Returned from military deployment
Z91.83 Wandering in diseases classified elsewhere
Code first underlying disorder such as:
Alzheimer's disease (G30.-)
autism or pervasive developmental disorder (F84.-)
intellectual disabilities (F70-F79)
unspecified dementia with behavioral disturbance (F03.9-)
Z91.89 Other specified personal risk factors, not elsewhere classified
Z92 Personal history of medical treatment
EXCLUDES2 *postprocedural states (Z98.-)*
Z92.0 Personal history of contraception
EXCLUDES1 *counseling or management of current contraceptive practices (Z30.-)*
long term (current) use of contraception (Z79.3)
presence of (intrauterine) contraceptive device (Z97.5)
Z92.2 Personal history of drug therapy
EXCLUDES2 *long term (current) drug therapy (Z79.-)*
Z92.21 Personal history of antineoplastic chemotherapy
Z92.22 Personal history of monoclonal drug therapy
Z92.23 Personal history of estrogen therapy
Z92.24 Personal history of steroid therapy
Z92.240 Personal history of inhaled steroid therapy
Z92.241 Personal history of systemic steroid therapy
Personal history of steroid therapy NOS
Z92.25 Personal history of immunosuppression therapy
EXCLUDES2 *personal history of steroid therapy (Z92.24)*
Z92.29 Personal history of other drug therapy
Z92.3 Personal history of irradiation
Personal history of exposure to therapeutic radiation
EXCLUDES1 *exposure to radiation in the physical environment (Z77.12)*
occupational exposure to radiation (Z57.1)
Z92.8 Personal history of other medical treatment
Z92.81 Personal history of extracorporeal membrane oxygenation (ECMO)
Z92.82 Status post administration of tPA (rtPA) in a different facility within the last 24 hours prior to admission to current facility
Code first condition requiring tPA administration, such as:
acute cerebral infarction (I63.-)
acute myocardial infarction (I21.-, I22.-)
AHA: Q4, 2013
Z92.83 Personal history of failed moderate sedation
Personal history of failed conscious sedation
EXCLUDES2 *failed moderate sedation during procedure (T88.52)*
● Z92.84 Personal history of unintended awareness under general anesthesia
EXCLUDES2 *unintended awareness under general anesthesia during procedure (T88.53)*
Z92.89 Personal history of other medical treatment
Z93 Artificial opening status
EXCLUDES1 *artificial openings requiring attention or management (Z43.-)*
complications of external stoma (J95.0-, K94.-, N99.5-)
Z93.0 Tracheostomy status
AHA: Q4, 2013
Z93.1 Gastrostomy status
Z93.2 Ileostomy status
Z93.3 Colostomy status
Z93.4 Other artificial openings of gastrointestinal tract status
Z93.5 Cystostomy status
Z93.50 Unspecified cystostomy status
Z93.51 Cutaneous-vesicostomy status
Z93.52 Appendico-vesicostomy status
Z93.59 Other cystostomy status
Z93.6 Other artificial openings of urinary tract status
Nephrostomy status
Ureterostomy status
Urethrostomy status
Z93.8 Other artificial opening status
Z93.9 Artificial opening status, unspecified
Z94 Transplanted organ and tissue status
INCLUDES *organ or tissue replaced by heterogenous or homogenous transplant*
EXCLUDES1 *complications of transplanted organ or tissue - see Alphabetical Index*
EXCLUDES2 *presence of vascular grafts (Z95.-)*
Z94.0 Kidney transplant status

Unspecified Code Other Specified Code Manifestation Code N Newborn P Pediatric M Maternity A Adult ♂ Male ♀ Female
● New Code ▲ Revised Code Title ►◄ Revised Text NOTES INCLUDES EXCLUDES1 Not coded here EXCLUDES2 Not included here
4th character required 5th character required 6th character required 7th character required
Extension 'X' Alert HAC Hospital-acquired condition (HAC) alert AHA AHA Coding Clinic©

Z94.1 Heart transplant status
EXCLUDES1 *artificial heart status (Z95.812)*
heart-valve replacement status (Z95.2-Z95.4)
Z94.2 Lung transplant status
Z94.3 Heart and lungs transplant status
Z94.4 Liver transplant status
Z94.5 Skin transplant status
Autogenous skin transplant status
Z94.6 Bone transplant status
Z94.7 Corneal transplant status
Z94.8 Other transplanted organ and tissue status
Z94.81 Bone marrow transplant status
Z94.82 Intestine transplant status
Z94.83 Pancreas transplant status
Z94.84 Stem cells transplant status
Z94.89 Other transplanted organ and tissue status
Z94.9 Transplanted organ and tissue status, unspecified

Z95 Presence of cardiac and vascular implants and grafts
EXCLUDES1 *complications of cardiac and vascular devices, implants and grafts (T82.-)*
Z95.0 Presence of cardiac pacemaker
Presence of cardiac resynchronization therapy (CRT-P) pacemaker
EXCLUDES1 *adjustment or management of cardiac device (Z45.0-)*
adjustment or management of cardiac pacemaker (Z45.0)
presence of automatic (implantable) cardiac defibrillator with synchronous cardiac pacemaker (Z95.810)
Z95.1 Presence of aortocoronary bypass graft
Presence of coronary artery bypass graft
Z95.2 Presence of prosthetic heart valve
Presence of heart valve NOS
Z95.3 Presence of xenogenic heart valve
Z95.4 Presence of other heart-valve replacement
Z95.5 Presence of coronary angioplasty implant and graft
EXCLUDES1 *coronary angioplasty status without implant and graft (Z98.61)*
Z95.8 Presence of other cardiac and vascular implants and grafts
Z95.81 Presence of other cardiac implants and grafts
Z95.810 Presence of automatic (implantable) cardiac defibrillator
Presence of automatic (implantable) cardiac defibrillator with synchronous cardiac pacemaker
Presence of cardiac resynchronization therapy defibrillator (CRT-D)
Presence of cardioverter-defibrillator (ICD)
Z95.811 Presence of heart assist device
Z95.812 Presence of fully implantable artificial heart
Z95.818 Presence of other cardiac implants and grafts
Z95.82 Presence of other vascular implants and grafts
Z95.820 Peripheral vascular angioplasty status with implants and grafts
EXCLUDES1 *peripheral vascular angioplasty without implant and graft (Z98.62)*
Z95.828 Presence of other vascular implants and grafts
Presence of intravascular prosthesis NEC
Z95.9 Presence of cardiac and vascular implant and graft, unspecified

Z96 Presence of other functional implants
EXCLUDES2 *complications of internal prosthetic devices, implants and grafts (T82-T85)*
fitting and adjustment of prosthetic and other devices (Z44-Z46)
Z96.0 Presence of urogenital implants
Z96.1 Presence of intraocular lens
Presence of pseudophakia
Z96.2 Presence of otological and audiological implants
Z96.20 Presence of otological and audiological implant, unspecified
Z96.21 Cochlear implant status
Z96.22 Myringotomy tube (s) status
Z96.29 Presence of other otological and audiological implants
Presence of bone-conduction hearing device
Presence of eustachian tube stent
Stapes replacement
Z96.3 Presence of artificial larynx
Z96.4 Presence of endocrine implants
Z96.41 Presence of insulin pump (external) (internal)
Z96.49 Presence of other endocrine implants
Z96.5 Presence of tooth-root and mandibular implants
Z96.6 Presence of orthopedic joint implants
Z96.60 Presence of unspecified orthopedic joint implant
Z96.61 Presence of artificial shoulder joint
Z96.611 Presence of right artificial shoulder joint
Z96.612 Presence of left artificial shoulder joint
Z96.619 Presence of unspecified artificial shoulder joint
Z96.62 Presence of artificial elbow joint
Z96.621 Presence of right artificial elbow joint
Z96.622 Presence of left artificial elbow joint
Z96.629 Presence of unspecified artificial elbow joint
Z96.63 Presence of artificial wrist joint
Z96.631 Presence of right artificial wrist joint
Z96.632 Presence of left artificial wrist joint
Z96.639 Presence of unspecified artificial wrist joint
Z96.64 Presence of artificial hip joint
Hip-joint replacement (partial) (total)
Z96.641 Presence of right artificial hip joint
Z96.642 Presence of left artificial hip joint
AHA: Q1, 2015
Z96.643 Presence of artificial hip joint, bilateral
Z96.649 Presence of unspecified artificial hip joint
Z96.65 Presence of artificial knee joint
Z96.651 Presence of right artificial knee joint
Z96.652 Presence of left artificial knee joint
Z96.653 Presence of artificial knee joint, bilateral
Z96.659 Presence of unspecified artificial knee joint
Z96.66 Presence of artificial ankle joint
Z96.661 Presence of right artificial ankle joint
Z96.662 Presence of left artificial ankle joint
Z96.669 Presence of unspecified artificial ankle joint
Z96.69 Presence of other orthopedic joint implants
Z96.691 Finger-joint replacement of right hand
Z96.692 Finger-joint replacement of left hand
Z96.693 Finger-joint replacement, bilateral
Z96.698 Presence of other orthopedic joint implants
Z96.7 Presence of other bone and tendon implants
Presence of skull plate
Z96.8 Presence of other specified functional implants
Z96.81 Presence of artificial skin
Z96.89 Presence of other specified functional implants
Z96.9 Presence of functional implant, unspecified

Z97 Presence of other devices
EXCLUDES1 *complications of internal prosthetic devices, implants and grafts (T82-T85)*
fitting and adjustment of prosthetic and other devices (Z44-Z46)
EXCLUDES2 *presence of cerebrospinal fluid drainage device (Z98.2)*
Z97.0 Presence of artificial eye
Z97.1 Presence of artificial limb (complete) (partial)

PDx Unacceptable principal diagnosis symbol per Medicare code edits; POA Code exempt from diagnosis present on admission requirement; Questionable admission; CC Complication or comorbidity; CC/MCC Exc CC/MCC exclusion; MCC Major complication or comorbidity; Principal diagnosis as its own CC; Principal diagnosis as its own MCC; Z code as first-listed diagnosis

Z97.10 Presence of artificial limb (complete) (partial), unspecified
Z97.11 Presence of artificial right arm (complete) (partial)
Z97.12 Presence of artificial left arm (complete) (partial)
Z97.13 Presence of artificial right leg (complete) (partial)
Z97.14 Presence of artificial left leg (complete) (partial)
Z97.15 Presence of artificial arms, bilateral (complete) (partial)
Z97.16 Presence of artificial legs, bilateral (complete) (partial)
Z97.2 Presence of dental prosthetic device (complete) (partial)
Presence of dentures (complete) (partial)
Z97.3 Presence of spectacles and contact lenses
Z97.4 Presence of external hearing-aid
Z97.5 Presence of (intrauterine) contraceptive device
EXCLUDES1 *checking, reinsertion or removal of ▶implantable subdermal contraceptive (Z30.46)◀*
checking, reinsertion or removal of intrauterine contraceptive device (Z30.43-)
Z97.8 Presence of other specified devices

Z98 Other postprocedural states
EXCLUDES2 *aftercare (Z43-Z49, Z51)*
follow-up medical care (Z08-Z09)
postprocedural complication - see Alphabetical Index
Z98.0 Intestinal bypass and anastomosis status
EXCLUDES2 *bariatric surgery status (Z98.84)*
gastric bypass status (Z98.84)
obesity surgery status (Z98.84)
Z98.1 Arthrodesis status
Z98.2 Presence of cerebrospinal fluid drainage device
Presence of CSF shunt
Z98.3 Post therapeutic collapse of lung status
Code first underlying disease
Z98.4 Cataract extraction status
Use additional code to identify intraocular lens implant status (Z96.1)
EXCLUDES1 *aphakia (H27.0)*
Z98.41 Cataract extraction status, right eye
Z98.42 Cataract extraction status, left eye
Z98.49 Cataract extraction status, unspecified eye
Z98.5 Sterilization status
EXCLUDES1 *female infertility (N97.-)*
male infertility (N46.-)
Z98.51 Tubal ligation status
Z98.52 Vasectomy status
Z98.6 Angioplasty status
Z98.61 Coronary angioplasty status
EXCLUDES1 *coronary angioplasty status with implant and graft (Z95.5)*
Z98.62 Peripheral vascular angioplasty status
EXCLUDES1 *peripheral vascular angioplasty status with implant and graft (Z95.820)*
Z98.8 Other specified postprocedural states
Z98.81 Dental procedure status
Z98.810 Dental sealant status
Z98.811 Dental restoration status
Dental crown status
Dental fillings status
Z98.818 Other dental procedure status
Z98.82 Breast implant status
EXCLUDES1 *breast implant removal status (Z98.86)*
Z98.83 Filtering (vitreous) bleb after glaucoma surgery status
EXCLUDES1 *Inflammation (infection) of postprocedural bleb (H59.4-)*
Z98.84 Bariatric surgery status
Gastric banding status
Gastric bypass status for obesity
Obesity surgery status
EXCLUDES1 *bariatric surgery status complicating pregnancy, childbirth, or the puerperium (O99.84)*
EXCLUDES2 *intestinal bypass and anastomosis status (Z98.0)*
Z98.85 Transplanted organ removal status
Transplanted organ previously removed due to complication, failure, rejection or infection
EXCLUDES1 *encounter for removal of transplanted organ -code to complication of transplanted organ (T86.-)*
Z98.86 Personal history of breast implant removal
Z98.87 Personal history of in utero procedure
Z98.870 Personal history of in utero procedure during pregnancy
EXCLUDES2 *complications from in utero procedure for current pregnancy (O35.7)*
supervision of current pregnancy with history of in utero procedure during previous pregnancy (O09.82-)
Z98.871 Personal history of in utero procedure while a fetus
Z98.89 Other specified postprocedural states
● Z98.890 Other specified postprocedural states
Personal history of surgery, not elsewhere classified
● Z98.891 History of uterine scar from previous surgery
EXCLUDES1 *Maternal care due to uterine scar from previous surgery (O34.2-)*

Z99 Dependence on enabling machines and devices, not elsewhere classified
EXCLUDES1 *cardiac pacemaker status (Z95.0)*
Z99.0 Dependence on aspirator
Z99.1 Dependence on respirator
Dependence on ventilator
Z99.11 Dependence on respirator [ventilator] status
AHA: Q1, 2015
Z99.12 Encounter for respirator [ventilator] dependence during power failure
EXCLUDES1 *mechanical complication of respirator [ventilator] (J95.850)*
Z99.2 Dependence on renal dialysis
Hemodialysis status
Peritoneal dialysis status
Presence of arteriovenous shunt for dialysis
Renal dialysis status NOS
EXCLUDES1 *encounter for fitting and adjustment of dialysis catheter (Z49.0-)*
EXCLUDES2 *noncompliance with renal dialysis (Z91.15)*
AHA: Q4, 2013
Z99.3 Dependence on wheelchair
Wheelchair confinement status
Code first cause of dependence, such as:
muscular dystrophy (G71.0)
obesity (E66.-)
Z99.8 Dependence on other enabling machines and devices
Z99.81 Dependence on supplemental oxygen
Dependence on long-term oxygen
AHA: Q4, 2013
Z99.89 Dependence on other enabling machines and devices
Dependence on machine or device NOS

Unspecified Code | Other Specified Code | Manifestation Code | N Newborn | P Pediatric | M Maternity | A Adult | ♂ Male | ♀ Female
● New Code | ▲ Revised Code Title | ▶◀ Revised Text | NOTES | INCLUDES | EXCLUDES1 Not coded here | EXCLUDES2 Not included here
4th character required | 5th character required | 6th character required | 7th character required
Extension 'X' Alert | HAC Hospital-acquired condition (HAC) alert | AHA AHA Coding Clinic®

This page intentionally left blank

Appendix A: Z Codes for Long-term Use of Drugs

The following Z codes/categories may only be reported as the principal/first-listed diagnosis, except when there are multiple encounters on the same day and the medical records for the encounters are combined:

Code	Code Descriptor	Brand Name Drug	Generic Drug Equivalent
Z79.01	Long term (current) use of anticoagulants	Arixtra®	fondaparinux
		Coumadin®	warfarin
		Eliquis®	apixaban
		Fragmin®	dalteparin
		Heparin Lock Flush®	heparin flush
		Heparin Sodium®	heparin
		Innohep®	tinzaparin
		Jantoven®	warfarin
		Lovenox®	enoxaparin
		Monoject Prefill Advanced®	heparin flush
		Orgaran®	danaparoid
		PosiFlush®	heparin flush
		Savaysa®	edoxaban
		Xarelto®	rivaroxaban
Z79.02	Long term (current) use of antithrombotics/ antiplatelets	Acova®	argatroban
		Angiomax®	bivalirudin
		Iprivask®	desirudin
		Pradaxa®	dabigatran
		Refludan®	lepirudin
Z79.1	Long term (current) use of non-steroidal anti-inflammatories (NSAID)	Actiprofen®	ibuprofen
		Addaprin®	ibuprofen
		Advil Children's®	ibuprofen
		Advil Infant's Concentrated Drops®	ibuprofen
		Advil Liqui-Gels®	ibuprofen
		Advil®	ibuprofen
		Aflaxen®	naproxen
		A-G Profen®	ibuprofen
		Aleve®	naproxen
		All Day Pain Relief®	naproxen
		All Day Relief®	naproxen
		Anaprox®	naproxen
		Anaprox-DS®	naproxen
		Ansaid®	flurbiprofen
		Arthrotec®	diclofenac/misoprostol
		Caldolor®	ibuprofen
		Cambia®	diclofenac
		Cataflam®	diclofenac
		Children's Motrin®	ibuprofen
		Clinoril®	sulindac
		Daypro®	oxaprozin
		Duexis®	famotidine/ibuprofen
		Dyloject®	diclofenac
		EC-Naprosyn®	naproxen
		Feldene®	piroxicam
		Fenortho®	fenoprofen
		Flanax Pain Reliever®	naproxen

Code	Code Descriptor	Brand Name Drug	Generic Drug Equivalent
Z79.1 *–Continued*		Genpril®	ibuprofen
		Haltran®	ibuprofen
		IBU®	ibuprofen
		IBU-200®	ibuprofen
		Ibu-4®	ibuprofen
		Ibu-6®	ibuprofen
		Ibu-8®	ibuprofen
		Ibu-Tab®	ibuprofen
		Indocin IV®	indomethacin
		Indocin SR®	indomethacin
		Indocin®	indomethacin
		Leader Naproxen Sodium®	naproxen
		Lodine XL®	etodolac
		Lodine®	etodolac
		Meclomen®	meclofenamate
		Midol Extended Relief®	naproxen
		Midol IB®	ibuprofen
		Mobic®	meloxicam
		Motrin Childrens®	ibuprofen
		Motrin IB®	ibuprofen
		Motrin Infant Drops®	ibuprofen
		Motrin Junior Strength®	ibuprofen
		Motrin®	ibuprofen
		Nalfon®	fenoprofen
		Naprelan®	naproxen
		Naprosyn®	naproxen
		NeoProfen®	ibuprofen
		Nuprin®	ibuprofen
		Orudis KT®	ketoprofen
		Orudis®	ketoprofen
		Oruvail®	ketoprofen
		Ponstel®	mefenamic acid
		Prevacid NapraPAC®	lansoprazole/naproxen
		Proprinal®	ibuprofen
		Q-Profen®	ibuprofen
		Relafen®	nabumetone
		Sprix®	ketorolac
		Tivorbex®	indomethacin
		Tolectin 600®	tolmetin
		Tolectin DS®	tolmetin
		Tolectin®	tolmetin
		Toradol IM®	ketorolac
		Toradol IV / IM®	ketorolac
		Toradol®	ketorolac
		Vimovo®	esomeprazole/naproxen
		Voltaren®	diclofenac
		Voltaren-XR®	diclofenac
		Zipsor®	diclofenac
		Zorvolex®	diclofenac

Code	Code Descriptor	Brand Name Drug	Generic Drug Equivalent
Z79.2	Long term (current) use of antibiotics	A / T / S®	erythromycin
		Akne-Mycin®	erythromycin
		Altabax®	retapamulin
		Antibiotic Plus Pain Relief®	neomycin/polymyxin b/pramoxine
		Avar Cleanser®	sulfacetamide sodium/sulfur
		Avar LS Cleanser®	sulfacetamide sodium/sulfur
		Avar®	sulfacetamide sodium/sulfur
		Avar-E Green®	sulfacetamide sodium/sulfur
		Avar-E LS®	sulfacetamide sodium/sulfur
		Avar-E®	sulfacetamide sodium/sulfur
		Baciguent®	bacitracin
		Bactroban Nasal®	mupirocin
		Bactroban®	mupirocin
		BP 10-Wash®	sulfacetamide sodium/sulfur
		Carmol Scalp Treatment Kit®	sulfacetamide sodium/urea
		Carmol Scalp Treatment®	sulfacetamide sodium/urea
		Carmol Scalp®	sulfacetamide sodium/urea
		Centany AT Kit®	mupirocin
		Centany®	mupirocin
		Cerisa Wash®	sulfacetamide sodium/sulfur
		Clarifoam EF®	sulfacetamide sodium/sulfur
		Clenia Emollient Cream®	sulfacetamide sodium/sulfur
		Duospore®	bacitracin/polymyxin b
		Dycill®	dicloxacillin
		Dynacin®	minocycline
		Dynapen®	dicloxacillin
		E.E.S. Granules®	erythromycin
		E.E.S.-400 Filmtab®	erythromycin
		E.E.S.-400®	erythromycin
		Emcin Clear®	erythromycin
		Emgel®	erythromycin
		Ery Pads®	erythromycin
		Eryc®	erythromycin
		Erycette®	erythromycin
		Eryderm®	erythromycin
		Erygel®	erythromycin
		Erymax®	erythromycin
		EryPed®	erythromycin
		Ery-Tab®	erythromycin
		Erythrocin Lactobionate®	erythromycin
		Erythrocin Stearate Filmtab®	erythromycin
		Erythrocin®	erythromycin
		Eryzole®	erythromycin/sulfisoxazole
		Flagyl 375®	metronidazole
		Flagyl ER®	metronidazole
		Flagyl IV®	metronidazole
		Flagyl®	metronidazole
		Fortaz®	ceftazidime
		Garamycin®	gentamicin
		Garimide®	sulfacetamide sodium/sulfur

Code	Code Descriptor	Brand Name Drug	Generic Drug Equivalent
Z79.2 *–Continued*		Geocillin®	carbenicillin
		Humatin®	paromomycin
		Ilosone®	erythromycin
		Invanz®	ertapenem
		Isoject Permapen®	penicillin G benzathine
		Kantrex®	kanamycin
		Keflex®	cephalexin
		Kefzol®	cefazolin
		Ketek Pak®	telithromycin
		Ketek®	telithromycin
		Kitabis Pak®	tobramycin
		Klaron®	sulfacetamide sodium
		Lincocin®	lincomycin
		Lorabid Pulvules®	loracarbef
		Lorabid®	loracarbef
		Maxipime®	cefepime
		Medi-Quik®	bacitracin/neomycin/polymyxin B
		Mefoxin®	cefoxitin
		Mepron®	atovaquone
		Merrem®	meropenem
		Metro®	metronidazole
		Mexar®	sulfacetamide sodium
		Minocin®	minocycline
		Monodox®	doxycycline
		Monurol®	fosfomycin
		Morgidox®	doxycycline
		Moxatag®	amoxicillin
		Moxilin®	amoxicillin
		Mycobutin®	rifabutin
		Myrac®	minocycline
		Nebcin®	tobramycin
		Nebupent®	pentamidine
		Neo-Fradin®	neomycin
		Neosporin Plus®	neomycin/polymyxin b/pramoxine
		Neosporin®	bacitracin/neomycin/polymyxin B
		Neo-Tab®	neomycin
		Neutrexin®	trimetrexate
		Ocudox®	doxycycline
		Omnicef Omni-Pac®	cefdinir
		Omnicef®	cefdinir
		Omnipen-N®	ampicillin
		Oracea®	doxycycline
		Oraxyl®	doxycycline
		Orbactiv®	oritavancin
		Ovace Plus®	sulfacetamide sodium
		Ovace®	sulfacetamide sodium
		Panixine®	cephalexin
		Paromycin®	paromomycin
		PC Pen VK®	penicillin V potassium
		PCE Dispertab®	erythromycin

Code	Code Descriptor	Brand Name Drug	Generic Drug Equivalent
Z79.2 *–Continued*		Pediazole®	erythromycin/sulfisoxazole
		Penicillin VK®	penicillin V potassium
		Pentam 300®	pentamidine
		Pentam®	pentamidine
		Periostat®	doxycycline
		Pfizerpen®	penicillin G potassium
		Pipracil®	piperacillin
		Plexion Cleansing Cloths®	sulfacetamide sodium/sulfur
		Plexion SCT®	sulfacetamide sodium/sulfur
		Plexion TS®	sulfacetamide sodium/sulfur
		Plexion®	sulfacetamide sodium/sulfur
		Polysporin®	bacitracin/polymyxin B
		Prascion Cleanser®	sulfacetamide sodium/sulfur
		Prascion FC Cloths®	sulfacetamide sodium/sulfur
		Prascion RA®	sulfacetamide sodium/sulfur
		Priftin®	rifapentine
		Primaxin IM®	cilastatin/imipenem
		Primaxin IV®	cilastatin/imipenem
		Principen®	ampicillin
		Raniclor®	cefaclor
		Rebetol®	ribavirin
		Relenza®	zanamivir
		RibaPak®	ribavirin
		Ribasphere®	ribavirin
		RibaTab®	ribavirin
		Rifadin IV®	rifampin
		Rifadin®	rifampin
		Rimactane®	rifampin
		Rocephin®	ceftriaxone
		Romycin®	erythromycin
		Rosac®	sulfacetamide sodium/sulfur
		Rosaderm Cleanser®	sulfacetamide sodium/sulfur
		Rosanil Cleanser®	sulfacetamide sodium/sulfur
		Rosula Cleanser®	sulfacetamide sodium/sulfur
		Rosula CLK®	sulfacetamide sodium/sulfur/urea
		Rosula NS®	sulfacetamide sodium/urea
		Rosula Wash®	sulfacetamide sodium/sulfur
		Rosula®	sulfacetamide sodium/sulfur
		Sebizon®	sulfacetamide sodium
		Seb-Prev®	sulfacetamide sodium
		Septra DS®	sulfamethoxazole/trimethoprim
		Septra®	sulfamethoxazole/trimethoprim
		Seromycin®	cycloserine
		Silvadene®	silver sulfadiazine
		Sivextro®	tedizolid
		SMZ-TMP DS®	sulfamethoxazole/trimethoprim
		Solodyn®	minocycline
		Spectracef®	cefditoren
		SSD AF®	silver sulfadiazine
		SSD®	silver sulfadiazine

Code	Code Descriptor	Brand Name Drug	Generic Drug Equivalent
Z79.2 *–Continued*		Staticin®	erythromycin
		Sulfacleanse 8 / 4®	sulfacetamide sodium/sulfur
		Sulfamylon®	mafenide
		Sulfatol C®	sulfacetamide sodium/sulfur
		Sulfatol Cleanser®	sulfacetamide sodium/sulfur/urea
		Sulfatol SS®	sulfacetamide sodium/sulfur
		Sulfatol®	sulfacetamide sodium/sulfur
		Sulfatrim Pediatric®	sulfamethoxazole/trimethoprim
		Sulfatrim®	sulfamethoxazole/trimethoprim
		Sumadan®	sulfacetamide sodium/sulfur
		Sumaxin Cleansing Pads®	sulfacetamide sodium/sulfur
		Sumaxin TS®	sulfacetamide sodium/sulfur
		Sumaxin®	sulfacetamide sodium/sulfur
		Sumycin®	tetracycline
		Suphera®	sulfacetamide sodium/sulfur
		Suprax®	cefixime
		Synercid®	dalfopristin/quinupristin
		Tazicef®	ceftazidime
		Teflaro®	ceftaroline
		Terramycin®	oxytetracycline
		Theramycin Z®	erythromycin
		Thermazene®	silver sulfadiazine
		Ticar®	ticarcillin
		Timentin®	clavulanate/ticarcillin
		TOBI Podhaler®	tobramycin
		Tobi®	tobramycin
		Topisulf®	sulfacetamide sodium/sulfur
		Totacillin-N®	ampicillin
		Trimox®	amoxicillin
		Triple Antibiotic®	bacitracin/neomycin/polymyxin B
		Trobicin®	spectinomycin
		T-Stat®	erythromycin
		Tygacil®	tigecycline
		Unasyn®	ampicillin/sulbactam
		Unipen®	nafcillin
		Uracil®	doxycycline
		Vancocin HCl Pulvules®	vancomycin
		Vancocin HCl®	vancomycin
		Vancocin®	vancomycin
		Vantin®	cefpodoxime
		Veetids®	penicillin V potassium
		Velosef®	cephradine
		Vibativ®	telavancin
		Vibramycin®	doxycycline
		Vibra-Tabs®	doxycycline
		Virazole®	ribavirin
		Virti-Sulf®	sulfacetamide sodium/sulfur
		Wycillin®	procaine penicillin
		Wymox®	amoxicillin
		Xifaxan®	rifaximin

Code	Code Descriptor	Brand Name Drug	Generic Drug Equivalent
Z79.2 *–Continued*		Ximino®	minocycline
		Zencia Wash®	sulfacetamide sodium/sulfur
		Zerbaxa®	ceftolozane/tazobactam
		Zetacet®	sulfacetamide sodium/sulfur
		Zinacef®	cefuroxime
		Zithromax®	azithromycin
		Zmax®	azithromycin
		Zosyn®	piperacillin/tazobactam
		Zyvox®	linezolid
Z79.3	Long term (current) use of hormonal contraceptives	Alesse®	ethinyl estradiol/levonorgestrel
		Altavera®	ethinyl estradiol/levonorgestrel
		Alyacen 1 / 35®	ethinyl estradiol/norethindrone
		Amethia Lo®	ethinyl estradiol/levonorgestrel
		Amethia®	ethinyl estradiol/levonorgestrel
		Amethyst®	ethinyl estradiol/levonorgestrel
		Apri®	desogestrel/ethinyl estradiol
		Aranelle®	ethinyl estradiol/norethindrone
		Ashlyna®	ethinyl estradiol/levonorgestrel
		Aubra®	ethinyl estradiol/levonorgestrel
		Aviane®	ethinyl estradiol/levonorgestrel
		Aygestin®	norethindrone
		Azurette®	desogestrel/ethinyl estradiol
		Balziva®	ethinyl estradiol/norethindrone
		Bekyree®	desogestrel/ethinyl estradiol
		Beyaz®	drospirenone/ethinyl estradiol/levomefolate calcium
		Brevicon®	ethinyl estradiol/norethindrone
		Briellyn®	ethinyl estradiol/norethindrone
		Camila®	norethindrone
		Camrese®	ethinyl estradiol/levonorgestrel
		CamreseLo®	ethinyl estradiol/levonorgestrel
		Caziant®	desogestrel/ethinyl estradiol
		Cesia®	desogestrel/ethinyl estradiol
		Chateal®	ethinyl estradiol/levonorgestrel
		Cryselle®	ethinyl estradiol/norgestrel
		Cyclafem 1 / 35®	ethinyl estradiol/norethindrone
		Cyclafem 7 / 7 / 7®	ethinyl estradiol/norethindrone
		Cyclessa®	desogestrel/ethinyl estradiol
		Cyred®	desogestrel/ethinyl estradiol
		Dasetta 1 / 35®	ethinyl estradiol/norethindrone
		Dasetta 7 / 7 / 7®	ethinyl estradiol/norethindrone
		Daysee®	ethinyl estradiol/levonorgestrel
		Delyla®	ethinyl estradiol/levonorgestrel
		Demulen®	ethinyl estradiol/ethynodiol
		Depo-Provera Contraceptive®	medroxyprogesterone
		Depo-Provera®	medroxyprogesterone
		depo-subQ provera 104®	medroxyprogesterone
		Desogen®	desogestrel/ethinyl estradiol
		Elinest®	ethinyl estradiol/norgestrel
		Emoquette®	desogestrel/ethinyl estradiol
		Enpresse®	ethinyl estradiol/levonorgestrel

Code	Code Descriptor	Brand Name Drug	Generic Drug Equivalent
Z79.3 *–Continued*		Enskyce®	desogestrel/ethinyl estradiol
		Errin®	norethindrone
		Estarylla®	ethinyl estradiol/norgestimate
		Estrostep Fe®	ethinyl estradiol/norethindrone
		Falmina®	ethinyl estradiol/levonorgestrel
		Femcon Fe®	ethinyl estradiol/norethindrone
		femhrt®	ethinyl estradiol/norethindrone
		Femynor®	ethinyl estradiol/norgestimate
		Generess Fe®	ethinyl estradiol/norethindrone
		Gianvi®	drospirenone/ethinyl estradiol
		Gildagia®	ethinyl estradiol/norethindrone
		Gildess 1 / 20®	ethinyl estradiol/norethindrone
		Gildess 1.5 / 30®	ethinyl estradiol/norethindrone
		Gildess Fe 1 / 20®	ethinyl estradiol/norethindrone
		Gildess Fe 1.5 / 30®	ethinyl estradiol/norethindrone
		Implanon®	etonogestrel
		Introvale®	ethinyl estradiol/levonorgestrel
		Jencycla®	norethindrone
		Jevantique®	ethinyl estradiol/norethindrone
		Jinteli®	ethinyl estradiol/norethindrone
		Jolessa®	ethinyl estradiol/levonorgestrel
		Jolivette®	norethindrone
		Juleber®	desogestrel/ethinyl estradiol
		Junel 1 / 20®	ethinyl estradiol/norethindrone
		Junel 1.5 / 30®	ethinyl estradiol/norethindrone
		Kariva®	desogestrel/ethinyl estradiol
		Kelnor 1 / 35®	ethinyl estradiol/ethynodiol
		Kimidess®	desogestrel/ethinyl estradiol
		Kurvelo®	ethinyl estradiol/levonorgestrel
		Larin Fe 1 / 20®	ethinyl estradiol/norethindrone
		Larin Fe 1.5 / 30®	ethinyl estradiol/norethindrone
		Larissia®	ethinyl estradiol/levonorgestrel
		Leena®	ethinyl estradiol/norethindrone
		Lessina®	ethinyl estradiol/levonorgestrel
		Levlen®	ethinyl estradiol/levonorgestrel
		Levlite®	ethinyl estradiol/levonorgestrel
		Levonest®	ethinyl estradiol/levonorgestrel
		Levonest-28®	ethinyl estradiol/levonorgestrel
		Levora®	ethinyl estradiol/levonorgestrel
		Liletta®	levonorgestrel
		Lo / Ovral®	ethinyl estradiol/norgestrel
		Lo Loestrin Fe®	ethinyl estradiol/norethindrone
		Lo Minastrin Fe®	ethinyl estradiol/norethindrone
		Loestrin 1 / 20®	ethinyl estradiol/norethindrone
		Loestrin 21 1.5 / 30®	ethinyl estradiol/norethindrone
		Loestrin 24 Fe®	ethinyl estradiol/norethindrone
		Loestrin Fe 1 / 20®	ethinyl estradiol/norethindrone
		Loryna®	drospirenone/ethinyl estradiol
		LoSeasonique®	ethinyl estradiol/levonorgestrel
		Low-Ogestrel-21®	ethinyl estradiol/norgestrel

Code	Code Descriptor	Brand Name Drug	Generic Drug Equivalent
Z79.3 *–Continued*		Lunelle®	estradiol/medroxyprogesterone
		Lutera®	ethinyl estradiol/levonorgestrel
		Lybrel®	ethinyl estradiol/levonorgestrel
		Lyza®	norethindrone
		Marlissa®	ethinyl estradiol/levonorgestrel
		Microgestin 1 / 20®	ethinyl estradiol/norethindrone
		Microgestin 1.5 / 30®	ethinyl estradiol/norethindrone
		Microgestin Fe 1 / 20®	ethinyl estradiol/norethindrone
		Minastrin 24 Fe®	ethinyl estradiol/norethindrone
		Mircette®	desogestrel/ethinyl estradiol
		Mirena®	levonorgestrel
		Modicon®	ethinyl estradiol/norethindrone
		Mono-Linyah®	ethinyl estradiol/norgestimate
		Mononessa®	ethinyl estradiol/norgestimate
		My Way®	levonorgestrel
		Myzilra®	ethinyl estradiol/levonorgestrel
		Natazia®	dienogest/estradiol
		Necon 1 / 35®	ethinyl estradiol/norethindrone
		Necon 1 / 50®	mestranol/norethindrone
		Necon 7 / 7 / 7®	ethinyl estradiol/norethindrone
		Nexplanon®	etonogestrel
		Next Choice®	levonorgestrel
		Nora-Be®	norethindrone
		Norinyl 1+50®	mestranol/norethindrone
		Nor-QD®	norethindrone
		Nortrel 1 / 35®	ethinyl estradiol/norethindrone
		NuvaRing®	ethinyl estradiol/etonogestrel
		Ocella®	drospirenone/ethinyl estradiol
		Ogestrel®	ethinyl estradiol/norgestrel
		Ogestrel-28®	ethinyl estradiol/norgestrel
		Orsythia®	ethinyl estradiol/levonorgestrel
		Ortho Cyclen®	ethinyl estradiol/norgestimate
		Ortho Evra®	ethinyl estradiol/norelgestromin
		Ortho Micronor®	norethindrone
		Ortho Tri-Cyclen Lo®	ethinyl estradiol/norgestimate
		Ortho Tri-Cyclen®	ethinyl estradiol/norgestimate
		Ortho-Cept®	desogestrel/ethinyl estradiol
		Ortho-Novum 1 / 35®	ethinyl estradiol/norethindrone
		Ortho-Novum 1 / 50®	mestranol/norethindrone
		Ortho-Novum 7 / 7 / 7®	ethinyl estradiol/norethindrone
		Ovcon 35®	ethinyl estradiol/norethindrone
		Philith®	ethinyl estradiol/norethindrone
		Pimtrea®	desogestrel/ethinyl estradiol
		Pirmella 1 / 35®	ethinyl estradiol/norethindrone
		Pirmella 7 / 7 / 7®	ethinyl estradiol/norethindrone
		Plan B One-Step®	levonorgestrel
		Plan B®	levonorgestrel
		Portia®	ethinyl estradiol/levonorgestrel
		Preven EC®	ethinyl estradiol/levonorgestrel
		Previfem®	ethinyl estradiol/norgestimate

Code	Code Descriptor	Brand Name Drug	Generic Drug Equivalent
Z79.3 *–Continued*		Provera®	medroxyprogesterone
		Quartette®	ethinyl estradiol/levonorgestrel
		Quasense®	ethinyl estradiol/levonorgestrel
		Reclipsen®	desogestrel/ethinyl estradiol
		Safyral®	drospirenone/ethinyl estradiol/levomefolate calcium
		Seasonale®	ethinyl estradiol/levonorgestrel
		Seasonique®	ethinyl estradiol/levonorgestrel
		Setlakin®	ethinyl estradiol/levonorgestrel
		Skyla®	levonorgestrel
		Solia®	desogestrel/ethinyl estradiol
		Sprintec®	ethinyl estradiol/norgestimate
		Sronyx®	ethinyl estradiol/levonorgestrel
		Syeda®	drospirenone/ethinyl estradiol
		Tilia Fe®	ethinyl estradiol/norethindrone
		Tri-Estarylla®	ethinyl estradiol/norgestimate
		Tri-Legest Fe®	ethinyl estradiol/norethindrone
		Tri-Legest®	ethinyl estradiol/norethindrone
		Tri-Linyah®	ethinyl estradiol/norgestimate
		Tri-Lo-Estarylla®	ethinyl estradiol/norgestimate
		Tri-Lo-Marzia®	ethinyl estradiol/norgestimate
		Tri-Lo-Sprintec®	ethinyl estradiol/norgestimate
		TriNessa Lo®	ethinyl estradiol/norgestimate
		TriNessa®	ethinyl estradiol/norgestimate
		Tri-Norinyl®	ethinyl estradiol/norethindrone
		Triphasil®	ethinyl estradiol/levonorgestrel
		Triphasil-21®	ethinyl estradiol/levonorgestrel
		Triphasil-28®	ethinyl estradiol/levonorgestrel
		Tri-Previfem®	ethinyl estradiol/norgestimate
		Tri-Sprintec®	ethinyl estradiol/norgestimate
		Trivora-28®	ethinyl estradiol/levonorgestrel
		Velivet®	desogestrel/ethinyl estradiol
		Vestura®	drospirenone/ethinyl estradiol
		Vienva®	ethinyl estradiol/levonorgestrel
		Viorele®	desogestrel/ethinyl estradiol
		Wera®	ethinyl estradiol/norethindrone
		Wymzya Fe®	ethinyl estradiol/norethindrone
		Yasmin®	drospirenone/ethinyl estradiol
		Yaz®	drospirenone/ethinyl estradiol
		Zarah®	drospirenone/ethinyl estradiol
		Zenchent Fe®	ethinyl estradiol/norethindrone
		Zenchent®	ethinyl estradiol/norethindrone
		Zeosa®	ethinyl estradiol/norethindrone
		Zovia 1 / 35®	ethinyl estradiol/ethynodiol
		Zovia 1 / 50®	ethinyl estradiol/ethynodiol
		Zovia®	ethinyl estradiol/ethynodiol
Z79.4	Long term (current) use of insulin	Afrezza®	insulin inhalation, rapid acting
		Apidra Solostar®	insulin glulisine
		Apidra®	insulin glulisine
		Basaglar®	insulin glargine
		Exubera®	insulin inhalation, rapid acting

Code	Code Descriptor	Brand Name Drug	Generic Drug Equivalent
Z79.4 *–Continued*		Humalog KwikPen®	insulin lispro
		Humalog Mix 50 / 50 KwikPen®	insulin lispro/insulin lispro protamine
		Humalog Mix 50 / 50®	insulin lispro/insulin lispro protamine
		Humalog Mix 75 / 25 KwikPen®	insulin lispro/insulin lispro protamine
		Humalog Mix 75 / 25®	insulin lispro/insulin lispro protamine
		Humalog Pen®	insulin lispro
		Humalog®	insulin lispro
		Humulin 70 / 30 Pen®	insulin isophane/insulin regular
		Humulin 70 / 30®	insulin isophane/insulin regular
		Humulin L®	insulin zinc
		Humulin N Pen®	insulin isophane
		Humulin N®	insulin isophane
		Humulin R®	insulin regular
		Humulin U®	insulin zinc extended
		Lantus Solostar®	insulin glargine
		Lantus®	insulin glargine
		Levemir®	insulin detemir
		Novolin 70 / 30®	insulin isophane/insulin regular
		Novolin N®	insulin isophane
		Novolin R®	insulin regular
		NovoLog FlexPen®	insulin aspart
		NovoLog Mix 70 / 30 FlexPen®	insulin aspart/insulin aspart protamine
		NovoLog Mix 70 / 30®	insulin aspart/insulin aspart protamine
		NovoLog PenFill®	insulin aspart
		Novolog®	insulin aspart
		Relion Novolin 70 / 30 Innolet®	insulin isophane/insulin regular
		Ryzodeg 70 / 30®	insulin aspart/insulin degludec
		Toujeo Solostar®	insulin glargine
		Toujeo®	insulin glargine
		Tresiba®	insulin degludec
Z79.51	Long term (current) use of inhaled steroids	Aerobid®	flunisolide
		Aerobid-M®	flunisolide
		Aerospan HFA®	flunisolide
		Alvesco®	ciclesonide
		Arnuity Ellipta®	fluticasone
		Asmanex HFA®	mometasone
		Asmanex Twisthaler®	mometasone
		Beclovent®	beclomethasone
		Flovent Diskus®	fluticasone
		Flovent HFA®	fluticasone
		Flovent Rotadisk®	fluticasone
		Flovent®	fluticasone
		Pulmicort Flexhaler®	budesonide
		Pulmicort Nebuamp®	budesonide
		Pulmicort Respules®	budesonide
		Pulmicort Turbuhaler®	budesonide
		Qvar®	beclomethasone
Z79.52	Long term (current) use of systemic steroids	A-Methapred®	methylprednisolone
		Aristocort For Injection®	triamcinolone
		Aristocort®	triamcinolone

Code	Code Descriptor	Brand Name Drug	Generic Drug Equivalent
Z79.52 *–Continued*		Aristospan®	triamcinolone
		AsmalPred Plus®	prednisolone
		Azmacort®	triamcinolone
		Baycadron®	dexamethasone
		Bubbli-Pred®	prednisolone
		Celestone Soluspan®	betamethasone
		Celestone®	betamethasone
		Clinacort®	triamcinolone
		Colocort®	hydrocortisone
		Cortef®	hydrocortisone
		Cortenema®	hydrocortisone
		Cortifoam®	hydrocortisone
		Cortone Acetate®	cortisone
		Cotolone®	prednisolone
		Decadron®	dexamethasone
		Deltasone®	prednisone
		Depo-Medrol®	methylprednisolone
		De-Sone LA®	dexamethasone
		Dexacen-4®	dexamethasone
		Dexamethasone Intensol®	dexamethasone
		Dexasone LA®	dexamethasone
		Dexasone®	dexamethasone
		Dexpak Taperpak®	dexamethasone
		Entocort EC®	budesonide
		Flo-Pred®	prednisolone
		Hydrocortone®	hydrocortisone
		Kenalog-10®	triamcinolone
		Kenalog-40®	triamcinolone
		Ken-Jec 40®	triamcinolone
		Medrol Dosepak®	methylprednisolone
		Medrol®	methylprednisolone
		Methylpred DP®	methylprednisolone
		MethylPREDNISolone Dose Pack®	methylprednisolone
		Millipred DP®	prednisolone
		Millipred®	prednisolone
		Orapred ODT®	prednisolone
		Orapred®	prednisolone
		PediaPred®	prednisolone
		Prednicot®	prednisone
		Prelone®	prednisolone
		Rayos®	prednisone
		Solu-Cortef®	hydrocortisone
		Solu-Medrol®	methylprednisolone
		Solurex LA®	dexamethasone
		Solurex®	dexamethasone
		Sterapred DS®	prednisone
		Sterapred®	prednisone
		TAC 3®	triamcinolone
		Triamcot®	triamcinolone
		Triam-Forte®	triamcinolone

Code	Code Descriptor	Brand Name Drug	Generic Drug Equivalent
Z79.52 *–Continued*		Triamonide 40®	triamcinolone
		Uceris®	budesonide
		U-Tri-Lone®	triamcinolone
		Veripred 20®	prednisolone
		Zema Pak®	dexamethasone
Z79.810	Long term (current) use of selective estrogen receptor modulators (SERMs)	Evista®	raloxifene
		Fareston®	toremifene
		Nolvadex®	tamoxifen
		Osphena®	ospemifene
		Soltamox®	tamoxifen
Z79.811	Long term (current) use of aromatase inhibitors	Arimidex®	anastrozole
		Aromasin®	exemestane
		Femara®	letrozole
		Teslac®	testolactone
Z79.818	Long term (current) use of other agents affecting estrogen receptors and estrogen levels	Eligard®	leuprolide
		Factrel®	gonadorelin
		Faslodex®	fulvestrant
		Lupron Depot 11.25 mg®	leuprolide
		Lupron Depot 3.75 mg®	leuprolide
		Lupron Depot®	leuprolide
		Lupron Depot-PED®	leuprolide
		Lupron®	leuprolide
		Megace ES®	megestrol
		Megace®	megestrol acetate
		Supprelin LA®	histrelin
		Synarel®	nafarelin
		Trelstar Depot®	triptorelin
		Trelstar LA®	triptorelin
		Trelstar®	triptorelin
		Vantas®	histrelin
		Viadur®	leuprolide
		Zoladex®	goserelin
Z79.82	Long term (current) use of aspirin	Arthritis Pain®	aspirin
		Ascriptin®	aspirin
		Aspir 81®	aspirin
		Aspir-Low®	aspirin
		Bayer Children's Aspirin®	aspirin
		Bufferin Low Dose®	aspirin
		Durlaza®	aspirin
		Ecotrin®	aspirin
		Ecpirin®	aspirin
		Fasprin®	aspirin
		Halfprin®	aspirin
		Miniprin®	aspirin

Code	Code Descriptor	Brand Name Drug	Generic Drug Equivalent
Z79.83	Long term (current) use of bisphosphonates	Aclasta®	zoledronic acid
		Actonel with Calcium®	calcium carbonate/risedronate
		Actonel®	risedronate
		Aredia®	pamidronate
		Atelvia®	risedronate
		Binosto®	alendronate
		Boniva®	ibandronate
		Didronel®	etidronate
		Fosamax®	alendronate
		Reclast®	zoledronic acid
		Skelid®	tiludronate
		Zometa®	zoledronic acid
Z79.84	Long term (current) use of oral hypoglycemic drugs	Actos®	pioglitazone (oral)
		Amaryl®	glimepiride
		Avandia®	rosiglitazone
		DiaBeta®	glyburide
		Fortamet®	metformin
		GlipiZIDE XL®	glipizide
		Glucophage®	metformin
		Glucophage XR®	metformin
		Glucotrol®	glipizide
		Glucotrol XL®	glipizide
		Glumetza®	metformin
		Glycet®	miglitol
		Glynase®	glyburide
		Micronase®	glyburide
		Orinase®	tolbutamide
		Orinase Diagnostic®	tolbutamide
		Precose®	acarbose
		PresTab®	glyburide
		Riomet®	metformin
		Tolinase®	tolazamide
		Tol-Tab®	tolbutamide
Z79.890	Hormone replacement therapy (postmenopausal)	Activella®	estradiol/norethindrone
		Alora®	estradiol
		Alyacen 1 / 35®	ethinyl estradiol/norethindrone
		Angeliq®	drospirenone/estradiol
		Aranelle®	ethinyl estradiol/norethindrone
		Balziva®	ethinyl estradiol/norethindrone
		Brevicon®	ethinyl estradiol/norethindrone
		Briellyn®	ethinyl estradiol/norethindrone
		Climara Pro®	estradiol/levonorgestrel
		Climara®	estradiol

Code	Code Descriptor	Brand Name Drug	Generic Drug Equivalent
Z79.890 *–Continued*		CombiPatch®	estradiol/norethindrone
		Covaryx HS®	esterified estrogens/methyltestosterone
		Covaryx®	esterified estrogens/methyltestosterone
		Cyclafem 1 / 35®	ethinyl estradiol/norethindrone
		Cyclafem 7 / 7 / 7®	ethinyl estradiol/norethindrone
		Dasetta 1 / 35®	ethinyl estradiol/norethindrone
		Dasetta 7 / 7 / 7®	ethinyl estradiol/norethindrone
		Delestrogen®	estradiol valerate
		Duavee®	bazedoxifene/conjugated estrogens
		EEMT DS®	esterified estrogens/methyltestosterone
		EEMT HS®	esterified estrogens/methyltestosterone
		EEMT®	esterified estrogens/methyltestosterone
		Ena®	estradiol/norethindrone
		Enjuvia®	synthetic conjugated estrogens, B
		Essian H.S.®	esterified estrogens/methyltestosterone
		Essian®	esterified estrogens/methyltestosterone
		Estraderm®	estradiol
		Estrasorb®	estradiol topical emulsion
		Estratest H.S.®	esterified estrogens/methyltestosterone
		Estratest®	esterified estrogens/methyltestosterone
		Estrostep Fe®	ethinyl estradiol/norethindrone
		Femcon Fe®	ethinyl estradiol/norethindrone
		femhrt®	ethinyl estradiol/norethindrone
		Femring®	estradiol acetate vaginal ring
		Generess Fe®	ethinyl estradiol/norethindrone
		Gildagia®	ethinyl estradiol/norethindrone
		Gildess 1 / 20®	ethinyl estradiol/norethindrone
		Gildess 1.5 / 30®	ethinyl estradiol/norethindrone
		Gildess Fe 1 / 20®	ethinyl estradiol/norethindrone
		Gildess Fe 1.5 / 30®	ethinyl estradiol/norethindrone
		Jevantique®	ethinyl estradiol/norethindrone
		Jinteli®	ethinyl estradiol/norethindrone
		Junel 1 / 20®	ethinyl estradiol/norethindrone
		Junel 1.5 / 30®	ethinyl estradiol/norethindrone
		Larin Fe 1 / 20®	ethinyl estradiol/norethindrone
		Larin Fe 1.5 / 30®	ethinyl estradiol/norethindrone
		Leena®	ethinyl estradiol/norethindrone
		Lo Loestrin Fe®	ethinyl estradiol/norethindrone
		Lo Minastrin Fe®	ethinyl estradiol/norethindrone
		Loestrin 1 / 20®	ethinyl estradiol/norethindrone
		Loestrin 21 1.5 / 30®	ethinyl estradiol/norethindrone
		Loestrin 24 Fe®	ethinyl estradiol/norethindrone
		Loestrin Fe 1 / 20®	ethinyl estradiol/norethindrone
		Menogen®	esterified estrogens/methyltestosterone
		Microgestin 1 / 20®	ethinyl estradiol/norethindrone
		Microgestin 1.5 / 30®	ethinyl estradiol/norethindrone
		Microgestin Fe 1 / 20®	ethinyl estradiol/norethindrone
		Mimvey®	estradiol/norethindrone
		Minastrin 24 Fe®	ethinyl estradiol/norethindrone
		Modicon®	ethinyl estradiol/norethindrone

Code	Code Descriptor	Brand Name Drug	Generic Drug Equivalent
Z79.890 *–Continued*		Necon 1 / 35®	ethinyl estradiol/norethindrone
		Necon 7 / 7 / 7®	ethinyl estradiol/norethindrone
		Nortrel 1 / 35®	ethinyl estradiol/norethindrone
		Ortho-Novum 1 / 35®	ethinyl estradiol/norethindrone
		Ortho-Novum 7 / 7 / 7®	ethinyl estradiol/norethindrone
		Ovcon 35®	ethinyl estradiol/norethindrone
		Philith®	ethinyl estradiol/norethindrone
		Pirmella 1 / 35®	ethinyl estradiol/norethindrone
		Pirmella 7 / 7 / 7®	ethinyl estradiol/norethindrone
		Prefest®	estradiol/norgestimate
		Premarin Intravenous®	conjugated estrogens
		Premarin Vaginal Cream®	conjugated estrogens
		Premarin®	conjugated estrogens
		Premphase®	conjugated estrogens/medroxyprogesterone
		Premphase®	conjugated estrogens/medroxyprogesterone acetate
		Prempro®	conjugated estrogens/medroxyprogesterone
		Tilia Fe®	ethinyl estradiol/norethindrone
		Tri-Legest Fe®	ethinyl estradiol/norethindrone
		Tri-Legest®	ethinyl estradiol/norethindrone
		Tri-Norinyl®	ethinyl estradiol/norethindrone
		Vivelle®	estradiol
		Vivelle-Dot®	estradiol
		Wera®	ethinyl estradiol/norethindrone
		Wymzya Fe®	ethinyl estradiol/norethindrone
		Zenchent Fe®	ethinyl estradiol/norethindrone
		Zenchent®	ethinyl estradiol/norethindrone
		Zeosa®	ethinyl estradiol/norethindrone
Z79.891	Long term (current) use of opiate analgesic	Avinza®	morphine sulfate extended-release
		Butrans®	buprenorphine
		Dolophine®	methadone hydrochloride
		Duragesic®	fentanyl
		Embeda®	morphine sulfate and naltrexone extended-release
		Exalgo®	hydromorphone hydrochloride extended-release
		Kadian ®	morphine sulfate extended-release
		MS Contin®	morphine sulfate controlled-release
		Nucynta ER®	tapentadol extended-release
		Opana ER®	oxymorphone hydrochloride extended-release
		OxyContin®	oxycodone hydrochloride controlled-release
		Palladone®	hydromorphone hydrochloride extended-release
Z79.899	Other long term (current) drug therapy	N/A	N/A

Note: This list of brand name drugs and their generic equivalents correspond by drug class to Z codes for long-term use of drugs. This comprehensive but not exhaustive list is provided solely as a reference and does not imply a guarantee of reimbursement. Check with individual payers to determine their billing, coding, and reimbursement guidelines.

Appendix B: Z Codes as First-listed Diagnosis

The following Z codes/categories may only be reported as the principal/first-listed diagnosis, except when there are multiple encounters on the same day and the medical records for the encounters are combined.

Codes	Descriptors
Z00	Encounter for general examination without complaint, suspected or reported diagnosis
Z00.0	Encounter for general adult medical examination
Z00.00	Encounter for general adult medical examination without abnormal findings
Z00.01	Encounter for general adult medical examination with abnormal findings
Z00.1	Encounter for newborn, infant and child health examinations
Z00.11	Newborn health examination
Z00.110	Health examination for newborn under 8 days old
Z00.111	Health examination for newborn 8 to 28 days old
Z00.12	Encounter for routine child health examination
Z00.121	Encounter for routine child health examination with abnormal findings
Z00.129	Encounter for routine child health examination without abnormal findings
Z00.2	Encounter for examination for period of rapid growth in childhood
Z00.3	Encounter for examination for adolescent development state
Z00.5	Encounter for examination of potential donor of organ and tissue
Z00.7	Encounter for examination for period of delayed growth in childhood
Z00.70	Encounter for examination for period of delayed growth in childhood without abnormal findings
Z00.71	Encounter for examination for period of delayed growth in childhood with abnormal findings
Z00.8	Encounter for other general examination
Z01	Encounter for other special examination without complaint, suspected or reported diagnosis
Z01.0	Encounter for examination of eyes and vision
Z01.00	Encounter for examination of eyes and vision without abnormal findings
Z01.01	Encounter for examination of eyes and vision with abnormal findings
Z01.1	Encounter for examination of ears and hearing
Z01.10	Encounter for examination of ears and hearing without abnormal findings
Z01.11	Encounter for examination of ears and hearing with abnormal findings
Z01.110	Encounter for hearing examination following failed hearing screening
Z01.118	Encounter for examination of ears and hearing with other abnormal findings
Z01.12	Encounter for hearing conservation and treatment
Z01.2	Encounter for dental examination and cleaning
Z01.20	Encounter for dental examination and cleaning without abnormal findings
Z01.21	Encounter for dental examination and cleaning with abnormal findings
Z01.3	Encounter for examination of blood pressure
Z01.30	Encounter for examination of blood pressure without abnormal findings
Z01.31	Encounter for examination of blood pressure with abnormal findings
Z01.4	Encounter for gynecological examination
Z01.41	Encounter for routine gynecological examination
Z01.411	Encounter for gynecological examination (general) (routine) with abnormal findings
Z01.419	Encounter for gynecological examination (general) (routine) without abnormal findings
Z01.42	Encounter for cervical smear to confirm findings of recent normal smear following initial abnormal smear
Z01.8	Encounter for other specified special examinations
Z01.81	Encounter for preprocedural examinations
Z01.810	Encounter for preprocedural cardiovascular examination
Z01.811	Encounter for preprocedural respiratory examination
Z01.812	Encounter for preprocedural laboratory examination
Z01.818	Encounter for other preprocedural examination
Z01.82	Encounter for allergy testing

Codes	Descriptors
Z01.83	Encounter for blood typing
Z01.84	Encounter for antibody response examination
Z01.89	Encounter for other specified special examinations
Z02	Encounter for administrative examination
Z02.0	Encounter for examination for admission to educational institution
Z02.1	Encounter for pre-employment examination
Z02.2	Encounter for examination for admission to residential institution
Z02.3	Encounter for examination for recruitment to armed forces
Z02.4	Encounter for examination for driving license
Z02.5	Encounter for examination for participation in sport
Z02.6	Encounter for examination for insurance purposes
Z02.7	Encounter for issue of medical certificate
Z02.71	Encounter for disability determination
Z02.79	Encounter for issue of other medical certificate
Z02.8	Encounter for other administrative examinations
Z02.81	Encounter for paternity testing
Z02.82	Encounter for adoption services
Z02.83	Encounter for blood-alcohol and blood-drug test
Z02.89	Encounter for other administrative examinations
Z02.9	Encounter for administrative examinations, unspecified
Z03	Encounter for medical observation for suspected diseases and conditions ruled out
Z03.6	Encounter for observation for suspected toxic effect from ingested substance ruled out
Z03.7	Encounter for suspected maternal and fetal conditions ruled out
Z03.71	Encounter for suspected problem with amniotic cavity and membrane ruled out
Z03.72	Encounter for suspected placental problem ruled out
Z03.73	Encounter for suspected fetal anomaly ruled out
Z03.74	Encounter for suspected problem with fetal growth ruled out
Z03.75	Encounter for suspected cervical shortening ruled out
Z03.79	Encounter for other suspected maternal and fetal conditions ruled out
Z03.8	Encounter for observation for other suspected diseases and conditions ruled out
Z03.81	Encounter for observation for suspected exposure to biological agents ruled out
Z03.810	Encounter for observation for suspected exposure to anthrax ruled out
Z03.818	Encounter for observation for suspected exposure to other biological agents ruled out
Z03.89	Encounter for observation for other suspected diseases and conditions ruled out
Z04	Encounter for examination and observation for other reasons
Z04.1	Encounter for examination and observation following transport accident
Z04.2	Encounter for examination and observation following work accident
Z04.3	Encounter for examination and observation following other accident
Z04.4	Encounter for examination and observation following alleged rape
Z04.41	Encounter for examination and observation following alleged adult rape
Z04.42	Encounter for examination and observation following alleged child rape
Z04.6	Encounter for general psychiatric examination, requested by authority
Z04.7	Encounter for examination and observation following alleged physical abuse
Z04.71	Encounter for examination and observation following alleged adult physical abuse
Z04.72	Encounter for examination and observation following alleged child physical abuse
Z04.8	Encounter for examination and observation for other specified reasons
Z04.9	Encounter for examination and observation for unspecified reason
Z31.81	Encounter for male factor infertility in female patient
Z31.83	Encounter for assisted reproductive fertility procedure cycle
Z31.84	Encounter for fertility preservation procedure

Codes	Descriptors
Z33.2	Encounter for elective termination of pregnancy
Z34	Encounter for supervision of normal pregnancy
Z34.0	Encounter for supervision of normal first pregnancy
Z34.00	Encounter for supervision of normal first pregnancy, unspecified trimester
Z34.01	Encounter for supervision of normal first pregnancy, first trimester
Z34.02	Encounter for supervision of normal first pregnancy, second trimester
Z34.03	Encounter for supervision of normal first pregnancy, third trimester
Z34.8	Encounter for supervision of other normal pregnancy
Z34.80	Encounter for supervision of other normal pregnancy, unspecified trimester
Z34.81	Encounter for supervision of other normal pregnancy, first trimester
Z34.82	Encounter for supervision of other normal pregnancy, second trimester
Z34.83	Encounter for supervision of other normal pregnancy, third trimester
Z34.9	Encounter for supervision of normal pregnancy, unspecified
Z34.90	Encounter for supervision of normal pregnancy, unspecified, unspecified trimester
Z34.91	Encounter for supervision of normal pregnancy, unspecified, first trimester
Z34.92	Encounter for supervision of normal pregnancy, unspecified, second trimester
Z34.93	Encounter for supervision of normal pregnancy, unspecified, third trimester
Z38	Liveborn infants according to place of birth and type of delivery
Z38.0	Single liveborn infant, born in hospital
Z38.00	Single liveborn infant, delivered vaginally
Z38.01	Single liveborn infant, delivered by cesarean
Z38.1	Single liveborn infant, born outside hospital
Z38.2	Single liveborn infant, unspecified as to place of birth
Z38.3	Twin liveborn infant, born in hospital
Z38.30	Twin liveborn infant, delivered vaginally
Z38.31	Twin liveborn infant, delivered by cesarean
Z38.4	Twin liveborn infant, born outside hospital
Z38.5	Twin liveborn infant, unspecified as to place of birth
Z38.6	Other multiple liveborn infant, born in hospital
Z38.61	Triplet liveborn infant, delivered vaginally
Z38.62	Triplet liveborn infant, delivered by cesarean
Z38.63	Quadruplet liveborn infant, delivered vaginally
Z38.64	Quadruplet liveborn infant, delivered by cesarean
Z38.65	Quintuplet liveborn infant, delivered vaginally
Z38.66	Quintuplet liveborn infant, delivered by cesarean
Z38.68	Other multiple liveborn infant, delivered vaginally
Z38.69	Other multiple liveborn infant, delivered by cesarean
Z38.7	Other multiple liveborn infant, born outside hospital
Z38.8	Other multiple liveborn infant, unspecified as to place of birth
Z39	Encounter for maternal postpartum care and examination
Z39.0	Encounter for care and examination of mother immediately after delivery
Z39.1	Encounter for care and examination of lactating mother
Z39.2	Encounter for routine postpartum follow-up
Z42	Encounter for plastic and reconstructive surgery following medical procedure or healed injury
Z42.1	Encounter for breast reconstruction following mastectomy
Z42.8	Encounter for other plastic and reconstructive surgery following medical procedure or healed injury
Z51.0	Encounter for antineoplastic radiation therapy
Z51.1	Encounter for antineoplastic chemotherapy and immunotherapy
Z51.11	Encounter for antineoplastic chemotherapy
Z51.12	Encounter for antineoplastic immunotherapy

Codes	Descriptors
Z52	Donors of organs and tissues
Z52.0	Blood donor
Z52.00	Unspecified blood donor
Z52.000	Unspecified donor, whole blood
Z52.001	Unspecified donor, stem cells
Z52.008	Unspecified donor, other blood
Z52.01	Autologous blood donor
Z52.010	Autologous donor, whole blood
Z52.011	Autologous donor, stem cells
Z52.018	Autologous donor, other blood
Z52.09	Other blood donor
Z52.090	Other blood donor, whole blood
Z52.091	Other blood donor, stem cells
Z52.098	Other blood donor, other blood
Z52.1	Skin donor
Z52.10	Skin donor, unspecified
Z52.11	Skin donor, autologous
Z52.19	Skin donor, other
Z52.2	Bone donor
Z52.20	Bone donor, unspecified
Z52.21	Bone donor, autologous
Z52.29	Bone donor, other
Z52.3	Bone marrow donor
Z52.4	Kidney donor
Z52.5	Cornea donor
Z52.6	Liver donor
Z52.8	Donor of other specified organs or tissues
Z52.81	Egg (Oocyte) donor
Z52.810	Egg (Oocyte) donor under age 35, anonymous recipient
Z52.811	Egg (Oocyte) donor under age 35, designated recipient
Z52.812	Egg (Oocyte) donor age 35 and over, anonymous recipient
Z52.813	Egg (Oocyte) donor age 35 and over, designated recipient
Z52.819	Egg (Oocyte) donor, unspecified
Z52.89	Donor of other specified organs or tissues
Z76.1	Encounter for health supervision and care of foundling
Z76.2	Encounter for health supervision and care of other healthy infant and child
Z99.12	Encounter for respirator [ventilator] dependence during power failure

Appendix C: Deleted Codes

The following codes have been deleted from the ICD-10-CM code set effective October 1, 2016. Asterisked codes now appear in this manual as categories, subcategories, or subclassifications.

D49.5*	Neoplasm of unspecified behavior of other genitourinary organs
E08.321*	Diabetes mellitus due to underlying condition with mild nonproliferative diabetic retinopathy with macular edema
E08.329*	Diabetes mellitus due to underlying condition with mild nonproliferative diabetic retinopathy without macular edema
E08.331*	Diabetes mellitus due to underlying condition with moderate nonproliferative diabetic retinopathy with macular edema
E08.339*	Diabetes mellitus due to underlying condition with moderate nonproliferative diabetic retinopathy without macular edema
E08.341*	Diabetes mellitus due to underlying condition with severe nonproliferative diabetic retinopathy with macular edema
E08.349*	Diabetes mellitus due to underlying condition with severe nonproliferative diabetic retinopathy without macular edema
E08.351*	Diabetes mellitus due to underlying condition with proliferative diabetic retinopathy with macular edema
E08.359*	Diabetes mellitus due to underlying condition with proliferative diabetic retinopathy without macular edema
E09.321*	Drug or chemical induced diabetes mellitus with mild nonproliferative diabetic retinopathy with macular edema
E09.329*	Drug or chemical induced diabetes mellitus with mild nonproliferative diabetic retinopathy without macular edema
E09.331*	Drug or chemical induced diabetes mellitus with moderate nonproliferative diabetic retinopathy with macular edema
E09.339*	Drug or chemical induced diabetes mellitus with moderate nonproliferative diabetic retinopathy without macular edema
E09.341*	Drug or chemical induced diabetes mellitus with severe nonproliferative diabetic retinopathy with macular edema
E09.349*	Drug or chemical induced diabetes mellitus with severe nonproliferative diabetic retinopathy without macular edema
E09.351*	Drug or chemical induced diabetes mellitus with proliferative diabetic retinopathy with macular edema
E09.359*	Drug or chemical induced diabetes mellitus with proliferative diabetic retinopathy without macular edema
E10.321*	Type 1 diabetes mellitus with mild nonproliferative diabetic retinopathy with macular edema
E10.329*	Type 1 diabetes mellitus with mild nonproliferative diabetic retinopathy without macular edema
E10.331*	Type 1 diabetes mellitus with moderate nonproliferative diabetic retinopathy with macular edema
E10.339*	Type 1 diabetes mellitus with moderate nonproliferative diabetic retinopathy without macular edema
E10.341*	Type 1 diabetes mellitus with severe nonproliferative diabetic retinopathy with macular edema
E10.349*	Type 1 diabetes mellitus with severe nonproliferative diabetic retinopathy without macular edema
E10.351*	Type 1 diabetes mellitus with proliferative diabetic retinopathy with macular edema
E10.359*	Type 1 diabetes mellitus with proliferative diabetic retinopathy without macular edema
E11.321*	Type 2 diabetes mellitus with mild nonproliferative diabetic retinopathy with macular edema
E11.329*	Type 2 diabetes mellitus with mild nonproliferative diabetic retinopathy without macular edema
E11.331*	Type 2 diabetes mellitus with moderate nonproliferative diabetic retinopathy with macular edema
E11.339*	Type 2 diabetes mellitus with moderate nonproliferative diabetic retinopathy without macular edema
E11.341*	Type 2 diabetes mellitus with severe nonproliferative diabetic retinopathy with macular edema
E11.349*	Type 2 diabetes mellitus with severe nonproliferative diabetic retinopathy without macular edema
E11.351*	Type 2 diabetes mellitus with proliferative diabetic retinopathy with macular edema
E11.359*	Type 2 diabetes mellitus with proliferative diabetic retinopathy without macular edema
E13.321*	Other specified diabetes mellitus with mild nonproliferative diabetic retinopathy with macular edema
E13.329*	Other specified diabetes mellitus with mild nonproliferative diabetic retinopathy without macular edema
E13.331*	Other specified diabetes mellitus with moderate nonproliferative diabetic retinopathy with macular edema
E13.339*	Other specified diabetes mellitus with moderate nonproliferative diabetic retinopathy without macular edema
E13.341*	Other specified diabetes mellitus with severe nonproliferative diabetic retinopathy with macular edema
E13.349*	Other specified diabetes mellitus with severe nonproliferative diabetic retinopathy without macular edema
E13.351*	Other specified diabetes mellitus with proliferative diabetic retinopathy with macular edema
E13.359*	Other specified diabetes mellitus with proliferative diabetic retinopathy without macular edema
E78.0*	Pure hypercholesterolemia
F32.8*	Other depressive episodes
F34.8*	Other persistent mood [affective] disorders
F42*	Obsessive-compulsive disorder
F50.8*	Other eating disorders
H34.811*	Central retinal vein occlusion, right eye
H34.812*	Central retinal vein occlusion, left eye

H34.813*	Central retinal vein occlusion, bilateral
H34.819*	Central retinal vein occlusion, unspecified eye
H34.831*	Tributary (branch) retinal vein occlusion, right eye
H34.832*	Tributary (branch) retinal vein occlusion, left eye
H34.833*	Tributary (branch) retinal vein occlusion, bilateral
H34.839*	Tributary (branch) retinal vein occlusion, unspecified eye
H35.31*	Nonexudative age-related macular degeneration
H35.32*	Exudative age-related macular degeneration
H40.11X0	Primary open-angle glaucoma, stage unspecified
H40.11X1	Primary open-angle glaucoma, mild stage
H40.11X2	Primary open-angle glaucoma, moderate stage
H40.11X3	Primary open-angle glaucoma, severe stage
H40.11X4	Primary open-angle glaucoma, indeterminate stage
I60.20	Nontraumatic subarachnoid hemorrhage from unspecified anterior communicating artery
I60.21	Nontraumatic subarachnoid hemorrhage from right anterior communicating artery
I60.22	Nontraumatic subarachnoid hemorrhage from left anterior communicating artery
I69.01*	Cognitive deficits following nontraumatic subarachnoid hemorrhage
I69.11*	Cognitive deficits following nontraumatic intracerebral hemorrhage
I69.21*	Cognitive deficits following other nontraumatic intracranial hemorrhage
I69.31*	Cognitive deficits following cerebral infarction
I69.81*	Cognitive deficits following other cerebrovascular disease
I69.91*	Cognitive deficits following unspecified cerebrovascular disease
I97.62*	Postprocedural hemorrhage and hematoma of a circulatory system organ or structure following other procedure
J98.5*	Diseases of mediastinum, not elsewhere classified
K04.0*	Pulpitis
K05.21*	Aggressive periodontitis, localized
K05.22*	Aggressive periodontitis, generalized
K05.31*	Chronic periodontitis, localized
K05.32*	Chronic periodontitis, generalized
K08.8*	Other specified disorders of teeth and supporting structures
K52.2*	Allergic and dietetic gastroenteritis and colitis
K55.0*	Acute vascular disorders of intestine
K59.3*	Megacolon, not elsewhere classified
K85.0*	Idiopathic acute pancreatitis
K85.1*	Biliary acute pancreatitis
K85.2*	Alcohol induced acute pancreatitis
K85.3*	Drug induced acute pancreatitis
K85.8*	Other acute pancreatitis
K85.9*	Acute pancreatitis, unspecified
K86.8*	Other specified diseases of pancreas
K90.4*	Malabsorption due to intolerance, not elsewhere classified
M26.60*	Temporomandibular joint disorder, unspecified
M26.61*	Adhesions and ankylosis of temporomandibular joint
M26.62*	Arthralgia of temporomandibular joint
M26.63*	Articular disc disorder of temporomandibular joint
M50.02*	Cervical disc disorder with myelopathy, mid-cervical region
M50.12*	Cervical disc disorder with radiculopathy, mid-cervical region
M50.22*	Other cervical disc displacement, mid-cervical region
M50.32*	Other cervical disc degeneration, mid-cervical region
M50.82*	Other cervical disc disorders, mid-cervical region
M50.92*	Cervical disc disorder, unspecified, mid-cervical region
N42.3*	Dysplasia of prostate
N50.8*	Other specified disorders of male genital organs

N61*	Inflammatory disorders of breast
N83.0*	Follicular cyst of ovary
N83.1*	Corpus luteum cyst
N83.20*	Unspecified ovarian cysts
N83.29*	Other ovarian cysts
N83.31*	Acquired atrophy of ovary
N83.32*	Acquired atrophy of fallopian tube
N83.33*	Acquired atrophy of ovary and fallopian tube
N83.4*	Prolapse and hernia of ovary and fallopian tube
N83.51*	Torsion of ovary and ovarian pedicle
N83.52*	Torsion of fallopian tube
N90.6*	Hypertrophy of vulva
N94.1*	Dyspareunia
O00.0*	Abdominal pregnancy
O00.1*	Tubal pregnancy
O00.2*	Ovarian pregnancy
O00.8*	Other ectopic pregnancy
O00.9*	Ectopic pregnancy, unspecified
O33.7*	Maternal care for disproportion due to other fetal deformities
O34.21*	Maternal care for scar from previous cesarean delivery
O70.2*	Third degree perineal laceration during delivery
Q25.2*	Atresia of aorta
Q25.4*	Other congenital malformations of aorta
Q52.12*	Longitudinal vaginal septum
Q66.2*	Congenital metatarsus (primus) varus
R31.2*	Other microscopic hematuria
R39.19*	Other difficulties with micturition
R40.241*	Glasgow coma scale score 13-15
R40.242*	Glasgow coma scale score 9-12
R40.243*	Glasgow coma scale score 3-8
R40.244*	Other coma, without documented Glasgow coma scale score, or with partial score reported
R82.7*	Abnormal findings on microbiological examination of urine
R93.4*	Abnormal findings on diagnostic imaging of urinary organs
R97.2*	Elevated prostate specific antigen [PSA]
S02.10XA	Unspecified fracture of base of skull, initial encounter for closed fracture
S02.10XB	Unspecified fracture of base of skull, initial encounter for open fracture
S02.10XD	Unspecified fracture of base of skull, subsequent encounter for fracture with routine healing
S02.10XG	Unspecified fracture of base of skull, subsequent encounter for fracture with delayed healing
S02.10XK	Unspecified fracture of base of skull, subsequent encounter for fracture with nonunion
S02.10XS	Unspecified fracture of base of skull, sequela
S02.3XXA	Fracture of orbital floor, initial encounter for closed fracture
S02.3XXB	Fracture of orbital floor, initial encounter for open fracture
S02.3XXD	Fracture of orbital floor, subsequent encounter for fracture with routine healing
S02.3XXG	Fracture of orbital floor, subsequent encounter for fracture with delayed healing
S02.3XXK	Fracture of orbital floor, subsequent encounter for fracture with nonunion
S02.3XXS	Fracture of orbital floor, sequela
S02.61XA	Fracture of condylar process of mandible, initial encounter for closed fracture
S02.61XB	Fracture of condylar process of mandible, initial encounter for open fracture
S02.61XD	Fracture of condylar process of mandible, subsequent encounter for fracture with routine healing
S02.61XG	Fracture of condylar process of mandible, subsequent encounter for fracture with delayed healing
S02.61XK	Fracture of condylar process of mandible, subsequent encounter for fracture with nonunion
S02.61XS	Fracture of condylar process of mandible, sequela
S02.62XA	Fracture of subcondylar process of mandible, initial encounter for closed fracture

S02.62XB	Fracture of subcondylar process of mandible, initial encounter for open fracture
S02.62XD	Fracture of subcondylar process of mandible, subsequent encounter for fracture with routine healing
S02.62XG	Fracture of subcondylar process of mandible, subsequent encounter for fracture with delayed healing
S02.62XK	Fracture of subcondylar process of mandible, subsequent encounter for fracture with nonunion
S02.62XS	Fracture of subcondylar process of mandible, sequela
S02.63XA	Fracture of coronoid process of mandible, initial encounter for closed fracture
S02.63XB	Fracture of coronoid process of mandible, initial encounter for open fracture
S02.63XD	Fracture of coronoid process of mandible, subsequent encounter for fracture with routine healing
S02.63XG	Fracture of coronoid process of mandible, subsequent encounter for fracture with delayed healing
S02.63XK	Fracture of coronoid process of mandible, subsequent encounter for fracture with nonunion
S02.63XS	Fracture of coronoid process of mandible, sequela
S02.64XA	Fracture of ramus of mandible, initial encounter for closed fracture
S02.64XB	Fracture of ramus of mandible, initial encounter for open fracture
S02.64XD	Fracture of ramus of mandible, subsequent encounter for fracture with routine healing
S02.64XG	Fracture of ramus of mandible, subsequent encounter for fracture with delayed healing
S02.64XK	Fracture of ramus of mandible, subsequent encounter for fracture with nonunion
S02.64XS	Fracture of ramus of mandible, sequela
S02.65XA	Fracture of angle of mandible, initial encounter for closed fracture
S02.65XB	Fracture of angle of mandible, initial encounter for open fracture
S02.65XD	Fracture of angle of mandible, subsequent encounter for fracture with routine healing
S02.65XG	Fracture of angle of mandible, subsequent encounter for fracture with delayed healing
S02.65XK	Fracture of angle of mandible, subsequent encounter for fracture with nonunion
S02.65XS	Fracture of angle of mandible, sequela
S02.67XA	Fracture of alveolus of mandible, initial encounter for closed fracture
S02.67XB	Fracture of alveolus of mandible, initial encounter for open fracture
S02.67XD	Fracture of alveolus of mandible, subsequent encounter for fracture with routine healing
S02.67XG	Fracture of alveolus of mandible, subsequent encounter for fracture with delayed healing
S02.67XK	Fracture of alveolus of mandible, subsequent encounter for fracture with nonunion
S02.67XS	Fracture of alveolus of mandible, sequela
S02.8XXA	Fractures of other specified skull and facial bones, initial encounter for closed fracture
S02.8XXB	Fractures of other specified skull and facial bones, initial encounter for open fracture
S02.8XXD	Fractures of other specified skull and facial bones, subsequent encounter for fracture with routine healing
S02.8XXG	Fractures of other specified skull and facial bones, subsequent encounter for fracture with delayed healing
S02.8XXK	Fractures of other specified skull and facial bones, subsequent encounter for fracture with nonunion
S02.8XXS	Fractures of other specified skull and facial bones, sequela
S03.0XXA	Dislocation of jaw, initial encounter
S03.0XXD	Dislocation of jaw, subsequent encounter
S03.0XXS	Dislocation of jaw, sequela
S03.4XXA	Sprain of jaw, initial encounter
S03.4XXD	Sprain of jaw, subsequent encounter
S03.4XXS	Sprain of jaw, sequela
S06.0X2A	Concussion with loss of consciousness of 31 minutes to 59 minutes, initial encounter
S06.0X2D	Concussion with loss of consciousness of 31 minutes to 59 minutes, subsequent encounter
S06.0X2S	Concussion with loss of consciousness of 31 minutes to 59 minutes, sequela
S06.0X3A	Concussion with loss of consciousness of 1 hour to 5 hours 59 minutes, initial encounter
S06.0X3D	Concussion with loss of consciousness of 1 hour to 5 hours 59 minutes, subsequent encounter
S06.0X3S	Concussion with loss of consciousness of 1 hour to 5 hours 59 minutes, sequela
S06.0X4A	Concussion with loss of consciousness of 6 hours to 24 hours, initial encounter
S06.0X4D	Concussion with loss of consciousness of 6 hours to 24 hours, subsequent encounter
S06.0X4S	Concussion with loss of consciousness of 6 hours to 24 hours, sequela
S06.0X5A	Concussion with loss of consciousness greater than 24 hours with return to pre-existing conscious level, initial encounter
S06.0X5D	Concussion with loss of consciousness greater than 24 hours with return to pre-existing conscious level, subsequent encounter
S06.0X5S	Concussion with loss of consciousness greater than 24 hours with return to pre-existing conscious level, sequela

S06.0X6A	Concussion with loss of consciousness greater than 24 hours without return to pre-existing conscious level with patient surviving, initial encounter
S06.0X6D	Concussion with loss of consciousness greater than 24 hours without return to pre-existing conscious level with patient surviving, subsequent encounter
S06.0X6S	Concussion with loss of consciousness greater than 24 hours without return to pre-existing conscious level with patient surviving, sequela
S06.0X7A	Concussion with loss of consciousness of any duration with death due to brain injury prior to regaining consciousness, initial encounter
S06.0X7D	Concussion with loss of consciousness of any duration with death due to brain injury prior to regaining consciousness, subsequent encounter
S06.0X7S	Concussion with loss of consciousness of any duration with death due to brain injury prior to regaining consciousness, sequela
S06.0X8A	Concussion with loss of consciousness of any duration with death due to other cause prior to regaining consciousness, initial encounter
S06.0X8D	Concussion with loss of consciousness of any duration with death due to other cause prior to regaining consciousness, subsequent encounter
S06.0X8S	Concussion with loss of consciousness of any duration with death due to other cause prior to regaining consciousness, sequela
T83.51XA	Infection and inflammatory reaction due to indwelling urinary catheter, initial encounter
T83.51XD	Infection and inflammatory reaction due to indwelling urinary catheter, subsequent encounter
T83.51XS	Infection and inflammatory reaction due to indwelling urinary catheter, sequela
T83.59XA	Infection and inflammatory reaction due to prosthetic device, implant and graft in urinary system, initial encounter
T83.59XD	Infection and inflammatory reaction due to prosthetic device, implant and graft in urinary system, subsequent encounter
T83.59XS	Infection and inflammatory reaction due to prosthetic device, implant and graft in urinary system, sequela
T83.6XXA	Infection and inflammatory reaction due to prosthetic device, implant and graft in genital tract, initial encounter
T83.6XXD	Infection and inflammatory reaction due to prosthetic device, implant and graft in genital tract, subsequent encounter
T83.6XXS	Infection and inflammatory reaction due to prosthetic device, implant and graft in genital tract, sequela
T84.040A	Periprosthetic fracture around internal prosthetic right hip joint, initial encounter
T84.040D	Periprosthetic fracture around internal prosthetic right hip joint, subsequent encounter
T84.040S	Periprosthetic fracture around internal prosthetic right hip joint, sequela
T84.041A	Periprosthetic fracture around internal prosthetic left hip joint, initial encounter
T84.041D	Periprosthetic fracture around internal prosthetic left hip joint, subsequent encounter
T84.041S	Periprosthetic fracture around internal prosthetic left hip joint, sequela
T84.042A	Periprosthetic fracture around internal prosthetic right knee joint, initial encounter
T84.042D	Periprosthetic fracture around internal prosthetic right knee joint, subsequent encounter
T84.042S	Periprosthetic fracture around internal prosthetic right knee joint, sequela
T84.043A	Periprosthetic fracture around internal prosthetic left knee joint, initial encounter
T84.043D	Periprosthetic fracture around internal prosthetic left knee joint, subsequent encounter
T84.043S	Periprosthetic fracture around internal prosthetic left knee joint, sequela
T84.048A	Periprosthetic fracture around other internal prosthetic joint, initial encounter
T84.048D	Periprosthetic fracture around other internal prosthetic joint, subsequent encounter
T84.048S	Periprosthetic fracture around other internal prosthetic joint, sequela
T84.049A	Periprosthetic fracture around unspecified internal prosthetic joint, initial encounter
T84.049D	Periprosthetic fracture around unspecified internal prosthetic joint, subsequent encounter
T84.049S	Periprosthetic fracture around unspecified internal prosthetic joint, sequela
T85.81XA	Embolism due to internal prosthetic devices, implants and grafts, not elsewhere classified, initial encounter
T85.81XD	Embolism due to internal prosthetic devices, implants and grafts, not elsewhere classified, subsequent encounter
T85.81XS	Embolism due to internal prosthetic devices, implants and grafts, not elsewhere classified, sequela
T85.82XA	Fibrosis due to internal prosthetic devices, implants and grafts, not elsewhere classified, initial encounter
T85.82XD	Fibrosis due to internal prosthetic devices, implants and grafts, not elsewhere classified, subsequent encounter
T85.82XS	Fibrosis due to internal prosthetic devices, implants and grafts, not elsewhere classified, sequela
T85.83XA	Hemorrhage due to internal prosthetic devices, implants and grafts, not elsewhere classified, initial encounter
T85.83XD	Hemorrhage due to internal prosthetic devices, implants and grafts, not elsewhere classified, subsequent encounter
T85.83XS	Hemorrhage due to internal prosthetic devices, implants and grafts, not elsewhere classified, sequela
T85.84XA	Pain due to internal prosthetic devices, implants and grafts, not elsewhere classified, initial encounter
T85.84XD	Pain due to internal prosthetic devices, implants and grafts, not elsewhere classified, subsequent encounter
T85.84XS	Pain due to internal prosthetic devices, implants and grafts, not elsewhere classified, sequela
T85.85XA	Stenosis due to internal prosthetic devices, implants and grafts, not elsewhere classified, initial encounter
T85.85XD	Stenosis due to internal prosthetic devices, implants and grafts, not elsewhere classified, subsequent encounter

T85.85XS	Stenosis due to internal prosthetic devices, implants and grafts, not elsewhere classified, sequela
T85.86XA	Thrombosis due to internal prosthetic devices, implants and grafts, not elsewhere classified, initial encounter
T85.86XD	Thrombosis due to internal prosthetic devices, implants and grafts, not elsewhere classified, subsequent encounter
T85.86XS	Thrombosis due to internal prosthetic devices, implants and grafts, not elsewhere classified, sequela
T85.89XA	Other specified complication of internal prosthetic devices, implants and grafts, not elsewhere classified, initial encounter
T85.89XD	Other specified complication of internal prosthetic devices, implants and grafts, not elsewhere classified, subsequent encounter
T85.89XS	Other specified complication of internal prosthetic devices, implants and grafts, not elsewhere classified, sequela
V47.01XA	Driver of sport utility vehicle injured in collision with fixed or stationary object in nontraffic accident, initial encounter
V47.01XD	Driver of sport utility vehicle injured in collision with fixed or stationary object in nontraffic accident, subsequent encounter
V47.01XS	Driver of sport utility vehicle injured in collision with fixed or stationary object in nontraffic accident, sequela
V47.02XA	Driver of other type car injured in collision with fixed or stationary object in nontraffic accident, initial encounter
V47.02XD	Driver of other type car injured in collision with fixed or stationary object in nontraffic accident, subsequent encounter
V47.02XS	Driver of other type car injured in collision with fixed or stationary object in nontraffic accident, sequela
V47.11XA	Passenger of sport utility vehicle injured in collision with fixed or stationary object in nontraffic accident, initial encounter
V47.11XD	Passenger of sport utility vehicle injured in collision with fixed or stationary object in nontraffic accident, subsequent encounter
V47.11XS	Passenger of sport utility vehicle injured in collision with fixed or stationary object in nontraffic accident, sequela
V47.12XA	Passenger of other type car injured in collision with fixed or stationary object in nontraffic accident, initial encounter
V47.12XD	Passenger of other type car injured in collision with fixed or stationary object in nontraffic accident, subsequent encounter
V47.12XS	Passenger of other type car injured in collision with fixed or stationary object in nontraffic accident, sequela
V47.31XA	Unspecified occupant of sport utility vehicle injured in collision with fixed or stationary object in nontraffic accident, initial encounter
V47.31XD	Unspecified occupant of sport utility vehicle injured in collision with fixed or stationary object in nontraffic accident, subsequent encounter
V47.31XS	Unspecified occupant of sport utility vehicle injured in collision with fixed or stationary object in nontraffic accident, sequela
V47.32XA	Unspecified occupant of other type car injured in collision with fixed or stationary object in nontraffic accident, initial encounter
V47.32XD	Unspecified occupant of other type car injured in collision with fixed or stationary object in nontraffic accident, subsequent encounter
V47.32XS	Unspecified occupant of other type car injured in collision with fixed or stationary object in nontraffic accident, sequela
V47.51XA	Driver of sport utility vehicle injured in collision with fixed or stationary object in traffic accident, initial encounter
V47.51XD	Driver of sport utility vehicle injured in collision with fixed or stationary object in traffic accident, subsequent encounter
V47.51XS	Driver of sport utility vehicle injured in collision with fixed or stationary object in traffic accident, sequela
V47.52XA	Driver of other type car injured in collision with fixed or stationary object in traffic accident, initial encounter
V47.52XD	Driver of other type car injured in collision with fixed or stationary object in traffic accident, subsequent encounter
V47.52XS	Driver of other type car injured in collision with fixed or stationary object in traffic accident, sequela
V47.61XA	Passenger of sport utility vehicle injured in collision with fixed or stationary object in traffic accident, initial encounter
V47.61XD	Passenger of sport utility vehicle injured in collision with fixed or stationary object in traffic accident, subsequent encounter
V47.61XS	Passenger of sport utility vehicle injured in collision with fixed or stationary object in traffic accident, sequela
V47.62XA	Passenger of other type car injured in collision with fixed or stationary object in traffic accident, initial encounter
V47.62XD	Passenger of other type car injured in collision with fixed or stationary object in traffic accident, subsequent encounter
V47.62XS	Passenger of other type car injured in collision with fixed or stationary object in traffic accident, sequela
V47.91XA	Unspecified occupant of sport utility vehicle injured in collision with fixed or stationary object in traffic accident, initial encounter
V47.91XD	Unspecified occupant of sport utility vehicle injured in collision with fixed or stationary object in traffic accident, subsequent encounter
V47.91XS	Unspecified occupant of sport utility vehicle injured in collision with fixed or stationary object in traffic accident, sequela
V47.92XA	Unspecified occupant of other type car injured in collision with fixed or stationary object in traffic accident, initial encounter
V47.92XD	Unspecified occupant of other type car injured in collision with fixed or stationary object in traffic accident, subsequent encounter
V47.92XS	Unspecified occupant of other type car injured in collision with fixed or stationary object in traffic accident, sequela
W45.1XXA	Paper entering through skin, initial encounter
W45.1XXD	Paper entering through skin, subsequent encounter
W45.1XXS	Paper entering through skin, sequela
W45.2XXA	Lid of can entering through skin, initial encounter
W45.2XXD	Lid of can entering through skin, subsequent encounter
W45.2XXS	Lid of can entering through skin, sequela
Z22.50	Carrier of unspecified viral hepatitis
Z22.51	Carrier of viral hepatitis B
Z22.52	Carrier of viral hepatitis C
Z22.59	Carrier of other viral hepatitis
Z98.89*	Other specified postprocedural states

Appendix D: Symbols for 7-character Codes

Adult

Age range is 18–124 years inclusive (e.g., senile delirium, mature cataract); based on Medicare's Outpatient Code Editor (OCE).

M80.00XA
M80.00XD
M80.00XG
M80.00XK
M80.00XP
M80.00XS
M80.011A
M80.011D
M80.011G
M80.011K
M80.011P
M80.011S
M80.012A
M80.012D
M80.012G
M80.012K
M80.012P
M80.012S
M80.019A
M80.019D
M80.019G
M80.019K
M80.019P
M80.019S
M80.021A
M80.021D
M80.021G
M80.021K
M80.021P
M80.021S
M80.022A
M80.022D
M80.022G
M80.022K
M80.022P
M80.022S
M80.029A
M80.029D
M80.029G
M80.029K
M80.029P
M80.029S
M80.031A
M80.031D
M80.031G
M80.031K
M80.031P
M80.031S
M80.032A
M80.032D
M80.032G
M80.032K
M80.032P
M80.032S
M80.039A
M80.039D
M80.039G
M80.039K
M80.039P
M80.039S
M80.041A
M80.041D
M80.041G
M80.041K
M80.041P
M80.041S
M80.042A
M80.042D
M80.042G
M80.042K
M80.042P
M80.042S
M80.049A
M80.049D
M80.049G
M80.049K
M80.049P
M80.049S
M80.051A
M80.051D
M80.051G
M80.051K
M80.051P
M80.051S
M80.052A
M80.052D
M80.052G
M80.052K
M80.052P
M80.052S
M80.059A
M80.059D
M80.059G
M80.059K
M80.059P
M80.059S
M80.061A
M80.061D
M80.061G
M80.061K
M80.061P
M80.061S
M80.062A
M80.062D
M80.062G
M80.062K
M80.062P
M80.062S
M80.069A
M80.069D
M80.069G
M80.069K
M80.069P
M80.069S
M80.071A
M80.071D
M80.071G
M80.071K
M80.071P
M80.071S
M80.072A
M80.072D
M80.072G
M80.072K
M80.072P
M80.072S
M80.079A
M80.079D
M80.079G
M80.079K
M80.079P
M80.079S
M80.08XA
M80.08XD
M80.08XG
M80.08XK
M80.08XP
M80.08XS
T74.01XA
T74.01XD
T74.01XS
T74.11XA
T74.11XD
T74.11XS
T74.21XA
T74.21XD
T74.21XS
T74.31XA
T74.31XD
T74.31XS
T74.91XA
T74.91XD
T74.91XS
T76.01XA
T76.01XD
T76.01XS
T76.11XA
T76.11XD
T76.11XS
T76.21XA
T76.21XD
T76.21XS
T76.31XA
T76.31XD
T76.31XS
T76.91XA
T76.91XD
T76.91XS

Complication or Comorbidity (CC)

Based on CMS data

H34.8110
H34.8111
H34.8112
H34.8120
H34.8121
H34.8122
H34.8130
H34.8131
H34.8132
H34.8190
H34.8191
H34.8192
M48.50XA
M48.51XA
M48.52XA
M48.53XA
M48.54XA
M48.55XA
M48.56XA
M48.57XA
M48.58XA
M80.00XA
M80.00XK
M80.00XP
M80.011A
M80.011K
M80.011P
M80.012A
M80.012K
M80.012P
M80.019A
M80.019K
M80.019P
M80.021A
M80.021K
M80.021P
M80.022A
M80.022K
M80.022P
M80.029A
M80.029K
M80.029P
M80.031A
M80.031K
M80.031P
M80.032A
M80.032K
M80.032P
M80.039A
M80.039K
M80.039P
M80.041A
M80.041K
M80.041P
M80.042A
M80.042K
M80.042P
M80.049A
M80.049K
M80.049P
M80.051A
M80.051K
M80.051P
M80.052A
M80.052K
M80.052P
M80.059A
M80.059K
M80.059P
M80.061A
M80.061K
M80.061P
M80.062A
M80.062K
M80.062P
M80.069A
M80.069K
M80.069P
M80.071A
M80.071K
M80.071P
M80.072A
M80.072K
M80.072P
M80.079A
M80.079K
M80.079P
M80.08XA
M80.08XK
M80.08XP
M80.80XA
M80.80XK
M80.80XP
M80.811A
M80.811K
M80.811P
M80.812A
M80.812K
M80.812P
M80.819A
M80.819K
M80.819P
M80.821A
M80.821K
M80.821P
M80.822A
M80.822K
M80.822P
M80.829A
M80.829K
M80.829P
M80.831A
M80.831K
M80.831P
M80.832A
M80.832K
M80.832P
M80.839A
M80.839K
M80.839P
M80.841A
M80.841K
M80.841P
M80.842A
M80.842K
M80.842P
M80.849A
M80.849K
M80.849P
M80.851A
M80.851K
M80.851P
M80.852A
M80.852K
M80.852P
M80.859A
M80.859K
M80.859P
M80.861A
M80.861K
M80.861P
M80.862A
M80.862K
M80.862P
M80.869A
M80.869K
M80.869P
M80.871A
M80.871K
M80.871P
M80.872A
M80.872K
M80.872P
M80.879A
M80.879K
M80.879P
M80.88XA
M80.88XK
M80.88XP
M84.30XK
M84.30XP
M84.311K
M84.311P
M84.312K
M84.312P
M84.319K
M84.319P
M84.321K
M84.321P
M84.322K
M84.322P
M84.329K
M84.329P
M84.331K
M84.331P
M84.332K
M84.332P
M84.333K
M84.333P
M84.334K
M84.334P
M84.339K
M84.339P
M84.341K
M84.341P
M84.342K
M84.342P
M84.343K
M84.343P
M84.344K
M84.344P
M84.345K
M84.345P
M84.346K
M84.346P
M84.350K
M84.350P
M84.351K
M84.351P
M84.352K
M84.352P
M84.353K
M84.353P
M84.359K
M84.359P
M84.361K
M84.361P
M84.362K
M84.362P
M84.363K
M84.363P
M84.364K
M84.364P
M84.369K
M84.369P
M84.371K
M84.371P
M84.372K
M84.372P
M84.373K
M84.373P
M84.374K
M84.374P
M84.375K
M84.375P
M84.376K
M84.376P
M84.377K
M84.377P
M84.378K
M84.378P
M84.379K
M84.379P
M84.38XK
M84.38XP
M84.40XA
M84.40XK
M84.40XP
M84.411A
M84.411K
M84.411P
M84.412A
M84.412K
M84.412P
M84.419A
M84.419K
M84.419P
M84.421A
M84.421K
M84.421P
M84.422A
M84.422K
M84.422P
M84.429A
M84.429K
M84.429P
M84.431A
M84.431K
M84.431P
M84.432A
M84.432K
M84.432P
M84.433A
M84.433K
M84.433P
M84.434A
M84.434K
M84.434P
M84.439A
M84.439K
M84.439P
M84.441A
M84.441K
M84.441P
M84.442A
M84.442K
M84.442P
M84.443A
M84.443K
M84.443P
M84.444A
M84.444K
M84.444P
M84.445A
M84.445K
M84.445P
M84.446A
M84.446K
M84.446P
M84.451A
M84.451K
M84.451P
M84.452A
M84.452K
M84.452P
M84.453A
M84.453K
M84.453P
M84.454A
M84.454K
M84.454P
M84.459A
M84.459K
M84.459P
M84.461A
M84.461K
M84.461P
M84.462A
M84.462K
M84.462P
M84.463A
M84.463K
M84.463P
M84.464A
M84.464K
M84.464P
M84.469A
M84.469K
M84.469P
M84.471A
M84.471K
M84.471P
M84.472A
M84.472K
M84.472P
M84.473A
M84.473K
M84.473P
M84.474A
M84.474K
M84.474P
M84.475A
M84.475K
M84.475P
M84.476A
M84.476K
M84.476P
M84.477A
M84.477K
M84.477P
M84.478A
M84.478K
M84.478P
M84.479A
M84.479K
M84.479P
M84.48XA
M84.48XK
M84.48XP
M84.50XA
M84.50XK
M84.50XP
M84.511A
M84.511K
M84.511P
M84.512A
M84.512K
M84.512P
M84.519A
M84.519K
M84.519P
M84.521A
M84.521K
M84.521P
M84.522A
M84.522K
M84.522P
M84.529A
M84.529K
M84.529P
M84.531A
M84.531K
M84.531P
M84.532A
M84.532K
M84.532P
M84.533A
M84.533K
M84.533P
M84.534A
M84.534K
M84.534P
M84.539A
M84.539K
M84.539P
M84.541A
M84.541K
M84.541P
M84.542A
M84.542K
M84.542P
M84.549A
M84.549K
M84.549P
M84.550A
M84.550K
M84.550P
M84.551A
M84.551K
M84.551P
M84.552A
M84.552K
M84.552P
M84.553A
M84.553K
M84.553P
M84.559A
M84.559K
M84.559P
M84.561A

Complication or Comorbidity (CC) (cont.)

Based on CMS data

M84.561K	M84.634K	M84.750K	O36.0114	O60.10X0	S02.400A	S02.621K	S04.02XA	S06.304A	S11.23XA
M84.561P	M84.634P	M84.750P	O36.0115	O60.10X1	S02.400B	S02.622A	S04.031A	S06.305A	S11.24XA
M84.562A	M84.639A	M84.751A	O36.0119	O60.10X2	S02.400K	S02.622B	S04.032A	S06.309A	S11.25XA
M84.562K	M84.639K	M84.751K	O36.0120	O60.10X3	S02.401A	S02.622K	S04.039A	S06.371A	S12.000A
M84.562P	M84.639P	M84.751P	O36.0121	O60.10X4	S02.401B	S02.630A	S04.041A	S06.372A	S12.000K
M84.563A	M84.641A	M84.752A	O36.0122	O60.10X5	S02.401K	S02.630B	S04.042A	S06.373A	S12.001A
M84.563K	M84.641K	M84.752K	O36.0123	O60.10X9	S02.402A	S02.630K	S04.049A	S06.374A	S12.001K
M84.563P	M84.641P	M84.752P	O36.0124	O60.20X0	S02.402B	S02.631A	S04.10XA	S06.375A	S12.01XA
M84.564A	M84.642A	M84.753A	O36.0125	O60.20X1	S02.402K	S02.631B	S04.11XA	S06.379A	S12.01XK
M84.564K	M84.642K	M84.753K	O36.0129	O60.20X2	S02.40AA	S02.631K	S04.12XA	S06.381A	S12.02XA
M84.564P	M84.642P	M84.753P	O36.0130	O60.20X3	S02.40AB	S02.632A	S04.20XA	S06.382A	S12.02XK
M84.569A	M84.649A	M84.754A	O36.0131	O60.20X4	S02.40AK	S02.632B	S04.21XA	S06.383A	S12.030A
M84.569K	M84.649K	M84.754K	O36.0132	O60.20X5	S02.40BA	S02.632K	S04.22XA	S06.384A	S12.030K
M84.569P	M84.649P	M84.754P	O36.0133	O60.20X9	S02.40BB	S02.63XA	S04.30XA	S06.385A	S12.031A
M84.571A	M84.650A	M84.755A	O36.0134	S01.101A	S02.40BK	S02.63XB	S04.31XA	S06.389A	S12.031K
M84.571K	M84.650K	M84.755K	O36.0135	S01.102A	S02.40CA	S02.63XK	S04.32XA	S06.811A	S12.040A
M84.571P	M84.650P	M84.755P	O36.0139	S01.109A	S02.40CB	S02.640A	S04.40XA	S06.812A	S12.040K
M84.572A	M84.651A	M84.756A	O36.0910	S02.0XXA	S02.40CK	S02.640B	S04.41XA	S06.813A	S12.041A
M84.572K	M84.651K	M84.756K	O36.0911	S02.0XXK	S02.40DA	S02.640K	S04.42XA	S06.814A	S12.041K
M84.572P	M84.651P	M84.756P	O36.0912	S02.101A	S02.40DB	S02.641A	S04.50XA	S06.815A	S12.090A
M84.573A	M84.652A	M84.757A	O36.0913	S02.101K	S02.40DK	S02.641B	S04.51XA	S06.819A	S12.090K
M84.573K	M84.652K	M84.757K	O36.0914	S02.102A	S02.40EA	S02.641K	S04.52XA	S06.821A	S12.091A
M84.573P	M84.652P	M84.757P	O36.0915	S02.102K	S02.40EB	S02.642A	S04.60XA	S06.822A	S12.091K
M84.574A	M84.653A	M84.758A	O36.0919	S02.109A	S02.40EK	S02.642B	S04.61XA	S06.823A	S12.100A
M84.574K	M84.653K	M84.758K	O36.0920	S02.109K	S02.40FA	S02.642K	S04.62XA	S06.824A	S12.100K
M84.574P	M84.653P	M84.758P	O36.0921	S02.110A	S02.40FB	S02.650A	S04.70XA	S06.825A	S12.101A
M84.575A	M84.659A	M84.759A	O36.0922	S02.110K	S02.40FK	S02.650B	S04.71XA	S06.829A	S12.101K
M84.575K	M84.659K	M84.759K	O36.0923	S02.111A	S02.411A	S02.650K	S04.72XA	S06.891A	S12.110A
M84.575P	M84.659P	M84.759P	O36.0924	S02.111K	S02.411B	S02.651A	S04.811A	S06.892A	S12.110K
M84.576A	M84.661A	M97.01XA	O36.0925	S02.112A	S02.411K	S02.651B	S04.812A	S06.893A	S12.111A
M84.576K	M84.661K	M97.02XA	O36.0929	S02.112K	S02.412A	S02.651K	S04.819A	S06.894A	S12.111K
M84.576P	M84.661P	M97.11XA	O36.0930	S02.113A	S02.412B	S02.652A	S04.891A	S06.895A	S12.112A
M84.58XA	M84.662A	M97.12XA	O36.0931	S02.113K	S02.412K	S02.652B	S04.892A	S06.899A	S12.112K
M84.58XK	M84.662K	M97.21XA	O36.0932	S02.118A	S02.413A	S02.652K	S04.899A	S06.9X1A	S12.120A
M84.58XP	M84.662P	M97.22XA	O36.0933	S02.118K	S02.413B	S02.66XA	S04.9XXA	S06.9X2A	S12.120K
M84.60XA	M84.663A	M97.31XA	O36.0934	S02.119A	S02.413K	S02.66XB	S05.20XA	S06.9X3A	S12.121A
M84.60XK	M84.663K	M97.32XA	O36.0935	S02.119K	S02.42XA	S02.66XK	S05.21XA	S06.9X4A	S12.121K
M84.60XP	M84.663P	M97.41XA	O36.0939	S02.11AA	S02.42XB	S02.670A	S05.22XA	S06.9X5A	S12.130A
M84.611A	M84.664A	M97.42XA	O36.4XX0	S02.11AK	S02.42XK	S02.670B	S05.30XA	S06.9X9A	S12.130K
M84.611K	M84.664K	M97.8XXA	O36.4XX1	S02.11BA	S02.5XXK	S02.670K	S05.31XA	S07.0XXA	S12.131A
M84.611P	M84.664P	M97.9XXA	O36.4XX2	S02.11BK	S02.600A	S02.671A	S05.32XA	S07.1XXA	S12.131K
M84.612A	M84.669A	O31.8X10	O36.4XX3	S02.11CA	S02.600B	S02.671B	S05.40XA	S07.8XXA	S12.14XA
M84.612K	M84.669K	O31.8X11	O36.4XX4	S02.11CK	S02.600K	S02.671K	S05.41XA	S07.9XXA	S12.14XK
M84.612P	M84.669P	O31.8X12	O36.4XX5	S02.11DA	S02.601A	S02.672A	S05.42XA	S09.0XXA	S12.150A
M84.619A	M84.671A	O31.8X13	O36.4XX9	S02.11DK	S02.601B	S02.672B	S05.50XA	S09.20XA	S12.150K
M84.619K	M84.671K	O31.8X14	O41.01X0	S02.11EA	S02.601K	S02.672K	S05.51XA	S09.21XA	S12.151A
M84.619P	M84.671P	O31.8X15	O41.01X1	S02.11EK	S02.602A	S02.69XA	S05.52XA	S09.22XA	S12.151K
M84.621A	M84.672A	O31.8X19	O41.01X2	S02.11FA	S02.602B	S02.69XB	S05.70XA	S09.301A	S12.190A
M84.621K	M84.672K	O31.8X20	O41.01X3	S02.11FK	S02.602K	S02.69XK	S05.71XA	S09.302A	S12.190K
M84.621P	M84.672P	O31.8X21	O41.01X4	S02.11GA	S02.609A	S02.80XA	S05.72XA	S09.309A	S12.191A
M84.622A	M84.673A	O31.8X22	O41.01X5	S02.11GK	S02.609B	S02.80XB	S05.8X1A	S09.311A	S12.191K
M84.622K	M84.673K	O31.8X23	O41.01X9	S02.11HA	S02.609K	S02.80XK	S05.8X2A	S09.312A	S12.200A
M84.622P	M84.673P	O31.8X24	O41.02X0	S02.11HK	S02.610A	S02.81XA	S05.8X9A	S09.313A	S12.200K
M84.629A	M84.674A	O31.8X25	O41.02X1	S02.19XA	S02.610B	S02.81XB	S05.91XA	S09.319A	S12.201A
M84.629K	M84.674K	O31.8X29	O41.02X2	S02.19XK	S02.610K	S02.81XK	S05.92XA	S09.391A	S12.201K
M84.629P	M84.674P	O31.8X30	O41.02X3	S02.2XXB	S02.611A	S02.82XA	S06.0X1A	S09.392A	S12.230A
M84.631A	M84.675A	O31.8X31	O41.02X4	S02.2XXK	S02.611B	S02.82XB	S06.0X9A	S09.399A	S12.230K
M84.631K	M84.675K	O31.8X32	O41.02X5	S02.30XA	S02.611K	S02.82XK	S06.2X1A	S11.10XA	S12.231A
M84.631P	M84.675P	O31.8X33	O41.02X9	S02.30XB	S02.612A	S02.91XA	S06.2X2A	S11.11XA	S12.231K
M84.632A	M84.676A	O31.8X34	O41.03X0	S02.30XK	S02.612B	S02.91XK	S06.2X3A	S11.12XA	S12.24XA
M84.632K	M84.676K	O31.8X35	O41.03X1	S02.31XA	S02.612K	S02.92XA	S06.2X4A	S11.13XA	S12.24XK
M84.632P	M84.676P	O31.8X39	O41.03X2	S02.31XB	S02.620A	S02.92XB	S06.2X5A	S11.14XA	S12.250A
M84.633A	M84.68XA	O36.0110	O41.03X3	S02.31XK	S02.620B	S02.92XK	S06.2X9A	S11.15XA	S12.250K
M84.633K	M84.68XK	O36.0111	O41.03X4	S02.32XA	S02.620K	S04.011A	S06.301A	S11.20XA	S12.251A
M84.633P	M84.68XP	O36.0112	O41.03X5	S02.32XB	S02.621A	S04.012A	S06.302A	S11.21XA	S12.251K
M84.634A	M84.750A	O36.0113	O41.03X9	S02.32XK	S02.621B	S04.019A	S06.303A	S11.22XA	S12.290A

Complication or Comorbidity (CC) (cont.)

Based on CMS data

S12.290K
S12.291A
S12.291K
S12.300A
S12.300K
S12.301A
S12.301K
S12.330A
S12.330K
S12.331A
S12.331K
S12.34XA
S12.34XK
S12.350A
S12.350K
S12.351A
S12.351K
S12.390A
S12.390K
S12.391A
S12.391K
S12.400A
S12.400K
S12.401A
S12.401K
S12.430A
S12.430K
S12.431A
S12.431K
S12.44XA
S12.44XK
S12.450A
S12.450K
S12.451A
S12.451K
S12.490A
S12.490K
S12.491A
S12.491K
S12.500A
S12.500K
S12.501A
S12.501K
S12.530A
S12.530K
S12.531A
S12.531K
S12.54XA
S12.54XK
S12.550A
S12.550K
S12.551A
S12.551K
S12.590A
S12.590K
S12.591A
S12.591K
S12.600A
S12.600K
S12.601A
S12.601K
S12.630A
S12.630K
S12.631A
S12.631K
S12.64XA
S12.64XK
S12.650A
S12.650K
S12.651A
S12.651K
S12.690A
S12.690K
S12.691A
S12.691K
S12.9XXA
S13.0XXA
S13.100A
S13.101A
S13.110A
S13.111A
S13.120A
S13.121A
S13.130A
S13.131A
S13.140A
S13.141A
S13.150A
S13.151A
S13.160A
S13.161A
S13.170A
S13.171A
S13.180A
S13.181A
S13.20XA
S13.29XA
S15.001A
S15.002A
S15.009A
S15.011A
S15.012A
S15.019A
S15.021A
S15.022A
S15.029A
S15.091A
S15.092A
S15.099A
S15.101A
S15.102A
S15.109A
S15.111A
S15.112A
S15.119A
S15.121A
S15.122A
S15.129A
S15.191A
S15.192A
S15.199A
S15.201A
S15.202A
S15.209A
S15.211A
S15.212A
S15.219A
S15.221A
S15.222A
S15.229A
S15.291A
S15.292A
S15.299A
S15.301A
S15.302A
S15.309A
S15.311A
S15.312A
S15.319A
S15.321A
S15.322A
S15.329A
S15.391A
S15.392A
S15.399A
S15.8XXA
S15.9XXA
S17.0XXA
S17.8XXA
S17.9XXA
S21.101A
S21.102A
S21.109A
S21.111A
S21.112A
S21.119A
S21.121A
S21.122A
S21.129A
S21.131A
S21.132A
S21.139A
S21.141A
S21.142A
S21.149A
S21.151A
S21.152A
S21.159A
S21.90XA
S21.91XA
S21.92XA
S21.93XA
S21.94XA
S21.95XA
S22.000A
S22.000K
S22.001A
S22.001K
S22.002A
S22.002K
S22.008A
S22.008K
S22.009A
S22.009K
S22.010A
S22.010K
S22.011A
S22.011K
S22.012A
S22.012K
S22.018A
S22.018K
S22.019A
S22.019K
S22.020A
S22.020K
S22.021A
S22.021K
S22.022A
S22.022K
S22.028A
S22.028K
S22.029A
S22.029K
S22.030A
S22.030K
S22.031A
S22.031K
S22.032A
S22.032K
S22.038A
S22.038K
S22.039A
S22.039K
S22.040A
S22.040K
S22.041A
S22.041K
S22.042A
S22.042K
S22.048A
S22.048K
S22.049A
S22.049K
S22.050A
S22.050K
S22.051A
S22.051K
S22.052A
S22.052K
S22.058A
S22.058K
S22.059A
S22.059K
S22.060A
S22.060K
S22.061A
S22.061K
S22.062A
S22.062K
S22.068A
S22.068K
S22.069A
S22.069K
S22.070A
S22.070K
S22.071A
S22.071K
S22.072A
S22.072K
S22.078A
S22.078K
S22.079A
S22.079K
S22.080A
S22.080K
S22.081A
S22.081K
S22.082A
S22.082K
S22.088A
S22.088K
S22.089A
S22.089K
S22.20XA
S22.20XK
S22.21XA
S22.21XK
S22.22XA
S22.22XK
S22.23XA
S22.23XK
S22.24XA
S22.24XK
S22.31XA
S22.31XK
S22.32XA
S22.32XK
S22.39XA
S22.39XK
S22.41XA
S22.41XK
S22.42XA
S22.42XK
S22.43XA
S22.43XK
S22.49XA
S22.49XK
S22.5XXK
S22.9XXA
S22.9XXK
S25.501A
S25.502A
S25.509A
S25.511A
S25.512A
S25.519A
S25.591A
S25.592A
S25.599A
S25.801A
S25.802A
S25.809A
S25.811A
S25.812A
S25.819A
S25.891A
S25.892A
S25.899A
S25.90XA
S25.91XA
S25.99XA
S26.00XA
S26.01XA
S26.09XA
S26.10XA
S26.11XA
S26.19XA
S26.90XA
S26.91XA
S26.99XA
S27.0XXA
S27.301A
S27.302A
S27.309A
S27.311A
S27.312A
S27.319A
S27.321A
S27.322A
S27.329A
S27.391A
S27.392A
S27.399A
S27.50XA
S27.51XA
S27.52XA
S27.53XA
S27.59XA
S27.60XA
S27.63XA
S27.69XA
S27.802A
S27.803A
S27.808A
S27.809A
S27.892A
S27.893A
S27.898A
S27.899A
S27.9XXA
S28.1XXA
S29.021A
S29.029A
S32.000A
S32.000K
S32.001A
S32.001K
S32.002A
S32.002K
S32.008A
S32.008K
S32.009A
S32.009K
S32.010A
S32.010K
S32.011A
S32.011K
S32.012A
S32.012K
S32.018A
S32.018K
S32.019A
S32.019K
S32.020A
S32.020K
S32.021A
S32.021K
S32.022A
S32.022K
S32.028A
S32.028K
S32.029A
S32.029K
S32.030A
S32.030K
S32.031A
S32.031K
S32.032A
S32.032K
S32.038A
S32.038K
S32.039A
S32.039K
S32.040A
S32.040K
S32.041A
S32.041K
S32.042A
S32.042K
S32.048A
S32.048K
S32.049A
S32.049K
S32.050A
S32.050K
S32.051A
S32.051K
S32.052A
S32.052K
S32.058A
S32.058K
S32.059A
S32.059K
S32.10XA
S32.10XK
S32.110A
S32.110K
S32.111A
S32.111K
S32.112A
S32.112K
S32.119A
S32.119K
S32.120A
S32.120K
S32.121A
S32.121K
S32.122A
S32.122K
S32.129A
S32.129K
S32.130A
S32.130K
S32.131A
S32.131K
S32.132A
S32.132K
S32.139A
S32.139K
S32.14XA
S32.14XK
S32.15XA
S32.15XK
S32.16XA
S32.16XK
S32.17XA
S32.17XK
S32.19XA
S32.19XK
S32.2XXA
S32.2XXK
S32.301A
S32.301K
S32.302A
S32.302K
S32.309A
S32.309K
S32.311A
S32.311K
S32.312A
S32.312K
S32.313A
S32.313K
S32.314A
S32.314K
S32.315A
S32.315K
S32.316A
S32.316K
S32.391A
S32.391K
S32.392A
S32.392K
S32.399A
S32.399K
S32.401K
S32.402K
S32.409K
S32.411K
S32.412K
S32.413K
S32.414K
S32.415K
S32.416K
S32.421K
S32.422K
S32.423K
S32.424K
S32.425K
S32.426K
S32.431K
S32.432K
S32.433K
S32.434K
S32.435K
S32.436K
S32.441K
S32.442K
S32.443K
S32.444K
S32.445K
S32.446K
S32.451K
S32.452K
S32.453K
S32.454K
S32.455K
S32.456K
S32.461K
S32.462K
S32.463K
S32.464K
S32.465K
S32.466K
S32.471K
S32.472K
S32.473K
S32.474K
S32.475K
S32.476K
S32.481K
S32.482K
S32.483K
S32.484K
S32.485K
S32.486K
S32.491K
S32.492K
S32.499K
S32.501A
S32.501K
S32.502A
S32.502K
S32.509A
S32.509K
S32.511A
S32.511K
S32.512A
S32.512K
S32.519A
S32.519K
S32.591A
S32.591K
S32.592A
S32.592K
S32.599A
S32.599K
S32.601A
S32.601K
S32.602A
S32.602K
S32.609A
S32.609K
S32.611A
S32.611K
S32.612A
S32.612K
S32.613A
S32.613K
S32.614A
S32.614K
S32.615A
S32.615K
S32.616A
S32.616K
S32.691A
S32.691K
S32.692A
S32.692K
S32.699A
S32.699K
S32.810A
S32.810K
S32.811A
S32.811K
S32.82XA
S32.82XK
S32.89XA
S32.89XK
S32.9XXA
S32.9XXK
S35.531A
S35.532A
S35.533A
S35.534A
S35.535A
S35.536A
S35.8X1A
S35.8X8A
S35.8X9A
S35.90XA
S35.91XA
S35.99XA
S36.00XA
S36.020A
S36.021A
S36.029A
S36.030A
S36.039A
S36.09XA
S36.112A
S36.113A
S36.114A
S36.118A
S36.119A
S36.122A
S36.123A
S36.128A
S36.129A
S36.13XA
S36.200A
S36.201A
S36.202A
S36.209A
S36.220A
S36.221A
S36.222A
S36.229A
S36.230A
S36.231A
S36.232A
S36.239A
S36.240A
S36.241A
S36.242A
S36.249A
S36.250A
S36.251A
S36.252A
S36.259A
S36.260A
S36.261A
S36.262A
S36.269A
S36.290A
S36.291A
S36.292A
S36.299A
S36.30XA
S36.32XA
S36.33XA
S36.39XA
S36.400A
S36.408A
S36.409A
S36.410A
S36.418A
S36.419A
S36.420A
S36.428A
S36.429A
S36.430A
S36.438A
S36.439A
S36.490A
S36.498A
S36.499A
S36.500A
S36.501A

Complication or Comorbidity (CC) (cont.)

Based on CMS data

S36.502A	S37.23XA	S42.023P	S42.124P	S42.192P	S42.249P	S42.301P	S42.345P	S42.413P	S42.447P
S36.503A	S37.29XA	S42.024B	S42.125B	S42.199B	S42.251A	S42.302A	S42.346A	S42.414A	S42.448A
S36.508A	S37.30XA	S42.024K	S42.125K	S42.199K	S42.251K	S42.302K	S42.346K	S42.414K	S42.448K
S36.509A	S37.32XA	S42.024P	S42.125P	S42.199P	S42.251P	S42.302P	S42.346P	S42.414P	S42.448P
S36.510A	S37.33XA	S42.025B	S42.126B	S42.201A	S42.252A	S42.309A	S42.351A	S42.415A	S42.449A
S36.511A	S37.39XA	S42.025K	S42.126K	S42.201K	S42.252K	S42.309K	S42.351K	S42.415K	S42.449K
S36.512A	S37.60XA	S42.025P	S42.126P	S42.201P	S42.252P	S42.309P	S42.351P	S42.415P	S42.449P
S36.513A	S37.62XA	S42.026B	S42.131B	S42.202A	S42.253A	S42.311A	S42.352A	S42.416A	S42.451A
S36.518A	S37.63XA	S42.026K	S42.131K	S42.202K	S42.253K	S42.311K	S42.352K	S42.416K	S42.451K
S36.519A	S37.69XA	S42.026P	S42.131P	S42.202P	S42.253P	S42.311P	S42.352P	S42.416P	S42.451P
S36.520A	S37.812A	S42.031B	S42.132B	S42.209A	S42.254A	S42.312A	S42.353A	S42.421A	S42.452A
S36.521A	S37.813A	S42.031K	S42.132K	S42.209K	S42.254K	S42.312K	S42.353K	S42.421K	S42.452K
S36.522A	S37.818A	S42.031P	S42.132P	S42.209P	S42.254P	S42.312P	S42.353P	S42.421P	S42.452P
S36.523A	S37.819A	S42.032B	S42.133B	S42.211A	S42.255A	S42.319A	S42.354A	S42.422A	S42.453A
S36.528A	S37.892A	S42.032K	S42.133K	S42.211K	S42.255K	S42.319K	S42.354K	S42.422K	S42.453K
S36.529A	S37.893A	S42.032P	S42.133P	S42.211P	S42.255P	S42.319P	S42.354P	S42.422P	S42.453P
S36.530A	S37.898A	S42.033B	S42.134B	S42.212A	S42.256A	S42.321A	S42.355A	S42.423A	S42.454A
S36.531A	S37.899A	S42.033K	S42.134K	S42.212K	S42.256K	S42.321K	S42.355K	S42.423K	S42.454K
S36.532A	S37.90XA	S42.033P	S42.134P	S42.212P	S42.256P	S42.321P	S42.355P	S42.423P	S42.454P
S36.533A	S37.92XA	S42.034B	S42.135B	S42.213A	S42.261A	S42.322A	S42.356A	S42.424A	S42.455A
S36.538A	S37.93XA	S42.034K	S42.135K	S42.213K	S42.261K	S42.322K	S42.356K	S42.424K	S42.455K
S36.539A	S37.99XA	S42.034P	S42.135P	S42.213P	S42.261P	S42.322P	S42.356P	S42.424P	S42.455P
S36.590A	S42.001B	S42.035B	S42.136B	S42.214A	S42.262A	S42.323A	S42.361A	S42.425A	S42.456A
S36.591A	S42.001K	S42.035K	S42.136K	S42.214K	S42.262K	S42.323K	S42.361K	S42.425K	S42.456K
S36.592A	S42.001P	S42.035P	S42.136P	S42.214P	S42.262P	S42.323P	S42.361P	S42.425P	S42.456P
S36.593A	S42.002B	S42.036B	S42.141B	S42.215A	S42.263A	S42.324A	S42.362A	S42.426A	S42.461A
S36.598A	S42.002K	S42.036K	S42.141K	S42.215K	S42.263K	S42.324K	S42.362K	S42.426K	S42.461K
S36.599A	S42.002P	S42.036P	S42.141P	S42.215P	S42.263P	S42.324P	S42.362P	S42.426P	S42.461P
S36.60XA	S42.009B	S42.101B	S42.142B	S42.216A	S42.264A	S42.325A	S42.363A	S42.431A	S42.462A
S36.61XA	S42.009K	S42.101K	S42.142K	S42.216K	S42.264K	S42.325K	S42.363K	S42.431K	S42.462K
S36.62XA	S42.009P	S42.101P	S42.142P	S42.216P	S42.264P	S42.325P	S42.363P	S42.431P	S42.462P
S36.63XA	S42.011B	S42.102B	S42.143B	S42.221A	S42.265A	S42.326A	S42.364A	S42.432A	S42.463A
S36.69XA	S42.011K	S42.102K	S42.143K	S42.221K	S42.265K	S42.326K	S42.364K	S42.432K	S42.463K
S36.81XA	S42.011P	S42.102P	S42.143P	S42.221P	S42.265P	S42.326P	S42.364P	S42.432P	S42.463P
S36.892A	S42.012B	S42.109B	S42.144B	S42.222A	S42.266A	S42.331A	S42.365A	S42.433A	S42.464A
S36.893A	S42.012K	S42.109K	S42.144K	S42.222K	S42.266K	S42.331K	S42.365K	S42.433K	S42.464K
S36.898A	S42.012P	S42.109P	S42.144P	S42.222P	S42.266P	S42.331P	S42.365P	S42.433P	S42.464P
S36.899A	S42.013B	S42.111B	S42.145B	S42.223A	S42.271A	S42.332A	S42.366A	S42.434A	S42.465A
S36.90XA	S42.013K	S42.111K	S42.145K	S42.223K	S42.271K	S42.332K	S42.366K	S42.434K	S42.465K
S36.92XA	S42.013P	S42.111P	S42.145P	S42.223P	S42.271P	S42.332P	S42.366P	S42.434P	S42.465P
S36.93XA	S42.014B	S42.112B	S42.146B	S42.224A	S42.272A	S42.333A	S42.391A	S42.435A	S42.466A
S36.99XA	S42.014K	S42.112K	S42.146K	S42.224K	S42.272K	S42.333K	S42.391K	S42.435K	S42.466K
S37.001A	S42.014P	S42.112P	S42.146P	S42.224P	S42.272P	S42.333P	S42.391P	S42.435P	S42.466P
S37.002A	S42.015B	S42.113B	S42.151B	S42.225A	S42.279A	S42.334A	S42.392A	S42.436A	S42.471A
S37.009A	S42.015K	S42.113K	S42.151K	S42.225K	S42.279K	S42.334K	S42.392K	S42.436K	S42.471K
S37.011A	S42.015P	S42.113P	S42.151P	S42.225P	S42.279P	S42.334P	S42.392P	S42.436P	S42.471P
S37.012A	S42.016B	S42.114B	S42.152B	S42.226A	S42.291A	S42.335A	S42.399A	S42.441A	S42.472A
S37.019A	S42.016K	S42.114K	S42.152K	S42.226K	S42.291K	S42.335K	S42.399K	S42.441K	S42.472K
S37.021A	S42.016P	S42.114P	S42.152P	S42.226P	S42.291P	S42.335P	S42.399P	S42.441P	S42.472P
S37.022A	S42.017B	S42.115B	S42.153B	S42.231A	S42.292A	S42.336A	S42.401A	S42.442A	S42.473A
S37.029A	S42.017K	S42.115K	S42.153K	S42.231K	S42.292K	S42.336K	S42.401K	S42.442K	S42.473K
S37.031A	S42.017P	S42.115P	S42.153P	S42.231P	S42.292P	S42.336P	S42.401P	S42.442P	S42.473P
S37.032A	S42.018B	S42.116B	S42.154B	S42.232A	S42.293A	S42.341A	S42.402A	S42.443A	S42.474A
S37.039A	S42.018K	S42.116K	S42.154K	S42.232K	S42.293K	S42.341K	S42.402K	S42.443K	S42.474K
S37.041A	S42.018P	S42.116P	S42.154P	S42.232P	S42.293P	S42.341P	S42.402P	S42.443P	S42.474P
S37.042A	S42.019B	S42.121B	S42.155B	S42.239A	S42.294A	S42.342A	S42.409A	S42.444A	S42.475A
S37.049A	S42.019K	S42.121K	S42.155K	S42.239K	S42.294K	S42.342K	S42.409K	S42.444K	S42.475K
S37.051A	S42.019P	S42.121P	S42.155P	S42.239P	S42.294P	S42.342P	S42.409P	S42.444P	S42.475P
S37.052A	S42.021B	S42.122B	S42.156B	S42.241A	S42.295A	S42.343A	S42.411A	S42.445A	S42.476A
S37.059A	S42.021K	S42.122K	S42.156K	S42.241K	S42.295K	S42.343K	S42.411K	S42.445K	S42.476K
S37.10XA	S42.021P	S42.122P	S42.156P	S42.241P	S42.295P	S42.343P	S42.411P	S42.445P	S42.476P
S37.12XA	S42.022B	S42.123B	S42.191B	S42.242A	S42.296A	S42.344A	S42.412A	S42.446A	S42.481A
S37.13XA	S42.022K	S42.123K	S42.191K	S42.242K	S42.296K	S42.344K	S42.412K	S42.446K	S42.481K
S37.19XA	S42.022P	S42.123P	S42.191P	S42.242P	S42.296P	S42.344P	S42.412P	S42.446P	S42.481P
S37.20XA	S42.023B	S42.124B	S42.192B	S42.249A	S42.301A	S42.345A	S42.413A	S42.447A	S42.482A
S37.22XA	S42.023K	S42.124K	S42.192K	S42.249K	S42.301K	S42.345K	S42.413K	S42.447K	S42.482K

Complication or Comorbidity (CC) (cont.)

Based on CMS data

S42.482P
S42.489A
S42.489K
S42.489P
S42.491A
S42.491K
S42.491P
S42.492A
S42.492K
S42.492P
S42.493A
S42.493K
S42.493P
S42.494A
S42.494K
S42.494P
S42.495A
S42.495K
S42.495P
S42.496A
S42.496K
S42.496P
S42.90XA
S42.90XK
S42.90XP
S42.91XA
S42.91XK
S42.91XP
S42.92XA
S42.92XK
S42.92XP
S43.201A
S43.202A
S43.203A
S43.204A
S43.205A
S43.206A
S43.211A
S43.212A
S43.213A
S43.214A
S43.215A
S43.216A
S43.221A
S43.222A
S43.223A
S43.224A
S43.225A
S43.226A
S45.101A
S45.102A
S45.109A
S45.111A
S45.112A
S45.119A
S45.191A
S45.192A
S45.199A
S45.201A
S45.202A
S45.209A
S45.211A
S45.212A
S45.219A
S45.291A
S45.292A
S45.299A
S45.301A
S45.302A
S45.309A
S45.311A
S45.312A
S45.319A
S45.391A
S45.392A
S45.399A
S45.801A
S45.802A
S45.809A
S45.811A
S45.812A
S45.819A
S45.891A
S45.892A
S45.899A
S45.901A
S45.902A
S45.909A
S45.911A
S45.912A
S45.919A
S45.991A
S45.992A
S45.999A
S46.021A
S46.022A
S46.029A
S46.121A
S46.122A
S46.129A
S46.221A
S46.222A
S46.229A
S46.321A
S46.322A
S46.329A
S46.821A
S46.822A
S46.829A
S46.921A
S46.922A
S46.929A
S48.011A
S48.012A
S48.019A
S48.021A
S48.022A
S48.029A
S48.111A
S48.112A
S48.119A
S48.121A
S48.122A
S48.129A
S48.911A
S48.912A
S48.919A
S48.921A
S48.922A
S48.929A
S49.001A
S49.001K
S49.001P
S49.002A
S49.002K
S49.002P
S49.009A
S49.009K
S49.009P
S49.011A
S49.011K
S49.011P
S49.012A
S49.012K
S49.012P
S49.019A
S49.019K
S49.019P
S49.021A
S49.021K
S49.021P
S49.022A
S49.022K
S49.022P
S49.029A
S49.029K
S49.029P
S49.031A
S49.031K
S49.031P
S49.032A
S49.032K
S49.032P
S49.039A
S49.039K
S49.039P
S49.041A
S49.041K
S49.041P
S49.042A
S49.042K
S49.042P
S49.049A
S49.049K
S49.049P
S49.091A
S49.091K
S49.091P
S49.092A
S49.092K
S49.092P
S49.099A
S49.099K
S49.099P
S49.101A
S49.101K
S49.101P
S49.102A
S49.102K
S49.102P
S49.109A
S49.109K
S49.109P
S49.111A
S49.111K
S49.111P
S49.112A
S49.112K
S49.112P
S49.119A
S49.119K
S49.119P
S49.121A
S49.121K
S49.121P
S49.122A
S49.122K
S49.122P
S49.129A
S49.129K
S49.129P
S49.131A
S49.131K
S49.131P
S49.132A
S49.132K
S49.132P
S49.139A
S49.139K
S49.139P
S49.141A
S49.141K
S49.141P
S49.142A
S49.142K
S49.142P
S49.149A
S49.149K
S49.149P
S49.191A
S49.191K
S49.191P
S49.192A
S49.192K
S49.192P
S49.199A
S49.199K
S49.199P
S52.001K
S52.001M
S52.001N
S52.001P
S52.001Q
S52.001R
S52.002K
S52.002M
S52.002N
S52.002P
S52.002Q
S52.002R
S52.009K
S52.009M
S52.009N
S52.009P
S52.009Q
S52.009R
S52.011A
S52.011K
S52.011P
S52.012A
S52.012K
S52.012P
S52.019A
S52.019K
S52.019P
S52.021K
S52.021M
S52.021N
S52.021P
S52.021Q
S52.021R
S52.022K
S52.022M
S52.022N
S52.022P
S52.022Q
S52.022R
S52.023K
S52.023M
S52.023N
S52.023P
S52.023Q
S52.023R
S52.024K
S52.024M
S52.024N
S52.024P
S52.024Q
S52.024R
S52.025K
S52.025M
S52.025N
S52.025P
S52.025Q
S52.025R
S52.026K
S52.026M
S52.026N
S52.026P
S52.026Q
S52.026R
S52.031K
S52.031M
S52.031N
S52.031P
S52.031Q
S52.031R
S52.032K
S52.032M
S52.032N
S52.032P
S52.032Q
S52.032R
S52.033K
S52.033M
S52.033N
S52.033P
S52.033Q
S52.033R
S52.034K
S52.034M
S52.034N
S52.034P
S52.034Q
S52.034R
S52.035K
S52.035M
S52.035N
S52.035P
S52.035Q
S52.035R
S52.036K
S52.036M
S52.036N
S52.036P
S52.036Q
S52.036R
S52.041K
S52.041M
S52.041N
S52.041P
S52.041Q
S52.041R
S52.042K
S52.042M
S52.042N
S52.042P
S52.042Q
S52.042R
S52.043K
S52.043M
S52.043N
S52.043P
S52.043Q
S52.043R
S52.044K
S52.044M
S52.044N
S52.044P
S52.044Q
S52.044R
S52.045K
S52.045M
S52.045N
S52.045P
S52.045Q
S52.045R
S52.046K
S52.046M
S52.046N
S52.046P
S52.046Q
S52.046R
S52.091K
S52.091M
S52.091N
S52.091P
S52.091Q
S52.091R
S52.092K
S52.092M
S52.092N
S52.092P
S52.092Q
S52.092R
S52.099K
S52.099M
S52.099N
S52.099P
S52.099Q
S52.099R
S52.101K
S52.101M
S52.101N
S52.101P
S52.101Q
S52.101R
S52.102K
S52.102M
S52.102N
S52.102P
S52.102Q
S52.102R
S52.109K
S52.109M
S52.109N
S52.109P
S52.109Q
S52.109R
S52.111A
S52.111K
S52.111P
S52.112A
S52.112K
S52.112P
S52.119A
S52.119K
S52.119P
S52.121K
S52.121M
S52.121N
S52.121P
S52.121Q
S52.121R
S52.122K
S52.122M
S52.122N
S52.122P
S52.122Q
S52.122R
S52.123K
S52.123M
S52.123N
S52.123P
S52.123Q
S52.123R
S52.124K
S52.124M
S52.124N
S52.124P
S52.124Q
S52.124R
S52.125K
S52.125M
S52.125N
S52.125P
S52.125Q
S52.125R
S52.126K
S52.126M
S52.126N
S52.126P
S52.126Q
S52.126R
S52.131K
S52.131M
S52.131N
S52.131P
S52.131Q
S52.131R
S52.132K
S52.132M
S52.132N
S52.132P
S52.132Q
S52.132R
S52.133K
S52.133M
S52.133N
S52.133P
S52.133Q
S52.133R
S52.134K
S52.134M
S52.134N
S52.134P
S52.134Q
S52.134R
S52.135K
S52.135M
S52.135N
S52.135P
S52.135Q
S52.135R
S52.136K
S52.136M
S52.136N
S52.136P
S52.136Q
S52.136R
S52.181K
S52.181M
S52.181N
S52.181P
S52.181Q
S52.181R
S52.182K
S52.182M
S52.182N
S52.182P
S52.182Q
S52.182R
S52.189K
S52.189M
S52.189N
S52.189P
S52.189Q
S52.189R
S52.201A
S52.201K
S52.201M
S52.201N
S52.201P
S52.201Q
S52.201R
S52.202A
S52.202K
S52.202M
S52.202N
S52.202P
S52.202Q
S52.202R
S52.209A
S52.209K
S52.209M
S52.209N
S52.209P
S52.209Q
S52.209R
S52.211A
S52.211K
S52.211P
S52.212A
S52.212K
S52.212P
S52.219A
S52.219K
S52.219P
S52.221A
S52.221K
S52.221M
S52.221N
S52.221P
S52.221Q
S52.221R
S52.222A
S52.222K
S52.222M
S52.222N
S52.222P
S52.222Q
S52.222R
S52.223A
S52.223K
S52.223M
S52.223N
S52.223P
S52.223Q
S52.223R
S52.224A
S52.224K
S52.224M
S52.224N
S52.224P
S52.224Q
S52.224R
S52.225A
S52.225K
S52.225M
S52.225N
S52.225P
S52.225Q
S52.225R
S52.226A
S52.226K
S52.226M
S52.226N
S52.226P
S52.226Q
S52.226R
S52.231A
S52.231K
S52.231M
S52.231N
S52.231P
S52.231Q
S52.231R
S52.232A
S52.232K
S52.232M
S52.232N
S52.232P
S52.232Q
S52.232R
S52.233A
S52.233K
S52.233M
S52.233N
S52.233P
S52.233Q
S52.233R
S52.234A
S52.234K
S52.234M
S52.234N
S52.234P
S52.234Q
S52.234R
S52.235A
S52.235K
S52.235M
S52.235N
S52.235P
S52.235Q
S52.235R
S52.236A
S52.236K
S52.236M
S52.236N
S52.236P
S52.236Q
S52.236R
S52.241A
S52.241K
S52.241M
S52.241N
S52.241P
S52.241Q
S52.241R
S52.242A
S52.242K
S52.242M
S52.242N
S52.242P
S52.242Q
S52.242R
S52.243A
S52.243K
S52.243M
S52.243N
S52.243P
S52.243Q
S52.243R
S52.244A
S52.244K
S52.244M
S52.244N
S52.244P
S52.244Q
S52.244R
S52.245A
S52.245K
S52.245M
S52.245N
S52.245P
S52.245Q
S52.245R
S52.246A
S52.246K
S52.246M

Complication or Comorbidity (CC) (cont.)

Based on CMS data

S52.246N
S52.246P
S52.246Q
S52.246R
S52.251A
S52.251K
S52.251M
S52.251N
S52.251P
S52.251Q
S52.251R
S52.252A
S52.252K
S52.252M
S52.252N
S52.252P
S52.252Q
S52.252R
S52.253A
S52.253K
S52.253M
S52.253N
S52.253P
S52.253Q
S52.253R
S52.254A
S52.254K
S52.254M
S52.254N
S52.254P
S52.254Q
S52.254R
S52.255A
S52.255K
S52.255M
S52.255N
S52.255P
S52.255Q
S52.255R
S52.256A
S52.256K
S52.256M
S52.256N
S52.256P
S52.256Q
S52.256R
S52.261A
S52.261K
S52.261M
S52.261N
S52.261P
S52.261Q
S52.261R
S52.262A
S52.262K
S52.262M
S52.262N
S52.262P
S52.262Q
S52.262R
S52.263A
S52.263K
S52.263M
S52.263N
S52.263P
S52.263Q
S52.263R
S52.264A
S52.264K
S52.264M
S52.264N
S52.264P
S52.264Q
S52.264R
S52.265A
S52.265K
S52.265M
S52.265N
S52.265P
S52.265Q
S52.265R
S52.266A
S52.266K
S52.266M
S52.266N
S52.266P
S52.266Q
S52.266R
S52.271K
S52.271M
S52.271N
S52.271P
S52.271Q
S52.271R
S52.272K
S52.272M
S52.272N
S52.272P
S52.272Q
S52.272R
S52.279K
S52.279M
S52.279N
S52.279P
S52.279Q
S52.279R
S52.281A
S52.281K
S52.281M
S52.281N
S52.281P
S52.281Q
S52.281R
S52.282A
S52.282K
S52.282M
S52.282N
S52.282P
S52.282Q
S52.282R
S52.283A
S52.283K
S52.283M
S52.283N
S52.283P
S52.283Q
S52.283R
S52.291A
S52.291K
S52.291M
S52.291N
S52.291P
S52.291Q
S52.291R
S52.292A
S52.292K
S52.292M
S52.292N
S52.292P
S52.292Q
S52.292R
S52.299A
S52.299K
S52.299M
S52.299N
S52.299P
S52.299Q
S52.299R
S52.301A
S52.301K
S52.301M
S52.301N
S52.301P
S52.301Q
S52.301R
S52.302A
S52.302K
S52.302M
S52.302N
S52.302P
S52.302Q
S52.302R
S52.309A
S52.309K
S52.309M
S52.309N
S52.309P
S52.309Q
S52.309R
S52.311A
S52.311K
S52.311P
S52.312A
S52.312K
S52.312P
S52.319A
S52.319K
S52.319P
S52.321A
S52.321K
S52.321M
S52.321N
S52.321P
S52.321Q
S52.321R
S52.322A
S52.322K
S52.322M
S52.322N
S52.322P
S52.322Q
S52.322R
S52.323A
S52.323K
S52.323M
S52.323N
S52.323P
S52.323Q
S52.323R
S52.324A
S52.324K
S52.324M
S52.324N
S52.324P
S52.324Q
S52.324R
S52.325A
S52.325K
S52.325M
S52.325N
S52.325P
S52.325Q
S52.325R
S52.326A
S52.326K
S52.326M
S52.326N
S52.326P
S52.326Q
S52.326R
S52.331A
S52.331K
S52.331M
S52.331N
S52.331P
S52.331Q
S52.331R
S52.332A
S52.332K
S52.332M
S52.332N
S52.332P
S52.332Q
S52.332R
S52.333A
S52.333K
S52.333M
S52.333N
S52.333P
S52.333Q
S52.333R
S52.334A
S52.334K
S52.334M
S52.334N
S52.334P
S52.334Q
S52.334R
S52.335A
S52.335K
S52.335M
S52.335N
S52.335P
S52.335Q
S52.335R
S52.336A
S52.336K
S52.336M
S52.336N
S52.336P
S52.336Q
S52.336R
S52.341A
S52.341K
S52.341M
S52.341N
S52.341P
S52.341Q
S52.341R
S52.342A
S52.342K
S52.342M
S52.342N
S52.342P
S52.342Q
S52.342R
S52.343A
S52.343K
S52.343M
S52.343N
S52.343P
S52.343Q
S52.343R
S52.344A
S52.344K
S52.344M
S52.344N
S52.344P
S52.344Q
S52.344R
S52.345A
S52.345K
S52.345M
S52.345N
S52.345P
S52.345Q
S52.345R
S52.346A
S52.346K
S52.346M
S52.346N
S52.346P
S52.346Q
S52.346R
S52.351A
S52.351K
S52.351M
S52.351N
S52.351P
S52.351Q
S52.351R
S52.352A
S52.352K
S52.352M
S52.352N
S52.352P
S52.352Q
S52.352R
S52.353A
S52.353K
S52.353M
S52.353N
S52.353P
S52.353Q
S52.353R
S52.354A
S52.354K
S52.354M
S52.354N
S52.354P
S52.354Q
S52.354R
S52.355A
S52.355K
S52.355M
S52.355N
S52.355P
S52.355Q
S52.355R
S52.356A
S52.356K
S52.356M
S52.356N
S52.356P
S52.356Q
S52.356R
S52.361A
S52.361K
S52.361M
S52.361N
S52.361P
S52.361Q
S52.361R
S52.362A
S52.362K
S52.362M
S52.362N
S52.362P
S52.362Q
S52.362R
S52.363A
S52.363K
S52.363M
S52.363N
S52.363P
S52.363Q
S52.363R
S52.364A
S52.364K
S52.364M
S52.364N
S52.364P
S52.364Q
S52.364R
S52.365A
S52.365K
S52.365M
S52.365N
S52.365P
S52.365Q
S52.365R
S52.366A
S52.366K
S52.366M
S52.366N
S52.366P
S52.366Q
S52.366R
S52.371A
S52.371K
S52.371M
S52.371N
S52.371P
S52.371Q
S52.371R
S52.372A
S52.372K
S52.372M
S52.372N
S52.372P
S52.372Q
S52.372R
S52.379A
S52.379K
S52.379M
S52.379N
S52.379P
S52.379Q
S52.379R
S52.381A
S52.381K
S52.381M
S52.381N
S52.381P
S52.381Q
S52.381R
S52.382A
S52.382K
S52.382M
S52.382N
S52.382P
S52.382Q
S52.382R
S52.389A
S52.389K
S52.389M
S52.389N
S52.389P
S52.389Q
S52.389R
S52.391A
S52.391K
S52.391M
S52.391N
S52.391P
S52.391Q
S52.391R
S52.392A
S52.392K
S52.392M
S52.392N
S52.392P
S52.392Q
S52.392R
S52.399A
S52.399K
S52.399M
S52.399N
S52.399P
S52.399Q
S52.399R
S52.501A
S52.501K
S52.501M
S52.501N
S52.501P
S52.501Q
S52.501R
S52.502A
S52.502K
S52.502M
S52.502N
S52.502P
S52.502Q
S52.502R
S52.509A
S52.509K
S52.509M
S52.509N
S52.509P
S52.509Q
S52.509R
S52.511A
S52.511K
S52.511M
S52.511N
S52.511P
S52.511Q
S52.511R
S52.512A
S52.512K
S52.512M
S52.512N
S52.512P
S52.512Q
S52.512R
S52.513A
S52.513K
S52.513M
S52.513N
S52.513P
S52.513Q
S52.513R
S52.514A
S52.514K
S52.514M
S52.514N
S52.514P
S52.514Q
S52.514R
S52.515A
S52.515K
S52.515M
S52.515N
S52.515P
S52.515Q
S52.515R
S52.516A
S52.516K
S52.516M
S52.516N
S52.516P
S52.516Q
S52.516R
S52.521A
S52.521K
S52.521P
S52.522A
S52.522K
S52.522P
S52.529A
S52.529K
S52.529P
S52.531A
S52.531K
S52.531M
S52.531N
S52.531P
S52.531Q
S52.531R
S52.532A
S52.532K
S52.532M
S52.532N
S52.532P
S52.532Q
S52.532R
S52.539A
S52.539K
S52.539M
S52.539N
S52.539P
S52.539Q
S52.539R
S52.541A
S52.541K
S52.541M
S52.541N
S52.541P
S52.541Q
S52.541R
S52.542A
S52.542K
S52.542M
S52.542N
S52.542P
S52.542Q
S52.542R
S52.549A
S52.549K
S52.549M
S52.549N
S52.549P
S52.549Q
S52.549R
S52.551A
S52.551K
S52.551M
S52.551N
S52.551P
S52.551Q
S52.551R
S52.552A
S52.552K
S52.552M
S52.552N
S52.552P
S52.552Q
S52.552R
S52.559A
S52.559K
S52.559M
S52.559N
S52.559P
S52.559Q
S52.559R
S52.561A
S52.561K
S52.561M
S52.561N
S52.561P
S52.561Q
S52.561R
S52.562A
S52.562K
S52.562M
S52.562N
S52.562P
S52.562Q
S52.562R
S52.569A
S52.569K
S52.569M
S52.569N
S52.569P
S52.569Q
S52.569R
S52.571A
S52.571K
S52.571M
S52.571N
S52.571P
S52.571Q
S52.571R
S52.572A
S52.572K
S52.572M
S52.572N
S52.572P
S52.572Q
S52.572R
S52.579A
S52.579K
S52.579M
S52.579N
S52.579P
S52.579Q
S52.579R
S52.591A
S52.591K
S52.591M
S52.591N
S52.591P
S52.591Q
S52.591R
S52.592A
S52.592K
S52.592M
S52.592N
S52.592P
S52.592Q
S52.592R
S52.599A
S52.599K
S52.599M
S52.599N
S52.599P
S52.599Q
S52.599R
S52.601A
S52.601K
S52.601M
S52.601N
S52.601P
S52.601Q
S52.601R
S52.602A
S52.602K
S52.602M
S52.602N

Complication or Comorbidity (CC) (cont.)

Based on CMS data

S52.602P
S52.602Q
S52.602R
S52.609A
S52.609K
S52.609M
S52.609N
S52.609P
S52.609Q
S52.609R
S52.611A
S52.611K
S52.611M
S52.611N
S52.611P
S52.611Q
S52.611R
S52.612A
S52.612K
S52.612M
S52.612N
S52.612P
S52.612Q
S52.612R
S52.613A
S52.613K
S52.613M
S52.613N
S52.613P
S52.613Q
S52.613R
S52.614A
S52.614K
S52.614M
S52.614N
S52.614P
S52.614Q
S52.614R
S52.615A
S52.615K
S52.615M
S52.615N
S52.615P
S52.615Q
S52.615R
S52.616A
S52.616K
S52.616M
S52.616N
S52.616P
S52.616Q
S52.616R
S52.621A
S52.621K
S52.621P
S52.622A
S52.622K
S52.622P
S52.629A
S52.629K
S52.629P
S52.691A
S52.691K
S52.691M
S52.691N
S52.691P
S52.691Q
S52.691R
S52.692A
S52.692K
S52.692M
S52.692N
S52.692P
S52.692Q
S52.692R
S52.699A
S52.699K
S52.699M
S52.699N
S52.699P
S52.699Q
S52.699R
S52.90XA
S52.90XK
S52.90XM
S52.90XN
S52.90XP
S52.90XQ
S52.90XR
S52.91XA
S52.91XK
S52.91XM
S52.91XN
S52.91XP
S52.91XQ
S52.91XR
S52.92XA
S52.92XK
S52.92XM
S52.92XN
S52.92XP
S52.92XQ
S52.92XR
S55.001A
S55.002A
S55.009A
S55.011A
S55.012A
S55.019A
S55.091A
S55.092A
S55.099A
S55.101A
S55.102A
S55.109A
S55.111A
S55.112A
S55.119A
S55.191A
S55.192A
S55.199A
S55.201A
S55.202A
S55.209A
S55.211A
S55.212A
S55.219A
S55.291A
S55.292A
S55.299A
S55.801A
S55.802A
S55.809A
S55.811A
S55.812A
S55.819A
S55.891A
S55.892A
S55.899A
S55.901A
S55.902A
S55.909A
S55.911A
S55.912A
S55.919A
S55.991A
S55.992A
S55.999A
S56.021A
S56.022A
S56.029A
S56.121A
S56.122A
S56.123A
S56.124A
S56.125A
S56.126A
S56.127A
S56.128A
S56.129A
S56.221A
S56.222A
S56.229A
S56.321A
S56.322A
S56.329A
S56.421A
S56.422A
S56.423A
S56.424A
S56.425A
S56.426A
S56.427A
S56.428A
S56.429A
S56.521A
S56.522A
S56.529A
S56.821A
S56.822A
S56.829A
S56.921A
S56.922A
S56.929A
S58.011A
S58.012A
S58.019A
S58.021A
S58.022A
S58.029A
S58.111A
S58.112A
S58.119A
S58.121A
S58.122A
S58.129A
S58.911A
S58.912A
S58.919A
S58.921A
S58.922A
S58.929A
S59.001A
S59.001K
S59.001P
S59.002A
S59.002K
S59.002P
S59.009A
S59.009K
S59.009P
S59.011A
S59.011K
S59.011P
S59.012A
S59.012K
S59.012P
S59.019A
S59.019K
S59.019P
S59.021A
S59.021K
S59.021P
S59.022A
S59.022K
S59.022P
S59.029A
S59.029K
S59.029P
S59.031A
S59.031K
S59.031P
S59.032A
S59.032K
S59.032P
S59.039A
S59.039K
S59.039P
S59.041A
S59.041K
S59.041P
S59.042A
S59.042K
S59.042P
S59.049A
S59.049K
S59.049P
S59.091A
S59.091K
S59.091P
S59.092A
S59.092K
S59.092P
S59.099A
S59.099K
S59.099P
S59.101K
S59.101P
S59.102K
S59.102P
S59.109K
S59.109P
S59.111K
S59.111P
S59.112K
S59.112P
S59.119K
S59.119P
S59.121K
S59.121P
S59.122K
S59.122P
S59.129K
S59.129P
S59.131K
S59.131P
S59.132K
S59.132P
S59.139K
S59.139P
S59.141K
S59.141P
S59.142K
S59.142P
S59.149K
S59.149P
S59.191K
S59.191P
S59.192K
S59.192P
S59.199K
S59.199P
S59.201A
S59.201K
S59.201P
S59.202A
S59.202K
S59.202P
S59.209A
S59.209K
S59.209P
S59.211A
S59.211K
S59.211P
S59.212A
S59.212K
S59.212P
S59.219A
S59.219K
S59.219P
S59.221A
S59.221K
S59.221P
S59.222A
S59.222K
S59.222P
S59.229A
S59.229K
S59.229P
S59.231A
S59.231K
S59.231P
S59.232A
S59.232K
S59.232P
S59.239A
S59.239K
S59.239P
S59.241A
S59.241K
S59.241P
S59.242A
S59.242K
S59.242P
S59.249A
S59.249K
S59.249P
S59.291A
S59.291K
S59.291P
S59.292A
S59.292K
S59.292P
S59.299A
S59.299K
S59.299P
S62.001B
S62.001K
S62.001P
S62.002B
S62.002K
S62.002P
S62.009B
S62.009K
S62.009P
S62.011B
S62.011K
S62.011P
S62.012B
S62.012K
S62.012P
S62.013B
S62.013K
S62.013P
S62.014B
S62.014K
S62.014P
S62.015B
S62.015K
S62.015P
S62.016B
S62.016K
S62.016P
S62.021B
S62.021K
S62.021P
S62.022B
S62.022K
S62.022P
S62.023B
S62.023K
S62.023P
S62.024B
S62.024K
S62.024P
S62.025B
S62.025K
S62.025P
S62.026B
S62.026K
S62.026P
S62.031B
S62.031K
S62.031P
S62.032B
S62.032K
S62.032P
S62.033B
S62.033K
S62.033P
S62.034B
S62.034K
S62.034P
S62.035B
S62.035K
S62.035P
S62.036B
S62.036K
S62.036P
S62.101B
S62.101K
S62.101P
S62.102B
S62.102K
S62.102P
S62.109B
S62.109K
S62.109P
S62.111B
S62.111K
S62.111P
S62.112B
S62.112K
S62.112P
S62.113B
S62.113K
S62.113P
S62.114B
S62.114K
S62.114P
S62.115B
S62.115K
S62.115P
S62.116B
S62.116K
S62.116P
S62.121B
S62.121K
S62.121P
S62.122B
S62.122K
S62.122P
S62.123B
S62.123K
S62.123P
S62.124B
S62.124K
S62.124P
S62.125B
S62.125K
S62.125P
S62.126B
S62.126K
S62.126P
S62.131B
S62.131K
S62.131P
S62.132B
S62.132K
S62.132P
S62.133B
S62.133K
S62.133P
S62.134B
S62.134K
S62.134P
S62.135B
S62.135K
S62.135P
S62.136B
S62.136K
S62.136P
S62.141B
S62.141K
S62.141P
S62.142B
S62.142K
S62.142P
S62.143B
S62.143K
S62.143P
S62.144B
S62.144K
S62.144P
S62.145B
S62.145K
S62.145P
S62.146B
S62.146K
S62.146P
S62.151B
S62.151K
S62.151P
S62.152B
S62.152K
S62.152P
S62.153B
S62.153K
S62.153P
S62.154B
S62.154K
S62.154P
S62.155B
S62.155K
S62.155P
S62.156B
S62.156K
S62.156P
S62.161B
S62.161K
S62.161P
S62.162B
S62.162K
S62.162P
S62.163B
S62.163K
S62.163P
S62.164B
S62.164K
S62.164P
S62.165B
S62.165K
S62.165P
S62.166B
S62.166K
S62.166P
S62.171B
S62.171K
S62.171P
S62.172B
S62.172K
S62.172P
S62.173B
S62.173K
S62.173P
S62.174B
S62.174K
S62.174P
S62.175B
S62.175K
S62.175P
S62.176B
S62.176K
S62.176P
S62.181B
S62.181K
S62.181P
S62.182B
S62.182K
S62.182P
S62.183B
S62.183K
S62.183P
S62.184B
S62.184K
S62.184P
S62.185B
S62.185K
S62.185P
S62.186B
S62.186K
S62.186P
S62.201B
S62.201K
S62.201P
S62.202B
S62.202K
S62.202P
S62.209B
S62.209K
S62.209P
S62.211B
S62.211K
S62.211P
S62.212B
S62.212K
S62.212P
S62.213B
S62.213K
S62.213P
S62.221B
S62.221K
S62.221P
S62.222B
S62.222K
S62.222P
S62.223B
S62.223K
S62.223P
S62.224B
S62.224K
S62.224P
S62.225B
S62.225K
S62.225P
S62.226B
S62.226K
S62.226P
S62.231B
S62.231K
S62.231P
S62.232B
S62.232K
S62.232P
S62.233B
S62.233K
S62.233P
S62.234B
S62.234K
S62.234P
S62.235B
S62.235K
S62.235P
S62.236B
S62.236K
S62.236P
S62.241B
S62.241K
S62.241P
S62.242B
S62.242K
S62.242P
S62.243B
S62.243K
S62.243P
S62.244B
S62.244K
S62.244P
S62.245B
S62.245K
S62.245P
S62.246B
S62.246K
S62.246P
S62.251B
S62.251K
S62.251P
S62.252B
S62.252K
S62.252P
S62.253B
S62.253K
S62.253P
S62.254B
S62.254K
S62.254P
S62.255B
S62.255K
S62.255P
S62.256B
S62.256K
S62.256P
S62.291B
S62.291K
S62.291P
S62.292B
S62.292K
S62.292P
S62.299B
S62.299K

Complication or Comorbidity (CC) (cont.)

Based on CMS data

S62.299P
S62.300B
S62.300K
S62.300P
S62.301B
S62.301K
S62.301P
S62.302B
S62.302K
S62.302P
S62.303B
S62.303K
S62.303P
S62.304B
S62.304K
S62.304P
S62.305B
S62.305K
S62.305P
S62.306B
S62.306K
S62.306P
S62.307B
S62.307K
S62.307P
S62.308B
S62.308K
S62.308P
S62.309B
S62.309K
S62.309P
S62.310B
S62.310K
S62.310P
S62.311B
S62.311K
S62.311P
S62.312B
S62.312K
S62.312P
S62.313B
S62.313K
S62.313P
S62.314B
S62.314K
S62.314P
S62.315B
S62.315K
S62.315P
S62.316B
S62.316K
S62.316P
S62.317B
S62.317K
S62.317P
S62.318B
S62.318K
S62.318P
S62.319B
S62.319K
S62.319P
S62.320B
S62.320K
S62.320P
S62.321B
S62.321K
S62.321P
S62.322B
S62.322K
S62.322P
S62.323B
S62.323K
S62.323P
S62.324B
S62.324K
S62.324P
S62.325B
S62.325K
S62.325P
S62.326B
S62.326K
S62.326P
S62.327B
S62.327K
S62.327P
S62.328B
S62.328K
S62.328P
S62.329B
S62.329K
S62.329P
S62.330B
S62.330K
S62.330P
S62.331B
S62.331K
S62.331P
S62.332B
S62.332K
S62.332P
S62.333B
S62.333K
S62.333P
S62.334B
S62.334K
S62.334P
S62.335B
S62.335K
S62.335P
S62.336B
S62.336K
S62.336P
S62.337B
S62.337K
S62.337P
S62.338B
S62.338K
S62.338P
S62.339B
S62.339K
S62.339P
S62.340B
S62.340K
S62.340P
S62.341B
S62.341K
S62.341P
S62.342B
S62.342K
S62.342P
S62.343B
S62.343K
S62.343P
S62.344B
S62.344K
S62.344P
S62.345B
S62.345K
S62.345P
S62.346B
S62.346K
S62.346P
S62.347B
S62.347K
S62.347P
S62.348B
S62.348K
S62.348P
S62.349B
S62.349K
S62.349P
S62.350B
S62.350K
S62.350P
S62.351B
S62.351K
S62.351P
S62.352B
S62.352K
S62.352P
S62.353B
S62.353K
S62.353P
S62.354B
S62.354K
S62.354P
S62.355B
S62.355K
S62.355P
S62.356B
S62.356K
S62.356P
S62.357B
S62.357K
S62.357P
S62.358B
S62.358K
S62.358P
S62.359B
S62.359K
S62.359P
S62.360B
S62.360K
S62.360P
S62.361B
S62.361K
S62.361P
S62.362B
S62.362K
S62.362P
S62.363B
S62.363K
S62.363P
S62.364B
S62.364K
S62.364P
S62.365B
S62.365K
S62.365P
S62.366B
S62.366K
S62.366P
S62.367B
S62.367K
S62.367P
S62.368B
S62.368K
S62.368P
S62.369B
S62.369K
S62.369P
S62.390B
S62.390K
S62.390P
S62.391B
S62.391K
S62.391P
S62.392B
S62.392K
S62.392P
S62.393B
S62.393K
S62.393P
S62.394B
S62.394K
S62.394P
S62.395B
S62.395K
S62.395P
S62.396B
S62.396K
S62.396P
S62.397B
S62.397K
S62.397P
S62.398B
S62.398K
S62.398P
S62.399B
S62.399K
S62.399P
S62.501B
S62.501K
S62.501P
S62.502B
S62.502K
S62.502P
S62.509B
S62.509K
S62.509P
S62.511B
S62.511K
S62.511P
S62.512B
S62.512K
S62.512P
S62.513B
S62.513K
S62.513P
S62.514B
S62.514K
S62.514P
S62.515B
S62.515K
S62.515P
S62.516B
S62.516K
S62.516P
S62.521B
S62.521K
S62.521P
S62.522B
S62.522K
S62.522P
S62.523B
S62.523K
S62.523P
S62.524B
S62.524K
S62.524P
S62.525B
S62.525K
S62.525P
S62.526B
S62.526K
S62.526P
S62.600B
S62.600K
S62.600P
S62.601B
S62.601K
S62.601P
S62.602B
S62.602K
S62.602P
S62.603B
S62.603K
S62.603P
S62.604B
S62.604K
S62.604P
S62.605B
S62.605K
S62.605P
S62.606B
S62.606K
S62.606P
S62.607B
S62.607K
S62.607P
S62.608B
S62.608K
S62.608P
S62.609B
S62.609K
S62.609P
S62.610B
S62.610K
S62.610P
S62.611B
S62.611K
S62.611P
S62.612B
S62.612K
S62.612P
S62.613B
S62.613K
S62.613P
S62.614B
S62.614K
S62.614P
S62.615B
S62.615K
S62.615P
S62.616B
S62.616K
S62.616P
S62.617B
S62.617K
S62.617P
S62.618B
S62.618K
S62.618P
S62.619B
S62.619K
S62.619P
S62.620B
S62.620K
S62.620P
S62.621B
S62.621K
S62.621P
S62.622B
S62.622K
S62.622P
S62.623B
S62.623K
S62.623P
S62.624B
S62.624K
S62.624P
S62.625B
S62.625K
S62.625P
S62.626B
S62.626K
S62.626P
S62.627B
S62.627K
S62.627P
S62.628B
S62.628K
S62.628P
S62.629B
S62.629K
S62.629P
S62.630B
S62.630K
S62.630P
S62.631B
S62.631K
S62.631P
S62.632B
S62.632K
S62.632P
S62.633B
S62.633K
S62.633P
S62.634B
S62.634K
S62.634P
S62.635B
S62.635K
S62.635P
S62.636B
S62.636K
S62.636P
S62.637B
S62.637K
S62.637P
S62.638B
S62.638K
S62.638P
S62.639B
S62.639K
S62.639P
S62.640B
S62.640K
S62.640P
S62.641B
S62.641K
S62.641P
S62.642B
S62.642K
S62.642P
S62.643B
S62.643K
S62.643P
S62.644B
S62.644K
S62.644P
S62.645B
S62.645K
S62.645P
S62.646B
S62.646K
S62.646P
S62.647B
S62.647K
S62.647P
S62.648B
S62.648K
S62.648P
S62.649B
S62.649K
S62.649P
S62.650B
S62.650K
S62.650P
S62.651B
S62.651K
S62.651P
S62.652B
S62.652K
S62.652P
S62.653B
S62.653K
S62.653P
S62.654B
S62.654K
S62.654P
S62.655B
S62.655K
S62.655P
S62.656B
S62.656K
S62.656P
S62.657B
S62.657K
S62.657P
S62.658B
S62.658K
S62.658P
S62.659B
S62.659K
S62.659P
S62.660B
S62.660K
S62.660P
S62.661B
S62.661K
S62.661P
S62.662B
S62.662K
S62.662P
S62.663B
S62.663K
S62.663P
S62.664B
S62.664K
S62.664P
S62.665B
S62.665K
S62.665P
S62.666B
S62.666K
S62.666P
S62.667B
S62.667K
S62.667P
S62.668B
S62.668K
S62.668P
S62.669B
S62.669K
S62.669P
S62.90XB
S62.90XK
S62.90XP
S62.91XB
S62.91XK
S62.91XP
S62.92XB
S62.92XK
S62.92XP
S65.001A
S65.002A
S65.009A
S65.011A
S65.012A
S65.019A
S65.091A
S65.092A
S65.099A
S65.101A
S65.102A
S65.109A
S65.111A
S65.112A
S65.119A
S65.191A
S65.192A
S65.199A
S65.201A
S65.202A
S65.209A
S65.211A
S65.212A
S65.219A
S65.291A
S65.292A
S65.299A
S65.301A
S65.302A
S65.309A
S65.311A
S65.312A
S65.319A
S65.391A
S65.392A
S65.399A
S65.401A
S65.402A
S65.409A
S65.411A
S65.412A
S65.419A
S65.491A
S65.492A
S65.499A
S65.500A
S65.501A
S65.502A
S65.503A
S65.504A
S65.505A
S65.506A
S65.507A
S65.508A
S65.509A
S65.510A
S65.511A
S65.512A
S65.513A
S65.514A
S65.515A
S65.516A
S65.517A
S65.518A
S65.519A
S65.590A
S65.591A
S65.592A
S65.593A
S65.594A
S65.595A
S65.596A
S65.597A
S65.598A
S65.599A
S65.801A
S65.802A
S65.809A
S65.811A
S65.812A
S65.819A
S65.891A
S65.892A
S65.899A
S65.901A
S65.902A
S65.909A
S65.911A
S65.912A
S65.919A
S65.991A
S65.992A
S65.999A
S66.021A
S66.022A
S66.029A
S66.120A
S66.121A
S66.122A
S66.123A
S66.124A
S66.125A
S66.126A
S66.127A
S66.128A
S66.129A
S66.221A
S66.222A
S66.229A
S66.320A
S66.321A
S66.322A
S66.323A
S66.324A
S66.325A
S66.326A
S66.327A
S66.328A
S66.329A
S66.421A
S66.422A
S66.429A
S66.520A
S66.521A
S66.522A
S66.523A
S66.524A
S66.525A
S66.526A
S66.527A
S66.528A
S66.529A
S66.821A
S66.822A
S66.829A
S66.921A
S66.922A
S66.929A
S68.411A
S68.412A
S68.419A
S68.421A
S68.422A
S68.429A
S68.711A
S68.712A
S68.719A
S68.721A
S68.722A
S68.729A
S72.001K
S72.001M
S72.001N
S72.001P
S72.001Q

Complication or Comorbidity (CC) (cont.)

Based on CMS data

S72.001R
S72.002K
S72.002M
S72.002N
S72.002P
S72.002Q
S72.002R
S72.009K
S72.009M
S72.009N
S72.009P
S72.009Q
S72.009R
S72.011K
S72.011M
S72.011N
S72.011P
S72.011Q
S72.011R
S72.012K
S72.012M
S72.012N
S72.012P
S72.012Q
S72.012R
S72.019K
S72.019M
S72.019N
S72.019P
S72.019Q
S72.019R
S72.021K
S72.021M
S72.021N
S72.021P
S72.021Q
S72.021R
S72.022K
S72.022M
S72.022N
S72.022P
S72.022Q
S72.022R
S72.023K
S72.023M
S72.023N
S72.023P
S72.023Q
S72.023R
S72.024K
S72.024M
S72.024N
S72.024P
S72.024Q
S72.024R
S72.025K
S72.025M
S72.025N
S72.025P
S72.025Q
S72.025R
S72.026K
S72.026M
S72.026N
S72.026P
S72.026Q
S72.026R
S72.031K
S72.031M
S72.031N
S72.031P
S72.031Q
S72.031R
S72.032K
S72.032M
S72.032N
S72.032P
S72.032Q
S72.032R
S72.033K
S72.033M
S72.033N
S72.033P
S72.033Q
S72.033R
S72.034K
S72.034M
S72.034N
S72.034P
S72.034Q
S72.034R
S72.035K
S72.035M
S72.035N
S72.035P
S72.035Q
S72.035R
S72.036K
S72.036M
S72.036N
S72.036P
S72.036Q
S72.036R
S72.041K
S72.041M
S72.041N
S72.041P
S72.041Q
S72.041R
S72.042K
S72.042M
S72.042N
S72.042P
S72.042Q
S72.042R
S72.043K
S72.043M
S72.043N
S72.043P
S72.043Q
S72.043R
S72.044K
S72.044M
S72.044N
S72.044P
S72.044Q
S72.044R
S72.045K
S72.045M
S72.045N
S72.045P
S72.045Q
S72.045R
S72.046K
S72.046M
S72.046N
S72.046P
S72.046Q
S72.046R
S72.051K
S72.051M
S72.051N
S72.051P
S72.051Q
S72.051R
S72.052K
S72.052M
S72.052N
S72.052P
S72.052Q
S72.052R
S72.059K
S72.059M
S72.059N
S72.059P
S72.059Q
S72.059R
S72.061K
S72.061M
S72.061N
S72.061P
S72.061Q
S72.061R
S72.062K
S72.062M
S72.062N
S72.062P
S72.062Q
S72.062R
S72.063K
S72.063M
S72.063N
S72.063P
S72.063Q
S72.063R
S72.064K
S72.064M
S72.064N
S72.064P
S72.064Q
S72.064R
S72.065K
S72.065M
S72.065N
S72.065P
S72.065Q
S72.065R
S72.066K
S72.066M
S72.066N
S72.066P
S72.066Q
S72.066R
S72.091K
S72.091M
S72.091N
S72.091P
S72.091Q
S72.091R
S72.092K
S72.092M
S72.092N
S72.092P
S72.092Q
S72.092R
S72.099K
S72.099M
S72.099N
S72.099P
S72.099Q
S72.099R
S72.101K
S72.101M
S72.101N
S72.101P
S72.101Q
S72.101R
S72.102K
S72.102M
S72.102N
S72.102P
S72.102Q
S72.102R
S72.109K
S72.109M
S72.109N
S72.109P
S72.109Q
S72.109R
S72.111K
S72.111M
S72.111N
S72.111P
S72.111Q
S72.111R
S72.112K
S72.112M
S72.112N
S72.112P
S72.112Q
S72.112R
S72.113K
S72.113M
S72.113N
S72.113P
S72.113Q
S72.113R
S72.114K
S72.114M
S72.114N
S72.114P
S72.114Q
S72.114R
S72.115K
S72.115M
S72.115N
S72.115P
S72.115Q
S72.115R
S72.116K
S72.116M
S72.116N
S72.116P
S72.116Q
S72.116R
S72.121K
S72.121M
S72.121N
S72.121P
S72.121Q
S72.121R
S72.122K
S72.122M
S72.122N
S72.122P
S72.122Q
S72.122R
S72.123K
S72.123M
S72.123N
S72.123P
S72.123Q
S72.123R
S72.124K
S72.124M
S72.124N
S72.124P
S72.124Q
S72.124R
S72.125K
S72.125M
S72.125N
S72.125P
S72.125Q
S72.125R
S72.126K
S72.126M
S72.126N
S72.126P
S72.126Q
S72.126R
S72.131K
S72.131M
S72.131N
S72.131P
S72.131Q
S72.131R
S72.132K
S72.132M
S72.132N
S72.132P
S72.132Q
S72.132R
S72.133K
S72.133M
S72.133N
S72.133P
S72.133Q
S72.133R
S72.134K
S72.134M
S72.134N
S72.134P
S72.134Q
S72.134R
S72.135K
S72.135M
S72.135N
S72.135P
S72.135Q
S72.135R
S72.136K
S72.136M
S72.136N
S72.136P
S72.136Q
S72.136R
S72.141K
S72.141M
S72.141N
S72.141P
S72.141Q
S72.141R
S72.142K
S72.142M
S72.142N
S72.142P
S72.142Q
S72.142R
S72.143K
S72.143M
S72.143N
S72.143P
S72.143Q
S72.143R
S72.144K
S72.144M
S72.144N
S72.144P
S72.144Q
S72.144R
S72.145K
S72.145M
S72.145N
S72.145P
S72.145Q
S72.145R
S72.146K
S72.146M
S72.146N
S72.146P
S72.146Q
S72.146R
S72.21XK
S72.21XM
S72.21XN
S72.21XP
S72.21XQ
S72.21XR
S72.22XK
S72.22XM
S72.22XN
S72.22XP
S72.22XQ
S72.22XR
S72.23XK
S72.23XM
S72.23XN
S72.23XP
S72.23XQ
S72.23XR
S72.24XK
S72.24XM
S72.24XN
S72.24XP
S72.24XQ
S72.24XR
S72.25XK
S72.25XM
S72.25XN
S72.25XP
S72.25XQ
S72.25XR
S72.26XK
S72.26XM
S72.26XN
S72.26XP
S72.26XQ
S72.26XR
S72.301K
S72.301M
S72.301N
S72.301P
S72.301Q
S72.301R
S72.302K
S72.302M
S72.302N
S72.302P
S72.302Q
S72.302R
S72.309K
S72.309M
S72.309N
S72.309P
S72.309Q
S72.309R
S72.321K
S72.321M
S72.321N
S72.321P
S72.321Q
S72.321R
S72.322K
S72.322M
S72.322N
S72.322P
S72.322Q
S72.322R
S72.323K
S72.323M
S72.323N
S72.323P
S72.323Q
S72.323R
S72.324K
S72.324M
S72.324N
S72.324P
S72.324Q
S72.324R
S72.325K
S72.325M
S72.325N
S72.325P
S72.325Q
S72.325R
S72.326K
S72.326M
S72.326N
S72.326P
S72.326Q
S72.326R
S72.331K
S72.331M
S72.331N
S72.331P
S72.331Q
S72.331R
S72.332K
S72.332M
S72.332N
S72.332P
S72.332Q
S72.332R
S72.333K
S72.333M
S72.333N
S72.333P
S72.333Q
S72.333R
S72.334K
S72.334M
S72.334N
S72.334P
S72.334Q
S72.334R
S72.335K
S72.335M
S72.335N
S72.335P
S72.335Q
S72.335R
S72.336K
S72.336M
S72.336N
S72.336P
S72.336Q
S72.336R
S72.341K
S72.341M
S72.341N
S72.341P
S72.341Q
S72.341R
S72.342K
S72.342M
S72.342N
S72.342P
S72.342Q
S72.342R
S72.343K
S72.343M
S72.343N
S72.343P
S72.343Q
S72.343R
S72.344K
S72.344M
S72.344N
S72.344P
S72.344Q
S72.344R
S72.345K
S72.345M
S72.345N
S72.345P
S72.345Q
S72.345R
S72.346K
S72.346M
S72.346N
S72.346P
S72.346Q
S72.346R
S72.351K
S72.351M
S72.351N
S72.351P
S72.351Q
S72.351R
S72.352K
S72.352M
S72.352N
S72.352P
S72.352Q
S72.352R
S72.353K
S72.353M
S72.353N
S72.353P
S72.353Q
S72.353R
S72.354K
S72.354M
S72.354N
S72.354P
S72.354Q
S72.354R
S72.355K
S72.355M
S72.355N
S72.355P
S72.355Q
S72.355R
S72.356K
S72.356M
S72.356N
S72.356P
S72.356Q
S72.356R
S72.361K
S72.361M
S72.361N
S72.361P
S72.361Q
S72.361R
S72.362K
S72.362M
S72.362N
S72.362P
S72.362Q
S72.362R
S72.363K
S72.363M
S72.363N
S72.363P
S72.363Q
S72.363R
S72.364K
S72.364M
S72.364N
S72.364P
S72.364Q
S72.364R
S72.365K
S72.365M
S72.365N
S72.365P
S72.365Q
S72.365R
S72.366K
S72.366M
S72.366N
S72.366P
S72.366Q
S72.366R
S72.391K
S72.391M
S72.391N
S72.391P
S72.391Q
S72.391R
S72.392K
S72.392M
S72.392N
S72.392P
S72.392Q
S72.392R
S72.399K
S72.399M
S72.399N
S72.399P
S72.399Q
S72.399R
S72.401A
S72.401K
S72.401M
S72.401N
S72.401P
S72.401Q
S72.401R
S72.402A
S72.402K
S72.402M
S72.402N
S72.402P
S72.402Q
S72.402R
S72.409A
S72.409K
S72.409M
S72.409N
S72.409P
S72.409Q
S72.409R
S72.411A
S72.411K
S72.411M
S72.411N
S72.411P
S72.411Q
S72.411R
S72.412A
S72.412K
S72.412M
S72.412N
S72.412P
S72.412Q
S72.412R

Complication or Comorbidity (CC) (cont.)

Based on CMS data

S72.413A
S72.413K
S72.413M
S72.413N
S72.413P
S72.413Q
S72.413R
S72.414A
S72.414K
S72.414M
S72.414N
S72.414P
S72.414Q
S72.414R
S72.415A
S72.415K
S72.415M
S72.415N
S72.415P
S72.415Q
S72.415R
S72.416A
S72.416K
S72.416M
S72.416N
S72.416P
S72.416Q
S72.416R
S72.421A
S72.421K
S72.421M
S72.421N
S72.421P
S72.421Q
S72.421R
S72.422A
S72.422K
S72.422M
S72.422N
S72.422P
S72.422Q
S72.422R
S72.423A
S72.423K
S72.423M
S72.423N
S72.423P
S72.423Q
S72.423R
S72.424A
S72.424K
S72.424M
S72.424N
S72.424P
S72.424Q
S72.424R
S72.425A
S72.425K
S72.425M
S72.425N
S72.425P
S72.425Q
S72.425R
S72.426A
S72.426K
S72.426M
S72.426N
S72.426P
S72.426Q
S72.426R
S72.431A
S72.431K
S72.431M
S72.431N
S72.431P
S72.431Q
S72.431R
S72.432A
S72.432K
S72.432M
S72.432N
S72.432P
S72.432Q
S72.432R
S72.433A
S72.433K
S72.433M
S72.433N
S72.433P
S72.433Q
S72.433R
S72.434A
S72.434K
S72.434M
S72.434N
S72.434P
S72.434Q
S72.434R
S72.435A
S72.435K
S72.435M
S72.435N
S72.435P
S72.435Q
S72.435R
S72.436A
S72.436K
S72.436M
S72.436N
S72.436P
S72.436Q
S72.436R
S72.441A
S72.441K
S72.441M
S72.441N
S72.441P
S72.441Q
S72.441R
S72.442A
S72.442K
S72.442M
S72.442N
S72.442P
S72.442Q
S72.442R
S72.443A
S72.443K
S72.443M
S72.443N
S72.443P
S72.443Q
S72.443R
S72.444A
S72.444K
S72.444M
S72.444N
S72.444P
S72.444Q
S72.444R
S72.445A
S72.445K
S72.445M
S72.445N
S72.445P
S72.445Q
S72.445R
S72.446A
S72.446K
S72.446M
S72.446N
S72.446P
S72.446Q
S72.446R
S72.451A
S72.451K
S72.451M
S72.451N
S72.451P
S72.451Q
S72.451R
S72.452A
S72.452K
S72.452M
S72.452N
S72.452P
S72.452Q
S72.452R
S72.453A
S72.453K
S72.453M
S72.453N
S72.453P
S72.453Q
S72.453R
S72.454A
S72.454K
S72.454M
S72.454N
S72.454P
S72.454Q
S72.454R
S72.455A
S72.455K
S72.455M
S72.455N
S72.455P
S72.455Q
S72.455R
S72.456A
S72.456K
S72.456M
S72.456N
S72.456P
S72.456Q
S72.456R
S72.461A
S72.461K
S72.461M
S72.461N
S72.461P
S72.461Q
S72.461R
S72.462A
S72.462K
S72.462M
S72.462N
S72.462P
S72.462Q
S72.462R
S72.463A
S72.463K
S72.463M
S72.463N
S72.463P
S72.463Q
S72.463R
S72.464A
S72.464K
S72.464M
S72.464N
S72.464P
S72.464Q
S72.464R
S72.465A
S72.465K
S72.465M
S72.465N
S72.465P
S72.465Q
S72.465R
S72.466A
S72.466K
S72.466M
S72.466N
S72.466P
S72.466Q
S72.466R
S72.471A
S72.471K
S72.471P
S72.472A
S72.472K
S72.472P
S72.479A
S72.479K
S72.479P
S72.491A
S72.491K
S72.491M
S72.491N
S72.491P
S72.491Q
S72.491R
S72.492A
S72.492K
S72.492M
S72.492N
S72.492P
S72.492Q
S72.492R
S72.499A
S72.499K
S72.499M
S72.499N
S72.499P
S72.499Q
S72.499R
S72.8X1K
S72.8X1M
S72.8X1N
S72.8X1P
S72.8X1Q
S72.8X1R
S72.8X2K
S72.8X2M
S72.8X2N
S72.8X2P
S72.8X2Q
S72.8X2R
S72.8X9K
S72.8X9M
S72.8X9N
S72.8X9P
S72.8X9Q
S72.8X9R
S72.90XK
S72.90XM
S72.90XN
S72.90XP
S72.90XQ
S72.90XR
S72.91XK
S72.91XM
S72.91XN
S72.91XP
S72.91XQ
S72.91XR
S72.92XK
S72.92XM
S72.92XN
S72.92XP
S72.92XQ
S72.92XR
S73.001A
S73.002A
S73.003A
S73.004A
S73.005A
S73.006A
S73.011A
S73.012A
S73.013A
S73.014A
S73.015A
S73.016A
S73.021A
S73.022A
S73.023A
S73.024A
S73.025A
S73.026A
S73.031A
S73.032A
S73.033A
S73.034A
S73.035A
S73.036A
S73.041A
S73.042A
S73.043A
S73.044A
S73.045A
S73.046A
S75.201A
S75.202A
S75.209A
S75.211A
S75.212A
S75.219A
S75.221A
S75.222A
S75.229A
S75.291A
S75.292A
S75.299A
S75.801A
S75.802A
S75.809A
S75.811A
S75.812A
S75.819A
S75.891A
S75.892A
S75.899A
S75.901A
S75.902A
S75.909A
S75.911A
S75.912A
S75.919A
S75.991A
S75.992A
S75.999A
S76.021A
S76.022A
S76.029A
S76.121A
S76.122A
S76.129A
S76.221A
S76.222A
S76.229A
S76.321A
S76.322A
S76.329A
S76.821A
S76.822A
S76.829A
S76.921A
S76.922A
S76.929A
S77.00XA
S77.01XA
S77.02XA
S77.10XA
S77.11XA
S77.12XA
S78.011A
S78.012A
S78.019A
S78.021A
S78.022A
S78.029A
S78.111A
S78.112A
S78.119A
S78.121A
S78.122A
S78.129A
S78.911A
S78.912A
S78.919A
S78.921A
S78.922A
S78.929A
S79.001K
S79.001P
S79.002K
S79.002P
S79.009K
S79.009P
S79.011K
S79.011P
S79.012K
S79.012P
S79.019K
S79.019P
S79.091K
S79.091P
S79.092K
S79.092P
S79.099K
S79.099P
S79.101A
S79.101K
S79.101P
S79.102A
S79.102K
S79.102P
S79.109A
S79.109K
S79.109P
S79.111A
S79.111K
S79.111P
S79.112A
S79.112K
S79.112P
S79.119A
S79.119K
S79.119P
S79.121A
S79.121K
S79.121P
S79.122A
S79.122K
S79.122P
S79.129A
S79.129K
S79.129P
S79.131A
S79.131K
S79.131P
S79.132A
S79.132K
S79.132P
S79.139A
S79.139K
S79.139P
S79.141A
S79.141K
S79.141P
S79.142A
S79.142K
S79.142P
S79.149A
S79.149K
S79.149P
S79.191A
S79.191K
S79.191P
S79.192A
S79.192K
S79.192P
S79.199A
S79.199K
S79.199P
S82.001A
S82.001B
S82.001C
S82.001K
S82.001M
S82.001N
S82.001P
S82.001Q
S82.001R
S82.002A
S82.002B
S82.002C
S82.002K
S82.002M
S82.002N
S82.002P
S82.002Q
S82.002R
S82.009A
S82.009B
S82.009C
S82.009K
S82.009M
S82.009N
S82.009P
S82.009Q
S82.009R
S82.011A
S82.011B
S82.011C
S82.011K
S82.011M
S82.011N
S82.011P
S82.011Q
S82.011R
S82.012A
S82.012B
S82.012C
S82.012K
S82.012M
S82.012N
S82.012P
S82.012Q
S82.012R
S82.013A
S82.013B
S82.013C
S82.013K
S82.013M
S82.013N
S82.013P
S82.013Q
S82.013R
S82.014A
S82.014B
S82.014C
S82.014K
S82.014M
S82.014N
S82.014P
S82.014Q
S82.014R
S82.015A
S82.015B
S82.015C
S82.015K
S82.015M
S82.015N
S82.015P
S82.015Q
S82.015R
S82.016A
S82.016B
S82.016C
S82.016K
S82.016M
S82.016N
S82.016P
S82.016Q
S82.016R
S82.021A
S82.021B
S82.021C
S82.021K
S82.021M
S82.021N
S82.021P
S82.021Q
S82.021R
S82.022A
S82.022B
S82.022C
S82.022K
S82.022M
S82.022N
S82.022P
S82.022Q
S82.022R
S82.023A
S82.023B
S82.023C
S82.023K
S82.023M
S82.023N
S82.023P
S82.023Q
S82.023R
S82.024A
S82.024B
S82.024C
S82.024K
S82.024M
S82.024N
S82.024P
S82.024Q
S82.024R
S82.025A
S82.025B
S82.025C
S82.025K
S82.025M
S82.025N
S82.025P
S82.025Q
S82.025R
S82.026A
S82.026B
S82.026C
S82.026K
S82.026M
S82.026N
S82.026P
S82.026Q
S82.026R
S82.031A
S82.031B
S82.031C
S82.031K
S82.031M
S82.031N
S82.031P
S82.031Q
S82.031R
S82.032A
S82.032B
S82.032C
S82.032K
S82.032M
S82.032N
S82.032P
S82.032Q
S82.032R
S82.033A
S82.033B
S82.033C
S82.033K
S82.033M
S82.033N
S82.033P
S82.033Q
S82.033R
S82.034A
S82.034B
S82.034C
S82.034K
S82.034M
S82.034N
S82.034P
S82.034Q
S82.034R
S82.035A
S82.035B
S82.035C
S82.035K
S82.035M
S82.035N
S82.035P
S82.035Q
S82.035R
S82.036A
S82.036B

S82.036C - S82.401M

Complication or Comorbidity (CC) (cont.)

Based on CMS data

S82.036C
S82.036K
S82.036M
S82.036N
S82.036P
S82.036Q
S82.036R
S82.041A
S82.041B
S82.041C
S82.041K
S82.041M
S82.041N
S82.041P
S82.041Q
S82.041R
S82.042A
S82.042B
S82.042C
S82.042K
S82.042M
S82.042N
S82.042P
S82.042Q
S82.042R
S82.043A
S82.043B
S82.043C
S82.043K
S82.043M
S82.043N
S82.043P
S82.043Q
S82.043R
S82.044A
S82.044B
S82.044C
S82.044K
S82.044M
S82.044N
S82.044P
S82.044Q
S82.044R
S82.045A
S82.045B
S82.045C
S82.045K
S82.045M
S82.045N
S82.045P
S82.045Q
S82.045R
S82.046A
S82.046B
S82.046C
S82.046K
S82.046M
S82.046N
S82.046P
S82.046Q
S82.046R
S82.091A
S82.091B
S82.091C
S82.091K
S82.091M
S82.091N
S82.091P
S82.091Q
S82.091R
S82.092A
S82.092B
S82.092C
S82.092K
S82.092M
S82.092N
S82.092P
S82.092Q
S82.092R
S82.099A
S82.099B
S82.099C
S82.099K
S82.099M
S82.099N
S82.099P
S82.099Q
S82.099R
S82.101A
S82.101K
S82.101M
S82.101N
S82.101P
S82.101Q
S82.101R
S82.102A
S82.102K
S82.102M
S82.102N
S82.102P
S82.102Q
S82.102R
S82.109A
S82.109K
S82.109M
S82.109N
S82.109P
S82.109Q
S82.109R
S82.111A
S82.111K
S82.111M
S82.111N
S82.111P
S82.111Q
S82.111R
S82.112A
S82.112K
S82.112M
S82.112N
S82.112P
S82.112Q
S82.112R
S82.113A
S82.113K
S82.113M
S82.113N
S82.113P
S82.113Q
S82.113R
S82.114A
S82.114K
S82.114M
S82.114N
S82.114P
S82.114Q
S82.114R
S82.115A
S82.115K
S82.115M
S82.115N
S82.115P
S82.115Q
S82.115R
S82.116A
S82.116K
S82.116M
S82.116N
S82.116P
S82.116Q
S82.116R
S82.121A
S82.121K
S82.121M
S82.121N
S82.121P
S82.121Q
S82.121R
S82.122A
S82.122K
S82.122M
S82.122N
S82.122P
S82.122Q
S82.122R
S82.123A
S82.123K
S82.123M
S82.123N
S82.123P
S82.123Q
S82.123R
S82.124A
S82.124K
S82.124M
S82.124N
S82.124P
S82.124Q
S82.124R
S82.125A
S82.125K
S82.125M
S82.125N
S82.125P
S82.125Q
S82.125R
S82.126A
S82.126K
S82.126M
S82.126N
S82.126P
S82.126Q
S82.126R
S82.131A
S82.131K
S82.131M
S82.131N
S82.131P
S82.131Q
S82.131R
S82.132A
S82.132K
S82.132M
S82.132N
S82.132P
S82.132Q
S82.132R
S82.133A
S82.133K
S82.133M
S82.133N
S82.133P
S82.133Q
S82.133R
S82.134A
S82.134K
S82.134M
S82.134N
S82.134P
S82.134Q
S82.134R
S82.135A
S82.135K
S82.135M
S82.135N
S82.135P
S82.135Q
S82.135R
S82.136A
S82.136K
S82.136M
S82.136N
S82.136P
S82.136Q
S82.136R
S82.141A
S82.141K
S82.141M
S82.141N
S82.141P
S82.141Q
S82.141R
S82.142A
S82.142K
S82.142M
S82.142N
S82.142P
S82.142Q
S82.142R
S82.143A
S82.143K
S82.143M
S82.143N
S82.143P
S82.143Q
S82.143R
S82.144A
S82.144K
S82.144M
S82.144N
S82.144P
S82.144Q
S82.144R
S82.145A
S82.145K
S82.145M
S82.145N
S82.145P
S82.145Q
S82.145R
S82.146A
S82.146K
S82.146M
S82.146N
S82.146P
S82.146Q
S82.146R
S82.151A
S82.151K
S82.151M
S82.151N
S82.151P
S82.151Q
S82.151R
S82.152A
S82.152K
S82.152M
S82.152N
S82.152P
S82.152Q
S82.152R
S82.153A
S82.153K
S82.153M
S82.153N
S82.153P
S82.153Q
S82.153R
S82.154A
S82.154K
S82.154M
S82.154N
S82.154P
S82.154Q
S82.154R
S82.155A
S82.155K
S82.155M
S82.155N
S82.155P
S82.155Q
S82.155R
S82.156A
S82.156K
S82.156M
S82.156N
S82.156P
S82.156Q
S82.156R
S82.161A
S82.161K
S82.161P
S82.162A
S82.162K
S82.162P
S82.169A
S82.169K
S82.169P
S82.191A
S82.191K
S82.191M
S82.191N
S82.191P
S82.191Q
S82.191R
S82.192A
S82.192K
S82.192M
S82.192N
S82.192P
S82.192Q
S82.192R
S82.199A
S82.199K
S82.199M
S82.199N
S82.199P
S82.199Q
S82.199R
S82.201A
S82.201K
S82.201M
S82.201N
S82.201P
S82.201Q
S82.201R
S82.202A
S82.202K
S82.202M
S82.202N
S82.202P
S82.202Q
S82.202R
S82.209A
S82.209K
S82.209M
S82.209N
S82.209P
S82.209Q
S82.209R
S82.221A
S82.221K
S82.221M
S82.221N
S82.221P
S82.221Q
S82.221R
S82.222A
S82.222K
S82.222M
S82.222N
S82.222P
S82.222Q
S82.222R
S82.223A
S82.223K
S82.223M
S82.223N
S82.223P
S82.223Q
S82.223R
S82.224A
S82.224K
S82.224M
S82.224N
S82.224P
S82.224Q
S82.224R
S82.225A
S82.225K
S82.225M
S82.225N
S82.225P
S82.225Q
S82.225R
S82.226A
S82.226K
S82.226M
S82.226N
S82.226P
S82.226Q
S82.226R
S82.231A
S82.231K
S82.231M
S82.231N
S82.231P
S82.231Q
S82.231R
S82.232A
S82.232K
S82.232M
S82.232N
S82.232P
S82.232Q
S82.232R
S82.233A
S82.233K
S82.233M
S82.233N
S82.233P
S82.233Q
S82.233R
S82.234A
S82.234K
S82.234M
S82.234N
S82.234P
S82.234Q
S82.234R
S82.235A
S82.235K
S82.235M
S82.235N
S82.235P
S82.235Q
S82.235R
S82.236A
S82.236K
S82.236M
S82.236N
S82.236P
S82.236Q
S82.236R
S82.241A
S82.241K
S82.241M
S82.241N
S82.241P
S82.241Q
S82.241R
S82.242A
S82.242K
S82.242M
S82.242N
S82.242P
S82.242Q
S82.242R
S82.243A
S82.243K
S82.243M
S82.243N
S82.243P
S82.243Q
S82.243R
S82.244A
S82.244K
S82.244M
S82.244N
S82.244P
S82.244Q
S82.244R
S82.245A
S82.245K
S82.245M
S82.245N
S82.245P
S82.245Q
S82.245R
S82.246A
S82.246K
S82.246M
S82.246N
S82.246P
S82.246Q
S82.246R
S82.251A
S82.251K
S82.251M
S82.251N
S82.251P
S82.251Q
S82.251R
S82.252A
S82.252K
S82.252M
S82.252N
S82.252P
S82.252Q
S82.252R
S82.253A
S82.253K
S82.253M
S82.253N
S82.253P
S82.253Q
S82.253R
S82.254A
S82.254K
S82.254M
S82.254N
S82.254P
S82.254Q
S82.254R
S82.255A
S82.255K
S82.255M
S82.255N
S82.255P
S82.255Q
S82.255R
S82.256A
S82.256K
S82.256M
S82.256N
S82.256P
S82.256Q
S82.256R
S82.261A
S82.261K
S82.261M
S82.261N
S82.261P
S82.261Q
S82.261R
S82.262A
S82.262K
S82.262M
S82.262N
S82.262P
S82.262Q
S82.262R
S82.263A
S82.263K
S82.263M
S82.263N
S82.263P
S82.263Q
S82.263R
S82.264A
S82.264K
S82.264M
S82.264N
S82.264P
S82.264Q
S82.264R
S82.265A
S82.265K
S82.265M
S82.265N
S82.265P
S82.265Q
S82.265R
S82.266A
S82.266K
S82.266M
S82.266N
S82.266P
S82.266Q
S82.266R
S82.291A
S82.291K
S82.291M
S82.291N
S82.291P
S82.291Q
S82.291R
S82.292A
S82.292K
S82.292M
S82.292N
S82.292P
S82.292Q
S82.292R
S82.299A
S82.299K
S82.299M
S82.299N
S82.299P
S82.299Q
S82.299R
S82.301B
S82.301C
S82.301K
S82.301M
S82.301N
S82.301P
S82.301Q
S82.301R
S82.302B
S82.302C
S82.302K
S82.302M
S82.302N
S82.302P
S82.302Q
S82.302R
S82.309B
S82.309C
S82.309K
S82.309M
S82.309N
S82.309P
S82.309Q
S82.309R
S82.311A
S82.311K
S82.311P
S82.312A
S82.312K
S82.312P
S82.319A
S82.319K
S82.319P
S82.391B
S82.391C
S82.391K
S82.391M
S82.391N
S82.391P
S82.391Q
S82.391R
S82.392B
S82.392C
S82.392K
S82.392M
S82.392N
S82.392P
S82.392Q
S82.392R
S82.399B
S82.399C
S82.399K
S82.399M
S82.399N
S82.399P
S82.399Q
S82.399R
S82.401K
S82.401M

Complication or Comorbidity (CC) (cont.)

Based on CMS data

S82.401N S82.401P S82.401Q S82.401R S82.402K S82.402M S82.402N S82.402P S82.402Q S82.402R S82.409K S82.409M S82.409N S82.409P S82.409Q S82.409R S82.421K S82.421M S82.421N S82.421P S82.421Q S82.421R S82.422K S82.422M S82.422N S82.422P S82.422Q S82.422R S82.423K S82.423M S82.423N S82.423P S82.423Q S82.423R S82.424K S82.424M S82.424N S82.424P S82.424Q S82.424R S82.425K S82.425M S82.425N S82.425P S82.425Q S82.425R S82.426K S82.426M S82.426N S82.426P S82.426Q S82.426R S82.431K S82.431M S82.431N S82.431P S82.431Q S82.431R S82.432K S82.432M S82.432N S82.432P S82.432Q S82.432R S82.433K S82.433M

S82.433N S82.433P S82.433Q S82.433R S82.434K S82.434M S82.434N S82.434P S82.434Q S82.434R S82.435K S82.435M S82.435N S82.435P S82.435Q S82.435R S82.436K S82.436M S82.436N S82.436P S82.436Q S82.436R S82.441K S82.441M S82.441N S82.441P S82.441Q S82.441R S82.442K S82.442M S82.442N S82.442P S82.442Q S82.442R S82.443K S82.443M S82.443N S82.443P S82.443Q S82.443R S82.444K S82.444M S82.444N S82.444P S82.444Q S82.444R S82.445K S82.445M S82.445N S82.445P S82.445Q S82.445R S82.446K S82.446M S82.446N S82.446P S82.446Q S82.446R S82.451K S82.451M S82.451N S82.451P S82.451Q S82.451R S82.452K S82.452M

S82.452N S82.452P S82.452Q S82.452R S82.453K S82.453M S82.453N S82.453P S82.453Q S82.453R S82.454K S82.454M S82.454N S82.454P S82.454Q S82.454R S82.455K S82.455M S82.455N S82.455P S82.455Q S82.455R S82.456K S82.456M S82.456N S82.456P S82.456Q S82.456R S82.461K S82.461M S82.461N S82.461P S82.461Q S82.461R S82.462K S82.462M S82.462N S82.462P S82.462Q S82.462R S82.463K S82.463M S82.463N S82.463P S82.463Q S82.463R S82.464K S82.464M S82.464N S82.464P S82.464Q S82.464R S82.465K S82.465M S82.465N S82.465P S82.465Q S82.465R S82.466K S82.466M S82.466N S82.466P S82.466Q S82.466R S82.491K S82.491M

S82.491N S82.491P S82.491Q S82.491R S82.492K S82.492M S82.492N S82.492P S82.492Q S82.492R S82.499K S82.499M S82.499N S82.499P S82.499Q S82.499R S82.51XB S82.51XC S82.51XK S82.51XM S82.51XN S82.51XP S82.51XQ S82.51XR S82.52XB S82.52XC S82.52XK S82.52XM S82.52XN S82.52XP S82.52XQ S82.52XR S82.53XB S82.53XC S82.53XK S82.53XM S82.53XN S82.53XP S82.53XQ S82.53XR S82.54XB S82.54XC S82.54XK S82.54XM S82.54XN S82.54XP S82.54XQ S82.54XR S82.55XB S82.55XC S82.55XK S82.55XM S82.55XN S82.55XP S82.55XQ S82.55XR S82.56XB S82.56XC S82.56XK S82.56XM S82.56XN S82.56XP S82.56XQ S82.56XR S82.61XB S82.61XC

S82.61XK S82.61XM S82.61XN S82.61XP S82.61XQ S82.61XR S82.62XB S82.62XC S82.62XK S82.62XM S82.62XN S82.62XP S82.62XQ S82.62XR S82.63XB S82.63XC S82.63XK S82.63XM S82.63XN S82.63XP S82.63XQ S82.63XR S82.64XB S82.64XC S82.64XK S82.64XM S82.64XN S82.64XP S82.64XQ S82.64XR S82.65XB S82.65XC S82.65XK S82.65XM S82.65XN S82.65XP S82.65XQ S82.65XR S82.66XB S82.66XC S82.66XK S82.66XM S82.66XN S82.66XP S82.66XQ S82.66XR S82.811K S82.811P S82.812K S82.812P S82.819K S82.819P S82.821K S82.821P S82.822K S82.822P S82.829K S82.829P S82.831K S82.831M S82.831N S82.831P S82.831Q S82.831R S82.832K S82.832M

S82.832N S82.832P S82.832Q S82.832R S82.839K S82.839M S82.839N S82.839P S82.839Q S82.839R S82.841B S82.841C S82.841K S82.841M S82.841N S82.841P S82.841Q S82.841R S82.842B S82.842C S82.842K S82.842M S82.842N S82.842P S82.842Q S82.842R S82.843B S82.843C S82.843K S82.843M S82.843N S82.843P S82.843Q S82.843R S82.844B S82.844C S82.844K S82.844M S82.844N S82.844P S82.844Q S82.844R S82.845B S82.845C S82.845K S82.845M S82.845N S82.845P S82.845Q S82.845R S82.846B S82.846C S82.846K S82.846M S82.846N S82.846P S82.846Q S82.846R S82.851B S82.851C S82.851K S82.851M S82.851N S82.851P S82.851Q S82.851R

S82.852B S82.852C S82.852K S82.852M S82.852N S82.852P S82.852Q S82.852R S82.853B S82.853C S82.853K S82.853M S82.853N S82.853P S82.853Q S82.853R S82.854B S82.854C S82.854K S82.854M S82.854N S82.854P S82.854Q S82.854R S82.855B S82.855C S82.855K S82.855M S82.855N S82.855P S82.855Q S82.855R S82.856B S82.856C S82.856K S82.856M S82.856N S82.856P S82.856Q S82.856R S82.861K S82.861M S82.861N S82.861P S82.861Q S82.861R S82.862K S82.862M S82.862N S82.862P S82.862Q S82.862R S82.863K S82.863M S82.863N S82.863P S82.863Q S82.863R S82.864K S82.864M S82.864N S82.864P S82.864Q S82.864R S82.865K S82.865M

S82.865N S82.865P S82.865Q S82.865R S82.866K S82.866M S82.866N S82.866P S82.866Q S82.866R S82.871B S82.871C S82.871K S82.871M S82.871N S82.871P S82.871Q S82.871R S82.872B S82.872C S82.872K S82.872M S82.872N S82.872P S82.872Q S82.872R S82.873B S82.873C S82.873K S82.873M S82.873N S82.873P S82.873Q S82.873R S82.874B S82.874C S82.874K S82.874M S82.874N S82.874P S82.874Q S82.874R S82.875B S82.875C S82.875K S82.875M S82.875N S82.875P S82.875Q S82.875R S82.876B S82.876C S82.876K S82.876M S82.876N S82.876P S82.876Q S82.876R S82.891B S82.891C S82.891K S82.891M S82.891N S82.891P S82.891Q S82.891R

S82.892B S82.892C S82.892K S82.892M S82.892N S82.892P S82.892Q S82.892R S82.899B S82.899C S82.899K S82.899M S82.899N S82.899P S82.899Q S82.899R S82.90XB S82.90XC S82.90XK S82.90XM S82.90XN S82.90XP S82.90XQ S82.90XR S82.91XB S82.91XC S82.91XK S82.91XM S82.91XN S82.91XP S82.91XQ S82.91XR S82.92XB S82.92XC S82.92XK S82.92XM S82.92XN S82.92XP S82.92XQ S82.92XR S85.101A S85.102A S85.109A S85.111A S85.112A S85.119A S85.121A S85.122A S85.129A S85.131A S85.132A S85.139A S85.141A S85.142A S85.149A S85.151A S85.152A S85.159A S85.161A S85.162A S85.169A S85.171A S85.172A S85.179A S85.181A S85.182A

S85.189A S85.201A S85.202A S85.209A S85.211A S85.212A S85.219A S85.291A S85.292A S85.299A S85.301A S85.302A S85.309A S85.311A S85.312A S85.319A S85.391A S85.392A S85.399A S85.401A S85.402A S85.409A S85.411A S85.412A S85.419A S85.491A S85.492A S85.499A S85.801A S85.802A S85.809A S85.811A S85.812A S85.819A S85.891A S85.892A S85.899A S85.901A S85.902A S85.909A S85.911A S85.912A S85.919A S85.991A S85.992A S85.999A S86.021A S86.022A S86.029A S86.121A S86.122A S86.129A S86.221A S86.222A S86.229A S86.321A S86.322A S86.329A S86.821A S86.822A S86.829A S86.921A S86.922A S86.929A S88.011A S88.012A

Complication or Comorbidity (CC) (cont.)

Based on CMS data

S88.019A
S88.021A
S88.022A
S88.029A
S88.111A
S88.112A
S88.119A
S88.121A
S88.122A
S88.129A
S88.911A
S88.912A
S88.919A
S88.921A
S88.922A
S88.929A
S89.001A
S89.001K
S89.001P
S89.002A
S89.002K
S89.002P
S89.009A
S89.009K
S89.009P
S89.011A
S89.011K
S89.011P
S89.012A
S89.012K
S89.012P
S89.019A
S89.019K
S89.019P
S89.021A
S89.021K
S89.021P
S89.022A
S89.022K
S89.022P
S89.029A
S89.029K
S89.029P
S89.031A
S89.031K
S89.031P
S89.032A
S89.032K
S89.032P
S89.039A
S89.039K
S89.039P
S89.041A
S89.041K
S89.041P
S89.042A
S89.042K
S89.042P
S89.049A
S89.049K
S89.049P
S89.091A
S89.091K
S89.091P
S89.092A
S89.092K
S89.092P
S89.099A
S89.099K
S89.099P
S89.101K
S89.101P
S89.102K
S89.102P
S89.109K
S89.109P
S89.111K
S89.111P
S89.112K
S89.112P
S89.119K
S89.119P
S89.121K
S89.121P
S89.122K
S89.122P
S89.129K
S89.129P
S89.131K
S89.131P
S89.132K
S89.132P
S89.139K
S89.139P
S89.141K
S89.141P
S89.142K
S89.142P
S89.149K
S89.149P
S89.191K
S89.191P
S89.192K
S89.192P
S89.199K
S89.199P
S89.201K
S89.201P
S89.202K
S89.202P
S89.209K
S89.209P
S89.211K
S89.211P
S89.212K
S89.212P
S89.219K
S89.219P
S89.221K
S89.221P
S89.222K
S89.222P
S89.229K
S89.229P
S89.291K
S89.291P
S89.292K
S89.292P
S89.299K
S89.299P
S89.301K
S89.301P
S89.302K
S89.302P
S89.309K
S89.309P
S89.311K
S89.311P
S89.312K
S89.312P
S89.319K
S89.319P
S89.321K
S89.321P
S89.322K
S89.322P
S89.329K
S89.329P
S89.391K
S89.391P
S89.392K
S89.392P
S89.399K
S89.399P
S92.001B
S92.001K
S92.001P
S92.002B
S92.002K
S92.002P
S92.009B
S92.009K
S92.009P
S92.011B
S92.011K
S92.011P
S92.012B
S92.012K
S92.012P
S92.013B
S92.013K
S92.013P
S92.014B
S92.014K
S92.014P
S92.015B
S92.015K
S92.015P
S92.016B
S92.016K
S92.016P
S92.021B
S92.021K
S92.021P
S92.022B
S92.022K
S92.022P
S92.023B
S92.023K
S92.023P
S92.024B
S92.024K
S92.024P
S92.025B
S92.025K
S92.025P
S92.026B
S92.026K
S92.026P
S92.031B
S92.031K
S92.031P
S92.032B
S92.032K
S92.032P
S92.033B
S92.033K
S92.033P
S92.034B
S92.034K
S92.034P
S92.035B
S92.035K
S92.035P
S92.036B
S92.036K
S92.036P
S92.041B
S92.041K
S92.041P
S92.042B
S92.042K
S92.042P
S92.043B
S92.043K
S92.043P
S92.044B
S92.044K
S92.044P
S92.045B
S92.045K
S92.045P
S92.046B
S92.046K
S92.046P
S92.051B
S92.051K
S92.051P
S92.052B
S92.052K
S92.052P
S92.053B
S92.053K
S92.053P
S92.054B
S92.054K
S92.054P
S92.055B
S92.055K
S92.055P
S92.056B
S92.056K
S92.056P
S92.061B
S92.061K
S92.061P
S92.062B
S92.062K
S92.062P
S92.063B
S92.063K
S92.063P
S92.064B
S92.064K
S92.064P
S92.065B
S92.065K
S92.065P
S92.066B
S92.066K
S92.066P
S92.101B
S92.101K
S92.101P
S92.102B
S92.102K
S92.102P
S92.109B
S92.109K
S92.109P
S92.111B
S92.111K
S92.111P
S92.112B
S92.112K
S92.112P
S92.113B
S92.113K
S92.113P
S92.114B
S92.114K
S92.114P
S92.115B
S92.115K
S92.115P
S92.116B
S92.116K
S92.116P
S92.121B
S92.121K
S92.121P
S92.122B
S92.122K
S92.122P
S92.123B
S92.123K
S92.123P
S92.124B
S92.124K
S92.124P
S92.125B
S92.125K
S92.125P
S92.126B
S92.126K
S92.126P
S92.131B
S92.131K
S92.131P
S92.132B
S92.132K
S92.132P
S92.133B
S92.133K
S92.133P
S92.134B
S92.134K
S92.134P
S92.135B
S92.135K
S92.135P
S92.136B
S92.136K
S92.136P
S92.141B
S92.141K
S92.141P
S92.142B
S92.142K
S92.142P
S92.143B
S92.143K
S92.143P
S92.144B
S92.144K
S92.144P
S92.145B
S92.145K
S92.145P
S92.146B
S92.146K
S92.146P
S92.151B
S92.151K
S92.151P
S92.152B
S92.152K
S92.152P
S92.153B
S92.153K
S92.153P
S92.154B
S92.154K
S92.154P
S92.155B
S92.155K
S92.155P
S92.156B
S92.156K
S92.156P
S92.191B
S92.191K
S92.191P
S92.192B
S92.192K
S92.192P
S92.199B
S92.199K
S92.199P
S92.201B
S92.201K
S92.201P
S92.202B
S92.202K
S92.202P
S92.209B
S92.209K
S92.209P
S92.211B
S92.211K
S92.211P
S92.212B
S92.212K
S92.212P
S92.213B
S92.213K
S92.213P
S92.214B
S92.214K
S92.214P
S92.215B
S92.215K
S92.215P
S92.216B
S92.216K
S92.216P
S92.221B
S92.221K
S92.221P
S92.222B
S92.222K
S92.222P
S92.223B
S92.223K
S92.223P
S92.224B
S92.224K
S92.224P
S92.225B
S92.225K
S92.225P
S92.226B
S92.226K
S92.226P
S92.231B
S92.231K
S92.231P
S92.232B
S92.232K
S92.232P
S92.233B
S92.233K
S92.233P
S92.234B
S92.234K
S92.234P
S92.235B
S92.235K
S92.235P
S92.236B
S92.236K
S92.236P
S92.241B
S92.241K
S92.241P
S92.242B
S92.242K
S92.242P
S92.243B
S92.243K
S92.243P
S92.244B
S92.244K
S92.244P
S92.245B
S92.245K
S92.245P
S92.246B
S92.246K
S92.246P
S92.251B
S92.251K
S92.251P
S92.252B
S92.252K
S92.252P
S92.253B
S92.253K
S92.253P
S92.254B
S92.254K
S92.254P
S92.255B
S92.255K
S92.255P
S92.256B
S92.256K
S92.256P
S92.301B
S92.301K
S92.301P
S92.302B
S92.302K
S92.302P
S92.309B
S92.309K
S92.309P
S92.311B
S92.311K
S92.311P
S92.312B
S92.312K
S92.312P
S92.313B
S92.313K
S92.313P
S92.314B
S92.314K
S92.314P
S92.315B
S92.315K
S92.315P
S92.316B
S92.316K
S92.316P
S92.321B
S92.321K
S92.321P
S92.322B
S92.322K
S92.322P
S92.323B
S92.323K
S92.323P
S92.324B
S92.324K
S92.324P
S92.325B
S92.325K
S92.325P
S92.326B
S92.326K
S92.326P
S92.331B
S92.331K
S92.331P
S92.332B
S92.332K
S92.332P
S92.333B
S92.333K
S92.333P
S92.334B
S92.334K
S92.334P
S92.335B
S92.335K
S92.335P
S92.336B
S92.336K
S92.336P
S92.341B
S92.341K
S92.341P
S92.342B
S92.342K
S92.342P
S92.343B
S92.343K
S92.343P
S92.344B
S92.344K
S92.344P
S92.345B
S92.345K
S92.345P
S92.346B
S92.346K
S92.346P
S92.351B
S92.351K
S92.351P
S92.352B
S92.352K
S92.352P
S92.353B
S92.353K
S92.353P
S92.354B
S92.354K
S92.354P
S92.355B
S92.355K
S92.355P
S92.356B
S92.356K
S92.356P
S92.401K
S92.401P
S92.402K
S92.402P
S92.403K
S92.403P
S92.404K
S92.404P
S92.405K
S92.405P
S92.406K
S92.406P
S92.411K
S92.411P
S92.412K
S92.412P
S92.413K
S92.413P
S92.414K
S92.414P
S92.415K
S92.415P
S92.416K
S92.416P
S92.421K
S92.421P
S92.422K
S92.422P
S92.423K
S92.423P
S92.424K
S92.424P
S92.425K
S92.425P
S92.426K
S92.426P
S92.491K
S92.491P
S92.492K
S92.492P
S92.499K
S92.499P
S92.501K
S92.501P
S92.502K
S92.502P
S92.503K
S92.503P
S92.504K
S92.504P
S92.505K
S92.505P
S92.506K
S92.506P
S92.511K
S92.511P
S92.512K
S92.512P
S92.513K
S92.513P
S92.514K
S92.514P
S92.515K
S92.515P
S92.516K
S92.516P
S92.521K
S92.521P
S92.522K
S92.522P
S92.523K
S92.523P
S92.524K
S92.524P
S92.525K
S92.525P
S92.526K
S92.526P
S92.531K
S92.531P
S92.532K
S92.532P
S92.533K

Complication or Comorbidity (CC) (cont.)

Based on CMS data

S92.533P	S95.809A	T17.808A	T22.391A	T23.749A	T25.799A	T34.42XA	T71.232A	T80.59XA	T81.596A
S92.534K	S95.811A	T17.810A	T22.392A	T23.751A	T26.20XA	T34.511A	T71.233A	T80.61XA	T81.597A
S92.534P	S95.812A	T17.818A	T22.399A	T23.752A	T26.21XA	T34.512A	T71.234A	T80.62XA	T81.598A
S92.535K	S95.819A	T17.820A	T22.70XA	T23.759A	T26.22XA	T34.519A	T71.29XA	T80.69XA	T81.599A
S92.535P	S95.891A	T17.828A	T22.711A	T23.761A	T26.70XA	T34.521A	T71.9XXA	T80.810A	T81.60XA
S92.536K	S95.892A	T17.890A	T22.712A	T23.762A	T26.71XA	T34.522A	T74.01XA	T80.818A	T81.61XA
S92.536P	S95.899A	T17.898A	T22.719A	T23.769A	T26.72XA	T34.529A	T74.02XA	T80.910A	T81.69XA
S92.591K	S95.901A	T20.30XA	T22.721A	T23.771A	T27.0XXA	T34.531A	T74.11XA	T80.911A	T81.710A
S92.591P	S95.902A	T20.311A	T22.722A	T23.772A	T27.1XXA	T34.532A	T74.12XA	T80.919A	T81.711A
S92.592K	S95.909A	T20.312A	T22.729A	T23.779A	T27.2XXA	T34.539A	T74.21XA	T80.A0XA	T81.718A
S92.592P	S95.911A	T20.319A	T22.731A	T23.791A	T27.3XXA	T34.60XA	T74.22XA	T80.A10A	T81.719A
S92.599K	S95.912A	T20.32XA	T22.732A	T23.792A	T27.4XXA	T34.61XA	T74.32XA	T80.A11A	T81.72XA
S92.599P	S95.919A	T20.33XA	T22.739A	T23.799A	T27.5XXA	T34.62XA	T74.4XXA	T80.A19A	T81.83XA
S92.811B	S95.991A	T20.34XA	T22.741A	T24.301A	T27.6XXA	T34.70XA	T74.91XA	T80.A9XA	T82.01XA
S92.811K	S95.992A	T20.35XA	T22.742A	T24.302A	T27.7XXA	T34.71XA	T74.92XA	T81.10XA	T82.02XA
S92.811P	S95.999A	T20.36XA	T22.749A	T24.309A	T28.1XXA	T34.72XA	T75.1XXA	T81.30XA	T82.03XA
S92.812B	S96.021A	T20.37XA	T22.751A	T24.311A	T28.2XXA	T34.811A	T76.01XA	T81.31XA	T82.09XA
S92.812K	S96.022A	T20.39XA	T22.752A	T24.312A	T28.6XXA	T34.812A	T76.02XA	T81.32XA	T82.110A
S92.812P	S96.029A	T20.70XA	T22.759A	T24.319A	T28.7XXA	T34.819A	T76.11XA	T81.33XA	T82.111A
S92.819B	S96.121A	T20.711A	T22.761A	T24.321A	T33.011A	T34.821A	T76.12XA	T81.4XXA	T82.118A
S92.819K	S96.122A	T20.712A	T22.762A	T24.322A	T33.012A	T34.822A	T76.21XA	T81.500A	T82.119A
S92.819P	S96.129A	T20.719A	T22.769A	T24.329A	T33.019A	T34.829A	T76.22XA	T81.501A	T82.120A
S92.901B	S96.221A	T20.72XA	T22.791A	T24.331A	T33.02XA	T34.831A	T76.32XA	T81.502A	T82.121A
S92.901K	S96.222A	T20.73XA	T22.792A	T24.332A	T33.09XA	T34.832A	T76.91XA	T81.503A	T82.128A
S92.901P	S96.229A	T20.74XA	T22.799A	T24.339A	T33.1XXA	T34.839A	T76.92XA	T81.504A	T82.129A
S92.902B	S96.821A	T20.75XA	T23.301A	T24.391A	T33.2XXA	T34.90XA	T78.00XA	T81.505A	T82.190A
S92.902K	S96.822A	T20.76XA	T23.302A	T24.392A	T33.3XXA	T34.99XA	T78.01XA	T81.506A	T82.191A
S92.902P	S96.829A	T20.77XA	T23.309A	T24.399A	T33.40XA	T67.0XXA	T78.02XA	T81.507A	T82.198A
S92.909B	S96.921A	T20.79XA	T23.311A	T24.701A	T33.41XA	T69.021A	T78.03XA	T81.508A	T82.199A
S92.909K	S96.922A	T21.30XA	T23.312A	T24.702A	T33.42XA	T69.022A	T78.04XA	T81.509A	T82.211A
S92.909P	S96.929A	T21.31XA	T23.319A	T24.709A	T33.511A	T69.029A	T78.05XA	T81.510A	T82.212A
S92.911K	S98.011A	T21.32XA	T23.321A	T24.711A	T33.512A	T70.3XXA	T78.06XA	T81.511A	T82.213A
S92.911P	S98.012A	T21.33XA	T23.322A	T24.712A	T33.519A	T71.111A	T78.07XA	T81.512A	T82.218A
S92.912K	S98.019A	T21.34XA	T23.329A	T24.719A	T33.521A	T71.112A	T78.08XA	T81.513A	T82.221A
S92.912P	S98.021A	T21.35XA	T23.331A	T24.721A	T33.522A	T71.113A	T78.09XA	T81.514A	T82.222A
S92.919K	S98.022A	T21.36XA	T23.332A	T24.722A	T33.529A	T71.114A	T78.2XXA	T81.515A	T82.223A
S92.919P	S98.029A	T21.37XA	T23.339A	T24.729A	T33.531A	T71.121A	T79.2XXA	T81.516A	T82.228A
S95.001A	S98.311A	T21.39XA	T23.341A	T24.731A	T33.532A	T71.122A	T79.7XXA	T81.517A	T82.310A
S95.002A	S98.312A	T21.70XA	T23.342A	T24.732A	T33.539A	T71.123A	T79.A0XA	T81.518A	T82.311A
S95.009A	S98.319A	T21.71XA	T23.349A	T24.739A	T33.60XA	T71.124A	T79.A11A	T81.519A	T82.312A
S95.011A	S98.321A	T21.72XA	T23.351A	T24.791A	T33.61XA	T71.131A	T79.A12A	T81.520A	T82.318A
S95.012A	S98.322A	T21.73XA	T23.352A	T24.792A	T33.62XA	T71.132A	T79.A19A	T81.521A	T82.319A
S95.019A	S98.329A	T21.74XA	T23.359A	T24.799A	T33.70XA	T71.133A	T79.A21A	T81.522A	T82.320A
S95.091A	S98.911A	T21.75XA	T23.361A	T25.311A	T33.71XA	T71.134A	T79.A22A	T81.523A	T82.321A
S95.092A	S98.912A	T21.76XA	T23.362A	T25.312A	T33.72XA	T71.141A	T79.A29A	T81.524A	T82.322A
S95.099A	S98.919A	T21.77XA	T23.369A	T25.319A	T33.811A	T71.143A	T79.A3XA	T81.525A	T82.328A
S95.101A	S98.921A	T21.79XA	T23.371A	T25.321A	T33.812A	T71.144A	T79.A9XA	T81.526A	T82.329A
S95.102A	S98.922A	T22.30XA	T23.372A	T25.322A	T33.819A	T71.151A	T80.1XXA	T81.527A	T82.330A
S95.109A	S98.929A	T22.311A	T23.379A	T25.329A	T33.821A	T71.152A	T80.211A	T81.528A	T82.331A
S95.111A	T17.400A	T22.312A	T23.391A	T25.331A	T33.822A	T71.153A	T80.212A	T81.529A	T82.332A
S95.112A	T17.408A	T22.319A	T23.392A	T25.332A	T33.829A	T71.154A	T80.218A	T81.530A	T82.338A
S95.119A	T17.410A	T22.321A	T23.399A	T25.339A	T33.831A	T71.161A	T80.219A	T81.531A	T82.339A
S95.191A	T17.418A	T22.322A	T23.701A	T25.391A	T33.832A	T71.162A	T80.22XA	T81.532A	T82.390A
S95.192A	T17.420A	T22.329A	T23.702A	T25.392A	T33.839A	T71.163A	T80.29XA	T81.533A	T82.391A
S95.199A	T17.428A	T22.331A	T23.709A	T25.399A	T33.90XA	T71.164A	T80.30XA	T81.534A	T82.392A
S95.201A	T17.490A	T22.332A	T23.711A	T25.711A	T33.99XA	T71.191A	T80.310A	T81.535A	T82.398A
S95.202A	T17.498A	T22.339A	T23.712A	T25.712A	T34.011A	T71.192A	T80.311A	T81.536A	T82.399A
S95.209A	T17.500A	T22.341A	T23.719A	T25.719A	T34.012A	T71.193A	T80.319A	T81.537A	T82.41XA
S95.211A	T17.508A	T22.342A	T23.721A	T25.721A	T34.019A	T71.194A	T80.39XA	T81.538A	T82.42XA
S95.212A	T17.510A	T22.349A	T23.722A	T25.722A	T34.02XA	T71.20XA	T80.40XA	T81.539A	T82.43XA
S95.219A	T17.518A	T22.351A	T23.729A	T25.729A	T34.09XA	T71.21XA	T80.410A	T81.590A	T82.49XA
S95.291A	T17.520A	T22.352A	T23.731A	T25.731A	T34.1XXA	T71.221A	T80.411A	T81.591A	T82.510A
S95.292A	T17.528A	T22.359A	T23.732A	T25.732A	T34.2XXA	T71.222A	T80.419A	T81.592A	T82.511A
S95.299A	T17.590A	T22.361A	T23.739A	T25.739A	T34.3XXA	T71.223A	T80.49XA	T81.593A	T82.512A
S95.801A	T17.598A	T22.362A	T23.741A	T25.791A	T34.40XA	T71.224A	T80.51XA	T81.594A	T82.513A
S95.802A	T17.800A	T22.369A	T23.742A	T25.792A	T34.41XA	T71.231A	T80.52XA	T81.595A	T82.514A

Complication or Comorbidity (CC) (cont.)

Based on CMS data

T82.515A
T82.518A
T82.519A
T82.520A
T82.521A
T82.522A
T82.523A
T82.524A
T82.525A
T82.528A
T82.529A
T82.530A
T82.531A
T82.532A
T82.533A
T82.534A
T82.535A
T82.538A
T82.539A
T82.590A
T82.591A
T82.592A
T82.593A
T82.594A
T82.595A
T82.598A
T82.599A
T82.6XXA
T82.7XXA
T82.817A
T82.818A
T82.827A
T82.828A
T82.837A
T82.838A
T82.847A
T82.848A
T82.855A
T82.856A
T82.857A
T82.858A
T82.867A
T82.868A
T82.897A
T82.898A
T82.9XXA
T83.010A
T83.020A
T83.030A
T83.090A
T83.110A
T83.111A
T83.112A
T83.113A
T83.118A
T83.120A
T83.121A
T83.122A
T83.123A
T83.128A
T83.190A
T83.191A
T83.192A
T83.193A
T83.198A
T83.21XA
T83.22XA
T83.23XA
T83.24XA
T83.25XA
T83.29XA
T83.410A
T83.411A
T83.418A
T83.420A
T83.421A
T83.428A
T83.490A
T83.491A
T83.498A
T83.510A
T83.511A
T83.512A
T83.590A
T83.591A
T83.592A
T83.593A
T83.61XA
T83.62XA
T83.69XA
T83.712A
T83.713A
T83.714A
T83.718A
T83.719A
T83.722A
T83.723A
T83.724A
T83.728A
T83.729A
T83.79XA
T83.81XA
T83.82XA
T83.83XA
T83.84XA
T83.85XA
T83.86XA
T83.89XA
T83.9XXA
T84.010A
T84.011A
T84.012A
T84.013A
T84.018A
T84.019A
T84.020A
T84.021A
T84.022A
T84.023A
T84.028A
T84.029A
T84.030A
T84.031A
T84.032A
T84.033A
T84.038A
T84.039A
T84.050A
T84.051A
T84.052A
T84.053A
T84.058A
T84.059A
T84.060A
T84.061A
T84.062A
T84.063A
T84.068A
T84.069A
T84.090A
T84.091A
T84.092A
T84.093A
T84.098A
T84.099A
T84.110A
T84.111A
T84.112A
T84.113A
T84.114A
T84.115A
T84.116A
T84.117A
T84.119A
T84.120A
T84.121A
T84.122A
T84.123A
T84.124A
T84.125A
T84.126A
T84.127A
T84.129A
T84.190A
T84.191A
T84.192A
T84.193A
T84.194A
T84.195A
T84.196A
T84.197A
T84.199A
T84.210A
T84.213A
T84.216A
T84.218A
T84.220A
T84.223A
T84.226A
T84.228A
T84.290A
T84.293A
T84.296A
T84.298A
T84.310A
T84.318A
T84.320A
T84.328A
T84.390A
T84.398A
T84.410A
T84.418A
T84.420A
T84.428A
T84.490A
T84.498A
T84.50XA
T84.51XA
T84.52XA
T84.53XA
T84.54XA
T84.59XA
T84.60XA
T84.610A
T84.611A
T84.612A
T84.613A
T84.614A
T84.615A
T84.619A
T84.620A
T84.621A
T84.622A
T84.623A
T84.624A
T84.625A
T84.629A
T84.63XA
T84.69XA
T84.7XXA
T84.81XA
T84.82XA
T84.83XA
T84.84XA
T84.85XA
T84.86XA
T84.89XA
T84.9XXA
T85.01XA
T85.02XA
T85.03XA
T85.09XA
T85.110A
T85.111A
T85.112A
T85.113A
T85.118A
T85.120A
T85.121A
T85.122A
T85.123A
T85.128A
T85.190A
T85.191A
T85.192A
T85.193A
T85.199A
T85.21XA
T85.22XA
T85.29XA
T85.310A
T85.311A
T85.320A
T85.321A
T85.390A
T85.391A
T85.41XA
T85.42XA
T85.43XA
T85.44XA
T85.49XA
T85.510A
T85.511A
T85.518A
T85.520A
T85.521A
T85.528A
T85.590A
T85.591A
T85.598A
T85.610A
T85.611A
T85.612A
T85.613A
T85.614A
T85.615A
T85.618A
T85.620A
T85.621A
T85.622A
T85.623A
T85.624A
T85.625A
T85.628A
T85.630A
T85.631A
T85.633A
T85.635A
T85.638A
T85.690A
T85.691A
T85.692A
T85.693A
T85.694A
T85.695A
T85.698A
T85.71XA
T85.72XA
T85.730A
T85.731A
T85.732A
T85.733A
T85.734A
T85.735A
T85.738A
T85.79XA
T85.810A
T85.810D
T85.820A
T85.820D
T85.830A
T85.830D
T85.840A
T85.840D
T85.850A
T85.850D
T85.860A
T85.860D
T85.890A
T85.890D
T88.0XXA
T88.1XXA
T88.2XXA
T88.3XXA
T88.6XXA

Complications or Comorbidities/Major Complications or Comorbidities (CC/MCC) Exclusions

Based on CMS data

E08.3211
E08.3212
E08.3213
E08.3219
E08.3291
E08.3292
E08.3293
E08.3299
E08.3311
E08.3312
E08.3313
E08.3319
E08.3391
E08.3392
E08.3393
E08.3399
E08.3411
E08.3412
E08.3413
E08.3419
E08.3491
E08.3492
E08.3493
E08.3499
E08.3511
E08.3512
E08.3513
E08.3519
E08.3521
E08.3522
E08.3523
E08.3529
E08.3531
E08.3532
E08.3533
E08.3539
E08.3541
E08.3542
E08.3543
E08.3549
E08.3551
E08.3552
E08.3553
E08.3559
E08.3591
E08.3592
E08.3593
E08.3599
E08.37X1
E08.37X2
E08.37X3
E08.37X9
E09.3211
E09.3212
E09.3213
E09.3219
E09.3291
E09.3292
E09.3293
E09.3299
E09.3311
E09.3312
E09.3313
E09.3319
E09.3391
E09.3392
E09.3393
E09.3399
E09.3411
E09.3412
E09.3413
E09.3419
E09.3491
E09.3492
E09.3493
E09.3499
E09.3511
E09.3512
E09.3513
E09.3519
E09.3521
E09.3522
E09.3523
E09.3529
E09.3531
E09.3532
E09.3533
E09.3539
E09.3541
E09.3542
E09.3543
E09.3549
E09.3551
E09.3552
E09.3553
E09.3559
E09.3591
E09.3592
E09.3593
E09.3599
E09.37X1
E09.37X2
E09.37X3
E09.37X9
E10.3211
E10.3212
E10.3213
E10.3219
E10.3291
E10.3292
E10.3293
E10.3299
E10.3311
E10.3312
E10.3313
E10.3319
E10.3391
E10.3392
E10.3393
E10.3399
E10.3411
E10.3412
E10.3413
E10.3419
E10.3491
E10.3492
E10.3493
E10.3499
E10.3511
E10.3512
E10.3513
E10.3519
E10.3521
E10.3522
E10.3523
E10.3529
E10.3531
E10.3532
E10.3533
E10.3539
E10.3541
E10.3542
E10.3543
E10.3549
E10.3551
E10.3552
E10.3553
E10.3559
E10.3591
E10.3592
E10.3593
E10.3599
E10.37X1
E10.37X2
E10.37X3
E10.37X9
E11.3211
E11.3212
E11.3213
E11.3219
E11.3291
E11.3292
E11.3293
E11.3299
E11.3311
E11.3312
E11.3313
E11.3319
E11.3391
E11.3392
E11.3393
E11.3399
E11.3411
E11.3412
E11.3413
E11.3419
E11.3491
E11.3492
E11.3493
E11.3499
E11.3511
E11.3512
E11.3513
E11.3519
E11.3521
E11.3522
E11.3523
E11.3529
E11.3531
E11.3532
E11.3533
E11.3539
E11.3541
E11.3542
E11.3543
E11.3549
E11.3551
E11.3552
E11.3553
E11.3559
E11.3591
E11.3592
E11.3593
E11.3599
E11.37X1
E11.37X2
E11.37X3
E11.37X9
E13.3211
E13.3212
E13.3213
E13.3219
E13.3291
E13.3292
E13.3293
E13.3299
E13.3311
E13.3312
E13.3313
E13.3319
E13.3391
E13.3392
E13.3393
E13.3399
E13.3411
E13.3412
E13.3413
E13.3419
E13.3491
E13.3492
E13.3493
E13.3499
E13.3511
E13.3512
E13.3513
E13.3519
E13.3521
E13.3522
E13.3523
E13.3529
E13.3531
E13.3532
E13.3533
E13.3539
E13.3541
E13.3542
E13.3543
E13.3549
E13.3551
E13.3552
E13.3553
E13.3559
E13.3591
E13.3592
E13.3593
E13.3599
E13.37X1
E13.37X2
E13.37X3
E13.37X9
H34.8110
H34.8111
H34.8112
H34.8120
H34.8121
H34.8122
H34.8130
H34.8131
H34.8132
H34.8190

Complications or Comorbidities/Major Complications or Comorbidities (CC/MCC) Exclusions (cont.)

Based on CMS data

H34.8191
H34.8192
H34.8310
H34.8311
H34.8312
H34.8320
H34.8321
H34.8322
H34.8330
H34.8331
H34.8332
H34.8390
H34.8391
H34.8392
M84.750A
M84.750K
M84.750P
M84.751A
M84.751K
M84.751P
M84.752A
M84.752K
M84.752P
M84.753A
M84.753K
M84.753P
M84.754A
M84.754K
M84.754P
M84.755A
M84.755K
M84.755P
M84.756A
M84.756K
M84.756P
M84.757A
M84.757K
M84.757P
M84.758A
M84.758K
M84.758P
M84.759A
M84.759K
M84.759P
M97.01XA
M97.02XA
M97.11XA
M97.12XA
M97.21XA
M97.22XA
M97.31XA
M97.32XA
M97.41XA
M97.42XA
M97.8XXA
M97.9XXA
S02.101A
S02.101B
S02.101K
S02.101S
S02.102A
S02.102B
S02.102K
S02.102S
S02.109A
S02.109B
S02.109K
S02.109S
S02.11AA
S02.11AB
S02.11AK
S02.11AS
S02.11BA
S02.11BB
S02.11BK
S02.11BS
S02.11CA
S02.11CB
S02.11CK
S02.11CS
S02.11DA
S02.11DB
S02.11DK
S02.11DS
S02.11EA
S02.11EB
S02.11EK
S02.11ES
S02.11FA
S02.11FB
S02.11FK
S02.11FS
S02.11GA
S02.11GB
S02.11GK
S02.11GS
S02.11HA
S02.11HB
S02.11HK
S02.11HS
S02.30XA
S02.30XB
S02.30XK
S02.30XS
S02.31XA
S02.31XB
S02.31XK
S02.31XS
S02.32XA
S02.32XB
S02.32XK
S02.32XS
S02.40AA
S02.40AB
S02.40AK
S02.40AS
S02.40BA
S02.40BB
S02.40BK
S02.40BS
S02.40CA
S02.40CB
S02.40CK
S02.40CS
S02.40DA
S02.40DB
S02.40DK
S02.40DS
S02.40EA
S02.40EB
S02.40EK
S02.40ES
S02.40FA
S02.40FB
S02.40FK
S02.40FS
S02.601A
S02.601B
S02.601K
S02.601S
S02.602A
S02.602B
S02.602K
S02.602S
S02.610A
S02.610B
S02.610K
S02.610S
S02.611A
S02.611B
S02.611K
S02.611S
S02.612A
S02.612B
S02.612K
S02.612S
S02.620A
S02.620B
S02.620K
S02.620S
S02.621A
S02.621B
S02.621K
S02.621S
S02.622A
S02.622B
S02.622K
S02.622S
S02.630A
S02.630B
S02.630K
S02.630S
S02.631A
S02.631B
S02.631K
S02.631S
S02.632A
S02.632B
S02.632K
S02.632S
S02.640A
S02.640B
S02.640K
S02.640S
S02.641A
S02.641B
S02.641K
S02.641S
S02.642A
S02.642B
S02.642K
S02.642S
S02.650A
S02.650B
S02.650K
S02.650S
S02.651A
S02.651B
S02.651K
S02.651S
S02.652A
S02.652B
S02.652K
S02.652S
S02.670A
S02.670B
S02.670K
S02.670S
S02.671A
S02.671B
S02.671K
S02.671S
S02.672A
S02.672B
S02.672K
S02.672S
S02.80XA
S02.80XB
S02.80XK
S02.80XS
S02.81XA
S02.81XB
S02.81XK
S02.81XS
S02.82XA
S02.82XB
S02.82XK
S02.82XS
S03.00XA
S03.01XA
S03.02XA
S03.03XA
S92.811A
S92.811B
S92.811K
S92.811P
S92.812A
S92.812B
S92.812K
S92.812P
S92.819A
S92.819B
S92.819K
S92.819P
T82.855A
T82.856A
T83.113A
T83.123A
T83.193A
T83.24XA
T83.25XA
T83.411A
T83.421A
T83.491A
T83.510A
T83.511A
T83.512A
T83.590A
T83.591A
T83.592A
T83.593A
T83.61XA
T83.62XA
T83.69XA
T83.712A
T83.713A
T83.714A
T83.719A
T83.722A
T83.723A
T83.724A
T83.729A
T83.79XA
T85.113A
T85.123A
T85.193A
T85.615A
T85.625A
T85.635A
T85.695A
T85.730A
T85.731A
T85.732A
T85.733A
T85.734A
T85.735A
T85.738A
T85.810A
T85.810D
T85.820A
T85.820D
T85.830A
T85.830D
T85.840A
T85.840D
T85.850A
T85.850D
T85.860A
T85.860D
T85.890A
T85.890D

Female

Based on Medicare's Outpatient Code Editor (OCE)

O31.00X0
O31.00X1
O31.00X2
O31.00X3
O31.00X4
O31.00X5
O31.00X9
O31.01X0
O31.01X1
O31.01X2
O31.01X3
O31.01X4
O31.01X5
O31.01X9
O31.02X0
O31.02X1
O31.02X2
O31.02X3
O31.02X4
O31.02X5
O31.02X9
O31.03X0
O31.03X1
O31.03X2
O31.03X3
O31.03X4
O31.03X5
O31.03X9
O31.10X0
O31.10X1
O31.10X2
O31.10X3
O31.10X4
O31.10X5
O31.10X9
O31.11X0
O31.11X1
O31.11X2
O31.11X3
O31.11X4
O31.11X5
O31.11X9
O31.12X0
O31.12X1
O31.12X2
O31.12X3
O31.12X4
O31.12X5
O31.12X9
O31.13X0
O31.13X1
O31.13X2
O31.13X3
O31.13X4
O31.13X5
O31.13X9
O31.20X0
O31.20X1
O31.20X2
O31.20X3
O31.20X4
O31.20X5
O31.20X9
O31.21X0
O31.21X1
O31.21X2
O31.21X3
O31.21X4
O31.21X5
O31.21X9
O31.22X0
O31.22X1
O31.22X2
O31.22X3
O31.22X4
O31.22X5
O31.22X9
O31.23X0
O31.23X1
O31.23X2
O31.23X3
O31.23X4
O31.23X5
O31.23X9
O31.30X0
O31.30X1
O31.30X2
O31.30X3
O31.30X4
O31.30X5
O31.30X9
O31.31X0
O31.31X1
O31.31X2
O31.31X3
O31.31X4
O31.31X5
O31.31X9
O31.32X0
O31.32X1
O31.32X2
O31.32X3
O31.32X4
O31.32X5
O31.32X9
O31.33X0
O31.33X1
O31.33X2
O31.33X3
O31.33X4
O31.33X5
O31.33X9
O31.8X10
O31.8X11
O31.8X12
O31.8X13
O31.8X14
O31.8X15
O31.8X19
O31.8X20
O31.8X21
O31.8X22
O31.8X23
O31.8X24
O31.8X25
O31.8X29
O31.8X30
O31.8X31
O31.8X32
O31.8X33
O31.8X34
O31.8X35
O31.8X39
O31.8X90
O31.8X91
O31.8X92
O31.8X93
O31.8X94
O31.8X95
O31.8X99
O32.0XX0
O32.0XX1
O32.0XX2
O32.0XX3
O32.0XX4
O32.0XX5
O32.0XX9
O32.1XX0
O32.1XX1
O32.1XX2
O32.1XX3
O32.1XX4
O32.1XX5
O32.1XX9
O32.2XX0
O32.2XX1
O32.2XX2
O32.2XX3
O32.2XX4
O32.2XX5
O32.2XX9
O32.3XX0
O32.3XX1
O32.3XX2
O32.3XX3
O32.3XX4
O32.3XX5
O32.3XX9
O32.4XX0
O32.4XX1
O32.4XX2
O32.4XX3
O32.4XX4
O32.4XX5
O32.4XX9
O32.6XX0
O32.6XX1
O32.6XX2
O32.6XX3
O32.6XX4
O32.6XX5
O32.6XX9
O32.8XX0
O32.8XX1
O32.8XX2
O32.8XX3
O32.8XX4
O32.8XX5
O32.8XX9
O32.9XX0
O32.9XX1
O32.9XX2
O32.9XX3
O32.9XX4
O32.9XX5
O32.9XX9
O33.3XX0
O33.3XX1
O33.3XX2
O33.3XX3
O33.3XX4
O33.3XX5
O33.3XX9
O33.4XX0
O33.4XX1
O33.4XX2
O33.4XX3
O33.4XX4
O33.4XX5
O33.4XX9
O33.5XX0
O33.5XX1
O33.5XX2
O33.5XX3
O33.5XX4
O33.5XX5
O33.5XX9
O33.6XX0
O33.6XX1
O33.6XX2
O33.6XX3
O33.6XX4
O33.6XX5
O33.6XX9
O35.0XX0
O35.0XX1
O35.0XX2
O35.0XX3
O35.0XX4
O35.0XX5
O35.0XX9
O35.1XX0
O35.1XX1
O35.1XX2
O35.1XX3
O35.1XX4
O35.1XX5
O35.1XX9
O35.2XX0
O35.2XX1
O35.2XX2
O35.2XX3
O35.2XX4
O35.2XX5
O35.2XX9
O35.3XX0
O35.3XX1
O35.3XX2
O35.3XX3
O35.3XX4
O35.3XX5
O35.3XX9
O35.4XX0
O35.4XX1
O35.4XX2
O35.4XX3
O35.4XX4
O35.4XX5
O35.4XX9
O35.5XX0
O35.5XX1
O35.5XX2
O35.5XX3
O35.5XX4
O35.5XX5
O35.5XX9
O35.6XX0
O35.6XX1
O35.6XX2
O35.6XX3
O35.6XX4
O35.6XX5
O35.6XX9
O35.7XX0
O35.7XX1
O35.7XX2
O35.7XX3
O35.7XX4
O35.7XX5
O35.7XX9
O35.8XX0
O35.8XX1
O35.8XX2
O35.8XX3
O35.8XX4
O35.8XX5
O35.8XX9
O35.9XX0
O35.9XX1
O35.9XX2

Female (cont.)

Based on Medicare's Outpatient Code Editor (OCE)

O35.9XX3
O35.9XX4
O35.9XX5
O35.9XX9
O36.0110
O36.0111
O36.0112
O36.0113
O36.0114
O36.0115
O36.0119
O36.0120
O36.0121
O36.0122
O36.0123
O36.0124
O36.0125
O36.0129
O36.0130
O36.0131
O36.0132
O36.0133
O36.0134
O36.0135
O36.0139
O36.0190
O36.0191
O36.0192
O36.0193
O36.0194
O36.0195
O36.0199
O36.0910
O36.0911
O36.0912
O36.0913
O36.0914
O36.0915
O36.0919
O36.0920
O36.0921
O36.0922
O36.0923
O36.0924
O36.0925
O36.0929
O36.0930
O36.0931
O36.0932
O36.0933
O36.0934
O36.0935
O36.0939
O36.0990
O36.0991
O36.0992
O36.0993
O36.0994
O36.0995
O36.0999
O36.1110
O36.1111
O36.1112
O36.1113
O36.1114
O36.1115
O36.1119
O36.1120
O36.1121
O36.1122
O36.1123
O36.1124
O36.1125
O36.1129
O36.1130
O36.1131
O36.1132
O36.1133
O36.1134
O36.1135
O36.1139
O36.1190
O36.1191
O36.1192
O36.1193
O36.1194
O36.1195
O36.1199
O36.1910
O36.1911
O36.1912
O36.1913
O36.1914
O36.1915
O36.1919
O36.1920
O36.1921
O36.1922
O36.1923
O36.1924
O36.1925
O36.1929
O36.1930
O36.1931
O36.1932
O36.1933
O36.1934
O36.1935
O36.1939
O36.1990
O36.1991
O36.1992
O36.1993
O36.1994
O36.1995
O36.1999
O36.20X0
O36.20X1
O36.20X2
O36.20X3
O36.20X4
O36.20X5
O36.20X9
O36.21X0
O36.21X1
O36.21X2
O36.21X3
O36.21X4
O36.21X5
O36.21X9
O36.22X0
O36.22X1
O36.22X2
O36.22X3
O36.22X4
O36.22X5
O36.22X9
O36.23X0
O36.23X1
O36.23X2
O36.23X3
O36.23X4
O36.23X5
O36.23X9
O36.4XX0
O36.4XX1
O36.4XX2
O36.4XX3
O36.4XX4
O36.4XX5
O36.4XX9
O36.5110
O36.5111
O36.5112
O36.5113
O36.5114
O36.5115
O36.5119
O36.5120
O36.5121
O36.5122
O36.5123
O36.5124
O36.5125
O36.5129
O36.5130
O36.5131
O36.5132
O36.5133
O36.5134
O36.5135
O36.5139
O36.5190
O36.5191
O36.5192
O36.5193
O36.5194
O36.5195
O36.5199
O36.5910
O36.5911
O36.5912
O36.5913
O36.5914
O36.5915
O36.5919
O36.5920
O36.5921
O36.5922
O36.5923
O36.5924
O36.5925
O36.5929
O36.5930
O36.5931
O36.5932
O36.5933
O36.5934
O36.5935
O36.5939
O36.5990
O36.5991
O36.5992
O36.5993
O36.5994
O36.5995
O36.5999
O36.60X0
O36.60X1
O36.60X2
O36.60X3
O36.60X4
O36.60X5
O36.60X9
O36.61X0
O36.61X1
O36.61X2
O36.61X3
O36.61X4
O36.61X5
O36.61X9
O36.62X0
O36.62X1
O36.62X2
O36.62X3
O36.62X4
O36.62X5
O36.62X9
O36.63X0
O36.63X1
O36.63X2
O36.63X3
O36.63X4
O36.63X5
O36.63X9
O36.70X0
O36.70X1
O36.70X2
O36.70X3
O36.70X4
O36.70X5
O36.70X9
O36.71X0
O36.71X1
O36.71X2
O36.71X3
O36.71X4
O36.71X5
O36.71X9
O36.72X0
O36.72X1
O36.72X2
O36.72X3
O36.72X4
O36.72X5
O36.72X9
O36.73X0
O36.73X1
O36.73X2
O36.73X3
O36.73X4
O36.73X5
O36.73X9
O36.80X0
O36.80X1
O36.80X2
O36.80X3
O36.80X4
O36.80X5
O36.80X9
O36.8120
O36.8121
O36.8122
O36.8123
O36.8124
O36.8125
O36.8129
O36.8130
O36.8131
O36.8132
O36.8133
O36.8134
O36.8135
O36.8139
O36.8190
O36.8191
O36.8192
O36.8193
O36.8194
O36.8195
O36.8199
O36.8210
O36.8211
O36.8212
O36.8213
O36.8214
O36.8215
O36.8219
O36.8220
O36.8221
O36.8222
O36.8223
O36.8224
O36.8225
O36.8229
O36.8230
O36.8231
O36.8232
O36.8233
O36.8234
O36.8235
O36.8239
O36.8290
O36.8291
O36.8292
O36.8293
O36.8294
O36.8295
O36.8299
O36.8910
O36.8911
O36.8912
O36.8913
O36.8914
O36.8915
O36.8919
O36.8920
O36.8921
O36.8922
O36.8923
O36.8924
O36.8925
O36.8929
O36.8930
O36.8931
O36.8932
O36.8933
O36.8934
O36.8935
O36.8939
O36.8990
O36.8991
O36.8992
O36.8993
O36.8994
O36.8995
O36.8999
O36.90X0
O36.90X1
O36.90X2
O36.90X3
O36.90X4
O36.90X5
O36.90X9
O36.91X0
O36.91X1
O36.91X2
O36.91X3
O36.91X4
O36.91X5
O36.91X9
O36.92X0
O36.92X1
O36.92X2
O36.92X3
O36.92X4
O36.92X5
O36.92X9
O36.93X0
O36.93X1
O36.93X2
O36.93X3
O36.93X4
O36.93X5
O36.93X9
O40.1XX0
O40.1XX1
O40.1XX2
O40.1XX3
O40.1XX4
O40.1XX5
O40.1XX9
O40.2XX0
O40.2XX1
O40.2XX2
O40.2XX3
O40.2XX4
O40.2XX5
O40.2XX9
O40.3XX0
O40.3XX1
O40.3XX2
O40.3XX3
O40.3XX4
O40.3XX5
O40.3XX9
O40.9XX0
O40.9XX1
O40.9XX2
O40.9XX3
O40.9XX4
O40.9XX5
O40.9XX9
O41.00X0
O41.00X1
O41.00X2
O41.00X3
O41.00X4
O41.00X5
O41.00X9
O41.01X0
O41.01X1
O41.01X2
O41.01X3
O41.01X4
O41.01X5
O41.01X9
O41.02X0
O41.02X1
O41.02X2
O41.02X3
O41.02X4
O41.02X5
O41.02X9
O41.03X0
O41.03X1
O41.03X2
O41.03X3
O41.03X4
O41.03X5
O41.03X9
O41.1010
O41.1011
O41.1012
O41.1013
O41.1014
O41.1015
O41.1019
O41.1020
O41.1021
O41.1022
O41.1023
O41.1024
O41.1025
O41.1029
O41.1030
O41.1031
O41.1032
O41.1033
O41.1034
O41.1035
O41.1039
O41.1090
O41.1091
O41.1092
O41.1093
O41.1094
O41.1095
O41.1099
O41.1210
O41.1211
O41.1212
O41.1213
O41.1214
O41.1215
O41.1219
O41.1220
O41.1221
O41.1222
O41.1223
O41.1224
O41.1225
O41.1229
O41.1230
O41.1231
O41.1232
O41.1233
O41.1234
O41.1235
O41.1239
O41.1290
O41.1291
O41.1292
O41.1293
O41.1294
O41.1295
O41.1299
O41.1410
O41.1411
O41.1412
O41.1413
O41.1414
O41.1415
O41.1419
O41.1420
O41.1421
O41.1422
O41.1423
O41.1424
O41.1425
O41.1429
O41.1430
O41.1431
O41.1432
O41.1433
O41.1434
O41.1435
O41.1439
O41.1490
O41.1491
O41.1492
O41.1493
O41.1494
O41.1495
O41.1499
O41.8X10
O41.8X11
O41.8X12
O41.8X13
O41.8X14
O41.8X15
O41.8X19
O41.8X20
O41.8X21
O41.8X22
O41.8X23
O41.8X24
O41.8X25
O41.8X29
O41.8X30
O41.8X31
O41.8X32
O41.8X33
O41.8X34
O41.8X35
O41.8X39
O41.8X90
O41.8X91
O41.8X92
O41.8X93
O41.8X94
O41.8X95
O41.8X99
O41.90X0
O41.90X1
O41.90X2
O41.90X3
O41.90X4
O41.90X5
O41.90X9
O41.91X0
O41.91X1
O41.91X2
O41.91X3
O41.91X4
O41.91X5
O41.91X9
O41.92X0
O41.92X1
O41.92X2
O41.92X3
O41.92X4
O41.92X5
O41.92X9
O41.93X0
O41.93X1
O41.93X2
O41.93X3
O41.93X4
O41.93X5
O41.93X9
O60.10X0
O60.10X1
O60.10X2
O60.10X3
O60.10X4
O60.10X5
O60.10X9
O60.12X0
O60.12X1
O60.12X2
O60.12X3
O60.12X4
O60.12X5
O60.12X9
O60.13X0
O60.13X1
O60.13X2
O60.13X3
O60.13X4
O60.13X5
O60.13X9
O60.14X0
O60.14X1
O60.14X2
O60.14X3
O60.14X4
O60.14X5
O60.14X9
O60.20X0
O60.20X1
O60.20X2
O60.20X3
O60.20X4
O60.20X5
O60.20X9
O60.22X0
O60.22X1
O60.22X2
O60.22X3
O60.22X4
O60.22X5
O60.22X9
O60.23X0
O60.23X1
O60.23X2
O60.23X3
O60.23X4
O60.23X5
O60.23X9
O64.0XX0
O64.0XX1
O64.0XX2
O64.0XX3
O64.0XX4
O64.0XX5
O64.0XX9
O64.1XX0
O64.1XX1
O64.1XX2
O64.1XX3
O64.1XX4
O64.1XX5
O64.1XX9
O64.2XX0
O64.2XX1
O64.2XX2
O64.2XX3
O64.2XX4
O64.2XX5
O64.2XX9
O64.3XX0
O64.3XX1
O64.3XX2
O64.3XX3
O64.3XX4
O64.3XX5
O64.3XX9
O64.4XX0
O64.4XX1
O64.4XX2
O64.4XX3
O64.4XX4
O64.4XX5
O64.4XX9
O64.5XX0
O64.5XX1
O64.5XX2
O64.5XX3
O64.5XX4

Female (cont.)

Based on Medicare's Outpatient Code Editor (OCE)

O64.5XX5
O64.5XX9
O64.8XX0
O64.8XX1
O64.8XX2
O64.8XX3
O64.8XX4
O64.8XX5
O64.8XX9
O64.9XX0
O64.9XX1
O64.9XX2
O64.9XX3
O64.9XX4
O64.9XX5
O64.9XX9
O69.0XX0
O69.0XX1
O69.0XX2
O69.0XX3
O69.0XX4
O69.0XX5
O69.0XX9
O69.1XX0
O69.1XX1
O69.1XX2
O69.1XX3
O69.1XX4
O69.1XX5
O69.1XX9
O69.2XX0
O69.2XX1
O69.2XX2
O69.2XX3
O69.2XX4
O69.2XX5
O69.2XX9
O69.3XX0
O69.3XX1
O69.3XX2
O69.3XX3
O69.3XX4
O69.3XX5
O69.3XX9
O69.4XX0
O69.4XX1
O69.4XX2
O69.4XX3
O69.4XX4
O69.4XX5
O69.4XX9
O69.5XX0
O69.5XX1
O69.5XX2
O69.5XX3
O69.5XX4
O69.5XX5
O69.5XX9
O69.81X0
O69.81X1
O69.81X2
O69.81X3
O69.81X4
O69.81X5
O69.81X9
O69.82X0
O69.82X1
O69.82X2
O69.82X3
O69.82X4
O69.82X5
O69.82X9
O69.89X0
O69.89X1
O69.89X2
O69.89X3
O69.89X4
O69.89X5
O69.89X9
O69.9XX0
O69.9XX1
O69.9XX2
O69.9XX3
O69.9XX4
O69.9XX5
O69.9XX9
S30.202A
S30.202D
S30.202S
S30.23XA
S30.23XD
S30.23XS
S30.814A
S30.814D
S30.814S
S30.816A
S30.816D
S30.816S
S30.824A
S30.824D
S30.824S
S30.826A
S30.826D
S30.826S
S30.844A
S30.844D
S30.844S
S30.846A
S30.846D
S30.846S
S30.854A
S30.854D
S30.854S
S30.856A
S30.856D
S30.856S
S30.864A
S30.864D
S30.864S
S30.866A
S30.866D
S30.866S
S30.874A
S30.874D
S30.874S
S30.876A
S30.876D
S30.876S
S30.95XA
S30.95XD
S30.95XS
S30.97XA
S30.97XD
S30.97XS
S31.40XA
S31.40XD
S31.40XS
S31.41XA
S31.41XD
S31.41XS
S31.42XA
S31.42XD
S31.42XS
S31.43XA
S31.43XD
S31.43XS
S31.44XA
S31.44XD
S31.44XS
S31.45XA
S31.45XD
S31.45XS
S31.502A
S31.502D
S31.502S
S31.512A
S31.512D
S31.512S
S31.522A
S31.522D
S31.522S
S31.532A
S31.532D
S31.532S
S31.542A
S31.542D
S31.542S
S31.552A
S31.552D
S31.552S
S35.531A
S35.531D
S35.531S
S35.532A
S35.532D
S35.532S
S35.533A
S35.533D
S35.533S
S35.534A
S35.534D
S35.534S
S35.535A
S35.535D
S35.535S
S35.536A
S35.536D
S35.536S
S37.401A
S37.401D
S37.401S
S37.402A
S37.402D
S37.402S
S37.409A
S37.409D
S37.409S
S37.421A
S37.421D
S37.421S
S37.422A
S37.422D
S37.422S
S37.429A
S37.429D
S37.429S
S37.431A
S37.431D
S37.431S
S37.432A
S37.432D
S37.432S
S37.439A
S37.439D
S37.439S
S37.491A
S37.491D
S37.491S
S37.492A
S37.492D
S37.492S
S37.499A
S37.499D
S37.499S
S37.501A
S37.501D
S37.501S
S37.502A
S37.502D
S37.502S
S37.509A
S37.509D
S37.509S
S37.511A
S37.511D
S37.511S
S37.512A
S37.512D
S37.512S
S37.519A
S37.519D
S37.519S
S37.521A
S37.521D
S37.521S
S37.522A
S37.522D
S37.522S
S37.529A
S37.529D
S37.529S
S37.531A
S37.531D
S37.531S
S37.532A
S37.532D
S37.532S
S37.539A
S37.539D
S37.539S
S37.591A
S37.591D
S37.591S
S37.592A
S37.592D
S37.592S
S37.599A
S37.599D
S37.599S
S37.60XA
S37.60XD
S37.60XS
S37.62XA
S37.62XD
S37.62XS
S37.63XA
S37.63XD
S37.63XS
S37.69XA
S37.69XD
S37.69XS
S38.002A
S38.002D
S38.002S
S38.03XA
S38.03XD
S38.03XS
S38.211A
S38.211D
S38.211S
S38.212A
S38.212D
S38.212S
T19.2XXA
T19.2XXD
T19.2XXS
T19.3XXA
T19.3XXD
T19.3XXS
T21.07XA
T21.07XD
T21.07XS
T21.17XA
T21.17XD
T21.17XS
T21.27XA
T21.27XD
T21.27XS
T21.37XA
T21.37XD
T21.37XS
T21.47XA
T21.47XD
T21.47XS
T21.57XA
T21.57XD
T21.57XS
T21.67XA
T21.67XD
T21.67XS
T21.77XA
T21.77XD
T21.77XS
T83.31XA
T83.31XD
T83.31XS
T83.32XA
T83.32XD
T83.32XS
T83.39XA
T83.39XD
T83.39XS
T83.711A
T83.711D
T83.711S
T83.721A
T83.721D
T83.721S

Hospital-acquired Condition (HAC)

Based on CMS data

S02.0XXA
S02.0XXB
S02.110A
S02.110B
S02.111A
S02.111B
S02.112A
S02.112B
S02.113A
S02.113B
S02.118A
S02.118B
S02.119A
S02.119B
S02.19XA
S02.19XB
S02.2XXB
S02.400A
S02.400B
S02.401A
S02.401B
S02.402A
S02.402B
S02.411A
S02.411B
S02.412A
S02.412B
S02.413A
S02.413B
S02.42XA
S02.42XB
S02.600A
S02.600B
S02.609A
S02.609B
S02.63XA
S02.63XB
S02.66XA
S02.66XB
S02.69XA
S02.69XB
S02.91XA
S02.91XB
S02.92XA
S02.92XB
S06.0X1A
S06.0X9A
S06.1X1A
S06.1X2A
S06.1X3A
S06.1X4A
S06.1X5A
S06.1X6A
S06.1X7A
S06.1X8A
S06.1X9A
S06.2X1A
S06.2X2A
S06.2X3A
S06.2X4A
S06.2X5A
S06.2X6A
S06.2X7A
S06.2X8A
S06.2X9A
S06.301A
S06.302A
S06.303A
S06.304A
S06.305A
S06.306A
S06.307A
S06.308A
S06.309A
S06.310A
S06.311A
S06.312A
S06.313A
S06.314A
S06.315A
S06.316A
S06.317A
S06.318A
S06.319A
S06.320A
S06.321A
S06.322A
S06.323A
S06.324A
S06.325A
S06.326A
S06.327A
S06.328A
S06.329A
S06.330A
S06.331A
S06.332A
S06.333A
S06.334A
S06.335A
S06.336A
S06.337A
S06.338A
S06.339A
S06.340A
S06.341A
S06.342A
S06.343A
S06.344A
S06.345A
S06.346A
S06.347A
S06.348A
S06.349A
S06.350A
S06.351A
S06.352A
S06.353A
S06.354A
S06.355A
S06.356A
S06.357A
S06.358A
S06.359A
S06.360A
S06.361A
S06.362A
S06.363A
S06.364A
S06.365A
S06.366A
S06.367A
S06.368A
S06.369A
S06.370A
S06.371A
S06.372A
S06.373A
S06.374A
S06.375A
S06.376A
S06.377A
S06.378A
S06.379A
S06.380A
S06.381A
S06.382A
S06.383A
S06.384A
S06.385A
S06.386A
S06.387A
S06.388A
S06.389A
S06.4X0A
S06.4X1A
S06.4X2A
S06.4X3A
S06.4X4A
S06.4X5A
S06.4X6A
S06.4X7A
S06.4X8A
S06.4X9A
S06.5X0A
S06.5X1A
S06.5X2A
S06.5X3A
S06.5X4A
S06.5X5A
S06.5X6A
S06.5X7A
S06.5X8A
S06.5X9A
S06.6X0A
S06.6X1A
S06.6X2A
S06.6X3A
S06.6X4A
S06.6X5A
S06.6X6A
S06.6X7A
S06.6X8A
S06.6X9A
S06.811A
S06.812A
S06.813A
S06.814A
S06.815A
S06.816A
S06.817A
S06.818A
S06.819A
S06.821A
S06.822A
S06.823A
S06.824A
S06.825A
S06.826A
S06.827A
S06.828A
S06.829A
S06.891A
S06.892A
S06.893A
S06.894A
S06.895A
S06.896A
S06.897A
S06.898A
S06.899A
S06.9X1A
S06.9X2A
S06.9X3A
S06.9X4A
S06.9X5A
S06.9X6A
S06.9X7A
S06.9X8A
S06.9X9A
S07.0XXA
S07.1XXA
S07.8XXA
S07.9XXA
S12.000A
S12.000B
S12.001A
S12.001B
S12.01XA
S12.01XB
S12.02XA
S12.02XB
S12.030A
S12.030B
S12.031A
S12.031B
S12.040A
S12.040B
S12.041A
S12.041B
S12.090A
S12.090B
S12.091A
S12.091B
S12.100A
S12.100B
S12.101A
S12.101B
S12.110A
S12.110B
S12.111A
S12.111B
S12.112A
S12.112B
S12.120A
S12.120B
S12.121A
S12.121B
S12.130A
S12.130B
S12.131A
S12.131B
S12.14XA
S12.14XB
S12.150A
S12.150B
S12.151A
S12.151B
S12.190A
S12.190B

Hospital-acquired Condition (HAC) (cont.)

Based on CMS data

S12.191A
S12.191B
S12.200A
S12.200B
S12.201A
S12.201B
S12.230A
S12.230B
S12.231A
S12.231B
S12.24XA
S12.24XB
S12.250A
S12.250B
S12.251A
S12.251B
S12.290A
S12.290B
S12.291A
S12.291B
S12.300A
S12.300B
S12.301A
S12.301B
S12.330A
S12.330B
S12.331A
S12.331B
S12.34XA
S12.34XB
S12.350A
S12.350B
S12.351A
S12.351B
S12.390A
S12.390B
S12.391A
S12.391B
S12.400A
S12.400B
S12.401A
S12.401B
S12.430A
S12.430B
S12.431A
S12.431B
S12.44XA
S12.44XB
S12.450A
S12.450B
S12.451A
S12.451B
S12.490A
S12.490B
S12.491A
S12.491B
S12.500A
S12.500B
S12.501A
S12.501B
S12.530A
S12.530B
S12.531A
S12.531B
S12.54XA
S12.54XB
S12.550A
S12.550B
S12.551A
S12.551B
S12.590A
S12.590B
S12.591A
S12.591B
S12.600A
S12.600B
S12.601A
S12.601B
S12.630A
S12.630B
S12.631A
S12.631B
S12.64XA
S12.64XB
S12.650A
S12.650B
S12.651A
S12.651B
S12.690A
S12.690B
S12.691A
S12.691B
S12.8XXA
S12.9XXA
S13.0XXA
S13.100A
S13.101A
S13.110A
S13.111A
S13.120A
S13.121A
S13.130A
S13.131A
S13.140A
S13.141A
S13.150A
S13.151A
S13.160A
S13.161A
S13.170A
S13.171A
S13.180A
S13.181A
S13.20XA
S13.29XA
S14.101A
S14.102A
S14.103A
S14.104A
S14.105A
S14.106A
S14.107A
S14.109A
S14.111A
S14.112A
S14.113A
S14.114A
S14.115A
S14.116A
S14.117A
S14.121A
S14.122A
S14.123A
S14.124A
S14.125A
S14.126A
S14.127A
S14.131A
S14.132A
S14.133A
S14.134A
S14.135A
S14.136A
S14.137A
S14.151A
S14.152A
S14.153A
S14.154A
S14.155A
S14.156A
S14.157A
S17.0XXA
S17.8XXA
S17.9XXA
S22.000A
S22.000B
S22.001A
S22.001B
S22.002A
S22.002B
S22.008A
S22.008B
S22.009A
S22.009B
S22.010A
S22.010B
S22.011A
S22.011B
S22.012A
S22.012B
S22.018A
S22.018B
S22.019A
S22.019B
S22.020A
S22.020B
S22.021A
S22.021B
S22.022A
S22.022B
S22.028A
S22.028B
S22.029A
S22.029B
S22.030A
S22.030B
S22.031A
S22.031B
S22.032A
S22.032B
S22.038A
S22.038B
S22.039A
S22.039B
S22.040A
S22.040B
S22.041A
S22.041B
S22.042A
S22.042B
S22.048A
S22.048B
S22.049A
S22.049B
S22.050A
S22.050B
S22.051A
S22.051B
S22.052A
S22.052B
S22.058A
S22.058B
S22.059A
S22.059B
S22.060A
S22.060B
S22.061A
S22.061B
S22.062A
S22.062B
S22.068A
S22.068B
S22.069A
S22.069B
S22.070A
S22.070B
S22.071A
S22.071B
S22.072A
S22.072B
S22.078A
S22.078B
S22.079A
S22.079B
S22.080A
S22.080B
S22.081A
S22.081B
S22.082A
S22.082B
S22.088A
S22.088B
S22.089A
S22.089B
S22.20XA
S22.20XB
S22.21XA
S22.21XB
S22.22XA
S22.22XB
S22.23XA
S22.23XB
S22.24XA
S22.24XB
S22.31XA
S22.31XB
S22.32XA
S22.32XB
S22.39XA
S22.39XB
S22.41XA
S22.41XB
S22.42XA
S22.42XB
S22.43XA
S22.43XB
S22.49XA
S22.49XB
S22.5XXA
S22.5XXB
S22.9XXA
S22.9XXB
S24.101A
S24.102A
S24.103A
S24.104A
S24.109A
S24.111A
S24.112A
S24.113A
S24.114A
S24.131A
S24.132A
S24.133A
S24.134A
S24.151A
S24.152A
S24.153A
S24.154A
S32.000A
S32.000B
S32.001A
S32.001B
S32.002A
S32.002B
S32.008A
S32.008B
S32.009A
S32.009B
S32.010A
S32.010B
S32.011A
S32.011B
S32.012A
S32.012B
S32.018A
S32.018B
S32.019A
S32.019B
S32.020A
S32.020B
S32.021A
S32.021B
S32.022A
S32.022B
S32.028A
S32.028B
S32.029A
S32.029B
S32.030A
S32.030B
S32.031A
S32.031B
S32.032A
S32.032B
S32.038A
S32.038B
S32.039A
S32.039B
S32.040A
S32.040B
S32.041A
S32.041B
S32.042A
S32.042B
S32.048A
S32.048B
S32.049A
S32.049B
S32.050A
S32.050B
S32.051A
S32.051B
S32.052A
S32.052B
S32.058A
S32.058B
S32.059A
S32.059B
S32.10XA
S32.10XB
S32.110A
S32.110B
S32.111A
S32.111B
S32.112A
S32.112B
S32.119A
S32.119B
S32.120A
S32.120B
S32.121A
S32.121B
S32.122A
S32.122B
S32.129A
S32.129B
S32.130A
S32.130B
S32.131A
S32.131B
S32.132A
S32.132B
S32.139A
S32.139B
S32.14XA
S32.14XB
S32.15XA
S32.15XB
S32.16XA
S32.16XB
S32.17XA
S32.17XB
S32.19XA
S32.19XB
S32.2XXA
S32.2XXB
S32.301A
S32.301B
S32.302A
S32.302B
S32.309A
S32.309B
S32.311A
S32.311B
S32.312A
S32.312B
S32.313A
S32.313B
S32.314A
S32.314B
S32.315A
S32.315B
S32.316A
S32.316B
S32.391A
S32.391B
S32.392A
S32.392B
S32.399A
S32.399B
S32.401A
S32.401B
S32.402A
S32.402B
S32.409A
S32.409B
S32.411A
S32.411B
S32.412A
S32.412B
S32.413A
S32.413B
S32.414A
S32.414B
S32.415A
S32.415B
S32.416A
S32.416B
S32.421A
S32.421B
S32.422A
S32.422B
S32.423A
S32.423B
S32.424A
S32.424B
S32.425A
S32.425B
S32.426A
S32.426B
S32.431A
S32.431B
S32.432A
S32.432B
S32.433A
S32.433B
S32.434A
S32.434B
S32.435A
S32.435B
S32.436A
S32.436B
S32.441A
S32.441B
S32.442A
S32.442B
S32.443A
S32.443B
S32.444A
S32.444B
S32.445A
S32.445B
S32.446A
S32.446B
S32.451A
S32.451B
S32.452A
S32.452B
S32.453A
S32.453B
S32.454A
S32.454B
S32.455A
S32.455B
S32.456A
S32.456B
S32.461A
S32.461B
S32.462A
S32.462B
S32.463A
S32.463B
S32.464A
S32.464B
S32.465A
S32.465B
S32.466A
S32.466B
S32.471A
S32.471B
S32.472A
S32.472B
S32.473A
S32.473B
S32.474A
S32.474B
S32.475A
S32.475B
S32.476A
S32.476B
S32.481A
S32.481B
S32.482A
S32.482B
S32.483A
S32.483B
S32.484A
S32.484B
S32.485A
S32.485B
S32.486A
S32.486B
S32.491A
S32.491B
S32.492A
S32.492B
S32.499A
S32.499B
S32.501A
S32.501B
S32.502A
S32.502B
S32.509A
S32.509B
S32.511A
S32.511B
S32.512A
S32.512B
S32.519A
S32.519B
S32.591A
S32.591B
S32.592A
S32.592B
S32.599A
S32.599B
S32.601A
S32.601B
S32.602A
S32.602B
S32.609A
S32.609B
S32.611A
S32.611B
S32.612A
S32.612B
S32.613A
S32.613B
S32.614A
S32.614B
S32.615A
S32.615B
S32.616A
S32.616B
S32.691A
S32.691B
S32.692A
S32.692B
S32.699A
S32.699B
S32.810A
S32.810B
S32.811A
S32.811B
S32.82XA
S32.82XB
S32.89XA
S32.89XB
S32.9XXA
S32.9XXB
S34.101A
S34.102A
S34.103A
S34.104A
S34.105A
S34.109A
S34.111A
S34.112A
S34.113A
S34.114A
S34.115A
S34.119A
S34.121A
S34.122A
S34.123A
S34.124A
S34.125A
S34.129A
S34.131A
S34.132A
S34.139A
S34.3XXA
S42.001B
S42.002B
S42.009B
S42.011B
S42.012B
S42.013B
S42.014B
S42.015B
S42.016B
S42.017B
S42.018B
S42.019B
S42.021B
S42.022B
S42.023B
S42.024B
S42.025B
S42.026B
S42.031B
S42.032B
S42.033B
S42.034B
S42.035B
S42.036B
S42.101B
S42.102B
S42.109B
S42.111B
S42.112B
S42.113B
S42.114B
S42.115B
S42.116B
S42.121B
S42.122B
S42.123B
S42.124B
S42.125B
S42.126B
S42.131B
S42.132B
S42.133B
S42.134B
S42.135B
S42.136B
S42.141B
S42.142B
S42.143B
S42.144B
S42.145B
S42.146B
S42.151B
S42.152B
S42.153B
S42.154B
S42.155B
S42.156B
S42.191B
S42.192B
S42.199B
S42.201A
S42.201B
S42.202A
S42.202B
S42.209A
S42.209B
S42.211A

Hospital-acquired Condition (HAC) (cont.)

Based on CMS data

S42.211B
S42.212A
S42.212B
S42.213A
S42.213B
S42.214A
S42.214B
S42.215A
S42.215B
S42.216A
S42.216B
S42.221A
S42.221B
S42.222A
S42.222B
S42.223A
S42.223B
S42.224A
S42.224B
S42.225A
S42.225B
S42.226A
S42.226B
S42.231A
S42.231B
S42.232A
S42.232B
S42.239A
S42.239B
S42.241A
S42.241B
S42.242A
S42.242B
S42.249A
S42.249B
S42.251A
S42.251B
S42.252A
S42.252B
S42.253A
S42.253B
S42.254A
S42.254B
S42.255A
S42.255B
S42.256A
S42.256B
S42.261A
S42.261B
S42.262A
S42.262B
S42.263A
S42.263B
S42.264A
S42.264B
S42.265A
S42.265B
S42.266A
S42.266B
S42.271A
S42.272A
S42.279A
S42.291A
S42.291B
S42.292A
S42.292B
S42.293A
S42.293B
S42.294A
S42.294B
S42.295A
S42.295B
S42.296A
S42.296B
S42.301A
S42.301B
S42.302A
S42.302B
S42.309A
S42.309B
S42.311A
S42.312A
S42.319A
S42.321A
S42.321B
S42.322A
S42.322B
S42.323A
S42.323B
S42.324A
S42.324B
S42.325A
S42.325B
S42.326A
S42.326B
S42.331A
S42.331B
S42.332A
S42.332B
S42.333A
S42.333B
S42.334A
S42.334B
S42.335A
S42.335B
S42.336A
S42.336B
S42.341A
S42.341B
S42.342A
S42.342B
S42.343A
S42.343B
S42.344A
S42.344B
S42.345A
S42.345B
S42.346A
S42.346B
S42.351A
S42.351B
S42.352A
S42.352B
S42.353A
S42.353B
S42.354A
S42.354B
S42.355A
S42.355B
S42.356A
S42.356B
S42.361A
S42.361B
S42.362A
S42.362B
S42.363A
S42.363B
S42.364A
S42.364B
S42.365A
S42.365B
S42.366A
S42.366B
S42.391A
S42.391B
S42.392A
S42.392B
S42.399A
S42.399B
S42.401A
S42.401B
S42.402A
S42.402B
S42.409A
S42.409B
S42.411A
S42.411B
S42.412A
S42.412B
S42.413A
S42.413B
S42.414A
S42.414B
S42.415A
S42.415B
S42.416A
S42.416B
S42.421A
S42.421B
S42.422A
S42.422B
S42.423A
S42.423B
S42.424A
S42.424B
S42.425A
S42.425B
S42.426A
S42.426B
S42.431A
S42.431B
S42.432A
S42.432B
S42.433A
S42.433B
S42.434A
S42.434B
S42.435A
S42.435B
S42.436A
S42.436B
S42.441A
S42.441B
S42.442A
S42.442B
S42.443A
S42.443B
S42.444A
S42.444B
S42.445A
S42.445B
S42.446A
S42.446B
S42.447A
S42.447B
S42.448A
S42.448B
S42.449A
S42.449B
S42.451A
S42.451B
S42.452A
S42.452B
S42.453A
S42.453B
S42.454A
S42.454B
S42.455A
S42.455B
S42.456A
S42.456B
S42.461A
S42.461B
S42.462A
S42.462B
S42.463A
S42.463B
S42.464A
S42.464B
S42.465A
S42.465B
S42.466A
S42.466B
S42.471A
S42.471B
S42.472A
S42.472B
S42.473A
S42.473B
S42.474A
S42.474B
S42.475A
S42.475B
S42.476A
S42.476B
S42.481A
S42.482A
S42.489A
S42.491A
S42.491B
S42.492A
S42.492B
S42.493A
S42.493B
S42.494A
S42.494B
S42.495A
S42.495B
S42.496A
S42.496B
S42.90XA
S42.90XB
S42.91XA
S42.91XB
S42.92XA
S42.92XB
S43.201A
S43.202A
S43.203A
S43.204A
S43.205A
S43.206A
S43.211A
S43.212A
S43.213A
S43.214A
S43.215A
S43.216A
S43.221A
S43.222A
S43.223A
S43.224A
S43.225A
S43.226A
S49.001A
S49.002A
S49.009A
S49.011A
S49.012A
S49.019A
S49.021A
S49.022A
S49.029A
S49.031A
S49.032A
S49.039A
S49.041A
S49.042A
S49.049A
S49.091A
S49.092A
S49.099A
S49.101A
S49.102A
S49.109A
S49.111A
S49.112A
S49.119A
S49.121A
S49.122A
S49.129A
S49.131A
S49.132A
S49.139A
S49.141A
S49.142A
S49.149A
S49.191A
S49.192A
S49.199A
S52.001B
S52.001C
S52.002B
S52.002C
S52.009B
S52.009C
S52.011A
S52.012A
S52.019A
S52.021B
S52.021C
S52.022B
S52.022C
S52.023B
S52.023C
S52.024B
S52.024C
S52.025B
S52.025C
S52.026B
S52.026C
S52.031B
S52.031C
S52.032B
S52.032C
S52.033B
S52.033C
S52.034B
S52.034C
S52.035B
S52.035C
S52.036B
S52.036C
S52.041B
S52.041C
S52.042B
S52.042C
S52.043B
S52.043C
S52.044B
S52.044C
S52.045B
S52.045C
S52.046B
S52.046C
S52.091B
S52.091C
S52.092B
S52.092C
S52.099B
S52.099C
S52.101B
S52.101C
S52.102B
S52.102C
S52.109B
S52.109C
S52.111A
S52.112A
S52.119A
S52.121B
S52.121C
S52.122B
S52.122C
S52.123B
S52.123C
S52.124B
S52.124C
S52.125B
S52.125C
S52.126B
S52.126C
S52.131B
S52.131C
S52.132B
S52.132C
S52.133B
S52.133C
S52.134B
S52.134C
S52.135B
S52.135C
S52.136B
S52.136C
S52.181B
S52.181C
S52.182B
S52.182C
S52.189B
S52.189C
S52.201A
S52.201B
S52.201C
S52.202A
S52.202B
S52.202C
S52.209A
S52.209B
S52.209C
S52.211A
S52.212A
S52.219A
S52.221A
S52.221B
S52.221C
S52.222A
S52.222B
S52.222C
S52.223A
S52.223B
S52.223C
S52.224A
S52.224B
S52.224C
S52.225A
S52.225B
S52.225C
S52.226A
S52.226B
S52.226C
S52.231A
S52.231B
S52.231C
S52.232A
S52.232B
S52.232C
S52.233A
S52.233B
S52.233C
S52.234A
S52.234B
S52.234C
S52.235A
S52.235B
S52.235C
S52.236A
S52.236B
S52.236C
S52.241A
S52.241B
S52.241C
S52.242A
S52.242B
S52.242C
S52.243A
S52.243B
S52.243C
S52.244A
S52.244B
S52.244C
S52.245A
S52.245B
S52.245C
S52.246A
S52.246B
S52.246C
S52.251A
S52.251B
S52.251C
S52.252A
S52.252B
S52.252C
S52.253A
S52.253B
S52.253C
S52.254A
S52.254B
S52.254C
S52.255A
S52.255B
S52.255C
S52.256A
S52.256B
S52.256C
S52.261A
S52.261B
S52.261C
S52.262A
S52.262B
S52.262C
S52.263A
S52.263B
S52.263C
S52.264A
S52.264B
S52.264C
S52.265A
S52.265B
S52.265C
S52.266A
S52.266B
S52.266C
S52.281A
S52.281B
S52.281C
S52.282A
S52.282B
S52.282C
S52.283A
S52.283B
S52.283C
S52.291A
S52.291B
S52.291C
S52.292A
S52.292B
S52.292C
S52.299A
S52.299B
S52.299C
S52.301A
S52.301B
S52.301C
S52.302A
S52.302B
S52.302C
S52.309A
S52.309B
S52.309C
S52.311A
S52.312A
S52.319A
S52.321A
S52.321B
S52.321C
S52.322A
S52.322B
S52.322C
S52.323A
S52.323B
S52.323C
S52.324A
S52.324B
S52.324C
S52.325A
S52.325B
S52.325C
S52.326A
S52.326B
S52.326C
S52.331A
S52.331B
S52.331C
S52.332A
S52.332B
S52.332C
S52.333A
S52.333B
S52.333C
S52.334A
S52.334B
S52.334C
S52.335A
S52.335B
S52.335C
S52.336A
S52.336B
S52.336C
S52.341A
S52.341B
S52.341C
S52.342A
S52.342B
S52.342C
S52.343A
S52.343B
S52.343C
S52.344A
S52.344B
S52.344C
S52.345A
S52.345B
S52.345C
S52.346A
S52.346B
S52.346C
S52.351A
S52.351B
S52.351C
S52.352A
S52.352B
S52.352C
S52.353A
S52.353B
S52.353C
S52.354A
S52.354B
S52.354C
S52.355A
S52.355B
S52.355C
S52.356A
S52.356B
S52.356C
S52.361A
S52.361B
S52.361C
S52.362A
S52.362B
S52.362C
S52.363A
S52.363B
S52.363C
S52.364A
S52.364B
S52.364C
S52.365A
S52.365B
S52.365C
S52.366A
S52.366B
S52.366C
S52.381A
S52.381B
S52.381C
S52.382A
S52.382B
S52.382C
S52.389A
S52.389B
S52.389C
S52.391A
S52.391B
S52.391C
S52.392A
S52.392B
S52.392C
S52.399A
S52.399B
S52.399C
S52.501A
S52.501B
S52.501C
S52.502A
S52.502B
S52.502C
S52.509A
S52.509B
S52.509C
S52.511A

Hospital-acquired Condition (HAC) (cont.)

Based on CMS data

S52.511B
S52.511C
S52.512A
S52.512B
S52.512C
S52.513A
S52.513B
S52.513C
S52.514A
S52.514B
S52.514C
S52.515A
S52.515B
S52.515C
S52.516A
S52.516B
S52.516C
S52.521A
S52.522A
S52.529A
S52.531A
S52.531B
S52.531C
S52.532A
S52.532B
S52.532C
S52.539A
S52.539B
S52.539C
S52.541A
S52.541B
S52.541C
S52.542A
S52.542B
S52.542C
S52.549A
S52.549B
S52.549C
S52.551A
S52.551B
S52.551C
S52.552A
S52.552B
S52.552C
S52.559A
S52.559B
S52.559C
S52.561A
S52.561B
S52.561C
S52.562A
S52.562B
S52.562C
S52.569A
S52.569B
S52.569C
S52.571A
S52.571B
S52.571C
S52.572A
S52.572B
S52.572C
S52.579A
S52.579B
S52.579C
S52.591A
S52.591B
S52.591C
S52.592A
S52.592B
S52.592C
S52.599A
S52.599B
S52.599C
S52.601A
S52.601B
S52.601C
S52.602A
S52.602B
S52.602C
S52.609A
S52.609B
S52.609C
S52.611A
S52.611B
S52.611C
S52.612A
S52.612B
S52.612C
S52.613A
S52.613B
S52.613C
S52.614A
S52.614B
S52.614C
S52.615A
S52.615B
S52.615C
S52.616A
S52.616B
S52.616C
S52.621A
S52.622A
S52.629A
S52.691A
S52.691B
S52.691C
S52.692A
S52.692B
S52.692C
S52.699A
S52.699B
S52.699C
S52.90XA
S52.90XB
S52.90XC
S52.91XA
S52.91XB
S52.91XC
S52.92XA
S52.92XB
S52.92XC
S59.001A
S59.002A
S59.009A
S59.011A
S59.012A
S59.019A
S59.021A
S59.022A
S59.029A
S59.031A
S59.032A
S59.039A
S59.041A
S59.042A
S59.049A
S59.091A
S59.092A
S59.099A
S59.201A
S59.202A
S59.209A
S59.211A
S59.212A
S59.219A
S59.221A
S59.222A
S59.229A
S59.231A
S59.232A
S59.239A
S59.241A
S59.242A
S59.249A
S59.291A
S59.292A
S59.299A
S62.001B
S62.002B
S62.009B
S62.011B
S62.012B
S62.013B
S62.014B
S62.015B
S62.016B
S62.021B
S62.022B
S62.023B
S62.024B
S62.025B
S62.026B
S62.031B
S62.032B
S62.033B
S62.034B
S62.035B
S62.036B
S62.101B
S62.102B
S62.109B
S62.111B
S62.112B
S62.113B
S62.114B
S62.115B
S62.116B
S62.121B
S62.122B
S62.123B
S62.124B
S62.125B
S62.126B
S62.131B
S62.132B
S62.133B
S62.134B
S62.135B
S62.136B
S62.141B
S62.142B
S62.143B
S62.144B
S62.145B
S62.146B
S62.151B
S62.152B
S62.153B
S62.154B
S62.155B
S62.156B
S62.161B
S62.162B
S62.163B
S62.164B
S62.165B
S62.166B
S62.171B
S62.172B
S62.173B
S62.174B
S62.175B
S62.176B
S62.181B
S62.182B
S62.183B
S62.184B
S62.185B
S62.186B
S62.201B
S62.202B
S62.209B
S62.231B
S62.232B
S62.233B
S62.234B
S62.235B
S62.236B
S62.241B
S62.242B
S62.243B
S62.244B
S62.245B
S62.246B
S62.251B
S62.252B
S62.253B
S62.254B
S62.255B
S62.256B
S62.291B
S62.292B
S62.299B
S62.300B
S62.301B
S62.302B
S62.303B
S62.304B
S62.305B
S62.306B
S62.307B
S62.308B
S62.309B
S62.310B
S62.311B
S62.312B
S62.313B
S62.314B
S62.315B
S62.316B
S62.317B
S62.318B
S62.319B
S62.320B
S62.321B
S62.322B
S62.323B
S62.324B
S62.325B
S62.326B
S62.327B
S62.328B
S62.329B
S62.330B
S62.331B
S62.332B
S62.333B
S62.334B
S62.335B
S62.336B
S62.337B
S62.338B
S62.339B
S62.340B
S62.341B
S62.342B
S62.343B
S62.344B
S62.345B
S62.346B
S62.347B
S62.348B
S62.349B
S62.350B
S62.351B
S62.352B
S62.353B
S62.354B
S62.355B
S62.356B
S62.357B
S62.358B
S62.359B
S62.360B
S62.361B
S62.362B
S62.363B
S62.364B
S62.365B
S62.366B
S62.367B
S62.368B
S62.369B
S62.390B
S62.391B
S62.392B
S62.393B
S62.394B
S62.395B
S62.396B
S62.397B
S62.398B
S62.399B
S62.501B
S62.502B
S62.509B
S62.511B
S62.512B
S62.513B
S62.514B
S62.515B
S62.516B
S62.521B
S62.522B
S62.523B
S62.524B
S62.525B
S62.526B
S62.600B
S62.601B
S62.602B
S62.603B
S62.604B
S62.605B
S62.606B
S62.607B
S62.608B
S62.609B
S62.610B
S62.611B
S62.612B
S62.613B
S62.614B
S62.615B
S62.616B
S62.617B
S62.618B
S62.619B
S62.620B
S62.621B
S62.622B
S62.623B
S62.624B
S62.625B
S62.626B
S62.627B
S62.628B
S62.629B
S62.630B
S62.631B
S62.632B
S62.633B
S62.634B
S62.635B
S62.636B
S62.637B
S62.638B
S62.639B
S62.640B
S62.641B
S62.642B
S62.643B
S62.644B
S62.645B
S62.646B
S62.647B
S62.648B
S62.649B
S62.650B
S62.651B
S62.652B
S62.653B
S62.654B
S62.655B
S62.656B
S62.657B
S62.658B
S62.659B
S62.660B
S62.661B
S62.662B
S62.663B
S62.664B
S62.665B
S62.666B
S62.667B
S62.668B
S62.669B
S62.90XB
S62.91XB
S62.92XB
S72.001A
S72.001B
S72.001C
S72.002A
S72.002B
S72.002C
S72.009A
S72.009B
S72.009C
S72.011A
S72.011B
S72.011C
S72.012A
S72.012B
S72.012C
S72.019A
S72.019B
S72.019C
S72.021A
S72.021B
S72.021C
S72.022A
S72.022B
S72.022C
S72.023A
S72.023B
S72.023C
S72.024A
S72.024B
S72.024C
S72.025A
S72.025B
S72.025C
S72.026A
S72.026B
S72.026C
S72.031A
S72.031B
S72.031C
S72.032A
S72.032B
S72.032C
S72.033A
S72.033B
S72.033C
S72.034A
S72.034B
S72.034C
S72.035A
S72.035B
S72.035C
S72.036A
S72.036B
S72.036C
S72.041A
S72.041B
S72.041C
S72.042A
S72.042B
S72.042C
S72.043A
S72.043B
S72.043C
S72.044A
S72.044B
S72.044C
S72.045A
S72.045B
S72.045C
S72.046A
S72.046B
S72.046C
S72.051A
S72.051B
S72.051C
S72.052A
S72.052B
S72.052C
S72.059A
S72.059B
S72.059C
S72.061A
S72.061B
S72.061C
S72.062A
S72.062B
S72.062C
S72.063A
S72.063B
S72.063C
S72.064A
S72.064B
S72.064C
S72.065A
S72.065B
S72.065C
S72.066A
S72.066B
S72.066C
S72.091A
S72.091B
S72.091C
S72.092A
S72.092B
S72.092C
S72.099A
S72.099B
S72.099C
S72.101A
S72.101B
S72.101C
S72.102A
S72.102B
S72.102C
S72.109A
S72.109B
S72.109C
S72.111A
S72.111B
S72.111C
S72.112A
S72.112B
S72.112C
S72.113A
S72.113B
S72.113C
S72.114A
S72.114B
S72.114C
S72.115A
S72.115B
S72.115C
S72.116A
S72.116B
S72.116C
S72.121A
S72.121B
S72.121C
S72.122A
S72.122B
S72.122C
S72.123A
S72.123B
S72.123C
S72.124A
S72.124B
S72.124C
S72.125A
S72.125B
S72.125C
S72.126A
S72.126B
S72.126C
S72.131A
S72.131B
S72.131C
S72.132A
S72.132B
S72.132C
S72.133A
S72.133B
S72.133C
S72.134A
S72.134B
S72.134C
S72.135A
S72.135B
S72.135C
S72.136A
S72.136B
S72.136C
S72.141A
S72.141B
S72.141C
S72.142A
S72.142B
S72.142C
S72.143A
S72.143B
S72.143C
S72.144A
S72.144B
S72.144C
S72.145A
S72.145B
S72.145C
S72.146A
S72.146B
S72.146C
S72.21XA
S72.21XB
S72.21XC
S72.22XA
S72.22XB
S72.22XC
S72.23XA
S72.23XB
S72.23XC
S72.24XA
S72.24XB
S72.24XC
S72.25XA
S72.25XB
S72.25XC
S72.26XA
S72.26XB
S72.26XC
S72.301A
S72.301B
S72.301C
S72.302A
S72.302B
S72.302C
S72.309A
S72.309B
S72.309C
S72.321A
S72.321B
S72.321C
S72.322A
S72.322B
S72.322C
S72.323A
S72.323B
S72.323C
S72.324A
S72.324B
S72.324C
S72.325A
S72.325B
S72.325C
S72.326A
S72.326B
S72.326C
S72.331A
S72.331B
S72.331C
S72.332A

Hospital-acquired Condition (HAC) (cont.)

Based on CMS data

S72.332B
S72.332C
S72.333A
S72.333B
S72.333C
S72.334A
S72.334B
S72.334C
S72.335A
S72.335B
S72.335C
S72.336A
S72.336B
S72.336C
S72.341A
S72.341B
S72.341C
S72.342A
S72.342B
S72.342C
S72.343A
S72.343B
S72.343C
S72.344A
S72.344B
S72.344C
S72.345A
S72.345B
S72.345C
S72.346A
S72.346B
S72.346C
S72.351A
S72.351B
S72.351C
S72.352A
S72.352B
S72.352C
S72.353A
S72.353B
S72.353C
S72.354A
S72.354B
S72.354C
S72.355A
S72.355B
S72.355C
S72.356A
S72.356B
S72.356C
S72.361A
S72.361B
S72.361C
S72.362A
S72.362B
S72.362C
S72.363A
S72.363B
S72.363C
S72.364A
S72.364B
S72.364C
S72.365A
S72.365B
S72.365C
S72.366A
S72.366B
S72.366C
S72.391A
S72.391B
S72.391C
S72.392A
S72.392B
S72.392C
S72.399A
S72.399B
S72.399C
S72.401A
S72.401B
S72.401C
S72.402A
S72.402B
S72.402C
S72.409A
S72.409B
S72.409C
S72.411A
S72.411B
S72.411C
S72.412A
S72.412B
S72.412C
S72.413A
S72.413B
S72.413C
S72.414A
S72.414B
S72.414C
S72.415A
S72.415B
S72.415C
S72.416A
S72.416B
S72.416C
S72.421A
S72.421B
S72.421C
S72.422A
S72.422B
S72.422C
S72.423A
S72.423B
S72.423C
S72.424A
S72.424B
S72.424C
S72.425A
S72.425B
S72.425C
S72.426A
S72.426B
S72.426C
S72.431A
S72.431B
S72.431C
S72.432A
S72.432B
S72.432C
S72.433A
S72.433B
S72.433C
S72.434A
S72.434B
S72.434C
S72.435A
S72.435B
S72.435C
S72.436A
S72.436B
S72.436C
S72.441A
S72.441B
S72.441C
S72.442A
S72.442B
S72.442C
S72.443A
S72.443B
S72.443C
S72.444A
S72.444B
S72.444C
S72.445A
S72.445B
S72.445C
S72.446A
S72.446B
S72.446C
S72.451A
S72.451B
S72.451C
S72.452A
S72.452B
S72.452C
S72.453A
S72.453B
S72.453C
S72.454A
S72.454B
S72.454C
S72.455A
S72.455B
S72.455C
S72.456A
S72.456B
S72.456C
S72.461A
S72.461B
S72.461C
S72.462A
S72.462B
S72.462C
S72.463A
S72.463B
S72.463C
S72.464A
S72.464B
S72.464C
S72.465A
S72.465B
S72.465C
S72.466A
S72.466B
S72.466C
S72.471A
S72.472A
S72.479A
S72.491A
S72.491B
S72.491C
S72.492A
S72.492B
S72.492C
S72.499A
S72.499B
S72.499C
S72.8X1A
S72.8X1B
S72.8X1C
S72.8X2A
S72.8X2B
S72.8X2C
S72.8X9A
S72.8X9B
S72.8X9C
S72.90XA
S72.90XB
S72.90XC
S72.91XA
S72.91XB
S72.91XC
S72.92XA
S72.92XB
S72.92XC
S73.001A
S73.002A
S73.003A
S73.004A
S73.005A
S73.006A
S73.011A
S73.012A
S73.013A
S73.014A
S73.015A
S73.016A
S73.021A
S73.022A
S73.023A
S73.024A
S73.025A
S73.026A
S73.031A
S73.032A
S73.033A
S73.034A
S73.035A
S73.036A
S73.041A
S73.042A
S73.043A
S73.044A
S73.045A
S73.046A
S77.00XA
S77.01XA
S77.02XA
S77.10XA
S77.11XA
S77.12XA
S79.001A
S79.002A
S79.009A
S79.011A
S79.012A
S79.019A
S79.091A
S79.092A
S79.099A
S79.101A
S79.102A
S79.109A
S79.111A
S79.112A
S79.119A
S79.121A
S79.122A
S79.129A
S79.131A
S79.132A
S79.139A
S79.141A
S79.142A
S79.149A
S79.191A
S79.192A
S79.199A
S82.001A
S82.001B
S82.001C
S82.002A
S82.002B
S82.002C
S82.009A
S82.009B
S82.009C
S82.011A
S82.011B
S82.011C
S82.012A
S82.012B
S82.012C
S82.013A
S82.013B
S82.013C
S82.014A
S82.014B
S82.014C
S82.015A
S82.015B
S82.015C
S82.016A
S82.016B
S82.016C
S82.021A
S82.021B
S82.021C
S82.022A
S82.022B
S82.022C
S82.023A
S82.023B
S82.023C
S82.024A
S82.024B
S82.024C
S82.025A
S82.025B
S82.025C
S82.026A
S82.026B
S82.026C
S82.031A
S82.031B
S82.031C
S82.032A
S82.032B
S82.032C
S82.033A
S82.033B
S82.033C
S82.034A
S82.034B
S82.034C
S82.035A
S82.035B
S82.035C
S82.036A
S82.036B
S82.036C
S82.041A
S82.041B
S82.041C
S82.042A
S82.042B
S82.042C
S82.043A
S82.043B
S82.043C
S82.044A
S82.044B
S82.044C
S82.045A
S82.045B
S82.045C
S82.046A
S82.046B
S82.046C
S82.091A
S82.091B
S82.091C
S82.092A
S82.092B
S82.092C
S82.099A
S82.099B
S82.099C
S82.101A
S82.101B
S82.101C
S82.102A
S82.102B
S82.102C
S82.109A
S82.109B
S82.109C
S82.111A
S82.111B
S82.111C
S82.112A
S82.112B
S82.112C
S82.113A
S82.113B
S82.113C
S82.114A
S82.114B
S82.114C
S82.115A
S82.115B
S82.115C
S82.116A
S82.116B
S82.116C
S82.121A
S82.121B
S82.121C
S82.122A
S82.122B
S82.122C
S82.123A
S82.123B
S82.123C
S82.124A
S82.124B
S82.124C
S82.125A
S82.125B
S82.125C
S82.126A
S82.126B
S82.126C
S82.131A
S82.131B
S82.131C
S82.132A
S82.132B
S82.132C
S82.133A
S82.133B
S82.133C
S82.134A
S82.134B
S82.134C
S82.135A
S82.135B
S82.135C
S82.136A
S82.136B
S82.136C
S82.141A
S82.141B
S82.141C
S82.142A
S82.142B
S82.142C
S82.143A
S82.143B
S82.143C
S82.144A
S82.144B
S82.144C
S82.145A
S82.145B
S82.145C
S82.146A
S82.146B
S82.146C
S82.151A
S82.151B
S82.151C
S82.152A
S82.152B
S82.152C
S82.153A
S82.153B
S82.153C
S82.154A
S82.154B
S82.154C
S82.155A
S82.155B
S82.155C
S82.156A
S82.156B
S82.156C
S82.161A
S82.162A
S82.169A
S82.191A
S82.191B
S82.191C
S82.192A
S82.192B
S82.192C
S82.199A
S82.199B
S82.199C
S82.201A
S82.201B
S82.201C
S82.202A
S82.202B
S82.202C
S82.209A
S82.209B
S82.209C
S82.221A
S82.221B
S82.221C
S82.222A
S82.222B
S82.222C
S82.223A
S82.223B
S82.223C
S82.224A
S82.224B
S82.224C
S82.225A
S82.225B
S82.225C
S82.226A
S82.226B
S82.226C
S82.231A
S82.231B
S82.231C
S82.232A
S82.232B
S82.232C
S82.233A
S82.233B
S82.233C
S82.234A
S82.234B
S82.234C
S82.235A
S82.235B
S82.235C
S82.236A
S82.236B
S82.236C
S82.241A
S82.241B
S82.241C
S82.242A
S82.242B
S82.242C
S82.243A
S82.243B
S82.243C
S82.244A
S82.244B
S82.244C
S82.245A
S82.245B
S82.245C
S82.246A
S82.246B
S82.246C
S82.251A
S82.251B
S82.251C
S82.252A
S82.252B
S82.252C
S82.253A
S82.253B
S82.253C
S82.254A
S82.254B
S82.254C
S82.255A
S82.255B
S82.255C
S82.256A
S82.256B
S82.256C
S82.261A
S82.261B
S82.261C
S82.262A
S82.262B
S82.262C
S82.263A
S82.263B
S82.263C
S82.264A
S82.264B
S82.264C
S82.265A
S82.265B
S82.265C
S82.266A
S82.266B
S82.266C
S82.291A
S82.291B
S82.291C
S82.292A
S82.292B
S82.292C
S82.299A
S82.299B
S82.299C
S82.301B
S82.301C
S82.302B
S82.302C
S82.309B
S82.309C
S82.311A
S82.312A
S82.319A
S82.391B
S82.391C
S82.392B
S82.392C
S82.399B
S82.399C
S82.401B
S82.401C
S82.402B
S82.402C
S82.409B
S82.409C
S82.421B
S82.421C
S82.422B
S82.422C
S82.423B
S82.423C
S82.424B
S82.424C
S82.425B
S82.425C
S82.426B
S82.426C
S82.431B
S82.431C
S82.432B
S82.432C
S82.433B
S82.433C
S82.434B
S82.434C
S82.435B
S82.435C
S82.436B
S82.436C
S82.441B
S82.441C
S82.442B
S82.442C
S82.443B
S82.443C
S82.444B
S82.444C
S82.445B
S82.445C
S82.446B
S82.446C
S82.451B
S82.451C
S82.452B
S82.452C
S82.453B
S82.453C
S82.454B

Hospital-acquired Condition (HAC) (cont.)

Based on CMS data

S82.454C
S82.455B
S82.455C
S82.456B
S82.456C
S82.461B
S82.461C
S82.462B
S82.462C
S82.463B
S82.463C
S82.464B
S82.464C
S82.465B
S82.465C
S82.466B
S82.466C
S82.491B
S82.491C
S82.492B
S82.492C
S82.499B
S82.499C
S82.51XB
S82.51XC
S82.52XB
S82.52XC
S82.53XB
S82.53XC
S82.54XB
S82.54XC
S82.55XB
S82.55XC
S82.56XB
S82.56XC
S82.61XB
S82.61XC
S82.62XB
S82.62XC
S82.63XB
S82.63XC
S82.64XB
S82.64XC
S82.65XB
S82.65XC
S82.66XB
S82.66XC
S82.831B
S82.831C
S82.832B
S82.832C
S82.839B
S82.839C
S82.841B
S82.841C
S82.842B
S82.842C
S82.843B
S82.843C
S82.844B
S82.844C
S82.845B
S82.845C
S82.846B
S82.846C
S82.851B
S82.851C
S82.852B
S82.852C
S82.853B
S82.853C
S82.854B
S82.854C
S82.855B
S82.855C
S82.856B
S82.856C
S82.871B
S82.871C
S82.872B
S82.872C
S82.873B
S82.873C
S82.874B
S82.874C
S82.875B
S82.875C
S82.876B
S82.876C
S82.891B
S82.891C
S82.892B
S82.892C
S82.899B
S82.899C
S82.90XB
S82.90XC
S82.91XB
S82.91XC
S82.92XB
S82.92XC
S89.001A
S89.002A
S89.009A
S89.011A
S89.012A
S89.019A
S89.021A
S89.022A
S89.029A
S89.031A
S89.032A
S89.039A
S89.041A
S89.042A
S89.049A
S89.091A
S89.092A
S89.099A
S92.001B
S92.002B
S92.009B
S92.011B
S92.012B
S92.013B
S92.014B
S92.015B
S92.016B
S92.021B
S92.022B
S92.023B
S92.024B
S92.025B
S92.026B
S92.031B
S92.032B
S92.033B
S92.034B
S92.035B
S92.036B
S92.041B
S92.042B
S92.043B
S92.044B
S92.045B
S92.046B
S92.051B
S92.052B
S92.053B
S92.054B
S92.055B
S92.056B
S92.061B
S92.062B
S92.063B
S92.064B
S92.065B
S92.066B
S92.101B
S92.102B
S92.109B
S92.111B
S92.112B
S92.113B
S92.114B
S92.115B
S92.116B
S92.121B
S92.122B
S92.123B
S92.124B
S92.125B
S92.126B
S92.131B
S92.132B
S92.133B
S92.134B
S92.135B
S92.136B
S92.141B
S92.142B
S92.143B
S92.144B
S92.145B
S92.146B
S92.151B
S92.152B
S92.153B
S92.154B
S92.155B
S92.156B
S92.191B
S92.192B
S92.199B
S92.201B
S92.202B
S92.209B
S92.211B
S92.212B
S92.213B
S92.214B
S92.215B
S92.216B
S92.221B
S92.222B
S92.223B
S92.224B
S92.225B
S92.226B
S92.231B
S92.232B
S92.233B
S92.234B
S92.235B
S92.236B
S92.241B
S92.242B
S92.243B
S92.244B
S92.245B
S92.246B
S92.251B
S92.252B
S92.253B
S92.254B
S92.255B
S92.256B
S92.301B
S92.302B
S92.309B
S92.311B
S92.312B
S92.313B
S92.314B
S92.315B
S92.316B
S92.321B
S92.322B
S92.323B
S92.324B
S92.325B
S92.326B
S92.331B
S92.332B
S92.333B
S92.334B
S92.335B
S92.336B
S92.341B
S92.342B
S92.343B
S92.344B
S92.345B
S92.346B
S92.351B
S92.352B
S92.353B
S92.354B
S92.355B
S92.356B
S92.901B
S92.902B
S92.909B
T20.30XA
T20.311A
T20.312A
T20.319A
T20.32XA
T20.33XA
T20.34XA
T20.35XA
T20.36XA
T20.37XA
T20.39XA
T20.70XA
T20.711A
T20.712A
T20.719A
T20.72XA
T20.73XA
T20.74XA
T20.75XA
T20.76XA
T20.77XA
T20.79XA
T21.30XA
T21.31XA
T21.32XA
T21.33XA
T21.34XA
T21.35XA
T21.36XA
T21.37XA
T21.39XA
T21.70XA
T21.71XA
T21.72XA
T21.73XA
T21.74XA
T21.75XA
T21.76XA
T21.77XA
T21.79XA
T22.30XA
T22.311A
T22.312A
T22.319A
T22.321A
T22.322A
T22.329A
T22.331A
T22.332A
T22.339A
T22.341A
T22.342A
T22.349A
T22.351A
T22.352A
T22.359A
T22.361A
T22.362A
T22.369A
T22.391A
T22.392A
T22.399A
T22.70XA
T22.711A
T22.712A
T22.719A
T22.721A
T22.722A
T22.729A
T22.731A
T22.732A
T22.739A
T22.741A
T22.742A
T22.749A
T22.751A
T22.752A
T22.759A
T22.761A
T22.762A
T22.769A
T22.791A
T22.792A
T22.799A
T23.301A
T23.302A
T23.309A
T23.311A
T23.312A
T23.319A
T23.321A
T23.322A
T23.329A
T23.331A
T23.332A
T23.339A
T23.341A
T23.342A
T23.349A
T23.351A
T23.352A
T23.359A
T23.361A
T23.362A
T23.369A
T23.371A
T23.372A
T23.379A
T23.391A
T23.392A
T23.399A
T23.701A
T23.702A
T23.709A
T23.711A
T23.712A
T23.719A
T23.721A
T23.722A
T23.729A
T23.731A
T23.732A
T23.739A
T23.741A
T23.742A
T23.749A
T23.751A
T23.752A
T23.759A
T23.761A
T23.762A
T23.769A
T23.771A
T23.772A
T23.779A
T23.791A
T23.792A
T23.799A
T24.301A
T24.302A
T24.309A
T24.311A
T24.312A
T24.319A
T24.321A
T24.322A
T24.329A
T24.331A
T24.332A
T24.339A
T24.391A
T24.392A
T24.399A
T24.701A
T24.702A
T24.709A
T24.711A
T24.712A
T24.719A
T24.721A
T24.722A
T24.729A
T24.731A
T24.732A
T24.739A
T24.791A
T24.792A
T24.799A
T25.311A
T25.312A
T25.319A
T25.321A
T25.322A
T25.329A
T25.331A
T25.332A
T25.339A
T25.391A
T25.392A
T25.399A
T25.711A
T25.712A
T25.719A
T25.721A
T25.722A
T25.729A
T25.731A
T25.732A
T25.739A
T25.791A
T25.792A
T25.799A
T26.20XA
T26.21XA
T26.22XA
T26.70XA
T26.71XA
T26.72XA
T27.0XXA
T27.1XXA
T27.2XXA
T27.3XXA
T27.4XXA
T27.5XXA
T27.6XXA
T27.7XXA
T28.1XXA
T28.2XXA
T28.6XXA
T28.7XXA
T33.011A
T33.012A
T33.019A
T33.02XA
T33.09XA
T33.1XXA
T33.2XXA
T33.3XXA
T33.40XA
T33.41XA
T33.42XA
T33.511A
T33.512A
T33.519A
T33.521A
T33.522A
T33.529A
T33.531A
T33.532A
T33.539A
T33.60XA
T33.61XA
T33.62XA
T33.70XA
T33.71XA
T33.72XA
T33.811A
T33.812A
T33.819A
T33.821A
T33.822A
T33.829A
T33.831A
T33.832A
T33.839A
T33.90XA
T33.99XA
T34.011A
T34.012A
T34.019A
T34.02XA
T34.09XA
T34.1XXA
T34.2XXA
T34.3XXA
T34.40XA
T34.41XA
T34.42XA
T34.511A
T34.512A
T34.519A
T34.521A
T34.522A
T34.529A
T34.531A
T34.532A
T34.539A
T34.60XA
T34.61XA
T34.62XA
T34.70XA
T34.71XA
T34.72XA
T34.811A
T34.812A
T34.819A
T34.821A
T34.822A
T34.829A
T34.831A
T34.832A
T34.839A
T34.90XA
T34.99XA
T67.0XXA
T69.021A
T69.022A
T69.029A
T70.3XXA
T71.111A
T71.112A
T71.113A
T71.114A
T71.121A
T71.122A
T71.123A
T71.124A
T71.131A
T71.132A
T71.133A
T71.134A
T71.151A
T71.152A
T71.153A
T71.154A
T71.161A
T71.162A
T71.163A
T71.164A
T71.191A
T71.192A
T71.193A
T71.194A
T71.20XA
T71.21XA
T71.29XA
T71.9XXA
T75.1XXA
T80.0XXA
T80.211A
T80.212A
T80.218A
T80.219A
T80.30XA
T80.310A
T80.311A
T80.319A
T80.39XA
T81.4XXA
T81.500A
T81.501A
T81.502A
T81.503A
T81.504A
T81.505A
T81.506A
T81.507A
T81.508A
T81.509A
T81.510A
T81.511A
T81.512A
T81.513A
T81.514A
T81.515A
T81.516A
T81.517A
T81.518A
T81.519A
T81.520A
T81.521A
T81.522A
T81.523A
T81.524A
T81.525A
T81.526A
T81.527A
T81.528A
T81.529A
T81.530A
T81.531A
T81.532A
T81.533A
T81.534A
T81.535A
T81.536A
T81.537A
T81.538A
T81.539A
T81.590A
T81.591A
T81.592A
T81.593A
T81.594A
T81.595A
T81.596A
T81.597A
T81.598A
T81.599A
T81.60XA
T81.61XA
T81.69XA
T82.6XXA
T82.7XXA
T84.60XA
T84.610A
T84.611A
T84.612A
T84.613A
T84.614A
T84.615A
T84.619A
T84.63XA
T84.69XA
T84.7XXA

Major Complication or Comorbidity (MCC)

Based on CMS data

O41.1010	O60.12X2	R40.2342	S06.336A	S06.6X3A	S12.24XB	S14.127A	S22.008B	S24.114A	S27.332A
O41.1011	O60.12X3	R40.2343	S06.337A	S06.6X4A	S12.250B	S14.128A	S22.009B	S24.131A	S27.339A
O41.1012	O60.12X4	R40.2344	S06.338A	S06.6X5A	S12.251B	S14.131A	S22.010B	S24.132A	S27.401A
O41.1013	O60.12X5	S02.0XXB	S06.339A	S06.6X6A	S12.290B	S14.132A	S22.011B	S24.133A	S27.402A
O41.1014	O60.12X9	S02.101B	S06.340A	S06.6X7A	S12.291B	S14.133A	S22.012B	S24.134A	S27.409A
O41.1015	O60.13X0	S02.102B	S06.341A	S06.6X8A	S12.300B	S14.134A	S22.018B	S24.141A	S27.411A
O41.1019	O60.13X1	S02.109B	S06.342A	S06.6X9A	S12.301B	S14.135A	S22.019B	S24.142A	S27.412A
O41.1020	O60.13X2	S02.110B	S06.343A	S06.816A	S12.330B	S14.136A	S22.020B	S24.143A	S27.419A
O41.1021	O60.13X3	S02.111B	S06.344A	S06.817A	S12.331B	S14.137A	S22.021B	S24.144A	S27.421A
O41.1022	O60.13X4	S02.112B	S06.345A	S06.818A	S12.34XB	S14.138A	S22.022B	S24.151A	S27.422A
O41.1023	O60.13X5	S02.113B	S06.346A	S06.826A	S12.350B	S14.141A	S22.028B	S24.152A	S27.429A
O41.1024	O60.13X9	S02.118B	S06.347A	S06.827A	S12.351B	S14.142A	S22.029B	S24.153A	S27.431A
O41.1025	O60.14X0	S02.119B	S06.348A	S06.828A	S12.390B	S14.143A	S22.030B	S24.154A	S27.432A
O41.1029	O60.14X1	S02.11AB	S06.349A	S06.896A	S12.391B	S14.144A	S22.031B	S25.00XA	S27.439A
O41.1030	O60.14X2	S02.11BB	S06.350A	S06.897A	S12.400B	S14.145A	S22.032B	S25.01XA	S27.491A
O41.1031	O60.14X3	S02.11CB	S06.351A	S06.898A	S12.401B	S14.146A	S22.038B	S25.02XA	S27.492A
O41.1032	O60.14X4	S02.11DB	S06.352A	S06.9X6A	S12.430B	S14.147A	S22.039B	S25.09XA	S27.499A
O41.1033	O60.14X5	S02.11EB	S06.353A	S06.9X7A	S12.431B	S14.148A	S22.040B	S25.101A	S27.812A
O41.1034	O60.14X9	S02.11FB	S06.354A	S06.9X8A	S12.44XB	S14.151A	S22.041B	S25.102A	S27.813A
O41.1035	O60.22X0	S02.11GB	S06.355A	S11.011A	S12.450B	S14.152A	S22.042B	S25.109A	S27.818A
O41.1039	O60.22X1	S02.11HB	S06.356A	S11.012A	S12.451B	S14.153A	S22.048B	S25.111A	S27.819A
O41.1210	O60.22X2	S02.19XB	S06.357A	S11.013A	S12.490B	S14.154A	S22.049B	S25.112A	S31.001A
O41.1211	O60.22X3	S02.91XB	S06.358A	S11.014A	S12.491B	S14.155A	S22.050B	S25.119A	S31.011A
O41.1212	O60.22X4	S06.1X0A	S06.359A	S11.015A	S12.500B	S14.156A	S22.051B	S25.121A	S31.021A
O41.1213	O60.22X5	S06.1X1A	S06.360A	S11.019A	S12.501B	S14.157A	S22.052B	S25.122A	S31.031A
O41.1214	O60.22X9	S06.1X2A	S06.361A	S11.021A	S12.530B	S14.158A	S22.058B	S25.129A	S31.041A
O41.1215	O60.23X0	S06.1X3A	S06.362A	S11.022A	S12.531B	S21.301A	S22.059B	S25.191A	S31.051A
O41.1219	O60.23X1	S06.1X4A	S06.363A	S11.023A	S12.54XB	S21.302A	S22.060B	S25.192A	S31.600A
O41.1220	O60.23X2	S06.1X5A	S06.364A	S11.024A	S12.550B	S21.309A	S22.061B	S25.199A	S31.601A
O41.1221	O60.23X3	S06.1X6A	S06.365A	S11.025A	S12.551B	S21.311A	S22.062B	S25.20XA	S31.602A
O41.1222	O60.23X4	S06.1X7A	S06.366A	S11.029A	S12.590B	S21.312A	S22.068B	S25.21XA	S31.603A
O41.1223	O60.23X5	S06.1X8A	S06.367A	S11.031A	S12.591B	S21.319A	S22.069B	S25.22XA	S31.604A
O41.1224	O60.23X9	S06.1X9A	S06.368A	S11.032A	S12.600B	S21.321A	S22.070B	S25.29XA	S31.605A
O41.1225	R40.2110	S06.2X6A	S06.369A	S11.033A	S12.601B	S21.322A	S22.071B	S25.301A	S31.609A
O41.1229	R40.2111	S06.2X7A	S06.370A	S11.034A	S12.630B	S21.329A	S22.072B	S25.302A	S31.610A
O41.1230	R40.2112	S06.2X8A	S06.376A	S11.035A	S12.631B	S21.331A	S22.078B	S25.309A	S31.611A
O41.1231	R40.2113	S06.306A	S06.377A	S11.039A	S12.64XB	S21.332A	S22.079B	S25.311A	S31.612A
O41.1232	R40.2114	S06.307A	S06.378A	S12.000B	S12.650B	S21.339A	S22.080B	S25.312A	S31.613A
O41.1233	R40.2120	S06.308A	S06.380A	S12.001B	S12.651B	S21.341A	S22.081B	S25.319A	S31.614A
O41.1234	R40.2121	S06.310A	S06.386A	S12.01XB	S12.690B	S21.342A	S22.082B	S25.321A	S31.615A
O41.1235	R40.2122	S06.311A	S06.387A	S12.02XB	S12.691B	S21.349A	S22.088B	S25.322A	S31.619A
O41.1239	R40.2123	S06.312A	S06.388A	S12.030B	S12.8XXA	S21.351A	S22.089B	S25.329A	S31.620A
O41.1410	R40.2124	S06.313A	S06.4X0A	S12.031B	S14.0XXA	S21.352A	S22.20XB	S25.391A	S31.621A
O41.1411	R40.2210	S06.314A	S06.4X1A	S12.040B	S14.101A	S21.359A	S22.21XB	S25.392A	S31.622A
O41.1412	R40.2211	S06.315A	S06.4X2A	S12.041B	S14.102A	S21.401A	S22.22XB	S25.399A	S31.623A
O41.1413	R40.2212	S06.316A	S06.4X3A	S12.090B	S14.103A	S21.402A	S22.23XB	S25.401A	S31.624A
O41.1414	R40.2213	S06.317A	S06.4X4A	S12.091B	S14.104A	S21.409A	S22.24XB	S25.402A	S31.625A
O41.1415	R40.2214	S06.318A	S06.4X5A	S12.100B	S14.105A	S21.411A	S22.31XB	S25.409A	S31.629A
O41.1419	R40.2220	S06.319A	S06.4X6A	S12.101B	S14.106A	S21.412A	S22.32XB	S25.411A	S31.630A
O41.1420	R40.2221	S06.320A	S06.4X7A	S12.110B	S14.107A	S21.419A	S22.39XB	S25.412A	S31.631A
O41.1421	R40.2222	S06.321A	S06.4X8A	S12.111B	S14.108A	S21.421A	S22.41XB	S25.419A	S31.632A
O41.1422	R40.2223	S06.322A	S06.4X9A	S12.112B	S14.111A	S21.422A	S22.42XB	S25.421A	S31.633A
O41.1423	R40.2224	S06.323A	S06.5X0A	S12.120B	S14.112A	S21.429A	S22.43XB	S25.422A	S31.634A
O41.1424	R40.2310	S06.324A	S06.5X1A	S12.121B	S14.113A	S21.431A	S22.49XB	S25.429A	S31.635A
O41.1425	R40.2311	S06.325A	S06.5X2A	S12.130B	S14.114A	S21.432A	S22.5XXA	S25.491A	S31.639A
O41.1429	R40.2312	S06.326A	S06.5X3A	S12.131B	S14.115A	S21.439A	S22.5XXB	S25.492A	S31.640A
O41.1430	R40.2313	S06.327A	S06.5X4A	S12.14XB	S14.116A	S21.441A	S22.9XXB	S25.499A	S31.641A
O41.1431	R40.2314	S06.328A	S06.5X5A	S12.150B	S14.117A	S21.442A	S24.0XXA	S26.020A	S31.642A
O41.1432	R40.2320	S06.329A	S06.5X6A	S12.151B	S14.118A	S21.449A	S24.101A	S26.021A	S31.643A
O41.1433	R40.2321	S06.330A	S06.5X7A	S12.190B	S14.121A	S21.451A	S24.102A	S26.022A	S31.644A
O41.1434	R40.2322	S06.331A	S06.5X8A	S12.191B	S14.122A	S21.452A	S24.103A	S26.12XA	S31.645A
O41.1435	R40.2323	S06.332A	S06.5X9A	S12.200B	S14.123A	S21.459A	S24.104A	S26.92XA	S31.649A
O41.1439	R40.2324	S06.333A	S06.6X0A	S12.201B	S14.124A	S22.000B	S24.111A	S27.1XXA	S31.650A
O60.12X0	R40.2340	S06.334A	S06.6X1A	S12.230B	S14.125A	S22.001B	S24.112A	S27.2XXA	S31.651A
O60.12X1	R40.2341	S06.335A	S06.6X2A	S12.231B	S14.126A	S22.002B	S24.113A	S27.331A	S31.652A

Major Complication or Comorbidity (MCC) (cont.)

Based on CMS data

S31.653A	S32.401A	S32.456B	S32.811B	S35.402A	S42.264B	S42.436B	S52.031C	S52.201B	S52.266C
S31.654A	S32.401B	S32.461A	S32.82XB	S35.403A	S42.265B	S42.441B	S52.032B	S52.201C	S52.271B
S31.655A	S32.402A	S32.461B	S32.89XB	S35.404A	S42.266B	S42.442B	S52.032C	S52.202B	S52.271C
S31.659A	S32.402B	S32.462A	S32.9XXB	S35.405A	S42.291B	S42.443B	S52.033B	S52.202C	S52.272B
S32.000B	S32.409A	S32.462B	S34.01XA	S35.406A	S42.292B	S42.444B	S52.033C	S52.209B	S52.272C
S32.001B	S32.409B	S32.463A	S34.02XA	S35.411A	S42.293B	S42.445B	S52.034B	S52.209C	S52.279B
S32.002B	S32.411A	S32.463B	S34.101A	S35.412A	S42.294B	S42.446B	S52.034C	S52.221B	S52.279C
S32.008B	S32.411B	S32.464A	S34.102A	S35.413A	S42.295B	S42.447B	S52.035B	S52.221C	S52.281B
S32.009B	S32.412A	S32.464B	S34.103A	S35.414A	S42.296B	S42.448B	S52.035C	S52.222B	S52.281C
S32.010B	S32.412B	S32.465A	S34.104A	S35.415A	S42.301B	S42.449B	S52.036B	S52.222C	S52.282B
S32.011B	S32.413A	S32.465B	S34.105A	S35.416A	S42.302B	S42.451B	S52.036C	S52.223B	S52.282C
S32.012B	S32.413B	S32.466A	S34.109A	S35.491A	S42.309B	S42.452B	S52.041B	S52.223C	S52.283B
S32.018B	S32.414A	S32.466B	S34.111A	S35.492A	S42.321B	S42.453B	S52.041C	S52.224B	S52.283C
S32.019B	S32.414B	S32.471A	S34.112A	S35.493A	S42.322B	S42.454B	S52.042B	S52.224C	S52.291B
S32.020B	S32.415A	S32.471B	S34.113A	S35.494A	S42.323B	S42.455B	S52.042C	S52.225B	S52.291C
S32.021B	S32.415B	S32.472A	S34.114A	S35.495A	S42.324B	S42.456B	S52.043B	S52.225C	S52.292B
S32.022B	S32.416A	S32.472B	S34.115A	S35.496A	S42.325B	S42.461B	S52.043C	S52.226B	S52.292C
S32.028B	S32.416B	S32.473A	S34.119A	S35.50XA	S42.326B	S42.462B	S52.044B	S52.226C	S52.299B
S32.029B	S32.421A	S32.473B	S34.121A	S35.511A	S42.331B	S42.463B	S52.044C	S52.231B	S52.299C
S32.030B	S32.421B	S32.474A	S34.122A	S35.512A	S42.332B	S42.464B	S52.045B	S52.231C	S52.301B
S32.031B	S32.422A	S32.474B	S34.123A	S35.513A	S42.333B	S42.465B	S52.045C	S52.232B	S52.301C
S32.032B	S32.422B	S32.475A	S34.124A	S35.514A	S42.334B	S42.466B	S52.046B	S52.232C	S52.302B
S32.038B	S32.423A	S32.475B	S34.125A	S35.515A	S42.335B	S42.471B	S52.046C	S52.233B	S52.302C
S32.039B	S32.423B	S32.476A	S34.129A	S35.516A	S42.336B	S42.472B	S52.091B	S52.233C	S52.309B
S32.040B	S32.424A	S32.476B	S34.131A	S35.59XA	S42.341B	S42.473B	S52.091C	S52.234B	S52.309C
S32.041B	S32.424B	S32.481A	S34.132A	S36.031A	S42.342B	S42.474B	S52.092B	S52.234C	S52.321B
S32.042B	S32.425A	S32.481B	S34.139A	S36.032A	S42.343B	S42.475B	S52.092C	S52.235B	S52.321C
S32.048B	S32.425B	S32.482A	S34.3XXA	S36.115A	S42.344B	S42.476B	S52.099B	S52.235C	S52.322B
S32.049B	S32.426A	S32.482B	S35.00XA	S36.116A	S42.345B	S42.491B	S52.099C	S52.236B	S52.322C
S32.050B	S32.426B	S32.483A	S35.01XA	S37.061A	S42.346B	S42.492B	S52.101B	S52.236C	S52.323B
S32.051B	S32.431A	S32.483B	S35.02XA	S37.062A	S42.351B	S42.493B	S52.101C	S52.241B	S52.323C
S32.052B	S32.431B	S32.484A	S35.09XA	S37.069A	S42.352B	S42.494B	S52.102B	S52.241C	S52.324B
S32.058B	S32.432A	S32.484B	S35.10XA	S37.091A	S42.353B	S42.495B	S52.102C	S52.242B	S52.324C
S32.059B	S32.432B	S32.485A	S35.11XA	S37.092A	S42.354B	S42.496B	S52.109B	S52.242C	S52.325B
S32.10XB	S32.433A	S32.485B	S35.12XA	S37.099A	S42.355B	S42.90XB	S52.109C	S52.243B	S52.325C
S32.110B	S32.433B	S32.486A	S35.19XA	S42.201B	S42.356B	S42.91XB	S52.121B	S52.243C	S52.326B
S32.111B	S32.434A	S32.486B	S35.211A	S42.202B	S42.361B	S42.92XB	S52.121C	S52.244B	S52.326C
S32.112B	S32.434B	S32.491A	S35.212A	S42.209B	S42.362B	S45.001A	S52.122B	S52.244C	S52.331B
S32.119B	S32.435A	S32.491B	S35.218A	S42.211B	S42.363B	S45.002A	S52.122C	S52.245B	S52.331C
S32.120B	S32.435B	S32.492A	S35.219A	S42.212B	S42.364B	S45.009A	S52.123B	S52.245C	S52.332B
S32.121B	S32.436A	S32.492B	S35.221A	S42.213B	S42.365B	S45.011A	S52.123C	S52.246B	S52.332C
S32.122B	S32.436B	S32.499A	S35.222A	S42.214B	S42.366B	S45.012A	S52.124B	S52.246C	S52.333B
S32.129B	S32.441A	S32.499B	S35.228A	S42.215B	S42.391B	S45.019A	S52.124C	S52.251B	S52.333C
S32.130B	S32.441B	S32.501B	S35.229A	S42.216B	S42.392B	S45.091A	S52.125B	S52.251C	S52.334B
S32.131B	S32.442A	S32.502B	S35.231A	S42.221B	S42.399B	S45.092A	S52.125C	S52.252B	S52.334C
S32.132B	S32.442B	S32.509B	S35.232A	S42.222B	S42.401B	S45.099A	S52.126B	S52.252C	S52.335B
S32.139B	S32.443A	S32.511B	S35.238A	S42.223B	S42.402B	S52.001B	S52.126C	S52.253B	S52.335C
S32.14XB	S32.443B	S32.512B	S35.239A	S42.224B	S42.409B	S52.001C	S52.131B	S52.253C	S52.336B
S32.15XB	S32.444A	S32.519B	S35.291A	S42.225B	S42.411B	S52.002B	S52.131C	S52.254B	S52.336C
S32.16XB	S32.444B	S32.591B	S35.292A	S42.226B	S42.412B	S52.002C	S52.132B	S52.254C	S52.341B
S32.17XB	S32.445A	S32.592B	S35.298A	S42.231B	S42.413B	S52.009B	S52.132C	S52.255B	S52.341C
S32.19XB	S32.445B	S32.599B	S35.299A	S42.232B	S42.414B	S52.009C	S52.133B	S52.255C	S52.342B
S32.2XXB	S32.446A	S32.601B	S35.311A	S42.239B	S42.415B	S52.021B	S52.133C	S52.256B	S52.342C
S32.301B	S32.446B	S32.602B	S35.318A	S42.241B	S42.416B	S52.021C	S52.134B	S52.256C	S52.343B
S32.302B	S32.451A	S32.609B	S35.319A	S42.242B	S42.421B	S52.022B	S52.134C	S52.261B	S52.343C
S32.309B	S32.451B	S32.611B	S35.321A	S42.249B	S42.422B	S52.022C	S52.135B	S52.261C	S52.344B
S32.311B	S32.452A	S32.612B	S35.328A	S42.251B	S42.423B	S52.023B	S52.135C	S52.262B	S52.344C
S32.312B	S32.452B	S32.613B	S35.329A	S42.252B	S42.424B	S52.023C	S52.136B	S52.262C	S52.345B
S32.313B	S32.453A	S32.614B	S35.331A	S42.253B	S42.425B	S52.024B	S52.136C	S52.263B	S52.345C
S32.314B	S32.453B	S32.615B	S35.338A	S42.254B	S42.426B	S52.024C	S52.181B	S52.263C	S52.346B
S32.315B	S32.454A	S32.616B	S35.339A	S42.255B	S42.431B	S52.025B	S52.181C	S52.264B	S52.346C
S32.316B	S32.454B	S32.691B	S35.341A	S42.256B	S42.432B	S52.025C	S52.182B	S52.264C	S52.351B
S32.391B	S32.455A	S32.692B	S35.348A	S42.261B	S42.433B	S52.026B	S52.182C	S52.265B	S52.351C
S32.392B	S32.455B	S32.699B	S35.349A	S42.262B	S42.434B	S52.026C	S52.189B	S52.265C	S52.352B
S32.399B	S32.456A	S32.810B	S35.401A	S42.263B	S42.435B	S52.031B	S52.189C	S52.266B	S52.352C

Major Complication or Comorbidity (MCC) (cont.)

Based on CMS data

S52.353B
S52.353C
S52.354B
S52.354C
S52.355B
S52.355C
S52.356B
S52.356C
S52.361B
S52.361C
S52.362B
S52.362C
S52.363B
S52.363C
S52.364B
S52.364C
S52.365B
S52.365C
S52.366B
S52.366C
S52.371B
S52.371C
S52.372B
S52.372C
S52.379B
S52.379C
S52.381B
S52.381C
S52.382B
S52.382C
S52.389B
S52.389C
S52.391B
S52.391C
S52.392B
S52.392C
S52.399B
S52.399C
S52.501B
S52.501C
S52.502B
S52.502C
S52.509B
S52.509C
S52.511B
S52.511C
S52.512B
S52.512C
S52.513B
S52.513C
S52.514B
S52.514C
S52.515B
S52.515C
S52.516B
S52.516C
S52.531B
S52.531C
S52.532B
S52.532C
S52.539B
S52.539C
S52.541B
S52.541C
S52.542B
S52.542C
S52.549B
S52.549C
S52.551B
S52.551C
S52.552B
S52.552C
S52.559B
S52.559C
S52.561B
S52.561C
S52.562B
S52.562C
S52.569B
S52.569C
S52.571B
S52.571C
S52.572B
S52.572C
S52.579B
S52.579C
S52.591B
S52.591C
S52.592B
S52.592C
S52.599B
S52.599C
S52.601B
S52.601C
S52.602B
S52.602C
S52.609B
S52.609C
S52.611B
S52.611C
S52.612B
S52.612C
S52.613B
S52.613C
S52.614B
S52.614C
S52.615B
S52.615C
S52.616B
S52.616C
S52.691B
S52.691C
S52.692B
S52.692C
S52.699B
S52.699C
S52.90XB
S52.90XC
S52.91XB
S52.91XC
S52.92XB
S52.92XC
S72.001A
S72.001B
S72.001C
S72.002A
S72.002B
S72.002C
S72.009A
S72.009B
S72.009C
S72.011A
S72.011B
S72.011C
S72.012A
S72.012B
S72.012C
S72.019A
S72.019B
S72.019C
S72.021A
S72.021B
S72.021C
S72.022A
S72.022B
S72.022C
S72.023A
S72.023B
S72.023C
S72.024A
S72.024B
S72.024C
S72.025A
S72.025B
S72.025C
S72.026A
S72.026B
S72.026C
S72.031A
S72.031B
S72.031C
S72.032A
S72.032B
S72.032C
S72.033A
S72.033B
S72.033C
S72.034A
S72.034B
S72.034C
S72.035A
S72.035B
S72.035C
S72.036A
S72.036B
S72.036C
S72.041A
S72.041B
S72.041C
S72.042A
S72.042B
S72.042C
S72.043A
S72.043B
S72.043C
S72.044A
S72.044B
S72.044C
S72.045A
S72.045B
S72.045C
S72.046A
S72.046B
S72.046C
S72.051A
S72.051B
S72.051C
S72.052A
S72.052B
S72.052C
S72.059A
S72.059B
S72.059C
S72.061A
S72.061B
S72.061C
S72.062A
S72.062B
S72.062C
S72.063A
S72.063B
S72.063C
S72.064A
S72.064B
S72.064C
S72.065A
S72.065B
S72.065C
S72.066A
S72.066B
S72.066C
S72.091A
S72.091B
S72.091C
S72.092A
S72.092B
S72.092C
S72.099A
S72.099B
S72.099C
S72.101A
S72.101B
S72.101C
S72.102A
S72.102B
S72.102C
S72.109A
S72.109B
S72.109C
S72.111A
S72.111B
S72.111C
S72.112A
S72.112B
S72.112C
S72.113A
S72.113B
S72.113C
S72.114A
S72.114B
S72.114C
S72.115A
S72.115B
S72.115C
S72.116A
S72.116B
S72.116C
S72.121A
S72.121B
S72.121C
S72.122A
S72.122B
S72.122C
S72.123A
S72.123B
S72.123C
S72.124A
S72.124B
S72.124C
S72.125A
S72.125B
S72.125C
S72.126A
S72.126B
S72.126C
S72.131A
S72.131B
S72.131C
S72.132A
S72.132B
S72.132C
S72.133A
S72.133B
S72.133C
S72.134A
S72.134B
S72.134C
S72.135A
S72.135B
S72.135C
S72.136A
S72.136B
S72.136C
S72.141A
S72.141B
S72.141C
S72.142A
S72.142B
S72.142C
S72.143A
S72.143B
S72.143C
S72.144A
S72.144B
S72.144C
S72.145A
S72.145B
S72.145C
S72.146A
S72.146B
S72.146C
S72.21XA
S72.21XB
S72.21XC
S72.22XA
S72.22XB
S72.22XC
S72.23XA
S72.23XB
S72.23XC
S72.24XA
S72.24XB
S72.24XC
S72.25XA
S72.25XB
S72.25XC
S72.26XA
S72.26XB
S72.26XC
S72.301A
S72.301B
S72.301C
S72.302A
S72.302B
S72.302C
S72.309A
S72.309B
S72.309C
S72.321A
S72.321B
S72.321C
S72.322A
S72.322B
S72.322C
S72.323A
S72.323B
S72.323C
S72.324A
S72.324B
S72.324C
S72.325A
S72.325B
S72.325C
S72.326A
S72.326B
S72.326C
S72.331A
S72.331B
S72.331C
S72.332A
S72.332B
S72.332C
S72.333A
S72.333B
S72.333C
S72.334A
S72.334B
S72.334C
S72.335A
S72.335B
S72.335C
S72.336A
S72.336B
S72.336C
S72.341A
S72.341B
S72.341C
S72.342A
S72.342B
S72.342C
S72.343A
S72.343B
S72.343C
S72.344A
S72.344B
S72.344C
S72.345A
S72.345B
S72.345C
S72.346A
S72.346B
S72.346C
S72.351A
S72.351B
S72.351C
S72.352A
S72.352B
S72.352C
S72.353A
S72.353B
S72.353C
S72.354A
S72.354B
S72.354C
S72.355A
S72.355B
S72.355C
S72.356A
S72.356B
S72.356C
S72.361A
S72.361B
S72.361C
S72.362A
S72.362B
S72.362C
S72.363A
S72.363B
S72.363C
S72.364A
S72.364B
S72.364C
S72.365A
S72.365B
S72.365C
S72.366A
S72.366B
S72.366C
S72.391A
S72.391B
S72.391C
S72.392A
S72.392B
S72.392C
S72.399A
S72.399B
S72.399C
S72.401B
S72.401C
S72.402B
S72.402C
S72.409B
S72.409C
S72.411B
S72.411C
S72.412B
S72.412C
S72.413B
S72.413C
S72.414B
S72.414C
S72.415B
S72.415C
S72.416B
S72.416C
S72.421B
S72.421C
S72.422B
S72.422C
S72.423B
S72.423C
S72.424B
S72.424C
S72.425B
S72.425C
S72.426B
S72.426C
S72.431B
S72.431C
S72.432B
S72.432C
S72.433B
S72.433C
S72.434B
S72.434C
S72.435B
S72.435C
S72.436B
S72.436C
S72.441B
S72.441C
S72.442B
S72.442C
S72.443B
S72.443C
S72.444B
S72.444C
S72.445B
S72.445C
S72.446B
S72.446C
S72.451B
S72.451C
S72.452B
S72.452C
S72.453B
S72.453C
S72.454B
S72.454C
S72.455B
S72.455C
S72.456B
S72.456C
S72.461B
S72.461C
S72.462B
S72.462C
S72.463B
S72.463C
S72.464B
S72.464C
S72.465B
S72.465C
S72.466B
S72.466C
S72.491B
S72.491C
S72.492B
S72.492C
S72.499B
S72.499C
S72.8X1A
S72.8X1B
S72.8X1C
S72.8X2A
S72.8X2B
S72.8X2C
S72.8X9A
S72.8X9B
S72.8X9C
S72.90XA
S72.90XB
S72.90XC
S72.91XA
S72.91XB
S72.91XC
S72.92XA
S72.92XB
S72.92XC
S75.001A
S75.002A
S75.009A
S75.011A
S75.012A
S75.019A
S75.021A
S75.022A
S75.029A
S75.091A
S75.092A
S75.099A
S75.101A
S75.102A
S75.109A
S75.111A
S75.112A
S75.119A
S75.121A
S75.122A
S75.129A
S75.191A
S75.192A
S75.199A
S79.001A
S79.002A
S79.009A
S79.011A
S79.012A
S79.019A
S79.091A
S79.092A
S79.099A
S82.101B
S82.101C
S82.102B
S82.102C
S82.109B
S82.109C
S82.111B
S82.111C
S82.112B
S82.112C
S82.113B
S82.113C
S82.114B
S82.114C
S82.115B
S82.115C
S82.116B
S82.116C
S82.121B
S82.121C
S82.122B
S82.122C
S82.123B
S82.123C
S82.124B
S82.124C
S82.125B
S82.125C
S82.126B
S82.126C
S82.131B
S82.131C
S82.132B
S82.132C
S82.133B
S82.133C
S82.134B
S82.134C
S82.135B
S82.135C
S82.136B
S82.136C
S82.141B
S82.141C
S82.142B
S82.142C
S82.143B
S82.143C
S82.144B
S82.144C
S82.145B
S82.145C
S82.146B
S82.146C
S82.151B
S82.151C
S82.152B
S82.152C
S82.153B
S82.153C
S82.154B
S82.154C
S82.155B
S82.155C
S82.156B
S82.156C
S82.191B
S82.191C
S82.192B
S82.192C
S82.199B
S82.199C
S82.201B
S82.201C
S82.202B
S82.202C
S82.209B
S82.209C

Major Complication or Comorbidity (MCC) (cont.)

Based on CMS data

S82.221B	S82.234C	S82.252B	S82.265C	S82.423B	S82.436C	S82.454B	S82.491C	S82.865B	S85.591A
S82.221C	S82.235B	S82.252C	S82.266B	S82.423C	S82.441B	S82.454C	S82.492B	S82.865C	S85.592A
S82.222B	S82.235C	S82.253B	S82.266C	S82.424B	S82.441C	S82.455B	S82.492C	S82.866B	S85.599A
S82.222C	S82.236B	S82.253C	S82.291B	S82.424C	S82.442B	S82.455C	S82.499B	S82.866C	T79.0XXA
S82.223B	S82.236C	S82.254B	S82.291C	S82.425B	S82.442C	S82.456B	S82.499C	S85.001A	T79.1XXA
S82.223C	S82.241B	S82.254C	S82.292B	S82.425C	S82.443B	S82.456C	S82.831B	S85.002A	T79.4XXA
S82.224B	S82.241C	S82.255B	S82.292C	S82.426B	S82.443C	S82.461B	S82.831C	S85.009A	T79.5XXA
S82.224C	S82.242B	S82.255C	S82.299B	S82.426C	S82.444B	S82.461C	S82.832B	S85.011A	T80.0XXA
S82.225B	S82.242C	S82.256B	S82.299C	S82.431B	S82.444C	S82.462B	S82.832C	S85.012A	T81.11XA
S82.225C	S82.243B	S82.256C	S82.401B	S82.431C	S82.445B	S82.462C	S82.839B	S85.019A	T81.12XA
S82.226B	S82.243C	S82.261B	S82.401C	S82.432B	S82.445C	S82.463B	S82.839C	S85.091A	T81.19XA
S82.226C	S82.244B	S82.261C	S82.402B	S82.432C	S82.446B	S82.463C	S82.861B	S85.092A	
S82.231B	S82.244C	S82.262B	S82.402C	S82.433B	S82.446C	S82.464B	S82.861C	S85.099A	
S82.231C	S82.245B	S82.262C	S82.409B	S82.433C	S82.451B	S82.464C	S82.862B	S85.501A	
S82.232B	S82.245C	S82.263B	S82.409C	S82.434B	S82.451C	S82.465B	S82.862C	S85.502A	
S82.232C	S82.246B	S82.263C	S82.421B	S82.434C	S82.452B	S82.465C	S82.863B	S85.509A	
S82.233B	S82.246C	S82.264B	S82.421C	S82.435B	S82.452C	S82.466B	S82.863C	S85.511A	
S82.233C	S82.251B	S82.264C	S82.422B	S82.435C	S82.453B	S82.466C	S82.864B	S85.512A	
S82.234B	S82.251C	S82.265B	S82.422C	S82.436B	S82.453C	S82.491B	S82.864C	S85.519A	

Male

Based on Medicare's Outpatient Code Editor (OCE)

S30.201A	S30.822S	S30.853D	S30.875A	S31.22XS	S31.33XD	S31.541A	S38.001S	S39.840D	T21.56XA
S30.201D	S30.823A	S30.853S	S30.875D	S31.23XA	S31.33XS	S31.541D	S38.01XA	S39.840S	T21.56XD
S30.201S	S30.823D	S30.855A	S30.875S	S31.23XD	S31.34XA	S31.541S	S38.01XD	T19.4XXA	T21.56XS
S30.21XA	S30.823S	S30.855D	S30.93XA	S31.23XS	S31.34XD	S31.551A	S38.01XS	T19.4XXD	T21.66XA
S30.21XD	S30.825A	S30.855S	S30.93XD	S31.24XA	S31.34XS	S31.551D	S38.02XA	T19.4XXS	T21.66XD
S30.21XS	S30.825D	S30.862A	S30.93XS	S31.24XD	S31.35XA	S31.551S	S38.02XD	T21.06XA	T21.66XS
S30.22XA	S30.825S	S30.862D	S30.94XA	S31.24XS	S31.35XD	S37.822A	S38.02XS	T21.06XD	T21.76XA
S30.22XD	S30.842A	S30.862S	S30.94XD	S31.25XA	S31.35XS	S37.822D	S38.221A	T21.06XS	T21.76XD
S30.22XS	S30.842D	S30.863A	S30.94XS	S31.25XD	S31.501A	S37.822S	S38.221D	T21.16XA	T21.76XS
S30.812A	S30.842S	S30.863D	S30.96XA	S31.25XS	S31.501D	S37.823A	S38.221S	T21.16XD	T83.410A
S30.812D	S30.843A	S30.863S	S30.96XD	S31.30XA	S31.501S	S37.823D	S38.222A	T21.16XS	T83.410D
S30.812S	S30.843D	S30.865A	S30.96XS	S31.30XD	S31.511A	S37.823S	S38.222D	T21.26XA	T83.410S
S30.813A	S30.843S	S30.865D	S31.20XA	S31.30XS	S31.511D	S37.828A	S38.222S	T21.26XD	T83.420A
S30.813D	S30.845A	S30.865S	S31.20XD	S31.31XA	S31.511S	S37.828D	S38.231A	T21.26XS	T83.420D
S30.813S	S30.845D	S30.872A	S31.20XS	S31.31XD	S31.521A	S37.828S	S38.231D	T21.36XA	T83.420S
S30.815A	S30.845S	S30.872D	S31.21XA	S31.31XS	S31.521D	S37.829A	S38.231S	T21.36XD	T83.490A
S30.815D	S30.852A	S30.872S	S31.21XD	S31.32XA	S31.521S	S37.829D	S38.232A	T21.36XS	T83.490D
S30.815S	S30.852D	S30.873A	S31.21XS	S31.32XD	S31.531A	S37.829S	S38.232D	T21.46XA	T83.490S
S30.822A	S30.852S	S30.873D	S31.22XA	S31.32XS	S31.531D	S38.001A	S38.232S	T21.46XD	
S30.822D	S30.853A	S30.873S	S31.22XD	S31.33XA	S31.531S	S38.001D	S39.840A	T21.46XS	

Maternity

For patients 12-55 years of age; based on Medicare's Outpatient Code Editor (OCE)

O31.00X0	O31.02X3	O31.10X9	O31.13X2	O31.21X5	O31.30X1	O31.32X4	O31.8X20	O31.8X93	O32.1XX9
O31.00X1	O31.02X4	O31.11X0	O31.13X3	O31.21X9	O31.30X2	O31.32X5	O31.8X21	O31.8X94	O32.2XX0
O31.00X2	O31.02X5	O31.11X1	O31.13X4	O31.22X0	O31.30X3	O31.32X9	O31.8X22	O31.8X95	O32.2XX1
O31.00X3	O31.02X9	O31.11X2	O31.13X5	O31.22X1	O31.30X4	O31.33X0	O31.8X23	O31.8X99	O32.2XX2
O31.00X4	O31.03X0	O31.11X3	O31.13X9	O31.22X2	O31.30X5	O31.33X1	O31.8X24	O32.0XX0	O32.2XX3
O31.00X5	O31.03X1	O31.11X4	O31.20X0	O31.22X3	O31.30X9	O31.33X2	O31.8X25	O32.0XX1	O32.2XX4
O31.00X9	O31.03X2	O31.11X5	O31.20X1	O31.22X4	O31.31X0	O31.33X3	O31.8X29	O32.0XX2	O32.2XX5
O31.01X0	O31.03X3	O31.11X9	O31.20X2	O31.22X5	O31.31X1	O31.33X4	O31.8X30	O32.0XX3	O32.2XX9
O31.01X1	O31.03X4	O31.12X0	O31.20X3	O31.22X9	O31.31X2	O31.33X5	O31.8X31	O32.0XX4	O32.3XX0
O31.01X2	O31.03X5	O31.12X1	O31.20X4	O31.23X0	O31.31X3	O31.33X9	O31.8X32	O32.0XX5	O32.3XX1
O31.01X3	O31.03X9	O31.12X2	O31.20X5	O31.23X1	O31.31X4	O31.8X10	O31.8X33	O32.0XX9	O32.3XX2
O31.01X4	O31.10X0	O31.12X3	O31.20X9	O31.23X2	O31.31X5	O31.8X11	O31.8X34	O32.1XX0	O32.3XX3
O31.01X5	O31.10X1	O31.12X4	O31.21X0	O31.23X3	O31.31X9	O31.8X12	O31.8X35	O32.1XX1	O32.3XX4
O31.01X9	O31.10X2	O31.12X5	O31.21X1	O31.23X4	O31.32X0	O31.8X13	O31.8X39	O32.1XX2	O32.3XX5
O31.02X0	O31.10X3	O31.12X9	O31.21X2	O31.23X5	O31.32X1	O31.8X14	O31.8X90	O32.1XX3	O32.3XX9
O31.02X1	O31.10X4	O31.13X0	O31.21X3	O31.23X9	O31.32X2	O31.8X15	O31.8X91	O32.1XX4	O32.4XX0
O31.02X2	O31.10X5	O31.13X1	O31.21X4	O31.30X0	O31.32X3	O31.8X19	O31.8X92	O32.1XX5	O32.4XX1

Maternity (cont.)

For patients 12-55 years of age; based on Medicare's Outpatient Code Editor (OCE)

O32.4XX2
O32.4XX3
O32.4XX4
O32.4XX5
O32.4XX9
O32.6XX0
O32.6XX1
O32.6XX2
O32.6XX3
O32.6XX4
O32.6XX5
O32.6XX9
O32.8XX0
O32.8XX1
O32.8XX2
O32.8XX3
O32.8XX4
O32.8XX5
O32.8XX9
O32.9XX0
O32.9XX1
O32.9XX2
O32.9XX3
O32.9XX4
O32.9XX5
O32.9XX9
O33.3XX0
O33.3XX1
O33.3XX2
O33.3XX3
O33.3XX4
O33.3XX5
O33.3XX9
O33.4XX0
O33.4XX1
O33.4XX2
O33.4XX3
O33.4XX4
O33.4XX5
O33.4XX9
O33.5XX0
O33.5XX1
O33.5XX2
O33.5XX3
O33.5XX4
O33.5XX5
O33.5XX9
O33.6XX0
O33.6XX1
O33.6XX2
O33.6XX3
O33.6XX4
O33.6XX5
O33.6XX9
O35.0XX0
O35.0XX1
O35.0XX2
O35.0XX3
O35.0XX4
O35.0XX5
O35.0XX9
O35.1XX0
O35.1XX1
O35.1XX2
O35.1XX3
O35.1XX4
O35.1XX5
O35.1XX9
O35.2XX0
O35.2XX1
O35.2XX2
O35.2XX3
O35.2XX4
O35.2XX5
O35.2XX9
O35.3XX0
O35.3XX1
O35.3XX2
O35.3XX3
O35.3XX4
O35.3XX5
O35.3XX9
O35.4XX0
O35.4XX1
O35.4XX2
O35.4XX3
O35.4XX4
O35.4XX5
O35.4XX9
O35.5XX0
O35.5XX1
O35.5XX2
O35.5XX3
O35.5XX4
O35.5XX5
O35.5XX9
O35.6XX0
O35.6XX1
O35.6XX2
O35.6XX3
O35.6XX4
O35.6XX5
O35.6XX9
O35.7XX0
O35.7XX1
O35.7XX2
O35.7XX3
O35.7XX4
O35.7XX5
O35.7XX9
O35.8XX0
O35.8XX1
O35.8XX2
O35.8XX3
O35.8XX4
O35.8XX5
O35.8XX9
O35.9XX0
O35.9XX1
O35.9XX2
O35.9XX3
O35.9XX4
O35.9XX5
O35.9XX9
O36.0110
O36.0111
O36.0112
O36.0113
O36.0114
O36.0115
O36.0119
O36.0120
O36.0121
O36.0122
O36.0123
O36.0124
O36.0125
O36.0129
O36.0130
O36.0131
O36.0132
O36.0133
O36.0134
O36.0135
O36.0139
O36.0190
O36.0191
O36.0192
O36.0193
O36.0194
O36.0195
O36.0199
O36.0910
O36.0911
O36.0912
O36.0913
O36.0914
O36.0915
O36.0919
O36.0920
O36.0921
O36.0922
O36.0923
O36.0924
O36.0925
O36.0929
O36.0930
O36.0931
O36.0932
O36.0933
O36.0934
O36.0935
O36.0939
O36.0990
O36.0991
O36.0992
O36.0993
O36.0994
O36.0995
O36.0999
O36.1110
O36.1111
O36.1112
O36.1113
O36.1114
O36.1115
O36.1119
O36.1120
O36.1121
O36.1122
O36.1123
O36.1124
O36.1125
O36.1129
O36.1130
O36.1131
O36.1132
O36.1133
O36.1134
O36.1135
O36.1139
O36.1190
O36.1191
O36.1192
O36.1193
O36.1194
O36.1195
O36.1199
O36.1910
O36.1911
O36.1912
O36.1913
O36.1914
O36.1915
O36.1919
O36.1920
O36.1921
O36.1922
O36.1923
O36.1924
O36.1925
O36.1929
O36.1930
O36.1931
O36.1932
O36.1933
O36.1934
O36.1935
O36.1939
O36.1990
O36.1991
O36.1992
O36.1993
O36.1994
O36.1995
O36.1999
O36.20X0
O36.20X1
O36.20X2
O36.20X3
O36.20X4
O36.20X5
O36.20X9
O36.21X0
O36.21X1
O36.21X2
O36.21X3
O36.21X4
O36.21X5
O36.21X9
O36.22X0
O36.22X1
O36.22X2
O36.22X3
O36.22X4
O36.22X5
O36.22X9
O36.23X0
O36.23X1
O36.23X2
O36.23X3
O36.23X4
O36.23X5
O36.23X9
O36.4XX0
O36.4XX1
O36.4XX2
O36.4XX3
O36.4XX4
O36.4XX5
O36.4XX9
O36.5110
O36.5111
O36.5112
O36.5113
O36.5114
O36.5115
O36.5119
O36.5120
O36.5121
O36.5122
O36.5123
O36.5124
O36.5125
O36.5129
O36.5130
O36.5131
O36.5132
O36.5133
O36.5134
O36.5135
O36.5139
O36.5190
O36.5191
O36.5192
O36.5193
O36.5194
O36.5195
O36.5199
O36.5910
O36.5911
O36.5912
O36.5913
O36.5914
O36.5915
O36.5919
O36.5920
O36.5921
O36.5922
O36.5923
O36.5924
O36.5925
O36.5929
O36.5930
O36.5931
O36.5932
O36.5933
O36.5934
O36.5935
O36.5939
O36.5990
O36.5991
O36.5992
O36.5993
O36.5994
O36.5995
O36.5999
O36.60X0
O36.60X1
O36.60X2
O36.60X3
O36.60X4
O36.60X5
O36.60X9
O36.61X0
O36.61X1
O36.61X2
O36.61X3
O36.61X4
O36.61X5
O36.61X9
O36.62X0
O36.62X1
O36.62X2
O36.62X3
O36.62X4
O36.62X5
O36.62X9
O36.63X0
O36.63X1
O36.63X2
O36.63X3
O36.63X4
O36.63X5
O36.63X9
O36.70X0
O36.70X1
O36.70X2
O36.70X3
O36.70X4
O36.70X5
O36.70X9
O36.71X0
O36.71X1
O36.71X2
O36.71X3
O36.71X4
O36.71X5
O36.71X9
O36.72X0
O36.72X1
O36.72X2
O36.72X3
O36.72X4
O36.72X5
O36.72X9
O36.73X0
O36.73X1
O36.73X2
O36.73X3
O36.73X4
O36.73X5
O36.73X9
O36.80X0
O36.80X1
O36.80X2
O36.80X3
O36.80X4
O36.80X5
O36.80X9
O36.8120
O36.8121
O36.8122
O36.8123
O36.8124
O36.8125
O36.8129
O36.8130
O36.8131
O36.8132
O36.8133
O36.8134
O36.8135
O36.8139
O36.8190
O36.8191
O36.8192
O36.8193
O36.8194
O36.8195
O36.8199
O36.8210
O36.8211
O36.8212
O36.8213
O36.8214
O36.8215
O36.8219
O36.8220
O36.8221
O36.8222
O36.8223
O36.8224
O36.8225
O36.8229
O36.8230
O36.8231
O36.8232
O36.8233
O36.8234
O36.8235
O36.8239
O36.8290
O36.8291
O36.8292
O36.8293
O36.8294
O36.8295
O36.8299
O36.8910
O36.8911
O36.8912
O36.8913
O36.8914
O36.8915
O36.8919
O36.8920
O36.8921
O36.8922
O36.8923
O36.8924
O36.8925
O36.8929
O36.8930
O36.8931
O36.8932
O36.8933
O36.8934
O36.8935
O36.8939
O36.8990
O36.8991
O36.8992
O36.8993
O36.8994
O36.8995
O36.8999
O36.90X0
O36.90X1
O36.90X2
O36.90X3
O36.90X4
O36.90X5
O36.90X9
O36.91X0
O36.91X1
O36.91X2
O36.91X3
O36.91X4
O36.91X5
O36.91X9
O36.92X0
O36.92X1
O36.92X2
O36.92X3
O36.92X4
O36.92X5
O36.92X9
O36.93X0
O36.93X1
O36.93X2
O36.93X3
O36.93X4
O36.93X5
O36.93X9
O40.1XX0
O40.1XX1
O40.1XX2
O40.1XX3
O40.1XX4
O40.1XX5
O40.1XX9
O40.2XX0
O40.2XX1
O40.2XX2
O40.2XX3
O40.2XX4
O40.2XX5
O40.2XX9
O40.3XX0
O40.3XX1
O40.3XX2
O40.3XX3
O40.3XX4
O40.3XX5
O40.3XX9
O40.9XX0
O40.9XX1
O40.9XX2
O40.9XX3
O40.9XX4
O40.9XX5
O40.9XX9
O41.00X0
O41.00X1
O41.00X2
O41.00X3
O41.00X4
O41.00X5
O41.00X9
O41.01X0
O41.01X1
O41.01X2
O41.01X3
O41.01X4
O41.01X5
O41.01X9
O41.02X0
O41.02X1
O41.02X2
O41.02X3
O41.02X4
O41.02X5
O41.02X9
O41.03X0
O41.03X1
O41.03X2
O41.03X3
O41.03X4
O41.03X5
O41.03X9
O41.1010
O41.1011
O41.1012
O41.1013
O41.1014
O41.1015
O41.1019
O41.1020
O41.1021
O41.1022
O41.1023
O41.1024
O41.1025
O41.1029
O41.1030
O41.1031
O41.1032
O41.1033
O41.1034
O41.1035
O41.1039
O41.1090
O41.1091
O41.1092
O41.1093
O41.1094
O41.1095
O41.1099
O41.1210
O41.1211
O41.1212
O41.1213
O41.1214
O41.1215
O41.1219
O41.1220
O41.1221
O41.1222
O41.1223
O41.1224
O41.1225
O41.1229
O41.1230
O41.1231
O41.1232
O41.1233
O41.1234
O41.1235
O41.1239
O41.1290
O41.1291
O41.1292
O41.1293
O41.1294
O41.1295
O41.1299
O41.1410
O41.1411
O41.1412
O41.1413
O41.1414
O41.1415
O41.1419
O41.1420
O41.1421
O41.1422
O41.1423
O41.1424
O41.1425
O41.1429
O41.1430
O41.1431
O41.1432
O41.1433
O41.1434
O41.1435
O41.1439
O41.1490
O41.1491
O41.1492
O41.1493
O41.1494
O41.1495
O41.1499
O41.8X10
O41.8X11
O41.8X12
O41.8X13
O41.8X14
O41.8X15
O41.8X19
O41.8X20
O41.8X21
O41.8X22
O41.8X23
O41.8X24
O41.8X25
O41.8X29
O41.8X30
O41.8X31
O41.8X32
O41.8X33
O41.8X34
O41.8X35
O41.8X39
O41.8X90
O41.8X91
O41.8X92
O41.8X93

Maternity (cont.)

For patients 12-55 years of age; based on Medicare's Outpatient Code Editor (OCE)

O41.8X94 O41.8X95 O41.8X99 O41.90X0 O41.90X1 O41.90X2 O41.90X3 O41.90X4 O41.90X5 O41.90X9 O41.91X0 O41.91X1 O41.91X2 O41.91X3 O41.91X4 O41.91X5 O41.91X9 O41.92X0 O41.92X1 O41.92X2 O41.92X3
O41.92X4 O41.92X5 O41.92X9 O41.93X0 O41.93X1 O41.93X2 O41.93X3 O41.93X4 O41.93X5 O41.93X9 O60.10X0 O60.10X1 O60.10X2 O60.10X3 O60.10X4 O60.10X5 O60.10X9 O60.12X0 O60.12X1 O60.12X2 O60.12X3
O60.12X4 O60.12X5 O60.12X9 O60.13X0 O60.13X1 O60.13X2 O60.13X3 O60.13X4 O60.13X5 O60.13X9 O60.14X0 O60.14X1 O60.14X2 O60.14X3 O60.14X4 O60.14X5 O60.14X9 O60.20X0 O60.20X1 O60.20X2 O60.20X3
O60.20X4 O60.20X5 O60.20X9 O60.22X0 O60.22X1 O60.22X2 O60.22X3 O60.22X4 O60.22X5 O60.22X9 O60.23X0 O60.23X1 O60.23X2 O60.23X3 O60.23X4 O60.23X5 O60.23X9 O64.0XX0 O64.0XX1 O64.0XX2 O64.0XX3
O64.0XX4 O64.0XX5 O64.0XX9 O64.1XX0 O64.1XX1 O64.1XX2 O64.1XX3 O64.1XX4 O64.1XX5 O64.1XX9 O64.2XX0 O64.2XX1 O64.2XX2 O64.2XX3 O64.2XX4 O64.2XX5 O64.2XX9 O64.3XX0 O64.3XX1 O64.3XX2 O64.3XX3
O64.3XX4 O64.3XX5 O64.3XX9 O64.4XX0 O64.4XX1 O64.4XX2 O64.4XX3 O64.4XX4 O64.4XX5 O64.4XX9 O64.5XX0 O64.5XX1 O64.5XX2 O64.5XX3 O64.5XX4 O64.5XX5 O64.5XX9 O64.8XX0 O64.8XX1 O64.8XX2 O64.8XX3
O64.8XX4 O64.8XX5 O64.8XX9 O64.9XX0 O64.9XX1 O64.9XX2 O64.9XX3 O64.9XX4 O64.9XX5 O64.9XX9 O69.0XX0 O69.0XX1 O69.0XX2 O69.0XX3 O69.0XX4 O69.0XX5 O69.0XX9 O69.1XX0 O69.1XX1 O69.1XX2 O69.1XX3
O69.1XX4 O69.1XX5 O69.1XX9 O69.2XX0 O69.2XX1 O69.2XX2 O69.2XX3 O69.2XX4 O69.2XX5 O69.2XX9 O69.3XX0 O69.3XX1 O69.3XX2 O69.3XX3 O69.3XX4 O69.3XX5 O69.3XX9 O69.4XX0 O69.4XX1 O69.4XX2 O69.4XX3
O69.4XX4 O69.4XX5 O69.4XX9 O69.5XX0 O69.5XX1 O69.5XX2 O69.5XX3 O69.5XX4 O69.5XX5 O69.5XX9 O69.81X0 O69.81X1 O69.81X2 O69.81X3 O69.81X4 O69.81X5 O69.81X9 O69.82X0 O69.82X1 O69.82X2 O69.82X3
O69.82X4 O69.82X5 O69.82X9 O69.89X0 O69.89X1 O69.89X2 O69.89X3 O69.89X4 O69.89X5 O69.89X9 O69.9XX0 O69.9XX1 O69.9XX2 O69.9XX3 O69.9XX4 O69.9XX5 O69.9XX9

Pediatrics

For patients 0-17 years of age; based on Medicare's Outpatient Code Editor (OCE)

T74.02XA T74.02XD T74.02XS T74.12XA
T74.12XD T74.12XS T74.22XA T74.22XD
T74.22XS T74.32XA T74.32XD T74.32XS
T74.4XXA T74.4XXD T74.4XXS T74.92XA
T74.92XD T74.92XS T76.02XA T76.02XD
T76.02XS T76.12XA T76.12XD T76.12XS
T76.22XA T76.22XD T76.22XS T76.32XA
T76.32XD T76.32XS T76.92XA T76.92XD
T76.92XS

Principal Diagnosis as its own Major Complication or Comorbidity (MCC)

Based on CMS data

S06.1X0A S06.1X1A S06.1X2A S06.1X3A S06.1X4A S06.1X5A S06.1X6A S06.1X7A S06.1X8A S06.1X9A

Unacceptable Principal Diagnosis

Based on Medicare code edits

H40.1210 H40.1211 H40.1212 H40.1213 H40.1214
H40.1220 H40.1221 H40.1222 H40.1223 H40.1224
H40.1230 H40.1231 H40.1232 H40.1233 H40.1234
H40.1290 H40.1291 H40.1292 H40.1293 H40.1294
H40.1310 H40.1311 H40.1312 H40.1313 H40.1314
H40.1320 H40.1321 H40.1322 H40.1323 H40.1324
H40.1330 H40.1331 H40.1332 H40.1333 H40.1334
H40.1390 H40.1391 H40.1392 H40.1393 H40.1394
O36.80X0 O36.80X1 O36.80X2 O36.80X3 O36.80X4
O36.80X5 O36.80X9 T81.12XA

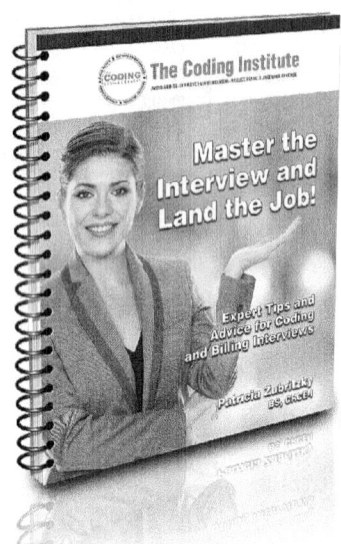

Notes